Comprehensive Clinical Nephrology

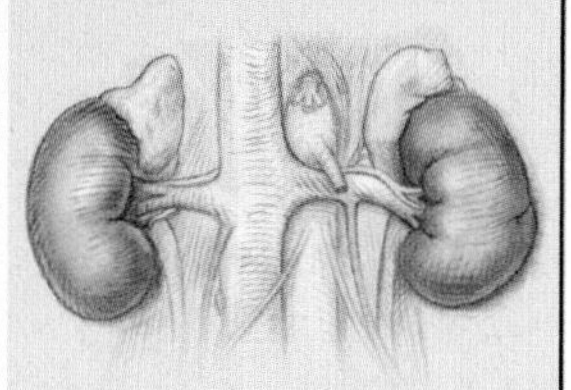

Comprehensive Clinical Nephrology

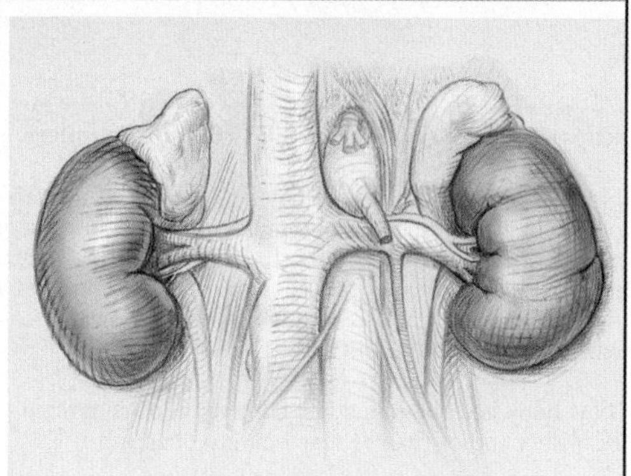

Fourth Edition

Jürgen Floege, MD
Medizinische Klinik II
RWTH University of Aachen
Aachen, Germany

Richard J. Johnson, MD
Professor of Medicine
Division Chief
Temple Hoyne Buell and NKF of Colorado Endowed Chair of Medicine
University of Colorado, Denver
Aurora, Colorado

John Feehally, DM, FRCP
Professor of Renal Medicine
The John Walls Renal Unit
Leicester General Hospital
Leicester, United Kingdom

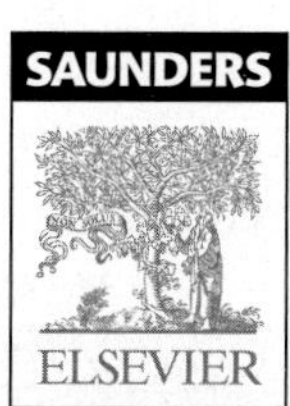

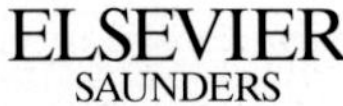

3251 Riverport Lane
St. Louis, Missouri 63043

COMPREHENSIVE CLINICAL NEPHROLOGY ISBN: 978-0-323-05876-6

Library of Congress Cataloging-in-Publication Data
Comprehensive clinical nephrology / [edited by] Jürgen Floege, Richard J. Johnson, John Feehally.—4th ed.
p. ; cm.
Includes bibliographical references and index.
ISBN 978-0-323-05876-6
1. Kidneys—Diseases. 2. Nephrology. I. Floege, Jürgen. II. Johnson, Richard J. (Richard Joseph). III. Feehally, John.
[DNLM: 1. Kidney Diseases. 2. Nephrology—methods. WJ 300 C7375 2010]
RC902.C55 2010
616.6′1—dc22

2009046367

Senior Acquisitions Editor: Kate Dimock
Developmental Editor: Joan Ryan
Publishing Services Manager: Anne Altepeter
Project Managers: Cindy Thoms/Vijay Antony Raj Vincent
Senior Book Designer: Ellen Zanolle

Printed in the United States of America

Last digit is the print number: 9 8 7 6 5 4 3 2 1

To our mentors in nephrology—especially Bill Couser, Stewart Cameron, and Karl M. Koch

To our colleagues and collaborators, as well as others, whose research continues to light the way

To our wives and families, who have once again endured the preparation of this fourth edition with unfailing patience and support

To our patients with renal disease, for whom it is a privilege to care

Jürgen Floege
Richard J. Johnson
John Feehally

CONTRIBUTORS

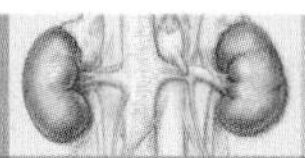

Sharon Adler, MD
Los Angeles Biomedical Research Institute at Harbor
University of California—Los Angeles
David Geffen School of Medicine
Torrance, California, USA
30: Prevention and Treatment of Diabetic Nephropathy

Horacio J. Adrogué, MD
Baylor College of Medicine
Methodist Hospital
Houston, Texas, USA
14: Respiratory Acidosis, Respiratory Alkalosis, and Mixed Disorders

Venkatesh Aiyagari, MBBS, DM
University of Illinois at Chicago
Chicago, Illinois, USA
40: Neurogenic Hypertension, Including Hypertension Associated with Stroke or Spinal Cord Injury

Robert J. Alpern, MD
Yale University School of Medicine
New Haven, Connecticut, USA
11: Normal Acid-Base Balance
12: Metabolic Acidosis

Charles E. Alpers, MD
University of Washington Medical Center
Seattle, Washington, USA
21: Membranoproliferative Glomerulonephritis, Dense Deposit Disease, and Cryoglobulinemic Glomerulonephritis

Gerald B. Appel, MD
Columbia University College of Physicians and Surgeons
New York Presbyterian Hospital
New York, New York, USA
18: Primary and Secondary (Non-Genetic) Causes of Focal and Segmental Glomerulosclerosis
25: Lupus Nephritis

Fatiu A. Arogundade, MBBS, FMCP, FWACP
Obafemi Awolowo University
Obafemi Awolowo University Teaching Hospitals Complex
Ile-Ife
Osun State, Nigeria
49: Sickle Cell Disease

Stephen R. Ash, MD, FACP
Clarian Arnett Health
Ash Access Technology, Inc.
HemoCleanse, Inc.
Lafayette, Indiana, USA
88: Diagnostic and Interventional Nephrology

Arif Asif, MD
University of Miami Miller School of Medicine
Miami, Florida, USA
88: Diagnostic and Interventional Nephrology

Pierre Aucouturier, PhD
Pierre and Marie Curie University
Paris, France
26: Renal Amyloidosis and Glomerular Diseases with Monoclonal Immunoglobulin Deposition

Phyllis August, MD, MPH
Weill Cornell Medical College
New York, New York, USA
42: Renal Complications in Normal Pregnancy

George L. Bakris, MD, FASN
University of Chicago Pritzker School of Medicine
Chicago, Illinois, USA
33: Primary Hypertension
36: Evaluation and Treatment of Hypertensive Urgencies and Emergencies

Adam D. Barlow, MB, ChB, MRCS
Leicester General Hospital
Leicester, England
99: Kidney Transplantation Surgery

Rashad S. Barsoum, MD, FRCP, FRCPE
Kasr El-Aini School of Medicine
Cairo University
Cairo, Egypt
54: The Kidney in Schistosomiasis
55: Glomerular Diseases Associated with Infection

Chris Baylis, PhD
University of Florida
Gainesville, Florida, USA
41: Renal Physiology in Normal Pregnancy

Aminu Bello, MD
Sheffield Kidney Institute
Sheffield, England
75: Epidemiology and Pathophysiology of Chronic Kidney Disease

Tomas Berl, MD
University of Colorado Denver
Aurora, Colorado, USA
8: Disorders of Water Metabolism

Suresh Bhat, MS, MCh (Urology)
Medical College
Kottayam, Kerala, India
52: Tuberculosis of the Urinary Tract

Gemma Bircher, BSC, RD, MSc
University Hospitals of Leicester NHS Trust
Leicestershire, England
83: Gastroenterology and Nutrition in Chronic Kidney Disease

Joseph V. Bonventre, MD, PhD
Brigham and Women's Hospital
Harvard Institutes of Medicine
Boston, Massachusetts, USA
68: Diagnosis and Clinical Evaluation of Acute Kidney Injury

Josée Bouchard, MD
University of California—San Diego
San Diego, California, USA
69: Prevention and Nondialytic Management of Acute Kidney Injury

Nicholas R. Brook, BSc, MSc, BM, MD, FRCS (Urol)
University of Adelaide
Royal Adelaide Hospital
Adelaide, South Australia
99: Kidney Transplantation Surgery

Christopher Brown, MD
Ohio State University Medical Center
Columbus, Ohio, USA
76: Retarding Progression of Kidney Disease

Mark A. Brown, MB, BS, MD
St. George Hospital
University of New South Wales
Sydney, Australia
43: Pregnancy with Preexisting Kidney Disease

Emmanuel A. Burdmann, MD, PhD
University of São Paulo Medical School
São Paulo, Brazil
55: Glomerular Diseases Associated with Infection
67: Acute Kidney Injury in the Tropics

David A. Bushinsky, MD
University of Rochester School of Medicine
University of Rochester Medical Center
Rochester, New York, USA
57: Nephrolithiasis and Nephrocalcinosis

Daniel C. Cattran, MD, FRCPC
University Health Network
Toronto General Hospital
Toronto, Ontario, Canada
20: Membranous Nephropathy

Matthew J. Cervelli, BPharm
Royal Adelaide Hospital
Adelaide, South Australia
73: Principles of Drug Therapy, Dosing, and Prescribing in Chronic Kidney Disease and Renal Replacement Therapy

Steven J. Chadban, BMed, PhD, FRACP
Royal Prince Alfred Hospital
Sydney Medical School
University of Sydney
Sydney, Australia
104: Recurrent Disease in Kidney Transplantation

Karen E. Charlton, MPhil (Epi), MSc, PhD
University of Wollongong
Wollongong, Australia
34: Nonpharmacologic Prevention and Treatment of Hypertension

Yipu Chen, MD
Beijing Anzhen Hospital
Capital Medical University
Beijing, People's Republic of China
6: Renal Biopsy

Ignatius K.P. Cheng, MBBS, PHD, FRCP, FRACP
The University of Hong Kong
Hong Kong, China
72: Hepatorenal Syndrome

John O. Connolly, PhD, FRCP
Royal Free Hospital
London, England
50: Congenital Anomalies of the Kidney and Urinary Tract

William G. Couser, MD
University of Washington
Seattle, Washington, USA
20: Membranous Nephropathy

Paolo Cravedi, MD
Mario Negri Institute for Pharmacological Research
Bergamo, Italy
28: Thrombotic Microangiopathies, Including Hemolytic Uremic Syndrome

Vivette D. D'Agati, MD
Columbia University College of Physicians and Surgeons
New York, New York, USA
18: Primary and Secondary (Non-Genetic) Causes of Focal and Segmental Glomerulosclerosis

Gabriel M. Danovitch, MD
University of California
Los Angeles David Geffen School of Medicine
Los Angeles, California, USA
101: Medical Management of the Kidney Transplant Recipient: Infections and Malignant Neoplasms
102: Medical Management of the Kidney Transplant Recipient: Cardiovascular Disease and Other Issues

Simon J. Davies, BSc, MD, FRCP
University Hospital of North Staffordshire
Staffordshire, England
93: Complications of Peritoneal Dialysis

John M. Davison, BSc, MD, MSc, FRCOG
Institute of Cellular Medicine
Reproductive and Vascular Biology Group
Medical School
Newcastle University and Royal Victoria Infirmary
Newcastle Upon Tyne
Tyne and Wear, England
41: Renal Physiology in Normal Pregnancy

Wayne Derman, MBChB, PhD, FACSM, FFIMS
University of Cape Town
Sport Science Institute of South Africa
Cape Town, South Africa
34: Nonpharmacologic Prevention and Treatment of Hypertension

Gerald F. DiBona, MD
University of Iowa College of Medicine
Iowa City, Iowa, USA
32: Normal Blood Pressure Control and the Evaluation of Hypertension

Tilman B. Drüeke, MD
Facultes de Medecine et de Pharmacie
Amiens, France
10: Disorders of Calcium, Phosphate, and Magnesium Metabolism

Jamie P. Dwyer, MD
Vanderbilt University Medical Center
Nashville, Tennessee, USA
64: Thromboembolic Renovascular Disease

Kai-Uwe Eckardt, MD
University of Erlangen-Nuremberg
Erlangen, Germany
79: Anemia in Chronic Kidney Disease

Jason Eckel, MD
Durham, North Carolina, USA
19: Inherited Causes of Nephrotic Syndrome

Frank Eitner, MD
RWTH University of Aachen
Aachen, Germany
85: Acquired Cystic Kidney Disease and Malignant Neoplasms

Mohsen El Kossi, MBBch, MSc, MD
Northern General Hospital
Sheffield, England
75: Epidemiology and Pathophysiology of Chronic Kidney Disease

Marlies Elger, PhD
University of Heidelberg
Heidelberg, Germany
1: Renal Anatomy

Elwaleed A. Elhassan, MD
University of Khartown
Khartown, Sudan
7: Disorders of Extracellular Volume

Pieter Evenepoel, MD, PhD
University Hospitals Leuven
Leuven, Belgium
84: Dermatologic Manifestations of Chronic Kidney Disease

June Fabian, MD
Charlotte Maxeke Johannesburg Hospital
University of the Witwatersrand
Johannesburg, South Africa
56: Human Immunodeficiency Virus Infection and the Kidney

Ronald J. Falk, MD
University of North Carolina-Chapel Hill
Chapel Hill, North Carolina, USA
24: Renal and Systemic Vasculitis

John Feehally, DM, FRCP
Leicester General Hospital
Leicester, England
15: Introduction to Glomerular Disease: Clinical Presentations
16: Introduction to Glomerular Disease: Histologic Classification and Pathogenesis
22: IgA Nephropathy and Henoch-Schönlein Nephritis

Evelyne A. Fischer, MD, PhD
Cochin Institute
Paris, France
60: Acute Interstitial Nephritis

Jonathan S. Fisher, MD, FACS
Scripps Clinic and Green Hospital
La Jolla, California, USA
106: Pancreas and Islet Transplantation

Jürgen Floege, MD
RWTH University of Aachen
Aachen, Germany
15: Introduction to Glomerular Disease: Clinical Presentations
16: Introduction to Glomerular Disease: Histologic Classification and Pathogenesis
22: IgA Nephropathy and Henoch-Schönlein Nephritis
81: Bone and Mineral Metabolism in Chronic Kidney Disease

Giovanni B. Fogazzi, MD
Fondazione IRCCS Ca' Granda
Ospedale Maggiore Policlinico
Milano, Italy
4: Urinalysis

John W. Foreman, MD
Duke University Medical Center
Durham, North Carolina, USA
48: Fanconi Syndrome and Other Proximal Tubule Disorders

Toshiro Fujita, MD
University of Tokyo
Tokyo, Japan
62: Chronic Interstitial Nephritis

F. John Gennari, MD
University of Vermont College of Medicine
Burlington, Vermont, USA
13: Metabolic Alkalosis

Evangelos G. Gkougkousis, MD
Leicester General Hospital
Leicester, England
59: Urologic Issues for the Nephrologist

Richard J. Glassock, MD, MACP
David Geffen School of Medicine
University of California Los Angeles
Los Angeles, California, USA
27: Other Glomerular Disorders and Antiphospholipid Syndrome

Philip B. Gorelick, MD
University of Illinois at Chicago
Chicago, Illinois, USA
40: Neurogenic Hypertension, Including Hypertension Associated with Stroke or Spinal Cord Injury

Barbara A. Greco, MD
Tufts University School of Medicine
Springfield, Massachusetts, USA
37: Renovascular Hypertension and Ischemic Renal Disease
64: Thromboembolic Renovascular Disease

Peter Gross, MD
University Medical Center
Dresden, Germany
47: Inherited Disorders of Sodium and Water Handling

Lisa M. Guay-Woodford, MD
University of Alabama at Birmingham
Birmingham, Alabama, USA
45: Other Cystic Kidney Diseases

Nabil Haddad, MD
Ohio State University College of Medicine
Columbus, Ohio, USA
76: Retarding Progression of Kidney Disease

Kevin P.G. Harris, MD
University of Leicester
University Hospitals of Leicester
Leicester, England
58: Urinary Tract Obstruction

Peter C. Harris, PhD
Mayo Clinic
Rochester, Minnesota, USA
44: Autosomal Dominant Polycystic Kidney Disease

Lee A. Hebert, MD
Ohio State University College of Medicine
Columbus, Ohio, USA
76: Retarding Progression of Kidney Disease

Peter Heduschka, MD
Universitatsklinikum Carl Gustav Carus
Dresden, Germany
47: Inherited Disorders of Sodium and Water Handling

Charles A. Herzog, MD
Hennepin County Medical Center
Cardiovascular Special Studies Center
University of Minnesota
Minneapolis, Minnesota, USA
78: Cardiovascular Disease in Chronic Kidney Disease

Thomas Hooton, MD
University of Miami Miller School of Medicine
Miami, Florida, USA
51: Urinary Tract Infections in Adults

Walter H. Hörl, MD, PhD, FRCP
University of Vienna
Vienna, Austria
80: Other Blood and Immune Disorders in Chronic Kidney Disease

Peter F. Hoyer, MD
Zentrum für Kinder und Jugendmedizin
Universitätsklinikum Essen
Essen, Germany
17: Minimal Change Nephrotic Syndrome

Jeremy Hughes, MA, MB, BS, PhD
The Queen's Medical Research Institute
University of Edinburgh
Edinburgh, Scotland, United Kingdom
58: Urinary Tract Obstruction

Christian Hugo, MD
University Erlangen-Nürnberg
Erlangen, Germany
65: Geriatric Nephrology

Enyu Imai, MD, PhD
Nagoya University Graduate School of Medicine
Nagoya, Japan
86: Approach to Renal Replacement Therapy

Ashley B. Irish, MBBS, FRACP
Royal Perth Hospital
University of Western Australia
Perth, Western Australia
63: Myeloma and the Kidney

Bertrand L. Jaber, MD, MS, FASN
Tufts University School of Medicine
St. Elizabeth's Medical Center
Boston, Massachusetts, USA
91: Acute Complications During Hemodialysis

Sunjay Jain, BSc, MBBS, MD, FRCS (Urol)
Spire Leeds Hospital
Leeds, England
59: Urologic Issues for the Nephrologist

David Jayne, MD, FRCP
Addenbrooke's Hospital Cambridge
Cambridge, England
25: Lupus Nephritis

J. Ashley Jefferson, MD, FRCP
University of Washington
Seattle, Washington, USA
66: Pathophysiology and Etiology of Acute Kidney Injury

J. Charles Jennette, MD
University of North Carolina
Chapel Hill, North Carolina, USA
24: Renal and Systemic Vasculitis

Vivekanand Jha, MD, DM, FRCP
Postgraduate Institute of Medical Education and Research
Chandigarh, India
67: Acute Kidney Injury in the Tropics

Richard J. Johnson, MD
University of Colorado, Denver
Aurora, Colorado, USA
16: Introduction to Glomerular Disease: Histologic Classification and Pathogenesis
33: Primary Hypertension
65: Geriatric Nephrology

Nigel S. Kanagasundaram, MB ChB, FRCP(UK), MD
Newcastle Upon Tyne Hospitals NHS Foundation Trust
Tyne and Wear, England
94: Dialytic Therapies for Drug Overdose and Poisoning

John Kanellis, MBBS (hons), PhD, FRACP
Monash Medical Centre
Clayton, Victoria, Australia
98: Evaluation and Preoperative Management of Kidney Transplant Recipient and Donor

S. Ananth Karumanchi, MD
Beth Israel Hospital
Harvard Medical School
Boston, Massachusetts, USA
42: Renal Complications in Normal Pregnancy

Clifford E. Kashtan, MD, FASN
University of Minnesota Medical School
University of Minnesota Amplatz Children's Hospital
Minneapolis, Minnesota, USA
46: Alport's, Fabry's, and Other Familial Glomerular Syndromes

Carol A. Kauffman, MD
University of Michigan Medical School
Ann Arbor, Michigan, USA
53: Fungal Infections of the Urinary Tract

Bisher Kawar, MD
Sheffield Kidney Institute
Sheffield, England
75: Epidemiology and Pathophysiology of Chronic Kidney Disease

Bryan Kestenbaum, MD, MS
University of Washington
Kidney Research Institute
Seattle, Washington, USA
10: Disorders of Calcium, Phosphate, and Magnesium Metabolism

Markus Ketteler, MD
Klinikum Coburg
Coburg, Germany
81: Bone and Mineral Metabolism in Chronic Kidney Disease

Jeffrey Kopp, MD
National Institute of Diabetes and Digestive and Kidney Diseases
National Institutes of Health
Bethesda, Maryland, USA
56: Human Immunodeficiency Virus Infection and the Kidney

Peter Kotanko, MD
Renal Research Institute
New York, New York, USA
89: Hemodialysis: Principles and Techniques
90: Hemodialysis: Outcomes and Adequacy

Wilhelm Kriz, MD
Medical Faculty Mannheim
University of Heidelberg
Heidelberg, Germany
1: Renal Anatomy

Martin K. Kuhlmann, MD
Vivantes Klinikum im Friedrichshain
Berlin, Germany
89: Hemodialysis: Principles and Techniques
90: Hemodialysis: Outcomes and Adequacy

Dirk R. Kuypers, MD, PhD
University Hospitals Leuven
Catholic University
Leuven, Belgium
84: Dermatologic Manifestations of Chronic Kidney Disease

Jonathan R.T. Lakey, PhD, MSM
University of California—Irvine
Irvine, California, USA
106: Pancreas and Islet Transplantation

Estelle V. Lambert, MD
University of Cape Town Sport Science
Institute of South Africa
Cape Town, South Africa
34: Nonpharmacologic Prevention and Treatment of Hypertension

William Lawton, MD
Roy J. and Lucille A. Carver College of Medicine
University of Iowa
Iowa City, Iowa, USA
32: Normal Blood Pressure Control and the Evaluation of Hypertension

Andrew S. Levey, MD
Tufts University School of Medicine
Boston, Massachusetts, USA
3: Assessment of Renal Function

Nathan W. Levin, MD
Renal Research Institute
New York, New York, USA
89: Hemodialysis: Principles and Techniques
90: Hemodialysis: Outcomes and Adequacy

Jeremy Levy, PhD, FRCP
Imperial College Kidney and Transplant Institute
Hammersmith Hospital
Imperial College Healthcare NHS Trust
London, England
95: Plasma Exchange

Andrew Lewington, BSc(Hons), MEd, MD, FRCP
St. James's University Hospital
Leeds, West Yorkshire, England
94: Dialytic Therapies for Drug Overdose and Poisoning

Julia B. Lewis, MD
Vanderbilt University School of Medicine
Nashville, Tennessee, USA
64: Thromboembolic Renovascular Disease

Felix F.K. Li, MD
The University of Hong Kong
Hong Kong, China
72: Hepatorenal Syndrome

Stuart L. Linas, MD
University of Colorado
Denver School of Medicine
Denver, Colorado, USA
9: Disorders of Potassium Metabolism

Friedrich C. Luft, MD, FACP, FRCP (Edin)
Experimental and Clinical Research Center
Berlin, Germany
32: Normal Blood Pressure Control and the Evaluation of Hypertension

Jan C. ter Maaten, MD, PhD
University Medical Center Groningen
Groningen, The Netherlands
49: Sickle Cell Disease

Iain C. Macdougall, BSc, MD, FRCP
King's College Hospital
Denmark Hill, London, England
79: Anemia in Chronic Kidney Disease

Etienne Macedo, MD
University of California—San Diego
San Diego, California, USA
69: Prevention and Nondialytic Management of Acute Kidney Injury

Nicolaos E. Madias, MD
Tufts University School of Medicine
Boston, Massachusetts, USA
14: Respiratory Acidosis, Respiratory Alkalosis, and Mixed Disorders

Colm C. Magee, MD, FRCPI, MPH
Beaumont Hospital
Dublin, Ireland
107: Kidney Disease in Liver, Cardiac, Lung, and Hematopoietic Cell Transplantation

Christopher L. Marsh, MD, FACS
Scripps Clinic and Green Hospital
La Jolla, California, USA
106: Pancreas and Islet Transplantation

Mark R. Marshall, MBChB, MPH(Hons), FRACP
South Auckland Clinical School
University of Auckland
Auckland, New Zealand
70: Dialytic Management of Acute Kidney Injury and Intensive Care Unit Nephrology

Kevin J. Martin, MB, BCh, FACP
Saint Louis University
Saint Louis, Missouri, USA
81: Bone and Mineral Metabolism in Chronic Kidney Disease

Philip D. Mason, BSc, PhD, M, BS, FRCP
Oxford Radcliffe Hospitals NHS Trust
Oxford, England
17: Minimal Change Nephrotic Syndrome

Ranjiv Mathews, MD, FAAP
Johns Hopkins School of Medicine
Brady Urological Institute
Baltimore, Maryland, USA
61: Primary Vesicoureteral Reflux and Reflux Nephropathy

Tej K. Mattoo, MD, DCH, FRCP (UK), FAAP
Wayne State University School of Medicine
Children's Hospital of Michigan
Detroit, Michigan, USA
61: Primary Vesicoureteral Reflux and Reflux Nephropathy

Ravindra L. Mehta, MD, FACP, FASN
University of California—San Diego
San Diego, California USA
69: Prevention and Nondialytic Management of Acute Kidney Injury

Herwig-Ulf Meier-Kriesche, MD
University of Florida
Gainesville, Florida, USA
105: Outcomes of Renal Transplantation

J. Kilian Mellon, MD, FRCS (Urol)
Leicester General Hospital
Leicestershire, England
59: Urologic Issues for the Nephrologist

M. Reza Mirbolooki, MD
University of California—Irvine
Irvine, California, USA
106: Pancreas and Islet Transplantation

Rebeca D. Monk, MD
Strong Memorial Hospital
Rochester, New York, USA
57: Nephrolithiasis and Nephrocalcinosis

Bruno Moulin, MD
Hopital de la Conception
Marseille, France
26: Renal Amyloidosis and Glomerular Diseases with Monoclonal Immunoglobulin Deposition

William R. Mulley, BMed(hons), FRACP, PhD
Monash University
Monash Medical Centre
Clayton, Victoria, Australia
98: Evaluation and Preoperative Management of Kidney Transplant Recipient and Donor

Meguid El Nahas, MD, PhD, FRCP
Sheffield Kidney Institute
Sheffield, England
75: Epidemiology and Pathophysiology of Chronic Kidney Disease

Saraladevi Naicker, MD, PhD
University of the Witwatersrand
Johannesburg, South Africa
56: Human Immunodeficiency Virus Infection and the Kidney

Masaomi Nangaku, MD, PhD
University of Tokyo School of Medicine
Tokyo, Japan
62: Chronic Interstitial Nephritis

Guy H. Neild, MD, FRCP, FRCPath
UCL Centre for Nephrology
Royal Free Campus
London, England
50: Congenital Anomalies of the Kidney and Urinary Tract

M. Gary Nicholls, MD
Christchurch School of Medicine and Health Sciences
Christchurch, New Zealand
39: Endocrine Causes of Hypertension

Michael L. Nicholson, MBBS, BMedSci, MD, FRCS, DSc
Leicester General Hospital
Leicester, England
99: Kidney Transplantation Surgery

Philip J. O'Connell, MBBS, FRACP, PhD
Centre for Transplant and Renal Research
Westmead Hospital
Westmead, Australia
103: Chronic Allograft Nephropathy

W. Charles O'Neill, MD
Emory University
Atlanta, Georgia, USA
88: Diagnostic and Interventional Nephrology

Biff F. Palmer, MD
University of Texas Southwestern Medical Center
Dallas, Texas, USA
11: Normal Acid-Base Balance
12: Metabolic Acidosis

Chirag Parikh, MD, PhD, FACP
Yale University
New Haven, Connecticut, USA
8: Disorders of Water Metabolism

Phuong-Chi T. Pham, MD
David Geffen School of Medicine
University of California Los Angeles
Olive View-University of California Los Angeles Medical Center
Sylmar, California, USA
101: Medical Management of the Kidney Transplant Recipient: Infections and Malignant Neoplasms

Phuong-Thu T. Pham, MD
David Geffen School of Medicine
University of California Los Angeles
Los Angeles, California, USA
101: Medical Management of the Kidney Transplant Recipient: Infections and Malignant Neoplasms
102: Medical Management of the Kidney Transplant Recipient: Cardiovascular Disease and Other Issues

Son V. Pham, MD, FACC
Bay Pines VA Medical Center
Bay Pines, Florida, USA
102: Medical Management of the Kidney Transplant Recipient: Cardiovascular Disease and Other Issues

Richard G. Phelps, MA, MB BChir, PhD, FRCP
Queen's Medical Research Institute
Edinburgh, Lothian, Great Britain
23: Antiglomerular Basement Membrane Disease and Goodpasture's Disease

Raimund Pichler, MD
University of Washington
Seattle, Washington, USA
65: Geriatric Nephrology

Tiina Podymow, MD
McGill University
Royal Victoria Hospital
Montreal, Quebec, Canada
42: Renal Complications in Normal Pregnancy

Wolfgang Pommer, MD
Vivantes Humboldt Klinikum
Berlin, Germany
31: Management of the Diabetic Patient with Chronic Kidney Disease

Charles D. Pusey, DSc, FRCP, FRCPath, FMedSci
Imperial College London
London, England
95: Plasma Exchange

Hamid Rabb, MD
Johns Hopkins University School of Medicine
Baltimore, Maryland, USA
96: Immunological Principles in Kidney Transplantation
97: Immunosuppresive Medications in Kidney Transplantation

Brian Rayner, MBChB, FCP, Mmed
Groote Schuur Hospital
University of Cape Town
Cape Town, South Africa
34: Nonpharmacologic Prevention and Treatment of Hypertension

Hugh C. Rayner, MD, FRCP, DipMedEd
Heart of England NHS Foundation Trust
Bordesley Green East
Birmingham, West Midlands, Great Britain
86: Approach to Renal Replacement Therapy

Giuseppe Remuzzi, MD, FRCP
Mario Negri Institute for Pharmacological Research
S. and T. Park Kilometro Rosso, Via Stezzano
Bergamo, Italy
28: Thrombotic Microangiopathies, Including Hemolytic Uremic Syndrome

A. Mark Richards, MBChB, MD, PhD, DSc
University of Otago, Christchurch
Christchurch, Canterbury, New Zealand
39: Endocrine Causes of Hypertension

Bengt Rippe, MD, PhD
University Hospital of Lund
Lund, Skane, Sweden
92: Peritoneal Dialysis: Principles, Techniques, and Adequacy

Eberhard Ritz, MD
Ruperto Carola University Heidelberg
Heidelberg, Germany
29: Pathogenesis, Clinical Manifestations, and Natural History of Diabetic Nephropathy

R. Paul Robertson, MD
University of Washington
Seattle, Washington, USA
106: Pancreas and Islet Transplantation

Bernardo Rodriguez-Iturbe, MD
Hospital Universitario de Maracaibo
Universidad del Zulia
Maracaibo, Zulia, Venezuela
33: Primary Hypertension
55: Glomerular Diseases Associated with Infection

Claudio Ronco, MD
St. Bortolo Hospital
Vicenza, Italy
71: Ultrafiltration Therapy for Refractory Heart Failure

Pierre M. Ronco, MD, PhD
Tenon Hospital
Université Pierre et Marie Curie
Paris, France
26: Renal Amyloidosis and Glomerular Diseases with Monoclonal Immunoglobulin Deposition

Edward A. Ross, MD
University of Florida
Gainesville, Florida, USA
71: Ultrafiltration Therapy for Refractory Heart Failure

Jerome A. Rossert, MD, PhD
Amgen
Thousand Oaks, California, USA
60: Acute Interstitial Nephritis

Piero Ruggenenti, MD
di Bergamo, Largo Barozzi
Bergamo, Italy
28: Thrombotic Microangiopathies, Including Hemolytic Uremic Syndrome

Sean Ruland, DO
University of Illinois at Chicago
Chicago, Illinois, USA
40: Neurogenic Hypertension, Including Hypertension Associated with Stroke or Spinal Cord Injury

Graeme R. Russ, MBBS, FRACP, PhD
Royal Adelaide Hospital
Adelaide, South Australia, Australia
73: Principles of Drug Therapy, Dosing, and Prescribing in Chronic Kidney Disease and Renal Replacement Therapy

Martin A. Samuels, MD, DSc(hon), FAAN, MACP, FRCP
Brigham and Women's Hospital
Harvard Medical School
Boston, Massachusetts, USA
82: Neurologic Complications of Chronic Kidney Disease

Pantelis A. Sarafidis, MD, MSc, PhD
AHEPA University Hospital
Thessaloniki, Greece
36: Evaluation and Treatment of Hypertensive Urgencies and Emergencies

F. Paolo Schena, MD
University of Bari
Bari, Italy
21: Membranoproliferative Glomerulonephritis, Dense Deposit Disease, and Cryoglobulinemic Glomerulonephritis

Jesse D. Schold, PhD
Cleveland Clinic
Cleveland, Ohio, USA
105: Outcomes of Renal Transplantation

Robert W. Schrier, MD
University of Colorado, Denver
Aurora, Colorado, USA
7: Disorders of Extracellular Volume
66: Pathophysiology and Etiology of Acute Kidney Injury

Victor F. Seabra, MD
St. Elizabeth's Medical Center
Boston, Massachusetts, USA
91: Acute Complications During Hemodialysis

Mark S. Segal, MD, PhD
University of Florida
Gainesville, Florida, USA
74: Herbal and Over-the-Counter Medicines and the Kidney

Julian Lawrence Seifter, MD
Brigham and Women's Hospital
Boston, Massachusetts, USA
82: Neurologic Complications of Chronic Kidney Disease

Shani Shastri, MD
Tufts University School of Medicine
Boston, Massachusetts, USA
3: Assessment of Renal Function

David G. Shirley, BSc, PhD
University College London Medical School
Royal Free Hospital
London, England
2: Renal Physiology

Visith Sitprija, MD, PhD
Queen Saovabha Memorial Institute
Bangkok, Thailand
67: Acute Kidney Injury in the Tropics

Titte R. Srinivas, MB, BS, MD
Cleveland Clinic
Cleveland, Ohio, USA
105: Outcomes of Renal Transplantation

Peter Stenvinkel, MD, PhD
Karolinska University Hospital at Huddinge Stockholm
Stockholm, Sweden
78: Cardiovascular Disease in Chronic Kidney Disease

Lesley A. Stevens, MD, MS
Tufts University School of Medicine
Boston, Massachusetts, USA
3: Assessment of Renal Function

Stephen C. Textor, MD
Mayo Clinic
Rochester, Minnesota, USA
37: Renovascular Hypertension and Ischemic Renal Disease

Joshua M. Thurman, MD
University of Colorado, Denver
Aurora, Colorado, USA
66: Pathophysiology and Etiology of Acute Kidney Injury

Li-Li Tong, MD
Harbor-University of California Medical Center
Torrance, California, USA
30: Prevention and Treatment of Diabetic Nephropathy

Peter S. Topham, MD, FRCP
Leicester General Hospital
Leicester, England
6: Renal Biopsy

Jan H.M. Tordoir, MD, PhD
Maastricht University Medical Center
Maastricht, The Netherlands
87: Vascular Access for Dialytic Therapies

Vicente E. Torres, MD, PhD
Mayo Clinic
Rochester, Minnesota, USA
44: Autosomal Dominant Polycystic Kidney Disease

Dace Trence, MD, FACE
University of Washington
Seattle, Washington, USA
31: Management of the Diabetic Patient with Chronic Kidney Disease

A. Neil Turner, PhD, FRCP
Queens Medical Research Institute
Little France Edinburgh, Scotland
23: Antiglomerular Basement Membrane Disease and Goodpasture's Disease

Robert J. Unwin, BM, PhD, FRCP, FSB
University College London Medical School
Royal Free Hospital, Hampstead
London, England
2: Renal Physiology

Henri Vacher-Coponat, MD
Hopital de la Conception
Marseille, France
104: Recurrent Disease in Kidney Transplantation

R. Kasi Visweswaran, MD, DM
Ananthapuri Hospitals and Research Institute
Trivandrum, Kerala, India
52: Tuberculosis of the Urinary Tract

Haimanot Wasse, MD, MPH
Emory University School of Medicine
Atlanta, Georgia, USA
88: Diagnostic and Interventional Nephrology

Moses D. Wavamunno, MD, PhD, FRACP
Westmead Hospital
Sydney, New South Wales, Australia
103: Chronic Allograft Nephropathy

I. David Weiner, MD
University of Florida College of Medicine
Gainesville, Florida, USA
9: Disorders of Potassium Metabolism
38: Endocrine Causes of Hypertension—Aldosterone

David C. Wheeler, MD, FRCP
University College London Medical School
London, England
77: Clinical Evaluation and Management of Chronic Kidney Disease

Bryan Williams, MD, FRCP, FAHA, FESC
University of Leicester
Glenfield Hospital
Leicester, England
35: Pharmacologic Treatment of Hypertension

John D. Williams, MD
Cardiff University
Heath Park
Cardiff, Wales
93: Complications of Peritoneal Dialysis

Charles S. Wingo, MD
University of Florida
Gainesville, Florida, USA
9: Disorders of Potassium Metabolism
38: Endocrine Causes of Hypertension—Aldosterone

Michelle Winn, MD
Duke University Medical Center
Durham, North Carolina, USA
19: Inherited Causes of Nephrotic Syndrome

Alexander C. Wiseman, MD
University of Colorado, Denver
Health Sciences Center
Aurora, Colorado, USA
100: Prophylaxis and Treatment of Kidney Transplant Rejection

Gunter Wolf, MD
University of Jena
Jena, Germany
29: Pathogenesis, Clinical Manifestations, and Natural History of Diabetic Nephropathy

Karl Womer, MD
Johns Hopkins University School of Medicine
Baltimore, Maryland, USA
96: Immunological Principles in Kidney Transplantation
97: Immunosuppresive Medications in Kidney Transplantation

Graham Woodrow, MBChB, MD, FRCP
St. James's University Hospital
Leeds, West Yorkshire, England
83: Gastroenterology and Nutrition in Chronic Kidney Disease

David C. Wymer, MD, FACR, FACNM
Randall Malcom VA Medical Center
University of Florida
Gainesville, Florida, USA
5: Imaging

Li Yang, MD
Peking University First Hospital
Beijing, People's Republic of China
68: Diagnosis and Clinical Evaluation of Acute Kidney Injury

Xueqing Yu, MD, PhD
First Affiliated Hospital
Sun Yat-Sen University
Guangzhou, Guangdong, China
74: Herbal and Over-the-Counter Medicines and the Kidney

PREFACE

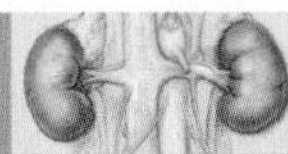

In the fourth edition of *Comprehensive Clinical Nephrology*, we continue to offer a text for fellows, practicing nephrologists, and internists that covers all aspects of the clinical work of the nephrologist, including fluid and electrolytes, hypertension, diabetes, dialysis, and transplantation. We recognize that this single volume does not compete with multivolume, highly referenced texts, and it remains our goal to provide "comprehensive" coverage of clinical nephrology yet also ensure that inquiring nephrologists can find the scientific issues and pathophysiology that underlie their clinical work.

For this edition all chapters have been extensively revised and updated in response to the advice and comments that we have received from many readers and colleagues. New features of the fourth edition include a chapter on inherited causes of nephrotic syndrome, an extended section on diabetic nephropathy, a revised section on infectious diseases and the kidney, a revised and extended section on acute kidney injury, a chapter on herbal and over-the-counter medicines and the kidney, and an extended section on medical management of the kidney transplant recipient.

By popular demand we continue to offer readers access to the images from the book that we are pleased to see used in lectures and seminars in many parts of the world.

This is the first edition that features access to a companion Expert Consult website, with fully searchable text, a downloadable image library, and links to PubMed.

JÜRGEN FLOEGE
RICHARD J. JOHNSON
JOHN FEEHALLY

CONTENTS

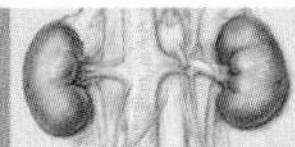

Section X: Urologic Disorders

Section XI: Tubulointerstitial and Vascular Diseases

Section XII: Geriatric Nephrology

Section XIII: Acute Kidney Injury

Section XIV: Drug Therapy in Kidney Disease

Section XV: Chronic Kidney Disease and the Uremic Syndrome

Section XVI: Dialytic Therapies

Section XVII: Transplantation

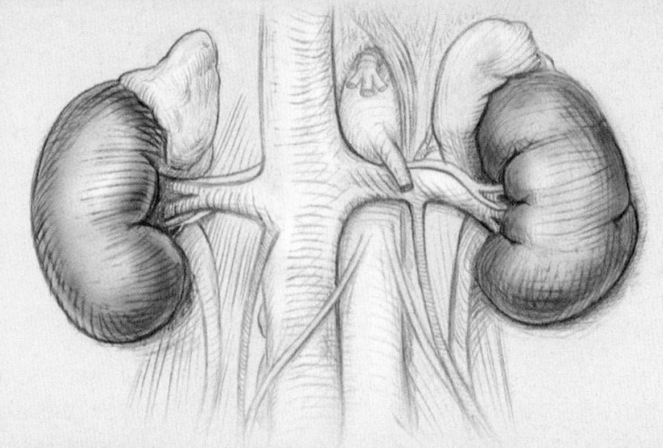

SECTION I

Essential Renal Anatomy and Physiology

CHAPTER 1

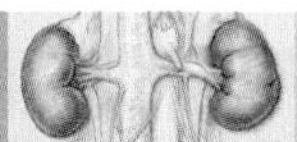

Renal Anatomy

Wilhelm Kriz, Marlies Elger

The complex structure of the mammalian kidney is best understood in the unipapillary form that is common to all small species. Figure 1.1 is a schematic coronal section through such a kidney with a cortex enclosing a pyramid-shaped medulla, the tip of which protrudes into the renal pelvis. The medulla is divided into an outer and an inner medulla; the outer medulla is further subdivided into an outer and an inner stripe.

STRUCTURE OF THE KIDNEY

The specific components of the kidney are the nephrons, the collecting ducts, and a unique microvasculature.[1] The multipapillary kidney of humans contains roughly one million nephrons; however, the number is quite variable. This number is already established during prenatal development; after birth, new nephrons cannot be developed, and a lost nephron cannot be replaced.

Nephrons

A nephron consists of a renal corpuscle (glomerulus) connected to a complicated and twisted tubule that finally drains into a collecting duct (Figs. 1.2 and 1.3). By the location of renal corpuscles within the cortex, three types of nephron can be distinguished: superficial, midcortical, and juxtamedullary nephrons. The tubular part of the nephron consists of a proximal tubule and a distal tubule connected by Henle's loop[2] (see later discussion). There are two types of nephron, those with long Henle's loops and those with short loops. Short loops turn back in the outer medulla or even in the cortex (cortical loops). Long loops turn back at successive levels of the inner medulla.

Collecting Ducts

A collecting duct is formed in the renal cortex when several nephrons join. A connecting tubule (CNT) is interposed between a nephron and a cortical collecting duct. Cortical collecting ducts descend within the medullary rays of the cortex. They traverse the outer medulla as unbranched tubes. On entering the inner medulla, they fuse successively and open finally as papillary ducts into the renal pelvis (see Figs. 1.2 and 1.3).

Microvasculature

The microvascular pattern of the kidney (Fig. 1.4; see also Fig. 1.1) is also similarly organized in mammalian species.[1,3] The renal artery, after entering the renal sinus, finally divides into the interlobar arteries, which extend toward the cortex in the space between the wall of the pelvis (or calyx) and the adjacent cortical tissue. At the junction between cortex and medulla, they divide and pass over into the arcuate arteries, which also branch. They give rise to the cortical radial arteries (interlobular arteries) that ascend radially through the cortex. No arteries penetrate the medulla.

Afferent arterioles generally arise from cortical radial arteries; they supply the glomerular tufts. Aglomerular tributaries to the capillary plexus are rarely found. As a result, the blood supply of the peritubular capillaries of the cortex and the medulla is exclusively postglomerular. Glomeruli are drained by efferent arterioles. Two basic types can be distinguished: cortical and juxtamedullary efferent arterioles. Cortical efferent arterioles, which derive from superficial and midcortical glomeruli, supply the capillary plexus of the cortex.

The efferent arterioles of juxtamedullary glomeruli represent the supplying vessels of the renal medulla. Within the outer stripe of the medulla, they divide into the descending vasa recta and then penetrate the inner stripe in cone-shaped vascular bundles. At intervals, individual vessels leave the bundles to supply the capillary plexus at the adjacent medullary level.

Ascending vasa recta drain the renal medulla. In the inner medulla, they arise at every level, ascending as unbranched vessels. They traverse the inner stripe within the vascular bundles. The ascending vasa recta that drain the inner stripe may either join the vascular bundles or ascend directly to the outer stripe between the bundles. All the ascending vasa recta traverse the outer stripe as individual wavy vessels with wide lumina interspersed among the tubules. Because true capillaries derived from direct branches of efferent arterioles are relatively scarce, it is the ascending vasa recta that form the capillary plexus of the outer stripe. Finally, the ascending vasa recta empty into arcuate veins.

The vascular bundles represent a countercurrent exchanger between the blood entering and that leaving the medulla. In addition, the organization of the vascular bundles results in a separation of the blood flow to the inner stripe from that to the inner medulla. Descending vasa recta supplying the inner medulla traverse the inner stripe within the vascular bundles. Therefore, blood flowing to the inner medulla has not been exposed previously to tubules of the inner or outer stripe. All ascending vasa recta originating from the inner medulla traverse the inner stripe within the vascular bundles; thus, blood that has perfused tubules of the inner medulla does not subsequently perfuse tubules of the inner stripe. However, the blood returning from either the inner medulla or the inner stripe afterward does perfuse the tubules of the outer stripe. It has been suggested that this arrangement in the outer stripe functions as the ultimate trap to prevent solute loss from the medulla.

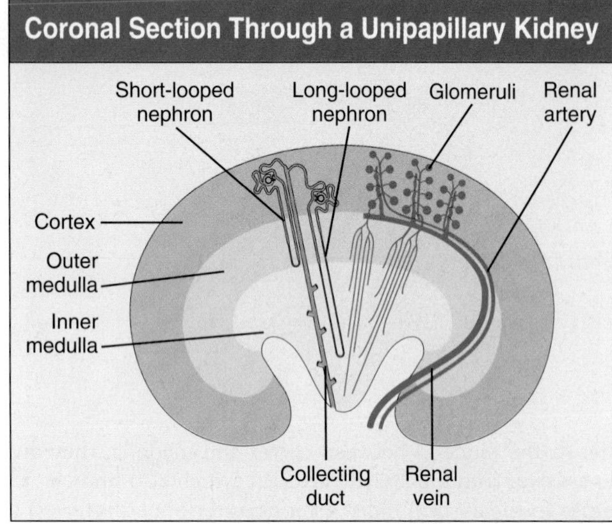

Figure 1.1 Coronal section through a unipapillary kidney.

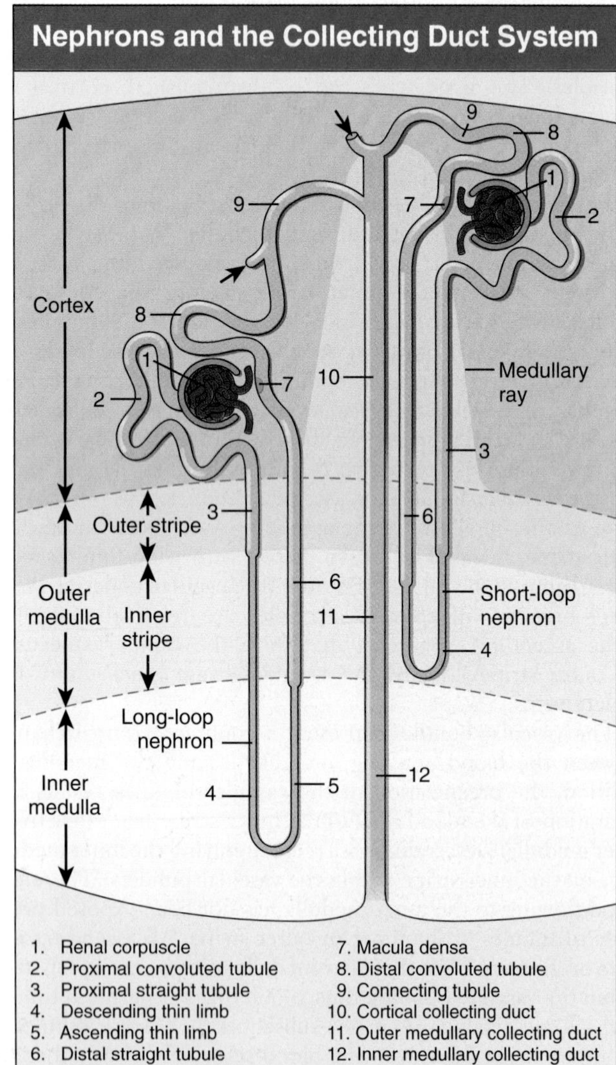

Figure 1.2 Nephrons and the collecting duct system. Shown are short-looped and long-looped nephrons, together with a collecting duct (not drawn to scale). *Arrows* denote confluence of further nephrons.

Subdivisions of the Nephron and Collecting Duct System

Section	Subsections
Nephron	
Renal corpuscle	Glomerulus: the term used most frequently to refer to the entire renal corpuscle Bowman's capsule
Proximal tubule	Convoluted part Straight part (pars recta) or thick descending limb of Henle's loop
Intermediate tubule	Descending part or thin descending limb of Henle's loop Ascending part or thin ascending limb of Henle's loop
Distal tubule	Straight part or thick ascending limb of Henle's loop: subdivided into a medullary and a cortical part; the latter contains in its terminal portion the macula densa Convoluted part
Collecting duct system	
Connecting tubule	Includes the arcades in most species
Collecting duct	Cortical collecting duct Outer medullary collecting duct subdivided into an outer and an inner stripe portion Inner medullary collecting duct subdivided into basal, middle, and papillary portions

Figure 1.3 Subdivisions of the nephron and collecting duct system.

The intrarenal veins accompany the arteries. Central to the renal drainage of the kidney are the arcuate veins, which, in contrast to arcuate arteries, do form real anastomosing arches at the corticomedullary border. They accept the veins from the cortex and the renal medulla. The arcuate veins join to form interlobar veins, which run alongside the corresponding arteries.

The intrarenal arteries and the afferent and efferent arterioles are accompanied by sympathetic nerve fibers and terminal axons representing the efferent nerves of the kidney.[1] Tubules have direct contact to terminal axons only when they are located around the arteries or the arterioles. As stated by Barajas,[4] "the tubular innervation consists of occasional fibers adjacent to perivascular tubules." The density of nerve contacts to convoluted proximal tubules is low; contacts to straight proximal tubules, thick ascending loops of the limbs of Henle, and collecting ducts (located in the medullary rays and the outer medulla) have never been encountered. The vast majority of tubular portions have no direct relationships to nerve terminals. Afferent nerves of the kidney are commonly believed to be sparse.[5]

NEPHRON

Renal Glomerulus (Renal Corpuscle)

The glomerulus comprises a tuft of specialized capillaries attached to the mesangium, both of which are enclosed in a pouch-like extension of the tubule, that is, Bowman's capsule (Figs. 1.5 and 1.6). The capillaries together with the mesangium

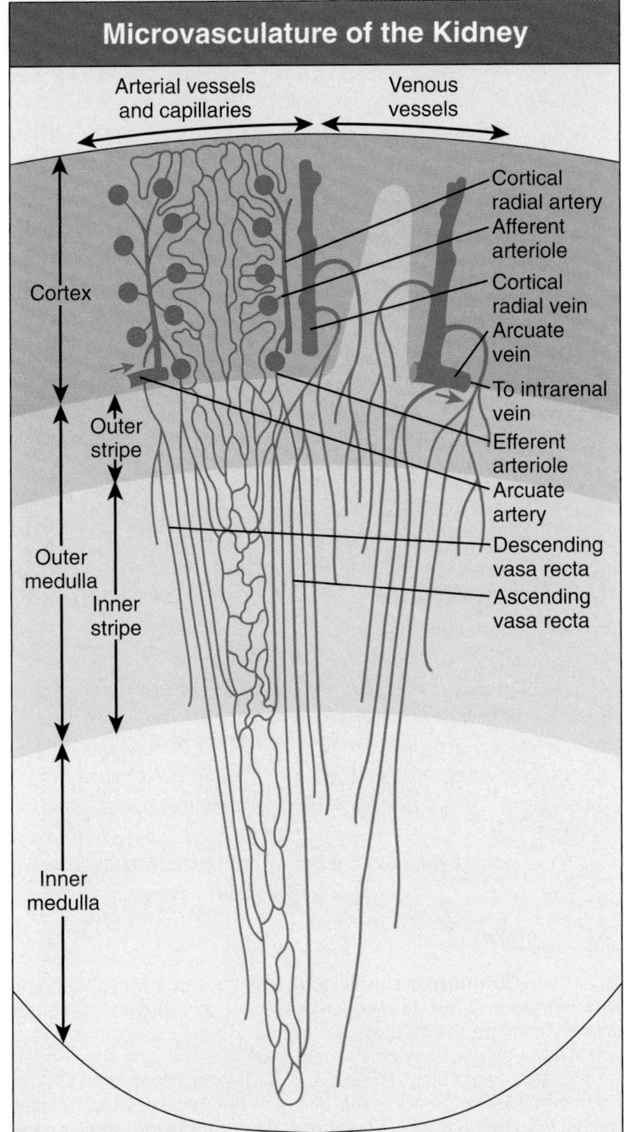

Figure 1.4 Microvasculature of the kidney. Afferent arterioles supply the glomeruli and efferent arterioles leave the glomeruli and divide into the descending vasa recta, which together with the ascending vasa recta form the vascular bundles of the renal medulla. The vasa recta ascending from the inner medulla all traverse the inner stripe within the vascular bundles, whereas most of the vasa recta from the inner stripe of the outer medulla ascend outside the bundles. Both types traverse the outer stripe as wide, tortuous channels.

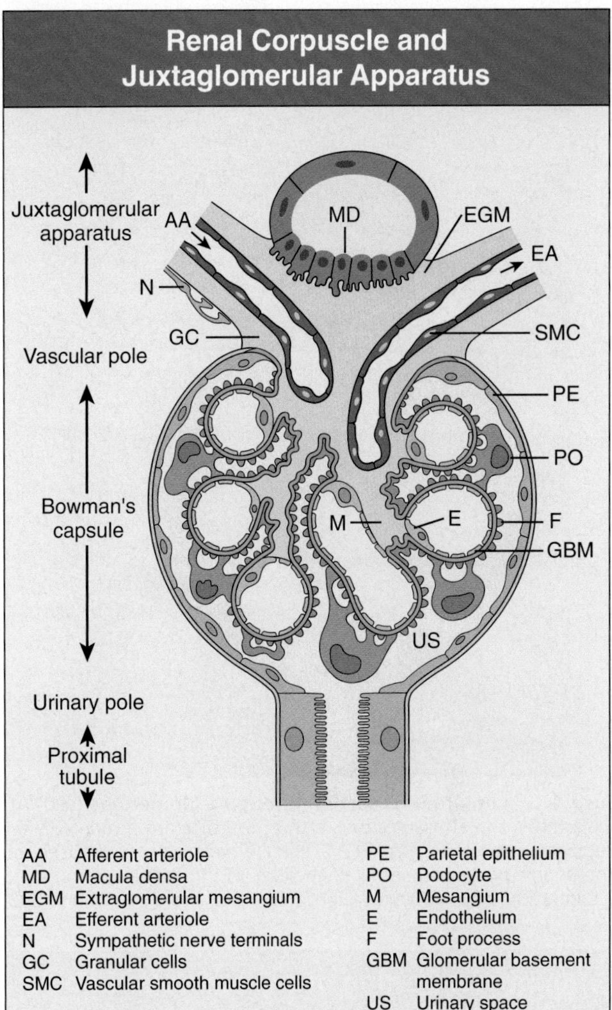

Figure 1.5 Renal corpuscle and juxtaglomerular apparatus. *(Modified with permission from reference 1.)*

are covered by epithelial cells (podocytes) forming the visceral epithelium of Bowman's capsule. At the vascular pole, this is reflected to become the parietal epithelium of Bowman's capsule. At the interface between the glomerular capillaries and the mesangium on one side and the podocyte layer on the other side, the glomerular basement membrane (GBM) is developed. The space between both layers of Bowman's capsule represents the urinary space, which at the urinary pole continues as the tubule lumen.

On entering the tuft, the afferent arteriole immediately divides into several (two to five) primary capillary branches, each of which gives rise to an anastomosing capillary network representing a glomerular lobule. In contrast to the afferent arteriole, the efferent arteriole is already established inside the tuft by confluence of capillaries from each lobule.[6] Thus, the efferent arteriole has a significant intraglomerular segment located within the glomerular stalk.

Glomerular capillaries are a unique type of blood vessel made up of nothing but an endothelial tube (Figs. 1.7 and 1.8). A small stripe of the outer aspect of this tube directly abuts the mesangium; a major part bulges toward the urinary space and is covered by the GBM and the podocyte layer. This peripheral portion of the capillary wall represents the filtration area. The glomerular mesangium represents the axis of a glomerular lobule to which the glomerular capillaries are attached.

Glomerular Basement Membrane

The GBM serves as the skeleton of the glomerular tuft. It represents a complexly folded sack with an opening at the glomerular hilum (see Fig. 1.5). The outer aspect of this GBM sack is completely covered with podocytes. The interior of the sack is filled with the capillaries and the mesangium. As a result, on its inner aspect, the GBM is in touch either with capillaries or with the mesangium. At any transition between these two locations, the GBM changes from a convex pericapillary to a concave perimesangial course; the turning points are called mesangial angles.

In electron micrographs of traditionally fixed tissue, the GBM appears as a trilaminar structure made up of a lamina densa

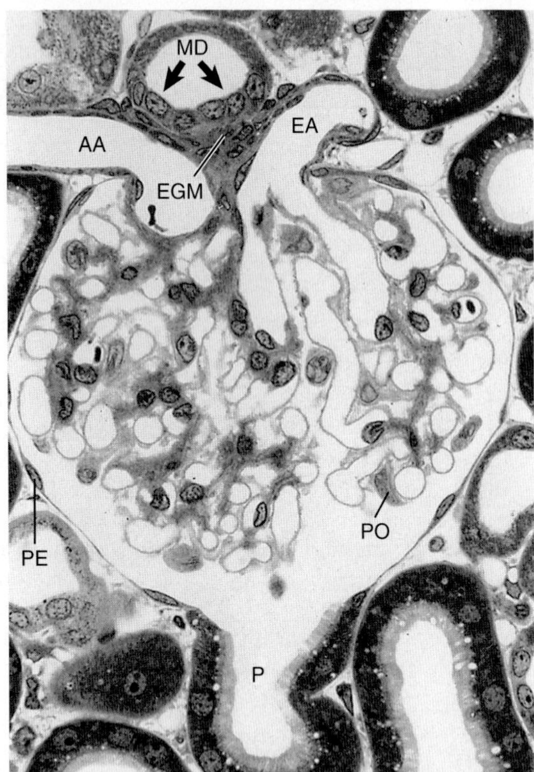

Figure 1.6 Longitudinal section through a glomerulus (rat). At the vascular pole, the afferent arteriole (AA), the efferent arteriole (EA), the extraglomerular mesangium (EGM), and the macula densa (MD) are seen. At the urinary pole, the parietal epithelium (PE) transforms into the proximal tubule (P). PO, podocyte. (Light microscopy; magnification ×390.)

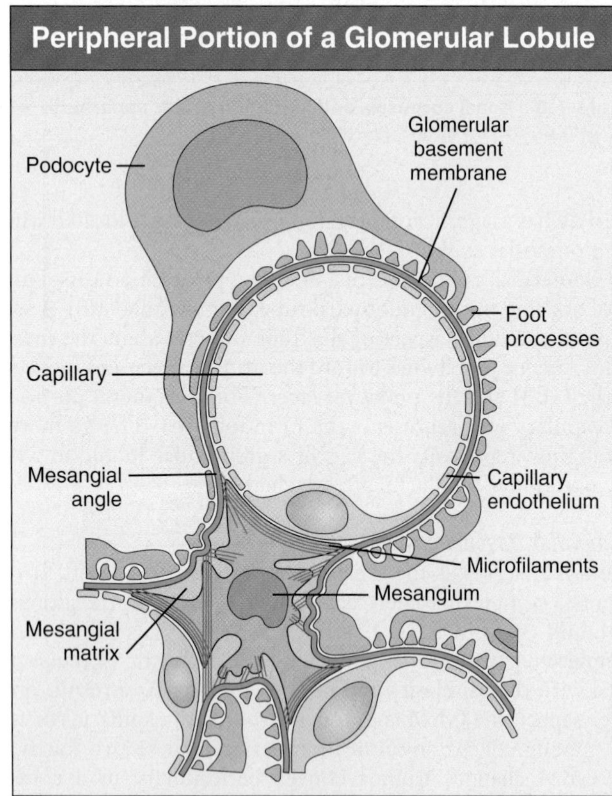

Figure 1.7 Peripheral portion of a glomerular lobule. This shows a capillary, the axial position of the mesangium, and the visceral epithelium (podocytes). At the capillary-mesangial interface, the capillary endothelium directly abuts the mesangium.

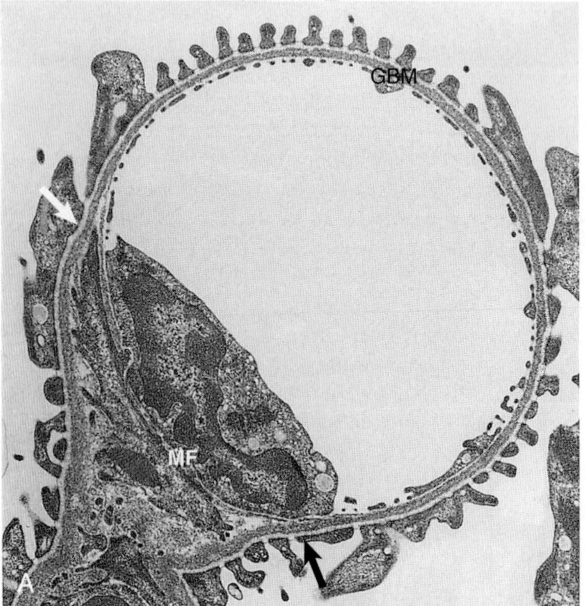

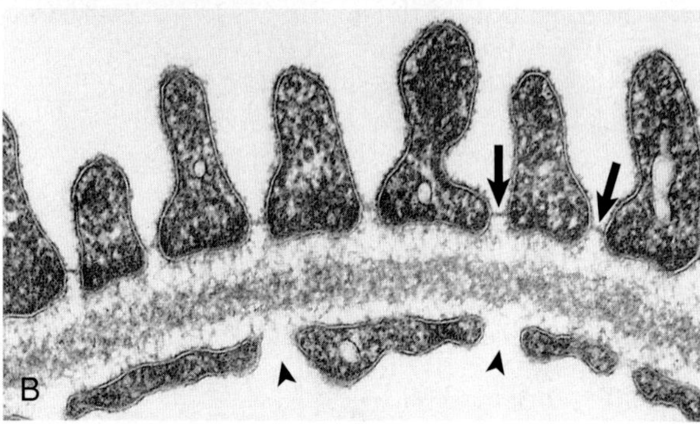

Figure 1.8 Glomerular capillary. A, The layer of interdigitating podocyte processes and the glomerular basement membrane (GBM) do not completely encircle the capillary. At the mesangial angles *(arrows)*, both deviate from a pericapillary course and cover the mesangium. Mesangial cell processes, containing dense bundles of microfilaments (MF), interconnect the GBM and bridge the distance between the two mesangial angles. **B,** Filtration barrier. The peripheral part of the glomerular capillary wall comprises the endothelium with open pores *(arrowheads)*, the GBM, and the interdigitating foot processes. The GBM shows a lamina densa bounded by the lamina rara interna and externa. The foot processes are separated by filtration slits bridged by thin diaphragms *(arrows)*. (Transmission electron microscopy; magnification: **A,** ×8770; **B,** ×50,440.)

bounded by two less dense layers: the lamina rara interna and externa (see Fig. 1.8). Studies using freeze techniques reveal only one thick dense layer directly attached to the bases of the epithelium and endothelium.[7]

The major components of the GBM include type IV collagen, laminin, and heparan sulfate proteoglycans, as in basement membranes at other sites. Types V and VI collagen and nidogen have also been demonstrated. However, the GBM has several unique properties, notably a distinct spectrum of type IV collagen and laminin isoforms. The mature GBM is made up of type IV collagen consisting of α3, α4, and α5 chains (instead of α1 and α2 chains of most other basement membranes) and of laminin 11 consisting of α5, β2, and γ1 chains.[8] Type IV collagen is the antigenic target in Goodpasture's disease (see Chapter 23), and mutations in the genes of the α3, α4, and α5 chains of type IV collagen are responsible for Alport's syndrome (see Chapter 46).

Current models depict the basic structure of the basement membrane as a three-dimensional network of type IV collagen.[7] The type IV collagen monomer consists of a triple helix of length 400 nm that has a large noncollagenous globular domain at its C-terminal end called NC1. At the N terminus, the helix possesses a triple helical rod of length 60 nm: the 7S domain. Interactions between the 7S domains of two triple helices or the NC1 domains of four triple helices allow type IV collagen monomers to form dimers and tetramers. In addition, triple helical strands interconnect by lateral associations through binding of NC1 domains to sites along the collagenous region. This network is complemented by an interconnected network of laminin 11, resulting in a flexible, nonfibrillar polygonal assembly that is considered to provide mechanical strength to the basement membrane and to serve as a scaffold for alignment of other matrix components.

The electronegative charge of the GBM mainly results from the presence of polyanionic proteoglycans. The major proteoglycans of the GBM are heparan sulfate proteoglycans, among them perlecan and agrin. Proteoglycan molecules aggregate to form a meshwork that is kept highly hydrated by water molecules trapped in the interstices of the matrix.

Mesangium

Three major cell types occur within the glomerular tuft, all of which are in close contact with the GBM: mesangial cells, endothelial cells, and podocytes. In the rat, the numerical ratio has been calculated to be 2:3:1. The mesangial cells together with the mesangial matrix establish the glomerular mesangium. In addition, some studies suggest that macrophages bearing HLA-DR/Ia-like antigens may also rarely be found in the normal mesangium.

Mesangial Cells Mesangial cells are quite irregular in shape with many processes extending from the cell body toward the GBM (see Figs. 1.7 and 1.8). In these processes, dense assemblies of microfilaments are found that contain actin, myosin, and α-actinin.[9] The processes are attached to the GBM either directly or through the interposition of microfibrils (see later discussion). The GBM represents the effector structure of mesangial contractility. Mesangial cell–GBM connections are especially prominent alongside the capillaries, interconnecting the two opposing mesangial angles of the GBM.

Mesangial Matrix The mesangial matrix fills the highly irregular spaces between the mesangial cells and the perimesangial GBM, anchoring the mesangial cells to the GBM.[6] The ultrastructural organization of this matrix is incompletely understood. In specimens prepared by a technique that avoids osmium tetroxide and uses tannic acid for staining, a dense network of elastic microfibrils is seen. A large number of common extracellular matrix proteins have been demonstrated within the mesangial matrix, including several types of collagens (IV, V, and VI) and several components of microfibrillar proteins (fibrillin and the 31-kd microfibril-associated glycoprotein). The matrix also contains several glycoproteins (fibronectin is most abundant) as well as several types of proteoglycans.

Endothelium

Glomerular endothelial cells consist of cell bodies and peripherally located, attenuated, and highly fenestrated cytoplasmic sheets (see Figs. 1.7 and 1.8). Glomerular endothelial pores lack diaphragms, which are encountered only in the endothelium of the final tributaries to the efferent arteriole.[6] The round to oval pores have a diameter of 50 to 100 nm. The luminal membrane of endothelial cells is negatively charged because of its cell coat of several polyanionic glycoproteins, including podocalyxin. In addition, the endothelial pores are filled with sieve plugs mainly made up of sialoglycoproteins.[10]

Visceral Epithelium (Podocytes)

The visceral epithelium of Bowman's capsule comprises highly differentiated cells, the podocytes (Fig. 1.9; see also Fig. 1.7). In the developing glomerulus, podocytes have a simple polygonal shape. In rats, mitotic activity of these cells is completed soon after birth together with the cessation of the formation of new nephron anlagen. In humans, this point is already reached during prenatal life. The differentiation of the adult podocyte phenotype with the characteristic cell process pattern (see later discussion) is associated with the appearance of several podocyte-specific proteins, including podocalyxin, nephrin, podocin, synaptopodin, and GLEPP1.[11,12] Differentiated podocytes are unable to replicate; therefore, in the adult, degenerated podocytes cannot be replaced. In response to an extreme mitogenic stimulation (e.g., by basic fibroblast growth factor 2), these cells may undergo mitotic nuclear division; however, the cells are unable to complete cell division, resulting in binucleated or multinucleated cells.[12]

Podocytes have a voluminous cell body that floats within the urinary space. The cell bodies give rise to long primary processes that extend toward the capillaries, to which they affix by their most distal portions and by an extensive array of foot processes.

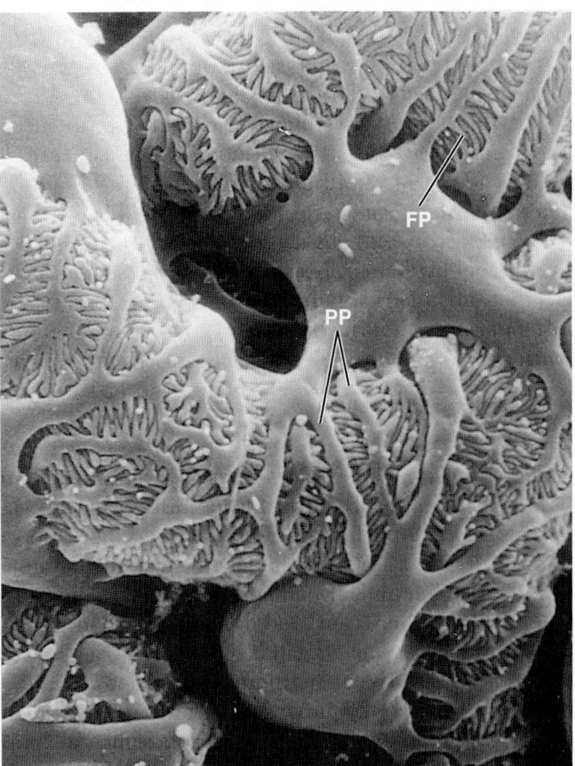

Figure 1.9 Glomerular capillaries in the rat. The urinary side of the capillary is covered by the highly branched podocytes. The interdigitating system of primary processes (PP) and foot processes (FP) lines the entire surface of the tuft, extending also beneath the cell bodies. The foot processes of neighboring cells interdigitate but spare the filtration slits in between. (Scanning electron microscopy; magnification ×2200.)

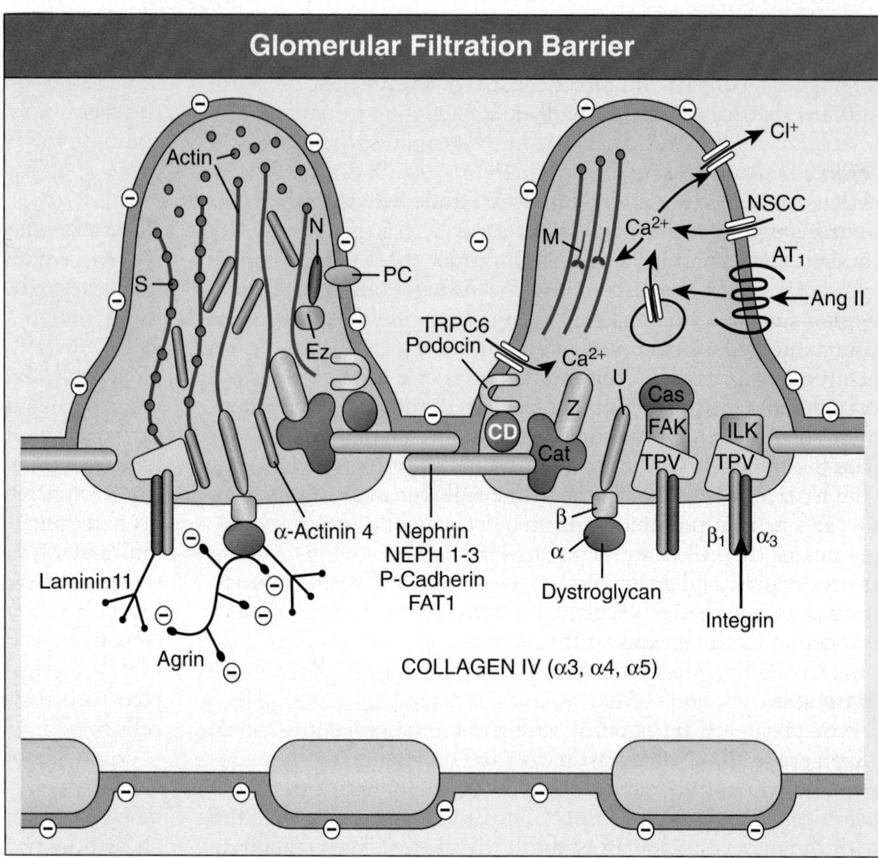

Figure 1.10 Glomerular filtration barrier. Two podocyte foot processes bridged by the slit membrane, the GBM, and the porous capillary endothelium are shown. The surfaces of podocytes and of the endothelium are covered by a negatively charged glycocalyx containing the sialoprotein podocalyxin (PC). The GBM is mainly composed of type IV collagen (α3, α4, and α5), laminin 11 (α5, β2, and γ1 chains), and the heparan sulfate proteoglycan agrin. The slit membrane represents a porous proteinaceous membrane composed of (as far as known) nephrin, NEPH1-3, P-cadherin, and FAT1. The actin-based cytoskeleton of the foot processes connects to both the GBM and the slit membrane. Regarding the connections to the GBM, $\beta_1\alpha_3$ integrin dimers specifically interconnect the TVP complex (talin, paxillin, vinculin) to laminin 11; the β- and α-dystroglycans interconnect utrophin to agrin. The slit membrane proteins are joined to the cytoskeleton by various adaptor proteins, including podocin, zonula occludens protein 1 (ZO-1; Z), CD2-associated protein (CD), and catenins (Cat). Among the nonselective cation channels (NSCC), TRPC6 associates with podocin (and nephrin, not shown) at the slit membrane. Only the angiotensin II (Ang II) type 1 receptor (AT_1) is shown as an example of the many surface receptors. Additional abbreviations: Cas, p130Cas; Ez, ezrin; FAK, focal adhesion kinase; ILK, integrin-linked kinase; M, myosin; N, NHERF2 (Na^+-H^+ exchanger regulatory factor); S, synaptopodin. *(Modified from reference 11.)*

The foot processes of neighboring podocytes regularly interdigitate with each other, leaving between them meandering slits (filtration slits) that are bridged by an extracellular structure, the slit diaphragm (Fig. 1.10; see also Figs. 1.7 to 1.9). Podocytes are polarized epithelial cells with a luminal and a basal cell membrane domain; the basal cell membrane domain corresponds to the sole plates of the foot processes that are embedded into the GBM. The border between basal and luminal membrane is represented by the slit diaphragm.[13]

The luminal membrane and the slit diaphragm are covered by a thick surface coat that is rich in sialoglycoproteins (including podocalyxin and podoendin) and is responsible for the high negative surface charge of the podocytes. By comparison, the abluminal membrane (i.e., the soles of podocyte processes) contains specific transmembrane proteins that connect the cytoskeleton to the GBM. Two systems are known; first, $\alpha_3\beta_1$ integrin dimers, which interconnect the cytoplasmic focal adhesion proteins vinculin, paxillin, and talin with the α3, α4, and α5 chains of type IV collagen; and second, β-α-dystroglycans, which interconnect the cytoplasmic adapter protein utrophin with agrin and laminin α5 chains in the GBM.[11] In addition, a subpodocyte space has also been recognized that can be altered by changes in ultrafiltration pressure and might theoretically be involved in the regulation of glomerular filtration.[12] Other membrane proteins, such as the C3b receptor and gp330/megalin, are present over the entire surface of podocytes.[13]

In contrast to the cell body (harboring a prominent Golgi system), the cell processes contain only a few organelles. A well-developed cytoskeleton accounts for the complex shape of the cells. In the cell body and the primary processes, microtubules and intermediate filaments (vimentin, desmin) dominate. Microfilaments form prominent U-shaped bundles arranged in the longitudinal axis of two successive foot processes in an overlapping pattern. Centrally, these bundles are linked to the microtubules of the primary processes; peripherally, they are linked to the GBM by integrins and dystroglycans (see previous discussion). α-Actinin 4 and synaptopodin establish the podocyte-specific bundling of the microfilaments.

The filtration slits (see Figs. 1.8 and 1.10) are the sites of convective fluid flow through the visceral epithelium. They have a constant width of about 30 to 40 nm. They are bridged by the slit diaphragm. This is a proteinaceous membrane whose molecular composition is presently not fully understood. Chemically fixed and tannic acid–treated tissue reveals a zipper-like structure with a row of pores approximately 14 nm^2 on either side of a central bar. At present, the following proteins are known to establish this membrane or to mediate its connection to the actin cytoskeleton of the foot processes: nephrin, P-cadherin, FAT1, NEPH1-3, and podocin.[14] However, how these molecules interact with each other to establish a size-selective porous membrane is unknown.

Parietal Epithelium

The parietal epithelium of Bowman's capsule consists of squamous epithelial cells resting on a basement membrane (see Figs. 1.5 and 1.6). The flat cells are filled with bundles of actin filaments running in all directions. The parietal basement membrane differs from the GBM in that it comprises several proteoglycan-dense layers that, in addition to type IV, contain type XIV collagen. The predominant proteoglycan of the parietal basement membrane is a chondroitin sulfate proteoglycan.[1] Whereas the parietal epithelial cell was historically viewed as simply composing the inside layer of Bowman's capsule, parietal epithelial cells were recently shown to represent endogenous stem cells, which can replace both podocytes and proximal tubular cells in health and in disease.[15]

Filtration Barrier

Filtration through the glomerular capillary wall occurs along an extracellular pathway including the endothelial pores, the GBM, and the slit diaphragm (see Figs. 1.8 and 1.10). All these components are quite permeable for water; the high permeability for water, small solutes, and ions results from the fact that no cell membranes are interposed. The hydraulic conductance of the individual layers of the filtration barrier is difficult to study. In a mathematical model of glomerular filtration, the hydraulic resistance of the endothelium was predicted to be small, whereas the GBM and filtration slits contribute roughly one half each to the total hydraulic resistance of the capillary wall.[16]

The barrier function of the glomerular capillary wall for macromolecules is selective for size, shape, and charge.[13] The charge selectivity of the barrier results from the dense accumulation of negatively charged molecules throughout the entire depth of the filtration barrier, including the surface coat of endothelial cells, and the high content of negatively charged heparan sulfate proteoglycans in the GBM. Polyanionic macromolecules, such as plasma proteins, are repelled by the electronegative shield originating from these dense assemblies of negative charges.

The crucial structure accounting for the size selectivity of the filtration barrier appears to be the slit diaphragm.[16] Uncharged macromolecules up to an effective radius of 1.8 nm pass freely through the filter. Larger components are more and more restricted (indicated by their fractional clearances, which progressively decrease) and are totally restricted at effective radii of more than 4 nm. Plasma albumin has an effective radius of 3.6 nm; without the repulsion from the negative charge, plasma albumin would pass through the filter in considerable amounts.

Stability of the Glomerular Tuft

The main challenge for the glomerular capillaries is to combine selective leakiness with stability. The walls of capillaries do not appear to be capable of resisting high transmural pressure gradients. Several structures and mechanisms are involved in counteracting the distending forces to which the capillary wall is constantly exposed. The locus of action of all these forces is the GBM.

Two systems appear to be responsible for the development of stabilizing forces. A basic system consists of the GBM and the mesangium. Cylinders of the GBM, in fact, largely define the shape of glomerular capillaries. These cylinders, however, do not completely encircle the capillary tube; they are open toward the mesangium. Mechanically, they are completed by contractile mesangial cell processes that bridge the gaps of the GBM between two opposing mesangial angles, permitting the development of wall tension.[17]

Podocytes act as a second structure-stabilizing system. Two mechanisms appear to be involved. First, in addition to mesangial cells, podocytes stabilize the folding pattern of glomerular capillaries by fixing the turning points of the GBM between neighboring capillaries (mesangial cells from inside, podocytes from outside).[17] Second, podocytes may contribute to structural stability of glomerular capillaries by a mechanism similar to that of pericytes elsewhere in the body. Podocytes are attached to the GBM by foot processes that cover almost entirely the outer aspect of the GBM. The foot processes possess a well-developed contractile system connected to the GBM. Because the foot processes are attached at various angles on the GBM, they may function as numerous small, stabilizing patches on the GBM, counteracting locally the elastic distention of the GBM.[9]

Renal Tubule

The renal tubule is subdivided into several distinct segments: a proximal tubule, an intermediate tubule, a distal tubule, a CNT, and the collecting duct (see Figs. 1.1 and 1.3).[1,2] Henle's loop comprises the straight part of the proximal tubule (representing the thick descending limb), the thin descending and the thin ascending limbs (both thin limbs together represent the intermediate tubule), and the thick ascending limb (representing the straight portion of the distal tubule), which includes the macula densa. The CNT and the various collecting duct segments form the collecting duct system.

The renal tubules are outlined by a single-layer epithelium anchored to a basement membrane. The epithelium is a transporting epithelium consisting of flat or cuboidal epithelial cells connected apically by a junctional complex consisting of a tight junction (zonula occludens), an adherens junction, and, rarely, a desmosome. As a result of this organization, two different pathways through the epithelium exist (Fig. 1.11): a transcellular pathway, including the transport across the luminal and the basolateral cell membrane and through the cytoplasm; and a paracellular pathway through the junctional complex and the lateral intercellular spaces. The functional characteristics of the paracellular transport are determined by the tight junction, which differs markedly in its elaboration in the various tubular segments. The transcellular transport is determined by the specific channels, carriers, and transporters included in the apical and basolateral cell membranes. The various nephron segments differ markedly in function, distribution of transport proteins, and responsiveness to hormones and drugs such as diuretics.

Proximal Tubule

The proximal tubule reabsorbs the bulk of filtered water and solutes (Fig. 1.12). The epithelium shows numerous structural

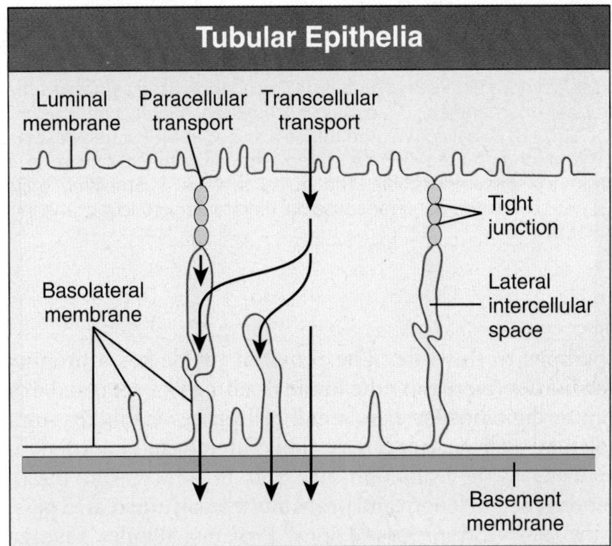

Figure 1.11 Tubular epithelia. Transport across the epithelium may follow two routes: transcellular across luminal and basolateral membranes and paracellular through the tight junction and intercellular spaces.

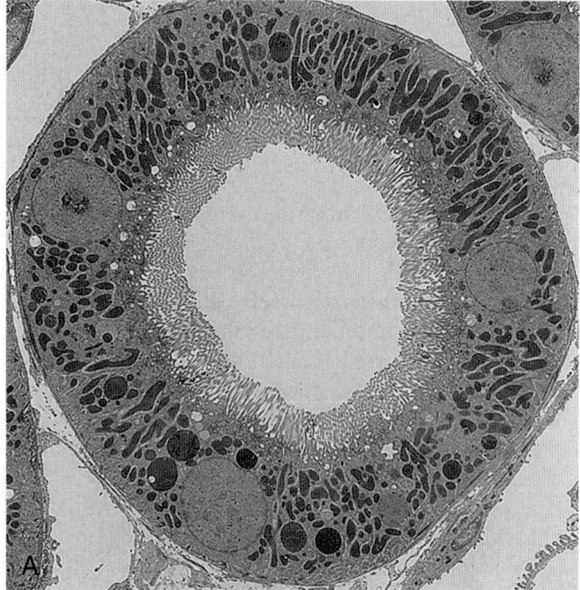

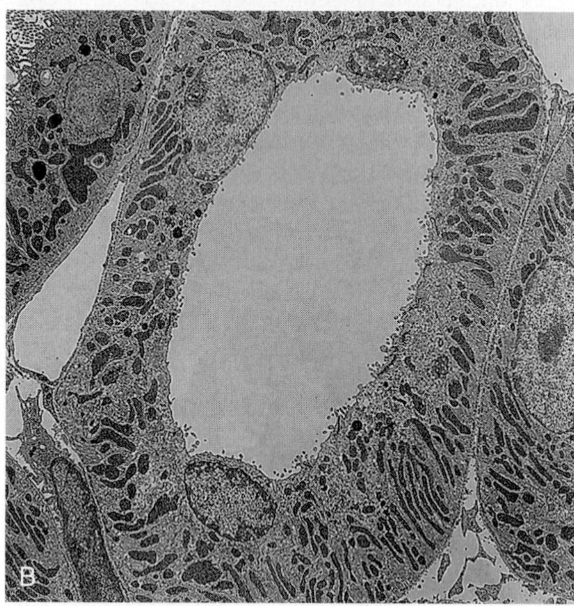

Figure 1.12 Tubules of the renal cortex. A, Proximal convoluted tubule is equipped with a brush border and a prominent vacuolar apparatus in the apical cytoplasm. The rest of the cytoplasm is occupied by a basal labyrinth consisting of large mitochondria associated with basolateral cell membranes. (Transmission electron microscopy; magnification ×1530.) **B,** Distal convoluted tubule also has interdigitated basolateral cell membranes intimately associated with large mitochondria; in contrast to the proximal tubule, the apical surface is amplified only by some stubby microvilli. (Transmission electron microscopy; magnification ×1830.)

adaptations to this role. The proximal tubule has a prominent brush border (increasing the luminal cell surface area) and extensive interdigitation by basolateral cell processes (increasing the basolateral cell surface area). This lateral cell interdigitation extends up to the leaky tight junction, thus increasing the tight junctional belt in length and providing a greatly increased passage for the passive transport of ions. Proximal tubules have large prominent mitochondria intimately associated with the basolateral cell membranes where the Na^+,K^+–adenosine triphosphatase (ATPase) is located; this machinery dominates the transcellular transport. The luminal transporter for Na^+ entry specific for the proximal tubule is the Na^+-H^+ exchanger. The high hydraulic permeability for water is rooted in abundant occurrence of the water channel protein aquaporin 1. A prominent lysosomal system is known as the apical vacuolar endocytotic apparatus and is responsible for the reabsorption of macromolecules (polypeptides and proteins such as albumin) that have passed through the glomerular filter. The proximal tubule is generally subdivided into three segments (known as S_1, S_2, S_3, or P_1, P_2, P_3) that differ considerably in cellular organization and, consequently, also in function.[18]

Henle's Loop

Henle's loop consists of the straight portion of the proximal tubule, the thin descending and (in long loops) thin ascending limbs, and the thick ascending limb (Fig. 1.13; see also Fig. 1.2). The thin descending limb, like the proximal tubule, is highly permeable for water (the channels are of aquaporin 1), whereas, beginning exactly at the turning point, the thin ascending limb is impermeable for water. The specific transport functions of the thin limbs contributing to the generation of the osmotic medullary gradient are under debate.

The thick ascending limb is often called the diluting segment. It is water impermeable but reabsorbs considerable amounts of salt, resulting in the separation of salt from water. The salt is trapped in the medulla, whereas the water is carried away into the cortex, where it may return into the systemic circulation. The specific transporter for Na^+ entry in this segment is the luminal Na^+-K^+-$2Cl^-$ cotransporter, which is the target of diuretics such as furosemide. The tight junctions of the thick ascending limb have a comparatively low permeability. The cells heavily interdigitate by basolateral cell processes, associated with large mitochondria supplying the energy for the transepithelial transport. The cells synthesize a specific protein, the Tamm-Horsfall protein, and release it into the tubular lumen. This protein is thought to be important later for preventing the formation of kidney stones. In contrast to the proximal tubule, the luminal membrane is only sparsely amplified by microvilli. Just before the transition to the distal convoluted tubule, the thick ascending limb contains the macula densa, which adheres to the parent glomerulus (see Juxtaglomerular Apparatus).

Distal Convoluted Tubule

The epithelium is fairly highly differentiated, exhibiting the most extensive basolateral interdigitation of the cells and the greatest density of mitochondria in all nephron portions (see Fig. 1.12). Apically, the cells are equipped with numerous microvilli. The specific Na^+ transporter of the distal convoluted tubule is the luminal Na^+-Cl^- cotransporter, which is the target of thiazide diuretics.

COLLECTING DUCT SYSTEM

The collecting duct system (see Fig. 1.2) includes the CNT and the cortical and medullary collecting ducts. Two nephrons may join at the level of the CNT, forming an arcade that, cytologically, is a CNT. Two types of cell line the CNT: the CNT cell, which is specific to the CNTs; and the intercalated (IC) cell, which also occurs later in the collecting duct. The CNT cells are similar to the collecting duct cells (CD cells) in cellular organization. Both cell types share sensitivity to vasopressin (antidiuretic hormone [ADH]; see later discussion); the CNT cell, however, lacks sensitivity to mineralocorticoids.

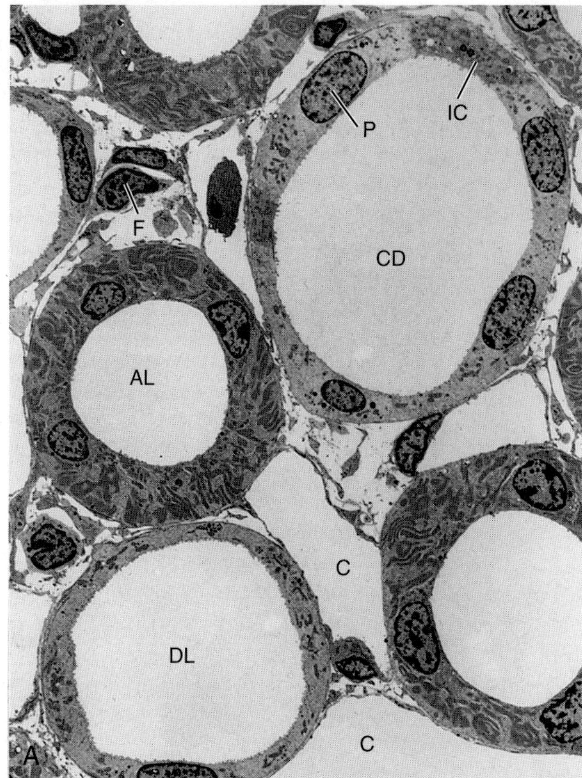

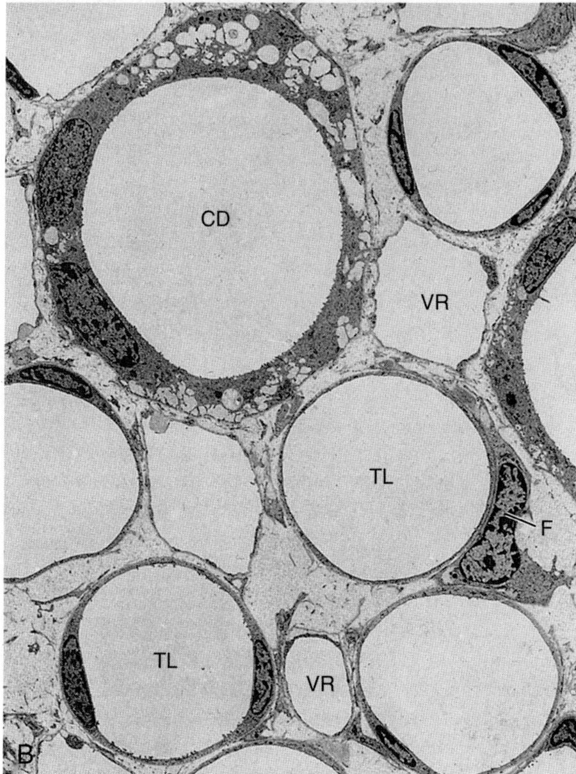

Figure 1.13 Tubules in the medulla. A, Cross section through the inner stripe of the outer medulla. A descending thin limb of a long loop (DL), the medullary thick ascending limbs (AL), and a collecting duct (CD) with principal cells (P) and intercalated cells (IC) are shown. C, peritubular capillaries; F, fibroblast. **B,** In the inner medulla cross section, thin descending and ascending limbs (TL), a collecting duct (CD), and vasa recta (VR) are seen. (Transmission electron microscopy; magnification: **A,** ×990; **B,** ×1120.)

Collecting Ducts

The collecting ducts (see Fig. 1.13) may be subdivided into cortical and medullary ducts, and the medullary ducts into outer and inner; the transitions are gradual. Like the CNT, the collecting ducts are lined by two types of cell: CD cells (principal cells) and IC cells. The IC cells decrease in number as the collecting duct descends into the medulla and are absent from the papillary collecting ducts.

The CD cells (Fig. 1.14A) are simple, polygonal cells increasing in size toward the tip of the papilla. The basal surface of these cells is characterized by invaginations of the basal cell membrane (basal infoldings). The tight junctions have a large apicobasal depth, and the apical cell surface has a prominent glycocalyx. Along the entire collecting duct, these cells contain a luminal shuttle system for aquaporin 2 under the control of vasopressin, providing the potential to switch the water permeability of the collecting ducts from zero (or at least from low) to permeable.[19] A luminal amiloride-sensitive Na^+ channel is involved in the responsiveness of cortical collecting ducts to aldosterone. The terminal portions of the collecting duct in the inner medulla express the urea transporter UTB1, which, in an ADH-dependent fashion, accounts for the recycling of urea, a process that is crucial in the urine-concentrating mechanism.[20]

The second cell type, the IC cell (Fig. 1.14B), is present in both the CNT and the collecting duct. There are at least two types of IC cells, designated A and B cells, distinguished on the basis of structural, immunocytochemical, and functional

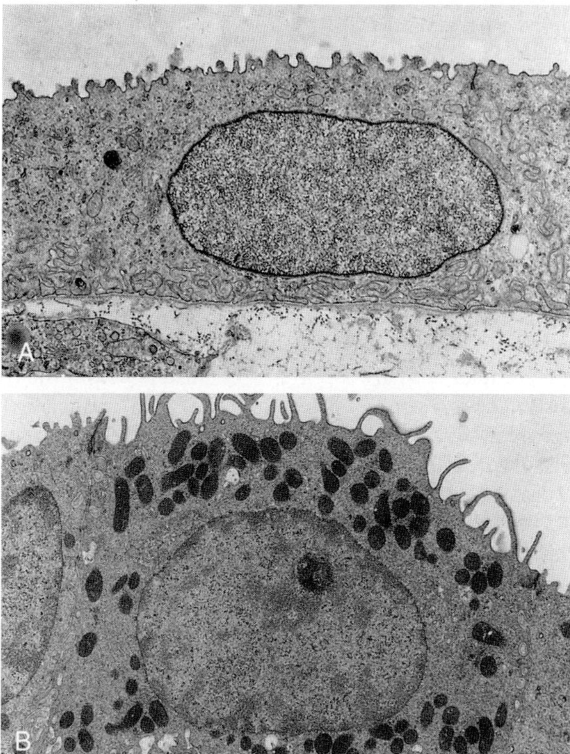

Figure 1.14 Collecting duct cells. A, Principal cell (CD cell) of a medullary collecting duct. The apical cell membrane bears some stubby microvilli covered by a prominent glycocalyx; the basal cell membrane forms invaginations. Note the deep tight junction. **B,** Intercalated cells, type A. Note the dark cytoplasm (dark cells) with many mitochondria and apical microfolds; the basal membrane forms invaginations. (Transmission electron microscopy; magnification: **A,** ×8720; **B,** ×6970.)

characteristics. Type A cells have been defined as expressing H^+-ATPase at their luminal membrane; they secrete protons. Type B cells express the H^+-ATPase at their basolateral membrane; they secrete bicarbonate ions and reabsorb protons.[21]

With these different cell types, the collecting ducts are the final regulators of fluid and electrolyte balance, playing important roles in the handling of Na^+, Cl^-, and K^+ as well as acid and base. The responsiveness of the collecting ducts to vasopressin enables an organism to live in arid conditions, allowing it to produce a concentrated urine and, if necessary, a dilute urine.

JUXTAGLOMERULAR APPARATUS

The juxtaglomerular apparatus (see Fig. 1.5) comprises the macula densa, the extraglomerular mesangium, the terminal portion of the afferent arteriole with its renin-producing granular cells (nowadays also often termed juxtaglomerular cells), and the beginning portions of the efferent arteriole.

The macula densa (Fig. 1.15A; see also Fig. 1.6) is a plaque of specialized cells in the wall of the thick ascending limb at the site where the limb attaches to the extraglomerular mesangium of the parent glomerulus. The most obvious structural feature is the narrowly packed cells with large nuclei, which account for the name macula densa. The cells are anchored to a basement membrane, which blends with the matrix of the extraglomerular mesangium.[1] The cells are joined by tight junctions with very low permeability and have prominent lateral intercellular spaces. The width of these spaces varies under different functional conditions.[1] The most conspicuous immunocytochemical difference between macula densa cells and any other epithelial cell of the nephron is the high content of neuronal nitric oxide synthase 1[22] and of cyclooxygenase 2.[23]

The basal aspect of the macula densa is firmly attached to the extraglomerular mesangium, which represents a solid complex of cells and matrix that is penetrated neither by blood vessels nor by lymphatic capillaries (see Figs. 1.5 and 1.15A). Like the mesangial cells proper, extraglomerular mesangial cells are heavily branched. Their processes, interconnected among each other by gap junctions, contain prominent bundles of microfilaments and are connected to the basement membrane of Bowman's capsule as well as to the walls of both glomerular arterioles. As a whole, the extraglomerular mesangium interconnects all structures of the glomerular entrance.[6]

The granular cells are assembled in clusters within the terminal portion of the afferent arteriole (Fig. 1.15B), replacing ordinary smooth muscle cells. Their name refers to the specific cytoplasmic granules in which renin, the major secretion product of these cells, is stored. They are the main site of the body where renin is secreted. Renin release occurs by exocytosis into the surrounding interstitium. Granular cells are connected to the extraglomerular mesangial cells, to adjacent smooth muscle cells, and to endothelial cells by gap junctions. They are densely innervated by sympathetic nerve terminals. Granular cells are modified smooth muscle cells; under conditions requiring enhanced renin synthesis (e.g., volume depletion or stenosis of the renal artery), additional smooth muscle cells located upstream in the wall of the afferent arteriole may transform into granular cells.

The structural organization of the juxtaglomerular apparatus suggests a regulatory function. There is agreement that some component of the distal urine (probably Cl^-) is sensed by the macula densa, and this information is used first to adjust the tone of the glomerular arterioles, thereby producing a change in glomerular blood flow and filtration rate. Even if many details of this mechanism are still subject to debate, the essence of this system has been verified by many studies, and it is known as the tubular glomerular feedback mechanism.[24] Second, this system determines the amount of renin that is released, through the interstitium, into the circulation, thereby acquiring great systemic relevance.

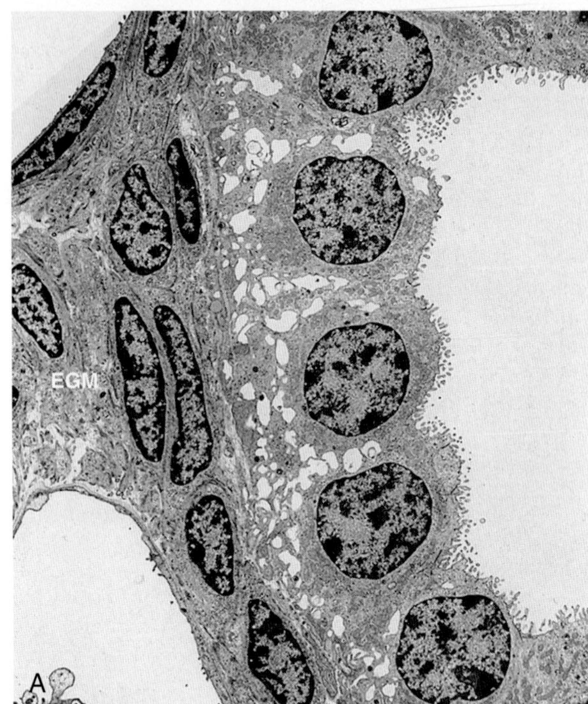

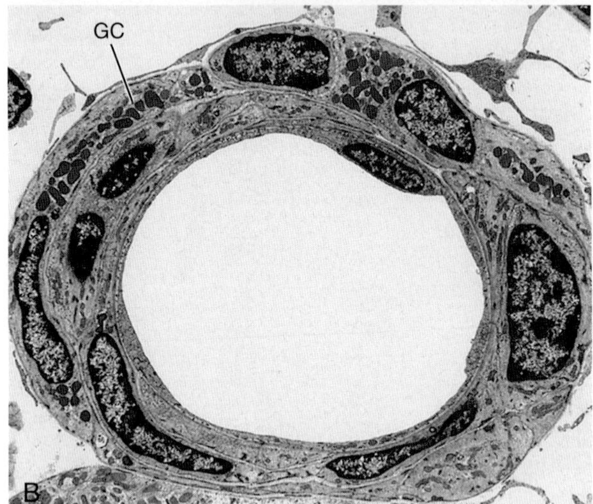

Figure 1.15 Juxtaglomerular apparatus. A, Macula densa of a thick ascending limb. The cells have prominent nuclei and lateral intercellular spaces. Basally, they attach to the extraglomerular mesangium (EGM). **B,** Afferent arteriole near the vascular pole. Several smooth muscle cells are replaced by granular cells (GC) containing accumulations of renin granules. (Transmission electron microscopy; magnification: **A,** ×1730; **B,** ×1310.)

RENAL INTERSTITIUM

The interstitium of the kidney is comparatively sparse. Its fractional volume in the cortex ranges from 5% to 7% (with a tendency to increase with age). It increases across the medulla from cortex to papilla: in the outer stripe, it is 3% to 4% (the lowest

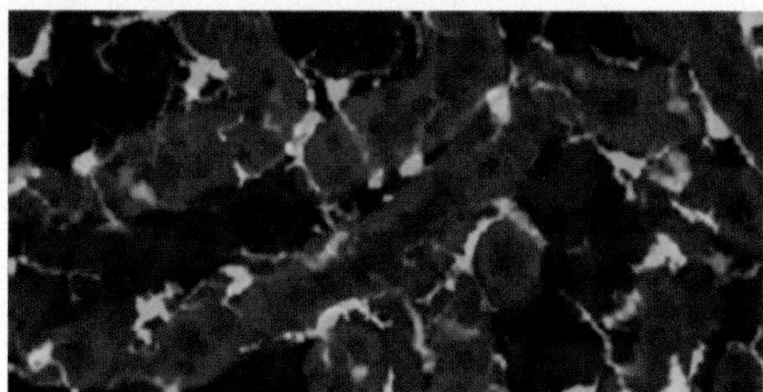

Figure 1.16 Renal dendritic cells. Dendritic cells (CX_3CR1^+ cells, *green*) surrounding tubular segments in the medulla of mice (three-dimensional reconstruction). *(Reprinted with permission from reference 26.)*

value of all kidney zones; this is interpreted as forming a barrier to prevent loss of solutes from a hyperosmolar medulla into the cortex); in the inner stripe, it is 10%; and in the inner medulla, it is up to ~30%. The cellular constituents of the interstitium are resident fibroblasts, which establish the scaffold frame for renal corpuscles, tubules, and blood vessels. In addition, there are varying numbers of migrating cells of the immune system, especially dendritic cells. The space between the cells is filled with extracellular matrix, namely, ground substance (proteoglycans, glycoproteins), fibrils, and interstitial fluid.[25]

From a morphologic point of view, fibroblasts are the central cells in the renal interstitium. They are interconnected by specialized contacts and adhere by specific attachments to the basement membranes surrounding the tubules, the renal corpuscles, the capillaries, and the lymphatics.

Renal fibroblasts are difficult to distinguish from interstitial dendritic cells on a morphologic basis because both may show a stellate cellular shape and both display substantial amounts of mitochondria and endoplasmic reticulum. They may, however, easily be distinguished by immunocytochemical techniques. Dendritic cells constitutively express the major histocompatibility complex class II antigen and may express antigens such as CD11c. Dendritic cells may have an important role in maintaining peripheral tolerance in the kidney (Fig. 1.16).[26] In contrast, fibroblasts in the renal cortex (not in the medulla) contain the enzyme ecto-5′-nucleotidase (5′-NT).[27] A subset of 5′-NT–positive fibroblasts of the renal cortex synthesize epoetin.[27] Under normal conditions, these fibroblasts are exclusively found within the juxtamedullary portions of the cortical labyrinth. When there is an increasing demand for epoetin, the synthesizing cells extend to more superficial portions of the cortical labyrinth and, to a lesser degree, to the medullary rays.[28]

Fibroblasts within the medulla, especially within the inner medulla, have a particular phenotype known as lipid-laden interstitial cells. The cells are oriented strictly perpendicularly toward the longitudinal axis of the tubules and vessels (running all in parallel) and contain conspicuous lipid droplets. These fibroblasts of the inner medulla produce large amounts of glycosaminoglycans and, possibly related to the lipid droplets, vasoactive lipids, in particular prostaglandin E_2.[26]

The intrarenal arteries are accompanied by a prominent sheath of loose interstitial tissue (Fig. 1.17); the renal veins are in apposition to this sheath but not included in it. Intrarenal nerve fibers and lymphatics run within this periarterial tissue. Lymphatics start in the vicinity of the afferent arteriole and leave the kidney running within the periarterial tissue sheath toward the hilum. Together with the lymphatics, the periarterial tissue constitutes a pathway for interstitial fluid drainage of the renal cortex; the renal medulla has no lymphatic drainage.

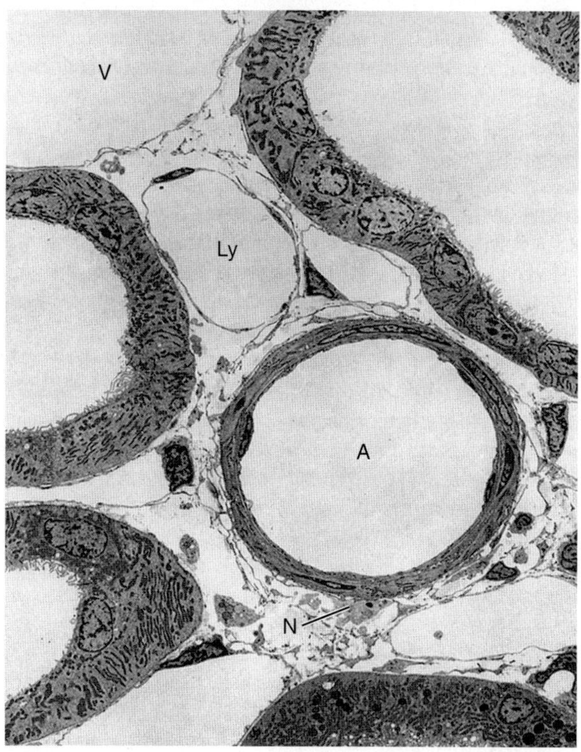

Figure 1.17 Intrarenal arteries in a periarterial connective tissue sheath. Cross section through a cortical radial artery surrounded by the sheath containing the renal nerves (N) and lymphatics (Ly). A vein lies outside the sheath. (Transmission electron microscopy; magnification ×830.)

REFERENCES

1. Kriz W, Kaissling B. Structural organization of the mammalian kidney. In: Seldin D, Giebisch G, eds. *The Kidney*. Philadelphia: Lippincott Williams & Wilkins; 2000:587-654.
2. Kriz W, Bankir L. A standard nomenclature for structure of the kidney. The Renal Commission of the International Union of Physiological Sciences (IUPS). *Pflugers Arch*. 1988;411:113-120.
3. Rollhäuser H, Kriz W, Heinke W. Das Gefässsystem der Rattenniere. *Z Zellforsch Mikrosk Anat*. 1964;64:381-403.
4. Barajas L. Innervation of the renal cortex. *Fed Proc*. 1978;37:1192-1201.
5. DiBona G, Kopp U. Neural control of renal function. *Physiol Rev*. 1997;77:75-197.
6. Elger M, Sakai T, Kriz W. The vascular pole of the renal glomerulus of rat. *Adv Anat Embryol Cell Biol*. 1998;139:1-98.
7. Inoue S. Ultrastructural architecture of basement membranes. *Contrib Nephrol*. 1994;107:21-28.
8. Miner J. Renal basement membrane components. *Kidney Int*. 1999;56:2016-2024.
9. Kriz W, Elger M, Mundel P, Lemley K. Structure-stabilizing forces in the glomerular tuft. *J Am Soc Nephrol*. 1995;5:1731-1739.
10. Rostgaard J, Qvortrup K. Electron microscopic demonstrations of filamentous molecular sieve plugs in capillary fenestrae. *Microvasc Res*. 1997;53:1-13.
11. Endlich K, Kriz W, Witzgall R. Update in podocyte biology. *Curr Opin Nephrol Hypertens*. 2001;10:331-340.
12. Neal CR, Crook H, Bell E, et al. Three-dimensional reconstruction of glomeruli by electron microscopy reveals a distinctive restrictive urinary subpodocyte space. *J Am Soc Nephrol*. 2005;16:1223-1235.
13. Pavenstadt H, Kriz W, Kretzler M. Cell biology of the glomerular podocyte. *Physiol Rev*. 2003;83:253-307.
14. Mundel P, Kriz W. Structure and function of podocytes: An update. *Anat Embryol*. 1995;192:385-397.

15. Appel D, Kershaw DB, Smeets B, et al. Recruitment of podocytes from glomerular parietal epithelial cells. *J Am Soc Nephrol*. 2009;20:333-343.
16. Drumond M, Deen W. Structural determinants of glomerular hydraulic permeability. *Am J Physiol*. 1994;266:F1-F12.
17. Kriz W, Endlich K. Hypertrophy of podocytes: A mechanism to cope with increased glomerular capillary pressures? *Kidney Int*. 2005;607:373-374.
18. Maunsbach A. Functional ultrastructure of the proximal tubule. In: Windhager E, ed. *Handbook of Physiology: Section on Renal Physiology*. New York: Oxford University Press; 1992:41-108.
19. Sabolic I, Brown D. Water channels in renal and nonrenal tissues. *News Physiol Sci*. 1995;10:12-17.
20. Bankir L, Trinh-Trang-Tan M. Urea and the kidney. In: Brenner B, ed. *The Kidney*. Philadelphia: WB Saunders; 2000:637-679.
21. Madsen K, Verlander J, Kim J, Tisher C. Morphological adaptation of the collecting duct to acid-base disturbances. *Kidney Int*. 1991;40(Suppl 33):S57-S63.
22. Mundel P, Bachmann S, Bader M, et al. Expression of nitric oxide synthase in kidney macula densa cells. *Kidney Int*. 1992;42:1017-1019.
23. Harris R, McKanna J, Akai Y, et al. Cyclooxygenase-2 is associated with the macula densa of rat kidney and increases with salt restriction. *J Clin Invest*. 1994;94:2504-2510.
24. Klamt B, Koziell A, Poulat F, et al. Frasier syndrome is caused by defective alternative splicing of WT1 leading to an altered ratio of WT1 +/−KTS splice isoforms. *Hum Mol Genet*. 1998;7:709-714.
25. Kaissling B, Hegyi I, Loffing J, Le Hir M. Morphology of interstitial cells in the healthy kidney. *Anat Embryol*. 1996;193:303-318.
26. Soos TJ, Sims TN, Barisoni L, et al. CX_3CR1^+ interstitial dendritic cells form a contiguous network throughout the entire kidney. *Kidney Int*. 2006;70:591-596.
27. Bachmann S, Le Hir M, Eckardt K. Co-localization of erythropoietin mRNA and ecto-5′-nucleotidase immunoreactivity in peritubular cells of rat renal cortex indicates that fibroblasts produce erythropoietin. *J Histochem Cytochem*. 1993;41:335-341.
28. Kaissling B, Spiess S, Rinne B, Le Hir M. Effects of anemia on the morphology of the renal cortex of rats. *Am J Physiol*. 1993;264:F608-F617.

CHAPTER 2

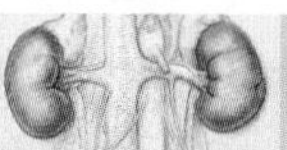

Renal Physiology

David G. Shirley, Robert J. Unwin

The prime function of the "kidneys" is to maintain a stable *milieu intérieur* by the selective retention or elimination of water, electrolytes, and other solutes. This is achieved by three processes: (1) filtration of circulating blood from the glomerulus to form an ultrafiltrate of plasma in Bowman's space; (2) selective reabsorption (from tubular fluid to blood) across the cells lining the renal tubule; and (3) selective secretion (from peritubular capillary blood to tubular fluid).

GLOMERULAR STRUCTURE AND ULTRASTRUCTURE

The process of urine formation begins by the production of an ultrafiltrate of plasma. Chapter 1 provides a detailed description of glomerular anatomy and ultrastructure; therefore, only the brief essentials for an understanding of how the ultrafiltrate is formed are given here. The pathway for ultrafiltration of plasma from the glomerulus to Bowman's space consists of the fenestrated capillary endothelium, the capillary basement membrane, and the visceral epithelial cell layer (podocytes) of Bowman's capsule; the podocytes have large cell bodies and make contact with the basement membrane only by cytoplasmic foot processes. Mesangial cells, which fill the spaces between capillaries, have contractile properties and are capable of altering the capillary surface area available for filtration.

Filtration is determined principally by the molecular size and shape of the solute and, to a much lesser extent, by its charge. The size cutoff is not absolute; resistance to filtration begins at an effective molecular radius of slightly less than 2 nm, and substances with an effective radius exceeding ~4 nm are not filtered at all. The fenestrations between capillary endothelial cells have a diameter of 50 to 100 nm, and the podocyte foot processes have gaps between them (filtration slits) with a diameter of 25 to 50 nm, but they are bridged by diaphragms (the slit diaphragms), which are themselves penetrated by small pores. The slit diaphragms constitute the main filtration barrier, although both the endothelium (by preventing the passage of blood cells) and the basement membrane contribute.[1] In addition, the podocytes and the endothelial cells are covered by a glycocalyx composed of negatively charged glycoproteins, glycosaminoglycans, and proteoglycans, and the basement membrane is rich in heparan sulfate proteoglycans. This accumulation of fixed negative charges further restricts the filtration of large negatively charged ions, mainly proteins (Fig. 2.1). This explains why albumin, despite an effective radius (3.6 nm) that would allow significant filtration based on size alone, is normally virtually excluded. If these fixed negative charges are lost, as in some forms of early or mild glomerular disease (e.g., minimal change nephropathy), albumin filterability increases and proteinuria results.

GLOMERULAR FILTRATION RATE

At the level of the single glomerulus, the driving force for glomerular filtration (the *net ultrafiltration pressure*) is determined by the net hydrostatic and oncotic (colloid osmotic) pressure gradients between glomerular plasma and the filtrate in Bowman's space. The rate of filtration (single-nephron glomerular filtration rate) is determined by the product of the net ultrafiltration pressure and the *ultrafiltration coefficient*, a composite of the surface area available for filtration and the hydraulic conductivity of the glomerular membranes. Therefore, the single-nephron glomerular filtration rate is

$$K_f[(P_{gc} - P_{bs}) - (\pi_{gc} - \pi_{bs})]$$

where K_f is the ultrafiltration coefficient, P_{gc} is glomerular capillary hydrostatic pressure (~45 mm Hg), P_{bs} is Bowman's space hydrostatic pressure (~10 mm Hg), π_{gc} is glomerular capillary oncotic pressure (~25 mm Hg), and π_{bs} is Bowman's space oncotic pressure (0 mm Hg). Thus, net ultrafiltration pressure is around 10 mm Hg at the afferent end of the capillary tuft. As filtration of protein-free fluid proceeds along the glomerular capillaries, π_{gc} increases (because plasma proteins are concentrated into a smaller volume of glomerular plasma) and, at a certain point toward the efferent end, π_{gc} may equal the net hydrostatic pressure gradient; that is, the net ultrafiltration pressure may fall to zero: so-called *filtration equilibrium* (Fig. 2.2). In humans, complete filtration equilibrium is approached but rarely if ever achieved.

The total rate at which fluid is filtered into all the nephrons (glomerular filtration rate [GFR]) is typically ~120 ml/min per 1.73 m^2 surface area, but the normal range is wide. GFR can be measured by use of renal clearance techniques. The renal clearance of any substance not metabolized by the kidneys is the volume of plasma required to provide that amount of the substance excreted in the urine per unit time; this virtual volume can be expressed mathematically as

$$C_y = U_y \times V / P_y$$

where C_y is the renal clearance of y, U_y is the urine concentration of y, V is the urine flow rate, and P_y is the plasma concentration of y. If a substance is freely filtered by the glomerulus and is not

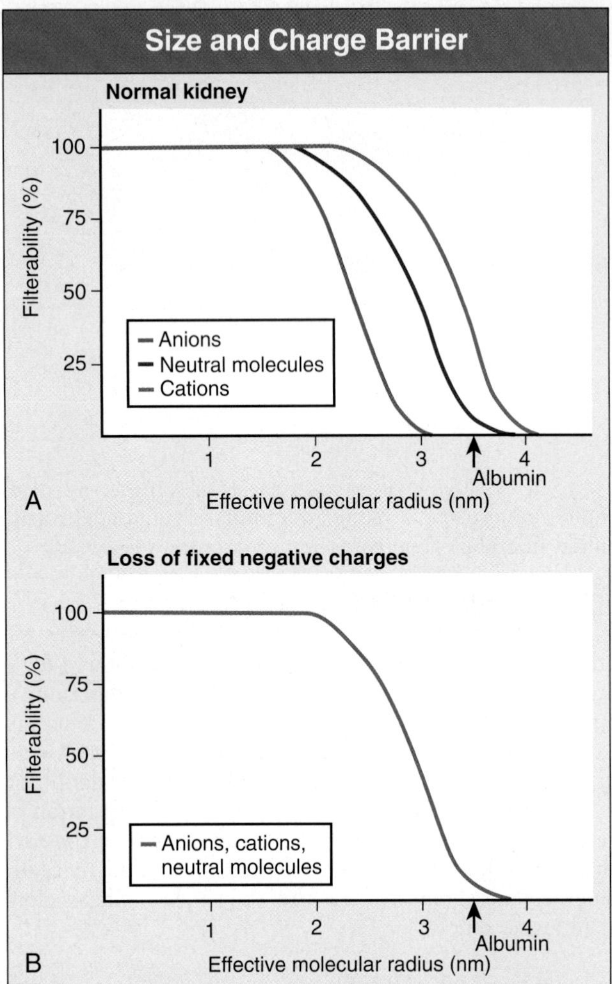

Figure 2.1 Size and charge barrier: effects of size and electrical charge on filterability. A, Normal kidney. **B,** Loss of fixed negative charges. A 100% filterability indicates that the substance is freely filtered, that is, its concentration in Bowman's space equals that in glomerular capillary plasma. For molecules and small ions (e.g., Na^+, Cl^-), charge has no effect on filterability; but for ions whose effective molecular radius exceeds ~1.6 nm, anions are filtered less easily than neutral molecules or cations. Thus, insignificant amounts of albumin (anion) are normally filtered. If the fixed negative charges of the glomerular basement membranes are lost, as in early minimal change nephropathy, charge no longer influences filterability; consequently, significant albumin filtration occurs.

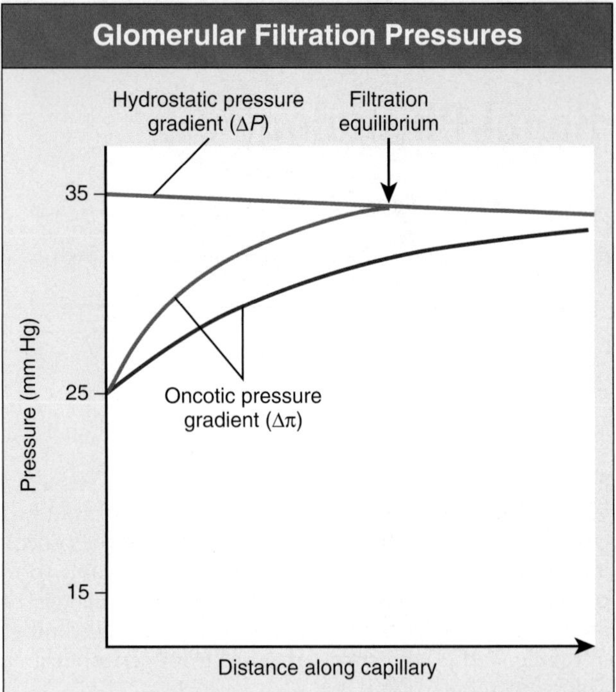

Figure 2.2 Glomerular filtration pressures along a glomerular capillary. The hydrostatic pressure gradient ($\Delta P = P_{gc} - P_{bs}$) is relatively constant along the length of a capillary, whereas the opposing oncotic pressure gradient ($\Delta\pi = \pi_{gc}$) increases as protein-free fluid is filtered, thereby reducing net ultrafiltration pressure. Two curves are shown, one where filtration equilibrium is reached and one where it is merely approached.

reabsorbed or secreted by the tubule, its renal clearance equals GFR; that is, it measures the volume of plasma filtered through the glomeruli per unit time. The various methods for measurement of GFR and their pitfalls are discussed in Chapter 3.

MEASUREMENT OF RENAL PLASMA FLOW

The use of the clearance technique and the availability of substances that undergo both glomerular filtration and virtually complete tubular secretion have made it possible to measure renal plasma flow (RPF; typically ~650 ml/min). *p*-Aminohippurate (PAH) is an organic acid that is filtered by the glomerulus and actively secreted by the proximal tubule. When the plasma concentration of PAH is lower than 10 mg/dl, most of the PAH reaching the peritubular capillaries is cleared by tubular secretion and little PAH appears in renal venous plasma. Under these circumstances, the amount of PAH transferred from the plasma to the tubular lumen through filtration and secretion (i.e., the amount found in the final urine) approximates the amount of PAH delivered to the kidneys in the plasma. Therefore,

$$\text{RPF} \times P_{\text{PAH}} = U_{\text{PAH}} \times V$$

or

$$\text{RPF} = (U_{\text{PAH}} \times V)/P_{\text{PAH}} = \text{PAH clearance}$$

where U_{PAH} and P_{PAH} are the concentrations of PAH in the urine and plasma, respectively, and V is the urine flow rate. Renal blood flow (RBF) can be calculated as

$$\text{RBF} = [\text{RPF}/(100 - \text{hematocrit})] \times 100$$

and is typically ~1200 ml/min.

The most important limitation of this method is the renal extraction of PAH, which is always less than 100%. At high plasma concentrations (>10 to 15 mg/dl), fractional tubular secretion of PAH declines and significant amounts appear in the renal veins; under these circumstances PAH clearance seriously underestimates RPF. There are also diseases that can produce either toxins or weak organic acids (e.g., liver and renal failure) that interfere with PAH secretion or cause tubular damage leading to inhibition of PAH transport. Finally, certain drugs, like probenecid, are organic acids and compete with PAH for tubular secretion, thereby reducing PAH clearance.

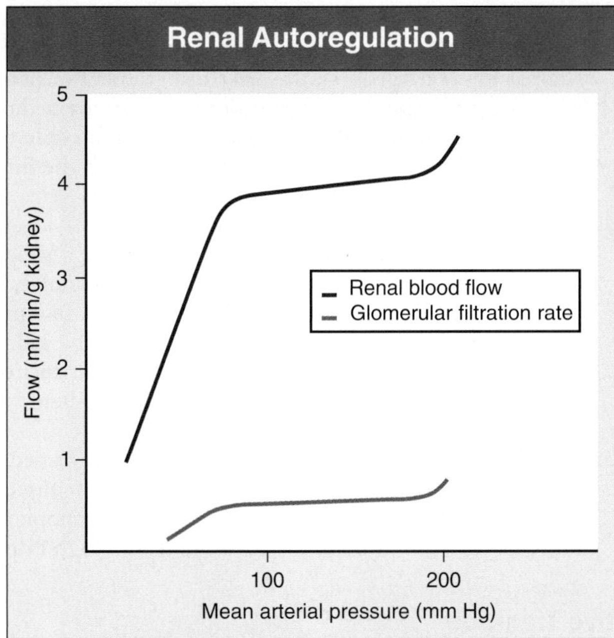

Figure 2.3 Renal autoregulation of renal blood flow and glomerular filtration rate. If mean arterial blood pressure is in the range of ~80 to 180 mm Hg, fluctuations in blood pressure have only marginal effects on renal blood flow and glomerular filtration rate. This is an intrinsic mechanism and can be modulated or overridden by extrinsic factors.

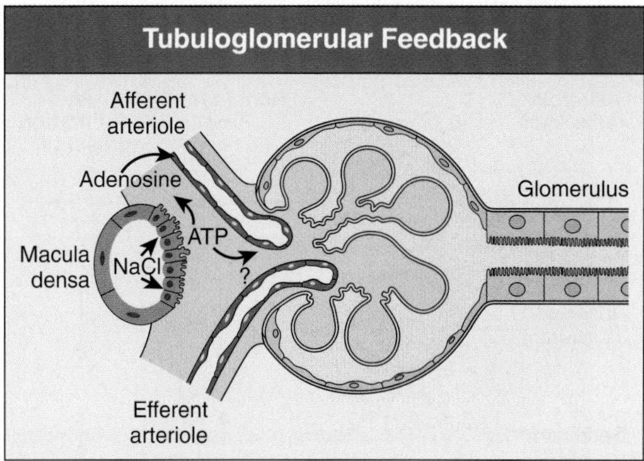

Figure 2.4 Tubuloglomerular feedback. Changes in the delivery of NaCl to the macula densa region of the thick ascending limb of the loop of Henle cause changes in the afferent arteriolar caliber. The response is mediated by adenosine or possibly adenosine triphosphate (ATP), and modulated by other locally produced agents, such as angiotensin II and nitric oxide. Increased macula densa NaCl delivery results in afferent arteriolar constriction, thereby reducing GFR.

AUTOREGULATION OF RENAL BLOOD FLOW AND GLOMERULAR FILTRATION RATE

Although acute variations in arterial blood pressure inevitably cause corresponding changes in RBF and GFR, they are short lived, and provided the blood pressure remains within the normal range, compensatory mechanisms come into play after a few seconds to return both RBF and GFR toward normal.[2] This is the phenomenon of *autoregulation* (Fig. 2.3). Autoregulation is effected primarily at the level of the afferent arterioles and is believed to result from a combination of two mechanisms:

1. a *myogenic reflex*, whereby the afferent arteriolar smooth muscle wall constricts automatically when renal perfusion pressure rises; and
2. *tubuloglomerular feedback* (TGF), whereby an increased delivery of NaCl to the macula densa region of the nephron (a specialized plaque of cells situated at the distal end of the loop of Henle), resulting from increases in renal perfusion pressure, causes vasoconstriction of the afferent arteriole supplying that nephron's glomerulus.

Because these mechanisms restore both RBF and P_{gc} toward normal, the initial change in GFR is also reversed. The TGF system is possible because of the *juxtaglomerular apparatus*, which consists of the macula densa region of each nephron and the adjacent glomerulus and afferent and efferent arterioles (Fig. 2.4). The primary mediator of TGF is adenosine triphosphate (ATP). Increased NaCl delivery to the macula densa leads to increased NaCl uptake by these cells, which triggers ATP release into the surrounding extracellular space.[3] It is thought that ATP has a direct vasoconstrictor effect, acting on $P2X_1$ purinoceptors on afferent arteriolar cells; but there is also good evidence that nucleotidases present in this region degrade ATP to adenosine, which, acting on afferent arteriolar A_1 receptors, can also cause vasoconstriction.[4] The sensitivity of TGF is modulated by locally produced angiotensin II (Ang II), nitric oxide, and certain eicosanoids (see later discussion).

Despite renal autoregulation, a number of extrinsic factors (nervous and humoral) can alter renal hemodynamics. Independent or unequal changes in the resistance of afferent and efferent arterioles, together with alterations in K_f (thought to result largely from mesangial cell contraction and relaxation), can result in disproportionate or even contrasting changes in RBF and GFR. In addition, within the kidney, changes in vascular resistance in different regions of the renal cortex can alter the distribution of blood flow, for example, diversion of blood from outer to inner cortex in hemorrhagic shock.[5] Figure 2.5 indicates how, in principle, changes in afferent and efferent arteriolar resistance will affect net ultrafiltration. Several important vasoactive factors that alter renal hemodynamics are listed in Figure 2.6 and discussed at the end of the chapter. In addition, studies suggest that disease of the renal afferent arteriole, such as occurs in hypertension and progressive kidney disease, may also interfere with renal autoregulatory mechanisms.

TUBULAR TRANSPORT

Vectorial transport, that is, net movement of substances from tubular fluid to blood (reabsorption) or vice versa (secretion), requires that the cell membrane facing the tubular fluid (*luminal* or *apical*) has properties different from those of the membrane facing the blood (*peritubular* or *basolateral*). In this polarized epithelium, certain transport proteins are located in one membrane, and others are located in the other, thus allowing the net movement of substances across the cell (transcellular route). The *tight junction*, which is a contact point close to the apical side of adjacent cells, limits water and solute movement between cells (paracellular route).

Solute transport across cell membranes uses either passive or active mechanisms.

Passive Transport

1. *Simple diffusion* always occurs down an electrochemical gradient, which is a composite of the concentration gradient

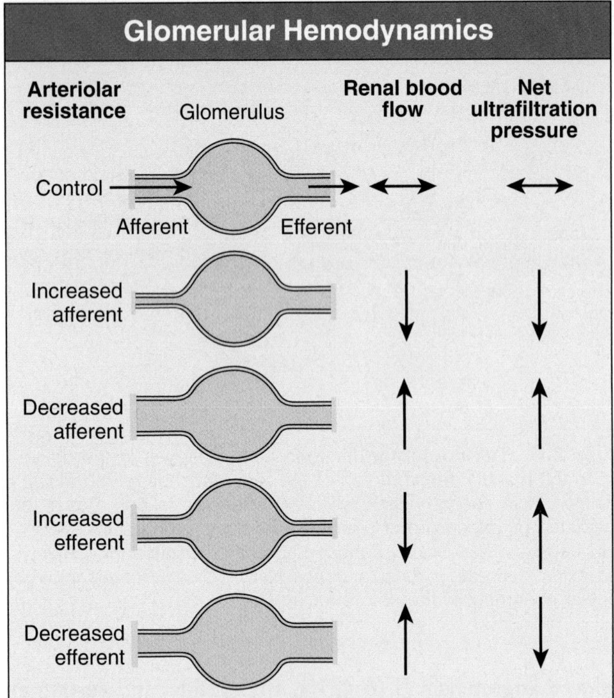

Figure 2.5 Glomerular hemodynamics. Changes in afferent or efferent arteriolar resistance will alter renal blood flow and (usually) net ultrafiltration pressure. However, the effect on ultrafiltration pressure depends on the relative changes in afferent and efferent arteriolar resistance. The overall effect on glomerular filtration rate will depend not only on renal blood flow and net ultrafiltration pressure, but also on the ultrafiltration coefficient (K_f; see Fig. 2.6).

and the electrical gradient. In the case of an undissociated molecule, only the concentration gradient is relevant; whereas for a charged ion, the electrical gradient must also be considered. Simple diffusion does not require a direct energy source, although an active transport process (see later discussion) is usually necessary to establish the initial concentration and electrical gradients.

2. *Facilitated diffusion* (or carrier-mediated diffusion) depends on an interaction of the molecule or ion with a specific membrane carrier protein that eases, or facilitates, its passage across the cell membrane's lipid bilayer. In almost all instances of carrier-mediated transport in the kidney, two or more ions or molecules share the carrier, one moiety moving down its electrochemical gradient, the other against (see later discussion).
3. *Diffusion through a membrane channel* (or pore) formed by specific integral membrane proteins is also a form of facilitated diffusion because it allows charged and lipophobic molecules to pass through the membrane at a high rate.

Active Transport

When an ion is moved directly against an electrochemical gradient ("uphill"), a source of energy is required, and this is known as active transport. In cells, this energy is derived from metabolism: ATP production and its hydrolysis. The most important active cell transport mechanism is the sodium pump, which extrudes Na^+ from inside the cell in exchange for K^+ from outside the cell.[6] In the kidney, it is confined to the basolateral membrane. It derives energy from the enzymatic hydrolysis of ATP, hence its more precise description as Na^+,K^+-ATPase. It exchanges $3Na^+$ ions for $2K^+$ ions, which makes it electrogenic

Physiologic and Pharmacologic Factors with Effects on Glomerular Hemodynamics

	Afferent Arteriolar Resistance	Efferent Arteriolar Resistance	Renal Blood Flow	Net Ultrafiltration Pressure	K_f	GFR
Renal sympathetic nerves	↑↑	↑	↓	↓	↓	↓
Epinephrine	↑	↑	↓	→	?	↓
Adenosine	↑	→	↓	↓	?	↓
Cyclosporine	↑	→	↓	↓	?	↓
NSAIDs	↑↑	↑	↓	↓	?	↓
Angiotensin II	↑	↑↑	↓	↑	↓	↓→
Endothelin 1	↑	↑↑	↓	↑	↓	↓
High-protein diet	↓	→	↑	↑	→	↑
Nitric oxide	↓	↓	↑	?	↑	↑(?)
Atrial natriuretic peptide (high dose)	↓	→	↑	↑	↑	↑
Prostaglandins E_2/I_2	↓	↓(?)	↑	↑	?	↑
Calcium channel blockers	↓	→	↑	↑	?	↑
ACE inhibitors/angiotensin receptor blockers	↓	↓↓	↑	↓	↑	?*

Figure 2.6 Physiologic and pharmacologic influences on glomerular hemodynamics. The overall effect on glomerular filtration rate (GFR) will depend on renal blood flow, net ultrafiltration pressure, and the ultrafiltration coefficient (K_f), which is controlled by mesangial cell contraction and relaxation. The effects shown are those seen when the agents are applied (or inhibited) in isolation; the actual changes that occur are dose-dependent and are modulated by other agents. *In clinical practice, GFR is usually either decreased or unaffected. ACE, angiotensin-converting enzyme; NSAIDs, nonsteroidal anti-inflammatory drugs.

because it extrudes a net positive charge from the cell. It is an example of a *primary* active transport mechanism. Other well-defined primary active transport mechanisms in the kidney are the proton-secreting H^+-ATPase, important in H^+ secretion in the distal nephron, and Ca^{2+}-ATPase, partly responsible for calcium reabsorption.

Activity of the basolateral Na^+,K^+-ATPase is key to the operation of all the passive transport processes outlined earlier. It ensures that the intracellular Na^+ concentration is kept low (10 to 20 mmol/l) and the K^+ concentration high (~150 mmol/l), compared with their extracellular concentrations (~140 and ~4 mmol/l, respectively). Sodium entry into tubular cells down the electrochemical gradient maintained by the sodium pump is either through Na^+ channels (in the distal nephron) or linked (coupled) through specific membrane carrier proteins to the influx (*cotransport*) or efflux (*countertransport*) of other molecules or ions. In various parts of the nephron, glucose, phosphate, amino acids, K^+, and Cl^- can all be cotransported with Na^+ entry, whereas H^+ and Ca^{2+} can be countertransported against Na^+ entry. In each case the non-sodium molecule or ion is transported against its electrochemical gradient by use of energy derived from the "downhill" movement of sodium. Their ultimate dependence on the primary active sodium pump makes them *secondary* active transport mechanisms.

TRANSPORT IN SPECIFIC NEPHRON SEGMENTS

Given a typical GFR, approximately 180 l of largely protein-free plasma is filtered each day, necessitating massive reabsorption by the nephron as a whole. Figure 2.7 shows the major transport mechanisms operating along the nephron (with the exception of the loop of Henle, which is dealt with separately).

Proximal Tubule

The proximal tubule is adapted for bulk reabsorption. The epithelial cells have microvilli (brush border) on their apical surface, providing a large absorptive area; the basolateral membrane is thrown into folds that similarly enhance surface area. The cells are rich in mitochondria (concentrated near the basolateral membrane) and lysosomal vacuoles, and the tight junctions between adjacent cells are relatively leaky. The proximal convoluted tubule (PCT; pars convoluta) makes up the first two thirds of the proximal tubule; the final third is the proximal straight tubule (pars recta).

On the basis of subtle structural and functional differences, the proximal tubule epithelium is subdivided into three types: S_1 makes up the initial short segment of the PCT; S_2, the remainder of the PCT and the cortical segment of the pars recta; and S_3, the medullary segment of the pars recta. The proximal tubule as a whole is responsible for the bulk of Na^+, K^+, Cl^-, and HCO_3^- reabsorption, and almost complete reabsorption of glucose, amino acids, and low-molecular-weight proteins (e.g., retinol-binding protein, α- and β-microglobulins) that have penetrated the filtration barrier. Most other filtered solutes are also reabsorbed to some extent in the proximal tubule (e.g., ~60% of calcium, ~80% of phosphate, ~50% of urea). The proximal tubule is highly permeable to water, so no quantitatively significant osmotic gradient can be established; thus, most filtered water (~65%) is also reabsorbed at this site. In the final section of the proximal tubule (late S_2 and S_3), there is some secretion of weak organic acids and bases, including most diuretics and PAH.

Loop of Henle

The loop of Henle is defined anatomically as comprising the pars recta of the proximal tubule (thick descending limb), the thin descending and ascending limbs (thin ascending limbs are present only in long-looped nephrons; see later), the thick ascending limb (TAL), and the macula densa. In addition to its role in the continuing reabsorption of solutes (Na^+, Cl^-, K^+, Ca^{2+}, Mg^{2+} [the TAL normally reabsorbs the bulk of filtered Mg^{2+}]), this part of the nephron is responsible for the kidney's ability to generate a concentrated or dilute urine and is discussed in detail later.

Distal Nephron

The distal tubule is made up of three segments: the distal convoluted tubule (DCT), where thiazide-sensitive NaCl reabsorption (through an apical cotransporter) occurs (see Fig. 2.7); the connecting tubule (CNT), whose function is essentially intermediate between that of the DCT and that of the next segment; and the initial collecting duct, which is of the same epithelial type as the cortical collecting duct. Two cell types make up the cortical collecting duct. The predominant type, the *principal cell* (see Fig. 2.7), is responsible for Na^+ reabsorption and K^+ secretion (as well as for water reabsorption; see later discussion). Sodium ions enter principal cells from the lumen through apical Na^+ channels (ENaC) and are extruded by the basolateral Na^+,K^+-ATPase. This process is electrogenic and sets up a lumen-negative potential difference. Potassium ions enter principal cells through the same basolateral Na^+,K^+-ATPase and leave through K^+ channels in both membranes; however, the smaller potential difference across the apical membrane (due to Na^+ entry) favors K^+ secretion into the lumen. The other cells in the late distal tubule and cortical collecting duct, the *intercalated cells*, are responsible for secretion of H^+ (by α-intercalated cells) or HCO_3^- (by β-intercalated cells) into the final urine (see Fig. 2.7). In the medullary collecting duct, there is a gradual transition in the epithelium. There are fewer and fewer intercalated cells while the "principal cells" are modified; although they reabsorb Na^+, they have no apical K^+ channels and therefore do not secrete K^+.

Figures 2.8 and 2.9 show the sites of Na^+ and K^+ reabsorption and secretion along the nephron. Figure 2.10 shows the pathophysiologic consequences of known genetic defects in some of the major transporters in the nephron (see Chapter 47 for a detailed account).

GLOMERULOTUBULAR BALANCE

Because the proportion of filtered sodium that is excreted in the urine is so small (normally <1%), it follows that without a compensatory change in reabsorption, even small changes in the filtered load would cause major changes in the amount excreted. For example, if GFR were to increase by 10% and the rate of reabsorption remained unchanged, sodium excretion would increase more than 10-fold. However, an intrinsic feature of tubular function is that the extent of sodium reabsorption in a given nephron segment is roughly proportional to the sodium delivery to that segment. This is the phenomenon of *glomerulotubular balance*. Perfect glomerulotubular balance would mean that both sodium reabsorption and sodium excretion change in exactly the same proportion as the change in GFR; but in reality, glomerulotubular balance is usually less than perfect. Most studies of glomerulotubular balance have focused on the proximal tubule. However, succeeding nephron segments exhibit the

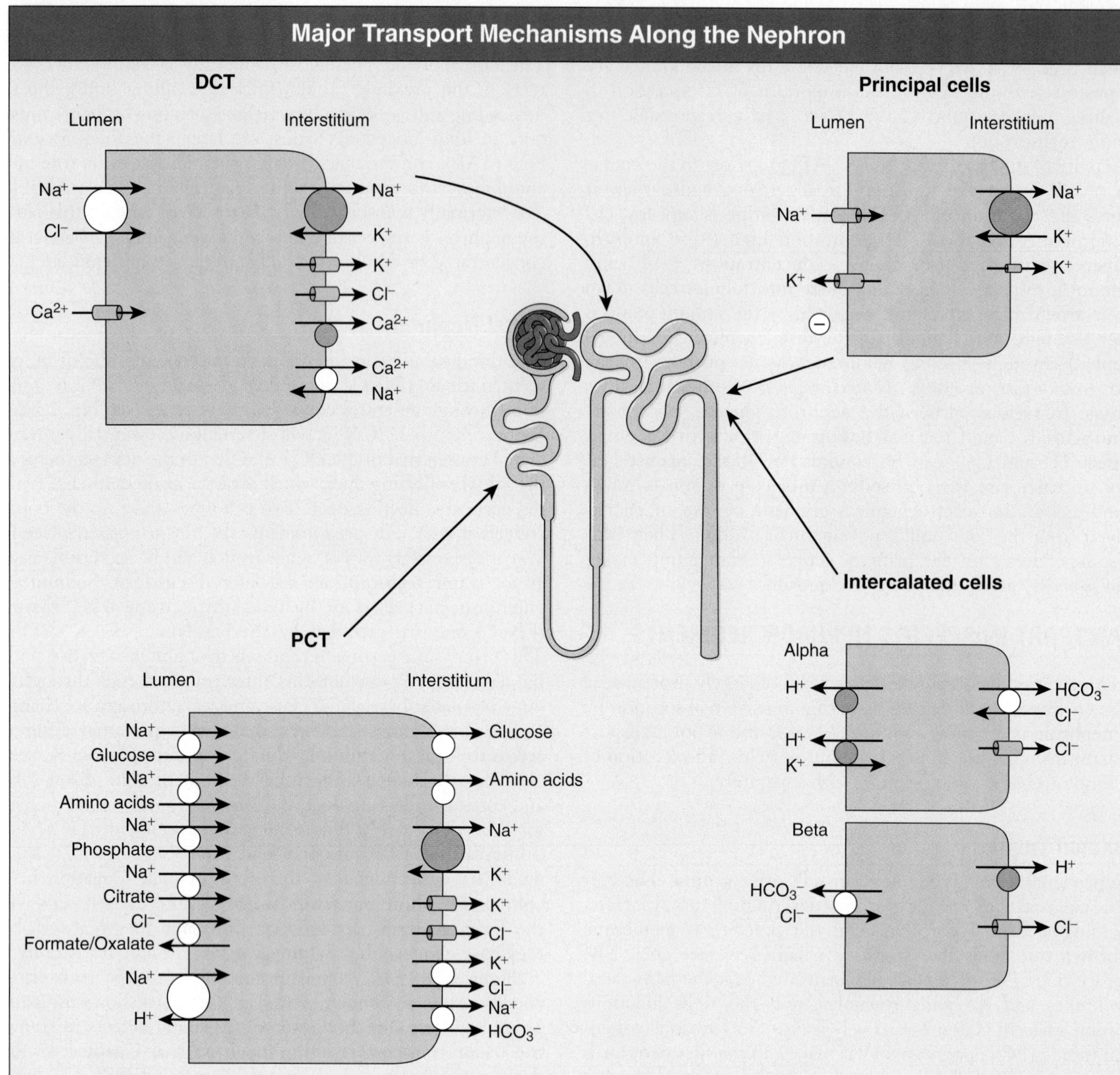

Figure 2.7 Major transport mechanisms along the nephron. Major transport proteins for solutes in the apical and basolateral membranes of tubular cells in specific regions of the nephron. Stoichiometry is not indicated; it is not 1:1 in all cases. *Red circles* represent primary active transport; *white circles* represent carrier-mediated transport (secondary active); *cylinders* represent ion channels. In the proximal convoluted tubule (PCT), Na^+ enters the cell through a Na^+-H^+ exchanger and a series of cotransporters; in the distal convoluted tubule (DCT), Na^+ enters the cell through the thiazide-sensitive Na^+-Cl^- cotransporter; and in the principal cells of the cortical collecting duct (CCD), Na^+ enters through a channel (ENaC). In all cases, Na^+ is extruded from the cells through the basolateral Na^+,K^+-ATPase. Transporters in the thick ascending limb of Henle are dealt with separately (see Fig. 2.12).

same property, so if the load to the loop of Henle or to the distal tubule is increased, some of the excess is mopped up. This is part of the reason that diuretics acting on the proximal tubule are relatively ineffective compared with those acting farther along the nephron; with the latter, there is less scope for buffering of their effects downstream. It is also the reason that combining two diuretics acting at different nephron sites causes a more striking diuresis and natriuresis.

The mechanism of glomerulotubular balance is not fully understood. As far as the proximal tubule is concerned, physical factors operating across peritubular capillary walls may be involved. Glomerular filtration of essentially protein-free fluid means that the plasma leaving the glomeruli in efferent arterioles and supplying the peritubular capillaries has a relatively high oncotic pressure, which favors uptake of fluid reabsorbed from the proximal tubules. If GFR were reduced in the absence of a change in RPF, peritubular capillary oncotic pressure would also be reduced and the tendency to take up fluid reabsorbed from the proximal tubule diminished. It is thought that some of this fluid might leak back through the leaky tight junctions, reducing net reabsorption (Fig. 2.11). However, this mechanism could work only if GFR changed in the absence of a corresponding change in

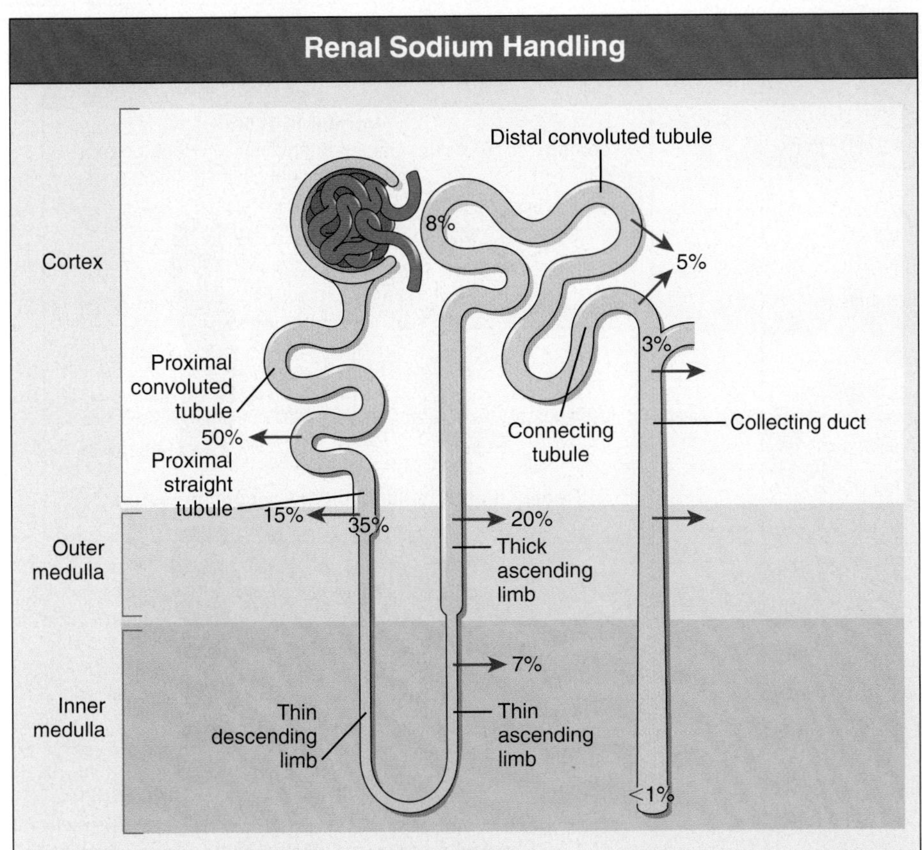

Figure 2.8 Renal sodium handling along the nephron. Figures outside the nephron represent the approximate percentage of the filtered load reabsorbed in each region. Figures within the nephron represent the percentages remaining. Most filtered sodium is reabsorbed in the proximal tubule and loop of Henle; normal day-to-day control of sodium excretion is exerted in the distal nephron.

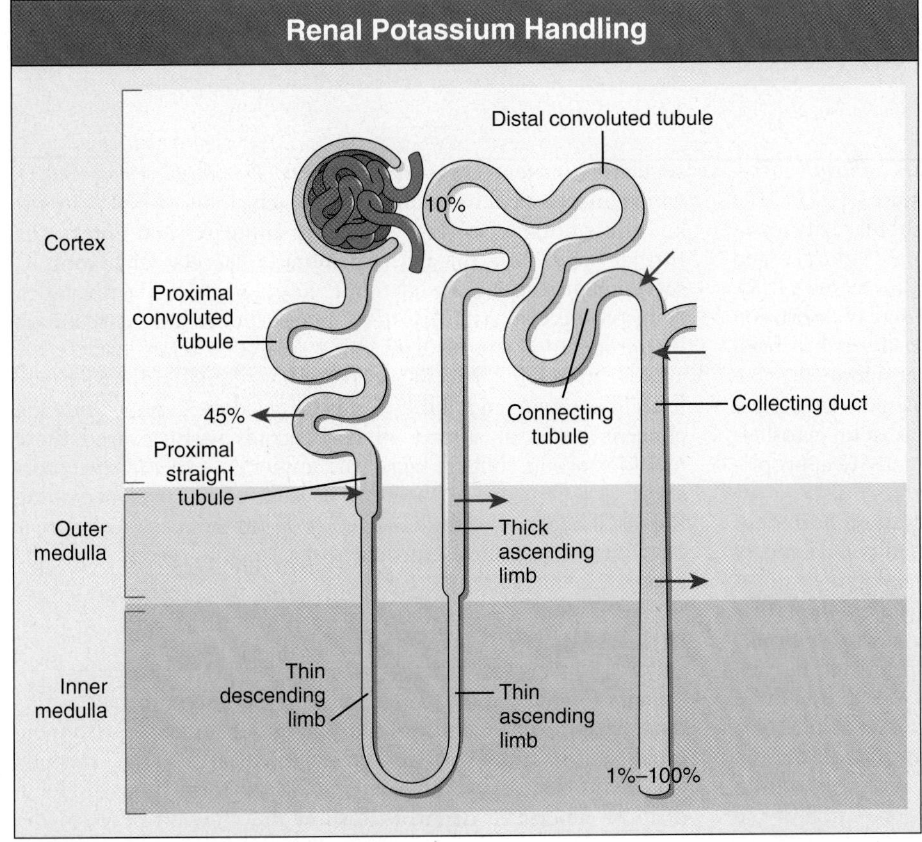

Figure 2.9 Renal potassium handling along the nephron. Figures are not given for percentages reabsorbed or remaining in every region because quantitative information is incomplete, but most filtered potassium is reabsorbed in the proximal convoluted tubule and thick ascending limb of Henle; approximately 10% of the filtered load reaches the early distal tubule. Secretion by connecting tubule cells and principal cells in the late distal tubule–cortical collecting duct is variable and is the major determinant of potassium excretion.

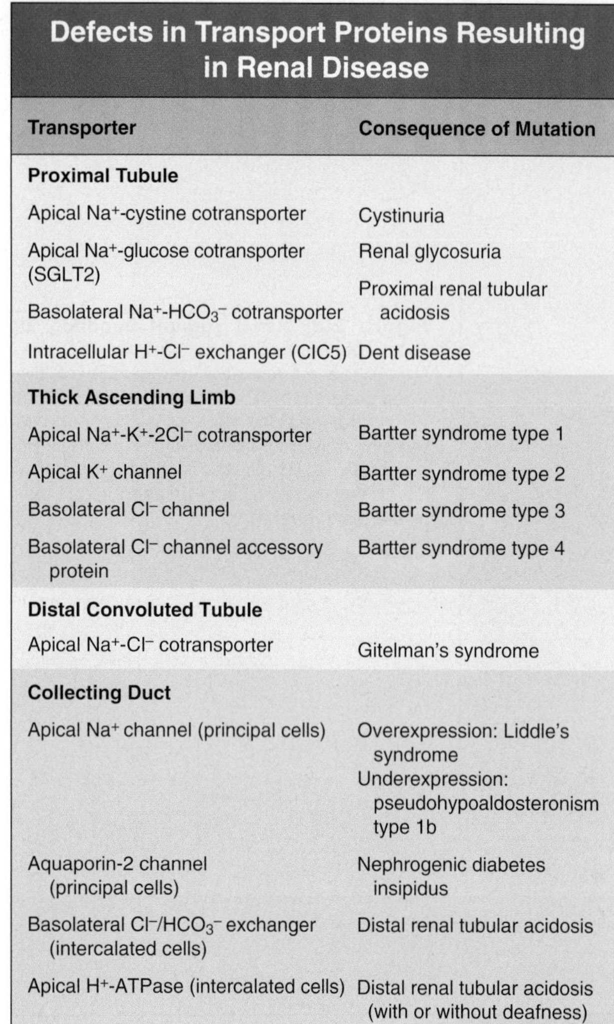

Defects in Transport Proteins Resulting in Renal Disease

Transporter	Consequence of Mutation
Proximal Tubule	
Apical Na^+-cystine cotransporter	Cystinuria
Apical Na^+-glucose cotransporter (SGLT2)	Renal glycosuria
Basolateral Na^+-HCO_3^- cotransporter	Proximal renal tubular acidosis
Intracellular H^+-Cl^- exchanger (ClC5)	Dent disease
Thick Ascending Limb	
Apical Na^+-K^+-$2Cl^-$ cotransporter	Bartter syndrome type 1
Apical K^+ channel	Bartter syndrome type 2
Basolateral Cl^- channel	Bartter syndrome type 3
Basolateral Cl^- channel accessory protein	Bartter syndrome type 4
Distal Convoluted Tubule	
Apical Na^+-Cl^- cotransporter	Gitelman's syndrome
Collecting Duct	
Apical Na^+ channel (principal cells)	Overexpression: Liddle's syndrome Underexpression: pseudohypoaldosteronism type 1b
Aquaporin-2 channel (principal cells)	Nephrogenic diabetes insipidus
Basolateral Cl^-/HCO_3^- exchanger (intercalated cells)	Distal renal tubular acidosis
Apical H^+-ATPase (intercalated cells)	Distal renal tubular acidosis (with or without deafness)

Figure 2.10 Genetic defects in transport proteins resulting in renal disease. For more detailed coverage of these clinical conditions, see Chapter 47.

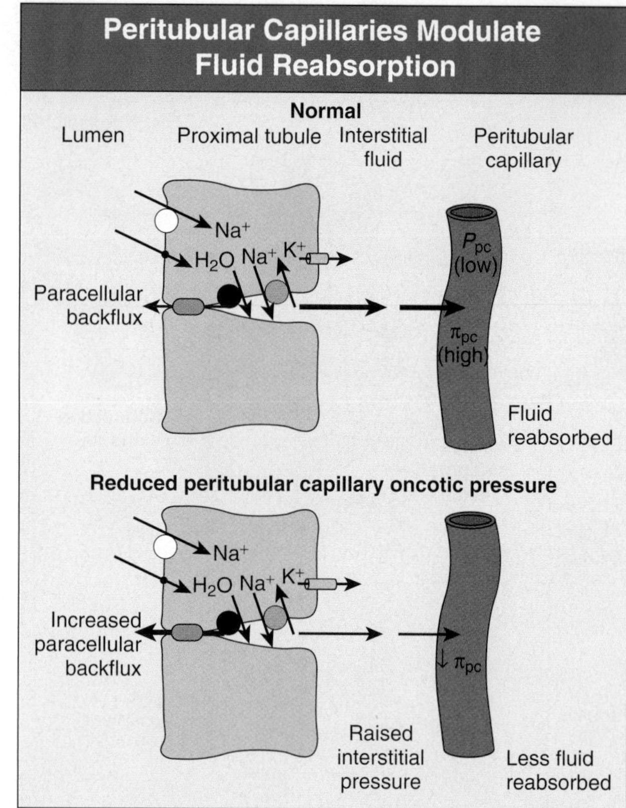

Figure 2.11 Physical factors and proximal tubular reabsorption. Influence of peritubular capillary oncotic pressure on net reabsorption in proximal tubules. Uptake of reabsorbate into peritubular capillaries is determined by the balance of hydrostatic and oncotic pressures across the capillary wall. Compared with those in systemic capillaries, the peritubular capillary hydrostatic (P_{pc}) and oncotic (π_{pc}) pressures are low and high, respectively, so that uptake of proximal tubular reabsorbate into the capillaries is favored. If peritubular capillary oncotic pressure decreases (or hydrostatic pressure increases), less fluid is taken up, interstitial pressure increases, and more fluid may leak back into the lumen paracellularly; net reabsorption in proximal tubules would therefore be reduced.

RPF; if the two change in parallel (i.e., unchanged *filtration fraction*), there would be no change in oncotic pressure.

A second contributory factor to glomerulotubular balance in the proximal tubule could be the filtered loads of glucose and amino acids; if their loads increase (because of increased GFR), the rates of sodium-coupled glucose and amino acid reabsorption in the proximal tubule will also increase. Finally, it has been proposed that the proximal tubular brush border microvilli serve a mechanosensor function, transmitting changes in torque (caused by altered tubular flow rates) to the cells' actin cytoskeleton, which can modulate tubular transporter activity appropriately (although the mechanisms are unknown).[7]

Although the renal sympathetic nerves and certain hormones can influence reabsorption in the proximal tubule and loop of Henle, the combined effects of autoregulation and glomerulotubular balance ensure that a relatively constant load of glomerular filtrate is delivered to the distal tubule under normal circumstances. It is in the final segments of the nephron that normal day-to-day control of sodium excretion is exerted. Evidence points toward important roles for the late DCT and the CNT, in addition to the collecting duct.[8] *Aldosterone*, secreted from the adrenal cortex, stimulates mineralocorticoid receptors within principal cells and CNT cells, which leads to generation of the regulatory protein *serum- and glucocorticoid-inducible kinase* (Sgk1), which increases the number of Na^+ channels (ENaC) in the apical membrane (see Fig. 2.7). This stimulates Na^+ uptake and further depolarizes the apical membrane, thereby facilitating K^+ secretion in the late distal tubule and cortical collecting duct. Aldosterone also stimulates Na^+ reabsorption and K^+ secretion by upregulating the basolateral Na^+,K^+-ATPase.

The mineralocorticoid receptors have equal affinity *in vitro* for aldosterone and adrenal glucocorticoids. The circulating concentrations of adrenal glucocorticoids vastly exceed those of aldosterone, but *in vivo*, the mineralocorticoid receptors show specificity for aldosterone because of the presence along the distal nephron of the enzyme *11β-hydroxysteroid dehydrogenase 2*, which inactivates glucocorticoids in the vicinity of the receptor.[9]

COUNTERCURRENT SYSTEM

A major function of the loop of Henle is the generation and maintenance of the interstitial osmotic gradient that increases from the renal cortex (~290 mOsm/kg) to the tip of the medulla (~1200 mOsm/kg). As indicated in Chapter 1, the loops of Henle of most superficial nephrons turn at the junction between the outer and inner medulla, whereas those of deep nephrons (long-looped nephrons) penetrate the inner medulla to varying degrees. The anatomic loops of Henle reabsorb approximately 40% of filtered Na^+ (mostly in the pars recta and TAL) and approximately 25% of filtered water (in the pars recta and in the thin descending limbs of deep nephrons). (Recent evidence suggests that the thin descending limb of superficial nephrons is relatively impermeable to water.[10]) Both the thin ascending limb (found only in deep nephrons) and the TAL are essentially impermeable to water; however, Na^+ is reabsorbed—passively in the thin ascending limb but actively in the TAL. Active Na^+ reabsorption in the TAL is again driven by the basolateral sodium pump, which maintains a low intracellular Na^+ concentration, allowing Na^+ entry from the lumen through the Na^+-$2Cl^-$-K^+ cotransporter (NKCC-2) and, to a much lesser extent, the Na^+-H^+ exchanger (Fig. 2.12). The apical NKCC-2 is unique to this nephron segment and is the site of action of loop diuretics like furosemide and bumetanide. Na^+ exits the cell through the sodium pump, and Cl^- and K^+ exit through basolateral ion channels and a K^+-Cl^- cotransporter. K^+ also re-enters the lumen (recycles) through apical membrane potassium channels. Re-entry of K^+ into the tubular lumen is necessary for normal operation of the Na^+-$2Cl^-$-K^+ cotransporter, presumably because the availability of K^+ is a limiting factor for the transporter (the K^+ concentration in tubular fluid being much lower than that of Na^+ and Cl^-). K^+ recycling is also partly responsible for generating the lumen-positive potential difference found in this segment. This potential difference drives additional Na^+ reabsorption through the paracellular pathway; for each Na^+ reabsorbed transcellularly, another one is reabsorbed paracellularly (see Fig. 2.12).[11] Other cations (K^+, Ca^{2+}, Mg^{2+}) are also reabsorbed by this route. The reabsorption of NaCl along the TAL in the absence of significant water reabsorption means that the tubular fluid leaving this segment is hypotonic; hence the name *diluting segment*.

The U-shaped, countercurrent arrangement of the loop of Henle, the differences in permeability of the descending and ascending limbs to Na^+ and water, and active Na^+ reabsorption in the TAL are the basis of *countercurrent multiplication* and generation of the medullary osmotic gradient (Fig. 2.13). Fluid

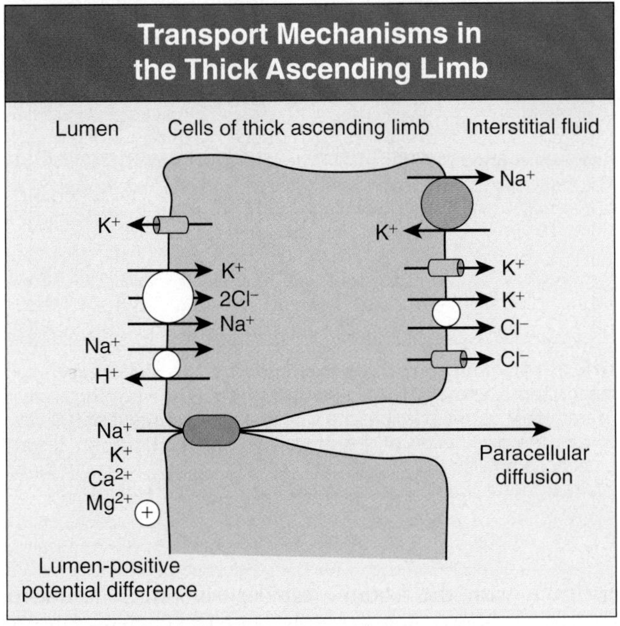

Figure 2.12 Transport mechanisms in the thick ascending limb of Henle. The major cellular entry mechanism is the Na^+-K^+-$2Cl^-$ cotransporter. The transepithelial potential difference drives paracellular transport of Na^+, K^+, Ca^{2+}, and Mg^{2+}.

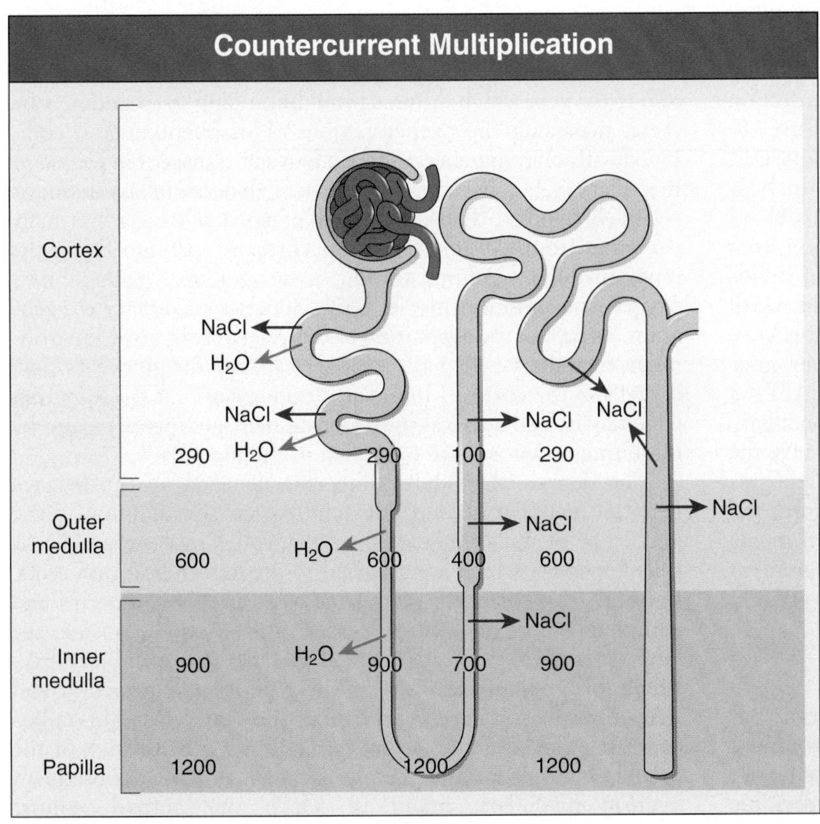

Figure 2.13 Countercurrent multiplication by the loop of Henle. The nephron drawn represents a deep (long-looped) nephron. Figures represent approximate osmolalities (mOsm/kg). Osmotic equilibration occurs in the thin descending limb, whereas NaCl is reabsorbed in the water-impermeable ascending limb; hypotonic fluid is delivered to the distal tubule. In the absence of vasopressin, this fluid remains hypotonic during its passage through the distal tubule and collecting duct, despite the large osmotic gradient favoring water reabsorption. A large volume of dilute urine is therefore formed. During maximal vasopressin secretion, water is reabsorbed down the osmotic gradient, so that tubular fluid becomes isotonic in the cortical collecting duct and hypertonic in the medullary collecting duct. A small volume of concentrated urine is formed.

entering the descending limb from the proximal tubule is isotonic (~290 mOsm/kg). On encountering the hypertonicity of the medullary interstitial fluid (which results from NaCl reabsorption in the water-impermeable ascending limb), the fluid in the descending limb comes into osmotic equilibrium with its surroundings, either by solute entry into the descending limb (superficial nephrons) or by water exit by osmosis (deep nephrons). These events, combined with continuing NaCl reabsorption in the ascending limb, result in a progressive increase in medullary osmolality from corticomedullary junction to papillary tip. A similar osmotic gradient exists in the thin descending limb, whereas at any level in the ascending limb, the osmolality is less than in the surrounding tissue. Thus, hypotonic (~100 mOsm/kg) fluid is delivered to the distal tubule. Ultimately, the energy source for countercurrent multiplication is active Na^+ reabsorption in the TAL. As indicated, Na^+ reabsorption in the thin ascending limb is passive, but how this comes about is not yet understood (see later discussion).

Role of Urea

The thin limbs of the loop of Henle are relatively permeable to urea (ascending > descending), but more distal nephron segments (TAL and beyond) are urea impermeable up to the final section of the inner medullary collecting duct. By this stage, vasopressin-dependent water reabsorption in the collecting ducts (see later discussion) has led to a high urea concentration within the lumen. Owing to vasopressin-sensitive urea transporters (UT-A1 and UT-A3) along the terminal segment of the inner medullary collecting duct, urea is reabsorbed (passively) into the inner medullary interstitium.[12] The interstitial urea exchanges with vasa recta capillaries (see later discussion), and some urea enters the S_3 segment of the pars recta and the descending and ascending thin limbs of the loop of Henle; it is then returned to the inner medullary collecting ducts to be reabsorbed. The net result of this urea recycling process is to add urea to the inner medullary interstitium, thereby increasing interstitial osmolality. The fact that the high urea concentration within the medullary collecting duct is balanced by a similarly high urea concentration in the medullary interstitium allows large quantities of urea to be excreted without incurring the penalty of an osmotic diuresis, as the urea in the collecting duct is rendered osmotically ineffective. Moreover, the high urea concentration in the medullary interstitium should also increase osmotic water abstraction from the thin descending limbs of deep nephrons, raising the intraluminal Na^+ concentration within the thin descending limbs. Until recently, it was thought that this process set the scene for passive Na^+ reabsorption from the thin ascending limbs. However, mice with genetic deletion of the urea transporters UT-A1 and UT-A3 have a much reduced urea concentration in the inner medullary interstitium but a normal interstitial NaCl gradient.[12] Thus, the mechanisms responsible for the inner medullary electrolyte gradient are still unclear. However, the ultimate driving force for countercurrent multiplication is active Na^+ reabsorption in the TAL, a fact underlined by the disruption of the osmotic gradient when loop diuretics are given.

Vasa Recta

The capillaries that supply the medulla also have a special anatomic arrangement. If they passed through the medulla as a more usual capillary network, they would soon dissipate the medullary osmotic gradient because of equilibration of the hypertonic interstitium with the isotonic capillary blood. This does not happen to any appreciable extent because the U-shaped arrangement of the *vasa recta* ensures that solute entry and water loss in the descending vasa recta are offset by solute loss and water entry in the ascending vasa recta. This is the process of *countercurrent exchange* and is entirely passive (Fig. 2.14).

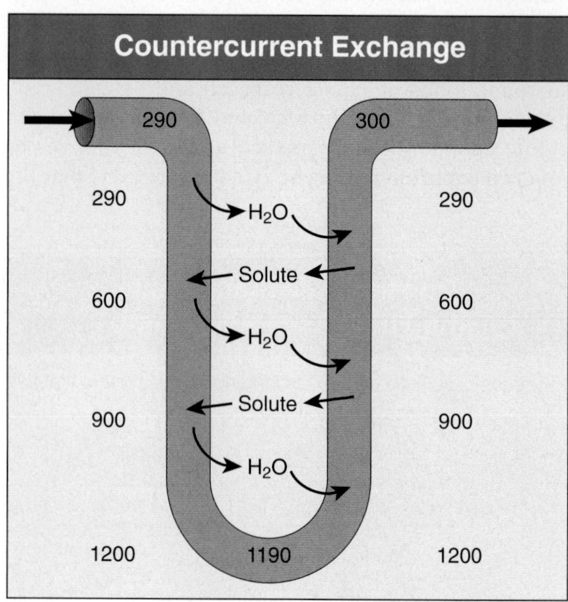

Figure 2.14 Countercurrent exchange by the vasa recta. Figures represent approximate osmolalities (mOsm/kg). The vasa recta capillary walls are highly permeable, but the U-shaped arrangement of the vessels minimizes the dissipation of the medullary osmotic gradient. Nevertheless, because equilibration across the capillary walls is not instantaneous, a certain amount of solute is removed from the interstitium.

Renal Medullary Hypoxia

Countercurrent exchange by the medullary capillaries applies also to oxygen, which diffuses from descending to ascending vasa recta, bypassing the deeper regions. This phenomenon, combined with ongoing energy-dependent salt transport in the outer medullary TAL, has the consequence that medullary tissue is relatively hypoxic. Thus, the partial pressure of oxygen normally decreases from ~50 mm Hg in the cortex to ~10 mm Hg in the inner medulla.[13] Administration of furosemide, which inhibits oxygen consumption in the TAL, increases medullary oxygenation. As part of the adaptation to this relatively hypoxic environment, medullary cells have a higher capacity for glycolysis than do cells in the cortex. Moreover, a number of *heat shock proteins*, which assist cell survival by restoring damaged proteins and by inhibiting apoptosis, are expressed in the medulla.[13]

The degree of medullary hypoxia depends on the balance between medullary blood flow and oxygen consumption in the TAL. The medullary blood flow is controlled by contractile cells called *pericytes*, which are attached to the descending vasa recta. In health, this balance is modulated by a variety of autocrine and paracrine agents (e.g., nitric oxide, eicosanoids, adenosine; see later discussion), several of which can increase medullary oxygenation by simultaneously reducing pericyte contraction and TAL transport. There is evidence that some cases of radiocontrast-induced nephropathy result from a disturbance of the balance between oxygen supply and demand, with consequent hypoxic medullary injury in which the normal cellular adaptations are overwhelmed, with subsequent apoptotic and necrotic cell death.

VASOPRESSIN (ANTIDIURETIC HORMONE) AND WATER REABSORPTION

Vasopressin, or antidiuretic hormone, is a nonapeptide synthesized in specialized neurons of the supraoptic and paraventricular nuclei. It is transported from these nuclei to the posterior pituitary and released in response to increases in plasma osmolality and decreases in blood pressure. Osmoreceptors are found in the hypothalamus, and there is also input to this region from arterial baroreceptors and atrial stretch receptors. The actions of vasopressin are mediated by three receptor subtypes: V_{1a}, V_{1b}, and V_2 receptors. V_{1a} receptors are found in vascular smooth muscle and are coupled to the phosphoinositol pathway; they cause an increase in intracellular Ca^{2+}, resulting in contraction. V_{1a} receptors have also been identified in the apical membrane of several nephron segments, although their role is not yet clear. V_{1b} receptors are found in the anterior pituitary, where vasopressin modulates adrenocorticotropic hormone release. V_2 receptors are found in the basolateral membrane of principal cells in the late distal tubule and the whole length of the collecting duct; they are coupled by a G_s protein to cyclic adenosine monophosphate generation, which ultimately leads to the insertion of water channels *(aquaporins)* into the apical membrane of this otherwise water-impermeable segment (Fig. 2.15). In the X-linked form of nephrogenic diabetes insipidus (the most common hereditary cause), the V_2 receptor is defective.[14]

Several aquaporins have been identified in the kidney.[15] Aquaporin 1 is found in apical and basolateral membranes of all proximal tubules and of thin descending limbs of long-looped nephrons; it is largely responsible for the permanently high water permeability of these segments. Aquaporin 3 is constitutively expressed in the basolateral membrane of CNT cells and cortical and outer medullary principal cells, and aquaporin 4 is constitutively expressed in the basolateral membrane of outer medullary principal cells and inner medullary collecting duct cells; but it is aquaporin 2 that is responsible for the variable water permeability of the late distal tubule and collecting duct. Acute vasopressin release causes shuttling of aquaporin 2 from intracellular vesicles to the apical membrane, while chronically raised vasopressin levels increase aquaporin 2 expression. The apical insertion of aquaporin 2 allows reabsorption of water, driven by the high interstitial osmolality achieved and maintained by the countercurrent system. Vasopressin also contributes to the effectiveness of this system by stimulating Na^+ reabsorption in the TAL (although this effect may be functionally significant only in rodents[16]) and urea reabsorption through the UT-A1 and UT-A3 transporters in the inner medullary collecting duct. In the rare autosomal recessive and even rarer autosomal dominant forms of nephrogenic diabetes insipidus, aquaporin 2 is abnormal or fails to translocate to the apical membrane.[15]

Aquaporin 2 dysfunction also appears to underlie the well-known urinary concentrating defect associated with hypercalcemia. Increased intraluminal Ca^{2+} concentrations, acting through an apically located calcium-sensing receptor, interfere with the insertion of aquaporin 2 channels in the apical membrane of the medullary collecting duct.[17] In addition, stimulation of a calcium receptor in the basolateral membrane of the TAL inhibits solute transport in this nephron segment (through inhibition of the apical NKCC-2 and potassium channels), thereby reducing the medullary osmotic gradient.[18]

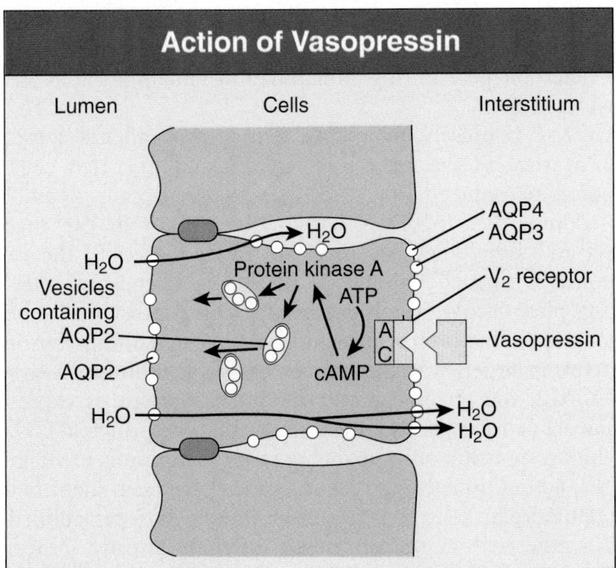

Figure 2.15 Mechanism of action of vasopressin (antidiuretic hormone). The hormone binds to V_2 receptors on the basolateral membrane of collecting duct principal cells and increases intracellular cyclic adenosine monophosphate (cAMP) production, causing, through intermediate reactions involving protein kinase A, insertion of preformed water channels (aquaporin 2 [AQP2]) into the apical membrane. The water permeability of the basolateral membrane, which contains aquaporins 3 and 4, is permanently high. Therefore, vasopressin secretion allows transcellular movement of water from lumen to interstitium. AC, adenylate cyclase.

INTEGRATED CONTROL OF RENAL FUNCTION

One of the major functions of the kidneys is the regulation of blood volume, through the regulation of *effective circulating volume*, an unmeasurable, conceptual volume that reflects the degree of fullness of the vasculature. This is achieved largely by control of the sodium content of the body. The mechanisms involved in the regulation of effective circulating volume are discussed in detail in Chapter 7. Some of the more important mediator systems are introduced here.

Renal Interstitial Hydrostatic Pressure and Nitric Oxide

Acute increases in arterial blood pressure lead to natriuresis *(pressure natriuresis)*. Because autoregulation is not perfect, part of this response is mediated by increases in RBF and GFR (see Fig. 2.3), but the main cause is reduced tubular reabsorption, which appears to result largely from an increase in *renal interstitial hydrostatic pressure* (RIHP). An elevated RIHP could reduce net reabsorption in the proximal tubule by increasing paracellular backflux through the tight junctions of the tubular wall (see Fig. 2.11). The increase in RIHP is thought to be dependent on intrarenally produced *nitric oxide*.[19] Moreover, increased nitric oxide production in macula densa cells (which contain the neuronal [type I] isoform of nitric oxide synthase [nNOS]) blunts the sensitivity of TGF, thereby allowing increased NaCl delivery to the distal nephron without incurring a TGF-mediated decrease in GFR.[20]

Another renal action of nitric oxide results from the presence of inducible (type II) nitric oxide synthase in glomerular mesangial cells: local production of nitric oxide counteracts the mesangial contractile response to agonists such as Ang II and endothelin (see later discussion). Furthermore, nitric oxide may have a role in the regulation of medullary blood flow. Locally synthesized nitric oxide offsets the vasoconstrictor effects of other agents on the pericytes of the descending vasa recta, and it reduces Na^+ reabsorption in the TAL; both actions will help protect the renal medulla from hypoxia. Finally, nitric oxide may promote natriuresis and diuresis through direct actions on the renal tubule. Thus, in addition to its effect on the TAL, locally produced nitric oxide inhibits Na^+ and water reabsorption in the collecting duct.[21]

Renal Sympathetic Nerves

Reductions in arterial pressure or central venous pressure result in reduced afferent signaling from arterial baroreceptors or atrial volume receptors, which elicits a reflex increase in renal sympathetic nervous discharge. This reduces urinary sodium excretion in at least three ways:

- Constriction of afferent and efferent arterioles (predominantly afferent), thereby directly reducing RBF and GFR, and indirectly reducing RIHP.
- Direct stimulation of sodium reabsorption in the proximal tubule and the TAL of the loop of Henle.
- Stimulation of *renin* secretion by afferent arteriolar cells (see later discussion).

Renin-Angiotensin-Aldosterone System

The renin-angiotensin-aldosterone system (RAAS) is central to the control of extracellular fluid volume (ECFV) and blood pressure. Renin is synthesized and stored in specialized afferent arteriolar cells that form part of the juxtaglomerular apparatus (see Fig. 2.4) and is released into the circulation in response to

- Increased renal sympathetic nervous discharge.
- Reduced stretch of the afferent arteriole after a reduction in renal perfusion pressure.
- Reduced delivery of NaCl to the macula densa region of the nephron.

Renin catalyzes the production of the decapeptide angiotensin I from circulating angiotensinogen (synthesized in the liver); angiotensin I is in turn converted to the octapeptide *Ang II* by the ubiquitous angiotensin-converting enzyme. Ang II has a number of actions pertinent to the control of ECFV and blood pressure:

- It causes general arteriolar vasoconstriction, including renal afferent and (particularly) efferent arterioles, thereby increasing arterial pressure but reducing RBF. The tendency of P_{gc} to increase is offset by Ang II–induced mesangial cell contraction and reduced K_f; thus, the overall effect on GFR is unpredictable.
- It directly stimulates sodium reabsorption in the proximal tubule.
- It stimulates aldosterone secretion from the zona glomerulosa of the adrenal cortex. As described earlier, aldosterone stimulates sodium reabsorption in the distal tubule and collecting duct.

Eicosanoids

Eicosanoids are a family of metabolites of arachidonic acid produced enzymatically by three systems: cyclooxygenase (of which two isoforms exist, COX-1 and COX-2, both expressed in the kidney), cytochrome P-450, and lipoxygenase. The major renal eicosanoids produced by the COX system are *prostaglandin* E_2 and *prostaglandin* I_2, both of which are renal vasodilators and act to buffer the effects of renal vasoconstrictor agents such as Ang II and norepinephrine; and *thromboxane* A_2, a vasoconstrictor. Under normal circumstances, prostaglandins E_2 and I_2 have little effect on renal hemodynamics; but during stressful situations such as hypovolemia, they help protect the kidney from excessive functional changes. Consequently, nonsteroidal anti-inflammatory drugs (NSAIDs), which are COX inhibitors, can cause dramatic falls in GFR. Prostaglandin E_2 also has tubular effects, inhibiting Na^+ reabsorption in the TAL of the loop of Henle and both Na^+ and water reabsorption in the collecting duct.[22] Its action in the TAL, together with a dilator effect on vasa recta pericytes, is another paracrine regulatory mechanism that helps protect the renal medulla from hypoxia. This may explain why inhibition of COX-2 can reduce medullary blood flow and cause apoptosis of medullary interstitial cells.

The metabolism of arachidonic acid by renal cytochrome P-450 enzymes yields *epoxyeicosatrienoic acids* (EETs), *20-hydroxyeicosatetraenoic acid* (20-HETE), and *dihydroxyeicosatrienoic acids* (DHETs). These compounds appear to have a multiplicity of autocrine, paracrine, and second-messenger effects on the renal vasculature and tubules that have not yet been fully unraveled.[23] Like prostaglandins, EETs are vasodilator agents, whereas 20-HETE is a potent renal arteriolar constrictor and may be involved in the vasoconstrictor effect of Ang II as well as the TGF mechanism. 20-HETE also constricts vasa recta pericytes and may be involved in the control of medullary blood flow. Some evidence suggests that locally produced 20-HETE and EETs can inhibit sodium reabsorption in the proximal tubule and TAL.[24] Indeed, cytochrome P-450 metabolites of arachidonic acid may contribute to the reduced proximal tubular reabsorption seen in pressure natriuresis.

The third enzyme system that metabolizes arachidonic acid, the lipoxygenase system, is activated (in leukocytes, mast cells, and macrophages) during inflammation and injury and is not considered here.

COX-2 is present in macula densa cells and has a critical role in the release of renin from juxtaglomerular cells in response to reduced NaCl delivery to the macula densa.[22] A low-sodium diet increases COX-2 expression in the macula densa and simultaneously increases renin secretion; the renin response is virtually abolished in COX-2 knockout mice or during pharmacologic inhibition of COX-2. It is likely, therefore, that the hyporeninemia observed during administration of NSAIDs is largely a consequence of COX-2 inhibition. As well as COX-2, the enzyme prostaglandin E synthase is expressed in macula densa cells, and it is thought that the principal COX-2 product responsible for enhancing renin secretion is prostaglandin E_2, acting on specific receptors that have been identified in juxtaglomerular cells; it is not clear whether prostaglandin I_2 is also synthesized in macula densa cells. As already indicated, nNOS (type I) is also present in macula densa cells and produces nitric oxide that blunts TGF.[25] Nitric oxide also has a permissive role in renin secretion, although the mechanism is not understood. The increase in macula densa COX-2 expression induced by a low-sodium diet is attenuated during administration of selective nNOS inhibitors, which has led to speculation that nitric oxide is responsible for the increase in COX-2 activity and the resulting increase in juxtaglomerular renin secretion.[26] The established and proposed roles of COX-2 and

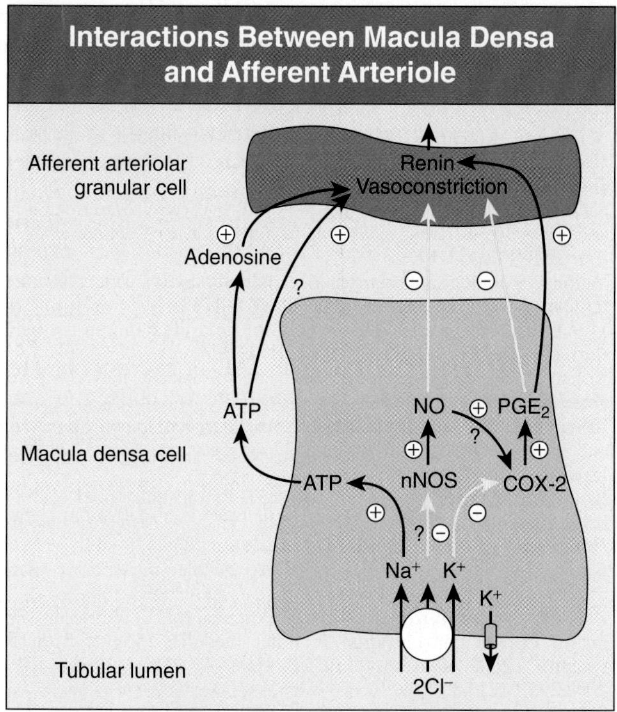

Figure 2.16 Interactions between macula densa and afferent arteriole: proposed mediators of renin secretion and tubuloglomerular feedback. Both cyclooxygenase 2 (COX-2) and neuronal nitric oxide synthase (nNOS) enzyme systems are present in macula densa cells. Increased NaCl delivery to the macula densa stimulates NaCl entry into the cells through the Na^+-K^+-$2Cl^-$ cotransporter. This causes afferent arteriolar constriction through adenosine or adenosine triphosphate (ATP), and also inhibits COX-2 activity; the latter effect might be mediated partly through inhibition of (nNOS-mediated) nitric oxide (NO) production. Generation of prostaglandin E_2 by COX-2 stimulates renin release. Prostaglandin E_2 (PGE_2) also modulates vasoconstriction, as does nitric oxide.

nNOS in the macula densa are shown diagrammatically in Figure 2.16.

Atrial Natriuretic Peptide

If blood volume increases significantly, the resulting atrial stretch stimulates the release of *atrial natriuretic peptide* from atrial myocytes. This hormone increases sodium excretion, partly by suppression of renin and aldosterone release and partly by a direct inhibitory effect on sodium reabsorption in the medullary collecting duct. Atrial natriuretic peptide may additionally increase GFR because high doses cause afferent arteriolar vasodilation and mesangial cell relaxation (thus increasing K_f; see Fig. 2.6).

Endothelins

Endothelins are potent vasoconstrictor peptides to which the renal vasculature is exquisitely sensitive.[27] They function primarily as autocrine or paracrine agents. The kidney is a rich source of endothelins, the predominant isoform being endothelin 1 (ET-1). ET-1 is generated throughout the renal vasculature, including afferent and efferent arterioles (where it causes vasoconstriction, possibly mediated by 20-HETE) and mesangial cells (where it causes contraction, i.e., decreases K_f). Consequently, renal ET-1 can cause profound reductions in RBF and GFR (Fig. 2.6).

In contrast to its effect on GFR, it is now clear that ET-1 can act on the renal tubule to increase urinary Na^+ and water excretion. ET-1 levels are highest in the renal medulla—in the TAL and, more prominently, the inner medullary collecting duct. The distribution of renal endothelin receptors (ET_A and ET_B receptors) reflects the sites of production; the predominant receptor in the inner medulla is ET_B.[28] Mice with collecting duct–specific deletions of either ET-1 or ET_B receptors exhibit salt-sensitive hypertension, whereas collecting duct–specific ET_A receptor deletion results in no obvious renal phenotype.[21] ET-1 knockout mice also show a greater sensitivity to vasopressin than do wild-type mice. There is mounting evidence that the natriuretic and diuretic effects of medullary ET_B receptor stimulation are mediated by nitric oxide.[21] Taken together with evidence that ET-1 can inhibit Na^+ reabsorption in the medullary TAL (also likely to be mediated by nitric oxide), these findings highlight the potential importance of ET-1 and nitric oxide interactions in the control of Na^+ and water excretion.

Purines

There is increasing evidence that extracellular *purines* (e.g., ATP, adenosine diphosphate [ADP], adenosine, uric acid) can act as autocrine or paracrine agents within the kidneys. Purinoceptors are subdivided into P1 and P2 receptors. The P1 receptors are responsive to adenosine and are more usually known as adenosine receptors (A_1, A_{2a}, A_{2b}, and A_3); the P2 receptors, responsive to nucleotides (e.g., ATP and ADP), are further subdivided into P2X (ligand-gated ion channels) and P2Y (metabotropic) receptors, each category having a number of subtypes. As indicated earlier, A_1 and $P2X_1$ receptors are found in afferent arterioles and mediate vasoconstriction. Purinoceptors are also found in the apical and basolateral membranes of renal tubular cells. Stimulation of A_1 receptors enhances proximal tubular reabsorption and inhibits collecting duct Na^+ reabsorption, whereas stimulation of P2 receptors generally has an inhibitory effect on tubular transport.[29] Thus, luminally applied nucleotides, acting on a variety of P2 receptor subtypes, can inhibit Na^+ reabsorption in the proximal tubule, distal tubule, and collecting duct[30]; and stimulation of $P2Y_2$ receptors in the collecting duct inhibits vasopressin-sensitive water reabsorption; an observation reinforced by the report of increased concentrating ability in $P2Y_2$ receptor knockout mice.[31] Despite these clear indications of tubular effects of nucleotides, further studies will be necessary before their roles in normal tubular physiology are clarified.

Finally, there is some evidence that the end product of purine metabolism, uric acid, may cause renal vasoconstriction, possibly by inhibiting endothelial release of nitric oxide and stimulation of renin.[32]

REFERENCES

1. Haraldsson B, Nyström J, Deen WM. Properties of the glomerular barrier and mechanisms of proteinuria. *Physiol Rev.* 2008;88:451-487.
2. Persson PB. Renal blood flow autoregulation in blood pressure control. *Curr Opin Nephrol Hypertens.* 2002;11:67-72.
3. Bell PD, Komlosi P, Zhang Z. ATP as a mediator of macula densa cell signalling. *Purinergic Signal.* 2009;5:461-471.
4. Inscho EW. ATP, P2 receptors and the renal microcirculation. *Purinergic Signal.* 2009;5:447-460.
5. Shirley DG, Walter SJ. A micropuncture study of the renal response to haemorrhage in rats: Assessment of the role of vasopressin. *Exp Physiol.* 1995;80:619-630.
6. Skou JC. The influence of some cations on an adenosine triphosphatase from peripheral nerves. *Biochim Biophys Acta.* 1957;23:394-401.
7. Du Z, Yan Q, Duan Y, et al. Axial flow modulates proximal tubule NHE3 and H-ATPase activities by changing microvillus bending moments. *Am J Physiol Renal Physiol.* 2006;290:F289-F296.

8. Meneton P, Loffing J, Warnock DG. Sodium and potassium handling by the aldosterone-sensitive distal nephron: The pivotal role of the distal and connecting tubule. *Am J Physiol Renal Physiol.* 2004;287:F593-F601.
9. Bailey MA, Unwin RJ, Shirley DG. In vivo inhibition of renal 11β-hydroxysteroid dehydrogenase in the rat stimulates collecting duct sodium reabsorption. *Clin Sci.* 2001;101:195-198.
10. Zhai X-Y, Fenton RA, Andreasen A, et al. Aquaporin-1 is not expressed in descending thin limbs of short-loop nephrons. *J Am Soc Nephrol.* 2007;18:2937-2944.
11. Greger R. Ion transport mechanisms in thick ascending limb of Henle's loop of mammalian nephron. *Physiol Rev.* 1985;65:760-795.
12. Fenton RA, Knepper MA. Mouse models and the urinary concentrating mechanism in the new millennium. *Physiol Rev.* 2007;87:1083-1112.
13. Neuhofer W, Beck F-X. Cell survival in the hostile environment of the renal medulla. *Annu Rev Physiol.* 2005;67:531-555.
14. Rosenthal W, Seibold A, Antaramian A, et al. Molecular identification of the gene responsible for congenital nephrogenic diabetes insipidus. *Nature.* 1992;359:233-235.
15. Nielsen S, Frøkiær J, Marples D, et al. Aquaporins in the kidney: From molecules to medicine. *Physiol Rev.* 2002;82:205-244.
16. Bankir L. Antidiuretic action of vasopressin: Quantitative aspects and interaction between V_{1a} and V_2 receptor–mediated effects. *Cardiovasc Res.* 2001;51:372-390.
17. Valenti G, Procino G, Tamma G, et al. Aquaporin 2 trafficking. *Endocrinology.* 2005;146:5063-5070.
18. Ward DT, Riccardi D. Renal physiology of the extracellular calcium-sensing receptor. *Pflugers Arch.* 2002;445:169-176.
19. Nakamura T, Alberola AM, Salazar FJ, et al. Effects of renal perfusion pressure on renal interstitial hydrostatic pressure and Na^+ excretion: Role of endothelium-derived nitric oxide. *Nephron.* 1998;78:104-111.
20. Thorup C, Persson AEG. Macula densa derived nitric oxide in regulation of glomerular capillary pressure. *Kidney Int.* 1996;49:430-436.
21. Pollock JS, Pollock DM. Endothelin and NOS1/nitric oxide signaling and regulation of sodium homeostasis. *Curr Opin Nephrol Hypertens.* 2008;17:70-75.
22. Hao C-M, Breyer MD. Physiological regulation of prostaglandins in the kidney. *Annu Rev Physiol.* 2008;70:357-377.
23. Maier KG, Roman RJ. Cytochrome P450 metabolites of arachidonic acid in the control of renal function. *Curr Opin Nephrol Hypertens.* 2001;10:81-87.
24. Sarkis A, Lopez B, Roman RJ. Role of 20-hydroxyeicosatetraenoic acid and epoxyeicosatrienoic acids in hypertension. *Curr Opin Nephrol Hypertens.* 2004;13:205-214.
25. Vallon V. Tubuloglomerular feedback in the kidney: Insights from gene-targeted mice. *Pflugers Arch.* 2003;445:470-476.
26. Welch WJ, Wilcox CS. What is brain nitric oxide doing in the kidney? *Curr Opin Nephrol Hypertens.* 2002;11:109-115.
27. Kohan DE. Endothelins in the normal and diseased kidney. *Am J Kidney Dis.* 1997;29:2-26.
28. Kohan DE. The renal medullary endothelin system in control of sodium and water excretion and systemic blood pressure. *Curr Opin Nephrol Hypertens.* 2006;15:34-40.
29. Bailey MA, Shirley DG, King BF, et al. Extracellular nucleotides and renal function. In: Alpern RJ, Hebert SC, eds. *The Kidney: Physiology and Pathophysiology.* 4th ed. Amsterdam: Elsevier; 2008:425-442.
30. Bailey MA, Shirley DG. Effects of extracellular nucleotides on renal tubular solute transport. *Purinergic Signal.* 2009;5:473-480.
31. Zhang Y, Sands JM, Kohan DE, et al. Potential role of purinergic signaling in urinary concentration in inner medulla: Insights from $P2Y_2$ receptor gene knockout mice. *Am J Physiol Renal Physiol.* 2008;295:F1715-F1724.
32. Sanchez-Lozada LG, Tapia E, Santamaria J, et al. Mild hyperuricemia induces severe cortical vasoconstriction and perpetuates glomerular hypertension in normal rats and in experimental chronic renal failure. *Kidney Int.* 2005;67:237-247.

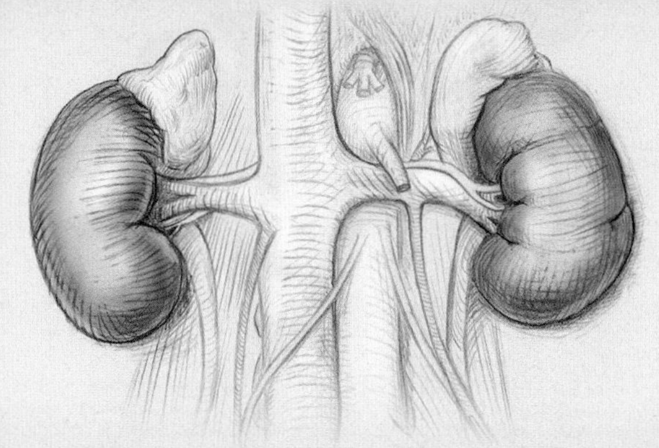

SECTION 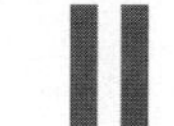

Investigation of Renal Disease

CHAPTER 3

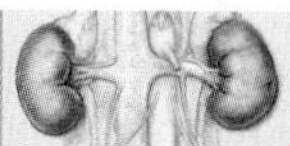

Assessment of Renal Function

Lesley A. Stevens, Shani Shastri, Andrew S. Levey

GLOMERULAR FILTRATION RATE

Glomerular filtration rate (GFR) is a product of the average filtration rate of each single nephron, the filtering unit of the kidneys, multiplied by the number of nephrons in both kidneys. The normal level for GFR is approximately 130 ml/min per 1.73 m^2 for men and 120 ml/min per 1.73 m^2 for women, with considerable variation among individuals according to age, sex, body size, physical activity, diet, pharmacologic therapy, and physiologic states such as pregnancy.[1] To standardize the function of the kidney for differences in kidney size, which is proportional to body size, GFR is adjusted for body surface area, computed from height and weight, and is expressed per 1.73 m^2 surface area, the mean surface area of young men and women. Even after adjustment for body surface area, GFR is approximately 8% higher in young men than in women and declines with age; the mean rate of decline is approximately 0.75 ml/min per year after the age of 40 years, but the variation is wide and the sources of variation are poorly understood. During pregnancy, GFR increases by about 50% in the first trimester and returns to normal immediately after delivery. GFR has a diurnal variation and is 10% lower at midnight compared with the afternoon. Within an individual, GFR is relatively constant over time but varies considerably among people, even after adjustment for the known variables.

Reductions in GFR can be due to either a decline in the nephron number or a decline in the single-nephron GFR (SNGFR) from physiologic or hemodynamic alterations. An increase in SNGFR due to increased glomerular capillary pressure or glomerular hypertrophy can compensate for a decrease in nephron number, and, therefore, the level of GFR may not reflect the loss of nephrons. As a result, there may be substantial kidney damage before GFR decreases.

MEASUREMENT OF THE GLOMERULAR FILTRATION RATE

GFR cannot be measured directly. Instead, it is measured as the urinary clearance of an ideal filtration marker.

Concept of Clearance

Clearance of a substance is defined as the volume of plasma cleared of a marker by excretion per unit of time. The clearance of substance x (C_x) can be calculated as $C_x = A_x / P_x$, where A_x is the amount of x eliminated from the plasma, P_x is the average plasma concentration, and C_x is expressed in units of volume per time. Clearance does not represent an actual volume; rather, it is a virtual volume of plasma that is completely cleared of the substance per unit of time. The value for clearance is related to the efficiency of elimination: the greater the rate of elimination, the higher the clearance. Clearance of substance x is the sum of the urinary and extrarenal clearance; for substances that are eliminated by renal and extrarenal routes, plasma clearance exceeds urinary clearance.

Urinary Clearance

The amount of substance x excreted in the urine can be calculated as the product of the urinary flow rate (V) and the urinary concentration (U_x). Therefore, urinary clearance is defined as follows:

$$C_x = (U_x \times V)/P_x$$

Urinary excretion of a substance depends on filtration, tubular secretion, and tubular reabsorption. Substances that are filtered but not secreted or reabsorbed by the tubules are ideal filtration markers because their urinary clearance can be used as a measure of GFR. For substances that are filtered and secreted, urinary clearance exceeds GFR; and for substances that are filtered and reabsorbed, urinary clearance is less than GFR.

Measurement of urinary clearance requires a timed urine collection for measurement of urine volume as well as urine and plasma concentrations of the filtration marker. Special care must be taken to avoid incomplete urine collections, which will limit the accuracy of the clearance calculation.

Plasma Clearance

There is an increasing interest in measurement of plasma clearance because it avoids the need for a timed urine collection. GFR is calculated from plasma clearance (C_x) after a bolus intravenous injection of an exogenous filtration marker, with the clearance (C_x) computed from the amount of the marker administered (A_x) divided by the plasma concentration (P_x), which is equivalent to the area under the curve of plasma concentration versus time.

$$C_x = A_x/P_x$$

The decline in plasma levels is secondary to the immediate disappearance of the marker from the plasma into its volume of distribution (fast component) and to renal excretion (slow component). Plasma clearance is best estimated by use of a two-compartment model that requires blood sampling early (usually two or three time points until 60 minutes) and late (one to three time points from 120 minutes onward). Like urinary clearance, plasma clearance of a substance depends on filtration, tubular secretion, and tubular reabsorption and, in addition, extrarenal elimination.

Exogenous Filtration Markers

Inulin, a 5200-d uncharged polymer of fructose, was the first substance described as an ideal filtration marker and remains the gold standard against which other markers are evaluated. The classic protocol for inulin clearance requires a continuous intravenous infusion to achieve a steady state and bladder catheterization with multiple timed urine collections. Because this technique is cumbersome, and inulin measurement requires a difficult chemical assay, this method has not been used widely in clinical practice and remains a research tool. Alternative exogenous substances include iothalamate, iohexol, ethylenediaminetetraacetic acid, and diethylenetriaminepentaacetic acid, often chelated to radioisotopes for ease of detection (Fig. 3.1). Alternative protocols to assess clearance have also been validated, including subcutaneous injection and spontaneous bladder emptying. There are advantages to alternative exogenous filtration markers and methods, but also limitations. Understanding of the strengths and limitations of each alternative marker and each clearance method will facilitate interpretation of measured GFR.[2]

Exogenous Filtration Markers for Estimation of GFR

Marker	Method of Administration	Comments
Inulin	Continuous IV	Gold standard
Iothalamate	Bolus IV or subcutaneous	Can be administered as radioactive compound with ^{125}I as the tracer or in nonradioactive form, with assay using HPLC methods. In radioactive form, potential problem of thyroid uptake of ^{125}I. Iothalamate is secreted, leading to overestimation of GFR
^{99m}Tc-DTPA	Bolus IV	Dissociation of ^{99m}Tc leads to plasma protein binding and under-estimation of GFR
^{51}Cr-EDTA	Bolus IV	10% lower clearance than inulin
Iohexol	Bolus IV	Low incidence of adverse effects Comparable to inulin Expensive and difficult to perform assay

Figure 3.1 Exogenous filtration markers for estimation of glomerular filtration rate. ^{51}Cr-EDTA, ^{51}Cr-labeled ethylenediaminetetraacetic acid; GFR, glomerular filtration rate; ^{99m}Tc-DTPA, ^{99m}Tc-labeled diethylenetriaminepentaacetic acid.

Endogenous Filtration Markers

Creatinine is the most commonly used endogenous filtration marker in clinical practice. Urea was widely used in the past, and cystatin C presently shows great promise. A comparison of these markers is outlined in Figure 3.2. For filtration markers that are excreted in the urine, urinary clearance can be computed from a timed urine collection and a single measurement of serum concentration. If the serum level is not constant during the urine collection, as in acute kidney disease or when residual kidney function is assessed in dialysis patients, it is also necessary to obtain additional blood samples during the urine collection to estimate the average serum concentration.

Estimation of GFR from Plasma Levels of Endogenous Filtration Markers

Figure 3.3 shows the relationship of plasma concentration of substance x to its generation (G_x) by cells and dietary intake, urinary excretion ($U_x \times V$), and extrarenal elimination (E_x) by gut and liver. The plasma level is related to the reciprocal of the level of GFR, but it is also influenced by generation, tubular secretion and reabsorption, and extrarenal elimination, collectively termed non-GFR determinants of the plasma level.

In the steady state, a constant plasma level of substance x is maintained because generation is equal to urinary excretion and extrarenal elimination. Estimating equations incorporate demographic and clinical variables as surrogates for the non-GFR determinants and provide a more accurate estimate of GFR than the reciprocal of the plasma level alone. Estimating equations are derived from regression of measured GFR on measured values of the filtration marker and observed values of the demographic and clinical variables. Estimated GFR may differ from measured GFR in a patient if there is a discrepancy between the true and average values for the relationship of the surrogate to the non-GFR determinants of the filtration marker. Other sources of errors include measurement error in the filtration marker (including failure to calibrate the assay for the filtration marker to the assay used in the development of the equation), measurement error in GFR in development of the equation, and regression to the mean. In principle, all these errors are likely to be greater at higher values for GFR.

CREATININE

Creatinine Metabolism and Excretion

Creatinine is a 113-d end product of muscle catabolism.[1] Advantages of creatinine include its ease of measurement and the low cost and widespread availability of assays. Disadvantages include the large number of non-GFR determinants (see Fig. 3.2), leading to a wide range of GFR for a given plasma creatinine level. For example, a serum creatinine level of 1.5 mg/dl (132 μmol/l) may correspond to a GFR from approximately 20 to 90 ml/min per 1.73 m^2.

Creatinine is derived by the metabolism of phosphocreatine in muscle as well as from dietary meat intake or creatine supplements. Creatinine generation is proportional to muscle mass, which can be estimated from age, gender, race, and body size. Figure 3.4 lists factors that can affect creatinine generation.

Creatinine is released into the circulation at a constant rate. It is not protein bound and is freely filtered across the glomerulus and secreted by the tubules. Several medications, such as cimetidine and trimethoprim, competitively inhibit creatinine

Comparison of Creatinine, Urea, and Cystatin C as Filtration Markers

Variable	Creatinine	Urea	Cystatin C
Molecular properties			
Weight	113 daltons	60 daltons	13,000 daltons
Structure	Amino acid derivative	Organic molecular product of protein metabolism	Nonglycosylated basic protein
Physiologic determinants of serum level			
Generation	Varies, according to muscle mass and dietary protein; lower in elderly persons, women, and Caucasians	Varies, according to dietary protein intake and catabolism	Thought to be constant by all nucleated cells; variation in cystatin levels, independent of GFR, may be due to generation
Handling by the kidney	Filtered, secreted, and excreted in the urine	Filtered, reabsorbed, and excreted in the urine	Filtered, reabsorbed, and catabolized
Extarenal elimination	Yes; increases at reduced GFR	Yes; increases at reduced GFR	Preliminary evidence of increases at reduced GFR
Use in estimating equations for GFR			
Demographic and clinical variables as surrogates for physiologic determinants	Age, sex, and race; related to muscle mass	Not applicable	Unknown
Accuracy	Accurate for GFR <60 ml/min/1.73 m^2	Not applicable	Unknown
Assay			
Method	Colorimetric or enzymatic	Direct measurement, enzymatic, colorimetric, and electrochemical	PENIA or PETIA
Assay precision	Very good except at low range	Precise throughout the range	Precise throughout the range
Clinical laboratory practice	Multiple assays; widely used nonstandard calibration	Multiple assays; enzymatic and colorimetric more commonly used	Not on most autoanalyzers; not standardized
Reference standard	IDMS	IDMS	None at present

GFR, glomerular filtration rate; IDMS, isotope dilution gas chromatography–mass spectroscopy; PENIA, particle-enhanced nephelometric immunoassay; PETIA, particle-enhanced turbidimetric immunoassay.

Figure 3.2 Comparison of creatinine, urea, and cystatin C as filtration markers. *(Modified from reference 3.)*

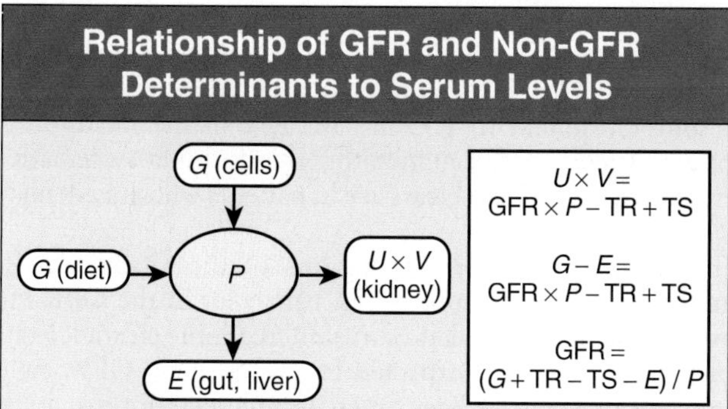

Figure 3.3 Relationship of GFR and non-GFR determinants to serum levels. G, generation; E, extrarenal elimination; TR, tubular reabsorption; TS, tubular secretion. *(Modified with permission from reference 4.)*

secretion and reduce creatinine clearance. These medications thus lead to a rise in the serum creatinine concentration without an effect on GFR (see Fig. 3.4).

In addition, creatinine is contained in intestinal secretions and can be degraded by bacteria. If GFR is reduced, the amount of creatinine eliminated through this extrarenal route is increased. Antibiotics can raise serum creatinine concentration by destroying intestinal flora, thereby interfering with extrarenal elimination, as well as by reduction of the GFR. The rise in serum creatinine concentration after inhibition of tubular secretion and extrarenal elimination is greater in patients with a reduced GFR. Clinically, it can be difficult to distinguish a rise in serum creatinine concentration due to inhibition of creatinine secretion or extrarenal elimination from a decline in GFR, but processes other than a decline in GFR should be suspected if serum urea concentration remains unchanged despite a significant change in serum creatinine concentration in a patient with an initially reduced GFR.

Factors Affecting Serum Creatinine Concentration

	Effect on Serum Creatinine	Mechanism/Comment
Age	Decrease	Reduced creatinine generation due to age-related decline in muscle mass
Female sex	Decrease	Reduced creatinine generation due to reduced muscle mass
Race		
African American	Increase	Higher creatinine generation due to higher average muscle mass in African Americans; not known how muscle mass in other races compares with that of African Americans or Caucasians
Diet		
Vegetarian diet	Decrease	Decrease in creatinine generation
Ingestion of cooked meats and creatinine supplements	Increase	Transient increase in creatinine generation; however, this may be blunted by transient increase in GFR
Body habitus		
Muscular	Increase	Increased muscle generation due to increased muscle mass ± increased protein intake
Malnutrition, muscle wasting, amputation	Decrease	Reduced creatinine generation due to reduced muscle mass ± reduced protein intake
Obesity	No change	Excess mass is fat, not muscle mass, and does not contribute to increased creatinine generation
Medications		
Trimethoprim, cimetidine, fibric acid derivatives other than gemfibrozil	Increase	Reduced tubular secretion of creatinine
Keto acids, some cephalosporins	Increase	Interference with alkaline picrate assay for creatinine

Figure 3.4 Factors affecting serum creatinine concentration. *(Reprinted with permission from reference 5.)*

Creatinine clearance is usually computed from the creatinine excretion in a 24-hour urine collection and single measurement of serum creatinine in the steady state. In a complete collection, creatinine excretion should be approximately 20 to 25 mg/kg per day and 15 to 20 mg/kg per day in healthy young men and women, respectively, and deviations from these expected values can give some indication of errors in timing or completeness of urine collection. Creatinine clearance systematically overestimates GFR because of tubular creatinine secretion. In the past, the amount of creatinine excreted by tubular secretion at normal levels of GFR was thought to be relatively small (10% to 15%), but with newer, more accurate assays for low values of serum creatinine, it appears that this difference may be substantially greater. At low values of GFR, the amount of creatinine excreted by tubular secretion may exceed the amount filtered.[6]

Creatinine Assay

Historically, the most commonly used assay for measurement of serum creatinine was the alkaline picrate (Jaffe) assay that generates a color reaction. Chromogens other than creatinine are known to interfere with the assay, giving rise to errors of up to approximately 20% in normal subjects.[4] Modern enzymatic assays do not detect non-creatinine chromogens and yield lower serum levels than with the alkaline picrate assays. Until recently, calibration of assays to adjust for this interference was not standardized across laboratories.

To address the heterogeneity in creatinine assays, the College of American Pathologists has prepared fresh-frozen serum pools with known creatinine levels that enable standardization of creatinine measurements and calibration of equipment.[7] Until standardization is complete globally, the variability in the calibration of creatinine assays will remain an important limitation of the use of GFR estimating equations, especially at higher levels of estimated GFR. This will affect the ability to compare the level of kidney function based on serum creatinine concentration reported by different laboratories, especially when the estimated GFR is more than 60 ml/min per 1.73 m^2. Standardization will reduce, but not completely eliminate, the error at higher levels of GFR.

Formulae for Estimating the Glomerular Filtration Rate from Serum Creatinine

GFR can be estimated from serum creatinine by equations that use age, sex, race, and body size as surrogates for creatinine generation. Despite substantial advances in the accuracy of estimating equations based on creatinine during the past several years, no equation can overcome the limitations of creatinine as a filtration marker. None of these equations is expected to work as well in patients with extreme levels for creatinine generation, such as amputees, large or small individuals, patients with muscle-wasting conditions, or people with high or low levels of dietary meat intake (see Fig. 3.4). Because of differences among racial and ethnic groups according to muscle mass and diet, it is unlikely that equations developed in one racial or ethnic group will be accurate in multiethnic populations.

Cockcroft-Gault Formula

The Cockcroft-Gault formula (Fig. 3.5) estimates creatinine clearance from age, sex, and body weight in addition to serum creatinine.[8] There is an adjustment factor for women that is based on a theoretical assumption of 15% lower creatinine generation due to lower muscle mass. Comparison to normal values for creatinine clearance requires computation of body surface area and adjustment to 1.73 m^2. Because of the inclusion of a term for weight in the numerator, this formula systematically overestimates creatinine clearance in patients who are edematous or obese.

There are three main limitations of the Cockcroft-Gault formula. First, it is not precise, in particular in the GFR range above 60 ml/min. Second, it estimates creatinine clearance rather than GFR; hence, it is expected to overestimate GFR. As discussed before, normal values for creatinine secretion are not well known. Third, it was derived by older assay methods for serum creatinine, which cannot be calibrated to newer assay methods, which would be expected to lead to a systematic bias in estimating creatinine clearance.

Importantly, before standardization of creatinine assays, the Cockcroft-Gault formula was widely used to assess

Equations for Estimating GFR

Cockroft-Gault formula[5]

Male $C_{cr}\text{ (ml/min)} = \dfrac{(140 - \text{age}) \times \text{weight}}{72 \times S_{cr}\text{(mg/dl)}}$ or $C_{cr}\text{ (ml/min)} = \dfrac{(140 - \text{age}) \times \text{weight}}{0.814 \times S_{cr}(\mu\text{mol/l})}$

Female $C_{cr}\text{ (ml/min)} = \dfrac{(140 - \text{age}) \times \text{weight} \times 0.85}{72 \times S_{cr}\text{(mg/dl)}}$ or $C_{cr}\text{ (ml/min)} = \dfrac{(140 - \text{age}) \times \text{weight} \times 0.85}{0.814 \times S_{cr}(\mu\text{mol/l})}$

MDRD study equation (four-variable equation)[7]

$\text{GFR (ml/min/1.73 m}^2) = 186 \times S_{cr}\text{ (mg/dl)}^{-1.154} \times \text{Age}^{-0.203} \times 0.742 \text{ (if female)} \times 1.210 \text{ (if black)}$

or

$\text{GFR (ml/min/1.73 m}^2) = 32{,}788 \times S_{cr}\ (\mu\text{mol/l})^{-1.154} \times \text{Age}^{-0.203} \times 0.742 \text{ (if female)} \times 1.210 \text{ (if black)}$

MDRD Study Equation for Use with Standardized Serum Creatinine (Four-variable equation)[7]

$\text{GFR (ml/min/1.73 m}^2) = 175 \times \text{Standardized } S_{cr}\text{(mg/dl)}^{-1.154} \times \text{age}^{-0.203} \times 0.742 \text{ (if female)} \times 1.210 \text{ (if black)}$

or

$\text{GFR (ml/min/1.73 m}^2) = 30{,}849 \times \text{Standardized } S_{cr}(\mu\text{mol/l})^{-1.154} \times \text{age}^{-0.203} \times 0.742 \text{ (if female)} \times 1.210 \text{ (if black)}$

CKD-EPI Equation for Use with Standardized Serum Creatinine[12]

$\text{GFR (ml/min/1.73 m}^2) = 141 \times \min(S_{cr}/\kappa, 1)^{\alpha} \times \max(S_{cr}/\kappa, 1)^{1.209} \times 0.993^{\text{Age}} \times 1.018 \text{ (if female)} \times 1.157 \text{ (if black)}$

where κ is 0.7 for females and 0.9 for males, α is −0.329 for females and −0.411 for males, min indicates the minimum of S_{cr}/κ or 1, and max indicates the maximum of S_{cr}/κ or 1.

Female	$\le 0.7 \rightarrow \text{GFR} = 144 \times (S_{cr}/0.7)^{-0.329}$	$\times (0.993)^{\text{Age}}$	$\times$ 1.157 (if black)
	$> 0.7 \rightarrow \text{GFR} = 144 \times (S_{cr}/0.7)^{-1.209}$		
Male	$\le 0.9 \rightarrow \text{GFR} = 141 \times (S_{cr}/0.9)^{-0.411}$		
	$> 0.9 \rightarrow \text{GFR} = 141 \times (S_{cr}/0.9)^{-1.209}$		

*Age in years, weight in kg, S_{cr}, serum creatinine

Figure 3.5 Equations for estimating glomerular filtration rate. The MDRD study equation calculator can also be found online at *http://www.kidney.org/professionals/kdoqi/gfr_calculator.cfm.*

pharmacokinetic properties of drugs in people with impaired kidney function, and it remains the standard for drug dosage adjustment in this setting. The accuracy of drug dosing recommendations based on the Cockcroft-Gault formula using creatinine values from modern assays remains an issue of debate. One study suggests that drug dosage adjustment guided by the Cockcroft-Gault formula is slightly less accurate than adjustments based on more accurate estimating equations.[9]

Modification of Diet in Renal Disease Study Equation

The Modification of Diet in Renal Disease (MDRD) study equation was originally expressed as a six-variable equation using serum creatinine, urea, and albumin concentrations in addition to age, sex, and race (African American versus Caucasian or other) to predict GFR as measured by urinary clearance of ^{125}I-iothalamate. The revised four-variable equation has now been re-expressed for use with standardized serum creatinine values (see Fig. 3.5).[10] This equation has been validated in African Americans, people with diabetic kidney disease, and kidney transplant recipients, three groups not included in large numbers in the original MDRD study. Its validity is independent of the etiology of kidney disease.[11] The equation appears to underestimate GFR in populations with higher levels of GFR, such as patients with type 1 diabetes without microalbuminuria and people undergoing kidney transplant donor evaluation (Fig. 3.6). It has not been validated in children, pregnant women, or the elderly (age >85 years). The MDRD study equation had greater precision and greater overall accuracy than the Cockcroft-Gault formula.

Many organizations now recommend GFR estimates as the primary method of clinical assessment of kidney function.[12] In 2004, the National Kidney Disease Education Program of the National Institute of Diabetes and Digestive and Kidney Diseases recommended that clinical laboratories in the United States report estimated GFR using the MDRD study equation when serum creatinine is reported.[13] A recent survey by the College of American Pathologists revealed that more than 70% of clinical laboratories in the United States now follow this practice.[6] Similarly, in 2006, the United Kingdom required hospital laboratories to report estimated GFR using the MDRD study equation with standardized creatinine measurement. Because of limitations in accuracy at higher levels, it has been recommended that GFR estimates be reported as a numerical value only if the GFR estimate is less than 60 ml/min per 1.73 m^2 and as "greater than 60 ml/min per 1.73 m^2" for higher values.

Modifications of the MDRD study equation have now been reported in racial and ethnic populations other than African American and Caucasian.[14] In general, these modifications improve the accuracy of the MDRD study equation in the study population, but there is some uncertainty because of inconsistencies between studies.[14]

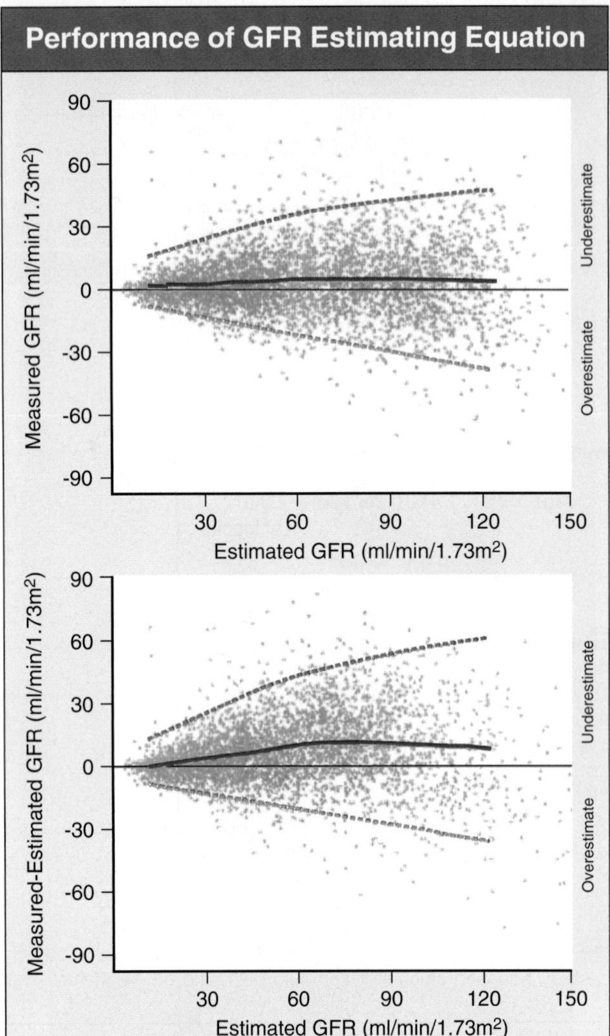

Figure 3.6 Comparison of performance of Chronic Kidney Disease Epidemiology Collaboration (CKD-EPI) and Modification of Diet in Renal Disease (MDRD) study equations. *Top,* Measured versus estimated GFR for the CKD-EPI equation. *Bottom,* Difference between measured and estimated versus estimated GFR for the MDRD study equation. Shown are smoothed regression line and 95% CI (computed by use of the lowest smoothing function in *R*), using quantile regression, excluding lowest and highest 2.5% of estimated GFR values. For the two equations, median bias (percentage of estimates within 30% of measured GFR [P_{30}]) is 2.5 (84) and 5.5 (81), respectively. To convert GFR from ml/min/1.73 m^2 to ml/s/m^2, multiply by 0.0167.

CKD-EPI Equation

A new estimating equation, the Chronic Kidney Disease Epidemiology Collaboration (CKD-EPI) equation (see Fig. 3.5), has been developed from a large database of subjects from research studies and patients from clinical populations with diverse characteristics, including people with and without kidney disease, diabetes, and a history of organ transplantation.[15] The equation is based on the same four variables as the MDRD study equation but uses a two-slope "spline" to model the relationship between GFR and serum creatinine, which partially corrects the underestimation of GFR at higher levels seen with the MDRD study equation. It also incorporates slightly different relationships for age, sex, and race. As a result, the CKD-EPI equation is as accurate as the MDRD study equation at estimated GFR below 60 ml/min per 1.73 m^2 and more accurate at higher levels (see Fig. 3.6). The CKD-EPI equation is more accurate than the MDRD study equation across a wide range of characteristics, including age, sex, race, body mass index, and presence or absence of diabetes or history of organ transplantation. With the CKD-EPI equation, it is now possible to report estimated GFR across the entire range of values without substantial bias. In our view, the CKD-EPI equation should replace the MDRD study equation for routine clinical use. However, GFR estimates are still limited by imprecision. As discussed later, it is likely that further improvements will require additional filtration markers.

UREA

The serum urea level has limited value as an index of GFR, in view of widely variable non-GFR determinants, primarily urea generation and tubular reabsorption (see Fig. 3.2).

Urea is a 60-d end product of protein catabolism by the liver. Factors associated with the increased generation of urea include protein loading from hyperalimentation and absorption of blood after a gastrointestinal hemorrhage. Catabolic states due to infection, corticosteroid administration, or chemotherapy also increase urea generation. Decreased urea generation is seen in severe malnutrition and liver disease.

Urea is freely filtered by the glomerulus and then passively reabsorbed in both the proximal and distal nephrons.[1] Owing to tubular reabsorption, urinary clearance of urea underestimates GFR. Reduced kidney perfusion in the setting of volume depletion and states of antidiuresis are associated with increased urea reabsorption. This leads to a greater decrease in urea clearance than the concomitant decrease in GFR. At GFR of less than approximately 20 ml/min per 1.73 m^2, the overestimation of GFR by creatinine clearance due to creatinine secretion is approximately equal to the underestimation of GFR by urea clearance due to urea reabsorption.

CYSTATIN C

Cystatin C Metabolism and Excretion

Cystatin C (see Fig. 3.2) is a 122–amino acid protein with a molecular mass of 13 kd. It has multiple biologic functions including extracellular inhibition of cysteine proteases, modulation of the immune system, exertion of antibacterial and antiviral activities, and modification of the body's response to brain injury.[16] The serum concentration of cystatin C remains constant from approximately 1 to 50 years of age. In analyses of the National Health and Nutrition Examination Survey (NHANES) III, the median and upper 99th percentile levels of serum cystatin C for people 20 to 39 years of age without history of hypertension and diabetes were 0.85 mg/l and 1.12 mg/l, respectively, with levels lower in women, higher in non-Hispanic whites, and increasing steeply with age.[17]

Cystatin C has been thought to be produced at a constant rate by a "housekeeping" gene expressed in all nucleated cells.[16] Cystatin C is freely filtered at the glomerulus because of its small size and basic pH.[16,18] After filtration, approximately 99% of the filtered cystatin C is reabsorbed by the proximal tubular cells, where it is almost completely catabolized, with the remaining uncatabolized form eliminated in the urine.[18] There is some evidence for the existence of tubular secretion as well as extrarenal elimination, which has been estimated to be between 15% and 21% of renal clearance.[16]

Because cystatin C is not excreted in the urine, it is difficult to study its generation and renal handling. Thus, understanding of determinants of cystatin C other than GFR relies on epidemiologic associations. There are suggestions that inflammation, adiposity, thyroid diseases, certain malignant neoplasms, and use of glucocorticoids may increase cystatin C levels. In two studies, key factors that led to higher levels of cystatin C after adjustment for creatinine clearance or measured GFR were older age, male gender, fat mass, white race, diabetes, higher C-reactive protein level and white blood cell count, and lower serum albumin level.[19,20] Altogether, these studies suggest that factors other than GFR must be considered in interpreting cystatin C levels.

Assay

There are currently two main automated methods for assay of cystatin C: immunoassays based on turbidimetry (particle-enhanced turbidimetric immunoassay, PETIA) and nephelometry (particle-enhanced nephelometric immunoassay, PENIA). The two methods result in different results.[16] International standardization of the assay is in process. The assays are considerably more expensive than those for creatinine determination.

Use as a Filtration Marker

Some studies show that elevations in cystatin C level are a better predictor of the risk of cardiovascular disease and total mortality than is an estimated GFR based on serum creatinine concentration. Whether this is due to its superiority as a filtration marker or to confounding by non-GFR determinants of cystatin C and creatinine remains to be determined.[1] Several studies have compared accuracy of serum cystatin C and creatinine in relation to measured GFR. The majority of studies have found serum cystatin C levels to be a better estimate of GFR than serum creatinine concentration is. However, cystatin C or equations based on cystatin C are not more accurate than creatinine-based estimating equations.[16] In studies of patients with chronic kidney disease, the combination of the two markers resulted in the most accurate estimate.[21] In certain populations, such as in children, elderly, transplant recipients, patients with neuromuscular diseases or liver disease, or those with higher levels of GFR, in whom serum creatinine–based equations are less accurate, cystatin C may result in a more accurate estimate, but this has not been rigorously evaluated.[16] In patients with acute kidney injury, serum cystatin C increases more rapidly than serum creatinine.[22] More data are required to establish whether it is a more sensitive indicator of rapidly changing kidney function than creatinine is.

In the future, GFR estimating equations using the combination of serum cystatin C and creatinine may have potential to provide more accurate estimates of GFR than do equations using serum creatinine. However, this is feasible only after standardization, widespread availability, and cost reductions of cystatin C assays as well as further investigation of non-GFR determinants of serum cystatin C.

CLINICAL APPLICATION OF ESTIMATED GLOMERULAR FILTRATION RATE

Chronic Kidney Disease

Estimation of GFR is necessary for the detection, evaluation, and management of chronic kidney disease (CKD). Current guidelines recommend testing of patients at increased risk of CKD for albuminuria as a marker of kidney damage or a reduced estimated GFR to assess kidney function and staging of the severity of CKD by the level of the estimated GFR. Use of serum creatinine alone as an index of GFR is unsatisfactory and can lead to delays in detection of CKD and misclassification of the severity of CKD. Use of estimating equations allows direct reporting of GFR estimates by clinical laboratories whenever serum creatinine is measured. Current estimating equations will be less accurate in people with factors affecting serum creatinine concentration other than GFR (see Fig. 3.4). In these situations, more accurate GFR estimates require a clearance measurement, by use of either an exogenous filtration marker or a timed urine collection for creatinine clearance.[2] In the future, improved estimating equations using creatinine and possibly cystatin C will allow more accurate GFR estimates.

Acute Kidney Injury

In the non-steady state, there is a lag before the rise in serum level due to the time required for retention of an endogenous filtration marker (Fig. 3.7). Conversely, after recovery of GFR, there is a lag before the excretion of the retained marker. During this time, neither the serum level nor the GFR estimated from the serum level accurately reflects the measured GFR. Nonetheless, a change in the estimated GFR in the non-steady state can be a useful indication of the magnitude and direction of the change in measured GFR. If the estimated GFR is falling, the decline in estimated GFR is less than the decline in measured GFR. Conversely, if the estimated GFR is rising, the rise in estimated GFR is greater than the rise in measured GFR. The more rapid the change in estimated GFR, the larger the change

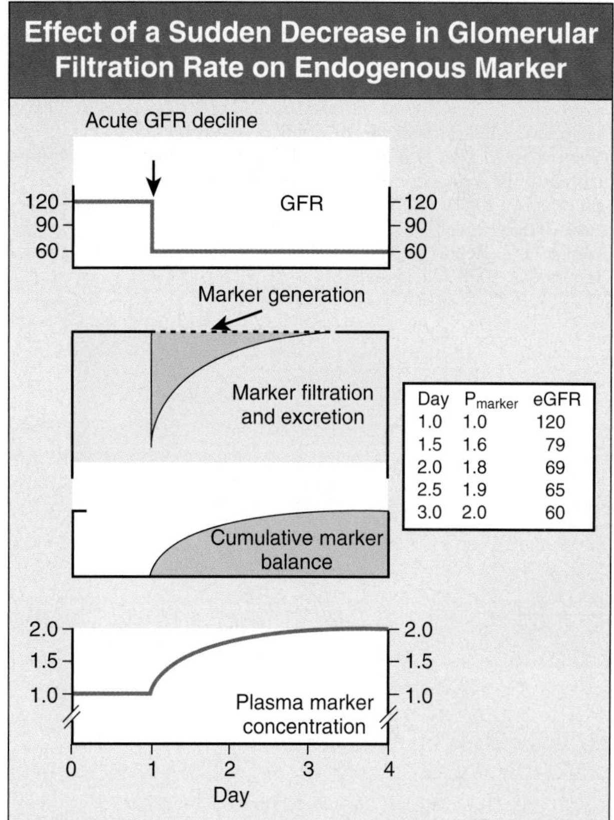

Figure 3.7 Effect of a sudden decrease in glomerular filtration rate on endogenous marker excretion, production, balance, and plasma marker concentration. *(Modified with permission from reference 4.)*

in measured GFR. When the estimated GFR reaches a new steady state, it more accurately reflects measured GFR.

MARKERS OF TUBULAR DAMAGE

Low-molecular-weight plasma proteins are readily filtered by the glomerulus and subsequently reabsorbed by the proximal tubule in normal subjects, with the result that only small amounts of the filtered proteins appear in the urine. The urinary excretion of these proteins rises when proximal tubular reabsorption is impaired. Because there is no distal tubular reabsorption, measurement of urinary low-molecular-weight proteins has been widely accepted as a marker of proximal tubular damage. Examples of low-molecular-weight proteins that could be measured in clinical practice are β_2-microglobulin (11,800 d), the light chain of the class I major histocompatibility antigens; α_1-macroglobulin (33,000 d), a glycosylated protein synthesized in the liver; and retinol-binding protein. β_2-Microglobulin is unstable in acidic urine (pH <6), leading to underestimation, whereas α_1-macroglobulin is stable and not readily affected by urine pH. Urine cystatin C and *N*-acetyl-β-glucosaminidase (NAG) have also been proposed as markers of tubular damage. Two more recently described markers of tubular damage are urinary kidney injury molecule 1 (KIM-1) and neutrophil gelatinase–associated lipocalin (NGAL).[23] These and other urinary markers of tubular damage under investigation are discussed further in Chapter 68.

REFERENCES

1. Stevens LA, Lafayette R, Perrone RD, Levey AS. *Laboratory Evaluation of Renal Function.* 8th ed. Philadelphia: Lippincott Williams & Wilkins; 2006.
2. Stevens LA, Levey A. Measured GFR as a confirmatory test for estimated GFR. *J Am Soc Nephrol.* 2009;20:2305-2313.
3. Stevens LA, Levey AS. Chronic kidney disease in the elderly—how to assess risk. *N Engl J Med.* 2005;352:2122-2124. Copyright © 2005 Massachusetts Medical Society. All rights reserved.
4. Stevens LA, Levey AS. Measured GFR as a confirmatory test for estimated GFR. *J Am Soc Nephrol.* 2009;20:2305-2313.
5. Stevens LA, Levey AS. Measurement of kidney function. *Med Clin North Am.* 2005;89:457-473.
6. Miller WG. Reporting estimated GFR: A laboratory perspective. *Am J Kidney Dis.* 2008;52:645-648.
7. Miller W, Myers G, Ashwood E, et al. Creatinine measurement: State of the art in accuracy and interlaboratory harmonization. *Arch Pathol Lab Med.* 2005;129:297-304.
8. Cockcroft DW, Gault MH. Prediction of creatinine clearance from serum creatinine. *Nephron.* 1976;16:31.
9. Stevens LA, Nolin T, Richardson M, et al. Comparison of drug dosing recommendations based on measured GFR and kidney function estimating equations. *Am J Kid Dis.* 2009;54:33-42.
10. Levey AS, Coresh J, Greene T, et al. Using standardized serum creatinine values in the Modification of Diet in Renal Disease study equation for estimating glomerular filtration rate. *Ann Intern Med.* 2006;145: 247-254.
11. Coresh J, Stevens LA. Kidney function estimating equations: Where do we stand? *Curr Opin Nephrol Hypertens.* 2006;15:276-284.
12. Levey AS, Schoolwerth AC, Burrows NR, et al. Comprehensive public health strategies for preventing the development, progression, and complications of CKD: Report of an expert panel convened by the Centers for Disease Control and Prevention. *Am J Kidney Dis.* 2009;53:522-535.
13. Myers GL, Miller WG, Coresh J, et al. Recommendations for improving serum creatinine measurement: A report from the Laboratory Working Group of the National Kidney Disease Education Program. *Clin Chem.* 2006;52:5-18.
14. Rule AD, Teo WB. Glomerular filtration rate estimation in Japan and China: What accounts for the difference? *Am J Kidney Dis.* 2009;53:932-935.
15. Levey A, Stevens LA, Schmid CH, et al. A new equation to estimate glomerular filtration rate. *Ann Intern Med.* 2009;150:604-612.
16. Madero M, Sarnak MJ, Stevens LA. Serum cystatin C as a marker of glomerular filtration rate. *Curr Opin Nephrol Hypertens.* 2006;15: 610-616.
17. Kottgen A, Selvin E, Stevens LA, et al. Serum cystatin C in the United States: The Third National Health and Nutrition Examination Survey (NHANES III). *Am J Kidney Dis.* 2008;51:385-394.
18. Tenstad O, Roald A, Grubb A, Aukland K. Renal handling of radiolabelled human cystatin C in the rat. *Scand J Clin Lab Invest.* 1996;56:409-414.
19. Knight EL, Verhave JC, Spiegelman D, et al. Factors influencing serum cystatin C levels other than renal function and the impact on renal function measurement. *Kidney Int.* 2004;65:1416-1421.
20. Stevens LA, Schmid CH, Greene T, et al. Factors other than glomerular filtration rate affect serum cystatin C levels. *Kidney Int.* 2009;75: 652-660.
21. Stevens LA, Coresh J, Schmid CH, et al. Estimating GFR using serum cystatin C alone and in combination with serum creatinine: A pooled analysis of 3,418 individuals with CKD. *Am J Kidney Dis.* 2008; 51:395-406.
22. Herget-Rosenthal S, Marggraf G, Husing J, et al. Early detection of acute renal failure by serum cystatin C. *Kidney Int.* 2004;66:1115-1122.
23. Coca SG, Parikh CR. Urinary biomarkers for acute kidney injury: Perspectives on translation. *Clin J Am Soc Nephrol.* 2008;3:481-490.

CHAPTER 4

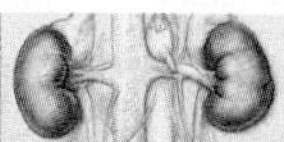

Urinalysis

Giovanni B. Fogazzi

DEFINITION

Urinalysis is one of the basic tests to evaluate kidney and urinary tract disease. When a patient is first seen by a nephrologist, urinalysis should always be performed. Dipsticks are the most widely used method for urinalysis, but the nephrologist should be aware of their limitations, especially in detecting urine proteins other than albumin. Urine microscopy should ideally be performed by trained nephrologists rather than by clinical laboratory personnel, who are often unable to identify important features[1,2] and are usually unaware of the clinical correlates of the findings.

URINE COLLECTION

The way urine is collected and handled can greatly influence the results (Fig. 4.1). Written instructions should be given to the patient as to how to perform a urine collection.[3] First, strenuous physical exercise (e.g., running, soccer match) must be avoided in the 72 hours preceding the collection to avoid exercise-induced proteinuria and hematuria or cylindruria. In women, urinalysis should also be avoided during menstruation because blood contamination can easily occur. The first or second morning urine specimen is recommended.[3]

After the washing of hands, women should spread the labia of the vagina and men withdraw the foreskin of the glans. The external genitalia are washed and wiped dry with a paper towel, and the "midstream" urine is collected after the first portion is discarded.[3] The same procedures can also be used for children; for small infants, bags for urine are often used, even though these carry a high probability of contamination. A suprapubic bladder puncture may occasionally be necessary. Urine can also be collected through a bladder catheter, although the catheter may cause hematuria. Permanent indwelling catheters are commonly associated with bacteriuria, leukocyturia, hematuria, and candiduria.

The container for urine should be provided by the laboratory or bought in a pharmacy. It should be clean, have a capacity of at least 50 to 100 ml, and have a diameter opening of at least 5 cm to allow easy collection. It should have a wide base to avoid accidental spillage and should be capped.[3] The label should identify the patient as well as the hour of urine collection.

Several elements (but especially leukocytes) can lyse rapidly after collection, and the best preservation method to minimize this is uncertain. Refrigeration of specimens at +2°C to +8°C assists preservation but may allow precipitation of phosphates or uric acids, which can hamper examination of the sample. Formaldehyde, glutaraldehyde, CellFIX (a formaldehyde-based fixative),[4] and tubes containing a lyophilized borate-formate-sorbitol powder[5] are good preservatives for the formed elements of urine.

PHYSICAL CHARACTERISTICS

Color

The color of normal urine ranges from pale to dark yellow and amber, depending on the concentration of the urochrome. Abnormal changes in color can be due to pathologic conditions, drugs, or foods.

The main pathologic conditions that can cause color changes of the urine are gross hematuria, hemoglobinuria, or myoglobinuria (pink, red, brown, or black urine); jaundice (dark yellow to brown urine); chyluria (white milky urine)[6]; massive uric acid crystalluria (pink urine); urinary infection due to some types of *Escherichia coli* (velvet urine); and porphyrinuria and alkaptonuria (red urine turning black on standing).

The main drugs responsible for abnormal urine color are rifampin (yellow-orange to red urine); phenytoin (red urine); chloroquine and nitrofurantoin (brown urine); triamterene, propofol, and blue dyes of enteral feeds (green urine); methylene blue (blue urine); and metronidazole, methyldopa, and imipenem-cilastatin (darkening on standing).

Among foods are beetroot (red urine), senna and rhubarb (yellow to brown or red urine), and carotene (brown urine).

Turbidity

Normal urine is transparent. Urine can be turbid because of an increased concentration of any urine particle. The most frequent causes of turbidity are urinary tract infection, heavy hematuria, and contamination from genital secretions. The absence of turbidity is not a reliable criterion by which to judge a urine sample because pathologic urine can be transparent.

Odor

A change in urine odor may be caused by the ingestion of some foods, such as asparagus. A pungent odor, due to the production of ammonia, is typical of most bacterial urinary tract infection, whereas there is often a sweet or fruity odor with ketones in the urine. Some rare conditions confer a characteristic odor to the urine. These include maple-syrup urine disease (maple syrup odor), phenylketonuria (musty or mousy odor), isovaleric

Procedures for Preparation and Examination of the Urine Sediment
Written instructions to the patients for urine collection
Collection in disposable containers of the second urine of the morning after discarding the first few milliliters of urine
Sample handling and analysis within 3 h from collection
Centrifugation of a 10 ml aliquot of urine at 400 g for 10 min
Removal by suction of 9.5 ml of supernatant urine
Gentle but thorough resuspension with a pipette of the sediment in the remaining 0.5 ml of urine
Transfer by a pipette of 50 μl of resuspended urine to a slide
Covering of sample with a 24 × 32-mm coverslip
Examination of the urine sediment by a phase contrast microscope at ×160 and ×400
Use of polarized light to identify doubtful lipids and crystals
Match the microscopic findings with dipstick for pH, specific gravity, hemoglobin, leukocyte esterase, nitrites, and albumin (the presence of albumin orients the examination of the sample toward a glomerular disease)
Cells expressed as lowest–highest number seen per high-power field, casts as number per low-power field, all the other elements (e.g., bacteria, crystals) on a scale from 0 to ++++

Figure 4.1 Procedures for preparation and examination of the urine sediment used in the author's laboratory.

acidemia (sweaty feet odor), and hypermethioninemia (rancid butter or fishy odor).

Relative Density

Relative density can be measured by a number of methods.

Specific gravity (SG) is a function of the number and weight of the dissolved particles and is influenced by urine temperature, proteins, glucose, and radiocontrast media. Historically, SG was measured by a urinometer, which is a weighted float marked with a scale from 1.000 to 1.060. Today, SG is most commonly measured by dry chemistry, which is incorporated into dipsticks. In the presence of cations, protons are released by a complexing agent and produce a color change in the indicator bromthymol blue from blue to blue-green to yellow. Underestimation occurs with urine pH above 6.5, whereas overestimation is found with urine protein concentration above 7.0 g/l. In addition, nonionized molecules, such as glucose and urea, are not detected. Not surprisingly, this method does not strictly correlate with the results obtained by osmolality[7] and refractometry.[8]

SG of 1.000 to 1.003 is consistent with marked urinary dilution, such as observed with diabetes insipidus or water intoxication. SG of 1.010 is often called isosthenuric urine because it is of similar SG (and osmolality) as plasma, so it is often observed in conditions in which urinary concentration is impaired, such as acute tubular necrosis (ATN) and chronic kidney disease. SG above 1.040 almost always indicates the presence of some extrinsic osmotic agent (such as contrast material).

Osmolality depends on the number of particles present and is measured by an osmometer. It is not influenced by urine temperature and protein concentrations. However, high glucose concentrations significantly increase osmolality (10 g/l of glucose = 55.5 mOsm/l).

Refractometry is based on measurement of the refractive index, which depends on the weight and the size of solutes per unit volume, and correlates well with osmolality.[7] Refractometers are simple to use and have the major advantage of requiring only one drop of urine. For these reasons, the use of refractometry rather than of SG is suggested, even though the factors that can interfere with SG can also interfere with refractometry.

CHEMICAL CHARACTERISTICS

Figure 4.2 summarizes the main false-negative and false-positive results that can occur with urine dipstick testing.

pH

The pH is determined by dipsticks that cover the pH range 5.0 to 8.5 or to 9.0. With use of dipsticks, significant deviations from true pH are observed for values below 5.5 and above 7.5. Therefore, a pH meter with a glass electrode is mandatory if an accurate measurement is necessary.[3]

Urine pH reflects the presence of hydrogen ions, but this does not necessarily reflect the overall acid load in the urine as most of the acid is excreted as ammonia. A low pH is often observed with metabolic acidosis (in which acid is secreted), with high-protein meals (which generate more acid and ammonia), and with volume depletion (in which aldosterone is stimulated, resulting in an acid urine). Indeed, low urine pH may help distinguish prerenal acute renal impairment from ATN (which is typically associated with a higher pH). High pH is often observed with renal tubular acidosis (especially distal, type 1; see Chapter 12), with vegetarian diets (due to minimal nitrogen and acid generation), and with infection with urease-positive organisms (such as *Proteus*) that generate ammonia from urea.

Measurement of urine pH is also needed for the interpretation of urinalysis (see later, Leukocyte Esterase and Urine Microscopy).

Hemoglobin

Hemoglobin is detected by a dipstick on the basis of the pseudoperoxidase activity of the heme moiety of hemoglobin, which catalyzes the reaction of a peroxide and a chromogen to produce a colored product. The presence of hemoglobin is shown as green spots, which are due to intact erythrocytes, or as a homogeneous diffuse green pattern, which is common with marked hematuria because of the high number of erythrocytes that cover the whole pad surface. It may also be observed if lysis of erythrocytes has occurred on standing or as a consequence of alkaline urine pH or a low specific gravity (especially <1.010).

The most important reasons for a positive test result in the absence of red cells are hemoglobinuria deriving from intravascular hemolysis, myoglobinuria deriving from rhabdomyolysis, and a high concentration of bacteria with pseudoperoxidase activity (Enterobacteriaceae, staphylococci, and streptococci).[9]

False-negative results are mainly due to ascorbic acid, a strong reducing agent, which can cause low-grade microscopic hematuria to be completely missed.[10]

Urine Dipstick Testing

Parameter	False-negative Results	False-positive Results
Specific gravity	Urine pH >6.5	Increased values in the presence of protein >7.0 g/l Ketoacids
pH	Reduced values in the presence of formaldehyde	—
Hemoglobin	Ascorbic acid Delayed examination High density of urine Formaldehyde (0.5 g/l)	Myoglobin Microbial peroxidases Oxidizing agents Hydrochloric acid
Glucose	Ascorbic acid Bacteria	Oxidizing detergents Hydrochloric acid
Albumin	Immunoglobulin light chains Tubular proteins Globulins Abnormally colored urine	Urine pH ≥ 9.0 Quaternary ammonium detergents Chlorhexidine Polyvinylpyrrolidone
Leukocyte esterase	High density of urine Vitamin C (intake: g/day) Protein >5.0 g/l, Glucose >20.0 g/l Cephalothin (+++), Tetracycline (+++), Cephalexin (++), Tobramycin (+)	Oxidizing detergents Formaldehyde (0.4 g/l) Sodium azide Abnormally colored urine due to beet
Nitrites	Bacteria that do not reduce nitrates to nitrites Short bladder incubation time No vegetables in diet	Abnormally colored urine
Ketones	Improper storage	Free sulfhydryl groups (e.g., captopril) Levodopa Abnormally colored urine

Figure 4.2 Urine dipstick testing. Main false-negative and false-positive results of urine dipsticks.

Detection of hemoglobin by dipstick has a high specificity and a low sensitivity.[11,12]

Glucose

Glucose is also commonly detected by dipstick. Glucose, with glucose oxidase as catalyst, is first oxidized to gluconic acid and hydrogen peroxide. Then, through the catalyzing activity of a peroxidase, hydrogen peroxide reacts with a reduced colorless chromogen to form a colored product. This test detects concentrations of 0.5 to 20 g/l. When more precise quantification of urine glucose is needed, enzymatic methods such as hexokinase must be used.

False-negative results occur in the presence of ascorbic acid and bacteria. False-positive findings may be observed in the presence of oxidizing detergents and hydrochloric acid.

Protein

Physiologic proteinuria does not exceed 150 mg/24 h for adults and 140 mg/m^2 for children. Three different approaches can be used for the evaluation of proteinuria.

Dipstick This relies on the fact that the presence of protein in a buffer causes a change of pH that is proportional to the concentration of protein itself. The dipstick changes its color (from pale green to green and blue) according to the pH changes induced by the protein. This method is highly sensitive for albumin (detection limit of approximately 0.20 to 0.25 g/l), whereas it has a very low sensitivity to other proteins such as tubular proteins and light-chain immunoglobulins.

Dipstick allows only a semiquantitative measurement of urine albumin, which is expressed on a scale from 0 to +++ or ++++. Although, in general, + albumin corresponds to 800 mg/l, ++ with 1450 mg/l, and +++ with 3000 mg/l, there is wide variance. Therefore, accurate quantification requires other methods, such as turbidimetric or dye-binding techniques (e.g., benzethonium chloride or pyrogallol red–molybdate colorimetric method).

The 24-Hour Protein Excretion This remains the reference (gold standard) method. It averages the variation of proteinuria due to the circadian rhythm and is the most accurate for monitoring of proteinuria during treatment, but it can be impractical in some settings (e.g., outpatients, elderly patients). Moreover, this method is subject to error due to overcollection or undercollection. One advantage is that 24-hour urine protein is usually measured by methods that quantify total protein rather than simply albumin, and hence this can result in detection of light chains in subjects with myeloma.

Protein-Creatinine Ratio on a Random Urine Sample This is a practical alternative to the 24-hour urine collection.[13] It is easy to obtain, it is not influenced by variation in water intake and rate of diuresis, and the same sample can also be used for microscopic investigation.

There is a strong correlation between the protein-creatinine ratio in a random urine sample and the 24-hour protein excretion.[14] However, although a normal protein-creatinine ratio is sufficient to rule out pathologic proteinuria, an elevated protein-creatinine ratio should be confirmed and quantified with a 24-hour collection. Moreover, the reliability of the protein-creatinine ratio for monitoring of proteinuria during treatment is still not proven. A discussion of how to measure and to monitor proteinuria in such patients is provided in Chapter 76.

Specific Protein Assays

A qualitative analysis of urine proteins can be performed by electrophoresis on cellulose acetate or agarose after protein concentration or by use of very sensitive stains, such as silver and gold. Sodium dodecyl sulfate–polyacrylamide gel electrophoresis (SDS-PAGE) can be used to identify the different urine proteins by molecular weight and to characterize the pattern of proteinuria.[15]

In some circumstances, measurement of a single specific protein may be informative, for example, neutrophil gelatinase-associated lipocalin for early detection of acute kidney injury (AKI).[16]

Bence Jones proteinuria can be suspected when the dipstick measurement for proteinuria is negative (because it mainly detects albumin) yet the 24-hour urine protein is elevated. Confirmation of free immunoglobulin light chains in the urine requires immunofixation.[17]

Selectivity of proteinuria in nephrotic syndrome can be assessed by the ratio of the clearance of IgG (molecular weight 160,000) to the clearance of transferrin (molecular weight 88,000).[18] Although it is not widely used, highly selective proteinuria (ratio <0.1) in nephrotic children suggests the diagnosis of minimal change disease and predicts corticosteroid responsiveness. Selectivity of proteinuria combined with SDS-PAGE and the excretion of low-molecular-weight proteins, such as α_1-microglobulin, is reported to predict the outcome and response to therapy in minimal change disease, focal segmental glomerulosclerosis, and membranous nephropathy.[19]

Leukocyte Esterase

This dipstick evaluates the presence of leukocytes on the basis of an indoxyl esterase activity released from lysed neutrophil granulocytes and macrophages. Leukocyte esterase may be positive when microscopy is negative when leukocytes are lysed because of low density, alkaline pH, or delay in sample handling and examination. The detection limit of the dipstick is 20×10^6 white blood cells per liter.

False-positive results are rare but may occur when formaldehyde is used as a urine preservative. False-negative results are more common from high glucose or protein concentrations (20 g/l and 5 g/l, respectively) or in the presence of cephalothin and tetracycline (strong inhibition), cephalexin (moderate inhibition), or tobramycin (mild inhibition). The sensitivity is also reduced by high specific gravity because this prevents leukocyte lysis. Sensitivity varies from 76% to 94% and specificity from 68% to 81%.[20,21]

Nitrites

The dipstick nitrites test detects bacteria that reduce nitrates to nitrites by nitrate reductase activity. This includes most gram-negative uropathogenic bacteria but not *Pseudomonas*, *Staphylococcus albus*, and *Enterococcus*. A positive test result also requires a diet rich in nitrates (vegetables), which form the substrate for nitrite production, and sufficient bladder incubation time. Thus, it is not surprising that the sensitivity of this test is low, whereas specificity is more than 90%.[22]

Bile Pigments

Measurements of urinary urobilinogen and bilirubin concentrations have lost their clinical value in the detection of liver disease after the introduction of serum tests of liver enzyme function.

Ketones

This dipstick tests for the presence of acetoacetate and acetone (but not β-hydroxybutyrate), which are excreted into urine during diabetic acidosis or during fasting, vomiting, or strenuous exercise. It is based on the reaction of the ketones with nitroprusside.

URINE MICROSCOPY

The urine sediment can contain cells, lipids, casts, crystals, organisms, and contaminants.

Methods

The first or second urine specimen of the morning should be collected, following the procedures described earlier (see Urine Collection and Fig 4.1). To avoid the lysis of elements, an aliquot of urine should be rapidly centrifuged and concentrated, after which a standardized volume of resuspended urine should be transferred to the slide and covered with a coverslip. The use of noncentrifuged samples greatly reduces sensitivity, especially for rare findings such as erythrocyte casts.

Phase contrast microscopy is recommended[3] because it improves the identification of particles, and polarized light is mandatory for the correct identification of lipids and crystals.[3] At least 10 microscopic fields, in different areas of the sample, should be examined at both low and high magnification.[3] More extensive examination may be required in certain clinical settings. For instance, for patients with isolated microscopic hematuria of unknown origin, always examine 50 low-power fields (×160) to search for erythrocyte casts.

For correct examination, both pH and specific gravity of the sample should be known. Both alkaline pH and low specific gravity (especially <1.010) favor the lysis of erythrocytes and leukocytes, which can cause discrepancies between dipstick readings and the microscopic examination (see earlier). Alkaline pH also impairs the formation of casts and favors the precipitation of phosphates.

The various elements observed are quantified as number per microscopic field, and if counting chambers are used, the elements are quantified as number per milliliter. Counting chambers allow a precise quantitation but are rarely used in everyday practice.

Cells

Erythrocytes

Erythrocytes have a diameter of 4 to 10 μm. There are two main types of urinary erythrocytes: isomorphic, with regular shapes and contours, derived from the urinary excretory system; and dysmorphic, with irregular shapes and contours, which are of glomerular origin (Fig. 4.3A, B).[23] Hematuria has been defined as nonglomerular when isomorphic erythrocytes predominate (>80% of total erythrocytes) and as glomerular when dysmorphic erythrocytes prevail (>80% of total erythrocytes).[24] Some diagnose glomerular hematuria when the two types of cells are in the same proportion (so-called mixed hematuria)[25] or when at least 5% of erythrocytes examined are acanthocytes,[26] a subtype of dysmorphic erythrocytes with a characteristic appearance that is due to the presence of one or more blebs protruding from a ring-shaped body (Fig. 4.3B, *inset*).

Glomerular hematuria is identified when there are 40% or more dysmorphic erythrocytes or 5% or more acanthocytes or one or more red cell casts in 50 low-power fields (×160 magnification). With this method in isolated microscopic hematuria, a good correlation between urinary and renal biopsy findings was found.[27]

The distinction between glomerular and nonglomerular hematuria aids in the evaluation of patients with isolated microscopic hematuria.[28] However, the evaluation of erythrocyte morphology is subjective and requires experience, which has limited its widespread introduction into clinical practice.

Erythrocyte dysmorphism is thought to result from deformation of the erythrocyte while it is passing through gaps of the glomerular basement membrane followed by physicochemical insults occurring while the erythrocyte passes through the tubular system.[29] In glomerulonephritis (GN), the number of urinary erythrocytes may also be of clinical significance; in proliferative GN, the number of erythrocytes is significantly higher than in patients with nonproliferative GN.[30]

Leukocytes

Neutrophils range from 7 to 15 μm in diameter and are the most frequently found leukocytes in the urine. They are identified by their granular cytoplasm and lobulated nucleus (Fig. 4.3C). Neutrophils often indicate lower or upper urinary tract infections but may result from genital secretions, especially in young women. They can also be found in proliferative or crescentic GN[30] and in acute or chronic interstitial nephritis.

Eosinophils, once considered a marker of acute allergic interstitial nephritis, are today seen as nonspecific particles because they may be present in various types of GN, prostatitis, chronic pyelonephritis, urinary schistosomiasis, and cholesterol embolism.[31,32] Eosinophiluria in the evaluation of acute interstitial nephritis is discussed further in Chapter 60.

Lymphocytes may indicate acute cellular rejection in renal allograft recipients, but their identification requires staining, and this technique is not widely used in clinical practice. Lymphocytes are also a typical finding in patients with chyluria.[6]

Macrophages have only recently been identified in urinary sediments. They are mononucleated or multinucleated cells of variable size (diameter, 13 to 95 μm) and variable appearance: granular (Fig. 4.3D), vacuolar, phagocytic (when cytoplasm contains bacterial debris, cell fragments, destroyed erythrocytes, crystals), or homogeneous (when cytoplasm does not contain granules or other particles). In patients with the nephrotic syndrome, macrophages may be engorged with lipid droplets, appearing as "oval fat bodies."[33] Macrophages have been found in the urine of patients with active GN,[33] including IgA nephropathy.[34] In our experience, macrophages are also present in the urine of transplant recipients with BK virus infection (see later discussion). However, urinary macrophages are not yet considered diagnostic of any specific condition.

Renal Tubular Epithelial Cells

These cells derive from the exfoliation of the tubular epithelium. In the urine, they can differ in size (diameter, ~9 to 25 μm) and shape (from roundish to rectangular or columnar; Fig. 4.3E). They are a marker of tubular damage and are not found in health but are found in AKI, acute interstitial nephritis, and acute cellular rejection of a renal allograft. In smaller numbers, they are also found in glomerular diseases.[30] In AKI, renal tubular epithelial cells are frequently damaged and necrotic; in other conditions, such as glomerular diseases, they usually have a normal appearance.

Renal tubular epithelial cells may be present in casts (epithelial casts), although the two are not always seen together.[30]

Uroepithelial Cells

These cells derive from the exfoliation of the uroepithelium, which lines the urinary tract from calyces to the bladder in women and to the proximal urethra in men. It is a multilayered epithelium, with small cells in the deep layers and larger cells in the superficial layers.

Cells of the deep layers (diameter, ~10 to 38 μm; Fig. 4.3F), when they are present in large numbers, reflect severe damage due to neoplasia, stones, or even ureteral stents.[35] Cells of the superficial layers (diameter, ~17 to 43 μm; Fig. 4.3G) are a common finding, especially in urinary tract infections.

Squamous Cells

These cells (diameter, 17 to 118 μm; Fig. 4.3H) derive from the urethra or from the external genitalia. In large numbers, they indicate urine contamination from genital secretions.

Lipids

Lipids may appear as spherical, translucent, or yellow drops of different size. They can be free in the urine (isolated or in clusters; Fig. 4.4A) or fill the cytoplasm of tubular epithelial cells or macrophages.[33] When they are entrapped within casts, lipids form fatty casts. Lipids can also appear as cholesterol crystals (see later, Crystals). Under polarized light, lipids have the appearance of Maltese crosses (Fig. 4.4B).

Lipids in the urine are typical of glomerular diseases associated with marked proteinuria, usually but not invariably in the nephrotic range. They can also be found in sphingolipidoses such as Fabry's disease. By electron microscopy, lipid particles in Fabry's disease differ from those in nephrotic syndrome by the appearance of intracellular and extracellular electron-dense lamellae and alternating dark and clear layers arranged in concentric whorls.[36]

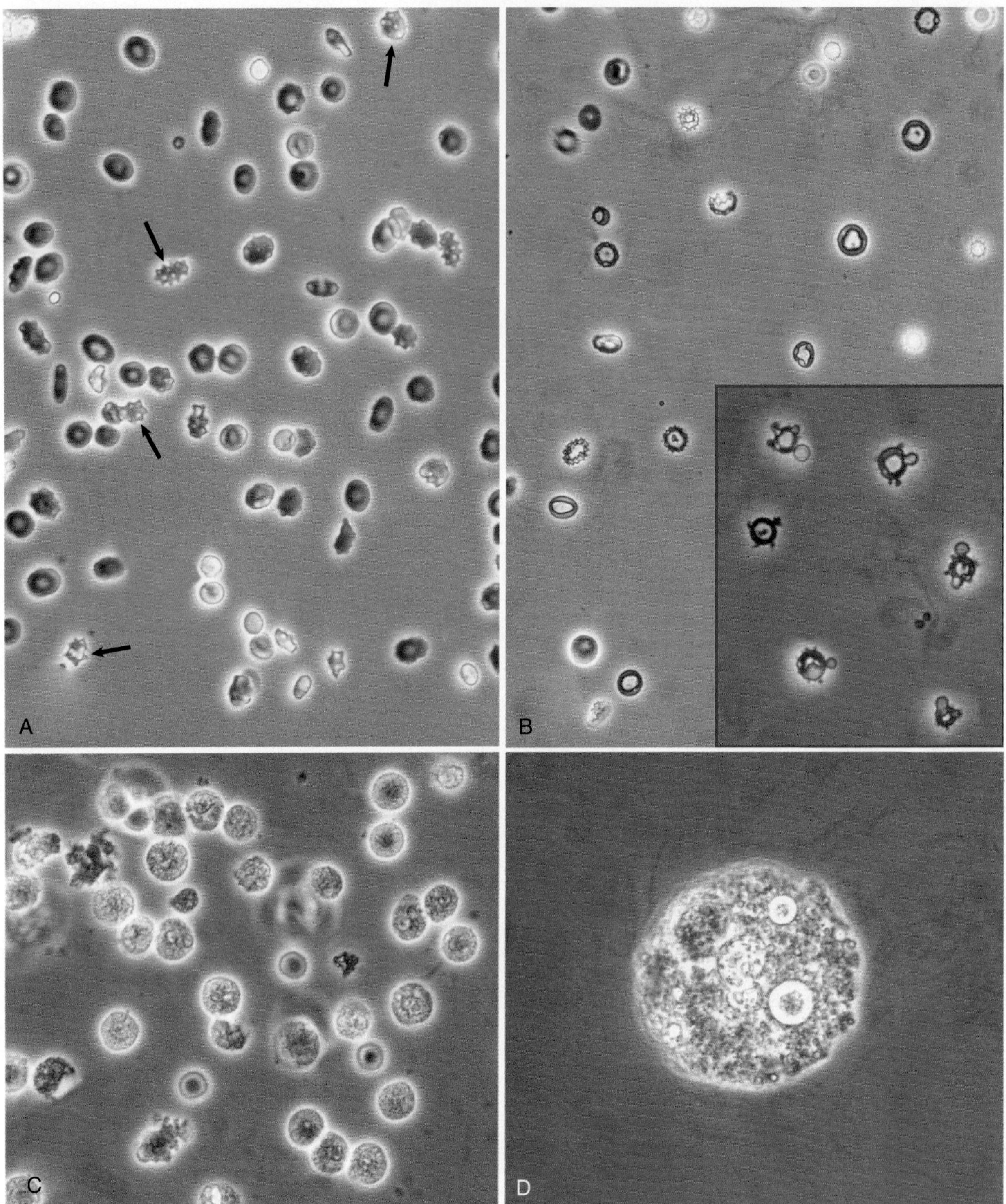

Figure 4.3 Urinary sediment cells. A, Isomorphic nonglomerular erythrocytes. The *arrows* indicate the so-called crenated erythrocytes, which are a frequent finding in nonglomerular hematuria. **B,** Dysmorphic glomerular erythrocytes. The dysmorphism consists mainly of irregularities of the cell membrane. *Inset,* Acanthocytes with their typical ring-formed cell bodies with one or more blebs of different sizes and shapes. **C,** Neutrophils. Note their typical lobulated nucleus and granular cytoplasm. **D,** A granular phagocytic macrophage (diameter about 60 μm).

Casts

Casts are cylindrical and form in the lumen of distal renal tubules and collecting ducts. Their matrix is due to Tamm-Horsfall glycoprotein (also called uromodulin), which is secreted by the cells of the thick ascending Henle's loop. Trapping of particles within the cast matrix results in casts with different appearances and clinical significance (Fig. 4.5). The trapping of cells within the matrix causes the appearance of erythrocytic, leukocytic, or renal tubular cell casts. Degradation can transform leukocyte or epithelial casts into coarse granular casts. Fine granular casts are mostly due to the trapping within the matrix of the casts of lysosomes containing serum ultrafiltered proteins.

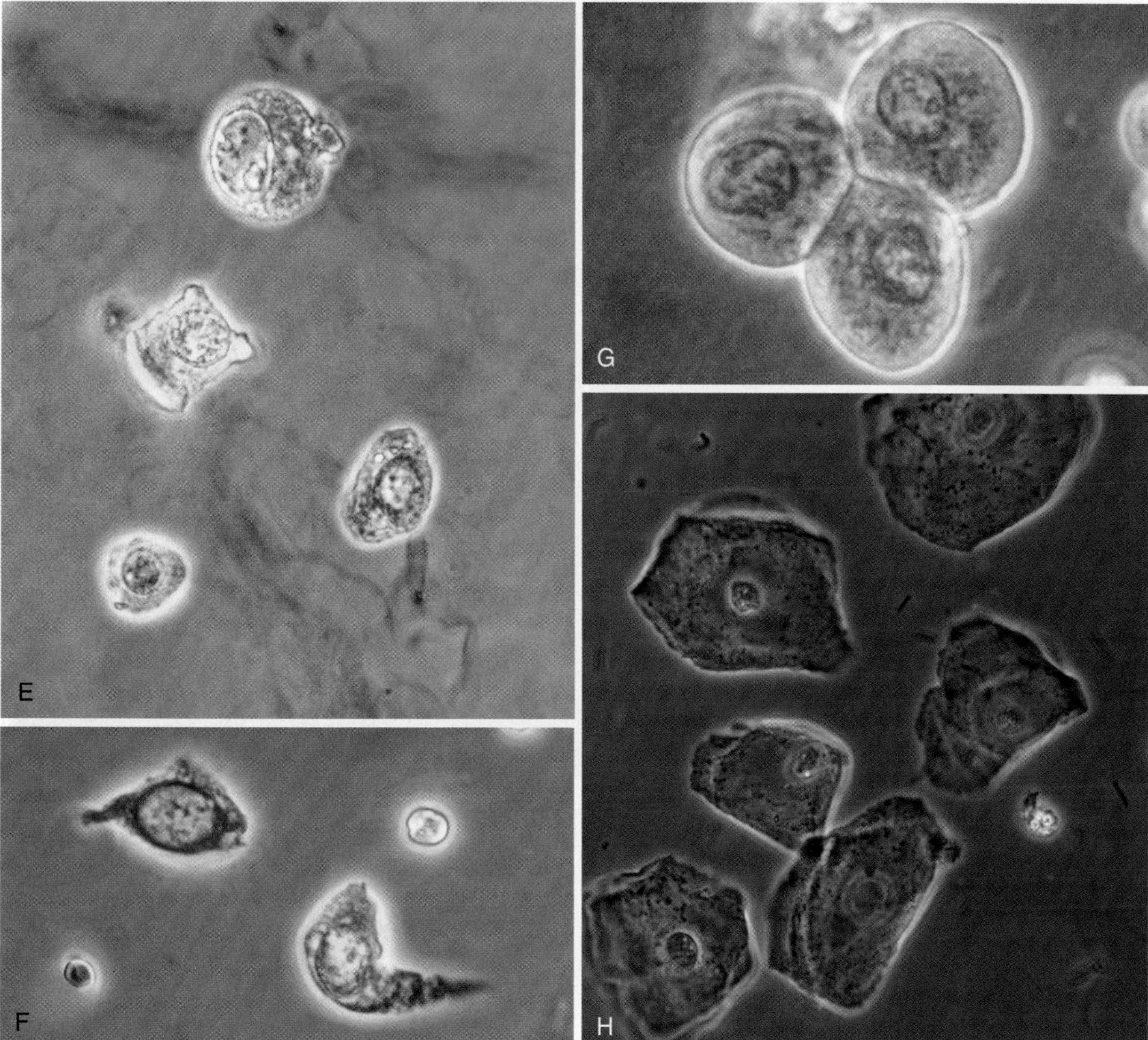

Figure 4.3, cont'd **E,** Different types of renal tubular cells. **F,** Two cells from the deep layers of the uroepithelium. **G,** Three cells from the superficial layers of the uroepithelium. Note the difference in shape and ratio of nucleus to cytoplasm existing between the two types of uroepithelial cells. **H,** Squamous cells. (All images by phase contrast microscopy; original magnification ×400.)

- *Hyaline casts* are colorless with a low refractive index (Fig. 4.6A). They are easily seen with phase contrast microscopy but can be overlooked when bright-field microscopy is used. Hyaline casts may occur in normal urine, especially in volume depletion, in which urine is concentrated and acidic (both favoring precipitation of Tamm-Horsfall protein). In patients with renal disease, they are usually associated with other types of casts.[30]
- *Hyaline-granular casts* contain granules within the hyaline matrix (Fig 4.6B). Rare but possible in normal individuals, they are common in GN.[30]
- *Granular casts* can be either finely granular (Fig. 4.6C) or coarsely granular. Both types are typical of renal disease but not more specific.
- *Waxy casts* derive their name from their appearance, which is similar to that of melted wax (Fig. 4.6D). The nature of waxy casts is still unknown. They are typical of patients with renal failure, and in our experience, they are also frequent in patients with rapidly progressive GN.
- *Fatty casts* contain variable amounts of lipid droplets, isolated, in clumps, or packed. They are typical of glomerular diseases associated with marked proteinuria or the nephrotic syndrome.
- *Erythrocyte (red cell) casts* may contain a few erythrocytes (Fig. 4.6E) or so many that the matrix of the cast cannot be identified. The finding of erythrocyte casts indicates hematuria of glomerular origin. Examination for erythrocyte casts is of particular importance in patients with isolated microscopic hematuria of unknown origin.[27]
- *Hemoglobin casts* have a brownish hue and often a granular appearance deriving from the degradation of erythrocytes entrapped within the casts (Fig.

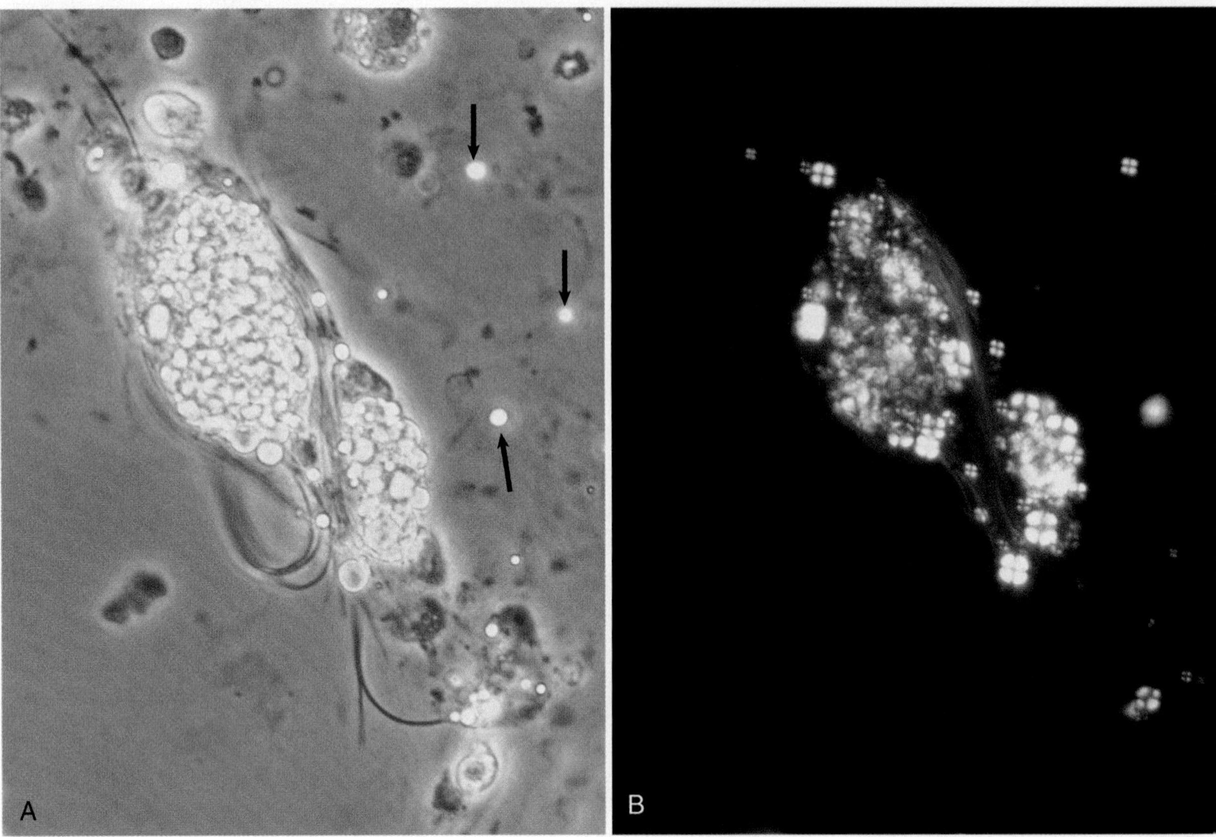

Figure 4.4 Two large aggregates of lipid droplets. Scattered in the specimen, there also are isolated fatty droplets *(arrows)*. **A,** As seen by phase contrast microscopy. **B,** Under polarized light, which shows the typical Maltese crosses with their symmetric arms. (Original magnification ×400.) For full morphologic details about these particles, see reference 36.

Figure 4.5 Main types of casts and their clinical significance.

Clinical Significance of Urinary Casts	
Cast	**Main Clinical Associations**
Hyaline	Normal subject and renal disease
Hyaline-granular	Normal subject and renal disease
Granular	Renal disease
Waxy	Renal impairment; rapidly progressive renal disease
Fatty	Marked proteinuria; nephrotic syndrome
Erythrocyte	Glomerular hematuria; proliferative or necrotizing glomerulonephritis
Hemoglobin	The same as the erythrocyte cast; hemoglobinuria due to intravascular hemolysis
Leukocyte	Acute interstitial nephritis; acute pyelonephritis; proliferative glomerulonephritis
Renal tubular epithelial cell (epithelial casts)	Acute tubular necrosis; acute interstitial nephritis; proliferative glomerulonephritis; nephrotic syndrome
Myoglobin	Rhabdomyolysis
Bacterial, fungal	Bacterial or fungal infection in the kidney

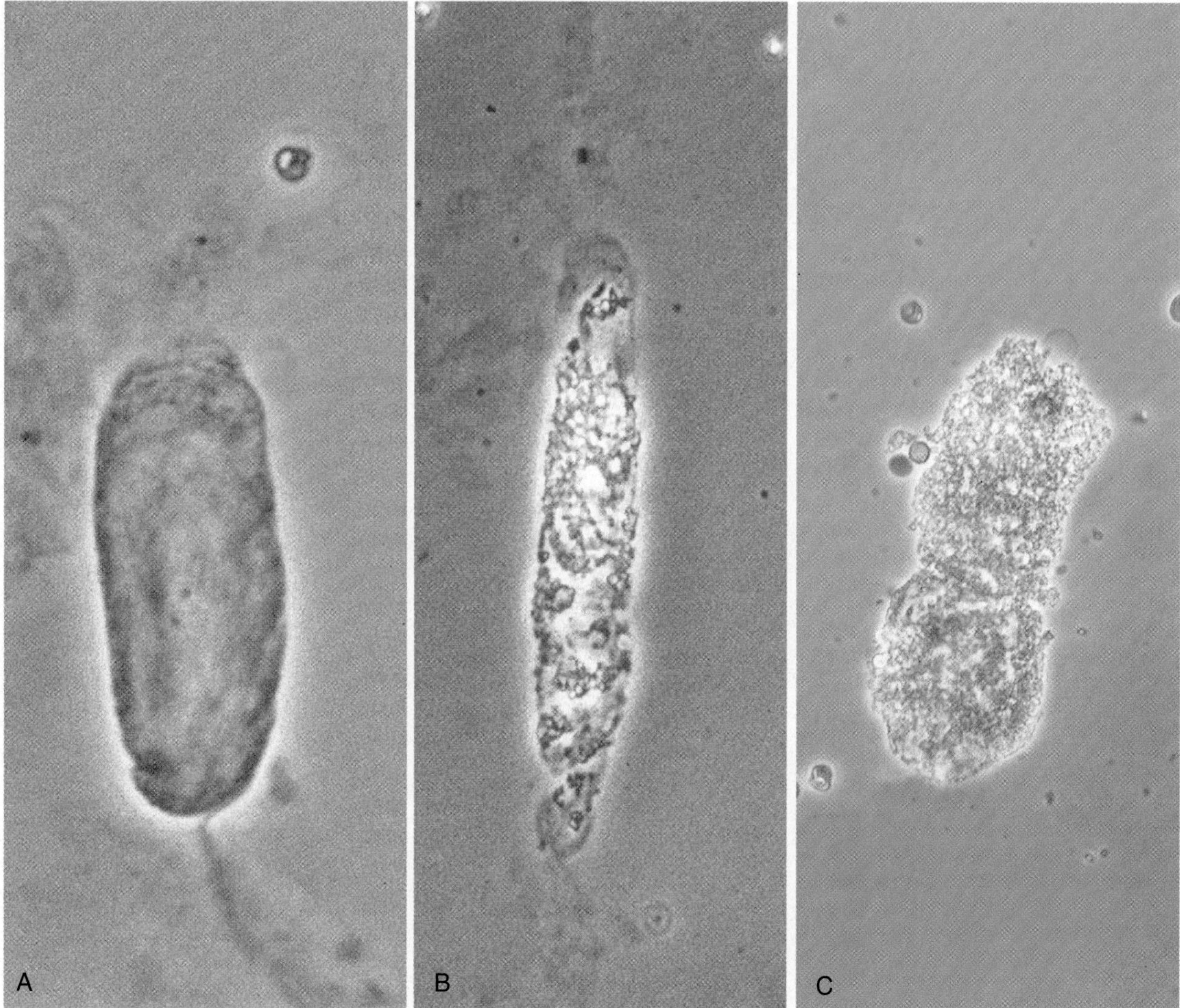

Figure 4.6 Casts. A, Hyaline cast. **B,** Hyaline-granular cast. **C,** Finely granular cast.

Continued

4.6F). Therefore, hemoglobin casts have the same clinical meaning as erythrocyte casts. However, they may also derive from free hemoglobinuria in patients with intravascular hemolysis.

- *Leukocyte casts* contain variable amounts of polymorphonuclear leukocytes (Fig. 4.6G). They are found in acute pyelonephritis and acute interstitial nephritis. In GN, they are the rarest type of cast.[30]
- *Epithelial casts* contain variable numbers of renal tubular cells, which can be identified by their prominent nucleus (Fig. 4.6H). Epithelial casts are a typical finding in ATN and acute interstitial nephritis. However, they are also frequent (even though in small numbers) in GN[30] and in the nephrotic syndrome.[35]
- *Myoglobin casts* contain myoglobin and may be similar to hemoglobin casts (Fig. 4.6F), from which they can be distinguished through knowledge of the clinical setting. They are observed in the urine of patients with AKI associated with rhabdomyolysis.
- *Casts containing microorganisms* (bacteria and yeasts) indicate renal infection.
- *Casts containing crystals* indicate that crystals derive from the renal tubules. They are an important diagnostic element in crystalluric forms of AKI, such as acute urate nephropathy.

Crystals

Correct identification of urine crystals requires knowledge of crystal morphologies, urine pH, and appearances under polarizing light.[37] Examination of the urine for crystals is informative in the assessment of patients with stone disease, with some rare inherited metabolic disorders, and with suspected drug nephrotoxicity. The following are the main crystals of the urine.

Uric Acid Crystals and Amorphous Uric Acids

Uric acid crystals have an amber color and a wide spectrum of appearances, including rhomboids and barrels (Fig. 4.7A). These crystals are found only in acid urine (pH ≤5.8) and are polychromatic under polarizing light.

Amorphous uric acids are tiny granules of irregular shape that also precipitate in acid urine. They are identical to amorphous phosphates, which, however, precipitate in alkaline pH. In addition, whereas uric acid crystals polarize light, phosphates do not.[35]

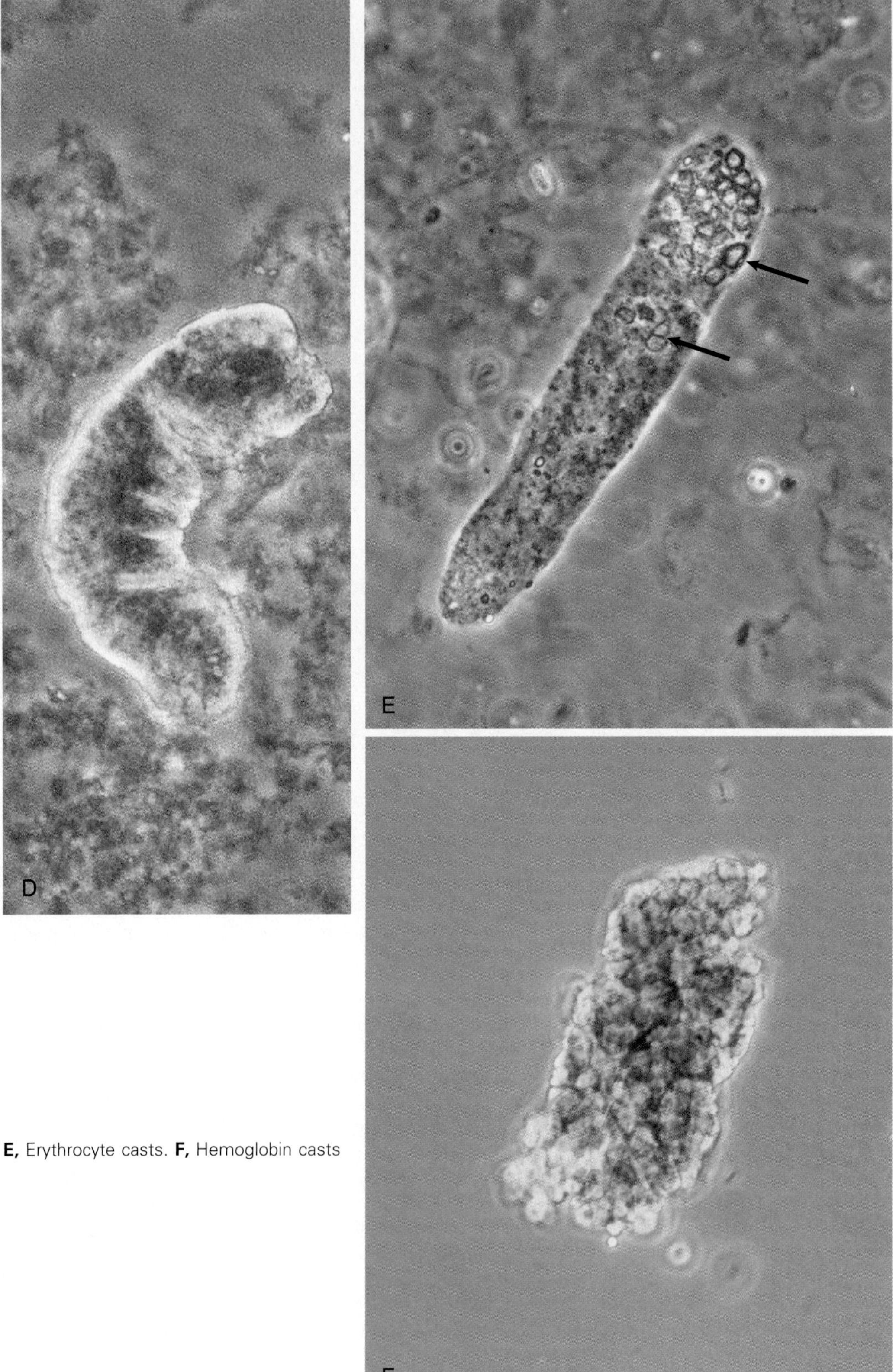

Figure 4.6, cont'd **D,** Waxy cast. **E,** Erythrocyte casts. **F,** Hemoglobin casts (note typical brownish hue).

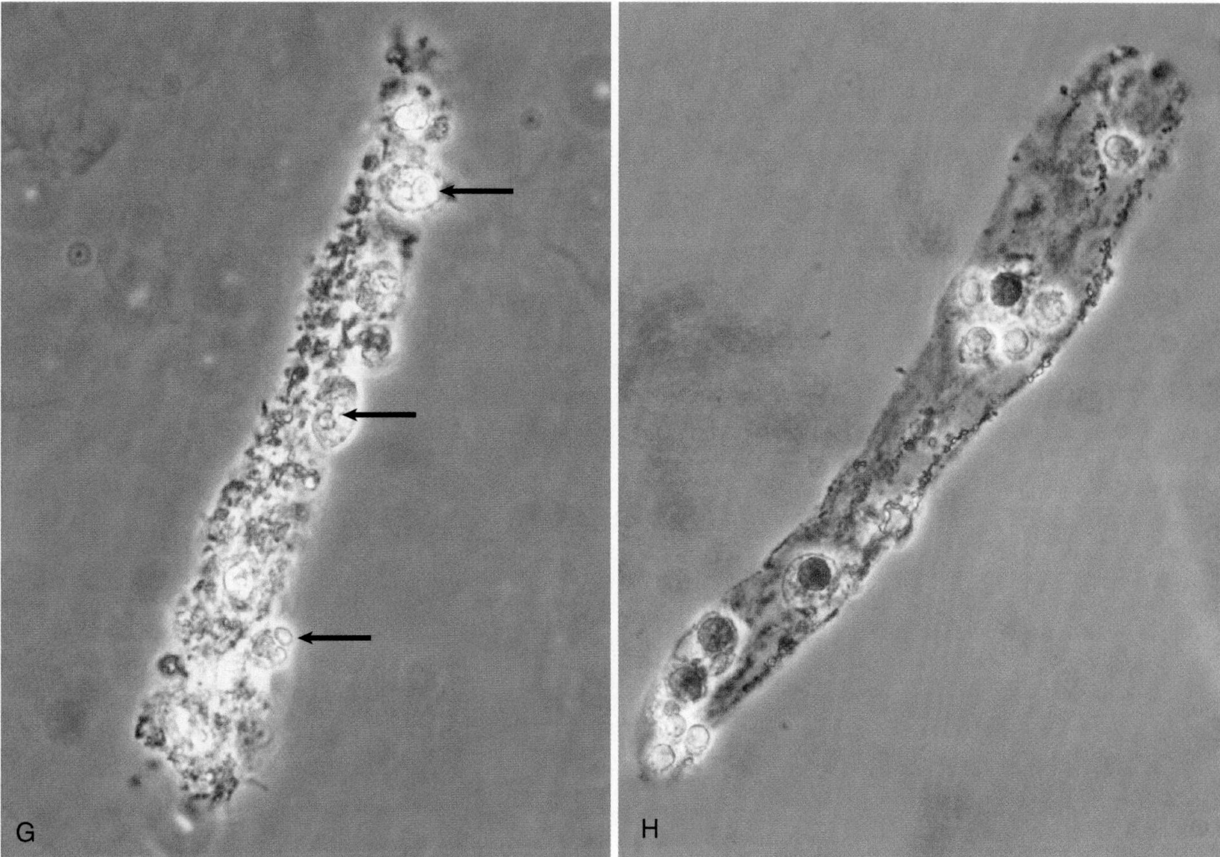

Figure 4.6, cont'd **G,** Leukocyte cast. The polymorphonuclear leukocytes are identifiable by their lobulated nucleus *(arrows)*. **H,** Epithelial cell casts. Renal tubular cells are identifiable by their large nucleus. (All images by phase contrast microscopy; original magnification ×400.) For full morphologic details about these particles, see reference 36.

Calcium Oxalate Crystals

There are two types of calcium oxalate crystals. Bihydrated (or weddellite) crystals most often have a bipyramidal appearance (Fig. 4.7B); monohydrated (or whewellite) crystals are ovoid, dumbbell shaped, or biconcave disks (Fig. 4.7C). Both types of calcium oxalate crystals precipitate at pH 5.4 to 6.7. Monohydrated crystals always polarize light, whereas bihydrated crystals usually do not.

Calcium Phosphate Crystals and Amorphous Phosphates

Calcium phosphate crystals are pleomorphic, appearing as prisms, star-like particles, or needles of various sizes and shapes (Fig. 4.7D). They can also appear as plates with a granular surface. These crystals precipitate in alkaline urine (pH ≥7.0) and, with the exception of plates, polarize light intensely.

Amorphous phosphates are tiny particles identical to amorphous uric acids. However, they precipitate at a pH of 7.0 or higher and do not polarize light.

Triple Phosphate Crystals

These crystals contain magnesium ammonium phosphate and in most instances have the appearance of "coffin lids" (Fig. 4.7E). They are found in alkaline urine (pH ≥7.0), polarize light strongly, and suggest the presence of a urease-splitting bacterium.

Cholesterol Crystals

They are transparent and thin plates, often clumped together, with sharp edges (Fig. 4.7F).

Cystine Crystals

These crystals occur in patients with cystinuria and are hexagonal plates with irregular sides that are often heaped one on the other (Fig. 4.7G). They precipitate only in acid urine, especially after the addition of acetic acid and after overnight storage at 4°C. Evaluation of their size can be used to predict the recurrence of cystine stones.[38]

2,8-Dihydroxyadenine Crystals

These are spherical, brownish crystals with radial striations from the center and polarize light strongly.[39,40] They are a marker of homozygotic deficiency of the enzyme adenine phosphoribosyltransferase. This rare condition causes crystalluria in about 96% of untreated patients, who frequently also suffer from radiolucent urinary stone formation, AKI, or even chronic kidney disease.[39,40]

Crystals Due to Drugs

Many drugs can cause crystalluria, especially in a setting of drug overdose, dehydration, or hypoalbuminemia in the presence of low urinary pH favoring drug crystallization. Examples include

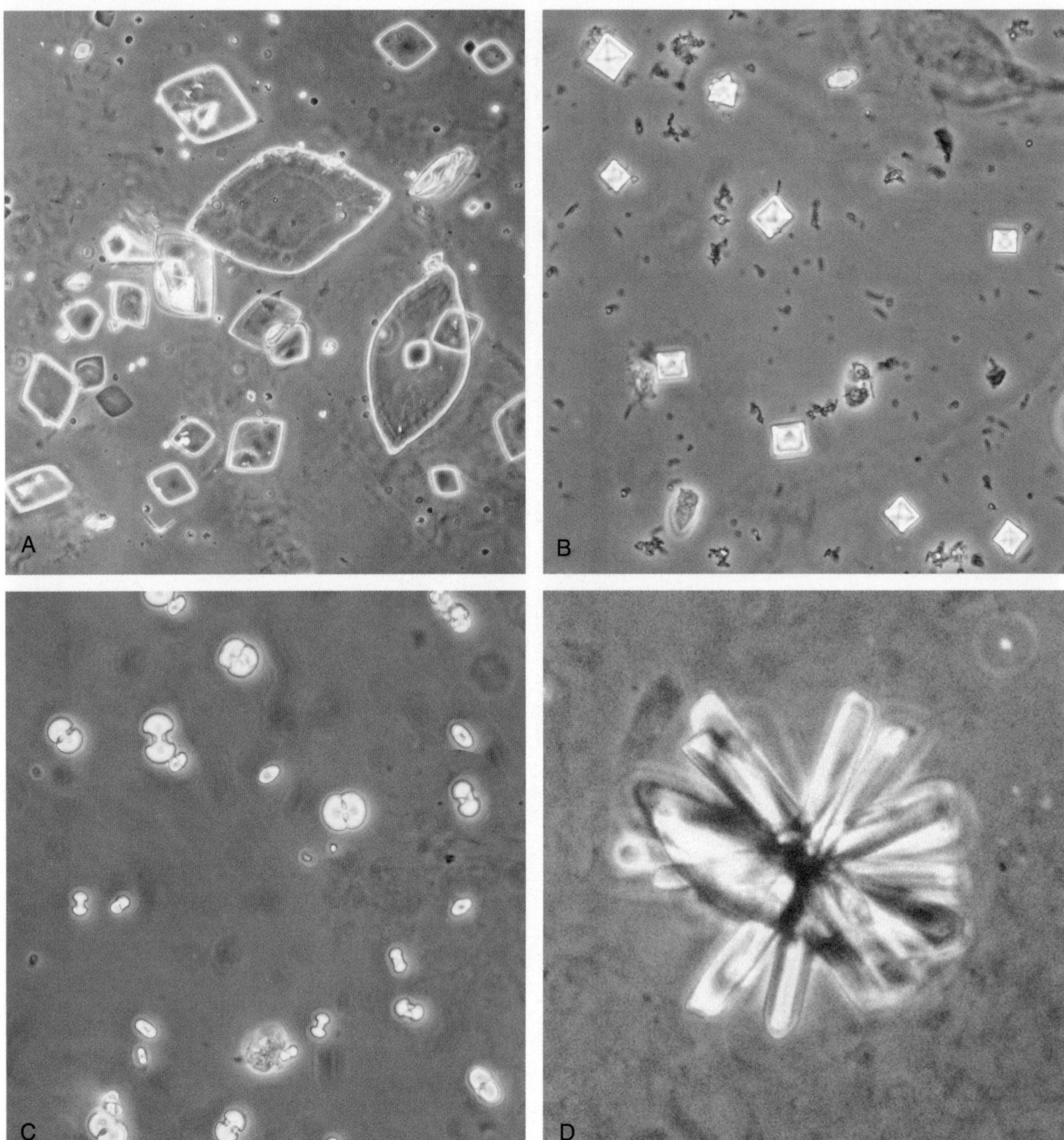

Figure 4.7 Crystals. A, Uric acid crystals. This rhomboid shape is the most frequent. **B,** Bihydrated calcium oxalate crystals with their typical appearance of a "letter envelope." **C,** Different types of monohydrated calcium oxalate crystals. **D,** A star-like calcium phosphate crystal.

the antibiotics sulfadiazine, amoxicillin (Fig 4.7H), and ciprofloxacin (Fig 4.7I)[41]; the antiviral agents acyclovir and indinavir (Fig. 4.7J); the vasodilators pyridoxylate and naftidrofuryl oxalate; the barbiturate primidone; the antiepileptic felbamate; the inhibitor of gastroenteric lipase orlistat; and intravenous vitamin C.[35]

Whereas most of these drugs cause crystals with unusual appearances, naftidrofuryl oxalate, orlistat, and vitamin C cause calcium oxalate crystals.

Clinical Significance of Crystals

Uric acid, calcium oxalate, and calcium phosphate crystals are common and may be without clinical importance because they can reflect transient supersaturation of the urine due to ingestion of some foods (e.g., meat for uric acid, spinach or chocolate for calcium oxalate, milk or cheese for calcium phosphate) or mild dehydration. However, the persistence of calcium oxalate or uric acid crystalluria may reflect hypercalciuria, hyperoxaluria, or hyperuricosuria. In calcium stone formers, crystalluria may be used to assess calcium stone disease activity.[37]

Large numbers of uric acid crystals may be associated with AKI due to acute urate nephropathy, whereas large numbers of monohydrated calcium oxalate crystals, especially with a spindle shape, may be associated with AKI from ethylene glycol intoxication. Triple phosphate crystals are often associated with urinary

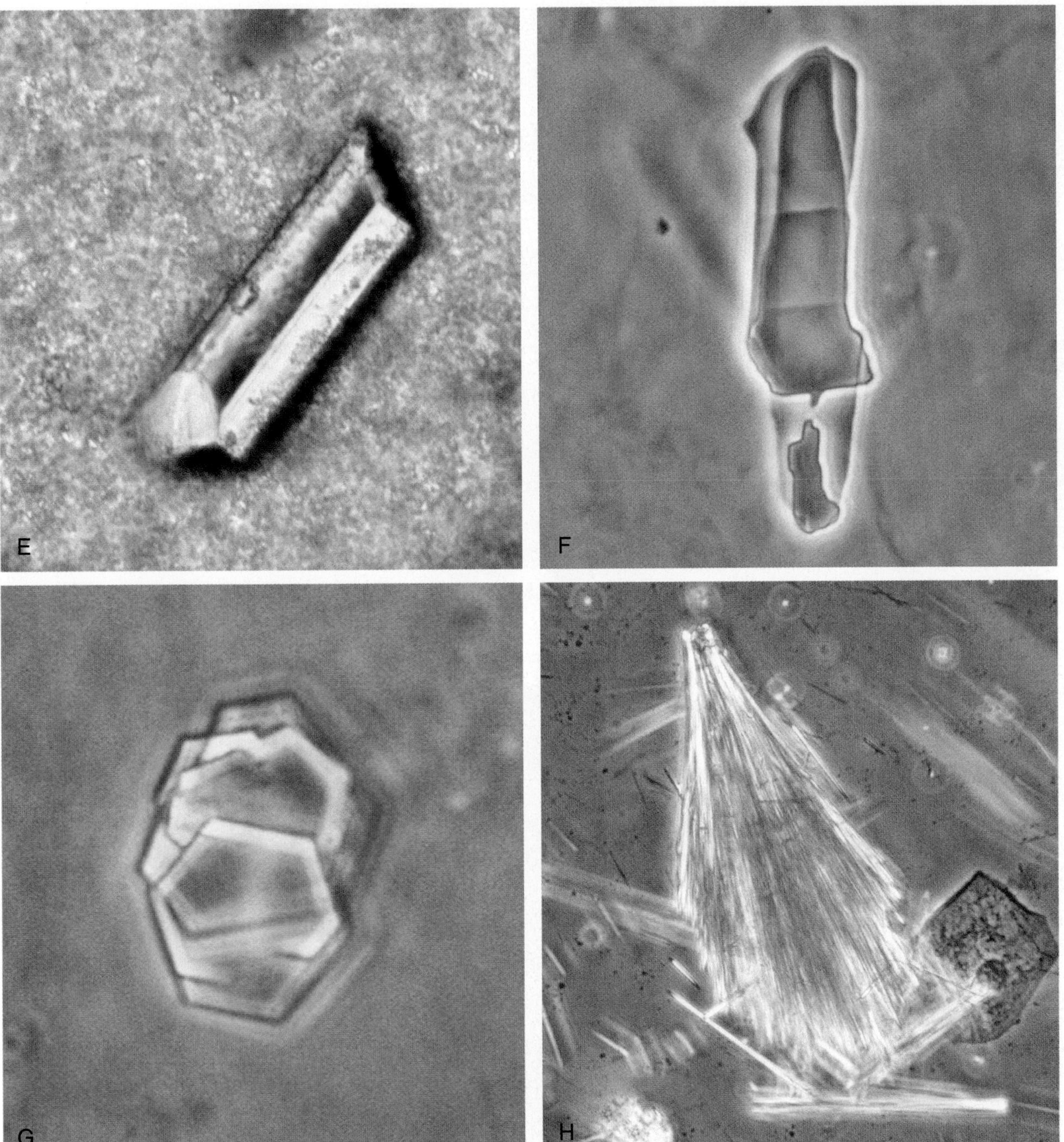

Figure 4.7, cont'd **E,** Triple phosphate crystal, on the background of a massive amount of amorphous phosphate particles. **F,** Cholesterol crystal. **G,** Cystine crystals heaped one on the other. **H,** Amoxicillin crystal resembling a branch of a broom bush.

Continued

tract infection caused by urea-splitting microorganisms such as *Ureaplasma urealyticum* and *Corynebacterium urealyticum*.

Some crystals are always pathologic. This is the case with cholesterol, which is found in patients with marked proteinuria; cystine, which is a marker of cystinuria; and 2,8-dihydroxyadenine.

When crystalluria is due to drugs, this may be the only urinary abnormality or it may be associated with hematuria, obstructive uropathy, or AKI due to the precipitation of crystals within the renal tubules. This last possibility has been described for almost all crystals due to drugs.[35]

Organisms

Bacteria are a frequent finding because urine is usually collected and handled under nonsterile conditions and examination is often delayed. Urine infection can be suspected only if bacteria are found in noncontaminated, freshly voided midstream urine, especially if numerous leukocytes are also present.[42]

Candida, *Trichomonas vaginalis*, and *Enterobius vermicularis* are mostly common contaminants derived from genital secretions.

Schistosoma haematobium is responsible for urinary schistosomiasis (see Chapter 54). In endemic areas, the examination of the

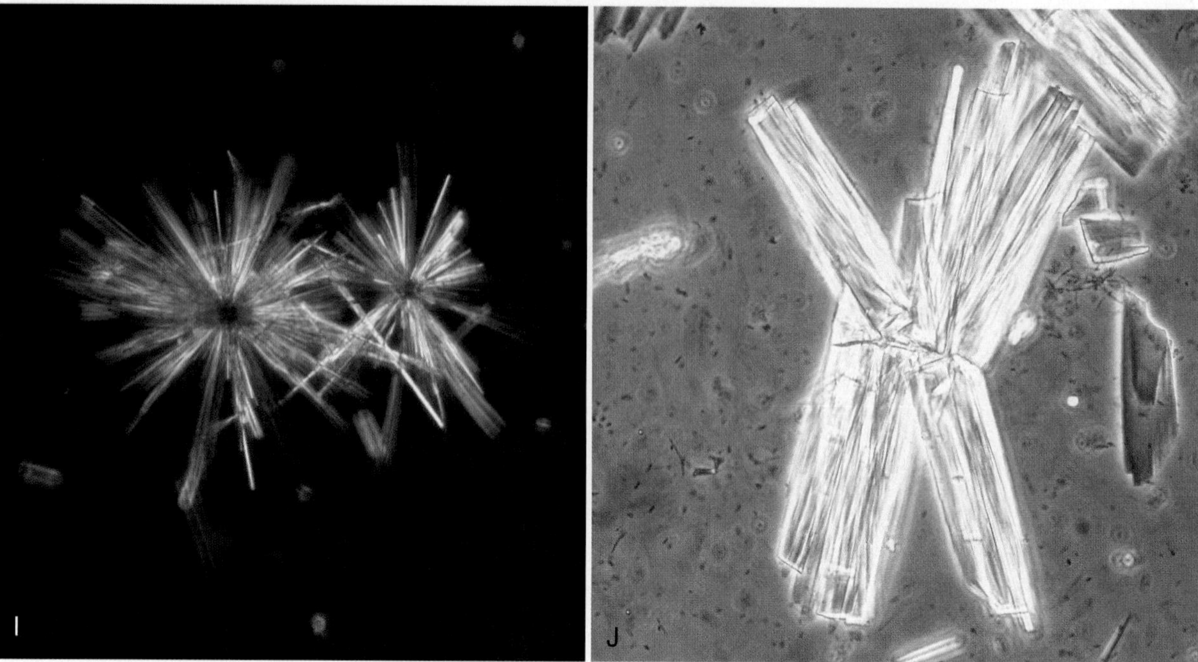

Figure 4.7, cont'd **I,** Star-like ciprofloxacin crystals as seen by polarized light. **J,** A large crystal of indinavir. (All images by phase contrast microscopy; original magnification ×400.)

urinary sediment is the most widely used method for diagnosis of this condition, which causes recurrent bouts of macroscopic hematuria and obstructive uropathy. The diagnosis is based on the finding of the parasite eggs, with their typical terminal spike (Fig. 4.8). The eggs are especially found between 10 AM and 2 PM and after strenuous exercise.

Contaminants

A large number of particles can contaminate urine. These may come from the patient (e.g., spermatozoa, erythrocytes from menstruation, leukocytes from vaginitis, cloth or synthetic fibers, creams or talcum), the laboratory (e.g., starch particles, glass fragments from coverslips), or the environment (e.g., pollens, plant cells, fungal spores).[36] Correct identification of these particles is important to avoid misinterpretations and false results.

INTERPRETATION OF THE MAIN URINE SEDIMENT FINDINGS

Examination of the urine sediment, coupled with the quantity of proteinuria and other urine and blood findings, results in urine sediment profiles that aid in the diagnosis of urinary tract diseases (Fig. 4.9).

Nephrotic Sediment

The typical nephrotic sediment contains lipids, casts, and tubular cells. Hyaline, hyaline-granular, granular, and fatty casts are seen; erythrocyte or hemoglobin casts, leukocyte casts, and waxy casts are rare or absent. Erythrocytes may be totally absent, especially in minimal change disease, or may be in moderate numbers, for example, in membranous nephropathy and focal segmental glomerulosclerosis. Leukocytes are usually not found.

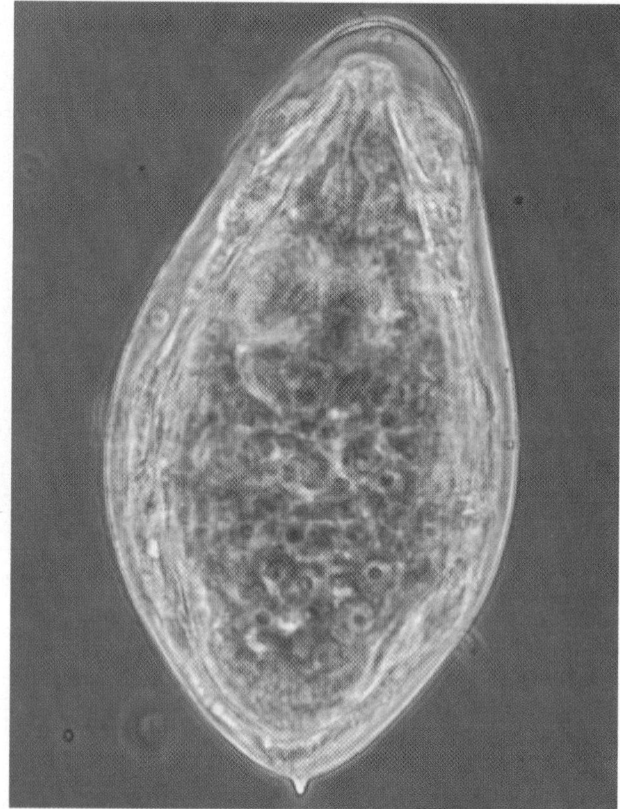

Figure 4.8 An egg of *Schistosoma haematobium*, containing the miracidium and with its typical terminal spike. (Phase contrast microscopy; original magnification ×400.)

Main Urinary Sediment Profiles

Renal Disease	Hallmark	Associated Findings
Nephrotic syndrome (proteinuria: ++++)	Lipiduria Marked cylindruria	Renal tubular epithelial cells (RTECs) RTEC casts Microscopic hematuria: absent to moderate
Nephritic syndrome (proteinuria: + → ++++)	Moderate to severe hematuria Erythrocyte/hemoglobin casts	Mild leukocyturia RTECs (low number) RTEC casts Waxy casts
Acute kidney injury (proteinuria: absent to trace)	RTECs either normal or damaged/necrotic RTEC casts Granular casts	Variable according to the cause of ATN (e.g., pigmented myoglobin casts in rhabdomyolysis; uric acid crystals in acute urate nephropathy)
Urinary tract infection (proteinuria: absent)	Bacteria Leukocytes	Superficial transitional epithelial cells Isomorphic erythrocytes Triple phosphate crystals (for infections due to urease-producing bacteria) Leukocyte casts (in renal infection)
Polyomavirus BK infection (proteinuria: absent)	Decoy cells	Macrophages

Figure 4.9 Main urinary sediment profiles. ATN, acute tubular necrosis.

Nephritic Sediment

Hematuria is the hallmark of the nephritic sediment. More than 100 erythrocytes per high-power field is not uncommon, especially in cases with extracapillary or necrotizing glomerular lesions. Mild leukocyturia is also frequent. Erythrocyte and hemoglobin casts are frequent. Leukocyte and waxy casts can also be observed.

The nephritic sediment may clear with treatment, but its reappearance usually indicates relapse of the disease, such as lupus nephritis[43] or systemic vasculitis.[44] In rare cases, there may be an active proliferative GN without a nephritic sediment.

In our experience, it is possible to distinguish proliferative from nonproliferative GN by the examination of the urine sediment with 80% sensitivity and 79% specificity. Proliferative GN is associated with higher numbers of erythrocytes, leukocytes, and tubular epithelial cells as well as with erythrocyte and epithelial cell casts.[31]

Sediment of Acute Kidney Injury

In AKI, the urine sediment contains variable numbers of renal tubular cells, either normal or damaged or necrotic, and a marked granular and epithelial cylindruria.[45] In addition, depending on the cause of the tubular damage, other elements can be seen. For instance, in rhabdomyolysis, myoglobin pigmented casts are found; in AKI due to intratubular precipitation of crystals (e.g., acute uric acid nephropathy, ethylene glycol poisoning, drugs), there may be massive crystalluria.

Sediment of Urinary Tract Infection

Bacteriuria and leukocyturia are the hallmarks of urinary tract infection, and superficial uroepithelial cells and isomorphic erythrocytes are common. Triple phosphate crystals are also present when the infection is caused by urease-producing bacteria, such as *U. urealyticum* or *C. urealyticum*. In the case of renal infection, leukocyte casts may be found.

The correlation between the urine sediment findings and the urine culture is usually good. False-positive results may occur as a consequence of urine contamination from genital secretions or bacterial overgrowth on standing. False-negative results may be due to misinterpretation of bacteria (especially with cocci) or the lysis of leukocytes.

BK Virus Infection

In this condition (see Chapter 101), the urinary sediment contains variable numbers of decoy cells. These are renal tubular cells with nuclear changes due to the cytopathic effect of the virus. There is nuclear enlargement ("ground glass appearance"), chromatin margination, abnormal chromatin patterns, and viral inclusion bodies of various sizes and shapes with or without a perinuclear halo. As a general rule, the higher the number, the more severe the infection. These cells can be seen by phase contrast microscopy in unstained samples (Fig. 4.10A),[46] even though they are usually identified by cytocentrifuged smears with the Papanicolaou stain (Fig. 4.10B).[47] Electron microscopy shows virus particles with mean diameter of 45 Å (Fig. 4.10C). In addition to decoy cells, macrophages are frequent and abundant. The finding of decoy cells in the urine is sufficient to diagnose reactivation of the viral infection; for the diagnosis of BK virus nephropathy, a renal biopsy is mandatory.

Nonspecific Urinary Abnormalities

Some urine sediments are less specific, such as variable numbers of nonspecific casts with or without mild erythrocyturia or leukocyturia, mild crystalluria, and small numbers of superficial

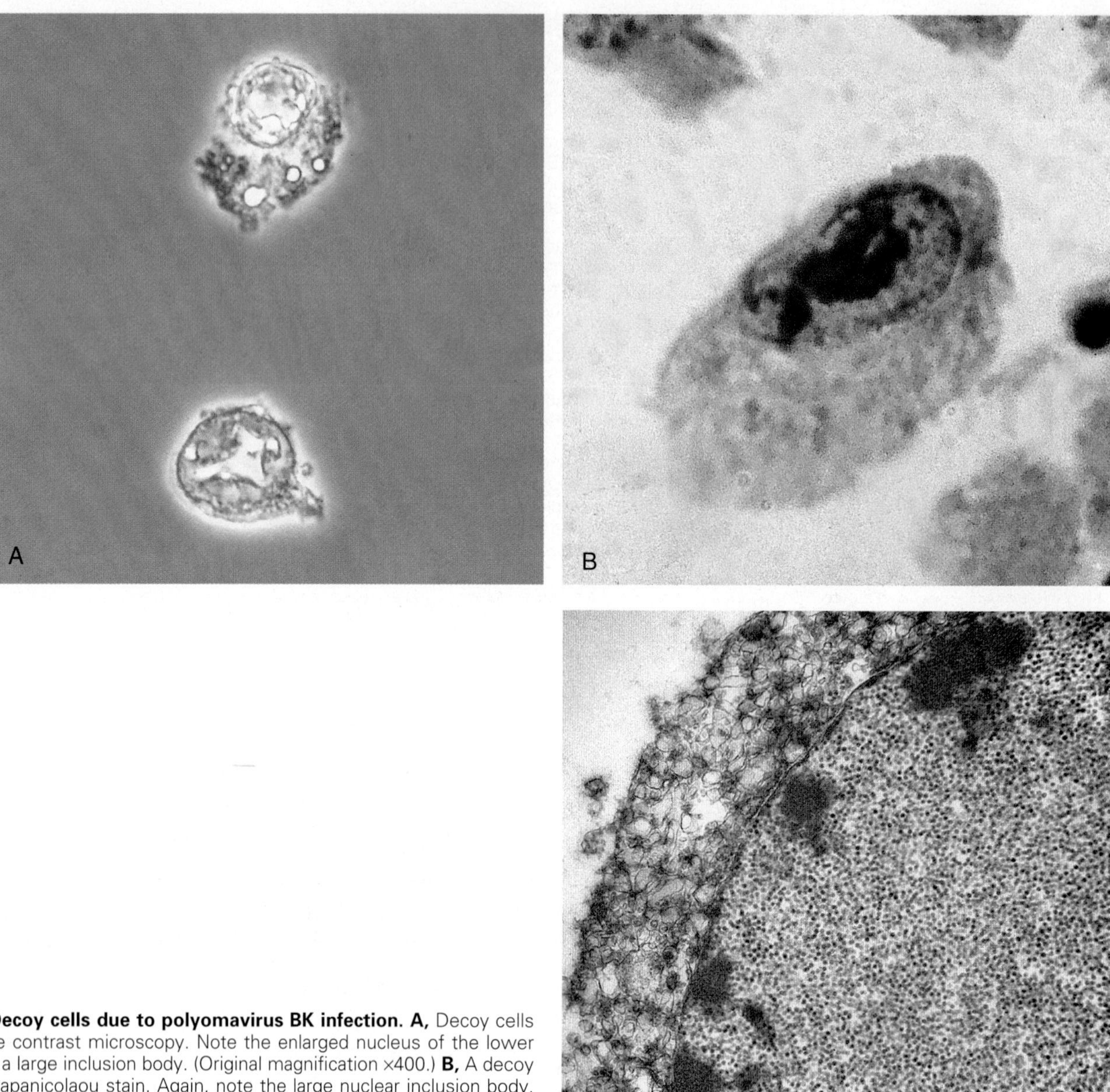

Figure 4.10 Decoy cells due to polyomavirus BK infection. A, Decoy cells as seen by phase contrast microscopy. Note the enlarged nucleus of the lower cell that contains a large inclusion body. (Original magnification ×400.) **B,** A decoy cell as seen by Papanicolaou stain. Again, note the large nuclear inclusion body. (Original magnification ×1000.) **C,** A decoy cell, as seen by transmission electron microscopy, whose nucleus is engorged with virus particles. (Original magnification ×30,000.) Also note various chromatin granules close to nuclear membrane (chromatin margination).

epithelial cells. In such cases, the correct interpretation of the urinary findings requires adequate clinical information and possibly renal biopsy.

AUTOMATED ANALYSIS OF THE URINE SEDIMENT

Instruments for the automated analysis of the urinary sediment are now available. These are based on flow cytometry or digital imaging. Flow cytometry uses stains for nucleic acid and cell membranes in uncentrifuged urine samples and so identifies cells, bacteria, and casts.[48] Accuracy is good for leukocytes and erythrocytes, even though the erythrocytes can be overestimated because of the interference from bacteria, crystals, and yeasts. As to casts, false-negative results are frequent, ranging from about 13% to 43%. Digital imaging systems supply black and white images of urine particles. Precision and accuracy are good for erythrocytes and leukocytes, but sensitivity for casts is relatively low.[49]

Today, automated instruments are used especially in large laboratories to screen large numbers of samples in a short time and to identify the samples that are normal or contain only minor changes. This approach greatly reduces the number of samples that require manual microscopy. However, these instruments do not recognize lipids, cannot distinguish between uroepithelial cells and renal tubular cells, and do not identify various types of casts and crystals, some of which are clinically important. Therefore, they cannot yet be used alone for the evaluation of the renal patient.

REFERENCES

1. Tsai JJ, Yeun JY, Kumar VA, Don BR. Comparison and interpretation of urinalysis performed by a nephrologist versus a hospital-based clinical laboratory. *Am J Kidney Dis*. 2005;46:820-829.
2. Fogazzi GB, Garigali G, Provano B, et al. How to improve the teaching of urine microscopy. *Clin Chem Lab Med*. 2007;45:407-412.
3. Kouri T, Fogazzi G, Gant V, et al. European urinalysis guidelines. *Scand J Clin Lab Med*. 2000;60(suppl 231):1-96.
4. Van der Snoek BE, Koene RAP. Fixation of urinary sediment. *Lancet*. 1997;350:933-934.
5. Kouri T, Vuotari L, Pohjavaara S, et al. Preservation of urine flow cytometric and visual microscopic testing. *Clin Chem*. 2002;48: 900-905.
6. Cheng JT, Mohan S, Nasr SH, et al. Chyluria presenting as milky urine and nephrotic-range proteinuria. *Kidney Int*. 2006;70:1518-1522.
7. Pradella M, Dorizzi RM, Rigolin F. Relative density of urine: Methods and clinical significance. *Crit Rev Clin Lab Sci*. 1988;26:195-242.
8. Dorizzi RM, Caputo M. Measurement of urine relative density using refractometer and reagent strips. *Clin Chem Lab Med*. 1998;36: 925-928.
9. Lam MO. False hematuria due to bacteriuria. *Arch Pathol*. 1995; 119:717-721.
10. Bridgen ML, Edgell D, McPherson M, et al. High incidence of significant urinary ascorbic acid concentration in a West Coast population—implication for routine analysis. *Clin Chem*. 1992;38:426-431.
11. Grienstead GF, Scott RE, Stevens BS, et al. The Ames Clinitek 200/ Multistix P urinalysis method compared with manual and microscopic method. *Clin Chem*. 1987;33:1660-1662.
12. Bank CM, Codrington JF, van Dieijen-Visser MP, Brombacher PJ. Screening urine specimen populations for normality using different dipsticks: Evaluation of parameters influencing sensitivity and specificity. *J Clin Chem Clin Biochem*. 1987;25:299-307.
13. National Kidney Foundation. K/DOQI Clinical Practice Guidelines for Chronic Kidney Disease: Evaluation, classification, and stratification. *Am J Kidney Dis*. 2002;39(suppl 1):S93-S102.
14. Price CP, Newall R, Boyd JC. Use of protein : creatinine ratio measurements on random urine samples for prediction of significant proteinuria: A systematic review. *Clin Chem*. 2005;51:1577-1586.
15. Bazzi C, Petrini C, Rizza V, et al. Characterization of proteinuria in primary glomerulonephritides. SDS-PAGE patterns: Clinical significance and prognostic value of low molecular weight ("tubular") proteins. *Am J Kidney Dis*. 1997;29:27-35.
16. Kuwabara T, Mori K, Mukoyama M, et al. Urinary neutrophil gelatinase-associated lipocalin levels reflect damage to glomeruli, proximal tubules, and distal nephrons. *Kidney Int*. 2009;75:284-294.
17. Graziani M, Merlini GP, Petrini C. IFCC Committee on Plasma Protein. Guidelines for the analysis of Bence Jones protein. *Clin Chem Lab Med*. 2003;41:338-346.
18. Cameron JS, Blandford G. The simple assessment of selectivity in heavy proteinuria. *Lancet*. 1966;2:242-247.
19. Bazzi C, Petrini C, Rizza V, et al. A modern approach to selectivity of proteinuria and tubulointerstitial damage in nephrotic syndrome. *Kidney Int*. 2001;58:1732-1741.
20. Kutter D, Figueiredo G, Klemmer L. Chemical detection of leukocytes in urine by means of a new multiple test strip. *J Clin Chem Clin Biochem*. 1987;25:91-94.
21. Skjold AC, Stover LR, Pendergrass JH, et al. New DiP-and-read test for determining leukocytes in urine. *Clin Chem*. 1987;33:1242-1245.
22. Lundberg JO, Carlsson S, Engstrand L, et al. Urinary nitrite: More than a marker of infection. *Urology*. 1997;50:189-191.
23. Fairley K, Birch DF. Hematuria: A simple method for identifying glomerular bleeding. *Kidney Int*. 1982;21:105-108.
24. Fasset RG, Horgan BA, Mathew TH. Detection of glomerular bleeding by phase contrast microscopy. *Lancet*. 1982;1:1432-1434.
25. Rizzoni G, Braggion F, Zacchello G. Evaluation of glomerular and nonglomerular hematuria by phase-contrast microscopy. *J Pediatr*. 1983;103:370-374.
26. Dinda AK, Saxena S, Guleria S, et al. Diagnosis of glomerular haematuria: Role of dysmorphic red cells, G1 cells and bright-field microscopy. *Scand J Clin Lab Invest*. 1997;57:203-208.
27. Fogazzi GB, Edefonti A, Garigali G, et al. Urine erythrocyte morphology in patients with microscopic haematuria caused by a glomerulopathy. *Pediatr Nephrol*. 2008;23:1093-1110.
28. Schramek P, Schuster FX, Georgopoulos M, et al. Value of urinary erythrocyte morphology in assessment of symptomless microhaematuria. *Lancet*. 1989;2:1314-1319.
29. Rath B, Turner C, Hartley B, Chantler C. What makes red cells dysmorphic in glomerular hematuria? *Paediatr Nephrol*. 1992;6:424-427.
30. Fogazzi GB, Saglimbeni L, Banfi G, et al. Urinary sediment features in proliferative and nonproliferative glomerular diseases. *J Nephrol*. 2005;18:703-710.
31. Nolan CR, Kelleher SP. Eosinophiluria. *Clin Lab Med*. 1988;8: 555-565.
32. Ruffing KA, Hoppes P, Blend D, et al. Eosinophils in urine revisited. *Clin Nephrol*. 1994;41:163-166.
33. Hotta O, Yusa N, Kitamura H, Taguma Y. Urinary macrophages as activity markers of renal injury. *Clin Chim Acta*. 2000;297:123-133.
34. Maruhashi Y, Nakajima M, Akazawa H, et al. Analysis of macrophages in urine sediments in children with IgA nephropathy. *Clin Nephrol*. 2004;62:336-343.
35. Fogazzi GB. *The Urinary Sediment. An Integrated View*. 3rd ed. Milano: Elsevier; 2009.
36. Praet M, Quatacker J, Van Loo A, et al. Non-invasive diagnosis of Fabry's disease by electronmicroscopic evaluation of urinary sediment. *Nephrol Dial Transplant*. 1995;10:902-903.
37. Daudon M, Jungers P. Clinical value of crystalluria and quantitative morphoconstitutional analysis of urinary calculi. *Nephron Physiol*. 2004;98:31-36.
38. Bouzidi H, Daudon M. Cystinurie: du diagnostic à la surveillance thérapeutique. *Ann Biol Clin*. 2007;65:473-481.
39. Edvarsson V, Palsson R, Olafsson I, et al. Clinical features and genotype of adenine phosphoribosyltransferase deficiency in Iceland. *Am J Kidney Dis*. 2001;38:473-480.
40. Bouzidi H, Lacour B, Daudon M. Lithiase de 2,8-dihydroxyadénine: du diagnostic à la prise en charge thérapeutique. *Ann Biol Clin*. 2007;65:585-592.
41. Fogazzi GB, Garigali G, Brambilla C, et al. Ciprofloxacin crystalluria. *Nephrol Dial Transplant*. 2006;21:2982-2983.
42. Vickers D, Ahmad T, Coulthard MG. Diagnosis of urinary tract infection in children: Fresh urine microscopy or culture? *Lancet*. 1991;338:767-770.
43. Hebert LA, Dillon JJ, Middendorf DF, et al. Relationship between appearance of urinary red blood cell/white blood cell casts and the onset of renal relapse in systemic lupus erythematosus. *Am J Kidney Dis*. 1995;26:432-438.
44. Fujita T, Ohi H, Endo M, et al. Levels of red blood cells in the urinary sediment reflect the degree of renal activity in Wegener's granulomatosis. *Clin Nephrol*. 1998;50:284-288.
45. Perazzella MA, Coca SG, Kanbai M, et al. Diagnostic value of urine microscopy for differential diagnosis of acute kidney injury in hospitalized patients. *Clin J Am Soc Nephrol*. 2008;3:1615-1619.
46. Fogazzi GB, Cantù M, Saglimbeni L: "Decoy cells" in the urine due to polyomavirus BK infection: Easily seen by phase-contrast microscopy. *Nephrol Dial Transplant*. 2001;16:1496-1498.
47. Drachemberg RC, Drachenberg CB, Papadimitriou JC, et al. Morphological spectrum of polyomavirus disease in renal allografts: Diagnostic accuracy of urine cytology. *Am J Transplant*. 2001;1:373-381.
48. Delanghe JR, Kouri TT, Huber AR, et al. The role of automated urine particles flow cytometry in clinical practice. *Clin Chim Acta*. 2000; 301:1-18.
49. Linko S, Kouri TT, Toivonen E, et al. Analytical performance of the Iris iQ200 automated urine microscopy analyzer. *Chim Clin Acta*. 2006;372:54-64.

CHAPTER 5

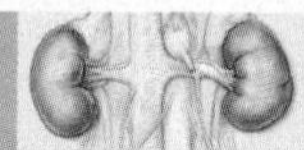

Imaging

David C. Wymer

DEFINITION

In recent years, there has been a significant change in imaging evaluation of patients with renal disease. Intravenous urography (IVU) is infrequently used and has mostly been replaced by ultrasound, computed tomography (CT), magnetic resonance imaging (MRI), and nuclear medicine scanning. There are major technologic advances in each of these modalities with the rapid changes in computer-based data manipulation. Three-dimensional and even four-dimensional (time-sensitive) image analysis is now available. "Molecular" imaging, in which biomarkers are used to visualize cellular function, is beginning to provide functional as well as anatomic information.

The American College of Radiology has published Appropriateness Criteria,[1] guidelines that suggest the choice of imaging to provide a rapid answer to the clinical question while minimizing cost and potential adverse effects to the patient, such as contrast-induced nephrotoxicity and radiation exposure. Relative radiation exposures are shown in Figure 5.1. First-choice imaging techniques in selected clinical scenarios are shown in Figure 5.2. Risks of imaging (Fig. 5.3) and cost need to be balanced against benefits.

ULTRASOUND

Ultrasound is relatively inexpensive and provides a rapid way to assess renal location, contour, and size without radiation exposure. Nephrologists are increasingly undertaking straightforward ultrasound examination; the practical techniques as well as the appropriate interpretative skills are discussed in Chapter 88. Portable ultrasound is available and is essential in the pediatric or emergency setting. Obstructing renal calculi can be readily detected, and renal masses can be identified as cystic or solid. In cases of suspected obstruction, the progression or regression of hydronephrosis is easily evaluated. Color Doppler imaging permits assessment of renal vascularity and perfusion. Unlike the other imaging modalities, ultrasound is highly dependent on operator skills. Limitations of ultrasound include lack of an acoustic window, body habitus, and poor cooperation of the patient.

Kidney Size

The kidney is imaged in transverse and sagittal planes and is normally 9 to 12 cm in length in adults. Differences in renal size can be detected with all imaging modalities. The common causes of enlarged and shrunken kidneys are shown in Figure 5.4.

Renal Echo Pattern

The normal cortex is hypoechoic compared with the fat-containing echogenic renal sinus (Fig. 5.5A). The cortical echotexture is defined as isoechoic or hypoechoic compared with the liver or spleen. In children, the renal pyramids are hypoechoic (Fig. 5.5B), and the cortex is characteristically hyperechoic compared with the liver and the spleen.[2] In adults, an increase in cortical echogenicity is a sensitive marker for parenchymal renal disease but is nonspecific (Fig. 5.6). Decreased cortical echogenicity can be found in acute pyelonephritis and acute renal vein thrombosis.

The normal renal contour is smooth, and the cortical mantle should be uniform and slightly thicker toward the poles. Two common benign pseudomasses that can be seen with ultrasound are the dromedary hump and the column of Bertin. The column of Bertin results from bulging of cortical tissue into the medulla; it is seen as a mass with an echotexture similar to that of the cortex, but it is found within the central renal sinus (Fig. 5.7). The renal pelvis and proximal ureter are anechoic. An extrarenal pelvis refers to the renal pelvis location outside the renal hilum. The ureter is not identified beyond the pelvis in nonobstructed patients.

Obstruction can be identified by the presence of hydronephrosis (Fig. 5.8). Parenchymal and pelvicalyceal nonobstructing renal calculi as well as ureteral obstructing calculi can be readily detected (Fig. 5.9). The upper ureter will also be dilated if obstruction is distal to the pelviureteral junction (see Fig. 5.8C). False-negative ultrasound examination findings with no hydronephrosis occasionally occur in early obstruction. Obstruction without ureteral dilation may also occur in retroperitoneal fibrosis and in transplanted kidneys as a result of periureteral fibrosis.

Renal Cysts

Cysts can be identified as anechoic lesions and are a frequent coincidental finding during renal imaging. Ultrasound usually readily identifies renal masses as cystic or solid (Figs. 5.10 and 5.11). However, hemorrhagic cysts can sometimes be mistakenly called solid because of increased echogenicity. Differentiation of cysts as simple or complex is required to plan intervention.

Simple Cysts

A simple cyst on ultrasound is anechoic, has a thin or imperceptible wall, and demonstrates through-transmission because of the relatively rapid progression of the sound wave through fluid compared with adjacent soft tissue.

Complex Cysts

Complex cysts contain calcifications, septations, and mural nodules. Instead of being anechoic, they may contain internal echoes representing hemorrhage, pus, or protein. Complex cysts may be benign or malignant; malignancy is strongly suggested

Relative Radiation Doses of Imaging Examinations	
Examination	**Effective Dose (mSv)**
Chest (PA film)	0.02
Lumbar spine	1.8
KUB (abdomen)	0.53
CT abdomen	10
CT chest	20–40
PET–CT	25
Ultrasound or MRI	0

Figure 5.1 Relative radiation doses of imaging examinations. *KUB,* kidney-ureter-bladder.

Risk Estimates in Diagnostic Imaging	
Cancer from 10 mSv of radiation (1 body CT)[3]	1 in 1000
Contrast-induced nephropathy in patient with renal impairment[4]	1 in 5
Nephrogenic systemic fibrosis[5,6]	1 in 25,000 to 30,000 (depends on gadolinium agent)
Death from iodine contrast anaphylaxis[7]	1 in 130,000
Death from gadolinium contrast anaphylaxis[8]	1 in 280,000

Figure 5.3 Risk estimates in diagnostic imaging. *(Modified from references 3-8.)*

Suggested Imaging in Renal Disease	
AKI or CKD	Ultrasound
Hematuria	Ultrasound or CT
Proteinuria, nephrotic syndrome	CT urography Ultrasound
Hypertension with normal renal function	Ultrasound *Consider* CT angiography or MR angiography
Hypertension with impaired renal function	Ultrasound with Doppler
Renal infection	CECT
Hydronephrosis seen by ultrasound	Nuclear renogram
Retroperitoneal fibrosis	CECT
Papillary or cortical necrosis	CECT
Renal vein thrombosis	CECT
Renal infarction	CECT
Nephrocalcinosis	CT

Figure 5.2 Suggested imaging in renal disease. These recommendations assume availability of all common imaging modalities. *CT,* computed tomography; *MR,* magnetic resonance; *CECT,* contrast enhanced CT. *(Modified from Appropriateness Criteria of the American College of Radiology.*[1]*)*

by cyst wall nodularity, septations, and vascularity. Complex cysts identified by ultrasound require further evaluation by contrast-enhanced CT (or MRI) to identify abnormal contrast enhancement of the cyst wall, mural nodule, or septum.

Bladder

Real-time imaging can be used to evaluate for bladder wall tumors and bladder stones. Color flow Doppler evaluation of the bladder in well-hydrated patients can be used to identify a ureteral jet. The jet is produced when peristalsis propels urine into the bladder, the incoming urine having a specific gravity higher relative to the urine already in the bladder (Fig. 5.12). Absence of the ureteral jet can indicate total ureteral obstruction.

Renal Vasculature

Color Doppler investigation of the kidneys provides a detailed evaluation of the renal vascular anatomy. The main renal arteries can be identified in most patients (Fig. 5.13). Power Doppler imaging is a more sensitive indicator of flow, but unlike color Doppler imaging, it does not provide any information about flow direction, and it cannot be used to assess vascular waveforms. It is, however, exquisitely sensitive for detection of renal parenchymal flow and has been used to identify cortical infarction.

Renal Artery Duplex Scanning

The role of gray-scale and color Doppler sonography in screening for renal artery stenosis is controversial.

The principle is that a narrowing in the artery will cause a velocity change commensurate with the degree of stenosis as well as a change in the normal renal arterial waveform downstream from the lesion. The normal renal arterial waveform demonstrates a rapid systolic upstroke and an early systolic peak (Fig. 5.14A). The waveform becomes dampened downstream from a stenosis. This consists of a slow systolic acceleration (tardus) and a decreased and rounded systolic peak (parvus; Fig. 5.14B). It also results in a decrease in the resistive index, defined as the end-diastolic velocity [EDV] subtracted from the peak systolic velocity [PSV] divided by PSV [(PSV – EDV)/PSV]. The normal resistive index is 0.70 to 0.72.

The entire length of the renal artery should be examined for the highest velocity signal. The origins of the renal arteries are important to identify because this is a common area affected by atherosclerosis, but they are often difficult to visualize because of overlying bowel gas. Within the kidney, medullary branches and cortical branches in the upper, middle, and lower thirds should be included to attempt detection of stenosis in accessory or branch renal arteries.

There are proximal and distal criteria for diagnosis of significant renal artery stenosis (usually defined as stenosis >60%). The proximal criteria detect changes in the Doppler signal at the site of stenosis and provide sensitivities and specificities ranging from 0% to 98% and 37% to 98%, respectively.[9,10] Technical failure rates are typically 10% to 20%.[11] Renal artery stenosis may also

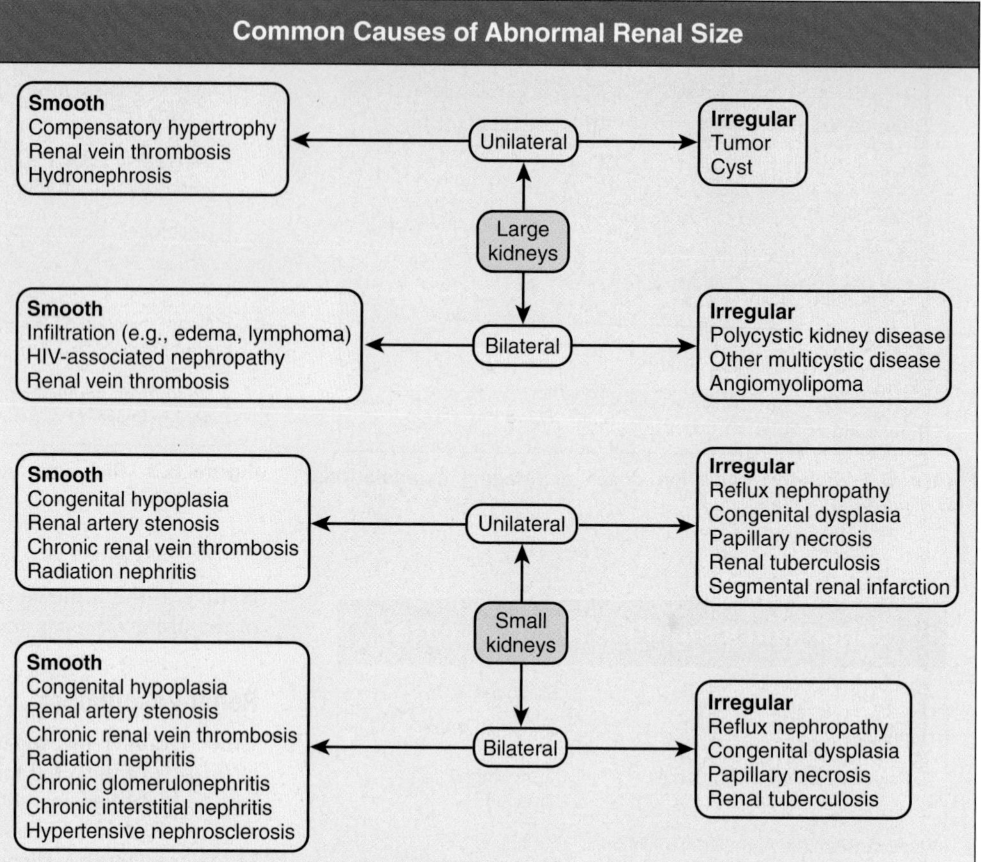

Figure 5.4 Common causes of abnormal renal size.

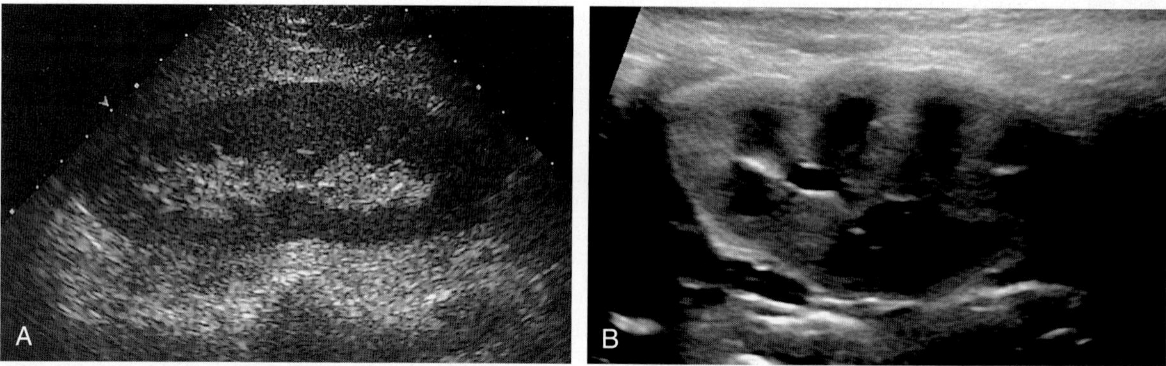

Figure 5.5 A, Normal sagittal renal ultrasound image. The cortex is hypoechoic compared with the echogenic fat containing the renal sinus. **B,** Normal infant renal ultrasound image. Note the hypoechoic pyramids.

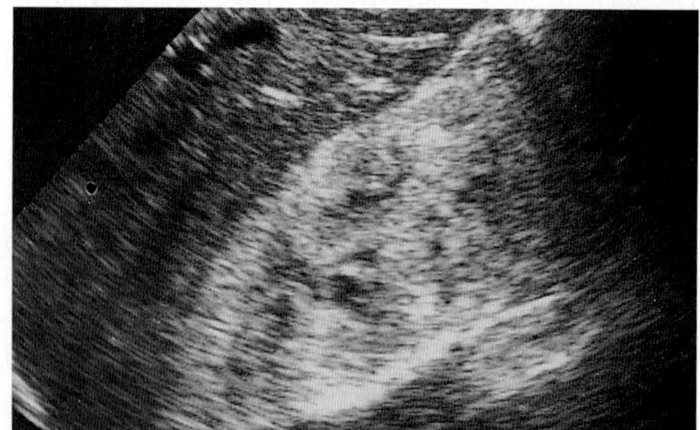

Figure 5.6 HIV-associated nephropathy. Enlarged echogenic kidney with lack of corticomedullary distinction. Bipolar length of kidney is 14.2 cm.

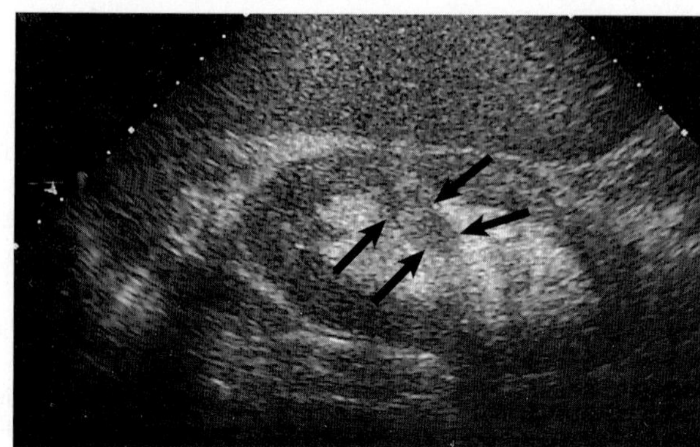

Figure 5.7 Sagittal renal ultrasound image. Column of Bertin is present *(arrows)* and is easily identified because of echotexture similar to that of the cortex.

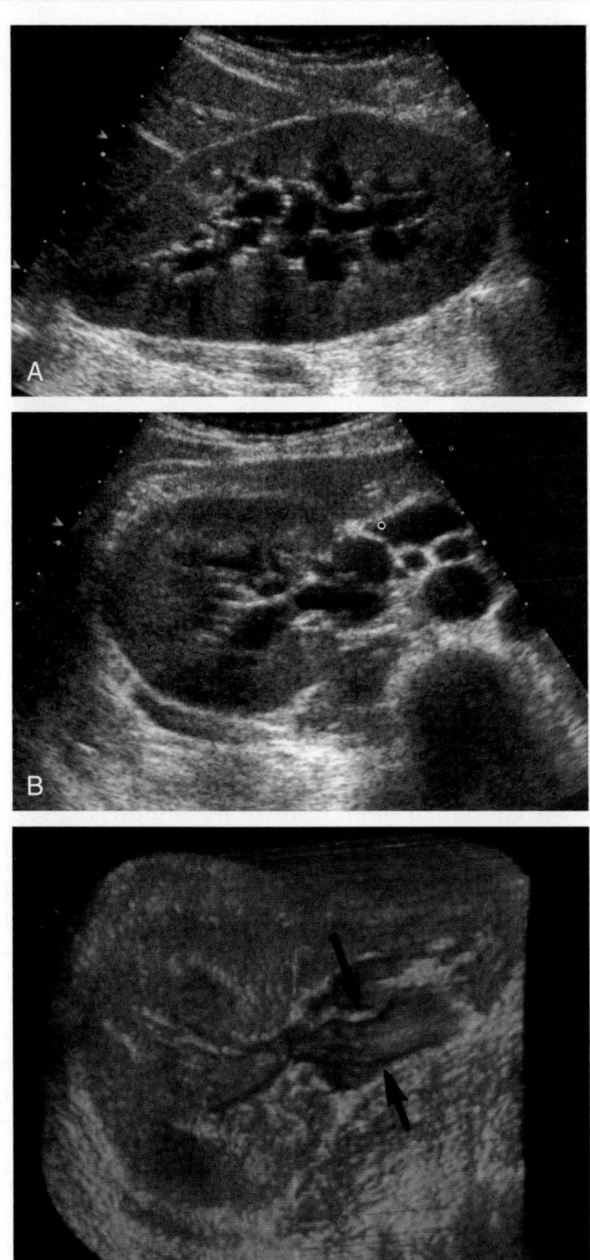

Figure 5.8 Renal ultrasound study demonstrating hydronephrosis. A, Sagittal image. **B,** Transverse image. **C,** Transverse three-dimensional surface-rendered image; *arrows* indicate the dilated proximal ureter.

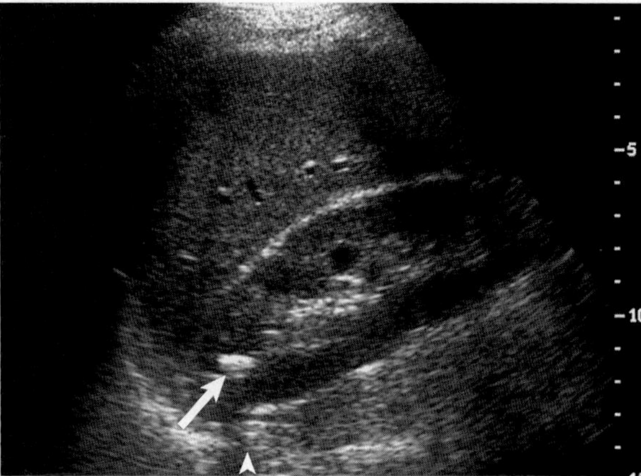

Figure 5.9 Sagittal ultrasound image showing an upper pole renal calculus *(arrow)*. Note the acoustic shadowing *(arrowhead)*.

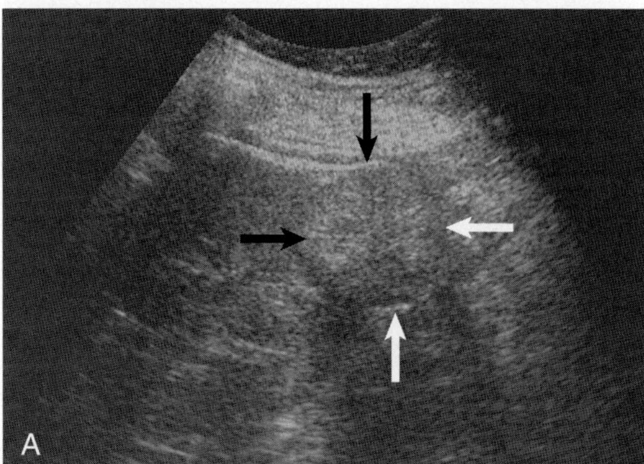

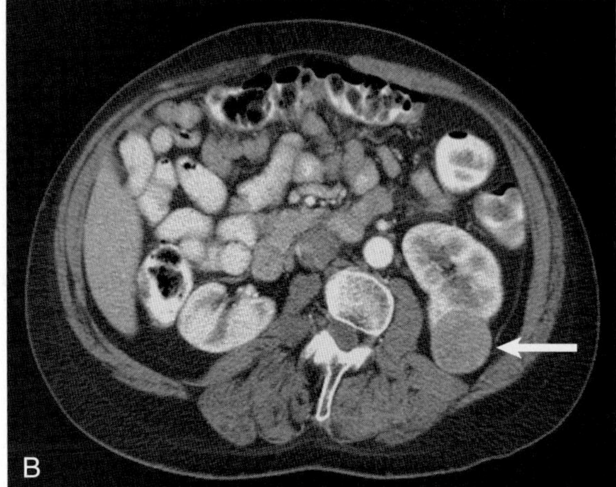

Figure 5.10 Evaluation of a renal mass. A, Sagittal ultrasound image showing a large hyperechoic mass arising from the lower pole *(arrows)*. **B,** Corresponding contrast-enhanced CT scan showing a renal cell carcinoma *(arrow)*.

be missed if PSV is low because of poor cardiac output or aortic stenosis. False-positive results can occur when renal artery velocity is increased because of high-flow states, such as hyperthyroidism or vessel tortuosity.[12] The distal criteria are related to detection of a tardus-parvus waveform distal to a stenosis; sensitivities and specificities of 66% to 100% and 67% to 94%, respectively, have been reported.[13,14] Technical failure is much lower than with proximal evaluation (<5%). False-negative results can occur from stiff poststenotic vessels, which will decrease the tardus-parvus effect.[15] The tardus-parvus effect may also be a result of aortic stenosis, low cardiac output, or collaterals in complete occlusion giving a false-positive result.

Combining the proximal and distal criteria improves the detection of stenoses. Sensitivity of 97% and specificity of 98% can be achieved when both the extrarenal and intrarenal arteries are examined.[16] When it is technically successful, Doppler ultrasound has a negative predictive value of more than 90%.[16] However, reliable results require a skilled and experienced sonographer and a long examination time. Notwithstanding these limitations,

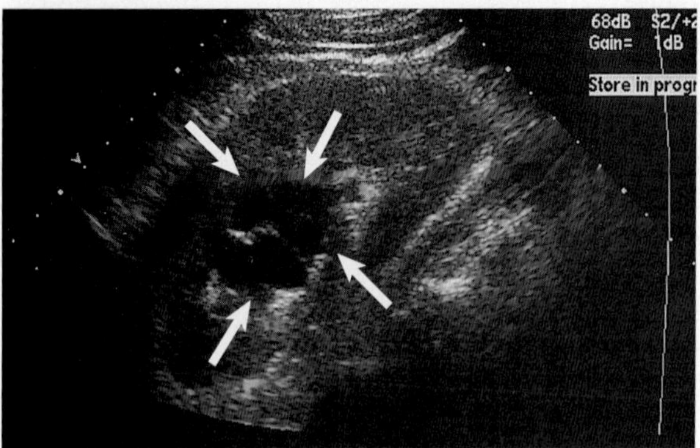

Figure 5.11 Sagittal renal ultrasound image showing a complex cyst *(arrows)*.

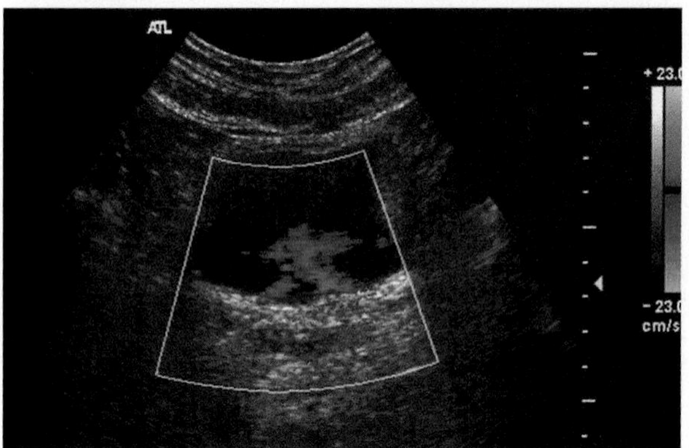

Figure 5.12 Bilateral ureteral jets in the bladder detected with color Doppler ultrasound study. This is a normal appearance.

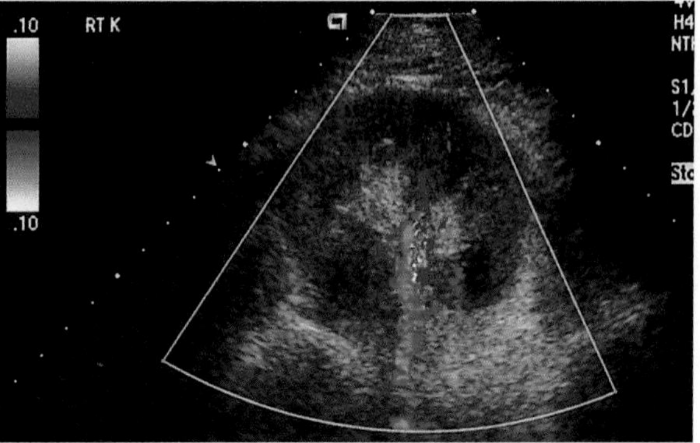

Figure 5.13 Transverse color Doppler ultrasound evaluation of the kidney. The artery is shown as *red,* the vein as *blue.*

Doppler studies also have several advantages. These studies are noninvasive, inexpensive, and widely available, and they allow structural and functional assessment of the renal arteries and image without exposure to radiation or nephrotoxic agents.

CT angiography (CTA) or magnetic resonance angiography (MRA) is preferred by some as a faster and more reliable screening tool, but at present, the choice should depend on local expertise and preference. For further discussion of the diagnosis and management of renovascular disease, see Chapters 37 and 64.

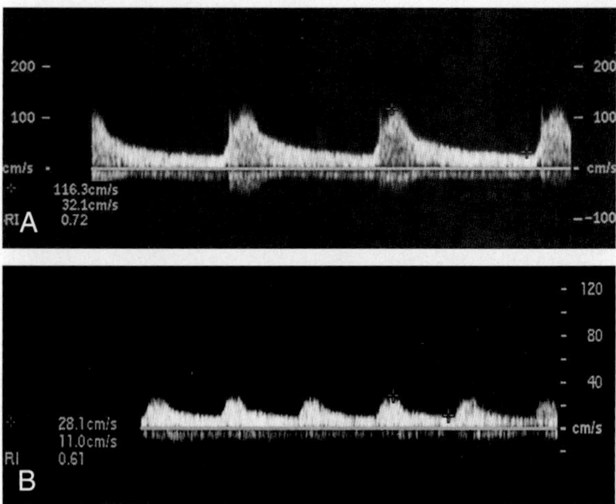

Figure 5.14 Renal artery color Doppler image and spectral tracing. A, Normal renal arterial tracing showing the rapid systolic upstroke and early systolic peak velocity (~100 cm/s). **B,** Tardus-parvus waveform demonstrating the slow systolic upstroke (acceleration) and decreased peak systolic velocity (~20 cm/s) associated with renal artery stenosis. Note different scales on vertical axis.

Contrast-Enhanced and Three-Dimensional Ultrasound

Ultrasound contrast agents, initially introduced to assess cardiac perfusion, are now being used to evaluate perfusion to other organs, such as the kidney. These intravenous agents are microbubbles that consist of a shell surrounding the echo-producing gas core; they are 1 to 4 μm in diameter, smaller than erythrocytes. The microbubbles oscillate in response to the ultrasound beam frequency and give a characteristic increased echo signal on the image. Preliminary studies evaluating renal perfusion in dysfunctional kidneys show reduced flow compared with normal kidneys and improved lesion detection (Fig. 5.15). However the clinical utility of microbubble imaging in the kidney remains uncertain, particularly given the general availability and robustness of CT and MRI.

Two-dimensional ultrasound images can be reconstructed into three-dimensional volume images by a process similar to three-dimensional reconstructions for MRI and CT. Although the current techniques are time-consuming, technical improvements should decrease reconstruction time. Potential applications include vascular imaging and fusion with MRI or positron emission tomography (PET).

PLAIN RADIOGRAPHY AND INTRAVENOUS UROGRAPHY

The use of IVU has receded as cross-sectional imaging by CT or MRI has become more widely applied to the urinary tract. Contrast urography now has few primary indications in many centers, but it may still be a key investigation in parts of the world where economic limitations mean that cross-sectional imaging is not available. However, plain radiography (often called a KUB—kidneys, ureter, bladder), still has an important role in the identification of soft tissue masses, bowel gas pattern, calcifications, and renal location.

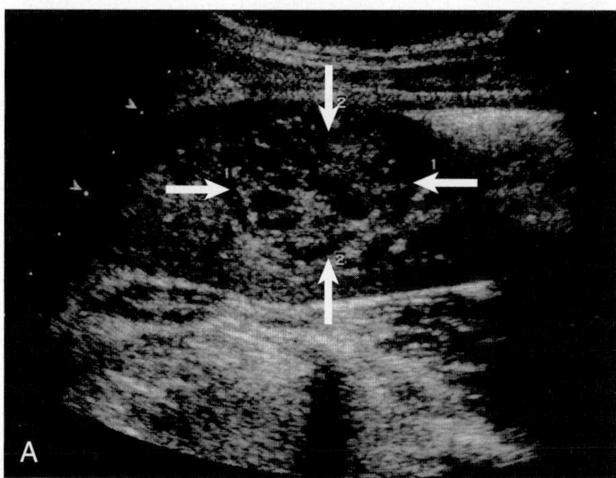
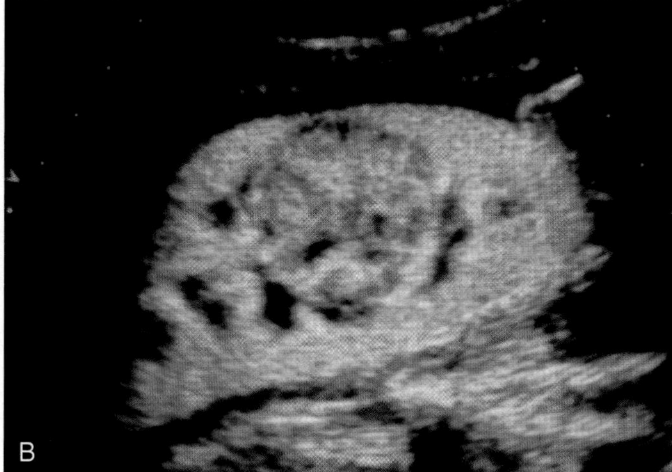

Figure 5.15 Contrast ultrasonography. A, Sagittal renal ultrasound image with a large central renal cell cancer *(arrows).* **B,** Central cancer better seen after injection of contrast material. *(Courtesy of Dr. Christoph F. Dietrich.)*

Renal Calcification

Most renal calculi are radiodense, although only ~60% of urinary stones detected on CT are visible on plain films.[17] CT demonstrates nonopaque stones, which include uric acid, xanthine, and struvite stones. However, neither CT nor plain films may detect calculi associated with protease inhibitor therapy.[18] Oblique films are sometimes obtained to confirm whether a suspicious upper quadrant calcification is renal in origin. Calculi that are radiolucent on plain films are usually detected as filling defects on IVU. Although IVU has a higher sensitivity compared with plain films, the sensitivity is lower compared with CT, which, if it is available, is the imaging modality of choice for detection of urinary calculi.[19]

Nephrocalcinosis may be medullary (Fig. 5.16A, B) or cortical (Fig. 5.16C) and is localized or diffuse. The common causes of nephrocalcinosis are shown in Figure 57.17.

Intravenous Contrast Urography

Before contrast material is administered, an abdominal compression device may be placed. It is placed to compress the mid ureters against the bony pelvis, retaining the excreted contrast material in the upper tract and distending the renal pelvis and calyces. The first film is usually performed at 30 seconds after injection of the contrast agent, when the renal parenchyma is at peak enhancement. Subtle renal masses are often detected only

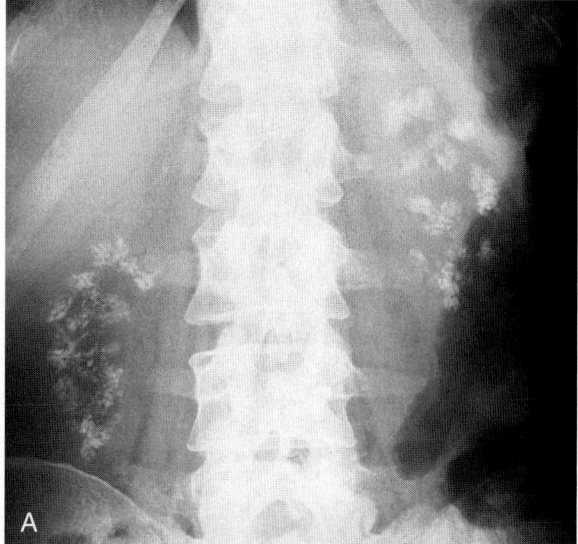
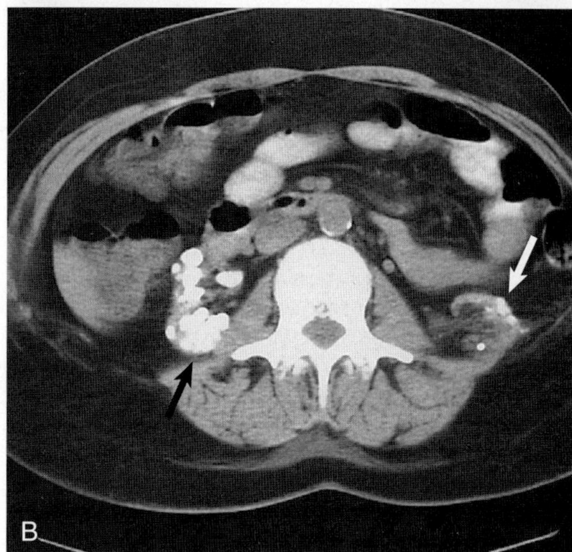
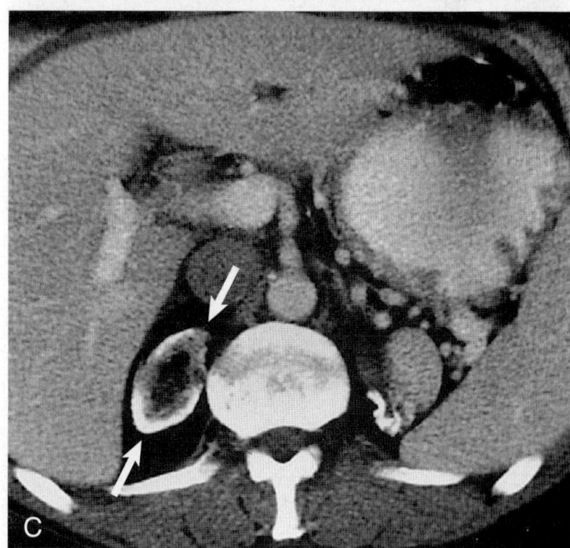

Figure 5.16 Nephrocalcinosis. A, Plain film showing bilateral medullary nephrocalcinosis in a patient with distal renal tubular acidosis. **B,** Non-contrast-enhanced CT scan in a patient with hereditary oxalosis and dense bilateral renal calcification *(arrows).* The left kidney is atrophic. **C,** Non-contrast-enhanced CT scan showing cortical nephrocalcinosis in the right kidney *(arrows)* after cortical necrosis.

on these early films. The compression device is then removed, and films of the entire abdomen are obtained at 5 minutes, when there is renal excretion of the contrast agent and the ureters are best evaluated. Prone films may be required to visualize the entirety of the ureter. A filled bladder film is obtained, and a postvoid film of the bladder assesses bladder emptying and is useful for evaluation of the distal ureters, which may be obscured by a distended contrast-filled bladder. IVU is contraindicated in patients with a history of allergic reactions to radiographic contrast agents. When the glomerular filtration rate (GFR) is below 60 ml/min, IVU yields increasingly poor images, and the risk of nephrotoxicity also increases.

Kidneys

Evaluation of the kidneys on IVU (and also on CT or MRI) should include their number, location, axis, size, contour, and degree of enhancement. Renal size is variable, but a normal kidney should be about three to four lumbar vertebral bodies in length. The renal outline should be smooth and sharply demarcated from the retroperitoneal fat. Renal enhancement after the administration of contrast material should be symmetric and progress centrally from the cortex, with excretion evident in the ureters by 5 minutes. Asymmetry of renal enhancement can be indicative of renal arterial disease.

Pelvicalyceal System

The pelvicalyceal system is best evaluated on the early postcontrast films. Normally, there are about 10 to 12 calyces per kidney. The calyces drain into the infundibula, which in turn empty into the renal pelvis (Fig. 5.17). The infundibulum and renal pelvis should have smooth contours without filling defects. There is a common variant wherein vessels can cross the pelvicalyceal system or ureters, causing extrinsic compression defects that should not be mistaken for tumors or other urothelial lesions. When more than one calyx drains into an infundibulum, it is known as a compound calyx, most frequently seen in the poles. The normal calyx is gently cupped. Calyceal distortion occurs with papillary necrosis and reflux nephropathy.

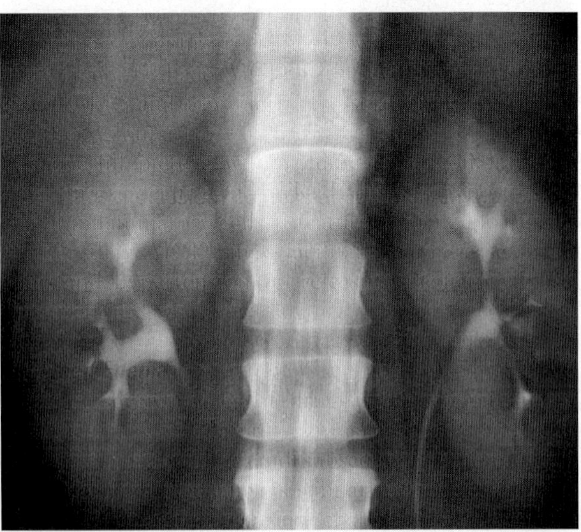

Figure 5.17 Normal parenchymal enhancement and normal renal excretion. Early postcontrast tomogram in intravenous urography.

Ureters

The ureters are often seen segmentally because of active peristalsis. The ureters should be free of filling defects and smooth. In the abdomen, the ureters lie in the retroperitoneum, passing anterior to the transverse processes of the vertebral bodies. In the pelvis, the ureters course laterally and posteriorly, eventually draining into the posteriorly located vesicoureteral junction. At the vesicoureteral junction, the ureters gently taper. Medial bowing or displacement of the ureter is often abnormal and can be seen secondary to ureter displacement from retroperitoneal masses, lymphadenopathy, and retroperitoneal fibrosis.

Bladder

The bladder should be rounded and smooth walled. Benign indentations on the bladder include the uterus, prostate gland, and bowel. In chronic bladder outlet obstruction and neurogenic bladder, there can be numerous trabeculations and diverticula around the bladder outline.

RETROGRADE PYELOGRAPHY

Retrograde pyelography is performed when the ureters are poorly visualized on other imaging studies or when samples of urine need to be obtained from the kidney for cytology or culture. Patients who have severe allergies to contrast agents or impaired renal function can be evaluated with retrograde pyelography. The examination is performed by placing a catheter through the ureteral orifice under cystoscopic guidance and advancing it into the renal pelvis. With use of fluoroscopy, the catheter is slowly withdrawn while radiographic contrast material is injected (see Figs. 58.4 and 58.13). This technique provides excellent visualization of the renal pelvis and ureter and can be used for cytologic sampling from suspect areas.

ANTEGRADE PYELOGRAPHY

Antegrade pyelography is performed through a percutaneous renal puncture and is resorted to when retrograde pyelography is not possible. Ureteral pressures can be measured, hydronephrosis evaluated, and ureteral lesions identified (see Fig. 58.16). The examination is often performed as a prelude to nephrostomy placement. Both antegrade and retrograde pyelography are invasive and should be performed only when other studies are inadequate.

ILEAL CONDUITS

After cystectomy, or bladder failure, there are numerous types of continent or incontinent urinary diversions that can be surgically created. One of the most common diversions is the ileal conduit: an ileal loop is isolated from the small bowel, and the ureters are implanted into the loop. This end of the loop is closed, and the other end exits through the anterior abdominal wall. This type of conduit can be evaluated by an excretory study or a retrograde study. The excretory or antegrade study is performed and monitored in the same way as an IVU. A retrograde examination, also referred to as a loop-o-gram, is obtained when the ureters and conduit are suboptimally evaluated on the excretory study. A Foley catheter is placed into the stoma, and contrast material is then slowly instilled. The ureters should fill by reflux

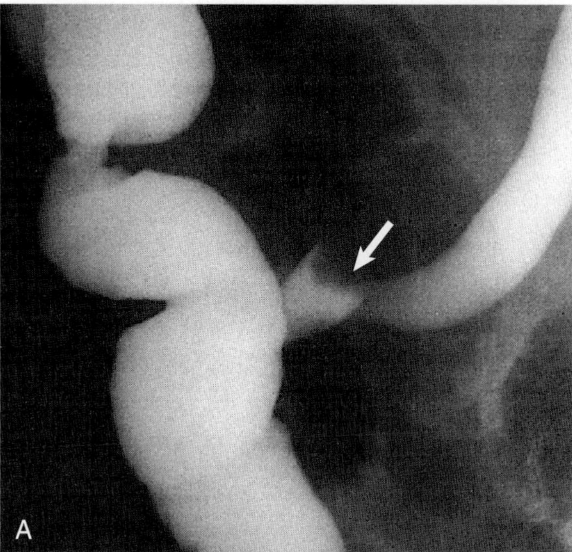

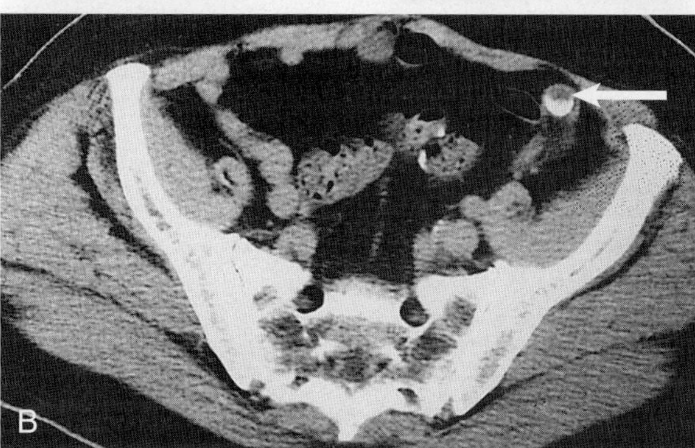

Figure 5.18 Imaging of an ileal conduit. A, Loop-o-gram. A recurrent transitional carcinoma is present in the reimplanted left ureter *(arrow)*. **B,** CT scan clearly showing the tumor as a filling defect in the anterior aspect of the opacified ureter *(arrow)*.

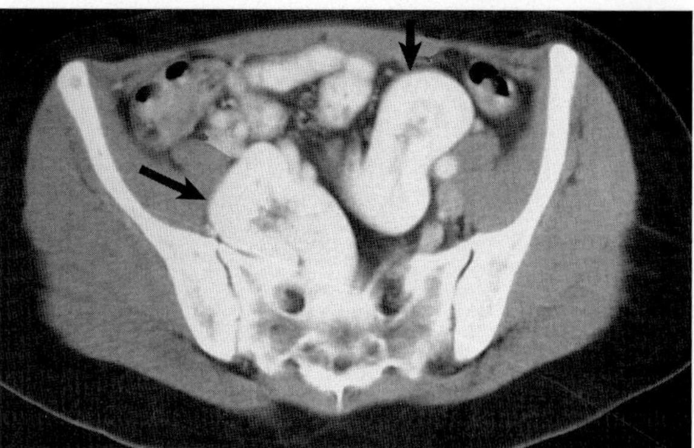

Figure 5.19 CT scan showing bilateral pelvic kidneys *(arrows)*.

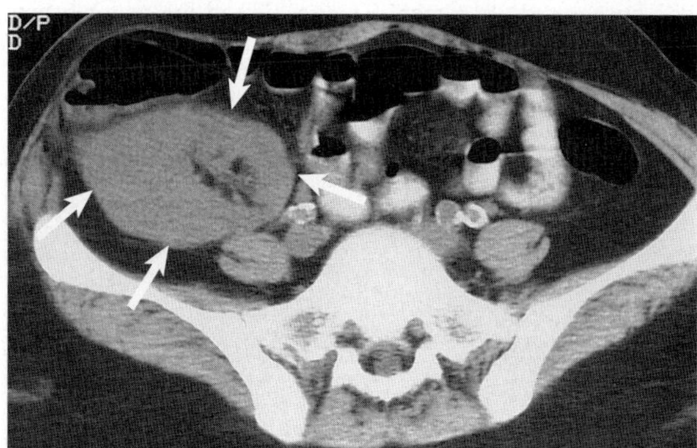

Figure 5.20 CT scan showing normal renal transplant *(arrows)*.

because the ureteral anastomoses are not of the antireflux variety (Fig. 5.18).

CYSTOGRAPHY

A cystogram is obtained when more detailed radiographic evaluation of the bladder is required. Voiding cystography is performed to identify ureteral reflux and to assess bladder function and urethral anatomy. A urethral catheter is placed into the bladder, and the urine is drained; contrast material is infused, and the bladder is filled under fluoroscopic guidance. Early supine frontal and oblique films are obtained while the bladder is filling. Ureteroceles are best identified on early films. When the bladder is full, multiple films are obtained with varying degrees of obliquity. Reflux may be seen on these films. To obtain a voiding cystogram, the catheter is removed, and the patient voids. The contrast material is followed into the urethra. On occasion, bladder diverticula are seen only on the voiding films. When the patient has completely voided, a final film is used to assess the amount of residual urine as well as the mucosal pattern. Radionuclide cystography is an alternative often used in children. It is useful in the diagnosis of reflux, but it does not provide the detailed anatomy that is seen with contrast cystography.

COMPUTED TOMOGRAPHY

CT examination of the kidneys is performed to evaluate suspect renal masses, to locate ectopic kidneys (Figs. 5.19 and 5.20), to investigate calculi, to assess retroperitoneal masses, and to evaluate the extent of parenchymal involvement in patients with acute pyelonephritis (Figs. 5.21 and 22). Helical CT scanners allow the abdomen and pelvis to be scanned at 3- to 5-mm intervals with one or two breath-held acquisitions, which eliminates motion artifact. Newer multidetector row CT results in multiple slices of information (currently 64-slice and now even 320-slice machines are becoming commonplace) being acquired simultaneously, allowing the entire abdomen and pelvis to be covered in one breath-hold, using even submillimeter intervals. However, the improved CT imaging comes at a price of significant radiation exposure to the patient. The CT data can be reconstructed in multiple planes and even in three dimensions for improved anatomic visualization and localization.

Tissue Density

The Hounsfield unit (HU) scale is a measurement of relative densities determined by CT. Distilled water at standard pressure and temperature is defined as 0 HU; the radiodensity of air is defined as −1000 HU. All other tissue densities are derived from this (Fig. 5.23). Tissues can vary in their exact HU measurements and will also change with contrast enhancement. Water, fat, and soft tissue can often look identical on the scan, depending on the window and level settings of the image, so actual HU measurement is essential to correctly characterize the tissues.

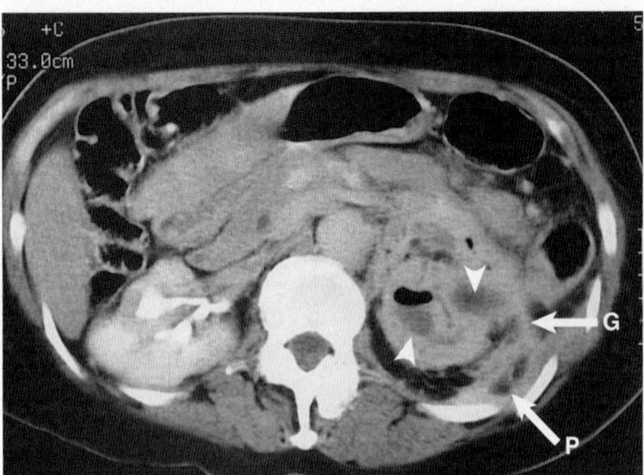

Figure 5.21 Emphysematous pyelonephritis. Contrast-enhanced CT scan showing gas *(arrowheads)* within an enlarged left kidney and marked enhancement of Gerota's fascia (G) and the posterior perirenal space (P) indicative of inflammatory involvement.

The Density of Common Substances Determined by CT

Substance	HU
Air	–1000
Fat	–120
Water	0
Muscle	+40
Bone	+400 or more

The Hounsfield unit (HU) scale is a measurement of relative densities compared with distilled water.

Figure 5.23 The density of common substances determined by CT.

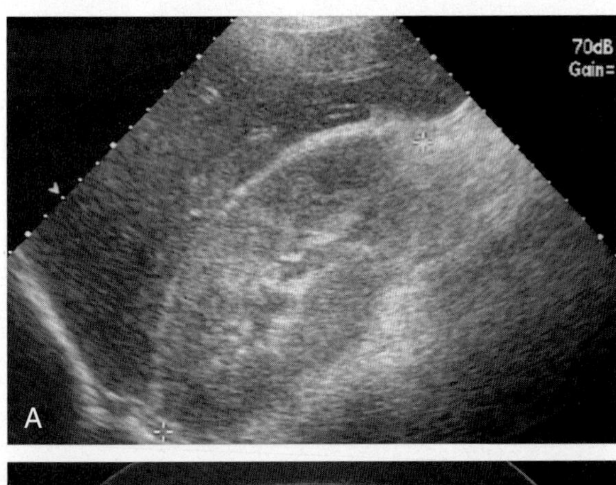

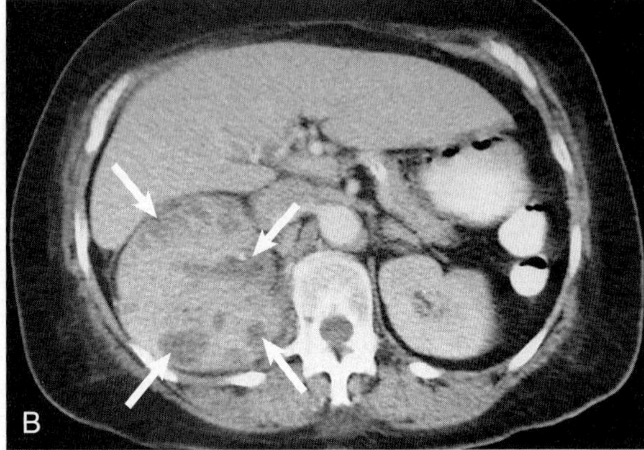

Figure 5.22 Acute pyelonephritis. A, Ultrasound image demonstrates an enlarged echogenic kidney. Bipolar length of kidney is 12.9 cm. **B,** CT scan with contrast enhancement obtained 24 hours later demonstrates multiple nonenhancing abscesses *(arrows)*.

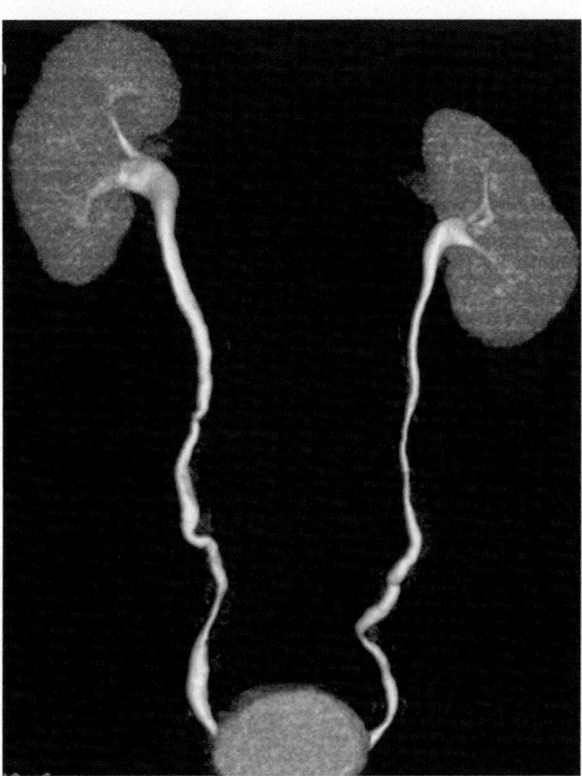

Figure 5.24 Computer-reformatted, volume-rendered CT urogram obtained from axial CT acquisition.

Contrast-Enhanced and Noncontrast Computed Tomography

CT examination of the kidneys can be performed with or without intravenous administration of contrast material. Noncontrast imaging allows the kidneys to be evaluated for the presence of calcium deposition and hemorrhage, which are obscured after the administration of contrast material.

Noncontrast CT (CT urography, CTU) is the examination of choice in patients with suspected nephrolithiasis and has replaced the KUB and intravenous urography in most situations.[20,21] The study consists of unenhanced images from the kidneys through the bladder for detection of calculi (Fig. 5.24). CTU has the advantage of being both highly sensitive (97% to 100%) and specific (94% to 96%) for diagnosis of urinary calculi.[19,22] It can identify a possible obstructing calculus as well as the extent of parenchymal and perinephric involvement.

In cases other than stone evaluation, the kidneys are imaged after the administration of contrast material. The kidneys are imaged in the corticomedullary phase for evaluation of the renal vasculature as well as in the nephrographic phase

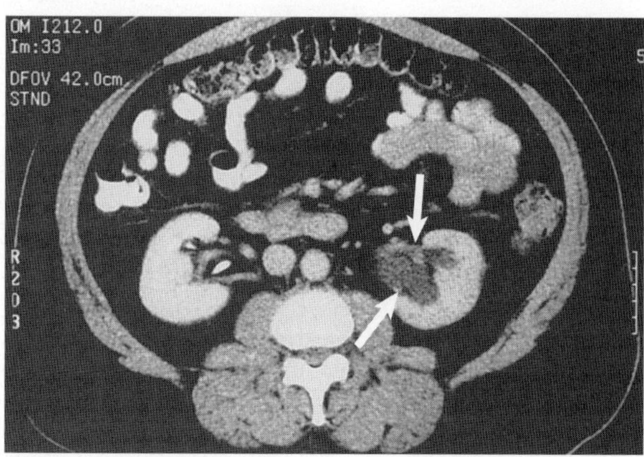

Figure 5.25 Delayed excretion in the left kidney secondary to a distal calculus. Contrast-enhanced CT scan showing dilated left renal pelvis *(arrows)*.

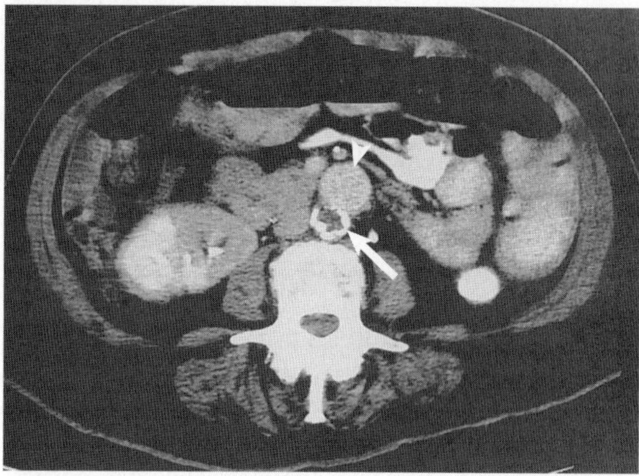

Figure 5.26 Renal infarction involving the medial half of the right kidney after aortic bypass surgery. CT scan shows densely calcified wall of the native aorta *(arrow)*. The aortic graft is anterior to the native aorta *(arrowhead)*.

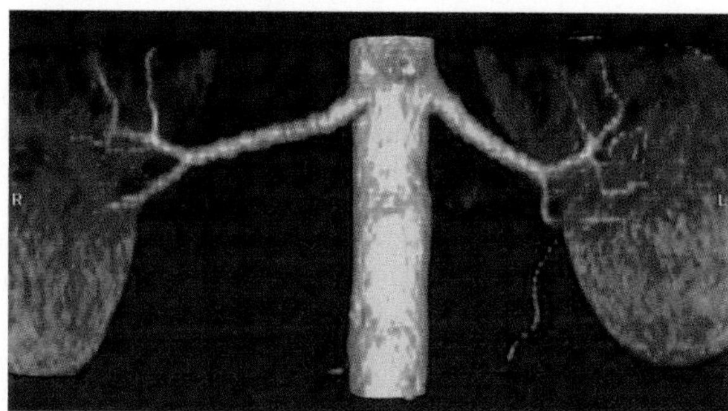

Figure 5.27 Three-dimensional reformatted CT angiogram of the normal renal arteries.

for evaluation of the renal parenchyma. The degree of enhancement can be assessed in both solid masses and complex cysts (see Fig. 58.11).

A compression device can be used as in IVU. Delayed images through the kidneys and bladder are performed for evaluation of the opacified and distended collecting system, ureters, and bladder.[23,24] Once the axial images have been obtained, they can be reformatted into coronal or sagittal planes to optimize visualization of the entire collecting system. The study can be tailored to the individual clinical scenario. For example, the corticomedullary phase can be eliminated to decrease the radiation dose if there is no concern about a vascular abnormality or no need for presurgical planning. A diuretic or saline bolus can be administered after the contrast agent to better distend the collecting system and ureters during the excretory phase.

The kidneys should be similar in size and show equivalent enhancement and excretion. During the cortical medullary phase, there is brisk enhancement of the cortex. The cortical mantle should be intact. Any disruption of the cortical enhancement requires further evaluation; it may be caused by acute pyelonephritis (see Fig. 5.22), scarring, mass lesions, or infarction (Fig. 5.26). During the excretory phase, the entire kidney and renal pelvis enhance. Delayed excretion and delay in pelvicalyceal appearance of contrast material can be findings in obstruction (see Fig. 5.25) but also in renal parenchymal disease such as acute tubular necrosis.

Computed Tomographic Angiography

Helical scanning facilitates CTA, which can produce images that are similar to those of conventional angiography, but it is less invasive. A bolus of contrast material is administered, and the images are obtained at 0.5- to 3-mm consecutive intervals. The contrast bolus is timed for optimal enhancement of the aorta. Thinner collimation of the CT beam allows higher resolution and better subsequent multiplanar reconstructions. The aorta and branch vessels are well demonstrated (Fig. 5.27). This technique is now widely used in living transplant donor evaluation (see Fig. 99.2), providing information not only on arterial and venous anatomy but also on size, number, and location of the kidneys as well as any ureteral anomalies of number or position.

CTA can also be used to screen for atheromatous renal artery stenosis, with sensitivity of 96% and specificity of 99% for the detection of hemodynamically significant stenosis compared with digital subtraction angiography.[25] Furthermore, CTA allows visualization of both the arterial wall and lumen, which helps in the planning of renal artery revascularization procedures. Another advantage of CTA is the depiction of accessory renal arteries as well as nonrenal causes of hypertension, such as adrenal masses. CTA can be used to diagnose fibromuscular dysplasia, but it has a much lower sensitivity (87%) than digital subtraction angiography.[26]

Limitations of Computed Tomography

There are some limitations of CT. The cradle that the patient lies on usually has an upper weight limit of 100 to 200 kg (300 to 400 pounds), but newer scanners can now accommodate up to 270 kg (600 pounds). Obese patients often have suboptimal scans because of weight artifact and need higher radiation exposures to adjust for x-ray attenuation. Contrast-enhanced CT studies are contraindicated in patients with an allergy to radiographic contrast dye and in patients with impaired renal function. To minimize contrast-induced nephropathy, contrast material should not be given to patients with GFR below 30 ml/min without carefully weighing the risks and benefits, and it should be used with caution with GFR of 30 to 60 ml/min.

CT is very sensitive to metal artifact and motion of the patient. Retroperitoneal clips and intramedullary rods will cause extensive streak artifact, which severely degrades the images. Patients who are unable to remain motionless will also have suboptimal or even nondiagnostic studies, and sometimes sedation or general anesthesia may be needed to obtain diagnostic scans, particularly in children. Intensive care unit and critically ill patients can be scanned by CT as long as they are stable enough to be transported to the CT suite. Ultrasound should be entertained as an alternative to CT in the seriously ill patient who cannot be safely transported.

MAGNETIC RESONANCE IMAGING

MRI should only rarely be the first examination used to evaluate the kidneys, but it is typically an adjunct to another imaging technique. The major advantage of MRI over the other imaging modalities is direct multiplanar imaging, whereas CT is limited to slice acquisition in the axial plane of the abdomen, and coronal and sagittal planes are acquired only by reconstruction, which can lead to loss of information.

Tissues contain an abundance of hydrogen, the nuclei of which are positively charged protons. These protons spin on their axis, producing a magnetic field (magnetic moment). When a patient is placed in a strong magnetic field in an MRI scanner, some of the protons align themselves with the field. When a radiofrequency pulse is applied, some of the protons aligned with the field will absorb energy and reverse their direction. This absorbed energy is given off as a radiofrequency pulse as the protons relax (return to their original alignment), producing a voltage in the receiver coil. The coil is the hardware that covers the region of interest. For renal imaging, a body coil or torso coil is used. Relaxation is a three-dimensional event giving rise to two parameters: T1 relaxation results in the recovery of magnetization in the longitudinal (spin-lattice) plane, whereas T2 results from the loss of transverse (spin-spin) magnetization. A rapid-sequence variant of T2 in common use is fast spin echo (FSE). Hydrogen ions move at slightly different rates in the different tissues. This difference is used to select imaging parameters that can suppress or aid in the detection of fat and water. Fluid, such as urine, is dark or low in signal on T1-weighted sequences and bright or high in signal on FSE sequences. Fat is bright on T1 and not as bright on FSE sequences (Fig. 5.28). The sequences and imaging planes selected must be tailored to the individual case. Diffusion-weighted imaging is a newer technique that evaluates the freedom of water molecules to diffuse in tissues; restriction of diffusion is imaged as bright areas on the scan and is seen in infection, neoplasia, inflammation, and ischemia.

Standard imaging usually includes T1, T2, or FSE sequences and often additional contrast-enhanced T1 images. The imaging plane varies according to the clinical concerns. Usually, at least one sequence is performed in the axial plane. Sagittal and coronal images cover the entire length of the kidney and can make some subtle renal parenchymal abnormalities more conspicuous (Fig. 5.29).

On T1-weighted sequences, the normal renal cortex is higher in signal than the medulla, producing a distinct corticomedullary differentiation, which becomes indistinct in parenchymal renal disease. It is analogous to the echogenic kidney seen on ultrasound. On FSE sequences, the corticomedullary distinction is not as sharp but should still be present.

Contrast-Enhanced Magnetic Resonance Imaging

As with CT, intravenous contrast material can be administered to allow further characterization of renal lesions. Gadolinium is a paramagnetic contrast agent that is frequently used in MRI and is much less nephrotoxic than iodinated contrast material.[27] Adverse reactions to gadolinium are discussed later (see Magnetic Resonance Contrast Agents). Paramagnetic contrast agents are currently being evaluated for measurement of glomerular function.

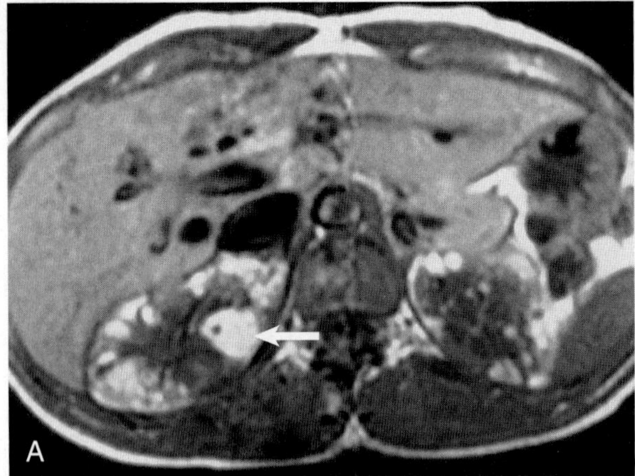

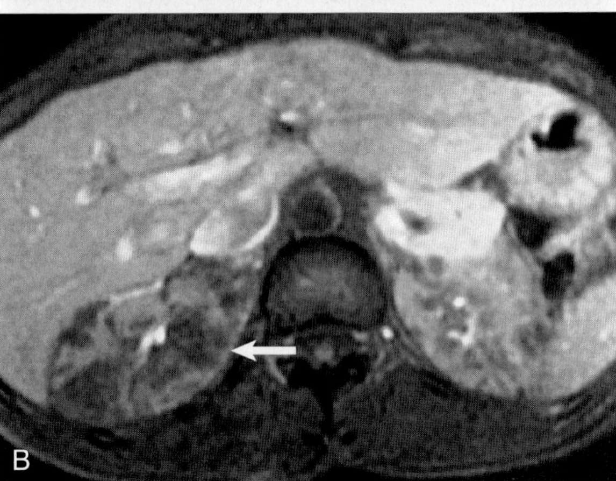

Figure 5.28 Magnetic resonance imaging of tuberous sclerosis. There are multiple renal angiomyolipomas. **A,** T1-weighted image. The tumors are high in signal on T1 because of their fat; the *arrow* shows the largest. **B,** T1-weighted image with fat suppression. The fat within the tumors is now low in signal *(arrow).*

After injection of gadolinium, the vessels appear high in signal, or white, on T1-weighted sequences. Multiple images can be obtained in a single breath-held acquisition. This technique is useful for lesion characterization in patients who cannot receive iodinated contrast material. As with contrast-enhanced CT, the kidneys initially show symmetric cortical enhancement, which progresses to excretion. A delay in enhancement can be seen with renal artery stenosis.

Magnetic Resonance Urography

There are two techniques for performing magnetic resonance urography (MRU).[28,29] The first technique is sometimes called static MRU. Because urine contains abundant water, it will demonstrate high signal on a T2-weighted image, so a heavily T2-weighted sequence accentuates the static fluid in the collecting system and ureters, which stands out against the darker background soft tissues. Static MRU can be performed rapidly, which is a benefit in imaging of children. A disadvantage is that any fluid in the abdomen or pelvis, such as fluid collections or fluid in small bowel, will demonstrate similar bright signal that

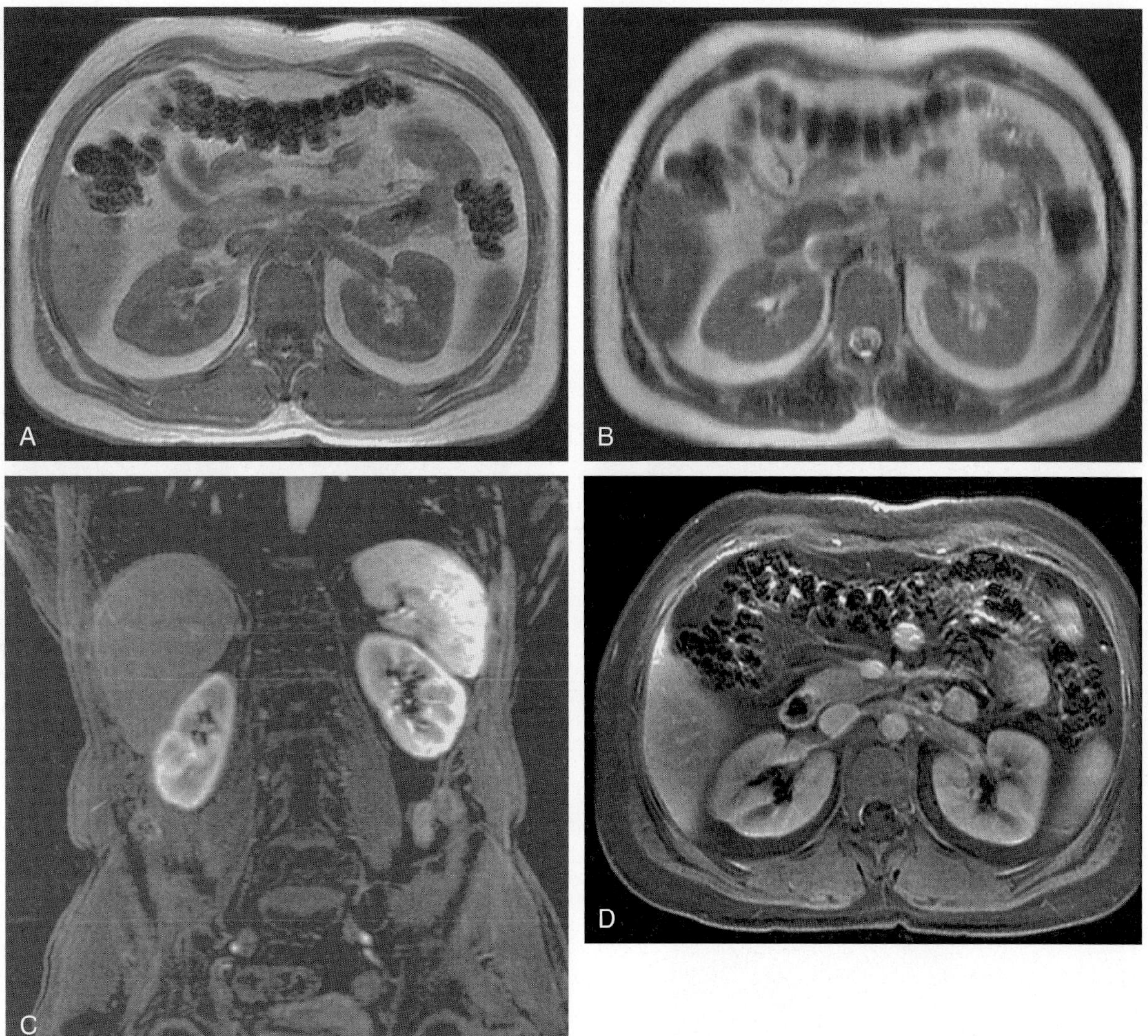

Figure 5.29 Normal magnetic resonance images through the kidneys. A, T1-weighted image. Note the distinct corticomedullary differentiation. **B,** Fast spin echo image. The urine within the collecting tubules causes the high signal within the renal pelvis on this sequence. **C,** Coronal T1-weighted, fat-suppressed image after administration of contrast material. **D,** Axial T1-weighted, fat-suppressed image after administration of contrast material.

can obscure superimposed structures. Also, the collecting system and ureters need to be distended for good images to be obtained.

The second technique, often referred to as excretory MRU, is similar to CTU. Intravenous administration of gadolinium is followed by T1-weighted imaging. This technique allows some assessment of renal function because the contrast material is filtered by the kidney and excreted into the urine (see Fig. 58.12). The opacified collecting system and ureters are well seen, and a diuretic can be administered to further dilate the renal pelvis and ureters if necessary. A limitation of MRU is in the detection of calculi because calcification is poorly visualized by MRI.

CTU and MRU are comparable examinations in identifying the cause and anatomic location of urinary obstruction, and the choice of modality is a matter of local preference. CTU is the better choice in the evaluation of urinary tract calculi. In patients with renal impairment because of obstruction, MRU is superior to CTU in identifying noncalculous causes of obstruction, whereas CTU is superior in identifying calculous causes of obstruction.[30,31] CTU is also more widely available, faster, and less expensive than MRU. MRU is better suited in patients with allergy to iodinated contrast agents and sometimes in children when radiation is an issue. MRU is also useful in depicting the anatomy in patients with urinary diversion to bowel conduits.

Magnetic Resonance Angiography

MRA can be performed with or without the intravenous administration of contrast material, although contrast provides better images. The aorta and branch vessels are beautifully demonstrated (Fig. 5.30). By adjustment of timing and type of sequences, the abdominal venous structures can be visualized (Fig. 5.31). MRA is performed to evaluate the renal arteries for stenosis and is less invasive than catheter angiography (Fig. 5.32; see also Fig. 64.18). Technical advances, including faster sequences, now give sensitivity of 97% and specificity of 93% compared with digital subtraction angiography for contrast-enhanced MRA in the detection of renal artery stenosis.[32] MRA without gadolinium has a lower sensitivity (53% to 100%) and specificity (65% to 97%) for detection of renal artery stenosis.[33] MRA has limited power to assess accessory renal arteries and therefore is not an ideal study to evaluate fibromuscular dysplasia. It has become the primary screening modality in patients with hypertension,

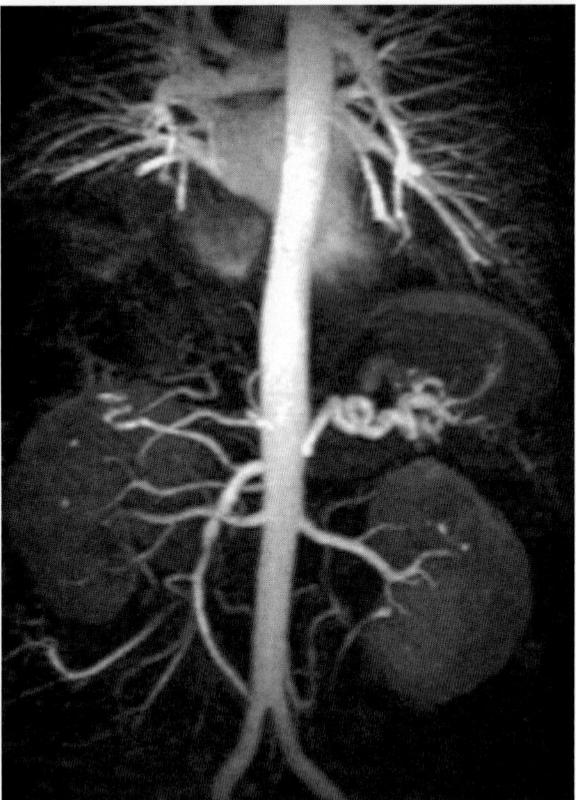

Figure 5.30 Magnetic resonance angiography. Coronal three-dimensional image after the administration of contrast material showing normal renal arteries.

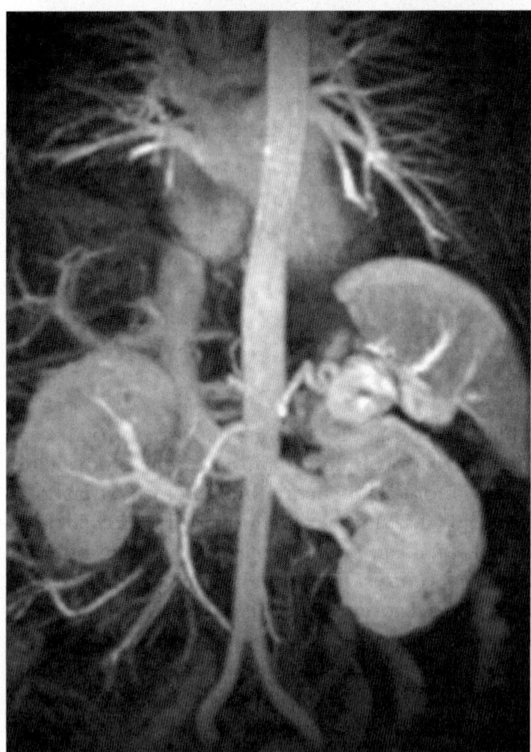

Figure 5.31 Magnetic resonance venography.

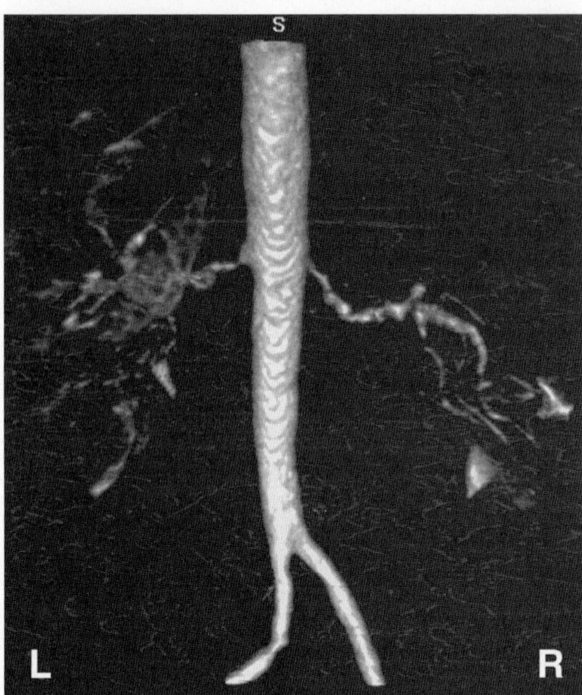

Figure 5.32 Magnetic resonance angiography. Coronal three-dimensional image showing fibromuscular dysplasia of the proximal right renal artery.

declining renal function, or allergy to iodinated contrast agents.[34] Where MRA is unavailable, Doppler ultrasound can be used.

Disadvantages of Magnetic Resonance Imaging

MRI, like CT, has some disadvantages. The table and gantry are confining, so claustrophobic patients may be unable to cooperate. Patients with some types of internal metallic hardware, such as pacemakers or cerebral aneurysm clips, cannot undergo MRI. Determination of in-stent stenosis is impossible as metallic artifact from renal artery stents completely obscures the lumen. Even with the new, fast imaging techniques, patients need to be able to cooperate with breath-holding instructions to minimize motion-related artifacts. Furthermore, MRI with gadolinium is contraindicated in patients with GFR below 30 ml/min per 1.73 m^2 because of the risk of nephrogenic systemic fibrosis (see Magnetic Resonance Contrast Agents).

MRI can be used in intensive care unit and critically ill patients only if they are stable enough to be transported to the MRI suite and have no implanted metallic devices. Ventilated patients can undergo MRI; however, specific MRI-compatible, nonferromagnetic ventilators and other life support devices must be used. Because of the confined nature of the MRI gantry, visualization and monitoring of the patient during the scan are compromised.

Incidental Findings on CT or MRI

With the growth of cross-sectional imaging, incidental renal lesions are being found with increasing frequency. Nearly 70% of renal cell carcinomas are discovered incidentally on imaging studies performed for other reasons. There is an age-dependent incidence of renal cysts from about 5% in patients younger than 30 years to nearly one third of patients older than 60 years.[35] The differentiation of solid and cystic lesions is the first mandate because as many as two thirds of solid lesions turn out to be malignant.[36] MRI is ideally suited for lesion evaluation and is often better than ultrasound, particularly in the case of complex cystic lesions. Parameters being characterized include solid versus cystic, overall lesion complexity, lesion enhancement, involvement of renal vasculature and collecting system, and extension into perirenal tissues and organs. Diffusion-weighted MRI sequences are now also being studied as a means of further differentiating benign and malignant solid lesions.

Measurement of Glomerular Filtration Rate with CT and MRI

Renal blood flow and split renal function can be evaluated by CT and MRI.[37-39] The attenuation of the accumulated contrast material within the kidney is directly proportional to the GFR. Taking into account the renal volume, the function of each kidney can be determined. Both modalities yield similar information; however, MRI is used more in pediatric patients and in those with allergy to contrast agents. This technique has not yet gained widespread acceptance, and renal scintigraphy remains the standard method for determination of renal function (discussed later).

ANGIOGRAPHY

Angiography is now most often performed for therapeutic intervention, such as embolotherapy or angioplasty and stenting, preceded by diagnostic angiography to evaluate the renal arteries for possible stenosis (Fig. 5.33). With improved resolution and scanning techniques, CTA and MRA have replaced conventional angiography, even for detection of accessory renal arteries, which are often small and bilateral but not infrequently a cause of hypertension. However, angiography remains the gold standard test for the diagnosis of renal artery stenosis and fibromuscular dysplasia. There also remains a role for diagnostic angiography in the evaluation of medium- and large-vessel vasculitis and detection of renal infarction.

The conventional angiogram is performed through arterial puncture followed by catheter placement in the aorta. An abdominal aortogram is obtained to identify the renal arteries. Selective renal artery catheterization can be performed as necessary. Contrast material is administered intra-arterially, and the images are obtained with conventional film or more commonly with digital subtraction angiography. Conventional angiography images are superior but require higher doses of contrast material and more radiation exposure. Digital subtraction angiography uses computer reconstruction and manipulation to generate the images, with the advantage that previously administered and excreted contrast material and bones can be digitally removed to better visualize the renal vasculature. As well as with the risk of contrast-induced nephropathy, angiography is associated with a risk of cholesterol embolization (see Chapter 64). Whereas pathology evidence of cholesterol embolization is frequent, clinically significant symptoms are very uncommon (1% to 2%).[40]

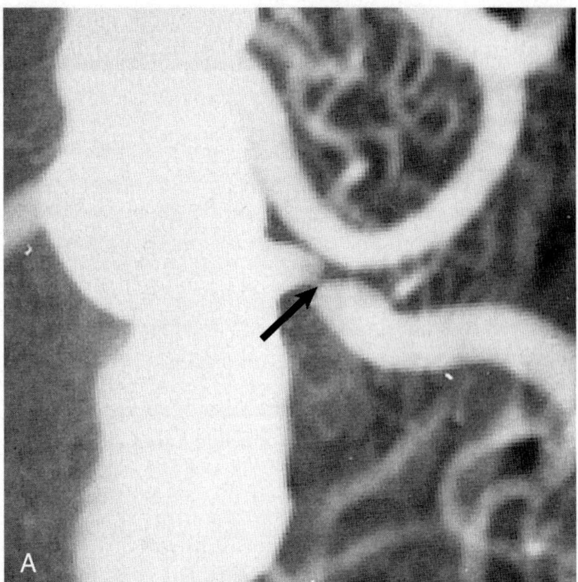

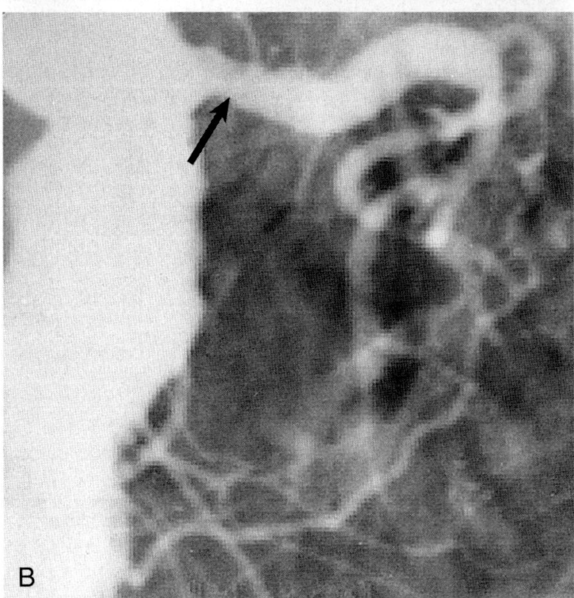

Figure 5.33 Left renal artery stenosis and angioplasty. A, Aortogram demonstrating a tight left renal artery stenosis *(arrow).* **B,** Postangioplasty image with marked improvement of the stenosis *(arrow).* *(Courtesy Dr. Harold Mitty.)*

RENAL VENOGRAPHY

Previously, catheter venography was used for evaluation of renal vein thrombosis, for evaluation of gonadal vein thrombosis, and for renal vein sampling to measure renin, but it has largely been replaced with Doppler ultrasound, followed by contrast-enhanced CT or MRI (see Fig. 5.31).

NUCLEAR MEDICINE

Nuclear scintigraphy evaluates function as well as the anatomy seen with other diagnostic imaging modalities. Radiotracers are designed to accumulate in tissues or organs on the basis of underlying functions unique to that organ. The gamma camera captures the photons from a radiotracer within the patient and generates an image. Single-photon emission computed tomography (SPECT) is a specialized type of imaging whereby the emitted photons are measured at multiple angles, similar to CT, and multiplanar or even three-dimensional images can be created. Three categories of radiotracers that differ in their mode of renal clearance are used in renal imaging: glomerular filtration, tubular secretion, and tubular retention agents (Fig. 5.34).

Choice of Radionuclide in Renal Imaging	
Glomerular filtration rate	^{99m}Tc-DTPA
Glomerular filtration rate with renal impairment	^{99m}Tc-MAG3, ^{131}I-OIH
Effective renal plasma flow	^{99m}Tc-MAG3, ^{131}I-OIH
Renal scarring	^{99m}Tc-DMSA, ^{99}Tc-GH
Renal pseudotumor	^{99m}Tc-DMSA
Upper renal tract obstruction	^{99m}Tc-DTPA
Upper renal tract obstruction with renal impairment	^{99m}Tc-MAG3

Figure 5.34 Choice of radionuclide in renal imaging.

Scintigraphy remains superior to the other imaging modalities in the evaluation of renal flow and function. It is the study of choice in the evaluation of renal transplants and for the evaluation of functional obstruction, especially when ultrasound evidence is equivocal.

It also provides an accurate assessment of renal function, which assists, for example, in estimating the reduction in renal function to be expected after nephron-sparing surgery. Although CT, MRI, and contrast-enhanced ultrasound are being assessed for the evaluation of renal function, scintigraphy remains the preferred modality. Both CTA and MRA have replaced nuclear scintigraphy in the evaluation of renal artery stenosis and in evaluation of benign renal masses, such as a column of Bertin. Nuclear medicine is still used to assess the functional significance of renal artery stenosis independent of anatomy.

Glomerular Filtration Agents

Glomerular filtration agents are cleared by the glomerulus and can be used to measure GFR. Technetium Tc 99m–labeled diethylenetriaminepentaacetic acid (^{99m}Tc-DTPA) is the most common glomerular agent used for imaging and can also be used for GFR calculation. In patients with poor renal function, renal imaging with tubular secretion agents such as mercaptoacetyltriglycine (^{99m}Tc-labeled MAG3) is superior to DTPA.[41,42]

Tubular Secretion Agents

^{99m}Tc-MAG3 is handled primarily by tubular secretion and can be used to estimate effective renal plasma flow. The clearance rate for ^{99m}Tc-MAG3 is 340 ml/min.[43]

Tubular Retention Agents

Tubular retention agents include ^{99m}Tc-labeled dimercaptosuccinate (DMSA) and less commonly ^{99m}Tc-labeled glucoheptonate (GH). These agents provide excellent cortical imaging and can be used in suspected renal scarring or infarction, in pyelonephritis, and for clarification of renal pseudotumors. These agents bind with high affinity to the sulfhydryl groups of the proximal tubules.

Renogram

A renogram is generated by scintigraphy and provides information about blood flow, renal uptake, and excretion. Time-activity graphs are produced that plot blood flow of the radiotracer into each kidney relative to the aorta. Peak cortical enhancement and pelvicalyceal clearance of the tracer are also plotted. DTPA or MAG3 can be used to generate the renogram. The relative radiotracer uptake can be measured and can provide split or differential information about renal function (Fig. 5.35).

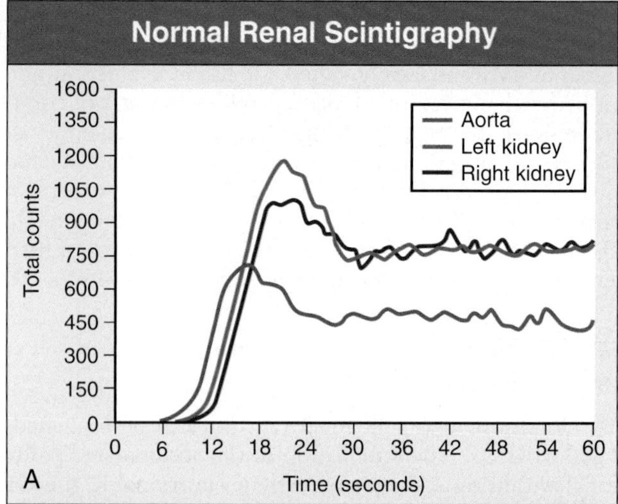

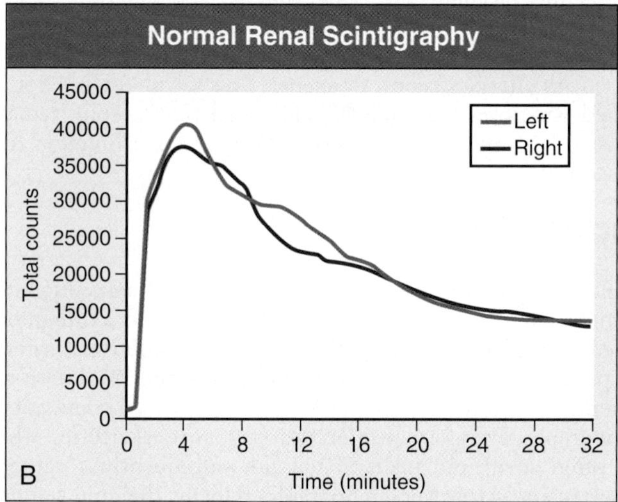

Figure 5.35 Normal ^{99m}Tc-labeled DTPA study: time-activity curves. A, Early (0-1 minute), showing renal blood flow. **B,** Later (0-30 minutes), showing renal uptake and excretion of tracer. *(Courtesy Dr. Chun Kim.)*

The blood pool or flow images are obtained after bolus injection of the radiotracers. Images are obtained with the gamma camera every few seconds for the first minute. The second component of the renogram evaluates renal function by measuring radiotracer uptake and excretion by the kidney. In normal patients, the peak renal cortical concentration occurs between 3 and 5 minutes after injection of tracer. Delayed transit of the isotope secondary to renal dysfunction (e.g., acute tubular necrosis or rejection) or obstructive uropathy will alter the curve of the renogram.

In cases of suspected obstructive uropathy, a diuresis renogram can be obtained. A loop diuretic is injected intravenously when radiotracer activity is present in the renal pelvis; a computer-generated washout curve is obtained. In patients with true obstruction, activity will remain in the renal pelvis, whereas it will quickly wash out in patients without an obstruction (Fig. 5.36; see also Figs. 50.21, 50.22, and 58.14).

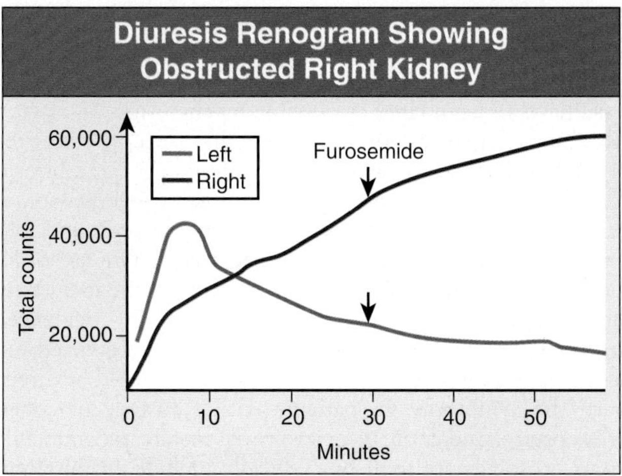

Figure 5.36 Diuresis renogram showing obstructed right kidney. Isotope continues to accumulate in the right kidney despite intravenous furosemide (given at ↓). Isotope excretion in the left kidney is normal.

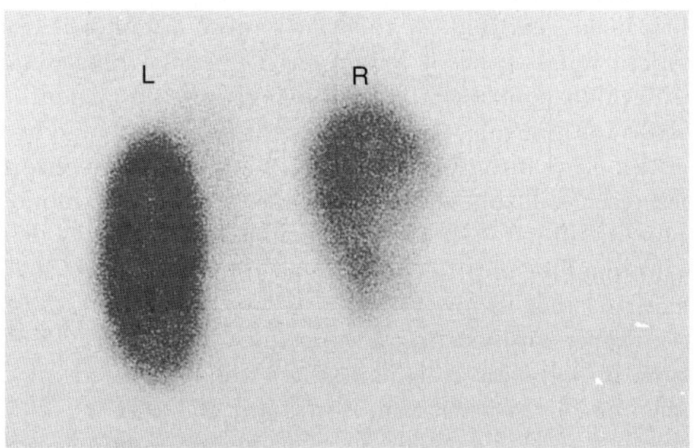

Figure 5.37 Renal infarct. ^{99m}Tc-DMSA scan in a newborn with a right lower pole infarct secondary to an embolus from an umbilical catheter. *(Courtesy Dr. Chun Kim.)*

Cortical Imaging

Renal cortical imaging is performed with tubular retention agents, usually ^{99m}Tc-DMSA. Information about renal size, location, and contour can be obtained (Fig. 5.37). The study is most commonly used for evaluation of renal scarring, particularly in children with reflux or chronic infections (see Chapter 61). It was formerly used for clarification of renal pseudotumors, such as a suspected column of Bertin, but this is now done with CT and MRI. Split renal function can also be determined from cortical imaging. Pinhole imaging (with a pinhole collimator, which magnifies the kidney to provide more anatomic detail than with planar imaging) and, more recently, SPECT imaging have been found useful for detection of cortical defects caused by inflammation or scarring. Cortical imaging may be better than ultrasound in the evaluation of the young patient with urinary tract infection.[44] Any infection, scar, or space-occupying lesion (tumor or cyst) will give a cortical defect, and correlation of the cortical defect site with other cross-sectional imaging should be performed to differentiate these entities.

Vesicoureteral Reflux

In children with suspected vesicoureteral reflux, a standard cystogram is obtained. If reflux is shown, follow-up is subsequently performed with radioisotope cystography, which exposes the child to a lower radiation dose and can be used to quantitate the bladder capacity when reflux occurs. The study is performed after instillation of technetium pertechnetate through a catheter into the bladder. Images are obtained during voiding.

Renal Transplant

Renal transplants are easily evaluated with scintigraphy. Because many transplant recipients develop declining renal function, ^{99m}Tc-MAG3 is the first-choice nuclide.

As with the normal kidneys, information about blood flow and function can be determined. Postoperative complications involving the artery, vein, or ureter are also well delineated. Nuclear imaging can help define acute tubular necrosis versus rejection in transplant patients with declining renal function. Ultrasound with Doppler evaluation of resistive index is often a complementary investigation, and choice of imaging modality in part depends on local expertise and preference.

Angiotensin-Converting Enzyme Inhibitor Renography

Angiotensin-converting enzyme (ACE) inhibitor renography was developed to detect renal artery stenosis. It relies on changes in scintigraphic findings that are exaggerated by administration of an ACE inhibitor, usually captopril. The limitation of captopril renography is poor sensitivity with impaired renal function and with bilateral renal artery stenosis. It has been almost completely replaced by CTA or MRA.[45,46]

POSITRON EMISSION TOMOGRAPHY

PET scanning uses radioactive positron emitters (most commonly ^{18}F-labeled fluorodeoxyglucose [FDG]). The FDG is intravenously injected and distributes in the body according to metabolic activity. Any process, such as tumor or infection, that causes increased metabolic activity will result in an area of increased uptake on the scan. These areas of abnormality need to be differentiated from normally hypermetabolic tissues, such as brain, liver, bone marrow, and to some extent heart and bowel (Fig. 5.38). Because FDG is cleared through the kidneys and excreted in the urine, PET scanning has a limited role in renal imaging, but it is useful in the staging and follow-up of metastatic renal cancer.[47,48]

MOLECULAR IMAGING

With molecular imaging, radiology is moving from the identification of generic anatomy and nonspecific enhancement patterns to assessment of specific molecular differences in tissues and disease processes. Nuclear imaging presently is molecular based but still nonspecific (e.g., FDG-PET, renal DTPA). The newer focus of molecular imaging studies dynamic processes like metabolic activity, cell proliferation, apoptosis, receptor status, and antigen modulation. Typically, this involves imaging of biochemical and physiologic processes. Techniques are being developed with use of optical scanning, MRI, and ultrasound as well as with radionuclides.

Applications are established in clinical practice, particularly in oncology (e.g., CD20 imaging in lymphoma), and work is under way for renal-specific molecular imaging. For example, MR renal cell imaging may soon be available to help differentiate acute

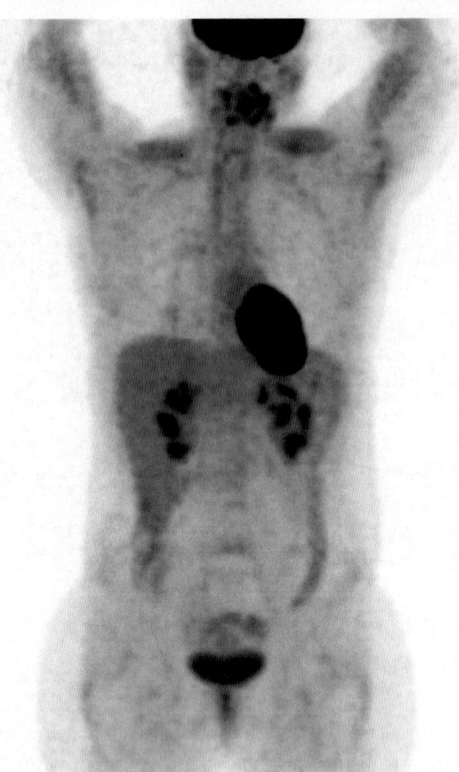

Figure 5.38 Normal PET scan. Note normal uptake in brain, heart, intestines, and liver with normal excretion in kidneys.

tubular necrosis from renal rejection and renal cell cancer from benign tumors.

RADIOLOGIC CONTRAST AGENTS

X-ray Contrast Agents

Contrast agents continue to have a role in many imaging techniques. A tri-iodinated benzene ring forms the chemical basis for CT intravascular contrast agents. Conventional contrast agents have high osmolality, about five times greater than plasma osmolality. They give excellent renal opacification, but this contributes to their toxicity. Modifications to the benzene ring have led to newer contrast agents, including low-osmolar and more recently iso-osmolar nonionic agents, which are less nephrotoxic.

Intravascular iodinated contrast material rapidly passes through the capillary pores into the interstitial, extracellular space and into the renal tubules through glomerular filtration.[49] In patients with normal renal function, the kidneys eliminate almost all of the contrast agent. Extrarenal routes of excretion include the liver and bowel wall and account for less than 1% of elimination but can increase when renal function is compromised. The half-time for elimination in patients with normal renal function is 1 to 2 hours, compared with 2 to 4 hours in dialysis patients.[50]

The overall incidence of contrast reactions for iodinated agents is 3.1% to 4.7%.[51-53] Twenty percent of patients who have a contrast reaction will experience a reaction on re-exposure that may be similar or worse. Contrast reactions can be anaphylactoid or chemotoxic reactions. The anaphylactoid reactions mimic an allergic response, whereas the chemotoxic reactions are believed to be mediated by direct toxic effects of the contrast material. The exact mechanism of contrast reaction is not known but is likely to be multifactorial. Formation of antigen-antibody complexes, complement activation, protein binding, and histamine release have all been cited as possible mechanisms.

Reactions may be minor, intermediate, or severe. Minor reactions include heat sensation, nausea, and mild urticaria. Intermediate reactions include vasovagal reaction, bronchospasm, and generalized urticaria. Severe reactions include profound hypotension, pulmonary edema, and cardiac arrest. The use of low-osmolar or iso-osmolar contrast agents reduces the incidence of minor and intermediate contrast reactions. The incidence of death related to high-osmolar contrast agents is reported to be 1 in 40,000. Immediate treatment of reactions should be directed toward the symptoms. In patients with a history of contrast allergy, pretreatment on re-exposure is usually recommended. Various protocols are used but typically include antihistamines and corticosteroids.

Contrast-Induced Nephropathy

Renal failure associated with the administration of contrast material has been reported as the third most common cause of in-hospital renal failure.[53] Patients with normal renal function rarely develop contrast-induced renal failure. In patients with GFR below 60 ml/min, iodinated contrast agents should be used with caution because the risk for contrast-induced nephropathy is increased. Nephrotoxicity ranges in severity from a nonoliguric transient fall in GFR to severe renal failure requiring dialysis. The combination of preexisting renal impairment and diabetes is the major risk factor. Other risk factors are cardiovascular disease, the use of diuretics, advanced age (>75 years), multiple myeloma in dehydrated patients, hypertension, uricosuria, and high dose of contrast material. Both ionic and nonionic contrast media can induce nephrotoxicity, although nonionic contrast material is significantly less nephrotoxic. In end-stage renal disease, fluid overload may follow the use of contrast material because of thirst provoked by the osmotic load.

The two major theories for the pathogenesis of contrast-induced nephropathy are renal vasoconstriction, perhaps mediated by alterations in nitric oxide, and direct nephrotoxicity of the contrast agent. Most underlying cellular events occur within the first 60 minutes after administration of the contrast agent, with the greatest risk in the first 10 minutes.

There is some evidence that people with diabetes and heart failure have altered nitric oxide metabolism, which may account for their increased risk for contrast-induced nephrotoxicity. Tubular injury produces oxygen free radicals, possibly as a result of the vasoconstriction. In animal studies, reduction in antioxidant enzymes associated with hypovolemia contributes to the injury.[54] Hydration is the mainstay of prevention, and hydration with intravenous sodium bicarbonate solution rather than with sodium chloride has been shown to give added benefit.[55] Acetylcysteine, a thiol-containing antioxidant given in conjunction with hydration, has not proved consistently to be protective.[56] In most patients, the renal failure is transient, and the patients recover without incident.

An important differential diagnosis for contrast-induced nephropathy in patients with vascular disease undergoing catheter angiography is cholesterol embolization (see Chapter 64).

In patients with GFR below 60 ml/min, low-osmolar or iso-osmolar contrast agents should be used and the doses reduced. Repetitive, closely performed contrast studies should be avoided. In high-risk patients, alternative imaging studies, ultrasound,

MRI, or noncontrast CT should always be considered. The prevention and management of contrast nephrotoxicity are discussed further in Chapter 64.

Magnetic Resonance Contrast Agents

There are two classes of MRI contrast agents: diffusion agents and nondiffusion agents. Diffusion agents, with appropriate timing of imaging sequences, can give delineation of vessels as well as of parenchymal tissues. Nondiffusion agents remain in the blood stream and are primarily useful for MRA. All of the contrast agents are based on the paramagnetic properties of gadolinium. Gadolinium itself is highly toxic and is given only when it is tightly chelated (e.g., Gd-DOTA, Gd-DTPA).

Minor reactions, such as headache and nausea, occur in 3% to 5% of patients; but severe life-threatening reactions and nephrotoxic reactions are rare. In patients with renal impairment, a rare severe reaction, nephrogenic systemic fibrosis, has been described (discussed further in Chapter 84), and therefore the use of gadolinium agents is generally contraindicated in patients with impaired renal function. In the United States, gadolinium is typically avoided at GFR below 30 ml/min.

REFERENCES

1. ACR Appropriateness Criteria. Available at: http://www.acr.org/ac.
2. O'Neill WC. Perianal anatomy. In: O'Neill WC, ed. *Atlas of Renal Ultrasonography*. Philadelphia: WB Saunders; 2001:3-10.
3. Committee on the Biological Effects of Ionizing Radiation Board on Radiation Effects Research Division on Earth and Life Studies National Research Council of the National Academies: Estimating Cancer Risk. Health Effects of Exposure to Low Levels of Ionizing Radiation: BEIR VII Phase 2. Washington, DC: National Academy Press; 2006:267-312.
4. Solomon R, Briguori C, Bettmann M. Selection of contrast media. *Kidney Int Suppl*. 2006;69:S39-S45.
5. Lauenstein TC, Salman K, Morreira R, et al. Nephrogenic systemic fibrosis: Center case review. *J Magn Reson Imaging*. 2007;26:1198-1203.
6. Wertman R, Altun E, Martin DR, et al. Risk of nephrogenic systemic fibrosis: Evaluation of gadolinium chelate contrast agents at four American universities. *Radiology*. 2008;248:799-806.
7. Bettman MA. Frequently asked questions: Iodinated contrast agents. *Radiographics*. 2004;24:S3-S10.
8. Murphy KJ, Brunberg JA, Cohan RH. Adverse reactions to gadolinium contrast media: A review of 36 cases. *AJR Am J Roentgenol*. 1996;167:847-849.
9. Berland LL, Koslin DB, Routh WD, Keller FS. Renal artery stenosis: Prospective evaluation of diagnosis with color duplex US compared with angiography. *Radiology*. 1990;174:421-423.
10. Olin JW, Piedmonte MR, Young JR, et al. The utility of ultrasound duplex scanning of the renal arteries for diagnosing significant renal artery stenosis. *Ann Intern Med*. 1995;122:833-838.
11. Spies KP, Fobbe F, El-Bedewi M, et al. Color-coded duplex sonography for noninvasive diagnosis and grading of renal artery stenosis. *Am J Hypertens*. 1995;8:1222-1231.
12. Lee HY, Grant EG. Sonography in renovascular hypertension. *J Ultrasound Med*. 2002;21:431-441.
13. Kliewer MA, Tupler RH, Carroll BA, et al. Renal artery stenosis: Analysis of Doppler waveform parameters and tardus-parvus pattern. *Radiology*. 1993;189:779-787.
14. Schwerk WB, Restrepo IK, Stellwaag M, et al. Renal artery stenosis: Grading with image-directed Doppler US evaluation of renal resistive index. *Radiology*. 1994;190:785-790.
15. Williams GJ, Macaskill P, Chan SF, et al. Comparative accuracy of renal duplex sonographic parameters in the diagnosis of renal artery stenosis: paired and unpaired analysis. *AJR Am J Roentgenol*. 2007;188:798-811.
16. Radermacher J, Chavan A, Schaffer J, et al. Detection of significant renal artery stenosis with color Doppler sonography: Combining extrarenal and intrarenal approaches to minimize technical failure. *Clin Nephrol*. 2000;53:333-343.
17. Mutgi A, Williams JW, Nettleman M. Renal colic: Utility of the plain abdominal roentgenogram. *Arch Intern Med*. 1991;151:1589-1592.
18. Blake SP, McNicholas MM, Raptopoulos V. Nonopaque crystal deposition causing ureteric obstruction in patients with HIV undergoing Indinavir therapy. *Am J Radiol*. 1998;171:717-720.
19. Niall O, Russell J, MacGregor R, et al. A comparison of noncontrast computerized tomography with excretory urography in the assessment of acute flank pain. *J Urol*. 1999;161:534-537.
20. Sommer FG, Jeffrey RB Jr, Rubin GD, et al. Detection of ureteral calculi in patients with suspected renal colic. Value of reformatted non-contrast helical CT. *Am J Radiol*. 1995;165:509-513.
21. Lanoue MZ, Mindell HJ. The use of unenhanced helical CT to evaluate suspected renal colic. *Am J Radiol*. 1997;169:1579-1584.
22. Smith RC, Verga M, McCarthy S, et al. Diagnosis of acute flank pain: Value of unenhanced helical CT. *AJR Am J Roentgenol*. 1996;166:97-101.
23. Joffe SA, Servaes S, Okon S, Horowitz M. Multi-detector row CT urography in the evaluation of hematuria. *Radiographics*. 2003;23:1441-1455.
24. Caoili EM, Cohan RH, Korobkin M, et al. Urinary tract abnormalities: Initial experience with CT urography. *Radiology*. 2002;222:353-360.
25. Wittenberg G, Kenn W, Tschammler A, et al. Spiral CT angiography of renal arteries: Comparison with angiography. *Eur Radiol*. 1999;9:546-551.
26. Beregi JP, Louvegny S, Gautier C, et al. Fibromuscular dysplasia of the renal arteries: Comparison of helical CT angiography and arteriography. *AJR Am J Roentgenol*. 1999;172:27-34.
27. Prince MR, Arnoldus C, Frisoli JK. Nephrotoxicity of high dose gadolinium compared with iodinated contrast. *J Magn Reson Imaging*. 1996;6:162-166.
28. Kawashima A, Glockner JF, King BF. CT urography and MR urography. *Radiol Clin North Am*. 2003;41:945-961.
29. Nolte-Ernsting CC, Staatz G, Tacke J, Gunther RW. MR urography today. *Abdom Imaging* 2003;28:191-209.
30. Shokeir AA, El-Diasty T, Eassa W, et al. Diagnosis of noncalcareous hydronephrosis: Role of magnetic resonance urography and noncontrast computed tomography. *Urology*. 2004;63:225-229.
31. Shokeir AA, El-Diasty T, Eassa W, et al. Diagnosis of ureteral obstruction in patients with compromised renal function: The role of noninvasive imaging modalities. *J Urol*. 2004;171:2303-2306.
32. Tan KT, van Beek EJR, Brown PWG, et al. Magnetic resonance angiography for the diagnosis of renal artery stenosis: A meta-analysis. *Clin Radiol*. 2002;51:617-624.
33. Grenier N, Trillaud H. Comparison of imaging methods for renal artery stenosis. *BJU Int*. 2000;86(suppl 1):84-94.
34. Marcos HB, Choyke PL. Magnetic resonance angiography of the kidney. *Semin Nephrol*. 2000;20:450-455.
35. Marumo K, Horiguchi Y, Nakagawa K, et al. Incidence and growth pattern of simple cysts of the kidney in patients with asymptomatic microscopic hematuria. *Int J Urol*. 2003;10:63-67.
36. Vasudevan A, Davies RJ, Shannon BA, Cohen RJ. Incidental renal tumours: The frequency of benign lesions and the role of preoperative core biopsy [comment in BJU Int 2006;98:465-466]. *BJU Int*. 2006;97:946-949.
37. Krier JD, Ritman EL, Bajzer Z, et al. Noninvasive measurement of concurrent single-kidney perfusion, glomerular filtration and tubular function. *Am J Physiol Renal Physiol*. 2001;281:F630-F638.
38. Nilsson H, Wadstrom J, Andersson LG, et al. Measuring split renal function in renal donors: Can computed tomography replace renography? *Acta Radiol*. 2004;45:474-480.
39. Lee VS, Rusinek H, Noz ME, et al. Dynamic three-dimensional MR renography for the measurement of single kidney function: Initial experience. *Radiology*. 2003;227:289-294.
40. Fukumoto Y, Tsutsui H, Tsuchihashi M, et al. The incidence and risk factors of cholesterol embolization syndrome. *J Am Coll Cardiol*. 2003;42:211-216.
41. Taylor A, Nally JV. Clinical applications of renal scintigraphy. *Am J Radiol*. 1995;64:31-41.
42. Taylor A Jr, Ziffer JA, Echima D. Comparison of Tc-99m MAG3 and Tc-99m DTPA in renal transplant patients with impaired renal function. *Clin Nucl Med*. 1990;15:371-378.
43. Taylor A, Eshima D, Christian PE, et al. A technetium-99m MAG3 kit formulation: Preliminary results in normal volunteers and patients with renal failure. *J Nucl Med*. 1988;29:616-662.

44. Mastin ST, Drane WE, Iravani A. Tc 99m DMSA SPECT imaging in patients with acute symptoms or history of UTI: Comparison with ultrasonography. *Clin Nucl Med*. 1995;20:407-412.
45. Soulez G, Oliva VL, Turpin S, et al. Imaging of renovascular hypertension: Respective values of renal scintigraphy, renal Doppler ultrasound, and MR angiography. *Radiographics*. 2000;20:1355-1368.
46. Eklof H, Ahlstrom H, Magnusson A, et al. A prospective comparison of duplex ultrasonography, captopril renography, MRA and CTA in assessing renal artery stenosis. *Acta Radiol*. 2006;47:764-774.
47. Kayani I, Groves AM. ^{18}F-Fluorodeoxyglucose PET/CT in cancer imaging. *Clin Med*. 2006;6:240-244.
48. Majhail NS, Urbain JL, Albani JM, et al. F-18 fluorodeoxyglucose positron emission tomography in the evaluation of distant metastases from renal cell carcinoma. *J Clin Oncol*. 2003;21:3995-4000.
49. Morris TW, Fischer HW. The pharmacology of intravascular radiocontrast media. *Annu Rev Pharmacol Toxicol*. 1986;26:143-160.
50. Bahlmann J, Kruskemper HL. Elimination of iodine containing contrast media by hemodialysis. *Nephron*. 1973;19:25-55.
51. Shehadi WH. Adverse reactions to intravascularly administered contrast media. *Am J Radiol*. 1975;124:145-152.
52. Katayama H, Yamaguchi K, Kozuka T, et al. Adverse reactions to ionic and nonionic contrast media: A report from the Japanese committee on the safety of contrast media. *Radiology*. 1990;175:616-618.
53. Cohan RH, Dunnick NR. Intravascular contrast media: Adverse reactions. *Am J Radiol*. 1987;149:665-670.
54. Yoshioka T, Fogo A, Beckman JK. Reduced activity of antioxidant enzymes underlies contrast media–induced renal injury in volume depletion. *Kidney Int*. 1992;41:1008.
55. Merten GJ, Burgess WP, Gray LV, et al. Prevention of contrast-induced nephropathy with sodium bicarbonate. *JAMA*. 2004;291:2328-2334.
56. Barrett BJ, Parfrey PS. Preventing nephropathy induced by contrast medium. *N Engl J Med*. 2006;354:379-386.

CHAPTER 6

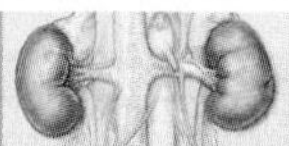

Renal Biopsy

Peter S. Topham, Yipu Chen

DEFINITION

Percutaneous renal biopsy was first described in the early 1950s by Iversen and Brun[1] and Alwall.[2] These early biopsies were performed with the patients in the sitting position by use of a suction needle and intravenous urography for guidance. An adequate tissue diagnosis was achieved in less than 40% of these early cases. In 1954, Kark and Muehrcke[3] described a modified technique in which the Franklin-modified Vim-Silverman needle was used, the patient lay in a prone position, and an exploring needle was used to localize the kidney before insertion of the biopsy needle. These modifications yielded a tissue diagnosis in 96% of cases, and no major complications were reported. Since then, the basic renal biopsy procedure has remained largely unchanged, although the use of real-time ultrasound and refinement of biopsy needle design have offered significant improvements. Renal biopsy is now able to provide a tissue diagnosis in more than 95% of cases with a life-threatening complication rate of less than 0.1%.

INDICATIONS FOR RENAL BIOPSY

The indications for renal biopsy are listed in Figure 6.1. Ideally, analysis of a renal biopsy sample should identify a specific diagnosis, reflect the level of disease activity, and provide information to allow informed decisions about treatment to be made. Although the renal biopsy is not always able to fulfill these criteria, it remains a valuable clinical tool and is of particular benefit in the following clinical situations.

Nephrotic Syndrome

Routine clinical and serologic examination of patients with nephrotic syndrome usually allows the clinician to determine whether a systemic disorder is present. In adults and adolescents beyond puberty without systemic disease, there is no reliable way to predict the glomerular pathologic process with confidence by noninvasive criteria alone; therefore, a renal biopsy should be performed. In children aged between 1 year and puberty, a presumptive diagnosis of minimal change disease can be made. Renal biopsy is reserved for nephrotic children with atypical features (microscopic hematuria, reduced serum complement levels, renal impairment, failure to respond to corticosteroids).

Acute Kidney Injury

In most patients with acute kidney injury (AKI) or AKI on a background of chronic kidney disease (CKD), the cause can be determined without a renal biopsy. Obstruction, reduced renal perfusion, and acute tubular necrosis can usually be identified from other lines of investigation. In a minority of patients, however, a confident diagnosis cannot be made. In these circumstances, a renal biopsy should be performed as a matter of urgency so that appropriate treatment can be started before irreversible renal injury develops. This is particularly the case if AKI is accompanied by an active urine sediment or if drug-induced or infection-induced acute interstitial nephritis is suspected.

Systemic Disease Associated with Renal Dysfunction

Patients with diabetes mellitus and renal dysfunction do not usually require a biopsy if the clinical setting is compatible with diabetic nephropathy (isolated proteinuria, diabetes of long duration, evidence of other microvascular complications). However, if the presentation is atypical (proteinuria associated with glomerular hematuria [acanthocytes], absence of retinopathy or neuropathy [in patients with type 1 diabetes], onset of proteinuria less than 5 years from documented onset of diabetes, uncharacteristic change in renal function or renal disease of acute onset, the presence of immunologic abnormalities), a renal biopsy should be performed.

Serologic testing for antineutrophil cytoplasmic antibodies (ANCA) and for anti–glomerular basement membrane antibodies has made it possible to make a confident diagnosis of renal small-vessel vasculitis or Goodpasture's disease without invasive measures in most patients. Nonetheless, a renal biopsy should still be performed to confirm the diagnosis and to clarify the extent of active inflammation versus chronic fibrosis and hence the potential for recovery. This information may be important in helping to decide whether to initiate or to continue immunosuppressive therapy, particularly in patients who may tolerate immunosuppression poorly.

Lupus nephritis can usually be diagnosed by noninvasive criteria (autoantibodies, urine protein excretion, renal function, and urine sediment abnormalities). Some experts argue that this information can be used to gauge the severity of renal involvement and to inform decisions about initial immunosuppressive treatment. However, a renal biopsy will clarify the underlying pathologic lesion, the level of acute activity, and the extent of chronic fibrosis, thereby providing robust guidance for evidence-based therapy.

The diagnosis of virus infection–related nephropathy, for example, hepatitis B virus–associated membranous nephropathy, is suggested by the presence of the expected glomerular lesion in association with evidence of active viral infection. However, the identification of virus-specific protein or DNA or RNA in the renal biopsy tissue by immunopathologic and molecular pathologic techniques (e.g., *in situ* hybridization) can ensure the diagnosis.

Indications for Renal Biopsy
Nephrotic Syndrome
Routinely indicated in adults; in prepubertal children, only if clinical features atypical of minimal change disease
Acute Kidney Injury
Indicated if obstruction, reduced renal perfusion, and acute tubular necrosis have been ruled out
Systemic Disease with Renal Dysfunction
Indicated in patients with small-vessel vasculitis, anti–glomerular basement-membrane disease, and systemic lupus; those with diabetes only if atypical features present
Non-nephrotic Proteinuria
May be indicated if proteinuria >1g/24h
Isolated Microscopic Hematuria
Indicated only in unusual circumstances
Unexplained Chronic Kidney Disease
May be diagnostic, (e.g., identify IgA nephropathy even in "end-stage kidney")
Familial Renal Disease
Biopsy of one affected member may give diagnosis and minimize further investigation of family members
Renal Transplant Dysfunction
Indicated if ureteral obstruction, urinary sepsis, renal artery stenosis, and toxic calcineurin inhibitor levels are not present

Figure 6.1 Indications for renal biopsy. See text for further discussion.

Other systemic diseases, such as amyloidosis, sarcoidosis, and myeloma, can be diagnosed with a renal biopsy. However, because these diagnoses can often be made by other investigative approaches, a renal biopsy is indicated only if the diagnosis remains uncertain or if knowledge of renal involvement would change management.

Renal Transplant Dysfunction

Renal allograft dysfunction in the absence of ureteral obstruction, urinary sepsis, renal artery stenosis, or toxic levels of calcineurin inhibitors requires a renal biopsy to determine the cause. In the early post-transplantation period, this is most useful in differentiating acute rejection from acute tubular necrosis and the increasingly prevalent BK virus nephropathy. Later, renal biopsy can differentiate late acute rejection from chronic allograft nephropathy, recurrent or *de novo* glomerulonephritis, and calcineurin inhibitor toxicity. The accessible location of the renal transplant in the iliac fossa facilitates biopsy of the allograft and allows repeated biopsies when indicated. This has encouraged many units to adopt a policy of protocol (surveillance) biopsies to detect subclinical acute rejection and renal scarring and to guide the choice of immunosuppressive therapy (see Chapter 100).

Non-nephrotic Proteinuria

The value of renal biopsy in patients with non-nephrotic proteinuria is debatable. All conditions that result in nephrotic syndrome can cause non-nephrotic proteinuria with the exception of minimal change disease. However, the benefit of specific treatment with corticosteroids and other immunosuppressive agents in this clinical setting probably does not justify the risk of significant drug-related side effects. In patients with proteinuria of more than 1 g/day, generic treatment with strict blood pressure control and angiotensin-converting enzyme (ACE) inhibitors and angiotensin receptor blockers (ARB) alone or in combination reduces proteinuria and reduces the risk for development of progressive renal dysfunction. Nonetheless, although the renal biopsy may not lead to an immediate change in management, it can be justified in these circumstances because it will provide prognostic information, may identify a disease for which a different therapeutic approach is indicated, and may provide clinically important information about the future risk of disease recurrence after renal transplantation.

Isolated Microscopic Hematuria

Patients with microscopic hematuria should initially be evaluated to identify structural lesions such as renal stones or renal and urothelial malignant neoplasms if they are older than 40 years. The absence of a structural lesion suggests that the hematuria may have a glomerular source. Biopsy studies have identified glomerular lesions in up to 75% of biopsies.[4] In all series, IgA nephropathy has been the most common lesion, followed by thin basement membrane nephropathy. In the absence of nephrotic proteinuria, renal impairment, or hypertension, the prognosis for these conditions is excellent, and because specific therapies are not available, renal biopsy in this setting is not necessary. Biopsy should be performed only if the result would provide reassurance to the patient, avoid repeated urologic investigations, or provide specific information (e.g., in the evaluation of potential living kidney donors, in familial hematuria, for life insurance and employment purposes).

Unexplained Chronic Kidney Disease

Renal biopsy can be informative in the patient with unexplained CKD with normal-sized kidneys because in contrast to AKI, it is often difficult to determine the underlying cause on the basis of clinical criteria alone. Studies have shown that in this setting, the biopsy will demonstrate disease that was not predicted in almost half of cases.[5] However, if both kidneys are small (<9 cm on ultrasound), the risks of the biopsy are increased, and the diagnostic information available from the biopsy may be limited by extensive glomerulosclerosis and tubulointerstitial fibrosis. In this setting, however, immunofluorescence studies may still be informative. For example, glomerular IgA deposition may be identified despite advanced structural damage.

Familial Renal Disease

A renal biopsy can be helpful in the investigation of patients with a family history of renal disease; and a biopsy performed on one affected family member may secure the diagnosis for the whole family and avoid the need for repeated investigation. Conversely, a renal biopsy may unexpectedly identify disease that has an inherited basis, thereby stimulating evaluation of other family members.

The Role of Repeated Renal Biopsy

In some circumstances, a repeated biopsy may be indicated. For example, the pathologic changes in lupus nephritis may evolve, and treatment adjustment may be necessary; minimal change disease that is corticosteroid resistant or dependent or frequently relapsing may actually represent a missed diagnosis of focal segmental glomerulosclerosis (FSGS), which may be detected on a repeated biopsy; and some nephrologists would argue that a repeated biopsy in patients who have had aggressive immunosuppressive treatment of crescentic glomerulonephritis can help in determining the most appropriate next line of therapy.

VALUE OF THE RENAL BIOPSY

Biopsy Adequacy

In the assessment of a renal biopsy, the number of glomeruli in the sample is the major determinant of whether the biopsy will be diagnostically informative.

For a focal disease such as FSGS, the diagnosis can potentially be made on a biopsy specimen containing a single glomerulus that contains a typical sclerosing lesion. However, the probability that FSGS is not present in a patient with nephrotic syndrome and minimal changes on the biopsy specimen is dependent on the actual proportion of abnormal glomeruli in the kidney and the number of glomeruli obtained in the biopsy specimen. For example, if 20% of glomeruli in the kidney have sclerosing lesions and five glomeruli are sampled, there is a 35% chance that all the glomeruli in the biopsy specimen will be normal and that the biopsy will miss the diagnosis. By contrast, in the same kidney, if 10 or 20 glomeruli are sampled, the chance of obtaining all normal glomeruli is reduced to 10% and less than 1%, respectively, and the biopsy is more discriminating. This argument assumes that any segmental lesions present in the biopsy specimen are actually identified; this requires the biopsy specimen to be sectioned at multiple levels.

Unless all glomeruli are affected equally, the probability that the observed involvement in the biopsy specimen accurately reflects true involvement in the kidney depends not only on the number of glomeruli sampled but also on the proportion of affected glomeruli. For example, in a biopsy specimen containing 10 glomeruli of which three are abnormal (30%), there is a 95% probability that the actual glomerular involvement is between 7% and 65%. In the same kidney, if the biopsy specimen contained 30 glomeruli with 30% being abnormal, the 95% confidence intervals are narrowed to 15% and 50%.

Therefore, the interpretation of the biopsy needs to take into account the number of glomeruli obtained. A typical biopsy sample will contain 10 to 15 glomeruli and will be diagnostically useful. Nonetheless, it must be appreciated that because of the sampling issue, a biopsy sample of this size will occasionally be unable to diagnose focal diseases and at best will provide imprecise guidance on the extent of glomerular involvement.

An adequate biopsy should also provide samples for immunohistology and electron microscopy. Immunohistology is provided by either immunofluorescence on frozen material or immunoperoxidase on fixed tissue, according to local protocols and expertise. It is helpful for the biopsy cores to be viewed under an operating microscope immediately after being taken to ensure that they contain cortex and that when the cores are divided, the immunohistology and electron microscopy samples both contain glomeruli.

If insufficient material for a complete pathologic evaluation is obtained, there should be a discussion with the pathologist about how best to proceed before the tissue is placed in fixative so that the material can be processed in a way that will provide maximum information for the specific clinical situation. For example, if the patient has heavy proteinuria, most information will be gained from electron microscopy because it is able to demonstrate podocyte foot process effacement, focal sclerosis, electron-dense deposits of immune complexes, and the organized deposits of amyloid.

If a sample is supplied for immunofluorescence microscopy but contains no glomeruli, it may be possible to reprocess the paraffin-embedded sample to identify immune deposits by either immunoperoxidase or immunofluorescence techniques.

Is Renal Biopsy a Necessary Investigation?

The role of the renal biopsy has been much debated. Early studies suggested that renal biopsy provided diagnostic clarity in the majority of cases but that this information did not alter management, with the exception of those with heavy proteinuria or systemic disease. More recent prospective studies have suggested that the renal biopsy identifies a diagnosis different from that predicted on clinical grounds in 50% to 60% of patients and leads to a treatment change in 20% to 50% of cases.[6] This is particularly apparent in patients with heavy proteinuria or AKI, in whom the biopsy findings alter management in more than 80% of cases.[7]

PREBIOPSY EVALUATION

This evaluation identifies issues that may compromise the safety and success of the procedure (Fig. 6.2). It will determine whether the patient has two normal-sized unobstructed kidneys, sterile urine, controlled blood pressure, and no bleeding diathesis. A thorough history should be taken to identify evidence of a bleeding diathesis, such as previous prolonged surgical bleeding, spontaneous bleeding, family history of bleeding, and ingestion of medication that increases bleeding risk (including antiplatelet agents and warfarin).

An ultrasound scan should be performed to assess kidney size and to identify significant anatomic abnormalities, such as solitary kidney, polycystic or simple cystic kidneys, malpositioned kidneys, horseshoe kidneys, small kidneys, or hydronephrosis.

The value of the bleeding time in patients undergoing renal biopsy is controversial. The predictive value of the bleeding time for postrenal biopsy bleeding has never been prospectively tested. Retrospective studies, however, demonstrated a threefold to fivefold increase in bleeding complications after renal biopsy in patients with prolonged bleeding times. Prospective studies of percutaneous liver biopsy patients showed a fivefold increase in bleeding complications in those with uncorrected bleeding times.[8] A consensus document concluded that the bleeding time is a poor predictor of postsurgical bleeding but that it does correlate with clinical bleeding episodes in uremic patients.[9]

Several approaches to the management of bleeding risk have been adopted: many centers measure the prebiopsy bleeding time and administer 1-desamino-8-D-arginine vasopressin (desmopressin or DDAVP) if the bleeding time is prolonged beyond 10 minutes; another preferred method is to no longer measure the bleeding time, but routinely administer DDAVP to those patients with significant renal impairment (blood urea nitrogen level >56 mg/dl [urea >20 mmol/l] or serum creatinine concentration >3 mg/dl [250 μmol/l]); in other centers, a platelet transfusion is used in preference to DDAVP. Platelet transfusion can also be used to reverse clopidogrel-induced platelet dysfunction when the renal biopsy is urgent.

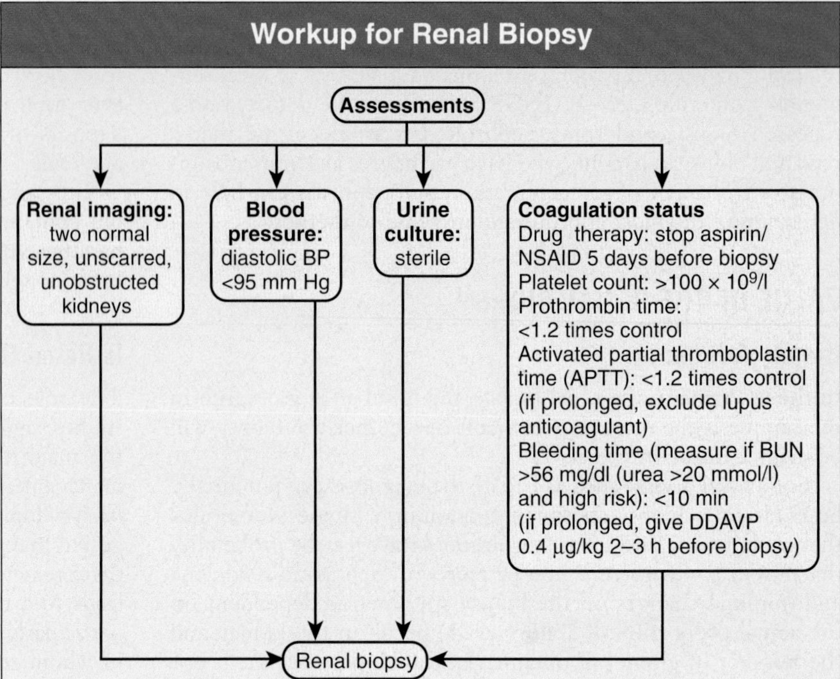

Figure 6.2 Workup for renal biopsy.

Contraindications to Renal Biopsy	
Kidney Status	**Patient Status**
Multiple cysts	Uncontrolled bleeding diathesis
Solitary kidney	Uncontrolled blood pressure
Acute pyelonephritis/ perinephric abscess	Uremia
Renal neoplasm	Obesity Uncooperative patient

Figure 6.3 Contraindications to renal biopsy. Most contraindications to renal biopsy are relative rather than absolute; when clinical circumstances necessitate urgent biopsy, they may be overridden, apart from uncontrolled bleeding diathesis.

The use of thromboelastography (TEG) has been described in the renal transplant biopsy setting.[10] TEG provides an overall measure of the coagulation, platelet, and fibrinolytic systems in one assay and therefore may be more predictive of clinical bleeding. In this study, most bleeding episodes were associated with normal clotting test results, but TEG was the only assay that was associated with an increased risk of postbiopsy bleeding. The role of TEG in native kidney renal biopsy requires further evaluation.

Contraindications to Renal Biopsy

The contraindications to percutaneous renal biopsy are listed in Figure 6.3. The major contraindication is a bleeding diathesis. If the disorder cannot be corrected and the biopsy is deemed indispensable, alternative approaches, such as open biopsy, laparoscopic biopsy, or transvenous (usually transjugular) biopsy, can be performed. Inability to comply with instructions during the biopsy is a further major contraindication to renal biopsy. Sedation or, in extreme cases, general anesthesia may be necessary.

Hypertension (>160/95 mm Hg), hypotension, perinephric abscess, pyelonephritis, hydronephrosis, severe anemia, large renal tumors, and cysts are relative contraindications to renal biopsy. When possible, they should be corrected before the biopsy is undertaken.

The presence of a solitary functioning kidney has been considered a contraindication to percutaneous biopsy, and it has been argued that the risk of biopsy is reduced by direct visualization at open biopsy. However, the postbiopsy nephrectomy rate of 1/2000 to 1/5000 is comparable to the mortality rate associated with the general anesthetic required for an open procedure. Therefore, in the absence of risk factors for bleeding, percutaneous biopsy of a solitary functioning kidney can be justified.

RENAL BIOPSY TECHNIQUE

Percutaneous Renal Biopsy

Native Renal Biopsy

In our center, the kidney biopsy is performed by nephrologists with continuous (real-time) ultrasound guidance and disposable automated biopsy needles. We use 16-gauge needles as a compromise between the greater tissue yield of larger needles and the trend to fewer bleeding complications of smaller needles. For most patients, premedication or sedation is not required. The patient is laid prone, and a pillow is placed under the abdomen at the level of the umbilicus to straighten the lumbar spine and to splint the kidneys. Figure 6.4 shows the anatomic relationships of the left kidney. Ultrasound is used to localize the lower pole of the kidney where the biopsy will be performed (usually the left kidney). An indelible pen mark is used to indicate the point of entry of the biopsy needle. The skin is sterilized with either

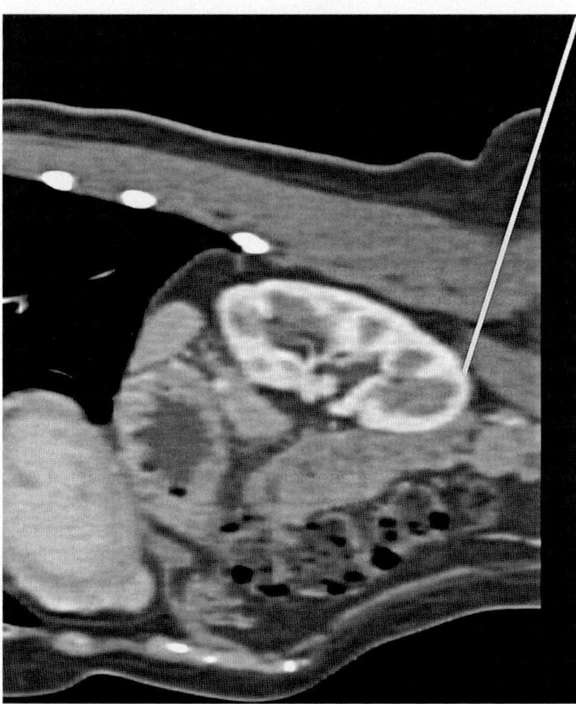

Figure 6.4 Computed tomography through the left kidney. The angle of approach of the needle is demonstrated. Note the relative adjacency of the lower pole of the kidney to other structures, particularly the large bowel.

povidone-iodine (Betadine) or chlorhexidine solution. A sterile fenestrated sheet is placed over the area to maintain a sterile field. Local anesthetic (2% lidocaine [lignocaine]) is infiltrated into the skin at the point previously marked. While the anesthetic takes effect, the ultrasound probe is covered in a sterile sheath. Sterile ultrasound jelly is applied to the skin, and under ultrasound guidance, a 10-cm, 21-gauge needle is guided to the renal capsule and further local anesthetic infiltrated into the perirenal tissues and then along the track of the needle on withdrawal. A stab incision is made through the dermis to ease passage of the biopsy needle. This is passed under ultrasound guidance to the kidney capsule (Fig. 6.5). As the needle approaches the capsule, the patient is instructed to take a breath until the kidney is moved to a position such that the lower pole rests just under the biopsy needle and then to stop breathing. The biopsy needle tip is advanced to the renal capsule, and the trigger mechanism is released, firing the needle into the kidney (Fig. 6.6). The needle is immediately withdrawn, the patient is asked to resume breathing, and the contents of the needle are examined (Fig. 6.7). We examine the tissue core under an operating microscope to ensure that renal cortex has been obtained (Fig. 6.8). A second pass of the needle is usually necessary to obtain additional tissue for immunohistology and electron microscopy. If insufficient tissue is obtained, further passes of the needle are made. However, in our experience, if the needle is passed more than four times, a modest increase in the postbiopsy complication rate is observed.

Once sufficient renal tissue has been obtained, the skin incision is dressed and the patient is rolled directly into bed for observation.

No single fixative has been developed that allows good-quality light microscopy, immunofluorescence, and electron microscopy to be performed on the same sample. In our center, therefore, the renal tissue is divided into three samples and placed in

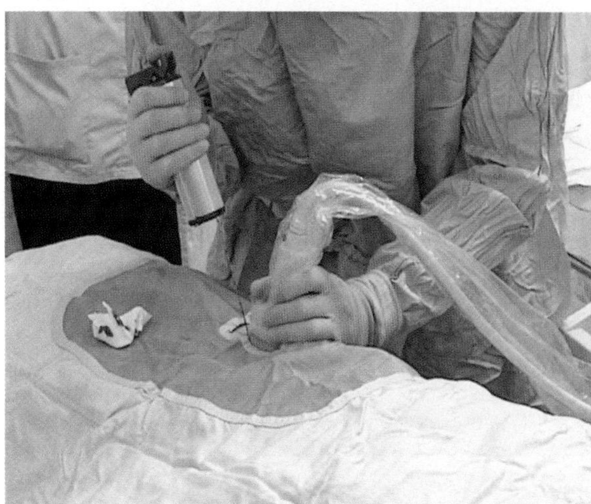

Figure 6.5 Renal biopsy procedure. The biopsy needle is introduced at an angle of approximately 70 degrees to the skin and is guided by continuous ultrasound. The operator is shown wearing a surgical gown. This is not strictly necessary; sterile gloves and maintenance of a sterile field are sufficient.

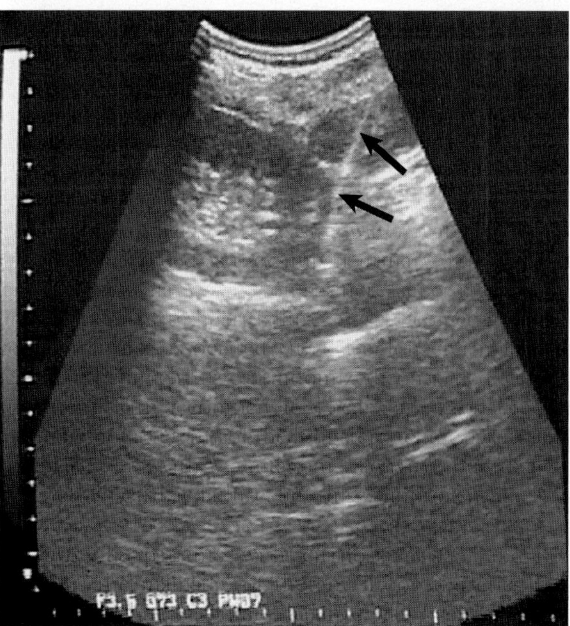

Figure 6.6 Renal biopsy. Ultrasound scan demonstrating the needle entering the lower pole of the left kidney. The *arrows* indicate the needle track, which appears as a fuzzy white line.

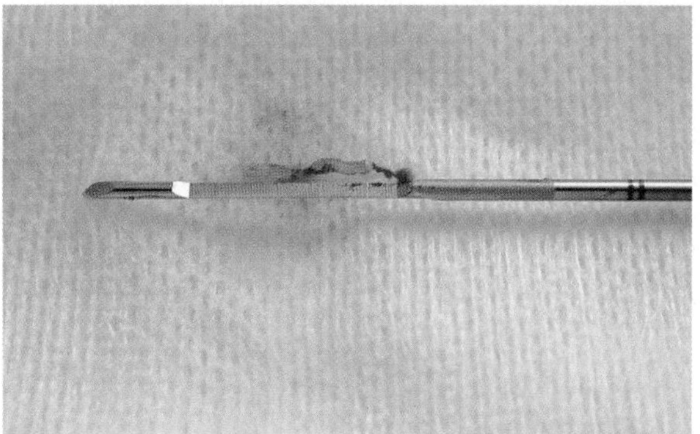

Figure 6.7 Renal biopsy. A core of renal tissue is demonstrated in the sampling notch of the biopsy needle.

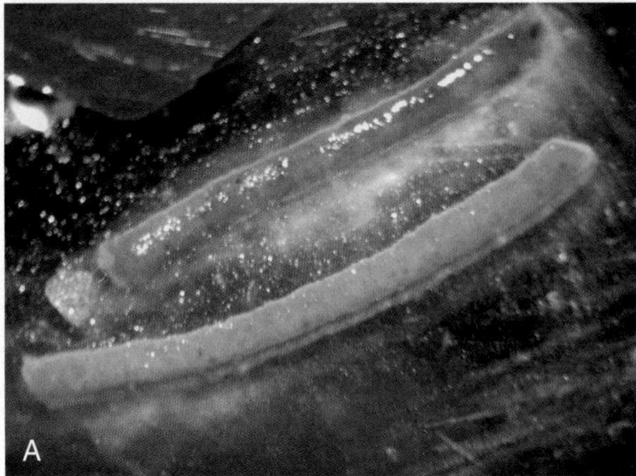

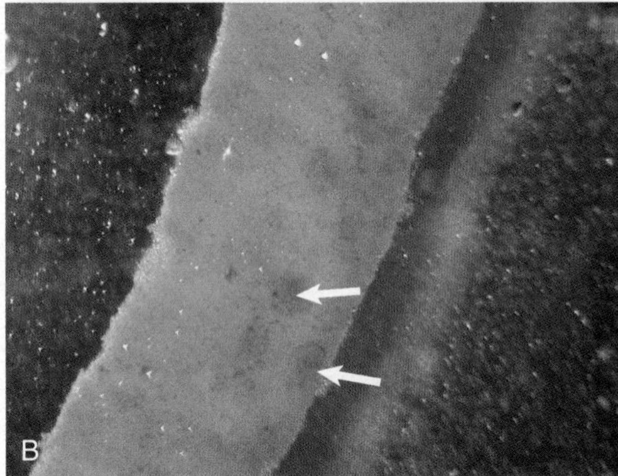

Figure 6.8 Renal biopsy. The appearance of renal biopsy material under the operating microscope. **A,** Low-power view showing two good-sized cores. **B,** Higher magnification view showing the typical appearance of glomeruli *(arrows).*

formalin for light microscopy, normal saline for subsequent snap-freezing in liquid nitrogen for immunofluorescence, and glutaraldehyde for electron microscopy.

There are a number of variations of the percutaneous renal biopsy technique. Whereas the majority of biopsies are guided by ultrasound, some operators choose to use it only to localize the kidney and to determine the depth and angle of approach of the needle, then performing the biopsy without further ultrasound guidance. The success and complication rates appear to be no different from those seen with continuous ultrasound guidance. For technically challenging biopsies, computed tomography can be used to guide the biopsy needle.

For obese patients and patients with respiratory conditions who find the prone position difficult, the supine anterolateral approach has recently been described.[11] Patients lie supine with the flank on the side to be sampled elevated by 30 degrees with towels under the shoulder and gluteus. The biopsy needle is inserted through Petit's triangle (bounded by latissimus dorsi muscle, 12th rib, and iliac crest). This technique provides good access to the lower pole of the kidney, is better tolerated than the prone position by such patients, and has a diagnostic yield and safety profile comparable to the standard technique.

Renal Transplant Biopsy

Biopsy of the transplant kidney is facilitated by the proximity of the kidney to the anterior abdominal wall and the lack of movement on respiration. It is performed under real-time ultrasound guidance with use of an automated biopsy needle. In most cases, the renal transplant biopsy is performed to identify the cause of acute allograft dysfunction. In these circumstances, the aim is to identify acute rejection, and therefore the diagnosis can be made on a formalin-fixed sample alone for light microscopy. If vascular rejection is suspected, a snap-frozen sample for C4d immunostaining should also be obtained. If recurrent or *de novo* glomerulonephritis is suspected in patients with chronic allograft dysfunction, additional samples for electron microscopy and immunohistology should be collected.

Postbiopsy Monitoring

After the biopsy, the patient is placed supine and subjected to strict bed rest for 6 to 8 hours. The blood pressure is monitored frequently, the urine is examined for macroscopic hematuria, and the skin puncture site is examined for excessive bleeding. If there is no evidence of bleeding after 6 hours following biopsy, the patient is sat up in bed and subsequently allowed to mobilize. If macroscopic hematuria develops, bed rest is continued until the bleeding settles.

Conventionally, patients have been kept in the hospital for 24 hours after a biopsy to be observed for complications. However, outpatient (day-case) renal biopsy with same-day discharge after 6 to 8 hours of observation has become increasingly popular for both native and renal transplant biopsies. This has been largely driven by the financial and resource implications of overnight hospital admission and has been justified by the perception that the significant complications of renal biopsy will become apparent during this shortened period of observation. This view has been challenged by a study of 750 native renal biopsies, which showed that only 67% of major complications (i.e., those that either required blood transfusion or an invasive procedure or resulted in urinary tract obstruction, septicemia, or death) were apparent by 8 hours after biopsy.[12] The authors concluded that the widespread application of an early discharge policy after renal biopsy is not in the patient's best interest and that a 24-hour period of observation is preferable.

In our center, approximately half of our renal biopsies are performed on an outpatient basis. The patient population is selected to avoid those with the highest risk of complications, for example, impaired renal function (creatinine concentration >3 mg/dl [250 μmol/l]), small kidneys, and uncontrolled hypertension. In addition, we require that the patient not be alone at home for at least one night after the biopsy. This selection policy has proved to be safe. Of the last 429 outpatient biopsies performed in our unit, 6% developed a self-limited postbiopsy complication within 6 hours that required a short hospital admission. Five patients returned after same-day discharge with biopsy-related complications, one with macroscopic hematuria 24 hours after the biopsy and four with loin pain between 3 and 5 days after biopsy. All patients recovered with conservative management. In our opinion, outpatient renal biopsy is acceptably safe when a low-risk patient group is selected.

A study has examined whether ultrasound 1 hour after biopsy is able to predict bleeding complications.[13] The absence of hematoma was predictive of an uncomplicated course, but the identification of hematoma was not reliably predictive of a significant biopsy complication (identification of hematoma at 1 hour had a 95% negative predictive value and 43% positive predictive value). The role of this practice in the wider clinical setting remains to be determined given the additional expense of the routine postbiopsy ultrasound scan.

Alternatives to the Percutaneous Approach

When the percutaneous approach is contraindicated, other approaches to renal biopsy have been described. The choice of technique depends on the safety, morbidity, recovery period, and adequacy of the technique, but probably above all on the local expertise that is available.

Transvenous (Transjugular or Transfemoral) Renal Biopsy

Transvenous sampling of the kidney is theoretically safer than the percutaneous approach because the needle passes from the venous system into the renal parenchyma and is directed away from large blood vessels. In addition, it is suggested that any bleeding that occurs should be directed back into the venous system, and if capsular perforation develops, significant bleeding points can be immediately identified and controlled by coil embolization. Others argue that coil embolization of the punctured vein is unhelpful because significant bleeding into either a perirenal hematoma or the urine indicates an arterial breach that requires selective angiography and arterial embolization.

Transvenous renal biopsy cannot be regarded as routine because it involves specialist skills and additional time and expense compared with the percutaneous approach. The main indication for this approach is an uncontrollable bleeding diathesis. It has also been advocated for use in a variety of other situations: patients receiving artificial ventilation in the intensive care unit; the need to obtain tissue from more than one organ, including the kidney, liver, or heart; large-volume ascites that precludes the prone position; uncontrolled hypertension; morbid obesity; severe respiratory insufficiency; solitary kidney; failed percutaneous approach; and coma.

The patient lies supine, and the right internal jugular vein is cannulated. A guide wire is passed into the inferior vena cava, and a catheter is passed over the guide wire and selectively into the right renal vein (the right renal vein is shorter and enters the vena cava at a more favorable angle than the left). A sheath is passed over the catheter to a suitable peripheral location in the kidney with the aid of contrast enhancement. Finally, the biopsy device (usually a side-cut biopsy needle system) is passed through the sheath and samples are taken. Contrast material is then injected into the biopsy track to identify capsular perforation, and embolization coils are inserted if brisk bleeding is identified.

The quality of renal tissue obtained by transjugular biopsy is variable, although studies report diagnostic yields of more than 90%.[14] The complication rate appears comparable to that seen with percutaneous renal biopsy, which is reassuring given that these are high-risk patients.

Open Renal Biopsy

This has been established as a safe alternative to percutaneous biopsy when uncorrectable contraindications exist. The largest study reported a series of 934 patients in which tissue adequacy was 100% with no major complications.[15] Nonetheless, although this is an effective approach with minimal postprocedure complications, the risk of general anesthesia and the delayed recovery time have prevented its widespread adoption. It may still, however, be performed when a renal biopsy is required in patients who are otherwise undergoing an abdominal surgical procedure.

Laparoscopic Renal Biopsy

This procedure requires general anesthesia and two laparoscopic ports in the posterior and anterior axillary lines to gain access to the retroperitoneal space. Laparoscopic biopsy forceps are used to obtain cortical biopsy samples, and the biopsy sites are coagulated with laser and packed to prevent hemorrhage. In the most recent and largest study, adequate tissue was obtained in 96% of the 74 patients included.[16] Significant bleeding occurred in three patients, the colon was injured in one, and a biopsy was performed inadvertently on the spleen and liver, respectively, in two others. This last complication was subsequently averted by the use of intraoperative ultrasound to define the anatomy in difficult cases.

Complications of Renal Biopsy

	1952–1977 (%)	1990 to Present (%)
Number	14,492	4,542
Hematoma	1	4.6
Gross hematuria	3	4.6
Arteriovenous fistula	0.1	0.18
Surgery	0.3	1 case
Death	0.12	1 case

Figure 6.9 Complications of renal biopsy. The data for 1952 to 1977 are taken from 20 series including 14,492 patients. (Data from reference 18.) The 1990 to present data are from eight series including 4542 patients. *(Data from references 12, 17, 19-25.)*

COMPLICATIONS OF RENAL BIOPSY

The complication rates compiled from large series of renal biopsies are shown in Figure 6.9.

Pain

A dull ache around the needle entry site is inevitable when the local anesthetic wears off, and patients should be warned about this. Simple analgesia with paracetamol or paracetamol-codeine combinations usually suffices. More severe pain in the loin or abdomen on the side of the biopsy raises the possibility of a significant perirenal hemorrhage. Opiates may be necessary for pain relief, and appropriate investigations to clarify the severity of the bleed should be performed. Patients with macroscopic hematuria may develop clot colic and describe the typical severe pain associated with ureteral obstruction.

Hemorrhage

A degree of perirenal bleeding accompanies every renal biopsy. The mean decrease in hemoglobin after a biopsy is approximately 1 g/dl.[17] Significant perirenal hematomas are almost invariably associated with severe loin pain. Both macroscopic hematuria and painful hematoma are seen in 3% of patients after biopsy. The initial management is strict bed rest and maintenance of normal coagulation indices. If bleeding is brisk and associated with hypotension or prolonged and fails to settle with bed rest, renal angiography should be performed to identify the source of bleeding. Coil embolization can be performed during the same procedure, and this has largely eliminated the need for open surgical intervention and nephrectomy.

Arteriovenous Fistula

Most postbiopsy arteriovenous fistulas are detected by Doppler ultrasound or contrast-enhanced computed tomography and, when looked for specifically, can be found in as many as 18% of patients. Because most are clinically silent and more than 95% resolve spontaneously within 2 years, they should not be routinely sought. In a small minority, they can lead to macroscopic hematuria (typically recurrent, dark red, and often with blood clots), hypertension, and renal impairment, in which case, embolization is indicated.

Other Complications

A variety of other rare complications have been reported, including biopsy inadvertently performed on other organs (liver, spleen, pancreas, bowel, and gallbladder), pneumothorax, hemothorax, calyceal-peritoneal fistula, dispersion of carcinoma, and the Page kidney. This last complication results from compression of the kidney by a perirenal hematoma leading to renin-mediated hypertension.

Death

Death resulting directly from renal biopsy has become much less common according to recent biopsy series compared with earlier reports. Most deaths are the result of uncontrolled hemorrhage in high-risk patients, particularly those with severe renal impairment.

REFERENCES

1. Iversen P, Brun C. Aspiration biopsy of the kidney. 1951. *J Am Soc Nephrol.* 1997;8:1778-1787; discussion 1778-1786.
2. Alwall N. Aspiration biopsy of the kidney, including i.a. a report of a case of amyloidosis diagnosed through aspiration biopsy of the kidney in 1944 and investigated at an autopsy in 1950. *Acta Med Scand.* 1952;143:430-435.
3. Kark RM, Muehrcke RC. Biopsy of kidney in prone position. *Lancet.* 1954;266:1047-1049.
4. Topham PS, Harper SJ, Furness PN, et al. Glomerular disease as a cause of isolated microscopic haematuria. *Q J Med.* 1994;87:329-335.
5. Kropp KA, Shapiro RS, Jhunjhunwala JS. Role of renal biopsy in end stage renal failure. *Urology.* 1978;12:631-634.
6. Turner MW, Hutchinson TA, Barre PE, et al. A prospective study on the impact of the renal biopsy in clinical management. *Clin Nephrol.* 1986;26:217-221.
7. Richards NT, Darby S, Howie AJ, et al. Knowledge of renal histology alters patient management in over 40% of cases. *Nephrol Dial Transplant.* 1994;9:1255-1259.
8. Boberg KM, Brosstad F, Egeland T, et al. Is a prolonged bleeding time associated with an increased risk of hemorrhage after liver biopsy? *Thromb Haemost.* 1999;81:378-381.
9. Peterson P, Hayes TE, Arkin CF, et al. The preoperative bleeding time test lacks clinical benefit: College of American Pathologists' and American Society of Clinical Pathologists' position article. *Arch Surg.* 1998;133:134-139.
10. Davis CL, Chandler WL. Thromboelastography for the prediction of bleeding after transplant renal biopsy. *J Am Soc Nephrol.* 1995;6:1250-1255.
11. Gesualdo L, Cormio L, Stallone G, et al. Percutaneous ultrasound-guided renal biopsy in supine antero-lateral position: A new approach for obese and non-obese patients. *Nephrol Dial Transplant.* 2008;23:971-976.
12. Whittier WL, Korbet SM. Timing of complications in percutaneous renal biopsy. *J Am Soc Nephrol.* 2004;15:142-147.
13. Waldo B, Korbet SM, Freimanis MG, Lewis EJ. The value of post-biopsy ultrasound in predicting complications after percutaneous renal biopsy of native kidneys. *Nephrol Dial Transplant.* 2009;24:2433-2439.
14. See TC, Thompson BC, Howie AJ, et al. Transjugular renal biopsy: Our experience and technical considerations. *Cardiovasc Intervent Radiol.* 2008;31:906-918.
15. Nomoto Y, Tomino Y, Endoh M, et al. Modified open renal biopsy: Results in 934 patients. *Nephron.* 1987;45:224-228.
16. Shetye KR, Kavoussi LR, Ramakumar S, et al. Laparoscopic renal biopsy: A 9-year experience. *BJU Int.* 2003;91:817-820.
17. Burstein DM, Korbet SM, Schwartz MM. The use of the automatic core biopsy system in percutaneous renal biopsies: A comparative study. *Am J Kidney Dis.* 1993;22:545-552.
18. Parrish AE. Complications of percutaneous renal biopsy: A review of 37 years' experience. *Clin Nephrol.* 1992;38:135-141.
19. Eiro M, Katoh T, Watanabe T. Risk factors for bleeding complications in percutaneous renal biopsy. *Clin Exp Nephrol.* 2005;9:40-45.
20. Fraser IR, Fairley KF. Renal biopsy as an outpatient procedure. *Am J Kidney Dis.* 1995;25:876-878.
21. Hergesell O, Felten H, Andrassy K, et al. Safety of ultrasound-guided percutaneous renal biopsy—retrospective analysis of 1090 consecutive cases. *Nephrol Dial Transplant.* 1998;13:975-977.
22. Manno C, Strippoli GF, Arnesano L, et al. Predictors of bleeding complications in percutaneous ultrasound-guided renal biopsy. *Kidney Int.* 2004;66:1570-1577.
23. Marwah DS, Korbet SM. Timing of complications in percutaneous renal biopsy: What is the optimal period of observation? *Am J Kidney Dis.* 1996;28:47-52.
24. Stiles KP, Hill C, LeBrun CJ, et al. The impact of bleeding times on major complication rates after percutaneous real-time ultrasound-guided renal biopsies. *J Nephrol.* 2001;14:275-279.
25. Stratta P, Canavese C, Marengo M, et al. Risk management of renal biopsy: 1387 cases over 30 years in a single centre. *Eur J Clin Invest.* 2007;37:954-963.

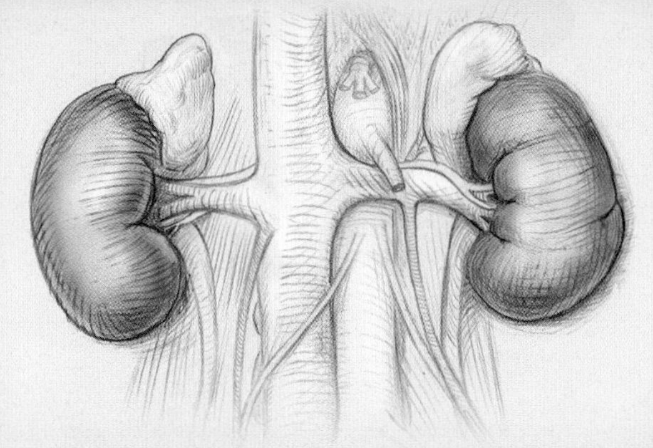

SECTION III

Fluid and Electrolyte Disorders

CHAPTER 7

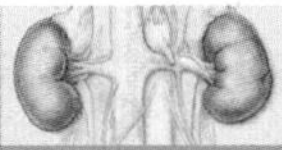

Disorders of Extracellular Volume

Elwaleed A. Elhassan, Robert W. Schrier

THE EXTRACELLULAR FLUID COMPARTMENT

Water is the predominant constituent of the human body. In healthy individuals, it makes up 60% of a man's body weight and 50% of a woman's body weight. Body water is distributed in two compartments, the intracellular fluid (ICF) compartment, containing 55% to 65%, and the extracellular fluid (ECF) compartment, containing the remaining 35% to 45%. The ECF is further subdivided into the interstitial space and the intravascular space. The interstitial space comprises approximately three fourths of ECF, whereas the intravascular space contains one fourth (Fig. 7.1).

Total body water diffuses freely between the intracellular space and the extracellular spaces in response to solute concentration gradients. Therefore, the amount of water in different compartments depends entirely on the quantity of solute in that compartment. The major solute in the ECF is sodium; potassium is the major intracellular solute. The maintenance of this distribution is fulfilled by active transport through the Na^+,K^+-ATP–dependent pumps on the cell membrane, and this determines the relative volume of different compartments. Because sodium is the predominant extracellular solute, the ECF is determined primarily by the sodium content of the body and the mechanisms responsible for maintaining it. The amount of sodium is therefore very tightly regulated by modulation of renal retention and excretion in situations of deficient and excess ECF, respectively.

Fluid movement between the intravascular and interstitial compartments of the ECF occurs across the capillary wall and is governed by the Starling forces, namely, the capillary hydrostatic pressure and colloid osmotic pressure. The transcapillary hydrostatic pressure gradient exceeds the corresponding oncotic pressure gradient, thereby favoring movement of plasma ultrafiltrate into the extravascular space. The return of fluid into the intravascular compartment occurs through lymphatic flow.

Maintaining the ECF volume determines the adequacy of the circulation and, in turn, the adequacy of delivery of oxygen, nutrients, and other substances needed for organ functions as well as for removal of waste products. This is achieved in spite of day-to-day variations in the intake of sodium and water, with the ECF volume varying by only 1% to 2%.

Effective Arterial Blood Volume

This term is used to describe the blood volume that is detected by the sensitive arterial baroreceptors in the arterial circulation. The effective arterial blood volume (EABV) can change independently of the total ECF volume and can explain the sodium and water retention in different health and disease clinical situations (see later discussion).

REGULATION OF EXTRACELLULAR FLUID HOMEOSTASIS

Circulatory stability depends on a meticulous degree of ECF homeostasis. The operative homeostatic mechanisms include an afferent sensing limb comprising several volume and stretch detectors distributed throughout the vascular bed and an efferent effector limb. Adjustments in the effector mechanisms occur in response to afferent stimuli by sensing limb detectors with the aim of modifying circulatory parameters. Disorders of either sensing or effector mechanisms can lead to failure of adjustment of sodium handling by the kidney with resultant hypertension or edema formation in the case of positive sodium balance or hypotension and hypovolemia in the case of negative sodium balance.

The Afferent (Sensor) Limb

Afferent limb sensing sites include low-pressure cardiopulmonary receptors (atrial, ventricular, and pulmonary stretch receptors), high-pressure arterial baroreceptors (carotid, aortic arch, and renal sensors), central nervous system (CNS) receptors, and hepatic receptors (Fig. 7.2). The cardiac atria possess the distensibility and the compliance needed to monitor changes in intrathoracic venous volume. An increase in left atrial pressure suppresses the release of the antidiuretic hormone arginine vasopressin (AVP). Atrial distention and a sodium load cause release into the circulation of atrial natriuretic peptide (ANP), a polypeptide normally stored in secretory granules within atrial myocytes. The closely related brain natriuretic peptide (BNP) is stored primarily in ventricular myocardium and is released when ventricular diastolic pressure rises. The atrial-renal reflexes aim to enhance renal sodium and water excretion on sensing of a distended left atrium.

The sensitive arterial stretch receptors in the carotid artery, aortic arch, and glomerular afferent arteriole respond to a decrease in arterial pressure. Information from these nerve endings is carried by the vagal and glossopharyngeal nerves to vasomotor centers in the medulla and brainstem. In the normal situation, the prevailing discharge from these receptors exerts a tonic restraining effect on the heart and circulation by inhibiting the sympathetic outflow and augmenting parasympathetic activity. In addition, changes in transmural pressure across the arterial vessels and the atria also influence the secretion of AVP and renin and the release of ANP. Activation of the arterial receptors signals the kidney to retain sodium and water by increases in the sympathetic activity and by increases in vasopressin release. Stimulation of the sympathetic nervous system also enhances the renin-angiotensin-aldosterone system (RAAS). A rise in arterial

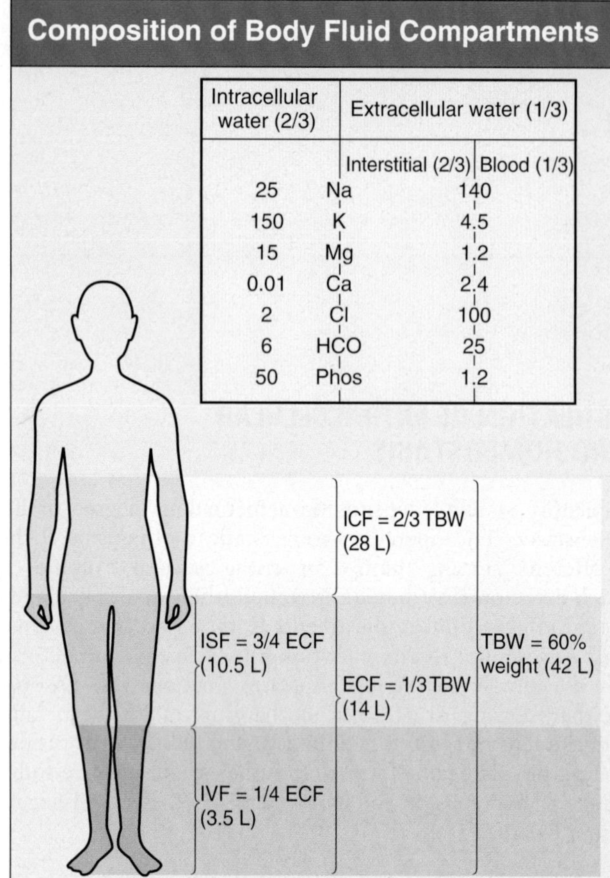

Figure 7.1 Composition of body fluid compartments. Schematic representation of body fluid compartments in humans. The shaded areas depict the approximate size of each compartment as a function of body weight. The figures indicate the relative sizes of the various fluid compartments and the approximate absolute volumes of the compartments (in liters) in a 70-kg adult. Intracellular electrolyte concentrations are in millimoles per liter and are typical values obtained from muscle. ECF, extracellular fluid; ICF, intracellular fluid; ISF, interstitial fluid; IVF, intravascular fluid; TBW, total body water. *(From reference 1. Reproduced with permission of Hodder Arnold.)*

pressure elicits the opposite response, resulting in decreased catecholamine release and natriuresis.

Renal sensing mechanisms include the juxtaglomerular apparatus, which is involved in the generation and release of renin from the kidney. Renin secretion is inversely related to perfusion pressure and directly related to intrarenal tissue pressure. Solute delivery to the macula densa is also an important determinant of renin release by way of the tubuloglomerular feedback (TGF) mechanism; an increase in chloride passage through the macula densa results in inhibition of renin release, whereas a decrease in concentration results in enhanced secretion of renin. Renal nerve stimulation through activation of β-adrenergic receptors of the juxtaglomerular apparatus cells directly stimulates renin release. Other receptors reside in the CNS and hepatic circulation but have been less well defined.

Efferent (Effector) Limb

The stimulation of the effector limb of the ECF volume homeostasis leads to activation of effector mechanisms (see Fig. 7.2). These effector mechanisms aim predominantly at modulation of renal sodium and water excretion to preserve circulatory stability.

Major Effector Homeostatic Mechanisms

Afferent	Efferent
Cardiopulmonary receptors Atrial Ventricular Pulmonary	Renal-angiotensin-aldosterone system
High-pressure baroreceptors Carotid Aortic Renal Glomerular afferent Juxtaglomerular apparatus	Prostaglandins
Central nervous system receptors	Arginine vasopressin
Hepatic receptors	Natriuretic peptides ANP BNP CNP Other hormones – NO Endothelin Kallikrein-kinin system

Figure 7.2 Major effector homeostatic mechanisms. ANP, atrial natriuretic peptide; BNP, brain natriuretic peptide; CNP, C-type natriuretic peptide; NO, nitric oxide.

Sympathetic Nervous System

Sympathetic nerves that originate in the prevertebral celiac and paravertebral ganglia innervate cells of the afferent and efferent arterioles, juxtaglomerular apparatus, and renal tubule. Sympathetic nerves alter renal sodium and water handling by direct and indirect mechanisms.[2] Increased nerve stimulation indirectly stimulates proximal tubular sodium reabsorption by altering preglomerular and postglomerular arteriolar tone, thereby influencing filtration fraction. Renal nerves directly stimulate proximal tubular fluid reabsorption through receptors on the basolateral membrane of the proximal convoluted tubule cells. These effects on sodium handling are further amplified by the ability of the sympathetic nerves to stimulate renin release, which leads to the formation of angiotensin II (Ang II) and aldosterone.

Renin-Angiotensin-Aldosterone System

Renin formation by the juxtaglomerular apparatus increases in response to the aforementioned ECF homeostatic afferent limb stimuli. Renin converts angiotensinogen to angiotensin I, which is then converted to Ang II by the action of angiotensin-converting enzyme (ACE); Ang II can subsequently affect circulatory stability and volume homeostasis. It is an effective vasoconstrictor and modulator of renal sodium handling mechanisms at multiple nephron sites. Ang II preferentially increases the efferent arteriolar tone and hence affects the glomerular filtration rate (GFR) and filtration fraction by altering Starling forces across the glomerulus, which leads to enhanced proximal sodium and water retention. Ang II also augments sympathetic neurotransmission and enhances the TGF mechanism. In addition to these indirect mechanisms, Ang II directly enhances proximal tubular volume reabsorption by activating apical membrane sodium-hydrogen exchangers. In addition to a nephron effect, Ang II enhances sodium absorption by stimulating the adrenal gland to secrete aldosterone, which in turn increases sodium reabsorption in the cortical collecting tubule.

Prostaglandins

Prostaglandins are proteins derived from arachidonic acid that modulate renal blood flow and sodium handling. Important renal prostaglandins include PGI_2, which mediates baroreceptor (but not β-adrenergic) stimulation of renin release. PGE_2 is stimulated by Ang II and has vasodilatory properties secondary to total blood volume or EABV contraction. Increased level of Ang II, AVP, and catecholamines stimulates synthesis of prostaglandins, which in turn act to dilate the renal vasculature, to inhibit sodium and water reabsorption, and further to stimulate renin release. By doing so, renal prostaglandins serve to dampen and counterbalance the physiologic effects of the hormones that elicit their production and so maintain renal function. Inhibition of prostaglandins by nonsteroidal anti-inflammatory drugs (NSAIDs) leads to magnification of the effect of vasoconstricting hormones and unchecked sodium and water retention.

Arginine Vasopressin

AVP is a polypeptide synthesized in supraoptic and paraventricular nuclei of the hypothalamus and is secreted by the posterior pituitary gland. Besides osmotic control of AVP release, a nonosmotic regulatory pathway sensitive to EABV exists.[3] AVP release is suppressed in response to ECF volume overload sensed by increased afferent impulses from arterial baroreceptors and atrial receptors, whereas decreased ECF volume has the opposite effect. AVP release leads to antidiuresis and, in high doses, to systemic vasoconstriction through the V_1 receptors.[4] The antidiuretic action of AVP is the result of the effect on the principal cell of the collecting duct through activation of the V_2 receptor. AVP increases the synthesis and provokes the insertion of aquaporin 2 water channels into the luminal membrane, thereby allowing water to be reabsorbed down the favorable osmotic gradient. AVP may also lead to enhanced reabsorption of sodium and the secretion of potassium. AVP appears to have synergistic effects with aldosterone on sodium transport in the cortical collecting duct.[5] AVP stimulates potassium secretion by the distal nephron, and this serves to preserve potassium balance during ECF depletion, when circulating levels of vasopressin are high and tubular delivery of sodium and fluid is reduced.

Natriuretic Peptides

ANP is a polypeptide hormone that stimulates diuresis, natriuresis, and vasorelaxation. ANP is primarily synthesized in the cardiac atria and released in response to a rise in atrial distention. ANP augments sodium and water excretion by increasing the GFR, possibly by dilating the afferent arteriole and constricting the efferent arteriole. Furthermore, it inhibits sodium reabsorption in the cortical collecting tubule and inner medullary collecting duct, reduces renin and aldosterone secretion, and opposes the vasoconstrictive effects of Ang II. BNP is another natriuretic hormone that is produced in the cardiac ventricles. It induces natriuretic, endocrine, and hemodynamic responses similar to those induced by ANP.[6] Circulating levels of ANP and BNP are elevated in congestive heart failure (CHF) and in cirrhosis with ascites, but not to levels sufficient to prevent edema formation. In addition, in those edematous states, there is resistance to the actions of natriuretic peptides.

C-type natriuretic peptide (CNP) is produced by endothelial cells, where it is believed to play a role in the local regulation of vascular tone and blood flow. However, its physiologic significance in the regulation of sodium and water balance in humans is not well defined.

Other Hormones

Several other hormones contribute to renal sodium handling and ECF volume homeostasis. They include nitric oxide, endothelin, and the kallikrein-kinin system. Nitric oxide is an endothelium-derived mediator that has been shown to participate in the natriuretic responses to increases in blood pressure or ECF volume expansion, so-called pressure natriuresis. Endothelins are natriuretic factors and kinins are potent vasodilator peptides whose physiologic roles are yet to be fully defined.

EXTRACELLULAR FLUID VOLUME CONTRACTION

ECF volume contraction refers to a decrease in ECF volume caused by sodium or water loss exceeding intake. Losses may be renal or extrarenal through the gastrointestinal tract, skin, and lungs or by sequestration in potential spaces in the body (e.g., abdomen, muscle) that are not in hemodynamic equilibrium with the ECF (Fig. 7.3). The reduction in ECF volume occurs simultaneously from both the interstitial and intravascular compartments and is determined by whether the volume loss is primarily solute-free water or a combination of sodium and water. The loss of solute-free water has a lesser effect on intravascular volume because of the smaller amount of water present in the ECF compared with the ICF and the free movement of water between fluid compartments.

Extrarenal Causes

Gastrointestinal Losses

Approximately 3 to 6 liters of fluids and digestive juices are secreted daily throughout the gastrointestinal tract, and most of this fluid is reabsorbed. Vomiting or nasogastric suction may cause volume loss that is usually accompanied by metabolic alkalosis, whereas diarrhea may result in volume depletion that is accompanied by metabolic acidosis.

Dermal Losses

Sweat production can be excessive in high ambient temperature or with prolonged exercise in hot, humid climates and may lead to volume depletion. Loss of the skin barrier with superficial burns and exudative skin lesions may lead to significant ECF volume depletion.

Third-Space Sequestration

Body fluid accumulation in potential spaces that are not in hemodynamic equilibrium with the ECF compartment can cause volume depletion. This pathologic accumulation is often referred to as third-space sequestration and includes ascites, hydrothorax, and intestinal obstruction, whereby fluid collects in the peritoneal cavity, pleural space, or intestines, respectively, and leads to significant ECF volume loss. Severe pancreatitis may result in retroperitoneal fluid collections.

Hemorrhage

Hemorrhage occurring internally, such as from bleeding esophageal varices, or externally as a result of trauma may lead to significant volume loss.

Renal Losses

In the normal individual, about 25,000 mmol of sodium is filtered every day, and a small amount of that quantity is excreted in the urine. The small quantities of sodium excreted in urine

Figure 7.3 Major causes of extracellular fluid volume depletion.

Major Causes of Extracellular Fluid Volume Depletion	
Renal	**Extrarenal**
Diuretic use	Gastrointestinal losses Vomiting or gastrointestinal suctioning Diarrhea Ileostomy or colostomy secretions
Tubular disorders Genetic Bartter and Gitelman's syndromes Pseudohypoaldosteronism type 1 Acquired tubular disorders: Acute kidney injury Recovery phase of oliguric kidney injury Release of urinary tract obstruction	Dermal losses Sweat Exudative skin disease
Hormonal and metabolic disturbances Mineralocorticoid deficiency or resistance Primary adrenal insufficiency (Addison's disease) Hyporeninemic hypoaldosteronism Diabetes mellitus Chronic interstitial renal diseases Solute diuresis	Third-space sequestration Ascites Pleural effusion, hydrothorax Intestinal obstruction Retroperitoneal collection
Renal water loss Diabetes insipidus	Hemorrhage Internal External

relative to the filtered load depend on intact tubular reabsorptive mechanisms to adjust urinary sodium excretion according to the degree needed to maintain ECF homeostasis. Impairment in the integrity of these sodium reabsorptive mechanisms can result in a significant sodium deficit and volume depletion.

Diuretic Use

Most of the widely used diuretic medications inhibit specific sites for sodium reabsorption at different segments of the nephron. These agents may cause renal sodium wasting, volume contraction, and metabolic acid-base disturbances if they are abused or inappropriately prescribed. Ingestion of osmotic diuretics results in obligatory renal sodium and water loss. Further discussion of diuretics is presented at the end of the chapter.

Genetic and Acquired Tubular Disorders

(see Chapters 47 and 48)

Tubular sodium reabsorption may be disrupted in several genetic disorders, such as Bartter syndrome and Gitelman's syndrome, which are autosomal recessive disorders caused by mutations of sodium transporters that are targets of diuretics or other transporters that are their essential cellular partners. Both conditions result in sodium wasting, volume contraction, and hypokalemic metabolic alkalosis.[7] Pseudohypoaldosteronism type 1 is a rare inherited disorder characterized by renal sodium wasting and hyperkalemic metabolic acidosis. Acquired tubular disorders that may be accompanied by sodium wasting include acute kidney injury during the recovery phase of oliguric acute kidney injury or urinary obstruction.

Hormonal and Metabolic Disturbances

Mineralocorticoid deficiency and resistance states often lead to sodium wasting. This may occur in the setting of primary adrenal insufficiency (Addison's disease) or with hyporeninemic hypoaldosteronism secondary to diabetes mellitus or other chronic interstitial renal diseases. Severe hyperglycemia or high levels of blood urea during release of urinary tract obstruction can lead to obligatory renal sodium and water loss secondary to glucosuria or urea diuresis, respectively.

Renal Water Loss

Diabetes insipidus represents a spectrum of diseases resulting from AVP deficiency or tubular resistance to the actions of AVP. In these disorders, the tubular reabsorption of solute-free water is impaired. This generally results in a lesser effect on ECF volume because a relatively smaller amount of the total body water, in contrast to sodium, exists in the ECF compartment compared with the ICF compartment.

Clinical Manifestations

The spectrum of the clinical manifestations of volume contraction depends on the amount and rate of volume loss as well as on the vascular and renal responses to that loss. An adequate history and physical examination are crucial to elucidate the cause of hypovolemia. Symptoms are usually nonspecific and can range from mild postural symptoms, thirst, muscle cramps, and weakness to drowsiness and disturbed mentation with profound volume loss. Physical examination may reveal tachycardia, cold clammy skin, postural or recumbent hypotension, and reduced urine output, depending on the degree of volume loss (Fig. 7.4). Reduced jugular venous pressure (JVP) noted at the base of the neck is a useful parameter of volume depletion and may roughly estimate the central venous pressure (CVP). However, an elevated CVP does not exclude hypovolemia in patients with underlying cardiac failure or pulmonary hypertension. The lack of symptoms or discernible physical findings does not preclude volume depletion in an appropriate clinical setting, and hemodynamic monitoring and administration of a fluid challenge may sometimes be necessary.

Clinical Evaluation of Extracellular Fluid Volume Depletion

Mild to moderate volume loss
- Thirst
- Delay in capillary refill
- Postural dizziness, weakness
- Dry mucous membranes and axillae
- Cool clammy extremities and collapsed peripheral veins
- Tachypnea
- Tachycardia with pulse rate >100 beats per minute or postural pulse increment of 30 beats/min or more
- Postural hypotension (systolic blood pressure decrease of >20 mm Hg with standing)
- Low jugular venous pulse
- Oliguria

Severe volume loss and hypovolemic shock
- Depressed mental status (or loss of consciousness)
- Peripheral cyanosis
- Reduced skin turgor (in young patients)
- Marked tachycardia, low pulse volume
- Supine hypotension (systolic blood pressure <100 mm Hg)

Figure 7.4 Clinical evaluation of extracellular fluid volume depletion.

Laboratory Indices

Laboratory parameters may assist in defining the underlying causes of volume depletion. Hemoconcentration and increased serum albumin concentration may be seen early with hypovolemia, but anemia or hypoalbuminemia caused by a concomitant disease may confound interpretation of these laboratory values. In healthy individuals, the blood urea nitrogen (BUN)/serum creatinine ratio is approximately equal to 10 mg/dl (40 mmol/l). In volume-contracted states, this ratio may significantly increase because of an associated differential increase in urea reabsorption in the collecting duct. Several clinical conditions affect this ratio. Upper gastrointestinal hemorrhage and administration of corticosteroids increase urea production, and hence the BUN/creatinine ratio increases. Malnutrition and underlying liver disease diminish urea production, and thus the ratio is less helpful to support volume depletion in such clinical settings.

Urine osmolality and specific gravity may be elevated in hypovolemic states but may be altered by an underlying renal disease that leads to renal sodium wasting, concomitant intake of diuretics, or a solute diuresis. Hypovolemia normally promotes avid renal sodium reabsorption, resulting in low urine sodium concentration and low fractional excretion of sodium. Urine chloride follows a similar pattern because sodium and chloride are generally reabsorbed together. Volume depletion with metabolic alkalosis (e.g., with vomiting) is an exception because of the need to excrete the excess bicarbonate in conjunction with sodium to maintain electroneutrality; in that case, the urine chloride concentration is a better index of sodium avidity. The fractional excretion of sodium (FE_{Na}) is calculated by the following formula:

$$FE_{Na} = [U_{Na} \times P_{creat} / U_{creat} \times P_{Na}] \times 100$$

where U_{Na} and U_{creat} are urinary sodium and creatinine concentrations, respectively, and P_{Na} and P_{creat} are serum sodium and creatinine concentrations, respectively. Elevated (>1) FE_{Na} is most helpful in the diagnosis of acute kidney injury; FE_{Na} of less than 1% is consistent with volume depletion.

Therapy for Extracellular Volume Contraction

The goals of treatment of ECF volume depletion are to replace the fluid deficit and to replace ongoing losses, in general, with a replacement fluid that resembles the lost fluid. The first step is estimating the magnitude of volume loss. Helpful tools include the clinical parameters for mild to moderate versus severe volume loss (see Fig 7.4), which can also be assessed by invasive monitoring when necessary. The initial replacement volume is then determined and delivered with an administration rate that is tailored as subsequently judged by frequent monitoring of clinical parameters. Mild volume contraction can usually be corrected through the oral route. In cases of hypovolemic shock with evidence of life-threatening circulatory collapse or organ dysfunction, intravenous fluid must be administered as rapidly as possible until clinical parameters improve. However, in most cases, a slow, more careful approach is warranted, particularly in the elderly and in patients with an underlying cardiac condition, to avoid overcorrection with subsequent pulmonary or peripheral edema. Crystalloid solutions with sodium as the principal cation are effective as they distribute primarily in the ECF. A third of an infusate of isotonic saline remains in and expands the intravascular compartment; two thirds distributes into the interstitial compartment. Colloid-containing solutions include human albumin (5% and 25% albumin) and hetastarch (6% hydroxyethyl starch). Because of large molecular size, these solutions remain within the vascular compartment, provided the transcapillary barrier is intact and not disrupted by capillary leak states, such as often occurs with multiorgan failure or systemic inflammatory response syndrome. They augment the plasma oncotic pressure and thus expand the plasma volume by counteracting the capillary hydraulic pressure. Studies have not shown an advantage for colloid-containing solutions in the treatment of hypovolemic states. A meta-analysis of 55 studies showed no outcome difference between critically ill patients who received albumin and those who received crystalloids.[8] Furthermore, a large multicenter trial that randomized medical and surgical critical patients to receive fluid resuscitation with 4% albumin or normal saline showed similar mortality, measured morbidity parameters, and hospitalization rates in the two groups.[9] Consequently, timely administration of a sufficient quantity of intravenous fluids is more important than the type of fluid chosen. However, because of the higher cost of colloids, these are best reserved for hemodynamically unstable patients in whom rapid correction is needed, such as trauma and burns victims. Otherwise, isotonic saline is usually the initial choice in volume-depleted patients with normal serum sodium concentration and most of those with low serum sodium concentration. Furthermore, isotonic saline is the preferred fluid to restore ECF volume in hypovolemic patients with hypernatremia. Once euvolemia is established, further fluid therapy should be delivered to gradually correct tonicity in the form of hypotonic (0.45%) saline. Administration of large volumes of isotonic saline may result in elevation of serum sodium above the normal range because it is slightly hypertonic (155 mmol/l) compared with plasma. If that happens, hypotonic saline can be continued instead, until volume is replete. Hypokalemia may be present initially or may subsequently ensue. It should be corrected by adding appropriate amounts of potassium chloride to replacement solutions.

Hypovolemic shock may be accompanied by lactic acidosis due to tissue hypoperfusion. Fluid resuscitation restores tissue oxygenation and will decrease the production of lactate. Correction of acidosis with sodium bicarbonate has the potential for increasing tonicity, expanding volume, worsening intracellular acidosis from increased carbon dioxide production, and not improving hemodynamics compared with isotonic saline. Use of sodium bicarbonate for correction of cardiac contractility coexisting with lactic acidosis has not been well documented by clinical studies. Therefore, its use to manage lactic acidosis in the setting of volume depletion is not recommended (unless the arterial pH is below 7.1).

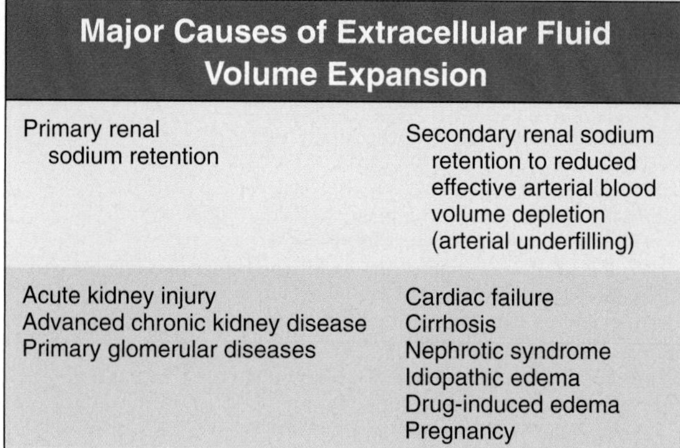

Major Causes of Extracellular Fluid Volume Expansion	
Primary renal sodium retention	Secondary renal sodium retention to reduced effective arterial blood volume depletion (arterial underfilling)
Acute kidney injury Advanced chronic kidney disease Primary glomerular diseases	Cardiac failure Cirrhosis Nephrotic syndrome Idiopathic edema Drug-induced edema Pregnancy

Figure 7.5 Major causes of extracellular fluid volume expansion.

EXTRACELLULAR FLUID VOLUME EXPANSION

Definition

ECF volume expansion refers to excess fluid accumulation in the ECF compartment, usually resulting from sodium and water retention by the kidneys. Generalized edema results when an apparent increase in the interstitial fluid volume takes place. It may occur in disease states most commonly in response to cardiac failure, cirrhosis with ascites, and the nephrotic syndrome. Weight gain of several liters usually precedes clinically apparent edema. Localized excess fluid may accumulate in the peritoneal and pleural cavities, giving rise to ascites and pleural effusion, respectively.

Pathogenesis

Renal sodium and water retention secondary to arterial underfilling leads to an alteration in capillary hemodynamics that favors fluid movement from the intravascular compartment into the interstitium. In general, these two processes account for edema formation.

Capillary Hemodynamic Disturbances

According to the Starling equation, the exchange of fluid between the plasma and the interstitium is determined by the hydrostatic and oncotic pressures in each compartment. Interstitial fluid excess results from a decrease in plasma oncotic pressure or an increase in capillary hydrostatic pressure. In other words, edema is a result of an increase of fluid movement from the intravascular compartment to the interstitial space, a decrease in fluid movement from the interstitial space to the intravascular compartment, or both. Thus, the degree of interstitial fluid accumulation as determined by the rate of fluid removal by the lymphatic vessels is a determinant of edema.

The capillary hydrostatic pressure is relatively insensitive to alterations in arterial pressure. The stability of the capillary pressure is due to variations in the precapillary sphincter, which governs how much arterial pressure is transmitted to the capillary, a response called autoregulation that is locally controlled. In contrast, the venous end is not similarly well regulated. Therefore, when the blood volume is expanded, such as in CHF and renal disease, capillary hydrostatic pressure increases and edema ensues. Venous obstruction works by the same mechanism to cause edema as exemplified, at least partially, by ascites formation in liver cirrhosis and by acute pulmonary edema after sudden impairment in cardiac function (as with myocardial infarction). In hepatic cirrhosis and nephrotic syndrome, another factor in edema formation is reduction in plasma oncotic pressure with a tendency for fluid transudation into the interstitial space. The balance of the Starling forces acting on the capillary favors the net filtration into the interstitium because capillary hydrostatic pressure exceeds the plasma colloid pressure, in several tissues, throughout the length of the capillary. In these tissues, a substantial amount of filtered fluid is returned to the circulation through lymphatics, which serve as a protective mechanism for minimizing edema formation.

Renal Sodium Retention

The mechanism for maintenance of ECF volume expansion and edema formation is renal sodium retention, which can be primary or secondary in response to reduction in EABV (Fig. 7.5).

Primary Renal Sodium Retention A primary defect in renal sodium excretion can occur with both acute and chronic renal failure and with glomerular disease. Patients with acute kidney injury have a limited ability to excrete sodium and water. Advanced chronic kidney disease may lead to sodium and water retention by GFR reduction secondary to a decrease in functioning nephrons. Some forms of glomerulonephritis are characterized by primary renal sodium retention. This happens by incompletely understood mechanisms in the presence of a relatively suppressed RAAS but frequently with a decreased GFR. States of mineralocorticoid excess or enhanced activity are associated with a phase of sodium retention. However, because of the phenomenon of "mineralocorticoid escape," the clinical manifestation is generally hypertension rather than hypervolemia. In normal subjects, administration of a high dose of mineralocorticoid initially increases renal sodium retention so that the volume of ECF is increased. However, renal sodium retention then ceases, spontaneous diuresis ensues, sodium balance is reestablished, and there is no detectable edema. This escape from mineralocorticoid-mediated sodium retention explains why edema is not a characteristic feature of primary hyperaldosteronism. The pathophysiologic mechanism of the mineralocorticoid escape phenomenon involves an increase in GFR and reduction of proximal tubular sodium and water reabsorption. This leads to an increase in sodium and water delivery to the distal nephron site of aldosterone action, which overrides the sodium reabsorption of aldosterone. Other mechanisms believed to account for this phenomenon involve decreased expression of distal tubular sodium transporters,[10] increased secretion of ANP induced by the hypervolemia,[11] and pressure natriuresis. Pressure natriuresis refers to the phenomenon whereby increasing renal perfusion pressure (due in part to systemic hypertension) enhances sodium excretion. These mechanisms act by decreasing tubular reabsorption at sites other than the aldosterone-sensitive cortical collecting duct.

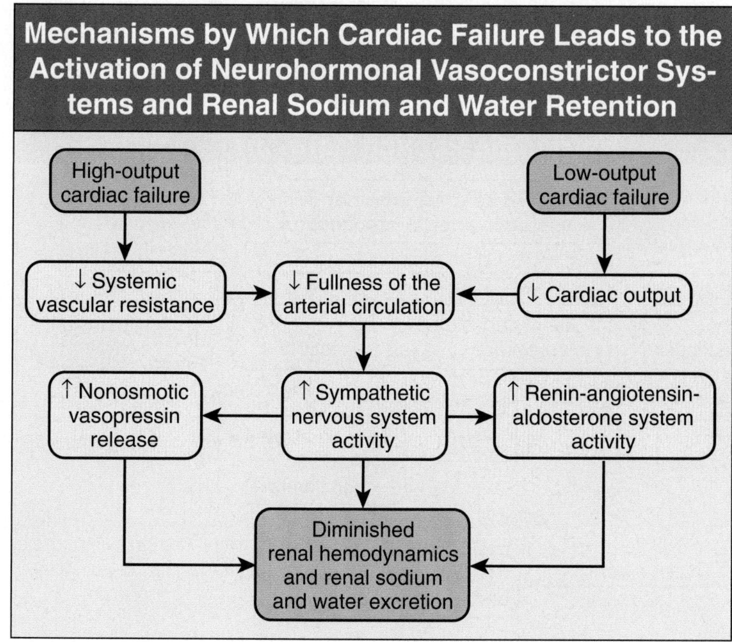

Figure 7.6 Mechanisms by which cardiac failure leads to the activation of neurohormonal vasoconstrictor systems and renal sodium and water retention. *(Modified from reference 12.)*

Renal Sodium Retention as a Compensatory Response to Effective Arterial Blood Volume Depletion (Arterial Underfilling)

PATHOPHYSIOLOGY OF ARTERIAL UNDERFILLING A unifying hypothesis elucidating the mechanisms by which the kidneys perceive arterial blood volume depletion and subsequently retain sodium and water in relevant clinical situations has been proposed and supported.[13] Estimates of blood volume distribution indicate that 85% of blood circulates on the low-pressure, venous side of the circulation, whereas an estimated 15% of blood is circulating in the high-pressure, arterial circulation. Thus, an increase in total blood volume could occur, even when there is underfilling of the arterial circulation, if the increase in total blood volume is primarily due to expansion of the venous compartment. Underfilling of the arterial circulation could occur secondary to either a decrease in cardiac output, as occurs in low-output cardiac failure, or systemic arterial vasodilation, which occurs early in cirrhosis as a result of diminished vascular resistance in the splanchnic circulation. This hypothesis proposes that the events triggered by arterial underfilling as a result of either a decrease in cardiac output or systemic arterial vasodilation (Fig. 7.6) are compensatory responses necessary to restore arterial circulatory integrity.

RENAL RESPONSE TO ARTERIAL UNDERFILLING If there is arterial underfilling, either due to a decrease in cardiac output or due to systemic arterial vasodilation, the underfilling is sensed by the arterial stretch receptors. This leads to activation of the efferent limb of body fluid volume homeostasis. Specifically, a decrease in glossopharyngeal and vagal tone from the carotid and aortic receptors to the CNS leads to a rapid increase in sympathetic activity with associated activation of the RAAS axis and nonosmotic release of vasopressin. The resultant increase in systemic vascular resistance and renal sodium and water retention attenuates the arterial underfilling and associated diminished arterial perfusion. The purpose of these concerted actions is to maintain the arterial circulatory integrity and restore the perfusion to the vital organs, which is mandatory for survival. Further discussion and explanation of how this mechanism operates in cardiac failure, cirrhosis, and pregnancy are now discussed.

Sodium and Water Retention in Cardiac Failure

The renal sodium and water retention that occurs in CHF involves several mediators.[14] Decreased cardiac output with arterial underfilling leads to reduced stretch of arterial baroreceptors. This results in increased sympathetic discharge from the CNS and resultant activation of the RAAS. Adrenergic stimulation and increased Ang II both activate receptors on the proximal tubular epithelium that enhance sodium reabsorption. The renal vasoconstriction of the glomerular efferent arteriole by Ang II in CHF also alters net Starling forces in the peritubular capillary in a direction to enhance sodium reabsorption.[15] Thus, angiotensin and α-adrenergic stimulation increase sodium reabsorption in the proximal tubule by a direct effect on the proximal tubule epithelium and secondarily by renal vasoconstriction. This subsequently leads to decreased sodium delivery to the collecting duct, which is the major site of action of aldosterone and the natriuretic peptides. CHF patients experience renal resistance to natriuretic effects of atrial and ventricular peptides. The resultant decreased sodium delivery to the distal nephron impairs the normal escape mechanism from the sodium-retaining effect of aldosterone and impairs the effect of natriuretic peptides; taken together, these effects explain at least partially why sodium retention and ECF expansion occur in CHF (Fig. 7.7). Accordingly, CHF patients have substantial natriuresis when spironolactone, a competitive mineralocorticoid receptor antagonist, is given in adequate doses to compete with increased endogenous aldosterone levels.[16]

Another outcome of the neurohumoral activation that occurs in cardiac failure is the baroreceptor-mediated nonosmotic release of AVP.[17] This nonosmotic AVP stimulation overrides the osmotic regulation of AVP and is the major factor leading to the hyponatremia associated with CHF.[18] AVP causes antidiuresis by activating vasopressin V_2 receptors on the basolateral surface of the principal cells in the collecting duct.[19] Activation of these receptors initiates a cascade of intracellular signaling events by means of the adenylyl cyclase–cyclic adenosine

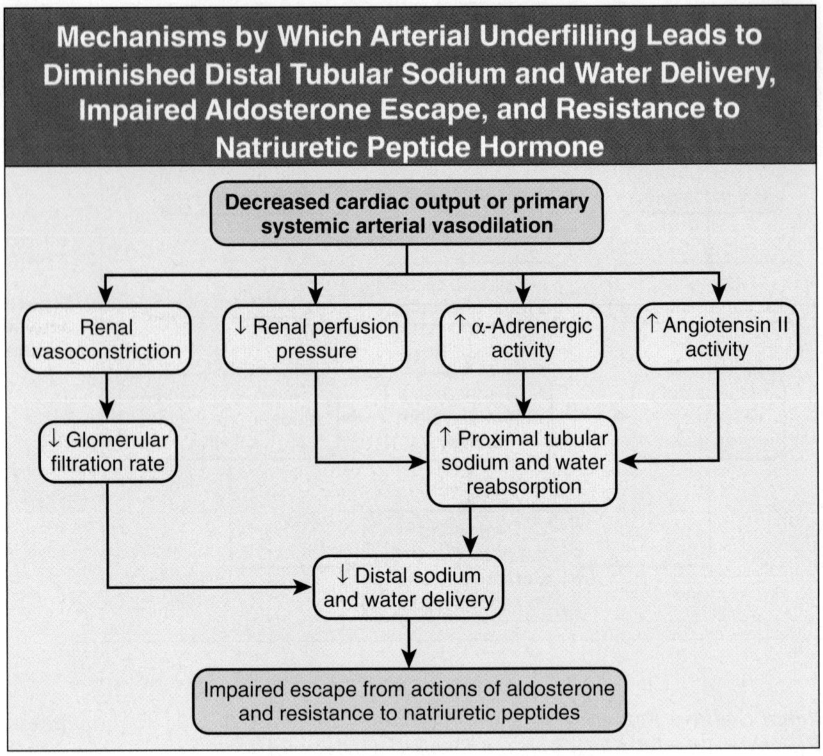

Mechanisms by Which Arterial Underfilling Leads to Diminished Distal Tubular Sodium and Water Delivery, Impaired Aldosterone Escape, and Resistance to Natriuretic Peptide Hormone

Decreased cardiac output or primary systemic arterial vasodilation

Renal vasoconstriction

↓ Renal perfusion pressure

↑ α-Adrenergic activity

↑ Angiotensin II activity

↓ Glomerular filtration rate

↑ Proximal tubular sodium and water reabsorption

↓ Distal sodium and water delivery

Impaired escape from actions of aldosterone and resistance to natriuretic peptides

Figure 7.7 Mechanisms by which arterial underfilling leads to diminished distal tubular sodium and water delivery, impaired aldosterone escape, and resistance to natriuretic peptide hormone. *(Modified from reference 21.)*

monophosphate pathway, leading to an increase in aquaporin 2 water channel protein expression and its trafficking to the apical membrane of the collecting duct. This sequence of events leads to increased water reabsorption and can cause hyponatremia, which is an ominous prognostic indicator in patients with heart failure.[20] Concurrently, increased nonosmotic AVP release stimulates V_1 receptors on vascular smooth muscle cells and thereby may increase systemic vascular resistance. This adaptive vasoconstrictive response may become maladaptive and contribute to cardiac dysfunction in patients with severe heart failure.

The atrial-renal reflexes, which normally enhance renal sodium excretion, are impaired during CHF because renal sodium and water retention occurs despite elevated atrial pressure. Moreover, in contrast to normal subjects, plasma levels of ANP were found not to increase further during a saline load in patients with dilated cardiomyopathy and mild heart failure, and the natriuretic response was also blunted. The attenuation of these reflexes on the low-pressure side of the circulation not only is attributable to a blunting of the atrial-renal reflexes but also may in part be caused by counteracting arterial baroreceptor-renal reflexes. Autonomic dysfunction and blunted arterial baroreceptor sensitivity in CHF occur and are associated with increased circulating catecholamines and increased renal sympathetic activity. There is also evidence for parasympathetic withdrawal in CHF in addition to the increase in sympathetic drive.

Sodium and Water Retention in Cirrhosis

In many aspects, there are similarities in the pathogenesis of sodium and water retention between cirrhosis and CHF (Fig. 7.8). The arterial underfilling in cirrhosis, however, occurs secondary to splanchnic arterial vasodilation, with resultant water and sodium retention. It is postulated that the initial event in ascites formation in cirrhotic patients is sinusoidal and portal hypertension.[22] In cirrhotic patients, this is a consequence of distortion of hepatic architecture, increased hepatic vascular tone, or increased splenohepatic flow. Decreased intrahepatic bioavailability of nitric oxide and increased production of vasoconstrictors such as angiotensin and endothelin also are responsible for increased resistance in the hepatic vasculature.[23] Portal hypertension due to increase in sinusoidal pressure activates vasodilatory mechanisms in the splanchnic circulation.[24] These mechanisms, mediated at least in part by nitric oxide and carbon monoxide overproduction, lead to splanchnic and peripheral arteriolar vasodilation. In advanced stages of cirrhosis, arteriolar vasodilation causes underfilling of the systemic arterial vascular space. This event, through a decrease in EABV, leads to a fall in arterial pressure. Consequently, baroreceptor-mediated activation of the RAAS, sympathetic nervous system stimulation, and nonosmotic release of antidiuretic hormone (ADH) occur to restore the normal blood volume homeostasis.[25] This involves compensatory vasoconstriction as well as renal sodium and water retention. However, splanchnic vasodilation also increases splanchnic lymph production, which exceeds the lymph transporting capacity, and thus lymph leakage into the peritoneal cavity occurs with ascites development.[26] Persistent renal sodium and water retention, along with increased splanchnic vascular permeability in addition to lymph leakage into the peritoneal cavity, plays the major role in a sustained ascites formation.

Sodium and Water Retention in Nephrotic Syndrome

Unlike CHF and liver cirrhosis, in which the kidneys are structurally normal, the nephrotic syndrome is characterized by diseased kidneys that are often functionally impaired. Nephrotic patients typically have a higher arterial blood pressure, higher GFR, and less impairment of sodium and water excretion than do patients with CHF and cirrhosis. Whereas edema is recognized as a major clinical manifestation of the nephrotic syndrome, its pathogenetic mechanism remains less clearly defined. Two possible explanations are the underfill and the overfill theories (Fig. 7.9). The underfill theory suggests that reduction in

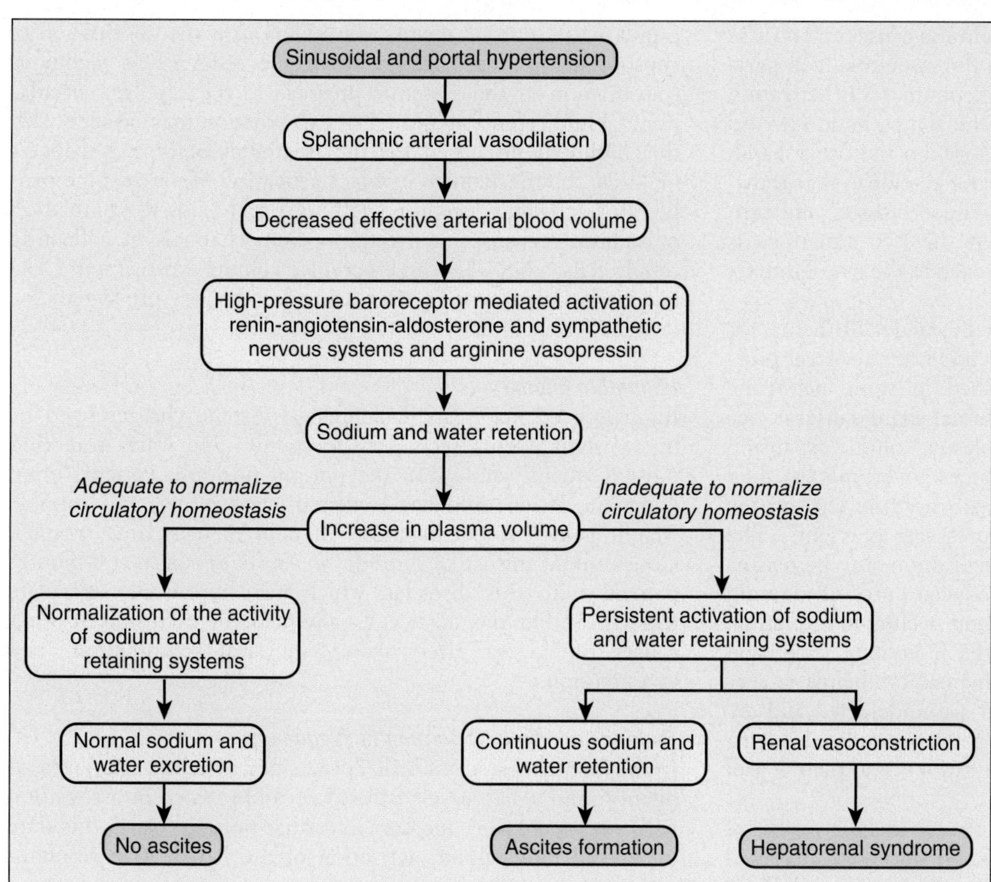

Figure 7.8 Pathogenesis of functional renal abnormalities and ascites formation in liver cirrhosis. *(Modified from reference 27.)*

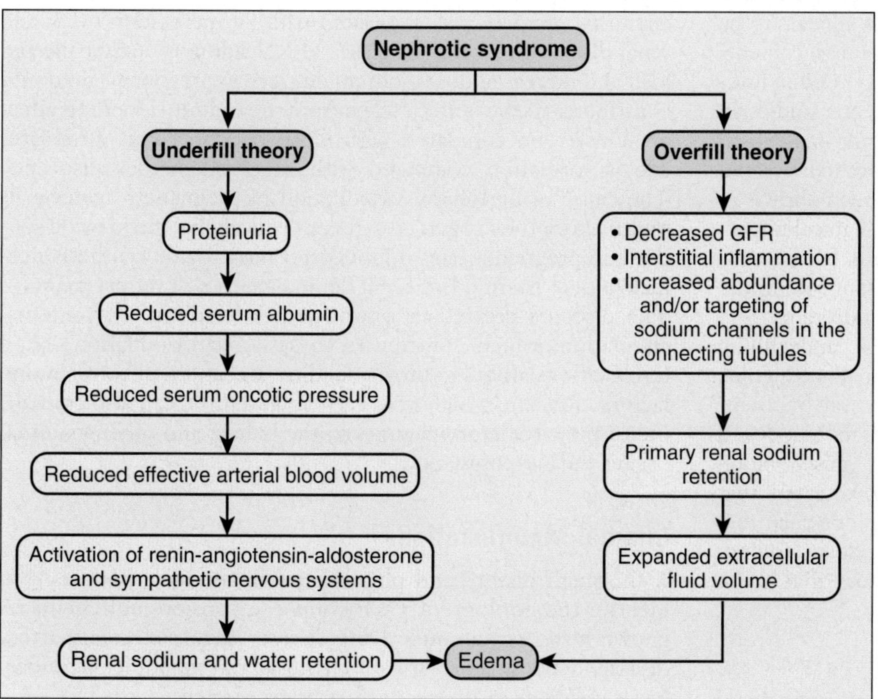

Figure 7.9 Pathogenesis of edema in the nephrotic syndrome.

the plasma oncotic pressure due to proteinuria causes an increase in fluid movement from the vascular to the interstitial compartment. The resultant arterial underfilling culminates in activation of homeostatic mechanisms involving the sympathetic nervous system and the RAAS. The overfill theory, on the other hand, implicates primary renal sodium and water retention that translates into elevated total plasma volume, hypertension, and suppressed RAAS. Distinguishing between the two situations is important because it influences the approach to the use of diuretics in nephrotic patients.

The following observations support the underfill theory for edema formation. Plasma volume, systemic arterial blood pressure, and cardiac output are diminished in some nephrotic patients, especially in children with minimal change disease (see Chapter 17), and can be corrected by plasma volume expansion with albumin infusion. The Starling forces governing the fluid movement across the capillary wall equal the difference of the hydrostatic pressure and the oncotic pressures gradients. The gradual fall in the plasma albumin concentration and the plasma oncotic pressure is mitigated by the reduced entry of albumin into the interstitial space and a concurrent decline in interstitial oncotic pressure. Consequently, less ECF volume expansion and edema formation is noted unless hypoalbuminemia is very severe.[28] Thus, nephrotic patients who are underfilled and are predisposed to acute kidney injury despite generalized edema generally have serum albumin concentrations less than 2 g/dl (20 g/l).

Observations supporting the overfill theory include studies of adults with minimal change disease (MCD) who have increased blood volume and blood pressure. After prednisone-induced remission, there are reductions in plasma volume and blood pressure decline with an increase in plasma renin activity. However, evaluation of intravascular volume is somewhat unreliable because the afferent stimulus for edema formation appears to be a dynamic process giving different results when measurements are taken at different phases of edema formation.[28] Other findings supporting primary renal sodium retention are studies in experimental animals with unilateral nephrotic syndrome, which demonstrate that sodium retention occurs secondary to increased reabsorption in the collecting tubules.[29] It has been shown in experimental animals that increased abundance and apical targeting of epithelial sodium channel (ENaC) subunits in the connecting tubule and collecting duct play an important role in the pathogenesis of sodium retention in nephrotic syndrome.[30]

In summary, nephrotic patients with arterial underfilling are more likely to have MCD with severe hypoalbuminemia, preserved GFR, and low blood pressure or postural hypotension. Other glomerular diseases are more often associated with an overfill picture with volume expansion, raised blood pressure, and a decline in GFR. It has been postulated that interstitial inflammatory cells, a feature of some glomerular diseases other than MCD, may facilitate an increase in sodium retention and hypertension by releasing mediators that cause vasoconstriction.[31]

Drug-Induced Edema

Ingestion of several types of drugs may generate peripheral edema. Systemic vasodilators such as minoxidil and diazoxide induce arterial underfilling and subsequent sodium with water retention, through mechanisms similar to those in CHF or cirrhosis. Dihydropyridine calcium channel blockers may cause peripheral edema, which is related to redistribution of fluid from the vascular space into the interstitium, possibly induced by capillary afferent sphincteric vasodilation in the absence of an appropriate microcirculatory myogenic reflex. This facilitates transmission of the systemic pressure to the capillary circulation.[32] Fluid retention and CHF exacerbation may be seen with thiazolidinediones, used for the treatment of type 2 diabetes mellitus; the mechanism involves activation of peroxisome proliferator-activated receptor γ (PPARγ) that leads to stimulation of sodium reabsorption by the sodium channels in collecting tubule cells.[33] NSAIDs can exacerbate volume expansion in CHF and cirrhotic patients by decreasing vasodilatory prostaglandins in the afferent arteriole of the glomerulus.

Idiopathic Edema

Idiopathic edema is an ill-defined syndrome characterized by intermittent edema secondary to sodium and water retention most frequently noted on the upright position. Patients often complain of face and hand edema, leg swelling, and variable weight gain.[34] It occurs most often in menstruating women. Concomitant misuse of diuretics or laxatives is also common in patients with this disorder, which may chronically stimulate the RAAS. The diagnosis is usually made by exclusion of other causes of edema after history, physical examination, and investigation.

Sodium and Water Retention in Pregnancy

In the first trimester of normal pregnancy, systemic arterial vasodilation and a decrease in blood pressure occur in association with a compensatory increase in cardiac output.[35] After this state of arterial underfilling, activation of the RAAS with resultant renal sodium and water retention occurs early in normal pregnancy. A decrease in plasma osmolality, stimulation of thirst, and persistent nonosmotic vasopressin release are other features of normal pregnancy. In contrast to disease states such as CHF and cirrhosis, pregnancy is associated with an increase in GFR and renal blood flow. The increased GFR, leading to higher filtered load and increased distal sodium delivery in pregnancy, no doubt contributes to the better escape from the sodium-retaining effect of aldosterone compared with CHF patients. This attenuates edema formation compared with other edematous disorders. The cause of peripheral vasodilation in pregnancy, however, is multifactorial. Estrogen upregulates endothelial nitric oxide synthase in pregnancy, and inhibitors of nitric oxide synthesis normalize the systemic and renal hemodynamics in rat pregnancy.[36] The placenta creates an arteriovenous fistula in the maternal circulation, which contributes to systemic vasodilation. High levels of vasodilating prostaglandins are another contributing factor.[37] Relaxin, which rises early in gestation, can also contribute to the circulatory changes in the kidney and other maternal organs during pregnancy.[38]

Clinical Manifestations

A thorough history and physical examination are important to identify the etiology of ECF volume expansion and edema. A known history of an underlying disease, such as coronary artery disease, hypertension, or liver cirrhosis, can pinpoint the underlying mechanism of edema formation. Patients with left-sided heart failure may present with exertional dyspnea, orthopnea, and paroxysmal nocturnal dyspnea; patients with right-sided heart failure or biventricular failure may exhibit weight gain and lower limb swelling. Physical examination reveals JVP elevation, pulmonary crackles, a third heart sound, or dependent peripheral edema that may be elicited in the ankles or sacrum.

Nephrotic patients classically present with periorbital edema because of their ability to lie flat during sleep. However, severe cases may exhibit marked generalized edema with anasarca. Cirrhotic patients present with ascites and lower limb edema consequent to portal hypertension and hypoalbuminemia. Physical examination may reveal stigmata of chronic liver disease and splenomegaly.

Diagnostic and Therapeutic Approach

Management of ECF volume expansion consists of recognizing and treating the underlying cause and attempting to achieve negative sodium balance by dietary sodium restriction and administration of diuretics. Before embarking on diuretic therapy in a congested patient, it is imperative to appreciate that ECF volume expansion may have occurred as a compensatory mechanism for arterial underfilling (e.g., in CHF and cirrhosis). Therefore, a judicious approach is necessary to avoid a precipitous fall in cardiac output and tissue perfusion. Rapid removal of excess fluid is generally necessary only in life-threatening situations, such as pulmonary edema and hypervolemia-induced hypertension, whereas a more gradual approach is warranted in less compromised patients.

Moderate dietary sodium restriction (2 to 3 g/day; 86 to 130 mmol/day) should be encouraged. If salt substitutes are used, it is important to consider that they contain potassium chloride, and therefore they should not be used for patients with advanced renal impairment or those who are concurrently taking potassium-sparing diuretics. Restriction of total fluid intake is usually necessary only for hyponatremic patients. Careful inquiry about concomitant medications that promote sodium restriction, such as NSAIDs, should be carried out, and they should be discontinued. Diuretics are the cornerstone of therapy to remove excess volume (see later discussion). Other measures can be employed when there is inadequate or lack of response to diuretics. In the case of liver cirrhosis, large-volume paracentesis with albumin infusion can be employed to remove large volumes of ascitic fluid. Interventional maneuvers to shunt ascitic fluid to a central vein can also be considered in refractory ascites, and they may result in improvement of the GFR and sodium excretion. Extracorporeal fluid removal by ultrafiltration can be used in patients with acute decompensated heart failure accompanied by renal insufficiency or diuretic resistance. Angiotensin-converting enzyme (ACE) inhibitors and angiotensin receptor blockers (ARBs) are adjunctive disease-modifying agents in cases of CHF and nephrotic syndrome. Additional aggressive therapies for cardiac failure include antiarrhythmic agents, positive inotropes, and mechanical assist devices such as intra-aortic balloon pump.

The treatment of suspected diuretic-induced edema, which is associated with persistent secondary hyperaldosteronism, is to withdraw diuretics for 3 to 4 weeks after warning the patient that edema may worsen initially. If the edema does not improve after 4 weeks, spironolactone can be instituted at a dose of 50 to 100 mg daily and increased to a maximum of 400 mg daily.

Diuretics

Principles of Action

Diuretics are the mainstay of therapy for edematous states. Diuretics can be classified into five classes on the basis of their predominant sites of action along the nephron (Fig. 7.10). As a group, most diuretics reach their luminal transport sites through tubular fluid secretion. All but osmotic agents have a high degree of protein binding, which limits glomerular filtration, traps them in the vascular spaces, and allows them to be delivered to the proximal convoluted tubule for secretion.[39] They act by inhibiting sodium reabsorption with an accompanying anion that is usually chloride. The resultant natriuresis decreases the ECF. In spite of the fact that administration of a diuretic causes a sustained net deficit in total body sodium, the time course of natriuresis is limited because renal mechanisms attenuate the sodium excretion. This phenomenon is known as diuretic braking, and its mechanism includes activation of the sympathetic nervous and RAAS systems, decreased systemic and renal arterial blood pressure, hypertrophy of the distal nephron cells with increased expression of epithelial transporters, and perhaps alterations in natriuretic hormones such as ANP.[41]

Adverse Effects

Many of the commonly used diuretics are derived from sulfanilamide and may therefore induce allergy in susceptible patients manifested as hypersensitivity reactions, usually as a rash or rarely acute interstitial nephritis. The most serious adverse effects of diuretics are electrolyte disturbances. By blocking sodium reabsorption in the loop of Henle and the distal tubule, loop and thiazide diuretics cause natriuresis and increased distal sodium delivery. The resultant negative sodium balance activates the RAAS. The effect of aldosterone to enhance distal potassium and hydrogen excretion can lead to hypokalemia and metabolic alkalosis. Patients should therefore be monitored, and oral supplementation or addition of a potassium-sparing diuretic may need to be considered. Loop diuretics impair tubular reabsorption by abolishing the transepithelial potential gradient and thus increase excretion of magnesium and calcium. Thiazide diuretics exert the same effect on magnesium, but contrary to loop diuretics, they decrease urinary calcium losses and are therefore preferred in the treatment of hypercalciuric states and in subjects with osteoporosis. Thiazide diuretics interfere with urine diluting mechanisms by blocking sodium reabsorption at the distal convoluted tubule, an effect that may pose a risk of hyponatremia. Acutely, loop and thiazide diuretics increase the excretion of uric acid, whereas chronic administration results in reduced uric acid excretion. The chronic effect may be due to enhanced transport in the proximal convoluted tubule secondary to volume depletion, leading to increased uric acid reabsorption, or competition between the diuretic and uric acid for secretion in the proximal tubule, leading to reduced uric acid secretion. Other adverse effects that may occur with large doses include ototoxicity with loop diuretics, particularly when an aminoglycoside is coadministered, and gynecomastia that may develop with spironolactone.

Diuretic Tolerance and Resistance

Long-term loop diuretic tolerance refers to the resistance of their action as a consequence of distal nephron segment hypertrophy and enhanced sodium reabsorption that follows increased exposure to solutes not absorbed proximally.[39] This problem can be addressed by combining loop and thiazide diuretics as the latter block those responsible distal nephron sites. Diuretic resistance refers to edema that is or has become refractory to a given diuretic. An algorithm for diuretic therapy in patients with edema caused by renal, hepatic, or cardiac disease is outlined in Figure 7.11. Diuretic resistance can be due to several causes. Chronic kidney disease is associated with a decreased tubular delivery and secretion of diuretics, which subsequently reduces their concentration at the active site in the tubular lumen. In

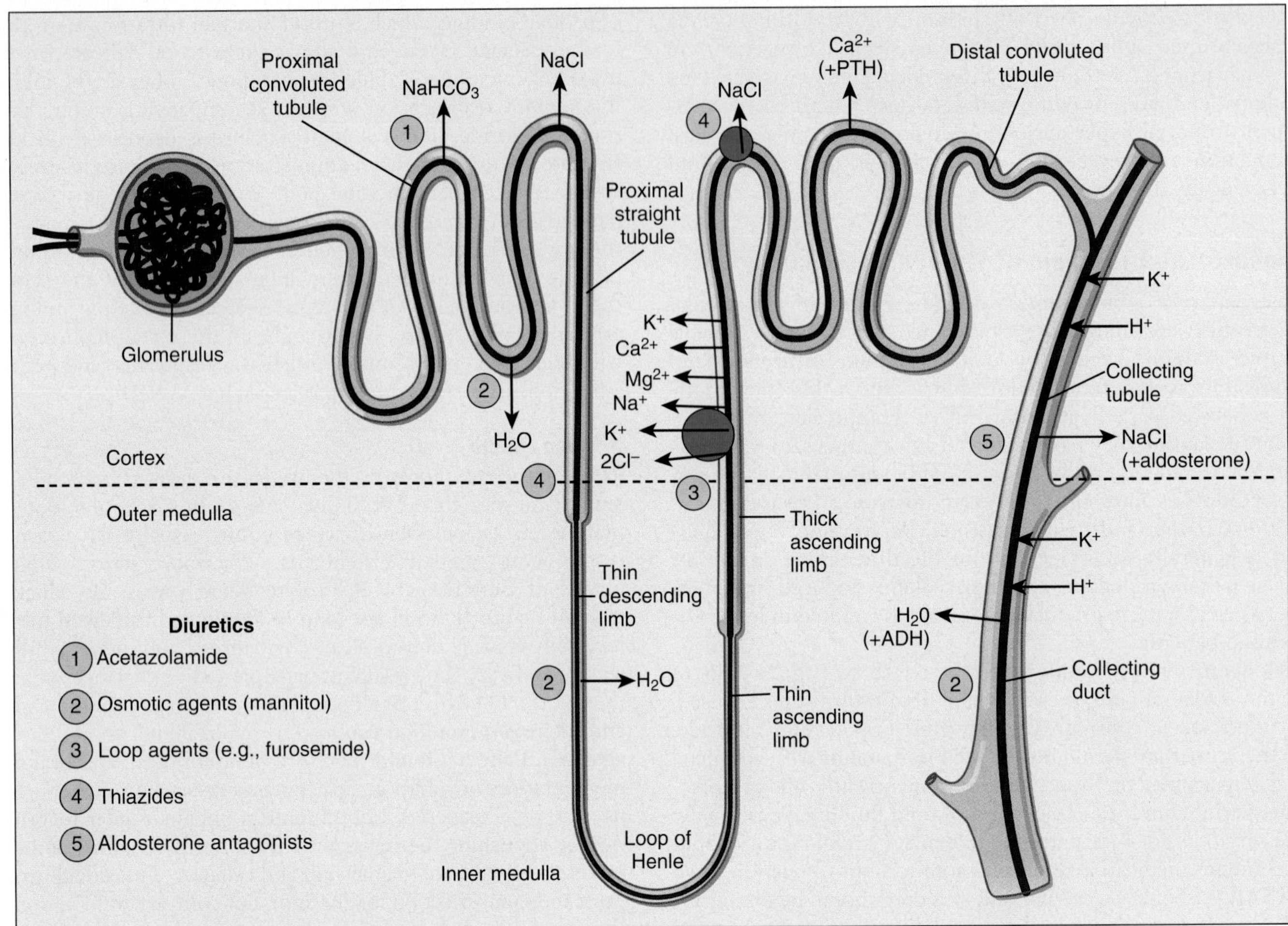

Figure 7.10 Tubule transport systems and sites of action of diuretics. *(Modified from reference 40.)*

nephrotic syndrome, it was once thought that the high protein content of tubular fluid increases protein binding of furosemide and other loop diuretics and therefore inhibits their action. However, recent data suggest that urinary protein binding does not affect the response to furosemide.[42] As explained earlier, arterial underfilling that takes place in cirrhosis and CHF is associated with diminished nephron responsiveness to diuretics because of increased proximal tubular sodium reabsorption, leading to decreased delivery of sodium to the distal nephron segment sites of diuretic action. NSAIDs block prostaglandin-mediated increases in renal blood flow and increase the expression of the sodium-potassium-chloride cotransporters in the thick ascending limb.

Salt restriction is the key approach to lessening postdiuretic sodium retention. Further approaches to antagonize diuretic resistance include increasing the dose of loop diuretic, administering more frequent doses, and using combination therapy to sequentially block more than one site in the nephron as that may result in a synergistic interaction between diuretics. Highly resistant edematous patients may be treated with ultrafiltration.

Loop Diuretics

This group includes furosemide, bumetanide, torsemide, and ethacrynic acid. They act by blocking the sodium-potassium-chloride cotransporters at the apical surface of the thick ascending limb cells, thereby diminishing net reabsorption. Loop diuretics are the most potent of all diuretics because of a combination of two factors. They are able to inhibit the reabsorption of 25% of filtered sodium that normally takes place at the thick ascending limb of the loop of Henle. Moreover, the nephron segment past the thick ascending limb does not possess the capacity to reabsorb completely the volume of fluid exiting the thick ascending limb. The oral bioavailability of furosemide varies between 10% and 100%; that of bumetanide and torsemide is comparatively higher. As a class, loop diuretics have short elimination half-lives, and consequently the dosing interval needs to be short to maintain adequate levels in the lumen. Excessive prolongation of dosing interval may lead to avid sodium reabsorption by the nephron, which may result in post-diuretic sodium retention.

The intrinsic potency of a diuretic is defined by its dose-response curve, which is generally sigmoid. The steep dose-response is the reason that loop diuretics are often referred to as threshold drugs. This is exemplified by furosemide, which can initiate diuresis in a subject with normal renal function with an intravenous dose of 10 mg, and a maximal effect is seen with 40 mg. Above this dose, little or no extra benefit occurs and side effects may increase. Furthermore, the effective diuretic dose is higher in patients with CHF, advanced cirrhosis, and renal failure (Fig. 7.12). In patients who have poor responses to intermittent doses of a loop diuretic, a continuous intravenous infusion can be tried; this enhances the response by virtue of maintaining an effective amount of the drug at the site of action.[43] The benefit of continuous infusion, however, was not confirmed

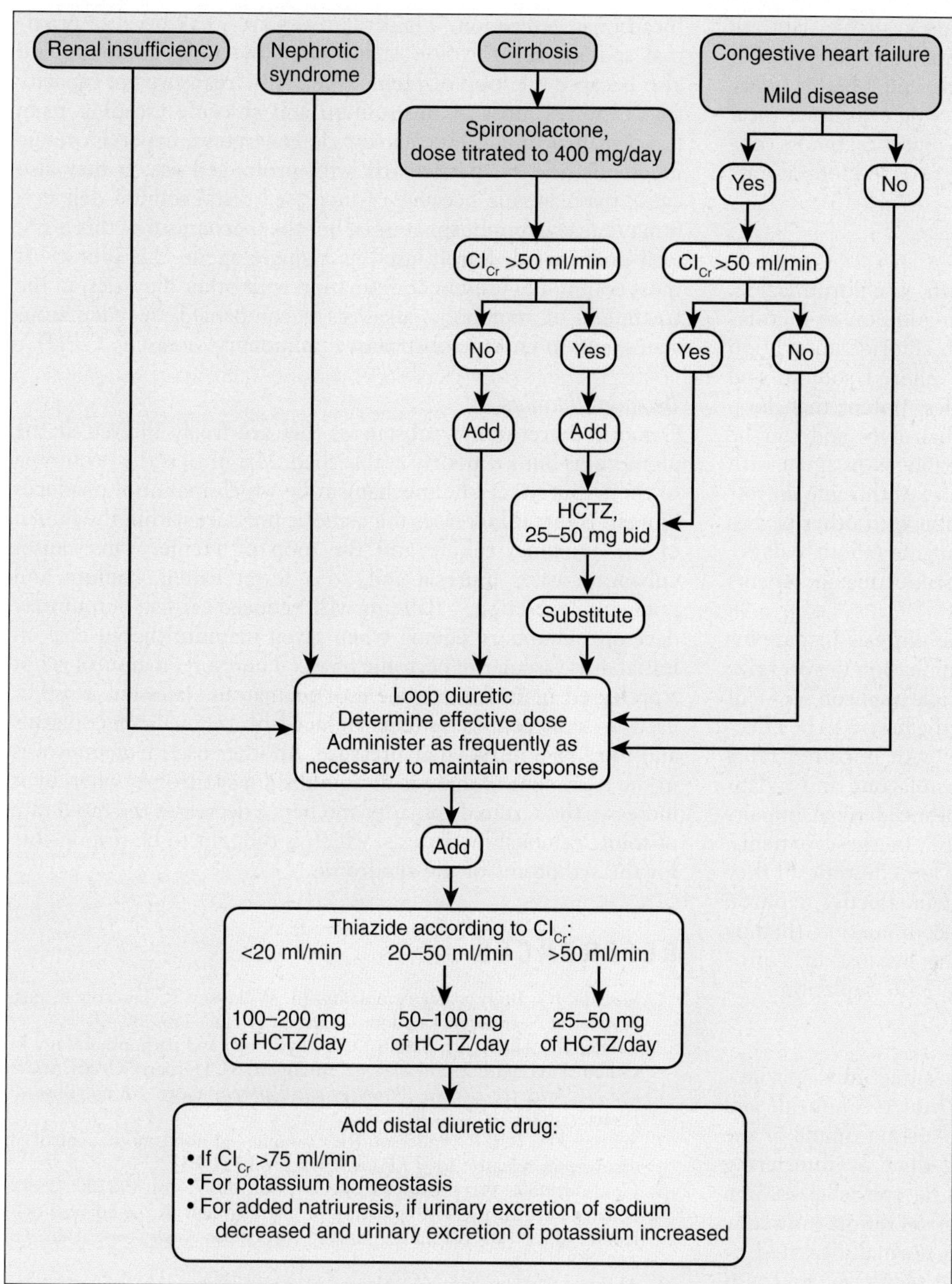

Figure 7.11 Algorithm for diuretic therapy in patients with edema caused by renal, hepatic, or cardiac disease. HCTZ, hydrochlorothiazide. *(Modified with permission from reference 39.)*

	Renal Insufficiency				Preserved Renal Function					
	Moderate		Severe		Nephrotic Syndrome		Cirrhosis		Congestive Heart Failure	
	PO	IV	PO	IV	PO	IV	PO	IV	PO	IV
Furosemide	80–160	80	240	200	240	120	80–160	40–80	160–240	40–80
Bumetanide	2–3	2–3	8–10	8–10	3	3	1–2	1	2–3	2–3
Torsemide	50	50	100	100	50	50	10–20	10–20	50	20–50

Figure 7.12 Therapeutic regimens for loop diuretics. *(Modified from reference 45.)*

in a Cochrane review, which concluded that available data are insufficient to confidently assess the merits of each approach (bolus or continuous) despite greater diuresis and a better safety profile of the continuous infusion.[44] Ethacrynic acid has typical pharmacologic characteristics of other loop diuretics, but its ototoxic potential is greater, and it is therefore reserved for patients allergic to other loop diuretics.

Distal Convoluted Tubule Diuretics

This group includes thiazide diuretics such as chlorothiazide, hydrochlorothiazide, and chlorthalidone in addition to metolazone and indapamide. They inhibit sodium chloride absorption in the distal tubule, where up to 5% of filtered sodium and chloride is reabsorbed, and are therefore less potent than loop diuretics. Thiazides have relatively long half-lives and can be administered once or twice per day. Metolazone is an agent with pharmacologic characteristics similar to those of thiazide diuretics. It is more commonly used in conjunction with other classes of diuretics. It has a longer elimination half-life (about 2 days); therefore, more rapidly acting and predictable thiazide agents may be preferred.

Thiazides may be used alone to induce diuresis in patients with mild CHF but more commonly in combination to synergize the effect of loop diuretics by blocking multiple nephron segment sites. Because thiazide diuretics must reach the lumen to be effective, higher doses are required in patients with impaired renal function. Thiazides (possibly excluding metolazone and indapamide) are ineffective in patients with advanced renal impairment (GFR is less than 30 to 40 ml/min). In these patients, thiazides can enhance the diuretic effect of loop diuretics if they are coadministered in sufficient doses to attain effective nephron lumen concentration. If it is used, such combination therapy should be initiated under close monitoring because of a pronounced risk of hypokalemia and excessive ECF depletion.

Collecting Duct Diuretics

Amiloride, triamterene, and the aldosterone antagonists spironolactone and eplerenone act on the collecting duct. Amiloride and triamterene act primarily in the cortical collecting tubule or the connecting tubule and cortical collecting duct by interfering with sodium reabsorption through the apical epithelial sodium channels (ENaC). They inhibit potassium secretion indirectly by dissipating the electronegative gradient normally created by sodium reabsorption that favors potassium secretion. Spironolactone and eplerenone are competitive antagonists of aldosterone and cause natriuresis and potassium retention. Potassium-sparing diuretics are considered to be weak diuretics because they block only a small part (about 3%) of the filtered sodium load reaching their site of action. Hence, they are most commonly used in combination with other diuretics to augment diuresis or to preserve potassium. Nevertheless, careful monitoring is essential if combinations therapy is employed to prevent dangerous hyperkalemia. Most vulnerable patients include those with underlying renal dysfunction, those with CHF, diabetic patients, and those concurrently taking ACE inhibitors, ARBs, NSAIDs, and β-blockers. Collecting duct diuretics are considered first-line agents in certain conditions, for example, spironolactone in liver cirrhosis with ascites and amiloride in the treatment of Liddle syndrome.

Proximal Tubule Diuretics

Acetazolamide is the prototype and acts by blocking the activity of the sodium-hydrogen ion exchanger, thus increasing sodium bicarbonate excretion. These diuretics are weak because proximal sodium reabsorption is mediated by other pathways and also because the loop of Henle has a large reabsorptive capacity that captures most of the sodium and chloride escaping from the proximal tubule. Acetazolamide generates a hyperchloremic metabolic acidosis particularly with prolonged use. It may also cause hypokalemia because of increased distal sodium delivery; it may cause hypophosphatemia, but the mechanism of this is not well understood. Rarely used as a single agent, this diuretic is most commonly used in combination with other diuretics, in the treatment of metabolic alkalosis accompanied by edematous states, and in chronic obstructive pulmonary disease (COPD).

Osmotic Diuretics

Osmotic diuretics are substances that are freely filtered at the glomerulus but are poorly reabsorbed. Mannitol is the prototype of these diuretics. The mechanism by which mannitol produces diuresis is that it increases the osmotic pressure within the lumen of the proximal tubule and the loop of Henle. This causes enhanced water diuresis and, to a lesser extent, sodium and potassium excretion.[46] Patients with reduced cardiac output may develop pulmonary edema when given mannitol because of an initial intravascular hypertonic phase. Therefore, mannitol is not a preferred agent for treatment of edematous states but is rather used to treat cerebral edema induced by trauma or neoplasms and to reduce intraocular pressure. Another use for mannitol is in the treatment of dialysis disequilibrium syndrome, whereby it increases the serum osmolality and hence decreases the rapid rate of solute removal by dialysis, which is thought to be responsible for the symptoms of the syndrome.

REFERENCES

1. Verbalis JG. Body water osmolality. In: Wilkinson R, Jamison R, eds. *Textbook of Nephrology*. London: Chapman & Hall; 1997:89-94.
2. Palmer BF, Alpern RJ, Seldin DW. Physiology and pathophysiology of sodium and retention and wastage. In: Alpern RJ, Herbert SC, eds. *Seldin and Giebisch's the Kidney: Physiology and Pathophysiology*. 4th ed. Boston: Elsevier; 2008:1005-1049.
3. Schrier RW, Berl T, Anderson RJ. Osmotic and nonosmotic control of vasopressin release. *Am J Physiol*. 1979;236:F321-F332.
4. Goldsmith SR. Vasopressin as a vasopressor. *Am J Med*. 1987;82:1213.
5. Schafer JA, Hawk CT. Regulation of Na^+ channels in the cortical collecting duct by AVP and mineralocorticoids. *Kidney Int*. 1992;41:255-268.
6. Akabane S, Matsushima Y, Matsuo H, et al. Effects of brain natriuretic peptide on renin secretion in normal and hypertonic saline–infused kidney. *Eur J Pharmacol*. 1991;198:143-148.
7. O'Shaughnessy KM, Karet FE. Salt handling and hypertension. *J Clin Invest*. 2004;113:1075-1081.
8. Wilkes MM, Navickis RJ. Patient survival after human albumin administration. A meta-analysis of randomized, controlled trials. *Ann Intern Med*. 2001;135:149-164.
9. Finfer S, Bellomo R, Boyce N, et al. A comparison of albumin and saline for fluid resuscitation in the intensive care unit. *N Engl J Med*. 2004;350:2247.
10. Wang XY, Masilamani S, Nielsen J, et al. The renal thiazide-sensitive Na-Cl cotransporter as mediator of the aldosterone-escape phenomenon. *J Clin Invest*. 2001;108:215-222.
11. Yokota N, Bruneau BG, Kuroski de Bold ML, de Bold AJ. Atrial natriuretic factor significantly contributes to the mineralocorticoid escape phenomenon. Evidence for a guanylate cyclase–mediated pathway. *J Clin Invest*. 1994;94:1938-1946.
12. Schrier RW, Abraham WT. Hormones and hemodynamics in heart failure. *N Engl J Med*. 1999;341:577-585.
13. Schrier RW. Body fluid volume regulation in health and disease: A unifying hypothesis. *Ann Intern Med*. 1990;113:155-159.
14. Schrier RW. Role of diminished renal function in cardiovascular mortality: Marker or pathogenetic factor? *J Am Coll Cardiol*. 2006;47:1-8.

15. Schrier RW, deWardener HE. Tubular reabsorption of sodium ion: Influence of factors other than aldosterone and glomerular filtration rate. *N Engl J Med*. 1971;285:1231-1242.
16. Hensen J, Abraham WT, Dürr J, Schrier RW. Aldosterone in congestive heart failure: Analysis of determinants and role in sodium retention. *Am J Nephrol*. 1991;11:441-446.
17. Schrier RW, Berl T. Nonosmolar factors affecting renal water excretion (first of two parts). *N Engl J Med*. 1975;292:81-88.
18. Szatalowicz VL, Arnold PE, Chaimovitz C, et al. Radioimmunoassay of plasma arginine vasopressin in hyponatremic patients with congestive heart failure. *N Engl J Med*. 1981;305:263-266.
19. Seibold A, Rosenthal W, Barberis C, Birnbaumer M. Cloning of the human type-2 vasopressin receptor gene. *Ann N Y Acad Sci*. 1993;689: 570-572.
20. Lee WH, Packer M. Prognostic importance of serum sodium concentration and its modification by converting-enzyme inhibition in patients with severe chronic heart failure. *Circulation*. 1986;73:257-267.
21. Schrier RW, Abraham WT. Hormones and hemodynamics in heart failure. *N Engl J Med*. 1999;341:577-585.
22. Ginès P, Schrier RW. Renal failure in cirrhosis. *N Engl J Med*. 2009;361:1279-1290.
23. Hernandez-Guerra M, Garcia-Pagan JC, Bosch J. Increased hepatic resistance: A new target in the pharmacologic therapy of portal hypertension. *J Clin Gastroenterol*. 2005;39:131-137.
24. Ginès P, Cardenas A, Arroyo V, Rodes J. Management of cirrhosis and ascites. *N Engl J Med*. 2004;350:1646-1654.
25. Schrier RW, Arroyo V, Bernardi M, et al. Peripheral arterial vasodilation hypothesis: A proposal for the initiation of renal sodium and water retention in cirrhosis. *Hepatology*. 1988;8:1151-1157.
26. Arroyo V, Ginès P, Gerbes AL, et al. Definition and diagnostic criteria of refractory ascites and hepatorenal syndrome in cirrhosis. International Ascites Club. *Hepatology*. 1996; 23:164-176.
27. Ginès P, Cardenas A, Schrier RW. Liver disease and the kidney. In: Schrier RW, ed. *Diseases of the Kidney and Urinary Tract*. 8th ed. Philadelphia: Lippincott Williams & Wilkins; 2006:2194.
28. Koomans HA, Kortlandt W, Geers AB, Dorhout Mees EJ. Lowered protein content of tissue fluid in patients with the nephrotic syndrome: Observations during disease and recovery. *Nephron*. 1985;40:391.
29. Ichikawa I, Rennke HG, Hoyer JR, et al. Role for intrarenal mechanisms in the impaired salt excretion of experimental nephrotic syndrome. *J Clin Invest*. 1983;71:91.
30. Kim SW, Frøkiaer J, Nielsen S. Pathogenesis of oedema in nephrotic syndrome: Role of epithelial sodium channel. *Nephrology (Carlton)*. 2007;12(Suppl 3):S8-S10.
31. Rodriguez-Iturbe B, Herrera-Acosta J, Johnson RJ. Interstitial inflammation, sodium retention, and the pathogenesis of nephrotic edema: A unifying hypothesis. *Kidney Int*. 2002;62:1379.
32. Gustafsson DJ. Microvascular mechanisms involved in calcium antagonist edema formation. *Cardiovasc Pharmacol*. 1987;10(Suppl 1):S121-S131.
33. Guan Y, Hao C, Cha DR, et al. Thiazolidinediones expand body fluid volume through PPARγ stimulation of ENaC-mediated renal salt absorption. *Nat Med*. 2005;11:861.
34. Streeten DH. Idiopathic edema. Pathogenesis, clinical features, and treatment. *Endocrinol Metab Clin North Am*. 1995;24:531-547.
35. Chapman AB, Abraham WT, Zamudio S, et al. Temporal relationships between hormonal and hemodynamic changes in early human pregnancy. *Kidney Int*. 1988;54:2056-2063.
36. Cadnapaphornchai MA, Ohara M, Morris KG, et al. Chronic nitric oxide synthase inhibition reverses systemic vasodilation and glomerular hyperfiltration in pregnancy. *Am J Physiol Renal Physiol*. 2001;280:F592-F598.
37. Whalen JB, Clancey CJ, Farley DB, Van Orden DE. Plasma prostaglandins in pregnancy. *Obstet Gynecol*. 1978;51:52-55.
38. Conrad KP, Jeyabalan A, Danielson LA, et al. Role of relaxin in maternal renal vasodilation of pregnancy. *Ann N Y Acad Sci*. 2005;1041:147-154.
39. Brater DC. Diuretic therapy. *N Engl J Med*. 1998;339:387-395.
40. Ives HE. Diuretic agents. In: Katzung BG, ed. *Basic and Clinical Pharmacology*. 10th ed. Columbus, Ohio: McGraw-Hill Medical; 2006:237.
41. Jackson EK. Diuretics. In: Brunton LL, ed. *Goodman & Gilman's the Pharmacological Basis of Therapeutics*. 11th ed. New York: McGraw-Hill; 2006: ebook accessed June 10, 2010 Chapter 28, Section V.
42. Agarwal R, Gorski JC, Sundblad K, Brater DC. Urinary protein binding does not affect response to furosemide in patients with nephrotic syndrome. *J Am Soc Nephrol*. 2000;11:1100-1105.
43. Rudy DW, Voelker JR, Greene PK, et al. Loop diuretics for chronic renal insufficiency: A continuous infusion is more efficacious than bolus therapy. *Ann Intern Med*. 1991;115:360-366.
44. Salvador D, Rey N, Ramos G, Punzalan F. Continuous infusion versus bolus injection of loop diuretics in congestive heart failure. Cochrane Database Syst Rev. 2004;1:CD003178.
45. Ellison D, Schrier RW. The edematous patient, cardiac failure, cirrhosis, and nephrotic syndrome. In: Schrier RW, ed. *Manual of Nephrology*. 6th ed. Philadelphia: Lippincott Williams & Wilkins; 2005:8.
46. Seely JF, Dirks JH. Micropuncture study of hypertonic mannitol diuresis in the proximal and distal tubule of the dog kidney. *J Clin Invest*. 1969;48:2330-2340.

CHAPTER 8

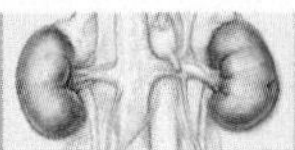

Disorders of Water Metabolism

Chirag Parikh, Tomas Berl

PHYSIOLOGY OF WATER BALANCE

The maintenance of the tonicity of body fluids within a narrow physiologic range is made possible by homeostatic mechanisms that control the intake and excretion of water. Vasopressin (also known as arginine vasopressin [AVP] or antidiuretic hormone [ADH]) governs the excretion of water by its effect on the renal collecting system. Osmoreceptors located in the hypothalamus control the secretion of vasopressin in response to changes in tonicity.

In the steady state, water intake matches water losses. Water intake is regulated by the need to maintain a physiologic serum osmolality of 285 to 290 mOsm/kg. Despite major fluctuations of solute and water intake, the total solute concentration (i.e., the tonicity) of body fluids is maintained virtually constant. The ability to dilute and to concentrate the urine allows a wide flexibility in urine flow (see Chapter 2). During water loading, the diluting mechanisms permit excretion of 20 to 25 liters of urine per day, and during water deprivation, the urine volume may be as low as 0.5 liter per day.[1,3]

VASOPRESSIN

Vasopressin plays a critical role in determining the concentration of urine. It is a cyclic peptide (1099 d) and is synthesized and secreted by the specialized supraoptic and paraventricular magnocellular nuclei in the hypothalamus. Vasopressin has a short half-life of about 15 to 20 minutes and is rapidly metabolized in the liver and the kidney.

Osmotic Stimuli for Vasopressin Release

Substances that are restricted to the extracellular fluid (ECF), such as hypertonic saline and mannitol, decrease cell volume by acting as effective osmoles and enhancing osmotic water movement from the cell. This stimulates vasopressin release; in contrast, urea and glucose cross cell membranes and do not cause any change in cell volume. The "osmoreceptor" cells, located close to the supraoptic nuclei in the anterior hypothalamus, are sensitive to changes in plasma osmolality as small as 1%. In humans, the osmotic threshold for vasopressin release is 280 to 290 mOsm/kg (Fig. 8.1). This system is so efficient that plasma osmolality usually does not vary by more than 1% to 2% despite wide fluctuations in water intake.

Nonosmotic Stimuli for Vasopressin Release

There are several other nonosmotic stimuli for vasopressin secretion. Decreased effective circulating volume (e.g., heart failure, cirrhosis, vomiting) causes discharge from parasympathetic afferent nerves in the carotid sinus baroreceptors and increases vasopressin secretion. Other nonosmotic stimuli include nausea, postoperative pain, and pregnancy. Much higher vasopressin levels can be achieved with hypovolemia than with hyperosmolality, although a large (7%) decrease in blood volume is required before this response is initiated.

Mechanism of Vasopressin Action

Vasopressin binds three types of receptors coupled to G proteins: the V_{1a} (vascular and hepatic), V_{1b} (anterior pituitary), and V_2 receptors. The V_2 receptor is primarily localized in the collecting duct and leads to an increase in water permeability (Fig. 8.2) through aquaporin 2 (AQP2), which is a member of a family of cellular water transporters.[4] AQP1 is localized in the apical and basolateral region of the proximal tubule epithelial cells and the descending limb of Henle and accounts for the high water permeability of these nephron segments. Because AQP1 is constitutively expressed, it is not subject to regulation by vasopressin. In contrast, AQP2 is found exclusively in apical plasma membranes and intracellular vesicles in the collecting duct principal cells. Vasopressin affects both the short- and long-term regulation of AQP2. The short-term regulation, also described as the shuttle hypothesis, explains the rapid and reversible increase (within minutes) in collecting duct water permeability that follows vasopressin administration. This involves the insertion of water channels from subapical vesicles into the luminal membrane. Long-term regulation involves vasopressin-mediated increased transcription of genes involved in AQP2 production and occurs if circulating vasopressin levels are elevated for 24 hours or more. The maximal water permeability of the collecting duct epithelium is increased as a consequence of an increase in the total number of AQP2 channels per cell. This process is not readily reversible.

AQP3 and AQP4 are located on the basolateral membranes of the collecting duct (see Fig. 8.2) and are probably involved in water exit from the cell. AQP3 is also urea permeable and under the stimulus of vasopressin increases the permeability of the collecting duct to urea, resulting in its movement into the interstitium. AQP4 is also in the hypothalamus and is a candidate osmoreceptor for the control of vasopressin release.

THIRST AND WATER BALANCE

Hypertonicity is the most potent stimulus for thirst, with a change of only 2% to 3% in plasma osmolality producing a strong desire to drink water. The osmotic threshold for thirst usually occurs at 290 to 295 mOsm/kg H_2O and is above the threshold for vasopressin release (see Fig. 8.1). It closely approximates the level at which maximal concentration of urine is achieved. Hypovolemia, hypotension, and angiotensin II (ANG II) are also stimuli for thirst. Between the limits imposed by the osmotic thresholds for thirst and vasopressin release, plasma osmolality may be regulated more precisely by small, osmoregulated adjustments in urine flow and water intake. The exact level at which balance occurs depends on various factors, for example, insensible losses through skin and lungs, the gains incurred from drinking water and eating, and water generated from metabolism. In general, overall intake and output come into balance at a plasma osmolality of 288 mOsm/kg.

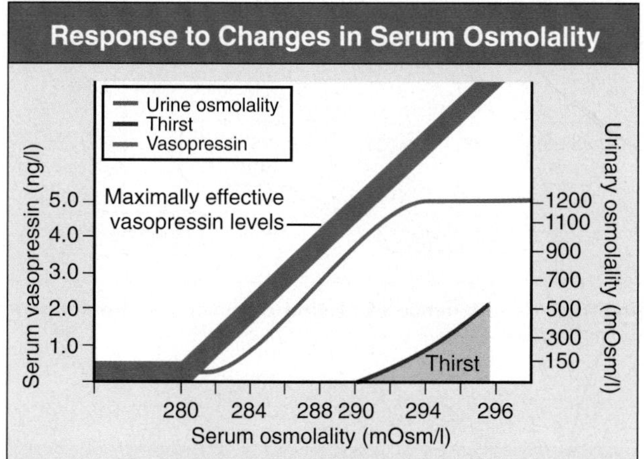

Figure 8.1 Mechanisms maintaining plasma osmolality. The response of thirst, vasopressin levels, and urinary osmolality to changes in serum osmolality. *(Modified from reference 2.)*

QUANTITATION OF RENAL WATER EXCRETION

Urine volume can be considered as having two components. The osmolar clearance (C_{osm}) is the volume needed to excrete solutes at the concentration of solutes in plasma. The free water clearance (C_{water}) is the volume of water that has been added to (positive C_{water}) or subtracted from (negative C_{water}) isotonic urine (C_{osm}) to create either hypotonic or hypertonic urine.

Urine volume flow (V) comprises the isotonic portion of urine (C_{osm}) plus the free water clearance (C_{water}).

$$V = C_{osm} + C_{water}$$

and, therefore,

$$C_{water} = V - C_{osm}$$

The term C_{osm} relates urine osmolality to plasma osmolality P_{osm} by

$$C_{osm} = \left(\frac{U_{osm} \times V}{P_{osm}}\right)$$

Therefore,

$$C_{water} = V - \left(\frac{U_{osm} \times V}{P_{osm}}\right) = V\left(1 - \frac{U_{osm}}{P_{osm}}\right)$$

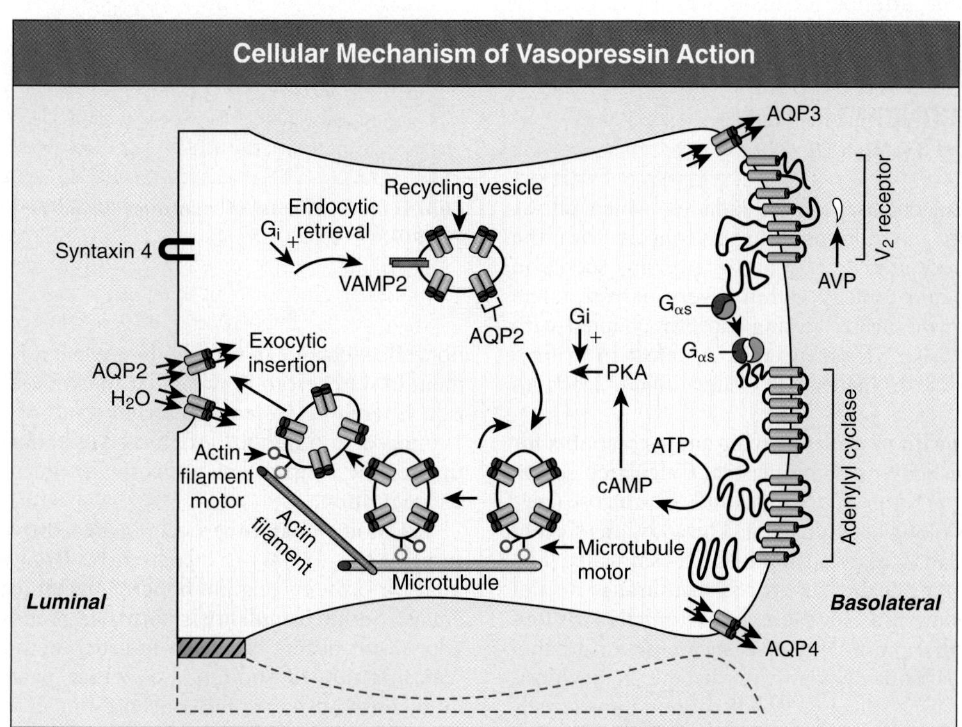

Figure 8.2 Cellular mechanism of vasopressin action. Vasopressin binds to V_2 receptors on the basolateral membrane and activates G proteins that initiate a cascade resulting in aquaporin 2 (AQP2) insertion in the luminal membrane. This then allows water uptake into the cell. ATP, adenosine triphosphate; AVP, arginine vasopressin; cAMP, cyclic adenosine monophosphate; PKA, protein kinase A; VAMP2, vesicle-associated membrane protein 2. *(Modified from reference 3.)*

This relationship determines that

1. in hypotonic urine ($U_{osm} < P_{osm}$), C_{water} is positive;
2. in isotonic urine ($U_{osm} = P_{osm}$), C_{water} is zero;
3. in hypertonic urine ($U_{osm} > P_{osm}$), C_{water} is negative (i.e., water is retained).

If excretion of free water in a polyuric patient is unaccompanied by water intake, the patient will become hypernatremic. Conversely, failure to excrete free water with increased water intake can cause hyponatremia.

A limitation of the equation is that it fails to predict clinically important alterations in plasma tonicity and serum Na^+ concentration because it factors in urea. Urea is an important component of urinary osmolality; however, because it crosses cell membranes readily, it does not establish a transcellular osmotic gradient and does not cause water movement between fluid compartments. Therefore, it does not influence serum Na^+ concentration or the release of vasopressin. As a result, changes in serum Na^+ concentration are better predicted by electrolyte free water clearance [$C_{water}(e)$]. The equation can be modified, replacing P_{osm} by plasma Na^+ concentration (P_{Na}) and the urine osmolality by urinary sodium and potassium concentrations ($U_{Na} + U_K$):

$$C_{water}(e) = V\left(1 - \frac{U_{Na} + U_K}{P_{Na}}\right)$$

If $U_{Na} + U_K$ is less than P_{Na}, then $C_{water}(e)$ is positive and the serum Na^+ concentration increases. If $U_{Na} + U_K$ is greater than P_{Na}, then $C_{water}(e)$ is negative and serum Na^+ concentration decreases. In the clinical setting, it is more appropriate to use the equation for electrolyte free clearance to predict if a patient's serum Na^+ concentration will increase or decrease in the face of the prevailing water excretion. For example, in a patient with high urea excretion, the original equation would predict negative water excretion and a decrease in serum Na^+ concentration; but in fact, serum Na^+ concentration increases, which is accurately predicted by the latter equation.

SERUM SODIUM CONCENTRATION, OSMOLALITY, AND TONICITY

The countercurrent mechanism of the kidneys, which allows urinary concentration and dilution, acts in concert with the hypothalamic osmoreceptors through vasopressin secretion to keep serum [Na^+] and tonicity within a very narrow range (Fig. 8.3). A defect in the urine-diluting capacity coupled with excess water intake leads to hyponatremia. A defect in urinary concentrating ability with inadequate water intake leads to hypernatremia.

Serum [Na^+] along with its accompanying anions accounts for nearly all the osmotic activity of the plasma. Calculated serum osmolality is given by 2[Na^+] + BUN (mg/dl)/2.8 + glucose (mg/dl)/18, where BUN is blood urea nitrogen. The addition of other solutes to ECF results in an increase in measured osmolality (Fig. 8.4). Solutes that are permeable across cell membranes do not cause water movement and do cause hypertonicity without causing cellular dehydration, for example, in uremia or ethanol intoxication. By comparison, a patient with diabetic ketoacidosis has an increase in plasma glucose, which cannot move freely across cell membranes in the absence of insulin and therefore causes water to move from the cells to the ECF, leading to cellular dehydration and lowering serum [Na^+]. This can be viewed as "translocational" at the cellular level, as the serum [Na^+] does not reflect change in total body water but rather reflects a movement of water from intracellular to extracellular space. A correction whereby a decrease in serum [Na^+] of 1.6 mmol/l for every 100 mg/dl (5.6 mmol/l) of glucose used may somewhat underestimate the impact of glucose to decrease serum sodium concentration.

Pseudohyponatremia occurs when the solid phase of plasma (usually 6% to 8%) is increased by large increments in either lipids or proteins (e.g., in hypertriglyceridemia and paraproteinemias). Serum osmolality is normal in pseudohyponatremia. This false result occurs because the usual method that measures the concentration of sodium uses whole plasma and not just the liquid phase, in which the concentration of sodium is 150 mmol/l. Many laboratories are now moving to direct ion-selective potentiometry, which will give the true aqueous sodium activity. In the absence of a direct-reading potentiometer, an estimate of plasma water can be obtained from the well-validated formula[6]

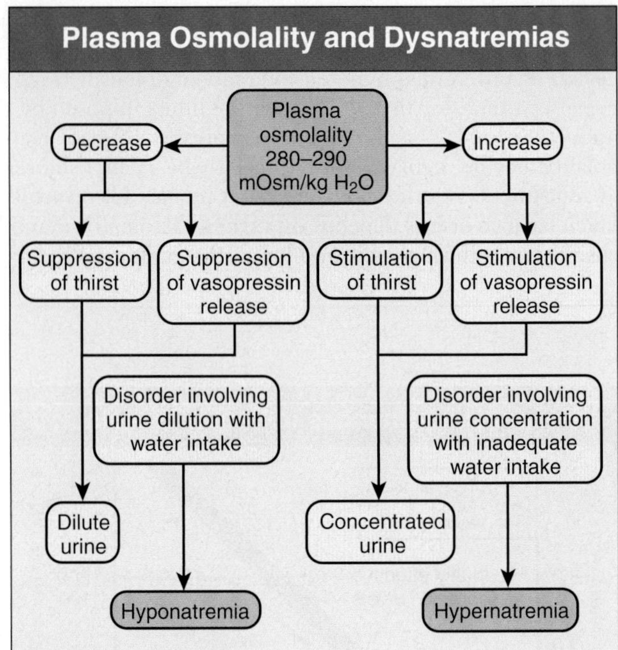

Figure 8.3 Maintenance of plasma osmolality and pathogenesis of dysnatremias. *(Modified with permission from reference 5.)*

Effects of Osmotically Active Substances on Serum Sodium Levels

Substances that increase osmolality without changing serum Na^+	Substances that increase osmolality and decrease serum Na^+ (translocational hyponatremia)
Urea	Glucose
Ethanol	Mannitol
Ethylene glycol	Glycine
Isopropyl alcohol	Maltose
Methanol	

Figure 8.4 Effects of osmotically active substances on serum sodium levels.

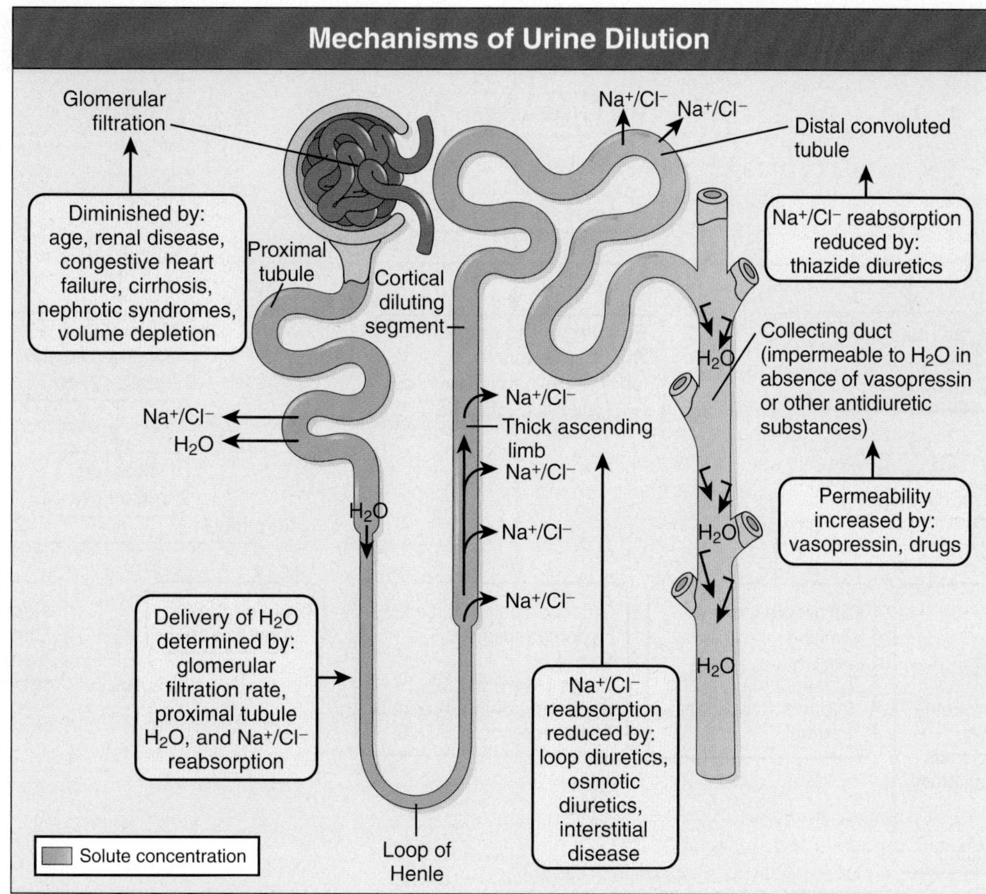

Figure 8.5 Mechanisms of urine dilution. Normal determinants of urinary dilution and disorders causing hyponatremia. *(Modified from reference 7.)*

$$\text{Plasma water content (\%)} = 99.1 - (0.1 \times L) - (0.07 \times P)$$

where L and P refer to the total lipid and protein concentration (in g/l), respectively. For example, if the formula reveals that plasma water is 90% of the plasma sample rather than the normal 93% (which yields a serum sodium concentration of 140 mmol/l as $150 \times 0.93 = 140$), the concentration of measured sodium would be expected to decrease to 135 mmol/l (150×0.90).

ESTIMATION OF TOTAL BODY WATER

In the normal man, total body water is approximately 60% of body weight (50% in women and obese individuals). With hyponatremia or hypernatremia, the change in total body water can be calculated from the serum Na^+ concentration by the following formula:

$$\text{Water excess} = 0.6W \times \left(1 - \frac{[Na^+]_{obs}}{140}\right)$$

$$\text{Water deficit} = 0.6W \times \left(\frac{[Na^+]_{obs}}{140} - 1\right)$$

where $[Na^+]_{obs}$ is observed sodium concentration (in mmol/l) and W is body weight (in kilograms). By use of this formula, a change of 10 mmol/l in the serum $[Na^+]$ in a 70-kg individual is equivalent to a change of 3 liters in free water.

HYPONATREMIC DISORDERS

Hyponatremia is defined as serum $[Na^+]$ of less than 135 mmol/l and equates with a low serum osmolarity once translocational hyponatremia and pseudohyponatremia are ruled out. True hyponatremia develops when normal urinary dilution mechanisms (Fig. 8.5) are disturbed. This may occur by three mechanisms. First, hyponatremia may result from intrarenal factors, such as a diminished glomerular filtration rate (GFR) and an increase in proximal tubular fluid and Na^+ reabsorption, which decrease distal delivery to the diluting segments of the nephron. Hyponatremia may also result from a defect in Na^+-Cl^- transport out of the water-impermeable segments of the nephrons (the thick ascending limb of Henle [TALH] or distal convoluted tubule). Most commonly, hyponatremia results from continued stimulation of vasopressin secretion by nonosmotic mechanisms despite the presence of serum hypo-osmolality.

Etiology and Classification of Hyponatremia

Once pseudohyponatremia and translocational hyponatremia are ruled out and the patient is established as truly hypo-osmolar, the next step is to classify the patient as hypovolemic, euvolemic, or hypervolemic (Fig. 8.6).

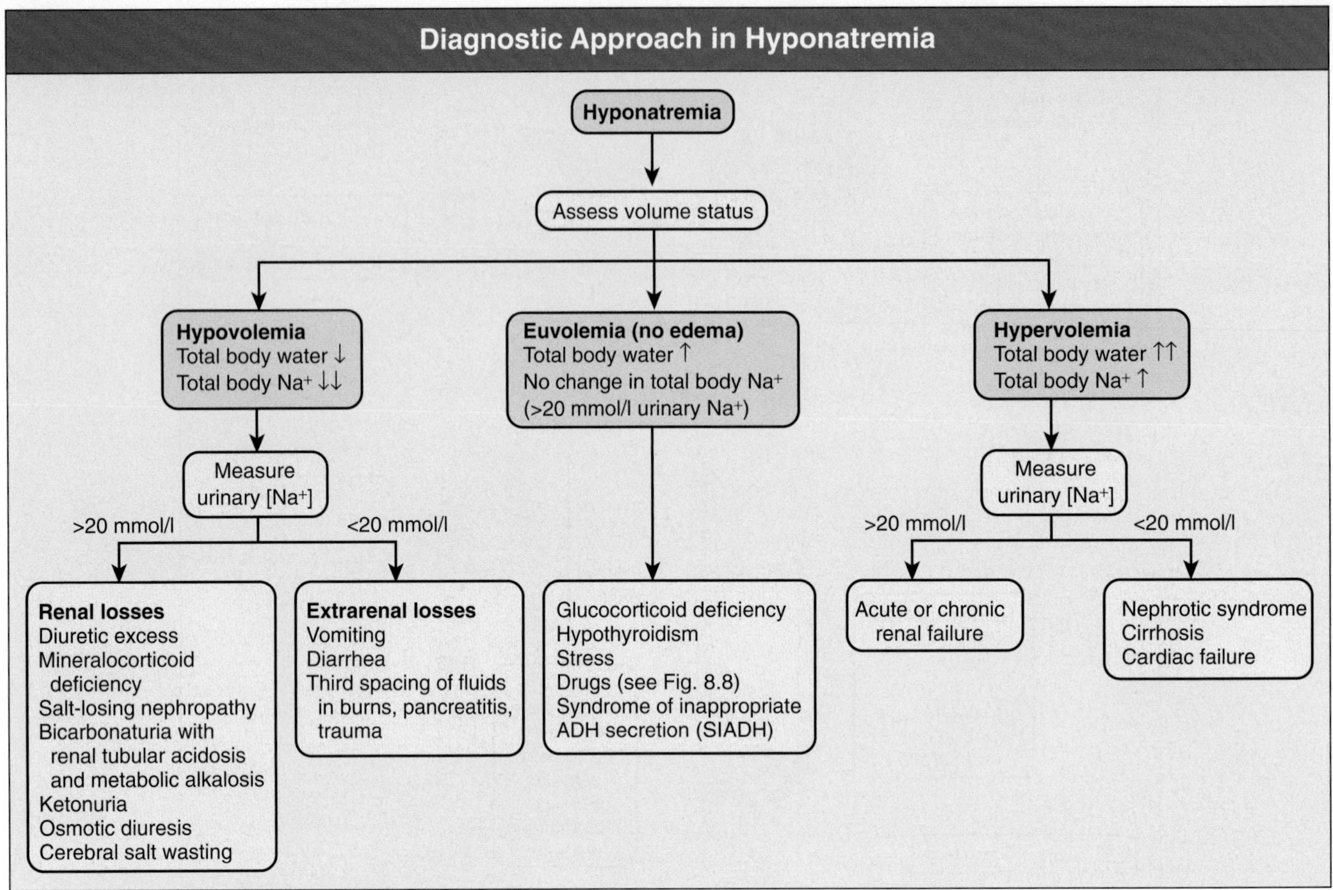

Figure 8.6 Diagnostic approach for the patient with hyponatremia. *(Modified with permission from reference 5.)*

Hypovolemia: Hyponatremia Associated with Decreased Total Body Sodium

A patient with hypovolemic hyponatremia has both a total body Na^+ and a water deficit, with the Na^+ deficit exceeding the water deficit. This occurs in patients with high gastrointestinal and renal losses of water and solute accompanied by free water or hypotonic fluid intake. The underlying mechanism is the nonosmotic release of vasopressin stimulated by volume contraction, which maintains vasopressin secretion despite the hypotonic state. Measurement of urinary Na^+ concentration is a useful tool in helping to diagnose these conditions (see Fig. 8.6).

Gastrointestinal and Third-Space Sequestered Losses In the setting of diarrhea or vomiting, the kidney responds to volume contraction by conserving Na^+ and Cl^-. A similar pattern is observed in burn patients and in patients with sequestration of fluids in third spaces, as in the peritoneal cavity with peritonitis or pancreatitis or in the bowel lumen with ileus. In all these situations, the urinary Na^+ concentration is usually less than 10 mmol/l and the urine is hyperosmolar. An exception to this is in patients with vomiting and metabolic alkalosis. Here, the increased HCO_3^- excretion requires simultaneous cation excretion such that urinary Na^+ concentration may be more than 20 mmol/l despite severe volume depletion and urinary Cl^- less than 10 mmol/l. Likewise, in chronic renal insufficiency, renal salt conservation is impaired and urine Na^+ concentration may be high.

Diuretics Diuretic use is one of the most common causes of hypovolemic hyponatremia associated with a high urine Na^+ concentration. Loop diuretics inhibit Na^+-Cl^- reabsorption in the TALH. This interferes with the generation of a hypertonic medullary interstitium. Therefore, even though volume contraction leads to increased vasopressin secretion, responsiveness to vasopressin is diminished and free water is excreted. In contrast, thiazide diuretics act in the distal tubule by interfering with urinary dilution rather than with urinary concentration, limiting free water excretion. Hyponatremia usually occurs within 14 days of initiation of therapy, although one third of cases present within 5 days. Underweight women and elderly patients appear to be most susceptible. Several mechanisms for diuretic-induced hyponatremia have been postulated, including:

- Hypovolemia-stimulated vasopressin release and decreased fluid delivery to the diluting segment.
- Impaired water excretion through interference with maximal urinary dilution in the cortical diluting segment.
- K^+ depletion, directly stimulating water intake by alterations in osmoreceptor sensitivity and increasing thirst.

Water retention can mask the physical findings of hypovolemia, thereby making the patients with diuretic-induced hyponatremia appear euvolemic.

Salt-Losing Nephropathy A salt-losing state sometimes occurs in patients with advanced chronic renal impairment (GFR

<15 ml/min), particularly due to interstitial disease. It is characterized by hyponatremia and hypovolemia. In proximal type 2 renal tubular acidosis, there is renal Na^+ and K^+ wastage despite only moderate renal impairment, and bicarbonaturia obligates urine Na^+ excretion.

Mineralocorticoid Deficiency Mineralocorticoid deficiency is characterized by hyponatremia with ECF volume contraction, urine [Na^+] above 20 mmol/l, and high serum K^+, urea, and creatinine. Decreased ECF volume provides the nonosmotic stimulus for vasopressin release.

Osmotic Diuresis An osmotically active, non-reabsorbable solute obligates the renal excretion of Na^+ and results in volume depletion. In the face of continuing water intake, the diabetic patient with severe glycosuria, the patient with a urea diuresis after relief of urinary tract obstruction, and the patient with mannitol diuresis all undergo urinary losses of Na^+ and water leading to hypovolemia and hyponatremia. Urinary [Na^+] is typically above 20 mmol/l. The ketone bodies β-hydroxybutyrate and acetoacetate also obligate urinary electrolyte losses and aggravate renal Na^+ wasting seen in diabetic ketoacidosis, starvation, and alcoholic ketoacidosis.

Cerebral Salt Wasting Cerebral salt wasting is a syndrome that has been described primarily in patients with subarachnoid hemorrhage. In this condition, the primary defect is salt wasting from the kidneys with subsequent volume contraction, which stimulates vasopressin release. The exact mechanism is not understood, but it is postulated that brain natriuretic peptide increases urine volume and Na^+ excretion. The diagnosis requires evidence of inappropriate sodium losses and reduced effective blood volume. These criteria are rarely fulfilled, suggesting that the entity is overdiagnosed.[8]

Hypervolemia: Hyponatremia Associated with Increased Total Body Sodium

In hypervolemia, if the total body Na^+ is increased more than total body water, there is hyponatremia. This occurs in congestive heart failure, nephrotic syndrome, and cirrhosis, all of which are associated with impaired water excretion (see Fig. 8.6). These pathophysiologic states are discussed in Chapter 7.

Congestive Heart Failure Edematous patients with heart failure have reduced effective intravascular volume due to lower systemic mean arterial pressure and cardiac output. This reduction is sensed by aortic and carotid baroreceptors activating non-osmotic pathways, and vasopressin is released. In addition, the relative "hypovolemic" state stimulates the renin-angiotensin axis and increases norepinephrine production, which in turn decreases GFR. The decrease in GFR leads to an increase in proximal tubular reabsorption and a decrease in water delivery to the distal tubule.

The neurohumorally mediated decrease in delivery of tubular fluid to the distal nephron and an increase in vasopressin secretion mediate hyponatremia by limiting Na^+-Cl^- and water excretion. In addition, low cardiac output and high ANG II levels are potent stimuli of thirst. There is also excessive intracellular targeting of AQP2 to the apical cell membrane of the collecting duct (Fig. 8.7). These effects are most likely a consequence of high circulating levels of vasopressin.

As cardiac function improves with afterload reduction, plasma vasopressin decreases with concomitant improvement in water excretion. The degree of hyponatremia has also been correlated with the severity of cardiac disease and with patient survival; serum Na^+ concentration of less than 125 mmol/l reflects severe heart failure.

Hepatic Failure Patients with cirrhosis and hepatic insufficiency also have increased extracellular volume (i.e., ascites, edema). Because of splanchnic venous dilation, they have an increased plasma volume. Unlike patients with congestive heart failure, cirrhotic patients have an increased cardiac output because of multiple arteriovenous fistulas in their alimentary tract and skin. Vasodilation and arteriovenous fistulas lead to a decrease in mean arterial blood pressure. As the severity of cirrhosis increases, there are progressive increases in plasma renin, norepinephrine, vasopressin, and endothelin. There is also an

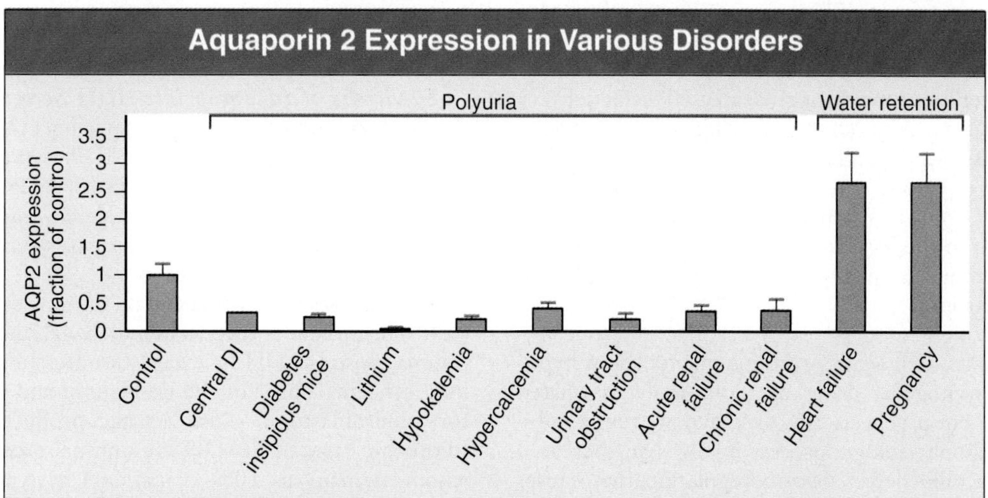

Figure 8.7 Changes in aquaporin 2 (AQP2) expression seen in association with different water balance disorders. Levels are expressed as a percentage of control levels (leftmost bar). AQP2 expression is reduced, sometimes dramatically, in a wide range of hereditary and acquired forms of diabetes insipidus (DI) characterized by different degrees of polyuria. Conversely, congestive heart failure and pregnancy are conditions associated with increased expression of AQP2 levels and excessive water retention. *(Modified from reference 9.)*

associated decline in mean arterial pressure and serum [Na^+]. In experimental models of cirrhosis, there is increased expression of vasopressin-regulated AQP2 in collecting ducts.[4]

Nephrotic Syndrome In some patients with nephrotic syndrome, especially children with minimal change disease, hypoalbuminemia and lowered plasma oncotic pressure alter Starling forces, leading to intravascular volume contraction. Most patients with nephrotic syndrome appear to have a renal defect in sodium excretion resulting in increased effective circulating volume. In experimental models of nephrotic syndrome, expression of AQP2 and AQP3 in the renal collecting ducts is downregulated.[4]

Advanced Chronic Renal Impairment Patients with advanced renal impairment, either acute or chronic, have a profound increase in fractional excretion of Na^+ to maintain normal salt balance given the overall decreased number of functioning nephrons. Edema usually develops when the Na^+ ingested exceeds the kidneys' capacity to excrete this load. Likewise, if water intake exceeds threshold, there is positive water balance and hyponatremia. At a GFR of 5 ml/min, only 7.2 liters of filtrate is formed daily. Approximately 30%, or 2.2 liters, of this filtered fluid will reach the diluting segment of the nephron, which is therefore the maximum solute-free water that can be excreted daily.

Euvolemia: Hyponatremia Associated with Normal Total Body Sodium

Euvolemic hyponatremia is the most commonly encountered dysnatremia in hospitalized patients. In these patients, no physical signs of increased total body Na^+ are detected.

Glucocorticoid Deficiency Glucocorticoid deficiency causes impaired water excretion in patients with primary and secondary adrenal insufficiency. Elevation of vasopressin accompanies the water-excretory defect resulting from anterior pituitary and adrenocorticotropic hormone deficiency. This can be corrected by physiologic doses of corticosteroids. In addition, implicated vasopressin-independent factors are impaired renal hemodynamics and decreased distal fluid delivery to the diluting segments of the nephron.

Hypothyroidism Hyponatremia occurs in patients with severe hypothyroidism, who usually meet the clinical criteria for myxedema coma. A decrease in cardiac output leads to nonosmotic release of vasopressin. A reduction in the GFR leads to diminished free water excretion through decreased distal delivery to the distal nephron. The exact mechanisms are unclear. Although a vasopressin-independent mechanism is suggested by normal suppression of vasopressin after water loading in patients with untreated myxedema, in advanced hypothyroidism, elevated levels of vasopressin in the basal state and after a water load are reported. Hyponatremia is readily reversed by treatment with levothyroxine (thyroxine).

Psychosis Patients with acute psychosis may develop hyponatremia. Some psychogenic drugs are commonly associated with hyponatremia, but psychosis can cause hyponatremia independently. The pathophysiologic process involves an increased thirst perception, a mild defect in osmoregulation that causes vasopressin to be secreted at lower osmolality, and an enhanced renal response to vasopressin. It has been suggested that subjects with self-induced water intoxication may also be more prone to development of rhabdomyolysis.[10]

Postoperative Hyponatremia Postoperative hyponatremia mainly occurs as a result of excessive infusion of electrolyte-free water (hypotonic saline or 5% dextrose in water) and the presence of vasopressin, which prevents its excretion. Hyponatremia can also occur despite near-isotonic saline infusion within 24 hours of induction of anesthesia, mostly through the generation of electrolyte-free water by the kidneys in the presence of vasopressin.[11] In young women, hyponatremia is rarely accompanied by cerebral edema, leading to seizures and hypoxia with catastrophic neurologic events, particularly after gynecologic surgery. The mechanism has not been fully elucidated, and the patients at highest risk cannot be prospectively identified. Nevertheless, hypotonic fluids should be avoided after surgery, isotonic fluids should be minimized, and serum [Na^+] concentration should be checked if there is any suspicion of hyponatremia (see later discussion).

Exercise-Induced Hyponatremia Hyponatremia is increasingly seen in long-distance runners. A study at a marathon race associated increased risk of hyponatremia with body mass index (BMI) below 20 kg/m^2, running time exceeding 4 hours, and greatest weight gain.[12] A study in ultramarathon runners showed elevated vasopressin despite normal or low serum sodium concentration.[13]

Drugs Causing Hyponatremia Drug-induced hyponatremia is becoming the most common cause of hyponatremia.[14] Thiazide diuretics are the most common cause, probably followed by selective serotonin reuptake inhibitors (SSRIs). Hyponatremia can be mediated by vasopressin analogues such as desmopressin (brand name DDAVP [1-desamino-D-arginine vasopressin]), drugs that enhance vasopressin release, and agents potentiating the action of vasopressin.[15] In other instances, the mechanism is unknown (Fig. 8.8). The increased use of desmopressin for nocturia in the elderly and enuresis in the young has resulted in a marked increase of reported cases of hyponatremia in these subjects.[16] With the increasing use of intravenous immune globulin (IVIG) as a therapeutic modality in many disorders, cases of hyponatremia associated with its use have been described.[17] The mechanism of IVIG-associated hyponatremia is multifactorial, involving pseudohyponatremia as the protein concentration increases, translocation because of the sucrose in the solution, and true dilutional hyponatremia related to retention of water, particularly in those with associated acute kidney injury.[16]

Syndrome of Inappropriate ADH Secretion Despite being the most common cause of hyponatremia in hospitalized patients, the syndrome of inappropriate ADH secretion (SIADH) is a diagnosis of exclusion. A defect in osmoregulation causes vasopressin to be inappropriately stimulated, leading to urinary concentration. The common causes of this syndrome are listed in Figure 8.9.

A few causes deserve special mention. Central nervous system (CNS) disturbances such as hemorrhage, tumors, infections, and trauma cause SIADH by excess vasopressin secretion. Small cell lung cancers, cancer of the duodenum and pancreas, and olfactory neuroblastoma cause ectopic production of vasopressin. Idiopathic cases of SIADH are unusual except in the elderly, in whom as many as 10% of patients have been found to have abnormal vasopressin secretion without known cause.[18]

Several patterns of abnormal vasopressin release have emerged from studies of patients with clinical SIADH.[1] In one third of patients with SIADH, vasopressin release varies appropriately

Drugs Associated with Hyponatremia*	
Vasopressin Analogues	**Drugs that Potentiate Renal Action of Vasopressin**
Desmopressin (DDAVP)	Chlorpropamide
Oxytocin	Cyclophosphamide
	Nonsteroidal anti-inflammatory drugs (NSADs)
	Acetaminophen
Drugs that Enhance Vasopressin Release	**Drugs that Cause Hyponatremia by Unknown Mechanisms**
Chlorpropamide	*Haloperidol*
Clofibrate	Fluphenazine
Carbamazepine-oxycarbazepine	Amitriptyline
Vincristine	Thioridazine
Nicotine	Fluoxetine
Narcotics	*Methamphetamine (MDMA or ecstasy)*
Antipsychotics/antidepressants (SSRI)	IVIG
Ifosfamide	

Figure 8.8 Drugs associated with hyponatremia. Terms in italics are the most common causes. *Not including diuretics. IVIG, intravenous immune globulin; SSRI, selective serotonin reuptake inhibitors. *(From reference 15.)*

with serum [Na+] but begins at a lower threshold of serum osmolality, implying a "resetting of the osmostat." Ingestion of free water then leads to water retention to maintain the serum [Na+] at a new lower level, usually 125 mmol/l to 130 mmol/l. In two thirds of patients, vasopressin release does not correlate with serum [Na+], but a solute-free urine cannot be excreted; therefore, ingested water is retained, giving rise to moderate nonedematous volume expansion and dilutional hyponatremia. In approximately 10% of patients, vasopressin levels are not measurable, suggesting that the syndrome of inappropriate antidiuresis (SIAD) is a more accurate term.[19] Such patients may have a nephrogenic syndrome of antidiuresis, and a gain-of-function mutation in the vasopressin receptor has been suggested as a possible mechanism.[20]

The diagnostic criteria for SIADH are summarized in Figure 8.10. Plasma vasopressin may be in the "normal" range (up to 10 ng/l), but this is inappropriate given the hypo-osmolar state. In clinical practice, the measurement of plasma vasopressin is rarely needed as the urinary osmolality provides an excellent surrogate bioassay. Thus, a hypertonic urine (>300 mOsm/kg) provides strong evidence for the presence of vasopressin in the circulation because such urinary tonicities are unattainable in its absence. Likewise, a urinary osmolality lower than 100 mOsm/kg reflects the virtual absence of the hormone. Urinary osmolalities in the range of 100 mOsm/kg to 300 mOsm/kg can occur in the presence or absence of the hormone.

Causes of the Syndrome of Inappropriate ADH Release (SIADH)			
Carcinomas	**Pulmonary Disorders**	**Nervous System Disorders**	**Other**
Bronchogenic carcinoma	*Viral pneumonia*	*Encephalitis (viral or bacterial)*	*AIDS–HIV*
Carcinoma of the duodenum	*Bacterial pneumonia*	*Meningitis (viral, bacterial, tuberculous, and fungal)*	*Idiopathic (elderly)*
Carcinoma of the pancreas	*Pulmonary abscess*	*Head trauma*	Prolonged exercise
Thymoma	*Tuberculosis*	*Brain abscess*	
Carcinoma of the stomach	Aspergillosis	*Brain tumors*	
Lymphoma	Positive pressure ventilation	Guillain-Barré syndrome	
Ewing's sarcoma	Asthma	Acute intermittent porphyria	
Carcinoma of the bladder	Pneumothorax	Subarachnoid hemorrhage or subdural hematoma	
Carcinoma of the prostate	Mesothelioma	Cerebellar and cerebral atrophy	
Oropharyngeal tumor	Cystic fibrosis	Carvernous sinus thrombosis	
Carcinoma of the ureter		Neonatal hypoxia Hydrocephalus Shy–Drager syndrome Rocky Mountain spotted fever Delirium tremens Cerebrovascular accident (cerebral thrombosis or hemorrhage) Acute psychosis Peripheral neuropathy Multiple sclerosis	

Figure 8.9 Causes of the syndrome of inappropriate ADH release (SIADH). Terms in italics are the most common causes. AIDS, acquired immunodeficiency syndrome; HIV, human immunodeficiency virus. *(From reference 15.)*

Diagnostic Criteria for the Syndrome of Inappropriate ADH Release
Essential Diagnostic Criteria
Decreased extracellular fluid effective osmolality (<270 mOsm/kg H_2O)
Inappropriate urinary concentration (>100 mOsm/kg H_2O)
Clinical euvolemia
Elevated urinary Na^+ concentration under conditions of normal salt and water intake
Absence of adrenal, thyroid, pituitary, or renal insufficiency or diuretic use
Supplemental Criteria
Abnormal water-load test (inability to excrete at least 90% of a 20-ml/kg water load in 4 hours and/or failure to dilute urine osmolality to <100mOsm/kg)
Plasma vasopressin level inappropriately elevated relative to the plasma osmolality
No significant correction of plasma Na^+ level with volume expansion, but improvement after fluid restriction

Figure 8.10 Diagnostic criteria for the syndrome of inappropriate ADH release (SIADH). *(Modified from reference 21.)*

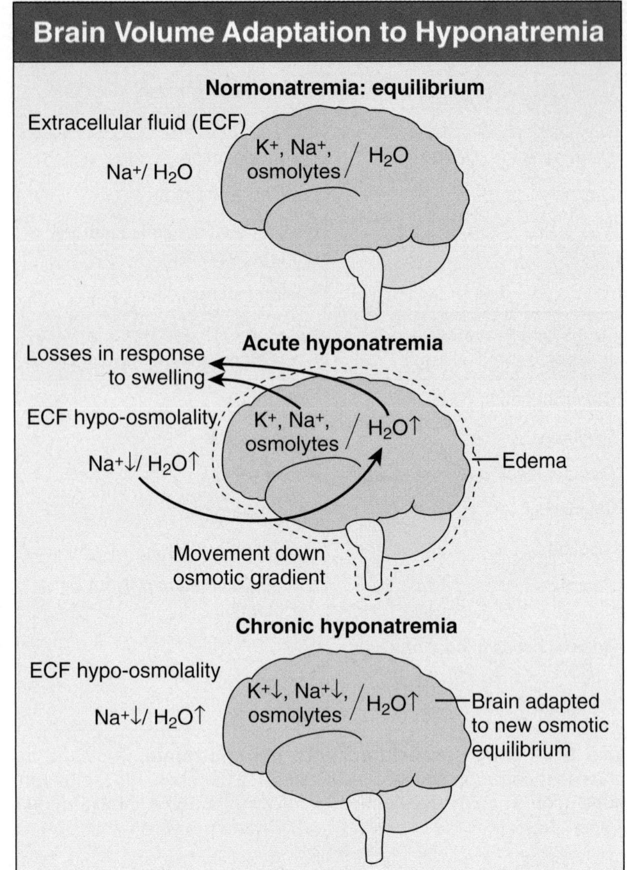

Figure 8.11 Brain volume adaptation to hyponatremia. Under normal conditions, brain osmolality and extracellular fluid (ECF) osmolality are in equilibrium. After the induction of ECF hypo-osmolality, water moves into the brain down osmotic gradients, producing brain edema. In response, the brain loses both extracellular and intracellular solutes (see text for details). As water losses accompany the losses of brain solute, the expanded brain volume then decreases back to normal. In chronic hyponatremia, the brain volume eventually normalizes completely, and the brain becomes fully adapted to the ECF hyponatremia. *(Modified from reference 24.)*

Clinical Manifestations of Hyponatremia

Most patients with a serum Na^+ concentration above 125 mmol/l are asymptomatic. Below 125 mmol/l, headache, yawning, lethargy, nausea, reversible ataxia, psychosis, seizures, and coma may occur as a result of cerebral edema. Rarely, hypotonicity leads to cerebral edema so severe that there is increased intracerebral pressure, tentorial herniation, respiratory depression, and death. Hyponatremia-induced cerebral edema usually occurs with rapid development of hyponatremia, typically in hospitalized postoperative patients receiving diuretics or hypotonic fluids. Untreated severe hyponatremia has a mortality up to 50%. Neurologic symptoms in a hyponatremic patient call for immediate attention and treatment.

The development of cerebral edema largely depends on the cerebral adaptation to hypotonicity. Decreases in extracellular osmolality cause movement of water into cells, increasing intracellular volume and causing tissue edema. The water channel AQP4 appears to play a key role in the movement of water across the blood-brain barrier, as knockout mice for AQP4 are protected from hyponatremic brain swelling,[22] whereas animals overexpressing the water channel have exaggerated brain swelling.[23] Cellular edema within the fixed confines of the cranium causes an increase in intracranial pressure, leading to the neurologic syndrome. In most patients with hyponatremia, mechanisms of volume regulation prevent cerebral edema.

Early in the course of hyponatremia (within 1 to 3 hours), a decrease in cerebral extracellular volume occurs by movement of fluid into the cerebrospinal fluid, which is then shunted back into the systemic circulation. This happens promptly and is evident by the loss of extracellular solutes Na^+ and Cl^- as early as 30 minutes after the onset of hyponatremia (Fig. 8.11). If hyponatremia persists for longer than 3 hours, the brain adapts by losing cellular osmolytes, including K^+ and organic solutes, which tend to lower the osmolality of the brain without substantial gain of water. Thereafter, if hyponatremia persists, other organic osmolytes, such as phosphocreatine, myoinositol, and amino acids (e.g., glutamine, taurine), are lost. The loss of these solutes markedly decreases cerebral swelling. It is because of these adaptations that some subjects, particularly the elderly, may have minimal symptoms despite severe ([Na^+] <125 mmol/l) hyponatremia.

Certain patients are at increased risk for development of acute cerebral edema in the course of hyponatremia (Fig. 8.12). For example, hospitalized premenstrual women with hyponatremia are more symptomatic and more likely to have complications of therapy than are postmenopausal women or men. This increased risk is independent of the rate of development or the magnitude of hyponatremia. The best management of these patients is to avoid the administration of hypotonic fluids in the postoperative setting. Hyponatremia may occur in the postoperative state even if isotonic fluid is being used if the concentration of Na^+ and K^+ in the urine exceeds that in the serum; the hyponatremia is mild and not associated with cerebral dysfunction.[11] Children are

Hyponatremic Patients at Risk for Neurologic Complications	
Acute Cerebral Edema	**Osmotic Demyelination Syndrome (Central Pontine Myelinolysis)**
Postoperative menstruating females	Liver transplant recipients
Elderly women taking thiazides	Alcoholics
Children	Malnourished patients
Polydipsia secondary to psychiatric disorders	Hypokalemic patients
Hypoxemic patients	Burn victims
Marathon runners	Elderly women taking thiazides
	Hypoxemic patients
	$[Na^+]$ <105 mmol/l

Figure 8.12 Hyponatremic patients at risk for neurologic complications. *(From reference 25.)*

particularly vulnerable to the development of acute cerebral edema, perhaps because of a relatively high ratio of brain to skull volume.

Another neurologic syndrome can occur in hyponatremic patients and is a complication of correction of hyponatremia. Osmotic demyelination most commonly affects the central pons of the brainstem and is therefore also termed central pontine myelinolysis. It occurs in all ages; those at most risk are shown in Figure 8.12. It is especially common after liver transplantation, with a reported incidence of 13% to 29% at autopsy. The risk of central pontine myelinolysis is related to the severity and chronicity of the hyponatremia. It rarely occurs with serum $[Na^+]$ above 120 mmol/l and if hyponatremia is acute in onset (<48 hours). The symptoms are biphasic. Initially, there is a generalized encephalopathy associated with rapid correction of serum $[Na^+]$. Two to 3 days after correction, there are behavioral changes, cranial nerve palsies, and progressive weakness culminating in quadriplegia and a locked in syndrome. On T2-weighted magnetic resonance imaging, there are nonenhancing and hyperintense pontine and extrapontine lesions. As these lesions may not appear until 2 weeks after development, a diagnosis of myelinolysis should not be excluded if the imaging is initially normal. The pathogenesis of this syndrome is uncertain; one suggestion is that sodium-coupled amino acid transporters (SNAT2) are downregulated by hypotonicity, thereby delaying the return of osmolytes to the brain, rendering it more sensitive to the correction of hyponatremia.[16] Although serum Na^+ and K^+ concentrations return to normal in a few hours, it takes several days for osmotically active solutes in the brain to reach normal levels. This temporary imbalance causes cerebral dehydration and can lead to a potential breakdown of the blood-brain barrier. Whereas central pontine myelinolysis was originally considered to be uniformly fatal, it is now evident that some neurologic recovery can occur and that milder forms of the disorder occur as well.

Treatment of Hyponatremia

Symptoms and duration of hyponatremia determine treatment. Acutely hyponatremic patients (hyponatremia developing within 48 hours) are at great risk for development of permanent neurologic sequelae from cerebral edema if the hyponatremia remains uncorrected. Patients with chronic hyponatremia are at risk for osmotic demyelination if the hyponatremia is corrected too rapidly.

Acute Symptomatic Hyponatremia

Acute symptomatic hyponatremia, especially associated with seizures or other neurologic manifestations, almost always develops in hospitalized patients receiving hypotonic fluids (Fig. 8.13). Treatment should be prompt as the risk of acute cerebral edema far exceeds the risk of osmotic demyelination. Serum $[Na^+]$ should be ideally corrected by 2 mmol/l per hour until symptoms resolve. It is not necessary to correct the serum $[Na^+]$ completely, although it does not appear to be unsafe to do so. Correction may be achieved by administration of hypertonic saline (3% NaCl) at the rate of 1 to 2 ml/h per kilogram of body weight.[25-26] The administration of a loop diuretic like furosemide enhances free water excretion and hastens the normalization of serum $[Na^+]$. If the patient presents with severe neurologic symptoms, such as seizures, obtundation, or coma, 3% NaCl may be infused at higher rates (4 to 6 ml/h per kilogram of body weight). Various formulas have been proposed to estimate an increase in serum $[Na^+]$ after administration of intravenous fluids,[19] but they tend to underestimate the rate of correction.[27] Therefore, during treatment with hypertonic saline, the patient should be monitored carefully for changes in neurologic and pulmonary status, and serum electrolytes should be checked frequently, approximately every 2 hours.

Chronic Symptomatic Hyponatremia

If the hyponatremia has taken more than 48 hours to evolve or if the duration is not known, correction should be undertaken with caution (see Fig. 8.13). Controversy exists as to whether it is the rate of correction or the magnitude of correction of hyponatremia that predisposes to neurologic complications. In clinical practice, it is difficult to dissociate these two variables because a rapid correction rate is usually accompanied by a greater absolute magnitude of correction during a given time. There are important principles to guide treatment:[25]

- Because cerebral water is increased only by approximately 10% in severe chronic hyponatremia, the goal is to increase the serum Na^+ level by 10% or by approximately 10 mmol/l.
- Do not exceed a correction rate of 1.0 to 1.5 mmol/l in any given hour.
- Do not increase the serum Na^+ level by more than 8 to 12 mmol/l per 24 hours.

It is important to take into account the rate and electrolyte content of infused fluids and the rate of production and electrolyte content of urine. Once the desired increment in serum Na^+ concentration is obtained, treatment should consist of water restriction.

If correction has proceeded more rapidly than desired (usually because of excretion of hypotonic urine), the risk of osmotic demyelination may be decreased by relowering serum Na^+ concentration with intravenous or subcutaneous desmopressin or administration of 5% dextrose.[28]

Chronic "Asymptomatic" Hyponatremia

Although many patients with chronic hyponatremia appear to be asymptomatic, formal neurologic testing frequently reveals subtle impairments, including gait disturbances comparable to those seen in subjects with toxic levels of alcohol that reverse with correction of the hyponatremia. This results in an increased

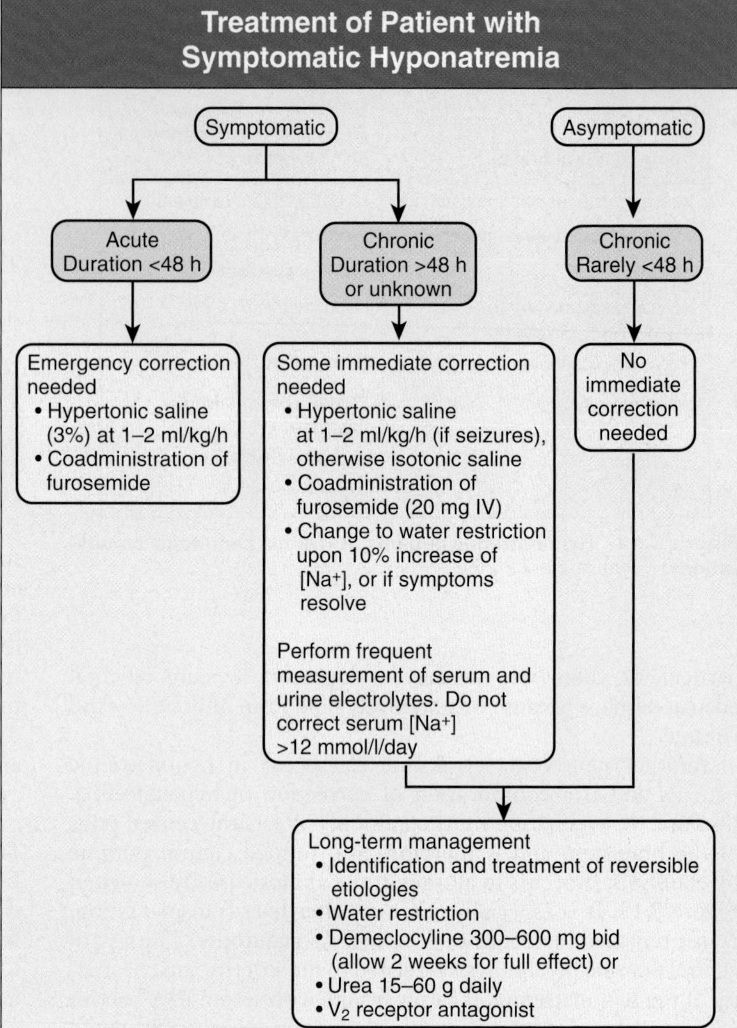

Figure 8.13 Treatment of patient with symptomatic hyponatremia. *(Modified from reference 25.)*

risk for falls and fractures.[29] Therefore, even "asymptomatic" patients should be treated in an attempt to restore serum sodium to nearly normal levels. These patients should be evaluated for hypothyroidism, adrenal insufficiency, and SIADH and have their medications reviewed.

Fluid Restriction Fluid restriction is the first-line therapy in patients with chronic asymptomatic hyponatremia (Fig. 8.14). This approach is usually successful if patients are compliant. It involves a calculation of the fluid restriction that will maintain a specific serum Na^+ concentration. The daily osmolar load (OL) and the minimal urinary osmolality $(U_{osm})_{min}$ determine a patient's maximal urine volume (V_{max}).

$$V_{max} = \frac{OL}{(U_{osm})_{min}}$$

The value of $(U_{osm})_{min}$ is a function of the severity of the diluting disorder. In the absence of circulating vasopressin, it can be as low as 50 mOsm. In a normal North American diet, the daily osmolar load is approximately 10 mOsm/kg (700 mOsm for a 70-kg person). Assuming that a patient with SIADH has a U_{osm} that cannot be lowered to less than 500 mOsm, the same osmolar load of 700 mOsm allows only 1.4 liters of urine to be excreted per day. Therefore, if the patient drinks more than 1.4 liters per day, the serum Na^+ concentration will decrease. Measurement of urine Na^+ and K^+ concentrations can indicate the degree of water restriction required in a given patient.[30] If the diluting defect is so severe that fluid restriction to less than 1 liter is necessary or if the patient's serum Na^+ concentration remains low (<130 mmol/l), an alternative approach to treatment, such as increasing solute excretion or pharmacologic inhibition of vasopressin, should be considered.

Maneuvers That Increase Solute Excretion If the patient remains unresponsive to fluid restriction, solute intake can be increased to facilitate an obligatory increase in excretion of solute and free water.[31] This can be achieved by increasing oral salt and protein intake in the diet to increase the C_{osm} of the urine. Loop diuretics combined with high sodium intake (2 to 3 g of additional salt) are effective in the management of hyponatremia. A single diuretic dose (40 mg furosemide) is usually sufficient but should be doubled if the diuresis induced in the first 8 hours is less than 60% of the total daily urine output.

The administration of urea increases urine flow by causing an osmotic diuresis. This permits a more liberal water intake

Treatment of Chronic Asymptomatic Hyponatremia				
Treatment	**Mechanism of Action**	**Dose**	**Advantages**	**Limitations**
Fluid restriction	Decreases availability of free water	Variable	Effective and inexpensive; not complicated	Noncompliance
Pharmacologic inhibition of vasopressin action				
Lithium	Inhibits the kidney's response to vasopressin	900–1200 mg/day	Unrestricted water intake	Polyuria, narrow therapeutic range, neurotoxicity
Demeclocyline	Inhibits the kidney's response to vasopressin	300–600 mg twice daily	Effective; unrestricted water intake	Neurotoxicity, polyuria, photosensitivity, nephrotoxicity
V_2 receptor antagonist	Antagonizes vasopressin action		Addresses underlying mechanisms	Limited clinical experience
Increased solute (salt) intake				
With furosemide	Increases free water clearance	Titrate to optimal dose; coadministration of 2–3g NaCl	Effective	Ototoxicity, K^+ depletion
With urea	Osmotic diuresis	30–60 g/day	Effective; unrestricted water intake	Polyuria, unpalatable, gastrointestinal symptoms

Figure 8.14 Treatment of patients with chronic asymptomatic hyponatremia.

without worsening the hyponatremia and without altering urinary concentration. The dose for urea is usually 30 to 60 g/day. The major limitations are gastrointestinal distress and unpalatability.

Pharmacologic Inhibition of Vasopressin Vaptans are novel oral V_2 receptor antagonists that block vasopressin binding to the collecting duct tubular epithelial cells and increase free water excretion without significantly altering electrolyte excretion. These agents are effective in the treatment of hyponatremia in euvolemic and hypervolemic patients.[32] Conivaptan, a V_2 and V_{1a} antagonist, is the only vaptan available for intravenous use.[33] It is used in the treatment of hyponatremia in hospitalized patients with transient SIADH, but treatment should be limited to 4 days because it is a potent CYP3A4 inhibitor. Tolvaptan, an oral V_2 antagonist, is now available in some countries at doses between 15 and 60 mg/day.

An alternative pharmacologic treatment is demeclocycline, 600 to 1200 mg daily given 1 to 2 hours after meals; calcium-, aluminum-, and magnesium-containing antacids should be avoided. Onset of action is usually 3 to 6 days after treatment is begun. Dose should be titrated to the minimum to keep the serum [Na^+] within the desired range with unrestricted water intake. Skin photosensitivity may develop and tooth or bone abnormalities may occur in children. Polyuria leads to noncompliance, and nephrotoxicity may occur, especially in patients with underlying liver disease. Lithium was previously used to block vasopressin action in the collecting duct but has been superseded by the vaptans and demeclocycline.

Hypovolemic Hyponatremia

When thiazides are prescribed, especially in elderly women, serum [Na^+] should be monitored and water intake restricted. If hyponatremia develops, the drug needs to be discontinued.

Neurologic syndromes directly related to hyponatremia are unusual in hypovolemic hyponatremia as both Na^+ and water loss limits any osmotic shifts in the brain. Restoration of ECF volume with crystalloids or colloids interrupts the nonosmotic release of vasopressin. Vasopressin antagonists should not be used in this clinical setting.

Hypervolemic Hyponatremia

Congestive Heart Failure In patients with heart failure, sodium and water restriction is critical. Patients may be treated with a combination of angiotensin-converting enzyme (ACE) inhibitors and diuretics. The increase in cardiac output that follows decreases the neurohumorally mediated processes that limit water excretion. Loop diuretics diminish the action of vasopressin on the collecting tubules, thereby decreasing water reabsorption. Thiazides should be avoided as they impair urinary dilution and may worsen hyponatremia. V_2 antagonists increase serum Na^+ concentration in patients with heart failure,[32,34] and correction of serum Na^+ concentration is associated with better long-term outcomes.[35] However, in the much larger randomized controlled EVEREST trial in patients with decompensated heart failure, treatment with tolvaptan did not alter any of the long-term clinical outcomes. In principle, a vaptan with V_1 antagonist activity could have additional benefit in cardiac failure, but this is unproven.

Cirrhosis In patients with cirrhosis, water and sodium restriction is the mainstay of therapy. Loop diuretics increase C_{water} once a negative sodium balance has been achieved. V_2 antagonists increase water excretion accompanied by an increase in serum Na^+ concentration.[34] In one study, satavaptan led to a mean increase in serum Na^+ concentration of 6.6. mmol/L.[36] The response to vaptans in cirrhosis is more attenuated than in patients with SIADH or heart failure, which suggests that vasopressin-independent mechanisms may also contribute to their hyponatremia.[32] The administration of V_2 antagonists to patients with liver failure is not associated with decrements in blood pressure. Combined V_1 and V_2 antagonists (e.g., conivaptan) should not be used in this population.

HYPERNATREMIC DISORDERS

Hypernatremia is defined as serum [Na^+] above 145 mmol/l and reflects serum hyperosmolarity. The renal concentrating mechanism represents the first defense mechanism against water depletion and hyperosmolarity. The components of the normal concentrating mechanism are shown in Figure 8.15. Disorders of urinary concentration may result from decreased delivery of

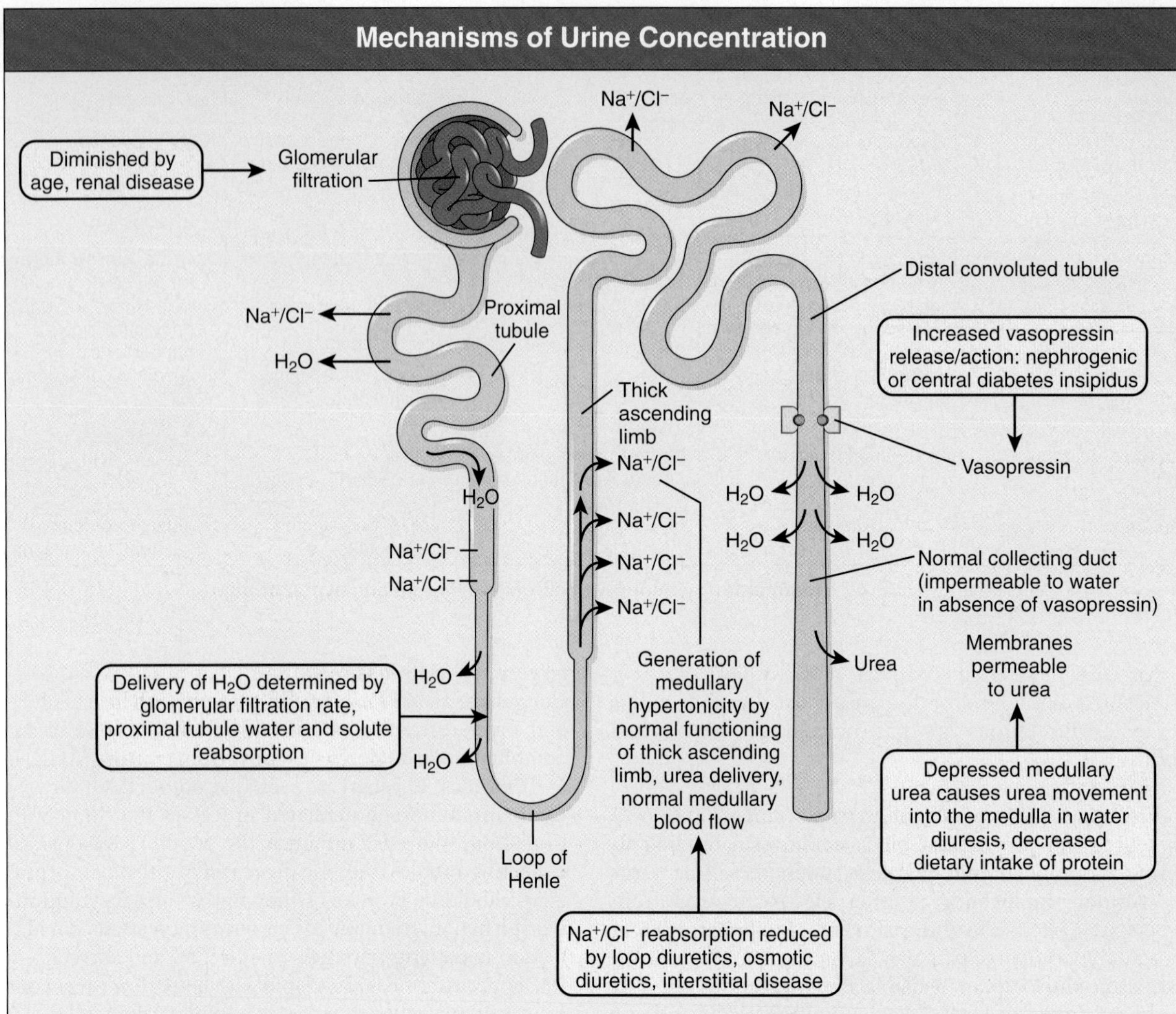

Figure 8.15 Urinary concentrating mechanisms. Determinants of normal urinary concentrating mechanism and disorders causing hypernatremia. *(Modified from reference 7.)*

solute (with decreasing GFR) or the inability to generate interstitial hypertonicity as a consequence of decreased Na^+ and Cl^- reabsorption in the ascending limb of the loop of Henle (loop diuretics), decreased medullary urea accumulation (poor dietary intake), or alterations in medullary blood flow. Hypernatremia may also result from failure to release or respond to AVP. Thirst is the first and most important defense mechanism in preventing hypernatremia.

Etiology and Classification of Hypernatremia

As with hyponatremia, patients with hypernatremia fall into three broad categories based on volume status.[15] A diagnostic algorithm is helpful in the evaluation of these patients (Fig. 8.16).

Hypovolemia: Hypernatremia Associated with Low Total Body Sodium

Patients with hypovolemic hypernatremia sustain losses of both Na^+ and water, but with a relatively greater loss of water. On physical examination, there are signs of hypovolemia such as orthostatic hypotension, tachycardia, flat neck veins, poor skin turgor, and sometimes altered mental status. Patients will generally have hypotonic water loss from the kidneys or the gastrointestinal tract; in the latter, the urinary [Na^+] will be low.

Hypervolemia: Hypernatremia Associated with Increased Total Body Sodium

Hypernatremia with increased total body Na^+ is the least common form of hypernatremia. It results from the administration of hypertonic solutions such as 3% NaCl given as intra-amniotic instillation for therapeutic abortion and $NaHCO_3$ for the treatment of metabolic acidosis, hyperkalemia, and cardiorespiratory arrest. It may also result from inadvertent dialysis against a dialysate with a high Na^+ concentration or from consumption of salt tablets. Therapeutic hypernatremia is also becoming common as hypertonic saline solutions have emerged as a preferable alternative to mannitol for treatment of increased intracranial pressure.[37] Hypernatremia is also increasingly recognized in hypoalbuminemic hospitalized patients with renal failure who are edematous and unable to concentrate their urine.

Euvolemia: Hypernatremia Associated with Normal Body Sodium

Most patients with hypernatremia secondary to water loss appear euvolemic with normal total body Na^+ because loss of

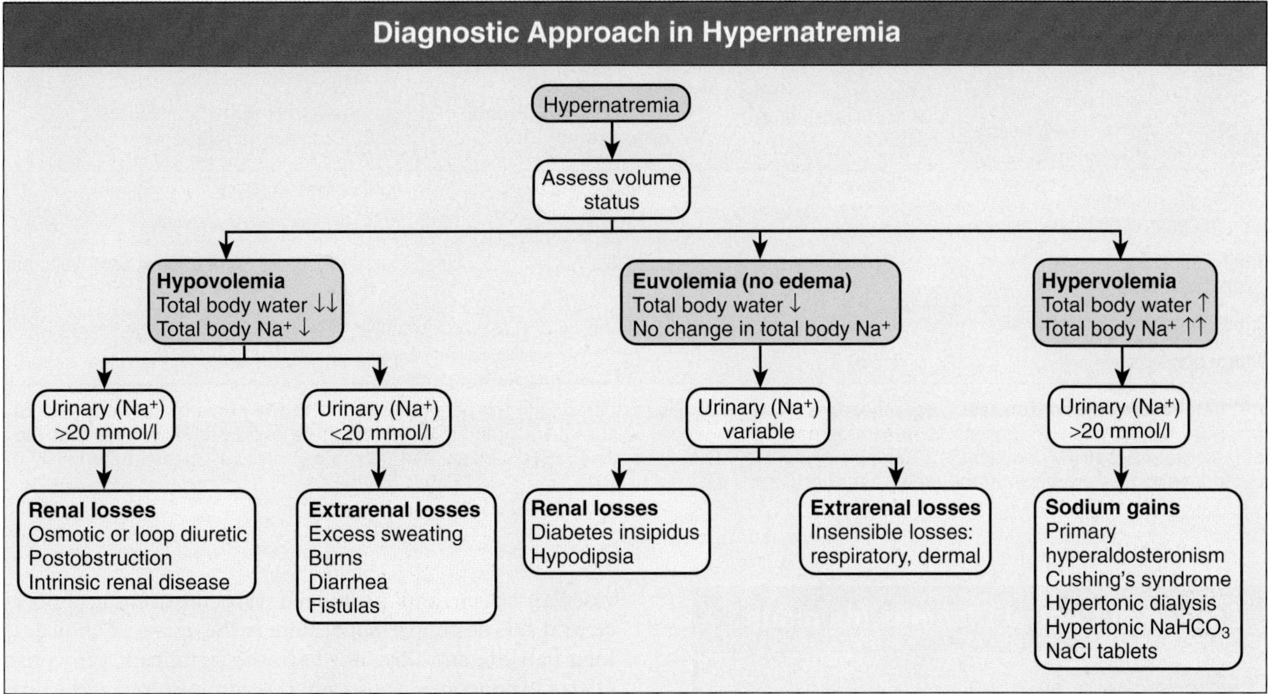

Figure 8.16 Diagnostic approach in hypernatremia. *(Modified with permission from reference 5.)*

water without Na^+ does not lead to overt volume contraction. Water loss *per se* need not result in hypernatremia unless it is unaccompanied by water intake. Because hypodipsia is uncommon, hypernatremia usually develops only in those who have no access to water and the very young and old, in whom there may be an altered perception of thirst. Extrarenal water loss occurs from the skin and respiratory tract in febrile or other hypermetabolic states and is associated with a high urine osmolality because the osmoreceptor-vasopressin-renal response is intact. The urine Na^+ concentration varies with the intake. Renal water loss leading to euvolemic hypernatremia results either from a defect in vasopressin production or release (central diabetes insipidus) or from a failure of the collecting duct to respond to the hormone (nephrogenic diabetes insipidus). Defense against the development of hyperosmolality requires the appropriate stimulation of thirst and the ability to respond by drinking water.

Polyuric disorders can result from either an increase in C_{osm} or an increase in C_{water}. An increase in C_{osm} occurs with diuretic use, renal salt wasting, excess salt ingestion, vomiting (bicarbonaturia), alkali administration, and administration of mannitol (as a diuretic, for bladder lavage, or for the treatment of cerebral edema). An increase in C_{water} occurs with excess ingestion of water (psychogenic polydipsia) or in abnormalities of the renal concentrating mechanism (diabetes insipidus).

Diabetes Insipidus Diabetes insipidus (DI) is characterized by polyuria and polydipsia and is caused by defects in vasopressin action. Patients with central and nephrogenic DI and primary polydipsia present with polyuria and polydipsia. The differentiation between these entities can be accomplished by clinical evaluation, with measurements of vasopressin levels and the response to a water deprivation test followed by vasopressin administration (Fig. 8.17).

Central Diabetes Insipidus

CLINICAL FEATURES Central DI usually has an abrupt onset. Patients have a constant need to drink, have a predilection for cold water, and commonly have nocturia. By contrast, the compulsive water drinker may give a vague history of the onset and has large variations in water intake and urine output. Nocturia is unusual in compulsive water drinkers. A plasma osmolality of more than 295 mOsm/kg suggests central DI, and a plasma osmolality of less than 270 mOsm/kg suggests compulsive water drinking.

CAUSES Central DI is caused by infection, tumors, granuloma, and trauma affecting the CNS in 50% of the cases; in the other 50%, it is idiopathic (Fig. 8.18). In a survey of 79 children and young adults, central DI was idiopathic in half the cases. The remainder had tumors and Langerhans cell histiocytosis; these patients had an 80% chance for development of anterior pituitary hormone deficiency compared with the patients with idiopathic disease.[38]

Autosomal dominant DI is caused by point mutations in a precursor gene for vasopressin that cause "misfolding" of the provasopressin peptide, preventing its release from the hypothalamic and posterior pituitary neurons.[39] Patients present with a mild polyuria and polydipsia in the first year of life. These children have normal physical and mental development. There is a rare autosomal recessive central DI associated with diabetes mellitus, optic atrophy, and deafness (Wolfram syndrome).[40] DI is usually partial and gradual in onset in Wolfram syndrome. It is linked to chromosome 4 and involves abnormalities in mitochondrial DNA.

A rare clinical entity is the combination of central DI and deficient thirst. It has been reported in a total of 70 patients in 41 studies.[41] When vasopressin secretion and thirst are both impaired, affected patients are vulnerable to recurrent episodes

Water Deprivation Test			
Condition	Urinary Osmolality with Water Deprivation (mOsm/kg H_2O)	Plasma Vasopressin after Dehydration (pg/ml)	Increase in Urinary Osmolality with Exogenous Vasopressin
Normal	>800	>2	Little or no increase
Complete central diabetes insipidus	<300	Undetectable	Substantially increased
Partial central diabetes insipidus	300–800	<1.5	Increase of >10% of urinary osmolality after water deprivation
Nephrogenic diabetes insipidus	<300–500	>5	Little or no increase
Primary polydipsia	>500	<5	Little or no increase

Figure 8.17 Water deprivation test. Test procedure: Water intake is restricted until the patient loses 3% to 5% of his or her body weight or until three consecutive hourly determinations of urinary osmolality are within 10% of each other. (Caution must be exercised to ensure that the patient does not become excessively dehydrated.) Aqueous vasopressin (5 U subcutaneously) is given, and urinary osmolality is measured after 60 minutes. The expected responses are given in the table. *(From reference 42.)*

Causes of Central Diabetes Insipidus
Congenital
Autosomal dominant
Autosomal recessive
Acquired
Post-traumatic
Iatrogenic (postsurgical)
Tumors (metastatic from breast, craniopharyngioma, pinealoma)
Histiocytosis
Granuloma (tuberculosis, sarcoid)
Aneurysm
Meningitis
Encephalitis
Guillain-Barré syndrome
Idiopathic

Figure 8.18 Causes of central diabetes insipidus. Entries in italics are the common causes.

of hypernatremia. Formerly called essential hypernatremia, the disorder is now called central DI with deficient thirst or adipsic DI.

DIFFERENTIAL DIAGNOSIS Measurement of circulating vasopressin by radioimmunoassay is preferred to the tedious water deprivation test. Under basal conditions, vasopressin levels are unhelpful because there is a significant overlap among the polyuric disorders. Measurement after a water deprivation test is more useful (see Fig. 8.17).

TREATMENT Central DI is treated with hormone replacement or pharmacologic agents (Fig. 8.19). In acute settings, when renal water losses are extensive, aqueous vasopressin (Pitressin) is useful. It has a short duration of action, allows careful monitoring, and avoids complications such as water intoxication. This drug should be used with caution in patients with underlying coronary artery disease and peripheral vascular disease as it may cause vascular spasm and prolonged vasoconstriction. For chronic central DI, desmopressin acetate is the agent of choice. It has a long half-life and does not have the significant vasoconstrictive effects of aqueous vasopressin. It is administered at the dose of 10 to 20 μg intranasally every 12 to 24 hours. It is tolerated well, safe to use in pregnancy, and resistant to degradation by circulating vasopressinase. Oral desmopressin (0.1 to 0.8 mg every 12 hours) is available as second-line therapy. In patients with partial DI, in addition to desmopressin itself, agents that potentiate the release of vasopressin may be used. These agents include chlorpropamide, clofibrate, and carbamazepine.

Congenital Nephrogenic Diabetes Insipidus Inherited forms of DI are due to mutations in genes for aquaporins or vasopressin receptors. Urine volumes are typically very high, and there is a risk for severe hypernatremia if patients do not have free access to water. These entities are discussed further in Chapter 47.

Acquired Nephrogenic Diabetes Insipidus Acquired nephrogenic DI is more common than and rarely as severe as congenital nephrogenic DI. In these patients, the ability to elaborate a maximal concentration of urine is impaired, but urinary concentrating mechanisms are partially preserved. For this reason, urinary volumes are less than 3 to 4 l/day, which contrasts with the much higher volumes seen in patients with congenital or central DI or compulsive water drinking. The causes and mechanisms of acquired nephrogenic DI are listed in Figure 8.20.

CHRONIC KIDNEY DISEASE A defect in urinary concentrating ability may develop in patients with chronic kidney disease of any etiology, but this defect is most prominent in tubulointerstitial diseases, particularly medullary cystic disease. Disruption of inner medullary structures and diminished medullary concentration are thought to play a role; alterations in V_2 receptor and AQP2 expression also contribute (see Fig. 8.7). To achieve daily osmolar clearance, an amount of fluid commensurate with the severity of the concentrating defect is necessary in patients who still make urine. Patients should be advised to maintain a fluid intake that matches their urine volume.

ELECTROLYTE DISORDERS Hypokalemia causes a reversible abnormality in urinary concentrating ability. Hypokalemia stimulates water intake and reduces interstitial tonicity, which relates

Treatment of Central Diabetes Insipidus			
Disease	**Drug**	**Dose**	**Interval**
Complete central diabetes insipidus	Desmopressin (DDAVP) Desmopressin (DDAVP)	10–20 μg intranasally 0.1–0.8 mg orally	12–24 h Every 12 h
Partial central diabetes insipidus	Desmopressin (DDAVP) Aqueous vasopressin Chlorpropamide Clofibrate Carbamazepine	10–20 μg intranasally 5–10 U subcutaneously 250–500 mg 500 mg 400–600 mg	12–24 h 4–6 h 24 h 6 or 8 h 24 h

Figure 8.19 Treatment of central diabetes insipidus.

Acquired Nephrogenic Diabetes Insipidus: Causes and Mechanisms				
Disease State	**Defect in Generation of Medullary Interstitial Tonicity**	**Defect in cAMP Generation**	**Downregulation of Aquaporin 2**	**Other**
Chronic renal insufficiency	Yes	Yes	Yes	Downregulation of V_2 receptor message
Hypokalemia	Yes	Yes	Yes	—
Hypercalcemia	Yes	Yes	—	—
Sickle cell disease	Yes	—	—	—
Protein malnutrition	Yes	—	Yes	—
Demeclocycline therapy	—	Yes	—	—
Lithium therapy	—	Yes	Yes	—
Pregnancy	—	—	—	Placental secretion of vasopressinase

Figure 8.20 Acquired nephrogenic diabetes insipidus: causes and mechanisms. cAMP, cyclic adenosine monophosphate.

to the decreased Na^+-Cl^- reabsorption in the TALH. Hypokalemia resulting from diarrhea, chronic diuretic use, and primary aldosteronism also decreases intracellular cyclic adenosine monophosphate accumulation and causes a reduction in vasopressin-sensitive AQP2 expression (see Fig. 8.7).

Hypercalcemia also impairs urinary concentrating ability, resulting in mild polydipsia. The pathophysiologic mechanism is multifactorial and includes a reduction in medullary interstitial tonicity caused by decreased vasopressin-stimulated adenylate cyclase in the TALH and a defect in adenylate cyclase activity with decreased AQP2 expression in the collecting duct.

PHARMACOLOGIC AGENTS Lithium is the most common cause of nephrogenic DI, occurring in up to 50% of patients receiving long-term lithium therapy. Lithium causes downregulation of AQP2 in the collecting duct; experimentally, it also increases cyclooxygenase 2 (COX-2) expression and urinary prostaglandins, which may contribute to the polyuria.[43] The concentrating defect of lithium may persist even when the drug is discontinued. The epithelial sodium channel, ENaC, is the entrance pathway for lithium into collecting duct principal cells. Amiloride inhibits lithium uptake through ENaC and has been used clinically to treat nephrogenic DI caused by lithium. Aldosterone administration dramatically increases urine production in experimental nephrogenic DI due to lithium[44] (an effect that is associated with decreased expression of AQP2 on luminal membranes of the collecting duct), whereas administration of the mineralocorticoid receptor blocker spironolactone decreased urine output and increased AQP2 expression.[45] It is not yet known if spironolactone is a useful treatment for humans with lithium-induced nephrogenic DI.

Other drugs impairing urinary concentrating ability include amphotericin, foscarnet, and demeclocycline, which reduces renal medullary adenylate cyclase activity, thereby decreasing the effect of vasopressin on the collecting ducts.

SICKLE CELL ANEMIA Patients with sickle cell disease and trait often have a urinary concentrating defect. In the hypertonic medullary interstitium, the "sickled" red cells cause occlusion of the vasa recta and papillary damage. The resultant medullary ischemia may impair Na^+-Cl^- transport in the ascending limb and diminish medullary tonicity. Although initially reversible, medullary infarcts occur with long-standing sickle cell disease and the concentrating defects become irreversible.

DIETARY ABNORMALITIES Extensive water intake or a marked decrease in salt and protein intake leads to impairment of maximal urinary concentrating ability through a reduction in medullary interstitial tonicity. On a low-protein diet with excessive water intake, there is a decrease in vasopressin-stimulated osmotic water permeability that is reversed with feeding.

Gestational Diabetes Insipidus In gestational DI, there is an increase in circulating vasopressinase, which is produced by the placenta. Patients are typically unresponsive to vasopressin but respond to desmopressin, which is resistant to vasopressinase.

Clinical Manifestations of Hypernatremia

Certain patients are at increased risk for development of severe hypernatremia (Fig. 8.21). Signs and symptoms mostly relate to the CNS and include altered mental status, lethargy, irritability, restlessness, seizures (usually in children), muscle twitching, hyperreflexia, and spasticity. Fever, nausea or vomiting, labored breathing, and intense thirst can also occur. In children, the mortality of acute hypernatremia ranges between 10% and 70%.

Patient Groups at Risk for Development of Severe Hypernatremia
Elderly patients or infants
Hospitalized patients receiving hypertonic infusions, tube feedings, osmotic diuretics, lactulose, mechanical ventilation
Altered mental status
Uncontrolled diabetes mellitus
Underlying polyuric disorders

Figure 8.21 Patient groups at risk for development of severe hypernatremia. *(From reference 25.)*

As many as two thirds of survivors have neurologic sequelae. In contrast, mortality in chronic hypernatremia is 10%. In adults, serum Na^+ concentrations above 160 mmol/l are associated with a 75% mortality, although this may reflect associated comorbidities rather than hypernatremia *per se*.

Treatment of Hypernatremia

Hypernatremia occurs in predictable clinical settings, allowing opportunities for prevention. Elderly and hospitalized patients are at high risk because of impaired thirst and inability to access free water independently.[46] Certain clinical situations, such as recovery from acute kidney injury, catabolic states, therapy with hypertonic solutions, uncontrolled diabetes, and burns, should prompt close attention to serum sodium concentration and increased administration of free water.

Hypernatremia always reflects a hyperosmolar state. The primary goal in the treatment of these patients is the restoration of serum tonicity. The treatment regimen depends on the volume status. Specific management options are outlined in Figure 8.22.[25]

The rapidity with which hypernatremia should be corrected is a matter of controversy. Some animal studies and case series in pediatric patients suggest that a correction rate of more than 0.5 mmol/l per hour in $[Na^+]$ can cause seizures. Cerebral edema also can be caused by rapid correction of hypernatremia by the net movement of water into the brain. Most clinicians believe that even in adults, correction should be achieved during 48 hours at a rate no greater than 2 mmol/l per hour.

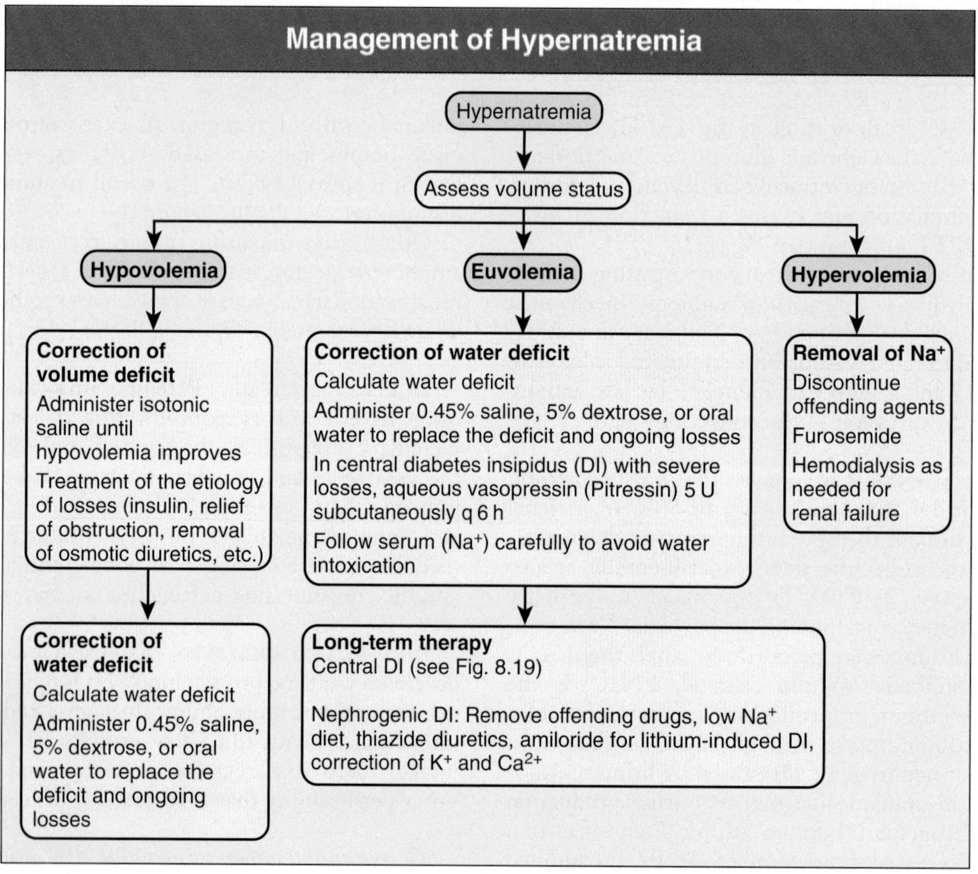

Figure 8.22 Management of hypernatremia. *(From reference 25.)*

REFERENCES

1. Verbalis J, Berl T. Disorders of water balance. In: Brenner BM, ed. *The Kidney*. 8th ed. Philadelphia: WB Saunders; 2008:459-504.
2. Narins RG, Krishna GC. Disorders of water balance. In: Stein JH, ed. *Internal Medicine*. Boston: Little, Brown; 1987, p 794.
3. Bichet D. Nephrogenic and central diabetes insipidus. In: Schrier R, ed. *Diseases of the Kidney and Urinary Tract*. Vol 3. 8th ed. Philadelphia: Lippincott Williams & Wilkins; 2007:2249-2269.
4. Nielsen S, Frøkiaer J, Marples D, et al. Aquaporins in the kidney: From molecules to medicine. *Physiol Rev*. 2002;82:205-244.
5. Halterman R, Berl T. Therapy of dysnatremic disorders. In: Brady H, Wilcox C, eds. *Therapy in Nephrology and Hypertension*. Philadelphia: WB Saunders; 1999, pp 257-269.
6. Nguyen MK, Ornekian V, Butch AW, et al. A new method for determining plasma water content: Application in pseudohyponatremia. *Am J Physiol*. 2007;292:F1652-F1656.
7. Cogan M. Normal water homeostasis. In: Cogan M, ed. *Fluid and Electrolytes*. Norwalk: CT, Lange; 1991, pp 98-106.
8. Sterns RH, Silver SM. Cerebral salt wasting versus SIADH: What difference? *J Am Soc Nephrol*. 2008;19:194-196.
9. Neilsen S, Schrier R, eds. *Diseases of the Kidney and Urinary Tract*, 8th ed. Philadelphia: Lippincott Williams & Wilkins; 2007.
10. Morita S, Inokuchi S, Yamamoto R, et al. Risk factors for rhabdomyolysis in self-induced water intoxication (SIWI) patients. *J Emerg Med*. 2008 Apr 23 [Epub ahead of print].
11. Steele A, Gowrishankar M, Abrahamson S, et al. Postoperative hyponatremia despite near-isotonic saline infusion: A phenomenon of desalination. *Ann Intern Med*. 1997;126:20-25.
12. Almond CS, Shin AY, Fortescue EB, et al. Hyponatremia among runners in the Boston Marathon. *N Engl J Med*. 2005;352:1550-1556.
13. Hew-Butler T, Jordaan E, Stuempfle KJ, et al. Osmotic and nonosmotic regulation of arginine vasopressin during prolonged endurance exercise. *J Clin Endocrinol Metab*. 2008;93:2072-2078.
14. Liamis G, Milionis H, Elisaf M. A review of drug-induced hyponatremia. *Am J Kidney Dis*. 2008;52:144-153.
15. Berl T, Schrier R. Disorders of water metabolism. In: Schrier R, ed. *Renal and Electrolyte Disorders*. 6th ed. Philadelphia: Lippincott Williams & Wilkins; 2010:1-44.
16. Palmer BF, Sterns RH. Fluid, electrolytes, and acid-base disturbances. *NephSAP*. 2009;8:70-167.
17. Daphnis E, Stylianou K, Alexandrakis M, et al. Acute renal failure, translocational hyponatremia and hyperkalemia following intravenous immunoglobulin therapy. *Nephron Clin Pract*. 2007;106:c143-148.
18. Miller M. Hyponatremia: Age related risk factors and therapy decisions. *Geriatrics*. 1998;53:32-33, 37-38, 41-42.
19. Ellison DH, Berl T. Clinical practice. The syndrome of inappropriate antidiuresis. *N Engl J Med*. 2007;356:2064-2072.
20. Decaux G, Vandergheynst F, Bouko Y, et al. Nephrogenic syndrome of inappropriate antidiuresis in adults: High phenotypic variability in men and women from a large pedigree. *J Am Soc Nephrol*. 2007;18:606-612.
21. Verbalis J. The syndrome of inappropriate antidiuretic hormone secretion and other hypo-osmolar disorders. In: Schrier R, ed. *Diseases of the Kidney and Urinary Tract*, 8th ed. Philadelphia: Lippincott Williams & Wilkins; 2007.
22. Papadopoulos MC, Verkman AS. Aquaporin-4 and brain edema. *Pediatr Nephrol*. 2007;22:778-784.
23. Yang B, Zador Z, Verkman AS. Glial cell aquaporin-4 overexpression in transgenic mice accelerates cytotoxic brain swelling. *J Biol Chem*. 2008;283:15280-15286.
24. Verbalis J. The syndrome of inappropriate antidiuretic hormone secretion and other hypo-osmolar disorders. In: Schrier R, ed. *Diseases of the Kidney and Urinary Tract*, 8th ed. Philadelphia: Lippincott Williams & Wilkins; 2007.
25. Thurman J, Berl T. Therapy of dysnatremic disorders. In: Wilcox C, ed. *Therapy in Nephrology and Hypertension*. 3rd ed. Philadelphia: WB Saunders; 2008:337-352.
26. Hew-Butler T, Ayus JC, Kipps C, et al. Statement of the Second International Exercise-Associated Hyponatremia Consensus Development Conference, New Zealand, 2007. *Clin J Sport Med*. 2008;18:111-121.
27. Mohmand HK, Issa D, Ahmad Z, et al. Hypertonic saline for hyponatremia: Risk of inadvertent overcorrection. *Clin J Am Soc Nephrol*. 2007;2:1110-1117.
28. Perianayagam A, Sterns RH, Silver SM, et al. DDAVP is effective in preventing and reversing inadvertent overcorrection of hyponatremia. *Clin J Am Soc Nephrol*. 2008;3:331-336.
29. Gankam Kengne F, Andres C, Sattar L, et al. Mild hyponatremia and risk of fracture in the ambulatory elderly. *QJM*. 2008;101:583-588.
30. Furst H, Hallows KR, Post J, et al. The urine/plasma electrolyte ratio: A predictive guide to water restriction. *Am J Med Sci*. 2000;319: 240-244.
31. Berl T. Impact of solute intake on urine flow and water excretion. *J Am Soc Nephrol*. 2008;6:1076-1078.
32. Schrier RW, Gross P, Gheorghiade M, et al. Tolvaptan, a selective oral vasopressin V_2-receptor antagonist, for hyponatremia. *N Engl J Med*. 2006;355:2099-2112.
33. Zeltser D, Rosansky S, van Rensburg H, et al. Assessment of the efficacy and safety of intravenous conivaptan in euvolemic and hypervolemic hyponatremia. *Am J Nephrol*. 2007;27:447-457.
34. Berl T, Schrier RW. Vasopressin antagonist in physiology and disease. In: Singh A, Williams G, eds. *Textbook of Nephro-Endocrinology*. San Diego: Academic Press; 2009:249-260.
35. Rossi J, Bayram M, Udelson JE, et al. Improvement in hyponatremia during hospitalization for worsening heart failure is associated with improved outcomes: Insights from the Acute and Chronic Therapeutic Impact of a Vasopressin Antagonist in Chronic Heart Failure (ACTIV in CHF) trial. *Acute Card Care*. 2007;9:82-86.
36. Ginès P, Wong F, Watson H, et al. Effects of satavaptan, a selective vasopressin V_2 receptor antagonist, on ascites and serum sodium in cirrhosis with hyponatremia: a randomized trial. *Hepatology*. 2008;48: 204-213.
37. Koenig MA, Bryan M, Lewin JL 3rd, et al. Reversal of transtentorial herniation with hypertonic saline. *Neurology*. 2008;70:1023-1029.
38. Maghnie M. Diabetes insipidus. *Horm Res*. 2003;59:42-54.
39. Phillips JA. Dominant-negative diabetes insipidus and other endocrinopathies. *J Clin Invest*. 2003;112:1641-1643.
40. Smith CJ, Crock PA, King BR, et al. Phenotype-genotype correlations in a series of Wolfram syndrome families. *Diabetes Care*. 2004; 27:2003-2009.
41. Mavrakis AN, Tritos NA. Diabetes insipidus with deficient thirst: Report of a patient and review of the literature. *Am J Kidney Dis*. 2008;51: 851-859.
42. Lanese D, Teitelbaum I. Hypernatremia. In: Jacobson HR, Striker GE, Klahr S, eds. *The Principles and Practice of Nephrology*, 2nd ed. St. Louis: Mosby; 1995, pp 893-898.
43. Rao R, Zhang MZ, Zhao M, et al. Lithium treatment inhibits renal GSK-3 activity and promotes cyclooxygenase 2 dependent polyuria. *Am J Physiol Renal Physiol*. 2005;288:F642-F649.
44. Bedford JJ, Weggery S, Ellis G, et al. Lithium-induced nephrogenic diabetes insipidus: Renal effects of amiloride. *Clin J Am Soc Nephrol*. 2008;3:1324-1331.
45. Nielsen J, Kwon TH, Frøkiaer J, et al. Lithium-induced NDI in rats is associated with loss of alpha-ENaC regulation by aldosterone in CCD. *Am J Physiol Renal Physiol*. 2006;290:F1222-F1233.
46. Polderman KH, Schreuder WO, van Schijndel RJ, et al. Hypernatremia in the intensive care unit: An indicator of quality of care? *Crit Care Med*. 1999;27:1105-1108.

CHAPTER 9

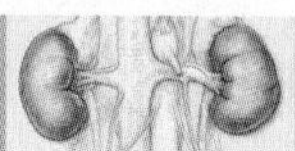

Disorders of Potassium Metabolism

I. David Weiner, Stuart L. Linas, Charles S. Wingo

DEFINITION

Potassium disorders are some of the most commonly encountered fluid and electrolyte abnormalities in clinical medicine. They can be asymptomatic or associated with symptoms ranging from mild weakness to sudden death. When the serum potassium concentration is verified as abnormal, correction is essential, but inappropriate treatment can worsen symptoms and even lead to death.

NORMAL PHYSIOLOGY OF POTASSIUM METABOLISM

Potassium Intake

Potassium is essential for many cellular functions, is present in most foods, and is excreted primarily by the kidney. The typical daily Western diet contains approximately 70 to 150 mmol potassium. The gastrointestinal tract efficiently absorbs potassium, and dietary potassium intake varies greatly with the composition of the diet. Figure 9.1 summarizes the potassium content of several foods high in potassium content.

Potassium Distribution

After absorption from the gastrointestinal tract, potassium distributes into the extracellular and intracellular fluid compartments. Potassium is the major intracellular cation, with values from ~100 to 120 mmol/l in the cytosol, and is distributed primarily intracellularly. Total intracellular potassium content is 3000 to 3500 mmol in healthy adults, which is distributed primarily in muscle (70%), with smaller amounts present in bone, red blood cells, liver, and skin (Fig. 9.2). Only 1% to 2% of total body potassium is present in the extracellular fluids. The electrogenic sodium pump, Na^+,K^+-ATPase, effects this asymmetric potassium distribution by active uptake, which occurs in virtually all cells. Na^+,K^+-ATPase transports two potassium ions into cells in exchange for extrusion of three sodium ions, which results in high intracellular potassium and low intracellular sodium activity. The ratio of intracellular to extracellular potassium concentration is a major determinant of cell membrane potential and intracellular electronegativity due to the action of potassium-selective ion channels. Normal maintenance of this ratio and membrane potential is critical for normal nerve conduction and muscle contraction.

Serum potassium concentration is tightly regulated through multiple mechanisms. Studies support a "feed forward" regulatory system involving gut or portal potassium sensors. This system adjusts renal potassium excretion through mechanisms independent of serum potassium and aldosterone.[1,2] This reflex system, which is still not understood fully, allows the kidney to "sense" dietary intake and to alter renal potassium excretion despite no discernible changes in plasma potassium or aldosterone concentration.

In addition, several hormones and factors can induce potassium shifts between the extracellular and intracellular potassium pools (Fig. 9.3). The most common causes include acid-base disorders, specific hormones, plasma osmolality, and exercise.

Acidosis due to inorganic anions, such as NH_4Cl and HCl, can cause hyperkalemia, but the mechanism is not fully understood. In contrast, organic acids (such as lactic acid), in general, do not cause transcellular potassium shifts. Insulin and β_2-adrenergic receptor activation induce cellular potassium uptake by stimulating Na^+,K^+-ATPase. Insulin directly stimulates the Na^+,K^+-ATPase pump through a mechanism separate from its stimulation of glucose entry. β_2-Adrenergic receptor activation increases intracellular cyclic adenosine monophosphate production, which stimulates Na^+,K^+-ATPase–mediated potassium uptake. α-Adrenergic activation opposes the effect of β_2-adrenergic receptor stimulation. The effects of insulin and β_2-adrenergic receptor activation are synergistic, as expected given the differing cellular mechanisms.

Aldosterone lowers serum potassium concentration by two major mechanisms. Aldosterone stimulates potassium movement into cells (redistribution), and it increases potassium excretion in the kidney and, to a lesser extent, in the gut. The primary renal action of aldosterone is to stimulate sodium reabsorption; but with ample sodium delivery to the late distal nephron and collecting duct, this promotes enhanced flow-dependent potassium excretion.

Hyperosmolality, if it is due to effective osmoles, can induce potassium shifts out of cells and result in hyperkalemia. The proposed mechanism is that increased plasma osmolality induces water movement out of the cells, which decreases cell volume and increases intracellular potassium concentrations. This is then thought to result in feedback inhibition of Na^+,K^+-ATPase, shifting potassium from the intracellular to the extracellular compartment and normalizing intracellular potassium concentration. The clinician should remember that this occurs only with effective osmoles, such as hyperglycemia in persons with diabetes or with mannitol. Both glucose, in a patient with intact insulin secretion, and urea are ineffective osmoles because they rapidly cross plasma membranes and therefore do not alter cell volume. Importantly, hyperglycemia in a nondiabetic patient, if it stimulates endogenous insulin secretion or if exogenous insulin is given, can cause insulin-induced cellular potassium uptake and resultant hypokalemia.

Exercise may result in hyperkalemia by α-adrenergic receptor activation that shifts potassium out of the skeletal muscle cells. The increased serum potassium induces arterial dilation, which

Potassium Content of Selected High-Potassium Foods

Food	Portion Size	mmol K^+
Artichoke, boiled	1, medium	27
Avocado	1, medium	38
Sirloin steak	8 oz	23
Hamburger, lean	8 oz	18
Cantaloupe, cut up	1 cup	13
Grapefruit juice	8 oz	10
Milk	8 oz	10
Orange juice	8 oz	12
Potato, baked	7 oz	22
Prunes	10	16
Raisins	2/3 cup	19
Squash	1 cup	15–20
Tomato paste	1/2 cup	31
Tomato juice	6 oz	10
Banana	Medium size	12

Figure 9.1 Potassium content of selected high-potassium foods. *(Data modified from Na-K-Phos Counter, published by the American Association of Kidney Patients, Inc., 1999.)*

Distribution of Total Body Potassium in Organs and Body Compartments

Organs and Compartments		Body Compartment Concentrations	
Muscle	2650 mmol	Intracellular concentration	150 mmol/l
Liver	250 mmol	Extracellular concentration	4 mmol/l
Interstitial fluid	35 mmol		
Red blood cells	35 mmol		
Plasma	15 mmol		

Figure 9.2 Distribution of total body potassium in organs and body compartments.

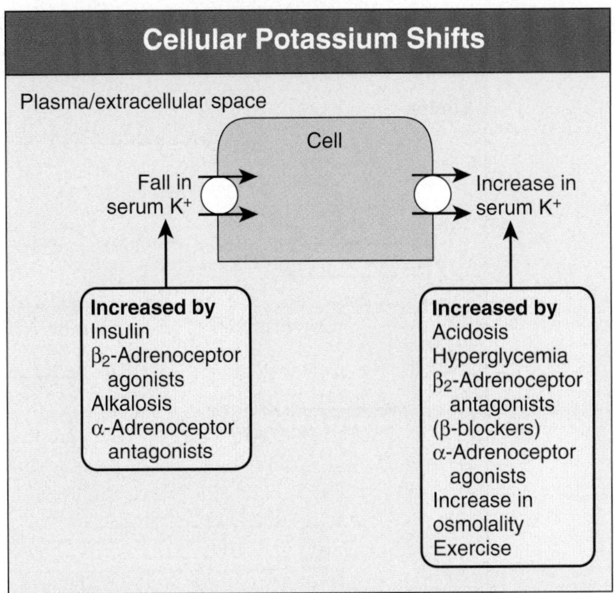

Figure 9.3 Regulation of extracellular-intracellular potassium shifts.

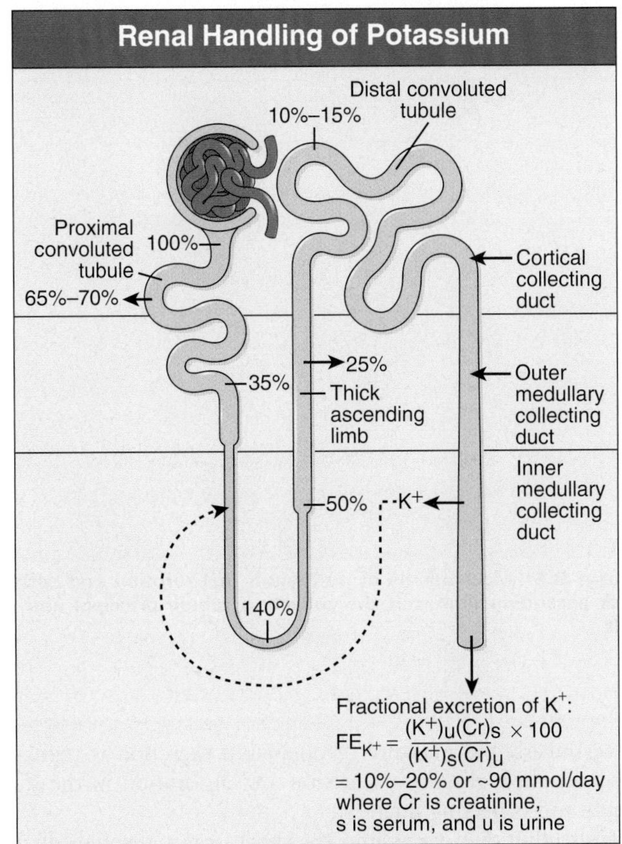

Figure 9.4 Renal handling of potassium.

increases skeletal muscle blood flow and acts as an adaptive mechanism during exercise. Simultaneous β_2-adrenergic receptor activation stimulates skeletal muscle cellular potassium uptake and minimizes the severity of exercise-induced hyperkalemia, but this can lead to hypokalemia after the cessation of exercise. In patients with preexisting potassium depletion, post-exercise hypokalemia may be severe and rhabdomyolysis may occur.[3]

Renal Potassium Handling with Normal Renal Function

Long-term potassium homeostasis is accomplished primarily through changes in renal potassium excretion and here almost entirely through regulated collecting duct potassium transport. Serum potassium is almost completely ionized, is not bound to plasma proteins, and is filtered efficiently by the glomerulus (Fig. 9.4). The proximal tubule reabsorbs the majority (~65% to 70%) of filtered potassium. Very little regulation occurs in response to changes in dietary potassium intake. Potassium is secreted by the descending loop of Henle, at least in deep nephrons, and is reabsorbed by the ascending loop of Henle through the action of the Na^+-K^+-$2Cl^-$ cotransporter (Fig. 9.5A). This results in modest net potassium reabsorption in the loop of Henle. This absorption can be reversed to secretion, however, by administration of a loop diuretic or by substantial potassium loading.

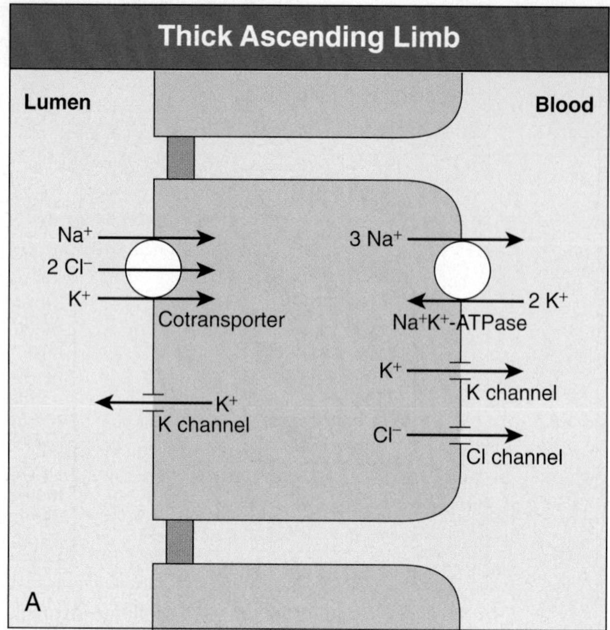

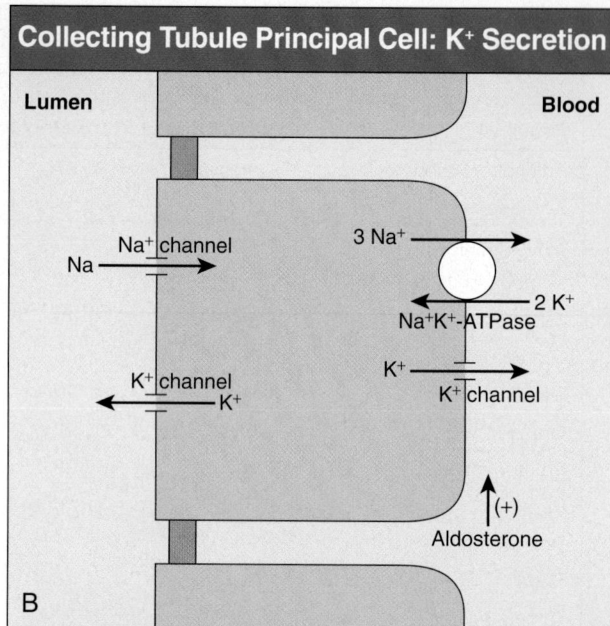

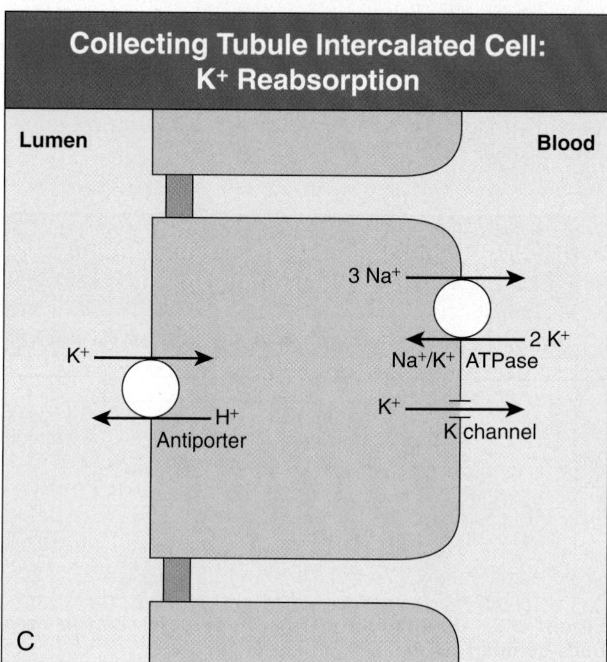

Figure 9.5 Mechanisms of potassium reabsorption and secretion in the thick ascending limb and the collecting tubule principal and intercalated cells.

Nevertheless, the majority of potassium excretion is regulated normally through active secretion and absorption in the distal tubule and collecting duct.

Collecting duct potassium transport occurs through distinct cell types that allow fine control of renal potassium excretion. The principal cell of the cortical collecting duct secretes potassium (Fig. 9.5B). Sodium reabsorption through the apical sodium channel (ENaC) stimulates basolateral Na^+,K^+-ATPase, and the active turnover of this pump maintains high intracellular potassium concentrations. Subsequent to basolateral potassium uptake, potassium is secreted into the luminal fluid by apical potassium channels and KCl cotransporters. Intercalated cells reabsorb potassium through an apical H^+,K^+-ATPase (Fig. 9.5C).[4] This protein actively secretes H^+ into the luminal fluid in exchange for potassium, resulting in potassium reabsorption. The presence of two separate potassium transport processes, secretion by principal cells and reabsorption by intercalated cells, enables effective regulation of renal potassium excretion.

Several factors regulate principal cell potassium secretion. In relative order of importance, these are luminal flow rate, distal sodium delivery, aldosterone, extracellular potassium, and extracellular pH. An increase in luminal flow rate reduces luminal potassium concentration, thereby increasing the concentration gradient across the apical membrane, which stimulates potassium secretion. In addition, flow rate directly influences cellular potassium secretion, possibly by modulating the activity of potassium channels. Conversely, reduced luminal flow, such as occurs in prerenal states or obstruction, may result in hyperkalemia. Decreased sodium reabsorption, whether from reduced luminal sodium delivery or from sodium channel inhibitors, decreases potassium secretion by altering electrochemical forces for potassium secretion. "Potassium-sparing diuretics," either directly or indirectly, reduce sodium reabsorption and thereby inhibit potassium secretion. Increased sodium delivery to the collecting duct, such as may occur with loop or thiazide diuretics, increases principal cell sodium reabsorption and causes a secondary increase in potassium secretion. Aldosterone has many effects that increase principal cell potassium secretion. These include increases in Na^+,K^+-ATPase expression and increased apical expression of the sodium channel ENaC. The net effect is increased potassium secretion. Increasing extracellular potassium directly stimulates Na^+,K^+-ATPase activity, leading to increased potassium secretion. Metabolic acidosis decreases potassium secretion both through direct effects on potassium channels and through changes in interstitial ammonia concentration, which then decreases potassium secretion.[5] Respiratory acid-base disorders in general have little effect on potassium secretion.

Potassium reabsorption, which decreases renal potassium excretion, occurs through the action of the active potassium-reabsorbing transporter H^+,K^+-ATPase. The major factors regulating H^+,K^+-ATPase expression and activity include potassium balance, aldosterone, and acid-base status. Potassium depletion increases H^+,K^+-ATPase expression, which then results in increased active potassium reabsorption and decreased potassium excretion. Aldosterone is a second factor that increases H^+,K^+-ATPase expression and activity. This may, by decreasing net potassium excretion, serve as a "counterbalancing factor" to minimize the hypokalemia that results generally from increased aldosterone. Metabolic acidosis has both direct and indirect (mediated through alterations of ammonia metabolism) effects that increase H^+,K^+-ATPase potassium transport. In some cases, this may contribute to the hyperkalemia that can occur with metabolic acidosis.

Intracellular kinases of a new class that are important for regulating renal potassium physiology in the distal nephron have recently been identified. The WNK (with no lysine) kinases are a family of proteins expressed in many cells of the body, including the kidney. Under basal conditions, several WNK kinases prevent sodium reabsorption (in part by downregulation of the Na^+-Cl^- cotransporter [NCC] and paracellular sodium flux) as well as potassium secretion (in part by inhibition of the renal outer medullary potassium channel [ROMK]). Genetic defects that inactivate several WNK kinases result in enhanced sodium reabsorption and reduced potassium secretion.

Renal Potassium Handling in Chronic Kidney Disease

Potassium homeostasis is relatively well preserved and serum potassium concentration usually remains in the normal range until glomerular filtration rate (GFR) is reduced substantially. This adaptation is due to increased potassium excretion per nephron in the connecting segment and the collecting duct. Both aldosterone and an increase in serum potassium may contribute to this adaptation. Intestinal potassium secretion increases also, although this is less important quantitatively.

Patients with chronic kidney disease (CKD) have more difficulty handling an acute potassium load, even when they have a normal serum potassium concentration. Because these patients have decreased nephron number, their maximal capacity for potassium secretion is limited. Patients with CKD are also routinely treated with medications that alter renal potassium handling, such as angiotensin-converting enzyme (ACE) inhibitors, angiotensin receptor blockers (ARBs), and β-adrenergic receptor blockers. These can decrease renal potassium sensitivity and result in higher serum potassium concentrations.

Patients with CKD generally tolerate hyperkalemia with fewer cardiac and electrocardiographic abnormalities than patients with normal renal function do. The mechanism of this adaptation is incompletely understood. Nevertheless, severe hyperkalemia (>6.0 mmol/l or the presence of electrocardiographic changes) can have lethal effects and should be treated aggressively.

HYPOKALEMIA

Epidemiology

The incidence of potassium disorders is strongly dependent on the patient population. Less than 1% of adults with normal renal function not receiving medicines develop hypokalemia or hyperkalemia; however, diets with large sodium and small potassium content may lead to potassium depletion. Thus, hypokalemia or hyperkalemia in a healthy adult not taking medicine should suggest an underlying disease. In contrast, hypokalemia frequently occurs in the setting of specific disease states and with the use of medicines that affect renal potassium handling. For example, hypokalemia may be present in up to 50% of patients using diuretics,[6] and it is present frequently in people with primary or secondary hyperaldosteronism.

Clinical Manifestations

Potassium deficiency alters the function of the heart and blood vessels, nerves, muscles, gut, and kidneys. Overall, children and young adults tolerate hypokalemia better than elderly individuals do. Prompt correction is warranted in the presence of ischemic heart disease or in patients receiving digitalis.

Cardiovascular

Epidemiologic studies link a low-potassium diet with an increased prevalence of hypertension. Hypokalemia has been shown experimentally to increase blood pressure modestly (5 to 10 mm Hg), and similarly, potassium supplementation can lower blood pressure.[7] Potassium deficiency probably increases blood pressure by stimulating sodium retention, with resultant intravascular volume expansion, and by sensitizing the vasculature to endogenous vasoconstrictors.[7] In part, sodium retention is related to decreased expression of the kidney-specific isoform of WNK1, which leads to increased NCC- and ENaC-mediated sodium reabsorption in the distal convoluted tubule and cortical collecting duct, respectively.[8]

Hypokalemia increases the risk for a variety of ventricular arrhythmias, including ventricular fibrillation.[9] Diuretic-induced hypokalemia is of particular concern, as sudden cardiac death may occur more commonly in those treated with thiazide diuretics.[9] Ventricular arrhythmias are also more common in hypokalemic patients receiving digoxin.

Hormonal

Hypokalemia impairs insulin release and also induces insulin resistance, resulting in worsened glucose control in diabetic patients.[10] Experimental studies have demonstrated that the insulin resistance observed with thiazide diuretics is due to endothelial dysfunction mediated by thiazide-induced hypokalemia and hyperuricemia.[11,12]

Muscular

Hypokalemia hyperpolarizes skeletal muscle cells, thereby impairing muscle contraction. Hypokalemia also reduces skeletal muscle blood flow, possibly by impairing local nitric oxide release, which can predispose patients to rhabdomyolysis during vigorous exercise.[13]

Renal

Hypokalemia leads to several important disturbances of renal function. These include reduced medullary blood flow and increased renal vascular resistance that may predispose to hypertension, tubulointerstitial and cystic changes, alterations in acid-base balance, and impairment of renal concentrating mechanisms.

Tubulointerstitial and Cystic Changes Potassium depletion causes tubulointerstitial fibrosis that is generally greatest in the outer medulla. Although usually reversible, it may result in renal failure. Experimental studies suggest that there is increased risk for irreversible renal injury in the neonatal period.[14] Potassium depletion also causes renal hypertrophy and predisposes to renal cyst formation, particularly when there is increased mineralocorticoid activity.

Acid-Base Metabolic alkalosis is a common acid-base consequence of potassium depletion and is due to increased renal net acid excretion.[15] Conversely, metabolic alkalosis may increase renal potassium excretion, resulting in potassium depletion. Severe hypokalemia can lead to respiratory muscle weakness and the development of respiratory acidosis.

Polyuria Severe hypokalemia also impairs concentrating ability, causing mild polyuria, typically 2 to 3 liters per day. Both increased thirst and mild nephrogenic diabetes insipidus contribute to the polyuria.[16]

Hepatic Encephalopathy

Hypokalemia increases renal ammonia production, approximately half of which returns to the systemic circulation through the renal veins and may worsen hepatic encephalopathy.[17]

Etiology

Hypokalemia results typically from one of four causes: pseudohypokalemia, redistribution, extrarenal potassium loss, and renal potassium loss. Of course, multiple causes may coexist in an individual person.

Pseudohypokalemia

Pseudohypokalemia refers to the condition in which serum potassium decreases, artifactually, after phlebotomy. The most common cause is acute myeloblastic leukemia, in which the large numbers of abnormal leukocytes take up potassium when the blood is stored in a collection vial for prolonged periods at room temperature. Rapid separation of plasma and storage at 4°C confirm this diagnosis and should be used for subsequent testing once pseudohypokalemia is diagnosed to avoid this artifact, leading to inappropriate treatment.

Redistribution

Because more than 98% of total body potassium is intracellular, small potassium shifts from the extracellular to the intracellular compartment can result in hypokalemia. As discussed before, many hormones, particularly insulin, aldosterone, and β_2-adrenergic agonists, stimulate transcellular potassium uptake.

Rarely, hypokalemia is due to hypokalemic periodic paralysis.[18] In this condition, attacks occur generally during the night or the early morning or after a carbohydrate-rich meal. Flaccid paralysis that persists typically for 6 to 24 hours characterizes these attacks. A genetic defect in a dihydropyridine-sensitive calcium channel has been identified in some cases[19]; other cases are associated with hyperthyroidism.

Nonrenal Potassium Loss

The skin and the gastrointestinal tract normally excrete small amounts of potassium. On occasion, excessive sweating or chronic diarrhea causes substantial potassium loss.[20] Vomiting or nasogastric suction may also result in loss of potassium, although gastric fluids typically contain only 5 to 8 mmol/l of potassium. However, the concomitant metabolic alkalosis and the intravascular volume depletion result in secondary hyperaldosteronism that can increase urinary potassium loss and contribute to the development of hypokalemia.[20]

Renal Potassium Loss

The most common cause of hypokalemia is renal potassium loss. This can occur from medications, endogenous hormone production, or, in rare conditions, intrinsic renal defects.

Medicines Both thiazide and loop diuretics increase urinary potassium excretion, and the incidence of diuretic-induced hypokalemia is both dose and treatment duration related. Adjusted for their natriuretic effect, thiazide diuretics cause more urinary potassium loss than loop diuretics do. Certain antibiotics increase urinary potassium excretion. Some penicillin analogues, such as carbenicillin, increase distal tubular delivery of a non-reabsorbable anion that obligates the presence of a cation such as potassium, thereby increasing urinary potassium excretion.[21] The antifungal agent amphotericin directly increases collecting duct potassium secretion.[22] Aminoglycosides may cause hypokalemia either with or without simultaneous nephrotoxicity. The mechanism is incompletely understood but may relate to magnesium depletion (see later discussion of magnesium sulfate). Cisplatin is a commonly used antineoplastic agent that can induce hypokalemia. Toluene exposure, from sniffing of certain glues, can also cause renal tubular acidosis with renal potassium wasting, leading to hypokalemia.[23] Finally, certain herbal products, including herbal cough mixtures, licorice tea, licorice root, and gan cao, contain glycyrrhizic and glycyrrhetinic acids, which have mineralocorticoid-like effects.[24]

Endogenous Hormones Endogenous hormones are important and common causes of hypokalemia. Aldosterone is the most important hormone regulating total body potassium homeostasis and causes hypokalemia both by stimulating potassium uptake into cells and by stimulating renal potassium excretion.

Other Rarely, genetic defects lead to excessive aldosterone production (see Chapter 47). In glucocorticoid-remediable aldosteronism, an adrenocorticotropic hormone (ACTH)–regulated promoter is linked to the gene for aldosterone synthase, the rate-limiting enzyme for aldosterone synthesis.[25] As a result, aldosterone synthase expression is regulated by ACTH, and hyperaldosteronism ensues. In congenital adrenal hyperplasia, there is persistent adrenal synthesis of 11-deoxycorticosterone, a potent mineralocorticoid.[26] This condition can be recognized by the associated effects on sex steroid production.

In another rare condition, glucocorticoid hormones activate the mineralocorticoid receptor. Under normal conditions, the enzyme 11β-hydroxysteroid dehydrogenase (11β-HSD) rapidly metabolizes cortisol to cortisone, thereby preventing inappropriate activation of mineralocorticoid receptors.[27] If this does not occur, glucocorticoid hormones are able to activate mineralocorticoid receptors. Some compounds, such as glycyrrhetinic acid, found in some chewing tobacco and licorice preparations, inhibit 11β-HSD, allowing cortisol to exert mineralocorticoid-like effects.[28] In severe Cushing's syndrome, circulating cortisol exceeds the metabolic capacity of 11β-HSDH and can cause hypokalemia.[29] Genetic deficiency of 11β-HSD (type 2) is rare but leads to severe hypertension and hypokalemia.

Magnesium Depletion

Magnesium deficiency inhibits renal potassium retention.[30] This is particularly true with diuretic-induced hypokalemia and in certain cases of aminoglycoside- and cisplatin-induced potassium wasting. This condition should be suspected in the individual in whom potassium replacement does not correct the hypokalemia.

Intrinsic Renal Defect

Intrinsic renal potassium transport defects leading to hypokalemia are rare but have led to important advances in our understanding of renal solute transport. Patients with Bartter syndrome have hypokalemia, reduced or normal blood pressure, hyperreninemia, metabolic alkalosis, and hypercalciuria. They typically present at a young age with severe volume depletion and growth retardation. Bartter syndrome results from genetic abnormalities in proteins involved in thick ascending limb of the loop of Henle sodium and potassium transport.[31] Gitelman's syndrome is similar to Bartter syndrome, except that patients have hypocalciuria, have milder clinical manifestations, and usually are diagnosed later in life. Gitelman's syndrome results from genetic abnormalities in the proteins involved in distal convoluted tubule sodium and potassium transport and causes clinical abnormalities similar to those seen with excessive thiazide diuretic use.[32]

Liddle syndrome is characterized by severe hypertension, hypokalemia, and suppressed renin and aldosterone levels. This condition is due to a mutation resulting in activation of the collecting duct epithelial sodium channel, leading to excessive sodium reabsorption, potassium excretion, volume expansion, and hypertension.[33]

Bicarbonaturia

Bicarbonaturia can result from metabolic alkalosis, distal renal tubular acidosis, or treatment of proximal renal tubular acidosis. In each case, the increased distal tubular bicarbonate delivery increases potassium secretion.

Diagnosis

The evaluation of hypokalemia is summarized in Figure 9.6. One should first exclude pseudohypokalemia or redistribution from the extracellular to the intracellular space. Insulin, aldosterone or its synthetic analogue fludrocortisone, and sympathomimetic agents, such as theophylline and β_2-adrenergic receptor agonists, are common causes of potassium redistribution.

If neither of these possibilities is present, the hypokalemia probably represents total body potassium depletion due to renal, gastrointestinal, or skin losses. Renal potassium loss is most frequently due to diuretics or metabolic alkalosis. Hypomagnesemia-induced hypokalemia causes renal potassium wasting and is frequently a complication of diuretic use. Rarer causes of renal potassium loss include renal tubular acidosis, diabetic ketoacidosis, and ureterosigmoidostomy. Primary aldosteronism, surreptitious diuretic use or vomiting, concomitant magnesium depletion, and Bartter or Gitelman's syndrome should be considered when the cause of the hypokalemia is not obvious. Finally, excessive potassium loss may result through the skin (excessive sweating) or from diarrhea, vomiting, nasogastric suction, or a gastrointestinal fistula. Patients are occasionally reluctant to admit to self-induced diarrhea, and the diagnosis may need to be confirmed by sigmoidoscopy or direct testing of the stool for cathartic agents.

Treatment

The risks associated with hypokalemia must be balanced against the risks of therapy. Usually, the primary short-term risks are cardiovascular arrhythmias and neuromuscular symptoms. In contrast, the primary risk of overaggressive replacement is acute hyperkalemia, which can cause ventricular fibrillation and sudden death.

Conditions requiring urgent therapy are rare. The clearest indications are hypokalemic periodic paralysis, severe hypokalemia in a patient requiring urgent surgery, and acute myocardial infarction in the patient with significant ventricular ectopy. In such cases, KCl can be given intravenously at a dose of 5 to 10 mmol during 15 to 20 minutes. This dose can be repeated as needed. Close, continuous monitoring of the serum potassium concentration and the electrocardiogram (ECG) is necessary to reduce the risk of hyperkalemia.

The body responds to chronic hypokalemia due to potassium losses by shifting potassium from the intracellular to the extracellular space. This minimizes the apparent magnitude of the hypokalemia, and the amount of potassium needed to replace the deficit is much greater than predicted by the change in extracellular potassium concentration and the extracellular fluid volume (Fig. 9.7). Potassium replacement can be given intravenously or orally, which is preferred if the patient can take oral medication and there is normal gastrointestinal tract function. When it is administered intravenously, replacement can be given safely at a rate of 10 mmol KCl per hour. Although significant variations can occur between patients, intravenous administration of 20 mmol KCl typically increases the serum potassium by ~0.25 mmol/l.[34] If more rapid replacement is necessary, 20 mmol/h can be administered through a central venous catheter, but simultaneous continuous ECG monitoring should be used under these circumstances.

The parenteral fluids used for potassium administration can affect the response. In patients without diabetes mellitus, dextrose administration increases serum insulin levels, which can cause redistribution of potassium from the extracellular to the intracellular space. As a result, if KCl is administered in dextrose-containing solutions (e.g., 5% dextrose in water), the dextrose load may actually stimulate cellular potassium uptake to an extent that exceeds the KCl replacement rate, resulting, paradoxically, in worsening of the hypokalemia.[35] Consequently, parenteral KCl should be administered in dextrose-free solutions.

The risk of hyperkalemia due to potassium replacement is less when it is given orally. This reflects several factors, most prominently gut sensors that minimize changes in serum potassium levels.

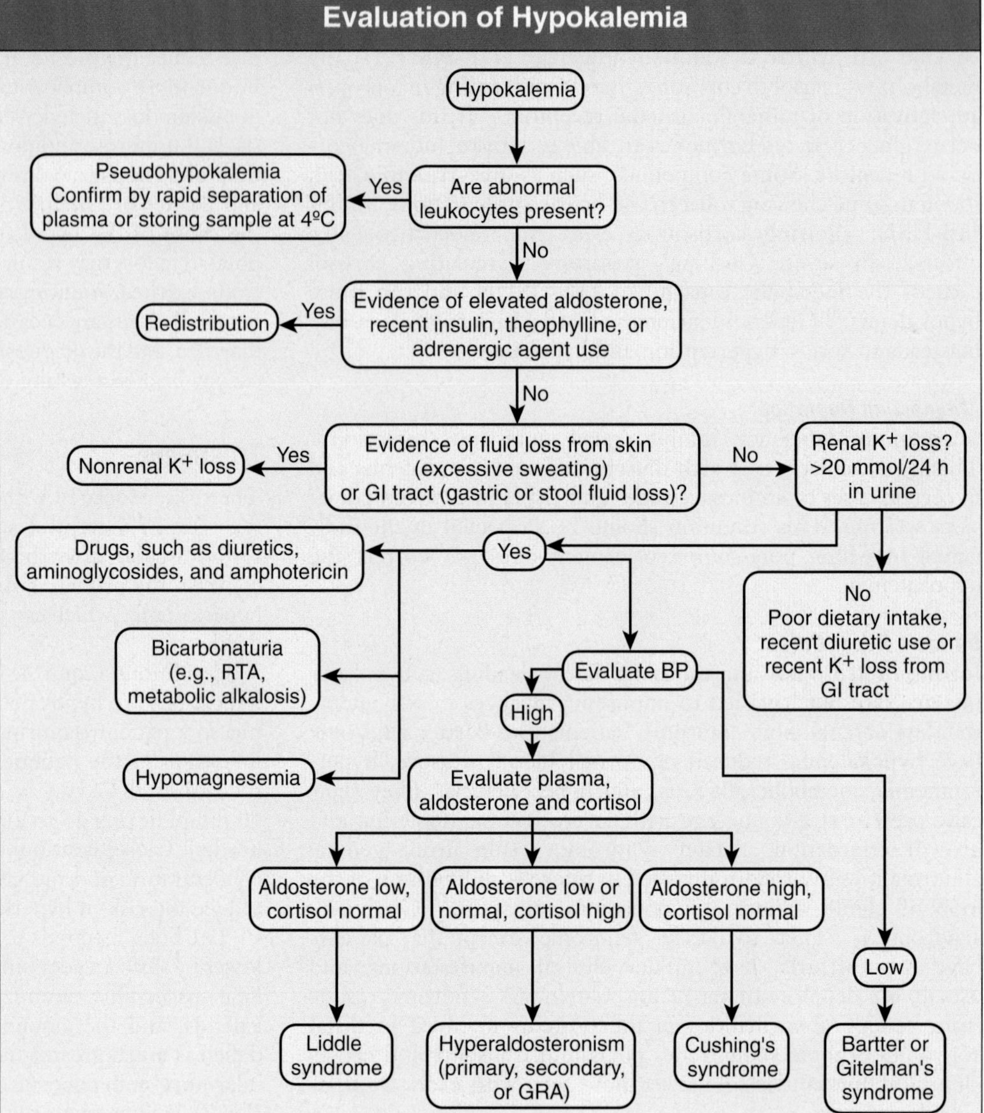

Figure 9.6 Diagnostic evaluation of hypokalemia. BP, blood pressure; GI, gastrointestinal; GRA, glucocorticoid-remediable aldosteronism; RTA, renal tubular acidosis.

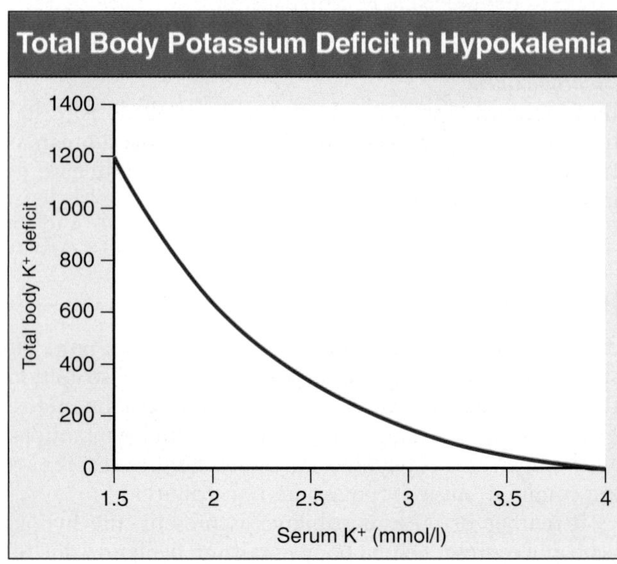

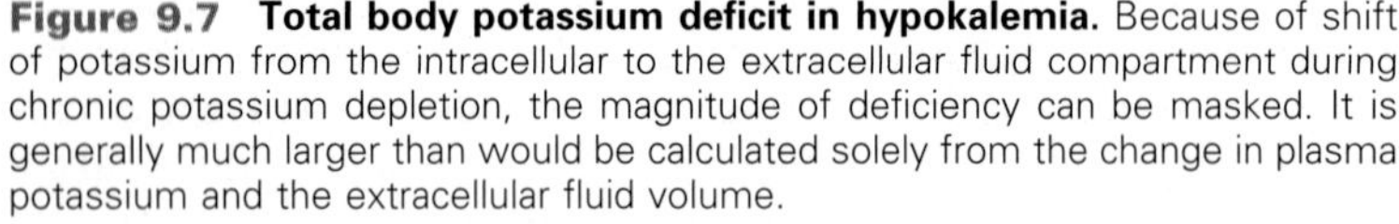

Figure 9.7 Total body potassium deficit in hypokalemia. Because of shift of potassium from the intracellular to the extracellular fluid compartment during chronic potassium depletion, the magnitude of deficiency can be masked. It is generally much larger than would be calculated solely from the change in plasma potassium and the extracellular fluid volume.

The underlying condition should be treated whenever possible. If patients with diuretic-induced hypokalemia still need diuretics, concomitant use of potassium-sparing diuretics may be considered. When oral replacement therapy is required, KCl is the preferred drug in all patients, except those with metabolic acidosis, in which potassium bicarbonate or potassium citrate may be considered a concomitant alkali source. If indicated for other reasons, β-blockers, ACE inhibitors, and ARBs can assist in maintaining serum potassium levels.

Hypomagnesemia can lead to refractoriness to potassium replacement because of inability of the kidneys to decrease potassium excretion.[30] Correction of the hypokalemia may not occur until the hypomagnesemia is corrected. Patients with unexplained hypokalemia or with diuretic-induced hypokalemia should have serum magnesium checked and, if indicated, magnesium replacement therapy instituted, usually with $MgSO_4$, and periodic measurement of serum [Mg^{2+}].

HYPERKALEMIA

Epidemiology

Hyperkalemia develops in less than 1% of normal healthy adults in the absence of significant underlying disease or medication use. This low frequency is a testament to the potent mechanisms for renal potassium excretion. Accordingly, hyperkalemia should suggest an underlying impairment of renal potassium excretion. Rarely, pseudohyperkalemia or conditions that shift potassium from the intracellular space to the extracellular space are present.

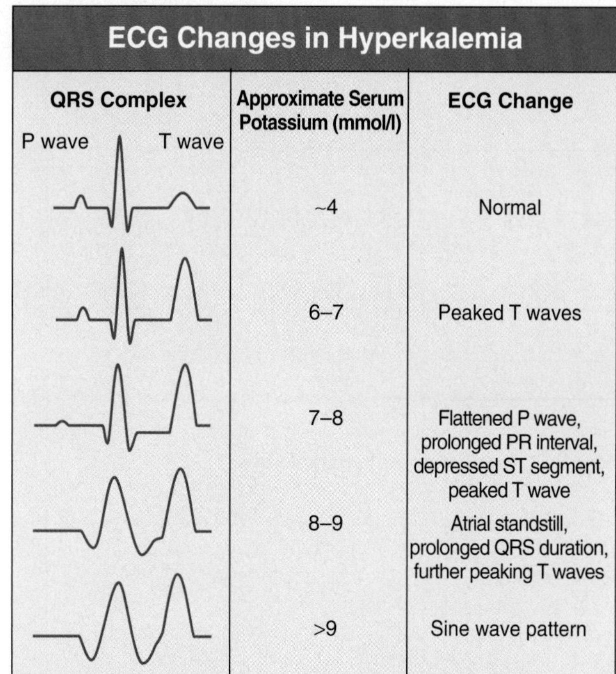

Figure 9.8 Electrocardiographic changes in hyperkalemia. Progressive hyperkalemia results in identifiable changes on the ECG. These include peaking of the T wave, flattening of the P wave, prolongation of the PR interval, ST-segment depression, prolongation of the QRS complex, and, eventually, progression to a sine wave pattern. Ventricular fibrillation may occur at any time during this progression.

Clinical Manifestations

Hyperkalemia may be asymptomatic but still life-threatening. The most prominent effect of hyperkalemia is alteration of cardiac conduction. This is demonstrable on the ECG (Fig. 9.8). The initial effect of hyperkalemia is a generalized increase in the height of the T waves, most evident in the precordial leads, which is known as tenting. More severe hyperkalemia is associated with delayed electrical conduction, resulting in increased PR and QRS intervals. This is followed by progressive flattening and eventual absence of the P waves. Under extreme conditions, the QRS complex widens sufficiently that it merges with the T wave, resulting in a sine wave pattern. Finally, an idioventricular rhythm followed by ventricular fibrillation develops. Although the ECG findings correlate generally with the degree of hyperkalemia, the rate of progression from mild to severe cardiac effects may be unpredictable and may not correlate well with changes in the plasma potassium concentration.

Hyperkalemia also affects muscle contraction. Skeletal muscle cells are particularly sensitive to hyperkalemia, causing weakness ("rubbery" or "spaghetti" legs). With severe hyperkalemia, respiratory failure may occur from paralysis of the diaphragm.

Etiology

Hyperkalemia can be due to pseudohyperkalemia, redistribution of potassium from the intracellular to the extracellular space, or imbalances between potassium intake and renal potassium excretion. A diagnostic approach is shown in Figure 9.9.

Pseudohyperkalemia

Serum potassium concentration may be artificially increased (pseudohyperkalemia) because of potassium release from erythrocyte hemolysis during collection or from cellular elements during clotting. The latter most commonly occurs in people with severe leukocytosis (>70,000/cm^3) or marked thrombocytosis. Approximately one third of patients with platelet counts of 500 to 1000 × 10^9/l exhibit pseudohyperkalemia. Ischemia from prolonged tourniquet time or exercise of the limb in the presence of a tourniquet can also lead to abnormally increased potassium values. Pseudohyperkalemia may also occur with hemolysis, which occurs in patients with rheumatoid arthritis or infectious mononucleosis, as well as in families that have abnormal red blood cell membrane potassium permeability.

Pseudohyperkalemia is diagnosed by showing that the serum potassium concentration is more than 0.3 mmol/l higher than in a simultaneous plasma sample. Once it is diagnosed, all further potassium levels should be measured in plasma to avoid inappropriate treatment.

Redistribution

Hyperkalemia may be observed in cases of severe hyperglycemia (due to effects of osmolarity), in association with severe nonorganic acidosis, and rarely with β-blockers. Patients who have received mannitol may also develop hyperosmolarity-induced hyperkalemia.

Excess Intake

Excessive potassium ingestion generally does not lead to hyperkalemia unless other contributing factors are present. Under normal conditions, the kidney can excrete hundreds of millimoles of potassium daily. However, if renal potassium excretion is impaired, for example, by drugs or renal impairment, excessive potassium intake can produce hyperkalemia.

Common causes of excess potassium intake are potassium supplements, salt substitutes, enteral nutrition products, and

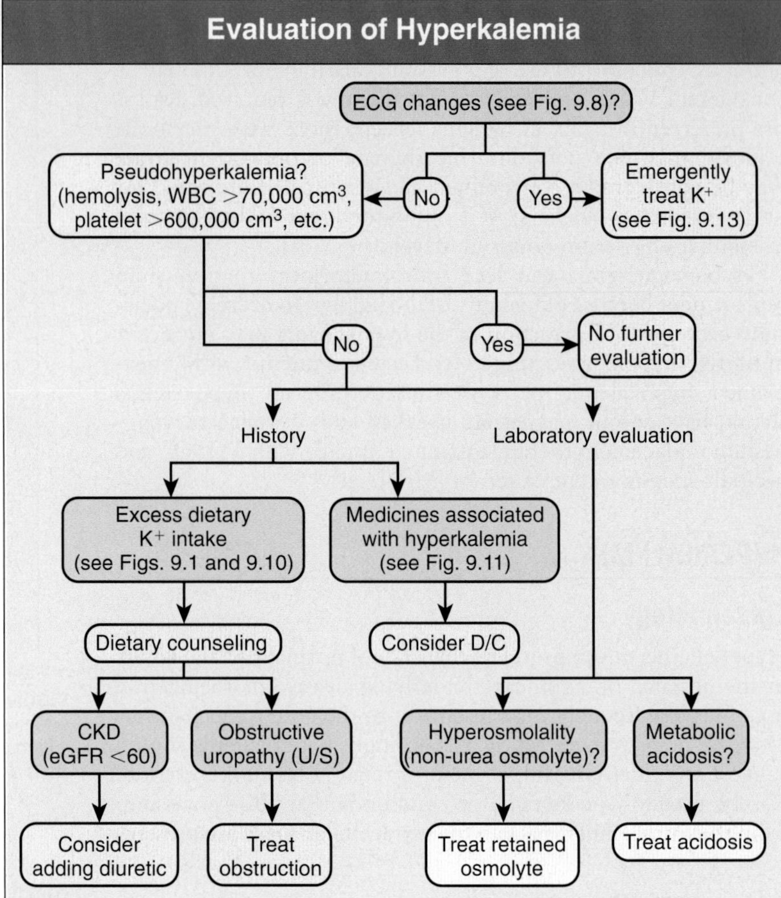

Figure 9.9 **Evaluation of hyperkalemia.**

Potassium Content of Common Enteral Products

	Calories/ml	Potassium (mmol/l)	Sodium (mmol/l)	Osmolality (mOsm/kg)
Ensure	1.06	40	37	470
Ensure Plus	1.50	54	49	690
Glucerna	1.00	40	40	375
Osmolite	1.06	26	27	300
Pulmocare	1.50	49	57	490
Suplena	2.00	29	34	615
Ultracal	1.06	41	41	310
Vivonex TEN	1.00	20	20	630

Figure 9.10 **Potassium content of common enteral products.**

common foods. As many as 4% of patients receiving potassium supplements develop hyperkalemia. Typical salt substitutes contain 10 to 13 mmol potassium/g, or 283 mmol/tablespoon. Many enteral nutrition products contain 40 mmol/l KCl or more; administration of 100 ml/h of such products can result in a potassium intake of ~100 mmol/day. Figure 9.10 summarizes the potassium content of many common enteral products. Finally, many food products are particularly high in potassium (see Fig. 9.1), and many pharmacies routinely label diuretic medicine bottles with suggestions for the patient to increase potassium intake from dietary sources, such as bananas and fresh fruits. Figure 9.1 summarizes the potassium content of some common foods.

Impaired Renal Potassium Secretion

The normal kidney possesses a remarkable ability to excrete potassium, so chronic hyperkalemia is difficult to produce unless renal potassium secretion is impaired. Factors that affect renal potassium excretion are classified into those due to reduced nephron number and those due to intrinsic impairment of renal potassium handling.

Because the kidney is the primary organ regulating potassium excretion, impaired renal function decreases maximal potassium excretion. In the absence of other contributing factors, renal potassium excretion is moderately well preserved until GFR is reduced to 10 to 20 ml/min. However, both CKD and acute kidney injury (AKI) limit maximal renal potassium excretion. This factor may be particularly important to consider in patients who are elderly, are cachectic, or have limb amputations, in whom low serum creatinine concentration leads to underestimation of the degree of renal impairment.

Obstructive uropathy leads frequently to hyperkalemia.[36] At least in part, it appears to be due to decreased Na^+,K^+-ATPase expression and activity.[37] In many cases, the hyperkalemia may persist for weeks after relief of the obstruction.

Specific Medicines The renin-angiotensin-aldosterone axis is the primary hormonal system regulating renal potassium excretion. Accordingly, medications that interfere with this system or that inhibit the cellular mechanisms of renal potassium

Medications Associated with Hyperkalemia		
Class	**Mechanism**	**Example**
Potassium-containing medicines	Increased potassium intake	KCl, PCN G, PolyCitra, PolyCitra K
β-Adrenergic receptor blockers	Inhibit renin release	Propranolol, metoprolol, atenolol
ACE inhibitor	Inhibit conversion of angiotensin I to Ang II	Captopril, lisinopril
Angiotensin receptor blocker (ARB)	Inhibit activation of AT_1 receptor by Ang II	Losartan, valsartan, irbesartan
Heparin	Inhibit aldosterone synthase, rate-limiting enzyme for aldosterone synthesis	Heparin sodium
Aldosterone receptor antagonist	Block aldosterone receptor activation	Spironolactone, eplerenone
Potassium-sparing diuretic	Block collecting duct apical sodium channel, decreasing gradient for potassium secretion	Amiloride, triamterene; certain antibiotics, specifically trimethoprim and pentamidine
NSAID and COX-2 inhibitors	Inhibit prostaglandin stimulation of collecting duct potassium secretion; inhibit renin release	Ibuprofen
Digitalis glycosides	Inhibit Na^+, K^+-ATPase necessary for collecting duct potassium secretion	Digoxin
Calcineurin inhibitors	Inhibit Na^+, K^+-ATPase necessary for collecting duct potassium secretion	Cyclosporine, tacrolimus

Figure 9.11 Medications associated with hyperkalemia. Ang II, angiotensin II.

Transtubular Potassium Gradient

TTKG is a measurement of net K^+ secretion by the distal nephron after correcting for changes in urinary osmolality and is often used to determine whether hyperkalemia is caused by aldosterone deficiency/resistance or whether the hyperkalemia is secondary to nonrenal causes. TTKG = $(K_u/K_s) \times (S_{osm}/U_{osm})$, where K_u and K_s are the concentration of K^+ in urine and serum, respectively, and U_{osm} and S_{osm} are the osmolalities of urine and serum, respectively.

TTKG Value		Indication
6–12		Normal
>10		Suggests normal aldosterone action and an extrarenal cause of hyperkalemia
<5–7		Suggests aldosterone deficiency or resistance
After 0.05 mg 9α-fludrocortisone		
	>10	Hypoaldosteronism is likely
	No change	Suggests a renal tubule defect from either K^+-sparing diuretics (amiloride, triamterene, spironolactone), aldosterone resistance (interstitial renal disease, sickle cell disease, urinary tract obstruction, pseudohypoaldosteronism type 1), or increased distal K^+ reabsorption (pseudohypoaldosteronism type 2, urinary tract obstruction)

Figure 9.12 Transtubular potassium gradient (TTKG).

excretion are frequent causes of hyperkalemia. Classes of medications that inhibit potassium secretion and their mechanism of action are summarized in Figure 9.11.

Intrinsic Renal Defect The rare genetic disorder pseudohypoaldosteronism type 2, also known as Gordon's syndrome, is characterized by hypertension, hyperkalemia, non–anion gap metabolic acidosis, and normal GFR.[38] Mutations in either of two proteins, WNK1 or WNK4, increase sodium absorption and inhibit potassium secretion in the distal convoluted tubule and collecting duct and lead to this phenotype.[8,39]

Distinguishing Renal and Nonrenal Mechanisms of Hyperkalemia

In most circumstances, a careful history and a 24-hour urine K^+ excretion rate will distinguish renal (K^+ <20 mmol/day) from extrarenal (K^+ >40 mmol/day) causes of hyperkalemia. Furthermore, in patients with a low urinary K^+ level, the administration of fludrocortisone may be used to distinguish aldosterone deficiency (urine K^+ increases to >40 mmol/day) from aldosterone resistance (K^+ remains <20 mmol/day). However, urinary K^+ measurements may be difficult to interpret because K^+ excretion is dependent on multiple factors; the most important are GFR, tubule lumen flow, and water reabsorption in the distal tubule and collecting duct. Fractional excretion of K^+ may help in differentiating renal from nonrenal causes of hyperkalemia because it normalizes K^+ excretion relative to GFR. When urine K^+ is equivocal, the transtubular K^+ gradient may be informative (Fig. 9.12).

Treatment

Therapies for hyperkalemia are divided into those that minimize the cardiac effects of hyperkalemia; those that induce potassium uptake by cells, resulting in a decrease in plasma potassium; and those that remove potassium from the body. Figure 9.13

Treatment of Hyperkalemia

Mechanism	Therapy	Dose	Onset	Duration
Antagonize membrane effects	Calcium	Calcium gluconate, 10% solution, 10 ml IV over 10 min	1–3 min	30–60 min
Cellular potassium uptake	Insulin	Regular insulin, 10 U IV, with dextrose, 50%, 50 ml if plasma glucose <250 mg/dl	30 min	4–6 h
	β_2-Adrenergic agonist	Nebulized albuterol, 10 mg	30 min	2–4 h
Potassium removal	Sodium polystyrene sulfonate	Kayexalate, 60 g PO, in 20% sorbitol, or 60 g in 250 ml water, per retention enema	1–2 h	4–6 h
	Hemodialysis	—	Immediate	Until dialysis completed

Figure 9.13 Treatment of hyperkalemia.

summarizes the available treatments, their mechanism of action, time at onset of action, and duration of action.

Treatment of hyperkalemia should not include $NaHCO_3$ therapy unless the patient is frankly acidotic (pH < 7.2) or unless substantial endogenous renal function is present. Administration of hypertonic $NaHCO_3$ can cause additional volume overload (a frequent issue in the patient with oliguric AKI), can cause acute hypernatremia, and, in general, has little effect on serum potassium concentration.[40]

Blocking Cardiac Effects

Intravenous calcium administration specifically antagonizes the effects of hyperkalemia on the myocardial conduction system and myocardial repolarization. Calcium is the most rapid way to stabilize the membrane voltage and to treat hyperkalemia; it should be given by the intravenous route if unambiguous ECG changes of hyperkalemia are present. All patients with prolonged PR interval, widened QRS complexes, or absence of P waves should receive intravenous calcium without delay. Responses can occur within 1 to 3 minutes and may last for 30 to 60 minutes. The dose may be repeated as needed if ECG changes persist or recur. If a delay in the institution of dialysis is anticipated, a calcium infusion should be considered because the effect of a calcium bolus is transient.

Intravenous calcium should not be administered in $NaHCO_3$-containing solutions because $CaCO_3$ precipitation can occur. Hypercalcemia, which occurs during rapid calcium infusion, can potentiate the myocardial toxicity of digoxin; patients taking digoxin, particularly if they have evidence of digoxin toxicity as a contributing cause of hyperkalemia, should be given calcium as a slow infusion lasting 20 to 30 minutes.

Cellular Potassium Uptake

The second most rapid way to treat hyperkalemia is to stimulate cellular potassium uptake, with either insulin or β_2-adrenergic agonist administration. Insulin rapidly stimulates cellular potassium uptake and should be administered intravenously to ensure predictable bioavailability. Effects on serum potassium concentration are generally seen within 10 to 20 minutes and will last for 4 to 6 hours. Glucose is generally coadministered to avoid hypoglycemia but may not be needed if hyperglycemia coexists, particularly because extracellular glucose in patients with diabetes mellitus can function as an "ineffective osmole" and can increase serum potassium concentration. If a delay in dialysis is anticipated, administration of a continuous infusion of insulin (4 to 10 U/h) with $D_{10}W$ (10% dextrose in water) may be beneficial; periodic monitoring of serum glucose and potassium concentrations is required.

β_2-Adrenergic receptor agonists directly stimulate cellular potassium uptake. These can be given through the intravenous, inhaled, or subcutaneous route. However, β_2-agonist therapy frequently induces substantial tachycardia, and as many as 25% of patients do not respond when it is given by nebulizer.[41] A frequent mistake in administering nebulized β_2-adrenergic receptor agonists is underdosage; the dose required is 2 to 8 times that usually given by nebulizer for bronchodilation and 50 to 100 times greater than the dose administered by metered dose inhalers.

Potassium Removal

Most cases of severe hyperkalemia are associated with increased extracellular fluid potassium content. Definitive treatment of these patients requires removal of potassium from the extracellular fluid.

In selected cases, treatment that focuses on increasing renal potassium elimination may be adequate. With chronic or mild hyperkalemia, loop or thiazide diuretics increase renal potassium excretion; loop diuretics may be the therapy of choice for patients with hyperkalemic renal tubular acidosis.[42] With life-threatening hyperkalemia, diuretics should be avoided because the rate of renal potassium excretion usually will not be adequate, and most patients will have renal impairment, which decreases the response to diuretic therapy. Whereas synthetic mineralocorticoids, such as fludrocortisone, increase renal potassium excretion, a relative contraindication to their use is the accompanying renal sodium retention, intravascular volume expansion, and increased blood pressure. Furthermore, mineralocorticoids can increase the rate of progression of CKD. If a rapidly reversible cause of renal failure is identified, such as obstructive uropathy or prerenal failure from volume depletion, treatment of the underlying condition along with close observation of plasma potassium concentration and continuous ECG observation may be adequate.

A second mode of potassium elimination is with cation exchange resins, such as sodium polystyrene sulfonate (Kayexalate). This resin exchanges sodium for potassium in the gastrointestinal tract, enabling potassium elimination. It can be administered either orally or per rectum as a retention enema. The rate of potassium removal is relatively slow, requiring about 4 hours for full effect, although administration as a retention enema results in more rapid onset of action. When it is given orally, sodium polystyrene sulfonate is generally administered with 20% sorbitol to avoid constipation. If it is given as an enema, sorbitol should be avoided because rectal administration of sodium polystyrene sulfonate with sorbitol can cause colonic perforation.[43]

Acute hemodialysis is the primary method of potassium removal when renal function is absent and hyperkalemia is persistent or severe. Serum potassium can decrease as much as 1.2 to 1.5 mmol/h with a potassium-free dialysate. In general, the more severe the hyperkalemia, the more rapid should be the reduction in plasma potassium and the lower the dialysate potassium concentration. However, care should be taken to avoid rapidly reducing the plasma potassium concentration in patients with ischemic heart disease or those predisposed to arrhythmias. In these patients, dialysis for a longer period with dialysate potassium of 3 to 3.5 mmol/l is better because serum potassium concentration can equilibrate to these levels during the dialysis. Continuous dialysis modalities, such as peritoneal dialysis and chronic venovenous hemodialysis, generally do not remove potassium sufficiently quickly for use in life-threatening hyperkalemia.

If dialysis is delayed, for example, because access to equipment or nursing support is not immediate or while vascular access is established, other therapies should be instituted and continued until hemodialysis is begun.

Specific therapies are available for certain causes of hyperkalemia. For example, digoxin-specific Fab fragments are beneficial in cases of severe digitalis toxicity.[44] Patients with acute urinary tract obstruction and hyperkalemia may be treated with relief of the urinary tract obstruction, but the rate of potassium excretion after relief of obstruction is variable, and frequent measurement of serum potassium concentration is necessary.

REFERENCES

1. Youn JH, McDonough AA. Recent advances in understanding integrative control of potassium homeostasis. *Annu Rev Physiol.* 2009;71:381-401.
2. Rabinowitz L, Aizman RI. The central nervous system in potassium homeostasis. *Front Neuroendocrinol.* 1993;14:1-26.
3. Aizawa H, Morita K, Minami H, et al. Exertional rhabdomyolysis as a result of strenuous military training. *J Neurol Sci.* 1995;132:239-240.
4. Milton AE, Weiner ID. Intracellular pH regulation in the rabbit cortical collecting duct A-type intercalated cell. *Am J Physiol.* 1997;273:F340-F347.
5. Hamm LL, Gillespie C, Klahr S. NH4Cl inhibition of transport in the rabbit cortical collecting tubule. *Am J Physiol.* 1985;248:F631-F637.
6. Bloomfield RL, Wilson DJ, Buckalew VM Jr. The incidence of diuretic-induced hypokalemia in two distinct clinic settings. *J Clin Hypertens.* 1986;2:331-338.
7. Barri YM, Wingo CS. The effects of potassium depletion and supplementation on blood pressure: a clinical review. *Am J Med Sci.* 1997;314:37-40.
8. Huang CL, Kuo E. Mechanisms of disease: WNK-ing at the mechanism of salt-sensitive hypertension. *Nat Clin Pract Nephrol.* 2007;3:623-630.
9. Siscovick DS, Raghunathan TE, Psaty BM, et al. Diuretic therapy for hypertension and the risk of primary cardiac arrest. *N Engl J Med.* 1994;330:1852-1857.
10. Knochel JP. Diuretic-induced hypokalemia. *Am J Med.* 1984;77:18-27.
11. Reungjui S, Pratipanawatr T, Johnson RJ, et al. Do thiazides worsen metabolic syndrome and renal disease? The pivotal roles for hyperuricemia and hypokalemia. *Curr Opin Nephrol Hypertens.* 2008;17:470-476.
12. Shafi T, Appel LJ, Miller III ER, et al. Changes in serum potassium mediate thiazide-induced diabetes. *Hypertension.* 2008;52:1022-1029.
13. Singhal PC, Abramovici M, Venkatesan J, et al. Hypokalemia and rhabdomyolysis. *Miner Electrolyte Metab.* 1991;17:335-339.
14. Ray PE, Suga S, Liu XH, et al. Chronic potassium depletion induces renal injury, salt sensitivity, and hypertension in young rats. *Kidney Int.* 2001;59:1850-1858.
15. Tizianello A, Garibotto G, Robaudo C, et al. Renal ammoniagenesis in humans with chronic potassium depletion. *Kidney Int.* 1991;40:772-778.
16. Berl T, Linas SL, Alisenbrye GA, et al. On the mechanism of polyuria in potassium depletion. The role of polydipsia. *J Clin Invest.* 1977;60:620.
17. Gabuzda GJ, Hall II. Relation of potassium depletion to renal ammonium metabolism and hepatic coma. *Medicine (Baltimore).* 1966;45:481-489.
18. Ahlawat SK, Sachdev A. Hypokalaemic paralysis. *Postgrad Med J.* 1999;75:193-197.
19. Antes LM, Kujubu DA, Fernandez PC. Hypokalemia and the pathology of ion transport molecules. *Semin Nephrol.* 1998;18:31-45.
20. Knochel JP, Dotin LN, Hamburger RJ. Pathophysiology of intense physical conditioning in a hot climate. I. Mechanisms of potassium depletion. *J Clin Invest.* 1972;51:242-255.
21. Gill MA, DuBe JE, Young WW. Hypokalemic, metabolic alkalosis induced by high-dose ampicillin sodium. *Am J Hosp Pharm.* 1977;34:528-531.
22. O'Regan S, Carson S, Chesney RW, et al. Electrolyte and acid-base disturbances in the management of leukemia. *Blood.* 1977;49:345-353.
23. Taher SM, Anderson RJ, McCartney R, et al. Renal tubular acidosis associated with toluene "sniffing." *N Engl J Med.* 1974;290:765-768.
24. Isnard Bagnis C, Deray G, Baumelou A, et al. Herbs and the kidney. *Am J Kidney Dis.* 2004;44: 1-11.
25. Lifton RP, Dluhy RG, Powers M, et al. A chimaeric 11β-hydroxylase/aldosterone synthase gene causes glucocorticoid-remediable aldosteronism and human hypertension. *Nature.* 1992;355:262-265.
26. White PC, New MI, Dupont B. Congenital adrenal hyperplasia. II. *N Engl J Med.* 1987;316:1580-1586.
27. Funder JW, Pearce PT, Smith R, et al. Mineralocorticoid action: Target tissue specificity is enzyme, not receptor, mediated. *Science.* 1988;242:583-585.
28. Farese RV Jr, Biglieri EG, Shackleton CH, et al. Licorice-induced hypermineralocorticoidism. *N Engl J Med.* 1991;325:1223-1227.
29. Ulick S, Wang JZ, Blumenfeld JD, et al. Cortisol inactivation overload: A mechanism of mineralocorticoid hypertension in the ectopic adrenocorticotropin syndrome. *J Clin Endocrinol Metab.* 1992;74:963-967.
30. Whang R. Magnesium deficiency: Pathogenesis, prevalence, and clinical implications. *Am J Med.* 1987;82:24-29.
31. Seyberth HW. An improved terminology and classification of Bartter-like syndromes. *Nat Clin Pract Nephrol.* 2008;4:560-567.
32. Riveira-Munoz E, Chang Q, Bindels RJ, et al. Gitelman's syndrome: Towards genotype-phenotype correlations? *Pediatr Nephrol.* 2007;22:326-332.
33. Schild L, Canessa CM, Shimkets RA, et al. A mutation in the epithelial sodium channel causing Liddle disease increases channel activity in the *Xenopus laevis* oocyte expression system. *Proc Natl Acad Sci USA.* 1995;92:5699-5703.
34. Kruse JA, Carlson RW. Rapid correction of hypokalemia using concentrated intravenous potassium chloride infusions. *Arch Intern Med.* 1990;150:613-617.
35. Kunin AS, Surawicz B, Sims EA. Decrease in serum potassium concentration and appearance of cardiac arrhythmias during infusion of potassium with glucose in potassium depleted patients. *N Engl J Med.* 1962;266:288.
36. Batlle DC, Arruda JA, Kurtzman NA. Hyperkalemic distal renal tubular acidosis associated with obstructive uropathy. *N Engl J Med.* 1981;304:373-380.
37. Kimura H, Mujais SK. Cortical collecting duct Na-K pump in obstructive nephropathy. *Am J Physiol.* 1990;258:F1320-F1327.
38. Gordon RD. Syndrome of hypertension and hyperkalemia with normal glomerular filtration rate. *Hypertension.* 1986;8:93-102.
39. Wilson FH, Disse-Nicodème S, Choate KA, et al. Human hypertension caused by mutations in WNK kinases. *Science.* 2001;293:1107-1112.
40. Allon M. Hyperkalemia in end-stage renal disease: Mechanisms and management. *J Am Soc Nephrol.* 1995;6:1134-1142.
41. Allon M, Dunlay R, Copkney C. Nebulized albuterol for acute hyperkalemia in patients on hemodialysis. *Ann Intern Med.* 1989;110:426-429.
42. Sebastian A, Schambelan M, Sutton JM. Amelioration of hyperchloremic acidosis with furosemide therapy in patients with chronic renal insufficiency and type 4 renal tubular acidosis. *Am J Nephrol.* 1984;4:287-300.
43. Gerstman BB, Kirkman R, Platt R. Intestinal necrosis associated with postoperative orally administered sodium polystyrene sulfonate in sorbitol. *Am J Kidney Dis.* 1992;20:159-161.
44. Smith TW, Butler VP Jr, Haber E, et al. Treatment of life-threatening digitalis intoxication with digoxin-specific Fab antibody fragments: Experience in 26 cases. *N Engl J Med.* 1982;307:1357-1362.

CHAPTER 10

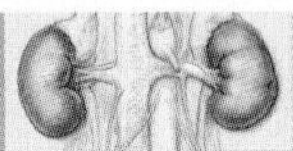

Disorders of Calcium, Phosphate, and Magnesium Metabolism

Bryan Kestenbaum, Tilman B. Drüeke

HOMEOSTASIS OF CALCIUM AND DISORDERS OF CALCIUM METABOLISM

Distribution of Calcium in the Organism and Calcium Homeostasis

Most calcium is bound and associated with bone structures (99%). The majority of free calcium, either in diffusible (ultrafilterable) nonionized form or in ionized form (Ca^{2+}), is found in the intracellular and extracellular fluid compartments. There is a steep concentration gradient of Ca^{2+} between the intracellular and the extracellular milieu as shown in Figure 10.1.

The plasma concentration of Ca^{2+} is tightly regulated by the actions of parathyroid hormone (PTH) and calcitriol (1,25-dihydroxycholecalciferol). The physiologic role of other calcium regulatory hormones, such as calcitonin, estrogens, and prolactin, is less clear. Figures 10.2 and 10.3 demonstrate the physiologic defense mechanisms used to counter changes in serum Ca^{2+} levels. Serum Ca^{2+} levels are also influenced by acid-base status; alkalosis causes a decrease in Ca^{2+}, and acidosis has the opposite effect.

Long-term maintenance of calcium homeostasis depends on the adaptation of intestinal Ca^{2+} absorption to the needs of the organism, on the balance between bone accretion and resorption, and on urinary excretion of calcium (see Fig. 10.3).

Intestinal, Skeletal, and Renal Handling of Calcium

Gastrointestinal calcium absorption is a selective process; only about 25% of total dietary calcium is absorbed. Ca^{2+} transport across the intestinal wall occurs in two directions: absorption and secretion. Absorption can be subdivided into transcellular and paracellular flow (Fig. 10.4).[1] Transcellular calcium flux takes place through the recently identified TRPV6 calcium channel. Calcitriol is its most important hormonal regulatory factor.[2] After binding to and activating the vitamin D receptor (VDR), calcitriol increases active transport by inducing the expression of TRPV6, calbindin D_{9k}, and Ca^{2+}-ATPase (PMCA1b) (see Fig. 10.4).[3] Other hormones, including estrogens, prolactin, growth hormone, and PTH, also stimulate Ca^{2+} absorption, either directly or indirectly. The amount of dietary calcium intake also regulates the proportion of calcium absorbed through the gastrointestinal tract (Fig. 10.5).

Cutaneous synthesis on exposure to UV light converts 7-dehydrocholesterol to vitamin D substrate (cholecalciferol). Cholecalciferol has minimal inherent biologic activity and requires two hydroxylation steps for full hormonal activity. 25-Hydroxylation occurs in the liver, is thought to be non–rate-limiting, and is widely accepted as a summary measure of vitamin D stores. Further hydroxylation to 1,25-dihydroxyvitamin D (calcitriol) occurs predominantly in the kidney, but also occurs in non-renal tissues.

Increased calcium absorption is required in puberty, pregnancy, and lactation. In all these states, calcitriol synthesis is increased. Intestinal Ca^{2+} absorption is also increased in vitamin D excess and acromegaly. Rarely, the ingestion of calcium and alkali in large quantities can overwhelm gastrointestinal checks on calcium absorption, resulting in hypercalcemia (milk-alkali syndrome); however, innate limitations on gastrointestinal calcium absorption prevent this condition from occurring in most individuals. A decrease in intestinal Ca^{2+} transport occurs in a low Ca^{2+}/phosphate ratio in the food, a high vegetable fiber and fat content of the diet, corticosteroid treatment, estrogen deficiency, advanced age, gastrectomy, intestinal malabsorption syndromes, diabetes mellitus, and renal failure. The decrease in Ca^{2+} absorption in the elderly probably results from multiple factors in addition to lower serum calcitriol and intestinal VDR levels.[4]

The net balance between Ca^{2+} entry and exit fluxes is positive during skeletal growth in children, zero in young adults, and negative in the elderly. Exchangeable skeletal Ca^{2+} contributes to maintenance of extracellular Ca^{2+} homeostasis. Several growth factors, hormones, and genetic factors participate in the differentiation from the mesenchymal precursor cell to the osteoblast and the maturation of the osteoclast from its granulocyte-macrophage precursor cell (Fig. 10.6). The regulation of bone formation and resorption involves a large number of hormones, growth factors, and mechanical factors (Fig. 10.7).[5]

The kidneys play a major role in the minute-by-minute regulation; the intestine and the skeleton ensure homeostasis in the mid and long term. To perform its task, the kidney uses a complex system of filtration and reabsorption (Fig. 10.8). The adjustment of blood Ca^{2+} is mainly achieved by modulation of tubular Ca^{2+} reabsorption in response to the body's needs, perfectly compensating minor increases or decreases in the filtered load of calcium at the glomerular level, which is normally about 220 mmol (8800 mg) in 24 hours (see Fig. 10.3). In the proximal tubule, most of the Ca^{2+} is reabsorbed by convective flow (as for Na^+ and water); in the distal segments of the tubule, the transport mechanisms are more complex. States of excess volume delivery to the kidney, such as a high-sodium diet, diminish the concentration gradient between proximal tubule and peritubular capillary, reducing calcium absorption and increasing calcium in the urine. This mechanism is thought to play a role in the pathogenesis of calcium-based kidney stones. On the other hand, volume depletion states increase salt, water, and (by convection) calcium reabsorption in the proximal tubule, exacerbating states of hypercalcemia. In the thick ascending loop, the transport of Ca^{2+} is primarily passive by the paracellular route, depending on the

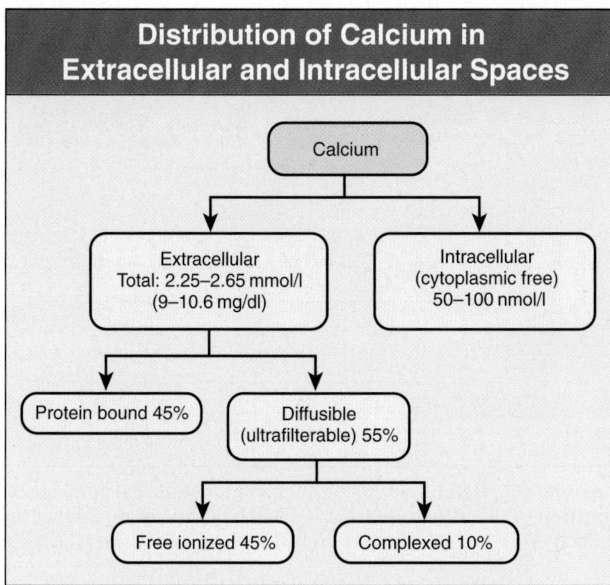

Figure 10.1 Distribution of calcium in extracellular and intracellular spaces.

electrical gradient, with the tubular lumen being positive, and also on the presence of claudin 16 in the tight junction. At this step, Ca^{2+} transport is enhanced by PTH, probably through an increase in paracellular permeability, but it is reduced by an increase in extracellular Ca^{2+} involving the Ca^{2+}-sensing receptor (CaR_G). Specifically, stimulation of CaR_G by elevated serum calcium levels decreases the activity of rectifying K^+ channels (ROMK), resulting in less Na^+-K^+-$2Cl^-$ cotransporter activity and less calcium reabsorption in this segment. In the distal tubule, Ca^{2+} transport is primarily active by the transcellular route, through TRPV5 located in the apical membrane and coupled with a specific basolateral Ca^{2+}-ATPase (PMCA1b) and a Na^+-Ca^{2+} exchanger (NCX1). Both PTH and calcitriol regulate distal tubular transport.

Numerous factors control the glomerular filtration and tubular reabsorption of Ca^{2+}.[3,6,7] Elevated renal blood flow and glomerular filtration pressure (during extracellular fluid volume expansion) lead to an increase in filtered load, as do changes in the ultrafiltration coefficient K_f and an increase in glomerular surface. True hypercalcemia also increases ultrafilterable calcium, whereas true hypocalcemia decreases it. PTH decreases glomerular K_f and thus reduces the ultrafiltered calcium load; it also increases Ca^{2+} reabsorption in the distal nephron. However, PTH and PTH-related peptide (PTHrP) also induce hypercalcemia, and because of the increase in serum calcium, the excretion of filtered calcium is elevated overall. Both extracellular Ca^{2+} and intracellular Ca^{2+} reduce tubular calcium reabsorption by activating CaR_G, and the effect of extracellular Ca^{2+} is enhanced by calcimimetics. Metabolic and respiratory acidoses lead to hypercalciuria, respiratory acidosis through an increase in plasma Ca^{2+} and metabolic acidosis through calcium release from bone and an inhibitory effect on tubular Ca^{2+} reabsorption. Conversely, alkali ingestion reduces renal excretion of calcium. The enhancing effect of phosphate depletion on urinary calcium elimination can partly occur through changes in PTH and calcitriol secretion. Dietary factors modify urinary excretion of calcium, mostly by their effects on intestinal Ca^{2+} absorption. Several classes of diuretics act directly on the tubules: loop

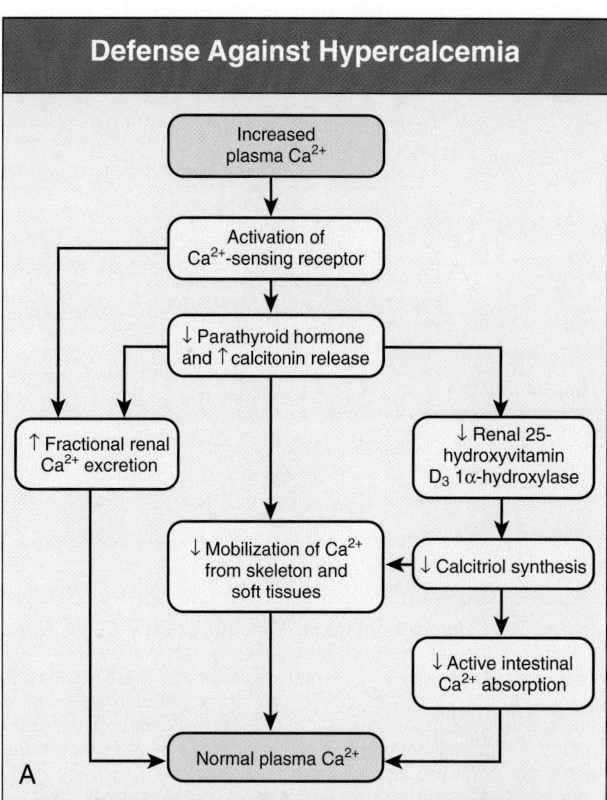

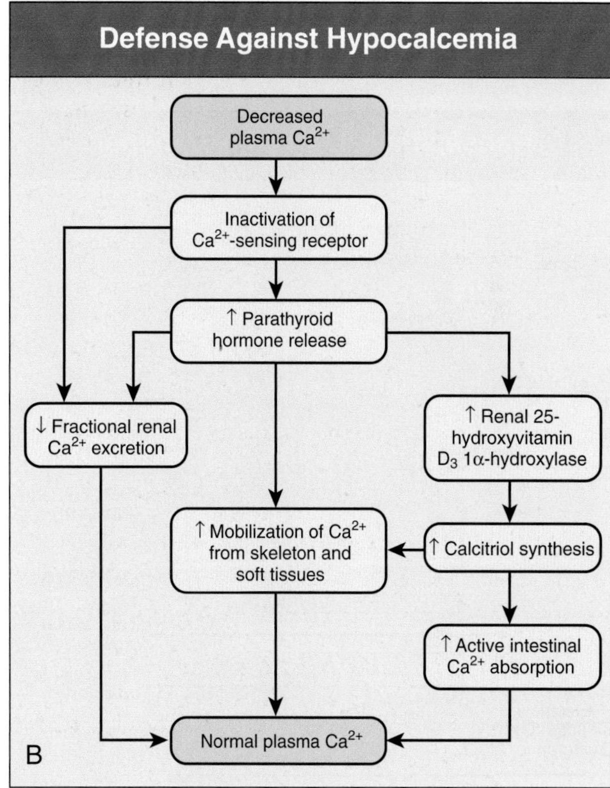

Figure 10.2 Physiologic defense mechanisms to counter changes in serum calcium. A, Hypercalcemia. **B,** Hypocalcemia. *(Modified from reference 8.)*

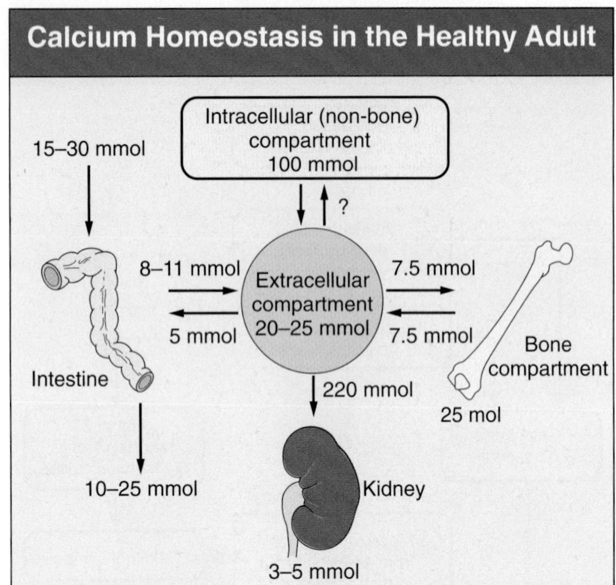

Figure 10.3 Calcium homeostasis in the healthy adult. Net zero Ca^{2+} balance is the result of net intestinal absorption (absorption minus secretion) and urinary excretion, which, by definition, are the same. After its passage into the extracellular fluid, Ca^{2+} enters the extracellular space, is deposited in bone, or is eliminated by the kidneys. Entry and exit fluxes between the extracellular and intracellular spaces (skeletal and nonskeletal compartments) are also of identical magnitude under steady-state conditions. Values linked to compartments respresent absolute amounts of calcium whereas values linked to the intestine and the kidney represent daily calcium entries and exits, and values between organs and compartments represent daily fluxes.

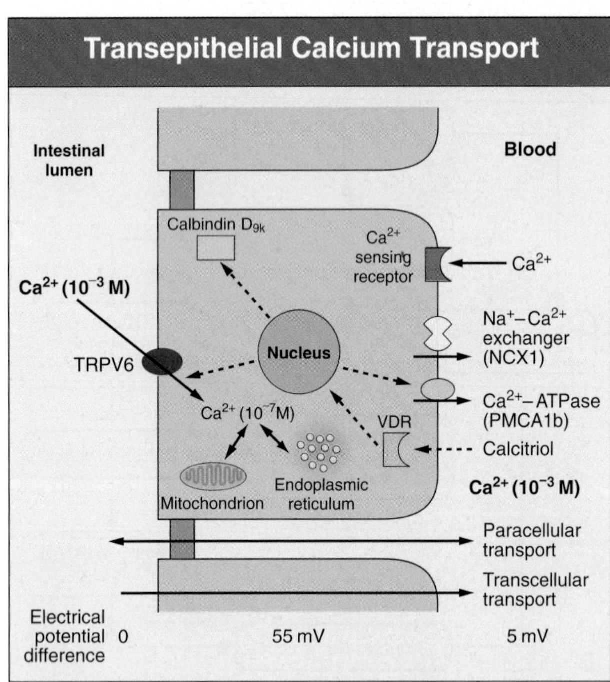

Figure 10.4 Transepithelial calcium transport in the small intestine. Calcium penetrates into the enterocyte by a recently discovered calcium channel (TRPV6) through the brush border membrane along a favorable electrochemical gradient. Under physiologic conditions, the cation is pumped out of the cell at the basolateral side against a steep electrochemical gradient by the adenosine triphosphate–consuming pump Ca^{2+}-ATPase. When there is a major elevation of intracytoplasmic Ca^{2+}, the cation leaves the cell using the Na^{+}-Ca^{2+} exchanger. Passive Ca^{2+} influx and efflux are sensitive to calcitriol, which binds the vitamin D receptor (VDR).

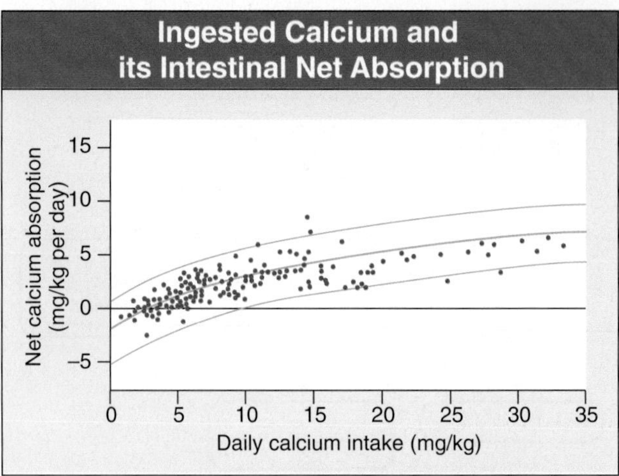

Figure 10.5 Relationship between ingested calcium and its absorption in the intestinal tract (net) in healthy young adults. *(From reference 9.)*

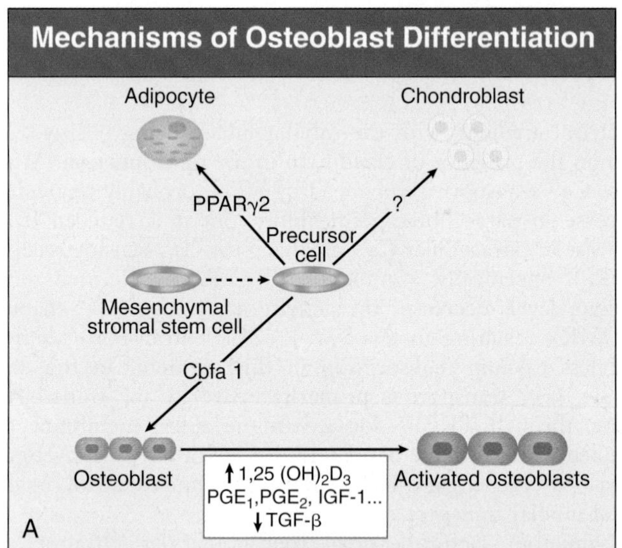

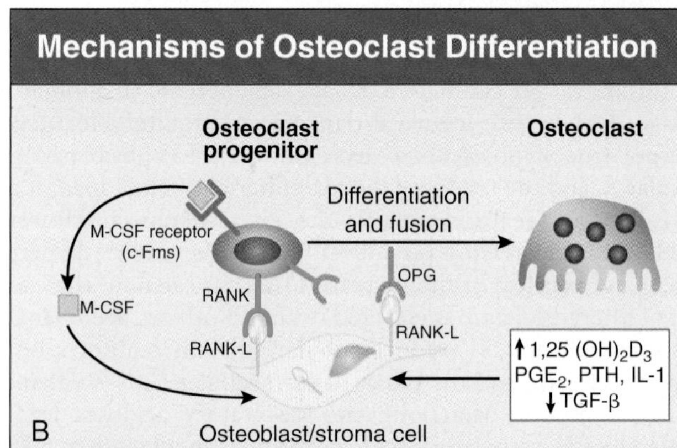

Figure 10.6 Mechanisms of osteoblast and osteoclast differentiation. A, The major growth factors and hormones controlling the differentiation from the mesenchymal precursor cell to the osteoblast. **B,** The major growth factors, cytokines, and hormones controlling osteoblast and osteoclast activity. IL, interleukin; M-CSF, macrophage colony-stimulating factor; OPG, osteoprotegerin; PGE_2, prostaglandin E_2; PPARγ2, peroxisome proliferator-activated receptor γ2; PTH, parathyroid hormone; RANK-L, receptor activator of nuclear factor-κB ligand; TGF-β, transforming growth factor β.

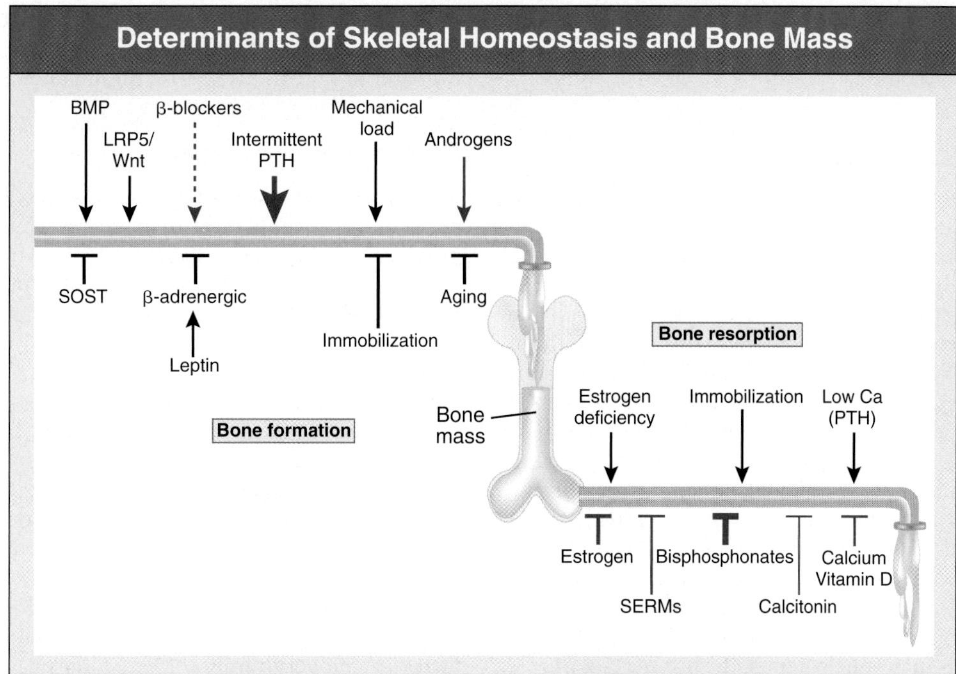

Figure 10.7 Determinants of skeletal homeostasis and bone mass. Physiologic *(black)* and pharmacologic *(red)* stimulators and inhibitors of bone formation and resorption are listed with the relative impact represented by the thickness of the *arrows*. BMP, bone morphogenetic protein; LRP5, low-density lipoprotein receptor–related protein 5; PTH, parathyroid protein; SERMs, selective estrogen receptor modulators; SOST, sclerostin. *(From reference 10.)*

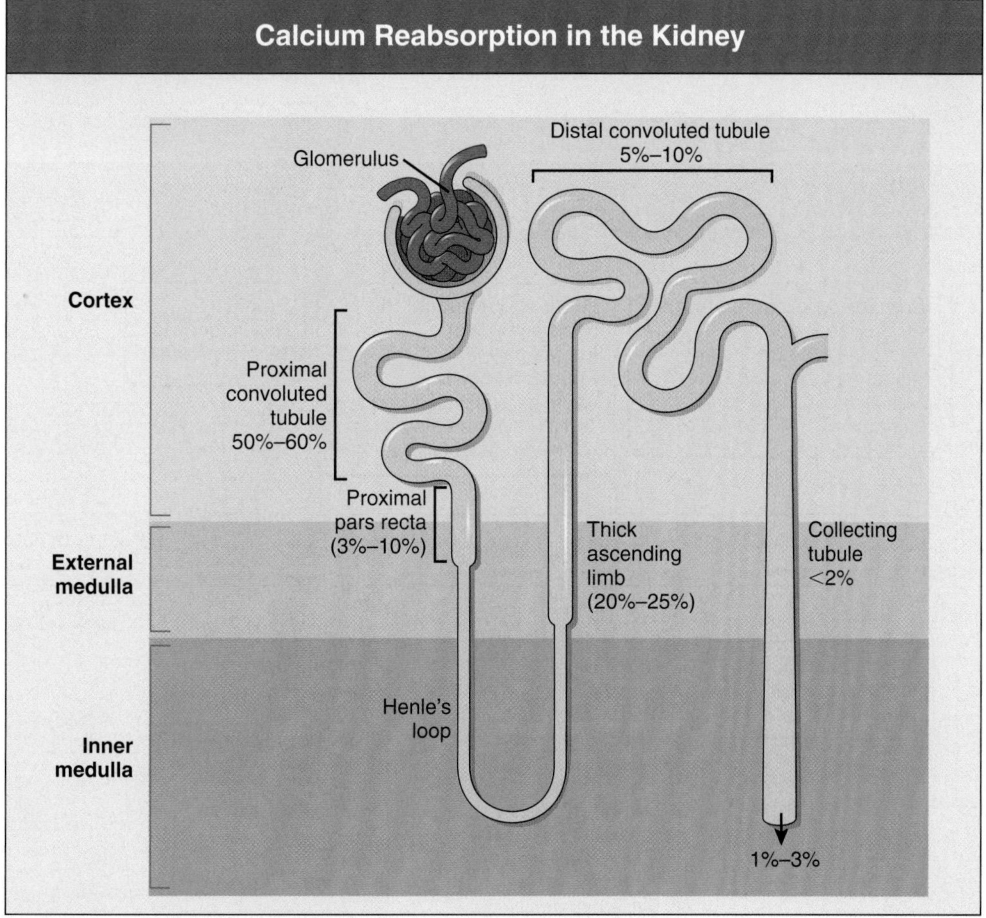

Figure 10.8 Sites of calcium reabsorption in various segments of the renal tubule. The percentage of Ca^{2+} absorbed in various segments after glomerular ultrafiltration is shown. *(Redrawn from reference 11.)*

diuretics and mannitol favor hypercalciuria, with a major impact on the thick ascending limb, whereas the thiazide diuretics and amiloride induce hypocalciuria.

HYPERCALCEMIA

Increased plasma total calcium concentration can result from an increase in plasma proteins (false hypercalcemia) or from an increase in plasma ionized Ca^{2+} (true hypercalcemia). Only the latter leads to clinically relevant hypercalcemia. When only the value for the total plasma calcium concentration is available rather than the free level ions, as is generally the case in clinical practice, plasma Ca^{2+} can be estimated by taking into account plasma albumin: an increase in albumin of 1.0 g/dl reflects a concomitant increase of 0.20 to 0.25 mmol/l (0.8 to 1.0 mg/dl) in plasma calcium. However, simple correction of total calcium for serum albumin may not be valid in patients with chronic kidney disease (CKD). A study of 691 individuals with CKD stages 3 to 5 demonstrated that the albumin-corrected total serum calcium concentration poorly correlated with the simultaneously measured ionized calcium concentration. Moreover, the two most common assays used to measure serum albumin yield discordant results in uremic patients, the bromcresol purple method providing lower albumin values than the bromcresol green method.

The recently cloned CaR_G has been identified in numerous tissues and its function well defined.[12] Mutations of the gene for CaR_G result in various clinical syndromes characterized either by hypercalcemia or by hypocalcemia (see later discussion). Several other Ca^{2+} receptors have been cloned subsequently. The precise functional properties of one of them, GPRC6A, which is expressed in osteoblasts and clearly distinct from CaR_G, have been characterized.[13] Its role in the regulation of osteoblast function and in human disease is still unknown.

Causes of Hypercalcemia

True hypercalcemia results from an increase in intestinal Ca^{2+} absorption, a stimulation of bone resorption, or a decrease in urinary Ca^{2+} excretion. Enhanced bone resorption is the predominant mechanism in most cases of hypercalcemia. The main causes of hypercalcemia are shown in Figure 10.9.

Malignant Neoplasias

The main cause of hypercalcemia is excessive bone resorption induced by neoplastic processes, usually solid tumors. Tumors of the breast, lung, and kidney are the most common, followed by hematopoietic neoplasias, particularly myeloma.

Most hypercalcemic tumors act on the skeleton either by direct invasion (metastases) or by producing factors that stimulate osteoclastic activity, including most commonly PTHrP as well as factors activating osteoclasts, transforming growth factors, prostaglandin E (PGE), rarely calcitriol and tumor necrosis factor α, and very rarely PTH, produced, for example, by parathyroid cancer.

Only 8 of the 13 first amino acids of PTHrP are identical with those of the N-terminal fragment of PTH, but the effects of both hormones on target cells are mostly the same. In addition to their common receptor, the PTH/PTHrP receptor, there is at least one other receptor, the PTH_2 receptor, which recognizes solely PTH, with similar or identical signal transduction systems. In pathologic conditions, most of the PTHrP in the body is

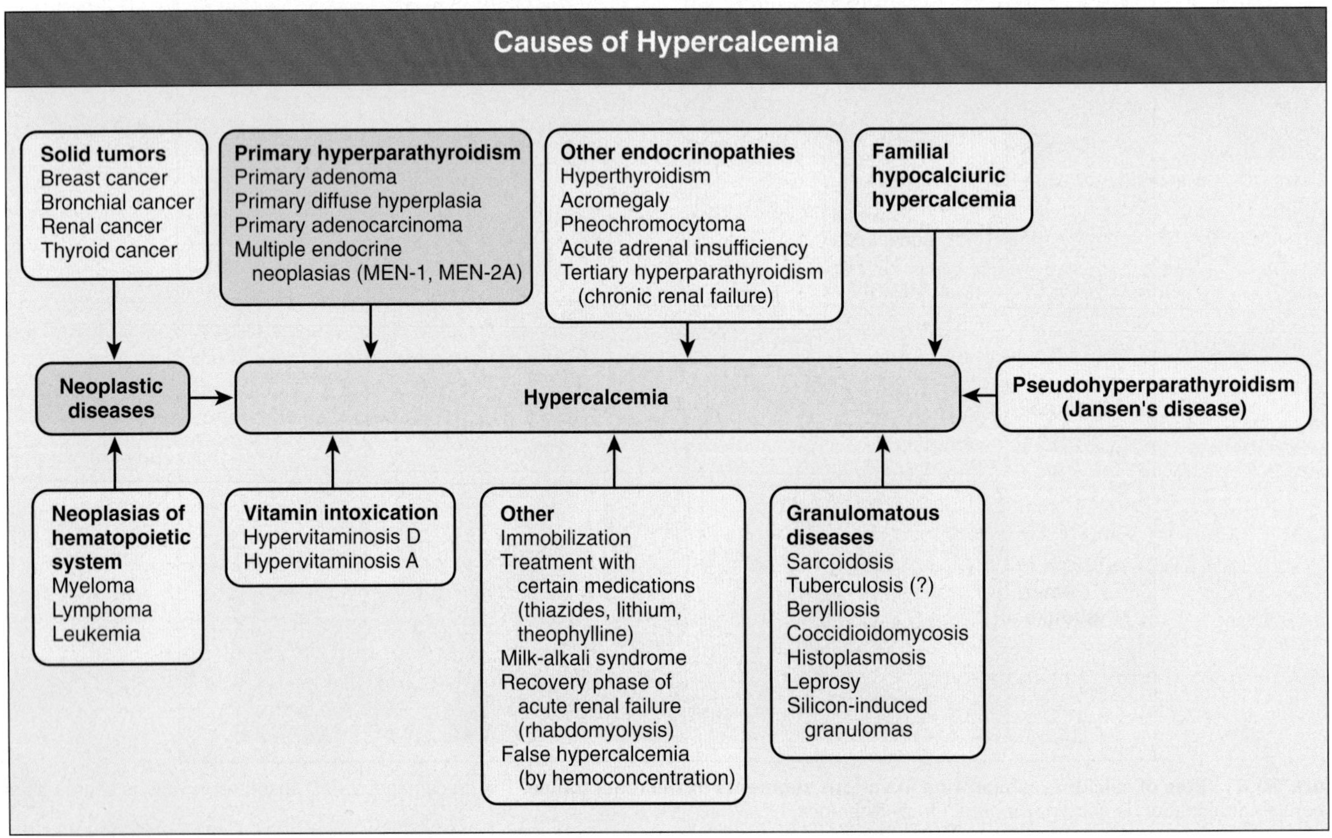

Figure 10.9 Causes of hypercalcemia. *Green boxes* indicate common causes of hypercalcemia. *(From reference 11.)*

synthesized by solid tumors. PTHrP stimulates osteoclastic activity and thus liberates excess quantities of calcium from the skeleton.

Osteoclast-activating factors secreted by myeloma plasmocytes and the lymphoblasts of malignant lymphomas include interleukins 1α, 1β, and 6 and also tumor necrosis factor α, which all stimulate osteoclast activity. Other osteoclast-activating factors are PGE_1 and PGE_2, which can be secreted in large amounts by some tumors (especially renal tumors). Some lymphoid tumors synthesize excess quantities of calcitriol. This capacity has been described in Hodgkin's disease, T-cell lymphoma, and leiomyoblastoma.

Primary Hyperparathyroidism

The second most common cause of hypercalcemia is primary hyperparathyroidism. Early diagnosis is achieved through the widespread use of routine plasma calcium determination. In more than 80% of cases, the disease is caused by adenoma of a single parathyroid gland; in 10% to 15%, there is diffuse hyperplasia of all glands, and in less than 5%, a parathyroid cancer. Primary hyperparathyroidism can be inherited either as diffuse hyperplasia of the parathyroid glands alone or as a component in multiple glandular hereditary endocrine disorders. Patients with multiple endocrine neoplasia type 1 (MEN-1) have various combinations of parathyroid, anterior pituitary, enteropancreatic, and other endocrine tumors, resulting in hypersecretion of prolactin and gastrin in addition to PTH. This disease is caused by inactivating germline mutations of a tumor-suppressor gene (the *MEN-1* gene) that is inherited as an autosomal dominant trait. In MEN-2A, the thyroid medulla and the adrenal medulla are involved with the parathyroid, resulting in hypersecretion of calcitonin and catecholamines. This disease is caused by activating mutations of the *RET* proto-oncogene. It is also inherited as an autosomal dominant trait. Not all patients with mildly elevated plasma PTH levels develop hypercalcemia; the development of hypercalcemia may depend on a concomitant elevation of plasma calcitriol.

Jansen's Disease

Jansen's disease is a rare hereditary form of short-limbed dwarfism characterized by severe hypercalcemia, hypophosphatemia, and metaphyseal chondrodysplasia.[14] It is the result of activating mutations of the gene for the PTH/PTHrP receptor, a particular form of pseudohyperparathyroidism.

Familial Hypocalciuric Hypercalcemia

Familial hypocalciuric hypercalcemia is a rare hereditary disease due to inactivating mutations in the gene for CaR_G[15] with autosomal dominant transmission. It is characterized by moderate chronic hypercalcemia associated with hypophosphatemia, hyperchloremia, and hypermagnesemia. Plasma PTH concentration is normal or moderately elevated, and the fractional excretion of calcium is lower than that observed in hyperparathyroidism. The fractional excretion of calcium is best assessed by calculating the calcium to creatinine clearance ratio:

$$\text{calcium to creatinine clearance ratio} = \frac{(\text{24-hour urine calcium}) \times (\text{serum creatinine})}{(\text{24-hour urine creatinine}) \times (\text{serum calcium})}$$

In familial hypocalciuric hypercalcemia, the urine calcium to creatinine clearance ratio is usually less than 0.01. In patients with this syndrome, hypercalcemia never leads to severe clinical signs (except during the neonatal period, in which malignant hypercalcemia can be observed in the context of severe hyperparathyroidism).

Other Endocrine Causes

Other endocrine disorders can be associated with moderate hypercalcemia, such as hyperthyroidism, acromegaly, and pheochromocytoma. In addition, acute adrenal insufficiency should also be considered in the differential diagnosis, although here hypercalcemia is usually false and results from hemoconcentration. Hypercalcemia can also occur in severe forms of the secondary hyperparathyroidism of CKD. However, this is relatively uncommon to date because low circulating calcitriol concentrations in CKD limit gastrointestinal calcium absorption[16] and because parathyroid overfunction is often treated at earlier stages.

Other Causes

Several other disorders sometimes induce hypercalcemia. Among the granulomatoses, sarcoidosis results in increased plasma Ca^{2+}, particularly in patients exposed to sunlight. The cause is uncontrolled production of calcitriol by macrophages (due to the presence of the 1α-hydroxylase in the macrophages within the granulomas). Tuberculosis, leprosy, berylliosis, and many other granulomatous diseases are sometimes (but much more rarely than sarcoidosis) the origin of hypercalcemia, probably through the same mechanism.

Hypercalcemia may also result from prolonged bed rest (especially in patients with preexisting high bone turnover rates, such as children, adolescents, and patients with Paget's disease). Recovery from acute renal failure secondary to rhabdomyolysis-induced renal failure has been associated with hypercalcemia in 25% of cases and is thought to occur as a consequence of mobilization of soft tissue calcium deposits and through increases in PTH and calcitriol. Other causes include intoxication by vitamin D or one of its derivatives, vitamin A overload, and treatment by thiazide diuretics. Large doses of calcium (5 to 10 g/day), especially when ingested with alkali (antacids), can also lead to hypercalcemia and nephrocalcinosis (milk-alkali syndrome).

Clinical Manifestations

The severity of clinical symptoms and signs caused by hypercalcemia depends not only on the degree but also on the velocity of its development. Severe hypercalcemia can be accompanied by few manifestations in some patients because of its slow, progressive development, whereas much less severe hypercalcemia can lead to major disorders if it develops rapidly.

In general, the first symptoms are increasing fatigue, muscle weakness, inability to concentrate, nervousness, increased sleepiness, and depression. Subsequently, gastrointestinal signs may occur, such as constipation, nausea and vomiting, and, rarely, peptic ulcer disease or pancreatitis. Renal-related signs include polyuria (secondary to nephrogenic diabetes insipidus), urinary tract stones and their complications, and occasionally tubulointerstitial disease with medullary and to a lesser extent cortical deposition of calcium (nephrocalcinosis). Neuropsychiatric manifestations include headache, loss of memory, somnolence, stupor, and, rarely, coma. Ocular symptoms include conjunctivitis from crystal deposition and, rarely, band keratopathy. Osteoarticular pain in primary hyperparathyroidism has become rare in Western countries because of earlier diagnosis of hypercalcemia. High blood pressure can be induced by hypercalcemia, but it is more frequently a chance association. Soft tissue calcifications can occur with long-standing hypercalcemia. Electrocardiography may show shortening of the QT interval and coving of the ST wave. Hypercalcemia may also increase cardiac contractility and can amplify digitalis toxicity.

Diagnosis

When the history and clinical examination are not helpful, primary hyperparathyroidism should be investigated first. Although this is only the second most frequent cause, its laboratory diagnosis is at present easier than that of tumoral involvement. In addition to total plasma calcium and ionized Ca^{2+}, plasma levels of albumin (or total protein), phosphate, creatinine, total alkaline phosphatase, and PTH and urinary concentrations of calcium and creatinine should be determined. Note that prolonged hypercalcemia is often associated with (reversible) increased serum creatinine. When plasma PTH is high or inappropriately normal with respect to the degree of hypercalcemia, the diagnosis is confirmed. Cervical ultrasonography and sestamibi isotope scanning may be performed to locate a parathyroid adenoma; but in general, experienced surgeons consider these examinations unnecessary before a first neck exploration. However, imaging is indispensable in recurrent hyperparathyroidism. If the plasma PTH level is low-normal or low, the possibility of a neoplastic disorder should be seriously considered. A low serum anion gap may be a clue to multiple myeloma (because occasionally the monoclonal IgG is positively charged). In addition to the usual examinations, such as serum protein electrophoresis, measurement of the plasma PTHrP level can now be done in specialized laboratories. Exogenous vitamin D overload is associated with increased serum 25-hydroxyvitamin D levels, and granulomatous diseases such as sarcoidosis are associated with elevated calcitriol levels and with increased serum angiotensin-converting enzyme activity.

Treatment

Treatment is aimed at the underlying cause. However, severe and symptomatic hypercalcemia requires rapid correction, whatever the cause. Initially, the patient must be rapidly rehydrated with isotonic saline for correction of the often marked volume depletion to reduce proximal tubule calcium reabsorption and to enhance calcium excretion. Only when euvolemia is established should loop diuretics be used (e.g., intravenous furosemide m every other hour) to facilitate urinary excretion of calcium; however, intravenous saline should be continued to prevent hypovolemia. Oral intake and intravenous administration of fluids and electrolytes should be carefully monitored and urinary and gastric excretions measured if excessive, especially those of potassium, magnesium, and phosphate. Acid-base balance should also be carefully monitored. Severe cardiac failure and CKD are contraindications to massive extracellular fluid volume expansion in conjunction with diuretics.

Bisphosphonates are the treatment of first choice, especially in hypercalcemia associated with cancer.[17] They inhibit bone resorption as well as calcitriol synthesis. They can be administered orally in less severe disease or intravenously in severe hypercalcemia. Frequently used bisphosphonates are clodronate (1600 to 3200 mg/day orally), pamidronate (15 to 90 mg intravenously during 1 to 3 days, once per month), and alendronate (10 mg/day orally). With intravenous administration, doses should be infused in 500 ml of isotonic saline or dextrose during at least 2 hours and up to 24 hours. Treatment of hypercalcemia with bisphosphonates may be complicated by concomitant renal impairment because of package warnings contraindicating bisphosphonate use in patients with kidney disease. However, there are virtually no clinical data to support these warnings, and bisphosphonates have been safely used in patients with CKD for the correction of hypercalcemia. A reasonable strategy is first to attempt correction of acute kidney injury (AKI) before a bisphosphonate is administered and to avoid repetitive dosing; a single 60 mg dose of pamidronate can maintain normal calcium concentrations for weeks. Calcitonin acts within hours, in particular after intravenous administration. Human, porcine, or salmon calcitonin can be given. However, calcitonin often has no effect or only a short-term effect because of the rapid development of tachyphylaxis.

Mithramycin is a cytostatic drug with a remarkable power to inhibit bone resorption. Administration of a single intravenous dose is generally followed by a rapid decline in plasma calcium within a few hours, and this effect lasts several days. However, its use is reserved for malignant hypercalcemia, and its cytotoxic effect and side effects (thrombocytopenia and liver function abnormalities) preclude prolonged administration. The maximal daily dose is 25 µg/kg.

Corticosteroids (0.5 to 1.0 mg/kg predniso(lo)ne daily) are mainly indicated in hypervitaminosis D of endogenous origin, such as sarcoidosis and tuberculosis, and of exogenous origin, such as vitamin D intoxication. Ketoconazole, an antifungal agent that can inhibit renal and extrarenal calcitriol synthesis, has also been proposed in hypervitaminosis D. Corticosteroids can also be tried in the treatment of hypercalcemia associated with some hematopoietic tumors, such as myeloma and lymphoma, and even for some solid tumors, such as breast cancer.

In rare cases of malignant hypercalcemia, treatment with prostaglandin antagonists, for example, indomethacin or aspirin, can be successful. Hyperkalemia and impaired renal function may occur with indomethacin. Hypercalcemia caused by thyrotoxicosis can rapidly resolve with intravenous administration of propranolol or less rapidly with oral administration.

In moderate and nonsymptomatic hypercalcemia of primary hyperparathyroidism, treatment with estrogens has been tried, at least in women. In patients with primary hyperparathyroidism, cinacalcet, the first of a new therapeutic class of CaR_G agonists (calcimimetics), can achieve normalization of serum Ca^{2+} concentration in most instances together with a reduction of serum PTH.[18] In dialysis patients with secondary and many cases of so-called tertiary uremic hyperparathyroidism, long-term administration of cinacalcet is superior to standard therapy in controlling serum PTH, calcium, and phosphorus concentrations.[19] Cinacalcet is also effective in patients with parathyroid carcinoma.

HYPOCALCEMIA

Like hypercalcemia, hypocalcemia can be secondary either to reduced plasma albumin (false hypocalcemia) or to a change in ionized Ca^{2+} (true hypocalcemia). False hypocalcemia can be excluded by direct measurement of plasma Ca^{2+}, by determination of plasma total protein or albumin levels, by the clinical context, or by other laboratory results. Acute hypocalcemia is often observed during acute hyperventilation and the respiratory alkalosis that follows, regardless of the cause of hyperventilation. Hyperventilation can occur secondary to cardiopulmonary or cerebral diseases.

After exclusion of false hypocalcemia linked to hypoalbuminemia, hypocalcemia can be divided into that associated with elevated and that associated with low plasma phosphate concentration.

Hypocalcemia Associated with Hyperphosphatemia

This form of hypocalcemia is caused by hypoparathyroid states that are idiopathic or acquired (after surgery or radiotherapy or secondary to amyloidosis). Sporadic cases of hypoparathyroidism can occasionally be seen in patients with pernicious anemia or adrenal insufficiency. Pseudohypoparathyroidism (Albright's hereditary osteodystrophy) is characterized by a particular phenotype including short neck, round face, and short metacarpals, with end-organ resistance to PTH. CKD, AKI in its oligoanuric phase (e.g., secondary to rhabdomyolysis), and massive phosphate administration can also lead to hypocalcemia with hyperphosphatemia. At least one form of inherited, familial hypocalcemia is linked to particular activating mutations of the CaR_G.[20]

Hypocalcemia Associated with Hypophosphatemia

Hypocalcemia with hypophosphatemia may occur from vitamin D–deficient states. This may result from insufficient sunlight exposure, dietary deficiency of vitamin D, decreased absorption after gastrointestinal surgery, intestinal malabsorption syndromes (steatorrhea), or hepatobiliary disease (primary biliary cirrhosis). Magnesium deficiency may also result in hypocalcemia, often in conjunction with hypokalemia, which may be due to inappropriate kaliuresis or diarrhea. The low serum Ca^{2+} concentration appears to result from decreased PTH release and end-organ resistance. AKI in the polyuric phase may also be associated with hypocalcemia and hypophosphatemia. The main causes of hypocalcemia are shown in Figure 10.10.

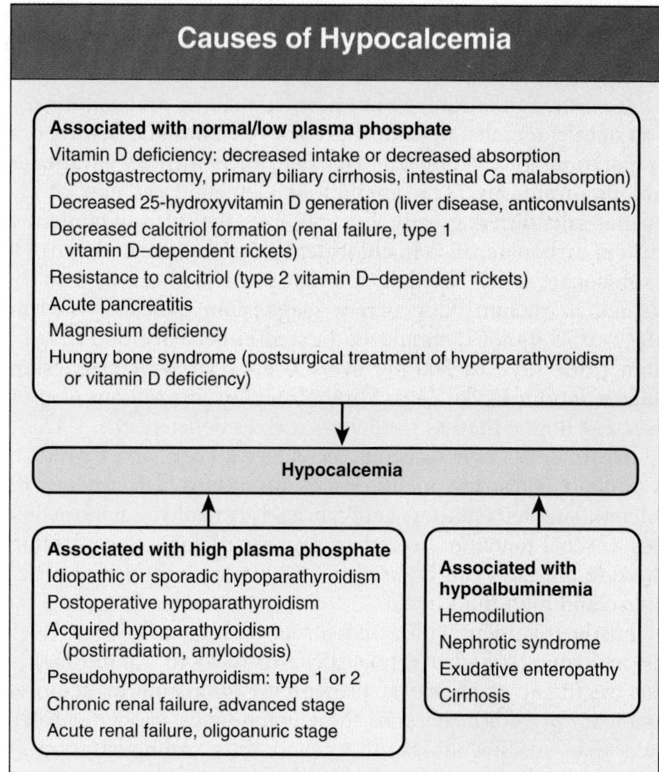

Figure 10.10 Causes of hypocalcemia.

Clinical Manifestations

As with hypercalcemia, the symptoms of hypocalcemia depend on the rate of its development and its severity. The most common manifestations, in addition to fatigue and muscle weakness, are increased irritability, loss of memory, a state of confusion, hallucination, paranoia, and depression. The best known clinical signs are Chovstek's sign (tapping of facial nerve branches leads to twitching of facial muscle) and Trousseau's sign (carpal spasm in response to forearm ischemia caused by sphygmomanometer cuff). In acute hypocalcemia, there may be paresthesias of the lips and the extremities, muscle cramps, and sometimes frank tetany, laryngeal stridor, or convulsions. Chronic hypocalcemia can be associated with cataracts, brittle nails with transverse grooves, dry skin, and decreased or even absent axillary and pubic hair, especially in idiopathic hypoparathyroidism, which is often of autoimmune origin.

Laboratory and Radiographic Signs

Plasma phosphate is elevated in hypoparathyroidism, pseudohypoparathyroidism, and advanced CKD, whereas it is decreased in steatorrhea, vitamin D deficiency, acute pancreatitis, and the polyuric phase during recovery from AKI. Plasma PTH is reduced in hypoparathyroidism and also during chronic magnesium deficiency, whereas it is normal or increased in pseudohypoparathyroidism and in CKD. Urinary calcium excretion is increased only in the treatment of hypoparathyroidism with calcium and vitamin D derivatives, in which it may lead to nephrocalcinosis; it is low in all other cases of hypocalcemia. Fractional urinary calcium excretion is, however, high in hypoparathyroidism, in the polyuric phase during recovery from AKI, and in severe CKD; it is low in all other cases of hypocalcemia. Urinary phosphate excretion is low in hypoparathyroidism, pseudohypoparathyroidism, and magnesium deficiency; it is high in vitamin D deficiency, steatorrhea, and CKD and during phosphate administration. Determination of serum 25-hydroxyvitamin D and calcitriol levels may also be useful.

Intracranial calcifications, notably of the basal ganglia, are observed radiographically in 20% of patients with idiopathic hypoparathyroidism but much less frequently in patients with postsurgical hypoparathyroidism or pseudohypoparathyroidism.

On electrocardiography, the corrected QT interval is frequently prolonged, and there are sometimes arrhythmias. Electroencephalography shows nonspecific signs, such as an increase in slow, high-voltage waves.

Treatment

The basic treatment is that of the underlying cause. Severe and symptomatic (tetany) hypocalcemia requires rapid treatment. Acute respiratory alkalosis, if present, should be corrected, if possible. When the cause is functional, the simple retention of carbon dioxide (e.g., by breathing into a paper bag) may suffice. In other cases and to obtain a prolonged effect, intravenous infusion of calcium salts is most often required. In the setting of seizures or tetany, calcium gluconate should be administered as an intravenous bolus (for instance, calcium gluconate, 10 ml 10% w/v [2.2 mmol of calcium], diluted in 50 ml of 5% dextrose or isotonic saline), followed by 12 to 24 g during 24 hours in 5%

dextrose or isotonic saline. Calcium gluconate is preferred to calcium chloride, which can lead to extensive skin necrosis in accidental extravasation.

Treatment of chronic hypocalcemia includes oral administration of calcium salts, thiazide diuretics, or vitamin D. Several oral preparations of calcium are available, each with its advantages and disadvantages. The amount of elemental calcium of the various salts differs greatly. For example, the calcium content is 40% in carbonate, 36% in chloride, 12% in lactate, and only 8% in gluconate salts. The daily amount prescribed can be 2 to 4 g elemental calcium. Concurrent magnesium deficiency (serum Mg^{2+} <0.75 mmol/l) should be treated either with oral magnesium oxide (250 to 500 mg every 6 days) or with magnesium sulfate: intramuscular (4 to 8 mmol/day) or intravenous (2 g i.v. over 2-4 hours, then as needed to correct deficiency).

Treatment of hypocalcemia secondary to hypoparathyroidism is difficult as urinary calcium excretion increases markedly with calcium supplementation and can lead to nephrocalcinosis and loss of renal function. To reduce urinary calcium concentration, thiazide diuretics can be used in association with restricted salt intake and high fluid intake.

Lastly, treatment with active forms of vitamin D, calcitriol or its analogue 1α-hydroxycholecalciferol (0.25 to 1.0 μg/day), is the treatment of choice at present for idiopathic or acquired hypoparathyroidism because these compounds are better tolerated than massive doses of calcium salts. Administration of vitamin D derivatives generally leads to hypercalciuria and, rarely, to nephrocalcinosis. It requires regular monitoring of the serum calcium concentration to avoid hypercalcemia.

PHOSPHATE HOMEOSTASIS

Distribution of Phosphate in the Organism

Phosphorus plays a crucial role in cell structure and metabolism. Phosphorus is found in the organism as both mineral phosphate and organic phosphate (phosphoric esters). Within cells, phosphate regulates enzymatic activity and serves as an essential component of nucleic acids and phospholipid membranes. Outside cells, phosphate resides in bone and teeth as hydroxyapatite; less than 1% circulates in serum. Phosphate circulates as HPO_4^{2-} and $H_2PO_4^-$, in a 4:1 ratio at normal pH of 7.4. Normal serum phosphate levels of 2.8 to 4.5 mg/dl (0.9 to 1.5 mmol/l) fluctuate in a circadian rhythm, with levels approximately 0.6 mg/dl higher in the afternoon compared with an 11 AM nadir. Figure 10.11 shows the distribution of phosphate in the extracellular and intracellular fluid compartments.

Figure 10.12 shows the balance of ingestion, body distribution, and excretion of phosphate in a healthy human. A young adult requires approximately 0.5 mmol/kg of phosphate daily. These needs are much higher in the child during growth. Phosphates are widely found in milk products, meat, eggs, and cereals and are used extensively as food additives.

Phosphate entrance into transport epithelia involves a secondary active Na^+-phosphate (Na^+-Pi) cotransport. Three different Na^+-Pi cotransporters have been identified and characterized.[21] The type 1 Na^+-Pi family is present in the renal tubule and may also have anion channel function. Type 2 Na^+-Pi cotransporters are the key players in phosphate homeostasis and include three members: NPT2a, NPT2b, and NPT2c. Two of them serve specific epithelial transport functions in the brush border of the proximal tubule (NPT2a, NPT2c) and of the small intestine (NPT2b), determining Na^+-dependent phosphate reabsorption. Type 3 Na^+-Pi cotransporters, Pit1 and Pit2, are ubiquitous. Phosphate entry into vascular smooth muscle cells through Pit1 is believed to be a necessary first step for initiation of pathologic smooth muscle calcification. The exit of phosphate at the basolateral side of the intestinal and renal tubular epithelium probably occurs by anionic exchange.

The transcellular transport of phosphate is controlled by metabolic, hormonal, and autocrine and paracrine factors, including calcitriol, growth hormone, insulin-like growth factor

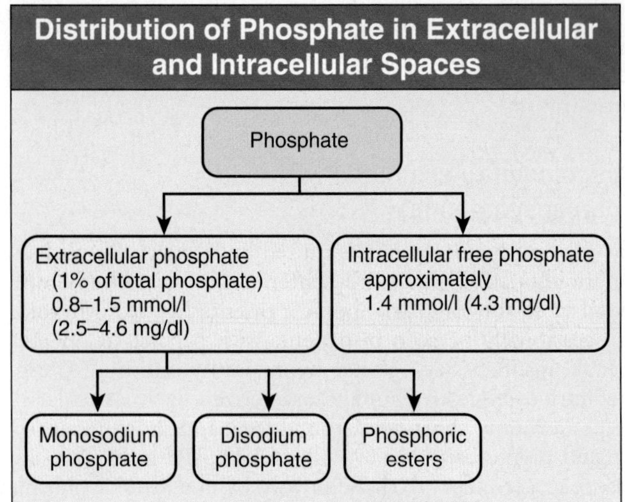

Figure 10.11 Distribution of phosphate in extracellular and intracellular spaces.

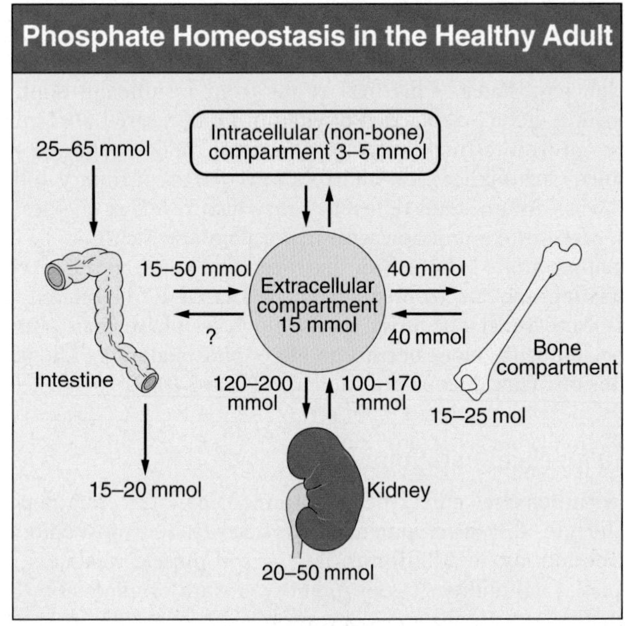

Figure 10.12 Phosphate homeostasis in healthy young adults. At net zero balance, identical net intestinal uptake (absorption minus secretion) and urinary loss occur. After its passage into the extracellular fluid, phosphate enters the intracellular space, is deposited in bone or soft tissue, or is eliminated by the kidneys. Entry and exit fluxes between the extracellular and intracellular spaces (skeletal and nonskeletal compartments) are also the same under steady-state conditions. Values linked to compartments represent absolute amounts of phosphate whereas values linked to the intestine and the kidney represent daily phosphate entries and exits, and values between organs and compartments represent daily fluxes.

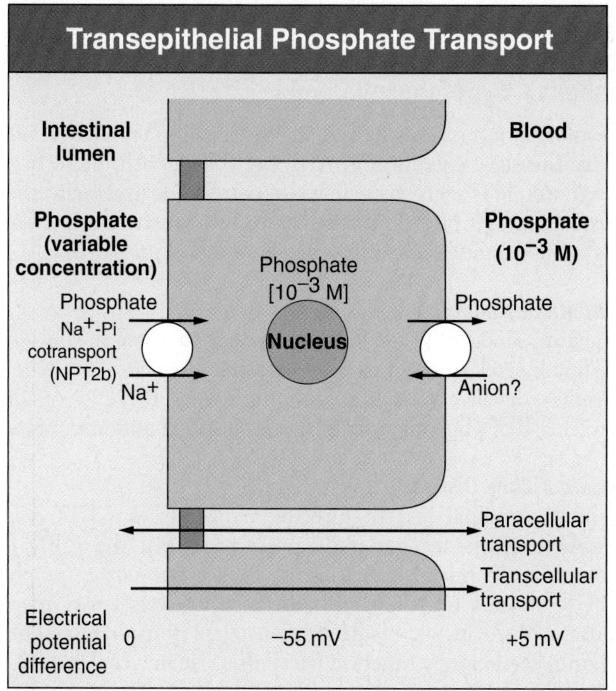

Figure 10.13 Transepithelial phosphate transport in the small intestine. Phosphate enters the enterocyte (influx) through the brush border membrane by the Na^+-Pi cotransport system, with a stoichiometry of 2:1, operating against an electrochemical gradient. Phosphate exit at the basolateral side possibly occurs by passive diffusion or (more probably) by anion exchange.

1, insulin, and thyroid hormone. In the kidney, PTH and fibroblast growth factor (FGF) 23 are major phosphaturic hormones that promote urinary phosphate excretion. Several other phosphatonins have also been identified subsequently, including secreted frizzled-related protein 4 (sFRP-4), matrix extracellular phosphoglycoprotein, and FGF-7.[22] The klotho protein participates directly in phosphate homeostasis by conferring specificity of the interaction of FGF-23 with its receptor FGF-R1. Deletion of *klotho* in the mouse induces a hyperphosphatemic phenotype. Of note, klotho also activates the calcium channel TRPV5.[23]

Intestinal, Renal, and Skeletal Handling of Phosphate

Phosphate transport across the intestinal wall occurs through both the transepithelial and the paracellular routes (Fig. 10.13). Absorption is a linear, nonsaturable function of phosphate intake (Fig. 10.14) and amounts to 60% to 75% of total phosphate intake (15 to 50 mmol/day). Calcitriol, which stimulates the NPT2b cotransporter, is the major hormonal determinant of intestinal phosphate absorption. Cations, such as calcium, magnesium, and aluminum, bind to phosphate in the gastrointestinal tract, limiting its absorption. In both animals and humans, ingestion of a high-phosphate meal results in the rapid excretion of phosphate in the urine, without detectable changes in serum phosphate levels.

The kidneys play a major role in controlling extracellular phosphate homeostasis.[24,25] Phosphate is freely filtered in the glomerulus and reabsorbed primarily in the proximal tubule of the kidney. Normally, the daily amount of phosphate excreted in urine equals that absorbed in the intestine, usually comprising 5% to 20% of the ultrafiltered phosphate load.

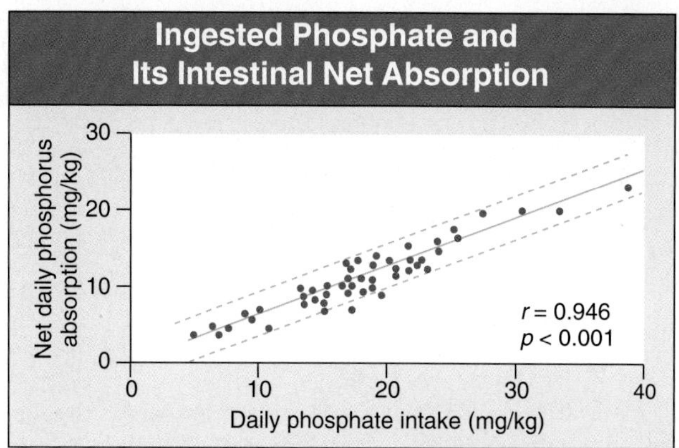

Figure 10.14 Relationship between ingested phosphate and that absorbed in the digestive tract (net absorption) in healthy young adults. *(From reference 9.)*

The amount of phosphate reabsorbed can be expressed in relation to the amount filtered as the urinary fractional excretion of phosphate (FE_{PO4}):

$$FE_{PO4} = (U_{PO4} \times S_{creat})/(S_{PO4} \times U_{creat})$$

where U_{PO4}, S_{PO4}, U_{creat}, and S_{creat} are urinary and serum phosphate and creatinine concentrations, respectively. Alternatively, the amount of phosphate reabsorbed can be expressed as the fraction (or percent) of filtered phosphate that is reabsorbed by the renal tubule (TRP, %). The maximal tubular reabsorption of phosphate (TmP) factored for GFR (TmP/GFR, Bijvoet index) represents the concentration above which most phosphate is excreted and below which most is reabsorbed. This can be calculated from the plasma phosphate concentration and tubular reabsorption of phosphate (Fig. 10.15).

After passage through the glomerulus, part of the filtered phosphate load is recovered by the tubule, depending on the body's needs. The major fraction of phosphate is reabsorbed in the proximal convoluted tubule through NPT2a, which is modulated by endocrine and metabolic factors.[25] Specifically, PTH, FGF-23, and hyperphosphatemia downregulate NPT2a, increasing urinary phosphate excretion, whereas hypophosphatemia upregulates NPT2a, decreasing urinary phosphate excretion.

Recent attention has focused on FGF-23 as a master regulator of phosphate metabolism. FGF-23 lowers serum phosphate concentrations by decreasing renal phosphate reabsorption and by inhibiting calcitriol production, thereby reducing phosphate absorption in the gut. Genetic disruption of FGF-23 in animals results in hyperphosphatemia, calcitriol toxicity, vascular calcification, and premature death. An identical phenotype is created by genetic disruption of *klotho*, which is needed for FGF-23 to bind its receptor in the renal proximal tubule and to enhance phosphate excretion. It has been proposed very recently that klotho could also have a direct phosphaturic action in the proximal tubule, independent of FGF23, via an enzymatic modification of apical membrane glycans.

Bone permanently exchanges phosphate with the surrounding milieu. Entry and exit of phosphate amount to approximately 100 mmol/day (slowly exchangeable phosphate), for a total skeleton content of approximately 20,000 mmol. The net balance is positive during growth, zero in the young adult, and negative in the elderly.

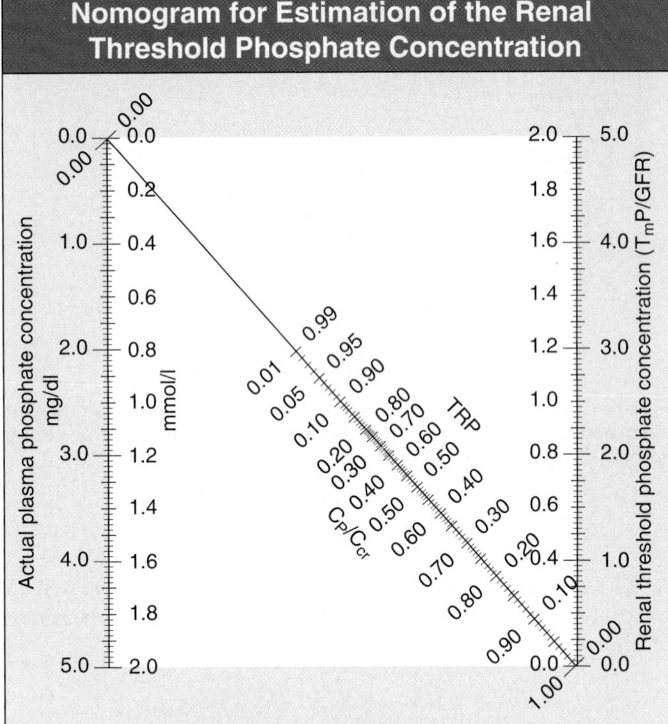

Figure 10.15 Nomogram for estimation of the renal threshold phosphate concentration (TmP/GFR) without any calculation. A straight line through the appropriate values of phosphate concentration and tubular reabsorption of phosphate (TRP, amount of phosphate reabsorbed) or C_P/C_{cr} (where C is clearance for phosphate [P] or creatinine [cr]) passes through the corresponding value of TmP/GFR. TRP = 1 – $FePO_4$ = 1 – (UPO_4 × Screat) (SPO_4 × Ucreat) *(From reference 26.)*

HYPERPHOSPHATEMIA

Causes of Hyperphosphatemia

The most common cause of increased serum phosphate levels is reduced urinary excretion in AKI and CKD.[27] Although hyperphosphatemia is seen particularly in conditions in which urinary phosphate excretion is perturbed, it can also be caused by increased exogenous or endogenous phosphate supply (Fig. 10.16).

Acute Kidney Injury

An acute reduction in GFR leads directly to a rise in the serum phosphate level, often in parallel with the serum creatinine level. Phosphate levels can be extremely high when there is concomitant release of phosphate from tissues, as in rhabdomyolysis.

Chronic Kidney Disease

Despite a gradual loss of filtering nephrons in CKD, serum phosphate levels are generally preserved until the GFR falls below about 35 ml/min per 1.73 m^2. Preservation of serum phosphate levels in CKD highlights the complex regulatory mechanisms involved in phosphate homeostasis. Phosphate retention with impaired kidney function parallels a rise in circulating levels of the phosphaturic hormones PTH and FGF-23, which defend serum phosphate levels by increasing urinary phosphate excretion. Both hormones downregulate NPT2a on the apical surface of the proximal tubule, increasing the fractional excretion of phosphate, which can exceed 60% in advanced CKD. However, there is a price paid for defending the serum phosphate level; FGF-23 potently suppresses 25-hydroxyvitamin D 1α-hydroxylase activity, possibly to limit further gastrointestinal absorption of phosphate, resulting in diminished calcium absorption and further stimulation of PTH. Eventually, reduced functional renal mass can no longer support further phosphate excretion, and serum phosphate levels rise. By this time, secondary hyperparathyroidism is usually evident, along with elevated levels of FGF-23 and lower levels of calcitriol and calcium.

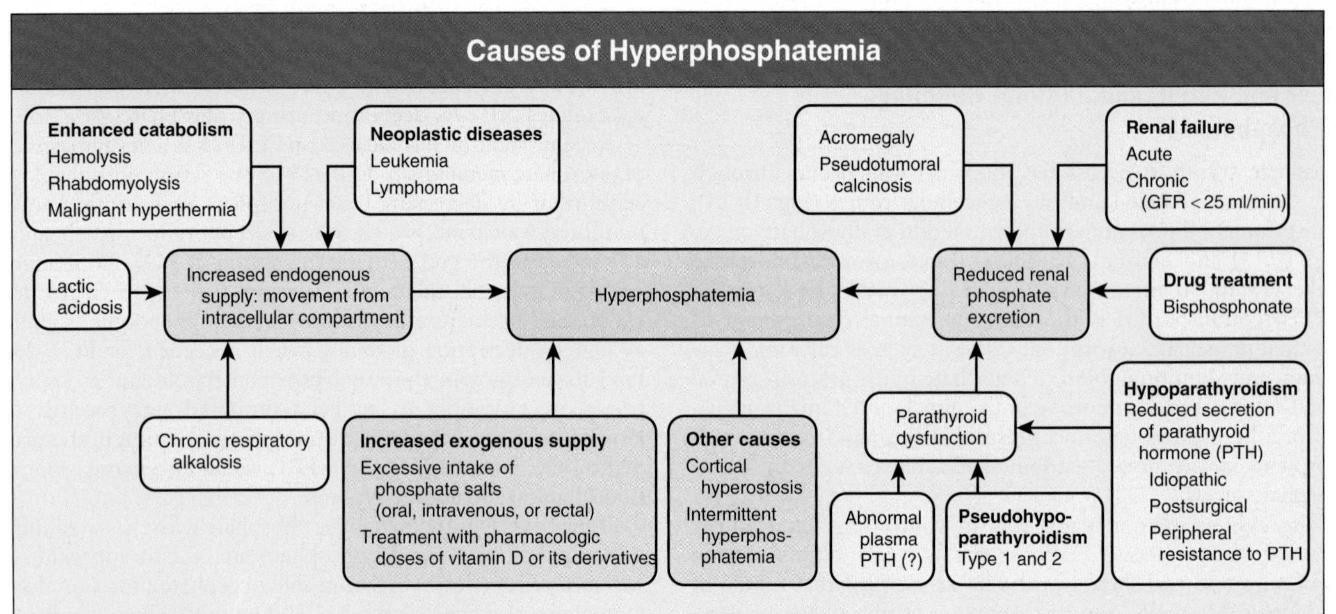

Figure 10.16 Causes of hyperphosphatemia.

Lytic States

Exaggerated phosphate loss by tissues can be observed in states of extreme cell lysis, particularly rhabdomyolysis (crush injury), or malignant neoplasms and their treatment (especially lymphomas and leukemias). The hyperphosphatemia of rhabdomyolysis is typically accompanied by hypocalcemia, myoglobinuria, and AKI. Severe hypercatabolic states during severe infection or in diabetic ketoacidosis can also cause hyperphosphatemia by increased cellular release of phosphate (which is usually accompanied with an acute reduction in GFR).

Treatment-Induced Hyperphosphatemia

A massive supply of phosphate, as may occur by phosphate-based laxative or enema use, can lead to hyperphosphatemia. Oral sodium phosphate solutions used to prepare for colonoscopy contain massive quantities of phosphate and can cause precipitation of calcium phosphate crystals within the renal tubules and AKI. Recovery from this condition is slow and often incomplete, with some cases resulting in permanent dialysis. For these reasons, bowel preparations other than those based on sodium phosphate salts should be used in patients with CKD. Bisphosphonates, in particular etidronate in Paget's disease, can sometimes increase serum phosphate levels, possibly through increased liberation of tissue phosphate or an increase in renal tubular reabsorption.

Hypoparathyroidism

PTH is a major phosphaturic hormone. In states of reduced PTH secretion (idiopathic or postsurgical hypoparathyroidism) or resistance to its peripheral action (pseudohypoparathyroidism), tubular excretion of phosphate is diminished. The resulting increase in plasma phosphate leads to an increase in the ultrafiltered load. This results in the regulation of plasma phosphate at a new steady-state level.

Chronic Hypocalcemia

Hyperphosphatemia is sometimes observed in association with chronic hypocalcemia with normal or high plasma PTH levels. In the absence of characteristic abnormalities of pseudohypoparathyroidism, the existence of an abnormal form of plasma PTH has been suggested, perhaps due to abnormal conversion of the prohormone to its secreted form.

Acromegaly

In this condition, hyperphosphatemia results from an increase in tubular reabsorption of phosphate due to stimulation by growth hormones or insulin-like growth factor 1.

Familial Tumoral Calcinosis

This rare, autosomal recessive disorder seen primarily in people of Middle Eastern or African ancestry is caused by inactivating or missense mutations in the *GALNT3*, FGF23 or klotho gene. Possibly the glycosyl transferase encoded by *GALNT3* is necessary for FGF-23 activity, thus resulting in a shared phenotype.[21] The lack of functional FGF-23 results in an exaggerated tubular phosphate reabsorption and uninhibited vitamin D activation, leading to hyperphosphatemia, an elevated serum calcium × phosphate product, high circulating levels of calcitriol, and metastatic soft tissue calcifications. Circulating PTH is not decreased.

Respiratory Alkalosis by Prolonged Hyperventilation

Respiratory alkalosis resulting from prolonged hyperventilation is characterized by resistance to the renal action of PTH, hyperphosphatemia, and hypocalcemia. There may also be functional pseudohypoparathyroidism because renal phosphate clearance is diminished, whereas plasma PTH is normal, despite hypocalcemia. There is no decrease in urinary calcium excretion.

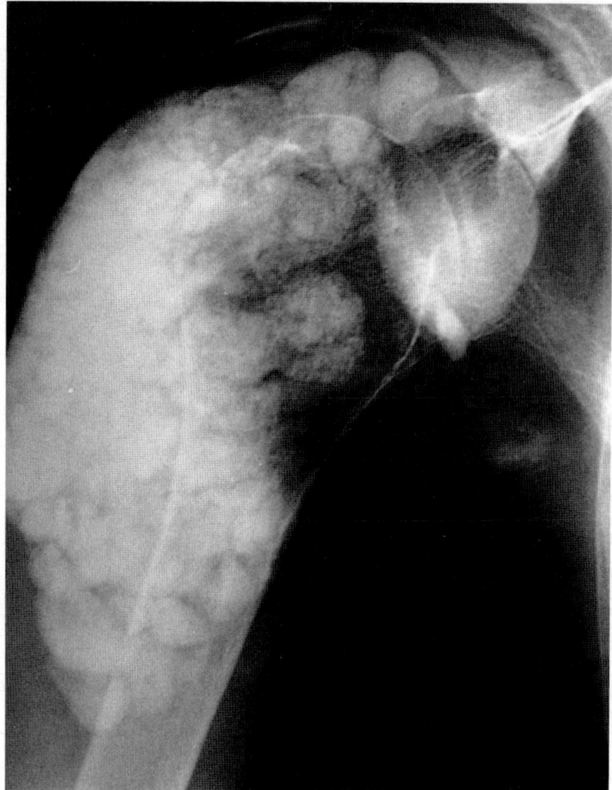

Figure 10.17 Tumor-like extraskeletal calcification in the shoulder.

Clinical Manifestations

Acute and severe hyperphosphatemia can induce hypocalcemia, which stimulates PTH but inhibits renal synthesis of calcitriol, which tends to further aggravate hypocalcemia. Chronic hyperphosphatemia is suspected to play a causal role in the pathogenesis of vascular calcification, particularly in CKD (see Chapter 78). In extreme cases, hyperphosphatemia can induce tumor-like soft tissue calcium phosphate deposits (Teutschländer's disease; Fig. 10.17) or extensive vascular calcification within the arteries of the skin (calciphylaxis or calcific uremic arteriolopathy; see Chapter 84).

Treatment

Treatment of acute hyperphosphatemia is usually targeted at improving phosphate excretion either by intravenous fluids or by renal replacement therapy in cases of severe AKI. Intravenous dextrose and insulin can also shift phosphate into cells, similar to its use for treatment of hyperkalemia. Treatment of chronic hyperphosphatemia typically requires the use of an oral phosphate binder, usually calcium acetate, calcium carbonate, sevelamer, or lanthanum carbonate, which complex with phosphate in the gastrointestinal tract and limit absorption (see Chapter 78).

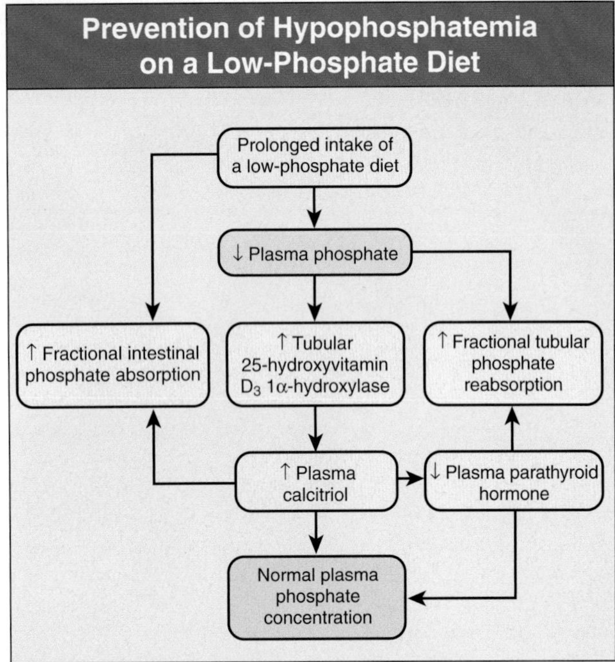

Figure 10.18 Compensatory mechanisms to prevent hypophosphatemia during a prolonged intake of a phosphate-poor diet.

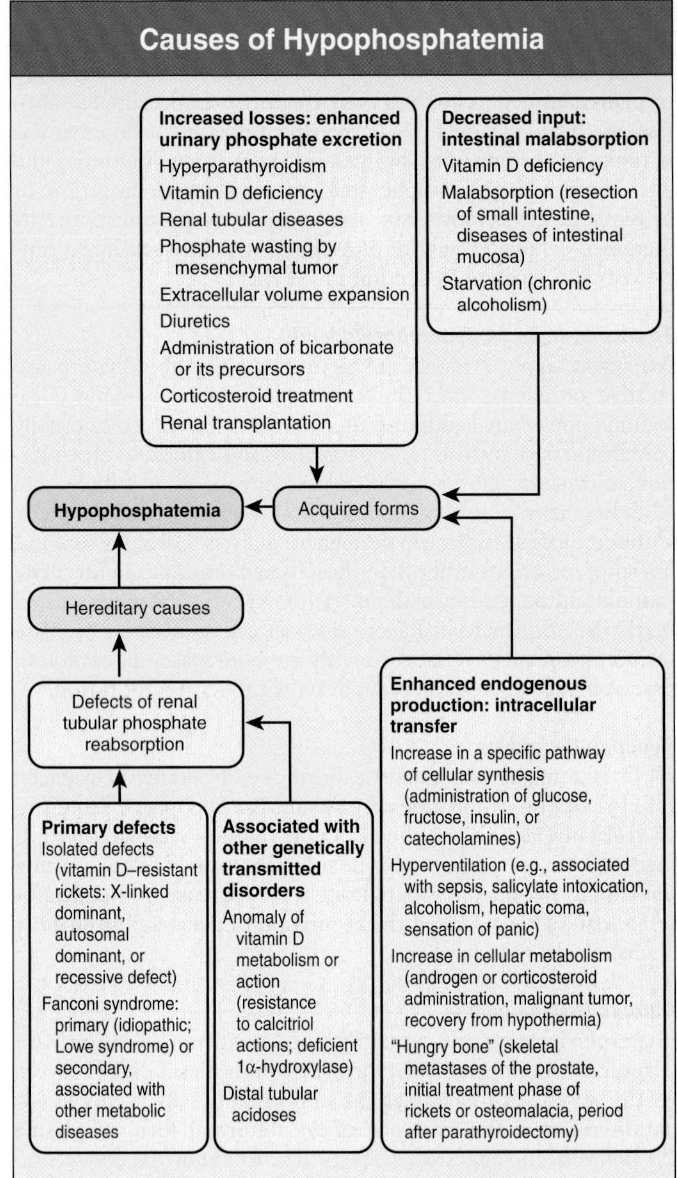

Figure 10.19 Causes of hypophosphatemia.

HYPOPHOSPHATEMIA

Decreased plasma phosphate levels may reflect phosphate deficiency. This can, theoretically, be observed during a prolonged decrease in phosphate intake. However, as shown in Figure 10.18, several defense mechanisms counter a decrease in plasma phosphate resulting from low intake. Moderately reduced plasma phosphate levels may also be seen with maldistribution between the intracellular and extracellular compartments during acute respiratory alkalosis.

Causes of Hypophosphatemia

Moderate hypophosphatemia can be caused by genetic diseases or by acquired conditions (Fig. 10.19).[32] The main acquired condition is malnutrition due to low food intake or anorexia during critical illness or alcoholism. Another cause is a shift of phosphate into cells, which can occur through various mechanisms, but especially with the administration of insulin. Although there are a large number of genetic diseases and syndromes, overall, these are rare. Severe forms of hypophosphatemia are all acquired.

Inherited Forms of Hypophosphatemia

Inherited diseases associated with chronic hypophosphatemia are generally diagnosed in childhood. Persistently low plasma phosphate usually leads to rickets or osteomalacia. Inherited hypophosphatemia results from primary defects that are either isolated or associated with tubular disorders (Fanconi syndrome) or defects secondary to another genetically transmitted disease, mainly metabolic disorders or disturbances in the action of vitamin D.

Autosomal Dominant Hypophosphatemic Rickets

Children with this phosphate-wasting disorder present with skeletal defects, including bowing of the long bones and widening of costochondral joints. The disease is linked to mutations in *FGF-23*, in which an aberrant form of the molecule is resistant to proteolytic cleavage.[28] Excess FGF-23 causes phosphate wasting by downregulation of NPT2a in the proximal renal tubule.

X-Linked Hypophosphatemic Rickets

This rare phosphate-wasting syndrome is characterized by skeletal deformities, short stature, and osteomalacia. The disease has been linked to various mutations in the *PHEX* gene (phosphate-regulating endopeptidase on the X chromosome). *PHEX* was believed to play a role in the proteolysis of FGF-23 but recent findings cast doubt on this hypothesis, so another mechanism needs to be identified.[29] *PHEX* mutations result in high circulating FGF-23 concentrations, renal phosphate wasting, and hypophosphatemia. Plasma calcium, calcitriol, and PTH levels are normal, and the alkaline phosphatase level is elevated.

Autosomal Recessive Hypophosphatemic Rickets

This disorder is caused by mutations in the gene encoding dentin matrix protein 1 (*DMP1*), which is believed to suppress FGF-23 secretion by bone.

Fanconi Syndrome and Proximal Renal Tubular Acidosis

Fanconi syndrome (see Chapter 48) is characterized by a complex transport defect of the proximal tubule that results in decreased reabsorption of glucose, amino acids, bicarbonate, and phosphate. Because 70% of the filtered phosphate load is typically reabsorbed in the proximal tubule, Fanconi syndrome can lead to phosphate wasting and hypophosphatemia. Causes of Fanconi syndrome can be primary (idiopathic, Lowe syndrome, Dent disease) or associated with other metabolic diseases (cystinosis, Wilson's disease, and others). In Dent disease and Lowe syndrome, a defective recycling of megalin to the apical cell surface of the proximal tubule has been found, implicating a role in abnormal tubular endocytic function.[30]

Fanconi syndrome with phosphate wasting can also occur as an acquired disorder in adults. Common causes are multiple myeloma and specific medications (tenofovir, ifosfamide, and carbonic anhydrase inhibitors).

In addition to a tubular defect causing phosphate wasting, the activity of renal 25-hydroxyvitamin D 1α-hydroxylase may be insufficient, resulting in decreased circulating calcitriol levels and bone disease such as rickets and osteomalacia. Functional disorders associated with the syndrome, such as polyuria and extracellular volume contraction, lead to hyperaldosteronism with hypokalemia and eventually to renal failure.

Hypophosphatemia Linked to Other Inherited Diseases

Several rare inherited diseases can be associated with hypophosphatemia, including vitamin D–dependent rickets type 1, caused by a defect of renal 25-hydroxyvitamin D 1α-hydroxylase, and type 2, caused by peripheral resistance to the action of calcitriol. Clinical signs are similar to those of vitamin D–deficient rickets, but alopecia also occurs in 50% of cases. In type 1, calcitriol levels are low, whereas in type 2, there is normal circulating 25-hydroxyvitamin D and high calcitriol. Low doses of calcitriol are sufficient for treatment of type 1, whereas extremely high doses of calcitriol or alfacalcidol are required for type 2.

Distal Renal Tubular Acidosis (Type 1)

Distal renal tubular acidosis (type 1; see Chapter 12) is associated with hypercalciuria and sometimes nephrocalcinosis because chronic acidosis enhances the reabsorption of citrate in the proximal tubule, preventing it from forming soluble calcium-citrate complexes in the urine. Chronic acidosis also causes increased calcium and phosphate release from bone. Hypophosphatemia is inconstant; it is possible that it results only when there is concomitant vitamin D deficiency.

Acquired Forms of Hypophosphatemia

The number of acquired diseases that can be associated with hypophosphatemia is even greater than the number of inherited diseases and includes hyperparathyroidism and vitamin D deficiency (see Fig. 10.19). True phosphate deficiency associated with total body depletion must be distinguished from enhanced influx of phosphate from the extracellular to the intracellular space or increased skeletal mineralization.

Alcoholism

Alcoholism is the most common cause of severe hypophosphatemia in Western countries. The causes are multiple, including prolonged insufficient food intake, excessive phosphate loss in urine secondary to hypomagnesemia, and phosphate transfer from the extracellular to the intracellular compartment secondary to hyperventilation or glucose infusion in subjects with post–alcoholic cirrhosis or in acute abstinence.

Hyperparathyroidism

PTH enhances urinary phosphate excretion by downregulation of the NPT2a cotransporter. Patients with primary hyperparathyroidism typically present with mild hypercalcemia and hypophosphatemia.

Post-Transplantation Hypophosphatemia

Renal phosphate wasting is exceedingly common in both cadaveric and living related renal transplant recipients. Most renal transplant patients develop hypophosphatemia at some point during their post-transplantation course, and in some instances, the condition may be prolonged. A number of explanations for this condition have been proposed, including residual hyperparathyroidism from chronic kidney failure; however, the best evidence implicates persistently high circulating levels of FGF-23 as the key factor responsible for post-transplantation urinary phosphate wasting.

Acute Respiratory Alkalosis

In intense and short-term hyperventilation, plasma phosphate can sometimes decrease considerably to values as low as 0.1 mmol/l (0.3 mg/dl). Such a decrease is never observed in acute metabolic alkalosis. Hypophosphatemia that follows acute and intense hyperventilation is probably the result of muscle sequestration of extracellular phosphate. However, prolonged chronic hyperventilation leads to hyperphosphatemia (see previous discussion).

Diabetic Ketoacidosis

During decompensated diabetes associated with acidosis provoked by accumulation of ketone bodies, glycosuria, and polyuria, plasma phosphate can be normal or high, even in the presence of hyperphosphaturia. Correction of this complication by insulin and refilling of the extracellular compartment leads to massive transfer of phosphate into the intracellular compartment, hypophosphatemia, and subsequently less urinary loss of phosphate. In general, plasma phosphate does not decrease to less than 0.3 mmol/l (0.9 mg/dl), except when there is preexisting phosphate deficiency.

Total Parenteral Nutrition

Hyperalimentation can also be associated with severe hypophosphatemia through the insulin-mediated shift of phosphate into cells, particularly if phosphate is omitted from the parenteral nutrition solution. Severe hypophosphatemia can also occur with acute feeding after starvation.

Oncogenic Hypophosphatemic Osteomalacia

Hypophosphatemia associated with tumor-induced osteomalacia results from renal phosphate wasting in patients with mesenchymal tumors (hemangiopericytomas, fibromas, angiosarcomas). The mechanism of hypophosphatemia is tumor secretion of phosphatonins (FGF-23, sFRP-4, matrix extracellular phosphoglycoprotein [MEPE], or FGF-7).[26] The condition resolves after tumor resection.

Drug-Induced Hypophosphatemia

Imatinib mesylate, a tyrosine kinase inhibitor, has been reported to cause hypophosphatemia and an elevation in PTH levels. The mechanism of action is not yet clear.

Clinical Manifestations

Clinical manifestations depend on the rate of onset of hypophosphatemia more than on its severity or the total body phosphate deficit. In practice, it is not clinically evident when serum phosphate concentration is more than 0.65 mmol/l (2.0 mg/dl). Manifestations include metabolic encephalopathy, red and white blood cell dysfunction, sometimes hemolysis, and thrombocytopenia. Reduced muscle strength and decreased myocardial contractility (with occasional rhabdomyolysis and cardiomyopathy, respectively) may occur.

Treatment

Phosphate deficiency is generally not an emergency. First, the mechanism involved should be defined to determine the most appropriate treatment.

When phosphate deficiency is diagnosed, oral treatment by milk products or phosphate salts should always be tried first whenever possible, except in the presence of nephrocalcinosis or nephrolithiasis with urinary phosphate wasting. In severe symptomatic deficiency, phosphate can also be infused intravenously, in divided doses during 24 hours. In patients undergoing parenteral nutrition, 10 to 25 mmol potassium phosphate should be given for each 1000 kcal, with care taken to avoid hyperphosphatemia because of the risk of inducing soft tissue calcifications. Dipyridamole (300 mg divided into four doses per day) has been shown to reduce the urinary excretion of phosphate in patients with a low renal phosphate threshold.

MAGNESIUM HOMEOSTASIS AND DISORDERS OF MAGNESIUM METABOLISM

Distribution of Magnesium in the Organism and Magnesium Homeostasis

Magnesium (Mg) is, after potassium, the second most abundant cation in the intracellular fluid in living organisms. Mg^{2+} is involved in the majority of metabolic processes. In addition, it plays a part in DNA and protein synthesis. It is involved in the regulation of mitochondrial function, inflammatory processes and immune defense, allergy, growth, and stress, and in the control of neuronal activity, cardiac excitability, neuromuscular transmission, vasomotor tone, and blood pressure. The distribution of Mg^{2+} within the intracellular and extracellular spaces is shown in Figure 10.20.

Figure 10.21 shows the balance of ingestion, body distribution, and excretion of Mg^{2+} in healthy humans. Mg^{2+} influx into and efflux out of cells are linked to carbohydrate-dependent active transport systems. The stimulation of β-adrenoceptors favors Mg^{2+} outflux, whereas insulin, calcitriol, and vitamin B_6 favor Mg^{2+} entry into cells.

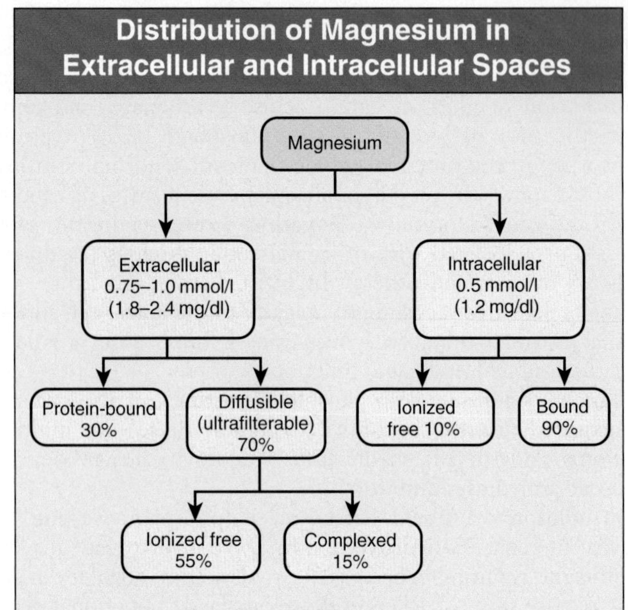

Figure 10.20 Distribution of magnesium in extracellular and intracellular spaces.

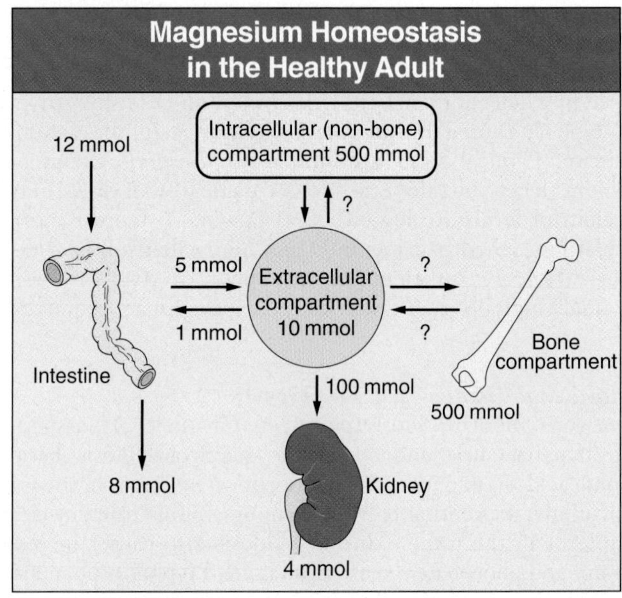

Figure 10.21 Magnesium homeostasis in the healthy young adult. Net zero balance results from net intestinal uptake (absorption minus secretion) equaling urinary loss. After its passage into the extracellular fluid, Mg^{2+} enters the intracellular space, is deposited in bone or soft tissue, or is eliminated by the kidneys. Entry and exit fluxes between the extracellular and intracellular spaces (skeletal and nonskeletal compartments) are also of identical magnitude; however, precise values of exchange are still debated. Values linked to compartments represent absolute amounts of magnesium whereas values linked to the intestine and the kidney represent daily magnesium entries and exits, and values between organs and compartments represent daily fluxes.

Intestinal and Renal Handling of Magnesium

The intestinal absorption of dietary magnesium occurs by both a saturable and a passive transport process, the major part being absorbed in the small intestine. The entry step in enterocyte brush border membrane is controlled by the magnesium channel TRPM6, which has been cloned recently and whose functional characterization is in progress.[3] Mg^{2+} absorption can vary by as much as 25% to 60%, with a mean absorption of approximately 30%. Intestinal transport does not change in response to chronic changes in dietary magnesium. However, TRPM6 is downregulated by an increase in intracellular Mg^{2+}.

Various factors modify intestinal Mg^{2+} absorption. High dietary phosphate intake is inhibitory, as is high phytate consumption. The effect of dietary calcium is complex, and vitamin D probably has an enhancing effect. Growth hormone

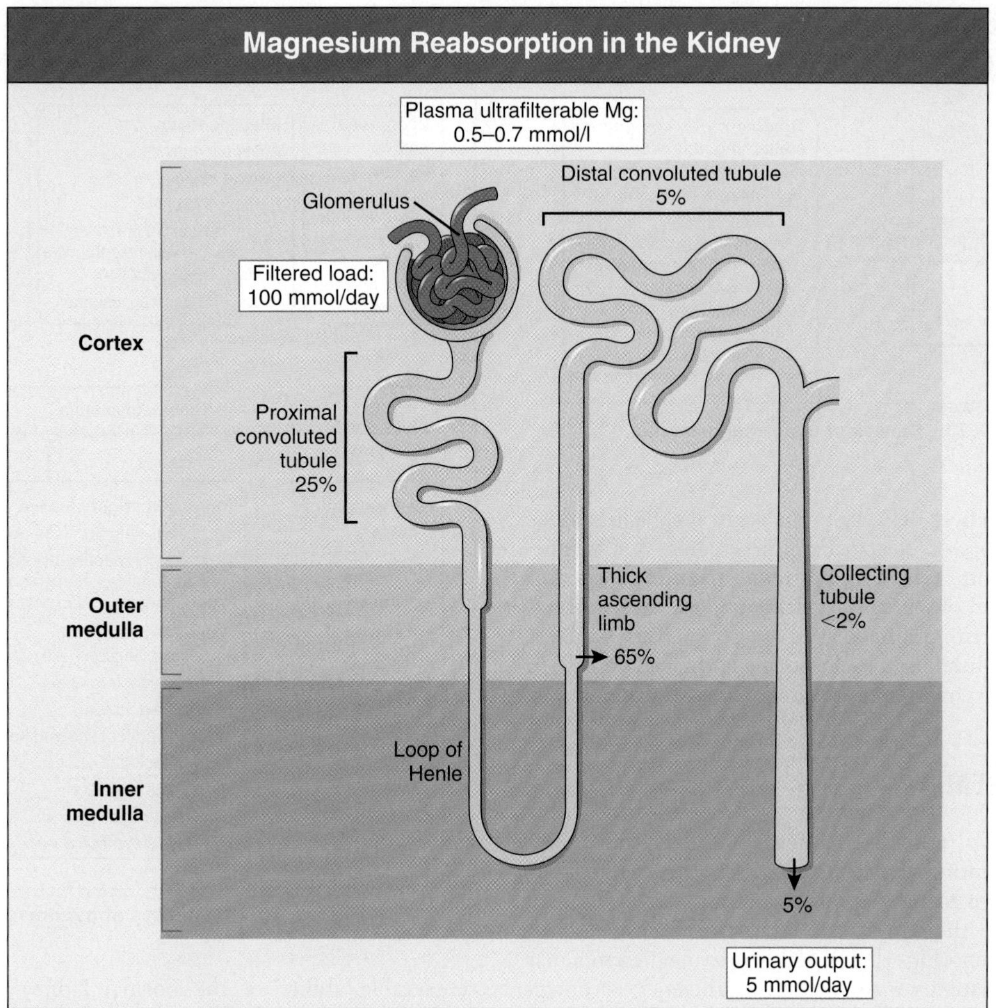

Figure 10.22 Sites of magnesium reabsorption in various segments of the renal tubule. The percentage absorbed in various segments from the glomerular ultrafiltrate is shown. *(Redrawn from reference 33.)*

slightly increases Mg^{2+} absorption, whereas aldosterone and calcitonin appear to reduce it. Vitamin B_6 has been reported to enhance it.

Mg^{2+} is eliminated by the kidney. Losses through intestinal secretion and sweat are negligible under normal conditions. With an ultrafilterable plasma magnesium concentration of 0.5 to 0.7 mmol/l (80% of total plasma magnesium), the filtered load of magnesium amounts to approximately 104 mmol (or 2500 mg) per day. The urinary output represents approximately 5% of the filtered load (4 to 5 mmol or 100 mg per day). The major portion of filtered magnesium is reabsorbed by the renal tubules (25% in the proximal tubule, 65% in the thick ascending loop of Henle, and 5% in the distal convoluted tubule) (Fig. 10.22).

Mg^{2+} transport in the thick ascending limb is primarily passive through the paracellular route. However, two conditions are necessary for normal Mg^{2+} reabsorption: first, the generation of an electrical, lumen-positive gradient induced by NaCl reabsorption that creates the driving force required for the reabsorption of divalent cations; and second, the expression of claudin 16 in the tight junction, which is responsible for the selectivity of the reabsorption of divalent cations. Different anomalies associated with NaCl reabsorption or with claudin 16 (formerly called paracellin) expression result in hypermagnesuria, for example, atypical cases of Bartter syndrome, which is defined by genetic defects related to NaCl transport in the thick ascending limb (see also later discussion).[34]

In the distal nephron, that is, the distal convoluted tubule and the connecting tubule, Mg^{2+} is reabsorbed through the transcellular route against an uphill electrochemical gradient. The molecular identity of the gatekeeper channel that controls Mg^{2+} entry into the tubular epithelium across the brush border membrane has been discovered recently as TRPM6.[3] It is identical to that of the intestine.

Tubular Mg^{2+} transport is modulated by serum Mg^{2+} and Ca^{2+} and extracellular fluid volume. An increase of plasma Mg^{2+} or Ca^{2+} concentration results in a depression of magnesium transport. Extracellular volume expansion produces a decrease in proximal tubular Mg^{2+} reabsorption, in parallel with that of Na^+ and Ca^{2+}. Dietary phosphate restriction results in marked hypercalciuria and hypermagnesuria and can thereby lead to overt hypomagnesemia. PTH, vasopressin, calcitonin, and glucagon increase tubular Mg^{2+} reabsorption, whereas acetylcholine, bradykinin, and atrial natriuretic peptide stimulate urinary Mg^{2+} excretion.

Finally, a number of drugs have been shown to increase renal Mg^{2+} excretion, including the loop diuretics such as furosemide and ethacrynic acid, distal diuretics such as thiazides, and osmotic diuretics such as mannitol and urea. Thiazide

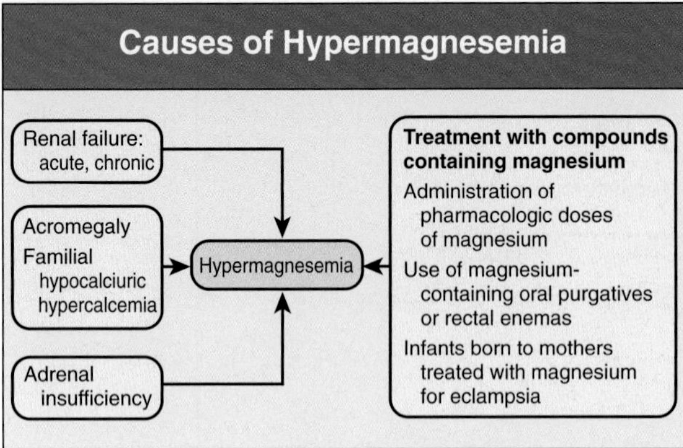

Figure 10.23 Causes of hypermagnesemia.

diuretics increase sodium delivery to the cortical collecting duct, dissipating the favorable electrochemical gradient for magnesium entry at this site. Furthermore, renal magnesium-wasting syndromes have been observed in patients treated with antibiotics such as gentamicin, antineoplastic agents such as cisplatin, and the calcineurin inhibitors cyclosporine and tacrolimus. The precise mechanisms of action of these agents are not well understood.

HYPERMAGNESEMIA

Elevated plasma Mg^{2+} is seen in patients with AKI and CKD, during the administration of pharmacologic doses of magnesium, in some infants born to mothers who received magnesium for eclampsia, and with the use of oral laxatives or rectal enemas containing magnesium (Fig. 10.23). Mild hypermagnesemia may also be present in patients with adrenal insufficiency, acromegaly, or familial hypocalciuric hypercalcemia.

Clinical Manifestations

Symptoms and signs are the result of the pharmacologic effects of increased Mg^{2+} concentrations on the nervous and cardiovascular systems. At Mg^{2+} concentrations up to 1.5 mmol/l (3.6 mg/dl), hypermagnesemia is asymptomatic. Deep tendon reflexes are usually lost when plasma Mg^{2+} concentration is greater than 3 mmol/l (7.2 mg/dl). Respiratory paralysis, hypotension, abnormal cardiac conduction, and loss of consciousness may occur as plasma levels of magnesium approach 5 mmol/l (12 mg/dl).

Treatment

Treatment consists of cessation of magnesium administration and the intravenous infusion of calcium salts. For the management of symptomatic hypermagnesemia, calcium gluconate may be given intravenously as 1 g in 10 ml during 5 to 10 minutes (each gram of calcium gluconate is equal to approximately 90 mg of elemental calcium).

HYPOMAGNESEMIA AND MAGNESIUM DEFICIENCY

Magnesium deficiency is defined as a decrease in total body magnesium content. Poor dietary intake of magnesium is usually not associated with marked magnesium deficiency because of the remarkable ability of the normal kidney to conserve Mg^{2+}. However, prolonged and severe dietary magnesium restriction of less than 0.5 mmol/day can produce symptomatic magnesium deficiency. Severe hypomagnesemia is usually associated with magnesium deficiency. Approximately 10% of patients admitted to a large city hospital in the United States were hypomagnesemic. The incidence may be as high as 65% in medical intensive care units.

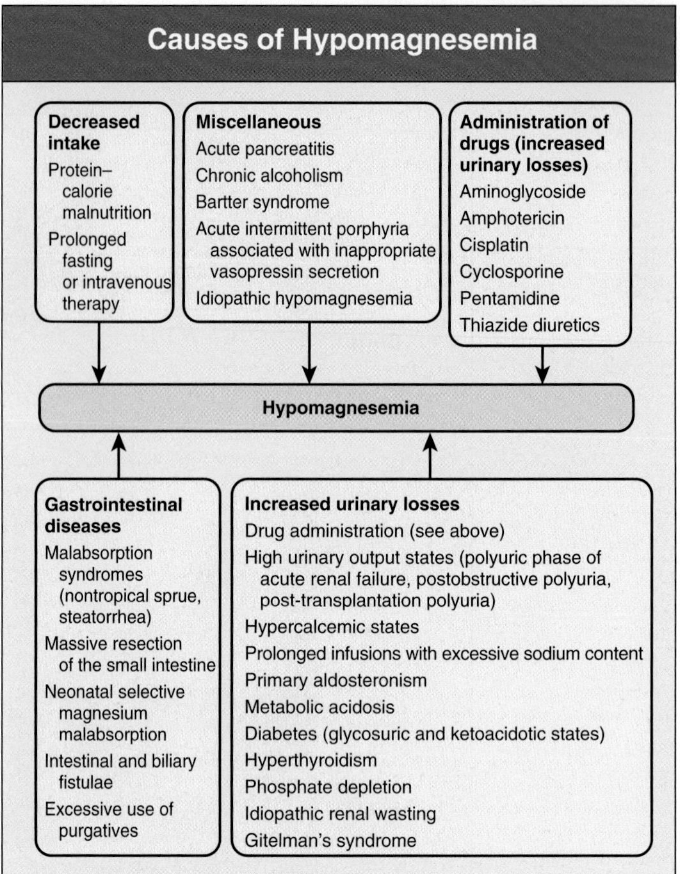

Figure 10.24 Causes of hypomagnesemia.

Underlying causes are usually diseases of the gastrointestinal tract, in particular malabsorption syndromes including nontropical sprue, and massive resection of the small intestine. Hypomagnesemia can also be induced by prolonged tube feeding without magnesium supplements and by the excessive use of laxatives (Fig. 10.24).

Hypomagnesemia is encountered in about 25% to 35% of patients with acute pancreatitis, is frequently observed in patients with chronic alcoholism, and can also be present in patients with poorly controlled diabetes mellitus. Hypomagnesemia can also be observed in patients with hypercalcemic disorders and in primary aldosteronism.

Excessive urinary loss of magnesium leads to hypomagnesemia and magnesium deficiency, even in the face of normal dietary intake. It may result from the overzealous use of diuretics; therefore, it is important to monitor plasma Mg^{2+} levels in patients with congestive heart failure who are treated with diuretic agents. Other drugs that may cause hypomagnesemia include gentamicin, cisplatin, and the calcineurin inhibitors cyclosporine and tacrolimus.

Several familial diseases are associated with hypermagnesuria, with or without hypomagnesemia. They are due to inactivating mutations of genes whose abnormal products are responsible for disturbed Mg^{2+} reabsorption in the thick ascending limb of Henle or in the distal nephron. Inactivating mutations of the genes of the Na-K-2Cl cotransporter, the rectifying K^+ channel (ROMK), or the basolateral Cl^- channel in Bartter syndrome are responsible for the abolition of the driving force for Mg^{2+} reabsorption. This can result in hypermagnesuria, which, however, is only rarely associated with hypomagnesemia. Inactivating mutations of the gene encoding CaR_G, whose protein product is a key regulator of NaCl reabsorption in the thick ascending limb through extracellular Ca^{2+} concentration, lead to hypermagnesuria and hypomagnesemia. A mutation of the gene encoding claudin 16 (previously paracellin 1) has been reported to induce a recessive disease characterized by hypomagnesemia, hypermagnesuria, hypercalciuria, and nephrocalcinosis. Mutations in the gene encoding TRPM6 induce profound hypomagnesemia by impaired intestinal Mg^{2+} absorption and renal Mg^{2+} wasting, with secondary hypocalcemia.[35]

In the distal convoluted tubule, inactivating mutations of the gene encoding the thiazide-sensitive, electroneutral Na^+-Cl^- cotransporter (NCCT) in Gitelman's syndrome are also responsible for selective renal magnesium wasting and hypomagnesemia.

Hypomagnesemia associated with inappropriate magnesuria has been reported in an autosomal dominant, isolated familial hypomagnesemia syndrome, which appears to be due to misrouting of the Na^+,K^+-ATPase γ subunit.[36]

Clinical Manifestations

Specific clinical manifestations of hypomagnesemia may be difficult to appreciate because of concomitant hypocalcemia and hypokalemia. The main clinical manifestations of moderate to severe magnesium depletion include general weakness and neuromuscular hyperexcitability with hyperreflexia, carpopedal spasm, seizure, tremor, and, rarely, tetany. Cardiac findings include a prolonged QT interval and ST depression. There is a predisposition to ventricular arrhythmias and potentiation of digoxin toxicity. The role of magnesium deficiency in the clinical development of seizures and cardiac arrhythmias is demonstrated by the treatment of these conditions with magnesium. In one large study of mothers with pregnancy-related hypertension, intravenous magnesium administration was more effective than phenytoin for prevention of eclamptic seizures. In several studies of patients with acute myocardial infarction and hypomagnesemia, magnesium repletion reduced the frequency of cardiac arrhythmias.

Magnesium deficiency can also be associated with hypocalcemia (decreased PTH release and end-organ responsiveness) and hypokalemia (urinary loss). In addition, intracellular K^+ is frequently decreased. Magnesium deficit constitutes a cardiovascular risk factor and also a risk factor in pregnancy for the mother and the fetus.

The diagnosis of moderate degrees of magnesium deficiency is not easy because clinical manifestations may be absent and blood Mg^{2+} levels may not reflect the state of body magnesium. Severe magnesium deficits, however, are associated with hypomagnesemia.

Treatment

Magnesium deficiency is managed with the administration of magnesium salts. Magnesium sulfate is generally used for parenteral therapy (1500 to 3000 mg [150 to 300 mg elemental magnesium] per day). A variety of magnesium salts are available for oral administration, including oxide, hydroxide, sulfate, lactate, chloride, carbonate, and pidolate. Oral magnesium salts often are not well tolerated. All of them may induce gastrointestinal intolerance, in particular diarrhea.

REFERENCES

1. Wasserman RH, Chandler JS, Meyer SA, et al. Intestinal calcium transport and calcium extrusion process at the basolateral membrane. *J Nutr.* 1992;122:662-671.
2. Wasserman RH, Fullmer CS. Vitamin D and intestinal calcium transport: Facts, speculations and hypotheses. *J Nutr.* 1995;125: 1971S-1979S.
3. Hoenderop JG, Bindels RJ. Epithelial Ca^{2+} and Mg^{2+} channels in health and disease. *J Am Soc Nephrol.* 2005;16:15-26.
4. Kinyamu HK, Gallagher C, Prahl JM, et al. Association between intestinal vitamin D receptor, calcium absorption, and serum 1,25 dihydroxyvitamin D in normal young and elderly women. *J Bone Miner Res.* 1997;12:922-928.
5. Martin T, Gooi JH, Sims NA. Molecular mechanisms in coupling of bone formation to resorption. *Crit Rev Eukaryot Gene Expr.* 2009;19: 73-88.
6. Mensenkamp AR, Hoenderop JG, Bindels RJ. Recent advances in renal tubular calcium reabsorption. *Curr Opin Nephrol Hypertens.* 2006; 15:524-529.
7. Boros S, Bindels RJ, Hoenderop JG. Active Ca^{2+} reabsorption in the connecting tubule. *Pflugers Arch.* 2009;458:99-109.
8. Kumar R. Vitamin D and calcium transport. *Kidney Int.* 1991;40: 1177-1189.
9. Wilkinson R. Absorption of calcium, phosphorus, and magnesium. In: Nordin BEC, ed. *Calcium and Magnesium Metabolism.* Edinburgh: Churchill Livingstone; 1976, pp 36-112.
10. Harada S, Rodan GA. Control of osteoblast function and regulation of bone mass. *Nature* 2003;423:349-355.
11. Puschett JB. Renal handling of calcium. In: Massry SG, Glassock RJ, eds. *Textbook of Nephrology.* Baltimore: Williams & Wilkins; 1989, pp 293-299.
12. Tfelt-Hansen J, Brown EM. The calcium-sensing receptor in normal physiology and pathophysiology: A review. *Crit Rev Clin Lab Sci.* 2005;42:35-70.
13. Pi M, Faber P, Ekema G, et al. Identification of a novel extracellular cation-sensing G-protein–coupled receptor. *J Biol Chem.* 2005; 280:40201-40209.
14. Schipani E, Langman CB, Parfitt AM, et al. Constitutively activated receptors for parathyroid hormone and parathyroid hormone–related peptide in Jansen's metaphyseal chondrodysplasia. *N Engl J Med.* 1996;335:708-714.
15. Thakker RV. Diseases associated with the extracellular calcium-sensing receptor. *Cell Calcium.* 2004;35:275-282.
16. Arnold A, Brown MF, Ureña P, et al. Monoclonality of parathyroid tumors in chronic renal failure and in primary parathyroid hyperplasia. *J Clin Invest.* 1995;95:2047-2054.
17. Stewart AF. Clinical practice. Hypercalcemia associated with cancer. *N Engl J Med.* 2005;352:373-379.
18. Peacock M, Bilezikian JP, Klassen PS, et al. Cinacalcet hydrochloride maintains long-term normocalcemia in patients with primary hyperparathyroidism. *J Clin Endocrinol Metab.* 2005;90:135-141.
19. Block GA, Martin KJ, de Francisco AL, et al. Cinacalcet for secondary hyperparathyroidism in patients receiving hemodialysis. *N Engl J Med.* 2004;350:1516-1525.
20. Egbuna OI, Brown EM. Hypercalcaemic and hypocalcaemic conditions due to calcium-sensing receptor mutations. *Best Pract Res Clin Rheumatol.* 2008;22:129-148.
21. Prié D, Beck L, Urena P, Friedlander G. Recent findings in phosphate homeostasis. *Curr Opin Nephrol Hypertens.* 2005;14:318-324.
22. Shaikh A, Berndt T, Kumar R. Regulation of phosphate homeostasis by the phosphatonins and other novel mediators. *Pediatr Nephrol.* 2008;23: 1203-1210.
23. Chang Q, Hoefs S, van der Kemp AW, et al. The beta-glucuronidase klotho hydrolyzes and activates the TRPV5 channel. *Science.* 2005; 310:490-493.

24. Murer H, Hernando N, Forster L, Biber J. Molecular mechanisms in proximal tubular and small intestinal phosphate reabsorption (plenary lecture). *Mol Membr Biol.* 2001;18:3-11.
25. Friedlander G. Autocrine/paracrine control of renal phosphate transport. *Kidney Int Suppl.* 1998;65:S18-S23.
26. Bijvoet OL. Relation of plasma phosphate concentration to renal tubular reabsorption of phosphate. *Clin Sci.* 1969;37:23-36.
27. Slatopolsky E, Brown A, Dusso A. Calcium, phosphorus and vitamin D disorders in uremia. *Contrib Nephrol.* 2005;149:261-271.
28. Shimada T, Muto T, Urakawa I, et al. Mutant FGF-23 responsible for autosomal dominant hypophosphatemic rickets is resistant to proteolytic cleavage and causes hypophosphatemia in vivo. *Endocrinology.* 2002;143:3179-3182.
29. Strom TM, Jüppner H. PHEX, FGF23, DMP1 and beyond. *Curr Opin Nephrol Hypertens.* 2008;17:357-362.
30. Norden AG, Lapsley M, Igarashi T, et al. Urinary megalin deficiency implicates abnormal tubular endocytic function in Fanconi syndrome. *J Am Soc Nephrol.* 2002;13:125-133.
31. Shimada T, Mizutani S, Muto T, et al. Cloning and characterization of FGF23 as a causative factor of tumor-induced osteomalacia. *Proc Natl Acad Sci USA.* 2001;98:6500-6505.
32. Prié D, Friedlander G. Genetic disorders of renal phosphate transport. *N Engl J Med.* 2010;362:2399-2409.
33. Quamme GA. Control of magnesium transport in the thick ascending limb. *Am J Physiol.* 1989;256:F197-F210.
34. Unwin RJ, Capasso G, Shirley DG. An overview of divalent cation and citrate handling by the kidney. *Nephron Physiol.* 2004;98:15-20.
35. Schlingmann KP, Sassen MC, Weber S, et al. Novel TRPM6 mutations in 21 families with primary hypomagnesemia and secondary hypocalcemia. *J Am Soc Nephrol.* 2005;16:3061-3069.
36. Meij IC, Koenderink JB, De Jong JC, et al. Dominant isolated renal magnesium loss is caused by misrouting of the Na^+,K^+-ATPase gamma-subunit. *Ann N Y Acad Sci.* 2003;986:437-443.

CHAPTER 11

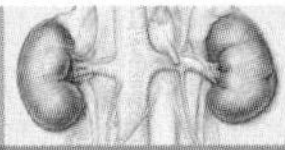

Normal Acid-Base Balance

Biff F. Palmer, Robert J. Alpern

DEFINITION

The acid-base status of the body is carefully regulated to maintain the arterial pH between 7.35 and 7.45 and the intracellular pH between 7.0 and 7.3. This regulation occurs in the setting of continuous production of acidic metabolites and is accomplished by intracellular and extracellular buffering processes in conjunction with respiratory and renal regulatory mechanisms. This chapter reviews the normal physiology of acid-base homeostasis.

NET ACID PRODUCTION

Both acid and alkali are generated from the diet. Lipid and carbohydrate metabolism result in production of CO_2, a volatile acid, at the rate of approximately 15,000 mmol/day. Protein metabolism yields amino acids, which can be metabolized to form nonvolatile acid and alkali. Amino acids such as lysine and arginine yield acid on metabolism, whereas the amino acids glutamate and aspartate and organic anions such as acetate and citrate generate alkali. Sulfur-containing amino acids (methionine and cysteine) are metabolized to sulfuric acid (H_2SO_4), and organophosphates are metabolized to phosphoric acid (H_3PO_4). In general, animal foods are high in proteins and organophosphates, thereby providing a net acid diet; plant foods are higher in organic anions and provide a net alkaline load. In addition to acid and alkali generated from the diet, there is a small daily production of organic acids including acetic acid, lactic acid, and pyruvic acid. Last, a small amount of acid is generated by the excretion of alkali into the stool. Under normal circumstances, daily net nonvolatile acid production is approximately 1 mmol hydrogen ions (H^+) per kilogram of body weight.

BUFFER SYSTEMS IN REGULATION OF pH

Intracellular and extracellular buffer systems minimize the change in pH during the addition of acid or base equivalents but do not remove acid or alkali from the body. The most important buffer system is that of the bicarbonate ion and carbon dioxide (HCO_3^--CO_2). In this system, [CO_2] is maintained at a constant level set by respiratory control. Addition of acid (HA) leads to conversion of HCO_3^- to CO_2 according to the reaction $HA + NaHCO_3 \rightarrow NaA + H_2O + CO_2$.

HCO_3^- is consumed, but [CO_2] does not change because this is maintained by respiration. The net result is that the acid load has been buffered and pH changes are minimal.

Whereas the HCO_3^--CO_2 buffer system is the most important of the buffers in extracellular fluid (ECF), other buffers such as plasma proteins and phosphate ions also participate in the maintenance of a stable pH. During metabolic acidosis, the skeleton becomes a major buffer source as acid-induced dissolution of bone apatite releases alkaline Ca^{2+} salts and HCO_3^- into the ECF. With chronic metabolic acidosis, this can result in osteomalacia and osteoporosis. The calcium released can result in hypercalciuria and an increased likelihood of renal stones. Within the intracellular compartment, pH is maintained by intracellular buffers such as hemoglobin, cellular proteins, organophosphate complexes, and HCO_3^- as well as by the H^+-HCO_3^- transport mechanisms that serve to transport acid and alkali in and out of the cell.

RESPIRATORY SYSTEM IN REGULATION OF pH

Removal of acid or alkali from the body is accomplished by the lungs and kidneys. The lungs regulate the CO_2 tension, and the kidneys regulate the serum HCO_3^- concentration. Although the HCO_3^--CO_2 buffer system is not the only buffer system, all extracellular buffer systems are in equilibrium. Because the serum HCO_3^- concentration is far greater than that of other buffers, changes in the HCO_3^--CO_2 buffer pair can easily titrate other buffer systems and thus set pH. The Henderson-Hasselbalch equation explains how the lungs and kidneys function in concert:

$$pH = 6.1 + \log\left[\frac{HCO_3^-}{(0.03 \times Paco_2)}\right]$$

As can be seen, pH is determined by the ratio of HCO_3^- to CO_2. Conditions associated with similar fractional changes in the concentrations of HCO_3^- and CO_2, such as when both are halved, will not change blood pH.

The lungs defend pH by altering alveolar ventilation, which alters the CO_2 excretion rate and thereby controls the $Paco_2$ of body fluids. Systemic acidosis stimulates the respiratory center, resulting in increased respiratory drive that lowers the $Paco_2$. As a result, the fall in blood pH is less than would have occurred in the absence of respiratory compensation. If the fractional change in CO_2 tension were similar to that in serum HCO_3^- concentration, blood pH would not change. However, respiratory compensation rarely normalizes blood pH, and thus the fractional change in CO_2 tension is less than the change in the serum HCO_3^- concentration. Quantitatively, the normal respiratory response in metabolic acidosis is a 1.2 mm Hg decrease in $Paco_2$ for every 1 mmol/l decrease in HCO_3^-; the increase in $Paco_2$ in response to metabolic alkalosis averages 0.7 mm Hg for every 1 mmol/L increase in HCO_3^- above baseline.[1]

RENAL REGULATION OF pH

Buffer systems and respiratory excretion of CO_2 help maintain normal acid-base balance, but the kidneys provide a critical role in acid-base homeostasis. The kidneys normally generate sufficient net acid excretion to balance nonvolatile acid produced from normal metabolism. Net acid excretion (NAE) has three components, titratable acids, ammonium, and bicarbonate, and is calculated by the following formula:

$$\text{NAE} = U_{\text{Am}}V + U_{\text{TA}}V - U_{\text{HCO}_3^-}V$$

where $U_{\text{Am}}V$ is the rate of NH_4^+ excretion, $U_{\text{TA}}V$ is the rate of titratable acid excretion, and $U_{\text{HCO}_3^-}V$ is the rate of HCO_3^- excretion. Under basal conditions, approximately 40% of net acid excretion is in the form of titratable acids and 60% is in the form of ammonia; urinary bicarbonate concentrations and excretion are essentially zero under normal conditions. When acid production increases, the increase in acid excretion is almost entirely due to an increase in excretion of NH_4^+.

RENAL TRANSPORT MECHANISMS OF HYDROGEN AND BICARBONATE IONS

Glomerulus

The glomerulus is not normally considered as participating in acid-base regulation. However, the glomerulus filters an amount of HCO_3^- equivalent to the serum HCO_3^- concentration multiplied by the glomerular filtration rate (GFR). Under normal circumstances, the filtered load of HCO_3^- averages approximately 4000 mmol/day. Normal acid-base homeostasis requires both the reabsorption of this filtered bicarbonate and the generation of "new" bicarbonate; the latter replenishes bicarbonate and other alkaline buffers consumed in the process of titrating endogenous acid production. From the standpoint of prevention of or correction of acidosis, GFR is not regulated by alterations in acid or base and therefore does not contribute to acid-base homeostasis.

Proximal Tubule

The proximal tubule reabsorbs approximately 80% of the filtered load of HCO_3^-. In addition, by titration of luminal pH from 7.4 down to approximately 6.7, the majority of phosphate, the major form of titratable acid, is titrated to its acid form. Lastly, ammonia synthesis occurs in the proximal tubule.

Figure 11.1 shows the acid-base transport mechanisms of the proximal tubule cell. HCO_3^- absorption from the tubular lumen is mediated by H^+ secretion across the membrane.[2] This H^+ secretion is active in that the electrochemical gradient favors H^+ movement from lumen to cell. Two mechanisms mediate active apical H^+ secretion. Approximately two thirds occurs through the apical membrane Na^+-H^+ antiporter NHE3.[3] This protein uses the inward Na^+ gradient to drive H^+ secretion. The Na^+-H^+ exchanger has a 1:1 stoichiometry and is electroneutral. In parallel with the Na^+-H^+ antiporter, there is an apical membrane H^+-ATPase that mediates approximately one third of basal proximal tubular HCO_3^- absorption.

Both of these H^+ transporters generate base in the cell, which must exit across the basolateral membrane to effect transepithelial transport. This primarily occurs through a basolateral Na^+-HCO_3^--CO_3^{2-} cotransporter. Because this protein transports the

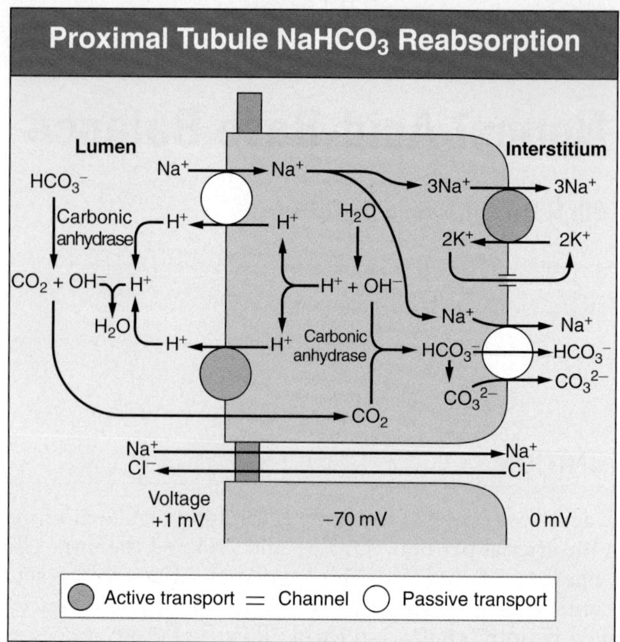

Figure 11.1 Proximal tubule $NaHCO_3$ reabsorption. The secretion of H^+ into the proximal tubule lumen involves a Na^+-H^+ antiporter and a H^+-ATPase. Apical membrane H^+ secretion generates OH^-, which reacts with CO_2 to form HCO_3^- and CO_3^{2-}, and these exit with a Na^+ on the basolateral membrane Na^+-HCO_3^--CO_3^{2-} cotransporter. The Na^+ absorbed by the Na^+-H^+ antiporter exits the cell on the basolateral membrane Na^+,K^+-ATPase and the Na^+-HCO_3^--CO_3^{2-} cotransporter. The K^+ that enters the cell on the Na^+,K^+-ATPase exits on a basolateral membrane K^+ channel. Carbonic anhydrase catalyzes the conversion of HCO_3^- to CO_2 and OH^- in the lumen and the reverse reaction in the cell. Electrogenic H^+ secretion generates a small lumen-positive voltage that generates a current flow across the paracellular pathway.

equivalent of two net negative charges, the negative cell voltage generated by the basolateral Na^+,K^+-ATPase provides a strong favorable driving force for base efflux. The Na^+ that is carried on this transporter is moved out of the cell energy free in that ATP is not required. The Na^+-3HCO_3^- cotransporter NBC1, encoded by the gene *SLC4A4*, mediates the majority of proximal tubule basolateral base exit.[4]

Carbonic anhydrase is present in the proximal tubular cell cytoplasm and on the apical and basolateral membranes. Carbonic anhydrase has a number of functions in the proximal tubule. Apical membrane carbonic anhydrase allows secreted H^+ ions to react with luminal HCO_3^-, forming H_2CO_3, which rapidly dissociates to CO_2 + H_2O. This CO_2 diffuses across the apical plasma membrane into the cell. There the process is reversed, with use of cytoplasmic carbonic anhydrase, generating intracellular H^+ and HCO_3^-. This H^+ "replenishes" the H^+ secreted across the apical membrane, resulting in net movement of the HCO_3^- from the luminal solution to the cell cytoplasm. The intracellular HCO_3^- is then secreted across the basolateral plasma membrane as described previously.

Thick Ascending Limb of the Loop of Henle

Tubular fluid arriving at the early distal tubule has a pH and serum HCO_3^- concentration similar to that in the late proximal tubule. Because there is significant water extraction in the loop of Henle, maintenance of a constant serum HCO_3^- concentration requires reabsorption of HCO_3^-. The majority of this HCO_3^- absorption occurs in the thick ascending limb

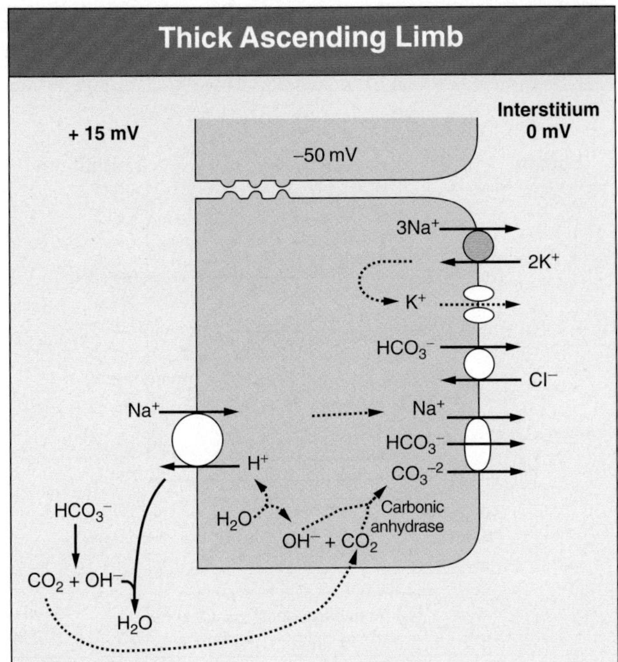

Figure 11.2 H^+ and HCO_3^- transport in the thick ascending limb. Apical H^+ secretion is mediated by a Na^+-H^+ antiporter. The low intracellular Na^+ concentration, maintained by the basolateral Na^+,K^+-ATPase, provides the primary driving force for the antiporter. Both Cl^--HCO_3^- exchange and Na^+-HCO_3^--CO_3^{2-} cotransport mediate base exit across the basolateral membrane.

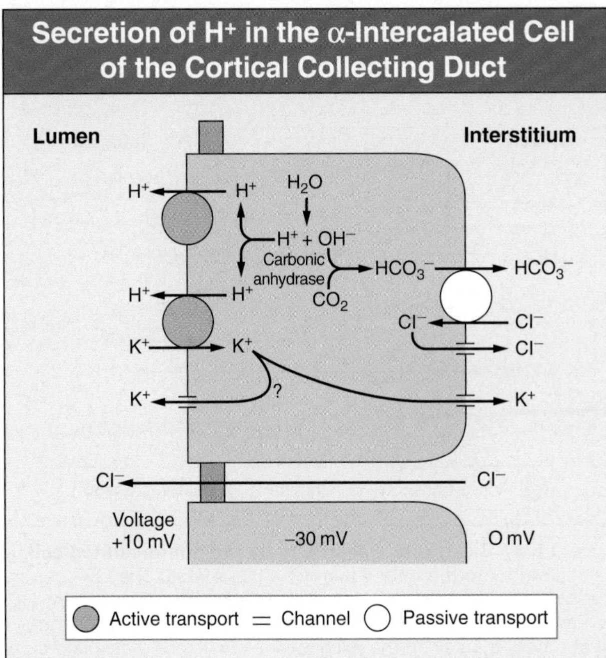

Figure 11.3 Secretion of H^+ in the α-intercalated cell. Secretion of H^+ into the lumen by a H^+-ATPase and a H^+,K^+-ATPase. Apical membrane H^+ secretion generates OH^-, which reacts with CO_2 to form HCO_3^-; this exits across the basolateral membrane on a Cl^--HCO_3^- exchanger. The Cl^- that enters the cell on the exchanger recycles across a basolateral membrane Cl^- channel. The K^+ that enters the cell on the H^+,K^+-ATPase appears to be able either to recycle across the apical membrane or to exit across the basolateral membrane, depending on the potassium balance of the individual. Carbonic anhydrase catalyzes the conversion of CO_2 and OH^- to HCO_3^- in the cell. Electrogenic H^+ secretion generates a lumen-positive voltage that generates a current flow across the paracellular pathway.

through mechanisms that are similar to those present in the proximal tubule (Fig. 11.2). The majority of apical membrane H^+ secretion is mediated by the Na^+-H^+ antiporter NHE3. As in the proximal tubule, the low intracellular Na^+ concentration maintained by the basolateral Na^+,K^+-ATPase provides the primary driving force for the antiporter. Base efflux across the basolateral membrane is mediated by a Cl^--HCO_3^- exchanger and a Na^+-HCO_3^--CO_3^{2-} cotransporter. These cells also possess a H^+-ATPase, but it is not clear what role it plays in acidification.

Distal Nephron

Approximately 80% of the filtered HCO_3^- is reabsorbed in the proximal tubule; most but not all of the remainder is absorbed in the thick ascending limb. One function of the distal nephron is to reabsorb the remaining 5% of filtered HCO_3^-. In addition, the distal nephron must secrete a quantity of H^+ equal to that generated systemically by metabolism to maintain acid-base balance.

The distal nephron is subdivided into several distinct portions that differ in their anatomy and acid secretory properties. Most of these segments transport H^+ and HCO_3^- into the luminal fluid, but the main segments appear to be in the collecting duct.[5] The segments of the collecting duct include the cortical collecting duct, the outer medullary collecting duct, and the inner medullary collecting duct. There are two distinct cell types in the cortical collecting duct that can be distinguished histologically: the principal cell and the intercalated cell. The principal cell reabsorbs Na^+ and secretes K^+ and is discussed further later. Depending on chronic acid-base status, the cortical collecting duct is capable of either H^+ or HCO_3^- secretion. These functions are mediated by two types of intercalated cells: the acid-secreting α-intercalated cell and the base-secreting β-intercalated cell. Both types of intercalated cells are rich in carbonic anhydrase.

Reabsorption of HCO_3^- in the distal nephron is mediated by apical H^+ secretion by the α-intercalated cell. Two transporters secrete H^+: a vacuolar H^+-ATPase and a H^+,K^+-ATPase (Fig. 11.3). The vacuolar H^+-ATPase is an electrogenic pump related to the H^+ pump present within lysosomes, the Golgi apparatus, and endosomes. The H^+,K^+-ATPase uses the energy derived from ATP hydrolysis to secrete H^+ into the lumen and to reabsorb K^+ in an electroneutral fashion. The activity of the H^+,K^+-ATPase increases in K^+ depletion and thus provides a mechanism by which K^+ depletion enhances both collecting duct H^+ secretion and K^+ absorption.

Active H^+ secretion by the apical membrane generates intracellular base that must exit the basolateral membrane. A basolateral Cl^--HCO_3^- exchanger is the mechanism by which this base exit occurs. The Cl^- that enters the cell in exchange for HCO_3^- exits the cell through a basolateral membrane Cl^- conductance channel (see Fig. 11.3).

The HCO_3^--secreting β-intercalated cell is a mirror image of the α-intercalated cell (Fig. 11.4). It possesses a H^+-ATPase on the basolateral membrane, which mediates active H^+ extrusion. Alkali that is generated within the cell then exits on an apical membrane Cl^--HCO_3^- exchanger. This Cl^--HCO_3^- exchanger is distinct from the basolateral Cl^--HCO_3^- exchanger present in the α-intercalated cell and functions as an anion exchanger or Cl^- channel in the luminal membrane of epithelial cells.[6] The SLC26A4 protein (pendrin) is a family member that mediates

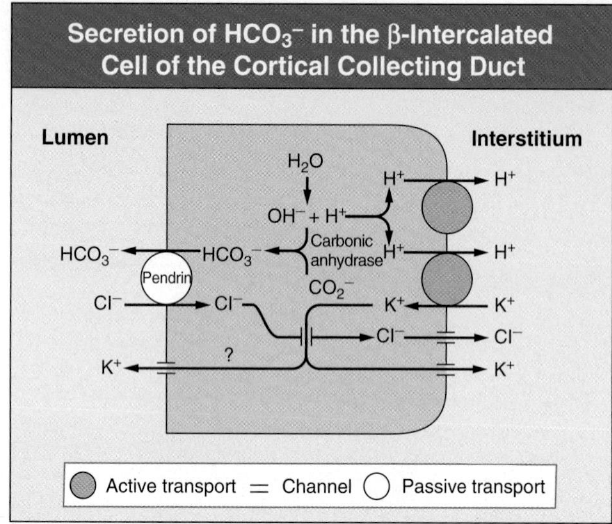

Figure 11.4 Bicarbonate secretion by the β-intercalated cell. Here H^+ is secreted into the interstitium by a H^+-ATPase. The OH^- generated by basolateral membrane H^+ secretion reacts with CO_2 to form HCO_3^-, which exits across the apical membrane on a Cl^--HCO_3^- exchanger. The Cl^- that enters the cell on the exchanger exits across a basolateral membrane Cl^- channel. Carbonic anhydrase catalyzes the conversion of CO_2 and OH^- to HCO_3^- in the cell.

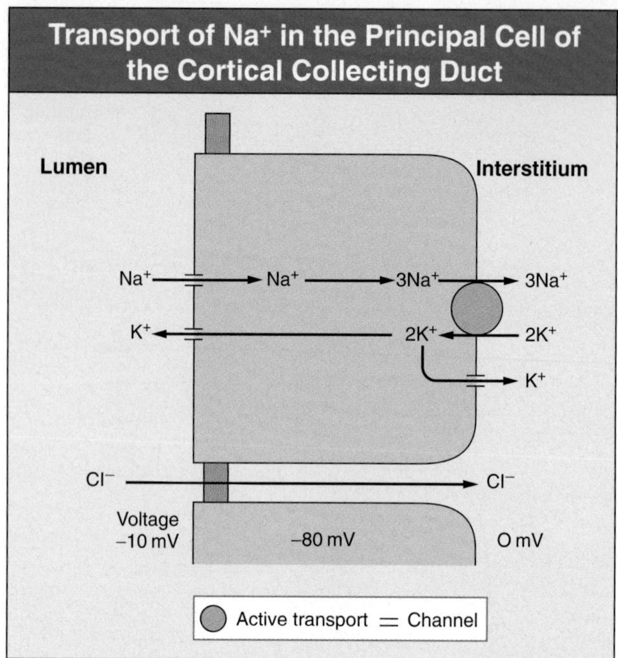

Figure 11.5 Transport of Na^+ in the principal cell of the cortical collecting duct. Electrogenic Na^+ absorption is mediated by a Na^+ channel. The Na^+ enters the cell across the apical membrane channel and exits the cell on the basolateral membrane Na^+,K^+-ATPase. The K^+ that enters the cell on the basolateral Na^+,K^+-ATPase can be secreted into the luminal fluid by an apical membrane K^+ channel. Electrogenic Na^+ absorption establishes a lumen-negative voltage that drives a paracellular current.

apical Cl^--HCO_3^- exchange in the β-intercalated cell of the kidney.

The other cortical collecting tubule cell type is the principal cell, and it too regulates acid-base transport, albeit indirectly. Principal cells mediate electrogenic Na^+ reabsorption that results in a net negative luminal charge (Fig. 11.5). The greater this negative charge is, the lesser the electrochemical gradient for electrogenic proton secretion and therefore the greater the rate of net proton secretion. Thus, factors that stimulate Na^+ reabsorption indirectly regulate the H^+ secretory rate.

The medullary collecting duct possesses mechanisms only for H^+ secretion. This H^+ secretion is mediated by α-intercalated cells but also by cells that appear morphologically distinct from intercalated cells yet are functionally similar.

Net Acid Excretion

For the kidney to generate net acid excretion, it must both reabsorb filtered HCO_3^- and excrete titratable acids and ammonia. Several weak acids, such as phosphate, creatinine, and uric acid, are filtered at the glomerulus and can buffer secreted protons. Of these, phosphate is the most important because of its favorable pK_a of 6.80 and its relatively high rate of urinary excretion (~25 to 30 mmol/day). However, the capacity of phosphate to buffer protons is maximized at a urine pH of 5.8, and acid-base disturbances do not, in general, induce substantial changes in urinary phosphate excretion. Other titratable acids, such as creatinine and uric acid, are limited by their lower excretion rates that are not dramatically changed in response to acid-base disturbances. As shown in Figure 11.6, titratable acid excretion is a minor component of the increase in net acid excretion in response to metabolic acidosis.

Ammonia Metabolism

Quantitatively, the most important component of net acid excretion is the NH_3/NH_4^+ system.[7] Unlike for titratable acids, the rate of ammonia production and excretion varies according to physiologic needs. Under normal circumstances, ammonia excretion accounts for approximately 60% of total net acid excretion, and in chronic metabolic acidosis, almost the entire increase in net acid excretion is due to increased ammonia metabolism. Ammonia metabolism involves an interplay between the proximal tubule, the thick ascending limb of the loop of Henle, and the collecting duct.

The proximal tubule is responsible for both ammonia production and luminal secretion. Ammonia is synthesized in the proximal tubule predominantly from glutamine metabolism through enzymatic processes in which phosphoenolpyruvate carboxykinase and phosphate-dependent glutaminase are the rate-limiting steps. This results in production of two NH_4^+ and two HCO_3^- ions from each glutamine ion. Ammonia is then preferentially secreted into the lumen. The primary mechanism for this luminal secretion appears to be NH_4^+ transport by the apical Na^+-H^+ antiporter NHE3.

Metabolic acidosis increases the mobilization of glutamine from skeletal muscle and intestinal cells. Glutamine is preferentially taken up by the proximal tubular cell through the Na^+- and H^+-dependent glutamine transporter SNAT3. This transporter is a member of the *SCL38* gene family of Na^+-coupled neutral amino acid transporters. SNAT3 expression increases severalfold in metabolic acidosis, and it is preferentially expressed on the cell's basolateral surface, where it is poised for glutamine uptake.[8] The increase in plasma glucocorticoids that typically accompanies metabolic acidosis plays a role in this transporter's upregulation.[9] Metabolic acidosis also causes increased expression and activity of phosphate-activated glutaminase and glutamate dehydrogenase.

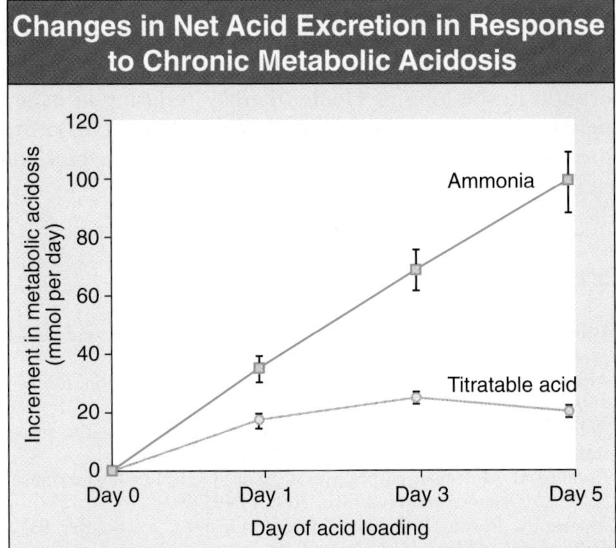

Figure 11.6 Changes in net acid excretion in response to chronic metabolic acidosis. Chronic metabolic acidosis increases net acid excretion dramatically during several days. This figure shows quantitatively the increases in the two major components of net acid excretion: titratable acids and ammonia. Titratable acid excretion increases slightly and predominantly in the first 24 to 48 hours. In contrast, urinary ammonia excretion progressively increases during a period of 7 days and is responsible for the majority of the increase in net acid excretion in chronic metabolic acidosis. *(Data plotted are redrawn from original data of reference 10.)*

Most of the ammonia that leaves the proximal tubule does not return to the distal tubule. Thus, there is transport of ammonia out of the loop of Henle. This transport appears to occur predominantly in the thick ascending limb of the loop of Henle and is mediated by at least three mechanisms. First, the lumen-positive voltage provides a driving force for passive paracellular NH_4^+ transport out of the thick ascending limb. Second, NH_4^+ can be transported out of the lumen by the furosemide-sensitive Na^+-K^+-$2Cl^-$ transporter. Last, NH_4^+ can leave the lumen across the apical membrane K^+ channel of the thick ascending limb cell. There is little information as to how NH_4^+ would then leave the cell across the basolateral membrane.

Finally, ammonia is secreted by the collecting duct. Although the traditional thought was that NH_3/NH_4^+ then enters the collecting duct by nonionic diffusion driven by the acid luminal pH, increasing evidence suggests that the nonerythroid glycoproteins Rhbg and Rhcg may be involved in collecting duct ammonia secretion.[11,12]

On the basis of the preceding discussion, ammonia excretion can be regulated by three mechanisms. First, ammonia synthesis in the proximal tubule can be regulated. Chronic acidosis and hypokalemia increase ammonia synthesis, whereas hyperkalemia suppresses ammonia synthesis. Second, ammonia delivery from the proximal tubule to the medullary interstitium can be regulated. In particular, chronic metabolic acidosis increases expression of both NHE3 and the loop of Henle Na^+-K^+-$2Cl^-$ cotransporter. Hyperkalemia can inhibit NH_4^+ reabsorption from the thick ascending limb. This may explain the low urinary [NH_4^+] found in hyperkalemic distal renal tubular acidosis (in addition to decreased synthesis of ammonia by hyperkalemia). In addition, any interstitial renal disease that destroys renal medullary anatomy may decrease medullary interstitial [NH_3/NH_4^+]. Last, mechanisms that regulate collecting duct H^+ secretion or ammonia transporter expression can regulate ammonia entry into the collecting duct and excretion. Importantly, the primary mechanisms require synthesis of new proteins to increase both ammonia production and transport. Accordingly, changes in ammonia excretion may be delayed, and the maximal renal response to chronic metabolic acidosis requires 4 to 7 days.

REGULATION OF RENAL ACIDIFICATION

The regulation of acid-base balance requires an integrated system that precisely regulates proximal tubular H^+-HCO_3^- transport, distal nephron H^+-HCO_3^- transport, and ammonia synthesis and transport.

Blood pH

The regulation of acid-base balance requires that net H^+ excretion increase in states of acidosis and decrease in states of alkalosis. This form of regulation involves both acute and chronic mechanisms. In the proximal tubule, acute decreases in blood pH increase the rate of HCO_3^- absorption, and acute increases in blood pH inhibit HCO_3^- absorption. These alterations in the rate of HCO_3^- absorption occur whether the change in pH is the result of changes in $Paco_2$ or serum HCO_3^- concentration. Similarly, in the collecting duct, acute changes in peritubular serum HCO_3^- concentration and pH regulate the rate of H^+ secretion.

In addition to acute regulation, mechanisms exist for chronic regulation. Chronic acidosis or alkalosis leads to parallel changes in the activities of the proximal tubule apical membrane Na^+-H^+ antiporter and basolateral membrane Na^+-HCO_3^--CO_3^{2-} cotransporter. Metabolic acidosis acutely increases the kinetic activity of NHE3 through direct pH effects and by phosphorylation; chronic acidosis increases the number of NHE3 transporters.[13,14] In addition, chronic acidosis increases proximal tubular ammonia synthesis by increasing the activities of the enzymes involved in ammonia metabolism.

The cortical collecting duct is also modified by chronic acid-base changes. Long-term increases in dietary acid lead to an increase in H^+ secretion, whereas long-term increases in dietary alkali lead to an increased capacity for HCO_3^- secretion.[15] This effect is mediated by changes in the relative number of α- and β-intercalated cells. For example, during metabolic acidosis, the number of α-intercalated cells increases while the number of β-intercalated cells decreases without a change in the total number of intercalated cells. Recent evidence suggests that the extracellular protein hensin may be involved in the switch between the predominant intercalated cell type.[16]

Mineralocorticoids, Distal Sodium Delivery, and Extracellular Fluid Volume

Mineralocorticoid hormones are key regulators of distal nephron and collecting duct H^+ secretion. Two mechanisms appear to be involved. First, mineralocorticoid hormone stimulates Na^+ absorption in principal cells of the cortical collecting duct (see Fig. 11.5). This leads to a more lumen-negative voltage that then stimulates H^+ secretion. This mechanism is indirect in that it requires the presence of Na^+ and of Na^+ transport.

A second mechanism is the direct activation of H^+ secretion by mineralocorticoids. This effect is chronic, requiring long exposure, and involves parallel increases in apical membrane H^+-ATPase and basolateral membrane Cl^--HCO_3^- exchanger activity.

Plasma Volume

Changes in plasma volume have important effects on acid-base homeostasis. This effect appears to be related to a number of factors. First, volume contraction is associated with a decreased GFR that lowers the filtered load of HCO_3^- and decreases the load placed on the tubules to maintain net acid excretion. Volume contraction also acutely decreases the paracellular permeability of the proximal tubule. This will decrease HCO_3^- backleak around cells, thereby increasing net bicarbonate reabsorption by the proximal tubule. Third, chronic volume contraction is associated with an adaptive increase in the activity of the proximal tubule apical membrane Na^+-H^+ antiporter NHE3. Because this transporter contributes to both $NaHCO_3$ and NaCl absorption, both of these capacities will be increased with chronic volume contraction. Last, volume contraction limits distal delivery of chloride. In the presence of chronic metabolic alkalosis, the cortical collecting duct is poised for HCO_3^- secretion. However, collecting duct HCO_3^- secretion requires luminal Cl^- and is inhibited by Cl^- deficiency.

Potassium

Potassium deficiency is associated with an increase in renal net acid excretion. This effect is multifactorial. First, chronic K^+ deficiency increases the proximal tubule apical membrane Na^+-H^+ antiporter and basolateral membrane Na^+-HCO_3^--CO_3^{2-} cotransporter activities. This effect is similar to that seen with chronic acidosis and may be due to intracellular acidosis. Chronic K^+ deficiency also increases proximal tubular ammonia production. Last, chronic K^+ deficiency leads to an increase in collecting duct H^+ secretion. This appears to be related to increased activity of the apical membrane H^+,K^+-ATPase. Such an effect increases the rate of H^+ secretion and the rate of K^+ reabsorption in the collecting duct. Finally, ammonia, whose production is stimulated by hypokalemia, has direct effects that stimulate collecting duct H^+ secretion. Counterbalancing these effects is that K^+ deficiency decreases aldosterone secretion, which can inhibit distal acidification. Thus, in normal individuals, the net effect of K^+ deficiency is typically a minor change in acid-base balance. However, in those in whom mineralocorticoid secretion is nonsuppressible (e.g., hyperaldosteronism, Cushing's syndrome), K^+ deficiency can markedly stimulate renal acidification and cause profound metabolic alkalosis.

Hyperkalemia appears to have opposite effects on renal acidification. The most notable effect of hyperkalemia is inhibition of ammonia synthesis in the proximal tubule and ammonia absorption in the loop of Henle, thereby resulting in inappropriately low levels of urinary ammonia excretion. This contributes to the metabolic acidosis seen in patients with hyperkalemic distal (type 4) renal tubular acidosis.

REFERENCES

1. Palmer BF. Approach to fluid and electrolyte disorders and acid-base problems. *Prim Care*. 2008;35:195-213.
2. Alpern RJ. Cell mechanisms of proximal tubule acidification. *Physiol Rev*. 1990;70:79-114.
3. Bobulescu A, Moe OW. Luminal Na^+/H^+ exchange in the proximal tubule. *Pflugers Arch*. 2009;458:5-21. Epub 2008 Oct 14.
4. Romero M. Molecular pathophysiology of SLC4 bicarbonate transporters. *Curr Opin Nephrol Hypertens*. 2005;14:495-501.
5. Alpern RJ, Preisig P. Renal acid base transport. In: Schrier RW, ed. *Diseases of the Kidney and Urinary Tract*. 8th ed. Philadelphia: Lippincott Williams and Wilkins; 2007:183-195.
6. Dorwart M, Shcheynikov N, Yang D, Muallem S. The solute carrier 26 family of proteins in epithelial ion transport. *Physiology (Bethesda)*. 2008;23:104-114.
7. Knepper MA, Packer R, Good DW. Ammonium transport in the kidney. *Physiol Rev*. 1989;69:179-249.
8. Moret C, Dave M, Schulz N, et al. Regulation of renal amino acid transporters during metabolic acidosis. *Am J Physiol Renal Physiol*. 2007;292:F555-F566.
9. Karinch A, Lin C, Meng Q, et al. Glucocorticoids have a role in renal cortical expression of the SNAT3 glutamine transporter during chronic metabolic acidosis. *Am J Physiol Renal Physiol*. 2007;292: F448-F455.
10. Elkinton JR, Huth EJ, Webster GD Jr, McCance RA. The renal excretion of hydrogen ion in renal tubular acidosis. I. Quantitative assessment of the response to ammonium chloride as an acid load. *Am J Med*. 1960;36:554-575.
11. Weiner ID. The Rh gene family and renal ammonium transport. *Curr Opin Nephrol Hypertens*. 2004;13:533-540.
12. Kim H, Verlander J, Bishop J, et al. Basolateral expression of the ammonia transporter family member Rh C glycoprotein in the mouse kidney. *Am J Physiol Renal Physiol*. 2009;296:F543-F555. Epub 2009 Jan 7.
13. Moe OW. Acute regulation of proximal tubule apical membrane Na/H exchanger NHE-3: Role of phosphorylation, protein trafficking, and regulatory factors. *J Am Soc Nephrol*. 1999;10:2412-2425.
14. Ambuhl P, Amemiya M, Danczkay M, et al. Chronic metabolic acidosis increases NHE3 protein abundance in rat kidney. *Am J Physiol*. 1996;271:F917-F925.
15. McKinney TD, Burg MB. Bicarbonate transport by rabbit cortical collecting tubules: Effect of acid and alkaline loads in vivo on transport in vitro. *J Clin Invest*. 1977;60:766-768.
16. Vijayakumar S, Erdjument-Bromage H, Tempst P, Al-Awqati Q. Role of integrins in the assembly and function of hensin in intercalated cells. *J Am Soc Nephrol*. 2008;19:1079-1091.

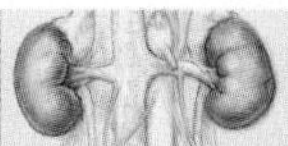

Metabolic Acidosis

Biff F. Palmer, Robert J. Alpern

DEFINITION

Metabolic acidosis is defined as a low arterial blood pH in conjunction with a reduced serum HCO_3^- concentration. Respiratory compensation results in a decrease in $Paco_2$. A low serum HCO_3^- concentration alone is not diagnostic of metabolic acidosis because it also results from the renal compensation to chronic respiratory alkalosis. Measurement of the arterial pH differentiates between these two possibilities. Figure 12.1 shows the expected compensatory responses for metabolic and respiratory acid-base disorders.[1]

After the diagnosis of metabolic acidosis is confirmed, the first step in the examination of metabolic acidosis is to calculate the serum anion gap. The anion gap is equal to the difference between the plasma concentrations of the major cation (Na^+) and the major measured anions (Cl^- and HCO_3^-) and is given by the following formula:

$$\text{anion gap} = [Na^+] - ([Cl^-] + [HCO_3^-])$$

In healthy individuals, the normal value of the anion gap is approximately 12 ± 2 mmol/l. Because many of the unmeasured anions consist of albumin, the normal anion gap is decreased by approximately 4 mmol/l for each 1 g/dl decrease in the serum albumin concentration below normal. The total number of cations must equal the total number of anions, so a decrease in the serum HCO_3^- concentration must be offset by an increase in the concentration of other anions. If the anion accompanying excess H^+ is Cl^-, the decrease in the serum HCO_3^- concentration is matched by an equal increase in the serum Cl^- concentration. This acidosis is classified as a "normal anion gap" or a "non–anion gap" or a hyperchloremic metabolic acidosis. By contrast, if excess H^+ is accompanied by an anion other than Cl^-, the decreased HCO_3^- is balanced by an increase in the concentration of the unmeasured anion. The Cl^- concentration remains the same. In this setting, the acidosis is said to be a "high anion gap" or "anion gap" metabolic acidosis.

The normal value for the anion gap has tended to fall over time because of changes in how serum Na^+ and Cl^- are measured.[2] Flame photometry for Na^+ measurement and a colorimetric assay for Cl^- have been replaced by the use of ion-selective electrodes, with which the serum Na^+ values have largely remained the same, whereas the serum Cl^- values have tended to be higher. As a result, the normal value for the anion gap has decreased to as low as 6 mmol/l in some reports. Recognizing this change, some laboratories have adjusted the calibration set point for Cl^- to return the normal value for the anion gap to the 12 ± 2 mmol/l range. It is important for the clinician to be aware that the average anion gap and range of normal values will vary among different facilities.

Figure 12.2 provides a recommended approach to a patient with metabolic acidosis and lists the common causes of metabolic acidosis according to the anion gap.

NON–ANION GAP (NORMAL ANION GAP) METABOLIC ACIDOSIS

A non–anion gap metabolic acidosis can result from either renal or extrarenal causes. Renal causes of metabolic acidosis occur when renal bicarbonate generation, which results from net acid excretion, does not balance the loss of bicarbonate and other alkali buffers consumed in the buffering of normal endogenous acid production. This failure of net acid excretion is termed renal tubular acidosis (RTA). Extrarenal causes occur when exogenous acid loads, endogenous acid production, or endogenous bicarbonate losses are elevated and exceed renal net acid excretion. The most common extrarenal cause of non–anion gap metabolic acidosis is chronic diarrhea.

Renal and extrarenal causes of metabolic acidosis can be distinguished by measuring urinary ammonia excretion.[3] The primary response of the kidney to metabolic acidosis is to increase urinary ammonia excretion, each millimole of urinary ammonia excreted resulting in the generation of 1 mmol of "new" bicarbonate. Thus, renal causes of metabolic acidosis are characterized by low urinary ammonia excretion rates. In contrast, in extrarenal metabolic acidosis, urinary ammonia excretion is elevated. Because most laboratories do not measure urinary ammonia, one can indirectly assess ammonia excretion by measuring the urinary anion gap (UAG):

$$\text{UAG} = (U_{Na^+} + U_{K^+}) - U_{Cl^-}$$

The UAG is normally a positive value, ranging from +30 to +50 mmol/l. A negative value for the UAG suggests increased renal excretion of an unmeasured cation (i.e., a cation other than Na^+ or K^+). One such cation is NH_4^+. With chronic metabolic acidosis due to extrarenal causes, urinary ammonia concentrations, in the form of NH_4Cl, can reach 200 to 300 mmol/l. As a result, the measured cation concentration will be less than the measured anion concentration, which includes the increased urinary Cl^-, and the UAG will be less than zero and frequently less than −20 mmol/l.

The UAG only indirectly reflects the urinary ammonia concentration and, if other unmeasured ions are excreted, can give misleading results. Examples include diabetic ketoacidosis, associated with substantial urinary excretion of sodium keto acid salts, and toluene exposure (discussed later), associated with increased urinary excretion of sodium hippurate and sodium

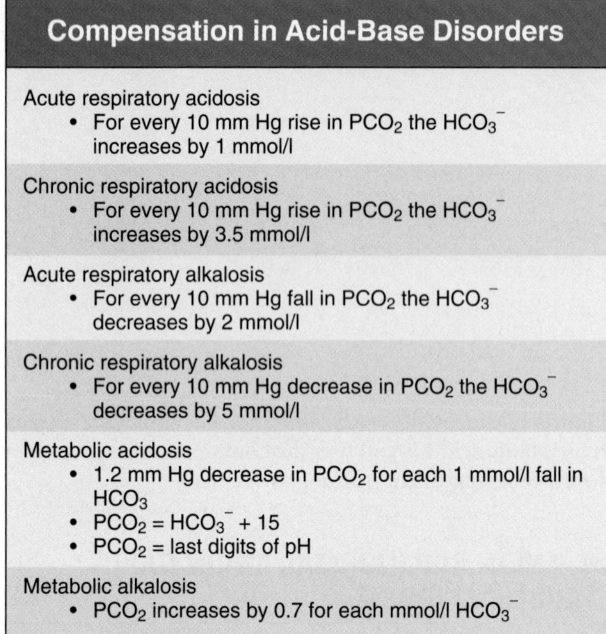

Figure 12.1 Expected compensatory responses to acid-base disorders.

benzoate. In these settings, the UAG value may remain positive despite an appropriate increase in urinary ammonia excretion because of the increased urinary excretion of Na^+ acid-anion salts. In most cases, these conditions are associated with an elevated anion gap metabolic acidosis, not a non–anion gap metabolic acidosis, and thus are easily distinguishable from diarrhea-induced metabolic acidosis.

Urine pH, in contrast to the UAG, does not reliably differentiate acidosis of renal origin from that of extrarenal origin. For example, an acid urine pH does not necessarily indicate an appropriate increase in net acid excretion. If renal ammonia metabolism is inhibited, as occurs with chronic hyperkalemia, there is decreased ammonia available in the distal nephron to serve as a buffer, and small amounts of distal H^+ secretion can lead to a significant urine acidification. In this setting, the urine pH is acid, but net acid excretion is low because of the low ammonia excretion. Similarly, alkaline urine does not necessarily imply a renal acidification defect. In conditions in which ammonia metabolism is stimulated, distal H^+ secretion can be massive and yet the urine remains relatively alkaline because of the buffering effects of ammonia.

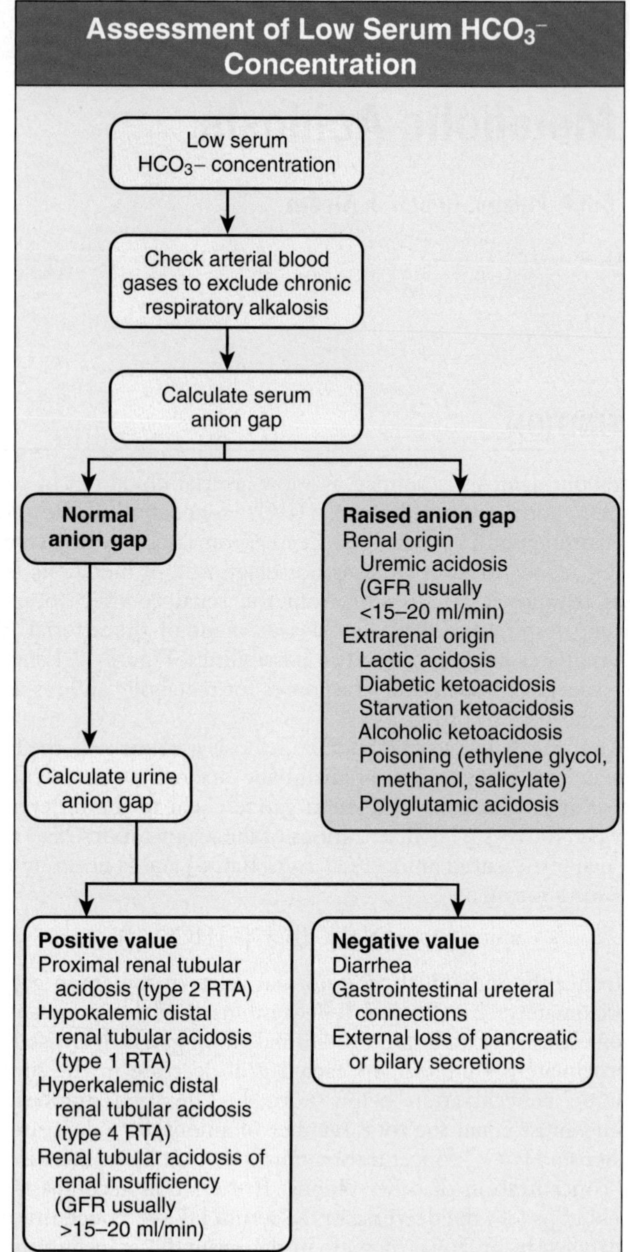

Figure 12.2 Approach to the patient with a low serum HCO_3^- concentration.

Metabolic Acidosis of Renal Origin

An overall approach for workup of metabolic acidosis of renal origin is shown in Figure 12.3.

Proximal Renal Tubular Acidosis (Type 2)

Normally 80% to 90% of the filtered load of HCO_3^- is reabsorbed in the proximal tubule. In proximal RTA, the proximal tubule has a decreased capacity to reabsorb filtered bicarbonate. When serum bicarbonate concentration is normal or nearly normal, the amount of bicarbonate filtered by the glomerulus exceeds proximal tubule bicarbonate reabsorptive capacity. When this happens, there is increased bicarbonate delivery to the loop of Henle and distal nephron that exceeds their capacity to reabsorb bicarbonate. As a result, some filtered bicarbonate appears in the urine. The net effect is that the serum HCO_3^- concentration decreases. Eventually, the filtered bicarbonate load decreases to the point at which the proximal tubule is able to reabsorb sufficient filtered bicarbonate that the bicarbonate load to the loop of Henle and the distal nephron is within their reabsorptive capacity. When this process occurs, no further bicarbonate is lost in the urine, net acid excretion normalizes, and a new steady-state serum bicarbonate concentration develops, albeit at a lower than normal level.

Hypokalemia is present in proximal RTA. Renal $NaHCO_3$ losses lead to intravascular volume depletion, which in turn activates the renin-angiotensin-aldosterone system. Distal Na^+ delivery is increased as a result of the impaired proximal reabsorption of $NaHCO_3$. Because of the associated hyperaldoste-

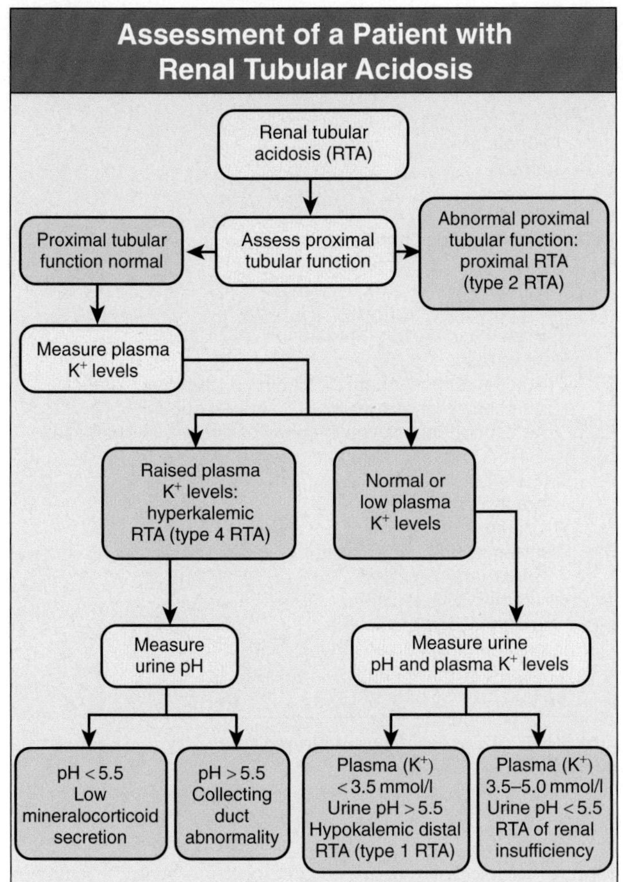

Figure 12.3 Approach to the patient with renal tubular acidosis (RTA).

ronism and increased distal nephron Na^+ reabsorption, there is increased K^+ secretion. The net result is renal potassium wasting and the development of hypokalemia. In the steady state, when virtually all the filtered HCO_3^- is reabsorbed in the proximal and distal nephron, renal potassium wasting is less and the degree of hypokalemia tends to be mild.

Proximal RTA may occur as an isolated defect in acidification, but it typically occurs in the setting of widespread proximal tubule dysfunction (Fanconi syndrome). In addition to decreased HCO_3^- reabsorption, patients with the Fanconi syndrome have impaired reabsorption of glucose, phosphate, uric acid, amino acids, and low-molecular-weight proteins. Various inherited and acquired disorders have been associated with the development of Fanconi syndrome and proximal RTA (Fig. 12.4). The most common inherited cause in children is cystinosis (see Chapter 48). Most adults with Fanconi syndrome have an acquired condition that is related to an underlying dysproteinemic condition, such as multiple myeloma.

Skeletal abnormalities are common in these patients. Osteomalacia can develop as a result of chronic hypophosphatemia due to renal phosphate wasting if Fanconi syndrome is present. These patients may also have a deficiency in the active form of vitamin D because of an inability to convert 25-hydroxyvitamin D_3 to 1,25-dihydroxyvitamin D in the proximal tubule.

In contrast to distal RTA, proximal RTA is not associated with nephrolithiasis or nephrocalcinosis. One exception is the use of topiramate,[4,5] an antiepileptic drug that is increasingly used to treat a variety of neurologic and metabolic disorders. The drug exerts an inhibitory effect on renal carbonic anhydrase

Causes of Proximal (Type 2) Renal Tubular Acidosis

- Not associated with Fanconi syndrome
  - Sporadic
  - Familial
  - Disorder of carbonic anhydrase
    - Drugs: acetazolamide, sulfanilamide, topiramate
    - Carbonic anhydrase II deficiency
- Associated with Fanconi syndrome
  - Selective (no systemic disease present)
    - Sporadic
    - Familial
      - Autosomal recessive proximal RTA with ocular abnormalities: Na^+-HCO_3^- cotransporter (NBCe1) defect
      - Autosomal recessive proximal RTA with osteopetrosis and cerebral calcification: carbonic anhydrase II defect
      - Generalized (systemic disorder present)
      - Genetic disorders
        - Cystinosis
        - Wilson's disease
        - Hereditary fructose intolerance
        - Lowe syndrome
        - Metachromatic leukodystrophy
    - Dysproteinemic states
      - Myeloma kidney
      - Light chain deposition disease
    - Primary and secondary hyperparathyroidism
    - Drugs and toxins
      - Outdated tetracycline
      - Ifosfamide
      - Gentamicin
      - Streptozocin
      - Lead
      - Cadmium
      - Mercury
    - Tubulointerstitial disease
      - Post-transplantation rejection
      - Balkan nephropathy
      - Medullary cystic disease
    - Others
      - Bone fibroma
      - Osteopetrosis
      - Paroxysmal nocturnal hemoglobinuria

Figure 12.4 Causes of proximal (type 2) renal tubular acidosis (RTA).

activity, resulting in a proximal acidification defect similar to that observed with acetazolamide. Use of the drug also is associated with hypocitraturia, hypercalciuria, and elevated urine pH, leading to an increased risk of kidney stone disease.

Proximal RTA should be suspected in a patient with a normal anion gap acidosis and hypokalemia who has an intact ability to acidify the urine to below 5.5 while in a steady state.[6] Proximal tubular dysfunction, such as euglycemic glycosuria, hypophosphatemia, hypouricemia, and mild proteinuria, helps support this diagnosis. The UAG is greater than zero, indicating the lack of increase in net acid excretion.

Treatment of proximal RTA is difficult. Administration of alkali increases the serum bicarbonate concentration, which increases urinary bicarbonate losses and thereby minimizes subsequent increases in the serum bicarbonate concentration. Moreover, the increased distal sodium load, in combination with increased circulating plasma aldosterone, results in increased renal potassium wasting and worsening hypokalemia. As a result, substantial amounts of alkali, often in the form of a potassium salt, such as potassium citrate, are required to prevent worsening hypokalemia. Children with proximal RTA should be aggressively treated to normalize their serum bicarbonate concentration to minimize growth retardation. These children may require large amounts of alkali therapy, typically 5 to 15 mmol/kg per day.

Adults with proximal RTA are frequently not treated as aggressively as children are because of the lack of systemic metabolic abnormalities or bone disease. Many clinicians administer alkali therapy if the serum bicarbonate concentration is less than 18 mmol/l to prevent severe acidosis. Whether more aggressive therapy to normalize the serum bicarbonate concentration is beneficial remains unknown. However, the large amounts of alkali required, approximately 700 to 1000 mmol/day for a 70-kg individual, makes this approach problematic.

Hypokalemic Distal Renal Tubular Acidosis (Type 1)

In contrast to proximal RTA, patients with distal RTA are unable to acidify their urine, either under basal conditions or in response to metabolic acidosis.[7,8] This disorder results from a reduction in net H^+ secretion in the distal nephron, which leads to continued urinary bicarbonate losses and prevents urinary acidification, thereby minimizing titratable acid excretion and urinary ammonia excretion. As a result, these patients are unable to match net acid excretion to endogenous acid production, and acid accumulation ensues. The subsequent metabolic acidosis stimulates reabsorption of bone matrix to release the calcium alkali salts present in bone. During prolonged periods, this can result in progressive osteopenia in adults and in osteomalacia in children.

Distal RTA can be caused by either impaired H^+ secretion (secretory defect) or an abnormally permeable distal tubule, resulting in increased backleak of normally secreted H^+ (gradient defect); it may be genetic or acquired. Certain medications, especially amphotericin, result in increased backleak of protons across the apical plasma membrane, thereby leading to a gradient defect form of distal RTA.

For patients with a secretory defect, the inability to acidify the urine below pH 5.5 results from abnormalities in any of the proteins involved in collecting duct H^+ secretion. Some patients may have an isolated defect in the H^+,K^+-ATPase that impairs H^+ secretion and K^+ reabsorption.[9] A defect confined to the vacuolar H^+-ATPase also results in renal potassium wasting.[10] The development of systemic acidosis tends to diminish net proximal fluid reabsorption with an increase in distal delivery, resulting in volume contraction and activation of the renin-aldosterone system. Increased distal Na^+ delivery coupled to increased circulating levels of aldosterone then leads to increased renal K^+ secretion. Defects in the basolateral anion exchanger (AE1) can also cause distal RTA. In this case, the lack of basolateral HCO_3^- exit leads to intracellular alkalinization, which inhibits apical proton secretion.

Patients with distal RTA have low ammonia secretion rates. The decreased secretion is caused by the failure to trap ammonia in the tubular lumen of the collecting duct as a result of the inability to lower luminal fluid pH. In addition, there is often impaired medullary transfer of ammonia because of interstitial disease. Interstitial disease is frequently present in such patients through an associated underlying disease or as a result of nephrocalcinosis or hypokalemia-induced interstitial fibrosis.

In contrast to proximal RTA, nephrolithiasis and nephrocalcinosis are common.[11] Urinary Ca^{2+} excretion is high secondary to acidosis-induced bone mineral dissolution. Luminal alkalinization also inhibits calcium reabsorption, resulting in further increases in urinary calcium excretion.[12] Calcium phosphate solubility is also markedly lowered at alkaline pH, and calcium phosphate stone formation is accelerated. Stone formation is further enhanced as a result of low urinary citrate excretion. Citrate is metabolized to HCO_3^-, and its renal reabsorption is stimulated by metabolic acidosis, thereby minimizing the severity of metabolic acidosis. Urinary citrate also chelates urinary calcium, thereby decreasing ionized calcium concentrations. Accordingly, the decreased citrate excretion that occurs in chronic metabolic acidosis due to distal RTA further contributes to both nephrolithiasis and nephrocalcinosis.

Causes of Hypokalemic Distal (Type 1) Renal Tubular Acidosis
Primary
Idiopathic
Familial
Secondary
Autoimmune disorders
Hypergammaglobulinemia
Sjögren's syndrome
Primary biliary cirrhosis
Systemic lupus erythematosus
Genetic diseases
Autosomal dominant RTA: anion exchanger 1 defect
Autosomal recessive: H^+-ATPase A4 subunit
Autosomal recessive with progressive nerve deafness: H^+-ATPase B1 subunit
Drugs and toxins
Amphotericin B
Toluene
Disorders with nephrocalcinosis
Hyperparathyroidism
Vitamin D intoxication
Idiopathic hypercalciuria
Tubulointerstitial disease
Obstructive uropathy
Renal transplantation

Figure 12.5 Causes of hypokalemic distal (type 1) renal tubular acidosis (RTA).

Distal RTA may be a primary disorder, either idiopathic or inherited, but it most commonly occurs in association with a systemic disease, of which one of the most common is Sjögren's syndrome (Fig. 12.5). Hypergammaglobulinemic states as well as drugs and toxins may also cause this disorder.

A common cause of acquired distal RTA is glue sniffing. Inhalation of toluene from the fumes of model glue, spray paint, and paint thinners can give rise to hypokalemic normal gap acidosis through multiple mechanisms. First, toluene inhibits collecting duct proton secretion. Second, metabolism of toluene produces the organic acids hippuric and benzoic acid. These are buffered by sodium bicarbonate, resulting in metabolic acidosis and the production of sodium hippurate and sodium benzoate. If plasma volume is normal, these salts are rapidly excreted in the urine, and a non–anion gap metabolic acidosis develops. If plasma volume is decreased, urinary excretion is limited, they accumulate, and an anion gap metabolic acidosis develops.

Distal RTA should be considered in all patients with a non–anion gap metabolic acidosis and hypokalemia who have an inability to lower the urine pH maximally. A urine pH above 5.5 in the setting of systemic acidosis is suggestive of distal RTA, and a UAG value greater than zero is confirmatory. Depending on the duration of the distal RTA, the metabolic acidosis can be either mild or very severe, with a serum bicarbonate concentration as low as 10 mmol/l. Urinary potassium losses lead to the

Factors Differentiating Type 1, Type 2 and Type 4 RTA

	Type 1 RTA	Type 2 RTA	Type 4 RTA
Serum K^+	Low	Low	High
Renal function	Normal or near normal	Normal or near normal	Stage 3, 4, or 5 chronic kidney disease
Urine pH during acidosis	High	Low	Low or high
Serum HCO_3^- (mmol/l)	10–20	16–18	16–22
Urine pCO_2 (mmHg)	<40	<40	>70
Urine citrate	Low	High	Low
Fanconi syndrome	No	May be present	No

Figure 12.6 Factors differentiating types 1, 2, and 4 renal tubular acidosis (RTA).

development of hypokalemia. Severe hypokalemia (<2.5 mmol/l) may result in musculoskeletal weakness and nephrogenic diabetes insipidus. The latter occurs because hypokalemia decreases AQP2 expression in the collecting duct, thereby minimizing the ability to concentrate urine. An abdominal ultrasound scan may reveal nephrocalcinosis.

In patients with minimal disturbances in blood pH and plasma HCO_3^- concentration, a test of urinary acidification is required. Traditionally, such a test involved oral NH_4Cl administration to induce metabolic acidosis with assessment of the renal response by serial measurement of urine pH. Many patients poorly tolerate NH_4Cl ingestion because of gastric irritation, nausea, and vomiting. An alternative way to test the capacity for distal acidification is to administer furosemide and the mineralocorticoid fludrocortisone simultaneously.[13] The combination of both increased distal Na^+ delivery and mineralocorticoid effect will stimulate distal H^+ secretion by both an increase in the luminal electronegativity and a direct stimulatory on H^+ secretion. Normal subjects will lower urine pH to values below 5.5 with either maneuver.

Correction of the metabolic acidosis in distal RTA can be achieved by administration of alkali in an amount only slightly greater than daily acid production (usually 1 to 2 mmol/kg per day). In patients with severe K^+ deficits, correction of the acidosis with HCO_3^-, particularly if it is done with sodium alkali salts such as sodium bicarbonate, can lower serum potassium concentration to dangerous levels. In this setting, potassium replacement should begin before the acidosis is corrected. In general, a combination of sodium alkali and potassium alkali is required for long-term treatment of distal RTA. For the patient with recurrent renal stone disease due to distal RTA, treatment of the acidosis increases urinary citrate excretion, which slows the rate of further stone formation and may even lead to stone dissolution.

Hyperkalemic Distal Renal Tubular Acidosis (Type 4)

Type 4 RTA is characterized by distal nephron dysfunction, resulting in impaired renal excretion of both H^+ and K^+ and causing a hyperchloremic normal gap acidosis and hyperkalemia.[14] The syndrome occurs most commonly with mild to moderate impairment in renal function; however, the magnitude of hyperkalemia and acidosis are disproportionately severe for the observed glomerular filtration rate (GFR). Whereas hypokalemic distal (type 1) RTA is also a disorder of distal nephron acidification, type 4 RTA is distinguished from type 1 RTA on the basis of several important characteristics (Fig. 12.6). Type 4 RTA is also a much more common form of RTA, particularly in adults.

Type 4 RTA results from either a deficiency in circulating aldosterone or abnormal cortical collecting duct function, or it can be related to hyperkalemia. In either case, a defect in distal H^+ secretion develops. Impaired Na^+ reabsorption by the principal cell leads to a decrease in the luminal electronegativity of the cortical collecting duct, which impairs distal acidification as a result of the decrease in driving force for H^+ secretion into the tubular lumen. The H^+ secretion is further impaired in this segment as well as in the medullary collecting duct as a result of either the loss of the direct stimulatory effect of aldosterone on H^+ secretion or an abnormality in the H^+ secreting cell.

A consequence of the decrease in luminal electronegativity in the cortical collecting duct is impaired renal K^+ excretion. In addition, a primary abnormality in the cortical collecting duct transport can also impair K^+ secretion. The development of hyperkalemia adds to the defect in distal acidification by decreasing the amount of ammonia available to act as a urinary buffer. Some studies suggest that hyperkalemia itself, through its effects on ammonia metabolism, is the primary mechanism by which the metabolic acidosis develops in type 4 RTA.

The etiology of type 4 RTA includes those conditions associated with decreased circulating levels of aldosterone and conditions associated with impaired function of the cortical collecting duct. The most common disease associated with type 4 RTA in adults is diabetes mellitus. In these patients, primary NaCl retention leads to volume expansion and suppression and atrophy of the renin-secreting juxtaglomerular apparatus. Several commonly used drugs, such as nonsteroidal anti-inflammatory agents (NSAIDs), angiotensin-converting enzyme (ACE) inhibitors, and high doses of heparin, as used for systemic anticoagulation, can lead to decreased mineralocorticoid synthesis. Impaired function of the cortical collecting duct can be a feature of structural damage to the kidney, as in interstitial renal diseases such as sickle cell nephropathy, urinary tract obstruction, and lupus; it may also result from use of drugs such as amiloride, triamterene, and spironolactone.[15]

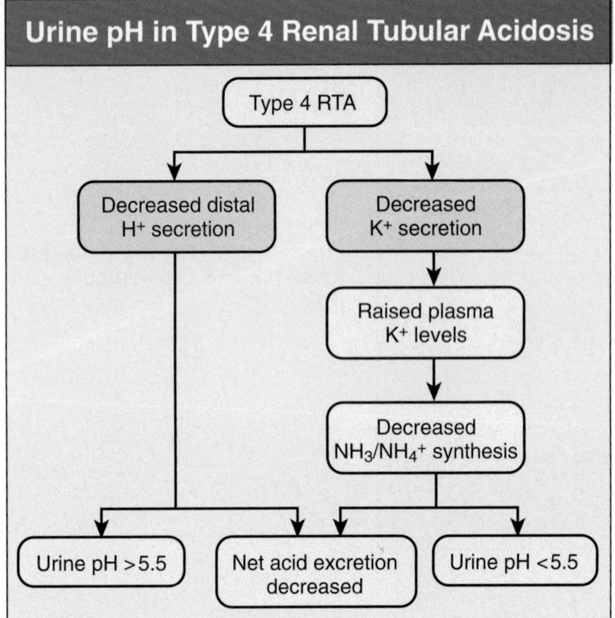

Figure 12.7 Urine pH in type 4 renal tubular acidosis (RTA). Net acid excretion is always decreased; however, the urine pH can be variable. In structural disease of the kidney, the predominant defect is usually decreased distal H^+ secretion, and the urine pH is above 5.5. In disorders associated with decreased mineralocorticoid activity, urine pH is usually below 5.5.

Causes of Hyperkalemic Distal (Type 4) Renal Tubular Acidosis

- Mineralocorticoid deficiency
  - Low renin, low aldosterone
    - Diabetes mellitus
    - Drugs
      - Nonsteroidal anti-inflammatory drugs (NSAIDs)
      - Cyclosporine, tacrolimus
      - β-Blockers
  - High renin, low aldosterone
    - Adrenal destruction
    - Congenital enzyme defects
    - Drugs
      - Angiotensin-converting enzyme (ACE) inhibitors
      - Angiotensin II receptor blockers (ARBs)
      - Heparin
      - Ketoconazole
- Abnormal cortical collecting duct
  - Absent or defective mineralocorticoid receptor
  - Drugs
    - Spironolactone, eplerenone
    - Triamterene
    - Amiloride
    - Trimethoprim
    - Pentamidine
  - Chronic tubulointerstitial disease

Figure 12.8 Causes of hyperkalemic distal (type 4) renal tubular acidosis (RTA).

Type 4 RTA should be suspected in a patient with a normal gap metabolic acidosis associated with hyperkalemia. The typical patient is in the fifth to seventh decade of life with a long-standing history of diabetes mellitus with a moderate reduction in the GFR. The plasma HCO_3^- concentration is usually in the range of 18 to 22 mmol/l and the serum K^+ concentration between 5.5 and 6.5 mmol/l. Most patients are asymptomatic; however, the hyperkalemia may occasionally be severe enough to cause muscle weakness or cardiac arrhythmias. The UAG value is slightly positive, indicating minimal ammonia excretion in the urine. Patients in whom the disorder is caused by a defect in mineralocorticoid activity typically have a urine pH below 5.5, reflecting a more severe defect in ammonia availability than in H^+ secretion (Fig. 12.7). In patients with structural damage to the collecting duct, the urine pH may be alkaline, reflecting both impaired H^+ secretion and decreased urinary ammonia excretion.

Treatment of type 4 RTA is directed at treatment of both the hyperkalemia and the metabolic acidosis. In many instances, lowering of the serum K^+ concentration will simultaneously correct the acidosis.[16] Correction of the hyperkalemia allows renal ammonia production to increase, thereby increasing the buffer supply for distal acidification. The first consideration in the treatment of patients is to discontinue any nonessential medication that might interfere in either the synthesis or activity of aldosterone or the ability of the kidneys to excrete potassium (Fig. 12.8). ACE inhibitors and angiotensin receptor blockers (ARBs) should usually be continued because of the beneficial effects on cardiovascular disease and their renoprotective benefits in patients with chronic kidney disease (CKD). In patients with aldosterone deficiency who are neither hypertensive nor fluid overloaded, administration of a synthetic mineralocorticoid such as fludrocortisone (0.1 mg/day) can be effective. In patients with hypertension or volume overload, particularly in association with CKD, administration of either a thiazide or a loop diuretic is frequently effective. Loop diuretics are required in patients with an estimated GFR below 30 ml/min. Loop and thiazide diuretics increase distal Na^+ delivery and, as a result, stimulate K^+ and H^+ secretion in the collecting duct. Alkali therapy (e.g., $NaHCO_3$) can also be used to treat the acidosis and hyperkalemia, but one must closely monitor the patient to avoid volume overload and worsening hypertension.

Renal Tubular Acidosis in Chronic Kidney Disease

Metabolic acidosis in advanced CKD is caused by failure of the tubular acidification process to excrete the normal daily acid load. As functional renal mass is reduced by disease, there is an adaptive increase in ammonia production and H^+ secretion by the remaining nephrons. Despite increased production of ammonia from each remaining nephron, overall production may be decreased secondary to the decrease in total renal mass. In addition, there is less delivery of ammonia to the medullary interstitium secondary to a disrupted medullary anatomy.[17] The ability to lower the urinary pH remains intact, reflecting the fact that the impairment in distal nephron H^+ secretion is less than that in ammonia secretion. Quantitatively, however, the total amount of H^+ secretion is small, and the acidic urine pH is the consequence of very little buffer in the urine. The lack of ammonia in the urine is reflected by a positive value for the UAG. Differentiation of RTA from type 4 RTA can be difficult as it is based on the clinician's determination of whether the severity of metabolic acidosis is out of proportion to the degree of renal dysfunction.

Patients with CKD may develop a hyperchloremic normal gap metabolic acidosis associated with normokalemia or mild hyperkalemia as GFR decreases to less than 30 ml/min. With more advanced CKD (GFR <15 ml/min), the acidosis may change to an anion gap metabolic acidosis, reflecting a progressive inability to excrete phosphate, sulfate, and various organic acids. At this stage, the acidosis is commonly referred to as uremic acidosis.

Correction of the metabolic acidosis in patients with CKD is achieved by treatment with $NaHCO_3$, 0.5 to 1.5 mmol/kg per day, beginning when the HCO_3^- level is less than 22 mmol/l. In some cases, non–sodium citrate formulations can be used. Loop diuretics are often used in conjunction with alkali therapy to prevent volume overload. If the acidosis becomes refractory to medical therapy, dialysis needs to be initiated. Recent evidence suggests that metabolic acidosis in the setting of CKD needs to be aggressively treated as chronic acidosis is associated with metabolic bone disease and may lead to an accelerated catabolic state in patients with chronic kidney disease.[18,19]

Extrarenal Origin

Diarrhea

Intestinal secretions from sites distal to the stomach are rich in HCO_3^-. Accelerated loss of this HCO_3^--rich solution can result in metabolic acidosis. The resultant volume loss signals the kidney to increase NaCl reabsorption; this combined with the intestinal $NaHCO_3$ losses generates a normal anion gap metabolic acidosis. The renal response is to increase net acid excretion by increasing urinary excretion of ammonia.[20] Hypokalemia, as a result of gastrointestinal losses, and the low serum pH both stimulate the synthesis of ammonia in the proximal tubule. The increase in availability of ammonia to act as a urinary buffer allows a maximal increase in H^+ secretion by the distal nephron.

The increase in urinary ammonia excretion associated with an extrarenal normal anion gap acidosis results in a negative UAG value. Urine pH can be misleading and in chronic diarrhea may be above 6.0 because of substantial increases in renal ammonia metabolism that result in increased urine pH from the buffering ability of the ammonia. Although the clinical history should distinguish between these two possibilities, in a patient with surreptitious laxative abuse, this may not be helpful because diarrhea may not be reported. Colonoscopy may be required to demonstrate characteristic findings of laxative abuse (such as melanosis coli), if this diagnosis is being considered.

Treatment of diarrhea-associated metabolic acidosis is based on treatment of the underlying diarrhea. If this is not possible, alkali treatment, possibly including potassium alkali to treat hypokalemia and metabolic acidosis simultaneously, is indicated.

Ileal Conduits

Surgical diversion of the ureter into an ileal pouch is used in the treatment of neurogenic bladder or after cystectomy. The procedure may rarely be associated with the development of a hyperchloremic normal anion gap metabolic acidosis. Acidosis in part is due to reabsorption of urinary NH_4Cl by the intestine. The ammonia is transported through the portal circulation to the liver or is metabolized to urea to prevent hyperammonemic encephalopathy. This metabolic process consumes equimolar amounts of bicarbonate and therefore can result in the development of metabolic acidosis. Metabolic acidosis may also develop because urinary Cl^- can be exchanged for HCO_3^- through activation of a Cl^--HCO_3^- exchanger on the intestinal lumen. In some patients, a renal defect in acidification can develop and exacerbate the degree of acidosis. Such a defect may result from tubular damage caused by pyelonephritis or high colonic pressures, secondarily causing urinary obstruction.

The severity of acidosis relates to the length of time the urine is in contact with the bowel and the total surface area of bowel exposed to urine. In patients with a ureterosigmoid anastomosis, these factors are increased and the acidosis tends to be more common and more severe than in those patients with an ileal conduit. The ileal conduit was designed to minimize the time and area of contact between urine and intestinal surface. Patients with surgical diversion of the ureter who develop metabolic acidosis should be examined for an ileal loop obstruction because this would lead to an increase in contact time between the urine and the intestinal surface.

ANION GAP METABOLIC ACIDOSIS

Lactic Acidosis

Lactic acid is the end product in the anaerobic metabolism of glucose and is generated by the reversible reduction of pyruvic acid by lactic acid dehydrogenase and NADH (reduced nicotinamide adenine dinucleotide), as shown in the following formula:

$$\text{pyruvate} + \text{NADH} + \text{H}^+ \leftrightarrow \text{lactate} + \text{NAD}^+$$

Under normal conditions, the reaction is shifted toward the right, and the normal lactate to pyruvate ratio is approximately 10:1. The reactants in this pathway are interrelated as shown in the following equation:

$$\text{lactate} = K[(\text{pyruvate})(\text{NADH})(\text{H}^+)]/(\text{NAD}^+)$$

where K is the equilibrium constant.

On the basis of this relationship, it is evident that lactate can increase for three reasons.[21] First, lactate can increase as a consequence of increased pyruvate production alone. In this situation, the normal 10:1 lactate to pyruvate ratio will be maintained. An isolated increase in pyruvate production can be seen in the setting of intravenous glucose infusions, intravenous administration of epinephrine, and respiratory alkalosis. Lactate levels in these conditions are minimally elevated, rarely exceeding 5 mmol/l. Second, lactate can increase as a result of an increased NADH/NAD$^+$ ratio. Under these conditions, the lactate to pyruvate ratio can increase to very high values. Finally, lactate can increase when there is a combination of increased pyruvate production with an increased NADH/NAD$^+$ ratio. This is common in severe lactic acidosis.

Lactic acidosis occurs whenever there is an imbalance between the production and use of lactic acid. The net result is an accumulation of serum lactate and the development of metabolic acidosis. The accumulation of the non–chloride anion lactate accounts for the increase in anion gap. Severe exercise and grand mal seizures are examples of when lactic acidosis can develop as a result of increased production. The short-lived nature of the acidosis in these conditions suggests that a concomitant defect in lactic acid use is present in most conditions of sustained and severe lactic acidosis.

A partial list of the disorders associated with the development of lactic acidosis is given in Figure 12.9. Type A lactic acidosis is characterized by underperfusion of tissue or acute hypoxia, such as hypotension, sepsis, acute tissue hypoperfusion, cardiopulmonary failure, severe anemia, hemorrhage, and carbon monoxide poisoning. Type B lactic acidosis occurs in the absence of overt hypoperfusion or hypoxia, such as with congenital defects in glucose or lactate metabolism, diabetes mellitus, liver disease, effects of drugs and toxins, and neoplastic diseases.[22-27] In clinical practice, many patients will often exhibit features of type A and type B lactic acidosis simultaneously.

Causes of Lactic Acidosis

Type A (tissue underperfusion or hypoxia)
- Cardiogenic shock
- Septic shock
- Hemorrhagic shock
- Acute hypoxia
- Carbon monoxide poisoning
- Anemia

Type B (absence of hypotension and hypoxia)
- Hereditary enzyme deficiency (glucose 6-phosphatase)
- Drugs or toxins
  - Phenformin, metformin
  - Cyanide
  - Salicylate, ethylene glycol, methanol
  - Propylene glycol[25]
  - Linezolid[22]
  - Propofol[24]
  - Nucleoside reverse transcriptase inhibitors: stavudine, didanosine[23]
  - Clenbuterol[26]
  - Isoniazid
- Systemic disease
  - Liver failure
  - Malignancy

Figure 12.9 Causes of lactic acidosis.

Therapy is aimed at correction of the underlying disorder. Restoration of tissue perfusion and oxygenation is attempted if they are compromised. The role of alkali in the treatment of lactic acidosis is controversial; some experimental models and clinical observations suggest that administration of HCO_3^- may depress cardiac function and exacerbate the acidemia. In addition, such therapy may be complicated by volume overload, hypernatremia, and rebound alkalosis after the acidosis has resolved. In general, HCO_3^- should be given when the systemic pH decreases to below 7.1, as hemodynamic instability becomes much more likely with severe acidemia. In such cases, alkali therapy should be directed at increasing the pH above 7.1; attempts to normalize the pH or $[HCO_3^-]$ should be avoided. Acute hemodialysis is rarely beneficial for lactic acidosis induced by tissue hypoperfusion. The hemodynamic instability that can occur with hemodialysis in these critically ill patients may worsen the underlying difficulty in tissue oxygenation.

Diabetic Ketoacidosis

Diabetic ketoacidosis results from the accumulation of acetoacetic acid and β-hydroxybutyric acid. The development of ketoacidosis is the result of insulin deficiency and a relative or absolute increase in glucagon.[28] These hormonal changes lead to increased fatty acid mobilization from adipose tissue and alter the oxidative machinery of the liver such that delivered fatty acids are primarily metabolized into keto acids. In addition, peripheral glucose use is impaired, and the gluconeogenic pathway in the liver is maximally stimulated. The resultant hyperglycemia causes an osmotic diuresis and volume depletion.

Ketoacidosis results when the rate of hepatic keto acid generation exceeds renal excretion, causing increased blood keto acid concentrations. The H^+ accumulation in the extracellular fluid decreases HCO_3^- concentration, whereas the keto acid anion concentration increases. An anion gap metabolic acidosis is the more common finding in diabetic ketoacidosis, but a normal gap metabolic acidosis can also be seen. In early stages of ketoacidosis, when the extracellular volume is nearly normal, keto acid anions that are produced are rapidly excreted by the kidney as Na^+ and K^+ salts. Excretion of these salts is equivalent to the loss of potential HCO_3^-. This loss of potential HCO_3^- in the urine at the same time that the kidney is retaining NaCl results in a normal gap metabolic acidosis. As volume depletion develops, renal keto acid excretion cannot match production rates, and keto acid anions are retained within the body, thus increasing the anion gap.

During treatment, the anion gap metabolic acidosis transforms once again into a normal gap acidosis. Treatment leads to a termination in keto acid production. As the extracellular fluid volume is restored, there is increased renal excretion of the Na^+ salts of the keto acid anions. The loss of this potential HCO_3^- combined with the retention of administered NaCl accounts for the redevelopment of the hyperchloremic normal gap acidosis. In addition, K^+ and Na^+ administered in solutions containing NaCl and KCl enter cells in exchange for H^+. The net effect is infusion of HCl into the extracellular fluid. The reversal of the hyperchloremic acidosis takes several days as the HCO_3^- deficit is corrected by the kidney.

Diabetic ketoacidosis can result in a severe metabolic acidosis with serum bicarbonate levels below 5 mmol/l. This diagnosis should be considered in patients with simultaneous metabolic acidosis and hyperglycemia. Diagnosis is confirmed by demonstration of retained keto acids with nitroprusside tablets or reagent strips. However, these tests detect only acetone and acetoacetate and not β-hydroxybutyrate. In the setting of lactic acidosis or alcoholic ketoacidosis, acetoacetate may be converted to β-hydroxybutyrate to an extent that depends on the NADH/NAD^+ ratio. With treatment of the diabetic ketoacidosis, acetoacetate is generated as the NADH/NAD^+ ratio falls, and the nitroprusside test result may suddenly become strongly positive.

The limitations of the nitroprusside test can be prevented by direct measurement of β-hydroxybutyrate. With uncontrolled diabetes, a serum β-hydroxybutyrate level above 3.0 and above 3.8 mmol/l in children and adults, respectively, confirms diabetic ketoacidosis.[29] Compared with urinary ketone measurements, capillary blood levels of β-hydroxybutyrate better correlate with both the degree of acidosis and the response to therapy.[30]

Treatment consists of insulin and intravenous fluids to correct volume depletion. Deficiencies in K^+, Mg^{2+}, and phosphate are common; therefore, these electrolytes are typically added to intravenous solutions. However, diabetic ketoacidosis typically presents with hyperkalemia due to the insulin deficiency. Potassium should be administered only as hypokalemia develops, usually during insulin treatment of diabetic ketoacidosis. If there is significant hypokalemia at presentation, potassium supplementation may be needed before insulin administration to avoid life-threatening worsening of hypokalemia. Alkali therapy is generally not required because administration of insulin leads to the metabolic conversion of keto acid anions to HCO_3^- and allows partial correction of the acidosis. However, HCO_3^- therapy may be indicated in those patients who present with severe acidemia (pH <7.1).[31]

D-Lactic Acidosis

D-Lactic acidosis is a unique form of metabolic acidosis that can occur in the setting of small bowel resections or in patients with a jejunoileal bypass. Such short bowel syndromes create a situation in which carbohydrates that are normally extensively reabsorbed in the small intestine are delivered in large amounts to the colon. In the presence of colonic bacterial overgrowth, these substrates are metabolized into D-lactate and absorbed into the systemic circulation. Accumulation of D-lactate produces an anion gap metabolic acidosis in which the serum lactate concentration is normal because the standard test for lactate is specific for L-lactate. These patients typically present after ingestion of a large carbohydrate meal with neurologic abnormalities consisting of confusion, slurred speech, and ataxia. Ingestion of low-carbohydrate meals and antimicrobial agents to decrease the degree of bacterial overgrowth are the principal treatments.

Starvation Ketosis

Abstinence from food can lead to a mild anion gap metabolic acidosis secondary to increased production of keto acids. The pathogenesis of this disorder is similar to that of diabetic ketoacidosis in that starvation leads to relative insulin deficiency and glucagon excess. As a result, there is increased mobilization of fatty acids while the liver is set to oxidize fatty acids to keto acids. With prolonged starvation, the blood keto acid level can reach 5 to 6 mmol/l. The serum [HCO_3^-] is rarely less than 18 mmol/l. More fulminant ketoacidosis is aborted by the fact that ketone bodies stimulate the pancreatic islets to release insulin and lipolysis is held in check. This break in the ketogenic process is notably absent in those with insulin-dependent diabetes. There is no specific therapy indicated in this disorder.

Alcoholic Ketoacidosis

Ketoacidosis develops in patients with a history of chronic ethanol abuse, decreased food intake, and often a history of nausea and vomiting. As with starvation ketosis, a decrease in the insulin to glucagon ratio leads to accelerated fatty acid mobilization and alters the enzymatic machinery of the liver to favor keto acid production. However, there are features unique to this disorder that differentiate it from simple starvation ketosis. First, the alcohol withdrawal combined with volume depletion and starvation markedly increases the levels of circulating catecholamines. As a result, the peripheral mobilization of fatty acids is much greater than that typically found with starvation alone. This sometimes massive mobilization of fatty acids can lead to marked keto acid production and severe metabolic acidosis. Second, the metabolism of ethanol leads to accumulation of NADH. The increase in the $NADH/NAD^+$ ratio is reflected by a higher β-hydroxybutyrate to acetoacetate ratio. As mentioned previously, the nitroprusside reaction may be diminished by this redox shift despite the presence of severe ketoacidosis. Treatment of this disorder is focused on glucose administration, which leads to the rapid resolution of the acidosis because stimulation of insulin release leads to diminished fatty acid mobilization from adipose tissue as well as decreased hepatic output of keto acids.

Ethylene Glycol and Methanol Intoxications

Ethylene glycol and methanol intoxications are characteristically associated with the development of a severe anion gap metabolic acidosis. Metabolism of ethylene glycol by alcohol dehydrogenase generates various acids, including glycolic, oxalic, and formic acids. Ethylene glycol is present in antifreeze and solvents and is ingested by accident or as a suicide attempt. The initial effects of intoxication are neurologic and begin with drunkenness but can quickly progress to seizures and coma. If left untreated, cardiopulmonary symptoms such as tachypnea, noncardiogenic pulmonary edema, and cardiovascular collapse may appear. Twenty-four to 48 hours after ingestion, patients may develop flank pain and acute kidney injury often accompanied by abundant calcium oxalate crystals in the urine (Fig. 12.10). A fatal dose is approximately 100 ml.

Ethylene Glycol and Methanol Poisoning

Time course of clinical symptoms and signs after ingestion
- Ethylene glycol
  - 0–12 hours: inebriation progressing to coma
  - 12–24 hours: tachypnea, noncardiogenic pulmonary edema
  - 24–36 hours: flank pain, renal failure, urinary calcium oxalate crystals
- Methanol
  - 0–12 hours: inebriation followed by asymptomatic period
  - 24–36 hours: pancreatitis, retinal edema progressing to blindness, seizures
  - >48 hours: putamen and white matter hemorrhage leading to Parkinson's disease–like state

Increased anion gap metabolic acidosis

Increased osmolar gap

Treatment
- Supportive care
  - Fomepizole (4-methylpyrazole) is agent of choice (competitor of alcohol dehydrogenase): 15 mg/kg IV loading dose, then 10 mg/kg every 12 hours for 48 hours; after 48 hours, increase dose to 15 mg/kg every 12 hours; increase frequency of dosing to 4 hours during hemodialysis
- Intravenous ethanol (5% or 10% solution) if fomepizole unavailable: loading dose of 0.6 g/kg followed by hourly maintenance dose of 66 mg/kg; increase maintenance dose when there is a history of chronic alcohol use and during hemodialysis
- Hemodialysis to accelerate removal of parent compound and metabolites
- Bicarbonate therapy to treat acidosis

Figure 12.10 Ethylene glycol and methanol poisoning.

Methanol is also metabolized by alcohol dehydrogenase and forms formaldehyde, which is then converted to formic acid. Methanol is found in a variety of commercial preparations, such as shellac, varnish, and de-icing solutions, and is also known as wood alcohol. Like ethylene glycol, methanol can be ingested either by accident or as a suicide attempt. Clinically, methanol ingestion is associated with an acute inebriation followed by an asymptomatic period lasting 24 to 36 hours. Abdominal pain caused by pancreatitis, seizures, blindness, and coma may develop. The blindness is due to direct toxicity of formic acid on the retina. Methanol intoxication is also associated with hemorrhage in the white matter and putamen, which can lead to the delayed onset of a Parkinson's disease–like syndrome (see Fig. 12.10). The lethal dose is between 60 and 250 ml. Lactic acidosis is also a feature of methanol and ethylene glycol poisoning and contributes to the elevated anion gap.

Together with an elevated anion gap, an osmolar gap is an important clue to the diagnosis of ethylene glycol and methanol poisoning. The osmolar gap is the difference between the measured and calculated osmolality. The formula for the calculated osmolality is as follows:

$$\text{calculated osmolality} = \frac{2 \times Na^+ + BUN}{2.8} + \frac{\text{glucose}}{18} + \frac{EtOH}{4.6}$$

where the blood urea nitrogen (BUN), glucose, and ethanol concentrations are in milligrams per deciliter. Inclusion of the ethanol concentration in this calculation is important as many patients who ingest either ethylene glycol or methanol do so while inebriated from ethanol ingestion. The normal value for the osmolar gap is less than 10 mOsm/kg. Each 100 mg/dl (161 mmol/l) of ethylene glycol will increase the osmolar gap by 16 mOsm/kg; methanol contributes 32 mOsm/kg for each 100 mg/dl (312 mmol/l).

In addition to supportive measures, ethylene glycol and methanol poisoning are treated with fomepizole (4-methylpyrazole), which inhibits alcohol dehydrogenase and prevents formation of toxic metabolites (see Fig.12.10).[32] If fomepizole is unavailable, intravenous ethanol can be used to prevent the formation of toxic metabolites. Ethanol has more than a 10-fold greater affinity for alcohol dehydrogenase than that of other alcohols. Ethanol has its greatest efficacy when levels of 100 to 200 mg/dl are obtained. In addition to both fomepizole and ethanol therapy, hemodialysis should be employed to remove both the parent compound and its metabolites. Finally, correction of the acidosis is accomplished with use of an HCO_3^--containing dialysate or by intravenous infusion of $NaHCO_3$.

Salicylate

Aspirin (acetylsalicylic acid) is associated with a large number of accidental or intentional poisonings. At toxic concentrations, salicylate uncouples oxidative phosphorylation and, as a result, leads to increased lactic acid production. In children, keto acid production may also be increased. The accumulation of lactic, salicylic, keto, and other organic acids leads to the development of an anion gap metabolic acidosis. At the same time, salicylate has a direct stimulatory effect on the respiratory center. Increased ventilation lowers the P_{CO_2}, contributing to the development of a respiratory alkalosis. Children primarily manifest an anion gap metabolic acidosis with toxic salicylate levels; a respiratory alkalosis is most evident in adults.

In addition to conservative management, the initial goals of therapy are to correct systemic acidemia and to increase the urine pH. By increasing systemic pH, the ionized fraction of salicylic acid will increase, and as a result, there will be less accumulation of the drug in the central nervous system. Similarly, an alkaline urine pH favors increased urinary excretion because the ionized fraction of the drug is poorly reabsorbed by the tubule. At serum concentrations above 80 mg/dl or in the setting of severe clinical toxicity, hemodialysis can be used to accelerate drug elimination.

Pyroglutamic Acidosis

Pyroglutamic acid, also known as 5-oxoproline, is an intermediate in glutathione metabolism. An anion gap acidosis due to pyroglutamic acid has been rarely described in critically ill patients receiving therapeutic doses of acetaminophen (Fig. 12.11).[33,34] Affected patients present with severe anion gap metabolic acidosis accompanied by alterations in mental status ranging from confusion to coma. High concentrations of pyroglutamic acid are found in the blood and urine. In this setting, glutathione levels are reduced because of the oxidative stress associated with critical illness and by the metabolism of acetaminophen. The reduction in glutathione secondarily leads to increased production of pyroglutamic acid. The diagnosis of pyroglutamic

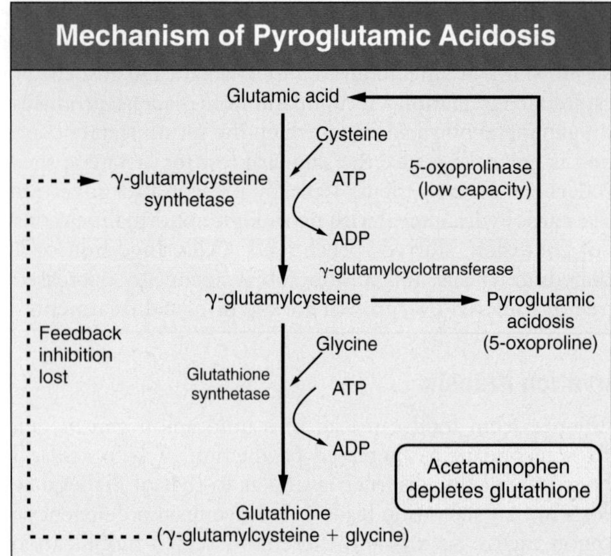

Figure 12.11 Mechanism of pyroglutamic acidosis. Glutathione is formed from γ-glutamylcysteine and glycine in the presence of glutathione synthetase. Glutathione normally regulates the activity of γ-glutamylcysteine synthetase through feedback inhibition. Depletion of glutathione results in increased formation of γ-glutamylcysteine, which in turn is metabolized to pyroglutamic acid (5-oxoproline) and cystine through γ-glutamylcyclotransferase. Pyroglutamic acid accumulates because the enzyme responsible for its metabolism (5-oxoprolinase) is low capacity. ADP, adenosine diphosphate; ATP, adenosine triphosphate.

acidosis should be considered in patients with unexplained anion gap metabolic acidosis and recent acetaminophen ingestion.

ALKALI TREATMENT OF METABOLIC ACIDOSIS

Treatment of metabolic acidosis usually involves either sodium bicarbonate or citrate (Fig. 12.12).[31] Sodium bicarbonate can be taken orally as tablets or powder or given intravenously as a hypertonic sodium bicarbonate bolus or an isotonic sodium bicarbonate infusion, which can be created by adding three ampules ("amps") of sodium bicarbonate (50 mmol/amp) to a liter of 5% dextrose in water (D_5W) solution. This solution is useful if treatment requires both volume expansion and alkali administration.

Citrate may be taken orally as a liquid, as sodium citrate, potassium citrate, or citric acid and as a combination of these. Many patients find citrate-containing solutions more palatable than oral sodium bicarbonate as a source of oral alkali therapy. Oral citrate therapy should not be combined with medications that include aluminum. Citrate, which has a −3 charge under normal conditions, can complex with aluminum (Al^{3+}) in the intestinal tract, resulting in an uncharged moiety that is rapidly absorbed across the intestinal tract and then can dissociate to release free aluminum. This can increase the rate of aluminum absorption dramatically and in some cases, particularly in patients with severe CKD, has resulted in acute aluminum encephalopathy.

The dose of alkali therapy that is administered is based on both the total body bicarbonate deficit and the desired rapidity of treatment. Under normal circumstances, the volume of distribution (V_D) for bicarbonate is approximately 0.5 l/kg total body weight. Thus, the bicarbonate deficit, in millimoles, can be estimated from the following formula:

Alkali Treatment Options			
	Route	Usual Dose per Unit	Comments
Sodium bicarbonate tablet	PO	650 mg = 8 mmol	May cause gastric gas
Sodium bicarbonate	IV	50 mmol in 50 ml	Hypertonic, may cause hypernatremia
D_5W with $NaHCO_3$	IV	150 mmol/l	Useful for simultaneous intravascular volume expansion and alkali administration
Sodium citrate/ citric acid (liquid)	PO	1 mmol of Na^+ and citrate per milliliter	1 mmol citrate equivalent to 1 mmol HCO_3^-. Avoid concomitant aluminum-containing medications such as antacids and sucralfate.
Potassium citrate (tablet)	PO	5 and 10 mmol per tablet	Useful for simultaneous K^+ and alkali therapy
Citric acid/potassium citrate/sodium citrate (liquid)	PO	1 mmol of Na^+ and K^+ and 2 mmol of citrate per milliliter	Avoid concomitant aluminum-containing medications
Potassium citrate (liquid)	PO	2 mmol of K^+ and 2 mmol of citrate per milliliter	Avoid concomitant aluminum-containing medications

Figure 12.12 Alkali treatment options.

$$\text{bicarbonate deficit} = (0.5 \times \text{LBW}_{\text{kg}}) \times (24 - \text{HCO}_3^-)$$

where LBW_{kg} is the lean body weight in kilograms and 24 is the desired resultant bicarbonate concentration.

Several caveats regarding this equation should be understood. First, edema fluid contributes to the volume of distribution of bicarbonate. Accordingly, an estimation of the amount of edema fluid should be included in this calculation. Second, the volume of distribution for bicarbonate increases as the severity of the metabolic acidosis worsens. When the serum bicarbonate concentration is 5 mmol/l or less, the volume of distribution may increase to 1 l/kg or more.

When acute treatment is desired, 50% of the bicarbonate deficit should be replaced during the first 24 hours. If hypertonic sodium bicarbonate is administered, the increase in serum bicarbonate concentration will be mirrored by an increase in serum sodium concentration. After the initial 24 hours of therapy, the response to therapy and the patient's current clinical condition are re-evaluated before future therapy is decided. Acute hemodialysis solely for the treatment of metabolic acidosis other than that associated with renal failure is rarely beneficial.

REFERENCES

1. Palmer BF. Approach to fluid and electrolyte disorders and acid-base problems. *Prim Care*. 2008;35:195-213.
2. Kraut J, Madias N. Serum anion gap: Its uses and limitations in clinical medicine. *Clin J Am Soc Nephrol*. 2007;2:162-174.
3. Halperin ML, Richardson RM, Bear R, et al. Urine ammonium: The key to the diagnosis of distal renal tubular acidosis. *Nephron*. 1988;50:1-4.
4. Vega D, Maalouf N, Sakhaee K. Increased propensity for calcium phosphate kidney stones with topiramate use. *Expert Opin Drug Saf*. 2007;6(5):547-557.
5. Welch B, Graybeal D, Moe O, et al. Biochemical and stone-risk profiles with topiramate treatment. *Am J Kidney Dis*. 2006;48(4):555-563.
6. Rodriguez S. Renal tubular acidosis: The clinical entity. *J Am Soc Nephrol*. 2002;13:2160-2170.
7. Kim S, Lee J, Park J, et al. The urine-blood Pco_2 gradient as a diagnostic index of H^+-ATPase defect distal renal tubular acidosis. *Kidney Int*. 2004;66:761-767.
8. Nicoletta J, Schwartz G. Distal renal tubular acidosis. *Curr Opin Pediatr*. 2004;16:194-198.
9. Codina J, DuBose T. Molecular regulation and physiology of the H^+,K^+-ATPases in kidney. *Semin Nephrol*. 2006;26:345-351.
10. Jefferies K, Cipriano D, Forgac M. Function, structure and regulation of the vacuolar H^+-ATPases. *Arch Biochem Biophys*. 2008;476:33-42.
11. Evan A, Lingeman J, Coe F, et al. Renal histopathology of stone-forming patients with distal renal tubular acidosis. *Kidney Int*. 2007;71(8):795-801.
12. Bonny O, Rubin A, Huang C, et al. Mechanism of urinary calcium regulation by urinary magnesium and pH. *J Am Soc Nephrol*. 2008;19:1530-1537.
13. Walsh S, Shirley D, Wrong O, Unwin R. Urinary acidification assessed by furosemide and fludrocortisone treatment: An alternative to ammonium chloride. *Kidney Int*. 2007;71:1310-1316.
14. DuBose TD. Hyperkalemic hyperchloremic metabolic acidosis: Pathophysiologic insights. *Kidney Int*. 1997;51:591-602.
15. Palmer BF. Managing hyperkalemia caused by inhibitors of the renin-angiotensin-aldosterone system. *N Engl J Med*. 2004;351:585-592.
16. Sebastian A, Schambelan M, Lindenfeld S, Morris RC. Amelioration of metabolic acidosis with fludrocortisone therapy in hyporeninemic hypoaldosteronism. *N Engl J Med*. 1977;297:576-583.
17. Buerkert J, Martin D, Trigg D, Simon E. Effect of reduced renal mass on ammonium handling and net acid formation by the superficial and juxtamedullary nephron of the rat. *J Clin Invest*. 1983;71:1661-1675.
18. Krieger N, Frick K, Bushinsky D. Mechanism of acid-induced bone resorption. *Curr Opin Nephrol Hypertens*. 2004;13:423-436.
19. Alpern RJ, Sakhaee K. The clinical spectrum of chronic metabolic acidosis: Homeostatic mechanisms produce significant morbidity. *Am J Kidney Dis*. 1997;29:291-302.
20. Garibotto G, Sofia A, Robaudo C, et al. Kidney protein dynamics and ammoniagenesis in humans with chronic metabolic acidosis. *J Am Soc Nephrol*. 2004;15:1606-1615.
21. Madias N. Lactic acidosis. *Kidney Int*. 1986;29:752-774.
22. Palenzuela L, Hahn N, Nelson R, et al. Does linezolid cause lactic acidosis by inhibiting mitochondrial protein synthesis? *Clin Infect Dis*. 2005;40:e113-e116.
23. Thoden J, Lebrecht D. Highly active antiretroviral HIV therapy–associated fatal lactic acidosis: Quantitative and qualitative mitochondrial DNA lesions with mitochondrial dysfunction in multiple organs. *AIDS*. 2008;22:1093-1094.
24. Fodale V, La Monaca E. Propofol infusion syndrome: An overview of a perplexing disease. *Drug Saf*. 2008;31(4):293-303.
25. Zar T, Yusufzai I, Sullivan A, Graeber C. Acute kidney injury, hyperosmolality and metabolic acidosis associated with lorazepam. *Nat Clin Pract Nephrol*. 2007;3(9):515-520.
26. Hoffman R, Kirrane B, Marcus S. A descriptive study of an outbreak of clenbuterol-containing heroin. *Ann Emerg Med*. 2008;52:548-553.
27. Creagh-Brown B, Ball J. An under-recognized complication of treatment of acute severe asthma. *Am J Emerg Med*. 2008;26(4):514.e1-514.e3.
28. Foster DW, McGarry JD. The metabolic derangements and treatment of diabetic ketoacidosis. *N Engl J Med*. 1983;309:159-169.
29. Sheikh-Ali M, Karon B, Basu A, et al. Can serum β-hydroxybutyrate be used to diagnose diabetic ketoacidosis? *Diabetes Care*. 2008;31(4):643-647.
30. Turan S, Omar A, Bereket A. Comparison of capillary blood ketone measurement by electrochemical method and urinary ketone in treatment of diabetic ketosis and ketoacidosis in children. *Acta Diabetol*. 2008;45:83-85.
31. Sabatini S, Kurtzman N. Bicarbonate therapy in severe metabolic acidosis. *J Am Soc Nephrol*. 2009;20:692-695. Epub 2008 Mar 5.

32. Kraut J, Kurtz I. Toxic alcohol ingestions: Clinical features, diagnosis, and management. *Clin J Am Soc Nephrol*. 2008;3(1):208-225.
33. Brooker G, Jeffery J, Nataraj T, et al. High anion gap metabolic acidosis secondary to pyroglutamic aciduria (5-oxoprolinuria): Association with prescription drugs and malnutrition. *Ann Clin Biochem*. 2007;44:406-409.
34. Fenves A, Kirkpatrick H, Patel V, et al. Increased anion gap metabolic acidosis as a result of 5-oxoproline (pyroglutamic acid): A role for acetaminophen. *Clin J Am Soc Nephrol*. 2006;1:441-447.

CHAPTER 13

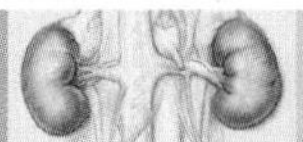

Metabolic Alkalosis

F. John Gennari

DEFINITION

Metabolic alkalosis is caused by retention of excess alkali and is manifested by an increase in venous [total CO_2] to greater than 30 mmol/l or in arterial [HCO_3^-] to greater than 28 mmol/l. The increase in pH that results from retained HCO_3^- induces hypoventilation, producing a secondary increase in arterial Pco_2. Thus, the disorder is characterized by coexisting elevations in serum [HCO_3^-], arterial pH, and Pco_2. Because the kidney normally responds to an increase in [HCO_3^-] by rapidly excreting the excess alkali, sustained metabolic alkalosis occurs only when some additional factor disrupts renal regulation of body alkali stores.

RENAL BICARBONATE TRANSPORT MECHANISMS

To examine the ways in which alkali balance is disrupted by metabolic alkalosis, a brief review of normal H^+ and HCO_3^- transport in the kidney is necessary. Bicarbonate ions are freely filtered across the glomerulus and must be completely recaptured from the tubule urine to conserve body alkali stores. In addition, acid excretion must occur to regenerate any HCO_3^- consumed in buffering of endogenously produced acids. Both tasks are accomplished by secretion of H^+ into the renal tubules.[1] Bicarbonate ions are recaptured when secreted H^+ combines with filtered HCO_3^- to produce CO_2 and water, removing HCO_3^- from the urine. At the same time, the secreted H^+ generates new HCO_3^- inside the cell that is then added to the peritubular blood.

Figure 13.1 illustrates the major apical membrane epithelial transporters and channels that participate in HCO_3^- reabsorption. In the proximal tubule and ascending limb of Henle's loop, H^+ is secreted through a Na^+-linked transporter (the Na^+-H^+ exchanger NHE3) and also by an H^+-ATPase. In the collecting duct, NHE3 is not present and H^+ secretion is accomplished primarily by an apical membrane H^+-ATPase. The activity of this H^+-ATPase is regulated by aldosterone and by the rate of Na^+ delivery to and reabsorption by the collecting duct. When body K^+ stores are low, an apical membrane H^+,K^+-ATPase is activated in the collecting duct, further promoting H^+ secretion driven by K^+ reabsorption.[2] If excess alkali is ingested, HCO_3^- can re-enter the tubule urine in the collecting duct through an apical membrane Cl^--HCO_3^- exchanger (pendrin).[3] This transporter is activated by alkalemia and requires Cl^- reabsorption in exchange for secreted HCO_3^-. The HCO_3^- secreted into the urine by this transporter can be recaptured again by H^+ secretion in the collecting duct, so that excretion of excess alkali requires both stimulation of the Cl^--HCO_3^- exchanger and suppression of the normally active collecting duct H^+-ATPase. As discussed later, abnormal stimulation of H^+-secreting transporters or changes in the activity of Na^+-linked Cl^- transporters in the loop of Henle and early distal tubule (see Fig. 13.1) can disrupt the renal regulation of body alkali stores and produce sustained metabolic alkalosis.

PATHOPHYSIOLOGY OF METABOLIC ALKALOSIS

Metabolic alkalosis can be produced by administration of HCO_3^- (or a HCO_3^- precursor) or by induction of either Cl^- or K^+ depletion. More rarely, sustained metabolic alkalosis is the result of primary abnormalities in the regulation of specific ion transporters in the loop of Henle, distal tubule, or collecting ducts. The most common clinical presentation of metabolic alkalosis is associated with Cl^- depletion. Although the term *contraction alkalosis* is often used as a synonym for Cl^- depletion alkalosis, this phrase is confusing because it implies that volume contraction is responsible for the disorder. The term refers specifically to the increase in serum [HCO_3^-] that follows only one type of extracellular fluid (ECF) volume contraction, that caused by selective Cl^- losses. Moreover, a sustained change in renal HCO_3^- reabsorption and acid excretion must occur for this increase to be maintained, and it remains unclear whether volume contraction is necessary or instrumental in inducing this change in renal function.[4,5] As is illustrated later, Cl^- and K^+ depletion are closely linked events in causing many forms of sustained metabolic alkalosis, and it is often difficult to determine which ion is the primary culprit. However, experimental depletion of either ion can be shown to induce sustained metabolic alkalosis.[5-7]

Potassium Depletion

Induction of net K^+ loss by severe restriction of dietary K^+ intake produces a small but significant increase in serum [HCO_3^-].[6] When dietary Cl^- intake is concomitantly restricted, however, the resultant alkalosis is four times as great, illustrating the complementary roles of Cl^- and K^+ in regulating renal HCO_3^- reabsorption. Depletion of body K^+ stores is probably the most important factor in producing and sustaining the rarer forms of metabolic alkalosis induced by mineralocorticoid excess or apparent mineralocorticoid excess (see later discussion).

Chloride Depletion

Selective Cl^- depletion, induced by vomiting or nasogastric suction, increases serum [HCO_3^-] (Fig. 13.2).[7] The degree of alkalosis generated is greater when H^+ loss also occurs, as in the example shown in Figure 13.2, but it may occur even when H^+ loss is minimized by administration of a proton pump inhibitor. In either setting, maintenance of the metabolic alkalosis is

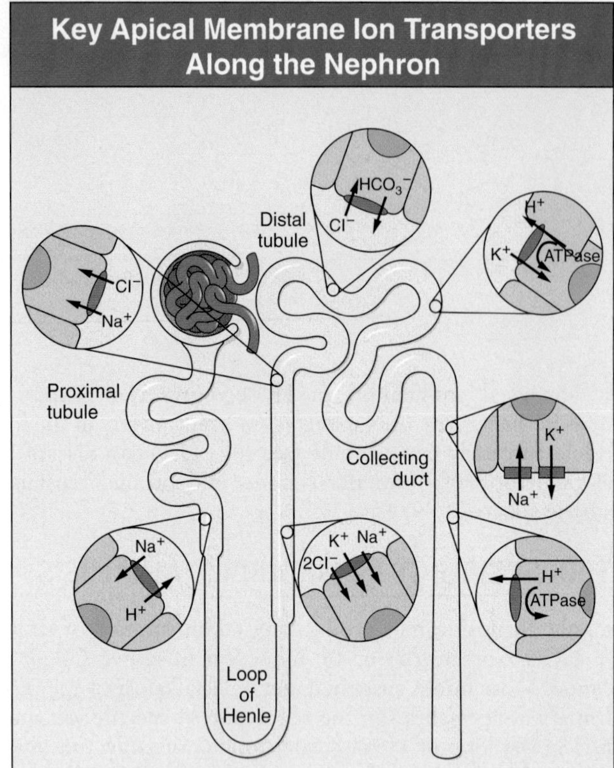

Figure 13.1 Key apical membrane ion transporters along the nephron. Bicarbonate ions (HCO_3^-) are recaptured by H^+ secretion throughout the renal tubules. In the proximal tubule and loop of Henle, H^+ secretion is directly linked to Na^+ reabsorption through the Na^+-H^+ exchanger. In addition, H^+ secretion occurs in these tubule segments through an apical membrane H^+-ATPase (not shown). In the collecting duct, H^+ secretion is indirectly coupled to Na^+ uptake through a Na^+ channel and parallel H^+-ATPase. Chloride-linked Na^+ reabsorption in the loop of Henle and early distal tubule affects H^+ secretion by determining Na^+ delivery to the collecting duct. Bicarbonate *secretion* occurs under conditions of alkalemia through a Cl^--linked exchanger. Potassium reabsorption in states of K^+ depletion is linked to H^+ secretion through a H^+,K^+-ATPase.

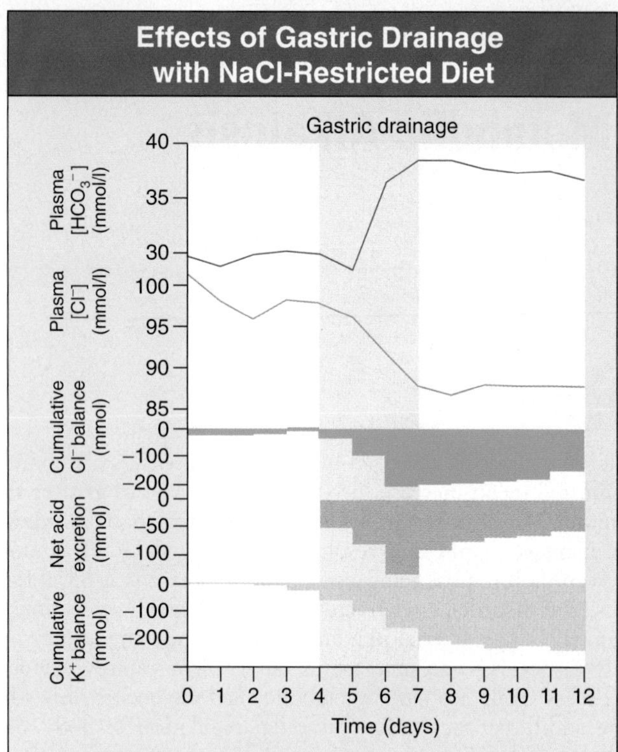

Figure 13.2 Effect of gastric drainage on plasma [HCO_3^-] and [Cl^-] and on the net balance of these two ions in the body in a normal individual ingesting a NaCl-restricted diet. Changes in net acid excretion are also shown. Gastric drainage on three consecutive nights in this subject increased plasma [HCO_3^-] by 9 mmol/l, a change that persisted after gastric drainage was stopped. Potassium depletion occurs as a result of renal K^+ losses during the period of gastric drainage. These losses are not regained, however, after the drainage is discontinued despite the continued daily ingestion of 70 mmol of K^+. Net acid excretion decreases transiently during the period of drainage but then returns to control levels despite sustained metabolic alkalosis. Chloride depletion is maintained by the low dietary intake of this ion.

dependent on sustaining the depletion of body Cl^- stores. Serum [HCO_3^-] returns to normal when sufficient Cl^- is given to replenish losses. Chloride-depletion metabolic alkalosis causes concomitant K^+ depletion through renal K^+ losses, but Cl^- administration corrects the alkalosis even if the K^+ deficit is deliberately maintained.[8] The role of Cl^- depletion, as opposed to ECF volume depletion, and the contribution of K^+ depletion in sustaining this form of metabolic alkalosis remain controversial.[4,8] Dissection of the contribution of each factor is of little importance in the clinic, however, as treatment is dictated by the particular clinical setting; some patients need NaCl to replenish extracellular volume, and most need KCl to treat K^+ depletion. A less severe Cl^--dependent metabolic alkalosis, without evident H^+ loss, is generated by the administration of thiazide or loop diuretics.

Interplay of K^+, Cl^-, and HCO_3^- Transport by the Kidney

When metabolic alkalosis is induced by Cl^- depletion and dietary Cl^- intake is restricted, a characteristic sequence of changes in renal electrolyte excretion occurs.[7] Sodium and HCO_3^- excretion increase transiently, then decrease rapidly to low levels, and K^+ excretion increases. The increase in K^+ excretion is also transient but nonetheless induces significant K^+ depletion (see Fig. 13.2). In the new steady state, urinary K^+ excretion matches intake despite persistent K^+ depletion. As a result, hypokalemia is a cardinal feature of metabolic alkalosis. Potassium depletion stimulates both H^+ secretion (through the H^+,K^+-ATPase; see Fig. 13.1) and may also stimulate HCO_3^- reabsorption in the ascending limb of the loop of Henle.[9] It also stimulates renal NH_4^+ production, facilitating the acid excretion needed to sustain metabolic alkalosis (Fig. 13.3). Although the Cl^--HCO_3^- exchanger is activated by metabolic alkalosis, continued secretion of aldosterone and collecting duct H^+ secretion appear to recapture all the secreted HCO_3^- and allow continued acid excretion. As a result, acid excretion matches net acid production in the steady state despite systemic alkalemia. When K^+ depletion is unusually severe, renal Cl^- reabsorption is also impaired, possibly by a limitation in Cl^- transport through the Na^+-K^+-$2Cl^-$ cotransporter (see Fig. 13.1), resulting in persistent Cl^- depletion despite intake or administration of this anion.[10]

Exogenous Alkali

The kidney responds rapidly to excess alkali by increasing HCO_3^- excretion, and thus metabolic alkalosis can be induced only transiently by alkali administration when renal function is

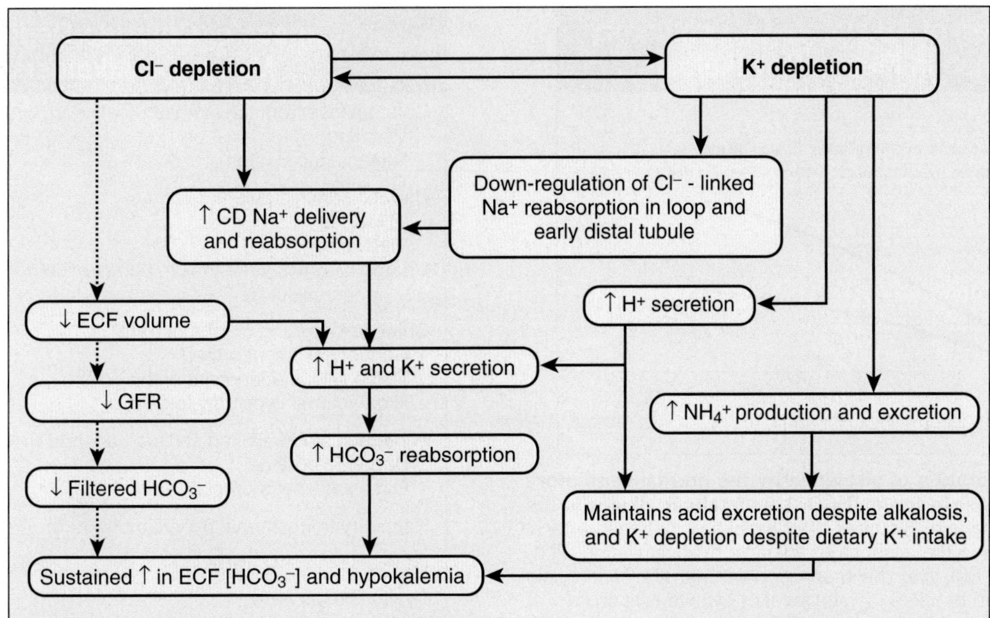

Figure 13.3 Pathophysiology of chloride-responsive metabolic alkalosis. Chloride depletion stimulates H^+ and K^+ secretion in the collecting duct as a result of disproportionate distal Na^+ delivery and reabsorption. The resultant K^+ depletion further stimulates H^+ secretion and promotes ammonium (NH_4^+) production and excretion as well as downregulating Na^+ reabsorption in the loop of Henle. These events all contribute to a sustained increase in serum [HCO_3^-]. Chloride depletion also reduces GFR and therefore HCO_3^- filtration, reducing potential alkali losses. As indicated by the *dashed lines*, the role of this effect in sustaining metabolic alkalosis remains controversial. CD, collecting duct.

normal. Even when supplemental $NaHCO_3$ is ingested daily, serum [HCO_3^-] does not increase unless dietary Cl^- intake is severely restricted.[11] If renal HCO_3^- excretion is impaired as a result of kidney failure, alkali administration can cause a sustained metabolic alkalosis independent of Cl^- intake.[12]

Primary Abnormalities in Renal Ion Transport

Acquired or inherited abnormalities in ion transport in the loop and distal tubule can cause metabolic alkalosis (Fig. 13.4). These forms of metabolic alkalosis account for less than 1% of all causes, and by far the most common of these is primary hyperaldosteronism.[13] In this disorder, persistently high and unregulated aldosterone secretion promotes Na^+ reabsorption and H^+ and K^+ secretion in the collecting duct by stimulating both the epithelial Na^+ channel and H^+-ATPase (see Figs. 13.1 and 13.4). The resultant K^+ depletion promotes NH_4^+ production and activates H^+,K^+ -ATPase activity, facilitating acid excretion. Sodium retention leads to hypertension and also ensures continued Na^+ delivery to the collecting duct, sustaining the cycle of increased reabsorption and increased K^+ and H^+ secretion. As a result of all these events, metabolic alkalosis is sustained despite normal Cl^- intake. Not surprisingly, the degree of alkalosis induced by primary hyperaldosteronism is modulated by both Cl^- and K^+ intake. More rarely, metabolic alkalosis is caused by genetic mutations in the regulation and function of specific transporters in the loop of Henle and distal nephron (see the section on etiology, Fig. 13.4, and Chapter 47).

Secondary Response to an Increase in Serum [HCO_3^-]

Regardless of the cause, blood pH increases in metabolic alkalosis and elicits secondary hypoventilation, increasing arterial Pco_2. The response is a potent one, occurring despite the concomitant

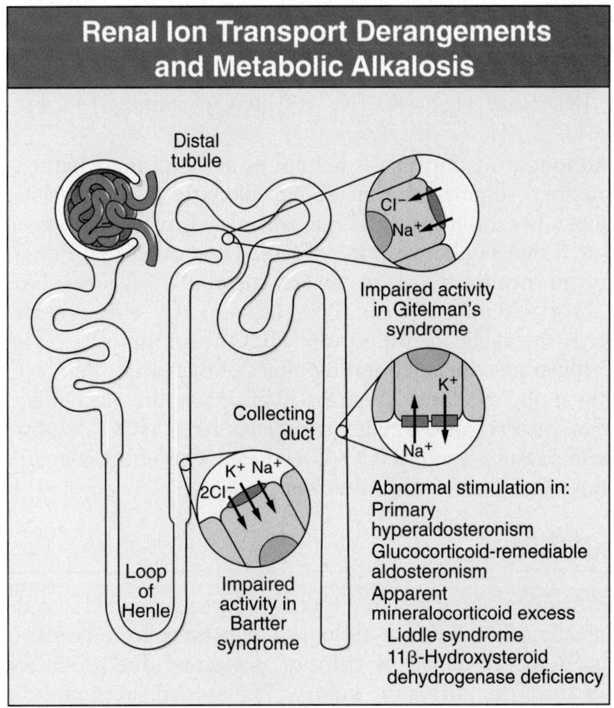

Figure 13.4 Primary derangements in renal ion transport that lead to sustained metabolic alkalosis. The epithelial Na^+ channel in the collecting duct is stimulated abnormally in primary hyperaldosteronism and in three defined genetic abnormalities. One of these causes aldosterone secretion to respond to adrenocorticotropic hormone rather than to angiotensin II (glucocorticoid-remediable aldosteronism); one blocks downregulation of the channel (Liddle syndrome), and one allows cortisol to act as a mineralocorticoid (11β-hydroxysteroid dehydrogenase deficiency). Bartter and Gitelman's syndromes are caused by genetic abnormalities that impede the activity of or inactivate Cl^--linked Na^+ reabsorption in two separate transporters in the nephron.

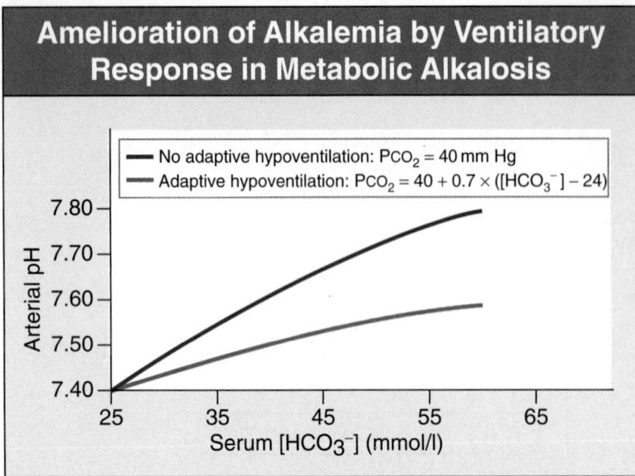

Figure 13.5 Amelioration of alkalemia by the normal ventilatory response to the increase in serum $[HCO_3^-]$ in metabolic alkalosis. The *red (upper) line* in the graph illustrates the relationship between arterial pH and serum $[HCO_3^-]$ in the absence of adaptive hypoventilation (PCO_2 maintained at 40 mm Hg), and the *green (lower) line,* the relationship when PCO_2 is increased by the expected level of hypoventilation.

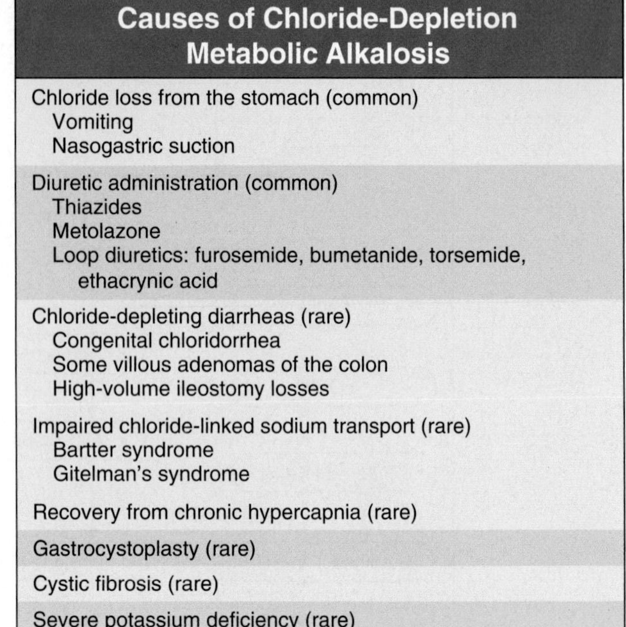

Causes of Chloride-Depletion Metabolic Alkalosis

Causes of Chloride-Depletion Metabolic Alkalosis
Chloride loss from the stomach (common) Vomiting Nasogastric suction
Diuretic administration (common) Thiazides Metolazone Loop diuretics: furosemide, bumetanide, torsemide, ethacrynic acid
Chloride-depleting diarrheas (rare) Congenital chloridorrhea Some villous adenomas of the colon High-volume ileostomy losses
Impaired chloride-linked sodium transport (rare) Bartter syndrome Gitelman's syndrome
Recovery from chronic hypercapnia (rare)
Gastrocystoplasty (rare)
Cystic fibrosis (rare)
Severe potassium deficiency (rare)

Figure 13.6 Causes of chloride-depletion metabolic alkalosis.

development of hypoxemia. On average, PCO_2 increases by 0.7 mm Hg (0.1 kP) for each 1 mmol/l increase in serum $[HCO_3^-]$. Assuming a normal $[HCO_3^-]$ and PCO_2 of 24 mmol/l and 40 mm Hg, respectively, the predicted PCO_2 for any given serum $[HCO_3^-]$ in metabolic alkalosis can be calculated as follows:

$$PCO_2(\text{mm Hg}) = 40 + 0.7 \times ([HCO_3^-](\text{mmol/l}) - 24)$$

Although this formula is helpful in determining whether the ventilatory response to metabolic alkalosis is appropriate, it implies a precision that does not exist in nature. Variations of up to 5 to 7 mm Hg between the observed and calculated PCO_2 may occur in health. Even in severe metabolic alkalosis (serum $[HCO_3^-]$ >50 mmol/l), the PCO_2 (in mm Hg) virtually always exceeds the value for the serum $[HCO_3^-]$ (in mmol/l).[14] Figure 13.5 illustrates the ameliorating effect of increasing PCO_2 on pH in metabolic alkalosis. Whereas it mitigates the alkalemia, the increase in PCO_2 also directly stimulates renal HCO_3^- reabsorption, increasing serum $[HCO_3^-]$ further.[15] This effect is small and unimportant in the clinical setting.

ETIOLOGY

The major causes of metabolic alkalosis are subdivided into three groups based on pathophysiology. The most common causes are induced and sustained by chloride depletion, due to abnormal losses from the gut or the kidney. The second subgroup, much rarer, includes the metabolic alkaloses induced and sustained by excess adrenal corticosteroids, or by collecting duct transport abnormalities that mimic excess mineralocorticoid activity. The third subgroup includes the causes of metabolic alkalosis caused by alkali administration or ingestion. This new classification replaces the traditional separation of causes based on treatment response (chloride-responsive and chloride-resistant) with a more straightforward and inclusive grouping. It also combines logically the causes of metabolic alkalosis that have the same pathophysiology (e.g., Bartter and Gitelman's syndrome and diuretic-induced metabolic alkalosis).

Chloride Depletion Metabolic Alkalosis

Figure 13.6 lists the causes of chloride depletion metabolic alkalosis.

Vomiting or Nasogastric Drainage

Loss of chloride from the upper gastrointestinal tract, often accompanied by concomitant H^+ losses, produces a metabolic alkalosis that is sustained until body Cl^- stores are replenished (see Fig. 13.2). With continued emesis or nasogastric suction and without replacement of Cl^- losses, serum $[HCO_3^-]$ may rise to very high levels (>45 mmol/l).[14]

Diuretic Administration

Diuretics that inhibit Cl^- transport proteins in the kidney are the most common cause of metabolic alkalosis (see Fig. 13.6). The thiazides and metolazone inhibit the Na^+-Cl^- cotransporter in the early distal tubule, and the loop diuretics inhibit the Na^+-K^+-$2Cl^-$ cotransporter in the ascending limb of the loop of Henle (see Fig. 13.1). These agents all impair Cl^- reabsorption, causing selective Cl^- depletion, and stimulate K^+ excretion by increasing Na^+ delivery to the collecting duct. The alkalosis produced is typically mild (serum $[HCO_3^-]$ <36 mmol/l), except in patients who continue to ingest excess salt and have extreme renal Na^+ avidity. Hypokalemia due to K^+ depletion is more prominent and is the major management problem.[16]

Impairment of Cl^--Linked Na^+ Transport

Bartter and Gitelman's syndromes are two hereditary disorders manifested by metabolic alkalosis and hypokalemia, but without hypertension (see Chapter 47). Bartter syndrome is caused by several mutations, all of which have the effect of impeding Cl^--associated Na^+ reabsorption in the ascending limb of the loop of Henle (through the Na^+-K^+-$2Cl^-$ cotransporter; see Fig. 13.4).[17,18] Patients with this syndrome usually become ill early in life with metabolic alkalosis and volume depletion, features similar to those seen in individuals abusing loop diuretic agents. Gitelman's syndrome is caused by genetic mutations that inactivate the

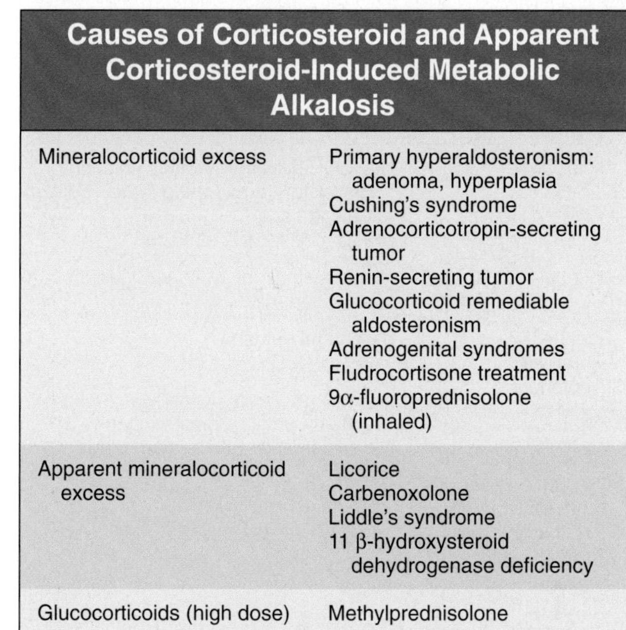

Causes of Corticosteroid and Apparent Corticosteroid-Induced Metabolic Alkalosis

Mineralocorticoid excess	Primary hyperaldosteronism: adenoma, hyperplasia Cushing's syndrome Adrenocorticotropin-secreting tumor Renin-secreting tumor Glucocorticoid remediable aldosteronism Adrenogenital syndromes Fludrocortisone treatment 9α-fluoroprednisolone (inhaled)
Apparent mineralocorticoid excess	Licorice Carbenoxolone Liddle's syndrome 11 β-hydroxysteroid dehydrogenase deficiency
Glucocorticoids (high dose)	Methylprednisolone

Figure 13.7 Causes of corticosteroid and apparent corticosteroid-induced metabolic alkalosis.

thiazide-sensitive Na^+-Cl^- cotransporter in the early distal tubule (see Fig. 13.4), leading to hypokalemia and metabolic alkalosis similar to that caused by thiazide diuretics.[18] Gitelman's syndrome becomes clinically apparent later in life and differs from Bartter syndrome in that hypomagnesemia and hypocalciuria are prominent features.[17]

Recovery from Chronic Hypercapnia

The renal response to sustained hypercapnia results in an increase in HCO_3^- reabsorption and a decrease in Cl^- reabsorption (see Chapter 14). As a result, serum [HCO_3^-] increases and body Cl^- stores are reduced. When P_{CO_2} is restored to normal, renal excretion of excess HCO_3^- requires repletion of the Cl^- losses incurred during adaptation. If these losses are not replaced, recovery from hypercapnia can result in a persistent metabolic alkalosis.

Congenital Chloridorrhea

This rare form of diarrhea is caused by an inactivating mutation in the "down-regulated in adenoma" (*DRA*) gene, an apical membrane Cl^--HCO_3^- exchanger in the small intestine.[19] The result is a large-volume diarrhea that is rich in Cl^-, causing selective loss of this ion as well as H^+ and K^+ losses. The resultant metabolic alkalosis is ameliorated by K^+ and Cl^- administration, but correction is difficult because of continuing losses. Interestingly, the volume of diarrhea is reduced dramatically by proton pump inhibition, which reduces gastric Cl^- secretion and presumably reduces Cl^- delivery to the small intestine.[20]

Other Causes of Excessive Chloride Losses

Villous adenomas occur in the distal colon and typically secrete 1 to 3 liters of fluid a day that is rich in Na^+, Cl^-, and K^+. Because the volume of secreted fluid is relatively low, these tumors are only occasionally associated with metabolic alkalosis, and the disorder, when it is present, is usually mild.[21] Cystic fibrosis is characterized by high sweat [Cl^-], and with excessive sweating, Cl^- losses can be large enough to cause metabolic alkalosis. In children and adolescents, this acid-base disorder can be the presenting symptom.[22] Patients with high-volume ileostomy losses can sometimes develop severe metabolic alkalosis.[23] In these cases, the fluid contains abnormally high concentrations of Na^+ and Cl^-. The use of gastric tissue to augment bladder size (gastrocystoplasty) can occasionally lead to transient metabolic alkalosis as a result of gastrin-induced Cl^- secretion into the urine.[24]

Severe K^+ Deficiency

In patients with severe K^+ depletion (serum [K^+] <2 mmol/l), metabolic alkalosis can be sustained despite Cl^- administration.[10] Chloride resistance in this setting is probably due to impairment of renal Cl^- reabsorption (see earlier discussion). Even partial repletion of K^+ stores rapidly reverses this problem and makes the alkalosis Cl^- responsive.

Corticosteroid and Apparent Corticosteroid-Induced Metabolic Alkalosis

Figure 13.7 lists the causes of these forms of metabolic alkalosis.

Mineralocorticoid Excess

Aldosterone and other mineralocorticoids cause metabolic alkalosis by stimulating both the H^+-ATPase and epithelial Na^+ channel (ENaC) in the collecting duct (see Figs. 13.1 and 13.4). The resultant Na^+ retention causes hypertension and also ensures continued delivery of Na^+ to the distal nephron, facilitating continued H^+ and K^+ secretion. The metabolic alkalosis is typically mild (serum [HCO_3^-] 30 to 35 mmol/l) and is associated with more severe hypokalemia (K^+ often <3 mmol/l) than is observed in most Cl^--responsive causes.[9,13] Primary hyperaldosteronism is by far the most common cause of this form of metabolic alkalosis (see Chapter 38), but it can also occur with rarer hereditary defects in cortisol synthesis or in the regulation of aldosterone secretion (see Fig. 13.7). Glucocorticoid-remediable aldosteronism (see Chapter 38) is caused by a mutation that results in stimulation of aldosterone secretion by adrenocorticotropic hormone (ACTH) rather than by angiotensin.[25] Fludrocortisone, an oral mineralocorticoid drug, as well as inhaled 9α-fluoroprednisolone can induce metabolic alkalosis if it is used inappropriately. Corticosteroids, when they are administered in very high doses, increase renal K^+ excretion nonspecifically and produce a mild increase in serum [HCO_3^-].

Apparent Mineralocorticoid Excess Syndromes

Several inherited abnormalities produce a metabolic alkalosis that is clinically indistinguishable from hyperaldosteronism but without measurable aldosterone (see Chapter 47). Liddle syndrome results from a genetic mutation that prevents the removal of epithelial Na^+ channels from the urinary membrane of collecting duct epithelial cells (see Fig. 13.4).[26] As a result, Na^+ reabsorption cannot be downregulated, causing the same cascade of events seen in hyperaldosteronism. Because continuous stimulation of Na^+ reabsorption expands ECF volume, however, aldosterone levels are vanishingly low. In another rare familial disorder, termed the syndrome of apparent mineralocorticoid excess, a mutation inactivates 11β-hydroxysteroid dehydrogenase, an enzyme adjacent to the mineralocorticoid receptor that rapidly converts cortisol to cortisone, minimizing cortisol binding to this receptor.[27] When the enzyme is inactivated, cortisol activates the receptor, stimulating Na^+ reabsorption and K^+ secretion and producing Cl^--resistant metabolic alkalosis and hypertension with low aldosterone levels. Glycyrrhizic acid (a component of natural licorice), carbenoxolone, and gossypol

Causes of Metabolic Alkalosis Associated with Alkali Administration	
Renal Status	**Causes**
Normal renal function (only in association with K^+ depletion or low NaCl intake)	Alkali intake: $NaHCO_3$, citrate, lactate, acetate, amino acid anions
Renal failure	Milk–alkali syndrome Alkali intake Aluminum hydroxide with K^+ exchange resin

Figure 13.8 Causes of metabolic alkalosis associated with alkali administration.

(an agent that inhibits spermatogenesis) inhibit the activity of 11β-hydroxysteroid dehydrogenase and can cause the same clinical picture.[9]

Alkali Administration

Exogenous alkali produces metabolic alkalosis in individuals with deficient body K^+ or Cl^- stores by impaired renal HCO_3^- excretion (Fig. 13.8; see earlier discussion).[11] In acute or chronic renal impairment, alkali administration or ingestion produces metabolic alkalosis independent of K^+ and Cl^- stores because the excess alkali cannot be excreted.[12] Milk-alkali syndrome is characterized by the concomitant presence of metabolic alkalosis and renal insufficiency, brought on by the ingestion of $NaHCO_3$ in combination with excess calcium (either in milk or as $CaCO_3$).[28,29] In this disorder, renal damage is caused by calcium deposition (facilitated by an alkaline urine). The renal damage in turn facilitates the development of metabolic alkalosis if alkali ingestion continues. Metabolic alkalosis is usually mild in these patients unless they develop concomitant vomiting. In hospitalized patients with renal failure, a wide variety of alkali sources or alkali precursors can cause metabolic alkalosis (Fig. 13.9). Although it is only rarely administered now, aluminum hydroxide in combination with sodium polystyrene sulfonate (Kayexalate) can cause metabolic alkalosis because aluminum binds to the resin in exchange for Na^+. As a result, the HCO_3^- normally secreted into the duodenum is not titrated by H^+ (which was neutralized by the aluminum hydroxide), nor does it form an insoluble salt with aluminum. Instead, it is completely reabsorbed from the gut, increasing serum [HCO_3^-].[30]

Other Causes

Refeeding after starvation causes an abrupt increase in serum [HCO_3^-] from the low levels characteristic of the fasting state. In some instances, serum [HCO_3^-] increases transiently above normal, causing a mild metabolic alkalosis. The causes are multiple, including HCO_3^- generation from metabolism of accumulated organic anions and K^+ and Cl^- depletion. Administration of vitamin D causes a small but significant increase in serum [HCO_3^-].[31,32] Hyperparathyroidism in the clinic, however, is not associated with metabolic alkalosis. Hypercalcemia and vitamin D intoxication have been associated with metabolic alkalosis, but in most instances, the alkalosis can be explained by the vomiting that characteristically accompanies these disorders. High aldosterone levels induced by hyperreninemia in renovascular or malignant hypertension are associated with hypokalemia and, occasionally, with very minor increases in serum [HCO_3^-].

Potential Sources of Alkali	
Alkali/Alkali Precursor	**Source**
Bicarbonate	$NaHCO_3$: pills, intravenous solutions Proprietary brands, e.g., Alka–Seltzer Baking soda $KHCO_3$: pills, oral solutions
Lactate	Ringer's solution, peritoneal dialysis solutions
Acetate Glutamate Propionate	Parenteral nutrition
Citrate	Blood products, plasma exchange, K^+ supplements, alkalinizing agents
Calcium compounds (alkalinizing effect minimal when given orally) Acetate Citrate Carbonate	Calcium supplements, phosphate binders

Figure 13.9 Potential sources of alkali.

CLINICAL MANIFESTATIONS

Mild to moderate metabolic alkalosis is well tolerated, with few clinically important adverse effects. Patients with serum [HCO_3^-] levels as high as 40 mmol/l are usually asymptomatic. The adverse effect of most concern is hypokalemia, which increases the likelihood of cardiac arrhythmias in patients with ischemic heart disease.[33] With more severe metabolic alkalosis (serum [HCO_3^-] >45 mmol/l), arterial Po_2 often decreases to less than 50 mm Hg (<6.65 kP) secondary to hypoventilation, and ionized calcium decreases (due to alkalemia). Patients with serum [HCO_3^-] greater than 50 mmol/l may develop seizures, tetany, delirium, or stupor. These changes in mental status are probably multifactorial in origin, due to alkalemia, hypokalemia, hypocalcemia, and hypoxemia.

DIAGNOSIS

Diagnosis of metabolic alkalosis involves three steps (Fig. 13.10). The first step, detection, is most often based on the finding of an elevated serum [total CO_2]. The second step is evaluation of the secondary response (hypoventilation), excluding the possibility that a respiratory acid-base abnormality is also present. This step requires measurement of arterial pH and Pco_2. The third step is determination of the cause.

Serum [total CO_2] above 30 mmol/l in association with hypokalemia is virtually pathognomonic of metabolic alkalosis. The only other cause of an elevated serum [HCO_3^-] is chronic respiratory acidosis, and hypokalemia is not a feature of this disorder (see Chapter 14). Because the diagnosis is usually evident and the disorder is almost always uncomplicated, one need not measure arterial pH and Pco_2 in most patients.

If the alkalosis is severe (serum [HCO_3^-] >40 mmol/l), if the cause of the elevated [HCO_3^-] is unclear, or if a mixed acid-base disorder is suspected, however, one should always measure pH

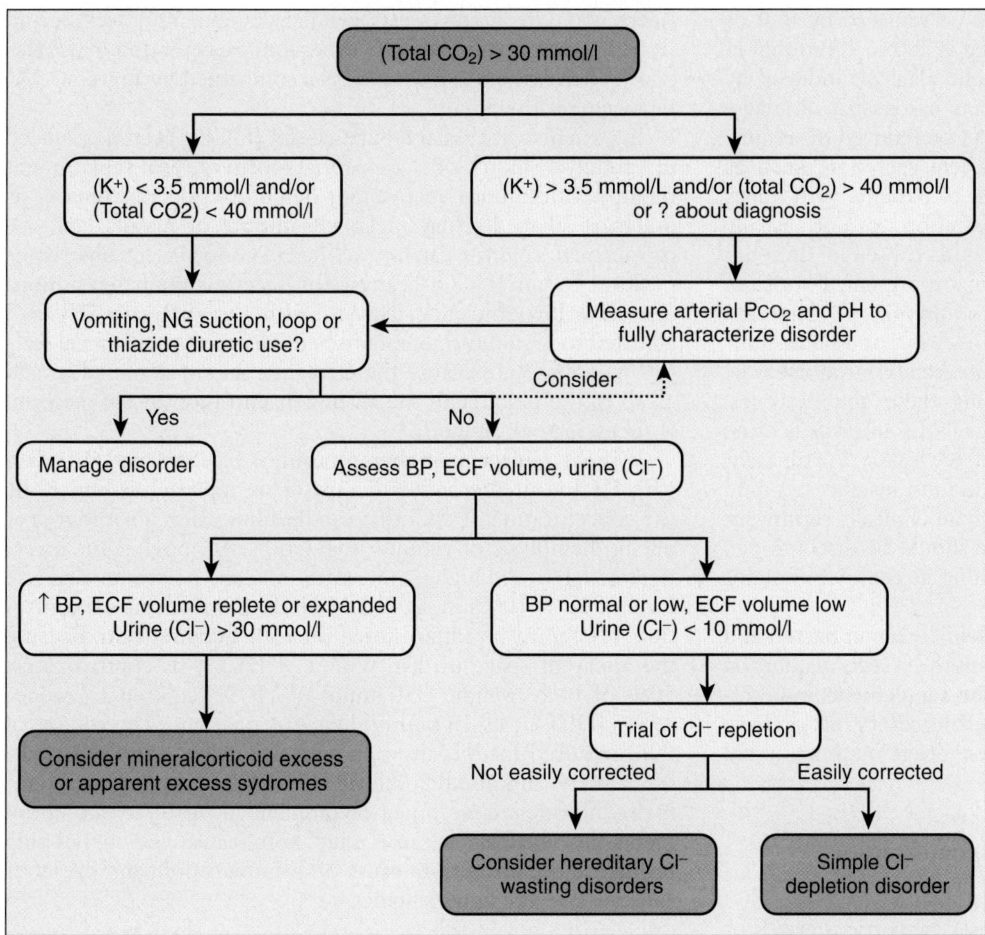

Figure 13.10 Approach to diagnosis of metabolic alkalosis. If the increase in [total CO_2] (or serum [HCO_3^-]) is mild and hypokalemia is present, arterial gas measurements are usually not necessary, and a simple algorithm can be used to diagnose Cl^--responsive and Cl^--resistant metabolic alkalosis. If hypokalemia is not present, if the increase in serum [total CO_2] is severe, or if there is a question about the diagnosis, arterial measurement of pH and Pco_2 is recommended to determine whether the condition is due to metabolic alkalosis, respiratory acidosis, or a mixed disorder. BP, blood pressure; ECF, extracellular fluid; NG, nasogastric.

and Pco_2 to fully characterize the disorder (see Fig. 13.10). These measurements confirm the presence of alkalosis and allow an estimation of whether the degree of hypoventilation is appropriate for the serum [HCO_3^-] (see earlier equation). A major deviation in Pco_2 from the expected value indicates the presence of a complicating respiratory acid-base disorder (either respiratory acidosis or alkalosis; see Chapter 14). The anion gap, [Na^+] – ([Cl^-] + [HCO_3^-]), is not increased in mild to moderate metabolic alkalosis, but it can be increased by as much as 3 to 5 mmol/l when alkalosis is severe. If the anion gap is more than 20 mmol/l, the disorder is most likely complicated by a superimposed metabolic acidosis (see Chapter 12).

In most instances, the third step, elucidation of the cause, is also straightforward. In more than 95% of cases, metabolic alkalosis is caused either by diuretic use or by Cl^- losses from the gastrointestinal tract. This is usually easily obtained from the history, and attention can be directed toward the appropriate treatment. If the cause is unclear from the history, measurement of urine [Cl^-] can help. Unless the patient has recently taken a diuretic agent, urine [Cl^-] should be less than 10 mmol/l if the metabolic alkalosis is due to Cl^- depletion. A confounding problem can be self-induced vomiting (bulimia) or the surreptitious use of diuretics, which presents the greater diagnostic dilemma because continued diuretic-induced Cl^- excretion may lead one to undertake an extensive workup for rarer forms of metabolic alkalosis. Urinary screens for specific diuretic compounds may be necessary to establish the correct diagnosis. In bulimic patients, urine Cl^- excretion should be low (spot urine [Cl^-] <10 mmol/l). If the cause is not apparent from this analysis, rarer forms of metabolic alkalosis caused by tubular transport abnormalities should be considered. In these forms of metabolic alkalosis, urine [Cl^-] is typically greater than 30 mmol/l.

In the patient with hypertension and adequate chloride intake, who is not taking any diuretic agents, the most common cause of metabolic alkalosis is primary hyperaldosteronism. Measurement of serum renin and serum or urine aldosterone levels can distinguish mineralocorticoid excess syndromes from the rarer syndromes of apparent mineralocorticoid excess (see Fig. 13.7). The details of such a workup are presented in Chapter 38. In the normotensive or hypotensive patient who is not taking any diuretic agents and has metabolic alkalosis despite adequate chloride intake, the diagnosis of either Bartter or Gitelman's syndrome should be considered. Aldosterone and renin levels are not helpful in making these diagnoses because the levels can be low or high, depending on the patient's ECF volume at the time of measurement. Familial genetic studies can establish these diagnoses with high specificity.

TREATMENT

Chloride Depletion Alkalosis

In the patient with metabolic alkalosis due to nasogastric drainage or vomiting, ECF volume depletion is always a concomitant feature, and treatment is straightforward. Administration of intravenous NaCl will correct both the alkalosis and the volume depletion. Potassium losses should also be replaced by oral or intravenous KCl. Typically, the K^+ deficit is 200 to 400 mmol in patients with mild to moderate metabolic alkalosis induced by upper gastrointestinal Cl^- losses. When nasogastric drainage must be continued, H^+ and Cl^- losses can be reduced by administration of drugs that inhibit gastric acid secretion, such as famotidine and omeprazole. In contrast to patients with upper gastrointestinal losses, NaCl administration is not usually required in patients with metabolic alkalosis caused by diuretics unless clinical signs of volume depletion are present. Potassium chloride supplements should be given to minimize K^+ depletion as well as the metabolic alkalosis. The addition of a potassium-sparing diuretic, such as amiloride, triamterene, spironolactone, or eplerenone, can assist in minimizing these abnormalities. Complete repair of diuretic-induced metabolic alkalosis is often difficult because of continued Cl^- and K^+ losses. Fortunately, such a therapeutic goal is not necessary in most instances. A mild metabolic alkalosis is well tolerated, with no clinically significant adverse effects. If possible, the diuretic should be discontinued and then the disorder will resolve so long as the diet contains adequate K^+ and Cl^-.

The metabolic alkalosis (and hypokalemia) seen in Bartter and Gitelman's syndromes is the most difficult to correct. In addition to oral KCl supplements (and magnesium supplements in Gitelman's syndrome), nonsteroidal anti-inflammatory drugs have been used with moderate success. These drugs minimize renal Cl^- losses.

Corticosteroid and Apparent Corticosteroid-Induced Metabolic Alkalosis

Management of metabolic alkalosis caused by corticosteroids or tubular transport abnormalities that mimic corticosteroid excess depends on the underlying cause. If the alkalosis is caused by an adrenal adenoma, the disorder is corrected by surgical removal of the tumor (see Chapter 38). In other forms of primary hyperaldosteronism, the alkalosis can be minimized by dietary NaCl restriction and by aggressive replacement of body K^+ stores with supplemental KCl. Spironolactone or eplerenone, competitive inhibitors of aldosterone, can also correct the disorder. In glucocorticoid-remediable aldosteronism, the disorder is corrected by dexamethasone administration, which suppresses ACTH secretion and thereby reduces aldosterone secretion. In the hereditary forms of apparent mineralocorticoid excess (Liddle syndrome and 11β-hydroxysteroid dehydrogenase deficiency), amiloride is the most effective treatment.

Alkali Ingestion

Treatment here is directed at identification and discontinuation of the offending alkali (see Fig. 13.9). In the intensive care unit, care should be taken to look for sources of exogenous alkali. A common offender is acetate used as a replacement for Cl^- in parenteral nutrition solutions.

SPECIAL PROBLEMS IN MANAGEMENT

Management of metabolic alkalosis is a more difficult undertaking in patients with severe congestive heart failure or renal failure. In patients with heart failure and fluid overload who still have renal function, acetazolamide can be used to reduce serum $[HCO_3^-]$. This carbonic anhydrase inhibitor blocks H^+-linked Na^+ reabsorption, leading to excretion of both Na^+ and HCO_3^-. Acetazolamide decreases extracellular volume and lowers serum $[HCO_3^-]$, but it stimulates K^+ excretion, exacerbating hypokalemia. When it is used, it should be accompanied by aggressive K^+ replacement therapy.

In patients with renal failure, serum $[HCO_3^-]$ can be reduced in a timely fashion by the appropriate form of renal replacement therapy. Continuous venovenous hemofiltration can remove as much as 20 to 30 l/day of an ultrafiltrate of plasma, and the replacement solution can be modified to control electrolyte composition. Serum $[HCO_3^-]$ can also be lowered rapidly by continuous slow low-efficiency dialysis, with the dialysate $[HCO_3^-]$ adjusted to 23 mmol/l. Standard hemodialysis or peritoneal dialysis is less useful because these treatments are designed to add alkali to the blood, and the alkali concentration in the dialysate is set at 35 to 40 mmol/l.

If renal replacement therapy cannot be instituted, titration with HCl is an alternative therapy. This approach is limited by the concentration of HCl that can be administered without producing hemolysis or venous coagulation. Although some investigators have used higher concentrations, the recommended safe level of H^+ is 100 mmol/l (0.1 N HCl). Even at this concentration, HCl must be administered through a central vein. Because the apparent space of distribution of HCO_3^- is approximately 50% of body weight, 350 mmol of H^+ is required to reduce serum $[HCO_3^-]$ by 10 mmol/l in a 70-kg patient. The volume of fluid required for this titration with use of HCl, unfortunately, is 3.5 liters. Ammonium chloride (NH_4Cl) and arginine monohydrochloride are no longer recommended for the treatment of metabolic alkalosis because they both cause life-threatening problems; the former can cause NH_3 intoxication, and the latter can cause severe hyperkalemia.

REFERENCES

1. Gennari FJ. Regulation of acid-base balance: Overview. In: Gennari FJ, Adrogue HJ, Galla JH, Madias NE, eds. *Acid-Base Disorders and Their Treatment*. Taylor & Francis: Boca Raton; 2005:177-208.
2. Ahn KY, Park KY, Kim KK, Kone BC. Chronic hypokalemia enhances expression of the H^+-K^+-ATPase α_2-subunit gene in renal medulla. *Am J Physiol*. 1996;271:F314-F321.
3. Royaux IE, Kim YH, Stanley L, et al. Pendrin, encoded by the Pendred syndrome gene, resides in the apical region of renal intercalated cells and mediates bicarbonate secretion. *Proc Natl Acad Sci U S A*. 2001; 98:4221-4226.
4. Jacobson HR, Seldin DW. On the generation, maintenance, and correction of metabolic alkalosis. *Am J Physiol*. 1983;245:F425-F432.
5. Galla JH. Chloride-depletion alkalosis. In: Gennari FJ, Adrogue HJ, Galla JH, Madias NE, eds. *Acid-Base Disorders and Their Treatment*. Taylor & Francis: Boca Raton; 2005:519-551.
6. Hernandez RE, Schambelan M, Cogan MG, et al. Dietary NaCl determines the severity of potassium depletion–induced metabolic alkalosis. *Kidney Int*. 1987;31:1356-1367.
7. Kassirer JP, Schwartz WB. The response of normal man to selective depletion of hydrochloric acid. *Am J Med*. 1966;40:10-18.
8. Kassirer JP, Schwartz WB. Correction of metabolic alkalosis in man without repair of potassium deficiency. *Am J Med*. 1966;40:19-26.
9. Soleimani M. Potassium-depletion metabolic alkalosis. In: Gennari FJ, Adrogue HJ, Galla JH, Madias NE, eds. *Acid-Base Disorders and Their Treatment*. Taylor & Francis: Boca Raton; 2005:553-584.
10. Garella S, Chazan JA, Cohen JJ. Saline resistant metabolic alkalosis or "chloride-wasting nephropathy." *Ann Intern Med*. 1970;73:31-38.
11. Cogan MG, Carneiro MW, Tatsumo J, et al. Normal diet NaCl variation can affect the set point for plasma pH-HCO_3^- maintenance. *J Am Soc Nephrol*. 1990;1:193-199.
12. Gennari FJ, Rimmer JM. Acid-base disorders in end-stage renal disease: Part II. *Semin Dial*. 1990;3:161-165.
13. Holland OB. Primary hyperaldosteronism. *Semin Nephrol*. 1995;15: 116-125.

14. Javaheri S, Nardell EA. Severe metabolic alkalosis: A case report. *Br Med J (Clin Res Ed)*. 1981;283:1016-1017.
15. Madias NE, Adrogue HJ, Cohen JJ. Maladaptive renal response to chronic metabolic alkalosis. *Am J Physiol*. 1980;238:F283-F289.
16. Gennari FJ. Hypokalemia. *N Engl J Med*. 1998;339:451-458.
17. Guay-Woodford LM. Bartter syndrome: Unraveling the pathophysiologic enigma. *Am J Med*. 1998;105:151-161.
18. Simon DB, Lifton RJ. The molecular basis of inherited hypokalemic alkalosis: Bartter and Gitelman syndromes. *Am J Physiol*. 1996;271:F961-F966.
19. Hoglund P, Haila S, Socha J, et al. Mutations of the down-regulated in adenoma (DRA) gene cause congenital chloride diarrhea. *Nat Genet*. 1996;14:316-319.
20. Aichbichler BW, Zerr CH, Santa Ana CA, et al. Proton-pump inhibition of gastric chloride secretion in congenital chloridorrhea. *N Engl J Med*. 1997;336:106-109.
21. Babior BM. Villous adenoma of the colon. Study of a patient with severe fluid and electrolyte disturbances. *Am J Med*. 1966;41:615-621.
22. Bates CM, Baum M, Quigley R. Cystic fibrosis presenting with hypokalemia and metabolic alkalosis in a previously healthy adolescent. *J Am Soc Nephrol*. 1997;8:352-356.
23. Weise WJ, Serrano FA, Fought J, Gennari FJ. Acute electrolyte and acid-base disorders in patients with ileostomies: A case series. *Am J Kidney Dis*. 2008;52:494-500.
24. DeFoor W, Minevich E, Reeves D, et al. Gastrocystoplasty: Long-term follow-up. *J Urol*. 2003;170:1647-1650.
25. Lifton RP, Dluhy RG, Powers M, et al. A chimaeric 11β-hydroxylase/aldosterone synthase gene causes glucocorticoid-remediable aldosteronism and human hypertension. *Nature*. 1992;355:262-265.
26. Tamura H, Schild L, Enomoto N, et al. Liddle disease caused by a missense mutation of β-subunit of the epithelial sodium channel gene. *J Clin Invest*. 1996;97:1780-1784.
27. Whorwood CB, Stewart PM. Human hypertension caused by mutations in the 11β-hydroxysteroid dehydrogenase gene: A molecular analysis of apparent mineralocorticoid excess. *J Hypertens*. 1996;14(suppl 5):S19-S24.
28. Orwoll ES. The milk-alkali syndrome: Current concepts. *Ann Intern Med*. 1982;97:242-248.
29. Beall DP, Scofield RH. Milk-alkali syndrome associated with calcium carbonate consumption. *Medicine (Baltimore)*. 1995;74:89-96.
30. Madias NE, Levey AS. Metabolic alkalosis due to absorption of "nonabsorbable" antacids. *Am J Med*. 1983;74:155-158.
31. Hulter HN, Sebastian A, Toto RD, et al. Renal and systemic effects of the chronic administration of hypercalcemia-producing agents: Calcitriol, PTH and intravenous calcium. *Kidney Int*. 1982;21:445-458.
32. Hulter HN, Peterson JC. Acid-base homeostasis during chronic PTH excess in humans. *Kidney Int*. 1985;28:187-192.
33. Schulman M, Narins RG. Hypokalemia and cardiovascular disease. *Am J Cardiol*. 1990;65:4E-9E.

CHAPTER 14

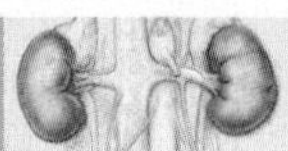

Respiratory Acidosis, Respiratory Alkalosis, and Mixed Disorders

Horacio J. Adrogué, Nicolaos E. Madias

Deviations of systemic acidity in either direction can have adverse consequences and, when severe, can be life-threatening. Therefore, it is essential for the clinician to recognize and properly diagnose acid-base disorders, to understand their impact on organ function, and to be familiar with their treatment and the potential complications of treatment.[1,2]

RESPIRATORY ACIDOSIS (PRIMARY HYPERCAPNIA)

Definition

Respiratory acidosis is the acid-base disturbance initiated by an increase in CO_2 tension of body fluids and in whole-body CO_2 stores. The secondary increment in plasma bicarbonate [HCO_3^-] observed in acute and chronic hypercapnia is an integral part of the respiratory acidosis.[3] The level of arterial CO_2 tension ($Paco_2$) is above 45 mm Hg (to convert values from mm Hg to kP, multiply by 0.1333) in patients with simple respiratory acidosis (measured at rest and at sea level). An element of respiratory acidosis may still occur with lower $Paco_2$ in patients residing at high altitude (e.g., 4000 m or 13,000 ft) or with metabolic acidosis, in whom a normal $Paco_2$ is inappropriately high for this condition.[4] Another special case of respiratory acidosis is the presence of arterial eucapnia, or even hypocapnia, occurring together with severe venous hypercapnia, in patients having an acute, profound decrease in cardiac output but relative preservation of respiratory function.[5,6] This disorder is known as pseudorespiratory alkalosis and is discussed under respiratory alkalosis.

Etiology and Pathogenesis

The ventilatory system is responsible for eucapnia by adjustment of alveolar minute ventilation ($\dot{V}_A$) to match the rate of CO_2 production. Its main elements are the respiratory pump, which generates a pressure gradient responsible for airflow, and the loads that oppose such action.

Carbon dioxide retention can occur from an imbalance between the strength of the respiratory pump and the extent of respiratory load (Fig. 14.1). When the respiratory pump is unable to balance the opposing load, respiratory acidosis develops. Respiratory acidosis may be acute or chronic (Figs. 14.2 and 14.3). Life-threatening acidemia of respiratory origin can occur during severe, acute respiratory acidosis or during respiratory decompensation in patients with chronic hypercapnia.

A simplified form of the alveolar gas equation at sea level and on breathing of room air (Fio_2, 21%) is as follows:

$$P_{AO_2} = 150 - 1.25\ Paco_2$$

where P_{AO_2} is alveolar O_2 tension (mm Hg). This equation demonstrates that patients breathing room air cannot reach $Paco_2$ levels much greater than 80 mm Hg (10.6 kP) because the hypoxemia that would occur at greater values is incompatible with life. Therefore, extreme hypercapnia occurs only during O_2 therapy, and severe CO_2 retention is often the result of uncontrolled O_2 administration.

Secondary Physiologic Response

Adaptation to acute hypercapnia elicits an immediate increment in plasma HCO_3^- concentration due to titration of non-HCO_3^- body buffers; such buffers generate HCO_3^- by combining with H^+ derived from the dissociation of carbonic acid:

$$CO_2 + H_2O \leftrightarrow H_2CO_3 \leftrightarrow HCO_3^- + H^+ \text{ and } H^+ + B^- \leftrightarrow HB$$

where B^- refers to the base component and HB refers to the acid component of non-HCO_3^- buffers. This adaptation is completed within 5 to 10 minutes from the increase in $Paco_2$, and assuming a stable level of hypercapnia, no further change in acid-base equilibrium is detectable for a few hours.[7] Moderate hypoxemia does not alter the adaptive response to acute respiratory acidosis. However, preexisting hypobicarbonatemia (whether it is caused by metabolic acidosis or chronic respiratory alkalosis) enhances the magnitude of the HCO_3^- response to acute hypercapnia; this response is diminished in hyperbicarbonatemic states (whether they are caused by metabolic alkalosis or chronic respiratory acidosis).[8,9]

The adaptive increase in plasma HCO_3^- concentration observed in acute hypercapnia is amplified greatly during chronic hypercapnia as a result of HCO_3^- generation by the kidney. In addition, the renal response to chronic hypercapnia includes a reduction in the rate of Cl^- reabsorption, resulting in depletion of body Cl^- stores. Complete adaptation to chronic hypercapnia requires 3 to 5 days.[7] Quantitative aspects of the secondary physiologic responses to acute and chronic hypercapnia are depicted in Figure 14.4. The renal response to chronic hypercapnia is not altered appreciably by dietary Na^+ or Cl^- restriction, moderate K^+ depletion, alkali loading, or moderate hypoxemia. However, recovery from chronic hypercapnia is crippled by a diet deficient in Cl^-; in this circumstance, despite correction of the level of $Paco_2$, plasma [HCO_3^-] remains elevated so long as the state of Cl^- deprivation persists, leading to posthypercapnic metabolic alkalosis.

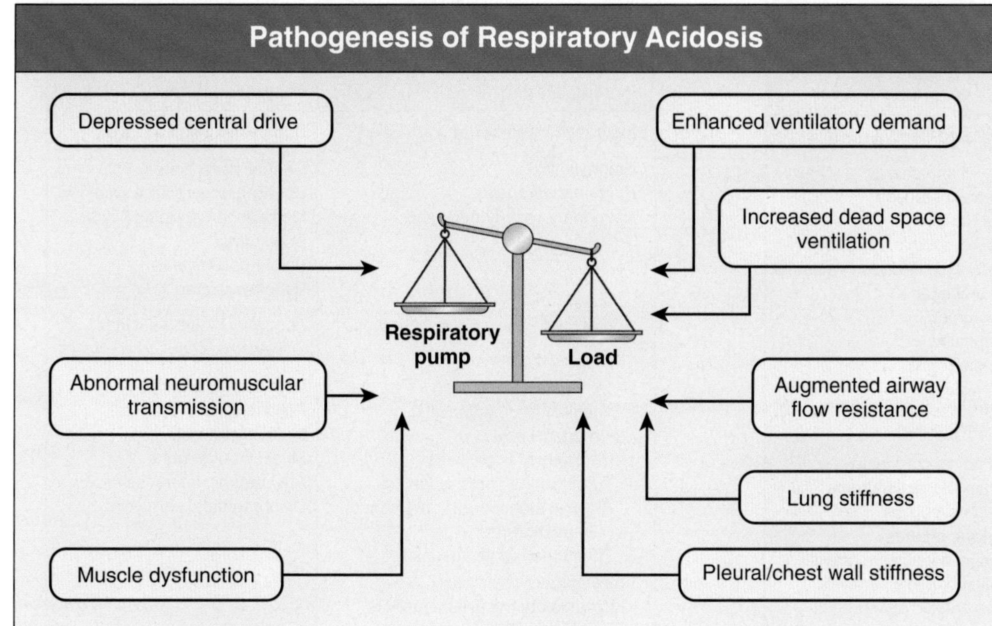

Figure 14.1 Pathogenesis of respiratory acidosis.

Clinical Manifestations

Because clinical hypercapnia almost always occurs in association with hypoxemia, it is often difficult to determine whether a specific manifestation is the consequence of the elevated $Paco_2$ or the reduced Pao_2. Nevertheless, one should bear in mind several characteristic manifestations of neurologic or cardiovascular dysfunction to diagnose the condition accurately and to treat it effectively.[4,7]

Neurologic Symptoms

Acute hypercapnia is often associated with marked anxiety, severe breathlessness, disorientation, confusion, incoherence, and combativeness. A narcotic-like effect is not uncommon in patients with chronic hypercapnia, and drowsiness, decreased alertness, inattention, forgetfulness, loss of memory, irritability, confusion, and somnolence can be observed. Motor disturbances, including tremor, myoclonic jerks, and asterixis, are frequently observed with both acute and chronic hypercapnia. Sustained myoclonus and seizure activity can also develop. Signs and symptoms of increased intracranial pressure (pseudotumor cerebri) are occasionally evident in patients with either acute or chronic hypercapnia, and they appear to be related to the vasodilating effects of CO_2 on cerebral blood vessels. Headache is a frequent complaint. Blurring of the optic discs and frank papilledema can be found when hypercapnia is severe. Hypercapnic coma characteristically occurs in patients with acute exacerbations of chronic respiratory insufficiency who are treated injudiciously with high-flow O_2.

Cardiovascular Symptoms

Acute hypercapnia of mild to moderate degree is usually characterized by warm and flushed skin, bounding pulse, sweating, increased cardiac output, and normal or increased blood pressure. By comparison, severe hypercapnia might be attended by decreases in both cardiac output and blood pressure. Cardiac arrhythmias occur frequently in patients with either acute or chronic hypercapnia, especially those receiving digoxin.

Renal Symptoms

Mild to moderate hypercapnia results in renal vasodilation, but acute increments in $Paco_2$ to levels above 70 mm Hg (9.3 kP) can induce renal vasoconstriction and hypoperfusion. Salt and water retention commonly attend sustained hypercapnia, especially in the presence of cor pulmonale. In addition to the effects of heart failure on the kidney, multiple other factors might be at play, including the prevailing stimulation of the sympathetic nervous system and the renin-angiotensin-aldosterone axis, the increased renal vascular resistance, and the elevated levels of antidiuretic hormone and cortisol.

Diagnosis

Whenever CO_2 retention is suspected, arterial blood gas values should be obtained.[10] If the patient's acid-base profile reveals hypercapnia in association with acidemia, at least an element of respiratory acidosis must be present. However, hypercapnia can be associated with a normal or even an alkaline pH if certain additional acid-base disorders are also present. Information from the patient's history, physical examination, and ancillary laboratory data should be used to assess whether part or all of the increase in $Paco_2$ reflects an adaptive response to metabolic alkalosis rather than being primary in origin.

Treatment

As previously noted, CO_2 retention, whether it is acute or chronic, is always associated with hypoxemia in patients breathing room air. Consequently, O_2 administration represents a critical element in the management of respiratory acidosis.[1,11] However, supplemental O_2 may lead to worsening hypercapnia, especially in patients with chronic obstructive pulmonary disease (COPD). Although a depressed respiratory drive in CO_2 retention seems to play a role, other factors might account for the worsening hypercapnia in response to supplemental O_2 therapy. These include an increase in dead space ventilation and

Causes of Acute Respiratory Acidosis

Increased Load	Depressed Pump
Enhanced Ventilatory Demand	**Depressed Central Drive**
High-carbohydrate diet High-carbohydrate dialysate (peritoneal dialysis) Sorbent-regenerative hemodialysis	General anesthesia Sedative overdose Head trauma Cerebrovascular accident Obesity-hypoventilation syndrome Cerebral edema Brain tumor Encephalitis Brainstem lesion
Increased Dead Space Ventilation	**Abnormal Neuromuscular Transmission**
Acute lung injury Multilobar pneumonia Cardiogenic pulmonary edema Pulmonary embolism Positive-pressure ventilation Supplemental oxygen	High spinal cord injury Guillain–Barré syndrome Status epilepticus Botulism, tetanus Crisis in myasthenia gravis Familial periodic paralysis Drugs or toxic agents (e.g., curare, succinylcholine, aminoglyosides, organophosphate poisoning)
Augmented Airway Flow Resistance	**Muscle Dysfunction**
Upper airway obstruction Coma-induced hypopharyngeal obstruction Aspiration of foreign body or vomitus Laryngospasm Angioedema Inadequate laryngeal intubation Laryngeal obstruction postintubation Lower airway obstruction Status asthmaticus Exacerbation of chronic obstructive pulmonary disease (COPD)	Fatigue Hyperkalemia Hypokalemia
Lung Stiffness	
Atelectasis	
Pleural/Chest Wall Stiffness	
Pneumothorax Hemothorax Flail chest Abdominal distention Peritoneal dialysis	

Figure 14.2 Causes of acute respiratory acidosis.

Causes of Chronic Respiratory Acidosis

Increased Load	Depressed Pump
Increased Dead Space Ventilation	**Depressed Central Drive**
Emphysema Pulmonary fibrosis Pulmonary vascular disease	Central sleep apnea Obesity-hypoventilation syndrome Methadone/heroin addiction Brain tumor Bulbar poliomyelitis Hypothyroidism
Augmented Airway Flow Resistance	**Abnormal Neuromuscular Transmission**
Upper airway obstruction Tonsillar and peritonsillar hypertrophy Paralysis of vocal cords Tumor of the cords or larynx Airways stenosis after prolonged intubation Thymoma, aortic aneurysm Lower airway obstruction Chronic obstructive pulmonary disease (COPD)	High spinal cord injury Poliomyelitis Multiple sclerosis Muscular dystrophy Amyotrophic lateral sclerosis Diaphragmatic paralysis
Lung Stiffness	**Muscle Dysfunction**
Severe chronic interstitial lung disease	Myopathic disease (e.g., polymyositis)
Pleural/Chest Wall Stiffness	
Kyphoscoliosis Thoracic cage disease Thoracoplasty Obesity	

Figure 14.3 Causes of chronic respiratory acidosis.

Secondary Response to Alterations in Acid-Base Status

Condition	Initiating Mechanism	Expected Response: Change in $[HCO_3^-]$ or $PaCO_2$	Maximal Level of Response
Respiratory acidosis	Increase in $PaCO_2$		
Acute		Increase in $[HCO_3^-] \approx 0.1\ PaCO_2$	30 mmol/l
Chronic		Increase in $[HCO_3^-] \approx 0.3\ PaCO_2$	45 mmol/l
Respiratory alkalosis	Decrease in $PaCO_2$		
Acute		Decrease in $[HCO_3^-] \approx 0.2\ PaCO_2$	16–18 mmol/l
Chronic		Decrease $[HCO_3^-] \approx 0.4\ PaCO_2$	12–15 mmol/l
Metabolic acidosis	Decrease in $[HCO_3^-]_p$	Decrease in $PaCO_2 \approx 1.2\ [HCO_3^-]$	10 mm Hg (1.3 kP)
Metabolic alkalosis	Increase in $[HCO_3^-]_p$	Increase in $PaCO_2 \approx 0.7\ [HCO_3^-]$	65 mm Hg (8.7 kP)

Figure 14.4 Secondary response to alterations in acid-base status.

ventilation/perfusion ($\dot{V}/\dot{Q}$) mismatch due to the loss of hypoxic pulmonary vasoconstriction and the Haldane effect (the decreased hemoglobin affinity for CO_2 in the presence of increased O_2 saturation), which mandates an increase in ventilation to eliminate the excess CO_2.[7]

The management of acute respiratory acidosis and chronic respiratory acidosis is presented in Figures 14.5 and 14.6. Whenever possible, treatment must be directed at removal or amelioration of the underlying cause. Immediate therapeutic efforts should focus on securing a patent airway and restoring adequate oxygenation by delivery of an O_2-rich inspired mixture. Supplemental oxygen can be administered to the spontaneously breathing patient with nasal cannulas, Venturi masks, or non-rebreathing masks. Oxygen flow rates up to 5 l/min can be used with nasal cannulas; each increment of 1 l/min increases the F_{IO_2} by

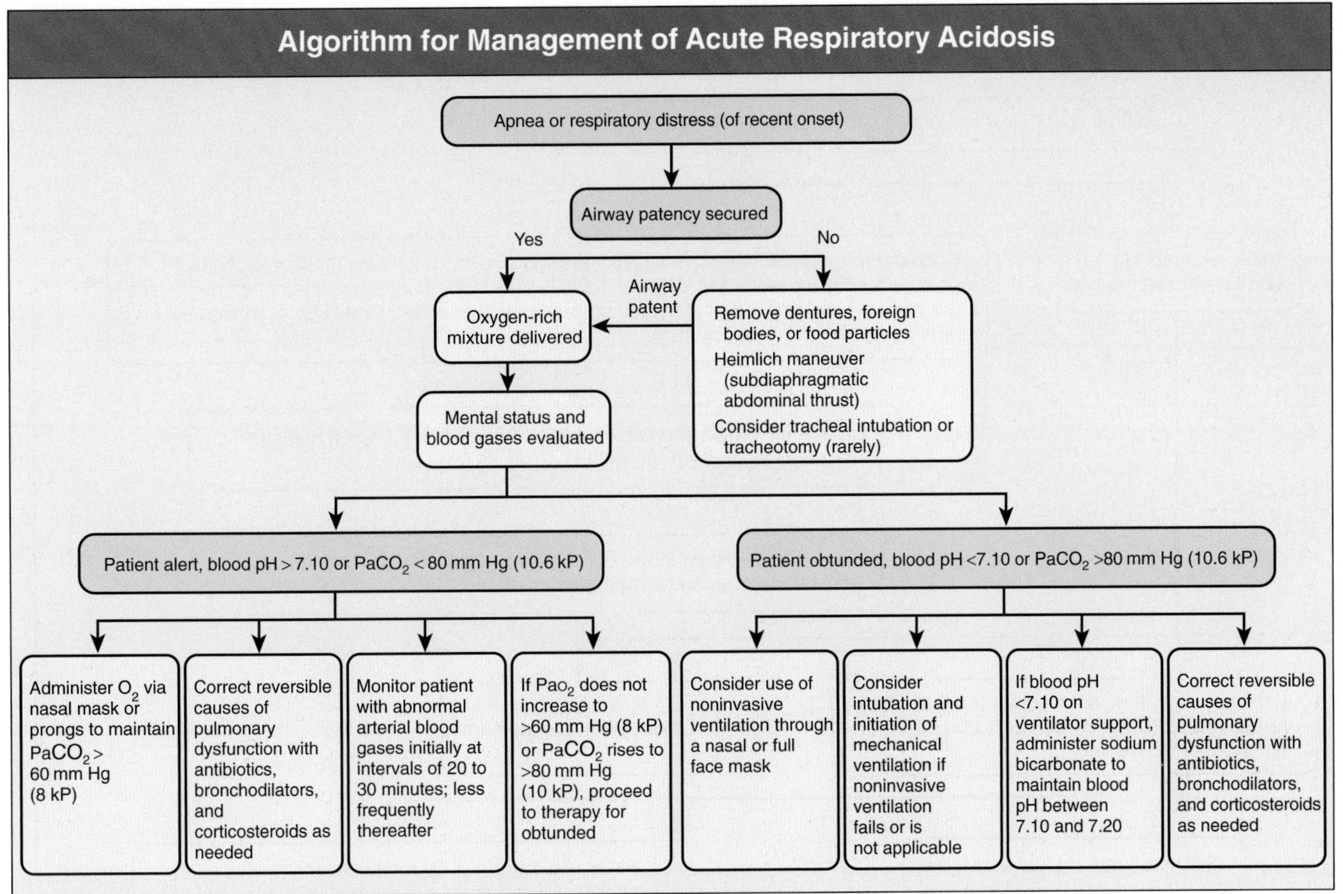

Figure 14.5 Algorithm for the management of acute respiratory acidosis.

approximately 4%. Venturi masks, calibrated to deliver FIO_2 between 24% and 50%, are most useful in patients with COPD because the PO_2 can be titrated, thus minimizing the risk of CO_2 retention. Oxygen saturation of hemoglobin of approximately 80% to 90% can be achieved with nonbreathing masks.

If the target PO_2 is not achieved with these measures and the patient is conscious, cooperative, hemodynamically stable, and able to protect the lower airway, a method of noninvasive ventilation through a mask can be used (e.g., bilevel positive airway pressure [BiPAP]). With BiPAP, the inspiratory-pressure support decreases the work of breathing, and the expiratory-pressure support improves gas exchange by preventing alveolar collapse.

Endotracheal intubation and mechanical ventilatory support should be initiated if adequate oxygenation cannot be secured by noninvasive measures, if progressive hypercapnia or obtundation develops, or if the patient is unable to cough and clear secretions. Minute ventilation should be raised so that the $PaCO_2$ gradually returns to near its long-term baseline and excretion of excess HCO_3^- by the kidneys is accomplished (assuming that Cl^- is provided). By contrast, overly rapid reduction in the $PaCO_2$ risks the development of posthypercapnic alkalosis, with potentially serious consequences. Should posthypercapnic alkalosis develop, it can be ameliorated by providing Cl^-, usually as the potassium salt, and administering the HCO_3^--wasting diuretic acetazolamide at doses of 250 to 500 mg once or twice daily. Vigorous treatment of pulmonary infections, bronchodilator therapy, and removal of secretions can offer considerable benefit. Naloxone will reverse the suppressive effect of narcotic agents on ventilation. Avoidance of tranquilizers and sedatives, gradual reduction of supplemental oxygen (aiming at a PaO_2 of about 60 mm Hg [8 kP]), and treatment of a superimposed metabolic alkalosis will optimize the ventilatory drive.

Mechanical ventilation with tidal volumes of 10 to 15 ml/kg body weight often leads to alveolar overdistention and volutrauma. Therefore, an alternative approach called permissive hypercapnia (or controlled mechanical hypoventilation) has been successfully applied to prevent barotrauma and cardiovascular collapse.[4,12] In this form of treatment, lower tidal volumes of less than 6 ml/kg body weight and lower peak inspiratory pressures are used. Further, $PaCO_2$ is allowed to increase but rarely exceeds 80 mm Hg, and blood pH can decrease to as low as 7.00 to 7.10, while adequate oxygenation is maintained. Because the patients commonly require neuromuscular blockade as well, accidental disconnection from the ventilator can cause sudden death. Contraindications to permissive hypercapnia include cerebrovascular disease, brain edema, increased intracranial pressure, convulsions, depressed cardiac function, arrhythmias, and severe pulmonary hypertension. Correction of acidemia attenuates the adverse hemodynamic effects of permissive hypercapnia.[13] It appears prudent, although still controversial, to keep the blood pH at approximately 7.30 by the administration of intravenous alkali when controlled hypoventilation is prescribed.[1,14]

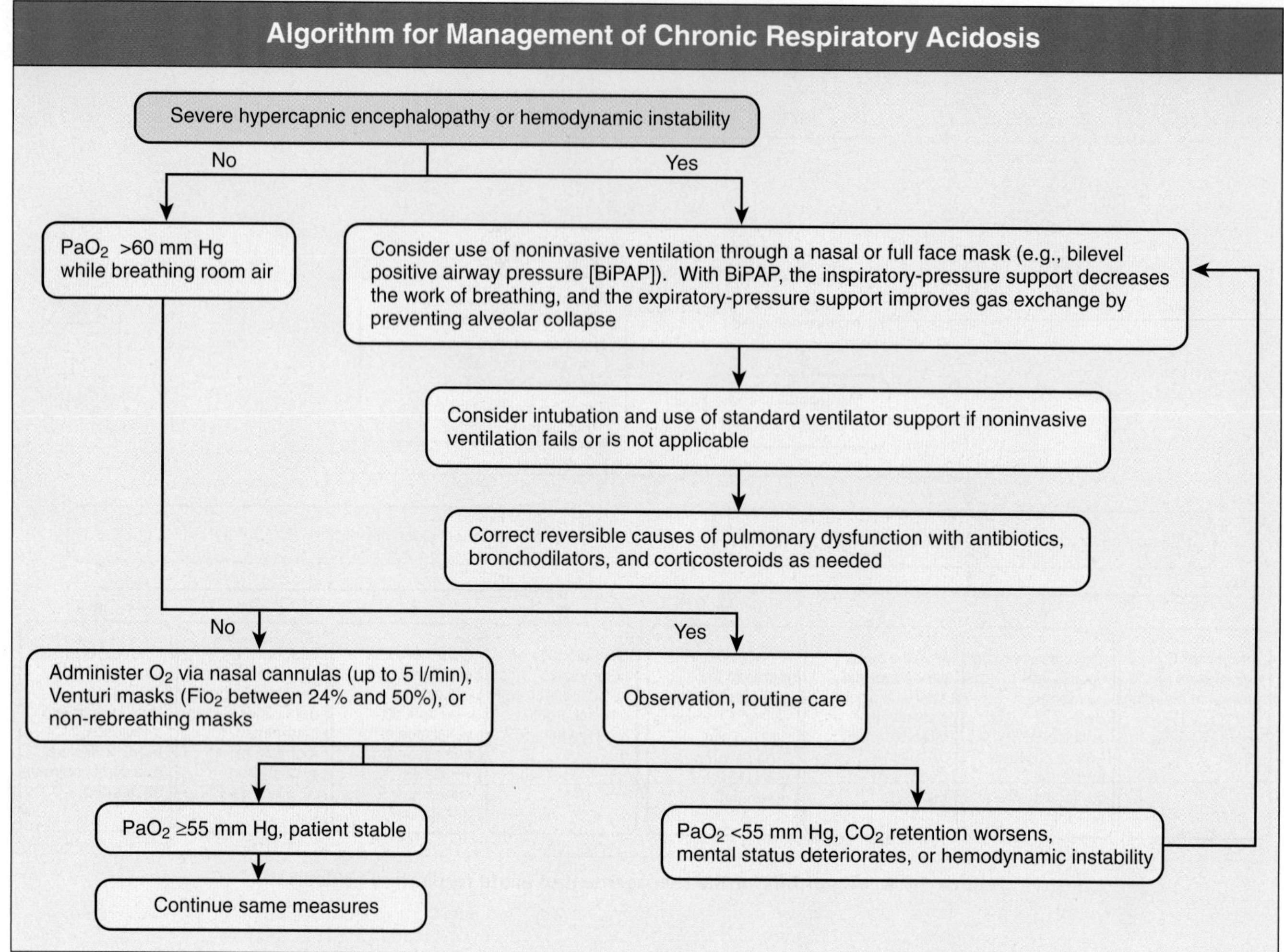

Figure 14.6 Algorithm for the management of chronic respiratory acidosis.

RESPIRATORY ALKALOSIS (PRIMARY HYPOCAPNIA)

Definition

Respiratory alkalosis is the acid-base disturbance initiated by a reduction in CO_2 tension of body fluids. The secondary decrease in plasma HCO_3^- concentration observed in acute and chronic hypocapnia is an integral part of the respiratory alkalosis. Whole-body CO_2 stores are decreased and $Paco_2$ is less than 35 mm Hg (4.7 kP) in patients with simple respiratory alkalosis who are at rest and at sea level. An element of respiratory alkalosis may still occur with higher levels of $Paco_2$ in patients with metabolic alkalosis, in whom a normal $Paco_2$ is inappropriately low for this primary metabolic disorder.

Etiology and Pathogenesis

Respiratory alkalosis is the most frequent acid-base disorder encountered because it occurs in normal pregnancy and with high-altitude residence.[2,15] It is also the most common acid-base abnormality in critically ill patients, occurring either as the simple disorder or as a component of mixed disturbances; indeed, in such patients, its presence may constitute a grave prognostic sign, especially if $Paco_2$ levels are below 20 to 25 mm Hg (2.7 to 3.3 kP). The presence of hypocapnia signifies transient or persistent alveolar hyperventilation relative to the prevailing CO_2 production, thus leading to negative CO_2 balance; primary hypocapnia might also originate from the extrapulmonary elimination of CO_2 by dialysis or other extracorporeal circulation (e.g., heart-lung machine).

Figure 14.7 gives the major causes of respiratory alkalosis.[6] In most patients, primary hypocapnia reflects alveolar hyperventilation due to increased ventilatory drive. This is a consequence of signals arising from the lung, the peripheral chemoreceptors (carotid and aortic), or the brainstem chemoreceptors or influences originating in other centers of the brain.

The response of the brainstem chemoreceptors to CO_2 can be augmented by systemic diseases (e.g., liver disease, sepsis), pharmacologic agents, and volition. Hypoxemia is a major stimulus of alveolar ventilation, but Pao_2 values below 60 mm Hg (8 kP) are required to elicit this effect consistently. Not uncommonly, alveolar hyperventilation is the result of maladjusted mechanical ventilators, psychogenic hyperventilation, and lesions involving the central nervous system.

In states of severe circulatory failure, arterial hypocapnia may coexist with venous and therefore tissue hypercapnia; under these conditions, the body CO_2 stores have been enriched so that there is respiratory acidosis rather than respiratory alkalosis. This entity, which we have termed pseudorespiratory alkalosis, develops in patients with profound depression of cardiac function and pulmonary perfusion but relative preservation of alveolar

Causes of Respiratory Alkalosis

Hypoxemia or Tissue Hypoxia	Drugs and Hormones
Decreased inspired O_2 tension High altitude Bacterial or viral pneumonia Aspiration of food, foreign body, or vomitus Laryngospasm Drowning Cyanotic heart disease Severe anemia Left shift deviation of HbO_2 curve Hypotension Severe circulatory failure Pulmonary edema Pseudorespiratory alkalosis	Respiratory stimulants (doxapram, nikethamide, ethamivan, progesterone, medroxyprogesterone) Salicylates Nicotine Xanthines Dinitrophenol Pressor hormones (epinephrine, norepinephrine, angiotensin II [ANG II])
Central Nervous System Stimulation	**Miscellaneous**
Voluntary Pain Anxiety–hyperventilation syndrome Psychosis Fever Subarachnoid hemorrhage Cerebrovascular accident Meningoencephalitis Tumor Trauma	Exercise Pregnancy Gram-positive septicemia Gram-negative septicemia Hepatic failure Mechanical hyperventilation Heat exposure Recovery from metabolic acidosis Hemodialysis with acetate dialysate
Pulmonary Diseases with Stimulation of Chest Receptors	
Pneumonia Asthma Pneumothorax Hemothorax Flail chest Acute respiratory distress syndrome Cardiogenic and noncardiogenic pulmonary edema Pulmonary embolism Pulmonary fibrosis	

Figure 14.7 Causes of respiratory alkalosis.

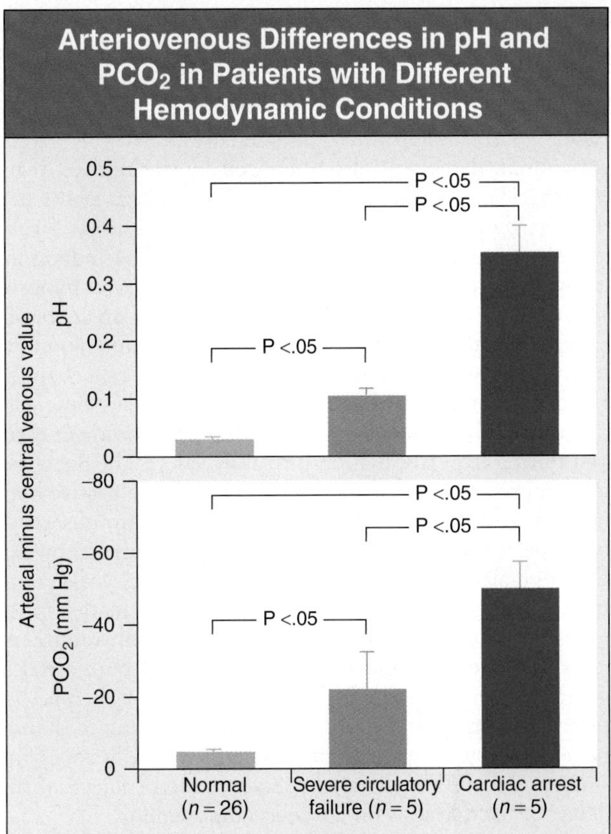

Figure 14.8 Arteriovenous differences in pH and PCO_2 in patients with different hemodynamic conditions.

ventilation, including patients with advanced circulatory failure and those undergoing cardiopulmonary resuscitation. The severely reduced pulmonary blood flow limits the CO_2 delivered to the lungs for excretion, thereby increasing the venous PCO_2. However, the increased ventilation/perfusion ratio causes a larger than normal removal of CO_2 per unit of blood traversing the pulmonary circulation, thereby giving rise to arterial eucapnia or frank hypocapnia. A progressive widening of the arteriovenous difference in pH and PCO_2 develops in two settings of cardiac dysfunction, circulatory failure and cardiac arrest (Fig. 14.8). In both situations, there is severe tissue O_2 deprivation, and it can be completely disguised by the reasonably preserved arterial O_2 values. Appropriate monitoring of acid-base composition and oxygenation in patients with advanced cardiac dysfunction requires mixed (or central) venous blood sampling in addition to the sampling of arterial blood.

Secondary Physiologic Response

Adaptation to acute hypocapnia is characterized by an immediate decrement in plasma HCO_3^- that results totally from nonrenal mechanisms and is explained principally by alkaline titration of the non-HCO_3^- body buffers (see second equation and Fig. 14.4). This adaptation is completed within 5 to 10 minutes of the onset of hypocapnia, and if there is no further change in $PaCO_2$, no additional detectable changes in acid-base equilibrium occur for a period of several hours.

Adaptation to chronic hypocapnia entails an additional, larger decrease in plasma HCO_3^- as a consequence of renal adjustments that reflect a dampening of H^+ secretion by the renal tubule.[7] Approximately 2 to 3 days are required for completion of the adaptation to chronic hypocapnia. Quantitative aspects of the secondary physiologic responses to acute and chronic hypocapnia are shown in Figure 14.4.

Clinical Manifestations

A rapid decrease in $PaCO_2$ to half normal values or lower is typically accompanied by numbness and paresthesias of the extremities, chest discomfort, circumoral numbness, lightheadedness, and mental confusion. Muscle cramps, increased deep tendon reflexes, carpopedal spasm, and generalized seizures occur infrequently. Cerebral vasoconstriction and reduced cerebral blood flow have been well documented during acute hypocapnia; in severe cases, cerebral blood flow might reach values below 50% of normal. Hypocapnia can have deleterious effects on the brain of premature infants; in patients with traumatic brain injury, acute stroke, or general anesthesia; and after sudden exposure to very high altitude.[16] Long-term neurologic sequelae can develop when immature brains are exposed to $PaCO_2$ levels below 15 mm Hg (2 kP) for even short periods. Furthermore, abrupt correction of hypocapnia in these patients leads to cerebral vasodilation, which might cause reperfusion injury or intraventricular hemorrhage.

Brain injury due to hypocapnia probably results from cerebral ischemia. Other factors include hypocapnia *per se*, alkalemia, pH-induced shift of the oxyhemoglobin dissociation curve, decrements in the levels of ionized calcium and potassium, depletion of the antioxidant glutathione by cytotoxic excitatory amino acids, increases in anaerobic metabolism, cerebral oxygen demand, neuronal dopamine, and seizure activity. If sepsis is present, brain damage is also enhanced by the release of lipopolysaccharide, interleukin-1β, and tumor necrosis factor α.[16]

The cardiovascular manifestations of respiratory alkalosis differ in passive and active hyperventilation. The induction of acute hypocapnia in anesthetized subjects (i.e., passive hyperventilation) results in a decrease in cardiac output, an increase in peripheral resistance, and a decrease in the systemic blood pressure. By contrast, active hyperventilation does not change or might even increase cardiac output and leaves systemic blood pressure virtually unchanged. The discrepant response of cardiac output during hyperventilation probably reflects the decrease in venous return caused by mechanical ventilation in passive hyperventilation and the reflex tachycardia consistently observed in active hyperventilation. Sustained hypocapnia induced by exposure to high altitude for several weeks results in a cardiac output equal to or higher than control values. Although acute hypocapnia does not lead to cardiac arrhythmias in normal volunteers, it appears that it contributes to the generation of both atrial and ventricular tachyarrhythmias in patients with ischemic heart disease; such arrhythmias are frequently resistant to standard forms of therapy. Chest pain and ischemic ST-T wave changes have been observed in acutely hyperventilating subjects with no evidence of fixed lesions on coronary angiography.

Diagnosis

Evaluation of the patient's history, physical examination, and ancillary laboratory data are required to establish the diagnosis of respiratory alkalosis.[10,15] Careful observation can detect abnormal patterns of breathing in some patients, yet marked hypocapnia can occur without a clinically evident increase in respiratory effort. Arterial blood gas determinations are required to confirm the presence of hyperventilation.

The diagnosis of respiratory alkalosis, especially the chronic form, is frequently missed; physicians often misinterpret the electrolyte pattern of hyperchloremic hypobicarbonatemia as indicative of normal anion gap metabolic acidosis. If the patient's acid-base profile reveals hypocapnia in association with alkalemia, at least an element of respiratory alkalosis must be present. Yet hypocapnia might be associated with a normal or an acidic pH because of the concomitant presence of additional acid-base disorders. One should also note that mild degrees of chronic hypocapnia leave blood pH within the high-normal range. The diagnosis of respiratory alkalosis can have important clinical implications; it often provides a clue to the presence of an unrecognized, serious disorder or signals the gravity of a known underlying disease.

Treatment

A synopsis of the management of respiratory alkalosis is presented in Figure 14.9. The widely held view that hypocapnia

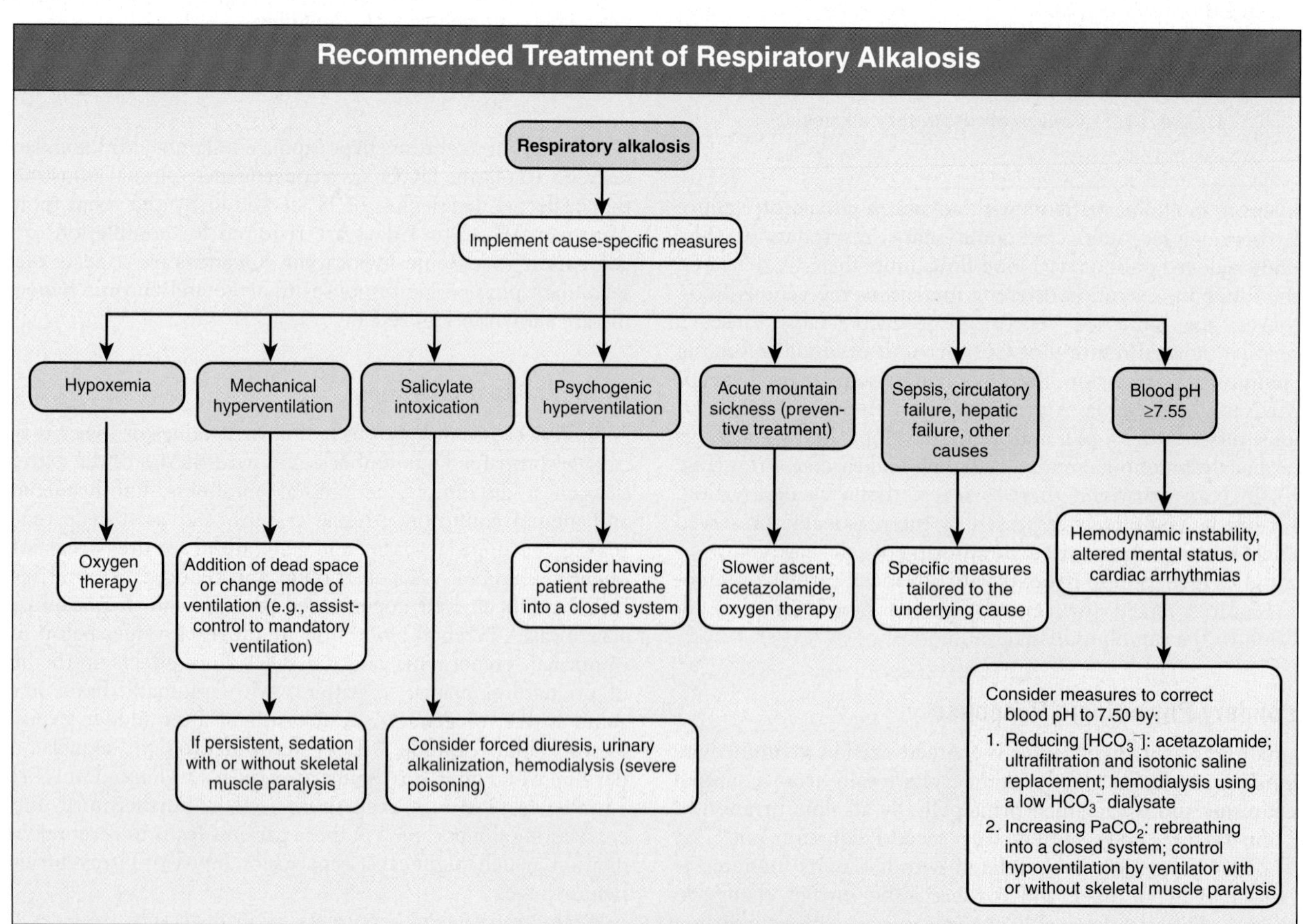

Figure 14.9 Recommended treatment of respiratory alkalosis.

poses little risk to health under most conditions is no longer considered accurate. In fact, substantial hypocapnia in hospitalized patients, whether it is spontaneous or deliberately induced, may result in transient or permanent damage in the brain as well as in the respiratory and cardiovascular systems.[16] Furthermore, rapid correction of severe hypocapnia leads to vasodilation of ischemic areas, resulting in reperfusion injury in the brain and lung. Consequently, severe hypocapnia in hospitalized patients must be prevented whenever possible, and if it is present, abrupt correction should be avoided. Severe alkalemia caused by acute primary hypocapnia requires corrective measures that depend on whether serious clinical manifestations are present. Such measures can be directed at reduction of plasma bicarbonate concentration, increase of $Paco_2$, or both. Even if baseline plasma bicarbonate concentration is moderately decreased, reducing it further can be particularly rewarding in this setting, as this maneuver combines effectiveness with relatively little risk. For patients with the anxiety-hyperventilation syndrome, in addition to reassurance or sedation, rebreathing into a closed system (e.g., a paper bag) might prove helpful by interrupting the vicious circle that can result from the reinforcing effects of the symptoms of hypocapnia.

Respiratory alkalosis resulting from severe hypoxemia requires O_2 therapy. The oral administration of 250 to 500 mg acetazolamide twice daily can be beneficial in the management of signs and symptoms of high-altitude sickness, a syndrome characterized by hypoxemia and respiratory alkalosis.[15] Of course, patients undergoing mechanical ventilation lend themselves to an effective correction of hypocapnia (whether it is caused by maladjusted ventilator or other factors) by resetting of the device.

MIXED ACID-BASE DISTURBANCES

Definition

Mixed acid-base disturbances are defined as the simultaneous presence of two or more acid-base disorders. Such association might include two or more simple acid-base disorders (e.g., metabolic acidosis and respiratory alkalosis), two or more forms of a simple disturbance having different time course or pathogenesis (e.g., acute and chronic respiratory acidosis or high anion gap and hyperchloremic metabolic acidosis, respectively), or a combination of these two forms.[17] The secondary or adaptive response to a simple acid-base disorder cannot be taken as one of the components of a mixed disorder.

Etiology and Pathogenesis

Mixed acid-base disturbances are commonly observed in hospitalized patients, especially those in critical care units.[18] Characterization of these disorders and proper identification of their pathogenesis can be challenging tasks and are a prerequisite for taking sound corrective action. Certain clinical settings are commonly associated with mixed acid-base disorders, including cardiorespiratory arrest, sepsis, drug intoxications, diabetes mellitus, and organ failure (especially renal, hepatic, and pulmonary failure). Patients with severe renal impairment or end-stage renal disease (ESRD) are prone to mixed acid-base disturbances of great complexity and severity.[19] Metabolic acidosis of the high anion gap type is frequently accompanied by a component of hyperchloremic acidosis, inability to mount an appropriate secondary response to chronic respiratory acidosis or alkalosis, inability to respond to a load of fixed acids (e.g., lactic acid) or a primary loss of alkali (e.g., diarrhea) with the expected increase in net acid excretion, and inability to respond to an alkali load with bicarbonaturia despite the presence of an increased plasma HCO_3^- concentration. As a result, these patients are particularly vulnerable to the development of both extreme acidemia and extreme alkalemia.

A practical classification of mixed acid-base disorders recognizes three main groups of disturbances in accordance with the preceding definition (Fig. 14.10). Representative examples are depicted in Figure 14.11, and some of these mixed disorders are reviewed.

Metabolic Acidosis and Respiratory Acidosis

The expected hypocapnia secondary to metabolic acidosis is estimated by $\Delta Paco_2/\Delta[HCO_3^-]$ equal to 1.2 mm Hg/mEq/l; if measured $Paco_2$ exceeds 5 mm Hg the estimated value, respiratory acidosis is also present. Clinical examples of metabolic

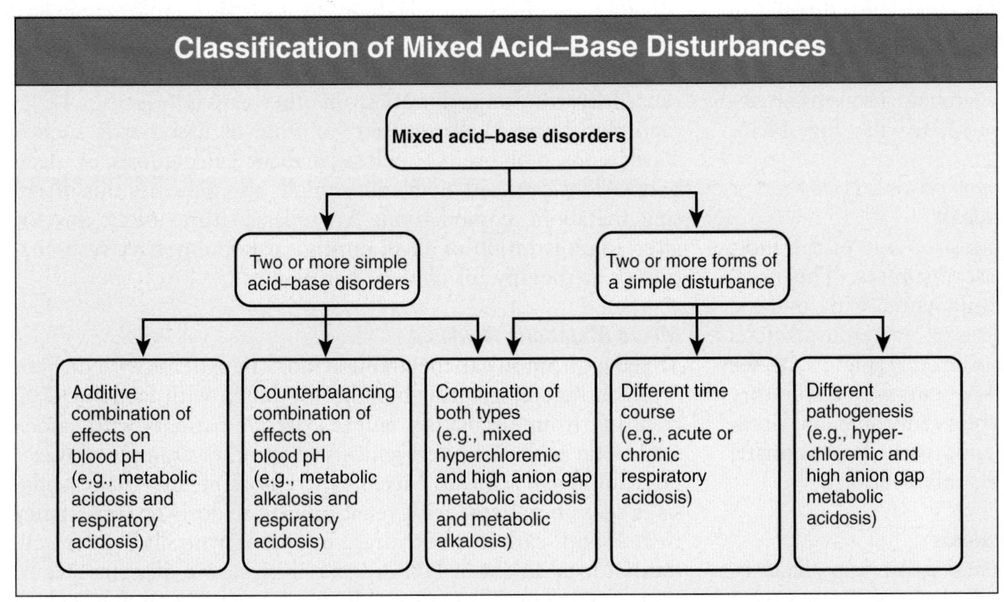

Figure 14.10 Classification of mixed acid-base disturbances.

Representative Examples of Mixed Acid-Base Disorders

Type of Mixed Disorder	Example No.	pH	Pa_{CO_2} (mm Hg)	HCO_3^- (mmol/l)	Na^+ (mmol/l)	K^+ (mmol/l)	Cl^- (mmol/l)	Anion gap (mmol/l)	Clinical Circumstances
Hyperchloremic and and high anion gap metabolic acidosis	1	7.12	16	5	137	3.6	114	18	Diabetic ketoacidosis with adequate salt and water balance
Mixed high anion gap metabolic acidosis and metabolic alkalosis	2	7.36	31	17	132	4.0	89	26	Alcoholic liver disease, vomiting, and lactic acidosis
	3	7.40	40	24	143	5.5	95	24	Diabetic ketoacidosis and lactic acidosis after bicarbonate therapy
Mixed high anion gap metabolic acidosis and respiratory acidosis	4	7.18	44	16	133	5.7	100	17	Hepatic, renal, and pulmonary failure
Metabolic alkalosis and respiratory acidosis	5	7.44	55	36	135	3.8	84	15	Chronic obstructive pulmonary disease (COPD) and diuretics
Metabolic alkalosis and respiratory alkalosis	6	7.60	40	38	131	3.6	77	16	Congestive heart failure and diuretics
Acute or chronic respiratory acidosis	7	7.22	80	32	141	4.3	99	10	Chronic obstructive pulmonary disease (COPD) and therapy with O_2-rich mixtures

Figure 14.11 Representative examples of mixed acid-base disorders. Anion gap is calculated as $[Na^+] - ([Cl^-] + [HCO_3^-])$.

acidosis combined with respiratory acidosis include untreated cardiopulmonary arrest, circulatory failure in patients with COPD, severe renal failure associated with hypercapnic respiratory failure, various intoxications, and hypokalemic (or less frequently hyperkalemic) paralysis of respiratory muscles in patients with diarrhea or renal tubular acidosis (Fig. 14.12; see also Fig. 14.11, example 4).

Metabolic Alkalosis and Respiratory Alkalosis

Metabolic alkalosis combined with respiratory alkalosis might be encountered in patients with primary hypocapnia associated with chronic liver disease who develop metabolic alkalosis from a variety of causes, including vomiting, nasogastric drainage, diuretics, profound hypokalemia, and alkali administration (e.g., absorption of antacids; infusion of lactated Ringer's solution, alimentation solutions, or citrated blood products), especially in the context of renal impairment. It also occurs in critically ill patients, particularly those undergoing mechanical ventilation, and in patients with respiratory alkalosis, caused by either pregnancy or heart failure, who experience metabolic alkalosis attributable to diuretics or vomiting (Fig. 14.13; see also Fig. 14.11, example 6).

Metabolic Alkalosis and Respiratory Acidosis

Metabolic alkalosis and respiratory acidosis is one of the most frequently encountered mixed acid-base disorders. The usual clinical setting involves COPD in conjunction with diuretic therapy, but it can occur with other causes of metabolic alkalosis (e.g., vomiting, administration of corticosteroids) (Fig. 14.14; see also Fig. 14.11, example 5). Critically ill patients with respiratory failure caused by acute respiratory distress syndrome and occasionally those with profound hypokalemia with diaphragmatic muscle weakness also might develop this mixed disorder.

Metabolic Acidosis and Respiratory Alkalosis

The combination of metabolic acidosis and respiratory alkalosis, like respiratory acidosis and metabolic alkalosis, is characterized by normal or nearly normal blood pH; its two components exert offsetting effects on systemic acidity (Fig. 14.15). This disorder is common in intensive care units and is generally associated with high mortality. Causes of the primary hypocapnia include fever, hypotension, gram-negative septicemia, pulmonary edema, hypoxemia, and mechanical hyperventilation. The component of metabolic acidosis, in turn, might be lactic acidosis (e.g., complicating shock, hepatic failure) or renal acidosis. Salicylate intoxication is another cause of this mixed acid-base disorder. Stimulation of the ventilatory center in the brainstem accounts for the respiratory alkalosis, whereas the accelerated production of organic acids (including pyruvic, lactic, and keto acids) and, to a small extent, the accumulation of salicylic acid itself are responsible for the metabolic acidosis.

Metabolic Acidosis and Metabolic Alkalosis

Metabolic acidosis and metabolic alkalosis are typically observed in patients with alcoholic liver disease who develop fasting ketoacidosis or lactic acidosis in conjunction with metabolic alkalosis caused by vomiting, diuretics, or other causes (see Fig. 14.11, examples 2 and 3). Protracted vomiting or nasogastric suction superimposed on uremic acidosis, diabetic ketoacidosis, or metabolic acidosis caused by diarrhea might also generate this offsetting metabolic combination. A similar picture might develop after administration of alkali during cardiopulmonary resuscitation or as therapy for diabetic ketoacidosis.

Mixed Metabolic Acidosis

Mixed high anion gap metabolic acidosis in patients with diabetic or alcoholic ketoacidosis may be combined with lactic acidosis resulting from circulatory failure. Uremic patients with associated lactic acidosis or ketoacidosis are another example of mixed high anion gap acidosis. Mixed hyperchloremic metabolic acidosis is seen in patients with renal tubular acidosis or those being treated with carbonic anhydrase inhibitors who also suffer substantial fecal losses of HCO_3^- caused by severe diarrhea. Coexistence of hyperchloremic and high anion gap metabolic acidosis

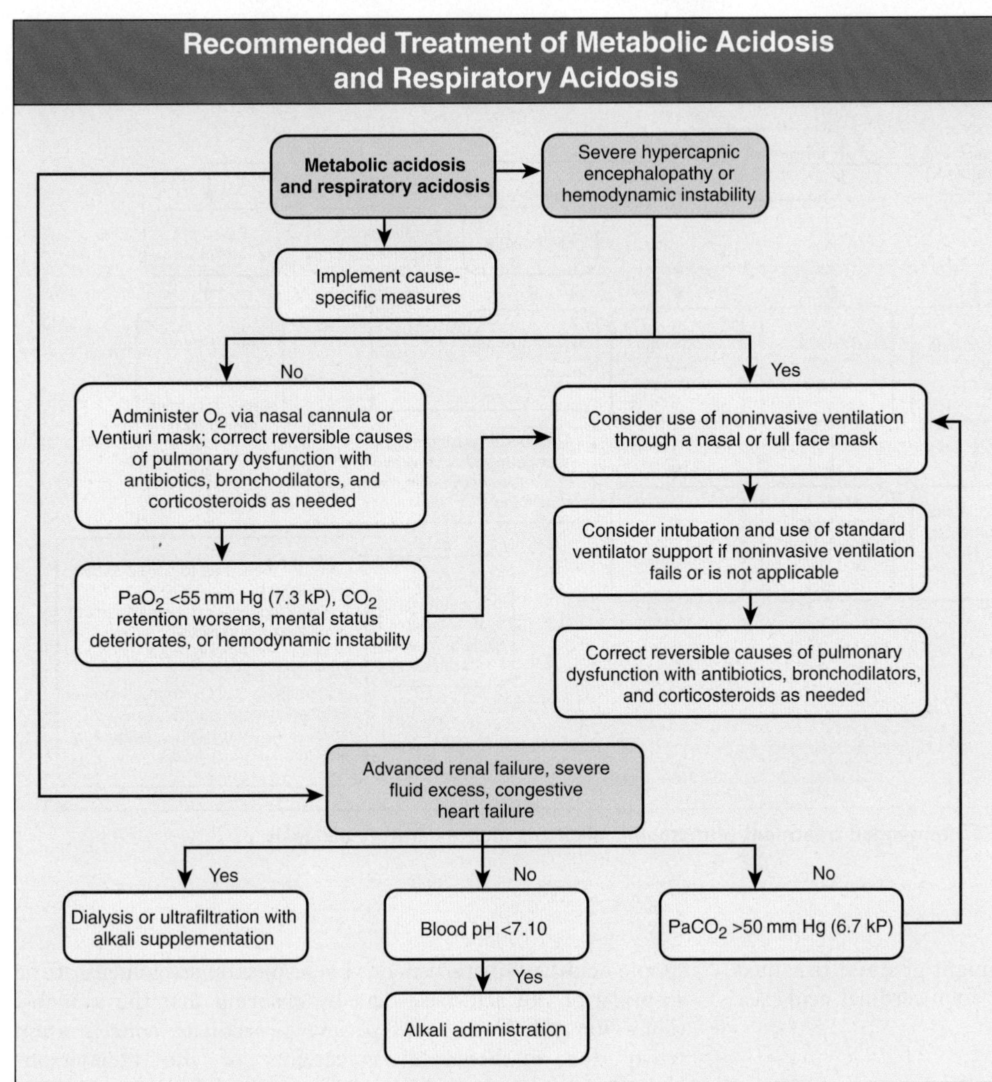

Figure 14.12 Recommended treatment of metabolic acidosis and respiratory acidosis.

occurs in patients with profuse diarrhea whose circulation becomes sufficiently compromised to generate, in turn, a high anion gap metabolic acidosis (as a result of renal failure or lactic acidosis). Patients with diabetic ketoacidosis, whose renal function is maintained at reasonable levels by adequate salt and water intake, might develop an element of hyperchloremic metabolic acidosis because of preferential excretion of ketone anions and conservation of Cl^- (see Fig. 14.11, example 1).[20]

Mixed Metabolic Alkalosis

The coincidence of several processes that each contribute to a primary increase in plasma HCO_3^- (including diuretic therapy, vomiting, mineralocorticoid excess, and severe potassium depletion) will give rise to mixed metabolic alkalosis.

Triple Disorders

The most frequent triple disorders comprise two cardinal metabolic disturbances in conjunction with either respiratory acidosis or respiratory alkalosis, for example, severely ill patients with COPD and CO_2 retention who simultaneously develop metabolic alkalosis (usually caused by diuretics and a Cl^--restricted diet) and metabolic acidosis (commonly lactic acidosis caused by hypoxemia, hypotension, or sepsis). This type of triple disorder also might be encountered during cardiopulmonary resuscitation when an element of metabolic alkalosis caused by alkali administration is superimposed on preexisting respiratory acidosis and metabolic (lactic) acidosis. Patients with respiratory alkalosis caused by advanced congestive heart failure also might have diuretic-induced metabolic alkalosis and lactic acidosis from tissue hypoperfusion. Such triple acid-base disorders can also be seen in patients with chronic alcoholism who develop metabolic alkalosis from vomiting, lactic acidosis from volume depletion or ethanol intoxication, and respiratory alkalosis from hepatic encephalopathy or sepsis.

Less common are triple disorders encompassing two cardinal respiratory disturbances in combination with either metabolic acidosis or metabolic alkalosis. The typical presentation involves critically ill patients with chronic respiratory acidosis who experience an abrupt reduction in $Pa{CO_2}$ because of mechanical ventilation and superimposed metabolic acidosis (usually lactic acidosis, reflecting circulatory failure) or metabolic alkalosis (e.g., as a result of gastric fluid loss, diuretics). In the last circumstance, extreme alkalemia might ensue because of the concomitant presence of hypocapnia and hyperbicarbonatemia. Even more

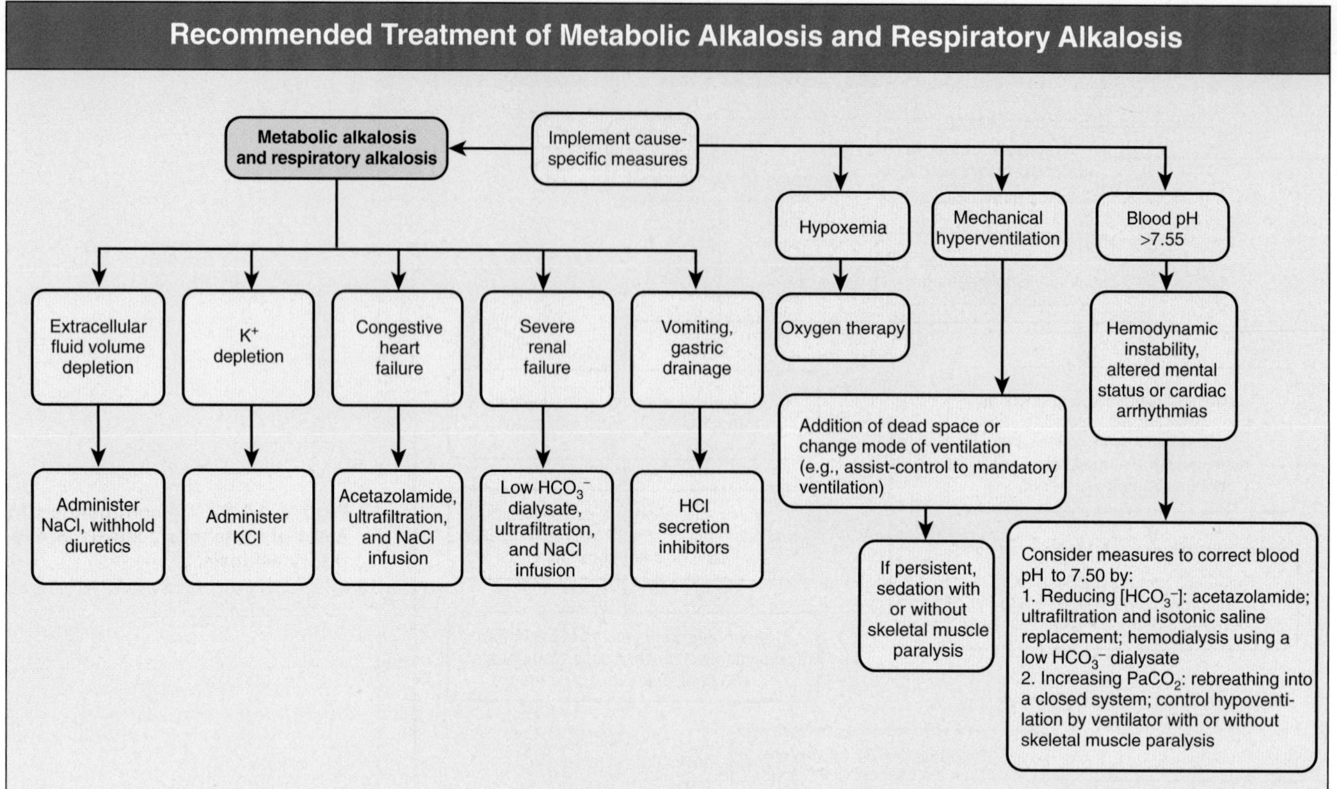

Figure 14.13 Recommended treatment of metabolic alkalosis and respiratory alkalosis.

infrequently, this same clinical setting might give rise to a quadruple acid-base disorder in which all four cardinal acid-base disturbances coexist.

Clinical Manifestations

The symptoms and signs of the underlying disease that give rise to the observed mixed acid-base disorder dominate the clinical picture, but the development of severe abnormalities in either $Paco_2$ (severe hypocapnia or hypercapnia) or systemic acidity (profound acidemia or alkalemia) might be responsible for the superimposition of additional clinical manifestations. On the one hand, profound hypocapnia might induce obtundation, generalized seizures, and occasionally even coma or death as a result of a critical reduction in cerebral blood flow and other mechanisms. Rarely, angina pectoris also might occur. On the other hand, severe hypercapnia might generate a profound encephalopathy with the classic features of pseudotumor cerebri, including headaches, obtundation, vomiting, and bilateral papilledema caused by increased intracranial pressure. Extreme acidemia results in depression of the central nervous system as well as the cardiovascular system.[7] Reduction in myocardial contractility and peripheral vascular resistance triggered by acidemia might result in severe hypotension. Finally, profound alkalemia might elicit paresthesias, tetany, cardiac dysrhythmias, or generalized seizures.

Diagnosis

The basic principles underlying the diagnosis of mixed acid-base disorders are identical to those required for the identification of simple acid-base disturbances. These include assessment of the accuracy of the acid-base data by ensuring that the available values for pH, $Paco_2$, and plasma bicarbonate concentration satisfy the mathematical constraints of the Henderson-Hasselbalch equation; obtainment of a careful history and performance of a complete physical examination; analysis of the plasma anion gap and other ancillary laboratory data; and knowledge of the quantitative aspects of the adaptive response to each of the four simple acid-base disturbances. Adherence to these principles cannot be overemphasized. Even experienced clinicians risk misdiagnosis of the prevailing acid-base status by bypassing this systematic approach.

Normality of the acid-base parameters is not in itself sufficient for diagnosis of normal acid-base status; indeed, normal acid-base values might be the fortuitous result of mixed acid-base disorders (e.g., high anion gap acidosis treated with alkali infusion, diarrhea-induced metabolic acidosis in conjunction with vomiting-induced metabolic alkalosis). A given set of acid-base parameters is never diagnostic of a particular acid-base disorder, whether it is simple or mixed in nature; rather, it is consistent with a range of acid-base abnormalities. What on the surface appears to be a clear-cut simple acid-base disorder might actually reflect the interplay of a number of coexisting acid-base disturbances. Information from the patient's history and findings from the physical examination frequently provide important insights into the prevailing acid-base status as well as useful clues to the differential diagnosis.

A critical component of the diagnostic process is the examination of the plasma anion gap (Fig. 14.16). This derived parameter provides important insights into the nature of the prevailing changes in plasma HCO_3^- concentration. An elevated plasma

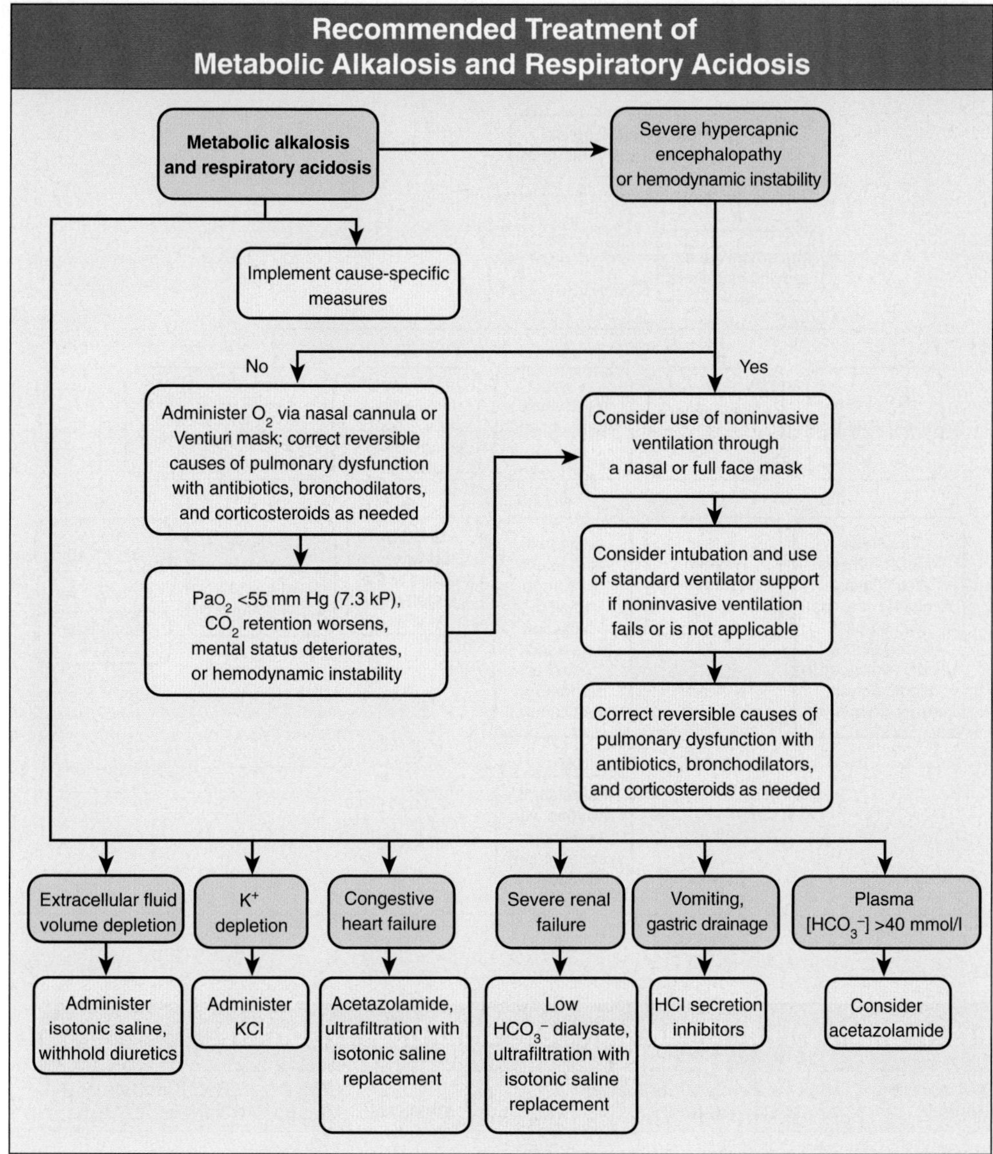

Figure 14.14 Recommended treatment of metabolic alkalosis and respiratory acidosis.

anion gap might offer the first clue to the presence of disordered acid-base status despite normal acid-base parameters. In the presence of a plasma HCO_3^- deficit ($\Delta[HCO_3^-]_p$), a normal or subnormal value for the plasma anion gap denotes that the entire decrease in HCO_3^- can be attributed to acidifying processes resulting in the loss of alkali (e.g., diarrhea, renal tubular acidosis) or to respiratory alkalosis. By comparison, with a high anion gap metabolic acidosis, there is usually a close reciprocal stoichiometry between the decrease in serum HCO_3^- and the increase in the anion gap, termed the Δ(anion gap). A reduction in serum HCO_3^- of 10 mmol/l is associated, therefore, with a Δ(anion gap) of 10 mmol/l. Addition of the value for the Δ(anion gap) to the prevailing level of serum HCO_3^- allows the derivation of the basal value of HCO_3^- existing before the development of the high anion gap metabolic acidosis. Appreciation of this reciprocal relationship between the $\Delta[HCO_3^-]_p$ and the Δ(anion gap) is important in distinguishing between a pure high anion gap metabolic acidosis and a mixed high and normal anion gap metabolic acidosis and in detecting a mixed high anion gap metabolic acidosis and metabolic alkalosis. Additional diagnostic insights are often obtained by examination of other laboratory data, including the serum potassium, glucose, urea nitrogen, and creatinine concentrations; semiquantitative measures for ketonemia or ketonuria; screening of blood or urine for toxins; and estimation of the serum osmolar gap.

Mild acid-base disorders pose particular diagnostic difficulty because of the overlap of values for the simple disturbances near the normal range. In such circumstances, any of several simple disorders or a variety of mixed disturbances might fully account for the acid-base data under evaluation. Again, careful correlation of all available clinical information should guide the diagnostic process.

Treatment

The management of mixed acid-base disturbances is aimed at restoration of the altered acid-base status by treatment of each simple acid-base disorder involved.[1,2,17,21] Recommendations for treatment of some common mixed acid-base disturbances are presented in Figures 14.12 to 14.15.

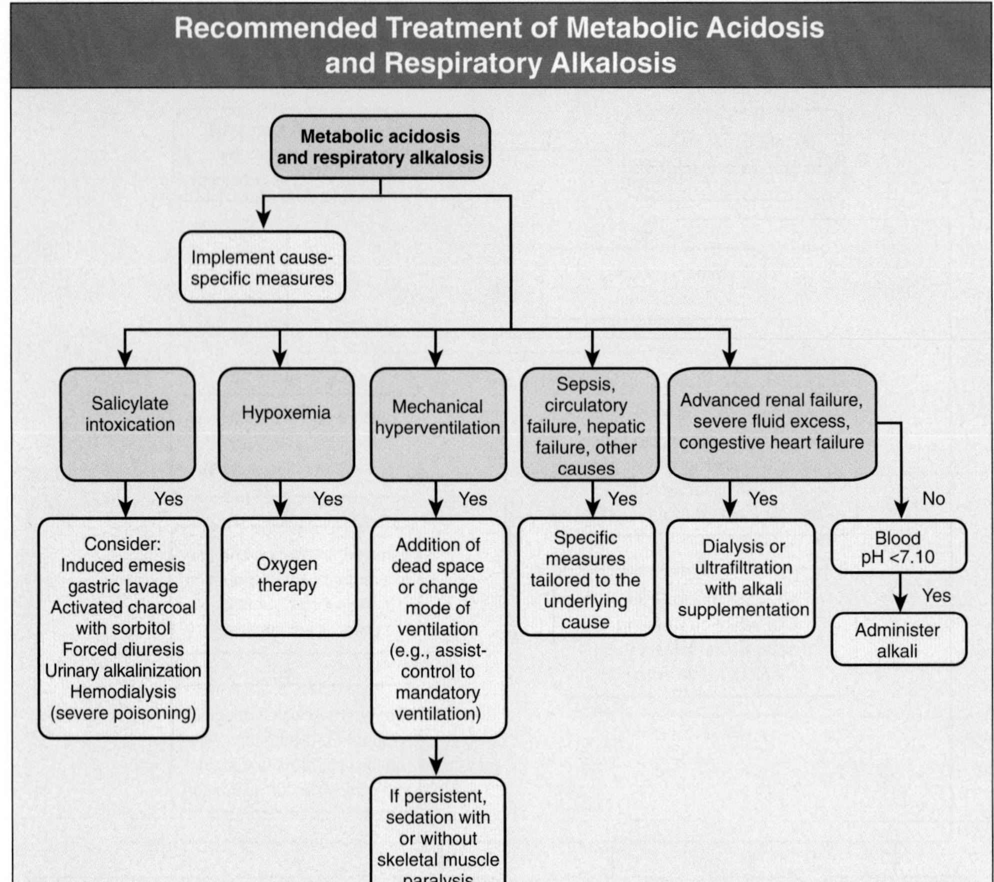

Figure 14.15 Recommended treatment of metabolic acidosis and respiratory alkalosis.

Blood Parameters in Diagnosis of Mixed Metabolic Acid-Base Disorders

Blood Composition	Normal	High Anion Gap Acidosis	High Anion Gap and Normal Anion Gap Acidosis	Metabolic Alkalosis	High Anion Gap Acidosis and Metabolic Alkalosis
pH	7.40	7.29	7.10	7.50	7.38
$PaCO_2$ (mm Hg)	40	30	20	45	35
Bicarbonate (mmol/l)	24	14	6	34	20
Anion gap (mmol/l)	10	20	20	12	26
Δ Bicarbonate	0	−10	−18	+10	−4
Δ Anion gap	0	+10	+10	+2	+16

Figure 14.16 Blood parameters in diagnosis of mixed metabolic acid-base disorders.

Given the variable response time to therapy of the individual components, it is crucial to be aware of the effect that graded correction might have on systemic acidity. The asynchronous reversal of the individual components might be used at times to therapeutic advantage; on other occasions, such a practice might prove catastrophic. For example, extreme acidemia caused by metabolic acidosis and respiratory acidosis or extreme alkalemia caused by metabolic alkalosis and respiratory alkalosis might be safely corrected by a rapid return of $Paco_2$ toward normal. By comparison, an asynchronous return of $Paco_2$ to normal in a patient with profound metabolic acidosis and superimposed respiratory alkalosis might prove disastrous. Similarly, extreme caution should be exercised in treating patients with respiratory acidosis and metabolic alkalosis, one of the most commonly encountered mixed acid-base disorders. Although therapeutic measures intended to improve alveolar ventilation should be instituted, an abrupt decrease in $Paco_2$ risks development of severe alkalemia. Therefore, aggressive measures should be taken to treat metabolic alkalosis, making certain that reversal of the metabolic component does not lag behind treatment of the respiratory element. In fact, because the ventilatory drive in patients with chronic respiratory acidosis depends in part on the prevailing acidemia, reversal of a complicating element of metabolic alkalosis regularly results in improved alveolar ventilation, and consequently a decrease in $Paco_2$ and an increase in Pao_2 are achieved.

REFERENCES

1. Adrogué HJ, Madias NE. Management of life-threatening acid-base disorders (part I). *N Engl J Med.* 1998;338:26-34.
2. Adrogué HJ, Madias NE. Management of life-threatening acid-base disorders (part II). *N Engl J Med.* 1998;338:107-111.
3. Adrogué HJ, Wesson DE. Overview of acid-base disorders. In: Adrogué HJ, Wesson DE, eds. *Blackwell's Basics of Medicine: Acid-Base.* Boston: Blackwell Science; 1994:49-133.
4. Epstein SK, Singh N. Respiratory acidosis. *Respir Care.* 2001;46: 366-383.
5. Adrogué HJ, Rashad MN, Gorin AB, et al. Assessing acid-base status in circulatory failure: Differences between arterial and central venous blood. *N Engl J Med.* 1989;320:1312-1316.
6. Adrogué HJ, Rashad MN, Gorin AB, et al. Arteriovenous acid-base disparity in circulatory failure: Studies on mechanism. *Am J Physiol.* 1989;257:F1087-F1093.
7. Madias NE, Adrogué HJ. Respiratory acidosis and alkalosis. In: Greenberg A, ed. *Primer on Kidney Diseases.* 5th ed. Philadelphia: Saunders Elsevier; 2009:91-97.
8. Madias NE, Adrogué HJ. Influence of chronic metabolic acid-base disorders on the acute CO_2 titration curve. *J Appl Physiol.* 1983;55: 1187-1195.
9. Adrogué HJ, Madias NE. Influence of chronic respiratory acid-base disorders on acute CO_2 titration curve. *J Appl Physiol.* 1985;58: 1231-1238.
10. Adrogué HJ, Madias NE. Arterial blood gas monitoring: Acid-base assessment. In: Tobin MJ, ed. *Principles and Practice of Intensive Care Monitoring.* New York: McGraw-Hill; 1998:217-241.
11. Adrogué HJ, Tobin MJ. Management of respiratory failure. In: Adrogué HJ, Tobin MJ, eds. *Blackwell's Basics of Medicine, vol 6. Respiratory Failure.* Boston: Blackwell Science; 1997:311-331.
12. Amato MBP, Barbas CSV, Medeiros DM, et al. Effect of a protective-ventilation strategy on mortality in the acute respiratory distress syndrome. *N Engl J Med.* 1998;338:347-354.
13. Cardenas VJ, Zwischenberger JB, Tao W, et al. Correction of blood pH attenuates changes in hemodynamics and organ blood flow during permissive hypercapnia. *Crit Care Med.* 1996;24:827-834.
14. Adrogué HJ, Brensilver J, Cohen JJ, Madias NE. Influence of steady-state alterations in acid-base equilibrium on the fate of administered bicarbonate in the dog. *J Clin Invest.* 1983;71:867-883.
15. Foster GT, Vaziri ND, Sassoon CSH. Respiratory alkalosis. *Respir Care.* 2001;46:384-391.
16. Laffey JG, Kavanagh BP. Hypocapnia. *N Engl J Med.* 2002;347:43-53.
17. Adrogué HJ, Madias NE. Mixed acid-base disorders. In: Jacobson HR, Striker GE, Klahr S, eds. *The Principles and Practice of Nephrology.* 2nd ed. Philadelphia: Decker; 1995:953-962.
18. Anderson LE, Henrich WL. Alkalemia-associated morbidity and mortality in medical and surgical patients. *South Med J.* 1987;80:729-733.
19. Madias NE, Perrone RD. Acid-base disorders in association with renal disease. In: Schrier SW, Gottschaid CW, eds. *Diseases of the Kidney.* 5th ed. Boston: Little, Brown; 1993:2669-2699.
20. Adrogué HJ, Wilson H, Boyd AE, et al. Plasma acid-base patterns in diabetic ketoacidosis. *N Engl J Med.* 1982;307:1603-1610.
21. Leung JM, Landow L, Franks M, et al. Safety and efficacy of intravenous Carbicarb in patients undergoing surgery: Comparison with sodium bicarbonate in the treatment of mild metabolic acidosis [erratum in Crit Care Med 1995;23:420]. *Crit Care Med.* 1994;22:1540-1549.

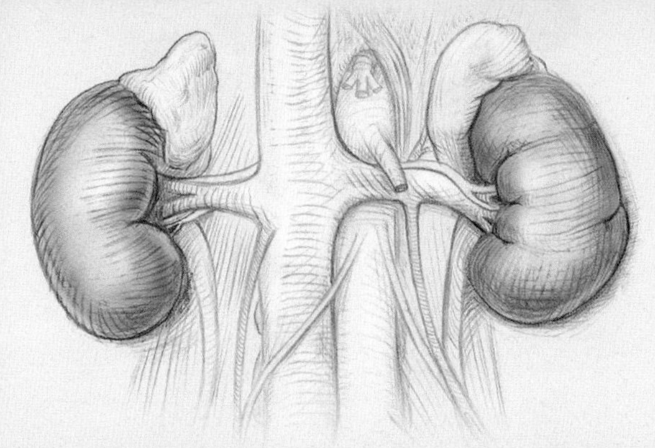

SECTION IV

Glomerular Disease

CHAPTER 15

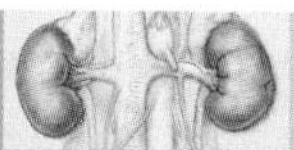

Introduction to Glomerular Disease: Clinical Presentations

Jürgen Floege, John Feehally

DEFINITION

Glomerular disease has clinical presentations that vary from the asymptomatic individual who is found to have hypertension, edema, hematuria, or proteinuria at a routine medical assessment to a patient with a fulminant illness with acute kidney injury (AKI) possibly associated with life-threatening extrarenal disease (Fig. 15.1). The most dramatic symptomatic presentations are uncommon. Asymptomatic urine abnormalities are much more common but less specific; they may also indicate a wide range of nonglomerular urinary tract disease.

CLINICAL EVALUATION OF GLOMERULAR DISEASE

The history, physical examination, and investigations are aimed at excluding nonglomerular disease, finding evidence of associated multisystem disease, and establishing renal function.

History

The majority of glomerular diseases do not lead to symptoms that patients will report. However, specific questioning may reveal edema, hypertension, foamy urine, or urinary abnormalities during prior routine testing (e.g., during routine medical examinations). Multisystem diseases associated with glomerular disease include diabetes, hypertension, amyloid, lupus, and vasculitis. Apart from the individual history suggestive of these diseases, a positive family history may also be obtained in some cases. Other causes of familial renal disease may include Alport's syndrome (especially if it is associated with hearing loss; see Chapter 46), uncommon familial forms of IgA nephropathy (see Chapter 22), focal segmental glomerulosclerosis (FSGS; see Chapters 18 and 19), hemolytic-uremic syndrome (HUS; see Chapter 28), and other rare conditions (see Chapter 27). Morbid obesity can be associated with FSGS. Certain drugs and toxins may cause glomerular disease; these include minimal change disease (MCD; nonsteroidal anti-inflammatory agents [NSAIDs] and interferon), membranous nephropathy (penicillamine; NSAIDs; mercury, for example, in skin-lightening creams), FSGS (pamidronate, heroin), and HUS (cyclosporine, tacrolimus, mitomycin C, oral contraceptives). Recent or persistent infection (especially streptococcal infection, infective endocarditis, and certain viral infections; see Chapters 21, 55, and 56) may also be associated with a variety of glomerular diseases.

Various malignant neoplasms are associated with glomerular disease. These include lung, breast, and gastrointestinal carcinoma (membranous nephropathy); Hodgkin's disease (MCD); non-Hodgkin's lymphoma (membranoproliferative glomerulonephritis [MPGN]); and renal carcinoma (amyloid; see Chapter 26). Patients will occasionally present with the renal disease as the first manifestation of a tumor.

Physical Examination

The presence of dependent pitting edema suggests the nephrotic syndrome, heart failure, or cirrhosis. In the nephrotic subject, edema is often periorbital in the morning (Fig. 15.2), whereas the face is not affected overnight in edema associated with heart failure (because of orthopnea resulting from pulmonary congestion) or cirrhosis (because the patient cannot lie flat owing to pressure on the diaphragm from ascites). As it progresses, edema of genitals and abdominal wall becomes apparent, and accumulation of fluid in body spaces leads to ascites and pleural effusions. Edema is unpleasant; it leads to feelings of tightness in the limbs and a bloated abdomen. There are practical problems of clothes and shoes no longer fitting. Yet surprisingly, edema may become massive in nephrotic syndrome before patients seek medical help; fluid gains of 20% of normal body weight are by no means unusual (Fig. 15.3). The edema becomes firm and stops pitting only when it is long-standing. In children, fluid retention may also be striking with nephritic syndrome. A useful clinical sign to help distinguish nephrotic from nephritic syndrome is Heyman's sign, the paper-thin, floppy ears typical of nephrotic syndrome. Chronic hypoalbuminemia is also associated with loss of normal pink color under the nails, resulting in white nails or white bands if the nephrotic syndrome is transient (Muehrcke's bands, Fig. 15.4). Xanthelasmas may also be present as a result of the hyperlipidemia associated with the nephrotic syndrome (Fig. 15.5).

The presence of pulmonary signs should suggest one of the pulmonary-renal syndromes (see Figs. 23.9 and 23.10). Palpable purpura may be seen in vasculitis, systemic lupus, cryoglobulinemia, or endocarditis.

Laboratory Studies

Assessment of renal function and careful examination of the urine (see Chapters 3 and 4) are critical. The quantity of urine protein and the presence or absence of dysmorphic red cells and casts will help classify the clinical presentation (see Fig. 15.1).

Certain serologic tests are also helpful. These include antinuclear and anti-DNA antibodies (lupus), cryoglobulins and rheumatoid factor (both suggestive of cryoglobulinemia), anti–glomerular basement membrane (anti-GBM) antibodies (Goodpasture's disease), antineutrophil cytoplasmic (ANCA) antibodies; vasculitis, and antistreptolysin O titer or streptozyme test (poststreptococcal glomerulonephritis [GN]). Serum and

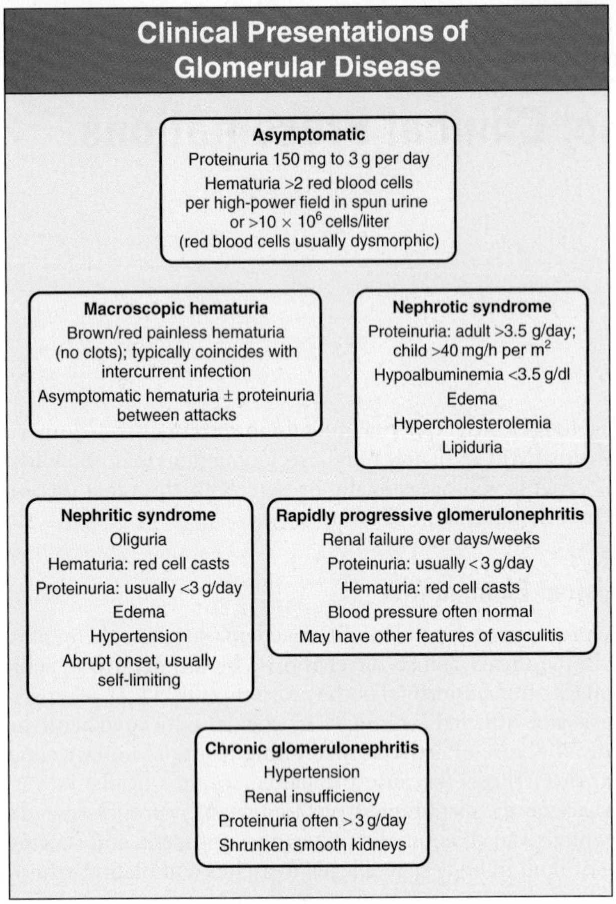

Clinical Presentations of Glomerular Disease

Asymptomatic
Proteinuria 150 mg to 3 g per day
Hematuria >2 red blood cells per high-power field in spun urine or >10 × 10^6 cells/liter (red blood cells usually dysmorphic)

Macroscopic hematuria
Brown/red painless hematuria (no clots); typically coincides with intercurrent infection
Asymptomatic hematuria ± proteinuria between attacks

Nephrotic syndrome
Proteinuria: adult >3.5 g/day; child >40 mg/h per m^2
Hypoalbuminemia <3.5 g/dl
Edema
Hypercholesterolemia
Lipiduria

Nephritic syndrome
Oliguria
Hematuria: red cell casts
Proteinuria: usually <3 g/day
Edema
Hypertension
Abrupt onset, usually self-limiting

Rapidly progressive glomerulonephritis
Renal failure over days/weeks
Proteinuria: usually < 3 g/day
Hematuria: red cell casts
Blood pressure often normal
May have other features of vasculitis

Chronic glomerulonephritis
Hypertension
Renal insufficiency
Proteinuria often > 3 g/day
Shrunken smooth kidneys

Figure 15.1 Clinical presentations of glomerular disease.

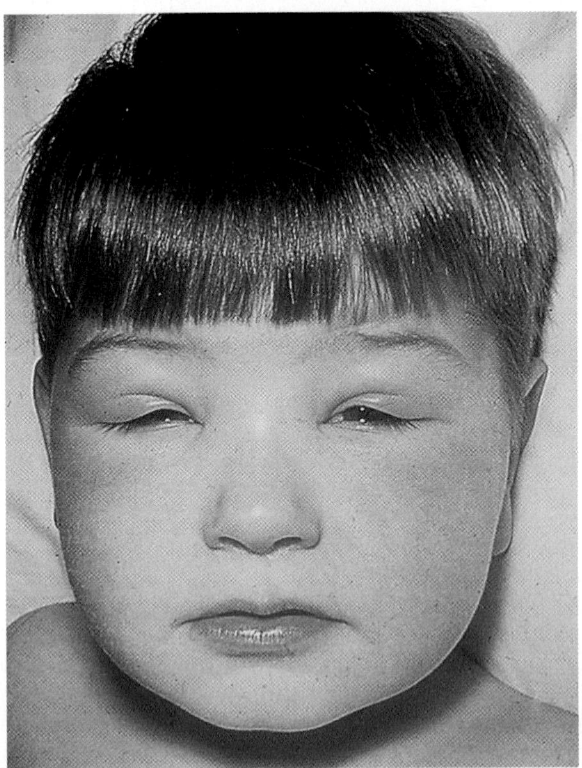

Figure 15.2 Nephrotic edema. Periorbital edema in the early morning in a nephrotic child. The edema resolves during the day under the influence of gravity.

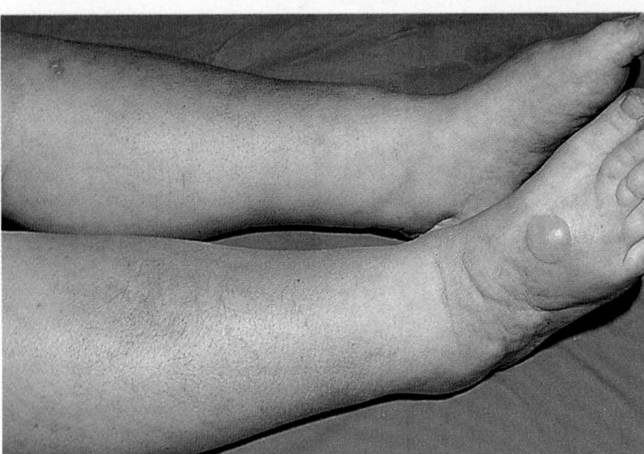

Figure 15.3 Nephrotic edema. Severe peripheral edema in nephrotic syndrome; note the blisters caused by intradermal fluid.

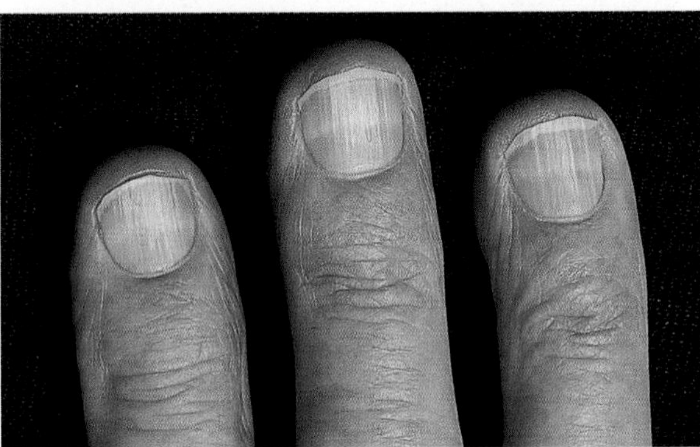

Figure 15.4 Muehrcke's bands in nephrotic syndrome. The white band grew during a transient period of hypoalbuminemia caused by the nephrotic syndrome.

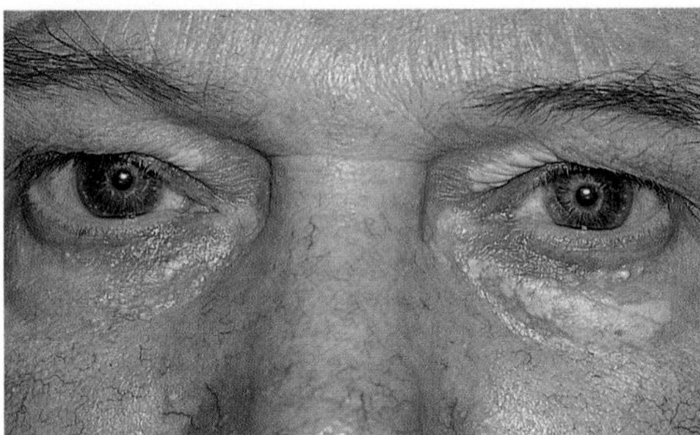

Figure 15.5 Xanthelasmas in nephrotic syndrome. These prominent xanthelasmas developed within a period of 2 months in a patient with recent onset of severe nephrotic syndrome and serum cholesterol level of 550 mg/dl (14.2 mmol/l).

urine electrophoresis will detect monoclonal light chains or heavy chains (myeloma-associated amyloid or light-chain deposition disease).

Testing for the presence of ongoing bacterial or viral infections is also useful. This includes blood cultures and testing for hepatitis B, hepatitis C, and human immunodeficiency virus (HIV) infection.

Measurement of systemic complement pathway activation by testing for serum C3, C4, and CH50 (50% hemolyzing dose of complement) is particularly helpful in limiting the differential diagnosis (Fig. 15.6).

Hypocomplementemia in Glomerular Disease

Pathway Affected	Complement Changes	Glomerular Diseases	Nonglomerular Diseases
Classical pathway activation	C3 ↓, C4 ↓, CH50 ↓	Lupus nephritis (especially class IV), mixed essential cryoglobulinemia	
	+ C4 nephritic factor	Membranoproliferative GN type 1	
Alternative pathway activation	C3 ↓, C4 normal, CH50 ↓	Poststreptococcal GN GN associated with other infection* Endocarditis, shunt nephritis, hepatitis B Hemolytic-uremic syndrome	Atheroembolic renal disease
	+ C3 nephritic factor	Membranoproliferative GN type II (Dense Deposit Disease)	
Reduced complement synthesis	Acquired		Hepatic disease Malnutrition
	Hereditary C2 deficiency Factor H deficiency	Lupus nephritis Familial hemolytic-uremic syndrome Membranoproliferative GN type II	

Figure 15.6 Hypocomplementemia in glomerular disease. *Glomerulonephritis (GN) with visceral abscesses is generally associated with normal or increased complement (elevations occur because complement components are acute-phase reactants). CH50, 50% hemolyzing dose of complement.

The emerging role for genetic evaluation in patients with FSGS is discussed in Chapter 19.

Imaging

Ultrasound scanning is recommended in the workup to ensure the presence of two kidneys, to rule out obstruction or anatomic abnormalities, and to assess kidney size. Renal size is often normal in GN, although large kidneys (>14 cm) are sometimes seen in nephrotic syndrome as sociated with diabetes, amyloid, or HIV infection. Large kidneys can also occasionally be seen with any acute severe GN. The occurrence of small kidneys (<9 cm) suggests chronic renal disease and should limit enthusiasm for renal biopsy or aggressive immunosuppressive therapies.

Renal Biopsy

Renal biopsy is generally required to establish the type of glomerular disease and to guide treatment decisions. The principles and practice of renal biopsy are discussed in Chapter 6. There are some situations, however, in which renal biopsy is not performed. If there are no unusual clinical features in nephrotic children, the probability of MCD is so high that corticosteroids can be initiated without biopsy (see Chapter 17). In acute nephritic syndrome, if all features point to poststreptococcal GN, especially in an epidemic, biopsy can be reserved for the minority who do not show early spontaneous improvement (see Chapter 55). In anti-GBM disease (see Chapter 23), the presence of lung hemorrhage and rapidly progressive renal failure with urinary red cell casts and high titers of circulating anti-GBM antibody establishes the diagnosis without the need for a biopsy, although a biopsy may still provide prognostic information. In patients with systemic features of vasculitis, a positive ANCA titer, negative blood cultures, and a tissue biopsy specimen from another site showing vasculitis are sufficient to secure a diagnosis of renal vasculitis. Again, however, renal biopsy may provide important clues to disease activity and chronicity. Biopsy is also not generally performed in long-standing diabetes with characteristic findings suggestive of diabetic nephropathy and other evidence of microvascular complications of diabetes (see Chapter 29). Biopsy may also not be indicated in many patients with mild glomerular disease presenting with asymptomatic urine abnormalities as the prognosis is excellent and histologic findings will not alter management.

ASYMPTOMATIC URINE ABNORMALITIES

Urine testing that detects proteinuria or microscopic hematuria is often the first evidence of glomerular disease. The random nature of urine testing in most communities inevitably means that much mild glomerular disease remains undetected. In some countries, symptomless individuals may have a urine test only if they require medical approval for some key life event: to obtain life insurance, to join the armed forces, or sometimes for employment purposes. In other countries, for example, Japan, urinalysis is performed routinely in school or for employment. These different practices may partly account for the apparently variable incidence of certain diseases, such as IgA nephropathy. Asymptomatic proteinuria and hematuria, and the combination of the two, increase in prevalence with age (Fig. 15.7).[1] Nevertheless, there is no evidence to justify routine population-wide screening for asymptomatic urine abnormalities as renal biopsy and therapeutic intervention are rarely required when renal function is preserved. Screening, in particular for microalbuminuria, may be indicated for high-risk populations, for example, patients with diabetes, hypertension, or cardiovascular disease, and those with a family history of renal disease.

Asymptomatic Microscopic Hematuria

Microscopic hematuria is defined as the presence of more than two red blood cells per high-power field in a spun urine sediment (3000 rpm for 5 minutes) or more than 10×10^6 red blood cells/liter.

Microscopic hematuria is common in many glomerular diseases, especially IgA nephropathy and thin basement membrane nephropathy, although there are many other causes of hematuria (discussed further in Chapter 46). A glomerular origin should especially be considered if more than 5% of the red cells are acanthocytes (see Chapter 4) or if the hematuria is accompanied by red cell casts or proteinuria (Fig. 15.8).

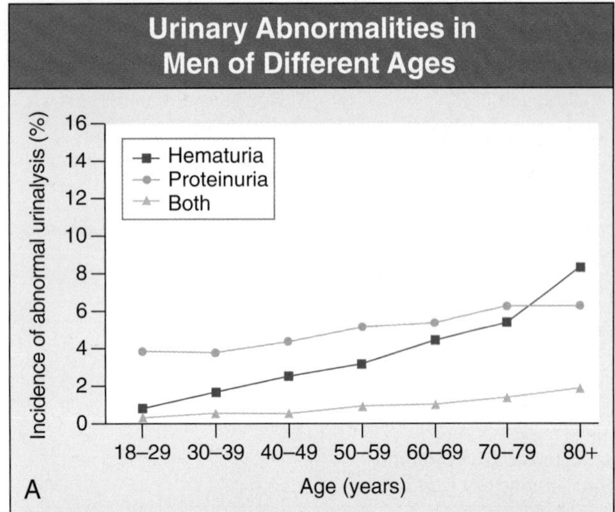

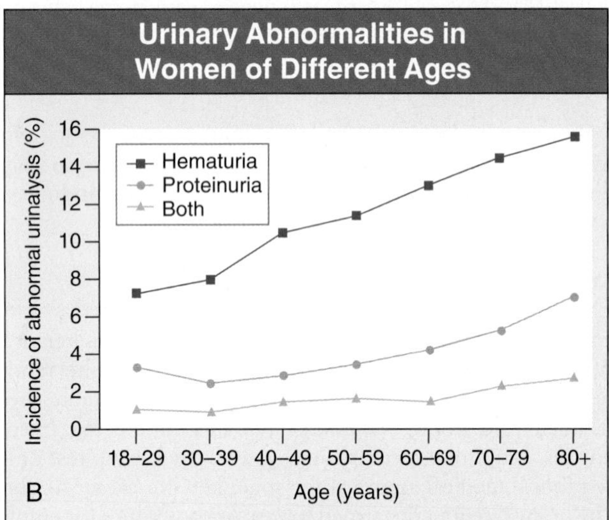

Figure 15.7 Prevalence of asymptomatic proteinuria and hematuria with age. Mass screening of a population of 107,192 adult men **A,** and women **B,** in Okinawa, Japan. Hematuria is more common in women. *(Modified from reference 1.)*

Pathogenesis

Glomerular hematuria is thought to result from small breaks in the GBM that allow extravasation of red blood cells into the urinary space. This may occur in the peripheral capillary wall but more commonly occurs in the paramesangial basement membrane, particularly in diseases in which there is injury to the mesangium (mesangiolysis).

Evaluation

The evaluation of microscopic hematuria, which is discussed further in Chapter 46, begins with a thorough history. Urine culture should exclude urinary or prostatic infection. Phase contrast microscopy should follow in cases of persistent microscopic hematuria to search for dysmorphic red cells and red cell casts. Any detectable proteinuria in the setting of asymptomatic microscopic hematuria virtually excludes "urologic" bleeding and strongly suggests a glomerular origin. If this evaluation is nondiagnostic, renal imaging is performed to exclude anatomic lesions such as polycystic kidneys, stones, tumors, and arteriovenous malformations.

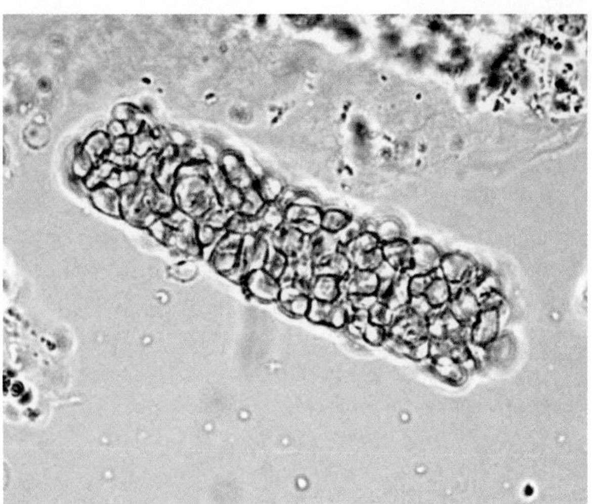

Figure 15.8 Red cell cast. A red cell cast typical of glomerular hematuria.

In those older than 40 years who have persistent isolated microscopic hematuria without evidence of a glomerular origin (see previous discussion), cystoscopy is mandatory to exclude uroepithelial malignant disease. In people younger than 40 years, such malignant disease is so rare that cystoscopy is not recommended. If all the prior study results are normal, a glomerular etiology is likely.[2] The glomerular etiology can be determined only by renal biopsy, but this is rarely done because the prognosis is excellent in the setting of normal renal function, normal blood pressure, and low-grade proteinuria (<0.5 g/day). However, repeated evaluation is mandatory.

Asymptomatic Non-nephrotic Proteinuria

The hallmark of glomerular disease is the excretion of protein in the urine. Normal urine protein excretion is less than 150 mg/24 h (consisting of 20 to 30 mg of albumin, 10 to 20 mg of low-molecular-weight proteins that undergo glomerular filtration, and 40 to 60 mg of secreted proteins such as Tamm-Horsfall protein and IgA). Proteinuria is identified and quantified by dipstick testing or by assay in timed urine collections. The interpretation of these methods is discussed in Chapter 4.

Microalbuminuria is defined as the excretion of 30 to 300 mg of albumin per day, equivalent to a urine albumin to creatinine (g/g) ratio of 0.03 to 0.3, and is detected by quantitative immunoassay or by special urine dipsticks as this is below the sensitivity of the normal dipstick. This measurement is primarily used to identify diabetic subjects at risk for development of nephropathy and to assess cardiovascular risk, for example, in patients with hypertension.

Non-nephrotic proteinuria is usually defined as a urine protein excretion of less than 3.5 g/24 h or a urine protein to creatinine (g/g) ratio of less than 3. Although nephrotic-range proteinuria is absolutely characteristic of glomerular disease, asymptomatic proteinuria (<3.5 g/24 h) is much less specific and may occur with a wide range of nonglomerular parenchymal diseases as well as with nonparenchymal renal and urinary tract conditions that must be excluded by clinical evaluation and investigation.

Increased urine protein excretion may result from alterations in glomerular permeability or tubulointerstitial disease, although only in glomerular disease will it be in the nephrotic range. It can also occur from increased filtration through normal glomeruli (overflow proteinuria).

Overflow Proteinuria

Overflow proteinuria is typical of urinary light-chain excretion. It is seen in myeloma but can occur in other settings (such as the release of lysozyme by leukemic cells) and should be suspected when the urine dipstick is negative for albumin despite detection of large amounts of proteinuria by other tests.

Tubular Proteinuria

Tubulointerstitial disease can also be associated with low-grade (usually <2 g/day) proteinuria. In addition to the loss of tubular proteins (such as α_1- or β_2-microglobulin), there will also be some albuminuria due to impaired tubular reabsorption of filtered albumin. Tubular proteinuria accompanying glomerular proteinuria is an adverse prognostic sign in various glomerular diseases as it usually indicates advanced tubulointerstitial damage.

Glomerular Proteinuria

Glomerular proteinuria is further classified into that which is transient or hemodynamic (functional), that which is present only during the day (orthostatic), and that which is persistent or fixed.

Functional Proteinuria Functional proteinuria refers to the transient non-nephrotic proteinuria that can occur with fever, exercise, heart failure, and hyperadrenergic or hyperreninemic states. Functional proteinuria is benign; it is usually assumed to be hemodynamic in origin and to be the consequence of increases in single-nephron flow or pressure.

Orthostatic Proteinuria In children and young adults, low-grade glomerular proteinuria may be orthostatic, meaning that proteinuria is absent when urine is generated in the recumbent position. If there is no proteinuria in early morning urine, the diagnosis of orthostatic proteinuria can be made. The mechanism of orthostasis is not understood. Total urine protein in orthostatic proteinuria is usually less than 1 g/24 h; hematuria and hypertension are absent. Renal biopsy usually shows normal morphology or occasionally mild glomerular change. The prognosis is uniformly good, and renal biopsy is not indicated.[3]

Fixed Non-nephrotic Proteinuria Fixed non-nephrotic proteinuria is usually caused by glomerular disease. If glomerular filtration rate (GFR) is preserved and proteinuria is less than 1 g/day, biopsy is not indicated but prolonged follow-up is necessary so long as significant proteinuria persists to rule out the possibility of disease progression. Previous studies indicate that the biopsy findings in these patients will be similar to those seen in nephrotic syndrome, although milder lesions are more common, particularly mesangial proliferative GN without immune deposits. In general, no treatment is necessary.

Although it is controversial, many nephrologists will perform a renal biopsy in patients with normal GFR if non-nephrotic proteinuria exceeds 1 g/day, in particular if it persists after initiation of angiotensin-converting enzyme (ACE) inhibitor or angiotensin receptor blocker (ARB) therapy.

The evaluation of isolated asymptomatic proteinuria is summarized in Figure 15.9.

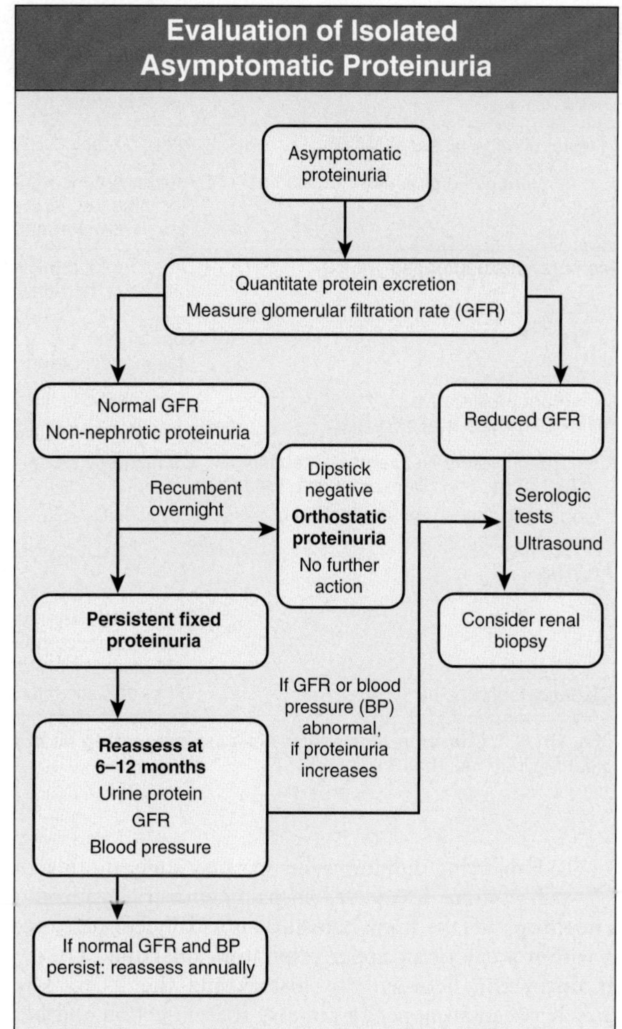

Figure 15.9 Evaluation of patients with isolated asymptomatic proteinuria.

Asymptomatic Proteinuria with Hematuria

When asymptomatic hematuria and proteinuria coincide, there is a much greater risk of significant glomerular injury, hypertension, and progressive renal dysfunction. Minor histologic changes are less common. Renal biopsy is indicated even if urine protein is only 0.5 to 1 g/24 h if there is also persistent microscopic hematuria with casts.

MACROSCOPIC HEMATURIA

Episodic painless macroscopic hematuria associated with glomerular disease is often brown or "smoky" rather than red, and clots are unusual. It must be distinguished from other causes of red or brown urine, including hemoglobinuria, myoglobinuria, porphyrias, consumption of food dyes (particularly beetroot), and intake of drugs (in particular rifampin).

Macroscopic hematuria caused by glomerular disease is observed primarily in children and young adults and is rare past the age of 40 years. Most cases are caused by IgA nephropathy, but hematuria may occur with other glomerular and nonglomerular renal diseases, including acute interstitial nephritis. Although macroscopic hematuria is typically painless, there may

Common Glomerular Diseases Presenting as Nephrotic Syndrome in Adults		
Disease	**Associations**	**Serologic Tests Helpful in Diagnosis**
Minimal change disease (MCD)	Allergy, atopy, NSAIDs, Hodgkin's disease	None
Focal segmental glomerulosclerosis (FSGS)	African Americans HIV infection Heroin, pamidronate	— HIV antibody —
Membranous nephropathy (MN)	Drugs: gold, penicillamine, NSAIDs Infections: hepatitis B, C; malaria Lupus nephritis Malignancy: breast, lung, gastrointestinal tract	— Hepatitis B surface antigen, anti–hepatitis C virus antibody Anti-DNA antibody —
Membranoproliferative glomerulonephritis (MPGN) (type I)	C4 nephritic factor	C3 ↓, C4 ↓
Membranoproliferative glomerulonephritis (MPGN) (type II) (Dense deposit disease)	C3 nephritic factor	C3 ↓, C4 normal
Cryoglobulinemic membranoproliferative glomerulonephritis	Hepatitis C	Anti-hepatitis C virus antibody, rheumatoid factor, C3 ↓, C4 ↓, CH50 ↓
Amyloid	Myeloma Rheumatoid arthritis, bronchiectasis, Crohn's disease (and other chronic inflammatory conditions), familial Mediterranean fever	Serum protein electrophoresis, urine immunoelectrophoresis —
Diabetic nephropathy	Other diabetic microangiopathy	None

Figure 15.10 Common glomerular diseases presenting as nephrotic syndrome in adults. HIV, human immunodeficiency virus; NSAIDs, nonsteroidal antiinflammatory drugs.

be an accompanying dull loin ache that may suggest other diagnoses, such as stone disease or loin-pain hematuria syndrome. In IgA nephropathy, the frank hematuria is usually episodic, occurring within a day of an upper respiratory infection. There is a clear distinction between this history and the 2- to 3-week latency between an upper respiratory tract infection and hematuria that is highly suggestive of postinfectious (usually poststreptococcal) GN; furthermore, in poststreptococcal disease, there will usually be other features of nephritic syndrome. Macroscopic hematuria requires urologic evaluation including cystoscopy at any age unless the history (as shown previously) is characteristic of glomerular hematuria.

NEPHROTIC SYNDROME

Definition

Nephrotic syndrome is pathognomonic of glomerular disease. It is a clinical syndrome with a characteristic pentad (see Fig. 15.1).[4] Patients may be nephrotic with preserved renal function, but in many circumstances, progressive renal failure will become superimposed when nephrotic syndrome is prolonged.

Independent of the risk of progressive renal failure, the nephrotic syndrome has far-reaching metabolic effects that can influence the general health of the patient. Fortunately, some episodes of nephrotic syndrome are self-limited, and a few respond completely to specific treatment (e.g., corticosteroids in MCD). However, for most patients, it is a chronic condition. Not all patients with proteinuria above 3.5 g/24 h will have a full nephrotic syndrome; some have a normal serum albumin concentration and no edema. This difference presumably reflects the varied response of protein metabolism; some patients sustain an increase in albumin synthesis in response to heavy proteinuria that may even normalize serum albumin.

Etiology

The major causes of nephrotic syndrome are shown in Figure 15.10. Proteinuria in the nephrotic range in the absence of edema and hypoalbuminemia has similar etiologies. The relative frequency of the different glomerular diseases varies with age (Fig. 15.11). Although it is predominant in childhood, MCD remains common at all ages.[5] There is an increased prevalence of FSGS in African Americans, and historical comparisons indicate that FSGS is becoming more common and MPGN less common in all adults.[6]

Hypoalbuminemia

Hypoalbuminemia is mostly a consequence of urinary losses. The liver responds by increasing albumin synthesis, but this compensatory mechanism appears to be blunted in nephrotic syndrome.[7] The end result is that serum albumin falls further. White bands in the nails (Muehrcke's bands) are a characteristic clinical sign of hypoalbuminemia (see Fig. 15.4). The increase in protein synthesis in response to proteinuria is not discriminating; as a result, proteins that are not being lost in the urine may actually increase in concentration in plasma. This is chiefly determined by molecular weight; large molecules will not spill into the urine and will increase in the plasma; smaller proteins, although synthesized to excess, will enter the urine and be diminished in the plasma. These variations in plasma proteins are clinically important in two areas: hypercoagulability and hyperlipidemia (see later discussion).

Edema

At least two major mechanisms are involved in the formation of nephrotic edema (Fig. 15.12; see Chapter 7).[8] In the first

Age-related Variations in Nephrotic Syndrome

	Prevalence (%)				
	Child	Young Adult		Middle and Old Age	
	(<15 years)	Whites	Blacks	Whites	Blacks
Minimal change disease (MCD)	78	23	15	21	16
Focal segmental glomerulosclerosis (FSGS)	8	19	55	13	35
Membranous nephropathy (MN)	2	24	26	37	24
Membranoproliferative glomerulonephritis (MPGN)	6	13	0	4	2
Other glomerulonephritis	6	14	2	12	12
Amyloid	0	5	2	13	11

Figure 15.11 Age-related variations in nephrotic syndrome. *(Data modified from references 5 and 6.)*

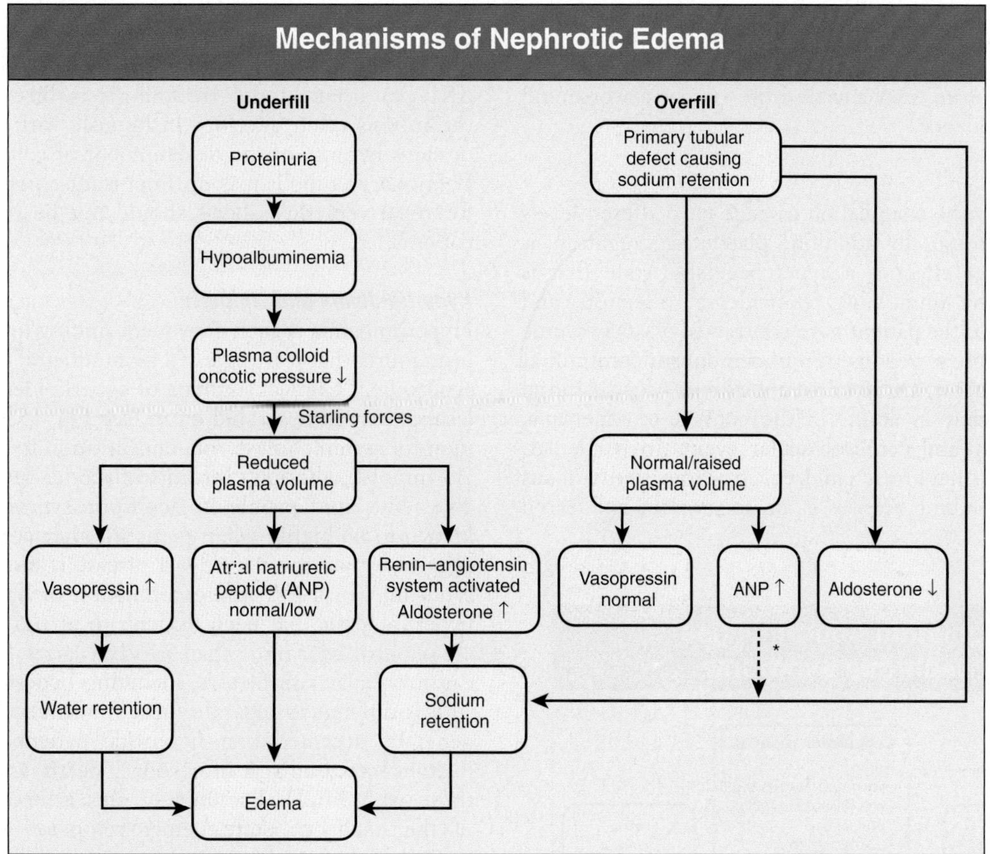

Figure 15.12 Mechanisms of nephrotic edema. *The kidney is relatively resistant to ANP in this setting, so ANP has little effect in countering sodium retention.

mechanism, which is more common in children with MCD, the edema appears to be the consequence of the low serum albumin producing a decrease in plasma oncotic pressure, which allows increased transudation of fluid from capillary beds into the extracellular space according to the laws of Starling. The consequent decrease in circulating blood volume (underfill) produces a secondary stimulation of the renin-angiotensin system, resulting in aldosterone-induced sodium retention in the distal tubule. This attempt to compensate for hypovolemia merely aggravates edema because the low oncotic pressure alters the balance of forces across the capillary wall in favor of hydrostatic pressure, forcing more fluid into the interstitial space rather than retaining it within the vascular compartment.

In many nephrotic patients, however, there appears to be a primary defect in the ability of the distal nephron to excrete sodium, possibly related to activation of the epithelial sodium channel (ENaC) by proteolytic enzymes that enter the tubular lumen in heavy proteinuria.[9] As a result, there is an increased blood volume, the suppression of renin-angiotensin and vasopressin, and a tendency to hypertension rather than to hypotension; the kidney is also relatively resistant to the actions of atrial natriuretic peptide. An elevated blood volume results (overfill), which, in association with the low plasma oncotic pressure, provokes transudation of fluid into the extracellular space and edema. The mechanism for the defect in sodium excretion remains unknown, although it has been hypothesized that inflammatory leukocytes in the interstitium, which are found in many glomerular diseases, may impair sodium excretion by producing angiotensin II and oxidants (the latter inactivate local nitric oxide, which is natriuretic).[10]

Metabolic Consequences of Nephrotic Syndrome

Negative Nitrogen Balance

The heavy proteinuria leads to marked negative nitrogen balance, usually measured in clinical practice by serum albumin. Nephrotic syndrome is a wasting illness, but the degree of muscle loss is masked by edema and not fully apparent until the patient is rendered edema free. Loss of 10% to 20% of lean body mass is not uncommon. Albumin turnover is increased in response to the tubular catabolism of filtered protein rather than merely to urinary protein loss. Increasing protein intake does not improve albumin metabolism because the hemodynamic response to an increased intake is a rise in glomerular pressure, producing enhanced urine protein losses. A low-protein diet in turn will reduce proteinuria but also reduces the albumin synthesis rate and, in the longer term, may increase the risk of a worsening negative nitrogen balance.

Hypercoagulability

Multiple proteins of the coagulation cascade have altered levels in nephrotic syndrome; in addition, platelet aggregation is enhanced.[11] The net effect is a hypercoagulable state that is enhanced further by immobility, coincidental infection, and hemoconcentration if the patient has a contracted plasma volume (Fig. 15.13). Not only is venous thromboembolism common at any site, but spontaneous arterial thrombosis may occur. Arterial thrombosis may occur in adults in the context of atheroma, promoting coronary and cerebrovascular events in particular; but it also occurs in nephrotic children, in whom spontaneous thrombosis of major limb arteries is an uncommon but feared complication. Up to 10% of nephrotic adults and 2% of children will have a clinical episode of thromboembolism. Individual levels of coagulation proteins are not helpful in assessing the risk of thromboembolism, and serum albumin is mostly used as a surrogate marker. Thromboembolic events increase markedly if the serum albumin concentration decreases to less than 2 g/dl.

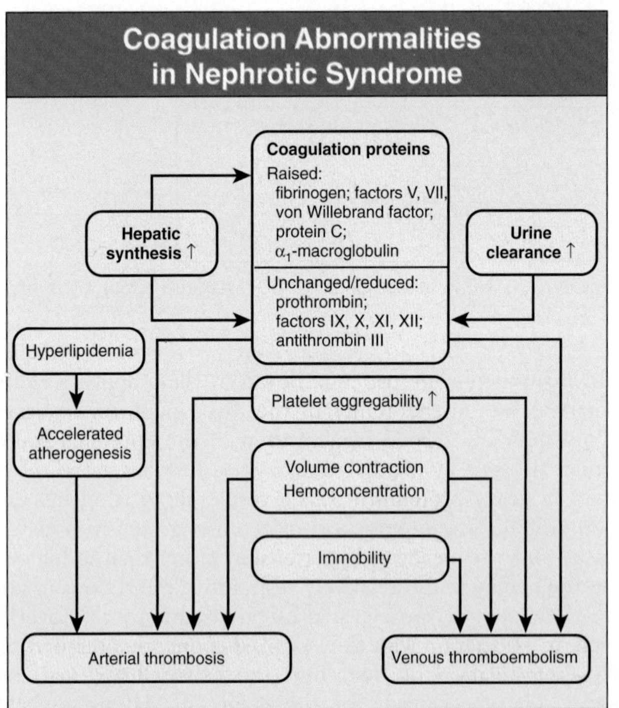

Figure 15.13 Coagulation abnormalities in nephrotic syndrome.

The hypoproteinemia and dysproteinemia produce an increase in erythrocyte sedimentation rate (ESR). Values up to 100 mm/h are not unusual, so ESR loses its clinical value as a marker of an acute-phase response in nephrotic patients.

Renal vein thrombosis (see Chapter 64) is an important complication of nephrotic syndrome. At one time, it was thought that renal vein thrombosis could cause nephrotic syndrome; this is no longer considered true. Renal vein thrombosis is reported clinically in up to 8% of nephrotic patients; but when it is sought systematically (by ultrasound or contrast venography), the frequency increases to 10% to 50%. It may be more common in membranous nephropathy than other disease patterns, although there is no explanation for this observation. Symptoms when the thrombosis is acute may include flank pain and hematuria; rarely, AKI can occur if the thrombosis is bilateral. However, the thrombosis often develops insidiously with minimal symptoms or signs because of the development of collateral blood supply. Pulmonary embolism is an important complication. Screening for renal vein thrombosis should not be routine in nephrotic patients.

Hyperlipidemia and Lipiduria

Hyperlipidemia is such a frequent finding in patients with heavy proteinuria that it is regarded as an integral feature of nephrotic syndrome.[12] Clinical stigmata of hyperlipidemia, such as xanthelasmas, may have a rapid onset (see Fig. 15.5). It is not uncommon for serum cholesterol concentration to be above 500 mg/dl (13 mmol/l), although serum triglyceride levels are highly variable. The lipid profile in nephrotic syndrome (Fig. 15.14) is known to be highly atherogenic in other populations. The presumption that coronary heart disease is increased in nephrotic syndrome, owing to the combination of hypercoagulation and hyperlipidemia, has been difficult to prove. Many patients who are nephrotic for more than 5 to 10 years will develop additional cardiovascular risk factors, including hypertension and uremia, so it is difficult to separate these influences. However, it is now generally accepted that nephrotic patients do carry about a fivefold increased risk of coronary death, with the exception of those with MCD. Presumably, this is because the transience of the nephrotic state before remission with corticosteroid treatment does not subject the patient with MCD to prolonged hyperlipidemia.

There is experimental evidence that hyperlipidemia contributes to progressive renal disease by various mechanisms, with protection afforded by lipid-lowering agents. However, clinical evidence to support a role of statins in retarding chronic kidney disease progression is inconclusive[13] as there are not yet adequate prospective clinical studies on this issue, and lipid-lowering drugs are chiefly indicated in nephrotic syndrome for cardiovascular reasons.

Several mechanisms account for the lipid abnormalities in nephrotic syndrome. These include increased hepatic synthesis of low-density lipoprotein (LDL), very low density lipoprotein (VLDL), and lipoprotein(a) secondary to the hypoalbuminemia; defective peripheral lipoprotein lipase activity resulting in increased VLDL; and urinary losses of high-density lipoprotein (HDL; see Fig. 15.14).

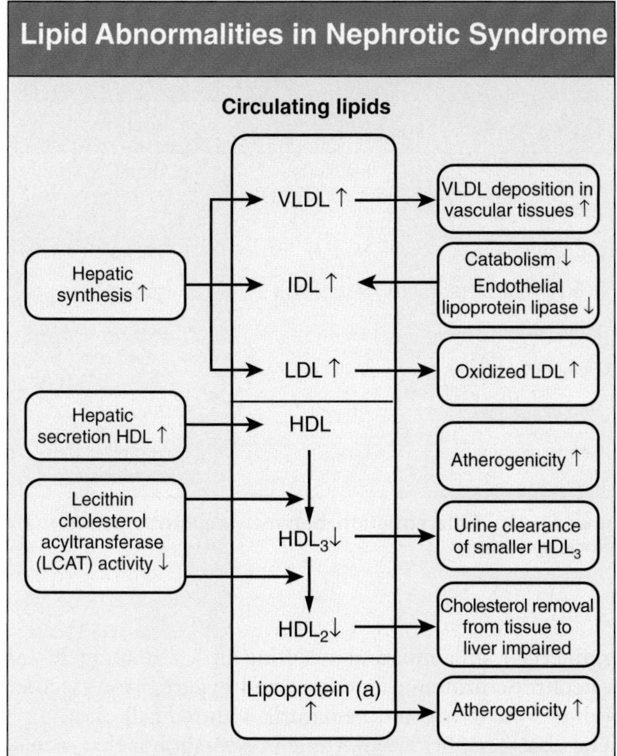

Figure 15.14 Lipid abnormalities in nephrotic syndrome. Changes in HDLs are more controversial than those in VLDLs. HDL, high-density lipoprotein; IDL, intermediate-density lipoprotein; VLDL, very low density lipoprotein.

Lipiduria, the fifth component of the nephrotic syndrome, is manifested by the presence of refractile accumulations of lipid in cellular debris and casts (oval fat bodies and fatty casts; Fig. 15.15). However, the lipiduria appears to be a consequence of the proteinuria and not of the plasma lipid abnormalities.

Other Metabolic Effects of Nephrotic Syndrome

Vitamin D–binding protein is lost in the urine, resulting in low plasma 25-hydroxyvitamin D levels, but plasma-free vitamin D is usually normal, and overt osteomalacia or uncontrolled hyperparathyroidism is very unusual in nephrotic syndrome in the absence of renal insufficiency. Thyroid-binding globulin is lost in the urine and total circulating thyroxine is reduced, but free thyroxine and thyroid-stimulating hormone are normal, and there are no clinical alterations in thyroid status. Occasional cases of copper, iron, or zinc deficiency have been described as a consequence of the loss of binding proteins in the urine.

Drug binding may be altered by the decrease in serum albumin. Although most drugs do not require dose modifications, one important exception is clofibrate, which at normal doses in nephrotic patients produces a severe myopathy. Reduced protein binding may also reduce the dose of warfarin (Coumadin) required to achieve adequate anticoagulation or the dose of furosemide required to achieve adequate fluid loss (see later discussion).

Infection

Nephrotic patients are prone to bacterial infection. Before corticosteroids were shown to be effective in childhood nephrotic syndrome, sepsis was the most common cause of death and remains a major problem in the developing world. Primary peritonitis, especially that caused by pneumococci, is particularly characteristic of nephrotic children. It is less common with increasing age; by the age of 20 years, most adults have antibodies against pneumococcal capsular antigens. Peritonitis caused by both β-hemolytic streptococci and gram-negative organisms occurs, but staphylococcal peritonitis is not reported. Cellulitis, especially in areas of severe edema, is also common, most frequently caused by β-hemolytic streptococci.

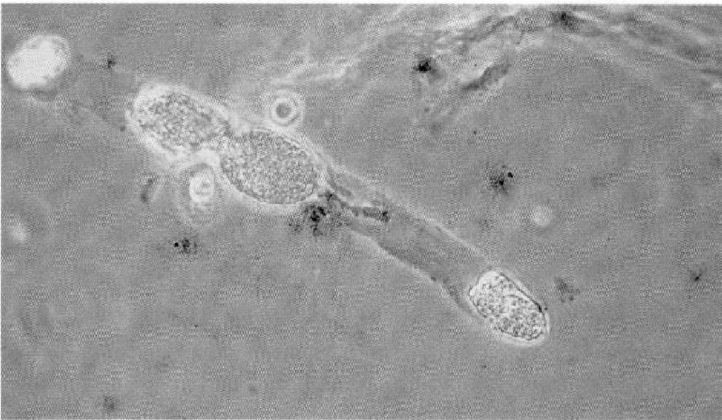

Figure 15.15 Fat in the urine. A hyaline cast containing oval fat bodies that are tubular epithelial cells full of fat. Oval fat bodies often appear brown.

There are several explanations for the increased risk of infection. Large fluid collections are sites for bacteria to grow easily; nephrotic skin is fragile, creating sites of entry; and edema may dilute local humoral immune factors. Loss of IgG and complement factor B (of the alternative pathway) in the urine impairs host ability to eliminate encapsulated organisms such as pneumococci. Zinc and transferrin are lost in the urine, and both are required for normal lymphocyte function. Neutrophil phagocytic function is impaired in nephrotic syndrome, and a number of *in vitro* T-cell dysfunctions are described, although their clinical significance is uncertain.

Acute and Chronic Changes in Renal Function in Nephrotic Syndrome

Acute Kidney Injury

Patients with nephrotic syndrome are also at risk for the development of AKI,[14] which can occur by a variety of mechanisms that are summarized in Figure 15.16. These include volume depletion or sepsis, resulting in either prerenal AKI or acute tubular necrosis[15]; transformation of the underlying disease (such as the development of crescentic nephritis in a patient with membranous nephropathy); development of bilateral renal vein thrombosis; increased disposition to azotemia from NSAIDs and ACE inhibitors or ARBs; and increased risk of allergic interstitial nephritis secondary to drugs, including diuretics. It has also been postulated that some patients develop AKI from intrarenal edema with compression of tubules; these patients, like nephrotic subjects with prerenal azotemia, may respond with diuresis to albumin infusions coupled with a loop diuretic.

Chronic Kidney Disease

With the exception of MCD, most causes of nephrotic syndrome are associated with some risk for the development of progressive renal failure. In this regard, one of the greatest risk factors for progression is the degree of proteinuria (see Chapter 76). Progression is uncommon if there is sustained proteinuria of less than 2 g/day. The risk increases in proportion to the severity of

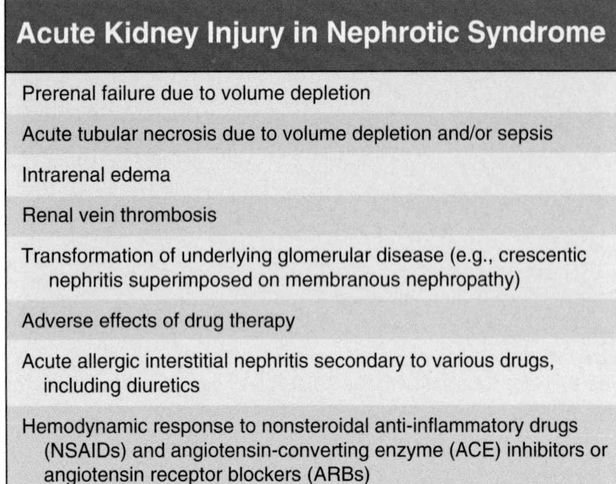

Acute Kidney Injury in Nephrotic Syndrome

Acute Kidney Injury in Nephrotic Syndrome
Prerenal failure due to volume depletion
Acute tubular necrosis due to volume depletion and/or sepsis
Intrarenal edema
Renal vein thrombosis
Transformation of underlying glomerular disease (e.g., crescentic nephritis superimposed on membranous nephropathy)
Adverse effects of drug therapy
Acute allergic interstitial nephritis secondary to various drugs, including diuretics
Hemodynamic response to nonsteroidal anti-inflammatory drugs (NSAIDs) and angiotensin-converting enzyme (ACE) inhibitors or angiotensin receptor blockers (ARBs)

Figure 15.16 Acute Kidney Injury in nephrotic syndrome. Problems to consider in the evaluation of acute deterioration in renal function in nephrotic syndrome.

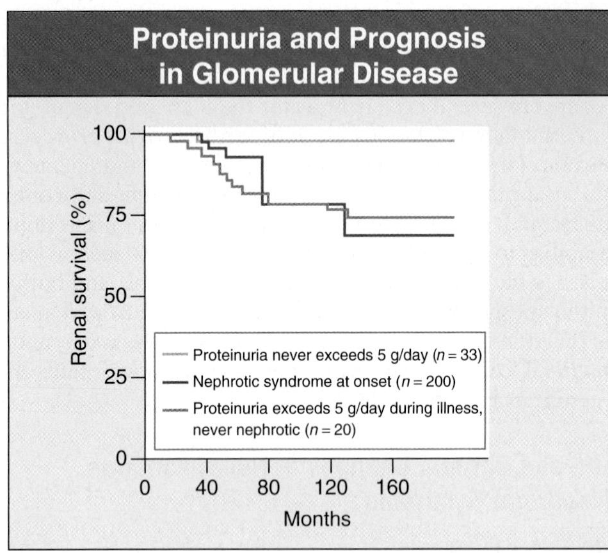

Figure 15.17 Proteinuria and prognosis in glomerular disease. The influence of heavy proteinuria on long-term renal function in 253 patients with primary glomerular disease at Manchester Royal Infirmary, United Kingdom. Heavy proteinuria at any time during long-term follow-up substantially worsens the prognosis even without frank nephrotic syndrome. *(Courtesy Dr. C. D. Short.)*

the proteinuria (Fig. 15.17), with marked risk of progression when protein excretion is more than 5 g/day. This may be because proteinuria identifies patients with severe glomerular injury, but there is also experimental and clinical evidence that proteinuria *per se* may be toxic, especially to the tubulointerstitium.[16] In several experimental models, measures that reduce proteinuria, such as the use of ACE inhibitors, also prevent tubulointerstitial disease and progressive renal failure.

NEPHRITIC SYNDROME

In nephrotic syndrome, the glomerular injury is manifested primarily as an increase in permeability of the capillary wall to protein. By contrast, in the nephritic syndrome, there is evidence of glomerular inflammation resulting in a reduction in GFR, non-nephrotic proteinuria, edema and hypertension (secondary to sodium retention), and hematuria with red cell casts.

Differentiation Between Nephrotic Syndrome and Nephritic Syndrome

Typical Features	Nephrotic	Nephritic
Onset	Insidious	Abrupt
Edema	++++	++
Blood pressure	Normal	Raised
Jugular venous pressure	Normal/low	Raised
Proteinuria	++++	++
Hematuria	May/may not occur	+++
Red cell casts	Absent	Present
Serum albumin	Low	Normal/slightly reduced

Figure 15.18 Differentiation between nephrotic syndrome and nephritic syndrome.

The classic nephritic syndrome presentation is that seen with acute poststreptococcal GN in children. These children usually present with rapid onset of oliguria, weight gain, and generalized edema during a few days. The hematuria results in brown rather than red urine, and clots are not seen. The urine contains protein, red cells, and red cell casts. Because proteinuria is rarely in the nephrotic range, serum albumin concentration is usually normal. Circulating volume increases with hypertension, and pulmonary edema follows without evidence of primary cardiac disease.

The distinction between typical nephrotic syndrome and nephritic syndrome is usually straightforward on clinical and laboratory grounds (Fig. 15.18), and the use of these clinical descriptions is particularly helpful in the approach to patients with suspected GN at first presentation, helping to narrow the differential diagnosis. However, the classification systems are imperfect, and patients with certain glomerular disease patterns, for example, MPGN, may present with either a nephrotic or a nephritic picture.

Etiology

The primary glomerular diseases associated with the nephritic syndrome and the serologic tests helpful in diagnosis are shown in Figure 15.19. The classification is even more challenging than for nephrotic syndrome as some diseases are identified by histology (IgA nephropathy), others by serology and histology (ANCA-associated vasculitis and lupus nephritis), and others by etiology (postinfectious GN).

RAPIDLY PROGRESSIVE GLOMERULONEPHRITIS

Rapidly progressive GN (RPGN) describes the clinical situation in which glomerular injury is so acute and severe that renal function deteriorates during days or weeks. The patient may present as a uremic emergency, with nephritic syndrome that is not self-limited but moves on rapidly to renal failure, or with rapidly deteriorating renal function when being investigated for

Common Glomerular Diseases Presenting as Nephritic Syndrome		
Disease	**Associations**	**Serologic Tests Helpful in Diagnosis**
Poststreptococcal glomerulonephritis	Pharyngitis, impetigo	ASO titer, streptozyme antibody
Other postinfectious disease		
Endocarditis	Cardiac murmur	Blood cultures, C3 ↓
Abscess	—	Blood cultures, C3, C4 normal or increased
Shunt	Treated hydrocephalus	Blood cultures, C3 ↓
IgA nephropathy	Upper respiratory or gastrointestinal infection	Serum IgA ↑
Systemic lupus	Other multisystem features of lupus	Antinuclear antibody, anti-double-stranded DNA antibody, C3 ↓, C4 ↓

Figure 15.19 Common glomerular diseases presenting as nephritic syndrome.

Common Glomerular Diseases Presenting as Rapidly Progressive Glomerulonephritis		
Disease	**Associations**	**Serologic Tests Helpful in Diagnosis**
Goodpasture's syndrome	Lung hemorrhage	Anti-glomerular basement membrane antibody (occasionally antineutrophil cytoplasmic antibodies [ANCA] present)
Vasculitis		
Wegener's granulomatosis	Upper and lower respiratory involvement	Cytoplasmic ANCA
Microscopic polyangiitis	Multisystem involvement	Perinuclear ANCA
Pauci-immune crescentic glomerulonephritis	Renal involvement only	Perinuclear ANCA
Immune complex disease		
Systemic lupus erythematosus	Other multisystem features of lupus	Antinuclear antibody, anti-double-stranded DNA antibody, C3 ↓, C4 ↓
Poststreptococcal glomerulonephritis	Pharyngitis, impetigo	ASO titer, streptozyme antibody, C3 ↓, C4 normal
IgA nephropathy/Henoch-Schönlein purpura	Characteristic rash ± abdominal pain in HSP	Serum IgA↑ (30%), C3 and C4 normal
Endocarditis	Cardiac murmur; other systemic features of bacteremia	Blood cultures, ANCA (occasionally) C3 ↓, C4 normal

Figure 15.20 Common glomerular diseases presenting as rapidly progressive glomerulonephritis. Note the overlap between these diseases and those in Figure 15.19. A number of glomerular diseases may present with either nephritic syndrome or rapidly progressive glomerulonephritis.

extrarenal disease (many of the patterns of GN associated with RPGN occur as part of a systemic immune illness).

The histologic counterpart of RPGN is crescentic GN. The proliferative cellular response seen outside the glomerular tuft but within Bowman's space is known as a crescent because of its shape on histologic cross section (see Fig. 16.9). Typically, the glomerular tuft also shows segmental necrosis, or focal segmental necrotizing GN; this is particularly characteristic of the vasculitis syndromes.

The term RPGN is therefore often used to describe acute deterioration in renal function in association with a crescentic nephritis. Unfortunately, not all patients with a nephritic urine sediment and acute kidney injury (AKI) will fit this syndrome. For example, AKI may also occur in milder forms of glomerular disease if it is complicated by accelerated hypertension, renal vein thrombosis, or acute tubular necrosis. This emphasizes the need to obtain histologic confirmation of the clinical diagnosis.

Etiology

The primary glomerular diseases associated with RPGN and helpful serologic tests are shown in Figure 15.20. As with nephritic syndrome, different assessment methods are useful for different diseases causing RPGN.

PROGRESSIVE CHRONIC KIDNEY DISEASE

In most types of chronic GN, a proportion of patients (often between 25% and 50%) will have slowly progressive renal impairment. If no clinical event early in the course of the disease brings them to medical attention, patients may present late with established hypertension, proteinuria, and renal impairment. In very long standing GN, the kidneys shrink (but remain smooth and symmetric). Renal biopsy at this stage is more hazardous and less likely to provide diagnostic material. Light microscopy often shows nonspecific features of end-stage kidney disease, consisting of focal or global glomerulosclerosis and dense tubulointerstitial fibrosis, and it may not be possible to define with confidence that a glomerular disease was the initiating renal injury, let alone define the pattern further. Immunofluorescence may be more helpful; in particular, mesangial IgA may be present in adequate amounts to allow a diagnosis of IgA nephropathy to be made. However, when renal imaging shows small kidneys, only rarely will biopsy be appropriate. For this reason, chronic GN has often been a presumptive diagnosis in patients presenting late with shrunken kidneys, proteinuria, and renal impairment. This is imprecise and in the past has led to an overestimate of the frequency of GN as a cause of end-stage renal disease in registry data. GN should be diagnosed only if there is confirmatory histologic evidence.

TREATMENT OF GLOMERULAR DISEASE

General Principles

Before any therapeutic decisions, it should always be ascertained that glomerular disease is primary and that no specific therapy is available. For example, treatment of an underlying infection or tumor may result in remission of GN. In the remaining cases, both general supportive treatment[17] (see Chapter 77) and disease-specific therapy should be considered. Supportive treatment includes measures to treat blood pressure, reduce proteinuria, control edema, and address other metabolic consequences of nephrotic syndrome. If successful, these relatively nontoxic therapies can prevent the need for immunosuppressive drugs, which have multiple potential side effects. Supportive therapy is usually not necessary in corticosteroid-sensitive MCD with rapid remission or in patients with IgA nephropathy, Alport's syndrome, or thin basement membrane nephropathy as long as they exhibit neither proteinuria nor hypertension.

Hypertension

Hypertension is very common in GN; it is virtually universal as chronic GN progresses toward end-stage renal disease and is the key modifiable factor in preserving renal function (see also Chapter 77). Sodium and water overload is an important part of the pathogenetic process, and high-dose diuretics with moderate dietary sodium restriction are usually an essential part of the treatment. As in other chronic renal diseases, the aim of blood pressure control is not only to protect against the cardiovascular risks of hypertension but also to delay progression of the renal disease. The ideal target blood pressure is not finally established, but in the Modification of Diet in Renal Disease (MDRD) study, patients with proteinuria (>1 g/day) had a better outcome if their blood pressure was reduced to 125/75 mm Hg rather than to the previous standard of 140/90 mm Hg.[18,19] There are strong theoretical and experimental reasons for ACE inhibitors and ARBs to be first-choice therapy, and this is now well documented in clinical studies.[20-22] Nondihydropyridine calcium channel blockers may also have a beneficial effect on proteinuria as well as on blood pressure. As in primary hypertension, lifestyle modification (salt restriction, weight normalization, regular exercise, and smoking cessation) should be an integral part of the therapy. If target blood pressure cannot be achieved with these measures, antihypertensive therapy should be stepped up according to current guidelines (see Chapter 35).

Treatment of Proteinuria

Besides hypertension, proteinuria represents the second key modifiable factor to preserve GFR (see also Chapter 77). Most studies suggest that the progressive loss of renal function observed in many glomerular diseases can largely be prevented if proteinuria can be reduced to levels below 0.5 g/day. This may be because many of the measures to reduce protein excretion, such as the use of ACE inhibitors or ARBs, also reduce glomerular hypertension, which contributes to progressive renal failure. However, there is also increasing evidence that proteinuria or factors present in proteinuric urine *per se* may be toxic to the tubulointerstitium.[16] Finally, in nephrotic patients, a reduction of proteinuria to a non-nephrotic range can induce serum proteins to rise, with alleviation of many of the metabolic complications of nephrotic syndrome.

Most of the agents used to reduce urinary protein excretion do so hemodynamically, either by blocking efferent arteriolar constriction (ACE inhibitors or ARBs) or by reducing preglomerular pressure (most other classes of antihypertensives). Some of the agents, such as ACE inhibitors and ARBs, may also have direct effects on reducing the increased glomerular capillary wall permeability. A consequence of this type of therapy is a reduction in GFR; however, in general, the decrease in GFR is of a lower magnitude than the decrease in protein excretion. The antiproteinuric agents of choice are ACE inhibitors and ARBs, which reduce proteinuria by an average of 40% to 50%, particularly if the patient is on dietary salt restriction. There is little clinical evidence to suggest that ACE inhibitors differ from ARBs in this respect. The combination of the two may result in additive antiproteinuric activity but increases the risk of AKI.[23] In addition, whereas other classes of antihypertensive agents will reduce proteinuria coincident with a decrease in systemic blood pressure (particularly the nondihydropyridine calcium channel blockers such as diltiazem), both ACE inhibitors and ARBs usually reduce proteinuria independent of blood pressure. If doses are increased slowly to minimize symptomatic hypotension, treatment with ACE inhibitors and ARBs is usually possible in the normotensive proteinuric patient. Increasing the dose of ACE inhibitors or ARBs may further reduce proteinuria without lowering blood pressure, which may indicate the inefficacy of other antihypertensive drugs in blocking the stimulated intrarenal renin-angiotensin system. Common side effects include hyperkalemia in patients with advanced renal failure, which may necessitate a loop diuretic but rarely should lead to cessation of ACE inhibitors and ARBs, and cough in the case of ACE inhibitors, in which case ARBs should be used instead. Because ACE inhibitors and ARBs lower GFR (see previous discussion), a 10% to 30% increase in serum creatinine concentration may be observed. Unless serum creatinine concentration continues to increase, this moderate increase reflects the therapeutic effect of these medications and should not prompt their withdrawal.

NSAIDs lessen proteinuria by reducing intrarenal prostaglandin production and dipyridamole through adenosine-mediated afferent arteriolar vasoconstriction. Given the safety of the therapies discussed previously, as well as the risk with NSAIDs of profound decreases in GFR, salt retention, and diuretic resistance, they are rarely used.

A low-protein diet will lessen proteinuria but must be advised with great care because of the risk of malnutrition. Adequate compensation must be made for urine protein losses,[24] and the patient must be carefully monitored for evidence of malnutrition (see Chapter 83). Whether a low-protein diet is still antiproteinuric in patients treated with a full-dose ACE inhibitor or ARB is not established.

Treatment of Hyperlipidemia

Treatment of hyperlipidemia in patients with glomerular disease should usually follow the guidelines that apply to the general population to prevent cardiovascular disease. It may also be that statin therapy protects from a decrease in GFR, although this is not firmly established. Dietary restriction alone has only modest effects on hyperlipidemia in glomerular disease, in particular in nephrotic syndrome. Side effects of some medications, for example, rhabdomyolysis provoked by fibrates, occur more frequently in patients with renal failure. The addition of bile acid sequestrants, such as cholestyramine, may lower LDL further and increase HDL but is usually not tolerated because of gastrointestinal effects.

Avoidance of Nephrotoxic Substances

Apart from NSAIDs, which may induce AKI, particularly in patients with preexisting renal impairment and dehydration, other nephrotoxic substances, such as radiocontrast agents, some cytotoxic drugs, and antibiotics (e.g., aminoglycoside antibiotics), should also be used with caution in patients with glomerular disease and renal impairment or nephrotic syndrome.

Special Therapeutic Issues in Patients with Nephrotic Syndrome

Treatment of Nephrotic Edema

In contrast to the lack of therapies in the past (Fig. 15.21), the mainstays of treatment nowadays are diuretics accompanied by moderate dietary sodium restriction (60 to 80 mmol/24 h). Nephrotic patients are diuretic resistant even if GFR is normal. Loop diuretics must reach the renal tubule to be effective, and transport from the peritubular capillary requires protein binding, which is reduced in hypoalbuminemia; once the drug reaches the renal tubule, it will become 70% bound to protein present in the urine and therefore be less effective. Oral diuretics with twice-daily administration are usually preferred, given the longer therapeutic effect compared with intravenous diuretics. However, in severe nephrosis, gastrointestinal absorption of the diuretic may be uncertain because of intestinal wall edema, and intravenous diuretic, by bolus injection or infusion, may be necessary to provoke an effective diuresis. Alternatively, combining a loop diuretic with a thiazide diuretic or with metolazone may overcome diuretic resistance. The characteristics of different diuretics are discussed in Chapter 7. Significant hypovolemia is not often a clinical problem, provided fluid removal is controlled and gradual. Daily weight is the best measurement of progress. Nephrotic children are much more prone to hypovolemic shock than adults are. A stepwise approach to diuretic use is required, aiming at fluid removal in adults of no more than 2 kg daily, moving on to the next drug level if this is not achieved (Fig. 15.22).

Correction of Hypoproteinemia

In view of the problems associated with either increased protein administration or dietary protein restriction in nephrotic patients (see previous discussion), adequate dietary protein should be ensured (0.8 to 1 mg/kg per day) with a high carbohydrate intake to maximize use of that protein. When there is very heavy proteinuria, the amount of urinary protein loss should be added to dietary protein intake.

In the rare setting in which proteinuria is so severe that the patient is dying of the complications of nephrotic syndrome, one may have to resort to nephrectomy to prevent continued protein losses. This may be done as a medical nephrectomy: the deliberate use of NSAIDs combined with ACE inhibitors and diuretic to lessen proteinuria by provoking AKI. If medical nephrectomy alone does not adequately reduce proteinuria, bilateral renal artery embolization can be considered. It may be a painful procedure and is not always as successful as might be expected (perhaps because of collateral arterial supply to the kidneys, which is not blocked by the embolization). A final alternative is bilateral nephrectomy, which carries significant mortality in these severely ill hypoproteinemic patients and is rarely used

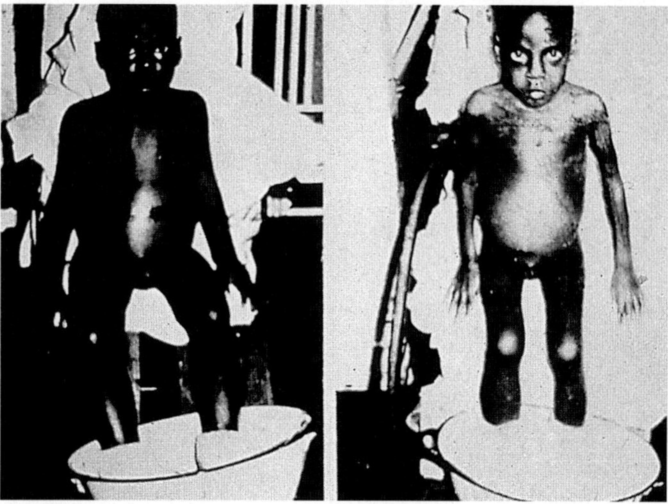

Figure 15.21 Treatment of nephrotic edema before the availability of diuretics. Edema in nephrotic syndrome was very difficult to treat. This child with anasarca, pictured in 1953, stands in a bowl while edema fluid drips out through small tubes placed through needles in the skin of the feet. This was nevertheless effective treatment. The two pictures of the same child were taken 4 days apart, during which time the child lost 4.5 kg (10 lb), or 18% of body weight. *(Courtesy Dr. Robert Vernier.)*

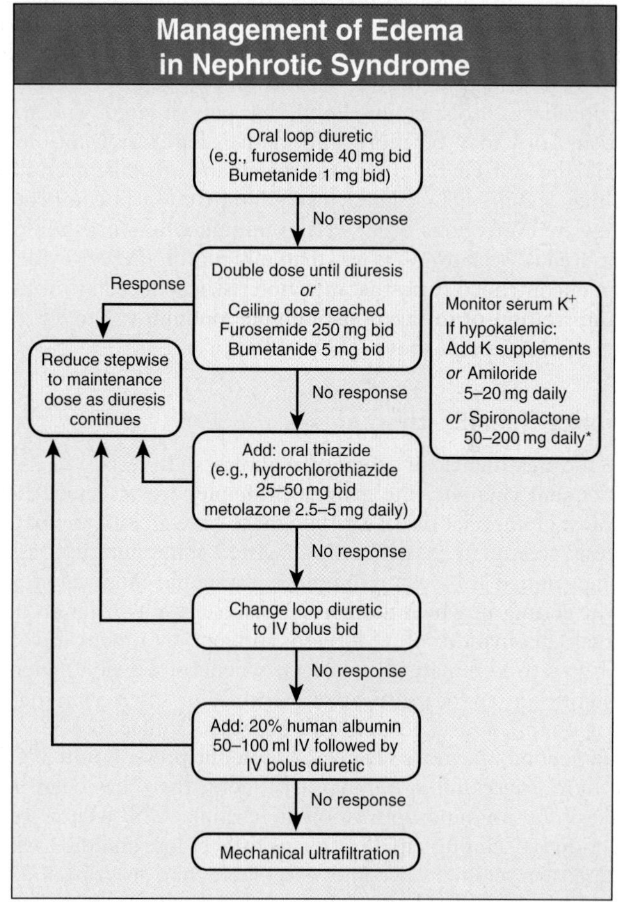

Figure 15.22 Management of edema in nephrotic syndrome. Edema is often diuretic resistant, but the response is not predictable. Therefore, stepwise escalation of therapy is appropriate until diuresis occurs. Even when there is anasarca, diuresis should not proceed faster than 2 kg/day in adults to minimize the risk of clinically significant hypovolemia. Mechanical ultrafiltration is rarely required for nephrotic edema unless there is associated renal insufficiency. *Spironolactone is less effective in nephrotic syndrome than in cirrhosis and is often poorly tolerated because of gastrointestinal side effects. Spironolactone should be used with great caution if the GFR is very low.

in adults, although it is a conventional part of management of infants with congenital nephrotic syndrome.

Treatment of Hypercoagulability

The risk of thrombotic events becomes progressively more important as serum albumin values decrease to less than 2.5 g/dl. Immobility as a consequence of edema or intercurrent illness further aggravates the risk. Prophylactic low-dose anticoagulation (e.g., heparin 5000 units subcutaneously twice daily) is indicated at times of high risk, such as relative immobilization in the hospital and albumin levels between 2 and 2.5 g/dl. Full-dose anticoagulation with low-molecular-weight heparin or warfarin should be considered if serum albumin decreases to less than 2 g/dl[11,25] and is mandatory if a thrombosis or pulmonary embolism is documented. Heparin is used for initial anticoagulation, but an increased dose may be needed because part of the action of heparin depends on antithrombin III, which is often reduced in the plasma in nephrotic patients. Warfarin (target international normalized ratio 2 to 3) is the long-term treatment of choice but should be manipulated with special care because of altered protein binding, which may require dose reductions.

Management of Infection

A high order of clinical suspicion for infection is vital in nephrotic patients. Especially in nephrotic children, ascitic fluid should be examined microscopically and cultured if there is any suspicion of systemic infection. Bacteremia is common even if clinical signs are localized. ESR is unhelpful, but an elevated C-reactive protein level may be more informative. Parenteral antibiotics should be started once culture specimens are taken, and the regimen should include benzylpenicillin (to cover pneumococci). If repeated infections occur, serum immunoglobulins should be measured. If serum IgG is less than 600 mg/dl, there is evidence in an uncontrolled study that infection risk is reduced by monthly administration of intravenous immune globulin (10 to 15 g) to keep the IgG levels above 600 mg/dl.[26]

Disease-Specific Therapies

Specific treatments for glomerular diseases are discussed in the subsequent chapters; the general principles are discussed here. As most glomerular disease is thought to have an immune pathogenesis, treatment has generally consisted of immunosuppressive therapy aimed at blocking of both the systemic and local effects. In the setting in which glomerular disease results from an ineffectual elimination of a foreign antigen, treatment involves measures to eliminate this antigen whenever possible (such as antibiotics in endocarditis-associated GN or interferon alfa for cryoglobulinemia associated with hepatitis C infection).

In general, the more severe and acute the presentation of GN, the more successful is immune treatment; there has been little success for immunosuppression in chronic GN. When renal function is declining rapidly, there is little to lose and the toxicity of intensive regimens becomes acceptable for a short period but would be unacceptable if prolonged. Furthermore, the nonspecific nature of most immune treatments results in widespread interruption of immune and inflammatory events at multiple levels. In the acute situation, this broad-based attack is a virtue; in more indolent disease, more specific treatment is needed but is unavailable. Despite great increases in the understanding of immune mechanisms in glomerular disease since the 1970s, immune therapies are not yet much more specific and precise. The mainstays of treatment remain agents that were available in the 1960s: corticosteroids, azathioprine, and cyclophosphamide. Other newer immunosuppressive agents developed for use in transplantation, including cyclosporine, tacrolimus, mycophenolate mofetil, and rapamycin, or those developed in oncology, including rituximab, have emerging indications in glomerular disease.

The use of immunosuppressive therapies to treat GN has certain drawbacks. In many diseases, treatment is based on small series, and good prospective controlled trials are lacking. Because of both the rarity and the variable natural history of GN, proof of efficacy for a particular therapy often requires a multicenter approach with prolonged follow-up, which is logistically difficult. If sufficient glomerular damage is present, proteinuria and progressive deterioration of renal function may occur by nonimmune pathways that may not be responsive to immunosuppressive therapies. Unfortunately, good noninvasive markers to assess disease activity are missing in most clinical circumstances. Given the frequent uncertainty of the response to immunosuppressive therapy, it becomes mandatory to weigh the potential benefits against the risks of therapy.

Immunosuppression may be associated with reactivation of tuberculosis and hepatitis B infection and can also lead to a hyperinfection syndrome in patients with *Strongyloides* species infection. Therefore, high-risk patients should be screened for these diseases before embarking on therapy.

Alkylating agents, such as cyclophosphamide and chlorambucil, have considerable toxicity. In the short term, leukopenia is common, as is alopecia, although hair will regrow within a few months of discontinuation of therapy. These agents can cause infertility (observed in adults with cumulative doses of cyclophosphamide >200 mg/kg and chlorambucil 10 mg/kg). There is also an increased incidence of leukemias (observed with total doses of cyclophosphamide >80 g and chlorambucil 7 g). Cyclophosphamide is also a bladder irritant, and treatment can result in hemorrhagic cystitis and bladder carcinoma, particularly after therapy lasting more than 6 months.[27] Irritation of the bladder is caused by a metabolite, acrolein. The effect can be minimized in patients receiving intravenous cyclophosphamide by enforcing a good diuresis and administering mesna. The dose of mesna (mg) should equal the dose of cyclophosphamide (mg); 20% is given intravenously with the intravenous cyclophosphamide, and the remaining 80% should be given in two equal oral doses at 2 and 6 hours by intravenous infusion at the same dose as the cyclophosphamide. Chlorambucil and cyclophosphamide also require dose reduction in the setting of renal insufficiency. Given all these concerns, oral treatment with these agents should ideally be limited to 12 weeks.

The modes of action and potential adverse effects of corticosteroids, azathioprine, and other immunosuppressives occasionally used in glomerular disease are discussed further in Chapter 97.

REFERENCES

1. Iseki K, Iseki C, Ikemiya Y, Fukiyama K. Risk of developing end-stage renal disease in a cohort of mass screening. *Kidney Int.* 1996;49:800-805.
2. Topham PS, Harper SJ, Furness PN, et al. Glomerular disease as a cause of isolated microscopic haematuria. *Q J Med.* 1994;87:329-336.
3. Springberg PD, Garrett LE, Thompson AL, et al. Fixed and reproducible orthostatic proteinuria. Results of a 20 year follow up study. *Ann Intern Med.* 1982;97:516-519.
4. Orth SR, Ritz E. The nephrotic syndrome. *N Engl J Med.* 1998;338:1201-1212.

5. Cameron JS. Nephrotic syndrome in the elderly. *Semin Nephrol.* 1996;16:319-329.
6. Haas M, Meehan SM, Karison TG, Spargo BH. Changing etiologies of unexplained adult nephrotic syndrome: A comparison of renal biopsy findings from 1976-1979 and 1995-1997. *Am J Kidney Dis.* 1997;30:621-631.
7. Kaysen G, Gambertoglio J, Felts J, Hutchison F. Albumin synthesis, albuminuria and hyperlipidemia in nephrotic syndrome. *Kidney Int.* 1987;31:1368-1376.
8. Humphreys MH. Mechanisms and management of nephrotic edema. *Kidney Int.* 1994;45:266-281.
9. Svenningsen P, Bistrup C, Friis UG, et al. Plasmin in nephrotic urine activates the epithelial sodium channel. *J Am Soc Nephrol.* 2009;20:299-310.
10. Rodriguez-Iturbe B, Herrera-Acosta J, Johnson RJ. Interstitial inflammation, sodium retention and the pathogenesis of nephrotic edema. *Kidney Int.* 2002;62:1379-1384.
11. Glassock RJ. Prophylactic anticoagulation in nephrotic syndrome: A clinical conundrum. *J Am Soc Nephrol.* 2007;18:2221-2225.
12. Wheeler DC, Bernard DB. Lipid abnormalities in nephrotic syndrome. *Am J Kidney Dis.* 1994;23:331-346.
13. Strippoli GFM, Navaneethan SD, Johnson DW, et al. Effects of statins in patients with chronic kidney disease: Meta-analysis and meta-regression of randomised controlled trials. *BMJ.* 2008;336:645-651.
14. Smith JD, Hayslett JP. Reversible renal failure in the nephrotic syndrome. *Am J Kidney Dis.* 1992;19:201-213.
15. Jennette JC, Falk RJ. Adult minimal change glomerulopathy with acute renal failure. *Am J Kidney Dis.* 1990;16:432-437.
16. Remuzzi G, Benigni A, Remuzzi A. Mechanisms of progression and regression of renal lesions of chronic nephropathies and diabetes. *J Clin Invest.* 2006;116:288-296.
17. Wilmer WA, Rovin BH, Hebert CJ, et al. Management of glomerular proteinuria: A commentary. *J Am Soc Nephrol.* 2003;14:3217-3232.
18. Klahr S, Levey AS, Beck GJ, et al. The effects of dietary protein restriction and blood pressure control on the progression of chronic renal disease. *N Engl J Med.* 1994;330:877-884.
19. Chobanian AV, Bakris GL, Black HR, et al. The Seventh Report of the Joint National Committee on Prevention, Detection, Evaluation, and Treatment of High Blood Pressure: The JNC 7 report. *JAMA.* 2003;289:2560-2572.
20. Maschio G, Alberti D, Janin G, et al. Effect of the angiotensin-converting-enzyme inhibitor, benazepril, on the progression of chronic renal insufficiency. *N Engl J Med.* 1996;334:939-945.
21. The GISEN Group. Randomised placebo-controlled trial of effect of ramipril on decline in glomerular filtration rate and risk of terminal renal failure in proteinuric, non-diabetic nephropathy. *Lancet.* 1997;349:1857-1863.
22. Jafar TH, Schmid CH, Landa M, et al. Angiotensin-converting enzyme inhibitors and progression of non-diabetic renal disease. A meta-analysis of patient-level data. *Ann Intern Med.* 2001;135:73-87.
23. Mann JF, Schmieder RE, McQueen M, et al. Renal outcomes with telmisartan, ramipril, or both, in people at high vascular risk (the ONTARGET study): A multicentre, randomised, double-blind, controlled trial. *Lancet.* 2008;372:547-553.
24. Maroni BJ, Staffield C, Young VR, et al. Mechanisms permitting nephrotic patients to achieve nitrogen equilibrium with a protein restricted diet. *J Clin Invest.* 1997;99:2479-2487.
25. Sarasin FP, Schifferli JA. Prophylactic oral anticoagulation in nephrotic patients with idiopathic membranous nephropathy. *Kidney Int.* 1994;45:578-585.
26. Ogi M, Yokoyama H, Tomosui N, et al. Risk factors for infection and immunoglobulin replacement therapy in adult nephrotic syndrome. *Am J Kidney Dis.* 1994;24:427-436.
27. Talar-Williams C, Hijazi C, Walther M, et al. Cyclophosphamide-induced cystitis and bladder cancer in patients with Wegener's granulomatosis. *Ann Intern Med.* 1996;124:477-484.

CHAPTER 16

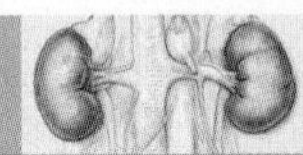

Introduction to Glomerular Disease: Histologic Classification and Pathogenesis

Richard J. Johnson, Jürgen Floege, John Feehally

HISTOLOGIC CLASSIFICATION

Glomerular disease may have a wide variety of causes and clinical presentations (see Chapter 15). Some glomerular diseases are given the generic title of glomerulonephritis (GN), which implies an immune or inflammatory pathogenesis. Although there are some situations in which specific diagnosis can be made on the basis of clinical presentation and laboratory tests, a renal biopsy is useful for both classification and prognosis in most cases. Ideally, the renal biopsy specimen should be examined by light microscopy, immunofluorescence, and electron microscopy. By use of this approach, a histologic pattern can be diagnosed. Some histologic patterns can be coupled with other laboratory test results to identify a specific etiology, but the condition is idiopathic in many cases. However, because treatments are often developed for specific histologic patterns, this approach is currently favored in the management of these disorders.

HISTOPATHOLOGY

The full assessment of a renal biopsy specimen requires light microscopy, electron microscopy, and examination for deposits of complement and immunoglobulin by immunofluorescence or immunoperoxidase techniques.

Light Microscopy

In GN, the dominant but not the only histologic lesions are in glomeruli (Fig. 16.1). GN is described as focal (only some glomeruli are involved) or diffuse. In any individual glomerulus, injury may be segmental (affecting only part of any glomerulus) or global. There is a potential for sampling error in a renal biopsy: the extent of a focal lesion may be misjudged in a small biopsy specimen, and sections through glomeruli may miss segmental lesions. Lesions may also be hypercellular due to either an increase in endogenous endothelial or mesangial cells (termed proliferative) or an infiltration of inflammatory leukocytes (termed exudative). Severe acute inflammation may produce glomerular necrosis, which is often segmental. The walls of the glomerular capillaries can also be thickened by a number of processes, which include an increase in glomerular basement membrane (GBM) material and immune deposits. Segmental sclerosis and scarring may also occur and are characterized by segmental capillary collapse with the accumulation of hyaline material and mesangial matrix and often with attachment of the capillary wall with Bowman's capsule (synechiae or adhesion formation).

The classic stains used in light microscopy include hematoxylin and eosin and the periodic acid–Schiff (PAS) reaction, which is particularly good for evaluating cellularity and matrix expansion. More specific stains include methenamine silver, which stains GBM and other matrix black. It may, for example, reveal a double contour to the GBM because of the interposition of cellular material, or it may show increased mesangial matrix not easily seen with other techniques. Trichrome staining is also useful to show areas of scarring (stains blue), whereas immune deposits stain red.

Crescents are inflammatory collections of cells in Bowman's space. Crescents develop when severe glomerular injury results in local rupture of the capillary wall or Bowman's capsule, allowing plasma proteins and inflammatory material to enter into Bowman's space. Crescents consist of proliferating parietal and visceral epithelial cells, infiltrating fibroblasts, and lymphocytes and monocytes-macrophages, often with local fibrin deposition. They are called crescents because of their appearance when the glomerulus is cut in one plane for histology. They are destructive and rapidly increasing in size and may lead to glomerular tuft occlusion (see Fig. 16.1). If the acute injury is stopped, the crescents may either resolve with restitution of normal morphology or heal by fibrosis, causing irreversible loss of renal function. Crescents are most commonly observed with vasculitis, in Goodpasture's disease, and in severe acute GN of any etiology.

Tubulointerstitial injury and fibrosis can also accompany GN and may play an important role in the prognosis (see Chapter 76).

Immunofluorescence and Immunoperoxidase Microscopy

Indirect immunofluorescence and immunoperoxidase staining are both used to identify immune reactants (Fig. 16.2). Examination consists of staining for immunoglobulins IgG, IgA, and IgM; for components of the complement system (usually C3, C4, and C1q); and for fibrin, which is commonly observed in crescents and in capillaries in thrombotic disorders (such as hemolytic-uremic syndrome and the antiphospholipid syndrome). Immune deposits may occur along the capillary loops or in the mesangium. They may be continuous (linear) or discontinuous (granular) along the capillary wall or in the mesangium.

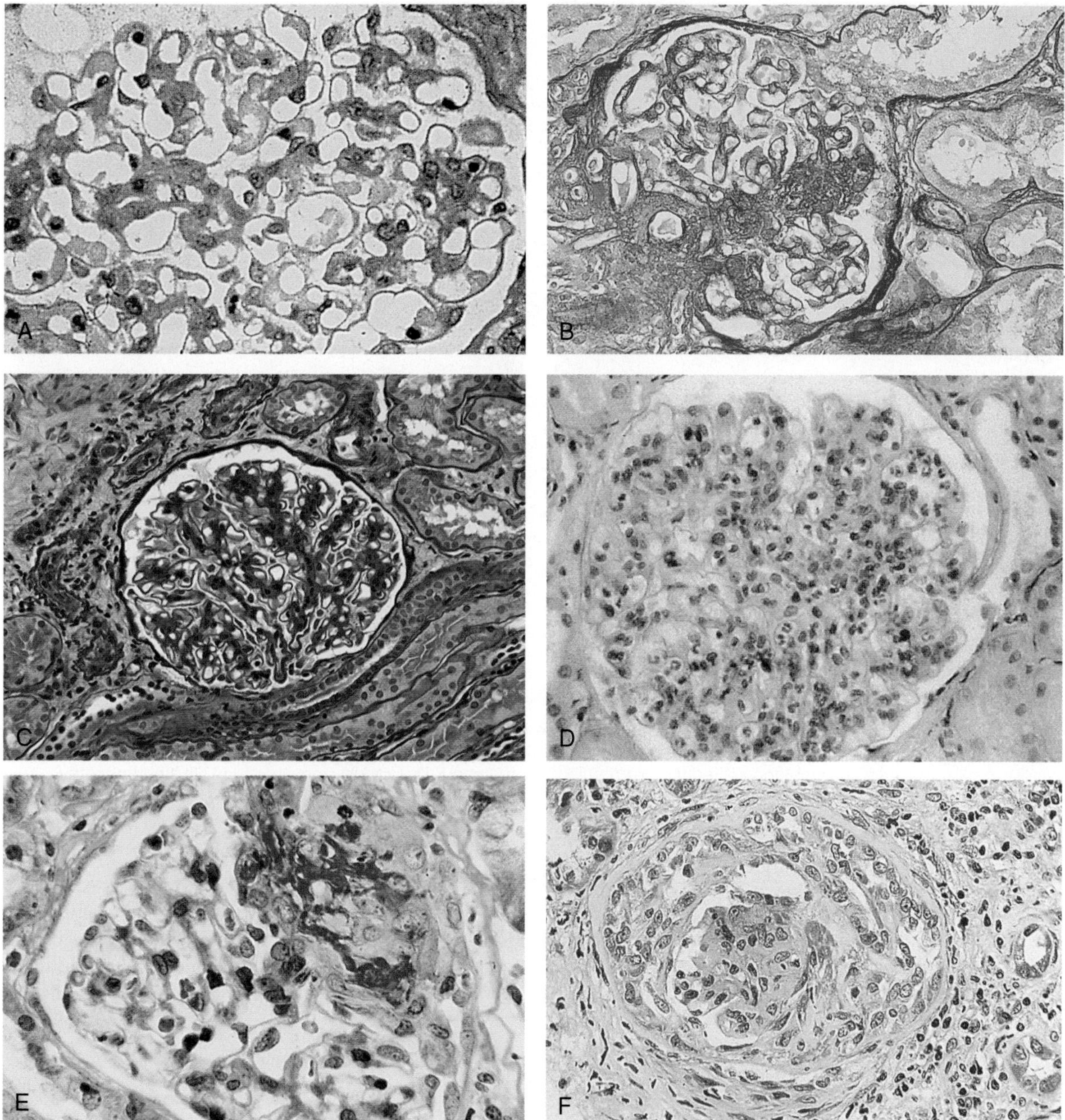

Figure 16.1 Pathology of glomerular disease: light microscopy. Characteristic patterns of glomerular disease illustrating the range of histologic appearances and the descriptive terms used. **A,** Normal glomerulus: minimal change disease. **B,** Segmental sclerosis: focal segmental glomerulosclerosis. **C,** Diffuse mesangial hypercellularity: IgA nephropathy. **D,** Diffuse endocapillary hypercellularity: poststreptococcal glomerulonephritis. **E,** Segmental necrosis: renal vasculitis. **F,** Crescent formation: anti–glomerular basement membrane disease. (**A** and **B,** Hematoxylin-eosin; **C, D,** and **F,** periodic acid–Schiff; **E,** trichrome.)

Electron Microscopy

Electron microscopy (EM) is valuable for defining the morphology of the basement membranes (abnormal in some forms of hereditary nephropathy, e.g., Alport's syndrome and thin basement membrane nephropathy [see Chapter 46]) and also for identifying fibrils (e.g., in amyloidosis) or tubuloreticular intracellular structures (e.g., in lupus nephritis). EM is also useful for localizing the site of immune deposits (which are usually homogeneous and electron dense; Fig. 16.3). Electron-dense deposits are seen in the mesangium or along the capillary wall on the subepithelial or subendothelial side of the GBM. Uncommonly, the electron-dense material lies linearly within the GBM. The sites of immune deposits are helpful in the classification of the types of GN.

GENERAL MECHANISMS OF GLOMERULAR INJURY

Proteinuria

Proteinuria is the hallmark of glomerular disease. Although there is some evidence that the endothelial glycocalyx, the GBM, and the podocytes may repel proteins in part through their highly negative charge (proteins are mostly negatively charged as well) from entering Bowman's space, a major barrier for protein is in

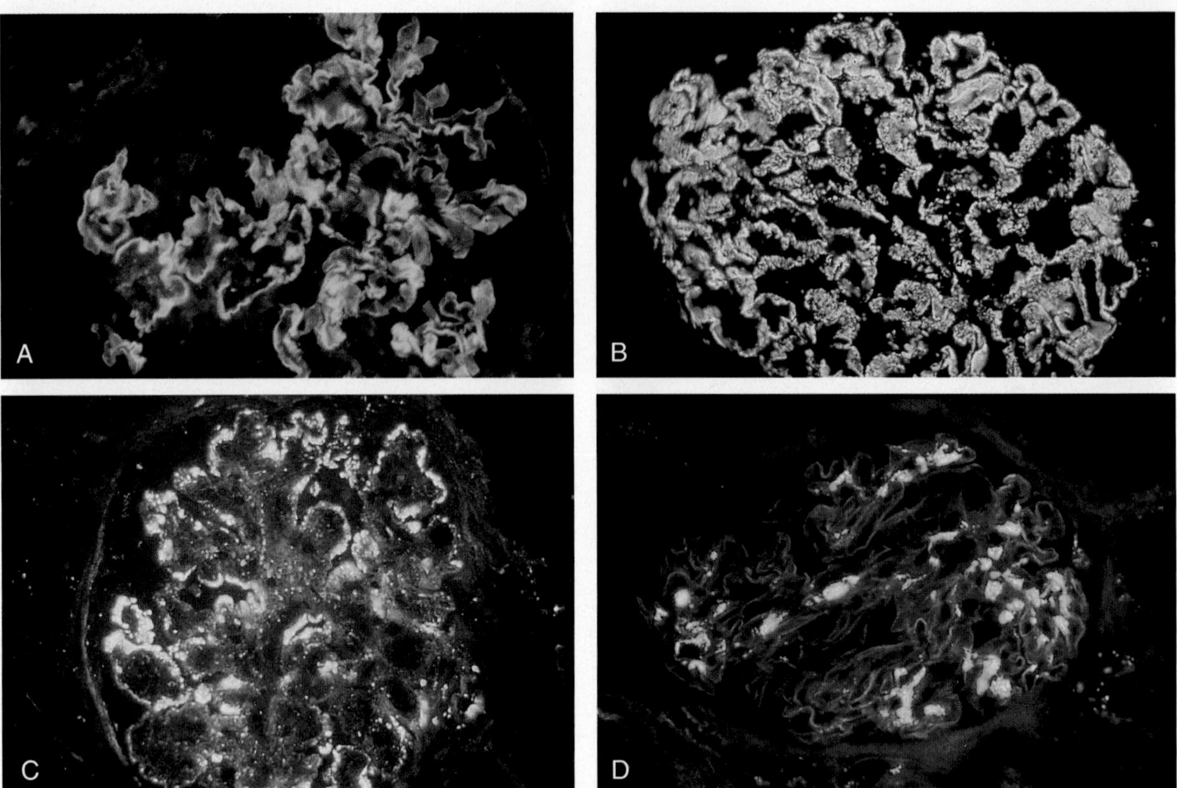

Figure 16.2 Pathology of glomerular disease: immunofluorescence microscopy. Common patterns of glomerular staining found by immunofluorescence. **A,** Linear capillary wall IgG: anti–glomerular basement membrane disease. **B,** Fine granular capillary wall IgG: membranous nephropathy. **C,** Coarse granular capillary wall IgG: membranoproliferative glomerulonephritis type I. **D,** Granular mesangial IgA: IgA nephropathy.

the slit diaphragm between the podocyte foot processes (Fig. 16.4).[1] The slit diaphragm consists of several transmembrane proteins that extend from adjacent interdigitating foot processes to form a zipper-like scaffold on the outer side of the GBM (Fig. 16.5).[1]

The importance of the slit diaphragm in proteinuric states has been documented in numerous hereditary types of nephrotic syndrome in which the mutations involve various slit diaphragm proteins (see Chapter 19).[2] These diseases usually present in childhood as a type of corticosteroid-resistant minimal change disease (MCD) or focal segmental glomerulosclerosis (FSGS). However, an exception is autosomal recessive corticosteroid-resistant nephrotic syndrome, in which the homozygous mutation in podocin (*NPHS2*) presents in childhood but the heterozygous mutation, when it coexists with the p.R229Q variant polymorphism, may be due to a mutation that under certain circumstances may not clinically manifest until young adulthood (20 to 40 years old).[3]

Whereas proteinuria may be the consequence of direct injury to the slit diaphragm, in most cases proteinuria may be due to injury to the podocyte. When the podocyte is injured, it will undergo shape change with swelling and loss or fusion of the foot processes. Filtration is actually reduced at sites where the foot processes fuse (which may account for the reduction of the filtration coefficient K_f seen in nephrotic syndrome), but there are gaps where the podocytes are detached from the GBM. It is at these sites that massive protein filtration occurs; structurally, the capillary wall defects are likely to correspond to the large pores noted in functional studies (Fig. 16.6).[4]

Podocyte immaturity can also result in nephrotic syndrome. Congenital nephrotic syndrome with mesangial sclerosis has recently been linked with mutations in phospholipase C epsilon gene (*PLCE1*), which is important in podocyte development.[5]

Antibody and Antigen

Many glomerular diseases are associated with positive staining for immunoglobulins, often with components of the complement system, and with the presence of electron-dense deposits by EM. These findings are thought to represent immune complexes. Experimentally, immune complexes can localize in glomeruli by two major mechanisms. In some conditions, such as mesangial proliferative GN, membranoproliferative GN (MPGN), and lupus nephritis, the immune complexes are thought to originate in the circulation and to be passively trapped in the mesangium or subendothelial areas. In contrast, circulating immune complexes cannot readily pass across the GBM, and the presence of IgG in membranous nephropathy is thought to be due to direct binding of antibody to antigens constitutively expressed on the podocyte or to an antigen that may first be "trapped" or bound at this site (*in situ* formation).[6] Complement activation can also occur in the absence of antigen (resulting in the ribbon deposits noted in patients with dense deposit disease (DDD, previously known as type II MPGN). Under some circumstances, antigens may also deposit that directly activate the alternative pathway of complement in the absence of IgG; this may occur in some forms of poststreptococcal GN (PSGN). Antibody with aberrant characteristics may also aggregate and activate complement in the

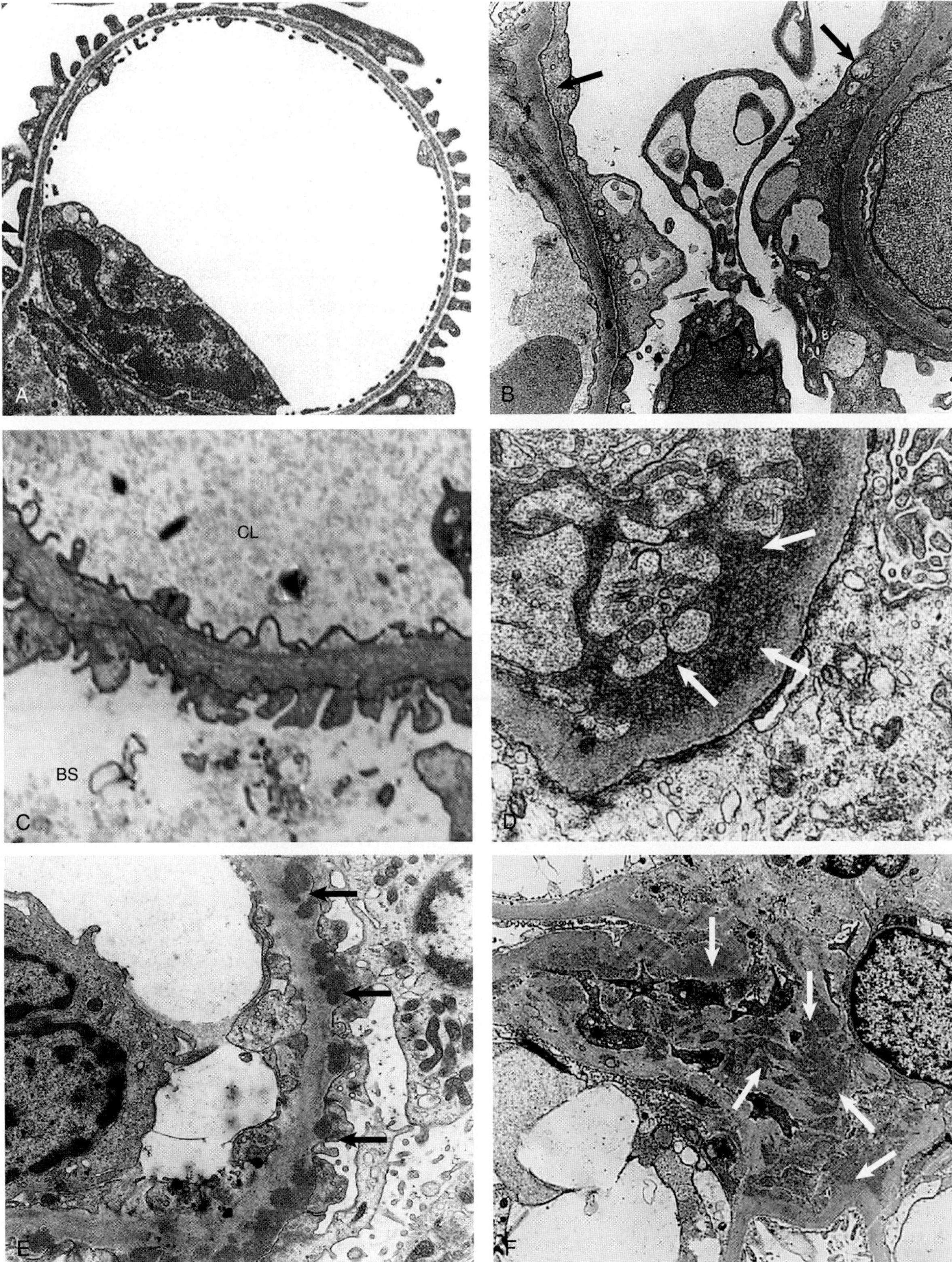

Figure 16.3 Ultrastructural pathology of glomerular disease. Some characteristic patterns of electron-dense deposits and GBM abnormalities seen in glomerular disease. **A,** Normal. **B,** Foot process effacement: minimal change disease *(arrows).* **C,** GBM thickening and splitting: Alport's syndrome. CL, capillary lumen; BS, Bowman's space. **D,** Subendothelial electron-dense deposits *(arrows):* membranoproliferative glomerulonephritis type I. **E,** Subepithelial electron-dense deposits *(arrows):* membranous nephropathy. **F,** Mesangial electron-dense deposits *(arrows):* IgA nephropathy.

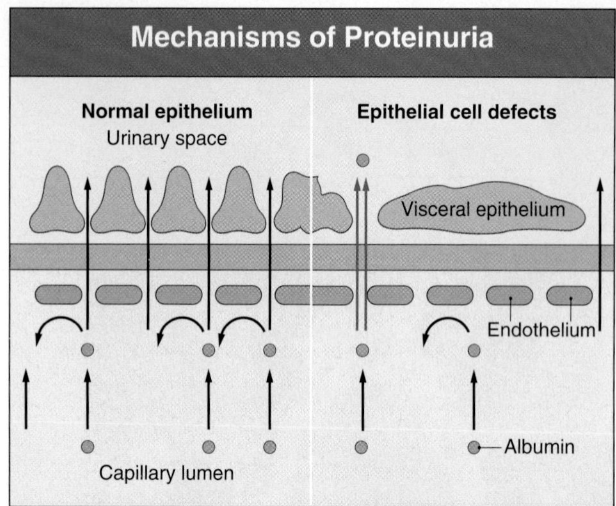

Figure 16.4 Mechanisms of proteinuria. Normally negatively charged proteins, such as albumin, are retarded by the negatively charged proteins in the endothelium (sialoglycoproteins) and basement membrane (heparan sulfate proteoglycans) as well as by a size barrier in the GBM and at the slit diaphragm. In most proteinuric states, the podocytes are injured, leading to foot process swelling and injury to the slit diaphragm; in these situations, protein (albumin) can pass through the GBM and the gaps between the fused foot processes.

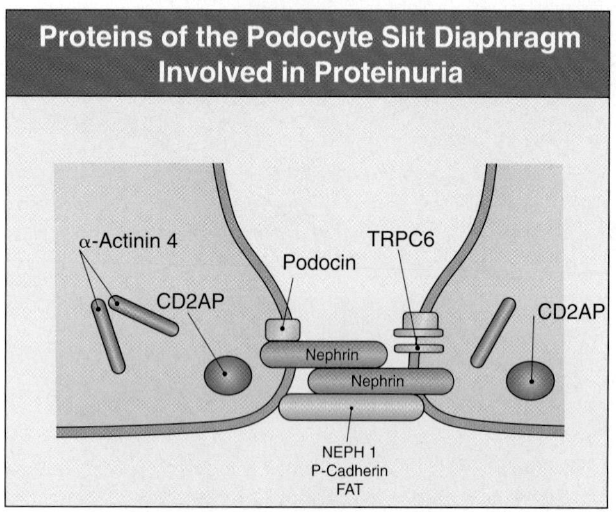

Figure 16.5 Proteins of the podocyte slit diaphragm involved in proteinuria. Several inherited glomerular diseases involve mutations of antigens associated with the slit diaphragm. These include nephrin (congenital nephrotic syndrome of the Finnish type), podocin (autosomal recessive FSGS), and α-actinin and TRPC6 (both associated with autosomal dominant FSGS). In addition, mutation of CD2-associated protein results in nephrotic syndrome in mice. *(Modified from reference 1.)*

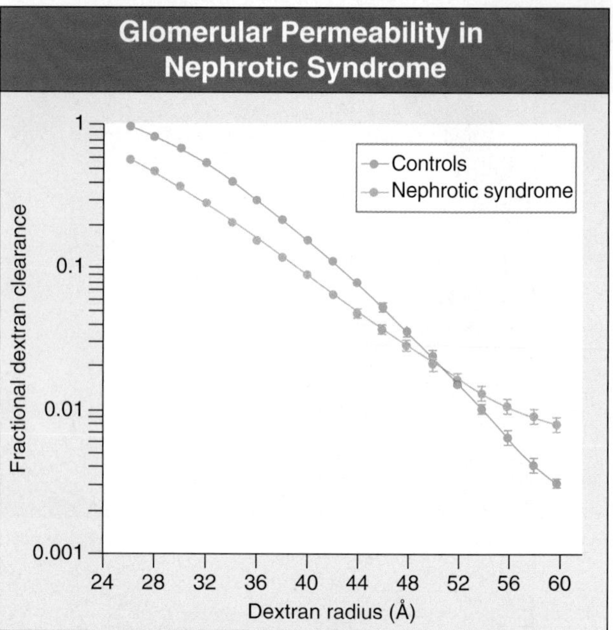

Figure 16.6 Glomerular permeability in nephrotic syndrome. A dextran sieving curve showing the relative glomerular permeability of different-sized dextrans in normal subjects and nephrotic patients with membranous nephropathy and minimal change disease. Nephrotic subjects actually have a lower fractional dextran clearance for small dextrans (26 to 48 Å [2.6 to 4.8 nm]) but have an increased clearance for dextrans of larger molecular weight (52 to 60 Å [5.2 to 6.0 nm]). This is consistent with large pores appearing in the GBM. *(Modified from reference 4.)*

absence of antigen (such as may occur in some cases of IgA nephropathy in which aberrantly glycosylated IgA may occur).[7]

Immune complexes are normally removed from the circulation by binding of the complex to the C3b receptors on erythrocytes; the immune complexes are then removed and degraded during transit of the erythrocytes in the liver and spleen. If antigenemia persists or clearance of complexes is impaired (such as in chronic liver disease), immune complexes may deposit in the glomerulus by binding to Fc receptors on mesangial cells or by passive deposition in the mesangium or subendothelial space. Physical characteristics of the complexes may also favor deposition, including avidity, charge, and size. Measurement of circulating immune complexes in patients with GN has not, however, shown close correlation with glomerular events and hence is not typically performed.

In some glomerular diseases, the target antigen has been identified (Fig. 16.7). Whereas the immune deposits may be associated with a specific antigen, glomerular diseases can also develop as a consequence of infection with organisms releasing superantigens that cause a polyclonal activation of B cells. The classic organism responsible for superantigen-associated GN is *Staphylococcus aureus*, and the pattern of immune deposits often includes the presence of both IgG and IgA. In other situations, infections may initiate an immune response that then results in cross-reaction with endogenous antigens. Studies suggest that this type of molecular mimicry may be responsible for both Goodpasture's syndrome and certain types of vasculitis (see Fig. 16.7).[8,9] Once an immune response is initiated, the local injury may lead to the release of additional antigens that may initiate an immune response (epitope spreading). In anti-GBM disease, in which the antigen is the α3 chain of type IV collagen, the antigen is present in the lung alveolar basement membrane but is normally sequestered. However, in tobacco smokers, the inhalation results in oxidative injury with exposure of the α3 chain, allowing the binding of antibody.[10] This may explain why lung involvement is almost exclusively observed in smokers in this disease.

Complement

The complement system is also often activated in glomerular disease (Fig. 16.8). Complement can be activated through three pathways. Classical activation involves the binding of C1q to the Fc region of antibody in IgG- and IgM-containing immune

Antigens Identified in Glomerulonephritis	
Poststreptococcal GN	Streptococcal pyrogenic exotoxin B (SPEB), plasmin receptor
Anti-GBM disease	α3 type IV collagen (likely induced by molecular mimicry)
IgA nephropathy	Possibly no antigen but rather polymerized polyclonal IgA (?superantigen driven)
Membranous nephropathy	Phospholipase A_2 receptor (idiopathic), neutral endopeptidase (NEP) in podocyte (congenital), HBeAg (hepatitis associated)
Staphylococcus aureus –associated GN	Staphylococcus superantigens induce polyclonal response; not necessarily antigen in glomeruli
Membranoproliferative GN	HCV and HBsAg in hepatitis-associated MPGN
ANCA-associated vasculitis	Proteinase 3 (c-ANCA) and myeloperoxidase (p-ANCA) in neutrophils; antibodies to lysosome-associated membrane protein 2 (LAMP-2) on endothelial cells (likely induced by molecular mimicry to fimbriated bacterial antigens)

Figure 16.7 Antigens identified in glomerulonephritis.

complexes and can result in reduced serum C4 and C3. This is common in lupus nephritis, type I MPGN, and cryoglobulinemic MPGN. Complement may also be activated by the alternative pathway, which is independent of immune complexes but triggered by polysaccharide antigens, polymeric IgA, injured cells, or endotoxins. This pathway appears to be activated in IgA nephropathy, DDD, and some cases of PSGN and membranous nephropathy. Serum complement levels are generally normal in both IgA nephropathy and membranous nephropathy; but in DDD and PSGN, the C3 is typically low, but C4 is normal. In DDD, the activation of the alternative pathway may not involve an antigen *per se* but rather may be due to an IgG autoantibody ("nephritic factor") that stabilizes the C3 convertase, resulting in its activation (see Chapter 21). Complement can also be activated through the mannose-binding pathway initiated by mannose-binding lectin, which has a similar structure to C1q. The role of the mannose-binding pathway in GN is emerging; it may be involved in some cases of IgA nephropathy.

Activation of the complement pathway has several consequences. Leukocyte recruitment is facilitated by the chemotactic factor C5a, and C3b binding is important in the binding and opsonization of the immune complexes by the infiltrating leukocytes. The terminal membrane attack complex of the cascade, C5b-9, inserts into cell membranes, where it can kill cells or activate them to secrete cytokines, oxidants, and extracellular matrix. C5b-9 is thought to be particularly important in mediating injury to the glomerular epithelial cell in membranous nephropathy, a disease in which immune deposits and complement activation occur in the subepithelial space. Complement can also be activated in proteinuric urine as a consequence of amidation of C3 by ammonia, and this may have a role in mediating tubulointerstitial injury even in conditions not associated with immune complex formation. Studies have emphasized the importance of local synthesis of complement components by the tubular cells as a mechanism that may augment this process.[11]

Activation of complement can occur easily, but it is usually tightly regulated by several complement regulatory proteins (see Fig. 16.8). It has recently been recognized that genetic absence or malfunction of factor H or other regulatory proteins can be associated with a hereditary form of MPGN or hemolytic-uremic syndrome.

Mechanisms of Immune Glomerular Injury

Two major mechanisms account for the presence of immune complexes in glomerular diseases. There may be ineffectual clearance of an antigen due to an impaired immune response, for example, in chronic viral infections such as hepatitis B and hepatitis C. Despite a strong humoral response, viral infection persists because the cell-mediated response required for elimination of these viruses from the liver is impaired. The consequence is a state of persistent antigenemia with circulating antigen-antibody complexes, which predisposes to glomerular injury. Eradication of the virus, for example, with interferon alfa therapy, can be associated with remission of the glomerular disease.

More commonly, glomerular disease may be due to autoimmunity. In health, a tension exists between the normal immune response to foreign antigen and tolerance, which is the cellular process that prevents an immune response to self antigen. Tolerance develops because self-reactive T and B cells are clonally deleted during fetal and neonatal life, although small numbers survive outside the thymus. Under certain conditions, these peripheral self-reactive T and B cells can be stimulated to generate a cellular and humoral response to a self antigen. Infection or toxins may play a role in initiating the response by releasing antigens from sequestered sites so they have access to T cells, by altering host proteins to make them more immunogenic, or by molecular mimicry, in which antibodies to an exogenous antigen (such as those present in an infecting organism) cross-react with a native protein. Activation of T cells may be further enhanced by the release of cytokines and lymphokines and the conversion of normally innocuous endogenous renal cells into antigen-presenting cells through the upregulated or *de novo* expression of HLA class II molecules.

A population of regulatory T cells ($CD4^+CD25^+$) has recently been shown to have a key role in controlling T cell responses and preventing the development of autoimmunity. These cells appear to be decreased in patients with anti-GBM disease at the time of presentation, which may play a role in the loss of tolerance. Indeed, in experimental anti-GBM nephritis, the administration of these cells can reduce glomerular damage by blocking T cell–dependent renal injury.[12]

Variations in HLA molecules and the T-cell receptor are under strong genetic influence. For that reason, immunogenetic associations, particularly between HLA expression and various patterns of GN, have been studied in great detail, but none of the reported associations is absolutely specific. For example, whereas HLA-DR2 identifies a powerful relative risk for the development of Goodpasture's disease, it is still possible for the disease to develop without HLA-DR2, and most individuals with HLA-DR2 never develop this rare disease. Furthermore, HLA associations often differ among racial groups that have different

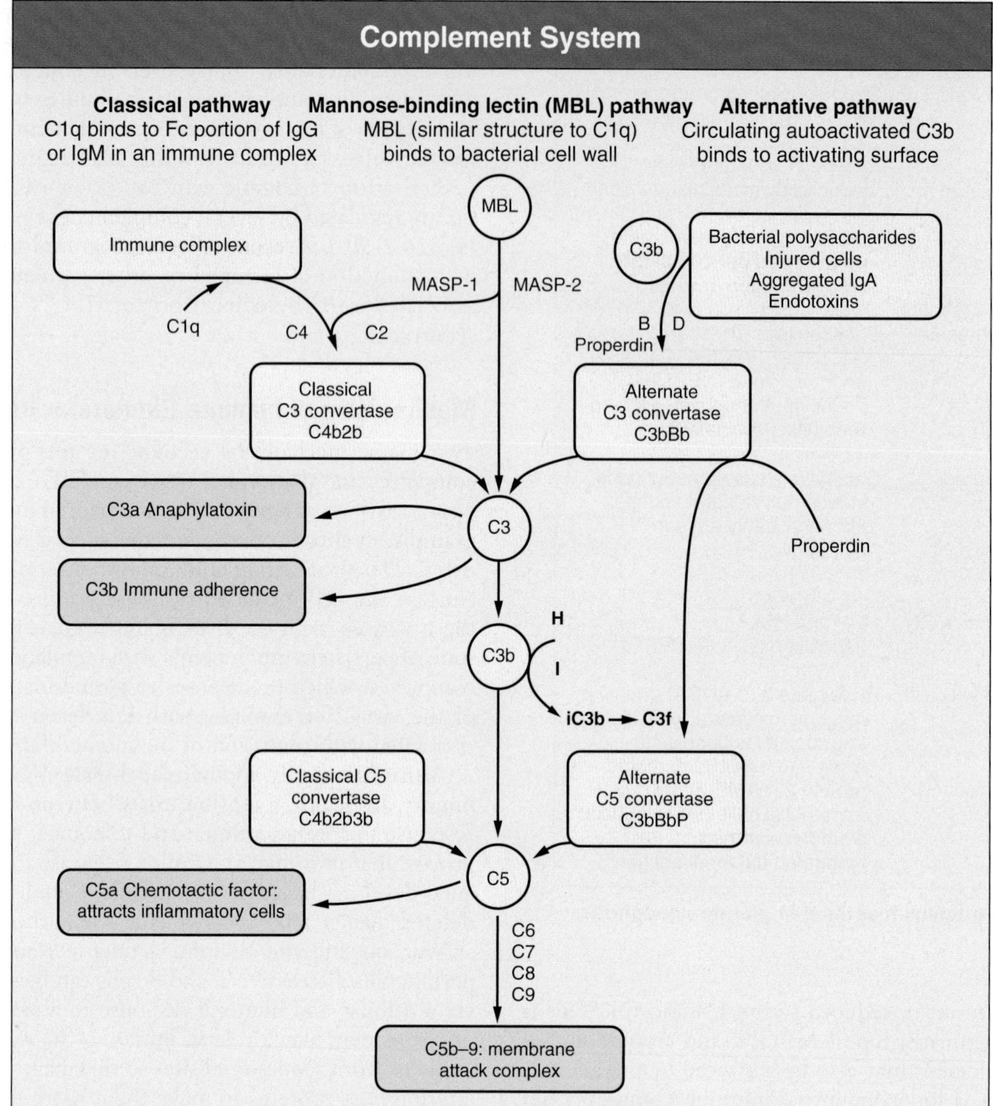

Figure 16.8 Complement system. The complement system is a self-amplifying cascade of proteins that generates a membrane attack complex, which is cytolytic; the cascade promotes inflammation by the activity of the fragments it produces. The amplifying cascades occur because activated fragments of the components combine to make convertase enzymes that degrade C3 and C5. The complement cascade is controlled in part by the very short active life of many of its components. There are also inhibitory regulatory proteins, most notably factors H and I inhibiting C3b. Activated fragments of any component are designated b (e.g., C3b); anaphylatoxic fragments are designated a (e.g., C5a). Inflammatory functions of complement components are shown in *green*. MASP, MBL-associated serine protease.

distributions of HLA. As yet, HLA associations have no practical diagnostic or therapeutic implications, and HLA typing is not needed in the clinical management of GN.

Inflammation

Infiltration by inflammatory cells is largely determined by the site of immune deposits. Immune deposits with direct access to the circulation (in particular those in subendothelial and basement membrane locations) are usually associated with a pronounced leukocyte accumulation. Mesangial deposits elicit an intermediate response, whereas immune deposits in the subepithelial space (such as in membranous nephropathy) generally are not associated with inflammatory cells.

In GN associated with subendothelial deposits, such as class IV lupus nephritis or MPGN, leukocyte infiltration is common. With acute injury, the predominant infiltrating cells are neutrophils, platelets, and monocytes; in chronic injury, the predominant cells are monocytes-macrophages and T cells. The primary mechanism for attracting these cells is the secretion of chemokines and the expression of leukocyte adhesion molecules by local endothelial and resident cells; local release of complement activation fragments (C5a) is also important.

In contrast to the immune complex mechanisms discussed previously, certain glomerular diseases develop primarily through cell-mediated immunity. For example, a direct role for T cells in mediating proteinuria and crescent formation has been shown in experimental crescentic nephritis.[13] It is thought that T cells in the glomeruli, sensitized to endogenous or exogenous antigen, recruit macrophages, resulting in a local delayed-type hypersensitivity reaction. In certain animal models, $CD8^+$ T cells have also been shown to mediate crescent formation, for example, through perforins (enzymes that act similarly to the complement membrane attack complex).

Proliferation, Apoptosis, and Fibrosis

Intrinsic glomerular cells (epithelial, mesangial, and endothelial) are also activated in various glomerular diseases. Mesangial cells, when activated, can become myofibroblast-like cells that proliferate and produce excessive extracellular matrix. Endothelial cells are a rich source of nitric oxide and other anti-inflammatory proteins, and injury to this cell population can result in the expression of leukocyte adhesion molecules and activation of the coagulation system. Podocytes are terminally differentiated cells; injury may result not only in proteinuria (see earlier discussion) but, when it is associated with apoptosis, also in glomerulosclerosis. Several key factors have been associated with glomerular injury, of which the most important appear to be transforming growth factor β that mediates matrix deposition, platelet-derived growth factor that mediates mesangial cell proliferation, and vascular endothelial growth factor required for endothelial health.

A particularly severe cellular response is the formation of crescents within Bowman's space. Crescent formation may be initiated by cytokine-driven proliferation of the parietal cells and possibly to a lesser extent the podocyte. Local breaks in the GBM or Bowman's capsule, mediated by activated leukocytes, are followed by macrophage infiltration, myofibroblast accumulation, and local fibrin deposition (Fig. 16.9). Most evidence suggests that crescent formation is a manifestation of cell-mediated rather than of humoral immune mechanisms.[13]

Glomerular scarring is often associated with proliferation of mesangial cells with loss of both endothelial cells and podocytes by apoptosis. Tubulointerstitial fibrosis also accompanies progressive glomerular disease and correlates with both renal function and prognosis. Proteinuria has been shown to activate tubular cells and induce toxicity, either directly or by the generation of oxidants (from iron proteins excreted in the urine) or complement activation (which can be shown in proteinuric urine). Tubulointerstitial ischemia may also be involved in the pathogenesis of renal fibrosis as a progressive loss of glomerular and peritubular capillaries can be shown in both experimental models and human disease. Finally, misdirected filtration (i.e., filtration of plasma ultrafiltrate into the peritubular space) as well as the formation of atubular glomeruli may contribute to progressive tubulointerstitial damage in the course of glomerular disease.

A detailed discussion of current mechanisms involved in glomerulosclerosis is presented in Chapter 76.

Specific pathogenic mechanisms in the different patterns of glomerular disease are discussed in the subsequent chapters in this section.

PATHOGENESIS OF SPECIFIC GLOMERULAR SYNDROMES

Minimal Change Disease

MCD is classically a corticosteroid-sensitive nephrotic syndrome in which the only structural abnormality is podocyte swelling and fusion of foot processes by EM (see Chapter 17). The disease is thought to be due to podocyte injury. The induction of CD80 (B7.1) in podocytes has been shown to cause rapid onset of proteinuria in experimental animals,[14] and CD80 has been recently identified in podocytes of patients with MCD. CD80 antigen is also present in the urine of subjects with MCD and correlates with disease activity. The mechanism of CD80 expression is unknown but could be mediated by viral or bacterial antigens or possibly by T-cell cytokines. T cells are activated in subjects with

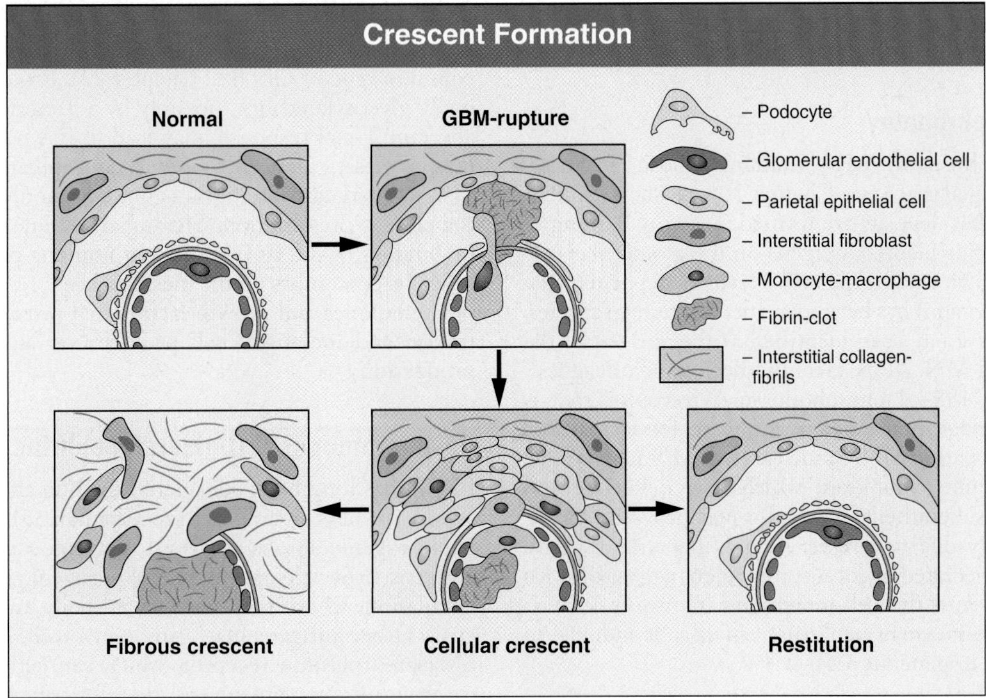

Figure 16.9 Crescent formation. In early crescent formation, cytokines and growth factors cross the GBM to initiate proliferation of the parietal epithelial cells. Small breaks in the GBM occur secondary to injury from oxidants and proteases from neutrophils and macrophages, thus allowing the macrophage to enter Bowman's space, where it can proliferate. Breaks in Bowman's capsule secondary to the periglomerular inflammation also occur, allowing the entrance of more inflammatory cells as well as fibroblasts. The proliferation of parietal and visceral epithelial cells and macrophages is associated with fibrin deposition, slowly choking the glomerular tuft until filtration becomes impossible. In the late stages, the crescent becomes fibrotic and the glomerulus end stage. Alternatively, in less severe cases, complete restitution of the glomerular tuft can occur.

MCD, and T-cell hybridomas from patients with MCD secrete a factor that provokes heavy proteinuria in rats.[15] Interleukin-13 is expressed by T cells in subjects with MCD, and overexpression of interleukin-13 induces CD80 in podocytes of rats with the development of nephrotic syndrome and histologic changes consistent with MCD. However, CD80 expression in podocytes can occur in the absence of T cells. In addition, proteinuria can be induced in immune-deficient mice by CD34-positive hematopoietic bone marrow cells of patients with MCD and recurrent FSGS but not by their T cells.[16] Thus, the role of T cells in this disorder remains to be clarified.

Focal Segmental Glomerulosclerosis

FSGS is a type of nephrotic syndrome that is often slowly responsive or nonresponsive to corticosteroids; there are no immune deposits, but there is foot process fusion by EM (see Chapter 18). However, the characteristic histologic lesion is of segmental sclerosis. Some cases of FSGS appear to be mediated by a soluble factor that is not yet fully defined. It is also not known if the pathogenesis overlaps with MCD.

A variant of FSGS is collapsing FSGS, in which there is proliferation of the normally quiescent podocyte, leading to collapse of the glomerular tuft, often in association with massive proteinuria. The pathogenesis may be due to production by the podocyte of growth factors (such as vascular endothelial growth factor) or local inhibition of cell cycle proteins that normally maintain the podocyte in a nonproliferative state.[17]

Focal sclerosing lesions in the absence of severe proteinuria can also occur in a wide variety of renal lesions besides nephrotic syndrome, including GN, chronic hypertension, and progressive renal disease of any etiology. These lesions are particularly common in African Americans; recent findings suggest that this susceptibility relates to increased frequency of a genetic polymorphism in *MYH9*, a gene coding for a nonmyosin protein in the podocyte that affects podocyte structure and function.[18]

Membranous Nephropathy

In membranous nephropathy (MN), immune deposits are localized to the subepithelial space (see Chapter 20). Most experimental studies suggest that deposits are formed *in situ* by binding of antibody to intrinsic or planted antigens on the glomerular epithelial cells. In animal studies (passive Heyman nephritis), the intrinsic antigen (megalin) has been identified. In human studies, neutral endopeptidase has been identified as the antigen in the very rare congenital MN. More recently, Beck and colleagues[19] have identified the 185-kd phospholipase A_2 receptor that is expressed on podocytes as the putative antigen for as many as 70% of cases of idiopathic MN. Some cases of MN may be due to low-avidity immune complexes, which may dissociate and then re-form at the subepithelial space; this may provide a mechanism for some MN due to viruses, such as hepatitis B virus. Podocyte injury is mediated by local complement activation with insertion of C5b-9 into the cell membrane. However, experimental MN (passive Heyman nephritis) can also be induced in rats that are unable to generate C5b-9.[20]

Membranoproliferative Glomerulonephritis

In MPGN type I, the immune deposits localize both to the mesangium and to the subendothelial space (see Chapter 21). A similar pattern is observed in cryoglobulinemic GN, in which the immune complexes contain a monoclonal IgM or polyclonal IgM that acts as a rheumatoid factor by binding to the IgG in the immune complex. In both cases, the disease is thought to occur by passive deposition from the circulation. When this pattern is seen in lupus nephritis, it may be facilitated by the binding of nucleosomes to the complexes (nucleosomes are cationic nuclear proteins that can interact with the negatively charged proteins within the glomerulus).

Studies in experimental models suggest that the intraglomerular immune complexes cause local complement activation with the generation of chemotactic factors (including C5a, chemokines, and leukotrienes). Leukocyte adhesion molecules on endothelial cells are upregulated (intracellular adhesion molecule 1) or expressed *de novo* (E- and P-selectins). Proinflammatory cytokines (interleukin-1 and tumor necrosis factor α) are generated locally and augment the inflammatory response. Neutrophils, platelets, and monocytes-macrophages then localize in the glomerulus and release oxidants (particularly hypohalous acids generated by neutrophil myeloperoxidase) and proteases (elastase, cathepsin G, and metalloproteinases) that cause local cellular injury and GBM degradation.

Dense Deposit Disease

In contrast to MPGN type I, immune complexes are absent in glomeruli of patients with DDD. Here, activation appears to derive from spontaneous intraglomerular activation of the alternative pathway of complement, for example, through mutations of the complement regulatory factor H.[21] In the case of factor H, the location of the mutation within the gene determines whether the disease is manifested as DDD or atypical hemolytic-uremic syndrome.[21]

Mesangial Proliferative Glomerulonephritis

IgA nephropathy, a mesangial proliferative GN, is the most common type of GN (see Chapter 22). Production of an abnormally glycosylated IgA, possibly by a bacterial superantigen[22] or aberrant T-cell response, may lead to IgA polymers that deposit in the mesangium; the glomerular capillary wall is relatively spared. Marked proteinuria is not commonly a major feature of the clinical presentation. Mesangial cell injury may be mediated by binding of the IgA-containing immune complexes to Fcα or other IgA receptors on the mesangial cell, resulting in the release of chemokines and growth factors that provokes leukocyte infiltration and mesangial cell proliferation and mesangial matrix production.

Poststreptococcal Glomerulonephritis

PSGN has long been considered the human equivalent of acute serum sickness in rabbits (see Chapter 55). It is thought that nephritogenic strains of group A streptococcus release specific antigens, especially streptococcal pyrogenic exotoxin B, into the circulation, where they bind to antibody and localize to glomeruli. Other antigens may also be involved, including nephritis-associated plasmin receptor, which can activate the alternative pathway of complement and therefore augment the inflammatory response independent of antibody. Activation of complement in the proximity of the endothelium leads to a brisk inflammatory reaction with local endothelial and mesangial cell proliferation and manifestations of the nephritic syndrome. Some deposits ("humps") also form in the subepithelial space and may represent the translocation of immune complexes across the GBM.

Goodpasture's Disease

Goodpasture's disease (anti-GBM disease) is due to an autoantibody to the $\alpha3$ chain of type IV collagen present in the GBM and alveolar basement membrane (see Chapter 23).[8] The autoantibody develops antigens in genetically susceptible individuals because of molecular mimicry between the type IV collagen antigens and certain bacterial antigens.[8] Binding of antibody results in complement activation with the infiltration of inflammatory cells that causes local capillary wall damage and proteinuria. Crescent formation also commonly occurs and may be mediated by both T cells and macrophages.

ANCA-Associated Vasculitis

A severe form of segmental necrotizing glomerular injury, often in association with crescents, can be observed with various types of vasculitis (see Chapter 24). The two most common types of vasculitis causing this type of injury are Wegener's granulomatosis and microscopic polyangiitis. Both are associated with circulating antibodies against neutrophil cytoplasmic antigens (ANCA); antibodies to proteinase 3 give a cytoplasmic pattern by staining (c-ANCA) in most patients with Wegener's granulomatosis, and antibodies to myeloperoxidase give a paranuclear staining pattern (p-ANCA) in subjects with microscopic polyangiitis. Whereas there is experimental evidence that ANCA are pathogenic by activating neutrophils within the vasculature, pathogenic autoantibodies to lysosome-associated membrane protein 2 (LAMP-2) present in endothelial cells have recently been identified in vasculitis.[9] LAMP antibodies appear to develop as a consequence of molecular mimicry with various bacteria and viruses and when injected into rats result in crescentic nephritis. The clinical value of measuring LAMP autoantibodies is not yet clear.

REFERENCES

1. Mundel P, Shankland SJ. Podocyte biology and response to injury. *J Am Soc Nephrol*. 2002;13:3005-3015.
2. Antignac C. Molecular basis of steroid-resistant nephrotic syndrome. *Nefrologia*. 2005;25(Suppl 2):25-28.
3. Machuca E, Hummel A, Nevo F, et al. Clinical and epidemiological assessment of steroid-resistant nephrotic syndrome associated with the NPHS2 R229Q variant. *Kidney Int*. 2009;75:727-735.
4. Myers BD, Guasch A. Mechanisms of proteinuria in nephrotic humans. *Pediatr Nephrol*. 1994;8:107-112.
5. Hinkes B, Wiggins RC, Gbadegesin R, et al. Positional cloning uncovers mutations in PLCE1 responsible for a nephrotic syndrome variant that may be reversible. *Nat Genet*. 2006;38:1397-1405.
6. Couser WG. Pathogenesis of glomerular damage in glomerulonephritis. *Nephrol Dial Transplant*. 1998;13(Suppl 1):10-15.
7. Suzuki H, Moldoveanu Z, Hall S, et al. IgA1-secreting cell lines from patients with IgA nephropathy produce aberrantly glycosylated IgA1. *J Clin Invest*. 2008;118:629-639.
8. Arends J, Wu J, Borillo J, et al. T cell epitope mimicry in antiglomerular basement membrane disease. *J Immunol*. 2006;176:1252-1258.
9. Kain R, Exner M, Brandes R, et al. Molecular mimicry in pauci-immune focal necrotizing glomerulonephritis. *Nat Med*. 2008;14:1088-1096.
10. Kalluri R, Cantley LG, Kerjaschki D, Neilson EG. Reactive oxygen species expose cryptic epitopes associated with autoimmune Goodpasture syndrome. *J Biol Chem*. 2000;275:20027-20032.
11. Sheerin NS, Risley P, Abe K, et al. Synthesis of complement protein C3 in the kidney is an important mediator of local tissue injury. *FASEB J*. 2008;22:1065-1072.
12. Wolf D, Hochegger K, Wolf AM, et al. $CD4^+CD25^+$ regulatory T cells inhibit experimental anti–glomerular basement membrane glomerulonephritis in mice. *J Am Soc Nephrol*. 2005;16:1360-1370.
13. Atkins RC, Nikolic-Paterson DJ, Song Q, Lan HY. Modulators of crescentic glomerulonephritis. *J Am Soc Nephrol*. 1996;7:2271-2278.
14. Reiser J, von Gersdorff G, Loos M, et al. Induction of B7-1 in podocytes is associated with nephrotic syndrome. *J Clin Invest*. 2004;113:1390-1397.
15. Koyama A, Fujisaki M, Kobayashi M, et al. A glomerular permeability factor produced by human T cell hybridomas. *Kidney Int*. 1991;40:453-460.
16. Sellier-Leclerc AL, Duval A, Riveron S, et al. A humanized mouse model of idiopathic nephrotic syndrome suggests a pathogenic role for immature cells. *J Am Soc Nephrol*. 2007;18:2732-2739.
17. Barisoni L, Kriz W, Mundel P, D'Agati V. The dysregulated podocyte phenotype: A novel concept in the pathogenesis of collapsing idiopathic focal segmental glomerulosclerosis and HIV-associated nephropathy. *J Am Soc Nephrol*. 1999;10:51-61.
18. Kopp JB, Smith MW, Nelson GW, et al. MYH9 is a major-effect risk gene for focal segmental glomerulosclerosis. *Nat Genet*. 2008;40:1175-1184.
19. Beck L, Bonegio R, Lambeau G, et al. Discovery of the phospholipase A_2 receptor as the target antigen in idiopathic membranous nephropathy [abstract]. *J Am Soc Nephrol*. 2008;19:104A.
20. Spicer ST, Tran GT, Killingsworth MC, et al. Induction of passive Heymann nephritis in complement component 6–deficient PVG rats. *J Immunol*. 2007;179:172-178.
21. Pickering MC, de Jorge EG, Martinez-Barricarte R, et al. Spontaneous hemolytic uremic syndrome triggered by complement factor H lacking surface recognition domains. *J Exp Med*. 2007;204:1249-1256.
22. Koyama A, Sharmin S, Sakurai H, et al. *Staphylococcus aureus* cell envelope antigen is a new candidate for the induction of IgA nephropathy. *Kidney Int*. 2004;66:121-132.

CHAPTER 17

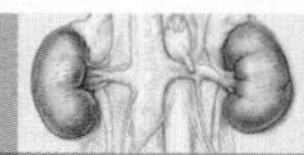

Minimal Change Nephrotic Syndrome

Philip D. Mason, Peter F. Hoyer

DEFINITION

Minimal change disease (MCD) is the cause of nephrotic syndrome in about 90% of children younger than 10 years, about 50% to 70% of older children, and 10% to 15% of adults. MCD is defined by the absence of histologic glomerular abnormalities, other than ultrastructural evidence of epithelial cell foot process fusion, in a patient presenting with nephrotic syndrome who is typically corticosteroid responsive. Corticosteroid-sensitive nephrotic syndrome is the term used to describe the disease occurring in children with nephrotic syndrome who respond to corticosteroids but who have not had a renal biopsy to provide the histologic proof of MCD. The presence of nephrotic syndrome is important because similar histologic findings may be seen in patients with proteinuria in the absence of nephrotic syndrome. Such patients may have different conditions with different prognoses and requirements for management.

Whereas MCD is classically associated with normal-appearing glomeruli and corticosteroid responsiveness, MCD appears to overlap with a variety of histologic variants that have a tendency to be less corticosteroid responsive. These conditions include focal segmental glomerulosclerosis (FSGS; see Chapter 18) and IgM nephropathy (see later discussion). It is possible that both MCD and FSGS have similar initial histologic appearances but that FSGS is less corticosteroid responsive and hence develops secondary sclerosing lesions over time. Whether this represents a continuum of the same disease in which some subjects are corticosteroid sensitive and others are not or whether they represent two distinct etiologies remains debated.

ETIOLOGY AND PATHOGENESIS

MCD is the most common cause of nephrotic syndrome in children aged 2 to 12 years. However, it is also relatively common in adults. Many patients have a history of allergy, including atopy, asthma, or eczema (Fig. 17.1). Most cases are idiopathic, but MCD has also been associated with certain cancers, especially Hodgkin's disease, in which it may be the presenting symptom. Finally, MCD has been associated with the use of certain drugs, such as interferon alfa and nonsteroidal anti-inflammatory drugs (NSAIDs) (see Fig. 17.1).

The primary abnormality in MCD is a defect in the glomerular filtration barrier to protein. In normal glomeruli, the barrier to protein filtration is provided by the glomerular basement membrane (GBM) and the slit diaphragm that extends between the podocyte foot processes. Size barriers and charge selectivity of GBM exclude neutral molecules larger than 4 to 4.5 nm from filtration; albumin molecules that are smaller than this are excluded because they are anionic and are repelled by the negative charge on the epithelial cells and GBM.

In MCD, FSGS, and other causes of nephrotic syndrome, the clearance of proteins becomes markedly enhanced, whereas the filtration of small molecules is actually reduced. Some authorities have attributed the reduction in small molecular clearance to the diffuse foot process fusion, which reduces overall slit diaphragm area and thereby may account for the reduction in the ultrafiltration coefficient (K_f, see Chapter 2) that is typically observed. In contrast, the albuminuria is thought to result from specific areas ("large pores") where the protein escapes into the urine.

Studies in nephrotic syndrome have implicated injury to the podocyte, and particularly the slit diaphragm, as the key factor leading to proteinuria. The importance of the slit diaphragm for nephrosis was first shown with the congenital nephrotic syndrome of the "Finnish type," in which the primary defect is a mutation in nephrin, a key protein in the slit diaphragm. In particular, this nephrotic syndrome can histologically and clinically appear identical to MCD, except that it typically begins shortly after birth and is corticosteroid resistant (see Chapter 19). Since the discovery of the etiology of this nephrotic syndrome, numerous other congenital causes of nephrotic syndrome have been identified that all have in common mutations in genes involved in the slit diaphragm (*NPHS1, NPHS2, NPHS3, WT1, LAMB2, LMXI2, ACTN4, CD2AP, TRPC6*; see Chapter 19).

Evidence for a primary podocyte abnormality contributing to MCD is beginning to emerge. For example, MCD is associated with expression of CD80 (B7.1) on the podocyte, and shed CD80 can be found in the urine of patients with MCD.[1] Experimental studies have shown that CD80 expression by podocytes results in shape change and the development of proteinuria. Reduced levels of dystroglycans (adhesion molecules believed to anchor podocytes to the GBM) have also been reported in MCD but not in FSGS, with normalization after corticosteroid treatment.[2]

Others have proposed that the permeability defect is due to alterations in the GBM, particularly a loss of negative charge. In this case, the podocyte changes could be secondary to the proteinuria. This would be consistent with observations of preserved foot processes in the early phase of some highly proteinuric states (e.g., recurrent FSGS after renal transplantation) and of podocyte foot process fusion in children with severe hypoalbuminemia, but not proteinuria, dying of kwashiorkor.[3]

There is also some evidence that there may be a circulating factor responsible for inducing the alteration in the capillary wall. Hemopexin, an acute-phase reactant extracted from human plasma, is capable of inducing proteinuria in rats,[4] and in one small study, plasma hemopexin activity was increased in MCD patients in relapse with some evidence of an altered isoform.[5] Evidence of a circulating factor in humans is also supported by the observation that proteinuria resolved within days after transplantation from a cadaveric donor with MCD.[6] Evidence for a T-cell abnormality includes the absence of immune deposits, the remarkable sensitivity of the disease to corticosteroids and cyclosporine, the relationship with Hodgkin's disease, and the reports that active measles infection (which depresses cell-mediated immunity) can rapidly induce remission. Studies have shown that T regulatory cells are abnormal in MCD and that there is generalized activation of T cells during active disease.

Some studies have also implicated interleukin (IL)–13 released from T cells in causing the proteinuria, as T-cell production of IL-13 is elevated and overexpression of IL-13 can induce nephrotic syndrome in rats.[7] Interestingly, the mechanism involved induction of CD80 in the podocyte. IL-13 is also a cytokine associated with allergic states, and MCD can be triggered by vaccination[8] or exposure to an allergen in sensitive individuals. As a result, patients with identified food allergies have been managed with exclusion diets with reported complete or partial remissions and with relapse after reintroduction of the offending food. However, even if the relationship is real, it is possible that the allergic events merely trigger relapse, as may infections.

Whereas a T-cell mechanism remains likely, there is also an interesting report in which proteinuria could be induced in experimental animals with use of $CD34^+$ stem cells from subjects with MCD.[9]

Finally, an association has been reported with HLA-DR7 (in some ethnic groups), at least in corticosteroid-responsive individuals.

Factors Associated with the Onset of Nephrotic Syndrome in Minimal Change Disease
Drugs
Nonsteroidal anti-inflammatory drugs (NSAIDs)
Interferon alfa
Lithium: rare (usually causes chronic interstitial nephritis)
Gold: rare (usually causes membranous nephropathy)
Allergy
Pollens
House dust
Insect stings
Immunizations
Malignancy
Hodgkin's disease
Mycosis fungoides
Chronic lymphocytic leukemia: uncommon (usually associated with membranoproliferative glomerulonephritis)

Figure 17.1 Factors associated with the onset of nephrotic syndrome in minimal change disease.

EPIDEMIOLOGY

MCD affects 2 to 7 per 100,000 children per year, with a prevalence of 15 per 100,000, most commonly presenting between 2 and 7 years of age. It is also an important cause of nephrotic syndrome in adults of all ages, although the incidence varies geographically. MCD is reported to be as low as 1 per million in the United Kingdom and up to 27 per million in the United States. It is more common in South Asians and Native Americans but is much rarer in African Americans, in whom nephrotic syndrome is much more likely to be due to FSGS and to be corticosteroid resistant. MCD is also relatively rare in developing countries, such as most countries in Africa and South America (Fig. 17.2).[10-12] Boys are twice as likely to be affected as are girls, but the sex incidence is equal in adolescents and adults. There are data suggesting that MCD has become less common in adults.[13]

CLINICAL MANIFESTATIONS

Patients typically present with edema that develops during days to weeks with fluid retention that often exceeds more than 3% of the body weight. Up to two thirds of initial presentations and relapses follow an infection, most commonly of the upper respiratory tract, but whether these are of causative significance is uncertain.

The clinical signs and symptoms are the same as those for nephrotic syndrome of any cause (see Chapter 15), although nephrotic syndrome is often of very rapid onset, increasing the risk of hypovolemia, particularly in children. Pleural effusions and ascites are common, particularly in children, who may present with abdominal pain, a symptom that may suggest peritonitis or herald hypovolemia. Pericardial effusions may occur infrequently (but rarely cause significant complications), and pulmonary edema is uncommon except after excessive treatment with albumin or with coexisting cardiac disease. Hepatomegaly is frequent in children but may be overlooked in the presence of

Frequency of Various Types of Nephrotic Syndrome in Children and Adults from Europe, the United States, and Africa

Histology	Children	Adults	Zimbabwe	Durban
MCD	76	20	9.2	14
FSGS	8	15	15.1	28
MN	7	40	15.1	41 (35 Hep B)
MPGN	4	7	33.6	9
Misc.	5	18	17.0	5

Figure 17.2 Frequency of various types of nephrotic syndrome (in annual incidence per million population) in children and adults from Europe, the United States, and Africa. MCD, minimal change disease; FSGS, focal and segmental glomerulosclerosis; MN, membranous nephropathy; MPGN, membranoproliferative glomerulosclerosis. *(Data from references 10-12.)*

ascites. The distribution of edema is gravitational, but facial puffiness is common and genital swelling may be very uncomfortable, especially in men. Gross edema may predispose to ulceration and infection of dependent skin; striae often appear even without corticosteroids, and lacerations or needlestick punctures weep fluid profusely. Edema of the bowel may cause diarrhea, rarely with significant albumin loss from the gut. Other clinical features include white nails, sometimes in bands (Muehrcke's bands) correlating with periods of clinical relapse (see Fig. 15.4). In adults, xanthomas may occasionally result in association with gross hyperlipidemia.

Microscopic hematuria is rare in MCD, and although hypertension is not typical in children, it has been observed at presentation in 30% of 89 adults in one study from the United Kingdom.[14] Higher blood pressure than normal has also been described in 14% to 21% of children, when comparisons are made with appropriate age- and sex-matched blood pressure reference ranges. This usually resolves during remission, especially in children. Hypertension is sometimes associated with expansion of the intravascular volume but may paradoxically be related to hypovolemia and stimulation of the renin-angiotensin system (RAS).

Before the introduction of corticosteroids, the morbidity and mortality of patients with MCD were high because of complications of nephrotic syndrome, particularly infection. Infection continues to be a serious problem, particularly in those presenting late,[15] and 6 of 389 children with MCD described by the International Study of Kidney Disease in Children (ISKDC) in 1984 died of sepsis.[16] Peritonitis remains a major cause of mortality in the developing world, mainly in children. *Streptococcus pneumoniae*, *Haemophilus influenzae*, and other encapsulated bacteria are commonly implicated. Children with frequently relapsing nephrotic syndrome should be immunized against *S. pneumoniae* and *H. influenzae* during remission and given prophylactic oral penicillin in relapse.[17] Peritonitis is rare in adults, who usually have protective antibodies against these bacteria, and prophylactic antibiotics are not indicated.

The risk of thromboembolism is increased in MCD, as in all subjects with nephrotic syndrome (see Chapter 15). Venous thromboembolism may occur in the lower extremities, renal veins, and other sites. Pulmonary embolism may be overlooked in children because of a lack of suspicion, even with pulmonary symptoms, and children may compensate better than adults do. Nephrotic children occasionally have other catastrophic events, such as intracerebral venous or sinus venous thrombosis. Arterial thrombosis is also a rare and feared complication that has been described in children almost exclusively and may result in loss of limbs.

Renal function is generally preserved, but the serum creatinine concentration is sometimes slightly elevated in adults. Acute kidney injury is a complication particularly seen in adults. It may follow hypovolemia, which should be avoided especially during intensive diuretic treatment, but it may also rarely occur in patients who are volume replete (see also Chapter 15).

Secondary MCD may mimic idiopathic MCD and may result from drugs or with cancer. The classic drugs associated with MCD are NSAIDS and particularly fenoprofen. This is an idiosyncratic reaction and is usually associated with chronic NSAID use that has occurred for several weeks or months. Unlike classic MCD, this syndrome is usually associated with massive nephrotic syndrome with impaired renal function, and renal biopsy shows MCD with features of an acute interstitial nephritis with T-cell infiltration. Other causes of secondary MCD, such as the use of interferon alfa or interferon beta, or MCD observed in Hodgkin's disease, may appear clinically identical to idiopathic MCD.

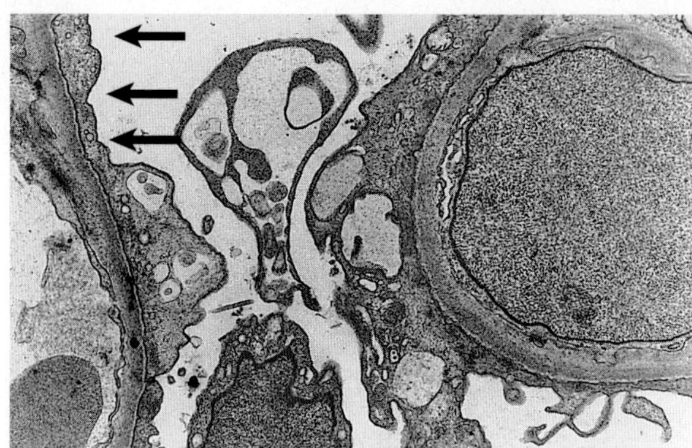

Figure 17.3 Podocyte foot process fusion in minimal change disease. The epithelial cells *(arrows)* are completely effaced along the glomerular basement membranes. (Electron micrograph; magnification ×6000.) The normal appearance of epithelial cell foot processes is shown in Figures 1.7 and 1.8 (see Chapter 1).

PATHOLOGY

Classically, MCD is associated with normal-appearing glomeruli by light microscopy and is negative for immunoglobulins and complement by immunofluorescence or other methodologies. Podocyte (epithelial cell) foot process effacement is observed with electron microscopy (Fig. 17.3) and is the only abnormality, but this is a nonspecific finding. The tubulointerstitium will show an absence of inflammation. Hyaline casts obstructing tubules, rare foam cells, and occasionally appearances consistent with acute tubular necrosis may be seen, especially if acute kidney injury is present at the time of biopsy.

Variants

Mild mesangial hypercellularity is an infrequent finding (3% to 5%), and small amounts of mesangial IgG, complement C3, and occasionally IgA may be observed in patients whose clinical course is indistinguishable from classic MCD.

The glomerular tip lesion describes structural segmental changes adjacent to the tubular pole of Bowman's capsule, with protrusion into the tubular lumen. This is observed more commonly in adults than in children. Whether this is a variant of MCD or should be considered a type of FSGS is controversial. Generally considered a benign lesion, it may also be rarely observed in membranoproliferative glomerulonephritis, IgA nephropathy, and renal allografts. The most important reason to recognize the lesion is to prevent a misdiagnosis of a proliferative glomerulonephritis.

The presence of mesangial hypercellularity in MCD may correlate with increased resistance to corticosteroid therapy.[18] Some consider mesangial hypercellularity to be an intermediate step in cases of evolution (progression) of MCD to FSGS (see Chapter 18).

IgM Nephropathy

Some patients presenting with nephrotic syndrome have mesangial deposits of IgM, often with a minor degree of mesangial hypercellularity. Patients are more likely to have microscopic (and occasionally macroscopic) hematuria and are also less likely to respond to corticosteroids (50% compared with 90% for minimal change nephrotic syndrome).[19] Whether this represents a distinct entity or is part of the spectrum observed with MCD and FSGS remains uncertain (see also Chapter 27).

Focal Segmental Glomerulosclerosis

Some patients who are considered to have MCD by renal biopsy may not respond to corticosteroids and on repeated biopsy are found to have FSGS. Others who initially are responsive to corticosteroids eventually become resistant and are discovered to have FSGS on a subsequent biopsy. This has led some to suggest that MCD and FSGS are part of a spectrum of the same disease process. However, it remains possible that the initial biopsies may have missed the sclerotic lesions of FSGS because they are focal.

DIAGNOSIS AND DIFFERENTIAL DIAGNOSIS

The clinical diagnosis of nephrotic syndrome is straightforward, with edema in the presence of heavy proteinuria, usually without microscopic hematuria on urine dipstick testing. Urine microscopy reveals hyaline casts and sometimes lipid casts. There is hypoalbuminemia (<2.5 g/dl) and nephrotic-range proteinuria (>3.5 g/24 h in adults or >1 g/m^2/24 h [=40 mg/m^2/h] in children) or a protein to creatinine ratio of more than 0.25 g/mmol (>2 mg protein/mg creatinine) on a spot urine sample. Hyperlipidemia is also a common laboratory finding. Hyponatremia and hemoconcentration may be seen, even before treatment. Elevated urea and creatinine concentrations occur more often in adults. Typically, serum IgG levels are low and IgM is increased. Serum complement levels are normal.

In children, corticosteroid-sensitive MCD is usually associated with selective proteinuria of smaller molecules, including albumin and transferrin, but not of larger molecules, such as immunoglobulins and ferritin. A selectivity index is usually derived from the ratio of IgG clearance to albumin clearance:

$$\text{Selectivity index} = [(\text{IgG})_u\,(\text{albumin})_s]/[(\text{IgG})_s\,(\text{albumin})_u]$$

where subscript *u* is concentration in urine and *s* is that in serum. If the selectivity index is less than 0.1, the proteinuria is highly selective, and if it is more than 0.2, it is nonselective. This is of limited clinical value because highly selective proteinuria is less common in adult MCD and does not influence the decision to treat with corticosteroids. However, highly selective proteinuria, when it is present, does indicate that MCD is more likely to be the diagnosis, and some argue that such patients should be given a trial of corticosteroids without a renal biopsy, especially if the risk of biopsy complications is high.

In children from the Northern Hemisphere aged 2 to 12 years, renal biopsy is unnecessary unless the patient does not respond to a standard prednisone treatment of 60 mg/m^2/day within 4 weeks. In Africa and South America, the prevalence is lower. In this setting, a trial of corticosteroids might depend on how common MCD is in this region and should also take into consideration the higher risk of infections.

In adults, in whom there is a wide differential diagnosis for nephrotic syndrome and corticosteroid responsiveness is less likely, a renal biopsy is required to establish the diagnosis.

On occasion, a renal biopsy may histologically appear like MCD, but there is another cause. In subjects with nephrotic syndrome, this may be due to FSGS in which the sclerotic glomeruli are not sampled. In young children, it could be due to a hereditary nephrotic syndrome resembling MCD (see Chapter 19). Rarely, early membranous nephropathy will have a light microscopic appearance of normal glomeruli, but immunofluorescence will reveal immune deposits. Early amyloidosis may also mimic MCD histologically in the adult. Finally, in non-nephrotic subjects, diseases such as thin basement membrane disease can appear histologically normal but can be diagnosed by demonstration of the thin GBM by electron microscopy.

NATURAL HISTORY

There is a tendency for patients with MCD to run a relapsing-remitting course, and this is more frequent in children. Those presenting younger are more likely to have more relapses and a longer disease course (Fig. 17.4).[20] Relapse is common, affecting more than two thirds of children, and nearly 50% will relapse more than four times, usually after corticosteroid cessation or reduction. If relapse occurs during corticosteroid reduction, the patient is described as corticosteroid dependent. Long-term remission can be expected in 75% of initial responders who do not relapse within 6 months; those who do relapse become nonrelapsing after an average of 3 years, and 84% are in long-term remission after 10 years.[21] Indeed, it is reassuring that less than 5% of children with MCD enter adulthood still having relapses, although the younger the age at the onset of the first attack, the longer the child is likely to continue having relapses.[20,22] In general, increasing time since last relapse reduces the risk of further relapse, but adults will occasionally have a relapse after an interval of 10 years or more.

MCD does not progress to renal failure. However, a number of adult patients, but fewer children, with an initial diagnosis of MCD are found to have FSGS on subsequent biopsies, and they may develop progressive renal failure. It is still unclear whether the focal nature of the disease caused the correct diagnosis to be missed on the initial biopsy or whether evolution from MCD to FSGS occurs in some individuals.

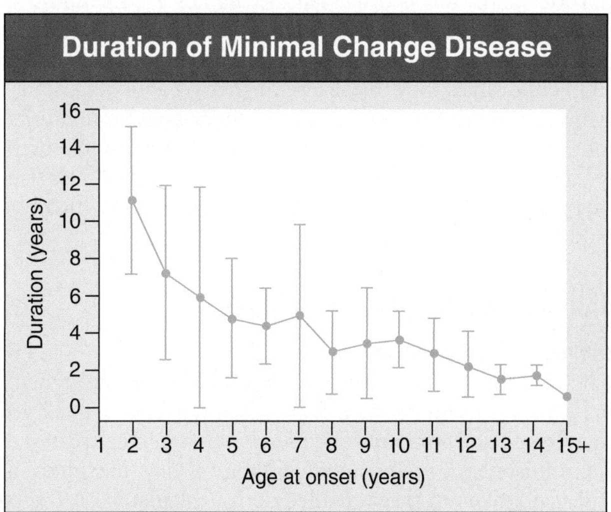

Figure 17.4 Long-term outcome in childhood-onset minimal change disease. The duration of disease is inversely related to the age at presentation. *(Modified from reference 20.)*

Nephrotic Syndrome: Definitions

Term	NS Definitions	
	Adult	Pediatric[14, 15]
Relapse	Proteinuria ≥35 g day^{-1} occurring after complete remission has been obtained for >1 month	Albu-stix 3+ or proteinuria >40 mgm^{-2}h^{-1} occurring on 3 days within 1 week
Frequently relapsing Complete remission	2+ relapses within 6 months Reduction of proteinuria to ≤0.20 g day^{-1} and serum albumin >35gl^{-1}	2+ relapses within 6 months <4 mg m^{-2}h^{-1} on at least 3 occasions within 7 days serum albumin >35 gl^{-1}
Partial remission	Reduction of proteinuria to between 0.21 g day^{-1} and 3.4 g day^{-1} ± decrease in proteinuria of ≥50% from baseline	Disappearance of edema. Increase in serum albumin >35 gl^{-1} and persisting proteinuria >4 mgm^{-2}h^{-1} or >100 mg m^{-2}day^{-1}
Steroid-resistant	Persistence of proteinuria despite prednisone therapy 1 mg kg^{-1} day^{-1} × 4 months	Persistence of proteinuria despite prednisone therapy 60 mg m^{-2} × 4 weeks[a]
Steroid-dependent—NS recurs when stop or decrease treatment	Two consecutive relapses occurring during therapy or within 14 days of completing steroid therapy[16]	Two relapses of proteinuria within 14 days after stopping or during alternate-day steroid therapy

Figure 17.5 Definition of terms used in idiopathic nephrotic syndrome in adults and children. The definitions were generated by a consensus of the International Society for Kidney Diseases in Children and the German Pediatric Nephrology Society. NS, nephrotic syndrome. [a]Or persistence of proteinuria despite prednisone therapy 60 mg m^{-2} × 4 weeks and three methylprednisolone pulses. *(Data from reference 23.)*

TREATMENT

Definitions That Guide Treatment

Figure 17.5 provides key definitions related to the clinical response of MCD to treatment that are used to guide therapy.[23] For example, subjects who relapse more than three times within a year are considered frequently relapsing, whereas subjects who respond to corticosteroids but relapse before discontinuation are considered corticosteroid dependent. Subjects who remain proteinuric despite a course of corticosteroids are considered corticosteroid resistant. Stratification of patients into their category can help in management (see later discussion).

Initial Treatment of Minimal Change Disease

Initial management of MCD includes standard management of nephrotic syndrome as discussed in Chapter 15, including low-sodium diet to control edema. Bed rest should be avoided because of the increased risk for thrombosis. Diuretics are infrequently used in children as they may cause further volume depletion, but they are often used to control extracellular volume in adults, in whom hypovolemia before treatment is less common. In those who remain with prolonged nephrotic syndrome, treatment of hyperlipidemia with statins and prophylaxis for thrombosis should be considered.

Childhood Minimal Change Disease

Treatment of First Episode

Corticosteroids are the initial treatment of choice (see algorithm, Fig. 17.6). According to the ISKDC, children (aged 2 to 12 years) with a first episode of nephrotic syndrome should be treated with oral prednisone (or prednisolone) 60 mg/m^2/day (maximum dose 80 mg/day) given in three divided doses (calculated on the basis of estimated dry weight). With this regimen, about 75% respond within 2 weeks, and almost all who are corticosteroid sensitive respond within 4 weeks (Fig. 17.7).[25,26] Those who do not respond within the period are regarded as nonresponders.[19]

Whereas the ISKDC recommendations proposed that the daily dose be continued for a total of 4 weeks, later studies argue for a duration of 6 weeks.[27] This daily dose should be followed by an alternate-day dose of 40 mg/m^2/48 h for an additional 4 weeks (ISKDC) or 6 weeks (recent data).[28] A meta-analysis of trials has demonstrated that extending the duration of corticosteroid treatment to at least 3 months reduces the 1- to 2-year risk of relapse (Fig. 17.8).[29]

The German Society for Pediatric Nephrology (Arbeitsgemeinschaft für Pädiatrische Nephrologie) recommends stopping corticosteroid treatment for the first episode after 12 weeks; others recommend tapering (e.g., reducing every 2 weeks by 15 mg/m^2 on alternate days). Although these two regimens have never been compared, we do not recommend tapering because of concerns of chronic corticosteroid use on growth.

Treatment of Relapses

The urine should be tested daily (usually by a parent) during and after treatment. The rationale is that relapses should be treated on the basis of proteinuria (usually requiring at least three or more positive dipstick measurements for 3 consecutive days) to initiate a further course of corticosteroids. The aim is to treat relapse early to avoid nephrosis-associated complications. The intensity of corticosteroid treatment for relapses has not been shown to have an impact on the probability of further relapses.

Our recommendation is oral prednisone 60 mg/m^2/day (maximum dose 80 mg/day) given daily in three divided doses until the urine is protein free for 3 days, followed by a course of alternate day prednisone 40 mg/m^2/48 h for 4 weeks, then stop. An alternative recommendation is to taper the alternate dose during weeks to months to define a relapse threshold. However, the acceptability of this approach depends on the corticosteroid threshold, and there is a risk of more corticosteroid toxicity with prolonged tapering.

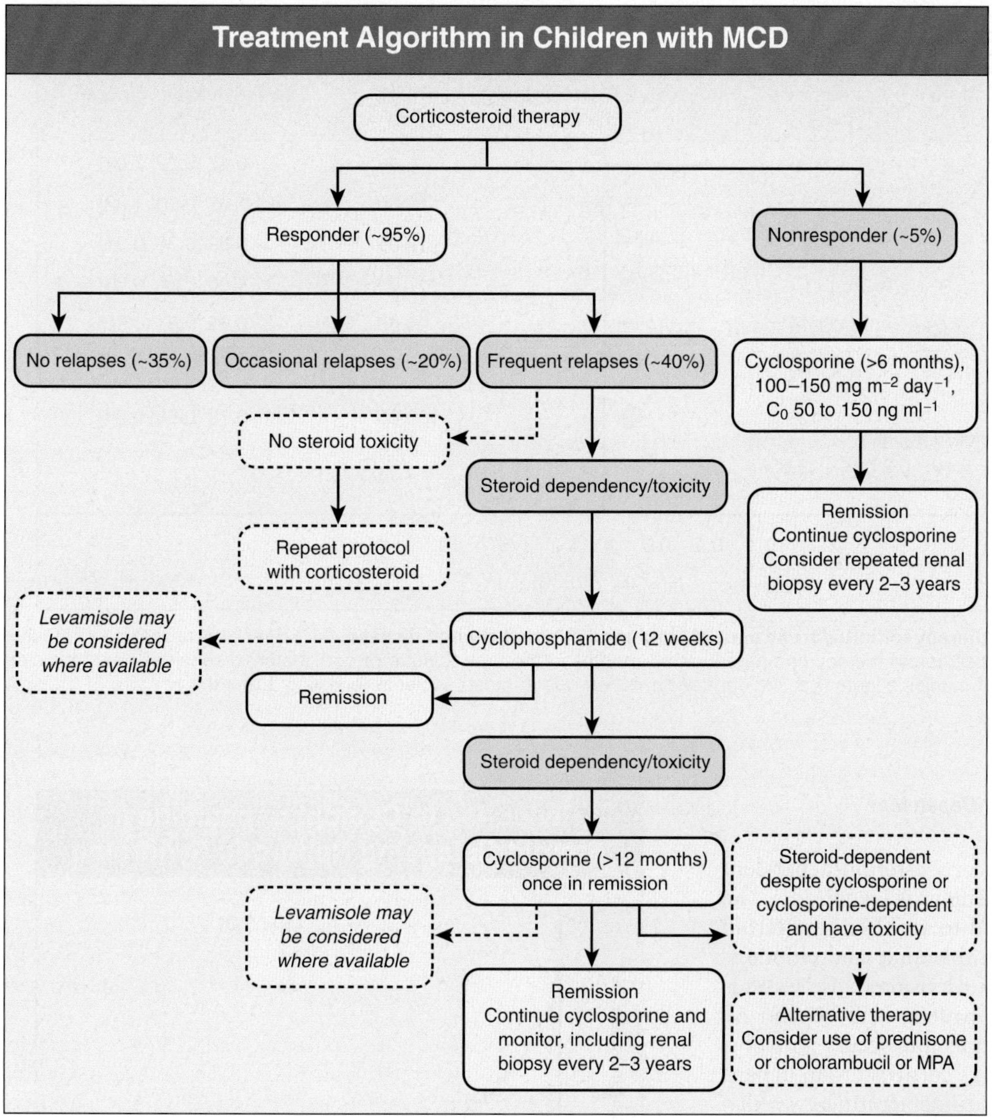

Treatment Algorithm in Children with MCD
Corticosteroid therapy
Responder (~95%)
Nonresponder (~5%)
No relapses (~35%)
Occasional relapses (~20%)
Frequent relapses (~40%)
Cyclosporine (>6 months), 100–150 mg m-2 day-1, C0 50 to 150 ng ml-1
No steroid toxicity
Steroid dependency/toxicity
Remission
Continue cyclosporine
Consider repeated renal biopsy every 2–3 years
Repeat protocol with corticosteroid
Levamisole may be considered where available
Cyclophosphamide (12 weeks)
Remission
Steroid dependency/toxicity
Cyclosporine (>12 months) once in remission
Steroid-dependent despite cyclosporine or cyclosporine-dependent and have toxicity
Levamisole may be considered where available
Remission
Continue cyclosporine and monitor, including renal biopsy every 2–3 years
Alternative therapy
Consider use of prednisone or cholorambucil or MPA

Figure 17.6 Algorithm for treatment of childhood minimal change disease (minimal change nephrotic syndrome). For definitions, see Figure 17.5. The patient or parents should be involved in the decision after the potential side effects of the second-line treatment are considered. In the rare patient who is a nonresponder to standard corticosteroid therapy and by definition corticosteroid resistant, a trial with cyclosporine may be considered.

Corticosteroid Response in Adults and Children with Minimal Change Disease
Urinary remission
Complete remission
Cumulative % of patients with urinary and complete remission
100
80
60
40
20
Pediatric patients receiving prednisone 60 mg/m2/day
Adult patients receiving 60 mg/day
0
10
20
30
40
50
60
90
294
Days of prednisone therapy

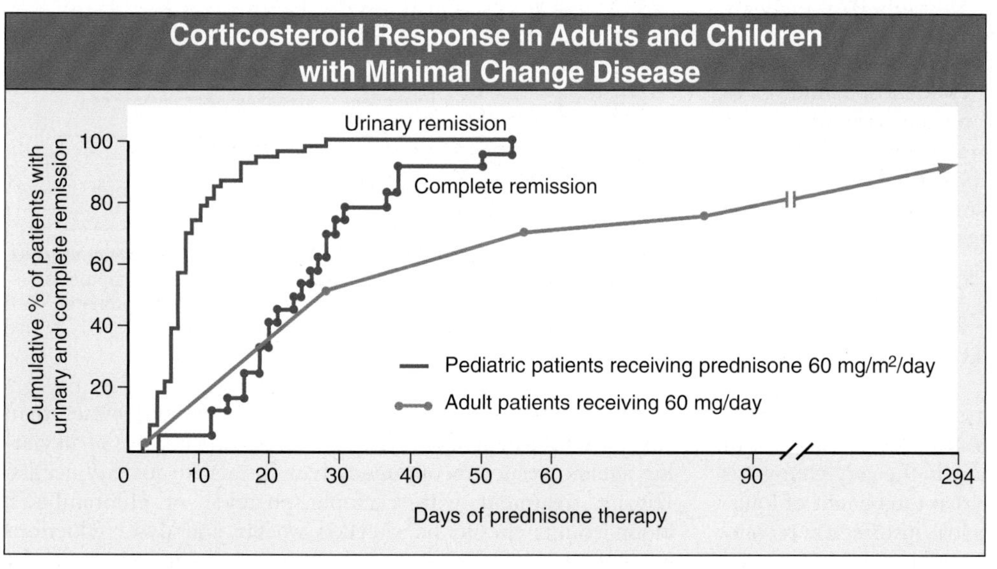

Figure 17.7 Corticosteroid response in adults and children with minimal change disease. Adults with the nephrotic syndrome and MCD take longer to respond than children do and are less likely to remit. The *orange line* shows the cumulative percentage of adults with complete remission (i.e., reduction of proteinuria ≤0.2 g/day and a serum albumin concentration >35 g/l). The *blue lines* show the cumulative percentage of pediatric patients with urinary remission and with complete remission. Urinary remission is defined by urine on dipstick negative or trace or proteinuria less than 4 mg/m²/day on at least 3 days; the definition of complete remission requires in addition to that a serum albumin concentration above 3.5 g/dl. *(Redrawn from data from references 25 and 26.)*

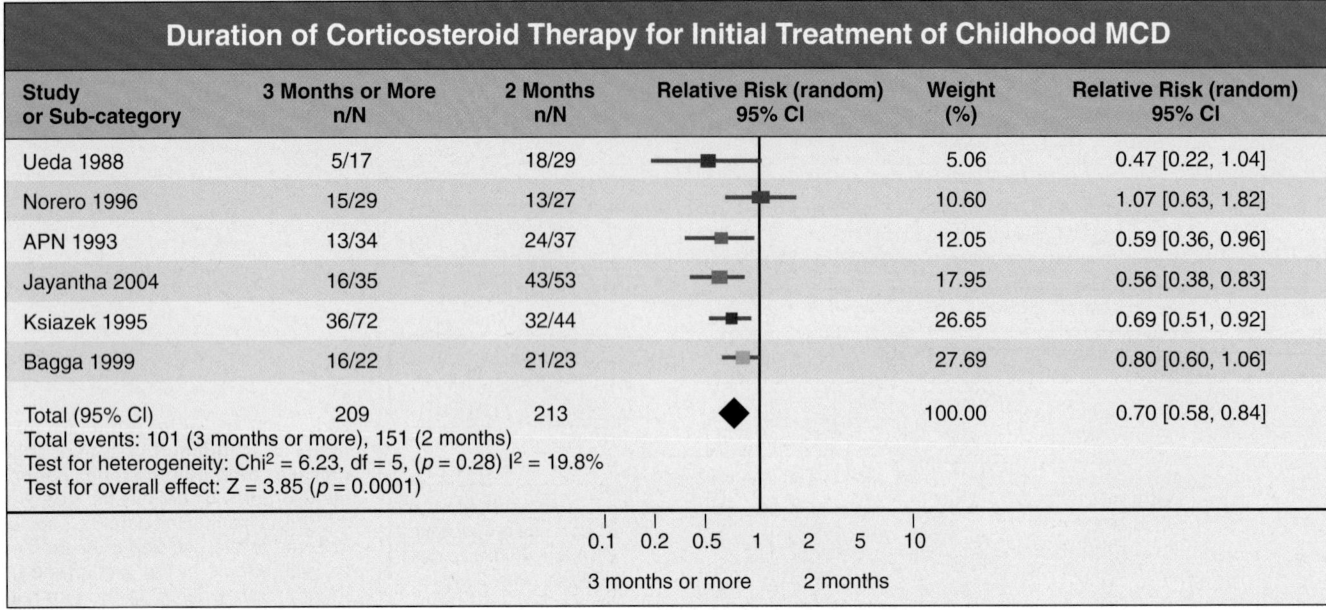

Duration of Corticosteroid Therapy for Initial Treatment of Childhood MCD

Study or Sub-category	3 Months or More n/N	2 Months n/N	Weight (%)	Relative Risk (random) 95% CI
Ueda 1988	5/17	18/29	5.06	0.47 [0.22, 1.04]
Norero 1996	15/29	13/27	10.60	1.07 [0.63, 1.82]
APN 1993	13/34	24/37	12.05	0.59 [0.36, 0.96]
Jayantha 2004	16/35	43/53	17.95	0.56 [0.38, 0.83]
Ksiazek 1995	36/72	32/44	26.65	0.69 [0.51, 0.92]
Bagga 1999	16/22	21/23	27.69	0.80 [0.60, 1.06]
Total (95% CI)	209	213	100.00	0.70 [0.58, 0.84]

Total events: 101 (3 months or more), 151 (2 months)
Test for heterogeneity: Chi² = 6.23, df = 5, (p = 0.28) I² = 19.8%
Test for overall effect: Z = 3.85 (p = 0.0001)

Figure 17.8 Duration of corticosteroid therapy for initial treatment of childhood minimal change disease. A Cochrane meta-analysis of studies supports a 12-week or longer course of corticosteroid therapy compared with 2 months in the first episode of corticosteroid-sensitive nephrotic syndrome to induce remission. The summary of studies suggests a 30% better remission rate in those subjects receiving 3 months or more of therapy. *(From reference 29.)*

Frequently Relapsing and Corticosteroid-Dependent Nephrotic Syndrome

For both frequently relapsing and corticosteroid-dependent nephrotic syndrome, second-line therapy is required. The second-line drugs most commonly used to avoid corticosteroid toxicity are alkylating agents (cyclophosphamide and chlorambucil), levamisole, and cyclosporine. The decision to use second-line therapy for chronically relapsing patients will depend on how quickly corticosteroid-induced remission occurs and how corticosteroids are tolerated. However, corticosteroid dependency is a clear indication for second-line treatment, which should be started before severe corticosteroid toxicity is apparent. The patient or parents usually are involved in the decision after the potential side effects of the second-line treatment are considered.

The alkylating agent cyclophosphamide is the recommended first choice of second-line therapy. Oral cyclophosphamide (2 to 2.5 mg/kg/day) is given for 12 weeks, on the basis of a study suggesting a lower 2-year remission rate compared with an 8-week course,[30] although these results have not been supported by all published data.[24] Cyclophosphamide can be associated with serious side effects (initially infection and alopecia and subsequently sterility,[31] hemorrhagic cystitis, bladder cancer, and hematologic malignant neoplasia). However, if therapy is limited to 12 weeks of treatment with 2 mg/kg/day or a total dose of 200 mg/kg body weight, the risks of these complications are low.

Although cyclophosphamide is often effective, it is less effective in children younger than 5.5 years in terms of duration of remission[32] (Fig. 17.9), so that this therapy in the very young has been questioned.[33] However, we believe that the benefit of long-term remission, even if the probability is low, justifies the recommendation to use this drug before the alternatives. Chlorambucil (0.2 mg/kg/day) for 2 months appears to be similar to cyclophosphamide in efficacy but has a greater frequency of adverse effects, including seizures, and therefore is not preferable.[34]

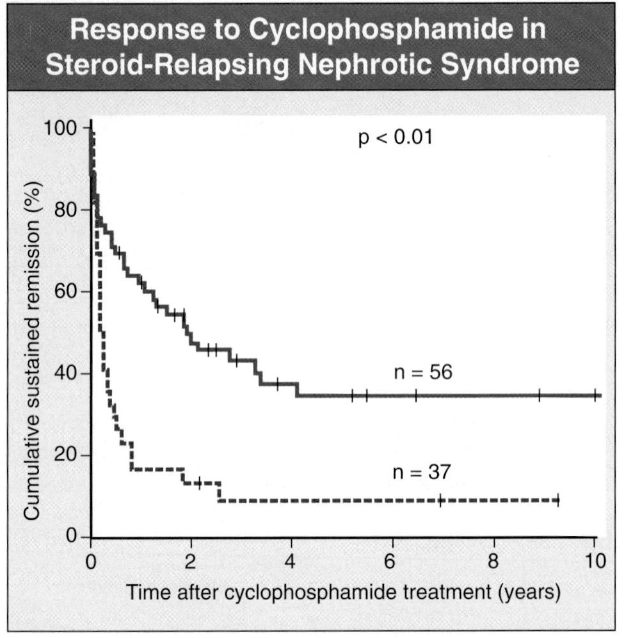

Figure 17.9 Response to cyclophosphamide in corticosteroid-relapsing nephrotic syndrome is dependent on age. Sustained remission is higher in children older than 5.5 years *(solid line)* compared with those younger *(dotted line)*. *(From reference 32.)*

In general, frequent relapsers tend to respond better than corticosteroid-dependent children do. Second courses of alkylating agents are not recommended as cumulative toxicity occurs. During treatment with cyclophosphamide or chlorambucil, blood counts should be checked weekly and dose reductions made if necessary. Primary varicella infection carries a particular risk for nonimmune children receiving immunosuppressive therapy, and these children should receive hyperimmune immunoglobulin and probably an anti-herpes agent such as valacyclovir if there is an unavoidable contact with active chickenpox or shingles infection.

An alternative medication to alkylating agents is cyclosporine. Cyclosporine (up to 150 mg/m^2 or 3 to 4 mg/kg/day with whole-blood trough levels of 50 to 150 ng/ml) is usually effective in children with both corticosteroid-dependent and frequently relapsing nephrotic syndrome.[32] However, relapse is almost invariable within 3 months of stopping treatment, and unfortunately, reintroduction of cyclosporine is often less effective once it has been interrupted. Therefore, cyclosporine is often used as long-term therapy.

If there is no response, increasing the dose of cyclosporine is sometimes effective, but there is a risk of cyclosporine nephrotoxicity even with low-dose regimens, and careful monitoring of blood levels, glomerular filtration rate (GFR), and blood pressure is required. The aim of therapy is to maintain remission without corticosteroids until the underlying disease remits. The optimal duration of cyclosporine therapy is not established, but early withdrawal is discouraged for children. Besides careful monitoring of renal function, kidney biopsies every 2 to 3 years are recommended to ensure safety of the therapy. Although cyclosporine-associated nephrotoxicity during long-term treatment has been reported, one study with careful follow-up suggested that whereas an initial drop in GFR was seen, no further deterioration occurred during the subsequent 5 to 10 years. More long-term studies are needed.

Cyclosporine is also an option in children with corticosteroid-resistant nephrotic syndrome, that is, those not responding to a standard corticosteroid treatment within 4 weeks (see Fig. 17.6).

Levamisole, an anthelmintic drug, has also been used successfully as a nontoxic alternative to corticosteroids (2.5 mg/kg on alternate days for 3 months),[35,36] but most patients relapse within 3 months of stopping the drug. It is used in the United States, Japan, and the United Kingdom, although it has been withdrawn from the rest of Europe. A clinical trial using levamisole in MCD is ongoing and may provide better insight if there is utility in this disease.

Azathioprine has no proven role in the management of children with MCD and was ineffective in a randomized trial.

Newer Agents

Patients with corticosteroid-sensitive nephrotic syndrome not responding to the established treatments are increasingly being tried on newer agents, including tacrolimus and mycophenolate mofetil (MMF). Tacrolimus is effective but does not have any advantages over cyclosporine. MMF is not nephrotoxic, and despite uncontrolled reports of benefit, a small randomized control trial suggested that the relapse under treatment might be inferior to cyclosporine, but more studies are needed before use of MMF can be recommended.

There have been recent case reports of a dramatic response of patients with childhood nephrotic syndrome to the anti-CD20 monoclonal antibody rituximab, which depletes B cells. The mechanism of the therapeutic effect is not known. In the largest reported multicenter series, 22 young patients (6 to 22 years) with severe corticosteroid- or cyclosporine-dependent nephrotic syndrome underwent remission after rituximab treatment, with one or more immunosuppressive drugs withdrawn in 85% of cases. Relapses occurred with reappearance of B cells. However, 45% reported adverse effects, including one death due to respiratory infection.[37] Careful indications and safety measures must be established before this therapy can be recommended.

Adult Minimal Change Disease

There are limited studies comparing different corticosteroid regimens in adults with MCD. As such, conventional treatment recommendations are extrapolated from successful approaches in children, although often with use of slightly lower doses of oral prednisolone (1 mg/kg/day, up to a maximum of 80 mg/day) (Fig. 17.10). There is no good evidence that alternate-day corticosteroids offer any clinical advantages over daily dosing.

Response is often delayed in comparison with children, and 25% fail to remit after 3 to 4 months (see Fig. 17.7).[14,25,38] The reasons for this are unclear. It has been suggested that many adults are often given a smaller dose of corticosteroids, or it may be that a greater proportion of adults have FSGS, missed on the original biopsy, which is more likely to be corticosteroid resistant.

The dose of prednisone should be reduced to a half-dose 1 week after remission (the absence of protein on urine dipstick testing) and continued for 4 to 6 more weeks, followed by tapering of the corticosteroids during an additional 4 to 6 weeks, aiming, as in children, for a total initial corticosteroid course of at least 3 months (although this principle is not evidence based).

Frequently Relapsing and Corticosteroid-Dependent Nephrotic Syndrome

Adults relapse less often than children (30% to 50%). Like children, some adults have transient non-nephrotic relapses. Treatment, initially a repeated course of corticosteroids, should await definitive evidence of relapse with more than 5 consecutive days of proteinuria (>2+ on urine dipstick testing) and a significant weight gain or the development of edema. Frequently relapsing and corticosteroid-dependent patients should be treated with a 12-week course of oral cyclophosphamide, which induces a permanent remission more often in adults than in children (75% and 66% at 2 and 5 years, respectively).[13] Although there are no satisfactory studies comparing 8- and 12-week courses in adults, the 12-week course is logical on the basis of the pediatric experience. If this treatment is selected, the opportunity for banking sperm or retrieval of eggs should be considered before treatment.

For patients who relapse after cyclophosphamide treatment, cyclosporine (4 to 6 mg/kg/day, aiming for trough whole-blood levels of 50 to 150 ng/ml for at least 12 months) is also effective, but relapse usually follows dose reduction or withdrawal. It is worth considering as a short- to medium-term management strategy because there is evidence that remission eventually occurs in 50% to 75% of patients even without treatment.[13] However, careful monitoring is required because nephrotoxicity is common after more than 1 year of treatment.[39] Some nephrologists prefer to try cyclosporine before cyclophosphamide, especially in younger adults. Tacrolimus appears to be similarly effective. Several uncontrolled reports suggest that MMF and rituximab may also have a place in management of corticosteroid- and cyclosporine-dependent patients,[40-42] but more data are needed before these could be widely recommended.

Minimal Change Disease with Non-nephrotic Proteinuria

In subjects with well-documented MCD who have the rare relapse in which the proteinuria is non-nephrotic, treatment does not require corticosteroids but rather can include

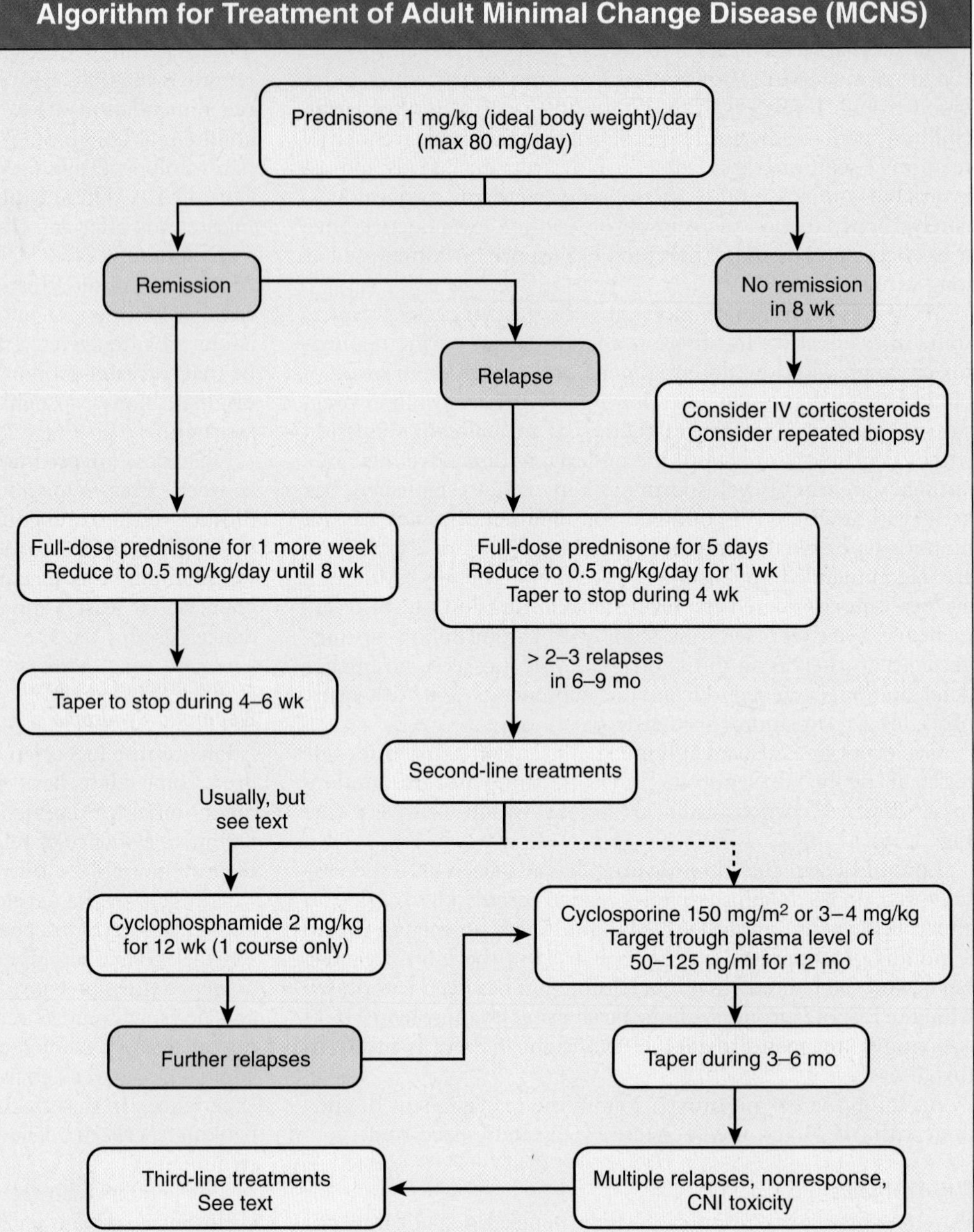

Figure 17.10 Algorithm for treatment of adult minimal change disease (minimal change nephrotic syndrome). CNI, calcineurin inhibitor.

angiotensin-converting enzyme (ACE) inhibitor or angiotensin receptor blocker (ARB) therapy. If there is any question as to diagnosis, repeated biopsy may be indicated because other conditions can mimic MCD (see differential diagnosis section).

Treatment of Secondary Minimal Change Disease

MCD secondary to NSAIDs requires discontinuation of the offending medication. Many subjects are treated with a course of corticosteroids for either MCD (higher dose) or for acute interstitial nephritis (see Chapter 60), but evidence that these treatments provide benefit is uncertain.

Secondary MCD from Hodgkin's disease usually responds to treatment of the lymphoma. Some subjects will also be treated with a regimen for MCD as an adjunctive treatment in addition to the chemotherapy directed at the tumor.

REFERENCES

1. Garin EH, Diaz LN, Mu W, et al. Urinary CD80 excretion increases in idiopathic minimal-change disease. *J Am Soc Nephrol.* 2009;20:260-266.
2. Regele HM, Fillipovic E, Langer B, et al. Glomerular expression of dystroglycans is reduced in minimal change nephrosis but not in focal segmental glomerulosclerosis. *J Am Soc Nephrol.* 2000;11:403-412.
3. Golden MH, Brooks SE, Ramdath DD, Taylor E. Effacement of glomerular foot processes in kwashiorkor. *Lancet.* 1990;336:1472-1474.
4. Cheung PK, Klok PA, Baller JF, Bakker WW. Induction of experimental proteinuria in vivo following infusion of human plasma hemopexin. *Kidney Int.* 2000;57:4512-4520.
5. Bakker WW, van Dael CM, Pierik LJ, et al. Altered activity of plasma hemopexin in patients with minimal change disease in relapse. *Pediatr Nephrol.* 2005;20:10410-10415.
6. Ali AA, Wilson E, Moorhead JF, et al. Minimal-change glomerular nephritis: Normal kidneys in an abnormal environment? *Transplantation.* 1994;58:849-852.

7. Lai KW, Wei CL, Tan LK, et al. Overexpression of interleukin-13 induces minimal-change-like nephropathy in rats. *J Am Soc Nephrol.* 2007;18:1476-1485.
8. Abeyagunawardena AS, Goldblatt D, Andrews N, Trompeter RS. Risk of relapse after meningococcal C conjugate vaccine in nephrotic syndrome. *Lancet.* 2003;362:449-450.
9. Sellier-Leclerc AL, Duval A, Riveron S, et al. A humanized mouse model of idiopathic nephrotic syndrome suggests a pathogenic role for immature cells. *J Am Soc Nephrol.* 2007;18:2732-2739.
10. Bhimma R, Coovadia HM, Adhikari M. Nephrotic syndrome in South African children: Changing perspectives over 20 years. *Pediatr Nephrol.* 1997;11:429-434.
11. Lewis MA, Baildom EM, Davies N, et al. Steroid-sensitive minimal change nephrotic syndrome. Long-term follow-up. *Contrib Nephrol.* 1988;67:226-228.
12. Barok M, Nathoo K, Gabriel R, Porter K. Clinicopathological features of Zimbabwean patients with sustained proteinuria. *Centr Afr Med* 1997,43:152-158.
13. Haas M, Meehan SM, Karrison TG, Spargo BH. Changing etiologies of unexplained adult nephrotic syndrome: A comparison of renal biopsy findings from 1976-1979 and 1995-1997. *Am J Kidney Dis.* 1997;30: 521-531.
14. Nolasco F, Cameron JS, Heywood EF, et al. Adult-onset minimal change nephrotic syndrome: A long term follow-up. *Kidney Int.* 1986;29:1215-1223.
15. Feinstein EI, Chesney RW, Zelikovic I. Peritonitis in childhood renal disease. *Am J Nephrol.* 1988;8:247-265.
16. Minimal change nephrotic syndrome in children: Deaths during the first 5 to 15 years' observation. Report of the International Study of Kidney Disease in Children. *Pediatrics.* 1984;73:497-501.
17. Overturf GD. American Academy of Pediatrics. Committee on Infectious Diseases. Technical report: Prevention of pneumococcal infections, including the use of pneumococcal conjugate and polysaccharide vaccines and antibiotic prophylaxis. *Pediatrics.* 2000;106:367-376.
18. Border WA. Distinguishing minimal change disease from mesangial disorders. *Kidney Int.* 1988;34:419-434.
19. The primary nephrotic syndrome in children: Identification of patients with minimal change nephrotic syndrome from initial response to prednisone. A report of the International Study of Kidney Disease in Children. *J Pediatr.* 1981;98:461-464.
20. Trompeter RS, Lloyd BW, Hicks J, et al. Long-term outcome for children with minimal change nephrotic syndrome. *Lancet.* 1985; 1:368-370.
21. Tarshish P, Tobin JN, Bernstein J, et al. Prognostic significance of the early course of minimal change nephrotic syndrome. Report of the International Study of Kidney Disease in Children. *J Am Soc Nephrol.* 1997;8:769-776.
22. Hoyer PF, Brodehl J. Initial treatment of idiopathic nephrotic syndrome in children: Prednisone versus prednisone plus cyclosporine A. A prospective, randomized trial. *J Am Soc Nephrol.* 2006;17:1151-1157.
23. Cattran DC, Alexopoulos E, Heering P, et al. Cyclosporin in idiopathic glomerular disease associated with the nephrotic syndrome: Workshop recommendations. *Kidney Int.* 2007;72:1429-1447.
24. Ueda N, Kuno K, Ito S. Eight and 12 week courses of cyclophosphamide in nephrotic syndrome. *Arch Dis Child.* 1990;65:1147-1150.
25. Nolasco F, Cameron JS, Heywood EF, et al. Adult-onset minimal change nephrotic syndrome: A long-term follow-up. *Kidney Int.* 1986;29:1215-1223.
26. Short versus standard prednisone therapy for initial treatment of idiopathic nephrotic syndrome in children. Arbeitsgemeinschaft für Pädiatrische Nephrologie. *Lancet.* 1988;1:380-383.
27. Ehrich JH, Brodehl J. Long versus standard prednisone therapy for initial treatment of idiopathic nephrotic syndrome in children. Arbeitsgemeinschaft für Pädiatrische Nephrologie. *Eur J Pediatr.* 1993;152:357-361.
28. Brodehl J. The treatment of minimal change nephrotic syndrome: Lessons learned from multicentre co-operative studies. *Eur J Pediatr.* 1991;150:380-387.
29. Hodson EM, Knight JF, Willis NS, Craig JC. Corticosteroid therapy for nephrotic syndrome in children. Cochrane Database Syst Rev. 2001;2:CD001533.
30. Cyclophosphamide treatment of steroid-dependent nephrotic syndrome: Comparison of eight week with 12 week course. Report of Arbeitsgemeinschaft für Padiatrische Nephrologie. *Arch Dis Child.* 1987;62:1102-1106.
31. Trompeter RS, Evans PR, Barratt TM. Gonadal function in boys with steroid-responsive nephrotic syndrome treated with cyclophosphamide for short periods. *Lancet.* 1981;1:1177-1179.
32. Durkan AM, Hodson EM, Willis NS, Craig JC. Immunosuppressive agents in childhood nephrotic syndrome: A meta-analysis of randomized controlled trials. *Kidney Int.* 2001;59:1919-1927.
33. Vester U, Kranz B, Zimmermann S, Hoyer PF. Cyclophosphamide in steroid-sensitive nephrotic syndrome: Outcome and outlook. *Pediatr Nephrol.* 2003;18:661-664.
34. Latta K, von Schnakenburg C, Ehrich JH. A meta-analysis of cytotoxic treatment for frequently relapsing nephrotic syndrome in children. *Pediatr Nephrol.* 2001;16:371-382.
35. British Association for Paediatric Nephrology. Levamisole for corticosteroid-dependent nephrotic syndrome in childhood. *Lancet.* 1991;337:1555-1557.
36. Al-Saran K, Mirza K, Al-Ghanam G, Abdelkarim M. Experience with levamisole in frequently relapsing, steroid-dependent nephrotic syndrome. *Pediatr Nephrol.* 2006;21:201-205.
37. Guigonis V, Dallocchio A, Baudouin V, et al. Rituximab treatment for severe steroid- or cyclosporine-dependent nephrotic syndrome: A multicentric series of 22 cases. *Pediatr Nephrol.* 2008;23:1269-1279.
38. Nakayama M, Katafuchi R, Yanase T, et al. Steroid responsiveness and frequency of relapse in adult-onset minimal change nephrotic syndrome. *Am J Kidney Dis.* 2002;39:503-512.
39. Melocoton TL, Vanni ES, Cohen AS, Fine RN. Long-term cyclosporin A treatment of steroid-resistant nephrotic and steroid-dependent nephrotic syndrome. *Am J Kidney Dis.* 1991;18:583-538.
40. Choi MJ, Eustace JA, Gimenez LF, et al. Mycophenolate mofetil treatment for primary glomerular diseases. *Kidney Int.* 2002;61:1098-1114.
41. Day CJ, Cockwell P, Lipkin GW, et al. Mycophenolate mofetil in the treatment of resistant idiopathic nephrotic syndrome. *Nephrol Dial Transplant.* 2002;17:2011-2113.
42. Bagga A, Hari P, Moudgil A, Jordan SC. Mycophenolate mofetil and prednisolone therapy in children with steroid-dependent nephrotic syndrome. *Am J Kidney Dis.* 2003;42:114-120.

CHAPTER 18

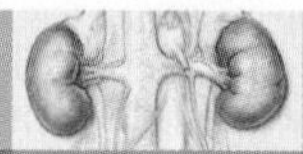

Primary and Secondary (Non-Genetic) Causes of Focal and Segmental Glomerulosclerosis

Gerald B. Appel, Vivette D. D'Agati

DEFINITION

Focal segmental glomerulosclerosis (FSGS), a histologic pattern of glomerular injury, defines a number of clinicopathologic syndromes that may be primary (idiopathic) or secondary to diverse etiologies (see also Chapter 19).[1-4] Early in the disease process, the pattern of glomerularsclerosis is focal, involving a minority of glomeruli, and segmental, involving a portion of the glomerular tuft.[4,5] Notably, alterations of podocyte cytoarchitecture identified by electron microscopy are relatively diffuse, underscoring the pathogenetic importance of podocyte injury. As the disease progresses, more diffuse and global glomerulosclerosis evolves. Although FSGS accounts for only a small percentage of cases of idiopathic nephrotic syndrome in children, it represents as many as 35% of cases in adults.[1] It is a major cause of progressive renal disease and end-stage renal disease (ESRD) in certain populations.[6]

Diverse pathogenetic mechanisms have been identified and often are manifested as particular histologic subtypes of disease. Through podocyte depletion or dysregulated proliferation, structural deterioration of the glomerular tuft leads to FSGS as a final common pathway.[5] Although primary (idiopathic) FSGS is potentially treatable and curable in many patients, the optimal type and duration of immunosuppressive therapy as well as adjunctive therapy remain controversial. For secondary FSGS, effective therapies exist to slow or to modify the disease course (see Chapter 76).

ETIOLOGY AND PATHOGENESIS

FSGS represents a common phenotypic expression of diverse clinicopathologic syndromes with distinct etiologies (Fig. 18.1). Causes are as varied as genetic mutations in podocyte proteins (see Chapter 19), circulating permeability factors, viral infections, drug toxicities, maladaptive responses to reduced number of functioning nephrons, and hemodynamic stress placed on an initially normal nephron population. In all these forms of FSGS, injury directed to or inherent within the podocyte is a central pathogenetic mediator.[2,7,8] These injuries promote altered cell signaling, reorganization of the actin cytoskeleton, and resulting foot process effacement. Critical levels of injury cause podocyte depletion through detachment or apoptosis. Stress placed on the remaining podocytes may lead to local propagation of damage (see also Chapter 75). Injury to podocytes may spread to adjacent podocytes by reduction in supportive factors (such as nephrin signaling) or increased toxic factors (such as angiotensin II [ang II] or mechanical strain on remnant podocytes).[9] Cell-to-cell spread of podocyte injury until the entire glomerular lobule is captured could explain the characteristic segmental nature of the sclerosing lesions.

Minimal Change Disease Versus Focal Segmental Glomerulosclerosis

By definition, the etiology of idiopathic or primary FSGS is unknown. Clinical data in some patients support etiologic factors similar to those operant in minimal change disease (MCD; see Chapter 17).[1] Some corticosteroid-responsive FSGS patients who exhibit MCD on initial biopsy subsequently relapse and display FSGS on repeated biopsy. In some, this may simply represent a sampling error in the initial biopsy. In others with well-documented repeated relapses of nephrotic syndrome and multiple biopsies over years, FSGS truly appears to have evolved from an initial MCD pattern. The relatedness of these two diseases is further supported by the observation that pathologic changes in the nonsclerotic glomeruli of idiopathic FSGS resemble glomeruli of MCD.[5] In addition, sequential biopsies of recurrent FSGS in the allograft have shown that it passes through an early stage that mimics MCD.[10] Thus, the spectrum of MCD and FSGS is often considered together under the rubric of podocytopathies. Recent studies suggest that FSGS and MCD may be distinguished based on the finding of elevated CD80 protein in the urine of corticosteroid sensitive MCD; further studies are necessary to confirm these findings.

As in MCD, in FSGS there is evidence that loss of the glomerular capillary wall charge barrier allows negatively charged albumin to leak into Bowman's space. The alterations in glomerular capillary wall permeability may occur in response to circulating humoral mechanisms that promote foot process effacement. Circulating permeability factors that enhance *in vitro* permeability of glomeruli to albumin have been found in the plasma of some FSGS patients.[11] The presence of such permeability factors has been used to predict the recurrence of FSGS in transplanted FSGS patients.[11] Some FSGS patients with recurrence of nephrotic syndrome after transplantation achieve remissions of nephrotic syndrome after plasma exchange or use of a protein A adsorption column, supporting the role of a circulating factor (see also Chapter 104).[12,13] A candidate protein for the permeability factor is cardiotrophin-like cytokine 1 (CLC1), a member of the IL-6 family of interleukins.[14] Receptors for this cytokine are present on podocytes and are upregulated in human recurrent FSGS.[14] The origin of the factor may be $CD34^+$ stem cells.[15] Induction of T regulatory cells attenuates the proteinuria in experimental FSGS, suggesting the capacity to block or to suppress the pathogenic cells.[16]

Etiologic Classification of Focal Segmental Glomerulosclerosis

Primary (Idiopathic) FSGS

Probably mediated by circulating/permeability factor(s)

Secondary FSGS

1. Familial/Genetic
   - Mutations in nephrin
   - Mutations in podocin
   - Mutations in α-actinin 4
   - Mutations in transient receptor potential cation 6 channel (TRPC6)
   - Mutations in WT1
   - Mutations in informin-2
   - Mutations in phospholipase C ε1
2. Virus Associated
   - HIV-1 ("HIV-associated nephropathy")
   - Parvovirus B19
   - SV40
   - CMV
3. Drug Induced
   - Heroin ("heroin-nephropathy")
   - Interferon
   - Lithium
   - Pamidronate
   - Sirolimus
4. Mediated by Adaptive Structural-Functional Responses (Postadaptive)
   - Reduced renal mass
     - Oligomeganephronia
     - Very low birth weight
     - Unilateral renal agenesis
     - Renal dysplasia
     - Reflux nephropathy
     - Sequela to cortical necrosis
     - Surgical renal ablation
     - Chronic allograft nephropathy
     - Any advanced renal disease with reduction in functioning nephrons
   - Initially normal renal mass
     - Hypertension
     - Atheroemboli or other acute vaso-occlusive processes
     - Obesity
     - Increased lean body mass
     - Anabolic steroids
     - Cyanotic congenital heart disease
     - Sickle cell anemia

Figure 18.1 Etiologic classification of focal segmental glomerulosclerosis (FSGS). WT, Wilms' tumor; HIV, human immunodeficiency virus; CMV, cytomegalovirus.

Whereas there are similarities between MCD and FSGS, the proteinuria in FSGS is often less selective, implying leakage of higher molecular weight macromolecules through "larger pores" in the glomerular basement membrane (GBM). In some toxin-induced animal models of FSGS, such as puromycin or doxorubicin (Adriamycin) nephrosis, nonselective proteinuria develops in conjunction with detachment of the visceral epithelial foot processes from the GBM. Rats injected with sera from patients with idiopathic collapsing FSGS developed proteinuria, glomerular tuft retraction, and podocyte damage, changes that were not seen in rats injected with sera from patients with other FSGS variants or normal controls.[17] The damage was lessened by removal of IgG from the FSGS sera.

Glomerular hypertrophy (or glomerulomegaly) may identify children with MCD at risk for development of FSGS. In early idiopathic FSGS and in many secondary forms of FSGS, such as obesity-related focal sclerosis, there is initially glomerular hypertrophy and a high glomerular filtration rate (GFR), supporting roles for hyperfiltration and increased intracapillary glomerular pressures as mediators of FSGS.[18] Similarly, in secondary forms of FSGS with reduced nephron numbers, maladaptive hemodynamic alterations may be associated with glomerular hyperfiltration and increased intraglomerular capillary pressures. Other factors, such as intraglomerular coagulation and abnormalities of lipid metabolism, may contribute to glomerulosclerosis in these patients (see Chapter 75).

Genetic Variants of Focal Segmental Glomerulosclerosis

Genetic and familial forms of FSGS are covered in detail in Chapter 19. Many cases of apparently primary FSGS may harbor unidentified mutations or polymorphisms in podocyte genes that go unrecognized because of lack of genetic testing and the absence of a heralding presentation with young-onset corticosteroid-resistant disease or familial inheritance. In primary FSGS, a genetic predisposition may underlie the susceptibility to a "second hit," whereby viral factors or other immune stimuli lead to the initiation of disease. Mutations in podocyte genes may also render a patient more susceptible to FSGS induced by such secondary causes as obesity, systemic hypertension, and infectious agents, allowing multifactorial podocyte stress. For example, mutations in myosin heavy chain 9 (*MYH9*) have been identified as a major risk factor for FSGS in patients of African ancestry.[19] Recent genetic mining of populations at risk for FSGS has identified APOL1 gene, rather than MYH9, as the major risk gene for FSGS and chronic hypertensive arterionephrosclerosis among patients of African descent.[19a] APOL1 encodes for apolipoprotein L-1. The gene is located along the same stretch of chromosome 22 and is in linkage disequilibrium with MYH9. G1 and G2 mutations in APOL1 are protective against infection by Trypanosoma brucei, the parasite spread in Africa by tsetse flies. Just as the gene for sickle cell disease conferred selective advantage against malaria, this appears to be an analogous situation where a genetic mutation became prevalent in a population because it was protective against an infectious pathogen, although it could predispose the host to other intrinsic disease. It remains unclear how sequence variations in APOL1 mechanistically cause glomerulosclerosis.

Viral Induction of Focal Segmental Glomerulosclerosis

Although a number of studies have noted a relationship between prior viral infection with parvovirus or other viruses and FSGS, in particular collapsing FSGS, the data have been far from consistent.[20] By contrast, the role of human immunodeficiency virus (HIV) infection in the pathogenesis is well established (see Chapter 56).

Drug-Induced Focal Segmental Glomerulosclerosis

A number of drugs and medications have been associated with the FSGS phenotype, including heroin, lithium, pamidronate, sirolimus, and interferon alpha, beta or gamma (see Fig. 18.1).[20a] The abuse of heroin has been associated with the nephrotic syndrome and an FSGS pattern on biopsy, although its incidence is decreasing in the modern era.[21] Pamidronate, a bisphosphonate used to prevent bone disease in myeloma and metastatic tumors, has been associated with both collapsing FSGS and MCD.[22] Stabilization of renal function and resolution of nephrotic syndrome may follow withdrawal of, for example, interferons, heroin or pamidronate. Longterm anabolic steroid abuse among bodybuilders has been associated with the development of FSGS. Many of these individuals also consume high protein diets and other potentially injurious supplements, including growth hormone. Mechanisms of glomerular injury include potential direct toxic effects of anabolic steroids on glomerular cells and adaptive responses to elevated lean body mass.[22a]

Structural Maladaptation Leading to Focal Segmental Glomerulosclerosis

Many secondary forms of FSGS are mediated by adaptive structural-functional responses.[1,7] These postadaptive forms include cases with congenital reduction in the number of functioning nephrons and acquired reduction of nephron numbers, whereas other secondary forms are associated with hemodynamic stress placed on an initially normal nephron population (see Fig. 18.1). Secondary FSGS resembling obesity-related glomerulopathy has been reported in nonobese, highly muscular patients with elevated body mass index due to bodybuilding.[23] Low birth weight associated with prematurity and reduced nephron endowment may also lead to secondary FSGS with glomerular hypertrophy in adolescence or adulthood.[24] Biopsy specimens with secondary postadaptive FSGS typically show glomerulomegaly and perihilar lesions of segmental sclerosis and hyalinosis. These conditions resemble experimental models of renal ablation in which the surgical reduction in renal mass causes functional hypertrophy of remnant nephrons with increased glomerular plasma flows and pressures. Whereas these changes are initially "adaptive," the resultant hyperfiltration and increased glomerular pressure become "maladaptive" and serve as mechanisms for progressive glomerular damage.[7,8]

Pathogenesis of Progressive Renal Failure in Focal Segmental Glomerulosclerosis

Although much attention has been focused on the pathogenetic basis for proteinuria in FSGS, it is clear that the segmental and eventual global glomerulosclerosis in association with interstitial fibrosis and tubular atrophy underlie the progression to renal failure. The etiology of glomerulosclerosis and its progressive nature are discussed in Chapter 75. Podocytes in some forms of FSGS, such as the collapsing variant, display a dysregulated phenotype with dedifferentiation, proliferation, and apoptosis.[25] Such biopsy samples have altered podocyte expression of cell cycle–related proteins.[26] In renal biopsy specimens of patients with FSGS, the expression levels of transforming growth factor (TGF) β1, thrombospondin 1, and TGF-β2 receptor proteins and mRNAs are all increased, as are podocyte markers of the phosphorylated Smad2/Smad3 signaling pathway.[27] Thus, pathways that promote podocyte depletion and overproduction of extracellular matrix converge to produce a sclerosing phenotype.

EPIDEMIOLOGY

Studies of patients who have had a kidney biopsy show an increasing prevalence of FSGS in both adults and children in a number of different countries on different continents.[28] In some countries, such as Brazil, FSGS is currently the most common primary renal disease.[29] An analysis of the prevalence of ESRD in the United States caused by FSGS during a 21-year period shows an increase from 0.2% in 1980 to 2.3% in 2000.[6] Although some of this change in prevalence may relate to changes in biopsy practice or disease classification, it is likely that there is a real increase in the frequency of FSGS.

Primary FSGS is slightly more common in males than in females, and the incidence in both children and adults is higher in blacks than in Caucasians.[1] In the United States, FSGS is the most common cause of idiopathic nephrotic syndrome in adult African Americans.[6] African Americans had a fourfold greater risk of ESRD from FSGS than Caucasians did. Nevertheless, even in an almost entirely Caucasian U.S. population, a clear major increase in the incidence of FSGS has been documented during a 20-year period in some but not all countries.[30,30a] The incidence of ESRD due to FSGS in males of all races is 1.5 to 2 times higher than in females. In the United States, idiopathic FSGS is the most common primary glomerular disease detected on renal biopsy that leads to ESRD in all races.[6]

CLINICAL MANIFESTATIONS

Most patients with idiopathic FSGS present with either asymptomatic proteinuria or full nephrotic syndrome.[1-3] In children, 10% to 30% of patients with asymptomatic proteinuria are most commonly detected on routine checkups and sports physical examinations; in adults, asymptomatic detection occurs at military induction examinations, obstetric checkups, and insurance or employment physical examinations. The incidence of nephrotic-range proteinuria at onset in children is 70% to 90%, whereas only 50% to 70% of adults with FSGS present with nephrotic syndrome. Edema is, by far, the most common manifestation of FSGS. Secondary forms of FSGS associated with hyperfiltration, such as remnant kidney and obesity-related glomerulopathy, typically have lower levels of proteinuria, and many such patients have subnephrotic proteinuria and a normal serum albumin concentration.[18,23]

Hypertension is found in 30% to 50% of children and adults with FSGS at the time of diagnosis. Microscopic hematuria is found in 25% to 75% of these patients, and a decreased GFR is noted at presentation in 20% to 30%.[1-3] Daily urinary protein excretion ranges from less than 1 to more than 30 g/day. Proteinuria is typically nonselective. Complement levels and other serologic test results are normal. Occasional patients will have glycosuria, aminoaciduria, phosphaturia, or a concentrating defect indicating functional tubular damage as well as glomerular injury.

When patients with the glomerular tip lesion were compared with cases of MCD and FSGS not otherwise specified (NOS), their clinical features were more similar to those of adults with MCD.[31] Those with tip lesion typically manifested abrupt clinical onset of full nephrotic syndrome (almost 90%), more severe proteinuria, and less chronic tubulointerstitial disease. These patients had a shorter time from onset of clinical disease to renal biopsy, suggesting that tip lesion is an earlier stage in the development of FSGS. The cellular variant also presents with greater proteinuria and incidence of nephrotic syndrome than FSGS NOS does. Patients with the collapsing variant of FSGS often present with greater proteinuria, more full-blown nephrotic syndrome, and lower GFR compared with those with FSGS NOS.[32,33]

DIAGNOSIS AND DIFFERENTIAL DIAGNOSIS

Before biopsy, patients with FSGS may be confused with any patient who has glomerular disease or nephrotic syndrome with negative serologic test results. In children with FSGS, the majority of whom present with nephrotic syndrome, the major differential will be between MCD and other variants of corticosteroid-resistant nephrotic syndrome. In adults with subnephrotic proteinuria, the differential includes almost all glomerular diseases without positive serologic test results. In adults with nephrotic syndrome, membranous nephropathy (MN) and MCD may present in an identical fashion, and only a renal biopsy will clarify the diagnosis. Focal sclerosing lesions due to other glomerulopathies (e.g., segmental scarring due to chronic glomerulonephritis [GN]) must be excluded. Moreover, because the defining glomerular lesion of FSGS is focal and may be confined to deeper juxtamedullary glomeruli early in the disease, it may not be sampled on renal biopsy. A large glomerular sample of more than 20 glomeruli for light microscopy increases the likelihood of identifying the diagnostic segmental lesions. Even after the diagnosis of FSGS is established, the primary (idiopathic) form must be distinguished from secondary forms by careful clinical-pathologic correlation (see Fig. 18.1). In general, many forms of postadaptive FSGS have lower levels of proteinuria than idiopathic FSGS does, a lower incidence of hypoalbuminemia, and, on biopsy, lesser degrees of foot process effacement. In patients younger than 25 years and in those with a family history of FSGS, genetic screening for mutations in podocin, nephrin, or other podocyte genes may be useful and should be performed more frequently now that these tests are becoming widely available.

PATHOLOGY

The pathologic manifestations of FSGS are heterogeneous, both qualitatively and with respect to the location of lesions within the glomerular tuft. A classification of FSGS by histologic variants has been proposed (Fig. 18.2).[34] This morphologic classification can be applied to both primary and secondary forms of FSGS listed in Figure 18.1. Subtypes include FSGS, classic or NOS; perihilar variant, in which more than 50% of glomeruli with segmental lesions display hyalinosis and sclerosis involving the vascular pole region; cellular variant, manifesting endocapillary hypercellularity; collapsing variant, in which at least one glomerulus has global collapse and overlying podocyte hyperplasia and hypertrophy; and tip variant, with segmental lesions involving the tubular pole. This working classification has been applied successfully to retrospective series of renal biopsies.

Morphologic Variants of Focal Segmental Glomerulosclerosis
1. FSGS, not otherwise specified (also known as classic FSGS)
2. FSGS, perihilar variant
3. FSGS, cellular variant
4. FSGS, collapsing variant (also known as collapsing glomerulopathy)
5. FSGS, tip variant

Figure 18.2 Morphologic variants of focal segmental glomerulosclerosis (FSGS).

Other more controversial histologic variants of FSGS include FSGS with diffuse mesangial hypercellularity and C1q nephropathy (see Chapter 27). Some believe that these are distinct disease entities with unique clinical-pathologic features; others believe that they are merely subgroups of FSGS.[35,36]

Classic Focal Segmental Glomerulosclerosis (Focal Segmental Glomerulosclerosis Not Otherwise Specified)

Classic FSGS, also called FSGS NOS, is the common generic form of FSGS. FSGS NOS requires exclusion of the other more specific subtypes described later. It is defined by accumulations of extracellular matrix that occlude glomerular capillaries, forming discrete segmental solidifications involving any portion of the tuft (Fig. 18.3).[34] There may be hyalinosis (plasmatic insudation of amorphous glassy material beneath the GBM), endocapillary foam cells, and wrinkling of the GBM (Fig. 18.4). Adhesions or synechiae to Bowman's capsule are common, and

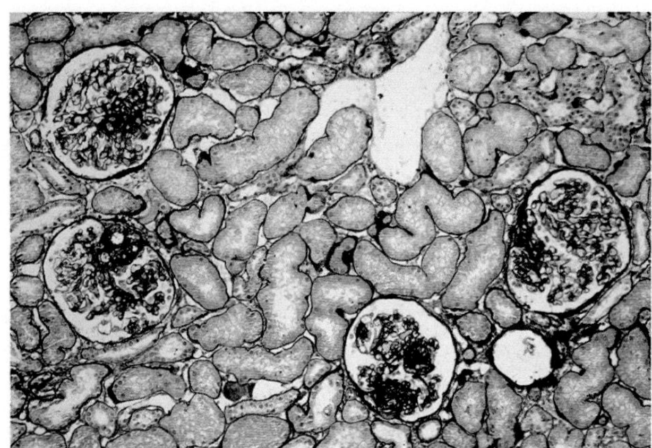

Figure 18.3 Focal segmental glomerulosclerosis, not otherwise specified (FSGS, NOS). A low-power view shows four glomeruli with discrete lesions of segmental sclerosis involving a portion of the tuft. The adjacent nonsclerotic capillaries are unremarkable. In this example, there is no evidence of tubulointerstitial injury. (Jones methenamine silver; magnification ×100.)

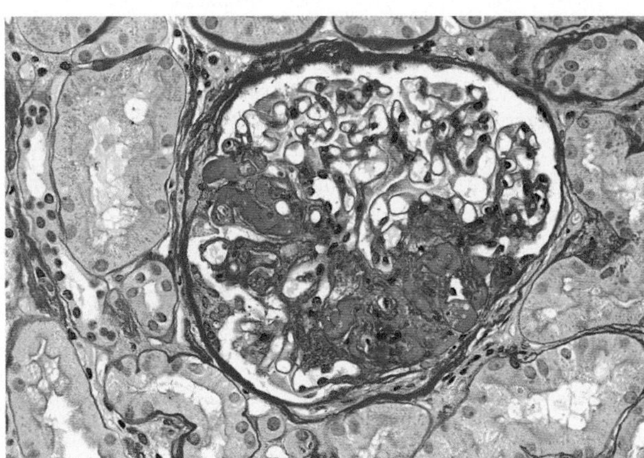

Figure 18.4 Focal segmental glomerulosclerosis, not otherwise specified (FSGS, NOS). The lesions of segmental sclerosis display increased extracellular matrix and hyalinosis. There is adhesion to Bowman's capsule without significant podocyte hypertrophy. The nonsclerotic capillaries have glomerular basement membranes of normal thickness and mild podocyte swelling. (Periodic acid–Schiff; magnification ×400.)

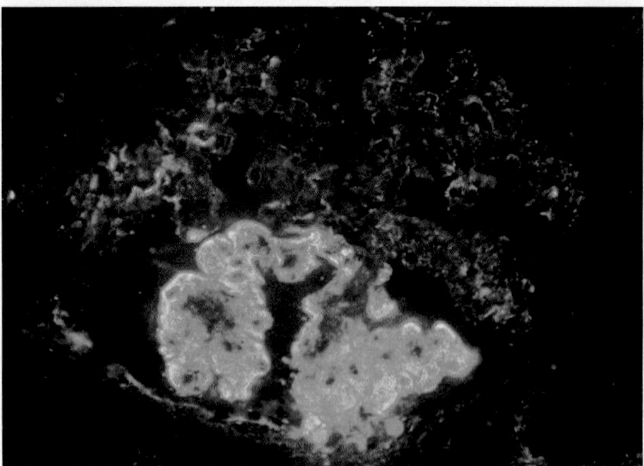

Figure 18.5 Focal segmental glomerulosclerosis, not otherwise specified. The lesions of segmental sclerosis contain deposits of IgM corresponding to areas of increased matrix and hyalinosis. Weaker staining for IgM is also seen in the adjacent mesangium. (Immunofluorescence micrograph; magnification ×400.)

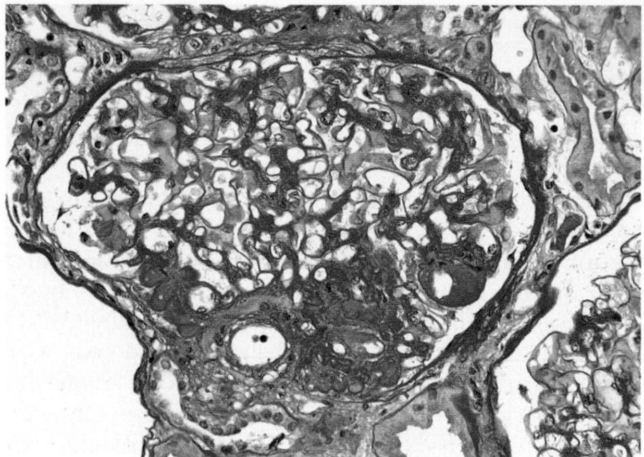

Figure 18.7 Focal segmental glomerulosclerosis, perihilar variant. A discrete lesion of segmental sclerosis and hyalinosis is located at the glomerular vascular pole (i.e., perihilar). The glomerulus is hypertrophied. The patient had secondary FSGS in the setting of solitary kidney due to contralateral renal agenesis. (Periodic acid–Schiff; magnification ×250.)

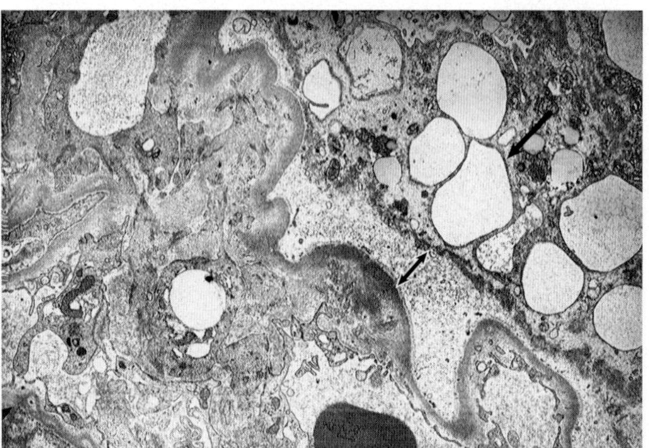

Figure 18.6 Focal segmental glomerulosclerosis, not otherwise specified. An electron micrograph illustrates the lesion of segmental sclerosis with obliteration of the glomerular capillaries by increased extracellular matrix with wrinkled and retracted glomerular basement membranes. The overlying podocytes are detached with complete effacement of foot processes *(double-headed arrow)* and numerous electron-lucent intracellular transport vesicles *(arrow)*. (Magnification ×2500.)

overlying visceral epithelial cells often appear swollen and form a cellular "cap" over the sclerosing segment. Glomerular lobules unaffected by segmental sclerosis appear normal by light microscopy except for mild podocyte swelling. Tubular atrophy and interstitial fibrosis are commensurate with the degree of glomerularsclerosis.

On immunofluorescence (IF), there is often focal and segmental granular deposition of IgM, C3, and more variably C1 in the distribution of the segmental glomerular sclerosis (Fig. 18.5). Nonsclerotic glomeruli may have weak mesangial staining for IgM and C3.

By electron microscopy (EM), segmental sclerotic lesions exhibit increased matrix, wrinkling and retraction of the GBM, accumulation of inframembranous hyaline, and resulting narrowing or occlusion of the glomerular capillary lumina (Fig. 18.6). No immune-type electron-dense deposits are found. Overlying the segmental sclerosis, there is usually complete effacement of foot processes and podocyte hypertrophy with focal microvillous transformation (the formation of slender cellular projections resembling villi along the surface of the podocytes). The adjacent nonsclerotic glomerular capillaries show only foot process effacement.

Perihilar Variant of Focal Segmental Glomerulosclerosis

The perihilar variant is defined as perihilar hyalinosis and sclerosis that involve more than 50% of glomeruli with segmental lesions.[34] This category requires that the cellular, tip, and collapsing variants be excluded. Podocyte hyperplasia is uncommon. IF reveals segmental deposits of IgM and C3 in areas of sclerosis and hyalinosis. There is variable foot process effacement. Although the perihilar variant may occur in primary FSGS, it is particularly common in secondary forms of FSGS mediated by adaptive structural-functional responses, in which it is typically accompanied by glomerular hypertrophy (Fig. 18.7). In this setting, the greater filtration pressures at the proximal end of the glomerular capillary bed may favor the development of lesions at the vascular pole.[7]

Cellular Variant of Focal Segmental Glomerulosclerosis

The cellular variant is characterized by focal and segmental endocapillary hypercellularity that may mimic a form of focal proliferative glomerulonephritis.[37] Glomerular capillaries are segmentally occluded by endocapillary hypercellularity, including foam cells, infiltrating leukocytes, karyorrhectic debris, and hyaline (Fig. 18.8). There is often hyperplasia of the visceral epithelial cells, which may appear swollen and crowded, sometimes forming pseudocrescents. This variant requires that tip lesions and collapsing lesions be excluded. IF microscopy again shows focal and segmental glomerular positivity for IgM and C3. EM reveals severe foot process effacement.

Collapsing Variant of Focal Segmental Glomerulosclerosis

The collapsing variant is defined by at least one glomerulus with segmental or global collapse and overlying hypertrophy and

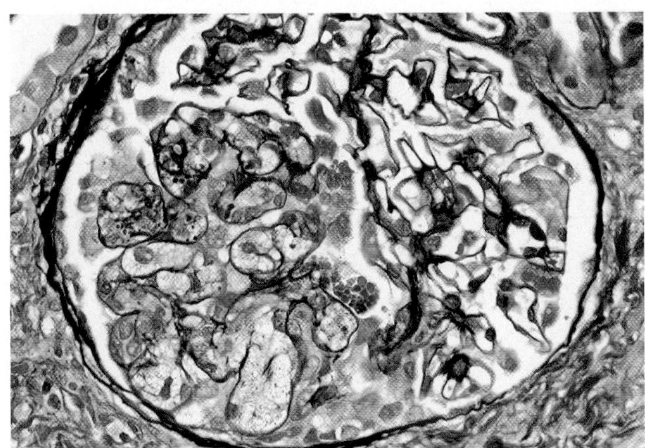

Figure 18.8 Focal segmental glomerulosclerosis (FSGS), cellular variant. The glomerular capillary lumina are segmentally occluded by endocapillary cells, including foam cells, infiltrating mononuclear leukocytes, and pyknotic debris. The findings mimic a proliferative glomerulonephritis because of the hypercellularity and absence of extracellular matrix material. There are hypertrophy and hyperplasia of the overlying podocytes, some of which contain protein resorption droplets. (Jones methenamine silver; magnification ×400.)

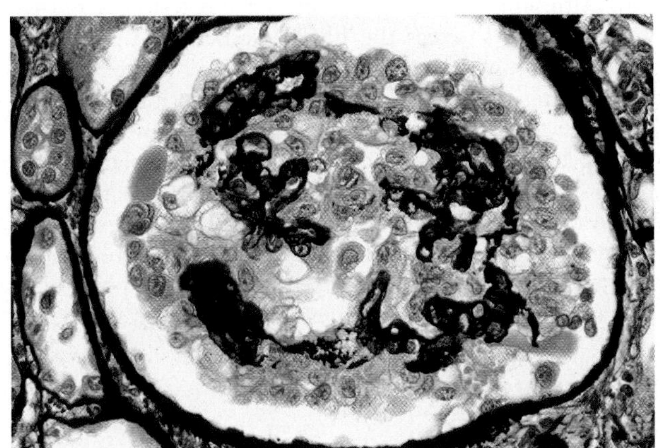

Figure 18.9 Focal segmental glomerulosclerosis (FSGS), collapsing variant. There is global implosive collapse of the glomerular tuft with obliteration of capillary lumina. The overlying podocytes appear hypertrophied and hyperplastic with enlarged nuclei and nucleoli. There are no adhesions to Bowman's capsule. (Jones methenamine silver; magnification ×400.)

hyperplasia of visceral epithelial cells (Fig. 18.9). In these areas, there is occlusion of glomerular capillary lumina by implosive wrinkling and collapse of the GBMs.[32,33] This lesion is more often global than segmental. Overlying podocytes display striking hypertrophy and hyperplasia and express proliferation markers. Podocytes often contain prominent intracytoplasmic protein resorption droplets and may fill Bowman's space, forming pseudocrescents (Figs. 18.10 and 18.11). Although podocyte hyperplasia is found in both the collapsing and cellular variants of FSGS, collapsing glomerulopathy is distinguished by the absence of endocapillary hypercellularity. In collapsing FSGS, there is prominent tubulointerstitial disease, including tubular atrophy, interstitial fibrosis, interstitial edema, and inflammation. A distinctive feature is the presence of dilated tubules forming microcysts that contain loose proteinaceous casts.

The collapsing lesions often have positivity for IgM and C3 by IF. On EM, there is typically severe foot process effacement affecting both collapsed and noncollapsed glomeruli (Fig. 18.12). Collapsing glomerulopathy may occur as a primary form of

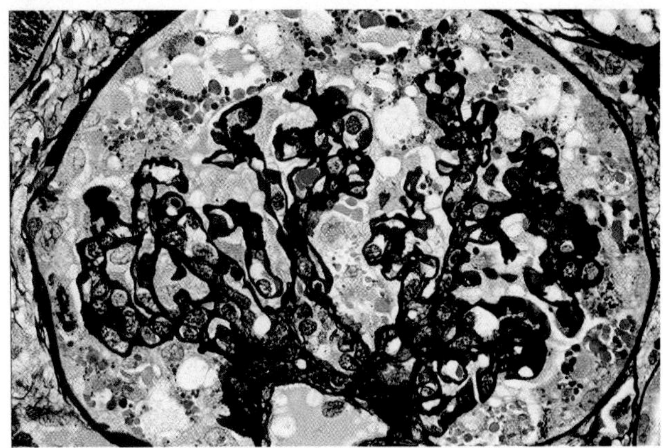

Figure 18.10 Focal segmental glomerulosclerosis (FSGS), collapsing variant. In this example, the exuberant proliferation of visceral epithelial cells forms a pseudocrescent that obliterates the urinary space. The pseudocrescent lacks the spindle cell morphology, ruptures of Bowman's capsule, or pericellular matrix typically seen in true inflammatory crescents of parietal epithelial origin. (Jones methenamine silver; magnification ×400.)

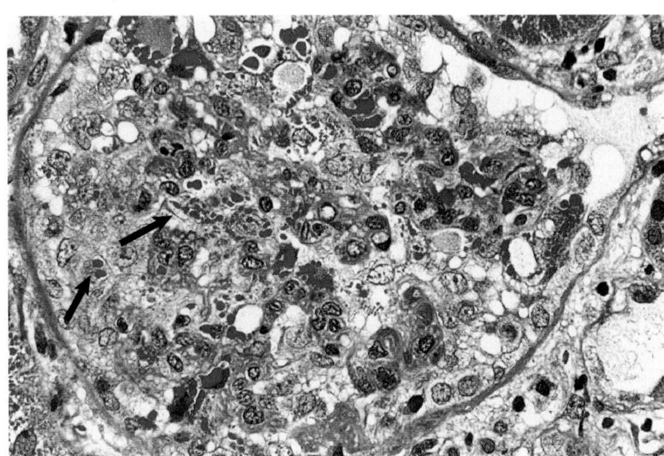

Figure 18.11 Focal segmental glomerulosclerosis (FSGS), collapsing variant. The crescent-like proliferation of glomerular epithelial cells contains numerous intracytoplasmic vacuoles and trichrome-red protein resorption droplets (arrows). (Masson trichrome; magnification ×400.)

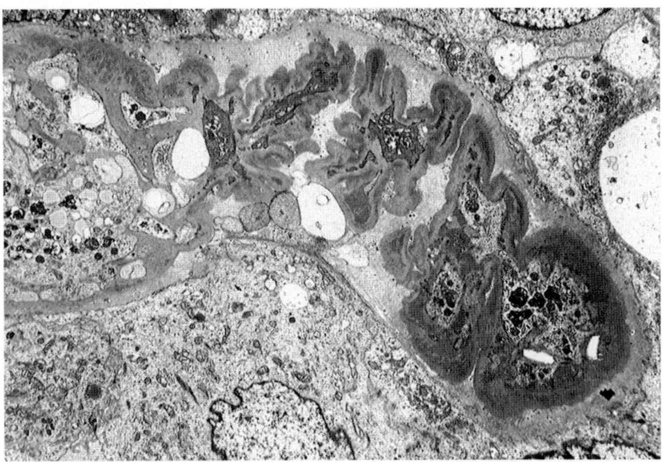

Figure 18.12 Focal segmental glomerulosclerosis, collapsing variant. On electron microscopy, there is tight collapse of the glomerular capillaries with corrugated glomerular basement membrane. The overlying podocytes appear detached and hypertrophied with complete loss of foot processes. (Magnification ×2500.)

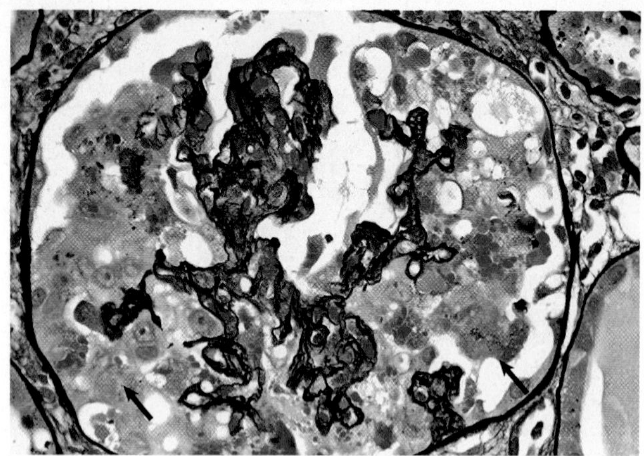

Figure 18.13 Focal segmental glomerulosclerosis (FSGS), collapsing variant, due to pamidronate toxicity. The glomerular tuft is retracted, without appreciable increase in matrix material. The overlying podocytes are enlarged and hyperplastic *(arrows)*, with numerous intracytoplasmic vacuoles and protein resorption droplets. (Jones methenamine silver; magnification ×400.)

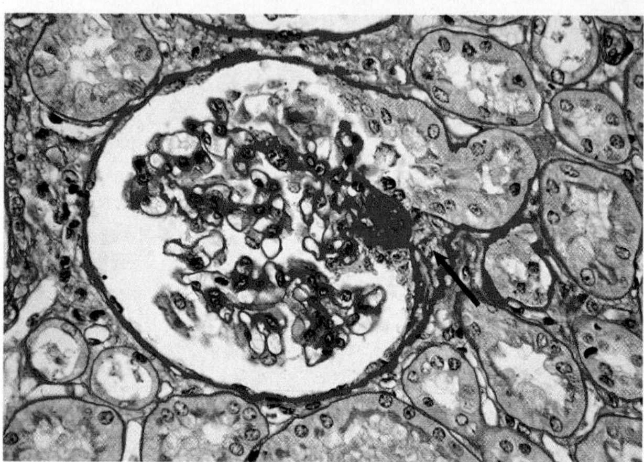

Figure 18.15 Focal segmental glomerulosclerosis (FSGS), tip lesion variant. A sclerosing tip lesion forms an adhesion to the tubular pole *(arrow)*. (Periodic acid–Schiff; magnification ×250.)

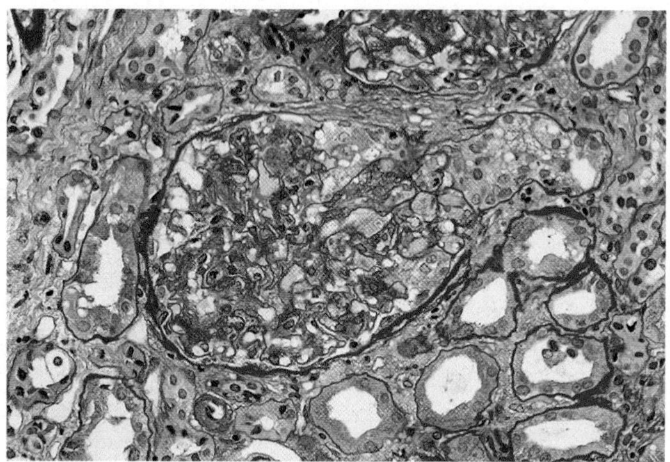

Figure 18.14 Focal segmental glomerulosclerosis (FSGS), tip lesion variant. A cellular tip lesion displays engorgement of glomerular capillaries by foam cells and adhesion of the involved segment to the origin of the proximal tubule (tubular pole). (Periodic acid–Schiff; magnification ×250.)

FSGS.[32,33] This pattern is also commonly observed in secondary FSGS due to HIV infection, parvovirus B19 infection, interferon therapy, and pamidronate toxicity (Fig. 18.13). The presence of endothelial tubuloreticular inclusions is helpful to identify collapsing glomerulopathy secondary to HIV-associated nephropathy or interferon therapy.

Tip Variant of Focal Segmental Glomerulosclerosis

This variant is defined by the presence of at least one segmental lesion involving the tip domain (i.e., the outer 25% of the tuft next to the origin of the proximal tubule).[31] There is either adhesion between the tuft and Bowman's capsule or confluence of swollen podocytes with parietal or tubular epithelial cells at the tubular lumen or neck. In some cases, the affected segment appears to herniate into the tubular lumen. The segmental lesions may be cellular or sclerosing in type (Figs. 18.14 and 18.15). Although initially peripheral, these lesions may evolve more centrally. Whereas the FSGS glomerular tip lesion may occur alone or with segmental lesions that are peripheral or indeterminate in location, the presence of perihilar sclerosis or collapsing sclerosis rules out the tip variant. In one study of FSGS tip lesions, biopsy specimens had glomerular tip lesions alone in 26% and glomerular tip lesions plus other peripheral FSGS lesions in the other 74%.[31] IF and EM findings are similar to those of other biopsies with FSGS. Most cases are idiopathic. Higher shear stress and tuft prolapse at the tubular pole are likely to play a role in the morphogenesis of this lesion.[7]

Other Variants of Focal Segmental Glomerulosclerosis

Two histologic variants often included within the FSGS spectrum are FSGS with diffuse mesangial hypercellularity and C1q nephropathy (see also Chapter 27).[5,35,36] FSGS with diffuse mesangial hypercellularity has lesions of FSGS on a background of generalized mesangial hypercellularity. By IF, there is diffuse mesangial positivity for IgM, with more variable mesangial staining for C3; by EM, there is extensive foot process effacement without glomerular electron-dense deposits. This variant occurs almost exclusively in young children.

C1q nephropathy is an idiopathic glomerulopathy defined by dominant or codominant IF staining for C1q, mesangial electron-dense deposits, and light microscopic findings resembling FSGS or MCD with variable mesangial hypercellularity. In one study, 17 patients had a light microscopic appearance of FSGS (including six collapsing and two cellular) and three of MCD.[35] In addition to C1q staining, biopsy specimens may show deposition of other immunoglobulins (particularly IgG) and complement components (C3), making exclusion of other clinical disease entities important (e.g., lupus nephritis, membranoproliferative glomerulonephritis [mPGN]). In C1q nephropathy, electron-dense deposits are typically located predominantly in the paramesangial region subjacent to the GBM reflection. There is variable foot process effacement. The largest series of C1q nephropathy supports that many cases represent a subgroup of primary FSGS or MCD, whereas others are an idiopathic immune complex–mediated glomerulonephritis.[36]

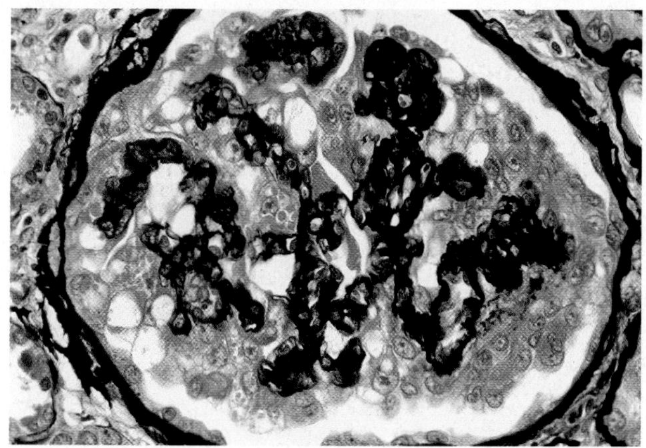

Figure 18.16 Human immunodeficiency virus–associated nephropathy. A globally collapsed glomerulus shows marked podocyte hypertrophy and hyperplasia. (Jones methenamine silver; magnification ×400.)

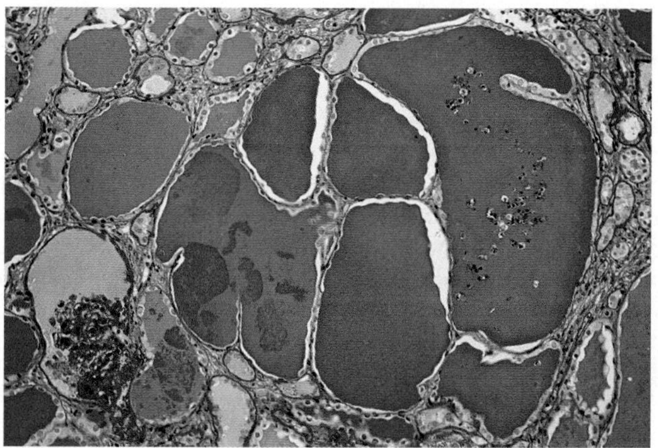

Figure 18.17 Human immunodeficiency virus–associated nephropathy. At low power, the renal parenchyma contains abundant tubular microcysts with proteinaceous casts. The glomerulus is collapsed with dilated urinary space. (Periodic acid–Schiff; magnification ×80.)

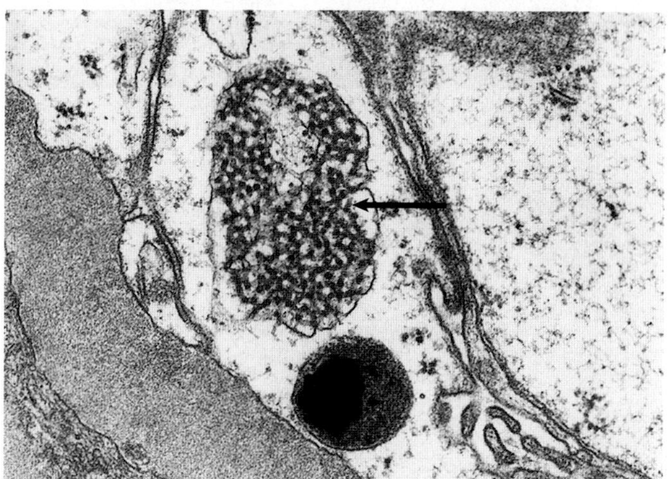

Figure 18.18 Human immunodeficiency virus–associated nephropathy. The glomerular endothelial cell pictured here contains a large intracytoplasmic tubuloreticular inclusion ("interferon footprint"; *arrow*) composed of interanastomosing tubular structures within a dilated cisterna of endoplasmic reticulum. (Electron micrograph; magnification ×15,000.)

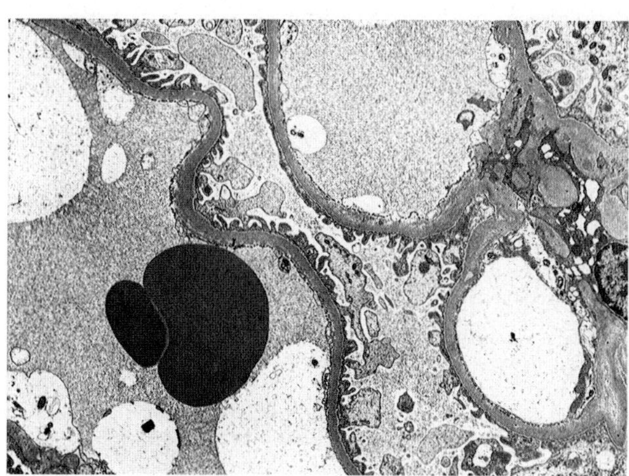

Figure 18.19 Secondary focal segmental glomerulosclerosis (FSGS) due to obesity. By light microscopy, this patient with morbid obesity had glomerular hypertrophy and predominantly perihilar lesions of segmental sclerosis and hyalinosis. The foot processes show mild effacement involving approximately 20% of the glomerular capillary surface area despite the presence of nephrotic-range proteinuria (electron micrograph). This mild degree of foot process effacement is less than that usually seen in primary FSGS. (Magnification ×2500.)

Distinguishing Pathologic Features of Secondary Focal Segmental Glomerulosclerosis

Although the pathology of some secondary forms of FSGS resembles closely that of primary FSGS, there are several noteworthy differences. Whereas the light microscopic findings in HIV-associated nephropathy are similar to those of idiopathic collapsing FSGS (Fig. 18.16), tubular microcysts are particularly common (Fig. 18.17).[38] By EM, a major difference is the abundance of tubuloreticular inclusions in the glomerular endothelial cells of HIV-associated nephropathy. These "interferon footprints" consist of 24-nm interanastomosing tubular structures located within dilated cisternae of endoplasmic reticulum (Fig. 18.18). Tubuloreticular inclusions have become less frequent in patients treated with highly active antiretroviral therapy.[38]

In secondary postadaptive forms of FSGS, renal biopsy typically shows glomerulomegaly and predominantly perihilar lesions of segmental sclerosis and hyalinosis. In secondary FSGS resulting from loss of renal mass (such as due to reflux nephropathy or hypertensive arterionephrosclerosis), FSGS is usually seen on a background of extensive global glomerulosclerosis, tubular atrophy, interstitial fibrosis, and arteriosclerosis. In secondary FSGS related to sickle cell disease, there is glomerular hypertrophy and sclerosis in association with capillary congestion by sickled erythrocytes and double contours of the GBM resembling those seen in chronic thrombotic microangiopathy. Importantly, in secondary postadaptive forms of FSGS, the degree of foot process effacement tends to be relatively mild, affecting less than 50% of the total glomerular capillary surface area, with correspondingly shorter foot process width (Fig. 18.19). In one study, a cutoff of more than 1500 nm for mean foot process width was able to distinguish primary from secondary (postadaptive) FSGS with high sensitivity and specificity.[39]

NATURAL HISTORY AND PROGNOSIS

The natural history of FSGS is varied.[1-3] Without therapy or response to therapy, the majority of patients with primary FSGS

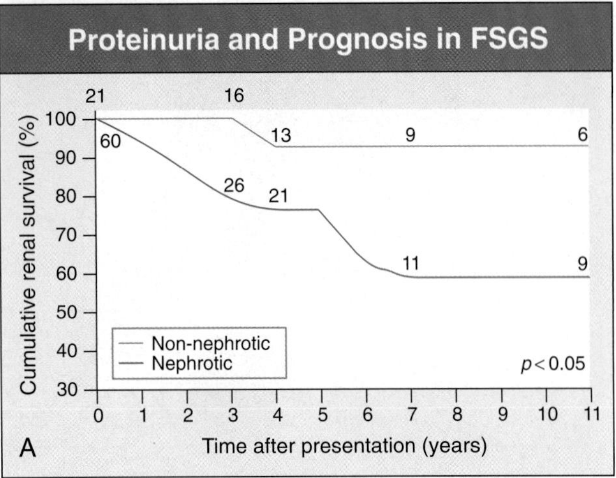

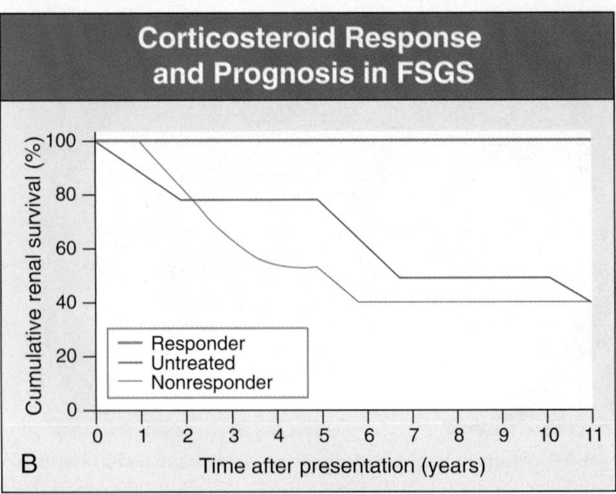

Figure 18.20 Prognosis in primary focal segmental glomerulosclerosis (FSGS). A, The risk for development of renal failure is related to the extent of proteinuria. Those with nephrotic-range proteinuria are much more likely to develop renal failure than are those with low-grade proteinuria. The figures indicate the number of at-risk patients at different time points. **B,** Corticosteroid-responsive patients are significantly less likely to develop renal failure than are nonresponders and untreated patients. *(Modified from reference 67.)*

Risk Factors for Progressive Renal Disease in Focal Segmental Glomerulosclerosis

Clinical features at time of biopsy
- Nephrotic-range proteinuria or massive proteinuria
- Elevated serum creatinine
- Black race

Histopathologic features at time of biopsy
- Collapsing variant
- Tubulointerstitial fibrosis

Clinical features during the course of FSGS
- Failure to achieve partial or complete remission

Figure 18.21 Risk factors for progressive renal disease in focal segmental glomerulosclerosis (FSGS).

will experience a progressive increase in proteinuria and progression to renal failure. Only 5% to 25% of patients undergo a spontaneous remission of proteinuria.[40] Both unresponsive children and adults have a similar course; most develop ESRD 5 to 20 years from presentation, with approximately 50% of such patients reaching ESRD by 10 years (Fig. 18.20).

Certain epidemiologic, clinical, and histologic findings at the time of diagnosis help predict the long-term course of FSGS patients (Fig. 18.21).[1-5] African Americans, even when controlled for degree of proteinuria, hypertension, and other features, experience a more rapid progression to renal failure. At biopsy, reduced GFR, greater degrees of proteinuria, and greater degrees of interstitial fibrosis predict a more progressive course.[1] The degree of glomerulosclerosis has been much less consistent as a prognostic finding.[1-5] Patients who experience a remission of proteinuria and the nephrotic syndrome have a far better renal survival than those who do not.[1,3,41,42] Even patients with a partial remission of nephrotic syndrome have a lower rate of long-term renal failure.[43]

There is a consensus that outcomes are best for tip variant and worst for collapsing variant of primary FSGS.[37,44,45] In a comparative series, the percentage of complete and partial remission was greatest for tip lesion (76%), lowest for collapsing variant (13%), and intermediate for cellular (44%), compared with 39% for FSGS NOS.[37] There was a strong inverse correlation between remission rates and progression to ESRD among these subgroups. Accordingly, the percentage ESRD was greatest for collapsing variant (65%), lowest for tip lesion (6%), and intermediate for cellular variant (28%), compared with 35% for FSGS NOS.[37]

TREATMENT

There is still considerable debate about the appropriate treatment of patients with FSGS[1-3,42] (Fig. 18.22). In part, this relates to confusion between primary and secondary forms of the disease, including unrecognized genetic variants. Even after biopsy, it is not always clear whether an obese person with glomerulomegaly and many segmentally sclerotic lesions has secondary or primary disease.[18] Moreover, the course of the disease is variable, and only recently have clear prognostic features been defined. Finally, although the disease is common in adults, there are many therapeutic options with few randomized, controlled trials on which to base judgment.

In early studies of FSGS, only 10% to 30% of those treated with corticosteroids for relatively short periods or other immunosuppressive agents experienced a remission of proteinuria, and the relapse rate was high.[1,42] Thus, many nephrologists considered FSGS to be a resistant disease and did not advocate immunosuppressive treatment. A classic study about 20 years ago documented that in Toronto, almost all children with FSGS were treated with immunosuppressives and that 44% experienced a remission.[41] Although the response rate for treated adults was similar (39%), most of the adults never received any immunosuppressive therapy.[41]

Use of Corticosteroids

In recent trials using longer (>6 months) courses of corticosteroids, the results have been much more promising. Therapy is usually with prednisone or prednisolone, 1 mg/kg/day or 1.5 to 2 mg/kg every other day for an initial period of 4 to 8 weeks, with subsequent tapering of the dose.[1,3,42] Initial response rates

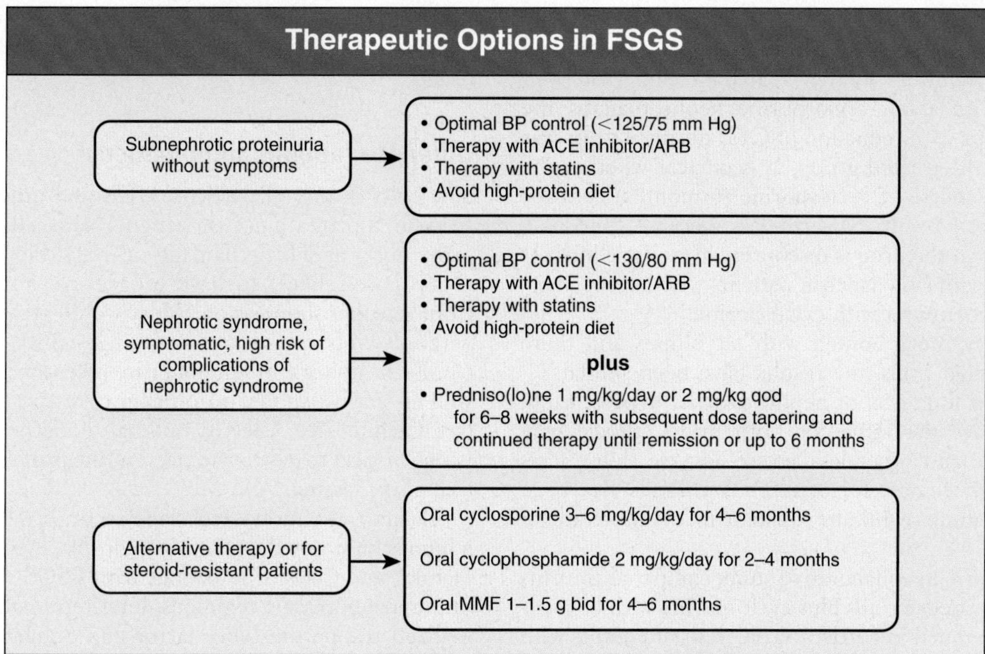

Figure 18.22 Therapeutic options in focal segmental glomerulosclerosis. For secondary FSGS treatment directed at the underlying cause (e.g., human immunodeficiency virus–associated nephropathy: treatment with highly active antiretroviral therapy; pamidronate nephrotoxicity: discontinue the medication; obesity-related glomerulopathy: weight loss). ACE, angiotensin-converting enzyme; ARB, angiotensin receptor blocker; BP, blood pressure; MMF, mycophenolate mofetil.

range from 40% to 80%. In children with biopsy-documented FSGS, 20% to 25% will have a complete remission with a short course of corticosteroids, but 50% will remit with more intensive therapy. In adults, although there are no large or randomized, controlled trials, more prolonged use of corticosteroids has led to much higher remission rates of nephrotic syndrome than in earlier studies.[1,3,42,46,47] The median duration of corticosteroid treatment for complete remission to be achieved is 3 to 4 months; most patients respond by 6 months. Most clinicians would treat all nephrotic FSGS patients and those at risk of progressive disease with a prolonged course (6 to 9 months) of daily or every-other-day corticosteroid therapy or other immunosuppressive medication in the hope of inducing a remission of nephrotic syndrome and preventing eventual ESRD. The corticosteroid dose should be tapered after 6 to 8 weeks to avoid cushingoid side effects.

Other Immunosuppressive Agents

For many years, either chlorambucil or cyclophosphamide combined with corticosteroids was the treatment of choice for children and for adults with corticosteroid-resistant FSGS.[1,48] One uncontrolled trial in children using combined intravenous pulse corticosteroids and long-term immunosuppression with corticosteroids and cytotoxics found a 60% complete remission rate and a 16% partial remission rate of the nephrotic syndrome and a low rate of progression to renal failure.[49] In adults with FSGS treated with either oral cyclophosphamide or chlorambucil, pooled data show a high response rate for patients with corticosteroid dependence or intolerance but a remission rate of only less than 20% for those who are corticosteroid resistant.[42]

A number of studies have used low-dose cyclosporine (3 to 6 mg/kg/day for 2 to 6 months) to treat corticosteroid-resistant FSGS (Fig. 18.23).[50,51] Complete plus partial remission rates of

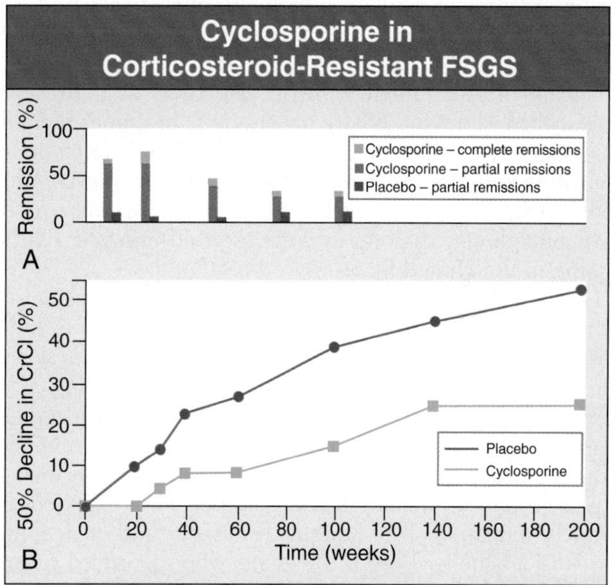

Figure 18.23 Cyclosporine in corticosteroid-resistant focal segmental glomerulosclerosis (FSGS). A randomized, controlled trial of 6 months of treatment with prednisolone and either cyclosporine or placebo. **A,** Cyclosporine induces a partial or complete remission significantly more often than placebo does. **B,** Cyclosporine treatment results in a lower rate of decline in renal function than with placebo even after 4 years. CrCl, creatinine clearance. *(Modified from reference 51.)*

60% to 70% have been achieved versus only 17% to 33% in the placebo groups. Adult North American FSGS patients randomized to either cyclosporine with low-dose corticosteroids or the same low dose of corticosteroids alone for a 6-month period exhibited a much higher remission rate (12% complete and >70% complete or partial) in the group treated with cyclosporine.[51] Despite relapses after the cyclosporine was discontinued, at the end of long-term follow-up, there were still significantly more remitters in the treated group. Moreover, despite initial worries about cyclosporine nephrotoxicity, the percentage of patients with reduction of GFR during 4 years was significantly less in the treated group. It is unclear whether the low dose and short course of cyclosporine (6 months) contributed to this beneficial result. Nevertheless, because there is a high relapse rate when the drug is discontinued, many clinicians use a 1-year course with slow taper in patients who have a favorable reduction of proteinuria with cyclosporine.[1,42]

Although data are more limited with tacrolimus and there are no large controlled trials, the results have been similar.[52,53] Because the major side effects of nephrotoxicity, hypertension, and hyperkalemia are the same for both drugs, choice may depend on cosmetic and other less severe adverse side effects (e.g., gum swelling, tremor, hirsutism). Tacrolimus has been effective in some patients who are resistant to or intolerant of cyclosporine.

A multicenter German collaborative study compared the efficacy and safety of corticosteroids plus cyclosporine with corticosteroids plus chlorambucil in corticosteroid-resistant adults with FSGS and nephrotic syndrome.[54] Total and partial remission rates were similar (about 20% full and 40% to 50% partial remission), and the addition of chlorambucil to the regimen did not improve outcome. Whether cyclosporine is equivalent or superior to corticosteroids as first-line therapy for FSGS has never been documented. However, some clinicians use cyclosporine as first-line therapy in patients at high risk of corticosteroid complications, such as those with concurrent diabetes or morbid obesity.

Mycophenolate mofetil (MMF) has been used in several uncontrolled series of FSGS patients.[55,56] In some, including those resistant to other therapies, there have been remissions of nephrotic syndrome and major reductions in proteinuria. A multicenter trial comparing cyclosporine and a regimen of oral MMF plus dexamethasone in corticosteroid-resistant FSGS is ongoing in the United States.

The use of sirolimus has been controversial since the drug was reported to induce proteinuria and FSGS lesions in kidney transplant patients. Sirolimus has been used in several small series of patients with glomerular disease including FSGS patients.[57,58] In one series, it was associated with worsening of renal function, episodes of acute renal failure, and no remissions of the nephrotic syndrome.[57] In another series, which included 21 corticosteroid-resistant FSGS patients, 19% experienced a complete remission, 38% a partial remission, and, hence, more than 50% a beneficial result.[58] Patients who responded to treatment had a shorter duration of FSGS than did resistant patients. Given the controversy about efficacy and toxicity, sirolimus should be considered experimental therapy until more data are available.

Rituximab has been used in small numbers of FSGS patients with anecdotal success. Most regimens have included other concomitant immunosuppressive therapies. A study found only three of eight corticosteroid-resistant adult patients with FSGS to benefit from such therapy.[59]

Plasma exchange, which is successful in treating some patients with recurrent FSGS in the renal allograft (see Chapter 104), has not proved useful in patients with disease in their native kidneys.[13] A study of low-density lipoprotein apheresis and prednisone in corticosteroid- and cyclosporine-resistant children with primary FSGS achieved a remission in 7 of 11 patients.[60] Unfortunately, the role of the individual components of treatment and the mechanisms of action are difficult to define in such uncontrolled trials.

Other Therapeutic Interventions

The role, if any, of corticosteroids and other immunosuppressives in the treatment of patients with subnephrotic levels of proteinuria and little damage on renal biopsy is unclear. This group is less likely to have progressive disease and to benefit from immunosuppression. Most would treat all FSGS patients without contraindications with angiotensin-converting enzyme (ACE) inhibitors or angiotensin receptor blockers (ARBs) as well as statins, similar to other progressive glomerular diseases (see Chapter 76). Clearly, optimal blood pressure control itself is also critical to slow or to prevent the progression of the disease (see also Chapter 76).

Galactose, a monosaccharide sugar, has been shown to have a high affinity for the cardiotrophin-like cytokine 1 permeability factor.[61] In at least one patient with FSGS resistant to multiple immunosuppressive regimens, long-term galactose therapy normalized the permeability factor and dramatically reduced proteinuria.[62] Recent data confirm that glomerular permeability can be improved in most FSGS patients with galactose, although the effects on proteinuria remain to be proved.

Another area of active research is the use of agents to prevent renal fibrosis in patients with FSGS. Pirfenidone, an oral TGF-β inhibitor, was used in 21 patients with FSGS and a declining GFR.[63] The drug slowed the loss of kidney function over time without altering either blood pressure or proteinuria. A study using an antibody to TGF-β is ongoing in FSGS patients.

For patients with secondary forms of FSGS, attempts to treat the primary cause of the FSGS should be the initial step in management. Patients with FSGS secondary to obesity and heroin nephropathy have had remissions of proteinuria after weight reduction or cessation of heroin use, respectively. In patients with HIV-associated nephropathy, therapy with highly active antiretroviral drugs and blockers of the renin-angiotensin system (RAS) has proved useful (see Chapter 56). The role of immunosuppressives has not yet been documented in controlled, randomized trials in any form of secondary FSGS. In all forms of secondary FSGS, supportive therapy as outlined in Chapter 76 is essential to prevent progressive renal disease in this population. In those patients with either primary idiopathic or secondary forms of FSGS who remain nephrotic, control of fluid retention and edema can be managed with salt restriction and diuretics (see Chapter 15).

TRANSPLANTATION

Idiopathic FSGS may recur in the transplanted kidney, in which it presents with severe proteinuria and nephrotic syndrome (see Chapter 104).[64] Children with FSGS and patients who manifest with more severe proteinuria and a more rapid course to renal failure in their native kidneys are at greater risk of recurrence in the allograft. Those who have lost a prior allograft because of recurrent FSGS are at highest risk of recurrence. Recurrence in the allograft may be seen immediately after transplantation, supporting the existence of a circulating factor, or years later. Interestingly, the histologic variant of recurrent FSGS was the same as that documented in the native kidney in 81% of cases, validating the fidelity of the histologic subclassification.[10] Plasma exchange has been used successfully to induce remissions of the proteinuria associated with recurrence, but the results are more favorable in children than in adults. Rituximab has been used in some patients for recurrent FSGS with varied outcomes.

Analysis of the outcomes of renal transplantation in children with FSGS shows a profound effect of race.[65] Among African American children with FSGS, allograft survival was not different from that of non-FSGS patients. Among non–African American children with FSGS, the risk of allograft failure was 1.3 times higher than for other causes of ESRD. Nevertheless, for non–African American children, a transplant from a living related donor gave a better allograft survival than that from a cadaveric donor. An analysis of all FSGS transplants in the United States Renal Data System (USRDS) database showed no risk of graft loss for zero-mismatched transplants in FSGS patients.[66] However, this analysis may have included patients with secondary forms of FSGS that would be unlikely to recur, thereby underestimating the overall risk of recurrence. Whereas most patients with genetic forms of FSGS have not experienced a recurrence in the allograft, this is not universally true, especially in those with compound heterozygous mutations.

REFERENCES

1. Aggarwal N, Appel GB. Focal segmental glomerulosclerosis. In: Greenberg A, ed. *Primer on Kidney Diseases*. 5th ed. Philadelphia: WB Saunders; 2009:165-170.
2. Meyrier A. Mechanisms of disease: focal segmental glomerulosclerosis. *Nat Clin Pract Nephrol.* 2005;1:44-54.
3. Chun MJ, Korbet SM, Schwartz MM, Lewis EJ. FSGS in nephrotic adults: Presentation, prognosis, and response to therapy of the histologic variants. *J Am Soc Nephrol.* 2004;15:2169-2177.
4. D'Agati V. Pathologic classification of focal segmental glomerulosclerosis. *Semin Nephrol.* 2003;23:117-135.
5. D'Agati VD. Focal segmental glomerulosclerosis. In: D'Agati V, Jennette JC, Silva FS, eds. *Atlas of Nontumor Pathology: Nonneoplastic Kidney Diseases*. Silver Spring, Md: American Registry of Pathology Press; 2005:125-159.
6. Kitiyakara C, Eggers P, Kopp JB. Twenty-one year trends in ESRD due to FSGS in the United States. *Am J Kidney Dis.* 2004;44:815-825.
7. D'Agati VD. The spectrum of focal segmental glomerulosclerosis: New insights. *Curr Opin Nephrol Hypertens.* 2008;17:271-281.
8. D'Agati VD. Podocyte injury in focal segmental glomerulosclerosis. Lessons from animal models. *Kidney Int.* 2008;73:399-406.
9. Ichikawa I, Ma J, Motojima M, Matsusaka T. Podocyte damage damages podocytes: Autonomous vicious cycle that drives local spread of glomerular sclerosis. *Curr Opin Nephrol Hypertens.* 2005;14:205-210.
10. Ijpelaar DH, Farris AB, Goemaere N, et al. Fidelity and evolution of recurrent focal segmental glomerulosclerosis in renal allografts. *J Am Soc Nephrol.* 2008;19:2219-2224.
11. Savin VJ, McCarthy ET, Sharma M. Permeability factors in FSGS. *Semin Nephrol.* 2003;23:147-161.
12. Dantal J, Bigot E, Bogers W, et al. Effect of plasma protein absorption on protein excretion in kidney-transplant recipients with recurrent nephrotic syndrome. *N Engl J Med.* 1994;330:7-11.
13. Matalon A, Markowitz GS, Joseph RE, et al. Plasmapheresis treatment of recurrent FSGS in adult transplant recipients. *Clin Nephrol.* 2001;56:271-278.
14 Savin VJ, Sharma M, McCarthy ET, et al. Cardiotrophin like cytokine-1: Candidate for the focal glomerular sclerosis permeability factor. *J Am Soc Nephrol.* 2008;19:59A.
15. Sellier-Leclerc AL, Duval A, Riveron S, et al. A humanized mouse model of idiopathic nephrotic syndrome suggests a pathogenic role for immature cells. *J Am Soc Nephrol.* 2007;18:2732-2739.
16. Le Berre L, Bruneau S, Naulet J, et al. Induction of T regulatory cells attenuates idiopathic nephrotic syndrome. *J Am Soc Nephrol.* 2009;20:57-67.
17. Del Carmen Avila-Casado M, Perez-Torres I, Auron A, et al. Proteinuria in rats induced by serum from patients with collapsing glomerulopathy. *Kidney Int.* 2004;66:133-143.
18. Kambham N, Markowitz GS, Valeri AM, et al. Obesity related glomerulomegaly: An emerging epidemic. *Kidney Int.* 2001;59:1498-1509.
19 Kopp JB, Smith MW, Nelson GW, et al. MYH9 is a major-effect risk gene for focal segmental glomerulosclerosis. *Nat Genet.* 2008;40:1175-1184.
19a. Genovese G, Friedman DJ, Ross MD, et al. Association of Trypanolytic ApoL1 Variants with Kidney Disease in African Americans. *Science* (in press, 2010).
20. Moudgil A, Nast CC, Bagga A, et al. Association of parvovirus B19 infection with idiopathic collapsing glomerulopathy. *Kidney Int.* 2001;59:2126-2133.
20a. Markowitz GS, Nasr SH, Stokes MB, D'Agati VD: Treatment with IFN-alpha, -beta, or -gamma is associated with collapsing focal segmental glomerulosclerosis. *Clin J Am Soc Nephrol.* 2010;5:607-615.
21. Kunis CL, Aggarwal N, Appel GB. Illicit drug abuse and renal disease. In: De Broe ME, Porter GA, eds. *Clinical Nephrotoxins*. 3rd ed. New York: Springer; 2008:595-617.
22. Markowitz G, Appel GB, Fine P, et al. Collapsing focal segmental glomerulosclerosis following treatment with high dose pamidronate. *J Am Soc Nephrol.* 2001;12:1164-1172.
22a. Herlitz LC, Markowitz GS, Farris AB, et al. Development of focal segmental glomerulosclerosis after anabolic steroid abuse. *J Am Soc Nephrol.* 2010;21:163-172.
23. Schwimmer JA, Markowitz GS, Valeri A, et al. Secondary FSGS in non-obese patients with increased muscle mass. *Clin Nephrol.* 2003;60:233-241.
24. Hodgin JB, Rasoulpour M, Markowitz GS, D'Agati VD. Very low birth weight is a risk factor for secondary focal segmental glomerulosclerosis. *Clin J Am Soc Nephrol.* 2009;4:71-76.
25. Barisoni L, Kriz W, Mundel P, D'Agati V. The dysregulated podocyte phenotype: A novel concept in the pathogenesis of collapsing idiopathic FSGS and HIV associated nephropathy. *J Am Soc Nephrol.* 1999;10:51-61.
26. Shankland SJ, Eitner F, Hudkins KL, et al. Differential expression of cyclin-dependent kinase inhibitors in human glomerular disease: Role in podocyte proliferation and maturation. *Kidney Int.* 2000;58:674-683.
27. Kim JH, Kim BK, Moon KC, et al. Activation of the TGF-β/Smad signaling pathway in focal segmental glomerulosclerosis. *Kidney Int.* 2003;64:1715-1721.
28. Haas M, Meehan S, Karrison TG, Spargo BH. Changing etiologies of unexplained adult nephrotic syndrome: A comparison of renal biopsy findings from 1976-1979 and 1995-1997. *Am J Kidney Dis.* 1997;30:621-631.
29. Bahiense-Oliveira M, Saldanha LB, Andrade Mota EL, et al. Primary glomerular disease in Brazil: 1979-1999. Is the frequency of FSGS increasing? *Clin Nephrol.* 2004;61:90-97.
30. Swaminathan S, Leung N, Lager DJ, et al. Changing incidence of glomerular disease in Olmsted County, Minnesota: A 30-year renal biopsy study. *Clin J Am Soc Nephrol.* 2006;1:483-487.
30a. Hanko JB, Mullan RN, O'Rourke DM, McNamee PT, Maxwell AP, Courtney AE. The changing pattern of adult primary glomerular disease. *Nephrol Dial Transplant.* 2009;24:3050-3054.
31. Stokes MB, Markowitz GSM, Lin J, et al. Glomerular tip lesion: A distinct entity within the minimal change/focal segmental glomerulosclerosis spectrum. *Kidney Int.* 2004;65:1690-1702.
32. Valeri A, Barisoni L, Appel GB, et al. Idiopathic collapsing FSGS: A clinicopathologic study. *Kidney Int.* 1996;50:1734-1746.
33. Schwimmer JA, Markowitz GS, Valeri A, Appel GB. Collapsing glomerulopathy. *Semin Nephrol.* 2003;23:209-219.
34. D'Agati VD, Fogo AB, Bruijn JA, Jennette JC. Pathologic classification of focal segmental glomerulosclerosis: A working proposal. *Am J Kidney Dis.* 2004;43:368-382.
35. Markowitz GS, Schwimmer JA, Stokes MB, et al. C1q nephropathy: A variant of focal segmental glomerulosclerosis. *Kidney Int.* 2003;64:1232-1240.
36. Vizjak A, Ferluga D, Rozic M, et al. Pathology, clinical presentations and outcomes of C1q nephropathy. *J Am Soc Nephrol.* 2008:19:2237-2244.
37. Stokes MB, Valeri AM, Markowitz GS, D'Agati VD. Cellular focal segmental glomerulosclerosis: Clinical and pathologic features. *Kidney Int.* 2006;70:1783-1792.
38. Wyatt CM, Klotman PE, D'Agati VD. HIV-associated nephropathy: Clinical presentation, pathology and epidemiology in the era of antiretroviral therapy. *Semin Nephrol.* 2008;28:513-522.
39. Deegens JKJ, Dijkman HB, Borm GF, et al. Podocyte foot process effacement as a diagnostic tool in focal segmental glomerulosclerosis. *Kidney Int.* 2008;74:1568-1576.

40. Stirling CM, Mathieson P, Bolton-Jones JM, et al. Treatment and outcome of adult patients with primary focal segmental glomerulosclerosis in five UK renal units. *Q J Med.* 2005;98:443-449.
41. Pei Y, Cattran D, Delmore T, et al. Evidence suggesting under-treatment of adults with idiopathic FSGS. *Am J Med.* 1987;82:938-944.
42. Matalon A, Valeri A, Appel GB. Treatment of focal segmental glomerulosclerosis. *Semin Nephrol.* 2000;20:309-317.
43. Troyanov S, Wall CA, Miller JA, et al. Focal and segmental glomerulosclerosis: Definition and relevance of a partial remission. *J Am Soc Nephrol.* 2005;16:1061-1068.
44. Thomas DB, Franceschini N, Hogan SL, et al. Clinical and pathologic characteristics of focal segmental glomerulosclerosis pathologic variants. *Kidney Int.* 2006;69:920-926.
45. Howie AJ, Pankhurst T, Sarioglu S, et al. Evolution of nephrotic-associated focal segmental glomerulosclerosis and relation to the glomerular tip lesion. *Kidney Int.* 2005;67:987-1001.
46. Ponticelli C, Villa M, Banfi G, et al. Can prolonged treatment improve the prognosis of FSGS? *Am J Kidney Dis.* 1999;34:618-625.
47. Korbet SM. Treatment of primary focal and segmental glomerulosclerosis. *Kidney Int.* 2002;62:2301-2310.
48. Ponticelli C, Passerini P. Other immunosuppressive agents for FSGS. *Semin Nephrol.* 2003;23:242-248.
49. Tune BM, Kirpekor R, Sibley R, et al. IV methylprednisolone and oral alkylating agent therapy of prednisone resistant pediatric FSGS: Long-term follow up. *Clin Nephrol.* 1995;43:83-88.
50. Lieberman KV, Tejani A, for the NY-NJ Pediatric Nephrology Study Group. A randomized double-blind trial of cyclosporine in steroid resistant FSGS in children. *J Am Soc Nephrol.* 1996;7:56-63.
51. Cattran D, Appel GB, Hebert L, et al. A randomized trial of cyclosporine in patients with steroid resistant focal segmental glomerulosclerosis: North America Nephrotic Syndrome Study Group. *Kidney Int.* 1999; 56:2220-2226.
52. Duncan N, Dhaygude A, Owen J, et al. Treatment of focal segmental glomerulosclerosis in adults with tacrolimus monotherapy. *Nephrol Dial Transplant.* 2004;19:3062-3063.
53. Loeffler K, Gowrishankar M, Yiu V. Tacrolimus therapy in pediatric patients with treatment resistant nephrotic syndrome. *Pediartr Nephrol.* 2004;19:281-287.
54. Heering P, Braun N, Mullejans R, et al. Cyclosporin A and chlorambucil in the treatment of idiopathic focal segmental glomerulosclerosis. *Am J Kidney Dis.* 2004;43:10-18.
55. Cattran DC, Wang MM, Appel GB, et al. Mycophenolate mofetil in the treatment of focal segmental glomerulosclerosis. *Clin Nephrol.* 2005; 62:405-412.
56. Appel AS, Appel GB. An update on the use of mycophenolate in lupus nephritis and other primary glomerular diseases. *Nat Clin Pract Nephrol.* 2009;5:132-142.
57. Fervenza F, Fitzpatrick PM, Mertz J, et al. Acute rapamycin nephrotoxicity in native kidneys in patients with chronic glomerulopathies. *Nephrol Dial Transplant.* 2004;19:1288-1292.
58. Tumlin JA, Miller D, Near M, et al. A prospective open-label trial of sirolimus in the treatment of focal segmental glomerulosclerosis. *Clin J Am Soc Nephrol.* 2006;1:109-117.
59. Fernandez-Fresnedo G, Segarra A, Gonzalez E, et al. Rituximab treatment of adult patients with steroid-resistant focal segmental glomerulosclerosis. *Clin J Am Soc Nephrol.* 2009;4:1317-1323.
60. Hattori M, Chikamoto H, Akioka Y, et al. A combined low-density lipoprotein apheresis and prednisone therapy for steroid-resistant primary focal segmental glomerulosclerosis in children. *Am J Kidney Dis.* 2003;42:1121-1130.
61. Savin VJ, McCarthy ET, Sharma R, et al. Galactose binds to focal segmental glomerulosclerosis permeability factor and inhibits its activity. *Transl Res.* 2008;151:288-292.
62. De Smet E, Rioux JP, Ammann H, et al. FSGS permeability factor–associated nephrotic syndrome: Remission after oral galactose therapy. *Nephrol Dial Transplant.* 2009;24:2938-2940.
63. Cho ME, Smith DC, Branton MH, et al. Pirfenidone slows renal function decline in patients with focal segmental glomerulosclerosis. *Clin J Am Soc Nephrol.* 2007;2:906-913.
64. Vincenti F, Ghiggeri GM. New insights into the pathogenesis and the therapy of recurrent FSGS. *Am J Transplant.* 2005;5:1179-1185.
65. Huang K, Ferris ME, Andreoni KA, Gipson DS. The differential effect of race among pediatric kidney transplant recipients with FSGS. *Am J Kidney Dis.* 2004;43:1082-1090.
66. Cibrik DM, Kaplan B, Campbell DA, Meier-Kriesche HU. Renal allograft survival in transplant recipients with focal glomerulosclerosis. *Am J Transplant.* 2003;3:64-67.
67. Rydel JJ, Korbet SM, Borok RZ, Schwartz MM. Focal segmental glomerular sclerosis in adults: Presentation, course, and response to treatment. *Am J Kidney Dis.* 1995;25:534-542.

CHAPTER 19

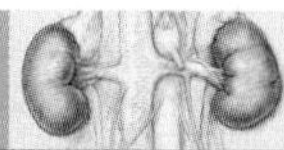

Inherited Causes of Nephrotic Syndrome

Jason Eckel, Michelle Winn

DEFINITION

Inherited nephrotic syndromes are rare diseases that present with nephrotic syndrome and varying degrees of renal impairment but at times may also present with subnephrotic proteinuria. They can be manifested *in utero* or shortly after birth, as in congenital nephrotic syndromes, or later in life with proteinuria and pathologic findings consistent with focal segmental glomerulosclerosis (FSGS). FSGS as the cause of nephrotic syndrome in adults is increasing according to biopsy studies in some but not all countries (see also Chapter 18). Some believe that up to 18% of cases of FSGS are due to hereditary disorders.[1] Autosomal dominant and recessive renal diseases result from defects in podocytes, the slit diaphragm, and the glomerular basement membrane (GBM). These primary renal disorders by definition do not recur after kidney transplantation. In children, syndromic conditions may be seen in which mutations in transcription factors involved in the development of multiple organ systems can also affect renal morphogenesis and result in glomerulopathy. Further insight into these hereditary diseases has been elucidated through animal models, in which mutations in corresponding proteins often result in FSGS and proteinuria. Understanding of these mechanisms not only provides better insight into abnormalities involved in idiopathic proteinuric kidney diseases but also allows the possible development of molecular drug targets that may improve the course of the renal disease and delay progression.[2-4]

AUTOSOMAL RECESSIVE DISEASES

Congenital Nephrotic Syndrome of the Finnish Type

In 1956, Hallman described a disorder of massive proteinuria *in utero* in the Finnish population. Congenital nephrotic syndrome of the Finnish type (CNF) or nephrotic syndrome type 1 (NPHS1) is an autosomal recessive disease. It has an incidence of 1 in 8200 births in Finland and has been reported less frequently in other ethnicities. The placenta is larger than the child at birth, and the baby is usually born prematurely. Affected children will have as much as 30 g of proteinuria per day, massive edema, hypoalbuminemia, and hyperlipidemia. By light microscopy, kidneys typically have cystic dilation of the proximal tubules and diffuse mesangial sclerosis (Fig. 19.1). Effacement of podocyte foot processes and loss of the glomerular slit diaphragm are seen with electron microscopy.[2]

Genome-wide linkage analysis localized the gene (*NPHS1*) to chromosome 19q13.1. The product of the *NPHS1* gene is specifically expressed in podocytes, localized to the slit diaphragm between podocyte foot processes, and is now named nephrin.[3] Nephrin is a transmembrane protein belonging to the immunoglobulin superfamily. The nephrin molecule has an intracellular, transmembrane, and extracellular domain. The extracellular domain forms the zipper-like structure of the slit diaphragm; the short intracellular domain interacts with the podocyte proteins podocin and CD2-associated protein (CD2AP). The most common mutations in nephrin are termed Fin-major and Fin-minor and account for 95% of the disease, but more than 50 other mutations in nephrin have also been reported.[4] The importance of nephrin in the function of the glomerular barrier has been demonstrated in mice; NPHS1 knockout mice have massive proteinuria, have absence of a slit diaphragm, and die within 24 hours of birth.[5]

CNF does not respond to cytotoxic therapy or corticosteroids. Angiotensin-converting enzyme (ACE) inhibitors and nonsteroidal anti-inflammatory drugs (NSAIDs) have no effect on reducing proteinuria in those with the Fin-major mutation, but there are some reports of efficacy of these agents in those with other mutations in nephrin. The ultimate goal of treatment of CNF is renal transplantation as mortality without this approach is nearly 100%. Because of overwhelming urinary loss of protein, affected infants without the Fin-major mutation may require medical nephrectomy with ACE inhibitors and NSAIDs followed by renal replacement therapy (RRT) before transplantation. There is a risk of recurrence of nephrotic syndrome in patients after transplantation, perhaps in as many as 20% to 25%. This is thought to be due to the introduction of a normal structural and functional nephrin in the transplanted kidney that sometimes leads to the production of anti-nephrin alloantibodies, which may be pathogenic.[2,4]

Corticosteroid-Resistant Nephrotic Syndrome

In children with nephrotic syndrome of unknown etiology, 90% of cases respond to corticosteroids. Of those who do not respond to corticosteroids, many have nephrotic syndrome type 2 (NPHS2), also known as corticosteroid-resistant nephrotic syndrome, an autosomal recessive disease seen mostly in children younger than 5 years.[6] Affected children have nephrotic-range proteinuria and rapid progression to end-stage renal disease (ESRD). As the disease name implies, patients do not respond to corticosteroids and suffer the extrarenal complications of massive proteinuria. By light microscopy, the renal lesions that have been seen vary along the spectrum of minimal change disease (MCD) to FSGS.[4] The gene *NPHS2* (nephrotic syndrome, type 2) was mapped to chromosome 1q25-q31 and determined to be the cause of corticosteroid-resistant nephrotic

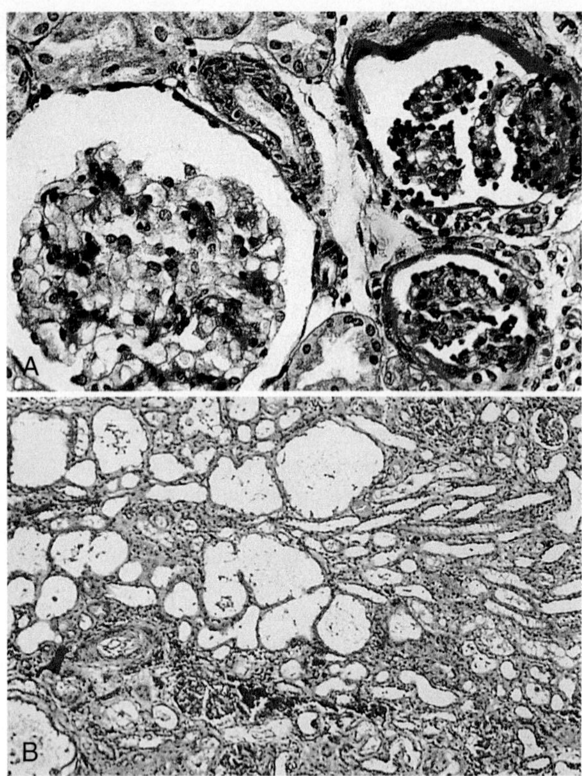

Figure 19.1 Congenital nephrotic syndrome, Finnish type. A, Diffuse mesangial thickening and partially collapsed glomeruli. (Periodic acid–Schiff; magnification ×260.) **B,** Microcystic dilation of the tubules. (Hematoxylin-eosin; magnification ×150.) *(Modified from reference 23.)*

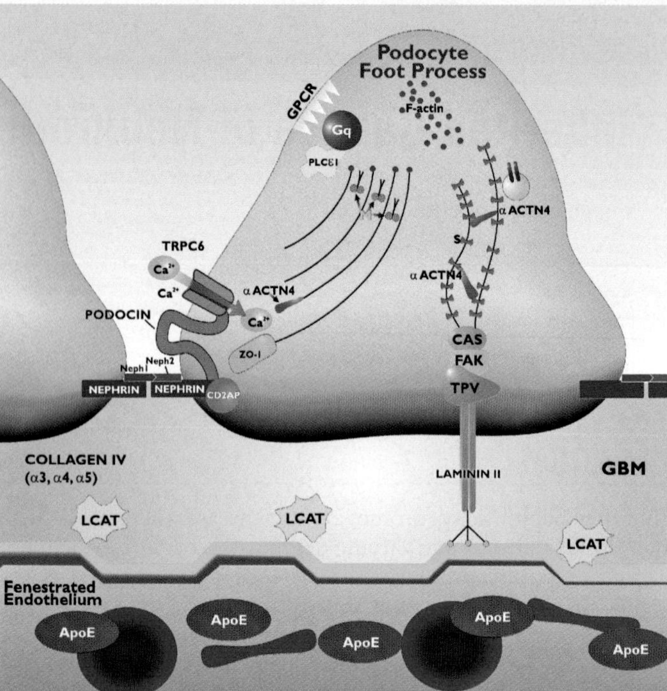

Figure 19.2 Podocyte foot process structure and proteins involved in hereditary nephrotic syndromes. The podocyte contains F-actin, myosin (M), and actin-binding proteins synaptopodin (S) and α-actinin-4 (αACTN4). αACTN4 is mutated in FSGS type 1. The slit diaphragm contains proteins that include nephrin, podocin, and CD2AP. Nephrin is mutated in congenital nephrotic syndrome of the Finnish type, and podocin in corticosteroid-resistant nephrotic syndrome. Zona occludens 1 (ZO-1) is a cell-to-cell junction protein. PLCε1 is an enzyme identified as a cause of diffuse mesangial sclerosis. Angiotensin receptor 1 is an example of a G protein–coupled receptor (GPCR) and can activate TRPC6. A TRPC6 mutation in FSGS type 2 results in increased calcium (Ca^{2+}) transients. INF2 (not shown) is mutated in FSGS type 5 and causes mislocalization of the INF2 protein. Talin, paxillin, and vinculin (TPV) are connected to laminin II through $\alpha_3\beta_1$ integrin dimers and are involved in anchoring of the podocyte to the glomerular basement membrane (GBM). The LAMB2 mutation is responsible for Pierson's syndrome and results in diffuse mesangial sclerosis. LCAT deficiency demonstrates lipid deposits in the GBM. Laminated apolipoprotein deposits (ApoE) are found in the capillaries in lipoprotein glomerulopathy. LMX1B and WT1 (not shown) are transcription factors mutated in syndromic proteinuric renal diseases. Catenins (CAT), p130Cas (CAS), and focal adhesion kinase (FAK) are structural proteins. *(Modified from reference 24.)*

syndrome.[7] Similar to the *NPHS1* gene product nephrin, the product of *NPHS2* is specifically expressed in podocytes in the kidney and is named podocin. Podocin is hairpin shaped and found along the podocyte membrane with both ends directed intracellularly (Fig. 19.2).[2] Podocin localizes to the foot processes and seems to be involved in podocyte structure as well as in intracellular signaling, with the recruitment of nephrin and CD2AP to microdomains along the slit diaphragm.[4]

The description of corticosteroid-resistant nephrotic syndrome attributed to the *NPHS2* mutation represents a condition seen in children between 3 months and 5 years of age. It appears that when the disease is manifested depends on the specific podocin mutation. The presence of at least one podocin mutation that codes for a stop codon or in patients homozygous for the R138Q mutation results in renal disease at around the age of 2 years. Two missense podocin mutations cause disease just before the age of 5 years. Furthermore, studies demonstrate podocin mutations in adult-onset forms of FSGS. This is seen around the end of the second decade. These patients must have two podocin mutations, one of which must be the podocin R229Q mutation.[8]

Isolated Diffuse Mesangial Sclerosis

Diffuse mesangial sclerosis is a pathologic finding in some cases of early-onset nephrotic syndrome. It is described as either syndromic, when it is associated with a particular clinical syndrome, or isolated, when the only manifestation is renal disease. The isolated disease presents as nephrotic syndrome in the first month of life with rapid progression to ESRD. By light microscopy, findings include podocyte hypertrophy, mesangial matrix expansion, thickened basement membranes, and decreased size of glomerular capillary lumina. In addition, some cases have shown response to cyclosporine.[9]

Diffuse mesangial sclerosis is inherited in an autosomal recessive pattern (Fig. 19.3). In 12 children with isolated diffuse mesangial sclerosis, the causative gene was mapped to chromosome 10q23. The gene *PLCE1* encodes phospholipase C epsilon 1 (PLCε1). PLCε1 is a phospholipase involved in the generation of diacylglycerol and inositol 1,4,5-trisphosphate, which are intracellular second messengers (see Fig. 19.2). Evidence of the role of PLCε1 in glomerular function was demonstrated in a *plc 1* knockout model in zebrafish. These animals had edema and pathologic characteristics of nephrotic syndrome during development. The mechanism of disease from the *PLCE1* mutation is not clear, but there is evidence that it interacts with a GTPase-activating protein involved in podocyte development and interaction with nephrin. *PLCE1* is not the only gene responsible for isolated diffuse mesangial sclerosis; more genetic causes are

Autosomal Recessive Nephrotic Syndromes				
Disease	**Gene**	**Protein**	**Clinical Presentation**	**Mechanism of Disease**
Congenital nephrotic syndrome of the Finnish type	*NPHSI*	Nephrin	Proteinuria *in utero* (sometimes >30 grams), large placenta, resistant to conventional therapy, transplant is the only treatment	Mutation in nephrin leads to loss or malfunction of the slit diaphragm
Steroid resistant nephrotic syndrome	*NPHS2*	Podocin	Various clinical manifestations and age of onset of proteinuria; resistant to steroids, generally progresses to FSGS	Mutation in podocin leads to loss or malfunction of the slit diaphragm
Isolated diffuse mesangial sclerosis	*PLCE1*	PLCε1	Nephrotic syndrome in the first year of life; rapid progression to ESRD	Unclear, but PLCε1 mutation results in abnormal podocyte differentiation potentially through nephrin; other mutations exist not attributed to *PLCE1*

Figure 19.3 Autosomal recessive nephrotic syndromes. ESRD, end-stage renal disease; FSGS, focal segmental glomerulosclerosis.

Autosomal Dominant Nephrotic Syndromes				
Disease	**Gene**	**Protein**	**Clinical Presentation**	**Mechanism of Disease**
FSGS type 1	*ACTN4*	α-actinin-4	Slow progression to ESRD; generally presents in adulthood with proteinuria	Mutation in α-actinin-4 results in abnormal assembly/disassembly of actin and podocyte structural abnormalities
FSGS type 2	*TRPC6*	TRPC6	Proteinuria seen in late adolescence to adulthood; 60% progress to ESRD by 10 years	Mutation in TRPC6 leads to increased calcium transients, which may result in disruption of podocyte structure or function
FSGS type 5	*INF2*	INF2	Moderate proteinuria seen in late adolescence to adult-hood; occasional microscopic hematuria and hypertension	Mutation in INF2 causes mis-localization of the protein

Figure 19.4 Autosomal dominant nephrotic syndromes. ESRD, end-stage renal disease; FSGS, focal segmental glomerulosclerosis.

under investigation, and further mechanisms as to the cause of this distinct clinicopathologic entity are yet to be defined.[9]

AUTOSOMAL DOMINANT DISEASES

Autosomal Dominant Familial Focal Segmental Glomerulosclerosis

In contrast to inherited nephrotic syndromes that present in childhood, there are familial proteinuric kidney diseases that are manifested in adolescence through adulthood. Most of these are inherited in an autosomal dominant fashion (Fig. 19.4). Typical pathology reveals the glomerular changes of FSGS, and there is variability in the rate of progression of renal impairment. Genetic mutations have been identified, and mechanisms of FSGS in sporadic forms can be elucidated from our increasing understanding of these familial cases.[10]

FSGS type 1 is an autosomal dominant form of FSGS caused by mutations in *ACTN4*, which has been mapped to chromosome 19q13.[2] The product of this gene is α-actinin 4, which is expressed in podocytes and cross-links with F-actin filaments in the foot processes (see Fig. 19.2). The mutation in *ACTN4* is believed to be a gain-of-function mutation, leading to increased cross-linking of F-actin with α-actinin 4, resulting in dysregulation of actin assembly and disassembly in the podocyte. It was recently found that the relaxation frequency from actin of mutant α-actinin 4 was an order of magnitude lower than wild-type α-actinin 4. The resultant structural abnormality is believed to be the reason for proteinuria, renal dysfunction, and subsequent glomerulosclerosis. This has been supported in mouse studies; those with mutated α-actinin 4 with high affinity for F-actin have an FSGS-like phenotype, and mice deficient in α-actinin 4 have abnormal podocytes and develop ESRD.[2,4] Patients with FSGS type 1 have variable age at onset and progression of renal disease.

The mutation responsible for FSGS type 2 was recently mapped to chromosome 11q21-22 in a New Zealand kindred and identified as transient receptor potential cation channel, subfamily C, member 6 (TRPC6).[10] TRP channels are involved in various biologic processes including cell growth, mechanosensation, vasoregulation, and cation entry into cells. The P112Q missense mutation involves the change of a proline (P) to a glutamine (Q) in a highly conserved region of the first ankyrin repeat of TRPC6 and results in a gain of function, with increased calcium influx presumably leading to glomerular dysfunction.[2,4] This is an autosomal dominant disease that is manifested in the third and fourth decades of life. As many as 60% of affected individuals will progress to ESRD in 10 years. In contrast to known mutations that result in structural podocyte and slit diaphragm abnormalities, such as podocin, nephrin, and α-actinin 4, this is the first ion channel to be implicated as a cause of hereditary nephrotic syndrome and FSGS. The importance of TRPC6 in normal podocyte function has been further supported through discovery of *TRPC6* mutations in additional families with hereditary FSGS, two of which also result in increased calcium influx.[11] Furthermore, there is increased expression of wild-type TRPC6 in human proteinuric kidney diseases, animal models of kidney injury, and cultured podocytes exposed to complement and anti-podocyte antibodies.[12]

CD2-associated protein (CD2AP), a widely expressed protein originally identified through its interaction with CD2 in T lymphocytes, has been implicated in proteinuric renal disease. Cd2ap-deficient mice die of renal failure at 6 to 7 weeks of age. On histologic examination, foot process effacement and glomerulosclerosis are seen. Furthermore, mice expressing Cd2ap only in the podocyte are protected from kidney disease, suggesting that the proteinuria is due to podocyte-specific loss of Cd2ap. A corresponding disease in humans due solely to *CD2AP* mutations has not been clearly established to this point, but mutations in *CD2AP* in two adults with FSGS have been reported.[13] CD2AP does localize to the slit diaphragm and has been shown to interact with nephrin and podocin (see Fig. 19.2).[4] Therefore, it is plausible that a *CD2AP* mutation in humans could result in glomerular disease.

Mutations in *INF2*, the formin gene cause FSGS type 5. Using linkage analysis, a locus was identified on chromosome 14q32 and nine non-conservative missense mutations were identified in eleven families.[13a] All mutations were located in the diaphanous inhibitory domain of *INF2*. Individuals in these families present in early adolescence or adulthood with moderate proteinuria that progresses to ESRD. Some individuals also presented with microscopic hematuria and hypertension. Pathology shows typical FSGS, however on electron microscopy, prominent actin bundles were also noted within the foot processes. INF2 is a member of the formin family. These proteins regulate actin and accelerate actin polymerization. INF2 is widely expressed throughout the body and also in podocytes. When mutant INF2 constructs were transfected into podocytes, they exhibited different localization patterns than wild-type INF2. The exact pathogenetic mechanism of *INF2* mutations remains to be elucidated.

SYNDROMIC PROTEINURIC RENAL DISEASE

Denys-Drash and Frasier Syndromes

The Denys-Drash syndrome (DDS) and the Frasier syndrome are rare diseases that are manifested with early onset of congenital nephrotic syndrome and male pseudohermaphroditism (Fig. 19.5). Both are associated with the development of urogenital tumors: nephroblastoma or Wilms' tumor in DDS, and gonadoblastoma in Frasier syndrome. Patients with DDS have a high incidence of severe hypertension and rapid progression to ESRD. The glomerular lesion of DDS is diffuse mesangial sclerosis, and patients progress to ESRD by the age of 3 years. In Frasier syndrome, male pseudohermaphrodites typically present as phenotypic females with amenorrhea or nephrotic syndrome or both. The nephrotic syndrome may be slowly progressive (usually during 10 years); it is typically corticosteroid resistant, and the pathologic lesion is FSGS. The patients develop ESRD in their second and third decades of life, with most cases occurring at puberty. There are cases that present in much younger children.[14] Rarely, an XX karyotype with a less severe phenotype may not be identified clinically as Frasier syndrome and presents only with renal disease.

The gene responsible for both Denys-Drash and Frasier syndromes has been localized to chromosome 11p13. The gene

Syndromic Proteinuric Renal Diseases

Disease	Inheritance	Gene	Protein	Clinical Presentation	Mechanism of Disease
Denys-Drasch and Frasier syndromes	AD	*WT1*	WT1	Male pseudo-hermaphroditisim, early nephropathy, and Wilms' tumor in Denys-Drasch; later onset of nephropathy, FSGS, and gonadoblastoma in Frasier syndrome	Mutation in *WT1* results in abnormal urogenital development
Nail-Patella syndrome	AD	*LMX1B*	LMX1B	Skeletal, nails, eyes, and renal abnormalities; variable renal disease from benign proteinuria to nephrotic syndrome	Mutation in *LMX1B* results in abnormal regulation of podocyte genes
Pierson's syndrome	AR	*LAMB2*	Laminin β2 chain	Microcoria, diffuse mesangial sclerosis, onset shortly after birth	Abnormal GBM due to mutations in adult form of laminin
Galloway-Mowat syndrome	AR	*Unknown*	Unknown	Microcephaly, abnormal cerebral gyral patterns, seizures, cranial dysmorphia, and glomerulopathy	Mechanism not known

Figure 19.5 Syndromic proteinuric renal diseases. AD, autosomal dominant; AR, autosomal recessive; FSGS, focal segmental glomerulosclerosis; GBM, glomerular basement membrane.

Glomerular Diseases Associated with Abnormalities in Lipid Metabolism

Disease	Inheritance	Gene	Protein	Clinical Presentation	Mechanism of Disease
Lipoprotein glomerulopathy	Unknown	*Unknown*	Apolipoprotein E	Type III hyperlipidemia, nephrotic syndrome, renal failure, and deposition of lipid thrombi in glomerular capillaries	Abnormal lipid metabolism and deposition in various tissues
LCAT deficiency	AR	*LCAT*	LCAT	Anemia, corneal opacities, low HDL, elevated LDL, proteinuria, and progressive renal failure	Abnormal lipid metabolism and deposition in various tissues

Figure 19.6 Glomerular diseases associated with abnormalities in lipid metabolism. AR, autosomal recessive; HDL, high-density lipoprotein; LCAT, lecithin–cholesterol acyltransferase; LDL, low-density lipoprotein.

product is the Wilms' tumor suppressor (WT1), which is a transcription factor involved in gonad and kidney development. WT1 seems to downregulate the expression of a number of genes involved in normal embryonic development of the urogenital system. Therefore, the decreased expression or lack of expression of WT1 seen in DDS and Frasier syndromes leads to the clinical manifestations of these diseases.[2,14] This has been supported in mouse studies as *Wt1* knockout mice lack kidneys and gonads.[14]

Nail-Patella Syndrome

Nail-Patella syndrome (hereditary onycho-osteodysplasia; Fong syndrome) is an autosomal dominant disease involving abnormalities of the skeleton, nails, eyes, and kidneys. Affected patients have nail dysplasia, absence of or poorly developed patellas, dysplasia of the iliac horns and elbows, cataracts, glaucoma, and glomerulopathy.[2] The syndrome is discussed in detail in Chapter 46.

Pierson's Syndrome

In 1963, Pierson and colleagues described cases of congenital nephrotic syndrome with distinct eye abnormalities.[15] Patients with Pierson's syndrome have hypoplasia of the ciliary body and iris resulting in fixed narrowing of the pupil (microcoria) as well as massive proteinuria at birth and rapid progression to ESRD. Most die before 2 months of age. Diffuse mesangial sclerosis exemplifies the renal pathology findings in Pierson's syndrome. The genetic defect has been isolated to chromosome 3p21, and the resultant mutation is in *LAMB2*, which codes for the laminin β2 chain. *LAMB2* is present in the normal GBM, and the mutation results in abnormal formation of the GBM as well as abnormal differentiation of podocyte foot processes (see Fig. 19.2). *Lamb2* knockout mice demonstrate congenital nephrosis with abnormalities of the retinal and neuromuscular junctions.[2,15]

Galloway-Mowat Syndrome

In 1968, two siblings with nephrotic syndrome, hiatal hernia, and abnormal development of the central nervous system were described by Galloway and Mowat.[16] By 2001, 31 more patients with similar clinical features had been described. The Galloway-Mowat syndrome is inherited in an autosomal recessive pattern. The currently recognized clinical features include microcephaly, abnormal cerebral gyral patterns, seizures, psychomotor retardation, cranial dysmorphia, and glomerulopathy. The renal disease generally presents as the nephrotic syndrome within the first few months of life with rapid progression to ESRD. Most affected children die before the age of 6 years. Based on the time of biopsy, various renal findings have been reported by light microscopy. These include diffuse mesangial sclerosis, mesangial proliferation, FSGS, cystic microdilation of tubules, and normal-appearing glomeruli. By electron microscopy, irregular thickening of the GBM and effacement of podocyte foot processes are seen. The genetic abnormality has not been found, but because of multiple reports of the same disease in siblings, it is presumed to be a familial disorder.[17]

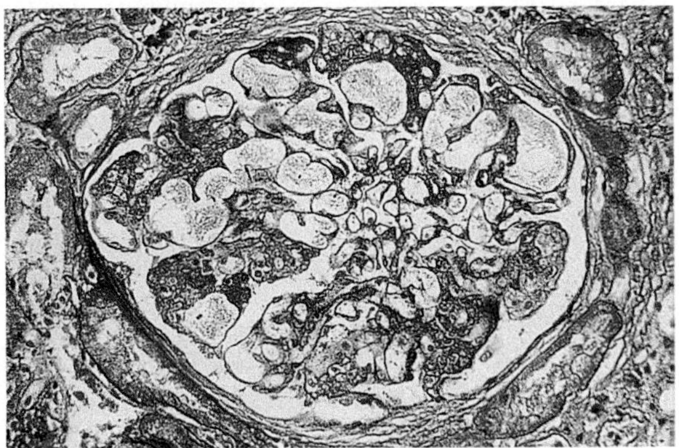

Figure 19.7 Lipoprotein glomerulopathy. Dilated capillary lumina containing a pale-stained, mesh-like or granular substance. (Trichrome stain; magnification ×260.) *(Modified from reference 23.)*

Glomerulopathy Associated with Abnormalities in Lipid Metabolism

Nephrotic-range proteinuria, edema, hypoalbuminuria, lipiduria, and hyperlipidemia are hallmarks of the nephrotic syndrome. Yet, the hyperlipidemia is thought to be a consequence of urinary losses of cholesterol and albumin, resulting in increased hepatic synthesis of low-density lipoproteins, very low density lipoproteins, and lipoprotein(a).[18] However, some rare proteinuric kidney diseases are due to abnormal metabolism of lipids, resulting in deposition of lipids in glomeruli and subsequent nephrotic syndrome (Fig. 19.6).

Lipoprotein glomerulopathy presents in adulthood with proteinuria and often nephrotic syndrome with rapid progression to renal failure. Light microscopy reveals extensive deposition of laminated lipid thrombi in glomerular capillaries (Fig. 19.7). The lipid deposits contain apolipoproteins A, B, and E (see Fig. 19.2). Because of studies of affected kindreds, particularly in Japan, it is thought to be a hereditary disease. The mutation is believed to be in apolipoprotein E as these patients also have a type III hyperlipidemia, characterized by elevated intermediate-density lipoproteins and apolipoprotein E. Treatment with lipid-lowering drugs, such as fibric acid derivatives, has shown some benefit.[19]

Lecithin–cholesterol acyltransferase (LCAT) deficiency is an autosomal recessive disease characterized by anemia, corneal opacities, low high-density lipoprotein level, elevated low-density lipoprotein level, proteinuria, and often nephrotic syndrome with progressive renal failure. The disease generally presents in adulthood and is slow in onset. Light microscopy reveals irregular thickening of the glomerular capillaries with "vacuolization" of the capillary basement membranes due to lipid droplets (Fig. 19.8). This is the "foamy" appearance characteristic of LCAT deficiency. Mesangial and basement membrane electron-dense lamellar structures are also seen and are unique to this disorder. The genetic mutation is in the *LCAT* gene on chromosome 16q22. LCAT deficiency responds poorly to treatment.[20]

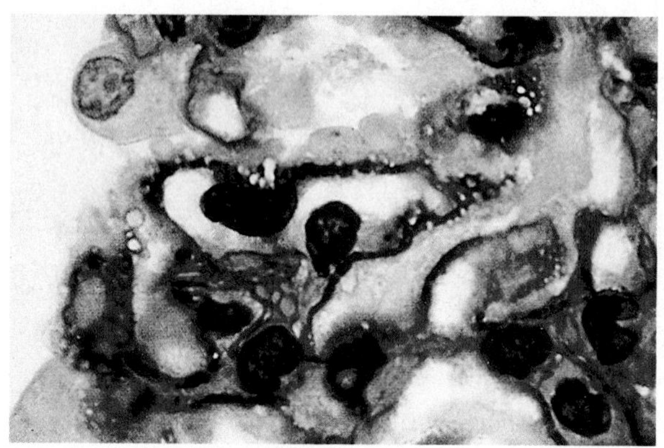

Figure 19.8 Lecithin–cholesterol acyltransferase deficiency. Note the irregular thickened glomerular capillary walls containing clear vacuoles, which are characteristic of the lesion. (Periodic acid–Schiff; magnification ×1000.) *(Modified from reference 23.)*

GENETIC TESTING

Children with a family history of corticosteroid-resistant nephrotic syndrome or after failure of an initial treatment course of corticosteroids should undergo renal biopsy and be considered for genetic testing. Mutations in the recessive genes that encode nephrin (*NPSH1*), podocin (*NPHS2*), phospholipase Cε1 (*PLCE1*), WT1 (*WT1*), and laminin β2 (*LAMB2*) cause proteinuric renal disorders in children. *NPHS1*, *NPHS2*, *LAMB2*, and *WT1* mutations are responsible for 85% of glomerular disease seen in the first 3 months of life and 66% in the first year, and these certainly should be the first tests sent in screening of children for inherited conditions.[8] Diffuse mesangial sclerosis is seen with mutations in *NPHS1*, *PLCE1*, *LAMB2*, and *WT1*. FSGS is seen with mutations in *NPHS2*. The Galloway-Mowat syndrome can have either diffuse mesangial sclerosis or FSGS-like changes, but the genetic defect is not known. Further testing will be determined by the patient's presentation. In most cases of syndromic disease, the clinical characteristics will dictate which genetic tests are necessary and may narrow the analysis to one or two genes. For example, in a patient with pseudohermaphroditism and renal disease, *WT1* mutations are likely, and *LAMB2* testing can be done in those with congenital nephrotic syndrome and microcoria.

Inherited nephrotic syndrome in adults generally presents as FSGS and is believed to be responsible for up to 18% of cases identified in those older than 18 years.[1] Genetic testing should be considered when there is a strong family history of disease. Autosomal dominant disease will exist in multiple family members in successive generations, and there will be male-to-male transmission. Known gene mutations to investigate include *ACTN4* and *TRPC6*. Young adults may have FSGS due to a combination of mutations in podocin, one of which is the R229Q mutation. This may be more difficult to identify because the inheritance pattern will not be as apparent (Fig. 19.9).[8]

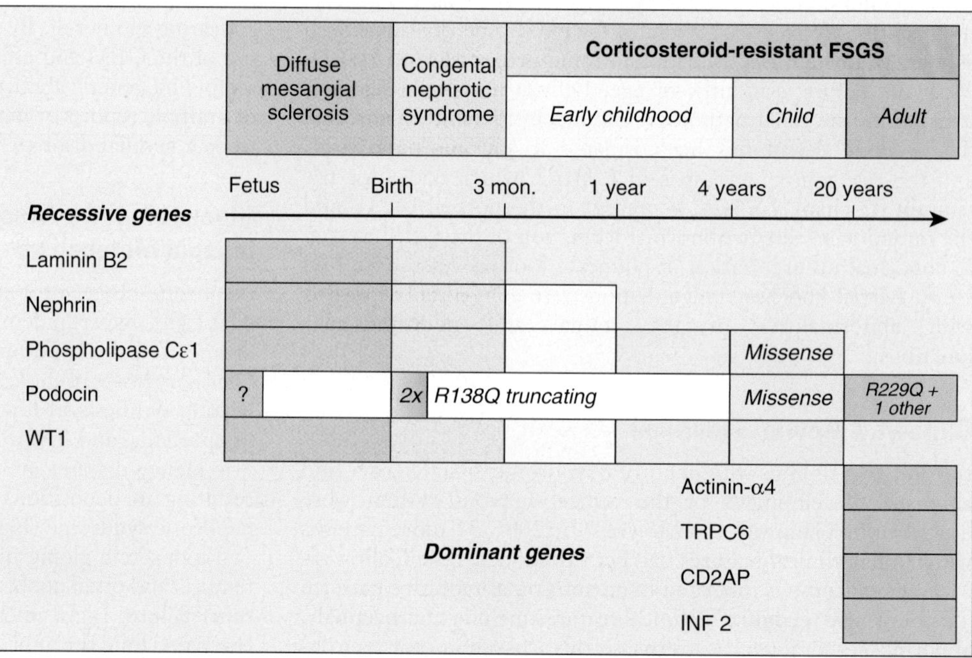

Figure 19.9 Inheritance patterns of nephrotic syndromes. Autosomal recessive diseases generally present early in life as diffuse mesangial sclerosis or congenital nephrotic syndrome. In early childhood, mutations in genes encoding nephrin, podocin, WT1, and phospholipase Cε1 will also cause disease. Podocin mutations result in disease at different times on the basis of the particular mutation, with disease in young adults as well (see text). Autosomal dominant conditions present later in life and have been described in families with FSGS with mutations in genes encoding α-actinin 4 and TRPC6. CD2AP mutations are suspected but have not been described as a sole cause of disease in humans. FSGS, focal segmental glomerulosclerosis. *(Modified from reference 8.)*

CLINICAL MANAGEMENT OF INHERITED NEPHROTIC SYNDROME

ACE inhibitors and angiotensin receptor blockers (ARBs) are appropriate medications for children with corticosteroid-resistant nephrotic syndrome. Cyclophosphamide, cyclosporine, tacrolimus, rituximab, and mycophenolate have been used with limited success in small studies. However, given the preponderance of side effects with these medications, they are generally not used in children.[21]

Adults with corticosteroid-resistant hereditary FSGS should be treated with ACE inhibitors and ARBs. Lipid-lowering medications are also recommended as adults with nephrotic syndrome have hyperlipidemia and may have increased risk of cardiovascular disease. Cyclosporine is generally used for initial treatment in FSGS not responsive to corticosteroids and may be appropriate in inherited forms as well. Mycophenolate can be substituted in those who do not respond to cyclosporine or have a contraindication to its use. Limited evidence is available for use of tacrolimus or sirolimus.[22]

As these disorders are due to inherited abnormalities in renal developmental or structural proteins, there should not be recurrence of the original condition after transplantation because the donor kidney presumably is from a patient without a genetic renal disease. However, the reported recurrence rate of nephrotic syndrome in those with inherited disorders is misleading as chronic allograft nephropathy can present with an FSGS-like phenotype. Similarly, reports of recurrence in patients with podocin mutations exist, but given the complex inheritance pattern, with some diseases manifesting in children and others in adults, it is difficult to interpret. More recent data suggest a recurrence rate of nephrotic syndrome in the transplant in those with *NPSH2* mutations to be very low.[8] Reappearance of the nephrotic syndrome in congenital nephrotic syndrome of the Finnish type is not truly a "recurrence" but thought to be due to anti-nephrin autoantibodies and not a *de novo* nephrin mutation in the transplanted kidney. Therefore, transplantation is not discouraged in those with congenital nephrotic syndromes, and their postsurgery management should not differ from usual clinical care; in fact, there are data to suggest that those with inherited nephrotic syndromes and FSGS may have better transplant survival outcomes than in those with idiopathic disease.

REFERENCES

1. Haas M, Meehan SM, Karrison TG, Spargo BH. Changing etiologies of unexplained adult nephrotic syndrome: A comparison of renal biopsy findings from 1976-1979 and 1995-1997. *Am J Kidney Dis*. 1997; 30:621-631.
2. Tryggvason K, Patrakka J, Wartiovaara J. Hereditary proteinuria syndromes and mechanisms of proteinuria. *N Engl J Med*. 2006;354: 1387-1401.
3. Kestila M, Lenkkeri U, Mannikko M, et al. Positionally cloned gene for a novel glomerular protein, nephrin, is mutated in congenital nephrotic syndrome. *Mol Cell*. 1998;1:575-582.
4. Daskalakis N, Winn MP. Focal and segmental glomerulosclerosis. *Cell Mol Life Sci*. 2006;63:2506-2511.
5. Putaala H, Soininen R, Kilpelainen P, et al. The murine nephrin gene is specifically expressed in kidney, brain, and pancreas: Inactivation of the gene leads to massive proteinuria and neonatal death. *Hum Mol Genet*. 2001;10:1-8.
6. Niaudet P. Podocin and nephrotic syndrome: Implications for the clinician. *J Am Soc Nephrol*. 2004;15:832-834.
7. Fuchshuber A, Jean G, Gribouval O, et al. Mapping a gene (SRN1) to chromosome 1q25-q31 in idiopathic nephrotic syndrome confirms a distinct entity of autosomal recessive nephrosis. *Hum Mol Genet*. 1995;4:2155-2158.
8. Hildebrandt F, Herringa SF. Specific podocin mutations determine the age of onset of nephrotic syndrome all the way into adult life. *Kidney Int*. 2009;75:669-671.
9. Hinkes B, Wiggins RC, Gbadegesin R, et al. Positional cloning uncovers mutations in PLCE1 responsible for a nephrotic syndrome variant that may be reversible. *Nat Genet*. 2006;12:1397-1405.
10. Winn MP, Conlon PJ, Lynn KL, et al. A mutation in the TRPC6 cation channel causes familial focal segmental glomerulosclerosis. *Science*. 2005;308:1801-1804.
11. Reiser J, Polu KR, Moller CC, et al. TRPC6 is a glomerular slit diaphragm–associated channel required for normal renal function. *Nat Genet*. 2005;37:739-744.
12. Moller CC, Wei C, Altintas MM, et al. Induction of TRPC6 channel in acquired forms of proteinuric kidney disease. *J Am Soc Nephrol*. 2007;18: 29-36.
13. Grunkemeyer JA, Kwoh C, Huber TB, Shaw AS. CD2-associated protein (CD2AP) expression in podocytes rescues lethality of CD2AP deficiency. *J Biol Chem*. 2005;280:29677-29681.

13a. Brown EJ, Schlondorff JS, Becker DJ, et al. Mutations in the formin gene *INF2* cause focal segmental glomerulosclerosis. *Nat Gen*. 2010;1:72-76.

14. Pritchard-Jones K, Fleming S, Davidson D, et al. The candidate Wilms' tumor gene is involved in genitourinary development. *Nature*. 1990;346: 194-197.
15. Pierson M, Cordier J, Hervouuet F, Rauber G. An unusual congenital and familial congenital malformative combination involving the eye and kidney. *J Genet Hum*. 1963;12:184-213.
16. Galloway WH, Mowat AP. Congenital microcephaly with hiatus hernia and nephrotic syndrome in two sibs. *J Med Genet*. 1968;5:319-321.
17. Lin CC, Tsai JD, Lin SP, et al. Galloway-Mowat syndrome: A glomerular basement membrane disorder? *Pediatr Nephrol*. 2001;16:653-657.
18. Wheeler DC, Bernard DB. Lipid abnormalities in nephrotic syndrome. *Am J Kidney Dis*. 1994 23:331-346.
19. Ieiri N, Hotta O, Taguma Y. Resolution of typical lipoprotein glomerulopathy by intensive lipid-lowering therapy. *Am J Kidney Dis*. 2003;41: 244-249.
20. Calabresi L, Pisciotta L, Constantin A, et al. The molecular basis of lecithin:cholesterol acyltranferase deficiency syndromes: A comprehensive study of molecular and biochemical findings in 13 unrelated Italian families. *Arterioscler Thromb Vasc Biol*. 2005;25:1972-1978.
21. Gregory MJ, Smoyer WE, Sedman A, et al. Long-term cyclosporine therapy for pediatric nephrotic syndrome: A clinical and histologic analysis. *J Am Soc Nephrol*. 1996;4:543-549.
22. Burgess E. Management of focal segmental glomerulosclerosis: Evidence-based recommendations. *Kidney Int*. 1999;70:S26-S32.
23. Churg J, Bernstein J, Glassock R, eds. *Renal Disease: Classification and Atlas of Glomerular Disease*. New York: Igaku-Shoin; 1995.
24. Mukerji N, Damodaran TV, Winn MP. TRPC6 and FSGS: The latest TRP channelopathy. *Biochim Biophys Acta*. 2007;1772:859-868.

CHAPTER 20

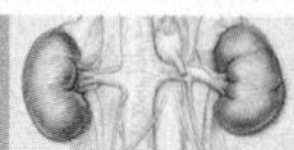

Membranous Nephropathy

William G. Couser, Daniel C. Cattran

DEFINITION

Membranous nephropathy (MN) is a glomerular disease in which immune deposits of IgG and complement components develop predominantly or exclusively beneath podocytes on the subepithelial surface of the glomerular capillary wall. Deposit formation is associated with a marked increase in glomerular permeability to protein, which is manifested clinically as nephrotic syndrome.[1] The disease occurs in association with a variety of conditions, some of which are likely to be causal and some of which probably represent only associations (Fig. 20.1).[2] However, most occurrences (two thirds) are without obvious initiating events. Idiopathic MN is the most common cause of primary nephrotic syndrome in older (>60 years) Caucasian adults and is rare in children.[3]

The term *membranous* refers to thickening of the glomerular capillary wall by light microscopy, but the entity now referred to as MN was defined when immunofluorescence and electron microscopy became routine tools in the study of renal biopsy specimens in the 1960s. These techniques demonstrated diffuse, finely granular immune deposits in the subepithelial space that are now regarded as pathognomonic of MN. Consequently, MN is a pathologic diagnosis made when glomeruli exhibit these deposits without associated hypercellularity or inflammatory changes.[1]

ETIOLOGY AND PATHOGENESIS

Etiology

The frequent occurrence of MN in autoimmune disorders (such as lupus and type 1 diabetes) and its remarkable similarity to a lesion induced in rats with antibody to antigens expressed on the foot processes of glomerular podocytes have fueled speculation that the disease is caused by deposits of autoantibody to fixed components of the podocyte membrane.[2,4] A large number of agents appear to be capable of initiating MN in genetically susceptible individuals (see Fig. 20.1). These include viruses such as hepatitis B (HBV) and hepatitis C (HCV); drugs, including gold, penicillamine, and nonsteroidal anti-inflammatory drugs (NSAIDs); environmental toxins, such as hydrocarbons and formaldehyde; and a variety of chronic immune disorders, such as lupus, thyroiditis, graft-versus-host disease, anti–glomerular basement membrane (anti-GBM) and antineutrophil cytoplasmic antibody (ANCA)–positive crescentic glomerulonephritis (GN), and the chronic immune response to renal allografts. In about two thirds of patients, however, no obvious etiologic agent or condition can be identified.

Mechanisms of Immune Deposit Formation

Regardless of the initiating events, MN appears to be mediated primarily by the Th2 humoral immune response, which leads to formation of deposits of IgG and complement on the outer surface of the glomerular capillary wall. Experimental evidence suggests that such deposits are produced by local or *in situ* immune complex formation involving antigens that could be exogenous or endogenous. Subepithelial immune complex deposits can form in three ways.[4] Antibodies can bind to exogenous antigens that localize on the subepithelial surface because of their cationic charge and small size; second, antigens and antibodies can be trapped as immune complexes on the inner surface of the capillary wall, dissociate, traverse the glomerular basement membrane (GBM), and reform in the subepithelial space; and finally, the antigens could be endogenous constituents of a fixed subepithelial structure, such as a podocyte membrane protein.[2,4] The absence of deposits at subendothelial (and mesangial) sites in idiopathic MN as well as the ability to exactly replicate the clinical and pathologic features of MN in rats with anti-podocyte antibodies (Heymann nephritis) strongly favors the third, or autoimmune, mechanism. In the Heymann nephritis models, the antigens responsible are components of the Heymann nephritis antigenic complex: a large (516-kd) glycoprotein, called megalin, bound to a smaller receptor-associated protein expressed in the clathrin-coated pits of the podocyte foot processes.[4] Whereas antibodies to small antigenic determinants on both molecules can form subepithelial immune complex deposits, additional antigen-antibody systems involving an unidentified glycolipid antigen that activates complement as well as antibodies that neutralize complement regulatory proteins are required to induce proteinuria in animals.[2,4] Once formed, these complexes of antigen and antibody are capped and shed from the cell surface, where they bind to underlying GBM, resist degradation, and persist for weeks or months as immune deposits detectable by immunofluorescence and electron microscopy (Fig. 20.2; see also Figs. 20.6 and 20.7).

Confirmation that a similar mechanism may be operative in idiopathic MN in humans has come from two sources. Several cases of congenital MN have been shown to be mediated by an antibody to neutral endopeptidase (NEP), an antigen expressed on the podocyte membrane.[2] In these cases, mothers with a hereditary absence of NEP become sensitized during pregnancy and passively transfer anti-NEP IgG to the infant, who is born with congenital nephrotic syndrome caused by MN through an alloimmune mechanism.[2] NEP has also been documented in glomerular deposits in some patients with *de novo* MN after renal transplantation but not in adult patients with idiopathic MN.[2] A particularly promising study in adults has identified antibody to

Conditions and Agents Associated with Membranous Nephropathy

Groups	Common	Uncommon
Immune diseases	Systemic lupus erythematosus, diabetes mellitus	Rheumatoid arthritis, Hashimoto's disease, Graves' disease, mixed connective tissue disease, Sjögren's syndrome, primary biliary cirrhosis, bullous pemphigoid, small bowel enteropathy syndrome, dermatitis herpetiformis, ankylosing spondylitis, graft-versus-host disease, Guillain-Barré syndrome, bone marrow and stem cell transplantation, anti-GBM and ANCA-positive crescentic GN
Infectious or parasitic diseases	Hepatitis B	Hepatitis C, syphilis, filariasis, hydatid disease, schistosomiasis, malaria, leprosy
Drugs and toxins	Gold, penicillamine, NSAIDs	Mercury, captopril, formaldehyde, hydrocarbons, bucillamine agents
Miscellaneous	Tumors, renal transplantation	Sarcoidosis, sickle cell disease, Kimura disease, angiofollicular lymph node hyperplasia

Figure 20.1 Conditions and agents associated with membranous nephropathy. The list excludes conditions for which only a single case has been reported or the lesions were atypical of membranous nephropathy. *(Modified with permission from reference 5.)*

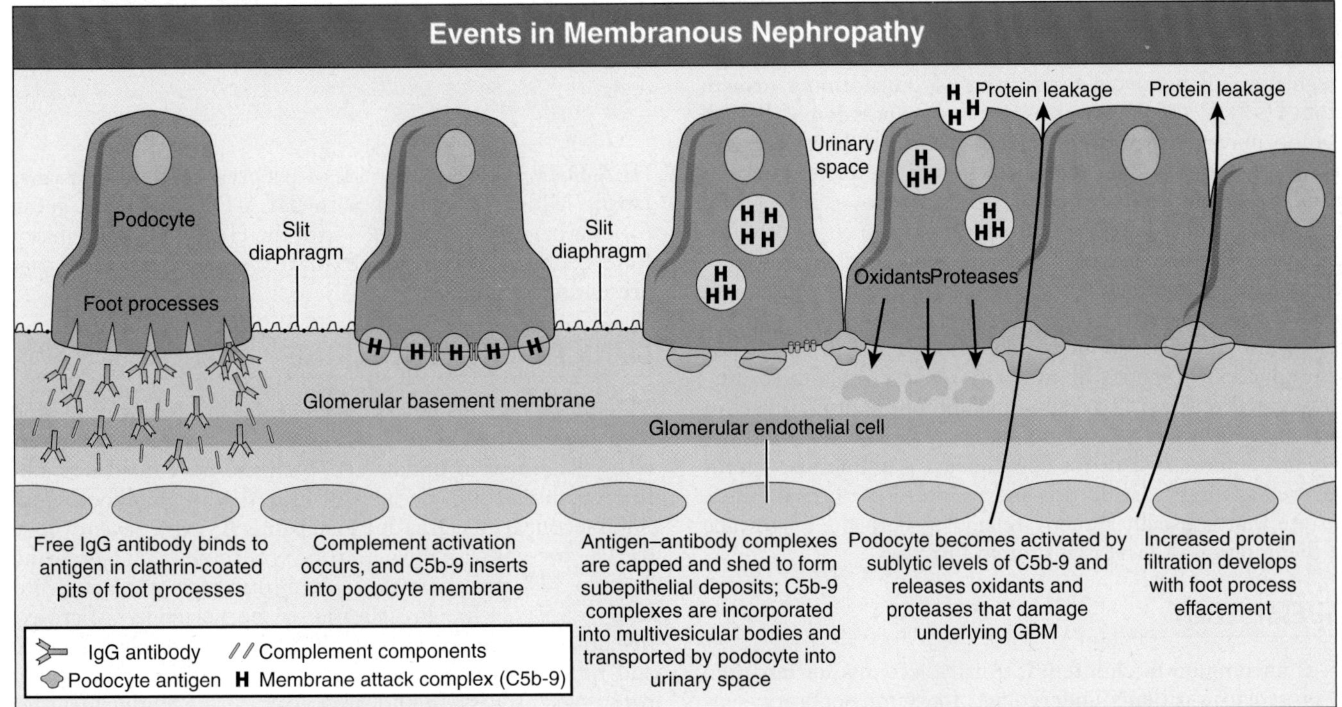

Figure 20.2 Events in a rat model of membranous nephropathy. Immune deposit formation, C5b-9 insertion, and podocyte activation lead to proteinuria (see text).

phospholipase A_2 receptor (PLAR), another antigen expressed on podocyte foot processes, in a majority of patients with active idiopathic MN and correlated antibody levels with disease activity and response to therapy.[6] This antibody has also been eluted from glomeruli of patients with MN. Anti-PLAR antibody has been identified only in primary idiopathic MN and not in MN secondary to other causes.

Mechanism of Glomerular Injury

Based entirely on studies in animal models, the mechanism of glomerular damage sufficient to cause proteinuria appears to involve sublytic effects of complement C5b-9 (a multimer comprising several complement components and also known as the membrane attack complex) on the podocyte,[4,7] although complement-independent mechanisms of proteinuria have also been described in some studies.[8] When complement activation occurs at the site of deposit formation, it leads to cleavage of C5, which generates C5a and C5b. C5b combines with C6 to form a lipophilic complex that inserts into the lipid bilayer of the podocyte, where C7, C8, and multiple C9 molecules are added to create a pore-forming complex, C5b-9. The podocyte is resistant to lysis and endocytoses the C5b-9, transporting the complex intracellularly in multivesicular bodies and extruding it into the urinary space. However, the membrane insertion of C5b-9, although insufficient to cause apoptosis or cell lysis, does induce cell activation and signal transduction. This results in increased production of multiple potentially nephritogenic molecules, including oxidants, proteases, cytokines, growth factors, vasoactive molecules, and extracellular matrix.[4,7] Current evidence is strongest for the role of podocyte-derived oxidants in producing the GBM damage that leads to increased protein filtration in MN. When antibody deposition, deposit formation, and complement activation are occurring, increased urinary excretion of C5b-9 and viable podocytes occurs.[9]

Consequences of Injury Induced by C5b-9

The glomerular injury mediated by C5b-9 induces a nonselective proteinuria through loss of both the size- and the charge-selective properties of the glomerular capillary wall. The subsequent reduction in glomerular filtration rate (GFR) that occurs in progressive MN has both glomerular and interstitial components. In the glomerulus, there is thickening of the GBM resulting from overproduction of several different extracellular matrix molecules that accumulate between and around the immune deposits to form the subepithelial "spikes" characteristic of this disease when a biopsy specimen is studied with silver methenamine staining (Fig. 20.5C). This appears to occur in part through upregulation of podocyte production of transforming growth factor (TGF) β2 and β3 as well as increased expression of TGF-β receptors in response to C5b-9.[7] Podocyte cell number decreases because of apoptosis and cell detachment as the glomerulus expands secondary to increased pressures and flows.[9] The podocyte itself has limited ability to proliferate and to cover denuded areas of GBM because of C5b-9–induced overexpression of cyclin kinase inhibitors and cell cycle arrest, and the consequent podocytopenia leads to progressive glomerulosclerosis. In the interstitium, there is an increased macrophage infiltrate and overproduction of matrix by interstitial myofibroblasts, leading to interstitial fibrosis,[3,10] a response common to all nonselective proteinuric disorders (see also Chapter 75). When nephrotic-range proteinuria persists, the consequence is glomerular sclerosis as well as interstitial fibrosis and progression to renal failure at a rate that is usually directly related to both the magnitude and the duration of increased protein filtration.

EPIDEMIOLOGY

MN is uncommon in children; it usually accounts for less than 5% of pediatric patients undergoing biopsy for nephrotic syndrome.[3] About 30% of all biopsy specimens for primary nephrotic syndrome reveal MN in adults and about 50% in older Caucasian adults.[1]

There is some variation in these figures among different countries, with slightly lower numbers in the United Kingdom and higher numbers in Greece and Macedonia. The United States Renal Data System in 2008 reported the incidence of end-stage renal disease (ESRD) due to MN from 2002 to 2006 at about 460 patients per year, which represents 0.4% of the total ESRD population.[11] Because only 20% of all patients with MN progress to ESRD, the real incidence of MN is approximately 2300 patients per year in the United States or about 8 patients per million population per year.

There is a threefold increased risk for MN in Caucasian patients with HLA-DR3, and associations with HLA-B8 and HLA-B18 have also been reported.[1] HLA-DR5, in addition to HLA-DR3, increases the risk of progression in Caucasians. In Japan, MN is associated with HLA-DR2. Some Caucasian patients have a deletion of C4 with the HLA-B8-DR3 haplotype. Rare examples of familial MN have also been reported, usually presenting in siblings.[3]

Clinical Features of Membranous Nephropathy
Rare in children – <5% of total cases of nephrotic syndrome
Common in adults – 15% to 50% of total cases of nephrotic syndrome, depending on age. Increasing frequency after age 40 years.
Males > females in all adults groups
Caucasians > Asians > African-Americans > Hispanics
Nephrotic syndrome in 60% to 70%
Normal or mildly elevated BP at presentation
"Benign" urinary sediment
Non-selective proteinuria
Tendency to thromboembolic disease (DVT, RVT, PE)
Secondary causes: infection, drugs, neoplasia, systemic lupus erythematosus

Figure 20.3 Clinical features of membranous nephropathy. BP, blood pressure; DVT, deep venous thrombosis; RVT, renal vein thrombosis; PE, pulmonary embolism.

CLINICAL MANIFESTATIONS

MN affects patients of all ages and races but is more common in men than in women by 2:1 (Fig. 20.3). Idiopathic MN is most often diagnosed in middle age, with the peak incidence during the fourth and fifth decades of life. MN in childhood is more often secondary (such as due to hepatitis B virus). Seventy percent to 80% present with the nephrotic syndrome.[12,13] The remaining 20% to 30% present with subnephrotic asymptomatic proteinuria (<3.5 g/24 h). Proteinuria is nonselective. Microscopic hematuria is common (30% to 40%), but macroscopic hematuria and red cell casts are rare and suggest a different glomerular pathologic process. In idiopathic MN, serum complement levels are normal despite evidence of intraglomerular complement activation, and serologic markers such as antinuclear antibodies, ANCA, and rheumatoid factor are normal or absent. At the time of diagnosis, only 10% to 20% have hypertension. Renal function is usually normal at presentation, with only a small fraction (<10%) presenting with renal impairment (Fig. 20.4). These presenting features can be modulated by age or preexisting hypertension; tubulointerstitial and vascular changes on biopsy may be related to these factors rather than to the severity of the MN.[14] This is supported by recent evidence that age *per se* does not influence the rate of progression in MN but does influence the GFR at presentation. Other complications related to the nephritic syndrome include dyslipidemia, which probably contributes to the increased cardiovascular risk, and a high prevalence (10% to 40%) of thromboembolic events including renal vein thrombosis.

Diagnosis and Management of Patients with Membranous Nephropathy

Patient Groups	Test
All patients	Blood pressure Renal function (serum creatinine and creatinine clearance) Urine protein excretion (24-h urine or urine protein to creatinine ratio) Serum albumin Serum cholesterol Urinalysis Renal biopsy
Associated disease	Hepatitis B (HBs antigen) Hepatitis C (HCV antibody) Antinuclear antibody (ANA), anti-double-stranded DNA (the hallmark of systemic lupus erythematosus) Complement C3, C4 (usually normal in idiopathic membranous nephropathy)
Selected Patients	
With suspected thromboembolic events, flank pain, hematuria, acute renal failure	Renal venous Doppler ultrasound Contrast CT, MRI
With sudden decrease in renal function, development of active urine sediment	Anti-GBM antibody ANCA Assess for interstitial nephritis
Suggestive symptoms or >50 years of age	Cancer screening (see text)

Figure 20.4 Diagnosis and management of patients with membranous nephropathy. ANCA, antineutrophil cytoplasmic antibody; anti-GBM, anti–glomerular basement membrane; CT, computed tomography; MRI, magnetic resonance imaging.

PATHOLOGY

The earliest pathologic feature of MN relates to the initial formation of subepithelial immune complexes of IgG and complement along the outer surface of the capillary wall in which glomeruli appear histologically normal and therefore may be mistaken for minimal change nephrotic syndrome if only light microscopy is performed. After immune complex formation, changes occur first in the podocyte, then in glomerular barrier function leading to proteinuria, then in the renal interstitium (probably as a consequence of the proteinuria), and finally in the GBM itself, which becomes thickened (membranous) through the accumulation of additional matrix material along the outer surface, often in an irregular or spike-like pattern.[2,13]

Light Microscopy

In the earliest stages of the disease, the glomeruli and interstitium appear normal by light microscopy, and the diagnosis is made by immunohistology and electron microscopy (Fig. 20.5A). The next stage of MN involves a homogeneous thickening of the capillary wall, seen with light microscopy in sections stained with hematoxylin and eosin or with periodic acid–Schiff reagent (Fig. 20.5B). By silver methenamine staining, early projections of the GBM between deposits may be detected in a characteristic spike-like configuration (see Fig. 20.5C). Later lucencies may develop in the GBM as immune deposits are resorbed, resulting in some areas of the GBM appearing as double contours by silver methenamine staining.

Leukocyte infiltration is absent in glomeruli in MN, probably because chemotactic products of complement activation follow filtration forces into the urinary space rather than diffusing backward into the capillary lumen, and the intervening GBM prevents immune adherence mechanisms from being operative. Although similar deposits at other sites may induce proliferation of glomerular endothelial and, particularly, mesangial cells, podocytes *in vivo* seem terminally differentiated and rarely proliferate.[6] As a result, the pathologic lesion of MN is characterized only by changes in podocytes and basement membrane without any associated glomerular hypercellularity.

The podocyte response to this form of injury includes effacement of foot processes visible only by electron microscopy. In general, there are no visible mesangial or endothelial cell abnormalities. The presence of significant mesangial hypercellularity suggests immune deposit formation in the mesangium and is more consistent with a secondary MN, such as class V lupus nephritis (see Chapter 25). In some patients with heavy proteinuria and progressive disease, glomeruli exhibit reduced podocyte numbers and areas of focal sclerosis that are similar to the appearance of idiopathic focal segmental glomerulosclerosis (FSGS) (see Chapter 18). These patients often have a more rapidly progressive course and a poor response to therapy. These sclerotic lesions may be a consequence of glomerular hypertrophy accompanied by an inability of the terminally differentiated podocytes to proliferate,[7] leading to areas of denuded GBM, attachment to Bowman's capsule, and subsequent capillary collapse (see Chapter 75).

As in all glomerular diseases, tubulointerstitial injury is common and correlates with both the renal function and the level of proteinuria. Some studies suggest that the long-term outcome correlates in general with the severity of the tubulointerstitial damage (see Chapter 75).

Immunohistology

The pattern of IgG staining in MN is characteristic and easily recognizable by immunohistology (Fig. 20.6). Positive staining for IgG marks the finely granular subepithelial deposits, which

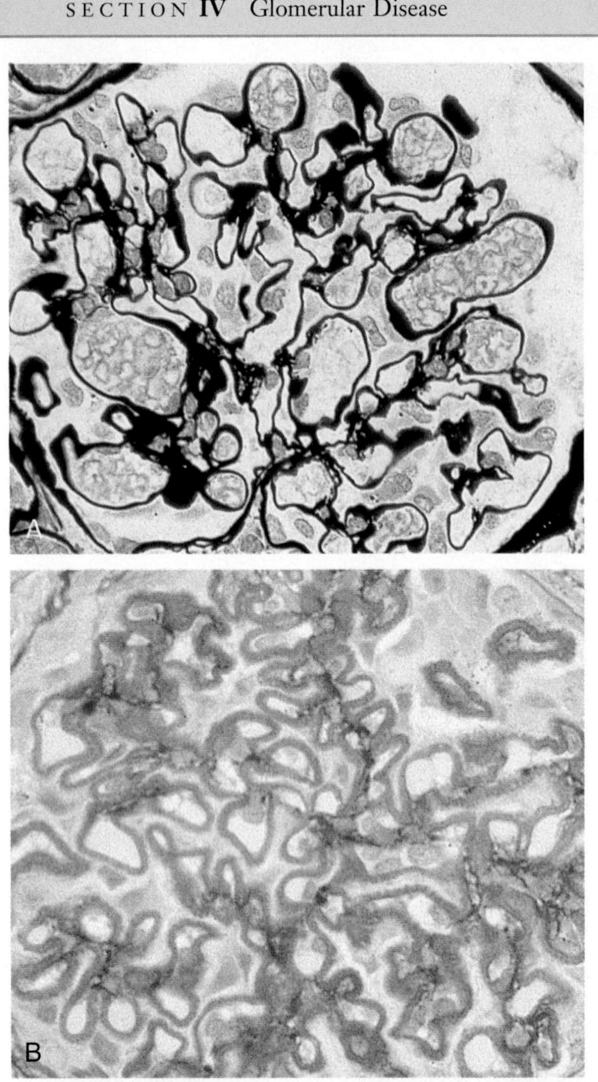

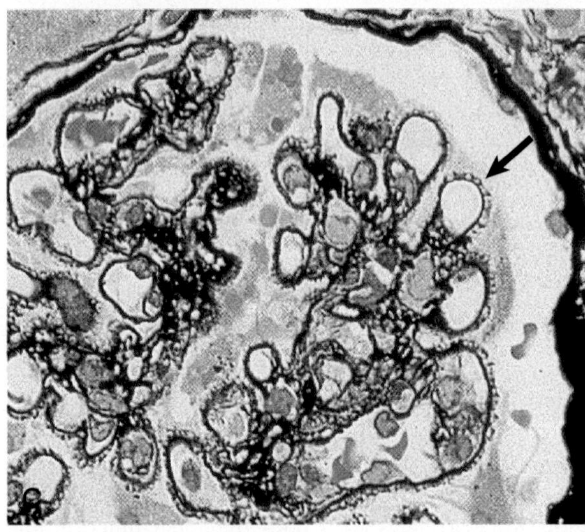

Figure 20.5 Light microscopy in membranous nephropathy. **A,** Early MN: a glomerulus from a patient with severe nephrotic syndrome and early MN exhibiting normal architecture and peripheral capillary basement membranes of normal thickness. (Silver methenamine; magnification ×400.) **B,** Morphologically advanced MN: uniform increase in the thickness of the glomerular capillary walls throughout the glomerulus without any increase in glomerular cellularity. (Periodic acid–Schiff; magnification ×400.) **C,** Morphologically more advanced MN (same patient as in **B**): discrete spikes of matrix emanating from the outer surface of the basement membrane *(arrow)* indicative of advanced MN are revealed by silver methenamine stain. (Magnification ×400.) *(Courtesy C. E. Alpers.)*

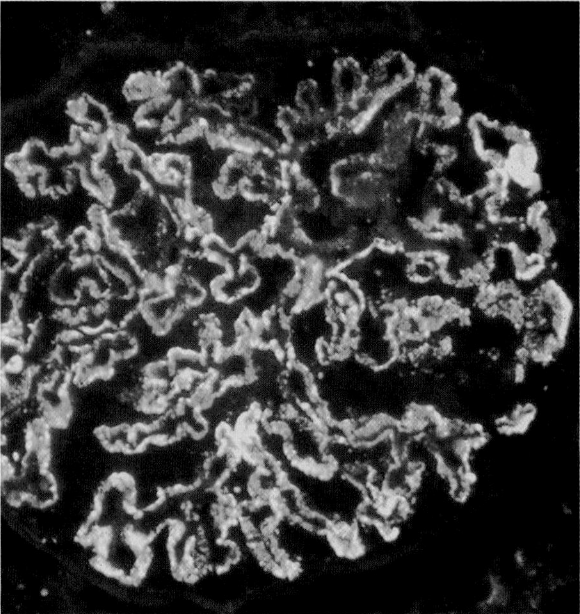

Figure 20.6 Immunofluorescence in membranous nephropathy. A glomerulus with diffuse, finely granular deposition of IgG along the outer surface of all capillary walls. The antibody is believed to represent autoantibody directed at some constituent of the podocyte membrane. (Original magnification ×400). *(Courtesy C. E. Alpers.)*

are present on the outer surface of all capillary walls.[2] The predominant IgG subclass in idiopathic MN is IgG4. Positive staining for IgG1 or IgG3, IgA, or IgM or significant staining in the glomerular mesangium suggests lupus as an underlying mechanism. Complement C3 is also present in about 50% of patients and usually reflects staining for C3c, a breakdown product of C3b that is rapidly cleared. Consequently, positive C3 staining probably reflects active, ongoing immune deposit formation and complement activation at the time of the biopsy, whereas the absence of C3 suggests that the process of forming deposits has ceased. When it is looked for, staining for C5b-9 is generally present as well, consistent with the proposed pathogenetic role of C5b-9 in this disease.[2,7] C1 and C4 are often absent, indicating activation of complement primarily through the alternative pathway as a consequence of podocyte damage or downregulation of complement regulatory proteins expressed on the podocyte membrane.

Electron Microscopy

The presence of subepithelial electron-dense deposits by electron microscopy parallels IgG staining. In idiopathic MN, immune deposit formation occurs in a subepithelial distribution, and deposits are not seen in mesangial or subendothelial sites. These deposits in early stages of the disease process are homogeneous and may even be confluent in some areas with overlying podocyte foot process effacement and little change in the underlying GBM (stage I). As the disease persists, there is projection of basement membrane material up between the deposits to form subepithelial spikes that can be detected by light microscopy with use of a silver methenamine stain and are easily visible by electron microscopy (stage II; Fig. 20.7A). Later, the spikes extend and the deposits may become surrounded by new basement membrane–like material (stage III; Fig. 20.7B). In stage IV disease, the basement membrane is overtly thickened, the

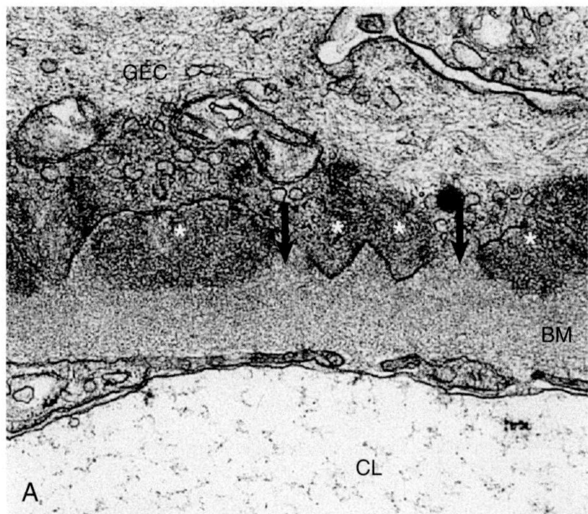

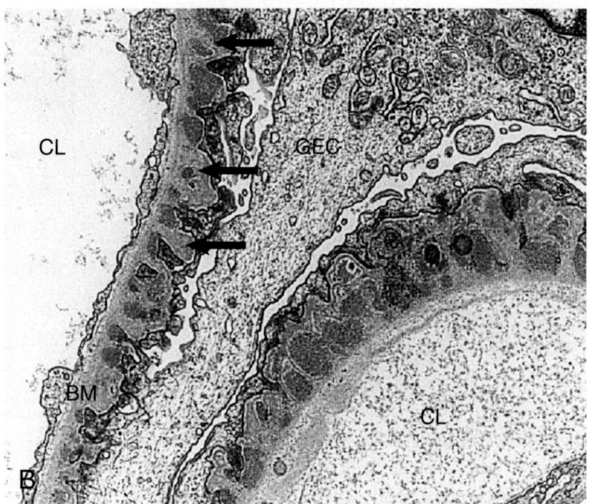

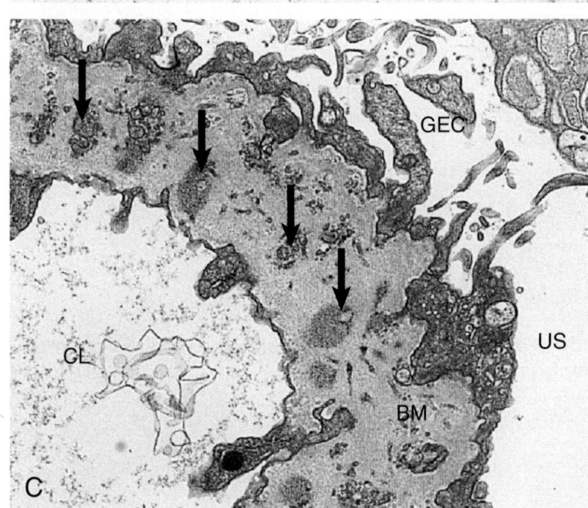

Figure 20.7 Electron microscopy in membranous nephropathy. A, Early (stage II) disease: glomerular capillary wall with discrete electron-dense deposits on the subepithelial surface of the basement membrane (BM) corresponding to granular deposits of IgG detected by immunofluorescence microscopy (corresponding to the light micrograph in Fig. 20.5B). There are diffuse, granular immune complex deposits *(asterisks)* along the outer surface of the capillary wall with effacement of overlying podocyte foot processes. Small extensions of BM between deposits *(arrows)* are also evident and represent the projections that are seen as spikes by light microscopy with silver methenamine staining. CL, capillary lumen; GEC, glomerular epithelial cell. **B,** More advanced disease (stage III): two glomerular capillary loops showing involvement of *(arrows)* the BM by the immune complex deposition. There is prominent membrane synthesis surrounding and incorporating these deposits into the BM (corresponding to the spikes seen on silver-stained histologic preparations). Overlying cells continue to demonstrate widespread effacement of foot processes. **C,** Morphologically advanced MN (stage IV): the capillary BM is diffusely thickened; scattered electron-dense immune deposits *(arrows)* are present throughout its thickness in addition to scattered subepithelial deposits. Overlying GECs continue to demonstrate effacement of foot processes. US, urinary space. (Original magnifications ×18,000.) *(Courtesy C. E. Alpers.)*

deposits incorporated in it become more lucent, and the spikes are less apparent (Fig. 20.7C). The extent to which individual patients will exhibit these stages as sequential changes depends on the duration of the underlying immunopathologic process and its severity. Although these changes clearly reflect the severity and duration of disease, they do not correlate well with clinical manifestations or outcome.

DIAGNOSIS AND DIFFERENTIAL DIAGNOSIS

When the initial presentation includes the nephrotic syndrome, the differential diagnosis includes minimal change disease (MCD), FSGS, membranoproliferative glomerulonephritis (MPGN) type I and dense deposit disease (DDD), amyloidosis, light-chain deposition disease, lupus nephritis, and diabetic nephropathy. In the 20% to 25% whose initial presentation is asymptomatic proteinuria, the differential is even more extensive.[15] Whereas clinical clues may increase the likelihood for one etiology over another, the etiology of the nephrotic syndrome is best determined by renal biopsy.

Patients presenting with clinical features including less than 3.5 g/day of proteinuria, no red cell casts, no hypertension, normal renal function, and no systemic features suggestive of a secondary cause have a relatively benign prognosis. If no renal biopsy is performed, these patients must be monitored because up to 50% may later develop nephrotic-range proteinuria, the majority within the first 2 years of presentation.

Secondary MN represents 20% to 30% of all cases (see Fig. 20.1); the most common causes are systemic lupus, hepatitis B, malignant neoplasms, and drugs. In addition to a careful history and physical examination, appropriate laboratory evaluation for potential secondary causes should include a complement profile, antinuclear antibodies, hepatitis serology, chest radiography, stool testing for occult blood, mammography in women, and prostate-specific antigen testing with or without digital rectal examination in men. In women between the ages of 20 and 50 years, a high index of suspicion is warranted for underlying lupus.[1] This diagnosis can be particularly difficult to make because the majority of these patients have no systemic symptoms and serologic markers of systemic lupus erythematosus are often absent. Membranous lupus accounts for 8% to 27% of cases of lupus nephritis (see Chapter 25).[1]

In adults, regardless of age, malignant neoplasia is the most common secondary cause of MN (see Fig. 20.1). The colon, kidney, and lung are the most common primary sites, and in some patients, the tumor may not have been discovered at the time the patient presents with renal disease. Although it is hypothesized that antigens derived from the tumor account for deposit formation and injury in glomeruli, very few tumor-related antigens have actually been demonstrated.

Hepatitis B (HBV)–associated MN is also a very common secondary cause in countries where HBV is endemic. It can affect both adults and children who are chronic carriers of HBV (positive HBsAg, HBcAg, and usually HBeAg).[16] This can occur with or without a history of overt liver disease. In children, HBV-associated MN most commonly presents as the nephrotic syndrome and usually follows a benign course.[3] In adults, progressive renal impairment is a more common outcome. Hypocomplementemia is present in approximately 50% of cases of MN with HBV.

MN secondary to drugs usually resolves after discontinuation of the offending agent.[17,18] The time to resolution, however, varies significantly from as early as 1 week (e.g., for NSAIDs) to several years for gold or D-penicillamine. Many other renal disorders have been seen in association with or superimposed on MN, including IgA nephropathy, FSGS, crescentic GN (anti-GBM disease, ANCA vasculitis), acute interstitial nephritis, and diabetic nephropathy.

CLINICAL COURSE, OUTCOMES, AND COMPLICATIONS

The clinical course of MN varies widely. Spontaneous remissions in proteinuria have been reported in up to 30% of cases. As the severity of proteinuria at presentation increases, the frequency of spontaneous remission appears to decrease. Female sex and lower grade (non-nephrotic) proteinuria at presentation are the only two features associated with a higher likelihood of spontaneous remission.[19] This is likely to produce a bias in renal survival because the majority of studies reporting 10-year outcomes in untreated patients have included those with subnephrotic proteinuria (<3.5 g/24 h). For example, one study reported a 72% renal survival at 8 years for 100 untreated patients, but 37% of the patients were non-nephrotic at presentation and more than 50% had less than 5 g/day.[20] In addition, deaths were excluded from the kidney survival analysis. Even so, there was a 25% ESRD rate by 8 years and almost 50% by 15 years.

In summary, although the majority of MN patients do reasonably well long term, MN is still the second or third leading cause of ESRD among subjects with primary GN. What is still missing from most MN survival data is the much higher than expected (standard incidence ratio) death rate due to cardiovascular disease or thromboembolic events seen in patients who remain nephrotic. When another renal condition is superimposed on MN, there is often an associated acceleration in the rate of deterioration in renal function. The most common conditions to consider in this setting are drug-induced interstitial nephritis, superimposed anti-GBM disease, and renal vein thrombosis.

Predictors of Poor Outcome

Given the wide variation in the natural history of MN and the current lack of a serologic marker of disease activity, other clinical markers that predict individual outcome would be valuable. A list of factors associated with progression and the strength of those associations is presented in Figure 20.8. Both age and sex influence outcome, with male sex and increasing age associated with a higher risk for renal failure. However, both have limitations.[21] Age seems to be related to the underlying pathologic process at the time of presentation rather than to the severity of disease because it does not influence rate of deterioration in function, and the sex of the patient seems more closely related

Factors Associated with Worse Renal Survival in Membranous Nephropathy

Factors	Predictor	Positive Predictive Value %
Clinical features		
Age	Older > younger	43
Sex	Male > female	30
HLA type	HLA/B18/DR 3/Bffl present	71
Hypertension	Present	39
Serum albumin	<1.5 g/dL	56
Serum creatinine	Above normal	61
Urine protein		
Nephrotic syndrome	Present	32
Proteinuria	>8 g for >6 months	66
IgG excretion	>250 mg/day	80
β2-Microglobulin excretion	>0.5 μg/min	79
C5b-9 excretion	>7 μg/mg creatinine	67
Biopsy changes		
Glomerular focal sclerosis	Present	34
Tubulointerstitial disease	Present	48
Electron microscopic stage III, IV	Present	67

Figure 20.8 Factors associated with worse renal survival in membranous nephropathy. Factors associated with increased likelihood of progression and their predictive value. (Positive predictive values modified from references 22 and 23.)

to the severity of proteinuria at presentation rather than representing an independent risk factor for progression. The severity of chronic changes seen on the biopsy specimen (i.e., degree of glomerulosclerosis, tubulointerstitial fibrosis, and vascular disease) has been associated with a poor prognosis but more closely reflects initial GFR than the subsequent rate of renal functional deterioration.[14] Other pathologic features, including the percentage of glomeruli with glomerulosclerosis and the configuration of the immune deposits (synchronic/single stage or heterogeneous/multistage) on electron microscopy, have also been suggested as predictors of both outcome and response to treatment but have not been validated in prospective studies. The degree of renal impairment at presentation has also been found to correlate with long-term renal survival, but a better and more sensitive predictor of long-term prognosis is the ongoing rate of renal function loss as measured by the decline of creatinine clearance over time.

One of the best models to calculate risk takes into consideration the initial creatinine clearance, the slope of the creatinine clearance during a fixed period, and the lowest level of proteinuria during that observation period (Fig. 20.9).[22] This risk score assessment has a reported sensitivity of 60% to 89%, specificity of 86% to 92%, and overall accuracy from 79% to 87%. The model predicts that patients with a normal creatinine clearance at presentation that remains stable during 6 months and with persistent proteinuria of less than 4 g/24 h have less than a 5% chance of progression, and only conservative treatment is recommended. In contrast, those patients with proteinuria that remains

Renal Disease Risk Categories		
Low Risk	**Medium Risk**	**High Risk**
Normal serum creatinine and creatinine clearance plus proteinuria <4 g/day over six months of observation	Normal or near normal creatinine clearance and persistent proteinuria ≥4 g/day to ≤8 g/day over 6 months despite maximum conservative treatment	Deteriorating renal function and/or persistent proteinuria ≥8 g/day for <3–6 months of observation

Figure 20.9 Risk categories of renal disease progression in membranous nephropathy.

above 4 g but less than 8 g/24 h during the same time frame have a 55% probability for development of chronic renal impairment; and those with persistent proteinuria above 8 g/24 h have a 66% to 80% probability of progression to chronic kidney disease within 10 years (see Fig. 20.9). Recently, other biomarkers including urinary α_1-microglobulin, β_2-microglobulin, IgM, and IgG have also been strongly associated with progression.[23] These markers measured together at a single time point have a higher positive predictive value than proteinuria alone, but none has yet been validated in an independent data set.

Relapse After Complete Remission or Partial Remission

Relapse from a complete remission occurs in approximately 25% to 40% of MN cases with an unpredictable time line. Relapses have been reported up to 20 years after the primary remission. However, the great majority of patients will relapse only with subnephrotic-range proteinuria and will maintain stable long-term kidney function with conservative management alone.[19] In contrast, the relapse rate is as high as 50% in those achieving only a partial remission. Achievement of either a complete or partial remission, however, significantly slows progression and increases renal survival. A recent review of 348 nephrotic MN patients documented a 10-year renal survival in patients with a complete remission of 100%; with partial remission, 90%; and with no remission, only 45%.[24]

TREATMENT

Nonimmunosuppressive Therapy

Conservative management is directed at control of edema, hypertension, hyperlipidemia, and proteinuria and is similar to that used for nephrotic syndrome of any etiology (see Chapter 15). Blood pressure control is important for both renal and cardiovascular protection. For patients with proteinuria of more than 1 g/day, the target for blood pressure is 125/75 mm Hg.[25] Numerous studies have shown that angiotensin-converting enzyme (ACE) inhibitors and angiotensin receptor blockers (ARBs) are cardioprotective and can reduce proteinuria and slow progression of renal disease in both diabetic and nondiabetic chronic nephropathy patients (see Chapter 76). A recent meta-analysis of the largest renal protection trials using ACE inhibitors showed that the degree of protection is closely correlated to the degree of proteinuria reduction. None of these studies has focused on the specific effect of renin-angiotensin system (RAS) blockade in MN. In secondary analyses, the number with MN has been small, and although the use of ACE inhibitors has been associated with significant improvement in some series, their antiproteinuric effect was modest (<30% reduction in proteinuria) in others.[26] When effective, the benefit of RAS blockade occurs early, usually within the first 3 months of initiation of treatment. Even patients at low risk for progression (proteinuria <4 g/24 h) should be treated with ACE inhibitors or ARBs because this may reduce proteinuria and offer additional renal protection with little chance of significant adverse effect. Patients must also follow a low-salt diet to achieve the maximum benefit from RAS blockade.

Proteinuria is also an independent risk factor for cardiovascular morbidity and mortality. When the proteinuria is in the nephrotic range, there is a clear increase in cardiovascular risk, with a threefold to fivefold increase in both coronary events and death rates in this population.[27] Patients with significant proteinuria almost always have elevated serum cholesterol and triglyceride levels. Although it is not proven, we recommend the use of statins to reduce low-density lipoprotein cholesterol to 100 mg/dl (2 mmol/l) or lower (see Chapters 76 and 78).[28,29]

It is recommended that both RAS blockade and lipid control be initiated early in the MN patients, although reaching a goal of complete remission or even partial remission in patients at higher risk of progression (with persistent proteinuria >5 g/24 h) with conservative treatment alone is unlikely. Dietary protein intake may be restricted to 0.8 g/kg body weight per day of high-quality protein[25] with additional dietary protein (gram per gram) to correct for urinary losses. Dietary protein restriction has been associated with reduced proteinuria (15% to 25%) and a slowing in renal disease progression but has never been shown to induce a complete remission or to add to effects obtained with RAS blockade. Protein restriction must be carefully monitored in nephrotic patients to avoid malnutrition.

Patients with severe nephrotic syndrome are at increased risk for thromboembolic complications, and prophylactic anticoagulation has been shown in retrospective reviews to be beneficial in reducing fatal thromboembolic episodes in nephrotic patients with MN without a concomitant increase in the risk of bleeding.[30] However, no randomized controlled trial has ever been done. Hence, there is no current consensus about prophylactic anticoagulation (see also Chapter 15) and no laboratory test that can predict with any accuracy such an event in any one patient. Certain clinical scenarios do have a higher likelihood of such an event and thus deserve more careful physician monitoring. These include patients with severe and persistent nephrotic syndrome (proteinuria >10 g/day and serum albumin <2.5 g/day). The majority of practicing nephrologists, however, will still wait until a primary thromboembolic event has occurred before using anticoagulants.

Other agents that have been tried with modest effects in small numbers of patients include probucol,[31] a lipid peroxidation scavenger, and high-dose intravenous immune globulin, an agent with multiple effects on antibody-mediated tissue injury.[32]

Immunosuppressive Therapy

Several regimens using a variety of immunosuppressive agents have been shown to be successful in reducing proteinuria in MN, but many questions remain unresolved: What should be the duration of conservative therapy while awaiting a spontaneous remission? How is it determined when to initiate immunosuppressive therapy? What is the most effective and safest of the available agents? and How long should treatment be given before futility is assessed?[33]

Corticosteroids

There have been three randomized controlled trials (RCTs) of corticosteroids in the treatment of idiopathic MN.[34,35] The overall consensus has been no significant long-term beneficial effect on proteinuria, rate of disease progression, or renal survival. The use of oral corticosteroids as a single agent for the treatment of MN is therefore not recommended. The one exception may be the Asian population, in which long-term observational studies have indicated improvement in both proteinuria and renal function preservation with use of corticosteroids as monotherapy.[36]

Cytotoxic Agents Combined with Corticosteroids

In patients at moderate risk of progression, a significant benefit has been described with the combination of a daily oral dose of a cytotoxic agent (either cyclophosphamide or chlorambucil) alternating monthly with corticosteroids (methylprednisolone pulses 3 × 1 g, intravenously, at months 1, 3, and 5; and oral prednisone, 0.5 mg/kg on alternate days for 6 months)[37-39]; complete or partial remission of the nephrotic syndrome was seen in close to 80% of treated patients, a threefold to fourfold increase compared with the control group. Both progression rate and renal survival were significantly improved. Both treatment regimens were remarkably safe, although relapses were seen within 2 years in 30% of the treatment group. Very similar results were obtained in an RCT (n = 93) using this same regimen to treat MN patients of Asian ethnicity.[40] Because the results of a cyclophosphamide-based regimen were similar to one based on chlorambucil,[40] cyclophosphamide is most commonly used because of a better safety profile.

The only RCT (n = 26) using cytotoxic agents in patients at high risk of progression (mean creatinine, 2.3 to 2.7 mg/day; proteinuria, 11 g/day) noted no statistical differences in proteinuria, remission rate, or rate of decline of renal function between the corticosteroid-alone and the combined treatment group.[41] However, this RCT employed monthly intravenous doses of cyclophosphamide rather than the oral regimen used in the Italian and Indian studies.

In older, smaller studies, these cytotoxic agents, even with appropriate adjustments in dose, have produced variable effects on outcome and significant adverse events in a high percentage of patients.[42-44] The most recent longer term studies in high-risk patients prospectively studied 65 patients with MN and serum creatinine concentration above 1.5 mg/dl treated with oral cyclophosphamide for 12 months and corticosteroids (same scheme as before).[45,46] Renal survival was 86% after 5 years and 74% after 7 years. Partial remission occurred in 56 patients. The relapse rate was similar to earlier cytotoxic-corticosteroid regimens, 30% at 5 years. Treatment-related complications were significant and occurred in two thirds of patients, mainly bone marrow suppression and infections. The majority of adverse events could be handled by dose reduction, although some required permanent discontinuation of treatment.

A recent meta-analysis showed that the use of alkylating agents was associated with higher remission rates (partial or complete remission), but no statistical benefit of cytotoxic drug therapy was demonstrated compared with placebo in rates of ESRD or death.[47] The difficulty with this type of analysis is that the endpoint of renal survival is far beyond the termination point of most clinical trials.

In summary, cyclophosphamide used in combination with corticosteroids appears to be effective in the treatment of patients with nephrotic-range proteinuria due to idiopathic MN, especially if renal function is well preserved at the time of initiation of therapy. This combination may work even in those with impaired renal function, but the supporting data are much less compelling, adverse effects are higher, and the likelihood of benefit is reduced, especially in patients with advanced renal failure (GFR <30 ml/min).[46] The favorable effects are maintained beyond the 1-year treatment period, but relapse rates approach 35% by 2 years. The adverse effects of cyclophosphamide when it is used long term are the major drawbacks to the universal application of this form of therapy. These include increased susceptibility to infections, anemia, thrombocytopenia, nausea, vomiting, sterility, and, in the long-term, malignant disease. Recent evidence suggests that the risk of cancer is accelerated at a much lower level of exposure than previously considered; the standardized incidence ratio was increased in a number of malignant neoplasms with total cyclophosphamide exposure as low as 36 g (approximately equivalent to 100 mg/day for 1 year).[48]

Calcineurin Inhibitors

Early uncontrolled studies using cyclosporine suggested an initial benefit but a high relapse rate. Cyclosporine may reduce proteinuria not only through its immunosuppressive effects but also by direct effects on the podocyte. In a single blind RCT, 51 patients with corticosteroid-resistant MN were treated for 6 months with cyclosporine (2 to 5 mg/kg) plus low-dose prednisone and compared with placebo plus prednisone.[49] Complete remission and partial remission were seen in 75% of cyclosporine-treated patients versus 22% of the placebo controls. Cyclosporine was well tolerated, and no adverse events requiring discontinuation of treatment were seen. However, relapses were common at 45% within 1 year after discontinuation of treatment. There has been only one RCT using cyclosporine in patients with high-grade proteinuria and progressive renal failure.[50] A reduction in both proteinuria and rate of loss of renal function was seen with cyclosporine compared with placebo that was sustained for up to 2 years after the drug was discontinued. Treatment with longer term cyclosporine (i.e., 12 months) has resulted in a higher rate of complete remission and partial remission (84%). In addition, persistence of remission was maintained with doses of cyclosporine as low as 1 to 2 mg/kg, although relapses were still common if the cyclosporine level fell below 100 ng/ml. Time to remission with use of cyclosporine varies from a few weeks to several months. This suggests that if no significant reduction in proteinuria (<40%) is noted within 3 to 4 months, a change in therapy may be warranted.

Significant adverse effects seen with this agent include hypertension, gingival hyperplasia, gastrointestinal complaints, muscle cramps, and, most important, nephrotoxicity, which is dose and duration of treatment dependent. Patients at particular risk are those with initial impaired renal function, especially if it is accompanied by extensive intrarenal vascular disease or chronic tubulointerstitial damage on biopsy.

In a recently completed 12-month RCT (n = 48), tacrolimus monotherapy was compared with a control group.[51] Proteinuria remission was 76% with tacrolimus versus 35% in the control group, and progression rate was also substantially slowed by the calcineurin inhibitor. The relapse rate after stopping of the drug, however, approached 50% by the end of 2 years of follow-up.

Mycophenolate Mofetil

Studies using mycophenolate mofetil (MMF) in MN have produced conflicting results. However, even in the most optimistic study, although initial response was high (used in combination with prednisone), the relapse rate within months approached 50%. The most pessimistic study (the only RCT), in comparison to conservative management only, showed no difference in remission rates.[52,53] Follow-up time was limited and the numbers in the latter study were small, but the reason behind the marked differences between these two trials is not obvious. In a small retrospective study in corticosteroid-resistant Asian MN patients, a higher response with MMF was observed, partial remission rate approaching 50%, possibly related to the ethnic characteristics of the population studied. The role of MMF in the treatment of MN is currently uncertain.

Rituximab

In several pilot studies, rituximab, despite substantial variations in the dose and timing of the drug, consistently reduced proteinuria by 60% to 70%.[54-56] The relapse rate, however, may be significantly less than with calcineurin inhibitor or cytotoxic-based regimens. The best predictor of which patients will respond to rituximab is unknown, although the absence of interstitial disease on the biopsy specimen may improve response rate. An RCT needs to be done before widespread use of this agent is advocated, given its very high cost and unknown long-term toxicity in this disease.

Eculizumab

Eculizumab is a humanized anti-C5 monoclonal antibody designed to prevent the cleavage of C5 into its proinflammatory byproducts. An RCT in 200 patients with MN that compared this agent with placebo during a total of 16 weeks showed no significant effect on proteinuria or renal function, but effective complement inhibition was not achieved.[57]

Adrenocorticotropic Hormone

Two small studies have reported the use of an intramuscular long-acting synthetic form of adrenocorticotropic hormone (ACTH) in MN.[58,59] The exact mechanism of action of this agent in MN is unknown but likely unrelated to corticosteroid effects because corticosteroids alone are not beneficial in MN. A dose escalation study showed prolonged remission in the majority of MN patients when they were treated with ACTH 1 to 2 mg weekly intramuscularly for a year. In a small RCT (n = 32), ACTH, with use of a similar dose regimen, was compared with a standard cytotoxic plus corticosteroids regimen. The remission rate was equal in the two groups, between 80% and 90%, but the relapse rate in the ACTH group was lower (14% versus 30%) after a follow-up of 1 year. Side effects of ACTH were few and included fluid retention, sleep disturbances, and bronze discoloration of the skin. Potassium supplementation was required in the majority of patients in one trial.[58]

Treatment Summary

Control of proteinuria, specifically achieving either a complete or partial remission of the nephrotic syndrome, is associated with prolonged renal survival and a slower rate of renal disease progression in MN. Supportive or conservative care should be given in all cases first and should include the use of diuretics, antihypertensive agents such as ACE inhibitors and ARBs (potentially renal protective), and lipid-lowering agents. In

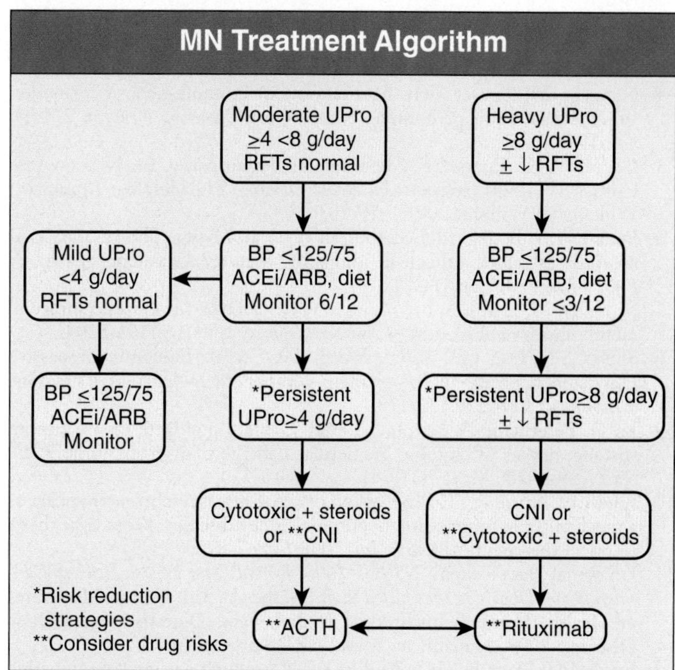

Figure 20.10 Algorithm for the treatment of membranous nephropathy. Details of possible therapies are discussed in the text. ACEi, ACE inhibitor; ACTH, adrenocorticotropic hormone; ARB, angiotensin receptor blocker; BP, blood pressure; CNI, calcineurin inhibitor; RFT, renal function test; UPro, urinary protein.

patients who require disease-specific therapy, the choice of agents remains controversial. A suggested management algorithm based on the level and persistence of proteinuria is outlined in Figure 20.10.

Both cytotoxic-corticosteroid combinations and calcineurin inhibitors have proved effective in reducing proteinuria in moderate or high-risk MN patients. The physician, in concert with the patient, must take into account all factors related to risk-benefit to arrive at the best decision about which of these therapies should be used first. These approaches are not mutually exclusive and can be used in sequence if the first one chosen does not succeed in inducing a remission or adverse effects are untenable. Ideally, one should leave 2 to 3 months between treatment regimens to help immune system recovery. Alternatively, a second course of the same immunosuppressive regimen could be used, but at the potential cost of cumulative toxicity, or a switch to another treatment regimen may be indicated if the patient's risk profile has changed. Preliminary evidence on the use of rituximab or long-acting ACTH suggests that both may be effective, and safer, than our current regimens, but both need to be assessed further before being widely recommended. Patients with severe renal impairment (GFR <30 ml/min) are less likely to benefit from immunosuppressive therapy, and the risks of treatment may favor conservative therapy as the best option for these patients

REFERENCES

1. Fervenza FC, Sethi S, Specks U. Idiopathic membranous nephropathy. Diagnosis and treatment. *Clin J Am Soc Nephrol.* 2008;3:905-919.
2. Ronco P, Debiec H. Target antigens and nephritogenic antibodies in membranous nephropathy: Of rats and men. *Semin Immunopathol.* 2007;4:445-458.

3. Jefferson AJ, Couser WG. Membranous nephropathy in the pediatric population. In: Avner E, Harmon W, Niaudet P, Yoshikawa N, eds. *Pediatric Nephrology*. 6th ed. Philadelphia: Springer; 2009:799-814.
4. Nangaku M, Couser WG. Mechanisms of immune-deposit formation and the mediation of immune renal injury. *Clin Exp Nephrol*. 2005;9: 183-191.
5. Couser WG, Alpers CE. Membranous nephropathy. In: Neilson EG, Couser WG, eds. *Immunologic Renal Diseases*. Philadelphia: Lippincott Williams & Wilkins; 2001:1029-1036.
6. Beck LH Jr, Bonegio RG, Lambeau G, et al. M-type phospholipase A_2 receptor as target antigen in idiopathic membranous nephropathy. *N Engl J Med*. 2009;361:11-21.
7. Nangaku M, Shankland SJ, Couser WG. Cellular response to injury in membranous nephropathy. *J Am Soc Nephrol*. 2005;16:1195-1204.
8. Spicer ST, Tran GT, Killingsworth MC, et al. Induction of passive Heymann nephritis in complement component 6–deficient PVG rats. *J Immunol*. 2007;179:172-178.
9. Yu D, Petermann A, Kunter U, et al. Urinary podocyte loss is a more specific marker of ongoing glomerular damage than proteinuria. *J Am Soc Nephrol*. 2005;16:1733-1741.
10. Fine LG, Norman JT. Progression of renal disease. Chronic hypoxia as a mechanism of progression of chronic kidney diseases: From hypothesis to novel therapeutics. *Kidney Int*. 2008;74:867-872.
11. US Renal Data System. *USRDS 2008 Annual Data Report. Atlas of End-Stage Renal Disease in the United States*. Bethesda, Md: National Institutes of Health, National Institute of Diabetes and Digestive and Kidney Diseases; 2008. Available at: www.USRDS.org/ref/htm.
12. Erwin DT, Donadio JV Jr, Holley KE. The clinical course of idiopathic membranous nephropathy. *Mayo Clin Proc*. 1973;48:697-712.
13. Gluck MC, Gallo G, Lowenstein J, Baldwin DS. Membranous glomerulonephritis. Evolution of clinical and pathologic features. *Ann Intern Med*. 1973;78:1-12.
14. Troyanov S, Roasio L, Pandes M, et al. Renal pathology in idiopathic membranous nephropathy: A new perspective. *Kidney Int*. 2006;69: 1641-1648.
15. Haas M, Meehan SM, Karrison TG, Spargo BH. Changing etiologies of unexplained adult nephrotic syndrome: A comparison of renal biopsy findings from 1976-1979 and 1995-1997. *Am J Kidney Dis*. 1997;30: 621-631.
16. Lai KN, Li PK, Lui SF, et al. Membranous nephropathy related to hepatitis B virus in adults. *N Engl J Med*. 1991;324:1457-1463.
17. Hall CL, Jawad S, Harrison PR, et al. Natural course of penicillamine nephropathy: A long term study of 33 patients. *Br Med J Clin Res Ed*. 1988;296:1083-1086.
18. Radford MG Jr, Holley KE, Grande JP, et al. Reversible membranous nephropathy associated with the use of nonsteroidal anti-inflammatory drugs. *JAMA*. 1996;276:466-469.
19. Ponticelli C, Passerini P, Altieri P, et al. Remissions and relapses in idiopathic membranous nephropathy. *Nephrol Dial Transplant*. 1992; 7(Suppl 1):85-90.
20. Schieppati A, Mosconi L, Perna A, et al. Prognosis of untreated patients with idiopathic membranous nephropathy. *N Engl J Med*. 1993; 329:85-89.
21. Cattran D, Reich H, Beanlands H, et al, for the Genes, Gender and Glomerulonephritis Group. The impact of sex in primary glomerulonephritis. *Nephrol Dial Transplant*. 2008;23:2247-2253.
22. Cattran DC, Pei Y, Greenwood CM, et al. Validation of a predictive model of idiopathic membranous nephropathy: Its clinical and research implications. *Kidney Int*. 1997;51:901-907.
23. Branten AJ, du Buf-Vereijken PW, Klasen IS, et al. Urinary excretion of β_2-microglobulin and IgG predict prognosis in idiopathic membranous nephropathy: A validation study. *J Am Soc Nephrol*. 2005;16: 169-174.
24. Troyanov S, Wall CA, Miller JA, et al. Idiopathic membranous nephropathy: Definition and relevance of a partial remission. *Kidney Int*. 2004;66:1199-1205.
25. Klahr S, Levey AS, Beck GJ, et al. The effects of dietary protein restriction and blood-pressure control on the progression of chronic renal disease. Modification of Diet in Renal Disease Study Group. *N Engl J Med*. 1994;330:877-884.
26. Rostoker G, Ben Maadi A, Remy P, et al. Low-dose angiotensin-converting-enzyme inhibitor captopril to reduce proteinuria in adult idiopathic membranous nephropathy: A prospective study of long-term treatment. *Nephrol Dial Transplant*. 1995;10:25-29.
27. Ordonez JD, Hiatt RA, Killebrew EJ, Fireman BH. The increased risk of coronary heart disease associated the nephrotic syndrome. *Kidney Int*. 1993;44:638-642.
28. Vidt DG, Cressman MD, Harris S, et al. Rosuvastatin-induced arrest in progression of renal disease. *Cardiology*. 2004;102:52-60.
29. Verhulst A, D'Haese PC, De Broe ME. Inhibitors of HMG-CoA reductase reduce receptor-mediated endocytosis in human kidney proximal tubular cells. *J Am Soc Nephrol*. 2004;15:2249-2257.
30. Sarasin F, Schifferli J. Prophylactic oral anticoagulation in nephrotic patients with idiopathic membranous nephropathy. *Kidney Int*. 1994;45: 578-585.
31. Haas M, Mayer G, Wirnsberger G, et al. Antioxidant treatment of therapy-resistant idiopathic membranous nephropathy with probucol: A pilot study. *Wien Klin Wochenschrift*. 2002;114:143-147.
32. Yokoyama H, Goshima S, Wada T, et al. The short- and long-term outcomes of membranous nephropathy treated with intravenous immune globulin therapy. Kanazawa Study Group for Renal Diseases and Hypertension. *Nephrol Dial Transplant*. 1999;14:2379-2386.
33. Cattran D. Management of membranous nephropathy: When and what for treatment. *J Am Soc Nephrol*. 2005;16:1188-1194.
34. Cameron JS, Healy MJ, Adu D. The Medical Research Council trial of short-term high-dose alternate day prednisolone in idiopathic membranous nephropathy with nephrotic syndrome in adults. The MRC Glomerulonephritis Working Party. *Q J Medicine*. 1990;74:133-156.
35. Cattran DC, Delmore T, Roscoe J, et al. A randomized controlled trial of prednisone in patients with idiopathic membranous nephropathy. *N Engl J Med*. 1989;320:210-215.
36. Shiiki H, Saiton T, Nishitani T, et al. Prognosis and risk factors for idiopathic membranous nephropathy with nephritic syndrome in Japan. *Kidney Int*. 2004;65:1400-1407.
37. Ponticelli C, Altieri P, Scolari F, et al. A randomized study comparing methylprednisolone plus chlorambucil versus methylprednisolone plus cyclophosphamide in idiopathic membranous nephropathy. *J Am Soc Nephrol*. 1998;9:444-450.
38. Ponticelli C, Zucchelli P, Passerini P, Cesana B. Methylprednisolone plus chlorambucil as compared with methylprednisolone alone for the treatment of idiopathic membranous nephropathy. The Italian Idiopathic Membranous Nephropathy Treatment Study Group. *N Engl J Med*. 1992;327:599-603.
39. Ponticelli C, Zucchelli P, Passerini P, et al. A 10-year follow-up of a randomized study with methylprednisolone and chlorambucil in membranous nephropathy. *Kidney Int*. 1995;48:1600-1604.
40. Jha V, Ganguli A, Saha TK, et al. A randomized, controlled trial of steroids and cyclophosphamide in adults with nephrotic syndrome caused by idiopathic membranous nephropathy. *J Am Soc Nephrol*. 2007;18:1899-1904.
41. Falk RJ, Hogan SL, Muller KE, Jennette JC. Treatment of progressive membranous glomerulopathy. A randomized trial comparing cyclophosphamide and corticosteroids with corticosteroids alone. The Glomerular Disease Collaborative Network. *Ann Intern Med*. 1992;116:438-445.
42. Torres A, Dominguez-Gil B, Carreno A, et al. Conservative versus immunosuppressive treatment of patients with idiopathic membranous nephropathy. *Kidney Int*. 2002;61:219-227.
43. Branten AJ, Reichert LJ, Koene RA, Wetzels JF. Oral cyclophosphamide versus chlorambucil in the treatment of patients with membranous nephropathy and renal insufficiency. *Q J Med*. 1998;91:359-366.
44. Warwick GL, Geddes CG, Boulton-Jones JM. Prednisolone and chlorambucil therapy for idiopathic membranous nephropathy with progressive renal failure. *Q J Med*. 1994;87:223-229.
45. du Buf-Vereijken PW, Branten AJ, Wetzels JF. Cytotoxic therapy for membranous nephropathy and renal insufficiency: Improved renal survival but high relapse rate. *Nephrol Dial Transplant*. 2004;19: 1142-1148.
46. du Buf-Vereijken PW, Wetzels JF. Efficacy of a second course of immunosuppressive therapy in patients with membranous nephropathy and persistent or relapsing disease activity. *Nephrol Dial Transplant*. 2004;19:2036-2043.
47. Perna A, Schieppati A, Zamora J, et al. Immunosuppressive treatment for idiopathic membranous nephropathy: A systematic review. *Am J Kidney Dis*. 2004;44:385-401.
48. Faurschour M, Sorensen IJ, Mellemkjaer L, et al. Malignancies in Wegener's granulomatosis: Incidence and relation to cyclophosphamide in a cohort of 293 patients. *J Rheumatol*. 2008;35:100-108.
49. Cattran DC, Appel GB, Hebert LA, et al. North America Nephrotic Syndrome Study Group, Cyclosporine in patients with steroid-resistant membranous nephropathy: A randomized trial. *Kidney Int*. 2001;59: 1484-1490.
50. Cattran DC, Greenwood C, Ritchie S, et al. A controlled trial of cyclosporine in patients with progressive membranous nephropathy. Canadian Glomerulonephritis Study Group. *Kidney Int*. 1995;47:1130-1135.

51. Praga M, Barrio V, Juárez GF, Luño J; Grupo Español de Estudio de la Nefropatía Membranosa. Tacrolimus monotherapy in membranous nephropathy: A randomized controlled trial. *Kidney Int.* 2007;71: 924-930.
52. Bertrand D, Morange S, Burtey S, et al. Mycophenolate mofetil monotherapy in membranous nephropathy: A 1-year randomized controlled trial. *Am J Kidney Dis.* 2008;52:699-705.
53. Branten AJ, du Buf-Vereijken PW, Vervloet M, Wetzels JF. Mycophenolate mofetil in idiopathic membranous nephropathy: A clinical trial with comparison to a historic control group treated with cyclophosphamide. *Am J Kidney Dis.* 2007;50:248-256.
54. Ruggenenti P, Chiurchiu C, Brusegan V, et al. Rituximab in idiopathic membranous nephropathy: A one-year prospective study. *J Am Soc Nephrol.* 2003;14:1851-1857.
55. Fervenza FC, Cosio FG, Erickson SB, et al. Rituximab treatment of idiopathic membranous nephropathy. *Kidney Int.* 2008;73:117-125.
56. Ruggenenti P, Chiurchiu C, Abbate M, et al. Rituximab for idiopathic membranous nephropathy: Who can benefit? Clin *J Am Soc Nephrol.* 2006;1:738-748.
57. Appel G, Nachman, P, Hogan S, et al. Eculizumab (C5 complement inhibitor) in the treatment of idiopathic membranous nephropathy [abstract]. *J Am Soc Nephrol.* 2002;13:668A.
58. Ponticelli C, Passerini P, Salvadori M, et al. A randomized pilot trial comparing methylprednisolone plus a cytotoxic agent versus synthetic adrenocorticotropic hormone in idiopathic membranous nephropathy. *Am J Kidney Dis.* 2006;47:233-240.
59. Berg A, Nilsson-Ehle P, Arnadottir M. Beneficial effects of ACTH on the serum lipoprotein profile and glomerular function in patients with membranous nephropathy. *Kidney Int.* 1999;56:1534-1543.

CHAPTER 21

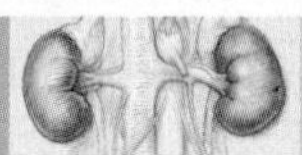

Membranoproliferative Glomerulonephritis, Dense Deposit Disease, and Cryoglobulinemic Glomerulonephritis

F. Paolo Schena, Charles E. Alpers

DEFINITION

Membranoproliferative glomerulonephritis (MPGN), or mesangiocapillary glomerulonephritis (GN), is characterized by diffuse proliferative lesions and widening of the capillary loops, often with a double-contoured appearance. MPGN may be idiopathic or secondary to chronic infections, cryoglobulinemia, or systemic autoimmune disorders that result in aberrant immune complex formation. Three types of MPGN have been described. Type I is characterized by immune deposits in the subendothelial space (capillary wall thickening) and in the mesangium. Type II, also known as dense deposit disease (DDD), is defined by dense deposits within the mesangium and in the basement membranes of the glomeruli, tubules, and Bowman's capsules. On the basis of its unique ultrastructural appearance and the varied morphologic patterns of injury, DDD is best considered a disease entity separate from MPGN. We include DDD in this chapter because of the extensive literature that identifies it as MPGN type II. Type III is a variant of type I, characterized by extensive subendothelial and subepithelial electron-dense deposits. This process is accompanied by alterations and remodeling of the lamina densa of the glomerular basement membrane (GBM) and newly elaborated lamina densa–like material.

ETIOLOGY AND PATHOGENESIS

Although it is frequently idiopathic, the histologic diagnosis of MPGN should provoke a search for secondary causes (Fig. 21.1).[1] In children and young adults (<30 years) with DDD (MPGN type II), the disease is often associated with the presence of nephritic factors, which are IgG or IgM autoantibodies that bind to and stabilize the C3 convertase of the alternative (C3bBb) or classical (C4b2b) pathway (Fig. 21.2), thus resulting in continued complement activation with a depletion of various complement components. In older adults (>30 years), MPGN type I is frequently associated with cryoglobulinemia and hepatitis C virus (HCV) infection.

MPGN type I is most likely to occur in the setting of chronic immune complex diseases, for example, when the host cannot eliminate a foreign antigen effectively despite a humoral response. This may account for the MPGN observed with chronic bloodborne viral (hepatitis C and hepatitis B), bacterial (endocarditis, infected ventriculoatrial shunt), and malarial infections (see Chapter 55). A histologic pattern resembling MPGN can also be observed in chronic immune complex diseases associated with autoimmune diseases such as lupus. Chronic immune complex disease and MPGN may also occur if the host has a defect in clearing immune complexes, as in complement deficiency, or when the reticuloendothelial system is impaired, as occurs with liver or splenic disease. Hereditary deficiencies of the classical pathway of complement (C1q, C2, C4) and of C3 are associated with the development of MPGN in addition to predisposing to lupus and bacterial infections. MPGN type I also is associated with some malignant neoplasms (especially chronic lymphocytic leukemia and lymphoma).

MPGN type I results from the glomerular deposition of immune complexes from the circulation or from circulating antigens and immunoglobulins that deposit in the glomerulus to form immune complexes *in situ*. These complexes preferentially localize in the mesangium and subendothelial space of the capillary walls. Once localized, the immune complexes typically activate complement through the classical pathway, leading to the generation of chemotactic factors (C5a), opsonins (C3b), and the membrane attack complex (C5b-9) as well as low C3 and C4 serum levels. In some patients, complement is activated by the C4 nephritic factor; in other cases, activation of complement may occur by the mannose-binding lectin pathway (see Fig. 21.2). Mannose-binding lectin, a lectin that binds IgG and activates complement, has been localized to the immune deposits of some patients with MPGN type I.[2] Complement activation results in the release of chemotactic factors that promote platelet and leukocyte accumulation (Fig. 21.3; see also Fig. 21.2). Leukocytes release oxidants and proteases, mediating capillary wall damage and proteinuria and a fall in the glomerular filtration rate. Cytokines and growth factors released by both exogenous and endogenous glomerular cells lead to mesangial proliferation and matrix expansion.

The pathogenesis of DDD is intricately linked to continual overactivation of the alternative pathway of complement (see Fig. 21.2). This can occur in humans through a dysfunctional constitutive inhibitor of alternative pathway activation (e.g., of factor H, see later discussion), such that there is unregulated and sustained activity of C3, or through the presence of an IgG or IgM autoantibody (C3 nephritic factor [C3Nef]) that binds the alternative pathway C3 convertase (C3bBb) and prevents its inactivation by factor H (see Fig. 21.2). The consequence is a low C3 level but normal circulating levels of C2 and C4 and terminal (C5 through C9) complement pathway components. The most commonly encountered defect in DDD is the C3Nef interaction with C3 convertase. C3Nef, although it is highly associated with DDD, is not specific for DDD and may also be encountered in some patients with MPGN type I and even in some healthy individuals.[3] The presence or absence of C3Nef therefore does not have clinical prognostic significance and does not independently predict recurrence of disease in allograft kidneys.[4-6] Likewise, C3 levels in serum also have no significant prognostic importance.

Etiology of Membranoproliferative Glomerulonephritis and Dense Deposit Disease

Type	Secondary Causes
MPGN Type I	
With mixed (type II or III) cryoglobulinemia	Hepatitis C virus (70%–90% of patients) Other infections: bacterial endocarditis, chronic hepatitis B viral infection Collagen vascular disease: systemic lupus erythematosus, Sjögren's syndrome Malignancy: chronic lymphocytic leukemia, non-Hodgkin's lymphoma
Without cryoglobulinemia	Bacterial infections: endocarditis, abscess, infected ventriculoatrial shunt Viral infections: hepatitis B, C, and G; human immunodeficiency virus; hantavirus Malarial (*Plasmodium malariae*) Collagen vascular disease (systemic lupus erythematosus–hypocomplementemic urticarial vasculitis) Hereditary complement deficiency (C1q, C2, C4, or C3) Acquired complement deficiency (presence of C4 nephritic factor) Chronic liver disease (especially associated with hepatitis B or C infection, chronic schistosomal infection, with splenorenal shunt for liver fibrosis, and with α_1-antitrypsin deficiency) Sickle cell disease Malignancy: chronic lymphocytic leukemia, lymphoma, thymoma, renal cell carcinoma
Dense Deposit Disease (MPGN Type II)	
Associated with C3 nephritic factor (C3 Nef)	With or without partial lipodystrophy and retinal abnormalities
Associated with factor H defect	Inherited mutations of factor H (deficiency) Autoantibodies to factor H
MPGN Type III	
	Secondary causes similar to MPGN type I (hepatitis C or B, and others)

Figure 21.1 Etiology of membranoproliferative glomerulonephritis and dense deposit disease.

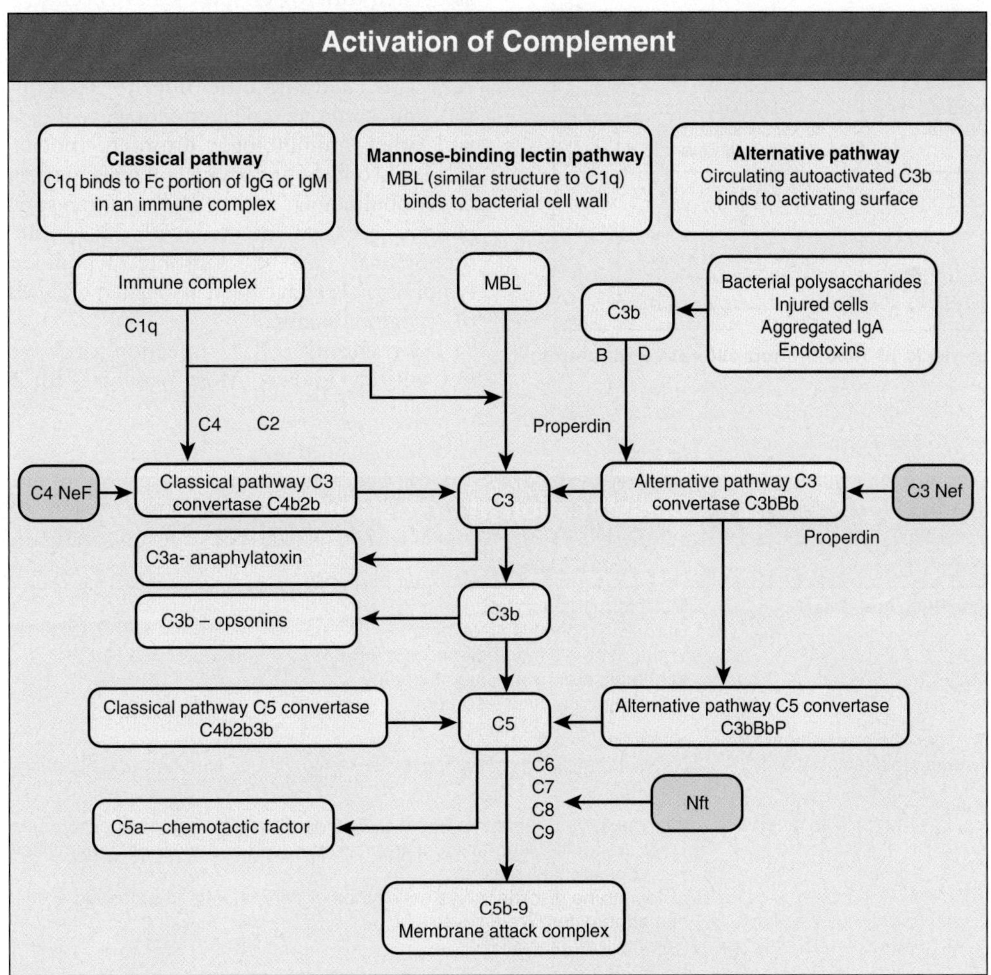

Figure 21.2 Mechanisms of activation of complement pathways including nephritic factors. See text for details. *NeF,* nephritic factor; *Nft,* nephritic factor of the terminal pathway.

Most patients with acquired partial lipodystrophy, an abnormality associated with DDD, also have circulating C3Nef and low serum C3 levels. The lipodystrophy results from complement-dependent loss of the adipocyte, mediated by activation of complement on the adipocyte surface due to both the presence of C3Nef and the overproduction by the adipocyte of adipsin, a protein that is identical to factor D of the alternative pathway (see Fig. 21.2).

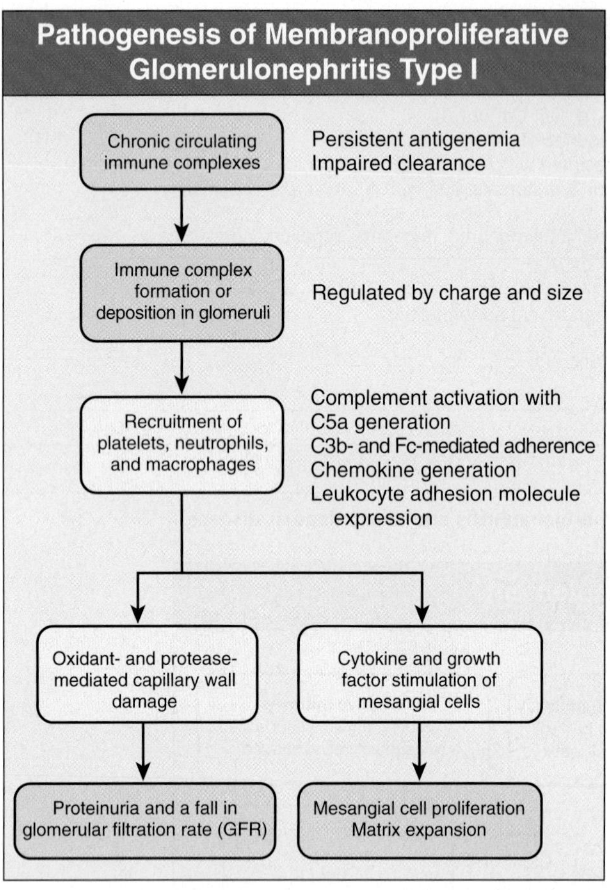

Figure 21.3 Pathogenesis of membranoproliferative glomerulonephritis type I.

Mutations in regulatory proteins of the alternative pathway also can lead to overactivity of C3 and DDD. Genetic mutations in factor H, a cofactor that normally inhibits continued activation of C3 convertase, have been found in patients with DDD and in a spontaneous porcine model of this disease. Factor H–deficient mice also develop GN with some features of DDD, which can be blocked by creation of additional mutations in components of the alternative pathway (e.g., factor B) that prevent further downstream activation of this pathway.[7] Although most patients with DDD do not have factor H gene mutations, genetic population studies show an association of DDD with individuals having several alleles of both complement factor H gene and the complement factor H–related 5 gene. One of these is the tyrosine-402-histidine (Y402H) polymorphism, which is present in both DDD and age-related macular degeneration, a condition characterized in part by ocular drusen bodies, which are also found in many patients with DDD (see Fig. 21.6B).[8-10]

The pathogenesis of MPGN type III is similar to that of MPGN type I, except that certain characteristics of the immune complexes may favor localization in the subepithelial space. MPGN type III patients exhibit depressed levels of properdin, C3, C5, and one or more of the other four terminal components and elevated levels of C5b-9. This rare disease was mapped to chromosome 1q31-32 in an Irish family.[11]

Cryoglobulins are immunoglobulins that precipitate in the cold. They are categorized as types I through III (Fig. 21.4). The mixed cryoglobulinemias (types II and III) are most commonly associated with MPGN; these have been strongly associated with chronic HCV infection in up to 80% to 90% of the patients with cryoglobulinemic vasculitis.[12] The non-HCV cases have been associated with other infections (chronic hepatitis B, bacterial endocarditis), collagen-vascular diseases (systemic lupus), and other immunologic disorders (notably poststreptococcal GN). Chronic lymphocytic leukemia may also be associated with cryoglobulinemia and MPGN; interestingly, some of these patients are also infected with HCV and have a circulating monoclonal IgM-κ. Chronic lymphocytic leukemia and lymphoma also have been associated with MPGN in the absence of cryoglobulinemia.[13]

How chronic HCV infection causes cryoglobulinemia is not entirely known. Most patients with HCV infection and

Classification of Cryoglobulins

Type	Composition	Associated Disease
I	Monoclonal IgG, IgA, or IgM	Multiple myeloma (IgG, IgM) Chronic lymphocytic leukemia Waldenström's macroglobulinemia (IgM) Idiopathic monoclonal gammopathy Lymphoproliferative disorders
II	Polyclonal IgG and monoclonal IgM (with rheumatoid factor activity)	Hepatitis C virus Neoplasms: chronic lymphocytic leukemia, diffuse lymphoma, B lymphocytic neoplasia Essential
III	Polyclonal IgG and polyclonal IgM	Infections: viral (hepatitis B and C, Epstein-Barr virus, cytomegalovirus), bacterial (endocarditis, leprosy, poststreptococcal glomerulonephritis), parasitic (schistosomiasis, toxoplasmosis, malaria) Autoimmune disorders: systemic lupus erythematosus, rheumatoid arthritis Lymphoproliferative disorders Chronic liver disease Essential

Figure 21.4 Classification of cryoglobulins.

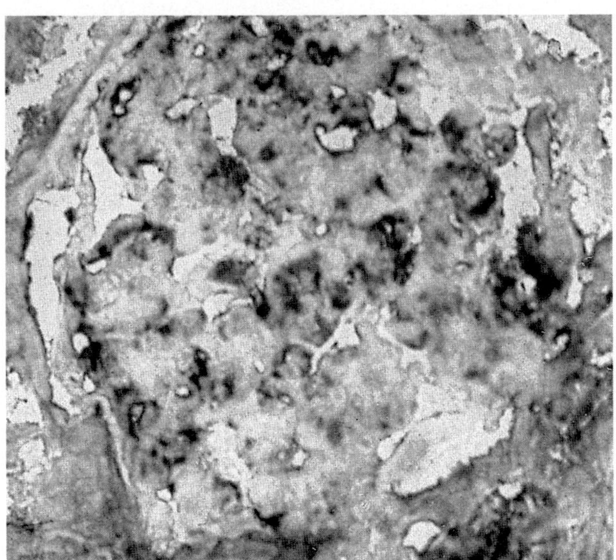

Figure 21.5 Hepatitis C virus–related antigen (c22-3) in the capillary wall of a glomerulus from a patient with cryoglobulinemic membranoproliferative glomerulonephritis (MPGN). (Light microscopy; magnification ×3100.)

cryoglobulinemia have an IgM-κ monoclonal antibody with rheumatoid factor activity. This rheumatoid factor can be found with anti-HCV IgG and HCV RNA in the cryoprecipitates. It has been postulated that the IgM is produced by dysregulated B cells infected with HCV. Cryoglobulinemia does not develop until many years (often >10 years) after HCV infection; but by the time chronic active hepatitis or cirrhosis develops, as many as 30% to 40% of patients will have circulating cryoglobulins or other evidence of cryoglobulinemia if it is searched for.[14] Most of these patients will not develop renal disease, but in some patients, possibly those in whom the cryoglobulins have an affinity for fibronectin, the cryoglobulins containing HCV antigens will deposit in glomeruli (Fig. 21.5).[15]

Specific HCV-related proteins have been detected in glomeruli, tubulointerstitium, and vessels in patients with cryoglobulinemic HCV-positive MPGN,[16] although difficulties with the antisera available to detect HCV render such findings controversial. In these studies, glomerular HCV deposits have displayed two different patterns: (1) a linear homogeneous deposition along glomerular capillary walls, including endothelial and subendothelial spaces; and (2) a granular appearance with distinct deposits in mesangial and paramesangial areas. IgG, IgM, and C3 deposits display features comparable to those of HCV RNA and core protein deposits, suggesting that in cryoglobulinemic HCV-positive MPGN, deposits consist of HCV containing immune complexes that may directly contribute to renal damage.[17] Further pathogenetic insight will likely be provided by new mouse models, including the transgenic thymic stromal lymphopoietin (TSLP) mouse, which develops mixed cryoglobulinemia and MPGN type I, and a DDD model, the factor H–deficient mouse.[18]

EPIDEMIOLOGY

In North America and Europe, MPGN (types I and III) and DDD constitute less than 5% of all primary glomerulonephritides. MPGN accounts for 5% to 10% of primary renal causes of nephrotic syndrome in children and adults.[19] It occurs equally in males and females and in the United States is relatively more common in Caucasians than in African Americans. MPGN presenting in childhood (primarily between the ages of 8 and 14 years) includes types I and III MPGN and DDD and is frequently idiopathic or associated with nephritic factors. By contrast, MPGN presenting in adults (typically older than 18 years) is usually type I or type III and is commonly associated with cryoglobulinemia and HCV infection (see Chapter 55).

The prevalence of MPGN type I is decreasing in Europe, presumably because some chronic infections are becoming less common. On the contrary, in the Middle East (Saudi Arabia), South America (Peru), and Africa (Nigeria), MPGN type I is still quite common because of its association with chronic bacterial, viral, and parasitic infections. The disease may be familial in rare cases, and different histologic lesions may occur in family members (i.e., type I in one member and type III in another).

DDD accounts for less than 20% of cases of MPGN in children and a very low percentage of cases in adults. It is estimated to affect two to three people per million.[20]

CLINICAL MANIFESTATIONS

MPGN and DDD may present as microscopic hematuria and non-nephrotic proteinuria (35%), as nephrotic syndrome with minimally depressed renal function (35%), as a chronically progressive GN (20%), or with rapidly deteriorating renal function with proteinuria and red cell casts (10%). Systemic hypertension is present in 50% to 80% of patients, and it may occasionally be so severe that the presentation may be confused with that of malignant hypertension.

Pediatric Population

MPGN type I in children and young adults is usually idiopathic and presents as a primary kidney disease without systemic manifestations. Asymptomatic Japanese children diagnosed as a consequence of a urinalysis screening program at school had lower blood pressure, proteinuria, and serum creatinine concentration compared with subjects who were diagnosed after presenting with symptoms.[21] Thus, early identification of the disease by urinary screening may allow early treatment.

DDD affects females slightly more frequently than males (3:2). It is usually diagnosed in children who are between 5 and 15 years old. Patients present with hematuria, proteinuria, hematuria plus proteinuria, acute nephritic syndrome, or nephrotic syndrome.[6]

Adult Population

MPGN in adults is also often limited to the kidney; but in patients with DDD, partial lipodystrophy that preferentially involves the face and upper body may be present (Fig. 21.6A). It may precede the renal disease by many years. Some patients with DDD will also have mild visual field and color defects and prolonged dark adaptation with mottled retinal pigmentation (drusen bodies; see Fig. 21.6B) and sometimes deterioration of vision. Eye examinations, including dark adaptation, electroretinography, and electro-oculography, should be performed on first presentation and annually thereafter. Indocyanine green angiography of the retina may reveal dense deposits in the ciliary epithelial basement membrane (abnormal fluorescent dots) and choroidal neovascularization.[22,23]

When MPGN is associated with systemic cryoglobulinemia, patients usually have chronic HCV infection and present with the

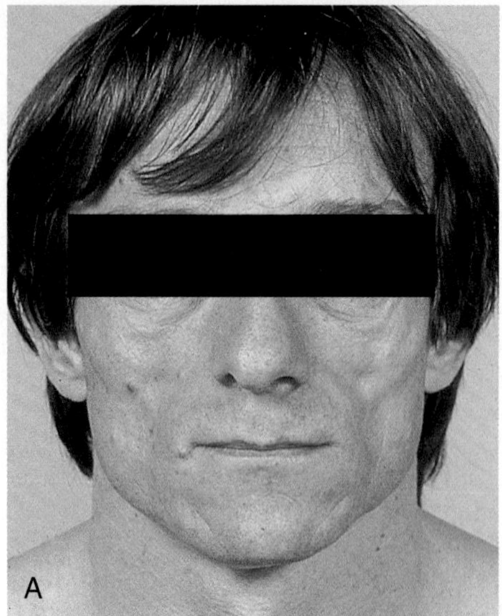

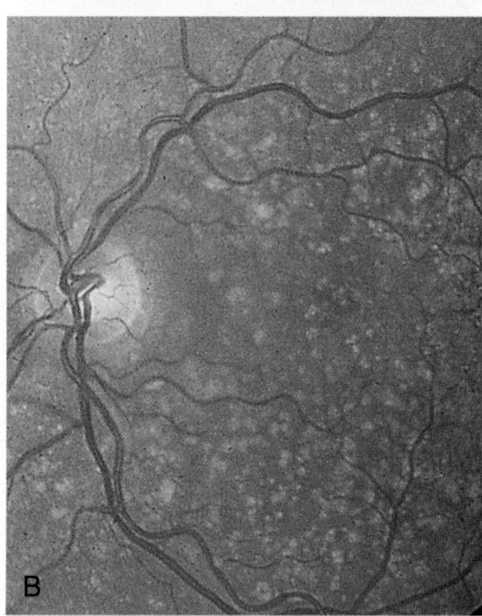

Figure 21.6 Dense deposit disease (MPGN type II). A, Partial lipodystrophy; note the absence of subcutaneous fat from the face. **B,** Drusen bodies in the retina. *(Courtesy Dr. C. D. Short, Manchester, UK.)*

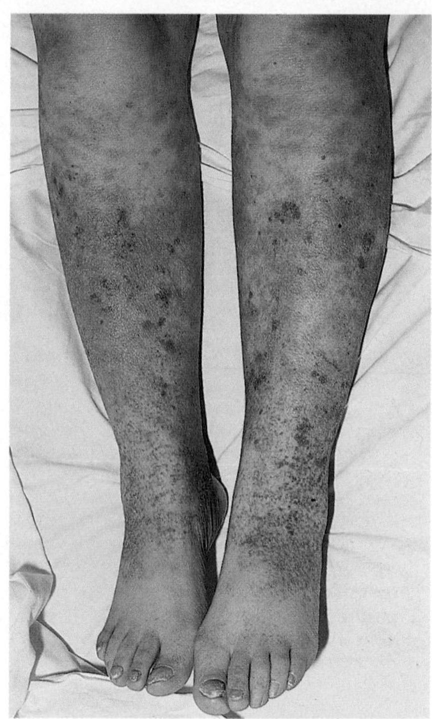

Figure 21.7 Purpura in a patient with hepatitis C virus–associated cryoglobulinemia. Raised purpuric lesions are present on the legs of this individual. The differential diagnosis of purpura and renal disease includes cryoglobulinemia, Henoch-Schönlein purpura, vasculitis, and endocarditis.

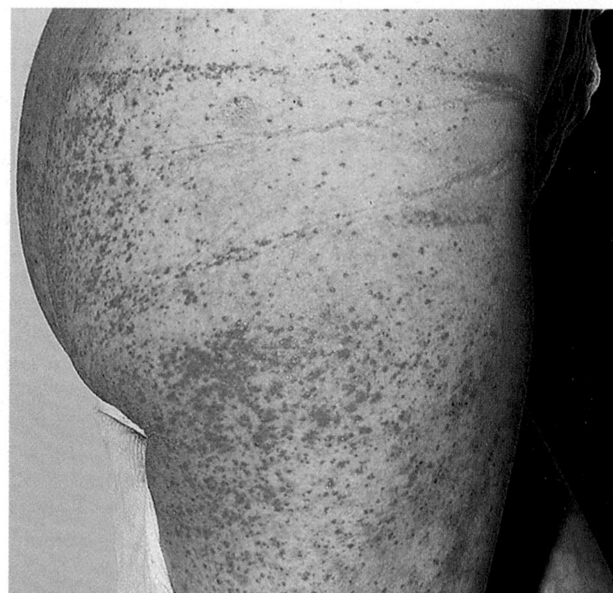

Figure 21.8 Purpura in a patient with hepatitis C virus–associated cryoglobulinemia. Purpuric lesions are present on the buttocks and thigh of the patient. Interestingly, note the purpuric lesions along the superior and inferior elastic border of the undergarment line.

triad of weakness, arthralgias, and purpura. The arthralgias are only rarely accompanied by arthritis, are usually symmetric, and classically involve the knees, hips, and shoulders. The purpura (Fig. 21.7) is usually painless, palpable, and nonpruritic; it occurs in "crops" that last 4 to 10 days and preferentially localizes to the extremities. Other manifestations may include ulcerative, vasculitic lesions that classically involve the lower extremities (see Fig. 21.7) and buttocks (Fig. 21.8), Raynaud's phenomenon, digital necrosis (Fig. 21.9), peripheral neuropathy, hepatomegaly, and, rarely, signs of cirrhosis (clubbing, spider angiomas, ascites). Although most patients with cryoglobulinemia have a chronic waxing and waning course, occasional patients may have a more fulminant presentation, with congestive heart failure (from an HCV-induced cardiomyopathy), infiltrates in the lung from deposition of cryoglobulins (Fig. 21.10), pulmonary hypertension, severe systemic hypertension, or mesenteric ischemia.

In view of the conditions associated with MPGN (see Fig. 21.1), signs of bacterial infection, viral infection, systemic lupus, malignant disease, and chronic liver disease should be sought.

Laboratory Findings

MPGN is often associated with depressed complement levels (C3 and total hemolytic complement [CH50]). In MPGN type I and in cryoglobulinemic MPGN, the classical pathway is often activated (low C3, low C4, and low CH50); in DDD, the

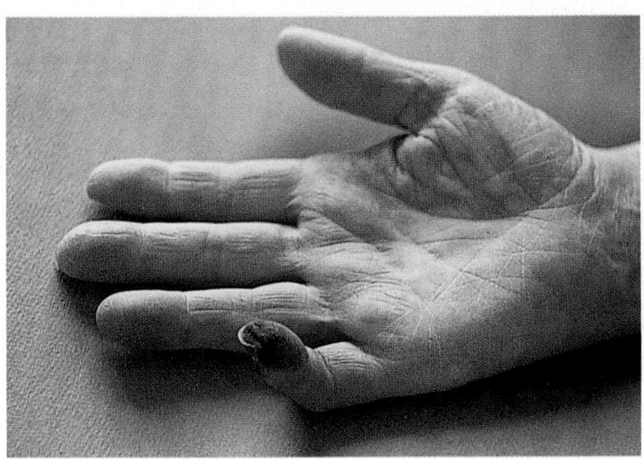

Figure 21.9 Necrosis of the distal portion of the little finger in a young woman with essential mixed cryoglobulinemia.

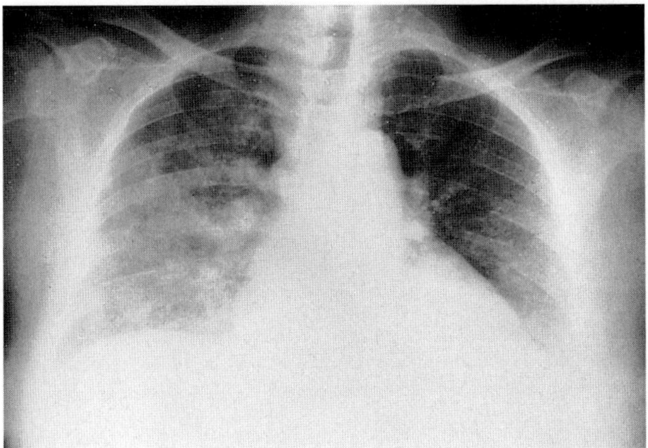

Figure 21.10 Chest radiograph showing nodular infiltrates in the lung secondary to cryoglobulinemic vasculitis in a patient with HCV infection.

alternative pathway is activated (low C3, normal C4, and low CH50); and in type III, C3 is generally low in association with a depression of terminal complement components (C5 through C9). C3Nef activity, strongly but not exclusively associated with DDD, is usually detected in plasma by the hemolytic test or the C3NeF IgG solid-phase assay.[24] The presence of rheumatoid factors or cryoglobulins should prompt testing for anti-HCV antibody and HCV RNA. However, MPGN can be associated with HCV infection in the absence of cryoglobulinemia or rheumatoid factors.[25] Failure to detect the cryoglobulins may result from improper handling of specimens or may occur because the cryoglobulinemia was transient; however, in some patients (especially in renal transplant recipients), test results for cryoglobulinemia may be persistently negative. Clinical or laboratory evidence of liver disease should prompt a search for causes of chronic liver disease, including hepatitis C, hepatitis B, and, if appropriate, rare entities such as schistosomiasis and α_1-antitrypsin deficiency.

PATHOLOGY

By light microscopy, MPGN type I is classically described as hypercellular because of both the influx of circulating leukocytes and intrinsic glomerular cell proliferation (typically mesangial cells), leading to a lobular appearance in some cases (Fig. 21.11A). Accumulation of extracellular material, predominantly matrix, contributes to the frequent mesangial expansion. The glomerular appearance can range from markedly hypercellular to predominantly sclerotic. In its most advanced form, sclerosis can be manifested as nodules indistinguishable from diabetic nodular mesangial sclerosis. Silver stain often shows a double contouring of the GBM ("tram tracks") as a result of the interposition of mesangial cells, leukocytes, or endothelial cells in the capillary wall with the synthesis of new basement membrane material (Fig. 21.12). Monocytes and macrophages are commonly present in the glomerulus and the periglomerular areas.[1,26]

DDD is characterized by dense deposits within the mesangium and the basement membranes of the glomeruli, tubules, and Bowman's capsules, often visible with eosin and periodic acid–Schiff stains but characteristically identified by electron microscopy. Whereas glomerular changes similar to those of MPGN type I were the most common histopathologic findings in a study in DDD,[27] another study identified a mesangial proliferative pattern of injury as most common (45% of patients).[28] Other histopathologic patterns identified in this latter series included MPGN (25%), acute proliferative and exudative GN (12%), and crescentic GN (18%); a few could not be readily classified (3%). This histologic heterogeneity of DDD, frequently manifested with a histopathologic pattern other than that of MPGN, and its unique ultrastructural appearance (described later) and unique pathogenesis provide the basis for separation of this entity from its historic classification as a type of MPGN. As in most glomerular diseases, the presence of a significant number of crescents portends a poor prognosis; the prognostic significance of the other glomerular injury patterns is unclear.

The hallmark of MPGN type III is the interruption of lamina densa associated with subendothelial and subepithelial deposits, often confluent, and interspersed with multilayers of new lamina densa. Type I and type III MPGN form a morphologic continuum and thus are not always separable by light microscopy.

Immunofluorescence in MPGN type I and type III frequently shows the deposition of IgM, IgG, and C3 in a granular capillary wall distribution (Fig. 21.11B), although the immunoglobulin deposits may be scant. Staining for C3 in a peripheral (lobular) pattern involving capillary walls and mesangial areas is the most constant and strongest pattern; staining for classical pathway complement components (C1q, C4) may also be seen in MPGN type I. In DDD, C3 but neither classical complement pathway components nor immunoglobulins are detected; this helps distinguish it from other types of injury with an MPGN pattern. The C3 stain is thought to bind to an unidentified substrate at the surface of the dense deposits, which occasionally gives an appearance of tram tracks or mesangial rings.

By electron microscopy, discrete immune deposits can be observed in the subendothelial portions of the capillary walls and mesangial regions in MPGN type I, often in association with platelet and leukocyte infiltration (Fig. 21.11C). The deposits are often discrete but may be confluent in their involvement of the capillary wall. They can be small and sparse or large and numerous such that they are visible by light microscopy. A separation of the endothelium from the GBM can occasionally be observed, usually with some synthesis of new basement membrane material under endothelial cells that have detached from the original basement membrane. Between these layers (old and new) of basement membranes, interposed cells of mesangial, endothelial, or leukocyte origin as well as immune deposits and matrix may be found.

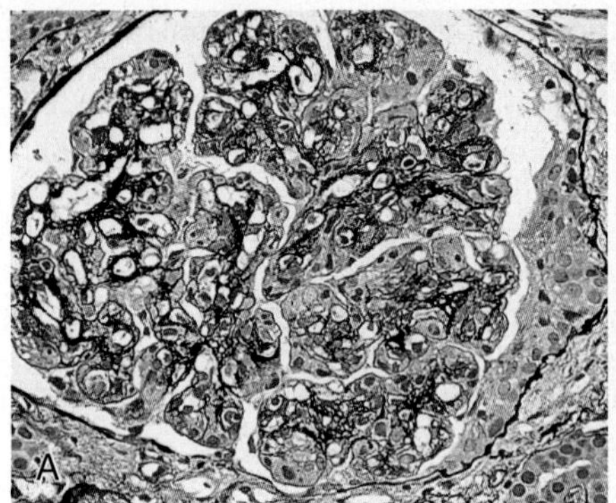

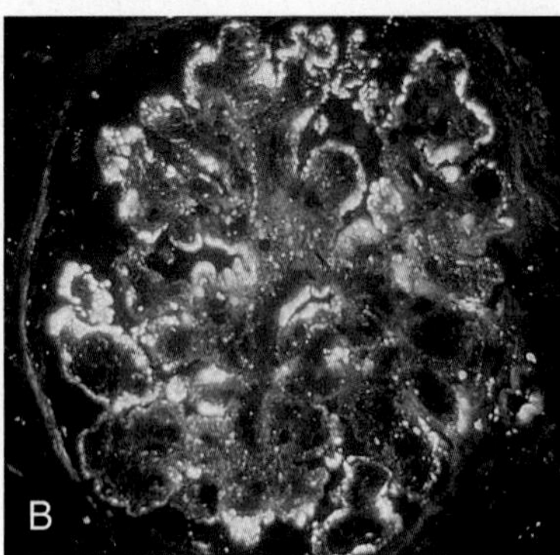

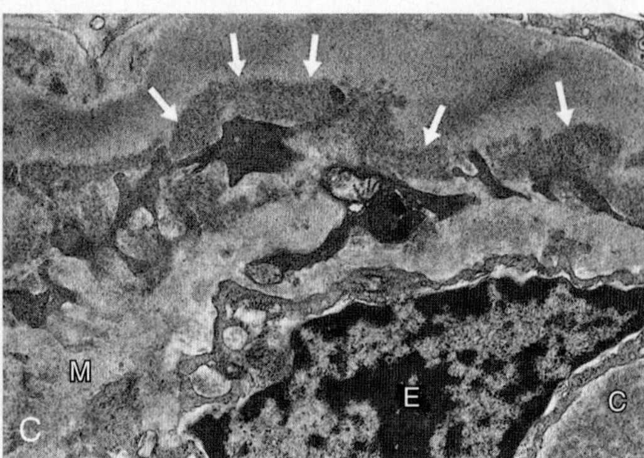

Figure 21.11 Pathology of membranoproliferative glomerulonephritis (MPGN) type I. A, Light microscopy shows a hypercellular glomerulus with accentuated lobular architecture and a small cellular crescent (methenamine silver). **B,** Immunofluorescence usually shows discrete, granular staining of the peripheral capillary wall for IgG (seen here) and C3 and occasionally for IgM and earlier complement components (C1q and C4). **C,** By electron microscopy, numerous subendothelial deposits are observed *(arrows)* between the duplicated basement membrane; these deposits extend into the mesangium (M). C, capillary lumen; E, endothelial cell nucleus.

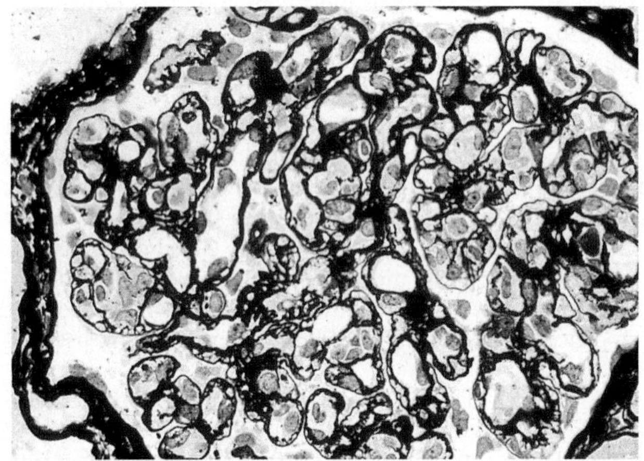

Figure 21.12 "Tram tracks" in membranoproliferative glomerulonephritis (MPGN) type I. By silver stain, a double contouring of the glomerular basement membrane (GBM) can be observed in MPGN type I, resembling tram tracks.

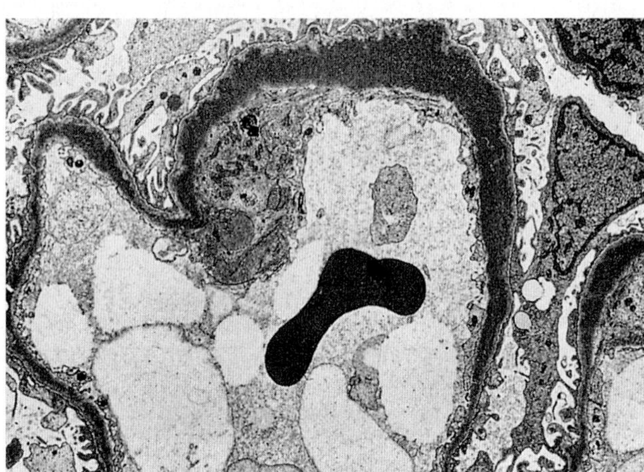

Figure 21.13 Electron microscopy of dense deposit disease. Dense material replaces sections of the glomerular basement membrane (GBM).

In DDD, electron microscopy shows replacement of large sections of the GBM with an extremely electron-dense band of homogeneous material, the identity of which remains unknown (Fig. 21.13). Involvement of mesangial regions, Bowman's capsules, and tubular basement membranes by the deposits is common.

Perhaps 15% of MPGN cases demonstrate both subendothelial and subepithelial deposits associated with minute disruptions of the lamina densa and newly elaborated lamina densa–like material (MPGN type III). There can be a continuum of subepithelial deposits in MPGN type I and type III from none or scanty to numerous, making it difficult to separate all cases into type I (scanty or no subepithelial deposits) or type III (numerous deposits) categories. After a number of years of normocomplementemia, the type III lesions can disappear, but this not inevitable.[29]

Cryoglobulinemic MPGN may appear histologically identical to MPGN type I. However, the cryoprecipitates can occasionally be observed by light microscopy as intracapillary hyaline-like deposits (Fig 21.14A), and there is often a more pronounced infiltration of macrophages within capillary lumina. Electron microscopy may also show highly organized microtubular or finely fibrillar structures consisting of the precipitated cryoglobulins (Fig. 21.14B).

DIAGNOSIS AND DIFFERENTIAL DIAGNOSIS

MPGN is diagnosed by renal biopsy in patients presenting with nephrotic or non-nephrotic proteinuria, especially when it is accompanied by microhematuria. By light microscopy, other entities may appear histologically similar, including poststreptococcal GN, the thrombotic microangiopathies, paraproteinemias, and fibrillary GN (Fig. 21.15). Immunofluorescence and electron microscopy are critical for separating these diseases. Systemic lupus usually can be eliminated by serologic testing.

Other useful tests are serum C3, C4, CH50, total hemolytic activity of the alternative complement pathway (APH50), and factor H levels. Low complement levels can also be observed in atheroembolic renal disease (low C3 with eosinophilia), in thrombotic microangiopathy, in chronic liver disease (because of decreased synthesis), and in several glomerular diseases including systemic lupus (low C3 and C4) and poststreptococcal GN (low C3). The detection of C3NeF activity in plasma suggests DDD, but C3NeF can also be identified in a significant proportion of patients with MPGN type I and even in healthy individuals. In cases of otherwise idiopathic DDD, screening for mutations of factor H gene is recommended.

Once MPGN is diagnosed, careful evaluation for secondary causes should be conducted (see Fig. 21.1 and Chapter 55).

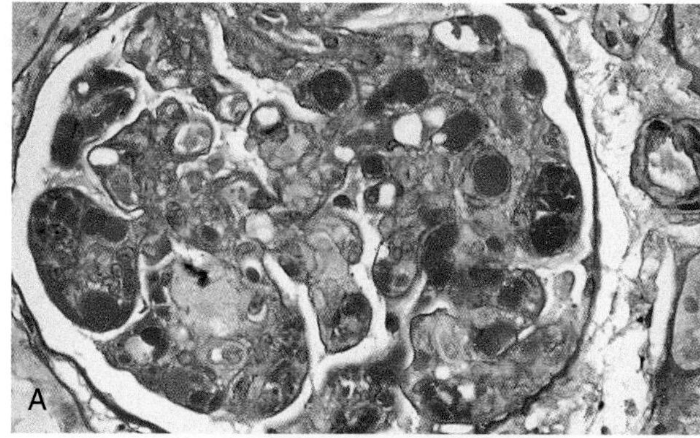

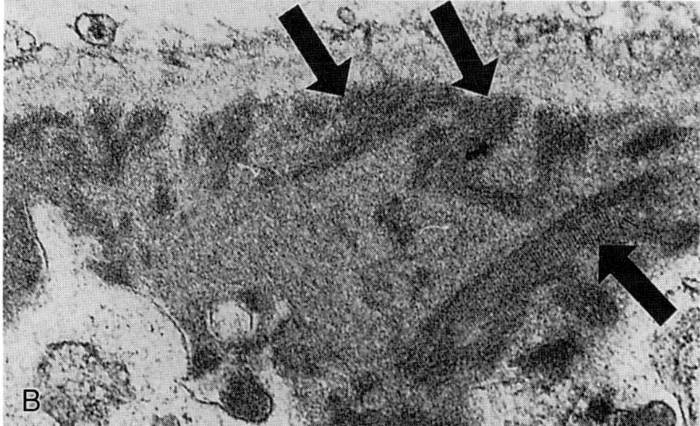

Figure 21.14 Pathology of cryoglobulinemic membranoproliferative glomerulonephritis (MPGN). A, Although cryoglobulinemic MPGN may histologically appear similar to MPGN type I (see Fig. 21.11), discrete precipitates of cryoglobulins may occasionally be found occluding individual capillary loops. **B,** In addition, electron microscopy shows organized fibrillar or tubular structures consistent with cryoglobulins *(arrows)*. *(**A** reprinted with permission from reference 30. **B** reprinted with permission from reference 31.)*

NATURAL HISTORY

Idiopathic MPGN in childhood has a relatively poor prognosis, with 40% to 50% of untreated patients progressing to renal failure during 10 years. Idiopathic MPGN in adults also carries an unfavorable prognosis. Five years after biopsy, 50% of patients either die or need renal replacement therapy (dialysis or transplantation). This proportion increases to 64% after 10 years. Risk of progression increases with elevated creatinine, nephrotic proteinuria, and severe hypertension or if a biopsy specimen shows more than 50% crescents or marked interstitial fibrosis.[32]

TRANSPLANTATION

The severity of crescent formation in native kidney biopsy specimens has predictive value for recurrence of disease in subsequent renal allografts.[33] For further discussion of recurrent MPGN and DDD, refer to Chapter 104. Systemic activation of the complement system makes recurrence more likely. HCV-associated MPGN can also occur *de novo* or recur in renal transplant recipients and after liver transplantation.

TREATMENT

The initial approach to MPGN aims at identification of the etiology, if possible, and initiation of supportive antiproteinuric and antihypertensive measures (see Chapter 76). Treatment

Diseases that Histologically Resemble Membranoproliferative Glomerulonephritis
Paraproteinemias: especially fibrillary glomerulonephritis, light-chain nephropathy
Thrombotic microangiopathies: hemolytic-uremic syndrome, scleroderma, radiation nephropathy, malignant hypertension
Glomerulosclerosis in liver diseases
Postinfectious glomerulonephritis
"Transplant" glomerulopathy
Rare diseases: collagen III glomerulopathy, C1q nephropathy, lipoprotein nephropathy

Figure 21.15 Diseases that histologically resemble membranoproliferative glomerulonephritis (MPGN).

plans for the various types of MPGN are discussed in the following sections (Fig. 21.16).

Idiopathic Membranoproliferative Glomerulonephritis in Childhood

Some studies that primarily used historical or nonrandomized controls demonstrated a benefit of alternate-day corticosteroids in childhood MPGN, particularly with administration in the first year of presentation. Although these data are not definitive, we recommend an initial corticosteroid treatment in this population. For children with MPGN with moderate proteinuria (<3 g/day) and normal renal function, we administer prednisone (40 mg/m^2) on alternate days for 3 months. In patients with nephrotic syndrome or impaired renal function, this dose of corticosteroids is administered for 2 years. In case of reduction of proteinuria or improvement of renal function, prednisone is tapered to a maintenance dose of 20 mg on alternate days for 3 to 10 years.[34] Treatment may be associated with a reduction in hematuria (80%), partial or complete reduction of proteinuria (25% to 40%), and better preservation of renal function (80% at 10 years versus 50% in historical controls). The most important side effects are exacerbation of hypertension, growth retardation, weight gain, and obesity. If no benefit is seen after 1 year of treatment, corticosteroids should be withdrawn and supportive therapy only continued. Responses to alternate-day corticosteroids are superior in children with type I MPGN, whereas children with type III MPGN are more likely to have a progressive reduction in renal function, slower reduction of serum C3, more persistent urinary abnormalities, and more frequent relapses.[35]

In children with DDD, corticosteroids and calcineurin inhibitors lack efficacy. Removal of C3NeF from the serum through plasma exchange improved serum creatinine in only a few cases.[36] The utility of immunosuppressive agents such as mycophenolate mofetil (MMF) has not been established. Plasma infusion with the use of fresh frozen plasma or recombinant factor H can be an effective therapy in patients with DDD secondary to pathologic mutations of factor H gene (*CFH*). This therapy replaces deficient factor H with normal factor H, correcting the complement defect.[6]

Idiopathic Membranoproliferative Glomerulonephritis in Adults

For patients with normal renal function and asymptomatic non-nephrotic–range proteinuria, no specific therapy is necessary.

Suggested Management of Membranoproliferative Glomerulonephritis	
Type	**Treatment**
All types	Supportive therapy following the recommendations discussed in Chapter 76
Idiopathic MPGN in children	Non-nephrotic proteinuria, normal renal function: follow with 3-month visits Normal renal function and moderate proteinuria (>3 g/day): prednisone 40 mg/m² on alternate days for 3 months Nephrotic or impaired renal function: prednisone 40 mg/m² on alternate days (80 mg maximum) for 2 years, tapering to 20 mg on alternate days for 3–10 years
Idiopathic MPGN in adults	Non-nephrotic, normal renal function: follow with 3-month visits Nephrotic or impaired renal function: 6-month course of corticosteroid with/without cyctotoxic agents (cyclophosphamide) or other drugs used: cyclosporine, tacrolimus, mycophenolate mofetil (MMF) Rapidly progressive renal failure with diffuse crescents: treat as for idiopathic rapidly progressive GN (see Chapter 24) In the presence of chronic renal failure or nephrotic proteinuria: ACE inhibitors
MPGN associated with HCV or cryoglobulinemia	Non-nephrotic, normal renal function: treat with interferon alpha (see Chapter 55) based on severity of liver disease (diagnosed by biopsy) Nephrotic syndrome, reduced renal function, or signs of cryoglobulinemia: pegylated interferon alfa-2b (1 μg/kg weekly) and ribavirin (15 mg/kg/day) for 12 months, followed by a short-term course of low-dose corticosteroids; if relapse occurs, consider high-dose interferon alfa (10 million U daily for 2 weeks, then every other day for 6 more weeks) Rapidly progressive renal failure or severe symptoms of vasculitis (heart failure, pulmonary disease): methylprednisolone 1 g daily for 3 days, followed by oral prednisone 60 mg/daily with slow taper during 2–3 months Cyclophosphamide (2 mg/kg/day with adjustment for renal function) and cryofiltration may be added as adjunctive therapy; when the prednisone is reduced to 20 mg/day and the cyclophosphamide is discontinued, add interferon alfa MPGN in the renal or liver transplant recipient: consider course of oral ribavirin (0.6–1 g/day)

Figure 21.16 Suggested management of membranoproliferative glomerulonephritis (MPGN).

Close follow-up every 3 to 4 months is recommended.[34] In patients with nephrotic syndrome and normal or impaired renal function, a 3- to 6-month course of corticosteroids (prednisone 1 mg/kg body weight per day) may be prescribed. If there is considerable reduction of proteinuria, corticosteroids may be continued at the minimal effective dose. If no response is observed within 3 months, corticosteroids should be stopped; treatment with cyclosporine, tacrolimus, or MMF has been recommended.[37]

Hepatitis B Virus–Associated Membranoproliferative Glomerulonephritis

In hepatitis B virus (HBV)–associated MPGN, treatment with antivirals aimed at eradication of HBV (interferon, lamivudine) is the recommended initial treatment. Immunosuppressive agents are discouraged because they promote further HBV replication and occasional deterioration of hepatic function (see Chapter 55).

Hepatitis C Virus–Associated Membranoproliferative Glomerulonephritis and Cryoglobulinemia

Treatment options in mixed cryoglobulinemia with renal involvement include corticosteroids, cytotoxic drugs such as cyclophosphamide, and parenteral administration of interferon alfa alone or in association with ribavirin. Parenteral interferon alfa often improves extrarenal manifestations in close association with reduced levels of viremia, but relapse is common after cessation of therapy. As also discussed in Chapter 55, the current treatment of choice in patients with HCV-associated MPGN or cryoglobulinemic MPGN with moderate proteinuria and nonrapid but progressive renal failure is standard interferon alfa (3 MU three times per week) or pegylated interferon alfa (1.5 μg/kg per week) and ribavirin, adapting the dose to the creatinine clearance or to a trough plasma concentration of 10 to 15 mmol/l. The anti-HCV therapy should be prolonged for 12 months.[38-41]

High-dose interferon alfa may cause severe influenza-like symptoms, depression or psychosis, the development of hypothyroidism, and, rarely, the development of proteinuria (with a minimal change type of lesion). The most frequent serious adverse side effect of ribavirin is hematopoietic toxicity as well as hemolytic anemia and teratogenic effect. Rituximab is a human-mouse chimeric monoclonal antibody that reacts with the CD20 antigen (thereby selectively targeting B cells). It seems to be as efficient as cyclophosphamide in blocking cryoglobulin production, is better tolerated, and does not enhance HCV replication. It should be administered at a dose of 375 mg/m² per week for 4 weeks.[42,43] Alternatively, oral cyclophosphamide may be used (2 mg/kg per day for 2 to 4 months).[41]

In patients with nephrotic-range proteinuria or progressive renal failure, the anti-HCV therapy is the same. Moreover, treatment may include plasma exchange (3 liters of plasma three times per week for 2 or 3 weeks) and methylprednisolone pulses (0.5 to 1 g/day for 3 consecutive days) followed by oral prednisone 60 mg/day with slow tapering during 2 to 3 months.[39] Cryofiltration, that is, double-filtration plasmapheresis with a cooling unit, has been introduced as a means to remove cryoglobulins.[44]

Other Types of Membranoproliferative Glomerulonephritis

MPGN associated with other infections may respond to effective treatment of the underlying pathogenic agent. MPGN associated with α_1-antitrypsin deficiency has been reported to be cured by liver transplantation, which cures the genetic defect. MPGN associated with malignant disease, such as B-cell lymphoma, may respond to effective treatment of the underlying cancer.

REFERENCES

1. Rennke HG. Secondary membranoproliferative glomerulonephritis (clinical conference). *Kidney Int.* 1995;47:643-656.
2. Lhotta K, Würzner R, König P. Glomerular deposition of mannose-binding lectin in human glomerulonephritis. *Nephrol Dial Transplant.* 1999;14:881-886.
3. Licht C, Fremeaux-Bacchi V. Hereditary and acquired complement dysregulation in membranoproliferative glomerulonephritis. *Thromb Haemost.* 2009;101:271-278.
4. Ohi H, Watanabe S, Fujita T, Yasugi T. Significance of C3 nephritic factor (C3 NeF) in non-hypocomplementaemic serum from patients with membranoproliferative glomerulonephritis (MPGN). *Clin Exp Immunol.* 1992;89:479-484.
5. Rodriguez de Cordoba S, Esparza-Gordillo J, Goicoechea de Jorge E, et al. The human complement factor H: Functional roles, genetic variations and disease associations. *Mol Immunol.* 2004;41:355-367.
6. Appel GB, Cook HT, Hageman G, et al. Membranoproliferative glomerulonephritis type II (dense deposit disease): An update. *J Am Soc Nephrol.* 2005;16:1392-1404.
7. Pickering MC, Cook HT. Translational mini-review series on complement factor H: Renal diseases associated with complement factor H: Novel insights from humans and animals. *Clin Exp Immunol.* 2008;151:210-230.
8. Smith RJ, Alexander J, Barlow PN, et al. New approaches to the treatment of dense deposit disease. *J Am Soc Nephrol.* 2007;18:2447-2456.
9. Noris M, Remuzzi G. Translational mini-review series on complement factor H: Therapies of renal diseases associated with complement factor H abnormalities: Atypical haemolytic uraemic syndrome and membranoproliferative glomerulonephritis. *Clin Exp Immunol.* 2008;151:199-209.
10. Berger SP, Daha MR. Complement in glomerular injury. *Semin Immunopathol.* 2007;29:375-384.
11. Neary JJ, Conlon PJ, Croke D, et al. Linkage of a gene causing familial membranoproliferative glomerulonephritis type III to chromosome 1. *J Am Soc Nephrol.* 2002;8:2052-2057.
12. Saadoun D, Landau DA, Calabrese LH, Cacoub PP. Hepatitis C–associated mixed cryoglobulinaemia: A crossroad between autoimmunity and lymphoproliferation. *Rheumatology.* 2007;46:1234-1242.
13. Alpers CE, Cotran RS. Neoplasia and glomerular injury. *Kidney Int.* 1986;30:465-473.
14. Alpers CE, Smith KD. Cryoglobulinemia and renal disease. *Curr Opin Nephrol Hypertens.* 2008;17:243-249.
15. Fornasieri A, Armelloni S, Bernasconi P, et al. High binding of immunoglobulin M kappa rheumatoid factor from type II cryoglobulins to cellular fibronectin: A mechanism for induction of in situ immune complex glomerulonephritis? *Am J Kidney Dis.* 1996;27:476-483.
16. Sansonno D, Gesualdo L, Manno C, et al. Hepatitis C virus–related proteins in kidney tissue from hepatitis C virus–infected patients with cryoglobulinemic membranoproliferative glomerulonephritis. *Hepatology.* 1997;24:1237-1244.
17. Sansonno D, Lauletta G, Montrone M, et al. Hepatitis C virus RNA and core protein in kidney glomerular and tubular structures isolated with laser capture microdissection. *Clin Exp Immunol.* 2005;140:498-506.
18. Smith KD, Alpers CE. Pathogenic mechanisms in membranoproliferative glomerulonephritis. *Curr Opin Nephrol Hypertens.* 2005;14:396-403.
19. Orth SR, Ritz E: The nephrotic syndrome. *N Engl J Med* 1998;338:1202-1211.
20. Smith RJ, Alexander J, Barlow PN, et al. New approaches to the treatment of dense deposit disease. *J Am Soc Nephrol.* 2007;18:2447-2456.
21. Kawasaki Y, Suzuki J, Nozawa R, Suzuki H. Efficacy of school urinary screening for membranoproliferative glomerulonephritis type I. *Arch Dis Child.* 2002;86:21-25.
22. Kim RY, Faktorovich EG, Kuo CY, Olson JL. Retinal function abnormalities in membranoproliferative glomerulonephritis type II. *Am J Ophthalmol.* 1997;123:619-628.
23. Parrat E, Arndt CF, Labalette P, et al. Retinochoroidal involvement of type II membranoproliferative glomerulonephritis: An angiographic study with indocyanine green. *J Fr Ophtalmol.* 1997;20:430-438.
24. Schwertz R, Rother U, Anders D, et al. Complement analysis in children with idiopathic membranoproliferative glomerulonephritis: A long-term follow-up. *Pediatr Allergy Immunol.* 2001;12:166-172.
25. Johnson RJ, Gretch DR, Couser WG, et al. Hepatitis C virus–associated glomerulonephritis. Effect of alpha-interferon therapy. *Kidney Int.* 1994;46:1700-1704.
26. Gesualdo L, Grandaliano G, Ranieri E, et al. Monocyte recruitment in cryoglobulinemic membranoproliferative glomerulonephritis: A pathogenetic role for monocyte chemotactic peptide-I. *Kidney Int.* 1997;51:155-163.
27. Nasr SH, Valeri AM, Appel GB, et al. Dense deposit disease: Clinicopathologic study of 32 pediatric and adult patients. *Clin J Am Soc Nephrol.* 2009;4:22-32.
28. Walker PD, Ferrario F, Joh K, Bonsib SM. Dense deposit disease is not a membranoproliferative glomerulonephritis. *Mod Pathol.* 2007;20:605-616.
29. West CD, McAdams AJ. Membranoproliferative glomerulonephritis type III: Association of glomerular deposits with circulating nephritic factor–stabilized convertase. *Am J Kidney Dis.* 1998;32:56-63.
30. Kim RY, Faktorovich EG, Kuo CY, Olson JL. Retinal function abnormalities in membranoproliferative glomerulonephritis type II. *Am J Ophthalmol.* 1997;123:619-628.
31. Johnson RJ, Gretch DR, Yamabe H, et al. Membranoproliferative glomerulonephritis associated with hepatitis C virus infection. *N Engl J Med.* 1993;328:465-470. Copyright © 1993 Massachusetts Medical Society. All rights reserved.
32. Schmitt H, Bohle A, Reincke T, et al. Long-term prognosis of membranoproliferative glomerulonephritis type I: Significance of clinical and morphological parameters: An investigation of 220 cases. *Nephron.* 1990;55:242-250.
33. Little MA, Dupont P, Campbell E, et al. Severity of primary MPGN, rather than MPGN type, determines renal survival and post-transplantation recurrence risk. *Kidney Int.* 2006;69:504-511.
34. Levin A. Management of membranoproliferative glomerulonephritis: Evidence-based recommendations. *Kidney Int.* 1999;55:S41-S46.
35. Braun MC, West CD, Strife CF. Differences between membranoproliferative glomerulonephritis types I and III in long-term response to an alternate-day prednisone regimen. *Am J Kidney Dis.* 1999;34:1022-1032.
36. McGinley E, Watkins R, McLay A, Bulton-Jones JM. Plasma exchange in the treatment of mesangiocapillary glomerulonephritis. *Nephron.* 1985;40:385-390.
37. Jones G, Juszczak M, Kingdon E, et al. Treatment of idiopathic membranoproliferative glomerulonephritis with mycophenolate mofetil and steroids. *Nephrol Dial Transplant.* 2004;12:3160-3164.
38. Rossi P, Bertani T, Baio P, et al. Hepatitis C virus–related cryoglobulinemic glomerulonephritis: Long-term remission after antiviral therapy. *Kidney Int.* 2003;63:2236-2241.
39. Bruchfeld A, Lindahl K, Stahle L, et al. Interferon and ribavirin treatment in patients with hepatitis C–associated renal disease and renal insufficiency. *Nephrol Dial Transplant.* 2003;18:1573-1580.
40. Alric L, Plaisier E, Thébault S, et al. Influence of antiviral therapy in hepatitis C virus–associated cryoglobulinemic MPGN. *Am J Kidney Dis.* 2004;43:617-623.
41. Kamar N, Rostaing L, Alric L. Treatment of hepatitis C-virus–related glomerulonephritis. *Kidney Int.* 2006;69:436-439.
42. Zaja F, De Vita S, Mazzaro C, et al. Efficacy and safety of rituximab in type II mixed cryoglobulinemia. *Blood.* 2003;101:3827-3834.
43. Roccatello D, Baldovino S, Rossi D, et al. Long-term effects of anti-CD20 monoclonal antibody treatment of cryoglobulinaemic glomerulonephritis. *Nephrol Dial Transplant.* 2004;19:3054-3061.
44. Kiyomoto H, Hitomi H, Hosotani Y, et al. The effect of combination therapy with interferon and cryofiltration on mesangial proliferative glomerulonephritis originating from mixed cryoglobulinemia in chronic hepatitis C virus infection. *Ther Apher.* 1999;3:329-333.

CHAPTER 22

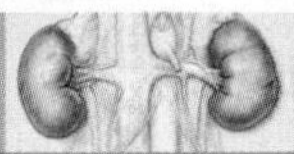

IgA Nephropathy and Henoch-Schönlein Nephritis

John Feehally, Jürgen Floege

DEFINITIONS

IgA Nephropathy

IgA nephropathy (IgAN) is a mesangial proliferative glomerulonephritis characterized by diffuse mesangial deposition of IgA. IgAN was first recognized when immunofluorescence techniques were introduced for the study of renal biopsy specimens. It was described in 1968 by a Parisian pathologist, Jean Berger (it has also been called Berger's disease). Although its most common clinical presentation is visible hematuria provoked by mucosal infection, this is neither universal nor necessary for the diagnosis. IgAN is unique among glomerular diseases in being defined by the presence of an immune reactant rather than by any other morphologic feature found on renal biopsy, and the light microscopic changes are variable. IgAN is the most prevalent pattern of glomerular disease seen in most Western and Asian countries where renal biopsy is widely practiced. At one time, the term *benign recurrent hematuria* was also used for IgAN, but it is now known to be an important cause of end-stage renal disease (ESRD). It is likely that IgAN is not a single entity but rather a common response to various injurious mechanisms.

Henoch-Schönlein Purpura

Henoch-Schönlein purpura (HSP) is a small-vessel vasculitis affecting the skin, joints, gut, and kidneys that predominantly affects children. It is defined by tissue deposition of IgA. HSP was described separately by Schönlein in 1837 and Henoch in 1874. Typically, there is clinical involvement in the skin, gut, and kidneys. The nephritis associated with HSP is also characterized by mesangial IgA deposition; indeed, the renal histologic features of Henoch-Schönlein (HS) nephritis are indistinguishable from those of IgAN. HS nephritis is differentiated from IgAN by the extrarenal manifestations.

ETIOLOGY AND PATHOGENESIS

Although infective episodes precede HSP in up to 50% of cases, there is no evidence of a role for any specific antigen. The clinical association of visible hematuria with upper respiratory tract infection in IgAN indicates that the mucosa may be a site of entry for foreign antigens. An infectious source has long been suspected, and there have been occasional reports of IgAN in association with microbial infection, both bacterial (including *Campylobacter*, *Yersinia*, *Mycoplasma*, and *Haemophilus*) and viral (including cytomegalovirus, adenovirus, coxsackievirus, and Epstein-Barr virus). A severe form of IgAN, which may be crescentic, has been reported in association with severe staphylococcal infection. None, however, has been consistently implicated by the finding of microbial antigen in glomerular deposits in typical cases of IgAN. Food antigens have also been proposed (particularly gliadin), but their involvement is not proven. The mesangial IgA may represent a common immune response to a variety of foreign antigens, the original antigen having disappeared from the deposits by the time of the biopsy. Alternatively, it may be an autoimmune disease directed against mesangial antigens, or it may develop through an antigen-independent mechanism such as altered IgA glycosylation.[1]

The regular recurrence of IgAN and HS nephritis after renal transplantation (see Chapter 104) strongly implies an abnormality in the host IgA immune system.

IgA Immune System

IgA is the most abundant immunoglobulin in the body and is chiefly concerned with mucosal defense. It has two subclasses, IgA1 and IgA2. Mucosal antigen challenge provokes polymeric IgA (pIgA) production by plasma cells of the mucosa-associated lymphoid tissue; the pIgA is then transported across epithelium into mucosal fluids, where it is released after coupling to secretory component as secretory IgA (sIgA). The function of circulating IgA is less clear; it is bone marrow derived and mostly monomeric IgA1 (mIgA1). Circulating IgA1 is cleared by the liver through hepatocyte asialoglycoprotein receptors and Kupffer cell Fcα receptors.

The mesangial IgA in IgAN is predominantly pIgA1. The clinical association with mucosal infection or superantigens from *Staphylococcus aureus* originally suggested that the mesangial pIgA1 comes from the mucosal immune system. In IgAN, however, pIgA1 production is downregulated in the mucosa and upregulated in the bone marrow. Moreover, the pIgA response to systemic immunization with common antigens is increased, whereas the response to mucosal immunization is impaired. Impaired mucosal IgA responses allowing enhanced antigen challenge to the marrow could be the primary abnormality in IgAN, although this remains unproven. Similarly attractive, yet still unproven, is the hypothesis that some mucosal IgA-producing plasma cells translocate to the bone marrow in IgAN; this could also explain the defective glycosylation of IgA1 in IgAN (see later discussion). Tonsillar pIgA1 production is also increased, although IgAN can occur after tonsillectomy, and the tonsil is a very minor source of IgA production compared with the mucosa or marrow. There are reports of sIgA in the mesangium, but this finding is not easily explained by current pathogenic concepts of IgAN. Hepatic clearance of IgA is reduced, possibly as a consequence of the altered molecular characteristics of IgA in IgAN (see later discussion).

Serum IgA levels are increased in one third of patients with IgAN and HSP. There are elevations in both mIgA and pIgA. High serum IgA *per se* is not, however, sufficient to cause IgAN; high circulating levels of monoclonal IgA (in myeloma) or polyclonal IgA (in acquired immunodeficiency syndrome [AIDS]) only infrequently provoke mesangial IgA deposition.

Circulating macromolecular IgA is characteristic of IgAN. It is often described as IgA immune complexes, although the antigen is only rarely identified. There are circulating IgA rheumatoid factors (IgA against the constant domain of IgG) in 30% of those with IgAN and 55% of those with HSP. Studies *in vitro* indicate that IgA production by mononuclear cells is exaggerated in IgAN and that these cells show abnormal patterns of cytokine production. The direct relevance of these observations to events *in vivo* is uncertain, however.

IgA Glycosylation

IgA1 carries distinctive *O*-linked sugars at its hinge region; IgA2 has no hinge and carries no such sugars. There is good evidence that circulating IgA1 in IgAN and HS nephritis has abnormal *O*-linked hinge-region sugars with reduced galactosylation because of altered IgA production in lymphocytes of patients with IgAN.[1] The pathogenic processes that lead to altered serum IgA1 *O*-glycosylation remain uncertain. There are some data pointing to defective function of the relevant glycosyltransferases that *O*-glycosylate IgA1, possibly with a genetic basis; other findings suggest that the primary abnormality may be that IgA of mucosal type, which has glycosylation patterns different from serum IgA1, reaches the circulation.[2]

Mesangial IgA1 in IgAN has the same abnormalities of *O*-glycosylation.[3,4] The altered glycosylation may lead to IgG anti-IgA autoantibodies and promote mesangial IgA1 deposition by predisposing to the formation of circulating IgA1 immune complexes or by directly modifying IgA1 interactions with matrix proteins and mesangial cell or monocyte Fc receptors.[5] It may also impair IgA1 clearance by inhibiting IgA1 interactions with hepatic and circulating myeloid cell IgA receptors. Some key elements involved in the pathogenesis of IgAN are summarized in Figure 22.1.

Glomerular Injury After IgA Deposition

Polymeric IgA deposition in the mesangium is typically followed by mesangial proliferative glomerulonephritis (GN). In animal models, codeposition of IgG and complement is necessary for inflammation, but this is not mandatory in human disease. Circulating antimesangial IgG has been associated with disease activity in IgAN; this remains unconfirmed, however. Complement deposits are usually C3 and properdin without C1q and C4. The extent to which IgA engages inflammatory cells in the circulation and especially in the kidney will also determine the

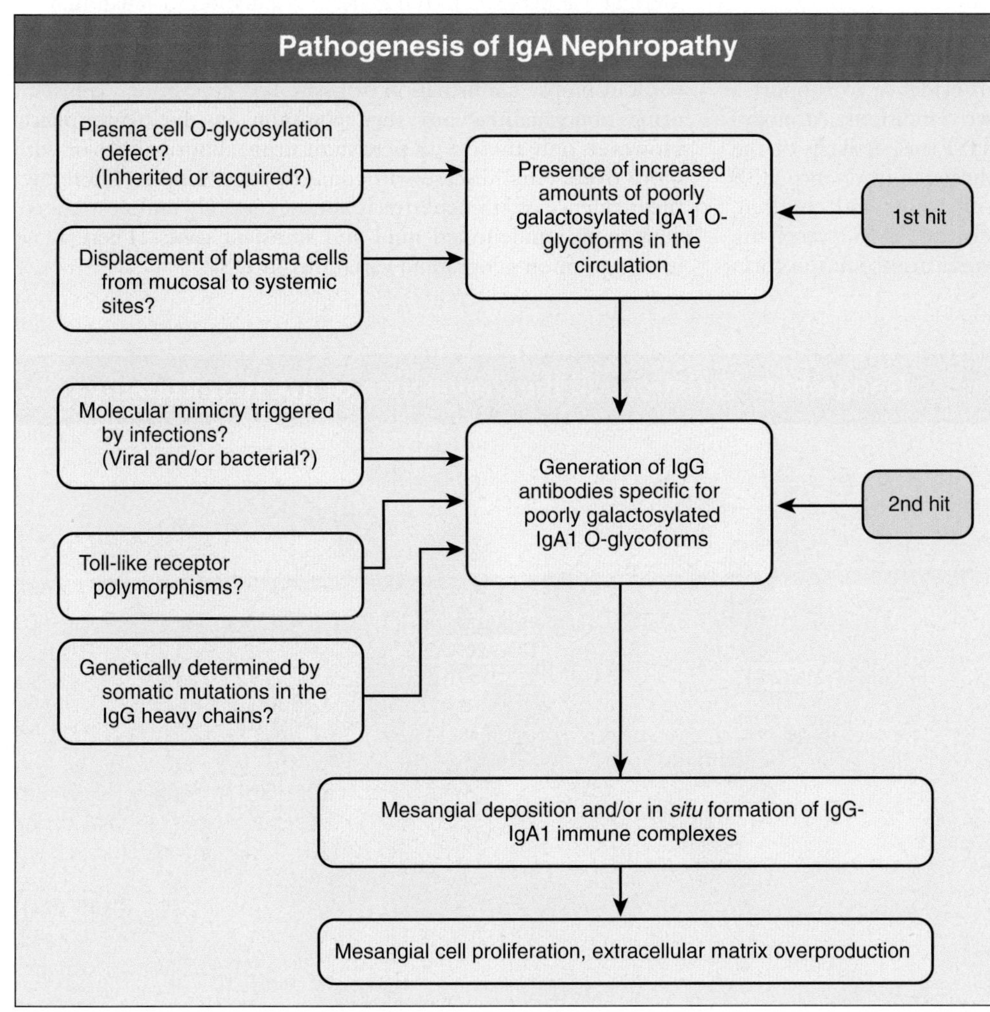

Figure 22.1 Pathogenesis of IgA nephropathy. Proposed mechanisms leading to mesangial deposition of abnormally glycosylated IgA1 and mesangial injury.

intensity of inflammation. Fc receptors for IgA (Fcα receptors) on myeloid and mesangial cells may play a key role.[6]

The mechanisms of mesangial proliferative GN have been studied in detail in animal models, particularly anti–Thy 1 nephritis in the rat. These studies have shown the key role of cytokines and growth factors in mesangial cell proliferation (particularly the B and D isoforms of platelet-derived growth factor[7] [PDGF]) and in the subsequent matrix production and sclerosis (particularly transforming growth factor β [TGF-β]). Studies of renal biopsy specimens in human IgAN also support a role for PDGF and TGF-β. These mechanisms are not unique to IgAN but are likely to be involved in all forms of mesangial proliferative GN, including those without IgA deposition. Clinical trials based on these pathogenetic insights, in particular with respect to PDGF, are being planned.[7]

Animal Models of IgA Nephropathy

Animal IgA does not have the same characteristics as human IgA1, and some animals also have IgA clearance mechanisms distinct from those in humans. It follows that animal models, even if they provoke mesangial IgA deposits, are not particularly informative about the mechanisms that underlie human mesangial pIgA1 deposition, although they have provided many insights into events after IgA deposits have developed. There is no animal model in existence for HSP.

Relationship Between IgA Nephropathy and Henoch-Schönlein Purpura

Despite some differences in age at onset and natural history of IgAN and HS nephritis,[8] there is much evidence to support a close pathogenetic link between the two conditions. Monozygotic twins who developed IgAN and HSP, respectively, at the same time have been described. The evolution of IgAN into HSP in the same patient is described in both adults and children, and HSP patients with, end-stage renal disease (ESRD) receiving a renal transplant may experience recurrent disease in the form of IgAN. Many of the abnormalities of IgA production and handling reported in IgAN are also detected in HSP.

IgA antineutrophil cytoplasmic antibodies (IgA-ANCA) have been proposed as a marker of the systemic features that differentiate HSP from IgAN. Circulating IgA-ANCA has been described in HSP, although findings are not consistent. IgA-ANCA is not found in IgAN.

EPIDEMIOLOGY

IgAN is the most prevalent pattern of glomerular disease in most countries where renal biopsy is widely used as an investigative tool. However, there is striking geographic variation (Fig. 22.2). Genetic variations may be important. For example, in North America, IgAN is less common in African Americans than in Caucasians of European origin. It is also very uncommon among black South Africans. In New Zealand, IgAN is much less common among Polynesians than among Caucasians of European origin, even though Polynesians have an increased prevalence of ESRD due to other renal diseases. Perceived prevalence of IgAN may also be influenced by attitudes to the investigation of microscopic hematuria. A country with an active program of routine urine testing will inevitably identify more individuals with urine abnormalities, but IgAN will be identified only if renal biopsy is performed. Even then, the prevalence of IgAN will be underestimated; a study of kidney donors suggests that the prevalence of IgAN with mesangial proliferative changes and glomerular C3 deposits in the general population in Japan may be 1.6%.[9]

In children, HSP is usually diagnosed on clinical grounds without biopsy confirmation of tissue IgA deposition. Transient urine abnormalities are very common in the acute phase. However, only those with persistent urine abnormalities or with more overt renal disease will come to renal biopsy. Therefore, the incidence of HS nephritis is almost certainly underestimated, with many unidentified mild and transient cases. There is no information on geographic variations in HSP.

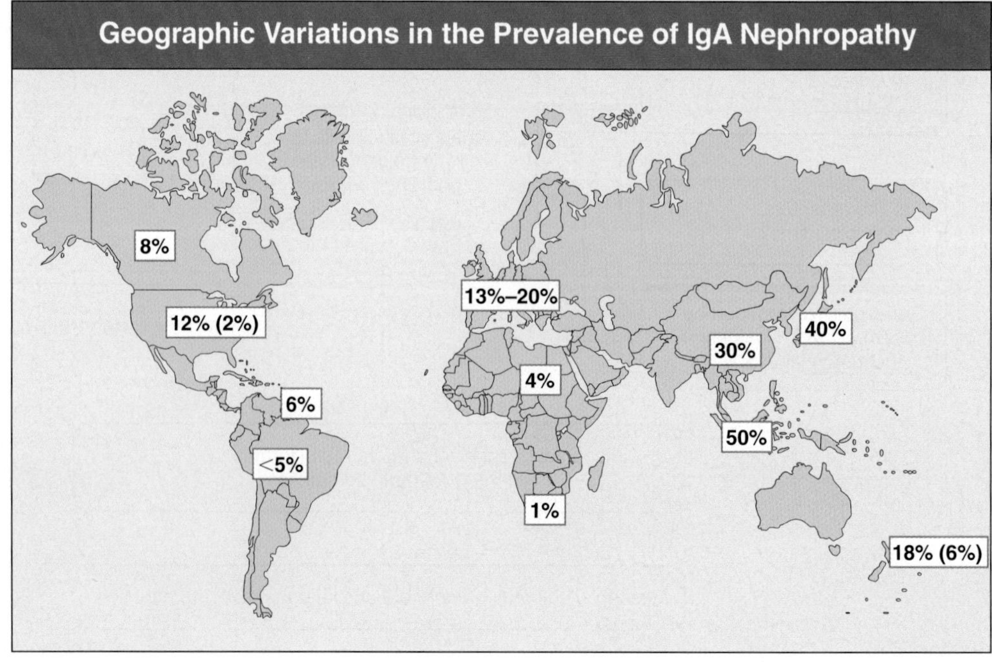

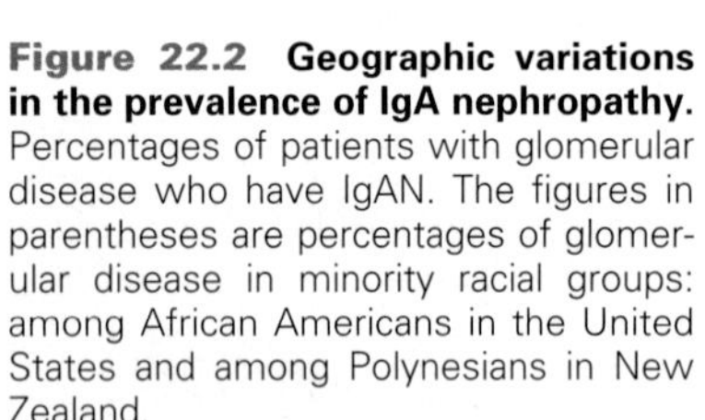
Figure 22.2 Geographic variations in the prevalence of IgA nephropathy. Percentages of patients with glomerular disease who have IgAN. The figures in parentheses are percentages of glomerular disease in minority racial groups: among African Americans in the United States and among Polynesians in New Zealand.

Genetic Basis of IgA Nephropathy

Urine abnormalities increase in frequency among the relatives of those with IgAN, although only in a few pedigrees is IgAN found in multiple generations. One very large pedigree has been described in Kentucky, and other large families have been found in Italy and Canada. However, more than 90% of all cases of IgAN appear to be sporadic.

In three different kindreds with IgAN, different regions of the genome are implicated in disease susceptibility, emphasizing the polygenic nature of this condition. Investigation of these genome regions has not yet yielded definitive candidate disease susceptibility genes.[10]

Many association studies have sought genes associated with disease in sporadic IgAN, so far without consistent findings.[10]

CLINICAL MANIFESTATIONS OF IgA NEPHROPATHY

The wide range of clinical presentations of IgAN varies in frequency with age (Fig. 22.3). No clinical pattern is pathognomonic of IgAN. In populations of Caucasian descent, it is more common in males than in females by a ratio of 3 : 1, whereas the ratio approaches 1 : 1 in most Asian populations.

Macroscopic Hematuria

In 40% to 50% of cases, the clinical presentation is episodic macroscopic hematuria, most frequently in the second and third decades of life. The urine is usually brown rather than red, and clots are unusual. There may be loin pain due to renal capsular swelling. Hematuria usually follows intercurrent mucosal infection, commonly in the upper respiratory tract (the term *synpharyngitic hematuria* has been used) or occasionally in the gastrointestinal tract. Hematuria is usually visible within 24 hours of the onset of the symptoms of infection, differentiating it from the 2- to 3-week delay between infection and subsequent hematuria in postinfectious (e.g., poststreptococcal) GN. The macroscopic hematuria resolves spontaneously in the course of a few days. There is persistent microscopic hematuria between attacks. Most patients have only a few episodes of frank hematuria. These become less frequent and resolve during a few years at most. Such episodes are sometimes associated with acute renal impairment.

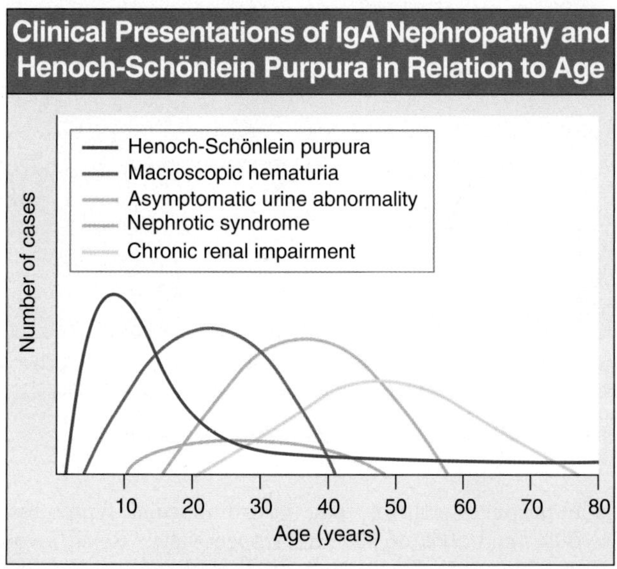

Figure 22.3 Clinical presentations of IgA nephropathy and Henoch-Schönlein purpura in relation to age at diagnosis. HSP is most common in childhood but may occur at any age. Macroscopic hematuria is very uncommon after the age of 40 years. The importance of asymptomatic urine abnormality as the presentation of IgAN will depend on attitudes to routine urine testing and renal biopsy. It is uncertain whether those presenting late with chronic renal impairment have a disease distinct from that of those presenting younger with macroscopic hematuria. Data from patients presenting in Leicester, United Kingdom, 1980 to 1995.

Asymptomatic Hematuria and Proteinuria

Asymptomatic urine testing identifies 30% to 40% of patients with IgAN in most reported series. Microscopic hematuria with or without proteinuria (usually <2 g/24 h) is noted. The number of patients identified in this way will depend on local attitudes to urine screening as well as on the use of renal biopsy in patients with isolated microscopic hematuria. Most patients with IgAN are asymptomatic and would be identified only when there is population-based urine screening.

Proteinuria and Nephrotic Syndrome

It is rare for proteinuria to occur without microscopic hematuria. Nephrotic syndrome is uncommon, occurring in only 5% of all patients with IgAN. Nephrotic syndrome may occur early in the course of the disease, with minimal glomerular change or with active mesangial proliferative GN. Alternatively, it may occur as a late manifestation of advanced chronic glomerular scarring.

Acute Kidney Injury

Acute kidney injury (AKI) is very uncommon in IgAN (<5% of all cases), although one study reports that it may be the presentation in up to 27% of those older than 65 years.[11] It develops by three distinct mechanisms. There may be acute severe immune and inflammatory injury with necrotizing GN and crescent formation (crescentic IgA nephropathy); this may be the first presentation of IgAN, or it may be superimposed on established, less aggressive disease. Rapid deterioration in IgAN in pregnancy may be due to crescentic transformation. Alternatively, acute renal failure can occur with mild glomerular injury when heavy glomerular hematuria leads to tubule occlusion by red cells. Finally, especially in elderly patients, chronic IgAN will predispose to AKI from a variety of incidental renal insults (see Chapter 66).

Chronic Kidney Disease

Some patients already have renal impairment and hypertension when they are first diagnosed. These patients tend to be older, and it is probable that they have long-standing disease that previously remained undiagnosed because the patient neither had frank hematuria nor underwent routine urinalysis. Hypertension is common as in other chronic glomerular disease; accelerated hypertension occurs in 5% of patients.

Clinical Associations with IgA Nephropathy

Although IgAN is clinically restricted to the kidney in most cases, there are case reports of associations with many other

Diseases Reported in Association with IgA Nephropathy

Disease	Common	Reported	Rare
Rheumatic and autoimmune disease	Ankylosing spondylitis Rheumatoid arthritis Reiter syndrome Uveitis	Behçet's syndrome* Takayasu's arteritis† Myasthenia gravis	Sicca syndrome
Gastrointestinal disease	Celiac disease	Ulcerative colitis	Crohn's disease Whipple's disease
Hepatic disease	Alcoholic liver disease Nonalcoholic cirrhosis Schistosomal liver disease		
Lung disease	Sarcoid		Pulmonary hemosiderosis
Skin disease	Dermatitis herpetiformis		
Malignancy		IgA monoclonal gammopathy	Bronchial carcinoma Renal carcinoma Laryngeal carcinoma Mycosis fungoides Sézary syndrome
Infection	Human immunodeficiency virus, hepatitis B (in endemic areas)	Brucellosis	Leprosy
Miscellaneous		Wiskott-Aldrich syndrome‡	

Figure 22.4 Diseases reported in association with IgA nephropathy: common, reported, and rare. Rare associations have been made in one or two reported cases only. In a disease as common as IgAN, it is therefore uncertain whether they are truly related. *Behçet's syndrome: a systemic vasculitis typified by orogenital ulceration and chronic uveitis. †Takayasu arteritis: a systemic vasculitis involving the aorta and its major branches, most often found in young women. ‡Wiskott-Aldrich syndrome: an X-linked disorder in which increased serum IgA is associated with the triad of recurrent pyogenic infection, eczema, and thrombocytopenia.

conditions, particularly with a number of immune and inflammatory diseases (Fig. 22.4). Their relationship to abnormalities of the IgA immune system is not always clear, and some may represent the coincidental development of unrelated but relatively common conditions.

Mesangial IgA deposition is a frequent finding in autopsy studies in chronic liver disease. Although it is particularly associated with alcoholic cirrhosis, it can occur in other chronic liver disease, including that caused by hepatitis B and schistosomiasis. It is thought to be a consequence of impaired clearance of IgA by the Kupffer cells (which express Fcα receptors) and hepatocytes (which express the asialoglycoprotein receptor). Clinical evidence of renal disease is more common than previously appreciated, and occasionally patients will develop ESRD.

A number of case reports have associated IgAN with human immunodeficiency virus/AIDS. It is not clear whether the polyclonal increase in serum IgA, which is a feature of AIDS, is the predisposing factor.

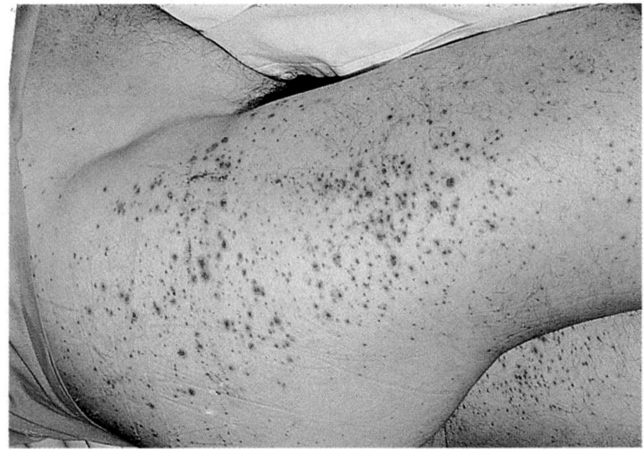

Figure 22.5 Henoch-Schönlein purpura. The rash is a palpable purpuric vasculitis on the lower limbs spreading on extensor surfaces to the buttocks and occasionally to the upper limbs. Histology shows leukocytoclastic vasculitis with IgA deposits in blood vessel walls.

CLINICAL MANIFESTATIONS OF HENOCH-SCHÖNLEIN PURPURA

HSP is most prevalent in the first decade of life but may occur at any age. A palpable purpuric rash, which may be recurrent, occurs on extensor surfaces (Fig. 22.5). There may be polyarthralgia (usually without joint swelling) and abdominal pain caused by gut vasculitis. This may be severe, with bloody diarrhea if intussusception develops. In practice, the diagnosis is made by clinical criteria in the great majority of children, in whom HSP is a self-limited illness. In adults, clinical features include purpura, arthritis, and gastrointestinal symptoms in 95%, 60%, and 50% of patients, respectively.[12] Renal involvement in adults with HSP is not different from isolated IgAN. Tissue confirmation of IgA deposition by renal or skin biopsy is necessary to establish the diagnosis.

Much renal involvement in HSP is transient. Urine abnormalities are noted during the acute presentation but may disappear. Of those referred to a nephrologist, asymptomatic urine abnormality is still the most frequent clinical manifestation. Nephrotic syndrome occurs in 20% to 30% of patients. AKI may develop as a result of crescentic GN.

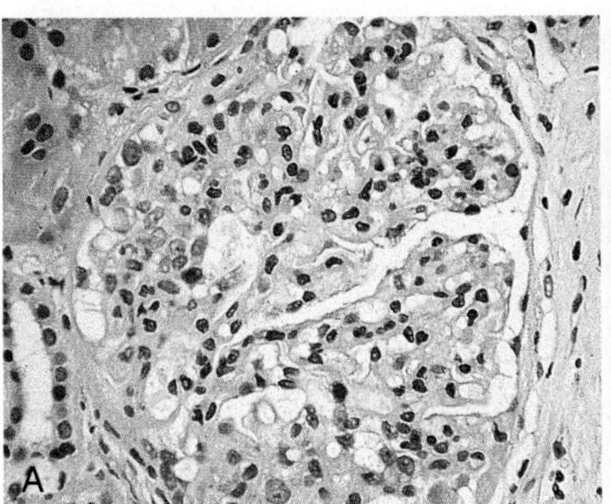

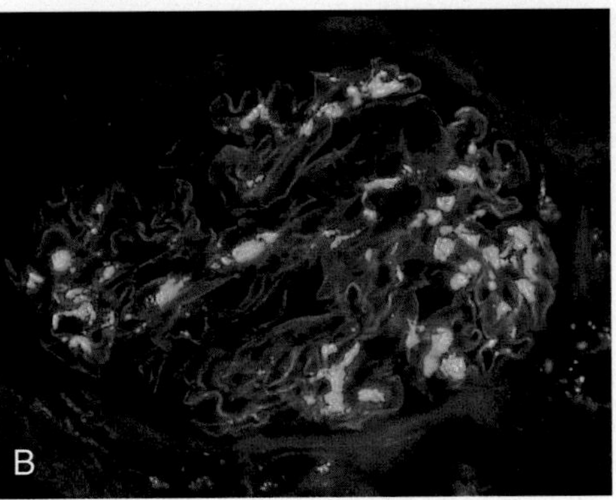

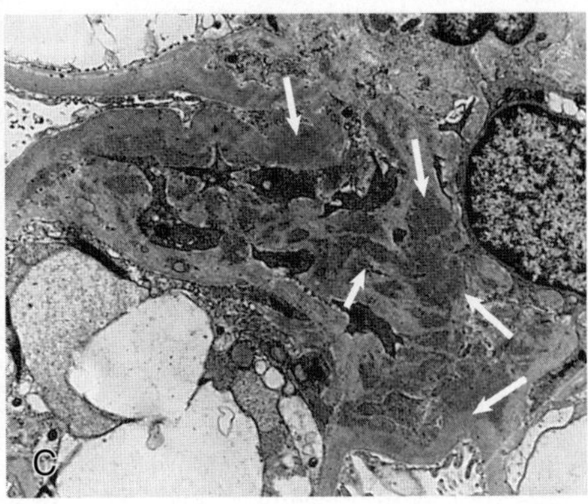

Figure 22.6 Renal pathology in IgA nephropathy. A, Light microscopy: diffuse mesangial hypercellularity. (Hematoxylin-eosin; magnification ×3300.) **B,** Immunofluorescence microscopy: diffuse mesangial IgA. (Indirect immunofluorescence with fluorescein isothiocyanate–anti-IgA; magnification × 3300.) **C,** Electron microscopy: mesangial electron-dense deposits. The deposits are shown by *arrows*. (Electron micrograph; magnification ×316,000.) *(**A** and **C** courtesy Prof. P. Furness.)*

PATHOLOGY

The renal histopathologic findings in IgAN and HS nephritis may be indistinguishable (Fig. 22.6).

Immune Deposits

Diffuse mesangial IgA, shown in Figure 22.6B, is the defining hallmark. C3 is codeposited in up to 90% of cases. IgG in 40% and IgM in 40% of cases may also be found in the same distribution. IgA also deposits sometimes along capillary loops (a pattern more common in HS nephritis); in IgAN, this pattern is associated with a worse prognosis. C5b-9 is found with properdin but not C4, indicating alternative complement pathway activation. Disappearance of IgA deposits after prolonged clinical remission has been documented in both children and adults. About one third of the patients also have deposits of sIgA in the mesangium and are characterized by more severe disease.[13]

Light Microscopy

Light microscopic changes are remarkably variable and do not correlate topographically with the IgA deposits. They can be almost normal glomerular architecture, diffuse mesangial proliferative GN (see Fig. 22.6A), focal segmental GN, or, in rare cases, focal segmental necrotizing GN with extracapillary proliferation. Typical cases are characterized by an increase in mesangial cells and mesangial matrix with normal-appearing capillary loops. Focal segmental or global glomerular sclerosis indicates that the disease has been ongoing for some time. In addition to glomerular changes, the preglomerular arterial vessels often exhibit wall hyalinosis and subintimal fibrosis even in cases of only mild arterial hypertension. In long-standing disease, tubulointerstitial inflammation leads to interstitial fibrosis and tubular atrophy in a pattern no different from other progressive glomerular disease. On occasion, IgAN and minimal change nephrotic syndrome coincide (see later under Nephrotic Syndrome), in which case light microscopy is normal but there are mesangial IgA deposits.

Morphology is of value in predicting prognosis in slowly progressive cases, although there has been no universal agreement until recently as to the ideal pathologic classification. However, the Oxford classification of IgAN is now being widely accepted.[14]

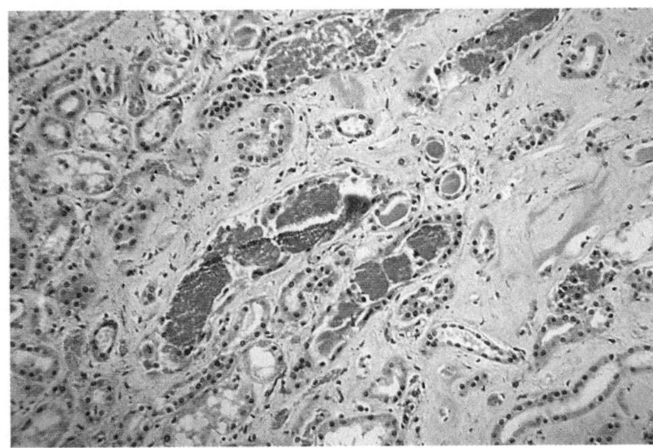

Figure 22.7 Acute kidney injury in IgA nephropathy. Tubular occlusion by red cells. (Hematoxylin-eosin; magnification ×300.) This appearance may be associated with only minor glomerular changes.

Two distinct patterns of injury are seen in AKI. There may be tubular occlusion by red cells with acute tubular epithelial injury in macrohematuria-associated AKI (Fig. 22.7). Alternatively, glomerular injury may be the cause of AKI with necrotizing GN and cellular crescent formation. Such crescentic IgAN may develop on a histologic background of established chronic renal injury due to IgAN or may be the first presentation of IgAN. It is not uncommon to see small numbers of crescents in patients with stable renal function and no other pathologic evidence of severe glomerular inflammation; the term *crescentic IgAN* should not be used for such cases, in which the prognosis is often favorable.

Electron Microscopy

Electron-dense deposits correspond to the mesangial (or capillary loop) IgA, as shown in Figure 22.6C. Typically, electron-dense deposits are confined to mesangial and paramesangial areas, but, in addition, subepithelial and subendothelial deposits can also be seen. Up to one third of patients will have some focal thinning of the glomerular basement membrane (GBM). On occasion, there will be extensive GBM thinning, suggesting a coincident diagnosis of thin membrane nephropathy (see Chapter 46).

Differential Diagnosis of IgA Nephropathy: Conditions Associated with Mesangial IgA Deposition

IgA nephropathy
Henoch-Schönlein nephritis
Lupus nephritis*
Alcoholic liver disease
IgA monoclonal gammopathy
Schistosomal nephropathy

Figure 22.8 Differential diagnosis of IgA nephropathy: conditions associated with mesangial IgA deposition. *Distinguishing lupus nephritis (especially International Society of Nephrology/Renal Pathology Society classes II and III) may cause difficulty. The finding of C1q deposition is useful. It indicates classical pathway involvement found in lupus nephritis but not in IgAN.

DIFFERENTIAL DIAGNOSIS

The diagnosis of IgAN or HS nephritis requires identification of mesangial IgA in the glomeruli. Therefore, it cannot be made without a renal biopsy, no matter how suggestive the clinical presentation may be. Serum IgA is often increased, and there may be IgA in cutaneous blood vessels in IgAN and in both affected and unaffected skin in HSP. Neither finding, however, is reliable enough to support the diagnosis without a renal biopsy. Serum complement components are normal.

Mesangial IgA occurs in other conditions (Fig. 22.8) that can usually be differentiated by clinical, serologic, and histologic criteria. None of the light microscopic features are of themselves diagnostic of IgAN.

Hematuria

Nonglomerular causes of hematuria, particularly stones and neoplasia, must be excluded by appropriate investigations (see Chapter 59). In its most characteristic clinical setting (recurrent macroscopic hematuria coinciding with mucosal infection in a man in the second or third decade of life), the diagnosis can be strongly suspected. Such a diagnosis, however, cannot be made without a biopsy because recurrent macroscopic hematuria also occurs in other glomerular diseases, particularly in children and young adults.

Nephrotic Syndrome

Patients with IgAN occasionally develop nephrotic syndrome, which is indistinguishable from that in minimal change disease (MCD). There is a sudden onset of nephrosis, with biopsy evidence of glomerular epithelial cell foot process effacement and a prompt complete remission of proteinuria in response to corticosteroids. Only hematuria and mesangial IgA deposits persist after treatment. This pattern occurs particularly in children. These patients are usually regarded as having two separate common glomerular diseases, IgAN and MCD.[15]

Other patients with IgAN may develop nephrotic syndrome with more structural glomerular damage and lack the response to corticosteroids. The clinical differential diagnosis includes common causes of nephrotic syndrome appropriate for the age of the patient (see Chapter 15).

Chronic Kidney Disease: Hypertension, Proteinuria, Renal Impairment

In this context, IgAN will be clinically indistinguishable from many forms of chronic kidney disease (CKD). The renal biopsy may be diagnostic by identifying mesangial IgA, even when structural damage is so advanced on light microscopy that it has the nonspecific features of ESRD.

Acute Kidney Injury

When AKI occurs in a patient known to have IgAN, renal biopsy should be performed unless there is rapid improvement in renal function after at least 5 days from the onset of kidney function worsening in response to supportive care and vigorous hydration. Renal biopsy may be required to differentiate the tubular occlusion and acute tubular necrosis that occasionally follow heavy glomerular hematuria from crescentic IgAN or other coincidental causes of AKI (see Fig. 22.7).

Differential Diagnosis of Henoch-Schönlein Purpura

In children, the diagnosis of HSP is usually made on the basis of clinical criteria. Confirmatory evidence of tissue IgA deposition will not be obtained unless persistence of renal disease results in a renal biopsy. In adults, the differential diagnosis is much wider and includes other forms of systemic vasculitis, requiring diagnosis by clinical, serologic, and histologic characteristics (see Chapter 24).

NATURAL HISTORY

Natural History of IgA Nephropathy

The overall prognosis of IgAN has now been defined in long-term natural history studies.[16] Although the evidence shows clinical remission (disappearance of hematuria and proteinuria) in up to one third of patients with mild disease, large studies with prolonged follow-up indicate a slow attrition. By 20 years, one fourth of patients will have ESRD, and a further 20% will have progressive impairment of renal function. It is important to appreciate that these natural history data are based on studies initiated more than 20 years ago; however, in a recent study from France, 7-year renal survival in IgAN was still only 82% despite widespread angiotensin-converting enzyme (ACE) inhibitor therapy.[17]

Although an active approach to the investigation of microscopic hematuria will increase the size of the cohort of patients found to have IgAN, it will include more with a good prognosis, thus altering the perceived risk of disease progression. Episodes of macroscopic hematuria do not confer a worse prognosis. This may indicate that such episodes occur only early in the natural history of the disease and that patients doing less well from the point of diagnosis in fact were identified at a later stage in their disease. This is also suggested by the adverse influence on outcome of advancing age at diagnosis.

The risk of ESRD is not uniform. As in any chronic glomerular disease, the presence of hypertension, proteinuria, and reduced glomerular filtration rate (GFR) at presentation, as well as histologic evidence of glomerular and interstitial fibrosis, identifies at the time of diagnosis those with a poor prognosis (Fig. 22.9).[14,16] Hyperuricemia and increased body mass index are also independent risk factors for progression. However, during

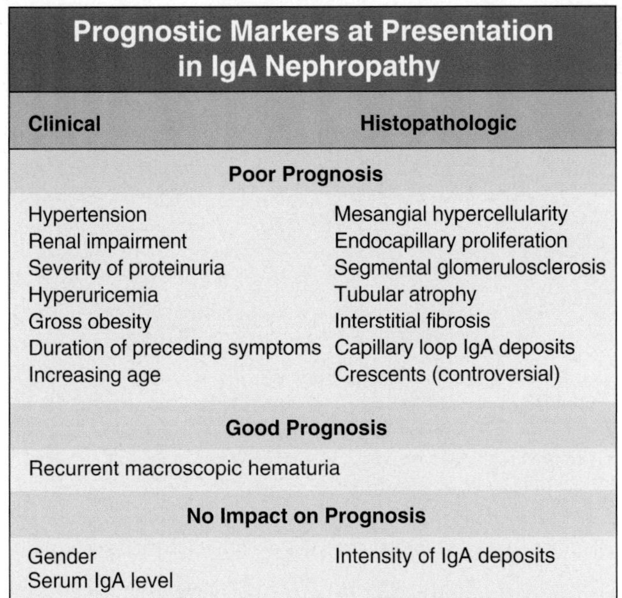

Prognostic Markers at Presentation in IgA Nephropathy

Clinical	Histopathologic
Poor Prognosis	
Hypertension	Mesangial hypercellularity
Renal impairment	Endocapillary proliferation
Severity of proteinuria	Segmental glomerulosclerosis
Hyperuricemia	Tubular atrophy
Gross obesity	Interstitial fibrosis
Duration of preceding symptoms	Capillary loop IgA deposits
Increasing age	Crescents (controversial)
Good Prognosis	
Recurrent macroscopic hematuria	
No Impact on Prognosis	
Gender	Intensity of IgA deposits
Serum IgA level	

Figure 22.9 Prognostic markers at presentation in IgA nephropathy. None of the clinical or histopathologic adverse features, except capillary loop IgA deposits, are specific to IgA nephropathy.

follow-up, only hypertension and proteinuria are reliable predictors of risk of progression.[18] Some evidence suggests geographic variation in risk of progression. A Canadian study indicates that risk of progression is negligible when proteinuria remains below 0.2 g/24 h with normal blood pressure (BP).[18] It also decreases very significantly if proteinuria can be reduced to less than 1 g/day by any therapeutic maneuver.[18] However, in contrast, a study from Hong Kong suggests that among those presenting with isolated microscopic hematuria, although up to 15% lost hematuria during follow-up, as many as 44% may subsequently develop proteinuria, hypertension, or renal impairment during a 7-year follow-up.[19]

Pathologic findings and clinical findings together inform prognosis. The Oxford classification of IgAN has shown that mesangial hypercellularity, endocapillary proliferation, and segmental sclerosis, as well as tubular atrophy and interstitial fibrosis, each add prognostic information even when clinical features (proteinuria, hypertension, GFR) are known at presentation and during follow-up.[14]

Natural History of Henoch-Schönlein Nephritis

This is less well defined than IgAN. Observations are restricted to those referred for renal biopsy. This therefore excludes the majority of patients with minor transient renal involvement who have an excellent prognosis. The renal prognosis is worse in adults than in children. In adults, up to 40% will have CKD or ESRD 15 years after biopsy. One series reports an increased mortality due to lung and gastrointestinal malignant disease.[12]

TRANSPLANTATION

Recurrent IgA Nephropathy

There is no evidence from transplant registry data that transplant outcome is inferior if IgAN is the primary renal disease (see also Chapter 104). Nevertheless, mesangial IgA deposits recur in the donor transplant kidney in up to 60% of patients with IgAN.[20] They may occur within days or weeks, but the risk increases with the duration of the transplant. The deposits seem benign in the short term and are not often associated initially with light microscopic changes. Graft failure due to recurrent IgAN, associated with proteinuria and hypertension, occurs in about 5% of cases within 5 years but significantly worsens the prognosis of grafts from 10 years onward or in case of repeated transplantation. In pooled series, recurrent IgAN is 30% in living related transplants versus 23% in cadaveric grafts,[21] but this does not affect graft survival, and living related donation should not be discouraged. However, any urinary abnormality in a potential related donor requires thorough evaluation, including, if necessary, a renal biopsy. Recurrence of crescentic IgAN with rapid graft failure occurs uncommonly and is generally resistant to treatment.

In a few unwitting experiments, cadaver kidneys with IgA deposits have been transplanted into recipients without IgAN. In all cases, the IgA rapidly disappeared, supporting the concept that abnormalities in IgAN lie in the IgA immune system and not in the kidney.

Recurrent Henoch-Schönlein Nephritis

HSP can recur as isolated IgA deposits in the graft (about 50% of transplants), as full-blown yet isolated IgAN, or rarely as a full recurrence of systemic involvement including a rash. The characteristics of renal recurrence are apparently similar to those of recurrent primary IgAN.[20] Delay of transplantation once ESRD is reached does not reduce the risk of recurrence.

TREATMENT

Although specific early treatment intervention might influence the IgA immune system abnormalities that underlie IgAN, the mechanisms of chronic disease progression are unlikely to be unique. It is probable, therefore, that studies of such IgAN patients will provide information applicable to many forms of chronic GN for which IgAN is the paradigm.

The balance of risk against benefit for immunosuppressive therapy is often unfavorable in IgAN, except in the unusual circumstance of crescentic IgAN.

The need for randomized controlled trials of adequate power to answer questions about the prevention of ESRD in IgAN is pressing. It is disappointing, despite the prevalence of IgAN and consensus about its definition and natural history, that there are so few such studies.[21,22] Patients with HSP have been excluded from almost all treatment studies, so it is uncertain whether any strategies developed for IgAN are applicable to HS nephritis.

TREATMENT OF IgA NEPHROPATHY

Treatment recommendations are summarized in Figure 22.10.

Reduction of IgA Production

Tonsillectomy reduces the frequency of episodic hematuria when tonsillitis is the provoking infection. A long-term retrospective study from Japan suggests that tonsillectomy may reduce the risk of renal failure,[23] but this is not supported by studies from Germany and China.[24] The lack of controlled trials is particularly important as the natural history is for macroscopic hematuria to become less frequent with time, independent of any

Treatment Recommendations for IgA Nephropathy
Recurrent macroscopic hematuria (preserved renal function) Aggressive hydration (no role for antibiotics or tonsillectomy)
Macroscopic hematuria with acute kidney injury Renal biopsy mandatory if persistent acute kidney injury (see text) Acute tubular necrosis: supportive measures only Crescentic IgAN Induction: Prednisolone 0.5–1 mg/kg/day for up to 8 weeks Cyclophosphamide 2 mg/kg/day for up to 8 weeks (no evidence favoring oral or intravenous route—follow local practice) Maintenance: Prednisolone in reducing dosage Azathioprine 2.5 mg/kg/day
Proteinuria <1 g/24 h (±microscopic hematuria) No specific treatment
Nephrotic syndrome with minimal change on light microscopy Prednisolone 0.5 1 mg/kg/day (children 60 mg/m²/day) for up to 8 weeks, then taper
Non-nephrotic proteinuria >1 g/24 h (±microscopic hematuria) ACE inhibitor and/or ARB (maximize dosage or combine to achieve target blood pressure and proteinuria<0.5 g/day); for additional measures, see Chapter 76 If proteinuria still >1 g/24 h on maximal supportive therapy and GFR <70 ml/min, consider fish oil—12 g/daily for 6 months. If further progression of renal failure, consider prednisolone (40 mg/day decreasing to 10 mg by 2 years)
Hypertension ACE inhibitors and ARB are agent of first choice—target blood pressure:130/80 mm Hg if proteinuria <1 g/24 h; 125/75 mm Hg if proteinuria >1 g/24 h
Transplantation No special measures required

Figure 22.10 Treatment recommendations for IgA nephropathy. ACE, angiotensin-converting enzyme; ARB, angiotensin receptor blocker.

specific treatment. Tonsillectomy may be indicated in the occasional patient with recurrent AKI with macroscopic hematuria induced by tonsillitis. There is no role for prophylactic antibiotics. Dietary gluten restriction, used to reduce mucosal antigen challenge, has not been shown to preserve renal function.

Prevention and Removal of IgA Deposits

The ideal treatment of IgAN would remove IgA from the glomerulus and prevent further IgA deposition. This remains a remote prospect while the pathogenesis remains incompletely understood.

Altering Immune and Inflammatory Events That Follow IgA Deposition

Rapidly Progressive Renal Failure Associated with Crescentic IgA Nephropathy

In this uncommon situation, the risk-benefit balance is most strongly placed in favor of intensive immunosuppressive therapy because, untreated, there will be rapid progression to ESRD. Treatment has often combined plasma exchange with prednisolone and cyclophosphamide.[25] Early clinical response is favorable, as in other crescentic nephritis. Medium-term results, however, are disappointing; in one half of the reported cases, patients have reached ESRD within 12 months.[25] A subset of patients with circulating IgG-ANCA may have a more favorable response to immunosuppressive therapy similar to that seen in other ANCA-positive crescentic nephritis.[26] There have been no controlled trials of treatment, so it is not possible to be certain which elements of the regimen (corticosteroids, cyclophosphamide, or plasma exchange) are mandatory.

Early Treatment with Immunosuppressive or Anti-inflammatory Regimens

Corticosteroids Corticosteroids were given in a short-term randomized, controlled trial in nephrotic adults.[27] Although the trial overall showed no benefit, there was a small group with very minor histologic changes that responded rapidly to treatment. Nephrotic syndrome may occur in this setting when MCD and IgAN coincide, in which case the nephrotic syndrome will be fully and promptly corticosteroid responsive. A trial of high-dose corticosteroid therapy is therefore justified in IgAN when there is nephrotic syndrome associated with minimal glomerular injury.

Uncontrolled data available for some years have favored the prolonged administration of alternate-day corticosteroids. This approach is further supported by a randomized, controlled trial indicating that 6 months of intravenous pulse methylprednisolone plus alternate-day corticosteroids in adults with low-grade proteinuria protects renal function during long-term follow-up.[28]

Another controlled trial using smaller doses of corticosteroids in patients with non-nephrotic proteinuria showed some reduction in protein excretion but no protection of renal function.[29]

It is unfortunate that these trials of corticosteroids were initiated before the importance was appreciated of rigorous BP control and the critical role of renin-angiotensin blockade in proteinuric glomerular disease. Variable achieved BP and inconsistent use of ACE inhibitors and angiotensin receptor blockers (ARBs) left uncertainty about the role of corticosteroids if tight BP control with renin-angiotensin blockade is maintained. However, two studies suggest significant benefits of 6 months of corticosteroids even when BP control and renin-angiotensin blockade are used in all patients[30,31]; this evidence is not yet definitive, and further trials are awaited.[32]

Cyclophosphamide Cyclophosphamide has been used in combination with warfarin and dipyridamole in two randomized, controlled trials, the results of which are not mutually consistent. Both showed modest reduction in proteinuria, but only one preserved renal function. Cyclophosphamide followed by azathioprine combined with prednisolone preserved renal function in a controlled trial in patients with a poor prognosis.[33] Many physicians regard the toxicity of cyclophosphamide as unacceptable in young adults with IgAN. In another recent study,[49] adding azathioprine to corticosteroids in proteinuric IgAN patients with a GFR >50 ml/min had no added benefit and only increased side effects.

Mycophenolate Mofetil Mycophenolate mofetil (MMF) has been used in several controlled trials in high-risk patients. Two trials in Caucasian patients failed to demonstrate any benefit, whereas a short-term study in Chinese patients noted reduced proteinuria. Whether racial effects indeed underlie these discrepant results remains to be clarified.[34] In another Chinese trial, four of 32 IgAN patients receiving MMF plus corticosteroids died of *Pneumocystis* pneumonia.[35]

Dipyridamole and Warfarin These have also been given in two controlled trials that showed mutually inconsistent results. There was no benefit in one and preserved renal function in the other.

Cyclosporine Cyclosporine has been used in one controlled trial. There was a reversible decrease in proteinuria. This went in parallel with a decrease in creatinine clearance, suggesting that the changes were a hemodynamic effect of cyclosporine rather than an immune-modulating effect.

Pooled Human Immunoglobulin Pooled human immunoglobulin has given encouraging preliminary results in IgAN with an aggressive clinical course: proteinuria lessened, deterioration of GFR slowed, and histologic activity lessened on repeated renal biopsies.[36] No controlled trial is available for this approach.

Treatment of Slowly Progressive IgA Nephropathy

There is little evidence to indicate that the events of progressive glomerular injury are unique to IgAN. Treatments available are nonspecific approaches for chronic glomerular disease (see also Chapter 77), of which IgAN is the most common and most easily defined.

Hypertension

There is compelling evidence of the benefit of lowering BP in the treatment of chronic progressive glomerular disease such as IgAN. In IgAN, there is also evidence that casual clinic BP readings underestimate BP load as judged by ambulatory BP monitoring and echocardiographic evidence of increased left ventricular mass.[37] Two prospective, controlled trials strongly support the use of ACE inhibitors in IgAN as first-choice hypotensive agents to minimize proteinuria as well as BP.[38,39] Low target BPs (<130/80 mm Hg if proteinuria is <1 g/24 h, 125/75 mm Hg if proteinuria is >1 g/24 h) are recommended from a number of large studies of chronic progressive renal disease. In a randomized study of IgAN, achieving a mean BP of 129/70 mm Hg prevented the decrease in renal function during 3 years seen in those achieving mean BPs of 136/76 mm Hg.[40]

Fish Oil

The favorable effects of supplementing the diet with omega-3 fatty acids in the form of fish oil include reductions in eicosanoid and cytokine production, changes in membrane fluidity and rheology, and reduced platelet aggregability. These features should significantly reduce the adverse influence of many mechanisms thought to affect progression of chronic glomerular disease.

A randomized, controlled trial provides convincing evidence of protection from 2 years of treatment with fish oil in patients with proteinuria and increasing serum creatinine.[41] It is, however, surprising that fish oil did not significantly reduce proteinuria, a major risk factor for progression. Another study showed no advantage for high- over low-dose fish oil.[42] However, other smaller controlled trials have shown no benefit,[43] although severity of renal impairment before treatment was not equivalent in all these studies. Fish oil treatment does not have the drawbacks associated with immunosuppressive treatment. It is safe apart from a decrease in blood coagulability, which is not usually a practical problem, and an unpleasant taste, with flatulence, which may make compliance difficult. Some fish oil preparations contain significant amounts of cholesterol, necessitating close surveillance if such treatment is initiated. A further confirmatory study of fish oil would be of great value.

Recommendation

The treatment of IgAN with proteinuria of more than 1 g/24 h remains controversial. Physicians are increasingly using corticosteroids when there is preserved renal function (GFR >70 ml/min) and fish oil when there is renal impairment (GFR <70 ml/min). Tight control of BP and proteinuria with ACE inhibitors or ARBs should be the first line of treatment, however. Fish oil or corticosteroids should be considered only if proteinuria above 1 g/24 h persists on maximal ACE inhibitor or ARB therapy with BP below 125/75 mm Hg. Azathioprine (or even cyclophosphamide) combined with corticosteroids should be reserved for desperate cases in which all other measures have failed, and this treatment option needs to be well balanced against its associated risks.

Transplant Recurrence

There is no evidence that newer immunosuppressive agents have modified the frequency of recurrent IgA deposits or are of value in recurrent disease. Most clinicians therefore just optimize supportive care in such instances. When crescentic IgAN recurs with rapidly deteriorating graft function, treatment as for primary crescentic IgAN has been used, although evidence of its success is sparse.

TREATMENT OF HENOCH-SCHÖNLEIN NEPHRITIS

Many patients have transient nephritis during the early phase of HSP, which spontaneously remits and requires no treatment. There are no prospective, randomized, controlled trials to guide the treatment of HS nephritis. Most therapeutic studies of IgAN

Treatment Recommendations for Henoch-Schönlein Nephritis

Crescentic nephritis: regimen as for crescentic IgA nephropathy (see Fig. 22.10)
All other Henoch-Schönlein nephritis (including nephrotic syndrome): no specific treatment, supportive measures only
Hypertension: ACE inhibitor and ARB — agents of first choice; target blood pressure: 130/80 mm Hg if proteinuria <1 g/24 h, 125/75 mm Hg if proteinuria >1 g/24 h
Transplantation: cadaveric donor may be preferable to living related donor in children (controversial)

Figure 22.11 Treatment recommendations for Henoch-Schönlein nephritis. ACE, angiotensin-converting enzyme; ARB, angiotensin receptor blocker.

exclude those with HSP, so it is uncertain whether a number of potential treatments have a role in HS nephritis. Treatment recommendations are summarized in Figure 22.11.

Rapidly Progressive Renal Failure Caused by Crescentic Nephritis

Crescentic nephritis is more common in HS nephritis than in IgAN, particularly early in the course of HSP. There is little specific information on treatment in adults or children, but regimens based on those for other forms of systemic vasculitis are widely used. These have included corticosteroids and cyclophosphamide, with the addition of plasma exchange or pulse methylprednisolone in some cases. There have been no controlled trials, and HS nephritis has usually been excluded from trials of severe nephritis in systemic vasculitis. It is not possible to define the best regimen on available evidence.

Active Henoch-Schönlein Nephritis Without Renal Failure

There is little information about less aggressive HS nephritis. Corticosteroids alone have never been shown to be beneficial. There is no evidence that early use of corticosteroids in HSP may prevent nephritis.[44] Promising findings with combination therapy of corticosteroids, cyclophosphamide, and antiplatelet agents have been reported in only small nonrandomized studies.[45] A nonrandomized study reported that prednisolone and azathioprine preserved renal function and improved histologic appearances but relied on historical controls.[46] There are very few patients with HS nephritis included in the promising studies of immunoglobulin.

Slowly Progressive Renal Failure

Whereas the renal histology and clinical course of slowly progressive HS nephritis and IgAN may be indistinguishable, patients with HS nephritis have not been included in studies of fish oil. Tight BP control with ACE inhibitors or ARBs is recommended for proteinuric HS nephritis as for IgAN.

Transplant Recurrence

No treatment is known to reduce the risk of recurrence. There is some evidence that recurrence is more common and more likely to lead to graft loss in children receiving kidneys from living rather than deceased donors, although this is not confirmed in adults.[47,48] If crescentic HS nephritis recurs, intensive immunosuppression may be justified as for primary disease. This, however, has not been thoroughly evaluated.

REFERENCES

1. Barratt J, Feehally J, Smith AC. Pathogenesis of IgA nephropathy. *Semin Nephrol.* 2004;24:197-217.
2. Barratt J, Eitner F, Feehally J, Floege J. Immune complex formation in IgA nephropathy: A case of the "right" antibodies in the "wrong" place at the "wrong" time? *Nephrol Dial Transplant.* 2009;24:3620-3623.
3. Allen AC, Bailey EM, Brenchley PEC, et al. Mesangial IgA1 in IgA nephropathy exhibits aberrant O-glycosylation: Observations in three patients. *Kidney Int.* 2001;60:969-973.
4. Hiki Y, Odani H, Takahashi M, et al. Mass spectrometry proves under-glycosylation of glomerular IgA1 in IgA nephropathy. *Kidney Int.* 2001;59:1077-1085.
5. Suzuki H, Fan R, Zhang Z, et al. Aberrantly glycosylated IgA1 in IgA nephropathy patients is recognized by IgG antibodies with restricted heterogeneity. *J Clin Invest.* 2009;119:1668-1677.
6. Moura IC, Benhamou M, Paunay P, et al. The glomerular response to IgA deposition in IgA nephropathy. *Semin Nephrol.* 2008;28:88-95.
7. Floege J, Eitner F, Alpers CE. A new look at platelet-derived growth factor in renal disease. *J Am Soc Nephrol.* 2008;19:12-23.
8. Davin JC, ten Berge IJ, Weening J. What is the difference between IgA nephropathy and Henoch-Schönlein purpura nephritis? *Kidney Int.* 2001;59:823-834.
9. Suzuki K, Honda K, Tanabe K, et al. Incidence of latent mesangial IgA deposition in renal allograft donors in Japan. *Kidney Int.* 2003;63: 2286-2294.
10. Hsu SI. Racial and genetic factors in IgA nephropathy. *Semin Nephrol.* 2008;28:48-57.
11. Rivera F, Lopez-Gomez JM, Perez-Brea MF, et al. Clinicopathologic correlations of renal pathology in Spain. *Kidney Int.* 2004;66:898-904.
12. Pillebout E, Thervet E, Hill G, et al. Henoch-Schönlein purpura in adults: Outcome and prognostic factors. *J Am Soc Nephrol.* 2002;13: 1271-1278.
13. Oortwijn BD, Eijgenraam JW, Rastaldi MP, et al. The role of secretory IgA and complement in IgA nephropathy. *Semin Nephrol.* 2008;28: 58-65.
14. Cattran D, Coppo R, Cook HT, et al, Working Group of the International IgA Nephropathy Network and the Renal Pathology Society. The Oxford classification of IgA nephropathy: Rationale, clinicopathological correlations, and classification. *Kidney Int.* 2009;76:534-545.
15. Clive DM, Galvanek EG, Silva FG. Mesangial immunoglobulin-A deposits in minimal change nephrotic syndrome: A report of an older patient and a review of the literature. *Am J Nephrol.* 1990;10:31-36.
16. D'Amico G. Natural history of IgA nephropathy and factors predictive of disease outcome. *Semin Nephrol.* 2004;24:179-196.
17. Moranne O, Watier L, Rossert J, et al. Primary glomerulonephritis: An update on renal survival and determinants of progression. *Q J Med.* 2008;101:215-224.
18. Reich HN, Troyanov S, Scholey JW. Remission of proteinuria improves prognosis in IgA nephropathy. *J Am Soc Nephrol.* 2007;18:3177-3183.
19. Szeto CC, Lai FM, To KF, et al. Natural history of immunoglobulin A nephropathy presenting with hematuria and minimal proteinuria. *Am J Med.* 2001;110:434-437.
20. Floege J. Recurrent IgA nephropathy after renal transplantation. *Semin Nephrol.* 2004;24:287-291.
21. Barratt J, Feehally J. IgA nephropathy & Henoch-Schonlein purpura. In: Wilcox CS, ed. *Therapy in Nephrology & Hypertension.* 3rd ed. Philadelphia: WB Saunders; 2008:172-186.
22. Floege J, Eitner F. Present and future treatment options in IgA-nephropathy. *J Nephrol.* 2005;18:354-361.
23. Hotta OF, Miyazaka M, Furuta T, et al. Tonsillectomy and steroid pulse therapy significantly impact on clinical remission in patients with IgA nephropathy. *Am J Kidney Dis.* 2001;38:36-43.
24. Rasche FM, Schwarz A, Keller F. Tonsillectomy does not prevent a progressive course in IgA nephropathy. *Clin Nephrol.* 1999;51: 147-152.
25. Roccatello D, Ferro G, Cesano D, et al. Steroid and cyclophosphamide in IgA nephropathy. *Nephrol Dial Transplant.* 2000;15:833-835.

26. Haas M, Jafri J, Bartosh SM, et al. ANCA-associated crescentic glomerulonephritis with mesangial IgA deposits. *Am J Kidney Dis.* 2000;36: 709-718.
27. Lai KN, Lai FM, Ho CP, et al. Corticosteroid therapy in IgA nephropathy with nephrotic syndrome: A long-term controlled trial. *Clin Nephrol.* 1986;26:174-180.
28. Pozzi C, Andrulli S, Del Vecchio L, et al. Corticosteroid effectiveness in IgA nephropathy: Long-term results of a randomized, controlled trial. *J Am Soc Nephrol.* 2004;15:157-163.
29. Katafuchi R, Ikeda K, Mizumasa T, et al. Controlled, prospective trial of steroid treatment in IgA nephropathy: A limitation of low-dose prednisolone therapy. *Am J Kidney Dis.* 2003;41:972-983.
30. Manno C, Torres DD, Rossini M, et al. Randomized controlled clinical trial of corticosteroids plus ACE-inhibitors with long-term follow-up in proteinuric IgA nephropathy. *Nephrol Dial Transplant.* 2009 Jul 23 [Epub ahead of print].
31. Lv J, Zhang H, Chen Y, et al. Combination therapy of prednisone and ACE inhibitor versus ACE-inhibitor therapy alone in patients with IgA nephropathy: A randomized controlled trial. *Am J Kidney Dis.* 2009;53:26-32.
32. Eitner F, Ackermann D, Hilgers RD, Floege J. Supportive Versus Immunosuppressive Therapy of Progressive IgA nephropathy (STOP) IgAN trial: Rationale and study protocol. *J Nephrol.* 2008;21:284-289.
33. Ballardie FW, Roberts IDS. Controlled prospective trial of prednisolone and cytotoxics in progressive IgA nephropathy. *J Am Soc Nephrol.* 2002;13:142-148.
34. Floege J. Mycophenolate mofetil alleviates persistent proteinuria in IgA nephropathy. *Nature Clin Pract Nephrol.* 2006;2:16-17.
35. Lv J, Zhang H, Cui Z, et al. Delayed severe pneumonia in mycophenolate mofetil–treated patients with IgA nephropathy. *Nephrol Dial Transplant.* 2008;23:2868-2872.
36. Rostoker G, Desvaux-Belghiti D, Pilatte Y, et al. High-dose immunoglobulin therapy for severe IgA nephropathy and Henoch-Schönlein purpura. *Ann Intern Med.* 1994;120:476-484.
37. Stefanski A, Schmidt KG, Waldherr R, Ritz E. Early increase in blood pressure and diastolic left ventricular malfunction in patients with glomerulonephritis. *Kidney Int.* 1995;54:926-931.
38. Praga M, Gutierrez E, Gonzalez E, et al. Treatment of IgA nephropathy with ACE inhibitors: A randomized and controlled trial. *J Am Soc Nephrol.* 2003;14:1578-1583.
39. Coppo R, Peruzzi L, Amore A, et al. IgACE: A placebo-controlled, randomized trial of angiotensin-converting enzyme inhibitors in children and young people with IgA nephropathy and moderate proteinuria. *J Am Soc Nephrol.* 2007;18:1880-1888.
40. Kanno Y, Okada H, Saruta T, Suzuki H. Blood pressure reduction associated with preservation of renal function in hypertensive patients with IgA nephropathy: A 3-year follow-up. *Clin Nephrol.* 2000;54: 360-365.
41. Donadio JV, Grande JP, Bergstralh EJ, et al. The long-term outcome of patients with IgA nephropathy treated with fish oil in a controlled trial. *J Am Soc Nephrol.* 1999;10:1772-1777.
42. Donadio JV, Larson TS, Bergstralh EJ, Grande JP. A randomized trial of high-dose compared with low-dose omega-3 fatty acids in severe IgA nephropathy. *J Am Soc Nephrol.* 2001;12:791-799.
43. Dillon JJ. Fish oil therapy for IgA nephropathy: Efficacy and interstudy variability. *J Am Soc Nephrol.* 1997;8:1739-1744.
44. Bayrakci US, Topaloglu R, Soylemezoglu O, et al. Effect of early corticosteroid therapy on development of Henoch-Schönlein nephritis. *J Nephrol.* 2007;20:406-409.
45. Oner A, Tinaztepe K, Erdogan O. The effect of triple therapy on rapidly progressive type of Henoch-Schönlein nephritis. *Pediatr Nephrol.* 1995;9:6-10.
46. Foster BJ, Bernard C, Drummond KN, Sharma AK. Effective therapy for Henoch-Schönlein purpura nephritis with prednisone and azathioprine: A clinical and histopathologic study. *J Pediatr.* 2000;136: 370-375.
47. Hasegawa A. Fate of renal grafts with recurrent Henoch-Schönlein purpura nephritis in children. *Transplant Proc.* 1989;21:2130-2133.
48. Meulders Q, Pirson Y, Cosyns J-P, et al. Course of Henoch-Schönlein nephritis after renal transplantation. *Transplantation.* 1994;48: 1179-1186.
49. Pozzi C, Andrulli S, Pani A, et al. Corticosteroids and azathioprine vs corticosteroids alone in IgA nephropathy. *J Am Soc Nephrol.* 2010 in press.

CHAPTER 23

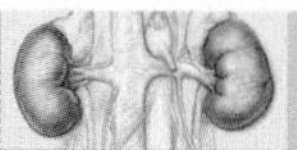

Antiglomerular Basement Membrane Disease and Goodpasture's Disease

Richard G. Phelps, A. Neil Turner

The syndrome of renal failure and lung hemorrhage was associated with the name of Ernest Goodpasture by Stanton and Tange in their description of nine cases in 1958.[1,2] All nine patients presented with lung hemorrhage and acute renal failure and died within hours or days. These features had been prominent in the case of a young man who died during the influenza pandemic of 1919, whose postmortem findings were memorably reported by Goodpasture[1]: "The lungs gave the impression of having been injected with blood through the bronchi so that all the air spaces were filled" (Fig. 23.1).

Several diseases are now recognized as being associated with alveolar hemorrhage and rapidly progressive glomerulonephritis (RPGN). Nevertheless, this remains a striking clinical entity with relatively few causes and few pathogenetic mechanisms.

Because the first recognized mechanism was anti–glomerular basement membrane (anti-GBM) antibody formation and deposition, Goodpasture's name is firmly associated with anti-GBM disease (Goodpasture's disease), even though this is responsible for only a proportion of patients with Goodpasture's syndrome of lung hemorrhage and RPGN. The terminology used in this chapter is defined in Figure 23.2.

ETIOLOGY AND PATHOGENESIS

Autoimmunity to a Component of the Glomerular Basement Membrane

Goodpasture's disease is caused by autoimmunity to the carboxyl terminal, noncollagenous (NC1) domain of a type IV collagen chain, α3(IV)NC1, also known as the Goodpasture antigen (Fig. 23.3).[3,4] Type IV collagen is an essential constituent of all basement membranes. In most tissues, it is composed of trimers comprising two α1 chains and one α2 chain, but there are also four tissue-specific chains, α3 through α6.[5,6] Three of these, α3 through α5, are found in GBM as well as in the basement membranes of the alveolus, the cochlea, parts of the eye (including corneal basement membrane and Bruch's membrane), the choroid plexus of the brain, and some endocrine organs.

All patients with RPGN, lung hemorrhage, and anti-GBM antibodies have antibodies to α3(IV)NC1, usually binding predominantly to a single or a very restricted set of epitopes. Some patients also have antibodies to other basement membrane constituents, including other collagen IV chains, usually in low titer.

Predisposing Factors

Both environmental and genetic factors appear to be important in etiology. There are strong associations between Goodpasture's disease and HLA class II alleles, including DRB1*1501 and DR4 alleles, whereas DR1 and DR7 confer strong and dominant protection.[7]

Precipitating Factors

The onset of acute disease has long been linked to various precipitating factors. Theories of pathogenesis include factors that alter antigen processing to generate peptides that are usually destroyed or hidden, and to which tolerance is therefore deficient[8,8a] and molecular mimicry.[9] None of these are proved. Reports of temporal and geographic clustering of cases suggest an environmental trigger,[10] but no specific infectious agent has been consistently identified. Hydrocarbon exposure has been linked to disease onset in several striking case reports; but in some cases, such exposure may simply trigger lung hemorrhage in patients who already have the disease. Furthermore, exposures of this kind are very common in the modern world. Similarly, cigarette smoking may precipitate lung hemorrhage in patients who already have circulating autoantibodies, but there is no evidence for a role in causation.

There are several instances in which renal trauma or inflammation (Fig. 23.4) has preceded the development of the disease. These may alter α3(IV)NC1 turnover and metabolism qualitatively or quantitatively, providing an opportunity for self tolerance to be broken. Qualitative changes in the basement membrane epitopes presented to T cells could be a result of overloading of the usual or recruitment of alternative processing pathways, such as extracellular processing by proteases released into inflamed glomeruli. The quantity of α3(IV)NC1 presented to T cells may be greater where there has been damage to the basement membrane, as occurs in systemic small-vessel vasculitis (see Chapter 24); some features suggest that an anti-GBM response may be a secondary phenomenon in some patients with vasculitis.[11,12] The association with membranous nephropathy is interesting as the thickened GBM in that disease contains increased amounts of the tissue-specific type IV collagen chains, including the Goodpasture antigen. The same could apply to a recently suggested possible association with long-standing type 1 diabetes mellitus.[13]

Mechanisms of Renal Injury

The α3(IV)NC1 autoantibodies (Fig. 23.5) are central in the pathogenesis of Goodpasture's disease.[14,15] Antibodies eluted from the kidneys of patients who had died of Goodpasture's disease rapidly bind to the GBM and cause glomerulonephritis (GN) when they are injected into monkeys.[16] Furthermore, the deposited antibodies are predominantly IgG1 and are complement fixing. Contributions to renal injury mediated by such antibodies come from complement and from neutrophil and macrophage infiltration. T cells are essential for driving autoantibody production by T cell–dependent B cells, and in experimental renal disease, they are critical in producing glomerular crescents,[14,17] which are a usual feature of Goodpasture's disease. Some experimental anti-GBM GN is clearly predominantly cell mediated.[14,17]

Agents that downregulate inflammation by inhibiting interleukin-1 or tumor necrosis factor α or that inhibit recruitment of inflammatory cells by blockade of adhesion molecules or chemoattractants suppress injury in experimental models of anti-GBM disease. There is supportive evidence in humans and in experimental animals that the severity of renal injury may be increased by proinflammatory cytokines or by stimuli likely to elicit them, such as bacteremia.[17] Crescent formation is seen in aggressive inflammatory GN. The mechanism by which it is believed to occur is described in Chapter 16 (see Fig. 16.9).

Lung Hemorrhage

Lung hemorrhage in Goodpasture's disease (but not in small-vessel vasculitis, the other major cause of Goodpasture's syndrome) occurs only if there is an additional insult to the lung, which is usually cigarette smoke. However, infection, fluid overload, toxicity from inhaled vapors or other irritants, and the systemic effects of some cytokines are also possibilities. This is probably because the alveolar capillary endothelial cell provides more of a barrier between circulating immunoglobulin and the underlying basement membrane than the diaphragm-free fenestrations of the glomerular capillary endothelial cell do. In the glomerulus, antibodies have direct access to the GBM because of the fenestrations of glomerular endothelium. Other sites at which the Goodpasture antigen is found are not involved in Goodpasture's disease, except possibly the choroid plexus, where the endothelium is again fenestrated, and more rarely the eye.

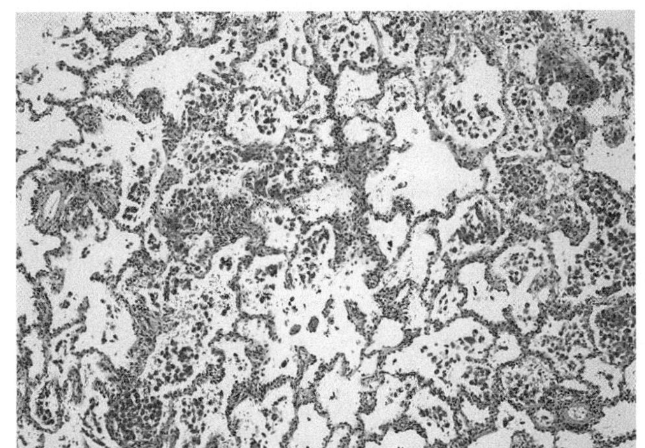

Figure 23.1 Alveolar hemorrhage in a patient with Goodpasture's disease. Open lung biopsy. *(Courtesy Dr. E. Mary Thompson, St Mary's Hospital, London, UK.)*

EPIDEMIOLOGY

Goodpasture's disease is rare, with a possibly increasing incidence in Caucasian populations approaching 1 case per million per annum.[13] The incidence in black and South Asian populations appears to be lower. The incidence in other racial groups is uncertain. There is a slight male predominance. Lung hemorrhage is more common in younger patients.

CLINICAL MANIFESTATIONS

Between 50% and 75% of patients present with acute symptoms of lung hemorrhage and are found to be in a state of advanced renal failure. Symptoms are usually confined to the preceding few weeks or months, but very rapid progression (during days) or much slower progression (during many months) may occur. A lack of systemic symptoms, other than those related to anemia, is typical, although it is common for an apparently minor infection to trigger the clinical presentation.

Lung Hemorrhage

Lung hemorrhage may occur with renal disease or in isolation. Presenting symptoms may include cough and hemoptysis, but hemorrhage into alveolar spaces may result in marked iron deficiency anemia and exertional dyspnea, even in the absence of hemoptysis. Depending on the degree and chronicity of lung hemorrhage, examination findings may include pallor, dry inspiratory crackles, signs of consolidation, or respiratory distress. Recent lung hemorrhage (Fig. 23.6) typically is shown on the

Definition of Terms

Term	Definition	Pathogenesis
Pulmonary renal syndrome	Renal and respiratory failure	Many causes (see Figure 23-10)
Goodpasture's syndrome	RPGN and alveolar hemorrhage	Several causes (see Figure 23-11)
Anti-GBM disease	Disease associated with antibodies specific for (any) components of the GBM	Most important are Goodpasture's syndrome and Alport's syndrome post-transplant anti-GBM disease
Goodpasture's disease	Disease associated with autoantibodies specific for α3(IV)NCI May include RPGN, lung hemorrhage, or both	Autoimmunity to α3(IV)NC1
Alport's syndrome post-transplant anti-GBM disease	Glomerulonephritis associated with anti-GBM antibodies developing after renal transplantation in patients with Alport's syndrome	Immunity to foreign collagen IV chains not expressed in Alport's syndrome patients usually α3 or α5 (IV)NCI

Figure 23.2 Definition of terms. GBM, glomerular basement membrane; RPGN, rapidly progressive glomerulonephritis.

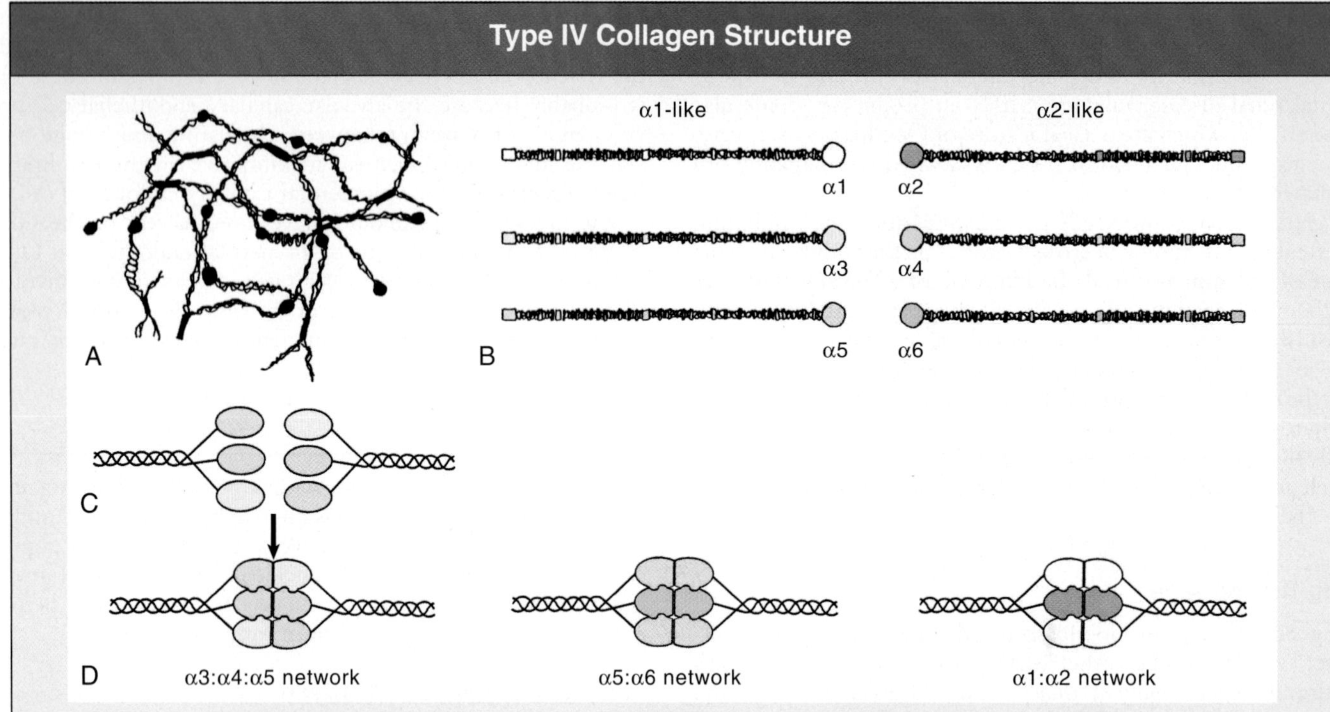

Figure 23.3 Type IV Collagen Structure. A, The type IV collagen network makes a "chicken wire" structure in the GBM. **B,** Six paired type IV collagen genes, *COL4A1* to *COL4A6*, encode type IV collagen monomers α1 to α6. These associate in two or three defined monomer types per protomer (carboxyl terminal domains of α3α4α5 shown in **C,** to form three recognized networks shown in **D,** α1α2 is present in almost all basement membranes; α3α4α5 is the major constituent of GBM and is a significant component of alveolar basement membrane and other locations (see text); and α5α6 is found in Bowman's capsule, skin, esophagus, and other locations.

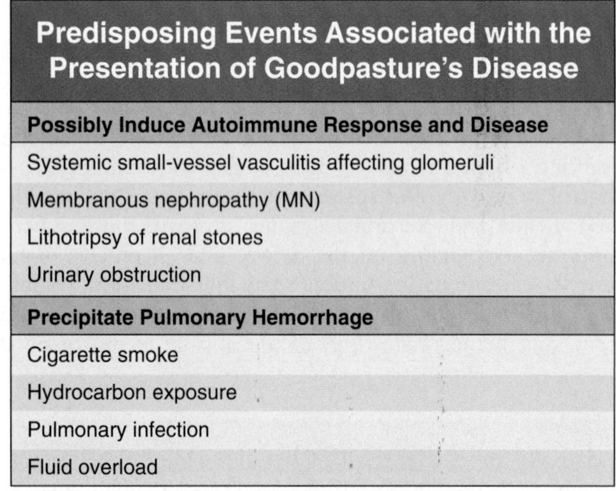

Predisposing Events Associated with the Presentation of Goodpasture's Disease
Possibly Induce Autoimmune Response and Disease
Systemic small-vessel vasculitis affecting glomeruli
Membranous nephropathy (MN)
Lithotripsy of renal stones
Urinary obstruction
Precipitate Pulmonary Hemorrhage
Cigarette smoke
Hydrocarbon exposure
Pulmonary infection
Fluid overload

Figure 23.4 Predisposing events associated with the presentation of Goodpasture's disease.

Figure 23.5 Autoantibodies to the Goodpasture antigen bound to a normal glomerulus. Shown by direct immunofluorescence in a patient with lung hemorrhage and hematuria. *(Courtesy Dr. Richard Herriot, Aberdeen Royal Infirmary, UK.)*

radiograph as central shadowing that may traverse fissures and give rise to the appearance of an air bronchogram. However, even lung hemorrhage sufficient to reduce the hemoglobin concentration may cause only minor or transient radiographic changes, and these cannot be confidently distinguished radiologically from other causes of alveolar shadowing (notably edema, infection). The most sensitive indicator of recent lung hemorrhage is an increased uptake of inhaled carbon monoxide (DLCO). Patients with lung hemorrhage are usually current cigarette smokers.

In isolated lung disease, progressive alveolar or fibrotic disease or pulmonary hemosiderosis may be suspected, although at least hematuria is usually present. This may continue for months or in rare cases recurrently for years before significant renal disease occurs.

Glomerulonephritis

Patients with GN may notice dark or red urine, but progression to oliguria is sometimes so rapid that this phase, if it occurs, is

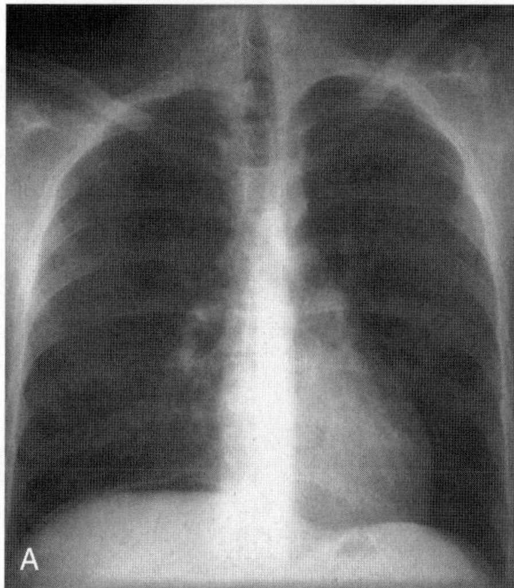

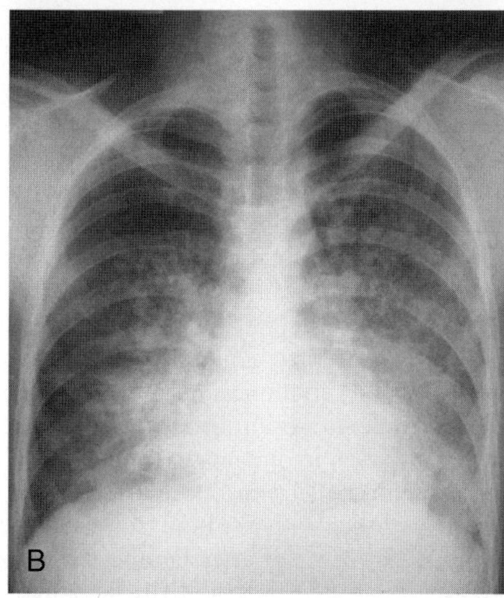

Figure 23.6 Lung hemorrhage. A, Patient with early pulmonary hemorrhage. The chest radiograph still appears normal. **B,** Radiograph taken 4 days later shows the evolution of alveolar shadowing caused by lung hemorrhage.

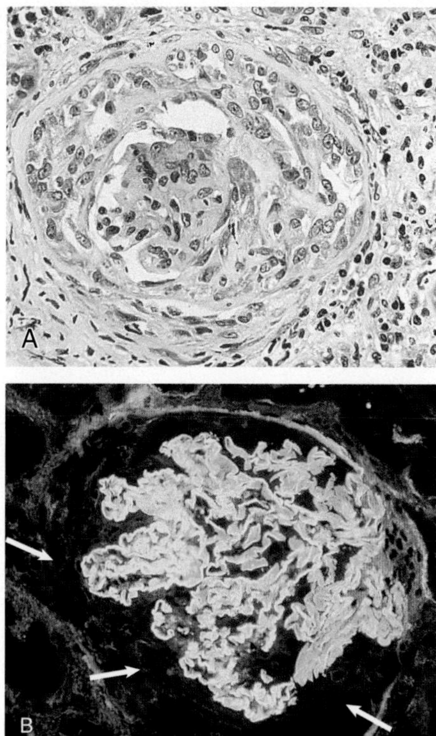

Figure 23.7 Renal biopsy in Goodpasture's disease. A, Glomerulus from a patient with Goodpasture's disease showing a recent, mostly cellular crescent. **B,** Direct immunofluorescence study showing ribbon-like linear deposition of IgG along the glomerular basement membrane (GBM). The glomerular tuft is slightly compressed by cellular proliferation (exhibiting no immunofluorescence), forming a crescent *(arrows). (Courtesy Dr. Richard Herriot, Aberdeen Royal Infirmary, UK.)*

missed. In one third to one half of patients, GN occurs in the absence of lung hemorrhage. In this subgroup, because systemic symptoms are generally not prominent, presentation is often late with renal failure.

Whatever the early pattern of disease, once significant renal impairment has occurred, further deterioration in renal function is usually rapid. Presentation at the time of or very shortly after acceleration of the disease process is common, and patients may demonstrate very rapid loss of renal function and life-threatening lung hemorrhage. Urinalysis always reveals hematuria (even in apparently isolated pulmonary disease), usually modest proteinuria, and dysmorphic red cells and red cell casts on microscopy. The kidneys are generally of normal size but may be enlarged. Hematuria may be substantial or associated with loin pain in acute disease.

PATHOLOGY

Renal biopsy is essential as it provides diagnostic and prognostic information. Typical appearances are of diffuse proliferative GN with variable degrees of necrosis, crescent formation, glomerulosclerosis, and tubular loss (Fig. 23.7). The degree of crescent formation and tubular loss correlates with renal prognosis. Characteristically, the crescents all appear to be of similar age and cellularity. When biopsy is performed earlier in the disease, changes may be limited to focal and segmental mesangial expansion, with or without necrosis. This progresses to hypercellularity and then to more general changes including fractures of the GBM and Bowman's capsule, neutrophils in the glomeruli, and glomerular capillary thrombosis.[18]

Immunohistology

In the presence of severe glomerular inflammation, linear deposition of immunoglobulin along the GBM is pathognomonic. The immunoglobulin is usually IgG, sometimes (10% to 15%) with IgA or IgM, but very rarely IgA alone is detected. Linear deposition of C3 is detectable in about 75% of biopsies. Linear immunofluorescence with anti-immunoglobulin reagents is occasionally seen in other conditions (Fig. 23.8), usually without glomerular inflammation. In most instances, the deposited immunoglobulin is less abundant than in Goodpasture's disease and is either nonspecifically deposited or bound to GBM components other than type IV collagen chains.

Circulating IgG anti-GBM antibodies are almost invariably present, even in the rare instances in which only IgM or IgA is demonstrated on the GBM. They may be detected and quantified by use of immobilized Goodpasture antigen in an immunoassay. The titer of anti-GBM antibody at presentation correlates

Conditions Associated with Linear Binding of Immunoglobulin to the GBM
Specific Binding to the GBM
Goodpasture's syndrome
Alport's syndrome after renal transplantation
Nonspecific Binding to the GBM
Diabetes
Cadaver kidneys
Light-chain disease
Fibrillary glomerulopathy
Systemic lupus erythematosus (possibly specific but not considered directly pathogenic)

Figure 23.8 Conditions associated with linear binding of immunoglobulin to the glomerular basement membrane (GBM).

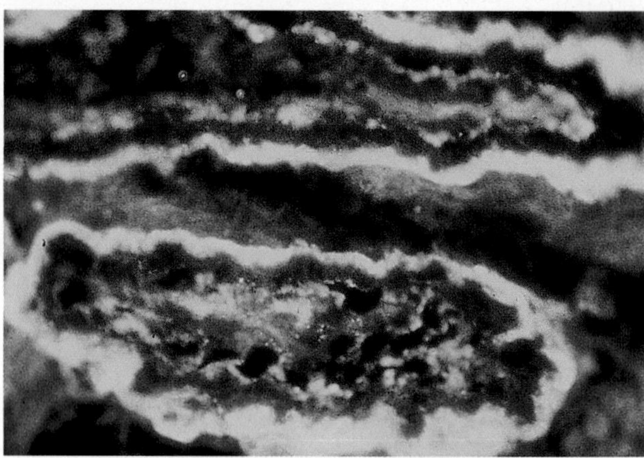

Figure 23.9 Direct immunofluorescence study showing binding of IgG to the choroid plexus of a patient who died of Goodpasture's disease. *(Courtesy Dr. Stephen Cashman, Imperial College, London, UK.)*

with the severity of nephritis. Treatment and relapse are often mirrored by changes in titer.

Pathology in Other Tissues

Pathologic changes in lung tissue can be difficult to interpret because the changes, including immunoglobulin deposition, are often patchy and may be missed. Frequently, the only findings are mild, chronic inflammation and hemosiderin-laden macrophages, which are consistent with other more common pathologic diagnoses. This makes negative bronchoscopic or open lung biopsy findings unhelpful in excluding the diagnosis.

Other tissues in which α3(IV)NC1 is expressed are rarely available for pathologic analysis, but if antibody is deposited in other sites, disease is rarely associated with it. A number of case reports describe neurologic syndromes, particularly convulsions, that might be related to antibody deposition in the choroid plexus (Fig. 23.9) but may have other explanations in patients with acute kidney injury. Other reports have described retinal detachment, in one instance with antibody deposition, but again this is rare.

DIFFERENTIAL DIAGNOSIS

Diagnosis of Goodpasture's disease in patients who present with Goodpasture's syndrome does not usually present difficulties once the possibility has been raised, although the urgency is often not appreciated. Direct immunofluorescence on renal tissue and assay for circulating anti-GBM antibodies are the most rapid techniques, and renal biopsy is always indicated. Diagnosis is often delayed when patients present with subacute disease affecting the lung or the kidney in isolation. Patients with subacute lung hemorrhage may never report hemoptysis and may present as cases of diffuse lung disease, of which there are many causes. Testing for hematuria is important.

Detection of Anti–Glomerular Basement Membrane Antibodies

Direct immunohistology using antibodies that are specific for different classes of immunoglobulin is very sensitive for detection of anti-GBM antibody production, as the GBM selectively adsorbs and concentrates low levels of circulating antibody. However, in some circumstances, GBM may also adsorb antibody nonspecifically (see Fig. 23.8). Detection of anti-GBM antibodies in serum requires solid-phase immunoassays based on preparations of human or animal GBM or recombinant antigen. The quality of these assays is variable. Confirmation of the specificity of anti-GBM antibodies may be obtained by Western blotting of serum onto solubilized human GBM or recombinant α3(IV)NC1, usually at a reference laboratory. Indirect immunohistology (putting patients' serum onto normal kidney sections) is too insensitive for reliable diagnostic use.

False-positive results may be encountered in sera from patients with inflammatory diseases that often exhibit increased nonspecific binding. This places greater emphasis on the purity of antigen used for anti-GBM assays. False-negative results are usually encountered in patients with low titers of antibodies in association with isolated lung disease or with very early or subacute renal disease. Low titers may also be associated with anti-GBM disease that occurs after renal transplantation in patients with Alport's syndrome (see later discussion).

In very advanced disease, linear antibody deposition may not be seen because of extensive destruction of GBM structure. Otherwise, deposited immunoglobulin remains detectable for some months after immunoassays have become negative.

Patients with Anti–Glomerular Basement Membrane Antibodies and Other Diseases

Antineutrophil Cytoplasmic Antibody and Systemic Small-Vessel Vasculitis

Anti-GBM antibodies are sometimes detected in patients with antineutrophil cytoplasmic antibodies (ANCA), especially ANCA with specificity for myeloperoxidase (see Chapter 24). Such "double-positive" patients may have a clinical course and response to treatment more typical of vasculitis than of Goodpasture's disease and have possibly developed anti-GBM antibodies secondary to vasculitic glomerular damage.[8-10] Anti-GBM titers tend to be lower in ANCA-positive anti-GBM antibody–positive patients than in patients with anti-GBM antibodies alone. Recovery of renal function may be more likely if ANCA are present, even if patients are dialysis dependent when treatment is started,

Non-Immune Causes of Pulmonary-Renal Syndrome
With Pulmonary Edema
Acute kidney injury with hypervolemia
Severe cardiac failure
Infective
Severe bacterial pneumonia (e.g., *Legionella*) with renal failure
Hantavirus infection
Opportunistic infections in the immunocompromised
Other
Acute respiratory distress syndrome with renal failure in multiorgan failure
Paraquat poisoning
Renal vein/inferior vena cava thrombosis with pulmonary emboli

Figure 23.10 Non-immune causes of pulmonary-renal syndrome.

Causes of Lung Hemorrhage and Rapidly Progressive Glomerulonephritis
Diseases Associated with Antibodies to the GBM (20%–40% of cases)
Goodpasture's disease (spontaneous anti-GBM disease)
Diseases Associated with Systemic Vasculitis (60%–80% of cases)
Wegener's granulomatosis (common)
Microscopic polyangiitis
Systemic lupus erythematosus
Churg-Strauss syndrome
Henoch-Schönlein purpura
Behçet's syndrome
Essential mixed cryoglobulinemia
Rheumatoid vasculitis
Drugs: penicillamine, hydralazine, propylthiouracil

Figure 23.11 Causes of lung hemorrhage and rapidly progressive glomerulonephritis. GBM, glomerular basement membrane.

although newer series have failed to detect the differences described in early reports.

Membranous Nephropathy

Anti-GBM antibodies are occasionally identified in patients with membranous nephropathy (MN), usually coincident with an accelerated decline in renal function and the formation of glomerular crescents.[5,13,19] In approximately two thirds of the two dozen or so published reports, there was evidence of evolution from preexisting nephrotic syndrome, and in about half, a previous kidney biopsy showed typical MN. Progression to end-stage renal disease (ESRD) has usually been rapid, but the diagnosis has rarely been made at an early enough stage to expect intensive treatment to be successful. Three patients with Goodpasture's disease later developed typical MN.

Differential Diagnosis of Goodpasture's Syndrome

A wide variety of conditions may cause simultaneous pulmonary and renal disease. The term *pulmonary-renal syndrome* implies failure of both organs, the most common cause being fluid overload in a patient with renal failure of any cause. This may resemble Goodpasture's syndrome, particularly if there is hematuria and preexisting cardiac dysfunction. However, a number of diseases may mimic Goodpasture's syndrome (lung hemorrhage with RPGN) to varying degrees by causing acute kidney injury (AKI) with acute lung disease (Fig. 23.10). Diseases associated with the syndrome fall into two pathogenetic classes: those characterized by systemic vasculitis and those associated with anti-GBM antibodies (Goodpasture's disease; Fig. 23.11).

These diseases can sometimes be differentiated clinically, but serology and renal biopsy are usually required. Renal biopsy also provides valuable prognostic information.

NATURAL HISTORY

There is some variability in the pattern of early disease. Most patients present acutely with lung hemorrhage or advanced renal failure and report that the illness developed during only weeks or a few months. However, there are several reports of patients presenting with mild respiratory symptoms or incidental microscopic hematuria with disease progressing much more slowly during months or years; some have abruptly developed the full acute syndrome.

Once RPGN has developed, renal function is rapidly and often irretrievably lost. Progression is often much more rapid than in RPGN occurring in other contexts, such as microscopic polyangiitis, perhaps because more glomeruli are simultaneously affected. Consequently, there is a much narrower window of opportunity for effective treatment.

Although a severe exacerbation of lung disease commonly coincides with deterioration of renal function, the natural history of isolated lung disease critically depends on continued exposure to irritants.

TREATMENT

Immunosuppressive Regimens

Before the introduction of immunosuppressive treatment, most patients died shortly after the development of renal impairment or lung hemorrhage.[17] Now lung hemorrhage can usually be arrested within 24 to 48 hours. Renal function can be protected if impairment is mild, and even severe renal impairment can be reversed in some circumstances. However, dialysis-dependent patients rarely recover kidney function despite immunosuppression and should probably be immunosuppressed only if lung hemorrhage occurs.

A chart recording treatment of a patient with Goodpasture's disease is shown in Figure 23.12. Recommended treatment for acute severe disease is shown in Figure 23.13. It was devised to reduce levels of circulating pathogenic antibodies as rapidly as possible and to curtail their contribution to the rapid glomerular destruction that can occur during acute severe disease, but almost certainly it is effective through a much broader range of mechanisms including T-cell depletion. Once the disease is controlled, immunosuppression can usually be tapered off during 3 months, and subsequent relapse is uncommon. The immune response is self-limited in the absence of immunosuppression, antibodies disappearing during 1 to 2 years. Spontaneous remissions and the effectiveness of relatively brief periods of immunosuppression are in striking contrast with the more prolonged immunosuppression generally required to prevent relapse of vasculitis and suggest that there is a greater capacity for the restoration of usual tolerance to α3(IV)NC1[20] than to targets in vasculitis.

In RPGN in which there is no evidence of an infective cause, immunosuppressive therapy should be started immediately, sometimes before the renal biopsy findings are available. If therapy is stopped after a few days, the patient will have incurred very little risk (as long as pulse high-dose corticosteroids are avoided) but sometimes has a great deal to gain from earlier treatment.

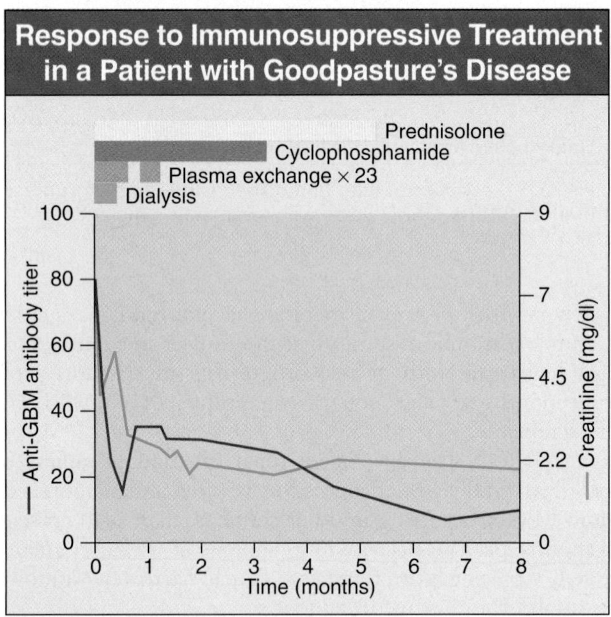

Figure 23.12 Response to immunosuppressive treatment in a patient with Goodpasture's disease. The patient required dialysis for renal disease but had no lung hemorrhage. The good response to treatment was unusual but not unique. The renal biopsy showed that 85% of glomeruli contained recent (mostly cellular) crescents, suggesting very acute disease, which may be indicative of a more favorable response to treatment.

Plasma Exchange and Immunosuppression

The regimen described in Figure 23.13 dramatically improved the outlook for patients when it was introduced in the 1970s. An early randomized trial[21] suggested some additional benefit of plasma exchange, but the interpretation was complicated by the fact that the recipient group had less severe disease at presentation. It showed that milder disease can be effectively treated with corticosteroids and cyclophosphamide alone, although the overall outcomes for all patients were not as good as have been described with more intensive regimens.[21] Historical evidence suggests that treatment with corticosteroids alone, or corticosteroids with azathioprine, is less effective. Plasma exchange is of value only if it is accompanied by adjunctive immunosuppressive therapy. Immunoadsorption to protein A also lowers anti-GBM antibodies rapidly; it does not deplete complement components or clotting factors, and a few reports suggest that it is as effective as plasma exchange. Information on the effectiveness of newer immunosuppressive agents such as mycophenolate mofetil (MMF) or anti-B cell antibodies (which tend to have only a slow effect on antibody production, but may affect antigen presentation), is lacking. Their use over proven therapy is rarely justifiable in this often very rapidly progressive disease. In contrast to advanced renal failure, in which treatment is unlikely to lead to recovery of renal function, even severe lung hemorrhage is likely to respond to treatment with full or nearly full recovery of lung function.

Lung hemorrhage occurring alone tends to be relapsing and remitting, so there have been many reports of treatments (including bilateral nephrectomy) that may help. Pulse methylprednisolone has been advocated, but high doses of corticosteroids fail to alter the underlying pathogenetic immune response and put the patient at increased risk of infective and other complications. We recommend treating seriously ill patients with moderate doses of corticosteroids plus plasma exchange and cyclophosphamide.

In other acute severe diseases, daily administration of cyclophosphamide has often been superseded by pulse administration. We still prefer to use daily oral administration because it is known to work and only 3 months of therapy is required. Patients

Treatment Regimen for Acute Goodpasture's Disease	
Prednisolone	1 mg/kg/24 h orally. Reduce at weekly intervals to achieve one sixth of this dose by 8 weeks. For a starting daily dose of 60 mg, use weekly reductions to 45, 30, 25, 20, and 15 mg; then 2 weekly to 12.5 and 10 mg. Maintain this dose to 3 months; then taper to stop by 4 months.
Cyclophosphamide	3 mg/kg/24 h orally, rounded down to the nearest 50 mg. Patients >55 years receive a reduced dose of 2.5 mg/kg.
Plasma exchange	Daily exchange of 1 volume of plasma for 5% human albumin for 14 days or until the circulating antibody is suppressed. In the presence of pulmonary hemorrhage or within 48 hours of an invasive procedure, 300 to 400 ml of fresh frozen plasma is given at the end of each treatment or according to coagulation tests.
Monitoring	Daily blood count during plasma exchange and while antibody titer remains elevated. At least twice weekly during first month, weekly thereafter. If white blood cell count decreases to <3.5×10^9/l, stop cyclophosphamide until the count recovers. Resume at lower dose if cessation has been necessary. Baseline DLCO, with further measurements as indicated. Daily coagulation tests during plasma exchange to monitor for significant depletion of clotting factors. Initially, daily checks of renal and hepatic function, glucose.
Prophylaxis against complications of treatment	Oral antifungal lozenges or rinse; proton pump inhibitor. Cotrimoxazole prophylaxis against *Pneumocystis carinii*. Avoid nonessential lines, catheters.

Figure 23.13 Treatment regimen for acute Goodpasture's disease.

Factors Influencing Decision to Treat or Not to Treat Aggressively in Goodpasture's Disease		
	Factors Favoring Aggressive Treatment	**Factors Against Aggressive Treatment**
Pulmonary hemorrhage	Present	Absent
Oliguria	Absent	Present
Creatinine	<5.5 mg/dl (approximately 500 µmol/l)	>5.5–6.5 mg/dl (approximately 500–600 µmol/l) and ANCA negative Severe damage on kidney biopsy No desire for early kidney transplantation
Other factors	Creatinine >5.5-6.5 mg/dl (approximately 500-600 µmol/l) *but* Rapid and recent progression ANCA positive Glomerular damage less severe than expected Crescents recent, nonfibrous Early renal transplantation desired	
Associated disease	Absent	Unusually high risk from immunosuppression

Figure 23.14 Factors influencing decision to treat or not to treat aggressively in Goodpasture's disease. ANCA, antineutrophil cytoplasmic antibody.

unable to take the drug orally can be given daily intravenous therapy at the usual oral dose. Dose does not need to be reduced in severe renal failure provided the white blood cell count is monitored closely, but reductions for older patients are important (see Fig. 23.13), and close monitoring of leukocyte counts is imperative in all patients. If pulsed therapy were chosen, the CYCLOPS regimen would be a reasonable if untested option (see Chapter 24).

Results from all series show that recovery of renal function is unlikely if, at the time treatment is commenced, the patient is oliguric, has a very high proportion of glomeruli with circumferential crescents, or has a serum creatinine level above 5.5 to 6.5 mg/dl (about 500 to 600 µmol/l).[22] This is a notably different experience from that encountered in systemic vasculitis or idiopathic RPGN (see Chapter 24), in which renal disease of apparently similar severity (judged by histology and serum creatinine level) can be salvaged by similar treatment protocols.[23] It has led to the suggestion that immunosuppressive treatment should be withheld from patients in whom the chance of recovery is slight (Fig 23.14 and see later).

Supportive Treatment

The most likely cause of death in the first few days is respiratory failure caused by lung hemorrhage. Lung hemorrhage may be precipitated or exacerbated by:

- Fluid overload.
- Smoking and other pulmonary irritants, possibly including high fractional inspired oxygen concentrations.
- Local or distant infection.
- Anticoagulation used during dialysis or plasma exchange.
- Thrombocytopenia, defibrination, and depletion of clotting factors as a consequence of plasma exchange.

It is therefore sensible to ensure correct fluid balance, to prohibit smoking, to use the lowest fractional inspired oxygen concentration that gives adequate oxygenation, and to minimize the use of heparin.

Plasma exchange should be monitored by daily blood counts, calcium concentration (if regional citrate anticoagulation is used), and coagulation tests. Diminished clotting factor levels should be replenished by administration of fresh frozen plasma or clotting factor preparations at the end of each plasma exchange session as required.

After the first few days, the major cause of morbidity and mortality is infection. Infection carries the added risk of potentiating glomerular and lung inflammation and injury, so precautions to reduce risk, such as minimizing indwelling cannulae, are important. If leukopenia below 3.5×10^9/l or neutropenia develops, cyclophosphamide should be discontinued and resumed at a lower dose when the neutrophil count recovers, if necessary with the assistance of granulocyte colony-stimulating factor.

Monitoring Effect of Treatment on Disease Activity

The effect of treatment on the renal disease is monitored by following serum creatinine values. Indicators of recent lung hemorrhage include hemoptysis, decreases in hemoglobin concentration, chest radiograph changes, and increases in the DLCO, the last being the most sensitive. Any worsening of symptoms during treatment may indicate inadequate immunosuppression, but it is frequently a consequence of intercurrent infection exaggerating immunologic injury or fluid overload or other factors precipitating lung hemorrhage.

Monitoring of anti-GBM titers during and particularly 24 hours after the last planned plasma exchange treatment is useful for confirming effective suppression of autoantibodies. They should be undetectable within 8 weeks, but even without treatment, they generally become undetectable by an average of 14 months.

Duration of Treatment and Relapses

Corticosteroid treatment may be gradually reduced and cyclophosphamide discontinued at 3 months. In contrast with the treatment of small-vessel vasculitis, it is not usually necessary to continue immunosuppression for longer than this. Longer treatment is appropriate for patients who are both anti-GBM antibody positive and ANCA positive (see later discussion). Late increases in anti-GBM level may predict clinical relapse, although antibodies are generally permanently suppressed in patients who have completed the immunosuppressive regimen. If there is recurrence, success has been achieved by treating as at first presentation.

Electing Not to Treat

Advanced renal failure, frequently already established at presentation, is generally not salvaged by any current treatment.[22,24,25] Furthermore, the immunosuppressive regimen outlined carries significant risks, and careful monitoring is required. For these reasons, it may be reasonable not to commence immunosuppression in patients who present with advanced renal failure without lung hemorrhage. The decision not to treat is strengthened if the renal biopsy specimen shows widespread glomerulosclerosis and tubular loss and the patient is dialysis dependent at presentation (see Fig. 23.14). The risk for development of late lung hemorrhage in these circumstances seems to be low but warrants particular care to avoid the major precipitating factors, smoking and pulmonary edema, in at least the first few months.

However, patients who are dialysis dependent should usually be treated if the renal histopathologic changes are unexpectedly mild or very recent (highly cellular crescents, even if 100% of glomeruli are involved, or acute tubular necrosis). Several reports describe good outcomes in these circumstances even after prolonged oliguria.

Treatment of Double-Positive Patients

Patients with both ANCA and anti-GBM antibodies may have other extrarenal disease requiring treatment (see Fig. 23.14). There is conflicting evidence as to whether their renal prognosis is the same as or better than that of other patients with anti-GBM antibodies. Earlier series suggested a better prognosis, but this was not confirmed in two later reports.[11,12] Because of the risk of serious disease in other organs, double-positive patients should usually receive an immunosuppressive regimen similar to that given for small-vessel vasculitis with continuing immunosuppression with azathioprine after 3 months of cyclophosphamide (see Chapter 24).

TRANSPLANTATION

Renal transplantation in patients who have had Goodpasture's disease carries the additional risk of disease recurrence. Recurrence with consequent loss of the graft has been reported and appears more likely when circulating anti-GBM antibodies are still detectable at the time of transplantation. For this reason, it is reasonable to delay transplantation until circulating anti-GBM antibodies have been undetectable for 6 months and to monitor graft function, urinary sediment, and circulating anti-GBM antibody levels to detect recurrent disease (see Chapter 104). Biopsies of well-functioning grafts sometimes show linear deposition of immunoglobulin on the GBM without clinical or histologic disease or apparently an adverse prognosis.

ALPORT'S SYNDROME POST-TRANSPLANT ANTI–GLOMERULAR BASEMENT MEMBRANE DISEASE

Patients with Alport's syndrome have mutations in a gene encoding one of the tissue-specific type IV collagen chains, usually α5. Because these chains assemble with each other during biosynthesis, the resulting phenotype in the case of most mutations often has all the tissue-specific chains (α3 through α5) missing from the basement membranes, where they are normally coexpressed. Altered expression may lead to absent or inadequate immunologic tolerance to these proteins and to the preservation of the capacity to mount a powerful (allo)immune response to the type IV collagen chains expressed in a normal donor kidney after renal transplantation. Most Alport's syndrome patients accommodate renal transplants with conventional immunosuppression without development of anti-GBM nephritis. However, the development of low titers of anti-GBM antibodies is shown by the fact that many such patients have linear deposition of IgG on the GBM of the transplanted kidney by direct immunofluorescence, without disease. This alone does not justify treatment.

Up to 5% of Alport patients develop RPGN in the transplanted kidney. It is clinically indistinguishable from Goodpasture's syndrome but without lung hemorrhage. This is more likely if they have a large gene deletion causing the disease rather than a point mutation, with the inference that their immune system has never been exposed to the mature protein. Typically, graft function is lost despite treatment for presumed acute rejection. Disease is usually encountered some months or longer after a first renal transplant, after weeks in a second, and after days in a third.[26] However, regrafting has been successful in two cases known to us and in two further cases in the literature. If the disease is recognized early, there are sound theoretical reasons for treating with the regimen recommended for Goodpasture's syndrome, but there are few data on its effectiveness.[26]

In contrast to spontaneous Goodpasture's syndrome, the specificity of anti-GBM antibodies in Alport's post-transplant anti-GBM disease is not always to α3(IV)NC1. In many patients, possibly in most, the autoantibodies are specific for α5(IV)NC1, encoded by the *COL4A5* gene usually implicated in causation of the disease.[27] This is important because immunoassays for anti-GBM antibodies are optimized for detection of the anti-α3(IV) NC1 antibodies of spontaneous Goodpasture's syndrome, and they may have low sensitivity for anti-α5(IV)NC1 antibodies. In the absence of widely available assays for these uncommon antibodies, renal biopsy with immunohistology is the only reliable method of diagnosis.

REFERENCES

1. Goodpasture EW. The significance of certain pulmonary lesions in relation to the etiology of influenza. *Am J Med Sci*. 1919;158:863-870.
2. Stanton MC, Tange JD. Goodpasture's syndrome (pulmonary haemorrhage associated with glomerulonephritis). *Aust N Z J Med*. 1958;7: 132-144.
3. Saus J, Wieslander J, Langeveld J, et al. Identification of the Goodpasture antigen as the a3(IV) chain of collagen IV. *J Biol Chem*. 1988; 263:13374-13380.
4. Turner N, Mason PJ, Brown R, et al. Molecular cloning of the human Goodpasture antigen demonstrates it to be the alpha 3 chain of type IV collagen. *J Clin Invest*. 1992;89:592-601.
5. Kashtan CE, Michael AF. Alport syndrome. *Kidney Int*. 1996;50: 1445-1463.
6. Aumailley M. Structure and supramolecular organization of basement membranes. *Kidney Int*. 1995;49:S4-S7.
7. Phelps RG, Rees AJ. The HLA complex in Goodpasture's disease: A model for analyzing susceptibility to autoimmunity. *Kidney Int*. 1999;56: 1638-1654.
8. Zou J, Henderson L, Thomas V, et al. Presentation of the Goodpasture autoantigen requires proteolytic unlocking steps that destroy prominent T cell epitopes *J Am Soc Nephrol*. 2007;18:771-779.

8a. Pedchenko V, Bondar O, Fogo AB, et al. Molecular architecture of the Goodpasture autoantigen in anti-GBM nephritis. *N Engl J Med*. 2010;363:343-354.

9. Arends J, Wu J, Borillo J, et al. T cell epitope mimicry in antiglomerular basement membrane disease. *J Immunol.* 2006;176:1252-1258.
10. Bolton WK. Goodpasture's syndrome. *Kidney Int.* 1996;50:1753-1766.
11. Rutgers A, Slot M, van Paassen P, et al. Coexistence of anti–glomerular basement membrane antibodies and myeloperoxidase-ANCAs in crescentic glomerulonephritis. *Am J Kidney Dis.* 2005;46:253-262.
12. Levy JB, Hammad T, Coulthart A, et al. Clinical features and outcome of patients with both ANCA and anti-GBM antibodies. *Kidney Int.* 2004;66:1535-1540.
13. Turner AN, Rees AJ. Antiglomerular basement membrane disease. In: Cameron JS, Davison AM, Grunfeld J-P, et al, eds. *Oxford Textbook of Nephrology*, 3rd ed. Oxford: Oxford University Press; 2005:579-600.
14. Ooi JD, Holdsworth SR, Kitching AR. Advances in the pathogenesis of Goodpasture's disease: From epitopes to autoantibodies to effector T cells. *J Autoimmun.* 2008;31:295-300.
15. Phelps RG, Turner AN. Goodpasture's syndrome: new insights into pathogenesis and clinical picture. *J Nephrol.* 1996;9:111-117.
16. Lerner R, Glassock R, Dixon F. The role of anti–glomerular basement membrane antibody in the pathogenesis of human glomerulonephritis. *J Exp Med.* 1967;126:989-1004.
17. Feehally J, Floege J, Savill J, Turner AN. Glomerular injury and glomerular response. In: Cameron JS, Davison AM, Grunfeld J-P, et al, eds. *Oxford Textbook of Nephrology*, 3rd ed. Oxford: Oxford University Press; 2005:363-388.
18. Heptinstall RH. Schönlein-Henoch syndrome: Lung hemorrhage and glomerulonephritis. In: Heptinstall RH, ed. *Pathology of the Kidney*. Boston: Little, Brown; 1983:761-791.
19. Thitiarchakul S, Lal SM, Luger A, Ross G. Goodpasture's syndrome superimposed on membranous nephropathy. A case report. *Int J Artif Organs.* 1995;18:763-765.
20. Cairns LS, Phelps RG, Bowie L, et al. The fine specificity and cytokine profile of T helper cells responsive to a glomerular autoantigen in Goodpasture's Disease. *J Am Soc Nephrol.* 2003;14:2801-2812.
21. Johnson JP, Moore JJ, Austin HA, et al. Therapy of anti–glomerular basement membrane antibody disease: Analysis of prognostic significance of clinical, pathologic and treatment factors. *Medicine (Baltimore).* 1985;64:219-227.
22. Levy JB, Turner AN, Rees AJ, Pusey CD. Long-term outcome of anti-glomerular basement membrane antibody disease treated with plasma exchange and immunosuppression. *Ann Intern Med.* 2001;134:1033-1042.
23. Hind CRK, Paraskevakou H, Lockwood CM, et al. Prognosis after immunosuppression of patients with crescentic nephritis requiring dialysis. *Lancet.* 1983;1:263-265.
24. Turner AN, Rees AJ. Anti–glomerular basement membrane antibody disease. In: Brady HR, Wilcox N, eds. *Therapy in Nephrology and Hypertension: A Companion to Brenner and Rector's The Kidney*, 3rd ed. Philadelphia: WB Saunders; 2008:197-204.
25. Flores JC, Taube D, Savage COS, et al. Clinical and immunological evolution of oliguric anti-GBM nephritis treated by haemodialysis. *Lancet.* 1986;1:5-8.
26. Browne G, Brown PA, Tomson CR, et al. Retransplantation in Alport post-transplant anti-GBM disease. *Kidney Int.* 2004;65:675-681.
27. Brainwood D, Kashtan C, Gubler MC, Turner AN. Targets of alloantibodies in Alport anti–glomerular basement membrane disease after renal transplantation. *Kidney Int.* 1998;53:762-766.

CHAPTER 24

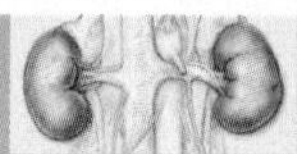

Renal and Systemic Vasculitis

J. Charles Jennette, Ronald J. Falk

DEFINITION

The kidneys are targets for a variety of systemic vasculitides, especially those that affect small vessels.[1-5] This is not surprising given the large number and variety of renal vessels. Vasculitis involving the kidneys can produce a wide variety of clinical manifestations, depending in large measure on the type of renal vessel affected. As demonstrated in Figures 24.1 to 24.3, vasculitides can be categorized as large-vessel vasculitis, medium-sized vessel vasculitis, and small-vessel vasculitis. The categorization of systemic vasculitides is controversial. For the purposes of the discussion in this chapter, the Chapel Hill Consensus Conference definitions are used (see Fig. 24.3).[4]

A number of the vasculitides listed in Figure 24.2 are covered elsewhere in the book and are not reviewed in detail here except in the context of differential diagnosis, for example, cryoglobulinemic vasculitis (see Chapter 55), Henoch-Schönlein purpura (HSP) (see Chapter 22), and anti–glomerular basement membrane (GBM) disease (see Chapter 23). Nephrologists most often encounter patients with small-vessel vasculitides because they often cause glomerulonephritis (GN); thus, these receive the most attention in this chapter.

Small-Vessel Vasculitis

Small-vessel vasculitis is necrotizing polyangiitis that affects predominantly vessels smaller than arteries, including capillaries, venules, and arterioles; however, arteries also may be involved. The most common renal targets for small-vessel vasculitides are the glomeruli, and therefore the most common clinical renal manifestations are those of GN.

Medium-Sized Vessel Vasculitis

Medium-sized vessel vasculitis is necrotizing arteritis that affects predominantly major visceral arteries. The interlobar arteries and arcuate arteries are affected most often, although the interlobular arteries and main renal artery may be affected. Inflammation and necrosis of arteries may result in thrombosis or rupture, which causes renal infarction and hemorrhage, respectively.

Large-Vessel Vasculitis

Large-vessel vasculitis is chronic granulomatous arteritis that affects predominantly the aorta and its major branches. When there is renal involvement, the ostia of the renal arteries and the main renal arteries are most often affected. The most common clinical renal manifestation is renovascular hypertension.

SMALL-VESSEL PAUCI-IMMUNE VASCULITIS

Wegener's granulomatosis, Churg-Strauss syndrome, and microscopic polyangiitis share an indistinguishable form of necrotizing small-vessel vasculitis that affects capillaries, venules, arterioles, and small arteries.[1-4] Some patients, however, have no evidence of involvement of arteries, even though they have involvement of glomerular capillaries, causing GN; pulmonary alveolar capillaries, causing pulmonary hemorrhage; or dermal venules, causing purpura. These so-called pauci-immune small-vessel vasculitides are distinguished from clinically and histologically similar forms of immune complex small-vessel vasculitis, such as cryoglobulinemic vasculitis and HSP, by the absence or paucity of immune complex deposits in vessel walls. The diagnosis for the specific subtypes of pauci-immune small-vessel vasculitides can be made on the basis of the accompanying syndrome.[4]

- Wegener's granulomatosis occurs in association with necrotizing granulomatous inflammation, which most often affects the respiratory tract.
- Churg-Strauss syndrome is vasculitis occurring in association with asthma, eosinophilia, and necrotizing granulomatous inflammation.
- Microscopic polyangiitis is pauci-immune systemic vasculitis occurring in the absence of evidence of Wegener's granulomatosis or Churg-Strauss syndrome, that is, in the absence of asthma and eosinophilia and with no evidence of necrotizing granulomatous inflammation.

Microscopic polyangiitis, Wegener's granulomatosis, and, less frequently, Churg-Strauss syndrome also share an indistinguishable pattern of GN that is the expression of the vasculitis in glomerular capillaries.[1,2] The GN usually has necrosis and crescent formation and an absence or paucity of immunoglobulin deposition and is often designated pauci-immune crescentic GN. When pauci-immune crescentic GN occurs in the apparent absence of systemic vasculitis, it is sometimes referred to as renal vasculitis, renal-limited vasculitis, or idiopathic rapidly progressive GN (RPGN).

Pathogenesis

Wegener's granulomatosis, microscopic polyangiitis, Churg-Strauss syndrome, and isolated pauci-immune crescentic GN are all associated with the presence in serum of autoantibodies

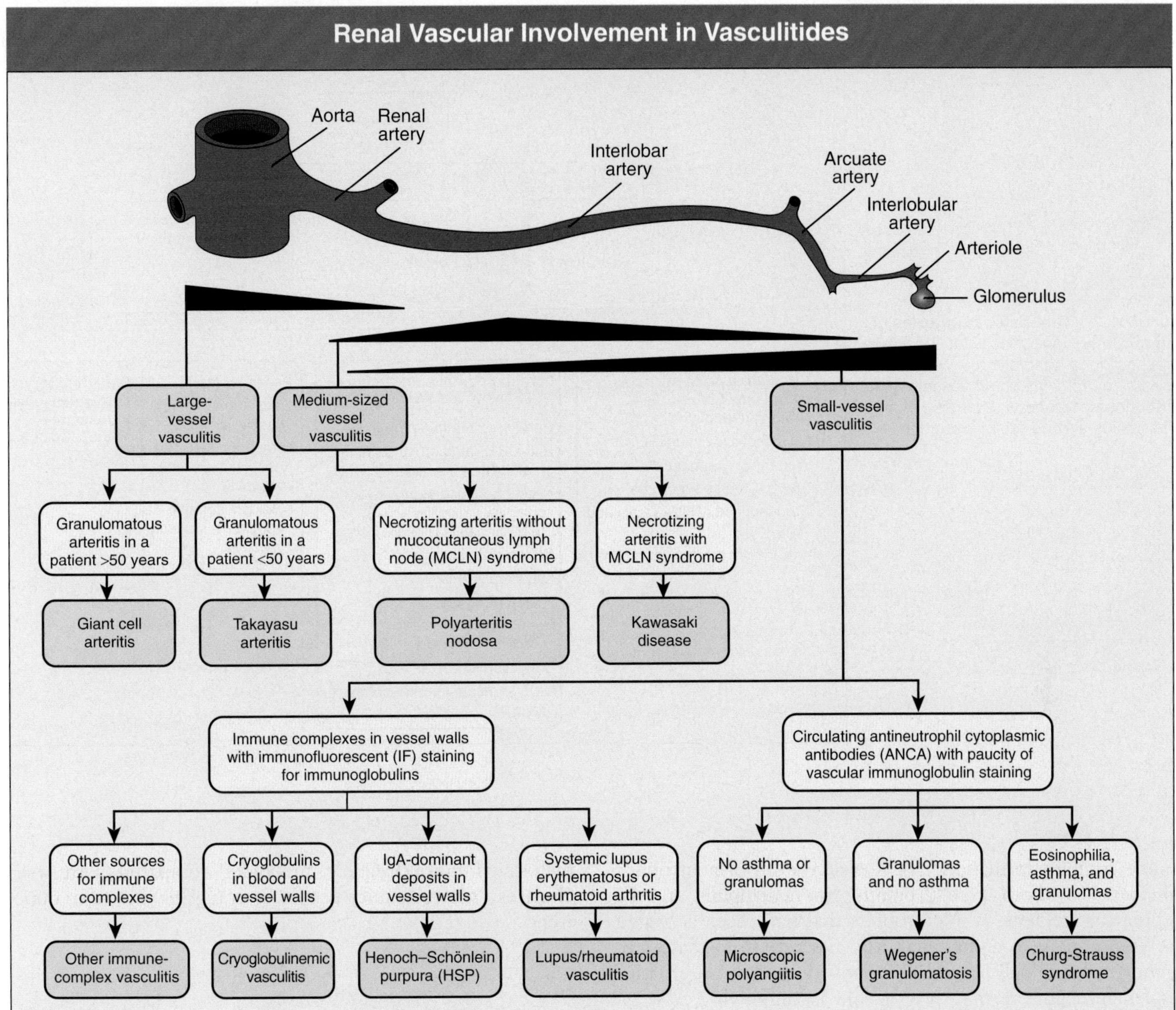

Figure 24.1 Renal vasculitis: the predominant distribution of renal vascular involvement by a variety of vasculitides. The heights of the trapezoids represent the relative frequency of involvement of different portions of the renal vasculature by the three major categories of vasculitis. *(Modified from reference 3.)*

against components of the cytoplasm of neutrophils: circulating antineutrophil cytoplasmic antibodies (ANCA).[6-9] The most common antigen specificities of ANCA in patients with vasculitis and GN are for proteinase 3 (PR3) and myeloperoxidase (MPO).

The strong association of ANCA with a distinctive form of small-vessel vasculitis raises the possibility that ANCA are involved in the pathogenesis.[6] The observation that ANCA titers correlate with disease activity is more suggestive; however, this is not a very tight correlation.[7,8] Even more supportive of a pathogenetic link is the observation that administration of certain drugs, such as propylthiouracil, hydralazine, and penicillamine, can induce ANCA in the circulation concurrent with the development of pauci-immune crescentic GN and small-vessel vasculitis.[10] Most compelling of all is the report of a neonate who developed GN and pulmonary hemorrhage apparently caused by transplacental passage of MPO-ANCA IgG.[11]

The ability of ANCA IgG to cause pauci-immune necrotizing and crescentic GN and vasculitis has been demonstrated in a mouse model. Wild-type or immunodeficient mice that receive anti-MPO antibodies intravenously develop pauci-immune focal necrotizing GN with crescents.[12] This GN is mediated by neutrophil activation and can be prevented by neutrophil depletion.[13] A rat model of pauci-immune necrotizing and crescentic GN has been developed by immunizing rats with human MPO, resulting in the development of antibodies that cross-react with rat MPO and are able to induce pauci-immune glomerular necrosis and crescents.[14]

A number of *in vitro* observations suggest mechanisms by which ANCA can cause vascular injury. Priming of neutrophils by cytokines, as would occur with a viral infection, causes neutrophils to increase expression of ANCA antigens on their surfaces, where they are accessible to interact with ANCA. Cytokine-primed neutrophils that are exposed to ANCA release IgG from granules, release toxic oxygen metabolites, and kill cultured endothelial cells.[6,15-17] ANCA-antigen complexes adsorb onto endothelial cells, where they could participate in *in situ*

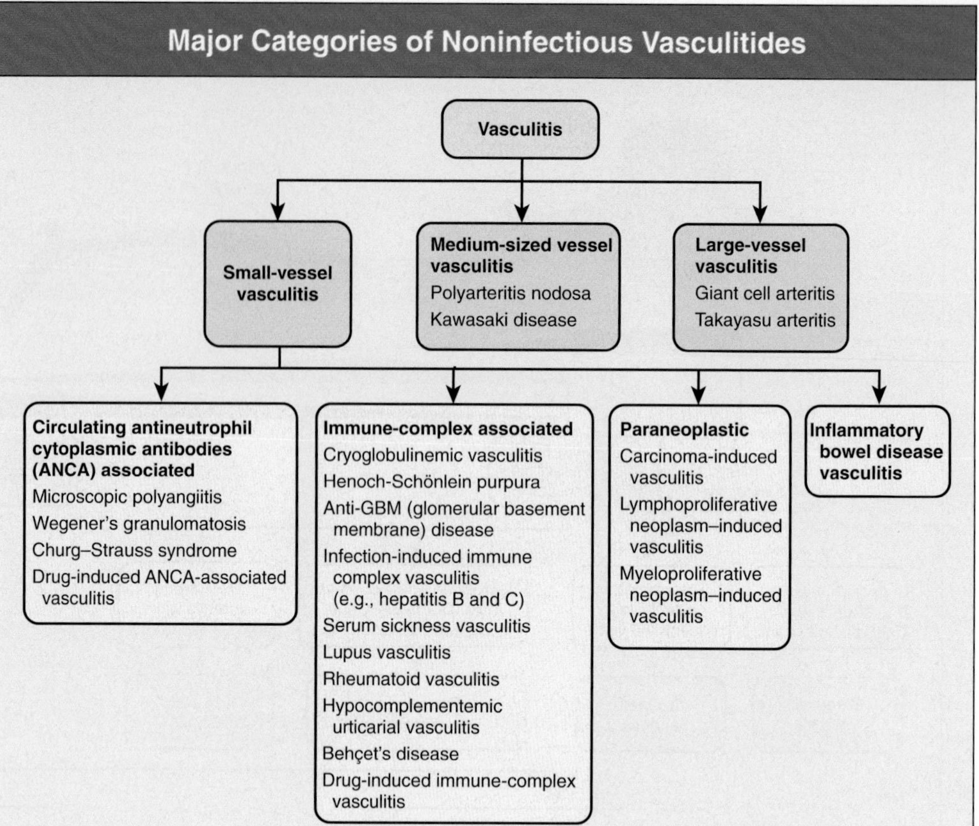

Figure 24.2 The major categories of noninfectious vasculitis. Not included are vasculitides that are known to be caused by direct invasion of vessel walls by infectious pathogens, such as rickettsial vasculitis and neisserial vasculitis.

immune complex formation.[18] ANCA activation of neutrophils is mediated by both $F(ab)'_2$ binding to neutrophils and Fc receptor engagement.[19,20] Neutrophils that have been activated by ANCA adhere to endothelial cells and release mediators of inflammation and cell injury.[14,16,17] Activation of the alternative complement pathway may play a role in amplifying ANCA-induced inflammation.[21] If these events occurred *in vivo*, they would lead to vasculitis as a result of neutrophils adhering to, penetrating, and destroying vessel walls (Fig. 24.4).[22]

Thus, the clinical and the experimental animal data support the hypothesis that ANCA can activate neutrophils and cause vasculitis, especially if there is a concurrent synergistic proinflammatory stimulus. The requirement for a synergistic inflammatory process may be reflected in the very frequent association of the onset of ANCA small-vessel vasculitis with an influenza-like syndrome.[23] An influenza-like syndrome is a manifestation of high levels of circulating cytokines that could serve as priming factors for neutrophils.

Epidemiology

Wegener's granulomatosis, microscopic polyangiitis, and Churg-Strauss syndrome usually begin during the fifth, sixth, and seventh decades of life, although they may occur at any age. There is a slight male predominance. The incidence is disproportionately greater in Caucasians than in African Americans. In Europe, microscopic polyangiitis has a prevalence of approximately 2.5/100,000; Wegener's granulomatosis, 2.5/100,000; and Churg-Strauss syndrome, 1/100,000.[24] Although it is not fully documented, there is a suspicion that Wegener's granulomatosis is more frequent in colder compared with warmer climates, whereas microscopic polyangiitis has the opposite trend.[24]

Clinical Manifestations

The clinical manifestations of Wegener's granulomatosis, microscopic polyangiitis, and Churg-Strauss syndrome are extremely varied because they are influenced by the sites of involvement and the activity versus the chronicity of involvement. All three categories of vasculitis share features caused by the small-vessel vasculitis, and patients with Wegener's granulomatosis and Churg-Strauss syndrome have the additional features that define each of these syndromes.[2,4,5,7,8,23,25,26]

Renal involvement is very common in Wegener's granulomatosis and microscopic polyangiitis and less frequent in Churg-Strauss syndrome (Fig. 24.5).[2] The most common renal manifestations are caused by glomerular involvement and include hematuria, proteinuria, and renal failure. The renal failure often has the characteristics of RPGN in patients with Wegener's granulomatosis and microscopic polyangiitis but usually is less severe in those with Churg-Strauss syndrome. Wegener's granulomatosis and microscopic polyangiitis also can present as a subacute or chronic nephritis. A cohort of more than 300 pauci-immune crescentic GN patients evaluated at the time of renal biopsy had a mean age of 56 ± 20 years (range, 2 to 92 years), male-to-female ratio of 1.0:0.9, mean serum creatinine concentration of 6.5 ± 4.0 mg/dl (range, 0.8 to 22.1 mg/dl), and proteinuria of 1.94 ± 2.95 g/dl (range, 0.11 to 18.00 g/dl).[27]

Names and Definitions of Vasculitis Adopted by the Chapel Hill Consensus Conference on the Nomenclature of Systemic Vasculitis

Category	Type	Definition
Large-vessel vasculitis	Giant cell (temporal) arteritis	Granulomatous arteritis of the aorta and its major branches, with a predilection for the extracranial branches of the carotid artery. Often involves the temporal artery. Usually occurs in patients older than 50 and often is associated with polymyalgia rheumatica.
	Takayasu arteritis	Granulomatous inflammation of the aorta and its major branches. Usually occurs in patients younger than 50.
Medium-sized vessel vasculitis	Polyarteritis nodosa (classic polyarteritis nodosa)	Necrotizing inflammation of medium-sized or small arteries without glomerulonephritis (GN) or vasculitis in arterioles, capillaries, or venules.
	Kawasaki disease	Arteritis involving large, medium-sized, and small arteries and associated with mucocutaneous lymph node syndrome. Coronary arteries are often involved. Aorta and veins may be involved. Usually occurs in children.
Small-vessel vasculitis	Wegener's granulomatosis	Granulomatous inflammation involving the respiratory tract and necrotizing vasculitis affecting small to medium-sized vessels (e.g., capillaries, venules, arterioles, and arteries. Necrotizing GN is common).
	Churg-Strauss syndrome	Eosinophil-rich and granulomatous inflammation involving the respiratory tract and necrotizing vasculitis affecting small to medium-sized vessels; associated with asthma and blood eosinophilia.
	Microscopic polyangiitis (microscopic polyarteritis)	Necrotizing vasculitis with few or no immune deposits affecting small vessels (i.e., capillaries, venules, arterioles). Necrotizing arteritis involving small and medium-sized arteries may be present. Necrotizing GN is very common. Pulmonary capillaritis often occurs.
	Henoch-Schönlein purpura	Vasculitis with IgA-dominant immune deposits affecting small vessels (i.e., capillaries, venules, arterioles). Typically involves skin, gut, and glomeruli and is associated with arthralgias or arthritis.
	Essential cryoglobulinemic vasculitis	Vasculitis with cryoglobulin immune deposits, affecting small vessels (i.e., capillaries, venules, arterioles); associated with cryoglobulins in serum. Skin and glomeruli are often involved.
	Cutaneous leukocytoclastic angiitis	Isolated cutaneous leukocytoclastic angiitis without systemic vasculitis or GN.

Figure 24.3 Names and definitions of vasculitis adopted by the Chapel Hill Consensus Conference on the nomenclature of systemic vasculitis. Note that all three categories affect arteries, but only small-vessel vasculitis has a predilection for vessels smaller than arteries. *(Modified from reference 22.)*

Generalized nonspecific manifestations of systemic inflammatory disease, such as fever, malaise, anorexia, weight loss, myalgias, and arthralgias, often are present. As noted earlier, many patients trace the onset of their disease to an influenza-like illness.[23]

Cutaneous involvement is frequent. Purpura is a common manifestation of Wegener's granulomatosis, microscopic polyangiitis, and Churg-Strauss syndrome (Fig. 24.6). The purpura is most common on the lower extremities and tends to occur as recurrent crops. The purpura may be accompanied by small areas of ulceration. Nodular cutaneous lesions are much more frequent in Wegener's granulomatosis and Churg-Strauss syndrome than in microscopic polyangiitis. Nodules can be caused by dermal or subcutaneous arteritis and by the necrotizing granulomatous inflammation.

Upper and lower respiratory tract involvement is most common in Wegener's granulomatosis and Churg-Strauss syndrome but also occurs in those with microscopic polyangiitis. All three categories can have pulmonary hemorrhage caused by hemorrhagic alveolar capillaritis. Wegener's granulomatosis and Churg-Strauss syndrome also can have pulmonary injury caused by necrotizing granulomatous inflammation, which may be detected radiographically as nodular or cavitating lesions. By definition, patients with microscopic polyangiitis do not have granulomatous respiratory tract lesions.[4]

Manifestations of upper respiratory tract disease include subglottic stenosis, sinusitis, rhinitis, otitis media, and ocular inflammation. These features are most common in Wegener's granulomatosis but may occur in Churg-Strauss syndrome and microscopic polyangiitis. The upper respiratory tract inflammation in microscopic polyangiitis is caused by angiitis alone, without granulomatous inflammation. Destruction of bone, for example, resulting in septal perforation and saddle nose deformity, appears to require necrotizing granulomatous inflammation and therefore does not occur in microscopic polyangiitis.

Cardiac disease is identified in approximately 50% of patients with Churg-Strauss syndrome but in less than 20% of patients with Wegener's granulomatosis or microscopic polyangiitis. Manifestations range from transient heart block and ventricular hypokinesis that respond to immunosuppressive treatment to infarction and severe life-threatening myocarditis. Pericarditis and endocarditis also may occur.

Peripheral neuropathy, usually with a mononeuritis multiplex pattern, is the most common neurologic manifestation and is most frequent in Churg-Strauss syndrome. Central nervous system involvement is less common and most often is manifested as vasculitis within the meninges. Gastrointestinal involvement typically causes abdominal pain and blood in the stool, with mesenteric ischemia and, rarely, intestinal perforation. Vasculitis

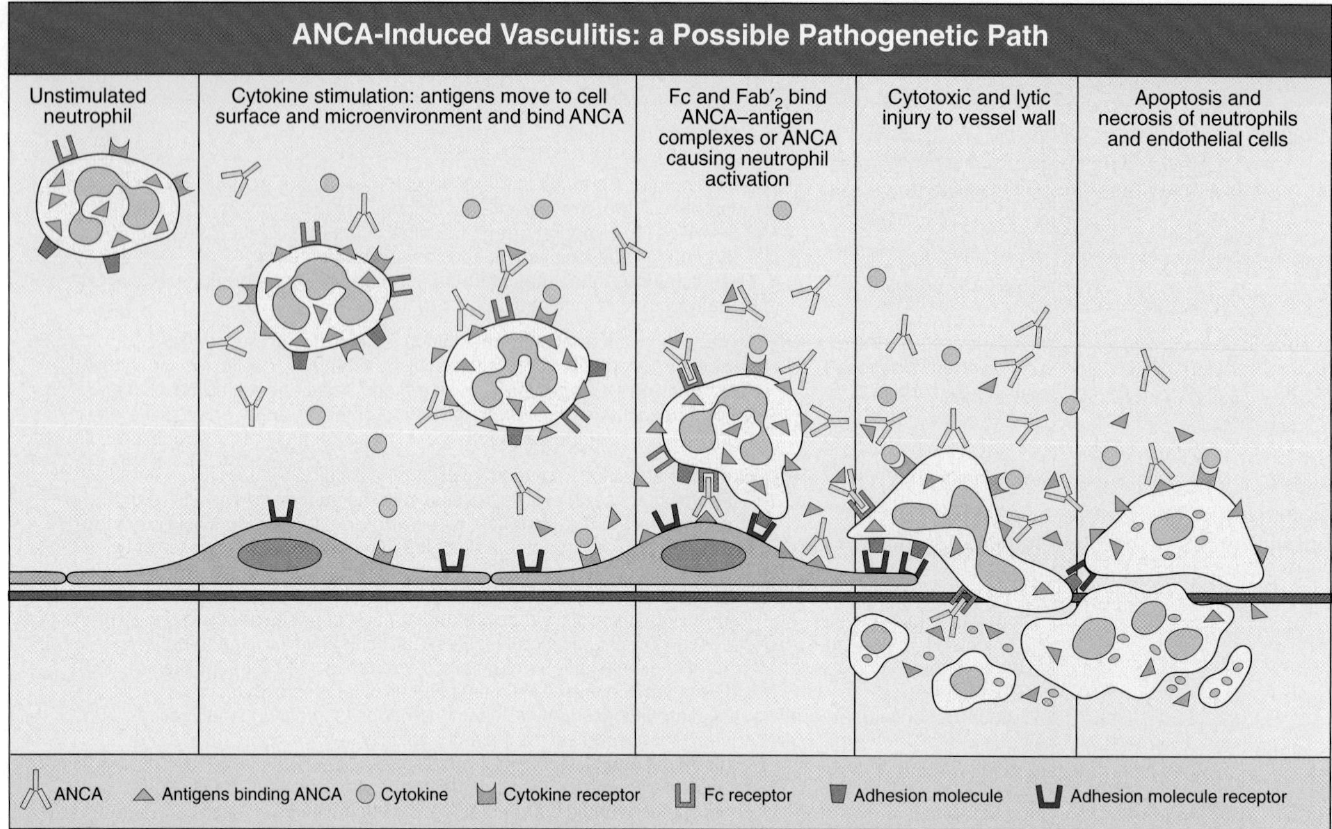

ANCA-Induced Vasculitis: a Possible Pathogenetic Path
Unstimulated neutrophil
Cytokine stimulation: antigens move to cell surface and microenvironment and bind ANCA
Fc and Fab′2 bind ANCA–antigen complexes or ANCA causing neutrophil activation
Cytotoxic and lytic injury to vessel wall
Apoptosis and necrosis of neutrophils and endothelial cells
ANCA
Antigens binding ANCA
Cytokine
Cytokine receptor
Fc receptor
Adhesion molecule
Adhesion molecule receptor

Figure 24.4 Vasculitis induced by antineutrophil cytoplasmic antibodies (ANCA): a hypothetical sequence of pathogenetic events. *(Modified from reference 22.)*

Organ System Involvement in Small-Vessel Vasculitis

	Frequency of Involvement (%)				
Organ System	**Microscopic Polyangiitis**	**Wegener's Granulomatosis**	**Churg-Strauss Syndrome**	**Henoch-Schönlein Purpura (HSP)**	**Cryoglobulinemic Vasculitis**
Kidney	90	80	45	50	55
Skin (cutaneous)	40	40	60	90	90
Lungs	50	90	70	>5	>5
Ear, nose, and throat	35	90	50	>5	>5
Musculoskeletal system	60	60	50	75	70
Neurologic system	30	50	70	10	40
Gastrointestinal system	50	50	50	60	30

Figure 24.5 Organ system involvement in small-vessel vasculitis. *(Modified from reference 2.)*

in the pancreas and liver can mimic pancreatitis and hepatitis symptomatically.

Antineutrophil Cytoplasmic Autoantibodies

Serologic testing for ANCA is a useful diagnostic procedure for pauci-immune small-vessel vasculitis and pauci-immune crescentic GN but should be interpreted in the context of other characteristics of the patient.[7,8,28-31] Laboratory testing for ANCA should include both indirect immunofluorescence microscopy assay (IFA) and enzyme immunoassay (EIA).[30]

IFA using normal human neutrophils as substrate produces two major staining patterns (Fig. 24.7): cytoplasmic (c-ANCA), in which staining occurs diffusely throughout the cytoplasm, and perinuclear (p-ANCA). By EIA, most c-ANCA have specificity for PR3 (PR3-ANCA), and most p-ANCA have specificity for MPO (MPO-ANCA). For adequate diagnostic accuracy, all serologic testing for ANCA should include an immunochemical analysis for antigen specificity, such as an EIA.[30] Although positive results are rare in completely healthy individuals, approximately one fourth of patients with other inflammatory renal diseases (especially lupus) will have a false-positive IFA result (usually with a p-ANCA pattern), and approximately 5% will have a false-positive EIA result (usually at low titer).[31]

ANCA testing has good sensitivity for pauci-immune small-vessel vasculitis and GN (80% to 90%). The specificity and predictive value depend on the population of patients.[29] Although ANCA are most frequent in patients with pauci-immune crescentic GN, approximately one fourth to one third of patients with anti-GBM crescentic GN and one fourth of patients with idiopathic immune-complex crescentic GN are ANCA positive.[27,32] Patients with concurrent ANCA and anti-GBM antibodies have a worse prognosis than that of patients with ANCA alone.

Figure 24.8 provides an estimate of the relative frequencies of PR3-ANCA/c-ANCA and MPO-ANCA/c-ANCA in the different clinical phenotypes of pauci-immune small-vessel vasculitis and crescentic GN. PR3-ANCA/c-ANCA are most prevalent in Wegener's granulomatosis, and MPO-ANCA/p-ANCA are most prevalent in renal-limited pauci-immune crescentic GN. Patients with microscopic polyangiitis have a more even distribution of PR3-ANCA/c-ANCA and MPO-ANCA/p-ANCA. Patients with Churg-Strauss syndrome have the lowest overall frequency of ANCA, but the frequency of ANCA is much higher in patients with GN (75%) compared with those with no GN (26%).[33] These data make it clear that ANCA antigen specificity cannot be used to determine the clinicopathologic phenotype of pauci-immune small-vessel vasculitis.

Changes in ANCA titers over time correlate to a degree with disease activity but are not infallible markers and thus must be interpreted with much caution.[7,8,30,34] In general, titers usually decrease with treatment and increase before or at the time of

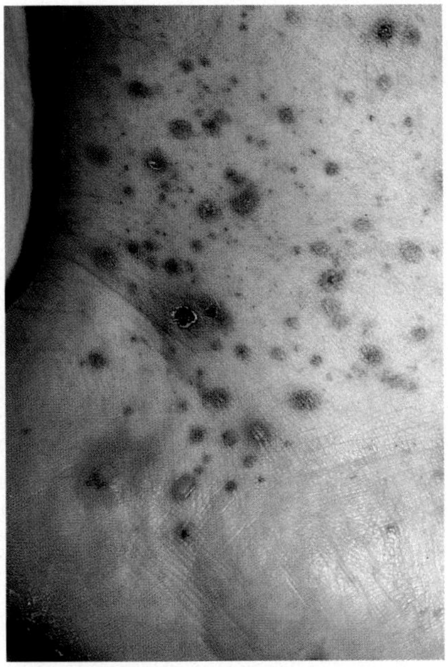

Figure 24.6 Cutaneous vasculitis. Ankle of a patient with small-vessel vasculitis, showing purpura and a few small ulcers.

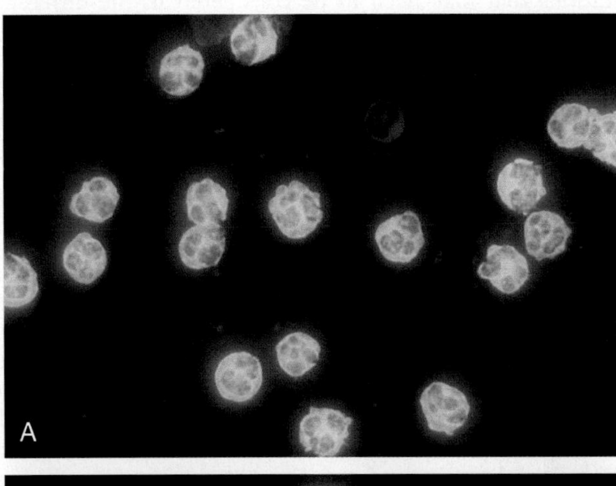

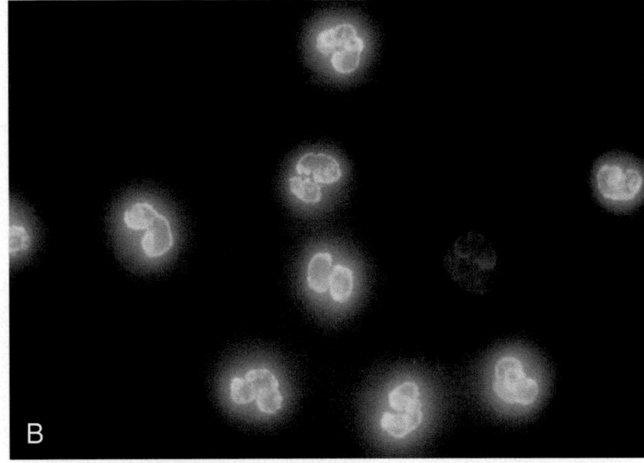

Figure 24.7 Indirect immunofluorescence for antineutrophil cytoplasmic antibodies (ANCA). Staining pattern of alcohol-fixed normal human neutrophils. **A,** Cytoplasmic pattern caused by ANCA with specificity for proteinase 3. **B,** Perinuclear pattern caused by ANCA with specificity for myeloperoxidase (anti-IgG). (Original magnification ×250.)

Antineutrophil Cytoplasmic Antibodies (ANCA) in Small-Vessel Vasculitis

	Frequency (%)		
	Proteinase 3 (PR3/c-ANCA)	Myeloperoxidase (MPO/p-ANCA)	Negative
Wegener's granulomatosis	70	25	5
Microscopic polyangiitis	40	50	10
Churg-Strauss syndrome	10	60	30
Pauci-immune glomerulonephritis (GN)	20	70	10

Figure 24.8 Antineutrophil cytoplasmic antibodies (ANCA) in small-vessel vasculitis. Approximate frequency of ANCA with specificity for proteinase 3 (PR3/c-ANCA) and for myeloperoxidase (MPO/p-ANCA) in patients with different categories of pauci-immune small-vessel vasculitis and crescentic glomerulonephritis.

disease recurrence. An increase in ANCA titer should prompt careful evaluation of the patient for corroborating evidence of exacerbation, but most physicians do not modify treatment on the basis of an increase in titer without accompanying clinical or laboratory evidence for increased disease activity.

Approximately 10% to 20% of patients with pauci-immune necrotizing and crescentic GN and small-vessel vasculitis will be ANCA negative. The clinical, pathologic, and outcome characteristics of these patients are no different from those of ANCA-positive patients.[35]

ANCA may sometimes be positive with other inflammatory conditions that may need to be considered in the differential diagnosis, including inflammatory bowel disease, rheumatoid disease, chronic inflammatory liver disease, bacterial endocarditis, and cystic fibrosis.[7] In this setting, specificity of the ANCA may not be against PR3 or MPO but against other neutrophil antigens, including lactoferrin, cathepsin G, and anti–bactericidal/permeability-increasing protein.

Pathology

The basic shared acute vascular lesion of the pauci-immune small-vessel vasculitides is segmental fibrinoid necrosis, often accompanied by leukocyte infiltration and leukocytoclasia (leukocyte fragmentation; Figs. 24.9 and 24.10).[1,2,36,37] The earliest vasculitic lesions have infiltrating neutrophils that are quickly replaced by predominantly mononuclear leukocytes. The acute necrotizing lesions evolve into sclerotic lesions and may be complicated by thrombosis.

These focal necrotizing lesions can affect many different vessels, thus causing many different signs and symptoms. For example, involvement of glomerular capillaries causes nephritis; of alveolar capillaries, pulmonary hemorrhage; of dermal venules, purpura; of upper respiratory tract mucosal venules, rhinitis and sinusitis; of abdominal visceral arteries, abdominal pain; and of epineural arteries, mononeuritis multiplex.

The shared glomerular lesion of the pauci-immune small-vessel vasculitides is a necrotizing GN, usually with resultant crescent formation (Figs. 24.11 and 24.12).[1,2,36,37] Early mild

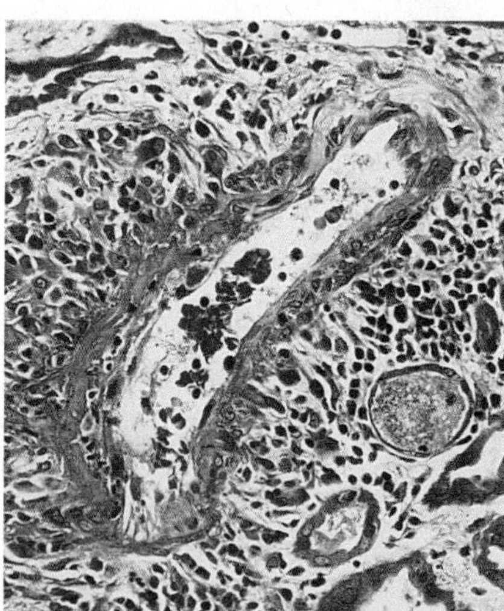

Figure 24.9 Necrotizing arteritis in an interlobular artery from a patient with antineutrophil cytoplasmic antibody (ANCA)–associated small-vessel vasculitis. There is segmental fibrinoid necrosis with adjacent perivascular leukocyte infiltration. (Hematoxylin-eosin; original magnification ×50.)

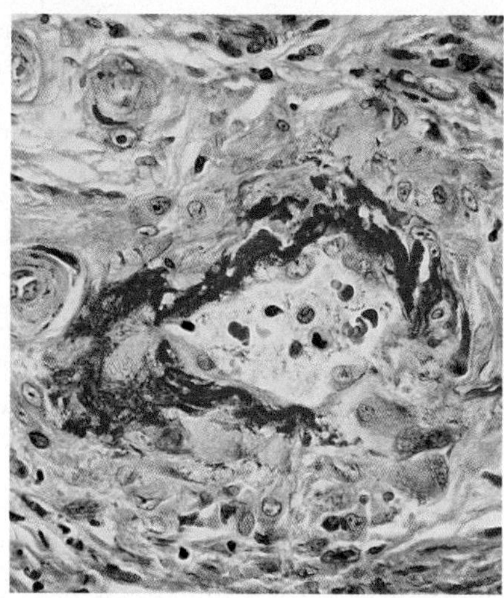

Figure 24.10 Necrotizing arteritis in an interlobular artery from a patient with antineutrophil cytoplasmic antibody (ANCA)–associated small-vessel vasculitis. The fibrinoid necrosis is accentuated by the red staining of the trichrome stain. (Masson trichrome; original magnification ×100.)

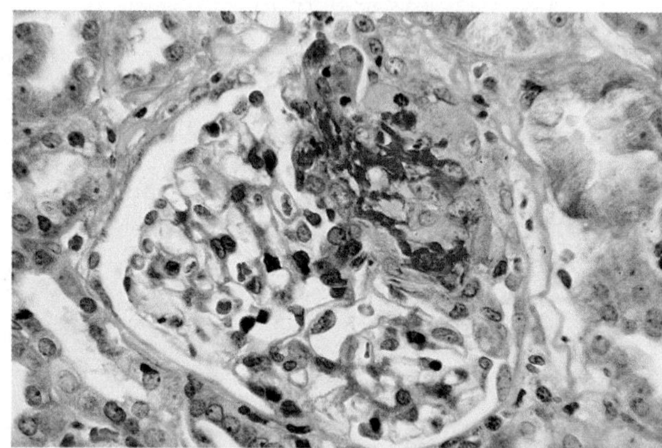

Figure 24.11 Segmental glomerular necrosis and crescent formation in a patient with antineutrophil cytoplasmic antibody (ANCA)–associated small-vessel vasculitis. The fibrinoid material is red. The uninvolved segments appear normal. (Masson trichrome; original magnification ×150.)

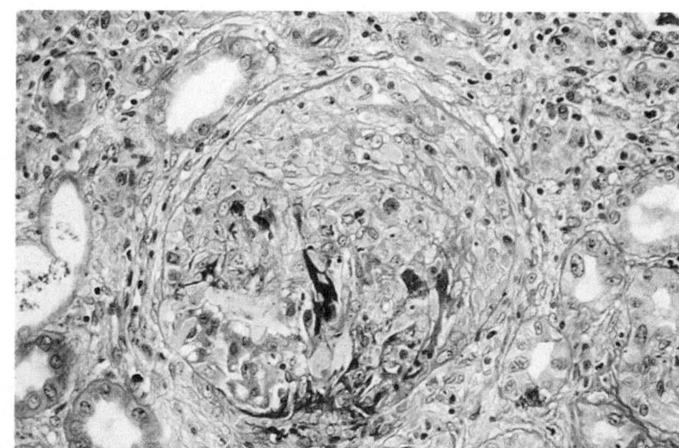

Figure 24.12 Global glomerular necrosis and circumferential crescent formation in a glomerulus from a patient with antineutrophil cytoplasmic antibody (ANCA)–associated small-vessel vasculitis. (Masson trichrome; original magnification ×150.)

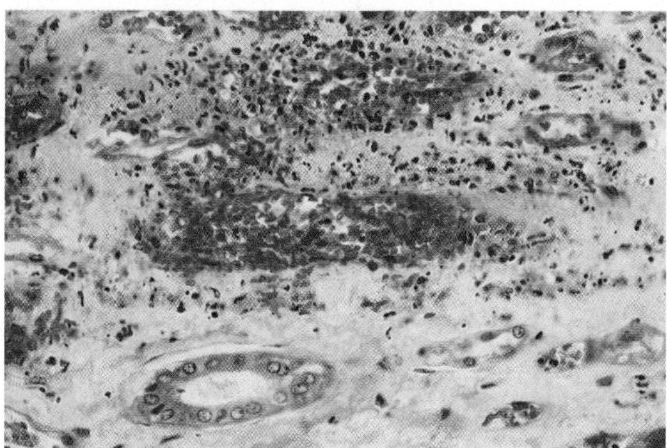

Figure 24.13 Medullary leukocytoclastic angiitis involving the vasa recta in a patient with Wegener's granulomatosis. (Hematoxylin-eosin; original magnification ×150.)

lesions have segmental fibrinoid necrosis with or without an adjacent small crescent (see Fig. 24.11). Severe acute lesions may have essentially global necrosis with large circumferential crescents (see Fig. 24.12). In a cohort of 181 renal biopsy specimens from patients with ANCA-associated GN, 89.5% had glomerular crescents that on average affected 49% of glomeruli, with half having crescents in more than 50% of glomeruli.[27] Non-necrotic segments within segmentally injured glomeruli (see Fig. 24.11) and glomeruli without necrosis typically have slight or no histologic abnormalities.

As mentioned previously, approximately one fourth of patients with anti-GBM crescentic GN and one fourth of patients with immune complex–mediated crescentic GN will be ANCA positive.[27] By contrast, less than 5% of patients with immune complex GN who do not have crescents will be ANCA positive. Therefore, even in patients with immune complex GN, the presence of ANCA is associated with an increased incidence of crescents (and also inflammation in vessels other than glomerular capillaries).

In addition to GN, patients with pauci-immune small-vessel vasculitis also may have renal arteritis, most often affecting interlobular arteries (see Figs. 24.9 and 24.10), and medullary angiitis affecting the vasa recta (Fig. 24.13).[1,2,36,37] The medullary angiitis may be severe enough to cause papillary necrosis, although this appears to be a rare complication.

Patients with Wegener's granulomatosis and Churg-Strauss syndrome have pathologic lesions in addition to the necrotizing small-vessel vasculitis that they have in common with microscopic polyangiitis patients.[1-4] The necrotizing granulomatous inflammation of Wegener's granulomatosis occurs most often in the respiratory tract and is characterized by zones of necrosis surrounded by mixed infiltrates of neutrophils, lymphocytes, monocytes, and macrophages, often including scattered multinucleated giant cells. Varying numbers of eosinophils may be present in the lesions of Wegener's granulomatosis, but these are more conspicuous in the necrotizing granulomatous inflammation of Churg-Strauss syndrome. Eosinophils also are typically conspicuous in the vasculitic lesions of Churg-Strauss syndrome, but this is not a pathognomonic observation because numerous eosinophils may be present in the vasculitic lesions of Wegener's granulomatosis, microscopic polyangiitis, polyarteritis nodosa, and other vasculitides.

Differential Diagnosis

ANCA-associated small-vessel vasculitis must be differentiated from other forms of small-vessel vasculitis that can produce the same signs and symptoms.[2] In addition, an attempt should be made to distinguish between microscopic polyangiitis, Wegener's granulomatosis, and Churg-Strauss syndrome, although sometimes this cannot be accomplished conclusively and is not required for initiation of therapy. Pathologic confirmation of the granulomatous inflammation that is seen in ANCA disease is particularly difficult because small biopsy specimens often show only nonspecific acute and chronic inflammation and necrosis. Thus, findings other than histologic lesions, such as nodular or cavitary lung lesions observed radiographically or destructive bone lesions in the nasal septum, often must be used as markers of necrotizing granulomatous inflammation to categorize patients. Because of the toxicity of the treatment, even in a patient with substantial clinical and serologic evidence of ANCA disease, pathologic confirmation of vasculitis is warranted. This can be accomplished with biopsy of many different involved sites, including skin, muscle, nerve, gut, and kidney. When there is substantial renal involvement, renal biopsy findings also can be useful for predicting the response to treatment and clinical outcome.[36-40]

All forms of small-vessel vasculitis listed in Figure 24.2 are capable of producing clinically indistinguishable overlapping features of disease, such as nephritis, purpura, peripheral neuropathy, myalgias, arthralgias, and abdominal pain. Figure 24.14 indicates a number of features that help discriminate between several important categories of small-vessel vasculitis.[2] Accurate differentiation among them is very important for proper patient management because the natural histories and appropriate treatments vary greatly. For example, a patient presenting with nephritis, arthralgias, and abdominal pain could have HSP, microscopic polyangiitis, cryoglobulinemic vasculitis, or a number of other small-vessel vasculitides. A number of serologic and pathologic observations are useful for reaching the correct diagnosis (see Fig. 24.14). A positive ANCA assay (confirmed by EIA to be MPO-ANCA or PR3-ANCA) supports a diagnosis of microscopic polyangiitis or one of the other pauci-immune small-vessel vasculitides. A negative ANCA assay and positive cryoglobulin assay (especially accompanied by hypocomplementemia and positive hepatitis C serology) support a diagnosis of cryoglobulinemic vasculitis. A negative ANCA assay, negative cryoglobulin assay, and normal complement levels support a diagnosis of HSP, especially in a patient younger than 21 years. The age of a patient influences the likelihood of a specific diagnosis. For example, approximately 80% of children younger than 10 years who have purpura, nephritis, and arthralgias will have HSP, whereas approximately 80% of adults older than 60 years with the same symptoms will have an ANCA-associated small-vessel vasculitis. However, each disease can occur at any age.

Exposure to drugs that may provoke ANCA vasculitis must be considered, including penicillamine, hydralazine, and propylthiouracil.[10] Cholesterol embolization (see Chapter 64) can also mimic the clinical features of small-vessel vasculitis, but ANCA assay is negative. The differential diagnosis of lung hemorrhage and nephritis is discussed further in Chapter 23.

Recently, autoantibodies to lysosomal membrane protein 2 (LAMP-2) were reportedly identified in the circulation of most patients with either MPO-ANCA or PR3-ANCA.[41] LAMP-2 has homology to the bacterial adhesin FimH, and thus

Features	Microscopic Polyangiitis	Wegener's Granulomatosis	Churg-Strauss Syndrome	Henoch-Schönlein Purpura (HSP)	Cryoglobulinemic Vasculitis
Vasculitic signs and symptoms*	+	+	+	+	+
IgA-dominant immune deposits	−	−	−	+	−
Cryoglobulins in blood and vessels	−	−	−	−	+
Antineutrophil cytoplasmic antibodies (ANCA) in blood	+	+	+	−	−
Necrotizing granulomas	−	+	+	−	−
Asthma and eosinophilia	−	−	+	−	−

Figure 24.14 Differential diagnostic features of selected forms of small-vessel vasculitis. *All these vessel vasculitides can manifest any of the shared features of small-vessel vasculitides, such as nephritis, purpura, abdominal pain, peripheral neuropathy, myalgias, and arthralgias. Each is distinguished by the presence and, just as important, by the absence of certain specific features. *(Modified from reference 2.)*

autoantibodies to LAMP-2 may arise by molecular mimicry secondary to infection with fimbriated gram-negative bacteria. Further, rats injected with anti–LAMP-2 or immunized with FimH develop pauci-immune focal necrotizing and crescentic GN. If these exciting observations are confirmed, anti–LAMP-2 antibodies will be a useful marker for pauci-immune small-vessel vasculitis but also may prove to be critically important in the pathogenesis of pauci-immune vasculitis and GN.

Natural History

Before the advent of immunosuppressive therapy, the survival of patients with Wegener's granulomatosis, microscopic polyangiitis, and Churg-Strauss syndrome was dismal, with most patients dying in less than a year. With adequate immunosuppressive therapy, 5-year renal and patient survival is 65% to 75%.[38] The likelihood of success of long-term maintenance of renal function is inversely correlated with the serum creatinine concentration when therapy begins, which indicates the importance of early diagnosis and prompt initiation of appropriate treatment. The likelihood of the patient's survival increases with early treatment of pulmonary hemorrhage and sepsis and avoidance of overimmunosuppression leading to life-threatening infections.[42] Older age, higher serum creatinine concentration at presentation, pulmonary hemorrhage, and especially dialysis-dependent renal failure correlate with an overall poor outcome.[38] However, even dialysis-dependent renal failure may resolve with aggressive early therapy. Respiratory tract disease and PR3-ANCA are predictors of higher relapse rates.[39,42] Pathologic features that correlate with renal outcome include histologically normal glomeruli, glomerular sclerosis, interstitial leukocyte infiltration, tubular necrosis, and tubular atrophy.[39] Glomerular filtration rate (GFR) at 18 months after diagnosis correlates with interstitial fibrosis and tubular atrophy, whereas the extent of recovery of renal function correlates with glomerular crescents and necrosis.[40] This suggests that active inflammatory lesions may be suppressed if not reversed by treatment, whereas chronic injury at the time that treatment is begun may be irreversible.

When severe GN is present, the renal prognosis is similar for patients with Wegener's granulomatosis, microscopic polyangiitis, Churg-Strauss syndrome, and isolated pauci-immune crescentic GN. Renal involvement, however, is not usually present or is mild in patients with Churg-Strauss syndrome. Cardiac involvement is the most frequent cause of death in patients with Churg-Strauss syndrome but only rarely causes mortality in microscopic polyangiitis or Wegener's granulomatosis. Wegener's granulomatosis has a broad spectrum of clinical manifestations, from very localized indolent disease to fulminant multisystem disease. For example, some patients have disease limited to the upper respiratory tract or to the upper and lower respiratory tract. Such limited disease may have a more benign natural history than systemic disease with substantial renal involvement and may warrant less aggressive treatment.

Patients with MPO-ANCA have a slightly better renal outcome than do those with PR3-ANCA even though they have more renal impairment and more chronic renal pathologic changes at presentation.[36-42] Patients with PR3-ANCA have more extrarenal organ manifestations (especially respiratory tract disease), higher chance for relapse, and higher mortality than MPO-ANCA patients do. Irrespective of the category of ANCA disease, the best clinical predictor of renal outcome is the GFR at the time of diagnosis, and the best pathologic predictor of response to treatment is the extent of active necrosis and cellular crescents in biopsy specimens.[40]

Treatment

This section focuses on patients with ANCA-associated small-vessel vasculitis affecting the kidneys. The goal should be not to overtreat mild disease and not to undertreat severe disease. GN that is severe enough to cause renal impairment is an indication for immunosuppressive treatment in patients with Wegener's granulomatosis, microscopic polyangiitis, Churg-Strauss syndrome, and isolated pauci-immune crescentic GN. Patients with ANCA-associated small-vessel vasculitis who have concurrent anti-GBM disease or concurrent immune complex disease should be treated similarly to patients with ANCA disease alone.

Treatment involves three phases: induction of remission, maintenance of remission, and treatment of relapse.[38,43]

Induction Therapy

The consensus is that corticosteroids alone are not as effective for induction therapy as are corticosteroids combined with a cytotoxic agent such as cyclophosphamide.[38,42-49] Combined treatment with corticosteroid and cyclophosphamide induces remission in approximately 75% of patients at 3 months and 90% at 6 months. The specifics of combined induction regimens vary with respect to agents, doses, route of administration, and duration. One induction approach is to begin with 7 mg/kg/day intravenous methylprednisolone for 3 days followed by oral prednisone 1 mg/kg/day, tapering to an alternate-day regimen and discontinuing within 3 to 4 months.[44] Alternatively, the corticosteroids can be administered as 1 mg/kg/day prednisolone tapered to 0.25 mg/kg/day by 3 months.[48] The corticosteroid treatment is combined with 2 mg/kg/day oral cyclophosphamide or intravenous cyclophosphamide at 0.5 g/m^2 per month adjusted upward to 1 g/m^2 on the basis of the leukocyte count after 2 weeks with a target nadir of 3000 cells/mm^3. The dose of oral cyclophosphamide can be reduced by 25 mg for patients older than 60 years.[48]

The role of plasma exchange as a component of induction therapy is becoming better defined. Plasma exchange may be of benefit in two specific populations: (1) those with life-threatening pulmonary hemorrhage[50] and (2) those who have dialysis-dependent renal failure at the time of presentation.[51] With respect to pulmonary hemorrhage, 20 of 20 patients treated with early plasma exchange had resolution of pulmonary bleeding compared with a 50% mortality rate in historical controls.[50] A trial by the European Vasculitis Study Group (MEPEX) evaluated the efficacy of intravenous methylprednisolone as induction therapy or plasma exchange in patients who had a serum creatinine concentration of more than 500 µmol/l.[51] Results from this study suggest that plasma exchange compared with pulse methylprednisolone in this population increases the rate of recovery from renal failure. Patient survival and adverse events were similar in patients who did or did not receive plasma exchange. Plasma exchange was associated with a 24% reduced risk of progression to end-stage renal disease (ESRD) (43% to 19% at 1 year). A subsequent study is being undertaken to more fully evaluate the role of plasma exchange in ANCA-positive patients.

Maintenance Therapy

The duration of induction therapy and the intensity of maintenance therapy should be reduced as much as possible to reduce toxic side effects. This is a difficult challenge because of the tendency of the pauci-immune small-vessel vasculitides to recur. A number of approaches have been used to reduce the cyclophosphamide dose, such as giving less cyclophosphamide through intravenous rather than oral schedules,[44,50] substituting a less toxic maintenance drug after 3 to 6 months,[48] and discontinuing therapy earlier in patients with lower risk of relapse. Intravenous cyclophosphamide regimens afford one third to one half of the total dose of cyclophosphamide given in oral regimens. A head-to-head comparison by the European Vasculitis Study Group (CYCLOPS trial) indicates that intravenous cyclophosphamide results in the same remission and relapse rates as oral cyclophosphamide does while reducing the total dose of cyclophosphamide.[52] Another approach to reducing cyclophosphamide dose is to convert to azathioprine after 3 to 6 months of therapy.[38,48] In the European Vasculitis Study Group CYCAZAREM trial, cyclophosphamide was replaced with 2 mg/kg/day azathioprine after 3 to 6 months with no change in the relapse rate at the end of the study.[48] Cyclophosphamide dose also could be reduced by alternative induction therapies. In a randomized trial of cyclophosphamide versus methotrexate in patients without critical organ damage and primarily ear, nose, and throat disease, methotrexate was less effective for inducing remission in patients who developed extensive disease and pulmonary involvement and was associated with more relapses than cyclophosphamide.[53] A study by the French Vasculitis Study Group has examined methotrexate compared with azathioprine as maintenance therapy in patients with Wegener's granulomatosis and microscopic polyangiitis. In this study, methotrexate was as effective as azathioprine for maintenance of remission, but methotrexate did not have fewer side effects.[54] An attractive alternative is to stop induction therapy at 6 to 12 months if the patient is in full remission, especially if the patient is at lower risk of relapse.[42]

Additional immunosuppressive agents that have been used for maintenance therapy in patients who have not responded well to more conventional treatment include anti–tumor necrosis factor α (anti-TNF α) (infliximab, etanercept), anti-CD20 (rituximab), and mycophenolate mofetil (MMF).[54-58] The results are not yet conclusive; however, MMF appears to be of some value at least as an adjunct to current immunosuppressive regimens.[57] There are a number of anecdotal and early randomized trial results with use of rituximab in therapy for small-vessel vasculitis. Whereas the initial reports appear encouraging, the full results of a true randomized control trial need to become available for the place of rituximab therapy to be more fully understood. The cost of this medication precludes its use at present, other than for those individuals who are refractory to other therapy and when leukopenia and infectious complications are problematic. In this population, there is evidence that rituximab can induce partial or complete remission.[54] The Wegener's Granulomatosis Etanercept Trial (WGET) examined the use of etanercept in addition to a methotrexate-based maintenance therapy.[58] This study was marked by a very low long-term remission rate of approximately 50% and a high rate of disease flares. Six patients treated with etanercept developed solid cancers. The investigators concluded that etanercept is not effective for the maintenance of remission in patients with Wegener's granulomatosis.[58]

The role of antimicrobial agents, such as trimethoprim-sulfamethoxazole, in maintenance of remission is controversial. Some studies have suggested a benefit, but others have not because of an increased likelihood of relapse.[59,60] Trimethoprim-sulfamethoxazole may be useful adjunct therapy, especially in patients with upper respiratory tract disease, but it should not be used in the absence of immunosuppressive drugs with more proven efficacy (e.g., cyclophosphamide, azathioprine) for induction or maintenance therapy for systemic vasculitis or GN.

Relapse Therapy

Approximately one fourth to one half of patients with pauci-immune small-vessel vasculitis and GN will experience a relapse within several years. Relapses are diagnosed on the basis of solid clinical and pathologic evidence of recurrent disease, not by an increase in ANCA titer alone.[33,34] However, an increase in ANCA titer increases the likelihood of a relapse, and there are some advocates for preemptive immunosuppressive therapy if the ANCA titer increases by at least fourfold.[34] We prefer to identify clear-cut clinical or pathologic evidence of relapse before increasing immunosuppressive therapy.[44]

The best treatment for relapses is unsettled. Reinstitution of treatment similar to an induction regimen is used most often, but less intensive or less toxic therapy may be adequate.[38,44,45] A number of therapies have been used, including cyclophosphamide, rituximab, intravenous immune globulin, and MMF in combination with methotrexate or azathioprine, and combinations of these drugs must be tailored to the individual patient with recalcitrant disease.

In some individuals, long-term therapy may not be required, especially if there is a very low risk of relapse. In prospective observational studies from the Glomerular Disease Collaborative, the relative risk of relapse was increased in those individuals who had PR3-ANCA and ear, nose, and throat disease and lung disease.[42] Patients had more than a threefold risk of relapse compared with those individuals with MPO-ANCA and without lung or ear, nose, and throat disease. In a follow-up study, this model of relapsing disease was investigated in a separate registry in France, in which PR3-ANCA in lung disease was the most important predictive marker.[61] Thus, it is possible that in those who have a much smaller risk of relapse, all therapy can be stopped, provided the patient and physician pursue a monitoring course in which the risk of early relapse is detected, for example, urinary dipstick testing in the home to monitor for the recurrence of hematuria. The risk of relapse is on the order of 10% to 15% even with remission maintenance therapy.

Transplantation

There are a few reports of recurrent disease in renal transplants given to patients with ESRD caused by pauci-immune crescentic GN, but they are not numerous enough to be a contraindication to transplantation. Although the data are limited, the frequency of recurrence appears to be approximately 20%, but graft loss caused by recurrence may be less than 5% (see Chapter 104). A positive ANCA titer at the time of transplantation does not increase the risk of recurrent disease in the transplant.[62,63] Recurrent ANCA GN in a renal transplant responds similarly to recurrent disease in native kidneys.[63] As with native kidney disease, an increase in ANCA titer and an active urine sediment should raise the possibility of recurrent GN, but the diagnosis requires pathologic confirmation.

POLYARTERITIS NODOSA

Polyarteritis nodosa is a systemic necrotizing arteritis that affects predominantly main visceral arteries and their intraparenchymal branches.[1,4,5,64] There is still much confusion about the relationship between polyarteritis nodosa and microscopic polyangiitis (which also has been referred to as microscopic polyarteritis). The Chapel Hill Nomenclature System limits the diagnosis of polyarteritis nodosa to patients who have only arteritis.[4] The presence of vasculitis in vessels other than arteries, such as capillaries, venules, or arterioles, excludes a diagnosis of polyarteritis nodosa and indicates some form of small-vessel vasculitis. Thus, GN excludes a diagnosis of polyarteritis nodosa. When polyarteritis nodosa is distinguished from microscopic polyangiitis by this approach, the two categories of vasculitis have not only different pathologic characteristics but also different clinical features and natural histories, which justifies the nosologic distinction between polyarteritis nodosa and microscopic polyangiitis.[5,64-68]

Pathogenesis

The etiology and pathogenesis of polyarteritis nodosa are unknown. When polyarteritis nodosa is separated from microscopic polyangiitis, the latter but not the former is associated with ANCA. An immune complex trigger for polyarteritis nodosa has been proposed but has not been confirmed as the major pathogenetic process. A minority of patients have hepatitis B virus infection, which has raised the possibility that the hepatitis B virus infection is producing immune complexes that are localizing in artery walls and inducing inflammation.[68] However, the evidence that hepatitis B virus infection is causing vascular immune complex deposition is stronger in certain forms of GN and small-vessel vasculitis than in polyarteritis nodosa.

Epidemiology

When it is defined by the Chapel Hill nomenclature system, polyarteritis nodosa has a prevalence of approximately 3/100,000 compared with 2.5/100,000 for microscopic polyangiitis, 2.5/100,000 for Wegener's granulomatosis, and 1/100,000 for Churg-Strauss syndrome.[24] This population study was carried out in an urban area in France, and the authors pointed out that this is a higher prevalence for polyarteritis nodosa compared with the ANCA-associated vasculitides than has been reported in other studies. They suggested that environmental factors may influence the prevalence of polyarteritis nodosa. Polyarteritis nodosa affects males and females equally and is found in all races. Onset is most frequent between the ages of 40 and 60 years.

Clinical Manifestations

The usual clinical presentation of polyarteritis nodosa includes nonspecific constitutional symptoms, such as fever, malaise, arthralgias, myalgias, and weight loss, as well as manifestations of arteritis.[64-68] Peripheral neuropathy, typically in the form of a mononeuritis multiplex, is a common manifestation. This is caused by inflammation of small epineural arteries and is clinically indistinguishable from the peripheral neuropathy caused by other forms of vasculitis that can affect epineural arteries, such as microscopic polyangiitis, Wegener's granulomatosis, and Churg-Strauss syndrome. Gastrointestinal involvement occurs in about half of patients, usually manifested as abdominal pain and blood in the stool. Bowel infarction is uncommon and perforation is rare. Renal involvement produces infarction and hemorrhage, which are indicated by flank pain and hematuria. Rupture of an arterial aneurysm with retroperitoneal or peritoneal hemorrhage is an uncommon but potentially lethal renal complication. Approximately one third of patients develop hypertension, which rarely reaches the malignant range. Red, tender inflammatory nodules are the most common cutaneous manifestation. Infarction, ulceration, and livedo reticularis may be present.

Arterial aneurysms may be detected by angiography in patients with polyarteritis nodosa (Fig. 24.15). This is not a completely specific determination because any necrotizing arteritis that affects arteries large enough to be seen by angiography can produce this finding.

Pathology

Any artery in the kidney can be affected by polyarteritis nodosa, from the main renal artery to the interlobular arteries, although the interlobar and arcuate arteries are affected most often.[1] Nodular inflammatory lesions and aneurysms (pseudoaneurysms) can be observed grossly when medium-sized arteries are involved. Inflammation in small arteries can be observed only by microscopy.

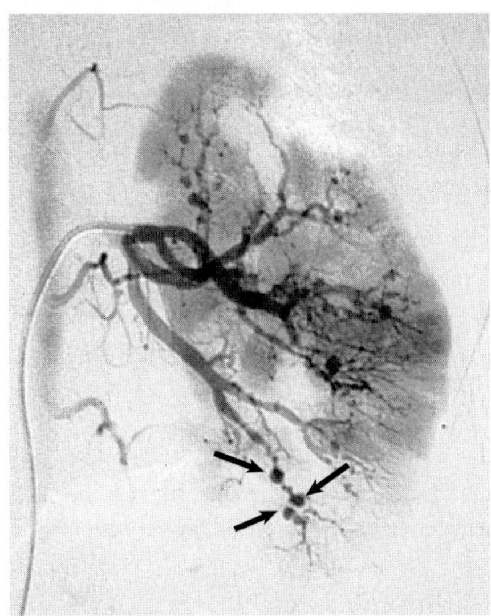

Figure 24.15 Renal angiogram in polyarteritis nodosa. Angiogram shows patchy renal perfusion defects and aneurysms *(arrows)*.

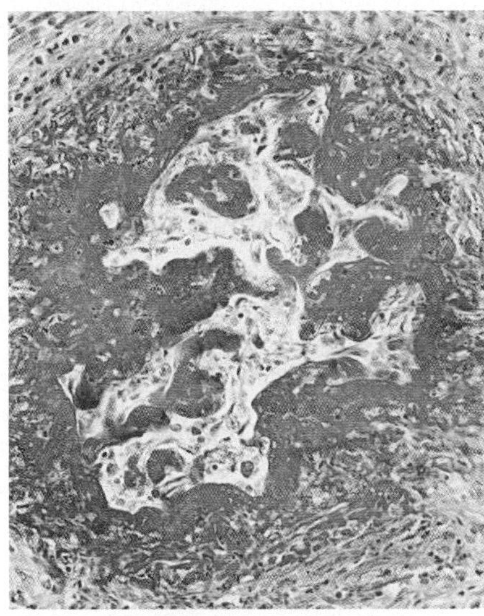

Figure 24.16 Necrotizing arteritis in an arcuate artery of a patient with polyarteritis nodosa. The lumen is partially occluded by thrombotic material that is continuous with the fibrinoid material that has replaced the entire wall of the artery. (Hematoxylin-eosin; original magnification ×50.)

The characteristic acute lesion is segmental transmural fibrinoid necrosis of arteries, usually accompanied by infiltrating leukocytes with leukocytoclasia (Fig. 24.16).[3,69] The earliest lesions have numerous neutrophils, and later lesions have predominantly mononuclear leukocytes. Acute lesions may be complicated by thrombosis or hemorrhage. Older lesions develop fibrosis and endarterial remodeling. The aneurysms of necrotizing arteritis are not true aneurysms but rather are inflammatory pseudoaneurysms. That is, the walls of the arteries are not dilated but rather have been eaten away by the necrotizing inflammation, which then erodes into the surrounding perivascular tissue to create an enlarged lumen at the site of inflammation. This explains the propensity for such lesions to induce thrombosis or to undergo rupture.

The necrotizing arteritis of polyarteritis nodosa cannot be distinguished by light microscopy from arteritis caused by other necrotizing vasculitides affecting arteries.[1,2] For example, necrotizing arteritis in a skeletal muscle biopsy specimen or a peripheral nerve biopsy specimen is histologically identical whether it is caused by polyarteritis nodosa, microscopic polyangiitis, Wegener's granulomatosis, or Churg-Strauss syndrome. For these vasculitides to be distinguished, additional clinical and serologic information is required.

Differential Diagnosis

Polyarteritis nodosa must be distinguished from other forms of vasculitis, especially other forms of necrotizing vasculitis that can affect arteries, such as microscopic polyangiitis. Lhote and Guillevin[67] have identified clinical features that assist in the differential diagnosis (Fig. 24.17).

A positive ANCA test result supports the presence of one of the ANCA-associated small-vessel vasculitides rather than polyarteritis nodosa. The presence of GN indicates some form of small-vessel vasculitis rather than polyarteritis nodosa. Vasculitic pulmonary disease is rare in polyarteritis nodosa but is frequent in microscopic polyangiitis, Wegener's granulomatosis, and Churg-Strauss syndrome. Peripheral neuropathy or muscle tenderness with arteritis in epineural or skeletal muscle arteries is not a useful differentiating feature because it is frequent in polyarteritis nodosa as well as in the ANCA-associated small-vessel vasculitides. Kawasaki disease causes necrotizing arteritis but is distinguished from polyarteritis nodosa by the presence of the mucocutaneous lymph node syndrome.

Natural History

The natural history of polyarteritis nodosa is difficult to determine because most of the early studies of outcome grouped polyarteritis nodosa together with microscopic polyangiitis. Polyarteritis nodosa with multisystem involvement has a very poor prognosis without therapy. Polyarteritis nodosa usually is treated with corticosteroids and cytotoxic drugs, such as cyclophosphamide.[66] The 10-year survival rate with appropriate treatment is approximately 80%. Approximately 15% of patients who enter remission develop a relapse, which is much less frequent than with microscopic polyangiitis. Relapse is more likely if treatment is delayed.

Treatment

Polyarteritis nodosa in patients with no evidence of hepatitis B virus infection is treated with corticosteroids and cytotoxic drugs, usually cyclophosphamide.[45,64-67] The regimens vary and include treatment approaches similar to those described earlier for microscopic polyangiitis and Wegener's granulomatosis. However, in patients with no risk factors for poor outcome (such as age older than 50 years, cardiac involvement, gut involvement, or renal involvement), corticosteroids alone may be adequate and are less toxic therapy than corticosteroids combined with cytotoxic agents.

Aggressive immunosuppressive therapy without initial antiviral therapy is contraindicated in patients with hepatitis B virus–associated polyarteritis nodosa because of potential adverse effects on the outcome of the hepatitis B virus infection. Short-term corticosteroid treatment combined with antiviral agents and possibly plasma exchange should precede more extensive immunosuppression in such patients.[65,68] The European League Against Rheumatism (EULAR) recommends initial treatment

Clinical Differences Between Polyarteritis Nodosa and Microscopic Polyangiitis		
Clinical Feature	**Polyarteritis Nodosa**	**Microscopic Polyangiitis**
Microaneurysms by angiography	Yes	No (?rare)
Rapidly progressive nephritis	No	Yes (very common)
Pulmonary hemorrhage	No	Yes
Renovascular hypertension	Yes (10%–33%)	No
Peripheral neuropathy	Yes (50%–80%)	Yes (10%–20%)
Positive hepatitis B serology	Uncommon	No
Positive antineutrophil cytoplasmic antibody	Rare	Frequent
Relapses	Rare	Frequent

Figure 24.17 Clinical differences between polyarteritis nodosa and microscopic polyangiitis. *(Modified from reference 26.)*

with high-dose corticosteroids tapered during 2 weeks followed by antiviral treatment.[45] The addition of plasma exchange may increase the likelihood of remission.

KAWASAKI DISEASE

Definition

Kawasaki disease is an acute febrile illness that usually occurs in young children, often younger than 1 year, and is characterized by the mucocutaneous lymph node (MCLN) syndrome (see later discussion).[4,70-72] Necrotizing arteritis is a complication of Kawasaki disease that is present in some but not all patients. Clinically significant renal involvement is very rare; therefore, Kawasaki disease is rarely encountered by nephrologists.

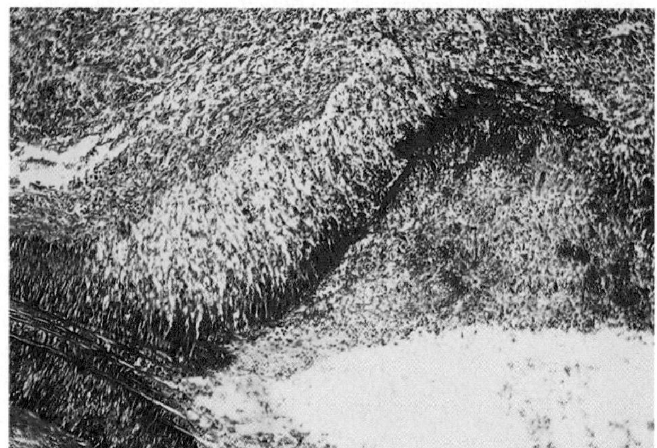

Figure 24.18 Kawasaki disease arteritis affecting a renal interlobar artery in a young child. The artery wall is intact on the far left. The remainder of the wall has extensive edema, infiltration by mononuclear leukocytes, and a band of fuchsinophilic (red) fibrinoid material roughly at the junction between the inflamed intima and muscularis. (Masson trichrome; original magnification ×25.)

Pathogenesis

The occasional occurrence of Kawasaki disease as an endemic or epidemic disease suggests that the cause may be an infectious agent or an environmental toxin. Both cell-mediated and antibody-mediated mechanisms have been incriminated, including a possible role for antiendothelial antibodies.[72] At the current time, the etiology and pathogenesis of Kawasaki disease are unproven.

Epidemiology

Kawasaki disease usually occurs in children younger than 5 years and has a peak incidence in the first year of life. It was first described in Japan, but it occurs worldwide. The disease is more common in Asians and Polynesians than in Caucasians and blacks. In Japan, the incidence is 50/100,000 children younger than 5 years, with 50% of the children younger than 2 years.[73] Kawasaki disease occasionally occurs in an endemic or epidemic pattern but usually is sporadic.

Clinical Manifestations

MCLV syndrome is the characteristic clinical manifestation of Kawasaki disease.[4,72] This includes fever (temperature of usually 38°C to 40°C), mucosal inflammation, swollen red tongue (strawberry tongue), polymorphous erythematous rash, indurative edema of the extremities, erythema of palms and soles, desquamation from the tips of digits, conjunctival injection, and enlarged lymph nodes.

The frequency of active arteritic lesions peaks during the first week of the illness and is markedly reduced after 1 month. Arteritis most often is manifested as cardiac disease. Thrombosis of inflamed coronary arteries in patients with Kawasaki disease is the most common cause of childhood myocardial infarction. Clinically significant renal disease is uncommon. This is somewhat surprising because autopsy reveals arteritis in renal vessels in up to three fourths of patients.[70]

Pathology

The arteritis of Kawasaki disease involves small and medium-sized arteries. The acute histologic lesion is necrotizing inflammation with less fibrinoid necrosis and more edema than is usually observed with polyarteritis nodosa (Fig. 24.18).[69] Aneurysm (pseudoaneurysm) formation and thrombosis may occur.

The most frequent site of arteritis is the coronary arteries, followed by the renal arteries.[70] Arteritis most often affects interlobar arteries, occasionally arcuate arteries, and only rarely interlobular arteries.

Differential Diagnosis

Kawasaki disease has sometimes been misdiagnosed as childhood polyarteritis nodosa. The differentiation of Kawasaki disease from polyarteritis nodosa is very important because corticosteroid treatment may increase the risk of coronary artery aneurysms in Kawasaki disease. Arteritis in a child younger than 5 years should always raise the possibility of Kawasaki disease. The presence or absence of the MCLN syndrome is the basis for distinguishing between Kawasaki disease and other forms of arteritis.[4]

Natural History

Kawasaki disease usually is self-limited with an uneventful recovery if it is treated promptly with intravenous gamma globulins.[71,72] Recurrence is rare. Only about 1% of patients develop severe arteritic complications, usually affecting the coronary arteries.

Treatment

Aspirin and intravenous gamma globulin are the standard therapy for Kawasaki disease.[71,72] Corticosteroid treatment may increase the risk of adverse coronary artery complications, although the data supporting this are limited.

TAKAYASU ARTERITIS AND GIANT CELL ARTERITIS

Takayasu arteritis and giant cell arteritis affect the aorta and its major branches.[4,69,74] Giant cell arteritis has a predilection for the extracranial branches of the carotid artery but can affect arteries in almost any organ. Takayasu arteritis has a predilection for major arteries supplying the extremities. Both diseases cause chronic vascular inflammation, often with a granulomatous appearance that may include multinucleated giant cells. Giant cell arteritis, but not Takayasu arteritis, is associated with polymyalgia rheumatica.

Pathogenesis

The etiology and pathogenesis of giant cell arteritis and Takayasu arteritis are unknown. Because of the histologic changes and the nature of the infiltrating leukocytes, cell-mediated immune mechanisms are incriminated. The inciting antigen or autoantigen has not been identified.

Epidemiology

Takayasu arteritis is seen most frequently in Asia. Giant cell arteritis is most frequent in individuals of northern European ancestry. Takayasu arteritis has a female-to-male ratio of approximately 9:1, and giant cell arteritis has a female-to-male ratio of 4:1. Takayasu arteritis usually is diagnosed in those between the ages of 10 and 20 years and is very rare after 50 years of age. Giant cell arteritis is very rare before the age of 50 years.

Clinical Manifestations

In addition to nonspecific constitutional symptoms, such as fever, arthralgias, and weight loss, the major clinical manifestations of Takayasu arteritis and giant cell arteritis are caused by arterial narrowing and resultant ischemia.[74]

The major clinical manifestations of Takayasu arteritis are reduced pulses (95% of patients), vascular bruits, claudication, and renovascular hypertension. Renovascular hypertension is a major cause of morbidity and mortality and results from renal ischemia caused by renal artery stenosis or aortic coarctation.[74,75] Reduced aortic elasticity and impairment of carotid artery baroreceptors also may play a role in some patients. EULAR recommends thorough imaging assessment of the entire major arterial tree when a diagnosis of Takayasu arteritis is suspected.[76]

Headache is the most common presenting symptom in patients with giant cell arteritis. Temporal artery tenderness, nodularity, or decreased pulsation is present in about half of patients. Additional common symptoms include blindness, deafness, jaw claudication, tongue dysfunction, extremity claudication, and reduced pulses. More than half of patients with giant cell arteritis have polymyalgia rheumatica, which is characterized by stiffness and aching in the neck and the proximal muscles of the shoulders and hips. Clinically significant renal disease is much rarer in giant cell arteritis than in Takayasu arteritis. There are case reports of necrotizing and crescentic GN associated with giant cell arteritis, but these may represent examples of Wegener's granulomatosis or microscopic polyangiitis with temporal artery involvement.

Pathology

The aortitis and arteritis of Takayasu arteritis and giant cell arteritis cannot be confidently distinguished from each other by pathologic examination.[69] Both are characterized in the active phase by inflammation with a predominance of mononuclear leukocytes, often with scattered multinucleated giant cells (Fig. 24.19). The chronic phase is characterized by progressive fibrosis that may cause severe narrowing of vessels, with resultant ischemia. Major renal arteries are often found to be involved at autopsy in both Takayasu arteritis and giant cell arteritis patients. However, clinically significant renal disease is relatively common in Takayasu arteritis but rare in giant cell arteritis. A glomerular lesion characterized by nodular mesangial matrix expansion and mesangiolysis may occasionally be a component of Takayasu arteritis.[77]

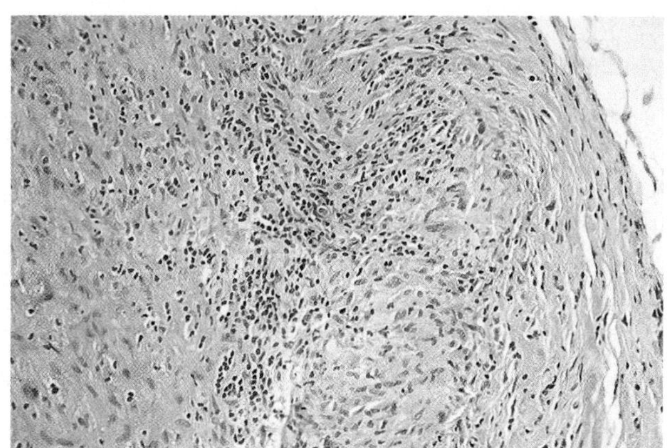

Figure 24.19 Severe giant cell arteritis affecting a main renal artery. This caused marked renal atrophy and renovascular hypertension. (Hematoxylin-eosin; original magnification ×50.)

Differential Diagnosis

There is a great deal of overlap between the clinical manifestations and pathologic features of Takayasu arteritis and giant cell arteritis. The age of the patient and the presence or absence of polymyalgia rheumatica are the best features for discriminating between these two vasculitides.

Giant cell arteritis also has been called temporal arteritis. This is a misleading designation because not all patients have temporal artery involvement, and patients with other types of vasculitis, such as polyarteritis nodosa, Wegener's granulomatosis, and microscopic polyangiitis, can have involvement of the temporal arteries. Some of the reported examples of necrotizing GN associated with temporal arteritis probably represent Wegener's granulomatosis or microscopic polyangiitis with temporal artery involvement.

Treatment

Corticosteroids are the usual treatment of giant cell arteritis and Takayasu arteritis.[76] EULAR recommends initial daily therapy with 1 mg/kg prednisolone for 1 month followed by tapering during several months.[76] More prolonged treatment may be dictated by persistent disease activity. Cytotoxic agents such as cyclophosphamide may be required in patients with recalcitrant disease. Patients with giant cell arteritis also should receive low-dose aspirin to protect against thrombotic vascular events.[76]

Management of renal disease is not an issue with typical giant cell arteritis, although rare patients have ischemic renal manifestations. Renovascular hypertension is the major renal problem caused by Takayasu arteritis.[74,75] When bilateral renal artery involvement occurs, angiotensin-converting enzyme (ACE) inhibitors may precipitate renal failure in patients with Takayasu arteritis.[78] When medical management fails, the renovascular hypertension in patients with Takayasu arteritis may be controlled by bypass surgery or angioplasty.[75] Reconstructive vascular surgery should be performed during a quiescent phase of the disease.[76] The management of renovascular hypertension is covered in Chapter 37.

REFERENCES

1. Jennette JC, Falk RJ. The pathology of vasculitis involving the kidney. *Am J Kidney Dis*. 1994;24:130-141.
2. Jennette JC, Falk RJ. Small vessel vasculitis. *N Engl J Med*. 1997;337: 1512-1523.
3. Jennette JC, Falk RJ. Renal involvement in systemic vasculitis. In: Greenberg A, Cheung AK, Coffman TM, et al, eds. *National Kidney Foundation Nephrology Primer*. 4th ed. Philadelphia: WB Saunders; 2005:226-233.
4. Jennette JC, Falk RJ, Andrassy K, et al. Nomenclature of systemic vasculitides: The proposal of an international consensus conference. *Arthritis Rheum*. 1994;37:187-192.
5. Samarkos M, Loizou S, Vaiopoulos G, Davies KA. The clinical spectrum of primary renal vasculitis. *Semin Arthritis Rheum*. 2005;35:95-111.
6. Jennette JC, Falk RJ. New insight into the pathogenesis of vasculitis associated with antineutrophil cytoplasmic autoantibodies. *Curr Opin Rheumatol*. 2008;20:55-60.
7. Savige J, Davies D, Falk RJ, et al. Antineutrophil cytoplasmic antibodies (ANCA) and associated diseases. *Kidney Int*. 2000;57:846-862.
8. Savage CO. ANCA-associated renal vasculitis. *Kidney Int*. 2001;60: 1614-1627.
9. Franssen CF, Stegeman CA, Kallenberg CG, et al. Antiproteinase 3- and antimyeloperoxidase-associated vasculitis. *Kidney Int*. 2000;57: 2195-2206.
10. Choi HK, Merkel PA, Walker AM, Niles JL. Drug-associated antineutrophil cytoplasmic antibody–positive vasculitis: Prevalence among patients with high titers of antimyeloperoxidase antibodies. *Arthritis Rheum*. 2000;43:405-413.
11. Schlieben DJ, Korbet SM, Kimura RE, et al. Pulmonary-renal syndrome in a newborn with placental transmission of ANCAs. *Am J Kidney Dis*. 2005;45:758-761.
12. Xiao H, Heeringa P, Hu P, et al. Antineutrophil cytoplasmic autoantibodies specific for myeloperoxidase cause glomerulonephritis and vasculitis in mice. *J Clin Invest*. 2002;110:955-963.
13. Xiao H, Heeringa P, Liu Z, et al. The role of neutrophils in the induction of glomerulonephritis by anti-myeloperoxidase antibodies. *Am J Pathol*. 2005;167:39-45.
14. Little MA, Smyth CL, Yadav R, et al. Antineutrophil cytoplasm antibodies directed against myeloperoxidase augment leukocyte-microvascular interactions in vivo. *Blood*. 2005;106:2050-2058.
15. Falk RJ, Terrell RS, Charles LA, Jennette JC. Anti-neutrophil cytoplasmic autoantibodies induce neutrophils to degranulate and produce oxygen radicals in vitro. *Proc Natl Acad Sci USA*. 1990;87:4115-4119.
16. Savage CO, Gaskin G, Pusey CD, Pearson JD. Myeloperoxidase binds to vascular endothelial cells, is recognized by ANCA and can enhance complement dependent cytotoxicity. *Adv Exp Med Biol*. 1993;336: 121-123.
17. Ewert BH, Jennette JC, Falk RJ. Anti-myeloperoxidase antibodies stimulate neutrophils to damage human endothelial cells. *Kidney Int*. 1992;41:375-383.
18. Vargunam M, Adu D, Taylor CM, et al. Endothelium myeloperoxidase-antimyeloperoxidase interaction in vasculitis. *Nephrol Dial Transplant*. 1992;7:1077-1081.
19. Kettritz R, Jennette JC, Falk RJ. Cross-linking of ANCA-antigens stimulates superoxide release by human neutrophils. *J Am Soc Nephrol*. 1997;8:386-394.
20. Williams JM, Ben Smith A, Hewins P, et al. Activation of the G_i heterotrimeric G protein by ANCA IgG F(ab')$_2$ fragments is necessary but not sufficient to stimulate the recruitment of those downstream mediators used by intact ANCA IgG. *J Am Soc Nephrol*. 2003;14:661-669.
21. Xiao H, Schreiber A, Heeringa P, et al. Alternative complement pathway in the pathogenesis of disease mediated by antineutrophil cytoplasmic autoantibodies. *Am J Pathol*. 2007;170:52-64.
22. Jennette JC, Falk RJ. Pathogenesis of the vascular and glomerular damage in ANCA-positive vasculitis. *Nephrol Dial Transplant*. 1998; 13(Suppl 1):16-20.
23. Falk RJ, Hogan S, Carey TS, Jennette JC. Clinical course of anti-neutrophil cytoplasmic autoantibody–associated glomerulonephritis and systemic vasculitis: The Glomerular Disease Collaborative Network. *Ann Intern Med*. 1990;113:656-663.
24. Mahr A, Guillevin L, Poissonnet M, Ayme S. Prevalences of polyarteritis nodosa, microscopic polyangiitis, Wegener's granulomatosis, and Churg-Strauss syndrome in a French urban multiethnic population in 2000: A capture-recapture estimate. *Arthritis Rheum*. 2004;51:92-99.
25. Duna GF, Galperin C, Hoffman GS. Wegener's granulomatosis. *Rheum Dis Clin North Am*. 1995;21:949-986.
26. Lhote F, Guillevin L. Polyarteritis nodosa, microscopic polyangiitis, and Churg-Strauss syndrome: Clinical aspects and treatment. *Rheum Dis Clin North Am*. 1995;21:911-947.
27. Jennette JC. Rapidly progressive crescentic glomerulonephritis. *Kidney Int*. 2003;63:1164-1177.
28. Hagen EC, Daha MR, Hermans J, et al. Diagnostic value of standardized assays for anti-neutrophil cytoplasmic antibodies in idiopathic systemic vasculitis: EC/BCR Project for ANCA Assay Standardization. *Kidney Int*. 1998;53:743-753.
29. Jennette JC, Wilkman AS, Falk RJ. Diagnostic predictive value of ANCA serology. *Kidney Int*. 1998;53:796-798.
30. Savige J, Gillis D, Davies D, et al. International consensus statement on testing and reporting of antineutrophil cytoplasmic antibodies (ANCA). *Am J Clin Pathol*. 1999;111:507-513.
31. Lim LC, Taylor JG III, Schmitz JL, et al. Diagnostic usefulness of antineutrophil cytoplasmic autoantibody serology: Comparative evaluation of commercial indirect fluorescent antibody kits and enzyme immunoassay kits. *Am J Clin Pathol*. 1999;111:363-369.
32. Rutgers A, Slot M, van Paassen P, et al. Coexistence of anti–glomerular basement membrane antibodies and myeloperoxidase-ANCAs in crescentic glomerulonephritis. *Am J Kidney Dis*. 2005;46:253-262.
33. Sinico RA, Di Toma L, Maggiore U, et al. Renal involvement in Churg-Strauss syndrome. *Am J Kidney Dis*. 2006;47:770-779.
34. Han WK, Choi HK, Roth RM, et al. Serial ANCA titers: Useful tool for prevention of relapses in ANCA-associated vasculitis. *Kidney Int*. 2003;63:1079-1085.

35. Eisenberger U, Fakhouri F, Vanhille P, et al. ANCA-negative pauci-immune renal vasculitis: Histology and outcome. *Nephrol Dial Transplant*. 2005;20:1392-1399.
36. Hauer HA, Bajema IM, Hagen EC, et al. Long-term renal injury in ANCA-associated vasculitis: An analysis of 31 patients with follow-up biopsies. *Nephrol Dial Transplant*. 2002;17:587-596.
37. Vizjak A, Rott T, Koselj-Kajtna M, et al. Histologic and immunohistologic study and clinical presentation of ANCA-associated glomerulonephritis with correlation to ANCA antigen specificity. *Am J Kidney Dis*. 2003;41:539-549.
38. Little MA, Pusey CD. Glomerulonephritis due to antineutrophil cytoplasm antibody–associated vasculitis: An update on approaches to management. *Nephrology*. 2005;10:368-376.
39. Bajema IM, Hagen EC, Hermans J, et al. Kidney biopsy as a predictor for renal outcome in ANCA-associated necrotizing glomerulonephritis. *Kidney Int*. 1999;56:1751-1758.
40. Hauer HA, Bajema IM, van Houwelingen HC, et al. Determinants of outcome in ANCA-associated glomerulonephritis: A prospective clinico-histopathological analysis of 96 patients. *Kidney Int*. 2002;62:732-742.
41. Kain R, Exner M, Brandes R, et al. Molecular mimicry in pauci-immune focal necrotizing glomerulonephritis. *Nat Med*. 2008;14:1088-1096.
42. Hogan SL, Falk RJ, Chin H, et al. Predictors of relapse and treatment resistance in ANCA small vessel vasculitis. *Ann Intern Med*. 2005;143: 621-631.
43. Bacon PA. Therapy of vasculitis. *J Rheumatol*. 1994;21:788-790.
44. Nachman PH, Hogan SL, Jennette JC, Falk RJ. Treatment response and relapse in ANCA-associated microscopic polyangiitis and glomerulonephritis. *J Am Soc Nephrol*. 1996;7:33-39.
45. Mukhtyar C, Guillevin L, Cid MC, et al. EULAR recommendations for the management of primary small and medium vessel vasculitis. *Ann Rheum Dis*. 2009;68:310-317.
46. Pusey CD, Rees AJ, Evans DJ, et al. Plasma exchange in focal necrotizing glomerulonephritis without anti-GBM antibodies. *Kidney Int*. 1991;40: 757-763.
47. Jayne DR, Davies MJ, Fox CJ, et al. Treatment of systemic vasculitis with pooled intravenous immunoglobulin. *Lancet*. 1991;337:1137-1139.
48. Jayne D, Rasmussen N, Andrassy K, et al. A randomized trial of maintenance therapy for vasculitis associated with antineutrophil cytoplasmic autoantibodies. *N Engl J Med*. 2003;349:36-44.
49. Guillevin L, Cordier JF, Lhote F, et al. A prospective, multicenter, randomized trial comparing steroids and pulse cyclophosphamide versus steroids and oral cyclophosphamide in the treatment of generalized Wegener's granulomatosis. *Arthritis Rheum*. 1997;40:2187-2198.
50. Klemmer PJ, Chalermskulrat W, Reif MS, et al. Plasmapheresis therapy for diffuse alveolar hemorrhage in patients with small-vessel vasculitis. *Am J Kidney Dis*. 2003;42:1149-1153.
51. Jayne DR, Gaskin G, Rasmussen N, et al. Randomized trial of plasma exchange or high-dosage methylprednisolone as adjunctive therapy for severe renal vasculitis. *J Am Soc Nephrol*. 2007;18:2180-2188.
52. De Groot K, Harper L, Jayne DR, et al. Pulse versus daily oral cyclophosphamide for induction of remission in antineutrophil cytoplasmic antibody–associated vasculitis: A randomized trial. *Ann Intern Med*. 2009;150:670-680.
53. De Groot K, Rasmussen N, Bacon PA, et al. Randomized trial of cyclophosphamide versus methotrexate for induction of remission in early systemic antineutrophil cytoplasmic antibody–associated vasculitis. *Arthritis Rheum*. 2005;52:2461-2469.
54. Lovric S, Erdbruegger U, Kümpers P, et al. Rituximab as rescue therapy in anti-neutrophil cytoplasmic antibody–associated vasculitis: A single-centre experience with 15 patients. *Nephrol Dial Transplant*. 2009;24: 179-185.
55. Booth A, Harper L, Hammad T, et al. Prospective study of TNFα blockade with infliximab in anti-neutrophil cytoplasmic antibody–associated systemic vasculitis. *J Am Soc Nephrol*. 2004;15:717-721.
56. Aries PM, Hellmich B, Both M, et al. Lack of efficacy of rituximab in Wegener's granulomatosis with refractory granulomatous manifestations. *Ann Rheum Dis*. 2006;65:853-858.
57. Joy MS, Hogan SL, Jennette JC, et al. A pilot study using mycophenolate mofetil in relapsing or resistant ANCA small vessel vasculitis. *Nephrol Dial Transplant*. 2005;20:2725-2732.
58. Wegener's Granulomatosis Etanercept Trial (WGET) Research Group. Etanercept plus standard therapy for Wegener's granulomatosis. *N Engl J Med*. 2005;352:351-361.
59. Stegeman CA, Cohen Tervaert JW, Sluiter WJ, et al. Association of chronic nasal carriage of *Staphylococcus aureus* and higher relapse rates in Wegener's granulomatosis. *Ann Intern Med*. 1994;120:12-17.
60. de Groot K, Reinhold-Keller E, Tatsis E, et al. Therapy for the maintenance of remission in sixty-five patients with generalized Wegener's granulomatosis. Methotrexate versus trimethoprim/sulfamethoxazole. *Arthritis Rheum*. 1996;39:2052-2061.
61. Pagnoux C, Mahr A, Hamidou MA, et al. Azathioprine or methotrexate maintenance for ANCA-associated vasculitis. *N Engl J Med*. 2008; 359:2790-2803.
62. Rostaing L, Modesto A, Oksman F, et al. Outcome of patients with antineutrophil cytoplasmic antibody–associated vasculitis following cadaveric kidney transplantation. *Am J Kidney Dis*. 1997;9:96-102.
63. Nachman PH, Segelmark M, Westman K, et al. Recurrent ANCA-associated small vessel vasculitis after transplantation: A pooled analysis. *Kidney Int*. 1999;56:1544-1550.
64. Gayraud M, Guillevin L, le Toumelin P, et al. Long-term followup of polyarteritis nodosa, microscopic polyangiitis, and Churg-Strauss syndrome: Analysis of four prospective trials including 278 patients. *Arthritis Rheum*. 2001;44:666-675.
65. Guillevin L, Lhote F, Leon A, et al. Treatment of polyarteritis nodosa related to hepatitis B virus with short term steroid therapy associated with antiviral agents and plasma exchanges: A prospective trial in 33 patients. *J Rheumatol*. 1993;20:289-298.
66. Guillevin L. Treatment of classic polyarteritis nodosa in 1999. *Nephrol Dial Transplant*. 1999;14:2077-2079.
67. Lhote F, Guillevin L. Polyarteritis nodosa, microscopic polyangiitis, and Churg-Strauss syndrome: Clinical aspects and treatment. *Rheum Dis Clin North Am*. 1995;21:911-947.
68. Janssen HL, van Zonneveld M, van Nunen AB, et al. Polyarteritis nodosa associated with hepatitis B virus infection: The role of antiviral treatment and mutations in the hepatitis B virus genome. *Eur J Gastroenterol Hepatol*. 2004;16:801-807.
69. D'Agati V, Jennette JC, Silva FG. Antineutrophil cytoplasmic autoantibody–associated pauci-immune glomerulonephritis and vasculitis, and other vasculitides. In *Non-Neoplastic Kidney Diseases. Atlas of Nontumor Pathology, First Series, Fascicle 4*. Washington, DC: American Registry of Pathology in collaboration with the Armed Forces Institute of Pathology; 2005:385-423.
70. Naoe S, Takahashi K, Masuda H, Tanaka N. Kawasaki disease. With particular emphasis on arterial lesions. *Acta Pathol Jpn*. 1991;41: 785-797.
71. Newburger JW, Takahashi M, Burns JC, et al. The treatment of Kawasaki syndrome with intravenous gammaglobulin. *N Engl J Med*. 1986;315:341-347.
72. Burns JC, Glode MP. Kawasaki syndrome. *Lancet*. 2004;364:533-544.
73. Watts RA, Scott DG. Epidemiology of the vasculitides. *Semin Respir Crit Care Med*. 2004;25:455-464.
74. Maksimowicz-McKinnon K, Hoffman GS. Large-vessel vasculitis. *Semin Respir Crit Care Med*. 2004;25:569-579.
75. Lagneau P, Michel JB. Renovascular hypertension and Takayasu's disease. *J Urol*. 1985;134:876-879.
76. Mukhtyar C, Guillevin L, Cid MC, et al. EULAR recommendations for the management of large vessel vasculitis. *Ann Rheum Dis*. 2009;68: 318-323.
77. Yoshimura M, Kida H, Saito Y, et al. Peculiar glomerular lesions in Takayasu's arteritis. *Clin Nephrol*. 1985;24:120-127.
78. Rapoport M, Averbukh Z, Chaim S, et al. Takayasu aortitis simulating bilateral renal-artery stenoses in patients treated with ACE inhibitors [letter]. *Clin Nephrol*. 1991;36:156.

CHAPTER 25

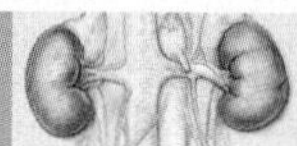

Lupus Nephritis

Gerald B. Appel, David Jayne

DEFINITION

Lupus nephritis (LN) is a common and serious feature of systemic lupus erythematosus (SLE).[1-4] SLE itself is defined by a combination of clinical and laboratory features. The American College of Rheumatology (ACR) criteria (Fig. 25.1) for the diagnosis of SLE have been widely used in both epidemiologic and treatment studies. However, many patients with "lupus-like" conditions or others who have as yet met fewer than four ACR criteria should still be recognized as requiring therapy.

EPIDEMIOLOGY

The incidence and prevalence of lupus and LN are influenced by age, gender, ethnicity, geographic region, diagnostic criteria employed, and method of ascertainment.[5] The peak incidence of lupus is 15 to 45 years, with females outnumbering males by 10:1. This gender predominance is less pronounced in children and older individuals. Among lupus patients, LN affects both genders equally and is more severe in children and men and less so in older adults. Both lupus and LN are three to four times more common in African Americans, Afro-Caribbeans, Asians, and Hispanic Americans than in Caucasians. Additional risk factors for renal disease include younger age, lower socioeconomic status, more ACR criteria for SLE, longer duration of disease, family history of SLE, and hypertension.

ETIOLOGY AND PATHOGENESIS

Genetics, Environment, and Animal Models

Multiple genes predispose to lupus.[3,5,6] This is supported by the clustering in families, the racial differences in susceptibility, the concordance of SLE in more than 25% of identical twins but in only 5% of fraternal twins, and the frequency of positive autoantibodies and other autoimmune disorders in family members of SLE patients. Homozygous deficiency of certain complement components (C1q, C2, C4) carries a high risk for development of SLE; this is also true for certain FcγRIII receptor polymorphisms. Genome-wide association studies have identified 17 loci associated with an increased risk of SLE that involve genes associated with B-cell signaling, Toll-like receptors, and neutrophil function.[7] Environmental factors also play a role in the onset of SLE and LN. Sun or ultraviolet light exposure and "sunburn" can precipitate and exacerbate SLE and LN.[3,5] Hormonal factors are evidenced by the strong female predisposition, the exacerbations during or shortly after pregnancy, and the role of hormonal treatment and ablation in animal models of LN. Whereas exposure to certain medications can produce SLE or a lupus-like syndrome, renal disease is infrequent in these patients. Conclusive evidence for a viral pathogenesis of SLE or LN has yet to be produced. Spontaneous and inducible models of SLE in mice include the NZB B/W F1 hybrid, the BXSB, and the MRL/lpr models.[3,6] Some of these models have defective apoptosis that may lead to defective clonal deletion and B-cell proliferation. SLE can be induced in animal models by injection of autoantibodies against DNA or phospholipids and by injection of peptides derived from Smith antigen.

Autoimmunity in Systemic Lupus Erythematosus

SLE patients typically develop a wide range of autoantibodies.[6-9] The disease process starts with a breakdown in self tolerance and autoantibody production. Subsequently, deposition of immune complexes and the inflammatory responses in various organs dictate the nature and extent of disease.[3] Many autoantibodies are directed against nucleic acids and proteins concerned with transcriptional and translational machinery, such as nucleosomes (DNA-histone), chromatin antigens, and small nuclear and cytoplasmic ribonuclear proteins. Polyclonal hyperactivity of B cells along with defective autoregulation of T cells is thought to underlie autoantibody production.[6-9] A number of mechanisms may contribute to this condition, including failure to remove or to silence autoreactive B and T cells, abnormal exposure to or presentation of self antigens, T-cell hyperactivity, increased B cell–stimulating cytokines, and B-cell hyperactivity.[6] The failure of apoptotic mechanisms to delete or to silence autoreactive cells (tolerance) may allow clonal expansion of such cells later in life, leading to autoreactive cells and autoantibody production. Abnormal exposure to self antigen may occur through nuclear autoantigens clustering on the blebs of apoptotic cells, which may be associated with germline mutations that lead to clonal expansion of autoreactive cells. Likewise, "antigen mimicry" may occur if exposure to viral or bacterial peptides containing sequences similar to native antigens leads to a similar induction of autoantibody-producing cell lines. The nature of antigen presentation may also be important, with certain nuclear antigens capable of triggering an immunogenic response through interactions with a variety of intracellular Toll-like receptors. In SLE, there is evidence that T-cell hyperactivity and failure of T-cell tolerance may allow autoreactive T cells to drive B-cell proliferations and the production of autoantibodies. Finally, proliferation of autoreactive B cells may occur through a variety of disturbances of positive and negative regulatory mechanisms (e.g., through stimulation by superantigens) in addition to the mechanisms mentioned. The end result is the loss of tolerance and production of a wide array of autoantibodies.[6-9]

American College of Rheumatology Criteria for the Diagnosis of Lupus
The presence of four or more of the following criteria gives 96% sensitivity and specificity for the diagnosis of lupus
1. Malar rash
2. Discoid rash
3. Photosensitivity
4. Oral ulcers
5. Nonerosive arthritis
6. Pleuropericarditis
7. Renal disease (proteinuria and/or cellular casts)
8. Neurologic disorder (seizures or psychosis in the absence of precipitating circumstances)
9. Hematologic disorder (hemolytic anemia, leukopenia/lymphopenia, thrombocytopenia)
10. Positive LE cell preparation, raised anti-DNA antibody, anti-Sm present, false-positive antitreponemal test)
11. Positive fluorescent antinuclear antibody test

Figure 25.1 American College of Rheumatology criteria for the diagnosis of lupus.

Pathogenesis of Lupus Nephritis

In SLE, some autoantibodies, such as those causing autoimmune hemolytic anemia, are directly pathogenic.[7] Other autoantibodies combine with antigen to produce immune complexes that if not adequately cleared may deposit in various organs, inciting inflammatory responses.[3,4] Complement components aid apoptotic clearance and removal of immune complexes, but they are also activated by and incorporated into the immune complexes and contribute to the inflammatory cascade. A hallmark of glomerular involvement in LN is the deposition of circulating immune complexes and the *in situ* formation of others. Although patients with LN have autoantibodies against double-stranded DNA (dsDNA), Sm antigen, C1q, and a variety of other antigens, the exact role of each in the immune complex formation seen in glomerular disease remains unclear. In proliferative LN, DNA and high-affinity complement-fixing antibodies are found. Immune complex deposition may also be facilitated by cationic histones that bind to the glomerular basement membrane. In general, mesangial and subendothelial immune deposits are derived from deposition of circulating immune complexes, whereas subepithelial complexes are often formed *in situ*. However, whether deposition of circulating complexes or *in situ* formation is the predominant pathogenic pathway in a given patient is not always clear. The localization of immune complexes within the glomerulus is influenced by size, charge, and avidity as well as by the clearing ability of the mesangium and local hemodynamics.[3,4] The localization of immune complexes in the glomerulus leads to complement activation and complement-mediated damage, activation of procoagulant factors, leukocyte infiltration with release of proteolytic enzymes, and activation of cytokines associated with cellular proliferation and matrix formation. Intraglomerular hypertension and activation of coagulation cascades may contribute to the glomerular injury especially in patients with antiphospholipid antibodies (APA). Additional components of extraglomerular renal damage in LN include vascular damage ranging from simple localization of immune complexes to rare necrotizing vasculitis and tubulointerstitial disease.

Renal Manifestations in Patients with Lupus	
Manifestation	**Prevalance**
Proteinuria	100%
• Nephrotic syndrome	45–65%
Hematuria	
• Microhematuria	80%
• Red cell casts	10%
• Macrohematuria	1–2%
Cellular casts	30%
Reduced renal function	40–80%
• RPGN	10–20%
• AKI	1–2%
Hypertension	15–50%
Hyperkalemia	15%
Tubular abnormalities (usually asymptomatic)	60–80%

Figure 25.2 Renal manifestations in patients with lupus. RPGN, rapidly progressive glomerulonephritis; AKI, acute kidney injury.

CLINICAL MANIFESTATIONS

SLE can affect virtually any organ of the body. The disease course of SLE is characterized by episodes of illness (flares) followed by episodes of relative quiescence (remissions). A number of reliable and reproducible scoring systems have been devised to follow the activity of an individual patient with SLE. These include the Systemic Lupus Erythematosus Disease Activity Index (SLEDAI), the British Isles Lupus Assessment Group (BILAG), and the Systemic Lupus Activity Measure (SLAM).

Renal Manifestations

From 30% to 50% of SLE patients will have clinically evident renal disease at presentation (Fig. 25.2).[1-4] During follow-up, renal involvement will occur in 60% of young adults and a greater percentage of young children. Renal involvement is manifested by proteinuria, active urinary sediment with microhematuria, dysmorphic erythrocytes and erythrocyte casts, and hypertension. In many cases with major renal involvement, the nephritic syndrome develops in association with proliferative glomerulonephritis (GN) and a decline in glomerular filtration rate (GFR). The clinical findings correlate well with histologic glomerular findings (see later discussion). Infrequently, renal disease in SLE patients presents with tubular disorders such as renal tubular acidosis with hypokalemia (type 1 RTA) or hyperkalemia (type 4 RTA) (see Chapter 12), thrombotic disorders associated with a secondary antiphospholipid syndrome (see Chapter 27), and fibrillary GN (see Chapter 26).

Extrarenal Manifestations

Patients with active SLE often present with nonspecific complaints of malaise, low-grade fever, poor appetite, and weight loss.[10] Other common features include patchy alopecia; oral or nasal ulcerations; arthralgias and nondeforming arthritis; and a variety of dermal findings, including photosensitivity, Raynaud's phenomenon, and the classic "butterfly" facial rash. Livedo reticularis is seen in up to 15% of cases and may be associated with miscarriages, thrombocytopenia, and the presence of APA.[11-14] Neuropsychiatric involvement presents with headache, nerve palsies, frank coma, and psychoses. Serositis, in the form of pleuritis or pericarditis, affects up to 40% of patients. Pulmonary hypertension can develop silently as a result of multiple pulmonary emboli or intravascular coagulation in association with APA or be caused by nonthrombotic pulmonary arterial disease. Libman-Sacks endocarditis and the far more common mitral valve prolapse can be detected either with clinical findings or by echocardiography. Splenomegaly and lymphadenopathy are present in about one fourth of patients. Hematologic abnormalities in SLE include anemia due to impaired erythropoiesis, autoimmune hemolysis, and bleeding. Thrombocytopenia and leukopenia may be part of the disease process or be due to complications of therapy. Thrombotic events should prompt a search for APA and other procoagulant abnormalities.

DIAGNOSIS AND DIFFERENTIAL DIAGNOSIS

Whereas the diagnosis of lupus may be obvious in a young female patient in the presence of classic manifestations and serologic markers, less typical presentations can result in multiple physician consultations and diagnostic delay.[14] This is due in part to the varied features of the disease, as the signs and symptoms in SLE evolve over time. Some patients, especially those with membranous LN, may present with renal disease as their initial manifestation without other systemic features. The presence of four or more ACR criteria (see Fig. 25.1) carries a 96% sensitivity and specificity for lupus. However, the ACR diagnostic criteria were developed for clinical studies and do not always prove useful in an individual patient. Other diseases mimicking SLE include fibromyalgia, Sjögren's syndrome, hematologic diseases such as thrombotic microangiopathies, and primary antiphospholipid syndrome (see Chapters 27 and 28).

Other autoimmune rheumatologic disorders, such as dermatomyositis and systemic sclerosis, can be confused with SLE. However, SLE may also present with overlapping features of other multisystem or organ-limited autoimmune syndromes. Nephritis has been reported in patients with mixed connective tissue disease when it is associated with the presence of anti-Ro and anti-La antibodies and the absence of anti-dsDNA antibodies. Rheumatoid arthritis can be associated with mesangial proliferative glomerulonephritis or renal disease due to AA amyloidosis. Some older lupus patients will present with joint deformities typical of rheumatoid arthritis.

A number of other common forms of glomerulonephritis must be distinguished from LN. Although Henoch-Schönlein purpura may present with a purpuric rash, systemic symptoms, arthritis, abdominal pain, and nephritis, the immune glomerular deposits show dominant or codominant IgA deposition. In LN, most active proliferative biopsy specimens will show a predominance of IgG and the presence of C1q and often "full house" staining with IgG, IgA, IgM, C3, and C1q present on biopsy. Pauci-immune rapidly progressive glomerulonephritis (RPGN) with antineutrophil cytoplasmic antibody (ANCA) positivity may be confused with lupus until the serologic or renal biopsy results are obtained (see Chapter 24). Patients who are seropositive for both ANCA and antinuclear antibody (ANA) or anti-dsDNA and who do not have immune deposits on renal biopsy should be treated like other pauci-immune GN patients. ANCA positivity by itself has no significance in a proven SLE patient, and false-positive MPO-ANCA assays may be seen in association with high binding levels of anti-dsDNA. Bacterial endocarditis and cryoglobulinemia (see Chapter 21) can also mimic lupus, especially because the serum complement levels may be low.

Immunologic Tests in Lupus

Because autoantibody production is a hallmark of SLE, a firm diagnosis of LN should not be made without the presence of some serum ANA.[7] ANA, being found in more than 90% of untreated patients, are a highly sensitive screen for SLE patients; however, they are nonspecific and are found in other rheumatologic and nonrheumatologic diseases. Some lupus-like patients with negative ANA test results will be found to have APA.[11-13] The presence of various patterns of ANA (diffuse, speckled) is not reliable in distinguishing lupus from similar rheumatologic diseases. Autoantibodies against dsDNA are far more specific, being present in about three fourths of untreated lupus patients, but they are a less sensitive marker. Whereas high titers of anti-dsDNA antibodies correlate with the presence of SLE and are often used to follow the course of LN, antibodies to single-stranded DNA (ssDNA) are found in many rheumatologic conditions and do not correlate with the course of LN. A variety of tests for anti-dsDNA antibodies are available, including the Farr radioimmunoassay, an immunofluorescent test directed against the DNA of the kinetoplast of *Crithidia luciliae*, and an enzyme-linked immunosorbent assay (ELISA). The ELISA is the most commonly used assay. Sm antibodies are strongly associated with the diagnosis of lupus and the presence of nephritis but are present in only about 25% to 30% of patients. Antibodies to C1q (anti-C1q) have been more closely associated with the activity of LN than anti-dsDNA antibodies and may have a prognostic role in the follow-up of patients with LN.[15]

Serum levels of total hemolytic complement and complement components C3 and C4 are often depressed in untreated lupus patients and especially those with LN. Either C3 and C4 are both depressed or the C4 is preferentially depressed in lupus patients, reflecting preferential activation of the classical complement pathway. In patients with postinfectious glomerulonephritis and idiopathic membranoproliferative glomerulonephritis, C3 is often preferentially depressed (see Chapter 21). Alternatively, low C4 with normal C3 may reflect genetic C4 deficiency in lupus patients (see earlier discussion).

One third to one half of lupus patients will have APA.[11-13] The misnomer "lupus anticoagulant" is based on the presence of APA, which prolong phospholipid-dependent coagulation studies *in vitro* (activated partial thromboplastin time [APTT] and kaolin clotting time [KCT]) but *in vivo* are associated with thrombosis. The prolonged APTT and KCT are not corrected by mixing with normal plasma. The exact mechanisms for the thrombotic tendency remain unclear but may include abnormal endothelial function, enhanced platelet aggregation, reduced production of prostacyclin and other endothelial anticoagulant factors, and activation of plasminogen.[11,12] APA have been associated with a multitude of primarily thrombotic events (see Chapter 27). APA are measured either as autoantibodies to cardiolipin or to β_2-glycoprotein 1 (both may be of IgG or IgM isotype) or as a transferable inhibitor of coagulation (the lupus anticoagulant), best assessed by prolongation of the dilute Russell's viper venom clotting time.

PATHOLOGY

Although LN may affect all structures of the kidney, glomerular involvement has been the best studied component, and it has been well correlated with the presentation, course, and treatment of the disease.[1-4] Adjacent glomeruli may show different degrees of involvement, and glomerular lesions may transform over time. For many years, the World Health Organization (WHO) classification of LN was used (Fig. 25.3). The 2004 modifications in the current International Society of Nephrology (ISN)/Renal Pathology Society (RPS) classification refine and clarify some of the deficiencies of the WHO classification (see Fig. 25.3).[16] As in the WHO classification, the ISN classification is based on light microscopy (LM), immunofluorescence (IF), and electron microscopy (EM) findings. Interobserver reproducibility and the predictive value have improved with the ISN/RPS system.[17,18]

ISN Classification of Lupus Nephritis

ISN class I (Fig. 25.4) denotes normal glomeruli by LM but with mesangial immune deposits. Class II (Fig. 25.5), mesangial proliferative LN, is defined as pure mesangial hypercellularity (more than three mesangial cells in areas away from the vascular pole in 3-μm-thick histologic sections) by LM with mesangial immune deposits. Class III (Fig. 25.6), focal LN, is defined as focal segmental or global endocapillary or extracapillary glomerulonephritis affecting less than 50% of the total glomeruli sampled. Class IV (Fig. 25.7), diffuse LN, has diffuse segmental or global endocapillary or extracapillary GN affecting 50% or more of glomeruli. Both class III and class IV have subendothelial immune deposits. Class IV is subdivided into diffuse segmental (IV-S) proliferation (i.e., >50% of affected glomeruli have segmental lesions) and diffuse global (IV-G) proliferation (i.e., >50% of affected glomeruli have global lesions). Both class III and class IV may have active (proliferative), inactive (sclerosing), or combined active and inactive lesions subclassified as A, C, and A/C, respectively. ISN class V (Fig. 25.8), membranous LN, is defined by subepithelial immune deposits. The membranous alterations may be present alone or on a background of mesangial hypercellularity and mesangial immune deposits. Patients with additional true focal or diffuse proliferative lesions and subendothelial immune complex deposits are no longer classified as Vc or Vd, as in the older WHO classification, but rather as V + III and V + IV under the ISN classification (see Fig. 25.3). ISN class VI, advanced sclerosing LN, is defined by global glomerular sclerosis affecting 90% or more of glomeruli.

On IF, IgG is almost always the dominant immunoglobulin, and early complement components such as C4 and especially C1q are usually present along with C3. The presence of all three immunoglobulins, IgG, IgA, and IgM, along with the two complement components, C1q and C3, is known as full house staining. It is highly suggestive of LN, as is strong C1q staining. Fibrin is often present in the glomerular tuft and especially in crescents.

By EM, the distribution of immune deposits corresponds to that of IF. Some electron-dense deposits have an organized substructure known as fingerprinting, corresponding to the presence of curvilinear microtubular or fibrillar structures composed of bands ranging from 10 to 15 nm in diameter. Tubuloreticular inclusions, 24 nm interanastomosing tubular structures located in the dilated cisternae of endoplasmic reticulum of renal endothelial cells, are often found in biopsy specimens of patients with LN.

Tubulointerstitial and Vascular Disease

Although LN classification is based on the degree of glomerular involvement, histologic and clinical involvement of other renal

Comparison of the WHO Classification (1995) of Lupus Nephritis with the ISN/RPS Classification (2004)

WHO, 1995		ISN/RPS, 2004	
Class	**Definition**	**Class**	**Definition**
I	Normal glomeruli (by LM, IF, EM)	I	Minimal mesangial LN Normal glomeruli by LM, but mesangial immune deposits by IF
II	Purely mesangial disease IIa: Normocellular mesangium by LM but mesangial deposits by IF and/or EM IIb: Mesangial hypercellularity with mesangial deposits by IF and/or EM	II	Mesangial proliferative LN Mesangial hypercellularity with mesangial immune deposits
III	Focal segmental proliferative glomerulonephritis (<50%)	III	Focal LN III (A): Purely active lesions: focal proliferative LN III (A/C): Active and chronic lesions: focal proliferative and sclerosing LN III (C): Chronic inactive lesions with glomerular scars: focal sclerosing LN
IV	Diffuse proliferative glomerulonephritis (≥50%)	IV	Diffuse LN IV-S (A) or IV-G (A): Purely active lesions: diffuse segmental (S) or global (G) proliferative LN IV-S (A/C) or IV-G (A/C): Active and chronic lesions: diffuse segmental or global proliferative and sclerosing LN IV-S (C) or IV-G (C): Inactive with glomerular scars: diffuse segmental or global sclerosing LN
V	Membranous glomerulonephritis Va: Pure membranous Vb: Associated mild mesangial proliferation Vc: Associated focal proliferative disease Vd: Associated diffuse proliferative disease	V	Membranous LN
		VI	Advanced sclerosing LN ≥90% of glomeruli globally sclerosed without residual activity

Figure 25.3 Comparison of the WHO classification (1995) of lupus nephritis (LN) with the ISN/RPS classification (2004). In the ISN/RPS classification, the distribution of hypercellularity is assessed as mesangial, endocapillary, or extracapillary (crescentic) and as focal (with <50% glomerular involvement) versus diffuse (with ≥50% glomeruli affected). The distribution of immune deposits by immunofluorescence (IF) and electron microscopy (EM) is judged as mesangial, subepithelial, or subendothelial. LM, light microscopy.

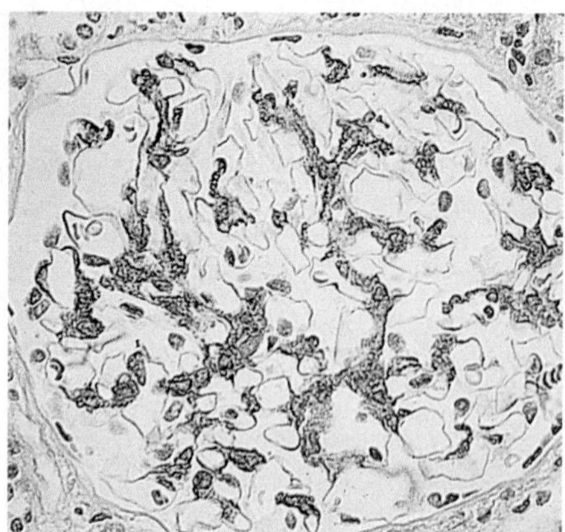

Figure 25.4 ISN/RPS class I: minimal mesangial lupus nephritis. Light microscopy is normal, but immunoperoxidase shows C1q localization (associated with IgG and C3) throughout the mesangial area.

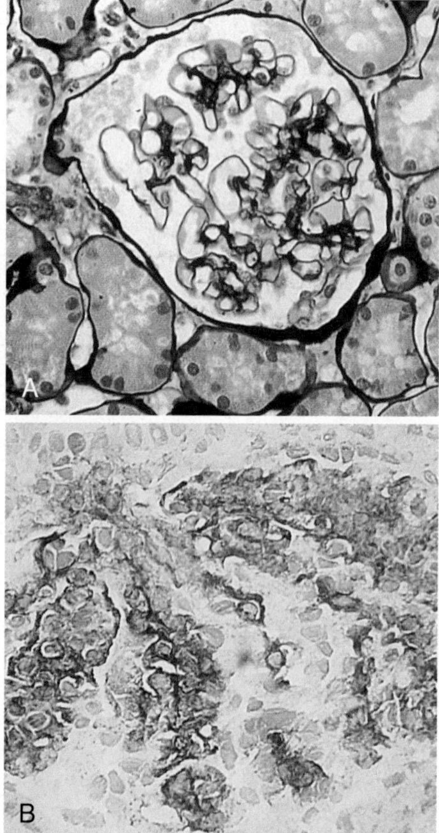

Figure 25.5 ISN/RPS class II: lupus nephritis (mesangial disease). **A,** Mesangial expansion but little increase in tuft cellularity, and the peripheral capillary walls are normal. (Silver methenamine stain.) **B,** Extensive mesangial IgG deposits shown by immunoperoxidase; the aggregates are just beginning to invade peripheral capillary walls.

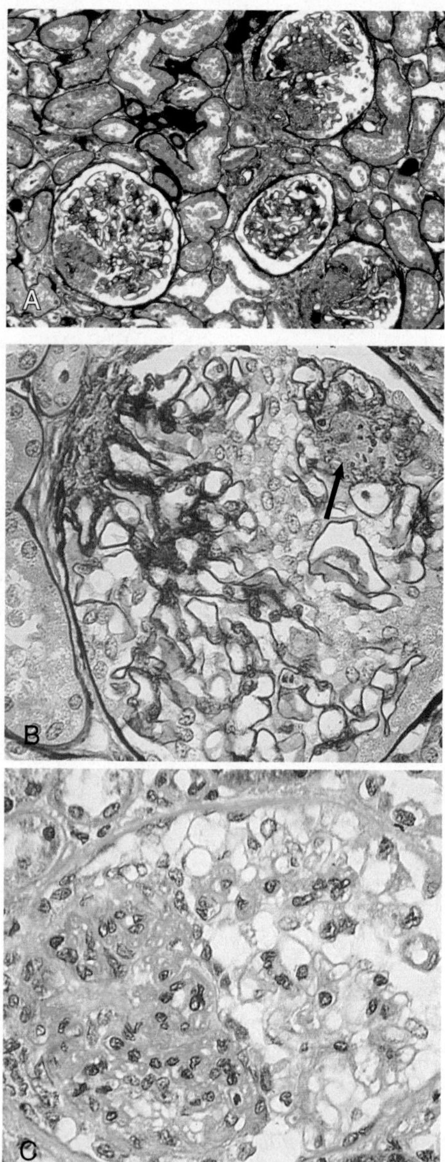

Figure 25.6 ISN/RPS class III: focal proliferative lupus nephritis. **A,** Low power showing focal and segmental proliferative lesion—active (class III A) with less than 50% of glomeruli affected. (Hematoxylin-eosin.) **B,** An area of focal necrosis containing cellular debris, karyorrhexis *(arrow),* is surrounded by an area of cellular proliferation. (Silver methenamine/hematoxylin-eosin.) **C,** A major focal and segmental proliferative lesion affecting almost half of the glomerular capillary tuft. (Hematoxylin/lissamine green.)

compartments is not rare in lupus patients.[3,4,19,20] In about 50% of patients with nephritis, predominantly those with proliferative glomerular lesions, immune aggregates are found along the tubular basement membranes. Interstitial infiltrates mainly of $CD4^+$ and $CD8^+$ T lymphocytes and monocytes are commonly found. In active disease, infiltration and invasion of the tubules (tubulitis) is found (Fig. 25.9); in chronic disease, the interstitium is expanded by fibrosis and sparser infiltrates. Interstitial inflammation has been correlated with renal dysfunction and hypertension, whereas immune deposition along the tubular basement membranes correlates better with the presence of high anti-dsDNA and depressed serum complement levels. Infrequently, tubulointerstitial nephritis is seen in the absence of glomerular disease and may produce acute renal failure or renal tubular acidosis.

A number of vascular lesions may be seen in lupus patients (Fig. 25.10).[20] True vasculitis is extremely rare. More commonly, there are vascular immune deposits seen by IF or EM, or a fibrinoid noninflammatory necrotizing lesion of the vessels in patients

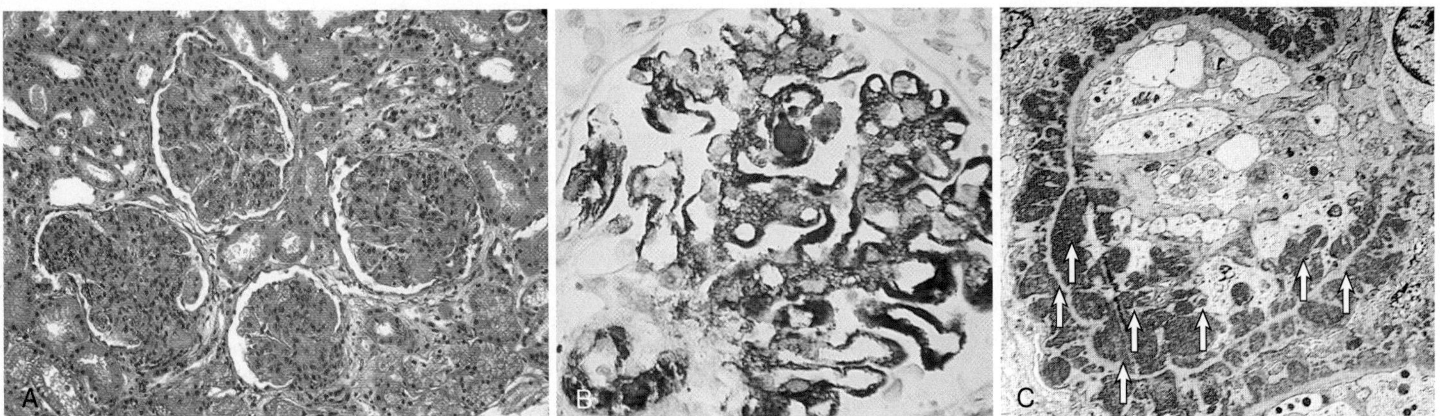

Figure 25.7 ISN/RPS class IV: lupus nephritis. A, Active diffuse proliferative lupus nephritis. **B,** By immunoperoxidase staining, there are dense irregular aggregates of IgG along the peripheral capillary walls. **C,** Electron microscopy reveals the immune aggregates as electron-dense deposits *(arrows)* predominantly in the subendothelial location.

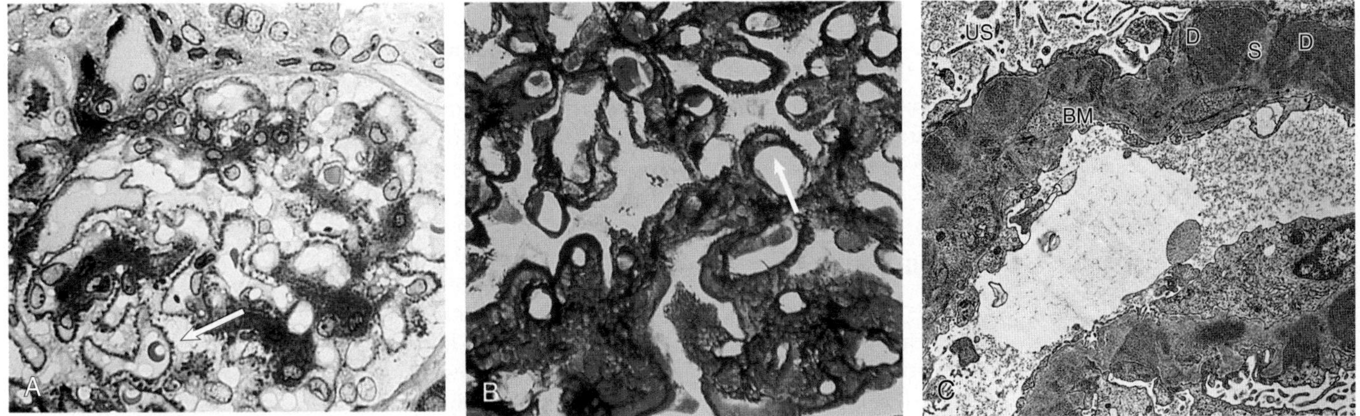

Figure 25.8 ISN/RPS class V: membranous lupus. A, A thick (~0.5 mm) araldite-embedded section stained with toluidine blue showing not only the extramembranous material in dark blue *(arrow)* but also the presence of mesangial deposits, which are common in lupus membranous nephropathy. **B,** A silver methenamine–stained section showing some double contouring of the silver-positive basement membrane *(arrow)* and subendothelium-deposited material as well as the characteristic silver-positive spikes of basement membrane–like material. **C,** An electron microphotograph showing the predominantly subepithelial electron-dense deposits (D) separated by protrusions of basement membrane material (spikes, S). BM, basement membrane; US, urinary space.

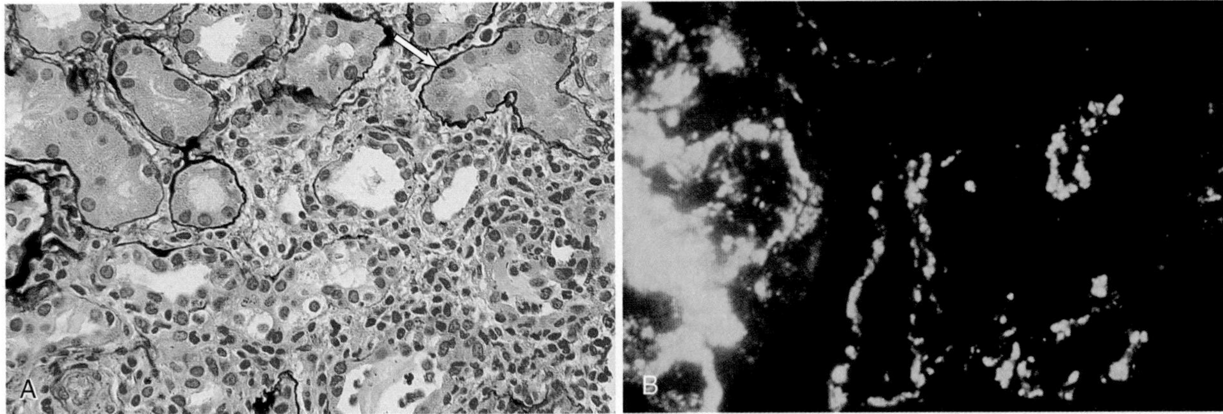

Figure 25.9 Interstitial lupus nephritis. A, Interstitial infiltrate invading and destroying tubules (tubulitis). The tubular basement membrane, stained black with silver *(arrow)*, is digested (see the lower half of **A**). **B,** Immunofluorescence showing aggregates of C3 in the tubular basement membrane *(right)* as well as within the glomerulus *(left)*. Such tubular basement membrane aggregates are common in lupus nephritis, being found in 60% to 65% of biopsy specimens overall and with increasing frequency from class II (20%) to class IV (75%).

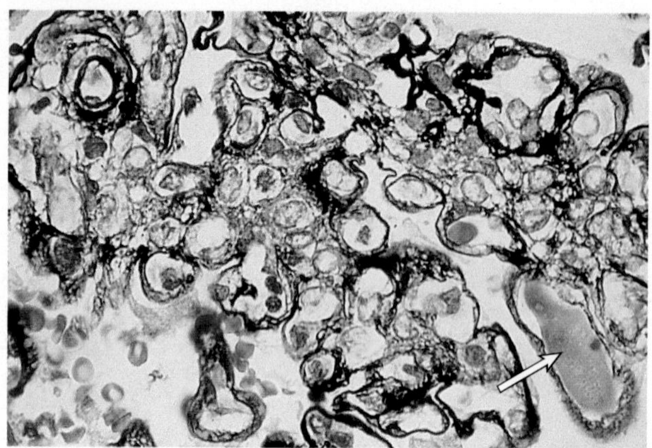

Figure 25.10 Vascular damage in lupus nephritis. Thrombus *(arrow)* occludes a glomerular capillary loop in this class IV biopsy specimen. Such a thrombus contains platelets and cross-linked fibrin as well as immunoglobulins and thus has some characteristics of true thrombus. Note also the subepithelial aggregates, spike formation, and double contouring of the capillary walls, all typical of class IV and active class III biopsy specimens. (Silver methenamine/hematoxylin.)

with severe proliferative nephritis, or a thrombotic microangiopathy. The last is most often found in patients who are APA positive with prior evidence of coagulation events and may occur in conjunction with a proliferative GN.[11-13]

Transformation of Histologic Appearance and "Silent" Lupus Nephritis

Serial biopsy specimens often show transformation from one to another histologic glomerular class.[4] Some patients with increased clinical activity will transform from a more benign or less proliferative class (ISN class II or class V) to a more active proliferative lesion (ISN class III or class IV). This is often heralded by increasing proteinuria and active urinary sediment. With successful treatment, other patients will transform from a proliferative class (ISN class III or class IV) to a more predominant membranous pattern (ISN class V).

Extremely uncommon are patients who have active proliferative LN on biopsy but no clinical or urinary sediment changes to indicate active disease and normal anti-dsDNA and serum complement levels, so-called silent LN or anephritic nephritis.[2] If the urine sediment is carefully checked, most patients with proliferative lesions will have microhematuria and often erythrocyte casts.

Clinical and Histopathologic Correlations and Other Correlates of Outcome

In general, the clinical correlates of the ISN and WHO classification systems are similar.[3,4] Patients assigned to ISN class I usually have no evidence of clinical renal disease. Likewise, patients in ISN class II may have elevated anti-dsDNA or low complement levels, but in general, their urinary sediment is inactive, hypertension is infrequent, the GFR is preserved, and proteinuria is rarely above 1 g/24 h. Patients with class I and class II biopsy findings have an excellent renal prognosis unless they transform to another pattern. An exception to this presentation are lupus patients who present with minimal change nephrotic syndrome or lupus podocytopathy.[21] They have the sudden onset of nephrotic syndrome with renal biopsy specimens showing no abnormalities on LM or class I or class II changes with extensive foot process effacement.

Patients with active ISN class III A or A/C often have microhematuria, hypertension, low complement levels, and proteinuria. From one quarter to one third of patients will have the nephrotic syndrome, and up to one in four will have an elevated serum creatinine concentration at renal biopsy. Patients with focal glomerular scarring (ISN class III C) usually have hypertension and reduced renal function but without active urinary sediment. Patients with mild proliferation in only a few glomeruli generally respond well to therapy, with less than 5% progressing to renal failure during 5 years of follow-up. Others with more glomerular involvement or with necrotizing features and crescent formation have a prognosis similar to that of class IV A patients. Whether patients with "severe" focal segmental proliferative class III have a worse prognosis than do those with diffuse proliferative class IV lesions is controversial.[22]

Patients with ISN class IV A classically have high serologic activity (low serum complement and high anti-dsDNA binding activity) along with active urinary sediment, hypertension, heavy proteinuria, and reduced GFR. Class IV diffuse proliferative disease carries the worst renal prognosis in most series, although this is greatly influenced by prognostic features such as racial background, socioeconomic factors, and renal features at presentation. Patients with segmental diffuse proliferative class IV S may fare worse than those with diffuse global involvement class IV G, although this remains controversial.[17]

ISN class V patients typically present with proteinuria and features of the nephrotic syndrome. However, at biopsy, up to 40% will have subnephrotic proteinuria, and up to 20% will have less than 1 g/24 h of proteinuria. Patients with ISN class V typically have less clinical renal and serologic activity. Some develop what appears to be idiopathic nephrotic syndrome before developing other features of lupus. ISN class V patients are predisposed to thrombotic complications, such as renal vein thrombosis and pulmonary emboli.[20] Ten-year renal survival rates are 75% to 85%.

Advanced sclerotic LN, ISN class VI, is usually the result of "burnt-out" class III or class IV LN. Many patients will nevertheless have persistent microhematuria and some proteinuria along with hypertension and a decreased GFR.

Other Histologic Prognostic Factors

Features of reversible (active) or irreversible (chronic) damage on biopsy may be able to predict the course of LN patients. Some[3,4] but not all[23] investigators have found that patients with a higher activity index or chronicity index* are more likely to progress to renal failure. Consistently, the renal prognosis is poor if biopsy specimens show extensive glomerulosclerosis or interstitial fibrosis.[1,3,4,19,24] Whereas there is disagreement about the value of the individual activity index or chronicity index, patients with high degrees of both activity and chronicity on biopsy (activity index >7 plus chronicity index >3) fare poorly, as do those with the combination of cellular crescents and interstitial fibrosis on biopsy. Finally, certain features found on repeated renal biopsy at 6 months predict 5-year progression to renal failure, including ongoing inflammation with cellular crescents and macrophages in the tubular lumina, persistent immune

*Calculated by grading on each biopsy specimen the various histologic features of activity [indicated by glomerular cellular proliferation, leukocyte infiltration, fibrinoid necrosis or karyorrhexis, cellular crescents, hyaline thrombi or wire loops, and tubulointerstitial mononuclear cell infiltrates] or chronicity [indicated by glomerulosclerosis, fibrous crescents, interstitial fibrosis, and tubular atrophy] and summing the scores.

Survival in Lupus and Lupus Nephritis			
	5-Year Survival (percent)*		
Period	All Lupus	Lupus Nephritis	Class IV Nephritis
1953–1969	49	44	17
1970–1979	82	67	55
1980–1989	86	82	80
1990–1995	92	82	82
2000–2010	95–100	95–100	90–95

Figure 25.11 Survival in lupus and lupus nephritis. Five-year actuarial survival for lupus, lupus nephritis, and World Health Organization class IV nephritis during the periods shown. *Weighted mean of published series. *(Modified from references 36,40,42).*

deposits (especially C3), and persistent subendothelial and mesangial deposits.[25] The finding of both crescents and interstitial fibrosis persisting on the 6-month biopsy specimen led to a very poor renal outcome.

NATURAL HISTORY

The natural history of LN in the modern era is unknown because virtually all patients with severe renal involvement receive therapy directed at their renal lesions. Fifty years ago, few patients with severe LN survived more than a few years, and half of those with even less severe forms of LN died within 5 years. Most patients today have a gratifying response to early treatment, followed by relatively quiescent disease under continuing immunosuppression that can be tapered off eventually (Fig. 25.11). Some patients will continue to have no disease activity; others will relapse with time. The frequency of relapse depends not only on the underlying disease severity but also on the intensity and duration of continued immunosuppression.

End-stage renal disease (ESRD) now affects 8% to 15% of patients with LN. Rare patients with progressive LN leading to dialysis may regain enough renal function to terminate dialysis. A renal biopsy is often useful to determine whether the disease is still active and potentially treatable or all chronic and irreversibly scarred.

In patients with active LN, fatal infections often associated with persistent extrarenal disease activity are the most common cause of death. Studies confirm that almost half of all lupus deaths are the result of excess cardiovascular mortality, often later in the course of the disease and particularly from premature myocardial ischemia (see the section on antiphospholipid antibodies and atherosclerotic and other complications).

Multiple factors have been associated with outcomes in LN, but the interaction between these factors has not been clearly elucidated. Epidemiologic predictors include race, with African Americans and Hispanic Americans faring worse[26-29]; those of Southeast Asian descent have more severe disease than other Asians or Caucasians do. Male gender, younger age (<24 years), and lower socioeconomic status, independent of race, are associated with a worse renal outcome.[28,29] Laboratory outcome predictors include the histologic features discussed before, higher baseline serum creatinine concentration or greater baseline proteinuria, hypertension, severe anemia, thrombocytopenia, and hypocomplementemia with elevated anti-dsDNA levels. Clinical management predictors include delay in the onset of therapy, degree of reduction of proteinuria with treatment, and nephritic relapse.

TREATMENT

It is useful to divide the treatment of patients with active proliferative LN into an induction phase and a maintenance phase. The induction phase deals with acute life- or organ-threatening disease, which often affects multiple organ systems. The maintenance phase focuses on the long-term management of chronic, more or less indolent disease and the management of nonhealing scars of disease and of increased cardiovascular and malignancy risk. Here, protection from the side effects of therapy and prevention of flares are more important.

Use of the ISN biopsy classification (see Fig. 25.3) can serve as a guide to initial therapy.[1-4,30] In general, patients assigned to ISN class I and class II need no therapy directed at the kidney. The majority of patients will have a benign long-term outcome, and the potential toxicity of any immunosuppressive regimen will negatively alter the risk-benefit ratio of treatment. An exception is the group of lupus patients with minimal change syndrome or lupus podocytopathy (see earlier discussion). These patients respond to a short course of high-dose corticosteroids in a fashion similar to patients with minimal change disease (MCD).[21] It is in patients with active focal proliferative LN (ISN class III A and III A/C), active diffuse proliferative LN (ISN class IV A and IV A/C), and membranous lupus (ISN class V) that combination corticosteroid and immunosuppressive therapy is most widely used.

The goal of induction therapy is to induce a renal remission. Studies have varied in their definition of remission, but this typically requires a reduction in proteinuria below 0.5 g/24 h or urine protein to creatinine ratio below 0.5 g/g, absence of glomerular hematuria or red cell casts, and normalization or at least stabilization of GFR. Subsequent flare is then defined by an isolated increase in proteinuria, typically at least doubling and above 1 g/24 h, as a proteinuric flare; or by the appearance of glomerular hematuria or red cell casts with proteinuria, with or without hypertension and a decline in GFR, as a nephritic flare.[31]

Evidence in support of different therapeutic agents and regimens has emerged from clinical trials conducted during the last 30 years. It is important to treat the conclusions of many of these trials with caution because many are of small size and have been uncontrolled or nonblinded, and LN is heterogeneous in its presentation and response to therapy. As toxicity of therapy is now a major factor in mortality and morbidity, claims of efficacy have to be carefully balanced against adverse events. Other factors, such as ethnicity, referral practice, center experience, and use of concomitant medications, vary between studies and over time, which reduces the generalizability of some study results. Consensus statements have addressed the methodology and terminology used in clinical studies of LN.[31]

The Treatment of Proliferative Lupus Nephritis: Induction Phase

Corticosteroids

Corticosteroids used in conjunction with other immunosuppressives are commenced at high dose: either predniso(lo)ne (1 mg/kg/day or 60 mg/day) or intravenous methylprednisolone infusions (0.5 to 1.0 g daily for 1 to 3 days), followed by oral prednisone (0.5 mg/kg/day). The oral dose is then reduced stepwise to approximately 10 mg/day by 3-6 months. Cosmetic effects, risk of gastrointestinal ulceration, hypertension, psychoses, and enhanced risk of infectious complications have led to attempts to minimize prolonged courses of high-dose corticosteroid therapy in lupus patients. Some small uncontrolled trials suggested that intravenous pulse therapy is either more effective or less toxic than high-dose oral therapy.

Cytotoxic Agents

Cytotoxic agents in conjunction with corticosteroids play a major role in many induction regimens for LN.[32-35] Cyclophosphamide is a powerful inhibitor of B cells as well as of other phases of the immune response. Both daily oral and intravenous pulses of cyclophosphamide have been effective in LN,[36] but intravenous therapy involves a lower cumulative exposure to cyclophosphamide and less frequent cytopenias, enables enhanced bladder protection, and avoids problems of nonadherence.

Studies of the U.S. National Institutes of Health initially established a role for every-third-month intravenous pulses of cyclophosphamide in preventing renal failure in patients with diffuse proliferative LN. Subsequent randomized, controlled trials in patients with severe proliferative LN[32] established that six pulses of intravenous cyclophosphamide at monthly intervals (0.5 to 1 g/m^2/hr) followed by pulses every 3 months along with low-dose corticosteroids were effective and prevented relapses better than a 6-month course alone did. A controlled trial established that pulse cyclophosphamide, when it is given with monthly pulses of methylprednisolone, led to better long-term GFR than did either regimen alone.[33] Follow-up of these patients showed that the regimen of intravenous pulse cyclophosphamide plus methylprednisolone had no more side effects than the regimen using pulses of cyclophosphamide alone. Nevertheless, side effects were significant (see later discussion) in both therapeutic arms of this study.[33] A study used intravenous cyclophosphamide to induce remissions in 59 patients with severe LN, almost half African American, with a mean serum creatinine concentration of 1.6 mg/dl and average urinary protein to creatinine ratio (g/g) of more than 5.[34] With six to eight monthly intravenous doses, 83% had a remission, with mean creatinine reduction from 1.59 to 0.97 mg/dl, mean urinary protein to creatinine ratio declining from 5.1 to 1.7, and correction of hypertension and serologic abnormalities. It is clear that this regimen of intravenous cyclophosphamide is effective in induction therapy, and most studies using newer regimens have focused on achieving this high induction response rate with fewer side effects.

A trial by the Euro–Lupus Group tried to decrease the risk of side effects from cyclophosphamide therapy without sacrificing efficacy.[35] This study randomized 90 predominantly Caucasian patients with diffuse or focal proliferative LN or membranous plus proliferative disease to receive either standard six monthly pulses of cyclophosphamide (0.5 to 1 g/m^2/month) followed by every-third-month infusions or a shorter treatment course consisting of 500 mg of intravenous cyclophosphamide every 2 weeks for six doses (total dose, 3 g), then switching to azathioprine maintenance therapy (2 mg/kg/day). Both regimens were equally effective in renal and extrarenal outcomes. The shorter regimen had less toxicity with significantly less severe and total infections as a complication of treatment. Subsequent reports after 5 and 10 years continued to find no differences in outcome between treatment groups.[36] Although this regimen has not yet been tested in significant populations of African Americans or Hispanics, it is being widely adopted in clinical practice as a method to avoid major cyclophosphamide side effects.

Mycophenolate Mofetil

Several recent controlled trials and subsequent meta-analyses have examined the role of mycophenolate mofetil (MMF) in the induction of remission of severe LN.[37-42] One evaluated 42 Chinese patients randomized to receive either 12 months of MMF or 6 months of oral cyclophosphamide followed by azathioprine for 6 months.[38] Both groups received concomitant tapering doses of corticosteroids. At 12 months, the number of complete or partial remissions and relapses was not different between the regimens. Infections were less in the MMF arm, and mortality was all in the cyclophosphamide group (0% versus 10%). Longer follow-up confirmed the benefits of the MMF group.[41] A second trial also in a Chinese population evaluated 46 patients treated with either pulse intravenous cyclophosphamide or MMF for 6 months.[39] Patients treated with MMF had greater reductions in proteinuria and greater improvement on renal biopsy.

Another trial examined 140 patients (>50% African Americans) with proliferative LN.[40] One half was randomized to intravenous cyclophosphamide monthly pulses and one half to MMF, each in conjunction with a fixed tapering dose of corticosteroids as induction therapy during 6 months. Complete and partial remissions at 6 months were significantly more common in the MMF arm. Side effect profile was better in the MMF group. At 3 years, rates of renal failure, ESRD, and mortality were similar.

A 370-patient international trial of induction therapy with either MMF or monthly intravenous cyclophosphamide yielded comparable rates of complete and partial remission as well as equivalent resolution or stability of all renal and extrarenal parameters after 6 months,[42] even in the subgroup presenting with a GFR below 30 ml/min.[43] Mortality was similar in both groups.

Given these recent induction trials, MMF is one of the recommended first-choice regimens for inducing a remission in severe active proliferative LN (Fig. 25.12).

Other Immunosuppressive Strategies

Azathioprine and cyclosporine have been used in combination with corticosteroids for the induction of remission in LN. A recent randomized trial comparing azathioprine with cyclophosphamide found no difference in eventual outcome but more relapses and more patients doubling their serum creatinine concentration in the azathioprine group.[44] One innovative approach is to use multitargeted therapy with three immunosuppressive agents, each with different toxicities. In a recent trial, the use of MMF along with tacrolimus and corticosteroids proved superior to intravenous cyclophosphamide plus corticosteroids in inducing remissions at both 6 months and longer in a group of patients with proliferative lesions superimposed on membranous LN.[45]

Plasma exchange has been added to other induction therapies (e.g., cyclophosphamide) in several controlled randomized trials. Although no trial demonstrated significant benefit in terms of renal or patient survival or in reduction of proteinuria or improvement of GFR, suggesting that the routine use of plasma exchange was not justified in LN, this procedure continues to be used for those with refractory or rapidly progressive renal disease in some centers. Intravenous gamma globulin has given encouraging results as adjunct therapy for patients with severe lupus and nephritis in preliminary studies. A major problem is that there is no standard accepted preparation of intravenous IgG, and a fall in GFR may be seen during administration that is not always reversible.

For patients with life-threatening resistant disease, small pilot studies have used total lymphoid irradiation and immunoablation

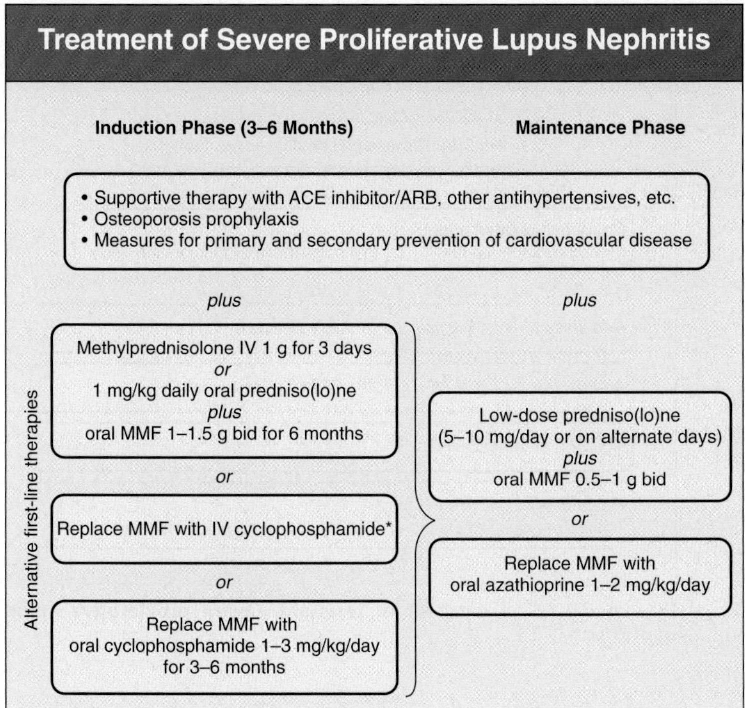

Treatment of Severe Proliferative Lupus Nephritis
Induction Phase (3–6 Months)
Maintenance Phase
• Supportive therapy with ACE inhibitor/ARB, other antihypertensives, etc.
• Osteoporosis prophylaxis
• Measures for primary and secondary prevention of cardiovascular disease
plus
plus
Methylprednisolone IV 1 g for 3 days or 1 mg/kg daily oral predniso(lo)ne plus oral MMF 1–1.5 g bid for 6 months
or
Replace MMF with IV cyclophosphamide*
or
Replace MMF with oral cyclophosphamide 1–3 mg/kg/day for 3–6 months
Low-dose predniso(lo)ne (5–10 mg/day or on alternate days) plus oral MMF 0.5–1 g bid
or
Replace MMF with oral azathioprine 1–2 mg/kg/day
Alternative first-line therapies

Figure 25.12 Treatment of severe proliferative lupus nephritis (ISN class III A or III A/C or ISN class IV A or IV A/C). ACE, angiotensin-converting enzyme; ARB, angiotensin receptor blocker; MMF, mycophenolate mofetil. *Use either 0.5-1 g/m^2 monthly for 6 months or follow the Euro-Lupus group protocol (see text).

by high-dose cyclophosphamide and antithymocyte globulin, with or without reconstitution with autologous stem cells. These approaches have led to sustained treatment-free remissions but are toxic and have a treatment-related mortality.[46,47] Their role in SLE therapy remains to be determined.

Biologic Agents

With respect to targeted biologic agents, early studies of monoclonal antibodies directed against B- and T-cell costimulation (anti-CD40 ligand) have proved unsuccessful, in part due to lack of efficacy and in part due to thrombotic complications. New trials using CTLA4Ig (abatacept) to block T- and B-cell costimulation are under way. In small pilot trials, rituximab, an anti-CD20 monoclonal antibody that depletes B cells, induced remissions in some patients with severe LN, including some who have failed cyclophosphamide or MMF therapy.[48] More recently, 140 patients with severe LN were randomized to rituximab versus placebo added to MMF and tapering dose of corticosteroids.[49] Both in this trial and in a trial in SLE patients without renal disease,[50] rituximab failed to add a major benefit in therapy. Whereas these results do not support the routine use of rituximab, the nature of the trial designs using rituximab in addition to conventional therapy and relatively short follow-up may have contributed to the negative results. Thus, the role of rituximab in the treatment of LN currently remains unclear. Inhibition of the B cell–stimulating cytokine (BLyS) by a monoclonal antibody, belimumab, has proved superior to placebo in extrarenal SLE. Other B-cell targeted therapies under investigation include a monoclonal antibody to CD22 (epratuzumab), a fully humanized anti-CD20 (ocrelizumab), and a soluble TACI (transmembrane activator and calcium-modulator and cyclophilin ligand interactor) receptor that inhibits B cell–stimulating cytokines (atacicept).[51]

Summary of Evidence of Induction Agents

Although corticosteroids are routinely recommended for LN induction therapy, their combination with MMF is emerging as the most attractive initial strategy because of the recent evidence supporting MMF and the desire to avoid toxicities associated with cyclophosphamide. However, approximately one third will not remit with MMF and corticosteroids, and a cascade of second- and third-line options needs to be considered when treatment is planned. Cyclophosphamide, azathioprine, cyclosporine, tacrolimus, and rituximab are alternatives in this setting. For the minority with progressive disease, the addition of intravenous corticosteroids, plasma exchange, and immunoglobulins is an option to be considered.

The Treatment of Proliferative Lupus Nephritis: Maintenance Therapy

In most patients, the acute renal disease will come under control by 3 months of therapy. By 6 months, almost all responders will have improving serologic markers (anti-DNA antibody levels, serum complement), improvement of GFR, and decline in proteinuria. Persistent but declining levels of proteinuria and some urinary sediment abnormalities at 6 months are not rare and do not indicate disease activity. The challenges once remission has been induced are to avoid flares of disease activity, to avoid smoldering activity leading to chronic irreversible renal scarring, and to prevent long-term side effects of therapy. A number of agents have been studied in maintenance regimens for LN patients once induction therapy has been completed.

Corticosteroids are a major component of treatment in the maintenance therapy for LN. To minimize the side effects of long-term corticosteroids, the dosage should be limited (e.g., predniso(lo)ne 5 to 15 mg/day), and osteoporosis prophylaxis should be given concomitantly (see Fig. 25.12). Both daily and alternate-day regimens have been used.

Meta-analyses unequivocally favor the additional benefit of using an immune suppressive agent during the maintenance therapy. During 10 to 15 years of follow-up, regimens of intravenous cyclophosphamide, oral cyclophosphamide, or oral cyclophosphamide plus oral azathioprine showed less progression of renal scarring than with either prednisone- or azathioprine-alone regimens.

Whereas oral cyclophosphamide has been used for induction therapy in a number of trials, its use for longer than 3 to 6 months should be avoided because of toxicities of alopecia, cystitis and bladder cancer, and gonadal damage with early menopause. Timing of the intravenous cyclophosphamide pulse in coordination with the menstrual cycle and the use of leuprolide acetate have been attempted, but infertility remains a major complication of all women older than 30 years and especially those receiving longer than a 6-month induction course.

Azathioprine in doses of 1 to 2.5 mg/kg/24 h has proved remarkably safe in the very long term. Macrocytosis, leukopenia, and interaction with allopurinol are all potential side effects along with the ever-present risk of infection from immunosuppression. Pancreatitis and hepatotoxicity are rare side effects. Azathioprine has a much lower oncogenic potential than cyclophosphamide, and pregnancy during maintenance azathioprine therapy may be relatively safer compared with other immunosuppressive agents (see later discussion). Two studies used azathioprine successfully as maintenance therapy after induction with a short or long course of cyclophosphamide or MMF.[34,35]

MMF has been used to maintain remission after MMF induction.[34,36] Both azathioprine and MMF have proved superior to continued every-third-month intravenous cyclophosphamide at maintaining remissions and preventing mortality or ESRD.[34] Major side effects were all significantly lower in the group receiving the oral agents. The teratogenicity of MMF complicates its long-term use in women whose lupus is in remission. A recent study of 227 patients who achieved remission of lupus nephritis after either IV cyclophosphamide or MMF induction therapy and were rerandomized to three years maintenance with either MMF or azathioprine showed clear superiority of the MMF at maintaining renal function, remisssions, and preventing ESRD.[51a]

Cyclosporine has been used with limited success as monotherapy for maintenance of remissions in patients with proliferative LN, with efficacy similar to that of azathioprine.[52] It has a greater role in the treatment of membranous lupus to reduce proteinuria and in combination with other medications to maintain remission of proliferative LN. Toxicity is discussed in Chapter 97. Tacrolimus has similar toxicities and is being used as an alternative to cyclosporine in recent trials in glomerular diseases.[45]

A summary of disease-specific treatment is given in Figure 25.12 for both induction and maintenance phases of treatment of severe proliferative LN. General renoprotective measures should follow the recommendations outlined in Chapter 76. Other agents used to treat extrarenal findings in lupus patients, including NSAIDs, antimalarials, androgens, and fish oil, have not shown benefit in terms of renal disease in SLE patients with the exception of a study with antimalarials.

The majority of patients will be maintained in remission by this treatment; but in a few cases, the initial disease is so severe that it does not come under control, or frequent early relapses are seen. An approach to the management of such patients is summarized in Figure 25.13.

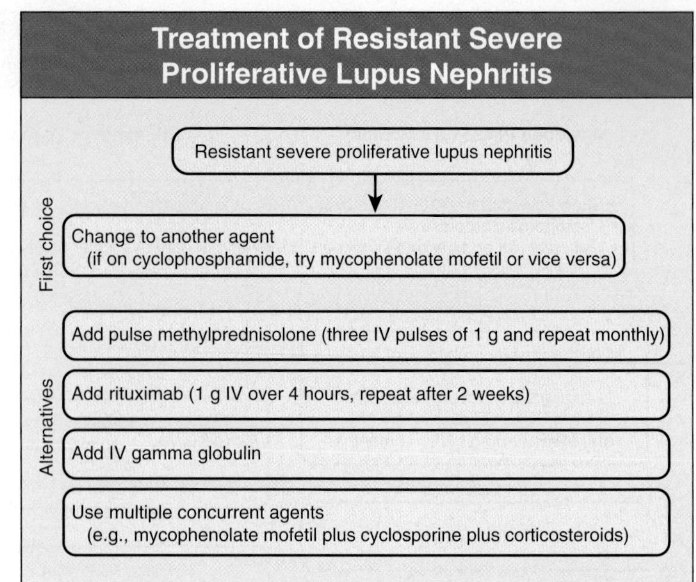

Figure 25.13 Treatment of resistant severe proliferative lupus nephritis.

Membranous Lupus Nephropathy

In the past, investigators reported different renal survival rates for different populations with membranous lupus nephropathy. In part, this was due to problems with the WHO classification, which included proliferative lesions superimposed on pure lupus membranous nephropathy (WHO class Vc and Vd) along with those with only predominantly membranous features (Va and Vb) (see Fig. 25.3).[17] Moreover, patients with subnephrotic proteinuria and pure membranous lupus nephropathy do extremely well regardless of treatment options, and no consensus of management has emerged yet for this group of patients.

In a controlled trial, 42 patients with lupus WHO class Va and Vb were randomized to receive monthly pulses of intravenous cyclophosphamide, oral cyclosporine, or oral prednisone for a year.[53] The patients had preserved GFR but a mean proteinuria of almost 6 g daily. At last follow-up, there were more complete and partial remissions in the cyclophosphamide and cyclosporine groups than in the prednisone group. Remissions occurred more quickly in the cyclosporine group, but there were fewer relapses in the cyclophosphamide group. Patients who relapsed or failed to respond to cyclosporine could subsequently be brought into remission with intravenous cyclophosphamide. Two recent trials of MMF versus intravenous cyclophosphamide induction in LN included 84 patients with pure membranous nephropathy among the 510 patients enrolled.[54] Remissions, relapses, and courses were similar in the patients treated with oral MMF and intravenous cyclophosphamide induction therapy. Azathioprine along with corticosteroids has also been successful in some populations of membranous LN.

Thus, for patients with membranous nephropathy who have subnephrotic levels of proteinuria and a preserved GFR, we recommend (Fig. 25.14) either conservative therapy with angiotensin-converting enzyme inhibitors or angiotensin receptor blockers and statins or a short course of corticosteroids or cyclosporine. For fully nephrotic patients and those at higher risk for progressive disease, there are multiple treatment options including a course of oral cyclosporine or tacrolimus, monthly intravenous pulses of cyclophosphamide, and MMF or azathioprine plus corticosteroids.[55] In all, the treatment regimen will have to be at least 6 months, and avoidance of side effects is paramount.

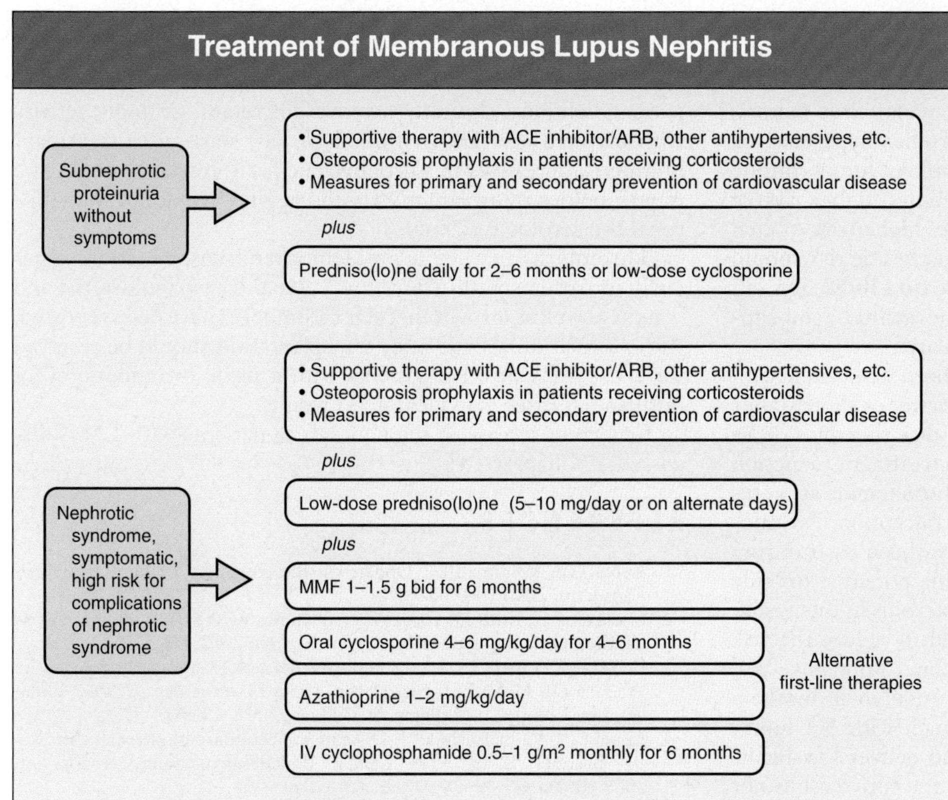

Treatment of Membranous Lupus Nephritis
Subnephrotic proteinuria without symptoms
• Supportive therapy with ACE inhibitor/ARB, other antihypertensives, etc.
• Osteoporosis prophylaxis in patients receiving corticosteroids
• Measures for primary and secondary prevention of cardiovascular disease
plus
Predniso(lo)ne daily for 2–6 months or low-dose cyclosporine
Nephrotic syndrome, symptomatic, high risk for complications of nephrotic syndrome
• Supportive therapy with ACE inhibitor/ARB, other antihypertensives, etc.
• Osteoporosis prophylaxis in patients receiving corticosteroids
• Measures for primary and secondary prevention of cardiovascular disease
plus
Low-dose predniso(lo)ne (5–10 mg/day or on alternate days)
plus
MMF 1–1.5 g bid for 6 months
Oral cyclosporine 4–6 mg/kg/day for 4–6 months
Azathioprine 1–2 mg/kg/day
IV cyclophosphamide 0.5–1 g/m2 monthly for 6 months
Alternative first-line therapies

Figure 25.14 Treatment of membranous lupus nephritis (ISN class V). ACE, angiotensin-converting enzyme; ARB, angiotensin receptor blocker; MMF, mycophenolate mofetil.

Remissions and Relapses and Stopping Therapy

Achieving a remission of LN predicts an improved long-term outcome. In one study, the 5-year patient and renal survival was 95% and 94%, respectively, for the group achieving remission and only 69% and 45%, respectively, for the group not achieving a remission.[56] Partial remission was also associated with improved outcomes compared with no remission. Predictors of remission included lower baseline serum creatinine concentration, lower baseline urinary protein excretion, better renal histologic class by the WHO or ISN system, lower chronicity index, stable GFR after 4 weeks of therapy, and Caucasian race.

The relapse rate for LN has ranged from 35% to almost 60%, depending on which population is studied, what criteria for relapse are used, and what maintenance therapy is used.[57-59] Elevation of anti-dsDNA and decline in serum complement levels may presage relapse. However, a number of patients maintain elevated anti-dsDNA levels for years without relapse, and most clinicians prefer not to treat "serologic" activity alone in the absence of clinical disease activity. A major value of a normal anti-dsDNA level is to indicate a lower risk of relapse after treatment reduction or withdrawal in the chronic phase of maintenance therapy.[60]

Monitoring of nephritis should include regular estimates of blood pressure, GFR, proteinuria, and urinary sediment. The role of repeated renal biopsy is controversial; routine follow-up biopsies have prognostic value and permit assessment of activity and progression of chronicity. Repeated biopsy at the time of flare will confirm the diagnosis of increased activity and will identify changes in histologic class, and repeated biopsy for a declining GFR will identify whether there are active lesions potentially modifiable by an increase in therapy. Although some patients will relapse many years after remission and disease quiescence, it is often possible to stop treatment entirely in many patients after 5 years or more, when the disease process has apparently "burned out." Stable GFR, lack of proteinuria, and normal immunologic test results predict successful discontinuation of immune suppressives. However, the longer corticosteroids and immunosuppressive drugs are continued, the lower the relapse rate, and it was notable in the 10-year follow-up of the Euro–Lupus study that 75% of patients were still receiving one of these interventions.[36]

Antiphospholipid Antibodies and Atherosclerotic and Other Complications

A significant percentage of lupus patients will have some form of APA detectable.[11-13] The risk of thrombotic episodes is highest with lupus anticoagulant and somewhat lower with anti–β_2-glycoprotein 1 and anticardiolipin antibodies. Disappearance of APA is unusual despite complete clinical remissions with immune suppressives and normalization of anti-dsDNA levels and other immunologic markers. There is an increased risk of hemorrhage after renal biopsy in the presence of the antiphospholipid syndrome, most likely caused by vascular damage to renal arteries that impedes hemostasis. Clinical manifestations and treatment of patients with APA are discussed further in Chapter 27.

Active organ involvement by lupus itself and infectious complications of treatment are being replaced by atherosclerotic complications as leading causes of morbidity and mortality.[61,62] Patients with lupus have increased risk of atherosclerotic complications compared with age-matched controls and greater atherosclerotic plaque burden. Young women with SLE have a risk of heart attack that is 50 times greater than that of healthy women, and even older women with SLE have 2.5 to 4 times the risk of myocardial infarction.[14] Many patients with active lupus have abnormalities of numerous cardiovascular risk factors, including hyperlipidemia, metabolic syndrome, hypertension, and systemic inflammation. Even after adjustment for all routine risk factors, SLE patients have a 7 to 10 times higher risk of nonfatal myocardial infarction and a 17 times higher risk of fatal myocardial infarction.[11] Reduction of atherosclerotic risk should be focused on tight control of blood pressure (to 130/80 mm Hg or lower), use of statins to correct lipid abnormalities, and suppression of active inflammatory disease activity.

Pregnancy in some lupus patients has been associated with flares of lupus activity either in the third trimester or shortly after delivery (see Chapter 43). It is important that therapy not be reduced in patients planning a pregnancy as treatment reduction increases the relapse risk. MMF and cyclophosphamide are teratogenic and should be withdrawn before conception. Azathioprine, cyclosporine, and corticosteroids have been used during pregnancy, although they are not without the potential for side effects. A short course of high-dose corticosteroids in the immediate postpartum period has been advocated to reduce the risk of flare at that time. The presence of immune suppressive and other drugs in breast milk needs to be considered in mothers planning to breast-feed. Compared to women with out lupus, SLE patients more commonly miscarry and deliver low-birth-weight babies. Studies suggest that oral contraceptive use is not associated with increased severe or mild to moderate flares of disease activity.[63] The use of hormone replacement therapy has been associated with only a small increase in the incidence of mild to moderate flares of disease in a study of more than 350 menopausal SLE patients.[64]

Osteoporosis and avascular necrosis of bone have become important long-term health issues for many lupus patients.[11] Women with SLE have five times higher fracture rates than normal women do. Minimizing the use of corticosteroids, especially the maintenance dose, and use of vitamin D and calcium supplements along with other agents to reduce bone loss are important.

End-Stage Renal Disease and Renal Transplantation

No more than 10% to 15% of lupus patients develop ESRD, and lupus represents only 1% to 2% of all patients with ESRD.[65] Many patients will have inactive burnt-out disease by the time they reach ESRD. Some who develop irreversible renal failure rapidly may still have active disease and require vigorous treatment while receiving renal replacement therapy. Survival of lupus patients on dialysis is comparable to that of other primary renal diseases.[65] Some patients with antiphospholipid syndrome require anticoagulation to prevent arteriovenous fistula or graft clotting.

Transplantation in lupus patients, whether from cadaveric or living donors, can be performed with only a few extra precautions. Outcomes in SLE patients undergoing transplantation are similar to those of patients with other diseases.[66,67] Crossmatching of donors with lupus patients may be difficult because the sera may contain antilymphocyte autoantibodies, rendering a false-positive "crossmatch." These can usually be "absorbed out" in testing and, in general, do not influence the course of the allograft. Immunosuppression, rejection episodes or graft loss, and infectious complications are similar to those of non-lupus patients.[67] Many clinicians prefer to wait until a patient has been maintained on 6 to 12 months of dialysis to be certain the lupus is not active at the time of transplantation. For those patients who are clinically inactive but retain serologic activity with elevated anti-DNA antibody levels, starting of transplant immunosuppressives in a prophylactic fashion several weeks to a month before transplantation with use of a live donor may suppress the serologic activity.

Thrombosis may be a problem after transplantation, especially in patients with APA.[11-13,20,68] Renal transplant arterial and venous as well as intraglomerular thromboses have been reported. Anticoagulation shortly after transplantation should be reserved for those APA-positive patients with a prior thrombotic event but in such cases may yield good results.

Recurrent disease in the allograft in patients with LN is discussed in Chapter 104.

REFERENCES

1. Appel GB, Waldman M. Update on the treatment of lupus nephritis. *Kidney Int*. 2006;70:1403-1412.
2. Contreras G, Roth D, Pardo V, et al. Lupus nephritis: A clinical review for the practicing nephrologist. *Clin Nephrol*. 2002;57:95-107.
3. D'Agati V, Appel GB. Lupus nephritis: Pathology and pathogenesis. In: Wallace DJ, Hahn BH, eds. *Dubois' Lupus Erythematosus*. 7th ed. Philadelphia: Lippincott Williams & Wilkins; 2007, Chapter 55.
4. Appel GB, Radhakrishnan J, D'Agati V. Secondary glomerular diseases. In: Brenner B, ed. *The Kidney*. Philadelphia: Saunders Elsevier; 2008:1067-1147.
5. Rus V, Maury EE, Hochberg MC. The epidemiology of systemic lupus erythematosus. In: Wallace DJ, Hahn BH, eds. *Dubois' Lupus Erythematosus*. 7th ed. Philadelphia: Lippincott Williams & Wilkins; 2007: 34-45.
6. Harley JB, Alarcon-Riquelme ME, Criswell LA, et al. Genome-wide association scan in women with systemic lupus erythematosus identifies susceptibility variants in ITGAM, PXK, KIAA1542 and other loci. *Nat Genet*. 2008;40:204-210.
7. Waldman M, Madaio MP. Pathogenic autoantibodies in lupus nephritis. *Lupus*. 2005;14:19-24.
8. Clatworthy MR, Smith KGC. Systemic lupus erythematosus: Mechansism. In: Mason JC, Pusey CD, eds. *The Kidney in Systemic Autoimmune Diseases*. Boston: Elsevier; 2008:285-309.
9. Rahman A, Isenberg DA. Systemic lupus erythematosus. *N Engl J Med*. 2008;358:929-959.
10. Wallace DJ. The clinical presentation of SLE. In: Wallace DJ, Hahn BH, eds. *Dubois' Lupus Erythematosus*. 7th ed. Philadelphia: Lippincott Williams & Wilkins; 2007:638-646.
11. Joseph R, Radhakrishnan J, Appel GB. Anticardiolipin antibodies and renal disease. *Curr Opin Hypertens Nephrol*. 2001;10:175-181.
12. Moroni G, Ventura D, Riva P, Panzeri P. Antiphospholipid antibodies are associated with an increased risk for chronic renal insufficiency in patients with lupus nephritis. *Am J Kidney Dis*. 2004;43:28-36.
13. D'Cruz D. Renal manifestations of the antiphospholipid syndrome. *Curr Rheumatol Rep*. 2009;11:52-60.
14. Manzi S. Lupus update: Perspective and clinical pearls. *Cleve Clin J Med*. 2009;76:137-142.
15. Moroni G, Radice A, Giammarresi G, et al. Are laboratory tests useful for monitoring the activity of lupus nephritis? A 6-year prospective study in a cohort of 228 patients with lupus nephritis. *Ann Rheum Dis*. 2009;68:234-237.
16. Weening JJ, D'Agati VD, Schwartz MM, et al. The classification of glomerulonephritis in systemic lupus nephritis revisited. *Kidney Int*. 2004;65:521-530.
17. Markowitz GS, D'Agati VD. The ISN/RPS classification of lupus nephritis: An assessment at 3 years. *Kidney Int*. 2007;71:491-495.
18. Furess PN, Taub N. Interobserver reproducibility and application of the ISN/RPS classification of lupus nephritis—a UK-wide study. *Am J Surg Pathol*. 2006;30:1030-1035.
19. Hill GS, Delahousse M, Nochy D, et al. Proteinuria and tubulointerstitial lesions in lupus nephritis. *Kidney Int*. 2001;60:1893-1903.
20. Sprangers B, Appel GB. Renal vascular involvement in SLE. In: Lewis EJ, Schwartz MM, Korbet SM, eds. *Lupus Nephritis*. New York: Oxford University Press; 1999:241-262.

21. Dube GK, Markowitz GS, Radhakrishnan J, et al. Minimal change disease in SLE. *Clin Nephrol.* 2002;57:120-126.
22. Najafi CC, Korbet SM, Lewis EJ, et al. Significance of histologic patterns of glomerular injury upon long-term prognosis in severe lupus glomerulonephritis. *Kidney Int.* 2001;59:2156-2163.
23. Schwartz MM. The Holy Grail: Pathological indices in lupus nephritis. *Kidney Int.* 2000;58:1354-1355.
24. Austin HA 3rd, Boumpas DT, Vaughan EM, Balow JE. High-risk features of lupus nephritis: Importance of race and clinical and histological factors in 166 patients. *Nephrol Dial Transplant.* 1995;10:1620-1628.
25. Hill GS, Delahousse M, Nochy D, et al. Predictive power of the second renal biopsy in lupus nephritis: Significance of macrophages. *Kidney Int.* 2001;59:304-316.
26. Korbet SM, Schwartz MM, Evans J, Lewis EJ. Severe lupus nephritis: Racial differences in presentation and outcome. *J Am Soc Nephrol.* 2007;18:244-254.
27. Alarcon GS, McGwin GJ, Petri M, et al. Time to renal disease and ESRD in PROFILE: A multiethnic lupus cohort. *PLoS Med.* 2006;3:e396.
28. Contreras G, Pardo V, Cely C, et al. Outcomes in African Americans and Hispanics with lupus nephritis. *Kidney Int.* 2006;69:1846-1851.
29. Barr RG, Seliger S, Appel GB, et al. Prognosis in proliferative lupus nephritis: The role of socio-economic status and race/ethnicity. *Nephrol Dial Transplant.* 2003;18:2039-2046.
30. Monahan M, Appel GB. Systemic lupus treatment. In: Mason JC, Pusey CD, eds. *The Kidney in Systemic Autoimmune Diseases.* Boston: Elsevier; 2008:323-333.
31. Gordon C, Jayne D, Pusey C, et al. European consensus statement on the terminology used in the management of lupus glomerulonephritis. *Lupus.* 2009;18:257-263.
32. Gourley MF, Austin HA 3rd, Scott D, et al. Methylprednisolone and cyclophosphamide, alone or in combination, in patients with lupus nephritis. A randomized, controlled trial. *Ann Intern Med.* 1996;125: 549-557.
33. Illei GG, Austin HA, Crane M, et al. Combination therapy with pulse cyclophosphamide plus pulse methylprednisolone improves long-term renal outcome without adding toxicity in patients with lupus nephritis. *Ann Intern Med.* 2001;135:248-257.
34. Contreras G, Pardo V, Leclercq B, et al. Sequential therapies for proliferative lupus nephritis. *N Engl J Med.* 2004;350:971-980.
35. Houssiau FA, Vasconcelos C, D'Cruz D, et al. Immunosuppressive therapy in lupus nephritis: The Euro–Lupus Nephritis Trial, a randomized trial of low-dose versus high-dose intravenous cyclophosphamide. *Arthritis Rheum.* 2002;46:2121-2131.
36. Houssiau FA, Vasconcelos C, D'Cruz D, et al. The 10-year follow-up data of the Euro–Lupus Nephritis Trial comparing low-dose versus high-dose intravenous cyclophosphamide. *Ann Rheum Dis.* 2010; 69:61-64.
37. Walsh M, James M, Jayne D, et al. Mycophenolate mofetil for induction therapy of lupus nephritis: A systematic review and meta-analysis. *Clin J Am Soc Nephrol.* 2007;2:968-975.
38. Chan TM, Li FK, Tang CS, et al. Efficacy of mycophenolate mofetil in patients with diffuse proliferative lupus nephritis. Hong Kong–Guangzhou Nephrology Study Group. *N Engl J Med.* 2000;343: 1156-1162.
39. Hu W, Liu Z, Chen H, et al. Mycophenolate mofetil vs cyclophosphamide therapy for patients with diffuse proliferative lupus nephritis. *Chin Med J (Engl).* 2002;115:705-709.
40. Ginzler EM, Dooley MA, Aranow C, et al. Mycophenolate mofetil or intravenous cyclophosphamide for lupus nephritis. *N Engl J Med.* 2005;353:2219-2228.
41. Chan TM, Tse KC, Tang CS, et al. Long-term study of mycophenolate mofetil as continuous induction and maintenance treatment for diffuse proliferative lupus nephritis. *J Am Soc Nephrol.* 2005;16:1076-1084.
42. Appel GB, Contreras G, Dooley MA, et al. Aspreva Lupus Management Study Group, Mycophenolate mofetil versus cyclophosphamide for induction treatment of lupus nephritis. *J Am Soc Nephrol.* 2009;20: 1103-1112.
43. Walsh M, Solomons N, Jayne D. MMF in lupus nephritis with poor renal function: Analysis of the ALMS data for the ALMS group. *J Am Soc Nephrol.* 2008;19:780A.
44. Grootscholten C, Ligtenberg G, Hagen EC, et al. Azathioprine/methylprednisolone versus cyclophosphamide in proliferative lupus nephritis. A randomized controlled trial. *Kidney Int.* 2006;70:732-742.
45. Bao H, Liu ZH, Xie HL, et al. Successful treatment of class V+IV lupus nephritis with multitarget therapy. *J Am Soc Nephrol.* 2008;19: 2001-2010.
46. Jayne D, Passweg J, Marmont A, et al. Autologous stem cell transplantation for systemic lupus erythematosus. *Lupus.* 2004;13:168-176.
47. Burt RK, Traynor A, Statkute L, et al. Nonmyeloablative hematopoietic stem cell transplantation for systemic lupus erythematosus. *JAMA.* 2006;295:527-535.
48. Lu TY, Ng KP, Cambridge G, et al. A retrospective seven-year analysis of the use of B cell depletion therapy in systemic lupus erythematosus at University College London Hospital: The first fifty patients. *Arthritis Rheum.* 2009;61:482-487.
49. Furie R, Looney RJ, Rovin B, et al. Efficacy and safety of rituximab in subjects with active proliferative lupus nephritis (LN): results from the randomised double-blind phase III Lunar study (abstract). *Arthritis Rheum.* 2009:60(Suppl 10):1149.
50. Merrill JT, Neuwelt CM, Wallace DJ, et al. Efficacy and safety of rituximab in moderately-to-severely active systemic lupus erythematosus: the randomized, double-blind, phase II/III systemic lupus erythematosus evaluation of rituximab trial. *Arthritis Rheum.* 2010;62:222-233.
51. Vincenti F, Cohen SD, Appel G. Novel B cell therapeutic targets in transplantation and immune mediated glomerular diseases. *Clin J Am Soc Nephrol.* 2010;5:142-151.
51a. Jayne DR, Appel G, Dooley MA, et al. Results of the ASPREVA Lupus Management Study (ALMS) maintenance phase (abstract). *J Am Soc Nephrol.* 2010:4380A.
52. Moroni G, Doria A, Mosca M, et al. A randomized pilot trial comparing cyclosporine and azathioprine for maintenance therapy in diffuse lupus nephritis over four years. *Clin J Am Soc Nephrol.* 2006;1:925-932.
53. Austin HA 3rd, Illei GG, Braun MJ, Balow JE. Randomized, controlled trial of prednisone, cyclophosphamide, and cyclosporine in lupus membranous nephropathy. *J Am Soc Nephrol.* 2009;20:901-911.
54. Radhakrishnan J, Solomons N, Ginzler E, Appel GB. Mycophenolate mofetil and intravenous cyclophosphamide are similar as induction therapy for class V lupus nephritis. *Kidney Int.* 2009 Nov 4 [Epub ahead of print].
55. Szeto CC, Kwan BC, Lai FM, et al. Tacrolimus for the treatment of systemic lupus erythematosus with pure class V nephritis. *Rheumatology (Oxford).* 2008;47:1678-1681.
56. Chen YE, Korbet SM, Katz RS, et al, Collaborative Study Group. Value of a complete or partial remission in severe lupus nephritis. *Clin J Am Soc Nephrol.* 2008;3:46-53.
57. Illei GG, Takada K, Parkin D, et al. Renal flares are common in patients with severe proliferative lupus nephritis treated with pulse immunosuppressive therapy: Long-term followup of a cohort of 145 patients participating in randomized controlled studies. *Arthritis Rheum.* 2002;46:995-1002.
58. Mosca M, Bencivelli W, Neri R, et al. Renal flares in 91 SLE patients with diffuse proliferative glomerulonephritis. *Kidney Int.* 2002;61: 1502-1509.
59. Ponticelli C, Moroni G. Flares in lupus nephritis: Incidence, impact on renal survival and management. *Lupus.* 1998;7:635-638.
60. Moroni G, Gallelli B, Quaglini S, et al. Withdrawal of therapy in patients with proliferative lupus nephritis: Long-term follow-up. *Nephrol Dial Transplant.* 2006;21:1541-1548.
61. Roman MJ, Shanker BA, Davis A, et al. Prevalence and correlates of accelerated atherosclerosis in systemic lupus erythematosus. *N Engl J Med.* 2003;349:2399-2406.
62. Bruce IN, Urowitz MB, Gladman DD, et al. Risk factors for coronary heart disease in women with systemic lupus erythematosus: The Toronto Risk Factor Study. *Arthritis Rheum.* 2003;48:3159-3167.
63. Petri M, Kim MY, Kalunian KC, et al. Combined oral contraceptives in women with SLE. *N Engl J Med.* 2005;353:2550-2558.
64. Buyon JP, Petri MA, Kim MY, et al. The effect of combined estrogen and progesterone hormone replacement therapy on disease activity in SLE: A randomized trial. *Ann Intern Med.* 2005;142:953-962.
65. Nossent HC. End-stage renal disease in the patient with SLE. In: Lewis EJ, Schwartz MM, Korbet SM, eds. *Lupus Nephritis.* New York: Oxford University Press; 2009:284-304.
66. Ward MM. Outcomes of renal transplantation among patients with ESRD caused by lupus nephritis. *Kidney Int.* 2000;57:2136.
67. Bunnapradist S, Chung P, Peng A, et al. Outcomes of renal transplantation in lupus nephritis: Analysis of the organ procurement and transplantation network data. *Transplantation.* 2006;82:612-618.
68. Stone JH, Amen WJ, Criswell LA. Antiphospholipid antibody syndrome in renal transplantation: Occurrence of clinical events in 96 consecutive patients with SLE. *Am J Kidney Dis.* 1999;34:1040.

CHAPTER 26

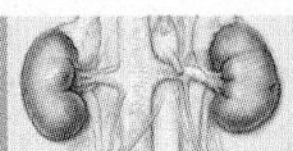

Renal Amyloidosis and Glomerular Diseases with Monoclonal Immunoglobulin Deposition

Pierre M. Ronco, Pierre Aucouturier, Bruno Moulin

The glomerular capillaries are a favorite site for the deposition of abnormal proteins. In most cases, the resulting diseases are caused by a monoclonal immunoglobulin subunit, and those can be classified into two categories by electron microscopy (Fig. 26.1). The first category includes diseases with fibril formation, mainly amyloidosis, and diseases with microtubule formation, including cryoglobulinemic (see Chapter 21) and immunotactoid glomerulonephritis (GN). The second category is characterized by nonorganized electron-dense granular deposits. They are localized along basement membranes in most tissues, especially in the kidney, and define a disease now termed monoclonal immunoglobulin deposition disease (MIDD). In some cases, monotypic immune complex–like deposits are observed in the setting of proliferative GN.

RENAL AMYLOIDOSIS

General Characteristics of Amyloidosis

Definition

Amyloidosis is a generic term for a family of diseases defined by morphologic criteria. The diseases are characterized by the deposition in extracellular spaces of a proteinaceous material. Amyloid deposits are composed of a felt-like array of 7.5- to 10-nm-wide rigid, linear, nonbranching, aggregated fibrils of indefinite length.[1] One amyloid fibril is made of two twisted 3-nm-wide filaments, each displaying the typical "cross-β" structure,[1] where antiparallel β-sheets are perpendicular to the filament axis.

Amyloid Precursor–Based Classification

Amyloidoses are classified by the type of precursor protein that composes the main component of fibrils (Fig. 26.2).[2] The amyloidogenic propensity is related to the ability of this precursor to form intermolecular β-sheets. Besides these structural properties, which may relate to genetically transmitted mutations, the amyloidogenic potential is enhanced by overproduction or impaired clearance of the precursor.

Renal amyloidoses mostly include immunoglobulin light chain (AL) and systemic secondary (AA) amyloidoses. Other precursors, such as transthyretin, fibrinogen, apolipoprotein A-I, and lysozyme, are responsible for rare familial cases.

Other Components of All Amyloid Fibrils

Glycosaminoglycans (GAGs) are tightly associated with amyloid fibrils. GAGs are polysaccharide chains made of repeating hyaluronic acid–hexosamine units normally linked to a protein core, thus forming proteoglycans. Proteoglycans, mostly of the heparan sulfate type, appear to induce and to stabilize the β-pleated amyloid structure.

Another constituent of all amyloid deposits is serum amyloid P component (SAP). SAP is resistant to proteolytic digestion, and coating of amyloid fibrils with SAP could result in their protection from catabolism. The high affinity of SAP toward amyloid was exploited for diagnosis, location, and monitoring of the extent of systemic amyloidosis by scintigraphy with [^{123}I]-SAP.

General Mechanisms of Fibrillogenesis

Amyloidogenesis involves a nucleation-dependent polymerization process. Formation of an ordered nucleus is the initial and thermodynamically limiting step, followed by addition of monomers and elongation of the fibrils.[3] Fibrillogenesis may involve several mechanisms of processing of the amyloid precursor, including partial proteolysis and conformational modifications. Conformational changes lead to a soluble, partially folded intermediate, whose subsequent ordered self-assembly results in fibril formation. Macrophages have a central role in AA amyloidosis by providing the intralysosomal processing of the precursor. In AL amyloidosis, the variable domain of the light chain V_L is the main component, which suggests a role of partial proteolysis of the light-chain precursor.

Pathology

On light microscopy, the deposits are extracellular, eosinophilic, and metachromatic. After Congo red staining, they appear faintly red (Fig. 26.3A) and show characteristic apple-green birefringence under polarized light (Fig. 26.3B). Metachromasia is also observed with crystal violet, which stains the deposits red.

The earliest lesions are located in the mesangium (see Fig. 26.3A), along the glomerular basement membrane (GBM), and in the blood vessels. Mesangial deposits are primarily in the mesangial matrix and spread from lobule to lobule until eventually the whole mesangial area is replaced. Amyloid deposits may also infiltrate the GBM or be localized on both sides of it. When subepithelial deposits predominate, spikes similar to those seen in membranous nephropathy (MN) may be observed. Advanced amyloid typically produces a nonproliferative, noninflammatory glomerulopathy and marked enlargement of the kidney. The amyloid deposits replace the normal glomerular architecture, with a consequent loss of cellularity. When glomeruli become massively sclerotic, the deposits may be difficult to demonstrate by Congo red staining. Electron microscopy may be helpful then and also in the very early stages, which may not be detected by

Glomerular Diseases with Tissue Deposition or Precipitation of Monoclonal Immunoglobulin Components

Immunoglobulin Deposits	Glomerular Disease
Organized	
Fibrillar	Amyloidosis (AL, AH)
Microtubular	Cryoglobulinemia; immunotactoid glomerulonephritis
Nonorganized: granular	Monoclonal immunoglobulin deposition disease: light-chain, heavy-chain, and light-plus heavy-chain deposition diseases
	Immune complex–like proliferative glomerulonephritis

Figure 26.1 Glomerular diseases with tissue deposition or precipitation of monoclonal immunoglobulin components.

light microscopy examination in patients presenting with the nephrotic syndrome. Amyloid deposits are characterized by randomly oriented, nonbranching fibrils with an 8- to 15-nm diameter (Fig. 26.4).

Except for fibrinogen amyloidosis, which characteristically does not affect renal vessels, the media of the blood vessels is prominently involved at early stages. Vascular involvement may predominate and occasionally occurs alone, particularly in AL amyloidosis. Deposits may also affect the tubules and the interstitium, leading to atrophy and disappearance of the tubular structures and to interstitial fibrosis.

Given the heterogeneity of amyloidoses, immunohistology should be routinely performed (Fig. 26.3C). Immunohistochemical classification of amyloid type is possible in most cases. Immunohistology with antibodies specific for immunoglobulin chains may be more difficult to interpret than that with anti-AA antiserum, perhaps because of the absence or inaccessibility of light-chain epitopes. A genetic cause should be sought in all patients with amyloidosis in whom confirmation of the amyloid precursor cannot be obtained by immunohistochemistry.[4]

Classification of Amyloidoses

Amyloid Protein	Precursor	Distribution	Type	Syndrome or Involved Tissues
AA	Serum amyloid A	Systemic	Acquired	Secondary amyloidosis, reactive to chronic infection or inflammation including hereditary periodic fever (FMF, TRAPS, HIDS, FCU, and MWS)
AApoAI	Apolipoprotein A-I	Systemic	Hereditary	Liver, kidney, heart
AApoAII	Apolipoprotein A-II	Systemic	Hereditary	Kidney, heart
Aβ	Aβ protein precursor	Localized	Acquired	Sporadic Alzheimer's disease, aging
		Localized	Hereditary	Prototypical hereditary cerebral amyloid angiopathy, Dutch type
Aβ2M	β_2-Microglobulin	Systemic	Acquired	Chronic hemodialysis
ABri	Abri protein precursor	Localized or systemic?	Hereditary	British familial dementia
ACys	Cystatin C	Systemic	Hereditary	Icelandic hereditary cerebral amyloid angiopathy
AFib	Fibrinogen Aα chain	Systemic	Hereditary	Kidney
AGel	Gelsolin	Systemic	Hereditary	Finnish hereditary amyloidosis
AH	Immunoglobulin heavy chain	Systemic or localized	Acquired	Primary amyloidosis, myeloma associated
AL	Immunoglobulin light chain	Systemic or localized	Acquired	Primary amyloidosis, myeloma associated
ALect2	Leukocyte chemotactic factor 2	Localized	Acquired ?	Kidney
ALys	Lysozyme	Systemic	Hereditary	Kidney, liver, spleen
APrP	Prion protein	Localized	Acquired	Sporadic (iatrogenic CJD, new variant CJD)
		Localized	Hereditary	Familial CJD, GSSD, FFI
ATTR	Transthyretin	Systemic	Hereditary Acquired	Prototypical FAP Senile heart, vessels

Figure 26.2 Classification of amyloidoses. Entries in bold type indicate amyloid types with kidney involvement. The following proteins may also cause amyloidosis: calcitonin, islet-amyloid polypeptides, atrial natriuretic factor, prolactin, insulin, lactadherin, keratoepithelin, and Danish amyloid protein (which comes from the same gene as ABri and has an identical N-terminal sequence). CJD, Creutzfeldt-Jakob disease; FAP, familial amyloidotic polyneuropathy; FCU, familial cold urticaria; FFI, fatal familial insomnia; FMF, familial Mediterranean fever; GSSD, Gerstmann-Sträussler-Scheinker disease; HIDS, hyper-IgD syndrome; MWS, Muckle-Wells syndrome; TRAPS, tumor necrosis factor receptor–associated periodic syndrome. *(Modified from references 5, 6.)*

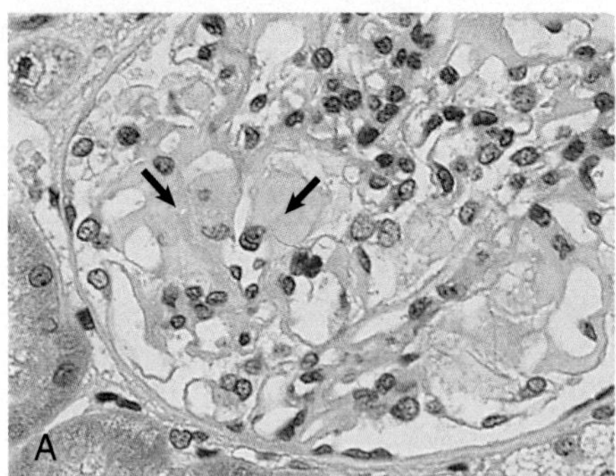

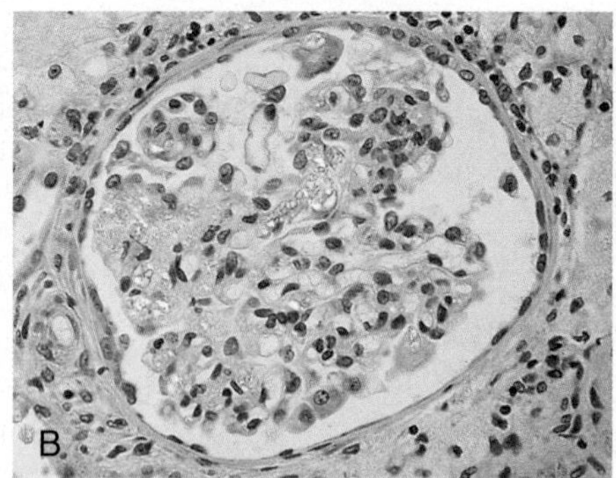

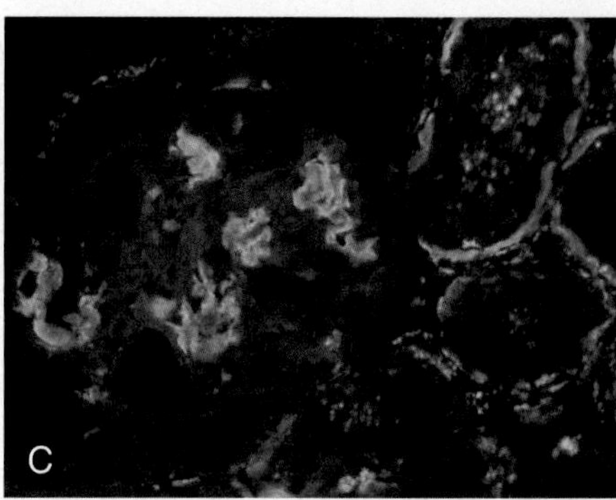

Figure 26.3 Amyloidosis. A, Amyloid deposits *(arrows)* in a glomerulus. (Hematoxylin-eosin; magnification ×312.) **B,** Congo red staining. Apple-green birefringence under polarized light. (Magnification ×312.) **C,** Immunofluorescence with anti-κ antibody. Note glomerular and tubular deposits. (Magnification ×312.) *(Courtesy Dr. Béatrice Mougenot, Paris, France.)*

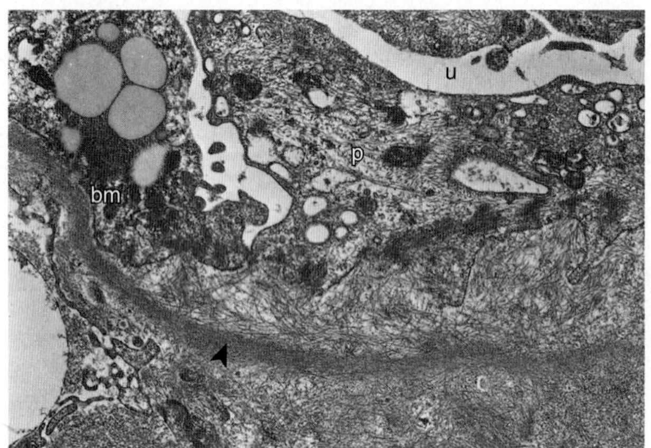

Figure 26.4 Electron micrograph of amyloid deposits invading glomerular basement membrane (GBM). Randomly oriented fibrils are located on both sides of the basement membrane (bm), and the lamina densa is attenuated *(arrowhead)*. (Magnification ×10,000.) p, podocyte; u, urinary space. *(Courtesy Dr. Béatrice Mougenot, Paris, France.)*

Immunoglobulin-Associated Amyloidosis (AL and AA)

Free immunoglobulin subunits, mostly light chains, secreted by a single clone of B cells, are the cause of the most frequent and severe amyloidosis affecting the kidney. Studies on the mechanisms of AL amyloidogenesis are made particularly difficult by the unique structural heterogeneity of the precursor: each monoclonal light chain is different from all others, so each patient is unique. The involvement of an immunoglobulin heavy chain in amyloidosis remains exceptional.[7]

Pathogenesis

Determinant factors are borne by the precursor light chain. In AL amyloidosis, there is a striking overrepresentation of the λ isotype, which is twofold to fourfold more frequent than the κ isotype. A rarely expressed homology family of light-chain variable regions, the $V_{\lambda VI}$ variability subgroup, is found only in amyloid-associated monoclonal immunoglobulins.

Amyloidogenicity is associated with physicochemical features including low-molecular-mass light-chain fragments in the urine, abnormal disulfide bonding of light chains, and low isoelectric point (pI). An analysis of nearly 200 light-chain sequences identified 12 positions in κ chains and 12 in λ chains where certain residues were associated with amyloidosis. Four structural risk factors were shown to define most fibril-forming κ light chains.[8] Because of their high dimerization constants, light chains from patients with AL amyloidosis may behave like antibodies with affinity for extracellular structures.

The tropism of organ involvement may be influenced both by the germline gene used for the light-chain variable region (V_L) and by somatic mutations occurring in the secreting clone.[9] Patients expressing a monoclonal light chain of the $V_{\lambda VI}$ subgroup are more likely to present with dominant renal involvement and less frequent cardiac and multisystem disease.[10] Patients with κ light chains are more likely to have dominant hepatic involvement. In addition, organ-specific environmental factors are also involved. For example, high intrarenal concentrations of urea enhance fibril formation by reducing the nucleation lag time.

Amyloid light chains may contribute directly to the pathogenesis, independent of extracellular fibril deposition. In the heart and the kidney at least, the infiltration alone does not correlate well with clinical manifestations. Light chains from amyloid patients incubated with mesangial cells induce a macrophage-like phenotype, whereas those from light-chain deposition disease patients induce a myofibroblast-like phenotype.[11]

Epidemiology

The incidence of AL amyloidosis is nine per million per year. Fewer than one of four patients with AL amyloidosis is considered to have an overt immunoproliferative disease, which usually is multiple myeloma, although other forms are seen, such as Waldenström's macroglobulinemia. Amyloid deposits are found in approximately 10% of all patients with myeloma and in 20% of those with pure light-chain myeloma. The apparent prevalence of myeloma depends on the diagnostic criteria used. Epidemiologic characteristics of primary amyloidosis, that is, amyloidosis without overt immunoproliferative disease, and myeloma are not significantly different. The median age at diagnosis is 64 years in patients with primary amyloidosis, with a slight predominance of male patients.[12]

Clinical Manifestations

The main clinical symptoms at presentation are weakness and weight loss (Fig. 26.5). Except for bone pain, the initial symptoms in patients with and without myeloma are similar. However, nephrotic syndrome, orthostatic hypotension, and peripheral neuropathy are more frequent in patients with AL amyloidosis without myeloma.[13] Amyloidosis is also different from many types of kidney disease in that the kidney is often enlarged and

Clinical and Laboratory Features at Presentation in 474 Patients with Proven AL-Amyloidosis

Features	Percentage
Initial symptoms	
Fatigue	62
Weight loss	52
Pain	5
Purpura	15
Gross bleeding	3
Physical findings	
Hepatomegaly	24
Palpable spleen	5
Lymphadenopathy	3
Macroglossia	9
Laboratory findings	
Increased plasma cells (bone marrow 6%)	56*
Anemia (hemoglobin <10 g/dl)	11
Elevated serum creatinine (1.3 mg/dl) (>113 μmol/l)	45
Elevated alkaline phosphatase	26
Hypercalcemia (>11 mg/dl) (>2.75 mmol/l)	2
Proteinuria (>1.0 g/24 h)	55
Urine light chain	73†
κ chain	23
λ chain	50

Figure 26.5 Clinical and laboratory features at presentation in 474 patients with proven light chain (AL) amyloidosis. *15% of patients having a myeloma. †Of 429 patients. *(From reference 12.)*

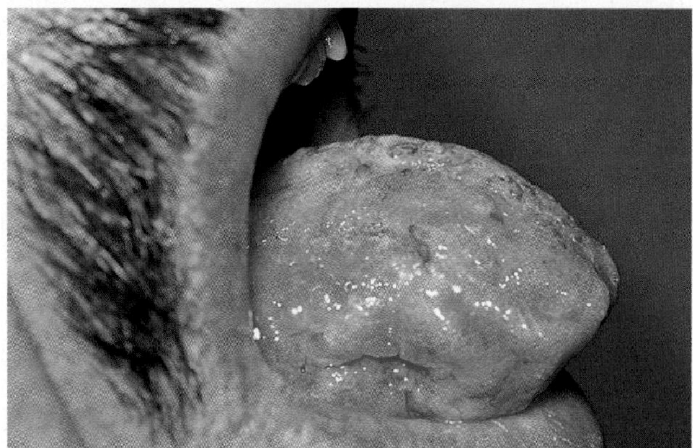

Figure 26.6 Macroglossia in a patient with AL amyloidosis. *(Courtesy Dr. S. Aractinji, Paris, France.)*

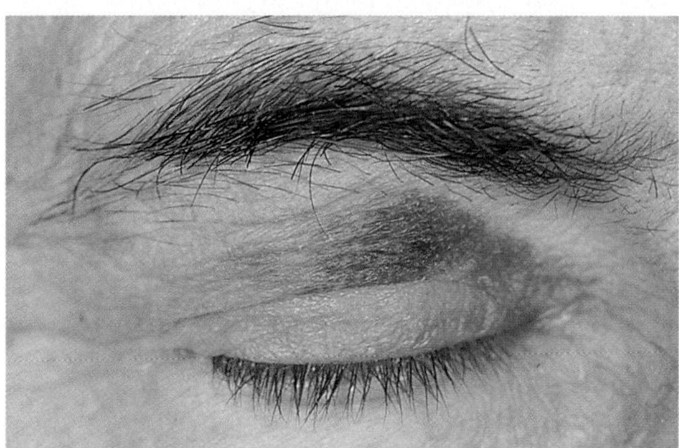

Figure 26.7 Skin involvement in AL amyloidosis. Noninfiltrated purpuric macule of the superior eyebrow, very typical of AL amyloidosis. *(Courtesy Dr. S. Aractinji, Paris, France.)*

hypertension is absent even when renal function is impaired. Proteinuria, mainly albuminuria, occurs in the absence of microscopic hematuria. Indeed, the presence of hematuria should prompt examination for a bleeding lesion in the urinary tract. Renal manifestations may also include renal tubular acidosis (mostly as a part of Fanconi syndrome; see Chapter 48) and polyuria-polydipsia (resulting from urinary concentration defect), when amyloid deposits occur around proximal tubules and Henle's loops (or collecting ducts), respectively.

AL amyloidosis may infiltrate almost any organ other than the brain and therefore can be responsible for a wide variety of clinical manifestations. Restrictive cardiomyopathy is found at presentation in up to one third of patients and causes death in about one half. Infiltration of the ventricular walls and the septum may be recognized by echocardiography. Amyloid may also induce arrhythmias and the sick sinus syndrome. Amyloid deposits in the coronary arteries may result in angina and myocardial infarction. Cardiac troponins and N-terminal pro–brain natriuretic peptide are sensitive markers of myocardial dysfunction and powerful predictors of overall survival in patients with AL amyloidosis.

Involvement of the gastrointestinal tract is common and can cause motility disturbances, malabsorption, hemorrhage, or obstruction. Macroglossia (Fig. 26.6) may interfere with eating and obstruct airways. Abnormalities of hepatic function are usually mild. Hyposplenism diagnosed by abnormal peripheral smear and liver spleen scan, commonly associated with splenomegaly, predisposes to fatal bacterial infections. Peripheral nerve involvement may result in a painful sensory polyneuropathy followed later by motor deficits. Autonomic neuropathy causing orthostatic hypotension, lack of sweating, gastrointestinal disturbances, bladder dysfunction, and impotence may occur alone or together with peripheral neuropathy. Orthostatic hypotension is one of the major hampering complications of AL amyloidosis, with some patients being bedridden. Skin involvement may take the form of purpura, characteristically around the eyes (Fig. 26.7), and ecchymoses, papules, nodules, and plaques, occurring usually on the face and upper trunk. AL amyloidosis may also infiltrate articular structures and mimic rheumatoid or an asymmetric seronegative synovitis. Infiltration of the shoulders may produce severe pain and swelling (shoulder pad sign).

A rare but potentially serious manifestation of AL amyloidosis is an acquired bleeding diathesis that may be associated with deficiency of factor X or factor IX or with increased fibrinolysis. It should be systematically sought before any biopsy of a deep organ. Widespread vascular deposits may also be responsible for bleeding. Prothrombin time and activated partial thromboplastin time measurements as well as determination of bleeding times are required to assess bleeding diathesis.

Monoclonal light chains can be detected by immunoelectrophoresis in 73% of the urine samples of patients with AL amyloidosis. The λ isotype is twice as frequent as the κ, contrasting with the 1:2 ratio of λ to κ observed in myeloma alone. With the use of more sensitive immunochemical techniques, a monoclonal immunoglobulin is found in the serum or the urine in nearly 90% of patients. The combination of immunochemical techniques and serum-free light-chain assay detects an abnormal result in 99% of patients.[14]

AL amyloidosis associated with IgM paraproteinemia characterizes a distinctive subset of patients who have a wider variety of underlying, often lymphoid clonal disorders (including 75% Waldenström's macroglobulinemia), usually low-level free light chains with a predominance of κ isotype, and higher prevalence of lymph node (31% versus 3%) and lung (17% versus 2%) involvement compared with patients with non-IgM monoclonal component.[15,16]

Diagnosis

AL amyloidosis should be considered in any patient who presents with nephrotic-range proteinuria with or without renal impairment, nondilated cardiomyopathy, peripheral neuropathy, hepatomegaly, or autonomic neuropathy, whether or not a paraprotein can be detected in the serum or urine (Fig. 26.8). Particular vigilance should be maintained in patients with multiple myeloma or monoclonal gammopathy of undetermined significance (MGUS), especially of the λ isotype. Initial investigation should confirm the diagnosis of amyloidosis on tissue biopsy, and this should be followed by investigations to establish the type of amyloid present and the extent of organ involvement.

All patients require immunofixation of serum and urine in an attempt to demonstrate the presence of a monoclonal light chain. A bone marrow specimen is necessary because 10% of patients will not have a demonstrable monoclonal light chain by immunofixation, and a clone of plasma cells detected in the bone marrow by immunohistochemistry is strong evidence of AL amyloidosis. Immunonephelometric quantitation of serum free light chains complements immunofixation because it shows remarkable specificity and sensitivity.[14]

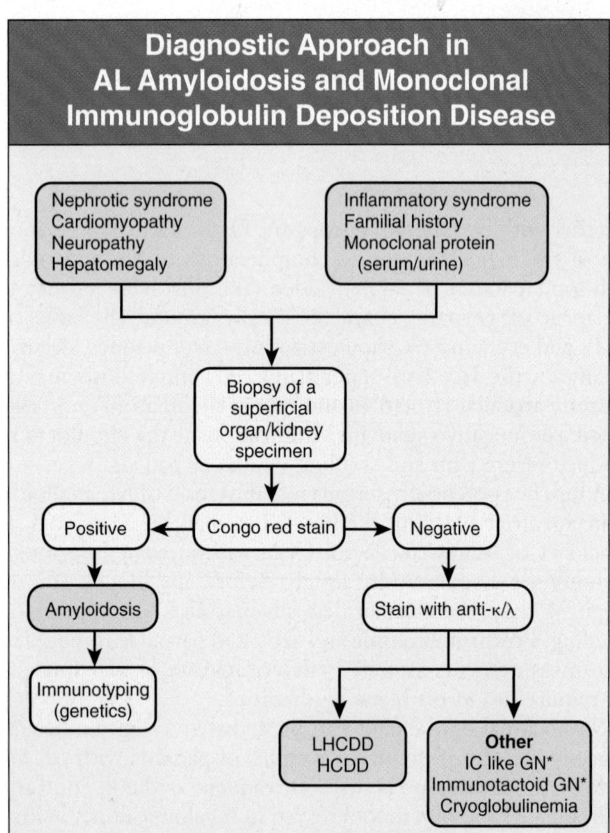

Figure 26.8 Algorithm of diagnostic procedures in light chain (AL) amyloidosis and monoclonal immunoglobulin deposition disease (MIDD). *No extrarenal manifestation. GN, glomerulonephritis; IC, immune complex; HCDD, heavy-chain deposition disease; LHCDD, light- and heavy-chain deposition disease.

Biopsy of an affected organ is usually diagnostic, but less invasive alternatives should be preferred first. Biopsies of salivary glands or subcutaneous abdominal fat yield positive results in 80% to 90% of cases. Rectal biopsy is diagnostic in more than 80% of cases, provided the biopsy specimen contains submucosal vessels in which early deposits are located. Bone marrow biopsy specimens should be stained with Congo red for the presence of amyloid, and involvement of the bone marrow (observed in about 50% of patients) is strongly suggestive of the AL type. Evaluation of adequate specimens in experienced laboratories is necessary to maintain high diagnostic sensitivity and specificity.

It is not always easy to be certain that amyloidosis is of the AL type because immunohistochemical staining for immunoglobulin light chains may not be diagnostic (because of loss of epitopes), and the presence of a monoclonal component is strong but not conclusive evidence of the AL type. Caution is required when patients have an intact monoclonal immunoglobulin in the serum without evidence of circulating free light chains in the serum or urine. In those cases, hereditary forms of amyloidosis should be considered because they may produce clinical syndromes indistinguishable from AL and coexist with MGUS.[4] In cases of doubt, DNA analysis or amyloid fibril sequencing by mass spectrometry may be necessary.

Natural History and Treatment

AL amyloidosis is among the most severe complications of plasma cell proliferative disorders. Median survival is about 10 months. Cardiac involvement responsible for congestive heart failure and arrhythmias account for at least 40% of deaths.

Therapy is aimed at annihilation of the plasma cell clone. All patients with AL amyloidosis deserve a trial of chemotherapy because of the improved survival of responders. In the responders, gradual regression of AL amyloid deposits is possible. However, the results of chemotherapy in AL amyloidosis are difficult to document because there is no easy way to measure amyloid load. Resolution of the nephrotic syndrome does not necessarily reflect loss of amyloid deposits, which can progress even with improved clinical and laboratory findings. Scintigraphy after the injection of [^{123}I]-SAP component may be helpful for monitoring the extent of systemic amyloidosis, but this technique is available in a few centers only. The definition of a response in amyloidosis should be hematologic and organ based. A complete hematologic response is defined by negativity of serum and urine for a monoclonal protein by immunofixation, normal free light-chain ratio by the serum free light-chain assay,[17] and less than 5% plasma cells in the bone marrow. There are consensus criteria for organ response and organ disease progression.[18]

Until 15 years ago, the only treatment of AL amyloidosis was melphalan with prednisone administered orally in repeated cycles during many months. This treatment had a modest impact on survival because of its delayed action and low rate of hematologic remission.[19] A more aggressive approach consisting of high-dose melphalan (HDM) administered in myeloablative doses (140 to 200 mg/m^2) followed by autologous stem cell transplantation (ASCT) started in the mid-1990s, with complete hematologic response and significant functional improvement in a substantial proportion of highly selected patients.[20-23] However, treatment-related mortality was consistently higher than in patients treated with ASCT for multiple myeloma or other malignant neoplasms. An alternative to HDM/ASCT consists of treatment with oral melphalan (10 mg/m²/day) together with dexamethasone administered at a high dosage (40 mg/day) in 4-day cycles each month (M/Dex). Early reports of M/Dex treatment described rapid eradication of light-chain production and rapid reduction in N-terminal brain natriuretic peptide.[24]

A recent trial randomly assigned 100 AL amyloidosis patients to HDM/ASCT or M/Dex.[25] Among the 65 patients for whom hematologic response could be evaluated, there was no significant difference in complete response, with 32% of those treated with M/Dex and 41% with HDM/ASCT responding. In an intention-to-treat analysis, median survival was 56.9 months in the M/Dex group compared with 22.2 months in the HDM/ASCT group (P = .04). The study investigators concluded that HDM/ASCT is not superior to M/Dex. Problems of the trial included that (1) only 37 of the patients who were randomly assigned to HDM/ASCT actually underwent the treatment and (2) treatment-related mortality in the HDM group (24%) was higher than that reported in single-center studies from amyloidosis referral centers (4% to 14%).[26] The high mortality was likely due to enrollment of patients who had severe organ dysfunction and would not be eligible for HDM/ASCT at many referral centers. However, a subset analysis of patients with low risk for an adverse outcome of intensive treatment also showed similar survival at 3 years of 80% in the M/Dex group and 58% in the HDM/ASCT group (P = 0.13). Furthermore, patients who survived for at least 6 months after randomization and who received their assigned treatment exhibited similar (20% to 30%) mortality rates.

On the basis of these findings, the following recommendations are proposed: (1) patients with severe organ dysfunction should receive M/Dex as first-line treatment; (2) patients with less severe disease are eligible for M/Dex or HDM/ASCT, still considered the reference treatment in experienced centers in the United States. Patients should be carefully monitored by assessment of free light chains. In those who do not show hematologic responses after 3 to 6 months (>50% decrease of free monoclonal light chain), treatment should be changed to alternatives such as lenalidomide- (or thalidomide-) or bortezomib-based regimens.

Dialysis and Transplantation

Most studies of the clinical course and outcome of dialysis patients include both AL and AA amyloidosis. The patient's survival rate is about 70% at 1 year and decreases to 30% to 44% at 5 to 6 years. Median survival is shorter in patients with AL amyloidosis (26 months) than with AA amyloidosis; sepsis and cardiac deaths are the main causes of mortality.[27]

Cardiac amyloid is the most important predictor of mortality in dialysis patients with AL amyloidosis.[27,28] The management of patients with AL amyloid on hemodialysis (HD) is often complicated by persistent hypotension, gastrointestinal hemorrhage, chronic diarrhea, and difficulties in the creation and maintenance of vascular access. It has therefore been suggested that peritoneal dialysis (PD) could have several advantages over HD in the management of end-stage renal amyloidosis, including avoidance of vascular access and deleterious effects on blood pressure; but PD may induce protein loss in the dialysate and thus enhance malnutrition. However, the survival rate of AL and AA amyloidosis patients treated with PD is similar to that of patients on HD.

Renal transplantation is limited by the severity of heart involvement and the recurrence of deposits in the transplanted kidney. There are a few cases and small series reported in the literature of renal transplantation in AL amyloidosis. Renal transplantation may be considered in patients whose underlying clonal plasma cell disease has remitted after chemotherapy. Heart transplantation can also be envisaged in specific cases as a tandem with HDM/ASCT or after remission.

AA Amyloidosis

Epidemiology

AA amyloidosis develops in 5% of patients with sustained elevation of serum amyloid A protein (SAA). Patients at risk are those with a long duration of chronic inflammatory disease (median, 17 years),[29] high magnitude of acute-phase SAA response, homozygosity for SAA1 isotype, familial Mediterranean fever (FMF) trait (heterozygosity for variant pyrin), and family history of AA amyloidosis.

An important epidemiologic aspect of AA amyloidosis is the changing spectrum of underlying diseases. Pyogenic and granulomatous infections, especially tuberculosis, account for far fewer cases today (15%) than previously.[29] Thus, antibiotic treatment efficiently prevents AA amyloidosis by suppressing its cause. In contrast, the prevalence of chronic inflammatory arthritis has increased dramatically (60%).[29] AA amyloidosis in patients with Hodgkin's disease has virtually disappeared with more efficient treatment of the hematologic disease. Hereditary AA amyloidoses associated with familial recurrent fever syndromes account for an increasing proportion of cases, about 10% in recent series.

Clinical Manifestations

Clinical manifestations of AA amyloidosis are shown in Figure 26.9.[29] The main target organ is the kidney, which is affected in almost all patients with AA amyloidosis. Presentation may be acute with nephrotic syndrome or very insidious. Proteinuria is absent in about 5% of cases. Gastrointestinal disturbances (including diarrhea, constipation, and malabsorption) and hepatosplenomegaly are the next most common manifestations. In contrast with AL amyloidosis, congestive heart failure, peripheral neuropathy, macroglossia, and carpal tunnel syndrome occur infrequently.

Diagnosis

A systematic search for amyloidosis is recommended in patients with active, long-lasting inflammatory arthritis, even in the absence of proteinuria and chronic kidney disease (CKD). Although findings on kidney biopsy are positive in almost 100% of symptomatic patients, less invasive biopsy procedures should be attempted first. Biopsies of accessory salivary glands, abdominal fat, and rectal mucosa yield positive results in 50% to 80% of patients. Immunohistochemical staining using antibodies to SAA is required to confirm that Congo red–positive amyloid deposits are of the AA type. SAP scintigraphy shows that bones are not affected (contrary to AL amyloidosis).

Natural History and Treatment

Survival time of patients with AA amyloidosis is 133 months, much longer than with AL amyloidosis.[29] Main causes of death are infections and dialysis-related complications but not cardiac complications. Amyloid load and clinical outcome relate to circulating concentrations of SAA.[29] The relative risk of death among patients with an SAA concentration below 4 mg/l is almost 18 times lower than among patients with an SAA concentration of 155 mg/l or greater. Even a very modest elevation in the SAA concentration of 4 to 9 mg/l is associated with a risk of death increased by a factor of 4. These data emphasize the importance of vigorous treatment of the underlying

Characteristics at Presentation of 374 Patients with Systemic AA Amyloidosis	
Age, yr (range)	50 (9-87)
Male sex, no. (%)	210 (56)
Race or ethnic group, no. (%)	
White	307 (82)
South Asian	27 (7)
Other	40 (11)
Duration of inflammatory disease at diagnosis (yr)	
Median	17
Range	0–68
Renal dysfunction	
Proteinuria >500 mg/day or serum creatinine >133 μmol/l, no. (%)	363 (97%)
End-stage renal failure no. (%)	41 (11%)
Proteinuria, g/day	
Median range	3.9 (0–26.0)
Liver involvement	
Hepatomegaly, no. (%)	35 (9%)
Deposits on SAP scintigraphy, no. (%)	85 (23%)
Splenic involvement	
Deposits on SAP scintigraphy, no. (%)	370 (99%)
Cardiac involvement	
Cardiac failure, no.	1
Cardiac infiltration, no.	2

Figure 26.9 Characteristics at presentation of 374 patients with systemic secondary (AA) amyloidosis. SAP, serum amyloid P component. *(From reference 29.)*

inflammatory disease. SAA (preferable to C-reactive protein) levels should be monitored monthly and maintained at a target value of less than 4 mg/l.[29]

Amyloid deposits regress in 60% of patients who have a median SAA concentration below 10 mg/l, and survival among these patients is superior to survival when amyloid deposits do not regress. Other factors associated with increased mortality are older age and end-stage renal disease (ESRD).

Eprodisate, a member of a new class of compounds interfering with interactions between amyloidogenic proteins and GAGs and thereby inhibiting polymerization of amyloid fibrils, slowed the decline of renal function in patients with AA amyloidosis.[30] However, eprodisate had no beneficial effect on proteinuria, ESRD, amyloid content of abdominal fat, or risk of death. Although eprodisate may be a promising treatment option for AA amyloidosis, emphasis should remain on treatment of the underlying inflammatory disorder.

Most described patients receiving renal transplantation in AA amyloidosis are those with rheumatic diseases. Amyloid deposits recur in about 10% of the grafts. Infection is the main cause of early death.

Familial Mediterranean Fever and Other Hereditary Recurrent Fever Syndromes

FMF represents a particular type of AA amyloidosis and the most frequent cause of familial amyloidosis. Colchicine has proved to be efficient in its prevention and treatment. FMF is usually transmitted as an autosomal recessive disorder and occurs most commonly in Sephardic Jews and Armenians. It is caused by mutations of the gene (*MEFV*) encoding a protein called pyrin or marenostrin.[31] Clinically, there are two independent phenotypes. In the first, brief, episodic, febrile attacks of peritonitis, pleuritis, or synovitis occur in childhood or adolescence and precede the renal manifestations. In the second, renal symptoms precede and may be the only manifestation of the disease for a long time. The attacks are accompanied by dramatic elevations of acute-phase reactants, including SAA. Amyloid deposits are responsible for severe renal lesions with prominent glomerular involvement, leading to ESRD at a young age, and for early deaths. Colchicine can prevent the development of proteinuria, may occasionally reverse the nephrotic syndrome, and may prevent the glomerular filtration rate (GFR) decline in patients with non-nephrotic proteinuria. It is less effective in preventing progression in patients with nephrotic syndrome or renal impairment. The minimal daily dose of colchicine for prevention of amyloidosis is 1 mg, and patients with clinical evidence of amyloidotic kidney disease should receive daily doses of 1.5 to 2 mg. However, about 10% of patients are unresponsive to colchicine. Interleukin-1 receptor antagonists are second-line agents. In patients with intolerance of colchicine, the drug should be stopped, then reintroduced at lower doses.

The recent identification of genes responsible for syndromes of periodic fever with amyloidosis has opened the way to a molecular diagnosis of hereditary AA amyloidosis. These syndromes include the tumor necrosis factor receptor–associated periodic syndrome, the Muckle-Wells syndrome, and the familial cold autoinflammatory syndrome. Only a few cases of systemic AA amyloidosis have been reported in the hyperimmunoglobulinemia D with periodic fever syndrome.

MONOCLONAL IMMUNOGLOBULIN DEPOSITION DISEASE

History and Definition

It was known from the late 1950s that nonamyloidotic forms of glomerular disease "resembling the lesion of diabetic glomerulosclerosis" could occur in multiple myeloma. Subsequently, monoclonal light chains were detected in these lesions.[32]

In clinical and pathologic terms, light-chain, light- and heavy-chain, and heavy-chain deposition disease (LCDD, LHCDD, and HCDD, respectively) are similar and may therefore be referred to as MIDD. They differ from amyloidosis in that the deposits lack affinity for Congo red and do not have a fibrillar organization. The distinction also relates to different pathophysiology of amyloid, which implicates one-dimensional elongation of a pseudocrystalline structure, and MIDD, which rather involves a one-step precipitation of immunoglobulin chains.

Epidemiology

LCDD is found in 5% of myeloma patients at autopsy, whereas the prevalence of AL amyloidosis is about 11%. LCDD and HCDD may occur in a wide range of ages (28 to 94 years) with a male preponderance (Fig. 26.10). More than 20 patients with HCDD have been described so far, but the disease is most likely underdiagnosed.

Pathogenesis

Light-chain deposition may require light chains with distinct properties that favor deposition in tissues. Various properties

Clinical, Histologic, and Laboratory Features in Patients with Monoclonal Immunoglobulin Deposition Disease

Characteristics	LCDD/LHCDD	HCDD
Male-to-female ratio	1.7	0.8
Age, yr (range)	57 (28–94)	57 (26–79)
Hypertension (%)	53	90
Renal failure (serum creatinine ≥130 μmol/l) (1.47 mg/dl)	93	83
Nephrotic syndrome* (%)	36	46
Hematuria (%)	45	89
Nodular glomerulosclerosis (%)	31–100	96
Multiple myeloma (%)	53	24
Monoclonal protein (blood or urine) (%)	88	58†

Figure 26.10 Clinical, histologic, and laboratory features in patients with monoclonal immunoglobulin deposition disease (MIDD). HCDD, heavy-chain deposition disease; LCDD, light-chain deposition disease; LHCDD, light- and heavy-chain deposition disease. *Proteinuria ≥3 g/day. †Including two cases with only free κ chain.

of light-chain variable domains may contribute to MIDD pathogenesis[33]:

1. Restricted usage of three κ germline genes, with an apparent overrepresentation of the rare $V_{\kappa IV}$ variability subgroup.
2. Size abnormalities of light chains, present in one third of patients.
3. Unusual amino acid substitutions in LCDD light chains may modify the light-chain conformation or be responsible for hydrophobic interactions between V domains or between V domains and extracellular matrix proteins.
4. When pathogenic light chains were absent in serum and urine, they seemed to be *N*-glycosylated, suggesting that glycosylation increases their propensity to precipitate in tissues. However, as in AL amyloidosis, extrinsic conditions may also contribute to aggregation of the light chain. The same light chain can form granular aggregates or amyloid fibrils, depending on the environment, and different partially folded intermediates of the light chain may be responsible for amorphous or fibrillar aggregation pathways.[34]

HCDD may also be associated with unique heavy chains. A deletion of the first constant domain C_H1 was found in deposited or circulating heavy chains in patients with γ-HCDD.[33,35] In the blood, the deleted heavy chain either was associated with light chains or circulated in small amounts as a free unassembled subunit.[36] It is likely that the C_H1 deletion facilitates the secretion of free heavy chains that are rapidly cleared from the circulation by organ deposition. The variable V_H domain also is likely to be required for tissue precipitation.

A striking feature of LCDD and HCDD is extracellular matrix accumulation. Nodules are made of normal matrix constituents. In cultured mesangial cells, LCDD light chains enhance the production of tenascin-C and of profibrotic cytokines, such as transforming growth factor β and platelet-derived growth factor.[37]

Clinical Manifestations

MIDD is a systemic disease with immunoglobulin chain deposition in a variety of organs leading to various clinical manifestations, but visceral immunoglobulin chain deposits may be totally asymptomatic and found only at autopsy.[33]

Renal Manifestations

Renal involvement is a constant feature of MIDD, and renal symptoms, mostly proteinuria and CKD, often dominate the clinical presentation (see Fig. 26.10).[33,35] In 18% to 53% of LCDD patients, albuminuria is associated with the nephrotic syndrome. However, in about one fourth, it is less than 1 g/day, and these patients exhibit mainly a tubulointerstitial syndrome. Albuminuria is not correlated with the presence of nodular glomerulosclerosis, at least initially, and may occur in the absence of significant light microscopic glomerular lesions. Hematuria is more frequent than one would expect for a nephropathy in which cell proliferation is usually modest.

The high prevalence, early appearance, and severity of CKD are other salient features of LCDD. In most cases, GFR declines rapidly, which is a main reason for referral. CKD occurs with comparable frequency in patients with either low or heavy protein excretion and may present in the form of a subacute tubulointerstitial nephritis or a rapidly progressive glomerulonephritis (RPGN), respectively. The prevalence of hypertension is variable, but it must be interpreted according to associated medical history. Renal features of patients with HCDD are basically similar to those seen in LCDD and LHCDD, with a higher prevalence of hypertension and hematuria; extrarenal manifestations are less frequent (see Fig. 26.10).

Extrarenal Manifestations

Liver and cardiac involvement occurs in about 25% of patients with LCDD and LHCDD. Liver deposits are constant. They are either discrete and confined to the sinusoids and basement membranes of biliary ductules without associated parenchymal lesions or massive with marked dilation and multiple ruptures of sinusoids, resembling peliosis. Hepatomegaly with mild alterations of liver function test results is the most common symptom, but patients may also develop life-threatening hepatic insufficiency and portal hypertension.

Cardiac involvement is also frequent and may be responsible for cardiomegaly and severe heart failure. Arrhythmias, conduction disturbances, and congestive heart failure are seen. Echocardiography and catheterization may reveal diastolic dysfunction and reduction in myocardial compliance similar to that found in cardiac amyloid.

Deposits may also occur along the nerve fibers and in the choroid plexus as well as in the lymph nodes, bone marrow, spleen, pancreas, thyroid gland, submandibular glands, adrenal glands, gastrointestinal tract, abdominal vessels, lungs, and skin. They may be responsible for peripheral neuropathy (20% of the reported cases), gastrointestinal disturbances, pulmonary nodules, amyloid-like arthropathy, and sicca syndrome. Extrarenal deposits are less common in patients with HCDD.

Hematologic Findings

Myeloma is diagnosed in about 50% of the patients with LCDD or LHCDD and in about 25% of those with HCDD. MIDD, like AL amyloidosis, is often the presenting disease that leads to the discovery of myeloma at an early stage. MIDD may occasionally complicate Waldenström's macroglobulinemia, chronic

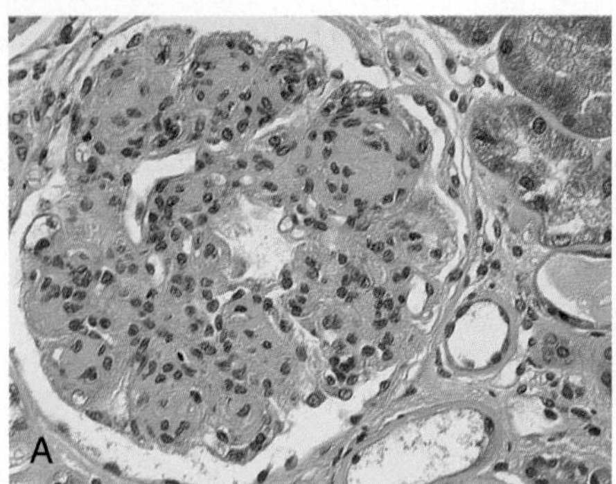

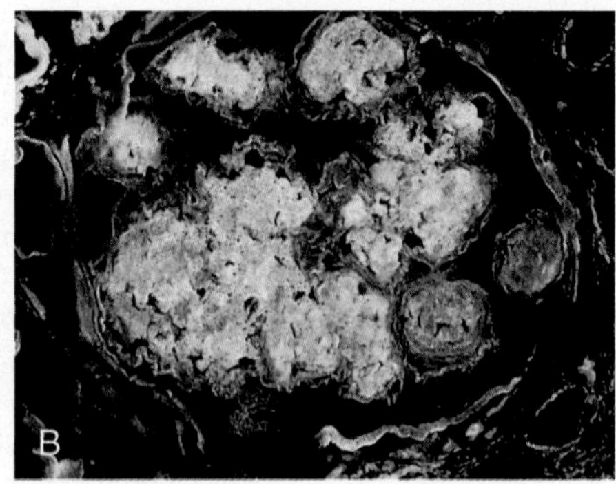

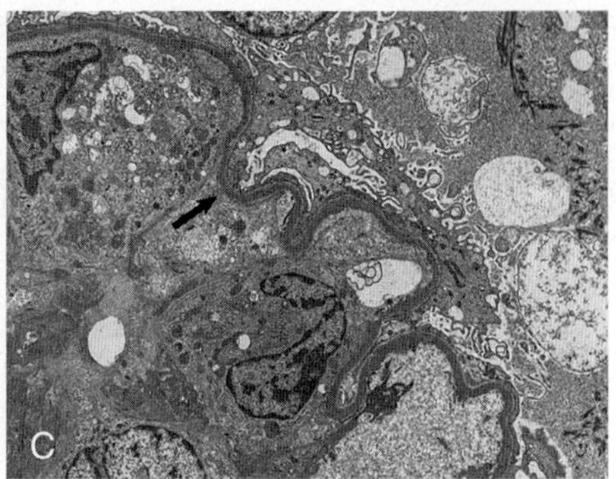

Figure 26.11 Light-chain deposition disease. A, Nodular glomerulosclerosis with mesangial matrix accumulation. (Masson trichrome; magnification ×312.) **B,** Staining of mesangial nodules and tubular basement membranes with anti-κ antibody. (Immunofluorescence; magnification ×312.) **C,** Electron micrograph showing a layer of dense granular deposits *(arrow)* under the endothelium along the glomerular basement membrane (GBM). (Magnification ×2500.) *(Courtesy Dr. Béatrice Mougenot, Paris, France.)*

lymphocytic leukemia, and nodal marginal zone lymphoma. It often occurs in the absence of a detectable malignant process, even after prolonged (>10 years) follow-up. A monoclonal bone marrow plasma cell population is then easily detectable by immunohistologic examination.

Pathology

Light Microscopy

MIDD is not only a glomerular disease, and tubular lesions may be more conspicuous than the glomerular damage. Tubular lesions are characterized by the deposition of a refractile, eosinophilic, periodic acid–Schiff (PAS)–positive, ribbon-like material along the outer part of the tubular basement membrane. The deposits predominate around the distal tubules, the loops of Henle, and, in some instances, the collecting ducts, whose epithelium is flattened and atrophied. Typical myeloma casts are only occasionally seen in pure forms of MIDD. In advanced stages, a marked interstitial fibrosis including refractile deposits is frequently associated with tubular lesions.

Glomerular lesions are heterogeneous. Nodular glomerulosclerosis is the most characteristic (Fig. 26.11A); it is found in 30% to 100% of patients with LCDD. Expansion of the mesangial matrix with nodular glomerulosclerosis characterizes HCDD. Mesangial nodules are composed of PAS-positive, membrane-like material and are often accompanied by mild mesangial hypercellularity. Lesions resemble diabetic nodular glomerulosclerosis. Distinctive characteristics include the following: the distribution of the nodules is fairly regular in a given glomerulus; the nodules are often poorly argyrophilic; and exudative lesions such as fibrin caps and extensive hyalinosis of the efferent arterioles are not observed. In occasional cases with prominent endocapillary cellularity and mesangial interposition, the glomerular features mimic membranoproliferative glomerulonephritis (MPGN). Milder forms of LCDD show increased mesangial matrix or cells and a modest basement membrane thickening, with abnormal brightness and rigidity. Glomerular lesions may be detectable only by immunostaining or ultrastructural examination in early stages or if they are induced by light chains with a weak pathogenic potential.

Arteries, arterioles, and peritubular capillaries all may contain PAS-positive deposits in close contact with their basement membranes. Deposits do not show the staining characteristics of amyloid, but Congo red–positive amyloid deposits co-occur in approximately 10% of patients.[35]

Immunohistology

Immunohistology is central in the diagnosis of the various forms of MIDD. A criterion required for the diagnosis of MIDD is monotypic light-chain (mostly κ; Fig. 26.11B) or heavy-chain fixation along tubular basement membranes. The tubular deposits stain strongly (see Fig. 26.11B) and predominate along the loops of Henle and the distal tubules, but they also often are detected along the proximal tubules. In contrast, glomerular immunohistology patterns display marked heterogeneity. In patients with nodular glomerulosclerosis, deposits of monotypic immunoglobulin chains are usually found along the peripheral GBM and, to a lesser extent, in the nodules themselves (Fig. 26.11B). Glomerular staining is typically weaker than that observed along the tubular basement membranes. This may not relate to the actual amount of deposited material because glomerular immunohistology may be negative despite prominent granular glomerular deposits observed by electron microscopy. Local modifications of deposited light chains thus might change their antigenicity. In patients without nodular lesions, glomerular staining occurs along the basement membrane and less frequently in the mesangium. A linear staining usually decorates Bowman's capsule. Deposits are frequent in vascular walls and interstitium.

In patients with HCDD, immunohistology with anti–light-chain antibodies is negative despite typical nodular glomerulosclerosis. Monotypic deposits of γ, α, or μ heavy chains may be identified. Any γ subclass may be observed. Analysis of the kidney biopsy specimen with monoclonal antibodies specific for the constant domains of the γ heavy chain allowed identification of a deletion of the C_H1 domain in all tested cases. In most cases of HCDD, especially when a γ1 or γ3 chain is involved, complement components including C1 could be demonstrated in a granular or pseudolinear pattern. Complement deposits were often associated with signs of complement activation in serum.[38]

Electron Microscopy

The most characteristic ultrastructural features are finely to coarsely granular electron-dense deposits along the outer (interstitial) aspect of the tubular basement membranes. In the glomerulus, they predominate in a subendothelial position along the GBM and are located mainly along and in the lamina rara interna (Fig. 26.11C). They can also be found in mesangial nodules, Bowman's capsule, and the wall of small arteries between the myocytes. Nonamyloid fibrils have been reported in a few patients with LCDD or HCDD.

Diagnosis

The diagnosis of MIDD must be suspected in any patient with the nephrotic syndrome or rapidly progressive tubulointerstitial nephritis or with echocardiographic findings indicating diastolic dysfunction and the presence of a monoclonal immunoglobulin component in the serum or the urine (see Fig 26.8). The same combination is also seen in AL amyloidosis, but AL amyloidosis is more often associated with the λ light-chain isotype. Because sensitive techniques including immunofixation fail to identify a monoclonal immunoglobulin component in 10% to 20% of patients with LCDD or LHCDD and about 40% of patients with HCDD (see Fig. 26.10), renal biopsy plays an essential role in the diagnosis of MIDD and the associated dysproteinemia.

The definitive diagnosis is made by the immunohistologic analysis of tissue from an affected organ, in most cases the kidney, with use of a panel of immunoglobulin chain–specific antibodies, including anti-κ and anti-λ light-chain antibodies to stain the non-congophilic deposits. When the biopsy specimen stains for a single heavy-chain isotype and does not stain for light-chain isotypes, the diagnosis of HCDD should be suspected.

The diagnosis of the plasma cell dyscrasia relies on bone marrow aspiration and bone marrow biopsy with cell morphologic evaluation and, if necessary, immunophenotyping with anti-κ and anti-λ antisera to demonstrate monoclonality.

Outcome

The outcome of MIDD remains uncertain, mainly because extrarenal deposits of light chains can be totally asymptomatic or cause severe organ damage leading to death. Survival from onset of symptoms varies from 1 month to 10 years. In the largest series of LCDD patients,[39] 36 of the 63 patients reached uremia, 37 of those patients died during follow-up, and patient survival was 66% at 1 year and 31% at 8 years, although most were treated by chemotherapy. By multivariate analysis, the only variables independently associated with renal survival were age and degree of chronic kidney disease (CKD) at presentation[39] or the time of renal biopsy.[35] Those variables independently associated with a worse patient survival were age, initial creatinine level, associated multiple myeloma, and extrarenal light-chain deposition.[33,37] Survival of the patients treated with dialysis was not different from that of the patients not reaching ESRD. Renal and patient survivals were significantly better in patients with pure MIDD (mean, 22 and 54 months, respectively) compared with those who presented with cast nephropathy (mean, 4 and 22 months, respectively).[35]

Treatment

As in AL amyloidosis, treatment should be aimed at reducing immunoglobulin production. Clearance of the light-chain deposits has been demonstrated in a few patients after intensive chemotherapy with syngeneic bone marrow transplantation or blood stem cell autografting. Nodular mesangial lesions and light-chain deposits are reversible, also disappearing after long-term chemotherapy.

In a retrospective study of 11 LHCDD patients (younger than 65 years) treated by high-dose therapy with the support of autologous blood stem cell transplantation, no treatment-related death occurred.[40] A decrease in the monoclonal immunoglobulin level was observed in eight patients, with complete disappearance from serum and urine in six cases. Clinical improvement was observed in six patients, and histologic regression was documented in cardiac, hepatic, and skin biopsy specimens. These results were confirmed in two small North American series.[41,42] Reversal of dialysis dependency and sustained improvement in renal function were also occasionally noted. Whether high-dose chemotherapy with blood stem cell transplantation provides benefits compared with conventional chemotherapy including high-dose dexamethasone, with or without bortezomib, remains to be established.

As with AL amyloidosis, monitoring of light-chain production should rely on serum free light-chain assay, particularly when a blood or urine monoclonal component cannot be detected by conventional methods.

Kidney transplantation in a few patients with MIDD usually led to recurrence of the disease and should therefore not be performed in LCDD patients unless measures have been taken to reduce light-chain production.[43]

Renal Diseases Associated with Monoclonal Immunoglobulin Deposition Disease

Myeloma Cast Nephropathy

The association of monoclonal light chain deposits, mostly along renal tubular basement membranes, with typical myeloma cast nephropathy is more frequent than reported initially. It was found in 11 of 34 patients with MIDD.[35] Nodular glomerulosclerosis is, however, infrequent (<10%), and some ribbon-like tubular basement membranes are seen in less than half of the patients. In addition, one third of the patients do not have granular dense deposits on electron microscopy.

AL Amyloidosis

Amyloid deposits are found in one or more organs in about 7% of LCDD patients. Because amyloid deposits are focal, their true incidence may be markedly underestimated. Although this association may result from peculiar light chains endowed with intrinsic properties that make them prone to form both fibrillar and nonfibrillar deposits, depending on the environment,[34] one cannot exclude the possibility that the coexisting diseases are induced by different variant clones.

NONAMYLOID FIBRILLARY AND IMMUNOTACTOID GLOMERULOPATHIES

Definition

Fibrillary and immunotactoid glomerulopathies are characterized, respectively, by fibrillar and microtubular deposits in the mesangium and the glomerular capillary loops (Fig. 26.12). These deposits do not have an amyloid-like cross-β structure and are readily distinguishable from amyloid by the larger thickness of fibrils and lack of Congo red staining. Whether fibrillary and immunotactoid glomerulopathies are totally distinct entities is debated. Some use immunotactoid glomerulopathy as a unifying term for glomerular deposition of either amyloid-like fibrils (12 to 22 nm) or larger microtubules (>30 nm) in patients for whom an associated systemic disease, including cryoglobulinemia and lymphoproliferative disorders, has been excluded.[44] For others, the distinction between nonamyloid fibrillary and immunotactoid glomerulopathy may be of great clinical and pathophysiologic interest in the context of plasma cell dyscrasias (see Fig. 26.12).[45-48]

Epidemiology

The incidence of glomerulopathy with nonamyloid deposition of fibrillar or microtubular material in a nontransplant adult biopsy population is estimated at around 1%. It is most likely underestimated because of the insufficient attention given to atypical reactions with histochemical amyloid stains and the frequent lack of immuno-ultrastructural studies.

Clinical Manifestations

The characteristics of fibrillary and immunotactoid glomerulopathies are described in Figure 26.12 in comparison to AL amyloidosis. Patients with immunotactoid and fibrillary glomerulopathies have a mean age of 55 to 60 years (extreme: 19 to 86 years). They usually present with the nephrotic syndrome, microscopic hematuria, and mild to severe CKD. In most recent series,[47,48] there was no significant difference between immunotactoid and fibrillary glomerulopathy patients in serum creatinine level, incidence of nephrotic syndrome, microscopic hematuria, hypertension, and CKD. Extrarenal manifestations are uncommon and may involve the lung, skin, and peripheral nervous system.

Pathology

Immunotactoid Glomerulopathy

Renal biopsy shows MN (often associated with segmental mesangial proliferation; Fig. 26.13) or lobular MPGN. Granular deposits of IgG and C3 are observed along capillary basement membranes and in mesangial areas. In a series of 23 patients in which diagnosis was based on ultrastructural appearance of the deposits, IgG deposits were monotypic in 13 of 14 patients with immunotactoid glomerulopathy (κ, seven cases; λ, six cases) and

Immunologic and Clinical Characteristics of Fibrillary and Immunotactoid Glomerulopathies

Characteristics	Amyloidosis (AL Type)	Fibrillary Glomerulopathy	Immunotactoid Glomerulopathy
Congo red staining	Yes	No	No
Composition	Fibrils	Fibrils	Microtubules
Fibril or microtubule size	8–15 nm	12–22 nm	>30 nm*
Organization in tissues	Random (β-pleated sheet)	Random	Parallel arrays
Immunoglobulin deposition	Monoclonal LC (mostly λ)	Usually polyclonal (mostly IgG4), occasionally monoclonal (IgG1, IgG4)	Usually monoclonal (IgGκ or IgGλ)
Glomerular lesions	Deposits spreading from the mesangium	MPGN, CGN, MP	Atypical MN, MPGN
Renal presentation	Severe NS, absence of hypertension and hematuria	NS with hematuria, hypertension; RPGN	NS with microhematuria and hypertension
Extrarenal manifestations (fibrillar deposits)	Systemic deposition disease	Pulmonary hemorrhage	Microtubular inclusions in leukemic lymphocytes
Association with LPD	Yes (myeloma)	Uncommon	Common (CLL, NHL, MGUS)
Treatment	Melphalan + dexamethasone; intensive therapy with blood stem cell autograft	Corticosteroids ± cyclophosphamide (crescentic GN)	Treatment of the associated LPD

Figure 26.12 Immunologic and clinical characteristics of fibrillary and immunotactoid glomerulopathies. CGN, crescentic glomerulonephritis; CLL, chronic lymphocytic leukemia; GN, glomerulonephritis; LC, light chain; LPD, lymphoproliferative disorder; MGUS, monoclonal gammopathy of undetermined significance; MN, membranous nephropathy; MP, mesangial proliferation; MPGN, membranoproliferative glomerulonephritis; NHL, non-Hodgkin's lymphoma; NS, nephrotic syndrome; RPGN, rapidly progressive glomerulonephritis. *Mean diameter of the substructures did not differ between fibrillary glomerulonephritis (15.8 ± 3.5 nm) and immunotactoid glomerulopathy (15.2 ± 7.3 nm) in the series of Bridoux and colleagues.[47]

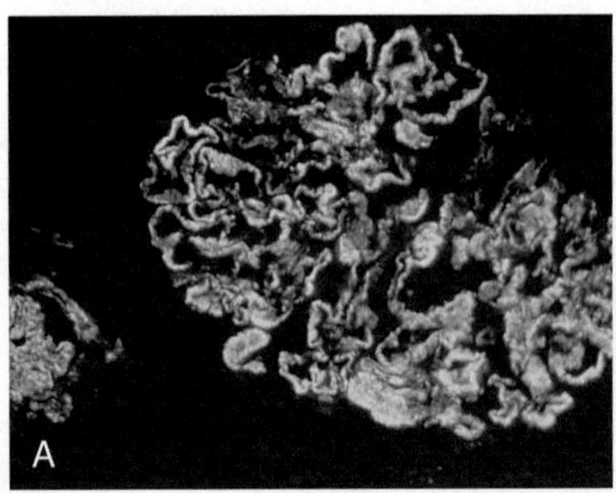

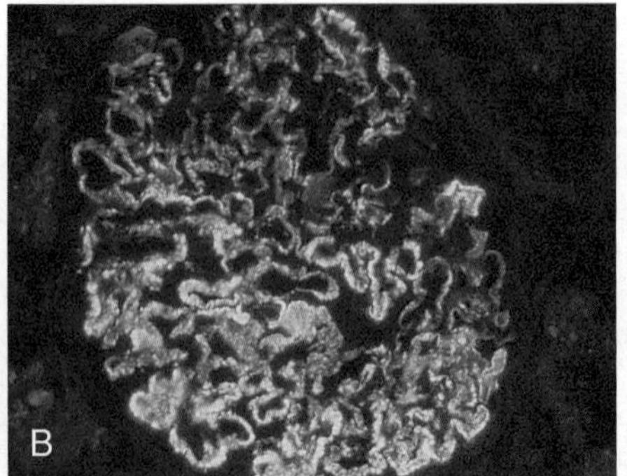

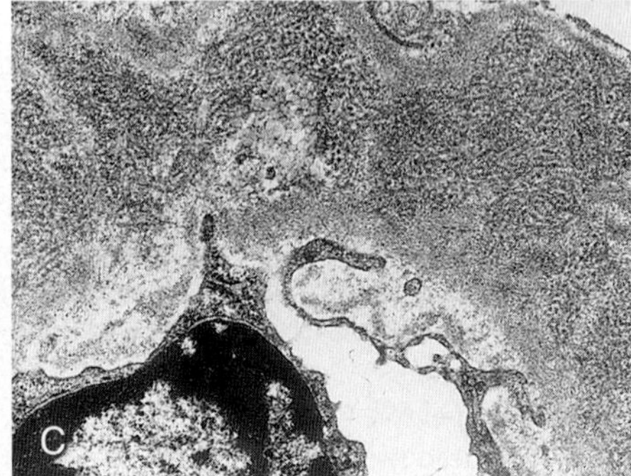

Figure 26.13 Immunotactoid glomerulopathy. Atypical membranous nephropathy showing exclusive staining of the deposits with anti-γ **A,** and anti-κ **B,** antibodies. (Immunofluorescence; magnification ×312.) **C,** Electron micrograph of glomerular basement membrane (GBM) showing microtubular structure of the subepithelial deposits. (Uranyl acetate and lead citrate; magnification ×20,000.) *(Courtesy Dr. Béatrice Mougenot, Paris, France.)*

in only one of nine patients with fibrillary glomerulopathy.[47] A circulating monoclonal immunoglobulin was detected in only six of the 14 patients with immunotactoid glomerulopathy. On electron microscopy, the distinguishing morphologic features of immunotactoid glomerulopathy are organized deposits of large, thick-walled microtubules (typically >30 nm in diameter), at times arranged in parallel arrays (Fig. 26.13C).

Of 14 patients with immunotactoid glomerulopathy,[47] six had chronic lymphocytic leukemia, one had a small lymphocytic B-cell lymphoma, and three had MGUS. Intracytoplasmic crystal-like immunoglobulin inclusions were found in four patients with chronic lymphocytic leukemia and in the lymphoma patient.[47] They showed the same microtubular organization and contained the same IgG subclass and light-chain isotype as renal deposits.

Fibrillary Glomerulopathy

Mesangial proliferation and aspects of MPGN are predominantly reported in series of fibrillary glomerulopathy. Glomerular crescents are present in about 30% of the biopsy specimens. Immunofluorescence studies mainly show IgG deposits of the γ4 isotype with a predominant mesangial localization. Monotypic deposits containing mostly IgGκ are detected in no more than 15% of patients. On electron microscopy, fibrils are randomly arranged, and their diameter varies between 12 and 22 nm. The fibril size alone is not sufficient to distinguish nonamyloidotic fibrillary GN from amyloid.[47]

Diagnosis

Diagnosis of immunotactoid and fibrillary glomerulopathies relies on electron microscopy, which must be performed in patients with atypical MN or MPGN as well as in those with monotypic deposits in glomeruli. Renal biopsy specimens from such patients with glomerular disease should be routinely examined with anti-κ and anti-λ light-chain antibodies. In patients with immunotactoid glomerulopathy, lymphoproliferative disease should be searched for. Association of immunotactoid and fibrillary glomerulopathy with hepatitis C or human immunodeficiency virus infection has also been reported.

Outcome and Treatment

Patients with fibrillary glomerulopathy usually respond poorly to corticosteroids and cytotoxic drugs, with an incidence of ESRD of 50%. Preliminary reports suggest that they may respond to rituximab.[49] By contrast, in patients with immunotactoid glomerulopathy, corticosteroids and chemotherapy were associated with partial or complete remission of the nephrotic syndrome in most cases, with a parallel improvement of the hematologic parameters.[47] Patient survival was found to be similar in both types of glomerulopathies, although the incidence of CKD and ESRD tended to be lower in the immunotactoid glomerulopathy group.[47] Renal transplantation has been performed in a few patients. Disease recurred in several, especially in those with a persistent monoclonal gammopathy.[50]

GLOMERULAR LESIONS ASSOCIATED WITH WALDENSTRÖM'S MACROGLOBULINEMIA

Symptomatic renal disease is much less common than in multiple myeloma. GN with intracapillary thrombi of aggregated IgM (intracapillary monoclonal deposit disease) is the most frequent renal morphologic finding, but it has become rare, probably because of increased efficacy of chemotherapy. This entity may also occur with other IgM-secreting monoclonal proliferations.[51] It is associated with variable degrees of proteinuria and altered renal function. It is characterized by PAS-positive, Congo red–negative intracapillary deposits, sometimes voluminous enough to occlude capillary lumina. By immunohistology, thrombi and deposits stain with anti-μ and with anti-κ. The deposits are electron dense and granular without any microtubular organization.[49] Some of these patients have strong activation of the classical complement pathway with or without cryoglobulinemia. Other patients have MPGN with a bright μ and κ staining along the glomerular capillaries, without cryoglobulinemia. Renal manifestations usually improve under chemotherapy. Renal amyloidosis (mostly AL) is uncommon but should be suspected in patients presenting with massive proteinuria. Because renal biopsy may be hazardous in patients with Waldenström's macroglobulinemia, who frequently have increased bleeding time, it is wise to search for amyloid deposits first by a less invasive tissue biopsy. Hematopoietic stem cell transplantation and purine analogues may represent the most effective therapies.[16]

OTHER TYPES OF GLOMERULONEPHRITIS

In some patients, glomerular deposition of monoclonal IgG can produce a proliferative GN that mimics immune complex GN on light and electron microscopy.[52] Proper recognition of this entity requires confirmation of monoclonality by immunostaining for the γ heavy chain subclasses. Tissue fixation of complement was observed in 90% of cases, and 40% of patients had hypocomplementemia. Clinical presentation included CKD in 80%, proteinuria in 100%, nephrotic syndrome in 44%, and microhematuria in 60%. A monoclonal serum protein with the same heavy- and light-chain isotype as that of the glomerular deposits was identified in 50% of cases. No patient had overt myeloma or lymphoma at presentation or during the course of follow-up.

REFERENCES

1. Glenner GG. Amyloid deposits and amyloidosis: The beta-fibrilloses. *N Engl J Med.* 1980;302:1283-1292.
2. Westermark P, Benson MD, Buxbaum JN, et al. Amyloid: Toward terminology clarification. Report from the Nomenclature Committee of the International Society of Amyloidosis. *Amyloid.* 2005;12:1-4.
3. Merlini G, Bellotti V. Molecular mechanisms of amyloidosis. *N Engl J Med.* 2003;349:583-596.
4. Lachmann HJ, Booth DR, Booth SE, et al. Misdiagnosis of hereditary amyloidosis as AL (primary) amyloidosis. *N Engl J Med.* 2002;346:1786-1791.
5. Westermark G, Benson MD, Buxbaum JN, et al. Amyloid fibril protein nomenclature. *Amyloid.* 2002;9:197-200.
6. Merlini G, Bellotti V. Molecular mechanisms of amyloidosis. *N Engl J Med.* 2003;349:583-596.
7. Eulitz M, Weiss DT, Solomon A. Immunoglobulin heavy-chain-associated amyloidosis. *Proc Natl Acad Sci USA.* 1990;87:6542-6546.
8. Stevens FJ. Four structural risk factors identify most fibril-forming kappa light chains. *Amyloid.* 2000;7:200-211.
9. Enqvist S, Sletten K, Stevens FJ, et al. Germ line origin and somatic mutations determine the target tissues in systemic AL-amyloidosis. *PLoS ONE.* 2007;2:e981.
10. Comenzo RL, Zhang Y, Martinez C, et al. The tropism of organ involvement in primary systemic amyloidosis: Contributions of Ig V_L germ line gene use and clonal plasma cell burden. *Blood.* 2001;98:714-720.
11. Keeling J, Teng J, Herrera GA. AL-amyloidosis and light-chain deposition disease light chains induce divergent phenotypic transformations of human mesangial cells. *Lab Invest.* 2004;84:1322-1338.

12. Kyle RA, Gertz MA. Primary systemic amyloidosis: Clinical and laboratory features in 474 cases. *Semin Hematol.* 1995;32:45-59.
13. Kyle RA, Greipp PR. Amyloidosis (AL): Clinical and laboratory features in 229 cases. *Mayo Clin Proc.* 1983;58:665-683.
14. Katzmann JA, Abraham RS, Dispenzieri A, et al. Diagnostic performance of quantitative kappa and lambda free light chain assays in clinical practice. *Clin Chem.* 2005;51:878-881.
15. Wechalekar AD, Lachmann HJ, Goodman HJ, et al. AL amyloidosis associated with IgM paraproteinemia: Clinical profile and treatment outcome. *Blood.* 2008;112:4009-4016.
16. Terrier B, Jaccard A, Harousseau JL, et al. The clinical spectrum of IgM-related amyloidosis: A French nationwide retrospective study of 72 patients. *Medicine (Baltimore).* 2008;87:99-109.
17. Lachmann HJ, Gallimore R, Gillmore JD, et al. Outcome in systemic AL amyloidosis in relation to changes in concentration of circulating free immunoglobulin light chains following chemotherapy. *Br J Haematol.* 2003;122:78-84.
18. Gertz MA, Comenzo R, Falk RH, et al. Definition of organ involvement and treatment response in immunoglobulin light chain amyloidosis (AL): A consensus opinion from the 10th International Symposium on Amyloid and Amyloidosis. *Am J Hematol.* 2005;79:319-328.
19. Kyle RA, Gertz MA, Greipp PR, et al. A trial of three regimens for primary amyloidosis: Colchicine alone, melphalan and prednisone, and melphalan, prednisone, and colchicine. *N Engl J Med.* 1997;336:1202-1207.
20. Comenzo RL, Vosburgh E, Falk RH, et al. Dose-intensive melphalan with blood stem-cell support for the treatment of AL (amyloid light-chain) amyloidosis: Survival and responses in 25 patients. *Blood.* 1998;91:3662-3670.
21. Dember LM, Sanchorawala V, Seldin DC, et al. Effect of dose-intensive intravenous melphalan and autologous blood stem-cell transplantation on AL amyloidosis–associated renal disease. *Ann Intern Med.* 2001;134:746-753.
22. Skinner M, Sanchorawala V, Seldin DC, et al. High-dose melphalan and autologous stem-cell transplantation in patients with AL amyloidosis: An 8-year study. *Ann Intern Med.* 2004;140:85-93.
23. Leung N, Dispenzieri A, Fervenza FC, et al. Renal response after high-dose melphalan and stem cell transplantation is a favorable marker in patients with primary systemic amyloidosis. *Am J Kidney Dis.* 2005;46:270-277.
24. Palladini G, Perfetti V, Obici L, et al. Association of melphalan and high-dose dexamethasone is effective and well tolerated in patients with AL (primary) amyloidosis who are ineligible for stem cell transplantation. *Blood.* 2004;103:2936-2938.
25. Jaccard A, Moreau P, Leblond V, et al. High-dose melphalan versus melphalan plus dexamethasone for AL amyloidosis. *N Engl J Med.* 2007;357:1083-1093.
26. Sanchorawala V. Light-chain (AL) amyloidosis: Diagnosis and treatment. *Clin J Am Soc Nephrol.* 2006;1:1331-1341.
27. Bollée G, Guery B, Joly D, et al. Presentation and outcome of patients with systemic amyloidosis undergoing dialysis. *Clin J Am Soc Nephrol.* 2008;3:375-381.
28. Gertz MA, Kyle RA, O'Fallon WM. Dialysis support of patients with primary systemic amyloidosis. A study of 211 patients. *Arch Intern Med.* 1992;152:2245-2250.
29. Lachmann HJ, Goodman HJ, Gilbertson JA, et al. Natural history and outcome in systemic AA amyloidosis. *N Engl J Med.* 2007;356:2361-2371.
30. Dember LM, Hawkins PN, Hazenberg BP, et al. Eprodisate for AA Amyloidosis Trial Group. Eprodisate for the treatment of renal disease in AA amyloidosis. *N Engl J Med.* 2007;356:2349-2360.
31. Dode C, Pecheux C, Cazeneuve C, et al. Mutations in the MEFV gene in a large series of patients with a clinical diagnosis of familial Mediterranean fever. *Am J Med Genet.* 2000;92:241-246.
32. Randall RE, Williamson WC Jr, Mullinax F, et al. Manifestations of systemic light chain deposition. *Am J Med.* 1976;60:293-299.
33. Ronco P, Plaisier E, Mougenot B, et al. Immunoglobulin light (heavy)–chain deposition disease: From molecular medicine to pathophysiology-driven therapy. *Clin J Am Soc Nephrol.* 2006;1:1342-1350.
34. Khurana R, Gillespie JR, Talapatra A, et al. Partially folded intermediates as critical precursors of light chain amyloid fibrils and amorphous aggregates. *Biochemistry.* 2001;40:3525-3535.
35. Lin J, Markowitz GS, Valeri AM, et al. Renal monoclonal immunoglobulin deposition disease: The disease spectrum. *J Am Soc Nephrol.* 2001;12:1482-1492.
36. Moulin B, Deret S, Mariette X, et al. Nodular glomerulosclerosis with deposition of monoclonal immunoglobulin heavy chains lacking C_H1. *J Am Soc Nephrol.* 1999;10:519-528.
37. Keeling J, Herrera GA. An in vitro model of light chain deposition disease. *Kidney Int.* 2009;75:634-645.
38. Kambham N, Markowitz GS, Appel GB, et al. Heavy chain deposition disease: The disease spectrum. *Am J Kidney Dis.* 1999;33:954-962.
39. Pozzi C, D'Amico M, Fogazzi GB, et al. Light chain deposition disease with renal involvement: Clinical characteristics and prognostic factors. *Am J Kidney Dis.* 2003;42:1154-1163.
40. Royer B, Arnulf B, Martinez F, et al. High dose chemotherapy in light chain or light and heavy chain deposition disease. *Kidney Int.* 2004;65:642-648.
41. Hassoun H, Flombaum C, D'Agati VD, et al. High-dose melphalan and auto-SCT in patients with monoclonal Ig deposition disease. *Bone Marrow Transplant.* 2008;42:405-412.
42. Lorenz EC, Gertz MA, Fervenza FC, et al. Long-term outcome of autologous stem cell transplantation in light chain deposition disease. *Nephrol Dial Transplant.* 2008;23:2052-2057.
43. Leung N, Lager DJ, Gertz MA, et al. Long-term outcome of renal transplantation in light-chain deposition disease. *Am J Kidney Dis.* 2004;43:147-153.
44. Korbet SM, Schwartz MM, Lewis EJ. Current concepts in renal pathology. The fibrillary glomerulopathies. *Am J Kidney Dis.* 1994;23:751-765.
45. Fogo A, Qureshi N, Horn RG. Morphologic and clinical features of fibrillary glomerulonephritis versus immunotactoid glomerulopathy. *Am J Kidney Dis.* 1993;22:367-377.
46. Alpers CE. Immunotactoid (microtubular) glomerulopathy: An entity distinct from fibrillary glomerulonephritis. *Am J Kidney Dis.* 1992;19:185-191.
47. Bridoux F, Hugue V, Coldefy O, et al. Fibrillary glomerulonephritis and immunotactoid (microtubular) glomerulopathy are associated with distinct immunologic features. *Kidney Int.* 2002;62:1764-1775.
48. Rosenstock JL, Markowitz GS, Valeri AM, et al. Fibrillary and immunotactoid glomerulonephritis: Distinct entities with different clinical and pathologic features. *Kidney Int.* 2003;63:1450-1461.
49. Collins M, Navaneethan SD, Chung M, et al. Rituximab treatment of fibrillary glomerulonephritis. *Am J Kidney Dis.* 2008;52:1158-1162.
50. Czarnecki PG, Lager DJ, Leung N, et al. Long-term outcome of kidney transplantation in patients with fibrillary glomerulonephritis or monoclonal gammopathy with fibrillary deposits. *Kidney Int.* 2009;75:420-427.
51. Audard V, Georges B, Vanhille P, et al. Renal lesions associated with IgM-secreting monoclonal proliferations: Revisiting the disease spectrum. *Clin J Am Soc Nephrol.* 2008;3:1339-1349.
52. Nasr SH, Satoskar A, Markowitz GS, et al. Proliferative glomerulonephritis with monoclonal IgG deposits. *J Am Soc Nephrol.* 2009;20:2055-2064.

CHAPTER 27

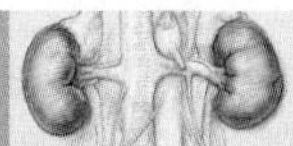

Other Glomerular Disorders and Antiphospholipid Syndrome

Richard J. Glassock

This chapter provides a description of several glomerular and vascular diseases, not necessarily related to each other. Each disorder must be recognized and differentiated from other more common glomerular disorders to estimate the prognosis, to determine whether a familial disorder is present, to plan appropriate therapy, or to determine the risk of a recurrence in the transplanted kidney.

MESANGIAL PROLIFERATIVE GLOMERULONEPHRITIS WITHOUT IgA DEPOSITS

Mesangial proliferative glomerulonephritis (MesPGN) encompasses a heterogeneous collection of disorders of diverse and largely unknown etiology and pathogenesis that have in common a histologic pattern by light microscopy of glomerular injury characterized by mesangial proliferation (Fig. 27.1).[1-3] MesPGN is noted for a diffuse and global increase in mesangial cells, often accompanied by an increase in mesangial matrix. Other cells (e.g., monocytes) may also contribute to the hypercellularity.

For the purpose of this discussion, other forms of cellular proliferation that occur within the mesangial zones but are more focally and segmentally distributed are not included. These focal and segmental forms of proliferative glomerulonephritis (GN) (often accompanied by areas of segmental necrosis of the glomerular tufts and very localized crescents) may be a part of the evolutionary stages of an initially pure MesPGN, but they very often signify the presence of systemic disease processes, including systemic lupus erythematosus (SLE), Henoch-Schönlein purpura and IgA nephropathy, infective endocarditis, microscopic polyangiitis, Wegener's granulomatosis, Goodpasture's disease, rheumatoid vasculitis, and mixed connective tissue disease. On occasion, a lesion of focal and segmental proliferative GN is discovered in the absence of any recognizable multisystem disease process and in the absence of IgA deposits (i.e., idiopathic focal and segmental proliferative GN). Such patients have a clinical presentation, course, and response to treatment that are similar to those described for pure MesPGN, but they are not discussed further in this section.

In "pure" MesPGN, the peripheral capillary walls are thin and delicate without obvious deposits, reduplication, focal disruptions, or cellular necrosis. The visceral and parietal epithelial cells, although occasionally enlarged, have not undergone proliferation. Crescents and segmental sclerosis should be absent in the pure disease. In addition, large deposits staining with periodic acid–Schiff or fuchsin in the mesangium should be absent, as they suggest IgA nephropathy (see Chapter 22) or lupus nephritis (see Chapter 25). The tubulointerstitium and vasculature are usually normal, unless reduced renal function or hypertension is present or the patient is of advanced age.

On immunofluorescence microscopy, a wide variety of patterns are observed (Fig. 27.2). Most commonly, diffuse and global IgM and C3 deposits are found scattered diffusely throughout the mesangium in a granular pattern (so-called IgM nephropathy), but isolated C3, C1q, or even IgG deposits may also be seen.[4] If IgA is the predominant immunoglobulin deposited, the diagnosis is IgA nephropathy. Not uncommonly, no immunoglobulin deposits are found at all.

On electron microscopy, the number of mesangial cells is increased, with an occasional infiltrating monocyte or polymorphonuclear leukocyte. The amount of mesangial matrix is commonly diffusely increased. Electron-dense deposits within the mesangium can be seen in many cases, particularly those with immunoglobulin (IgG, IgM, or IgA) deposits on immunofluorescence microscopy. Very large mesangial or paramesangial electron-dense deposits suggest IgA nephropathy even if immunofluorescence microscopy is not available. Subendothelial and subepithelial deposits are not seen. If present, they suggest a postinfectious etiology or underlying lupus nephritis. Deposits of multiple immunoglobulin classes identified by immunohistology and large numbers of tubuloreticular inclusions on electron microscopy suggest underlying lupus nephritis.

The clinical presentation of MesPGN is varied, although persistent or recurring microscopic or macroscopic hematuria with mild proteinuria is most common. Nephrotic syndrome with heavy proteinuria is a less frequent initial presentation but is seen more frequently in association with diffuse mesangial IgM deposits (IgM nephropathy)[2] or C1q deposits (C1q nephropathy).[4,5] Pure MesPGN is a rather uncommon lesion (<5%) in patients diagnosed with idiopathic nephrotic syndrome.[2,3] Renal function and blood pressure are usually normal, at least initially. Serologic studies are generally unrewarding. Serum C3 and C4 complement components and hemolytic complement activity (CH50) are normal. Assay results for antinuclear antibody (ANA), antineutrophil cytoplasmic autoantibody (ANCA), anti–glomerular basement membrane (anti-GBM) autoantibody, and cryoimmunoglobulins are negative. Nevertheless, these studies should be performed in most patients to exclude known causes. MesPGN can also be a finding in resolving postinfectious (poststreptococcal) GN. Isolated C3 deposits with scanty subendothelial or subepithelial (hump-like) deposits on electron microscopy may be seen in this situation.

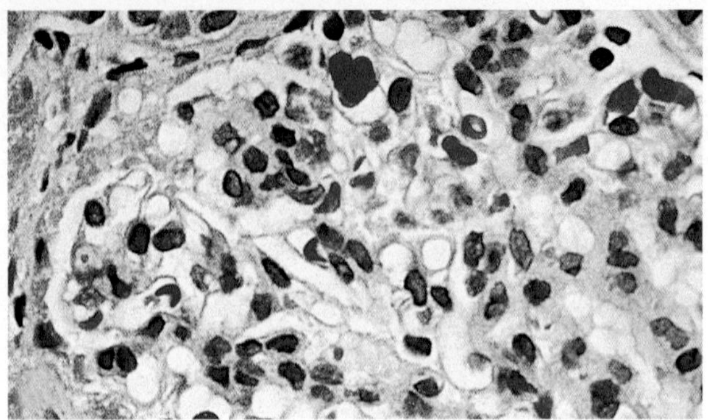

Figure 27.1 Pure mesangial proliferative glomerulonephritis (MesPGN). Note the increase in mesangial cellularity, the delicate peripheral capillary walls, and the absence of sclerosis or parietal epithelial cell proliferation. (Hematoxylin-eosin; magnification ×410.) *(Modified from reference 1.)*

Immunofluorescence Microscopy Patterns in Mesangial Proliferative Glomerulonephritis

Pattern	Associated Disorders
Predominantly mesangial IgA deposits	IgA nephropathy (± IgM, C3)
Predominantly mesangial IgG deposits	Often associated with systemic lupus (± IgM, C3)
Predominantly mesangial IgM deposits	IgM nephropathy (± C3)
Mesangial C1q deposits	C1q nephropathy (± IgG, IgM, C3)
Isolated mesangial C3 deposits	Often associated with resolving poststreptococcal GN
Negative for immunoglobulin or complement deposits	Idiopathic MesPGN

Figure 27.2 Immunofluorescence microscopy patterns in mesangial proliferative glomerulonephritis (MesPGN).

IgM Nephropathy

IgM nephropathy[2] is characterized by diffuse and generalized glomerular deposits of IgM often accompanied by C3. Mesangial electron-dense deposits are also observed. On light microscopy, a picture of pure MesPGN is observed. Patients may present with recurring macroscopic hematuria and proteinuria, the latter in the nephrotic range in as many as 50% of patients. Persisting abnormalities and a poor response to corticosteroids or immunosuppressive therapy are often seen. As many as 50% of patients will eventually progress to typical focal and segmental glomerulosclerosis and, if unresponsive to corticosteroids, will slowly develop chronic kidney disease (CKD) and end-stage renal disease (ESRD). The etiology and pathogenesis are unknown.

C1q Nephropathy

C1q nephropathy is characterized by diffuse deposits of C1q, often accompanied by IgG, IgM, or both.[4,5] C3 deposits are observed less frequently. These immunopathologic features resemble those seen in lupus nephritis; however, these patients have none of the clinical features of SLE and do not develop SLE even after prolonged follow-up.[5] In addition to MesPGN, other morphologic lesions, including focal and segmental glomerulosclerosis, are commonly observed by light microscopy. Nephrotic-range proteinuria, often with hematuria, is observed. Males predominate, and African Americans are commonly affected. Serum C3 components, ANA, and anti–double-stranded DNA antibodies are consistently normal or negative. The response to treatment is poor, and progression to ESRD may occur. The existence of both entities, that is, IgM nephropathy and C1q nephropathy, is disputed by some renal pathologists.

Mesangial Proliferative Glomerulonephritis Associated with Minimal Change Disease

MesPGN may also be a part of the spectrum of minimal change disease (MCD)–focal segmental glomerulosclerosis (FSGS) lesions (see also Chapters 17 to 19). Distinct mesangial hypercellularity superimposed on a lesion of MCD (diffuse foot process effacement seen on electron microscopy) may point to a greater likelihood for corticosteroid unresponsiveness and an eventual evolution to the FSGS lesion.

Natural History of Mesangial Proliferative Glomerulonephritis

The natural history of MesPGN is quite varied, undoubtedly the result of etiologic heterogeneity. In many patients, a benign course ensues, especially if hematuria and scant proteinuria (<1 g/day) are the principal features. Persisting nephrotic syndrome has a less favorable prognosis, and such patients may evolve into FSGS (see Chapter 18) and accompanying progressive CKD.[3]

Treatment of Mesangial Proliferative Glomerulonephritis

The treatment of pure MesPGN, unaccompanied by other underlying diseases or lesions such as SLE, C1q nephropathy, IgM nephropathy, minimal change lesion, or IgA nephropathy, has not been well defined.[2,3] No prospective, randomized, controlled trials have been performed because of the uncommon nature of the disorder. As the prognosis for patients with isolated hematuria or hematuria combined with mild proteinuria (<500 mg/day) is generally benign, no treatment other than management of hypertension is needed. For those patients with nephrotic syndrome, with or without impaired renal function, a more aggressive approach is often recommended, especially in the presence of diffuse IgM deposits, because many such patients will eventually progress to FSGS. Even in the absence of controlled trials, an initial course of corticosteroid therapy may be justified in most patients with nephrotic-range proteinuria (e.g., prednisone 60 mg/day or 120 mg every other day for 2 to 3 months followed by lowered doses, on an alternate-day regimen, for 2 to 3 additional months). About 50% of patients so treated will experience a decrease in proteinuria to subnephrotic levels. Complete remissions occasionally occur. However, relapses of proteinuria are common when corticosteroids are tapered or discontinued. Such relapsing, partially corticosteroid responsive patients might benefit from the addition of cyclophosphamide, chlorambucil, or even cyclosporine or mycophenolate mofetil (MMF) to the regimen, although information on the therapeutic efficacy and safety of these agents in pure MesPGN is limited.

Collagen-Vascular (Rheumatic) Diseases Associated with Glomerular Lesions
SLE (see Chapter 25)
Rheumatoid arthritis
Mixed connective tissue disease
Rheumatic fever
Ankylosing spondylitis
Reiter's syndrome
Dermatomyositis/polymyositis
Scleroderma
Relapsing polychondritis
Systemic or renal limited polyangiitis (see Chapter 24)

Figure 27.3 Collagen-vascular (rheumatic) diseases associated with glomerular lesions. SLE, systemic lupus erythematosus.

Patients with persistent treatment-unresponsive nephrotic syndrome will almost invariably progress to ESRD during a period of several years. Whereas transplantation is not contraindicated, those patients who do progress to ESRD rapidly and who develop superimposed FSGS may have a high risk of recurrence of proteinuria and FSGS in the transplanted kidney.

Renal Disease in Rheumatoid Arthritis
Glomerular Lesions that May Be Direct Complications of the Disease
MN
MesPGN (± IgA or IgM deposits)
Diffuse proliferative GN Necrotizing and crescentic GN (rheumatoid vasculitis)
Amyloidosis (AA type)
Glomerular Lesions Associated with Agents Used in the Treatment of Rheumatoid Arthritis
Gold: MN, MCD acute tubular necrosis
Penicillamine: MN, crescentic GN, MCD
NSAIDs: acute tubulointerstitial nephritis (TIN) with MCD, acute tubular necrosis, MCD without TIN
Cyclosporine: chronic vasculopathy and TIN, focal and segmental glomerulosclerosis (?)
Azathioprine/6-mercaptopurine: acute interstitial nephritis
Pamidronate: focal segmental glomerulosclerosis

Figure 27.4 Renal disease in rheumatoid arthritis. MCD, minimal change disease; MesPGN, mesangial proliferative glomerulonephritis; MN, membranous nephropathy; NSAIDs, nonsteroidal antiinflammatory agents; TIN, tubulointerstitial nephropathy.

GLOMERULONEPHRITIS WITH RHEUMATIC DISEASE

Several so-called collagen-vascular diseases other than SLE may be complicated by GN (Fig. 27.3). This section covers the glomerulonephritides that accompany rheumatoid arthritis, mixed connective tissue disease,[6] polymyositis and dermatomyositis, acute rheumatic fever, scleroderma, and relapsing polychondritis. IgA nephropathy may also be seen in association with the seronegative spondyloarthropathies.

Rheumatoid Arthritis

A wide variety of glomerular, tubulointerstitial, and vascular lesions of the kidney may complicate rheumatoid arthritis (Fig. 27.4). Clinical abnormalities, including abnormal urinalyses (hematuria, leukocyturia, proteinuria), and reduced renal function are common in patients with rheumatoid arthritis, particularly those with severe or long-standing disease. Membranous nephropathy (MN) (see Chapter 20) is the most common glomerular lesion encountered. This may be due to the underlying disease itself or its therapy (parenteral or oral gold or penicillamine). The presence of HLA-DR3 increases the risk for development of MN in a patient with rheumatoid arthritis.

The course of MN in association with rheumatoid arthritis, in the absence of drugs, is similar to that of the idiopathic disease, although spontaneous remissions appear less likely to occur. By comparison, MN associated with drugs used to treat rheumatoid arthritis is most likely to remit after discontinuance of the drug therapy.[7] Such remissions may take many months to occur. Nevertheless, 60% to 80% of patients with drug-induced MN in a setting of rheumatoid arthritis will remit within a year of stopping treatment.

Secondary (AA) amyloidosis is found in 5% to 20% of patients with rheumatoid arthritis undergoing renal biopsy. Nephrotic syndrome and progressive renal failure are common. AA amyloidosis is discussed in detail in Chapter 26.

The use of nonsteroidal anti-inflammatory drugs (NSAIDs) may also produce tubulointerstitial nephritis or MCD (see also Chapters 60 and 17).[8] A severe, necrotizing polyangiitis may sometimes complicate the course of long-standing rheumatoid arthritis (rheumatoid vasculitis).[8] The patients may have profound reduction in C3 levels, striking elevation of rheumatoid factors, and marked polyclonal hypergammaglobulinemia. Renal involvement in rheumatoid vasculitis is relatively uncommon for poorly understood reasons.

Mixed Connective Tissue Disease

Mixed connective tissue disease is characterized by features that overlap with those of SLE, scleroderma, and polymyositis. Typically, the serum of such patients contains high-titer autoantibodies to extractable nuclear antigens (ribonucleoprotein-extractable nuclear antigen, U1 ribonucleoprotein antigen). Low titers of anti–double-stranded DNA antibody may also be found. Renal disease, originally thought to be quite rare, is found in 10% to 50% of patients, most frequently MN and MesPGN.[9] Treatment with corticosteroids is generally effective, but some patients exhibit progressive CKD. Patients with severe GN may respond to treatment regimens similar to those used in the treatment of lupus nephritis (see Chapter 25).

Polymyositis and Dermatomyositis

These related collagen-vascular diseases are characterized by inflammatory lesions in muscle and variable skin lesions and often include Raynaud's phenomenon.[10] On occasion, patients develop proteinuria and hematuria secondary to MesPGN with IgM deposits. Acute kidney injury (AKI) may rarely supervene when severe muscle injury and myoglobinuria are present. Treatment with corticosteroids may, at least in part, ameliorate the renal manifestations in concert with improvement in the muscle and skin manifestations.

Acute Rheumatic Fever

Acute rheumatic fever secondary to a pharyngeal infection with a rheumatogenic strain of group A β-hemolytic streptococci is seldom accompanied by renal disease (see Chapter 55).[11] Poststreptococcal GN and acute rheumatic fever almost never coexist because of the distinct difference between nephritogenic and rheumatogenic strains of streptococci. In addition, cutaneous streptococcal infections are never associated with acute rheumatic fever sequelae. Nevertheless, on rare occasions, MesPGN has been associated with acute rheumatic fever.[11] It usually is manifested with hematuria with scant proteinuria and often resolves with appropriate treatment and control of acute rheumatic fever.

Ankylosing Spondylitis and Reiter's Syndrome (Seronegative Spondyloarthropathies)

The seronegative spondyloarthropathies and oligoarticular arthropathies may from time to time be associated with mesangial IgA deposition and MesPGN. Clinical manifestations are usually mild and nonprogressive. AA amyloidosis may complicate long-standing ankylosing spondylitis.

Scleroderma (Systemic Sclerosis)

Scleroderma is a heterogeneous disorder of unknown etiology and pathogenesis characterized by uncontrolled expansion of connective tissue in the skin and other visceral organs. There is also a marked tendency to produce vascular thickening and narrowing. Clinical manifestations vary from increased connective tissue in localized patches of skin (morphea) to diffuse and generalized disease (systemic sclerosis). The latter pattern leads to thickening of the skin of the face and hands, telangiectasia, Raynaud's phenomenon, tendon friction rubs, and sclerodactyly. A characteristic pattern of blood vessel abnormalities is seen in the nail beds. Visceral involvement in the systemic form causes interstitial pulmonary fibrosis, loss of esophageal and other gastrointestinal motility, restrictive cardiomyopathy, and renal disease. Limited forms of the disease (CREST syndrome: calcinosis, Raynaud's phenomenon, esophageal dysmotility, sclerodactyly, and telangiectasia) also occur but are seldom associated with renal disease. The disorder is seen more frequently in females, with an onset usually in young adults. Approximately 90% of patients will have a speckled pattern of fluorescent ANA; 20% will have detectable antibody to topoisomerase I (Scl-70). Anticentromere antibody is strongly associated with the CREST syndrome. Anti-DNA polymerase is associated with a poor prognosis and a high prevalence of renal involvement. Rarely, the visceral abnormalities may occur in the absence of cutaneous lesions (scleroderma sine scleroderma).

Renal involvement in scleroderma can be quite varied, from a low-grade proteinuria and slight impairment of glomerular filtration rate (GFR), to a more marked reduction in renal blood flow leading to a greatly elevated filtration fraction due to a mild MesPGN, to severe AKI. The last is referred to as scleroderma renal crisis and consists of severe (hyperreninemic) hypertension, encephalopathy, systolic and diastolic congestive heart failure, and AKI. There is often an accompanying microangiopathic hemolytic anemia with schistocytes in the peripheral blood film and greatly elevated serum lactate dehydrogenase levels. On occasion, AKI may develop in the absence of hypertension. AKI results from primary involvement of the arcuate and interlobular arteries (Fig. 27.5) and may be superimposed on lesions of hypertensive emergencies (malignant hypertension, such as fibrinoid necrosis of the afferent arterioles) and ischemic glomerular changes, such as wrinkling of the capillary wall and thickening of the basal lamina. The prognosis of scleroderma crisis has remarkably improved with the use of angiotensin-converting enzyme (ACE) inhibitors. In one study, ACE inhibitor treatment was associated with better patient survival at 1 year (75% versus 15%) and with significant preservation or recovery of renal function.[12] Transplantation may be a reasonable treatment option, but progression of disease in other visceral organs may limit life expectancy.

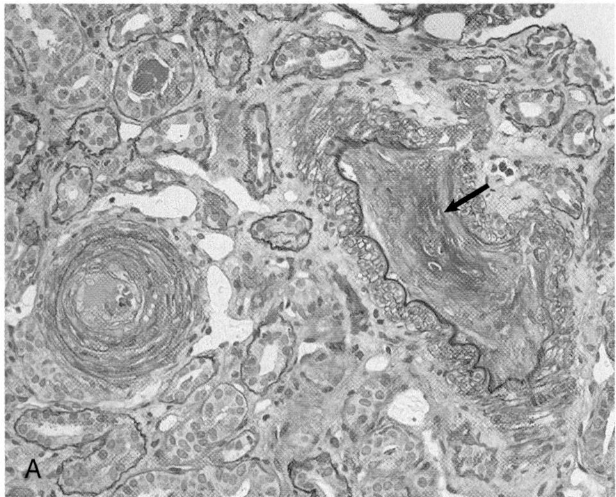

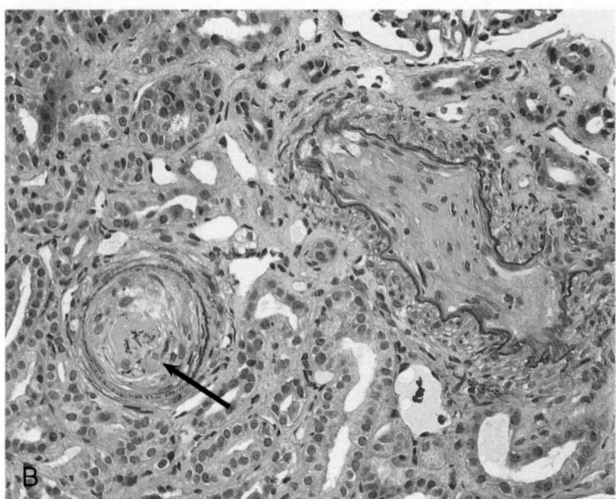

Figure 27.5 Scleroderma. A, Two interlobular arteries, one transversely and one tangentially cut, show a pronounced subendothelial thickening with weakly periodic acid–Schiff–positive mucinous material and myofibroblasts *(arrow)*. **B,** Fragmented erythrocytes (schistocytes) can be seen in the Goldner elastica stain in red *(arrow)*. The process is limited to the intima as the lamina elastica interna is preserved. Surrounding tubules are collapsed and have atrophic epithelia due to postarteriolar ischemia. *(Courtesy H. J. Groene, Heidelberg, Germany.)*

Relapsing Polychondritis

Polychondritis is a chronic relapsing disorder characterized by destructive inflammation of cartilage (ear, nose, trachea, costal cartilage) and may be associated with crescentic GN, MesPGN, or MN. Lesions of cartilage may lead to deformities (saddle nose, floppy ears, tracheal collapse or stenosis), and the renal disease may be severe and progressive, leading to renal failure. Aggressive management of progressive disease with corticosteroids and cytotoxic agents (cyclophosphamide) is indicated to control both the systemic and renal manifestations.

ANTIPHOSPHOLIPID ANTIBODY SYNDROME

The antiphospholipid antibody syndrome (aPLA syndrome) is a prothrombotic disorder characterized by venous and arterial thrombosis and by the presence of circulating autoantibodies to phospholipid-protein complexes, including those of the coagulation cascade.[13,14] The syndrome was first recognized by Hughes in 1983 and in the succeeding quarter-century has been described to have protean manifestations ranging from migraine headaches to multiple thrombosis and multiorgan failure ("catastrophic" aPLA syndrome). The clinical features are quite varied, and a high degree of clinical suspicion is required for early diagnosis. Neurologic symptoms and signs are common, including transient cerebral ischemic attacks (TIA), strokes, migraine, seizures, myelitis, and balance and sensory disturbances (often resembling multiple sclerosis). Cardiovascular problems, such as pulmonary hypertension, premature atheromatous disease, renal artery stenosis, and myocardial infarction, are common. Livedo reticularis is an important diagnostic clue (Fig. 27.6). Adrenal infarction or hepatic venous thrombosis may lead to acute adrenal insufficiency or Budd-Chiari syndrome, respectively. Visual loss, field defects, anosmia, aseptic bone necrosis, fracture, spinal claudication, and autonomic dystrophy are other less well described complications. Repeated pregnancy loss (two or more) is observed often. The kidneys are frequently involved with a form of thrombotic microangiopathy (see Chapter 28).

The aPLA syndrome may occur as a "primary" form without any known systemic disease or may accompany SLE (see also Chapter 25). The aPLA syndrome (primary or SLE related) should always be suspected whenever a history of migraine, headache, TIA or stroke, multiple pregnancy loss, or arterial or venous thrombosis or a family history of autoimmune disease is elicited.

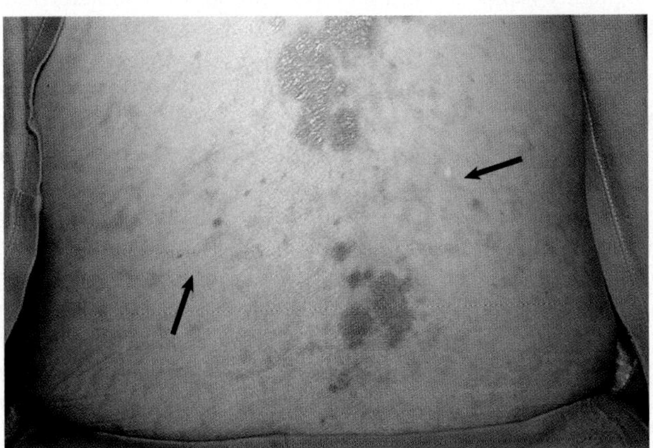

Figure 27.6 Livedo racemosa in a patient with antiphospholipid syndrome. Note reticulated skin changes *(arrows)* in addition to psoriasis lesions. *(Courtesy J. Floege, Aachen, Germany.)*

Laboratory testing will commonly reveal an autoantibody to phospholipids (anticardiolipin, anti–β_2-glycoprotein 1, or prothrombin), but "antibody-negative" aPLA syndrome has been described.[13-15] False-positive test results for syphilis and a "lupus anticoagulant" are frequent. A prolonged prothrombin or partial thromboplastin time that does not correct when plasma is diluted 1:1 with normal plasma is found in such circumstances. Antiphospholipid antibodies may also cross-react with platelet factor 4–heparin complex and thus may be associated with a "false positive" for antibody in heparin-induced thrombocytopenia,[16] giving rise to significant clinical confusion. Mild thrombocytopenia is common (platelet counts around 100,000/mm^3, but usually not less than 80,000/mm^3). This may be an *in vitro* phenomenon related to the effect of the aPLA antibody on platelet membrane biology. A mild hemolytic anemia (Coombs negative or positive) may coexist, giving rise to confusion with thrombotic thrombocytopenic purpura, hemolytic-uremic syndrome, and Evans syndrome. A frank microangiopathic hemolytic anemia is relatively uncommon.

In the primary aPLA syndrome, overt renal manifestations are generally mild (proteinuria, hematuria, hypertension, reduced renal function) and are frequently absent. Nephrotic syndrome is relatively rare. In aPLA syndrome associated with SLE, the renal manifestations are determined largely by the severity of the underlying glomerular lesions, but the coexistence of the aPLA syndrome adds a dimension of vascular disease (microangiopathy) that contributes to a worsened prognosis and to a multiplicity of extrarenal manifestations (neurologic, cardiovascular, osseous, ophthalmologic, hepatic, visceral, and obstetric) (see also Chapter 25).

The therapy for aPLA syndrome is difficult. Immunosuppressive agents, such as corticosteroids or cytotoxic agents, even when they are used to control SLE, have yielded disappointing results. Symptomatic patients are best treated with anticoagulation. Aspirin (or clopidogrel) can be used routinely in mild cases. Combinations of aspirin and low-dose warfarin might be effective, but the risk of bleeding may be increased. Warfarin is the mainstay of treatment in severe cases, with the international normalized ratio (INR) adjusted to a level depending on symptoms; INR between 2.0 and 3.5 may be required. Low-molecular-weight heparin (subcutaneous or intravenous) is the treatment of choice for pregnancy complicated by aPLA syndrome and is also useful in alleviating migraine headache. High-dose intravenous IgG can have dramatic beneficial effects, especially in acutely evolving disease associated with SLE. The benefits of newer immunomodulating agents, such as rituximab and MMF, have not been adequately evaluated in aPLA syndrome. Intensive plasma exchange (plus immunosuppression) may rarely be effective in pregnancy[17] but has not been fully evaluated in other circumstances, such as in aPLA syndrome associated with SLE.

GLOMERULONEPHRITIS ASSOCIATED WITH MALIGNANT DISEASE

Many malignant disorders and their treatment may be complicated by the development of glomerular lesions.[18] Furthermore, the treatment of glomerular disease with certain agents may give rise to neoplasia. Malignant neoplasms may also be associated with a wide variety of fluid, electrolyte, acid-base, divalent ion, tubulointerstitial, and vascular disorders, including direct invasion of the renal parenchyma by neoplastic cells.

Major Glomerular Lesions Associated with Neoplastic Disease	
Glomerular Disease	**Commonly Associated Malignancy**
MN	Colon, breast, stomach, and lung cancer
MCD	Hodgkin's lymphoma, pancreatic cancer, mesothelioma, prostate cancer
FSGS	Leukemia, lymphoma
MPGN	Chronic lymphocytic leukemia, lymphoma (some associated with HCV)
IgA nephropathy	Lung carcinoma
Crescentic GN/systemic vasculitis	Lung carcinoma
Systemic amyloidosis AL type	Multiple myeloma, Waldenström's macroglobulinemia
Systemic amyloidosis AA type	Carcinoma (especially renal)
Cryoglobulinemic GN	Chronic lymphocytic leukemia (often hepatitis C associated)
Light-chain nephropathy	Lymphoma, myeloma
Fibrillary (immunotactoid) GN	Lymphoma
Hemolytic-uremic syndrome	Gastric cancer, mucin-producing cancer

Figure 27.7 Major glomerular lesions associated with neoplastic disease. FSGS, focal segmental glomerulosclerosis; HCV, hepatitis C virus; MCD, minimal change disease; MN, membranous nephropathy; MPGN, membranoproliferative glomerulonephritis.

The glomerular lesions commonly observed in association with neoplastic processes are listed in Figure 27.7. MN is the most common lesion (see also Chapter 20). Approximately 7% to 20% of patients with MN will be found to have an underlying malignant neoplasm. Most patients are adults older than 50 years; however, despite the increasing frequency of malignant disease with age in the general population, epidemiologic studies support the notion that the prevalence of malignant disease is higher in patients with MN than in age-matched controls.[19] In addition, remissions (albeit temporary) can be achieved by surgical removal or chemotherapy of the neoplastic disease, and relapses may develop with recurrence of tumor. Furthermore, tumor neoantigens or antibodies have been detected within the glomerular deposits, suggesting an immune complex pathogenesis. In about one third of patients, the neoplastic disorder is already evident before the development of glomerular lesions; in about one third, it is discovered concomitantly with the onset of glomerular disease; and in about one third, the neoplastic process is detected after the diagnosis of glomerular disease. MN occurring with an underlying malignant neoplasm can closely resemble the idiopathic disease both clinically and morphologically, so it is prudent to undertake an exploration for possible malignant disease in any patient older than 50 years who presents with an apparent "idiopathic" MN. This can consist of a careful physical examination, several stool specimens for occult blood, colonoscopy, computed tomographic (CT) scan of the chest (especially in smokers), mammography (in women), and prostate-specific antigen determination (in men). Some studies have also suggested that prominent IgG1 and IgG2 instead of IgG4 deposits in the glomeruli are suggestive of a malignant cause or underlying lupus nephritis. The role of searching for specific autoantibodies in MN remains relatively unexplored territory.

Less frequent lesions observed in patients with neoplasia include minimal change, FSGS, proliferative GN (including crescentic GN), thrombotic microangiopathy, monoclonal immunoglobulin deposition diseases (MIDD), and amyloidosis. MCD may be associated with lymphoma (particularly Hodgkin's disease) and certain other cancers (pancreas, mesothelioma, prostate). Membranoproliferative GN (MPGN) may be associated with chronic lymphocytic leukemia and lymphoma. FSGS may also occasionally be encountered in patients with underlying malignant disease, including leukemia and lymphoma. IgA nephropathy and crescentic GN may be associated with lung cancer. Vasculitis accompanied by crescentic GN, often resembling Henoch-Schönlein purpura, has been reported with several malignant neoplasms, most notably lung cancer.

Systemic amyloidosis (AL type) may affect the kidney and produce nephrotic syndrome and renal failure in 10% to 15% of patients with multiple myeloma and rarely in association with Waldenström's macroglobulinemia (see Chapter 26). Carcinomas, including renal cell carcinoma, are also rarely complicated by amyloidosis, which is usually of the AA variety. MIDD (see Chapter 26) may accompany lymphomas and leukemias. Light-chain nephropathy, in which deposits of either κ or γ light chain are found in the glomerular capillaries and tubular basement membranes, may occur in association with a variety of neoplastic lymphoproliferative states (see also Chapter 26).

Thrombotic microangiopathy, producing renal cortical necrosis or glomerular lesions resembling MPGN, may be seen in association with disseminated cancer (carcinoma of the stomach) and other mucin-producing carcinomas. It may also appear secondary to treatment with certain antineoplastic agents, especially mitomycin (mitomycin C; see also Chapter 28).

Interferon treatment, used in the management of certain malignant neoplasms, may rarely cause MCD, often in association with interstitial nephritis; rarely it may also cause focal segmental glomerulosclerosis (FSGS) (see Chapter 18).

OTHER UNCOMMON DISORDERS

Lipoprotein Glomerulopathy

Lipoprotein glomerulopathy is believed to be caused by an abnormality in lipoprotein metabolism[20] and is characterized by extensive deposits of apolipoproteins A, B, and E in the glomeruli (mostly apolipoprotein E), leading to greatly expanded capillaries filled with a pale-staining, mesh-like substance having the appearance of lipid "thrombi" (Fig. 27.8). Clinically, there may be heavy proteinuria with nephrotic syndrome. Apolipoprotein B and E levels are increased in plasma in association with a type III hyperlipoproteinemia. The apolipoprotein E usually shows a heterozygous E2/E3 or E2/E4 phenotype, but homozygosity for apolipoprotein E2 or E3 has also been observed. Homozygous apolipoprotein E2 is also seen in familial type III hyperlipoproteinemia. Low low-density lipoprotein receptor binding and high heparin affinity may explain some of the pathogenetic processes in lipoprotein glomerulopathy. The disease can be associated with psoriasis[21]; otherwise, there are no distinctive clinical features. Familial cases have strongly suggested a hereditary abnormality. The disorder may recur in the renal transplant. Treatment with bezafibrate or fenofibrate may be effective.[22,23]

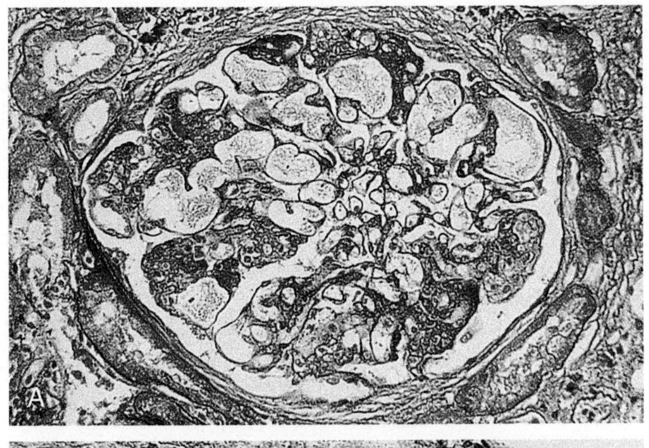

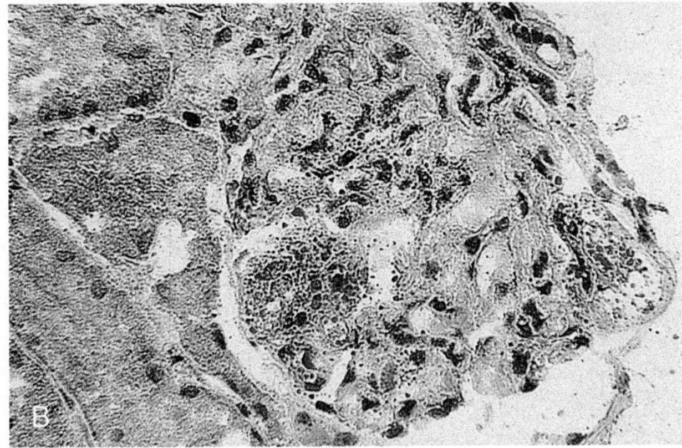

Figure 27.8 Lipoprotein glomerulopathy. A, Dilated capillary lumina containing a pale-stained, mesh-like or granular substance. (Trichrome stain; magnification ×260.) **B,** The granules stain positively with oil red O and antilipoprotein E antisera. (Oil red O; magnification ×260.) *(Modified from reference 1.)*

Lecithin–Cholesterol Acyltransferase Deficiency

Lecithin–cholesterol acyltransferase (LCAT) deficiency is an autosomal recessive disorder.[24] The mutations are on the *LCAT* gene located on chromosome 16q22.[25] The clinical characteristics include corneal opacities (misty deposits, also known as "fish eye"), normocytic normochromic anemia, premature atherosclerosis, low high-density lipoprotein and α-lipoprotein levels, and elevated low-density lipoproteins. Proteinuria (including the nephrotic syndrome), hypertension, and progressive renal failure are the main renal manifestations. On light microscopy, the glomeruli reveal foam cells, intimal hyperplasia, and thickening of the basement membrane with effacement of the foot processes (Fig. 27.9). Progressive renal failure is the rule; however, it is of slow and insidious onset and is usually first detected by the fourth decade of life. Treatment is generally ineffective, but theoretically, an inhibitor of hepatic acyl coenzyme A–cholesterol acyltransferase activity might be of benefit.[25]

Collagen III Glomerulopathy

Collagen III glomerulopathy (also known as collagenofibrotic glomerulopathy) is an autosomal recessive systemic disorder with prominent renal manifestations that may be a *forme fruste* of nail-patella syndrome (see Chapter 46) because the glomerular abnormalities are similar.[26,27] Nevertheless, patients with collagen III glomerulopathy lack the typical skeletal abnormalities observed in the nail-patella syndrome. Clinically, patients present

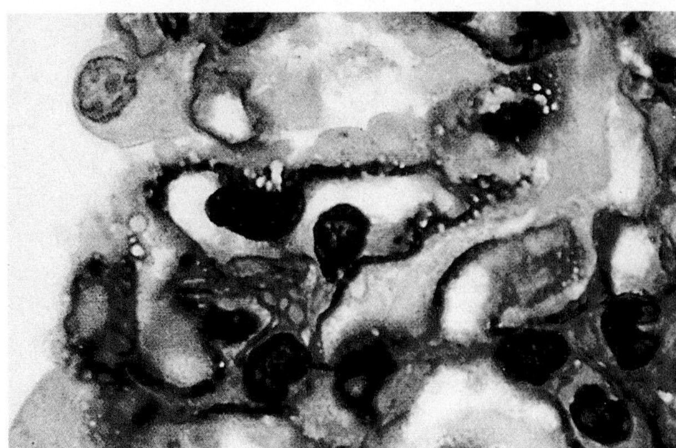

Figure 27.9 Lecithin–cholesterol acyltransferase deficiency. Note the irregular thickened glomerular capillary walls containing clear vacuoles, which are characteristic of the lesion. (Periodic acid–Schiff; magnification ×1000.) *(Modified from reference 1.)*

with proteinuria and slowly progressive renal failure. Patients may be of any age, and males predominate. On light microscopy, the glomeruli are enlarged with a marked expansion of the mesangial matrix by material weakly positive for staining with periodic acid–Schiff (Fig. 27.10). Conventional immunofluorescence microscopy is negative, but antisera to collagen type III will strongly react with the glomerular deposits. Electron microscopy shows bundles spirally arranged and frayed fibrillar deposits (Congo red negative) with periodicity characteristic of collagen. Similar deposits may be found in the spleen, liver, myocardium, and thyroid in fatal cases. No treatment is effective, and there are no data yet on recurrent disease after renal transplantation, but because of the systemic nature of the disease, such recurrences would be likely.

Fibronectin Glomerulopathy

Fibronectin glomerulopathy is a rare, autosomal dominant, nonamyloid, fibrillary glomerular disease with onset usually in early adolescence with proteinuria, microhematuria, hypertension, distal (type 4) renal tubular acidosis, and slowly progressive renal failure.[28,29] The gene responsible for the disorder maps to chromosome 1q32 near markers D1S2872 and D1S2891.[30] Most patients reach ESRD between the second and sixth decades of life. The renal pathology usually reveals enlarged, hyperlobular, and normocellular glomeruli with a homogeneous or fibrillar material (on periodic acid–Schiff staining) in the mesangium and subendothelium (Congo red negative). Electron microscopy shows randomly oriented fibrils (12 to 16 nm wide and 120 to 170 nm long). Immunofluorescence is negative for antibody and complement components but will stain brightly with use of an antifibronectin antibody. The pathogenesis of the disease is unknown, although mice "knocked out" for uteroglobin develop a similar lesion. However, studies in humans have not documented any linkage to genes for uteroglobin or fibronectin. The differential diagnosis includes other disorders associated with fibril deposition (see Chapter 26). There is no known effective treatment.

Nephropathic Cystinosis

Late-onset adult cystinosis is a variant of typical pediatric cystinosis in which the mutations in the *CTNS* gene result in a milder

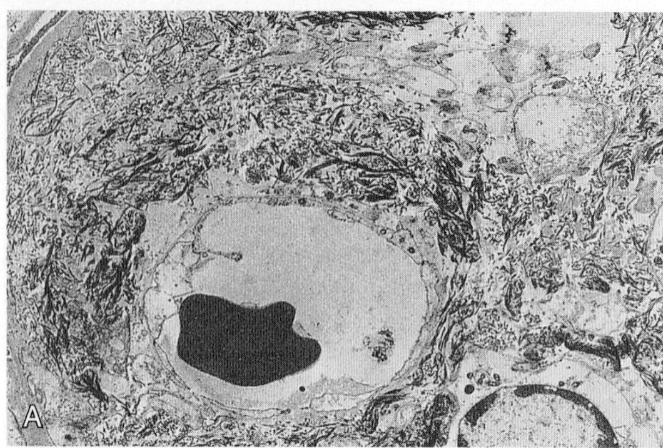

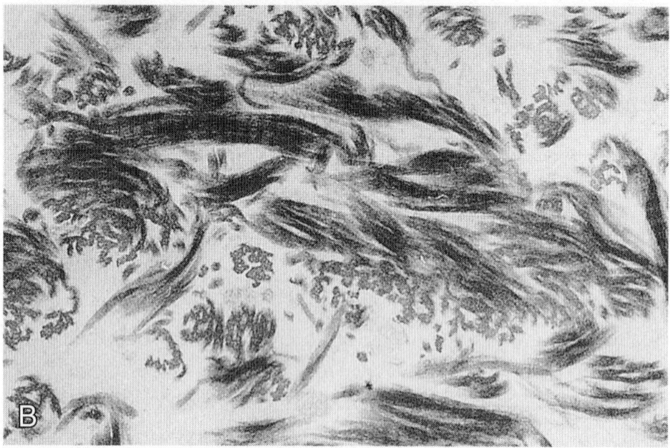

Figure 27.10 Electron microscopy of collagen III glomerulopathy (collagenofibrotic glomerulopathy). A, Fine fibrils occur in the mesangial and subendothelial areas. (Magnification ×3000). **B,** These fibrils are randomly oriented with typical periodicity and average 30 nm in diameter. The fibrils are strongly positive for staining with periodic acid–Schiff stain and react with anticollagen III antibodies. (Magnification ×15,000.) *(Modified from reference 1.)*

phenotype. These patients may present with glomerular disease during the teenage years. Nephrotic syndrome may occur, and the glomerular lesions resemble FSGS except that crystals of cystine are found in glomerular and tubular epithelial cells.[3,31] Patients with cystinosis may also have blond hair, photophobia, hypothyroidism, corneal deposits, rickets, and Fanconi syndrome (see also Chapter 48).

Miscellaneous Storage Diseases and Other Unusual Glomerular Lesions

A variety of diseases associated with storage of abdominal lipids or carbohydrates in tissue may provoke glomerular lesions; these include Hurler's syndrome (type I mucopolysaccharidoses), von Gierke's disease (glycogen storage disease), Gaucher's disease, Refsum's disease, nephrosialidosis, and I-cell disease (mucolipidosis type II). Juvenile malabsorption of vitamin B_{12} with megaloblastic anemia (Imerslund syndrome) can be associated with prolonged glomerular proteinuria, but progressive renal disease does not develop. Asphyxiating thoracic dystrophy (Jeune's syndrome) is associated with glomerular, tubular, and interstitial abnormalities. Hereditary osteolysis causing arthralgias and deformities of wrists and ankles can be accompanied by chronic GN. The nail-patella syndrome and Fabry's disease are discussed in Chapter 46.

"Idiopathic" Nodular Glomerulosclerosis

An intercapillary nodular expansion of the mesangium encroaching on the glomerular capillary lumina is characteristically called the Kimmelstiel-Wilson lesion and is most commonly associated with diabetes mellitus and proliferative diabetic retinopathy (see Chapter 29). However, in recent years, a small group of patients have been described in whom a similar or identical lesion is seen in the absence of any overt features of diabetes mellitus or disordered glucose metabolism or other known causes of a similar lesion (such as κ light-chain nephropathy [see Chapter 26], chronic thrombotic microangiopathy, monoclonal immunoglobulin deposition diseases, fibrillary GN, and fibronectin glomerulopathy). Thus, idiopathic nodular glomerulosclerosis is a diagnosis of exclusion. The first examples of this new disorder were recognized in 1989,[32] and approximately 50 additional cases have subsequently been reported.[33-35] Whereas some of these patients may have had intermittent manifestation of diabetes or only mild abnormalities of glucose homeostasis, such as an abnormal glucose tolerance test result, most have not had any features conventionally used to define the presence of diabetes mellitus (i.e., normal fasting blood glucose concentration and hemoglobin A_{1c} measurements). Thus, the intercapillary nodular lesion does not appear to require prolonged abnormal glucose homeostasis for its generation.

The clinical features are nonspecific and nondiagnostic. Patients with idiopathic nodular glomerulosclerosis are usually older (average age of about 70 years), and nephrotic syndrome is a common presentation. A heavy smoking history and long-standing hypertension are frequently present, but the role of these abnormalities in the pathogenesis of the lesion is unknown.

The pathology includes typical intercapillary nodular glomerulosclerosis with thickening of the GBM and varying degrees of arteriolonephrosclerosis and hyalinosis identical to the diabetes-associated Kimmelstiel-Wilson lesions. No electron-dense or organized deposits are seen on electron microscopy. The GBM and tubular basement membrane may "stain" with IgG and albumin on immunofluorescence. Neovascularization can be seen within the nodules.

The prognosis is poor and relates to the persistence of nephrotic-range proteinuria. Most patients will progress to ESRD, sometimes quite rapidly. The 50% renal survival point in those who continue to smoke heavily is about 1 year after diagnosis. There is no known effective therapy, other than angiotensin inhibition to reduce the proteinuria. Stopping smoking may be beneficial and should be urged for all patients with this diagnosis.

REFERENCES

1. Churg J, Bernstein J, Glassock R, eds. *Renal Disease: Classification and Atlas of Glomerular Disease*. New York: Igaku-Shoin; 1995.
2. Cohen AH, Border WA, Glassock R. Nephrotic syndrome with glomerular mesangial IgM deposits. *Lab Invest*. 1978;38:610-619.
3. Alexopoulos E, Papagianni A, Stangou M, et al. Adult onset idiopathic nephrotic syndrome associated with pure diffuse mesangial hypercellularity. *Nephrol Dial Transplant*. 2000;15:981-987.
4. Jennette C, Falk R. C1q nephropathy. In: Massry S, Glassock R, eds. *Textbook of Nephrology*. 3rd ed. Baltimore: Williams & Wilkins; 1995: 749-752.
5. Sharman A, Furness P, Feehally J. Distinguishing C1q nephropathy from lupus nephritis. *Nephrol Dial Transplant*. 2004;19:1420-1426.
6. Samuels B, Lee JC, Engleman EP, Hopper J. Membranous nephropathy in patients with rheumatoid arthritis: relationship to gold therapy. *Medicine (Baltimore)*. 1978;57:319-327.

7. Cohen IM, Swerdlin AHR, Steenberg S, Stone RA. Mesangial proliferative GN in mixed connective tissue disease. *Clin Nephrol.* 1980; 13:93-96.
8. Whelton A. Nephrotoxicity of nonsteroidal anti-inflammatory drugs: Physiological functions and clinical implications. *Am J Med.* 1999;106: 13S-24S.
9. Geirsson AJ, Sturfelt G, Truedsson L. Clinical and serological features of severe vasculitis in rheumatoid arthritis: Prognostic implications. *Ann Rheum Dis.* 1987;46:727-733.
10. Valenzuela OF, Reiser W, Porush JG. Idiopathic polymyositis and glomerulonephritis. *J Nephrol.* 2001;14:120-124.
11. Gibney R, Reinecke H, Bannayan G, Stein J. Renal lesions in rheumatic fever. *Ann Intern Med.* 1981;94:322-326.
12. Steen VD, Constantino JP, Shapiro AP, Medsger TA. Outcome of renal crisis in systemic sclerosis: Relation to availability of angiotensin converting enzyme inhibitors. *Ann Intern Med.* 1991;114:249-250.
13. Hughes GRV. Hughes syndrome (the antiphospholipid syndrome): Ten clinical lessons. *Autoimmun Rev.* 2008;7:262-266.
14. D'Cruz DP. Renal manifestations of the antiphospholipid syndrome. *Lupus.* 2005;14:45-48.
15. Shovman O, Gilburd B, Barzilai O, et al. Novel insights into associations of antibodies against cardiolipin and β -glycoprotein I with clinical features of antiphospholipid syndrome. *Clin Rev Allergy Immunol.* 2007;32: 145-152.
16. Bourhim M, Darnige I, Legallais C, et al. Anti–β_2-glycoprotein I antibodies recognizing platelet factor 4–heparin complex in antiphospholipid syndrome in a patient with mouse model. *J Mol Recognit.* 2003; 16:125-130.
17. Ruffatti A, Marson P, Pengo V, et al. Plasma exchange in the management of high-risk pregnant patients with primary antiphospholipid syndrome. A report of 9 cases and a review of the literature. *Autoimmun Rev.* 2007;6:196-202.
18. Alpers CE, Cotran R. Neoplasia and glomerular injury. *Kidney Int.* 1986;30:465-473.
19. Lefaucher C, Stengel B, Nochy D, et al; GN-PROGRESS Study Group. Membranous nephropathy and cancer: Epidemiologic evidence and determinants of high-risk cancer association. *Kidney Int.* 2006;70: 1510-1517.
20. Saito T, Oikawa S, Sato H, et al. Lipoprotein glomerulopathy: Renal lipoidosis induced by novel apolipoprotein E variants. *Nephron.* 1999;83: 193-201.
21. Chang CF, Lin CC, Chen JY, et al. Lipoprotein glomerulopathy associated with psoriasis vulgaris: A report of 2 cases with apolipoprotein E3/3. *Am J Kidney Dis.* 2003;42:E18-E23.
22. Arai T, Yamashita S, Yamane M, et al. Disappearance of intraglomerular lipoprotein thrombi and marked improvement of nephrotic syndrome by benzafibrate treatment in a patient with lipoprotein glomerulopathy. *Atherosclerosis.* 2003;169:293-299.
23. Ieiri N, Hotta O, Taguma Y. Resolution of typical lipoprotein glomerulopathy by intensive lipid-lowering therapy. *Am J Kidney Dis.* 2003;41: 244-249.
24. Calabresi L, Pisciotta L, Costantin A, et al. The molecular basis of lecithin:cholesterol acyltransferase deficiency syndromes: A comprehensive study of molecular and biochemical findings in 13 unrelated Italian families. *Arterioscler Thromb Vasc Biol.* 2005;25:1972-1978.
25. Vaziri N, Liang K. ACAT inhibition reverses LCAT deficiency and improves plasma HDL in chronic renal failure. *Am J Physiol Renal Physiol.* 2004;287:F1038-F1043.
26. Ikeda K, Yokayama H, Tomosugi N, et al. Primary glomerular fibrosis: A new nephropathy caused by diffuse intraglomerular increase in atypical collagen III fibers. *Clin Nephrol.* 1990;33:155-159.
27. Yasuda T, Imai H, Nakamoto Y, et al. Collagenofibrotic glomerulopathy: A systemic disease. *Am J Kidney Dis.* 1999;33:123-127.
28. Strøm EH, Banfi G, Krapf R, et al. Glomerulopathy associated with predominant fibronectin deposits: A newly recognized hereditary disease. *Kidney Int.* 1995;48:163-170.
29. Gemperle O, Neuweiler J, Reutter FW, et al. Familial glomerulopathy with giant fibrillar (fibronectin-positive) deposits: A 15 year follow-up in a large kindred. *Am J Kidney Dis.* 1996;28:668-675.
30. Vollmer M, Jung M, Ruschendorf F, et al. The gene for human fibronectin glomerulopathy maps to 1q32, in the region of the regulation of complement activation gene cluster. *Am J Hum Genet.* 1998;63: 1724-1731.
31. Pabico RC, Panner BJ, McKenna BA, Bryson MF. Glomerular lesions in patients with late onset cystinosis with massive proteinuria. *Renal Physiol.* 1980;3:347-354.
32. Alpers CE, Biava CG. Idiopathic lobular glomerulonephritis (nodular mesangial sclerosis). A distinct diagnostic entity. *Clin Nephrol.* 1989;32: 68-74.
33. Herzenberg AM, Holden JK, Singh S, Magil AB. Idiopathic nodular glomerulosclerosis. *Am J Kidney Dis.* 1999;34:560-564.
34. Markowitz GS, Lin J, Valeri AM, et al. Idiopathic nodular glomerulosclerosis as a distinct clinicopathologic entity linked to hypertension and smoking. *Hum Pathol.* 2002;33:826-835.
35. Navaneethan DS, Singh S, Choudry W. Nodular glomerulosclerosis in a non-diabetic patient: Case report and review of the literature. *J Nephrol.* 2005;18:613-615.

CHAPTER 28

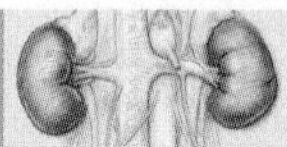

Thrombotic Microangiopathies, Including Hemolytic Uremic Syndrome

Piero Ruggenenti, Paolo Cravedi, Giuseppe Remuzzi

DEFINITIONS

Thrombotic microangiopathy (TMA) is characterized by an acute syndrome of microangiopathic hemolytic anemia, thrombocytopenia, and variable signs of organ injury due to platelet thrombosis in the microcirculation.[1] Depending on the predominant distribution of the lesions—kidney or central nervous system (CNS)—two pathologically identical but clinically distinct entities are described: hemolytic-uremic syndrome (HUS) and thrombotic thrombocytopenic purpura (TTP). HUS usually affects young children and is characterized by acute kidney injury (AKI) and absent or minimal neurologic abnormalities. TTP occurs in adults and is characterized by severe neurologic involvement in most cases and variable renal involvement. In some patients, features of HUS and TTP may coexist. Injury to the endothelial cell is the central and likely inciting factor in the sequence of events leading to TMA. Loss of physiologic thromboresistance, leukocyte adhesion to damaged endothelium, complement consumption, abnormal von Willebrand factor (vWF) release and fragmentation, and increased vascular shear stress may then sustain and amplify the microangiopathic process. Toxins, autoantibodies, pregnancy, systemic diseases, and drugs have been associated with TMA (Fig. 28.1). In most of these cases, early recognition and treatment of the underlying condition are therefore of paramount importance for remission to be achieved.[1]

CLINICAL AND LABORATORY SIGNS

TMA is characterized by thrombocytopenia (often with purpura but rarely with severe bleeding), microangiopathic hemolytic anemia, AKI that may be associated with anuria, neurologic deficits, and fever. Thrombocytopenia and hemolytic anemia are the key laboratory abnormalities. Thrombocytopenia is caused by platelet aggregation in the microcirculation; hemolytic anemia is due to mechanical fragmentation of erythrocytes during their passage through the narrowed vessels. Thrombocytopenia is usually more severe in TTP than in HUS. At the onset of TTP, platelet counts may be less than 20×10^9 cells/l. In HUS, values between 30×10^9 and 100×10^9 cells/l are frequent; however, values can be normal. Anemia is usually severe, with hemoglobin concentrations below 6.5 mg/dl in about 40% of cases. Hyperbilirubinemia (mainly indirect), reticulocytosis, circulating free hemoglobin, and low haptoglobin levels are typical. The serum lactate dehydrogenase (LDH) level is extremely high, reflecting hemolysis but also, in some patients, diffuse tissue infarction. Platelet count and serum LDH level are useful parameters for both diagnosis and response to treatment. Fragmented red blood cells (schistocytes) with the typical appearance of a helmet in the peripheral smear (Fig. 28.2) and a negative Coombs test result (with the exception of neuraminidase-associated TMA) are needed to confirm the microangiopathic nature of hemolysis. There is often leukocytosis with a left shift in Shiga toxin (Stx)–associated HUS, whereas leukocytes are usually normal in atypical HUS (aHUS) and TTP. Hypocomplementemia (low serum C3 levels) is occasionally present. Prothrombin time and partial thromboplastin time, factor V, factor VIII, and fibrinogen are normal in most cases. Determination of total hemolytic activity (CH50) usually does not help the diagnosis. AKI is usually associated with mild proteinuria (usually 1 to 2 g/day) and few red blood cells and casts in the urinary sediment. Seizure and coma may occur in TTP and, much less frequently, in HUS, often in the setting of severe or refractory hypertension.

DIAGNOSIS AND DIFFERENTIAL DIAGNOSIS

The diagnosis of TMA is based on the preceding clinical and laboratory findings. Renal biopsy is indicated when the diagnosis is uncertain and thrombocytopenia is not severe. In case of thrombocytopenia, microangiopathic hemolytic anemia, and AKI, the differential diagnosis includes systemic vasculitis, hypertensive emergency, disseminated intravascular coagulation (DIC), and endemic Hantavirus infection. Other conditions that can cause an HUS-like picture include scleroderma and radiation injury. Vasculitis is usually characterized by other systemic symptoms, such as cutaneous rash (palpable purpura) and arthralgias; the platelet count is usually normal, and neurologic involvement is predominantly peripheral rather than central. Patients with hypertensive emergencies have a history of high blood pressure, very high systolic/diastolic blood pressure at the time of evaluation, and typical retinal lesions. DIC is usually associated with sepsis, shock, and obstetric complications; patients typically have consumption of all the components of the coagulation cascade, including fibrinogen, factor V, and factor VIII, with subsequent prolongation of prothrombin time and partial thromboplastin time. Hantavirus infection causes high fever, lumbar pain, AKI, and thrombocytopenia but usually no hemolysis.

PATHOLOGY

The diagnostic histologic lesions of TMA consist of widening of the subendothelial space and microvascular thrombosis. Electron microscopy best identifies the characteristic lesions of swelling and detachment of the endothelial cells from the basement membrane and the accumulation of fluffy material in the subendothelium (Fig. 28.3), intraluminal platelet thrombi, and partial or

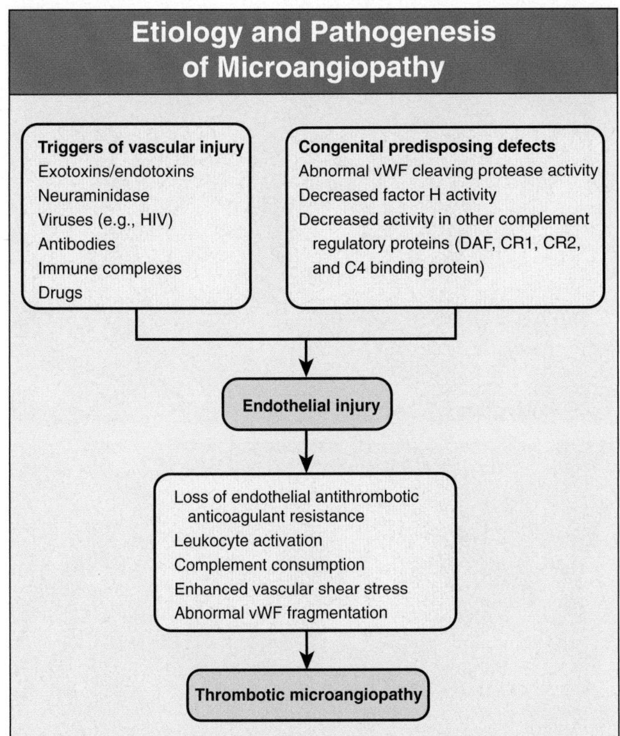

Etiology and Pathogenesis of Microangiopathy
Triggers of vascular injury
Exotoxins/endotoxins
Neuraminidase
Viruses (e.g., HIV)
Antibodies
Immune complexes
Drugs
Congenital predisposing defects
Abnormal vWF cleaving protease activity
Decreased factor H activity
Decreased activity in other complement regulatory proteins (DAF, CR1, CR2, and C4 binding protein)
Endothelial injury
Loss of endothelial antithrombotic anticoagulant resistance
Leukocyte activation
Complement consumption
Enhanced vascular shear stress
Abnormal vWF fragmentation
Thrombotic microangiopathy

Figure 28.1 A suggested sequence of events leading to thrombotic microangiopathy (TMA) in predisposed subjects exposed to triggers of endothelial injury. HIV, human immunodeficiency virus; vWF, von Willebrand factor.

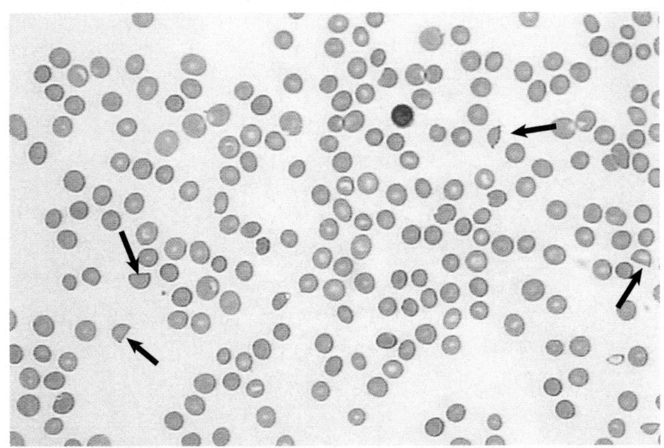

Figure 28.2 Peripheral blood smear from a patient with hemolytic-uremic syndrome (HUS). The presence of fragmented red blood cells with the appearance of a helmet *(arrows)* is pathognomonic for microangiopathic hemolysis in patients with no evidence of heart valvular disease.

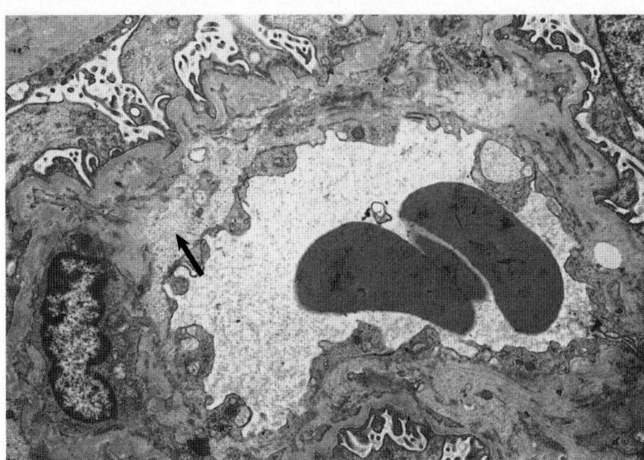

Figure 28.3 Electron micrograph of a glomerular capillary in hemolytic-uremic syndrome (HUS). The endothelium is detached from the glomerular basement membrane (GBM); the subendothelial space is widened and occupied by electron-lucent fluffy material and cell debris *(arrow)*. Beneath the endothelium is a thin layer of newly formed GBM.

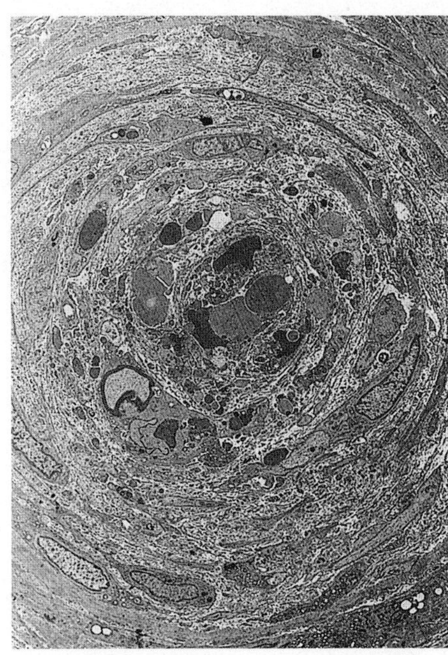

Figure 28.4 Electron micrograph of a renal arteriole in hemolytic-uremic syndrome (HUS). The vascular lumen is completely occluded by thrombi. There is marked intimal edema with consequent separation of myointimal cells.

complete obstruction of vessel lumina (Fig. 28.4). These lesions are similar to those seen in other renal diseases, such as scleroderma, malignant nephrosclerosis, chronic transplant rejection, and calcineurin inhibitor (CNI) nephrotoxicity. In HUS, microthrombi are present primarily in the kidneys; in TTP, they mainly involve the brain, where thrombi may repeatedly form and resolve, producing intermittent neurologic deficits. In pediatric patients, particularly in those younger than 2 years, and in those with HUS secondary to gastrointestinal infection with Stx-producing strains of *Escherichia coli*, the glomerular injury is predominant (Figs. 28.5 and 28.6). Thrombi and infiltration by leukocytes are common in the early phases of the disease and usually resolve after 2 to 3 weeks. Patchy cortical necrosis may be present in severe cases; crescent formation is uncommon. In idiopathic and familial forms and in adults, the injury mostly involves arteries and arterioles (Fig. 28.7), with secondary glomerular ischemia and retraction of the glomerular tuft (Fig. 28.8). The prognosis is good in the patients with predominant glomerular involvement, but it is more severe in those with predominant preglomerular injury. Focal segmental glomerulosclerosis (FSGS) may be a long-term sequela of acute cases of HUS and is usually seen in children with long-lasting hypertension and progressive chronic renal function deterioration.

The typical pathologic change of TTP involves occlusion of capillaries and arterioles in many organs and tissues by thrombi.

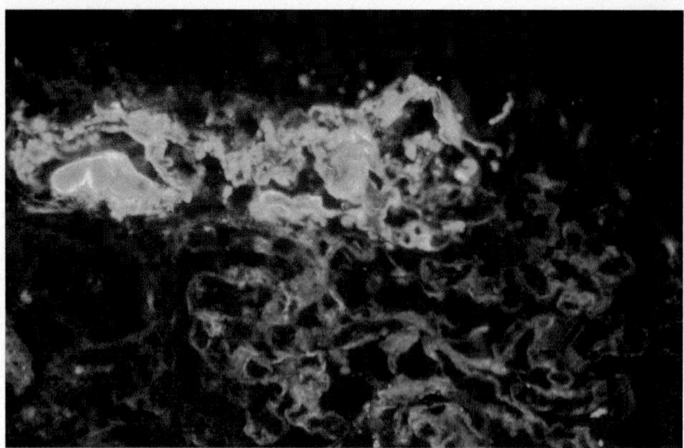

Figure 28.5 Glomerulus with its vascular pole from a patient with Shiga toxin–associated hemolytic-uremic syndrome (Stx-associated HUS). Strong staining with fluorescein-labeled antifibrinogen antibody occurs in the glomerulus and in the arteriolar wall.

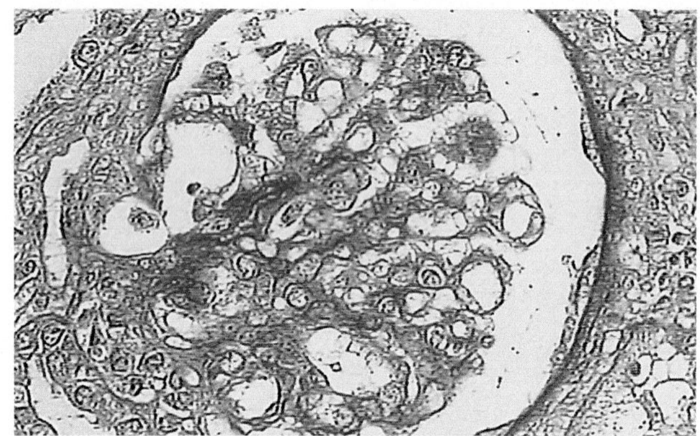

Figure 28.6 Glomerulus from a patient with Shiga toxin–associated hemolytic-uremic syndrome (Stx-associated HUS). A marked thickening of the glomerular capillary wall occurs with many double contours.

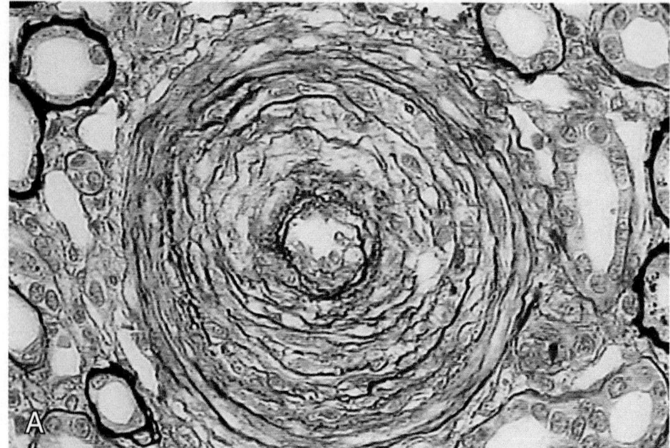

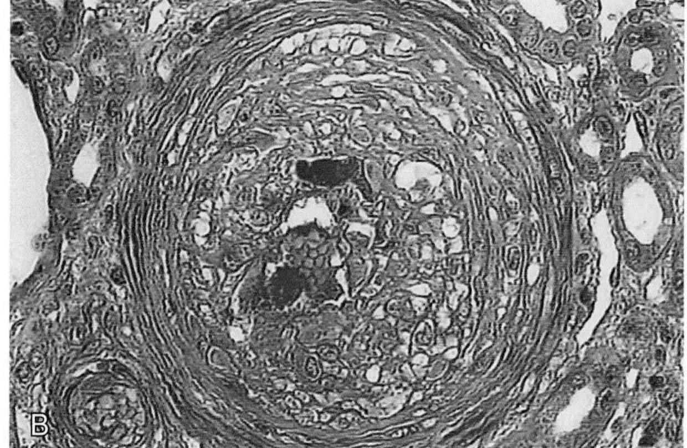

Figure 28.7 Interlobular artery in a case of hemolytic-uremic syndrome (HUS) with severe vascular involvement. A, The vascular lumen is almost completely occluded. Changes include myointimal proliferation and reduplication of the lamina elastica. **B,** Thrombotic material and erythrocytes can be seen in the lumen and within the vascular wall.

These thrombi consist of fibrin and platelets, and their distribution is widespread. They are most commonly detected in kidneys, pancreas, heart, adrenals, and brain. Compared with HUS, pathologic changes of TTP are more extensively distributed, probably reflecting the more systemic nature of the disease.

CLINICAL FEATURES, MECHANISMS, AND MANAGEMENT OF SPECIFIC FORMS OF THROMBOTIC MICROANGIOPATHY

Differentiation of the various forms of TMA is important to predict disease outcome and to establish the correct therapeutic approach based on different clinical presentations (Figs. 28.9 to 28.11).

Thrombotic Microangiopathy Associated with Infectious Diseases

Shiga Toxin–Associated Hemolytic-Uremic Syndrome

Stx-associated HUS is the most frequent form of TMA.[1] It is associated with infection by certain strains of *E. coli* (mostly O157:H7 serotype) or *Shigella dysenteriae* type 1 that produce a powerful exotoxin. The human disease is caused by two distinct *E. coli* exotoxins, Stx1 and Stx2, almost identical to the toxin produced by *S. dysenteriae* type 1. It is also referred to as D$^+$ HUS because AKI is preceded by diarrhea.

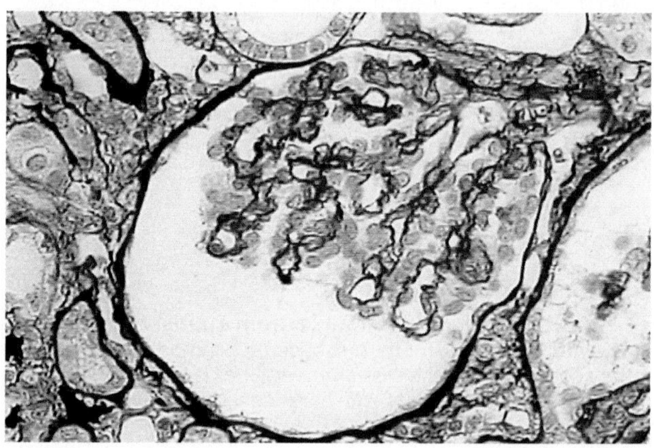

Figure 28.8 Glomerulus from a patient with atypical hemolytic-uremic syndrome (aHUS) with predominant vascular involvement. Severe ischemic changes have occurred. Note the shrinkage of the glomerular tuft and marked thickening and wrinkling of the capillary wall.

The overall incidence is estimated to be 2.1 cases per 100,000 persons per year, with a peak incidence in children younger than 5 years (6.1/100,000 per year), although no age group is exempt. *E. coli* O157:H7 infection is most frequent in the warm summer months. Illness follows infection with Stx-producing *E. coli* a few

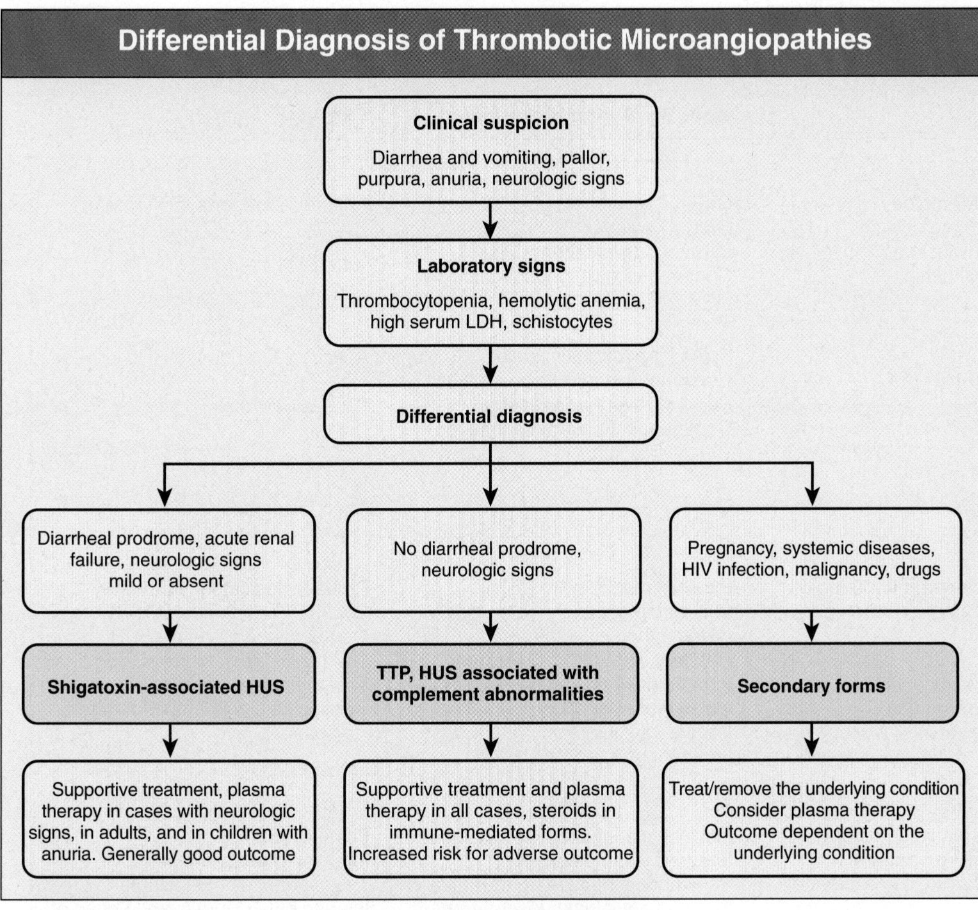

Figure 28.9 Algorithm for the differential diagnosis of thrombotic microangiopathies (TMAs). Patients with suggestive symptoms should be investigated for specific signs of microangiopathic hemolysis. In adults, secondary forms of the disease must be ruled out. Early diagnosis may help establish the most appropriate therapy. Specific therapies should be considered in children with anuria or neurologic signs, in cases without prodromal diarrhea, and in adult forms regardless of clinical presentation. In secondary forms, treatment or removal of the underlying disease is fundamental. HUS, hemolytic-uremic syndrome; LDH, lactate dehydrogenase; TTP, thrombotic thrombocytopenic purpura; HIV, human immunodeficiency virus.

Classification of Thrombotic Microangiopathies

TMA associated with infectious disease
- Shigatoxin-associated HUS
- Neuraminidase (pneumococcal)-associated TMA
- HIV infection

TTP associated with genetic or immune-mediated ADAMTS13 abnormalities

HUS associated with genetic or immune-mediated abnormalities of the complement system
- Genetically determined factor H deficiency
- Genetic membrane cofactor protein abnormalities
- Complement factor I deficiency
- Gain-of-function mutations of complement factor B
- Complement C3 mutations
- Immune-mediated factor H deficiency

Pregnancy-associated TMA
- TTP
- HELLP syndrome
- Postpartum HUS

Systemic disease-associated TMA
- Antiphospholipid, scleroderma, malignant hypertension
- Malignancy

Drug associated

Transplant associated
- *De novo* HUS
- Recurrent post-transplantation HUS

Figure 28.10 Classification of thrombotic microangiopathies (TMAS). HELLP, hemolysis, elevated liver enzymes and low platelet; HIV, human immunodeficiency virus; HUS, hemolytic-uremic syndrome; TMA, thrombotic microangiopathy; TTP, thrombotic thrombocytopenic purpura.

days later. HUS complicates enteric infection with *E. coli* O157:H7 in about 3% to 7% of sporadic cases and in 20% or more of the epidemic form. Mean onset of HUS is 6 days after the onset of diarrhea. Humans may be infected from contaminated milk and meat and fecally contaminated water or by contact with infected animals or human excretions.[2] Cattle represent the major natural reservoir of *E. coli* O157:H7. The most important route of Stx transmission is contaminated food (mainly undercooked ground beef including meat patties, roast beef, ham, turkey, cheese, potatoes, unpasteurized milk, and water). Secondary person-to-person contact is an important route of spread in institutional centers, particularly daycare centers and nursing homes. In these cases, the most important preventive measure is hand washing.

After oral ingestion of contaminated food or water, *E. coli* reaches the gut, closely binds to the gastrointestinal mucosa, and causes cell death. In non–Stx-producing *E. coli* strains, this normally results in nonbloody diarrhea. Strains producing a large amount of Stx may damage the mucosal vasculature, causing hemorrhagic colitis. Once the toxin reaches the systemic circulation, microvascular damage develops at target organs, giving rise to the clinical manifestations of HUS or, less frequently, TTP. Stx1 and Stx2 bind to different epitopes of the specific glycolipidic receptors (Gb3 molecules) and also differ in binding affinity and kinetics.[2]

High concentrations of Stx block protein synthesis and destroy endothelial cells. If endothelial cells are exposed to sublethal Stx doses, which exert a minimal influence on protein synthesis only, a nuclear factor-κB–mediated proinflammatory

Specific Therapies Used in Thrombotic Microangiopathy, Doses, Modalities of Administration, and Effectiveness			
Therapy	**Dosing**	**Modality of Administration**	**Efficacy**
Antiplatelet agents			
Aspirin	325–1300 mg/day	Oral	Anecdoctal reports In TTP forms
Dipyridamole	400–600 mg/day	Oral	" "
Dextran 70	500 mg twice/day	Intravenous injection	" "
Prostacyclln	4–20 ng/kg/mln	Continuous intravenous infusion	" "
Antithrombotic agents			
Heparin	5000 U 750–1000 U/hour	Pulse intravenous injectlon Continuous intravenous infusion	Anecdoctal reports In HUS
Streptokinase	250,000 U 100,000 U/hour	Pulse intravenous injection Continuous intravenous infusion	" "
Antioxidant agents			
Vitamin E	1000 mg/m²/day	Oral	Anecdoctal reports In HUS
Immunosuppressive agents			
Prednisone / prednisolone	200 mg tapered to 60 mg/day Then 5-mg reduction per week	Intravenous or oral during active disease then continue with oral	Probably indicated in patients with TTP and antl-ADAMTS13 autoantibodies or in aHUS with anti-factor H autoantibodies and in forms associated with autoimmune diseases
Immunoglobulins	400 mg/kg/day	Intravenous infusion	
Vincristine	1.4 mg/m² on day 1 1 mg every 4 days Intravenous	Intravenous injection Intravenous injection up to 4 doses	
Rituximab	375 mg/m²/week for 4 weeks	Intravenous injection	
Fresh frozen plasma			
Exchange	1–2 plasma volumes/day	Intravenous infusion, up to remission	First-line therapy
Infusion	20–30 ml/kg on day 1 10–20 ml/kg/day thereafter	Intravenous Infusion Intravenous infusion up to remission	First-line therapy if plasma exchange is not available
Cryosupernatant	See plasma infusion/exchange	See plasma infusion/exchange	Instead of whole plasma in case of plasma resistance or sensitization
Solvent detergent treated	See plasma infusion/exchange	See plasma infusion/exchange	Instead of whole plasma to limit the risk of infections
Others			
Liver transplant			To cure complement genetic defect (factor H)
Eculizumab	600 mg weekly for the first 4 weeks 900 mg every 14 days thereafter up to 6 months	Intravenous infusion	Reported efficacy in cases of aHUS due to factor H mutations and of aHUS recurrence after kidney transplant

Figure 28.11 Treatment options for thrombotic microangiopathies (TMAs). aHUS, atypical hemolytic-uremic syndrome; TTP, thrombotic thrombocytopenic purpura. ADAMTS13, a disintegrin and metalloprotease with thrombospondin type 1 domain 13.

response is induced, favoring leukocyte-dependent inflammation.[2] Stx also induces loss of thromboresistance in endothelial cells. Thus, human microvascular endothelial cells pre-exposed to Stx1 at high shear stress induce early platelet activation and adhesion, followed by formation of organized thrombi dependent on endothelial P-selectin and platelet–endothelial cell adhesion molecule 1. Finally, higher than normal levels of plasminogen activator inhibitor type 1 indicate that fibrinolysis is substantially inhibited.[2]

Clinical findings typically include abdominal cramps and nonbloody diarrhea; diarrhea usually becomes bloody within a few days. Vomiting occurs in about 30% to 60% of cases and fever in 30%. Leukocytosis is usually present. Dialysis is required in 50% of cases and red blood cell transfusions in 75%; neurologic signs including stroke, seizure, and coma occur in 25%. Pancreatitis occurs in about 20% of cases. HUS is usually considered a benign disease because about 90% of patients fully recover from the acute syndrome. However, 3% to 5% of patients die during the acute phase, and up to 5% have severe renal and extrarenal sequelae. Moreover, up to 40% of those recovering from the acute disease may develop during several years a form of progressive chronic kidney disease (CKD).

Age younger than 2 years, severe gastrointestinal prodromes, elevated white cell count, anuria early in the course of the disease, and cortical necrosis or involvement of more than 50% of glomeruli at renal biopsy are predictors of poor outcome. Anuria for more than 10 days or need for dialysis in the acute phase and proteinuria at 12-month follow-up are associated with an increased risk of chronic renal failure (CRF) in the long term. Diagnosis rests on detection of *E. coli* O157:H7 or, much less frequently, other *E. coli* serotypes in stool culture samples that may be present for several weeks even after symptoms. Analysis of bacterial serotypes should be limited to patients with diarrhea, however. Serologic tests for antibodies to Stx and O157 lipopolysaccharide can be performed in research laboratories, and tests are being developed for rapid detection of *E. coli* O157:H7 and Stx in stools. Utility of anti-Stx antibody monitoring has never been proved in clinical practice, however.

In general, children with cramping or bloody diarrhea exposed to an identified case of Stx-associated HUS should receive a rapid stool test. Early etiologic diagnosis and hospitalization of children with acute Stx-producing *E. coli* colitis may prevent spreading of the pathogen and secondary cases.

Treatment

SUPPORTIVE THERAPY In children, Stx-associated HUS usually resolves spontaneously. Early diagnosis and improved supportive management of renal failure, anemia, hypertension, and fluid-electrolyte imbalance have played a major role in the significant reduction of mortality rates during the past decades. In infants, early peritoneal dialysis (PD) prevents fluid overload and uremic symptoms and may remove procoagulant substances from the plasma. Blood transfusions are often needed for symptomatic anemia. Bowel rest is important for the enterohemorrhagic colitis but is not needed in less severe cases with nonbloody diarrhea. In patients with Stx–*E. coli* gastrointestinal infection, antibiotics should be avoided unless the patient presents with severe systemic bacteremia.[2] Although a recent meta-analysis of 26 reports failed to show a higher risk of HUS with antibiotic use,[2] there is no reason to prescribe antibiotics because they do not improve the outcome of colitis, and bacteremia is only exceptionally found in Stx-HUS sustained by *E. coli* O157:H7 infection. On the contrary, they are recommended in Stx-HUS precipitated by *S. dysenteriae* type 1, in which bacteremia is common and patients eventually progress to death if antibiotics are not started early enough. Antimotility agents are contraindicated because they may exacerbate HUS by decreasing fecal excretion of *E. coli* and its toxins. A new agent to prevent organ exposure to Stx, SYNSORB-Pk, composed of silicon particles linked to globotriaosylceramide, given orally, failed to improve outcome over placebo.[2] In those HUS patients who suffer chronic renal damage, treatment should follow the general recommendations that apply to all patients with CKD (see Chapter 76).

PLASMA THERAPY AND OTHER SPECIFIC TREATMENTS In children with Stx-associated HUS, the long-term renal outcome and patient survival are not appreciably improved by plasma therapy.[3,4] Two prospective controlled trials found that plasma infusion may limit short-term renal lesions but does not affect long-term renal outcome and survival of patients.[3,4] Corticosteroids are ineffective and should be avoided because they increase the risk of colonic perforation in patients with active colitis. Heparin and antithrombotic agents increase the risk of bleeding and should be avoided. In adults with Stx-associated HUS, uncontrolled studies suggest that plasma exchange (up to 16 procedures, with 2.0 to 2.4 liters of plasma exchanged with fresh frozen plasma [FFP]) significantly lowers mortality rate and the risk of end-stage renal disease (ESRD).[5,6] Moreover, comparative analyses of two large series of patients treated or not with plasma suggest that plasma therapy may decrease overall mortality of Stx–*E. coli* O157:H7–associated HUS. Thus, even if no prospective, randomized trial has definitely established so far whether plasma infusion or exchange may offer some specific benefit compared with supportive treatment alone in adults with HUS, plasma infusion or exchange should be considered in adult patients, in particular in those with severe renal insufficiency and CNS involvement. Hence, we suggest its use in adult patients, in whom renal and neurologic involvement is usually more severe and sequelae more frequent than in children.

BILATERAL NEPHRECTOMY Very rare cases characterized by severe changes in the renal microvasculature may be complicated by refractory hypertension, persistent thrombocytopenia, and major neurologic dysfunction that expose the patient to an imminent risk of death. In these life-threatening situations, after all other therapeutic approaches have failed, bilateral nephrectomy may induce complete clinical and hematologic remission within 2 weeks.[7] It is possible that removal of the kidneys eliminates a major site of vWF fragmentation, thus limiting platelet activation and further spread of microvascular lesions.

KIDNEY TRANSPLANTATION Kidney transplantation is effective and safe for those children with Stx-HUS who progress to ESRD. The recurrence rates range from 0% to 10%, and graft survival at 10 years is even better than in pediatric transplant recipients with other primary renal disease.[2]

Neuraminidase-Associated Thrombotic Microangiopathy This is a rare but potentially fatal complication of pneumonia or, less frequently, meningitis caused by *Streptococcus pneumoniae*.[1] Neuraminidase is a protease produced by this bacterium that exposes a specific cryptic antigen, Thomsen-Friedenreich, present on platelets and endothelial cell surface, to preformed circulating IgM antibodies with subsequent platelet aggregation and endothelial injury. The clinical picture is usually severe, with respiratory distress, anuria, neurologic involvement, and coma. The outcome is strongly dependent on the effectiveness of antibiotic therapy. The role of plasma therapy is controversial. In theory, plasma should be contraindicated in the adult because it contains antibodies against the Thomsen-Friedenreich antigen that may accelerate polyagglutination and hemolysis.[8] However, in some cases, plasma therapy, in combination with corticosteroids, induces recovery. Leukocyte-poor erythrocyte preparations should be used to reduce the risk of allosensitization that might prevent a future kidney transplant.

Thrombotic Thrombocytopenic Purpura Associated with Genetic or Immune-Mediated ADAMTS13 Abnormalities

Studies suggest that most patients with TTP have a specific pathogenetic defect characterized by the inability to cleave ultra-large vWF (ULvWF). Normally, ULvWF multimers are synthesized in endothelial cells and are rapidly degraded by a specific protease as soon as they are secreted into the circulation.[9] ULvWF multimers accumulate in patients with TTP and can attach to activated platelets, promoting their aggregation. They are normally cleaved by a metalloprotease, ADAMTS13 (a disintegrin and metalloprotease with thrombospondin type 1 domain 13).[10] Low ADAMTS13 activity can result from a constitutive deficiency or circulating acquired IgG autoantibodies to different antigenic regions of the ADAMTS13 molecule in patients with acute TTP.[11] The pathogenetic role of this autoantibody is supported by its disappearance from the circulation when remission is achieved by effective treatment, and this occurs in parallel with the normalization of plasma vWF-cleaving protease activity. Autoantibodies against ADAMTS13 have also been observed in patients developing TTP during treatment with antiplatelet drugs such as ticlopidine and clopidogrel.[11]

The differential diagnosis of TTP associated with genetic or immune-mediated ADAMTS13 abnormalities is important to predict disease outcome and to guide specific treatments. Disease related to genetic defects may affect relatives and tends to recur in the same individual. Immune-mediated disease does not cluster in families, may unmask an underlying autoimmune disease or follow the exposure to certain drugs, and may have a chronic, relentless course that parallels the production of the ADAMTS13 autoantibody. The rationale of treatment is also different (see later discussion). Monitoring of the severity of ADAMTS13 deficiency and the levels of the autoantibodies is also important to monitor the patient's response to treatment. Levels of ADAMST13 activity below 10% to 15% are characteristic of an active disease. Levels between 20% and 50% may not be associated with TTP and can frequently be found in patients with liver disease or in uremic patients.

Treatment

Plasma Exchange or Infusion The most effective treatment of genetic defects in ADAMST13 is exchange of plasma (plasma exchange) or plasma infusion, whereas corticosteroids or rituximab combined with plasma exchange might lead to long-lasting clearance of anti-ADAMST13 antibodies in patients with acquired defects (see Fig. 28.11). More generally, plasma exchange has the practical advantage over plasma infusion of allowing larger amounts of plasma to be provided, avoiding the risk of volume overload, which may be of major concern in patients with kidney failure or cardiac dysfunction. The overall response rate to plasma exchange is 90% in recent series with FFP as replacement therapy. Patients who respond to plasma therapy usually have a good prognosis if the patient survives the acute episode.[12,13] Infusion of cryosupernatant of plasma (i.e., plasma devoid of vWF multimers, fibrinogen, and fibronectin, which remain in the cryoprecipitate) may induce remission in patients who do not respond to repeated plasma exchanges with FFP.[14] Patients who do not respond to plasma therapy usually have a very poor prognosis, but occasional responses to splenectomy or vincristine have been reported. However, the results of delayed splenectomy are possibly biased by selection of patients.

Most of these series, however, were reported before measurements of ADAMTS13 activity and autoantibodies were available. Thus, outcome data are difficult to interpret because patients with genetic or autoimmune disease were most likely considered together.

New Rationale for Established Treatments Better understanding of the pathogenetic mechanisms may help explain the heterogeneous responses to treatment in apparently similar diseases. Patients with genetically determined ADAMTS13 deficiency may benefit from both plasma infusion and exchange (with plasma replacement) because both may replace the defective activity. Those with immune-mediated deficiency benefit the most from the exchange procedure, which in addition to supplying fresh protease that may saturate the autoantibody activity may also remove the autoantibody from the circulation. The same considerations apply to the use of corticosteroids, vincristine, immunoglobulins, immunosuppressants, and splenectomy. Corticosteroids have yielded inconsistent results in patients with so-called idiopathic TTP. This is likely to be due to the fact that in immune forms, these treatments may aim to inhibit the production of the autoantibody and, combined with plasma exchange, may result in effective clearance of the autoantibody from the circulation. On the contrary, they have no role in the treatment of genetic forms. Trials considering the two forms together invariably diluted the potential benefits of corticosteroids or immunosuppressive therapy in subjects with immune-mediated disease. Novel studies should probably focus on the role of corticosteroids as first-line therapy for immune-mediated forms and on vincristine, high-dose immunoglobulins, or other immunosuppressants as second-line therapy, with splenectomy considered as rescue therapy for those patients with refractory disease and life-threatening thrombocytopenia or neurologic involvement.

Rituximab, a humanized monoclonal antibody directed against the B-cell antigen CD20, induces a rapid and prolonged depletion of B cells that usually lasts 6 to 9 months. To date, more than 70 patients with severe TTP refractory to standard treatment have been treated with high response rates.[15]

Patients with TTP due to anti-ADAMTS13 autoantibodies have a high rate of relapse,[16] and in recurrent cases, death and neurologic sequelae are common outcomes. The ideal treatment should retard or prevent relapses, but the response to these immunosuppressive treatments is variable and often inconclusive.[17] Contrasting results have also been obtained with splenectomy.[17]

In patients who exhibited persistently undetectable ADAMTS13 activity and high titers of autoantibodies but who were in clinical remission, preemptive treatment with rituximab maintained remission for up to 29 months in three patients, whereas two relapsed after 51 and 13 months.[18]

Thrombotic Microangiopathy Associated with Genetic or Immune-Mediated Abnormalities of the Complement System

Factor H

Human glomerular endothelial cells and glomerular basement membrane (GBM) are rich in polyanionic molecules, which normally bind the factor H (FH) molecules deposited on their surface, providing an efficient shield against complement attack. Various mutations have been detected in the FH gene in familial cases of aHUS but also in patients with no familial history.[19] The FH mutants are functionally inactive but normally secreted and detectable in immunoassays. Moreover, because not all patients have a persistent reduction in C3 levels, the diagnosis of FH-related aHUS cannot be excluded on the basis of normal C3 and FH serum concentrations. Genetic counseling of families with recognized genetic mutations allows the prenatal identification of affected offspring.

Plasma infusion or exchange has been used in patients with HUS and FH mutations, with the rationale of providing normal plasma FH activity.[2] Plasma exchange is first-line therapy during acute disease because defective FH may antagonize the function of normal FH provided with the infused plasma, and its removal may accelerate disease recovery. Weekly infusion of plasma may be required to raise FH plasma levels enough to maintain remission.[2] One patient regained normal renal function, and plasma therapy could be stopped after 1 year.[20] The rate of recurrence after kidney transplantation alone is 30% to 100%, occurring within 1 month after surgery in most cases. The role of simultaneous kidney and liver transplantation in such patients is discussed later.

Membrane Cofactor Protein

A rare cause of aHUS is a heterozygous mutation in membrane cofactor protein (MCP), a widely expressed transmembrane glycoprotein that regulates complement activation. MCP is highly expressed in the kidney and plays a major role in regulating glomerular C3 activation. When there is reduced expression of MCP, complement-activating stimuli may lead to microvascular cell damage. Fever accompanies the other clinical features of aHUS.[21] The outcome is usually poor. Plasma infusion or exchange still remains a valid therapy that may have some effect.

As the graft has normal MCP expression, the risk of post-transplantation recurrence is logically expected to be negligible. Unexpectedly, of 10 MCP-mutated patients who received renal allografts with (theoretically) normal MCP, two had recurrences. One of these two patients probably had a mutation in another regulator of the complement alternative pathway, whereas in the other patient, endothelial microchimerism was proposed as the explanation of recurrence.[21]

Other Complement Factors

More than 30 cases of complement factor I (CFI) deficiency have been described since 1970.[22] CFI is a plasma glycoprotein predominantly synthesized in the liver that inactivates C3b and C4b, prevents the formation of the C3 and C5 convertases, and thus inhibits the alternative and the classical complement pathways. The clinical signs often begin in early childhood and include increased susceptibility to recurrent infection, in particular with *Neisseria meningitides* and *Streptococcus pneumoniae*. Plasma therapy appears to represent the most reasonable approach, although experience is very limited so far. Recurrence after kidney transplantation alone is extremely high; thus, combined liver-kidney transplantation seems preferable.[23]

Additional genetic mutations have been recently associated with HUS, including heterozygous gain-of-function missense mutations in factor B and mutations in C3 factor. Moreover, rare cases of immune-mediated aHUS have been described. IgG antibodies to FH were detected in the plasma of three of 48 children with recurrent HUS after transplantation. FH plasma activity was decreased, whereas plasma FH antigenic levels and FH gene analysis were normal.[24]

Screening and Diagnosis of Atypical Hemolytic-Uremic Syndrome In parallel with the improving understanding of the genetic basis of aHUS and its implications for patient management, in particular in the perspective of kidney transplantation for those who progress to ESRD, the demand for genetic screening has been progressively increasing. However, a full analysis for mutations in the four complement proteins so far recognized to be involved in the disease is extremely expensive and time-consuming. To optimize cost-effectiveness of genetic studies and to guarantee timely delivery of the results, an initial screen based on protein levels (either serum levels or surface expression) appears to be a rational approach for rapid identification of the likely gene involved (Fig. 28.12). When complement regulatory protein levels are normal, both the titer of anti-CFH antibodies and possibly involved genes should be studied according to the expected frequency of mutations. Thus, analysis should be considered first for the gene encoding CFH because it can be mutated in about 30% of cases, followed by the genes encoding MCP and CFI, which can be mutated in about 10% and 2% to 5% of cases, respectively. (For a list of laboratories performing the analyses, refer to reference 36.)

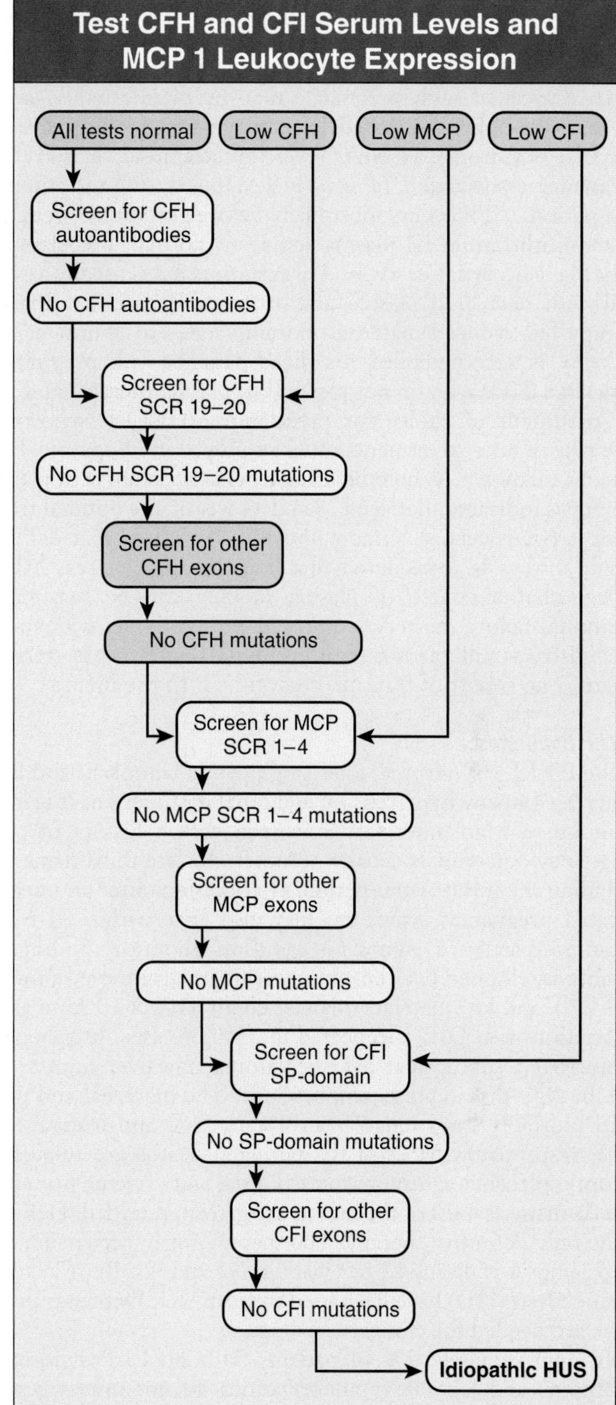

Figure 28.12 Flow diagram of the steps suggested to optimize the cost-effectiveness of screening for genetic defects in patients with non–Stx-associated HUS and genetically determined abnormalities in complement regulatory proteins. CFH, complement factor H; CFI, complement factor I; HUS, hemolytic-uremic syndrome; MCP, membrane cofactor protein; SCR, short consensus repeats. *(From reference 25.)*

Pregnancy-Associated Thrombotic Microangiopathy

TMA associated with pregnancy may be manifested as acute TTP; as hemolysis, elevated liver enzymes, and low platelets (HELLP) syndrome, a form of severe preeclampsia; or as HUS.[26] Pregnancy-associated TTP usually develops during the antepartum period. TTP occurs most likely before gestational week 28, when antithrombin III plasma activity is normal; preeclampsia most likely occurs after week 34 of gestation and is usually associated with decreased plasma antithrombin III activity. Plasma therapy has reduced maternal mortality rates to almost zero.[27] Delivery is recommended for those patients with pregnancy-associated TTP who do not respond to plasma therapy, and it is the treatment of choice for preeclampsia/HELLP syndrome. The role of other treatments often employed in idiopathic TTP remains unknown. When the disease persists, a course of plasma therapy is indicated. Between 28 and 34 weeks, the optimal treatment is controversial. Some authorities have held that delivery should always be considered first-line therapy, whereas others believe that a course of plasma therapy can be reasonably attempted before delivery is induced if there is no evidence of fetal distress and plasma antithrombin III activity is normal. There is no report of transmission of TTP to the infant.

HELLP Syndrome

In the HELLP syndrome, microangiopathic hemolysis and liver injury accompany hypertension and renal dysfunction. It is most common in white multiparous women with a history of poor pregnancy outcome. It usually occurs in the late third trimester, including the intrapartum period. On occasion, after an uncomplicated pregnancy, symptoms may also arise within 24 to 48 hours postpartum. Diagnosis is based on laboratory findings of hemolysis, elevated liver enzymes (serum aspartate transaminase >70 U/l), and low platelets (platelet count $<100 \times 10^3/mm^3$). An association with DIC is reported in 25% of cases. Intrahepatic hemorrhage, subcapsular liver hematoma, and liver rupture are rare but life-threatening complications. The maternal and perinatal mortality rates range from 0% to 24% and from 8% to 60%, respectively. Most of the perinatal deaths are related to abruptio placentae, intrauterine asphyxia, and extreme prematurity. As many as 44% of the infants are growth retarded. Delivery is the only definitive therapy. The therapy for hypertension and preeclampsia is discussed in Chapters 42 and 43. Both PD and hemodialysis (HD) have been used to treat AKI. Platelet transfusions are needed for clinical bleeding.

In approximately 5% of patients with HELLP syndrome, symptoms and laboratory abnormalities do not improve after delivery. These more often include CNS abnormalities associated with renal and cardiopulmonary dysfunction and activation of coagulation. Uncontrolled studies suggest that plasma exchange may help recovery in patients with persistent evidence of disease 72 hours or longer after delivery. Plasma therapy is ineffective during pregnancy and may increase fetal and maternal risk when it is used to delay delivery. Preliminary evidence suggested that corticosteroids may hasten disease recovery postpartum and postpone delivery and reduce the mother's need for blood products antepartum. However, the benefit of corticosteroids in postpartum HELLP syndrome was not confirmed in a randomized placebo-controlled trial of 105 women with postpartum HELLP syndrome. There was no difference in maternal morbidity, duration of hospital stay, need for rescue scheme, or use of blood products between the groups, nor was there any difference with respect to the pattern of platelet counts, recovery, aspartate transaminase, LDH, hemoglobin, or diuresis.[28]

Postpartum Hemolytic-Uremic Syndrome

Postpartum HUS is manifested within 6 months from normal delivery. The clinical course is usually fulminant. Supportive care, including dialysis, transfusions, and careful fluid management, remains the most important form of treatment. Whether plasma therapy improves survival or limits renal sequelae has not been established. Antiplatelet agents, heparin, and antithrombotic therapy may enhance the risk of bleeding and have no proven efficacy. Full recovery of renal function is very uncommon. The mortality rate ranged from 50% to 60%. Surviving patients have residual renal dysfunction and hypertension.

Systemic Disease–Associated Thrombotic Microangiopathy

Antiphospholipid Syndrome, Scleroderma, Hypertensive Emergencies

Plasma therapy should always be attempted in TMA associated with systemic diseases even though its efficacy is poorly defined.[29] In the antiphospholipid syndrome (see also Chapter 27), oral anticoagulation remains the only treatment of proven efficacy to prevent and to treat microvascular and macrovascular thrombosis, even if concomitant thrombocytopenia may increase the risk of bleeding. Preliminary reports suggest a potential efficacy of rituximab therapy, but further controlled studies are needed.[30] Blood pressure control is fundamental in TMA associated with scleroderma crisis and hypertensive emergencies.

Human Immunodeficiency Virus

HUS and TTP are both possible complications of acquired immunodeficiency syndrome (AIDS) that may account for as much as 30% of hospitalized TMA patients in cities where AIDS is epidemic.[31] Plasma therapy is the only feasible approach in these forms, although the prognosis is poor. Uncontrolled series show that the survival rate of human immunodeficiency virus (HIV)–infected patients with TTP and without AIDS is comparable to that of idiopathic TTP.

Malignant Disease

Spontaneous TMA complicates almost 6% of cases of metastatic gastric carcinoma, which in turn accounts for about 50% of all malignant disease–associated TMA. The prognosis is extremely poor. Therapy is minimally effective. Administration of blood products to correct symptomatic anemia often results in exacerbation of the syndrome.[1,2]

Drugs

Drugs associated with TMA[32] include mitomycin C, ticlopidine, clopidogrel, quinine, interferon, CNIs, and estrogen-containing oral contraceptives (Fig. 28.13). Discontinuation of the offending drug is fundamental. The efficacy of plasma therapy is unclear; it seems ineffective with some drugs, such as mitomycin C, and very important with others, such as quinine.

Mitomycin and Anticancer Drugs TMA, more commonly resembling HUS, is described in 2% to 10% of cancer patients treated with mitomycin C. Renal dysfunction rarely occurs in patients given a cumulative dose lower than 30 mg/m^2. Patients who develop mitomycin C–associated TMA are usually in

Drug-Associated Thrombotic Microangiopathy
Drugs Used in Cancer Therapy
Mitomycin C*
Tamoxifen*
Bleomycin*
Cisplatin*
Gemcitabine
Deoxycorfomycin
Methyl-CCNU
Daunorubicin
Cytosine arabinoside
Neocarcinostatin
Other Drugs
Ticlopidine/clopidogrel*
Quinine*
Interferon-α*
Calcineurin inhibitors*
OKT3*
Oral contraceptives
Penicillin
Rifampin
Metronidazole

Figure 28.13 Drug-associated thrombotic microangiopathy (TMA). *Drugs most commonly involved in drug-associated TMA.

remission from their malignant disease. The fatality rate is about 70%, and median time to death is about 4 weeks. Patients surviving the acute phase often remain on chronic dialysis or die later of recurrence of the tumor or metastases. The possibility of preventing the disease by giving corticosteroids during mitomycin treatment has been suggested and needs to be confirmed. Plasma exchange is usually attempted, but its effectiveness is unproven. Platinum- and bleomycin-containing combinations have also been reported to induce HUS.

Antiplatelet Drugs TMA occurs in one case per 1600 to 5000 patients treated with ticlopidine. Induction of autoantibodies against ADAMTS13 may be involved in the pathogenesis. Neurologic abnormalities dominate the clinical picture and usually occur within a few weeks of treatment. The overall survival rate is 67% and is improved by early treatment withdrawal and plasma therapy, which result in recovery of ADAMTS13 activity. Eleven cases have been reported during treatment with clopidogrel, mostly within 2 weeks of therapy.[33] All patients had neurologic involvement. After plasma exchange, most patients recovered. Half the patients were concomitantly treated with cholesterol-lowering drugs, and clinicians should be aware of this possible complication.

Quinine Quinine is one of the most common drugs associated with TMA.[34] It is generally used to treat muscle cramps but is also contained in beverages and nutrition health products (e.g., tonic water, herbal preparations). TMA typically occurs in patients sensitized by prior exposure to quinine and rapidly follows re-exposure to the drug. Quinine-dependent platelet, erythrocyte, granulocyte, lymphocyte, and endothelial antibodies may contribute to the pathogenesis. Severe renal impairment is frequent, and HD is required in most cases. Recent outcome data show a high rate of death and chronic renal failure.[34] Quinine cessation and plasma therapy should be initiated rapidly. Avoidance of future quinine use is necessary.

Interferon Alfa TMA associated with interferon alfa is characterized by predominant renal impairment. Recovery of the disease is common in cases of early discontinuation of the drug and prompt supportive therapy. However, kidney prognosis is usually poor, with ESRD reported in about 42% of cases. The effectiveness of specific therapies, such as plasma exchange or infusion, is unknown.

Organ Transplantation–Associated Hemolytic-Uremic Syndrome

Post-transplantation HUS is reported increasingly.[35] In renal transplants, HUS may develop *de novo* after transplantation or may recur in patients whose primary cause of ESRD was HUS. Treatment of post-transplantation HUS is based on relief of symptoms, removal of the inciting factors, and plasma therapy. No other approach has proved effective.

De Novo Post-Transplantation Hemolytic-Uremic Syndrome

This form affects both renal and nonrenal transplant recipients and is usually triggered by immunosuppressive drugs, such as CNIs and OKT3, or less frequently by viral infections (HIV, parvovirus B19) and in renal transplant recipients by acute vascular rejection.[35] A particular form of *de novo* post-transplantation HUS may affect the recipients of a bone marrow transplant, usually in cases of graft-versus-host disease (GVHD) or of intensive GVHD prophylaxis, including total body irradiation. Drug withdrawal or dose reduction and plasma therapy achieved a high success rate (84%) in *de novo* cyclosporine- and tacrolimus-associated forms. A similar response rate, but in smaller studies, has been described with intravenous IgG infusion given with the rationale of neutralizing hypothetical circulating cytotoxic or platelet agglutinating factors. Once remission is achieved, possible immunosuppression treatments may include a decreased dose of cyclosporine or tacrolimus, a change from cyclosporine to tacrolimus or vice versa, and the avoidance of CNIs by use of mycophenolate mofetil or sirolimus. However, some cases of HUS have also been reported with sirolimus. Monoclonal anti–interleukin-2 receptor antagonists may also be a valid option to maintain adequate immunosuppression while avoiding the toxic effects of CNIs. The outcome of *de novo* forms occurring in the setting of viral infection is strongly influenced by the response to the treatment of the underlying disease. The outcome of *de novo* forms complicating bone marrow transplantation is very poor, with a mortality rate close to 90%.[35] In addition to the severity of HUS, infection, progressive GVHD, or relapse of the underlying disease may account for these discouraging outcomes.

Recurrent Post-Transplantation Hemolytic-Uremic Syndrome

Mutations in circulating complement factors H, I, B, and C3, all of which are mainly produced by the liver, will persist after kidney transplantation, resulting in post-transplantation recurrence in 80% of patients with mutations in the gene encoding complement factor F or I. Recurrence rates in patients with complement factor B or C3 mutations are less well established.[36]

Liver transplantation in addition to a renal allograft corrects the complement abnormality and prevents disease recurrence in such patients. Whereas this procedure appeared effective in preventing disease recurrence in early attempts, it was also associated with irreversible liver failure secondary to uncontrolled complement activation. Subsequently, the pivotal modification to avoid liver failure was to exchange large quantities of plasma before transplantation with further plasma supplementation during the procedure. This both increased the bioavailability of functional factor H during the critical period needed for the liver graft to recover synthetic functions and, at the same time, removed the endogenous mutant factor H, preventing possible antagonism of normal factor H supplied with plasma.[37] Patients also empirically received low-molecular-weight heparin (LMWH) and low-dose aspirin. Of the first seven patients treated this way, six patients were successfully treated and did not display any recurrence, whereas one died. At present, there is consensus that this procedure, with proper consideration of individual risks and benefits, offers the best opportunity for long-term transplant success.[36]

Other less invasive treatment strategies to prevent recurrence of aHUS after kidney transplantation in patients with factor H mutations include intensified plasma exchange and C5 blockade. Intensive plasma exchange given before and long lasting after a single kidney transplantation and followed by chronic weekly plasma infusion[38] prevented HUS recurrences in five of six patients. Problems associated with chronic plasma treatment as well as the development of plasma resistance limit the feasibility of this approach.

Eculizumab is a humanized monoclonal antibody against complement C5, thereby inhibiting its cleavage to C5a and C5b and preventing the generation of C5b-9. It has been approved for the treatment of paroxysmal nocturnal hemoglobinuria and displays an excellent safety profile.[39] Eculizumab (Fig. 28.11) so far has been given to two patients with aHUS, one of them with recurrent aHUS in a renal allograft.[39,40] In both, treatment resulted in reversal of hemolysis and partial recovery of renal function.[39,40]

REFERENCES

1. Ruggenenti P, Noris M, Remuzzi G. Thrombotic microangiopathy, hemolytic uremic syndrome, and thrombotic thrombocytopenic purpura. *Kidney Int.* 2001;60:831-846.
2. Noris M, Remuzzi G. Hemolytic uremic syndrome. *J Am Soc Nephrol.* 2005;16:1035-1050.
3. Rizzoni G, Claris-Appiani A, Edefonti A. Plasma infusion for hemolytic uremic syndrome in children: Results of a multicenter controlled trial. *J Pediatr.* 1988;112:284-290.
4. Loirat C, Sonsino E, Hinglais N, et al. Treatment of the childhood haemolytic uraemic syndrome with plasma. A multicentre randomized controlled trial. The French Society of Paediatric Nephrology. *Pediatr Nephrol.* 1988;2:279-285.
5. Dundas S, Murphy J, Soutar RL, et al. Effectiveness of therapeutic plasma exchange in the 1996 Lanarkshire *Escherichia coli* O157:H7 outbreak. *Lancet.* 1999;354:1327-1330.
6. Carter AO, Borczyk AA, Carlson JA, et al. A severe outbreak of *Escherichia coli* O157:H7–associated hemorrhagic colitis in a nursing home. *N Engl J Med.* 1987;317:1496-1500.
7. Remuzzi G, Galbusera M, Salvadori M, et al. Bilateral nephrectomy stopped disease progression in plasma-resistant hemolytic uremic syndrome with neurological signs and coma. *Kidney Int.* 1996;49: 282-286.
8. McGraw ME, Lendon M, Stevens RF, et al. Haemolytic uraemic syndrome and the Thomsen Friedenreich antigen. *Pediatr Nephrol.* 1989;3:135-139.
9. Furlan M, Robles R, Lammle B. Partial purification and characterization of a protease from human plasma cleaving von Willebrand factor to fragments produced by in vivo proteolysis. *Blood.* 1996;87:4223-4234.
10. Lammle B, Kremer Hovinga J, Studt JD. Thrombotic thrombocytopenic purpura. *Hematol J.* 2004;5:S6-S11.
11. Moake JL. Thrombotic microangiopathies. *N Engl J Med.* 2002;347:589-600.
12. Bell WR, Braine HG, Ness PM, Kickler TS. Improved survival in thrombotic thrombocytopenic purpura–hemolytic uremic syndrome. Clinical experience in 108 patients. *N Engl J Med.* 1991;325:398-403.
13. Rock GA, Shumak KH, Buskard NA, et al. Comparison of plasma exchange with plasma infusion in the treatment of thrombotic thrombocytopenic purpura. Canadian Apheresis Study Group. *N Engl J Med.* 1991;325:393-397.
14. Byrnes JJ, Moake JL, Klug P, Periman P. Effectiveness of the cryosupernatant fraction of plasma in the treatment of refractory thrombotic thrombocytopenic purpura. *Am J Hematol.* 1990;34:169-174.
15. Garvey B. Rituximab in the treatment of autoimmune haematological disorders. *Br J Haematol.* 2008;141:149-169.
16. Vesely SK, George JN, Lammle B, et al. ADAMTS13 activity in thrombotic thrombocytopenic purpura–hemolytic uremic syndrome: Relation to presenting features and clinical outcome in a prospective cohort of 142 patients. *Blood.* 2003;102:60-68.
17. Yomtovian R, Niklinski W, Silver B, et al. Rituximab for chronic recurring thrombotic thrombocytopenic purpura: A case report and review of the literature. *Br J Haematol.* 2004;124:787-795.
18. Bresin E, Gastoldi S, Daina E, et al. Rituximab as pre-emptive treatment in patients with thrombotic thrombocytopenic purpura and evidence of anti-ADAMTS13 autoantibodies. *Thromb Haemost.* 2009;101: 233-238.
19. Noris M, Ruggenenti P, Perna A, et al. Hypocomplementemia discloses genetic predisposition to hemolytic uremic syndrome and thrombotic thrombocytopenic purpura: Role of factor H abnormalities. Italian Registry of Familial and Recurrent Hemolytic Uremic Syndrome/Thrombotic Thrombocytopenic Purpura. *J Am Soc Nephrol.* 1999;10: 281-293.
20. Stratton JD, Warwicker P. Successful treatment of factor H–related haemolytic uraemic syndrome. *Nephrol Dial Transplant.* 2002;17: 684-685.
21. Noris M, Brioschi S, Caprioli J, et al. Familial haemolytic uraemic syndrome and an MCP mutation. *Lancet.* 2004;362:1542-1547.
22. Alper CA, Abramson N, Johnston RB Jr, et al. Increased susceptibility to infection associated with abnormalities of complement mediated functions and of the third component of complement (C3). *N Engl J Med.* 1970;282:350-354.
23. Zheng XL, Sadler JE. Pathogenesis of thrombotic microangiopathies. *Annu Rev Pathol.* 2008;3:249-277.
24. Dragon-Durey MA, Loirat C, Cloarec S, et al. Anti–factor H autoantibodies associated with atypical hemolytic uremic syndrome. *J Am Soc Nephrol.* 2005;16:555-563.
25. Brady HR, Wilcox CS, eds. *Therapy in Nephrology and Hypertension: A Companion to Brenner and Rector's The Kidney.* 3rd ed. Philadelphia: Saunders Elsevier; 2008.
26. Weiner CP. Thrombotic microangiopathy in pregnancy and the postpartum period. *Semin Hematol.* 1987;24:119-129.
27. Martin JN Jr, Bailey AP, Rehberg JF, et al. Thrombotic thrombocytopenic purpura in 166 pregnancies: 1955-2006. *Am J Obstet Gynecol* 2008;199:98-104.
28. Katz L, de Amorim MM, Figueiroa JN, et al. Postpartum dexamethasone for women with hemolysis, elevated liver enzymes, and low platelets (HELLP) syndrome: A double-blind, placebo-controlled, randomized clinical trial. *Am J Obstet Gynecol.* 2008;198:1-8.
29. Ruggenenti P, Galli M, Remuzzi G. Hemolytic uremic syndrome, thrombotic thrombocytopenic purpura, and antiphospholipid antibody syndromes. In: Neilson EG, Couser WG, eds. *Immunologic Renal Diseases.* 2nd ed. Philadelphia: Lippincott Williams & Wilkins; 2001: 1179-1208.
30. Adamson R, Sangle S, Kaul A, et al. Clinical improvement in antiphospholipid syndrome after rituximab therapy. *J Clin Rheumatol.* 2008;14:359-360.
31. Thompson CE, Damon LE, Ries CA, et al. Thrombotic microangiopathies in the 1980s: Clinical features, response to treatment, and the impact of the human immunodeficiency virus epidemic. *Blood.* 1992;80: 1890-1895.

32. Pisoni R, Ruggenenti P, Remuzzi G. Drug-induced thrombotic microangiopathy: Incidence, prevention and management. *Drug Saf.* 2001;24:491-501.
33. Bennett CL, Connors JM, Carwile JM, et al. Thrombotic thrombocytopenic purpura associated with clopidogrel. *N Engl J Med.* 2000;342:1773-1777.
34. Kojouri K, Vesely SK, George JN. Quinine-associated thrombotic thrombocytopenic purpura–hemolytic uremic syndrome: Frequency, clinical features, and long-term outcomes. *Ann Intern Med.* 2001;135:1047-1051.
35. Ruggenenti P. Post-transplant hemolytic-uremic syndrome. *Kidney Int.* 2002;62:1093-1104.
36. Saland JM, Ruggenenti P, Remuzzi G. Liver-kidney transplantation to cure atypical hemolytic uremic syndrome. *J Am Soc Nephrol.* 2009;20:940-949.
37. Saland JM, Emre SH, Shneider BL, et al. Favorable long-term outcome after liver-kidney transplant for recurrent hemolytic uremic syndrome associated with factor H mutation. *Am J Transplant.* 2006;6:1948-1952.
38. Davin JC, Strain L, Goodship TH. Plasma therapy in atypical haemolytic uremic syndrome: Lessons from a family with a factor H mutation. *Pediatr Nephrol.* 2008;23:1517-1521.
39. Gruppo RA, Rother RP. Eculizumab for congenital atypical hemolytic-uremic syndrome. *N Engl J Med.* 2009;360:544-546.
40. Nuernberger J, Witzke O, Saez AO, et al. Eculizumab for atypical hemolytic-uremic syndrome. *N Engl J Med.* 2009;360:542-544.

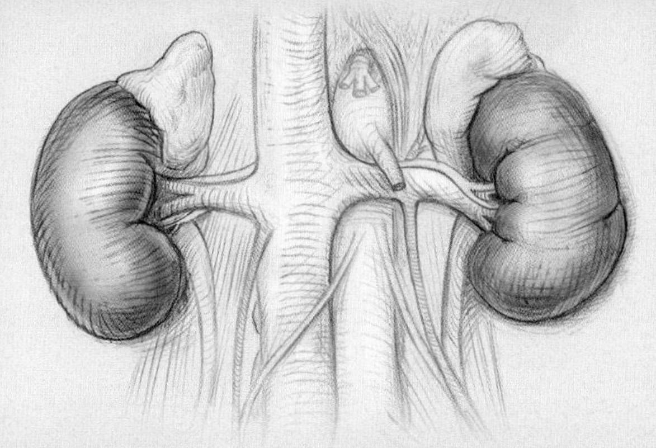

SECTION V

Diabetic Nephropathy

CHAPTER 29

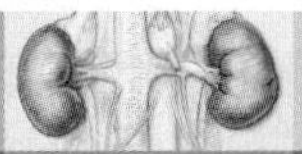

Pathogenesis, Clinical Manifestations, and Natural History of Diabetic Nephropathy

Eberhard Ritz, Gunter Wolf

DEFINITIONS

Diabetic nephropathy (DN) is the leading cause of end-stage renal disease (ESRD) in most Western societies. It can develop in the course of both type 1 and type 2 diabetes and as a consequence of other forms of diabetes mellitus (DM).

Type 1 diabetes is an autoimmune disease characterized by antibody- and cell-mediated destruction of pancreatic islets. Type 1 diabetes may occur at any age but is common in childhood, usually presenting before the age of 30 years.

Type 2 diabetes is characterized by a combination of insulin resistance and insulin deficiency. The metabolic syndrome (insulin resistance, visceral obesity, hypertension, hyperuricemia, and dyslipidemia with high triglyceride levels and low amounts of high-density lipoprotein [HDL]) is often followed by type 2 diabetes. For a long period, insulin resistance is compensated by increased insulin secretion, but a gradual decline in pancreatic β-cell function finally culminates in hyperglycemia and ultimately insulin requirement in 40% to 50% of patients with type 2 diabetes. Type 2 diabetes was typically a disease of mostly elderly adults, but recently it is increasingly seen in adolescents and even in children. In addition, there are several other types of DM (e.g., different types of maturity-onset diabetes of the young, gestational diabetes, diabetes secondary to various metabolic disorders or the consequence of corticosteroid treatment).

PATHOGENESIS OF DIABETIC NEPHROPATHY

Genetic Factors

The risk of nephropathy is strongly determined by polygenetic factors, and only approximately 30% to 40% of patients with either type 1 or type 2 diabetes will ultimately develop nephropathy. The risk for development of DN is equal in type 1 and type 2 diabetes. The prevalence of nephropathy among diabetic patients varies between different racial and ethnic groups such that it is relatively increased in African Americans, Native Americans, Mexican Americans, Polynesians, Australian aborigines, and urbanized Indo-Asian immigrants in the United Kingdom compared with Caucasians. Although barriers to care seem likely to account for some of these interpopulation differences, genetic factors are also likely to contribute. Familial clustering of DN has been reported in both type 1 and type 2 diabetes and in both Caucasian and non-Caucasian populations. In a type 1 diabetic patient who has a first-degree relative with diabetes and nephropathy, the risk for development of DN is 83%. The frequency is only 17% if there is a first-degree relative with diabetes but without nephropathy.[1] In type 2 diabetes, familial clustering has been well documented in Pima Indians,[2] and a familial determinant is also suggested by the observation that albumin excretion rates are higher in offspring of type 2 diabetic patients with nephropathy. The risk is particularly high in the offspring if the mother had been hyperglycemic during pregnancy, presumably because this causes reduced formation of nephrons ("nephron underdosing") in the offspring,[3] as shown in experimental studies.[4] Low birth weight and nephron underdosing are also associated with hypertension, metabolic syndrome, and, although the data are somewhat controversial on this point, DN. The hypothesis has been proposed that nephron underdosing[5] leads to compensatory glomerular hypertrophy and increased single-nephron glomerular filtration rate (GFR), thus aggravating glomerular injury if a renal insult such as diabetes occurs.

There is ongoing research to identify genetic loci for DN susceptibility through genomic screening and candidate gene approaches. The major problem is that there is no simple mendelian inheritance, and several genes are presumably involved. Whole genome scans searching the entire genome for chromosomal regions that are linked with DN identified several susceptibility loci, for example, on chromosomes 3q, 7p, and 18q. At present, the pathophysiologic function of such genetic regions is unknown. Gene polymorphisms may also contribute to familial clustering. A study suggested a genetic predisposition to DN due to a polymorphism in the carnosinase gene, causing accumulation of carnosine with antioxidant properties.[6] Several studies also suggested some detrimental effect of the double deletion (DD) polymorphism of the angiotensin-converting enzyme (ACE) genotype on disease progression,[7] although the finding has not been uniformly confirmed.[8,9]

Hemodynamic Changes

Hyperfiltration is common in early diabetes but can be corrected with good glycemic control. Increased GFR involves glucose-dependent effects causing afferent arteriolar dilation, mediated by a range of vasoactive mediators (insulin-like growth factor 1 [IGF-1], transforming growth factor beta [TGF-β1], vascular endothelial growth factor [VEGF], nitric oxide [NO], prostaglandins, and glucagon) (Fig. 29.1). Renal injury in DN is caused not only by hemodynamic disturbances (e.g., hyperfiltration, hyperperfusion) but also by disturbed glucose homeostasis, and the two pathways interact. For example, shear stress increases glucose transport into mesangial cells by upregulation of the specific glucose transporter. Furthermore, shear stress and mechanical strain resulting from altered glomerular

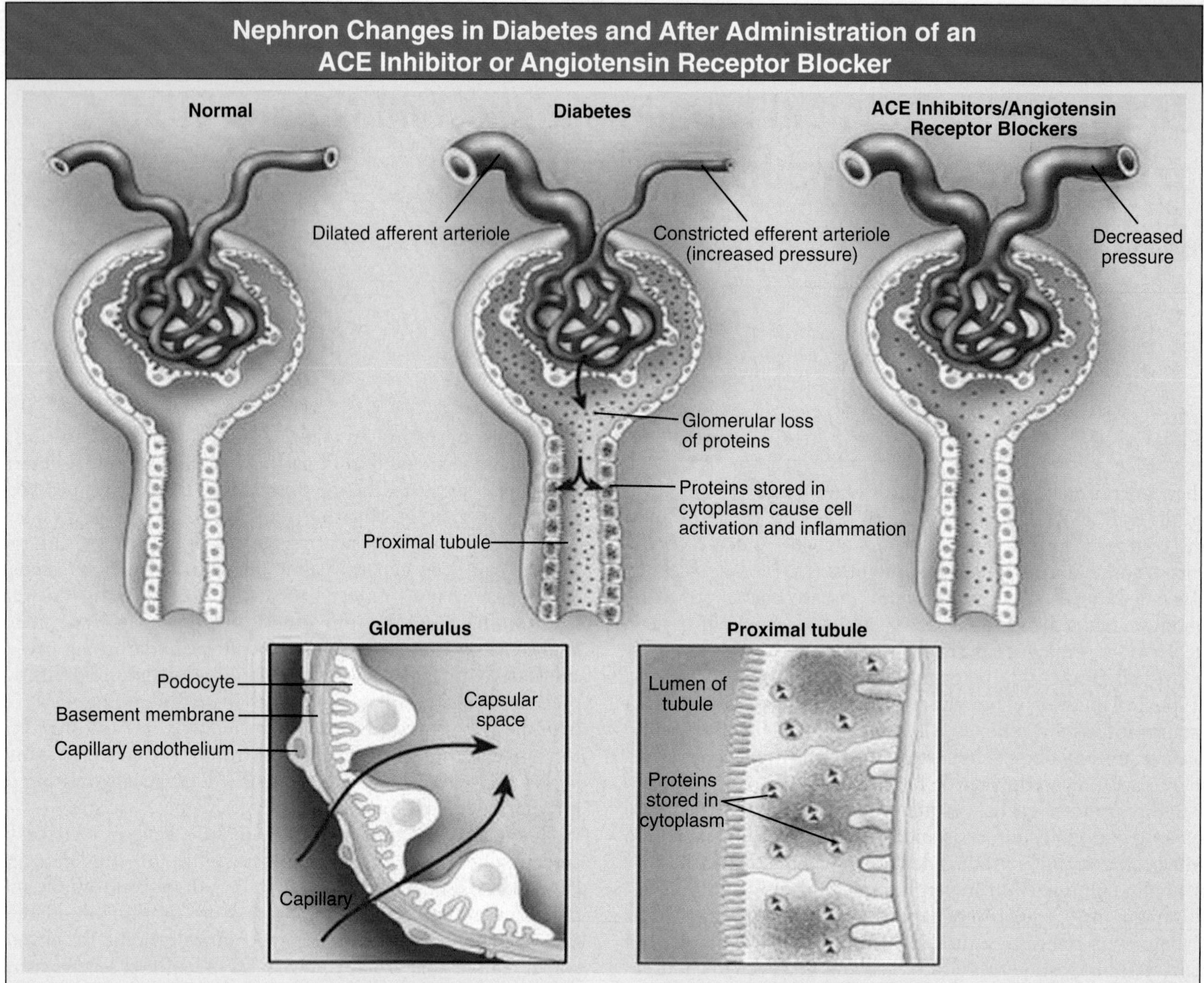

Figure 29.1 Schematic comparison of a normal nephron, a nephron in diabetic nephropathy (DN), and a nephron in DN after administration of angiotensin-converting enzyme (ACE) inhibitor/angiotensin receptor blocker (ARB). Note afferent vasodilation and efferent angiotensin II (Ang II)–mediated vasoconstriction in diabetes causing glomerular hypertension, which is relieved by ACE inhibitor/ARB treatment. Note also protein leakage into the filtrate and tubular loading with endocytosed protein causing an inflammatory reaction that promotes interstitial fibrosis. This is reversed by ACE inhibitor/ARB treatment.

hemodynamics trigger autocrine and paracrine release of cytokines and growth factors in the glomerulus.

There are also tubular abnormalities (e.g., increased tubular reabsorption of sodium). Hyperfiltration increases the colloid osmotic pressure in postglomerular capillaries, thus facilitating reabsorption of sodium in the proximal tubule. In the presence of hyperglycemia, increased proximal sodium reabsorption may also result from increased activity of the glucose- sodium cotransporter. Finally, there appears to be a role for angiotensin II (Ang II) causing hypertrophic proximal tubular growth and increased sodium reabsorption.[10]

Renal Hypertrophy

Renal growth is seen early after the onset of diabetes. The size of the kidney may increase by several centimeters. Glomerular enlargement is associated with an increase in the number of mesangial cells and of capillary loops, thus enhancing the filtration surface area. Enlargement of the glomeruli is the result of cellular hypertrophy, whereas the tubular epithelial cells undergo both proliferation and hypertrophy.

In animal experiments, avoidance of hyperglycemia prevents renal hypertrophy. Elevated plasma glucose levels cause hypertrophy by stimulating growth factors in the kidney, including IGF-1, epidermal growth factor (EGF), platelet-derived growth factor (PDGF), VEGF, TGF-β, and Ang II. The molecular mechanisms involved in glycemia-induced hypertrophy include induction of cell cycle inhibitors such as $p27^{Kip1}$. TGF-β stimulates protein synthesis (hypertrophy) but prevents cell proliferation and division by induction of cell cycle inhibitors. It is overexpressed in the glomeruli and the tubulointerstitium both in experimental and in human DN. Glucose as well as glucose-derived advanced glycation end products (AGEs) and Ang II stimulate the production of TGF-β in mesangial cells, podocytes, and tubular epithelial cells. Hyperglycemia also induces the expression of thrombospondin, a potent activator of latent TGF-β. Treatment of diabetic mice with neutralizing anti–TGF-β antibodies attenuated diabetes-related renal hypertrophy and extracellular matrix accumulation and preserved renal function, but it had little influence on proteinuria. Similarly, inhibition of VEGF prevented glomerular hypertrophy in models of DN and also reduced albuminuria.

Mesangial Expansion and Nodule Formation

The hallmarks of DN are mesangial expansion, nodular diabetic glomerulosclerosis (the acellular Kimmelstiel-Wilson lesion), and diffuse glomerulosclerosis. The early mesangial lesion is characterized by a variable increase in mesangial cell number and size associated with an increased deposition of extracellular matrix. In later stages, a general loss of mesangial cells occurs. Increasing evidence suggests that local NO deficiency contributes to these histologic lesions, in particular nodule formation. Indeed, endothelial cell nitric oxide synthase (NOS)–deficient mice made diabetic with streptozotocin represent one of the most promising models for DN.

Mesangial expansion is mediated by both glucose and glucose-derived AGEs. In experimental models, mesangial changes can largely be prevented by tight glycemic control or the use of AGE inhibitors such as aminoguanidine. The effects are presumably mediated by TGF-β.

Inflammation and Diabetic Nephropathy

Inflammatory processes and immune cells are involved in the development and progression of DN.[11] Glomerular and interstitial infiltration by monocytes-macrophages and activated T lymphocytes is observed both in human biopsy specimens and in animal models of DN. An inflammatory state is also suggested by the common elevation of serum levels of acute-phase proteins and elevated neutrophil counts. Chemokines and their receptors, in particular monocyte chemoattractant protein 1 (MCP-1/CCL2), as well as adhesion molecules seem to contribute to this.[11] Possibly fractalkine/CX3CL1 functions as an arrest chemokine in monocyte-macrophage adhesion before migration into the kidney. T-lymphocyte recruitment is the consequence of glomerular and tubulointerstitial upregulation of RANTES/CCL5 structures as well as tubulointerstitial upregulation of IP-10/CXCL10 (Fig. 29.2).

Mechanisms Underlying Proteinuria

Widening of the glomerular basement membrane (GBM) is associated with accumulation of type IV collagen and net reduction in negatively charged heparin sulfate. However, the latter cannot be the key factor underlying proteinuria as selective reduction of GBM proteoglycans unexpectedly reduced rather than increased proteinuria.[12] This supports the notion that the podocyte is more important in the genesis of proteinuria.[12] Biopsies in patients with DN documented a correlation between the degree of proteinuria and podocyte pathology, specifically the width of the foot processes. The expression of one permeability-controlling protein, nephrin, is abnormally low in DN.[12] The transcription of nephrin is suppressed by Ang II and restored by inhibitors of the renin-angiotensin system (RAS). In addition, in DN, apoptosis of podocytes is triggered by various factors including Ang II and TGF-β. Finally, migration of podocytes is reduced by AGE-induced suppression of neuropilin 1, preventing surviving podocytes from covering denuded areas of basement membrane, thus causing formation of synechia and development of focal glomerulosclerosis (FSGS).

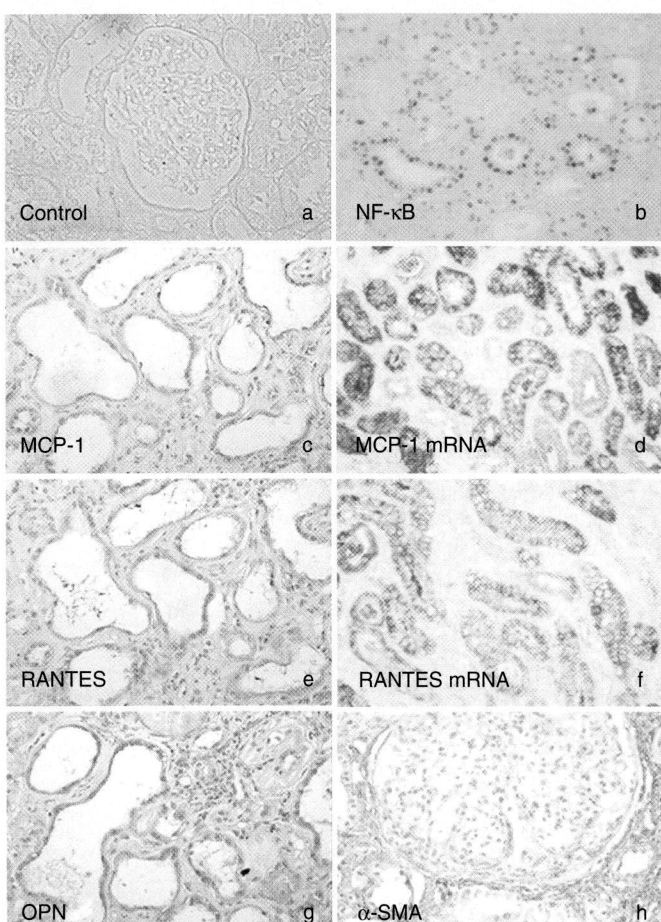

Figure 29.2 Activated nuclear factor (NF)-κB and overexpression of related chemokines in human diabetic nephropathy (DN). Overexpression of chemokines (MCP-1, RANTES), osteopontin (OPN), and activated NF-κB in human DN (**a,** normal, non-diabetic kidney; **b-h,** DN) indicating the inflammatory nature of DN. α-SMA, α-smooth muscle actin. *(From reference 13.)*

There is crosstalk between glomerular endothelial cells and podocytes, and this involves activated protein C (APC). APC formation is regulated by endothelial thrombomodulin and is reduced in diabetic mice.[14] In DN, thrombomodulin-dependent APC formation inhibits podocyte apoptosis (Fig. 29.3).[14]

In cultured podocytes, adiponectin administration reduced the permeability to albumin and caused podocyte dysfunction. Because adiponectin levels are low in patients with the metabolic syndrome or type 2 diabetes, lack of adiponectin may further contribute to proteinuria.

In advanced stages of DN, high-molecular-weight serum proteins are able to escape across basal membranes with disrupted texture, gaps, and holes (nonselective proteinuria).

Tubulointerstitial Fibrosis and Tubular Atrophy

Tubulointerstitial pathology is seen early[15] in DN and correlates with prognosis. The pathomechanisms underlying tubulointerstitial fibrosis and tubular atrophy are similar to or identical with those in nondiabetic progressive renal disease (see Chapter 75): release of growth factors, in particular TGF-β, and other cytokines from the glomerulus and direct or indirect effects of proteinuria. Under the influence of mediators such as TGF-β and

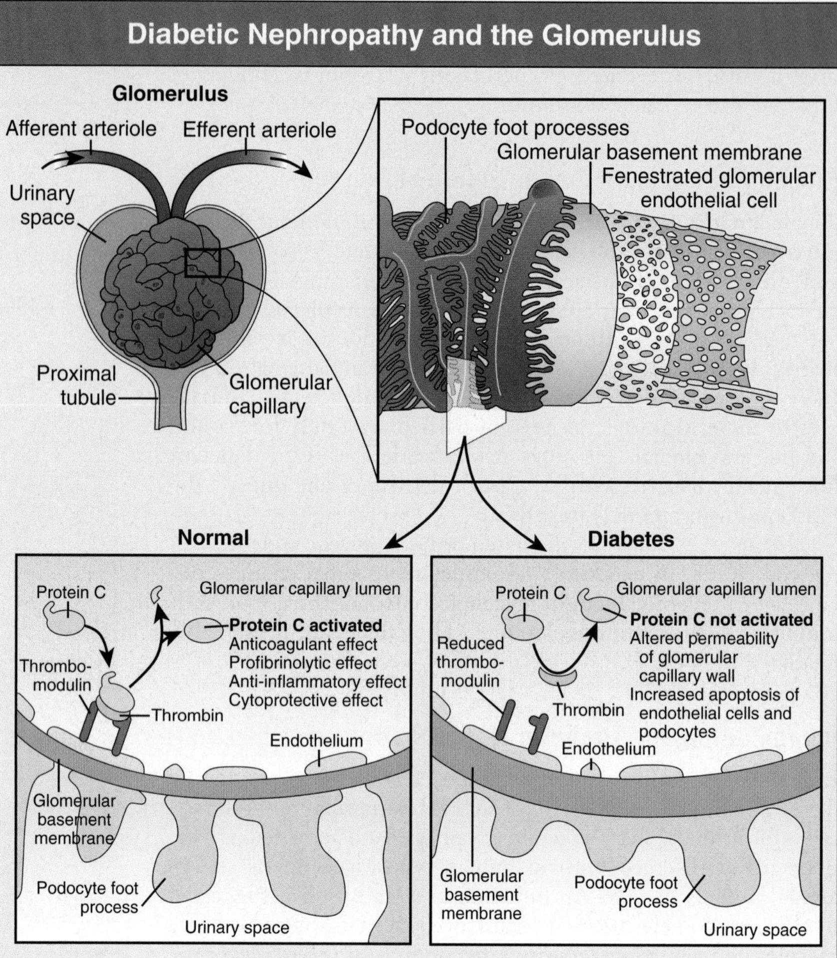

Figure 29.3 Crosstalk between endothelial cells and podocytes involving protein C. Under physiologic conditions, protein C is activated by the binding of thrombin to its receptor, called thrombomodulin, on glomerular endothelial cells. The formed complex catalyzes the conversion of protein C to its catalytically activated form, which has potent anticoagulant, profibrinolytic, anti-inflammatory, and cytoprotective effects. In diabetic nephropathy (DN), the production of activated protein C in the glomerulus is reduced because of suppression of thrombomodulin expression. Decreased functional activity of activated protein C affects the permeability of the glomerular capillary wall and enhances apoptosis of glomerular endothelial cells and podocytes. *(From reference 16.)*

Ang II, tubular cells change their phenotype and become fibroblasts.[14] High glucose concentration and AGEs further stimulate this process. Proapoptotic genes are expressed by tubular cells in DN, and this is promoted by Ang II.

Clinical studies provided evidence that even mild anemia (hemoglobin level <13.8 g/dl) increases the risk of progression of DN. Treatment of anemia early in renal failure with erythropoietin (EPO) may slow the decline of renal dysfunction in DN. Anemia presumably causes renal hypoxia.[15] Moreover, hypoxia is further amplified by the progressive hyalinosis of the afferent and efferent arterioles and loss of peritubular capillaries.[17] In experimental models of chronic renal injury, hypoxia is an important factor aggravating interstitial fibrosis, partly by the induction of factors such as TGF-β and VEGF. The transition of tubular epithelial cells into fibroblasts is stimulated by cellular hypoxia. The induction of growth factors and cytokines is mediated by hypoxia-inducing factor 1, and Ang II can aggravate this.

Hyperglycemia and Diabetic Nephropathy

Role of Glucose Control

Evidence of the role of tight glycemic control in retarding the development of DN includes the following:

- Studies suggest that with good glycemic control (reflected by an average HbA_{1c} level of 7.0%), only 9% of type 1 diabetic subjects will develop ESRD after 25 years as opposed to the historical prevalence of 40%.[18]
- Results from the Diabetes Control and Complications Trial (DCCT) showed a remarkable reduction in progression from normoalbuminuria to microalbuminuria and other microvascular complications, specifically retinopathy, in patients with type 1 diabetes with tight glycemic control.[19] At least for cardiovascular (CV) sequelae, the benefit of early aggressive reduction of glycemia persisted despite later deterioration of the glycemic control.[20]
- Euglycemia that followed isolated transplantation of the pancreas was associated with a regression of the diabetic glomerulosclerosis after 10 years.[21]
- Evidence from the United Kingdom Diabetes Prospective Study (UKPDS) showed that reducing the HbA_{1c} level by ~0.9% in subjects with type 2 diabetes reduces the risk for development of microvascular complications, including nephropathy.[22]
- The ADVANCE study randomly assigned 11,140 patients with type 2 diabetes to either intensive glucose control or standard glucose control. At the end of follow-up of 5 years, the HbA_{1c} level was 6.5% in the intensive group and 7.3% in the standard therapy group. Intensive glucose control was associated with a significant reduction in renal events and new-onset microalbuminuria. The trial did not show a significant effect of intensive control on major macrovascular events.[24]

The mechanisms by which hyperglycemia induces DN are complex and may involve not only effects of elevated glucose

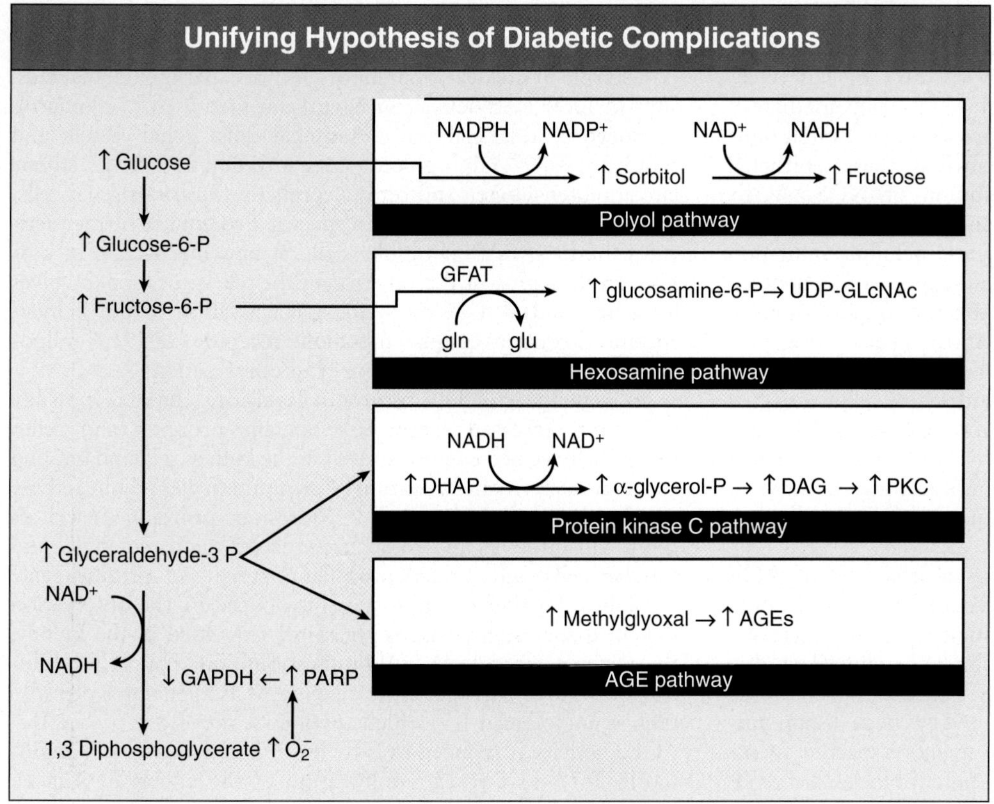

Figure 29.4 Unifying hypothesis of diabetic complications. Mitochondrial overproduction of superoxide activates four major pathways of hyperglycemic damage by inhibiting GAPDH. DHAP, dihydroxyacetone phosphate; DAG, diacylglycerine (an activator of protein kinase C, PKC, and of triose phosphates to methylglyoxal), the main intracellular advanced glycation endproduct (AGE) precursor. Increased flux of fructose-6-phosphate to UDP-N-acetylglucosamine increases modification of proteins by O-linked N-acetylglucosamine (GlcNAc) and increased glucose flux through the polyol pathway consumes nicotinamide adenine dinucleotide phosphate (NADPH) and depletes glutathione (GSH). NAD, nicotinamide adenine dinukleotide; UDP, uridine diphosphate; GAPDH, glycerinaldehyde-3-phosphate-dehydrogenase; GFAT, glutamine fructose-6-phosphate amidotransferase; gln, glutamine; glu, glutaminic acid; PARP, poly [ADP-ribose] polymerase; P, phosphate. *(From reference 23.)*

levels *per se* but also the generation of AGEs and alcohol sugars (polyols) as a consequence of hyperglycemia.

Brownlee proposed a unifying mechanism of how hyperglycemia leads to diabetic complications including DN (Fig. 29.4). An increase in intracellular glucose concentrations stimulates glucose oxidation in the tricarboxylic acid cycle, pushing more electron donors (NADH, $FADH_2$) into the electron transport chain.[25] When a critical threshold is reached and electrons are donated to molecular oxygen, superoxide is generated. This mitochondrial overproduction of superoxide activates four major pathways that are involved in DN.

Protein Kinase C (PKC) Pathway Many of the adverse effects of hyperglycemia have been attributed to activation of PKC, a family of serine-threonine kinases that regulate diverse vascular functions. The activity of PKC, especially the membrane-bound form, is increased in the retina, aorta, heart, and glomeruli of diabetic animals. In short- and long-term studies of diabetic rats, an orally effective PKC-β–selective inhibitor ameliorated glomerular hyperfiltration, albuminuria, and renal TGF-β overexpression as well as extracellular matrix accumulation. PKC-α may represent an additional therapeutic target because albuminuria was virtually absent in diabetic PKC-α knockout mice.

Advanced Glycation End Products Pathway Chronic hyperglycemia can lead to nonenzymatic glycation of amino acids and proteins (Maillard or browning reaction) (Fig. 29.5).[26] Over time, these products undergo rearrangement, including cross-linking, to become irreversible AGEs. Both circulating and tissue proteins as well as lipids and nucleic acids may thus be glycated. Although primarily observed in diabetes, AGEs also accumulate in aging and in renal failure.[26]

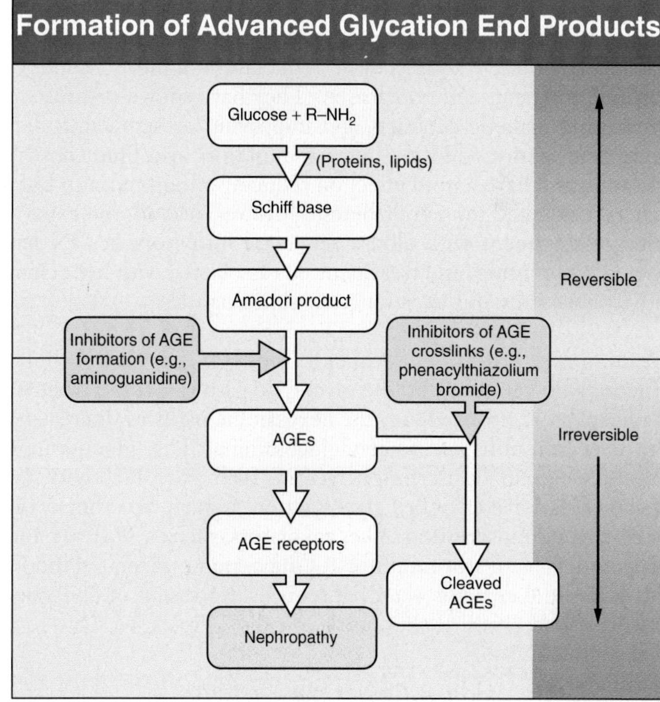

Figure 29.5 Mechanism of formation of advanced glycation end products (AGEs).

The concentration of AGEs is increased in the sera of DN patients. AGEs have also been localized to diabetic glomeruli by immunohistochemistry. AGEs bind to a variety of cell types, including macrophages and mesangial cells. They mediate a variety of cellular actions, including expression of adhesion molecules, cell hypertrophy, extracellular matrix synthesis, epithelial to mesenchymal transition, and inhibition of NOS. AGEs injected *in vivo* induce albuminuria and glomerulosclerosis.[23] AGEs have profound effects on podocytes, including induction of hypertrophy followed by apoptosis and suppression of nephrin synthesis. Among several binding sites, the most important is the putative receptor RAGE (receptor for AGE), a pattern recognition receptor. It is present in tubular cells and podocytes. Ang II stimulates upregulation of RAGE on podocytes.[27] This effect is mediated by angiotensin$_2$ (AT_2) receptors not blocked by sartanes.[27] One of the actions of RAGE is activation of nuclear factor (NF)-κB. sRAGE, the soluble extracellular domain of RAGE, acts as a decoy receptor and experimentally ameliorates the renal lesions in diabetes.[28]

Administration of aminoguanidine, an inhibitor of AGE formation, to animals with diabetes reduces AGE deposition, mesangial matrix expansion, and albuminuria but has inconsistent effects on GBM thickening. Preliminary clinical studies suggest beneficial effects on retinopathy, lipids, and proteinuria. The clinical experience with this compound has been disappointing and riddled with side effects. Newer, more specific agents have been developed that may be more potent blockers of AGE formation. Phenacylthiazolium bromide is a novel compound that cleaves covalent, AGE-derived protein cross-links and provides a conceptual basis for the reversal of AGE-mediated tissue damage, which until now has been regarded as irreversible.

Polyol Pathway The role of polyols in diabetic complications has been assessed with aldose reductase inhibitors, such as sorbinil, tolrestat, and ponalrestat. They have shown promise in preventing diabetic cataracts and improving or stabilizing diabetic neuropathy. Aldose reductase inhibitors also blunt hyperfiltration and have a mild effect on reducing albuminuria in both experimental and human diabetes. However, overall, the experience of treatment with aldose reductase inhibitors in DN has been disappointing, and treatment was associated with hypersensitivity reactions and liver function abnormalities.

Hexosamine Pathway Although most of the intracellular glucose is metabolized by the glycolytic pathway, some fructose 6-phosphate is diverted into the hexosamine pathway, increasing the concentrations of *N*-acetylglucosamine. This glucosamine modifies certain transcription factors, such as Sp1 activity, by post-translational *O*-linked glycosylation. In turn, Sp1 then leads to enhanced transcription of key mediators, such as TGF-β1 and plasminogen activator inhibitor 1. Glucosamine-mediated modification of the enzyme Akt/PKB reduces expression of endothelial NOS and promotes apoptosis of cells.

Renin-Angiotensin-Aldosterone System and Diabetic Nephropathy

Studies in patients with type 1 and type 2 diabetes as well as in various animal models of diabetes suggest that ACE inhibitors or angiotensin receptor blockers (ARBs) retard progression of DN (see Chapter 30).

Although plasma renin activity is low in DN, it is inappropriate in relation to increased extracellular volume and exchangeable sodium, suggesting activation of the RAS.[29] This has raised the possibility that activation of the intrarenal RAS may play a critical role in the development of DN. In experimental diabetes, sites of local RAS activation have been identified in glomeruli (podocytes, mesangial and endothelial cells), renal vessels, and tubular cells.[28,29] High glucose concentration and AGEs stimulate angiotensinogen and renin expression in various renal cells, mainly through reactive oxygen species. Proteinuria further activates the local RAS of tubular cells. A new mechanism of how high levels of glucose directly trigger the release of renin involves local accumulation of succinate and activation of the kidney-specific G protein–coupled metabolic receptor GPR91.[30] Adipocytes are another source of Ang II in obese patients.

In patients with DN, prorenin levels are elevated, possibly reflecting increased synthesis.[31] Specific prorenin and renin receptors have been demonstrated in the kidney[31]; ligand binding causes nonenzymatic activation of prorenin to yield renin activity and locally produced Ang II.[31] Moreover, prorenin as well as renin can directly bind to specific receptors on mesangial and tubular cells and induce proinflammatory and profibrogenic cytokines. Further complexity is introduced by the observation that in diabetes, chymase is strikingly expressed in the kidney; this enzyme generates Ang II but is not inhibited by ACE inhibitors.[32] On the other hand, the enzyme ACE2 generates peptides such as angiotensin 1-7, which antagonize the effects of Ang II.[28] ACE2 activity is reduced in DN, leading to a decrease in angiotensin 1-7 and further amplification of the effects of Ang II. Interestingly, 1,25-dihydroxyvitamin D_3 suppresses the RAS. Thus, in diabetics with advancing chronic kidney disease (CKD), decreasing calcitriol production further activates the RAS.

Ang II has many nonhemodynamic effects and mediates cell proliferation, hypertrophy, matrix expansion, and cytokine (TGF-β, VEGF) synthesis.[29] Therefore, ACE inhibitors and ARBs presumably act by hemodynamic as well as by nonhemodynamic actions.

Aldosterone accelerates progression in renal damage models independently of Ang II. In DN, aldosterone escape has been linked to progression of proteinuria (see Chapter 30). Aldosterone synthesis is stimulated in DN, and this steroid hormone stimulates the synthesis of other proinflammatory and profibrogenic cytokines (MCP-1, TGF-β).

Other vasoactive agents may also be involved in the pathogenesis of DN, including alterations in systemic or intrarenal production of endothelin, NO, the kallikrein-kinin system, and natriuretic peptides.

Uric Acid and Fructose

Experimental and clinical studies have suggested that uric acid may contribute to the development of hypertension and kidney disease. Uric acid stimulates mitogen-activated kinases (p38 and ERK) and nuclear transcription factors (NF-κB and activator protein [AP] 1), resulting in PDGF-dependent proliferation, cyclooxygenase 2–dependent thromboxane production, MCP-1 and C-reactive protein synthesis, and stimulation of Ang II in renal cells.[33] Clinical studies indicate that uric acid level early after onset of type 1 diabetes is independently associated with the risk for later development of DN.[34]

It has been proposed that excessive fructose intake (>50 g/day) may be one of the underlying causes of metabolic syndrome and type 2 diabetes. The primary sources of fructose are sugar (sucrose) and high-fructose corn syrup. The ingestion of excessive fructose induces features of metabolic syndrome in both

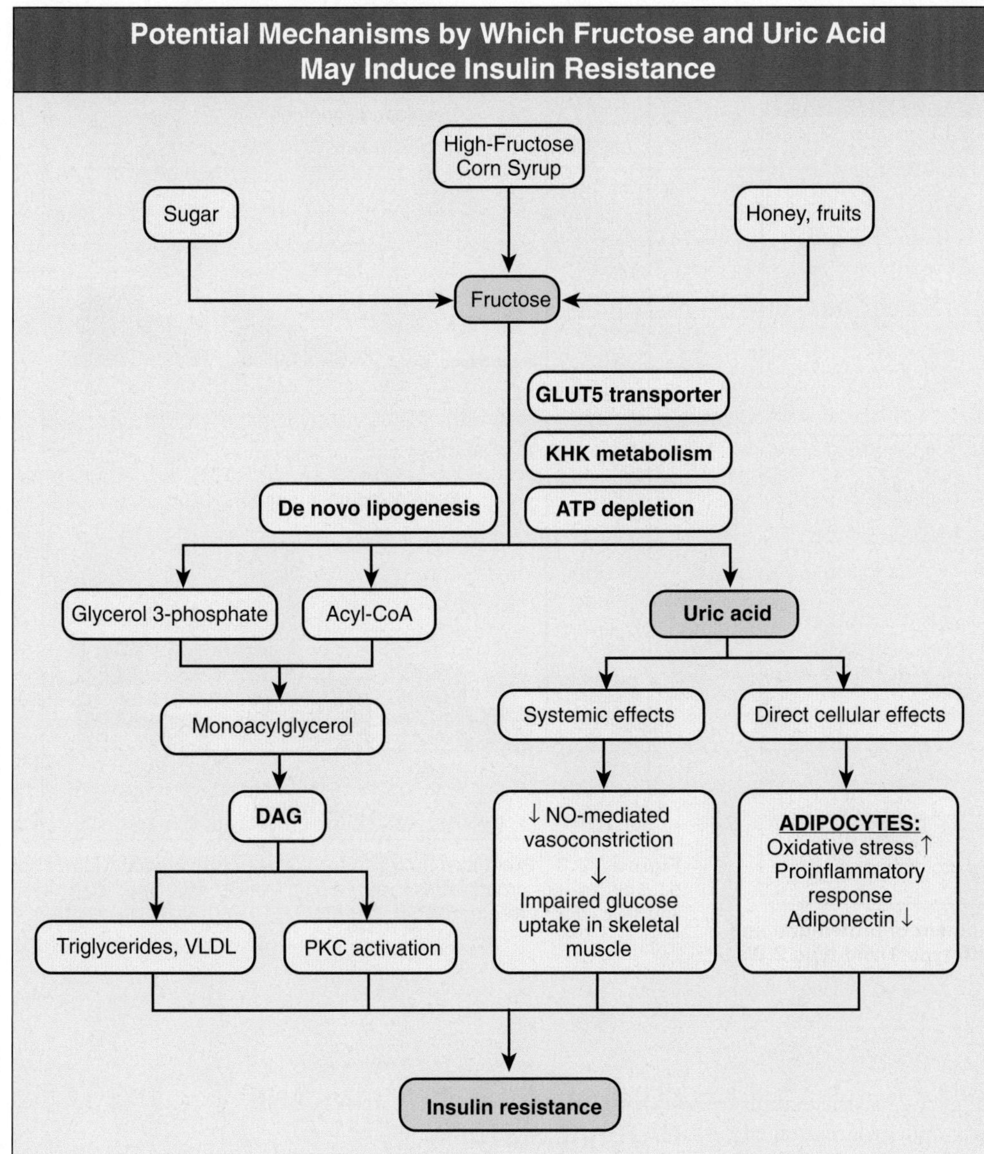

Figure 29.6 Potential role of fructose and uric acid in mediating insulin resistance. Fructose enters the cell through the GLUT5 transporter and is metabolized by fructokinase (ketohexokinase [KHK]). As part of this metabolism, ATP depletion may occur, generating uric acid with systemic effects that block insulin-dependent nitric oxide (NO)–mediated vascular dilation as well as direct cellular effects on the adipocyte. Fructose also causes *de novo* lipogenesis, which can lead to intracellular triglycerides that can also induce insulin resistance. ATP, adenosine triphosphate; DAG, diacylglycerol; HFCS, high-fructose corn syrup; PKC, protein kinase C; VLDL, very low density lipoprotein. *(From reference 30.)*

laboratory animals and humans. Interestingly, fructose appears to mediate the metabolic syndrome in part by raising uric acid.[33] Fructose and uric acid also mediate insulin resistance (Fig. 29.6). Thus, excessive fructose intake in concert with uric acid may foster the development and progression of DN.

EPIDEMIOLOGY

In most Western countries, DN has become the leading cause of ESRD. According to the U.S. Renal Data System (*www.USRDS.org*), in 2006, DN was the most frequent primary diagnosis with 159 per million population per year. The proportion of diabetics among patients with ESRD varies considerably between countries but had consistently been on the rise in all countries until recently, when the incidence figures have stabilized. In patients admitted for renal replacement therapy (RRT), we found diabetes in 49%, but classic features of DN were observed in only 60% of these (i.e., large kidneys, proteinuria exceeding 1 g/24 h with or without retinopathy); 13% exhibited an atypical presentation with ischemic nephropathy, and in 27% of the cases, a known primary renal disease (e.g., polycystic kidney disease [PKD], analgesic nephropathy, glomerulonephritis [GN]) coexisted with diabetes.[35] An important mode of presentation has become irreversible acute kidney injury (AKI), for example, after administration of radiocontrast media, cardiac events, and septicemia. Often, the diagnosis of diabetes had not been made at the time of admission because hyperglycemia may disappear when patients lose weight secondary to anorexia from renal failure (so-called DN without diabetes). This may explain why at least 5% of patients develop apparent *de novo* diabetes after the start of dialysis.

The great majority (in our experience, >90%) of patients entering ESRD with diabetes as a comorbid condition suffer from type 2 diabetes. In the past, few type 2 diabetic patients had a chance to live long enough to develop nephropathy. Today, with better treatment of hypertension and of coronary heart disease, an increasing proportion of type 2 diabetic patients survive and are exposed to the risk for development of DN and ESRD. The proportion of type 1 and type 2 diabetic patients who develop proteinuria and elevated serum creatinine concentration is related

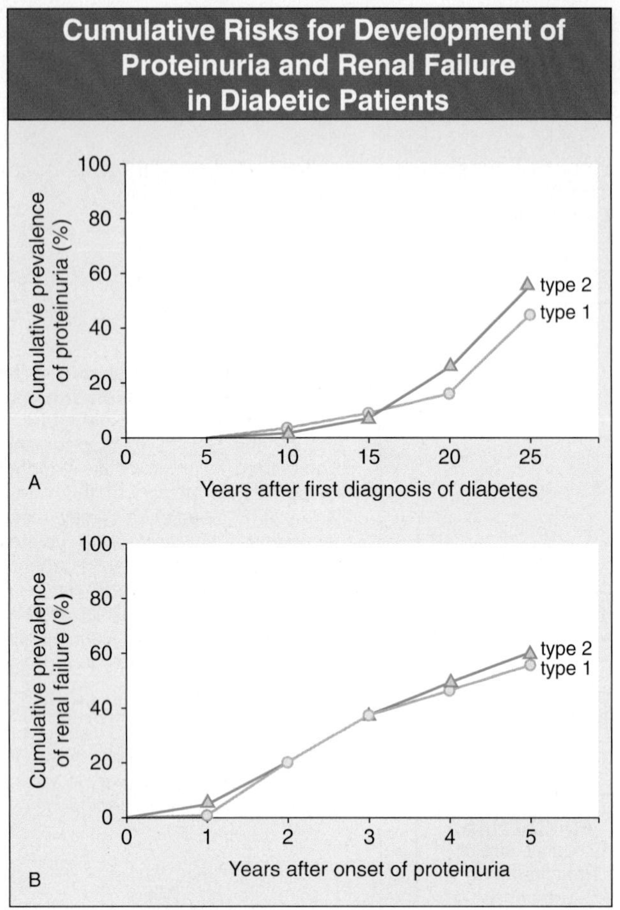

Figure 29.7 Cumulative risks for development of proteinuria and progression to renal failure in patients with type 1 and type 2 diabetes. *(From reference 35.)*

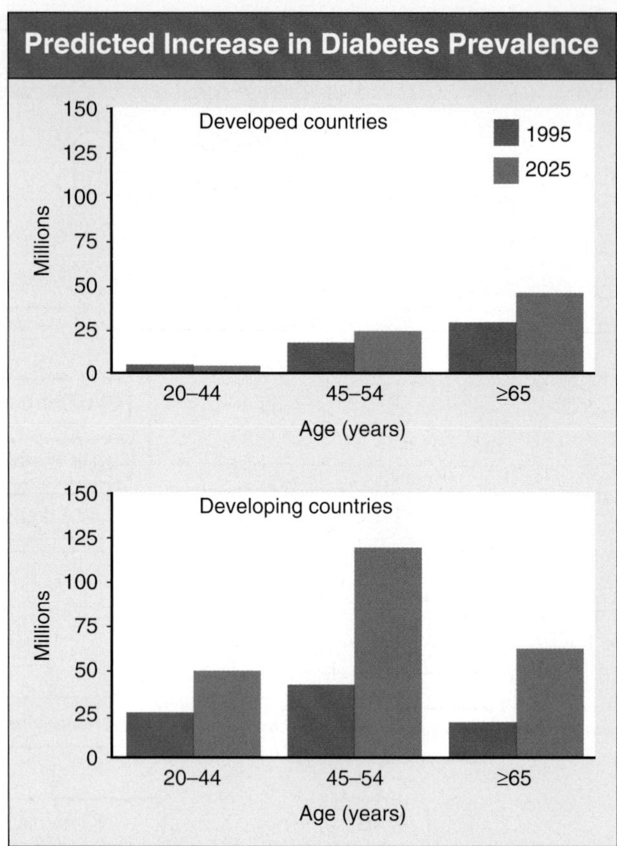

Figure 29.8 Predicted increase in diabetes prevalence. Number of patients by age group, region (developing versus developed countries), and year. *(From reference 39.)*

to the duration of diabetes. As shown in Figure 29.7, the cumulative risks for development of proteinuria and progression are practically superimposable in type 1 and type 2.[32] Diabetes-related deaths amounted to almost 3 million, equivalent to 5% of world all-cause mortality in 2000. There is a major increase in the prevalence of type 2 diabetes in the developing world compared with the developed world (Fig. 29.8). For example, in Asia, the excess death from diabetes is most prominent in the age group between 50 and 60 years, which translates to a reduction in life expectancy of more than a decade. Up to 60% of Asian diabetic patients have microalbuminuria or macroalbuminuria, compared with 30% to 40% reported in Western diabetic populations in cross-sectional surveys.[36] One explanation for this ethnic disparity in renal risk may be that longer survival in Asians provides greater opportunity for the evolution of renal complication. In addition, several polymorphisms have been discovered to independently predict DN in Chinese patients.[37]

There is also a difference in the incidence of diabetes-associated ESRD in Western countries, with very high numbers of patients in the United States.[38] The reasons for this fact are certainly complex and may include genetic variability, differences in lifestyle, different national health systems with variable access to screening programs, and other factors.[40] A targeted screening program may help in the early identification of individuals at high risk for DN.[38]

CLINICAL MANIFESTATIONS AND NATURAL HISTORY

DN constitutes part of a generalized microvascular syndrome that is accompanied by macrovascular disease.

Obesity, The Metabolic Syndrome, and Renal Disease

The metabolic syndrome—defined as having at least three of the five parameters of increased waist circumference, elevated triglycerides, decreased high-density lipoproteins, elevated blood pressure, and elevated fasting blood glucose concentration—is increasingly being recognized not only as a major contributor to cardiovascular diseases but also as an influence on renal function. The recognition that the metabolic syndrome is strongly associated with kidney disease has been appreciated only recently.[41] Obese individuals (body mass index >30) have large kidneys and glomerulomegaly. These patients have increased renal blood flow, increased filtration fraction, and glomerular hyperfiltration.[42] Obese patients exhibit microalbuminuria even in the absence of concomitant hypertension. The resemblance of obesity-related kidney disease to the early features of diabetic kidney disease is striking. In addition, sleep apnea, which is common in obese individuals, leading to hypoxic episodes, may also contribute to kidney impairment. Visceral adipocytes are a potent source of deleterious factors[43] that could have an impact on renal function (Ang II, leptin, tumor necrosis factor [TNF] α). Thus, renal changes may occur years before the manifestation of type 2 diabetes during obesity and the development of the metabolic syndrome.

Evolution of Diabetic Nephropathy

One of the earliest changes of renal function in diabetes is an increase in GFR, or hyperfiltration, which is observed in patients with type 1 and also many with type 2 diabetes. It is paralleled by an increase in renal size. The next observable change is the development of albuminuria. Somewhat arbitrarily, albumin excretion rates between 0 and 30 mg/day are called normoalbuminuria, and between 30 and 300 mg/day, microalbuminuria. Diabetic patients with persistent microalbuminuria are at markedly increased risk for development of overt DN, which is heralded by the development of proteinuria (albuminuria >300 mg/day), on average 15 years after disease onset, with progressive increase in proteinuria and BP as well as development of progressive CKD.

Mogensen[44] proposed a scheme of the different stages of DN (Fig. 29.9) that is valid in type 1 diabetes but less reliable in type 2 diabetes, in which CKD may occur in the absence of microalbuminuria, possibly the result of microvascular disease.

Hypertension and Diabetic Nephropathy

If hypertension develops in a patient with type 1 diabetes, it is almost always of renal parenchymal origin. However, today, type 1 diabetics survive longer, and a minority of elderly type 1 diabetics develop primary hypertension with no evidence of nephropathy. In patients with type 2 diabetes, hypertension often precedes the onset of diabetes by many years and decades as a feature of the metabolic syndrome. At the time when type 2 diabetes is diagnosed, an abnormal BP and an abnormal circadian BP profile are found in 80% of patients. Prediabetic hypertension increases the risk of onset and progression of DN. If patients with type 2 diabetes ultimately develop nephropathy, the prevalence of hypertension increases further and the degree of BP elevation is greater, but the relationship between hypertension and nephropathy is generally much less close than in type 1 diabetes. The pathogenesis of hypertension in type 2 diabetes is complex and involves activation of the RAS, direct sympathicus activation, and macrovascular changes.[45] Furthermore, there is evidence that genetic factors defining primary hypertension as well as diabetes are clustered (Fig. 29.10).

In DN, it has been well documented that the nocturnal BP decrease is frequently attenuated (nondipping), and nondipping even precedes the onset of microalbuminuria.[46] Furthermore, the BP response to exercise tends to be exaggerated, even when the BP is normal under basal conditions. Diminished compliance of the central arteries with stiffening of the aorta increases the peak systolic pressure and decreases the diastolic pressure, resulting in increased BP amplitude. The great BP amplitude explains why isolated systolic hypertension is so common in patients with type 2 diabetes.[47] Low diastolic pressure increases the risk of coronary events because coronary perfusion occurs during diastole only. Ambulatory pulse pressure and impaired nocturnal BP decline are independent predictors of nephropathy progression in type 2 diabetic patients (Fig. 29.11).

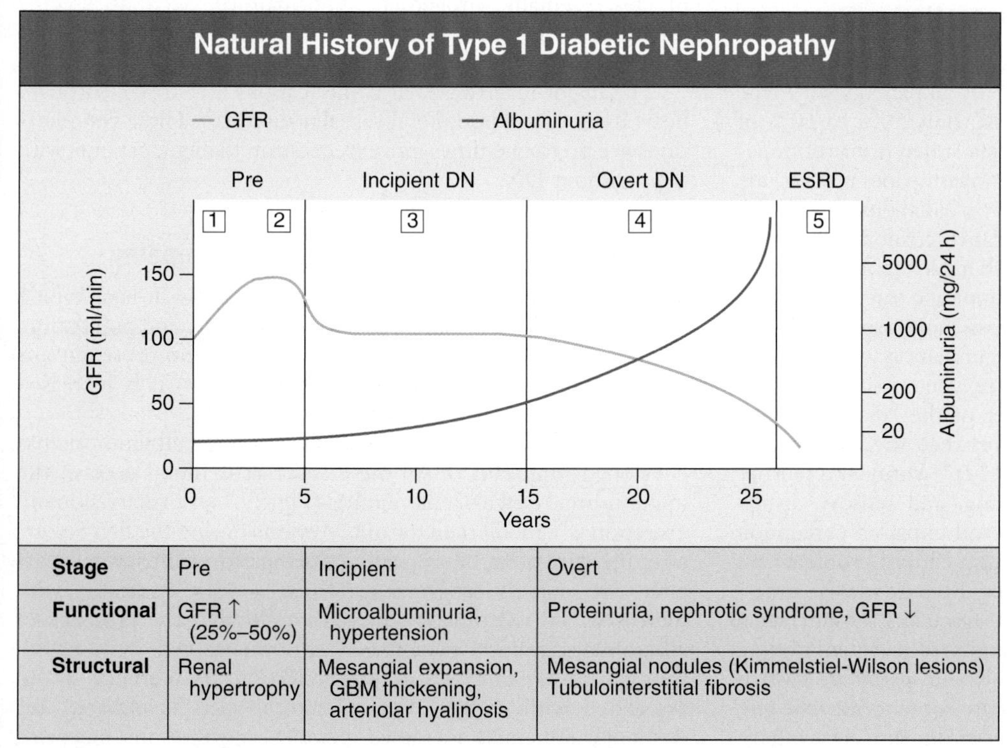

Stage	Pre	Incipient	Overt
Functional	GFR ↑ (25%–50%)	Microalbuminuria, hypertension	Proteinuria, nephrotic syndrome, GFR ↓
Structural	Renal hypertrophy	Mesangial expansion, GBM thickening, arteriolar hyalinosis	Mesangial nodules (Kimmelstiel-Wilson lesions) Tubulointerstitial fibrosis

Figure 29.9 Natural history of type 1 diabetic nephropathy (DN). Functional and structural manifestations of DN. Numbers 1 through 5 indicate the stages of nephropathy defined by Mogensen. DN, diabetic nephropathy; ESRD, end-stage renal disease; GBM, glomerular basement membrane; GFR, glomerular filtration rate. *(From reference 44.)*

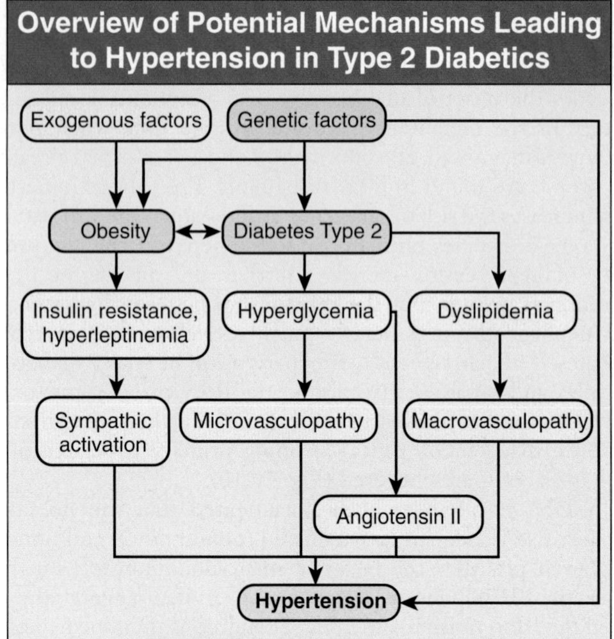

Figure 29.10 Overview of potential mechanisms leading to hypertension in type 2 diabetics. Genetic susceptibility factors for primary hypertension and diabetes may be clustered so that an individual patient may have a higher incidence of both diseases. Obesity and the metabolic syndrome lead to insulin resistance and hyperleptinemia associated with sympathic nerve activation. Hyperglycemia directly activates the renin-angiotensin system (RAS) and, in addition, through renal microvasculopathy stimulates development of hypertension. Dyslipidemia leads through macrovasculopathic alteration to stiffness of vessels and hypertension.

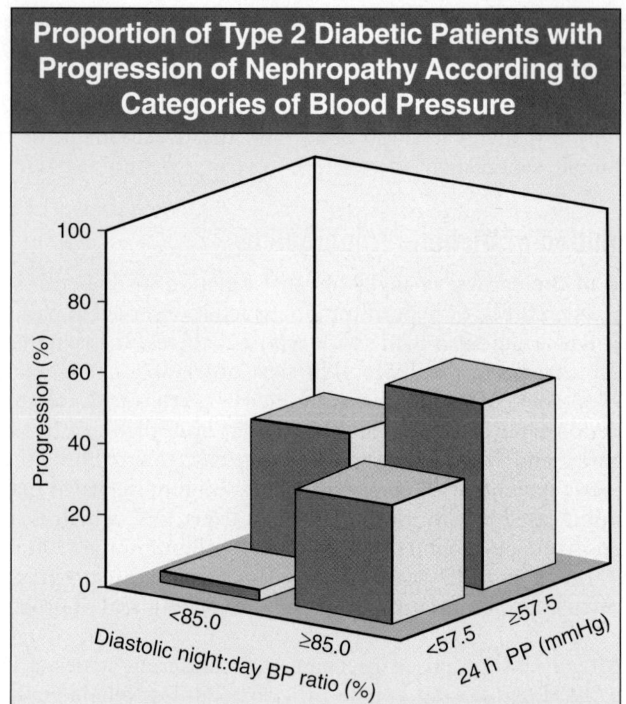

Figure 29.11 Proportion of type 2 diabetic patients with progression of nephropathy according to categories of blood pressure. Progression risk according to categories of night:day diastolic BP (median value <85% or >85%), and 24 hour ambulatory pulse pressure (PP) (median value <57.5% or >57.%). *(From reference 51.)*

Extrarenal Microvascular and Macrovascular Complications Associated with Diabetic Nephropathy

Diabetic retinopathy is present in virtually all patients with type 1 diabetes and nephropathy. In contrast, only 50% to 60% of proteinuric patients with type 2 diabetes suffer from retinopathy.[48] Consequently, the absence of retinopathy does not exclude the diagnosis of DN in patients with type 2 diabetes.[49] The risk of blindness because of severe proliferative retinopathy is substantially higher in diabetic patients with nephropathy, but it has become rare today with better ophthalmologic care. In patients with DN, retinopathy tends to progress more rapidly so that yearly or half-yearly ophthalmologic examination is indicated.

Many patients with DN also have polyneuropathy. Sensory polyneuropathy is an important aspect of the "diabetic foot." There is a strong inverse correlation between the incidence of diabetic foot and renal function (Fig. 29.12).[50] Motor and sensory neuropathy may cause areflexia, wasting, and sensory disturbances such as paresthesia, anesthesia, and impaired perception of vibration and pain, but the most vexing clinical problems are the results of autonomic polyneuropathy. Because cardiac innervation is defective, pain and angina are frequently absent when the patient has ischemic heart disease and myocardial infarction. Further consequences of autonomic polyneuropathy are gastroparesis, that is, delayed emptying of gastric contents into the gut, and diarrhea or constipation (often alternating with each other). These problems are caused by impaired intestinal innervation, often complicated by intestinal bacterial overgrowth because of stasis. Finally, urogenital abnormalities, such as erectile impotence or detrusor paresis with delayed and incomplete emptying of the bladder, are frequent.

The major macrovascular complications are stroke, coronary heart disease, and peripheral vascular disease.[52] These complications are up to five times more frequent in diabetic patients with than without DN.

Survival in Patients with Diabetic Nephropathy

The presence of DN greatly increases mortality in both type 1 and type 2 diabetes. Compared with the background population, mortality in patients with type 1 diabetes and no proteinuria is elevated only twofold to threefold; in contrast, it is increased 20- to 200-fold in patients with proteinuria.[53]

The major increase in risk starts when microalbuminuria has developed (Fig. 29.13). An increased risk is found even in the upper normal range of albuminuria (Fig. 29.14). Urinary albumin excretion is a good predictor of CV events during the first 5 years after measurement, but repeating the measurement several years later also detects progression, which is also associated with increased CV risk.[54] It is widely thought that the presence of albuminuria reflects generalized endothelial cell dysfunction, thus increasing the risk of atherosclerosis. Its presence is also associated with many CV risk factors, such as elevated BP, dyslipoproteinemia, increased platelet aggregation, increased C-reactive protein concentration, and others. An added risk

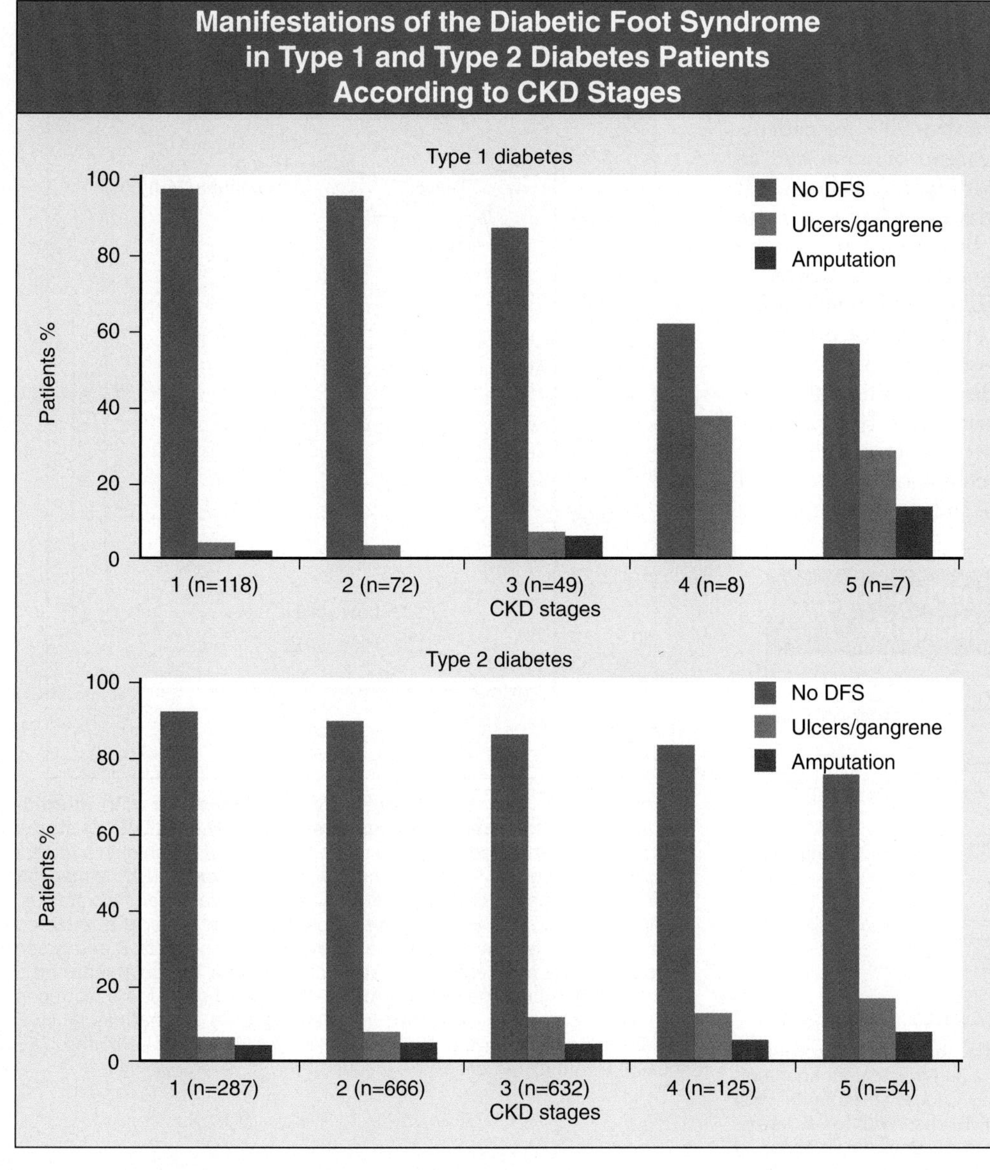

Figure 29.12 Association between manifestations of the diabetic foot syndrome (DFS) in type 1 and 2 diabetes patients classified according to chronic kidney disease (CKD) stages. Only patients with albuminuria were studied. All patients in a CKD stage were considered 100%. DFS increases with higher CKD stages. *(From reference 55.)*

factor is presumably the association with autonomic polyneuropathy, the presence of which predicts death from myocardial infarction or arrhythmia (sudden death).

RENAL PATHOLOGY

After the onset of diabetes, kidney weight increases by an average of 15%. Renal size remains increased until overt nephropathy is established. In most patients with type 1 diabetes, there is a sustained increase in glomerular volume and glomerular capillary luminal volume. Although atrophic ischemic glomeruli are present, some of the nonfunctioning glomeruli fill up with material staining with periodic acid–Schiff (PAS), thus preserving their increased dimensions. These changes are accompanied by hypertrophy of the interstitium.

In patients with a duration of diabetes of more than 10 years irrespective of whether nephropathy is present, GBM thickening up to three times the normal range of 270 to 359 nm is an almost universal feature (Fig. 29.15). In advancing DN, there is a consistent correlation between GBM thickness and fractional mesangial volumes with the urinary albumin excretion rate.

Nodular glomerular intercapillary lesions in advanced DN were described in 1936 by Kimmelstiel and Wilson (Fig. 29.16C). The nodules are located in the central regions of peripheral glomerular lobules as well-demarcated eosinophilic and PAS-positive masses (Fig. 29.16C and D). When they are not acellular, they contain pyknotic nuclei. It is suggested that they result from microaneurysmal dilation of the associated capillary followed by mesangiolysis and laminar organization of the mesangial debris with lysis of the center of the lobule. Foam cells often surround the nodules. These appearances are pathognomonic for diabetes but are reported in only 10% to 50% of biopsy specimens in both type 1 and type 2 diabetes. Nodules are also seen in membranoproliferative glomerulonephritis (MPGN) (see Chapter 21), in amyloidosis and light-chain deposition disease (LCDD) (see Chapter 26), and very rarely without diabetes (see Chapter 27); specific stains and immunofluorescence (IF) findings, respectively, will clarify the diagnosis. When there are no nodules seen, specific staining should be used to exclude amyloid.

The diffuse glomerular lesion is more frequent than the nodular lesion, with an incidence of more than 90% for patients with type 1 diabetes longer than 10 years in duration and an incidence of 25% to 50% in patients with type 2 diabetes.[56] It comprises an increase of mesangial matrix extending to involve the capillary loops (see Fig. 29.16B). In contrast to nodular lesions, which are of little functional significance, the degree of diffuse glomerulosclerosis correlates with the clinical manifestations of worsening renal function. Accumulation of mesangial matrix is the feature most consistently associated with progression.[57] In more severe disease, the capillary wall thickening and mesangial expansion lead to capillary narrowing (Fig. 29.15B) and hyalinization, with accompanying periglomerular fibrosis.

Podocytes are involved early in the course of DN in type 1 and type 2 diabetes mellitus (Fig. 29.17), and an increase in foot

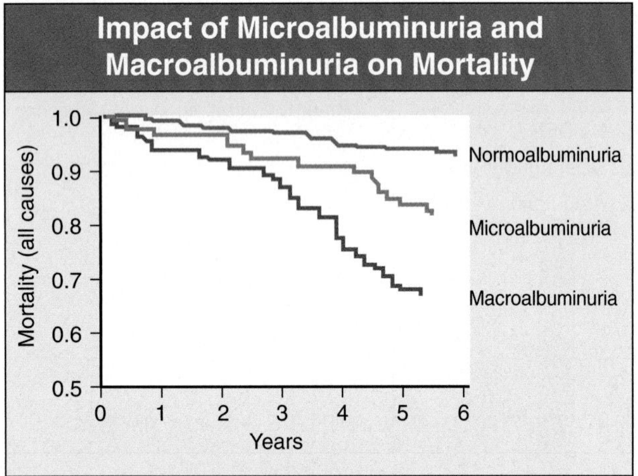

Figure 29.13 Impact of microalbuminuria and macroalbuminuria on mortality. The impact of microalbuminuria and macroalbuminuria on mortality was evaluated prospectively in 328 Caucasian patients with non–insulin-dependent diabetes mellitus (DM) observed for 5 years. Microalbuminuria and macroalbuminuria led to a significant increase in total mortality compared with patients who remained normoalbuminuric. *(From reference 53.)*

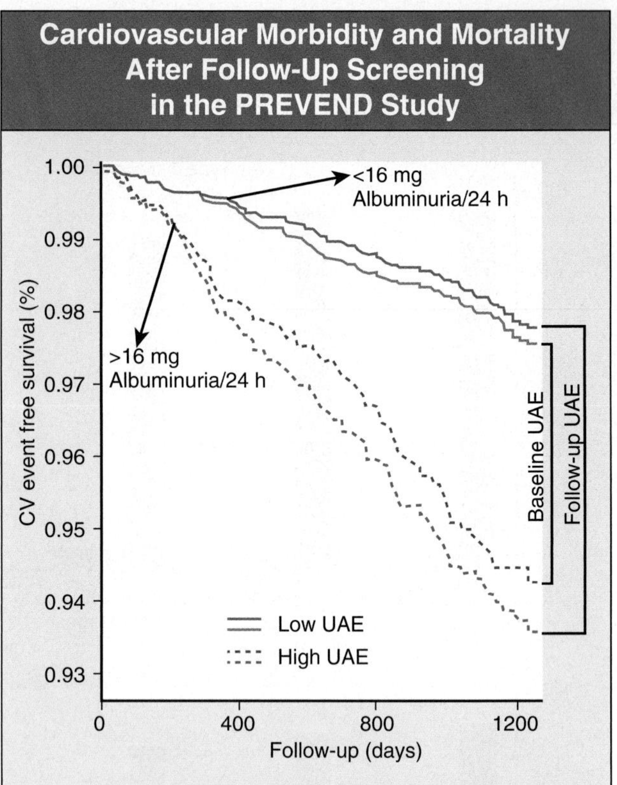

Figure 29.14 Event-free survival for cardiovascular (CV) morbidity and mortality after follow-up screening in the PREVEND study. Individuals are stratified according to the presence of a high or low urinary albumin excretion (UAE). High and low UAE are defined by either the UAE measurement from the baseline screening *(orange and violet lines)* of approximately 4.2 years before follow-up screening or the repeated UAE measurement at time of the follow-up screening *(blue and green lines)*. To allow comparison, the survival curves for the 6800 individuals with either the baseline or follow-up measurement of UAE are plotted in the same graph. A high UAE *(dashed lines)* is defined as a UAE ≥16.2 mg/24 h, being the 75th percentile of UAE with use of the UAE measurement of the baseline screening. *(From reference 54.)*

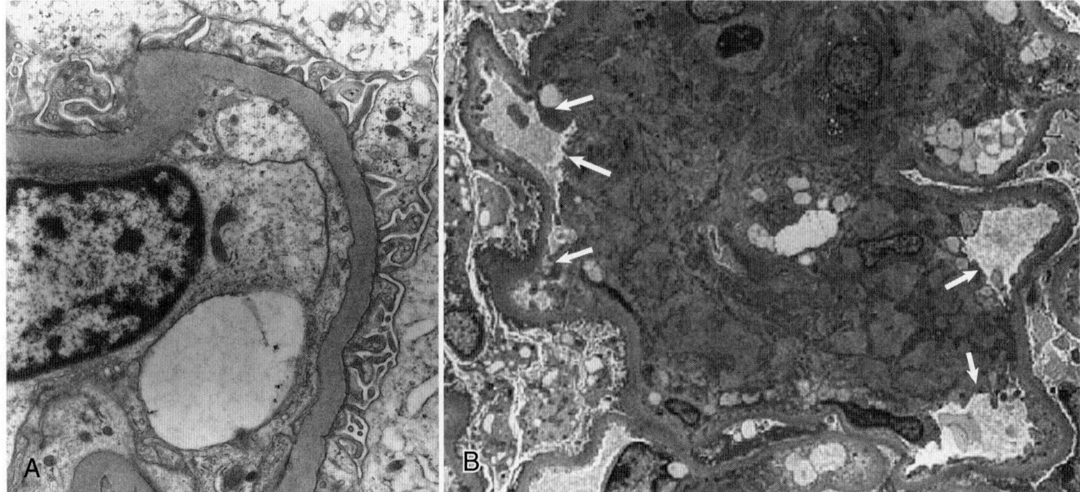

Figure 29.15 Electron microscopy of structural changes in diabetic nephropathy (DN). A, Glomerular basement membranes (GBMs) are diffusely thickened. **B,** The expanded mesangium encroaches on the capillary spaces *(arrows)*.

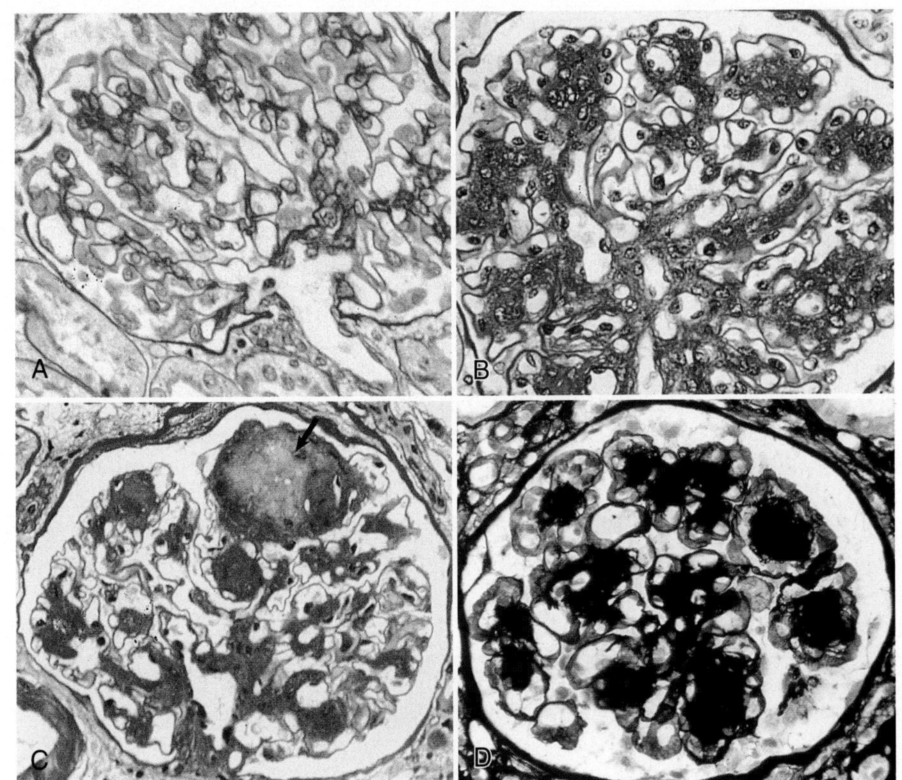

Figure 29.16 Light microscopy of structural changes in diabetic nephropathy (DN). A, Normal glomerulus (periodic acid–Schiff). **B,** Diffuse glomerular lesion: widespread mesangial expansion (periodic acid–Schiff). **C,** Nodular lesion as well as mesangial expansion; there is a typical Kimmelstiel-Wilson nodule at the top of the glomerulus *(arrow)* (periodic acid–Schiff). **D,** Nodular lesion: methenamine silver staining showing the marked nodular expansion of mesangial matrix.

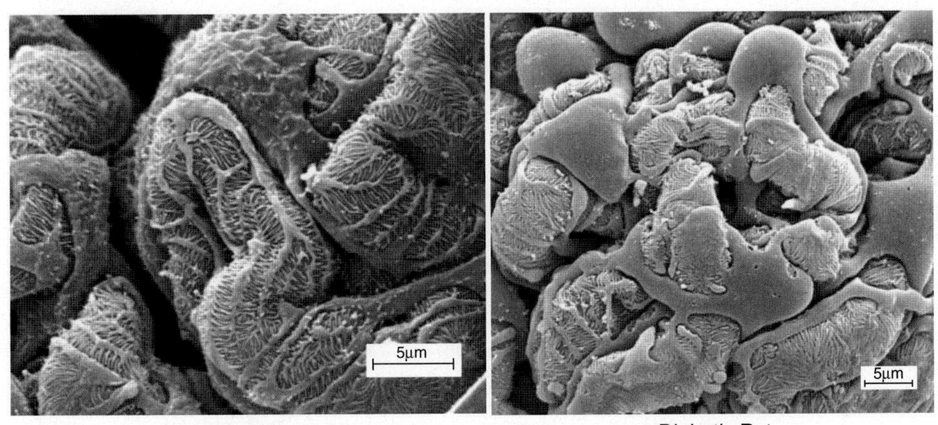

Figure 29.17 Electron micrograph of the external surface of glomerular tufts from rats after removal of Bowman's capsule by freeze-fracture. *Left,* A normal rat kidney with podocyte cell body; the primary processes and terminal foot processes resting on the glomerular capillary basement membrane are clearly seen. *Right,* The decrease in the density of foot processes and the denuded glomerular capillary basement membrane are apparent. *(From reference 59)*

process width is already observed in microalbuminuric type 1 diabetics.[58] Longitudinal studies in DN demonstrated a reduction in podocyte number that closely correlated with proteinuria. Renal biopsy specimens from Pima Indians with type 2 diabetes showed a broadening in podocyte foot processes and a concomitant reduction in the number of podocytes per glomerulus.[60]

Arteriolar lesions are prominent in diabetes. Hyaline material progressively replaces the entire wall structure and involves both the afferent and efferent vessels, which is highly specific for diabetes.

The tubules and the interstitium may show a variety of changes, including tubular cell vacuolization and tubulointerstitial fibrosis.[61] In patients with glycemia above 500 mg/dl and severe glycosuria, Armani-Ebstein lesions can be found (Fig. 29.18). They consist of deposits of glycogen in the tubular epithelial cells (pars straight of proximal convoluted tubule and loop of Henle) but are very rarely seen today. Tubulointerstitial leukocyte infiltration is often found in DN. Tubulointerstitial fibrosis and tubular atrophy are presumably the best pathologic correlates for the progressive decline in GFR. Tubulointerstitial fibrosis and renal arteriosclerosis are more prevalent in type 2 than in type 1 diabetics. Renal structure is, in fact, heterogeneous in type 2 diabetic patients; only a subset has typical diabetic glomerulopathy, whereas a substantial proportion has more advanced tubulointerstitial and vascular rather than glomerular lesions or has normal or nearly normal renal structure.[62] In a proportion of patients with type 2 diabetes, the kidney has an appearance that is more suggestive of glomerular ischemia or tubulointerstitial disease.

DIAGNOSIS

The diagnosis of DN is based on the detection of proteinuria. In addition, most patients also have hypertension and retinopathy. The main diagnostic procedures in the patient with suspected DN include:

- Measurement of urinary albumin or protein
- Measurement of serum creatinine concentration and estimation of GFR
- Measurement of BP
- Ophthalmologic examination.

Measurement of Albuminuria or Proteinuria

Microalbuminuria is arbitrarily defined as the excretion of 30 to 300 mg/24 h albumin in at least two of three consecutive nonketotic sterile urine samples (Fig. 29.19). There is substantial intraindividual day-to-day variation of albumin excretion (coefficient of variation, 30% to 50%) and also between day and night collections (Fig. 29.20). Even in the upper quantiles of so-called normoalbuminuria, however, the risk of progression and of CV events is definitely elevated. In this range of albumin concentrations, albumin is normally not detected by nonspecific tests for protein (e.g., Biuret reaction). Albumin can be detected, however, by use of specific techniques such as dipstick, enzyme-linked immunosorbent assay, nephelometry, and radioimmunoassay. Instead of difficult to obtain 24-hour urine collections, the albumin concentration can be determined in spot urine or, better, first-void morning urine samples. The normal range is 20 to 200 μg/min or 20 to 200 μg/ml.

The detection of urinary albumin is a specific indicator of DN only if confounding factors such as fever, physical exercise, urinary tract infection (UTI), nondiabetic renal disease, hematuria from other causes, heart failure, uncontrolled hypertension, and uncontrolled hyperglycemia have been excluded.

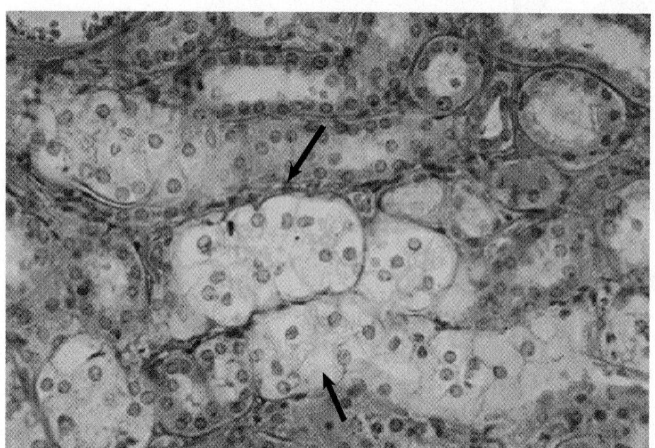

Figure 29.18 Armani-Ebstein lesions of tubular cells *(arrows)* that occur during very high hyperglycemia and massive glucosuria. These lesions consist of deposits of glycogen and are rarely seen today.

Urinary Albumin Excretion Rate

	UAER	
Condition	**24 hr (mg/day)**	**Overnight (μg/min)**
Normoalbuminuria	>30	>20
Microalbuminuria	30–300	20–200
Overt nephropathy	>300	>200

Figure 29.19 Urinary albumin excretion rate (UAER). Levels of 24 hour and overnight UAE are diagnostic for microalbuminuria and overt diabetic nephropathy (DN).

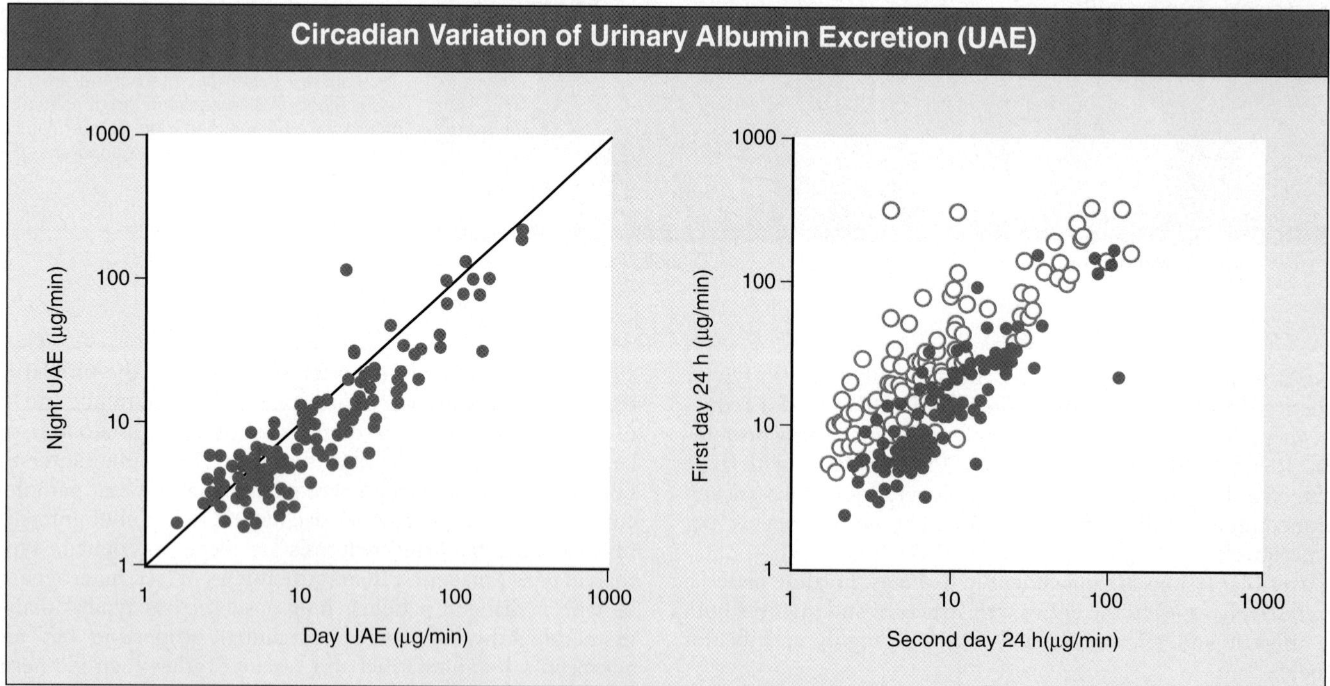

Figure 29.20 Circadian variation of urinary albumin excretion (UAE). UAE is lower in resting conditions at night than during daytime activity. Relationship between UAE assessed on two different days 1 week apart in patients with type 1 diabetes *(open circles)* and primary hypertension *(closed circles)*. There is substantial intraindividual day-to-day variation of albumin excretion and also between day and night collections. *(From reference 63.)*

The main advantage of searching for microalbuminuria early in the course of diabetes is that it predicts a high renal and CV risk and thus allows targeted intervention. The American Diabetes Association *(www.diabetes.org)* and other societies recommend annual screening of all diabetic patients.

By definition, clinically overt DN (macroalbuminuria) is present if the rate of albumin excretion exceeds 300 mg/day. At this point, usually serum proteins other than albumin are excreted in the urine as well (nonselective proteinuria).

Measurement of Blood Pressure

In measuring the BP in a diabetic patient, one should be aware of several problems:

- In overweight patients with type 2 diabetes, the size of the cuff has to be adapted to the upper arm circumference. When this exceeds 32 cm, cuffs of 18-cm width are indicated.
- Patients with severe autonomic polyneuropathy tend to develop orthostatic hypotension, namely, a decrease of systolic BP by more than 20 mm Hg in the upright position. It is therefore advisable to measure BP in the upright position at regular intervals.
- The circadian BP profile tends to be abnormal in early stages, and even a paradoxical increase in the nighttime BP is not rare. In the diabetic patient with nephropathy, it has been shown that a nighttime increase in BP is independently associated with a 20-fold higher mortality and a higher risk of renal failure. Occasional measurements of ambulatory BP are particularly useful to assess the efficacy of antihypertensive treatment.
- In diabetic patients with sclerosis or calcification of the radial and brachial arteries, pseudohypertension may occasionally occur, that is, spuriously elevated BP values despite normotension by intra-arterial BP measurements. Suspicion of this condition should be raised if a discrepancy is found between modest target organ damage, for example, left ventricular hypertrophy, and very high measured BP values. Such patients tend to develop marked hypotension even with relatively modest antihypertensive medication.

Measurement of Serum Creatinine and Estimation of Glomerular Filtration Rate

In clinical practice, the serum creatinine concentration is most frequently used to assess renal function, but it may be grossly misleading in wasted patients when muscle mass is low. This problem is particularly frequent in elderly female patients with type 2 diabetes. Therefore, the Kidney Disease Outcome Quality Initiative (KDOQI) guidelines recommend that the GFR be estimated according to the Modification of Diet in Renal Disease (MDRD) study equation (see Chapter 3).

Differential Diagnoses

Although hematuria has been considered one of the atypical features indicating the presence of nondiabetic renal disease among patients with diabetes, the clinical significance of hematuria in the overall course of DN suggests that hematuria could be a sign of DN. Moreover, a study identified hematuric patients with pathologically defined DN, and they all had a significantly lower renal function than nonhematuric patients with DN.[64] The prevalence of nephrotic syndrome and retinopathy was significantly higher in the cases with hematuric diabetic glomerulosclerosis than in the cases with nonhematuric diabetic glomerulosclerosis.

On the other hand, non-DN is not an uncommon entity in type 2 diabetes. Younger patients with diabetes, shorter duration of diabetes, and the association of proteinuria with the absence of retinopathy strongly suggest renal disease of nondiabetic genesis.[65] Nondiabetic renal disease is a heterogeneous group. Membranous nephropathy (MN), FSGS, acute interstitial nephritis, postinfectious GN, and IgA nephropathy have been described in type 2 diabetic patients in whom DN was suspected on clinical grounds (Fig. 29.21).

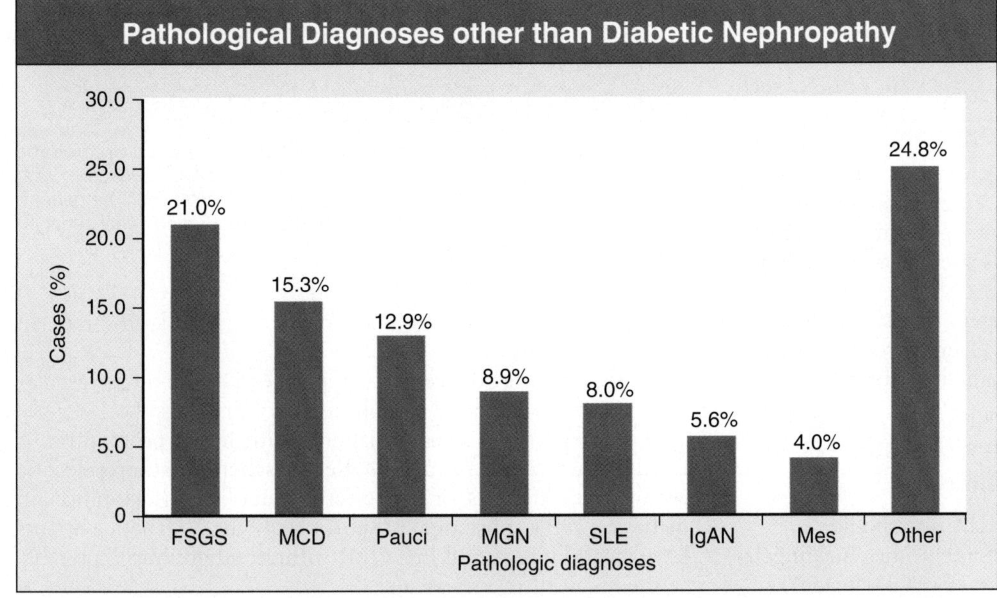

Figure 29.21 Pathologic diagnoses other than diabetic nephropathy are found in more than half of patients with type 2 diabetes with proteinuria. A total of 233 patients were studied; 53.2% (124 patients) had a diagnosis of nondiabetic renal diseases. FSGS, focal segmental glomerulosclerosis; IgAN, IgA nephropathy; MCD, minimal change disease; Mes, mesangial immune complex glomerulonephritis; MGN, membranous nephropathy; Pauci, ANCA-positive pauci-immune glomerulonephritis; SLE, systemic lupus erythematosus. *(From reference 65.)*

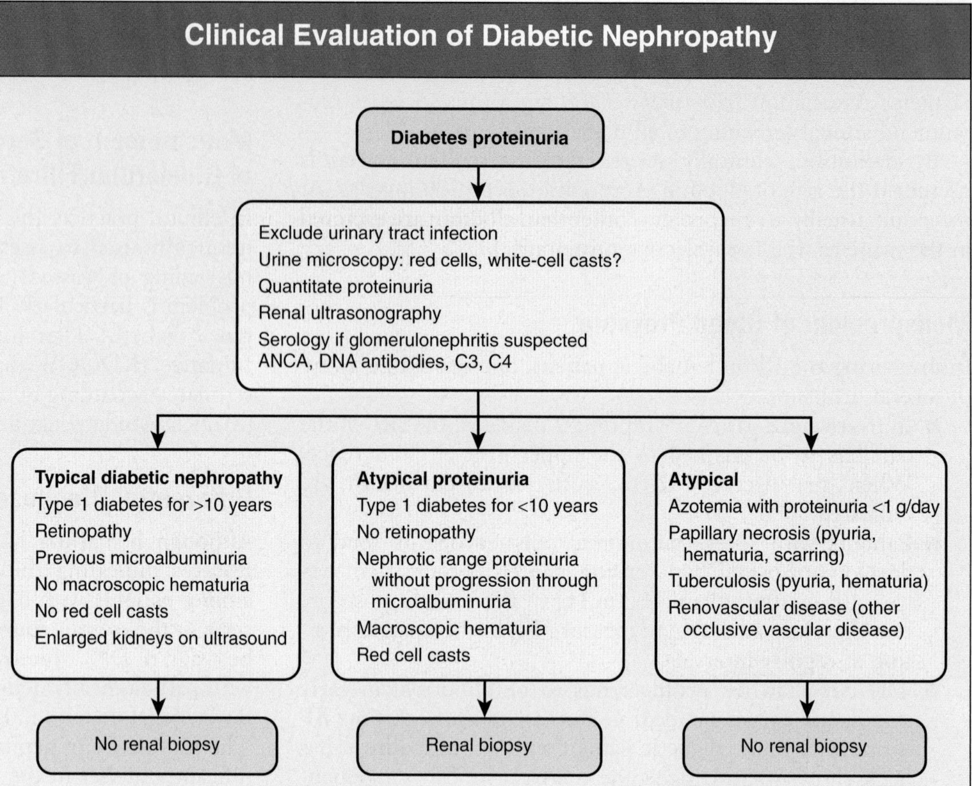

Figure 29.22 Clinical evaluation of diabetic renal disease. ANCA, antineutrophil cytoplasmic antibody.

Indications for Renal Biopsy

Further investigation including a renal biopsy should be considered (Fig. 29.22):

- If retinopathy is not present in type 1 diabetes with proteinuria or moderately impaired renal function (absence of retinopathy does not exclude DN in type 2 diabetes).
- If the onset of proteinuria has been sudden and rapid, particularly in type 1 diabetes, and if the duration of type 1 diabetes has been less than 5 years or if the evolution has been atypical, for example, without transition through the usual stages, particularly the development of nephrotic syndrome without previous microalbuminuria.
- If macroscopic hematuria is present or an active nephritic urinary sediment is found that is suggestive of GN, such as acanthocytes and red cell casts; the sediment in DN typically is unremarkable apart from some occasional erythrocytes.
- If the decline of renal function is exceptionally rapid or if renal dysfunction is found without significant proteinuria (first, of course, renovascular disease must be excluded Fig. 29.23).

If renal ultrasound reveals small kidneys or a size difference, it is prudent not to perform biopsy. Overall, renal biopsy is indicated only in a small minority of diabetic patients.

Points to Consider in Dealing with a Diabetic Patient with Impaired Renal Function

When seeing a diabetic patient with CKD, one should:

- Assess the cause of CKD (acute versus chronic renal impairment; DN versus alternative causes of renal damage).

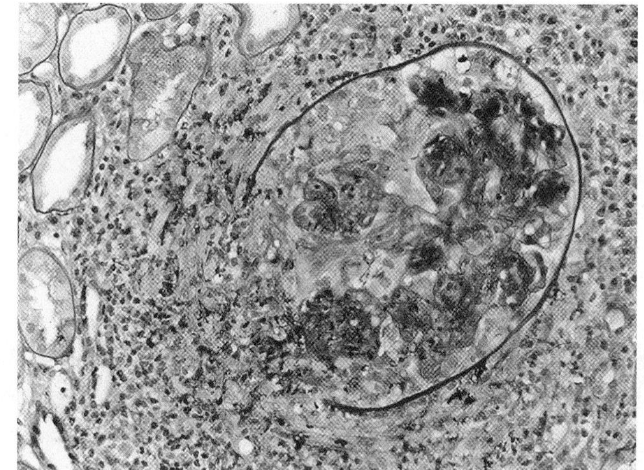

Figure 29.23 Glomerulonephritis (GN) superimposed on diabetic nephropathy (DN). A glomerulus showing a cellular crescent with rupture of Bowman's capsule superimposed on nodular DN. The patient, known to have DN, presented with rapidly deteriorating renal function and red cell casts in the urine.

- Assess the magnitude of proteinuria and the rate of progression.
- Search for evidence of the typical extrarenal microvascular and macrovascular complications of diabetes.

The majority of diabetic patients with heavy proteinuria or renal failure suffer from DN. Renal ischemia (atherosclerotic renal artery stenosis or cholesterol embolism) is common in diabetics, and a substantial proportion of type 2 diabetic patients have small kidneys and low GFR without albuminuria, possibly as the result of macrovascular disease.

If UTIs occur, they are more severe in the diabetic compared with the nondiabetic patient. Purulent papillary necrosis and intrarenal abscess formation, however, have become rare nowadays.

Diabetic patients with nephropathy are particularly prone to development of AKI after administration of nonsteroidal anti-inflammatory drugs (NSAIDs) or radiocontrast media or after CV events or septicemia. Preventive measures are discussed in Chapter 69 . AKI superimposed on preexisting DN carries a very poor prognosis.

REFERENCES

1. Seaquist ER, Goetz FC, Rich S, Barbosa J. Familial clustering of diabetic kidney disease. Evidence for genetic susceptibility to diabetic nephropathy. *N Engl J Med*. 1989;320:1161-1165.
2. Nelson RG, Knowler WC, Pettitt DJ, et al. Diabetic kidney disease in Pima Indians. *Diabetes Care*. 1993;16:335-341.
3. Nelson RG, Morgenstern H, Bennett PH. Intrauterine diabetes exposure and the risk of renal disease in diabetic Pima Indians. *Diabetes*. 1998;47:1489-1493.
4. Amri K, Freund N, Van Huyen JP, et al. Altered nephrogenesis due to maternal diabetes is associated with increased expression of IGF-II/mannose-6-phosphate receptor in the fetal kidney. *Diabetes*. 2001;50:1069-1075.
5. Zandi-Nejad K, Luyckx VA, Brenner BM. Adult hypertension and kidney disease: The role of fetal programming. *Hypertension*. 2006;47:502-508.
6. Janssen B, Hohenadel D, Brinkkoetter P, et al. Carnosine as a protective factor in diabetic nephropathy: Association with a leucine repeat of the carnosinase gene CNDP1. *Diabetes*. 2005;54:2320-2327.
7. Marre M, Jeunemaitre X, Gallois Y, et al. Contribution of genetic polymorphism in the renin-angiotensin system to the development of renal complications in insulin-dependent diabetes: Genetique de la Nephropathie Diabetique (GENEDIAB) study group. *J Clin Invest*. 1997;99:1585-1595.
8. Ruggenenti P, Bettinaglio P, Pinares F, Remuzzi G. Angiotensin converting enzyme insertion/deletion polymorphism and renoprotection in diabetic and nondiabetic nephropathies. *Clin J Am Soc Nephrol*. 2008;3:1511-1525.
9. Schmidt S, Ritz E. Angiotensin I converting enzyme gene polymorphism and diabetic nephropathy in type II diabetes. *Nephrol Dial Transplant*. 1997;12(Suppl 2):37-41.
10. Satriano J, Vallon V. Primary kidney growth and its consequences at the onset of diabetes mellitus. *Amino Acids*. 2006;31:1-9.
11. Ruster C, Wolf G. The role of chemokines and chemokine receptors in diabetic nephropathy. *Front Biosci*. 2008;13:944-955.
12. Wolf G, Ziyadeh FN. Cellular and molecular mechanisms of proteinuria in diabetic nephropathy. *Nephron Physiol*. 2007;106:26-31.
13. Mezzano S, Aros C, Droguett A, et al. NF-κB activation and overexpression of regulated genes in human diabetic nephropathy. *Nephrol Dial Transplant*. 2004;19:2505-2512.
14. Isermann B, Vinnikov IA, Madhusudhan T, et al. Activated protein C protects against diabetic nephropathy by inhibiting endothelial and podocyte apoptosis. *Nat Med*. 2007;13:1349-1358.
15. Simonson MS. Phenotypic transitions and fibrosis in diabetic nephropathy. *Kidney Int*. 2007;71:846-854.
16. Gilbert RE, Marsden PA. Activated protein C and diabetic nephropathy. *N Engl J Med*. 2008;358:1628-1630.
17. Nangaku M. Chronic hypoxia and tubulointerstitial injury: A final common pathway to end-stage renal failure. *J Am Soc Nephrol*. 2006;17:17-25.
18. Krolewski AS, Laffel LM, Krolewski M, et al. Glycosylated hemoglobin and the risk of microalbuminuria in patients with insulin-dependent diabetes mellitus. *N Engl J Med*. 1995;332:1251-1255.
19. The effect of intensive treatment of diabetes on the development and progression of long-term complications in insulin-dependent diabetes mellitus. The Diabetes Control and Complications Trial Research Group. *N Engl J Med*. 1993;329:977-986.
20. Nathan DM, Cleary PA, Backlund JY, et al. Intensive diabetes treatment and cardiovascular disease in patients with type 1 diabetes. *N Engl J Med*. 2005;353:2643-2653.
21. Fioretto P, Steffes MW, Sutherland DE, et al. Reversal of lesions of diabetic nephropathy after pancreas transplantation. *N Engl J Med*. 1998;339:69-75.
22. Intensive blood-glucose control with sulphonylureas or insulin compared with conventional treatment and risk of complications in patients with type 2 diabetes (UKPDS 33). UK Prospective Diabetes Study (UKPDS) Group. *Lancet*. 1998;352:837-853.
23. Brownlee M. Biochemistry and molecular cell biology of diabetic complications. *Nature*. 2001;414:813-820.
24. Patel A, MacMahon S, Chalmers J, et al. Intensive blood glucose control and vascular outcomes in patients with type 2 diabetes. *N Engl J Med*. 2008;358:2560-2572.
25. Brownlee M. The pathobiology of diabetic complications: A unifying mechanism. *Diabetes*. 2005;54:1615-1625.
26. Bohlender JM, Franke S, Stein G, Wolf G. Advanced glycation end products and the kidney. *Am J Physiol Renal Physiol*. 2005;289:F645-F659.
27. Rüster C, Bondeva T, Franke S, et al. Angiotensin II upregulates RAGE expression on podocytes: Role of AT2 receptors. *Am J Nephrol*. 2009;29:538-550.
28. Ribeiro-Oliveira A Jr, Nogueira AI, Pereira RM, et al. The renin-angiotensin system and diabetes: An update. *Vasc Health Risk Manag*. 2008;4:787-803.
29. Wolf G. Renal injury due to renin-angiotensin-aldosterone system activation of the transforming growth factor-beta pathway. *Kidney Int*. 2006;70:1914-1999.
30. Toma I, Kang JJ, Sipos A, et al. Succinate receptor GPR91 provides a direct link between high glucose levels and renin release in murine and rabbit kidney. *J Clin Invest*. 2008;118:2526-2534.
31. Nguyen G, Danser AH. Prorenin and (pro)renin receptor: A review of available data from in vitro studies and experimental models in rodents. *Exp Physiol*. 2008;93:557-563.
32. Huang XR, Chen WY, Truong LD, Lan HY. Chymase is upregulated in diabetic nephropathy: Implications for an alternative pathway of angiotensin II–mediated diabetic renal and vascular disease. *J Am Soc Nephrol*. 2003;14:1738-1747.
33. Johnson RJ, Perez-Pozo SE, Sautin YY, et al. Hypothesis: Could excessive fructose intake and uric acid cause type 2 diabetes? *Endocr Rev*. 2009;30:96-116.
34. Hovind P, Rossing P, Tarnow L, et al. Serum uric acid as a predictor for development of diabetic nephropathy in type 1 diabetes—an inception cohort study. *Diabetes*. 2009;58:1668-1671.
35. Hasslacher C, Ritz E, Wahl P, Michael C. Similar risks of nephropathy in patients with type I or type II diabetes mellitus. *Nephrol Dial Transplant*. 1989;4:859-863.
36. Parving HH, Lewis JB, Ravid M, et al; DEMAND investigators: Prevalence and risk factors for microalbuminuria in a referred cohort of type II diabetic patients: A global perspective. *Kidney Int*. 2006;69:2057-2063.
37. So WY, Ma RC, Ozaki R, et al. Angiotensin-converting enzyme (ACE) inhibition in type 2, diabetic patients—interaction with ACE insertion/deletion polymorphism. *Kidney Int*. 2006;69:1438-1443.
38. Whaley-Connell A, Sowers JR, McCullough PA, et al. Diabetes mellitus and CKD awareness: The Kidney Early Evaluation Program (KEEP) and National Health and Nutrition Examination Survey (NHANES). *Am J Kidney Dis*. 2009;4(Suppl 1):S11-S21.
39. King H, Aubert RE, Herman WH. Global burden of diabetes, 1995-2025: Prevalence, numerical estimates, and projections. *Diabetes Care*. 1998;21:1414-1431.
40 Nguyen NT, Magno CP, Lane KT, et al. Association of hypertension, diabetes, dyslipidemia, and metabolic syndrome with obesity: Findings from the National Health and Nutrition Examination Survey, 1999 to 2004. *J Am Coll Surg*. 2008;207:928-934.
41. Wolf G. After all those fat years: Renal consequences of obesity. *Nephrol Dial Transplant*. 2003;18:2471-2474.
42. Chagnac A, Herman M, Zingerman B, et al. Obesity-induced glomerular hyperfiltration: Its involvement in the pathogenesis of tubular sodium reabsorption. *Nephrol Dial Transplant*. 2008;23:3946-3952.
43. Rasouli N, Kern PA. Adipocytokines and the metabolic complications of obesity. *J Clin Endocrinol Metab*. 2008;93(Suppl 1):S64-S73.
44. Mogensen CE. How to protect the kidney in diabetic patients with special reference to NIDDM. *Diabetes*. 1997;56(Suppl 2):104-111.
45. Mourad JJ, Le Jeune S. Blood pressure control, risk factors and cardiovascular prognosis in patients with diabetes: 30 years of progress. *J Hypertens*. 2008;26:S7-S13.
46. Muxfeldt ES, Cardoso CR, Salles GF. Prognostic value of nocturnal blood pressure reduction in resistant hypertension. *Arch Intern Med*. 2009;169:874-880.

47. Winer N, Sowers JR. Diabetes and arterial stiffening. *Adv Cardiol.* 2007;44:245-251.
48. Girach A, Vignati L. Diabetic microvascular complications—can the presence of one predict the development of another? *J Diabetes Complications.* 2006;20:228-237.
49. Wolf G, Müller N, Mandecka A, Müller UA. Association of diabetic retinopathy and renal function in patients with types 1 and 2 diabetes mellitus. *Clin Nephrol.* 2007;68:81-86.
50. Margolis DJ, Hofstad O, Feldman HI. Association between renal failure and foot ulcer of lower-extremity amputation in patients with diabetes. *Diabetes Care.* 2008;31:1331-1336.
51. Knudsen ST, Laugesen E, Hansen KW, et al. Ambulatory pulse pressure, decreased nocturnal blood pressure reduction and progression of nephropathy in type 2 diabetic patients. *Diabetologia.* 2009;52:698-704.
52. Krentz AJ, Clough G, Byrne CD. Interactions between microvascular and macrovascular disease in diabetes: Pathophysiology and therapeutic implications. *Diabetes Obes Metab.* 2007;9:781-791.
53. Gall MA, Borch-Johnsen K, Hougaard P, et al. Albuminuria and poor glycemic control predict mortality in NIDDM. *Diabetes.* 1995;44:1303-1309.
54. Brantsma AH, Bakker SJ, de Zeeuw D, et al. PREVEND Study Group: Extended prognostic value of urinary albumin excretion for cardiovascular events. *J Am Soc Nephrol.* 2008;19:1785-1791.
55. Wolf G, Müller N, Busch M, et al. Diabetic foot syndrome and renal function in type 1 and 2 diabetes mellitus show close association. *Nephrol Dial Transplant.* 2009;24:1896-1901.
56. Fioretto P, Mauer M, Brocco E, et al. Patterns of renal injury in NIDDM patients with microalbuminuria. *Diabetologia.* 1996;39:1569-1576.
57. Fioretto P, Steffes MW, Sutherland DE, Mauer M. Sequential renal biopsies in insulin-dependent diabetic patients: Structural factors associated with clinical progression. *Kidney Int.* 1995;48:1929-1935.
58. Wolf G, Chen S, Ziyadeh FN. From the periphery of the glomerular capillary wall toward the center of disease: Podocyte injury comes of age in diabetic nephropathy. *Diabetes.* 2005;54:1626-1634.
59. Marshall SM. The podocyte: A major player in the development of diabetic nephropathy? *Horm Metab Res.* 2005;37(Suppl 1):9-16.
60. Pagtalunan ME, Miller PL, Jumping-Eagle S, et al. Podocyte loss and progressive glomerular injury in type II diabetes. *J Clin Invest.* 1997;99:342-348.
61. Ziyadeh FN. Significance of tubulointerstitial changes in diabetic renal disease. *Kidney Int.* 1996;54:S10-S13.
62. Musso C, Javor E, Cochran E, et al. Spectrum of renal diseases associated with extreme forms of insulin resistance. *Clin J Am Soc Nephrol.* 2006;1:616-622.
63. Redon J. Measurement of microalbuminuria—what the nephrologist should know. *Nephrol Dial Transplant.* 2006;21:573-576.
64. Akimoto T, Ito C, Saito O, et al. Microscopic hematuria and diabetic glomerulosclerosis—clinicopathological analysis of type 2 diabetic patients associated with overt proteinuria. *Nephron Clin Pract.* 2008;109:c119-c126.
65. Pham TT, Sim JJ, Kujubu DA, et al. Prevalence of nondiabetic renal disease in diabetic patients. *Am J Nephrol.* 2007;27:322-328.

CHAPTER 30

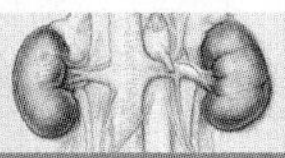

Prevention and Treatment of Diabetic Nephropathy

Li-Li Tong, Sharon Adler

Nephropathy in patients with diabetes, primarily type 2, remains the leading cause of end-stage renal disease (ESRD) in the Western world. Examination of trends in ESRD attributed to diabetic nephropathy (DN) in the United States suggests a possible plateau in incidence in recent years.[1] The implementation of renoprotective therapy in the past 2 decades may have contributed to this phenomenon.

Classically, DN evolves through several clinical stages based on the values of urine albumin excretion (UAE): normoalbuminuria, microalbuminuria, and macroalbuminuria or overt nephropathy. The level of UAE has predictive importance for both renal outcome and cardiovascular (CV) morbidity and mortality and affects the choice of therapeutic intervention. Although difficult, normoalbuminuria is the ideal treatment goal. Understanding of the pathogenesis of hypertension in DN is important for rational selection of therapeutic agents:

- The important role of sodium retention and hypervolemia explains why dietary sodium restriction and diuretics are so effective.
- The activation of the intrarenal renin-angiotensin-aldosterone system (RAS) explains the efficacy of angiotensin-converting enzyme (ACE) inhibitors and angiotensin II receptor blockers (ARBs).
- The activation of the sympathetic nervous system and its role in the genesis of renal hypertension presumably explain why β-blockers are effective in retarding progression.

This chapter reviews the current preventive and therapeutic strategies that promote renoprotection and cardioprotection in diabetic patients. A summary of these strategies is shown in Figure 30.1. In general, the treatment principles for established DN are similar to those adopted for the prevention of DN, although multiple and more intensive strategies may be required for treatment. Special considerations are indicated in the management of the diabetic patient with advanced chronic kidney disease (CKD) (see Chapter 31). Many therapeutic issues discussed here are not specific for DN and thus are also relevant for CKD in general (see Chapter 76).

PREVENTION OF DIABETIC NEPHROPATHY

Prevention and early detection of nephropathy improve patient outcome. General measures for prevention of DN include glycemic control and blood pressure control. Because diabetes is associated with increased risk for CV morbidity and mortality, treatment of dyslipidemia as well as diet and lifestyle modifications, including physical activity and weight reduction as appropriate and smoking cessation, can significantly lower the CV risks.

Glycemic Control

In type 1 diabetic patients, strict glycemic control decreased the risk for microalbuminuria. The Diabetes Control and Complications Trial (DCCT) (Fig. 30.2) compared the effects of intensive glucose control with conventional treatment on the development and progression of the long-term complications of type 1 diabetes. During a 9-year period, patients receiving intensive therapy (mean HbA_{1c} 7%) had a 35% to 45% lower risk for development of microalbuminuria compared with the control group (mean HbA_{1c} 9%).[2] Renoprotection can persist even after a return to less intensive therapy.[3]

For type 2 diabetes, several major studies have demonstrated a lower risk of nephropathy with stricter glycemic control. In a study design similar to the DCCT, the Kumamoto study found a 60% reduction in the rate of microalbuminuria in relatively young nonobese type 2 diabetic patients receiving intensive glycemic treatment (HbA_{1c} 7.1%) compared with conventional treatment (HbA_{1c} 9.4%).[4] In the U.K. Prospective Diabetes Study (UKPDS) trial, newly diagnosed patients with type 2 diabetes were randomly assigned to intensive management (HbA_{1c} 7.0%) with a sulfonylurea or insulin or to conventional management (HbA_{1c} 7.9%) with diet alone. After 9 years of intensive therapy, relative risk reduction for the development of microalbuminuria was 24%.[5] After termination of the study, patients were observed for a further 10 years. The differences in HbA_{1c} were lost within 1 year, but a 24% lower risk of microvascular disease and myocardial infarction (–15%) persisted. All-cause mortality (–13%) was also reduced. This suggests glycemic memory ("legacy effect"), that is, long-lasting beneficial effects of good glycemic control explained by long-lasting modification of transcription of genes relevant in the genesis of complications. This observation underlies the importance of early glycemic control before complications have set in.

Three major trials testing whether glycemic control reduced cardiovascular disease (CVD) risk in type 2 diabetics have considerably increased our knowledge of and refined our approach to establishing glycemic goals. The Action in Diabetes and Vascular Disease, Perindopril and Indapamide Controlled Evaluation (ADVANCE) study showed that intensive blood glucose control (HbA_{1c} 6.5% versus 7.3%) yielded a 10% relative reduction in the combined outcome of major macrovascular and microvascular events, primarily as a consequence of a 21%

Management of Type 1 Diabetes	
Stage	**Management**
Normoalbuminuria/ Normotensive	Optimize glycemic control (target HbA_{1c} <7%)
Normoalbuminuria/ Hypertensive	Consider ACE inhibitor or ARB as antihypertensive agent (target BP <130/80 mm Hg); dietary sodium restriction +/– diuretic therapy
Microalbuminuria/ Normotensive	Start ACE inhibitor or ARB, titrate dose as tolerated to normoalbuminuria
Microalbuminuria/ Hypertensive	Titrate ACE inhibitor or ARB as tolerated; consider addition of selective aldosterone receptor antagonist (e.g., spironolactone, eplerenone), nondihydropyridine calcium channel blockers (e.g., diltiazem, verapamil), direct renin inhibitor (e.g., aliskiren); dietary sodium restriction +/– loop or thiazide diuretic; treat to normoalbuminuria and BP <130/80 mm Hg
Overt proteinuria	Continue management as above with aggressive BP control; treat cardiovascular risks and consider aspirin therapy, statin therapy, smoking cessation, weight reduction as appropriate
Declining glomerular filtration rate (GFR)	Provide nutrition counseling regarding sodium, potassium, and phosphorus restriction; avoid protein-calorie malnutrition; treat anemia; prepare for dialysis or transplantation when GFR is <20 ml/min

Figure 30.1 Management of type 1 diabetes. A similar strategy can be used in patients with type 2 diabetes with increased emphasis on management of cardiovascular risk factors. In considering the management of patients with diabetic and chronic kidney disease (CKD), a global perspective is required, which includes therapy that retards progression of kidney disease as well as therapy that minimizes cardiovascular risk and addresses other major diabetic complications, including coronary artery disease, peripheral vascular disease, retinopathy, neuropathy, gastroparesis, and dyslipidemia. ACE, angiotensin-converting enzyme; ARB, angiotensin II receptor blocker; BP, blood pressure.

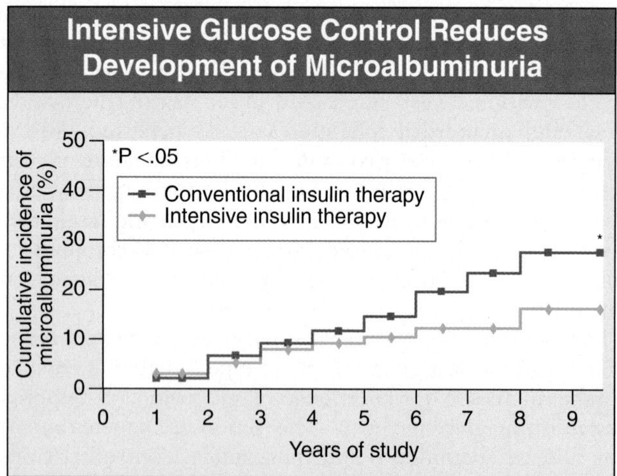

Figure 30.2 Diabetes Control and Complications Trial. Intensive glucose control was associated with a decreased risk for the subsequent development of microalbuminuria in type 1 diabetes. *(Modified from reference 2.)*

relative reduction in nephropathy.[6] However, the Food and Drug Administration recently halted one of the arms of the Action to Control Cardiovascular Risk in Diabetes (ACCORD) trial when it became apparent that very tight glycemic control (lowering of HbA_{1c} to a median of 6.4% versus 7.5% with conventional control) was associated with a higher mortality (increase in risk by 22%; $P = .04$).[7] A third major study of tight glucose control in type 2 diabetics, the Veterans Affairs Diabetes Trial (VADT), found no significant reduction in CV deaths or events during 7.5 years in high-risk patients treated aggressively for glycemic control (median HbA_{1c} 6.9%) compared with standard therapy (median HbA_{1c} 8.4%).[8]

It is apparent that glycemic control in type 2 diabetic patients must be individualized and take into account the patient's duration of diabetes, presence of CVD, and microvascular risks and complications as well as previous glycemic control and susceptibility to and awareness of hypoglycemia. In patients with recently diagnosed diabetes and no prior CVD events, strict glycemic control can reduce the risk of nephropathy and other microvascular complications. In patients with long-standing diabetes and known CVD, data do not support strict glycemic control in reducing the risk of further CVD events or mortality. The National Kidney Foundation's Kidney Disease Outcomes Quality Initiative (KDOQI) guideline recommends lowering of HbA_{1c} levels to 7.0% for both type 1 and type 2 diabetic patients.[9] At even lower glycemic targets, any potential renoprotective effects of tight glucose control must be counterbalanced by the possibility of more frequent hypoglycemic episodes.

Antihypertensive Therapy

Hypertension is present in about 40% of type 1 and 70% of type 2 diabetic patients with normoalbuminuria.[10] Higher blood pressure level is associated with an increased risk for the development of nephropathy; and in patients with established nephropathy, it is associated with more rapid progression and increased risk of kidney failure.[11] The National Kidney Foundation, the Seventh Report of the Joint National Committee on Prevention, Detection, Evaluation, and Treatment of High Blood Pressure (JNC 7), and the American Diabetes Association recommend a target blood pressure value of below 130/80 mm Hg in diabetic patients.[12]

Renin-Angiotensin-Aldosterone System Blockade

The role of RAS blockade in normotensive, normoalbuminuric diabetic patients for the primary prevention of DN is controversial. Most patients with diabetes do not develop DN, even after long periods of uncontrolled hyperglycemia, and there are potential risks and side effects with the use of RAS blocking drugs, including their potential teratogenicity in pregnancy. In a recent post hoc analysis of three randomized controlled trials conducted as part of the multicenter Diabetic Retinopathy Candesartan Trials (DIRECT) program, which included normotensive and normoalbuminuric type 1 diabetics and normoalbuminuric type 2 diabetics with or without hypertension, the ARB candesartan was found to have no effect on the development of microalbuminuria.[13]

In hypertensive diabetic patients, an ACE inhibitor or an ARB is effective as a first-line antihypertensive agent. The Bergamo Nephrologic Diabetes Complications Trial (BENEDICT), which randomized hypertensive normoalbuminuric type 2 diabetic patients to placebo, verapamil, trandolapril, or a combination of verapamil plus trandolapril, showed less progression to microalbuminuria in patients receiving trandolapril either alone or in combination with verapamil.[14] Verapamil alone was not different from placebo. There were similar findings in smaller studies with other RAS inhibitors, implicating a class effect.[15] Very long term studies would be required to demonstrate the effects of RAS blockade on the clinically important outcomes of death, dialysis, and doubling of serum creatinine level in normoalbuminuric patients. It is likely that therapy for the prevention of DN will be guided exclusively by studies using albuminuria as a surrogate.

Treatment of Dyslipidemia

There are few clinical data concerning the effects of lipid lowering alone in preventing DN. In the Diabetes Atherosclerosis Intervention Study (DAIS), type 2 diabetic patients taking fenofibrate had a significantly lower rate of progression from normoalbuminuria to microalbuminuria at 3 years compared with placebo.[16] Current guidelines recommend a goal for low-density lipoprotein (LDL) cholesterol of below 100 mg/dl (2.57 mmol/l) for diabetic patients in general and below 70 mg/dl (1.81 mmol/l) for diabetic patients with CVD.[17]

Nonpharmacologic Interventions

For all diabetics, emphasis should be placed on lifestyle modification to lower the risk of CV events, including dietary restriction of salt and saturated fat, weight reduction and exercise as appropriate, and smoking cessation. Smoking in particular is an independent risk factor for the development of nephropathy in type 2 diabetes and is associated with an accelerated loss of renal function.[18]

TREATMENT OF DIABETICS WITH MICROALBUMINURIA OR OVERT NEPHROPATHY

For diabetic patients with incipient or established DN, the optimal therapeutic approach to reduce the rate of progression of nephropathy and to minimize the risk for CV events involves aggressive management of hypertension with emphasis on a RAS blocker combined with management of dyslipidemia, hyperglycemia, and albuminuria as well as diet modification, exercise, and smoking cessation. Such multifactorial therapy in the Steno type 2 trial in type 2 diabetics included management of hyperglycemia and of hypertension, ACE inhibition, statins, aspirin, reduction of fat intake, light to moderate exercise, and cessation of smoking.[19,20] Impressive lowering of the risk of CV disease, nephropathy, retinopathy, and autonomic polyneuropathy was noted after 7.7 years, and even a delayed reduction of mortality was seen.

In general, patients with DN require multiple antihypertensive agents (including RAS blocking agents) to achieve blood pressure goal, intensive insulin therapy in type 1 diabetes, two or more drugs for glucose control in type 2 diabetes, at least one lipid-lowering agent, and an aspirin or other antiplatelet agent for CV protection. One obstacle to achieving adherence is the number of medicines and the complexity of these regimens. Therefore, treatment of patients with DN needs to be individualized and requires considerations of the cost, side effects, and convenience of the drug regimen. Regular monitoring of UAE and serum creatinine concentration to assess response to therapy and progression of disease is required.

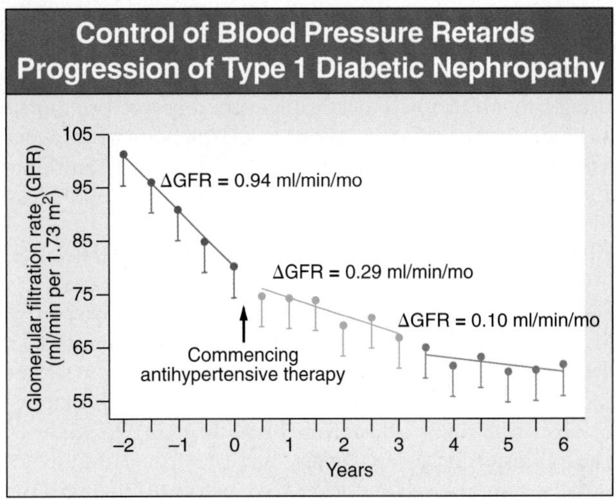

Figure 30.3 Control of blood pressure reduces the risk for progression in type 1 diabetic nephropathy. *(Modified from reference 21.)*

Antihypertensive Therapies

In type 1 and type 2 diabetic patients with established DN, hypertension is an almost universal finding and is associated with volume expansion and salt sensitivity. The absence of hypertension in an untreated patient with overt nephropathy should raise suspicion for underlying cardiac problems. Uncontrolled hypertension is associated with more rapid progression of DN[11] and increased risk of fatal and nonfatal CV events.[22] Thus, effective treatment of systemic hypertension is arguably the single most important strategy in the treatment of established DN (Fig. 30.3). Some have suggested that the overall effect of lowering blood pressure may be more important than the type of antihypertensive agent used.[23] Antihypertensive therapies, irrespective of the agent used, reduce UAE, delay progression of nephropathy, postpone renal insufficiency, and improve survival in both type 1 and type 2 diabetics with DN.[24]

The current recommended blood pressure target for all diabetics is below 130/80 mm Hg, but even lower systolic pressures may be more beneficial in diabetic patients with established nephropathy. In a secondary analysis of the Irbesartan Diabetic Nephropathy Trial (IDNT), progressive lowering of systolic blood pressure to 120 mm Hg was associated with improved renal and patient survival, an effect independent of baseline renal function.[25] However, mortality increased with systolic blood pressure below 120 mm Hg, although a cause and effect relationship cannot be inferred from the data. The optimal lower limit for systolic blood pressure, therefore, remains unclear. From a safety perspective, diastolic pressure is also important. Low diastolic pressures are poorly tolerated, and the incidence of myocardial infarction and mortality increases at values below 70 mm Hg, at least in patients with coronary heart disease, presumably because coronary perfusion occurs only during diastole. Indeed, in the IDNT study, CV mortality increased not only with higher systolic pressures but also with low diastolic pressure.

Renin-Angiotensin-Aldosterone System Blockade in Diabetic Nephropathy

In diabetic patients with established DN, RAS blockade with ACE inhibitors or ARBs confers renoprotection that is independent of blood pressure reduction. Intraglomerular hemodynamic and nonhemodynamic renal effects of angiotensin II, some of which are probably mediated by the fibrotic agent transforming growth factor β, best explain the observed renoprotection. In support of this hypothesis is a large body of evidence in *in vitro* models of DN showing cellular effects of RAS inhibition that are consistent with benefit independent of blood pressure effects (see Chapter 29).

Although many studies have demonstrated a beneficial effect of ACE inhibitors and ARBs in retarding progressive renal disease, they did not differentiate between the relative contributions of the RAS blockade versus aldosterone system blockade. In fact, plasma aldosterone levels are elevated in a subset of patients despite ACE inhibitor and ARB therapy (also known as aldosterone escape or aldosterone breakthrough). In studies that defined aldosterone escape as any increase from an individual's baseline serum aldosterone level (i.e., before ACE inhibitor or ARB therapy), the incidence ranged from 40% during 10 months to 53% during 12 months.[26] In addition to its classic effects of promoting sodium retention and enhancing potassium and magnesium excretion, aldosterone promotes tissue inflammation and fibrosis.[27] Small studies have demonstrated considerably faster decline in glomerular filtration rate (GFR) in patients who experienced aldosterone escape (median, 5.0 ml/min per year) than in those who did not (median, 2.4 ml/min per year). Aldosterone blockade, independent of RAS blockade, reduces proteinuria and retards progression of nephropathy. Current evidence is not strong enough to support widespread screening for aldosterone escape. However, in selected patients, additional aldosterone blockade may represent optimal therapy for patients who show aldosterone escape during treatment with an ACE inhibitor or an ARB and who no longer show maximal antiproteinuric effects with these agents.

RAS Blockade in Type 1 Diabetics

In type 1 diabetics with microalbuminuria, ACE inhibitors reduce the risk of progression to overt nephropathy.[28,29] In a meta-analysis of 12 placebo-controlled trials in 698 normotensive patients with type 1 diabetes and microalbuminuria treated with ACE inhibitors, the majority for more than 2 years, treatment was associated with a 60% reduction in progression to macroalbuminuria and a threefold increase in regression to normoalbuminuria.[30] Changes in blood pressure cannot entirely explain the antiproteinuric effect of ACE inhibitors.

In patients with macroalbuminuria or overt nephropathy, the Collaborative Study Group trial demonstrated that captopril reduced albuminuria, slowed the decrement in GFR, and delayed the onset of kidney failure compared with placebo.[31] The beneficial effect of captopril was greater in patients with reduced GFR at baseline largely because the end point, a doubling of baseline serum creatinine level, is achieved more quickly in these patients.

There are insufficient data and no large long-term clinical trials to demonstrate the efficacy of ARBs in type 1 DN. Nevertheless, based on the shared properties of ACE inhibitors and ARBs in inhibiting the RAS, there is reason to believe that both are effective in the treatment of type 1 DN.

RAS Blockade in Type 2 Diabetics

In type 2 diabetics, there are more data available on the renoprotective effect of ARBs compared with ACE inhibitors. In the stage of microalbuminuria, the IRMA 2 study showed that the ARB irbesartan reduces progression to overt nephropathy by 70% in hypertensive type 2 diabetic patients during a 2-year follow-up period.[32] In the MARVAL trial, the ARB valsartan (80 mg/day) produced a greater reduction in UAE than did amlodipine (44% versus 8%) with the same degree of blood pressure reduction, suggesting that the antiproteinuric effect of ARBs is blood pressure independent.[33]

In type 2 diabetic patients with macroalbuminuria and decreased GFR, large randomized controlled trials (IDNT and RENAAL) have demonstrated that ARBs are effective in lowering proteinuria and decreased the relative risk of reaching the composite end point of death, dialysis, and doubling of serum creatinine level.[34,35] However, the risk reduction for reaching the composite end point was only 18% to 20% in these studies in patients with type 2 diabetes and nephropathy, compared with the more robust risk reduction of ~50% in patients with type 1 diabetes receiving captopril. ARBs did not decrease CV death in these trials but did decrease the incidence of heart failure.

Compared with ARBs, data on the efficacy of ACE inhibitors in type 2 DN are less strong, largely because the studies were underpowered by small sample size or short follow-up. Nevertheless, some studies did show that ACE inhibitor use results in greater reduction in albuminuria and slower decrease in GFR compared with other antihypertensive agents. Whereas both ACE inhibitors and ARBs are probably effective for treatment of DN in patients with type 2 diabetes, few studies have directly compared their efficacy. In a small randomized controlled trial of type 2 diabetes and early nephropathy with 5 years of follow-up, the ARB telmisartan was not inferior to the ACE inhibitor enalapril in providing long-term renoprotection.[36] Some pharmaceutical companies marketing both ACE inhibitors and ARBs have attempted to make the argument that particular characteristics of individual agents within these classes, such as differences in tissue levels or differential effects on the metabolic syndrome, confer some with special beneficial properties. To date, there have not been high-quality prospective randomized trials proving such superiority for any particular agent for DN.

Combination Therapy of RAS Antagonists in Diabetic Nephropathy

ACE inhibitors and ARBs have been used simultaneously for therapeutic synergy in patients with nondiabetic renal disease (COOPERATE trial),[37] but doubts about the data have led to a formal retraction of the paper.[38] In both type 1 and type 2 diabetics with nephropathy, results of several earlier small trials suggested that the combination of an ACE inhibitor and an ARB is more effective in reducing blood pressure and proteinuria than is either drug alone.[39,40] However, there were no data from these trials on the effect of combined therapy on kidney disease progression. The recent ONTARGET study, which included diabetic and nondiabetic patients with CV risk, failed to show improved CV outcomes from a combination of an ACE inhibitor and an ARB. Instead, it showed increased renal functional decline, a trend toward an increase in the development of ESRD that fell just short of statistical significance, and a possible increase in mortality.[41] Whereas most of the ONTARGET study population did not have overt DN, the data nevertheless suggest caution in the use of these agents in combination, which is presumably not superior to dose escalation of the monotherapies. ACE inhibitors and ARBs have also been studied in combination with aldosterone receptor antagonists (e.g., spironolactone, eplerenone)[42] and a direct renin inhibitor (aliskiren)[43]; further reductions in proteinuria have been reported with these combinations compared with the ACE inhibitor or ARB alone. However, no studies with these combinations have yet been reported in which the primary end point has been death, dialysis, or doubled serum creatinine level.

Dosing and Adverse Effects Associated with ACE Inhibitors and ARBs

The antiproteinuric effect of ACE inhibitors and ARBs is at least in part independent of blood pressure reduction, and in individual patients, proteinuria may continue to respond to dose escalations beyond those recommended for blood pressure control.[44] Unfortunately, maximal dosing of ACE inhibitors or ARBs may be limited by side effects, including hyperkalemia, hypotension, and reduced GFR. In women of reproductive age, counseling about pregnancy prevention and contraceptive use should begin before an ACE inhibitor or an ARB is started.

An increase in serum creatinine concentration of up to 30% may occur in proteinuric patients with renal impairment after an ACE inhibitor is started. This rise in creatinine is associated with long-term renoprotection, and therefore the ACE inhibitor should not necessarily be stopped in these patients.[45] Increases in serum creatinine concentration above 30% after initiation of an ACE inhibitor should raise the suspicion of renal artery stenosis. Aggressive dose increments of ACE inhibitors or ARBs, especially in conjunction with diuresis, can precipitate acute kidney injury. In advanced CKD, although ACE inhibitors and ARBs are not contraindicated, the introduction of these agents or injudicious dose increments may precipitate the need for dialysis prematurely, so some caution is appropriate.

Other Antihypertensive Agents in Diabetic Nephropathy

Diuretics

The antiproteinuric effects of RAS blockade are enhanced by sodium restriction. Thus, patients receiving ACE inhibitors or ARBs should be instructed to take a low-sodium diet (e.g., less than 2 g of sodium per day). The combination of a loop diuretic or a thiazide diuretic with agents that block the RAS may be more effective than either type of treatment alone for lowering blood pressure. Selective aldosterone receptor antagonists (e.g., spironolactone, eplerenone) also reduce proteinuria when they are used alone and have an additive effect on proteinuria when they are used in combination with an ACE inhibitor or ARB.[42] As discussed earlier, aldosterone blockade may be especially beneficial in patients demonstrating aldosterone escape. The risk of hyperkalemia, however, frequently limits the use of combined aldosterone receptor antagonists with ACE inhibitors or ARBs, especially in patients with reduced GFR.

Calcium Channel Blockers

Nondihydropyridine calcium channel blockers (e.g., diltiazem, verapamil) have been shown in some studies to have antiproteinuric effects.[46] In type 2 diabetic patients with normoalbuminuria, however, nondihydropyridine calcium channel blockers did not reduce the incidence of microalbuminuria relative to placebo,[14] nor do they enhance the effect of ACE inhibitors in preventing microalbuminuria.

Dihydropyridine calcium channel blockers (e.g., nisoldipine, nifedipine, amlodipine) may be used as additional antihypertensive agents, but they have not been shown to reduce albuminuria or to slow the progression of renal disease.[47] In the Appropriate Blood Pressure Control in Diabetes (ABCD) trial, the long-acting calcium antagonist nisoldipine was compared with the ACE inhibitor enalapril as first-line antihypertensive therapy in 470 hypertensive type 2 diabetic patients. The incidence of fatal and nonfatal myocardial infarctions was significantly higher among those receiving nisoldipine compared with those receiving enalapril during a 5-year study period.[48] In a meta-analysis, patients with diabetes treated with dihydropyridine calcium channel blockers had more severe proteinuria and a more rapid decline in renal function than did those treated with other antihypertensive agents.[49]

β-Blockers

Classic β-blockers have adverse metabolic effects and are therefore undesirable in diabetics, but this is no longer true for the modern β-blockers carvedilol and nebivolol. Despite insufficient controlled evidence, β-blockade with these novel blockers appears to be useful because of the extremely high CV risk in diabetic patients with nephropathy.

Direct Renin Inhibitors

Aliskiren is the first orally active direct renin inhibitor approved for treatment of hypertension. In the AVOID trial, the addition of aliskiren produced greater reduction in UAE compared with placebo in type 2 diabetic patients with hypertension and nephropathy receiving the maximum recommended dose of losartan (100 mg daily).[43] The major side effects of aliskiren relate to its inhibition of the RAS, including hyperkalemia, hypotension, and reduced GFR. Its effect on long-term renal outcomes remains to be seen.

Glycemic Control

Most of the evidence favoring strict glycemic control comes from studies of patients with normoalbuminuria or early stages of DN. Fewer studies addressed intensive glycemic control in patients with advanced stages of DN, in which it may be difficult to show a benefit because the results are confounded by the effects of concomitant hypertension and CVD. Even so, for type 1 diabetic patients with overt nephropathy, there is evidence to support glycemic control in reducing the risk of worsening albuminuria and renal functional decline.[50,51] Strict glycemic control may also improve renal histology. Renal biopsy specimens from pancreatic transplant recipients in whom true euglycemia is restored showed stabilized glomerular structure at 5 years of follow-up and improved glomerular and tubular structure at 10 years after transplantation.[52]

For type 2 diabetics with established DN, strict glycemic control may provide some renoprotection but does not protect against macrovascular complications. In the Kumamoto study, there was a reduction in the rate of conversion from microalbuminuria to macroalbuminuria in type 2 diabetic patients receiving intensive glycemic treatment (HbA_{1c} 7.1% with intensive treatment compared with HbA_{1c} 9.4% with conventional treatment).[4] The ADVANCE study recently confirmed the predicted reductions in new-onset microalbuminuria and nephropathy in patients with nearly normal glycemic control (HbA_{1c} 6.5% versus 7.3%).[6] In contrast, studies have failed to show a lower rate of major CV events in patients prescribed strict glycemic control. Furthermore, there was a troubling finding from the ACCORD trial, in which type 2 diabetic patients with either established CVD or additional CV risk factors had increased mortality when given intensive glycemic treatment (lowering of HbA_{1c} to a median of 6.4% versus 7.5% with conventional control).[7]

The most appropriate target for glycated hemoglobin for patients with DN is 7.0%, especially for high-risk patients with established CVD. Lower individualized targets may be appropriate when the focus is the treatment of microvascular disease such as nephropathy, but the potential renal benefits need to be balanced with the increased rates of adverse events such as hypoglycemia, especially in patients with declining GFR due to decreased clearance of insulin or oral hypoglycemic agents.

The most plausible conclusion is that glucose-lowering treatment must be individualized in type 2 diabetes. It should be more aggressive in young patients with short duration of diabetes, high life expectancy, and low risk of hypoglycemia. A more cautious approach is sensible in the elderly patient who has long-standing diabetes, has preexisting CV problems, gains weight with insulin, and is susceptible to hypoglycemic episodes. Type 2 diabetes is a progressive disease with progressive loss of endogenous insulin secretion so that ultimately insulin will often become necessary. The American Diabetes Association and the European Association for the Study of Diabetes guidelines recommend lifestyle intervention first and suggest the addition of basal insulin (most effective), sulfonylurea (least expensive), or thiazolidinediones (no hypoglycemia) if HbA_{1c} values still exceed 7%.

Treatment of Dyslipidemia

Most patients with DN have dyslipidemia, characterized by low levels of high-density lipoprotein (HDL) cholesterol, high triglyceride (TG) levels, and a shift from larger toward smaller LDL cholesterol.[53] Dyslipidemia in diabetic patients may contribute to the development of glomerulosclerosis and progressive renal disease.[54,55]

In type 2 diabetic patients with non–dialysis dependent DN, treatment with statins provides substantial CV benefit.[56,57] In contrast, statin therapy in ESRD may come too late to translate into improved CV outcomes (see Chapters 31 and 78).

Current guidelines recommend a goal for LDL cholesterol of below 100 mg/dl (2.57 mmol/l) for diabetic patients in general and below 70 mg/dl (1.81 mmol/l) for diabetic patients with CVD.[17] However, LDL cholesterol is not the sole lipid that defines CV risk. As major statin trials have demonstrated, lowering of LDL cholesterol does not prevent the majority of adverse CV events and does not bring the CV risk in diabetics down to the level of nondiabetic patients. This has been referred to as residual CV risk. Atherogenic dyslipidemia, specifically elevated TG, low HDL cholesterol, elevated apolipoprotein β, and elevated apolipoprotein C-III, are thought to be key factors associated with residual CV risk in diabetic patients.[58] In the UKPDS, elevated TG was independently associated with albuminuria in type 2 diabetic patients. Thus, interventions aimed at improving all lipid targets are required. However, the lack of clinical trial data on the use of combined lipid-altering treatment presents a therapeutic dilemma because it is not known whether this is best achieved by intensification of statin therapy or by supplementation of statin therapy with a fibrate, niacin, or omega-3 fatty acid.

Nonpharmacologic Interventions

Dietary protein restriction may alleviate uremic symptoms in patients at or approaching ESRD. However, it is of uncertain benefit in the treatment of DN. Small trials have shown low-protein diet (0.8 g/kg per day) to significantly reduce proteinuria with an increase in plasma albumin in macroalbuminuric type 2 diabetic patients.[59] A recent meta-analysis, however, concluded that although low-protein diet improved proteinuria, it is also associated with lower serum albumin concentrations and was not associated with a significant improvement of renal function in patients with either type 1 or type 2 DN.[60] Nutritionist counseling is advised for all patients with advanced CKD to avoid protein-calorie malnutrition before renal replacement therapy, which has been shown to be a strong predictor for subsequent increased morbidity and mortality during maintenance dialysis. Furthermore, all patients with DN should be given counseling on salt, potassium, and phosphate restriction as well as choice of carbohydrates and fats.

Lifestyle modifications such as smoking cessation and weight reduction can provide additive renal benefits and lower the risk of CV events in patients with established DN. There is evidence that smoking cessation ameliorates progression of microalbuminuria to macroalbuminuria and improves renal prognosis.[61] Weight reduction may also improve renal outcome. In a small randomized trial of obese (body mass index >27 kg/m^2) diabetic and nondiabetic patients with proteinuric renal disease, patients who lost weight through dieting had marked improvement in proteinuria compared with those who lost no weight.[62]

NEWER TREATMENTS OF DIABETIC NEPHROPATHY

Peroxisome proliferator-activated receptors (PPAR) are ligand-activated transcription factors involved in regulating adipogenesis, insulin sensitivity, inflammation, and blood pressure; they may have a role in the development of nephropathy in type 2 diabetics. Thiazolidinediones (e.g., pioglitazone, rosiglitazone) are PPARγ agonists with insulin-sensitizing actions. Pioglitazone in combination with the ARB losartan seems to offer greater renoprotection than does losartan alone in short-term studies.[63] Currently, it is premature to suggest routine therapy with a thiazolidinedione in DN. The glycosaminoglycan sulodexide has recently been shown to have no benefit for microalbuminuric or overtly proteinuric DN. Serum uric acid is predictive of the development and progression of DN in type 1 diabetic subjects, and experimental lowering of uric acid is protective in experimental DN. These observations suggest that future studies examining the effect of lowering uric acid as a potential therapy are needed. Several other agents, including avosentan (an endothelin A receptor blocker), protein kinase C inhibitors, fenofibrate, pirfenidone, monoclonal anti–connective tissue growth factor antibody, mycophenolate mofetil (MMF), and fish oil, have been evaluated for proteinuric renal disease including DN. There are insufficient data on any of these agents at this time for their use to be advocated in the prevention or treatment of DN. New insights into the molecular mechanisms that underlie the origin and progression of DN are emerging from large-scale genetic and molecular studies in experimental models and humans. It is anticipated that strategies for the prevention and treatment of DN will continue to improve as newer agents become available.

REFERENCES

1. U.S. Renal Data System. *USRDS 2008 Annual Data Report: Atlas of End-Stage Renal Disease in the United States*. Bethesda, Md: National Institutes of Health, National Institute of Diabetes and Digestive and Kidney Diseases; 2008.
2. The Diabetes Control and Complications Trial Research Group. The effect of intensive treatment of diabetes on the development and progression of long-term complications in insulin-dependent diabetes mellitus. *N Engl J Med*. 1993;329:977-986.

3. Writing Team for the Diabetes Control and Complications Trial/ Epidemiology of Diabetes Interventions and Complications Research Group. Sustained effect of intensive treatment of type 1 diabetes mellitus on development and progression of diabetic nephropathy: The Epidemiology of Diabetes Interventions and Complications (EDIC) study. *JAMA*. 2003;290:2159-2167.
4. Shichiri M, Kishikawa H, Ohkubo Y, Wake N. Long-term results of the Kumamoto Study on optimal diabetes control in type 2 diabetic patients. *Diabetes Care*. 2000;23(Suppl 2):B21-B29.
5. U.K. Prospective Diabetes Study (UKPDS) Group. Intensive blood-glucose control with sulphonylureas or insulin compared with conventional treatment and risk of complications in patients with type 2 diabetes (UKPDS 33). *Lancet*. 1998;352:837-853.
6. The ADVANCE Collaborative Group. Intensive blood glucose control and vascular outcomes in patients with type 2 diabetes. *N Engl J Med*. 2008;358:2560-2572.
7. The Action to Control Cardiovascular Risk in Diabetes Study Group. Effects of intensive glucose lowering in type 2 diabetes. *N Engl J Med*. 2008;358:2545-2559.
8. Duckworth W, Abraira C, Moritz T, et al. Glucose control and vascular complications in veterans with type 2 diabetes. *N Engl J Med*. 2009; 360:129-139.
9. KDOQI Clinical Practice Guidelines and Clinical Practice Recommendations for Diabetes and Chronic Kidney Disease. *Am J Kidney Dis*. 2007;49:S12-S154.
10. Tarnow L, Rossing P, Gall MA, et al. Prevalence of arterial hypertension in diabetic patients before and after the JNC-V. *Diabetes Care*. 1994;17: 1247-1251.
11. Bakris GL, Williams M, Dworkin L, et al. Preserving renal function in adults with hypertension and diabetes: A consensus approach. National Kidney Foundation Hypertension and Diabetes Executive Committees Working Group. *Am J Kidney Dis*. 2000;36:646-661.
12. American Diabetes Association Clinical Practice Recommendations 2001. *Diabetes Care*. 2001;24(Suppl 1):S1-S133.
13. Bilous R. DIRECT-Renal: The effect of the angiotensin type 1 receptor blocker candesartan on the development of microalbuminuria in type 1 and type 2 diabetes. American Society of Nephrology's (ASN) 41st Annual Meeting and Scientific Exposition; Philadelphia; 2008.
14. Ruggenenti P, Fassi A, Ilieva AP, et al. Preventing microalbuminuria in type 2 diabetes. *N Engl J Med*. 2004;351:1941-1951.
15. Kvetny J, Gregersen G, Pedersen RS. Randomized placebo-controlled trial of perindopril in normotensive, normoalbuminuric patients with type 1 diabetes mellitus. *QJM*. 2001;94:89-94.
16. Ansquer JC, Foucher C, Rattier S, et al. Fenofibrate reduces progression to microalbuminuria over 3 years in a placebo-controlled study in type 2 diabetes: Results from the Diabetes Atherosclerosis Intervention Study (DAIS). *Am J Kidney Dis*. 2005;45:485-493.
17. Grundy SM, Cleeman JI, Merz CN, et al. Implications of recent clinical trials for the National Cholesterol Education Program Adult Treatment Panel III guidelines. *Circulation*. 2004;110:227-239.
18. Ritz E, Ogata H, Orth SR. Smoking: A factor promoting onset and progression of diabetic nephropathy. *Diabetes Metab*. 2000;26(Suppl 4):54-63.
19. Gaede P, Vedel P, Parving HH, Pedersen O. Intensified multifactorial intervention in patients with type 2 diabetes mellitus and microalbuminuria: The Steno type 2 randomised study. *Lancet*. 1999;353: 617-622.
20. Gaede P, Vedel P, Larsen N, et al. Multifactorial intervention and cardiovascular disease in patients with type 2 diabetes. *N Engl J Med*. 2003;348:383-393.
21. Parving HH, Andersen AR, Smidt VM, et al. Effect of anti-hypertensive treatment on kidney function in diabetic nephropathy. *BMJ*. 1987;294: 1443-1447.
22. Hansson L, Zanchetti A, Carruthers SG, et al. Effects of intensive blood-pressure lowering and low-dose aspirin in patients with hypertension: Principal results of the Hypertension Optimal Treatment (HOT) randomised trial. HOT Study Group. *Lancet*. 1998;351:1755-1762.
23. Ismail N, Becker B, Strzelczyk P, Ritz E. Renal disease and hypertension in non–insulin-dependent diabetes mellitus. *Kidney Int*. 1999;55:1-28.
24. Mogensen CE. Microalbuminuria and hypertension with focus on type 1 and type 2 diabetes. *J Intern Med*. 2003;254:45-66.
25. Pohl MA, Blumenthal S, Cordonnier DJ, et al. Independent and additive impact of blood pressure control and angiotensin II receptor blockade on renal outcomes in the irbesartan diabetic nephropathy trial: Clinical implications and limitations. *J Am Soc Nephrol*. 2005;16: 3027-3037.
26. Bomback AS, Klemmer PJ. The incidence and implications of aldosterone breakthrough. *Nat Clin Pract Nephrol*. 2007;3:486-492.
27. Hollenberg NK. Aldosterone in the development and progression of renal injury. *Kidney Int*. 2004;66:1-9.
28. The Microalbuminuria Captopril Study Group. Captopril reduces the risk of nephropathy in IDDM patients with microalbuminuria. *Diabetologia*. 1996;39:587-593.
29. The EUCLID Study Group. Randomised placebo-controlled trial of lisinopril in normotensive patients with insulin-dependent diabetes and normoalbuminuria or microalbuminuria. *Lancet*. 1997;349:1787-1792.
30. Should all patients with type 1 diabetes mellitus and microalbuminuria receive angiotensin-converting enzyme inhibitors? A meta-analysis of individual patient data. *Ann Intern Med*. 2001;134:370-379.
31. Lewis EJ, Hunsicker LG, Bain RP, Rohde RD. The Collaborative Study Group: The effect of angiotensin-converting-enzyme inhibition on diabetic nephropathy. *N Engl J Med*. 1993;329:1456-1462.
32. Parving HH, Lehnert H, Brochner-Mortensen J, et al. The effect of irbesartan on the development of diabetic nephropathy in patients with type 2 diabetes. *N Engl J Med*. 2001;345:870-878.
33. Viberti G, Wheeldon NM. Microalbuminuria reduction with valsartan in patients with type 2 diabetes mellitus: A blood pressure–independent effect. *Circulation*. 2002;106:672-678.
34. Brenner BM, Cooper ME, de Zeeuw D, et al. Effects of losartan on renal and cardiovascular outcomes in patients with type 2 diabetes and nephropathy. *N Engl J Med*. 2001;345:861-869.
35. Lewis EJ, Hunsicker LG, Clarke WR, et al. Renoprotective effect of the angiotensin-receptor antagonist irbesartan in patients with nephropathy due to type 2 diabetes. *N Engl J Med*. 2001;345:851-860.
36. Barnett AH, Bain SC, Bouter P, et al. Angiotensin-receptor blockade versus converting-enzyme inhibition in type 2 diabetes and nephropathy. *N Engl J Med*. 2004;351:1952-1961.
37. Nakao N, Yoshimura A, Morita H, et al. Combination treatment of angiotensin-II receptor blocker and angiotensin-converting-enzyme inhibitor in non-diabetic renal disease (COOPERATE): A randomised controlled trial. *Lancet*. 2003;361:117-124.
38. Retraction—Combination treatment of angiotensin-II receptor blocker and angiotensin-converting-enzyme inhibitor in non-diabetic renal disease (COOPEPATE): a randomisid controlled trial. *Lancet*. 2009; 374:1226.
39. Mogensen CE, Neldam S, Tikkanen I, et al. Randomised controlled trial of dual blockade of renin-angiotensin system in patients with hypertension, microalbuminuria, and non–insulin dependent diabetes: The candesartan and lisinopril microalbuminuria (CALM) study. *BMJ*. 2000; 321:1440-1444.
40. Jacobsen P, Rossing K, Parving HH. Single versus dual blockade of the renin-angiotensin system (angiotensin-converting enzyme inhibitors and/or angiotensin II receptor blockers) in diabetic nephropathy. *Curr Opin Nephrol Hypertens*. 2004;13:319-324.
41. The ONTARGET Investigators. Telmisartan, ramipril, or both in patients at high risk for vascular events. *N Engl J Med*. 2008;358: 1547-1559.
42. Epstein M, Williams GH, Weinberger M, et al. Selective aldosterone blockade with eplerenone reduces albuminuria in patients with type 2 diabetes. *Clin J Am Soc Nephrol*. 2006;1:940-951.
43. Parving HH, Persson F, Lewis JB, et al; the AVOID Study Investigators. Aliskiren combined with losartan in type 2 diabetes and nephropathy. *N Engl J Med*. 2008;358:2433-2446.
44. Rossing K, Schjoedt KJ, Jensen BR, et al. Enhanced renoprotective effects of ultrahigh doses of irbesartan in patients with type 2 diabetes and microalbuminuria. *Kidney Int*. 2005;68:1190-1198.
45. Bakris GL, Weir MR. Angiotensin-converting enzyme inhibitor–associated elevations in serum creatinine: Is this a cause for concern? *Arch Intern Med*. 2000;160:685-693.
46. Bakris GL, Weir MR, Secic M, et al. Differential effects of calcium antagonist subclasses on markers of nephropathy progression. *Kidney Int*. 2004;65:1991-2002.
47. Koshy S, Bakris GL. Therapeutic approaches to achieve desired blood pressure goals: Focus on calcium channel blockers. *Cardiovasc Drugs Ther*. 2000;14:295-301.
48. Estacio RO, Schrier RW. Antihypertensive therapy in type 2 diabetes: Implications of the appropriate blood pressure control in diabetes (ABCD) trial. *Am J Cardiol*. 1998;82:9R-14R.
49. Weidmann P, Schneider M, Bohlen L. Therapeutic efficacy of different antihypertensive drugs in human diabetic nephropathy: An updated meta-analysis. *Nephrol Dial Transplant*. 1995;10(Suppl 9):39-45.
50. Mulec H, Blohme G, Grande B, Bjorck S. The effect of metabolic control on rate of decline in renal function in insulin-dependent diabetes

mellitus with overt diabetic nephropathy. *Nephrol Dial Transplant.* 1998;13:651-655.

51. Alaveras AE, Thomas SM, Sagriotis A, Viberti GC. Promoters of progression of diabetic nephropathy: The relative roles of blood glucose and blood pressure control. *Nephrol Dial Transplant.* 1997;12(Suppl 2):71-74.
52. Fioretto P, Sutherland DE, Najafian B, Mauer M. Remodeling of renal interstitial and tubular lesions in pancreas transplant recipients. *Kidney Int.* 2006;69:907-912.
53. Jenkins AJ, Lyons TJ, Zheng D, et al. Lipoproteins in the DCCT/EDIC cohort: Associations with diabetic nephropathy. *Kidney Int.* 2003;64: 817-828.
54. Krolewski AS, Warram JH, Christlieb AR. Hypercholesterolemia—a determinant of renal function loss and deaths in IDDM patients with nephropathy. *Kidney Int Suppl.* 1994;45:S125-S131.
55. Tonolo G, Velussi M, Brocco E, et al. Simvastatin maintains steady patterns of GFR and improves AER and expression of slit diaphragm proteins in type II diabetes. *Kidney Int.* 2006;70:177-186.
56. Colhoun HM, Betteridge DJ, Durrington PN, et al. Primary prevention of cardiovascular disease with atorvastatin in type 2 diabetes in the Collaborative Atorvastatin Diabetes Study (CARDS): Multicentre randomised placebo-controlled trial. *Lancet.* 2004;364:685-696.
57. Tonelli M, Keech A, Shepherd J, et al. Effect of pravastatin in people with diabetes and chronic kidney disease. *J Am Soc Nephrol.* 2005;16: 3748-3754.
58. Fruchart JC, Sacks F, Hermans MP, et al. The Residual Risk Reduction Initiative: A call to action to reduce residual vascular risk in patients with dyslipidemia. *Am J Cardiol.* 2008;102:1K-34K.
59. Giordano M, Lucidi P, Ciarambino T, et al. Effects of dietary protein restriction on albumin and fibrinogen synthesis in macroalbuminuric type 2 diabetic patients. *Diabetologia.* 2008;51:21-28.
60. Pan Y, Guo LL, Jin HM. Low-protein diet for diabetic nephropathy: A meta-analysis of randomized controlled trials. *Am J Clin Nutr.* 2008;88:660-666.
61. Phisitkul K, Hegazy K, Chuahirun T, et al. Continued smoking exacerbates but cessation ameliorates progression of early type 2 diabetic nephropathy. *Am J Med Sci.* 2008;335:284-291.
62. Morales E, Valero MA, Leon M, et al. Beneficial effects of weight loss in overweight patients with chronic proteinuric nephropathies. *Am J Kidney Dis.* 2003;41:319-327.
63. Jin HM, Pan Y. Renoprotection provided by losartan in combination with pioglitazone is superior to renoprotection provided by losartan alone in patients with type 2 diabetic nephropathy. *Kidney Blood Press Res.* 2007;30:203-211.

CHAPTER 31

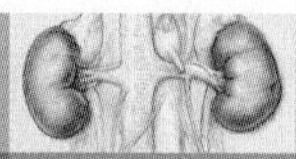

Management of the Diabetic Patient with Chronic Kidney Disease

Dace Trence, Wolfgang Pommer

Diabetic patients with chronic kidney disease (CKD) are the fastest growing population in renal care and dialysis (Fig. 31.1). Many of these patients present to nephrologists with advanced stages of CKD. Renal disease in these subjects may not be due solely to diabetic nephropathy (DN) but may be secondary to hypertensive or vascular disease and in some cases glomerular or tubulointerstitial diseases unrelated to diabetes mellitus (DM). Thus, the initial approach is to identify, if possible, the etiology of the underlying kidney disease to guide specific treatment (see Chapter 29).

The main focus of therapeutic intervention in stage 3 to stage 5 CKD is:

- Prevention of or retarding further progression of CKD.
- Timely treatment of secondary complications of CKD (i.e., Hypertension, acid-base and electrolyte disturbances, anemia, hyperparathyroidism).
- Improvement of the patient's survival by aggressive therapy of coexisting disease, in particular cardiovascular disease (CVD).
- Timely institution of and correct choice of renal replacement therapy (RRT).

Prevention of cardiac death in CKD and retarding progression to end-stage renal disease (ESRD) are the most pressing long-term issues in the diabetic patient with renal disease. Diabetic patients with CKD benefit from a multidisciplinary therapeutic approach involving general practitioners, nephrologists, diabetologists, interventional cardiologists, podiatrists, dietitians, and special renal and diabetes nurse specialists.[1] Although the value of such a multifactorial approach in diabetics with CKD is generally accepted,[2] it is controversial when to refer to the nephrologist. This is in part constrained by availability of nephrologists and socioeconomic conditions of different health care systems. CKD patients with type 2 DM ideally should be referred to the nephrologist as early as kidney disease has been diagnosed to exclude nondiabetic kidney disease requiring specific treatment. Regular follow-up is recommended, minimally yearly to ideally quarterly per year if CKD continues to progress (Fig. 31.2). However, with the shortage of nephrologists in many countries, if nephrologists were dedicated just to DM patients, lack of care for other renal disease patients would easily result if these recommendations were enforced. Consequently, general care providers often have to compensate for the lack of nephrologists. This includes knowledge of the medical issues involved in DM at each stage of CKD and the therapeutic interventions required (Fig. 31.3).

METABOLIC CONTROL

Glycemic control has a beneficial impact on prevention of CKD and preservation of renal function in type 1 DM as well as in type 2 DM (see Chapter 30). However, advancing CKD causes insulin resistance, impaired glucose tolerance, and hyperglycemia because a circulating factor interferes with the action of insulin. Because the insulin inhibitor is dialyzable, insulin resistance diminishes after the start of dialysis. At the same time, the half-life of insulin is prolonged. Furthermore, the potential for hypoglycemia with both oral agents and insulin increases in the presence of CKD (with the exception of gliquidone and glimepiride). Self-monitoring of blood glucose concentration is therefore imperative.

Ideally, reversal of DN through euglycemia and restoration of normal insulin secretion and action should be the goal. Thus, in type 1 DM, a pancreas transplant alone can induce regression of moderate DN lesions in native kidneys, but only during a period of 10 years after transplantation.[3] Pancreas transplantation at the time of renal transplantation has been shown to prevent or to slow the development of DN in the transplanted kidney.

The choice of therapeutic approaches to glycemic control depends on the CKD stage (Fig. 31.4), the risk for hypoglycemia, and the patient's personal choice. Metformin has been used in low doses in patients with glomerular filtration rate (GFR) as low as 30 to 60 ml/min. It should not be used at a GFR below 30 ml/min, given the risk for lactic acidosis. As renal function can deteriorate abruptly, it is better to avoid metformin once serum creatinine concentration rises above 1.5 mg/dl (132 μmo/l) in men and above 1.3 mg/dl (117 μmol/l) in women. Insulin secretagogues (sulfonylurea and meglitinides) can be associated with hypoglycemia, with occurrence rates reported from 10% to 35%. These can be severe and long lasting in those receiving sulfonylureas, requiring hospitalization for treatment. Glycosidase inhibitors are short acting; because they interfere with the absorption of sucrose or starch; patients taking these agents need to use dextrose tablets or glucose gels to treat hypoglycemia. Glycosidase inhibitors are contraindicated in renal failure. Thiazolidinediones are associated with weight gain, in part from fluid retention but also due to nonfluid gains. In patients at risk for congestive heart failure, these should be avoided. There is also concern about increased bone fracture rates in patients using thiazolidinediones, which could potentiate CKD-related bone disease.[4]

Insulin regimens are the most commonly used to control glycemia in CKD. Given the increasing half-life of insulin as

Percentage of Incident Patients with End-Stage Renal Disease Due to Diabetes, By Year					
	2002	2003	2004	2005	2006
Argentina	-	-	31	35	34
Australia	27	26	30	31	32
Austria	35	34	33	34	33
Belgium, Dutch speaking	22	24	24	24	22
Belgium, French speaking	23	25	27	24	23
Bosnia & Herzegovina	-	23	20	21	28
Canada	34	34	34	35	-
Croatia	29	27	29	30	-
Denmark	26	23	22	24	24
Finland	39	35	33	35	35
France	-	-	-	23	35
Germany	36	36	34	35	34
Greece	27	28	28	29	30
Hong Kong	47	40	41	42	41
Hungary	26	26	30	26	28
Iceland	10	0	4	16	33
Israel	39	38	41	39	40
Italy	16	16	16	18	-
Jalisco (Mexico)	51	51	56	60	50
Japan	39	41	41	42	43
Luxembourg	-	-	-	-	28
Malaysia	50	52	55	52	58
Netherlands	17	17	17	16	16
New Zealand	45	41	41	42	42
Norway	12	16	17	13	16
Pakistan	40	40	-	36	38
Philippines	29	33	34	37	39
Rep. of Korea	41	43	43	39	42
Romania	-	-	-	11	12
Russia	9	11	-	11	14
Scotland	19	19	18	22	22
Spain	-	-	18	23	23
Sweden	24	24	25	26	26
Taiwan	39	37	38	41	42
Turkey	46	23	27	30	23
UK. (England, Wales, & N. Ireland)	-	-	-	19	19
United States	45	45	45	44	44
Uruguay	20	30	28	30	17

Figure 31.1 Percentage of incident patients with end-stage renal disease (ESRD) due to diabetes, by year. Diabetes was the primary cause of end-stage renal disease (ESRD) in 58% of new patients in Malaysia in 2006 and 50% of those in Mexico. In a majority of reporting countries, 20% to 44% of new patients have this primary diagnosis. Countries with the lowest reported rates of ESRD due to diabetes include Romania, Russia, the Netherlands, Norway, Uruguay, and the United Kingdom (England, Wales, and N. Ireland), each with 12% to 19%. *(Source: USRDS slides 2008.)*

CKD progresses, the risk for hypoglycemia increases. Consequently, multiple daily injections or continuous insulin infusion per pump, by which insulin doses can be more closely regulated, would seem optimal. However, ideal insulin therapies remain undefined in CKD, given a paucity of pharmacokinetic studies that could guide insulin adjustment on the basis of GFR. It is also unclear whether intermediate or longer acting insulins should be avoided and rapid-acting analogues used instead. The rapidly acting insulin analogues lispro and aspart exhibit similar pharmacokinetics in CKD patients as in patients with normal GFR. The same is true for detemir, but so far no clinical data on its use in CKD patients are available.[5] Glargine has been shown to reduce hypoglycemia in hemodialysis (HD) patients.

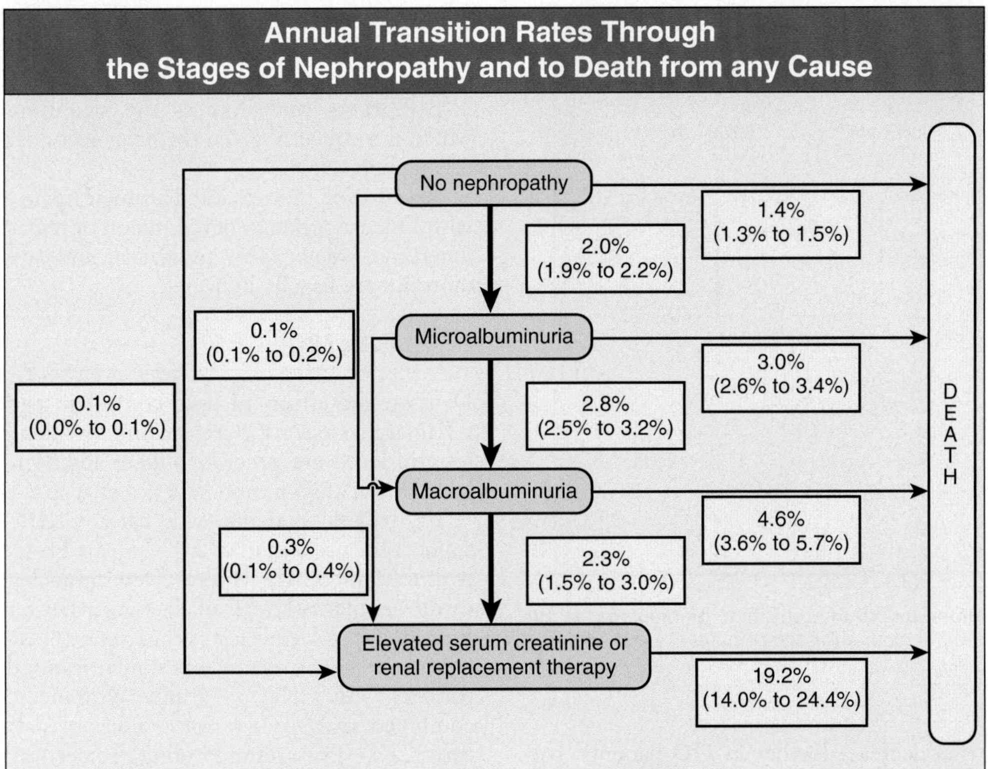

Figure 31.2 Annual transition rates with 95% confidence intervals through the stages of nephropathy and to death from any cause. *(Modified from reference 6.)*

Standard Care and Target Values Proposed for CKD Patients with Diabetes Mellitus

Parameter	CKD 3/4	CKD 5 and 5D
Metabolic control		
glycosylated hemoglobin	> 6.5 – 7.5 g%	> 7.0-8.0 g%
preferred agents	meglitinides/sulfonyl ureas/insulin	insulin
Blood pressure	130/80 mmHg	
preferred agents	ACE/ARB's	np/Betablockers
Lipid treatment		
LDL cholesterol	<100 mg/dl	np
preferred agents	statins	np/ns
Anemia treatment		
Hemoglobin level	11.0 – 12.0 g/dl	11.0 – 12.0 g/dl (avoid >13)
preferred agents	iron/ESA	ESA/iron
Vitamin D supplements	Vit. D3/1.25-OHD	1.25 OHD/Vit. D3
Supportive treatment		
Smoking cessation	++	np
hypoglyemia awareness	++	+++
Lowdose aspirin	++	+/np
Exercise (daily/weekly)	+	+
Foot care	+++	+++
Prevention of falls	+	+++

Figure 31.3 Standard care and target values proposed for CKD patients with diabetes mellitus. For details, see text. ACE, angiotensin-converting enzyme; ARB, angiotensin receptor blocker; ESA, erythropoiesis-stimulating agent; LDL, low-density lipoprotein; NP, not proven; NS, not significant; +/++/+++, moderately/very/highly indicated.

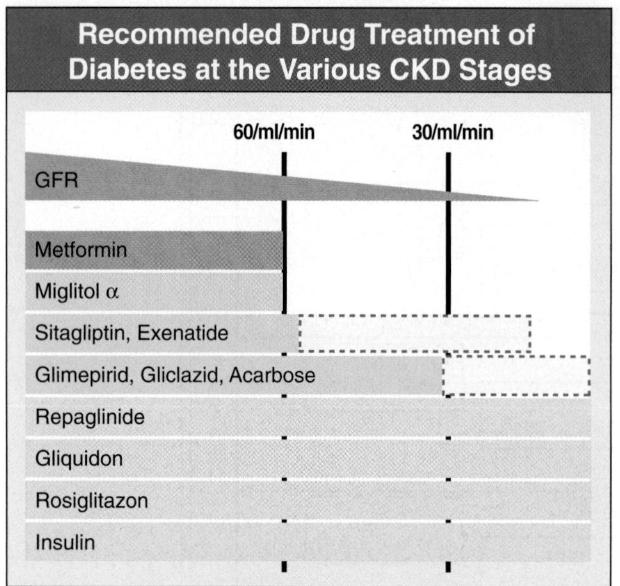

Figure 31.4 Recommended drug treatment of diabetes at the various CKD stages. GFR, glomerular filtration rate. Hatched green boxes indicate missing data.

Insulin requirements decrease further in HD patients, particularly in those with residual diuresis (<500 ml/day), insulin requirement often decreases by 30%. Two doses of an intermediate-acting insulin plus one preprandial rapidly acting insulin dose can usually achieve reasonable control. In peritoneal dialysis (PD) patients, intraperitoneal insulin is more physiologic than subcutaneous, as portal absorption of insulin may better mimic the endogenous insulin effect. Insulin requirements typically increase by 200% to 300% in this situation.[5]

BLOOD PRESSURE CONTROL

Blood pressure control is critical for primary and secondary prevention of renal disease and CVD in DM. At any given level of GFR, blood pressure tends to be higher in diabetic than in nondiabetic patients with CKD. Generally recommended blood pressure targets are 130/80 mm Hg, with recognition that in specific ethnic groups, 120/70 mm Hg may be a more appropriate target for decreasing renal disease progression. In diabetics with CKD, it will typically take three or four drugs to accomplish this, starting with an angiotensin-converting enzyme (ACE) inhibitor or angiotensin receptor blocker (ARB), then a diuretic, calcium channel blocker, β-blocker, or the recently licensed renin inhibitors.[7]

As discussed in Chapter 30, ACE inhibitors or ARBs are obligatory unless there are contraindications (e.g., an acute increase in serum creatinine of 50% or more; renal artery stenosis; hypovolemia; congestive heart failure; or hyperkalemia resistant to corrective maneuvers, such as administration of loop diuretics, dietary potassium restriction, or correction of metabolic acidosis). An increase in serum creatinine of 10% to 20% is expected and should not deter the administration of ACE inhibitors or ARBs. However, in patients with CKD stage 5, administration of ACE inhibitors may lower GFR to such an extent that dialysis becomes necessary. At this stage, these drugs are therefore no longer the first choice. However, if a patient is already established on an ACE inhibitor or ARB, these drugs should be continued in advanced renal failure unless there has been an abrupt recent increase in serum creatinine. For example, in the Irbesartan in Diabetic Nephropathy Trial (IDNT),[8] administration of ARBs extended the time until patients required dialysis.

β-Blockers can suppress the symptoms of hypoglycemia, which is a concern, given the propensity of diabetics with CKD for hypoglycemia.

Because of their marked propensity to retain salt, patients with DN are prone to development of hypervolemia and edema. Therefore, dietary salt restriction and administration of loop diuretics are usually indicated.

LIPID CONTROL

Data on the effects of lipid control in patients with DM and CKD are sparse. Triglyceride and low-density lipoprotein cholesterol levels are generally higher and high-density lipoprotein levels lower than in nondiabetics in type 2 DM.[9]

In diabetic patients with early CKD, secondary analyses support the use of statins. In the Heart Protection Study, patients with DM and CKD who received statins had a 23% decrease in cardiovascular risk with an absolute event reduction of 80%.[10] In the Cholesterol And Recurrent Events (CARE) study, risk reduction for coronary events was similar in nondiabetic and diabetic patients with CKD (creatinine clearances <75 ml/min).[11,12] A combined analysis of various studies of statins in diabetics with early CKD (Pravastatin Pooling Project, CARE, and Long-term Intervention with Pravastatin in Ischemic Disease [LIPID]) showed that the risk reduction for cardiovascular events was 6.5% and thus exceeded that observed in diabetics without CKD or nondiabetics.[9]

In HD patients with type 2 DM, the addition of 20 mg of atorvastatin did not decrease cardiovascular death, nonfatal myocardial infarction, or stroke despite a 40% decrease in low-density lipoprotein cholesterol levels.[13] If strokes were omitted from the analyses, there was a significant decrease in cardiac events. Observational data in dialysis patients also suggest that statins decrease total and cardiovascular mortality.[8,14] However, these studies were not limited to diabetics; 60%[14] and 43%[8] of the patients receiving statins were diabetic.

As metabolism of different statins varies, the need to modify doses as GFR changes should be kept in mind. Atorvastatin can be given in doses up to 80 mg/day for those on HD and PD. Fluvastatin can also be given in doses up to 80 mg/day. Pravastatin should be limited to 10 mg, as active metabolites can accumulate, although in the Pravastatin Pooling Project, doses of up to 40 mg were safely used down to GFR of 30 ml/min per 1.73 m^2. Simvastatin, 20 mg/day, can be safely used, with 40-mg daily doses in the Heart Protection Study used safely even in stage 3 CKD. Rosuvastatin should be limited to not more than 10 mg daily when GFR falls below 30 ml/min per 1.73 m^2. Ezetimibe can be safely used in renal impairment, as can bile acid sequestrants, but the potential effect on absorption of other prescriptive drugs, particularly with the bile acid sequestrants, should be kept in mind. Fenofibrate doses should be reduced by one third in CKD stage 2, reduced by two thirds in CKD stages 3 and 4, and avoided in CKD stage 5. Gemfibrozil can be safely used, although in PD, elevated CPK levels have been reported at usual doses. Sustained-release niacin should be decreased by 50% at CKD stage 5.[9]

DIET AND MALNUTRITION

Diabetic patients with renal failure are often severely catabolic and tend to develop malnutrition (see Chapter 83). This risk is particularly high during periods of intercurrent illness and fasting but may also be the result of ill-advised recommendations to restrict protein intake. Anorectic obese patients with type 2 diabetes and advanced CKD often undergo massive weight loss, leading to normalization of fasting glucose concentration and even of hyperglycemia after a glucose load. Low muscle mass because of wasting is an important reason for misjudging the severity of renal failure, leading, for example, to delayed start of RRT. Therefore, creatinine clearance should be measured, or at least an estimate of GFR by use of the Cockcroft-Gault or the Modification of Diet in Renal Disease (MDRD) study formula should be obtained rather than relying on serum creatinine.

ANEMIA

Anemia occurs at an earlier stage of CKD in DM patients and is often more severe.[15,16] However, confounding these data is the fact that in diabetes, anemia can develop even at a normal GFR. At GFR of 30 to 60 ml/min, 20% of diabetics are anemic.[17] If a hemoglobin cutoff of 11 g/dl is used, 20% to 31% of patients with diabetes and CKD stage 3 or higher are anemic; at GFR below 50 ml/min per 1.73 m^2, this increases to 27% to 42%.[17]

In a meta-analysis of several community longitudinal studies, anemia was found to be a risk factor for adverse cardiovascular outcomes as well as for all-cause mortality in those with diabetes and CKD.[18] In the Atherosclerosis Risk In Communities (ARIC) study, anemia alone was a risk factor; but when anemia and CKD were both present, a synergistic risk for stroke and coronary disease was found, compared with each risk factor alone. In those with DM, microvascular as well as macrovascular disease of the coronary circulation or more severe left ventricular hypertrophy could increase susceptibility to ischemia induced by anemia.[19] Erythropoietin-dependent anemia is also associated with autonomic neuropathy, which itself is a risk factor for a cardiovascular event. It is also associated with impaired sleep, impaired cognitive function, decreased exercise tolerance, and a general decrease in quality of life. Finally, anemia predicts a faster rate of progression of renal disease.[16]

Small studies have suggested that treatment with erythropoietin (EPO) can effectively treat anemia associated with CKD in diabetes, but in higher dosages compared with nondiabetic patients. Quality of life and well-being improve. The recent TREAT-study randomly assigned 2012 diabetics with CKD stage 3 to 4 to darbepoetin alfa to achieve a hemoglobin level of approximately 13 g per deciliter and 2026 patients to placebo, with rescue darbepoetin alfa when the hemoglobin level was less than 9.0 g per deciliter. The higher target hemoglobin failed to reduce death, cardiovascular or renal events and was associated with an increased risk of stroke, supporting a target hemoglobin of 11-12 g/dl in such patients (see also Chapter 79).[20]

MINERAL AND BONE DISEASE

Diabetic patients with CKD develop secondary hyperparathyroidism at a slower rate than nondiabetics do and are predisposed to low-turnover (adynamic) bone disease (see Chapter 81). Adynamic bone disease in turn is a recognized risk factor for cardiovascular calcification (see Chapters 78 and 81), as is diabetes itself. Thus, it is not surprising that CKD and diabetes appear to exert additive effects on cardiovascular calcification. At GFR of about 50 ml/min, 100% of diabetics exhibit coronary calcification and 20% have calcification of the aortic wall.

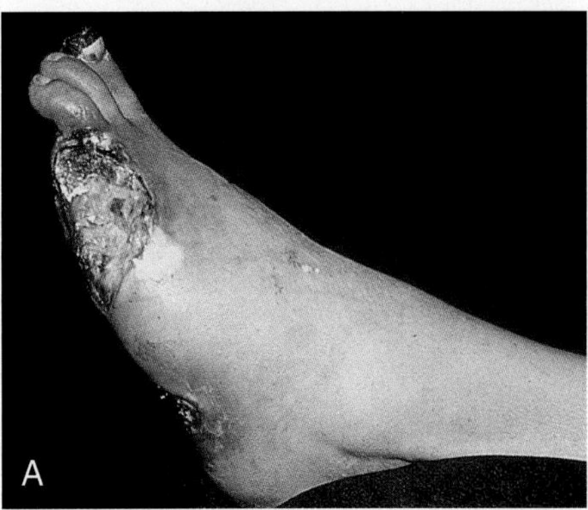

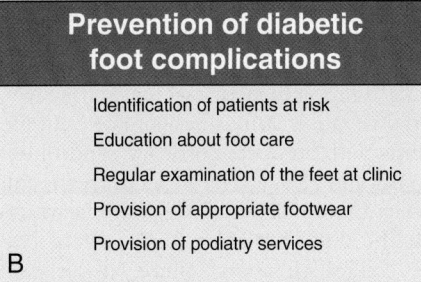

Prevention of diabetic foot complications

- Identification of patients at risk
- Education about foot care
- Regular examination of the feet at clinic
- Provision of appropriate footwear
- Provision of podiatry services

B

Figure 31.5 The diabetic foot. A, Gangrenous ulcers in a diabetic caused by a combination of large- and small-vessel disease and neuropathy. **B,** Prevention of diabetic foot complications.

Preventive and therapeutic approaches to CKD-related bone and mineral disease do not differ substantially between diabetics and nondiabetics (see Chapter 81). However, given the increased prevalence of low-turnover bone disease in diabetics with CKD, care should be taken to avoid calcium loading. These patients also appear to accumulate aluminum more readily and are more susceptible to aluminum-induced bone disease. Aluminum-containing phosphate binders should always be avoided in the diabetic patient with advanced CKD.

EXTRARENAL COMPLICATIONS CAUSED BY MICROANGIOPATHY AND MACROANGIOPATHY

Even the asymptomatic diabetic patient with advanced CKD must be monitored at regular intervals for timely detection of microvascular and macrovascular complications (ophthalmologic examination at half-yearly intervals; cardiac and angiologic status including imaging of the carotid artery yearly; foot inspection preferably at each visit). In particular, problems related to the diabetic foot are a major cause of hospital admission and nontraumatic amputation (Fig. 31.5A). Diabetic microangiopathy of the foot is frequently complicated by diabetic and uremic polyneuropathy, both of which respond poorly to conventional treatments (see Chapter 82). The situation is further aggravated by an increased risk of diabetics for infections, in particular staphylococcal infection.

Measures to prevent diabetic foot complications are shown in Figure 31.5B.

PREVENTION AND TREATMENT OF CARDIAC DISEASE

In diabetics, the likelihood of death due to cardiovascular events far exceeds that of reaching ESRD, and thus the population of diabetics on dialysis represents a "positive selection."[21] In type 2 DM, the annual transition rate through the various stages of nephropathy was far lower than the annual mortality rate (see Fig. 31.2).[22] Similar observations have been made in the Diabetes Control and Complications Trial/Epidemiology of Diabetes Interventions and Complications (DCCT/EDIC) trial in type 1 diabetics[23] and in particular in the Steno-2 population, in which 27 deaths (14 due to CVD) occurred during a mean follow-up of 7.8 years, whereas mean GFR decreased by about 30 ml/min per 1.73 m^2 and no subject reached ESRD.[24] Two studies designed to evaluate the effect of intensive treatment on vascular complications, the Action to Control Cardiovascular Risk in Diabetes (ACCORD) and Action in Diabetes and Vascular Disease: Preterax and Diamicron MR Controlled Evaluation (ADVANCE) trials, substantiate the high incidence of fatal cardiovascular events compared with the low progress to advanced renal failure.[25,26] Once a diabetic has reached ESRD, the cardiovascular mortality rate is still excessive. For example, in diabetic dialysis patients with an acute coronary syndrome, mortality is 42% after 1 year and 75% after 5 years of treatment.[27] This may relate to the fact that in diabetics, coronary heart disease is often amplified by the coexistence of more severe left ventricular hypertrophy, congestive heart failure, disturbed sympathetic innervation, and microvascular disease.

How and when best to intervene in the progressive course of CVD in diabetics with CKD has not been precisely defined. Recent American Diabetes Association recommendations underline the role of smoking cessation, lifestyle changes, and medical treatment in patients with diabetes and known CVD.[28] These risk factors may be even more critical in advanced CKD, given the multiple consequences of a single risk factor such as smoking on blood pressure, lipids, and glucose, which further amplify the independent risks of these factors in patients with both diabetes and CKD.

In the absence of data, recommendations for the formal workup of coronary heart disease in diabetic patients with CKD should be no different from those for nondiabetic CKD patients (see also Chapter 78).[29] The rate of all coronary revascularization procedures in the ESRD population has risen in the last 10 years.[21] In nondialysis patients, both coronary intervention and bypass surgery can be associated with significant risk of acute renal deterioration, which must be weighed against the potential outcome benefits in the individual patient. In general, to preserve residual renal function, bypass grafting might be favored in nondialysis CKD stages, whereas interventional stenting procedures might be assumed to be more appropriate for dialysis patients with limited life span, if risks of cerebrovascular complications are assessed and treated adequately. For further discussion of whether to use coronary stenting or bypass grafting in diabetics with CKD, refer to Chapter 78.

RENAL REPLACEMENT THERAPY

As discussed in Chapter 86, whereas the mean estimated GFR at the start of dialysis is 7 to 8 ml/min per 1.73 m^2 in most dialysis populations, a higher threshold is usually used in diabetics (serum creatinine >6 mg/dl [530 µmol/l] or estimated GFR <15 ml/min) as they tend to tolerate uremia poorly and are frequently troubled by sodium retention and fluid overload.

Selection of the mode of dialysis is discussed in Chapter 86; advantages and disadvantages of each technique are outlined in Figure 31.6. Death rates of diabetic patients on HD and PD have decreased substantially but remain higher than rates of nondiabetics on both modalities.[30] Younger diabetics treated with peritoneal dialysis have a significantly lower risk of death than do those treated with hemodialysis during early years of dialysis. Technique failure is higher in diabetics compared with nondiabetics and in peritoneal dialysis compared with hemodialysis. Patients with diabetes have higher rates of hospital admission than do nondiabetics on hemodialysis or peritoneal dialysis, with significantly higher rates in peritoneal dialysis compared with hemodialysis.[30] Peritoneal dialysis–associated glucose loading in diabetics can be overcome by replacing glucose solutions in part by amino acid solutions and polyglucose. Loss of solute and water transport often limits long-term use of peritoneal dialysis to 3 to 5 years. Switching to hemodialysis should be considered before volume overload or uremic symptoms occur. In diabetics on peritoneal dialysis, maltose and polyglucose, present in dialysis solutions, affect glucose dehydrogenase–based glucose meters. Glucose meters for home blood glucose monitoring should be changed to those using a glucose oxidase test method.[31]

Comparison of Dialysis Options for the Diabetic Patient

	Peritoneal Dialysis		Hemodialysis	
Parameters	Advantages	Disadvantages	Advantages	Disadvantages
Technique	No need for vascular access, better preservation of residual renal function	Low technique survival rate, high hospitalization rate, higher rate of infections	Better technique survival rate, lower hospitalization and infection rate	Frequent difficulty in obtaining good vascular access
Blood pressure	Good control, slow ultrafiltration, and fewer episodes of cardiovascular instability			Difficult control, more frequent hypotensive episodes (in particular, in patients with autonomic neuropathy)
Nutritional factors	Fewer dietary restrictions	Excessive weight gain, poor nutrition		Difficulty with fluid and dietary restrictions
Biochemical and metabolic control	Steady-state biochemical parameters	Worsening of blood glucose control and hyperlipidemia, increased insulin requirements	Efficient solute and water extraction	
Social factors	Maintains independence		Better medical surveillance	In most diabetics, cannot be performed at home

Figure 31.6 Comparison of dialysis options for the diabetic patient.

Higher levels of comorbidity predict excess mortality in diabetic dialysis patients.[32] Because infectious complications are the leading cause of hospitalization and the second most frequent cause of death in diabetes, prevention of fistula infections and the diabetic foot syndrome is essential. Vaccination should be considered to prevent pneumonia and influenza (see Chapter 80). Protection from falls may lower risk of fractures and their fatal consequences.

Diabetics with ESRD of all age groups significantly benefit from kidney transplantation, although only a minority of older diabetics will be eligible for transplantation, cardiovascular comorbidity being the most common reason for exclusion.[33] If renal transplantation is not immediately available, peritoneal dialysis is an option for bridging to transplantation. Peritoneal dialysis is associated with longer protection of residual renal function, better blood pressure control, and higher level of quality of life, and it preserves blood vessels for future vascular access.[34]

Finally, there is evidence that ESRD rates may be stabilizing in diabetics and that efforts to reduce progression may start to show benefits.[35]

REFERENCES

1. Rastogi A, Linden A, Nissenson AR. Disease management in chronic kidney disease. *Adv Chronic Kidney Dis.* 2008;15:1-28.
2. KDOQI Clinical Practice Guidelines and Clinical Practice Recommendations for Diabetes and Chronic Kidney Disease. *Am J Kidney Dis.* 2007;49(Suppl 2):S12-S154.
3. Fioretto P, Steffes MW, Sutherland DE, et al. Reversal of lesions of diabetic nephropathy after pancreas transplantation. *N Engl J Med.* 1998;339:69-75.
4. Yale J-F. Oral hypoglycemia agents and renal disease: New agents, new concepts. *J Am Soc Nephrol.* 2005;16:S7-S10.
5. Iglesias P, Diez JJ. Insulin therapy in renal disease. *Diabetes Obes Metab.* 2008;10:811-823.
6. KDOQI Clinical Practice Guidelines and Clinical Recommendations for Diabetes and Chronic Kidney Disease. *Am J Kidney Dis* 2007;49[Suppl 2]:S28.
7. Vijan S, Hayward RA. Treatment of hypertension in type 2 diabetes mellitus: Blood pressure goals, choice of agents, and setting priorities in diabetes care. *Ann Intern Med.* 2003;138:593-602.
8. Mason NA, Bailie GR, Satayathum S, et al. HMG-CoA reductase inhibitor use is associated with mortality reduction in hemodialysis patients. *Am J Kidney Dis.* 2005;45:119-126.
9. Molitch M. Management of dyslipidemias in patients with diabetes and chronic kidney disease. *Clin J Am Nephrol.* 2006;1:1090-1099.
10. Collins R, Armitage J, Parish S, et al; Heart Protection Study Collaborative Group. MRC/BHF Heart Protection Study of cholesterol-lowering with simvastatin in 5963 people with diabetes: A randomised placebo-controlled trial. *Lancet.* 2003;361:2005-2016.
11. Tonelli M, Moyé L, Sacka FM, et al. Pravastatin for secondary prevention of cardiovascular events in persons with mild chronic renal insufficiency. *Ann Intern Med.* 2003;138:98-104.
12. Tonelli M, Keech A, Shepard J, et al. Effect of pravastatin in people with diabetes and chronic kidney disease. *J Am Soc Nephrol.* 2005;16: 3748-3754.
13. Wanner C, Krane V, Marz W, et al. Atorvastatin in patients with type 2 diabetes mellitus undergoing hemodialysis. *N Engl J Med.* 2005;353:238-248.
14. Seliger SL, Weiss NS, Gillen DL, et al. HMG-CoA reductase inhibitors are associated with reduced mortality in ESRD patients. *Kidney Int.* 2002; 61:297-304.
15. Deray G, Heurtier A, Grimaldi A, et al. Anemia and diabetes. *Am J Nephrol.* 2004;24:522-526.
16. Thomas S, Rampersad M. Anaemia in diabetes. *Acta Diabetol.* 2004; 41(Suppl 1):S13-S17.
17. New JP, Aung T, Baker PG, et al. The high prevalence of unrecognized anaemia in patients with diabetes and chronic kidney disease: A population-based study. *Diabet Med.* 2008;25:564-569.
18. Vlagopoulos PT, Tighiouart H, Weiner D, et al. Anemia as a risk factor for cardiovascular disease and all-cause mortality in diabetes: The impact of chronic kidney disease. *J Am Soc Nephrol.* 2005;16:3403-3410.
19. Abramson JL, Jurkovitz CT, Vaccarino V, et al. Chronic kidney disease, anemia, and incident stroke in a middle-aged, community-based population: The ARIC Study. *Kidney Int.* 2003;64:610-615.
20. Pfeffer MA, Burdmann EA, Chen CY, et al. A trial of darbepoetin alfa in type 2 diabetes and chronic kidney disease. *N Engl J Mod.* 2009;361: 2019-2032.
21. http://www.usrds.org/2008/view/default.asp.
22. Adler AI, Stevens RJ, Manley SE, et al. Development and progression of nephropathy in type 2 diabetes: The United Kingdom Prospective Study (UKPDS 64). *Kidney Int.* 2003;63:225-232.
23. The Diabetes Control and Complications Trial/Epidemiology of Diabetes Interventions and Complications (DCCT/EDIC) Study Research Group. Intensive diabetes treatment and cardiovascular disease in patients with type 1 diabetes. *N Engl J Med.* 2005;353:2643-2653.
24. Gaede P, Vedel P, Larsen N, et al. Multifactorial intervention and cardiovascular disease in patients with type 2 diabetes. *N Engl J Med.* 2003;348:383-393.
25. The ADVANCE Co orative Group. Intensive blood glucose control and vascular outcomes in patients with type 2 diabetes. *N Engl J Med.* 2008;358:2560-2572.
26. Duckworth W, Abraira C, Moritz T, et al. Glucose control and vascular complications in veterans with type 2 diabetes. *N Engl J Med.* 2009;360:129-139.
27. Herzog CA, Ma JZ, Collins AJ. Poor long-term survival after acute myocardial infarction among patients on long-term dialysis. *N Engl J Med.* 1998;339:799-805.
28. American Diabetes Association (ADA), Executive summary. Standards of medical care in diabetes—2008. *Diabetes Care.* 2008;31:S5-S11.
29. KDOQI Clinical Practice Guidelines for Cardiovascular Disease in Dialysis Patients. 2005. Available at: http://www.kidney.org/professionals/kdoqi/guidelines_cvd/index.htm.
30. Lee HB, Chung SH, Chu WS, et al. Peritoneal dialysis in diabetic patients. *Am J Kidney Dis.* 2001;38(Suppl 1):S200-S203.
31. Tang Z, Du X, Louie RF, Kost GJ. Effects of drugs on glucose measurement with handheld glucose meters and a portable glucose analyzer. *Am J Clin Pathol.* 2000;113:75-86.
32. Zoccali C, Tripepi G, Mallamaci F. Predictors of cardiovascular death in ESRD. *Semin Nephrol.* 2005;25:358-362.
33. Wolfe RA, Ashby VB, Milford EL. Comparison of mortality in all patients on dialysis, patients on dialysis awaiting transplantation, and recipients of a first cadaveric transplant. *N Engl J Med.* 1999;341: 1725-1730.
34. Yao Q, Lindholm B, Heimberger O. Peritoneal dialysis prescription for diabetic patients. *Perit Dial Int.* 2005;25(Suppl 3):S76-S79.
35. Kiberd B. The chronic kidney disease epidemic: Stepping back and looking forward. *J Am Soc Nephrol.* 2006;17:2967-2973.

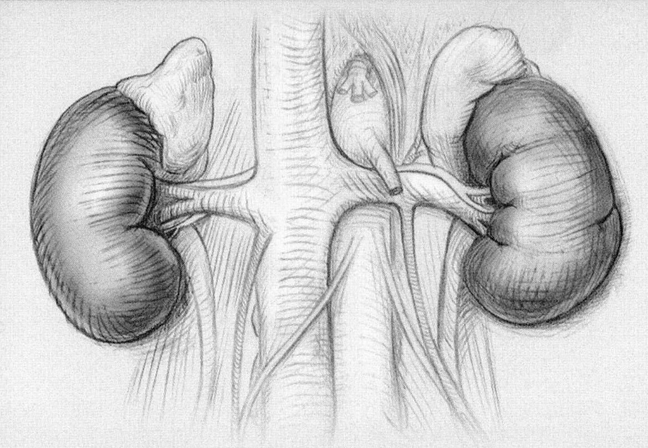

SECTION VI

Hypertension

CHAPTER 32

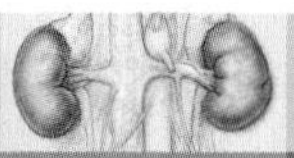

Normal Blood Pressure Control and the Evaluation of Hypertension

William J. Lawton, Friedrich C. Luft, Gerald F. DiBona

NORMAL BLOOD PRESSURE CONTROL

Systemic arterial blood pressure (BP), or the pressure of the blood within the arteries exerted against the arterial wall, is produced by the contraction of the left ventricle (producing blood flow) and the resistance of the arteries and arterioles. Systolic blood pressure (SBP), or maximum BP, occurs during left ventricular systole. Diastolic blood pressure (DBP), or minimum BP, occurs during ventricular diastole. The difference between SBP and DBP is the pulse pressure.[1] The mean arterial pressure (MAP) is clinically defined as the DBP plus one third of the pulse pressure.

Blood flow (Q) is defined by Ohm's law and varies directly with the change in pressure (P) across a blood vessel and inversely with the resistance R (defined as $Q = P/R$). Rearrangement shows that pressure varies directly with blood flow and resistance ($P = QR$). Ohm's law suffices for an overall view of the circulation. However, for a more detailed picture of the resistance to flow in any given vessel, the relationship of Hagen-Poiseuille should be applied:

$$Q = \Delta P \times (\pi r^4/8L) \times (1/\eta)$$

Here, r is the radius of the pipe, L is its length, and η is the coefficient of viscosity. Thus, as the lumen of a vessel decreases, the pressure will increase to the fourth power of the radius for the same blood flow. In other words, a 50% reduction in radius will require a 16-fold increase in pressure to maintain equivalent flow.

Normal BP is controlled by cardiac output and the total peripheral resistance and is dependent on the heart, the blood vessels, the extracellular volume, the kidneys, the nervous system, humoral factors, and cellular events at the membrane and within the cell (Fig. 32.1). Cardiac output is determined by the stroke volume (liters/minute) and the heart rate. In turn, stroke volume is dependent on intravascular volume regulated by the kidneys as well as on myocardial contractility. Myocardial contractility is a complex function involving sympathetic and parasympathetic control of heart rate, intrinsic activity of the cardiac conduction system, complex membrane transport and cellular events requiring influx of calcium that lead to myocardial fiber shortening and relaxation, and effects of humoral substances (e.g., catecholamines) on stimulating heart rate and myocardial fiber tension.

Total peripheral resistance is regulated by complex interactive mechanisms, including baroreflexes and sympathetic nervous system activity, response to neurohumoral substances and endothelial factors, myogenic responses, and intercellular events mediated by receptors and mechanisms for signal transduction.[2] For example, there are two major neural reflex arcs. Baroreflexes are derived from (1) high-pressure baroreceptors in the aortic arch and carotid sinus and (2) low-pressure cardiopulmonary baroreceptors in ventricles and atria. These receptors respond to stretch (high pressure) or filling pressures (low pressure) and send tonic inhibitory signals to the brainstem (nucleus tractus solitarius). If BP increases and tonic inhibition increases, inhibition of sympathetic efferent outflow occurs and decreases vascular resistance and heart rate. However, if BP decreases, less tonic inhibition ensues from the baroreflexes and both heart rate and peripheral vascular resistance increase, thereby increasing BP.

The brainstem cardiovascular centers are localized in the dorsomedial medulla. Neural afferents from cranial nerves IX and X are integrated in the nucleus tractus solitarius (NTS). From here, vasoconstriction and increased heart rate are mediated through the caudal and rostral ventrolateral medulla by the sympathetic nervous system. Also, NTS efferents communicate with the nucleus ambiguus (vagal nucleus) to decrease heart rate through the vagus nerve. In addition, the neural control of renal function produces alterations in renal blood flow, glomerular filtration rate (GFR), excretion of sodium and water, and release of renin and other vasoactive substances. These factors, in turn, have effects on the regulation of intravascular volume, vascular resistance, and BP.[3]

Numerous vasoactive substances have effects on blood vessels, the heart, the kidneys, and the central nervous system and often counterbalance one another. Some of these substances and membrane and cellular events are shown in Figures 32.2 and 32.3. The renin-angiotensin system (RAS) and aldosterone are extremely important effector systems that regulate both volume and peripheral vascular resistance as shown in Figure 32.4. Angiotensin II (Ang II) constricts vascular smooth muscle; stimulates aldosterone secretion; potentiates sympathetic nervous system activity; stimulates salt and water reabsorption in the proximal tubule; stimulates prostaglandin, nitric oxide, and endothelin release; increases thirst; and is a growth factor. When it is present in excess, Ang II can induce remodeling, inflammation, and vasculopathy. The kallikrein-kinin system produces vasodilator kinins that in turn may stimulate prostaglandins and nitric oxide and counterbalance the RAS (see Fig. 32.4). Aldosterone mediates changes in sodium channels in distal renal tubular epithelium, leading to sodium retention and potassium excretion. The hormone also functions as a growth factor and exerts complex nongenomic and genomic events through the mineralocorticoid receptor in vascular cells and in the heart.

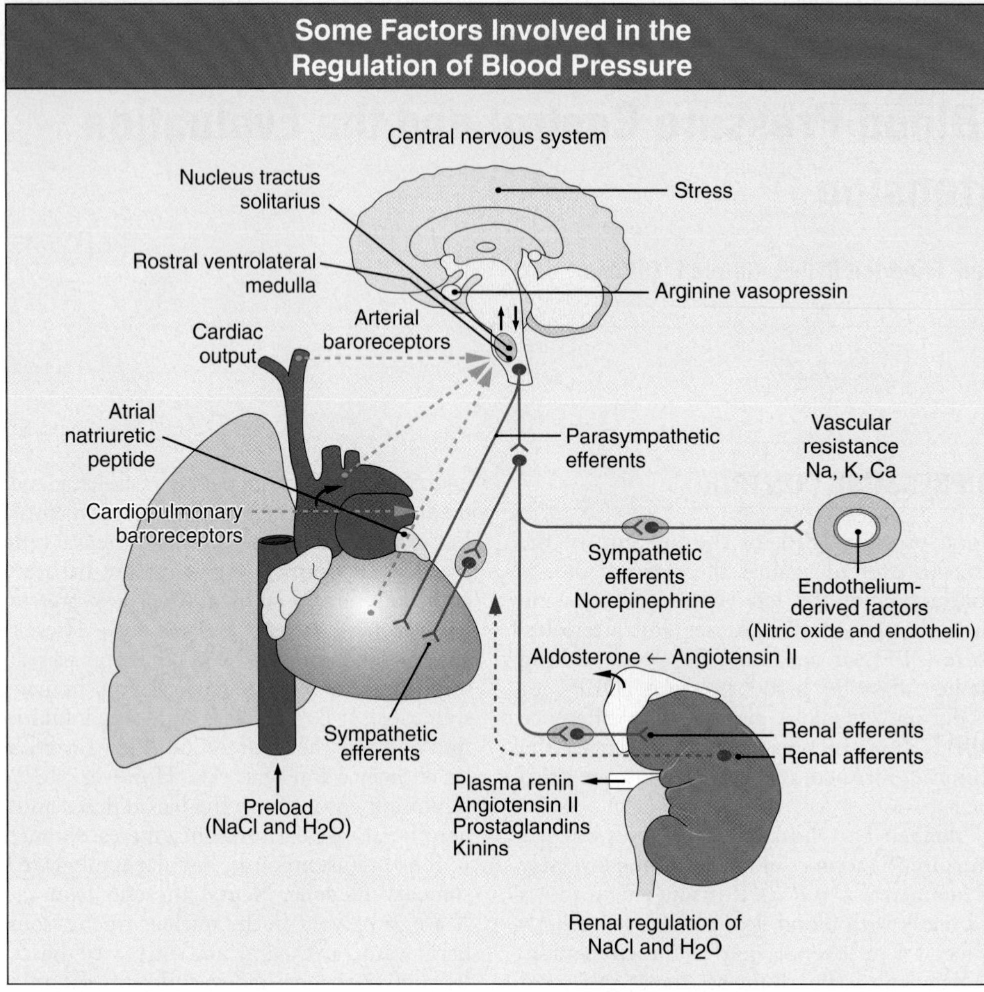

Figure 32.1 Some factors involved in the regulation of blood pressure.

Plasma concentrations of renin and aldosterone are both inversely related to salt intake and are influenced by various medications. Aldosterone is measured by radioimmunoassay. Plasma renin is measured as plasma renin activity based on the generation of angiotensin in the presence of angiotensin–degrading enzyme inhibitors or as plasma renin concentration by immunoassay.

A second major effector system is the sympathetic nervous system. Nerve endings release norepinephrine. This potent neurotransmitter is a vasoconstrictor through α-adrenergic receptor–mediated mechanisms. Vascular cells, renal cells, and many other cells (e.g., adipocytes) are innervated. Epinephrine increases heart rate, stroke volume, and SBP through α- and β-adrenoceptors. The hormone is released from the adrenal medulla. There is compelling evidence that increased sympathetic tone has long-term influences on cardiovascular regulation and that disturbed sympathetic tone may cause hypertension. In the kidneys, sympathetic nerves are important mediators of renin release. Furthermore, innervation of each individual nephron has an important bearing on sodium reabsorption. Thus, the sympathetic nervous system regulates both effective circulating fluid volume and peripheral vascular resistance.

Prostaglandin E and prostacyclin act to counterbalance vasoconstriction by Ang II and norepinephrine. Two endothelium-derived factors have opposite effects on the blood vessels: nitric oxide is a vasodilator, whereas the endothelins are vasoconstrictors. Natriuretic peptides induce vasodilation, and natriuresis and inhibit other vasoconstrictors (RAS, sympathetic nervous system, and endothelin). Renalase is a recently discovered flavin adenine dinucleotide–dependent amine oxidase that is secreted by the kidney, circulates in the blood, and modulates cardiac function and systemic BP. It acts by metabolizing catecholamines, and its discovery should further our understanding of sympathetic regulation.[4,5] Urotensin II is a cyclic vasoactive peptide expressed in many organ systems and is inversely related to norepinephrine and brain natriuretic peptide. High plasma levels of urotensin II, a cyclic vasoactive peptide predict reduced cardiovascular complications in patients with chronic kidney disease (stages 2 to 5).[6] Heme oxygenase (HO) has recently been found to suppress arachidonic acid metabolism and to decrease BP in several models of hypertension. The HO system may have an important role in regulating BP and kidney function.[7]

Postreceptor intracellular signaling events also regulate peripheral vascular resistance. For instance, the small guanosine triphosphatase Rho and its effector, Rho-associated kinase (Rho-kinase) are important in Ca^{2+}-independent regulation of smooth muscle contraction. The Rho,Rho-kinase pathway modulates the level of phosphorylation of the myosin light chain of myosin II, mainly through inhibition of myosin phosphatase, and contributes to agonist-induced Ca^{2+} sensitization in smooth muscle contraction. Rho,Rho-kinase mechanisms also participate in a variety

Vasoactive Substances that Modulate Blood Pressure

Vasoactive Substances		
Group	**Compound**	**Cellular Effects**
Catecholamines	Norepinephrine, epinephrine, dopamine	Adrenergic receptors (α_1, α_2, β_1, β_2) causing protein phosphorylation and increased intracellular calcium via G proteins linked to ion channels or second messengers (cyclic nucleotides, phosphoinositide hydrolysis)
Renin-angiotensin system (RAS)	Angiotensin II (Ang II)	Angiotensin receptors (AT_1, AT_2, AT_4) causing increased intracellular calcium and protein phosphorylation via second messenger, phosphoinositide hydrolysis, and activated protein kinases Aldosterone stimulation
Mineralocorticoids	Aldosterone	Genomic: Binds to cytoplasmic mineralocorticoid receptor (MR), translocates to nucleus, modulates gene expression, signals transduction and effectors (S_gK, CHIF, K_i-Ras) which increases transport proteins (increasing ENaC number and open probability) Non-Genomic: Effects via separate membrane or cytosolic proteins
Kallikrein–kinin system	Bradykinin	Bradykinin receptors (B_1, B_2), B_2-G protein coupling cause activation of phospholipase C, increased inositol phophates, and intracellular calcium
Arachidonic acid products	Prostaglandins: prostaglandin E, prostacyclin, thromboxanes Lipoxygenase enzyme products: leukotrienes, hydroxyeicosatetraenoates	Nine prostaglandin receptors coupled to G proteins: (e.g., PGI_2 [Receptor IP], PGE_2 [Receptors EP_1, EP_2]); $PGF_{2\alpha}$ (Receptor FP)
Endothelium-derived factors	Endothelium-derived relaxing factor (nitric oxide) Endothelins (ET-1, ET-2, ET-3)	Increased levels of cylic guanosine monophosphate cause activation of protein kinases G proteins activate phospholipase C and L-type calcium channels Class 2 G protein–coupled receptor
Natriuretic peptides (NPs)	Atrial, brain, and C-type NPs	Activation of three receptor types; further effects mediated by cGMP
Posterior pituitary hormones	Arginine vasopressin	Vasopressin receptors (AVPR 1A; AVPR 1B) mediated by second messenger system, phosphatidyl, inositol/calcium; AVPR2 effects via adenylate cyclase (cAMP)
Other substances	Acetylcholine, adenosine, insulin, neuropeptide Y, serotonin, sex hormones (estrogens, progesterone, androgens), glucocorticoids, other mineralocorticoids, substance P, vasopressin, renalase, heme oxygenase 1	

Figure 32.2 Vasoactive substances that modulate blood pressure.

Cellular Events Linked to the Activity of Vasoactive Substances

Membrane sodium transport: Epithelial Na channel; Na^+, K^+-ATPase
Na^+-H^+ exchange; Na^+-Ca^{2+} exchange; Na^+-K^+-2Cl^- transport; Na^+–Cl^-; CO–transport, passive Na^+ transport; Na^+-organic solutes; Na^+-inorganic anion CO-transport
Potassium channels
Cell volume and intracellular pH changes
Calcium channels
Signal transduction via G proteins, cyclic nucleotides, inositol phosphates and intracellular calcium, diacylglycerol and protein kinases
Rho, Rho-kinase signaling

Figure 32.3 Cellular events linked to the activity of vasoactive substances.

of the cellular functions of nonmuscle cells, such as stress fiber formation, cytokinesis, and cell migration. A specific pharmacologic Rho-kinase inhibitor (fasudil) has been developed that may have utility in treating cerebral artery spasm and other forms of severe vascular constriction.[8]

Guyton and Hall[1] have analyzed the temporal sequence for adjustment of BP. In their analysis, central nervous system mechanisms (e.g., baroreflexes) provide regulation of the circulation within seconds to minutes. Other mechanisms, such as the renin-angiotensin-aldosterone system and fluid shifts, occur during minutes to hours. It was once considered that only the kidneys have the ability for long-term adjustments in BP, predominantly through regulation of extracellular volume[1] (Fig. 32.5); but recent evidence indicates that long-term afferent baroreflex stimulation by an electrical device can lower BP chronically in several different animal models.[9] The critical role for the kidney in the long-term control of BP received strong support from kidney cross-transplantation experiments. Nevertheless, precisely such experiments have recently shown that both intrarenal and extrarenal mechanisms are involved.[10]

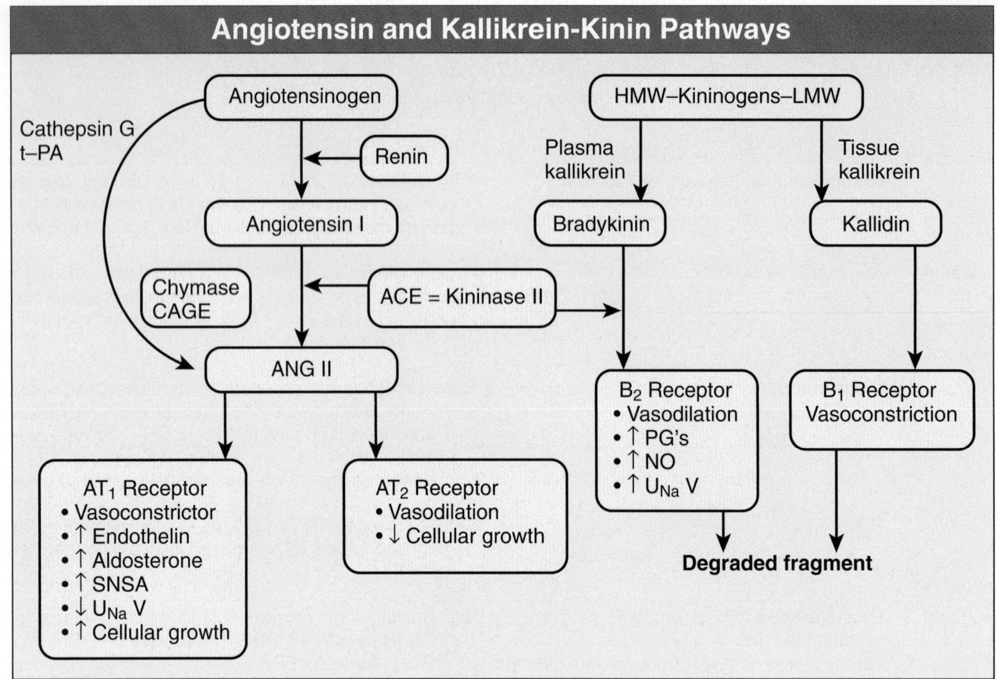

Figure 32.4 Interactions and functions of the renin-angiotensin and kallikrein-kinin systems. ACE, angiotensin I converting enzyme; ANG II, angiotensin II; CAGE, chymostatin-sensitive angiotensin II–generating enzyme; HMW, high molecular weight; LMW, low molecular weight; PG, prostaglandins; NO, nitric oxide; SNSA, sympathetic nervous system activity; t-PA, tissue plasminogen activator; $U_{Na}V$, urinary sodium excretion.

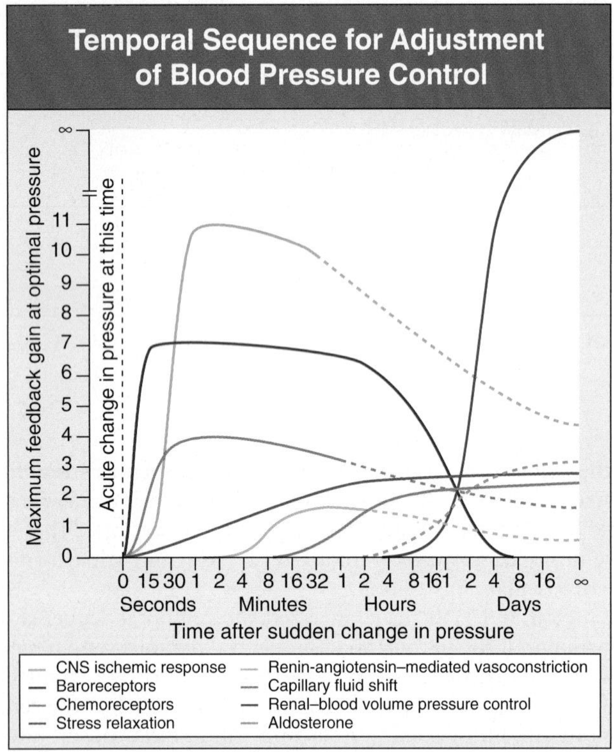

Figure 32.5 Temporal sequence for adjustment of blood pressure control. Degree of activity, expressed as feedback gain, of several arterial pressure control systems at various times after a sudden change in arterial pressure. Note the infinite gain of the renal-volume mechanism for pressure control. CNS, central nervous system. *(Reprinted with permission from reference 1.)*

DEFINITION OF HYPERTENSION

Concepts

BP is normally distributed in the general population. Thus, any definition of hypertension is arbitrary. Hypertension is usually asymptomatic; patients are more typically symptomatic from the sequelae of hypertension or its treatment. Hypertension may be defined by its associated morbidity and mortality, as increases over arbitrary cutoff points, or by thresholds defining therapeutic benefit.

Blood Pressure in Relation to Morbidity and Mortality

The first approach defines hypertension by relating BP levels to the risk of morbidity and mortality. The association of SBP and DBP with cardiovascular and renal complications is continuous over the entire BP range.[11] Observational studies involving more than 1 million individuals have found that death from both ischemic heart disease and stroke increases progressively and linearly from BP as low as 115 mm Hg SBP and 75 mm Hg DBP upward (Figs. 32.6 and 32.7). The increased risks are present in all age groups ranging from 40 to 89 years. For every increase of 20 mm Hg SBP or 10 mm Hg DBP, the mortality from both ischemic heart disease and stroke doubles. On the basis of these data, the Joint National Committee (JNC) 7 report introduced a new classification that includes the term *prehypertension* for those with BP ranging from 120 to 139 mm Hg SBP or 80 to 89 mm Hg DBP.[12] The designation prehypertensive identifies persons in whom early intervention (lifestyle) could reduce BP or avoid further increases. Since JNC 7, the Writing Group of the American Society of Hypertension (WG-ASH) has proposed a new definition of hypertension not based on BP values alone but considering hypertension as a complex cardiovascular disorder. The new definition includes target organ damage, early disease markers, and cardiovascular risk factors (Fig. 32.8).[13] Although it is not uniformly agreed on, the risk-based approach

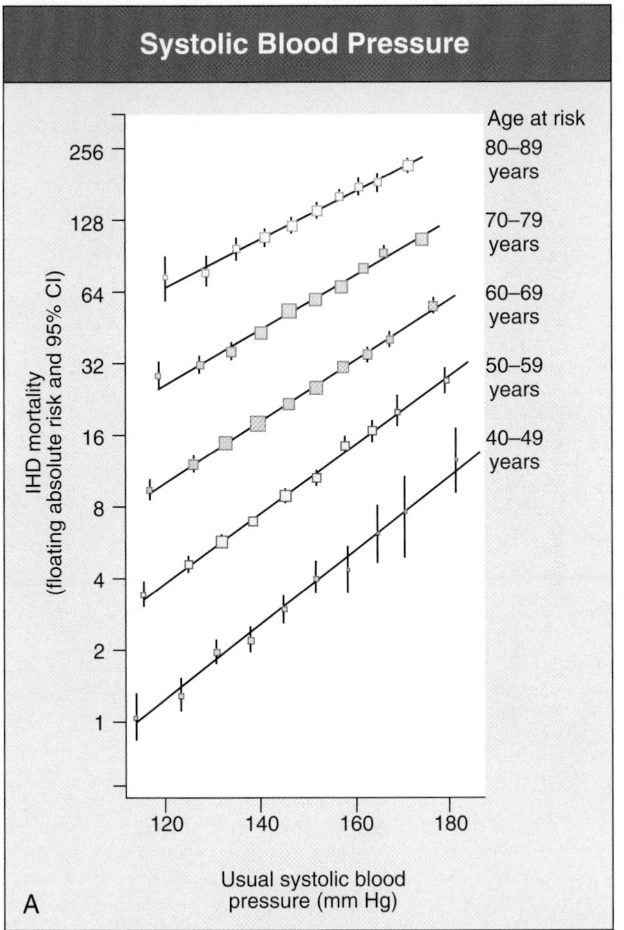

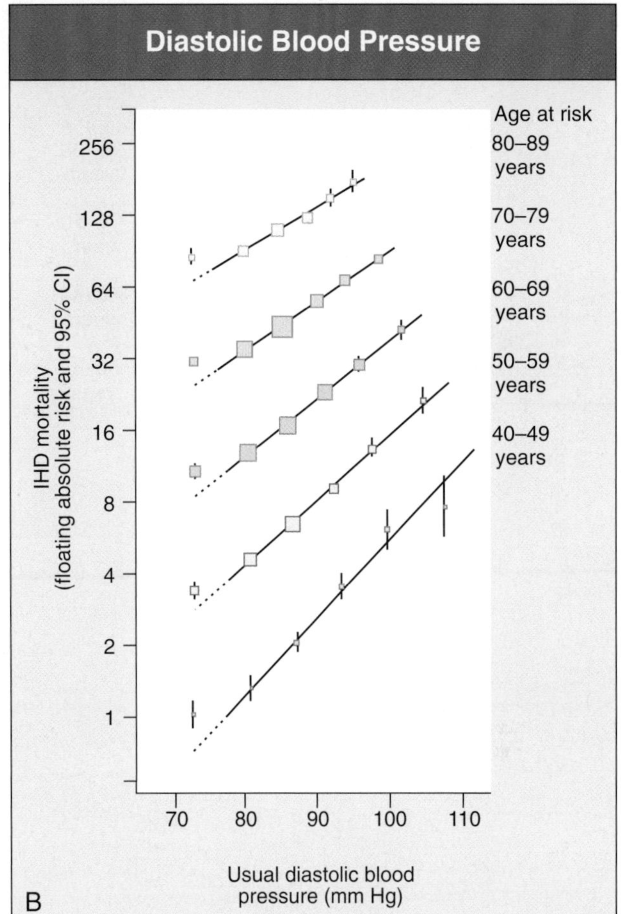

Figure 32.6 Ischemic heart disease (IHD) mortality rate in each decade of age versus usual blood pressure at the start of that decade. **A,** Systolic blood pressure. **B,** Diastolic blood pressure. Floating absolute risk corrects for the absolute death rate within a particular community. The size of the squares correlates inversely with the variance of the data collected for that data point. CI, confidence interval. *(Reprinted with permission from reference 11.)*

seeks to identify individuals with an increased likelihood of future cardiovascular events at any BP level. The WG-ASH stage 1 can include the "prehypertension" in JNC 7.

Elevation of Blood Pressure by Arbitrary Cut Points

A second approach defines hypertension by the frequency distribution within a population. This statistical approach will arbitrarily designate values above a certain percentile as hypertensive. This method is used in defining hypertension in children. The values defining hypertension will vary according to age, gender, body size, and race.[14] This frequency distribution method is not helpful for determining a value for initiation of antihypertensive treatment but is useful in epidemiologic studies, for example, defining the prevalence of hypertension in various age groups or the changing prevalence of hypertension in a given population over time. The prevalence of hypertension in adults in the United States, defined as BP of 140/90 mm Hg or higher, has increased progressively from 11% of the population in 1939 to 29.3% in 2004.[15] The prevalence of hypertension in six European countries has been reported at 44%, and it is 66.3% in those older than 60 years.[16]

Threshold of Therapeutic Benefit

The third concept for defining hypertension is derived from randomized trials that have demonstrated reductions in mortality and morbidity. As a result of these clinical trials, consensus has been reached on intervention levels for moderate and severe hypertension but not for lower levels of hypertension. The Hypertension Optimal Treatment (HOT) study showed benefits of lowering BP to 138/83 mm Hg in hypertensive subjects in the absence of diabetes mellitus, chronic kidney disease, coronary artery disease risk, or target organ damage. For subjects with these complications, a treatment goal below 130/80 mm Hg is recommended (JNC 7).

Operational Definitions

The European Society of Hypertension (ESH) divides normotension into three categories (optimum, normal, and high-normal) and describes hypertension as mild, moderate, or severe (Fig. 32.9).[17,18] The ESH also gave values for automated 24-hour BP measurements, divided into daytime and nighttime.

In the United States, the JNC 7 defined hypertension for individuals 18 years of age and older.[12] The Committee settled on normal, prehypertension, and stage 1 and stage 2 hypertension (Fig. 32.10). For children, the JNC considers that BP at the 95th percentile or higher at each age is elevated.

Clinicians evaluate hypertensive patients and treatment goals on the basis of overall cardiovascular risk factors, not by BP alone. Age, gender, and ethnicity cannot be altered and are

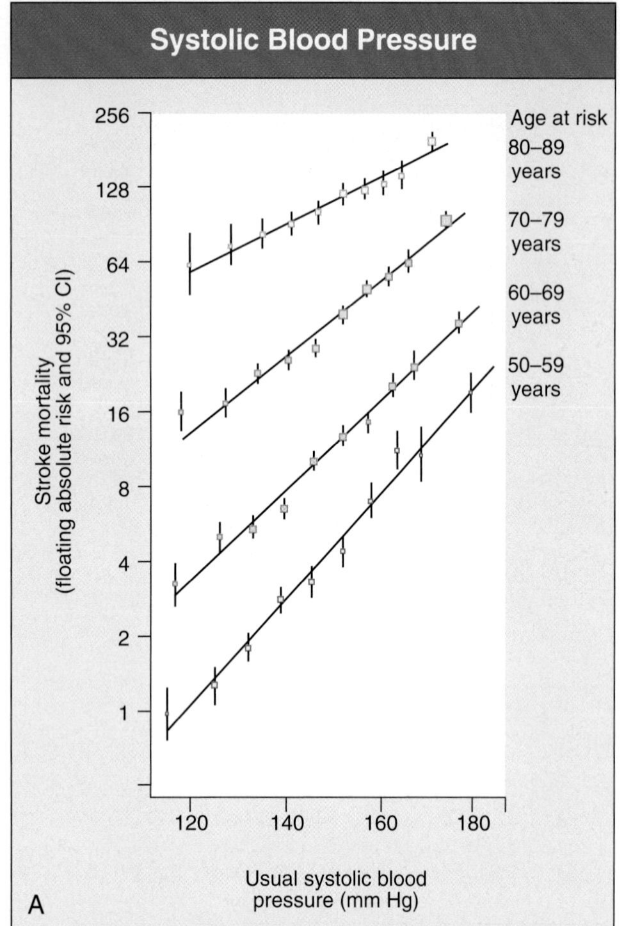

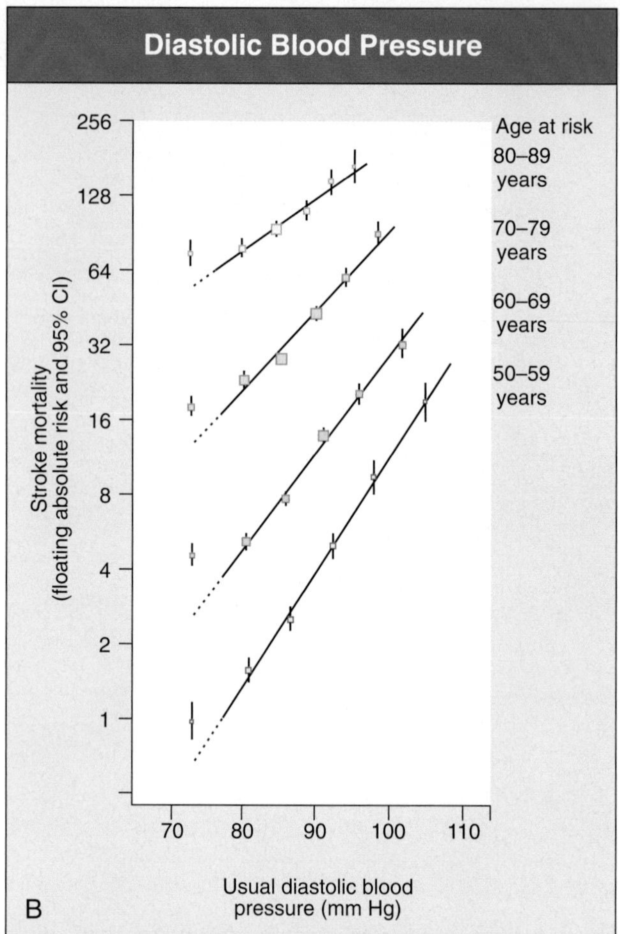

Figure 32.7 Stroke mortality rate in each decade of age versus usual blood pressure at the start of that decade. A, Systolic blood pressure. **B,** Diastolic blood pressure. Floating absolute risk corrects for the absolute death rate within a particular community. The size of the squares correlates inversely with the variance of the data collected for that data point. CI, confidence interval. *(Reprinted with permission from reference 11.)*

WG-ASH Definition and Classification of Hypertension

Classification	Blood Pressure Elevations		Cardiovascular Disease*	Cardiovascular Risk Factors	Early Disease Markers	Target Organ Disease
Normal	Normal or rare	or	None	None or few	None	None
Hypertension						
Stage 1	Occasional interrmittent	or	Early	Several	Usually present	None
Stage 2	Sustained	or	Progressive	Many	Overtly present	Early signs present
Stage 3	Marked and sustained	or	Advanced	Many	Overtly present with progression	Overtly present with or without cardiovascular disease events

Figure 32.8 Working Group–American Society of Hypertension (WG-ASH) definition and classification of hypertension. *Determined by constellation of risk factors, early disease markers, and target organ disease.

European Society of Hypertension Consensus Classification

Conventional Blood Pressure Measurement*		Ambulatory Blood Pressure Measurement†			
Category	**Boundaries**	**Measurement**	**P95‡**	**Normotension**	**Hypertension**
Normotension		Ambulatory			
Optimum	<120/<80	24-h	132/82	<130/<80	>135/85
Normal	120–129/80–84	Daytime	138/87	>135/<85	>140/90
High-normal	130–139/85–89	Nighttime	123/74	<120/<70	>125/75
Hypertension		Self-recorded			
Grade I (mild)	140–159/90–99	Morning	136/85	<135/85	>140/90
Subgroup borderline	140–149/90–94	Evening	138/86	<135/85	>140/90
Grade II (moderate)	160–179/100–109	Both	137/85	<135/85	>140/90
Grade III (severe)	>180/>110				
Isolated systolic hypertension	>140/<90				
Subgroup borderline	140–149/<90				

Figure 32.9 European Society of Hypertension consensus classification. Blood pressure readings are in millimeters of mercury (mm Hg). *Consensus classification proposed by the European Society of Hypertension/European Society of Cardiology guidelines (see reference 17). †Classification proposed at the Eighth International Consensus Conference on Ambulatory Blood Pressure Measurement (Sendai, Japan, October 2001). ‡Mean of 95th percentiles in subjects who on conventional blood pressure measurement were normotensive in large-scale studies.

JNC 7 Classification of Blood Pressure for Adults (2003)

BP Classification	SBP (mm Hg)	DBP (mm Hg)
Normal	<120	and <80
Prehypertension	120–139	or 80–89
Stage 1 hypertension	140–159	or 90–99
Stage 2 hypertension	≥160	or ≥100

Figure 32.10 The Joint National Committee (JNC) 7 classification of blood pressure for adults (2003). BP, blood pressure; DBP, diastolic blood pressure; SBP, systolic blood pressure.

important risk factors. However, cholesterol, high-density lipoprotein (HDL) cholesterol, smoking, control of diabetes, obesity, and left ventricular hypertrophy are potentially modifiable (Fig. 32.11).[18] The cluster of risk factors that increase cardiovascular risk and are often associated with hypertension is termed the metabolic syndrome (Fig. 32.12). Decreased renal function is also recognized as an independent cardiovascular risk factor.[19] The same is true for proteinuria, starting with the barely detectable amount of more than 6 mg/day albumin. Figure 32.13 gives the JNC 7 recommendations for follow-up of BP findings in a given individual.

Special Definitions

Prehypertension (High-Normal or Borderline Hypertension) Despite lack of uniform agreement, prehypertension is most usefully defined as BP of 130 to 139/85 to 89 mm Hg (also called stage 2 prehypertension; stage 1 prehypertension, 120 to 129/80 to 84 mm Hg). An older definition of "borderline hypertension" defined individuals whose BP was sometimes above 140/90 mm Hg but would decrease to levels below this with rest. Estimates of prehypertension or borderline hypertension have ranged between 12% and 30% of the adult population. Individuals with prehypertension (stage 2) have a threefold greater likelihood for development of sustained hypertension. During a 20-year follow-up, weight gains of 15 to 20 pounds (6.8 to 9.1 kg) in this group may be associated with a higher risk for development of sustained hypertension. Some of these individuals have a high cardiac output and increased catecholamine turnover. Borderline hypertension may represent an exaggeration of normal physiologic responses to stress. Individuals with prehypertension may have a greater frequency of obesity, abnormal lipids, and other cardiovascular risk factors, with twice the cardiovascular events compared with those with BP below 120/80 mm Hg.[20] Because all BP is "labile" (variable) and generally varies on a diurnal cycle, the term *labile hypertension* is not helpful and should not be used.

White Coat Hypertension White coat hypertension is defined as BP that is normal during usual daily activities but is hypertensive in a clinical setting. Normal pressures outside the physician's office are determined by measurement with standard techniques or by ambulatory BP recordings. White coat hypertension can be seen at all ages, including the elderly. The white coat phenomenon is seen less frequently when a nurse or technician takes the BP rather than a physician. White coat hypertension is present in approximately 20% of hypertensive persons. Guidelines are available to assist in assessing patients with isolated clinic hypertension or isolated ambulatory hypertension.[21]

The significance and prognosis of white coat hypertension are unclear. Some studies show that the office- or clinic-induced increase in BP is benign. Other studies report that white coat hypertension is characterized by increases in left ventricular mass index at levels intermediate between normotensive and persistently hypertensive persons.[22] White coat hypertensive patients have impaired diastolic function and higher levels of catecholamines, plasma renin activity, aldosterone, and low-density lipoprotein (LDL) cholesterol. There is also some evidence that subjects with white coat hypertension may be at increased risk for development of persistent hypertension.[22] Thus, each patient with white coat hypertension needs evaluation for cardiovascular risk factors and correction of these, if present, as well as continued follow-up.

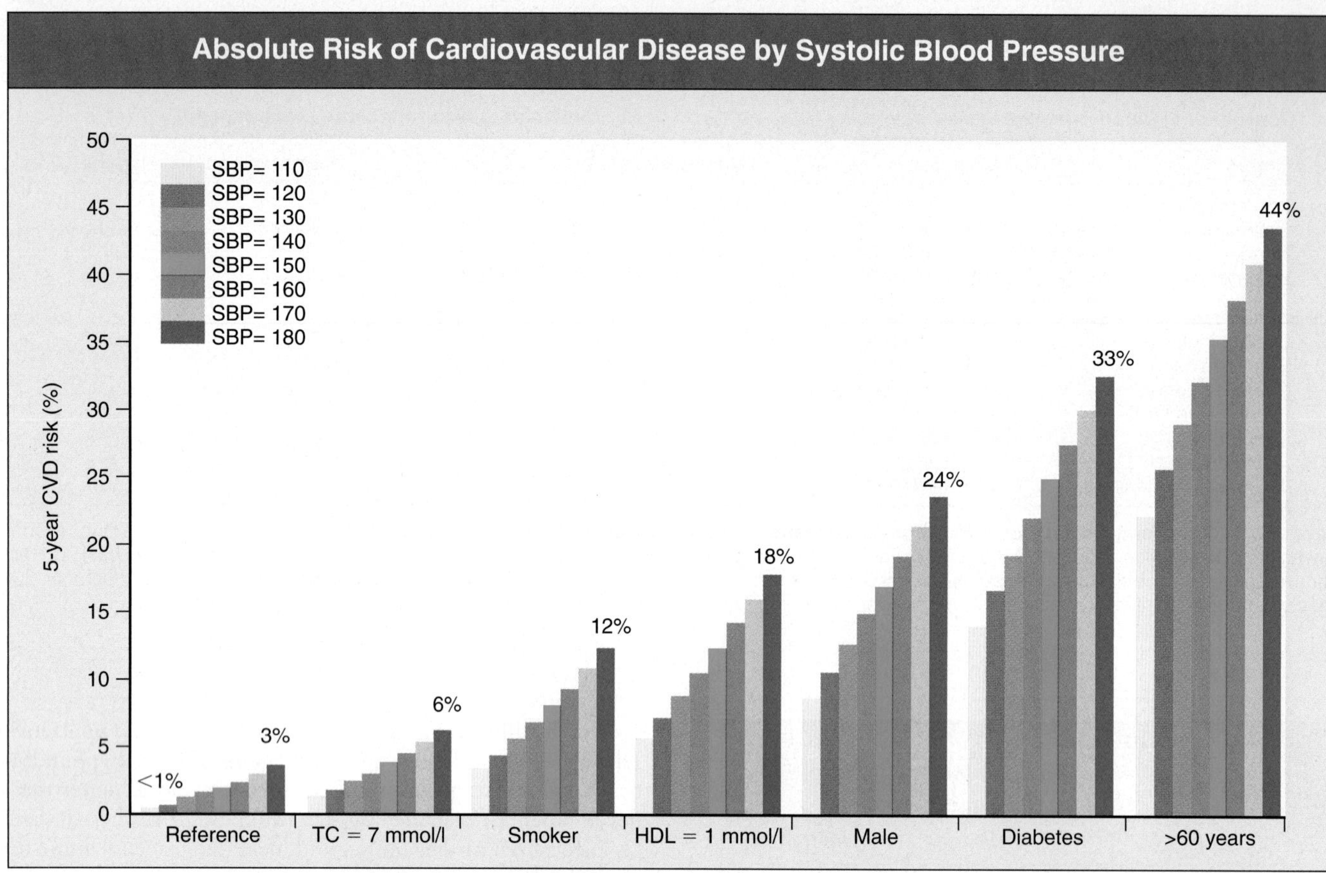

Figure 32.11 Absolute risk of cardiovascular disease during 5 years in patients by systolic blood pressure at specified levels of other risk factors. Reference category is a nondiabetic, nonsmoking woman aged 50 years with total cholesterol (TC) level of 4 mmol/l (155 mg/dl) and high-density lipoprotein (HDL) level of 1.6 mmol/l. Risks are given for systolic blood pressure (SBP) levels of 110, 120, 130, 140, 150, 160, 170, and 180 mm Hg. In the other categories, additional risk factors are added consecutively, for example, the diabetes category is a diabetic 50-year-old male cigarette smoker with a total cholesterol level of 7 mmol/l (270 mg/dl) and HDL level of 1 mmol/l (39 mg/dl). CVD, cardiovascular disease. *(Reprinted with permission from reference 18.)*

Common Definitions for Metabolic Syndrome

Criterion	NCEP ATP III (3 or more criteria)
Abdominal obesity	Waist circumferance
Men	>40 inches (>102 cm)
Women	>35 inches (>88 cm)
Hypertriglyceridemia	>150 mg/dL (≥1.7 mmol/l)
Low HDL	
Men	<40 mg/dL (<1.03 mmol/l)
Women	<50 mg/dL (<1.30 mmol/l)
Hypertension	≥130/85 mm Hg or on antihypertensive medication
Impaired fasting glucose or diabetes	>100 mg/dl (5.6 mmol/l) or taking insulin or hypoglycemic medication

Figure 32.12 Common definitions for the metabolic syndrome. *(From reference 23.)*

Recommendations for Follow-Up Based on the Initial Blood Pressure Measurements for Adults

Initial Blood Pressure (mm Hg)*		
Systolic	Diastolic	Follow-Up Recommended
>130	>85	Recheck in 1 year
130–139	85–89	Recheck in 1 year; provide information about lifestyle modification
140–159	90–99	Confirm within 2 months
160–179	100–109	Evaluate or refer to source of care within 1 month
≥180	≥110	Evaluate or refer to source of care immediately or within 1 week, depending on clinical situation

Figure 32.13 Recommendations for follow-up based on the initial blood pressure measurements for adults. *If systolic and diastolic categories are different, follow recommendations for the shorter time for follow-up. The schedule for follow-up should be modified according to reliable information about past blood pressure measurements, other cardiovascular risk factors, or target organ disease.

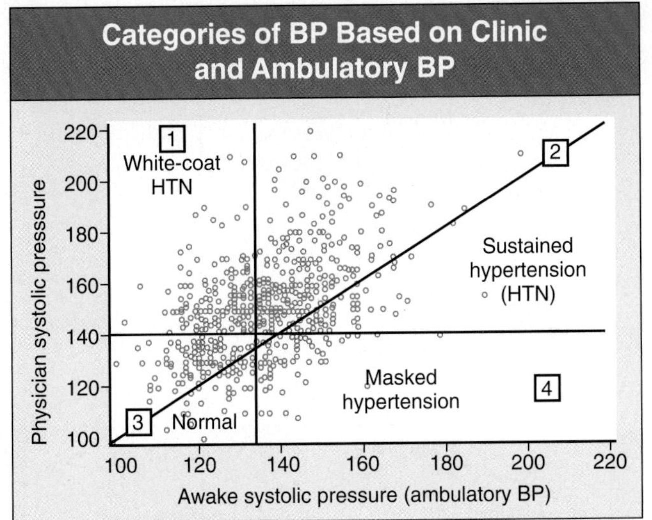

Figure 32.14 Plot of clinic systolic and daytime ambulatory blood pressure to define four groups: normal, white coat hypertension, sustained hypertension, and masked hypertension. *(From reference 24.)*

Masked Hypertension Masked hypertension is defined as BP that is lower in the office or clinic compared with ambulatory BP. In one study, the 10-year risk of stroke and cardiovascular mortality in subjects with masked hypertension was similar to that of patients with sustained hypertension (Fig. 32.14).[22]

Sustained Hypertension Sustained hypertension, also called persistent hypertension, defines individuals whose BP levels are elevated both inside and outside the clinic setting, including at home and during usual daily activities. Office BP readings are frequently higher in sustained hypertensives compared with their ambulatory BP.

Pseudohypertension Pseudohypertension is defined as "a condition in which the cuff pressure is inappropriately higher when compared to the intra-arterial pressure because of excessive atheromatosis and/or medial hypertrophy in the arterial tree."[25] Pseudohypertension can be suspected by the "Osler maneuver," in which the BP cuff is inflated above the SBP (detected by auscultation). If either the brachial or radial artery remains palpable, when pulseless, the patient is considered to be Osler maneuver positive. In general, patients with pseudohypertension have intra-arterial DBP measurements 10 to 15 mm Hg below indirect BP cuff diastolic measurements. None of the definitions specifically addresses the SBP. If a patient is suspected of having pseudohypertension, confirmation by intra-arterial pressure measurement may be considered, with decision for treatment goals based on the intra-arterial findings.

Isolated Systolic Hypertension Arteriosclerosis, characterized by remodeling and stiffening of large elastic arteries, is the most significant manifestation of vascular aging.[26] The increased stiffening is believed to originate from a gradual mechanical senescence of the elastic network, alterations in cross-linking of extracellular matrix components, fibrosis, and calcification of elastic fibers. Stiffening of large arteries reduces their capacitance and accelerates pulse wave velocity, thus contributing to a widening of pulse pressure and to the increased prevalence of isolated systolic hypertension (ISH) with age. Perhaps as a consequence, the increase in SBP continues throughout life, in contrast to DBP, which increases until the age of 50 years and decreases later in life (Fig. 32.15). Diastolic hypertension is more common before the age of 50 years, either alone or in combination with elevated SBP. After the age of 50 years, SBP is more important than DBP.

ISH is defined as SBP of 140 mm Hg or higher and DBP of 90 mm Hg or lower. The prevalence of ISH increases with age and affects most individuals older than 60 years. In the Framingham study, elevations in SBP determined a greater risk of both heart attacks and strokes compared with elevations of DBP. Indeed, JNC 7 assigned SBP a higher level of importance than DBP.[12] Several clinical trials have clearly demonstrated that treatment of ISH reduces the cardiovascular event rate.[27] Nevertheless, controversy exists as to the choice of antihypertensive agents. Elderly hypertensive patients should be treated aggressively to the same target BPs identified for younger patients. However, it is appropriate to initiate treatment with lower doses of antihypertensive agents and to bring the pressure down more slowly, monitoring for orthostatic hypotension, impaired cognition, and electrolyte abnormalities.

Resistant Hypertension Resistant hypertension is defined as BP that is not at treatment goal despite optimal doses of three antihypertensive drugs, including a diuretic. Although it is not well quantified, some clinical trials suggest that resistant hypertension may occur in 30% of hypertensive subjects. Older age and obesity are strong risk factors. Secondary hypertension is more common in resistant hypertension, with primary aldosteronism reported in 18% to 23% of patients.[28]

Accelerated Hypertension/Hypertensive Urgencies and Emergencies Accelerated hypertension is severe diastolic hypertension (usually >120 mm Hg) in the presence of grade III retinopathy (arteriolosclerotic changes of arteriolar narrowing and nicking plus hypertensive changes of flame-shaped hemorrhages and soft exudates).[29] In the past, "malignant" hypertension referred to severe diastolic hypertension and grade IV retinopathy (grade III plus papilledema). Because the prognosis for untreated severe hypertension with grade III or IV retinopathy is so poor, there is little clinical rationale for using the two terms separately. More recently, accelerated hypertension with hypertensive retinopathy is defined as a hypertensive urgency if treatment is required to decrease BP within hours, whereas hypertensive emergencies are clinical conditions in which severe hypertension must be lowered within minutes. Emergencies include acute dissection of the aorta, acute left ventricular failure, intracerebral hemorrhage, and crises caused by pheochromocytoma, drug abuse, and eclampsia (see Chapter 36).

Hypertension in Children Hypertension in children is defined by average SBP or DBP at or above the 95th percentile for gender and age, measured on at least three occasions. The reported causes of hypertension in children vary. Most prepubertal hypertension is thought to have renal causes, although some children may have BP levels above the 95th percentile because of an earlier growth spurt and large size. In postpubertal children, mild hypertension is likely to be primary hypertension, whereas more severe hypertension is usually of renal cause. Primary aldosteronism and thyroid disease seem rare.

Hypertension in Pregnancy Hypertension may occur in more than 5% of all pregnancies and in approximately 5% of women

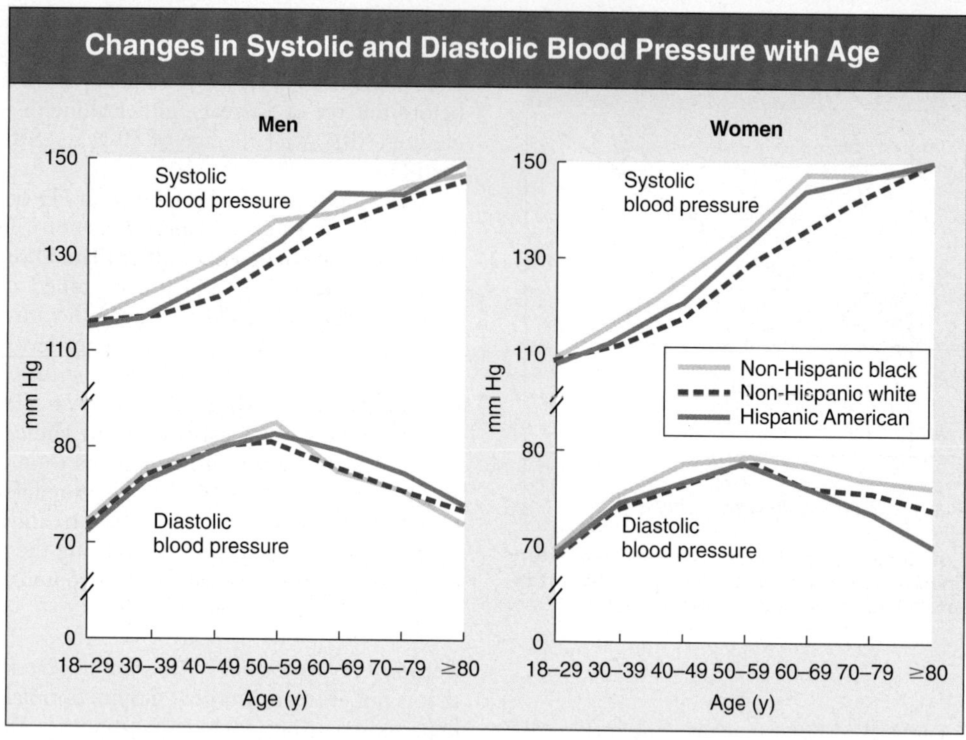

Figure 32.15 Changes in systolic and diastolic blood pressure with age. Systolic blood pressure and diastolic blood pressure by age and race or ethnicity for men and women older than 18 years in the U.S. population. Data from NHANES III, 1988 to 1991. *(From reference 30.)*

taking oral contraceptives. Definitions and implications of hypertension in pregnancy are discussed in Chapters 42 and 43.

Classification by Cause of Hypertension

Although a large number of causes are recognized for hypertension, the etiology in 90% to 95% of patients with hypertension is unknown. These patients are considered to have primary (or essential) hypertension (see Chapter 33). Figure 32.16 shows the more common causes of secondary hypertension. These include renal parenchymal disease (2% to 6% of all hypertensives), renovascular hypertension (1% to 4%), and all endocrine hypertension (traditionally thought to be 1%, including primary aldosteronism, pheochromocytoma, Cushing's syndrome, and others). More recent studies have shown an increasing prevalence of primary aldosteronism, ranging from 2% to 13% in stage 1 to stage 3 hypertension. Other causes include coarctation of the aorta (0.1% to 1.0%) and obstructive sleep apnea and obesity. An often overlooked cause of hypertension is drug induced (1%), including oral contraceptives, decongestants or sympathomimetic agents, and nonsteroidal anti-inflammatory drugs (NSAIDs).

EVALUATION OF HYPERTENSION

Proper Measurement of Blood Pressure

Arterial BP is usually measured in the brachial artery by use of the cuff-based sphygmomanometer, in which the arterial pressure is recorded by detecting sounds that are generated (auscultatory method) or by recording vascular pulsations (oscillometric method) after decompression of a compressed artery. Guidelines for BP measurement are given in Figure 32.17. Unfortunately, if it is not properly used, the method can be unreliable and inaccurate. The most common reason for inaccuracy is an inappropriate cuff size as the accuracy of these measurements is influenced by the size of the inflatable bladder relative to the girth of the compressed limb. To provide uniform compression of the underlying artery, the length of the bladder should be at least 80% of the upper arm circumference, and the width of the bladder should be at least 40% of the upper arm circumference. A simple bedside maneuver to check the appropriateness of the cuff size consists of aligning the cuff so that its long axis is parallel to the long axis of the arm. The bladder width should then be sufficient to encircle half of the upper arm circumference. If the bladder width encompasses less than half of the upper arm, a larger cuff must be selected. No change in cuff size is necessary if the cuff width encircles more than half the upper arm because large cuffs on thin limbs do not produce considerable errors in the BP measurement. For purists, accepted bladder dimensions for varying arm sizes are given in Figure 32.18. Another potential error relates to the auscultatory method, which relies on the ability to hear the Korotkoff sounds. The human ear has a sound threshold of about 16 Hz. The Korotkoff sounds occur at slightly above this level (25 to 50 Hz). Thus, the human ear is almost deaf to the sounds it must hear to measure BP. The bell-shaped stethoscope head should be used to measure BP. Interestingly, many physicians and most nurses are not equipped with a bell-shaped stethoscope head.

The oscillometric method is based on the principle of plethysmography to detect pulsatile pressure changes in a nearby artery. When an arm cuff is inflated, pulsatile pressure changes in an underlying artery produce periodic pressure changes in the inflated cuff. The oscillometric method thus measures periodic pressure changes, oscillations, in an inflated cuff as an indirect measure of pulsatile pressure in an underlying artery.

There are three types of sphygmomanometer in use worldwide. Because of environmental concerns, the standard mercury manometer has been abandoned in some areas.[31] The second type

Common Causes of Secondary Hypertension	
Condition/Disorder	**Diseases: Comments**
Renal disorders	Renal parenchymal disease: acute and chronic glomerular diseases, chronic tubulointerstitial disease, PKD, obstructive uropathy Renovascular disease: renal artery stenosis caused by atherosclerosis or fibromuscular dysplasia; arteritis; extrinsic compression of the renal artery Other renal causes: renin-producing tumors, renal sodium retention (Liddle syndrome)
Endocrine disorders	Adrenocortical disorders: primary aldosteronism, congenital adrenal hyperplasia, Cushing's syndrome Adrenomedullary tumors: pheochromocytoma (also extra-adrenal chromaffin tumor) Thyroid disease: hyperthyroidism, hypothyroidism Hyperparathyroidism: hypercalcemia Acromegaly Carcinoid tumors
Exogenous medications and drugs	Oral contraceptives, sympathomimetics, glucocorticoids, mineralocorticoids, NSAIDs, calcineurin inhibitors, tyramine-containing foods and monoamine oxidase inhibitors, EPO, ergot alkaloids, amphetamines, herbal remedies, licorice (mimics primary aldosteronism), ethanol, cocaine and other illicit drugs, abrupt withdrawal of clonidine
Pregnancy	Preeclampsia and eclampsia
Coarctation of the aorta	
Neurologic disorders	Sleep apnea Increased intracranial pressure: brain tumors Affective disorders Spinal cord injury: quadriplegia, paraplegia, Guillain-Barré syndrome Baroreflex dysregulation
Psychosocial factors	
Intravascular volume overload	
Systolic hypertension	Loss of elasticity of aorta and great vessels Hyperdynamic cardiac output: hyperthyroidism, aortic insufficiency, anemia, arteriovenous fistula, beri-beri, Paget's disease of the bone
Obesity	White adipose tissue has endocrine function: leptins; adiponectin; cytokines; chemokines; Ang II; other adipokines

Figure 32.16 Common causes of secondary hypertension. Ang II, angiotensin II; EPO, erythropoietin; NSAIDs, nonsteroidal antiinflammatory drugs; PKD, polycystic kidney disease.

in wide use is the aneroid manometer. There are also numerous semiautomatic oscillometric electronic recording manometers. The manufacturers must ensure accuracy, and in many countries, the local hypertension societies have arranged for certification of these devices. The technical capabilities of the devices have increased greatly. Physicians must be aware that many patients purchase devices and measure their own BP. These devices should be inspected and checked by the physician.

Variability of Blood Pressure

Wake-Sleep Cycle and Office Versus Home Blood Pressure

BP varies considerably in individual subjects and may vary significantly throughout the day. This variation causes considerable difficulties in identifying individuals who are hypertensive, especially in terms of the preceding classification schemes. The differing BP values are due to both biologic variation (variations of pressures within a given individual) and variation in the measurement itself. Errors in measurement can be minimized by attention to the proper technique for recording BP, as noted previously. Biologic variation is addressed by repeated BP measurement at a given visit (at least two pressures taken at least 30 seconds apart or additional BP measurements if there is a difference of 5 mm Hg between repeated measures). In addition, in most patients with milder forms of hypertension, repeated measurements during different clinic visits over time are recommended to approach the true BP.

Readings of BP at home, and outside the clinic or office setting, are recommended to assess the severity and frequency of hypertension and BP control during treatment. The instruments used at home must be checked against a standard on a regular basis, and the techniques for correct BP measurement must be taught to the patient. This includes having the brachial artery at the level of the heart when BP is measured. Levels measured at home are generally lower than those measured in the clinic or office. Patients should be discouraged from very frequent home BP measurement and from frequent adjustment of medications, which may result in unnecessary emergency department visits and hospital admissions for symptomatic hypotension or uncontrolled hypertension. It is worthwhile to ask the patient to keep a daily calendar and to measure BP under controlled conditions two or three times daily, for instance, while sitting quietly in the mornings, afternoons, and evenings. If three fourths of the measurements achieve goal or better, office control is generally also achieved.

Biologic variation during the day is related to physical and mental activity and emotional factors. There is also diurnal variation, with a decrease in BP during sleep (averaging 20%) secondary to a decrease in sympathetic activity; similar reductions in BP occur after hospital admission and bed rest. The normal diurnal pattern includes an increase in BP before awakening that

Guidelines for Measurement of Blood Pressure	
Factors	**Important Features**
Patient factors	Caffeine should not be taken for up to 1 hour before the blood pressure measurement. Cigarettes should not be smoked for at least 15 minutes prior to the blood pressure reading. The standard measurement should be made with the patient seated comfortably, arm supported, and the cuff must be at the level of the heart; the arm should be bared. On an initial examination, blood pressure should also be checked in the supine position after 5 minutes of rest, in the standing position after 2 minutes, and in both arms in patients who are diabetic, older than 65 years, or receiving antihypertensive therapy. Use the higher value if the arms have differing blood pressures. If sequential pressures are taken in the same position, at least 30 seconds must elapse between blood pressure readings. In patients younger than 30 years, check blood pressure in one leg. To establish a diagnosis of hypertension, obtain blood pressure readings on three different occasions, at least 1 week apart.
Equipment	The length of the bladder with the cuff should encircle at least 80% of the arm. The width of the cuff should be equal to two thirds of the distance from the antecubital space to the axilla and be 40% of the arm circumference. The best cuff for most adults is the 15-cm-wide cuff with a bladder of 33–35 cm in length. The distal edge of the cuff should be 2.5 cm above the antecubital fossa. For leg BP, thigh cuff length should encircle 80% of the thigh, and width should be 40% of the thigh circumference. For leg BP, the patient should be prone and popliteal artery sounds measured by auscultation. For automated equipment, the sensor should be over the brachial (or radial or popliteal) artery. In extremely obese patients, blood pressure may be more accurate when measured in the forearm, palpating and auscultating the radial artery. For infants, ultrasound equipment may need to be used. The bell of the stethoscope is preferred.
Technique	The initial systolic blood pressure should be checked by palpating the disappearance of the radial or brachial pulse prior to auscultation and the cuff then deflated. The second blood pressure check requires cuff inflation 20–30 mm Hg above the palpable systolic level. Deflate the cuff at a rate of 2–4 mm Hg per second. Record the Korotkoff sound I (appearance of sound) as the systolic pressure and record the Korotkoff sound V (the last sound before complete disappearance of sound) as the more reproducible diastolic pressure. If the sounds do not disappear, record the muffled sound (phase IV) as the diastolic. The sounds may be augmented by having the patient raise the arm and by opening and closing the hand 10 times before inflating the pressure. Do not stop between systolic and diastolic readings; deflate the cuff, wait at least 30 seconds, and then reinflate. On each occasion, record at least two readings. If the readings vary by more than 5 mm Hg, take additional readings until two are within 5 mm Hg. In children, the same standards apply for cuff size; Korotkoff sound V should be used. If the child is uncooperative, the systolic blood pressure may be determined by palpation.

Figure 32.17 Guidelines for measurement of blood pressure.

Accepted Bladder Dimensions for Varying Arm Sizes			
Patient	**Arm Circumference Range at Midpoint (cm)**	**Bladder Width (cm)**	**Bladder Length (cm)**
Newborn	6	3	6
Infant*	6–15	5	15
Child*	16–21	8	21
Small adult	22–26	10	24
Adult	27–34	13	30
Large adult	35–44	16	38
Adult thigh	45–52	20	42

Figure 32.18 Accepted bladder dimensions for varying arm sizes. *To approximate a bladder width to arm circumference ratio of 0.4 more closely in children, additional cuffs are available. There is some overlap in the recommended ranges for arm circumference to limit the number of cuffs. It is suggested that the larger cuff be used if it is available. *(From reference 32.)*

has been associated with increased incidence of myocardial infarction, stroke, and sudden death in the first few hours after awakening. Those with the usual pattern of BP decrease during sleep are known as nocturnal "dippers." Those whose BP does not fall during sleep are called "nondippers." The failure to decrease BP during sleep has been associated with increased incidence of left ventricular hypertrophy and raises the possibility of secondary hypertension.

Ambulatory Blood Pressure

Because of the variability in BP that occurs throughout the day, home BP and ambulatory BP monitoring are used to define BP more clearly. Home BP monitoring is advised for all patients and may help identify white coat hypertension and borderline hypertension and may also help monitor response to therapy, including identification of hypotension as well as hypertension. The instructions to each patient must be individualized, but home BP monitoring may be advised two or three times per day while the patient is awake. These BP values must be self-recorded and reviewed. The prognostic value of ambulatory and home BP compared with office BP in the general population was recently reported from the Pressioni Arteriose Monitorate e Loro Associazioni (PAMELA) study.[33] A total of 2051 persons were observed for 10 years; risk of death increased more with a given

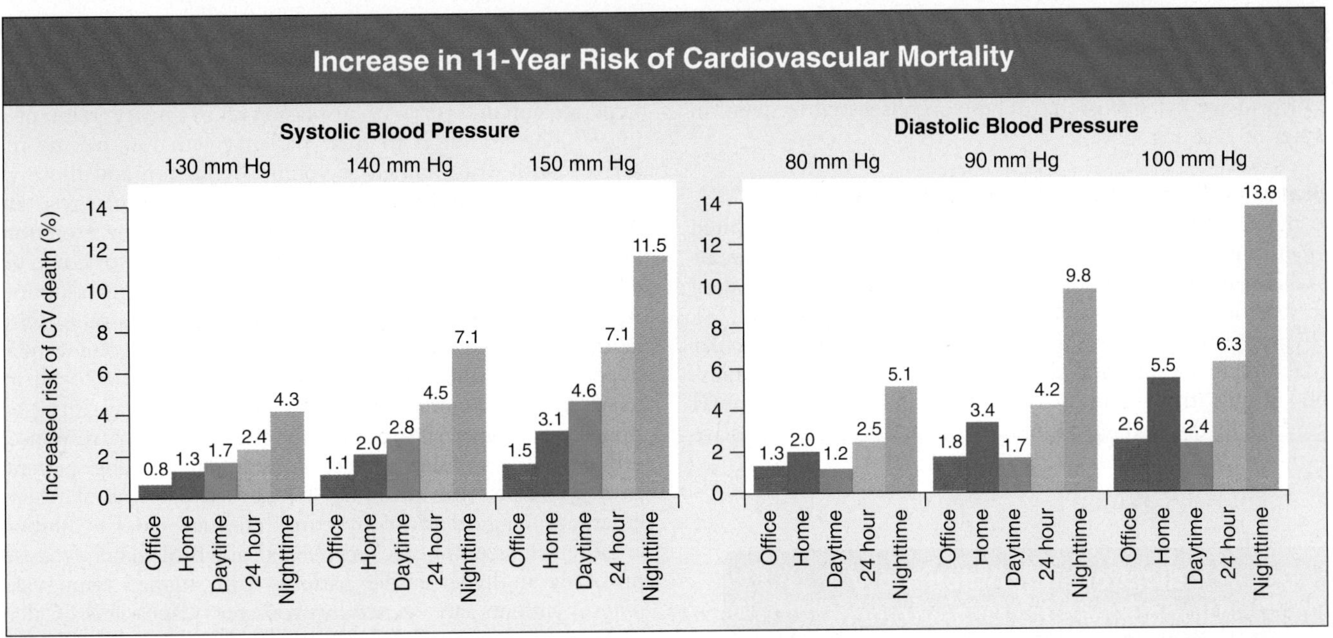

Figure 32.19 Increase in 11-year risk of cardiovascular (CV) mortality for 10 mm Hg increase in office, home, and ambulatory blood pressure (BP) at various initial BP values. *(Reprinted with permission from reference 33.)*

increase in home or ambulatory BP than in office BP. The overall ability to predict death, however, was not greater for home and ambulatory than for office BP, although it was somewhat increased by the combination of office and outside-of-office values. SBP was almost invariably superior to DBP, and night BP was superior to day BP (Fig. 32.19).

Ambulatory BP monitoring is recommended for certain indications beyond the information available from home BP recording (Fig. 32.20). Ambulatory BP monitoring uses a noninvasive system. The BP is determined by auscultation with use of either oscillometry, which measures variations in pressure within the cuff, or a microphone placed under the cuff and over the brachial artery. The ambulatory BP device can be programmed to record at frequent intervals during the daytime (e.g., every 10 minutes) and less frequently at night during sleep (e.g., every 30 minutes). The ambulatory BP equipment might not provide accurate readings in patients with large upper arms due to obesity or increased musculature, and the equipment may be inaccurate during vigorous activity. The equipment generally records BP during a 24-hour period. Although most patients adjust to the repetitive measurements throughout the day, some patients may have a startle response with each BP recording. Most patients are able to sleep, although some have their sleep disturbed by the BP recording, and therefore determination of nocturnal fall in BP is inaccurate. Indications for ambulatory BP determinations are shown in Figure 32.21.[34]

There are disadvantages to use of the ambulatory BP equipment. Trained personnel must place the monitoring equipment. Calibration of ambulatory BP equipment with a mercury manometer must be recorded at the beginning and end of the ambulatory BP session. Three to six readings must be taken at each time, and the SBP and DBP measurements must both agree within 5 mm Hg. The end calibration is critical to ensure proper functioning of the ambulatory BP monitor throughout the 24-hour period. The cuff inflation may interfere with activities, work, or sleep. The cuff may cause discomfort or skin irritation, or it may malfunction and fail to deflate, causing pain and interruption of recording. The data correlating ambulatory BP with target organ disease are limited. Standards for assessment of data and their use in decisions for therapy are limited. In addition, equipment is expensive and its use is limited by lack of reimbursement by health insurance systems in a number of countries, including the United States and some European countries.

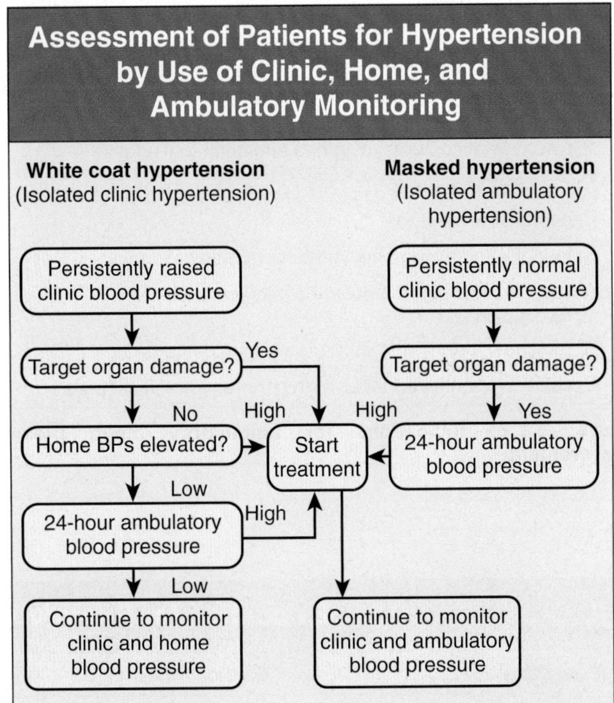

Figure 32.20 Guidelines for assessment of patients by use of clinic, home, and ambulatory monitoring of blood pressure.

Risk Factors for Hypertension

A number of factors are known to be associated with an increased risk of primary hypertension.[35] These are discussed in detail in Chapter 33 (see Fig. 33.8).

Evaluation for Primary Versus Secondary Hypertension

The medical history, the physical examination, and a limited number of laboratory tests provide critical information in deciding which individuals require further evaluation for secondary hypertension and target organ disease (Figs. 32.22 and 32.23). All hypertensive persons should be assessed for cardiovascular risk factors, including total cholesterol, HDL and LDL cholesterol, fasting triglycerides, renal function, and proteinuria (according to the Kidney Disease Outcomes Quality Initiative classification), and for the presence of diabetes mellitus or the metabolic syndrome.

Some authorities advocate assessment of patients with primary hypertension in terms of their plasma renin activity (renin profiling).[36] The notion is to treat patients with low plasma renin activity with drugs aimed at volume reduction and those with higher values with drugs aimed at peripheral vascular resistance. Although a 24-hour urine collection for sodium excretion is helpful information, the collection is not mandatory, nor must all medication be discontinued before a renin measurement. According to renin profiling, patients with plasma renin activity below 0.65 ng/ml/h are more likely to have volume-related hypertension, whereas those with values above 0.65 ng/ml/h have more predominant vasoconstriction. Systematic drug rotation studies have shown that the rank order of response to different drugs indeed varies substantially among patients.[37] In support of renin profiling, two broad patterns of response emerged. Angiotensin-converting enzyme (ACE) inhibitors, angiotensin receptor blockers (ARBs), and β-blockers were useful primarily in hypertensive patients with higher renin values. These patients are generally younger Caucasians. Calcium channel blockers and diuretics were more useful in low-renin hypertension, which is commonly observed in Afro-Caribbeans, African Americans, and older Caucasians.

If the history, physical examination, or screening laboratory studies suggest secondary hypertension, additional studies are warranted. If renal parenchymal disease is suspected, quantitative studies to assess GFR and urinary protein excretion should be performed. Renal ultrasound is useful to evaluate renal size and echogenicity (to help assess chronicity) and to evaluate for obstructive uropathy. Renal artery stenosis should be suspected by the presence of severe hypertension with abnormal renal function or with asymmetric renal size. If primary aldosteronism is suspected because of hypokalemia, the ratio of plasma aldosterone to plasma renin activity may be useful. If the ratio is above 25 to 30 and plasma aldosterone concentration is more than 20 ng/dl, the diagnosis should be pursued further. The extended results of patients undergoing operation have been published.[38] Resolution of hypertension after adrenalectomy for primary aldosteronism was independently associated with a lack of family history of hypertension and preoperative use of two or fewer antihypertensive agents. Further evaluation for other forms of secondary hypertension is listed in Figure 32.23.

Indications for Ambulatory Blood Pressure Measurement
White coat hypertension
Evaluation of apparent drug resistance
Hypotensive symptoms
Autonomic dysfunction
Episodic hypertension
Evaluation of nocturnal decreases in blood pressure as a prognostic factor for target organ disease (left ventricular hypertrophy, ischemic optic neuropathy)
Evaluation of blood pressure changes in patients with paroxysmal nocturnal dyspnea and nocturnal angina
Carotid sinus syncope
Pacemaker syndromes
Safety of withdrawing antihypertensive medication
Assess 24-hour blood pressure control on once-daily medication
Borderline hypertension with target organ damage
Evaluation of antihypertensive drug therapy in clinical trials

Figure 32.21 Indications for ambulatory blood pressure measurement.

Evaluation for Primary Versus Secondary Hypertension			
Classification	**Medical History**	**Physical Examination**	**Laboratory Studies**
General information and evaluation of target organs	Duration and course of hypertension Prior workup and treatment Diet/lifestyle: salt intake, tobacco, caffeine	Evaluation of volume status, optic fundi, heart, lungs, peripheral vessels, and nervous system	Complete blood count, fasting glucose, lipid profile (includes HDL, LDL, cholesterol, triglyceride), uric acid Consider echocardiogram
Primary (essential or idiopathic) or secondary?	Family history: hypertension, cardiovascular and renal diseases Symptoms of target organ disease (related to eyes, central nervous system, cardiorespiratory, and peripheral vascular)	See Figure 32.23 for signs suggestive of secondary hypertension	See Figure 32.23 for additional laboratory studies to rule out secondary hypertension

Figure 32.22 Evaluation for primary versus secondary hypertension. HDL, high-density lipoprotein; LDL, low-density lipoprotein.

Evaluation of Secondary Hypertension			
Target Organ/System	**Medical History**	**Physical Examination**	**Laboratory Studies**
Kidney			
Renal parenchymal	History of renal disease (including glomerulonephritis, nephrotic syndrome, calculi, urinary tract infection) Symptoms include nocturia, frequency, dysuria, hesitancy, urgency, incomplete emptying, dribbling, hematuria, pyuria, flank pain	Tenderness in costovertebral angles; palpable kidneys	BUN, serum creatinine; urinalysis, urine culture if indicated; 24-h urine for protein and creatinine clearance if indicated; consider microalbuminuria measurement, or random urine protein to creatinine ratio
Renovascular hypertension		Epigastric bruit; other vascular bruits	Renal ultrasonography with duplex Doppler flow study; consider angiography or magnetic resonance angiography
Endocrine			
Primary aldosteronism	Muscle weakness, cramps		Serum potassium: consider serum aldosterone to plasma renin activity ratio; 24-h urine aldosterone, Na, K, creatinine
Cushing's syndrome	Weight gain, cosmetic changes	Body habitus: body fat, striae	Morning serum cortisol after dexamethasone suppression
Pheochromocytoma	Headaches; vasomotor symptoms, (inappropriate sweating, pallor); cardiac symptoms (awareness, tachycardia, palpitations)	Paroxysmal or intermittent hypertension (50% of patients)	Single voided urine for metanephrine and creatinine; consider 24-h urine for VMA, metanephrines; and catecholamines; if positive, proceed with magnetic resonance imaging or thin-section computed tomography of the adrenals
Carcinoid	Flushing		24-h urine 5-hydroxyindoleacetic acid excretion
Hyperthyroidism	Weight loss, tachycardia, palpitations, sweating, heat intolerance	Palpable thyroid	Total and free thyroxine
Hypothyroidism	Weight gain, dry skin, cold intolerance, hair loss		Thyroid-stimulating hormone, total and free thyroxine
Hyperparathyroidism	Nausea, vomiting, bone pain, nephrolithiasis		Serum calcium, intact parathyroid hormone
Acromegaly	Change in size of head, hands, or feet (adult)	Appearance	GH level (see Figure 39-10)
Medication	Review of prescribed and over-the-counter medications (especially oral contraceptives, NSAIDs, sympathomimetic agents [cold and allergy drugs], illicit or recreational drugs, including alcohol, herbal remedies)		
Coarctation of the aorta	Onset or detection of hypertension in childhood or adolescence	Simultaneous palpation of radial and femoral arteries to detect pulse lag in femorals; leg blood pressure	Chest radiograph for heart size, configuration of aorta, rib notching; consider aortography
Neurologic disorders			
Sleep apnea	Obesity; weight gain; daytime somnolence; snoring, poor sleep habits (frequent awakening, not rested on arising); early morning headache	Obesity; narrowed airway in hypopharynx; redundant pharyngeal tissue	Formal sleep study (polysomnography)
Increased intracranial pressure	Headache; neurologic symptoms	Papilledema	↑Cerebrospinal fluid pressure
Affective disorders†			
Spinal cord injury†			
Psychosocial factors	Family and support structure, occupation, education, stressors		
Volume overload	Excess salt and water intake (may be iatrogenic with excess parenteral fluid)	Increased jugular venous distention, pulmonary rales, presacral and peripheral edema, hepatomegaly	Chest radiograph
Isolated systolic hypertension		Pseudohypertension (positive Olser's maneuver); cardiac and vascular examination (evaluate for aortic insufficiency, arteriovenous fistula)	

Figure 32.23 History, physical examination, and initial laboratory evaluation for secondary hypertension. A more detailed discussion is provided in other relevant chapters. Pregnancy-associated hypertension is discussed in Chapters 42 and 43. †Medical history, physical examination and laboratory tests are either obvious or beyond the scope of the discussion. BUN, blood urea nitrogen; NSAIDs, nonsteroidal antiinflammatory drugs.

REFERENCES

1. Guyton AC, Hall JE. Dominant role of the kidneys in long-term regulation of arterial pressure and in hypertension: The integrated system for pressure control. In: Guyton AC, Hall JE, eds. *Textbook of Medical Physiology*. 10th ed. Philadelphia: WB Saunders; 2000:221-234.
2. Izzo JL Jr, Black HR, eds. *Hypertension Primer*. 3rd ed. Dallas: Council on High Blood Pressure Research, American Heart Association; 2003:3-78.
3. DiBona GF. Functionally specific renal sympathetic nerve fibers: Role in cardiovascular regulation. *Am J Hypertens*. 2001;14:163S-170S.
4. Xu J, Li G, Wang P, et al. Renalase is a novel, soluble monoamine oxidase that regulates cardiac function and blood pressure. *J Clin Invest*. 2005;115:1275-1280.
5. Zhao Q, Fan Z, He J, et al. Renalase gene is a novel susceptibility gene for essential hypertension. *J Mol Med*. 2007;85:877-885.
6. Ravani P, Tripepi G, Pecchini P, et al. Urotensin II is an inverse predictor of death and fatal cardiovascular events in chronic kidney disease. *Kidney Int*. 2008;73:95-101.
7. Botros FT, Navar LG. Heme oxygenase in regulation of renal function and blood pressure. *Curr Hypertens Rev*. 2009;5:13-23.
8. Fukata Y, Amano M, Kaibuchi K. Rho–Rho-kinase pathway in smooth muscle contraction and cytoskeletal reorganization of non-muscle cells. *Trends Pharmacol Sci*. 2001;22:32-39.
9. Lohmeier TE, Hildebrandt DA, Warren S, et al. Recent insights into the interactions between the baroreflex and the kidneys in hypertension. *Am J Physiol Regul Integr Comp Physiol*. 2005;288:R828-R836.
10. Crowley SD, Gurley SB, Oliverio MI, et al. Distinct roles for the kidney and systemic tissues in blood pressure regulation by the renin-angiotensin system. *J Clin Invest*. 2005;115:1092-1099.
11. Lewington S, Clarke R, Qizilbash N, et al. Prospective Studies Collaboration: Age-specific relevance of usual blood pressure to vascular mortality: A meta-analysis of individual data for one million adults in 61 prospective studies. *Lancet*. 2002;360:1903-1913.
12. Chobanian AV, Bakris GL, Black HR, et al. Joint National Committee on Prevention, Detection, Evaluation, and Treatment of High Blood Pressure; National Heart, Lung, and Blood Institute; National High Blood Pressure Education Program Coordinating Committee: Seventh report of the Joint National Committee on Prevention, Detection, Evaluation, and Treatment of High Blood Pressure. *Hypertension*. 2003;42: 1206-1252.
13. Giles T. New definition of hypertension proposed. Available at: http://www.medscape.com/viewarticle/505745. Accessed March 1, 2009.
14. Cruickshank JK, Mzayek F, Liu L, et al. Origins of the "black/white" difference in blood pressure: Roles of birth weight, postnatal growth, early blood pressure, and adolescent body size: The Bogalusa Heart Study. *Circulation*. 2005;111:1932-1937.
15. Ong KL, Cheung BM, Man YB, et al. Prevalence, awareness, treatment, and control of hypertension among United States adults 1994-2004. *Hypertension*. 2007;49:69-75.
16. Wolf-Maier K, Cooper R, Banegas J, et al. Hypertension prevalence and blood pressure levels in 6 European countries, Canada, and the United States. *JAMA*. 2003;289:2363-2369.
17. ESH '07: New Consensus Hypertension Guidelines from the European Society of Hypertension/European Society of Cardiology (ESH/ESC). Available at: http://www.medscape.com/viewarticle/560317. Accessed March 1, 2009.
18. Jackson R, Lawes CM, Bennett DA, et al. Treatment with drugs to lower blood pressure and blood cholesterol based on an individual's absolute cardiovascular risk. *Lancet*. 2005;365:434-441.
19. Klausen K, Borch-Johnsen K, Feldt-Rasmussen B, et al. Very low levels of microalbuminuria are associated with increased risk of coronary heart disease and death independently of renal function, hypertension, and diabetes. *Circulation*. 2004;110:32-35.
20. Egan B, Nesbitt S, Julius S. Prehypertension: Should we be treating with pharmacologic therapy? *Ther Adv Cardiovasc Dis*. 2008;2:305-314.
21. Pickering TG, Gerin W, Schwartz AR. What is the white-coat effect and how should it be measured? *Blood Press Monit*. 2002;7:293-300.
22. Ohkubo T, Kikuya M, Metoki H, et al. Prognosis of "masked" hypertension and "white-coat" hypertension detected by 24-h ambulatory blood pressure monitoring 10-year follow-up from the Ohasama study. *J Am Coll Cardiol*. 2005;46:508-515.
23. NCEP ATP III, National Cholesterol Education Program (NCEP) Adult Treatment Panel III (ATP III). *JAMA*. 2001;285:2486-2497 and Diabetes Care 2003;26:3160-3167.
24. Pickering TG. The ninth Sir George Pickering memorial lecture. Ambulatory monitoring and the definition of hypertension. *J Hypertens*. 1992;10:401-409.
25. Mansoor GA. A practical approach to persistent elevation of blood pressure in the hypertension clinic. *Blood Press Monit*. 2003;8:97-100.
26. Dao HH, Essalihi R, Bouvet C, Moreau P. Evolution and modulation of age-related medial elastocalcinosis: Impact on large artery stiffness and isolated systolic hypertension. *Cardiovasc Res*. 2005;66:307-317.
27. Sander GE. Hypertension in the elderly. *Curr Hypertens Rep*. 2004;6: 469-476.
28. Epstein M. Resistant hypertension: Prevalence and evolving concepts. *J Clin Hypertens (Greenwich)*. 2007;9(Suppl 1):2-6.
29. Elliot WJ. Clinical features and management of selected hypertensive emergencies. *J Clin Hypertens (Greenwich)*. 2004;6:587-592.
30. Burt VL, Whelton P, Roccella EJ, et al. Prevalence of hypertension in the US adult population: Results from the Third National Health and Nutrition Examination Survey, 1988-1991. *Hypertension*. 1995;23: 305-313.
31. Jones DW, Frohlich ED, Grim CM, et al. Mercury sphygmomanometers should not be abandoned: An advisory statement from the Council for High Blood Pressure Research, American Heart Association. *Hypertension*. 2001;37:185-186.
32. Perloff D, Grim C, Flack J, et al. Human blood pressure determination by sphygmomanometry. *Circulation*. 1993;88:2460-2470.
33. Sega R, Facchetti R, Bombelli M, et al. Prognostic value of ambulatory and home blood pressures compared with office blood pressure in the general population: Follow-up results from the Pressioni Arteriose Monitorate e Loro Associazioni (PAMELA) study. *Circulation*. 2005;111: 1777-1783.
34. O'Brien E, Asmar R, Beilin L, et al. European Society of Hypertension Working Group on Blood Pressure Monitoring: Practice guidelines of the European Society of Hypertension for clinic, ambulatory and self blood pressure measurement. *J Hypertens*. 2005;23:697-701.
35. Franklin SS, Pio JR, Wong ND, et al. Predictors of new-onset diastolic and systolic hypertension: The Framingham Heart Study. *Circulation*. 2005;111:1121-1127.
36. Laragh JH, Sealey JE. Relevance of the plasma renin hormonal control system that regulates blood pressure and sodium balance for correctly treating hypertension and for evaluating ALLHAT. *Am J Hypertens*. 2003;16:407-415.
37. Mackenzie IS, Brown MJ. Genetic profiling versus drug rotation in the optimisation of antihypertensive treatment. *Clin Med*. 2002;2: 465-473.
38. Sawka AM, Young WF, Thompson GB, et al. Primary aldosteronism: Factors associated with normalization of blood pressure after surgery. *Ann Intern Med*. 2001;135:258-261.

CHAPTER 33

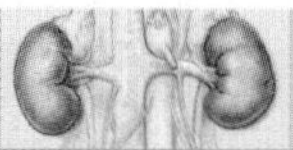

Primary Hypertension

Richard J. Johnson, Bernardo Rodriguez-Iturbe, George L. Bakris

DEFINITION

Primary (also known as essential) hypertension is defined as a blood pressure (BP) above 140/90 mm Hg without an identifiable cause. Several readings on different occasions and times are necessary to document that the BP is elevated because of substantial variability in BP. This variability in BP results from a circadian rhythm that generates the most significant increase in BP in early morning hours (6:00 to 10:00). BP falls at bedtime with recumbency or sleep, secondary to a decrease in sympathetic nervous system tone and reduced activity of other neuroendocrine systems. There are also minute-to-minute variations in BP (Fig. 33.1). Transient elevations in BP, reaching 150 mm Hg systolic, occur in the majority of normotensive subjects on any given day.[1] However, BP that is repeatedly 140/90 mm Hg or greater is considered elevated. Details on the method and interpretation of BP measurements, including the use of ambulatory BP monitoring, can be found in Chapter 32.

Hypertension is classified according to severity (Fig. 33.2).[2] Stages in hypertension have been adapted by both the Joint National Committee (JNC 7) and the European Society of Hypertension and European Society of Cardiology (ESH/ESC) guidelines to allow a prognosis to be associated with different levels of BP elevation. The prognosis has been adapted from epidemiologic studies that demonstrate a linear relationship between the risk of cardiovascular events and sustained elevations of arterial pressure.

If only the systolic BP is elevated (systolic BP >140 mm Hg and diastolic BP <90 mm Hg), it is called isolated systolic hypertension. The former terms borderline hypertension and high-normal hypertension (defined as BP of 130 to 139/85 to 89 mm Hg) are now classified as prehypertension (defined as BP ≥120 to 139/80 to 89 mm Hg). White coat hypertension is an elevation of more than 20 mm Hg in systolic pressure noted only in the physician's office above that seen at home or in another setting. In contrast, masked hypertension is BP that is normal in the office but elevated by more than 20 mm Hg when it is measured by ambulatory BP monitoring.

Other terms used to describe specific clinical presentations include hypertensive emergencies, which are associated with acute end-organ damage requiring immediate treatment, usually in the intensive care unit, and hypertensive urgencies, which need correction in hours or a few days (see Chapter 36). In hypertensive crises, the reduction of BP will halt, prevent, or reverse falling glomerular filtration rate (GFR). These terms have replaced malignant hypertension and accelerated hypertension. Resistant hypertension is defined as hypertension that remains above 140/90 mm Hg despite use of three maximally dosed antihypertensive medications of different classes.

ETIOLOGY AND PATHOGENESIS

The kidney has a key role in the pathogenesis of hypertension. Guyton proposed that the kidney in subjects with hypertension has a physiologic defect in sodium excretion. Whereas an increase in sodium intake is associated with a rise in pressure and prompt excretion of the salt load in most subjects, this pressure-natriuresis relationship is abnormal in the hypertensive subject[3] (Fig. 33.3). In some hypertensive subjects, especially those younger than 40 years, the response to a salt load is similar to that of normal subjects but is just shifted rightward such that higher pressures are required for a specific salt load (salt-resistant hypertension). In contrast, some hypertensive subjects, and especially older subjects and African Americans, have both a rightward shift and a change in the slope such that BP increases more for the same sodium load (i.e., salt-sensitive hypertension). Additional evidence in support of a renal defect in sodium handling comes from the observation that kidney transplantation can transfer the susceptibility for hypertension in response to salt in various rat strains. Epidemiologic studies have also documented that dietary sodium content correlates with the prevalence of hypertension in various populations, and intervention studies with salt restriction or loading have shown that the BP response in many hypertensive patients is salt sensitive. The basis for this renal defect in hypertension remains controversial, but three major hypotheses have been proposed.

Genetic (Polygene) Hypothesis

Pickering and later Lifton proposed that hypertension results from the expression of multiple genetic polymorphisms (polygene hypothesis) that favor sodium retention by the kidney in a westernized society in which there is often excessive intake (>10 g/day) of salt. The observation that numerous monogenic forms of both hypertension and hypotension are mediated by specific mutations involving sodium transport, especially involving the epithelial sodium channel (see Chapter 47), supports this hypothesis (Fig. 33.4).[4] Indeed, more than 20 genes have been identified in which mutations or polymorphisms can strongly influence BP.[4] Many of these involve sodium transport in the distal tubule or the collecting duct. Interestingly, some heterozygous mutations (such as the Na-K-2Cl cotransporter *SLC12A1* or the inward rectifier K^+ channel *KCNJ1*) that are carrier states for Gitelman's syndrome and the heterozygous mutation of the Na-Cl cotransporter *SLC12A3* that is a carrier state for Bartter syndrome actually confer protection from hypertension.[5] Whereas genetic polymorphisms clearly have an important influence on BP, many studies suggest that genetic mechanisms can account for only 20% to 30% of cases of primary hypertension,

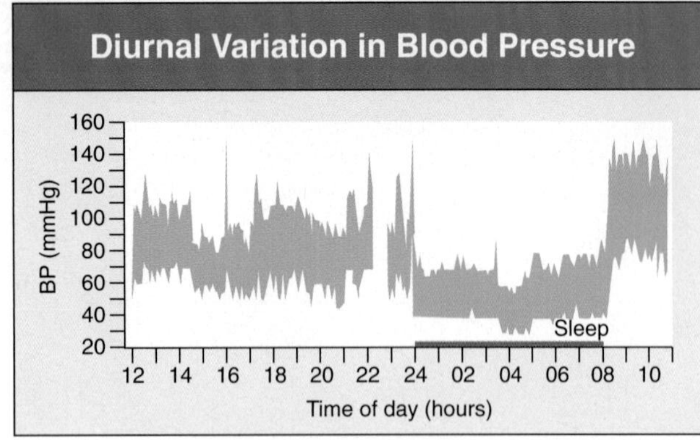

Figure 33.1 Blood pressure variability in a normotensive individual. In most normal individuals, systolic blood pressure reaches 150 mm Hg at least once per day. *(Reprinted with permission from reference 1.)*

Classification of Blood Pressure

BP Classification	Systolic BP (mmHg)		Diastolic BP (mmHg)
Normal	<120	and	<80
Prehypertension	120–139	or	80–89
Stage 1 hypertension	140–159	or	90–99
Stage 2 hypertension	≥160	or	≥100

Figure 33.2 Classification of blood pressure. Shown is the BP classification according to the seventh report of the Joint National Committee on Prevention, Detection, and Treatment of High Blood Pressure: the JNC 7 report. *(From reference 2.)*

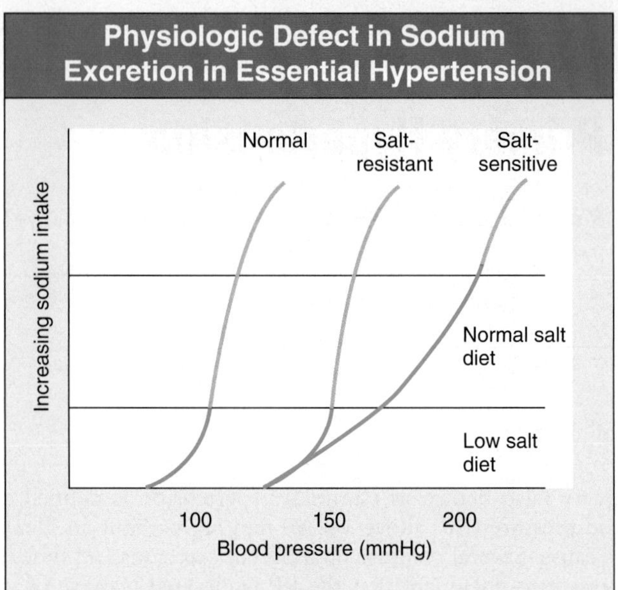

Figure 33.3 A physiologic defect in sodium excretion in primary hypertension. Evidence suggests that in patients with primary hypertension, a higher blood pressure is required to excrete an individual sodium load. In salt-resistant hypertension, the pressure-natriuresis curve has a rightward but parallel shift; with salt-sensitive hypertension, it is a shift to the right as well as a change in slope. *(Modified from reference 4.)*

Monogenic Diseases Associated with Alterations in Blood Pressure

Condition	Gene	Inheritance	Site	Manifestations
Glucocorticoid-remediable aldosteronism (GRA)	Chimeric ACTH-responsive promoter with aldosterone synthase	AD	Collecting duct	Hypertension, metabolic alkalosis
Mendelian hypertension exacerbated by pregnancy	Gain-of-function of mineralocorticoid receptor (MR)	AD	Collecting duct	Hypertension, worsened by pregnancy (progesterone)
Liddle syndrome	Gain-of-function of β or γ subunit of epithelial sodium channel (ENaC)	AD	Collecting duct	Hypertension, metabolic alkalosis
Pseudohypoaldosteronism type 1 (PHA1)	ENaC loss of function MR loss of function	AR AD	Collecting duct	Neonatal hypotension, acidosis, salt wasting
Gitelman's syndrome	Na-Cl cotransporter (NCC) Loss of function	AR	Distal convoluted tubule (DCT)	Low BP, salt wasting, metabolic alkalosis
Bartter syndrome	4 gene mutations: Na-K-2Cl, K channel, C1 channel, Barttin	AD or AR	Thick ascending limb	Low BP, salt wasting, metabolic alkalosis
Metabolic syndrome	Mitochondrial tRNA	Maternal	?	Hypertension, hypercholesterolemia, hypomagnesemia
Pseudohypoaldosteronism type 2 (PHA 2) or Gordon's syndrome	WNK1 and WNK4 serine threonine kinases	AD	DCT and Collecting duct	Hypertension, ↑K, metabolic acidosis

Figure 33.4 Monogenic diseases associated with alterations in blood pressure. ACTH, adrenocorticotropic hormone; AD, autosomal dominant; AR, autosomal recessive; BP, blood pressure.

indicating that other mechanisms are also likely to be operative.

Congenital (The Low Nephron Number) Hypothesis

In 1989, Barker reported an increased risk for hypertension, obesity, and diabetes in subjects with low birth weights.[6] Mothers of low-birth-weight infants frequently have hypertension, obesity, preeclampsia, or malnutrition, and these maternal factors are also associated with an increased risk for hypertension in the progeny. Brenner and colleagues[7] independently postulated that hypertension might be predisposed by being born with kidneys with a lower nephron number, which commonly occurs in low-birth-weight infants. Consistent with this hypothesis, experimental studies have demonstrated that maternal malnutrition predisposes to small babies, a low nephron number, and the future predisposition for hypertension. Furthermore, a study reported that Caucasians with primary hypertension have nearly 50% fewer nephrons than do age- and sex-matched controls.[8] However, more recent studies in the African American population could not confirm the relationship between low nephron number and hypertension. In addition, low birth weight cannot be the primary risk factor. For example, one study found that although low-birth-weight infants have a 25% risk for development of hypertension as adults, high-birth-weight infants have a 20% risk.[9] Thus, other mechanisms are also likely contributory in the pathogenesis of hypertension.

Acquired Renal Injury Hypothesis

Primary hypertension is commonly associated with renal arteriolosclerosis and hyalinosis with variable degrees of glomerulosclerosis and ischemic tubular injury. Whereas renal function is often normal or only slightly depressed, renal vascular resistance is high due to intense vasoconstriction of the afferent arteriole. It is likely that overt structural changes are the consequence of hypertension; yet experimental induction of microvascular disease and renal inflammation in normal rats also results in the development of salt-sensitive hypertension.

Salt-sensitive hypertension can be induced by a variety of means that usually involve renal vasoconstriction (Fig. 33.5). Renal microvascular injury leads to oxidative stress, resulting in an influx of macrophages and T cells, activation of the local renin-angiotensin system (RAS), and a decrease in local nitric oxide. Some studies suggest that the local T cells may be reacting with *de novo* expressed antigens, such as heat shock protein 70, to cause the hypertensive response. These data are consistent with accumulating evidence that T cells may have a role in the pathogenesis of hypertension. Indeed, blocking of T cells and macrophage accumulation in the kidney with mycophenolate mofetil (MMF) can prevent hypertension in various experimental models of salt-sensitive hypertension. Interestingly, rats born with low nephron number also develop renal microvascular disease and intrarenal T-cell accumulation, and administration of MMF also reduces BP in these animals. MMF has also been reported to lower BP in humans with psoriasis and primary hypertension.

How Does Renal Injury Lead to Sodium Retention?

Renal tubulointerstitial inflammation, local oxidative stress with inactivation of nitric oxide, and local angiotensin II (Ang II) activity maintain intrarenal vasoconstriction and sodium retention. Afferent arteriole remodeling results from the

Mechanisms that can Induce Salt-Sensitive Hypertension in Experimental Animals
Angiotensin II infusion
Inhibition of nitric oxide synthesis (treatment with L-NAME)
Catecholamine infusion
Diet-induced hypokalemia
Hyperuricemia induced by uricase inhibition
Reduced nephron number via maternal malnutrition
Induction of nephrotic syndrome with use of bovine serum albumin
Page kidney
Lead-induced hypertension
Cyclosporine nephropathy
Genetic models of hypertension (Dahl salt-sensitive rat, spontaneously hypertensive rat)

Figure 33.5 Mechanisms that can induce salt-sensitive hypertension in experimental animals. All experimental models involve the development of renal microvascular injury and interstitial inflammation.

increased BP as well as from a direct stimulation of smooth muscle cell proliferation by Ang II and other mediators. Whereas the renal arteriolar disease is mild, a given sodium gain is met with a rise in systemic and renal perfusion pressures, and the pressure-natriuresis relationship maintains the same slope as in the normal response, resulting in a salt-resistant form of hypertension. As progressive renal arteriosclerosis develops, there is uneven blood perfusion of the kidney, with underperfused areas distal to regions with severe arteriolar disease and overperfused areas distal to areas with preserved arteriolar structure. The consequence of this condition is renal ischemia with a right shift of the pressure-natriuresis curve with a change of the slope, characteristic of salt-sensitive hypertension (Fig. 33.6).[10]

What Pathogenic Mechanisms Are Driving the Current Epidemic of Hypertension?

As discussed later (see Epidemiology), there has been a marked rise in the prevalence of hypertension in the last century. There is evidence that the marked rise in hypertension corresponds with the introduction of Western diet and lifestyle and with the dramatic increase in obesity. Obesity may cause hypertension through multiple mechanisms, including subtle renal injury, the effects of hyperleptinemia or hyperinsulinemia, the coexistence of endothelial dysfunction, and the activation of the sympathetic nervous system (SNS).[11] However, a recent hypothesis suggests that the rapid increase in sugar intake (and in particular fructose) may have a direct role in driving the obesity and hypertension epidemic.[12] Fructose is unique among sugars in being rapidly phosphorylated within the cell, resulting in local adenosine triphosphate (ATP) depletion and uric acid generation. In turn, uric acid has been shown to induce endothelial dysfunction, to activate the local and systemic RAS, to stimulate aldosterone, and possibly to activate the SNS. Experimentally induced hyperuricemia also causes hypertension with afferent arteriolar disease and tubulointerstitial inflammation similar to that observed with other vasoconstrictive agents.

Studies in humans and experimental animals suggest that fructose can raise BP by a uric acid–dependent mechanism. Uric acid levels have risen in the last century in parallel with increased

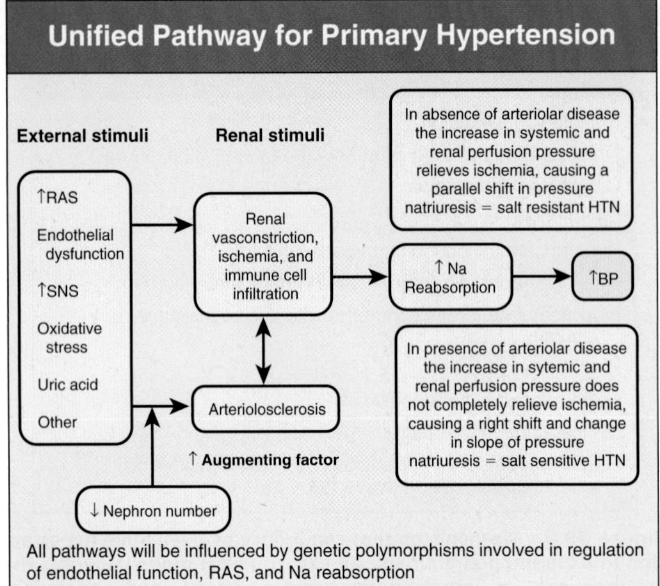

Figure 33.6. Unified pathway for primary hypertension. Hypertension may be hypothesized as occurring in two phases. The first phase is mediated by renal vasoconstriction due to stimuli such as a hyperactive sympathetic nervous system (SNS), hyperuricemia, endothelial dysfunction, or an activated renin-angiotensin system (RAS). This results in a salt-resistant form of hypertension. Whereas hypertension may remain salt resistant, we hypothesize that progressive renal microvascular disease and tubulointerstitial inflammation will develop in many subjects, with a switch to a salt-sensitive phenotype and an increased risk for microalbuminuria. BP, blood pressure; HTN, hypertension.

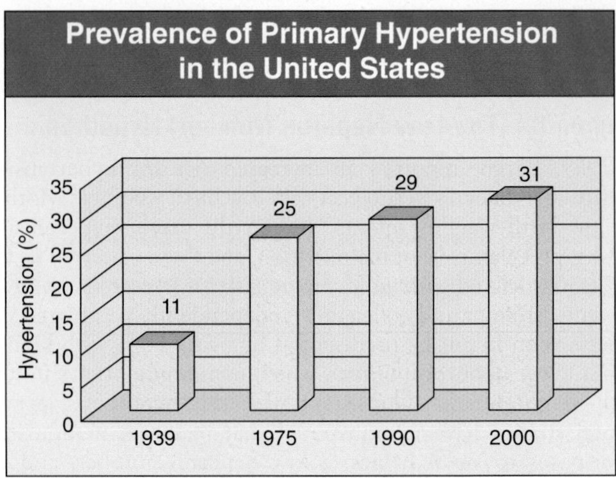

Figure 33.7 Prevalence of primary hypertension in the United States. The prevalence of primary hypertension (defined as BP >140/90 mm Hg) in the United States has been rising from a prevalence of 11% in 1939 to 31% today.

fructose intake and the rise in hypertension and obesity. In one study of newly diagnosed hypertension in obese adolescents, an elevated uric acid level was observed in nearly 90% of cases. In a small double-blind placebo-controlled study, the lowering of uric acid levels to below 5.0 mg/dl resulted in normal BP in 86% of subjects compared with 3% of controls.[13] While exciting, further studies are needed before lowering of uric acid can be recommended for treatment or prevention of hypertension or cardiovascular disease.

A hyperactive SNS is also commonly involved in early hypertension, particularly in young or borderline hypertensive patients.[14] Postulated mechanisms include a defect in baroreceptor sensitivity and an increase in SNS response to emotional or work-related stress. Activation of either the systemic or local RAS is also common in hypertension. Whereas plasma renin activity is elevated in 20% of patients, renin activity is either normal (50%) or low (30%) in the majority. However, normal renin activity may be inappropriately high in relation to the total body sodium. Finally, some hypertensive subjects will have elevated plasma aldosterone, especially if the RAS is inhibited with angiotensin-converting enzyme (ACE) inhibitors or angiotensin receptor blockers (ARBs).[15,16] Typically, such subjects are obese and have hyperinsulinemia or some degree of endothelial dysfunction. In these subjects, the aldosteronism is driven by a mechanism other than Ang II or hyperkalemia, and some studies suggest that it may be due to the presence of circulating oxidized fatty acids (especially linoleic acid) or uric acid.

How Does Salt Retention Lead to Hypertension?

An acute infusion of saline administered to animals with experimentally induced hypertension will initially raise blood volume and cardiac output, but the increase in cardiac output is transient and is replaced by a rise in the systemic vascular resistance, a process that Guyton and associates[3] termed autoregulation because they postulated that the vasoconstriction is an adaptive response resulting from the need to reduce unnecessary increments in tissue perfusion. Several mechanisms may account for the rise in systemic vascular resistance. First, volume expansion is known to increase circulating Na^+,K^+-ATPase inhibitors (such as ouabain from the adrenal gland) that raise intracellular sodium and facilitate sodium-calcium exchange in the vascular smooth muscle cell.[17] This would lead to a rise in intracellular calcium concentration and stimulate vascular smooth muscle contraction, vasoconstriction, and the rise in vascular resistance. Circulating nitric oxide synthase (NOS) inhibitors have also been documented in some patients with primary hypertension. A small increase in serum sodium concentration may also occur in hypertensive subjects and may stimulate the release of vasoconstrictive substances such as vasopressin, which may have a role particularly in African Americans.[18] Activation of the SNS may also occur in salt-sensitive hypertension in response to a salt load.[19] A possible explanation is that in the setting of tubulointerstitial injury and intrarenal ischemia, the salt load will trigger an intense tubuloglomerular feedback (TGF) signal with activation of the renal afferent SNS, which activates central nervous system (CNS) sympathetic activity.[19] Other mechanisms that could contribute to increased systemic vascular resistance are loss of vasodilatory substances from the kidney, such as kallikrein and medullipin, or the loss of systemic capillaries (microvascular rarefaction).

EPIDEMIOLOGY

Primary hypertension is epidemic. In the United States, the prevalence has increased from 5% to 11% of the population in the early 1900s to 31% (65 million people) today (Fig. 33.7).[20] The increase in prevalence, which has also been observed in Europe, is not completely accounted for by the increasing life expectancy in the population. Similarly, hypertension was virtually absent outside Europe and North America until the 1930s, but it has subsequently increased to prevalence rates of 20% to 30% in conjunction with adaptation of the Western diet and lifestyle. By 2025, an estimated 1.56 billion people will have primary hypertension. The increase in hypertension

Risk Factors for Primary Hypertension	
Genetic	Family history Polymorphisms (adducin, endothelial nitric oxide synthase, angiotensinogen, β2-adrenoceptor, human G protein β3 subunit)
Congenital	Low birth weight, low nephron number, maternal hypertension, maternal preeclampsia, maternal malnutrition
Physical	Obesity, older age, African American, African Caribbean, increased heart rate (>83 beats/min), increased emotional stress
Diet/toxin	Increased sodium intake, low potassium intake, low dairy products intake, heavy alcohol intake, low level lead or cadmium intoxication
Metabolic (laboratory-based parameters)	Elevated uric acid, insulin resistance, elevated hematocrit
Other	Low socioeconomic status, urban vs rural

Figure 33.8 Major risk factors for primary hypertension.

correlates with increasing frequencies of obesity, type 2 diabetes, and chronic kidney disease (CKD), suggesting a strong interrelationship.

There are several major risk factors for hypertension (Fig. 33.8). First, the risk for primary hypertension increases with age, with a 65% prevalence in the population at the age of 65 years and 75% at 75 years.[21] This age-related increase in prevalence of hypertension has been observed in most Western countries but has not been uniformly observed in all populations. Second, hypertension is more common in men, although the prevalence in women may surpass that in men in the postmenopausal years. Certain racial groups are also at increased risk, particularly African Americans and Filipino Americans in the United States and various minority populations throughout the world (such as the Pima Indians, Australian aborigines, and the Maoris). Risk factors for hypertension include obesity, insulin resistance, hyperuricemia or gout, sleep apnea, low socioeconomic status, and increased stress at work. Certain physical features, such as elevated heart rate or an increased BP response to exercise, are also predictive, as is elevated hematocrit.

Genetic factors also contribute (see Etiology/Pathogenesis). Although the inheritance patterns do not follow classic mendelian genetics for a single gene locus, there is evidence that as much as 30% of hypertension may have a genetic basis because of the cumulative effect of multiple susceptibility genes (the polygene hypothesis). An increased risk for hypertension has been associated with genetic polymorphisms involving the immune system and oxidative stress mechanisms (heat shock protein 70 variants and extracellular superoxide dismutase), vasoactive mediators (angiotensinogen, endothelial NOS, prostacyclin synthase, β_2-adrenoceptor, 20-HETE synthase [*CYP4F2* gene], and G protein β3), mediators of vascular smooth muscle tone (calcium-dependent potassium channel [*KCNMA*]), or mediators controlling renal sodium transport (α-adducin and 11β-hydroxysteroid dehydrogenase type 2, aldosterone synthase, WNK kinases).[19]

Hypertension is more likely to occur if the mother has a history of hypertension, obesity, preeclampsia, or malnutrition. These risk factors are all associated with intrauterine growth retardation and low birth weight, both of which predispose to future hypertension as well as diabetes and obesity.

Dietary and other environmental factors may contribute to the risk for hypertension. Obesity (with or without features of insulin resistance and the metabolic syndrome) is a major risk factor for hypertension. Obesity is increasing in both developing and industrialized countries and parallels the rise in hypertension in these countries. Epidemiologic and interventional studies have linked salt intake with hypertension, although the relationship is best demonstrated in older subjects and in African Americans. Diets low in calcium and dairy products or potassium are also associated with a higher prevalence of hypertension. Increasing potassium intake lowers BP in both experimental and human studies. Finally, certain toxins, most notably low-level lead or cadmium intoxication, are associated with increased frequency of hypertension.

CLINICAL MANIFESTATIONS

Evaluation of a patient with hypertension includes a careful history and physical examination, an evaluation of risk factors for hypertension, a search for potential secondary causes of hypertension, and an evaluation for end-organ damage.

BP should be repeatedly measured on at least three occasions to confirm persistent hypertension by the techniques described in Chapter 32. Home BP monitoring or 24-hour ambulatory BP monitoring (see Chapter 32) is recommended to determine if the hypertension occurs only in the physician's office (white coat hypertension) and rarely to identify masked hypertension, in which elevations in BP occur only outside the physician's office. Because white coat and masked hypertension can be associated with end-organ disease (including left ventricular hypertrophy and microalbuminuria), diagnosis should be followed by assessment of cardiovascular risk factors and frequent re-evaluation of BP.

The history should investigate the onset and duration of hypertension and the presence of a family history of hypertension or cardiorenal disease. The history should identify risk factors for hypertension (obesity, diabetes, physical activity, alcohol, smoking, diet, emotional or work-related stress, and over-the-counter and prescribed medications) and any hypertension-related morbidity. Hypertension is often considered asymptomatic, but there is increasing evidence that it can be associated with reduction in memory and mental performance, and hypertension remains a major risk factor for vascular dementia. Good BP control may both improve mental performance and decrease the risk for development of dementia.[22,23]

Hypertension, especially stage 2 (see Fig. 33.2), may also be associated with headache (classically occipital and pulsatile). In hypertension emergency, encephalopathy may rarely occur with an acute decrease in mental status or seizures. Rarely, patients may lose vision from papilledema. Severe hypertension may also place individuals at acute risk for myocardial infarction, congestive heart failure with pulmonary edema, aortic dissection, stroke, and renal failure.

Physical examination should include measurement of BP in both arms and a careful cardiac examination. Attention should be focused on both the large vessels (by both palpation and listening for bruits) and the retina to grade the severity of disease in the microvasculature (Fig. 33.9).

Laboratory tests should include hematocrit, electrolyte values, creatinine concentration, calcium and phosphate concentrations, fasting lipid profile (cholesterol and triglycerides), uric acid level, C-reactive protein level, and urinalysis, including a spot urine albumin to creatinine ratio for microalbuminuria. Chest radiography and electrocardiography should also be performed to assess cardiac size and the presence of left ventricular hypertrophy and to look for aortic dilation.

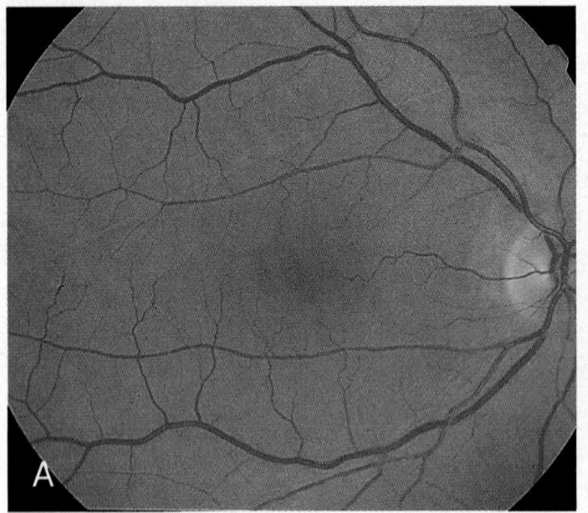

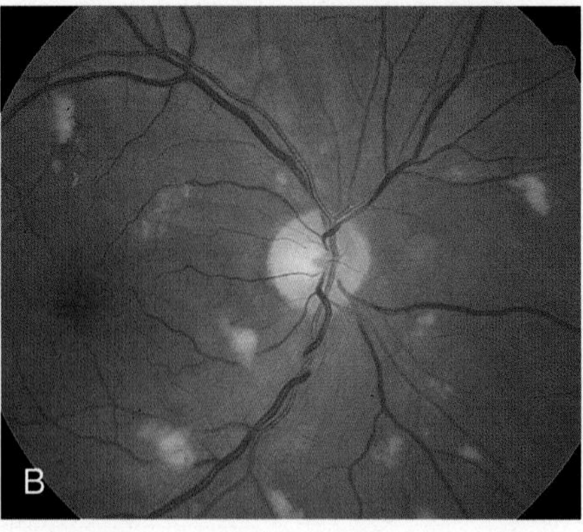

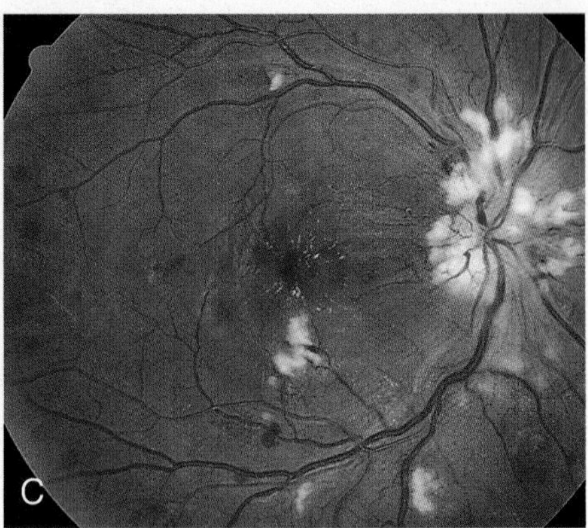

Figure 33.9 Different grades of hypertensive retinopathy. A, Mild hypertensive retinopathy, with arteriolar narrowing and arteriovenous nicking. **B,** Moderate hypertensive retinopathy, with cotton wool spots (nerve fiber layer infarcts) and arteriovenous nicking. **C,** Malignant hypertension with papilledema, cotton-wool spots, macular yellow exudates (star formation pattern), and retinal hemorrhages. *(Gift J. Kinyoun, Seattle, Washington, USA.)*

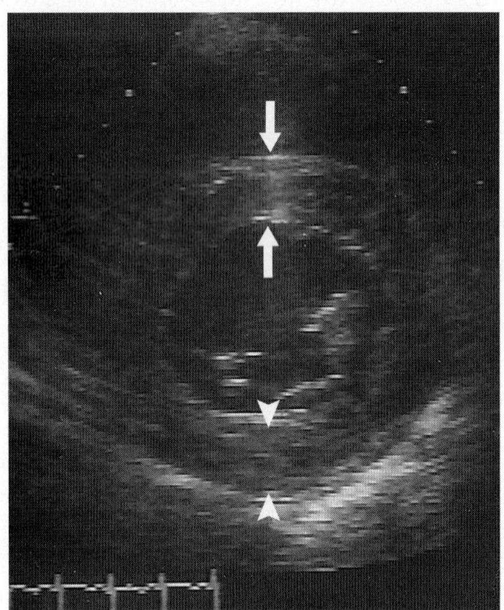

Figure 33.10 Echocardiogram showing concentric left ventricular hypertrophy. Septal thickness *(between large arrows)* and posterior wall thickness *(between arrowheads)* are increased (to 16 mm) in a patient with primary hypertension (normal is 11 mm or less). *(Gift of A. Pearlman, Seattle, Washington, USA.)*

Additional tests that may be helpful include an estimated GFR and, under certain circumstances, a 24-hour urine sodium and potassium determination. Urinary excretion will correlate closely with intake if the patient is in steady state (the desirable values are <100 mmol/l Na^+ and >100 mmol/l K^+ in 24 hours). A spot urine albumin to creatinine ratio and an echocardiogram may uncover additional evidence of end-organ damage (Fig. 33.10). Note that a spot urine albumin to creatinine ratio is recommended only for those with diabetes or stage 2 or higher CKD. Echocardiography is not recommended for routine use in people with hypertension because of its cost, although it is appropriate for people with cardiac problems.

PATHOLOGY

Primary hypertension has characteristic renal pathology in which there is preferential involvement of the preglomerular arterial vessels, primarily the afferent arteriole and interlobular artery. The classic vascular lesion, seen in 90% of cases, is arteriolosclerosis, in which smooth muscle cells of the media in the afferent arteriole are replaced by connective tissue (Fig. 33.11).[24] The arteriolar lesions are often associated with the accumulation of hyaline material (plasma proteins) in the subintima (hyalinosis). In addition, there is often evidence of glomerular and tubulointerstitial ischemia with shrinkage of the glomerular tuft, tubular atrophy, and interstitial fibrosis. On occasion, glomerulosclerosis and severe tubulointerstitial injury are seen. In cases of hypertensive emergency, there is a proliferative arteriolopathy, occasionally with fibrinoid necrosis. Concentric layers of connective tissue and cells may give an onion-skin appearance to the intima, which may progress to a total obliteration of the lumen.

DIAGNOSIS AND DIFFERENTIAL DIAGNOSIS

The diagnosis of primary hypertension requires the elimination of secondary causes, of which the more common include medication (nonsteroidal agents, corticosteroids, sympathomimetics, oral contraceptives), drugs (excessive alcohol intake, cocaine), intrinsic renal parenchymal disease, renovascular disease, and primary aldosteronism from adrenal hyperplasia or tumors. Hyperuricemia may also be a cause of some forms of primary hypertension, especially in the adolescent. A more complete list along with the recommended evaluation for secondary causes is provided in Chapter 32.

NATURAL HISTORY

The major long-term risk of hypertension is cardiovascular disease, which can be separated into pressure-related (stroke, heart failure), atherosclerotic (myocardial infarction), and renal (CKD) etiologies. Hypertension is the most common cause of stroke and congestive heart failure, and the risk increases linearly with BP (Fig. 33.12).[25] Other pressure-related morbidities include aortic dissection and cerebral and aortic aneurysms. Increased systolic, diastolic, and pulse pressure all confer risk, although the systolic BP and the pulse pressure are the more important determinants of risk for the pressure-related morbidities. This increased risk is dependent on age (increases with age), sex (greater in males), ethnic origin (greater in African Americans), and other associated risk factors (e.g., diabetes).

Hypertensive heart disease begins with concentric left ventricular hypertrophy associated with supernormal systolic function. Over time, impaired diastolic dysfunction may occur, as

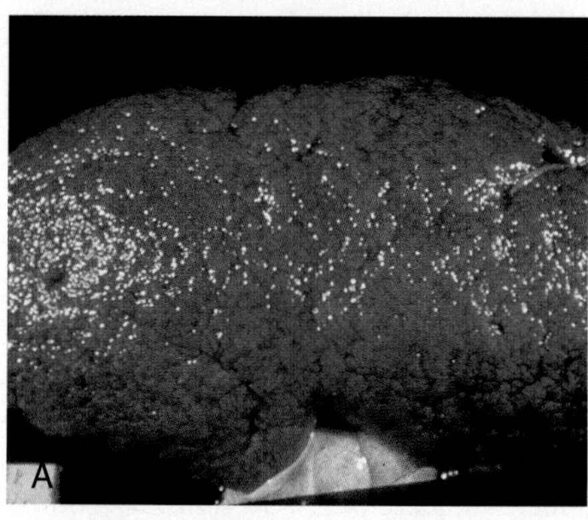

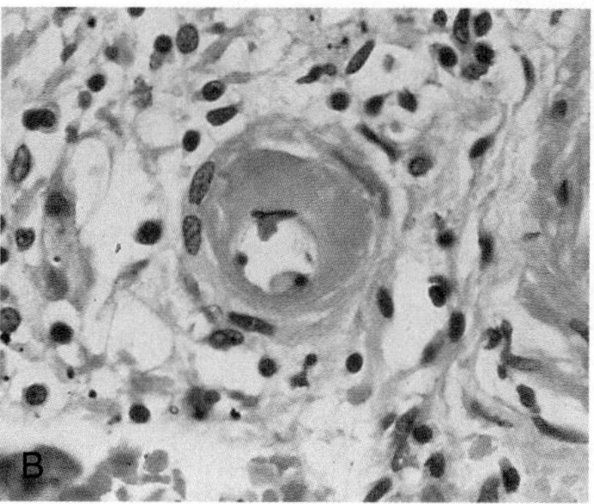

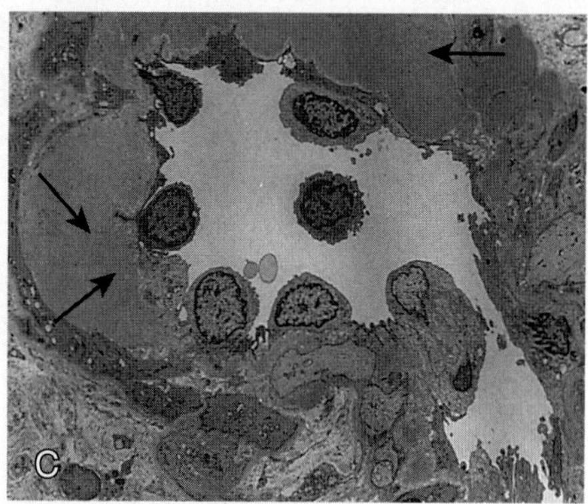

Figure 33.11 Renal pathology in primary hypertension. A, A granular pitted kidney of benign nephrosclerosis. **B,** Arteriolosclerosis with subintimal hyalinosis. **C,** Electron micrograph showing hyalinosis with the accumulation of insudative plasma proteins in the subendothelium of an arteriole. *(**A,** gift of Harvard Medical School; **B** and **C** from C. E. Alpers, Seattle, Washington, USA.)*

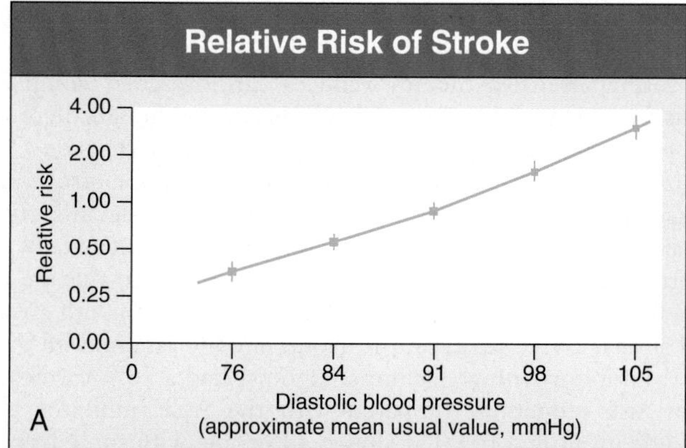

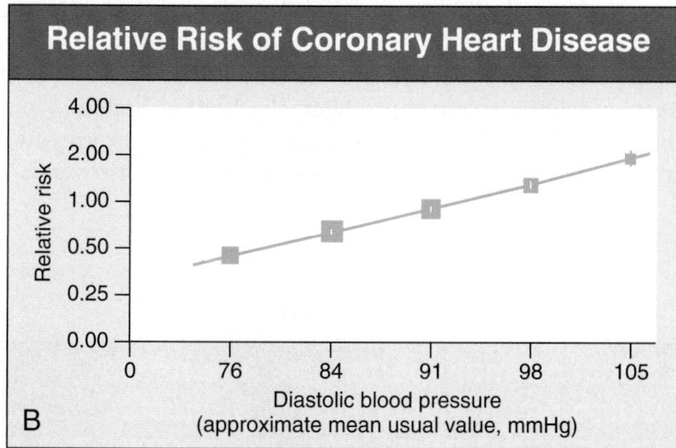

Figure 33.12 Relative risks for stroke (A) and coronary heart disease (B) increase with higher diastolic blood pressure. The stroke data are from seven prospective observational studies and 843 events; the coronary heart disease data are from nine studies and 4856 events. Size of squares is proportional to the number of events in each category; the vertical lines indicate 95% confidence intervals. *(Modified with permission from reference 25.)*

manifested by slow diastolic filling, which reflects decreased diastolic relaxation. This may progress to congestive heart failure. Nearly 90% of patients with heart failure have a history of hypertension.

Hypertension also confers risk for atherosclerotic-associated morbidities, including coronary heart disease,[25] peripheral vascular disease, and carotid atherosclerosis with or without cerebral emboli. In addition to an increased prevalence of hypertension, African Americans also have a 50% greater risk for heart disease.

Kidney Disease

Most patients with newly diagnosed primary hypertension will have normal renal function or stage 1 (GFR >90 ml/min per 1.73 m^2 with microalbuminuria) or stage 2 (GFR 60 to 90 ml/min per 1.7 3 m^2) CKD with elevated renal vascular resistance.[20] Despite relatively normal renal function, renal biopsy, if it is done, usually shows arteriolosclerosis and hyalinosis (see Fig. 33.11).

Before effective antihypertensive agents, proteinuria developed in up to 40% of patients, and as many as 18% developed renal insufficiency over time. Currently, microalbuminuria, which is a marker of vascular disease and cardiovascular risk, occurs in 15% to 30% of patients, and fewer patients develop non-nephrotic or, rarely, nephrotic-range proteinuria.[26] The development of microalbuminuria is associated with salt sensitivity, with the loss of nocturnal dipping in BP, and with increased target organ damage (especially left ventricular hypertrophy). Elevations in serum creatinine develop in 10% to 20% of patients with poorly controlled BP, and the risk is greater in African Americans, in the elderly, and in those with higher systolic BP (systolic BP >160 mm Hg).[27,28] In 2% to 5% with poorly controlled systolic BP (i.e., >160 mm Hg), progression to renal failure will occur during the subsequent 10 to 15 years (Figs. 33.13 and 33.14). Despite the relative infrequency for progression of hypertension to end-stage renal disease (ESRD), hypertension is recorded as the second most common cause of ESRD after diabetes in the United States and Europe. Furthermore, almost all patients with diabetes have hypertension when they start dialysis.

The incidence of ESRD secondary to hypertension is fourfold to sixfold greater in African Americans.[29] Renal biopsy specimens of African Americans with hypertension tend to show more severe forms of hypertensive injury, with more prominent vascular changes and increased frequency of segmental and global glomerulosclerosis. Whereas some of these vascular changes may relate to the presence of certain transforming growth factor β polymorphisms or higher uric acid levels that are common in this population, studies suggest that the increased frequency of glomerulosclerosis may be due to polymorphisms in the gene encoding apolipoprotein L-1 (APOL-1), which became prevalent in the African population since it confers protection from African sleeping sickness (trypanosomiasis) but which has the disadvantage of increasing the risk for focal segemental glomerulosclerosis (FSG) in the presence of hypertension.[30,31] The

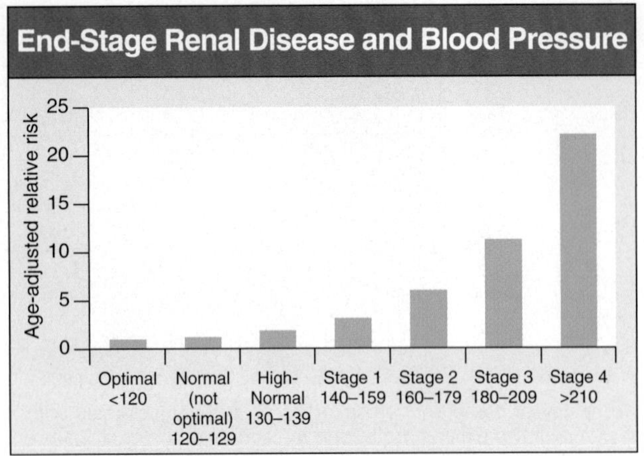

Figure 33.13 End-stage renal disease and blood pressure (ESRD). Incidence of ESRD related to baseline blood pressure in the MRFIT study. Mean follow-up was 16 years. *(From reference 27.)*

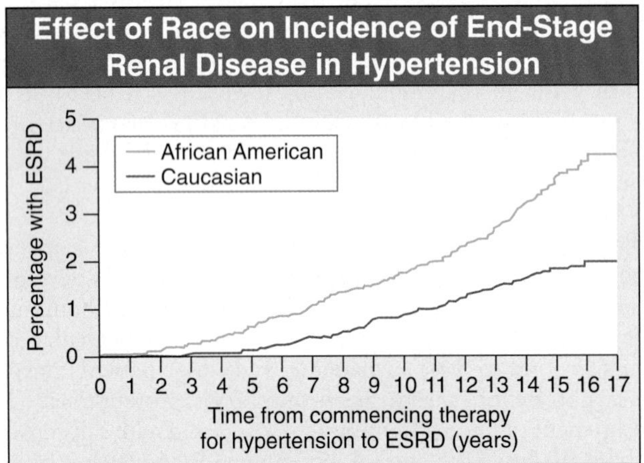

Figure 33.14 Effect of race on incidence of end-stage renal disease (ESRD) in hypertension. The rate of ESRD in African American and Caucasian hypertensive veterans. (Kaplan-Meier estimates). *(From reference 28.)*

observation that much of the increased risk for renal failure in the African American may be accounted for by APOL-1 polymorphisms raises the question of how often stage 1 hypertension itself may cause ESRD in this cohort.

Effect of Antihypertensive Therapy on the Natural History of Hypertensive Cardiovascular Disease and Kidney Disease Progression

According to a recent report, only 59% of subjects with hypertension in the United States are receiving treatment, and only 34% have their BP under adequate (<140/90 mm Hg) control.[2] Although there has been significant reduction in the age-adjusted death rate for stroke and coronary artery disease since the early 1980s as a result of better BP control (and better treatment of other risk factors, such as hyperlipidemia), heart disease and stroke remain the first and third leading causes of death in the United States. This emphasizes the importance of identifying and treating patients with hypertension.

Antihypertensive therapy reduces cardiovascular complications in patients with stage 2 hypertension, although there are far fewer data to support this for stage 1 hypertension (Fig. 33.15).[32] The reduced risk is most significant for stroke and congestive heart failure but also occurs for myocardial infarction. In all trials, to date, it is the group with the best overall BP control that has the best result.[33] One exception to this are the data from the recent ACCOMPLISH trial, in which both groups had similar BP control, yet the group initially randomized to an ACE inhibitor with a calcium antagonist had a 20% cardiovascular risk reduction compared with the ACE inhibitor plus diuretic group.[34] Note that almost all people with some level of kidney disease will require two or more medications. Diuretics are better initially for lowering BP and required in those with renal insufficiency but are not considered initial agents of choice by any guidelines except those from the United States.

The effect of antihypertensive therapy on the progression of renal disease secondary to hypertension is more controversial. In

Meta-Analysis of Effect of Antihypertensive Agents On Cardiovascular Outcomes in Hypertensive Subjects

Outcome	No. of Trials	Effects Model	RR (95% CI)	*P* Value for Heterogeneity
Coronary heart disease	24	Fixed	0.86 (0.80-0.93)	.55
		Random	0.87 (0.80-0.94)	.55
Stroke	23	Fixed	0.69 (0.64-0.74)	.004
		Random	0.68 (0.61-0.76)	.004
CHF	7	Fixed	0.54 (0.45-0.66)	.66
		Random	0.60 (0.49-0.74)	.80
Major CVD events	28	Fixed	0.78 (0.74-0.81)	<.001
		Random	0.73 (0.62-0.87)	<.001
CVD mortality	23	Fixed	0.84 (0.78-0.90)	.10
		Random	0.84 (0.78-0.90)	.10
Total mortality	25	Fixed	0.90 (0.85-0.95)	.58
		Random	0.90 (0.85-0.95)	.59

Figure 33.15 Meta-analysis of effect of antihypertensive agents on cardiovascular outcomes in hypertensive subjects. The analysis was based on 42 clinical trials that included 192,478 patients randomized to seven major treatment strategies, including placebo. CHF, congestive heart failure; CI, confidence interval; CVD, cardiovascular disease; RR, relative risk. *The no treatment comparison group includes placebo-treated controls, participants not treated in open trials, and participants receiving usual care. *(Reprinted with permission from reference 32.)*

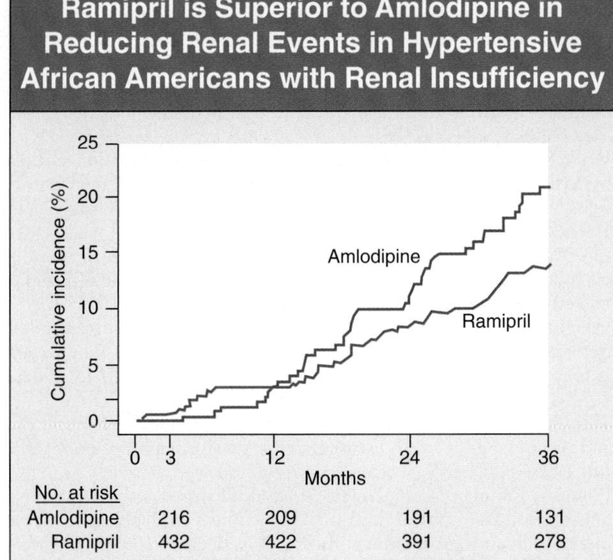

Figure 33.16 Ramipril is superior to amlodipine in reducing renal events in hypertensive African Americans with mild to moderate renal insufficiency. The ACE inhibitor ramipril resulted in fewer renal end points (proteinuria, decline in renal function, ESRD, or death) compared with the dihydropyridine calcium channel blocker amlodipine in the African American Study of Kidney Disease. ACE, angiotensin-converting enzyme; ESRD, end-stage renal disease. *(Reprinted with permission from reference 36.)*

the Multiple Risk Factor Intervention Trial (MRFIT), in which diuretics and β-blockers were primarily used to control BP, slowing or stabilization of renal function was observed only in nonblack as opposed to African American men.[35] In the African American Study of Kidney Disease, the use of an ACE inhibitor (ramipril) was found to be more effective at slowing renal progression compared with either the dihydropyridine calcium channel blocker amlodipine (Fig. 33.16) or metoprolol.[36,37] However, both this study and others have failed to show superior protection with tight BP control compared with conventional BP targets in subjects with renal disease secondary to hypertension.[37,38] Masked hypertension may be a confounder to these results; a subanalysis of ambulatory BP showed inadequate 24-hour BP control in more than 70% of the cohort. Masked hypertension and nondipping (i.e., the lack of fall in BP with sleep) were the two most common reasons for poor BP control.[39] Further studies regarding the dosing and timing of antihypertensive treatment are being performed to evaluate changes in overall BP control. In contrast, *post hoc* analyses of trials show that subjects with diabetic renal disease or with proteinuric (>300 mg/day) renal disease, including that due to hypertension, do appear to benefit from lower BP goals in terms of renal protection. On the basis of current evidence, achieved BP levels should be below 140 mm Hg systolic for nonproteinuric hypertensive renal disease and below 130/80 mm Hg in those with diabetes and hypertensive subjects with proteinuria.[40]

Finally, a number of studies suggest that thiazide diuretics are associated with worsening of renal function in subjects with hypertension. In the European Working Party on High Blood Pressure in the Elderly trial, a significantly higher incidence of impaired renal function was found in those receiving diuretics compared with placebo.[41] In the Systolic Hypertension in the Elderly trial, serum creatinine increased significantly in the subjects treated with thiazide diuretics compared with placebo.[42] In the Antihypertensive and Lipid-Lowering Treatment to Prevent Heart Attack Trial (ALLHAT), the chlorthalidone-treated group showed a statistically worse renal function than either the amlodipine- or lisinopril-treated group at both the 2- and 4-year end points.[43] Whereas this could probably be accounted for by volume depletion in many cases, diuretics have been shown to induce mild renal injury in various animal models, possibly as a consequence of hypokalemia, hyperuricemia, and stimulation of the renin-angiotensin-aldosterone system related to the reduction in renal perfusion pressure.[44]

Can Primary Hypertension Spontaneously Remit?

Before the age of 60 years, as many as 15% to 20% of patients with prehypertension may become normotensive spontaneously. Furthermore, in patients with established hypertension who have good BP control for 5 years with treatment, as many as 20% to 40% can be withdrawn from therapy successfully, especially if they have stage 1 hypertension and adhere to salt restriction and weight reduction. This suggests that the processes that mediate hypertension are at times reversible.

REFERENCES

1. Bevan AT, Honour AJ, Stott FH. Direct arterial pressure recording in unrestricted man. *Br Heart J.* 1969;31:387-388.
2. Chobanian AV, Bakris GL, Black HR, et al. The Seventh Report of the Joint National Committee on Prevention, Detection, Evaluation, and Treatment of High Blood Pressure: The JNC 7 report. *JAMA.* 2003;289:2560-2572.
3. Guyton AC, Coleman TG, Cowley AV Jr, et al. Arterial pressure regulation. Overriding dominance of the kidneys in long-term regulation and in hypertension. *Am J Med.* 1972;52:584-594.
4. Lifton RP. Genetic dissection of human blood pressure variation: Common pathways from rare phenotypes. *Harvey Lect.* 2004;100:71-101.
5. Ji W, Foo JN, O'Roak BJ, et al. Rare independent mutations in renal salt handling genes contribute to blood pressure variation. *Nat Genet.* 2008;40:592-599.
6. Barker DJ, Osmond C, Golding J, et al. Growth in utero, blood pressure in childhood and adult life, and mortality from cardiovascular disease. *BMJ.* 1989;298:564-567.
7. Brenner BM, Garcia DL, Anderson S. Glomeruli and blood pressure. Less of one, more the other? *Am J Hypertens.* 1988;1:335-347.
8. Keller G, Zimmer G, Mall G, et al. Nephron number in patients with primary hypertension. *N Engl J Med.* 2003;348:101-108.
9. Eriksson J, Forsen T, Tuomilehto J, et al. Fetal and childhood growth and hypertension in adult life. *Hypertension.* 2000;36:790-794.
10. Johnson RJ, Rodriguez-Iturbe B, Kang DH, et al. A unifying pathway for essential hypertension. *Am J Hypertens.* 2005;18:431-440.
11. Wofford MR, Hall JE. Pathophysiology and treatment of obesity hypertension. *Curr Pharm Des.* 2004;10:3621-3637.
12. Johnson RJ, Segal MS, Sautin Y, et al. Potential role of sugar (fructose) in the epidemic of hypertension, obesity and the metabolic syndrome, diabetes, kidney disease, and cardiovascular disease. *Am J Clin Nutr.* 2007;86:899-906.
13. Feig DI, Soletsky B, Johnson RJ. Effect of allopurinol on the blood pressure of adolescents with newly diagnosed essential hypertension. *JAMA.* 2008;300:922-930.
14. Julius S. The evidence for a pathophysiologic significance of the sympathetic overactivity in hypertension. *Clin Exp Hypertens.* 1996;18:305-321.
15. Schjoedt KJ, Andersen S, Rossing P, et al. Aldosterone escape during blockade of the renin-angiotensin-aldosterone system in diabetic nephropathy is associated with enhanced decline in glomerular filtration rate. *Diabetologia.* 2004;47:1936-1939.
16. Ubaid-Girioli S, Ferreira-Melo SE, Souza LA, et al. Aldosterone escape with diuretic or angiotensin-converting enzyme inhibitor/angiotensin II receptor blocker combination therapy in patients with mild to moderate hypertension. *J Clin Hypertens (Greenwich).* 2007;9:770-774.

17. Hamlyn JM, Ringel R, Schaeffer J, et al. A circulating inhibitor of (Na^+ + K^+)ATPase associated with essential hypertension. *Nature*. 1982; 300:650-652.
18. Bakris G, Bursztyn M, Gavras I, et al. Role of vasopressin in essential hypertension: Racial differences. *J Hypertens*. 1997;15:545-550.
19. DiBona GF, Kopp UC. Neural control of renal function. *Physiol Rev*. 1997;77:75-197.
20. Johnson RJ, Segal MS, Srinivas T, et al. Essential hypertension, progressive renal disease, and uric acid: A pathogenetic link? *J Am Soc Nephrol*. 2005;16:1909-1919.
21. Burt VL, Whelton P, Roccella EJ, et al. Prevalence of hypertension in the US adult population. Results from the Third National Health and Nutrition Examination Survey, 1988-1991. *Hypertension*. 1995;25: 305-313.
22. Forette F, Seux ML, Staessen JA, et al. Prevention of dementia in randomised double-blind placebo-controlled Systolic Hypertension in Europe (Syst-Eur) trial. *Lancet*. 1998;352:1347-1351.
23. Goldstein G, Materson BJ, Cushman WC, et al. Treatment of hypertension in the elderly: II. Cognitive and behavioral function. Results of a Department of Veterans Affairs Cooperative Study. *Hypertension*. 1990; 15:361-369.
24. Sommers SC, Relman AS, Smithwick RH. Histologic studies of kidney biopsy specimens from patients with hypertension. *Am J Pathol*. 1958;34:685-715.
25. MacMahon S, Peto R, Cutler J, et al. Blood pressure, stroke, and coronary heart disease. Part 1, Prolonged differences in blood pressure: Prospective observational studies corrected for the regression dilution bias. *Lancet*. 1990;335:765-774.
26. Bakris GL. *Microalbuminuria: Marker of Kidney and Cardiovascular Disease*. London: Current Medicine Group; 2007.
27. Klag MJ, Whelton PK, Randall BL, et al. Blood pressure and end-stage renal disease in men. *N Engl J Med*. 1996;334:13-18.
28. Perry HM Jr, Miller JP, Fornoff JR, et al. Early predictors of 15-year end-stage renal disease in hypertensive patients. *Hypertension*. 1995;25: 587-594.
29. Sarafidis PA, Li S, Chen SC, et al. Hypertension awareness, treatment, and control in chronic kidney disease. *Am J Med*. 2008;121:332-340.
30. Genovese G, Friedman DJ, Ross MD, et al. Association of Trypanolytic ApoL1 Variants with Kidney Disease in African-Americans. *Science*. 2010 in press.
31. Tzur S, Rosset S, Shemer R, et al. Missense mutations in the *APOL1* gene are highly associated with end stage kidney disease risk previously attributed to the *MYH9* gene. *Human Genetics*. 2010 (in press).
32. Psaty BM, Lumley T, Furberg CD, et al. Health outcomes associated with various antihypertensive therapies used as first-line agents: A network meta-analysis. *JAMA*. 2003;289:2534-2544.
33. Turnbull F, Neal B, Ninomiya T, et al. Effects of different regimens to lower blood pressure on major cardiovascular events in older and younger adults: Meta-analysis of randomised trials. *BMJ*. 2008;336: 1121-1123.
34. Jamerson K, Weber MA, Bakris GL, et al. Benazepril plus amlodipine or hydrochlorothiazide for hypertension in high-risk patients. *N Engl J Med*. 2008;359:2417-2428.
35. Walker WG, Neaton JD, Cutler JA, et al. Renal function change in hypertensive members of the Multiple Risk Factor Intervention Trial. Racial and treatment effects. The MRFIT Research Group. *JAMA*. 1992;268:3085-3091.
36. Agodoa LY, Appel L, Bakris GL, et al. Effect of ramipril vs amlodipine on renal outcomes in hypertensive nephrosclerosis: A randomized controlled trial. *JAMA*. 2001;285:2719-2728.
37. Wright JT Jr, Bakris G, Greene T, et al. Effect of blood pressure lowering and antihypertensive drug class on progression of hypertensive kidney disease: Results from the AASK trial. *JAMA*. 2002;288: 2421-2431.
38. Toto RD, Mitchell HC, Smith RD, et al. "Strict" blood pressure control and progression of renal disease in hypertensive nephrosclerosis. *Kidney Int*. 1995;48:851-859.
39. Pogue V, Rahman M, Lipkowitz M, et al. Disparate estimates of hypertension control from ambulatory and clinic blood pressure measurements in hypertensive kidney disease. *Hypertension*. 2009;53:20-27.
40. KDOQI Clinical Practice Guidelines and Clinical Practice Recommendations for Diabetes and Chronic Kidney Disease. *Am J Kidney Dis*. 2007;49:S12-S154.
41. Fletcher A, Amery A, Birkenhager W, et al. Risks and benefits in the trial of the European Working Party on High Blood Pressure in the Elderly. *J Hypertens*. 1991;9:225-230.
42. Savage PJ, Pressel SL, Curb JD, et al. Influence of long-term, low-dose, diuretic-based, antihypertensive therapy on glucose, lipid, uric acid, and potassium levels in older men and women with isolated systolic hypertension: The Systolic Hypertension in the Elderly Program. SHEP Cooperative Research Group. *Arch Intern Med*. 1998;158: 741-751.
43. Major outcomes in high-risk hypertensive patients randomized to angiotensin-converting enzyme inhibitor or calcium channel blocker vs diuretic: The Antihypertensive and Lipid-Lowering Treatment to Prevent Heart Attack Trial (ALLHAT). *JAMA*. 2002;288:2981-2997.
44. Reungjui S, Hu H, Mu W, et al. Thiazide-induced subtle renal injury not observed in states of equivalent hypokalemia. *Kidney Int*. 2007;72: 1483-1492.

CHAPTER 34

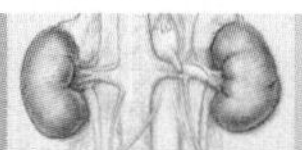

Nonpharmacologic Prevention and Treatment of Hypertension

Brian Rayner, Karen E. Charlton, Estelle V. Lambert, Wayne Derman

Lifestyle changes, including a combination of increased fat and refined carbohydrate intake and reduced physical activity, have resulted in an epidemic of obesity, type 2 diabetes mellitus, and hypertension. The epidemic is evident worldwide and often is greatest in underserved and indigenous populations.

Adoption of healthy lifestyles is critical for both the prevention of high blood pressure (BP) and its management. According to the Seventh Report of the Joint National Committee on Prevention, Evaluation, and Treatment of High Blood Pressure (JNC 7),[1] lifestyle interventions lower BP, enhance efficacy of antihypertensive medication, and lower overall cardiovascular risk. The lifestyle changes that are widely agreed to lower BP and cardiovascular risk are (1) smoking cessation, (2) weight reduction, (3) moderation of alcohol intake, (4) physical exercise, (5) reduction of salt intake, (6) increase in fruit and vegetable intake, and (7) decrease in saturated and total fat intake.[1]

Interventions may have efficacy similar to that of single-drug therapy (Fig. 34.1). However, lifestyle changes should not delay the initiation of drug therapy in patients at higher cardiovascular risk.

PREVENTION

The importance of primary prevention has been underscored by the recognition that the treatment of hypertension is expensive, the control of BP in hypertensive individuals does not restore cardiovascular risk to normal, and the majority of hypertensive individuals do not reach goal BP. The most important subjects to target are those with prehypertension (defined by JNC 7 as 120 to 139/80 to 89 mm Hg; see Chapter 33).[1] Individuals with prehypertension have an increased prevalence of early vascular damage, an increased risk of incident hypertension, and an increased risk of cardiovascular events compared with those with optimal levels (<120/80 mm Hg).[2] The JNC 7 recommends lifestyle changes in all patients with prehypertension to prevent hypertension and to reduce their cardiovascular risk.[1]

The contribution of body weight, physical inactivity, and dietary factors to the prevalence of hypertension in Europe and the United States has been quantified in a meta-regression analysis.[3] Being overweight made the largest contribution to hypertension, with population-attributable risk percentages (PAR%) between 11% (Italy) and 25% (United States). PAR% was 5% to 13% for physical inactivity, 9% to 17% for high sodium intake, 4% to 17% for low potassium intake, and 4% to 8% for low magnesium intake. The impact of alcohol was small (2% to 3%) in all populations. PAR% varied among populations for inadequate intake of calcium (2% to 8%), coffee (0% to 9%), and fish fatty acids (3% to 16%).

WEIGHT LOSS

Obesity is epidemic throughout the world, and 65% of the adult population in the United States is either overweight (body mass index [BMI], 25.0 to 29.9) or obese (BMI ≥30).[4] Obese individuals have a threefold increased prevalence of hypertension. Possible mechanisms for obesity-induced hypertension include overactivity of the sympathetic nervous system (RAS), hyperinsulinemia (which may increase renal sodium reabsorption), hyperuricemia, activation of the renin-angiotensin system, and sleep apnea. Abdominal or visceral obesity is a greater predictor of both hypertension and cardiovascular risk than is a predominant lower body fat distribution. Abdominal obesity is defined as a waist circumference of more than 88 cm (35 inches) in women and more than 102 cm (40 inches) in men. These reference values were developed in Caucasian populations, and differing criteria may be more appropriate for other ethnic groups.

In obese hypertensives or those with high-normal BP, weight loss of as little as 4 to 5 kg is often associated with a significant reduction in BP. Weight loss is one of the most effective nonpharmacologic interventions to reduce BP.[5] A meta-analysis has demonstrated that a weight reduction of 5.1 kg reduced systolic BP by 4.44 mm Hg and diastolic BP by 3.57 mm Hg.[6] A rule of thumb is that for every kilogram lost, there is a reduction of 1 mm Hg in both systolic and diastolic BP. To minimize the risk of relapse and to maintain sustainability of the weight loss program, the initial target should be 5% to 10% of current weight, or 1 to 2 BMI units. Marked oscillations in weight should be avoided because this increases the risk for development of hypertension in obese, normotensive subjects.[7] A randomized trial of the effectiveness of four popular diets on sustained weight loss and cardiovascular disease risk reduction concluded that a variety of diets can similarly reduce weight and BP, but only a minority of individuals can sustain high dietary adherence. High-protein diets such as the Atkins diet, often advocated for weight loss by the media and lay public, have no place in hypertensive patients with renal disease.

Weight reduction should be accompanied by recommendations to increase physical activity unless it is contraindicated. Bariatric surgery, pharmacologic interventions for weight loss (e.g., sibutramine, orlistat), and very low calorie (liquid) diets or meal replacement diets may be useful to achieve weight loss in some patients, but always as an adjunct to rather than a substitute for lifestyle modification.

PHYSICAL ACTIVITY

Physical inactivity is associated with at least a 1.5- to 2-fold higher risk of hypertension and coronary heart disease.[8] Regular

Lifestyle Modifications for the Prevention and Management of Hypertension (Joint National Committee 7 Guidelines[1])		
Modification	**Recommendation**	**Average Systolic BP Reduction Range Achieved with Intervention***
Weight reduction	Maintain normal body weight (BMI = 18.5–24.9 kg/m^2)	5–20 mmHg/10 kg
DASH eating plan	Adopt a diet rich in fruits, vegetables, and low-fat dairy products with reduced content of saturated and total fat	8–14 mmHg
Dietary sodium restriction	Reduce dietary sodium intake to 100 mmol/day (2.4 g sodium or 6 g sodium chloride)	2–8 mmHg
Aerobic physical activity	Regular aerobic physical activity (e.g., brisk walking) at least 30 min/day, most days of the week	4–9 mmHg
Moderation of alcohol consumption	Men: limit to 2 drinks† per day; women and lighter-weight persons: limit to 1 drink per day	2–4 mmHg

Figure 34.1 Lifestyle modifications for the prevention and management of hypertension (Joint National Committee 7 guidelines[1]). BMI, body mass index; BP, blood pressure; DASH, Dietary Approaches to Stop Hypertension. *Effects are dose and time dependent. †One drink = ½ oz or 15 ml ethanol (e.g., 12 oz of beer, 5 oz of wine, 1.5 oz of 80-proof whiskey).

physical activity is known to lower the risk of all-cause morbidity and mortality and provides the basis for public health recommendations to exercise at least 30 minutes per day.

Exercise Training Dose Response

In a meta-analysis of studies involving more than 1500 patients, exercise training in normotensive subjects has been shown to reduce systolic and diastolic BP by 3.0 ± 1 and 1.7 ± 1 mm Hg, respectively.[9] In hypertensive subjects, the effect of exercise training is even more marked (a reduction of 7.8 ± 3.5 and 5.8 ± 2.0 mm Hg for systolic and diastolic BP, respectively). Studies in hypertensive subjects have shown that the benefit of exercise on BP is maximal with 90 minutes of exercise per week, after which there was no further improvement.[10] Furthermore, only a modest amount of exercise was needed to reduce BP in patients with hypertension (>30 min/wk).

Fagard[9] found no benefit of increasing exercise intensity on BP reduction with exercise training, as long as intensity ranged between 40% and 70% of maximal, age-predicted heart rate. This contrasts with the acute effects of exercise on the attenuation of postexercise BP. Exercise of higher intensity (75% maximum) was associated with a more marked and prolonged reduction in BP in the postexercise window compared with lower intensity exercise (50% maximum).[11] In addition, regular exercise prevents the development of left ventricular hypertrophy that is independent of BP in young stage 1 hypertensive subjects.[12]

Mechanisms

In the acute postexercise period, the reduction in BP has been linked to a sympathetic inhibition and increased release of vasodilator substances.[13] The mechanisms by which chronic exercise lowers BP are less well understood but include reductions in systemic vascular resistance secondary to neurohumoral and structural adaptations. Chronic exercise is also associated with a loss of weight and a reduction of serum uric acid levels, both of which could potentially lead to a reduction in BP.

Antihypertensive Medication and Guidelines for Exercise

Exercise guidelines for patients with hypertension are shown in Figure 34.2.[14] β-Blockers decrease exercise tolerance. β-Blockers and diuretics may also alter thermoregulation in hot environments and provoke hypoglycemia. Patients using these medications should be educated about exercising in the heat, clothing, the role of adequate hydration, and methods to prevent hypoglycemia.[15,16] Angiotensin-converting enzyme (ACE) inhibitors, angiotensin receptor blockers (ARBs), and calcium channel blockers may be better suited for patients who exercise frequently or athletes with hypertension.

For patients undergoing supervised exercise training, the monitoring of postexercise BP may be helpful so that medications may be adjusted appropriately, considering the likelihood of postexercise hypotension. Particular care should be taken with patients planning to exercise in a hot environment.

DIET

Salt Intake

Epidemiologic studies have demonstrated that the prevalence of hypertension is directly related to the dietary salt intake in societies throughout the world in whom the intake is above 50 to 100 mmol/day or 3 to 6 g sodium chloride (Fig. 34.3).[17] Where daily intake is below that range, hypertension is rare. Salt intake also plays an important role in the age-related increase in BP (Fig. 34.4).[18]

Not all individuals respond similarly to high salt intake. Salt sensitivity describes a group of individuals who significantly decrease or increase their BP during periods of salt restriction or loading, respectively. Conversely, salt-resistant subjects have minimal BP response to changes in salt intake,[19] and it has been argued that a high salt intake may not be detrimental in salt-resistant subjects and that salt restriction should not be universally recommended. However, a prospective study of 1173 men and 1263 women in Finland found that coronary heart disease,

Practical Guidelines for Exercise in Patients with Hypertension
All apparently healthy individuals should undergo pre-exercise screening to determine health risk status. The American College of Sports Medicine (ACSM) recognizes that two or more of the following risk factors increase the risk associated with exercise, and individuals should undergo pre-exercise graded exercise testing. Risk factors include male gender (older than age 45 years) or female gender (older than 55 years); serum cholesterol concentrations >5.2 mmol/l; impaired glucose tolerance or diabetes mellitus; smoking; obesity (BMI≥30); inactivity; and family history of cardiovascular disease.
Patients with uncontrolled hypertension should embark on exercise training only after evaluation and initiation of therapy. Furthermore, patients should not participate in an exercise training session if resting systolic blood pressure is >200 mmHg or diastolic blood pressure is >115 mmHg.
Many patients with hypertension are overweight and should therefore be encouraged to follow a program that combines both exercise training and restricted calorie intake.[14]
Type of exercise: this should be predominantly endurance physical activity including walking, jogging, cycling, swimming, or dancing. This should be supplemented by resistance exercise that can be prescribed according to the ACSM or American Heart Association guidelines.[15]
Frequency of exercise: most or preferably every day.
Intensity of exercise: moderate intensity at 40%–60% of VO_2 peak.
Duration of exercise: >30 minutes of continuous or accumulated moderate physical activity daily.

Figure 34.2 Practical guidelines for exercise in patients with hypertension. BMI, body mass index. *(Modified from references 14 and 15.)*

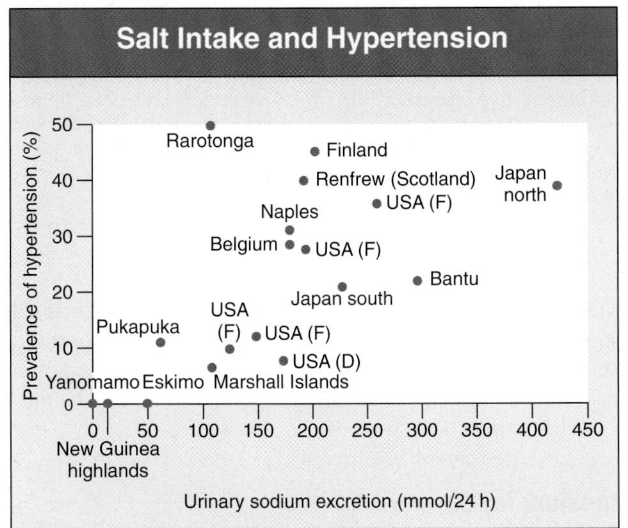

Figure 34.3 Relationship of salt intake with frequency of hypertension in different populations. D, data from Dahl. F, data from the Framingham study. *(Modified from reference 17.)*

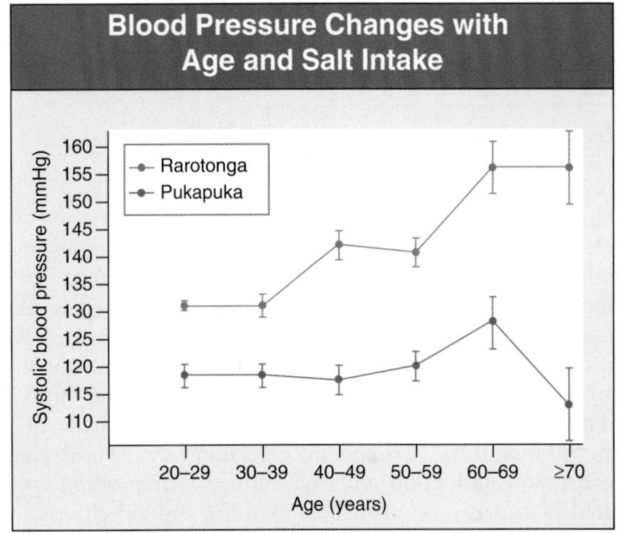

Figure 34.4 Blood pressure changes with age and salt intake. The increase in systolic blood pressure with age correlates with a higher salt intake in two Polynesian populations. In men of Rarotonga Island in Polynesia, where the sodium intake averages 130 mmol/day, systolic blood pressure increases with age. In contrast, it remains constant in men from Pukapuka Island, where the sodium intake averages 50 to 70 mmol/day. *(Modified from reference 18.)*

cardiovascular disease, and all-cause mortality increased significantly with increasing 24-hour urinary sodium excretion, independently of BP and other cardiovascular risk factors.[20] In a combined analysis of the Trials of Hypertension Prevention (TOHP) I and II, salt restriction not only reduced BP but also resulted in a 25% reduction in cardiovascular events.[21] Experimental studies in mice suggest that salt intake accelerates atherosclerosis by the intravascular generation of angiotensin II.[22]

There is no easy way to identify a patient with salt sensitivity, but a suppressed plasma renin activity may be a useful marker. Several studies have shown a higher frequency of salt sensitivity in the following groups of patients:

- African Americans;
- elderly people;
- obese subjects (not in all studies);
- type 1 and 2 diabetics;
- patients treated with calcineurin inhibitors; and
- patients with chronic kidney disease.

Salt sensitivity is observed in 75% of hypertensive African Americans compared with about 50% of Caucasian hypertensives[19] and increases with age in both normotensive and hypertensive populations (Fig. 34.5).[23] There is convincing reason to recommend universal salt restriction in all older people. A randomized, controlled trial in British people aged 60 to 78 years who were not receiving antihypertensive medication found that a modest salt restriction from 5 g to 10 g per day resulted in an impressive reduction of BP of 7.2/3.2 mm Hg during a 4-week period.[5,24] Importantly, unlike in studies of younger subjects, similar decreases in BP were seen for both normotensive and hypertensive subjects. These findings are consistent with predictions that a reduction in sodium intake of 50 mmol/day (about 3 g of salt) in older people would lower systolic BP by an average

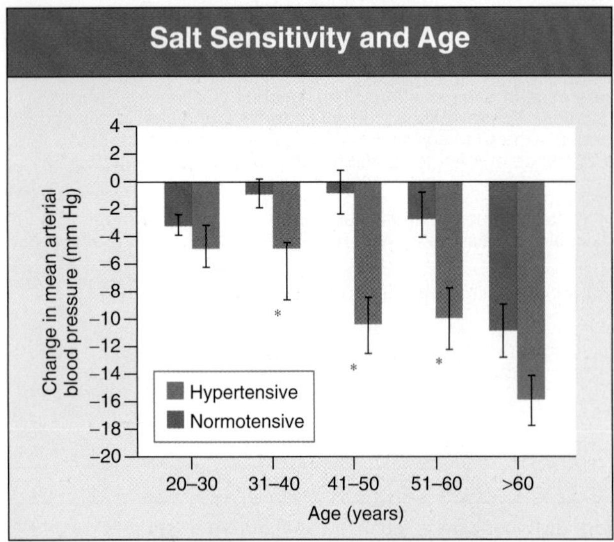

Figure 34.5 Increase in magnitude of salt sensitivity with increasing age. Salt sensitivity (determined by a standardized test evaluating the change in blood pressure from a volume-expanded to a contracted state) increases proportionately with age in both hypertensive and normotensive subjects (bars indicate standard error of the mean; $*P < .05$). *(Modified from reference 19.)*

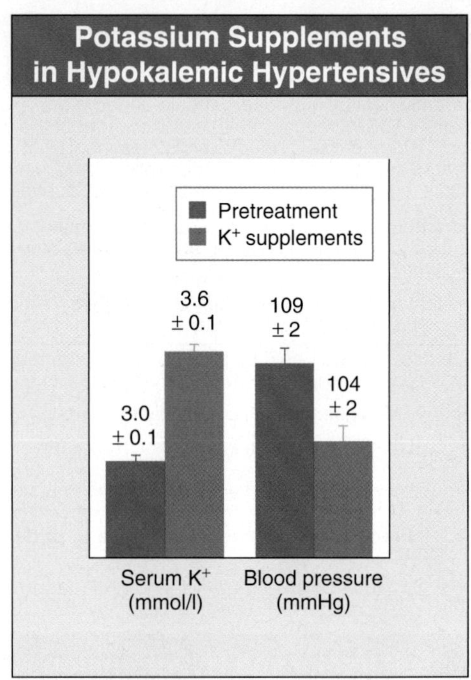

Figure 34.6 Potassium supplementation lowers blood pressure in hypokalemic hypertensive patients. Treatment with potassium chloride (60 mmol/day potassium for 6 weeks) resulted in an increase in serum potassium concentration and a decrease in mean arterial pressure in hypertensive patients taking thiazide diuretics. *(Redrawn from reference 31.)*

of 5 mm Hg,[25] which is estimated to reduce stroke by 36% during 5 years.

Putative mechanisms for salt sensitivity are alterations in circulating levels of (or renal responses to) atrial natriuretic factor, kallikrein, prostaglandins, and nitric oxide; increased levels of norepinephrine; abnormal suppression of both renin and aldosterone; genetic mechanisms; congenital reduction in nephron number; and acquired renal microvascular and tubular injury.[19,26]

The JNC 7 guidelines recommend a sodium intake of less than 100 mmol/day (6 g sodium chloride)[1]; the World Health Organization and Food and Agriculture Organization of the United Nations recommend less than 5 g sodium chloride per day as a population goal, while ensuring that the salt is iodized.[27] Avoidance of added salt and salt-rich processed foods can reduce intake from 9 g to about 6 g/day. Further reduction in salt requires specialized dietary counseling. Despite these recommendations, long-term studies have reported only small reductions in BP associated with salt restriction (an average of only 1.1/0.6 mm Hg).[28] These results undoubtedly reflect limited compliance, but this can be improved by regular contact with the patient, dietetic counseling, and educational sessions. Measurement of 24-hour urinary sodium is useful to check adherence with salt restriction (calculated as urine sodium [mmol/day] × 0.0585 = grams NaCl/day).

Population-Based Strategies to Lower Salt Intake

One of the most cost-effective ways to lower salt intake in the general population is to reduce salt in processed foods. This approach was effective in lowering the BP in drug-treated hypertensives in a low-income community setting in South Africa through the modification of the salt content of a small number of commonly consumed foods, including bread.[29] In Belgium, the reduction in the salt content of bread between the mid-1960s and the early 1980s was accompanied by marked reductions in 24-hour urinary sodium excretion. In recognition of the need for a concerted global effort to reduce population-wide salt intake, a World Health Organization Forum and Technical meeting in 2006 recommended an integrated approach incorporating a commitment by the food industry to product reformulation, increased consumer awareness, and social marketing around salt and health issues.[30]

Potassium Intake

One of the confounding factors of the relationship of salt and BP has been the inverse relationship between the intake of salt and potassium. Typically, diets with a high salt intake are relatively deficient in potassium (and calcium); but in those who consume little salt, the potassium (and calcium) intake is high. These disparate groups also differ in other factors, such as physical activity, industrialization of the society, and racial and genetic characteristics.

In normotensive subjects with an average potassium intake above 1.95 g/day (50 mmol/day), potassium supplementation has no significant effect on BP. However, among hypertensive subjects who are potassium deficient because of diuretic treatment or low potassium intake, potassium supplementation lowers BP (Fig. 34.6).[31] The Dietary Approaches to Stop Hypertension (DASH) diet lowers BP and is high in potassium because of the high fruit and vegetable content and inclusion of low-fat dairy products (Fig. 34.7).[32] However, the synergistic effect of the various food groups in the DASH diet makes it difficult to ascertain the contribution of the individual nutritional components. The mechanisms by which a low-potassium diet may contribute to hypertension are complex and poorly understood. They may relate to stimulation of intrarenal angiotensin (Ang) II, oxidants, and endothelin; inhibition of intrarenal nitric oxide and prostaglandins; and induction of renal ischemia.

Dietary Approaches to Stop Hypertension (DASH) Diet*

Food Group	Daily Servings	Serving Sizes	Examples and Notes	Significance to the DASH Diet Pattern
Grains and grain products	7–8	1 slice bread 1/2 cup dry cereal 1/2 cup cooked rice, pasta, or cereal	Whole-wheat bread, muffin, pita bread, bagel, cereals, oatmeal	Major sources of energy and fiber
Vegetables	4–5	1 cup raw, leafy vegetables 1/2 cup cooked vegetables 6 oz vegetable juice	Tomatoes, potatoes, carrots, peas, squash, broccoli, turnip greens, kale, spinach, artichokes, green beans, sweet potatoes	Rich sources of potassium, magnesium, and fiber
Fruits	4–5	1 medium fruit 1/4 cup dried fruit 6 oz fruit juice 1/2 cup fresh, frozen, or canned fruit	Apricots, bananas, dates, oranges, orange juice, grapefruit, grapefruit juice, mangoes, melons, peaches, pineapples, prunes, raisins, strawberries, tangerines	Important sources of potassium, magnesium, and fiber
Low-fat or nonfat dairy foods	2–3	8 oz milk 1 cup yogurt 1.5 oz cheese	Skim or low-fat (2%) milk, skim or low-fat buttermilk, nonfat or low-fat yogurt, nonfat or low-fat cheeses	Major sources of calcium and protein
Meats, poultry, and fish	≤2	3 oz cooked meats, poultry, or fish	Select only lean meats; trim away visible fats; broil, roast, or boil instead of frying; remove skin from poultry	Rich sources of protein and magnesium
Nuts, seeds, and legumes	4–5 wk	1.5 oz 1/3 cup nuts 1/2 oz or 2 tablespoons seeds 1/2 cup cooked legumes	Almonds, mixed nuts, peanuts, walnuts, sunflower seeds, kidney beans, lentils, split peas	Rich sources of energy, magnesium, potassium, protein, and fiber

Figure 34.7 Dietary Approaches to Stop Hypertension (DASH) diet. *The DASH eating plan shown is based on 2000 kcal/day (8400 kJ/day). Depending on energy needs, the number of daily servings in a food group may vary from those listed. *(Modified from the Sixth Report of the Joint National Committee on Prevention, Detection, Evaluation, and Treatment of High Blood Pressure.)*

In the TOHP I and II trials, a higher sodium to potassium excretion ratio (implying a high-salt and low-potassium intake) was more strongly associated with subsequent cardiovascular events than either urinary sodium or potassium excretion alone.[33] Overall, it appears to be beneficial to optimize potassium intake in hypertensive humans to minimize hypokalemia, being careful to avoid the risk of hyperkalemia in subjects with renal impairment or in other susceptible individuals. If renal function is normal, optimal potassium intake is 80 to 120 mmol/day.

Calcium and Dairy Food Intake

Cross-sectional population surveys of self-reported nutrient intake suggest an inverse relationship between calcium intake and BP. The relationship is more convincing at low levels of calcium consumption (<300 to 600 mg/day). There may be a threshold of 700 to 800 mg/day, above which any further reduction in BP is attenuated. A meta-analysis of randomized calcium supplementation trials (mostly with 1 or 1.5 g calcium/day) has demonstrated reductions in systolic BP (–0.9 to –1.7 mm Hg) that are of little clinical importance.[34] Although calcium in milk may contribute to BP lowering, dairy products may lower BP by other mechanisms. Biologically active peptides formed during the milk fermentation process, such as the casein-derived tripeptides isoleucine-proline-proline and valine-proline-proline, have ACE-inhibiting properties. These milk-derived tripeptides have been shown to reduce BP by 4.8 mm Hg and 2.2 mm Hg for systolic and diastolic BP, respectively.[35] Vitamin D, which is often added to milk, may also help reduce BP by reducing renin expression. At present, the American Heart Association and JNC 7 do not recognize dairy consumption as a dietary approach to the prevention and management of hypertension. Nevertheless, low-fat dairy products are recommended as an integral part of the DASH diet.

Magnesium Intake

A weak inverse relationship has been reported between dietary intake of magnesium and BP. Nevertheless, in a meta-analysis of 20 randomized clinical trials,[36] magnesium supplementation had an insignificant effect on BP. Magnesium has been shown to influence cardiac function and rhythm; therefore, JNC 7 has recommended an adequate intake of magnesium pending more definitive information.[1] The optimal levels of magnesium intake are not yet established.

Other Micronutrients and Bioactive Food Components

The inverse association between fruit and vegetable intake and BP and other cardiovascular risk factors is well established. The biologic effects of certain flavonoids and related phenolic compounds present in these foods are receiving increasing attention. Regular consumption of flavanol-rich foods, such as cocoa products, tea, and red wine, has been shown to be associated with decreased BP. Foods rich in garlic may also have beneficial effects on BP.[37]

Dietary Fats and Sugars

High intake of fructose present in table sugar and high fructose corn syrup has been correlated with the epidemics of obesity, hypertension, metabolic syndrome, and diabetes. In animals, the intake of fructose but not of glucose or starch can rapidly induce features of the metabolic syndrome. In an experimental study, an intake of 200 g fructose per day in healthy overweight adult men caused a significant increase in systolic and diastolic BP, a rise in plasma triglycerides, a fall in high-density lipoprotein (HDL) cholesterol, and an increase in relative insulin resistance. Other studies have shown that a diet rich in fructose can increase intra-abdominal fat and cause insulin resistance, particularly in subjects who are already overweight. The pathogenesis of the hypertension may be related to the unique ability of fructose as a sugar to cause intracellular ATP depletion and uric acid generation. Allopurinol has been found to block the BP rise to fructose in both humans and rats.[38] These studies suggest that excessive sugar intake could have a role in the metabolic syndrome and that reduction of sugar intake could be beneficial. Interestingly, whole fruits, which also contain fructose, do not appear to cause metabolic syndrome, probably because of the lower fructose content and the presence of numerous antioxidants (such as vitamin C) that block the effect of fructose to induce insulin resistance.

In epidemiologic studies, substantial red meat intake (mean 103 g/day) is associated with a rise in systolic BP of 1.25 mm Hg.[39] Red meat intake has also been associated with an increased risk for diabetes. The mechanisms are unknown but may be related to the production of oxidants, inflammatory cytokines, or uric acid.

Supplementation with omega-3 fatty acids reduces the risk of myocardial infarction and sudden cardiac death,[40] but their effect on BP is small. In a recent meta-analysis, omega-3 supplementation significantly reduced diastolic BP by a mean of 1.8 mm Hg but had no effect on systolic BP, fibrinogen level, or heart rate.[41] About ten portions of oily fish per week or nine or ten fish oil capsules per day are required, and this is not tolerated by most subjects because of belching and fishy taste. Concerns about the cholesterol content as well as dioxin and polychlorinated biphenyl content (environmental pollutants that have carcinogenic potential and, being fat soluble, can accumulate in the body) of some fish oil supplements also raise questions about the safety of very large doses.

Dietary Approaches to Stop Hypertension (DASH) Diet

The DASH randomized, controlled trial provided unequivocal evidence that nonpharmacologic methods can reduce BP.[32] Subjects fed a diet rich in fruit and vegetables for 8 weeks had a greater reduction in systolic and diastolic BP (2.8 and 1.1 mm Hg, respectively) than did subjects on a typical American control diet. Subjects randomized to the DASH diet, rich in fruit, vegetables, and low-fat dairy products and with a reduced sugar and saturated and total fat intake (see Fig. 34.7), had an even greater reduction in both systolic and diastolic BP (5.5 and 3.0 mm Hg, respectively). The effects of the 8-week DASH diet were greatest in hypertensive African Americans, in whom the BP reduction was 13.2/6.1 mm Hg. Increased efficacy of the DASH diet in African Americans may reflect a greater response to the higher potassium, calcium, and magnesium content of the diet in subjects who have habitually low intake of these nutrients.

The follow-up DASH and low-salt diet study investigated the additional benefits of salt restriction over and above the DASH diet.[42] Reduction of sodium intake from a high (150 mmol/day or 9 g NaCl) to either an intermediate (100 mmol/day or 6 g NaCl) or a low (65 mmol/day or 4 g NaCl) intake resulted in a stepwise reduction in BP, which was approximately twice as great in subjects on the control than on the DASH diet (Fig. 34.8). In those following the DASH diet, the addition of salt restriction resulted in a relatively small additional decrease in BP (3.0 and 1.6 mm Hg for systolic and diastolic BP, respectively). Thus, the greatest benefits of salt restriction are seen in those with a poor diet (i.e., typical westernized high-fat, low-nutrient diet).

SMOKING

Cigarette smoking is a well-established major risk factor for cardiovascular disease, but its role in the development of hypertension is not well elucidated and not routinely included in recommendations for prevention and treatment of hypertension.[1] The relationship with hypertension may be confounded by changes in weight during and after the cessation of smoking. In a large epidemiologic study of middle-aged and older men from the United States, smoking was associated with a modest but important risk for development of hypertension; but in a study of Turkish adults, current smoking carried a borderline protective effect, whereas former smokers with abdominal obesity had a higher risk of incident hypertension.[43,44] Nevertheless, smoking increases overall noncardiovascular and cardiovascular morbidity and mortality, and all smokers should be advised to quit.

ALCOHOL

There is a linear relationship between alcohol consumption, BP levels, and the prevalence of hypertension in populations.[45] In Japan, alcohol intake above 300 g/wk (about three drinks per day) was associated with significantly greater increases of BP during a 7-year period, and baseline BP was higher in drinkers consuming 200 g/wk, with the effects more marked in men.[46,47] Heavy drinking is associated with increased risk of stroke, increase in BP after alcohol withdrawal, and attenuation of antihypertensive efficacy. Paradoxically, alcohol has a J-shaped relationship with coronary heart disease, with moderate consumption (1 to 2 drinks per day) having the lowest risk. In a large epidemiologic study, modest alcohol consumption was protective against first myocardial infarction.[48] Alcohol may increase BP through activation of the sympathetic nervous system, whereas its protective effects include increasing HDL cholesterol, lowering fibrinogen, and inhibiting platelet activation. The JNC 7 guidelines recommend limiting alcohol consumption to no more than two drinks per day (24 oz of beer, 10 oz of wine, or 3 oz of 80-proof whiskey) in most men and no more than one drink per day in women or lighter weight men (see Fig. 34.1).

CAFFEINE

Caffeine is the most widely used psychoactive substance worldwide. Caffeine stimulates the cardiovascular system through the blockade of vascular adenosine receptors.[49] In a meta-analysis of randomized, controlled studies of caffeine tablet and coffee ingestion, BP increases appeared to be greater for caffeine tablets (systolic, 4.16 mm Hg; diastolic, 2.41 mm Hg) than for coffee (systolic, 1.22 mm Hg; diastolic, 0.49 mm Hg), despite similar caffeine (total gram) intake.[50] Coffee may also increase cardiovascular risk in smokers,[51] whereas paradoxically it may reduce the risk for metabolic syndrome and diabetes. The JNC 7 guidelines are silent on the issue of caffeine, but it seems reasonable to propose that modest coffee consumption is safe, at least in

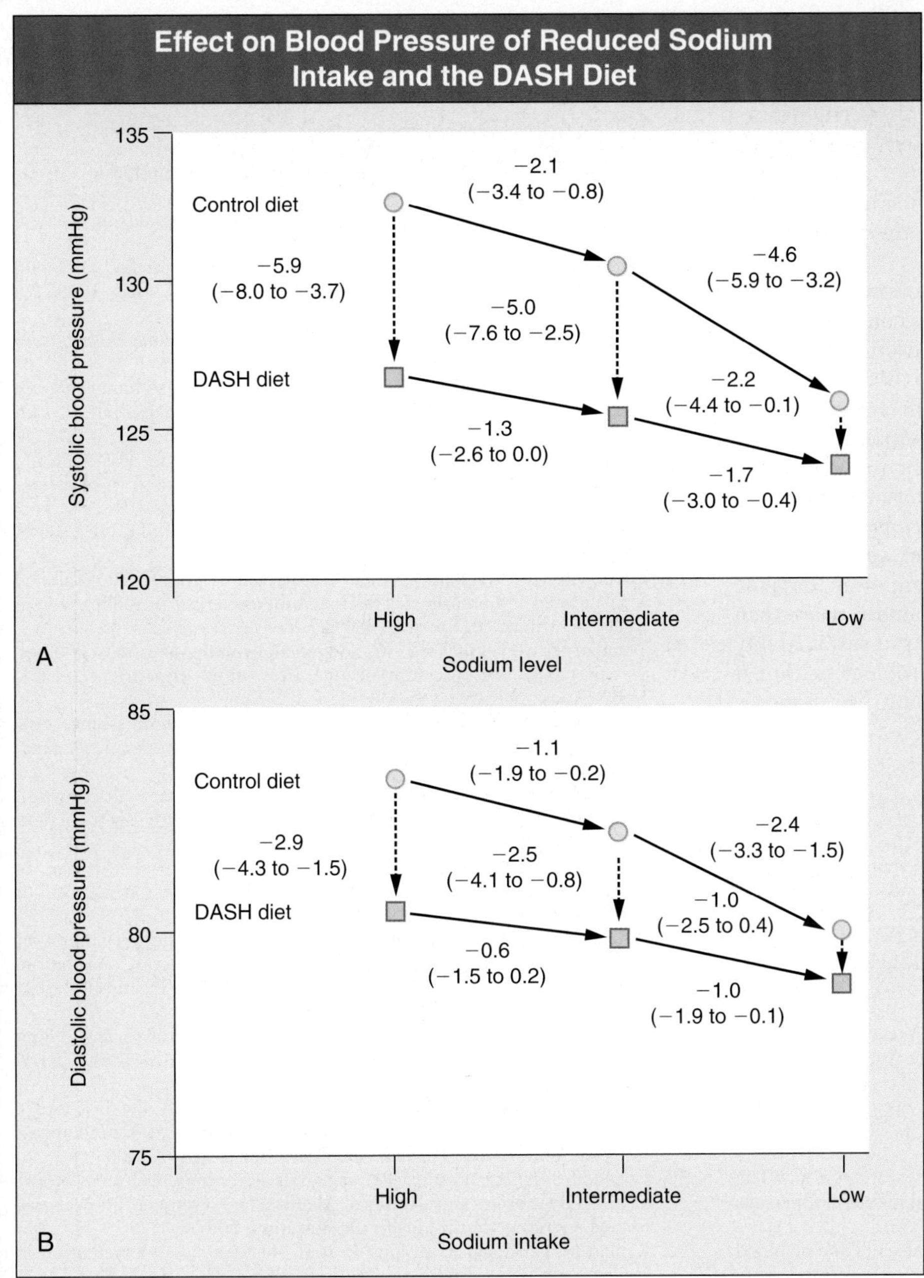

Figure 34.8 Reduced sodium intake and the DASH diet. The effect on systolic blood pressure **A,** and diastolic blood pressure **B.** *(Redrawn from reference 42.)*

nonsmokers, but that pharmacologic ingestion of caffeine and the use of "smart drinks" (which are supplemented with caffeine) should be avoided.

PSYCHOLOGICAL STRESS

Chronic psychosocial stress is an important contributor to the development and maintenance of hypertension. Men exposed to job strain had a 10.7 mm Hg and 15.4 mm Hg higher work and home ambulatory systolic BP than did controls, respectively.[52] The INTERHEART study showed that psychosocial stress was associated with a twofold increase in the risk of the first myocardial infarction.[48] Nevertheless, stress reduction approaches have shown either negative or heterogeneous effects on BP.[53] As a result, JNC 7 does not recommend stress reduction techniques for the sole management of hypertension.[1] However, evidence suggests that transcendental meditation and control of respiration may have beneficial effects on BP as an adjunct to pharmacologic therapy.[54]

ADOPTING LIFESTYLE MODIFICATIONS

Compliance with lifestyle changes has always been a concern. The Prevention of Myocardial Infarction Early Remodeling (PREMIER) trial evaluated the effects of implementing JNC 7 lifestyle recommendations and the DASH diet.[55] Adults with prehypertension or untreated stage 1 hypertension were randomly assigned to one of three groups for 6 months: advice only; JNC recommendations; and JNC recommendations plus DASH diet. At 6 months, the JNC and JNC plus DASH groups had significantly reduced BP in comparison with the advice-only group, but there was little additional benefit of adding the DASH diet to JNC recommendations. However, participants purchased their own foods in the PREMIER study, instead of being provided with foods as in the DASH[32] and DASH low-salt diet[42] studies. Similarly, in the DASH low-salt diet study, the BP-lowering effect attributable to salt reduction was −6.7/−3.5 mm Hg; whereas in meta-analyses of 40 salt restriction trials in which participants prepared their own low-salt meals, this effect was only −2.54/−1.96 mm Hg.[56] Thus, in the outpatient setting, even highly motivated individuals usually cannot meet DASH dietary goals unless their meals are provided.

In the TOHP II study, the problems of sustainability of dietary intervention and the need for regular counseling were demonstrated.[57] The effect of adding salt restriction to weight loss appeared to offer no further decrease in BP. Assessed by urinary sodium excretion, adherence to lower dietary sodium was poor in the long term. At 36 months of follow-up, mean urinary sodium was 40.4 mmol/24 h lower than baseline in the sodium-restricted group, and only 21% achieved the target of less than 80 mmol/24 h. A higher attendance at counseling sessions was associated with a greater reduction in urinary sodium. At 36 months, a decrease of 84 mmol/day of sodium from baseline levels could be achieved only in those who attended more than 80% of the counseling sessions. In summary, the sustainability of long-term lifestyle interventions remains problematic, but it appears that regular and long-term counseling can improve adherence.

REFERENCES

1. Chobanian A, Bakris GL, Black HR, et al. The seventh report of the Joint National Committee on Prevention, Detection, Evaluation, and Treatment of High Blood Pressure. The JNC 7 report. *JAMA*. 2003;289:2560-2582.
2. Vasan RS, Larson MG, Leip EP, et al. Impact of high-normal blood pressure on the risk of cardiovascular disease. *N Engl J Med*. 2001;345:1291-1297.
3. Geleijnse JM, Kok FJ, Grobbee DE. Impact of dietary and lifestyle factors on the prevalence of hypertension in Western populations. *Eur J Public Health*. 2004;14:235-239.
4. Hedley AA, Ogden CL, Johnson CL, et al. Overweight and obesity among US children, adolescents, and adults, 1999-2002. *JAMA*. 2004;291:2847-2850.
5. Trials of Hypertension Prevention Collaboration Research Group. The effects of nonpharmacologic interventions on blood pressure of persons with high normal levels. *JAMA*. 1992;267:1213-1220.
6. Neter JE, Stam BE, Kok FJ, et al. Influence of weight reduction on blood pressure. A meta-analysis of randomized controlled trials. *Hypertension*. 2003;42:878-884.
7. Schulz M, Liese AD, Boeing H, et al. Associations of short-term weight changes and weight cycling with incidence of essential hypertension in the EPIC-Potsdam Study. *J Hum Hypertens*. 2005;19:61-67.
8. Farrell SW, Kampert JB, Kohl HW 3rd, et al. Influences of cardiorespiratory fitness levels and other predictors on cardiovascular disease mortality in men. *Med Sci Sports Exerc*. 1998;30:899-905.
9. Fagard RH. Exercise characteristics and the blood pressure response to dynamic physical training. *Med Sci Sports Exerc*. 2001;33:S484-S492.
10. Ishikawa-Takata K, Ohta T, Tanaka H. How much exercise is required to reduce blood pressure in essential hypertensives: A dose-response study. *Am J Hypertens*. 2003;16:629-633.
11. Quinn J. Twenty-four hour, ambulatory blood pressure responses following acute exercise: Impact of exercise intensity. *Hum Hypertens*. 2000;14:547-553.
12. Palatini P, Visentin P, Dorigatti F, et al, HARVEST Study Group. Regular physical activity prevents development of left ventricular hypertrophy in hypertension. *Eur Heart J*. 2009;30:225-232.
13. Halliwill J. Mechanisms and clinical implications of post-exercise hypotension in humans. *Exerc Sports Sci Rev*. 2001;29:65-70.
14. Pescatello LS, Franklin BA, Farquhar WB, et al, American College of Sports Medicine. American College of Sports Medicine position stand. Exercise and hypertension. *Med Sci Sports Exerc*. 2004;36:533-553.
15. Pollock ML, Franklin BA, Balady GJ, et al. AHA Science Advisory. Resistance exercise in individuals with and without cardiovascular disease: Benefits, rationale, safety, and prescription: An advisory from the Committee on Exercise, Rehabilitation, and Prevention, Council on Clinical Cardiology, American Heart Association. *Circulation*. 2000;101:828-833.
16. Franklin BA, Gordon S, Timmis GC. Exercise prescription for hypertensive patients. *Ann Med*. 1991;23:279-287.
17. MacGregor GA. Sodium is more important than calcium in essential hypertension. *Hypertension*. 1985;7:628-637.
18. Prior IAM, Evans JG, Harvey HB, et al. Sodium intake and blood pressure in two Polynesian populations. *N Engl J Med*. 1968;279:515-520.
19. Weinberger MH. Salt sensitivity of blood pressure in humans. *Hypertension*. 1996;27:481-490.
20. Tuomilehto J, Jousilahti P, Rastenyte D, et al. Urinary sodium excretion and cardiovascular mortality in Finland: A prospective study. *Lancet*. 2001;357:848-851.
21. Cook NR, Cutler JA, Obarzanek E, et al, Trials of Hypertension Prevention Collaborative Research Group. Long term effects of dietary sodium reduction on cardiovascular disease outcomes: Observational follow-up of the trials of hypertension prevention (TOHP). *BMJ*. 2007;334:885.
22. Johansson ME, Bernberg E, Andersson IJ, et al. High salt diet combined with elevated angiotensin II accelerates atherosclerosis in apolipoprotein E–deficient mice. *J Hypertens*. 2009;27:41-47.
23. Weinberger MH, Fineberg NS. Sodium and volume sensitivity of blood pressure: Age and pressure change over time. *Hypertension*. 1991;18:67-71.
24. Cappuccio FP, Markandu ND, Carney C, et al. Double-blind randomised trial of modest salt restriction in older people. *Lancet*. 1997;350:850-854.
25. Law MR, Frost CD, Wald NJ. By how much does dietary salt reduction lower blood pressure? III. Analysis of data from trials of salt reduction. *BMJ*. 1991;302:819-824.
26. Johnson RJ, Herrera-Acosta J, Schreiner GF, Rodriguez-Iturbe B. Mechanisms of disease: Subtle acquired renal injury as a mechanism of salt-sensitive hypertension. *N Engl J Med*. 2002;346:913-923.
27. World Health Organization. Diet, nutrition and the prevention of chronic diseases. Report of a Joint WHO/FAO Expert Consultation. Geneva, World Health Organization, 2003. WHO Technical Report Series No. 916.
28. Hooper L, Bartlett C, Smith GD, Ebrahim S. Systematic review of long term effects of advice to reduce dietary salt intake in adults. *BMJ*. 2002;325:628-637.
29. Charlton KE, Steyn K, Levitt NS, et al. A food-based dietary strategy lowers blood pressure in a low socio-economic setting: A randomised study in South Africa. *Public Health Nutr*. 2008;11:1397-1406.
30. World Health Organization. Reducing salt intake in populations. Report of a WHO Forum and Technical Meeting; 5-7 October. 2006; Paris, France. Geneva, World Health Organization, 2007.
31. Kaplan N, Carnegie A, Risking P, et al. Potassium supplementation in hypertensive patients with diuretic-induced hypokalemia. *N Engl J Med*. 1985;312:746-749.
32. Appel L, Moore T, Obarzanek E, et al. A clinical trial of the effects of dietary patterns on blood pressure. *N Engl J Med*. 1997;336:1117-1124.
33. Cook NR, Obarzanek E, Cutler JA, et al, Trials of Hypertension Prevention Collaborative Research Group. Joint effects of sodium and potassium intake on subsequent cardiovascular disease: The Trials of Hypertension Prevention follow-up study. *Arch Intern Med*. 2009;169:32-40.
34. Griffith LE, Guyatt GH, Cook RJ, et al. The influence of dietary and nondietary calcium supplementation on blood pressure: An updated meta-analysis of randomized controlled trials. *Am J Hypertens*. 1999;12:84-92.
35. Xu JY, Qin LQ, Wang PY, et al. Effect of milk tripeptides on blood pressure: A meta-analysis of randomized controlled trials. *Nutrition*. 2008;24:933-940.
36. Jee SH, Miller ER, Guallar E, et al. The effect of magnesium supplementation on blood pressure: A meta-analysis of randomized clinical trials. *Am J Hypertens*. 2002;15:691-696.
37. Reid K, Frank OR, Stocks NP, et al. Effect of garlic on blood pressure: A systematic review and meta-analysis. *BMC Cardiovasc Disord*. 2008;8:13.
38. Perez-Pozo SE, Schold J, Nakagawa T, et al. Excessive fructose intake induces the features of metabolic syndrome in healthy adult men: role

of uric acid in the hypertensive response. *Int J Obes (Lond)*. 2010:34: 454-461.
39. Tzoulaki I, Brown IJ, Chan Q, et al. Relation of iron and red meat intake to blood pressure: Cross sectional epidemiological study. *BMJ*. 2008; 337:a258.
40. Mozaffarian D. Fish and n-3 fatty acids for the prevention of fatal coronary heart disease and sudden cardiac death. *Am J Clin Nutr*. 2008; 87:1991S-1996S.
41. Hartweg J, Farmer AJ, Holman RR, Neil HA. Meta-analysis of the effects of n-3 polyunsaturated fatty acids on haematological and thrombogenic factors in type 2 diabetes. *Diabetologia*. 2007;50:250-258.
42. Sacks FM, Svetkey LP, Vollmer WM, et al, DASH-Sodium Collaborative Research Group. Effects on blood pressure of reduced dietary sodium and the dietary approaches to stop hypertension (DASH) diet. *N Engl J Med*. 2001;344:3-10.
43. Halperin RO, Gaziano JM, Sesso HD. Smoking and the risk of incident hypertension in middle-aged and older men. *Am J Hypertens*. 2008;21:148-152.
44. Onat A, U ur M, Hergenc G, et al. Lifestyle and metabolic determinants of incident hypertension, with special reference to cigarette smoking: A longitudinal study. *Am J Hypertens*. 2009;22:156-162.
45. Puddey IB, Beilin LJ, Rakey V. Alcohol, hypertension, and the cardiovascular system: A critical appraisal. *Addict Biol*. 1997;2:159-170.
46. Yoshita K, Miura K, Morikawa Y, et al. Relationship of alcohol consumption to 7-year blood pressure change in Japanese men. *J Hypertens*. 2005;23:1485-1490.
47. Wakabayashi I. Influence of gender on the association of alcohol drinking with blood pressure. *Am J Hypertens*. 2008;21:1310-1317.
48. Yusuf S, Hawken S, Ôunpuu S, et al, INTERHEART Study Investigators. Effect of potentially modifiable risk factors associated with myocardial infarction in 52 countries (the INTERHEART study): Case-control study. *Lancet*. 2004;364:937-950.
49. Smits P, Boekema P, de Abreu R, et al. Evidence for an antagonism between caffeine and adenosine in the human cardiovascular system. *J Cardiovasc Pharmacol*. 1987;10:136-143.
50. Noordzij M, Uiterwaal CS, Arends LR, et al. Blood pressure response to chronic intake of coffee and caffeine: A meta-analysis of randomized controlled trials. *J Hypertens*. 2005;23:921-928.
51. Klatsky AL, Koplik S, Kipp H, Friedman GD. The confounded relation of coffee to coronary artery disease. *Am J Cardiol*. 2008;101:825-827.
52. Schnall PL, Schwartz JE, Landsbergis PA, et al. A longitudinal study of job strain and ambulatory blood pressure: Results from a three-year follow-up. *Psychosom Med*. 1998;60:697-706.
53. Ebrahim S, Smith G. Lowering blood pressure: A systematic review of sustained effects of non-pharmacological interventions. *J Public Health Med*. 1998;20:441-448.
54. Anderson JW, Liu C, Kryscio RJ. Blood pressure response to transcendental meditation: A meta-analysis. *Am J Hypertens*. 2008;21:310-316.
55. Writing Group of the PREMIER Collaborative Research Group. Effects of comprehensive lifestyle modification on blood pressure control: Main results of the PREMIER clinical trial. *JAMA*. 2003;289:2083-2093.
56. Geleijnse JM, Kok FJ, Grobbee DE. Blood pressure response to changes in sodium and potassium intake: A metaregression analysis of randomised trials. *J Hum Hypertens*. 2003;17:471-480.
57. Kumanyika SK, Cook NR, Cutler JA, et al. Sodium reduction for hypertension prevention in overweight adults: Further results from the Trials of Hypertension Prevention Phase II. *J Hum Hypertens*. 2005; 19:33-45.

CHAPTER 35

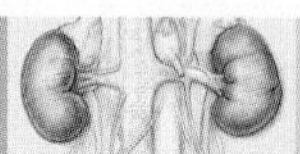

Pharmacologic Treatment of Hypertension

Bryan Williams

TODAY'S PHARMACOLOGIC TREATMENT OF HYPERTENSION IN PERSPECTIVE

Successful lifestyle interventions can delay the development of hypertension (see Chapter 34), but the majority of patients with confirmed hypertension require lifelong drug treatment, often with more than one drug. This has resulted in a billion-dollar industry, in which numerous pharmacologic agents have been introduced (Fig. 35.1). In turn, this creates complexity for clinicians in trying to decide which drugs would be the most effective option for specific patient groups. The following sections review who should receive pharmacologic treatment, what target blood pressures to attain, and how to decide on what pharmacologic agent to use.

DEFINING WHO SHOULD RECEIVE PHARMACOLOGIC TREATMENT

Definitions of Hypertension from the Perspective of Treatment

Blood pressure (BP) is normally distributed within populations, and thus "hypertension" is an arbitrarily defined, moving target with diagnostic thresholds subject to change as new evidence from clinical trials emerges. From a practical perspective, hypertension is best defined as *that level of blood pressure at which treatment to lower blood pressure results in significant clinical benefit*. This statement highlights the conundrum in defining hypertension because the risk associated with BP is a continuum and the level of pressure at which treatment results in "significant clinical benefit" for any individual will depend on the absolute cardiovascular (CV) risk.[1-3] This varies because some people will be more vulnerable than others to end-organ damage at a given level of pressure. Defining that vulnerability case by case remains impractical, and so differential BP targets and thresholds have emerged that group patients into categories defining their threshold BP for therapeutic intervention and optimal BP goals. In addition, specific drug classes have been given "compelling indications" and "compelling contraindications" for specific groups of patients. This has been useful in tailoring therapy from a wide range of drug classes but has sometimes been misinterpreted as indicating that the specific drug is more important than the achieved BP, which is not the case. The primary objective of therapy must always be to lower BP as effectively as possible.[4-6]

Blood Pressure Thresholds for Intervention (Office Blood Pressure)

There is substantial evidence that treating a seated "office" BP above a systolic pressure of 160 mm Hg or a diastolic pressure above 100 mm Hg reduces strokes, myocardial infarction, heart failure, and mortality.[4-10] There is also evidence that treating pressures above 140/90 mm Hg, especially in higher risk patients, is beneficial. Consequently, most guidelines define hypertension as an office BP of 140/90 mm Hg or higher.[7-10] Various grades of hypertension are also specified (Fig. 35.2). Guidelines from the United States also include a category of prehypertension to highlight those with borderline hypertension.[7] This was designed to encourage lifestyle change because the risk of progression from prehypertension to overt hypertension is very high. Furthermore, data from the Framingham Heart Study have shown that patients with a high-normal BP experience a doubling of risk of CV complications (Fig. 35.3).[11] Thus, prehypertension is not benign, the cardiovascular disease (CVD) risk of these people is already elevated, and they are almost certain to develop more severe hypertension without a change in lifestyle or intervention with drug therapy.

Clinical Dilemma of End-Organ Damage and a "Normal" Blood Pressure

Debate exists with relation to treating people with prehypertension who already have evidence of end-organ damage (e.g., left ventricular hypertrophy [LVH]) or microalbuminuria. One wonders if this is an example of the insensitivity of the defined thresholds for diagnosis of hypertension; clearly, such a patient who has developed hypertensive LVH or microalbuminuria has a BP that is causing damage but one that is considered below the usual threshold for intervention. Thus, clinical understanding of the disease process is critical to enable the optimal use of guidelines for treatment decisions. There remains considerable uncertainty in the evidence base, and clinical judgment should not and indeed cannot be replaced by guidelines.

Blood Pressure Thresholds for Intervention (Ambulatory and Home Blood Pressure Monitoring)

Diagnostic thresholds for hypertension vary according to the method of measurement. Ambulatory BP monitoring and home BP monitoring are increasingly advocated and used. When they are used to classify hypertension, the diagnostic thresholds are lower.

The diagnostic thresholds for hypertension according to different methods of measurement are summarized in Figure 35.4 (see also Chapter 32).

WHAT ARE THE BLOOD PRESSURE TREATMENT GOALS?

An area of the greatest uncertainty is identifying BP treatment goals. As suggested before, the optimal goal of treatment is likely

The Development of Therapeutic Strategies for Hypertension	
Year	**Non-Drug Treatments**
1920s	Strict low-sodium diet
1929	Lumbar sympathectomy
1944	Kempner rice diet
Year	**Drug Treatments**
1930s	Veratrum alkaloids
1940s	Thiocyanates
1948	Reserpine, phenoxybenzamine
1950	Ganglion blockers
1951	Monoamine oxidase inhibitors
1958	Thiazide diuretics (chlorthiazide)
1960s	Central α-2 receptor agonists, nondihydropyridine calcium channel blockers and β-blockers
1970s	ACE inhibitors, α-1 receptor blockers
1980s	Dihydropyridine calcium channel blockers
1990s	Angiotensin receptor blockers
2000s	Direct renin inhibitors

Figure 35.1 The development of therapeutic strategies for hypertension. ACE, angiotensin-converting enzyme.

to be patient specific, but guidelines must be generalizable to populations. This means that guidelines, in my view, should be conservative, be pragmatic, curb the zeal of specialists to advocate ever lower BP goals, and confine their recommendations to those supported by solid evidence. Herein lies a problem. Currently, there are two internationally endorsed BP targets for people with hypertension: less than 140/90 mm Hg for those with "uncomplicated hypertension" and a lower target of less than 130/80 mm Hg for those at higher risk, that is, those with diabetes, established CV or cerebrovascular disease, and chronic kidney disease (CKD).[7-10] To define such goals, ideally there should be trials that have randomized different groups of patients to different BP treatment targets (i.e., "more versus less" BP control) to determine whether the more aggressive BP target is appropriate; but despite the firm consensus on BP targets outlined before, there have been no such large-scale trials targeting more versus less systolic BP lowering and only a small number of trials targeting more versus less diastolic BP lowering.[12,13] In an attempt to obtain more data with regard to systolic BP lowering, the Cardio-Sis study[14] showed that targeting treatment to a systolic BP of less than 130 mm Hg versus less than 140 mm Hg was more effective at preventing the development of electrocardiographically defined LVH and a composite CV outcome. However, this is a single, relatively small study (N = 1111), and more substantial data are needed to support the recommended lower (<130/80 mm Hg) BP target (Fig. 35.5). A recent analysis of the baseline and in-treatment BP levels of patients at high CVD risk in the ONTARGET trial suggests that for people with hypertension at baseline (i.e., systolic BP ≥140 mm Hg), the risk of major CV events and of stroke in particular was reduced with progressive BP lowering.[15] However, for those with a systolic BP of 130 mm Hg or less at baseline, there was much less evidence of benefit with further BP lowering and a signal of possible harm. The recent ACCORD trial tested the more (<120 mm Hg) versus less (<140 mm Hg) systolic BP lowering hypothesis in a high risk population with type 2 diabetes.[16] The study failed to provide conclusive evidence that the more intensive BP treatment strategy reduced a composite of major cardiovascular events, although of interest, stroke rates were significantly reduced. This study looked underpowered to definitively test this hypothesis. For the moment, a BP target of below 140/90 mm Hg should be the goal for most people with hypertension, with a more conservative target of below 150/90 mm Hg for those 80 years of age or older based on recent data from the HYVET study.[17] Lower BP targets may be appropriate in higher risk patients, on a case-by-case basis, depending on the patient's ability to tolerate lower levels of treated BP, with the caveat that the evidence supporting such a strategy is limited.

GUIDE TO SELECTION OF ANTIHYPERTENSIVE AGENTS

Key Principles from Clinical Trials

Aside from the limitations of the evidence defining optimal BP treatment targets, the pharmacologic treatment of hypertension has the most impressive evidence base in medicine to guide treatment decisions. BP lowering undoubtedly reduces morbidity and mortality, but we do not know how low to go. Many large randomized controlled trials have compared different classes of active treatments with placebo and different treatment strategies with each other (see references 4 to 6 for overviews). Figure 35.6 summarizes a recent systematic review and analysis conducted for the National Institute for Health and Clinical Excellence (NICE) hypertension guideline development group in the United Kingdom,[10] which compared and ranked the effectiveness of different classes of BP-lowering medication with regard to major CV events. The differences between the various drug classes on clinical outcomes are primarily driven by differences in the quality of BP control. Analysis of these trials has provided some important guiding principles with regard to treatment strategies for hypertension:

1. Effective BP lowering is overwhelmingly important in reducing the risk of major CV events in people with hypertension. Thus, the first priority in treatment is to control BP.
2. Early studies focused primarily on diastolic BP as the treatment target, but systolic BP is invariably more difficult to control and more closely linked to CV outcomes and should now be the main focus of treatment.
3. Monotherapy is rarely sufficient to control BP, and many patients will require more than one drug as part of their treatment strategy.
4. The response to any class of BP-lowering medication is heterogeneous, that is, some patients will respond better than others.
5. Some trials have indicated that certain comorbidities (e.g., diabetes) and target organ damage (e.g., LVH, CKD) provide compelling indications for inclusion of specific classes of drug therapy in the treatment regimen, but this consideration should not override the importance of BP control *per se*.
6. There are inadequate clinical outcome data for treatment studies of younger patients. Most studies, especially the

Classification of Hypertension according to Current Hypertension Guidelines

European Society of Hypertension Classification of Hypertension (circa 2007)

Category	Systolic (mm Hg)		Diastolic (mm Hg)
Optimal	<120	and	<80
Normal	120–129	and/or	80–84
High–normal	130–139	and/or	85–89
Grade 1 hypertension	140–159	and/or	90–99
Grade 2 hypertension	160–179	and/or	100–109
Grade 3 hypertension	≥180	and/or	≥110
Isolated systolic hypertension	≥140	and	<90

JNC 7 Classification of Hypertension (circa 2003)

BP Category	SBP* (mm Hg)	DBP* (mm Hg)	Lifestyle Modification	Initial Drug Therapy: Without Compelling Indications	Initial Drug Therapy: With Compelling Indications
Normal	<120	and <80	Encourage	No antihypertensive drug indicated	Drug(s) for compelling indications‡
Prehypertension	120–139	or 80–89	Yes		
Stage 1 hypertension	140–159	or 90–99	Yes	Thiazide-type diuretics for most. May consider ACE inhibitor, ARB, BB, CCB, or combination	Drug(s) for the compelling indications‡ Other anti-hypertensive drugs (diuretics, ACE inhibitor, ARB, BB, CCB) as needed
Stage 2 hypertension	≥160	or ≥100	Yes	Two-drug combination for most† (usually thiazide-type diuretic and ACE inhibitor or ARB or BB or CCB)	

Figure 35.2 Classification of hypertension according to current hypertension guidelines. Hypertension grades or stages replace the older terminology of mild, moderate, and severe. DBP, diastolic blood pressure; SBP, systolic blood pressure. Drug abbreviations: ACE, angiotensin-converting enzyme inhibitor; ARB, angiotensin receptor blocker; BB, β-blocker; CCB, calcium channel blocker. *Treatment determined by highest blood pressure (BP) category. †Initial combined therapy should be used cautiously in those at risk for orthostatic hypotension. ‡Treat patients with chronic kidney disease (CKD) or diabetes to BP goal of less than 130/80 mm Hg.

more recent, have been conducted in patients older than 55 years and typically with a mean age of more than 65 years.

7. On average, lowering of BP by 20/10 mm Hg will reduce the risk of major CV events by half.
8. The reduction in stroke risk appears to follow the predicted reduction in risk based on the epidemiologic association between stroke and BP.
9. There appears to be a shortfall in the reduction in risk of ischemic heart disease with BP lowering compared with epidemiologic predictions, which is best addressed by attention to concomitant risk factors.
10. Importantly, the risk reduction associated with BP lowering appears to be continuous across a wide range of BPs; thus, the absolute benefit from treatment is greatest in those with the highest absolute CVD risk. This provides the rationale for advocating the use of complementary strategies to reduce CVD risk (e.g., statins and antiplatelet therapy in those with established vascular disease, with target organ damage, or at high calculated CVD risk, i.e., ≥20% during 10 years).

Selection of Drug Therapy

The major classes of BP-lowering therapies are summarized here. International guidelines recommend certain indications and contraindications for the use of specific classes of BP-lowering therapy in specific clinical situations, and these are detailed in Figures 35.7 and 35.8. These lists are not comprehensive and are subject to change as new evidence emerges. The more common adverse effects associated with the major classes of BP-lowering drug therapies are shown in Figure 35.9. The sites of mechanism of action of the various classes of BP-lowering drugs discussed are shown in Figure 35.10.

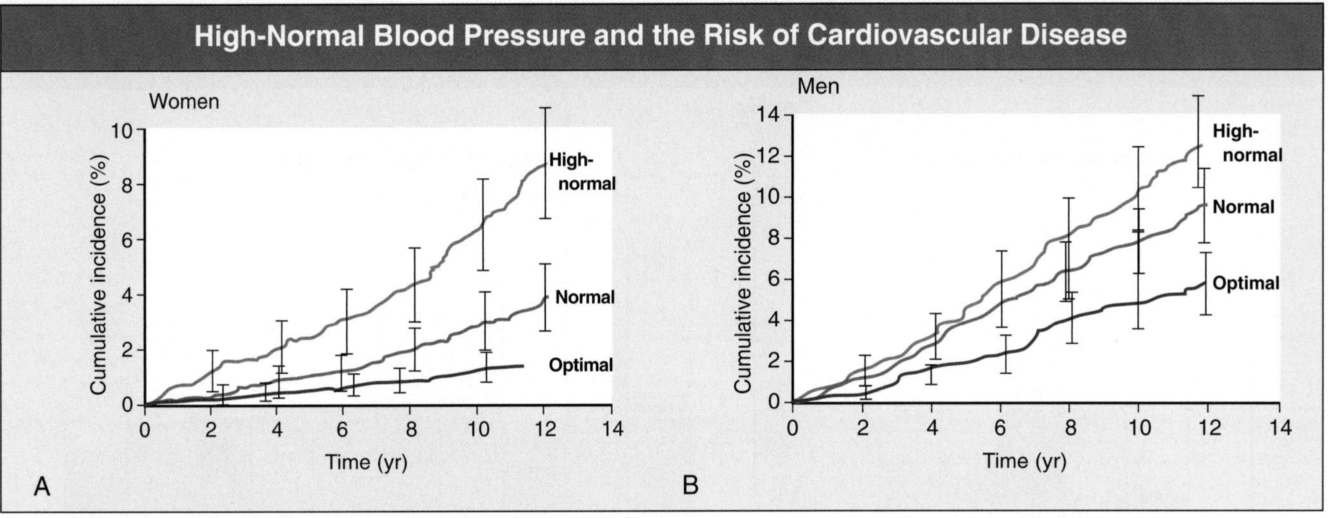

Figure 35.3 High-normal blood pressure (BP) and the risk of cardiovascular disease (CVD). Cumulative incidence of CV events in women **A,** and men **B,** without hypertension, according to BP category at the baseline examination, showing 95% confidence intervals. For this analysis, **optimal BP** was defined as systolic pressure of less than 120 mm Hg and diastolic pressure of less than 80 mm Hg; **normal BP** as systolic pressure of 120 to 129 mm Hg or diastolic pressure of 80 to 84 mm Hg; and **high-normal BP** as systolic pressure of 130 to 139 mm Hg or diastolic pressure of 85 to 89 mm Hg. *(Modified from reference 11.)*

Diagnostic Thresholds for Hypertension According to Different Methods of Measurement

	Systolic BP	Diastolic BP
Office or clinic	140	90
24-hour	125–130	80
Day	130–135	85
Night	120	70
Home	130–135	85

Figure 35.4 Diagnostic thresholds for hypertension according to different methods of measurement. SBP, systolic blood pressure (in mm Hg); DBP, diastolic blood pressure (in mm Hg); 24-hour, day, and night refer to average blood pressures in those time periods recorded by ambulatory blood pressure monitoring; home refers to an average of 7 days of seated blood pressure monitoring at home, usually twice per day (i.e., an average of ~14 readings).

Thiazide-Type Diuretics

Thiazide-type diuretics were the first major class of drug used to treat hypertension on a large scale and remain a major therapeutic option for the treatment of primary hypertension. They are referred to here as thiazide-type diuretics because these drugs do not have a common structure. Commonly used examples are chlorthalidone, hydrochlorothiazide, indapamide, and bendroflumethiazide. They all act primarily by inhibiting the Na^+Cl^- cotransporter in the distal tubule of the kidney, promoting sodium excretion, which is integral to their antihypertensive effect. The early changes in salt and water balance are often accompanied by counteractivation of several vasoconstrictor mechanisms, including the renin-angiotensin-aldosterone system, which may transiently raise peripheral vascular resistance and attenuate BP lowering. Subsequently, a gradual reduction in peripheral vascular resistance and a new steady state of reduced total body sodium and BP are established, usually after about 2 months of treatment.

The sustained actions of thiazide-type diuretics on the kidney make them preferable to loop diuretics for the control of BP. Although loop diuretics are more potent with regard to promoting acute sodium and water loss, they are shorter acting, and there is usually compensatory sodium retention during the latter part of the dosing interval, thereby reducing their BP-lowering efficacy. Loop diuretics have no place in the routine management of primary hypertension in patients with a well-preserved glomerular filtration rate (GFR). However, thiazide-type diuretics lose efficacy in patients with a GFR below 30 ml/min. In such patients, loop diuretics are often required for effective BP lowering, especially when there is clinical evidence of sodium and water retention.

The main adverse effects of thiazide-type diuretics are hypokalemia, hyponatremia (less commonly), impaired glucose tolerance, and small increments in blood levels of low-density lipoprotein (LDL) cholesterol and triglycerides. Thiazide-type diuretics also elevate serum uric acid levels and should be avoided in patients predisposed to gout and also in those receiving lithium because of a high risk of lithium toxicity. Lithium is reabsorbed like sodium through the proximal tubule, and thus distal sodium loss due to thiazides can promote proximal reabsorption of sodium and lithium; as lithium has a narrow therapeutic window, this can lead to lithium toxicity. An incidental advantage of thiazide-type diuretics may be reduction in osteoporosis as a result of calcium retention.

There has been a trend during recent years to reduce the recommended dose of thiazide-type diuretics to minimize their adverse metabolic effects. The dose-response to thiazide-type diuretics is flat (unlike the adverse effect profile), and this has been used to justify the low-dose strategy. However, some patients respond well to higher doses of thiazide-type diuretics, which they tolerate. Moreover, when thiazides are combined with drugs that block the RAS (e.g., angiotensin-converting

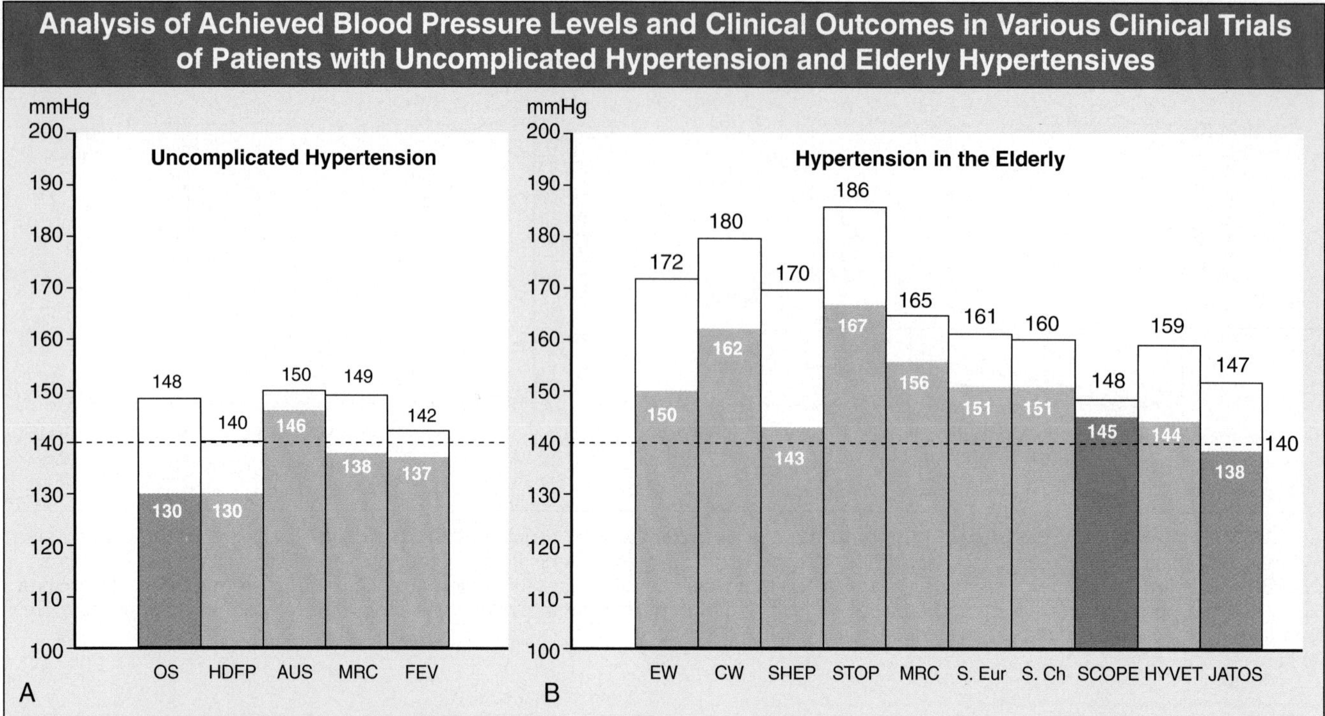

Figure 35.5 Analysis of achieved blood pressure (BP) levels and clinical outcomes in various clinical trials of patients with uncomplicated hypertension A, and elderly hypertensives B. The abbreviations on the base axis refer to the trials for the source data. *Open rectangles* show less active BP lowering; *solid rectangles* show more active BP lowering. The achieved systolic BP values are shown; *orange rectangles,* no significant benefit of more active treatment; *blue,* significant benefit of more active treatment on major cardiovascular outcomes; *purple bar,* significant benefit limited to some secondary outcomes. Numbers refer to achieved mean systolic BP for less active versus more active treatment for each study. The *dotted line* shows the currently recommended systolic BP treatment target. Details are available from the source text. *(Modified from reference 13.)*

Relative Risk and Benefit of Drugs Used to Treat Hypertension

Outcome	Thiazide-Type Diuretics (D)	Calcium-Channel Blockers (C)	Beta-Blockers (B)	ACE Inhibitor/ ARB (A)
Unstable angina	0.893	0.881	0.984	0.970
MI	0.780	0.796	0.855	0.816
Diabetes	0.985	0.808	1.137	0.720
Stroke	0.690	0.656	0.851	0.731
Heart failure	0.530	0.731	0.761	0.642
Death	0.910	0.883	0.939	0.902

Figure 35.6 Relative risk and benefit of drugs used to treat hypertension. The figure shows effectiveness of drugs: 1.0 = no benefit or harm; <1.0 = benefit; >1 = potential harmful effect. Modified from a meta-analysis of major BP-lowering trials conducted for the NICE hypertension guideline development group, 2006. Note that angiotensin-converting enzyme (ACE) inhibitors and angiotensin receptor blockers (ARB) were grouped as a single class for the purposes of this analysis. MI, myocardial infarction. *(Modified from data in http://www.nice.org.uk/CG034guidance.)*

enzyme [ACE] inhibitors or angiotensin receptor blockers [ARBs]), the dose-response is steeper, and higher doses (e.g., hydrochlorothiazide 25 to 50 mg or chlorthalidone 25 mg) may be especially effective in patients with more resistant hypertension.

Potassium-Retaining Diuretics (e.g., Spironolactone, Amiloride, Eplerenone) Spironolactone is an aldosterone receptor antagonist that acts in the renal distal tubule and collecting ducts, decreasing the reabsorption of sodium and water and decreasing the excretion of potassium. The main action of spironolactone is to decrease the tubular expression of epithelial sodiun channel (ENaC) and renal outer medullary K (ROMK) channels, and thus it has a relatively slow onset and offset of action. Because its main site of action is on sodium and water handling in distal tubule and collecting ducts, it is a relatively weak diuretic. Nevertheless, it is effective as a BP-lowering agent but currently rarely used for the routine treatment of hypertension. Spironolactone has the advantage over thiazide-type diuretics that it does not cause hypokalemia or hyperuricemia, and it does not impair

Clinical Indications Favoring the Use of Specific Classes of Blood Pressure-Lowering Medications in Hypertensive Patients

Thiazide diuretics
- Isolated systolic hypertension (elderly)
- Heart failure
- Hypertension in blacks

ACE inhibitors
- Heart failure
- LV dysfunction
- Post–myocardial infarction
- Diabetic nephropathy
- Nondiabetic nephropathy
- LV hypertrophy
- Carotid atherosclerosis
- Proteinuria/microalbuminuria
- Atrial fibrillation
- Metabolic syndrome

β-Blockers
- Angina pectoris
- Post–myocardial infarction
- Heart failure
- Tachyarrhythmias
- Glaucoma
- Pregnancy

ARBs
- Heart failure
- Post–myocardial infarction
- Diabetic nephropathy
- Proteinuria/microalbuminuria
- LV hypertrophy
- Atrial fibrillation
- Metabolic syndrome
- ACE inhibitor-induced cough

Calcium antagonists (dihydropyridines)
- Isolated systolic hypertension (elderly)
- Angina pectoris
- LV hypertrophy
- Carotid/coronary atherosclerosis
- Pregnancy
- Hypertension in blacks

Diuretics (antialdosterone)
- Heart failure
- Post–myocardial infarction

Calcium antagonists (verapamil, diltiazem)
- Angina pectoris
- Carotid atherosclerosis
- Supraventricular tachycardia

Loop diuretics
- ESRD
- Heart failure

Figure 35.7 Clinical indications favoring the use of specific classes of BP-lowering medications in hypertensive patients. ACE, angiotensin-converting enzyme; ARBs, angiotensin receptor blockers; ESRD, end-stage renal disease; LV, left ventricle.

Compelling and Possible Contraindications to Specific Classes of Blood Pressure-Lowering Therapies

	Compelling	Possible
Thiazide diuretics	Gout	Metabolic syndrome Glucose intolerance Pregnancy
β-blockers	Asthma A-V block (grade 2 or 3)	Peripheral artery disease Metabolic syndrome Glucose intolerance Athletes and physically active patients Chronic obstructive pulmonary disease
Calcium antagonists (dihydropiridines)		Tachyarrhythmias Heart failure
Calcium antagonists (verapamil, diltiazem)	A-V block (grade 2 or 3) Heart failure	
ACE inhibitors	Pregnancy Angioneurotic edema Hyperkalemia Bilateral renal artery stenosis	
ARBs	Pregnancy Hyperkalemia Bilateral renal artery stenosis	
Diuretics (antialdosterone)	Renal failure Hyperkalemia	
DRIs	Pregnancy Hyperkalemia Bilateral renal artery stenosis	

Figure 35.8 Compelling and possible contraindications to specific classes of blood pressure (BP) lowering therapies. A-V, atrioventricular; ACE, angiotensin-converting enzyme; ARBs, angiotensin receptor blockers; DRIs, direct renin inhibitors.

Drug Class	Side Effects
ACE inhibitors	Cough, hyperkalemia
ARBs	Much less frequent hyperkalemia compared to ACE inhibitors
CCBs	
DHPCCB	Pedal edema, headache
Non-DHPCCB	Constipation (verapamil), headache (diltiazem)
Diuretics	Frequent urination, hyperglycemia, hyperlipidemia, hyperuricemia, sexual dysfunction
Central α-agonists	Sedation, dry mouth, rebound hypertension, sexual dysfunction
α-Blockers	Pedal edema, orthostatic hypotension, dizziness
β-Blockers	Fatigue, bronchospasm, hyperglycemia, sexual dysfunction
[K$^+$] Channel openers	Hypertrichosis (minoxidil); lupus-like reactions, pedal edema (hydralazine)

Figure 35.9 Common side effects associated with various classes of antihypertensive drugs. ACE, angiotensin-converting enzyme; ARBs, angiotensin receptor blockers; CCBs, calcium channel blockers; DHPCCB, dihydropyridine calcium channel blocker; non-DHPCCB, nondihydropyridine calcium channel blocker.

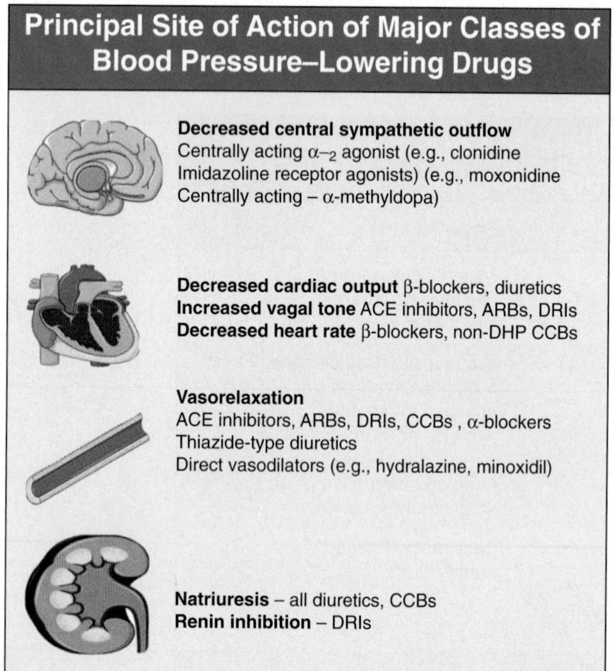

Figure 35.10 Principal site of action of major classes of blood pressure (BP)–lowering drugs. ACE, angiotensin-converting enzyme; ARBs, angiotensin receptor blockers; CCBs, calcium channel blockers; DRIs, direct renin inhibitors; non-DHP CCBs, nondihydropyridine calcium channel blockers.

glucose tolerance. However, spironolactone has antiandrogen activity by binding to the androgen receptor and preventing it from interacting with dihydrotestosterone. Consequently, it can cause nipple tenderness and gynecomastia in some patients, which is dose dependent and can limit its use. Another concern with potassium-sparing diuretics, in general, is the risk of hyperkalemia in people with substantially reduced GFR (see later discussion).

Eplerenone is more selective for the aldosterone receptor than spironolactone is, thereby avoiding the antiandrogen effects of spironolactone. There is very limited experience of eplerenone for the routine management of hypertension. Empirically, milligram per milligram, eplerenone appears less potent than spironolactone. Amiloride is an antagonist of the ENaC in the distal convoluted tubules and collecting ducts of the kidney, decreasing sodium and water reabsorption and promoting potassium excretion. Previously, amiloride was a popular treatment of primary hypertension, when, like spironolactone, it was often used in combination with thiazide-type diuretics. It is less used today even though it shares the advantage of spironolactone over thiazide-type diuretics of not causing hypokalemia, hyperuricemia, or impaired glucose tolerance.

The reason for the decline in popularity of potassium-sparing diuretics for the initial treatment of primary hypertension is not clear; it may reflect the emergence of ACE inhibitors or ARBs. These RAAS blockers are increasingly used for the routine management of hypertension, and there is an increased risk of hyperkalemia when they are combined with spironolactone or amiloride, especially in patients with renal impairment. Spironolactone and amiloride are increasingly used as additional diuretic therapy in patients as part of a multidrug strategy for the treatment of resistant hypertension.[18-20]

β-Adrenoceptor Blocking Drugs (β-Blockers)

β-Blockers reduce BP and CV events in patients with hypertension. Most β-blockers, with the exception of those with strong intrinsic sympathomimetic activity, reduce cardiac output by their negative chronotropic and inotropic effects. As with diuretics, short-term hemodynamic responses can be offset by counteractivation of vasoconstrictor mechanisms, which may limit initial BP lowering. Longer term reduction in arterial pressure during days occurs because of restoration of vascular resistance to pretreatment levels. Partial blockade of renin release from the kidney may contribute to the later hemodynamic response.

β-Blockers differ in their duration of action, selectivity for β_1 receptors, lipophilicity, and partial agonist activity. Side effects include lethargy, aches in the limbs on exercise, impaired concentration and memory, aggravation of depression and psoriasis, erectile dysfunction, vivid dreams, and exacerbation of symptoms of peripheral vascular disease and Raynaud's syndrome. They are contraindicated in asthma and can cause adverse metabolic effects, including impaired glucose tolerance and worsening of dyslipidemia, notably reduced high-density lipoprotein (HDL) cholesterol and raised triglyceride levels. There is accumulating evidence that β-blockers increase the likelihood of new-onset diabetes, particularly in combination with thiazide-type diuretics.[21,22] Moreover, recent meta-analyses suggest that there is a shortfall in CV protection with β-blocker–based treatment of hypertension (especially in stroke reduction) compared with treatment with other major drug classes (see Fig. 35.6).[10,23-25] As a consequence, the recent U.K. guidelines suggested that β-blockers are no longer preferred as an initial therapy for routine hypertension and should be used only when there is a compelling indication other than BP control (e.g., in patients with hypertension and angina or chronic heart failure).[10] One caveat is in younger women of childbearing potential, in whom β-blockers are often effective at lowering BP, perhaps because of higher renin levels in younger people, and are safer than ACE inhibitors or ARBs in those anticipating pregnancy.

Calcium Channel Blockers

Calcium channel blockers (CCBs) are effective at reducing BP and have an extensive evidence base supporting their use for the treatment of hypertension.[4,6] In addition to their BP-lowering properties, they are also effective antianginal agents. They appear to be metabolically neutral with regard to glucose tolerance. An interesting aspect of the BP response to CCBs is that it is largely determined by the magnitude of BP elevation, perhaps more so than with other drugs. Thus, those with higher baseline BP levels experience greater BP lowering with CCBs, whereas those with only modest elevations of BP experience much smaller falls in BP.

There are two main groups of CCBs, the dihydropyridines (e.g., amlodipine, nifedipine) and the nondihydropyridines (e.g., diltiazem, verapamil). The dihydropyridine CCBs act mainly by inducing relaxation of arterial smooth muscle by blocking L-type calcium channels, thereby inducing peripheral vascular relaxation with a fall in vascular resistance and arterial pressure. Nondihydropyridine CCBs block calcium channels in cardiac muscle and reduce cardiac output. Verapamil has an additional antiarrhythmic action through its effects on the atrioventricular node.

The earlier formulations of some dihydropyridine CCBs, such as capsular nifedipine, had a rapid onset and short duration of action, with unpredictable effects on BP. These responses were often accompanied by reflex sympathetic stimulation and tachycardia. The shorter acting oral preparations of CCBs have no place in the routine management of hypertension. More modern, longer acting formulations of dihydropyridine CCBs produce more predictable responses.

Side effects of dihydropyridine CCBs include dose-dependent peripheral edema, which is not due to fluid retention but results from transudation of fluid from the vascular compartments into the dependent tissues because of precapillary arteriolar dilation. This edema does not respond to diuretic therapy but is alleviated by limb elevation. There is emerging evidence that this edema may also be reduced by coadministration of an ACE inhibitor or ARB because of their effects on venous capacitance. Gum hypertrophy can occur with dihydropyridine CCBs but is rarely seen with nondihydropyridine CCBs. Nondihydropyridine CCBs cause less peripheral edema but are negatively inotropic and negatively chronotropic and should therefore be avoided in patients with compromised left ventricular function and in combination with β-blockers. Verapamil use is commonly accompanied by constipation.

Blockade of the Renin-Angiotensin System

RAAS has become a popular target for drug development to treat hypertension. Inhibition of RAAS is predictably effective at lowering BP by inhibiting the various central and peripheral pressor effects of angiotensin II (Ang II). Blockade of RAAS may also lower BP by other mechanisms involving improvements in endothelial function, vagal tone, and baroreceptor function and through inhibition of the renal tubular reabsorption of sodium. In addition, inhibition of RAAS has been popularized by clinical trial evidence showing reduced morbidity and mortality in patients with heart failure, delayed progression of renal disease, and reduced CV events in patients at high CV risk with treatment strategies that involve inhibition of RAAS.[6] Three classes of drugs are now available that directly target RAAS (Fig. 35.11): ACE inhibitors, ARBs, and a new class, the direct renin inhibitors (DRIs).[26]

Angiotensin-Converting Enzyme Inhibitors ACE inhibitors were the first effective strategy to inhibit RAAS and have been used to treat hypertension since the late 1970s. ACE inhibitors block the conversion of Ang I to Ang II by inhibiting ACE. The resulting reduction in levels of Ang II leads to vasodilation and a fall in BP. Ang II has many additional actions that are potentially harmful to the CV system and has been implicated in the pathogenesis of structural changes in the heart, blood vessels, and kidneys in hypertension. Sharp falls in BP after the introduction of ACE inhibitors may occur when the RAS is activated, for example, in patients who are dehydrated, in heart failure, or with

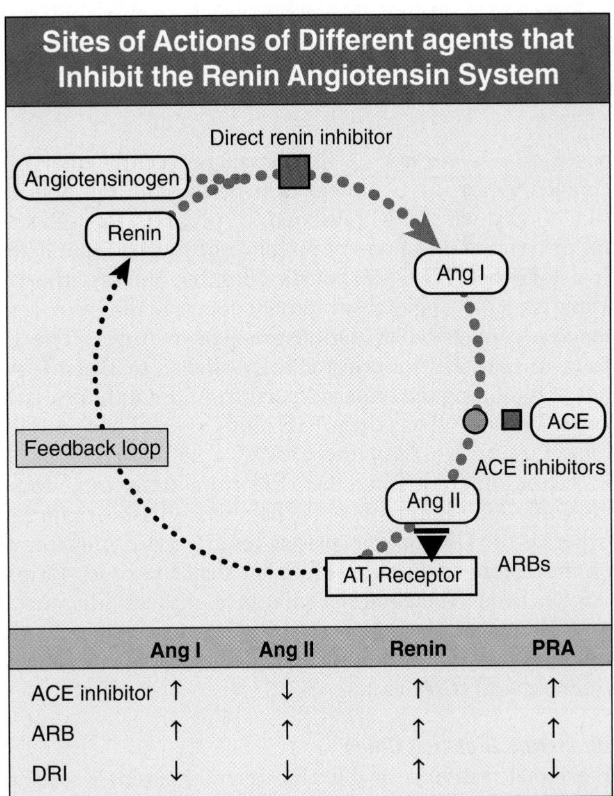

	Ang I	Ang II	Renin	PRA
ACE inhibitor	↑	↓	↑	↑
ARB	↑	↑	↑	↑
DRI	↓	↓	↑	↓

Figure 35.11 Sites of actions of different agents that inhibit the renin-angiotensin system. The resulting neurohumoral profile is also shown. ACE, angiotensin-converting enzyme; Ang, angiotensin; ARB, angiotensin receptor blocker; DRI, direct renin inhibitor; PRA, plasma renin activity.

accelerated hypertension. This is rarely a problem when therapy is initiated in uncomplicated hypertensive patients.

Side effects of ACE inhibitors include the development of a persistent dry cough in about 20% of users. This is more common in women and in people from the Far East and Pacific Rim. The cough disappears only after discontinuation of the drug. Another rare but important complication is angioedema, which occurs in ~1% and is much more common in the black population (~4%). ACE inhibitors should be avoided in women of childbearing potential because of the danger of fetal malformation. They should not be used in patients with significant bilateral renal artery disease because they may precipitate deterioration in renal function and renal failure. Careful monitoring of renal function and serum potassium concentration is also required in patients with more advanced renal impairment of any cause because of the risk of hyperkalemia.

Angiotensin Receptor Blockers In the 1990s, ARBs emerged as an alternative to ACE inhibition. ARBs are highly selective inhibitors of the Ang II type 1 receptor (AT_1). In common with ACE inhibitors, ARBs inhibit the actions of Ang II on the CV system and kidney. ARBs reduce BP as effectively as ACE inhibitors but generally have a longer duration of action than ACE inhibitors. When ACE inhibitors and ARBs have been compared "head to head," they appear to be equally effective in reducing albuminuria and preserving GFR[27] as well as similar in efficacy for preventing major CV events in people with established CVD.[28] Because of their selectivity and specificity for the AT_1 receptor, the ARBs are well tolerated by patients, with a placebo-like adverse effect profile. Moreover, cough and angioedema are much less likely to occur with ARBs than with ACE inhibitors, and most guidelines recommend switching patients to an ARB when an ACE-induced cough occurs. Cautions and contraindications are similar to those outlined for ACE inhibitors.

Direct Renin Inhibition A third strategy recently emerged to inhibit RAAS for the treatment of hypertension: the first nonpeptide, orally active DRI (aliskiren).[26] Aliskiren has high specificity for renin and is a potent inhibitor of plasma renin activity with a long half-life (~24 hours). Aliskiren inhibits the rate-limiting step in angiotensin production, notably the renin-dependent conversion of angiotensinogen to Ang I. The DRI appears to have BP-lowering efficacy similar to that of other means of inhibiting the renin system (i.e., ACE inhibitors, ARBs) but with less side effects than ACE inhibitors.[26] The contraindications to use are similar to those for ACE inhibitors, ARBs. The main factor differentiating the DRI from ACE inhibitors or ARBs is that ACE inhibitors or ARBs activate plasma renin activity, whereas the DRI inhibits plasma renin activity. Aliskiren also has a much longer duration of action than the other forms of RAAS blockade. The clinical significance of these differences in mode of action will be uncovered by an extensive ongoing clinical trial program that will ultimately define the role for DRIs in the hierarchy of treatment.

α-Adrenergic Blocking Drugs

The original members of this class (e.g., prazosin) were short-acting drugs that blocked the activation of α_1-adrenoceptors in the vasculature, leading to vasodilation. Initially, the recommended dosage was too high, and postural hypotension and syncope proved serious problems that retarded the acceptance of this class of drugs, although the use of lower doses and the development of longer acting agents (e.g., doxazosin) have largely overcome this problem. Blockade of sphincteric receptors improves symptoms in patients with benign prostatic hypertrophy. On occasion, these same sphincteric effects can worsen symptoms of stress incontinence in women. Uniquely among antihypertensive drugs, the α_1-antagonists produce modest favorable changes in plasma lipids, with a reduction in total and LDL cholesterol and triglyceride levels and an increase in HDL cholesterol.

Centrally Acting Sympatholytic Drugs

Some of the earliest drugs developed to treat hypertension targeted the activation of the sympathetic nervous system (SNS) at various levels, including the CV regulatory nuclei in the brainstem, the peripheral autonomic ganglia, and the postganglionic sympathetic neuron. Few of these agents have any residual role to play in the modern treatment of hypertension because side effects are common and their use has been superseded by classes of drugs with a more tailored mechanism of action.

Methyldopa reduces sympathetic outflow from the brainstem. It was originally developed in the late 1950s, and it was one of the mainstays of antihypertensive therapy for many years. However, it frequently causes sedation, impaired psychomotor performance, dry mouth, and erectile dysfunction. Its unfavorable impact on quality of life caused it to be gradually replaced by more effective drugs, although it is still extensively used in the management of hypertension of pregnancy, which is now its main indication.

Clonidine is now rarely used because of its short duration of action and risks of a withdrawal syndrome, which occurs when sudden discontinuation results in a rebound rise in catecholamines with features that may resemble pheochromocytoma, such as severe hypertension, tachycardia, and sweating. This is exacerbated when patients are also receiving nonselective β-blockers such as propranolol. The syndrome is treated by readministration of the drug and then gradual discontinuation or the intravenous infusion of labetalol in an emergency. Clonidine is still used and can be effective in some patients with drug-resistant hypertension. Longer acting preparations of clonidine are being developed and may find a place in the management of resistant hypertension.

Moxonidine, a newer centrally acting agent that is an imidazoline receptor agonist, reduces sympathetic outflow and BP. It has a lower incidence of side effects and is better tolerated than other centrally acting agents. It has no clinical trial evidence to support its use as a preferred first-line agent but is used in patients with more resistant hypertension.

Direct Vasodilators

Hydralazine was previously extensively used as part of the original "stepped care" treatment regimens for hypertension. The main disadvantages were sympathetic activation and the development of a lupus-like syndrome, particularly in patients with the slow acetylator genotype. There was also the need for multiple daily dosage. Hydralazine is no longer recommended as a first-line agent for hypertension management. It is still occasionally used in severe hypertension and hypertension associated with pregnancy.

Minoxidil is a potent vasodilator, and its use is largely confined to specialist centers for the treatment of severe and resistant hypertension. This is because of its side effect profile, which is unenviable and includes stimulation of body hair growth; tachycardia and severe fluid retention reflect its potent vasodilator action and concomitant reflex activation of the SNS. For this reason, minoxidil is usually combined with a potent loop diuretic and a β-blocker as part of a triple-therapy approach to severe hypertension. Long-term use can be associated with insidious development of peritoneal and pericardial effusions (especially in subjects with impaired renal function). These necessitate and respond to treatment withdrawal.

Treatment Strategies

Given the multiple drug classes for the treatment of hypertension, there is a need for a treatment strategy that identifies the preferred drugs for initial therapy and preferred combinations for those requiring more than monotherapy to control their BP. The use of drug therapy to lower BP should usually follow a period of observation and repeated measures of BP to ensure that there is a sustained elevation of BP that merits treatment. The duration of the observation period is inversely related to the severity of hypertension. This ranges from immediate treatment to repeated measurement during days or months.

Lifestyle interventions (discussed in Chapter 34) should be initiated during this period of observation and continued even if treatment with drug therapy is initiated. This is important because the actions of drug therapy can often be potentiated by concomitant lifestyle changes (especially body weight reduction and reduction in dietary sodium intake).[29] Furthermore, lifestyle changes are also important to improve the overall health and CV risk profile of the patient, beyond their impact on BP. Another key aspect of the initial assessment of patients is to identify concomitant risk factors, comorbidities, and target organ damage, all of which might influence the selection of drug therapies to improve BP control.

Initial Drug Therapy

Current practice is to initiate treatment with a single drug. Depending on the BP level at baseline, monotherapy will on average reduce systolic pressure by 7 to 13 mm Hg and diastolic pressure by 4 to 8 mm Hg; the greater reductions will generally be observed in those with the highest baseline BP.[30] It is emphasized that these are "average BP responses," and there can be marked heterogeneity in response among individual patients and with different classes of drugs in individual patients. Treatment should normally commence with a low dose of the drug selected. If this is inadequate, there are a range of options:

1. If BP responds to low-dose monotherapy and is not yet controlled but is likely to be controlled with monotherapy (i.e., BP within ~10/5 mm Hg of BP goal), the dose of the initial drug should be titrated upward.
2. If the BP response to the initial low dose is inadequate and the patient's BP remains well short of the target BP, a more appropriate action is to add a second drug, either separately or as a combination tablet, because the majority will require two or more drugs to control their BP.
3. If the initial drug produced a weak response or no response at all and the patient could conceivably achieve the BP goal with monotherapy, the first drug could be discontinued and replaced with another class of antihypertensive agent.

Choice of Initial Therapy There is wide variation in the international guidelines with regard to the preferred initial therapy for primary hypertension.

The U.S. guideline, based on the recommendations of the U.S. Joint National Committee 7 (JNC 7), recommends low-dose thiazide diuretic as initial therapy for all patients (unless contraindicated), reflecting a view that the most important driver of benefit is BP control and that the low-dose diuretic is the most cost-effective way to deliver that.[7] It will be of interest to see whether there is deviation from this stance in the forthcoming JNC 8 guidance due to be published in 2010.

The European guideline positions itself at the other extreme from JNC 7 in suggesting that five major classes of BP-lowering drugs (ACE inhibitors, ARBs, β-blockers, CCBs, and diuretics) are suitable as initial therapy. The choice in part reflects the physician's assessment of concomitant conditions and specific indications and contraindications for different drug classes in an individual patient.[8]

The British Hypertension Society and U.K. NICE guideline have adopted a different and perhaps more pragmatic approach. Their analysis of the data suggested that a CCB (C) or alternatively a thiazide-type diuretic (D) would most likely deliver the most effective initial BP lowering in older people (i.e., ≥55 years), whereas an ACE inhibitor or an ARB (A) would be the preferred initial therapy for younger patients (<55 years), with the caveat that C or D would be the preferred therapy for people of black African origin at any age (Fig. 35.12).[10] The rationale for this recommendation was founded on the observation that plasma renin levels fall as people age and are lower in blacks at any age. Therefore, drugs that target the renin system are more likely to be more effective initial therapy in the younger patients with higher renin activity, whereas the converse is true with aging.

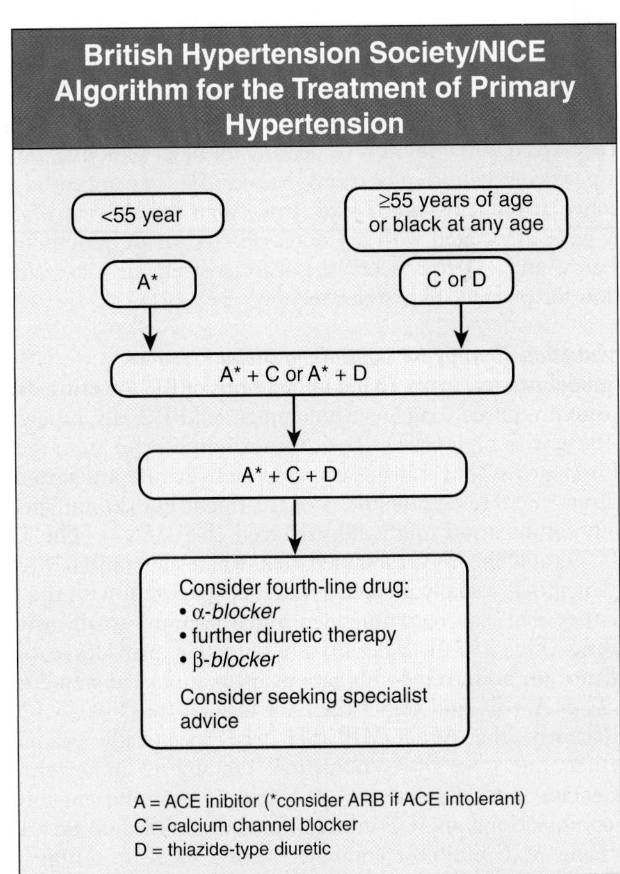

Figure 35.12 British Hypertension Society/NICE algorithm for the treatment of primary hypertension. ACE, angiotensin-converting enzyme; ARB, angiotensin receptor blocker. *(Modified from the NICE hypertension guideline, reference 10.)*

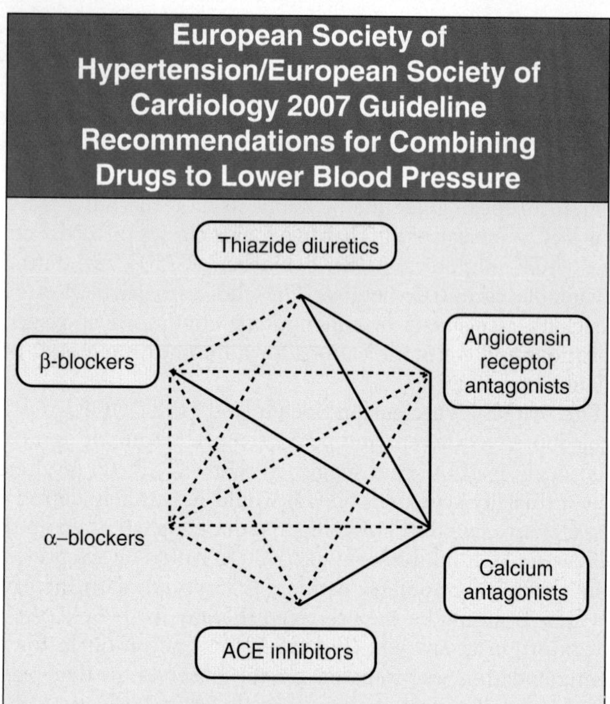

Figure 35.13 European Society of Hypertension/European Society of Cardiology 2007 guideline recommendations for combining drugs to lower blood pressure. The preferred combinations in the general hypertensive population are represented as *thick lines*. Classes of agents proven to be beneficial in controlled intervention trials are enclosed in boxes. ACE, angiotensin-converting enzyme. *(From reference 8.)*

These guidelines also recommended against the use of β-blockers as a preferred initial therapy (especially for older patients), unless there are compelling indications, because (1) they appeared less effective at reducing the risk of stroke than the alternatives, (2) they were associated with an increased risk for development of diabetes, and (3) they were the least cost-effective treatment option for primary hypertension.[10,25]

Combination Therapy for Controlling Blood Pressure

All guidelines recognize that combinations of BP-lowering drugs are often required to achieve recommended BP goals, especially for those with high CVD risk or comorbidities who are targeted to lower goals. The European guidelines provide a diagram to illustrate suitable combinations of treatment but do not specify which combination might be preferred (Fig. 35.13). The U.S. JNC 7 guideline recommended that whatever combination is used, it should usually include a diuretic, consistent with the fact that they had also recommended initial therapy usually with a diuretic (Fig. 35.14). The British guideline provides explicit guidance on preferred combinations of treatment at step 2 (i.e., A + C or A + D) and step 3 (i.e., A + C + D) (see Fig. 35.12).

Recently, the ACCOMPLISH trial specifically evaluated whether the type of combination therapy is important in influencing clinical outcomes by comparing two different single-pill combinations, an ACE inhibitor plus a thiazide diuretic versus the same ACE inhibitor combined with a CCB, in a high-risk group of patients.[31] There was a significant (~20%) reduction in the primary endpoint in favor of the ACE-CCB treatment group, and all components showed this trend. This difference does not appear to be due to differences in BP control between groups. Whatever the explanation for the difference in primary outcomes between treatment groups, the ACCOMPLISH study has established that combining a CCB with ACE inhibitor or presumably other forms of RAAS blockade is an effective treatment option for high-risk patients with hypertension. This result should not lead to a downgrading of diuretic therapy as a preferred component of two-drug combinations. Physicians still need choices—not every patient will tolerate a CCB or a diuretic. Most physicians would choose some form of RAAS blockade (ACE inhibitor, ARB, or DRI) as part of the preferred treatment strategy for hypertension. The data from ACCOMPLISH, alongside a wealth of data with diuretics, provide two excellent evidence-based options to combine with RAAS blockade, a diuretic or a CCB, and perhaps both in those with more resistant hypertension.

Initial Therapy with a Two-Drug Combination "Low-dose" two-drug combination therapy has been recommended in the European and American hypertension guidelines for the treatment of patients whose BP is more than 20/10 mm Hg above their goal BP and therefore unlikely to be controlled with monotherapy (see Fig. 35.12). The concept of initial therapy with a two-drug combination has in part been driven by concern that the upward titration of treatment in people at high risk may be too slow and leave them at risk for too long. A two-drug combination is also logical because the response to a single drug is often limited by counteractivation of pressor systems that limit the effectiveness of monotherapy. This also explains why many BP-lowering drugs in monotherapy have a relatively flat dose-response. For example, sodium and water loss due to diuretics or vasodilation with CCBs will activate RAAS, which limits the BP lowering. Thus, low-dose two-drug combination therapy is likely (1) to produce much greater BP lowering, (2) to reduce heterogeneity in the BP-lowering response, and (3) to have a more effective dose-response to upward titration of either component. The main concern has been safety and tolerability with regard to potentially large initial BP falls in treatment-naive patients. It seems inevitable that low-dose combinations will become more popular as an initial therapy option for a greater proportion of patients, with the preferred combinations likely to be RAAS blockade plus diuretic and RAAS blockade plus CCB.

Combining RAS Blockade?

The popular view that RAAS blockade is an important way of preventing or regressing hypertension-mediated structural and functional damage led to suggestions that different strategies to block RAAS should be combined to deliver more effective RAAS blockade. The recent ONTARGET trial demonstrated that an ACE inhibitor plus ARB combination was no more effective than ACE inhibitor alone at preventing major CV events in a high-risk population of patients.[28] This suggests that this combination of ACE inhibitor plus ARB should not be routinely used for the management of patients with primary hypertension or patients at high CV risk in general. Further studies are required to better define the place for alternative options for dual RAS blockade (e.g., ACE inhibitor or ARB plus direct renin inhibition). Such studies are ongoing.

Resistant Hypertension

Resistant hypertension has been defined as BP that remains above goal in spite of the concurrent use of three antihypertensive agents of different classes. The U.S. guidance suggests that one of the three agents should be a diuretic and all agents should be prescribed at optimal doses.[19] The definition could have been

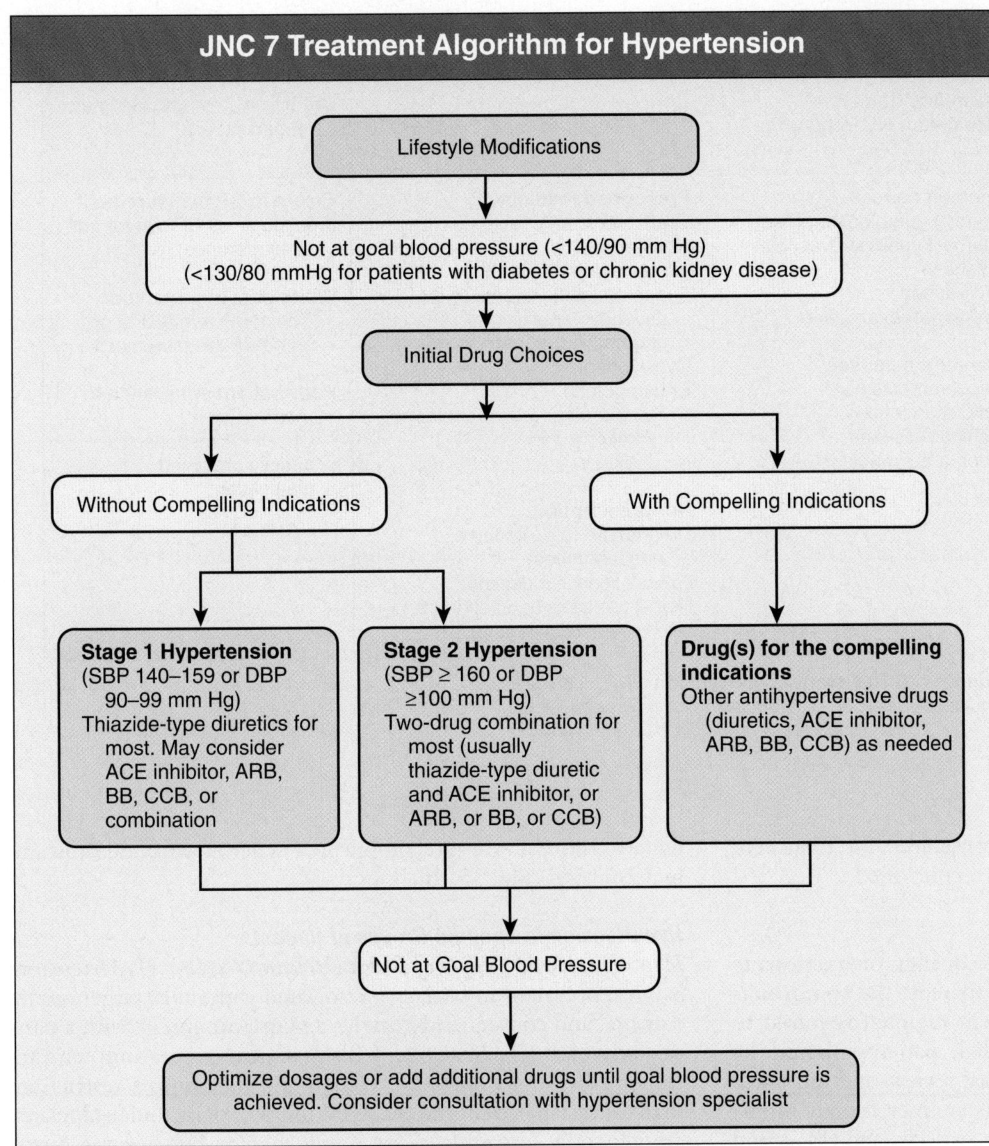
JNC 7 Treatment Algorithm for Hypertension
Lifestyle Modifications
Not at goal blood pressure (<140/90 mm Hg)
(<130/80 mmHg for patients with diabetes or chronic kidney disease)
Initial Drug Choices
Without Compelling Indications
With Compelling Indications
Stage 1 Hypertension
(SBP 140–159 or DBP 90–99 mm Hg)
Thiazide-type diuretics for most. May consider ACE inhibitor, ARB, BB, CCB, or combination
Stage 2 Hypertension
(SBP ≥ 160 or DBP ≥100 mm Hg)
Two-drug combination for most (usually thiazide-type diuretic and ACE inhibitor, or ARB, or BB, or CCB)
Drug(s) for the compelling indications
Other antihypertensive drugs (diuretics, ACE inhibitor, ARB, BB, CCB) as needed
Not at Goal Blood Pressure
Optimize dosages or add additional drugs until goal blood pressure is achieved. Consider consultation with hypertension specialist

Figure 35.14 JNC 7 treatment algorithm for hypertension. DBP, diastolic blood pressure; SBP, systolic blood pressure. Drug abbreviations: ACEI, angiotensin-converting enzyme inhibitor; ARB, angiotensin receptor blocker; BB, β-blocker; CCB, calcium channel blocker. *(From reference 7.)*

even more prescriptive by suggesting that the three drugs would usually comprise A + C + D in best tolerated doses. Most of these people will be older, often obese, and invariably with evidence of target organ damage. In the absence of evidence of target organ damage, white coat hypertension should be excluded by 24-hour ambulatory monitoring. Other causes of resistant hypertension should also be considered (Fig. 35.15).[16]

The evidence base from which to define the optimal treatment of resistant hypertension is limited. Most patients with drug-resistant hypertension are likely to be retaining sodium and will respond to further diuretic therapy. This can be achieved by further increasing the dose of the thiazide diuretic or using low-dose spironolactone (e.g., 25 mg/day) or amiloride (10 to 20 mg/day), with careful monitoring of electrolytes. Recent data suggest that a selective endothelin type A receptor antagonist (darusentan) is effective at reducing BP in people with resistant hypertension but should be avoided in people with a prior history of heart failure or left ventricular dysfunction.[32] For some patients with severe drug-resistant hypertension, it may be necessary to use a combination of minoxidil, loop diuretic, and β-blocker to improve BP control. Beyond drug therapy, a novel approach to treatment of patients with resistant hypertension by use of radiofrequency ablation of renal sympathetic nerves was recently reported and requires further evaluation.[33]

Medication to Reduce Cardiovascular Risk

BP should not be treated in isolation, and treatment should be considered part of a more comprehensive strategy to reduce CVD risk. Patients at high risk, that is, those with established CVD, target organ damage, or diabetes, and those with a calculated CVD risk that is elevated (e.g., ≥20% during 10 years) should be considered for additional interventions to reduce risk.[34] These include reinforcement of lifestyle advice, especially smoking cessation, and treatment with statin therapy to further reduce the risk of stroke and coronary disease. In recent studies, routine use of statins to reduce total cholesterol values by 40 mg/dl (~1 mmol/l) has been associated with a reduction in the risk of ischemic heart disease events by about one third and of stroke by about one fifth, over and above the benefit already accrued from BP lowering.[34,35] Moreover, the relative risk reduction associated with statin therapy in higher risk hypertensive patients was not dependent on a high baseline cholesterol value. Higher risk

Considerations in the Patient with Resistant Hypertension	Secondary Causes of Resistant Hypertension	Concomitant Drugs that May Raise BP and Counter Antihypertensive Agent Effects	Causes of "Pseudoresistant Hypertension"
Demographics Older age; especially >75 yrs Obesity Women> men More common in blacks Excess dietary sodium High baseline BP and chronicity of uncontrolled hypertension **Concomitant disease** Target organ damage: LVH or CKD Diabetes Atherosclerotic vascular disease Aortic stiffening	**Common causes** Primary hyperaldosteronism Atherosclerotic renovascular disease Sleep apnea Chronic kidney disease **Uncommon causes:** Pheochromoctoma Aortic coarctation Cushing's disease Hyperparathyroidism	**Prescribed medicines** Oral contraceptives Nonsteroidal anti-inflammatory drugs Sypathomimetic agents (e.g., decongestants in proprietary cold remedies) Cyclosporine Erthyropoietin Corticosteroids (e.g., prednisone, hydrocortisone) **Nonprescription:** Drug abuse (e.g., cocaine, amphetamines) Excess licorice ingestion Herbal remedies (e.g., ephedra, also known as mahuang)	**Errors in BP measurement** (i.e., too small BP cuff for arm circumference) **White coat hypertension** Check BP with ABPM or home BP measurements **Poor patient adherence to medications** Check BP response to directly observed medication

Figure 35.15 Considerations in the Patient with Resistant Hypertension. BP, blood pressure; ABPM, ambulatory blood pressure monitoring; CKD, chronic kidney disease; LVH, left ventricular hypertrophy. *(Modified from reference 18.)*

hypertensive patients should also be considered for treatment with antiplatelet drugs once BP has been controlled.

Follow-up

In the early stages of treatment, the frequency of monitoring will be determined by the response to therapy, the comorbidities, and the complexity of the treatment regimen required to control the BP. Once BP is controlled, patients should be re-evaluated at least annually for a formal review, and most will be re-evaluated every 6 months. Patients are increasingly monitoring their own BP in the intervening periods, and this trend is likely to increase.

Withdrawal of Therapy

Most patients with hypertension require lifelong therapy. Some with grade 1 hypertension who make major adjustments to their lifestyle may obtain sufficient fall in their BP to warrant safe withdrawal of monotherapy. However, patients with target organ damage or those at high CVD risk should not usually have their therapy withdrawn unless there is a compelling clinical reason to do so.[9] In patients with previously severe hypertension that has subsequently been well controlled, treatment withdrawal may not always result in an immediate increase in BP. After treatment withdrawal, BP can sometimes take many months to progressively rise back to dangerously high pretreatment values. Any patient who discontinues therapy must remain under review with regular monitoring of BP. All but a very few will require treatment again.

Indications for Specialist Referral

Referral to a specialist center is sometimes indicated for the management of hypertension. Indications include uncertainty about the decision to treat, investigations to exclude secondary hypertension, severe and complicated hypertension, and resistant hypertension (Fig. 35.16).

Hypertension in Specific Groups of Patients

Hypertension in People of Black African Origin Hypertension is more prevalent in blacks, is associated with more target organ damage, and consequently carries a worse prognosis, with a particularly high risk of stroke.[37] Black patients as a group tend to respond better to diuretics, CCBs, and dietary salt restriction than caucasian patients do. ACE inhibitors, ARBs, and β-blockers are generally less effective as initial therapy but become more effective in combination with diuretics or CCBs.

Hypertension in Older People If a BP of 140/90 mm Hg or higher is used to define hypertension, then more than 70% of people older than 60 years will be hypertensive, the majority of these patients having isolated systolic hypertension.[38] Surveys suggest that physicians consistently underestimate the risks and undertreat hypertension in older people. There are, however, some important considerations in treating older people.

1. The arterial wall stiffening that gives rise to systolic hypertension and increased pulse pressure (isolated systolic hypertension) is also associated with impaired baroreflex sensitivity with increased risk of orthostatic hypotension. Thus, it is important to record lying and standing BP in the elderly.
2. Estimated GFR declines with age, and renal conservation of sodium and fluid in the face of depletion is impaired. Elderly patients are therefore more subject to volume depletion as a result of diuretic therapy.
3. Clearance of drugs and their active metabolites is decreased as a result of declining hepatic and renal function.
4. Cardiac function and reserve are often reduced, and patients are therefore much more likely to develop cardiac failure. This explains why endpoint trials of hypertension

Indications for Specialist Referral for Patients with Hypertension

Urgent treatment needed
Accelerated hypertension (severe hypertension with grade III–IV retinopathy)
Particularly severe hypertension (>220/120 mm Hg)
Impending complications (e.g., transient ischemic attack, left ventricular failure)

Possible underlying cause
Any clue in history or examination of a secondary cause (e.g., hypokalemia with increased or high–normal plasma sodium)
Elevated serum creatinine
Proteinuria or hematuria
Sudden onset or worsening of hypertension
Resistance to multidrug regimen (i.e., ≥ 3 drugs)
Young age (any hypertension <20 years; needing treatment <30 years)

Therapeutic problems
Multiple drug intolerance
Multiple drug contraindications
Persistent nonadherence or noncompliance

Special situations
Unusual blood pressure variability
Possible white coat hypertension
Hypertension in pregnancy

Figure 35.16 Indications for specialist referral for patients with hypertension.

treatment have consistently shown reductions in morbidity and mortality from cardiac failure.

5. Comorbidity is much more common.
6. Communication and adherence with therapy may be more difficult with decline in cognitive function. Some evidence from clinical trials suggests that this decline may be retarded by antihypertensive treatment.

Despite these considerations, the elderly tolerate BP-lowering medications well, and the benefits of BP reduction are impressive with regard to reductions in morbidity and mortality due to stroke, ischemic heart disease, and heart failure. As a general rule, drug regimens should be as simple as possible and dosages increased more gradually. The greatest danger results from lowering of pressure too rapidly. Until recently, there was uncertainty about the risks and benefits of treating hypertension in the very elderly, that is, those older than 80 years. The HYVET study[17] in this age group confirmed that treatment is well tolerated and associated with impressive reductions in the risk of stroke, heart failure, and mortality. Thus, there is no reason to manage very elderly patients any differently from those who are not as old. Biologic rather than chronologic age should be the deciding factor in initiating antihypertensive treatment.

REFERENCES

1. Lewington S, Clarke R, Qizilbash N, et al. Age-specific relevance of usual blood pressure to vascular mortality: A meta-analysis of individual data for one million adults in 61 prospective studies. *Lancet*. 2002;360: 1903-1913.
2. Lawes CM, Vander Hoorn S, Rodgers A. Global burden of blood-pressure-related disease, 2001. *Lancet*. 2008;371:1513-1518.
3. Asia Pacific Cohort Studies Collaboration (APCSC). Joint effects of systolic blood pressure and serum cholesterol on cardiovascular disease in the Asia Pacific region. *Circulation*. 2005;112:3384-3390.
4. Blood Pressure Lowering Treatment Trialists' Collaboration. Effects of different blood-pressure-lowering regimens on major cardiovascular events: Results of prospectively-designed overviews of randomised trials. *Lancet*. 2003;362:1527-1545.
5. Staessen JA, Wang JG, Thijs L, et al. Cardiovascular prevention and blood pressure reduction: A quantitative overview updated until 1st March 2003. *J Hypertens*. 2003;21:1055-1076.
6. Williams B. Recent hypertension trials: Implications and controversies. *J Am Coll Cardiol*. 2005;45:813-827.
7. Chobanian AV, Bakris GL, Black HR, et al. The Seventh Report of the Joint National Committee on Prevention, Detection, Evaluation and Treatment of High Blood Pressure: The JNC 7 report. *JAMA*. 2003;289: 2560-2572.
8. The Task Force for the Management of Arterial Hypertension of the European Society of Hypertension (ESH) and of the European Society of Cardiology (ESC). 2007 Guidelines for the Management of Arterial Hypertension. *J Hypertens*. 2007;25:1105-1187.
9. Williams B, Poulter NR, Brown MJ, et al. Guidelines for management of hypertension: Report of the fourth working party of the British Hypertension Society, 2004—BHS IV. *J Hum Hypertens*. 2004;18: 139-185.
10. Higgins B, Williams B, Guideline Development Group. Pharmacological management of hypertension. *Clin Med*. 2007;7:612-616.
11. Vasan RS, Larson MG, Leip EP, et al. Impact of high-normal BP on the risk of cardiovascular disease. *New Engl J Med*. 2001;345: 1291-1297.
12. Arguedas JA, Perez MI, Wright JM. Treatment blood pressure targets for hypertension. Cochrane Database Syst Rev. 2009;3:CD004349.
13. Zanchetti A, Grassi G, Mancia G. When should antihypertensive drug treatment be initiated and to what levels should systolic blood pressure be lowered? A critical reappraisal. *J Hypertens*. 2009;27:923-934.
14. Verdecchia P, Staessen JA, Angeli F, et al. Cardio-Sis investigators. Usual versus tight control of systolic blood pressure in non-diabetic patients with hypertension (Cardio-Sis): An open-label randomised trial. *Lancet*. 2009;374:525-533.
15. Sleight P, Redon J, Verdecchia P, et al. Prognostic value of blood pressure in patients with high vascular risk in the Ongoing Telmisartan Alone and in combination with Ramipril Global Endpoint Trial study. *J Hypertens*. 2009;27:1360-1369.
16. ACCORD study Group. Effects of intensive blood pressure control in type 2 diabetes mellitus. *New Eng J Med*. 2010;362:1575-1585.
17. Beckett NS, Peters R, Fletcher AE, et al. Treatment of hypertension in patients 80 years of age or older. *N Engl J Med*. 2008;358: 1887-1898.
18. Williams B. Resistant hypertension: An unmet treatment need. *Lancet*. 2009;374:1396-1398.
19. Calhoun DA, Jones D, Textor S, et al. Resistant hypertension: Diagnosis, evaluation and treatment. A scientific statement from the American Heart Association Professional Education Committee of the Council for High Blood Pressure Research. *Hypertension*. 2008;51:1403-1419.
20. Chapman N, Dobson J, Wilson S, et al. Anglo-Scandinavian Cardiac Outcomes Trial Investigators. Effect of spironolactone on blood pressure in subjects with resistant hypertension. *Hypertension*. 2007;49: 839-845.
21. Pepine CJ, Cooper-DeHoff RM. Cardiovascular therapies and risk of the development of diabetes. *J Am Coll Cardiol*. 2004;44:609-612.
22. Mason JM, Dickinson HO, Nicolson DJ, et al. The diabetogenic potential of thiazide-type diuretic and beta-blocker combinations in patients with hypertension. *J Hypertens*. 2005;23:1777-1781.
23. Lindholm LH, Carlberg B, Samuelsson O. Should β blockers remain first choice in the treatment of primary hypertension? A meta-analysis. *Lancet*. 2005;366:1545-1553.
24. Wiysonge C, Bradley H, Myose B, et al. Beta-blockers for hypertension. Cochrane Database Syst Rev. 2007;1:CD002003.
25. Williams B. Beta-blockers and the treatment of hypertension. *J Hypertens* 2007;25:1351-1353.
26. Brown MJ. Aliskiren. *Circulation*. 2008;118:773-784.
27. Barnett AH, Bain SC, Bouter P, et al. Diabetics Exposed to Telmisartan and Enalapril Study Group. Angiotensin Receptor Blockade versus converting enzyme inhibition in type 2 diabetes with nephropathy. *N Engl J Med*. 2004;351:1952-1961.
28. ONTARGET Study Investigators. Telmisartan, ramipril, or both in patients at high risk for vascular events. *N Engl J Med*. 2008;358: 1547-1559.
29. Dickinson HO, Mason JM, Nicolson DJ, et al. Lifestyle interventions to reduce raised blood pressure: A systematic review of randomized controlled trials. *J Hypertens*. 2006;24:215-233.

30. Law MR, Wald NJ, Morris JK, Jordan RE. Value of low dose combination treatment with blood pressure lowering drugs: Analysis of 354 randomised trials. *BMJ*. 2003;326:1427.
31. Jamerson K, Weber MA, Bakris GL, et al. Benazepril plus amlodipine or hydrochlorothiazide for hypertension in high-risk patients. *N Engl J Med*. 2008;359:2417-2428.
32. Weber MA, Black H, Bakris G, et al. A selective endothelin-receptor antagonist to reduce blood pressure in patients with treatment-resistant hypertension: A randomised, double-blind, placebo-controlled trial. *Lancet*. 2009;374:1423-1431.
33. Krum H, Schlaich M, Whitbourn R, et al. Catheter-based renal sympathetic denervation for resistant hypertension: A multicentre safety and proof-of-principle cohort study. *Lancet*. 2009;373:1275-1281.
34. Mendis S, Lindholm LH, Mancia G, et al. World Health Organization (WHO) and International Society of Hypertension (ISH) risk prediction charts: Assessment of cardiovascular risk for prevention and control of cardiovascular disease in low and middle-income countries. *J Hypertens*. 2007;25:1578-1582.
35. Sever PS, Dahlof B, Poulter NR, et al. ASCOT Investigators. Prevention of coronary and stroke events with atorvastatin in hypertensive patients who have average or lower-than-average cholesterol concentrations, in the Anglo-Scandinavian Cardiac Outcomes Trial–Lipid Lowering Arm (ASCOT-LLA): A multicentre randomised controlled trial. *Lancet*. 2003;361:1149-1158.
36. Emberson J, Whincup P, Morris R, et al. Evaluating the impact of population and high-risk strategies for the primary prevention of CVD. *Eur Heart J*. 2004;25:484-491.
37. Douglas JG, Bakris GL, Epstein M, et al, the Hypertension in African Americans Working Group. Management of high blood pressure in African Americans. *Arch Intern Med*. 2003;163:525-541.
38. Chobanian AV. Isolated systolic hypertension in the elderly. *N Engl J Med*. 2007;357:789-796.

CHAPTER 36

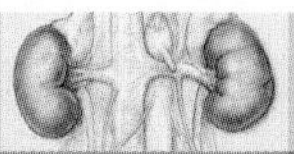

Evaluation and Treatment of Hypertensive Urgencies and Emergencies

Pantelis A. Sarafidis, George L. Bakris

The term *malignant hypertension* first appeared in 1928[1] to describe patients with very high blood pressure (BP) values. "Malignant" was used to compare the prognosis of these patients with that of most cancers because they had such rapid target organ deterioration, such as retinal hemorrhages or exudates and papilledema, usually associated with encephalopathy, acute renal failure, and microangiopathic hemolytic anemia.[2,3] Dramatic advancements of both in-hospital and outpatient treatment of hypertensive emergencies, however, have led to an improved prognosis, that is, decrease in 1-year mortality from 80% in 1928 to 50% in 1955 and 10% in 1989.[4] Thus, terms such as *malignant* and *accelerated* hypertension have been replaced by the terms *hypertensive emergency* and *hypertensive urgency*.

Marked elevations in systolic and diastolic BP, usually above 180/120 mm Hg, can be classified as either emergencies or urgencies. A hypertensive emergency is defined as marked elevation in BP complicated by evidence of acute life-threatening target organ damage, such as coronary ischemia, dissecting aortic aneurysm, pulmonary edema, hypertensive encephalopathy, cerebral hemorrhage, and eclampsia. In this clinical condition, BP should be reduced by at least 20 to 40 mm Hg within 10 to 30 minutes with parenteral drug therapy in an intensive care unit. Hypertensive urgency is a clinical setting of significant BP elevation, generally above 180/110 mm Hg, *without* life-threatening target organ dysfunction (i.e., papilledema, evidence of early heart failure, acute renal failure), although some evidence of target organ damage is usually present (hemorrhages and exudates in fundi, headaches). The approach to hypertensive urgency is a gradual BP reduction within hours, usually with oral medications.[4-6]

ETIOLOGY AND PATHOGENESIS

Both hypertensive emergencies and urgencies can develop *de novo* in normotensive individuals or complicate patients with underlying primary or secondary hypertension.[3,4] Some hypertensive emergencies have acute BP elevations through increased activity of the renin-angiotensin system (RAS), for example, acute glomerulonephritis, renal crisis in patients with systemic sclerosis, or renal artery stenosis. In others, acutely elevated BP is the result of excess catecholamine release, such as from pheochromocytoma, monoamine oxidase inhibitor crisis, cocaine intoxication, or spinal cord injury. Occult renal artery stenosis is a frequent cause of elevated BP resulting in acute left ventricular failure or pulmonary edema. It may be difficult to differentiate whether BP elevation is the cause or the result of a hypertensive emergency. Thus, a careful diagnostic evaluation of hypertensive emergencies and urgencies is essential to guide proper treatment.

The most common clinical setting for a hypertensive urgency is the chronic, often untreated or poorly controlled hypertensive patient whose usual BP is above 180/110 mm Hg. In many of these patients, chronically elevated BP does not affect target organ perfusion because of autoregulation. Autoregulation is the ability of blood vessels to dilate or to constrict in response to changes in perfusion pressure and thereby to maintain normal organ perfusion.[7] This mechanism is present in the brain and kidneys and involves L-type calcium channels.[7] Arteries from normotensive individuals can maintain flow over a wide range (80 to 150 mm Hg) of mean arterial pressures. Chronic elevations in BP cause compensatory functional and structural changes in the arteriolar circulation and shift the autoregulatory curve to the right, which allows hypertensive patients to maintain normal perfusion and to avoid excessive blood flow at higher BP levels.[3,8] These features are established for the cerebral and renal circulation (Fig. 36.1).[7,9]

Target organ damage associated with hypertensive emergency results from the inability of autoregulatory mechanisms to maintain normal perfusion pressures in vascular beds of the brain and kidney when BP rises to values above the autoregulatory range.[8] This causes endothelial injury that results in increased vascular wall permeability, cell proliferation, and activation of platelets and the coagulation cascade, leading to further vascular damage and tissue ischemia. This is coupled with activation of hormonal systems and release of vasoactive substances (RAS, catecholamines, endothelin, vasopressin) that maintain a vicious circle between elevated BP and vascular injury.[10] Other mechanisms that contribute to impaired autoregulation include progressive disease of arterioles, observed in both cerebral and renal circulations as well as when autoregulation is pharmacologically inhibited (such as with dihydropyridines or furosemide). In most cases, the development of a hypertensive emergency occurs in the presence of chronic hypertension and relates to the disease status of the arterioles that already have some impaired autoregulation.

The structural changes associated with hypertensive emergencies are fibrinoid necrosis of small arteries and arterioles in the brain and kidney (Fig. 36.2), coupled with findings of injury of the afflicted organs (e.g., cerebral edema).[8,11]

EPIDEMIOLOGY

The exact incidence of hypertensive emergencies and urgencies as well as their demographic distribution is not known. One

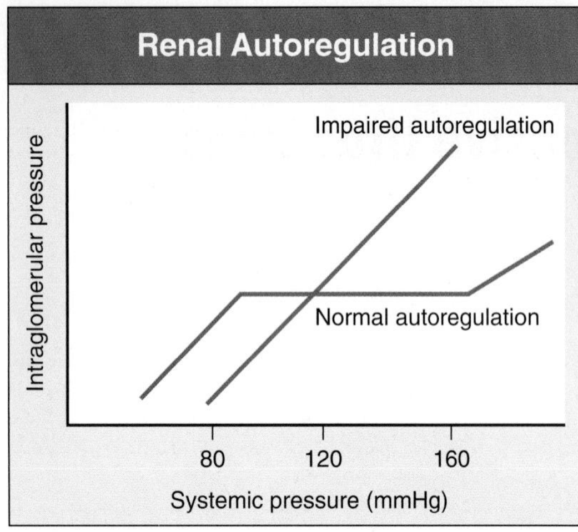

Figure 36.1 Renal autoregulation. Relationship of systemic to glomerular pressure in the setting of normal or abnormal renal autoregulation.

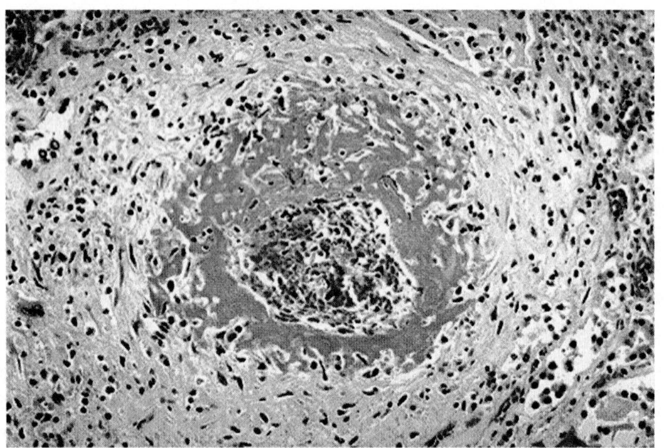

Figure 36.2 Fibrinoid necrosis, noted as a pink homogeneous material, in the renal interlobar artery of a patient with severe hypertensive emergency.

Diagnostic Evaluation for Hypertensive Emergencies and Urgencies

History	Previous diagnosis and treatment of hypertension Symptoms, previous diagnoses and treatment of cardiac, cerebral, and visual damage Intake of pressor agents: sympathomimetrics, illicit substances
Repeated blood pressure measurements (first measurement in both arms)	
Physical examination	Cardiac Vascular Pulmonary Neurologic Optic fundi
Laboratory studies	Full blood count, urinanalysis, creatinine, urea, electrolytes Plasma renin activity, aldosterone, and catecholamines if secondary hypertension is suspected
Electrocardiography	
Chest radiograph	
Further investigations (according to the clinical presentation)	Brain CT scan or MRI Echocardiography (transthoracic, transesophageal) Thoracoabdominal CT scan or MRI Abdominal ultrasonography

Figure 36.3 Diagnostic evaluation for hypertensive emergencies and urgencies. CT, computed tomography; MRI, magnetic resonance imaging.

study with more than 14,000 emergency department visits during 12 months showed that hypertensive urgencies accounted for 76% and emergencies for 24% of hypertension-related visits.[12] In this study, the most common presentations of hypertensive emergencies were associated with cerebral infarction (24.5%), acute pulmonary edema (22%), hypertensive encephalopathy (16%), and acute heart failure (14%), followed by myocardial infarction (12%), cerebral hemorrhage (5%), eclampsia (5%), and aortic dissection (2%). Note that scleroderma can also present as a hypertensive emergency but is rare. In a different series of 435 hypertensive emergency department visits, 40% were hypertensive urgencies, almost all with some degree of preexisting kidney disease, and 60% were emergencies.[13] Hospitalization for hypertensive emergency occurs at a rate of 1 to 2 cases per million per year in the United States.[8]

In developed countries, widespread use of antihypertensive agents has reduced the incidence of hypertensive emergencies. This hypothesis is supported from several indirect observations.[8,10] Use of any antihypertensive drug reduces the risk of hypertensive emergencies because poor treatment compliance and outpatient BP control are predictors of subsequent hypertensive crises. In a series of 100 patients hospitalized for severe hypertension, 93% had previously stopped prescribed antihypertensive drugs or were unable to access health care resources. Further, hospitalization for hypertensive emergency is more common in developing countries, ethnic minorities (African Americans and Hispanics in the United States), and individuals with low socioeconomic status.[14]

DIAGNOSIS

The primary goal of the diagnostic process is differentiation of a true hypertensive emergency from urgency, as the respective therapeutic approaches are different. The second goal is quick assessment of the type and the severity of ongoing target organ damage. In some hypertensive emergencies, information from history (acute head trauma, preeclampsia, scleroderma) or overt symptoms and signs (chest or back pain, dyspnea, throbbing abdominal mass) may guide the diagnosis; whereas in other cases (severe hypertension with altered mental status), the evaluation is more protracted.

The diagnostic approach begins with the patient's history, with attention to duration, severity, and treatment of preexisting hypertension and associated conditions (Fig. 36.3).[6,10] BP measurements should be performed in both arms (if possible, in both sitting and standing positions) and a leg according to current guidelines (see Chapter 32).[2,5] A careful cardiac, pulmonary, peripheral vessel, and neurologic examination with assessment of mental status should follow, coupled with a thorough funduscopic examination for hemorrhages, exudates, and papilledema. Secondary hypertension should not be missed in this initial examination. For example, an abdominal bruit suggests renovascular hypertension, a palpable abdominal mass suggests abdominal aneurysm or polycystic kidneys, a radial-femoral pulse delay suggests aortic coarctation, abdominal striae are observed with central obesity and Cushing's syndrome, and exophthalmos suggests hyperthyroidism.

The basic laboratory studies in a hypertensive emergency include a complete blood count with peripheral smear, urinalysis, creatinine concentration, urea concentration, and electrolyte values.[6,10] Assessment of kidney function and, if possible, comparison with a patient's recent measurement is very important. Severe hypertension accompanied by acute deterioration in kidney function, microscopic hematuria, or nephritic urine sediment suggests acute glomerulonephritis. If a secondary form of hypertension is suspected, samples for plasma renin activity, aldosterone concentration, and 24-hour urine metanephrine values should also be drawn *before* initiation of treatment. Testing should be performed with the patient supine, and ideally the patient should not be receiving β-blockers, especially labetalol, as they will give false-positive readings of metanephrine values. Electrocardiography to rule out myocardial ischemia and left ventricular strain or hypertrophy as well as chest radiography should be performed in every patient.[6]

Neurologic syndromes associated with hypertension (subarachnoid hemorrhage, intracerebral hemorrhage, thrombotic stroke, and hypertensive encephalopathy) are difficult to distinguish from one another. Computed tomography (CT) or magnetic resonance imaging (MRI) provides a definite diagnosis of a hemorrhagic or thrombotic stroke. Echocardiography, thoracoabdominal CT or MRI, or abdominal ultrasound may be needed in suspected aortic dissection or pheochromocytoma.[6]

TREATMENT

General Principles for Management of Hypertensive Emergencies

Although therapy with parenteral antihypertensive agents may be initiated in the emergency department, patients with a hypertensive emergency should be admitted to an intensive care unit for continuous BP monitoring, clinical surveillance, and continued parenteral administration of an appropriate agent (Figs. 36.4 and 36.5). Specific BP levels do not determine the severity and the emergency of the situation because the autoregulatory structural and functional changes may vary between individuals, such that some individuals may develop target organ damage at lower BP. Understanding of autoregulation is crucial for therapeutic decisions; sudden lowering of BP into a "normal" range could lead to inadequate tissue perfusion.[8] There is evidence that abrupt lowering of BP is harmful. For example, the use of sublingual nifedipine may precipitate stroke or shunt blood away from the penumbra of the brain, resulting in cognitive dysfunction.[15] Thus, the goal of antihypertensive therapy is not to rapidly normalize BP but to prevent target organ damage by gradually reducing BP while minimizing the risk of hypoperfusion.

For most hypertensive emergencies, the mean BP should be reduced by no more than 20% to 25% within the first few minutes to an hour.[5,6] A diastolic BP target between 100 and 110 mm Hg or a reduction of 25% compared with the initial baseline, whichever is higher, is appropriate to be achieved within the next 2 to 6 hours. Reduction of BP diastolic pressure to less than 90 mm Hg or by 35% or more of the initial mean BP has been associated with major organ dysfunction, coma, and death.

If the level of BP reduction is well tolerated and the patient clinically stable, further gradual reductions toward levels below 140/90 mm Hg should be implemented within the next 24 to 48 hours. Typically, a long-acting oral calcium channel blocker (CCB) is given along with either an α- and β-blocker like carvedilol or nebivolol or RAS blocker, and the intravenous medication is gradually reduced during 1 to 2 hours.[8]

An important consideration before initiation of intravenous therapy is assessment of the patient's volume status. Because of pressure natriuresis, patients with hypertensive emergencies may be volume depleted, and restoration of intravascular volume may help restore organ perfusion and prevent a precipitous fall in BP.[16]

Major exceptions to these treatment recommendations include (1) patients with acute stroke, in whom there is no clear evidence to support immediate BP lowering and a more cautious approach is needed (see Chapter 40); (2) patients with aortic dissection, who should have their systolic BP lowered to below 100 mm Hg if tolerated; and (3) patients in whom BP should be lowered to enable the use of thrombolytic agents.[5,6,16]

A systematic review of four hypertensive emergency and 15 urgency studies suggested that several medications are effective for lowering BP in a hypertensive emergency (see Fig. 36.4). However, the authors concluded that because of the lack of large randomized controlled trials, questions including appropriate duration of follow-up and whether any of the agents provide mortality or morbidity benefits remain unanswered.[17] A recent meta-analysis of 15 trials[18] showed some minor differences in the degree of BP lowering when one class of antihypertensive drug was compared with another, but the clinical significance is unknown.

Specific Aspects of Antihypertensive Drug Use for Hypertensive Emergencies (see Fig. 36.5)

For several years, sodium nitroprusside was considered the first-choice drug for all hypertensive emergencies. It is easily titrated, is inexpensive, and has a long record of effectiveness in treating hypertensive emergencies of nearly all types.[6,8,10,19] Limitations of nitroprusside use include the need for invasive BP monitoring and its metabolic products (thiocyanate and cyanide), which contraindicate its use in pregnancy and limit the time used (48 hours) in patients with renal or hepatic dysfunction. Nitroprusside is reported to increase intracranial pressure in high doses, to obliterate cerebral autoregulation, and to reduce regional coronary blood flow, which could limit its usefulness in patients with neurologic complications or acute coronary syndromes. Nitroprusside infusion typically begins at 0.3 μg/kg/min and increases by 0.2 to 1.0 μg/kg/min every 3 to 5 minutes until BP reaches the target range. Because of the toxicity issues, some authors suggest that nitroprusside be used only when alternative drug choices are not available and not exceed a dose of 2 μg/kg/min.[16]

Two other drugs approved in the United States for hypertensive emergencies are increasingly used. Nicardipine is a dihydropyridine CCB with intermediate onset and duration of effect, prolonged half-life, and strong cerebral and coronary vasodilatory activity. It is useful for most hypertensive emergencies, especially in patients with coronary artery disease. Nicardipine interacts with inhalant anesthetics.[8,16,19] Fenoldopam mesylate is a selective agonist of dopaminergic 1 receptors located mainly in the renal and splanchnic arteries with lesser density in the coronary and cerebral arteries.[8,10,19] Intravenous fenoldopam does not cross the blood-brain barrier and has no central nervous system activity because it is a poorly lipid soluble molecule. In clinical trials compared with sodium nitroprusside, fenoldopam demonstrated similar BP-lowering efficacy and beneficial renal effects (increased diuresis, natriuresis, and creatinine clearance, and it has a very short half-life).[20] Thus, fenoldopam is mostly useful for BP

Treatment of Hypertensive Emergencies

Drug	Mechanism of Action	Dose	Onset of Action	Duration of Action	Adverse Effects*	Special Indications
Vasodilators						
Sodium nitroprusside	↑ Cyclic GMP, blocks intracellular Ca^{2+} increase	0.25–10 µg/kg/min IV infusion†	Immediate	1–2 min	Nausea, vomiting, muscle twitching, sweating, thiocyanate and cyanide intoxication	Most hypertensive emergencies; caution with high intracranial pressure, hepatic or renal failure
Nicardipine hydrochloride	Calcium channel blocker	5–15 mg IV every hour	5–10 min	15–30 min, may exceed 4 h	Tachycardia, headache, flushing, nausea, vomiting, local phlebitis	Most hypertensive emergencies except acute heart failure; caution with coronary ischemia
Fenoldopam mesylate	Dopamine 1 receptor agonist	0.1–0.3 µg/kg/min IV infusion	>5 min	30 min	Tachycardia, headache, nausea, flushing	Most hypertensive emergencies; caution with glaucoma
Nitroglycerin	↑ Nitrate receptors	5–100 µg/min IV infusion	2–5 min	5–10 min	Headache, vomiting, methemoglobinemia, tachyphylaxis, tolerance with prolonged use	Coronary ischemia, pulmonary edema
Hydralazine hydrochloride	Opens K+ channels	10 IV	10–20 min	1–4 h	Tachycardia, flushing, headache, vomiting, aggravation of angina	Eclampsia
Enalaprilat	ACE inhibitor	1.25–5 mg every 6 h IV	15–30 min	6–12 h	Precipitous fall in BP in high-renin states, variable response, acute renal failure	Acute left ventircular failure; avoid in acute myocardial infarction
Diazoxide	Direct-acting vasodilator	50–150 mg every 5 min IV or 15–30 mg/min IV infusion	1–5 min	4–12 h	Nausea, flushing, reflex sympathetic stimulation, aggravation of angina, sodium retention, hyperglycemia	Avoid in angina, acute myocardial infarction, aortic dissection
Clevidipine butyrate	CCB	1–2 mg/h IV infusion Increase every 5–10 min up to 16 mg/h	2–4 min	5–15 min	Tachycardia, headache, flushing, heart failure deterioration	Most hypertensive emergencies except acute heart failure; caution with severe aortic stenosis
Adrenergic inhibitors						
Labetalol hydrochloride	α_1, β-Blocker	20–80 mg IV bolus every 10 min or 0.5– 2 mg/min IV infusion	5–10 min	3–6 h	Nausea, vomiting, scalp tingling, bronchoconstriction, dizziness, heart block, congestive heart failure	Most hypertensive emergencies except acute heart failure
Esmolol hydrochloride	β_1-Blocker	0.5–2.0 mg/min IV infusion or 250–500 µg/kg/ min IV bolus, then 50–100 µg/kg/ min by infusion May repeat bolus after 5 min or increase infusion to 300 µg/min	1–2 min	10–30 min	Nausea, asthma, first-degree heart block, heart failure, thrombophlebitis	Aortic dissection, perioperative
Urapidil	α_1-Blocker	12.5–25 mg IV bolus followed by 5–40 mg/h IV infusion	3–5 min	4–6 h	Headache, dizziness	Perioperative
Phentolamine	α-Blocker	5–15 mg IV bolus	1–2 min	10–30 min	Tachycardia, flushing, headache	Catecholamine excess

Treatment of Hypertensive Urgencies

Drug	Mechanism of Action	Dose	Onset of Action	Duration of Action	Adverse Effects*	Special Indications
Captopril	ACE inhibitor	12.5–25 mg per os every 1–2 h	15–30 min	4–6 h	Angioedema, cough, acute renal failure	
Clonidine	Central α_2-agonist	0.1–0.2 mg per os every 1–2 h	30–60 min	6–8 h	Sedation, dry mouth, bradycardia, rebound hypertension after withdrawal	
Labetalol	α_1,β-Blocker	200–400 mg per os every 2–3 h	30–120 min	6–8 h	Bronchoconstriction, heart block, congestive heart failure	
Furosemide	Loop diuretic	20–40 mg per os every 2–3 h	30–60 min	8-12 h	Volume depletion, hyponatriemia, hypokaliemia	
Isradipine	CCB	5–10 mg per os every 4–6 h	30–90 min	8-16 h	Headache, tachycardia, flushing, peripheral edema	

*Hypotension may occur with all agents
†Requires light-resistant delivery system

Figure 36.4 Pharmacologic agents for treatment of hypertensive emergencies and urgencies. *Hypotension may occur with all agents. †Requires light-resistant delivery system. ACE, angiotensin-converting enzyme; BP, blood pressure; CCB, calcium channel blocker; GMP, guanosine monophosphate.

Management of Specific Types of Hypertensive Emergencies				
Type of Emergency	**First Choice of Drug(s)**	**Second Choice/Additional Drug(s)**	**Drugs to Be Avoided**	**Aim of BP Reduction**
Neurological				
Hypertensive encephalopathy	Nicardipine, fenoldopam, labetalol	Esmolol, urapidil, nitroprusside*		20–25% reduction in mean BP over 1–2 hours
Ischemic stroke	Nicardipine, labetolol, nitroprusside*	Esmolol, urapidil		Reduction of BP if above 220/120 mmHg (mean BP >130 mmHg) by no more than 10%–15% within the first 24 hours to avoid impairing cerebral blood flow in the penumbra.
Intracerebral hemorrhage	Nicardipine, labetolol, nitroprusside*	Esmolol, urapidil, nimodipine for subarachnoid haemorrhage		Decrease in BP below 185/110 mmHg to prevent further bleeding and hypoperfusion. For subarachnoid haemorrhage in normotensive patients reduction to systolic BP 130–160 mmHg.
Cardiac				
Coronary ischemia/infarction	Nitroglycerin or nitroprusside*	Nicardipine; labetalol, esmolol if heart failure absent	Diazoxide, hydralazine	Improvement in cardiac perfusion
Heart failure/ pulmonary edema	Nitroglycerin or nitroprusside* or fenoldopam	Enalaprilat; diuretics	Diazoxide, hydralazine; β-blockers	Decrease in afterload
Aortic dissection	Labetalol or combination of esmolol with fenoldopam or nicardipine	Nitroprusside*	Diazoxide, hydralazine	Decrease of aortic wall stress with systolic BP reduction <100–120 mmHg in 20 minutes (if possible)
Renal				
Acute glomerulonephritis, collagen-vascular renal disease, or renal artery stenosis	Fenoldopam	Nicardipine, labetalol; diuretics for volume overload	Sodium nitroprusside; RAS blockers (use initially for scleroderma but after renal function stabilizes for other conditions)	Reduction in vascular resistance and volume overload without compromise of renal blood flow or GFR
Catecholamine Excess States				
Pheochromocytoma	Phentolamine or labetalol	β-blocker in the presence of phentolamine	Diuretics	Control of BP paroxysms from sympathetic stimulation
Ingestion of cocaine or other sympathomimetic	Phentolamine or labetalol	β-blocker in the presence of phentolamine	Diuretics	Control of BP paroxysms from sympathetic stimulation
Perioperative/Postoperative Hypertension				
Coronary artery surgery	Nitroglycerin	Esmolol, labetalol, sodium nitroprusside*, fenoldopam, nicardipine, urapidil, clevidipine		Protection against target organ damage and surgical complications (keep BP <140/90 or mean BP 105 mmHg)
Non-cardiac surgery	Esmolol, labetalol, nitroprusside, fenoldopam, nicardipine, urapidil, nitroglycerin, clevidipine			Protection against target organ damage and surgical complications
Pregnancy-related				
Eclampsia	Hydralazine, labetalol, long-acting nifedipine	$MgSO_4$, methyldopa	Nitroprusside*, ACE inhibitors, ARBs	Control of BP (typically <90 mmHg diastolic but often lower) and protect placental blood flow

Figure 36.5 Management of specific types of hypertensive emergencies. *Nitroprusside obliterates cerebral autoregulation, fenoldopam does not and hence is preferred if cost not prohibitive. Nimodipine has also been shown to be effective in ischemic strokes. ACE, angiotensin-converting enzyme; ARBs, angiotensin receptor blockers; BP, blood pressure; RAS, renin-angiotensin system.

reduction in patients with renal impairment, those with heart failure, and those undergoing vascular surgery. Fenoldopam infusion typically begins at 0.1 μg/kg/min and is increased at 20-minute intervals by 0.1 to 0.2 μg/kg/min, with a maximum dose of 1.5 μg/kg/min. Fenoldopam must be administered with caution, if at all, to patients with glaucoma, as it increases intraocular pressures. In relation to nitroprusside, nicardipine and fenoldopam appear much safer, but they are both more expensive.

Labetalol is a nonselective α_1- and β-blocker (in the ratio of 1:7, given intravenously) that can be used in many hypertensive emergencies as it has rapid onset of action, potent and sustained effect, and low toxicity. It reduces peripheral vascular resistance without a reflex increase in systolic volume. Its main indications are aortic dissection, acute coronary syndromes, hypertensive encephalopathy, and adrenergic crisis. It is contraindicated in patients with heart failure, heart block, and chronic obstructive pulmonary disease.[6,10,16]

A newer agent that may provide a useful alternative for the treatment of hypertensive crises is clevidipine, a third-generation dihydropyridine CCB, developed for use in clinical settings in which tight BP control is crucial. Clevidipine is a short-acting selective arteriolar vasodilator that reduces peripheral resistance without affecting cardiac filling pressures. Its metabolism is not affected by renal or hepatic function.[16] Recent trials demonstrate clevidipine to be effective and safe in the control of postoperative hypertension[21] as well as in hypertensive emergencies.[22] Clevidipine butyrate was approved in the United States at mid-2008 for BP reduction when oral therapy is not feasible or not desirable.

In hypertensive emergencies due to catecholamine excess states (pheochromocytoma, monoamine oxidase inhibitor crisis, cocaine intoxication), the use of diuretics should be avoided as these patients are usually volume depleted.

Treatment of Hypertensive Urgencies

There is no proven benefit from rapid BP reduction in asymptomatic patients without evidence of acute target organ damage; thus, all authorities agree that BP lowering should occur during a longer time than for a hypertensive emergency. BP reduction to levels within the range below 160/100 mm Hg may be accomplished within 2 to 4 hours in the emergency department with orally administered drugs.[5,6] In short, the most important aspect of treatment of a hypertensive urgency is not achievement of BP goal but ensuring adequate follow-up, within a week, generally.[5,8]

All agents that may be used to manage such conditions are listed in Figure 36.4. The choice of drugs for treatment of hypertensive urgency is much broader than for emergencies because almost all antihypertensive drugs lower BP effectively in a reasonable time. Captopril, clonidine, labetalol, and other short-acting antihypertensive drugs have been mostly used for this condition (see Fig. 36.4).[5,6] Short-acting nifedipine, although once commonly used, is now contraindicated secondary to a higher incidence of stroke, myocardial infarctions, and deaths related to precipitous hypotensive episodes.[23]

Oral clonidine (0.1 to 0.2 mg) is one of the most commonly used short-acting agents in this setting. However, patients should not be routinely discharged with clonidine if they have a history of nonadherence to drug regimens because of the risk of rebound hypertension if clonidine is abruptly stopped.

Furosemide can effectively lower BP if elevated pressure is related to volume, which is uncommon. A common physiologic response of the kidney to elevated pressures is a natriuresis; hence, many such patients may be volume depleted. Longer acting CCBs, such as nifedipine XL, amlodipine, and sustained-release isradipine, also have a key role in longer term maintenance of this condition.[6] Their disadvantage is that they inhibit renal autoregulation; thus, they should not be used as initial agents when BP is very high for routine management of hypertension. Because of their delayed onset of action, they also do not have a role in management of hypertensive emergencies.

REFERENCES

1. Keith NM, Wagener HP, Kernohan JW. The syndrome of malignant hypertension. *Arch Intern Med.* 1928;41:141-153.
2. Mancia G, De Backer G, Dominiczak A, et al. 2007 Guidelines for the Management of Arterial Hypertension: The Task Force for the Management of Arterial Hypertension of the European Society of Hypertension (ESH) and of the European Society of Cardiology (ESC). *J Hypertens.* 2007;25:1105-1187.
3. Moser M, Izzo JL Jr, Bisognano J. Hypertensive emergencies. *J Clin Hypertens (Greenwich).* 2006;8:275-281.
4. Elliott WJ. Clinical features and management of selected hypertensive emergencies. *J Clin Hypertens (Greenwich).* 2004;6:587-592.
5. Chobanian AV, Bakris GL, Black HR, et al. Seventh report of the Joint National Committee on Prevention, Detection, Evaluation, and Treatment of High Blood Pressure. *Hypertension.* 2003;42:1206-1252.
6. Agabiti-Rosei E, Salvetti M, Farsang C. European Society of Hypertension Scientific Newsletter: Treatment of hypertensive urgencies and emergencies. *J Hypertens.* 2006;24:2482-2485.
7. Palmer BF. Renal dysfunction complicating the treatment of hypertension. *N Engl J Med.* 2002;347:1256-1261.
8. Elliott WJ. Clinical features in the management of selected hypertensive emergencies. *Prog Cardiovasc Dis.* 2006;48:316-325.
9. Bidani AK, Griffin KA. Pathophysiology of hypertensive renal damage: Implications for therapy. *Hypertension.* 2004;44:595-601.
10. Vaughan CJ, Delanty N. Hypertensive emergencies. *Lancet.* 2000;356: 411-417.
11. Escande M, Diadema B, Icard MC, Peyre JP. [Hypertensive emergencies]. *Ann Cardiol Angeiol (Paris).* 2007;56:174-182.
12. Zampaglione B, Pascale C, Marchisio M, Cavallo-Perin P. Hypertensive urgencies and emergencies. Prevalence and clinical presentation. *Hypertension.* 1996;27:144-147.
13. Martin JF, Higashiama E, Garcia E, et al. Hypertensive crisis profile. Prevalence and clinical presentation. *Arq Bras Cardiol.* 2004;83: 131-136.
14. Bennett NM, Shea S. Hypertensive emergency: Case criteria, sociodemographic profile, and previous care of 100 cases. *Am J Public Health.* 1988;78:636-640.
15. Messerli FH, Eslava DJ. Treatment of hypertensive emergencies: Blood pressure cosmetics or outcome evidence? *J Hum Hypertens.* 2008;22: 585-586.
16. Marik PE, Varon J. Hypertensive crises: Challenges and management. *Chest.* 2007;131:1949-1962.
17. Cherney D, Straus S. Management of patients with hypertensive urgencies and emergencies: A systematic review of the literature. *J Gen Intern Med.* 2002;17:937-945.
18. Perez MI, Musini VM. Pharmacological interventions for hypertensive emergencies: A Cochrane systematic review. *J Hum Hypertens.* 2008; 22:596-607.
19. Feldstein C. Management of hypertensive crises. *Am J Ther.* 2007; 14:135-139.
20. Pilmer BL, Green JA, Panacek EA, et al. Fenoldopam mesylate versus sodium nitroprusside in the acute management of severe systemic hypertension. *J Clin Pharmacol.* 1993;33:549-553.
21. Aronson S, Dyke CM, Stierer KA, et al. The ECLIPSE trials: Comparative studies of clevidipine to nitroglycerin, sodium nitroprusside, and nicardipine for acute hypertension treatment in cardiac surgery patients. *Anesth Analg.* 2008;107:1110-1121.
22. Noviawaty I, Uzun G, Qureshi AI. Drug evaluation of clevidipine for acute hypertension. *Expert Opin Pharmacother.* 2008;9:2519-2529.
23. Grossman E, Messerli FH, Grodzicki T, Kowey P. Should a moratorium be placed on sublingual nifedipine capsules given for hypertensive emergencies and pseudoemergencies? *JAMA.* 1996;276:1328-1331.

CHAPTER 37

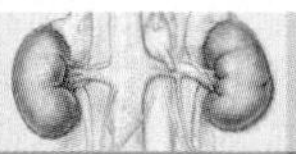

Renovascular Hypertension and Ischemic Renal Disease

Stephen C. Textor, Barbara A. Greco

Renovascular disease with reduced perfusion of the kidney can produce several clinical syndromes, most commonly a rise in arterial pressure designated renovascular hypertension (RVH), with or without associated ischemic and hypertensive renal injury. RVH is usually caused by renal artery stenosis, and it is among the most common secondary forms of hypertension. Recognition that reduction of renal perfusion pressure activates a series of hormonal and neuronal responses that raise systemic arterial pressure remains one of the seminal observations in blood pressure (BP) regulation. Not surprisingly, high blood pressure in patients with renal artery stenosis frequently leads to the assumption that the stenosis is the cause of the hypertension. However, there are several clinical scenarios for patients with renal artery stenosis and hypertension: (1) true RVH, in which renal artery stenosis is the sole cause of the hypertension; (2) pure primary hypertension, in which renal artery stenosis is present but does not contribute to the hypertension at all; (3) primary hypertension with superimposed RVH due to renal artery stenosis; and (4) renal artery stenosis in concert with other causes of renal parenchymal damage in which the elevated arterial pressure may be driven by the pathophysiologic factors characteristic of renal injury. Final proof that a patient has RVH rests with the demonstration that the hypertension is improved or eliminated by removal of the stenosis by surgical or endovascular revascularization or by removal of the kidney distal to the stenosis.

The term *ischemic nephropathy* or ischemic renal disease (IRD) refers to the reduced glomerular filtration rate (GFR) associated with reduced renal blood flow beyond the level of renal autoregulatory compensation.[1] Over time, IRD can lead to renal atrophy and progressive renal impairment. As with RVH, establishment of the causal relationship between proximal renal artery stenosis and the development and progression of chronic kidney disease (CKD) is often difficult. Collateral renal blood supply can preserve renal viability in the face of proximal atherosclerotic renovascular occlusive disease, whereas small-vessel and parenchymal disease often coexist with main renovascular disease, particularly from atherosclerosis. Attempts to revascularize ischemic kidneys sometimes succeed in recovering renal function, but results are often disappointing. There are few predictors to guide therapeutic choices in these patients, who are often at high risk for complications of interventions.

Management of renovascular disease has been changing in recent years. New antihypertensive drug regimens are well tolerated and more effective. Endovascular procedures allowing percutaneous restoration of blood flow for atherosclerotic lesions are also more widely available and safer than ever before.[2] Whereas a decade ago, most clinicians would have favored immediate revascularization for threatened kidneys, recent prospective trials have failed to demonstrate major advantages to revascularization compared with intensive medical therapy alone.[3] As a result, there is justifiable uncertainty as to the optimal timing and intervention for many such patients. As with most vascular disease, the issue is most often one of timing, rather than simply deciding whether to rely on one therapy or another indefinitely.

DEFINITION, ETIOLOGY, AND EPIDEMIOLOGY

RVH is defined as a syndrome of elevated BP (systolic or diastolic) produced by a variety of conditions that interfere with arterial circulation to the kidneys. The majority of patients with RVH have significant main renal artery stenosis with concomitant reduced renal perfusion pressure. Most conditions arise with reduced perfusion to one kidney, while a second "contralateral" kidney is exposed to elevated systemic pressures, so-called two-kidney hypertension by analogy to experimental models of "two-kidney, one-clip hypertension" (see later discussion). Figure 37.1 provides a list of conditions that can produce the syndrome of RVH by impairing renal blood supply. Many of these are rare, but all have in common a significant reduction in renal perfusion pressure. Other rarely encountered clinical conditions associated with the syndrome of RVH include unilateral renal trauma with associated intrarenal or perirenal hematoma (identified as a Page kidney), unilateral ureteral obstruction, atrophic pyelonephritis, and congenitally hypoplastic kidney. In some circumstances, both kidneys are affected (such as may happen with atheroembolic disease) or a solitary functioning kidney is affected, leading to a syndrome without a contralateral kidney, designated one-kidney RVH (see Fig. 37.1). Of the conditions that may produce the syndrome of RVH, main renal artery stenosis is by far the most common. The two major causes of main renal artery disease are fibromuscular dysplasia (FMD) and atherosclerotic renal vascular disease (ASRVD).

Fibromuscular Dysplasia

FMD produces aberrancies in luminal diameter of large and medium-sized renal arteries due to nonatherosclerotic arteriopathies. The lesions usually involve the mid to distal vessel beyond the first 2 cm from the aorta (Fig. 37.2). Clinical manifestations of renal artery FMD are summarized in Figure 37.3A. The prevalence of clinically apparent renovascular FMD is estimated at

Renovascular Hypertension: Classification

"Two-Kidney Hypertension" (implies that a contralateral, nonaffected kidney is present)
- Unilateral fibromuscular dysplasia
- Unilateral atherosclerotic renovascular disease
- Renal artery aneurysm
- Renal artery embolism
- Traumatic arterial occlusion
- Arteriovenous fistula
- Renal artery dissection or thrombosis
- Aortic dissections with compromise to renal ostium
- Page kidney (i.e., post-traumatic perirenal fibrosis)
- Metastatic tumor compressing renal parenchyma
- Pheochromocytoma compressing renal artery
- Phakomatosis pigmentovascularis type II b
- Neurofibromatosis
- Behçet's disease
- Covering of origin of renal artery by aortic stent graft
- Renal artery spasm

"One-Kidney Hypertension" (implies that the entire renal mass is beyond the vascular lesion, either bilateral disease or a solitary functioning kidney)
- Stenosis to solitary kidney
- Bilateral arterial stenosis
- Coarctation of the aorta
- Vasculitis involving renal arteries
- Congenital vascular anomalies
- Atheroembolic renal disease

Figure 37.1 Renovascular Hypertension: Classification. Examples of renovascular disease with associated renovascular hypertension or ischemic renal disease.

4/1000, with a lower prevalence of cerebrovascular involvement of 1/1000.[4] Data from screening angiography in potential kidney donors suggest that the prevalence may be higher, with FMD observed in 3% to 6% of normotensive individuals. FMD is most common among young females and usually presents as early-onset hypertension between the ages of 15 and 50 years. Because FMD is commonly asymptomatic for many years, FMD can be discovered at any age, sometimes as an incidental finding during angiography. Familial FMD occurs in approximately 10% of cases and tends to involve both renal arteries.[4] It has also been associated with subclinical evidence of carotid flow abnormalities in first-degree relatives, consistent with an autosomal dominant inheritance pattern.[5] FMD may also complicate other hereditary conditions, such as Ehlers-Danlos and Marfan syndromes (Fig. 37.3B).

Renal arteries are involved with FMD in 65% to 70% of cases, whereas only 25% to 30% of cases involve cerebral arteries. Both sites are involved in approximately 15% of patients. Hence, young patients presenting with spontaneous carotid artery dissection or occlusion should be considered at risk for FMD of the kidney and vice versa.

The molecular etiology of FMD is unknown. Multiple candidate genes have been proposed, but no specific genetic mutations have been identified. These lesions are disruptions of vascular wall components with abnormal deposition of collagen in bands and, in some cases, disruption of elastic membrane. Several subtypes of FMD have been described on the basis of the predominant layers of the arterial wall involved, but these are not mutually exclusive. The three main types of FMD are medial fibroplasia, which is the most common, and intimal and periadventitial fibroplasia.

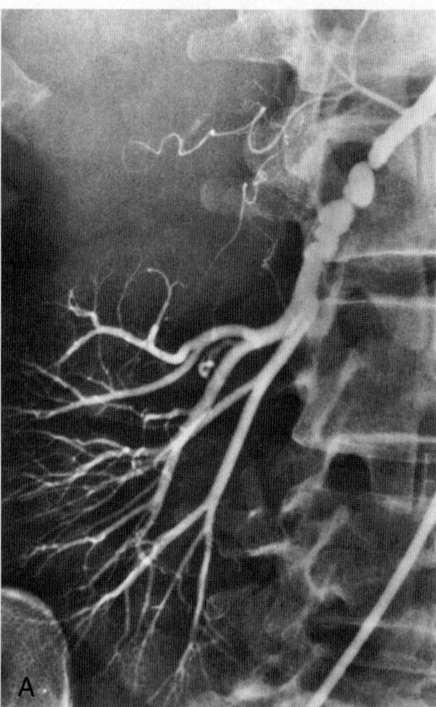

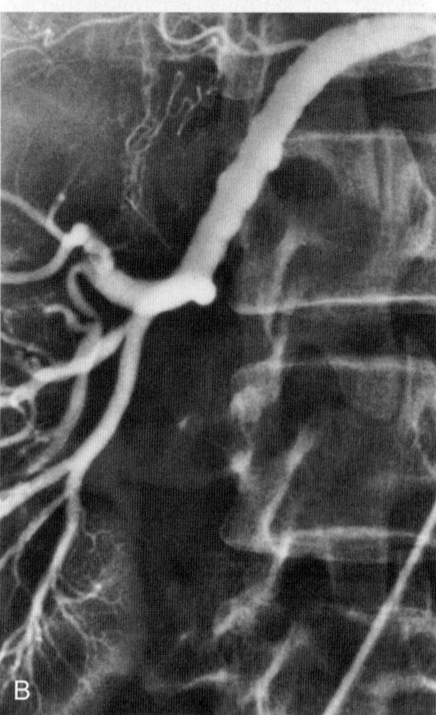

Figure 37.2 Fibromuscular dysplasia. A, Selective renal arteriogram illustrating the beaded appearance of fibromuscular dysplasia with multiple webs characteristic of medial fibroplasia in a 39-year-old woman. **B,** Selective injection of the same renal artery after technically successful percutaneous transluminal renal angioplasty. *(Courtesy Michael McKusick, MD, Mayo Clinic, Rochester, Minnesota, USA.)*

The histologic features coincide with the arteriographic "phenotype" outlined in Figure 37.4. Medial fibroplasia is most common and is manifested as a "string of beads" appearance of alternating stenoses with apparent luminal dilations. Other lesions appear as focal or elongated vascular narrowing, sometimes with diffuse attenuation of branch or distal vessels. Unlike ASRVD, FMD generally appears in the middle or distal

Clinical Manifestations and Disorders Associated with Fibromuscular Dysplasia
Clinical Manifestations
Incidental finding (e.g., living kidney donors)
Renovascular hypertension
Renal infarction
Loin or flank pain
Hematuria
Retroperitoneal hemorrhage
Cerebrovascular accident
Disorders
Tuberous sclerosis
Marfan syndrome
Ehler's-Danlos syndrome
Cystic medial necrosis
Coarctation of the aorta
Alport's syndrome
Renal agenesis or dysgenesis
α 1-Antitrypsin deficiency
Medullary sponge kidney
Pheochromocytoma
Infantile myofibromatosis
Ergotamine preparation, methysergide
Cigarette smoking
Collagen III glomerulopathy
Atherosclerotic renovascular disease

Figure 37.3 Clinical manifestations and disorders associated with fibromuscular dysplasia.

portions of the renal artery or branch vessels. Renal artery aneurysms occur in up to 50% of cases of FMD and can cause vessel occlusion or dissection. Arteriovenous fistulas and thrombosis can also occur.

Atherosclerotic Renovascular Disease

Atherosclerotic narrowing of the renal arteries generally occurs in older patients (>50 years of age) and is associated with systemic atherosclerosis. Younger patients with premature atherosclerosis are also at risk. ASRVD is the most common cause of RVH and can contribute to loss of renal function leading to end-stage renal disease (ESRD) (Fig. 37.5). Atherosclerotic plaque often arises in the first or second centimeter of the renal artery or may extend from the aorta into the renal ostium. Aortic and renal vascular calcification is often present. ASRVD is a manifestation of systemic atherosclerotic disease and is associated with coronary, cerebrovascular, peripheral vascular, and aortic disease.[6] The prevalence of ASRVD appears to be increasing. This probably reflects the fact that more people are surviving to ages when atherosclerotic vascular disease in the visceral abdominal vessels can reach critical levels, producing RVH when the kidney is affected. In patients undergoing angiography of the peripheral or coronary circulation, ASRVD is found in 11% to 42%.[7] Predictors of ASRVD include a history of hypertension, presence of renal functional impairment, coexisting vascular or coronary artery disease, presence of abdominal bruits, and history of smoking. Renal artery lesions are bilateral in 20% to 40% of such patients.

Estimates of the prevalence of ASRVD depend on the population screened. One population-based study of a cohort of 870 patients older than 65 years screened with renal artery duplex sonography found a 6.8% prevalence of ASRVD, defined as greater than 60% stenosis. No differences were detected between African Americans and Caucasians.[8] Autopsy series report an overall prevalence of 4% to 20%, with progressively higher rates

Histologic Classifications of Fibromuscular Dysplasia and Angiographic Phenotypes

Type	Frequency	Histology	Angiographic Apperance
Medial			
Medial fibroplasia	85%-100% most common	Alternating ridges of collagen /loss of elastic membrane	"String of beads" Medial: bead diameter is larger than lumen diameter
Perimedial fibroplasia	Rarer (10%–15%)		Perimedial: bead diameter is smaller than lumen diameter
Medial hyperplasia	Rarest	True smooth muscle hyperplasia: no fibrosis	Medial hyperplasia: smooth stenosis without beads
Intimal	<10%	Circumferential deposition of collagen in intima: fragmented or duplicated internal elastic lamina	Concentric smooth stenosis: long smooth narrowing
Adventitial	<1%	Dense collagen replaces fibrous tissue in adventitia and surrounding tissue	Smooth stenosis or diffuse attenuation of vessel lumen

Figure 37.4 Histologic classifications of fibromuscular dysplasia and angiographic phenotypes.

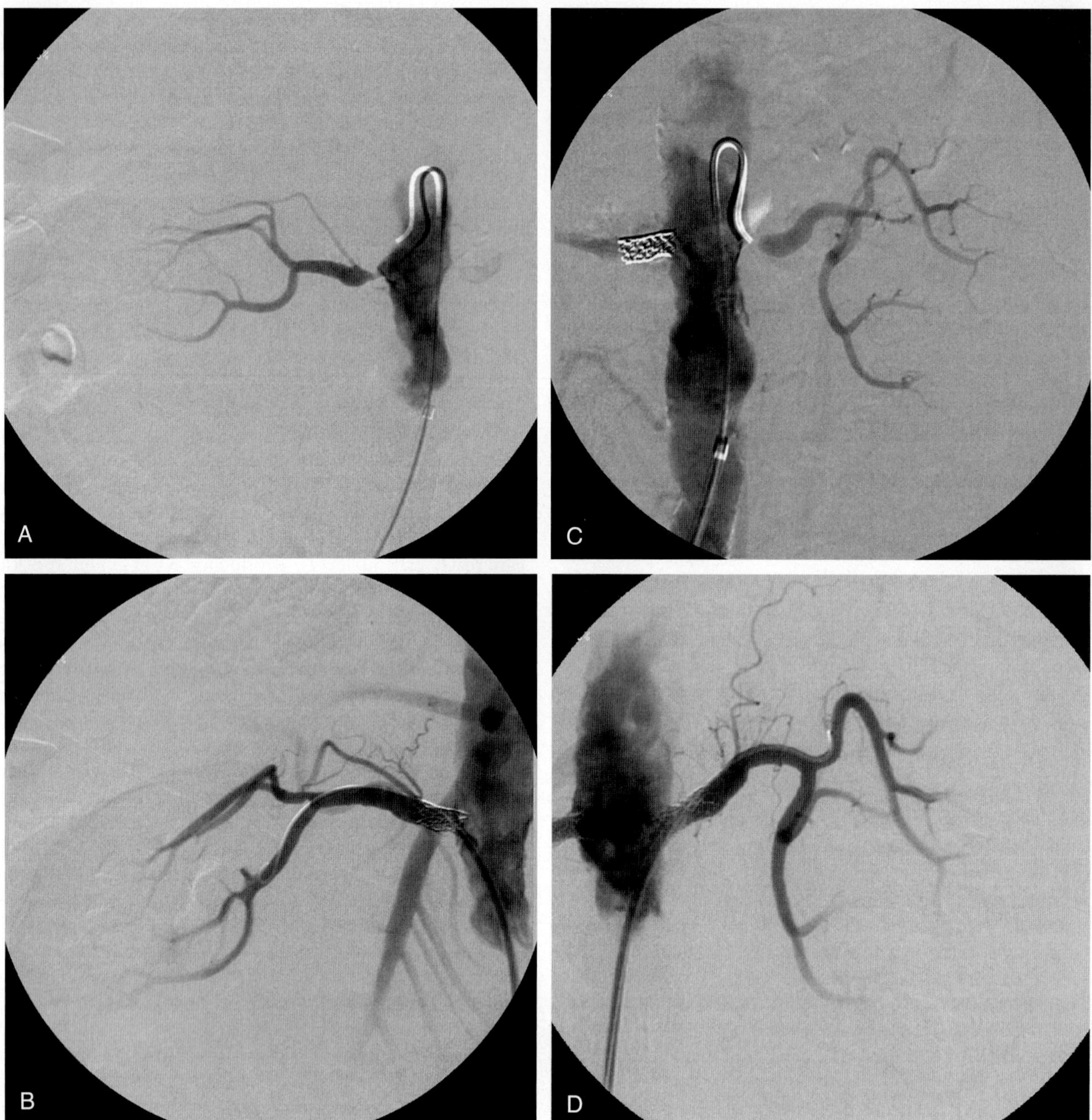

Figure 37.5 Angiogram of atherosclerotic renal artery stenosis. A, Proximal, high-grade stenosis near the ostium. **B,** Restoration of vessel patency by endovascular stent placement. **C,** Image of contralateral, high-grade stenosis of the left kidney. **D,** Improved flow after endovascular stenting.

for those older than 60 years (25% to 30%) and 75 years (40% to 60%). These studies suggest that ASRVD leading to renal artery stenosis is the single most common cause of secondary hypertension in patients older than 50 years. It is also commonly a resistant form of hypertension and can be associated with systolic hypertension with wide pulse pressures. Furthermore, renal artery stenosis from ASRVD has been reported to contribute to the decline in renal function in 15% to 22% of patients reaching ESRD.

PATHOPHYSIOLOGY

Renovascular occlusive disease from any cause can activate pressor pathways that tend to restore renal artery perfusion pressures. Most notable among these is activation of the renin-angiotensin-aldosterone system (RAS). Activation of plasma renin occurs only after poststenotic pressures fall by at least 10% to 20% compared with aortic pressures.[9] Luminal occlusion of less than 60% (cross-sectional area) rarely produces any measurable decrements in either pressure or flow. Hence, a fall in renal perfusion pressure sufficient to initiate RVH occurs only when luminal occlusion is relatively severe, usually in the 70% to 80% cross-sectional occlusion range (Fig. 37.6).

When critical stenosis develops and reduces renal perfusion pressure, multiple mechanisms are activated in the kidney to restore renal blood flow. Central to this process is the release of renin from the juxtaglomerular apparatus, leading to activation of the RAS. This is mediated in part by stimulation of neuronal

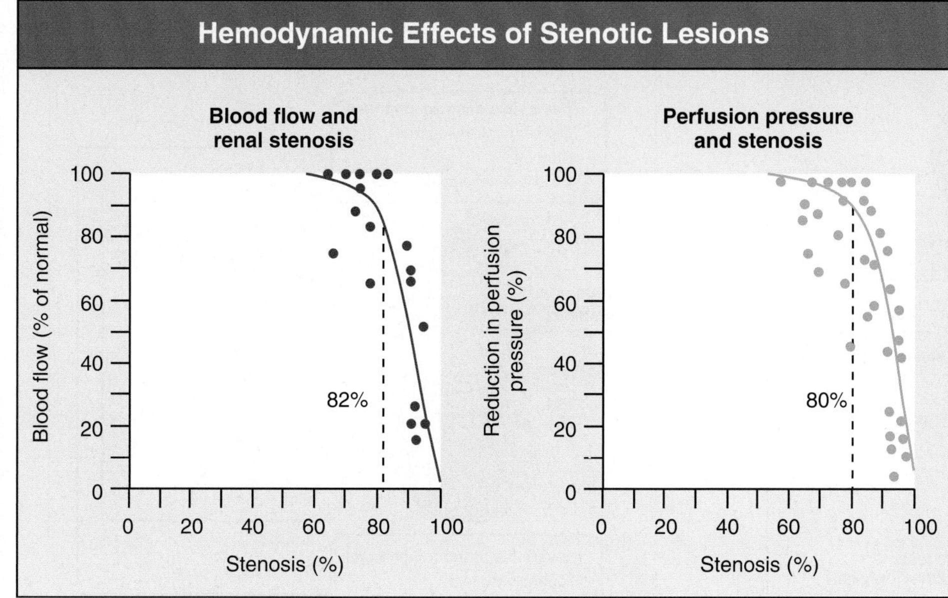

Figure 37.6 Hemodynamic effects of stenotic lesions. Changes in blood flow and arterial pressure across a carefully quantitated arterial lesion are barely detectable until cross-sectional area diminishes by 75% to 80%. *(From reference 10.)*

nitric oxide synthase (NOS) and cyclooxygenase 2 in the macula densa. Blockade of the RAS at the time an experimental renal artery lesion is created prevents the development of hypertension. Studies in transgenic mice without receptors to angiotensin confirm that development of RVH requires an intact RAS.[11] In the absence of RAS blockade, systemic arterial pressures increase until renal perfusion is restored. Studies in both experimental models and humans indicate that additional mechanisms contribute to long-term elevation of BP in the presence of renal artery stenosis, including activation of the sympathetic nervous system (SNS), impairment of nitric oxide (NO) generation, and release of endothelin as well as hypertensive microvascular injury to the nonstenosed kidney.[12]

Mechanisms responsible for sustained RVH differ according to whether one or both kidneys are affected by significant stenoses, either pathologically or created in animal models with use of clips (Fig. 37.7). The nomenclature distinguishes between a situation in which one clip is present with a normal contralateral or unclipped kidney (so-called one-clip, two-kidney hypertension) and a situation in which the entire renal mass is affected with no contralateral kidney (one-clip, one-kidney hypertension). Both of these situations depend on impaired renal perfusion and initial activation of the RAS with sodium retention. However, the presence of a normal contralateral kidney allows pressure natriuresis to occur (see Chapter 2), in which the elevated perfusion pressure mediates natriuresis in the nonstenotic kidney. Because the nonstenotic kidney functions to eliminate the excess sodium, the level of perfusion to the stenotic side remains reduced, leading to sustained activation of the renal artery stenosis. This sequence of events producing angiotensin II (Ang II)–dependent hypertension and secondary aldosterone excess with hypokalemia is summarized in Figure 37.7.

By contrast, one-clip, one-kidney hypertension represents a model in which the entire renal mass is exposed to reduced pressures beyond a stenosis. There is no normal or nonstenotic kidney to counteract increased systemic pressures. As a result, sodium is retained and blood volume expanded, which eventually feeds back to inhibit the RAS (Fig. 37.7B). Therefore, one-clip, one-kidney hypertension is typically not angiotensin dependent unless removal of volume is achieved that reduces renal perfusion pressure and activates the RAS.

The fundamental differences between these forms of RVH have clinical implications. Many diagnostic studies used to evaluate the functional significance of renal artery lesions depend on comparisons of the different physiologic response of the two kidneys, which may give a false impression if both kidneys are involved. Furthermore, diagnostic tests that depend on differences in responses to alterations in sodium status (such as measurement of renal vein renin levels after sodium depletion or individual kidney sodium reabsorption) may be problematic, as high levels of Ang II and aldosterone stimulate sodium reabsorption in both the stenotic and nonstenotic kidney. This accounts in part for the less frequent use of such tests in recent years.

Variations in the natural history of RVH complicate understanding of primary pathogenic mechanisms. Rarely is it known exactly when critical levels of stenosis develop. In experimental models, the relative importance of pressor mechanisms, including measurable activation of the RAS, changes with time. Levels of circulating plasma renin activity decrease, as does the responsiveness of BP to short-term blockade of the renin system. Several mechanisms have been proposed to explain such changes, including a slowly developing pressor action of Ang II, a transition to alternative pressor mechanisms, and intrinsic renal injury to the nonstenotic kidney, which ultimately sustains hypertension despite reversal of the vascular lesion. In experimental models, this translates into a time limit for reversibility of RVH.

There are several clinical correlates of variable time course. First, it is not known how best to identify when revascularization will fail to improve BP control, although a brief duration of hypertension suggests a more favorable response to intervention. As a result, many of the diagnostic studies that depend on lateralization of effects have only modest predictive value when results are negative. As a general rule, they are most reliable when results are positive, meaning that high-grade lateralization accurately predicts improvement after revascularization. A negative test result, however, may also be associated with a beneficial outcome. Second, coexistent intrarenal disease, such as arteriolosclerosis with glomerulosclerosis, is usually associated with persistent hypertension despite correction of renal artery

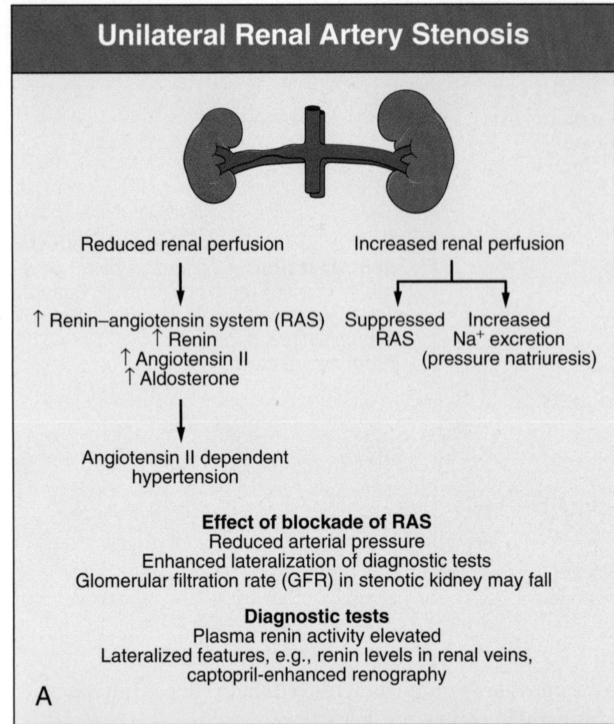

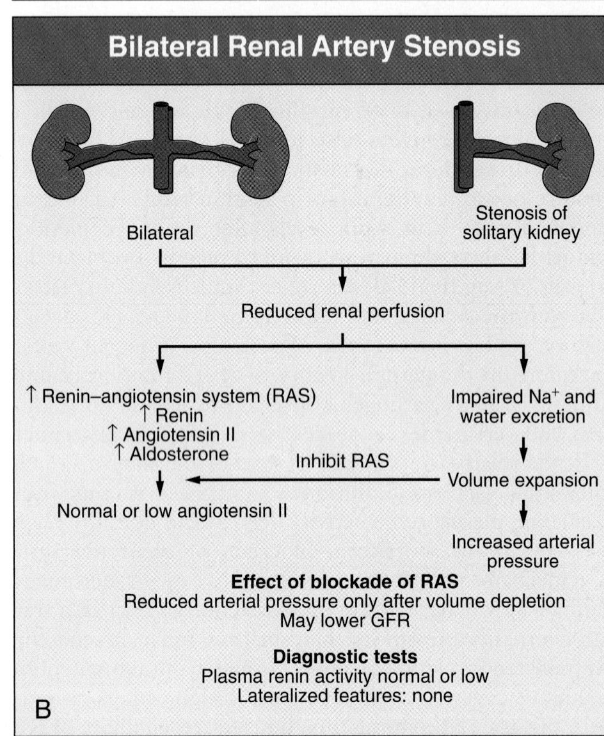

Figure 37.7 Pathogenesis of renovascular hypertension in one-kidney versus two-kidney model. A, In unilateral stenosis with two kidneys, opposing forces between the stenotic kidney, which has reduced perfusion pressures, and the nonstenotic contralateral kidney, which has increased perfusion pressures, result in laboratory and clinical features of angiotensin-dependent hypertension. **B,** In unilateral stenosis with a solitary functioning kidney or in a patient with bilateral critical renal artery stenosis, reduced perfusion pressure to the stenotic kidney in the absence of a normal kidney excreting sodium leads to sodium and volume retention, ultimately associated with hypertension without persistent activation of the RAS.

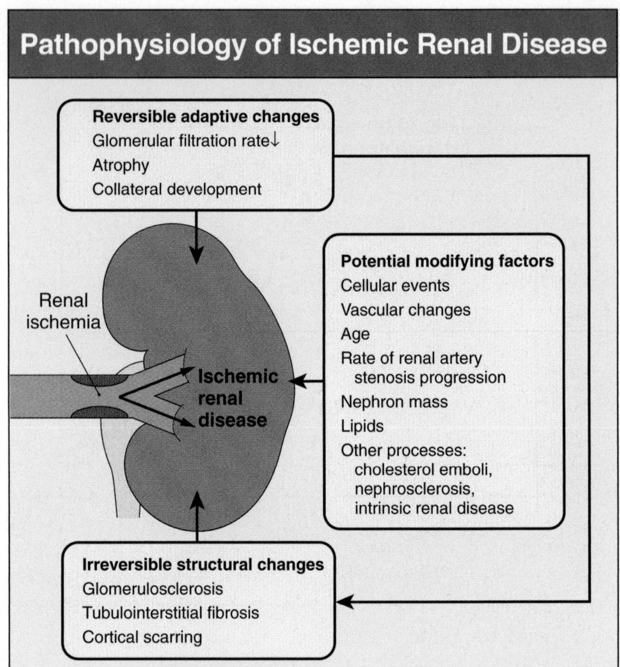

Figure 37.8 Pathophysiology of ischemic renal disease. Chronic ischemia of the kidney is associated with reversible functional involution and atrophy as well as with irreversible structural changes. A number of external factors influence the renal response to chronic ischemia. *(Modified from reference 14.)*

stenosis, particularly for patients with ASRVD.[13] In these patients, a long duration of hypertension allows the development of arteriolosclerotic lesions and renal injury in the contralateral kidney (Fig. 37.7A). Thus, older age and a long duration of hypertension, for example, more than 3 to 5 years, predict a poorer outcome of intervention in this population of patients. Most of these elderly patients with ASRVD also have impaired renal function related to the renal injury in addition to main renal artery stenosis.

Relationship to Ischemic Renal Disease

Activation of pressor mechanisms producing RVH can occur without loss of renal size or function. However, the more common clinical scenario involves both increasing severity of hypertension and deteriorating renal function, often with loss of renal size. Hence, the decision to consider renal revascularization most commonly combines consideration of both the likelihood of salvage or preservation of function and the benefits regarding BP control. Mechanisms underlying parenchymal renal damage may differ from those responsible for generating hypertension. Improved BP control after revascularization sometimes may be achieved without appreciable improvement in kidney function.

The sequence of events underlying the transition from "reversible" loss of function beyond a vascular lesion to "irreversible" tissue fibrosis is not well understood. Renal blood flow differs from many other organs in being vastly greater than needed for metabolic needs alone. Basal energy requirements are met with less than 10% of blood flow, consistent with its filtration function. Nonetheless, reduced renal perfusion activates multiple mechanisms of tissue injury. A general scheme by which vasoactive and inflammatory pathways are activated is summarized in Figure 37.8. Atherosclerotic and inflammatory pathways sometimes lead to arteriolar disease, often with abnormal endothelial function that may parallel tissue injury and accelerate cytokine signaling pathways.[15] At some phase, microvascular rarefaction occurs that accompanies a fall in tissue oxygenation and activation of fibrogenic pathways.[16] Irreversible loss of viable microcirculation may explain some of the limitations observed after restoration of large-vessel patency (e.g., with renal revascularization).

Activation of the RAS and endothelial systems, such as endothelin and oxidative stress pathways, has been demonstrated with renal artery stenosis models.[15] These systems are known to modulate both inflammatory and fibrogenic pathways that lead to tissue scarring. The term "ischemic" renal disease is speculative; studies of renal vein oxygen levels and erythropoietin (EPO) secretion do not support the premise of whole-kidney oxygen deprivation. Measurements of cortical and medullary deoxyhemoglobin by use of blood oxygen level–dependent magnetic resonance (MR) in most patients with renal arterial disease fail to demonstrate oxygen desaturation under most chronic conditions.[17] Medullary oxygen levels are normally substantially lower than those in the cortex and are heavily dependent on the level of solute transport. Under acute conditions of reduced blood flow with persistent filtration and tubular function, levels of deoxygenated hemoglobin representing medullary ischemia rise.[18]

At some level of sustained vascular occlusion, pathways of cytokine and cell signaling activate tissue fibrogenesis and breakdown of intact tubular structures. Glomeruli are usually well preserved, although collapsed.

Sodium Retention and Flash Pulmonary Edema

Some subjects with bilateral renal artery stenosis will develop severe hypertension and extracellular fluid volume excess due to impaired pressure natriuresis. Under such conditions, there can be the sudden ("flash") onset of pulmonary edema in association with rapid development of circulatory congestion. Diuresis can result in exaggerated swings in BP, circulatory congestion, and renal function.[19] Case series suggest that renal revascularization can facilitate fluid volume management, reduce hospitalization, and occasionally improve cardiac function independent of interventional procedures for the heart itself.[20]

CLINICAL MANIFESTATIONS

Renovascular Hypertension

In the 1970s, a cooperative study of RVH compared clinical characteristics of patients with surgically proven RVH with those of patients with primary hypertension. Some of these were statistically more prevalent in RVH, such as the presence of an abdominal bruit, hypokalemia, and absence of a family history of hypertension. Recent studies suggest that for any level of blood pressure, patients with RVH may have higher nocturnal pressures (nondipper) and have more severe target organ manifestations, including left ventricular hypertrophy (Fig. 37.9).[21] Series of individuals with treatment-resistant hypertension indicate that elevated cholesterol, impaired renal function, lower body mass index (BMI), and smoking offer positive clues. In practical terms, none of these features is sufficiently sensitive or specific to offer diagnostic precision. Recent reports indicate that RVH rarely may be associated with nephrotic-range proteinuria, which can regress with correction of the vascular lesions.[22]

Clinical Manifestations of Renovascular Hypertension

Features of Renovascular Hypertension
- Activation of renin-angiotensin-aldosterone system (RAS) - early
- Paroxysmal symptoms: sympathetic nervous system activation
- Abnormal circadian rhythm: loss of nocturnal pressure fall
- Accelerated target organ damage
  - Left ventricular hypertrophy
  - Microvascular disease
  - Renal injury: fibrosis

Clinical Syndromes Associated with Atherosclerotic Renal Artery Stenosis
- "Incidental lesion": no hemodynamic effect
- Renovascular hypertension (see above)
  - New-onset hypertension
  - Acceleration in previously hypertensive patient
- Acute renal dysfunction
  - ACE or ARB-induced acute renal failure
  - Acute or chronic renal insufficiency
- Unexplained chronic kidney disease: especially in the elderly
- Circulatory congestion: "flash pulmonary edema"

Figure 37.9 Clinical manifestations of renovascular hypertension. ACE, angiotensin-converting enzyme; ARB, angiotensin receptor blocker.

Blood pressure elevations from RVH vary widely. Acute renal artery occlusion may only gradually produce an increase in pressure or it may produce a rapid increase in hypertension that may precipitate a hypertensive urgency or emergency (see Chapter 36). Before the current era of antihypertensive agents, 30% of Caucasian patients appearing in an emergency department with hypertensive urgency (defined as grade III or IV hypertensive retinopathy) were ultimately found to have RVH. Syndromes of polydipsia and accelerated hypertension with hyponatremia and hypokalemia, sometimes attributed to the dipsogenic actions of Ang II, also have been observed.

Current antihypertensive medications have changed the clinical presentation of RVH. Recent consensus documents emphasize the need for effective population-wide BP control while limiting the number and expense of diagnostic studies. As a result, most patients with hypertension simply are treated and subjected to few laboratory investigations. For those who reach acceptable BP control without adverse effects, no further studies are performed. Hence, many if not most cases of true RVH are not detected (Fig. 37.10) unless hypertension becomes more difficult to treat or renal dysfunction ensues.

An additional reason that RVH is less frequently detected is the availability of orally active antihypertensive agents that block the RAS. Early studies beginning with captopril indicated that satisfactory BP control can be achieved in more than 86% of patients with RVH compared with less than 50% with previously available drugs. In recent years, widespread application of angiotensin-converting enzyme (ACE) inhibitors and angiotensin receptor blockers (ARBs) for indications other than hypertension, for example, congestive cardiac failure, diabetic nephropathy, and other proteinuric renal diseases, increases the exposure of individuals with undetected renal artery stenosis to these drugs.[23]

One result of these changes has been the emergence of distinctive clinical syndromes that merit evaluation in patients at

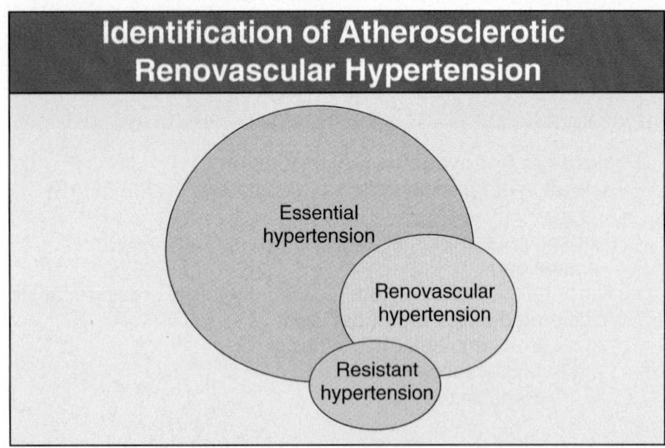

Figure 37.10 Identification of atherosclerotic renovascular hypertension. Venn diagram indicates that many patients with renovascular hypertension are indistinguishable from patients with primary hypertension. A subset develops problematic or resistant hypertension, which brings them to clinical attention and consideration for renal revascularization.

risk for ASRVD (see Fig. 37.9). As a result, patients who typically undergo diagnostic evaluation and renal revascularization are a subset of the population of patients with RVH. This subset is characterized generally by more severe hypertension, decreasing renal function, propensity for rapid volume accumulation manifested as flash pulmonary edema, and, occasionally, advanced renal failure.

Ischemic Renal Disease

The diagnosis of IRD should be considered in several clinical settings as summarized in Figure 37.9.

Renal Impairment in Patients with Renovascular Hypertension or in the Atherosclerotic Age Range

IRD should be excluded in the atherosclerotic age group, particularly when other vascular disease is detected. Many but not all will have a history of hypertension. It remains difficult to separate primary vascular disease from renal parenchymal injury associated with nephrosclerosis from other vascular insults. Clues to IRD include asymmetry of renal size and recent deterioration of renal function, as opposed to slowly progressive CKD. An asymmetrically small kidney in an adult older than 50 years has a 70% chance of being associated with ipsilateral renal artery stenosis.

The development of renal impairment in patients treated medically for long-standing hypertension should raise suspicion for possible IRD. Given the high frequency of bilateral renal artery stenosis (between 30% and 50%), the possibility of IRD should always be considered in patients with known prior RVH. The most common presentation of atherosclerotic renal artery stenosis is unilateral involvement in a patient with CKD associated with long-standing hypertension. In this instance, renal impairment cannot be attributed solely to IRD because the renal artery stenosis affects only one kidney. The kidney supplied by the stenotic vessel may be ischemic, resulting in diminished GFR, RVH, and atrophy. The contralateral kidney with the patent renal vessel often hypertrophies and compensates with hyperfiltration. However, over time, this kidney develops parenchymal injury. Much of the time, the kidney with the patent renal artery has worse renal function than the poststenotic kidney.[24]

Acute Kidney Injury After Starting of Antihypertensive Medications or RAS Blockade

Patients with hemodynamically significant renal artery stenosis to the entire functioning nephron mass are at risk for the development of "functional" acute kidney injury (AKI) after institution of ACE inhibitors or ARBs. The sudden reduction in systemic BP, in the setting of critical renal artery stenosis, may reduce renal artery pressure below the levels needed to sustain glomerular filtration by autoregulation, estimated to be about 60 mm Hg. This can occur with reduction in BP by any antihypertensive agent. With medications that block the production or action of Ang II, alterations in glomerular hemodynamics may result in acute worsening in GFR that is independent of effects on systemic blood pressure.[25] Normally, activation of Ang II causes efferent arteriolar vasoconstriction, which preserves transcapillary filtration pressures at the glomerulus when preglomerular pressures are reduced, thereby maintaining GFR. The loss of this compensatory mechanism induced by agents that inhibit or block the RAS can result in functional AKI. This typically occurs within a few days from the start of antihypertensive therapy and is usually but not always reversible.

Most patients with renal vascular disease who are treated with ACE inhibitors or ARBs do not develop AKI. This probably reflects minimal dependence on Ang II because those with unilateral stenosis have preserved function in the nonstenosed kidney and those with bilateral renovascular disease often have sodium retention that suppresses the RAS. ACE inhibitors and ARBs are more likely to precipitate renal failure in patients with bilateral renal vascular disease if the patients are volume depleted or taking diuretics, producing circumstances that increase Ang II dependence of the GFR. Conversely, AKI can occur with the use of ACE inhibitors without IRD. This most commonly occurs in patients with cardiac or hepatic dysfunction or in patients with intravascular volume depletion because, in these settings, GFR is also Ang II dependent. For this reason, it is imperative to recheck kidney function within 2 weeks of institution of therapy with medications that block the RAS.[26] In a prospective study, the observation of 20% increase in serum creatinine or more after administration of an ACE inhibitor detected most cases of bilateral severe renal artery stenosis.[27]

Flash Pulmonary Edema

IRD may present as recurrent episodes of flash pulmonary edema. These episodes can be unpredictable, sudden, and life-threatening and may be associated with low, normal, or very high BP at the time of presentation. Renal revascularization can reverse the cyclical flash pulmonary edema and improve pulmonary function even in those patients with poor preoperative cardiopulmonary status.[28] In one series, 41% of subjects with bilateral renal artery stenosis had a history of pulmonary edema compared with 12% with unilateral renovascular disease. Seventy-seven percent of the patients with bilateral renal artery stenosis had no further pulmonary edema after renal artery stent placement in one or both arteries. The patients who did have recurrent pulmonary edema all had evidence of stent thrombosis or restenosis.[29] The mechanisms of pulmonary edema reflect combinations of diastolic or systolic ventricular dysfunction occurring in association with chronic reduction in GFR and sodium retention. These may coincide with superimposed episodes of severe hypertension or further increases in sodium retention. There are no prospective clinical studies specifically examining the effect of optimal medical therapy for BP and volume status on the frequency of events in these patients. Initial reports from prospective, randomized clinical studies, such as the Angioplasty and Stenting for Renal Artery Lesions (ASTRAL) study, demonstrated no differences in hospitalizations or episodes of congestive heart failure (CHF) in intensively treated subjects with or without renal artery stenting.[30]

Acute Oligoanuric Renal Failure Superimposed on Chronic Kidney Disease

Patients with high-grade renal artery stenosis are at risk for renal artery occlusion. When renal artery stenosis is bilateral or unilateral in the setting of a single functioning kidney, progression to total occlusion can present as oligoanuric acute renal failure, sometimes associated with a hypertensive emergency. A clinical clue to this diagnosis is abrupt-onset oligoanuria. In this setting, the kidney parenchyma may be viable despite lack of filtration; in some patients, collateral vessels maintain renal viability in the face of proximal renal artery occlusion. Clues to renal viability include preserved renal length and evidence of renal contrast enhancement ("renal blush") seen on delayed or venous-phase images during renal angiography. When these factors are present and the clinical course is consistent with recent occlusion, there is a chance of retrieval of renal function if revascularization is feasible clinically and anatomically. In this setting, urgent vascular surgical consultation should be sought, and it should be assumed that the kidneys may be viable for weeks to months.

Incidental Renal Artery Stenosis

As mentioned, ASRVD is highly correlated with disease in both the coronary and peripheral vasculature. It is commonly identified incidentally at the time of angiography or computed tomographic (CT) imaging for other indications. Most of these patients with coexisting ASRVD and coronary artery disease have only moderate degrees of renal artery stenosis (50% to 75%) of minimal hemodynamic impact. The use of screening renal aortography at the time of coronary angiography has been proposed for some situations. Whereas the addition of aortography to the coronary procedure adds only minimal risk, it does incur expense. One follow-up study of patients with incidentally detected renal artery lesions during coronary angiography found that the presence of renal artery lesions is an independent risk factor for mortality, which may reach 30% during 4 years in high-risk groups.[31] This does not mean, however, that revascularization of renal artery stenosis in these patients reverses this risk. Indeed, renal artery revascularization for such patients should be reserved for those with firm indications for intervention.

NATURAL HISTORY

Disease Progression

The risk of progressive vascular occlusion is a central issue in management of renovascular disease. As well as the risk of progressive renal atrophy and progression to advanced kidney failure, there are also associated risks for cardiovascular events. The natural history of fibromuscular disease differs from that of ASRVD.

Fibromuscular Dysplasia

The natural history of FMD is variable, but angiographic progression can occur. This can be manifested as the development of new focal lesions within the same arterial bed, worsening arterial luminal diameter narrowing within a specific lesion, involvement of a new vascular territory, or development of arteriovenous fistulas or aneurysms or enlargement of existing ones. Most studies of the natural history of FMD show a decline in progression with age, with few patients developing new or progressive lesions after the age of 50 years. From a renal standpoint, FMD rarely causes ischemic renal failure, but the attendant hypertension can be associated with renal cortical atrophy.[32] FMD can also rarely lead to thrombosis or dissection of the renal vessel with renal infarction.

Atherosclerotic Renal Artery Stenosis

The natural history of atherosclerotic renal artery stenosis includes risk for progressive vascular occlusion that clinically translates into stability of BP control, kidney size and function, and cardiovascular risk. Retrospective serial angiographic studies (1980s) suggested that renal artery stenosis commonly progresses during a 2- to 5-year period. Progression is usually defined as a greater than 25% luminal diameter narrowing or progression from severe stenosis to vascular occlusion. During a 4- to 5-year period, between 6% and 16% of stenoses proceed to occlusion. Prospective studies between 1990 and 1997 using Doppler ultrasound in patients with atherosclerotic renal artery lesions indicated that hemodynamic progression overall approaches 31% during 3 years, varying by the degree of initial stenosis. In this series, only nine of 295 vessels (3%) resulted in total occlusion.[33] Measurable loss of renal length (more than 1 cm) is less common but accompanies progressive vascular occlusion. Changes in serum creatinine concentration are often minimal.[34]

The predictors of progressive disease relate primarily to the degree of initial stenosis, being most likely in those with more than 60% stenosis. Progressive renovascular disease often occurs without changes in BP control. Dyslipidemias associated with atherosclerosis have not been shown to be independent predictors of progression. However, therapy with statins appears to reduce the risk of progression and even to induce regression of atherosclerotic renal artery stenosis.[35] Statins also appear to attenuate renal parenchymal injury associated with experimental ASRVD.[36]

Follow-up studies of patients with incidentally detected, high-grade renal artery stenosis (>70%) treated medically indicate that less than 10% required later revascularization for intractable hypertension.[37] Another report noted that few patients with incidental renal artery stenosis progressed to ESRD during a follow-up period between 8 and 9 years.[38] In patients observed after simultaneous renal angiography at the time of cardiac catheterization, no difference in serum creatinine concentration was noted between those with and those without renal artery stenosis at follow-up.

Mortality

ASRVD and IRD are associated with limited long-term survival, consistent with widespread atherosclerotic disease. Recent retrospective analyses report 3- to 5-year mortality rates between 30% and 35% in patients with renal artery stenosis largely due to cardiovascular events or stroke. In follow-up of a large cohort of more than 1200 patients who underwent coronary and renal angiography, patients with renal artery stenosis were found to have a 65% 4-year survival rate versus 85% for those without renal artery stenosis at the time of catheterization. Five- and 10-year survival rates for patients reaching ESRD due to IRD are as low as 18% and 5%, respectively.[39]

Relative Value of Imaging Methods for Evaluating the Renal Vasculature					
Methods	**Images of Vessels**	**Tissue Perfusion**	**Function (GFR)**	**Advantages**	**Disadvantages**
Spiral computed tomographic angiography	+++	+	±	Provision of three types of images, examination of venous structures, might be useful for evaluating transplant donors	High contrast requirement
Contrast angiography	+++	++	±	Nephrography estimates volume of viable tissue; gold standard	Risk of catheter-induced injuries and contrast nephropathy
Captopril renography	–	+++	++	Change in GFR might estimate reversibility of the lesion; widely available, noninvasive; totally normal renogram effectively excludes significant vascular disease	
Duplex ultrasonography	++	++	–	Precise measurement of flow velocity, suitable for serial studies, relatively inexpensive	Produces little functional information; is not suitable for accessory vessels
Magnetic resonance angiography	++	++	±	No radiation exposure	Gadolinium contrast not used for eGFR <30ml/mg concern for nephrogenic systemic fibrosis

Figure 37.11 Relative value of imaging methods for evaluating the renal vasculature. The available techniques vary in their ability to image the renal vessels, to assess tissue perfusion, and to measure glomerular filtration rate (GFR).

Whether renal revascularization improves survival in atherosclerotic renal artery stenosis is controversial.[40] In one study, those patients with bilateral ASRVD who were treated medically actually had better follow-up renal function than did those who had undergone revascularization, and there was no difference in survival.[41] However, other studies suggest that intervention directed at improving renal function may improve survival in this group of patients with diffuse atherosclerotic disease. Watson and colleagues[42] reported 2-year survival rates of 80% among patients with ischemic nephropathy who underwent endovascular stenting. Yet, the increased mortality risk of worsening renal function complicating endovascular interventions has to be considered in the risk-benefit analysis of interventions.[43] Randomized trials currently in progress are addressing whether intervention confers quality of life and mortality benefit from interventions or medical therapy alone.

DIAGNOSIS

Several screening laboratory tests have been proposed over the years to identify patients with RVH. Some of these depend on identifying activation of the RAS, such as renin-sodium profiling, and many depend on side-to-side comparisons of kidneys, assuming that one kidney is unaffected. Under the best of circumstances, these studies are rarely more than 80% sensitive or specific. As a result, their value as predictors depends greatly on the pretest probability of renovascular disease.[13] Furthermore, functional tests related to activation of the RAS depend heavily on the test conditions, including sodium intake and concurrent antihypertensive medications, many of which affect levels of plasma renin activity. As a result, many clinicians no longer use these tests extensively.

Diagnosis of RVH requires demonstration of a critical stenotic vascular lesion affecting the renal artery. Conventional angiography remains the reference standard to define the anatomy of the renal vasculature, but it is usually performed only after a less invasive procedure has increased the level of probability that such a lesion is present. Angiography is often performed at the same procedure with an endovascular intervention such as angioplasty with or without stenting. Several characteristics of commonly used noninvasive imaging procedures are summarized in Figure 37.11.

The goal of noninvasive testing is to allow the physician to limit further invasive testing. The most commonly employed noninvasive vascular studies include nuclear renal scan (usually captopril- or enalapril-enhanced renography), renal artery duplex ultrasonography, CT angiography, and magnetic resonance angiography (MRA) (see Chapter 5). These methods provide different information and may vary between institutions as regards both availability and reliability. Figure 37.12 illustrates an example of a captopril-enhanced renogram in a patient with renal artery stenosis. This examination provides no direct image of the renal vessel but does provide a view of the rate of isotope appearance and washout, reflecting the sequence of renal blood flow and filtration. The study provides functional information about the size and excretory capacity of the kidney as well as emphasizing the role of Ang II in maintaining GFR. This test has a high negative predictive value when it is completely normal. Several studies suggest that a completely normal captopril renogram effectively excludes hemodynamically significant renal artery stenosis.[44] The fact that many intrinsic renal abnormalities unrelated to the main renal artery may change these curves limits its value in the presence of reduced GFR (serum creatinine concentration >2.0 mg/dl or 176 μmol/l).

Renal artery duplex scanning is applied widely to identify and to follow hemodynamic effects of vascular lesions serially. It is relatively inexpensive and requires no administration of contrast material. It is most effective in detecting lesions of the main renal artery near the ostium, making it a better screening test for ASRVD than for FMD. However, the reliability of this method depends on the skill and patience of the ultrasonographer and on the body habitus of the patient. Duplex ultrasound provides little functional information about the kidney beyond the vascular lesion, although many important structural features, including the size of the kidney and presence

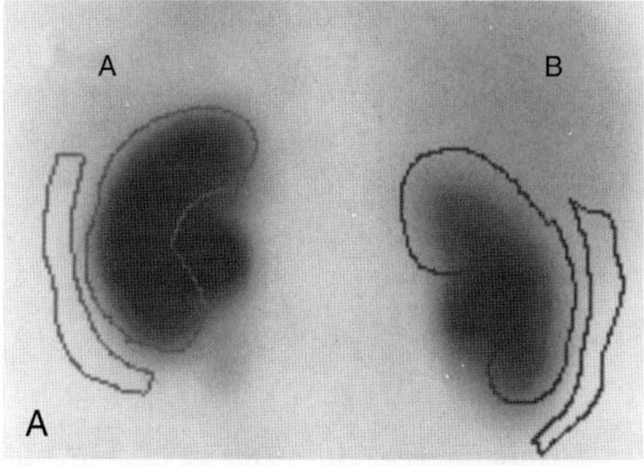

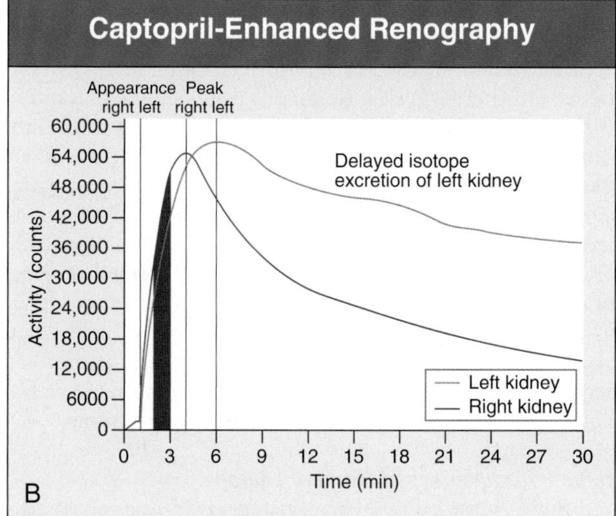

Figure 37.12 Captopril-enhanced renography. A, Scan in a patient with newly developing hypertension. **B,** Renogram demonstrates delayed arrival and excretion of isotope (MAG3) in the affected left kidney.

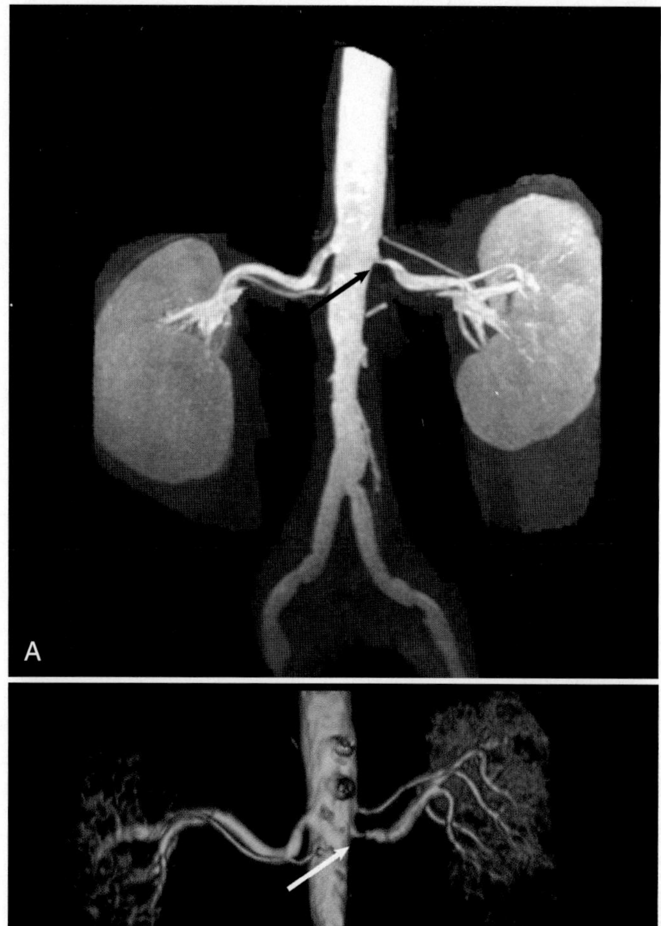

Figure 37.13 Magnetic resonance angiogram with and without gadolinium contrast enhancement. A, High-grade stenosis affecting the left inferior renal artery is evident, with functioning kidney tissue as reflected by gadolinium nephrogram *(arrow)*. Concerns about the role of gadolinium in the development of nephrogenic systemic fibrosis have greatly reduced the use of this contrast agent. **B,** As a result, methods to image the vasculature without contrast material are being developed that produce excellent reconstructed images *(arrow)*.

of ureteral obstruction, may be determined. The diagnostic criteria for hemodynamically significant renal artery stenosis by duplex sonography include acceleration of blood flow through the area of stenosis that exceeds that in the aorta and abnormal waveforms representing blood flow in the affected vessel (see Chapter 5).

MRA offers the potential to provide both structural vascular imaging and functional information. MRA with gadolinium contrast enhancement gives excellent imaging of the main renal arteries but is now less used because of the association of nephrogenic systemic fibrosis with gadolinium exposure in patients with reduced GFR and ESRD. Other limitations of MRA include interobserver variability, a recognized tendency to overestimate luminal narrowing, and limited sensitivity for mid and distal vascular lesions associated with FMD. Studies are under way to improve the sensitivity and negative predictive value of non-gadolinium-enhanced MRA in the detection of renal artery stenosis (Fig. 37.13).

CT angiography (CTA) with vascular reconstruction achieves image qualities nearly equivalent to those of angiography but requires more iodinated contrast material. It is becoming the noninvasive study of choice in those patients whose risk of contrast-associated nephrotoxicity is minimal. Yet, CTA also can overestimate the degree of stenosis with an estimated false-positive rate that varies according to reconstruction protocols and regional differences in experience. It is highly sensitive for identification of lesions associated with FMD and is a good screening test for these patients who generally have good kidney function (Fig. 37.14).[45]

Angiography remains the gold standard for defining the degree of stenosis associated with ASRVD and for identification of FMD. Aortography provides important anatomic and functional information in cases of tight stenosis or occlusion, including the demonstration of delayed perfusion of the kidney and distal reconstitution of the proximally occluded renal vessel. This is important in consideration of surgical revascularization for retrieval of renal function. In experienced hands, diagnostic renal arteriography to identify significant renal artery stenosis can be performed with as little as 20 ml of iodinated contrast material. In very high risk cases, carbon dioxide can be used in place of contrast material to assess the renal ostium and proximal vessel, where atherosclerosis commonly develops.

Renal vein renin measurements can be helpful in predicting the BP response to renal revascularization.[46] Previous studies indicated that lateralization of renal vein levels (a ratio of more than 1.5:1 between stenotic and nonstenotic kidneys) predicts a favorable blood pressure response for more than 90% of patients.

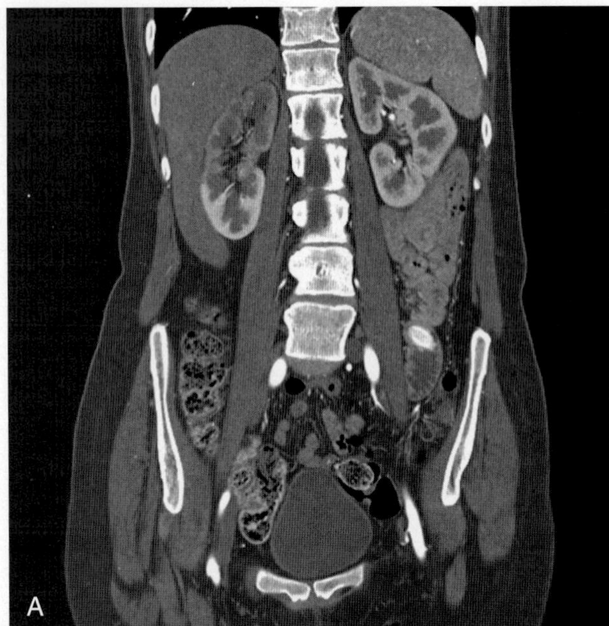

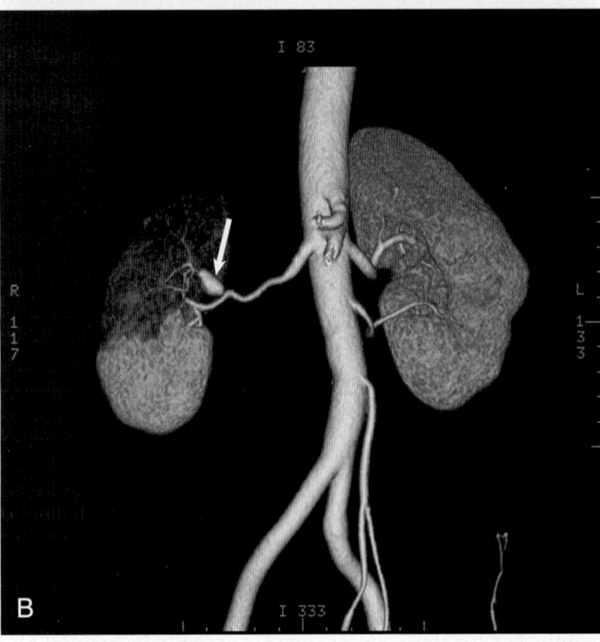

Figure 37.14 Computed tomographic angiogram illustrating a renal artery aneurysm with an area of renal infarction in right kidney. Coronal image **A,** demonstrates area of intact tissue with no blood perfusion within the kidney parenchyma. Image **B,** illustrates reconstructed view with vascular aneurysm *(arrow)* and minimal flow in the distribution beyond this segment, consistent with nearly total occlusion. This case presented as accelerated renovascular hypertension treated primarily with blockade of the RAS (see text).

Because failure to lateralize also carried a favorable response in nearly half, the negative predictive value is limited. Some clinicians use these measurements to verify the role of a pressor kidney before undertaking nephrectomy.

TREATMENT OF RENOVASCULAR DISEASE

The Joint National Committee (JNC 7) stated goal of hypertension therapy is to reduce morbidity and mortality "by the least intrusive means possible." In RVH, this entails balancing the risks and benefits of several modalities ranging from medical therapy to surgical or endovascular repair. Whether renal revascularization improves outcomes in the era of effective medical therapy is currently the subject of several prospective randomized trials, including ASTRAL and the Cardiovascular Outcomes in Renal Atherosclerotic Lesions (CORAL) study in the United States.

Medical Therapy

Most patients with RVH are treated initially with conventional antihypertensive medications (see Chapter 35). Treatment should address modifiable cardiovascular risk factors (promotion of weight loss, smoking cessation) and include low-dose aspirin and control of hyperlipidemia with statin therapy. Current guidelines for BP control recommend target levels below 140/90 mm Hg or below 130/80 mm Hg for patients with CKD, diabetes, or other high risk. Regimens using agents that interfere with the RAS, such as ACE inhibitors, ARBs, and renin inhibitors as well as the dihydropyridine class of calcium channel blockers, allow achievement of target BP levels in most patients. Based on the benefits of blocking of neurohormonal signals associated with accelerated atherosclerotic disease risk, blockade of the RAS is considered fundamental. Successful renal revascularization rarely leads to withdrawal of all antihypertensive medications in the current era. Hence, it may be questioned whether the costs and risks of renal revascularization are warranted for patients whose blood pressures and kidney function are stable on an acceptable regimen of antihypertensive medications.

Adverse Consequences of Medical Therapy

When there is critical renal artery stenosis, reduction of arterial pressure has the potential for reduction of renal blood flow below levels needed to sustain glomerular filtration. Renal artery pressures beyond the stenosis may decrease below those needed for autoregulation of blood flow and GFR, estimated to be 60 mm Hg in humans.[25] Such a reduction in blood flow can develop with any antihypertensive drugs, including β-blockers and sodium nitroprusside. Under these circumstances, renal blood flow may decrease such that thrombotic occlusion may develop.

Antihypertensive agents that interrupt the RAS have an important additional effect: they remove the vasoconstrictive action of Ang II at the efferent arteriole. When preglomerular pressures are reduced for any reason, Ang II preserves glomerular transcapillary filtration pressures by constricting the efferent arteriole preferentially. This allows continued urine formation despite marginal blood flow. Removal of Ang II under these conditions can lead to abrupt cessation of glomerular filtration and urine formation. This decrease in filtration produces a syndrome of "functional acute renal insufficiency," first described clinically with ACE inhibitors.[47] The decrease in GFR is apparent clinically under conditions in which the entire renal mass is affected, for example, bilateral renal artery stenosis or stenosis to a solitary functioning kidney. These principles are particularly relevant in nephrology because removal of the efferent actions of Ang II and reduction of transcapillary filtration pressure are advantageous in renal diseases characterized by glomerular hypertension, such as diabetic nephropathy.

Whether the overall effects of ACE inhibitors and ARBs on GFR in renovascular hypertensive patients are beneficial or detrimental has been a matter of controversy. Some diagnostic studies to identify functionally important renal artery stenosis employ ACE inhibitors to magnify differences in GFR between kidneys, for example, captopril-enhanced renography and

Guidelines for Limiting Renal Toxicity with ACE Inhibitors	
Recognize predisposing condition	Widespread atherosclerotic disease Associated renal artery stenosis Impaired pretreatment renal function Solitary functioning kidney Activated renin angiotensin system Low sodium intake Diuretic therapy Other volume losses: vomiting, diarrhea Vasodilator administration Low cardiac function: hypotension, hyponatremia Other agents affecting kidney function (e.g., nonsteroidal anti-inflammatory agents)
Monitor effects of initiating ACE inhibitor therapy	Serum creatinine: measure over the first days and at weeks 2 and 4, especially in high-risk patients Elevated serum potassium: withhold potassium supplements, withhold potassium-sparing agents, and use low-potassium diet
Manage volume	Temporarily withhold diuretics Dose titrate both diuretics and ACE inhibitor Liberalize sodium intake/replace volume, consider rechallenge with ACE inhibitor after volume repletion

Figure 37.15 Guidelines for limiting renal toxicity with ACE inhibitors. ACE, angiotensin-converting enzyme.

Technical Success and Clinical Effect of Percutaneous Transluminal Renal Angioplasty (PTRA)		
	1989–1995 (%)	**1981–1987 (%)**
Patients	1359	691
Arteries	1664	—
Fibromuscular disease		
Cured	42	53
Improved	36	38
Cured plus improved	78	91
Failed	21	8
Atherosclerotic renovascular disease		
Cured	14	18
Improved	51	48
Cured plus improved	65	67
Failed	34	32

Figure 37.16 Technical success and clinical effect of percutaneous transluminal renal angioplasty (PTRA). Summary of 17 reports of PTRA comprising more than 2000 patients, beginning in 1981. *(Modified from references 51 and 52.)*

captopril-stimulated renal vein renin determinations. It may be argued that identifying a decrease in GFR with an ACE inhibitor allows early detection of critical stenotic lesions in time for renal revascularization. Conversely, some have proposed that administration of an ACE inhibitor to patients with renal artery stenosis poses the hazard of a "pharmacologic nephrectomy," with the potential for inducing irreversible renal parenchymal injury through ischemia.[48] Although the functional decrease in GFR induced by ACE inhibitors is usually reversible, patients occasionally do not recover renal function. Hence, ACE inhibitors are a double-edged sword in RVH. They have unique properties, allowing more effective BP control than previously possible, but at the same time, this class of medication has the potential for early loss of filtration pressure in patients with critical levels of renal artery stenosis.

Clinical experience with ACE inhibitors is, however, reassuring. Monitoring studies both in clinical use and in large, prospective trials of patients at high risk for undetected renal artery stenosis, such as the trials of CHF, indicate that clinically important loss of GFR is not common. Most of these trials excluded patients with significant renal dysfunction, however. Postmarketing surveys of more than 15,000 prescriptions in the United Kingdom after the release of enalapril indicated few but important adverse experiences. Most often, these occurred in patients with preexisting renal dysfunction who were taking potassium-sparing diuretics and had other known atherosclerotic disease.[25] The clinician caring for patients with complex hypertension should recognize both hyperkalemia and increasing creatinine values during treatment with ACE inhibitors or ARBs (Fig. 37.15) as a sign of potentially critical renal artery stenosis, which may dictate alternative therapy or renal revascularization.

Further diagnostic and therapeutic maneuvers may be warranted in patients with resistant hypertension in which BP remains unsatisfactorily controlled despite three drugs or more. As noted previously, these patients are likely to have associated cardiovascular disease and other comorbid risk. Such patients may benefit from renal revascularization regarding both level of BP control and stabilization of renal function.

Renal Revascularization

Restoration of the renal blood supply is a rational goal of treating hypertension related to renovascular disease. In a young person with FMD, a permanent cure of hypertension is sometimes achieved. Revascularization offers such a patient relief from a lifelong regimen of antihypertensive medications and cardiovascular risk associated with high BP. In practice, however, cures are infrequent. More often, renal revascularization allows improved BP control and stabilization of the kidney circulation.

Percutaneous Transluminal Renal Angioplasty and Stenting

Fibromuscular Dysplasia The current standard of care in most centers for treatment of hypertension associated with FMD is percutaneous transluminal renal angioplasty (PTRA). Approximately 75% of patients require less antihypertensive medication after technically successful PTRA. Complete cure, defined as normal arterial pressure without medications, is uncommon but can occur. Predictors of hypertensive response include lower levels of preintervention systolic BP, younger age of the patient, shorter duration of hypertension, and positive result of simplified captopril test.[49] Figure 37.16 summarizes 17 reported series assessing technical success and clinical effect of PTRA in patients with RVH due to FMD.[50] Although primary technical success rates for PTRA are high (>90%) for FMD, clinicians need to be aware of the potential for restenosis due to either inadequate initial treatment or recurrent fibrosis. This can be treated by repeated PTRA if needed.

When FMD is associated with large aneurysmal dilations exceeding 1.5 cm in diameter, surgical revascularization has been the standard of care. Recent reports indicate that endovascular management of renal artery aneurysms sometimes can

Renal Function Outcomes after Endovascular Stenting

Year	Author	No. of Patients	Follow-up	Renal Function Outcome (%) Improved	Stable	Worse	Restenosis (%)
1991	Rees	100*	7 mo	36	36	28	25
1994	Hennequin	100*	32 mo	17	50	33	20
1995	van de Ven	92*	6 mo	36	64	0	13
1996	Iannone	86*	10 mo	36	45	19	14
1997	Boisclair	100*	13 mo	41	35	24	ND
1997	Harden	100*	6 mo	34	34	32	13
1998	Shannon	100*	9 mo	43	29	28	0
1998	Dorros	163*	6–48 mo		66–75§	25–33	
2000	Baumgartner	107†	12 mo	33	42	25	21
2000	Watson	25	8 mo	72	28	0	ND
2000	Burket	37†/127*	15 mo	43	24	33	ND
2001	Bush	69	20 mo	22	48	25	ND
2001	Beutler	63	23 mo	12	68	19	17–19

Figure 37.17 Renal function outcomes after endovascular stenting. ND, not done. *Includes patients with and without renal insufficiency. †Patients with renal insufficiency. §Includes those with stable or improved renal function at last follow-up; the 75% and 25% values represent those stented for bilateral renal artery stenosis. *(Modified from reference 54.)*

be achieved by use of "covered" stent grafts to exclude the aneurysm.

Atherosclerotic Disease: Endovascular Stents Primary endovascular renal artery stenting has become standard for the interventional treatment of atherosclerotic renal artery stenosis in most centers. Comparisons between PTRA alone and PTRA with stent placement establish superior immediate and long-term results with stents.[53] With current techniques, target vessel patency rates regularly exceed 95%. Some centers use platelet inhibitors (e.g., clopidogrel) for several months, although the benefits of this approach are unproven.

Functional changes and BP changes may develop during weeks and months, when antihypertensive medications can be adjusted. A rise in BP should raise the question of vessel restenosis, which occurs in between 14% and 30% of subjects during the first year. Most occur within 6 months of revascularization and are more common for smaller vessels.

Figure 37.17 summarizes results from observational reports of more than 1000 patients undergoing renal artery stent placement for either hypertension or renal function preservation. BP control rates were improved in 50%, with 68% of patients experiencing "stabilization" or "improvement" in renal function during a mean of 17 months.[54] The effects of renal artery stenting on the course of renal impairment in patients with renal artery stenosis remain ambiguous. In nearly all studies reporting renal function outcome after stenting, the percentage of patients experiencing improvement in renal function is offset by a group with worsening renal function. Those whose renal function improves the most tend to be those whose renal function was actively deteriorating during the preceding year.[55] Patients with deterioration of renal function after stenting likely experience complications such as cholesterol embolization or contrast nephropathy.

Diabetic patients form an important subgroup of those with IRD. Surgical revascularization in this group is associated with similar renal functional responses but an inferior rate of BP responses and a higher postoperative risk for death or eventual dialysis dependence.

Complications Reviews of PTRA and stenting vary widely regarding the incidence of minor and major complications. Common complications are shown in Figure 37.18 and include contrast nephrotoxicity, which is usually reversible, and atheroembolism, from which patients commonly do not recover. Recent reviews suggest that between 7.5% and 9% of individuals have a major complication related to the procedure.[54] These include local arterial dissection, aortic dissection, and segmental renal infarction.

Surgical Revascularization

Before the introduction of PTRA with stents, surgical revascularization was the standard treatment of RVH and IRD. A summary of results of surgical revascularization for RVH is shown in Figure 37.19. Such procedures involve major vascular surgery and carry considerable risk, cost, and morbidity. Risks are reduced with preoperative screening and treatment of associated coronary and carotid disease. As a result, surgical intervention for renovascular disease now is reserved for patients refractory to medical therapy, for whom endovascular therapy fails or does not offer adequate therapy for associated aortic disease.[56] Despite these caveats, successful surgical revascularization in well-selected cases provides durable restoration of kidney blood supply and long-term survival (81% at 5 years).[57]

Some patients with IRD who are dialysis dependent experience recovery of renal function after surgical revascularization.[59] The best predictor of successful and sustained withdrawal from dialysis is a rapid and recent preoperative decline in GFR, often

Complications of Percutaneous Transluminal Renal Angioplasty

Type (Frequency)	Complications
Total (63/691 or 9.1%)	—
Fatal (3/691)	Cholesterol embolism Cerebral hemorrhage Bowel infarction
Most frequent	Cholesterol embolism Contrast-associated nephrotoxicity Renal artery dissection Renal artery thrombosis/occlusion Segmental renal infarction Hematoma at puncture site
Classified as indirect	Cerebrovascular accident Myocardial infarction Anterior spinal artery thrombosis Branchial artery thrombosis Bowel infarction

Figure 37.18 Complications of percutaneous transluminal renal angioplasty (PTRA). *(Modified from reference 58.)*

Blood Pressure Outcome for Surgical Revascularization in Renovascular Hypertension

Outcome (%)	Fibromuscular Disease (N = 575)	Atherosclerosis of Renal Arteries (N = 631)
Cured	62	37
Improved	26	46
Cured plus improved	89	84
Failed	10	15

Figure 37.19 Blood pressure outcome for surgical revascularization in renovascular hypertension. A summary of results for more than 1200 patients. Follow-up procedures and definitions of blood pressure cure varied greatly between series. Surgical mortality was 1.3% to 5.8% in patients with stenosis from atherosclerosis and nil in those with fibromuscular disease. *(Modified from reference 60.)*

associated with occlusion of a critically stenotic main renal artery and a kidney with preserved size and extensive collateral supply.

Some patients develop RVH associated with total occlusion of a preexisting renal artery stenosis, resulting in nonfunction of that kidney. Hypertension in these cases may be improved by nephrectomy, which can be undertaken with a laparoscopic procedure. Results from a recent series indicate that improved blood pressures can be obtained in such instances without important loss of renal function. Estimates of renal function in this group were 11% in the removed kidney and 89% in the contralateral kidneys.[61]

Realistic Outcomes of Renal Revascularization

For some patients, technically successful renal revascularization leads to better BP control and improved kidney function. Antihypertensive medication requirements decrease, although rarely are they eliminated entirely. Most series report stabilization of renal function, meaning that average serum creatinine levels do not change. This interpretation may be misleading. Some patients experience a marked improvement in renal function, whereas others have a clinically significant loss of renal function. In most series, this occurs in up to 18% to 20% of patients treated with either PTRA or surgery. Although group average values do not change, some patients experience adverse effects on renal function that should be considered for management decisions.

The benefits of modestly improved BP control and reduced antihypertensive drug requirements should not be understated. Treatment trials in primary hypertension based on BP differences of 10 to 15 mm Hg between treatment and placebo groups established major differences in cardiovascular endpoints, including overall mortality. Age and the likely ability of patients to adhere to antihypertensive drug therapy may be important considerations.

The limited prospective data comparing medical therapy with renal revascularization in the current era have demonstrated only modest benefit regarding cardiovascular outcomes for atherosclerotic disease. Each of three small, randomized trials could identify only minor differences in BP and renal outcomes.[62-64] Recent larger trials are only now being reported; initial data from the United Kingdom regarding the ASTRAL study demonstrate no differences in renal functional, BP, CHF, or mortality endpoints during several years.[30] This study enrolled patients on the basis of the "uncertainty" of the clinicians (i.e., including those patients for whom benefit was not certain). No definition of certainty was provided, making it unclear exactly how these results can be generalized to wider groups. A small, randomized trial extending more than 9 years failed to detect a mortality benefit with surgical revascularization.[65] Retrospective observational reports are frequently limited by poorly standardized methods of BP measurement and drug therapy. Despite relatively few prospective trials, the application of endovascular renal artery stenting in the United States rose more than fourfold between 1996 and 2005.[66] This trend prompted the Center for Medicare and Medicaid Services to commission a formal review of the published outcome data by the Agency for Healthcare Research and Quality.[40] These authors concluded that "available evidence does not clearly support one treatment approach over another for atherosclerotic renal artery stenosis." Among the few prospective, randomized trials, the largest was the Dutch Renal Artery Stenosis Intervention Cooperative (DRASTIC) study. It included 106 patients with relatively resistant hypertension randomized to either medical therapy or PTRA. The lack of difference in BP after 1 year between patients treated with PTRA and patients treated medically led the authors to conclude that "angioplasty has little advantage over antihypertensive drug therapy."[64] The results of this study were analyzed under "intention-to-treat" statistical rules but were confounded by 22 of 50 patients assigned to medical therapy (44%) who crossed over to the PTRA arm because of uncontrolled BP levels at 3 months. Despite their inclusion in the medical arm, many authorities reviewing these data argue that this group offers compelling evidence of medical treatment failure in some instances and the benefit of renal revascularization for such individuals. Clinicians caring for such patients will need to consider each case individually.

An Integrated Approach to Treatment of Renovascular Disease

Aging demographics in the United States and other Western countries favor development of critical levels of renal artery stenosis in more patients than ever before. Critical to the

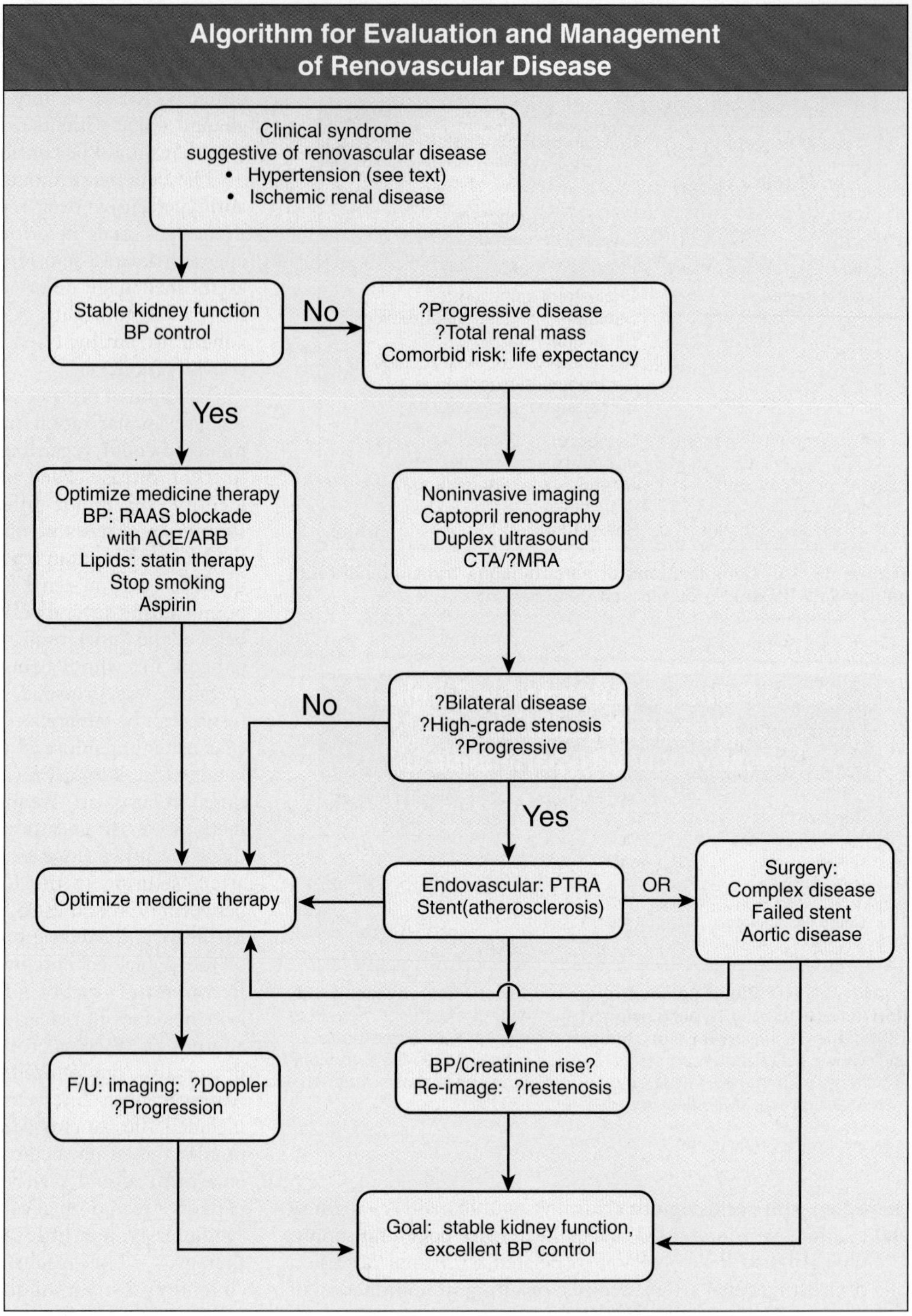

Algorithm for Evaluation and Management of Renovascular Disease

Clinical syndrome suggestive of renovascular disease
- Hypertension (see text)
- Ischemic renal disease

Stable kidney function
BP control

No

?Progressive disease
?Total renal mass
Comorbid risk: life expectancy

Yes

Optimize medicine therapy
BP: RAAS blockade with ACE/ARB
Lipids: statin therapy
Stop smoking
Aspirin

Noninvasive imaging
Captopril renography
Duplex ultrasound
CTA/?MRA

No

?Bilateral disease
?High-grade stenosis
?Progressive

Yes

Optimize medicine therapy

Endovascular: PTRA
Stent(atherosclerosis)

OR

Surgery:
Complex disease
Failed stent
Aortic disease

F/U: imaging: ?Doppler
?Progression

BP/Creatinine rise?
Re-image: ?restenosis

Goal: stable kidney function, excellent BP control

Figure 37.20 Algorithm for evaluation and management of renovascular disease. The intensity of imaging and revascularization depends on both the level of kidney function and blood pressure, in addition to the comorbid disease risks for the individual subject. The overall goal should focus on stable kidney function and blood pressure levels. As with any other vascular disease, monitoring for disease progression and recurrence is an important element of long-term management. ACE, angiotensin-converting enzyme; ARB, angiotensin receptor blocker; BP, blood pressure; CTA, computed tomographic angiography; F/U, follow-up; MRA, magnetic resonance angiography; PTRA, percutaneous transluminal renal angioplasty; RAAS, renin-angiotensin-aldosterone system.

management of such patients is the recognition of distinctive clinical syndromes of renovascular disease, linking acceleration of hypertension with deteriorating renal function and, occasionally, episodic circulatory congestion (flash pulmonary edema). Most patients can be managed effectively by medical means, including vigorous measures to prevent atherosclerotic progression with statin therapy, and smoking cessation. Long-term care of such patients is an ongoing process that should be reviewed at regular intervals. When progressively more complex antihypertensive regimens become required or renal function deteriorates, consideration should be given to identification and correction of critical vascular lesions affecting the kidneys.

Figure 37.20 illustrates a general algorithm by which such patients can be managed. This scheme emphasizes the need to evaluate whether the patient is a candidate for renal revascularization based on clinical features including age, other diseases, and whether stable BP and kidney function can be achieved with medical therapy. If the patient is well-controlled or is not a candidate for revascularization, there is little to be gained from extensive diagnostic studies. Conversely, if BP control and stable renal function are not achieved with medical therapy, beginning a systematic evaluation of the renal vasculature with the objective of vascular intervention is justified. The decision to undertake renal revascularization remains a highly individual judgment based on comorbid disease risk, age, and refractoriness to therapy. In cases of atherosclerotic disease, invasive angiography now is limited mainly to patients for whom revascularization is anticipated, often at the same procedure. This approach limits the hazards of vessel instrumentation and contrast nephrotoxicity to a single procedure. Since the widespread introduction of endovascular stent procedures, surgical reconstruction is often limited to patients with technically challenging vascular lesions or associated aortic disease. Even after successful revascularization, medical therapy and follow-up remain essential. Balancing the potential risks and benefits of medical therapy versus primary revascularization remains a complex challenge.

REFERENCES

1. Garovic V, Textor SC. Renovascular hypertension and ischemic nephropathy. *Circulation*. 2005;112:1362-1374.
2. White CJ. Catheter-based therapy for atherosclerotic renal artery stenosis. *Circulation*. 2006;113:1464-1473.
3. Textor SC, Lerman L, McKusick M. The uncertain value of renal artery interventions: Where are we now? *JACC Cardiovasc Interv*. 2009;2: 175-182.
4. Slovut DP, Olin JW. Current concepts: Fibromuscular dysplasia. *N Engl J Med*. 2004;350:1862-1871.
5. Perdu J, Boutouyrie P, Bourgain C, et al. Inheritance of arterial lesions in renal fibromuscular dysplasia. *J Hum Hypertens*. 2007;21: 393-400.
6. Novick AC. Management of renovascular disease: A surgical perspective. *Circulation*. 1991;83(Suppl I):I167-I171.
7. Fisher JEE, Olin JW. Renal artery stenosis: Clinical evaluation. In Creager MA, Loscalzo J (eds): *Vascular Medicine: A Companion to Braunwald's Heart Disease*. Philadelphia, Saunders Elsevier, 2006, pp 335-347.
8. Hansen KJ, Edwards MS, Craven TE, et al. Prevalence of renovascular disease in the elderly: A population based study. *J Vasc Surg*. 2002;36: 443-451.
9. De Bruyne B, Manoharan G, Pijls NHJ, et al. Assessment of renal artery stenosis severity by pressure gradient measurements. *J Am Coll Cardiol*. 2006;48:1851-1855.
10. Textor SC. Pathophysiology of renovascular hypertension. *Urol Clin North Am*. 1984;11:373-381.
11. Crowley SD, Gurley SB, Oliverio MI, et al. Distinct roles for the kidney and systemic tissues in blood pressure regulation by the renin-angiotensin system. *J Clin Invest*. 2005;115:1092-1099.
12. Lerman LO, Nath KA, Rodriguez-Porcel M, et al. Increased oxidative stress in experimental renovascular hypertension. *Hypertension*. 2001;37: 541-546.
13. Safian RD, Madder RD. Refining the approach to renal artery revascularization. *JACC Cardiovasc Interv*. 2009;2:161-174.
14. Greco BA, Breyer JB. Atherosclerotic ischemic renal disease. *Am J Kidney Dis*. 1997;29:167-187.
15. Chade AR, Rodriguez-Porcel M, Grande JP, et al. Mechanisms of renal structural alterations in combined hypercholesterolemia and renal artery stenosis. *Aterioscler Thromb Vasc Biol*. 2003;23:1295-1301.
16. Lerman LO, Chade AR. Angiogenesis in the kidney: A new therapeutic target? *Curr Opin Nephrol Hypertens*. 2009;18:160-165.
17. Textor SC, Glockner JF, Lerman LO, et al. The use of magnetic resonance to evaluate tissue oxygenation in renal artery stenosis. *J Am Soc Nephrol*. 2008;19:780-788.
18. Juillard L, Lerman LO, Kruger DG, et al. Blood oxygen level–dependent measurement of acute intra-renal ischemia. *Kidney Int*. 2004;65: 944-950.
19. Messina LM, Zelenock GB, Yao KA, Stanley JC. Renal revascularization for recurrent pulmonary edema in patients with poorly controlled hypertension and renal insufficiency: A distinct subgroup of patients with arteriosclerotic renal artery occlusive disease. *J Vasc Surg*. 1992;15: 73-82.
20. Gray BH, Olin JW, Childs MB, et al. Clinical benefit of renal artery angioplasty with stenting for the control of recurrent and refractory congestive heart failure. *Vasc Med*. 2002;7:275-279.
21. Losito A, Fagugli RM, Zampi I, et al. Comparison of target organ damage in renovascular and essential hypertension. *Am J Hypertens*. 1996;9:1062-1067.
22. Chen R, Novick AC, Pohl M. Reversible renin mediated massive proteinuria successfully treated by nephrectomy. *J Urol*. 1995;153: 133-134.
23. Hackam DG, Duong-Hua ML, Mamdani M, et al. Angiotensin inhibition in renovascular disease: A population-based cohort study. *Am Heart J*. 2008;156:549-555.
24. Wright JR, Shurrab AE, Cheung C, et al. A prospective study of the determinants of renal functional outcome and mortality in atherosclerotic renovascular disease. *Am J Kidney Dis*. 2002;39:1153-1161.
25. Textor SC. Renal failure related to ACE inhibitors. *Semin Nephrol*. 1997;17:67-76.
26. Schoolwerth AC, Sica DA, Ballermann BJ, Wilcox CS. Renal considerations in angiotensin converting enzyme inhibitor therapy. *Circulation*. 2001;104:1985-1991.
27. van de Ven PJG, Beutler JJ, Kaatee R, et al. Angiotensin converting enzyme inhibitor–induced renal dysfunction in atherosclerotic renovascular disease. *Kidney Int*. 1998;53:986-993.
28. Missouris CG, Buckenham T, Vallance PJT, MacGregor GA. Renal artery stenosis masquerading as congestive heart failure. *Lancet*. 1993;341:1521-1522.
29. Bloch MJ, Trost DW, Pickering TG, et al. Prevention of recurrent pulmonary edema in patients with bilateral renovascular disease through renal artery stent placement. *Am J Hypertens*. 1999;12:1-7.
30. Wheatley K, Kalra PA, Moss J, et al. Lack of benefit of renal artery revascularization in atherosclerotic renovascular disease (ARVD): Results of the ASTRAL trial. *J Am Soc Nephrol*. 2008;19:47A.
31. Conlon PJ, Little MA, Pieper K, Mark DB. Severity of renal vascular disease predicts mortality in patients undergoing coronary angiography. *Kidney Int*. 2001;60:1490-1497.
32. Schreiber MJ, Pohl MA, Novick AC. The natural history of atherosclerotic and fibrous renal artery disease. *Urol Clin North Am*. 1984;11: 383-392.
33. Caps MT, Perissinotto C, Zierler RE, et al. Prospective study of atherosclerotic disease progression in the renal artery. *Circulation*. 1998;98: 2866-2872.
34. Caps MT, Zierler RE, Polissar NL, et al. Risk of atrophy in kidneys with atherosclerotic renal artery stenosis. *Kidney Int*. 1998;53:735-742.
35. Cheung CM, Patel A, Shaheen N, et al. The effects of statins on the progression of atherosclerotic renovascular disease. *Nephron Clin Pract*. 2007;107:c35-c42.
36. Lerman LO, Chade AR. Atherosclerotic process, renovascular disease and outcomes from bench to bedside. *Curr Opin Nephrol Hypertens*. 2006;15:583-587.
37. Chabova V, Schirger A, Stanson AW, et al. Outcomes of atherosclerotic renal artery stenosis managed without revascularization. *Mayo Clin Proc*. 2000;75:437-444.
38. Leertouwer TC, Pattynama PMT, van den Berg-Huysmans A. Incidental renal artery stenosis in peripheral vascular disease: A case for treatment? *Kidney Int*. 2001;59:1480-1483.
39. Crowley JJ, Santos R, Peter RH, et al. Progression of renal artery stenosis in patients undergoing cardiac catheterization. *Am Heart J*. 1998;136:913-918.
40. Balk E, Raman G, Chung M, et al. Effectiveness of management strategies for renal artery stenosis: A systematic review. *Ann Intern Med*. 2006;145:901-912.
41. Pillay WR, Kan YM, Crinnion JN, Wolfe JH. Prospective multicentre study of the natural history of atherosclerotic renal artery stenosis in patients with peripheral vascular disease. *Br J Surg*. 2002;89: 737-740.
42. Watson PS, Hadjipetrou P, Cox SV, et al. Effect of renal artery stenting on renal function and size in patients with atherosclerotic renovascular disease. *Circulation*. 2001;102:1671-1677.
43. Davies MG, Saad WE, Peden EK, et al. Implications of acute functional injury following percutaneous renal artery intervention. *Ann Vasc Surg*. 2008;22:783-789.
44. Wilcox CS. Non-invasive evaluation of renovascular disease. *Tech Vasc Intervent Radiol*. 1999;2:60-64.
45. Sabharwal R, Vladica P, Coleman P. Multidetector spiral CT renal angiography in the diagnosis of renal artery fibromuscular dysplasia. *Eur J Radiol*. 2007;61:520-527.
46. Postma CT, van Oijen AH, Barentsz JO, et al. The value of tests predicting renovascular hypertension in patients with renal artery stenosis treated by angioplasty. *Arch Intern Med*. 1991;151:1531-1535.
47. Hricik DE, Browning PJ, Kopelman R, et al. Captopril-induced functional renal insufficiency in patients with bilateral renal-artery stenosis or renal-artery stenosis in a solitary kidney. *N Engl J Med*. 1983;308: 377-381.

48. Jackson B, Franze L, Sumithran E, Johnston CI. Pharmacologic nephrectomy with chronic angiotensin converting enzyme inhibitor treatment in renovascular hypertension in the rat. *J Lab Clin Med.* 1990;115:21-27.
49. Davidson RA, Barri Y, Wilcox CS. Predictors of cure of hypertension in fibromuscular renovascular disease. *Am J Kidney Dis.* 1996;28:334-338.
50. Aurell M, Jensen G. Treatment of renovascular hypertension. *Nephron.* 1997;75:373-383.
51. Aurell M, Jensen G. Treatment of renovascular hypertension. *Nephron.* 1997;75:373-383.
52. Ramsey LE, Waller PC. Blood pressure response to percutaneous transluminal angioplasty for renovascular hypertension: An overview of published series. *BMJ.* 1990;300:569-572.
53. van de Ven PJ, Kaatee R, Beutler JJ, et al. Arterial stenting and balloon angioplasty in ostial atherosclerotic renovascular disease: A randomised trial. *Lancet.* 1999;353:282-286.
54. Leertouwer TC, Gussenhoven EJ, Bosch JP, et al. Stent placement for renal arterial stenosis: Where do we stand? A meta-analysis. *Radiology.* 2000;21:78-85.
55. Muray S, Martin M, Amoedo ML, et al. Rapid decline in renal function reflects reversibility and predicts the outcome after angioplasty in renal artery stenosis. *Am J Kidney Dis.* 2002;39:60-66.
56. Hallett JW, Textor SC, Kos PB, et al. Advanced renovascular hypertension and renal insufficiency: Trends in medical comorbidity and surgical approach from 1970 to 1993. *J Vasc Surg.* 1995;21:750-759.
57. Steinbach F, Novick AC, Campbell S, Dykstra D. Long-term survival after surgical revascularization for atherosclerotic renal artery disease. *J Urol.* 1997;158:38-41.
58. Ramsey LE, Waller PC. Blood pressure response to percutaneous transluminal angioplasty for renovascular hypertension: An overview of published series. *BMJ.* 1990;300:569-572.
59. Hansen KJ, Cherr GS, Craven TE, et al. Management of ischemic nephropathy: Dialysis-free survival after surgical repair. *J Vasc Surg.* 2000;32:472-482.
60. Stanley JC, David M, Hume Memorial Lecture. Surgical treatment of renovascular hypertension. *Am J Surg.* 1997;174:102-110.
61. Kane GC, Textor SC, Schirger A, Garovic VD. Revisiting the role of nephrectomy for advanced renovascular disease. *Am J Med.* 2003;114:729-735.
62. Webster J, Marshall F, Abdalla M, et al. Randomised comparsion of percutaneous angioplasty vs continued medical therapy for hypertensive patients with atheromatous renal artery stenosis. *J Hum Hypertens.* 1998;12:329-335.
63. Plouin PF, Chatellier G, Darne B, Raynaud A. Blood pressure outcome of angioplasty in atherosclerotic renal artery stenosis: A randomized trial. *Hypertension.* 1998;31:822-829.
64. van Jaarsveld BC, Krijnen P, Pieterman H, et al. The effect of balloon angioplasty on hypertension in atherosclerotic renal-artery stenosis. *N Engl J Med.* 2000;342:1007-1014.
65. Uzzo RG, Novick AC, Goormastic M, et al. Medical versus surgical management of atherosclerotic renal artery stenosis. *Transplant Proc.* 2002;34:723-725.
66. Textor SC. Atherosclerotic renal artery stenosis: Overtreated, but underrated? *J Am Soc Nephrol.* 2008;19:656-659.

CHAPTER 38

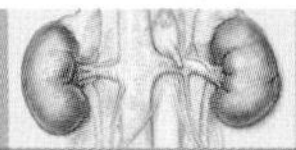

Endocrine Causes of Hypertension—Aldosterone

I. David Weiner, Charles S. Wingo

Recent advances in the diagnosis of aldosterone-induced hypertension have led to the recognition that primary hyperaldosteronism is more common than previously thought. Effective diagnostic strategies are available, and treatment regimens are highly effective.

ETIOLOGY AND PATHOGENESIS

Aldosterone is a steroid hormone produced normally by the zona glomerulosa of the adrenal glands. Figure 38.1 shows the biochemical pathway of aldosterone production. Aldosterone synthase, which is encoded by the gene *CYP11B2*, is the rate-limiting enzyme in adrenal aldosterone production.

Figure 38.2 summarizes factors known either to stimulate or to inhibit aldosterone synthesis by the adrenal gland. Aldosterone exhibits a circadian change in plasma concentrations, greatest in the late morning and with peak values ~50% greater than the average concentration. The factors accepted as physiologically important regulators of aldosterone production include angiotensin II (Ang II), which stimulates aldosterone production through activation of the AT_1 receptor, and atrial natriuretic peptide (ANP) and chronic hypokalemia, which inhibit aldosterone production.[1]

Aldosterone regulates blood pressure by several mechanisms (Fig. 38.3). These include effects on the kidneys, vasculature, central nervous system (CNS), and other endocrine hormones. No single effect is sufficient to explain the hypertension that occurs in primary hyperaldosteronism; taken together, these mechanisms explain why primary hyperaldosteronism causes refractory hypertension. Aldosterone has multiple renal effects that regulate blood pressure. First, aldosterone stimulates renal sodium chloride retention by increasing expression of the thiazide-sensitive sodium-chloride cotransporter in the distal convoluted tubule, the amiloride-sensitive epithelial sodium channel (ENaC) in the collecting duct, and the chloride-reabsorbing protein pendrin in the cortical collecting duct.[3-5] Aldosterone also has acute effects on sodium reabsorption in these segments through mechanisms that do not require protein synthesis.[6]

Second, aldosterone alters blood pressure through generation of hypokalemia. The increased sodium reabsorption enhances potassium secretion. In addition, aldosterone increases extrarenal cellular potassium uptake by stimulating the ubiquitous Na^+,K^+-ATPase, further decreasing extracellular potassium.[7] As discussed in Chapter 9, potassium depletion predisposes to hypertension through a variety of mechanisms.

Aldosterone has multiple effects on the vasculature. Aldosterone increases both basal vascular tone and vascular reactivity to circulating vasoconstrictors, including norepinephrine, epinephrine, Ang II, and vasopressin.[8,9] It decreases flow-mediated vasodilation perhaps by decreased nitric oxide (NO) production resulting from decreased endothelial nitric oxide synthase expression (NOS).[10] In the CNS, aldosterone stimulates CNS–mediated sympathetic nervous tone, which further increases blood pressure.[11] Finally, aldosterone causes perivascular fibrosis and increases vascular expression of endothelin.[12]

Aldosterone mediates its physiologic and pathophysiologic effects predominantly by activating the mineralocorticoid receptor.[13] The mineralocorticoid receptor is located in the inactive state in the cytoplasm; aldosterone binding to the mineralocorticoid receptor promotes a conformational change and translocation to the nucleus, where it regulates gene transcription.

Cortisol is a naturally synthesized glucocorticoid with an affinity for the mineralocorticoid receptor similar to that of aldosterone, but it is present in plasma at ~100-fold greater levels than aldosterone. The enzyme 11β-hydroxysteroid dehydrogenase type 2 is expressed in the aldosterone-sensitive distal nephron and collecting duct; it metabolizes cortisol to cortisone, which binds to the mineralocorticoid receptor poorly, thereby preventing glucocorticoid-dependent activation of the mineralocorticoid receptor.[14] Either the genetic deficiency or the ingestion of inhibitors of 11β-hydroxysteroid dehydrogenase can result in excessive activation of the mineralocorticoid receptor and the development of severe hypertension (see Chapter 47).[14] Aldosterone also has nongenomic effects, but their role in mineralocorticoid-dependent blood pressure regulation remains unclear.[15,16]

Primary hyperaldosteronism may result from either unilateral or bilateral adrenal disease. Typically, unilateral disease results from adenoma and bilateral disease from hyperplasia. This association is not absolute, and ~10% of those with primary hyperaldosteronism exhibit either bilateral aldosterone-producing adenoma, which may be microscopic, or unilateral hyperplasia.

EPIDEMIOLOGY

The exact incidence of primary hyperaldosteronism varies with the patient population and the diagnostic criteria used. Early studies, which recognized only severe cases, suggested that primary hyperaldosteronism was rare, with an incidence of less than 1% to 2%.[17] More accurate diagnosis has led to the recognition that primary hyperaldosteronism is relatively common. Patients with treatment-resistant hypertension (i.e., inadequately controlled hypertension despite treatment with three medications at appropriate dosages including a diuretic)

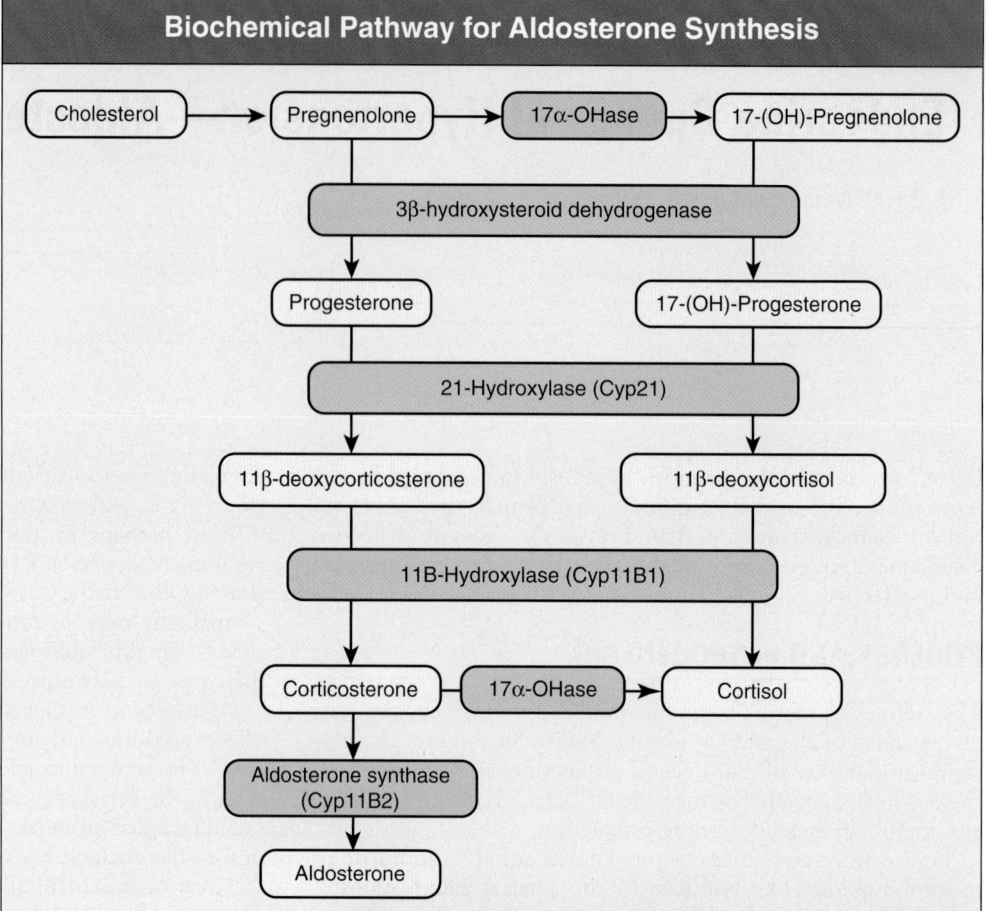

Figure 38.1 Biochemical pathway for aldosterone synthesis.

Factors that Regulate Aldosterone Release

Stimulatory	Inhibitory
Angiotensin II	*Atrial natriuretic peptide*
Adrenocorticotropic hormone	*Hypokalemia*
Acetylcholine	Calcitonin gene-related peptide
Adenosine triphosphate	Dopamine
Bradykinin	Nitric oxide
Cholecystokinin	Platelet-derived growth factor
β-Endorphin	Somatostatin
Endothelin	Unsaturated fatty acids
Enkephalins	Transforming growth factor β
Epidermal growth factor	
Hyperkalemia	
Melanocyte stimulating hormone	
Neuropeptide Y	
Neurotensin	
Norepinephrine	
Parathyroid hormone	
Prolactin	
Serotonin	
Substance P	
Vasoactive intestinal peptide	
Vasopressin	

Figure 38.2 Factors that regulate aldosterone release. Those stimuli that exert significant effects on aldosterone release under the majority of clinical circumstances are noted in italics. Stimuli listed in italic are those that are clinically most relevant; otherwise these stimuli are listed in alphabetical order. *(Data from references 1 and 2.)*

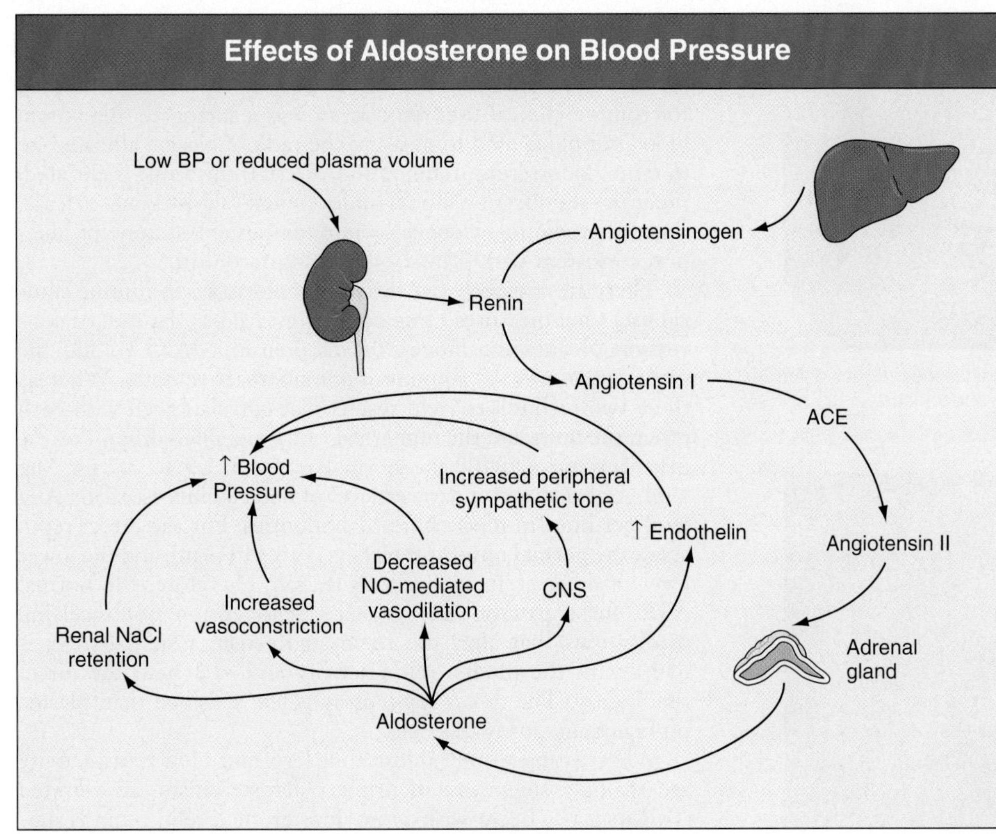

Figure 38.3 Effects of aldosterone on blood pressure. ACE, angiotensin-converting enzyme; BP, blood pressure; CNS, central nervous system; NO, nitric oxide.

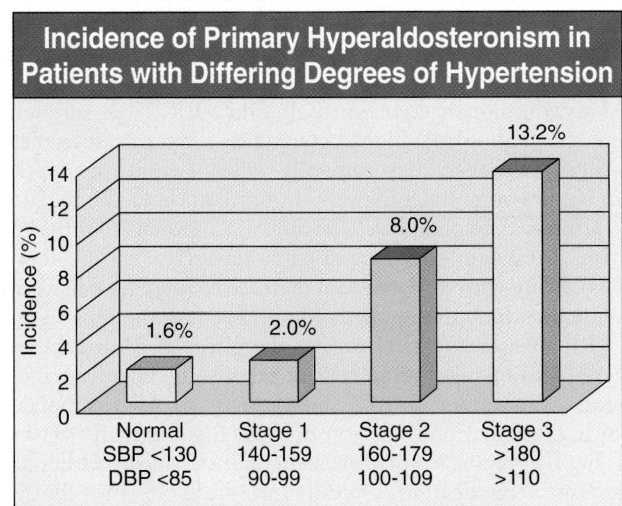

Figure 38.4 Incidence of primary hyperaldosteronism in patients with differing degrees of hypertension. *(From reference 19.)*

Typical Characteristics at Time of Diagnosis of Primary Hyperaldosteronism

Sex (female/male)	4/6
Age, yr (range)	52 +/– 1 (29–74)
Hypertension duration (yrs)	10 ± 1.4
Number (range) of hypertensive medications	2.4 ± 0.1 (0–4)
Percentage requiring ≥3 medications	53.7%
Blood pressure controlled on current medical regimen	20.4%
Neither hypokalemic nor uncontrolled on 3 or more medications	52%
Plasma aldosterone (ng/dl)	
<15	37%
15–40	54%
>40	9%
Plasma renin activity (ng Ang I/ml/hr)	0.3 ± 0.04

Figure 38.5 Typical characteristics at time of diagnosis of primary hyperaldosteronism. *(Data from reference 20.)*

have a high likelihood of having primary hyperaldosteronism; rates are typically 20% to 40% and as high as 67% in some studies.[18] Some studies (Fig. 38.4) have found a 1% to 2% incidence of hyperaldosteronism in normotensive patients, with the incidence increasing as blood pressure increases.[19]

CLINICAL MANIFESTATIONS

Patients with primary hyperaldosteronism frequently have characteristics suggestive of secondary hypertension, such as onset of hypertension between the ages of 20 and 39 years or onset in the elderly, worsening hypertension control, and the need for multiple medications for blood pressure control. It may also present in the 40- to 50-year-old age range and may escape diagnosis for many years because of the slow worsening of hypertension. Figure 38.5 summarizes characteristics of those with primary hyperaldosteronism. Because of improved screening techniques, hypokalemia and metabolic alkalosis are no longer considered

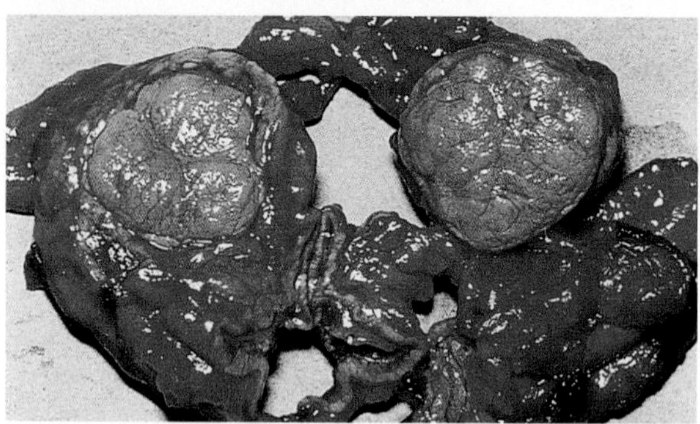

Figure 38.6 Adrenal adenoma. An aldosterone-producing adrenal adenoma with typical cholesterol-rich yellow appearance.

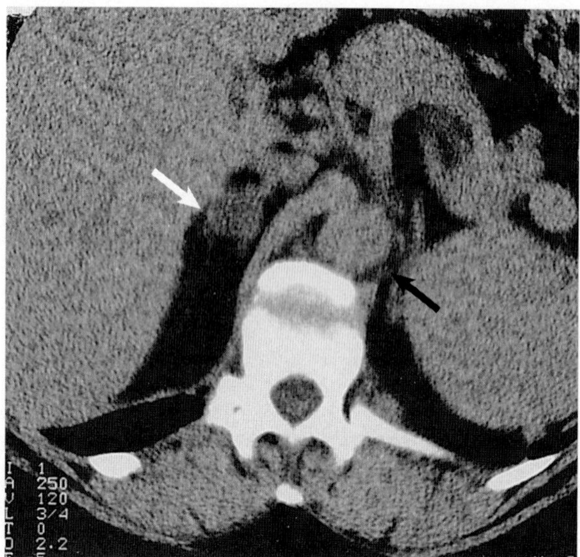

Figure 38.7 Adrenal adenoma by CT scan. A normal linear image of the left adrenal *(black arrow)* and expansion of the right adrenal with a 2-cm aldosterone-producing adenoma *(white arrow)*.

hallmarks of primary hyperaldosteronism and in fact are absent in the majority of patients.

PATHOLOGY

Primary hyperaldosteronism can result either from an aldosterone-producing adenoma (Fig. 38.6) or from hyperplasia of the zona glomerulosa. Most aldosterone-producing adenomas are unilateral and are large enough (>1 cm) to be identified by computed tomography (CT) scanning (Fig. 38.7). However, aldosterone-producing adenoma may also be microscopic and may be bilateral. Hyperplasia is typically bilateral but may develop asynchronously in the two adrenal glands, and it may be unilateral. The factors that lead to either aldosterone-producing adenoma or hyperplasia are not well understood.

DIAGNOSIS AND DIFFERENTIAL DIAGNOSIS

Evaluation of the patient with suspected primary hyperaldosteronism is directed at identifying those who have autonomous aldosterone release, then at identifying whether treatment should be based on a medical or a surgical approach. A diagnostic algorithm is shown in Figure 38.8.

Evidence of Ang II–independent aldosterone release is used to indicate autonomous aldosterone production and therefore primary hyperaldosteronism. Because Ang II cannot be assayed for routine clinical use, renin is used as a surrogate. A random blood sample is used to measure the ratio of plasma aldosterone to renin (aldosterone-renin ratio [ARR]). If this value is elevated, there is significant Ang II–independent aldosterone release, thereby providing evidence of autonomous aldosterone production consistent with primary hyperaldosteronism.

There are currently two different renin assays in routine clinical use. One measures renin activity, assayed as the rate of conversion of angiotensinogen to angiotensin I (Ang I), and the second measures the amount of immunoreactive renin. Whereas these two techniques yield results that correlate well with each other, the units and the numerical values obtained differ. For the plasma renin activity, the normal range is 1.9 to 3.7 ng Ang I/ml per hour, and the lower level of detectability is 0.2 ng Ang I/ml per hour in most clinical laboratories. For the direct renin assay, the normal range is typically 13 to 44 IU/ml, and the lower level of detectability is ~6 to 8 IU/ml. Therefore, the normal ARR, for a patient with primary hypertension not receiving medications that alter the renin-angiotensin system (RAS), is ~10:1 with the plasma renin activity and ~1:1 with the direct renin assay. The direct renin assay is less sensitive than plasma renin activity at lower values.

Whereas an elevated aldosterone level and a low renin activity are strongly suggestive of primary aldosteronism, an elevated ARR may also occur with a low aldosterone level if renin is suppressed. Combining an elevated ARR with "nonsuppressed" aldosterone levels decreases the rate of "false-positive" screening for primary hyperaldosteronism. The lowest plasma aldosterone value that may still be associated with aldosteronism is unclear; we suggest a minimum diagnostic value of 10 ng/dl.

Many common medicines may alter the ARR.[21,22] β-Adrenergic receptor antagonists (β-blockers) suppress renin release, typically by ~50%. However, they generally will not result in complete renin suppression and generally do not confound the diagnosis of primary hyperaldosteronism.[22] Angiotensin-converting enzyme (ACE) inhibitors and angiotensin receptor blockers (ARBs), along with diuretics, can increase renin release in normal individuals, which theoretically might decrease the sensitivity of the ARR measurement. However, the effect of ACE inhibitors and ARBs to increase renin release can also be an advantage; in patients using either an ACE inhibitor or an ARB, suppressed renin in combination with nonsuppressed aldosterone (>10 ng/dl) is highly specific for primary hyperaldosteronism. Other antihypertensive medications typically have little effect on the ARR measurement.

An elevated ARR alone, although it is sensitive for detection of primary hyperaldosteronism, is not highly specific. In unselected populations or populations with only mild or moderate hypertension, as many as 50% of patients with elevated ARR do not have primary hyperaldosteronism. Current recommendations therefore suggest confirmatory testing to establish the diagnosis of primary hyperaldosteronism.[23,24] Figure 38.9 summarizes the various confirmatory testing methods in routine use.

Once primary hyperaldosteronism is diagnosed, the clinician should determine whether unilateral aldosterone release is present, in which case adrenalectomy may be curative. If the patient is not a surgical candidate, this evaluation is not necessary. Because ~90% of patients with unilateral aldosterone release have an aldosterone-producing adenoma, an adrenal imaging protocol CT scan is the next diagnostic step; this uses

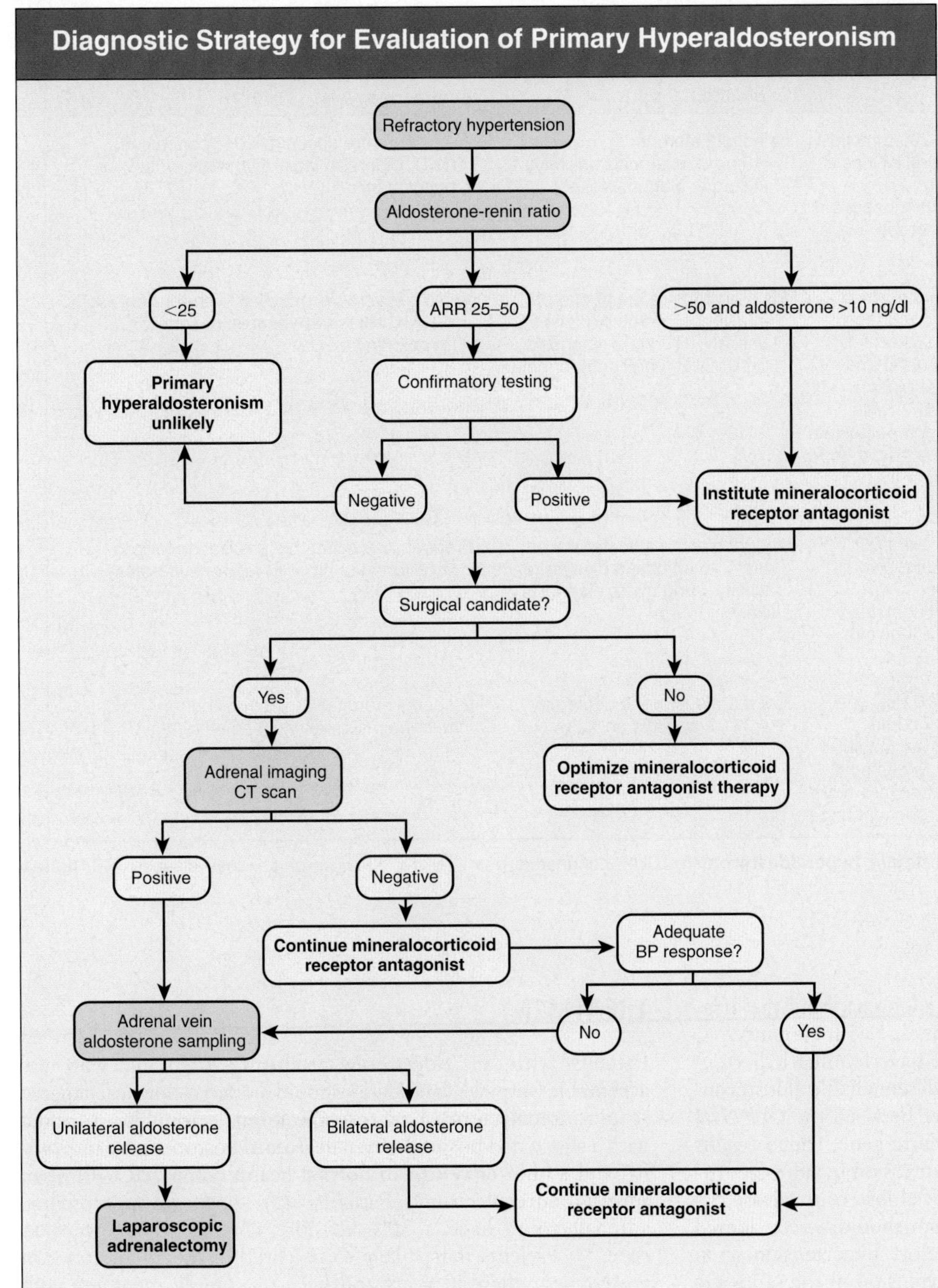

Figure 38.8 Diagnostic strategy for evaluation of primary hyperaldosteronism. ARR, aldosterone-renin ratio; BP, blood pressure; CT, computed tomography.

3-mm slices, whereas a conventional abdominal CT scan using 10-mm slices may fail to identify small adrenal adenomas.

The next step is to determine by adrenal vein sampling whether an identified adenoma is aldosterone producing or a nonfunctional adenoma ("incidentaloma"), which is present in ~5% of the adult population.

Occasionally patients will have unilateral aldosterone release but will not have an adenoma detectable on CT imaging. These patients may have either unilateral adrenal hyperplasia or micronodular aldosterone-producing adenoma. This diagnosis should be considered when the response to mineralocorticoid receptor antagonists (such as spironolactone and eplerenone) is small. Despite a normal CT scan, adrenal vein sampling is used to identify whether the patient has surgically treatable unilateral autonomous adrenal aldosterone release.

Many other diagnostic tests have been suggested in the evaluation of primary hyperaldosteronism, but none has widespread acceptance. The postural stimulation test may help differentiate bilateral adrenal hyperplasia from an aldosterone-producing adenoma. All medicines that affect the RAS, including diuretics, β-blockers, ACE inhibitors, and ARBs, must be discontinued before testing, but the difficulty in controlling blood pressure in these patients without medicines often limits the utility of this test. Its main role is in the evaluation of patients with an adrenal adenoma and unsuccessful adrenal vein sampling.[23] Assessment of 18-hydroxysteroid metabolites may also be helpful; if elevated,

Confirmatory Testing for Diagnosis of Primary Hyperaldosteronism

Test	Method	Evaluation	Limitations
Oral NaCl loading	Oral NaCl intake >200 mmol/d for 3 days, with oral KCl as needed to prevent hypokalemia, with subsequent 24–h urine aldosterone measurement	Urine aldosterone <10 µg/d, diagnosis unlikely; >12 µg/d, diagnosis likely	Avoid if severe uncontrolled hypertension, CKD, CHF, cardiac arrhythmias, or severe hypokalemia
Saline infusion test	Patient in recumbent position for 1 h before testing and then throughout entire test Begin test between 8:00 and 9:30 am. Measure plasma aldosterone, plasma renin activity, cortisol, and potassium at beginning of test and then after infusion of 2 L/NS IV during 4 h	Plasma aldosterone at end of infusion <5 ng/dl, diagnosis unlikely; <10 ng/dl diagnosis likely; 5–10 ng/dl, indeterminate	Avoid if severe uncontrolled hypertension, CKD, CHF, cardiac arrhythmias, or severe hypokalemia
Fludrocortisone suppression test	Fludrocortisone, 0.1 mg PO every 6 h for 4 days, plus oral NaCl, 30 mmol 3x/d, and high-salt diet combined with sufficient KCl to avoid hypokalemia	Upright plasma aldosterone on day 4 >6 ng/dl and plasma renin activity <1 ng/ml/hr, diagnosis likely	Frequently requires hospitalization for patient monitoring of blood pressure and potassium
Captopril challenge test	Oral captopril, 20–50 mg, with plasma aldosterone and plasma renin activity obtained immediately before captopril and then 1–2 h afterward, with patient seated throughout test	Plasma aldosterone decrease >30%, diagnosis unlikely	Probably more false-positive and false-negative results than other tests

Figure 38.9 Confirmatory testing for primary hyperaldosteronism. CHF, congestive heart failure; CKD, chronic kidney disease; NS, normal saline. *(From reference 23.)*

they suggest an aldosterone-producing adenoma,[25] but the diagnostic accuracy is inadequate to plan therapy with certainty.

Rare patients with an elevated ARR have familial hypertension type 1, also known as glucocorticoid-remediable aldosteronism. In this condition, there is crossover between the *CYP11B1* and *CYP11B2* genes, producing a chimeric gene, which results in regulation of aldosterone synthase expression by adrenocorticotropic hormone (ACTH) and excessive aldosterone release.[26,27] Glucocorticoid-remediable aldosteronism should be considered in children or young adults with refractory hypertension or in whom there is a family history of hypertension in the same age range or history of premature hemorrhagic stroke.[23] If it is suspected, genetic testing is now the preferred diagnostic approach because of improved sensitivity and specificity over measurement of corticosteroid metabolites or dexamethasone suppression testing.[23,24] If glucocorticoid-remediable aldosteronism is identified, administration of glucocorticoids in the minimal dose necessary to suppress ACTH release can dramatically improve blood pressure control (see Chapter 47).

NATURAL HISTORY

The natural history of untreated primary hyperaldosteronism is uncertain. Although there are case reports of remission of primary hyperaldosteronism, these all followed adrenal venography and may reflect complications related to the venography. Therefore, treatment is universally recommended.

TREATMENT

Patients with an aldosterone-producing adenoma who are acceptable surgical candidates should undergo surgical laparoscopic adrenalectomy. Laparoscopic adrenalectomy is associated with a shortened hospital stay, a decreased postoperative morbidity, and a quicker return to normal health compared with open surgical adrenalectomy. Patients who undergo laparoscopic adrenalectomy have a 30% to 60% chance of hypertension cure.[28-30] Patients most likely to be cured of their hypertension are younger than 50 years and have few family members with primary hypertension. Those not cured have a more than 95% chance of improvement in their blood pressure.[29,30] The lack of complete cure may reflect intrarenal microvascular disease that developed as a consequence of the poorly controlled hypertension.

Those who are not candidates for surgical adrenalectomy or who have bilateral aldosterone production should be treated with mineralocorticoid receptor antagonists. Figure 38.10 summarizes characteristics of the two major mineralocorticoid receptor antagonists currently available, spironolactone and eplerenone. Both are highly effective, and their major difference relates to their side effect profiles and their costs. Spironolactone has partial affinity for both androgenic and progesterone receptors, resulting in dose-related side effects. For example, gynecomastia occurs in ~7% of men treated with 50 mg daily or less but in more than 50% of those treated with 150 mg or more daily.[31]

Comparison of Currently Available Aldosterone-Receptor Antagonists

Medication	Dose Range (mg/day)	Common Side Effects
Spironolactone	25–400	Gynecomastia Breast pain (mastodynia) Impotence Decreased libido Menstrual irregularities
Eplerenone	25–200	Generally well tolerated Gynecomastia or abnormal vaginal bleeding in <2%

Figure 38.10 Comparisons of the different mineralocorticoid receptor antagonists.

Eplerenone has affinity for the mineralocorticoid receptor similar to that of spironolactone but ~100-fold less affinity for androgenic and progesterone receptors than spironolactone.[32] Accordingly, the incidence of side effects related to androgenic or progesterone receptor activation, such as gynecomastia, gynecodynia (breast pain), vaginal bleeding, and impotence, is greatly reduced. Eplerenone use may be limited because of greater cost.

Treatment with a mineralocorticoid receptor antagonist usually results in dramatically improved blood pressure control. Many patients will respond to a low dose, 25 to 50 mg daily, as initial therapy. Both systolic and diastolic blood pressure frequently decrease by ~25 mm Hg during a period of a few weeks to months. Dosage of the mineralocorticoid receptor antagonists can be increased as necessary but generally should not be changed more frequently than every 2 to 4 weeks. Hypokalemia and metabolic alkalosis, if present, improve. Potassium supplements can be tapered rapidly with improvement of hypokalemia. With time, blood pressure can be controlled in many patients with a mineralocorticoid receptor antagonist and a single alternative agent. We typically use ACE inhibitors because renin activity, which is suppressed initially, typically increases after mineralocorticoid receptor antagonist therapy is started. Synergistic use of an ACE inhibitor may prevent development of a renin-stimulated, Ang II–dependent component of hypertension. However, many antihypertensive combinations can be used successfully with the mineralocorticoid receptor antagonist.

Aldosterone Breakthrough

RAS inhibition is widely used to slow the progression of chronic kidney disease (CKD) and to decrease cardiovascular mortality in patients with congestive heart failure. These treatment regimens usually involve either ACE inhibitors or ARBs, which, by blocking Ang II–dependent stimulation of aldosterone production, should decrease plasma aldosterone levels. However, many patients develop "aldosterone breakthrough," in which the initial decrease in plasma aldosterone is followed by a later rise in aldosterone levels to greater than before ACE inhibitor or ARB treatment. Aldosterone breakthrough is associated with faster loss of glomerular filtration rate (GFR) in patients with CKD, reduced exercise capacity and reduced venous compliance in patients with congestive heart failure, and adverse effects on left ventricular mass index in hypertensive patients.[33,34] Patients with CKD who develop aldosterone breakthrough have a greater rate of loss of GFR, and treatment of these patients with low doses of mineralocorticoid receptor antagonists, such as spironolactone, 25 mg orally once a day, appears to decrease proteinuria, predicting a renoprotective benefit.[35]

REFERENCES

1. Quinn SJ, Williams GH. Regulation of aldosterone secretion. *Annu Rev Physiol.* 1988;50:409-426.
2. Spat A, Hunyady L. Control of aldosterone secretion: A model for convergence in cellular signaling pathways. *Physiol Rev.* 2004;84:489-539.
3. Verlander JW, Hassell KA, Royaux IE, et al. Deoxycorticosterone upregulates PDS (Slc26a4) in mouse kidney: Role of pendrin in mineralocorticoid-induced hypertension. *Hypertension.* 2003;42:356-362.
4. Kim GH, Masilamani S, Turner R, et al. The thiazide-sensitive Na-Cl cotransporter is an aldosterone-induced protein. *Proc Natl Acad Sci USA.* 1998;95:14552-14557.
5. Blazer-Yost BL, Liu X, Helman SI. Hormonal regulation of ENaCs: Insulin and aldosterone. *Am J Physiol.* 1998;274:C1373-C1379.
6. Wingo CS, Kokko JP, Jacobson HR. Effects of in vitro aldosterone on the rabbit cortical collecting tubule. *Kidney Int.* 1985;28:51-57.
7. Bia MJ, DeFronzo RA. Extrarenal potassium homeostasis. *Am J Physiol.* 1981;240:F257-F268.
8. Finch L, Haeusler G. Vascular resistance and reactivity in hypertensive rats. *Blood Vessels.* 1974;11:145-158.
9. Berecek KH, Stocker M, Gross F. Changes in renal vascular reactivity at various stages of deoxycorticosterone hypertension in rats. *Circ Res.* 1980;46:619-624.
10. Nishizaka MK, Zaman MA, Green SA, et al. Impaired endothelium-dependent flow-mediated vasodilation in hypertensive subjects with hyperaldosteronism. *Circulation.* 2004;109:2857-2861.
11. Gomez-Sanchez EP. Brain mineralocorticoid receptors: Orchestrators of hypertension and end-organ disease. *Curr Opin Nephrol Hypertens.* 2004;13:191-196.
12. Gumz ML, Popp MP, Wingo CS, Cain BD. Early transcriptional effects of aldosterone in a mouse inner medullary collecting duct cell line. *Am J Physiol Renal Physiol.* 2003;285:F664-F673.
13. Fuller PJ, Young MJ. Mechanisms of mineralocorticoid action. *Hypertension* 2005;46:1227-1235.
14. Rogerson FM, Fuller PJ. Mineralocorticoid action. *Steroids.* 2000;65:61-73.
15. Funder JW. Non-genomic actions of aldosterone: Role in hypertension. *Curr Opin Nephrol Hypertens.* 2001;10:227-230.
16. Funder JW. The nongenomic actions of aldosterone. *Endocr Rev.* 2005;26:313-321.
17. Ganguly A. Primary aldosteronism. *N Engl J Med.* 1998;339:1828-1834.
18. Eide IK, Torjesen PA, Drolsum A, et al. Low-renin status in therapy-resistant hypertension: A clue to efficient treatment. *J Hypertens.* 2004;22:2217-2226.
19. Mosso L, Carvajal C, Gonzalez A, et al. Primary aldosteronism and hypertensive disease. *Hypertension.* 2003;42:161-165.
20. Stowasser M, Gordon RD, Gunasekera TG, et al. High rate of detection of primary aldosteronism, including surgically treatable forms, after "non-selective" screening of hypertensive patients. *J Hypertens.* 2003;21:2149-2157.
21. Seiler L, Rump LC, Schulte-Monting J, et al. Diagnosis of primary aldosteronism: Value of different screening parameters and influence of antihypertensive medication. *Eur J Endocrinol.* 2004;150:329-337.
22. Mulatero P, Rabbia F, Milan A, et al. Drug effects on aldosterone/plasma renin activity ratio in primary aldosteronism. *Hypertension.* 2002;40:897-902.
23. Funder JW, Carey RM, Fardella C, et al. Case detection, diagnosis, and treatment of patients with primary aldosteronism: An endocrine society clinical practice guideline. *J Clin Endocrinol Metab.* 2008;93:3266-3281.
24. Young WF. Primary aldosteronism: Renaissance of a syndrome. *Clin Endocrinol (Oxf).* 2007;66:607-618.
25. Ulick S, Blumenfeld JD, Atlas SA, et al. The unique steroidogenesis of the aldosteronoma in the differential diagnosis of primary aldosteronism. *J Clin Endocrinol Metab.* 1993;76:873-878.

26. Lifton RP, Dluhy RG, Powers M, et al. A chimaeric 11β-hydroxylase/aldosterone synthase gene causes glucocorticoid-remediable aldosteronism and human hypertension. *Nature*. 1992;355:262-265.
27. Pascoe L, Curnow KM, Slutsker L, et al. Glucocorticoid-suppressible hyperaldosteronism results from hybrid genes created by unequal crossovers between CYP11B1 and CYP11B2. *Proc Natl Acad Sci USA*. 1992;89:8327-8331.
28. Weinberger MH, Grim CE, Hollifield JW, et al. Primary aldosteronism. Diagnosis, localization, and treatment. *Ann Intern Med*. 1979;90:386-395.
29. Sawka AM, Young WF Jr, Thompson GB, et al. Primary aldosteronism: Factors associated with normalization of blood pressure after surgery. *Ann Intern Med*. 2001;135:258-261.
30. Meyer A, Brabant G, Behrend M. Long-term follow-up after adrenalectomy for primary aldosteronism. *World J Surg*. 2005;29:155-159.
31. Jeunemaitre X, Chatellier G, Kreft-Jais C, et al. Efficacy and tolerance of spironolactone in essential hypertension. *Am J Cardiol*. 1987;60:820-825.
32. Lim PO, Young WF, Macdonald TM. A review of the medical treatment of primary aldosteronism. *J Hypertens*. 2001;19:353-361.
33. Epstein M. Aldosterone blockade: An emerging strategy for abrogating progressive renal disease. *Am J Med*. 2006;119:912-919.
34. Lakkis J, Lu WX, Weir MR. RAAS escape: A real clinical entity that may be important in the progression of cardiovascular and renal disease. *Curr Hypertens Rep*. 2003;5:408-417.
35. Sato A, Hayashi K, Naruse M, Saruta T. Effectiveness of aldosterone blockade in patients with diabetic nephropathy. *Hypertension*. 2003;41:64-68.

CHAPTER 39

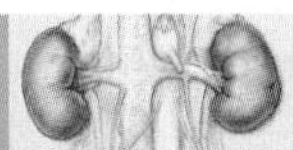

Endocrine Causes of Hypertension

A. Mark Richards, M. Gary Nicholls

The true incidence and prevalence of hypertension with endocrine etiology are unknown. However, primary aldosteronism, the most common form, is reported in 2% to 12% of patients with newly diagnosed hypertension. Overall, an endocrine contribution to high blood pressure may be present in more than 10% of cases. Endocrine hypertension often remains undiagnosed because physicians consider it rare and therefore unlikely, and access to the required specialized tests is limited.

Endocrine hypertension may occur in the absence of readily observed signs, symptoms, or abnormalities in routine biochemical tests. However, certain features should trigger a simple screen (Fig. 39.1), such as a family history of inherited conditions, including pheochromocytoma, neurofibromatosis, multiple endocrine neoplasia, and aldosteronism. Refractory hypertension (i.e., blood pressure resistant to administration of three antihypertensive drugs of different classes) mandates consideration of secondary hypertension, provided iatrogenic factors and noncompliance have been ruled out. The differential diagnoses will include endocrine, renal, and renovascular disease.

Symptoms and signs may be present. Severe hypokalemia may cause weakness, polyuria, and cardiac arrhythmia. Hyperadrenergic symptoms occur with pheochromocytoma. Changes in temperature tolerance, body weight, hair and skin condition, and bowel habit are clues in thyroid dysfunction or hypercortisolism. Thyroid disease, Cushing's syndrome, and acromegaly are associated with typical changes in body habitus. Abnormal sweating occurs in pheochromocytoma, thyrotoxicosis, and acromegaly.

Hypokalemia and diabetes mellitus are hallmarks of endocrine pathologic processes in hypertension. Hypokalemia in the absence of diuretic use should suggest diagnoses such as primary aldosteronism, pseudoaldosteronism, renin-secreting tumor, Cushing's disease, and accelerated hypertension of any cause. Therefore, concurrent high blood pressure and hypokalemia should prompt consideration of endocrine hypertension. Hyperglycemia is common to Cushing's syndrome, pheochromocytoma (especially when epinephrine levels are increased), acromegaly, and primary aldosteronism.

Diagnosis of endocrine forms of hypertension often offers the chance of cure, of altering an otherwise catastrophic natural history (e.g., in pheochromocytoma), and of applying specific and effective therapies that ameliorate other elements of the disease beyond control of blood pressure. Aldosteronism is addressed in Chapter 38. The following sections address other types of endocrine hypertension.

CUSHING'S SYNDROME

Definition

This syndrome of sustained glucocorticoid excess is most commonly secondary to production of adrenocorticotropic hormone (ACTH) by a pituitary adenoma (Cushing's disease). Less frequently, it is the result of cortisol overproduction from an adrenal adenoma or carcinoma, and rarely it may be secondary to ectopic ACTH or corticotropin secretion.[1] It can also result from exogenous corticosteroid administration. The incidence of endogenous Cushing's syndrome is 5 to 10 cases per million population per year. Cushing's disease and cortisol-secreting adrenal tumors are four times more common in women than in men. Approximately 0.5% of patients with bronchogenic carcinoma (more common in men than in women) develop ectopic ACTH syndrome.

Etiology, Pathogenesis, and Epidemiology

Hypertension is present in 80% of patients with Cushing's syndrome (less often when it is due to exogenous synthetic glucocorticoid administration) and results from an increase in both cardiac output and total peripheral resistance. The mechanisms underlying these hemodynamic changes are complex.[2] In some subjects, it may be due to concurrent overproduction of mineralocorticoids (aldosterone, 11-deoxycorticosterone, or corticosterone). Cortisol, although it is capable of binding the mineralocorticoid receptor, usually does not. This is because of the renal enzyme 11β-hydroxysteroid dehydrogenase type 2 (β-HSD2), which inactivates cortisol to corticosterone, thereby preventing its binding to the mineralocorticoid receptor. However, in the setting in which β-HSD2 activity is low or in which cortisol levels are extremely high (such as in ectopic ACTH syndrome), there may be sufficient excess cortisol that binding to the mineralocorticoid receptor occurs. Inhibition of the vasodilator nitric oxide (NO) by cortisol may also contribute to the hypertension, along with enhanced pressor responsiveness to catecholamines and angiotensin II (Ang II), heightened cardiac inotropic sensitivity to β-adrenergic stimulation, and increased plasma volume.[2] The sympathetic nervous and the renin-angiotensin systems are, if anything, suppressed even though circulating levels of renin substrate are increased. The possibility that elevated levels of vasoconstrictor hormones (vasopressin,

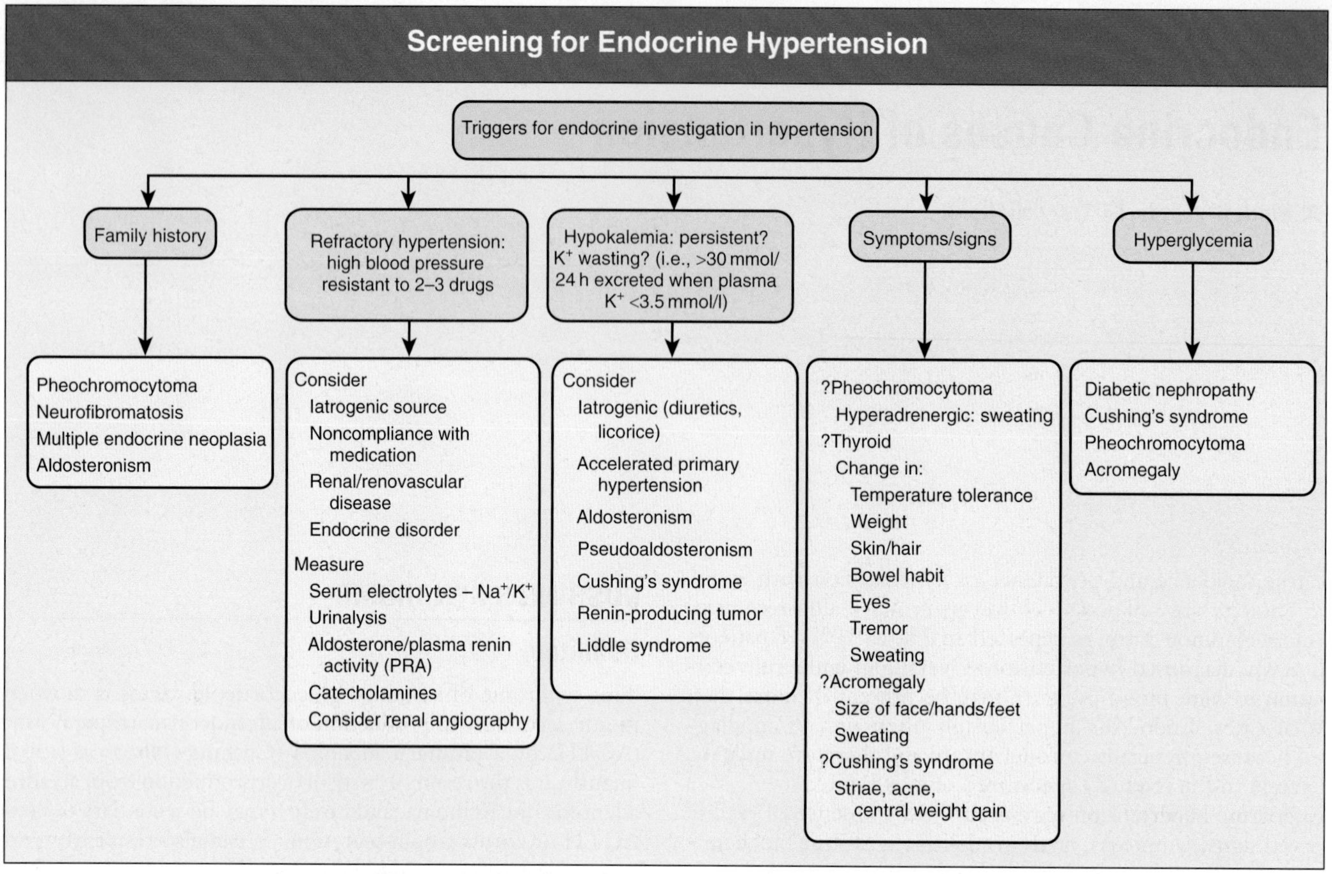

Screening for Endocrine Hypertension

Triggers for endocrine investigation in hypertension

- **Family history**
  - Pheochromocytoma
  - Neurofibromatosis
  - Multiple endocrine neoplasia
  - Aldosteronism
- **Refractory hypertension: high blood pressure resistant to 2–3 drugs**
  - Consider
    - Iatrogenic source
    - Noncompliance with medication
    - Renal/renovascular disease
    - Endocrine disorder
  - Measure
    - Serum electrolytes – Na^+/K^+
    - Urinalysis
    - Aldosterone/plasma renin activity (PRA)
    - Catecholamines
    - Consider renal angiography
- **Hypokalemia: persistent? K^+ wasting? (i.e., >30 mmol/24 h excreted when plasma K^+ <3.5 mmol/l)**
  - Consider
    - Iatrogenic (diuretics, licorice)
    - Accelerated primary hypertension
    - Aldosteronism
    - Pseudoaldosteronism
    - Cushing's syndrome
    - Renin-producing tumor
    - Liddle syndrome
- **Symptoms/signs**
  - ?Pheochromocytoma
    - Hyperadrenergic: sweating
  - ?Thyroid
    - Change in:
      - Temperature tolerance
      - Weight
      - Skin/hair
      - Bowel habit
      - Eyes
      - Tremor
      - Sweating
  - ?Acromegaly
    - Size of face/hands/feet
    - Sweating
  - ?Cushing's syndrome
    - Striae, acne, central weight gain
- **Hyperglycemia**
  - Diabetic nephropathy
  - Cushing's syndrome
  - Pheochromocytoma
  - Acromegaly

Figure 39.1 Screening for endocrine hypertension. Clinical observations suggesting endocrine investigation in hypertension.

endothelin 1, thromboxane, erythropoietin [EPO], and insulin) or subnormal concentrations of vasodilator systems (kallikrein-kinins and prostaglandins) contribute to the hypertension of Cushing's syndrome has been raised, but the evidence is frail.[2] The vasodilator atrial natriuretic peptide (ANP) is elevated in Cushing's syndrome, although biologic responses to ANP are impaired; in theory, ANP resistance could also contribute to the hypertension.[3] Successful treatment of Cushing's disease or removal of an underlying adrenal adenoma usually results in a reduction of blood pressure and partial return of the previously impaired nocturnal fall in arterial pressure, although hypertension persists in a sizable minority of patients.

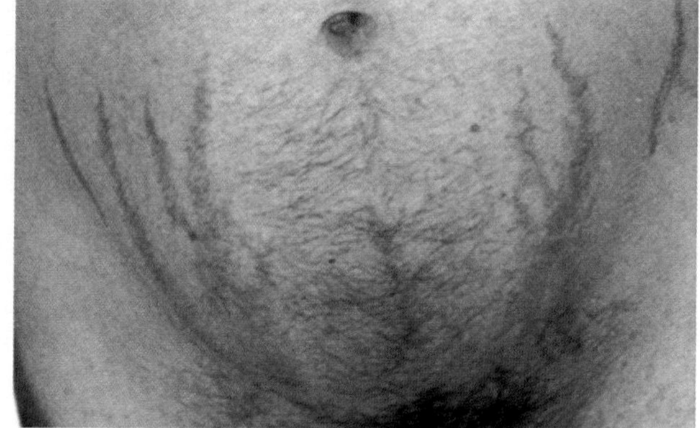

Figure 39.2 Striae and central obesity of Cushing's syndrome.

Clinical Manifestations

Clinical features in Cushing's disease result from elevated circulating levels of pro-opiomelanocortin hormones including ACTH (increased pigmentation) and cortisol (central adiposity, muscle wasting and weakness, plethoric facies, purple striae [Fig. 39.2], easy bruising, osteoporosis, psychological problems). In some patients, androgen effects are observed (hirsutism, acne, virilization), and these may be striking in those with adrenal adenoma or carcinoma. Ectopic ACTH syndrome due to small cell bronchogenic carcinoma or other tumors (e.g., bronchial or thymic carcinoid) presents typically as a wasting disease often with hyperpigmentation and hypokalemia. Hypertension is often associated with left ventricular hypertrophy, which can be disproportionate to the blood pressure, and frank cardiac failure is occasionally the presenting feature.[4]

Differential Diagnosis

Pseudo-Cushing's syndrome can occur with a sustained high intake of alcohol (by inducing augmented cortisol secretion and reduced cortisol metabolism due to hepatic damage); in depression; and in obesity, in which the plasma clearance rate of cortisol is increased, leading to a slightly elevated production rate of cortisol, but plasma levels of the hormone are normal. A careful physical examination differentiates obesity from Cushing's syndrome in all but a few patients.

Diagnosis

An elevated urinary free cortisol excretion (or early morning cortisol to creatinine ratio) and absence of suppression of 8 AM plasma cortisol after a low dose of dexamethasone (1 mg at midnight) are the commonly used initial tests.

Further key investigations include computed tomography (CT) and magnetic resonance imaging (MRI) of the pituitary and adrenals (and also the thorax, abdomen, and pelvis when ACTH-producing carcinoid tumors are suspected), plasma ACTH (which is suppressed in cortisol-secreting adrenal tumors but elevated in the ectopic ACTH syndrome), high-dose dexamethasone test (which partially suppresses ACTH in cases of pituitary tumors but not with ectopic ACTH), corticotropin-releasing hormone test, and simultaneous bilateral inferior petrosal sinus sampling for ACTH measurements. The last test is useful in differentiating Cushing's disease from ectopic ACTH syndrome when the previously listed tests give equivocal results.

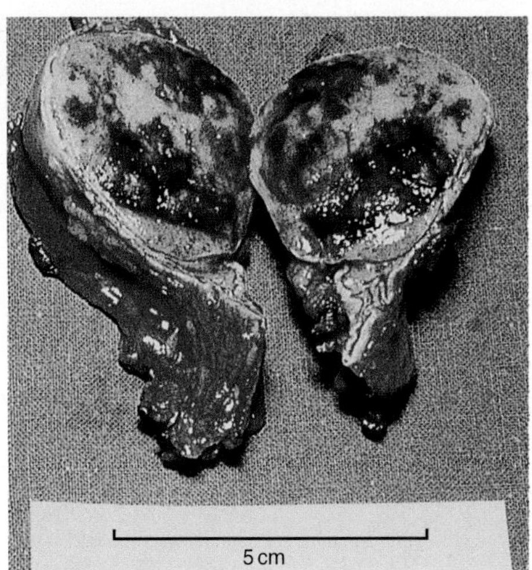

Figure 39.3 Large adrenal pheochromocytoma with areas of hemorrhagic necrosis.

Treatment and Prognosis

Untreated, Cushing's syndrome has a 50% 5-year mortality due to cardiovascular risk from hypertension along with glucose intolerance and insulin resistance, hyperlipidemia, obesity, and elevated fibrinogen levels.[5]

Cure rates in treatment of Cushing's disease are 80% to 90% by selective removal of a pituitary microadenoma and 50% for pituitary macroadenomas. Cushing's syndrome due to an adrenal adenoma is almost always cured by unilateral adrenalectomy. However, when the underlying lesion is adrenal carcinoma, most patients succumb within 2 years. The prognosis is also poor when Cushing's syndrome results from ectopic ACTH syndrome due to small cell bronchogenic carcinoma. If the ACTH-producing tumor is benign and can be located, however, removal usually leads to cure. After cure of Cushing's syndrome, approximately 30% of patients have persistent hypertension.[6]

In managing the hypertension due to Cushing's syndrome, there is no good evidence to support the use of any class of antihypertensive drug over another. Potassium-losing diuretics can exacerbate both hypokalemia and glucose intolerance, whereas potassium-sparing diuretics, usually in combination with other antihypertensive agents, may correct hypokalemia and reduce edema while lowering the blood pressure.

PHEOCHROMOCYTOMA

Definition

This disorder has challenged and fascinated clinicians since its first description by Frankel in 1886. Clinical manifestations can mimic a wide spectrum of other disorders; hence, the diagnosis is frequently delayed or missed altogether, sometimes with fatal consequences.[7]

Pheochromocytoma refers to a dusky tumor whose cells stain brown with chromium salts. Such tumors arise most commonly within the adrenal glands (Fig. 39.3), but approximately 10% are extra-adrenal (paraganglioma). Although the majority are benign, around 10% metastasize to regional lymph nodes and beyond. Histologic features are not a reliable guide to malignant behavior. The tumors can secrete a wide variety of hormones but most characteristically produce norepinephrine, epinephrine, and dopamine, with patterns differing between patients. Few paragangliomas produce epinephrine. Very high dopamine production is associated with malignant disease or a large tumor mass.

Etiology, Pathogenesis, and Epidemiology

The prevalence of pheochromocytoma in patients with hypertension in general medical outpatient clinics is 0.1% to 0.6%.[8] Because as many people die with unsuspected pheochromocytoma as with a firm diagnosis, however, the prevalence may be considerably higher.[9]

Pheochromocytomas can be sporadic or familial. Whereas sporadic cases are usually unicentric and unilateral, familial pheochromocytomas are often multicentric and bilateral. Familial pheochromocytomas are the result of a germline mutation in one of five genes: the *RET* gene leading to multiple endocrine neoplasia type 2; the von Hippel–Lindau (*VHL*) gene, which causes the von Hippel–Lindau syndrome; the neurofibromatosis type 1 (*NF1*) gene resulting in von Recklinghausen's disease; and the genes encoding the B and D subunits of mitochondrial succinate dehydrogenase (*SDHB* and *SDHD*), which are associated with familial paragangliomas and pheochromocytomas. Clinical features of syndromes associated with pheochromocytoma are described in Figure 39.4. For patients with apparently sporadic pheochromocytomas, an underlying germline mutation of the genes mentioned may be present in around 20% of cases and should be considered in younger patients (<50 years) and those with multifocal or extra-adrenal tumors.[8,10] Patients found to harbor a germline mutation need to be identified for appropriate guidance of medical management for them and their families.

Clinical Manifestations

Clinical features reflect episodic or continuous overproduction of catecholamines and depend in part on which catecholamine dominates. Symptoms include headache, sweating, palpitations, anxiety, and pallor (Fig. 39.5).[11] Hypertension or diabetes mellitus, with or without symptoms, may be the initial manifestation. Alternatively, pheochromocytoma may present as a tumor mass, usually an enlarging primary lesion in the abdomen or a paraganglioma in the neck, ear, thorax, or abdomen. On occasion, a metastatic lesion may be the presenting sign. Physical examination may reveal labile (66%) or persistent (33%) hypertension,

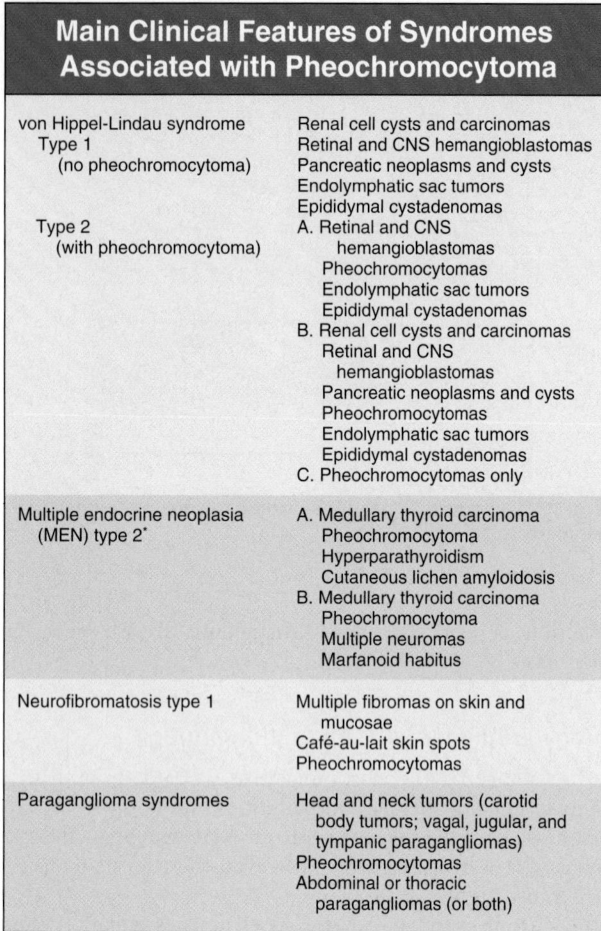

Main Clinical Features of Syndromes Associated with Pheochromocytoma

Syndrome	Features
von Hippel-Lindau syndrome Type 1 (no pheochromocytoma)	Renal cell cysts and carcinomas Retinal and CNS hemangioblastomas Pancreatic neoplasms and cysts Endolymphatic sac tumors Epididymal cystadenomas
Type 2 (with pheochromocytoma)	A. Retinal and CNS hemangioblastomas Pheochromocytomas Endolymphatic sac tumors Epididymal cystadenomas B. Renal cell cysts and carcinomas Retinal and CNS hemangioblastomas Pancreatic neoplasms and cysts Pheochromocytomas Endolymphatic sac tumors Epididymal cystadenomas C. Pheochromocytomas only
Multiple endocrine neoplasia (MEN) type 2*	A. Medullary thyroid carcinoma Pheochromocytoma Hyperparathyroidism Cutaneous lichen amyloidosis B. Medullary thyroid carcinoma Pheochromocytoma Multiple neuromas Marfanoid habitus
Neurofibromatosis type 1	Multiple fibromas on skin and mucosae Café-au-lait skin spots Pheochromocytomas
Paraganglioma syndromes	Head and neck tumors (carotid body tumors; vagal, jugular, and tympanic paragangliomas) Pheochromocytomas Abdominal or thoracic paragangliomas (or both)

Figure 39.4 Main clinical features of syndromes associated with pheochromocytoma. CNS, central nervous system. *A third type of MEN type 2 consists of familial medullary thyroid carcinoma only (without pheochromocytoma).

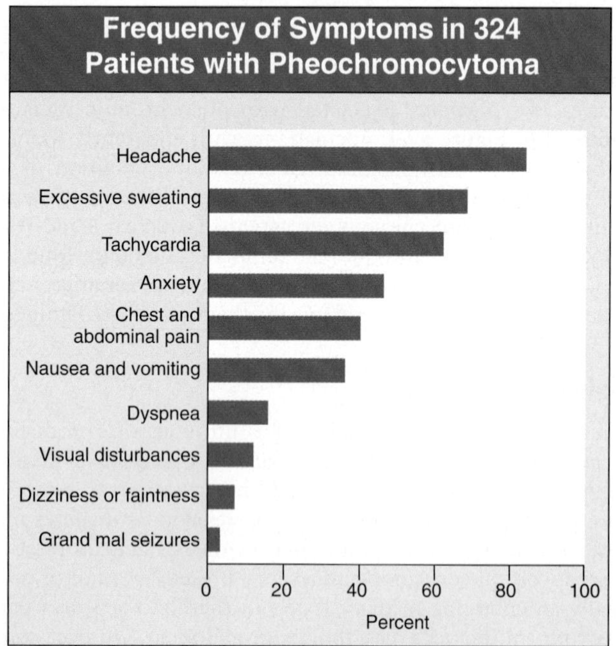

Figure 39.5 Frequency of symptoms in 324 patients with pheochromocytoma. *(Modified from reference 11.)*

sometimes with reciprocal changes in blood pressure and heart rate when the tumor secretes norepinephrine predominantly.[12] The patient may have cool, mottled extremities and a low-grade fever with tachycardia and postural hypotension. Patients may also present as an emergency with severe hypertension with or without heart failure and a variety of symptoms attributable to high plasma catecholamines. This can occur after minor or major trauma, at the time of delivery, or apparently spontaneously owing to sudden release of catecholamines from or hemorrhage into the tumor. Pheochromocytoma in pregnancy presents particular difficulties in diagnosis and management.[13]

Diagnosis

Diagnosis of pheochromocytoma is based on clinical suspicion but demands biochemical confirmation (Fig. 39.6). Current evidence is that plasma free metanephrines provide the best

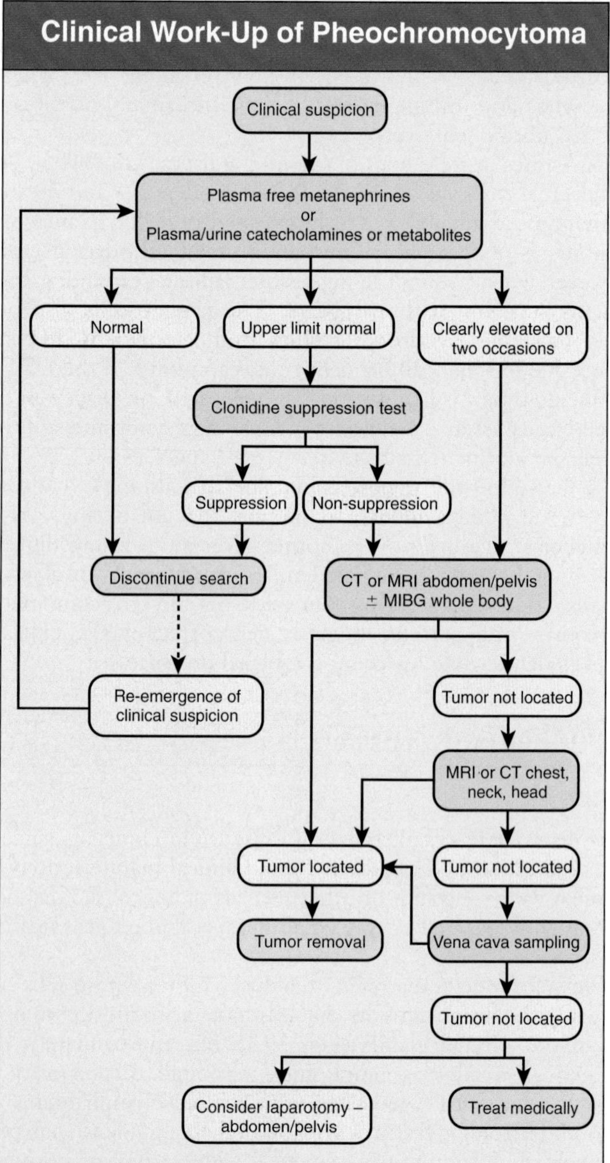

Figure 39.6 Clinical work-up of pheochromocytoma. CT, computed tomography; MIBG, metaiodobenzylguanidine; MRI, magnetic resonance imaging.

biochemical test for diagnosis or exclusion of pheochromocytoma, and the levels are relatively independent of renal function while also providing some guidance for tumor size and location.[14-16] When plasma free metanephrines are not available, plasma or urinary catecholamines or their other metabolites may be used and typically are 5- to 10-fold greater than normal. When catecholamine levels are at the upper limits of normal, a suppression test with clonidine (which suppresses plasma norepinephrine into the normal range if there is no pheochromocytoma but fails to do so in patients harboring a pheochromocytoma) is useful.[17]

Once a firm biochemical diagnosis is secured, the lesion must be localized (see Fig. 39.6). Imaging of a pheochromocytoma requires realization that the tumor, like the clinical syndrome itself, may mimic other lesions.[18] MRI or CT scan of the abdomen and pelvis, concentrating first on the adrenals, is successful in most patients, but additional investigations may be required if no lesion is detected. Such investigations may include selective venous sampling to detect a step-up in catecholamine levels, metaiodobenzylguanidine (MIBG) scanning, indium In 111–labeled octreotide scanning, measurements of plasma free metanephrines coupled with vena caval sampling, and positron emission tomography (PET) scanning.[19] Removal of a pheochromocytoma-containing adrenal can result in compensatory medullary hyperplasia in the contralateral adrenal, giving a false-positive MIBG scan; hence, interpretation must be cautious.[20]

Treatment

Once the tumor has been localized, the patient should be prepared for surgery with a collaborative team approach by the surgeon, anesthesiologist, and physician. Blockade of α-adrenoceptors, usually with phenoxybenzamine, with the later addition of β-blockade if it is necessary to control blood pressure and tachycardia, should be implemented for some weeks before surgery. β-Blockade monotherapy is contraindicated because of the risk of unopposed α-adrenergic stimulation leading to catastrophic hypertensive crisis. Alternative drugs that have been used successfully before surgery include prazosin (α-blocker) and labetalol (combined α- and β-blocker).

A laparoscopic approach to surgical removal of adrenal pheochromocytomas and some extra-adrenal tumors has gained widespread acceptance, but the laparoscopic approach should be converted to open adrenalectomy for difficult dissection, invasion, adhesions, or surgical inexperience.[21] Laparoscopic surgery has also been used successfully for hereditary bilateral or recurrent pheochromocytoma. Agents used to achieve intraoperative blood pressure control include phentolamine, sodium nitroprusside, and magnesium sulfate.

Hypotension and hypoglycemia are potential postoperative problems. In most cases, surgical removal of pheochromocytoma normalizes plasma catecholamine levels and previously suppressed central sympathetic outflow. Whereas blood pressure often improves with removal of the pheochromocytoma, it remains elevated in some patients, especially in those whose hypertension had been persistent as opposed to episodic. These subjects require long-term antihypertensive therapy.

For malignant pheochromocytoma, consideration should be given to aggressive surgical resection, particularly when there is a single metastatic lesion. Symptoms should be controlled with α- and β-blocking agents as needed, and irradiation can be useful for bone metastases. Chemotherapy, usually with cyclophosphamide, vincristine, and dacarbazine, should be considered for those with surgically inaccessible metastases producing symptoms that cannot be controlled by α- and β-blockade. Progression of malignant pheochromocytoma is extremely variable, with survival for decades in some cases. Median survival is approximately 5 years.

ADRENAL INCIDENTALOMA

Definition and Epidemiology

"Incidentaloma" refers to the incidental discovery of an adrenal mass in the course of investigation for other conditions in the absence of any prior suspicion of adrenal disease.[22] The increasing use and sophistication of abdominal imaging for a wide range of indications frequently leads to the incidental discovery of an adrenal mass. Current prevalence of unsuspected adrenal masses is reported at between 1% and 5% (less than 1% in those younger than 30 years, rising to 7% in those older than 70 years). Hypertension is more common in those with incidentalomas (40%) than in the general population. In a substantial series of more than 1000 incidentalomas, about 75% proved to be nonsecretory benign adenomas. However, an important minority (approximately 20%) showed endocrine activity, including aldosteronoma (1.4%, frequently normokalemic), pheochromocytoma (4.2%, with half normotensive), and cortisol-secreting tumors (9.2%, frequently with subclinical cortisol excess).[22]

Importantly, adrenal carcinoma, although rare at 0.6 to 2.0 cases per million population, accounted for 4% of cases in a large and well-documented series of incidentalomas. Adrenal carcinoma is more likely with increasing size of the adrenal mass (2% of masses up to 4 cm in diameter, 6% of masses 4 to 6 cm in diameter, and 25% of tumors larger than 6 cm). Adrenal carcinomas may or may not be functional. The prognosis is poor, with a 5-year survival of less than 20%. The differential diagnosis of incidentalomas includes metastases, myelolipoma, ganglioneuromas, cysts, hemorrhage, and infections.

Management

Incidentalomas mandate a careful history, directed at possible symptoms of endocrine hypertension; physical examination; and initial screening for pheochromocytoma (urine free metanephrines), glucocorticoid excess (urinary free cortisol to creatinine ratio and early morning plasma cortisol concentration after 1 mg dexamethasone), or primary aldosteronism (plasma and 24-hour urinary potassium levels and plasma renin to aldosterone ratio) as outlined in the relevant sections of this chapter and the chapter on primary aldosteronism.

RENIN-SECRETING TUMOR

Definition

Primary renin-secreting tumors are rare. Diagnostic criteria include an elevated plasma renin or prorenin level, which decreases on removal of the tumor, and demonstration of renin within the tumor. Most cases are due to benign renal juxtaglomerular cell tumors ranging from 5 mm to 6 cm in diameter, but they occasionally occur with nephroblastomas, renal cell carcinomas, and extrarenal neoplasms (bronchial or pancreatic carcinoma, ovarian tumors, carcinoma of ileum or colon, soft tissue sarcomas, orbital hemangiopericytoma).

Etiology and Pathogenesis

Autonomous hypersecretion of renin results in high circulating levels of Ang II, which increase arterial pressure. Secondary hyperaldosteronism, giving rise to hypokalemia, results from stimulation of the adrenal glomerulosa by Ang II. High Ang II levels also induce hyponatremia in a minority of patients (by stimulation of thirst and antidiuretic hormone secretion together with a direct renal water-retaining action of the peptide) and may also cause proteinuria.[23]

Clinical Manifestations

Cases show slight female predominance; 75% of patients are younger than 30 years, presenting usually with severe, occasionally paroxysmal hypertension (average 206/131 mm Hg), hypokalemia (<3.0 mmol/l in approximately 70% of cases), proteinuria (>0.4 g/day in around 50% of patients), and, in a minority, hyponatremia.[24] Glomerular filtration rate (GFR) is normal or high. Blood pressure may decrease substantially with the first dose of angiotensin-converting enzyme (ACE) inhibitor or angiotensin receptor blocker (ARB).

Pathology

Renin-secreting tumors are encapsulated and tan or grayish yellow, with scattered hemorrhages. They consist largely of polygonal or spindle cells in close contact with capillary and sinusoidal vessels and contain cytoplasmic renin granules.[24]

Diagnosis and Differential Diagnosis

Patients presenting with hypertension and hypokalemia together with elevated renin (and prorenin) and aldosterone levels may harbor a renin-secreting tumor, among which a renal juxtaglomerular cell tumor is most common. Renal artery stenosis or occlusion must first be ruled out by CT or MRI angiography or renal arteriography. These investigations also might reveal a radiolucent, relatively avascular, usually peripheral juxtaglomerular cell tumor (Fig. 39.7).[25] CT and MRI scans showing an isodense or hypodense lesion with little or no enhancement after injection of contrast material have proved helpful in the provisional localization of these tumors. Bilateral, simultaneous renal vein sampling may enable lateralization of the tumor. Because renal blood flow to the culprit kidney is not impaired, however, a renin ratio of more than 1.2:1 between the two renal veins may not be present, in contrast to the situation of unilateral renal artery stenosis, in which reduced blood flow to the stenosed kidney and renin oversecretion contribute to an often high renal vein renin ratio. Selective segmental renal vein renin sampling may help localize the tumor. When no renal lesion can be visualized and lateralization of renin secretion is not evident, an extrarenal renin-secreting lesion must be considered and sought by appropriate radiographic investigations and venous sampling for renin measurements.

Apart from renal artery stenosis or occlusion, it may be necessary to exclude other renin-producing lesions including Wilms' tumor, renal carcinoma, neuroblastoma, hepatocellular carcinoma, and pheochromocytoma, which can either themselves secrete renin or, alternatively, stimulate renal renin production. A careful clinical history and physical examination together with selected radiography and, occasionally, selective venous sampling for measurements of renin should, in most instances, differentiate these disorders from a juxtaglomerular cell tumor.

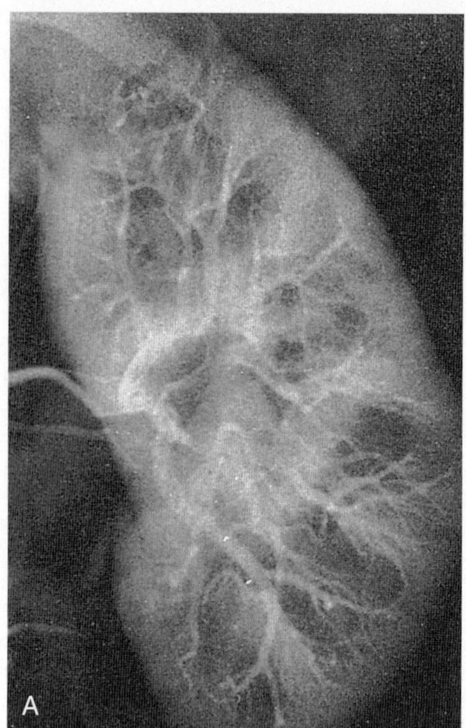

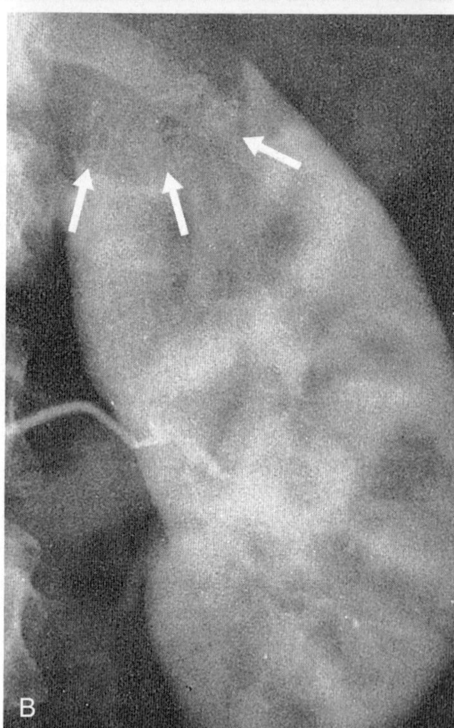

Figure 39.7 Renin-secreting tumor. Left renal angiography arterial **(A)** and nephrogram **(B)** phases revealing a 2.5-cm juxtaglomerular cell tumor with a circumscribed and relatively avascular appearance at the upper pole *(arrows)*. *(Modified from reference 25.)*

Treatment

Preoperative control of arterial pressure is based on an ACE inhibitor or ARB, introduced with caution to avoid first-dose hypotension. For juxtaglomerular cell tumors, local excision, where possible, is advisable to preserve nephrons. When doubt exists, an intraoperative frozen section will differentiate a benign juxtaglomerular cell tumor from malignant lesions and guide surgery. Removal of a juxtaglomerular cell tumor results in the return of renin and aldosterone levels to normal. Blood pressure decreases rapidly, but not always to normal if there is a background of primary hypertension or when there is hypertensive vascular damage.

ACROMEGALY

Definition and Epidemiology

Acromegaly is caused by excessive circulating growth hormone (GH), usually from a pituitary tumor. It is rare, with a prevalence of 40 cases per million. Hypertension is more common in acromegaly than in the general population, with an estimated 35% of subjects with a diastolic blood pressure above 100 mm Hg and higher frequencies in female and older patients. Uncertainty about the prevalence (between 17.5% and 57% in more than 20 different reports) reflects variation in definitions of hypertension and the stage of the disease.[26] Acromegalic patients who have additional hypopituitarism or advanced cardiac disease may have blood pressure reduction masking prior hypertension.

The pathogenesis of hypertension in acromegaly is complex but reflects sodium retention and volume expansion associated with an inappropriate response of hormonal systems to counteract these effects. Total exchangeable sodium, total body water, and extracellular fluid volume are increased. Volume expansion should suppress plasma renin levels, but although levels are low, they are not consistent with the sodium status. Aldosterone levels are also normal or only slightly suppressed. Plasma ANP, which should be elevated in the volume-expanded state, remains normal in acromegaly. The kidneys are enlarged and GFR is increased, but sodium balance is not corrected unless the acromegaly is cured. Other mechanisms contributing to hypertension may include the presence of circulating endogenous Na^+,K^+-ATPase (digoxin-like substances), GH-induced vascular hypertrophy resulting in decreased vascular compliance, effects on the sympathetic nervous system (SNS), and undefined genetic factors.

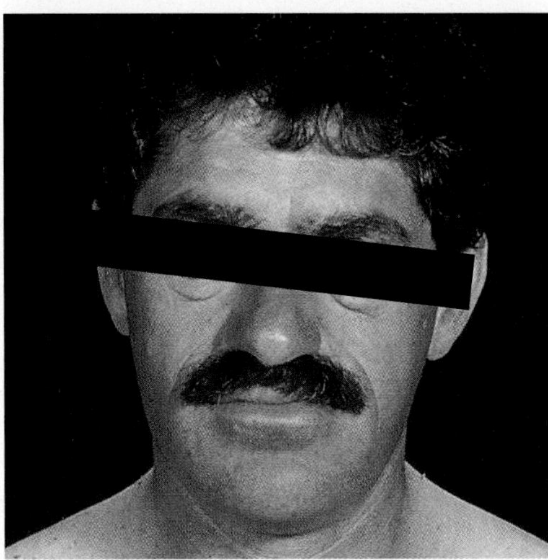

Figure 39.8 Facial features of acromegaly with enlargement of brow, nose, and jaw.

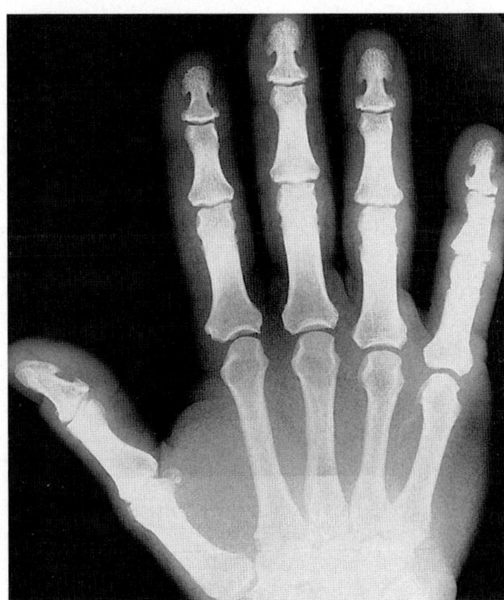

Figure 39.9 Radiograph of the hand in acromegaly. "Arrowhead" distal phalanges, expanded joint spaces, and increased soft tissue can be seen.

Clinical Manifestations

Acromegaly is characterized by enlargement of the skull (Fig. 39.8), hands (Fig. 39.9), and feet. Other symptoms result from local effects of an expanding pituitary tumor and include visual field defects and headache. Signs and symptoms include headache (40%), excessive sweating (50%), loss of libido (35%), amenorrhea (45%), carpal tunnel syndrome (25%), diabetes mellitus (19%), and visual field defects (5%).[27,28] Thyroid enlargement occurs in 50% of subjects and thyrotoxicosis in 6%. Hirsutism occurs in 24% of women and galactorrhea in 10%.

Diagnosis

Clinical suspicion should be raised by symptoms and signs. Figure 39.10 indicates appropriate tests. Elevated plasma GH, especially in response to an oral glucose tolerance test, is strongly suggestive of the diagnosis. Visual field assessment and MRI of the pituitary fossa are necessary to define the tumor and to exclude supratentorial extension. Most patients with acromegaly have a GH-secreting pituitary adenoma. Rarely, pancreatic or

Tests for Acromegaly
Plasma growth hormone
Plasma growth hormone responses to glucose tolerance test
Plasma insulin-like growth factor I
Lateral skull X-ray
Magnetic resonance imaging of the pituitary fossa
Visual field measurements
Assessment of other pituitary functions (e.g., thyroid function tests, thyroid-stimulating hormone, prolactin level, ACTH, and cortisol)

Figure 39.10 Tests for acromegaly.

hypothalamic tumors release GH-releasing hormone with secondary GH excess. Breast and bronchial tumors can also produce GH.

Treatment

Transsphenoidal adenomectomy is the treatment of choice. Irradiation and drug therapy are valuable when complete removal of tumor tissue is not possible (one third of cases) and when surgery is contraindicated. Dopaminergic agents, such as bromocriptine and cabergoline, and the somatostatin analogue octreotide reduce plasma GH in acromegaly. Bromocriptine may induce tumor shrinkage and improve diabetes. Radiation therapy may not exert its full effect for months or years. Hypopituitarism may occur late after treatment and necessitate endocrine replacement for ACTH, thyroid-stimulating hormone (TSH), or gonadotropin deficiency. Hence, regular monitoring of pituitary function is required after treatment.

Management of Hypertension in Acromegaly

Surgical removal of the pituitary adenoma with normalization of GH levels may reduce blood pressure to some extent, but the majority of patients will continue to require antihypertensive therapy.

Antihypertensive treatment requires a diuretic, given the volume-expanded state. Additional antihypertensive agents are frequently required, and both calcium channel blockers and ACE inhibitors may be effective. β-Blockers may also be used, although theoretically such agents may increase GH hormone concentration.

HYPOTHYROIDISM

Definition and Epidemiology

Hypothyroidism results from deficient production of thyroid hormones, whether through inadequate TSH secretion (from hypothalamic or pituitary lesions) or by impaired functioning of the thyroid itself (loss or atrophy of the gland, autoimmune destruction, iodine deficiency, antithyroid agents, or hereditary defects in hormone synthesis).[29] It is estimated that hypertension is 1.5 to 2 times more common in hypothyroid patients than in the general population.[30]

The pathogenesis of the hypertension is multifactorial and associated with both increased total body sodium and increased peripheral vascular resistance. Even within euthyroid subjects, serum free thyroxine index (FTI) is lower and TSH is higher in hypertensive than in normotensive subjects, and FTI also independently predicts the blood pressure response to increments in dietary sodium in both normotensive and hypertensive subjects.[31] Hypothyroidism is associated with increased aortic stiffness, which is reversed by hormone replacement therapy.[32] Observations of short-term hypothyroidism have confirmed increases in arterial pressure, plasma catecholamines, aldosterone, and cortisol, all reversible with thyroid hormone treatment.[33] The relationship between plasma catecholamine levels and blood pressure is steepened in hypothyroidism. The catecholamine levels of hypothyroid subjects also show more variability associated with more variability in blood pressure. This suggests underdamping of swings in sympathetic activity in the hypothyroid state.[34] Hypertension develops despite a low cardiac output. Thyroid replacement therapy corrects the electrolyte, hemodynamic, and hormone changes and cures the hypertension in most patients.

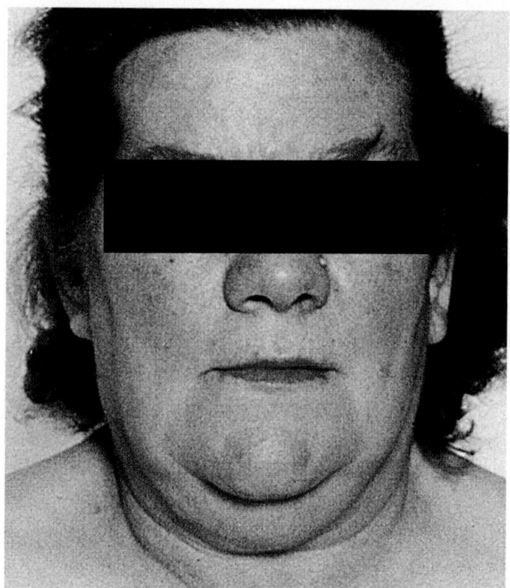

Figure 39.11 **Hypothyroid facies.**

Clinical Features

Any organ system can be affected in primary hypothyroidism. Symptoms and signs can be protean. The onset of clinical abnormalities is usually gradual, and diagnosis may not be made until gross hypothyroidism is established. Common clinical features include weakness, dry skin, lethargy, slow slurred speech, sensitivity to cold, thick tongue, facial puffiness (Fig. 39.11), coarse hair, failing memory, constipation, and weight gain with reduced appetite. Coronary heart disease is common, with contributions from dyslipidemia and hypertension accelerating the atherogenic process.

Diagnosis

Hypothyroidism should be considered in any patient with hypertension. Because the clinical manifestations of hypothyroidism are often difficult to elicit, especially in the elderly, thyroid function tests, including TSH when FTI is equivocal, should be performed. In patients with primary hypothyroidism in whom normotension is not achieved by full thyroxine replacement therapy, it is likely that primary hypertension is a concomitant disorder. For those with gross or long-standing hypothyroidism, replacement thyroxine therapy should be cautious to minimize the chances of exacerbating myocardial ischemia.

HYPERTHYROIDISM

Definition and Epidemiology

Hyperthyroidism and thyrotoxicosis may result from Graves' disease and less commonly toxic multinodular goiter, toxic adenoma, high iodine intake, trophoblastic tumor, and (rarely) excessive pituitary TSH secretion. Hypertension is common in hyperthyroidism, with a prevalence of 60% in toxic adenoma and approximately 30% in Graves' disease.

Clinical Features

The clinical features depend on the underlying cause of the hyperthyroidism, severity of the disorder, rapidity of onset, age of the patient, and concomitant disease. Abnormalities may be evident in the cardiovascular system (tachyarrhythmias, heart failure), skin (increased sweating, increasing pigmentation with vitiligo), eyes (lid lag, exophthalmos), nervous system (hypertension, nervousness), alimentary system (increased appetite yet weight loss, diarrhea), and muscles (proximal weakness).

Hypertension in hyperthyroidism is associated with elevated systolic blood pressure and normal or low diastolic pressure. It may be observed in both postpartum thyrotoxicosis and neonatal thyrotoxicosis. Elevation of diastolic pressure is unusual unless there is concomitant primary hypertension.

The hemodynamic characteristics in hypertension of thyrotoxicosis are an increased cardiac output, increased myocardial contractility, tachycardia, decreased peripheral vascular resistance, and expanded blood volume. These indices return to normal in most patients on achieving the euthyroid state. Interestingly, catecholamine levels tend to be low (inversely to hypothyroid hypertension), and there is no heightened activity of the sympathetic system. The renin-angiotensin system (RAS) tends to be activated and the aldosterone levels increased in hyperthyroidism, and this may contribute to the development of systolic hypertension.

Suspicion of hyperthyroidism should be high in the elderly patient with hypertension and a high pulse pressure, particularly if there is also atrial fibrillation. Such patients are liable to develop cardiac failure, in which case the increased systolic arterial pressure will diminish, masking previous hypertension. Hypertension with a high pulse pressure, although typical of hyperthyroidism, is observed in many elderly primary hypertensives because of the loss of the compliance of the aorta with aging.

Diagnosis and Treatment

Diagnosis of hyperthyroidism is confirmed by thyroid function tests, including measurement of TSH. β-Blockers are often effective first-line therapy for hyperthyroidism-associated hypertension. Treatment of hyperthyroidism, whether by antithyroid drugs, surgery, or radioiodine, will often normalize the increased systolic arterial pressure, although this is by no means invariable in the elderly, in whom there may be concomitant primary hypertension.

REFERENCES

1. Stewart PM. The adrenal cortex. In: Larsen PR, Kronenberg HM, Melmed S, Polonsky KS, eds. *Williams Textbook of Endocrinology*, 10th ed. Philadelphia: WB Saunders; 2003:491-551.
2. Whitworth JA, Williamson PM, Mangos G, Kelly JL. Cardiovascular consequences of cortisol excess. *Vasc Health Risk Manag*. 2005;1:291-299.
3. Sala C, Ambrosi B, Morganti A. Blunted vascular and renal effects of exogenous atrial natriuretic peptide in patients with Cushing's disease. *J Clin Endocrinol Metab*. 2001;86:1957-1961.
4. Sugihara N, Shimizu M, Kita Y, et al. Cardiac characteristics and postoperative courses in Cushing's syndrome. *Am J Cardiol*. 1992;69:1475-1480.
5. Mancini T, Kola B, Mantero F, et al. High cardiovascular risk in patients with Cushing's syndrome according to 1999 WHO/ISH guidelines. *Clin Endocrinol*. 2004;61:768-777.
6. Baid S, Nieman LK. Glucocorticoid excess and hypertension. *Curr Hypertens Rep*. 2004;6:493-499.
7. Manger WM, Gifford RW, eds. *Clinical and Experimental Pheochromocytoma*. Cambridge: Blackwell Science; 1996.
8. Lenders JWM, Eisenhofer G, Mannelli M, et al. Phaeochromocytoma. *Lancet*. 2005;366:665-675.
9. McNeil AR, Blok BH, Koelmeyer TD, et al. Phaeochromocytomas discovered during coronial autopsies in Sydney, Melbourne and Auckland. *Aust N Z J Med*. 2000;30:648-652.
10. Neumann HPH, Bausch B, McWhinney SR, et al. Germ-line mutations in nonsyndromic pheochromocytoma. *N Engl J Med*. 2002;346:1459-1466.
11. Ross ZJ, Griffith DN. The clinical presentation of phaeochromocytoma. *Q J Med*. 1989;71:485-494.
12. Richards AM, Nicholls MG, Espiner EA, et al. Arterial pressure and hormone relationships in phaeochromocytoma. *J Hypertens*. 1983;1:373-379.
13. Manger WM. The vagaries of pheochromocytomas. *Am J Hypertens*. 2005;18:1266-1270.
14. Lenders JW, Pacak K, Walther MM, et al. Biochemical diagnosis of pheochromocytoma. Which test is best? *JAMA*. 2002;287:1427-1434.
15. Eisenhofer G, Huysmans F, Pacak K, et al. Plasma metanephrines in renal failure. *Kidney Int*. 2005;67:668-677.
16. Eisenhofer G, Lenders JW, Goldstein DS, et al. Pheochromocytoma catecholamine phenotypes and prediction of tumor size and location by use of plasma free metanephrines. *Clin Chem*. 2005;51:735-744.
17. Bravo EL, Tarazi RC, Fouad FM, et al. Clonidine-suppression test. A useful aid in the diagnosis of pheochromocytoma. *N Engl J Med*. 1981;305:623-626.
18. Blake MA, Kalra MK, Maher MM, et al. Pheochromocytoma: An imaging chameleon. *Radiographics*. 2004;24(Suppl 1):S87-S99.
19. Pacak K, Goldstein DS, Doppman JL, et al. A "pheo" lurks: Novel approaches for locating occult pheochromocytoma. *J Clin Endocrinol Metab*. 2001;86:3641-3646.
20. Burt MG, Allen B, Conaglen JV. False positive ^{131}I-metaiodobenzylguanide scan in the postoperative assessment of malignant phaeochromocytoma secondary to medullary hyperplasia. *N Z Med J*. 2002;115:18.
21. Shen WT, Sturgeon C, Clark OH, et al. Should pheochromocytoma size influence surgical approach? A comparison of 90 malignant and 60 benign pheochromocytomas. *Surgery*. 2004;136:1129-1137.
22. Cicala MV, Sartorato P, Mantero F. Incidentally discovered masses in hypertensive patients. *Best Pract Res Clin Endocrinol Metab*. 2006;20:451-466.
23. Robertson PW, Klidjian A, Harding LK, et al. Hypertension due to a renin-secreting tumor. *Am J Med*. 1967;43:963-976.
24. Lindop GBM, Leckie BJ, Mimran A. Renin-secreting tumors. In: Robertson JIS, Nicholls MG, eds. *The Renin-Angiotensin System*. London: Gower Medical; 1993:54.1-54.12.
25. Lam ASC, Bédard YC, Buckspan MB, et al. Surgically curable hypertension associated with reninoma. *J Urol*. 1982;128:572-575.
26. Vitale G, Pivonello R, Auriemma RS, et al. Hypertension in acromegaly and in the normal population: Prevalence and determinants. *Clin Endocrinol*. 2005;63:470-476.
27. Nabarro JDM. Acromegaly. *Clin Endocrinol*. 1987;26:481-512.
28. Jadresic A, Banks LM, Child DG, et al. The acromegaly syndrome. *Q J Med*. 1982;51:189-204.
29. Larsen PR, Ingbar SH. The thyroid gland. In: Wilson JD, Foster DW, eds. *Williams Textbook of Endocrinology*. Philadelphia: WB Saunders; 1992:357-487.
30. Bing RF. Thyroid disease and hypertension. In: Robertson JIS, ed. *Handbook of Hypertension: Clinical Hypertension*. Amsterdam: Elsevier; 1992:576-593.
31. Gumieniak O, Perlstein TS, Hopkins PN, et al. Thyroid function and blood pressure homeostasis in euthyroid subjects. *J Clin Endocrinol Metab*. 2004;89:3455-3461.
32. Dernellis J, Panaretou M. Effects of thyroid replacement therapy on arterial blood pressure in patients with hypertension and hypothyroidism. *Am Heart J*. 2002;143:718-724.
33. Fommei E, Iervasi G. The role of thyroid hormone in blood pressure homeostasis: Evidence from short-term hypothyroidism in humans. *J Clin Endocrinol Metab*. 2002;87:1996-2000.
34. Richards AM, Nicholls MG, Espiner EA, et al. Hypertension in hypothyroidism: Arterial pressure and hormone relationships. *Clin Exp Hypertens*. 1985;7:1499-1514.

CHAPTER 40

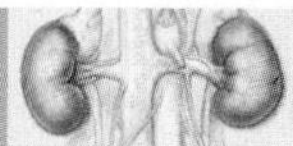

Neurogenic Hypertension, Including Hypertension Associated with Stroke or Spinal Cord Injury

Venkatesh Aiyagari, Sean Ruland, Philip B. Gorelick

An intimate relationship exists between the nervous system and blood pressure (BP).[1] The role of the sympathetic nervous system in both the short- and long-term regulation of BP is becoming increasingly appreciated. The sympathetic nervous system also has an important role in hypertension after neurologic injury. In this chapter, we discuss the physiology and management of hypertension in such injury.

PHYSIOLOGY AND PATHOPHYSIOLOGY

Neural Control of Blood Pressure

The brainstem, especially the ventral medulla, has a key role in the maintenance of BP (Fig. 40.1). BP is controlled by the nucleus tractus solitarius, which receives inhibitory baroreceptor afferents, and the rostral ventrolateral medulla and rostral ventromedial medulla, which are the source of excitatory descending bulbospinal pressor pathways. In addition, a depressor center in the caudal ventrolateral medulla composed of γ-aminobutyric acid (GABA)–containing neurons receives afferents from the nucleus tractus solitarius and projects to the rostral ventral medulla. These inhibitory GABA-containing neurons are tonically active, and reduced activity of these neurons leads to hypertension.[2-4]

The ultimate effector units are the sympathetic neurons located in the intermediolateral cell column of the spinal cord and the parasympathetic neurons found in the dorsal motor nucleus of the vagus and nucleus ambiguus located in the medulla. In addition, impulses from the limbic system, cerebral cortex, and hypothalamus also directly or indirectly project to the intermediolateral cell column of the spinal cord and influence BP regulation.

Cerebrovascular Autoregulation

Under normal conditions, cerebral blood flow (CBF) of the adult brain is 50 ml/100 g/min. CBF is regulated by the relationship between cerebral perfusion pressure (CPP) and cerebrovascular resistance (CVR):

$$\text{CBF} = \text{CPP}/\text{CVR}$$

Cerebral perfusion pressure is defined as the difference between the mean arterial blood pressure (MAP) and the intracranial pressure (ICP). If ICP is increased, systemic BP needs to be higher to maintain CPP and CBF.

Cerebrovascular autoregulation maintains a constant blood flow over a wide range of CPP. Normally, changes in CPP have little effect on CBF because of compensatory changes in CVR. An increase in CPP produces vasoconstriction and a decrease produces vasodilation, thus keeping the CBF constant (Fig. 40.2). Autoregulation is effective for a range of CPP from about 60 to 150 mm Hg. In chronically hypertensive individuals, the cerebral arterioles develop medial hypertrophy and lose the ability to dilate effectively at lower pressures. This leads to a shift of the autoregulatory curve to the right.[5] In these individuals, a rapid reduction of BP may lead to a drop in CBF even though the BP might still be within the "normal" range. With effective control of hypertension for several months, the normal range for autoregulation can be reestablished.[6]

Above the upper limit of autoregulation, there is breakthrough vasodilation leading to damage of the blood-brain barrier and cerebral edema and possibly cerebral hemorrhage. Below the lower limit of autoregulation, decreases in CPP lead to a decrease in CBF. Under these circumstances, increased extraction of oxygen and glucose maintains normal cerebral metabolism and brain function. When the CBF decreases to less than 20 ml/100 g/min, the increase in oxygen extraction is no longer able to supply the metabolic needs of the brain, leading to impairment of brain function.

SPECIFIC SYNDROMES

Hypertension After Stroke

Epidemiology

Hypertension is the most important modifiable risk factor for stroke, and reduction in BP is effective in the primary prevention of stroke, improves outcomes in patients who have had an ischemic stroke, and may be especially beneficial for lowering risk of stroke among those with a history of intracerebral brain hemorrhage.[7] Combined data from 40 trials of antihypertensive agents have demonstrated that a 10% reduction in systolic blood pressure (SBP) lowers stroke risk by one third.[8] A 5-mm lower diastolic pressure together with a 9-mm lower systolic pressure confers a 33% lower risk of stroke, and a 10-mm lower diastolic pressure together with an 18- to 19-mm lower systolic pressure confers more than a 50% reduction in stroke risk.[9] In patients who have had a stroke, the Perindopril Protection Against Recurrent Stroke Study (PROGRESS) showed that a reduction of BP was associated with a significant reduction of total stroke recurrence by 28% and a reduction of major coronary

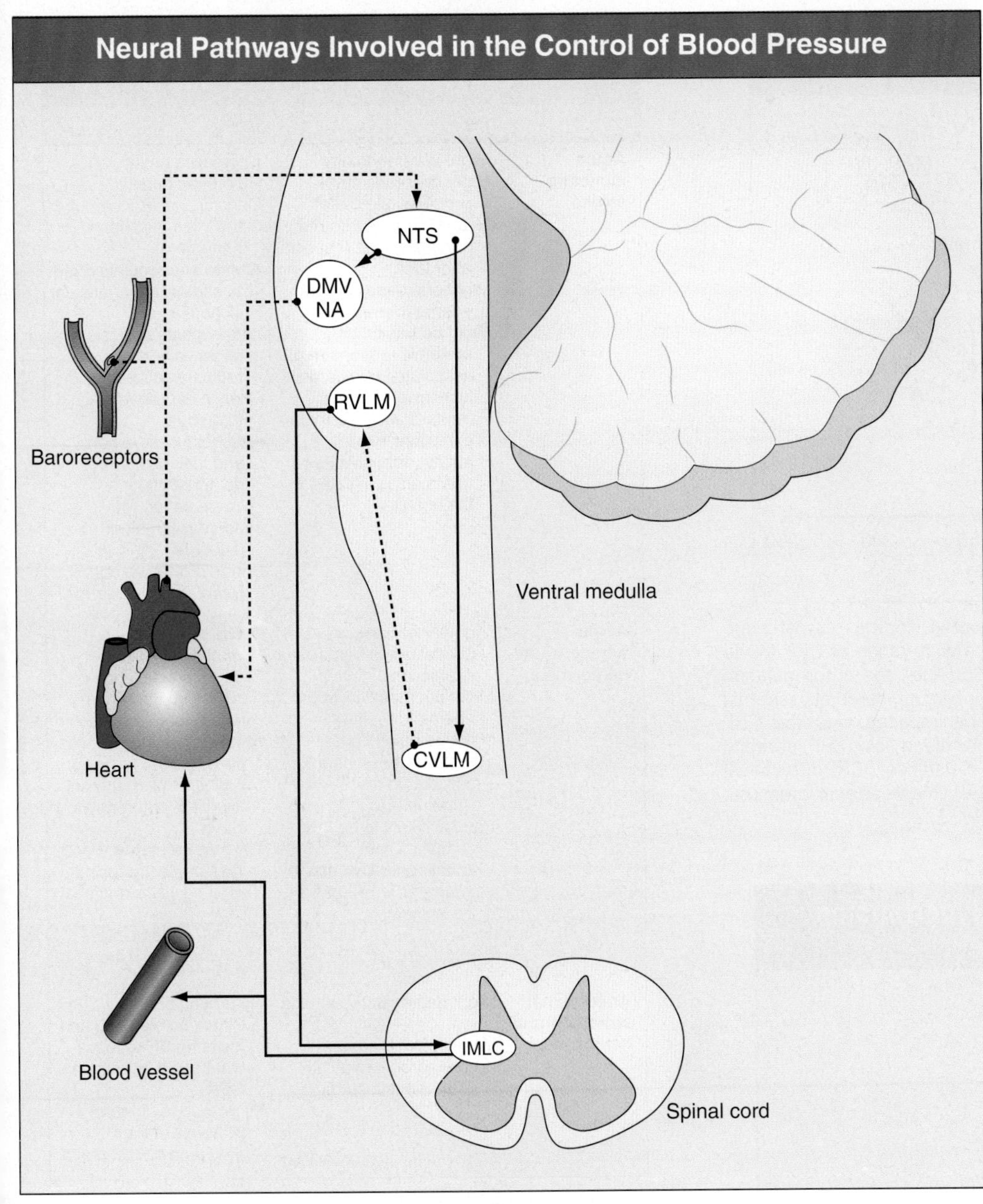

Figure 40.1 Neural pathways involved in the control of blood pressure. The ventral medulla has a key role in generating both excitatory *(solid line)* and inhibitory *(dotted line)* pathways, largely through the rostral ventrolateral medullary neurons (RVLM) and nucleus tractus solitarius (NTS), respectively. Ultimate effector control is provided by sympathetic activation originating in the intermediolateral cell column (IMLC) and parasympathetic action through the nucleus ambiguus (NA) and dorsal motor nucleus of the vagus nerve (DMV). CVLM, caudal ventrolateral medullary neurons.

and vascular events by 26%, even in subjects with a normal initial BP.[10]

However, the management of BP in the immediate aftermath of a stroke is controversial.[11] A high proportion of patients have elevated BP immediately after a stroke, and BP has been shown to spontaneously decrease during 1 to 2 weeks to the prestroke baseline in most patients. Some of the postulated causes of elevated BP are listed in Figure 40.3. An increased BP after stroke is associated with a higher mortality. Nonetheless, it is uncertain whether the increased BP directly contributes to poor outcome and whether immediate lowering of BP will lead to better outcomes.

Pathophysiology

An understanding of cerebrovascular pathophysiology is essential to understand the pros and cons of treating hypertension in these patients (Fig. 40.4).

In patients with an ischemic stroke, vascular occlusion leads to a central region of irreversibly ischemic brain surrounded by an ischemic zone where blood flow is reduced but brain tissue is still viable. After 2 or 3 days, the ischemic areas either recover completely or undergo infarction. In the first few days, perfusion in this zone is marginal, and a further decrease in blood flow might lead to infarction. Because cerebral autoregulation is impaired with acute ischemic stroke, a fall in BP could lower blood flow and extend infarction, and a very high BP could lead to hemorrhagic transformation, especially if thrombolytic agents have been given.

At times, it can be difficult to distinguish between hypertensive encephalopathy, in which lowering of BP is clearly indicated, and ischemic stroke with hypertension. The level of consciousness, the presence of focal neurologic deficits, and the funduscopic examination can help in making this distinction. Hypertensive encephalopathy is a syndrome of global neurologic dysfunction, usually with papilledema, and focal neurologic deficits are usually less prominent. In acute ischemic stroke, the focal neurologic deficit is more prominent, and alterations of consciousness are less common except with brainstem strokes or when there is “malignant” brain edema due to a massive hemispheric infarction.

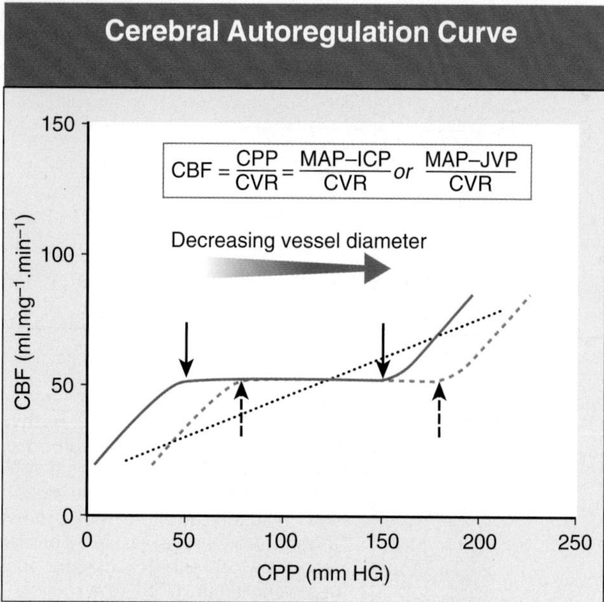

Figure 40.2 Cerebral autoregulation curve. In the normal state *(solid line)*, the CBF is held constant across a wide range of CPP (60 to 150 mm Hg). In chronic hypertension *(dashed line)*, the autoregulation curve shifts to the right. In the presence of acute cerebral ischemia *(dotted line)*, cerebral autoregulation may be impaired, and the CBF becomes dependent on the CPP. CBF, cerebral blood flow; CPP, cerebral perfusion pressure; CVR, cerebral venous resistance; ICP, intracranial pressure; JVP, jugular venous pressure; MAP, mean arterial pressure. *(Reproduced with permission from reference 12.)*

Postulated Causes of Hypertension After Stroke
Preexisting hypertension
White coat effect
Stress of hospitalization
Cushing reflex*
Catecholamine and cortisol release
Lesion of brainstem or hypothalamus
Nonspecific response to brain damage

Figure 40.3 Postulated causes of hypertension after stroke. *A hypothalamic response to raised intracranial pressure or ischemia consisting of hypertension with bradycardia.

Pros and Cons of Acute Treatment of Hypertension in Stroke

	Pros	Cons
Acute ischemic stroke	Might lower mortality Might decrease stroke progression Might decrease hemorrhagic transformation (especially after t-PA) Might decrease cerebral edema formation Might be helpful for systemic reasons (e.g., associated myocardial ischemia) Patients likely to be more compliant with antihypertensive use if treatment is initiated in the hospital	Decreases on its own No proven benefit Ongoing ischemia around the infarct (ischemic penumbra) Altered autoregulation due to chronic hypertension, ischemia Large-vessel stenosis might have resulted in reduction of perfusion Chance of propagating thrombus Anecdotal case reports and trial results demonstrating deterioration with decrease in blood pressure Principle of do no harm *(primum non nocere)*
Acute intracerebral hemorrhage	Might lower mortality Might decrease hematoma expansion Might decrease cerebral edema formation Might be helpful for systemic reasons (e.g., associated myocardial ischemia) Patients likely to be more compliant with antihypertensive use if treatment is initiated in the hospital	Decreases on its own No proven benefit There may be a zone of ischemia around an intracerebral hematoma Chronically hypertensive patients require higher perfusion pressure due to shift of autoregulatory curve ICP may be elevated and lowering BP reduces what could be marginal CPP Principle of do no harm *(primum non nocere)*
Aneurysmal subarachnoid hemorrhage	Might decrease rebleeding rate Might help if there is cardiac ischemia (stunned myocardium)	No proven benefit ICP may be elevated and lowering BP reduces what could be marginal CPP Might lead to cerebral ischemia in the presence of vasopasm

Figure 40.4 Pros and cons of acute treatment of hypertension in stroke. BP, blood pressure; CPP, cerebral perfusion pressure; ICP, intracranial pressure; t-PA, tissue plasminogen activator.

In patients with intracerebral hemorrhage (ICH), the considerations are different. Hematoma expansion occurs in one third of patients with ICH in the first 24 hours.[13] Therefore, BP is often lowered in these patients in the hope that this might decrease hematoma expansion. However, the evidence does not support a clear association between high BP and hematoma expansion.[14] On the other hand, some patients with ICH might have increased ICP due to the hematoma volume or associated hydrocephalus. In such a situation, lowering of BP is not warranted as it might critically lower CPP. Monitoring of ICP and CPP may be helpful in these circumstances.

In patients with aneurysmal subarachnoid hemorrhage (SAH), there is a significant risk of rebleeding; tight BP control is recommended to decrease the rebleeding risk. Some patients with SAH have associated myocardial dysfunction ("stunned myocardium"), in which case high BP might worsen myocardial function. As described before, in patients with hydrocephalus or an associated ICH, ICP and CPP monitoring can help guide BP management. In the latter half of the first week and in the second week after SAH, many patients develop vasospasm of the intracranial arteries. Reduction of BP may lead to worsening of cerebral ischemia in this situation. Therefore, once the aneurysmal rupture has been adequately treated with surgical clipping or coiling, BP is usually maintained at a normal or slightly elevated level in these patients.

Diagnosis and Treatment

Large studies adequately powered to assess the benefits and risks of BP lowering after ischemic and hemorrhagic stroke have not yet been performed. A recent Cochrane review on this topic concluded that there is insufficient evidence to evaluate the effect of altering BP on outcome during the acute phase of stroke.[15] The available evidence is summarized here.

A broad overview of recommendations for treating BP in different clinical situations is outlined in Figure 40.5.

Acute Ischemic Stroke The Acute Candesartan Cilexetil Evaluation in Stroke Survivors (ACCESS) trial studied early or late treatment with candesartan after a stroke in patients who were conscious, had a motor paresis, and were hypertensive. The combined endpoint of total mortality, cerebral complications, and cardiovascular complications at the end of 3 months was reduced by 48% for patients treated with candesartan (4 to 16 mg) initiated within 72 hours after stroke compared with those in whom it was instituted 7 days later. However, this difference in outcome was not associated with any difference in BP.[16]

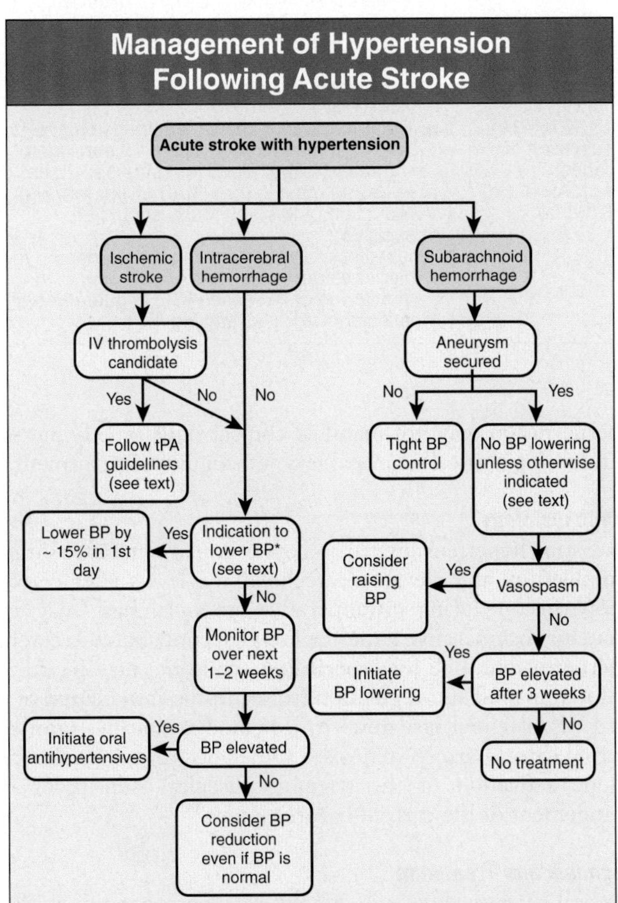

Figure 40.5 Management of hypertension after acute stroke. BP, blood pressure; t-PA, tissue plasminogen activator. *Indication for treatment includes systolic BP above 220 mm Hg or diastolic BP above 120 mm Hg for ischemic stroke, the presence of associated conditions such as aortic dissection or myocardial infarction, and, in cases of cerebral hemorrhage, systolic BP above 180 mm Hg or mean arterial pressure above 130 mm Hg.

In the Controlling Hypertension and Hypotension Immediately Post-Stroke (CHHIPS) trial, hypertensive patients with an ischemic or hemorrhagic stroke were randomized within the first 36 hours to labetalol, lisinopril, or placebo, titrated to a systolic BP goal of 145 to 155 mm Hg or a systolic BP reduction of 15 mm Hg from the BP at randomization. The primary outcome of death or dependency at 2 weeks in the treated group was not significantly different from that of the placebo group; however, mortality was halved at 3 months in the treatment groups compared with placebo.[17]

Early decrease in BP had no effect on outcome in the Glycine Antagonist in Neuroprotection (GAIN Americas) trial. In the Intravenous Nimodipine West European Stroke Trial (INWEST), a more than 20% reduction of diastolic BP on day 2 was associated with a worse outcome.[18,19]

The currently recommended guidelines of the American Heart Association/American Stroke Association and the European Stroke Organization for BP management in acute ischemic stroke are summarized in Figure 40.6.[20,21]

Intracerebral Hemorrhage A small controlled study of 14 hypertensive patients with a small- to moderate-sized ICH within 24 hours showed that treatment with nicardipine or labetalol to reduce MAP by 15% to a lower MAP limit of ~120 mm Hg produced no change in cerebral blood flow.[22] In contrast, a decrease in MAP by more than 20% or a SBP below 110 mm Hg in patients with ICH has been shown to lower blood flow.[23]

The Antihypertensive Treatment in Acute Cerebral Hemorrhage (ATACH) study used intravenous nicardipine infusion for 18 to 24 hours in patients with ICH with a SBP above 200 mm Hg presenting within 6 hours of symptoms. Patients with small hematomas (mean volume <20 ml) were treated to three different SBP goals (170 to 200, 140 to 170, and 110 to 140 mm Hg) with no difference in 3-month mortality between the groups.[24]

The Intensive Blood Pressure Reduction in Acute Cerebral Hemorrhage Trial (INTERACT) randomized hypertensive patients within 6 hours of symptom onset to achieve a target of

Guidelines for Blood Pressure Management after Acute Ischemic Stroke

AHA/ASA	ESO

• For patients eligible for thrombolytic therapy
  • Before treatment with thrombolytics
    • Lower BP if SBP >185 mm Hg or DBP >110 mmHG
  • After treatment with thrombolytics:
    • Lower BP if SBP >180 mm HG or DBP >105 mm Hg
• For patients not eligible for thrombolytic therapy
  • Patients with markedly elevated BP may have their BP lowered
  • Lowering BP by ~15 % in these patients is reasonable
  • Antihypertensives should be withheld unless SBP is > 220 mm Hg or DBP is >120 mm Hg
	• Routine BP lowering is not recommended
	• Cautious BP lowering is recommended in patients with extremely high BPs (>220/120 mm Hg) on repeated measurements, or with severe cardiac failure, aortic dissection, or hypertensive encephalopathy
	• Abrupt BP lowering should be avoided
	• BP must be below 185/110 mm Hg before, and for the first 24h after, thrombolysis

Figure 40.6 Guidelines of the American Heart Association/American Stroke Association (AHA/ASA) and the European Stroke Organization (ESO) for blood pressure management after acute ischemic stroke. BP, blood pressure; SBP, systolic blood pressure; DBP, diastolic blood pressure.

Figure 40.7 Guidelines of the American Heart Association/American Stroke Association (AHA/ASA) and the European Stroke Initiative (EUSI) for blood pressure management after acute cerebral hemorrhage. BP, blood pressure; SBP, systolic blood pressure; DBP, diastolic blood pressure, MAP mean arterial pressure; ICP, intracranial pressure; CPP, cerebral perfusion pressure.

Guidelines for Blood Pressure Management after Acute Cerebral Hemorrhage

AHA/ASA	EUSI

• If SBP is >200 mmHG or MAP is >150 mm Hg, then consider aggressive reduction of blood pressure
• If SBP is >180 mmHg or MAP is >130 mmHg and there is evidence of or suspicion of elevated ICP, then consider monitoring ICP and reducing blood pressure to keep cerebral perfusion pressure > 60 to 80 mm Hg
• If SBP is >180 mm Hg or MAP is >130 mm Hg and there is not evidence of or suspicion of elevated ICP, then consider a modest reduction of blood pressure (e.g., MAP of 110 mm Hg target blood pressure of 160/90 mm Hg)
	• Routine BP lowering is not recommended
	• Treatment is recommended in:
	  • Patients with known history of hypertension or signs (ECG, retina) of chronic hypertension: SBP >180 mmHg or DBP >105 mm Hg. If treated, target blood pressure should be 170/100 mm Hg (or a MAP of 125 mm Hg)
	  • Patients without known hypertension: SBP >160 mm Hg and/or DBP >95 mm Hg. If treated, target blood pressure should be 150/90 mm Hg (or a MAP of 110 mm Hg)
	• A reduction of MAP by >20% should be avoided
	• These limits and targets should be adapted to higher values in patients undergoing monitoring of increased ICP, to guarantee a sufficient CPP >70 mm Hg

140 or 180 mm Hg. Treatment was for 7 days or until hospital discharge. The lower BP target resulted in less hematoma expansion at 24 hours, but this difference was not significant after adjustment for initial hematoma volume and time from onset of ICH to computed tomographic CT scan. There was no significant difference in adverse event rate or outcome at 90 days.[25]

Although neither ATACH nor INTERACT was powered to detect a difference in clinical outcome, the results indicate that acute BP reduction in ICH may be safe.

The currently recommended guidelines of the American Heart Association/American Stroke Association and the European Stroke Initiative for BP management in acute ICH are summarized in Figure 40.7.[26,27]

Subarachnoid Hemorrhage Before definitive treatment of the ruptured aneurysm, SBP is usually kept below 140 to 160 mm Hg, although there is no conclusive evidence that higher BPs increase rebleeding rate. In patients with suspected elevation of ICP, it is important to monitor ICP and to keep the CPP above 70 mm Hg. The recently published American Heart Association/American Stroke Association guidelines recommend monitoring and control of BP to balance the risk of stroke, hypertension-related bleeding, and maintenance of CPP, but no absolute treatment thresholds or goals are specified.[28] After the ruptured aneurysm has been secured, aggressive treatment of BP should be avoided, and in the setting of cerebral vasospasm, BP is usually elevated until the neurologic deficits resolve, generally up to a SBP of 200 to 220 mm Hg.

Hypertension After Carotid Endarterectomy and Endovascular Procedures

Definition and Epidemiology

Hemodynamic disturbances such as hypotension, bradycardia, and hypertension are common (10% to 40%) after carotid endarterectomy and endovascular procedures such as angioplasty and stenting. In addition, 10% of patients develop the "carotid hyperperfusion (or reperfusion) syndrome." This syndrome occurs in the first week after surgery or angioplasty-stenting and is manifested as transient or permanent contralateral neurologic signs, ipsilateral pulsatile headache, seizures, ICH, or reversible cerebral edema.[29-31] Some subjects with post-revascularization cerebral hyperperfusion may not manifest clinical signs acutely but may later develop cortical neuronal loss and cognitive impairment.[32]

Pathophysiology

Preexisting hypertension, baroreceptor impairment after surgical manipulation, and elevated catecholamine levels after cerebral hypoperfusion during intraoperative cross-clamping may contribute to postoperative hypertension that contributes to cerebral hyperperfusion. The hyperperfusion syndrome may be due, in part, to impaired autoregulation from chronic vasodilation of the distal vascular bed ipsilateral to a hemodynamically significant internal carotid artery stenosis.[33] Other postulated mechanisms include activation of the trigeminovascular axon reflex and derangement of the carotid baroreceptors.[34]

Diagnosis and Treatment

Cerebral hyperperfusion is defined as a postoperative increase in CBF of more than 100% compared with preoperative flow. However, this increase in blood flow may be only approximately 20% compared with the contralateral side.[35] Subjects at risk for development of this syndrome are those with extensive microvascular disease, preoperative hypoperfusion and impaired autoregulation, or postoperative hyperperfusion.

Because of the risk for development of carotid hyperperfusion syndrome after carotid endarterectomy or stenting, all patients should have continuous intraoperative and postoperative BP monitoring. Most authors advocate strict BP control (SBP <120 mm Hg) from the time of intraoperative internal carotid artery unclamping or angioplasty, particularly in high-risk subjects.[36] Elevated BP should be treated with intravenous labetalol or clonidine. Vasodilators such as nitroglycerin and sodium nitroprusside should be avoided.

Hypertension After Spinal Cord Injury

Definition and Epidemiology

Autonomic dysreflexia occurs in up to 70% of subjects after spinal injury. It is defined as an increase in SBP by at least 20%, associated with a change in heart rate and accompanied by at least one sign (sweating, piloerection, facial flushing) or symptom (headache, blurred vision, stuffy nose).[37] If it is unrecognized, it can result in serious sequelae, such as posterior leukoencephalopathy, ICH, SAH, seizures, arrhythmia, pulmonary edema, retinal hemorrhage, and rarely coma or death.[38]

Pathophysiology and Diagnosis

The spinal cord lesion is typically at or above the sixth thoracic spinal nerve level. Immediately after the injury, there is initial loss of supraspinal sympathetic control similar to the initial period of muscle flaccidity. This often leads to hypotension and bradycardia (spinal shock). After a few weeks to months, there is extrajunctional sprouting of the α-receptors, denervation hypersensitivity, and impaired presynaptic uptake of norepinephrine. In addition, there may be derangement of spinal glutaminergic interneurons. Noxious stimuli below the neurologic level of the lesion trigger a spinal reflex arc that results in increased sympathetic tone and hypertension.[39] The most common inciting events are urinary overdistention and fecal impaction. However, it may be secondary to precipitants including sympathomimetic medications and sildenafil citrate used for sperm retrieval.[40]

Clinical symptoms include pulsatile headache, blurred vision, nasal congestion, nausea, and sweating above the spinal nerve level. The flushed sweaty skin above the lesion level is due to brainstem parasympathetic activation. At and below the lesion, the skin remains pale, cool, and dry. Heart rate can be quite variable from bradycardia to tachycardia. The hallmark physical finding is elevated BP. However, as BP may normally be quite low after spinal cord injury, baseline BP readings may be within the normal range but elevated for a given individual, making clinical suspicion and reliance on other clinical signs and symptoms paramount in the diagnosis if baseline BP is not known.[39]

Treatment

Vigilant preventive measures for autonomic dysreflexia include proper bowel, bladder, and skin care. However, expeditious treatment of elevated BP is critical to avoid the potentially severe consequences. Placement of the patient upright to precipitate orthostatic BP lowering and removal of any possible noxious stimuli, such as binding clothing and devices, are the initial treatment steps. Checking for fecal impaction and urinary overdistention and changing, flushing, or insertion of a new catheter if the patient receives intermittent catheterization are important.

Pharmacologic treatment with rapid-acting, short-lived agents may be indicated for SBP elevation of 150 mm Hg or more that persists after the preceding interventions. To avoid precipitating hypotension, nitrate-containing agents should not be given for 24 hours before the use of sildenafil or similar agents. If the bladder is empty and the BP is below 150 mm Hg, fecal disimpaction with topical anesthetic should be attempted. If dysreflexia is refractory or associated with severe clinical presentation, other precipitants should be sought and hospitalization may be indicated.[41]

Up to 90% of pregnant women with upper spinal cord injury experience autonomic dysreflexia during labor and delivery. Appropriate epidural or spinal anesthesia techniques can ameliorate the risk.[42]

Cerebrovascular Effects of Antihypertensive Agents

Different classes of antihypertensive agents have different direct effects on the CBF, ICP, and autoregulation. The ideal drug would not increase ICP or decrease blood flow to ischemic regions. In addition, in treatment of hypertension in the acute setting, drugs that can be given intravenously, have a short half-life, and do not cause sedation are preferable. In the chronic phase after a stroke, there is no clear evidence favoring one class of antihypertensive agent over another.

The advantages and disadvantages of various classes of antihypertensive agents in the acute stroke setting are summarized in Figure 40.8.

β-Adrenergic antagonists (e.g., esmolol) and combined α- and β-adrenergic receptor antagonists (e.g., labetalol) do not increase ICP or affect cerebral autoregulation. They are suitable for treatment of hypertension in the setting of cerebral ischemia or

Preferred Antihypertensive Agents in the Treatment of Stroke-Associated Hypertension

Drug	Mechanism of Action	Intravenous Dose	Advantages	Disadvantages
Labetalol	α_1-, β_1-, and β_2-receptor antagonist	Test dose 5 mg, then 20- to 80-mg bolus every 10 min up to 300 mg; IV infusion 0.5–2 mg/min	Does not lower CBF Does not increase ICP	May exacerbate bradycardia
Esmolol	β_1-receptor antagonist	500-µg/kg bolus, then 50–300 mg/kg/min	Does not lower CBF Does not increase ICP	May exacerbate bradycardia
Sodium nitroprusside	Vasodilator	0.25–10 µg/kg/min	Potent antihypertensive	May increase ICP Can cause cerebral steal Potential for cyanide toxicity
Nitroglycerin	Vasodilator	5–100 µg/kg/min	Can be helpful for concomitant cardiac ischemia	May increase ICP Can cause cerebral steal
Hydralazine	Vasodilator	2.5- to 10-mg bolus	Can be given as IV bolus when labetalol is contraindicated due to bradycardia	May increase ICP Can cause cerebral steal
Nicardipine	L-type CCB	5–15 mg/h	Does not decrease CBF	May increase ICP Long duration of action
Enalaprilat	ACE inhibitor	0.625–1.25 mg every 6 hr	Does not decrease CBF	Variable response Long duration of action

Figure 40.8 Preferred antihypertensive agents in the treatment of stroke-associated hypertension. ACE, angiotensin-converting enzyme; CBF, cerebral blood flow; CCB, calcium channel blocker; ICP, intracranial pressure.

increased ICP. However, bradycardia secondary to increased ICP is a relative contraindication.

Vasodilators (e.g., hydralazine, sodium nitroprusside, nitroglycerin) cause cerebral arterial dilation and venodilation and can theoretically increase ICP and cause a cerebral steal phenomenon in patients with cerebral ischemia. However, they may be used in patients with small and moderate-sized ICH and in patients with SAH if increased ICP is not a concern.

Calcium channel blockers (CCB) have varying effects on cerebral autoregulation. Nifedipine can lead to severe reduction in BP and is not recommended. Nimodipine is used routinely in patients with SAH as it has been shown to improve outcome, possibly due to a neuroprotective effect. Nicardipine has been used in patients with acute ICH without any change in CBF and is often used in patients with SAH.

Angiotensin-converting enzyme (ACE) inhibitors and the angiotensin receptor blocker (ARB) candesartan have been used in patients with cerebral ischemia and have no effect on CBF. However, short-acting parenteral forms of these drugs are not available. ACE inhibitors and ARBs shift the lower limit of cerebral autoregulation toward lower BP in rats and humans. However, these agents have a long half-life, which is not desirable in treatment of hypertension in the acute phase.

Similarly, because of its long half-life and sedative effect, the α_2-adrenergic agonist clonidine is not preferred.

REFERENCES

1. Qureshi AI. Acute hypertensive response in patients with stroke: pathophysiology and management. *Circulation*. 2008;118:176-187.
2. Chalmers J. Volhard Lecture. Brain, blood pressure and stroke. *J Hypertens*. 1998;16(pt 2):1849-1858.
3. Colombari E, Sato MA, Cravo SL, et al. Role of the medulla oblongata in hypertension. *Hypertension*. 2001;38(pt 2):549-554.
4. Talman WT. Cardiovascular regulation and lesions of the central nervous system. *Ann Neurol*. 1985;18:1-13.
5. Strandgaard S, Olesen J, Skinhoj E, Lassen NA. Autoregulation of brain circulation in severe arterial hypertension. *Br Med J*. 1973;1:507-510.
6. Strandgaard S. Autoregulation of cerebral blood flow in hypertensive patients. The modifying influence of prolonged antihypertensive treatment on the tolerance to acute, drug-induced hypotension. *Circulation*. 1976;53:720-727.
7. Pedelty L, Gorelick PB. Chronic management of blood pressure after stroke. *Hypertension*. 2004;44:1-5.
8. Lawes CM, Bennett DA, Feigin VL, Rodgers A. Blood pressure and stroke: an overview of published reviews. *Stroke*. 2004;35:1024.
9. MacMahon S, Peto R, Cutler J, et al. Blood pressure, stroke, and coronary heart disease. Part 1, prolonged differences in blood pressure: prospective observational studies corrected for the regression dilution bias. *Lancet*. 1990;335:765-774.
10. PROGRESS Collaborative Group. Randomised trial of a perindopril-based blood-pressure-lowering regimen among 6,105 individuals with previous stroke or transient ischaemic attack. *Lancet*. 2001;358: 1033-1041.
11. Aiyagari V, Gorelick PB. Management of blood pressure for acute stroke and recurrent stroke. *Stroke*. 2009;40:2251-2256.
12. Testai FD, Aiyagari V. Acute hemorrhagic stroke pathophysiology and medical interventions: blood pressure control, management of anticoagulant-associated brain hemorrhage and general management principles. *Neurol Clin*. 2008;26:963-985.
13. Brott T, Broderick J, Kothari R, et al. Early hemorrhage growth in patients with intracerebral hemorrhage. *Stroke*. 1997;28:1-5.
14. Jauch EC, Lindsell CJ, Adeoye O, et al. Lack of evidence for an association between hemodynamic variables and hematoma growth in spontaneous intracerebral hemorrhage. *Stroke*. 2006;37:2061-2065.
15. Geeganage C, Bath PM. Interventions for deliberately altering blood pressure in acute stroke. *Cochrane Database Syst Rev*. 2008;4: CD000039.
16. Schrader J, Luders S, Kulschewski A, et al; Acute Candesartan Cilexetil Therapy in Stroke Survivors Study Group. The ACCESS Study: evaluation of acute candesartan cilexetil therapy in stroke survivors. *Stroke*. 2003;34:1699-1703.
17. Potter JF, Robinson TG, Ford GA, et al. Controlling hypertension and hypotension immediately post-stroke (CHHIPS): a randomised, placebo-controlled, double-blind pilot trial. *Lancet Neurol*. 2009;8:48-56.
18. Aslanyan S, Fazekas F, Weir CJ, et al; GAIN International Steering Committee and Investigators. Effect of blood pressure during the acute period of ischemic stroke on stroke outcome: a tertiary analysis of the GAIN International Trial. *Stroke*. 2003;34:2420-2425.
19. Ahmed N, Nasman P, Wahlgren NG. Effect of intravenous nimodipine on blood pressure and outcome after acute stroke. *Stroke*. 2000;31:1250-1255.
20. Adams HP Jr, del Zoppo G, Alberts MJ, et al; American Heart Association, American Stroke Association Stroke Council, Clinical Cardiology Council, Cardiovascular Radiology and Intervention Council, Atherosclerotic Peripheral Vascular Disease and Quality of Care Outcomes in Research Interdisciplinary Working Groups. Guidelines for the early management of adults with ischemic stroke: a guideline from the American Heart Association/American Stroke Association Stroke Council, Clinical Cardiology Council, Cardiovascular Radiology and Intervention Council, and the Atherosclerotic Peripheral Vascular Disease and Quality of Care Outcomes in Research Interdisciplinary Working Groups: the American Academy of Neurology affirms the value of this guideline as an educational tool for neurologists. *Stroke*. 2007;38:1655-1711.
21. European Stroke Organisation (ESO) Executive Committee, ESO Writing Committee. Guidelines for management of ischaemic stroke and transient ischaemic attack 2008. *Cerebrovasc Dis*. 2008;25:457-507.
22. Powers WJ, Zazulia AR, Videen TO, et al. Autoregulation of cerebral blood flow surrounding acute (6 to 22 hours) intracerebral hemorrhage. *Neurology*. 2001;57:18-24.
23. Kuwata N, Kuroda K, Funayama M, et al. Dysautoregulation in patients with hypertensive intracerebral hemorrhage. A SPECT study. *Neurosurg Rev*. 1995;18:237-245.
24. Qureshi AI. Acute blood pressure management—the North American perspective. Update on cerebral hemorrhage trials session. Presented at the International Stroke Conference; New Orleans; February 20, 2008. Available at: http://www.scienceondemand.org/stroke2008/sessions/player.html?sid=08020172.758. Accessed July 4, 2008.
25. Anderson CS, Huang Y, Wang JG, et al; INTERACT Investigators. Intensive blood pressure reduction in acute cerebral haemorrhage trial (INTERACT): a randomised pilot trial. *Lancet Neurol*. 2008;7: 391-399.
26. Broderick J, Connolly S, Feldmann E, et al; American Heart Association, American Stroke Association Stroke Council, High Blood Pressure Research Council, Quality of Care and Outcomes in Research Interdisciplinary Working Group. Guidelines for the management of spontaneous intracerebral hemorrhage in adults: 2007 update: a guideline from the American Heart Association/American Stroke Association Stroke Council, High Blood Pressure Research Council, and the Quality of Care and Outcomes in Research Interdisciplinary Working Group. *Stroke*. 2007;38:2001-2023.
27. Steiner T, Kaste M, Forsting M, et al. Recommendations for the management of intracranial haemorrhage—part I: spontaneous intracerebral haemorrhage. The European Stroke Initiative Writing Committee and the Writing Committee for the EUSI Executive Committee. *Cerebrovasc Dis*. 2006;22:294-316.
28. Bederson JB, Connolly ES Jr, Batjer HH, et al; American Heart Association. Guidelines for the management of aneurysmal subarachnoid hemorrhage: A statement for healthcare professionals from a special writing group of the Stroke Council, American Heart Association. *Stroke*. 2009;40:994-1025.
29. Qureshi AI, Luft AR, Sharma M, et al. Frequency and determinants of postprocedural hemodynamic instability after carotid angioplasty and stenting. *Stroke*. 1999;30:2086-2093.
30. Wade JG, Larson CP Jr, Hickey RF, et al. Effect of carotid endarterectomy on carotid chemoreceptor and baroreceptor function in man. *N Engl J Med*. 1970;282:823-829.
31. Wong JH, Findlay JM, Suarez-Almazor ME. Hemodynamic instability after carotid endarterectomy: risk factors and associations with operative complications. *Neurosurgery*. 1997;41:35-41; discussion 41-43.
32. Chida K, Ogasawara K, Suga Y, et al. Postoperative cortical neural loss associated with cerebral hyperperfusion and cognitive impairment after carotid endarterectomy: ^{123}I-iomazenil SPECT study. *Stroke*. 2009;40: 448-453.
33. Yoshimoto T, Houkin K, Kuroda S, et al. Low cerebral blood flow and perfusion reserve induce hyperperfusion after surgical revascularization:

case reports and analysis of cerebral hemodynamics. *Surg Neurol.* 1997;48:132-138; discussion 138-139.

34. van Mook WN, Rennenberg RJ, Schurink GW, et al. Cerebral hyperperfusion syndrome. *Lancet Neurol.* 2005;4:877-888.
35. Karapanayiotides T, Meuli R, Devuyst G, et al. Postcarotid endarterectomy hyperperfusion or reperfusion syndrome. *Stroke.* 2005;36:21-26.
36. Abou-Chebl A, Reginelli J, Bajzer CT, Yadav JS. Intensive treatment of hypertension decreases the risk of hyperperfusion and intracerebral hemorrhage following carotid artery stenting. *Catheter Cardiovasc Interv.* 2007;69:690-696.
37. Furlan JC, Fehlings MG. Cardiovascular complications after acute spinal cord injury: pathophysiology, diagnosis, and management. *Neurosurg Focus.* 2008;25:E13.
38. Valles M, Benito J, Portell E, Vidal J. Cerebral hemorrhage due to autonomic dysreflexia in a spinal cord injury patient. *Spinal Cord.* 2005;43:738-740.
39. Blackmer J. Rehabilitation medicine: 1. Autonomic dysreflexia. *CMAJ.* 2003;169:931-935.
40. Sheel AW, Krassioukov AV, Inglis JT, Elliott SL. Autonomic dysreflexia during sperm retrieval in spinal cord injury: influence of lesion level and sildenafil citrate. *J Appl Physiol.* 2005;99:53-58.
41. Consortium for Spinal Cord Medicine. Acute management of autonomic dysreflexia: individuals with spinal cord injury presenting to health-care facilities. *J Spinal Cord Med.* 2002;25(suppl 1):S67-S88.
42. Ribes Pastor MP, Vanarase M. Peripartum anaesthetic management of a parturient with spinal cord injury and autonomic hyperreflexia. *Anaesthesia.* 2004;59:94.

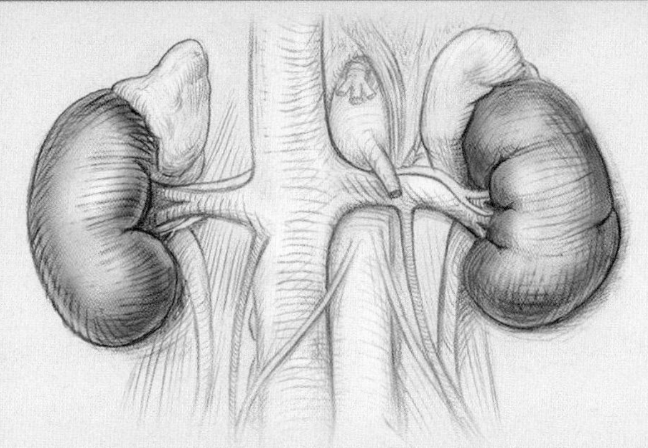

SECTION VII

Pregnancy and Renal Disease

CHAPTER 41

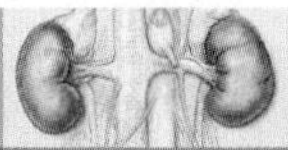

Renal Physiology in Normal Pregnancy

Chris Baylis, John M. Davison

There are profound changes in renal function in normal pregnancy that lead to marked alterations from the nonpregnant physiologic norm. An appreciation and understanding of these alterations are essential to recognize both normal and compromised pregnancies.

ANATOMY

The kidneys increase 1 to 2 cm in length and in volume by up to 70% in normal pregnancy because of increases in both vascular and interstitial fluid compartments. The most striking anatomic change is dilation of the calyces, renal pelvis, and ureter (more prominent on the right side), and by the third trimester, about 80% of women show evidence of hydronephrosis (Fig. 41.1).[1] A consequence of the ureteral dilation is urinary stasis, which predisposes pregnant women with asymptomatic bacteriuria to development of symptomatic ascending infection (acute pyelonephritis). Rarely, the anatomic changes may be extreme and precipitate the overdistention syndrome, with massive dilation, recurrent severe flank pain, increasing serum creatinine, hypertension, or even reversible acute kidney injury.[2]

SYSTEMIC HEMODYNAMICS

There are significant alterations in systemic hemodynamics in normal pregnancy. A plasma (and extracellular fluid) volume expansion occurs while red cell volume also increases, leading to a large increase in blood volume that correlates with clinical outcome and birth weight. Interestingly, subsequent pregnancies tend to be more successful than the first, with bigger babies and larger plasma volume increases. Women with twins and triplets have proportionately greater increments, and those with poorly growing fetuses, as in preeclampsia or when there is a history of poor reproductive performance, have correspondingly poor plasma volume responses. The increase in plasma volume (maximum increase ~1.25 liters) takes place progressively up to 32 to 34 weeks, after which there is little further change. The plasma volume expansion has a hemodilutional effect, causing decreases in hematocrit: the physiologic anemia of normal pregnancy.[3]

Cardiac output is significantly increased by the fifth gestational week, initially caused by a 10% to 20% increase in heart rate (80 to 90 beats per minute), with stroke volume increased by more than 20% the eighth week. Cardiac output increases of 40% to 50% are well established by the 24th week. Left atrial and left ventricular end-diastolic dimensions increase, suggesting an associated increase in venous return. There is also a progressive increase in aortic valve orifice area. Despite the 40% to 50% increase in cardiac output, systemic blood pressure substantially decreases in normal pregnancy (representative values are shown in Figs. 41.2 and 41.3).[4] The physiologic decrease in blood pressure results from a profound reduction in systemic vascular resistance of unknown cause, although the loss of responsiveness to vasoconstrictor agents (e.g., angiotensin II, arginine vasopressin) certainly contributes.[5] Inhibition of angiogenic factors in preeclampsia causes vasoconstriction, suggesting that these factors, such as vascular endothelial growth factor, may contribute importantly to normal gestational vasodilation through stimulation of endothelial nitric oxide and prostaglandins.[6] The combination of increased cardiac output and peripheral vasodilation means that organ blood flow increases in pregnancy, with the most dramatic changes occurring in the kidney and skin circulation throughout gestation and in the uterus in the second part of the pregnancy.[4] In the third trimester, the enlarged uterus compresses surrounding tissues and can influence hemodynamic measurements, so that attention should be paid to maternal posture during hemodynamic monitoring. In the supine position, there is partial obstruction of the inferior vena cava and decreased venous return, reducing cardiac output and causing a decrease in blood pressure, the supine hypotensive syndrome of pregnancy. It is important to be aware of these postural effects in measuring blood pressure in late pregnancy.[4]

RENAL HEMODYNAMICS

There are striking changes in renal hemodynamics in normal pregnancy, with an increase in glomerular filtration rate (GFR) and consequent decrease in serum creatinine detectable very early.[7] The GFR increases ~25% by 4 weeks after the last menstrual period, and a robust early increase in GFR (see Fig. 41.3) is invariably associated with a good obstetric outcome. Longitudinal studies in normal pregnant women show that GFR (measured by inulin or 24-hour creatinine clearance) increases by a maximum of ~50% by mid-pregnancy, which is maintained until the last few weeks of the pregnancy, when values begin to decrease but remain above the nonpregnant level (Fig. 41.4; see also Fig. 41.2).[8] These marked increases in GFR mean that serum creatinine decreases to ~0.4 to 0.5 mg/dl (36 to 45 μmol/l),[9] and values considered normal for nonpregnant conditions of 0.7 to 0.8 mg/dl (63 to 72 μmol/l) are a cause for concern in normal pregnancy (see Fig. 41.3). The increase in renal plasma flow (RPF) of ~60% is slightly more pronounced than the increase in GFR (see Fig. 41.2), so that the filtration fraction (FF) decreases (see later discussion). At the end of pregnancy, the RPF decreases

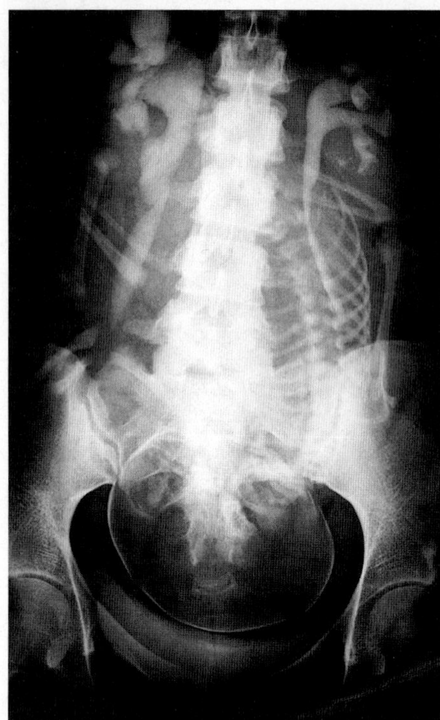

Figure 41.1 Hydronephrosis in normal pregnancy. Intravenous urogram at 36 weeks' gestation. Note bilateral hydronephrosis, more marked on the right side.

Changes in Some Common Indices During Pregnancy

	Nonpregnant	Pregnant
Hematocrit (%)	41	33
Plasma protein (g/dl)	7.0	6.0
Plasma osmolality (mOsm/kg)	285	275
Plasma sodium (mmol/l)	140	135
Plasma creatinine (mg/dl, μmol/l)	0.8 (73)	0.5 (45)
Blood urea nitrogen (mg/dl)	12.7	9.3
Plasma urea (mmol/l)	4.5	3.3
pH units	7.40	7.44
Arterial PCO_2 (mm Hg)	40	30
Plasma bicarbonate (mmol/l)	25	20
Plasma uric acid (mg/dl, μmol/l)	4.0 (240)	3.2 (190) early 4.3 (260) late
Systolic BP (mm Hg)	115	105
Diastolic BP (mm Hg)	70	60

Figure 41.3 Changes in some common indices during pregnancy. BP, blood pressure. *(Mean values compiled from references 7-9, 16, 27.)*

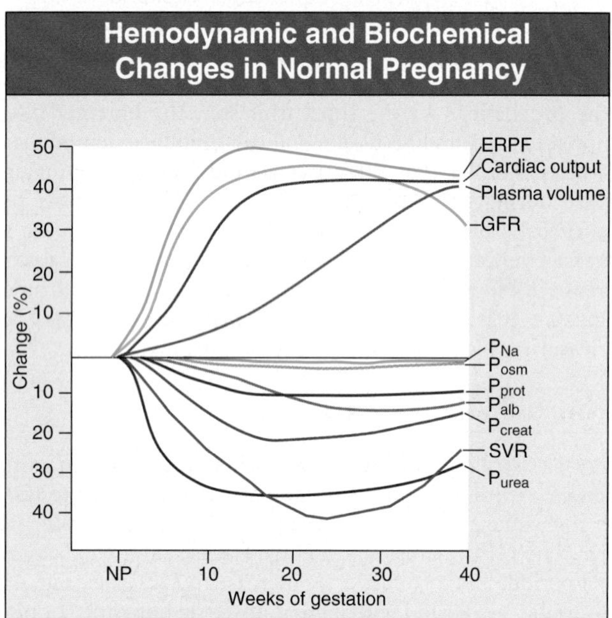

Figure 41.2 Hemodynamic alterations induced by normal pregnancy. Increments and decrements in hemodynamic and biochemical parameters shown as percentage of change from nonpregnant baseline. ERPF, effective renal plasma flow; GFR, glomerular filtration rate; NP, nonpregnant; SVR, systemic vascular resistance.

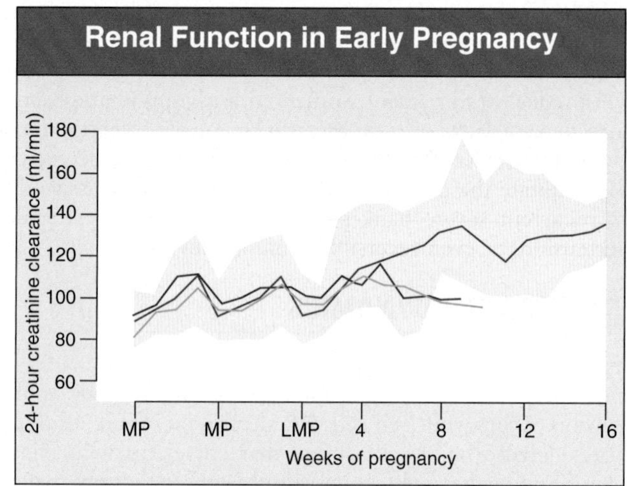

Figure 41.4 Renal function in early pregnancy. Changes in 24-hour creatinine clearance measured weekly before conception and through pregnancy. There was uncomplicated spontaneous abortion in two women *(red and green colored lines)*. The *blue line* represents the mean and the *yellow area* shows the range for nine women with successful obstetric outcome. LMP, last menstrual period; MP, menstrual period. *(Modified from references 7, 8, and 16.)*

proportionally more than the GFR, so that FF increases to the nonpregnant value.[8,10]

A similar pattern of renal hemodynamic change occurs during pregnancy in some animals, including the rat, in which GFR increases to a maximum of 30% to 40% above the virgin value by midterm, with a late return toward the nonpregnant value close to term (22 days). Glomerular micropuncture studies have shown that the increase in GFR is paralleled by increases in single-nephron GFR secondary to increased glomerular plasma flow.[11] Because the preglomerular and postglomerular resistance vessels dilate in parallel, glomerular plasma flow increases without a change in glomerular blood pressure. As shown in Figure 41.5, the glomerular blood pressure remains unchanged throughout the pregnancy despite marked alterations in preglomerular vascular resistance. Similar conclusions have been reached by an indirect modeling approach in normal pregnant

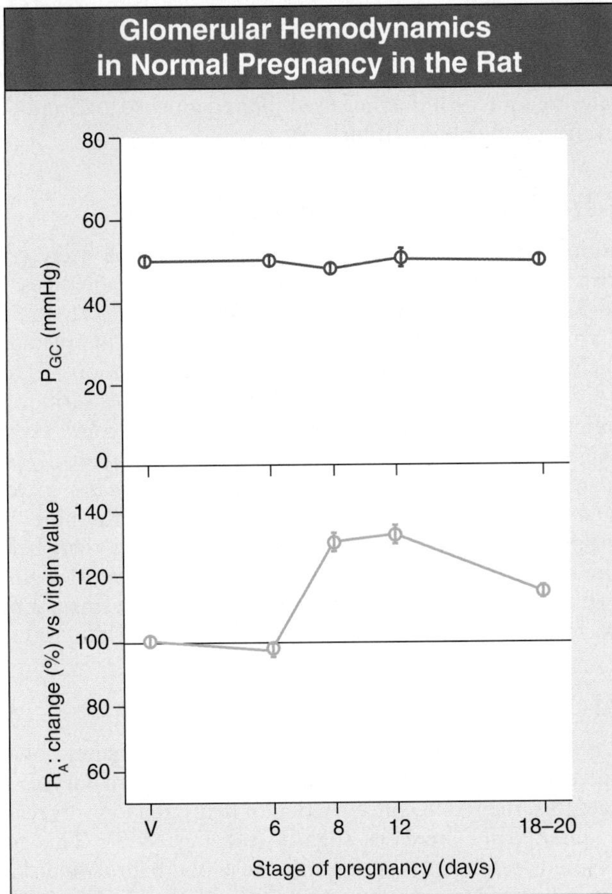

Figure 41.5 Glomerular hemodynamics in normal pregnancy in the rat. Summary of mean glomerular capillary blood pressure (P_{GC}, *upper panel*) and preglomerular arteriolar resistance (R_A, *lower panel*) in Munich Wistar rats in the virgin state (V) and throughout normal pregnancy.[11,12]

women measuring whole-kidney GFR, RPF, and plasma protein concentrations; in addition, polydisperse neutral dextran was infused for determination of dextran sieving curves.[7,10] This approach allows (with certain reasonable assumptions) modeling of glomerular hemodynamics. In pregnant women, there is a decrease in plasma protein concentration that contributes slightly to the increased GFR. As in the rat, the majority of the gestational increase in GFR in normal women is due to increased RPF with no change in glomerular blood pressure. The constancy of glomerular blood pressure during sustained renal vasodilation has important implications for the long-term effects of pregnancy on renal function, as discussed later.

It is often assumed that a change in FF reflects a change in glomerular blood pressure, but this is not always the case because FF is also determined by K_f, the product of water permeability of the glomerular wall and total glomerular capillary surface area.[8] Both glomerular wall water permeability and filtration pressure are very high, and thus filtration proceeds rapidly. In some situations, not all the available filtration surface area is used, so that filtration ceases (because the driving pressure is exhausted) before the end of the glomerulus. This state is known as filtration pressure equilibrium. When plasma flow increases during filtration pressure equilibrium, a proportional increase in GFR occurs with no change in FF. This is seen in the normal pregnant rat.[11] In contrast, FF decreases during normal pregnancy in women as RPF is increasing.[8] Most likely this reflects the fact that humans are closer than rats to filtration pressure disequilibrium, a situation in which the entire glomerular capillary surface area available for filtration is used, leaving a positive driving pressure at the end of the glomerulus. At filtration pressure disequilibrium, GFR becomes less dependent on plasma flow; thus, an increase in plasma flow (with no change in the other determinants of filtration) leads to a disproportionately smaller increase in GFR, with a decrease in FF (see reference 12 for a fuller explanation).

Despite the prolonged renal vasodilation, the renal vasculature remains fully responsive to various stimuli during pregnancy. For example, in the rat, the intrinsic renal autoregulatory ability remains intact,[13] and the tubuloglomerular feedback component of renal autoregulation is reset to recognize the elevated GFR as normal.[14] Both pregnant rats and women exhibit a marked additional renal vasodilation in response to amino acid infusion,[15,16] demonstrating substantial renal vasodilatory reserve in normal pregnancy. The cause of the gestational increase in GFR remains uncertain, although studies in the pseudopregnant rat have shown that the fetoplacental unit is not necessary,[17] indicating that a maternal stimulus must initiate the gestational renal hemodynamic changes. A number of vasoactive factors have been evaluated as possible mediators of the renal vasodilation,[11] and although there are no clinical data, animal studies have implicated a role for nitric oxide.[18-20] Studies have suggested a key role for the ovarian hormone relaxin, which may signal increased renal nitric oxide production in pregnancy, possibly through an endothelin type B receptor mechanism.[21,22] The renal vasodilatory signal of pregnancy is remarkably robust because women with single kidneys (organ donors) and renal transplant recipients who have already undergone significant compensatory renal hypertrophy and vasodilation can produce further increases in RPF and GFR in pregnancy.[7,8] Furthermore, in the human, the signal is not solely relaxin as there is still a gestational increase in GFR, albeit blunted, in infertile women who lack ovarian function and who conceive from ovum donation and assisted conception techniques.[23]

Glomerular hypertension associated with renal vasodilation is considered a primary pathogenic stimulus to progressive renal injury in chronic kidney disease.[24] As discussed before, normal pregnancy is also a state of chronic renal vasodilation; however, glomerular blood pressure remains normal. This may account for the findings that repetitive pregnancies in women and rats with normal renal function have no long-term adverse effects on glomerular function or structure.[25] Pregnancy will increase the rate of loss of renal function in some women with underlying renal disease (see Chapter 43), but the available evidence suggests that this is not by a hemodynamically mediated action.[7,25]

Formulae that use serum creatinine in relation to age, height, and weight to calculate GFR (e.g., the Cockcroft-Gault formula) should not be used in pregnancy because body weight or size does not reflect kidney size. The use of estimated GFR (eGFR) from the Modification of Diet in Renal Disease (MDRD) study equation, whereby serum creatinine is adjusted for age, gender, and race, cannot be recommended in pregnancy because it significantly underestimates GFR.[26]

Abnormal Renal Hemodynamics

A woman may lose up to 50% of her renal function and still maintain serum creatinine concentration below 1.5 mg/dl (130 μmol/l) because of hyperfiltration in remaining nephrons; but if there is more severe compromise, further glomerular damage will cause serum creatinine to increase.[7,26,27] Pregnancy in the presence of impaired renal function has a marked adverse effect on obstetric outcome as well as increased risk of an accelerated decline in renal function, as mentioned before (discussed in Chapter 43).[28]

In preeclampsia, both RPF and GFR decrease, although absolute values may remain above the nonpregnant range. A decrease in ultrafiltration coefficient (K_f) of around 50% in combination with reduced RPF is the most likely mechanism for the hypofiltration.[27] The endothelium is targeted at an early stage in preeclampsia and the glomerulus is not spared, with the vascular endothelial cell dysfunction (glomerular endotheliosis) resulting in so-called swollen bloodless glomeruli and the loss of glomerular barrier size and charge selectivities (see Chapter 42). Glomerular endotheliosis is considered by most to be merely characteristic, not pathognomonic, of preeclampsia, whereas others believe this not to be the case because renal biopsy also reveals the lesion in healthy controls,[29] but in a study in which there are concerns about qualitative histologic grading as well as ethical issues.[30]

RENAL TUBULAR FUNCTION IN PREGNANCY

There is an enormous plasma volume expansion in normal pregnancy and resultant small decrements in plasma concentration of many solutes (see Fig. 41.2). Nevertheless, the large increase in GFR means that the filtered load of most plasma constituents will increase during pregnancy.[7,8] Increments in excretion are seen for some substances, but this is limited by increases in tubular reabsorption, preventing depletion. Intake also often increases, with net retention leading to positive balance for many of the key constituents. The renal handling of a number of solutes is altered in normal pregnancy.

Uric Acid

Uric acid, an endpoint of purine metabolism, is freely filtered at the glomerulus, extensively reabsorbed in the proximal tubule with further downstream reabsorption and possibly some active secretion, such that only ~10% of filtered load is excreted. Plasma uric acid concentration decreases during early pregnancy by ~25% (see Fig. 41.3), which may reflect a decrease in net tubular reabsorption.[8] As the pregnancy advances, fractional excretion of uric acid decreases, leading to an increasing plasma uric acid concentration, attaining levels close to the nonpregnant mean. Serum uric acid concentrations are significantly higher in preeclamptic pregnancy, and above a critical level of 6 mg/dl (350 µmol/l), there is excess perinatal mortality in hypertensive patients (see Chapter 42). It must be borne in mind, however, that physiologic variability is such that some healthy women have high plasma uric acid levels without problems, so that uric acid values must be interpreted in the clinical context.

Glucose

Excretion of glucose increases soon after conception to approximately 10 times the nonpregnant value and remains high throughout pregnancy, although glycosuria is variable.[8] The glycosuria is not related to changes in plasma glucose concentration and reflects decreased tubular reabsorption. In the nonpregnant individual, there is usually complete renal reabsorption of glucose, mostly in the proximal tubule, where there is a very high capacity for glucose transport. This maximum transport capacity (T_{max}) is not usually reached until plasma glucose increases to values in excess of ~200 mg/dl (11 mmol/l). The glycosuria of pregnancy is due to a decrease in T_{max} or the inability of the renal tubules to cope with the increased filtered glucose load and does not reflect a metabolic disturbance.

Water-Soluble Vitamins and Amino Acids

Nicotinic acid, ascorbic acid, and folic acid are all excreted in increased amounts during pregnancy,[7] which emphasizes the need for adequate vitamin supplementation.

Urinary excretion of most amino acids increases in pregnancy, probably as a result of decreased tubular reabsorption.[31] There are distinct patterns. Glycine, histidine, threonine, serine, and alanine excretion increases early, and values remain elevated throughout pregnancy. Excretion of lysine, cystine, taurine, phenylalanine, valine, leucine, and tyrosine also increases in early pregnancy but later declines. Glutamic acid, methionine, and ornithine are excreted in slightly greater amounts than before pregnancy, isoleucine excretion is unchanged, and arginine excretion decreases, consistent with decreases in plasma arginine in normal pregnancy.

Acid-Base Balance

The generation of hydrogen ions increases in pregnancy because of an increased basal metabolism and greater food intake, but despite this, the blood concentration of hydrogen ions decreases; thus, plasma pH increases slightly (see Fig. 41.3). This mild alkalemia is respiratory in origin because pregnant women normally hyperventilate, leading to a primary decrease in arterial Pco_2 and secondary compensatory decreases in plasma bicarbonate concentration (see Fig. 41.3). A mild chronic respiratory alkalosis is a feature of normal pregnancy.

Potassium

Potassium excretion decreases, and there is a slow cumulative net potassium retention in pregnancy that is distributed between the enlarging maternal tissues and the developing fetus. The decrease in potassium excretion occurs in spite of the mild alkalosis and high aldosterone values of normal pregnancy and is at least partly due to the potent anti-mineralocorticoid action of progesterone (see later discussion).[32]

Calcium

Calcium excretion increases two to three times during pregnancy because of the increased filtered load and despite some increase in tubular reabsorption. This could predispose to the formation of calcium stones, but increased magnesium and citrate, acidic glycoproteins, and nephrocalcin serve to inhibit calcium oxalate stone formation so that the incidence of stone formation is not increased in normal pregnancy.[33]

Protein

Increased urinary total protein excretion in pregnancy should not be considered abnormal until it exceeds 500 mg in 24 hours,[7,8,16,19] although many classifications and definitions of the hypertensive disorders of pregnancy still define more than 300 mg/24 h as abnormal.[34] There is usually a small increment in albumin excretion during the third trimester. Increased total protein and albumin excretion may continue into the puerperium, with nonpregnant levels not restored until 5 to 6 months after delivery. The gestational changes may be related to alterations in glomerular permeability and charge selectivity as well as tubular function. In clinical practice, urine protein above 300 mg/24 h roughly correlates with 30 mg/dl in a random urine sample, but given the problems with dipstick tests, many still prefer a 24-hour or some timed quantitative determination. Use of a random urine protein-creatinine ratio is, however, a clinically useful alternative, with a threshold value of 30 mg/mmol creatinine (0.3 mg/mg) a reasonable cutoff for defining significant proteinuria.[8,34,35]

Sodium

A massive, cumulative volume expansion occurs during pregnancy with an associated gradual retention of sodium of ~900 mmol, distributed between the products of conception and maternal extracellular space. This positive sodium balance develops despite a ~30% increase in filtered load and reflects an increase in tubular reabsorption that allows net additional sodium retention of ~2 to 3 mmol/day.[3] Nevertheless, it is normal for sodium excretion to increase in pregnancy, reflecting the marked increase in sodium intake. Lithium clearance studies in women have indicated enhanced sodium reabsorption in the proximal tubule and distal nephron segments in late pregnancy, whereas animal studies have been contradictory.[36] The reason for the net renal sodium retention in pregnancy is not known. As shown in Figure 41.6, there are many factors operating both to increase and to decrease sodium excretion, and exactly how the normal balance of net retention is achieved remains a mystery. Several antinatriuretic systems are activated in normal pregnancy.[37] Renin, angiotensin, and aldosterone levels are all markedly increased, and the renin-angiotensin system (RAS) can be appropriately regulated around these new set points when changes occur in extracellular fluid volume. In addition to stimulating aldosterone release, physiologic levels of angiotensin II act directly on the proximal tubule to increase sodium reabsorption. However, a marked refractoriness develops to the vascular actions of angiotensin II in normal pregnancy,[37] which may blunt angiotensin II–dependent net sodium retention. The high aldosterone levels of pregnancy will certainly promote renal sodium retention in the distal tubule and collecting duct. The very high levels of deoxycorticosterone (from 21-hydroxylation of progesterone) may also exert mineralocorticoid actions to promote sodium retention.[38] Estrogens increase markedly during human pregnancy and may directly induce renal sodium retention or act indirectly by enhancing the conversion of progesterone to deoxycorticosterone.[38] In addition to hormonal factors, the increased ureteral pressure and the decrease in systemic blood pressure both decrease sodium excretion.

Factors Influencing Sodium Excretion During Pregnancy

Antinatriuretic	Natriuretic
Aldosterone	↑ Glomerular filtration rate
Angiotensin II	Progesterone
Estrogen	Atrial natriuretic peptide
Deoxycorticosterone	Nitric oxide
Supine posture	Prostaglandins
Upright posture	
Decreased blood pressure	
Increased ureteral pressure	
Placental shunting	

Figure 41.6 Factors influencing sodium excretion during pregnancy.

The concentrations of several natriuretic agents also increase in pregnancy. Progesterone increases by 10 to 100 times, and these levels exert a marked anti-mineralocorticoid action by competing with aldosterone for the mineralocorticoid receptor.[38] Plasma atrial natriuretic peptide (ANP) levels are also moderately elevated,[39] as is nitric oxide.[20] In addition to natriuretic factors, the large increase in GFR leads to increased filtration of sodium (despite the small decrease in plasma sodium concentration), which will also increase sodium excretion. Decreases in plasma albumin concentration and the increment in effective renal plasma flow during pregnancy will also enhance sodium excretion by inhibiting sodium reabsorption.[10] Animal studies have suggested that there is a generalized loss in pregnancy of natriuretic responsiveness to cGMP-dependent signals[20] due to increased inner medullary phosphodiesterase V activity.

Despite the many conflicting stimuli, net sodium retention and marked plasma volume expansion are normal in pregnancy. In the normal nonpregnant steady state, plasma volume expansion and renal sodium retention cannot coexist. However, pregnancy is not a steady state, and the volume sensing and regulatory systems are dramatically readjusted throughout pregnancy to accommodate and to maintain the volume expansion (see later discussion).

OSMOREGULATION

There is a very early decrease in plasma osmolality (P_{osm}) by ~10 mOsm/kg below the nonpregnant norm due to a reduction in plasma sodium and associated anions (see Fig. 41.3). Whereas a decrease in P_{osm} of this magnitude would completely suppress release of the antidiuretic hormone arginine vasopressin (AVP) in nonpregnant individuals, in pregnancy, the osmotic thresholds for AVP release as well as for thirst are reduced to recognize the reduced plasma osmolality as normal.[40] Figure 41.7 demonstrates the resetting of the relationship between plasma AVP and P_{osm} during normal pregnancy. The placental hormone human chorionic gonadotropin (which stimulates the release of ovarian relaxin)[41] may have a role in this reduction in the osmotic threshold for AVP release.[40] Plasma volume status is a separate, nonosmotic determinant of AVP release, and this system is also reset to recognize the massively expanded plasma volume as normal. The metabolic clearance rate of AVP has increased four times by mid-pregnancy because of the release of cystine aminopeptidase (vasopressinase) from the placenta,[40] so the rate of AVP production must also be accelerated. Despite these marked alterations, the urinary concentrating and diluting capacity remain good, although there is a slight reduction in the maximum urine concentration in the second part of pregnancy.[40]

VOLUME REGULATION

As discussed previously, there is a continual sodium retention and cumulative volume expansion in pregnancy that reflects

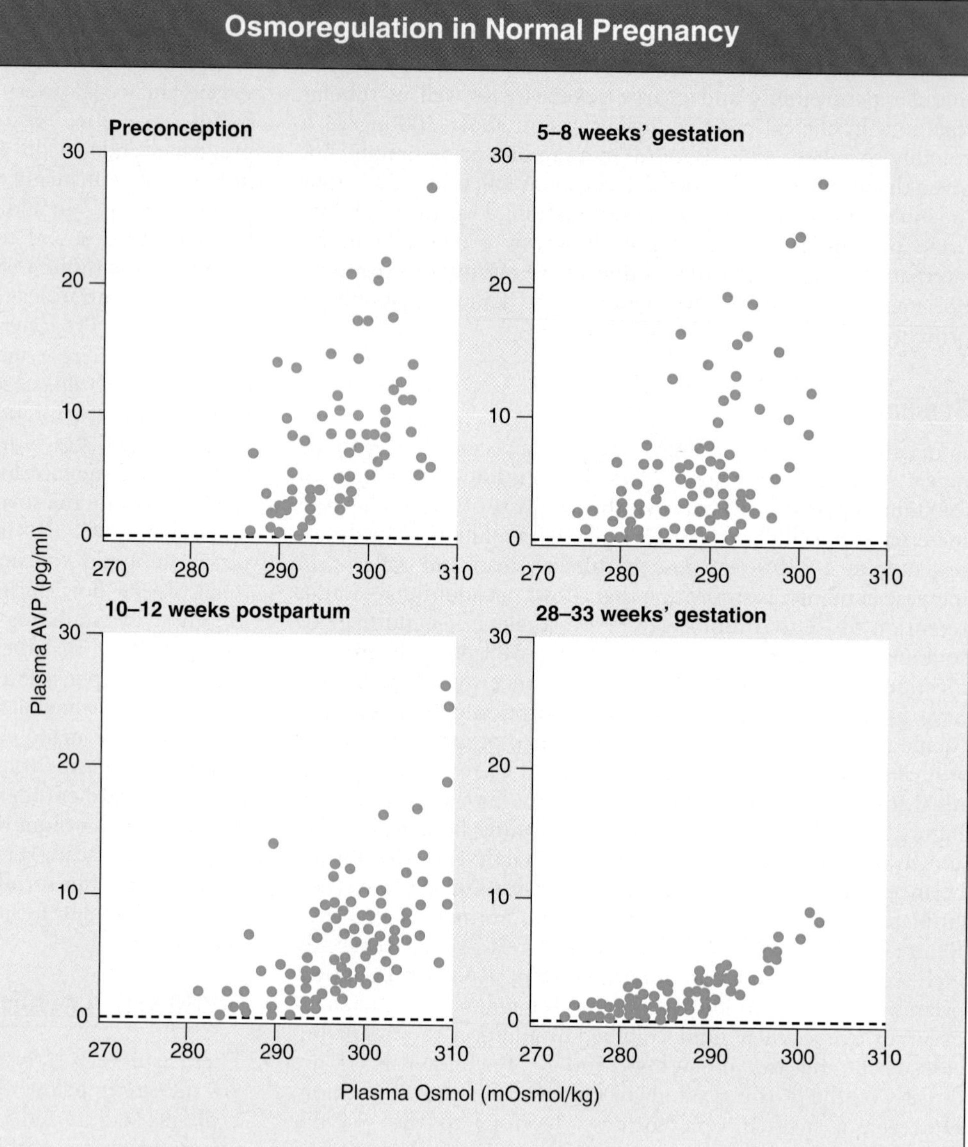

Figure 41.7 Osmoregulation in normal pregnancy. Relationship between plasma arginine vasopressin concentration (AVP) and plasma osmolarity (Osmol) during several 5% saline infusions in eight women before and during pregnancy. Each point represents an individual plasma measurement. There is a marked decrease in osmotic threshold for AVP release during pregnancy. Values for the osmotic threshold for thirst (not shown) were always 2 to 5 mOsmol/kg above AVP release thresholds and 10 mOsmol/kg lower in pregnancy.[7,40]

complex readjustments of the various volume regulatory systems. These readjustments also permit volume expansion without increases in blood pressure; in fact, blood pressure decreases substantially as pregnancy proceeds (see Fig. 41.3). What happens to volume perception and regulatory systems in pregnancy can be considered in terms of the effective circulating volume.[42,43] The RAS is an antinatriuretic system activated by volume depletion, and the increase in plasma renin activity and angiotensin and aldosterone concentrations of normal pregnancy suggests an underfill signal, despite the absolute increase in plasma volume. It has been suggested that the primary event in pregnancy is peripheral vasodilation that generates an underfill signal that leads to renal sodium retention.[42] In contrast to the RAS, as discussed previously, both osmotic and nonosmotic control of AVP release is reset in a manner indicating that the expanded volume of pregnancy is sensed as normal.[40] The tubuloglomerular feedback system is suppressed by volume expansion in the nonpregnant state but is reset in pregnant rats to recognize the expanded volume and increased GFR as normal.[14] Plasma ANP increases slightly in late pregnant women, but this is unlikely to reflect a physiologic response to volume expansion because even greater increases in ANP are seen in volume-contracted, preeclamptic pregnancies.[39] Thus, volume regulation in pregnancy remains an enigma.

IMPACT OF MATERNAL HEMODYNAMIC CHANGES ON FETAL PROGRAMMING

There is strong evidence that women with normal pregnancies who have suboptimal increases in plasma volume are more likely to deliver babies small for gestational age. Fetal growth restriction is often seen in preeclamptic pregnancies in which volume contraction usually occurs.[44] Reductions in uterine blood flow (as occur in preeclampsia or when volume expansion is inadequate) and maternal (and thence fetal) malnutrition have been implicated in the pathogenesis of fetal growth restriction. There is considerable epidemiologic as well as animal evidence suggesting that adverse events *in utero* that lead to fetal growth restriction can program the offspring for the later development of hypertension, other cardiovascular events, and chronic kidney disease, at least in part due to reduction in nephron number.[45,46] Thus, optimal maternal systemic and renal hemodynamic changes have a huge impact not only on fetal well-being but on the long-term health of the offspring.

REFERENCES

1. Jeyabalan A, Lain KY. Anatomic and functional changes of the upper urinary tract during pregnancy. *Urol Clin North Am*. 2007;34:1-6.
2. Khauna N, Nguyn H. Reversible acute renal failure in association with bilateral ureteral obstruction and hydronephrosis in pregnancy. *Am J Obstet Gynecol*. 2001;184:239-240.
3. Brown M, Gallery EDM. Volume homeostasis in normal pregnancy and preeclampsia: Physiology and clinical implications. *Clin Obstet Gynecol*. 1994:8:287-310.
4. de Swiet M. The cardiovascular system. In: Chamberlain G, Broughton Pipkin F, eds. *Clinical Physiology in Obstetrics*, 3rd ed. Oxford: Blackwell Science; 1998:33-70.
5. Magness RR, Gant NF. Normal vascular adaptations in pregnancy. Potential clues for understanding pregnancy induced hypertension. In: Walker JJ, Gant NF, eds. *Hypertension in Pregnancy*. London: Chapman & Hall Medical; 1997:5-26.
6. Maynard SE, Min J-Y, Merchan J, et al. Excess placental soluble fms-like tyrosine kinase (sFlt1) may contribute to endothelial dysfunction, hypertension and proteinuria in preeclampsia. *J Clin Invest*. 2003;111: 649-658.
7. Lindheimer MD, Davison JM, Katz AI. The kidney and hypertension in pregnancy: Twenty exciting years. *Semin Nephrol*. 2001;21:173-189.
8. Baylis C, Davison JM. The renal system. In: Chamberlain, G, Broughton Pipkin F, eds. *Clinical Physiology in Obstetrics*, 3rd ed. Oxford: Blackwell Science; 1998:263-307.
9. Larsson A, Palm M, Hansson L-O, Axelsson O. Reference values for clinical chemistry tests during normal pregnancy. *Br J Obstet Gynaecol*. 2008;115:874-881.
10. Roberts M, Lindheimer MD, Davison JM. Altered glomerular permselectivity to neutral dextran and heteroporous membrane modeling in human pregnancy. *Am J Physiol*. 1996;270:F338-F343.
11. Baylis C. Glomerular filtration and volume regulation in gravid animal models. *Clin Obstet Gynecol*. 1994;8:235-264.
12. Baylis C. Glomerular filtration dynamics. In: Lote CJ, ed. *Advances in Renal Physiology*. London: Croom Helm; 1986:33-83.
13. Reckelhoff JF, Yokota S, Baylis C. Renal autoregulation in mid-term and late pregnant rats. *Am J Obstet Gynecol*. 1992;166:1546-1550.
14. Baylis C, Blantz RC. Tubuloglomerular feedback activity in virgin and pregnant rats. *Am J Physiol*. 1985;249:F169-F173.
15. Baylis C. Effect of amino acid infusion as an index of renal vasodilatory capacity in pregnant rats. *Am J Physiol*. 1988;254:F650-F656.
16. Milne JE, Lindheimer MD, Davison JM. Glomerular heteroporous membrane modeling in third trimester and postpartum before and during amino acid infusion. *Am J Physiol Renal Physiol*. 2002;282: F170-F175.
17. Baylis C. Glomerular ultrafiltration in the pseudopregnant rat. *Am J Physiol*. 1982;243:F300-F305.
18. Danielson LA, Conrad KP. Nitric oxide mediates renal vasodilation and hyperfiltration during pregnancy in chronically instrumented, conscious rats. *J Clin Invest*. 1995;96:482-490.
19. Baylis C, Engels K. Adverse interactions between pregnancy and a new model of systemic hypertension produced by chronic blockade of EDRF in the rat. *Clin Exp Hypertens*. 1992;B11:117-129.
20. Baylis C. Recent advances in renal disease in pregnancy. In: Davison JM, Nelson-Piercy C, Kehoe S, Baker P, eds. *Renal Disease in Pregnancy*. London: RCOG Press; 2008:3-18.
21. Danielson LA, Sherwood OD, Conrad KP. Relaxin is a potent renal vasodilator in conscious rats. *J Clin Invest*. 1999;103:525-533.
22. Conrad KP, Jeyabalan A, Danielson LA, et al. Role of relaxin in the maternal renal vasodilation of pregnancy. *Ann N Y Acad Sci*. 2005;1041: 147-154.
23. Smith MC, Murdoch AP, Danielson LA, et al. Relaxin has a role at establishing a renal response in pregnancy. *Fertil Steril*. 2006;86: 253-255.
24. Brenner BM. Nephron adaptation to renal injury or ablation. *Am J Physiol*. 1985;249:F324-F337.
25. Baylis C. Glomerular filtration rate (GFR) in normal and abnormal pregnancies. *Semin Nephrol*. 1999;9:133-139.
26. Smith MC, Moran P, Ward MK, Davison JM. Assessment of glomerular filtration rate in pregnancy using the MDRD formula. *Br J Obstet Gynaecol*. 2008;115:109-112.
27. Moran P, Lindheimer MD, Davison JM. The renal response to preeclampsia. *Semin Nephrol*. 2004;24:588-595.
28. Williams D, Davison JM. Chronic kidney disease in pregnancy. *BMJ*. 2008;336:211-215.
29. Strevens H, Wide-Swensson D, Hansen A, et al. Glomerular endotheliosis in normal pregnancy and preeclampsia. *Br J Obstet Gynaecol*. 2003;110:831-836.
30. Brunskill NJ. Renal biopsy in pregnancy. In: Davison JM, Nelson-Piercy C, Kehoe S, Baker P, eds. *Renal Disease in Pregnancy*. London: RCOG Press; 2008:201-206.
31. Hytten FE, Cheyne GA. The aminoaciduria of pregnancy. *J Obstet Gynaecol Br Commonw*. 1972;79:424-432.
32. Lindheimer MD, Richardson DA, Ehrlich EN, Katz AI. Potassium homeostasis in pregnancy. *J Reprod Med*. 1987;32:517-520.
33. Olsburgh J. Urological problems in pregnancy. In: Davison JM, Nelson-Piercy C, Kehoe S, Baker P, eds. *Renal Disease in Pregnancy*. London: RCOG Press; 2008:209-220.
34. Roberts JM, Pearson GD, Cutler, JA, Lindheimer MD. Summary of NHLBI Group on Research on Hypertension during Pregnancy. *Hypertens Pregnancy*. 2003;22:109-127.
35. Chappell LC, Shennan AH. Assessment of proteinuria in pregnancy. *BMJ*. 2008;336:968-969.
36. Atherton JC, Beilinska A, Davison JM, et al. Sodium and water reabsorption in the proximal and distal nephron in conscious pregnant rats and third trimester women. *J Physiol*. 1988;396:457-470.
37. August P, Lindheimer M. Pathophysiology of preeclampsia. In: Laragh JH, Brenner BM, eds. *Hypertension: Pathophysiology, Diagnosis and Management*, 2nd ed. New York: Raven Press, 1995:2407-2426.
38. MacDonald PC, Cutter S, MacDonald SC, et al. Regulation of extra-adrenal steroid 21-hydroxylase activity: Increased conversion of plasma progesterone during estrogen treatment of women pregnant with a dead fetus. *J Clin Invest*. 1982;69:469-474.
39. Irons DW, Baylis PH, Davison JM. Effect of atrial natriuretic peptide on renal hemodynamics and sodium excretion during human pregnancy. *Am J Physiol*. 1996;271:F239-F242.
40. Lindheimer MD, Davison JM. Osmoregulation, the secretion of arginine vasopressin and its metabolism during pregnancy [minireview]. *Eur J Endocrinol*. 1995;132:133-143.
41. Randeva HS, Jackson A, Karteris E, Hillhouse EW. hCG production and activity during pregnancy. *Fetal Matern Med Rev*. 2001;12: 191-208.
42. Schrier RW. Pathogenesis of sodium and water retention in high-output and low-output cardiac failure, nephrotic syndrome, cirrhosis and pregnancy. Part 2. *N Engl J Med*. 1988;319:1127-1134.
43. Durr JA, Lindheimer MD. Control of volume and body tonicity. In: Lindheimer MD, Roberts JM, Cunningham FG, eds: *Chesley's Hypertensive Disorders in Pregnancy*, 2nd ed. Stamford, CT: Appleton & Lange; 1999:103-166.
44. Chesley LC, Lindheimer MD. Renal hemodynamics and intravascular volume in normal and hypertensive pregnancy. In: Rubin PC, ed. *Hypertension: Hypertension in Pregnancy*. Amsterdam: Elsevier; 1988:10-38.
45. Zandi-Nejad K, Luyckx VA, Brenner BM. Adult hypertension and kidney disease: The role of fetal programming. *Hypertension*. 2006;47: 502-508.
46. Godfrey KM, Barker DJ. Fetal programming and adult health. *Public Health Nutr*. 2001;4:611-624.

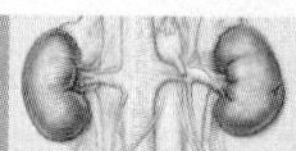

CHAPTER 42

Renal Complications in Normal Pregnancy

S. Ananth Karumanchi, Phyllis August, Tiina Podymow

This chapter discusses kidney disease that develops for the first time during pregnancy, particularly disorders specific to pregnancy, including preeclampsia, hypertensive disorders, and acute kidney injury. In addition, pregnant women are at risk for any of the renal diseases that occur in young women, which may develop coincidentally for the first time during pregnancy. Because many young women undergo urinalysis and blood pressure measurement for the first time during pregnancy, this means that previously undetected kidney disease may be identified. The management of pregnancy with preexisting kidney disease is discussed in Chapter 43. Urinary tract infection and stone disease present particular risks and management issues in pregnancy and are also discussed in Chapter 43.

URINALYSIS

For many young women, pregnancy is the first occasion that they have urinalysis and urine microscopy performed. Hematuria, proteinuria, and pyuria may be detected, either related to or coincidental to the pregnancy.

Hematuria

Microscopic hematuria can be detected at some time during pregnancy in about 20% of women, but it is persistent in only half of those and usually disappears after delivery, when it can be investigated further if it is still present. Persistent microscopic hematuria with normal blood pressure may be present in lupus nephritis, sickle cell trait, thin basement membrane nephropathy, IgA nephropathy, or polycystic kidneys and with renal calculi. The most common cause of gross hematuria in pregnancy is hemorrhagic bacterial cystitis; a less common cause is renal calculi, and rarely it may be bladder or renal neoplasms.

Proteinuria

The urinary excretion of protein rises during pregnancy because of an increase in glomerular filtration rate (GFR) (see Chapter 41), so that the 24-hour excretion of protein, normally below 150 mg/day, may reach 300 mg/day. The pregnancy-induced increase in GFR usually produces more substantial increases in protein excretion in patients with preexisting proteinuria. Patients with a history of glomerulonephritis in whom prepregnant levels of protein excretion are less than 1 g/24 h may excrete 2 to 6 g/24 h during a normal pregnancy because of glomerular hyperperfusion, without any other sign of exacerbation of the nephritis. In such women, plasma uric acid levels are unchanged if preeclampsia is not present.

The development of new and significant proteinuria during pregnancy is almost always associated with the development of preeclampsia and therefore needs thorough investigation, including the measurement of blood pressure, liver function tests, and determination of serum uric acid level. In the absence of urinary tract infection or preeclampsia, isolated proteinuria in pregnancy usually reflects new-onset glomerular disease, for example, primary glomerulonephritis such as IgA nephropathy or focal segmental glomerulosclerosis, or a systemic disease such as systemic lupus. If proteinuria is persistently detected by dipstick testing (≥1+ [100 mg/dl]), the urine protein-creatinine ratio in a random urine sample should be measured. A ratio above 0.3 (mg protein/mg creatinine) that corresponds to a protein excretion of more than 300 mg/24 h is needed to confirm proteinuria.

Pyuria

Isolated leukocyturia (pyuria) is common in normal pregnancy because of contamination by vaginal secretions. It requires no action other than ensuring that it disappears by 3 months postpartum.

RENAL BIOPSY

Percutaneous renal biopsy is usually avoided during pregnancy because of the fear of bleeding from the biopsy site, but it is not clear that the risk of hemorrhage is actually greater than in the nonpregnant state.[1] Renal biopsy is not usually required for the diagnosis and management of preeclampsia. Renal biopsy is indicated, however, if there is reason to suspect a renal disorder that may be treated successfully, especially in early pregnancy, while permitting the pregnancy to continue; this is discussed further in Chapter 43. Diseases in this category include lupus nephritis, minimal change nephrotic syndrome, immune-mediated interstitial nephritis, crescentic glomerulonephritis, and vasculitis. Percutaneous biopsy of the kidney may be performed with ultrasound localization in the usual prone position or with the woman lying on her right side.

KIDNEY SIZE AND HYDRONEPHROSIS

The volume, weight, and size of the kidneys increase in gestation; renal lengths increase by about 1 cm measured by ultrasound.[2] The collecting systems of both kidneys are normally dilated during pregnancy (see Chapter 41, Fig. 41.1), most marked on the right. The dilation is probably caused by hormonal changes of pregnancy and also by ureteral obstruction by the pregnant uterus. Because ureteral dilation is so common during normal gestation, it may be difficult to diagnose frank urinary obstruction. An unusual syndrome of late pregnancy is characterized by abdominal pain, marked hydronephrosis, and a variable increase in serum creatinine, managed successfully by the placement of ureteral stents.[2] Because "physiologic hydronephrosis" is so common, pregnant women are particularly susceptible to ascending pyelonephritis as a result of bladder infections. In the immediate puerperium, a rare occurrence is massive hematuria, usually from the right ureter, which subsides spontaneously and has been attributed to decompression of the partially obstructed right collecting system.

Organisms Most Commonly Responsible for Asymptomatic Bacteriuria in Pregnancy
Escherichia coli (>70% of infections)
Klebsiella species
Proteus species (particularly in diabetic women or urinary tract obstruction)
Enterococci
Staphylococci, especially *Staphyloccocus saprophyticus*
Pseudomonas
Streptococci

Figure 42.1 Organisms most commonly responsible for asymptomatic bacteriuria in pregnancy.

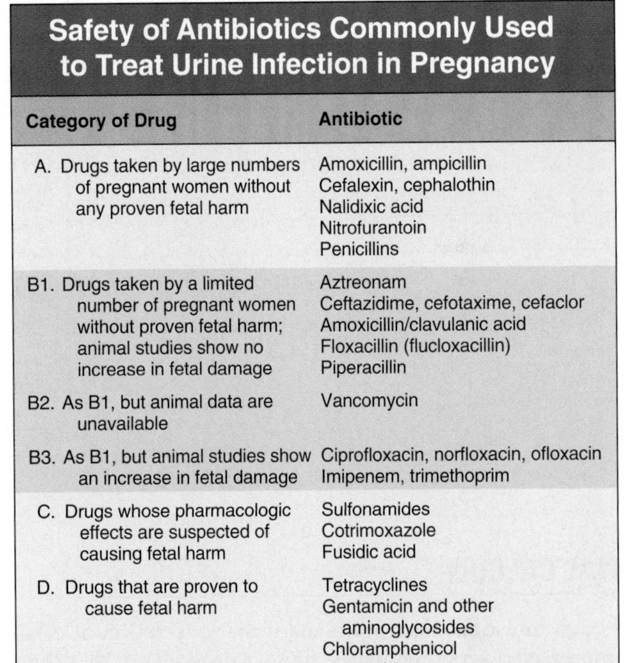

Safety of Antibiotics Commonly Used to Treat Urine Infection in Pregnancy

Category of Drug	Antibiotic
A. Drugs taken by large numbers of pregnant women without any proven fetal harm	Amoxicillin, ampicillin Cefalexin, cephalothin Nalidixic acid Nitrofurantoin Penicillins
B1. Drugs taken by a limited number of pregnant women without proven fetal harm; animal studies show no increase in fetal damage	Aztreonam Ceftazidime, cefotaxime, cefaclor Amoxicillin/clavulanic acid Floxacillin (flucloxacillin) Piperacillin
B2. As B1, but animal data are unavailable	Vancomycin
B3. As B1, but animal studies show an increase in fetal damage	Ciprofloxacin, norfloxacin, ofloxacin Imipenem, trimethoprim
C. Drugs whose pharmacologic effects are suspected of causing fetal harm	Sulfonamides Cotrimoxazole Fusidic acid
D. Drugs that are proven to cause fetal harm	Tetracyclines Gentamicin and other aminoglycosides Chloramphenicol

Figure 42.2 Safety of antibiotics commonly used to treat urinary tract infection in pregnancy.

URINARY INFECTION AND ASYMPTOMATIC BACTERIURIA

Urinary frequency, sometimes accompanied by dysuria, is common during the latter half of pregnancy, even when the urine is not infected, because of pressure on the bladder from an enlarged pregnant uterus.

Urinary Tract Infection

Urinary tract infections that may present as cystitis or acute pyelonephritis complicates 1% to 2% of pregnancies. Urinary stasis and anatomic displacement of the ureters during pregnancy contribute to pathogenesis. In pregnancy, quantitative urine cultures should be obtained in women with persistent leukocyturia (more than two or three white blood cells per high-power field in spun sediment) or symptoms of cystitis. If there are more than 10^5 bacteria of a single species per milliliter of urine, significant bacteriuria is present. Acute pyelonephritis or cystitis can be diagnosed even with 10^2 bacteria/ml if it is accompanied by clinical symptoms. Acute pyelonephritis is a serious complication during pregnancy and usually presents between 20 and 28 weeks of gestation with fevers, loin pain, and dysuria. Bacteremia, usually accompanying pyelonephritis, can progress to endotoxic shock, disseminated intravascular coagulation, and acute renal failure. Pregnant women with acute pyelonephritis should be admitted to the hospital and treated with intravenous antibiotics and hydration. The intravenous administration of cephalosporins or gentamicin for 24 to 48 hours or until the patient is afebrile is followed by oral antibiotics for 10 to 14 days. Antibiotic regimens for treatment of urinary tract infection in pregnancy are shown in Figure 43.6.

Asymptomatic Bacteriuria

Asymptomatic bacteriuria complicates 2% to 10% of pregnancies and may occur without pyuria. It is frequently associated with a reduction in the concentrating ability of the kidney. The organisms associated with asymptomatic bacteriuria are shown in Figure 42.1. Reagent strip testing for asymptomatic bacteriuria is associated with a high false-negative rate, and quantitative urine culture should be performed to rule out significant bacteriuria.

Asymptomatic bacteriuria has been associated with an increased risk of premature delivery and low birth weight. Treatment of asymptomatic bacteriuria during pregnancy reduces these complications and improves perinatal morbidity and mortality.[3] Without treatment, asymptomatic bacteriuria will persist in more than 80% of women and may progress to symptomatic urinary tract infection or acute pyelonephritis. Screening for asymptomatic bacteriuria with a urine culture is recommended during the first prenatal visit and is repeated only in high-risk women, such as those with a history of recurrent urinary infections or urinary tract anomalies. If asymptomatic bacteriuria is found, prompt treatment is warranted, usually with a cephalosporin, for 3 days; a single dose of fosfomycin can also be used (see Fig. 43.6). Antibiotics useful in treating urinary infections during pregnancy are listed in Figure 42.2. Trimethoprim-sulfamethoxazole (cotrimoxazole) is contraindicated in early pregnancy because of its association with birth defects. Tetracycline and chloramphenicol are also contraindicated. Use of quinolones is discouraged during pregnancy because of some evidence of teratogenicity in animals. Women treated for asymptomatic bacteriuria should have a repeated urine culture 2 weeks after therapy to ensure that bacteriuria has been eradicated. Suppressive therapy with nitrofurantoin or cephalexin is recommended for those patients with bacteriuria that persists after two courses of therapy. Prolonged suppressive treatment of bacteriuria reduces the incidence of pyelonephritis.[4]

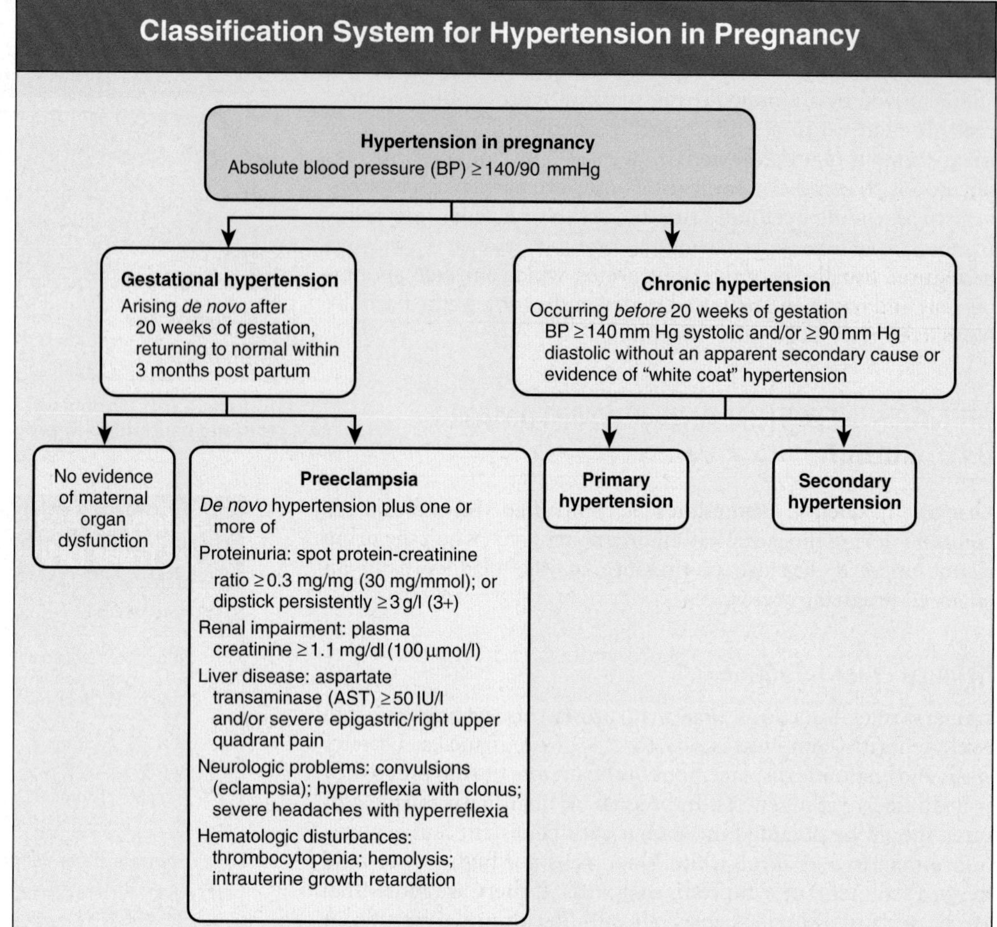

Figure 42.3 Classification of hypertension in pregnancy.

RENAL CALCULI

Although intestinal absorption and urinary excretion of calcium are increased during pregnancy, there is no evidence that the risk of nephrolithiasis is increased. Women who have had kidney stones can be reassured that pregnancy is not likely to increase stone formation. The management of symptomatic stone disease in pregnancy is discussed further in Chapter 43.

HYPERTENSIVE DISORDERS OF PREGNANCY

Hypertensive disorders of pregnancy can be considered in three categories:

1. gestational hypertension, including preeclampsia and eclampsia;
2. chronic or preexisting hypertension of any cause; and
3. preeclampsia superimposed on chronic hypertension.

Figure 42.3 illustrates the various hypertensive disorders of pregnancy and the criteria used to make the distinction. Preeclampsia (pure or superimposed, categories 1 and 3) poses the greatest threat to fetal survival and is the disorder most often associated with severe maternal complications (including fatalities) (Fig. 42.4). The majority of women in the second category have primary hypertension, and their pregnancies usually remain uncomplicated and end successfully. On occasion, however, the high blood pressure is due to specific causes, including pheochromocytoma, Cushing's syndrome, renal artery stenosis,

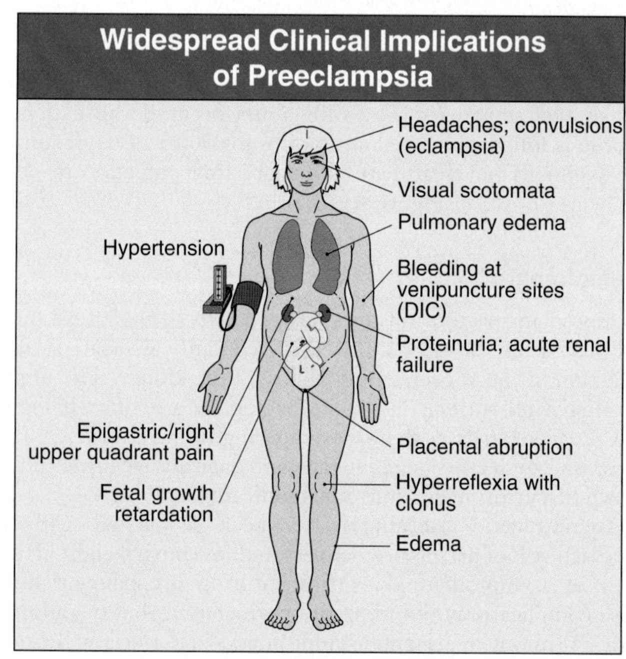

Figure 42.4 Widespread clinical implications of preeclampsia. DIC, disseminated intravascular coagulation.

and primary renal disease,[5,6] and some of these women with secondary forms of hypertension do poorly during gestation. Thus, pheochromocytoma, although rare, may present for the first time during gestation and is especially lethal when it is unsuspected; whereas when it is diagnosed, it can be managed to a successful outcome, either surgically or pharmacologically (with α-blockade), depending on the stage of pregnancy.[5] Cushing's syndrome has been associated with exacerbations of hypertension during pregnancy and poor fetal outcomes. Finally, both angioplasty and stent placement have been successfully performed in pregnant women with renal artery stenosis.[5]

GESTATIONAL HYPERTENSION

Pregnant women with blood pressure above 140/90 mm Hg, without proteinuria, and whose blood pressure was lower before pregnancy are described as having gestational hypertension. There are a range of possible causes. Some women, usually with a strong family history of primary hypertension, have a normal blood pressure throughout most of pregnancy, but at the end of the third trimester, blood pressure tends to rise to approach the higher pre-pregnant level. Usually there is no protein in the urine, and the serum uric acid is not elevated. There is evidence that transient hypertension of pregnancy occurs in women destined to have primary hypertension later in life (analogous to women with gestational hyperglycemia who eventually develop type 2 diabetes).

A substantial proportion of women (approximately 30%) with gestational hypertension have an early phase of preeclampsia, in which proteinuria has not yet appeared. This subgroup of patients may have some evidence of glomerular endotheliosis on renal biopsy (Fig. 42.5).[7] On occasion, the elevated blood pressure has a psychiatric cause, such as an anxiety or panic disorder. A rare group of patients have activating mineralocorticoid receptor mutations that result in an exaggerated sensitivity to the usually weak mineralocorticoid effect of progesterone.[8] They manifest salt-sensitive hypertension, accompanied by hypokalemia, but virtually undetectable aldosterone levels, most marked during pregnancy as progesterone levels rise. The administration of large amounts of intravenous saline during a cesarean section can sometimes result in postpartum hypertension and edema that disappear in a few days when the large salt load is excreted.

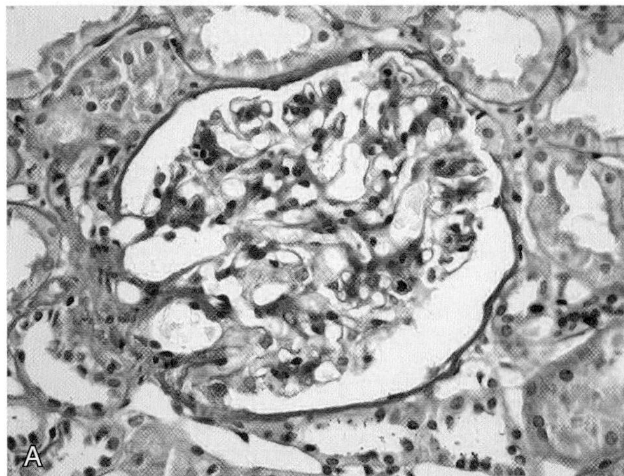

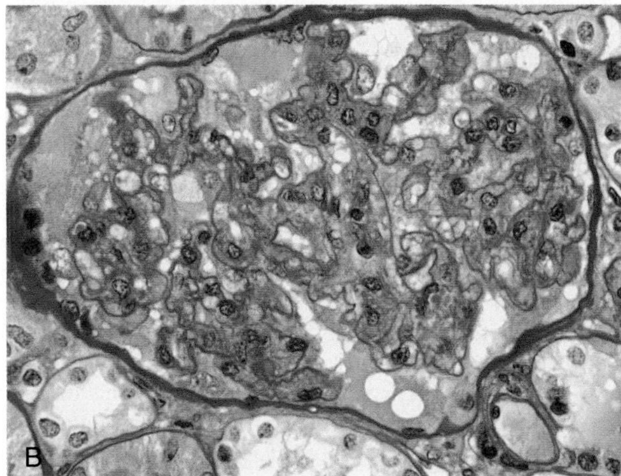

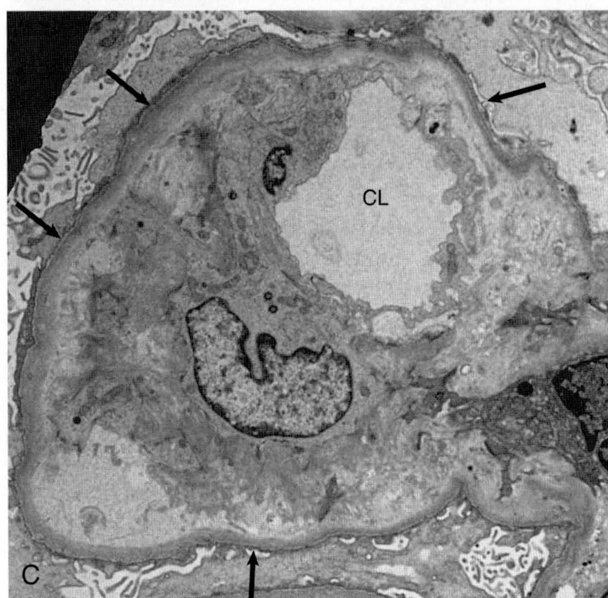

Figure 42.5 Glomerular endotheliosis. A, Normal glomerulus. (Light microscopy, periodic acid–Schiff stain; magnification ×40.) **B,** Glomerulus from a patient with preeclampsia. (Light microscopy, periodic acid–Schiff stain; magnification ×40.) Note occlusion of capillary lumina by swollen endothelial cells. **C,** Electron microscopy. Note glomerular basement membrane *(arrows)* and marked reduction of capillary lumen (CL) due to swollen endothelial cell cytoplasm. (Original magnification ×7500.) *(Courtesy Prof. P. Furness, University of Leicester, UK)*

PREECLAMPSIA

Definition

Preeclampsia is the most frequently encountered renal complication of pregnancy. It is characterized by the new onset of hypertension and proteinuria, usually after 20 weeks of pregnancy, and is commonly associated with edema and hyperuricemia. Blood pressure of 140/90 mm Hg or higher during pregnancy is required for the diagnosis.[9] It was previously recommended that a rise in systolic blood pressure of more than 30 mm Hg or in diastolic blood pressure of more than 15 mm Hg from baseline values was sufficient to define hypertension; however, epidemiologic data indicate that outcomes are similar whatever the magnitude of the rise, provided blood pressure remains below 140/90 mm Hg. Nevertheless, the U.S. National High Blood Pressure Education Program still recommends that women with blood pressure below 140/90 mm Hg who have experienced an increase of 30 or 15 mm Hg in systolic or diastolic levels, respectively, should be managed as high-risk patients. Proteinuria is

Criteria for the Diagnosis of Severe Preeclampsia
In patients with preeclampsia, **severe preeclampsia** can be diagnosed if any one of the following criteria is present:
Blood pressure 160 mm Hg systolic or 110 mmHg diastolic or higher on two separate occasions at least 6 hours apart
Proteinuria Random urine protein-creatinine ratio ≥ 5 mg/mg (500mg/mmol) *or* proteinuria > 5 g/24 h
Oliguria < 500 ml in 24 hours
Cerebral or visual disturbances such as cerebrovascular accident, seizures, or visual loss
Pulmonary edema
Epigastric or right upper quadrant pain
Hepatocellular injury (serum transaminases at least twice normal)
Serum lactate dehydrogenase: > 600 IU/l
Thrombocytopenia < 100 × 10^9/l
Fetal growth restriction (birth weight less than 10th percentile for the gestational age)

Figure 42.6 Criteria for the diagnosis of severe preeclampsia. *(Modified from reference 9.)*

Risk Factors for the Development of Preeclampsia
Preeclampsia in prior pregnancy
Family history of preeclampsia
Nulliparity
Multiple gestation
Molar pregnancies
Older maternal age
Obesity
Preexisting hypertension
Preexisting chronic kidney disease
Diabetes mellitus
Thrombotic vascular disease (antithrombin III deficiency, protein C or S deficiency, factor V Leiden, antiphospholipid antibody syndrome)
Trisomy 13 fetus
Fetal hydrops
High altitude

Figure 42.7 Risk factors for the development of preeclampsia.

defined as urine protein-creatinine ratio above 0.3 mg/mg (30 mg/mmol), which is sufficiently reliable to avoid the need for 24-hour urine collection. Finally, although serum uric acid is not included in the formal definition of preeclampsia, uric acid level above 5.5 mg/dl (325 μmol/l) may point to a diagnosis of preeclampsia, especially in patients with preexisting renal disease or hypertension although other causes of hyperuricemia should always be considered (see Chapter 43). Preeclampsia is considered severe with urine protein-creatinine ratio above 5, with blood pressure of 160/110 mm Hg or higher, with evidence of the HELLP syndrome (hemolysis, elevated liver enzymes, low platelet count) or central nervous system dysfunction, or with the presence of intrauterine fetal growth restriction (Fig. 42.6).

Epidemiology

Preeclampsia complicates approximately 5% of all pregnancies. It is about twice as common in first pregnancies as in multigravidas. Preeclampsia is also slightly more common in multigravidas who have a new partner, suggesting that prior exposure to paternal antigens may be protective.[10] However, recent evidence from a large Norwegian birth registry suggests that prolonged interpregnancy interval, rather than primipaternity, may account for this increase in risk, for reasons that are unclear. Other predisposing factors include preexisting hypertension, chronic renal disease, obesity, diabetes mellitus, thrombophilias (factor V Leiden, antiphospholipid syndrome, and antithrombin III deficiency), and multiple gestation (Fig. 42.7). It occurs more frequently in women whose mothers had preeclampsia and in women whose fathers were products of a preeclamptic pregnancy, perhaps because the placenta itself is a creation of both the mother and the father.[10] The incidence of preeclampsia is also higher in women who live in high altitudes, suggesting that hypoxia may contribute to the development of the syndrome.

Pathogenesis

Preeclampsia occurs only in the presence of the placenta, even when there is no fetus (as in hydatidiform mole) and usually remits when the placenta is delivered. The placenta in preeclampsia is often abnormal, with evidence of hypoperfusion and ischemia. Preeclampsia is characterized by widespread systemic vascular endothelial dysfunction and microangiopathy in the mother but not in the fetus. It is currently thought that preeclampsia is due to a circulating factor or factors produced by the diseased placenta that induce maternal vascular endothelial dysfunction.[11]

Abnormal Placentation in Preeclampsia

The characteristic placental lesion in preeclampsia is a diminution in endovascular invasion by cytotrophoblasts and a decrease in remodeling of the uterine spiral arterioles.[12] The hypothesis that defective trophoblastic invasion with accompanying uteroplacental hypoperfusion may lead to preeclampsia is supported by animal and human studies. Placentas from pregnancies with advanced preeclampsia often have numerous placental infarcts and sclerotic narrowing of arterioles.[10] Uteroplacental blood flow is usually diminished and uterine vascular resistance increased in preeclamptic women. Placental ischemia induced by mechanical constriction of the uterine arteries or aorta produces hypertension, proteinuria, and, variably, glomerular endotheliosis in several animal species.[13] However, placental ischemia alone, as seen in many cases of intrauterine growth restriction, does not appear to be sufficient to produce preeclampsia.

The Preeclampsia Factors

There has been an intense search for circulating factors that may cause the maternal syndrome of preeclampsia. Increased sensitivity to the vasopressor effects of angiotensin is a feature of preeclampsia, perhaps due to increased plasma concentrations of angiotensin AT_1–bradykinin B_2 receptor heterodimers.[10] Circulating concentrations of agonistic antibodies to the angiotensin AT_1 receptor have been reported in women with preeclampsia[14] and are also encountered in other examples of vascular injury, such as vascular rejection, suggesting that they may be secondary to the generalized microangiopathy of preeclampsia. Reactive free oxygen radicals may have a causal role in preeclampsia.[11] In some but not all studies, markers of oxidative stress are elevated in women with preeclampsia. Decreased intake of the antioxidant vitamin C and low circulating ascorbic acid levels are associated with an increased risk of preeclampsia. However, a randomized therapeutic trial of antioxidants (vitamins C and E) in pregnant women did not prevent preeclampsia, suggesting that oxidant stress is unlikely to be the primary mediator.[15]

"Export" of fragments of trophoblastic material from the diseased placenta into the circulation has also been suggested as a possible cause for the generalized microangiopathy of preeclampsia.[11]

Circulating Antiangiogenic Factors

sFlt-1 (soluble fms-like tyrosine kinase 1, also referred to as sVEGFR-1) production is increased in the placenta in preeclamptic women.[16] sFlt-1 is a secreted protein, a splice variant of the vascular endothelial growth factor (VEGF) receptor Flt-1 lacking the transmembrane cytoplasmic domain of the membrane-bound receptor. It is a potent circulating antagonist to VEGF and placental growth factor (PlGF) (Fig. 42.8). Both VEGF and PlGF are made by the placenta and circulate in high concentration during pregnancy. VEGF is also synthesized by glomerular podocytes and vascular endothelial cells. Circulating sFlt-1 levels are greatly increased in women with established preeclampsia and before onset of clinical symptoms, whereas free PlGF levels are decreased.[17] When it is administered to pregnant and non-pregnant rats, sFlt-1 produces hypertension, proteinuria, and glomerular endotheliosis resembling the human syndrome of preeclampsia. The glomerular lesion in these experimental animals, consisting of severe glomerular endothelial swelling and loss of endothelial fenestrae with relatively preserved foot processes in association with heavy proteinuria, is striking in its resemblance to human preeclampsia (see Fig. 42.5).[16,18]

The concentration of circulating sFlt-1 starts to rise near the end of the second trimester in women destined to have preeclampsia, 4 to 5 weeks before clinical manifestations such as hypertension and proteinuria are first detected.[17] By the time clinically overt preeclampsia has developed, plasma sFlt-1 is two to four times higher than in normal pregnancy at the same stage of gestation. The concentration of sFlt-1 in plasma is higher in patients with severe preeclampsia than in those with milder disease.[19] There is also a modest but significant decrease in circulating free PlGF levels in the first trimester in women who later develop preeclampsia, but from mid-pregnancy on, the concentration of PlGF in plasma falls at the time when sFlt-1 levels are rising.[19] Because unbound PlGF is freely filtered, urinary PlGF levels may prove to be a predictor of subsequent preeclampsia.[19] Women carrying trisomy 13 fetuses have an increased risk of preeclampsia and high circulating concentrations of sFlt-1, perhaps not surprising because the gene for Flt-1/sFlt-1 is located on chromosome 13.[20]

The possibility that an antagonist of VEGF and PlGF might play a role in preeclampsia has a sound physiologic basis. As well as being potent promoters of angiogenesis, VEGF and PlGF are known to induce the synthesis of nitric oxide and vasodilating prostacyclins in endothelial cells, decreasing vascular tone and blood pressure. VEGF, synthesized in large amounts by glomerular podocytes, may be important in maintaining the health and healing of glomerular vascular endothelial cells, so that its absence induces proteinuria and glomerular endotheliosis.[21] The organs targeted in preeclampsia, such as the glomerulus and the hepatic sinusoids, have fenestrated endothelia. VEGF induces endothelial fenestrae *in vitro*, and even a 50% decrease in VEGF production in the glomerulus in mice leads to glomerular endotheliosis and loss of glomerular endothelial fenestrae.[21] Antagonists of VEGF, used in cancer therapy, sometimes produce hypertension, proteinuria, and reversible posterior leukoencephalopathy—hallmarks of preeclampsia and eclampsia.[10] Furthermore, exogenous VEGF and PlGF can reverse the

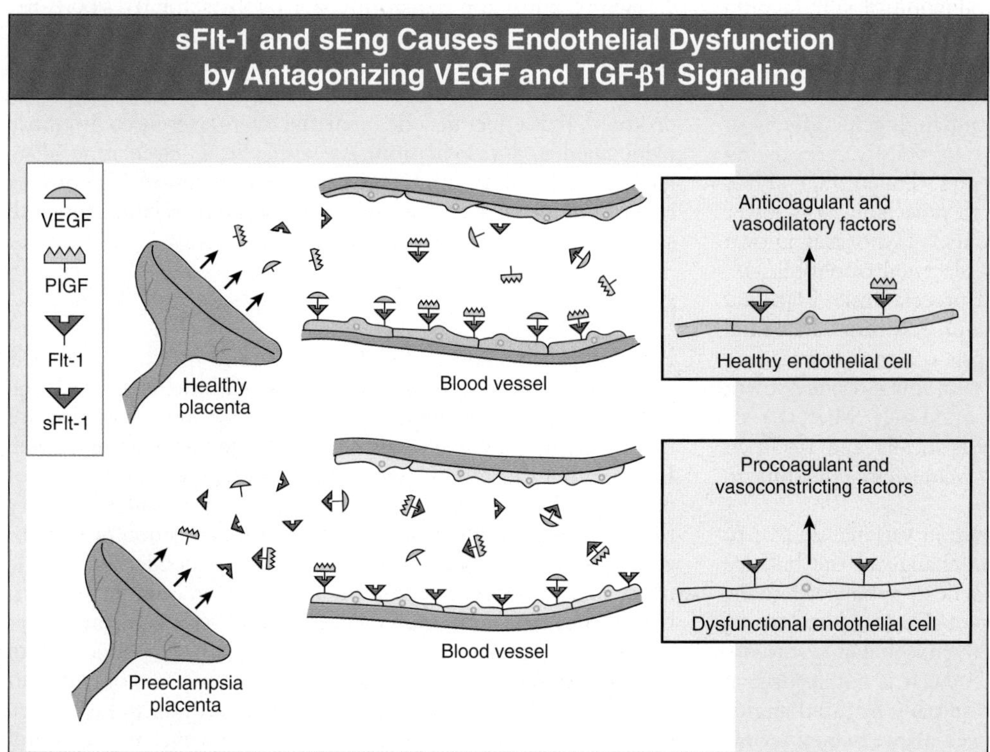

Figure 42.8 sFlt-1 and sEng cause endothelial dysfunction by antagonizing VEGF and TGF-β1 signaling. There is mounting evidence that vascular endothelial growth factor (VEGF) and transforming growth factor β1 (TGF-β1) are required to maintain endothelial health in several tissues, including the kidney and perhaps the placenta. During normal pregnancy, vascular homeostasis is maintained by physiologic levels of VEGF and TGF-β1 signaling in the vasculature. In preeclampsia, excess placental secretion of sFlt-1 and sEng (two endogenous circulating antiangiogenic proteins) inhibits VEGF and TGF-β1 signaling, respectively, in the vasculature. This results in endothelial cell dysfunction, including decreased prostacyclin, nitric oxide production, and release of procoagulant proteins. PlGF, placental growth factor. *(Reproduced with permission from reference 48.)*

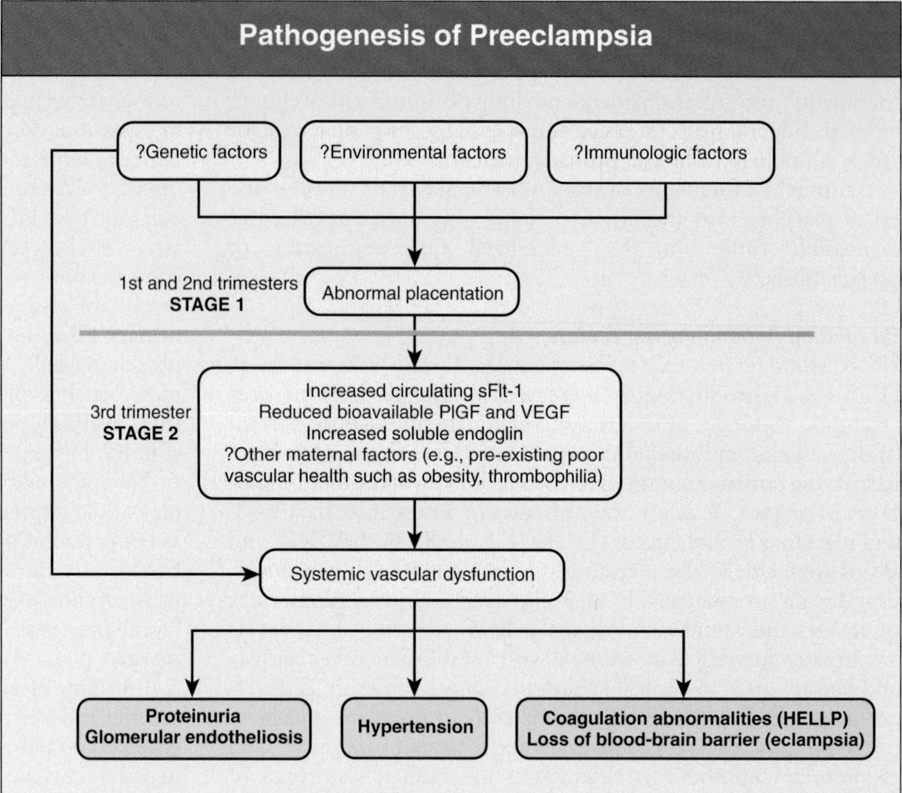

Figure 42.9 Summary of the pathogenesis of preeclampsia. PlGF, placental growth factor; sFlt-1, soluble fms-like tyrosine kinase 1; VEGF, vascular endothelial growth factor.

antiangiogenic effects of preeclamptic blood *in vitro*.[16] Thus, the antiangiogenic effects of sFlt-1 may account for many of the manifestations of preeclampsia, including the unique glomerular changes.

The likely role of sFlt-1 in the pathogenesis of preeclampsia is summarized in Figure 42.9. Overproduction of sFlt-1 could explain susceptibility to preeclampsia in multiple gestation, hydatidiform mole, trisomy 13, and possibly first pregnancy. Alternatively, preeclampsia could follow sensitization of the maternal vascular endothelium to the antiangiogenic effects of sFlt-1. Such sensitization might occur in obesity, preexisting hypertension or renal disease, and diabetes. The average sFlt-1 level in the serum of obese patients with preeclampsia is lower than that in thinner preeclamptic patients.[17] Hypoxia is known to increase the production of sFlt-1 by placental trophoblasts,[10] so that placental ischemia might trigger preeclampsia. Placental ischemia is common but not universal in preeclampsia. Placental infarction unaccompanied by preeclampsia is a common finding in mothers with sickle cell anemia and with intrauterine growth restriction. Placental overproduction of sFlt-1, whatever its cause, might itself decrease angiogenesis locally and result in placental ischemia, thereby initiating a vicious circle leading to even more sFlt-1 production.

These three factors may all contribute in variable degree to the pathogenesis of preeclampsia: (1) a change in the balance of circulating factors controlling angiogenesis-antiangiogenesis, attributable to placental overproduction of sFlt-1 and underproduction of PlGF; (2) increased vascular endothelial sensitivity to such factors[22]; and (3) placental ischemia. It is not surprising that in human pregnancy, characterized initially by rapid angiogenesis localized to the placenta, followed as pregnancy terminates by regression of blood vessel growth, there should sometimes occur systemic manifestations of a derangement of this process.

Another antiangiogenic protein, soluble endoglin (sEng), is also upregulated in preeclampsia in a pattern similar to that of sFlt-1. sEng is a truncated form of endoglin (CD105), a cell surface receptor for transforming growth factor β1 (TGF-β1) (see Fig. 42.8). Soluble endoglin amplifies the vascular damage mediated by sFlt-1 in pregnant rats, inducing a severe preeclampsia-like syndrome with features of the HELLP syndrome.[23] This effect may be mediated by interference with nitric oxide–mediated vasodilation. As with sFlt-1, circulating sEng levels are elevated weeks before preeclampsia onset.[24] The precise role of soluble endoglin in preeclampsia and its relationship with sFlt-1 are currently being explored.

Pathology

Preeclampsia is associated with a unique and specific glomerular appearance referred to as glomerular endotheliosis (see Fig. 42.5). By light microscopy, the glomerular capillary lumina are narrowed and appear bloodless, and the glomeruli are enlarged. Unlike other thrombotic microangiopathies, the endotheliosis of preeclampsia is usually not accompanied by prominent capillary thrombi. Immunofluorescence may reveal deposition of fibrinogen derivatives, especially when signs of systemic thrombotic microangiopathy are prominent. There are no immune deposits in the glomeruli, and serum complement levels are normal. Electron microscopy shows relative preservation of the podocyte foot processes despite heavy proteinuria, but there is loss of endothelial fenestrae, and endothelial cells become swollen and separated from the basement membrane by electron-lucent material.[18] Mild glomerular endotheliosis has been noted in up to 30% of patients with pregnancy-induced hypertension without proteinuria,[7,25] suggesting that some cases of pregnancy-induced hypertension may reflect an earlier or milder form of preeclampsia. The glomerular changes usually disappear within 8 weeks of delivery, coinciding with resolution of the hypertension and proteinuria. Focal segmental glomerulosclerosis is said to accompany the generalized glomerular endotheliosis of preeclampsia in up to 50% of cases.[10] Although this change has been taken by some to suggest that there was kidney disease before pregnancy, it seems possible that it is the consequence of the preeclamptic process itself because similar changes may develop rapidly when glomerular endotheliosis is induced in animals.[21]

Clinical Manifestations

Preeclampsia is the most frequently encountered renal complication of pregnancy. It is characterized by the new onset of hypertension and proteinuria, usually during the last trimester of pregnancy, and is commonly associated with edema and hyperuricemia. Preeclampsia is characterized by widespread vascular endothelial dysfunction and microangiopathy in the mother but not in the fetus. The predominant target organ may be the brain (seizures or eclampsia), the liver (HELLP syndrome), or the kidney (glomerular endotheliosis and proteinuria) (see Fig. 42.4). Severe preeclampsia is also associated with intrauterine growth restriction and small for gestational age babies.

Hypertension

During normal pregnancy, peripheral vascular resistance and systemic arterial blood pressure are decreased; but in preeclampsia, these changes are reversed. Increased peripheral vascular resistance rather than increased cardiac output is the chief cause of hypertension.[10] As in other forms of hypertension, sympathetic activation is prominent, and there is an exaggerated response to infusions of angiotensin II and other hypertensive stimuli.[10]

In preeclampsia, the renin-angiotensin-aldosterone system (RAS) is suppressed,[26] suggesting that vasoconstriction, increased peripheral vascular resistance, and renal sodium and water retention are initial events, resulting in an increased effective circulating blood volume and subsequent RAS suppression. This is consistent with the observation that although total plasma volume is slightly decreased, the hypertension of preeclampsia is exacerbated by salt loading and at least partly ameliorated by diuretics and salt deprivation.[10] A comparable decrease in total plasma volume with an increase in peripheral vascular resistance and arterial blood pressure can be produced by the infusion into normal subjects of norepinephrine and other vasoconstrictors. The vasoconstriction of preeclampsia appears to be mediated by alterations in several vasoactive molecules, including the vasoconstrictors norepinephrine, endothelin, and perhaps thromboxane and the vasodilators prostacyclin and perhaps nitric oxide.

Edema

Sudden weight gain, with edema of the feet, hands, and face, is a common presenting symptom in preeclampsia. Women with preeclampsia excrete a much smaller percentage of an intravenous saline load than do normal pregnant women.[10] Because there is RAS suppression, this implies primary renal retention of salt and water. The edema of preeclampsia thus resembles the "overfill" edema of acute glomerulonephritis or of acute ischemic renal failure with volume overload.

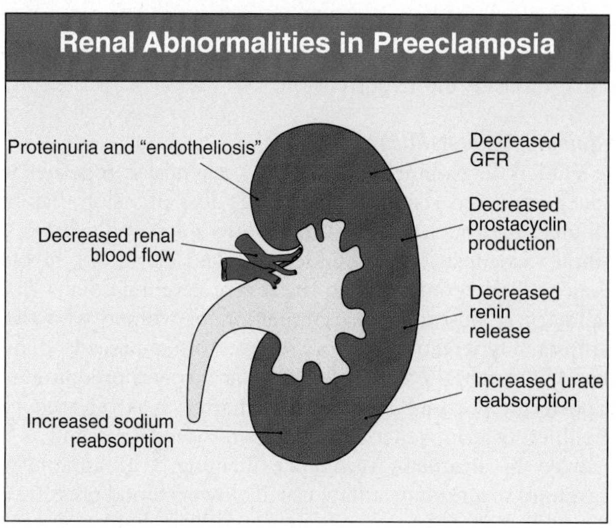

Figure 42.10 Renal abnormalities in preeclampsia. GFR, glomerular filtration rate.

A generalized increase in capillary permeability is unlikely to explain preeclamptic edema because the concentration of protein in interstitial fluid from preeclamptic patients is not elevated.[10] Hypoalbuminemia is common, and it may contribute to edema formation in some patients.

Renal Function, Proteinuria, and the Urinary Sediment

Abnormalities of renal function in preeclampsia are summarized in Figure 42.10. GFR and renal plasma flow are uniformly decreased, compared with the increases in normal pregnancy. Blood urea nitrogen and serum creatinine concentrations often remain in the nonpregnant normal range, despite a significant decrease in GFR from the elevated levels of normal pregnancy. Simultaneous measurements of GFR and renal plasma flow indicate that the filtration fraction is lower during preeclampsia than in normal women during the last trimester of pregnancy.[18,27]

The urinary sediment is usually "bland" in preeclampsia, with few leukocytes, erythrocytes, or cellular casts. Hyaline casts may be present when proteinuria is heavy. The presence of many erythrocytes or erythrocyte casts suggests glomerulonephritis. The proteinuria of preeclampsia is "nonselective," that is, whereas most of the urinary protein is albumin, high-molecular-weight proteins are present as well.[27] After delivery, proteinuria usually disappears within 7 to 10 days; in a few women, it may persist, although gradually diminishing, for 3 to 6 months.

Uric Acid

A disproportionate fall in uric acid clearance is a key feature of preeclampsia. The serum uric acid concentration rises as preeclampsia progresses; a level above 5.5 mg/dl (325 μmol/l) is a strong indicator of preeclampsia, and a level above 7.8 mg/dl (460 μmol/l) is associated with significant maternal morbidity. The degree of uric acid elevation correlates with the severity of proteinuria and renal pathologic changes and with fetal demise.[10] Often, the elevation of uric acid precedes the onset of proteinuria and changes in GFR. Lowering of serum uric acid by the administration of probenecid does not alter the hypertension and proteinuria of preeclampsia, so it is likely that hyperuricemia is a secondary rather than a primary phenomenon, analogous to the disproportionate fall in urate clearance produced in normal human subjects by vasoconstrictors like angiotensin II and norepinephrine.[10] Nevertheless, rodent studies suggest that hyperuricemia may play a pathogenic role by contributing to the vascular damage and hypertension.[28]

Neurologic Abnormalities

The sudden development of seizures (eclampsia), together with headache, blurred vision, or temporary loss of vision, has been attributed to brain edema, thrombotic microangiopathy, and cerebral vasoconstriction. Sudden, marked elevations of blood pressure usually contribute to the severe cerebral edema that is a hallmark at postmortem examination of women who die of eclampsia. Hyperactive tendon reflexes often precede convulsions. The cerebral edema of eclampsia involves predominantly the posterior portions of the white matter; it is referred to as reversible posterior leukoencephalopathy syndrome and is best visualized by magnetic resonance imaging.[29] Treatment with intravenous magnesium sulfate usually lowers blood pressure and reduces central nervous system irritability, but it does not improve renal function. On occasion, seizures occur postpartum, usually within 4 days but very rarely as long as 3 to 4 weeks after delivery in women in whom preeclampsia, although probably present, was not detected during the pregnancy.

HELLP Syndrome

This term is applied to patients with preeclampsia in whom the clinical picture is dominated by hemolysis, elevated liver enzymes, and low platelet count, all occurring as a result of the generalized maternal vascular dysfunction of preeclampsia.[30] Very occasionally, subcapsular liver hemorrhage or liver rupture may develop. HELLP syndrome occurs in 10% to 20% of patients with preeclampsia and is one of its most severe forms. Symptoms and signs usually disappear promptly after delivery, although laboratory measures may transiently worsen in the first 24 hours but improve within 7 days after delivery. Thrombocytopenia is a consequence of consumption coagulopathy. It does not respond to exchange transfusion but usually disappears by 1 week postpartum.

Natural History

After delivery, the hypertension and proteinuria of preeclampsia usually disappear within a few days to weeks, but complete resolution may occasionally take longer. In exceptional cases, proteinuria lingers up to 6 months after delivery. Renal biopsy is indicated if proteinuria persists more than 6 months or earlier if the proteinuria is accompanied by an active urine sediment or rapidly deteriorating renal function.

Considerable evidence suggests that preeclampsia predisposes women to late vascular disease.[31,32] Fifteen years after an episode of preeclampsia, the incidence of hypertension is five times that found in women with normal pregnancies who never had preeclampsia (37% versus 7%).[33] This tendency to later hypertension appears to be the result of preeclampsia rather than inherited factors because the same risk is not found in the siblings of preeclamptic patients.[33] Epidemiologic studies suggest that preeclampsia predicts remote cardiovascular deaths.[34] Preeclampsia is also a marker for increased risk of subsequent end-stage renal disease, although the absolute risk is low.[35]

Prevention

Because preeclampsia occurs more frequently in women with chronic hypertension, it is thought that if high blood pressure is controlled in such women, the risk of preeclampsia is lowered, but this is not yet known with certainty. Low-dose aspirin (75-150 mg daily) is said to reduce the incidence of preeclampsia, but this has not been demonstrated in large prospective studies.[36] A meta-analysis suggested that antiplatelet agents have a modest benefit, with a relative risk of preeclampsia of 0.81 for aspirin-treated patients.[37] Because the benefits of aspirin prophylaxis are modest, it should be used only in high-risk women, such as those with underlying renal disease or preexisting hypertension. Oral calcium supplements may reduce the likelihood of preeclampsia in women whose calcium intake is extremely low.[38] Vitamin C and vitamin E do not protect against preeclampsia.[15]

Management of Preeclampsia

Clinical Problem	Management
Assess indications for delivery	Always review whether an indication for delivery is present by clinical and laboratory monitoring
Control blood pressure (BP)	Acute treatment if BP ≥170/110 mmHg Chronic treatment if BP ≥140/90 mmHg
Eclampsia prophylaxis or treatment	Diazepam 10–20 mg IV to terminate convulsions Magnesium sulfate for persistent neurologic signs (also an indication for delivery): 4 g IV over 20 min, then 1.5 g/h for 48 h
Supportive therapies (sometimes required)	Platelet infusion if count < 20–40 ×10⁹/l Fresh-frozen plasma for microangiopathy or for reduced clotting factors Dialysis for established acute kidney injury
Progressive decline in renal, hepatic, or clotting function or of fetal growth	Delivery

Figure 42.11 Management of preeclampsia.

Treatment

Figure 42.11 lists the key management options for patients with preeclampsia. The most reliable treatment of preeclampsia is delivery. Removal of the placenta usually produces prompt improvement, although in a few cases in which the disease has been explosive, symptoms may progress for several days, even after delivery. Unexpected uterine hemorrhage may produce shock and cortical necrosis, and excessive saline infusions given to prevent that eventuality may trigger pulmonary edema or exacerbate hypertension.

The hypertension of preeclampsia usually responds to pharmacologic treatment. Prompt lowering of the blood pressure is important to reduce the risk of cerebral edema, cerebral hemorrhage, and eclampsia. Blood pressure should be maintained below 140/90 mm Hg; however, it is important to not lower the blood pressure below 120/80 mm Hg as relative hypotension may further compromise the fetoplacental blood flow.[39] Figure 42.12 summarizes the recommended pharmacologic treatments of hypertension in pregnancy and preeclampsia. Angiotensin-converting enzyme inhibitors and angiotensin receptor blockers interfere with renal development in the fetus and should not be used in pregnancy. Although proteinuria may lessen as the blood pressure falls, renal function usually does not improve, and the mother remains at risk for development of the HELLP syndrome and the fetus for intrauterine death or placental abruption. Abrupt falls in blood pressure produced by medication may produce renal cortical necrosis.

Common Medications Used in the Treatment of Hypertension in Preeclampsia

Type of Hypertension	Drug	Treatment Regimen
Acute	Hydralazine	5-mg 1V bolus every 20–30 min to maximum of 20 mg, then infusion at 5–10 mg/h
	Labetalol	50 mg 1V every 20 min to maximum 300 mg
	Nifedipine SR	20 mg oral
Chronic		
First-line choice	Methyldopa	500–2000 mg/day PO
	Clonidine	0.2–0.8 mg/day PO
	Oxprenolol	80–480 mg/day PO
	Labetalol	200–1200 mg/day PO
	Atenolol	50–100 mg/day PO
Second-line choice	Hydralazine	25–200 mg/day PO
	Prazosin	1–10 mg/day PO
	Nifedipine SR	40–100 mg/day PO

Figure 42.12 Common medications in the treatment of hypertension in preeclampsia. Diuretics and propranolol are not recommended. Angiotensin-converting enzyme inhibitors and angiotensin receptor blockers are contraindicated. SR, sustained release.

Comparison of Clinical and Laboratory Characteristics of TTP/HUS, HELLP and AFLP

Clinical Feature	HUS/TTP	HELLP	AFLP
Hemolytic anemia	+++	++	+/–
Thrombocytopenia	+++	++	+/–
Coagulopathy	–	+/–	+
CNS symptoms	++	+/-	+/–
Renal failure	+++	+	++
Hypertension	+/–	+++	+/–
Proteinuria	+/–	++	+/–
Elevated AST	+/–	++	+++
Elevated bilirubin	++	+	+++
Anemia	++	+	+/–
Blood ammonia	Normal	Normal	High
Effect of delivery on disease	None	Recovery	Recovery
Management	Plasma exchange	Supportive care, delivery	Supportive care, delivery

Figure 42.13 Comparison of clinical and laboratory characteristics of HUS-TTP, HELLP, and AFLP. AFLP, acute fatty liver of pregnancy; AST, aspartate transaminase; CNS, central nervous system; HELLP, syndrome of hemolysis, elevated liver enzymes, and low platelet count; HUS, hemolytic-uremic syndrome; TTP, thrombotic thrombocytopenic purpura.

Infusions of magnesium sulfate are effective in preventing epileptic seizures and lowering blood pressure. At high concentrations, magnesium ions depress the respiratory center, and magnesium infusions should not be given if the deep tendon reflexes (e.g., patellar reflex) cannot be elicited. Intravenous dexamethasone is suggested to hasten recovery in HELLP syndrome, but this has not been confirmed by larger studies.[40] Platelet transfusions are indicated if there is significant maternal bleeding or if platelet counts are less than 20×10^9/l.

ACUTE KIDNEY INJURY IN PREGNANCY

Acute kidney injury (AKI) in association with pregnancy, a rare complication in developed countries, is also decreasing in incidence in the developing world.[41] Recent estimates suggest that the incidence of AKI from obstetric causes is less than 1 in 20,000 pregnancies.[42] When AKI occurs early in pregnancy (12 to 18 weeks), it is usually in association with septic abortion or volume depletion due to hyperemesis gravidarum. Pregnancy confers a peculiar susceptibility to the vascular effects of gram-negative endotoxin (Shwartzman phenomenon). Perhaps because of the physiologic increase in procoagulant factors that occurs in normal pregnancy, the thrombotic microangiopathy and renal cortical necrosis that characterize septic shock, especially with gram-negative organisms, are particularly pronounced during pregnancy. Renal cortical necrosis is a common complication, for example, of septic abortion.

Most cases of AKI in pregnancy occur between gestational week 35 and the puerperium and are primarily due to preeclampsia and bleeding complications associated with placental abruption or other causes of obstetric hemorrhage. HELLP is also an important cause of AKI in pregnancy,[43] especially if it is not treated promptly by delivery. On occasion, nonsteroidal anti-inflammatory agents, used for postpartum analgesia, may precipitate AKI in patients who are volume depleted from hemorrhage, decreased fluid intake, or both. In severe cases of obstetric hemorrhage, acute cortical necrosis with associated disseminated intravascular coagulation may be present, and ultrasound or computed tomography may demonstrate hyperechoic or hypodense areas in the renal cortex.

General Management of Acute Kidney Injury in Pregnancy

The key issue in management of AKI in pregnancy is restoration of fluid volume deficits and, in later pregnancy, delivery of the baby and placenta as quickly as possible. No specific therapy is effective in acute cortical necrosis. Most patients with acute cortical necrosis ultimately require dialysis that may be permanent, but 20% to 40% have partial recovery of renal function. Both peritoneal dialysis and hemodialysis have been used during pregnancy, but peritoneal dialysis carries the risk of impairing uteroplacental blood flow.

Hemolytic-Uremic Syndrome and Thrombotic Thrombocytopenic Purpura

Although rare, thrombotic microangiopathy due to hemolytic-uremic syndrome (HUS) or thrombotic thrombocytopenic purpura (TTP) is an important cause of pregnancy-associated AKI, with considerable morbidity. Thrombotic microangiopathy shares several clinical and laboratory features of pregnancy-specific disorders, such as the HELLP variant of preeclampsia and acute fatty liver of pregnancy; thus, distinction of these syndromes is important for therapeutic and prognostic reasons.

Features that may be helpful in making the correct diagnosis include timing of onset and the pattern of laboratory abnormalities (Fig. 42.13). HELLP syndrome typically develops in the third trimester; only a few cases have developed in the postpartum period, usually within a few days of delivery. In contrast, the symptoms of HUS-TTP may begin antepartum, but most cases are diagnosed postpartum. Preeclampsia–HELLP syndrome is much more common than HUS-TTP, and it is usually preceded by hypertension and proteinuria. Renal failure is unusual in women with HELLP syndrome, even with severe cases, unless significant bleeding or hemodynamic instability or marked disseminated intravascular coagulation occurs. HELLP syndrome recovers with delivery, whereas HUS-TTP is often associated with persistent renal impairment and hypertension, with many requiring dialysis or transplantation long term.[44] Another laboratory feature of preeclampsia–HELLP syndrome that is not usually associated with HUS-TTP is marked elevation in liver enzymes. The presence of fever is more consistent with a diagnosis of TTP than of preeclampsia or HUS. Treatment of HUS-TTP includes plasma infusion or exchange and other modalities used in nonpregnant patients with these disorders. The management is discussed further in Chapter 28.

ACUTE FATTY LIVER OF PREGNANCY

Acute fatty liver of pregnancy (AFLP) is an extremely rare complication characterized by rapidly progressive liver failure that is estimated to occur in about 1 in 10,000 pregnancies. Women usually present with nausea, vomiting, and anorexia, and many have clinical and laboratory features that overlap with preeclampsia or HELLP syndrome (see Fig. 42.13). In addition to marked elevations in bilirubin, alanine transaminase, and aspartate transaminase, other frequently observed abnormalities include hypofibrinogenemia, prolonged partial thromboplastin time, hypoglycemia, anemia, and low platelet count. AKI occurs more commonly in AFLP than in the HELLP syndrome.[45] Because a defect in mitochondrial fatty acid oxidation due to mutations in the long-chain 3-hydroxyacyl-CoA dehydrogenase has recently been hypothesized as a risk factor for the development of fatty liver of pregnancy,[46] it is possible that the kidney dysfunction associated with AFLP reflects inhibition of β-oxidation of fats in the kidney. The histologic abnormalities are swollen hepatocytes filled with microvesicular fat and minimal hepatocellular necrosis. Delivery is urgently required, and most patients improve shortly afterward. This disorder was formerly associated with a more ominous outcome, which may have been a consequence of late diagnosis, although maternal mortality was two of six cases in a recent case series.[47]

REFERENCES

1. Packham D, Fairley KF. Renal biopsy: Indications and complications in pregnancy. *Br J Obstet Gynaecol.* 1987;94:935-939.
2. Lindheimer MD, Davison JM. Renal disorders. In: Barron WM, Lindheimer MD, eds. *Medical Disorders During Pregnancy.* St. Louis: Mosby–Year Book; 1990:42-72.
3. Smaill F. Antibiotics for asymptomatic bacteriuria in pregnancy. Cochrane Database Syst Rev. 2001;2:CD000490.
4. Rouse DJ, Andrews WW, Goldenberg RL, Owen J. Screening and treatment of asymptomatic bacteriuria of pregnancy to prevent pyelonephritis: A cost-effectiveness and cost-benefit analysis. *Obstet Gynecol.* 1995; 86:119-123.
5. August P, Lindheimer MD. Chronic hypertension and pregnancy. In: Laragh JH, Brenner BM, eds. *Chesley's Hypertensive Disorders in Pregnancy.* 2nd ed. Stamford, CT: Appleton & Lange; 1999:••.
6. Lindheimer MD, Richardson DA, Ehrlich EN, Katz AI. Potassium homeostasis in pregnancy. *J Reprod Med.* 1987;32:517-522.
7. Strevens H, Wide-Swensson D, Hansen A, et al. Glomerular endotheliosis in normal pregnancy and pre-eclampsia. *BJOG.* 2003;110: 831-836.
8. Geller DS, Farhi A, Pinkerton N, et al. Activating mineralocorticoid receptor mutation in hypertension exacerbated by pregnancy. *Science.* 2000;289:119-123.
9. ACOG practice bulletin. Diagnosis and management of preeclampsia and eclampsia. Number 33, January 2002. *Obstet Gynecol.* 2002;99: 159-167.
10. Karumanchi SA, Maynard SE, Stillman IE, et al. Preeclampsia: A renal perspective. *Kidney Int.* 2005;67:2101-2113.
11. Redman CW, Sargent IL. Latest advances in understanding preeclampsia. *Science.* 2005;308:1592-1594.
12. Red-Horse K, Zhou Y, Genbacev O, et al. Trophoblast differentiation during embryo implantation and formation of the maternal-fetal interface. *J Clin Invest.* 2004;114:744-754.
13. Podjarny E, Baylis C, Losonczy G. Animal models of preeclampsia. *Semin Perinatol.* 1999;23:2-13.
14. Wallukat G, Homuth V, Fischer T, et al. Patients with preeclampsia develop agonistic autoantibodies against the angiotensin AT_1 receptor. *J Clin Invest.* 1999;103:945-952.
15. Poston L, Briley AJ, Seed PT, et al. Vitamin C and vitamin E in pregnant women at risk for pre-eclampsia (VIP trial): Randomised placebo-controlled trial. *Lancet.* 2006;367:1145-1154.
16. Maynard SE, Min JY, Merchan J, et al. Excess placental soluble fms-like tyrosine kinase 1 (sFlt1) may contribute to endothelial dysfunction, hypertension, and proteinuria in preeclampsia. *J Clin Invest.* 2003;111: 649-658.
17. Levine RJ, Maynard SE, Qian C, et al. Circulating angiogenic factors and the risk of preeclampsia. *N Engl J Med.* 2004;350:672-683.
18. Lafayette RA, Druzin M, Sibley R, et al. Nature of glomerular dysfunction in pre-eclampsia. *Kidney Int.* 1998;54:1240-1249.
19. Lam C, Lim KH, Karumanchi SA. Circulating angiogenic factors in the pathogenesis and prediction of preeclampsia. *Hypertension.* 2005;46: 1077-1085.
20. Bdolah Y, Palomaki GE, Yaron Y, et al. Circulating angiogenic proteins in trisomy 13. *Am J Obstet Gynecol.* 2006;194:239-245.
21. Eremina V, Sood M, Haigh J, et al. Glomerular-specific alterations of VEGF-A expression lead to distinct congenital and acquired renal diseases. *J Clin Invest.* 2003;111:707-716.
22. Thadhani R, Ecker JL, Mutter WP, et al. Insulin resistance and alterations in angiogenesis: Additive insults that may lead to preeclampsia. *Hypertension.* 2004;43:988-992.
23. Venkatesha S, Toporsian M, Lam C, et al. Soluble endoglin contributes to the pathogenesis of preeclampsia. *Nat Med.* 2006;12:642-649.
24. Levine RJ, Lam C, Qian C, et al. Soluble endoglin and other circulating antiangiogenic factors in preeclampsia. *N Engl J Med.* 2006;355: 992-1005.
25. Fisher KA, Luger A, Spargo BH, Lindheimer MD. Hypertension in pregnancy: Clinical-pathological correlations and remote prognosis. *Medicine (Baltimore).* 1981;60:267-276.
26. August P, Lenz T, Ales KL, et al. Longitudinal study of the renin-angiotensin-aldosterone system in hypertensive pregnant women: Deviations related to the development of superimposed preeclampsia. *Am J Obstet Gynecol.* 1990;163:1612-1621.
27. Moran P, Baylis PH, Lindheimer MD, Davison JM. Glomerular ultrafiltration in normal and preeclamptic pregnancy. *J Am Soc Nephrol.* 2003;14:648-652.
28. Kang DH, Finch J, Nakagawa T, et al. Uric acid, endothelial dysfunction and pre-eclampsia: Searching for a pathogenetic link. *J Hypertens.* 2004;22:229-235.
29. Hinchey J, Chaves C, Appignani B, et al. A reversible posterior leukoencephalopathy syndrome. *N Engl J Med.* 1996;334:494-500.
30. Sibai BM. Diagnosis, controversies, and management of the syndrome of hemolysis, elevated liver enzymes, and low platelet count. *Obstet Gynecol.* 2004;103:981-991.
31. Sibai BM, el-Nazer A, Gonzalez-Ruiz A. Severe preeclampsia-eclampsia in young primigravid women: Subsequent pregnancy outcome and remote prognosis. *Am J Obstet Gynecol.* 1986;155:1011-1016.
32. Irgens HU, Reisaeter L, Irgens LM, Lie RT. Long term mortality of mothers and fathers after pre-eclampsia: Population based cohort study. *BMJ.* 2001;323:1213-1217.
33. Epstein FH. Late vascular effects of toxemia of pregnancy. *N Engl J Med.* 1964;271:391-395.
34. Funai EF, Friedlander Y, Paltiel O, et al. Long-term mortality after preeclampsia. *Epidemiology.* 2005;16:206-215.
35. Vikse BE, Irgens LM, Leivestad T, et al. Preeclampsia and the risk of end-stage renal disease. *N Engl J Med.* 2008;359:800-809.
36. Caritis S, Sibai B, Hauth J, et al. Low-dose aspirin to prevent preeclampsia in women at high risk. *N Engl J Med.* 1998;338:701-705.

37. Duley L, Henderson-Smart DJ, Meher S, King JF. Antiplatelet agents for preventing pre-eclampsia and its complications. Cochrane Database Syst Rev. 2007;2:CD004659.
38. Villar J, Abdel-Aleem H, Merialdi M, et al. World Health Organization randomized trial of calcium supplementation among low calcium intake pregnant women. *Am J Obstet Gynecol.* 2006;194:639-649.
39. Podymow T, August P. Update on the use of antihypertensive drugs in pregnancy. *Hypertension.* 2008;51:960-969.
40. Fonseca JE, Mendez F, Catano C, Arias F. Dexamethasone treatment does not improve the outcome of women with HELLP syndrome: A double-blind, placebo-controlled, randomized clinical trial. *Am J Obstet Gynecol.* 2005;193:1591-1598.
41. Prakash J, Kumar H, Sinha DK, et al. Acute renal failure in pregnancy in a developing country: Twenty years of experience. *Ren Fail.* 2006;28: 309-313.
42. Gammill HS, Jeyabalan A. Acute renal failure in pregnancy. *Crit Care Med.* 2005;33:S372-S384.
43. Khoury JC, Miodovnik M, LeMasters G, Sibai B. Pregnancy outcome and progression of diabetic nephropathy. What's next? *J Matern Fetal Neonatal Med.* 2002;11:238-244.
44. Dashe JS, Ramin SM, Cunningham FG. The long-term consequences of thrombotic microangiopathy (thrombotic thrombocytopenic purpura and hemolytic uremic syndrome) in pregnancy. *Obstet Gynecol.* 1998; 91:662-668.
45. Vigil-De Gracia P. Acute fatty liver and HELLP syndrome: Two distinct pregnancy disorders. *Int J Gynaecol Obstet.* 2001;73:215-220.
46. Ibdah JA, Bennett MJ, Rinaldo P, et al. A fetal fatty-acid oxidation disorder as a cause of liver disease in pregnant women. *N Engl J Med.* 1999;340:1723-1731.
47. Fesenmeier MF, Coppage KH, Lambers DS, et al. Acute fatty liver of pregnancy in 3 tertiary care centers. *Am J Obstet Gynecol.* 2005;192: 1416-1419.
48. Karumanchi SA, Epstein FH. Placental ischemia and soluble fms-like tyrosine kinase 1: Cause or consequence of preeclampsia? *Kidney Int.* 2007;71:959-961.

CHAPTER 43

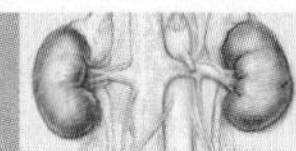

Pregnancy with Preexisting Kidney Disease

Mark A. Brown

Historically, renal disease was considered a contraindication to pregnancy, but now many pregnant women with chronic kidney disease (CKD) have successful outcomes. Accordingly, nephrologists and obstetricians need to be skilled in the management and counseling of such women.

THE ADVERSE EFFECTS OF CHRONIC KIDNEY DISEASE ON PREGNANCY

Up to 3% to 10% of women of childbearing age have CKD stages 3 to 5.[1] Available data on pregnancy outcomes are mainly from studies published 10 to 20 years ago[2-4] and probably overestimate risk compared with outcomes achieved with modern care, particularly with improvements in neonatal intensive care. The key pre-pregnancy factors predicting outcome include:

- Degree of renal impairment.
- Control of hypertension before pregnancy.
- Degree of proteinuria.

In most circumstances, these features are more important than the mother's specific renal disease in predicting outcome.

Most women with mild renal impairment (serum creatinine concentration <1.5 mg/dl [130 μmol/l]) and controlled hypertension have a successful pregnancy outcome. Preexisting hypertension is probably the main predictor of pregnancy outcome in women with mild renal impairment.

In contrast, those with moderate (serum creatinine concentration of 1.5 to 2.5 mg/dl [130 to 220 μmol/l]) to severe (>2.5 mg/dl [220 μmol/l]) renal impairment, particularly when it is accompanied by hypertension and heavy proteinuria, have a lower chance of having a live baby and a greater risk for maternal complications, including progression of the renal disease (Fig. 43.1).

Control of Hypertension

A retrospective analysis of 358 pregnant women with CKD in the United Kingdom found an association between diastolic blood pressure (BP) above 90 mm Hg (treated or untreated) and neonatal death. This relatively mild degree of hypertension also compounded the risk of preterm birth that arises from renal impairment alone.[5]

Progression of Chronic Kidney Disease

The risk of progression of renal disease during pregnancy likewise depends less on the specific renal disorder but more on:

- Baseline serum creatinine concentration.
- Control of hypertension.
- Increasing proteinuria or the onset of superimposed preeclampsia.

The natural history of most CKD is that accelerated deterioration during a pregnancy is unlikely, the main exception being systemic lupus, which can flare, leading to worsening renal disease during the pregnancy. However, 50% of women with moderate renal impairment (serum creatinine >1.5 mg/dl [130 μmol/l]) have a significant rise in serum creatinine in the third trimester or early postpartum, and if this occurs, almost one in five progresses to end-stage renal disease within 6 months after delivery.

Prematurity or Fetal Growth Restriction

Prematurity, fetal growth restriction, and stillbirth are the major concerns for pregnancies of women with renal impairment, particularly if superimposed preeclampsia develops. Uncontrolled hypertension at conception is a poor prognostic feature in terms of fetal outcome (Fig. 43.2).

Fertility

Fertility rate is reduced in women with moderate to severe renal impairment, but there are no precise estimates. Because even women on dialysis may become pregnant, all should be advised to use contraception unless planning a pregnancy.

MANAGEMENT COMMON TO ALL PREGNANCY WITH PREEXISTING KIDNEY DISEASE

The principles of management of pregnancy in women with CKD are summarized in Figure 43.3.

Pre-Pregnancy Counseling

Any woman with CKD stages 3 to 5 should receive pre-pregnancy counseling. So should women with CKD stages 1 and 2 if they have hypertension, significant proteinuria, poor obstetric history, recurrent urine infections, inheritable renal disease, or diseases (e.g., systemic lupus) likely to worsen during pregnancy. Issues that should be covered in counseling are shown in Figure 43.4.

Excretory Renal Function

Glomerular filtration rate (GFR) rises by about 50% during normal pregnancy, typically apparent by the end of the first trimester (see Chapter 41). Serum creatinine above 1 mg/dl (88 μmol/l) in a pregnant woman generally indicates reduced

Renal Outcomes According to Pre-Pregnancy Serum Creatinine

Creatinine < 1.5 mg/dl (130 μmol/l)
- Permanent loss of GFR in <10% of women
- Major determinant of ESRD progression is hypertension

Creatinine 1.5–2.5 mg/dl (130–220 μmol/l)
- Decline or permanent loss of GFR in 30% of women
- Increased to 50% if uncontrolled hypertension
- 10% ESRD soon after pregnancy

Creatinine > 2.5 mg/dl (220 μmol/l)
- Progression to ESRD highly likely during or soon after pregnancy

Figure 43.1 Renal outcomes according to pre-pregnancy serum creatinine. ESRD, end-stage renal disease; GFR, glomerular filtration rate.

Fetal Outcomes According to Maternal Serum Creatinine Before Pregnancy

Outcomes after accounting for first-trimester miscarriage

Creatinine < 1.5 mg/dl (130 μmol/l)
- Live births in >90% of women

Creatinine 1.5–2.5 mg/dl (130–220 μmol/l)
- Live births in about 85% of women unless uncontrolled hypertension (MAP >105) at conception
- 60% prematurity - mainly iatrogenic (preeclampsia/fetal growth restriction)

Creatinine > 2.5 mg/dl (220 μmol/l)
- Fetal loss high - estimates uncertain

Figure 43.2 Fetal outcomes according to maternal serum creatinine before pregnancy. MAP, mean arterial pressure.

Principles of Antenatal Care with Preexisting CKD

- Management of hypertension aiming for BP 110-140/80-90 mm Hg
- Use aspirin (75–150 mg/day) if creatinine ≥ 1.5 mg/dl (130 μmol/l)
- Correct interpretation and management of changes in serum creatinine
- Measurement, interpretation, and management of proteinuria, including nephrotic syndrome – use heparin prophylaxis if nephrotic
- Identification and management of urinary tract infection
- Clinical assessment and maintenance of volume homeostasis
- Consideration of appropriate "renal" and antihypertensive medications throughout pregnancy – cease statins, ACEI, and ARB
- Identification of superimposed preeclampsia
- Assessment of fetal well-being – review at each visit whether there are indications for delivery (see fig 43.5)
- Consideration of the primary underlying renal disease and its peculiar problems

Figure 43.3 Principles of antenatal care with preexisting CKD. ACEI, angiotensin-converting enzyme inhibitor; ARB, angiotensin receptor blocker; BP, blood pressure; GFR, glomerular filtration rate.

Pre-pregnancy Counseling in CKD

Maternal risks
Accelerated decline in GFR, sometimes precipitating dialysis during pregnancy or soon after
Severe maternal hypertension
Superimposed preeclampsia with renal, hepatic, thrombotic, or bleeding and neurologic risks
Nephrotic syndrome with risks of thrombosis or sepsis

Fetal risks
Fetal growth restriction or intrauterine fetal death due to placental insufficiency
Prematurity
Complications of drug therapy for renal disease during pregnancy
Inheritance of a renal disorder

Figure 43.4 Pre-pregnancy counseling in CKD. Issue that should be discussed at pre-pregnancy counseling for women with CKD. GFR, glomerular filtration rate.

GFR. The Modification of Diet in Renal Disease (MDRD) study equation or other formulae that estimate GFR are not valid for pregnancy. Measurement of creatinine clearance requires 24-hour urine collection, which is cumbersome; and even when it is conducted diligently, it may be inaccurate because of ureteral dilation, which results in pooling of urine and an incomplete collection. Serum cystatin C is being evaluated, but serum creatinine remains the standard for assessment of GFR during pregnancy.

The limited outcome data for pregnancy with kidney disease are mainly derived from studies using serum creatinine.

Blood Urea Nitrogen

Increments in blood urea nitrogen (BUN) and creatinine may indicate deteriorating GFR and point to the need for initiation of dialysis if the pregnancy is to have any chance of success (see later, Dialysis in Pregnancy). However, a rising BUN concentration, particularly when it is accompanied by rising hemoglobin or hematocrit, may represent intravascular contraction, typically seen in preeclampsia.

Serum Electrolytes, Albumin, and Volume Homeostasis

Plasma sodium and bicarbonate are slightly reduced, potassium is at the lower end of the normal range, and albumin and urate are lower than in the nonpregnant state. Increases in plasma sodium to levels of nonpregnant women should raise the possibility of (reversible) pregnancy-specific diabetes insipidus (due to excess placental vasopressinase). In general, this is a mild disorder, but DDAVP should be given if plasma sodium rises above 150 mmol/l.

Adequate intravascular volume is essential to preservation of GFR and good pregnancy outcome for mother and baby. Clinically, it is difficult to assess maternal volume homeostasis. Edema is an unhelpful sign in pregnancy, so hematocrit should be measured in women with underlying CKD at the initial first-trimester visit, along with serum albumin. Both measures should fall slightly as pregnancy progresses. A rise in either value strongly suggests intravascular volume contraction, although there is no absolute discriminant value. Conversely, a significant fall in either value does not by itself diagnose excessive volume expansion because the hematocrit depends on other factors, and serum albumin may fall in patients with nephrotic syndrome, who in turn may have reduced intravascular volume.

In practice, volume excess, provided there is no respiratory compromise and BP can be controlled, is more favorable than volume depletion for maternal renal function and fetal growth.

When there is concern about fetal growth or deteriorating GFR in women with CKD and reduced intravascular volume is suggested by the change in hematocrit and albumin from baseline, a trial of intravenous normal saline (no more than 1 liter) under observation in the hospital is a reasonable clinical approach.

Urinalysis

A dipstick test result of "negative" or "trace" protein in most (but not all) cases excludes true proteinuria. Any woman with 1+ (0.3 g/l) proteinuria or above should have formal quantification of protein excretion with either a spot urine protein to creatinine (PC) ratio or a 24-hour urine collection.

Glycosuria may be normal and is not diagnostic of diabetes mellitus. However, when glycosuria is detected in early pregnancy in a woman with CKD, a formal 75-g oral glucose tolerance test should be arranged.

Dipstick hematuria during pregnancy is common and often resolves after delivery. Provided there is no urinary tract infection, urine sediment is inactive, and serum creatinine concentration is normal, this is not associated with adverse maternal or fetal outcomes during pregnancy and can be investigated if it is persistent postpartum.[6] Pregnancy may be the first time a woman's urine is examined, so previously undetected renal disorders may be diagnosed.

Proteinuria and Nephrotic Syndrome

In the nonpregnant woman, daily protein excretion is generally less than 150 mg/day, composed of up to 20 mg/day albumin and the remainder of other proteins, often of tubular origin.[7] Albumin excretion during normal pregnancy is unchanged, but total protein excretion is increased in normal pregnancy, predominantly because of an increase in the porosity of the glomerular basement membrane, through unknown mechanisms.[7] The upper limit of normal protein excretion during pregnancy is defined as 300 mg/day. In a midstream specimen of urine, a PC ratio above 30 mg/mmol (0.3 mg/mg) correlates with proteinuria of more than 300 mg/day.[8]

New-Onset Proteinuria

Isolated non-nephrotic proteinuria may develop *de novo* during pregnancy.[9] In these cases, in which GFR is normal, one of three scenarios usually unfolds:

1. Preeclampsia is subsequently evident.
2. No pregnancy complications occur, and the proteinuria disappears postpartum.
3. Intrinsic glomerular disease has developed and remains postpartum. In my experience, this is an uncommon event.

Preexisting Proteinuria

Although the spot urine PC ratio in pregnancy is a reasonably reliable method of determining whether protein excretion is abnormal, there have been no studies to date to show that serial measurements of urine PC ratio reliably predict *changes* in proteinuria. A practical approach is to measure 24-hour urinary protein and creatinine excretion and to determine the PC ratio at the early pregnancy visit; subsequent PC ratios will give a guide to that woman's protein excretion.

When there is a true increase in protein excretion during pregnancy in women with underlying renal disease, there are few therapeutic options apart from ensuring BP control (see later).

Nephrotic Syndrome

The one situation in which 24-hour urinary protein excretion should be measured in these women is to diagnose nephrotic syndrome. Because serum albumin concentration falls in most pregnancies because of volume expansion and is often below 30 g/l, this is not a reliable indicator of nephrotic syndrome. A spot urine PC ratio above 230 mg/mmol indicates that protein excretion is above 3 g/day,[10] and this should be confirmed with measurement of 24-hour urinary protein. These women will generally have edema, but this is unhelpful as it occurs in two thirds of normal pregnancies. Although a rise in serum cholesterol level is typical of nephrotic syndrome, this may occur during normal pregnancy.

Confirmation of true nephrotic syndrome has important implications in pregnancy. There will be urinary loss of vitamin D–binding protein, transferrin, immunoglobulins, and antithrombin III (accompanied by increased hepatic synthesis of clotting factors) and a propensity for intravascular volume contraction. These changes can result in calcium deficiency, iron deficiency, increased likelihood of infection, thrombosis and reduced uteroplacental blood flow with fetal growth restriction or death,[11] and sometimes reduced renal blood flow with worsening renal function. Treatment requires oral calcium, vitamin D, and iron supplementation and subcutaneous heparin for thrombosis prophylaxis, ensuring adequate fetal growth and amniotic fluid by ultrasound and reassessment of maternal serum creatinine concentration on a regular basis. If nephrotic syndrome occurs early in pregnancy, I add vitamin D for prophylaxis against osteoporosis, although there are no controlled trials to test this practice.

Hypertension

Hypertension in pregnancy is defined as BP above 140/90 mm Hg, and this is generally the threshold for treatment, with an acceptable range on treatment of 110 to 140/80 to 90 mm Hg. This range of treatment is not based on solid pregnancy outcome data but is thought to be the range that reduces maternal risk for severe hypertension while providing sufficient systemic BP to maintain placental perfusion. Because the target BP for nonpregnant women with CKD is less than 130/80 mm Hg (or <125/75 mm Hg with proteinuria >1 g/day), a woman with CKD may have a period of 40 weeks or so when BP is above usual target, which may contribute to progressive renal impairment after the pregnancy. Nevertheless, if a pregnant woman develops BP below 110/80 mm Hg, it is my practice to reduce antihypertensives to avoid the risk of fetal hypoperfusion.

Most pregnant women with CKD will not exhibit the usual early fall in BP, and in many, BP increases as the pregnancy progresses. Why this occurs is not entirely clear. Normal pregnancy is accompanied by significant volume expansion that does not usually induce hypertension. However, in CKD, there is often inability to excrete a sodium load with accompanying hypertension, and it is likely that this mechanism contributes in pregnancy. Other factors almost certainly playing a role in this hypertension include stimulation of the renin-angiotensin and sympathetic nervous systems; alterations in endothelial factors, such as prostacyclin, nitric oxide, and endothelin; and particularly in transplant patients, the drugs used, such as calcineurin inhibitors and corticosteroids. Regardless of its cause, persistence of hypertension is an adverse factor in pregnancy outcome.[12] Fear of using antihypertensives in pregnancy has been associated with poorer pregnancy outcomes, at least in women with renal transplants.[13]

BP will often rise significantly soon after delivery. Therefore, BP measurement and treatment should be undertaken diligently in the early postpartum period.

Control of BP is imperative to successful pregnancy outcome in women with underlying renal disease. Diuretics are not recommended during pregnancy as any reduction in maternal plasma volume may have adverse effects on uteroplacental or renal perfusion. Angiotensin-converting enzyme (ACE) inhibitors or angiotensin receptor blockers (ARBs) must be discontinued, preferably before pregnancy but certainly as soon as pregnancy is diagnosed because of increased risks of fetal growth restriction, oligohydramnios, neonatal renal failure, and probably cardiac and neurologic development abnormalities. Aldosterone antagonists should also be avoided. Atenolol has been associated with fetal growth restriction. Suitable antihypertensives include methyldopa, labetalol, oxprenolol, hydralazine, and nifedipine, and they may all be used in conventional doses. Diltiazem may also have a small benefit.

Superimposed Preeclampsia

Preeclampsia (see Chapter 42) is a placental disorder of unknown etiology that has several predisposing risk factors, one of which is CKD. The maternal renal effects of preeclampsia include a reduction in renal blood flow, increased sodium and uric acid reabsorption, reduced circulating renin and aldosterone concentrations, proteinuria, and impaired GFR.[14]

Superimposed preeclampsia in a woman with underlying renal impairment will lead to worsening renal function; exaggerated hypertension and proteinuria with risks of nephrotic syndrome; short-term and long-term risks to maternal renal function; and increased risks for fetal growth restriction, prematurity, and perinatal mortality.

However, it is difficult to diagnose superimposed preeclampsia in a woman who begins her pregnancy with renal impairment or proteinuria. An increase in BP, decline in GFR, increased serum urate, or increasing protein excretion can all be due to progression of the underlying renal disorder rather than superimposed preeclampsia, and as yet there is no definitive diagnostic test. However, when these features are accompanied by neurologic signs such as hyperreflexia with clonus or by abnormal liver transaminases or new-onset thrombocytopenia (except in systemic lupus), it is highly likely that superimposed preeclampsia has developed. Typically, these changes occur after 20 weeks of gestation.

Diagnosis of superimposed preeclampsia is to some extent an academic exercise as clinicians managing the woman with underlying renal disease should be vigilant for changes in maternal and fetal condition in all cases, and the indications for delivery in women with preeclampsia are broadly the same as those in women with progressive underlying renal disease (Fig. 43.5).

Limited studies suggest that aspirin is of benefit in reducing superimposed preeclampsia and perinatal death in women with

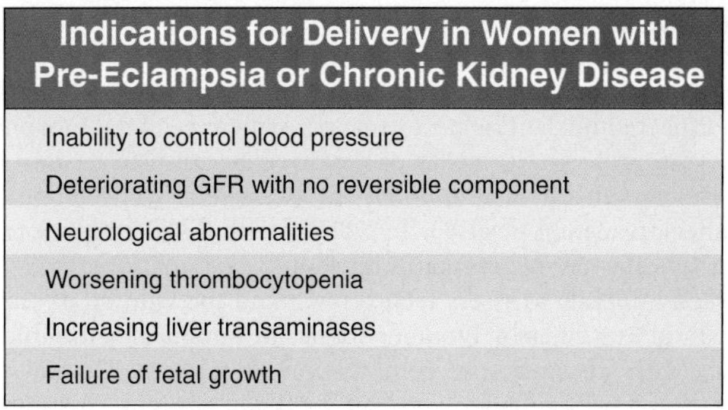

Indications for Delivery in Women with Pre-Eclampsia or Chronic Kidney Disease
Inability to control blood pressure
Deteriorating GFR with no reversible component
Neurological abnormalities
Worsening thrombocytopenia
Increasing liver transaminases
Failure of fetal growth

Figure 43.5 Indications for delivery in women with preeclampsia or CKD. GFR, glomerular filtration rate.

underlying renal disease; the number needed to treat was between 9 and 57 for prevention of preeclampsia and between 42 and 357 to prevent perinatal death.[15] The PARIS study also found that aspirin reduced superimposed preeclampsia in women with underlying renal disease (RR 0.63, 0.38-1.06), but only 450 women were included in this analysis.[16] My practice is to use low-dose aspirin (150 mg/day) for all women with CKD and serum creatinine above 1.5 mg/dl (130 μmol/l) or for those with lower serum creatinine who have had early-onset severe preeclampsia or fetal loss in a previous pregnancy; the effects of this dose of aspirin on renal function are minimal, and this is generally a safe approach.

RENAL BIOPSY IN PREGNANCY

It is rare for renal biopsy to be required in pregnancy. After 32 weeks of gestation, if the renal state has changed so much that biopsy is considered necessary to guide treatment, it is better to deliver the baby and to manage the renal disease outside of pregnancy. Situations in which biopsy may provide information that could have a significant impact on the pregnancy outcome for mother and baby are the following:

1. *De novo* onset of nephrotic-range proteinuria or unexplained impaired GFR with abnormal urine sediment before fetal viability, that is, before 24 weeks of gestation. Nephrotic syndrome after this stage can generally be managed conservatively until delivery usually at about 32 weeks. Most such cases are due to preeclampsia.
2. Before 32 weeks of gestation when the clinician and patient have agreed that immunosuppression or plasma exchange will be used if necessary while prolonging the pregnancy to about 32 weeks: rapidly declining GFR without any apparent reversible cause in women with underlying primary glomerulonephritis; acute kidney injury with active urine sediment; and declining GFR or increasing proteinuria in a woman with lupus nephritis or lupus without previously known nephritis.
3. Deteriorating GFR before 32 weeks of gestation without obvious cause in a woman with a kidney transplant to exclude acute rejection.

The usual technique of renal biopsy (see Chapter 6) can be applied in pregnancy, although the sitting position rather than the supine position is better tolerated in the second trimester onward. Complication rates of renal biopsy in pregnancy are similar to those in general nephrology practice.[17]

ASSESSMENT OF FETAL WELL-BEING

An early pregnancy ultrasound is invaluable in accurately dating the expected birth. The next usual assessment is a fetal morphology scan at 18 to 20 weeks of gestation to confirm gestational age, to screen for fetal anomaly, to assess fetal well-being, and to check placental position. In women with CKD stages 3 to 5, this is followed by regular ultrasound examinations at 2- to 4-week intervals to assess fetal growth and the volume of amniotic fluid as well as by Doppler studies of umbilical artery blood flow. More recently, the combination of tests at 12 weeks of gestation for pregnancy-associated plasma protein A, inhibin, human chorionic gonadotropin, and alpha-fetoprotein with measurement of uterine artery pulsatility index at 20 weeks of gestation has provided a good negative predictive test for fetal outcome in women with high-risk pregnancies, although these studies are not specific for women with underlying renal disease.

Asymmetric intrauterine growth restriction [IUGR], in which the abdominal measurements are more decreased than the fetal head and femur measurements, is characteristic of IUGR related to maternal CKD.

Amniotic fluid volume correlates well with perinatal outcome, and a low amniotic fluid index helps distinguish babies small because of IUGR from those that are constitutionally small. Mid-trimester severe oligohydramnios is associated with very poor outcome; it indicates nonfunctioning fetal kidneys and usually also leads to pulmonary hypoplasia and limb contractures.

Absent end-diastolic flow on umbilical artery velocimetry is usually an indication for delivery, depending on gestation. The development of reversed end-diastolic flow flags a high risk of fetal hypoxia, acidosis, and death.

Fetal assessment by one or more of these means should be carried out regularly throughout pregnancy and particularly in the third trimester.

TIMING OF DELIVERY

In women with stable CKD and no evidence of fetal compromise, pregnancies can be continued to term and spontaneous labor awaited. The method of delivery, either vaginal or by cesarean section, is normally determined by other issues (such as previous cesarean section, presentation, or previous poor obstetric history) rather than by the presence of CKD *per se*. The usual indications for delivery are listed in Figure 43.5.

The goal is to time delivery such that the risks of delivery (to both mother and fetus) are less than the risks if the pregnancy continues. This is often a difficult and individual decision requiring consultation among nephrologist or obstetric medicine physician, obstetrician, midwife, and neonatologist. The following issues need to be considered:

1. Gestational age is the most important determinant of outcome. Decisions are difficult to make at the borderlines of viability (23 to 25 weeks of gestation). Although outcome data vary from country to country, approximate survival rates increase from 30% at 23 weeks to 65% at 25 weeks to 95% at 30 weeks of gestation. Babies born before 30 weeks of gestation have significant risks of long-term morbidity, including chronic lung disease and cerebral palsy.
2. The most common problem faced by preterm babies is respiratory distress syndrome. Maternally administered antenatal corticosteroids, generally intramuscular betamethasone (11.4 mg, two doses 12 hours apart), have been shown to reduce respiratory distress syndrome by 50%. For best effect, the corticosteroids need to be administered at least 24 hours before delivery.
3. There is less neonatal morbidity and mortality if babies are born in hospitals where there is appropriate neonatal care rather than being transferred after delivery. Thus, if preterm delivery is likely, transfer of the mother to an appropriate unit before delivery should be considered.

Whereas these pregnancies are certainly high risk compared with the normal pregnant woman, it is important for clinicians and midwives to remember that the final pregnancy outcome in most cases is successful for both mother and baby. Clinicians can take a positive approach, at all times emphasizing the need for diligence and assessment for potential complications but highlighting that the end result in most cases will be good, in turn helping to relieve some of the stress that accompanies pregnancy for these women.

MANAGEMENT OF SPECIFIC RENAL DISORDERS DURING PREGNANCY

The most common chronic kidney diseases predating pregnancy are primary glomerulonephritis (usually IgA nephropathy or focal segmental glomerulosclerosis), diabetic nephropathy, lupus nephritis, and reflux nephropathy.

IgA Nephropathy

Long-term follow-up of childhood IgA nephropathy showed that later pregnancy was complicated by hypertension in half the cases and prematurity in one third,[18] but these outcomes are not peculiar to this renal disease. Rare cases are familial, in which case the pregnant woman should be advised to have her child screened by urinalysis in the first few years of life. Macroscopic hematuria is no more likely during pregnancy unless there is intervening respiratory or gastrointestinal tract infection. IgA nephropathy should be managed like other CKD during pregnancy.

Diabetic Nephropathy

Recent data in the United Kingdom found that 8% of pregnant women with type 1 diabetes and 5% of those with type 2 diabetes had nephropathy.[19] Diabetes *per se* increases risks for preterm birth, cesarean section, and perinatal mortality. The presence of overt nephropathy more than doubles the risk of fetal death after 20 weeks. There is an added risk for congenital abnormalities if blood glucose concentration was not adequately controlled at the time of conception.

The Diabetes Control and Complications Trial and the EURODIAB study both concluded that pregnancy does not increase the progression of diabetes to early diabetic nephropathy (microalbuminuria).[20,21] Whereas microalbuminuria alone did not correlate with increased perinatal risk, both prematurity and superimposed preeclampsia rates were higher than in type 1 diabetics without microalbuminuria.

The outcome of established diabetic nephropathy during pregnancy depends on the usual factors of preexisting renal impairment and control of hypertension. Meticulous control is required of both blood glucose concentration and BP during pregnancy in women with early or overt diabetic nephropathy. One study showed that failure to achieve mean arterial pressure of less than 100 mm Hg was associated with increased risk of early delivery even after adjustment for glucose control.[22] Ideally, ACE inhibitors should be introduced soon after delivery for prevention of progression of diabetic nephropathy; at least captopril is safe during breast-feeding.

Lupus Nephritis

Women with lupus nephritis should have quiescent disease at conception to offer the best chance of a successful pregnancy outcome. Those with active disease at conception have a higher likelihood for development of acute lupus nephritis during pregnancy, which is then associated with high fetal risk. Ideally, women with lupus should be in remission for about 12 months before conception and on maintenance corticosteroids in doses less than prednisolone 20 mg/day. In such women, the prior histologic class of lupus nephritis has no influence on pregnancy outcome. Hydroxychloroquine may be continued during pregnancy.

New onset or a flare of lupus nephritis, evidenced by increasing proteinuria, active urine sediment, and rising serum creatinine concentration, is a major concern, and such cases have sometimes been associated with maternal death. These women, with new onset or a flare of lupus nephritis, should be treated by increasing doses of prednisolone with the early introduction of azathioprine. Some prefer to undertake renal biopsy at this point to confirm the histologic changes before introducing immunosuppression. Either approach is reasonable, but my approach is to introduce corticosteroids and azathioprine and to reserve biopsy for after delivery.

Other women with known lupus nephritis in remission before conception should remain on their low-dose prednisolone and azathioprine throughout pregnancy. Cyclophosphamide is contraindicated in pregnancy because of teratogenicity; although it has been used successfully in a few cases of lupus nephritis, its use is not recommended.

Lupus nephritis may develop or flare in the postpartum period, but prophylactic corticosteroid therapy in those who have not had a flare during the pregnancy is not indicated. The major cause of maternal death in lupus nephritis is sepsis, and immunosuppression should be used with care in pregnant women.[23]

Reflux Nephropathy

As for other renal disorders, the outcome of pregnancies in women with reflux nephropathy depends on the preexisting renal function and control of BP rather than on the disorder itself. Approximately one in four may develop preeclampsia, and about 40% of offspring have vesicoureteral reflux. These women are more predisposed to urinary tract infection throughout pregnancy, as are women who have had surgically corrected reflux in childhood.[24] Around 20% of women with reflux nephropathy will develop urinary tract infection in pregnancy,[25] with about 6% of these due to acute pyelonephritis. Significant urinary tract infection can be associated with premature labor or spontaneous rupture of membranes. Regular urine culture should be obtained throughout pregnancy in women with underlying reflux nephropathy.

Inherited Renal Disorders

Inherited renal disorders are likely to have been diagnosed before the pregnancy, and the specific implications of this for the offspring will have been discussed. The most common is autosomal dominant polycystic kidney disease. Others include Alport's syndrome and familial hyperuricemic nephropathy.

Reflux nephropathy is not inherited by specific mendelian traits but tends to cosegregate within families, and the pregnant woman needs to be aware of this.

Fetal renal anomalies are usually identified at the time of routine ultrasound screening or during evaluation of a fetus from a family with a known hereditary renal disorder. Invasive procedures, such as chorionic villus sampling for DNA analysis, are rarely informative and should be undertaken only after advice from a clinical geneticist.

RECURRENT URINARY TRACT INFECTION

Urinary tract infection during pregnancy develops more readily into acute pyelonephritis and is generally of greater consequence than in the nonpregnant state.

Asymptomatic bacteriuria occurs in 2% to 10% of pregnancies and is associated with preterm labor, IUGR, and perinatal mortality. In the normal nongravid woman, asymptomatic bacteriuria rarely progresses to cystitis. In pregnancy, however, the chance for development of overt infection is much greater, with rates of acute pyelonephritis complicating asymptomatic bacteriuria reported as high as 40%. If asymptomatic bacteriuria is treated in pregnant women, this risk is reduced to below 10%. The range of organisms causing urinary tract infection in pregnancy does not differ from that outside of pregnancy; *Escherichia coli* causes approximately 90% of infections.

Standard antenatal care should include culture of a midstream specimen of urine early in the pregnancy. In those with abnormal urinary tract structure, a history of recurrent urinary tract infection, CKD, or diabetes, further regular cultures are required. Women who have threatened premature labor should have further urine cultures even without symptoms suggestive of urinary tract infection. Treatment of bacteriuria has been proved beneficial in a number of randomized controlled studies[26]; 3 days of treatment is recommended for treating and eradicating bacteriuria. Amoxicillin resistance is relatively common; it should be replaced by cephalexin, amoxicillin–clavulanic acid, trimethoprim, or nitrofurantoin (Fig. 43.6).

Women with a history of recurrent urinary tract infection should have monthly urine cultures. For those with a predictable history of postcoital cystitis, postcoital single-dose cephalexin (250 mg) or nitrofurantoin (50 mg) can significantly reduce the likelihood of infection. For others with recurrent urinary tract infection before pregnancy, low-dose first-generation cephalosporins at night may help suppress further infections and therefore reduce the risks of pyelonephritis and premature labor. Any woman who has recurrent urinary tract infection before pregnancy should undergo ultrasound of the urinary tract before conception or in early pregnancy to exclude structural disease.

Prophylactic antibiotics should also be given to women with recurrent asymptomatic bacteriuria or infection during pregnancy. Nighttime cephalexin (250 mg) or nitrofurantoin (50 mg) is usually sufficient to prevent infection. Breakthrough infections should be treated with a 7-day course of antibiotics.

Pyelonephritis is usually uncomplicated but can cause bacteremia, anemia, respiratory insufficiency, renal impairment, and premature labor. In pregnancy, pyelonephritis should be managed initially in the hospital with intravenous fluids and intravenous antibiotics. Empiric antibiotics should include a cephalosporin and gentamicin added if this proves unsuccessful.

Antibiotic Regimens for Treatment of Urinary Tract Infections in Pregnancy

Acute Cystitis			
Amoxicillin	500 mg	Three times daily	3–7 days
Nitrofurantoin	100 mg	Twice daily	3–7 days
Cephalexin	500 mg	Two-three times daily	3–7 days
Asymptomatic Bacteriuria			
Cephalexin	500 mg	Three times daily	3 days
Amoxicillin	500 mg	Three times daily	3 days
Amoxicillin–clavulanic acid	500 mg	Three times daily	3 days
Nitrofurantoin	50 mg	Four times daily	3 days
Fosfomycin	3 g	Single dose	
Recurrent Bacteriuria or Cystitis			
Cephalexin		250 mg nighttime (or postcoital)	
Nitrofurantoin		50 mg nighttime (or postcoital)	
Amoxicillin		250 mg nighttime (or postcoital)	
Pyelonephritis (inital IV therapy)			
Ceftriaxone		1 g daily	
Ampicillin (with gentamicin)		1 g q6h	
Gentamicin		3 mg/kg daily	
Ticarcillin		3.2 g q8h	
Piperacillin		4 g q8h	

Figure 43.6 Antibiotic regimens for treatment of urinary tract infections in pregnancy. Local bacteriologic patterns and sensitivity results should influence which antibiotics are used.

Pregnant women should continue oral antibiotic treatment after discharge for a further 10 to 14 days, then take a low-dose "suppressive" antibiotic until after delivery (see Fig. 43.6). In all cases of urinary tract infection in pregnancy, a follow-up urine culture 1 to 2 weeks after the antibiotic course is mandatory to exclude recurrent or persistent infection.

Cephalosporins, amoxicillin, trimethoprim, and nitrofurantoin are safe for treatment of urine infection during pregnancy, although trimethoprim can occasionally induce hyperkalemia in some women.

Gentamicin should be reserved for the treatment of severe pyelonephritis with systemic sepsis. It has been the practice to avoid quinolones because of teratogenic risks in animals, but data in humans suggest that they are safe and can be used when there is a compelling microbiologic reason.[27] Information on safety of antibiotics in pregnancy is also shown in Figure 42.2.

RENAL CALCULI IN PREGNANCY

Women with a history of metabolic abnormalities causing stone formation before pregnancy need their treatment modified during pregnancy. I advocate simply the adherence to a fluid intake of 2.5 to 3 liters per day and recommend that thiazides (for hypercalciuria), allopurinol (for hyperuricosuria), or captopril or penicillamine (for cystinuria) be discontinued. Fortunately, normal pregnancy is accompanied by increased urine pH, and this may help reduce uric acid or cystine stone formation.

Despite relative hypercalciuria and urinary stasis in pregnancy, pregnant women may be protected against renal calculi by the simultaneous increase in endogenous inhibitors of stone formation, such as urinary thiosulfate, which parallels hypercalciuria during gestation and returns to normal postpartum.

Because of concerns about irradiation from computed tomographic scanning and the uncertain utility of magnetic resonance imaging in this setting, ultrasound is the preferred investigation for renal colic in pregnancy, despite its poor sensitivity and specificity for stone diagnosis (on the order of 30% to 60%).

Definitive management of a calculus is usually best left until after delivery. Because ultrasound will almost always show pelviureteral dilation, which is a feature of normal pregnancy, systemic infection and acute kidney injury are the only indications for urgent decompression of an obstructed system by percutaneous nephrostomy. Conservative therapy with analgesia and hydration will result in spontaneous passage of a stone in the majority of cases. Extracorporeal shock wave lithotripsy is contraindicated as it is potentially deleterious to fetal hearing. If a surgical procedure is necessary, ureteroscopy with YAG laser lithotripsy has been used and is considered relatively safe in pregnancy.

THROMBOTIC MICROANGIOPATHIES

Thrombotic microangiopathies that can develop in pregnancy (i.e., thrombotic thrombocytopenic purpura, hemolytic-uremic syndrome, and the HELPP syndrome) are discussed in Chapters 28 and 42.

DIALYSIS IN PREGNANCY

There has been significant recent improvement in the outcome of pregnant women with renal disease requiring dialysis during pregnancy. Such pregnancies (mostly in women already on dialysis) now have a one in two chance of fetal survival, albeit with about 80% chance of prematurity.[28] These improved outcomes have been associated with more intensive dialysis regimens, and advances in neonatal care also allow survival for more premature and growth-restricted infants. Recommendations for managing hemodialysis during pregnancy are listed in Figure 43.7.

Initiating Dialysis for Progressive Chronic Kidney Disease

A key question is when to initiate dialysis in women who have advanced CKD but are not yet on dialysis at the time of

Managing Hemodialysis During Pregnancy

Pre-pregnancy
- Advise risks of pregnancy (miscarriage, fetal death, prematurity, fetal growth restriction, preeclampsia)
- Cease ACE inhibitors, ARB, or atenolol; ensure that any other medications are safe in pregnancy
- Use aspirin (75–150 mg/day)
- Folate 5 mg daily

During Pregnancy
- A minimum of 20 hours per week dialysis during a minimum of 4 sessions, aiming for predialysis BUN < 40 mg/dl (serum urea ~ 15 mmol/l)
- Maintenance of serum calcium with additional oral calcium and vitamin D and increased calcium dialysate, monitored with frequent calcium measures as occasionally placental production of vitamin D–like substances and PTHrP may lead to increased serum calcium
- Dietitian advice about adequate protein and nutrient intake
- Supplement with oral phosphate or increased dialysate phosphate if necessary
- Less aggressive use of oral and dialysate bicarbonate to maintain serum bicarbonate in the usual pregnancy range of 18 to 22 mmol/l
- Intravenous iron as required to ensure adequate iron stores
- ESAs at doses generally higher than needed before pregnancy to maintain hemoglobin 10–11 g/dl, with increased surveillance of blood pressure
- Dialysis heparin requirements are often increased because of the hypercoagulable state of pregnancy; this is not the situation for every pregnant woman and is assessed by monitoring dialysis adequacy and dialyser clotting

After Delivery
- Return to usual dialysis schedule immediately
- Readjust dry weight and antihypertensives weekly for 6 weeks

Figure 43.7 Managing hemodialysis during pregnancy. ACE, angiotensin-converting enzyme; ARB, angiotensin receptor blocker; ESAs, erythropoiesis-stimulating agents; PTHrP, parathyroid hormone–related peptide.

conception. It is generally recommended to commence dialysis at estimated GFR 20 ml/min or BUN 50 mg/dl (serum urea 18 mmol/l) and to aim for predialysis BUN < 40 mg/dl (serum urea 15 mmol/l).[2,29] The available data suggest that dialysis initiated during pregnancy is associated with greater likelihood of successful pregnancy than is continuation of maintenance dialysis, probably because of the benefits of residual renal function.

Women Already Needing Regular Dialysis

Women of childbearing age undergoing dialysis have around 1 in 20 chance of conceiving throughout their years on dialysis.[30] Women of childbearing age on maintenance dialysis therefore need to be counseled about adequate contraception, particularly in view of the fairly poor outcomes of these pregnancies.

Dialysis Regimens in Pregnancy

Reports of successful pregnancy outcomes, albeit with high rates of preterm delivery and polyhydramnios, generally include intensified hemodialysis or peritoneal dialysis schedules. Daily hemodialysis may be necessary to achieve the biochemical goal of predialysis BUN < 40 mg/dl (serum urea 15 mmol/l). Nocturnal hemodialysis may allow improved dialysis clearances with greater hemodynamic stability.

More intensive dialysis improves phosphate control, phosphate binders become unnecessary, and additional oral phosphate or increased dialysate phosphate may be needed because of the intensified dialysis and the fetal requirements for phosphate.

There is little information concerning specific requirements of women on peritoneal dialysis during pregnancy. There is no need to switch from peritoneal dialysis to hemodialysis even as the uterus enlarges. Dialysis adequacy can be maintained throughout pregnancy, although a major risk is that peritonitis may provoke premature labor or premature rupture of membranes.

Other management necessary for a successful pregnancy outcome includes the following:

- Control of maternal BP, generally to 110 to 140/80 to 90 mm Hg. This is difficult to achieve in many cases. Despite minimal or even lack of endogenous renal function, there still appears to be volume expansion in women on maintenance hemodialysis who become pregnant, as evidenced by their anemia and fall in serum albumin. There are no data yet in pregnancy on newer means of assessing volume status in dialysis patients, such as ultrasound measurement of inferior vena cava diameter or bioimpedance measurements.
- Active management of anemia with iron and erythropoiesis-stimulating agents. Target hemoglobin level should be 10 to 11 g/dl.
- Detection and early treatment of sepsis, which in turn precipitates premature labor or premature rupture of membranes. For those with residual renal function, repeated urine cultures are justified to detect and to treat asymptomatic bacteriuria.
- There are ongoing trials concerning the potential benefit of progesterone or its metabolites for the prevention of preterm labor, although not specifically in dialysis patients. Reports of changes in serum progesterone during dialysis vary widely, from significant reduction even to an increase.

At least weekly surveillance of pregnant women on dialysis is required to optimize outcome; dialysis intensity should be increased as far as practically possible if biochemical goals are not achieved. Fetal monitoring should include at least 2- to 4-week ultrasound scanning from the time of fetal viability, around 24 weeks of gestation.

RENAL TRANSPLANTATION AND PREGNANCY

Successful renal transplantation is an excellent way of restoring fertility in women with end-stage renal disease. The key questions in relation to management of women with a renal transplant in pregnancy are whether the pregnancy will have any effects on graft survival and whether the fetus will suffer as a result of the transplant or the immunosuppressive drugs.

Women should be advised to wait 12 months after a successful renal transplantation before embarking on pregnancy to ensure stable transplant function and maintenance immunosuppression. This interval is not based on solid pregnancy outcome data but is a practical time for ensuring clinical stability after transplantation, having optimal BP control and stable immunosuppression.

Immunosuppressive drugs considered safe in the transplant patient[31] include prednisolone, azathioprine, and cyclosporine.

Tacrolimus has been associated with neonatal hyperkalemia, but recent data support its safety.[32] Mycophenolate is associated with embryotoxic effects and must be avoided in pregnancy.

A favorable view of pregnancy in women who have undergone successful renal transplantation is supported by observations in more than 3000 pregnancies from 2000 women mostly receiving azathioprine and prednisone.[33] About 15% of these pregnancies miscarried spontaneously, and of those going past the first trimester, pregnancy was successful in more than 90% of cases, provided hypertension or a decline in renal function had not occurred before 28 weeks of gestation, in which case successful pregnancy outcome was reduced to about 70%. Women with preconception serum creatinine below 1.4 mg/dl (125 μmol/l) had 96% pregnancy success, whereas those with higher serum creatinine level had a 75% success rate. In keeping with the data for all women with CKD, long-term decline in renal function occurred significantly more often (27%) in those with preconception serum creatinine above 1.4 mg/dl (125 μmol/l).

Hypertension, either accelerated from preexisting hypertension or *de novo* during pregnancy, is present in 58% to 72% of cases. Even with these relatively good outcomes, somewhere between 30% and 70% of women will have hypertension requiring treatment as the pregnancy progresses (sometimes superimposed preeclampsia). Fetal growth restriction occurs in 40% to 50% of cases, and preterm delivery occurs in as many as two thirds, with attendant long-term risks of prematurity.[34] Cesarean section is necessary in approximately half of cases.

The United States National Transplantation Pregnancy Registry[32] reported in 2004 on the outcomes of 1125 women who had received kidney-alone transplants. As this is a voluntary registry, however, there is potential for reporting bias. The majority of women were taking cyclosporine or tacrolimus. The mean preconception serum creatinine was 1.4 mg/dl (125 μmol/l). Spontaneous abortion rates ranged from 12% to 24%, and 40% to 50% of surviving pregnancies were of low birth weight and 50% born preterm; 4% of babies had a birth defect. Graft loss within 2 years ranged from 4% to 13%. Twenty-four pregnancies were reported in women taking mycophenolate or sirolimus, 12 of which resulted in spontaneous abortion, raising concern about women taking these agents in pregnancy. Fetal risks for pregnancy in women with a renal transplant are summarized in Figure 43.8.

Graft and patient survivals are similar in those with and without any pregnancy as long as 15 years of follow-up. A post-pregnancy increase in serum creatinine concentration has been associated with cyclosporine use, possibly because cyclosporine doses were increased during pregnancy as plasma levels fell, presumably due to the associated plasma volume expansion of pregnancy. It remains controversial whether cyclosporine or tacrolimus doses should be increased during pregnancy. It is not my practice to make dose adjustments unless there are marked deviations from the baseline blood level during pregnancy.

Acute transplant rejection is uncommon, reported in less than 1 in 20 cases. Presentation as acute graft dysfunction is not different in pregnancy; renal biopsy is required to confirm the diagnosis.

There is an increased risk of infection (20% to 35%), particularly urinary tract infection but also cytomegalovirus infection with attendant maternal and fetal risks. The consequences of any infection can include premature labor and preterm rupture of membranes.

Gestational diabetes occurs in 3% to 12% of these pregnancies, no more common in tacrolimus-treated women than in those receiving cyclosporine.

Recommendations remain uncertain about breast-feeding for women taking immunosuppressive agents. Only about 25 to 30 reports of breast-feeding have been documented, none with any known adverse effects. The decision to breast-feed must be an individual one, informing the woman that effects on the baby remain largely unknown but that breast-feeding may have considerable advantages, particularly in premature and growth-restricted babies.

Recommendations for management of pregnancy in women with a renal transplant are summarized in Figure 43.9.

Outcomes of pregnancies fathered by male transplant recipients showed that mean gestational age and mean birth weight were similar to those of the general population.

Fetal Risks in Renal Transplant Pregnancies

- Spontaneous miscarriage of about 1 in 5 to 10 cases
- Prematurity in almost half of cases
- Fetal growth restriction in almost half of cases
- Birth defects, probably no more common than in the general population
- Long-term consequences of prematurity, although most babies have normal postnatal growth and development

Figure 43.8 Fetal risks in renal transplant pregnancies. Data derived from studies of women with pre-pregnancy serum creatinine concentrationin in the range 1.1-1.6 mg/dl (100-140 μmol/l); some studies reported patients with higher pre-pregnancy creatinine levels.[32]

PREGNANCY IN THE RENAL DONOR

Whereas it remains true that being a renal donor does not adversely affect future pregnancy outcomes in terms of fetal birth weight, stillbirth, or prematurity, studies suggest that there may be an increased risk of preeclampsia in these women in pregnancies after organ donation than before.[35] The key message is that all such women should be treated as "at-risk" pregnancies and have a higher number of clinical reviews, focusing on maternal BP and urinalysis and fetal growth, than in normal low-risk pregnancies.

COURSE OF CHRONIC KIDNEY DISEASE AFTER PREGNANCY

In a review of 49 women with stages 3 to 5 CKD before conception and whose pregnancy proceeded beyond 20 weeks, GFR was lower after pregnancy than before conception, and this fall was predicted by the combination of preconception GFR below 40 ml/min and proteinuria of more than 1 g/day, but not by GFR alone.[1]

The course of renal disease postpartum is unpredictable. Even some women with stable renal function throughout their pregnancy develop an acute deterioration postpartum.[36] Of women with moderate renal impairment (serum creatinine >1.5 mg/dl [130 μmol/l]), 50% have a significant rise in serum creatinine in the third trimester or early postpartum, and if this occurs, almost one in five progresses to end-stage renal disease within 6 months after delivery.[33]

General Management of Renal Transplants During Pregnancy

Pre-Pregnancy
- Graft function should be stable, with at least a one year interval from the time of transplantation.
- Discuss potential risks with transplant recipient and her partner. Although pregnancy outcomes are generally favorable, this is not always the case, and the impact of fetal death or graft loss is enormous.
- Best pregnancy outcome will occur if:
    1. Pre-pregnancy serum creatinine is less than 1.4 mg/dl (125 µmol/l).
    2. Proteinuria is less than 500 mg/day.
    3. Blood pressure is below 140/190 mmHg.
    4. Aspirin (75-150 mg) is used if serum creatinine > 1.5 mg/dl (130 µmol/l).
- Explain that it is sometimes prudent to delay pregnancy while using ACE inhibitors to control blood pressure and to reduce proteinuria, then switch to other drugs that are safe to use for treatment of hypertension during pregnancy, such as oxprenolol, methyldopa, or prazosin.
- Ensure that urinary tract infections are eradicated before pregnancy; prophylactic antibiotics are indicated for women who have had recurrent urine infections since their transplant to prevent pregnancy complications, such as spontaneous rupture of membranes and allograft dysfunction.
- Cyclosporine or tacrolimus blood levels should be stable.
- Diabetes should be tested for and controlled in advance of a pregnancy.

During Pregnancy
- The pregnant woman should be seen alternately between her nephrologist and obstetrician so that 2 week visits are undertaken up until 24 weeks of gestation (i.e., the time of fetal viability), and thereafter weekly visits.
- Assess fetal growth by ultrasound at least every 4 weeks, and possible more often, from 24 weeks, gestation.
- Do not adjust CNI dose during pregnancy unless there are extreme variations from stable pre-pregnancy levels.
- Screen for gestational diabetes at 28 weeks of gestation with 1–hour 50 g glucose challenge test.
- At each visit, assess BP (aim 110–140/80-90 mm Hg), proteinuria (dipstick, then PC ratio if result is dipstick result is positive), urine culture (if history of recurrent UTI, otherwise at 24, 28, and 32 weeks of gestation), electrolytes, creatinine and full blood count, CNI level, fetal growth.
- Reassess at each visit whether there is an impending indication for delivery (see fig. 43.5).

During Delivery
- Vaginal delivery is usually possible despite pelvic kidney.
- Prophylactic antibiotics are not required routinely.

Postpartum
- Monitor CNI and creatinine levels daily in hospital.
- Breast-feeding appears safe with CNI drugs, azathioprine, and corticosteroids, but discuss individual case with neonatologist.

Figure 43.9 General management of renal transplants during pregnancy. ACE, angiotensin-converting enzyme; BP, blood pressure; CNI, calcineurin inhibitor; PC ratio, protein-creatinine ratio; UTI, urinary tract infection.

Managing Women with Preexisting Renal Disease During Pregnancy

1. Women with CKD should be managed by a team comprising obstetrician, renal or obstetric medicine physician, and experienced midwife, preferably in a high-risk pregnancy clinic or day assessment unit.
2. GFR should be measured by serum creatinine in pregnancy, proteinuria as changes in spot urine protein to creatinine ratio after calculation of the initial ratio on a 24-hour urine collection, and blood pressure by sphygmomanometry or else a validated automated blood pressure recorder.
3. Women with CKD should receive low-dose aspirin for the prevention of preeclampsia or perinatal death if there is no obvious contraindication and should receive subcutaneous heparin if nephrotic syndrome develops.
4. The main determinants of a successful pregnancy outcome are the pre-pregnancy degree of proteinuria and GFR. This should be the focus in counseling women about their pregnancy risks.
5. The primary issues during pregnancy are control of maternal hypertension, regular assessment of GFR, watching for features of emerging preeclampsia, and regular assessment of fetal well-being. All of this allows optimal timing of delivery.

Figure 43.10 Managing women with preexisting renal disease during pregnancy. CKD, chronic kidney disease; GFR, glomerular filtration rate.

Surveillance by the nephrologist therefore needs be just as diligent in the first 3 months postpartum as during pregnancy. ACE inhibitors or ARB should be commenced soon after delivery for their antiproteinuric effect if GFR is stable.

SUMMARY

There are a number of factors to be considered in managing a pregnant woman with renal disease (Fig 43.10). Attention to these issues from preconception to postpartum can result in good pregnancy outcomes with preservation of maternal health.

REFERENCES

1. Imbasciati E, Gregorino G, Cabiddu G, et al. Pregnancy in CKD stages 3 to 5: Fetal and maternal outcomes. *Am J Kidney Dis.* 2007;49:753-762.
2. Lindheimer MD, Greenfeld JP, Davison JM. Renal disorders. In: Barron WM, Lindheimer MD, eds. *Medical Disorders in Pregnancy*. St. Louis: Mosby; 2000:39-70.
3. Lindheimer MD, Katz AI. Gestation in women with kidney disease: Prognosis and management. *Baillieres Clin Obstet Gynaecol.* 1994;8:387-404.
4. Ramin SM, Vidaeff AC, Yeomans ER, Gilstrap LC. Chronic renal disease in pregnancy. *Obstet Gynecol.* 2006;108:1531-1539.

5. Kilby M, Lipkin GW. Management of hypertension in renal disease in pregnancy. In: Davison JM, Nelson-Piercy C, Kehoe S, Baker P, eds. *Renal Disease in Pregnancy*. London: RCOG Press; 2008:149-165.
6. Brown MA, Holt JL, Mangos GJ, et al. Microscopic hematuria in pregnancy: Relevance to pregnancy outcome. *Am J Kidney Dis*. 2005;45: 667-673.
7. Roberts M, Lindheimer MD, Davison JM. Altered glomerular permselectivity to neutral dextrans and heteroporous membrane modeling in human pregnancy. *Am J Physiol*. 1996;270:F338-F343.
8. Saudan PJ, Brown MA, Farrell T, Shaw L. Improved methods of assessing proteinuria in hypertensive pregnancy. *Br J Obstet Gynaecol*. 1997;104:1159-1164.
9. Holston AM, Qian C, Yu KF, et al. Circulating angiogenic factors in gestational proteinuria without hypertension. *Am J Obstet Gynecol*. 2009;200:392.e1-392.e10.
10. Lane C, Brown M, Dunsmuir W, et al. Can spot urine protein/creatinine ratio replace 24 h urine protein in usual clinical nephrology? *Nephrology*. 2006;11:245-249.
11. Newman MG, Robichaux AG, Stedman CM, et al. Perinatal outcomes in preeclampsia that is complicated by massive proteinuria. *Am J Obstet Gynecol*. 2003;188:264-268.
12. Chakravarty EF, Colon I, Langen ES, et al. Factors that predict prematurity and preeclampsia in pregnancies that are complicated by systemic lupus erythematosus. *Am J Obstet Gyneol*. 2005;192:1897-1904.
13. Galdo T, Gonzalez F, Espinoza M, et al. Impact of pregnancy on the function of transplanted kidneys. *Transplant Proc*. 2005;37:1577-1579.
14. Brown MA, Whitworth JA. The kidney in hypertensive pregnancies—victim and villain. *Am J Kidney Dis*. 1992;20:427-442.
15. Coomarasamy A, Honest H, Papaioannou S, et al. Aspirin for prevention of preeclampsia in women with historical risk factors: A systematic review. *Obstet Gynecol*. 2003;101:1319-1332.
16. Askie LM, Duley L, Henderson-Smart DJ, Stewart LA; PARIS Collaborative Group. Antiplatelet agents for prevention of preeclampsia: A meta-analysis of individual patient data. *Lancet*. 2007;369:1791-1798.
17. Brunskill N. Renal biopsy in pregnancy. In: Davison JM, Nelson-Piercy C, Kehoe S, Baker P, eds. *Renal Disease in Pregnancy*. London: RCOG Press; 2008:201-206.
18. Ronkainen J, Ala-Houhala M, Autio-Harmainen H, et al. Long-term outcome 19 years after childhood IgA nephritis: A retrospective cohort study. *Pediatr Nephrol*. 2006;21:1266-1273.
19. Confidential Enquiry into Maternal and Child Health. *Diabetes in pregnancy: Are we providing the best care? Findings of a national enquiry: England, Wales and Northern Ireland*. London: CEMACH; 2007.
20. The Diabetes Control and Complications Trial Research Group: Effect of pregnancy on microvascular complications in the diabetes control and complications trial. *Diabetes Care*. 2000;23:1084-1091.
21. Verier-Mine O, Chaturvedi N, Webb D, et al. Is pregnancy a risk factor for microvascular complications? The EURODIAB Prospective Complications Study. *Diabetes Med*. 2005;22:1503-1509.
22. McCarthy A. Diabetic nephropathy in pregnancy. In: Davison JM, Nelson-Piercy C, Kehoe S, Baker P, eds. *Renal Disease in Pregnancy*. London: RCOG Press; 2008:111-125.
23. Venning M, Patel M. Lupus and connective tissue disease in pregnancy. In: Davison JM, Nelson-Piercy C, Kehoe S, Baker P, eds. *Renal Disease in Pregnancy*. London: RCOG Press; 2008:95-109.
24. Mor Y, Leibovitch I, Zalts R, et al. Analysis of the long-term outcome of surgically corrected vesico-ureteric reflux. *BJU Int*. 2003;92:97-100.
25. Brunskill NJ. Reflux nephropathy in pregnancy. In: Davison JM, Nelson-Piercy C, Kehoe S, Baker P, eds. *Renal Disease in Pregnancy*. London: RCOG Press; 2008:89-93.
26. Smaill F, Vazquez JC. Antibiotics for asymptomatic bacteriuria in pregnancy. Cochrane Database Syst Rev. 2007;2:CD000490. DOI: 10.1002/14651858.CD000490.pub2.
27. Loebstein R, Addis A, Ho E, et al. Pregnancy outcome following gestational exposure to fluoroquinolones: A multicenter prospective controlled study. *Antimicrob Agents Chemother*. 1998;42:1336-1339.
28. Hou S. Historical perspective of pregnancy in chronic kidney disease. 2007. *Adv Chronic Kidney Dis*. 2007;14:116-118.
29. Asamiya Y, Otsubo S, Matsuda Y, et al. The importance of low blood urea nitrogen levels in pregnant patients undergoing hemodialysis to optimize birth weight and gestational age. *Kidney Int*. 2009;75; 1217-1222.
30. Plant L. Pregnancy and dialysis. In: Davison JM, Nelson-Piercy C, Kehoe S, Baker P, eds. *Renal Disease in Pregnancy*. London: RCOG Press; 2008:61-68.
31. Bar J, Stahl B, Hod M, et al. Is immunosuppression therapy in renal allograft recipients teratogenic? A single-center experience. *Am J Med Genet*. 2003;116:31-36.
32. Armenti VT, Radomski JS, Moritz MJ, et al. Report from the National Transplantation Pregnancy Registry (NTPR): Outcomes of pregnancy after transplantation. *Clin Transpl*. 2006:57-70.
33. Davison JM. Pregnancy in renal allograft recipients: Problems, prognosis and practicalities. *Baillieres Clin Obstet Gynaecol*. 1994;8:501-525.
34. Carr S. Pregnancy and the renal transplant recipient. In: Davison JM, Nelson-Piercy C, Kehoe S, Baker P, eds. *Renal Disease in Pregnancy*. London: RCOG Press; 2008:69-87.
35. Nevis IF, Garg AX. Maternal and fetal outcomes after living kidney donation. *Am J Transplant*. 2009;9:661-668.
36. Jones DC, Hayslett JP. Outcomes of pregnancy in women with moderate or severe renal insufficiency. *N Engl J Med*. 1996;335:226-232.

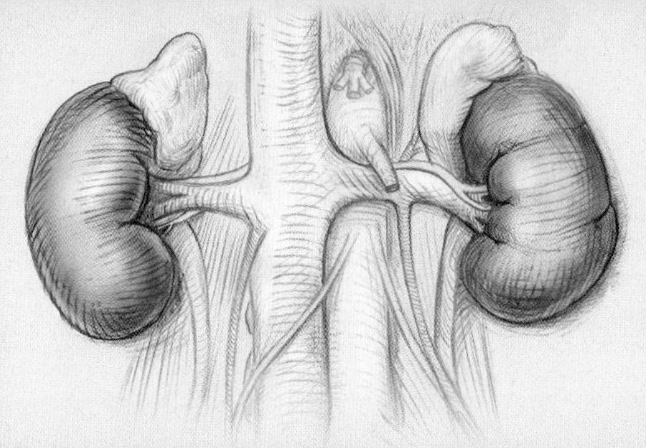

SECTION VIII

Hereditary and Congenital Diseases of the Kidney

CHAPTER 44

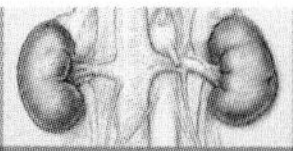

Autosomal Dominant Polycystic Kidney Disease

Vicente E. Torres, Peter C. Harris

DEFINITION

Autosomal dominant polycystic kidney disease (ADPKD) is a multisystem disorder characterized by multiple, bilateral renal cysts associated with cysts in other organs, such as liver, pancreas, and arachnoid membranes.[1,2] It is a genetic disorder mediated primarily by mutations in two different genes and is expressed in an autosomal dominant pattern, with variable expression. Although benign renal cysts are common, multiple bilateral cysts are not. Therefore, an underlying inherited disease should be considered in patients with normal renal function and multiple bilateral renal cysts.

ETIOLOGY AND PATHOGENESIS

The polycystic kidney disease (PKD) proteins now known as polycystin 1 and polycystin 2 play a critical role in the normal function of the primary cilium that is essential to maintaining the differentiated phenotype of tubular epithelium. Disordered function of polycystins is the basis for cyst formation in PKD by permitting a less differentiated tubular epithelial phenotype.

Genetic Mechanisms

ADPKD is genetically heterogeneous with two genes identified (Fig. 44.1), *PKD1* (chromosome 16p13.3) and *PKD2* (4q21). Autosomal dominant polycystic liver disease (ADPLD) also exists as an independent entity and is genetically heterogeneous; the first two genes identified (*PRKCSH* in chromosome 19 and *SEC63* in chromosome 6) account for about one third of isolated ADPLD cases.

Evidence from animal models of ADPKD and analysis of cystic epithelia have shown that renal cysts may develop from loss of functional polycystin with somatic inactivation of the normal allele, which is consistent with a "two-hit" mechanism. However, cysts can develop even if the protein is not completely lost. Furthermore, transgenic rodents overexpressing either *Pkd1* or *Pkd2* develop renal cystic disease resembling human ADPKD, which suggests that multiple genetic mechanisms that cause an imbalance in the expression of polycystins can affect their function and lead to development of cysts.[2]

Polycystic Kidney Disease Proteins

Polycystin 1 (PC1) and polycystin 2 (PC2) belong to a subfamily of transient receptor potential (TRP) channels.

PC1 (TRPP1; ~460 kd) has the structure of a receptor or adhesion molecule and contains a large extracellular N region, 11 transmembrane regions, and a short intracellular C region (see Fig. 44.1). It interacts with PC2 through a coiled-coil domain in the C-terminal portion and with multiple other proteins at different extracellular and intracellular sites. PC1 is found in the primary cilia, cytoplasmic vesicles, plasma membrane at focal adhesions, desmosomes, adherens junctions, and possibly endoplasmic reticulum and nuclei. PC1 may regulate the mechanical strength of adhesion between cells by controlling the formation of stabilized, actin-associated adherens junctions.[3]

PC2 (TRPP2; ~110 kd) contains a short N-terminal cytoplasmic region with a ciliary targeting motif, six transmembrane domains, and a short C-terminal portion. PC2 is localized predominantly to the endoplasmic reticulum but also to the plasma membrane, primary cilium, centrosome, and mitotic spindles in dividing cells.

Mechanisms of Cyst Formation

Experimental data indicate that the timing of ciliary loss or *Pkd1* inactivation determines the rate of development of cystic disease. Early inactivation results in rapidly progressive cystic disease.[4] Cysts also develop rapidly in the corticomedullary region (pars recta and thick ascending limbs of Henle) of adult mouse kidneys subjected to renal ischemia or reperfusion injury to stimulate cell proliferation.[5] Analysis of pre-cystic tubules shows that the loss of cilia results in aberrant planar cell polarity manifested by abnormalities in the orientation of cell division. The age dependence, location, and induction of the cysts by ischemia or reperfusion injury suggest that cyst formation is associated with increased rates of cell proliferation.

The polycystins are involved in the detection of extracellular cues at primary cilia, cell-cell contacts, and cell-matrix contacts and are essential to maintain the differentiated phenotype of the tubular epithelium. Reduction in one of the polycystins below a critical threshold results in a phenotypic switch characterized by inability to maintain planar polarity, increased rates of proliferation and apoptosis, expression of a secretory phenotype, and remodeling of the extracellular matrix. The molecular mechanisms include alterations of intracellular calcium homeostasis and activation of cyclic nucleotide, tyrosine kinase receptor, canonical Wnt, and other intracellular signaling pathways (Fig. 44.2).[2]

Beyond the loop of Henle, tubular epithelial cells have the capacity to secrete as well as to reabsorb solutes and fluid. Normally, absorptive flux exceeds secretory flux. Sodium chloride reabsorption in cortical collecting duct principal cells, arguably the main origin of the cysts in ADPKD, is driven by

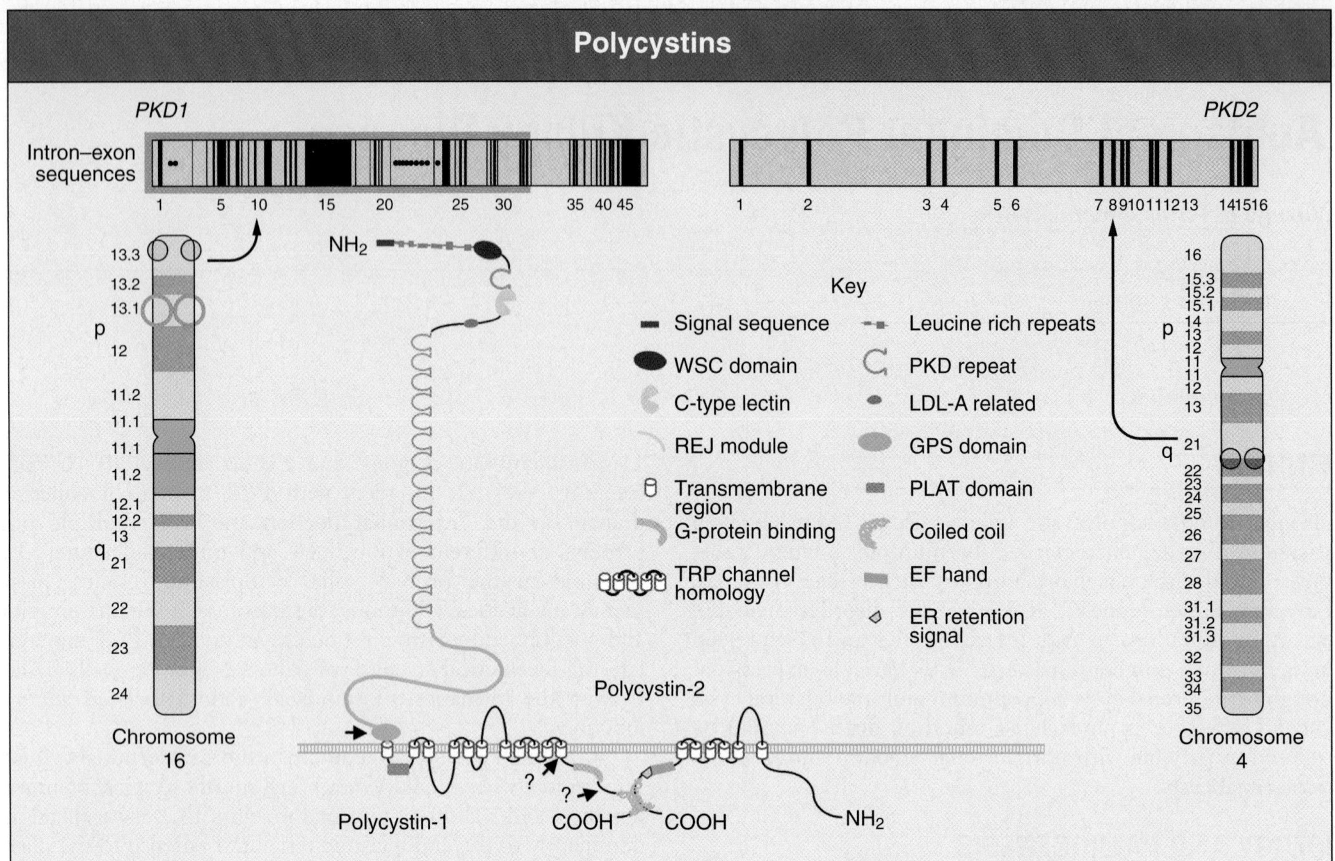

Figure 44.1 Polycystins: genes, mRNAs, and proteins. Diagrammatic representation of chromosome 16 *(left)* and chromosome 4 *(right)*. Intron-exon sequences of *PKD1 (upper left)* and *PKD2 (upper right)*. Diagram of proposed structural features of the polycystin 1 and polycystin 2 proteins *(center)*.

low intracellular sodium concentration generated by basolateral Na^+,K^+-ATPase. Sodium chloride enters the luminal membrane through epithelial sodium and chloride channels. Apical recycling of potassium occurs through renal outer medullary K (ROMK) channels. Water enters the cells across the luminal membrane through vasopressin-sensitive aquaporin 2 channels. Cystic epithelial cells are markedly different from normal cortical collecting duct principal cells. Chloride enters across basolateral Na^+-K^+-$2Cl^-$ cotransporters, driven by the sodium gradient generated by basolateral Na^+,K^+-ATPase, and exits across apical protein kinase A–stimulated cystic fibrosis transmembrane conductance regulator (CFTR). Basolateral recycling of potassium may occur through KCa3.1.[2,6]

In tubular epithelial cells, the primary cilium projects into the lumen and is thought to have a sensory role. The PC1-PC2 complex acts as a sensor on cilia that translates mechanical or chemical stimulation into calcium influx through PC2 channels. This in turn induces calcium release from intracellular stores.

A common finding in animal models of PKD is increased levels of cyclic adenosine monophosphate (cAMP), not only in the kidney but also in the liver, vascular smooth muscle, and choroid plexus. It has been suggested that alterations in intracellular calcium homeostasis account for the accumulation of cAMP, which in turn contributes to the development and progression of PKD by stimulating CFTR-driven chloride and fluid secretion and cell proliferation. Whereas cAMP inhibits MAP kinase signaling and cell proliferation under normal conditions, it stimulates cell proliferation in PKD or in conditions of calcium deprivation, probably linked to the alterations in intracellular calcium. Cell proliferation may be further enhanced by stimulation of epidermal growth factor–like factors present in cyst fluid, increased insulin-like growth factor 1 in cystic tissues, and activation of mTOR.

Upregulation of the vasopressin V_2 receptor and high circulating vasopressin levels may contribute to the increased cAMP levels.

Liver Cyst Development

Liver cysts arise by excessive proliferation and dilation of biliary ductules and peribiliary glands. Scanning electron microscopy has shown that the cyst epithelium displays heterogeneous features, being normal in small cysts (<1 cm), characterized by rare or shortened cilia in 1- to 3-cm cysts, and exhibiting absence of both primary cilia and microvilli in large cysts (>3 cm).[7] Estrogen receptors, insulin-like growth factor 1 (IGF1), IGF1 receptors, and growth hormone receptor are expressed in the epithelium lining the hepatic cysts, and estrogens and IGF1 stimulate hepatic cyst–derived cell proliferation.[7] Cyst growth is also promoted by growth factors and cytokines secreted into the cyst fluid.

Hypertension

Hypertension is a major clinical manifestation and predictor of outcome in ADPKD (see Clinical Manifestations). Several factors contribute to the development of hypertension in

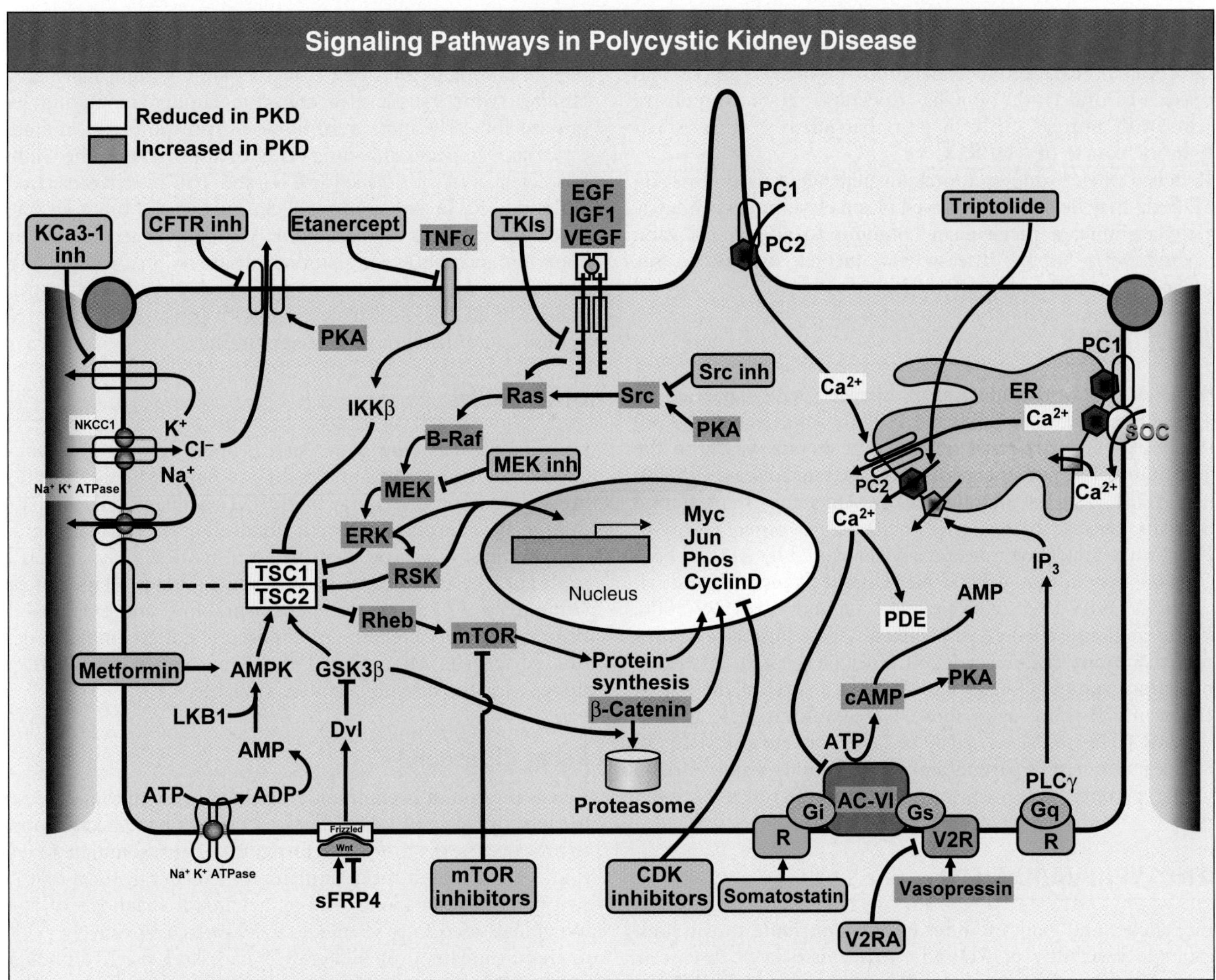

Figure 44.2 Signaling pathways in polycystic kidney disease. Pathways that are upregulated or downregulated in polycystic kidney disease and rationale for potential therapies *(green boxes)*.

Dysregulation of intracellular cAMP, mislocalization of ErbB receptors, and upregulation of epidermal growth factor (EGF), insulin-like growth factor 1 (IGF1), vascular endothelial growth factor (VEGF), and tumor necrosis factor α (TNFα) occur in cells and kidneys bearing PKD mutations.

Increased accumulation of cAMP in polycystic kidneys may result from (1) disruption of the polycystin complex because PC1 may act as a G_i protein–coupled receptor; (2) stimulation of calcium inhibitable AC-VI or inhibition of calcium-dependent PDE1 by a reduction in intracellular calcium; (3) increased circulating vasopressin due to an intrinsic concentrating defect; and (4) upregulation of vasopressin V_2 receptors. Increased cAMP levels contribute to cystogenesis by stimulating chloride and fluid secretion. In addition, cAMP stimulates mitogen-activated protein kinase/extracellularly regulated kinase (MAPK/ERK) signaling and cell proliferation in a Src- and Ras-dependent manner in cyst-derived cells or in wild-type tubular epithelial cells treated with calcium channel blockers or in a low Ca^{2+} medium. Activation of tyrosine kinase receptors by ligands present in cystic fluid also contributes to the stimulation of MAPK/ERK signaling and cell proliferation. Phosphorylation of tuberin by ERK (or inadequate targeting to the plasma membrane due to defective interaction with polycystin 1) may lead to the dissociation of tuberin and hamartin and the activation of Rheb and mTOR. Upregulation of TNFα or downregulation of AMPK signaling may also stimulate mTOR signaling through inhibition of the tuberin-hamartin complex. Activation of MAPK may also blunt cystogenesis through inhibition of CFTR and ERK. Upregulation of Wnt signaling stimulates mTOR and β-catenin signaling. ERK and mTOR activation promotes G_1/S transition and cell proliferation through regulation of cyclin D1, phosphorylation of retinoblastoma protein (RB) by CDK4/6–cyclin D and CDK2–cyclin E, and release of E2F transcription factor.

AC-VI, adenylate cyclase 6; AMPK, AMP kinase; CDK, cyclin-dependent kinase; ER, endoplasmic reticulum; MAPK, mitogen-activated protein kinase; mTOR, mammalian target of rapamycin; PC1, polycystin 1; PC2, polycystin 2; PDE, phosphodiesterase; PKA, protein kinase A; R, somatostatin sst_2 receptor; TSC, tuberous sclerosis proteins tuberin (TSC2) and hamartin (TSC1); V2R, vasopressin V_2 receptor; V2RA, vasopressin V_2 receptor antagonists. *(Modified with permission from reference 2.)*

ADPKD. Activation of the intrarenal renin-angiotensin system (RAS) may play an important role, but there is controversy whether the circulating RAS is inappropriately activated.[8] PC1 and PC2 are expressed in vascular smooth muscle and endothelium, along with enhanced vascular smooth muscle contractility[9] and impaired endothelium-dependent vasorelaxation, suggesting that disruption of polycystin function contributes to hypertension. PC1 in the primary cilia plays a role in the translation of physiologic changes in fluid shear stress into cytosolic calcium and nitric oxide signals. Other factors include increased sympathetic nerve activity and plasma endothelin 1 levels and insulin resistance.

Endothelial vasodilation and constitutive nitric oxide synthase activity are reduced in subcutaneous resistance vessels from patients with ADPKD and normal glomerular filtration rate (GFR). Flow-induced vasodilation of the brachial artery is inconsistently impaired,[10,11] whereas pulse wave reflection is amplified, suggesting a predominant involvement of small resistance vessels.[12] Reduced coronary flow velocity reserve and increased carotid intima-media thickness in normotensive patients with normal GFR suggest that atherosclerosis starts early in the course of ADPKD.[13]

Reduced nitric oxide endothelium-dependent vasorelaxation in ADPKD may be due to increased plasma levels of asymmetric dimethylarginine, a mechanism common to all hypertension associated with kidney disease (for further discussion, see Chapter 78).

EPIDEMIOLOGY

ADPKD occurs worldwide and in all races, with a prevalence estimated to be between 1:400 and 1:1000.[1] Approximately 2100 ADPKD patients start renal replacement therapy yearly in the United States. The percentage of end-stage renal disease (ESRD) due to ADPKD is less among African Americans than among Caucasians because of a higher incidence of other causes of ESRD. Yearly incidence rates for ESRD caused by ADPKD are 8.7 and 6.9 per million (1998-2001, United States), 7.8 and 6.0 per million (1998-1999, Europe), and 5.6 and 4.0 (1999-2000, Japan) in men and women, respectively. Age-adjusted sex ratios greater than unity (1.2-1.3) suggest more progressive disease in men than in women. Consistent with this, a survival analysis of 1391 parent-offspring pairs showed a significant male gender effect (HR, 1.424; 95% CI, 1.180 to 1.719) on age at ESRD (58 and 57 years for female parents and offspring and 54 and 54 years for male parents and offspring), but no difference between pairs.[14]

PHENOTYPIC VARIABILITY

Genic, allelic, and gene modifier effects contribute to the high phenotypic variability of ADPKD. *PKD1*-associated disease is more severe than *PKD2*-associated disease (age at ESRD, 54 years versus 74 years for *PKD1* and *PKD2*, respectively). The greater severity of *PKD1* is due to the development of more cysts at an early age, not to faster cyst growth.[15] Both *PKD1* and *PKD2* can be associated with severe polycystic liver disease and vascular abnormalities. Because of the lesser severity of the renal involvement, the prevalence of *PKD2*-associated disease has likely been underestimated in clinical studies.

PKD1 and *PKD2* mutations are highly variable and usually private (unique to a kindred). The ADPKD Mutation Database (*http://pkdb.mayo.edu*) lists 333 truncating *PKD1* mutations identified in 417 families with a total of 869 variants including missense mutations and silent polymorphisms. Ninety-five *PKD2* truncating mutations are listed in 178 families, with a total of 128 different variants.

The influence of allelic factors (mutation type or location) on the severity of ADPKD is limited. Patients with mutations in the 5′ region of *PKD1* have more severe disease (19% versus 40% with adequate renal function at 60 years) and are more likely to have intracranial aneurysms and aneurysm ruptures than are patients with 3′ mutations. There are no clear correlations with mutation type in *PKD1* or *PKD2* or with mutation type or position in *PKD2*. Recently, however, hypomorphic or incompletely penetrant *PKD1* or *PKD2* alleles have been described.[16] These alleles alone may result in mild cystic disease; two such alleles cause typical to severe disease and in combination with an inactivating allele may be associated with early-onset disease.

The large intrafamilial variability of ADPKD highlights a role for genetic background in disease presentation. Age at clinical manifestations in ADPKD is less variable within than between families, which suggests a common familial modifying background for early and severe disease expression (e.g., mutations or variants in genes encoding other cystoproteins). The contiguous deletion of the adjacent *PKD1* and *TSC2* is characterized by childhood PKD with additional clinical signs of tuberous sclerosis complex. Other modifying loci are likely to account for more common and subtle intrafamilial variability, but studies of candidate loci, selected because of presumed relevance to the pathogenesis of ADPKD or association with prognosis in other renal diseases, have been mostly disappointing.

DIAGNOSIS

Only individuals who have been properly informed about the advantages and disadvantages of screening should be offered presymptomatic screening. If ADPKD is diagnosed, the patient can receive appropriate genetic counseling, and risk factors such as hypertension can be identified and treated early. If ADPKD is absent, the patient can be reassured. Disadvantages of presymptomatic screening relate to insurability and employability. Presymptomatic screening of children is not recommended, but this advice can be expected to change when more effective therapy for the disease becomes available.

Renal Ultrasound

Renal ultrasound is commonly used for presymptomatic testing because of cost and safety. Revised criteria have been proposed to improve the diagnostic performance of ultrasound in ADPKD (Fig. 44.3). At least three (unilateral or bilateral) renal cysts and two cysts in each kidney are sufficient for diagnosis of at-risk individuals aged 15 to 39 and 40 to 59 years, respectively.[17] Three or more (unilateral or bilateral) cysts have a positive predictive

Ultrasound Criteria for the Diagnosis of ADPKD

Age (years)	Criteria	PPV	NPV
Original Ravine's PKD1 diagnostic criteria			
15–29	≥2 cysts, unilateral or bilateral	99.2	87.7
30–39	≥2 cysts in each kidney	100	87.5
40–59	≥2 cysts in each kidney	100	94.8
≥60	≥4 cysts in each kidney	100	100
Revised unified diagnostic criteria			
15–29	≥3 cysts, unilateral or bilateral	100	85.5
30–39	≥3 cysts, unilateral or bilateral	100	86.4
40–59	≥2 cysts in each kidney	100	94.8
≥60	≥4 cysts in each kidney	100	100
Revised criteria for exclusion of diagnosis			
15–29	≥1 cyst	96.6	90.8
30–39	≥1 cyst	94.0	98.3
40–59	≥2 cysts	96.7	100
≥60	≥3 cysts in each kidney	100	100

Figure 44.3 Ultrasound criteria for diagnosis of ADPKD. NPV, negative predictive value; PPV, positive predictive value. *(Reprinted with permission from reference 33.)*

value of 100% in the younger age group and minimize false-positive diagnoses because 2.1% and 0.7% of the genetically unaffected individuals younger than 30 years have one and two renal cysts, respectively. For at-risk individuals 60 years of age and older, four or more cysts in each kidney are required.

Whereas the overall specificity and positive predictive value of ultrasound are high by use of these criteria, their sensitivity and negative predictive value when applied to 15- to 59-year-old *PKD2* patients are low. This is a problem in the evaluation of potential kidney donors, in which exclusion of the diagnosis is important.[17] Different criteria have therefore been proposed to exclude a diagnosis of ADPKD in an individual at risk from a family with an unknown genotype. An ultrasound scan finding of normal kidneys or one renal cyst in an individual aged 40 years or older has a negative predictive value of 100%. The absence of any renal cyst provides near certainty that ADPKD is absent in at-risk individuals aged 30 to 39 years, with a false-negative rate of 0.7% and a negative predictive value of 98.7%. A normal or indeterminate ultrasound scan does not exclude ADPKD with certainty in an at-risk individual younger than 30 years; a normal magnetic resonance (MR) or contrast-enhanced computed tomography (CT) scan provides further assurance, but there are insufficient data to quantify its predictive accuracy.

Genetic Testing

Genetic testing can be performed when a precise diagnosis is needed and the results of imaging testing are indeterminate. However, there are limitations to genetic testing, by either linkage or mutation analysis. Linkage analysis requires accurate diagnosis and the availability and willingness of sufficient affected family members to be tested; it is feasible in less than 50% of families. *De novo* mutations can also complicate interpretation of results. Molecular testing by direct DNA sequencing is now possible in ~85% of patients.[18] However, as most mutations are unique and up to one third of *PKD1* changes are missense, the pathogenicity of some changes is difficult to prove.

In preimplantation genetic diagnosis, genetic analysis is carried out on single blastomeres from preimplantation embryo biopsy specimens obtained after in vitro fertilization, and only embryos unaffected by the disease under investigation are selected for transfer. Preimplantation genetic diagnosis for ADPKD has been performed in very few cases; it is complicated by the genetic heterogeneity of the disease and by the large size and complex structure of the *PKD1* gene.

DIFFERENTIAL DIAGNOSIS

Renal cystic disease can be a manifestation of many other systemic diseases. Conditions to keep in mind when renal cystic disease is detected but the presentation is not typical of ADPKD include autosomal recessive PKD, tuberous sclerosis complex, von Hippel–Lindau disease, and orofaciodigital syndrome type I as well as medullary sponge kidney and simple renal cysts. These are discussed further, including differential diagnosis, in Chapter 45. If the patient has ESRD, acquired cystic disease should also be considered (see Chapter 85).

CLINICAL MANIFESTATIONS

ADPKD is a multisystem disorder. Multiple renal and extrarenal manifestations of ADPKD have been described that cause significant complications.

Renal manifestations of ADPKD
Functional Manifestations
Concentrating defect
Reduced urine NH_4 relative to pH
Reduced renal blood flow
Hypertension → Target Organ Damage
Cardiac
Cerebrovascular
Arteriolosclerosis and glomerulosclerosis
Peripheral vascular disease
Pain, Caused by
Cyst hemorrhage
Gross hematuria
Nephrolithiasis
Infection
Renal enlargement
Renal Failure, Possibly Due to
Interstitial inflammation
Apoptosis of tubular epithelial cells
Hypertensive glomerulosclerosis
Compression atrophy

Figure 44.4 Renal manifestations of ADPKD.

Renal Manifestations

A number of clinical features that result from renal damage can be identified (Fig. 44.4). Reduction in urinary concentrating capacity and glomerular hyperfiltration are early functional abnormalities that can be observed in some children and adolescents with ADPKD.

Renal Size

Renal size increases with age, and renal enlargement eventually occurs in 100% of patients with ADPKD. The severity of structural abnormality correlates with the manifestations of ADPKD, such as pain, hematuria, hypertension, and renal impairment.[19] Massive renal enlargement can lead to compression of local structures, resulting in such complications as inferior vena cava compression and digestive symptoms. Most manifestations are directly related to the development and enlargement of renal cysts. The Consortium for Radiologic Imaging Studies of Polycystic Kidney Disease (CRISP), a prospective study of 241 patients by annual magnetic resonance imaging (MRI), has shown that total kidney volume and cyst volumes increased exponentially.[19] Rates of growth were relatively constant, averaging 5.3% per year, but highly variable from patient to patient. Baseline total kidney volume predicted the subsequent rate of increase in renal volume and was associated with declining GFR in patients with baseline total kidney volume above 1500 ml.

Pain

Episodes of acute renal pain are seen frequently; causes include cyst hemorrhage, infection, stone, and rarely tumor, and these must be investigated thoroughly. A few ADPKD patients with renal enlargement and structural distortion develop chronic flank pain without specifically identifiable etiology.

Hematuria and Cyst Hemorrhage

Visible hematuria may be the initial presenting symptom and occurs in up to 40% of ADPKD patients at some time during the course of the disease. Many have recurrent episodes. Differential diagnosis includes cyst hemorrhage, stone, infection, and tumor. Cyst hemorrhage is a frequent complication and produces gross hematuria when the cyst communicates with the collecting system. Frequently, the cyst does not communicate with the collecting system, and flank pain without hematuria occurs. It can present with fever, raising the possibility of cyst infection. On occasion, a hemorrhagic cyst will rupture, resulting in a retroperitoneal bleed that can be significant, potentially requiring transfusion. In most patients, cyst hemorrhage is self-limited, resolving within 2 to 7 days. If symptoms of hematuria or flank pain last longer than 1 week or if the initial episode of hematuria occurs after the age of 50 years, investigation to exclude neoplasm should be undertaken.

Urinary Tract Infection and Cyst Infection

Urinary tract infection is common in ADPKD, but its incidence may have been overestimated because sterile pyuria is common in these patients. Urinary tract infection presents as cystitis, acute pyelonephritis, cyst infection, and perinephric abscesses. As in the general population, females are affected more frequently than males. Most infections are caused by *Escherichia coli*, *Klebsiella* species, *Proteus* species, and other Enterobacteriaceae. The route of infection in acute pyelonephritis and cyst infection is usually retrograde from the bladder; therefore, cystitis should be promptly treated to prevent complicated infections.

CT and MRI are both sensitive to detect complicated cysts and to provide anatomic definition, but the findings are not specific for infection. Nuclear imaging, especially indium-labeled white blood cell scanning, is useful, but both false-negative and false-positive results are possible. [^{18}F]Fluorodeoxyglucose (FDG) positron emission tomography (PET) has recently been used for detection of infected cysts.[20] FDG is taken up by inflammatory cells because of their high metabolic rate but is filtered by the kidneys, not reabsorbed, and appears in the collecting system, which may limit its use in diagnosis of renal cyst infections; its present role is for diagnosis of infected liver cysts. FDG PET is expensive and not yet widely available, but it provides rapid imaging with high spatial resolution, high target to background ratio, low radiation burden, and high interobserver agreement.

When there is fever and flank pain with suggestive diagnostic imaging but blood and urine cultures are negative, cyst aspiration under ultrasound or CT guidance should be undertaken to culture the organism and to assist in selection of antimicrobial therapy.

Nephrolithiasis

Renal stone disease occurs in about 20% of patients with ADPKD. Most stones are composed of uric acid, calcium oxalate, or both. Uric acid stones are more common in ADPKD than in stone formers without ADPKD. Urinary stasis secondary to distorted renal anatomy possibly plays a role in the pathogenesis of nephrolithiasis. Predisposing metabolic factors include decreased ammonia excretion, low urinary pH, and low urinary citrate concentration.[21]

Stones can be difficult to diagnose on imaging in ADPKD because of cyst wall and parenchymal calcification. The distorted anatomy can cause difficulty in localizing stones to the collecting system on plain films. Intravenous urography has the advantage of specifically localizing stone material to the collecting system and may provide clues to stone composition. Intravenous urography can also detect pericalyceal tubular ectasia, found in 15% of ADPKD patients. CT scanning is more sensitive in detecting small or radiolucent stones and for differentiating stones from tumor, clot, and cyst wall or parenchymal calcification. Dual-energy CT is increasingly used to distinguish between calcium and uric acid stones.

Hypertension

Hypertension is the most common manifestation of ADPKD and a major contributor to renal disease progression (Fig. 44.5) and cardiovascular morbidity and mortality. Microalbuminuria, proteinuria, and hematuria, which are independent risk factors for renal functional decline, are more common in hypertensive patients with ADPKD. Hypertension may also increase morbidity from valvular heart disease and intracranial aneurysms, which are common in ADPKD.

Ambulatory blood pressure monitoring of children or young adults without diagnosed hypertension often reveals elevated blood pressure, attenuated nocturnal blood pressure dipping, and exaggerated blood pressure response during exercise. A study stratified 65 children by blood pressure into three cohorts: hypertensive (≥95th percentile), borderline hypertensive (75th to 95th percentile), and normotensive (≤75th percentile).[22] Both the hypertensive and borderline hypertensive children had significantly higher left ventricular mass indices than normotensive children did. Among normotensive children, indices were significantly higher in those within the upper quartile of the normal blood pressure. These observations suggest that target organ damage develops early in ADPKD and that antihypertensive treatment may be indicated in children with ADPKD and borderline hypertension.

End-Stage Renal Disease

In most patients, renal function is maintained within the normal range, despite relentless growth of cysts, until the fourth to sixth

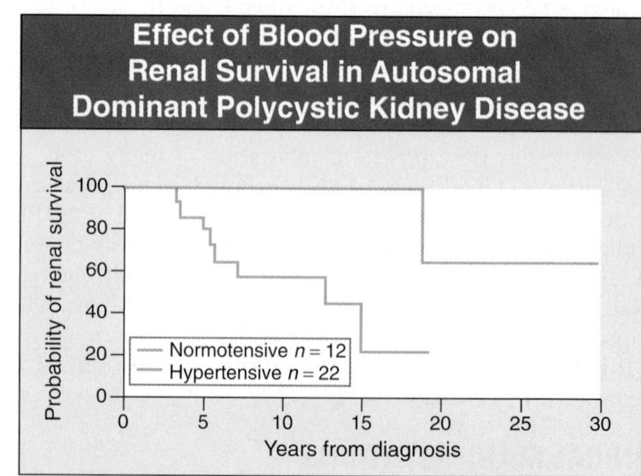

Figure 44.5 Patients with polycystic kidney disease and hypertension at diagnosis have less probability of renal survival than those with normal blood pressure. *(Reprinted with permission from reference 47.)*

decade of life. By the time renal function starts declining, the kidneys usually are markedly enlarged and distorted with little recognizable parenchyma on imaging studies. At this stage, the average rate of GFR decline is 4.4 to 5.9 ml/min per year. Nevertheless, ESRD is not inevitable in ADPKD. Up to 77% of patients are alive with preserved renal function at age 50 years, and 52% at age 73 years. Men tend to progress to renal failure more rapidly and require renal replacement therapy at a younger age than do women. Other risk factors for renal failure include black race, diagnosis of ADPKD before the age of 30 years, first episode of hematuria before the age of 30 years, onset of hypertension before the age of 35 years, hyperlipidemia, low high-density lipoprotein cholesterol level, and sickle cell trait.[23]

Several mechanisms account for renal function decline. The CRISP study has confirmed that kidney and cyst volumes are the strongest predictors of renal functional decline.[19] CRISP also found that renal blood flow (or vascular resistance) is an independent predictor.[24] This points to the importance of vascular remodeling in the progression of the disease and may account for cases in which the decline of renal function seems to be out of proportion to the severity of the cystic disease. Other factors, such as heavy use of analgesics, may contribute to chronic kidney disease progression in some patients.

Extrarenal Manifestations

Polycystic Liver Disease

Polycystic liver disease (PLD) is the most common extrarenal manifestation of ADPKD. It is associated with both *PKD1* and *PKD2* genotypes. In addition, PLD also occurs as a genetically distinct disease in the absence of renal cysts. Most simple hepatic cysts are solitary, and PLD should be suspected when four or more cysts are present in the hepatic parenchyma. The liver in PLD contains multiple microscopic or macroscopic cysts that result in hepatomegaly (Fig. 44.6), but typically there is preservation of normal hepatic parenchyma and liver function.

Hepatic cysts are exceedingly rare in children with ADPKD. Their frequency increases with age and may have been underestimated by ultrasound and CT studies. Their prevalence by MRI scanning in the CRISP study is 58%, 85%, and 94% in 15- to 24-year-old, 25- to 34-year-old, and 35- to 46-year-old participants.[25] Women develop more cysts, at an earlier age than men do. Women who have multiple pregnancies or who have used oral contraceptive agents or estrogen replacement therapy postmenopausally have worse disease, supporting the importance of estrogen exposure in hepatic cyst growth.

Typically, PLD is asymptomatic, but reported symptoms have become more frequent as the life span of ADPKD patients is prolonged with dialysis and transplantation. Symptoms result from mass effect or from complications related to the cysts themselves. Symptoms typically caused by massive enlargement of the liver or by mass effect from a single or a limited number of dominant cysts include dyspnea, orthopnea, early satiety, gastroesophageal reflux, mechanical low back pain, uterine prolapse, and even rib fracture. Other complications caused directly by mass effect include hepatic venous outflow obstruction, inferior vena cava compression, portal vein compression, and bile duct compression presenting as obstructive jaundice. Hepatic venous outflow obstruction is an uncommon condition caused by severe extrinsic compression of the intrahepatic inferior vena cava and hepatic veins by cysts, rarely with superimposed thrombosis. Symptomatic cyst complications include cyst hemorrhage, which occurs less frequently than renal cyst hemorrhage; cyst infection; and the rare occurrence of torsion or rupture of cysts. Hepatic cyst infection can be a serious complication and typically presents with localized pain, fever, leukocytosis, elevated sedimentation rate, and often elevated alkaline phosphatase. Enterobacteriaceae are the most common microorganisms causing cyst infection. The same imaging techniques discussed for the investigation of renal cyst infections may be useful for the localization of infected cysts in the liver.

Intracranial Aneurysms

Intracranial aneurysms occur in about 8% of those with ADPKD. There is some familial clustering; intracranial aneurysms occur in 6% of patients with a negative family history and 16% of those with a positive family history.[26] Most are asymptomatic. Focal findings, such as cranial nerve palsy and seizure, may result from compression of local structures by an enlarging aneurysm (Fig. 44.7). Yearly rupture rates increase with size, ranging from less than 0.5% for aneurysms smaller than 5 mm in diameter to 4% for aneurysms larger than 10 mm in diameter. Rupture carries a 35% to 55% risk for combined severe morbidity and mortality. The mean age at rupture in ADPKD is 39 years (compared with 51 years in the general population), with a range of 15 to 69 years. Most patients have normal renal function, and up to 29% have normal blood pressure at the time of rupture.

Screening is not indicated for all people with ADPKD because most intracranial aneurysms found by presymptomatic screening are small, have a low risk for rupture, and require no treatment because the risks of intervention exceed any risk of rupture.[27] Indications for screening in patients with a good life expectancy

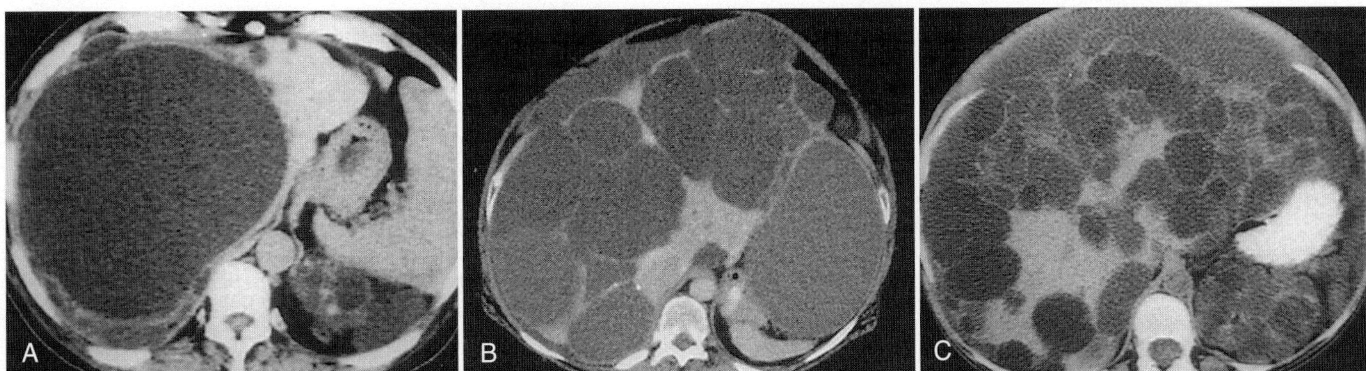

Figure 44.6 Variable presentation of symptomatic polycystic liver disease. A, Hepatomegaly caused by a very large, isolated, dominant cyst. **B,** Hepatomegaly caused by several large cysts. **C,** Hepatomegaly caused by multiple smaller cysts throughout the hepatic parenchyma.

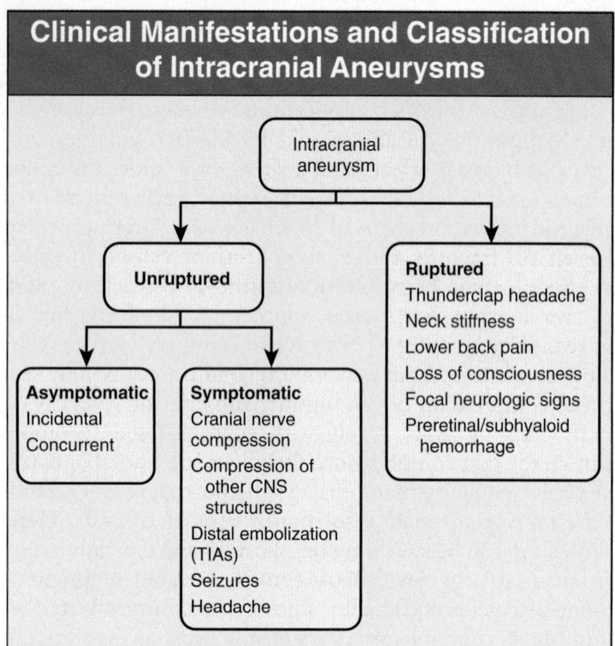

Figure 44.7 Intracranial aneurysms. Clinical manifestations and classification. CNS, central nervous system; TIAs, transient ischemic attacks.

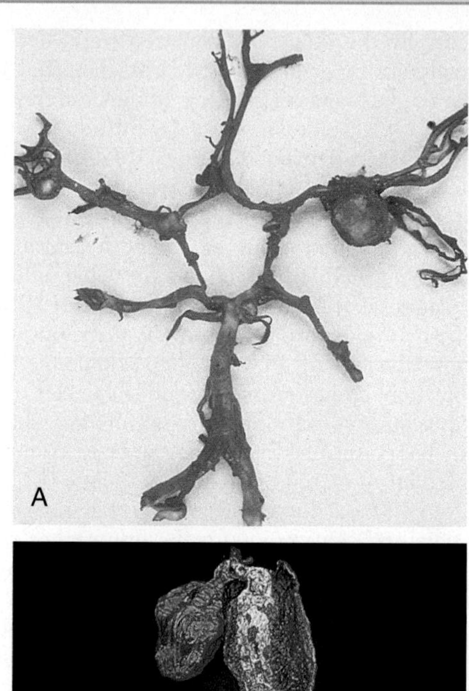

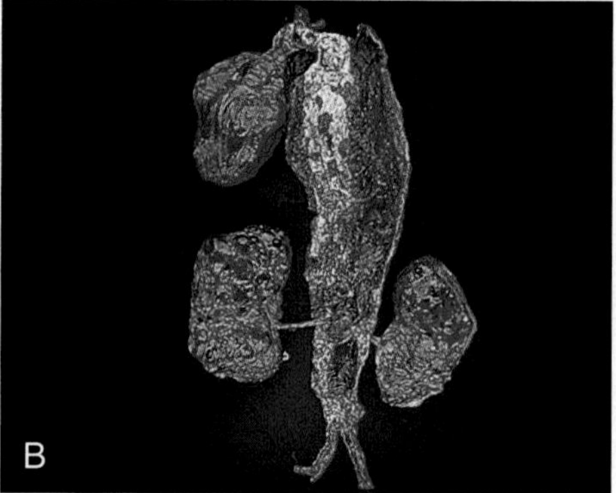

Figure 44.8 Vascular manifestations of ADPKD. A, Gross specimen demonstrating bilateral aneurysms of the middle cerebral arteries. **B,** Gross specimen demonstrating a thoracic aortic dissection extending into the abdominal aorta in a patient with ADPKD.

include family history of intracranial aneurysm or subarachnoid hemorrhage, previous aneurysmal rupture, preparation for elective surgery with potential hemodynamic instability, high-risk occupations (e.g., airline pilots), and significant anxiety on the part of the patient despite adequate information about the risks. MR angiography is the diagnostic imaging modality of choice for presymptomatic screening because it is noninvasive and does not require the intravenous administration of contrast material. CT angiography is a satisfactory alternative if there is no contraindication to the intravenous administration of contrast material.

Other Vascular Abnormalities

In addition to intracranial aneurysms, ADPKD has been associated with other vascular abnormalities, such as thoracic aortic and cervicocephalic arterial dissections, coronary artery aneurysms, and retinal artery and vein occlusions (Fig. 44.8). Thoracic aortic dissection is seven times more common in ADPKD than in the general population in autopsy series, but reported cases are rare. Rare patients with coronary aneurysms can present with cardiac ischemia and thrombus in the aneurysm in the absence of atherosclerotic disease. Several case reports describe abdominal aortic aneurysms in ADPKD. However, a prospective ultrasound study showed neither a wider aortic diameter nor a higher prevalence of abdominal aortic aneurysms in ADPKD patients compared with unaffected kindred in any age group. On pathologic examination, tissues from arterial aneurysms and dissections demonstrate disruption of elastic tissue. Polycystin 1 and polycystin 2 are both expressed in the myocytes of elastic and large distributive arteries, suggesting a direct pathogenetic role for ADPKD-related mutations in the arterial complications of this disease.

Valvular Heart Disease and Other Cardiac Manifestations

Mitral valve prolapse is the most common valvular abnormality and has been demonstrated in up to 25% of ADPKD patients by echocardiography. Mitral regurgitation, tricuspid regurgitation, and tricuspid prolapse also occur more frequently in ADPKD than in unaffected kindred. Aortic regurgitation may be associated with dilation of the aortic root. On histologic examination, valvular tissue shows myxoid degeneration with disruption of collagen, as seen in Marfan and Ehlers-Danlos syndromes. Although the lesions may progress with time, they rarely require valve replacement. Screening echocardiography is not indicated unless a murmur is detected on physical examination. Small, hemodynamically insignificant pericardial effusion can be detected by CT scanning in up to 35% of ADPKD patients.[28]

Other Associated Conditions

Cyst formation has been described in such diverse organs as the pancreas, seminal vesicles, and arachnoid membrane (Fig. 44.9). Seminal vesicle cysts, usually multiple and bilateral, are found in 40% of ADPKD compared with 2% of nonaffected males. Ovarian cysts are not associated with ADPKD. Pancreas and arachnoid membrane cysts are present in 5% and 8% of patients, respectively. Pancreatic cysts are almost always asymptomatic, with very rare occurrences of recurrent pancreatitis and possibly chance associations of intraductal papillary mucinous tumor or carcinoma. Epididymal and prostate cysts may also occur with increased frequency. Sperm abnormalities with defective motility are common in ADPKD and rarely may be a cause of male infertility.[29] Spinal meningeal diverticula may occur with

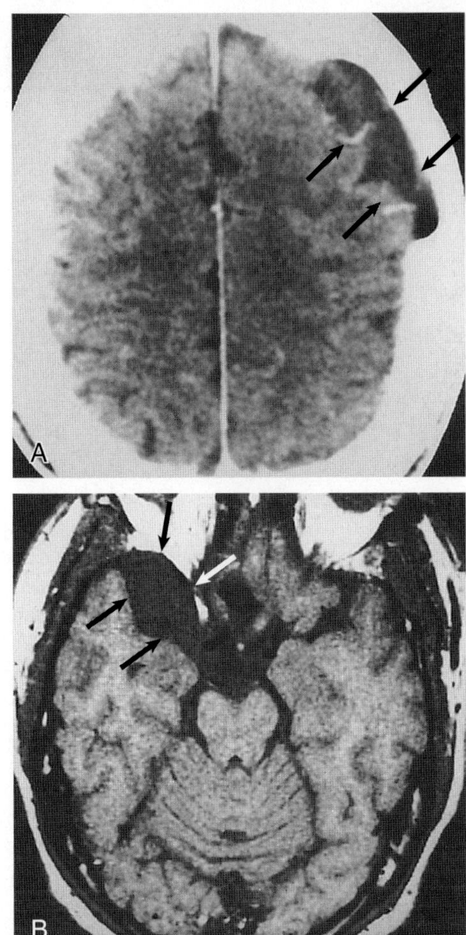

Figure 44.9 Extrarenal manifestations of ADPKD. Arachnoid cysts *(arrows)* demonstrated by CT **(A)** and MRI **(B)**.

increased frequency and rarely present with intracranial hypotension (orthostatic headache, diplopia, hearing loss, ataxia) due to cerebrospinal fluid leak.[30] The prevalence of colonic and duodenal diverticula may also be increased.[31]

PATHOLOGY

Polycystic kidneys are diffusely cystic and enlarged (Fig. 44.10). Size varies from normal to weighing more than 4 kg. The outer and cut surfaces show numerous spherical cysts of varying size, which are distributed evenly between cortex and medulla. The collecting system typically is distorted. The epithelium lining the cysts is characterized by hyperplastic changes, including flat nonpolypoid hyperplasia, polypoid hyperplasia and microscopic adenomas (Fig. 44.11), and increased rates of cell proliferation and apoptosis. Despite the frequency of hyperplastic lesions and microscopic adenomas, the incidence of renal cell carcinoma is not increased.

Cysts arise from focal dilation of existing renal tubules, arising from all segments of the nephron and collecting ducts. As they grow, they dissociate from the parent tubule and eventually become isolated, fluid-filled sacs. There is no agreement on whether the cysts originate preferentially from particular tubular segments. Cysts with fluid sodium, chloride, potassium, and urea concentrations similar to those of plasma (nongradient cysts) are thought to be derived from proximal tubules, whereas cysts with low sodium and chloride and high potassium and urea concentrations are considered to be distally derived. Histochemical studies provide inconsistent evidence about the site of origin within the tubule. Most studies indicate that cysts are predominantly of distal nephron and collecting duct origin. Studies in advanced renal disease showing proximal tubular cysts may be confounded by the effects of obstruction and acquired renal cystic disease. A study has shown that most claudin isoforms expressed in ADPKD cysts are of distal nephron and collecting duct origin and that claudin 2, normally expressed in proximal tubules, is absent from the cysts.[32]

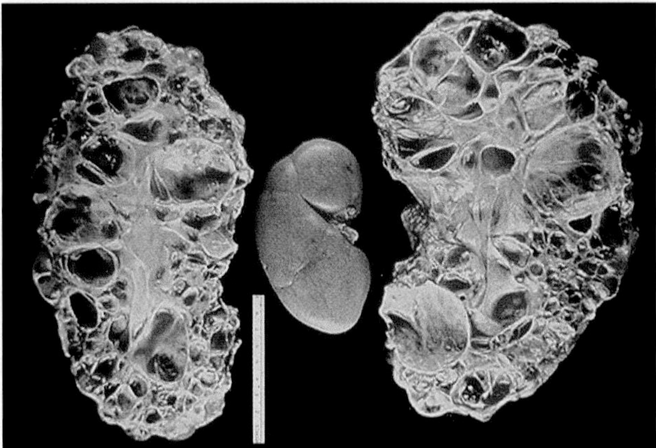

Figure 44.10 Polycystic kidneys. Markedly enlarged polycystic kidneys from a patient with ADPKD in comparison to a normal kidney in the middle.

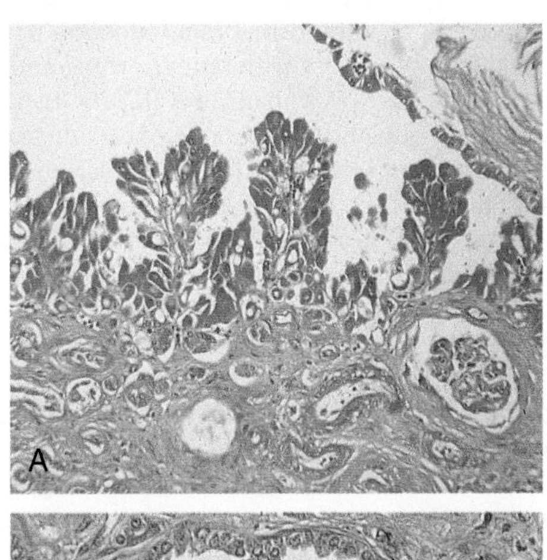

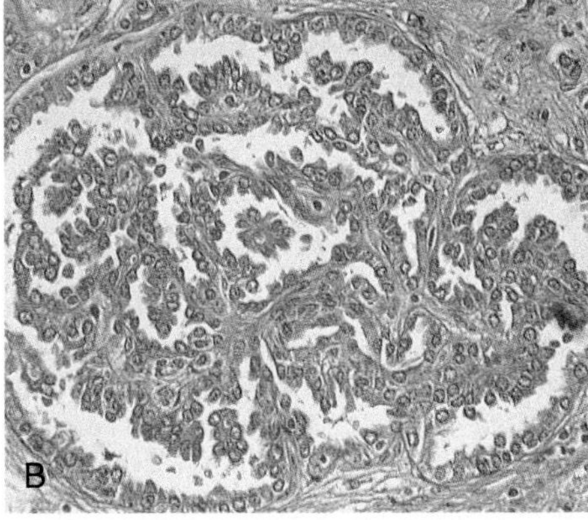

Figure 44.11 Renal cyst histology in ADPKD. A, Papillary hyperplasia of cyst epithelium. **B,** Papillary microscopic adenoma in an ADPKD kidney. (Magnification ×200.)

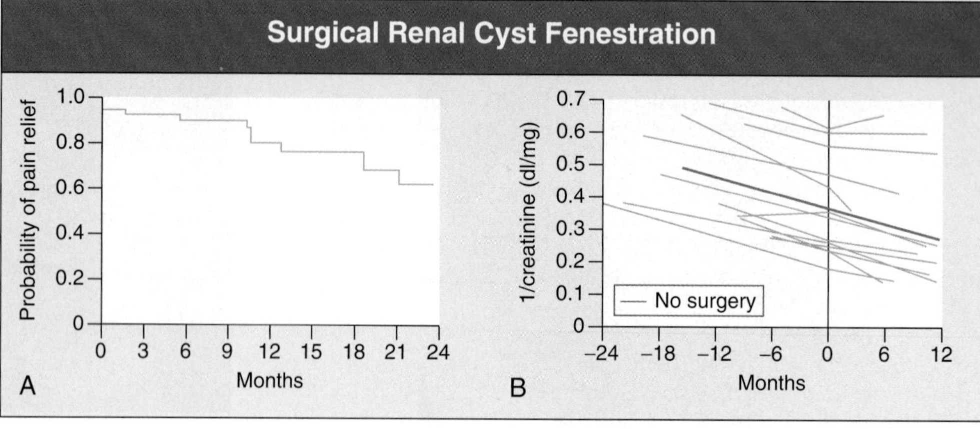

Figure 44.12 Surgical cyst fenestration for symptomatic ADPKD. A, Effects on relief of pain. **B,** Rate of decline of renal function. *Orange lines* indicate the course of renal function in individual patients who underwent cyst fenestration at month 0. *(Reprinted with permission from reference 48.)*

Polycystic kidneys demonstrate advanced sclerosis of preglomerular vessels, interstitial fibrosis, and tubular epithelial hyperplasia, even in patients with normal renal function or early renal failure.[33] Sclerosis involves both afferent arterioles and interlobular arteries. This is more prominent in ADPKD than in patients with glomerular disease and comparable renal function and may be attributable to hypertension and the activation of the RAS demonstrated in ADPKD. Interstitial fibrosis is also prominent, even in early disease. It is associated with an interstitial infiltrate of macrophages and lymphocytes.

TREATMENT

Current therapy is directed toward the renal and extrarenal complications of the disease in an effort to limit morbidity and mortality. Advances in the understanding of the genetics of ADPKD and mechanisms of cyst development and growth have raised hopes for treatments specifically directed toward limiting the development and progression of the disease, and some of these treatments are now being evaluated in clinical trials (see later, Novel Therapies).

Flank Pain

Causes of flank pain that may require intervention, such as infection, stone, and tumor, should be excluded. Care should be taken to avoid long-term administration of nephrotoxic agents, such as combination analgesics and nonsteroidal anti-inflammatory drugs. Narcotic analgesics should be reserved for the management of acute pain. Patients with chronic kidney pain are at risk for narcotic and analgesic dependence, and a psychological evaluation and a supportive attitude on the part of the physician are essential. Reassurance, lifestyle modification, and avoidance of aggravating activities may be helpful. Tricyclic antidepressants are helpful as in other chronic pain syndromes, with a generally well tolerated side-effect profile. Splanchnic nerve blockade with local anesthesia or corticosteroids results in pain relief prolonged beyond the duration of the local anesthetic.

When distortion of the kidneys by large cysts is deemed responsible for the pain and conservative measures fail, cyst decompression should be considered. Cyst aspiration, under ultrasound or CT guidance, is a relatively simple procedure; to prevent the reaccumulation of cyst fluid, sclerosing agents such as 95% ethanol or acidic solutions of minocycline are commonly used, with a success rate of greater than 90%. Minor complications include microscopic hematuria, localized pain, transient fever, and systemic absorption of the alcohol. More serious complications, such as pneumothorax, perirenal hematoma, arteriovenous fistula, urinoma, and infection, are rare. Complications from aspiration of centrally located cysts are more common, and the morbidity of the procedure is proportional to the number of cysts treated.

If multiple cysts are contributing to pain, laparoscopic or surgical cyst fenestration may be of benefit. Surgical decompression is effective in 80% to 90% of patients at 1 year, and 62% to 77% have sustained pain relief for more than 2 years (Fig. 44.12A). Surgical intervention does not accelerate the decline in renal function, as once thought, but does not appear to preserve declining renal function either (Fig. 44.12B). Laparoscopic fenestration is as effective as open surgical fenestration in short-term follow-up in patients with limited disease, and there is a shorter, less complicated recovery period compared with open surgery. Previous abdominal surgery with possible adhesion formation is a relative contraindication to the procedure.

There are a number of other interventions for the management of pain in ADPKD whose roles have not been fully defined. Laparoscopic renal denervation has been used in combination with cyst fenestration and may be considered, particularly in polycystic kidneys without large cysts. A nonrandomized, open label, uncontrolled trial of videothoracoscopic sympatho-splanchnicectomy is under way (*www.clinicaltrials.gov*, NCT00571909). Laparoscopic and retroperitoneoscopic nephrectomy and arterial embolization have been used to treat symptomatic polycystic kidneys in ADPKD patients with ESRD.

Cyst Hemorrhage

Episodes of cyst hemorrhage are self-limited and respond well to conservative management with bed rest, analgesics, and adequate fluid intake to prevent obstructing clots. Rarely, bleeding is more severe, with extensive subcapsular or retroperitoneal hematoma causing significant decrease in hematocrit and hemodynamic instability. This requires hospitalization and transfusion. In cases of unusually severe or persistent hemorrhage, segmental arterial embolization can be successful. If not, surgery may be required to control bleeding.

Urinary Tract and Cyst Infection

Because most renal cyst infections begin as cystitis, prompt treatment of symptomatic cystitis and asymptomatic bacteriuria is indicated to prevent retrograde seeding of the renal parenchyma. Antibiotics that require glomerular filtration, such as highly polar aminoglycosides, are not effective for upper urinary tract infection in severe renal impairment. Cyst infection is often difficult to treat despite prolonged therapy with an antibiotic to which the organism is susceptible. Treatment failure occurs if antibiotics do not penetrate the cyst epithelium and achieve therapeutic concentrations within the cysts. With gradient cysts, the epithelium lining the cyst has functional and ultrastructural characteristics of the distal tubule epithelium. Penetration is through tight junctions, allowing only lipid-soluble agents access. Nongradient cysts, which are more common, allow solute access through diffusion, suggesting that water-soluble agents should gain entry to the cysts. However, kinetic studies indicate that these agents penetrate nongradient cysts slowly and irregularly, giving rise to unreliable drug concentrations within the cysts. Lipophilic agents have been shown to penetrate both gradient and nongradient cysts equally and reliably and have a pK_a that allows favorable electrochemical gradients into acidic cyst fluid. Therapeutic agents of choice include trimethoprim-sulfamethoxazole and fluoroquinolones, both of which have shown favorable intracystic therapeutic concentration gradients at physiologic pH in gradient and nongradient cysts.

If fever persists after 1 to 2 weeks of appropriate antimicrobial therapy, percutaneous or surgical drainage of infected cysts should be undertaken. In the case of end-stage polycystic kidneys, nephrectomy should be considered. If fever recurs after stopping of antibiotics, complicating features such as obstruction, perinephric abscess, and stone should be excluded. If no such complicating features are identified, the antibiotic course should be extended and may require several months to fully eradicate infection.

Nephrolithiasis

Treatment of nephrolithiasis in patients with ADPKD is not different from that in patients without ADPKD. Potassium citrate is the treatment of choice in the three stone-forming conditions associated with ADPKD: uric acid lithiasis, hypocitraturic calcium oxalate nephrolithiasis, and distal acidification defects. Extracorporeal shock wave lithotripsy and percutaneous nephrostolithotomy are reported to be 82% and 80% successful, respectively, without significant complication.[34]

Hypertension

Control of hypertension is essential because uncontrolled hypertension accelerates the decline in renal function and aggravates extrarenal complications. Antihypertensive agents of choice and optimal blood pressure targets in ADPKD have not been established. Angiotensin-converting enzyme (ACE) inhibitors or angiotensin receptor blockers (ARBs) increase renal blood flow in ADPKD, have a low side effect profile, and may have renoprotective properties that go beyond blood pressure control. Although studies have failed to demonstrate a beneficial effect of ACE inhibitors on the progression of ADPKD,[35-38] these studies have been limited by the use of low drug dosages, small numbers of patients, short duration of follow-up, and inclusion of patients with widely different renal function. An extended follow-up of ADPKD patients in the Modification of Diet in Renal Disease (MDRD) study showed a delayed onset of kidney failure and lower composite outcome of kidney failure and all-cause mortality in the low blood pressure group (51% of them taking ACE inhibitors) compared with those in the usual blood pressure group (32% of them taking ACE inhibitors).[39] An ongoing study (HALT PKD) is designed to determine whether combined therapy with an ACE inhibitor and an ARB is superior to an ACE inhibitor alone in delaying the progression of the cystic disease in patients with preserved renal function or in slowing the decline of renal function in patients with chronic kidney disease stage 3. HALT PKD will also determine whether a low blood pressure target is superior to a standard blood pressure target in patients with preserved renal function. Although these definitive studies are needed, on available evidence, we recommend tight blood pressure control to 125/75 mm Hg with a regimen that includes ACE inhibitors or ARBs.

Progressive Renal Failure

General strategies to delay progression of chronic kidney disease are discussed in Chapter 76. A subgroup analysis of the MDRD trial, however, showed no beneficial effect on renal function in ADPKD of strict compared with standard blood pressure control and marginal benefit of a very low protein diet. Because these interventions were introduced late in that study (GFR 13 to 55 ml/min per 1.73 m^2), these results do not exclude a beneficial effect of earlier interventions. The benefit of avoiding high fluid intake in ADPKD remains controversial.[40]

ADPKD patients do better on dialysis than patients with ESRD from other causes. Women appear to do better than men. The good outcome in ADPKD may be due to higher endogenous erythropoietin production and better maintenance of hemoglobin, or lower comorbidity. Rarely, hemodialysis can be complicated by intradialytic hypotension if there is inferior vena cava compression by a medially located renal cyst. Despite renal size, peritoneal dialysis can usually be performed in ADPKD, although there is increased risk for inguinal and umbilical hernias, which require surgical repair.

Polycystic Liver Disease

PLD is usually asymptomatic and requires no treatment. When it is symptomatic, therapy is directed toward reducing cyst volume and hepatic size. Noninvasive measures include avoiding ethanol, other hepatotoxins, and possibly cAMP agonists (e.g., caffeine), which have been shown to stimulate cyst fluid secretion *in vitro*. Histamine H_2 blockers and somatostatin have been suggested to reduce secretion of secretin and secretory activity of cyst walls. Estrogens are likely to contribute to cyst growth, but the use of oral contraceptive agents and postmenopausal estrogen replacement therapy are contraindicated only if the liver is significantly enlarged and the risk for further hepatic cyst growth outweighs the benefits of estrogen therapy. Rarely, symptomatic PLD may require invasive measures to reduce cyst volume and hepatic size. Options include percutaneous cyst aspiration and sclerosis, laparoscopic fenestration, and open surgical fenestration. Cyst aspiration is the procedure of choice if symptoms are caused by one or a few dominant cysts or by cysts that are easily accessible to percutaneous intervention. To prevent the reaccumulation of cyst fluid, sclerosis with minocycline or 95% ethanol is often successful. Laparoscopic fenestration can be considered for large cysts that are more likely to recur after ethanol sclerosis or if several cysts are present that would require multiple percutaneous passes to be treated adequately. Partial hepatectomy with cyst fenestration is an option because PLD often spares a part of the liver with adequate preservation of hepatic parenchyma and liver function (see Fig. 44.13). In the rare case in which no segments are spared, liver transplantation may be necessary.[41]

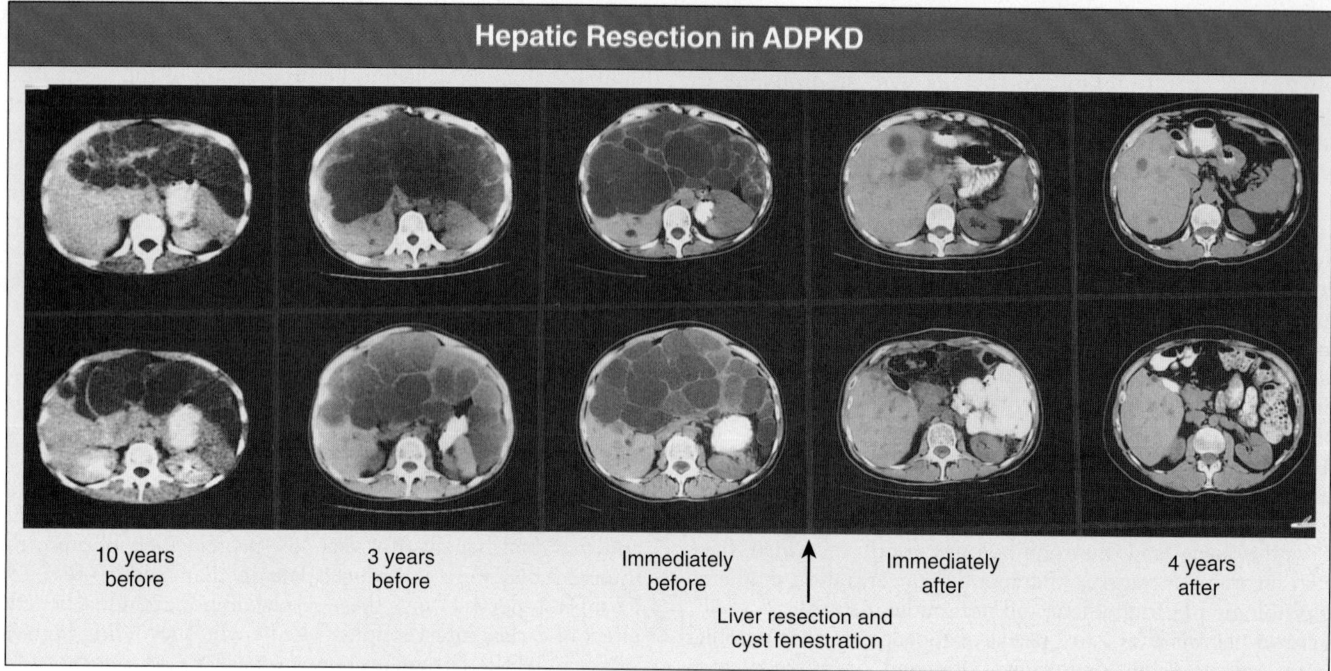

Figure 44.13 Hepatic resection in ADPKD. CT scans of the abdomen 10 years before (column 1), 3 years before (column 2), immediately before (column 3), immediately after (column 4), and 4 years after (column 5) liver resection and cyst fenestration demonstrating long-term, sustained reduction in liver size after the procedure. *(Reprinted with permission from reference 49.)*

When a hepatic cyst infection is suspected, any cyst with unusual appearance on an imaging study should be aspirated for diagnostic purposes. The best management is percutaneous cyst drainage in combination with antibiotic therapy. Long-term oral antibiotic suppression or prophylaxis should be reserved for relapsing or recurrent cases. Antibiotics of choice are trimethoprim-sulfamethoxazole and the fluoroquinolones, which are effective against the typical infecting organisms and concentrate in the biliary tree and cysts.

Intracranial Aneurysm

Ruptured or symptomatic intracranial aneurysm requires surgical clipping of the neck of the aneurysm. Asymptomatic aneurysms measuring less than 5 mm, diagnosed by presymptomatic screening, can be observed with repeated MR angiography at 6 months, then annually and less frequently after stability of the aneurysm has been established. If the size increases, surgery is indicated. Definitive management of aneurysms between 6 and 9 mm remains controversial. Surgical intervention is usually indicated for all unruptured aneurysms 10 mm in diameter or larger. For patients with high surgical risk or with technically difficult lesions, endovascular treatment with detachable platinum coils may be indicated.

NOVEL THERAPIES

A better understanding of the pathophysiology and the availability of animal models have facilitated the development of promising candidate drugs for clinical trials (see Fig. 44.2).

Vasopressin Antagonists

The effect of vasopressin, through V_2 receptors, on cAMP levels in the collecting duct, the major site of cyst development in ADPKD, and the role of cAMP in cystogenesis provided the rationale for successful preclinical trials of vasopressin V_2 receptor antagonists.[2] High water intake by itself also exerted a protective effect on the development of PKD in PCK rats, probably because of suppression of vasopressin.[42] Genetic elimination of arginine vasopressin in these rats yielded animals born with normal kidneys that remained relatively free of cysts unless an exogenous V_2 receptor agonist was administered.[43] Phase II clinical trials with tolvaptan have been completed, and a phase III clinical trial is ongoing (NCT00428948).

Somatostatin Analogues

Somatostatin acting on sst_2 receptors inhibits cAMP accumulation not only in the kidney but also in the liver. Octreotide, a metabolically stable somatostatin analogue, halted the expansion of hepatic cysts from PCK rats *in vitro* and *in vivo*. Similar effects were observed in the kidneys. Clinical trials of octreotide and lanreotide for PKD and PLD are currently active (NCT00309283, NCT00426153, NCT00565097).

mTOR Inhibitors

The mammalian target of rapamycin (mTOR) is activated in animal models of PKD. Patients with the contiguous *PKD1/TSC2* gene syndrome exhibit a more severe form of PKD than do those with ADPKD alone. This observation suggests a convergence of signaling pathways downstream from PC1 and the TSC proteins tuberin and hamartin that control the activity of mTOR. Studies in three rodent models of PKD have shown that the mTOR inhibitors sirolimus and everolimus significantly retard cyst expansion and protect renal function.[44] Small retrospective studies of ADPKD patients after transplantation have shown a significant reduction in the volume of the polycystic kidneys or polycystic liver in patients treated with sirolimus compared with patients treated with calcineurin inhibitors.[45,46] However randomized trials using everolimus and sirolimus for 18-24 months have not consistently delayed the increase in kidney size nor slowed the decline in progressive renal impairment.[50,51]

Other strategies targeting molecular mechanisms that are altered in PKD have shown promising results in animal studies but have not yet been assessed in clinical studies. These include activators of the polycystin 2 calcium channel (triptolide) and AMP-activated protein kinase (metformin) and inhibitors or antagonists of transporters and channels required for chloride secretion (CFTR inhibitors). Other promising agents are inhibitors of recycling of potassium out of the cell (KCa3.1 inhibitor), tyrosine kinase receptors (ErbB1, ErbB2, VEGF), tumor necrosis factor receptor, Src, MEK, cyclin-dependent kinases, cyclooxygenase 2, E-prostanoid 2 receptor, 20-hydroxyeicosatetraenoic acid synthesis, and caspases (see Fig. 44.2).[2]

TRANSPLANTATION

Transplantation is the treatment of choice for ESRD in ADPKD. There is no difference in patient or graft survival between ADPKD patients and other ESRD populations. Living donor transplants also have graft survival no different from that of non-ADPKD populations. However, living related transplantation has only recently been widely practiced in the ADPKD population. In 1999, 30% of kidney transplants for ADPKD patients were from living donors, compared with 12% in 1990.

Complications after transplantation are no greater in the ADPKD population than in the general population, and specific complications directly related to ADPKD are rare. Cyst infection is not increased after transplantation, and there is no significant increase in the incidence of symptomatic mitral valve prolapse or hepatic cyst infection. One study showed an increased rate of diverticulosis and bowel perforation in ADPKD. Whether ADPKD increases the risk for development of new-onset diabetes mellitus after transplantation is controversial.

Although practiced routinely in the past, pretransplantation nephrectomy has fallen out of favor. Indications for nephrectomy include a history of infected cysts, frequent bleeding, severe hypertension, and massive renal enlargement with extension into the pelvis. There is no evidence for an increased risk for development of renal cell carcinoma in native ADPKD kidneys after transplantation. When nephrectomy is indicated, hand-assisted laparoscopic nephrectomy is associated with less intraoperative blood loss, less postoperative pain, and faster recovery compared with open nephrectomy and is increasingly being used.

REFERENCES

1. Torres VE, Harris PC, Pirson Y. Autosomal dominant polycystic kidney disease. *Lancet*. 2007;369:1287-1301.
2. Torres VE, Harris PC. Autosomal dominant polycystic kidney disease: The last three years. *Kidney Int*. 2009;76:149-168.
3. Boca M, D'Amato L, Distefano G, et al. Polycystin-1 induces cell migration by regulating phosphatidylinositol 3-kinase–dependent cytoskeletal rearrangements and GSK3β-dependent cell-cell mechanical adhesion. *Mol Biol Cell*. 2007;18:4050-4061.
4. Piontek K, Menezes LF, Garcia-Gonzalez MA, et al. A critical developmental switch defines the kinetics of kidney cyst formation after loss of Pkd1. *Nat Med*. 2007;13:1490-1495.
5. Patel V, Li L, Cobo-Stark P, et al. Acute kidney injury and aberrant planar cell polarity induce cyst formation in mice lacking renal cilia. *Hum Mol Genet*. 2008;17:1578-1590.
6. Alper SL. Let's look at cysts from both sides now. *Kidney Int*. 2008;74:699-702.
7. Alvaro D, Onori P, Alpini G, et al. Morphological and functional features of hepatic cyst epithelium in autosomal dominant polycystic kidney disease. *Am J Pathol*. 2008;172:321-332.
8. Doulton TW, Saggar-Malik AK, He FJ, et al. The effect of sodium and angiotensin-converting enzyme inhibition on the classic circulating renin-angiotensin system in autosomal-dominant polycystic kidney disease patients. *J Hypertens*. 2006;24:939-945.
9. Qian Q, Hunter LW, Du H, et al. Pkd2$^{+/-}$ vascular smooth muscles develop exaggerated vasocontraction in response to phenylephrine stimulation. *J Am Soc Nephrol*. 2007;18:485-493.
10. Clausen P, Feldt-Rasmussen B, Iversen J, et al. Flow-associated dilatory capacity of the brachial artery is intact in early autosomal dominant polycystic kidney disease. *Am J Nephrol*. 2006;26:335-339.
11. Turgut F, Oflaz H, Namli S, et al. Ambulatory blood pressure and endothelial dysfunction in patients with autosomal dominant polycystic kidney disease. *Ren Fail*. 2007;29:979-984.
12. Borresen ML, Wang D, Strandgaard S. Pulse wave reflection is amplified in normotensive patients with autosomal-dominant polycystic kidney disease and normal renal function. *Am J Nephrol*. 2007;27:240-246.
13. Turkmen K, Oflaz H, Uslu B, et al. Coronary flow velocity reserve and carotid intima media thickness in patients with autosomal dominant polycystic kidney disease: From impaired tubules to impaired carotid and coronary arteries. *Clin J Am Soc Nephrol*. 2008;3:986-991.
14. Reed BY, McFann K, Bekheirnia MR, et al. Variation in age at ESRD in autosomal dominant polycystic kidney disease. *Am J Kidney Dis*. 2008;51:173-183.
15. Harris PC, Bae KT, Rossetti S, et al. Cyst number but not the rate of cystic growth is associated with the mutated gene in autosomal dominant polycystic kidney disease. *J Am Soc Nephrol*. 2006;17:3013-3019.
16. Rossetti S, Kubly V, Consugar M, et al. Incompletely penetrant PKD1 alleles suggest a role for gene dosage in cyst initiation in polycystic kidney disease. *Kidney Int*. 2009;75:848-855. Epub 2009 Jan 21.
17. Pei Y, Obaji J, Dupuis A, et al. Unified criteria for ultrasonographic diagnosis of ADPKD. *J Am Soc Nephrol*. 2009;20:205-212.
18. Rossetti S, Consugar MB, Chapman AB, et al. Comprehensive molecular diagnostics in autosomal dominant polycystic kidney disease. *J Am Soc Nephrol*. 2007;18:2143-2160.
19. Grantham JJ, Chapman AB, Torres VE. Volume progression in autosomal dominant polycystic kidney disease: The major factor determining clinical outcomes. *Clin J Am Soc Nephrol*. 2006;1:148-157.
20. Bleeker-Rovers CP, Vos FJ, Corstens FH, et al. Imaging of infectious diseases using [^{18}F] fluorodeoxyglucose PET. *Q J Nucl Med Mol Imaging*. 2008;52:17-29.
21. Torres VE, Wilson DM, Hattery RR, et al. Renal stone disease in autosomal dominant polycystic kidney disease. *Am J Kidney Dis*. 1993;22:513-519.
22. Cadnapaphornchai MA, McFann K, Strain JD, et al. Increased left ventricular mass in children with autosomal dominant polycystic kidney disease and borderline hypertension. *Kidney Int*. 2008;74:1192-1196.
23. Johnson A, Gabow P. Identification of patients with autosomal dominant polycystic kidney disease at highest risk for end-stage renal disease. *J Am Soc Nephrol*. 1997;8:1560-1567.
24. Torres VE, King BF, Chapman AB, et al. Magnetic resonance measurements of renal blood flow and disease progression in autosomal dominant polycystic kidney disease. *Clin J Am Soc Nephrol*. 2007;2:112-120.
25. Bae KT, Zhu F, Guay-Woodford LM, et al. Magnetic resonance imaging evaluation of hepatic cysts in early autosomal dominant polycystic kidney disease. *Clin J Am Soc Nephrol*. 2006;1:64-69.
26. Pirson Y, Chauveau D, Torres VE. Management of cerebral aneurysms in autosomal dominant polycystic kidney disease: Unruptured asymptomatic intracranial aneurysms. *J Am Soc Nephrol*. 2002;13:269-276.
27. Torres VE, Pirson Y, Wiebers DO. Cerebral aneurysms. *N Engl J Med*. 2006;355:2703-2704; author reply 2705.
28. Qian Q, Hartman RP, King BF, et al. Increased occurrence of pericardial effusion in patients with autosomal dominant polycystic kidney disease. *Clin J Am Soc Nephrol*. 2007;2:1223-1227.
29. Torra R, Sarquella J, Calabia J, et al. Prevalence of cysts in seminal tract and abnormal semen parameters in patients with autosomal dominant polycystic kidney disease. *Clin J Am Soc Nephrol*. 2008;3:790-793.
30. Schievink WI, Palestrant D, Maya MM, Rappard G. Spontaneous spinal cerebrospinal fluid leak as a cause of coma after craniotomy for clipping of an unruptured intracranial aneurysm. *J Neurosurg*. 2009;110:521-524.

31. Kumar S, Adeva M, King BF, et al. Duodenal diverticulosis in autosomal dominant polycystic kidney disease. *Nephrol Dial Transplant*. 2006;21: 3576-3578.
32. Yu AS, Kanzawa SA, Usorov A, et al. Tight junction composition is altered in the epithelium of polycystic kidneys. *J Pathol*. 2008;216: 120-128.
33. Zeier M, Fehrenbach P, Geberth S, et al. Renal histology in polycystic kidney disease with incipient and advanced renal failure. *Kidney Int*. 1992;42:1259-1265.
34. Torres VE, Wilson DM, Hattery RR, et al. Renal stone disease in autosomal dominant polycystic kidney disease. *Am J Kidney Dis*. 1993;22: 513-519.
35. Ecder T, Chapman A, Brosnahan G, et al. Effect of antihypertensive therapy on renal function and urinary albumin excretion in hypertensive patients with autosomal dominant polycystic kidney disease. *Am J Kidney Dis*. 2000;35:427-432.
36. Jafar T, Schmid C, Landa M, et al. Angiotensin-converting enzyme inhibitors and progression of nondiabetic renal disease: A meta-analysis of patient-level data. *Ann Intern Med*. 2001;135:73-87.
37. Schrier R, McFann K, Johnson A, et al. Cardiac and renal effects of standard versus rigorous blood pressure control in autosomal-dominant polycystic kidney disease: Results of a seven-year prospective randomized study. *J Am Soc Nephrol*. 2002;13:1733-1739.
38. Schrier RW, McFann KK, Johnson AM. Epidemiological study of kidney survival in autosomal dominant polycystic kidney disease. *Kidney Int*. 2003;63:678-685.
39. Sarnak MJ, Greene T, Wang X, et al. The effect of a lower target blood pressure on the progression of kidney disease: Long-term follow-up of the modification of diet in renal disease study. *Ann Intern Med*. 2005;142:342-351.
40. Torres VE, Bankir L, Grantham JJ. A case for water in the treatment of polycystic kidney disease. *Clin J Am Soc Nephrol*. 2009;4:1140-1150.
41. Schnelldorfer T, Torres VE, Zakaria S, et al. Polycystic liver disease: A critical appraisal of hepatic resection, cyst fenestration, and liver transplantation. *Ann Surg*. 2009;250:112-118.
42. Nagao S, Nishii K, Katsuyama M, et al. Increased water intake decreases progression of polycystic kidney disease in the PCK rat. *J Am Soc Nephrol*. 2006;17:2220-2227.
43. Wang X, Wu Y, Ward CJ, et al. Vasopressin directly regulates cyst growth in the PCK rat. *J Am Soc Nephrol*. 2008;19:102-108.
44. Edelstein CL. Mammalian target of rapamycin and caspase inhibitors in polycystic kidney disease. *Clin J Am Soc Nephrol*. 2008;3:1219-1226.
45. Shillingford JM, Murcia NS, Larson CH, et al. The mTOR pathway is regulated by polycystin-1, and its inhibition reverses renal cystogenesis in polycystic kidney disease. *Proc Natl Acad Sci U S A*. 2006;103: 5466-5471.
46. Qian Q, Du H, King BF, et al. Sirolimus reduces polycystic liver volume in ADPKD patients. *J Am Soc Nephrol*. 2008;19:631-638.
47. Iglesias CG, Torres VE, Offord KP, et al. Epidemiology and ADPKD. Olmsted County, Minnesota: 1935-1980. *Am J Kidney Dis*. 1983;2: 630-639.
48. Elzinga LW, Barry JM, Torres VE, et al. Cyst decompression surgery for autosomal dominant polycystic kidney disease. *J Am Soc Nephrol*. 1992;2:1219-1226.
49. Que F, Nagorney DM, Gross JB, Torres VE. Liver resection and cyst fenestration in the treatment of severe polycystic liver disease. *Gastroenterology*. 1995;108:487-494.
50. Walz G, Budde K, Mannaa M, et al. Everolimus in Patients with Autosomal Dominant Polycystic Kidney Disease. *N Engl J Med*. 2010 Jun 26. [Epub ahead of print].
51. Serra AL, Poster D, Kistler AD, et al. Sirolimus and Kidney Growth in Autosomal Dominant Polycystic Kidney Disease. *N Engl J Med*. 2010 Jun 26. [Epub ahead of print].

CHAPTER 45

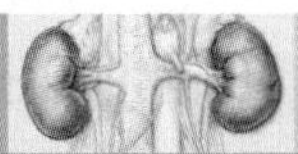

Other Cystic Kidney Diseases

Lisa M. Guay-Woodford

In addition to autosomal dominant polycystic kidney disease (ADPKD), there are numerous other disorders that share renal cysts as a common feature (Fig. 45.1).[1] These disorders may be inherited or acquired; their manifestations may be confined to the kidney or expressed systemically. They may present at a wide range of ages, from the perinatal period to old age (Fig. 45.2). The renal cysts may be single or multiple, and the associated renal morbidity may range from clinical insignificance to progressive parenchymal destruction with resultant renal impairment.

The clinical context often helps distinguish these renal cystic disorders from one another. Echogenic, enlarged kidneys in a neonate or infant should raise suspicion about autosomal recessive polycystic kidney disease (ARPKD), ADPKD, tuberous sclerosis complex, or one of the many congenital syndromes associated with renal cystic disease. Renal impairment in an adolescent suggests juvenile nephronophthisis–medullary cystic disease complex and ARPKD as possible causes. The finding of a solitary cyst in a 5-year-old may indicate a calyceal diverticulum, whereas this finding in a 50-year-old is most compatible with a simple renal cyst. Renal stones occur in ADPKD and medullary sponge kidneys. For those disorders with systemic manifestations, such as ADPKD, tuberous sclerosis complex, and von Hippel–Lindau disease, the associated extrarenal features may provide other important differential diagnostic clues.

For an increasing number of conditions, genetic testing is available in expert laboratories around the world. These are listed at *http://www.genetests.org*.

AUTOSOMAL RECESSIVE POLYCYSTIC KIDNEY DISEASE

Definition

ARPKD is an inherited malformation complex with varying degrees of renal collecting duct dilation, biliary ductal ectasia, and associated fibrosis.[2]

Genetic Basis of ARPKD

All typical forms of ARPKD are caused by mutations in a single gene, *PKHD1* (polycystic kidney and hepatic disease), which encodes multiple alternatively spliced isoforms predicted to form both membrane-bound and secreted proteins.[3] The largest protein product of *PKHD1*, termed fibrocystin/polyductin complex (FPC), contains one membrane spanning domain and an intracellular C-terminal tail. FPC localizes, at least in part, to the primary cilium and the centrosome in renal epithelial cells.[4] The basic defects observed in ARPKD suggest that FPC mediates the terminal differentiation of the collecting duct and biliary tract. However, the exact function of the numerous isoforms has not been defined, and the widely varying clinical spectrum of ARPKD may depend, in part, on the nature and number of splice variants that are disrupted by specific *PKHD1* mutations.

Pathogenesis

ARPKD typically begins *in utero*, and the renal cystic lesion appears to be superimposed on a normal developmental sequence. The tubular abnormality primarily involves fusiform dilation of the collecting ducts. Detailed microdissection studies have excluded tubular obstruction as a primary pathogenic mechanism. The biliary lesion appears to involve defective remodeling of the ductal plate *in utero*. As a result, primitive bile duct configurations persist and progressive portal fibrosis evolves.[5] The remainder of the liver parenchyma develops normally. The defect in ductal plate remodeling is accompanied by abnormalities in the branching of the portal vein. The resulting histopathologic pattern is referred to as congenital hepatic fibrosis.

The primary cilium plays a central role in the pathogenesis of hepatorenal fibrocystic diseases.[6] The weight of the experimental evidence from human ARPKD and animal model studies suggests that ciliary dysfunction contributes to a maturational arrest in both renal and biliary tubuloepithelial differentiation.

Epidemiology

The estimated incidence of ARPKD is 1 per 20,000 live births.[7] It occurs more frequently in Caucasians than in other ethnic populations.

Clinical Manifestations

The clinical spectrum of ARPKD is variable and depends on the age at presentation. The majority of cases are identified either *in utero* or at birth. The most severely affected fetuses have enlarged echogenic kidneys and oligohydramnios due to poor fetal urine output. These fetuses develop the Potter phenotype, with pulmonary hypoplasia, a characteristic facies, and deformities of the spine and limbs. At birth, these neonates often have a critical degree of pulmonary hypoplasia that is incompatible with survival. The estimated perinatal mortality is about 30%. Renal function, although frequently compromised, is rarely a cause of neonatal death.

For those who survive the first month of life, the reported mean 5-year patient survival rate is 85% to 90%.[2,8] Morbidity

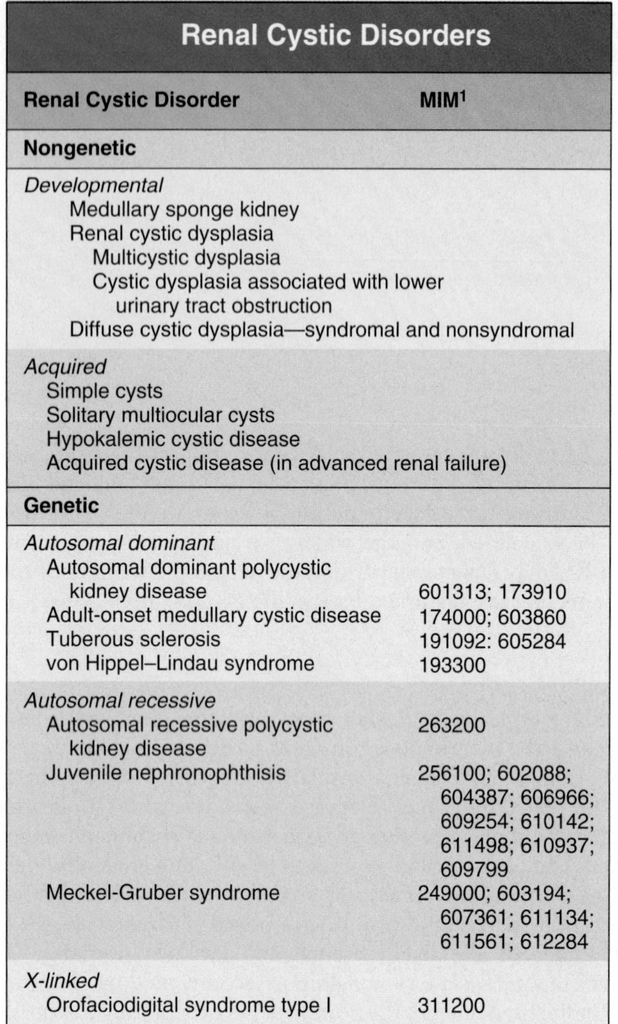

Renal Cystic Disorders

Renal Cystic Disorder	MIM[1]
Nongenetic	
Developmental	
Medullary sponge kidney	
Renal cystic dysplasia	
Multicystic dysplasia	
Cystic dysplasia associated with lower urinary tract obstruction	
Diffuse cystic dysplasia—syndromal and nonsyndromal	
Acquired	
Simple cysts	
Solitary multiocular cysts	
Hypokalemic cystic disease	
Acquired cystic disease (in advanced renal failure)	
Genetic	
Autosomal dominant	
Autosomal dominant polycystic kidney disease	601313; 173910
Adult-onset medullary cystic disease	174000; 603860
Tuberous sclerosis	191092: 605284
von Hippel–Lindau syndrome	193300
Autosomal recessive	
Autosomal recessive polycystic kidney disease	263200
Juvenile nephronophthisis	256100; 602088; 604387; 606966; 609254; 610142; 611498; 610937; 609799
Meckel-Gruber syndrome	249000; 603194; 607361; 611134; 611561; 612284
X-linked	
Orofaciodigital syndrome type I	311200

Figure 45.1 Renal cystic disorders.[1] Mendelian Inheritance in Man (*http://www.ncbi.nlm.nih.gov/entrez/query.fcgi?db=OMIM*).

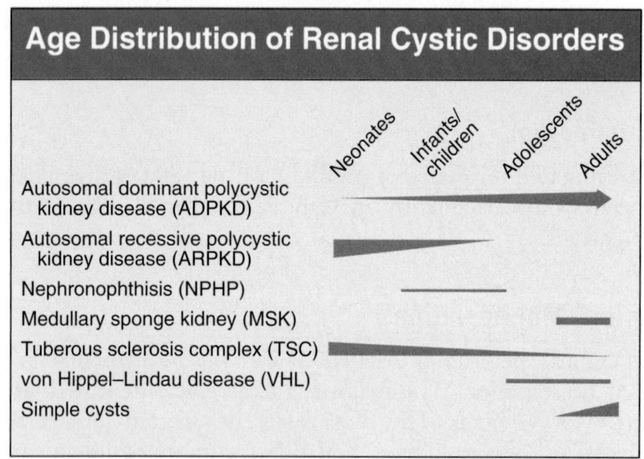

Figure 45.2 Age distribution of renal cystic disorders.

and mortality result from severe systemic hypertension, renal impairment, and portal hypertension due to portal tract hyperplasia and fibrosis.[2,8,9] Hypertension usually develops in the first few months and ultimately affects 70% to 80% of patients. ARPKD patients have defects in both urinary diluting capacity and concentrating capacity. Newborns can have hyponatremia. Whereas net acid excretion may be reduced, metabolic acidosis is not a significant clinical feature. Abnormal urinalysis is common in both infants and older children.[2] Microscopic or gross hematuria, proteinuria, and sterile pyuria have all been reported. Two retrospective studies have noted an increased incidence of culture-confirmed urinary tract infections.

In the first 6 months of life, ARPKD infants may have a transient improvement in glomerular filtration rate (GFR) due to renal maturation. Subsequently, a progressive but variable decline in renal function occurs, with some patients not progressing to end-stage renal disease (ESRD) until adolescence or early adulthood. With advances in effective therapy for ESRD, prolonged survival is common, and the hepatic complications become the dominant clinical issue for many patients.

On average, those infants with serum creatinine values above 2.2 mg/dl (200 μmol/l) progress to ESRD within 5 years, but this is highly variable. In longitudinal studies, the probability of renal survival without ESRD is ~85% at 1 year, ~70% at 10 years, ~65% at 15 years, and ~40% at 20 years.[8,9]

In children who present later in childhood or in adolescence, portal hypertension is frequently the predominant clinical abnormality, with hepatosplenomegaly and bleeding esophageal or gastric varices as well as hypersplenism with consequent thrombocytopenia, anemia, and leukopenia. Hepatocellular function is usually preserved. Ascending suppurative cholangitis is a serious complication and can cause fulminant hepatic failure.[10]

Pathology

Kidney

The renal involvement is invariably bilateral and largely symmetric. The histopathology varies according to the age at presentation and the extent of cystic involvement (Fig. 45.3A, B).

In the affected neonate, the kidneys can be 10 times normal size but retain their reniform configuration. Dilated, fusiform collecting ducts extend radially through the cortex. In the medulla, the dilated collecting ducts are more often cut tangentially or transversely. Up to 90% of the collecting ducts are involved. Associated interstitial fibrosis is minimal in neonates and infants but increases with progressive disease.

In patients diagnosed later in childhood, the kidney size and extent of cystic involvement tend to be more limited. Cysts can expand up to 2 cm in diameter and assume a more spherical configuration. Progressive interstitial fibrosis is probably responsible for secondary tubular obstruction. In older children, medullary ductal ectasia is the predominant finding.

Cysts are lined with a single layer of nondescript cuboidal epithelium. The glomeruli and nephron segments proximal to the collecting ducts are initially structurally normal but are often crowded between ectatic collecting ducts or displaced into subcapsular wedges. The presence of cartilage or other dysplastic elements indicates a diagnosis other than ARPKD, such as cystic dysplasia.

Liver

The liver lesion in ARPKD is characterized by ductal plate malformation.[5] The liver can be either normal in size or somewhat enlarged. Bile ducts are dilated (biliary ectasia), and marked cystic dilation of the entire intrahepatic biliary system (Caroli's disease) has been described. In neonatal ARPKD, the bile ducts are increased in number, tortuous in configuration, and often located around the periphery of the portal tract. In older children, the biliary ectasia is accompanied by increasing portal tract

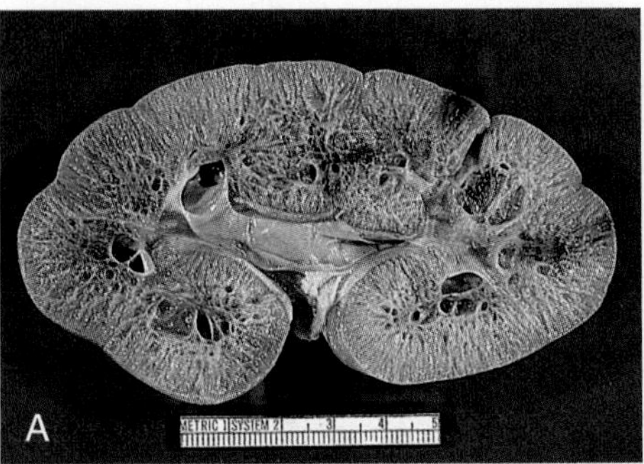
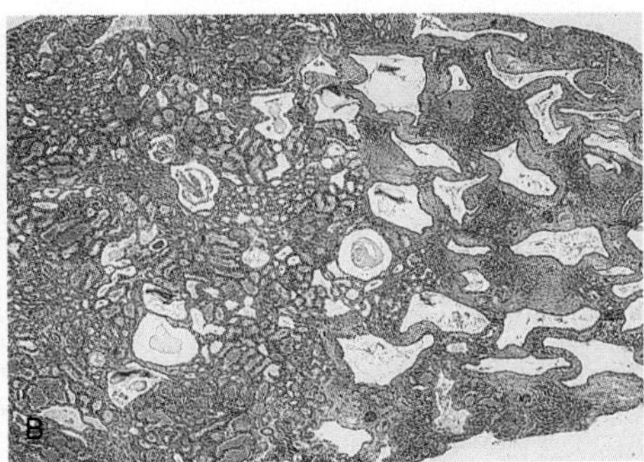
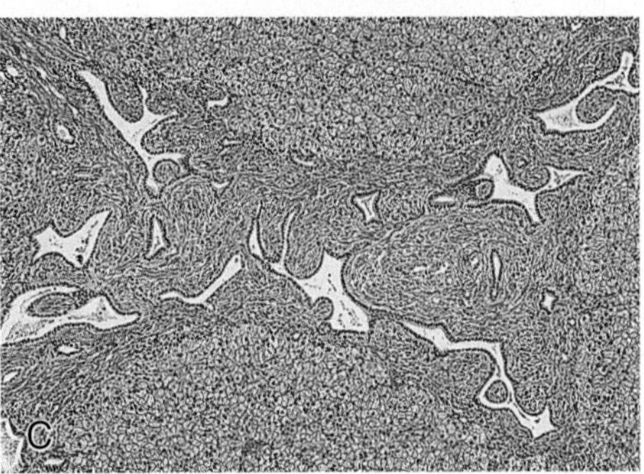

Figure 45.3 Pathologic features of ARPKD. A, Cut section: ARPKD kidney from 1-year-old child reveals discrete medullary cysts and dilated collecting ducts. **B,** Light microscopy: later-onset ARPKD kidney with prominent medullary ductal ectasia. (Hematoxylin and eosin; magnification ×10.) **C,** Light microscopy: congenital hepatic fibrosis. There is extensive fibrosis of the portal area with ectatic, tortuous bile ducts and hypoplasia of the portal vein. (Hematoxylin and eosin; magnification ×40.)

fibrosis and hypoplasia of the small portal vein branches (Fig. 45.3C). The hepatic parenchyma may be intersected by delicate fibrous septa that link the portal tracts, but the hepatocytes themselves are seldom affected.

Diagnosis

ARPKD must be differentiated from a range of other pediatric renal cystic disorders (Fig. 45.4).

Imaging

In the past decade, clinical diagnosis has increasingly relied on imaging instead of histopathologic analysis.

ARPKD belongs to a group of disorders described as hepatorenal fibrocystic diseases.[11] Whereas most of these disorders are characterized by large, echogenic kidneys in the fetus and neonate, studies indicate that to a large extent they can be distinguished by ultrasound.[12]

ARPKD kidneys *in utero* are hyperechogenic and display *decreased* corticomedullary differentiation because of the hyperechogenic medulla (Fig. 45.5A). With high-resolution ultrasound, the radial array of dilated collecting ducts may be imaged. In comparison, ADPKD kidneys *in utero* tend to be moderately enlarged with a hyperechogenic cortex and relatively hypoechogenic medulla, causing *increased* corticomedullary differentiation.

Kidney size typically peaks at 1 to 2 years of age, then gradually declines relative to the child's body size and stabilizes by 4 to 5 years. As patients age, there is increased medullary echogenicity with scattered small cysts, measuring less than 2 cm in diameter. These cysts and progressive fibrosis can alter the reniform contour, causing ARPKD in some older children to be mistaken for ADPKD. Contrast-enhanced computed tomography (CT) can be useful in delineating the renal architecture in these children (Fig. 45.5B). Bilateral pelvicaliectasis and renal calcifications have been reported in 25% and 50% of ARPKD patients, respectively.[9,13] In adults with medullary ectasia alone, the cystic lesion may be confused with medullary sponge kidney.

The liver may be either normal in size or enlarged. It is usually less echogenic than the kidneys. Prominent intrahepatic bile duct dilation suggests associated Caroli's disease. With age, the portal fibrosis tends to progress, and in older children, ultrasound typically shows hepatosplenomegaly and a patchy increase in hepatic echogenicity.

Genetic Testing

With the identification of *PKHD1* as the principal disease gene in ARPKD, genetic testing is available as a clinical diagnostic tool. The mutation detection rate is 80% to 87%. Current diagnostic algorithms include gene-based analysis and haplotype-based genotyping in informative families (*http://www.genetests.org/*). Genetic testing is primarily applied in the context of prenatal testing[14] and preimplantation genetic diagnosis.[15] To date, there is limited evidence for genotype-phenotype correlations, although patients with two truncating mutations have a higher risk of perinatal demise.[16,17] There is a high percentage of unique, missense changes in *PKHD1*, which can complicate the unequivocal interpretation of gene-based testing. Moreover, about 20% of ARPKD siblings have discordant clinical phenotypes.[8] These data potentially complicate genetic counseling, and caution must be exercised in predicting the clinical outcome of future affected children.

Treatment

The survival of ARPKD neonates has improved significantly in the last two decades because of advances in mechanical ventilation for neonates and other supportive measures. Aggressive interventions, such as unilateral or bilateral nephrectomies and continuous hemofiltration, have been advocated in neonatal management, but prospective, controlled studies have yet to be performed.

For those children who survive the perinatal period, careful blood pressure monitoring is required. Angiotensin-converting enzyme (ACE) inhibitors, calcium channel blockers, β-blockers, and loop diuretics are effective antihypertensive agents. The management of ARPKD children with declining GFR should follow the standard guidelines established for chronic kidney disease (CKD) in children.[18]

Given the relative urinary concentrating defect, ARPKD children should be monitored for dehydration during intercurrent illnesses associated with fever, tachypnea, nausea, vomiting, or diarrhea. In those infants with severe polyuria, thiazide diuretics may be used to decrease distal nephron solute and water delivery. Acid-base balance should be closely monitored and supplemental bicarbonate therapy initiated as needed.

Close monitoring for portal hypertension is warranted in all ARPKD patients. The severity of portal hypertension and its progression can be followed by serial ultrasound and Doppler flow studies. Hematemesis or melena suggests the presence of

Clinical Characteristics of Pediatric Renal Cystic Disease						
	ARPKD	NPHP	Meckel-Gruber[1]	GCKD[2]	ADPKD	TSC
Clinical onset (years)	Perinatal	NPHP2: 0–5 NPHP: 10–18	Perinatal infancy	Infancy, older children	Infancy[3], older children	Infancy[3], older children
Enlarged kidneys	Yes	NPHP2: yes NPHP3: some cases NPHP: no	Yes	No	Occurs	Occurs
Renal pathology	Multiple cysts	NPHP2: multiple cysts NPHP: few cysts at C-M junction	Multiple cysts	Multiple cortical cysts	Multiple cysts	Few to multiple cysts; angiomyolipoma
Cyst infection	Uncommon	No	Uncommon	No	Occurs	Uncommon
BP	Normal/increased	NPHP2: increased NPHP: normal	Normal	Normal/ increased	Normal/ increased	Normal/ increased
Renal function	Normal/impaired	Normal/impaired	Normal/impaired	Normal	Normal	Normal
Nephrocalcinosis/ nephrolithiasis	Nephrocalcinosis up to 25%	No	No	No	Nephrolithiases occur	No
CHF	Yes	Rare	Yes	No	10%–15%infantile ADPKD	No
Pancreas lesions	No	No	No	MODY5	No	No
CNS involvement	No	(Joubert)[4]	Encephalocele; mental retardation	No	No	Seizures, mental retardation
Genetics of Pediatric Renal Cystic Disease						
Disease gene	PKHD1	NPHP1-NPHP4	MSK1-MSK6	PKD1 TCF2	PKD1 PKD2	TSC1 TSC2
Genetic testing[5]	Yes	Yes	No	Yes	Yes	Yes

Figure 45.4 Features of pediatric renal cystic disease.[1] Meckel-Gruber syndrome is a severe, often lethal, autosomal recessive disorder characterized by bilateral renal cystic dysplasia, biliary ductal dysgenesis, bilateral postaxial polydactyly, and variable central nervous system malformations. The triad of renal cystic disease, occipital encephalocele, and polydactyly is most common. [2]Glomerulocystic kidney disease (GCKD) can occur as the infantile manifestation of ADPKD. Familial hypoplastic GCKD, due to mutations in *TCF2*, the gene encoding hepatocyte nuclear factor 1β, can be associated with maturity-onset diabetes of the young, type 5 (MODY5). [3]A contiguous germline deletion of both the *PKD1* and *TSC2* genes (the PKTS contiguous gene syndrome) occurs in a small group of patients with features of TSC as well as massive renal cystic disease reminiscent of ADPKD, severe hypertension, and a progressive decline in renal function with the onset of ESRD in the second or third decade of life. [4]Joubert syndrome (JBTS; MIM 213300) is a genetically heterogeneous (JBTS1-7), autosomal recessive disorder characterized by developmental defects in the cerebellum (cerebellar vermis aplasia) and the eye (coloboma) as well as retinitis pigmentosa, congenital hypotonia, and either ocular motor apraxia or irregularities in breathing patterns during the neonatal period. The disease can be associated with NPHP, and mutations in *NPHP1* have been described in a small subset of patients (JBTS4). Disease genes have been identified for JBTS3 and JBTS5-7. [5]Listed at GeneTests (*http://www.genetests.org*). ADPKD, autosomal dominant polycystic kidney disease; ARPKD, autosomal recessive polycystic kidney disease; BP, blood pressure; CHF, congestive heart failure; CNS, central nervous system; NPHP, nephronophthisis; TSC, tuberous sclerosis complex.

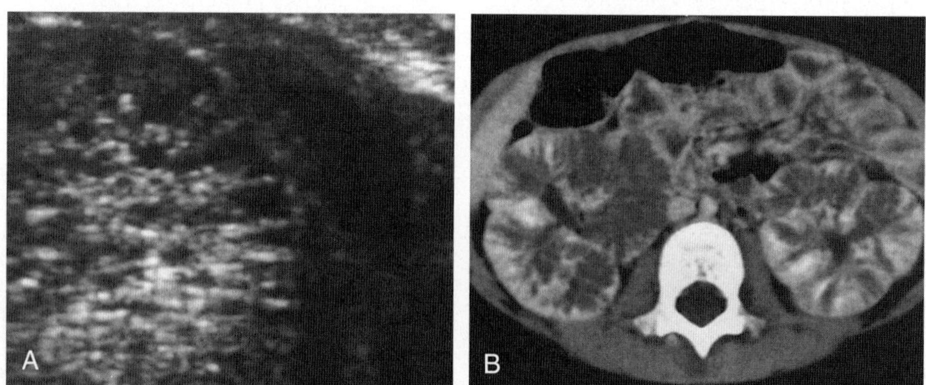

Figure 45.5 Radiologic findings associated with ARPKD. A, ARPKD in a neonate. High-resolution ultrasound reveals radially arrayed dilated collecting ducts. **B,** ARPKD in a symptomatic 4-year-old girl. Contrast-enhanced CT shows a striated nephrogram and prolonged corticomedullary differentiation.

esophageal varices. Medical management may include sclerotherapy, variceal banding, or transjugular intrahepatic portosystemic shunt. Surgical approaches, such as portocaval or splenorenal shunting, may be indicated in some patients. Although hypersplenism occurs fairly commonly, splenectomy is seldom warranted. Unexplained fever with or without elevated transaminase levels suggests bacterial cholangitis and requires meticulous evaluation, sometimes including a percutaneous liver biopsy, to make the diagnosis and to guide aggressive antibiotic therapy.

Effective management of systemic and portal hypertension, coupled with successful renal replacement therapy, has allowed long-term patient survival. Therefore, the prognosis in ARPKD, particularly for those children who survive the first month of life, is far less bleak than popularly thought, and aggressive medical therapy is warranted.

Transplantation

A prolonged period of dialysis in childhood has been associated with both cognitive and educational impairment. Therefore, renal transplantation is the treatment of choice for ESRD in ARPKD patients, and at least one report advocates preemptive nephrectomy in neonates with markedly enlarged kidneys.[19] Because ARPKD is a recessive disorder, either parent may be a suitable kidney donor. Native nephrectomies may be warranted in patients with massively enlarged kidneys to allow allograft placement.

In some patients, combined kidney-liver transplantation is appropriate.[20] Indications include the combination of renal failure and either recurrent cholangitis or significant complications of portal hypertension (e.g., recurrent variceal bleeding, refractory ascites, and the hepatopulmonary syndrome). In addition, liver transplantation may be a reasonable option for patients with a single episode of cholangitis in the context of marked abnormalities in the biliary system (Caroli's syndrome).[21]

JUVENILE NEPHRONOPHTHISIS–MEDULLARY CYSTIC DISEASE COMPLEX

Definitions

Juvenile nephronophthisis (NPHP) and medullary cystic kidney disease share the same triad of histopathologic features: tubular basement membrane irregularities, tubular atrophy with cyst formation, and interstitial cell infiltration with fibrosis. These histopathologically similar disorders differ only in their mode of transmission, age at onset, and genetic defects. Juvenile NPHP is an autosomal recessive disorder that presents in childhood. Medullary cystic disease is an autosomal dominant disorder that occurs in adults. The inclusive term *juvenile nephronophthisis–medullary cystic disease complex* has been used to describe these disorders. However, juvenile NPHP is far more common than medullary cystic disease and has been reported both as an isolated renal disease and in association with retinitis pigmentosa, congenital hepatic fibrosis, oculomotor apraxia, and skeletal anomalies. Therefore, these entities are considered separately.

Autosomal Recessive Juvenile Nephronophthisis

Genetic Basis of Nephronophthisis

Nine genes (*NPHP1-NPHP9*) involved in juvenile NPHP have been identified.[22] Defects in *NPHP1* account for 21% of NPHP, with large, homozygous deletions detected in 80% of affected family members and in 65% of sporadic cases. Mutations in each of the remaining NPHP genes cause no more than 3% of NPHP-related disease. Clinical disease expression seems to be exacerbated by oligogenic inheritance, that is, patients carrying two mutations in a single NPHP gene as well as a single-copy mutation in an additional NPHP gene. In addition, multiple allelism, or distinct mutations in a single gene, appears to explain the continuum of multiorgan phenotypic abnormalities observed in NPHP, Meckel syndrome, and Joubert syndrome.

The *NPHP1* and *NPHP3-5* genes encode novel cytosolic proteins that are collectively called the nephrocystins. The *NPHP2* gene, involved in infantile NPHP, encodes inversin, a protein that localizes in a cell cycle–dependent manner to different subcellular locations. When it is expressed at the basal body of the primary cilium, inversin has been shown to regulate the Wnt signaling pathway. The gene products encoded by *NPHP6/CEP290*, *NPHP8/RPGRIP1L*, and *NPHP9/NEK8* are all expressed in or at the base of primary cilia in renal epithelial cells. The *NPHP7/GLIS2* gene encodes the transcription factor Gli-similar protein 2, thus implicating the hedgehog signaling pathway in the pathogenesis of renal cystic diseases.

All of the proteins encoded by *NPHP1-9* are expressed in or at the base of primary cilia in renal epithelial cells, giving rise to a unifying theory that defines cystic kidney diseases as "ciliopathies."[22] However, the subcellular localization of these proteins is not confined to the cilium. For example, nephrocystin and nephrocystin 4 have also been localized to cell junctions and shown to interact with components of cell-cell and cell-matrix interaction complexes. These observations suggest that NPHP proteins may have multiple functions, depending on their localization in different cell compartments and their association with distinct protein complexes.

Clinical Manifestations

Renal Disease NPHP accounts for 5% to 15% of ESRD in children and adolescents. Three distinct forms of the disease (infantile, juvenile, and adolescent) have been described on the basis of the age at onset of ESRD. However, further clinical, pathologic, and genetic analyses indicate that the adolescent and juvenile forms are virtually indistinguishable and should be described with the single designation juvenile NPHP.[23] In juvenile NPHP (the most common form), ESRD occurs at a mean age of 13 years; in the infantile form, the onset of ESRD consistently occurs before 5 years of age.

Decreased urinary concentrating capacity is invariable in NPHP and usually precedes the decline in renal function, with onset between 4 and 6 years of age. Polyuria and polydipsia are common. Salt wasting develops in most patients with renal impairment, and sodium supplementation is often required until the onset of ESRD. One third of patients become anemic before the onset of renal impairment, and this has been attributed to a defect in the functional regulation of erythropoietin production by peritubular fibroblasts.[24] Growth retardation, out of proportion to the degree of renal impairment, is a common finding.

Slowly progressive decline in renal function is typical of juvenile NPHP. Whereas symptoms can be detected after the age of 2 years, they may progress insidiously, such that 15% of affected patients are recognized only after ESRD has developed. There is no specific treatment. The disease is not known to recur in renal allografts.

Children with the infantile variant develop symptoms in the first few months of life and rapidly progress to ESRD, usually before the age of 2 years but invariably by 5 years of age. Severe hypertension is common in this disorder. This disorder is a distinct genetic entity with a characteristic renal histopathology and has not been reported in sibships with classic juvenile NPHP.[25]

Unlike patients with polycystic kidney disease or medullary sponge kidney, NPHP patients rarely develop flank pain, hematuria, hypertension, urinary tract infections, or renal calculi.

Associated Extrarenal Abnormalities Extrarenal abnormalities have been described in approximately 10% to 15% of juvenile NPHP patients.[23] The most frequently associated anomaly is retinal dystrophy due to tapetoretinal degeneration (Senior-Loken syndrome). Severely affected patients present with coarse nystagmus, early blindness, and a flat electroretinogram (Leber amaurosis); those with moderate retinal dystrophy typically have mild visual impairment and retinitis pigmentosa. Other extrarenal anomalies include oculomotor apraxia (Cogan syndrome), cerebellar vermis aplasia (Joubert syndrome), and cone-shaped epiphyses of the bones. Congenital hepatic fibrosis occurs occasionally in NPHP patients, but the associated bile duct proliferation is mild and qualitatively different from that found in ARPKD.

Pathology

In juvenile NPHP, the kidneys are moderately contracted with parenchymal atrophy, causing a loss of corticomedullary demarcation. Histopathologic findings include tubular atrophy with thickened tubular basement membrane, diffuse and severe interstitial fibrosis, and cysts of variable size distributed in an irregular pattern at the corticomedullary junction and in the outer medulla. However, up to 25% of NPHP kidneys have no grossly visible cysts.

In the typical NPHP renal lesion, clusters of atrophic tubules alternate either with groups of viable tubules showing dilation or with marked compensatory hypertrophy or with groups of collapsed tubules. Multilayered thickening of tubular basement membranes is a prominent histopathologic feature (Fig. 45.6). Whereas this histopathologic pattern is not unique, the abrupt transition from one type of tubular profile to another is suggestive of NPHP. Moderate interstitial fibrosis, usually without a significant inflammatory cell infiltrate, is interspersed among the atrophic tubules. Spherical, thin-walled cysts lined with a simple cuboidal epithelium may be evident at the corticomedullary junction, in the medulla, and even in the papillae. Microdissection studies indicate that these cysts arise from the loop of Henle, distal convoluted tubules, and collecting ducts. Glomeruli may be normal, although some may be completely sclerosed; others may show periglomerular fibrosis, and still others dilation of Bowman's space.

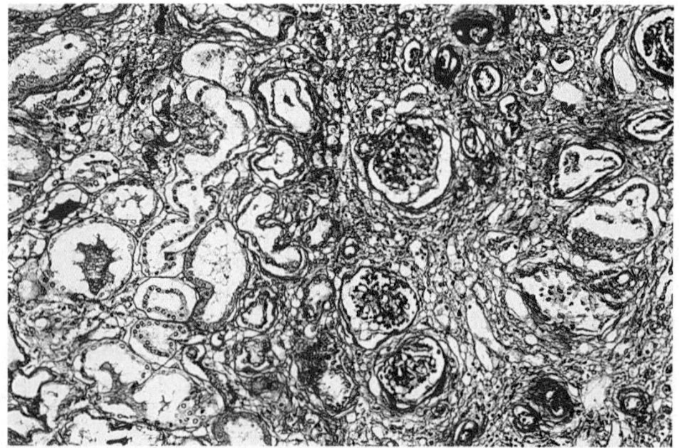

Figure 45.6 Renal pathology in juvenile nephronophthisis. Light microscopy: tubulointerstitial nephropathy. Atrophic tubules with irregularly thickened basement membranes are surrounded by interstitial fibrosis. Dilated tubules are evident at the corticomedullary junction. (Hematoxylin and eosin; magnification ×40.)

In comparison, the infantile form has features of both juvenile NPHP (such as tubular cell atrophy, interstitial fibrosis, and tubular cysts) and polycystic kidney disease, including enlarged kidneys and widespread cystic involvement.[26]

Diagnosis and Differential Diagnosis

In a child with NPHP and renal impairment, ultrasound reveals normal-sized or small kidneys with increased echogenicity and loss of corticomedullary differentiation. On occasion, cysts can be detected at the corticomedullary junction or in the medulla. Thin-section CT scanning may be more sensitive than ultrasound in detecting these cysts.

The pathologic findings in NPHP are not unique; hence, in the early stages of the disease, neither renal imaging nor histopathology can confirm the clinical diagnosis. As an alternative strategy, molecular testing has become increasingly useful in establishing the diagnosis of NPHP, with use of an algorithm for gene-based diagnosis[27] that addresses four critical diagnostic issues: (1) detection of the classic homozygous deletion of *NPHP1;* (2) detection of rare, smaller homozygous deletions of *NPHP1;* (3) testing for a heterozygous deletion; and (4) potential exclusion of linkage to *NPHP1*. Genetic testing is currently available for *NPHP1*-related disease (*http://www.genetests.org/*). As new genes are identified and their relative contribution to the NPHP disease spectrum is determined, mutational algorithms will be expanded to include analyses of these NPHP genes.

Autosomal Dominant Medullary Cystic Kidney Disease

Medullary cystic kidney disease is an autosomal dominant condition that is much rarer than autosomal recessive NPHP but histopathologically indistinguishable. Some patients have had phenotypically unaffected parents but an affected second- or third-degree relative, suggesting that the disease is poorly recognized in affected family members or that there is variable penetrance.

Clinically, medullary cystic kidney disease is distinguished from NPHP by its dominant mode of inheritance, later age at onset, progression to ESRD in the third to fourth decade of life, and lack of associated growth retardation and extrarenal manifestations.

Genetic linkage analyses indicate that defects in at least two loci (*MCKD1* and *MCKD2*) can cause medullary cystic kidney disease. Uremia occurs after 60 years of age in MCKD1; whereas in MCKD2, progression to ESRD occurs around 30 years of age. Mutations in the gene *UMOD*, which encodes uromodulin or Tamm-Horsfall protein, have been identified in MCKD2 patients. Subsequently, *UMOD* mutations have also been identified in families with familial juvenile hyperuricemic nephropathy (FJHN; MIM 162000), a dominantly transmitted disorder characterized by medullary cystic kidney disease, hyperuricemia, and gout,[28] as well as familial glomerulocystic disease with hyperuricemia (MIM 609886).[29]

The diagnosis can usually be made on the basis of the family history, the clinical associations of hyperuricemia and gout, and the ultrasound finding of medullary cysts. Genetic testing is available for *UMOD*-related disease (*http://www.genetests.org/*).

MEDULLARY SPONGE KIDNEY

Definition

Medullary sponge kidney (MSK) is a relatively common disorder characterized by dilated medullary and papillary collecting ducts that give the renal medulla a "spongy" appearance.[30]

Etiology and Pathogenesis

The occasional presence of embryonal tissue in the affected papillae and coexistence of other urinary tract anomalies suggest that MSK results from a developmental defect in the medullary pyramids. In addition, MSK occurs more frequently in individuals with other congenital defects, (e.g., congenital hemihypertrophy, Beckwith-Wiedemann syndrome, Ehlers-Danlos syndrome, and Marfan syndrome).[30]

Less than 5% of cases are familial, and a clear genetic basis for MSK has not been established.

Epidemiology

In the general population, the frequency of MSK may be underestimated because some affected individuals remain entirely asymptomatic. Up to 20% of patients with nephrolithiasis have at least a mild degree of MSK, but excretory urography in *unselected* patients indicates a disease frequency of approximately 1 in 5000 individuals.

Clinical Manifestations

MSK disease is asymptomatic unless it is complicated by nephrolithiasis, hematuria, or infection. Symptoms typically begin between the fourth and fifth decades of life, but adolescent presentations have been reported. Stones and granular debris in MSK patients are composed of either pure apatite (calcium phosphate) or a mixture of apatite and calcium oxalate. Several factors appear to contribute to stone formation, including urinary stasis within the ectatic ducts, hypercalciuria, and hyperoxaluria. Hyperparathyroidism has also been reported.

Hematuria, unrelated to either coexisting stones or infection, may be recurrent. The bleeding is usually asymptomatic, unless gross hematuria causes clot-related colic. Urinary tract infection may occur in association with nephrolithiasis or as an independent event. In those patients with stones, infections are more likely to occur in females than in males.

Approximately one third to one half of MSK patients have hypercalcemia,[30] but the mechanism has not been established. Decreased renal concentrating ability and impaired urinary acidification have been reported. In most patients, the acidification defect is not associated with systemic acidosis.

Pathology

The pathologic changes are confined to the renal medullary and intrapapillary collecting ducts. Multiple spherical or oval cysts measuring 1 to 8 mm may be detected in one or more papillae. These cysts may be isolated or may communicate with the collecting system. The cysts are frequently bilateral and often contain spherical concretions composed of apatite. The affected pyramids and associated calyces are usually enlarged, and nephromegaly can result when many pyramids are involved. The renal cortex, medullary rays, calyces, and pelvis appear normal, unless complications, such as pyelonephritis or urinary tract obstruction, become superimposed.

Diagnosis

Abdominal plain radiographs often reveal radiopaque concretions in the medulla (Fig. 45.7A). The diagnosis is established by intravenous urography (Fig. 45.7B). Retention of contrast media by the ectatic collecting ducts appears either as spherical cysts or more commonly as diffuse linear striations, which impart a

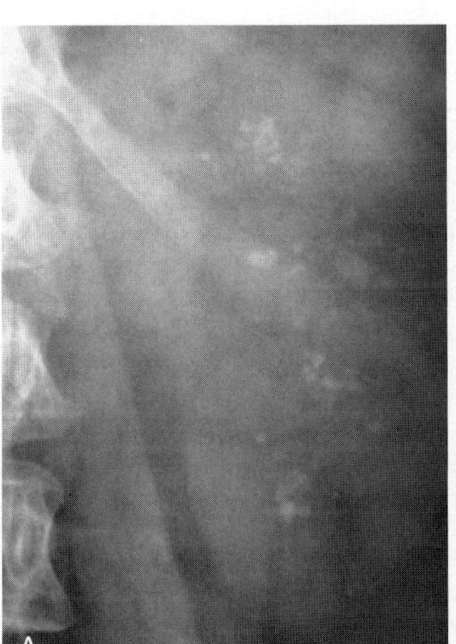

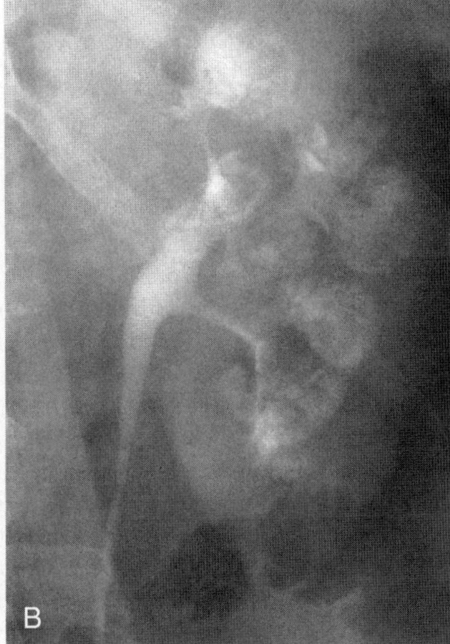

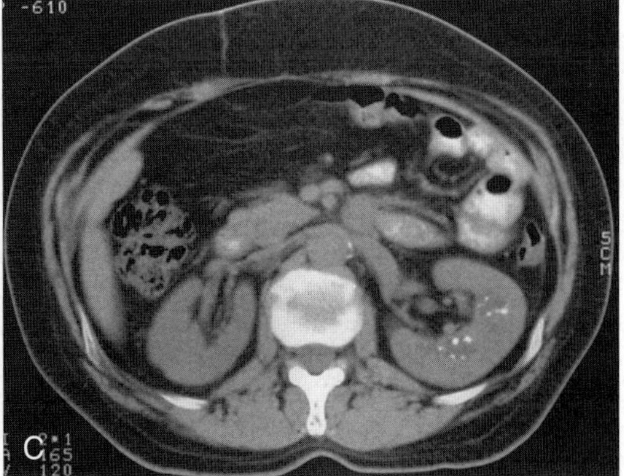

Figure 45.7 Radiologic findings associated with medullary sponge kidney. MSK in a 52-year-old symptomatic woman. **A,** Preliminary film shows medullary nephrolithiases. **B,** Ten-minute film from excretory urography shows clusters of rounded densities in the papillae amid discrete linear opacities (paintbrush appearance). **C,** Nonenhanced CT reveals densely echogenic foci in the medulla.

characteristic blush-like pattern to the papillae, the so-called bouquet of flowers or paintbrush appearance. CT is usually not necessary, but nonenhanced CT may help distinguish MSK from papillary necrosis or even ADPKD (Fig. 45.7C).

Treatment

Asymptomatic patients in whom MSK is detected as an incidental finding require no therapy. Hematuria in the absence of stones or infection requires no intervention. If the tubular ectasia is unilateral and segmental, partial nephrectomy may alleviate recurrent nephrolithiasis and urinary tract infection. However, for the majority of patients who have bilateral disease, medical management is sufficient.

Hypercalciuria is the predominant cause of nephrolithiasis in MSK. The mainstay of treatment is high fluid intake to increase urine output and to reduce the precipitation of calcium salts in ectatic ducts. Patients with documented hypercalciuria may benefit from thiazide diuretics. If thiazides are poorly tolerated or contraindicated, inorganic phosphate therapy may be useful. To avoid struvite stone formation, oral phosphates should *not* be used in patients with previous urinary tract infections caused by urease-producing organisms. Patients who form and pass stones recurrently may require lithotripsy or surgical intervention (see Chapter 57).

Urinary tract infection should be treated with standard antibiotic regimens, and for some patients, prolonged therapy may be warranted. Urease-producing organisms, such as coagulase-negative staphylococcus, are particularly problematic as urinary pathogens in MSK. Positive urine cultures, even with relatively insignificant colony counts, must be vigorously pursued.

With proper management of the clinical complications, the long-term prognosis is excellent. Progression to renal impairment is unusual.

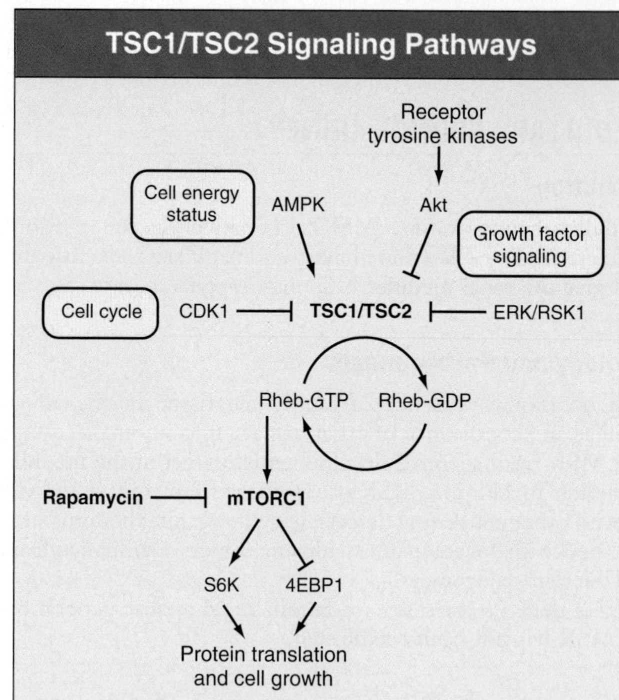

Figure 45.8 TSC1/TSC2 signaling pathways. Hamartin (TSC1) and tuberin (TSC2) integrate cues from extracellular growth factor binding (through Akt and ERK/RSK1), the intracellular energy status (through AMPK), and the cell cycle (through CDK1) to direct signaling pathways that regulate cellular proliferation, differentiation, and migration.[34,36] Tuberin contains a GTPase-activating protein (GAP) domain in its carboxyl terminus, and when it forms a complex with hamartin (TSC1/TSC2 complex), the small GTPase Rheb is converted from its active GTP-bound state to an inactive GDP-bound state. Rheb is an activator of the mTORC1 kinase, which regulates a number of processes linked to protein synthesis and cell growth (through the ribosomal S6 kinases and the eukaryotic initiation factor 4E-binding protein [4EBP1]). mTORC1 is activated physiologically in response to growth factor signaling, which causes phosphorylation of tuberin, dissociation of the TSC1/TSC2 complex, and increased levels of Rheb-GTP. Inactivation of the TSC1/TSC2 complex through mutations in *TSC1* or *TSC2* leads to inappropriate activation of mTORC1. Rapamycin is an mTOR inhibitor. *(Modified with permission from reference 34.)*

TUBEROUS SCLEROSIS COMPLEX

Definition

Tuberous sclerosis complex (TSC) is an autosomal dominant, tumor-suppressor gene syndrome in which tumor-like malformations, called hamartomas, develop in multiple organ systems, including the kidneys, brain, heart, lungs and skin.

Genetic Basis of Tuberous Sclerosis Complex

TSC results from inactivating mutations in one of two genes, *TSC1* on chromosome 9q32-q34[31] and *TSC2* on chromosome 16p13, adjacent to the *PKD1* gene.[32] Large deletions involving both *PKD1* and *TSC2* can result in the PKD1/TSC2 (PKTS) contiguous gene deletion syndrome.[33]

The focal nature of TSC-associated disease and the variability of disease expression even within families have suggested that *TSC1* and *TSC2* function as tumor-suppressor genes.[34] The tumor-suppressor gene paradigm hypothesizes that two successive mutations are necessary to inactivate a tumor-suppressor gene and to cause tumor formation. The first mutation, inherited and therefore present in all cells, is necessary but not sufficient to produce tumors. A second mutation occurs after fertilization and is required to induce tumor transformation. The inactivating germline mutations identified in *TSC1* and *TSC2* as well as the loss of heterozygosity detected in 50% of *TSC2*-associated hamartomas and ~10% of *TSC1*-associated hamartomas support the hypothesis that both *TSC1* and *TSC2* function as tumor-suppressor genes.

The *TSC2* gene product tuberin interacts with hamartin, the product of the *TSC1* gene. As described in Figure 45.8, the hamartin/tuberin (TSC1/TSC2) complex functions in multiple cellular pathways, primarily by inhibiting the kinase activity of mTOR, the mammalian target of rapamycin. mTOR functions in a protein complex (mTORC1) to regulate nutrient uptake, cell cycle progression, cell growth, and protein translation.[35,36]

The *PKD1* gene product polycystin 1 plays a key role in regulating mTORC1 activity by complexing with tuberin and mTOR, thereby inhibiting the mTOR pathway.[37] In normal adult kidney, mTOR is inactive. With loss of function of either polycystin 1 or tuberin, mTOR activity is upregulated, contributing to dysregulated cell growth and cystogenesis. In addition, hamartin appears to function through TORC1-independent pathways to regulate the structural integrity of the primary cilium, suggesting that ciliary dysfunction is an additional mechanism in TSC pathogenesis.[38]

Epidemiology

TSC affects 1 in 6000 individuals.[35] The disease penetrance is quite variable. About two thirds of TSC patients are sporadic cases with no family history, and the disease apparently results from new mutational events. Among patients with sporadic disease, mutations in *TSC2* are approximately five times more common than mutations in *TSC1*, whereas the ratio is 1:1 in familial cases. *TSC1*-related disease is milder, apparently because of a reduced rate of second hits.

Clinicopathologic Manifestations

The clinical features of *TSC1*- and *TSC2*-linked disease are similar, although *TSC2*-linked disease tends to be more severe. The most common clinical manifestations are seizures, mental retardation or autism, skin lesions, interstitial lung disease, and tumors in the brain, retina, kidney, and heart. In affected individuals older than 5 years, the most common skin lesions are facial angiofibromas (Fig. 45.9), hypomelanotic macules, and ungual fibromas.[39]

Kidney involvement occurs frequently in TSC; one large study reported renal lesions in 57% of TSC patients.[40] The principal manifestations include angiomyolipomas (85%), cysts (45%), and renal malignant neoplasms (4%). Some of the malignant tumors originally thought to be renal cell carcinoma (RCC) are now regarded as malignant epithelioid angiomyolipomas.[41] Other renal neoplasms, interstitial fibrosis with focal segmental glomerulosclerosis (FSGS), glomerular microhamartomas, and peripelvic and perirenal lymphangiomatous cysts have also been observed in TSC patients. Renal involvement in TSC often progresses insidiously but can result in considerable morbidity, including retroperitoneal hemorrhage, renal impairment (~1%), and death. Renal complications are the most frequent cause of death in TSC.[36]

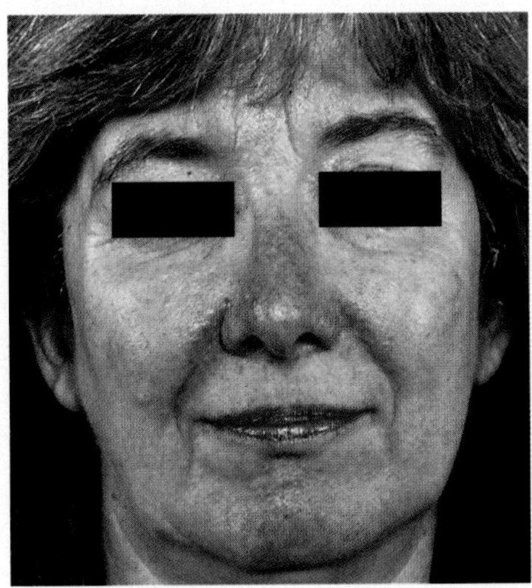

Figure 45.9 Facial angiofibromas in a 49-year-old patient with tuberous sclerosis complex.

Renal Angiomyolipomas

Angiomyolipomas are hamartomatous structures composed of abnormal, thick-walled vessels and varying amounts of smooth muscle–like cells and adipose tissue (Fig. 45.10A, B). These are the most common renal lesion in TSC patients, evident in ~80% of TSC patients by age 10 years.[34] Whereas solitary angiomyolipomas are found in the general population, particularly among older women, TSC-associated angiomyolipomas are multiple and bilateral with a young age at onset. Angiomyolipomas rarely occur before 5 years of age but increase in frequency and size with age.[42] These tumors can be locally invasive, extending into the perirenal fat or, more rarely, the collecting system, renal vein, and even the inferior vena cava and right atrium. Lymph node and splenic involvement probably represents multifocal origin rather than metastasis.

Clinical manifestations are due to hemorrhage (intratumoral or retroperitoneal) or mass effects (abdominal or flank masses and tenderness, hypertension, renal impairment). Women tend to have more numerous and larger angiomyolipomas than men. Pregnancy appears to increase the risk of rupture and hemorrhage.

Renal Cystic Disease

Renal cysts occur less frequently than angiomyolipoma in TSC patients (47% versus 80%[42]). However, like angiomyolipomas, renal cysts tend to increase in size and number over time. The concurrence of cysts and angiomyolipomas, easily detected by CT, is strongly suggestive of TSC.

The cysts in TSC can develop from any nephron segment. When limited in number and size, TSC-related cysts are predominantly cortical. In some cases, glomerular cysts predominate. The epithelial lining of the cysts is distinctive and appears to be unique to TSC, with large and acidophilic epithelia containing large hyperchromatic nuclei with occasional mitotic

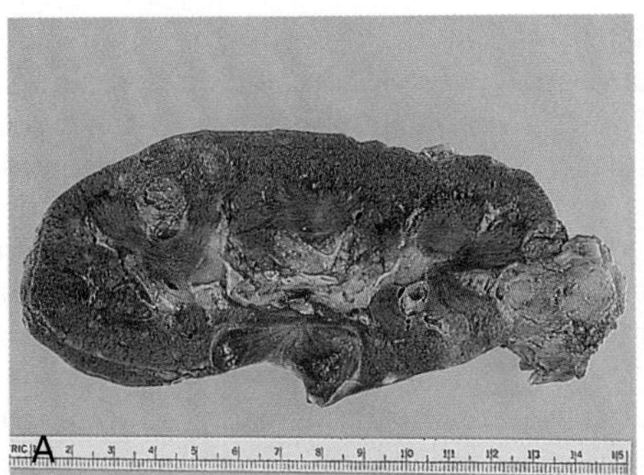

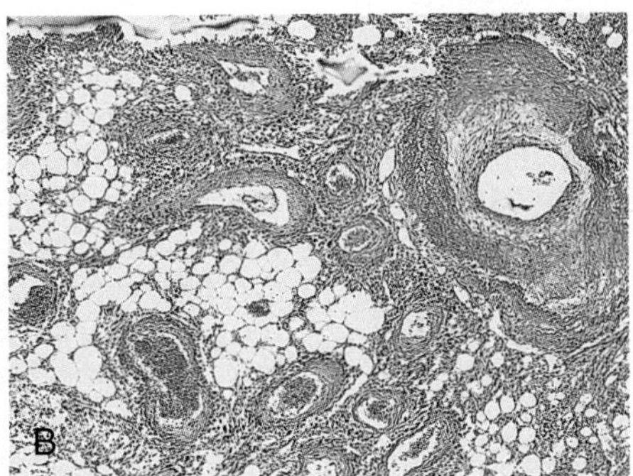

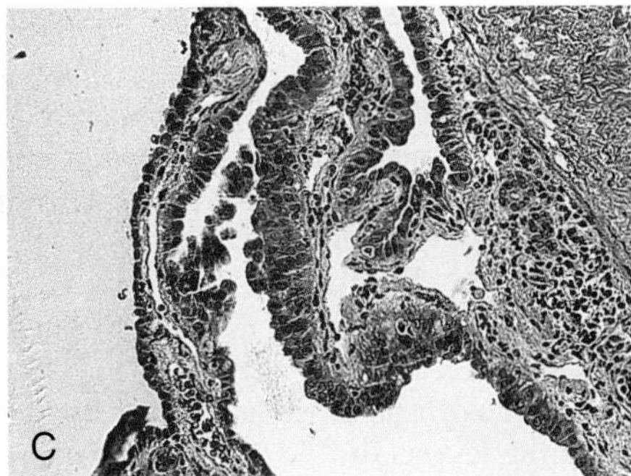

Figure 45.10 Renal pathology in tuberous sclerosis complex. A, Cut section: multiple angiomyolipomas in the kidney of a 60-year-old symptomatic woman. **B,** Light microscopy: angiomyolipoma containing adipose tissue and spindle smooth muscle–like cells interspersed between abnormal vessels with thickened walls. (Hematoxylin and eosin; magnification ×16.) **C,** Light microscopy: TSC cysts lined with distinctive epithelia consisting of large, acidophilic cells with hyperchromatic nuclei. (Hematoxylin and eosin; magnification ×65.)

Clinical Diagnostic Criteria for Tuberous Sclerosis Complex (TSC)*

Major:
- Facial angiofibromas or forehead plaque
- Nontraumatic ungual or periungual fibroma
- Hypomelanotic macules (>3)
- Shagreen patch (connective tissue nevus)
- Multiple retinal nodular hamartomas
- Cortical tubers
- Subependymal nodule
- Subependymal giant cell astrocytoma
- Cardiac rhabdomyomas (≥1)
- Lymphangioleiomyomatosis
- Renal angiomyolipoma

Minor:
- Multiple, random dental pits
- Hamartomatous gastrointestinal or rectal polyps
- Bone cysts
- White matter radial migration lines
- Gingival fibromas
- Nonrenal hamartoma
- Retinal achromic patch
- "Confetti" skin lesions
- Multiple renal cysts

Figure 45.11 Clinical diagnostic criteria for tuberous sclerosis complex (TSC). *Two major features or one major feature with two minor features indicates definite TSC; one major feature and one minor feature indicate probable TSC; and one major feature or two minor features indicate possible TSC. *(Modified with permission from reference 39.)*

figures (Fig. 45.10C). Associated papillary hyperplasia and adenomas are common.

A small subset of affected infants can present with massive renal cystic disease reminiscent of ADPKD, severe hypertension, and a progressive decline in renal function with the onset of ESRD in the second or third decade of life. The majority of these patients have a contiguous germline deletion involving both the *TSC2* and *PKD1* genes, the PKTS contiguous gene syndrome (MIM 600273).[43] Early detection, strict blood pressure control, and prompt therapy for the associated infantile spasms may have a favorable impact on the overall prognosis.

Renal Neoplasms

Many cases of benign epithelial tumors, such as papillary adenomas and oncocytomas, have been reported in TSC patients. However, despite the multiplicity of benign tumors, neoplastic transformation is rare.[44]

TSC-associated renal neoplasms are primarily clear cell RCC, but there is pathologic heterogeneity, with papillary and chromophobe carcinomas reported.[41] The prognosis of TSC-associated renal carcinomas compared with sporadic renal carcinomas in the general population is unknown. The lifetime risk for development of RCC in the context of TSC is 2% to 3%.[44]

Diagnosis

TSC is a pleiotropic disease in which the size, number, and location of the lesions can be variable, even among members of the same family. Major and minor criteria (Fig. 45.11) have been developed to guide the diagnostic approach in TSC. The diagnosis is made when two major features or one major and two minor ones can be demonstrated.[39] Imaging is the mainstay for diagnosis of TSC-associated renal lesions. The presence of small cysts and fat-containing angiomyolipomas is strongly suggestive of TSC. Whereas the median age at presentation for both renal cysts and angiomyolipomas is 9 years, these lesions have been detected in patients as young as 16 days and 4 months, respectively.[42]

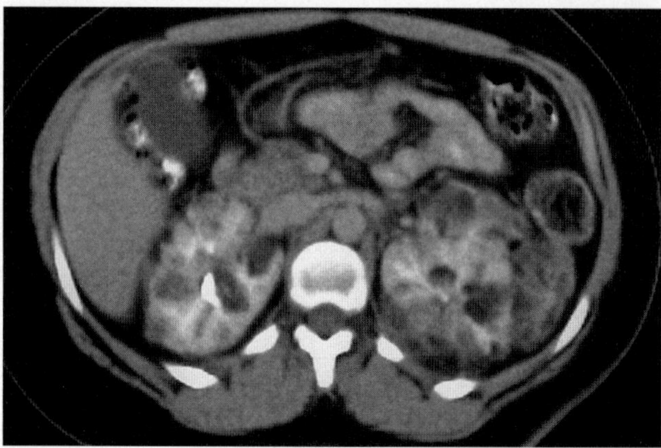

Figure 45.12 Radiologic findings associated with tuberous sclerosis complex. Contrast-enhanced CT scan showing bilateral angiomyolipomas in a 34-year-old symptomatic woman.

Annual renal imaging is advised for TSC patients. Ultrasound may be more sensitive than CT for detection of small angiomyolipomas because fatty tissue is highly echogenic. Conversely, CT may be superior for detection of small angiomyolipomas in diffusely hyperechoic kidneys and for differentiation of small angiomyolipomas from perinephric or renal sinus fat (Fig. 45.12). On occasion, the distinction between an angiomyolipoma and carcinoma cannot be reliably established by imaging, and biopsy is indicated.

TSC-associated renal cysts can radiologically mimic simple cysts and, when numerous, ADPKD. In the absence of angiomyolipomas, TSC-related renal cystic disease is suggested by the limited number of cysts compared with ADPKD and the absence of associated hepatic cysts. Although 10% of TSC patients have hepatic angiomyolipomas, hepatic cysts are rare.

Gene-based diagnosis is currently available for *TSC1*- and *TSC2*-related disease as well as to detect large-scale deletions associated with the PKTS contiguous gene syndrome (*http://www.genetests.org/*).

Treatment

Renal Angiomyolipomas

Renal angiomyolipomas are benign lesions and often require no treatment. However, given the potential for growth and associated complications, such as pain, bleeding, and hypertension, annual re-evaluation with ultrasound or CT is recommended. Larger angiomyolipomas frequently develop microaneurysms and macroaneurysms, and the risk of serious hemorrhage correlates with aneurysms of more than 5 mm in diameter.[36] Therefore, these large angiomyolipomas require preemptive treatment with either surgical removal in a nephron-sparing procedure or embolization.[34] In addition to size and complications such as pain and hemorrhage, the inability to exclude an associated renal carcinoma is an indication for intervention. When an associated malignant neoplasm cannot be excluded, renal-sparing surgery, such as enucleation or partial nephrectomy, is preferred.

The increased frequency and size of the angiomyolipomas in women and the reports of hemorrhagic complications during pregnancy suggest that female sex hormones may accelerate the growth of these lesions. Therefore, it is prudent to caution patients with multiple angiomyolipomas about the potential risks of pregnancy and estrogen administration.

As noted, defective mTORC1 signaling is a central feature of TSC. A small clinical trial of sirolimus (rapamycin), an mTOR inhibitor, has demonstrated regression of astrocytomas, angiofibromas, and angiomyolipomas as well as improved pulmonary function in TSC patients.[45] The efficacy of everolimus, another mTOR inhibitor, is now being assessed in a clinical trial in TSC patients with angiomyolipomas (*http://clinical trials.gov*).

Renal Cystic Disease

The mainstay of treatment of the cystic disease associated with TSC is strict control of the hypertension. Surgical decompression of these cystic kidneys has been suggested, but no significant beneficial effect has been established.

Renal Carcinoma

Renal carcinoma should be suspected in enlarging, fat-poor lesions or when intratumoral calcifications are present. In these cases, biopsy is indicated. Because renal carcinoma is frequently bilateral in TSC, renal-sparing surgery should be performed whenever possible.

Transplantation

CKD, although rare in tuberous sclerosis, can occur by several different mechanisms, including angiomyolipoma-related parenchymal destruction, progressive renal cystic disease, interstitial fibrosis, and FSGS. A survey of 260 French dialysis centers indicated that the approximate prevalence of tuberous sclerosis–associated ESRD is 0.7 case per million and that of ESRD in tuberous sclerosis is 1 per 100.[46] CKD in tuberous sclerosis was more frequent in females (63%) and was diagnosed at a mean age of 29 years. Renal impairment was the first TSC manifestation in about half the cases. Renal tumors were frequent, with angiomyolipomas in 23%, cysts in 18%, and both in 54%, although malignant neoplasms were observed in only 14%. All but one of the 48 patients with ESRD were treated by dialysis; 20 were transplanted, with good results. Therefore, both dialysis and renal transplantation provide an adequate means of survival, but the risk of renal hemorrhage related to angiomyolipomas and malignant degeneration in TSC poses special problems. Therefore, it is advisable that patients with TSC and ESRD undergo bilateral nephrectomy when renal replacement therapy is initiated.

VON HIPPEL–LINDAU DISEASE

Definition

von Hippel–Lindau disease (VHL) is a dominantly transmitted, multisystem cancer predisposition syndrome associated with tumors of the eyes, cerebellum, spinal cord, adrenal glands, pancreas, and epididymis as well as renal and pancreatic cysts.[47]

Genetic Basis of von Hippel–Lindau Disease

VHL results from germline mutations in the *VHL* tumor-suppressor gene. In approximately 80% of patients, VHL is familial, and disease in ~20% of cases results from *de novo* mutations. Moreover, *VHL* mutations have been identified in the germline of VHL patients as well as in sporadic clear cell RCCs, implying that *VHL* plays an important role in the pathogenesis of clear cell RCC.

The VHL protein (pVHL) plays a critical role as a negative regulator of hypoxia-inducible genes.[36,48] In the normal physiologic state, pVHL functions in a multiprotein complex that directs the α subunits of the transcription factor hypoxia-inducible factor (HIF-α) for destruction through the ubiquination pathway. In cells that lack pVHL, HIF-α subunits are stabilized and bind to HIF-β family member proteins. The heterodimer then translocates to the nucleus, leading to overexpression of HIF target genes, which encode proteins that regulate glucose uptake, metabolism, extracellular pH, angiogenesis (vascular endothelial growth factor and platelet-derived growth factor B), and mitogenesis (transforming growth factor β and erythropoietin). This transcriptional dysregulation promotes the pathologic growth and survival of endothelial cells, pericytes, and stromal cells and ultimately their malignant transformation.[47,48]

Clinical Manifestations

VHL has an incidence of 1 in 36,000 newborns and has been observed in all ethnic groups.[47] Biallelic *VHL* inactivation leads to increased risk of central nervous system (CNS) and retinal hemangioblastomas, clear cell RCCs, pheochromocytomas, pancreatic islet cell tumors, endolymphatic sac tumors, and papillary cystadenomas of the broad ligament (females) and epididymis (males). In addition, cystic changes can occur in the kidney and pancreas.[48]

VHL-associated disease appears to cluster into two disease complexes (Fig. 45.13). In the initial stratification, VHL patients can be subclassified on the basis of a low risk (type 1) or high risk (type 2) for development of pheochromocytoma. Type 2 patients can be further subtyped according to the risk for development of RCC—low in type 2A and high in type 2B. In type 2C, patients present with familial pheochromocytoma without the other VHL-associated malignant neoplasms. Deletions and protein-truncating mutations are associated with the VHL type

Classification of VHL Based on Tumor Spectrum

VHL Subtype	Tumor Manifestations
Type 1	Hemangioblastoma (CNS, retina), renal cell carcinoma Low risk for pheochromocytoma and pancreatic endocrine tumors
Type 2A	Hemangioblastoma (CNS, retina), pheochromocytoma, pancreatic endocrine tumors Low risk for renal cell carcinoma
Type 2B	Hemangioblastoma (CNS, retina), renal cell carcinoma, pheochromocytoma, pancreatic endocrine tumors
Type 2C	Predominantly pheochromocytoma Very limited risks for hemangioblastoma and renal cell carcinoma

Figure 45.13 Classification of VHL based on tumor spectrum. CNS, central nervous system. *(Modified with permission from reference 48.)*

1 phenotype, whereas type 2 disease primarily involves missense mutations.[47,48]

RCCs are typically multiple and bilateral. Whereas RCC may present with hematuria or back pain, more often detection occurs as an incidental finding on unrelated imaging studies or when VHL families are screened for occult renal disease. The mean age at presentation is 35 to 40 years, although patients have been diagnosed in adolescence. In VHL, men and women are equally affected with RCC, in contrast to the male predominance in sporadic RCC. VHL-associated RCC metastasizes to the lymph nodes, liver, lungs, and bones and accounts for about 50% of VHL deaths.

In VHL, renal cysts arise from tubular cells that have undergone somatic loss of the wild-type allele. Renal cysts occur in about 60% of patients and are commonly bilateral; deterioration of renal function due to cystic kidney disease has been reported but is exceptional. However, some of these cysts become malignant over time, presumably because of mutations affecting other loci.[36]

Pathology

RCC is one of the most common tumors in VHL, occurring in up to 75% of patients by age 60 years.[47] VHL-associated RCCs are mostly of the clear cell type and usually bilateral and multifocal in distribution. Detailed microscopic examination of VHL-associated renal cystic lesions often reveals small foci of carcinoma; these RCCs tend to have low-grade histology and a better 10-year survival than sporadic RCC. More advanced RCCs do metastasize, and metastatic disease is a major cause of death in VHL patients.

Diagnosis

The minimal clinical criteria for the diagnosis of VHL in an at-risk individual include the presence of a single retinal or cerebellar hemangioblastoma, or RCC, or pheochromocytoma. As many as 50% of affected family members may manifest only one feature of the syndrome. In presumed sporadic cases, the clinical diagnosis requires two or more retinal or CNS hemangioblastomas or a single hemangioblastoma and a characteristic visceral tumor.

Molecular analysis of the VHL gene is indicated in patients with known or suspected VHL or in at-risk children from VHL families, given that unsuspected, untreated tumors can cause significant morbidity.[47] Presymptomatic genotyping can be useful in determining the phenotypic classification of VHL and be used to direct monitoring for a specific subset of tumors. In addition, genotyping can be useful in distinguishing whether a pheochromocytoma has occurred in the context of VHL type 2 or in multiple endocrine neoplasia type 2 or is nonsyndromic.[47,48] Genetic testing information is available at *http://www.genetests.org/*.

In proven gene carriers or those at-risk individuals who cannot be evaluated at the molecular level, regular surveillance for occult disease manifestations is indicated. A comprehensive screening program, typically initiated at age 18 years and performed annually, includes gadolinium-enhanced magnetic resonance imaging (MRI) of the brain and spinal cord, detailed ophthalmologic examination, and a CT or MRI scan of the abdomen and pelvis to screen for visceral manifestations.[36] About 40% of patients with VHL develop radiographically apparent renal cancers, which may appear as simple or complex cysts or solid renal masses. Comparison of images before and after the administration of contrast material distinguishes whether lesions are enhancing. Ultrasound can be helpful in the further characterization of indeterminate renal lesions but should not be the primary mode of diagnostic imaging. For individuals with VHL type 2 mutations, annual surveillance for pheochromocytoma should include a 24-hour urine collection for metanephrines and catecholamines, abdominal magnetic resonance tomography, or *m*-iodobenzylguanidine (MIBG) scintigraphy.[47]

Germline mutations in the VHL gene have been detected in some families who do not meet the clinical criteria for VHL. Such families should be considered to have VHL and be managed like typical VHL families, including periodic clinical screening. For those at-risk individuals who do not inherit the mutant gene, further clinical surveillance is not necessary.

Differential Diagnosis

The differential diagnosis of VHL-associated renal lesions includes several conditions, most notably ADPKD and TSC (Fig. 45.14). Like VHL, ADPKD affects both sexes with a similar mean age at presentation. However, kidney involvement in VHL is characterized by a few bilateral cysts (Fig. 45.15A), RCC, normal kidney size, normal blood pressure, and usually normal renal function. Cyst infection, a frequent finding in ADPKD, is uncommon in VHL. RCC is an infrequent complication of ADPKD. Cysts in the liver are frequent in ADPKD and rare in VHL. Pancreatic cysts are rare in ADPKD but can be numerous and scattered through the pancreas in VHL (Fig. 45.15A). The CNS in ADPKD is affected by arterial aneurysms, whereas hemangioblastomas are the CNS manifestation of VHL (Fig. 45.15B).

TSC should be considered in the differential diagnosis of multiple renal tumors. In both TSC and VHL, multiple renal cysts occur. However, the TSC-associated renal tumor is usually an angiomyolipoma, and extrarenal lesions readily distinguish VHL and TSC.

Treatment

At present, surgery is the mainstay for RCC therapy in VHL patients. Optimal management requires surgical intervention before renal vein invasion and distant metastases occur because metastatic lesions respond poorly to chemotherapy and radiation therapy. Nephron-sparing surgery is the procedure of choice when possible. Repeated surgical intervention may be required as tumors continue to develop. Laparoscopic surgery may have a role in the future management of these patients.

Bilateral nephrectomy and renal transplantation may be an acceptable alternative to repeated nephron-sparing surgery in patients with VHL-associated RCC. It remains to be determined whether post-transplantation immunosuppression enhances the growth of the retinal and CNS hemangioblastomas and other lesions found in patients with VHL.

In terms of medical management, drugs that inhibit HIF-α, or its downstream targets, could be therapeutically useful in pVHL-related hemangioblastomas and clear cell RCCs.[48] Whereas DNA-binding transcription factors such as HIF have not proved to be tractable as drug targets *per se*, agents such as mTOR inhibitors that downregulate HIF-α protein levels are attractive as therapeutic agents; preclinical studies indicate that pVHL-defective cells are quite sensitive to mTOR inhibitors. Antibodies directed against vascular endothelial growth factor have shown significant efficacy in RCC in terms of tumor

Clinical and Genetic Features of Adult Renal Cystic Disease

	Simple Cysts	ADPKD	MSK	VHL	TSC	Acquired Cystic Disease
Clinical onset (years)	>40	30–40	20–40	30–40	10–30	Chronic renal failure
Cysts	Single, multiple	Multiple	Multiple	Few, bilateral	Multiple	Multiple
Cyst infection	Uncommon	Common	Common	Uncommon	Uncommon	Uncommon
Tumors	No	Rare	No	RCC, often bilateral	AML/RCC	Common
BP	Normal, increased	Increased	Normal	Normal/ increased	Normal/ increased	Normal/ increased
Renal function	Normal	Normal/impaired	Normal	Normal	Normal/impaired	Impaired/ESRD
Nephrolithiasis	No	Common	Common	No	No	No
Liver cysts	No	Common	No	Rare	No	No
Pancreas cysts	No	Few	No	Multiple	No	No
CNS involvement	No	Aneurysms	No	Hemangioblastomas	Seizures, mental retardation	No
Skin lesions	No	No	No	No	See Fig. 45.9	No
Genetics of adult renal cystic disease						
Disease gene	No	*PKD1* *PKD2*	*MKS1-MSK6*	*VHL*	*TSC1* *TSC2*	No
Genetic testing[1]	No	Yes	Yes	Yes	Yes	No

Figure 45.14 Features of adult renal cystic disease. ADPKD, autosomal dominant polycystic kidney disease; AML, angiomyolipoma; BP, blood pressure; CNS, central nervous system; ESRD, end-stage renal disease; MSK, medullary sponge kidney; TSC, tuberous sclerosis complex; VHL, von Hippel–Lindau disease; RCC, renal cell carcinoma. [1]Listed at GeneTests (*http://www.genetests.org*).

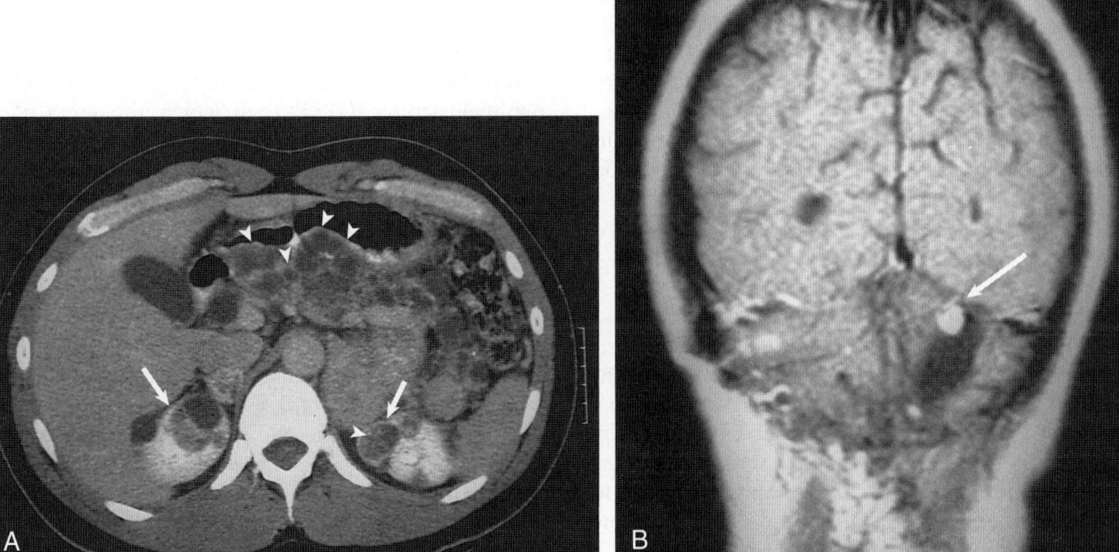

Figure 45.15 Radiologic findings associated with VHL. A, Non–contrast-enhanced CT image shows massive cystic involvement of the pancreas *(arrowheads)* and bilateral renal cysts *(arrows)*. **B,** Contrast-enhanced MR image shows a right cerebellar hemangioblastoma with a small enhancing mass *(arrow)*.

shrinkage and disease stabilization.[48] A number of clinical trials are in progress (*http://clinical trials.gov*).

SIMPLE CYSTS

Definition

Simple renal cysts are the most commonly acquired renal cystic lesion and occur twice as frequently in men as in women. Simple cysts are usually unilateral and may be either solitary or multiple. They occur rarely in children but become increasingly common with age.[49] In one large ultrasound study, unilateral cysts were detected in 1.7% of patients 30 to 49 years of age, 11% of patients 50 to 70 years of age, and 22% to 30% of patients older than 70 years.[50] This age-related increase in cyst incidence has been corroborated by MR studies.[51]

Etiology and Pathogenesis

Simple renal cysts likely originate from the distal convoluted tubule or collecting ducts and may arise from renal tubular diverticula, but the pathogenic mechanism is unknown. Focal tubular obstruction and renal parenchymal ischemia have both been suggested as etiologic processes. Less likely is the possibility that simple cysts arise from calyceal diverticula because simple cysts are often found in the renal cortex and their frequency increases with age.

In addition to age, smoking, renal dysfunction, and hypertension[52] have been implicated as risk factors in the occurrence of simple cysts. However, these associations may be coincidental, given that the studies were largely retrospective, the cohorts had variable reasons for diagnostic referral, and the observations were not optimally controlled for age of the patient.[49]

Clinical Manifestations

Simple cysts are typically asymptomatic. On occasion, patients present with hypertension, hematuria, abdominal or back pain due to bleeding, palpable abdominal mass, evidence of infection, or obstruction of the collecting system. Clinical symptoms are more common with neoplasms than with simple cysts. Therefore, the onset of symptoms should raise the possibility of an associated malignant neoplasm and prompt additional diagnostic studies.[49,53]

Pathology

Whether unilateral or bilateral, simple cysts are usually spherical and unilocular. They may be solitary or multiple. On average, simple cysts measure 0.5 to 1.0 cm in diameter, but 3- to 4-cm cysts are not uncommon. Simple cysts can occur in the cortex (where they often protrude from the cortical surface), the corticomedullary junction, or the medulla. By definition, they do not communicate with the renal pelvis. The cyst walls are typically thin and transparent, lined with a single layer of flattened epithelium. Cyst fluid is essentially an ultrafiltrate of plasma. In the wake of infection, cyst walls can become thickened, fibrotic, and even calcified.

Diagnosis

Simple cysts are most often detected as incidental findings during abdominal imaging studies. They are occasionally discovered during radiologic evaluation of palpable abdominal masses, pyelonephritis, or hematuria following abdominal trauma.

The critical clinical issue is to distinguish single or multiple simple cysts from cysts associated with ADPKD, other cystic diseases, or RCC. This distinction can usually be made on the basis of the patient's age, family history, and renal imaging patterns.[49,54]

The ultrasound features of simple cysts include smooth walls, no septa, and no intracystic debris. If the ultrasound pattern is indeterminate, CT scanning should be performed. A classification system for renal cysts based on their appearance and enhancement on CT, described by Bosniak, is widely used (see Fig. 59.11).[54] Benign cysts (class I) have homogeneous attenuation, no contrast enhancement, thin and smooth cyst walls, and no associated calcifications unless prior infection has occurred.

Treatment

Simple cysts associated with pain or renin-dependent hypertension can be punctured with ultrasound guidance and drained, and a sclerosing agent is instilled into the cyst cavity. Laparoscopic or retroperitoneoscopic cyst unroofing may be more appropriate for large cysts containing volumes in excess of 100 ml. Infection with Enterobacteriaceae, staphylococci, and *Proteus* has been reported in simple cysts, and operative or percutaneous drainage is often required in addition to antibiotic treatment.

SOLITARY MULTILOCULAR CYSTS

Solitary multilocular cysts are generally benign neoplasms that arise from the metanephric blastema.[55] These solitary cysts have also been designated multilocular cystic nephroma, benign cystic nephroma, and papillary cystadenoma. By definition, the cystic structures are unilateral, solitary, and multilocular. The cystic locules do not communicate with each other or with the renal pelvis. These locules are lined with a simple epithelium, and the interlocular septa do not contain differentiated renal epithelia structures.

Multilocular cysts represent a spectrum[56]; at one end is cystic nephroma, and at the other end is cystic partially differentiated nephroblastoma (CPDN), in which the septa contain foci of blastemal cells. It is not certain whether a multilocular cyst represents a congenital abnormality in nephrogenesis, a hamartoma, a partially or completely differentiated Wilms' tumor, or a benign variant of Wilms' tumor.

A bimodal age distribution has been described[55]; approximately half the cases occur in children younger than 4 years, and half the cases are detected in adults. The childhood cases (mostly CPDN) are usually found in boys, whereas multilocular cysts presenting in adulthood (mostly cystic nephroma) occur more commonly in women. An abdominal or flank mass is the most common clinical feature, as these cysts are typically quite large and often replace an entire pole. Associated hematuria, calculi, urinary tract obstruction, and infection occur in rare instances. Diagnosis can be made by either ultrasound or CT (Fig. 45.16).

Almost all multilocular cysts are Bosniak class III (see Fig. 59.11), complex renal cysts suggestive of malignancy.[54] CPDN in children may contain blastema and incompletely differentiated metanephric tissue but usually has a benign course.[57] In adults, associated foci of RCC or sarcoma must be excluded; partial nephrectomy is usually required. However, the typical prognosis of solitary multilocular cysts is excellent.

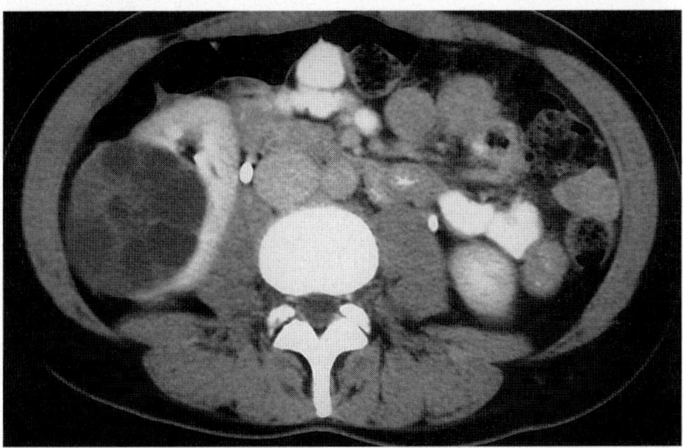

Figure 45.16 Solitary multilocular cyst. Contrast-enhanced CT image shows a solitary, septated, and well-circumscribed renal cystic lesion in the right kidney.

RENAL LYMPHANGIOMATOSIS

Renal lymphangiomatosis is a rare, generally benign disorder characterized by developmental malformation of renal lymphatic channels.[58] It has also been referred to as hilar, pericalyceal, paracalyceal, peripelvic, or parapelvic lymphangiectasis.

The cystic phenotype is widely variable and the underlying pathogenesis is unclear. The dilation may involve a single lymphatic channel or multiple channels. The lymphangiectasis may be unilateral or bilateral, may be limited to the hilar region, or may extend into the renal parenchyma to the corticomedullary junction. On occasion, renal lymphangiomatosis may be very extensive and simulate ADPKD. The thin-walled cysts are lined by lymphatic endothelium, and the cyst fluid is quite distinct from that in ADPKD cysts as it contains lymphatic constituents such as albumin and lipid.

The characteristic ultrasound or CT findings include multiple, bilateral small peripelvic cysts that splay the renal hilum as well as capsular cysts in the perirenal space, both separated by thin septations.[59] Renal lymphangiomas are most often asymptomatic and require no treatment. However, the condition may be exacerbated by pregnancy, resulting in large perinephric lymph collections and ascites that may require percutaneous drainage.[60]

GLOMERULOCYSTIC KIDNEY DISEASE

Cystic glomeruli are evident in three different clinical contexts: (1) isolated glomerulocystic kidney disease (GCKD); (2) glomerulocystic kidneys associated with heritable malformation syndromes, such as tuberous sclerosis, Meckel syndrome, medullary cystic kidney disease, orofaciodigital syndrome type I, trisomy 9, trisomy 13, trisomy 18, the short-rib polydactyly syndromes, and Zellweger cerebrohepatorenal syndrome; and (3) glomerular cysts present in dysplastic kidneys.[61]

GCKD can occur as a sporadic condition, a familial disorder, or the infantile manifestation of ADPKD. On pathologic examination, the kidney architecture is normal, with no dysplastic elements in the cortex and no evidence of urinary tract obstruction. Cystic dilation predominantly involves Bowman's space and the initial proximal tubule; it is defined as a twofold to threefold dilation of Bowman's space versus the normal glomerular dimension.[61] Glomerular cysts can be distributed from the subcapsular zone to the inner cortex. The typical ultrasound pattern in GCKD involves increased echogenicity of the renal cortex with minute cysts, smaller than those evident in ADPKD. Young infants with either familial or sporadic forms of GCKD may also have renal medullary dysplasia and biliary dysgenesis.[61]

GCKD is usually transmitted as an autosomal dominant trait. It is usually discovered in infants with a familial history of ADPKD. In these infants, the kidneys are bilaterally enlarged and diffusely cystic. In addition, familial GCKD has been observed in infants, older children, and adults in whom the disease locus is not linked to *PKD1* or *PKD2*, but the specific causative gene has yet to be identified.[62] In these non–ADPKD-associated GCKD families, the kidneys are typically normal in size, although enlarged kidneys are occasionally observed. Finally, several sporadic cases of nonsyndromal GCKD have been described, suggesting either new spontaneous mutations or a recessively transmitted disorder.[63]

Familial hypoplastic GCKD (MIM 137920) is probably a different type of GCKD. The kidneys are smaller than normal and often associated with medullocalyceal abnormalities. The disease is pleiotropic among affected family members with variable associations of hypoplastic GCKD, gynecologic abnormalities, and maturity-onset diabetes of the young, type 5, which results from mutations in *TCF2*, the gene encoding hepatocyte nuclear factor 1β.[64]

ACQUIRED CYSTIC DISEASE

Hypokalemic Cystic Disease

Renal cysts are often seen in association with chronic hypokalemia due to primary hyperaldosteronism or other renal potassium-wasting disorders. Nearly 50% of patients with idiopathic adrenal hyperplasia and 60% of patients with adrenal tumors have been found to have renal cysts, which were distributed primarily in the renal medulla. These cysts typically regress after adrenalectomy.[65]

Hilar Cysts

Hilar cysts are spherical accumulations of clear, fat droplet–containing fluid within the renal sinus. These cystic structures are not lined by epithelia. They are most commonly seen in debilitated patients and may represent atrophy of the renal sinus fat.

Perinephric Pseudocysts

Perinephric pseudocysts are also unlined cavities. They typically occur under the renal capsule or in the perirenal fascia as a result of urine extravasation from a renal cyst after traumatic or spontaneous rupture or as the posterior extension of a pancreatic pseudocyst. Surgical intervention is indicated for associated urinary tract obstruction. Otherwise, treatment is directed to the underlying cause.

ACQUIRED CYSTIC DISEASE IN RENAL FAILURE

Acquired cystic disease is a significant complication of prolonged renal failure. It should be considered in the differential diagnosis of cystic disease presenting with long-standing chronic renal failure (see Fig. 45.14). Acquired cystic disease is discussed further in Chapter 85.

REFERENCES

1. Fick G, Gabow P. Hereditary and acquired cystic disease of the kidney. *Kidney Int*. 1994;46:951-964.
2. Guay-Woodford L, Desmond R. Autosomal recessive polycystic kidney disease (ARPKD): The clinical experience in North America. *Pediatrics*. 2003;111:1072-1080.
3. Onuchic L, Furu L, Nagasawa Y, et al. PKHD1, the polycystic kidney and hepatic disease 1 gene, encodes a novel large protein containing multiple IPT domains and PbH1 repeats. *Am J Hum Genet*. 2002;70:1305-1317.
4. Menezes F, Cai Y, Nagasawa Y, et al. Polyductin, the PKHD1 gene product, comprises isoforms expressed in plasma membrane, primary cilium and cytoplasm. *Kidney Int*. 2004;66:1345-1355.
5. Desmet V. Pathogenesis of ductal plate abnormalities. *Mayo Clin Proc*. 1998;73:80-89.
6. Yoder B. Role of primary cilia in the pathogenesis of polycystic kidney disease. *J Am Soc Nephrol*. 2007;18:1381-1388.
7. Zerres K, Becker J, Muecher G, et al. Haplotype-based prenatal diagnosis in autosomal recessive polycystic kidney disease (ARPKD). *Am J Med Genet*. 1998;76:137-144.
8. Bergmann C, Senderek J, Windelen E, et al. Clinical consequences of PKHD1 mutations in 164 patients with autosomal recessive polycystic kidney disease (ARPKD). *Kidney Int*. 2005;67:829-848.
9. Adeva M, El-Youssef M, Rossetti S, et al. Clinical and molecular characterization defines a broadened spectrum of autosomal recessive polycystic kidney disease (ARPKD). *Medicine (Baltimore)*. 2006;85:1-21.
10. Davis ID, Ho M, Hupertz V, Avner ED. Survival of childhood polycystic kidney disease following renal transplantation: The impact of advanced hepatobiliary disease. *Pediatr Transplant*. 2003;7:364-369.
11. Kerkar N, Norton K, Suchy F. The hepatic fibrocystic diseases. *Clin Liver Dis*. 2006;10:55-71.
12. Chaumoitre K, Brun M, Cassart M, et al. Differential diagnosis of fetal hyperechogenic cystic kidneys unrelated to renal tract anomalies: A multicenter study. *Ultrasound Obstet Gynecol*. 2006;28:911-917.
13. Capisonda R, Phan V, Traubuci J, et al. Autosomal recessive polycystic kidney disease: Clinical course and outcome, a single center experience. *Pediatr Nephrol*. 2003;18:119-126.
14. Zerres K, Senderek J, Rudnik-Schoneborn S, et al. New options for prenatal diagnosis in autosomal recessive polycystic kidney disease by mutation analysis of the PKHD1 gene. *Clin Genet*. 2004;66:53-57.
15. Gigarel N, Frydman N, Burlet P, et al. Preimplantation genetic diagnosis for autosomal recessive polycystic kidney disease. *Reprod Biomed Online*. 2008;16:152-158.
16. Sharp A, Messiaen L, Page G, et al. Comprehensive genomic analysis for PKHD1 mutations in ARPKD cohorts. *J Med Genet*. 2005;42:336-349.
17. Rossetti S, Harris PC. Genotype-phenotype correlations in autosomal dominant and autosomal recessive polycystic kidney disease. *J Am Soc Nephrol*. 2007;18:1374-1380.
18. Seikaly M, Ho P, Emmett L, et al. Chronic renal insufficiency in children: The 2001 Annual Report of the NAPRTCS. *Pediatr Nephrol*. 2003;18:796-804.
19. Beaunoyer M, Snehal M, Li L, et al. Optimizing outcomes for neonatal ARPKD. *Pediatr Transplant*. 2007;11:267-271.
20. Sutherland SM, Alexander SR, Sarwal MM, et al. Combined liver-kidney transplantation in children: Indications and outcome. *Pediatr Transplant*. 2008;12:835-846.
21. Shneider B, Magid M. Liver disease in autosomal recessive polycystic kidney disease. *Pediatr Transplant*. 2005;9:634-649.
22. Hildebrandt F, Attanasio M, Otto E. Nephronophthisis: Disease mechanisms of a ciliopathy. *J Am Soc Nephrol*. 2009;20:23-35.
23. Saunier S, Salomon R, Antignac C. Nephronophthisis. *Curr Opin Genet Dev*. 2005;15:324-331.
24. Ala-Mello S, Kivivuori S, Ronnholm K, et al. Mechanism underlying early anemia in children with familial juvenile nephronophthisis. *Pediatr Nephrol*. 1996;10:578-581.
25. Otto E, Schermer B, Obara T, et al. Mutations in INVS encoding inversin cause nephronophthisis type 2, linking renal cystic disease to the function of primary cilia and left-right axis determination. *Nat Genet*. 2003;34:413-420.
26. Salomon R, Gubler M, Antignac C. Nephronophthisis. In: Davidson A, Cameron J, Grunfeld J, et al, eds. *Oxford Text Book of Clinical Nephrology*. Oxford: Oxford University Press; 2005:2325-2334.
27. Heninger E, Otto E, Imm A, et al. Improved strategy for molecular genetic diagnostics in juvenile nephronophthisis. *Am J Kidney Dis*. 2001;37:1131-1139.
28. Scolari F, Caridi G, Rampoldi L, et al. Uromodulin storage diseases: Clinical aspects and mechanisms. *Am J Kidney Dis*. 2004;44:987-999.
29. Lens XM, Banet JF, Outeda P, Barrio-Lucia V. A novel pattern of mutation in uromodulin disorders: Autosomal dominant medullary cystic kidney disease type 2, familial juvenile hyperuricemic nephropathy, and autosomal dominant glomerulocystic kidney disease. *Am J Kidney Dis*. 2005;46:52-57.
30. Yendt E. Medullary sponge kidney. In: Gardner K, Bernstein J, eds. *The Cystic Kidney*. Dordrecht, Netherlands: Kluwer; 1990:379-391.
31. The European Chromosome 16 Tuberous Sclerosis Consortium. Identification and characterization of the tuberous sclerosis gene on chromosome 16. *Cell*. 1993;75:1305-1315.
32. van Slegtenhorst M, de Hoogt R, Hermans C, et al. Identification of the tuberous sclerosis gene TSC1 on chromosome 9q34. *Science*. 1997;277:805-808.
33. Consugar MB, Wong WC, Lundquist PA, et al. Characterization of large rearrangements in autosomal dominant polycystic kidney disease and the PKD1/TSC2 contiguous gene syndrome. *Kidney Int*. 2008;74:1468-1479.
34. Henske E. Tuberous sclerosis and the kidney: From mesenchyme to epithelium and beyond. *Pediatr Nephrol*. 2005;20:854-857.
35. Curatolo P, Bombardieri R, Jozwiak S. Tuberous sclerosis. *Lancet*. 2008;372:657-668.
36. Siroky BJ, Czyzyk-Krzeska MF, Bissler JJ. Renal involvement in tuberous sclerosis complex and von Hippel–Lindau disease: Shared disease mechanisms? *Nat Clin Pract Nephrol*. 2009;5:143-156.
37. Shillingford J, Murcia N, Larson C, et al. The mTOR pathway is regulated by polycystin-1, and its inhibition reverses renal cystogenesis in polycystic kidney disease. *Proc Natl Acad Sci U S A*. 2006;103:5466-5471.
38. Hartman TR, Liu D, Zilfou JT, et al. The tuberous sclerosis proteins regulate formation of the primary cilium via a rapamycin-insensitive and polycystin 1–independent pathway. *Hum Mol Genet*. 2009;18:151-163.
39. Roach ES, Gomez MR, Northrup H. Tuberous sclerosis complex consensus conference: Revised clinical diagnostic criteria. *J Child Neurol*. 1998;13:624-628.
40. Rakowski SK, Winterkorn EB, Paul E, et al. Renal manifestations of tuberous sclerosis complex: Incidence, prognosis, and predictive factors. *Kidney Int*. 2006;70:1777-1782.
41. Pea M, Bonetti F, Martignoni G, et al. Apparent renal cell carcinomas in tuberous sclerosis are heterogeneous: The identification of malignant epithelioid angiomyolipoma. *Am J Surg Pathol*. 1998;22:180-187.
42. Casper K, Donnelly LF, Chen B, Bissler JJ. Tuberous sclerosis complex: Renal imaging findings. *Radiology*. 2002;225:451-456.
43. Sampson J, Maheshwar M, Aspinwall R, et al. Renal cystic disease in tuberous sclerosis: Role of the polycystic kidney disease 1 gene. *Am J Hum Genet*. 1997;61:843-851.
44. Kwiatkowski D, Manning B. Tuberous sclerosis: A GAP at the crossroads of multiple signaling pathways. *Hum Mol Genet*. 2005;14:R1-R8.
45. Bissler JJ, McCormack FX, Young LR, et al. Sirolimus for angiomyolipoma in tuberous sclerosis complex or lymphangioleiomyomatosis. *N Engl J Med*. 2008;358:140-151.
46. Schillinger F, Montagnac R. Chronic renal failure and its treatment in tuberous sclerosis. *Nephrol Dial Transplant*. 1996;11:481-485.
47. Joerger M, Koeberle D, Neumann H, Gillessen S. Von Hippel–Lindau disease—a rare disease important to recognize. *Onkologie*. 2005;28:159-163.
48. Kaelin WG. Von Hippel–Lindau disease. *Annu Rev Pathol*. 2007;2:145-173.
49. Eknoyan G. A clinical view of simple and complex renal cysts. *J Am Soc Nephrol*. 2009;20:1874-1876.
50. Ravine D, Gibson RN, Donlan J, Sheffield LJ. An ultrasound renal cyst prevalence survey: Specificity data for inherited renal cystic diseases. *Am J Kidney Dis*. 1993;22:803-807.
51. Nascimento AB, Mitchell DG, Zhang XM, et al. Rapid MR imaging detection of renal cysts: Age-based standards. *Radiology*. 2001;221:628-632.
52. Chin HJ, Ro H, Lee HJ, et al. The clinical significances of simple renal cyst: Is it related to hypertension or renal dysfunction? *Kidney Int*. 2006;70:1468-1473.
53. Terada N, Arai Y, Kinukawa N, Terai A. The 10-year natural history of simple renal cysts. *Urology*. 2008;71:7-11; discussion 11-12.
54. Isreal G, Bosniak M. An update of the Bosniak renal cyst classification system. *Urology*. 2005;86:484-488.
55. Novick A, Campbell S. Renal tumors. In: Walsh P, Retik A, Vaughan E, Wein AJ, eds. *Campbell's Urology*. 8th ed. Philadelphia: WB Saunders; 2002:2672-2731.

56. Silver IM, Boag AH, Soboleski DA. Best cases from the AFIP: Multilocular cystic renal tumor: Cystic nephroma. *Radiographics*. 2008;28:1221-1225; discussion 1225-1226.
57. Josh, VV, Beckwith JB. Multilocular cyst of the kidney (cystic nephroma) and cystic, partially differentiated nephroblastoma. Terminology and criteria for diagnosis. *Cancer*. 1989;64:466-479.
58. Honma I, Takagi Y, Shigyo M, et al. Lymphangioma of the kidney. *Int J Urol*. 2002;9:178-182.
59. Varela JR, Bargiela A, Requejo I, et al. Bilateral renal lymphangiomatosis: US and CT findings. *Eur Radiol*. 1998;8:230-231.
60. Ozmen M, Deren O, Akata D, et al. Renal lymphangiomatosis during pregnancy: Management with percutaneous drainage. *Eur Radiol*. 2001; 11:37-40.
61. Bernstein J. Glomerulocystic kidney disease—nosological considerations. *Pediatr Nephrol*. 1993;7:464-470.
62. Sharp C, Bergman S, Stockwin J, et al. Dominantly-inherited glomerulocystic kidney disease: A distinct genetic entity. *J Am Soc Nephrol*. 1997;8:77-84.
63. Bisceglia M, Galliani C, Senger C, et al. Renal cystic diseases: A review. *Adv Anat Pathol*. 2006;13:26-56.
64. Bingham C, Hattersley A. Renal cysts and diabetes syndrome resulting from mutations in hepatocyte nuclear factor-1b. *Nephrol Dial Transplant*. 2004;19:2703-2708.
65. Torres V, Young W, Offord K, Hattery R. Association of hypokalemia, aldosteronism, and renal cysts. *N Engl J Med*. 1990;322:345-351.
66. Friedrich C. Genotype-phenotype correlations in von Hippel-Lindau syndrome. *Hum Mol Genet*. 2001;10:763-767.

CHAPTER 46

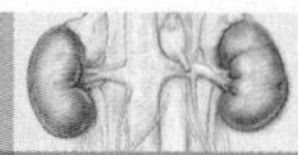

Alport's and Other Familial Glomerular Syndromes

Clifford E. Kashtan

ALPORT'S SYNDROME

Definition

Alport's syndrome (AS) is a generalized, inherited disorder of basement membranes due to mutations affecting specific proteins of the type IV (basement membrane) collagen family. The major features of AS are hematuria, progressive nephritis with proteinuria and declining renal function, sensorineural deafness, and ocular abnormalities. The course of AS is gender dependent; affected males typically have severe disease, whereas the manifestations of AS in women are usually mild. In 1902, Guthrie provided the first description of familial hematuria.[1] Later studies of Guthrie's family by Hurst[2] and Alport[3] revealed the progressive nature of the nephropathy, its association with deafness, and the poorer prognosis in affected males. In the 1970s, the glomerular basement membrane (GBM) was recognized as the site of the primary abnormality in AS.[4-6] Indirect evidence of abnormalities in type IV collagen[7,8] was followed by mapping of the major AS locus to the X chromosome,[9] cloning of a new type IV collagen gene (*COL4A5*) and its assignment to the same X-chromosomal region,[10] and identification of the first *COL4A5* mutations in patients with X-linked AS.[11]

Etiology and Pathogenesis

Type IV Collagen

Type IV collagen is a major constituent of basement membranes. The type IV collagen family of proteins comprises six isomeric chains, designated α1(IV) to α6(IV). Each of these chains has a major collagenous domain of about 1400 residues containing the repetitive triplet sequence glycine (Gly)–X–Y, in which X and Y represent a variety of other amino acids; a C-terminal noncollagenous (NC1) domain of about 230 residues; and a noncollagenous N-terminal sequence of 15 to 20 residues.

Each type IV collagen molecule is a heterotrimer composed of three α chains. Formation of these heterotrimers is initiated by C-terminal NC1 domain interactions, accompanied by folding of the collagenous domains into triple helices. There is evidence for at least three types of type IV collagen heterotrimer: $\alpha1(IV)_2$–α2(IV), α3(IV)–α4(IV)–α5(IV), and $\alpha5(IV)_2$–α6(IV). Type IV collagen triple helices form open, nonfibrillar networks that associate with laminin assemblies through interactions mediated by nidogen to form basement membranes.

The six type IV collagen genes are arranged in pairs on three chromosomes (Fig. 46.1). The 5′ ends of each gene pair are adjacent to each other, separated by sequences of varying length that contain motifs involved in the regulation of transcriptional activity.

Tissue Distribution of Type IV Collagen There are several distinct type IV collagen networks in basement membranes: a ubiquitous network comprising the α1(IV) and α2(IV) chains; and other networks, restricted in distribution, composed of α3(IV), α4(IV), and α5(IV) chains, or α5(IV) and α6(IV) chains. GBM contains separate α1–α2(IV) and α3–α4–α5(IV) networks, whereas epidermal basement membranes contain separate networks of α1–α2(IV) chains and α5–α6(IV) chains. It is likely that these networks have different functional characteristics and interact differently with other matrix components and with adjacent cells.

Genetics

Three forms of AS have been established on a molecular genetic basis: an X-linked form resulting from mutations at the *COL4A5* locus, primarily affecting the α5(IV) chain; an autosomal recessive form arising from mutations at the *COL4A3* locus or the *COL4A4* locus, affecting the α3(IV) and α4(IV) chains, respectively; and an autosomal dominant form due to heterozygous mutations in *COL4A3* or *COL4A4* (Fig. 46.2).

X-Linked Alport's Syndrome X-linked Alport's syndrome (XLAS) is the predominant form of the disease, accounting for about 80% of patients. Several hundred *COL4A5* mutations have been described, mostly missense mutations, splice-site mutations, and deletions of fewer than 10 base pairs.[12,13] A common missense mutation involves replacement of a glycine residue in the collagenous domain of the α5(IV) chain by another amino acid. Such mutations are thought to interfere with the normal folding of the α5(IV) chain into triple helices with other α(IV) chains.

Male patients with *COL4A5* deletions consistently progress to end-stage renal disease (ESRD) during the second or third decade of life and have deafness[14]; this phenotype is associated with most of the missense, nonsense, and splicing mutations of *COL4A5* described so far. Several missense mutations of *COL4A5* have been associated with late-onset (after the third decade) ESRD and with late development of deafness or normal hearing. The severity of disease in a female heterozygous for a *COL4A5* mutation probably depends primarily on the relative activities of the mutant and normal X chromosomes in renal, cochlear, and ocular tissues.

Autosomal Recessive Alport's Syndrome Autosomal recessive Alport's syndrome (ARAS) arises from mutations affecting both alleles of *COL4A3* or *COL4A4*.[15,16] ARAS should be suspected when an individual exhibits the typical clinical and pathologic features of the disease but lacks a positive family history, especially when a young female has findings indicative of severe

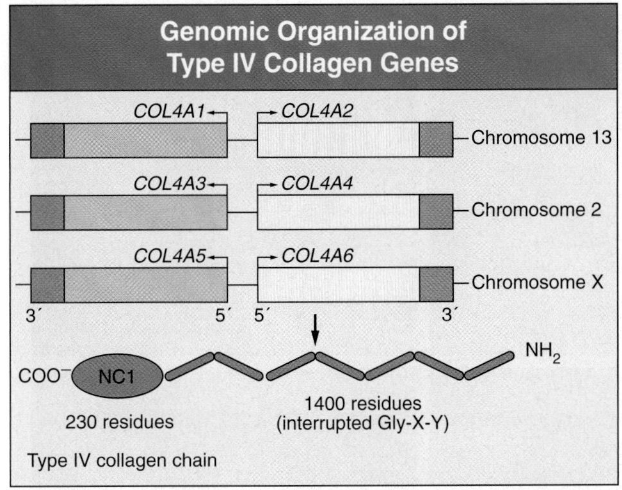

Figure 46.1 Genomic organization of type IV collagen genes.

Molecular Genetics of Alport's Syndrome

Inheritance	Affected Locus	Gene Product
X-linked (XLAS)	*COL4A5*	α5(IV)
X-linked + leiomyomatosis	*COL4A5* + *COL4A6*	α5(IV) + α6(IV)
Autosomal recessive (ARAS)	*COL4A3* *COL4A4*	α3(IV) α4(IV)
Autosomal dominant	*COL4A3* *COL4A4*	α3(IV) α4(IV)

Figure 46.2 Molecular genetics of Alport's syndrome.

disease, such as deafness, nephrotic syndrome, and impaired renal function, However, sporadic cases of AS may represent *de novo* mutations at the *COL4A5* locus or a germline *COL4A5* mutation in the proband's mother. Most patients with ARAS develop ESRD and deafness before the age of 30 years, regardless of gender.

Autosomal Dominant Alport's Syndrome Heterozygous mutations in *COL4A3* or *COL4A4* typically result in asymptomatic hematuria[15,16] but in some families may also be associated with progressive nephropathy, that is, autosomal dominant Alport's syndrome (ADAS).[17,18] ADAS patients tend to have a slower course to ESRD than do those with XLAS or ARAS.[19]

Type IV Collagen in Alport's Basement Membranes

The GBMs and tubular basement membranes of males with XLAS usually fail to stain for the α3(IV), α4(IV), and α5(IV) chains but do express the α1(IV) and α2(IV) chains (Fig. 46.3).[20] Women with XLAS frequently exhibit mosaicism of GBM expression of the α3(IV), α4(IV), and α5(IV) chains, whereas expression of the α1(IV) and α2(IV) chains is preserved (see Fig. 46.3). Most males with XLAS show no epidermal basement membrane expression of α5(IV), whereas female heterozygotes frequently display mosaicism (Fig. 46.4). Lens capsules of some males with XLAS do not express the α3(IV), α4(IV), or α5(IV) chains, whereas expression of these chains appears normal in other patients.

In most patients with ARAS, GBM shows no expression of the α3(IV), α4(IV), or α5(IV) chains, but α5(IV) and α6(IV) are expressed in Bowman's capsule, distal tubular basement membrane, and epidermal basement membrane (Fig. 46.5).[20] Therefore, XLAS and ARAS may be differentiated by immunohistochemical analysis. Basement membrane expression of type IV collagen α chains appears to be normal in patients with ADAS.

These observations indicate that a mutation affecting one of the chains involved in the α3–α4–α5(IV) network can prevent GBM expression not only of that chain but also of the other two chains. Most observational and experimental evidence supports the hypothesis that these effects reflect post-translational events. Some mutant chains are unable to participate in the formation of trimers; as a result, the normal chains that are prevented from forming trimers undergo degradation. Other mutations may allow formation of abnormal trimers that are degraded before deposition in basement membranes can occur.

Clinical Manifestations

Renal Defects

Hematuria is the cardinal finding of AS. Affected males have persistent microscopic hematuria. Many also have episodic gross hematuria, precipitated by upper respiratory infections, usually during the first two decades of life. Hematuria has been discovered in the first year of life in affected boys, in whom it is probably present from birth. Boys who are free of hematuria during the first 10 years of life are unlikely to be affected.

More than 90% of females with XLAS have persistent or intermittent microscopic hematuria, but about 7% of obligate heterozygotes never manifest hematuria.[21] Hematuria appears to be persistent in both males and females with ARAS. About 50% of carriers of *COL4A3* or *COL4A4* mutations have hematuria.[15,16]

Proteinuria is usually absent early in life but develops eventually in all males with XLAS and in both males and females with ARAS. Proteinuria increases progressively with age and may result in the nephrotic syndrome. Proteinuria develops eventually in most heterozygous females.[21] Hypertension also increases in incidence and severity with age. Similar to proteinuria, hypertension is more likely to occur in affected males than in affected females with XLAS, but there are no gender differences in the hypertension frequency in ARAS.

ESRD develops in all affected males with XLAS, at a rate determined primarily by the nature of the underlying *COL4A5* mutation.[14] Thus, the rate of progression is fairly constant among affected males within a particular family, but there is significant interkindred variability. Significant intrakindred variability in the rate of progression to ESRD has been reported in some families with missense *COL4A5* mutations.

Progression to ESRD in females with XLAS was, until recently, considered an unusual event. However, a study of several hundred XLAS females found that 12% developed ESRD before the age of 40 years (compared with 90% of XLAS males), increasing to 30% by age 60 years and 40% by age 80 years.[21] The risk for ESRD was significantly increased in heterozygotes with proteinuria. The outcome of XLAS in females is presumed to be dependent on the relative activities of the normal and mutant X chromosomes, but this has yet to be proved. Gross hematuria in childhood, nephrotic syndrome, and the finding of diffuse GBM thickening by electron microscopy are risk factors for chronic kidney disease in affected females.[22] Sensorineural deafness and anterior lenticonus are also indicative of an unfavorable outcome in affected women. Both males and females with

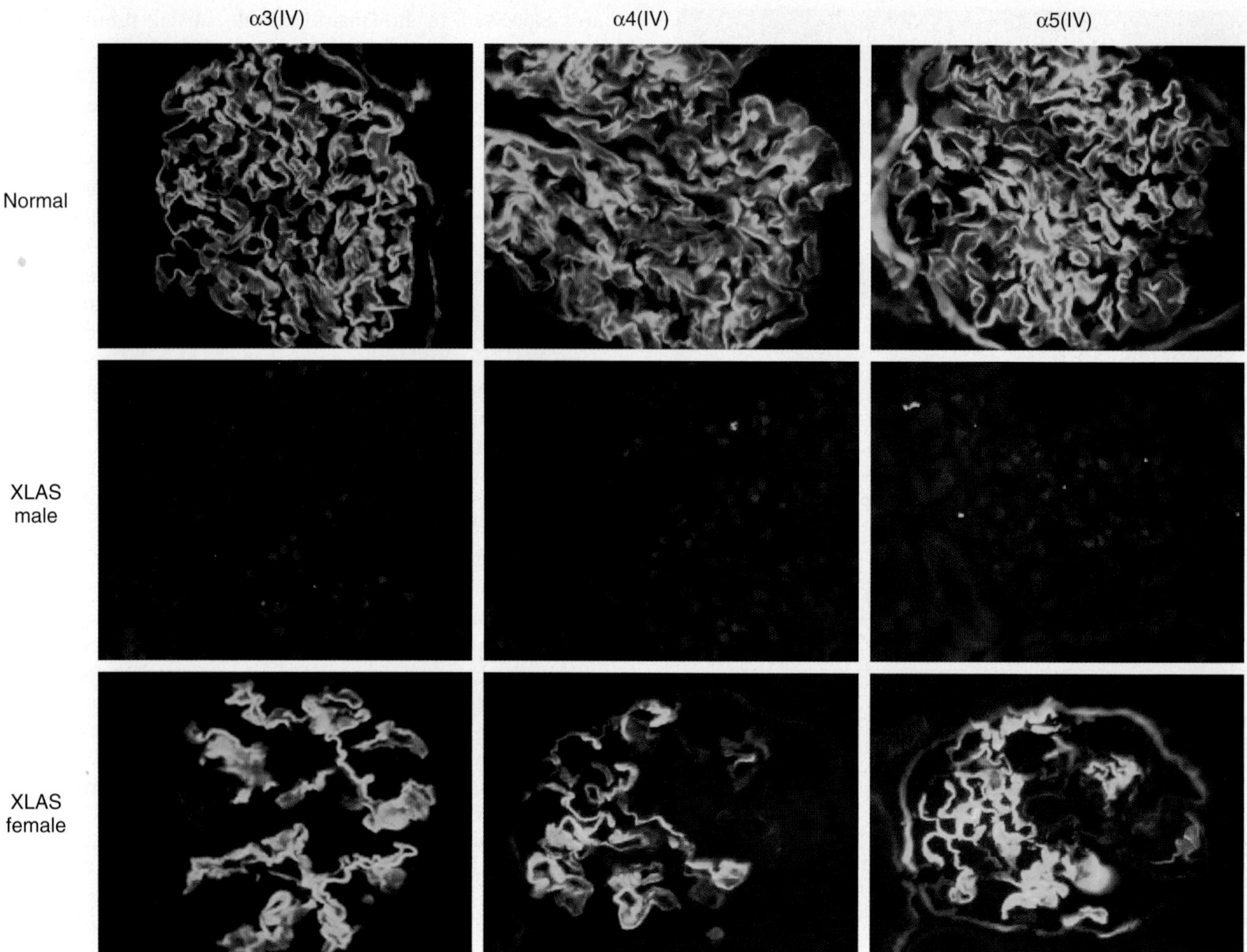

Figure 46.3 Immunohistochemistry of glomerular basement membrane (GBM) in X-linked Alport's syndrome. In a normal individual, GBM stains strongly for the α3(IV), α4(IV), and α5(IV) chains of type IV collagen. Staining of GBM of an affected male is negative for each of these chains, whereas an affected female shows mosaic immunoreactivity.

ARAS appear likely to progress to ESRD during the second or third decade of life.

Cochlear Defects

Deafness is frequently but not universally associated with the Alport's renal lesion, occurring in about 80% of males and 25% to 30% of females with the disease.[14,21] In some families with Alport's nephropathy and apparently normal hearing, deafness may occur late and be very slowly progressive.

Hearing loss in AS is never congenital and usually becomes apparent by late childhood to early adolescence in boys with XLAS and in both boys and girls with ARAS. Hearing impairment in members of families with AS is always accompanied by evidence of renal involvement. There is no convincing evidence that deaf males lacking renal disease can transmit AS to their offspring. In its early stages, the hearing deficit is detectable only by audiometry, with bilateral reduction in sensitivity to tones in the range 2000 to 8000 Hz. In affected males, the deficit extends progressively to other frequencies, including those of conversational speech.

Ocular Defects

Ocular defects occur in 30% to 40% of XLAS males and in about 15% of XLAS females.[14,21] Anterior lenticonus, which is virtually pathognomonic of AS, occurs in about 15% of XLAS males and is almost entirely restricted to AS families with progression to ESRD before the age of 30 years and deafness.[14] Anterior lenticonus is absent at birth, usually appearing during the second to third decade of life, and is bilateral in 75% of patients (Fig. 46.6A). The spectrum and frequencies of ocular lesions appear to be similar in XLAS and ARAS.[23]

Another common ocular manifestation of AS is a maculopathy, which consists of whitish or yellowish flecks or granulations in a perimacular distribution (Fig. 46.6B) and occurs in 15% to 30% of patients. The maculopathy does not appear to be associated with any visual abnormalities.

Corneal endothelial vesicles (posterior polymorphous dystrophy) have been observed in AS and may indicate defects in Descemet's membrane, the basement membrane underlying the corneal endothelium. Recurrent corneal erosion in AS has been attributed to alterations of the corneal epithelial basement membrane.

Leiomyomatosis

The association of AS with leiomyomatosis of the esophagus and tracheobronchial tree has been reported in about 30 families.[13] Affected females typically exhibit genital leiomyomas as well, with clitoral hypertrophy and variable involvement of the labia

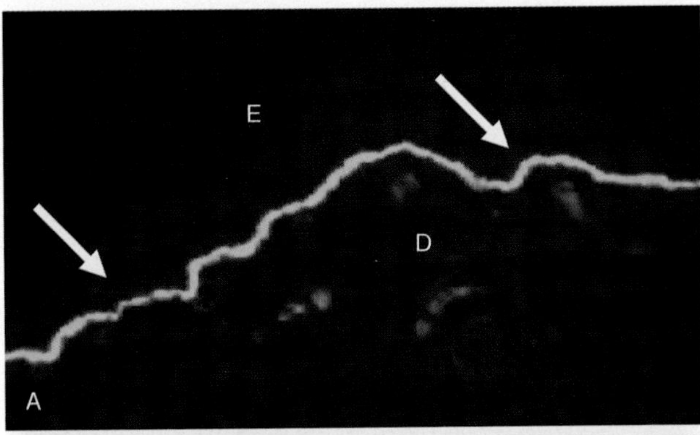

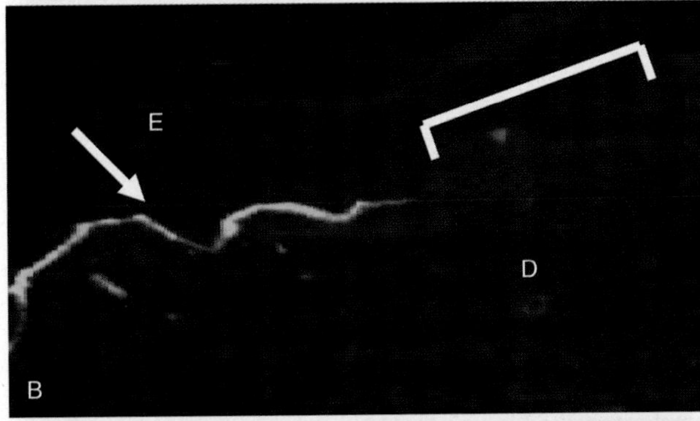

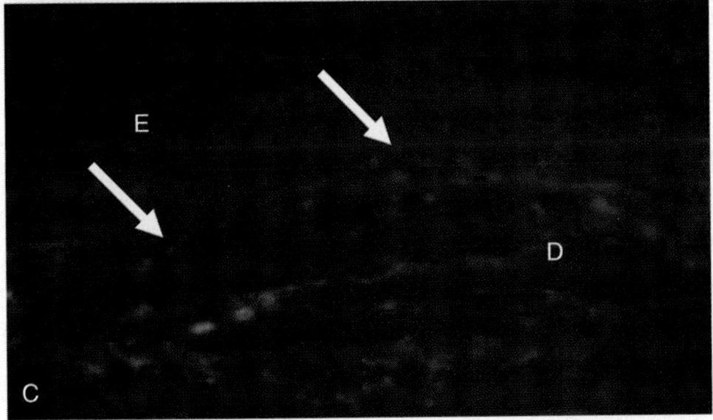

Figure 46.4 Immunohistochemistry of epidermal basement membrane (EBM) in X-linked Alport's syndrome. A, In a normal male, EBM shows strong staining for α5(IV) at the dermoepidermal junction *(arrows)* between dermis (D) and epidermis (E). **B,** In an affected female, EBM shows mosaic staining *(arrow);* the bracket identifies a length of EBM negative for α5(IV). **C,** In affected males, staining of EBM *(arrows)* for α5(IV) is absent.

majora and uterus. Bilateral posterior subcapsular cataracts also occur frequently in affected individuals. Symptoms usually appear in late childhood and include dysphagia, postprandial vomiting, retrosternal or epigastric pain, recurrent bronchitis, dyspnea, cough, and stridor. All patients with AS–diffuse leiomyomatosis complex have been found to have deletions that encompass the 5′ ends of *COL4A5* and *COL4A6*.

Hematologic Defects

An autosomal dominant syndrome of hereditary nephritis, deafness, and megathrombocytopenia, Epstein's syndrome, has been described in a handful of families. Families with Fechtner's syndrome exhibit these features as well as leukocyte inclusions (May-Hegglin anomaly). Both Epstein's and Fechtner's syndromes arise from mutations in non-muscle myosin heavy chain IIA.[24] Basement membranes of these patients do not exhibit abnormalities in expression of type IV collagen α chains. Therefore, Epstein's and Fechtner's syndromes are best considered distinct forms of hereditary nephritis rather than variants of AS.

Pathology

There are no pathognomonic lesions by light microscopy or direct immunofluorescence in AS. Indirect immunofluorescence of type IV collagen α-chain expression in renal or skin basement membranes can be diagnostic (see earlier discussion) and is increasingly available in specialized laboratories around the world.

Electron microscopy frequently reveals diagnostic abnormalities. The cardinal fine structural feature of the kidney that occurs in most patients with AS is the variable thickening, thinning, basket weaving, and lamellation of the GBM (Fig. 46.7). The thick segments measure up to 1200 nm in depth, usually have irregular outer and inner contours, and are found more commonly in males than in females. The lamina densa is transformed into a heterogeneous network of membranous strands, which enclose clear electron-lucent areas that may contain round granules of variable density measuring 20 to 90 nm in diameter. There are variable degrees of epithelial foot process fusion.

Not all Alport's kindreds demonstrate these characteristic ultrastructural features. Thick, thin, normal, and nonspecifically altered GBM have all been described. Affected young males, heterozygous females at any age, and, on occasion, affected adult males may have diffusely attenuated GBM measuring as little as 100 nm or less in thickness rather than the pathognomonic lesion. Although diffuse attenuation of GBM has been considered the hallmark of thin basement membrane nephropathy (as discussed elsewhere in this chapter), some patients with this abnormality are members of kindreds with a history of progression to renal failure. Therefore, the significance of an ultrastructural finding of thin GBM must be considered in the context of the family history, basement membrane expression of type IV collagen α chains, and, if it is available, molecular genetic information.

Diagnosis and Differential Diagnosis

A summary of the evaluation of patients with hematuria and a positive family history is given in Figure 46.8. AS should be included in the initial differential diagnosis of patients with persistent microscopic hematuria, once structural abnormalities of the kidneys or urinary tract have been excluded. The presence on electron microscopy of diffuse thickening and multilamellation of the GBM predicts a progressive nephropathy, regardless of family history. However, in a patient with a negative family history, electron microscopy cannot differentiate *de novo* XLAS from ARAS. In some patients, the biopsy findings may be ambiguous, particularly in females and young patients of either sex. Furthermore, families with progressive nephritis and *COL4A5* mutations in association with GBM thinning have been described, indicating that the classic Alport's GBM lesion is not present in all Alport's kindreds.

It is not unusual to see a patient with hematuria and to discover that multiple relatives also have hematuria, although none has ever undergone kidney biopsy. Who should undergo biopsy in such instances? The natural history of the AS renal lesion suggests that older, male subjects are more likely to exhibit diagnostic ultrastructural GBM abnormalities. In families in which a firm diagnosis of AS has been established, evaluation of individuals with newly recognized hematuria can be limited to ultrasound

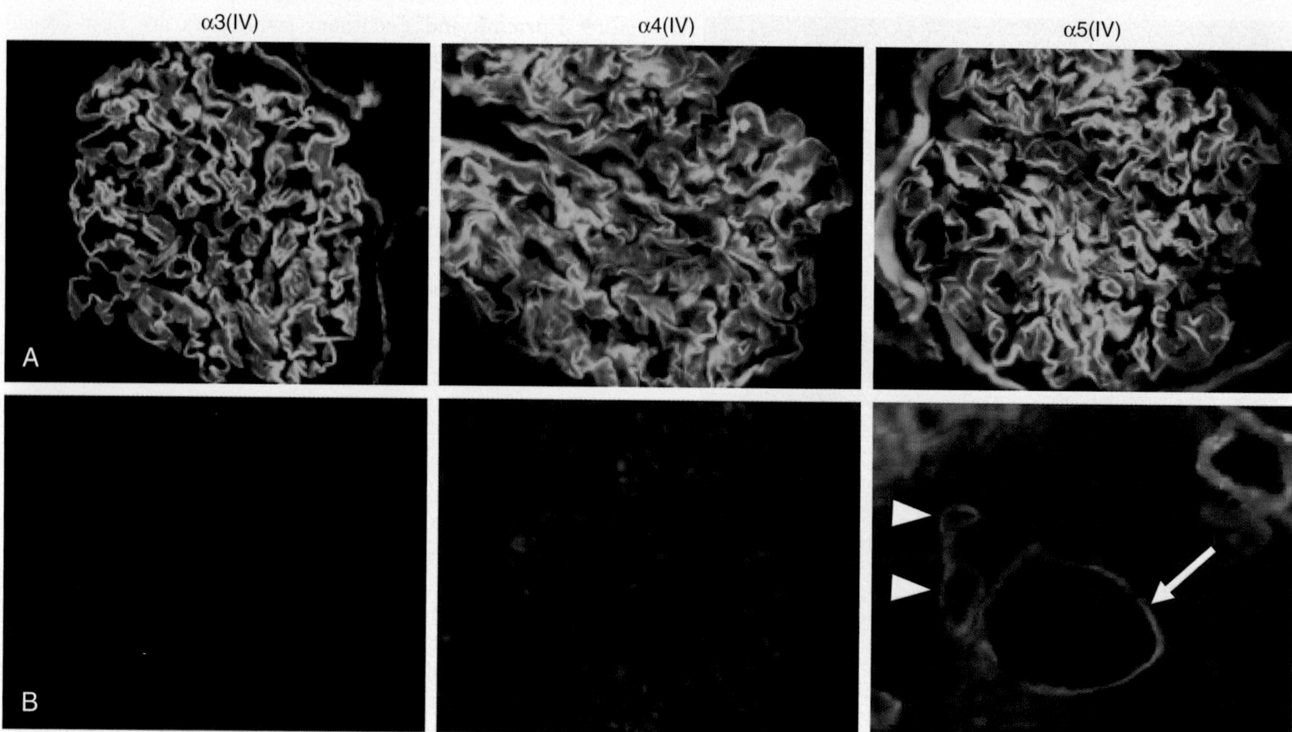

Figure 46.5 Immunohistochemistry of the kidney in a patient with autosomal recessive Alport's syndrome. A, Normal GBM and Bowman's capsule staining for α3(IV), α4(IV), and α5(IV). **B,** Patient shows no GBM staining, but it is present in Bowman's capsule *(arrow)* and distal tubular basement membranes *(arrowheads)*.

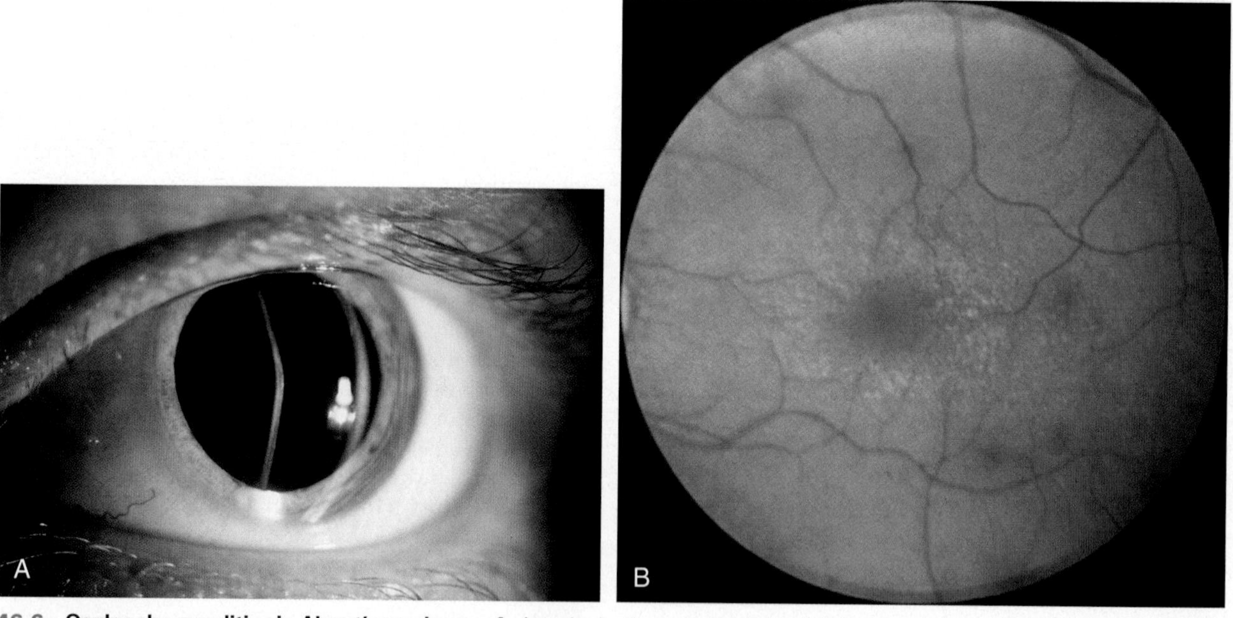

Figure 46.6 Ocular abnormalities in Alport's syndrome. A, Anterior lenticonus shown by slit-lamp ophthalmoscopy. **B,** Perimacular flecks. *(From Flinter FA: Disorders of the basement membrane: Hereditary nephritis. In Morgan SH, Grunfeld J-P [eds]: Inherited Disorders of the Kidney. Oxford, Oxford University Press, 1998.)*

of the kidneys and urinary tract to exclude coincidental tumor or structural anomalies of the urinary tract.

Absence of the α3, α4, and α5 chains of type IV collagen from GBM and distal tubular basement membrane has not been described in any condition other than AS, making this a diagnostic finding on kidney biopsy (Fig. 46.9). Examination of skin biopsy specimens by immunofluorescence for expression of α5(IV) in the epidermal basement membrane may be informative, but apparently normal expression of type IV collagen α chains in basement membranes does not exclude the diagnosis of AS. Mosaic expression of α5(IV) is frequent in heterozygous females. Although mosaic expression of α5(IV) is diagnostic of the carrier state, a normal result does not exclude heterozygosity. A female member of an Alport's kindred who does not have

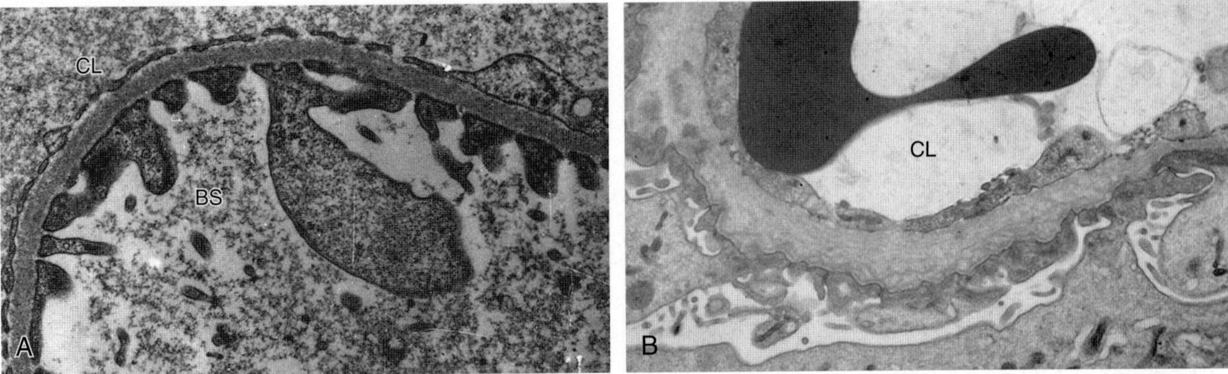

Figure 46.7 Renal biopsy in Alport's syndrome. A, A normal glomerular capillary wall is shown. **B,** Glomerular capillary wall from a patient with Alport's syndrome, at the same magnification. Note the thickening of the GBM, the splitting of the lamina densa into multiple strands, and the marked irregularity of the epithelial aspect of the GBM in the patient with Alport's syndrome. BS, Bowman's space; CL, capillary lumen.

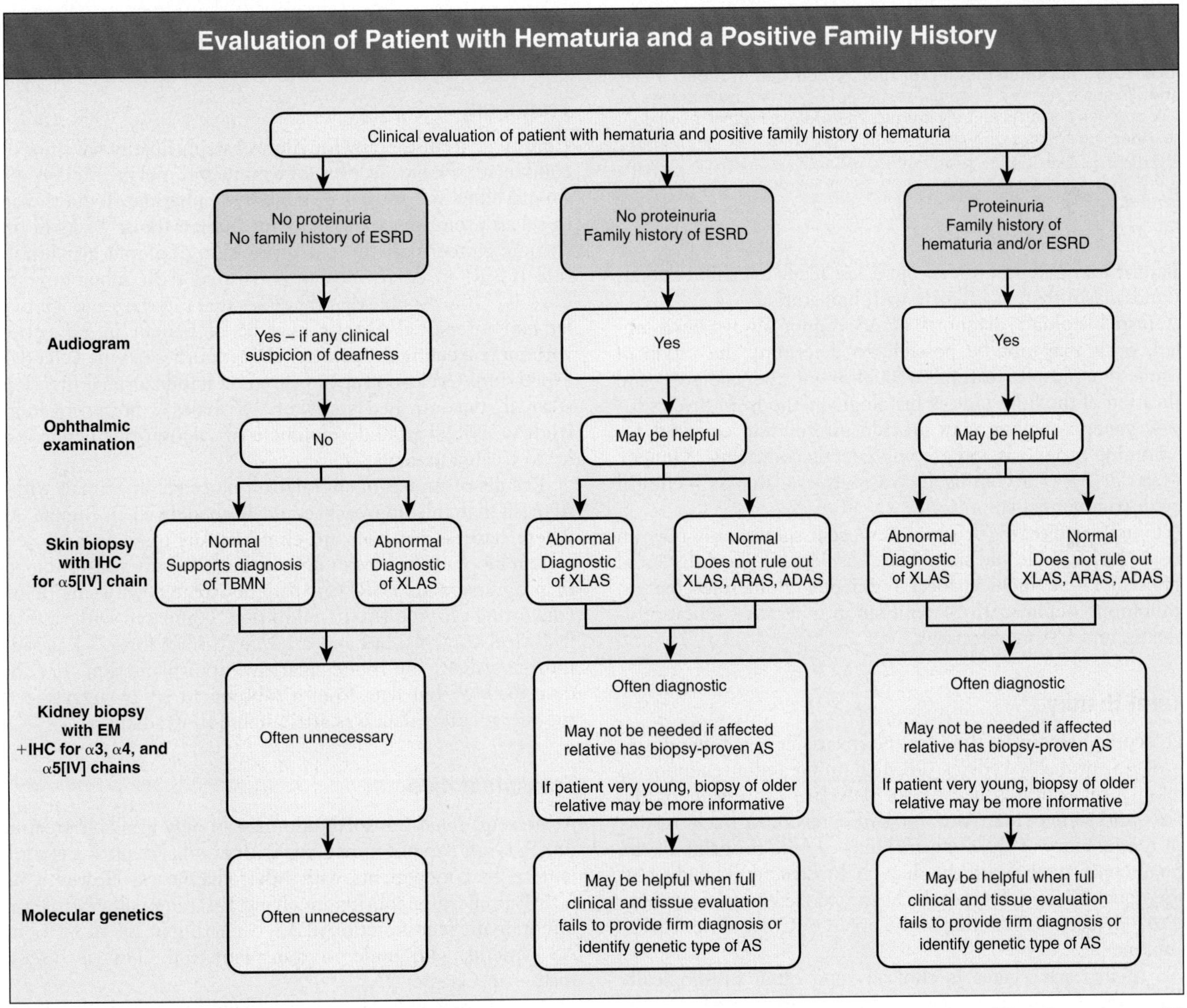

Evaluation of Patient with Hematuria and a Positive Family History

Clinical evaluation of patient with hematuria and positive family history of hematuria

	No proteinuria No family history of ESRD	No proteinuria Family history of ESRD	Proteinuria Family history of hematuria and/or ESRD
Audiogram	Yes – if any clinical suspicion of deafness	Yes	Yes
Ophthalmic examination	No	May be helpful	May be helpful
Skin biopsy with IHC for α5[IV] chain	Normal: Supports diagnosis of TBMN Abnormal: Diagnostic of XLAS	Abnormal: Diagnostic of XLAS Normal: Does not rule out XLAS, ARAS, ADAS	Abnormal: Diagnostic of XLAS Normal: Does not rule out XLAS, ARAS, ADAS
Kidney biopsy with EM +IHC for α3, α4, and α5[IV] chains	Often unnecessary	Often diagnostic May not be needed if affected relative has biopsy-proven AS If patient very young, biopsy of older relative may be more informative	Often diagnostic May not be needed if affected relative has biopsy-proven AS If patient very young, biopsy of older relative may be more informative
Molecular genetics	Often unnecessary	May be helpful when full clinical and tissue evaluation fails to provide firm diagnosis or identify genetic type of AS	May be helpful when full clinical and tissue evaluation fails to provide firm diagnosis or identify genetic type of AS

Figure 46.8 Evaluation of the patient with hematuria and a positive family history. ADAS, autosomal dominant Alport's syndrome; ARAS, autosomal recessive Alport's syndrome; AS, Alport's syndrome; EM, electron microscopy; ESRD, end-stage renal disease; IHC, immunohistochemistry; TBMN, thin basement membrane nephropathy; XLAS, X-linked Alport's syndrome.

Immunostaining for Type IV Collagen in Alport's Syndrome

Type IV Collagen Group	Glomerular Basement Membranes	Bowman's Capsules	Distal Tubular Basement Membrane	Epidermal Basement Membrane
Normal (males and females)				
α3(IV)	Present	Present	Present	Absent
α4(IV)	Present	Present	Present	Absent
α5(IV)	Present	Present	Present	Present
X-linked (males)*				
α3(IV)	Absent	Absent	Absent	Absent
α4(IV)	Absent	Absent	Absent	Absent
α5(IV)	Absent	Absent	Absent	Absent
X-linked (females)†				
α3(IV)	Mosaic			Absent
α4(IV)	Mosaic			Absent
α5(IV)	Mosaic			Mosaic
Autosomal recessive (males and females)*				
α3(IV)	Absent	Absent	Absent	Absent
α4(IV)	Absent	Absent	Absent	Absent
α5(IV)	Absent	Present	Present	Present

Figure 46.9 Immunostaining for type IV collagen in Alport's syndrome. *In some Alport's kindreds, staining of basement membranes for type IV collagen chains is entirely normal. Therefore, a normal result does not exclude a diagnosis of X-linked Alport's syndrome. †Some heterozygous females have normal basement membrane immunoreactivity for type IV collagen chains. Therefore, a normal result does not exclude the carrier state.

hematuria may still be a carrier but is less likely to exhibit detectable mosaicism than is a female with hematuria.

A firm histologic diagnosis of AS cannot always be established, or it may not be possible to determine the mode of transmission, despite careful evaluation of the pedigree and application of the full range of histologic methods. In these situations, genetic analysis may provide information essential for determining prognosis and guiding genetic counseling. Genetic analysis for AS is becoming increasingly available as a clinical assay in commercial laboratories.

Glomerular diseases that typically occur sporadically may on occasion be heritable and should be considered in the differential diagnosis. These include focal segmental glomerulosclerosis, membranous nephropathy, membranoproliferative glomerulonephritis, and IgA nephropathy.

Natural History

Microscopic hematuria, the first and invariable renal manifestation of AS, probably reflects GBM thinning and a tendency to develop focal ruptures because of defective expression of the α3–α4–α5(IV) network. Anterior lenticonus most likely results from the inability of the abnormal lens capsule to maintain the normal conformation of the lens. Ultrastructural studies of Alport's cochleae suggest that the hearing deficit may be attributable to a defect in adherence of the organ of Corti to the basilar membrane.[25]

AS in its early stages is clinically and often histologically indistinguishable from thin basement membrane nephropathy, which typically has a benign outcome. GBM attenuation is therefore an insufficient explanation for the divergent natural histories of the two conditions. What factors initiate and drive the progression of Alport's nephropathy to ESRD? Reduction in the quantity of α3(IV), α4(IV), and α5(IV) chains in GBM, as likely occurs in thin basement membrane nephropathy, probably has consequences different from complete loss of these chains, as occurs in most males with XLAS and most patients with ARAS. There is increasing information about the molecular events that occur consequent to the loss of the α3(IV)–α4(IV)–α5(IV) network. In the GBM, the normal transition from the $\alpha1(IV)_2$–$\alpha2(IV)_1$ network of nascent glomeruli to the α3(IV)–α4(IV)–α5(IV) network of mature glomeruli fails to occur, and α1(IV) and α2(IV) chains accumulate in Alport's glomeruli as the disease progresses.[26,27] Alport's GBM shows overexpression of other matrix proteins that are normally absent from GBM or present in scant quantities, including type V collagen, type VI collagen, laminin α2 chain, and fibronectin. These alterations in GBM composition are unique to AS.[26,28] Both glomerular endothelial cells and podocytes appear to contribute to the accumulation of these proteins in Alport's GBM. Alterations in glomerular extracellular matrix are accompanied by changes in glomerular cell behavior, including expression of transforming growth factor β1, integrins, and matrix metalloproteinases.[29] Activation of fibrogenic pathways in the renal interstitium presumably represents a downstream consequence of glomerular disease.

Treatment

Clinical trials of therapy for Alport's nephropathy have not been conducted. The availability of canine and murine models of AS should allow the testing of genetic or pharmacologic therapies to select promising treatments for human trials.[30,31] As in other chronic glomerulopathies, deterioration of glomerular filtration rate (GFR) in AS is closely correlated with tubulointerstitial fibrosis.[32] It is possible that therapies that interfere with glomerular and interstitial fibrosis may be of benefit in AS patients, without correcting the primary abnormalities of type IV collagen expression. Cyclosporine appeared to stabilize renal function in a small, uncontrolled study of AS males[33]; however, another study described rapid development of cyclosporine nephrotoxicity in treated patients.[34]

Results of studies of angiotensin blockade in animals with AS suggest that this approach could be beneficial in human AS.[35] There have as yet been no clinical trials of renin-angiotensin system blockade in human AS, although a study suggesting delay in progression to ESRD in patients treated with angiotensin-converting enzyme (ACE) inhibition, compared with untreated historical controls, has appeared in abstract form.[36] Reversal of murine ARAS by bone marrow transplantation has been described,[37,38] but data from a subsequent study suggested that the therapeutic effect was attributable to irradiation.[39]

Transplantation

At present, renal transplantation is the only available treatment of AS. Graft survival in patients with familial nephritis is equivalent to that in patients with other diagnoses. However, anti-GBM glomerulonephritis involving the renal allograft is a rare but dramatic manifestation of AS, occurring in 2% to 3% of male AS patients who undergo transplantation. This is discussed further in Chapter 23.

Are women who are heterozygous for *COL4A5* mutations suitable kidney donors? Clearly, those with proteinuria, hypertension, or reduced GFR should not donate, and the same applies if there is any hearing loss. What about heterozygotes with hematuria but normal renal function and hearing? There is no long-term follow-up information on the impact of uninephrectomy in such women. But given the recent finding that 30% to

40% of heterozygous women may eventually develop ESRD, the risk that a heterozygous donor will ultimately develop significant renal impairment must be higher than for the usual kidney donor.

However, a common clinical scenario is a mother wishing to donate to her son with AS, and the wishes of the whole family should be thoughtfully considered.

THIN BASEMENT MEMBRANE NEPHROPATHY: FAMILIAL AND SPORADIC

Definition

Isolated glomerular hematuria may occur as a familial or sporadic condition and is often associated with a renal biopsy finding of excessively thin GBM. The term *benign familial hematuria* was used in the past to describe disease kindreds in which multiple individuals in several generations have isolated hematuria without progression to ESRD. More recently, thin basement membrane nephropathy (TBMN) has been used to identify both familial and sporadic isolated hematuria associated with attenuated GBM. It is likely that several disorders that differ at the molecular level are associated with GBM thinning, and in some instances, it is probably a normal variant. In general, the discussion that follows applies to both familial and sporadic TBMN.

Similar to AS, familial TBMN is an inherited GBM disorder manifested by chronic hematuria, but it differs clinically from AS in several important respects: (1) extrarenal abnormalities are rare; (2) proteinuria, hypertension, and progression to ESRD are unusual; (3) gender differences in expression of TBMN are not apparent; and (4) transmission is autosomal dominant. TBMN and early AS may be difficult to differentiate histologically because diffuse GBM attenuation is characteristic of both. However, the GBM of patients with TBMN remains attenuated over time, rather than undergoing the progressive thickening and multilamellation that occurs in AS.

Etiology and Pathogenesis

TBMN is an autosomal dominant condition, but a negative family history may not be reliable because patients are frequently unaware that they have relatives with hematuria. Familial TBMN has been localized to *COL4A3* or *COL4A4* in numerous kindreds[40,41]; 50% or more of heterozygous carriers of a *COL4A3* or *COL4A4* mutation have hematuria.[15,16] However, linkage to *COL4A3* and *COL4A4* has been excluded in other families with isolated hematuria, indicating that TBMN is a genetically heterogeneous condition.

Immunohistologic studies of type IV collagen in GBM of patients with TBMN have found no abnormalities in the distribution of any of the six α chains. Immunohistologic evaluation of GBM type IV collagen may therefore be useful in the differentiation of TBMN from AS (see later discussion).

Clinical Manifestations

It has been estimated that 20% to 25% of patients referred to a nephrologist for evaluation of persistent hematuria will prove to have thin GBM on renal biopsy. Individuals with TBMN typically have persistent microscopic hematuria that is first detected in childhood. In some patients, microscopic hematuria is intermittent and may not be detected until adulthood. Episodic macroscopic hematuria, often in association with upper respiratory infections, is not unusual. The hematuria of TBMN appears to be lifelong.

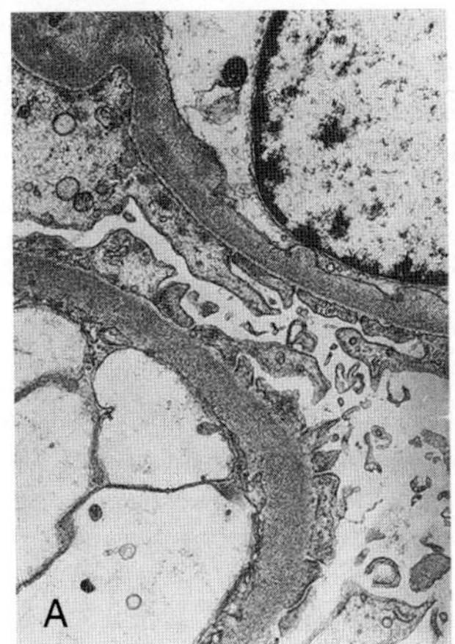

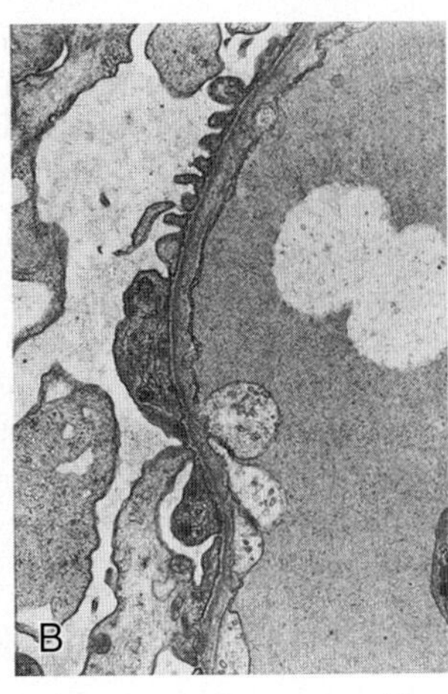

Figure 46.10 Thin basement membrane nephropathy. Electron micrographs of renal biopsy specimens. **A,** Normal glomerular capillary wall. **B,** Thin basement membrane nephropathy at the same magnification. Note the diffuse and uniform attenuation of the GBM and the lamina densa. *(From Warrell DA, Cox TM, Firth JD, Benz EJ Jr [eds]: Oxford Textbook of Medicine. Oxford, Oxford University Press, 2003, p 322.)*

Overt proteinuria and hypertension are unusual in TBMN but have been reported. Some of these patients may have actually had AS, in which the predominant abnormality of GBM was attenuation rather than thickening and multilamellation. Other glomerular disorders, such as IgA nephropathy and focal or global glomerulosclerosis, may occur concurrently with TBMN.

Pathology

Light and immunofluorescence microscopy are unremarkable in typical cases of TBMN. Most patients exhibit diffuse thinning of the whole GBM and of the lamina densa (Fig. 46.10). GBM width is age and gender dependent in normal individuals. Both the lamina densa and the GBM increase rapidly in thickness between birth and 2 years of age, followed by gradual thickening into adulthood. GBM thickness in adult men (373 ± 42 nm) exceeds that in adult women (326 ± 45 nm).[31] Each electron microscopy laboratory should establish a consistent technique for measuring GBM thickness and determine its own reference range for GBM width to make comparisons with published data meaningful. Typically, a value of 250 nm will accurately separate adults with normal GBM from those with TBMN.[42] For children, the cutoff is in the range of 200 to 250 nm. Intraglomerular variability in GBM width is small in individuals with TBMN.

Diagnosis and Differential Diagnosis

If the family history indicates autosomal dominant transmission of hematuria, if there is no history of chronic renal failure, and if kidney and urinary tract imaging studies are normal, a presumptive diagnosis of TBMN can often be made without kidney biopsy (see Fig. 46.8). When family history is negative or unknown or there are atypical coexisting features, such as proteinuria and deafness, renal biopsy may be very informative. A finding of thin GBM may be further characterized by examining the distribution of type IV collagen α chains in the kidney. Normal distribution of these chains provides supportive although not conclusive evidence for a diagnosis of TBMN. Marked variability in GBM width within a glomerulus in a patient with persistent microhematuria should raise suspicion of AS, although focal lamina densa splitting has been described in TBMN. Genetic analysis may confirm a heterozygous mutation in *COL4A3* or *COL4A4*.

Treatment

Patients with TBMN should be reassured but not lost to follow-up examination. The risk for chronic renal impairment is small but real. Urinalysis and measurement of blood pressure and renal function are recommended every 1 to 2 years.

FABRY'S DISEASE (ANDERSON-FABRY DISEASE)

Definition

Fabry's disease comprises the clinical and pathologic manifestations of hereditary deficiency of the enzyme α-galactosidase A (α-Gal A), resulting in the intracellular accumulation of neutral glycosphingolipids with terminal α-linked galactosyl moieties (globotriaosylceramide; Fig. 46.11). Anderson[43] and Fabry[44] each described the characteristic skin lesions of this condition in 1898 and noted the association of proteinuria with the skin lesion, for which Fabry coined the term *angiokeratoma corporis diffusum*.

Etiology and Pathogenesis

More than 100 mutations causing Fabry's disease have been identified in the gene for α-Gal A, which is located on the X chromosome. Most of the described mutations are associated with the classic Fabry phenotype, in which there is multisystem involvement. Certain missense mutations have been identified in patients with a mild phenotype limited to cardiac abnormalities.[45]

Deficiency of α-Gal A leads to progressive intracellular accumulation of neutral glycosphingolipids, particularly those with α-galactosyl moieties, the most abundant of which is globotriaosylceramide (Gb3). Glycosphingolipids are normal constituents of the plasma membrane, the membranes of intracellular organelles, and circulate in association with apolipoproteins. The glycosphingolipids that accumulate in Fabry's disease are identical to those found in normal tissue. All tissues except red blood cells accumulate Gb3, with the highest concentrations found in the diseased kidney.

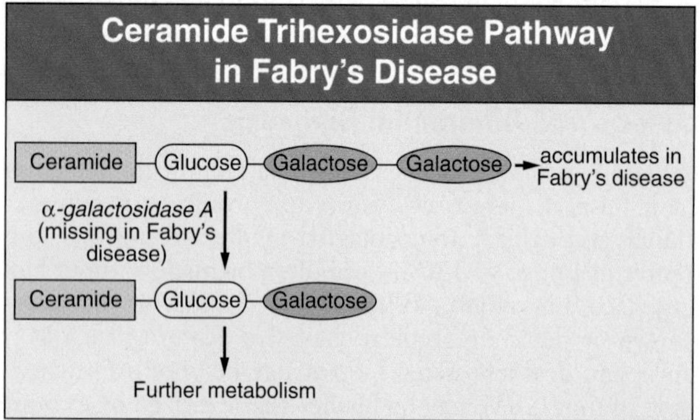

Figure 46.11 The ceramide trihexosidase pathway in Fabry's disease. α-Galactosidase A deficiency leads to tissue accumulation of trihexosylceramide.

Clinical Manifestations and Pathology

Classic Fabry's disease is a multisystem disorder, with prominent and potentially devastating involvement of the kidneys, heart, and peripheral and central nervous system. As expected for an X-linked disorder, severe clinical manifestations occur in hemizygous males, whereas heterozygous females exhibit a variable but typically less severe course. In affected males, the initial features of the disease are seen in childhood and early adolescence and consist of paresthesias and pain in the hands and feet with episodic pain crises. The course of the disease is variable but usually leads to ESRD in the third to sixth decade. Myocardial or cerebral infarctions are typical terminal events. Severe Fabry's disease in a female reflects extensive inactivation of the X chromosome carrying the normal α-Gal A allele.

Renal Defects

Although the earliest manifestation of renal involvement is a concentrating defect, the nephropathy of Fabry's disease typically is manifested as mild to moderate proteinuria, sometimes with microscopic hematuria, beginning in the third decade of life. Nephrotic syndrome is unusual. Urinary oval fat bodies, with a Maltese cross configuration when viewed with a polarizing microscope, are a result of the large amounts of glycosphingolipid in the urine (see Chapter 4, Fig. 4.4B). Deterioration of renal function is gradual, with hypertension and ESRD developing by the fourth or fifth decade of life. Heterozygous women typically display mild renal involvement but may develop ESRD.

Light microscopy shows striking glomerular changes (Fig. 46.12) with additional abnormalities of tubular epithelium and vessels. Glomerular visceral epithelial cells are enlarged and packed with small, clear vacuoles, which represent glycosphingolipid material that has been extracted during processing. Vacuoles may also be seen in parietal epithelial cells and the epithelial cells of the distal convoluted tubule and loop of Henle but only rarely in mesangial cells, glomerular endothelial cells, or proximal tubular epithelial cells. There is progressive segmental and global glomerulosclerosis. Vacuoles are also observed in endothelial cells and smooth muscle cells of arterioles and arteries.

On electron microscopy, there are abundant inclusions within lysosomes, particularly within visceral epithelial cells (Fig. 46.13). The inclusions (myelin figures) are typically round, comprising concentric layers of dense material separated by clear spaces. The layers may be arranged in parallel (zebra bodies).

Detachment of visceral epithelial cells from the underlying basement membrane may be observed. Inclusions are also observed in heterozygous females, although usually in smaller numbers than in affected males. Typical inclusions may be noted in excreted renal tubular cells.

The progression of Fabry's nephropathy to ESRD probably reflects two parallel processes. Visceral epithelial cell dysfunction, which results in proteinuria, is followed by visceral epithelial cell detachment and necrosis leading to capillary loop collapse and segmental sclerosis. Simultaneously, progressive impairment of arteriolar flow may develop, as enlarging endothelial cells impinge on vascular lumina, resulting in ischemic glomerular damage.

Heart Defects

Glycosphingolipid accumulation in coronary arterial endothelial cells and in the myocardium results in coronary artery narrowing, which may lead to angina, myocardial infarction, or congestive heart failure. Arrhythmias and valvular lesions have been

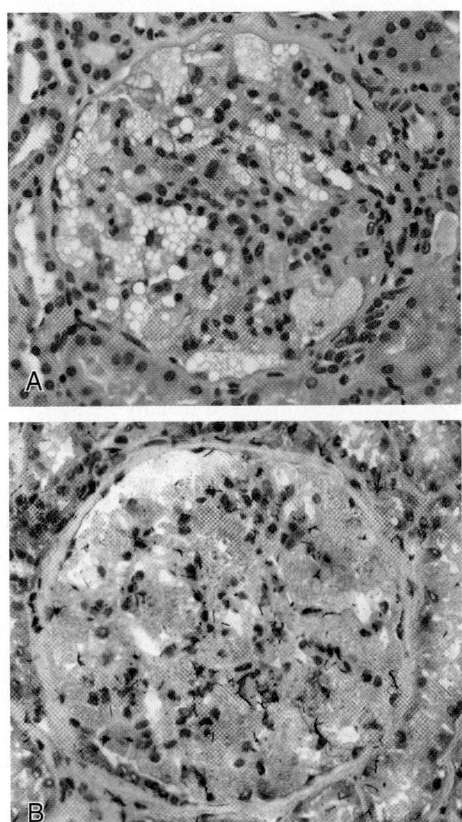

Figure 46.12 Light microscopy of a renal biopsy specimen in Fabry's disease. Glomerular epithelial cell glycosphingolipid deposition demonstrated by **(A)** vacuolation on hematoxylin and eosin staining (magnification ×20) and **(B)** oil red O staining (magnification ×20). *(Courtesy Dr. Paolo Menè and Dr. Antonella Stoppacciaro, University of Rome.)*

identified. Certain missense mutations affecting α-Gal A may present as isolated left ventricular hypertrophy.[45]

Nervous System

Autonomic dysfunction is a prominent feature of Fabry's disease, commonly manifested by hypohidrosis, acral paresthesias, and altered intestinal motility. Cerebrovascular symptoms tend to appear during the fourth decade of life and include hemiparesis, vertigo, diplopia, dysarthria, nystagmus, nausea and vomiting, headache, ataxia, and memory loss. The vertebrobasilar circulation is preferentially involved. Symptoms are often recurrent. Life-threatening intracerebral hemorrhage and infarction are not unusual. Dementia arising from glycosphingolipid accumulation in small cerebral blood vessels has also been described.

Skin

Angiokeratomas usually appear during the second decade of life, presenting as dark red macules or papules of variable size (Fig. 46.14). Typical locations include the lower trunk, buttocks, hips, genitalia, and upper thighs. The number of lesions varies from none up to 40. On histologic examination, angiokeratomas consist of dilated small veins in the upper dermis, covered by hyperkeratotic epidermis. Telangiectasias may be noted, especially behind the ears.

Eyes

Characteristic corneal opacities are common in both men and women with Fabry's disease. These lesions, termed verticillata,

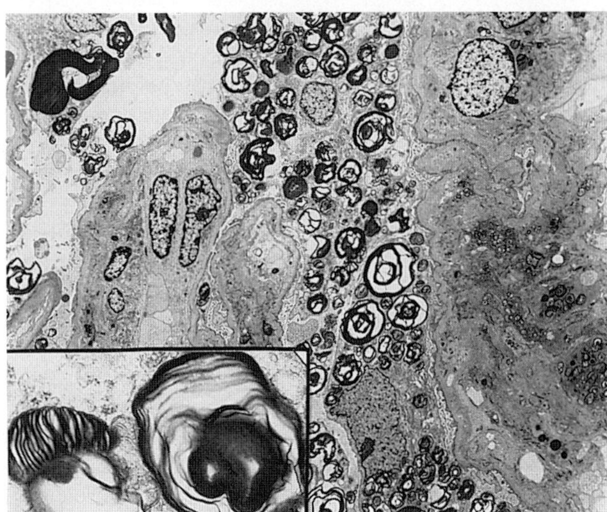

Figure 46.13 Electron micrograph of a renal biopsy specimen in Fabry's disease. Glycosphingolipid is deposited in cytoplasmic vacuoles in glomerular visceral epithelial cells. *Inset:* Cytoplasmic vacuoles contain electron-dense material in parallel arrays (zebra bodies) and in concentric whorls (myelin figures). *(Courtesy Dr. J. Carlos Manivel.)*

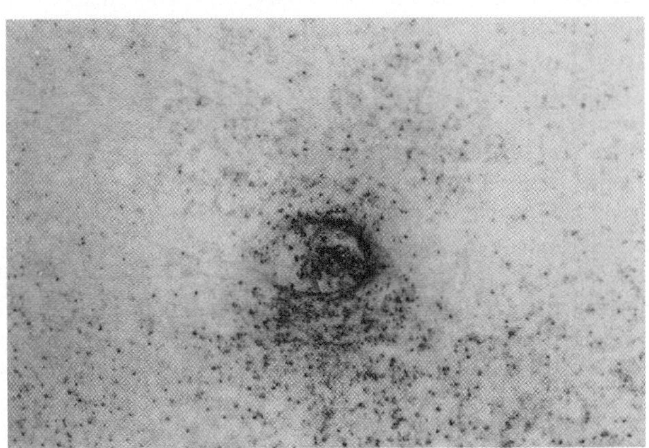

Figure 46.14 Angiokeratoma in Fabry's disease. Note the multiple periumbilical angiokeratomas. *(Courtesy Dr. S. Waldek.)*

are identified by slit-lamp examination and are whorls of whitish discoloration that radiate from the center of the cornea. Cataracts and dilated conjunctival or retinal vessels may be observed.

Lungs

Dyspnea and cough are common in men with Fabry's disease, often with airflow limitation on spirometry. This may be a consequence of fixed narrowing of the airways due to glycosphingolipid accumulation.

Diagnosis

Diagnosis of affected males can usually be made on clinical grounds with the additional information from slit-lamp examination of the eye. The diagnosis should be confirmed by demonstrating decreased or absent α-Gal A activity in serum, leukocytes, cultured skin fibroblasts, or tissue. Atypical variants may have enzyme activity up to 35% of normal. Heterozygous females have intermediate levels of α-Gal A activity, but values may be in the low-normal range, making measurement of enzyme activity an insensitive way of diagnosing carriers. Alternatives include careful slit-lamp eye examination, measurement of urinary ceramide digalactoside and trihexoside, and molecular techniques using restriction fragment length polymorphisms of either the α-Gal A gene or closely linked markers on the X chromosome. Identification of carriers is particularly relevant when family members are being considered as living kidney donors.

Fabry's disease should be considered in patients with unexplained ESRD,[46] especially if left ventricular hypertrophy is present or there is a history of stroke.[47]

Treatment

Until recently, clinicians could offer little beyond palliative, symptomatic care, but the introduction of enzyme replacement therapy with recombinant human α-Gal A (agalsidase) has transformed the treatment of Fabry's disease. Randomized clinical trials showed that agalsidase administration during 5 to 6 months resulted in reduced plasma and urine Gb3; amelioration of neuropathic pain; enhanced quality of life; clearing of Gb3 deposits from kidney, heart, and skin; and improved cerebral blood flow.[48,49] A multicenter longitudinal study showed that agalsidase stabilized renal function in patients with mild to moderate renal impairment at baseline and reduced left ventricular mass in those with left ventricular hypertrophy at baseline during 1 to 2 years of treatment.[50] In patients with ESRD, agalsidase infusion may be combined with hemodialysis because there is little clearance of the enzyme by dialysis.[51] Agalsidase therapy has been recommended for all affected males and symptomatic carrier females.[52]

Renal transplantation is an effective treatment of advanced Fabry's nephropathy but does not ameliorate the extrarenal manifestations. Transplanted kidneys from deceased donors or unaffected living donors may develop glycosphingolipid inclusions, but these are generally infrequent and clinically insignificant. Fabry heterozygotes should not become kidney donors. Coronary artery and cerebrovascular disease are the major causes of death in patients with Fabry's disease who have undergone renal transplantation. Renal allograft recipients with Fabry's disease are candidates for agalsidase treatment.[52]

Fabry's Disease in Childhood

Because it is often not appreciated that the signs and symptoms of Fabry's disease, particularly pain crises, acroparesthesias, angiokeratomas, and corneal opacities, typically have their onset in childhood, the diagnosis is frequently delayed until well into adult life.[53] Symptomatic children with Fabry's disease are potential candidates for agalsidase therapy, and treatment trials in children are now under way.

NAIL-PATELLA SYNDROME

Definition

Nail-patella syndrome (NPS) is an autosomal dominant condition characterized by hypoplasia or absence of the patellae, dystrophic nails, dysplasia of the elbows and iliac horns, and renal disease.

Etiology and Pathogenesis

The NPS locus was identified in 1998 as the LIM homeodomain transcription factor *LMX1B*.[54,55] A variety of mutations in *LMX1B* have been found in NPS patients, including missense, splicing, insertion or deletion, and nonsense alterations. The results of *in vitro* studies of the transcriptional effects of mixing wild-type and mutant *LMX1B* suggest that NPS results from haploinsufficiency of *LMX1B*, rather than a dominant-negative effect.[56] Although *LMX1B* appears to be important for normal limb and kidney development, the precise mechanisms for the renal effects of *LMX1B* mutations remain under investigation.

Clinical Manifestations

Renal Defects

Clinically apparent renal disease occurs in less than half of NPS patients. The nephropathy is usually benign, with about a 10% risk for progression to ESRD. The clinical signs of NPS nephropathy appear in adolescence or young adulthood and typically include microscopic hematuria and mild proteinuria, although some patients develop nephrotic syndrome and mild hypertension. The severity of the renal manifestations may differ substantially in related individuals.

Skeletal Defects

The patellae are absent or hypoplastic in more than 90% of patients with NPS (Fig. 46.15) and may be associated with effusions and osteoarthritis of the knees. In about 80% of patients, there are osseous processes projecting posteriorly from the iliac wings (iliac horns), which are pathognomonic (Fig. 46.16). Anomalies of the elbows include aplasia, hypoplasia, and posterior processes at the distal ends of the humeri.

Nails

Nail abnormalities occur in about 90% of patients and are typically bilateral and symmetric. Fingernails are more commonly affected than toenails. The nails may be absent or dystrophic with discoloration, koilonychia, longitudinal ridges, or triangular lunulae.

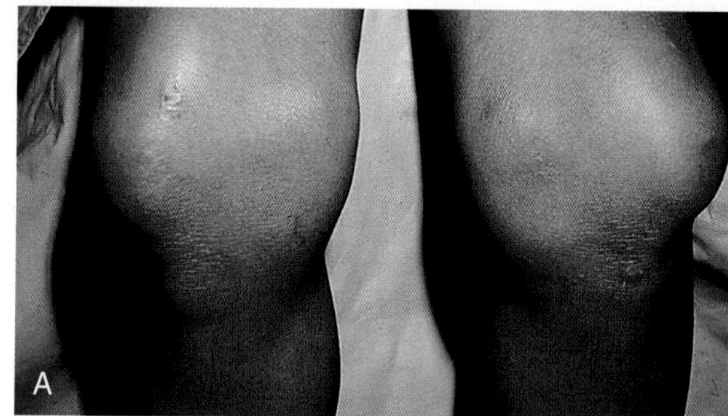

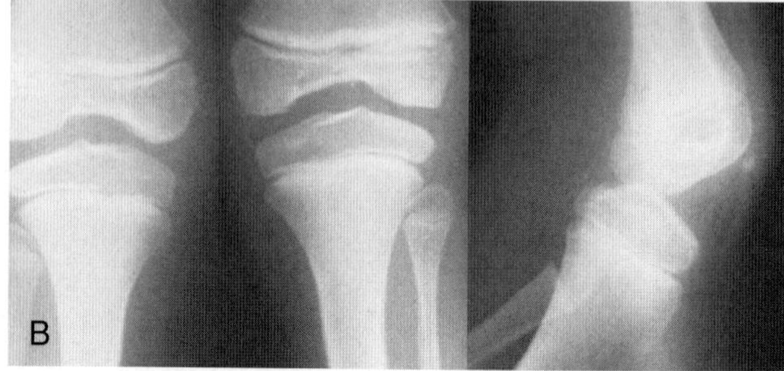

Figure 46.15 Nail-patella syndrome. Clinical **(A)** and radiologic **(B)** appearance of absence of the patellae. *(Courtesy Dr. R. Vernier.)*

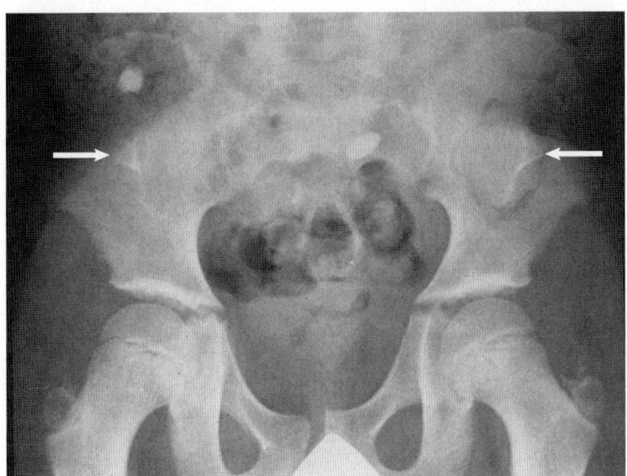

Figure 46.16 Nail-patella syndrome. Iliac horns *(arrows)*. *(Courtesy Dr. R. Vernier.)*

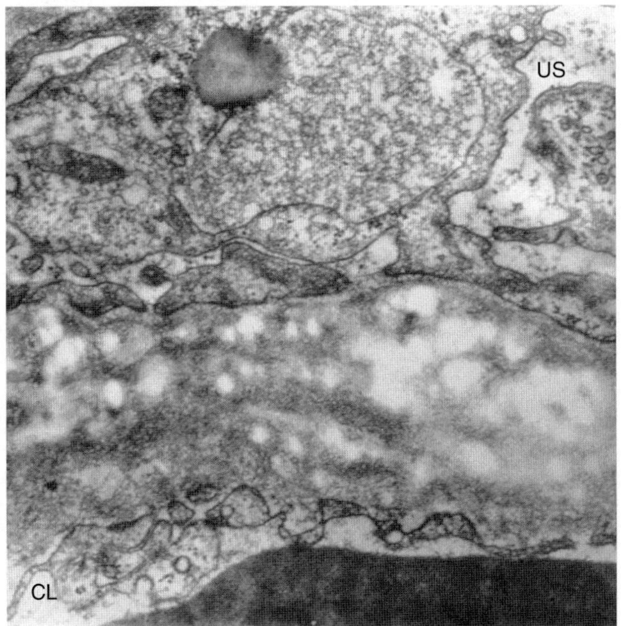

Figure 46.17 Electron micrograph of renal biopsy specimen in nail-patella syndrome. The GBM appears moth-eaten on routine staining. CL, capillary lumen; US, urinary space. *(Courtesy Dr. R. Vernier.)*

Pathology

The only specific features of the NPS renal lesion are ultrastructural; electron microscopy shows multiple irregular lucencies of the GBM, giving it a moth-eaten appearance (Fig. 46.17). Such lucencies may also be observed in the mesangium. These lucent areas sometimes contain cross-banded collagen fibrils, which are more easily observed after staining with phosphotungstic acid (Fig. 46.18). The fibrils, which are type III collagen,[57] tend to be arranged in clusters, and the surrounding GBM is often thickened. They may be observed in the kidneys in the absence of clinically evident renal disease, but they have not been found in extraglomerular basement membranes. Cross-banded fibrils of type III collagen have been seen in GBM of patients with glomerular disease who lack nail or skeletal abnormalities, sometimes as a familial condition with autosomal recessive inheritance (collagen type III glomerulopathy; see Chapter 27). It is uncertain whether there is a pathogenetic relationship between collagen type III glomerulopathy and NPS.

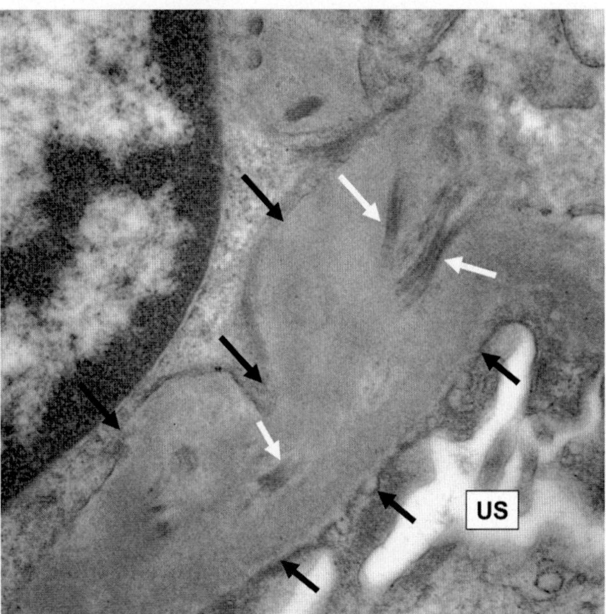

Figure 46.18 Electron micrograph of renal biopsy specimen in nail-patella syndrome stained with phosphotungstic acid. *Black arrows* show margins of irregular GBM. Staining with phosphotungstic acid reveals fibrillar collagen *(white arrows)*. US, urinary space.

Treatment

There is no specific therapy for the nephropathy of NPS. There has been no reported recurrence in transplanted kidneys. Because NPS is an autosomal dominant disorder, careful evaluation of potential living related kidney donors for features of the disease is essential.

REFERENCES

1. Guthrie LG. "Idiopathic," or congenital, hereditary and familial hematuria. *Lancet.* 1902;1:1243-1246.
2. Hurst AF. Hereditary familial congenital haemorrhagic nephritis occurring in sixteen individuals in three generations. *Guys Hosp Rec.* 1923; 3:368-370.
3. Alport AC. Hereditary familial congenital haemorrhagic nephritis. *BMJ.* 1927;1:504-506.
4. Spear GS, Slusser RJ. Alport's syndrome: Emphasizing electron microscopic studies of the glomerulus. *Am J Pathol.* 1972;69:213-222.
5. Hinglais N, Grunfeld J-P, Bois LE. Characteristic ultrastructural lesion of the glomerular basement membrane in progressive hereditary nephritis (Alport's syndrome). *Lab Invest.* 1972;27:473-487.
6. Churg J, Sherman RL. Pathologic characteristics of hereditary nephritis. *Arch Pathol.* 1973;95:374-379.
7. McCoy RC, Johnson HK, Stone WJ, Wilson CB. Absence of nephritogenic GBM antigen(s) in some patients with hereditary nephritis. *Kidney Int.* 1982;21:642-652.
8. Kashtan C, Fish AJ, Kleppel M, et al. Nephritogenic antigen determinants in epidermal and renal basement membranes of kindreds with Alport-type familial nephritis. *J Clin Invest.* 1986;78:1035-1044.
9. Atkin CL, Hasstedt SJ, Menlove L, et al. Mapping of Alport syndrome to the long arm of the X chromosome. *Am J Hum Genet.* 1988;42: 249-255.
10. Hostikka SL, Eddy RL, Byers MG, et al. Identification of a distinct type IV collagen α chain with restricted kidney distribution and assignment of its gene to the locus of X chromosome–linked Alport syndrome. *Proc Natl Acad Sci U S A.* 1990;87:1606-1610.

11. Barker DF, Hostikka SL, Zhou J, et al. Identification of mutations in the COL4A5 collagen gene in Alport syndrome. *Science*. 1990;248:1224-1227.
12. Lemmink HH, Schröder CH, Monnens LAH, Smeets HJM. The clinical spectrum of type IV collagen mutations. *Hum Mutat*. 1997;9:477-499.
13. Antignac C, Heidet L. Mutations in Alport syndrome associated with diffuse esophageal leiomyomatosis. *Contrib Nephrol*. 1996;117:172-182.
14. Jais JP, Knebelmann B, Giatras I, et al. X-linked Alport syndrome: Natural history in 195 families and genotype-phenotype correlations in males. *J Am Soc Nephrol*. 2000;11:649-657.
15. Boye E, Mollet G, Forestier L, et al. Determination of the genomic structure of the COL4A4 gene and of novel mutations causing autosomal recessive Alport syndrome. *Am J Hum Genet*. 1998;63:1329-1340.
16. Heidet L, Arrondel C, Forestier L, et al. Structure of the human type IV collagen gene COL4A3 and mutations in autosomal Alport syndrome. *J Am Soc Nephrol*. 2001;12:97-106.
17. van der Loop FTL, Heidet L, Timmer EDJ, et al. Autosomal dominant Alport syndrome caused by a COL4A3 splice site mutation. *Kidney Int*. 2000;58:1870-1875.
18. Ciccarese M, Casu D, Ki Wong F, et al. Identification of a new mutation in the α4(IV) collagen gene in a family with autosomal dominant Alport syndrome and hypercholesterolaemia. *Nephrol Dial Transplant*. 2001;16:2008-2012.
19. Pochet JM, Bobrie G, Landais P, et al. Renal prognosis in Alport's and related syndromes: Influence of the mode of inheritance. *Nephrol Dial Transplant*. 1989;4:1016-1021.
20. Kashtan CE, Kleppel MM, Gubler MC. Immunohistologic findings in Alport syndrome. *Contrib Nephrol*. 1996;117:142-153.
21. Jais JP, Knebelmann B, Giatras I, et al. X-linked Alport syndrome: Natural history and genotype-phenotype correlations in girls and women belonging to 195 families: A "European Community Alport Syndrome Concerted Action" study. *J Am Soc Nephrol*. 2003;14:2603-2610.
22. Grunfeld J-P, Noel LH, Hafez S, Droz D. Renal prognosis in women with hereditary nephritis. *Clin Nephrol*. 1985;23:267-271.
23. Colville D, Savige J, Morfis M, et al. Ocular manifestations of autosomal recessive Alport syndrome. *Ophthalmic Genet*. 1997;18:119-128.
24. Heath KE, Campos-Barros A, Toren A, et al. Nonmuscle myosin heavy chain IIA mutations define a spectrum of autosomal dominant macrothrombocytopenias: May-Hegglin anomaly and Fechtner, Sebastian, Epstein and Alport-like syndromes. *Am J Hum Genet*. 2001;69:1033-1045.
25. Merchant SN, Burgess BJ, Adams JC, et al. Temporal bone histopathology in Alport syndrome. *Laryngoscope*. 2004;114:1609-1618.
26. Kashtan CE, Kim Y. Distribution of the α1 and α2 chains of collagen IV and of collagens V and VI in Alport syndrome. *Kidney Int*. 1992;42:115-126.
27. Kalluri R, Shield CF, Todd P, et al. Isoform switching of type IV collagen is developmentally arrested in X-linked Alport syndrome leading to increased susceptibility of renal basement membranes to endoproteolysis. *J Clin Invest*. 1997;99:2470-2478.
28. Kashtan CE, Kim Y, Lees GE, et al. Abnormal glomerular basement membrane laminins in murine, canine, and human Alport syndrome: Aberrant laminin α2 deposition is species independent. *J Am Soc Nephrol*. 2001;12:252-260.
29. Rao VH, Lees GE, Kashtan CE, et al. Increased expression of MMP-2, MMP-9 (type IV collagenases/gelatinases), and MT1-MMP in canine X-linked Alport syndrome (XLAS). *Kidney Int*. 2003;63:1736-1748.
30. Kashtan CE. Animal models of Alport syndrome. *Nephrol Dial Transplant*. 2002;17:1359-1362.
31. Rheault MN, Kren SM, Thielen BK, et al. Mouse model of X-linked Alport syndrome. *J Am Soc Nephrol*. 2004;15:1466-1474.
32. Kashtan CE, Gubler MC, Sisson-Ross S, Mauer M. Chronology of renal scarring in males with Alport syndrome. *Pediatr Nephrol*. 1998;12:269-274.
33. Callis L, Vila A, Carrera M, Nieto J. Long-term effects of cyclosporine A in Alport's syndrome. *Kidney Int*. 1999;55:1051-1056.
34. Charbit M, Gubler MC, Dechaux M, et al. Cyclosporin therapy in patients with Alport syndrome. *Pediatr Nephrol*. 2007;22:57-63.
35. Gross O, Schulze-Lohoff E, Koepke ML, et al. Antifibrotic, nephroprotective potential of ACE inhibitor vs AT1 antagonist in a murine model of renal fibrosis. *Nephrol Dial Transplant*. 2004;19:1716-1723.
36. Gross O, Reinhardt J, Brinckmann S, et al. Interim report of the European Alport Registry and its implications for a prospective trial. American Society of Nephrology Annual Meeting; Philadelphia, Pa; November 7, 2008.
37. Sugimoto H, Mundel TM, Sund M, et al. Bone-marrow-derived stem cells repair basement membrane collagen defects and reverse genetic kidney disease. *Proc Natl Acad Sci U S A*. 2006;103:7321-7326.
38. Prodromidi EI, Poulsom R, Jeffery R, et al. Bone marrow–derived cells contribute to podocyte regeneration and amelioration of renal disease in a mouse model of Alport syndrome. *Stem Cells*. 2006;24:2448-2455.
39. Katayama K, Kawano M, Naito I, et al. Irradiation prolongs survival of Alport mice. *J Am Soc Nephrol*. 2008;19:1692-1700.
40. Lemmink HH, Nillesen WN, Mochizuki T, et al. Benign familial hematuria due to mutation of the type IV collagen α4 gene. *J Clin Invest*. 1996;98:1114-1118.
41. Savige J, Rana K, Tonna S, et al. Thin basement membrane nephropathy. *Kidney Int*. 2003;64:1169-1178.
42. Steffes MW, Barbosa J, Basgen JM, et al. Quantitative glomerular morphology of the normal human kidney. *Lab Invest*. 1983;49:82-86.
43. Anderson W. A case of "angio-keratoma." *Br J Dermatol*. 1898;10:113-117.
44. Fabry J. Ein Beitrag zur Kenntniss der Purpura haemorrhagica nodularis (Purpura papulosa haemorrhagica Hebrae). *Arch Dermatol Syph*. 1898;43:187-200.
45. Nakao S, Takenaka T, Maeda M, et al. An atypical variant of Fabry's disease in men with left ventricular hypertrophy. *N Engl J Med*. 1995;333:288-293.
46. Ichinose M, Nakayama M, Ohashi T, et al. Significance of screening for Fabry disease among male dialysis patients. *Clin Exp Nephrol*. 2005;9:228-232.
47. Rolfs A, Bottcher T, Zschiesche M, et al. Prevalence of Fabry disease in patients with cryptogenic stroke. *Lancet*. 2005;366:1794-1796.
48. Eng CM, Banikazemi M, Gordon RE, et al. A phase 1/2 clinical trial of enzyme replacement in Fabry disease: Pharmacokinetic, substrate clearance, and safety studies. *Am J Hum Genet*. 2001;68:711-722.
49. Schiffmann R, Kopp JB, Austin HA, et al. Enzyme replacement therapy in Fabry disease: A randomized controlled trial. *JAMA*. 2001;285:2743-2749.
50. Beck M, Ricci R, Widmer U, et al. Fabry disease: Overall effects of agalsidase alpha treatment. *Eur J Clin Invest*. 2004;34:838-844.
51. Kosch M, Koch HG, Oliveira JP, et al. Enzyme replacement therapy administered during hemodialysis in patients with Fabry disease. *Kidney Int*. 2004;66:1279-1282.
52. Desnick RJ, Brady R, Barranger J, et al. Fabry disease, an underrecognized multisystemic disorder: Expert recommendations for diagnosis, management, and enzyme replacement therapy. *Ann Intern Med*. 2003;138:338-346.
53. Desnick RJ, Brady RO. Fabry disease in childhood. *J Pediatr*. 2004;144:S20-S26.
54. Chen H, Lun Y, Ovchinnikov D, et al. Limb and kidney defects in Lmx1b mutant mice suggest an involvement of LMX1B in human nail patella syndrome. *Nat Genet*. 1998;19:51-55.
55. Dreyer SD, Zhou G, Baldini A, et al. Mutations in LMX1B cause abnormal skeletal patterning and renal dysplasia in nail patella syndrome. *Nat Genet*. 1998;19:47-50.
56. Dreyer SD, Morello R, German MS, et al. LMX1B transactivation and expression in nail-patella syndrome. *Hum Mol Genet*. 2000;9:1067-1074.
57. Heidet L, Bongers EM, Sich M, et al. In vivo expression of putative LMX1B targets in nail-patella syndrome kidneys. *Am J Pathol*. 2003;163:145-155.

CHAPTER 47

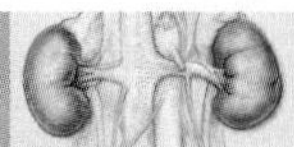

Inherited Disorders of Sodium and Water Handling

Peter Gross, Peter Heduschka

Glomerular filtration yields about 150 l of water, 21,000 mmol of Na^+, and 750 mmol of K^+ in a healthy individual in 24 hours, yet only minute fractions of these quantities are excreted eventually as urine. This remarkable volume reduction is accomplished by highly active tubular transport. Inherited defects of tubular transport proteins may thus lead to major fluid and electrolyte derangements. This chapter describes disorders arising in the thick ascending limb of Henle's loop and thereafter; proximal tubular disorders are described in Chapter 48 and disturbances of acidification in Chapter 12.

Genetic studies have unraveled the molecular basis of most of the inherited tubular disorders, establishing specific diagnoses more clearly and explaining the corresponding pathogenesis more reliably than was possible before. It is hoped that improved therapies will be developed in time. Diagnostic genetic testing is available for a number of the disorders discussed in this chapter (see *www.genetests.org*).

PHYSIOLOGY OF SODIUM AND WATER REABSORPTION

Sodium Reabsorption

In all tubular epithelial cells, a basolateral energy requiring Na^+,K^+-ATPase will ensure that intracellular Na^+ is kept at low levels while K^+ is high. The resulting concentration gradients of Na^+ across the apical cell membrane drive passive Na^+ reabsorption from the tubular lumen to the cell interior. Apical Na^+ channels and transport proteins serve to regulate the Na^+ reabsorption, and the proteins involved differ from one tubular segment to the next.

In the proximal tubule, an apical Na^+-H^+ exchange protein (NHE3) facilitates most of the Na^+ reabsorbed. It is inhibitable by acetazolamide. The thick ascending limb has an apical Na^+-K^+-$2Cl^-$ cotransporter (NKCC2; Fig. 47.1) that can be blocked by furosemide and bumetanide. For efficient Na^+ reabsorption by NKCC2, it is required that K^+ be returned through a K^+ channel called ROMK from the cell to the low K^+ tubular fluid (see Fig. 47.1). It is also important that sodium transport by this segment is dependent on a basolateral Cl^- channel (ClC-Kb) and an accessory protein of ClC-Kb called barttin (see Fig. 47.1).

The distal convoluted tubule reabsorbs Na^+ by a unique apical Na^+-Cl^- cotransporter (NCCT). The protein is specifically inhibited by thiazides (Fig. 47.2). A basolateral ClC-Kb chloride channel is also necessary for efficient sodium reabsorption.

In the collecting duct, an apical Na^+ channel called ENaC regulates Na^+ reabsorption. Amiloride and triamterene specifically block ENaC, whereas the mineralocorticoid aldosterone upregulates ENaC (Fig. 47.3). An overview of tubular proteins of Na^+ reabsorption and their corresponding inheritable disorders is provided in Figure 47.4.

Water Reabsorption

In most nephron segments, water follows NaCl passively through aquaporins, constitutively open water transport proteins in apical and basolateral tubular cell membranes. However, the collecting duct is different. It is equipped with apical aquaporin 2, which is the sole water channel in the kidney that can be regulated on a short-term basis by vasopressin. In this way, the collecting duct provides for eventual fine-tuning of water reabsorption or excretion (Fig. 47.5).

DISORDERS OF SODIUM HANDLING

An overview of inherited disorders of Na^+ transport is shown in Figure 47.6. On clinical grounds, it is possible to broadly distinguish four different phenotypes:

1. Hypokalemia and normal blood pressure (Bartter syndrome, Gitelman's syndrome).
2. Hypokalemia and high blood pressure (Liddle syndrome, apparent mineralocorticoid excess, glucocorticoid-remediable hyperaldosteronism, adrenal 17α-hydroxylase deficiency, adrenal 11β-hydroxylase deficiency).
3. Hyperkalemia and normal blood pressure (pseudohypoaldosteronism, adrenal 21-hydroxylase deficiency, adrenal aldosterone synthase deficiency).
4. Hyperkalemia and high blood pressure (Gordon's syndrome).

Some of the disorders are caused by mutated renal transport proteins (e.g., Gitelman's syndrome). In others, the genetic defect resides in the adrenals, and the changes of adrenal mineralocorticoids and glucocorticoids bring about the renal phenotype.

CONDITIONS WITH HYPOKALEMIA, METABOLIC ALKALOSIS, AND NORMAL BLOOD PRESSURE

Bartter Syndrome

Bartter syndrome is rare and is manifested in childhood or in the perinatal period with severe hypokalemia, metabolic alkalosis, and low-normal blood pressure, all of which are caused by tubular wasting of Na^+ and Cl^-.[1] In contrast, Gitelman's syndrome is mostly a disorder of adults, and hypomagnesemia is a defining feature.[2]

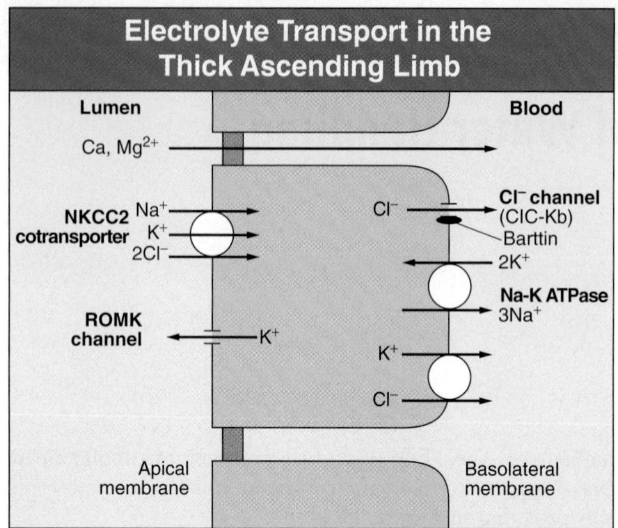

Figure 47.1 Electrolyte transport in the thick ascending limb of the loop of Henle. The furosemide-sensitive Na^+-K^+-$2Cl^-$ (NKCC2) cotransporter is driven by low intracellular Na^+ and Cl^- concentrations produced by the Na^+,K^+-ATPase pump, the K^+-Cl^- cotransporter, and the basolateral Cl^- channel (ClC-Kb). The β subunit (barttin) is crucial for normal functioning of the ClC-Kb channels. Apical K^+ recycling through the low-conductance, ATP-sensitive renal medullary K^+ (ROMK) channel ensures the efficient functioning of the NKCC2 cotransporter.

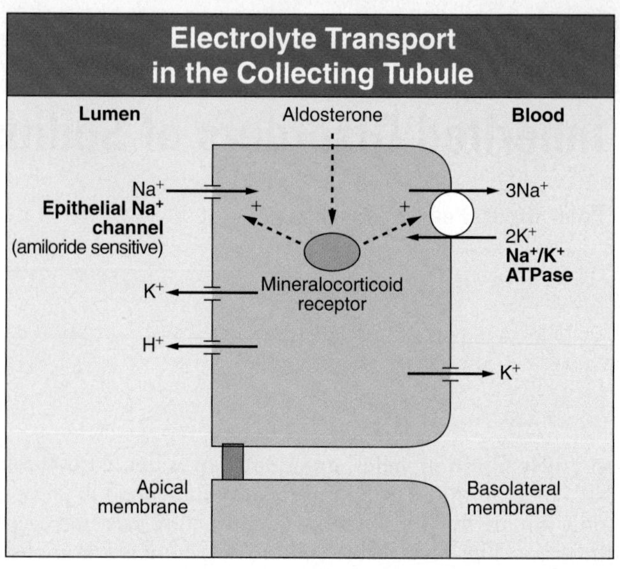

Figure 47.3 Electrolyte transport in the principal cell of the collecting tubule. Reabsorption of Na^+ occurs through the amiloride-sensitive epithelial Na^+ channel (ENaC). Its uptake is coupled to K^+ and H^+ secretion. Aldosterone increases the activity of ENaC and Na^+,K^+-ATPase, which increases Na^+ reabsorption and K^+ and H^+ secretion, resulting in hypokalemic alkalosis. Cortisol is also a ligand for the mineralocorticoid receptor but is normally removed by oxidation by 11β-hydroxysteroid dehydrogenase to cortisone.

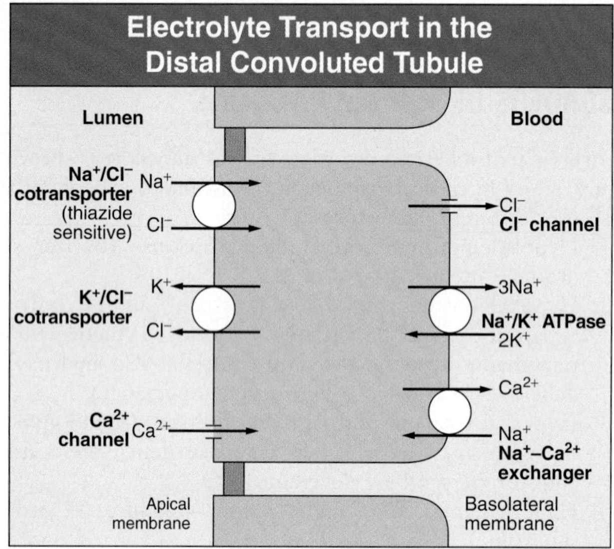

Figure 47.2 Electrolyte transport in the distal convoluted tubule. Reabsorption of Na^+ and Cl^- occurs across the apical membrane by the thiazide-sensitive Na^+-Cl^- cotransporter (NCCT), and these ions leave the cell through the Cl^- channels and through the Na^+,K^+-ATPase pump. Calcium ions enter the cell through the Ca^{2+} channels and exit through the Na^+-Ca^{2+} exchanger.

Pathogenesis

Bartter syndrome is due to dysfunction of the thick ascending limb and is caused by inactivating mutations of each of its major transport proteins (NKCC2, Bartter syndrome type 1; ROMK, type 2; ClC-Kb, type 3; barttin, type 4) (Fig. 47.7; see also Fig. 47.1).[3-6] The pathogenic consequences of these mutations are broadly similar in all four varieties except that the more severe phenotypes (types 1, 2, and 4) are manifested earlier in life.

Loss of function of any one of the four transport proteins will impair NaCl reabsorption by the thick ascending limb, increasing the delivery of salt to the distal nephron. NaCl reabsorption is stimulated in those segments but compensates only partially for the salt wasting; it is associated with distal secretion of K^+ and H^+. The net loss of NaCl from the nephron will cause plasma volume contraction, low-normal blood pressure, and secondary hyperaldosteronism. The loss of K^+ and H^+ will be followed by severe hypokalemia and metabolic alkalosis. Hypokalemia and increased angiotensin II also stimulate prostaglandin E_2 production.

Reduced Cl^- absorption in the loop of Henle inhibits voltage-driven paracellular absorption of Ca^{2+}, causing hypercalciuria, an important feature of Bartter syndrome that may be associated with nephrocalcinosis.

Inactivating mutations of barttin also cause deafness because barttin-dependent chloride transport is crucial to endolymph production in the inner ear.[6] In some individuals with mutation of ClC-Kb (type 3), there is a mixed Bartter and Gitelman's syndrome.[7] In these patients, the features of Bartter syndrome are associated with hypomagnesemia and hypocalciuria. Age at presentation is 1 month to 29 years. This mixed syndrome may be explained by the overlapping distribution of ClC-Kb, which is also expressed in the distal tubule, the site affected in Gitelman's syndrome.[7] Finally, gain-of-function mutations in the extracellular calcium ion–sensing receptor also cause a Bartter-like syndrome.[8] The receptor is normally expressed in the thick ascending limb, and its activation inhibits salt reabsorption similar to furosemide; in addition, this syndrome is associated with hypocalcemia.[8]

Clinical Manifestations

Bartter syndrome from mutations in NKCC2, ROMK, or barttin has a more severe phenotype than that caused by mutations of ClC-Kb. The more severe phenotype typically presents in the perinatal period and is called antenatal Bartter syndrome. The milder variety is called classic Bartter syndrome.

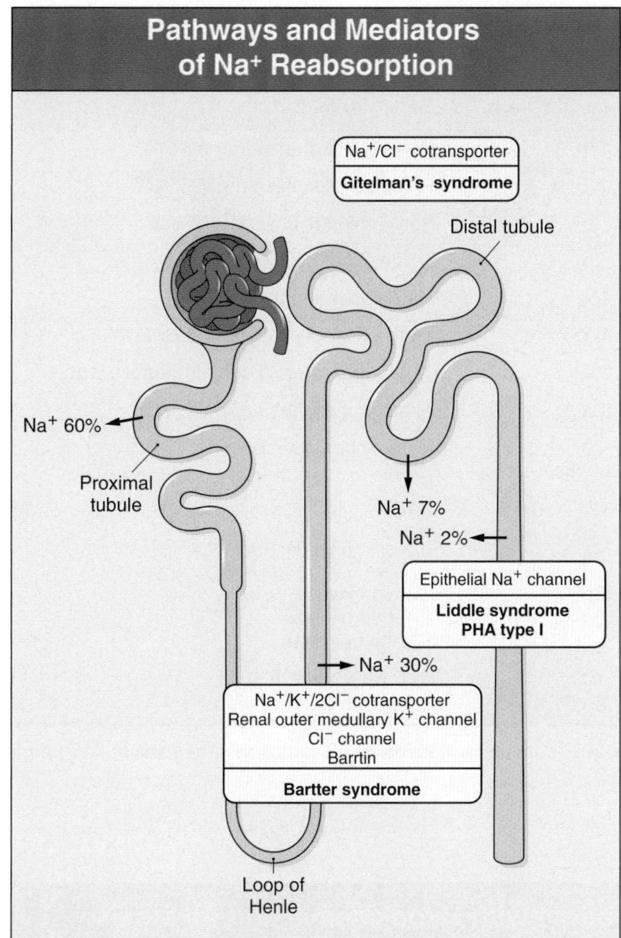

Figure 47.4 Pathways and mediators involved in Na⁺ reabsorption. Almost 60% of the filtered Na⁺ is reabsorbed in the proximal tubule. The distal portions of the nephron reabsorb the remainder. The chief mediators involved in Na⁺ reabsorption and disorders resulting from their mutations are shown in boxes. PHA, pseudohypoaldosteronism.

The clinical features of antenatal Bartter syndrome include hypokalemia and metabolic alkalosis in a newborn with vomiting and failure to thrive. There may also be a history of polyhydramnios and premature delivery. Polyuria, hypercalciuria, and high urinary chloride concentrations are characteristic. Nephrocalcinosis may be manifested later in life. A prenatal diagnosis of Bartter syndrome may be made by demonstration of high Cl^- concentrations in amniotic fluid.

Patients with classic Bartter syndrome develop normally during the first 2 to 5 years of life. Thereafter, vomiting, polyuria, recurrent episodes of dehydration, and fever may become apparent. Carpopedal spasms and fatigue are common. Many children show developmental delay. The blood pressure is low normal. The laboratory features are comparable to those described previously, but nephrocalcinosis is usually absent.

Diagnosis

A newborn or a young child with vomiting, dehydration, low-normal blood pressure, severe hypokalemia, and metabolic alkalosis is likely to have Bartter syndrome if there is high urinary Cl^- and K^+. The suspected diagnosis will receive further support if supplements of K^+ and Cl^- are inefficient in correcting the severe hypokalemia and the blood pressure. Diuretics will not be found in the urine. Hypomagnesemia and hypocalciuria are

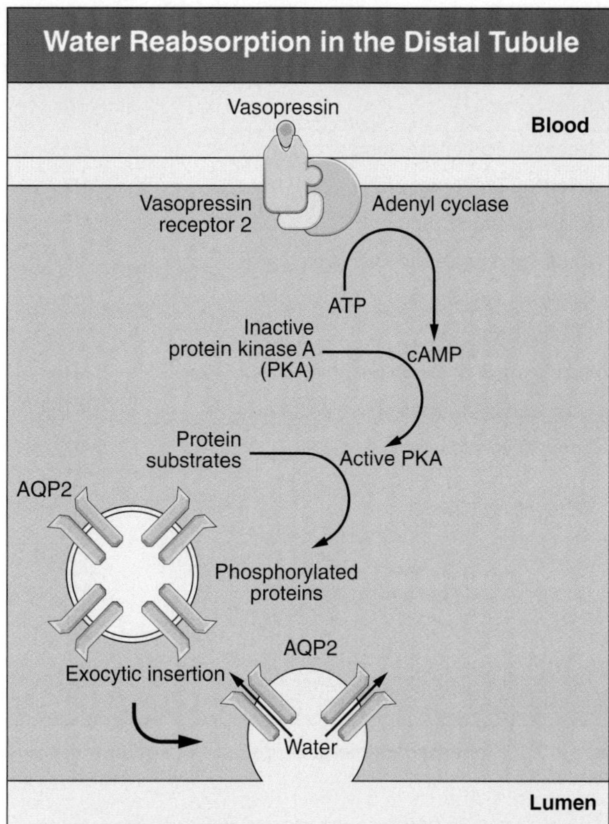

Figure 47.5 Water reabsorption in the distal tubule. The aquaporin AQP2, which is exclusively present in the principal cells of the collecting tubules and ducts, is the chief vasopressin-regulated water channel. Activation of cAMP-dependent protein kinase A mediates protein phosphorylation that triggers exocytic insertion of AQP2 channels into the apical membrane. These channels increase the water permeability of the apical membrane, facilitating water transport.

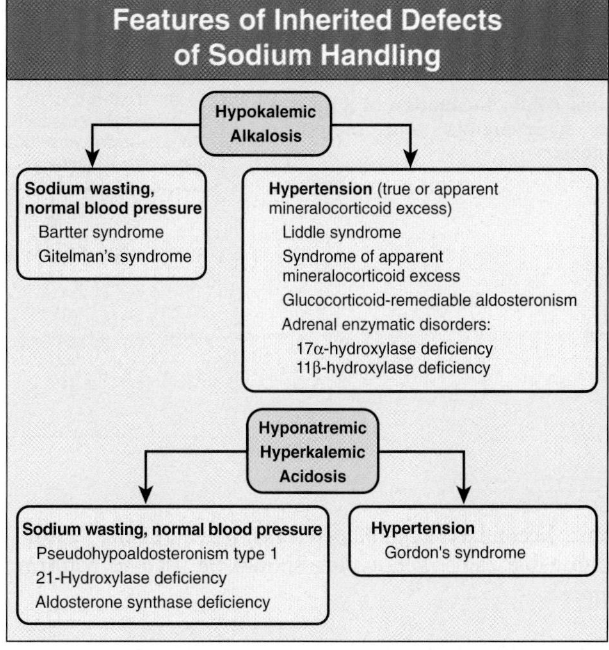

Figure 47.6 Features of inherited defects of sodium handling.

Inherited Single Gene Defects of Sodium and Water Handling

Syndrome	Inheritance	Gene Localization	Gene Product
Neonatal Bartter syndrome	AR	15q	Na-K-2C1 cotransporter *NKCC2*
Neonatal Bartter syndrome	AR	11q	Renal potassium channel *ROMK*
Classic Bartter syndrome	AR	Ip	Renal chloride channel *CIC-Kb*
Bartter syndrome with deafness	AR	Ip	β-Subunit of CIC-Kb *Barttin*
Gitelman's syndrome	AR	16q	NaCl cotransporter *NCCT*
Liddle syndrome	AD	16p	Epithelial sodium channel *ENaC*
Syndrome of apparent mineralocorticoid excess	AR	16q	11β-hydroxysteroid dehydrogenase type II
Glucocorticoid-remediable aldosteronism	AD	8q	Aldosterone synthase *CYP11B2*
Pseudohypoaldosteronism type I	AD AR	4p 12p, 16p	Mineralocorticoid receptor *ENaC*
Gordon's syndrome	AD	12p 17q 1q	WNK1 WNK4 Not identified
Congenital adrenal hyperplasia	AR AR AR	6p 8q 10q	21 hydroxylase 11β-hydroxylase 17α-hydroxylase
Nephrogenic diabetes insipidus	X-linked AR	Xq 12q	AVP receptor 2 Aquaporin 2

Figure 47.7 Inherited single-gene defects of sodium and water handling. AD, autosomal dominant; AR, autosomal recessive; AVP, arginine vasopressin.

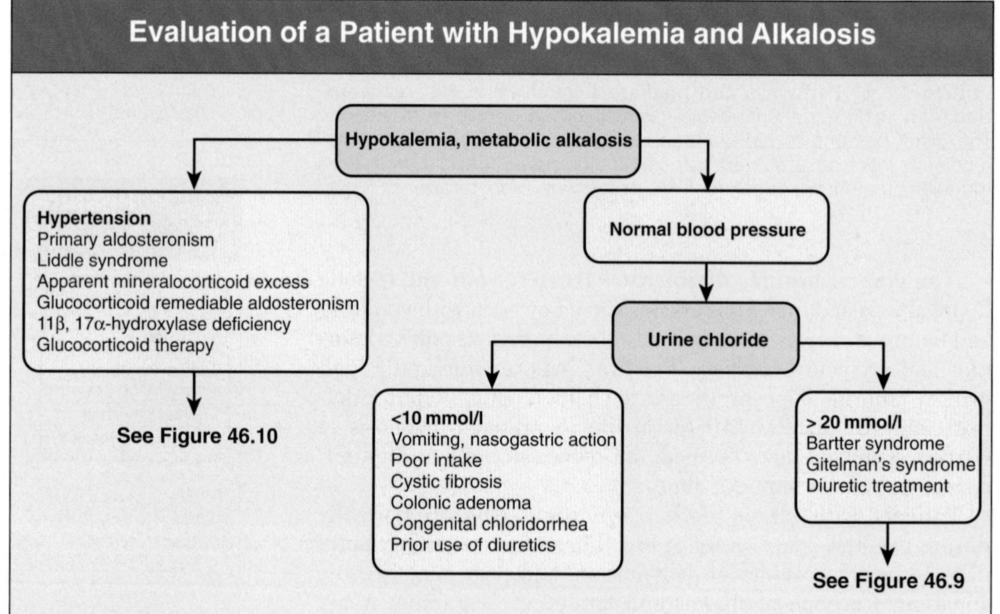

Figure 47.8 Evaluation of a patient with hypokalemia and metabolic alkalosis.

absent. Secondary hyperaldosteronism is a regular feature. In questionable cases, genotyping should be used to confirm the diagnosis.

Differential Diagnosis

In syndromes of chronic severe hypokalemia with metabolic alkalosis, the differential diagnosis may be facilitated greatly by taking into consideration the associated blood pressure and the urinary chloride concentration (Fig. 47.8).

If there is hypertension, this points to disorders related to hyperaldosteronism. If, however, the syndrome is associated with a normal or low-normal blood pressure, extrarenal or renal Cl^- and Na^+ losses are the culprits. Extrarenal loss of sodium occurs in diarrhea, vomiting, or burns. It is characterized by very low Cl^- concentrations in the urine, often as low as 1 mmol/l. By contrast, renal loss of salt with high urinary Cl^- and Na^+ is typical of Bartter syndrome, Gitelman's syndrome, and diuretic use. The absence of hypomagnesemia and hypocalciuria will then

Features Differentiating Bartter and Gitelman's Syndromes

Features	Neonatal Bartter Syndrome	Classic Bartter Syndrome	Gitelman's Syndrome
Age at onset	Neonatal period	Infancy/childhood	Childhood/later
Maternal hydramnios	Common	Rare	Absent
Polyuria, polydipsia	Marked	Present	Rare
Dehydration	Present	Often present	Absent
Tetany	Absent	Rare	Present
Growth retardation	Present	Present	Absent
Urinary calcium	Very high	Normal or high	Low
Nephrocalcinosis	Present	Rare	Absent
Serum magnesium	Normal	Occasionally low	Low
Urine prostaglandins (PGE_2)	Very high	High or normal	Normal
Response to indomethacin (improvement of hypokalemia and renal salt wasting)	Good	Good	Rare

Figure 47.9 Features differentiating Bartter and Gitelman's syndromes. In addition to these clinical and laboratory features, molecular diagnosis is now possible (see text). PGE_2, prostaglandin E_2.

argue against Gitelman's syndrome (Fig. 47.9). Genotyping is recommended to diagnose overlap of Bartter and Gitelman's syndromes.

Treatment

Patients with the neonatal form of Bartter syndrome have marked fluid and electrolyte disturbances that need to be corrected carefully. Saline infusion may be required in the neonatal period. Potassium chloride supplementation is always necessary.[9] Addition of spironolactone or triamterene may be useful in correcting hypokalemia, but the effect of these drugs is usually transient. Angiotensin-converting enzyme (ACE) inhibitors have been used for correction of hypokalemia, with conflicting results. Magnesium deficiency may aggravate renal K^+ wasting and, if present, should be corrected.

The efficacy of long-term treatment with prostaglandin synthase inhibitors, such as indomethacin (1 to 3 mg/kg per 24 hours) or ibuprofen, is well established.[9] They act by reducing cortical perfusion and decreasing delivery of Na^+ and Cl^- to the distal nephron, ameliorating many of the features of the disease. The amplifying effect of prostaglandins on the renal tubules is also neutralized. Treatment results in reduction of polyuria and polydipsia, restitution of normal growth and activity, and correction of hypokalemia; serum K^+, however, rarely exceeds 3.5 mmol/l. Plasma levels of renin and aldosterone reduce to the normal range.

Outcome

If not treated, patients may succumb to episodes of dehydration, electrolyte disturbance, or intercurrent infection. With appropriate therapy, most children improve clinically and show catch-up growth; pubertal and mental developments are usually normal. Lifelong therapy is needed. Chronic tubulointerstitial nephropathy due to persistent hypokalemia, hypercalciuria, and nephrocalcinosis may lead to progressive decline in renal function. There are anecdotal reports of renal transplantation in patients with end-stage renal disease. The biochemical parameters return to normal after transplantation.

Gitelman's Syndrome

Gitelman's syndrome is an autosomal recessive condition also characterized by hypokalemic metabolic alkalosis but with hypocalciuria and hypomagnesemia.

Pathogenesis

The similarity between the features of Gitelman's syndrome and those caused by thiazide administration originally suggested that the defect might be in the distal convoluted tubule. The condition has now been linked to inactivating mutations in the gene for NCCT (see Figs. 47.2 and 47.4).[10] Loss of NCCT function results in Na^+ and Cl^- wasting from this segment, leading to hypovolemia with secondary activation of the renin-aldosterone system. The resulting increase in collecting tubule Na^+ reabsorption is, however, counterbalanced by K^+ and H^+ excretion, causing hypokalemic alkalosis. The distal convoluted tubule normally reabsorbs only 7% to 8% of the filtered Na^+ and Cl^- load. The degree of volume contraction, the stimulation of the renin-angiotensin system, and the amount of K^+ loss are therefore not substantial enough to stimulate prostaglandin E_2 production.

The hypocalciuria is due to the associated plasma volume contraction. The renal magnesium wasting is caused by down-regulation of the epithelial Mg^{2+} channel TRPM6 in distal convoluted tubules.

Clinical Manifestations and Diagnosis

Most adults believed to have Bartter syndrome will be found to suffer from Gitelman's syndrome, and this diagnosis is not very rare. The severity of symptoms varies widely. More severely affected patients complain of generalized and muscle weakness, inability to work for extended periods, salt craving, and a preference for licorice. Cardiac disturbances, muscle cramps, and tetany are only exceptionally present. Chondrocalcinosis of the knees does occur later in life; it is a consequence of hypomagnesemia. Laboratory evaluation will show moderate hypomagnesemia, severe hypokalemia, hypocalciuria, high urinary chloride concentration, and absence of thiazides from the urine. The

Features of Liddle Syndrome, Apparent Mineralocorticoid Excess, and Glucocorticoid-Remediable Aldosteronism

Features	Liddle Syndrome	AME	GRA
Inheritance	Autosomal dominant	Autosomal recessive	Autosomal dominant
Chief features	Significant hypertension, polyuria, growth retardation	Low birth weight, early-onset hypertension, polyuria, growth retardation	Significant hypertension, hemorrhagic stroke
Plasma aldosterone	Reduced	Reduced	Elevated
Plasma renin activity	Reduced	Reduced	Reduced
Urinary mineralocorticoid metabolites	Normal	Elevated ratios of THF + alloTHF to THE; free cortisol to cortisone	Elevated cortisol C-18 oxidation products
Response of the hypertension to			
Glucocorticoids	No	Satisfactory	Satisfactory
Triamterene	Satisfactory	Satisfactory	Satisfactory
Spironolactone	No	Satisfactory	Satisfactory

Figure 47.10 Features of Liddle syndrome, apparent mineralocorticoid excess (AME), and glucocorticoid-remediable aldosteronism (GRA). These syndromes are all characterized by hypokalemia, metabolic alkalosis, and hypertension. THE, tetrahydrocortisone; THF, tetrahydrocortisol.

blood pressure will be in the low-normal range. These findings establish the diagnosis. Genotyping should be performed in questionable or incomplete syndromes.

Treatment

There is no consensus on the best mode of treatment. Magnesium aspartate (5 to 15 mmol Mg^{2+}/day), magnesium oxide, and potassium supplements are usually given to improve muscle weakness or cramps. However, dosing may be limited by diarrhea and abdominal discomfort. In exceptional cases, parenteral Mg^{2+} has been infused. Indomethacin, cyclooxygenase 2 inhibitors, and spironolactone are usually not helpful. The long-term prognosis for cardiac and renal function as well as for general health is good.

CONDITIONS WITH HYPOKALEMIA, METABOLIC ALKALOSIS, AND HYPERTENSION

Conditions with hypokalemia, metabolic alkalosis, and hypertension all have true or apparent mineralocorticoid excess.

Liddle Syndrome (Pseudohyperaldosteronism)

Liddle syndrome is an autosomal dominant syndrome of hypertension and variable degrees of hypokalemic metabolic alkalosis. The patients resemble those with primary hyperaldosteronism, but levels of mineralocorticoid hormones are not increased. Renin and aldosterone are suppressed, and there is no response to spironolactone.[11] However, triamterene and amiloride, aldosterone-independent inhibitors of distal Na^+ transport, correct hypertension, renal K^+ loss, and hypokalemia.[12]

Pathogenesis

Liddle syndrome is related to mutations of the β or γ subunit of the collecting duct sodium channel ENaC.[13] The mutations result in truncations of the cytoplasmic C-terminal tail of the affected subunits. Collecting duct sodium reabsorption is dependent on the channel density present in the apical cell membrane. Channel density is regulated by removal of ENaC from the cell membrane, ubiquitination, and degradation. In Liddle syndrome, the mutated ENaC protein cannot be recognized by NEDD4, a ubiquitin ligase protein; hence, the channels remain in the cell membrane for prolonged periods.[12] This action results in enhanced sodium reabsorption, hypertension, and hypokalemic alkalosis (see Fig. 47.3).

Clinical Manifestations and Diagnosis

Liddle syndrome is a rare disorder of hypertension in teenage children[12] that is associated with hypokalemic metabolic alkalosis and low blood levels of renin and aldosterone. The original patient developed renal failure from an unknown cause and eventually underwent transplantation.[14] Thereafter, her blood pressure normalized, and renin and aldosterone responded normally to provocative measures.

This condition should be differentiated from primary hyperaldosteronism, apparent mineralocorticoid excess, and glucocorticoid-remediable aldosteronism (Fig. 47.10) as well as 11β-hydroxylase (steroid 11β-monooxygenase) or 17α-hydroxylase (steroid 17α-monooxygenase) deficiency. Activating mutations of the mineralocorticoid receptor have been reported and should also be differentiated.[15]

Treatment

Therapy consists of sodium restriction and K^+ supplements. Triamterene directly inhibits apical Na^+ channels, resulting in increased urinary Na^+ and decreased K^+ excretion and resolution of hypertension. Amiloride also normalizes the blood pressure and K^+ levels. However, most patients continue to have growth retardation. Because the pathogenetic disorder is not correctable with age, lifelong therapy is required.

Apparent Mineralocorticoid Excess

Pathogenesis

Apparent mineralocorticoid excess (AME) is an autosomal recessive condition resulting from deficiency of the type II (renal and placental) isoform of the enzyme 11β-hydroxysteroid dehydrogenase. Clinical features of this condition closely mimic those of Liddle syndrome.[16]

In normal conditions, aldosterone is the chief mineralocorticoid regulating electrolyte and water balance, through its effects on distal renal tubules and cortical collecting ducts. After binding to the mineralocorticoid receptor, aldosterone increases synthesis of various proteins, chiefly Na^+,K^+-ATPase on the basolateral surface and ENaC on the apical surface. These proteins increase Na^+ reabsorption and K^+ secretion in the distal tubules (see Fig. 47.3). Cortisol is also a ligand for the mineralocorticoid receptor and shows potent sodium-retaining activity. Cortisol is, however, normally metabolized by 11β-hydroxysteroid dehydrogenase to cortisone, which lacks such an action.

Loss-of-function mutations in the gene encoding 11β-hydroxysteroid dehydrogenase have been detected in patients with the inherited form of AME.[17,18] As a consequence, in the kidney, intracellular metabolic clearance of cortisol is severely impaired. The accumulation of cortisol causes nonspecific stimulation of the mineralocorticoid receptor. This will be followed by increased sodium reabsorption together with K^+ and H^+ secretion.

The 11β-hydroxysteroid dehydrogenase is also expressed in the placenta. Reduced placental 11β-hydroxysteroid dehydrogenase activity might be related to the low birth weight that is characteristic of AME patients.

Carbenoxolone and glycyrrhizic acid (found in licorice compounds) are potent inhibitors of this enzyme. Consumption of these agents may be associated with features similar to AME.

Clinical Manifestations and Diagnosis

AME is characterized by an onset of hypertension in childhood, hypokalemia, metabolic alkalosis, very low plasma levels of renin and aldosterone, and increased metabolites of cortisol in the urine. There may be a history of low birth weight and subsequent failure to thrive.

The diagnosis of AME is made by finding, on gas chromatography or mass spectroscopy, elevated urinary levels of hydrogenated metabolites of cortisol (tetrahydrocortisol plus allotetrahydrocortisol) compared with cortisone (tetrahydrocortisone). The ratio of urinary free cortisol to cortisone is also increased.[19] Heterozygotes may occasionally show hypertension, normal serum K^+, suppressed plasma renin and aldosterone, and moderately elevated urinary cortisol to cortisone metabolite ratio. A variant of AME, called AME type 2, has similar clinical features but a milder urinary steroid profile.[20]

Treatment

Treatment with oral dexamethasone (0.75 to 5 mg/day) suppresses cortisol secretion, resulting in reduced Na^+ reabsorption and amelioration of hypertension and hypokalemia. Urinary concentrations of metabolites of cortisol and cortisone are only moderately affected. As in Liddle syndrome, patients respond to treatment with K^+ supplements combined with triamterene or amiloride. Spironolactone is effective in AME although not in Liddle syndrome. Renal transplantation is followed by normalization of cortisol metabolism, biochemical abnormalities, and hypertension.[21]

Glucocorticoid-Remediable Aldosteronism

Glucocorticoid-remediable aldosteronism (GRA) appears to be the most common monogenic form of human hypertension. It is an autosomal dominant condition. Patients present with typical features of primary hyperaldosteronism: hypertension, suppressed plasma renin activity, and hypokalemia. Unlike primary hyperaldosteronism (due to aldosterone-producing adrenal adenoma), hypersecretion of aldosterone in GRA can be reversed by the administration of corticosteroids. Affected individuals have early-onset hypertension. There is a high prevalence of hemorrhagic stroke, largely as a result of ruptured intracranial aneurysms. Hypokalemia is typically mild but becomes more pronounced if diuretics are given. Potassium levels may occasionally be normal.

Pathogenesis

Patients with GRA have adrenocorticotropic hormone (ACTH)–sensitive aldosterone production occurring in the zona fasciculata of the adrenal gland, which is usually responsible only for cortisol synthesis. Normal subjects synthesize aldosterone in the zona glomerulosa. Two isoenzymes of 11β-hydroxylase are involved in the biosynthesis of aldosterone and cortisol: steroid 11β-hydroxylase (CYP11B1) and aldosterone synthase (CYP11B2), respectively (Fig. 47.11). The genes for these isoenzymes are located close to each other on the long arm of chromosome 8. Unequal meiotic crossovers may produce hybrid genes by fusion of the promoter end of *CYP11B1* with the coding sequence of *CYP11B2*, so that *CYP11B2* encoding aldosterone synthase is inappropriately regulated by ACTH, as is *CYP11B1*.[16] Abnormal expression of this chimeric gene in the adrenal zona fasciculata has been shown by *in situ* hybridization.

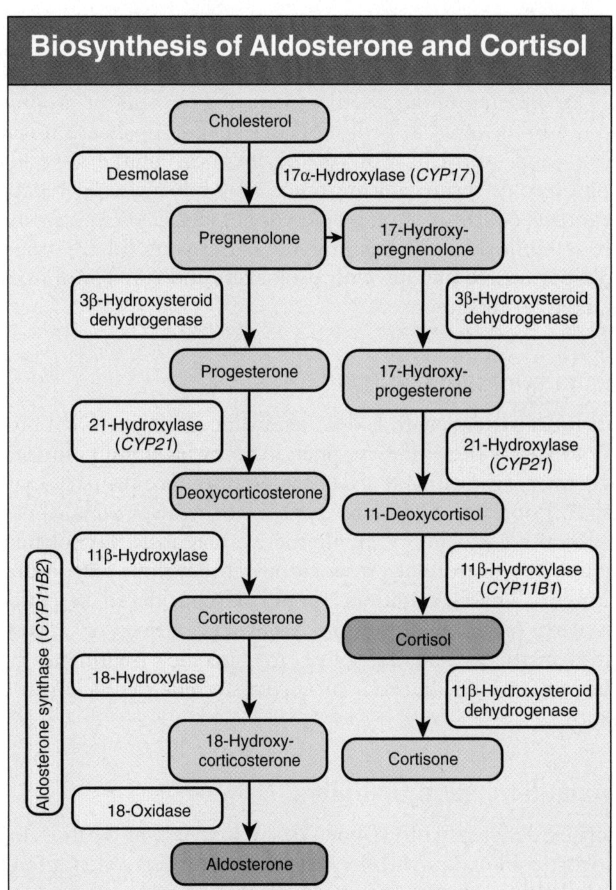

Figure 47.11 Biosynthesis of aldosterone and cortisol. Although cortisol and aldosterone both require 11β-hydroxylation of precursors, these steps are catalyzed by different isoenzymes: steroid 11β-hydroxylase (CYP11B1) and aldosterone synthase (CYP11B2), respectively. Aldosterone synthase also mediates two further conversions. Common enzyme deficiencies leading to derangement in sodium and water balance are shown in boxes. Cortisol is converted peripherally by 11β-hydroxysteroid dehydrogenase to cortisone.

Diagnosis

Patients are often misdiagnosed as having primary hypertension. Hypertensive subjects with early-onset hypertension, early cerebral hemorrhage (<40 years), hypokalemia after treatment with diuretics, and refractoriness to standard antihypertensive medication are candidates for GRA testing. Similar to other genetic forms of hypertension (Liddle syndrome, AME, Gordon's syndrome), plasma renin activity is low. Although the mean aldosterone levels are high, determination of serum aldosterone has poor sensitivity as a screening test. In GRA, the aldosterone to renin ratio is elevated (>300), whereas in primary hypertension, AME, and Liddle syndrome, it is not.

The biochemical hallmark of GRA is overproduction and excretion of cortisol C-18 oxidation products, reflecting the action of aldosterone synthase on cortisol in the zona fasciculata. Large amounts of the so-called hybrid steroids (18-hydroxycortisol and 18-oxocortisol) can be found in the urine by specialized steroid laboratories.

Dexamethasone leads to suppression of blood aldosterone levels. When 0.5 mg of dexamethasone is given every 6 hours for 2 days, it suppresses aldosterone to undetectable levels (<4 ng/dl).

Direct screening for the hybrid gene *CYP11B1/CYP11B2* can also be performed and confirms the diagnosis (test can be obtained by *www.brighamandwomens.org/gra/introduction.aspx*).[22]

Treatment

Treatment with low-dose corticosteroid is effective. Typically, 0.125 to 0.25 mg of dexamethasone or 2.5 to 5 mg of prednisolone is administered at bedtime. Therapeutic goals are normotension and normalization of biochemical markers (urinary 18-oxosteroid, serum aldosterone). Mineralocorticoid receptor antagonists (spironolactone, eplerenone) and ENaC antagonists such as amiloride and triamterene are also useful treatments. Antihypertensive therapy with β-blockers and ACE inhibitors is less likely to be effective.

Incomplete Phenotypes

Occasional patients with Liddle syndrome, AME, or GRA either do not express the complete phenotype or have mild clinical or biochemical features and are considered to have primary hypertension. Poor blood pressure control with conventional therapy should raise suspicion of an alternative diagnosis. Hypokalemia may not be a feature at presentation but develops with diuretic treatment. These conditions should be considered in patients with early-onset hypertension, failure to thrive, or a strong family history. The response to specific treatment with potassium-sparing diuretics or corticosteroids may suggest the diagnosis.

Adrenal Enzymatic Disorders

Inherited deficiency of 11β- or 17α-hydroxylase also causes mineralocorticoid excess with hypertension and hypokalemic metabolic alkalosis (see Fig. 47.11).

Deficiency of 17α-hydroxylase (CYP17) impairs normal production of cortisol and adrenal androgens, resulting in pseudohermaphroditism in genetic males and primary amenorrhea in females. Cortisol deficiency results in increased ACTH secretion, low levels of renin and aldosterone, hypokalemia, metabolic alkalosis, and hypertension. Diagnosis is confirmed by finding excessive levels of deoxycorticosterone and corticosterone in the urine. Administration of corticosteroids corrects the mineralocorticoid excess state.

Deficiency of 11β-hydroxylase (CYP11B1) also impairs cortisol production but results in excessive androgens. Genetic females show pseudohermaphroditism, whereas males have virilization. The cortisol deficiency results in high blood levels of ACTH, deoxycortisol, and deoxycorticosterone; corticosterone levels are normal. Hypokalemia is variable. Diagnosis is confirmed by measurement of high levels of tetrahydro-11-deoxycortisol in the urine. Hypokalemia is variable. Treatment with corticosteroids corrects hypertension and hypokalemia; renin levels increase, but aldosterone remains low because of the biosynthetic defect.

CONDITIONS WITH HYPONATREMIA, HYPERKALEMIA, METABOLIC ACIDOSIS, AND NORMAL BLOOD PRESSURE

Conditions with hyponatremia, hyperkalemia, metabolic acidosis, and normal blood pressure have features of mineralocorticoid deficiency either because of a synthetic defect or because of end-organ resistance.

Pseudohypoaldosteronism

Pseudohypoaldosteronism (PHA) is a state of renal tubular (and other tissue) unresponsiveness to the action of aldosterone.[23] Symptoms start in early infancy with marked salt wasting and failure to thrive. PHA type 1 includes at least two major entities, with either renal or multiple target organ defects; the former is more common.

The inheritance of renal PHA type 1 is autosomal dominant but may be sporadic. Loss-of-function mutations of the gene for the mineralocorticoid receptor (located on 4p) have been identified.[24]

Multiple end-organ PHA type 1 is a severe autosomal recessive disorder with multiple target organ resistance to the action of mineralocorticoids and is associated with inactivating mutations of α, β, or γ subunits of ENaC.[25] Differences between the two major types are shown in Figure 47.12.

Aldosterone Biosynthetic Defects

Patients with defects in aldosterone biosynthesis show salt wasting with hyponatremia, hyperkalemia, hypovolemia, and elevated plasma renin activity.[26]

The enzymes cholesterol desmolase, 3β-hydroxysteroid dehydrogenase, and 21-hydroxylase are required for synthesis of cholesterol and aldosterone, whereas aldosterone synthase is selectively responsible for aldosterone production in the adrenal cortex (see Fig. 47.11). Characteristics of diseases with aldosterone biosynthetic defects are shown in Figure 47.13.

Deficiency of 21-Hydroxylase

Mutations in the gene encoding 21-hydroxylase (*CYP21*) result in two major forms of the disease: a virilizing form and the more common salt-wasting type.[27] Patients with signs only of androgen excess are said to have the virilizing form. Female infants show varying degrees of pseudohermaphroditism, whereas affected males have normal or precocious sexual development. The salt-wasting type presents with hyponatremia, hyperkalemia, and moderate to severe volume depletion.

The diagnosis of 21-hydroxylase deficiency should be suspected in any newborn with genital ambiguity, salt wasting, or hypotension. Blood levels of progesterone, 17-hydroxyprogesterone, and dehydroepiandrosterone are raised several-fold above normal.

Features of Renal-Limited and Multisystem Forms of Pseudohypoaldosteronism Type I

Feature	Renal-limited Form	Multisystem Form
Underlying defect	Mineralocorticoid receptor	Epithelial sodium channel
Affected organs	Kidney only	Kidney, sweat, salivary glands, distal colon
Inheritance	Autosomal dominant	Autosomal recessive
Salt wasting	Variable	Severe
Blood renin, aldosterone	Very high	Very high aldosterone
Sweat, salivary Na^+	Normal	High
Clinical features	Salt wasting variable, during stress	Severe salt wasting, often life-threatening (e.g., hyperkalemia, infections of the skin), often respiratory tract (mimics cystic fibrosis) destabilization
Treatment	Sodium chloride supplements for 1–3 years Carbenoloxone is effective in some patients (creates situation akin to AME)	Lifelong sodium chloride supplements, strict potassium restriction, prophylactic antibiotics to prevent skin sepsis, no response to carbenoloxone
Prognosis	Improvement usually by 6–8 years, need for salt supplement diminishes	Improvement rare with age

Figure 47.12 Features of renal-limited and multisystem forms of pseudohypoaldosteronism type 1. AME, apparent mineralocorticoid excess.

Patients with electrolyte imbalance and shock require resuscitation with intravenous fluids and salt supplements. Replacement therapy with oral hydrocortisone and 9α-fludrocortisone is required long term. Some amelioration of the tendency to salt wasting may be seen with age because of the ability of children to regulate their dietary salt intake and maturation of proximal tubular function.

Reconstructive genital surgery may be required in females with genital ambiguity. Fetal DNA analysis and demonstration of elevated 17-hydroxyprogesterone in amniotic fluid allow prenatal detection of affected female infants. Treatment of the mother with dexamethasone from early in gestation reduces virilization of genitalia of the affected female fetus.

CONDITIONS WITH HYPERKALEMIA, METABOLIC ACIDOSIS, AND HYPERTENSION

Pseudohypoaldosteronism Type 2 (Gordon's Syndrome)

Gordon's syndrome is the clinical inverse of Gitelman's syndrome. It is an autosomal dominant condition characterized by hypertension, hyperkalemia, and mild hyperchloremic metabolic acidosis.

Pathogenesis

Two responsible genes have been identified.[28] They encode two members of the with-no-lysine kinase family: WNK1 and WNK4. The WNK kinases are both expressed in the kidney within the convoluted tubule and the collecting ducts.

WNK4 acts as a negative regulator of thiazide-sensitive Na^+-Cl^- cotransporter (NCCT) function (see Fig 47.2), reducing cell surface expression of NCCT. WNK4 also downregulates the potassium channel ROMK and epithelial chloride flux.

Mutations in WNK4 are missense mutations and cause loss of function, so that WNK4 loses its ability to suppress NCCT and ROMK. Transporter overactivity consequently leads to sodium and potassium retention.

WNK1 prevents WNK4 from interacting with NCCT. Mutations in WNK1 are intronic deletions that increase WNK1

Aldosterone Biosynthesis Defects

Defective enzyme	21-hydroxylase	3β-hydroxysteroid dehydrogenase	Cholesterol desmolase	Aldosterone synthase
Incidence	Most common (1:11,000–23,000)	Rare	Rare	Rare
Aldosterone	Deficient	Deficient	Deficient	Deficient
Cortisol production	Deficient	Deficient	Deficient	Normal cortisol
ACTH	Loss of feedback inhibition	Loss of feedback inhibition	Loss of feedback inhibition	Normal feedback inhibition
Adrenal hyperplasia	Yes	Yes	Yes	No
Genital ambiguity	In females	In females	In females	No
Clinical features	Children with failure to thrive; hyponatremia, hyperkalemia, acidosis, and hypotension			
Elevated metabolites	17-Hydroxyprogesterone	Dehydroepiandrosterone	Dehydroepiandrosterone	Corticosterone
Therapy	Oral hydrocortisone and 9α-fludrocortisone			9α-fludrocortisone

Figure 47.13 Characteristics of diseases with aldosterone biosynthetic defects. ACTH, adrenocorticotropic hormone.

expression. WNKs are intriguing targets for novel antihypertensive agents.

Clinical Manifestations and Diagnosis

Hyperkalemia may be present from birth, but as in GRA, hypertension may not be manifested until later in life. Patients show hyperchloremic metabolic acidosis; plasma renin and aldosterone are reduced to variable degrees.

Treatment

As specific inhibitors of the NCCT, thiazides are able to correct completely the clinical and biochemical features of Gordon's syndrome.

NEPHROGENIC DIABETES INSIPIDUS

Congenital nephrogenic diabetes insipidus (NDI) is a rare polyuric disorder identified by the failure to concentrate urine despite normal or elevated levels of vasopressin. Glomerular filtration rate (GFR) and solute excretion rate are normal. Congenital NDI is due to mutations in key proteins controlling water reabsorption in the distal tubule (see Fig. 47.5). Acquired diabetes insipidus is much more common, and its diagnosis and management are discussed in Chapter 8.

Pathogenesis

More than 90% of patients have X-linked recessive NDI with mutations in *AVPR2*, the gene at Xq28 coding for the arginine vasopressin receptor (AVPR). Mutant proteins are conformationally different, resulting in intracellular trapping of the receptor, which is retained in the endoplasmic reticulum. On occasion, the receptor may be expressed on the cell surface but is unable to bind vasopressin or to trigger an appropriate cyclic adenosine monophosphate (cAMP) response.[29] In less than 10% of the families, congenital NDI has an autosomal recessive inheritance, and mutations have been identified in the gene for aquaporin 2 located on chromosome 12q13. Similar to X-linked NDI, most autosomal recessive AQP2 mutations are held back in the endoplasmic reticulum. A rare autosomal dominant form of NDI, also caused by mutation in *AQP2*, has been reported. These mutations lead to mistransporting of AQP2 mutant proteins to the basolateral membrane instead of the apical membrane.[30] Reduced expression of AQP2 may result in acquired NDI secondary to lithium or demeclocycline therapy.

Clinical Features

Manifestations of congenital NDI appear within the first weeks of life. Males with *AVPR2* mutations have marked polyuria and excessive thirst, which is often not recognized in early infancy. Unless the condition is suspected early, children have recurrent episodes of severe hypernatremic dehydration, occasionally complicated by convulsions.[31] Delayed development and mental retardation are possible consequences of these episodes. Cranial computed tomography may occasionally show dystrophic calcification in the basal ganglia and the cerebral cortex.

A reduced intake of calories because of the large quantities of water that are ingested leads to growth failure beginning in early childhood. Increased urine volumes may result in dilation of the lower urinary tract. Renal cortical damage, because of recurrent episodes of severe dehydration, may result in impairment of renal function. Heterozygous females may show variable degrees of polyuria and polydipsia. The onset and severity of clinical features of autosomal recessive NDI are similar to those of the X-linked form.

Diagnosis

Episodes of dehydration are marked by hypernatremia, hyperchloremia, and occasionally elevated levels of urea and creatinine. Polyuria with low urine osmolality (<200 mOsm/kg) and hypernatremia with plasma Na^+ concentration above 150 mmol/l and plasma osmolality above 300 mOsm/kg are highly suggestive of either vasopressin deficiency (central diabetes insipidus) or resistance to its action (NDI). Central diabetes insipidus is more common than NDI. Primary polydipsia resembles true diabetes insipidus in that compulsive water drinking results in polyuria with low urine osmolality; however, the plasma osmolality in primary polydipsia is normal or borderline low.

To confirm the lack of renal concentrating ability and to distinguish NDI from central diabetes insipidus and primary polydipsia, a vasopressin test is performed. Desamino-8-D-arginine vasopressin (DDAVP) is administered nasally (5 to 10 μg in neonates and infants, 20 μg in children) or by an intramuscular injection (0.4 to 1.0 μg in infants and young children, 2 μg in older children). Hourly urine collection is done during the next 6 hours. After administration of DDAVP, patients with NDI fail to show a rise of urine osmolality, from 200 to 300 mOsm/kg (normal, >800 mOsm/kg). Those with central diabetes insipidus and primary polydipsia concentrate urine appropriately.

Persistence of polyuria for years may result in a washout of the medullary countercurrent concentration mechanism. Several days of treatment with DDAVP may be required to elicit an appropriate response in these patients. In patients in whom the diagnosis of primary polydipsia is strongly suspected, supervised reduction of fluid intake during several days may restore normal sensitivity to DDAVP.

Differential Diagnosis

Patients with central diabetes insipidus show hypernatremia with inappropriately dilute urine, no primary renal disease, and a rise in urine osmolality after administration of vasopressin or its analogues. Central diabetes insipidus usually results from posterior pituitary neuronal damage, which may be secondary to tumors (craniopharyngioma, optic glioma, metastasis), Langerhans cell histiocytosis, trauma (e.g., fracture of base of skull), or infections (meningitis, encephalitis). Deficiency of vasopressin may also be familial, with an autosomal dominant inheritance. Mutations of AVP-NPII, the gene for vasopressin–neurophysin II, have been reported.[32] The onset of vasopressin deficiency in the familial form may not be apparent until after the first few years of life. Central diabetes insipidus may also occur with the autosomal recessive syndrome of diabetes insipidus, diabetes mellitus, optic atrophy, and deafness (DIDMOAD, or Wolfram syndrome), which is autosomal recessive.

Many patients with central diabetes insipidus or NDI have a partial defect in vasopressin secretion or action. They are therefore able to concentrate urine to varying degrees after DDAVP administration, making precise diagnosis difficult. Measurement of plasma vasopressin in relation to plasma osmolality after an osmotic stimulus, such as fluid restriction, allows differentiation in these patients. Patients with severe or partial central diabetes insipidus always show subnormal vasopressin levels relative to plasma osmolality. In contrast, the values from patients with NDI or psychogenic polydipsia are always within or above the normal range.

Magnetic resonance imaging of the brain produces a bright spot on T1-weighted images of the posterior pituitary in normal individuals and also those with NDI or primary polydipsia. This signal is absent in most patients with central diabetes insipidus.

The differential response of clotting factors and urine osmolality to DDAVP is useful in differentiating X-linked (*AVPR2* abnormalities) from autosomal recessive (*AQP2* mutations) NDI. Patients with *AQP2* abnormalities show normal increases in factor VIII and von Willebrand factor after DDAVP infusion; this response is absent in those with an *AVPR2* defect.[31,33] Sequencing of *AVPR2* and *AQP2* is useful in identification of the molecular defect underlying NDI. Congenital NDI should also be differentiated from acquired forms of NDI (see Chapter 8).

Treatment

Appropriate management of patients with NDI prevents episodes of dehydration, allowing normal physical growth and development. Patients must have adequate water intake to prevent dehydration. The renal solute load is minimized by restriction of dietary protein and salt intake. Adequate energy and nutrients, depending on the age, should be provided to promote normal growth and development.

Thiazide diuretics, such as hydrochlorothiazide (1 to 2 mg/kg every 12 hours), when combined with reduction of salt intake, are effective in reducing urine output. Thiazides inhibit salt reabsorption in distal convoluted tubules, which leads to mild volume depletion. Hypovolemia stimulates fluid reabsorption in the proximal tubules, thereby diminishing water delivery to vasopressin-sensitive sites in the collecting ducts. The antipolyuric effect can be enhanced by combination therapy with amiloride (0.1 to 0.2 mg/kg every 8 to 12 hours).

Because prostaglandins normally antagonize the action of vasopressin, prostaglandin synthase inhibitors are also effective in reducing urine volume and free water clearance. Not all nonsteroidal anti-inflammatory drugs are equally potent in inhibiting renal prostaglandin synthesis. Indomethacin (1 mg/kg every 12 hours) is most commonly used but may reduce GFR and cause gastrointestinal side effects.

REFERENCES

1. Bartter FC, Pronove P, Gill J, MacCardle R. Hyperplasia of the juxtaglomerular complex with hyperaldosteronism and hypokalemic alkalosis. *Am J Med*. 1962;33:811-828.
2. Gitelman HJ, Graham JB, Welt LG. A new familial disorder characterized by hypokalemia and hypomagnesemia. *Trans Assoc Am Physicians*. 1966;79:221-235.
3. Shaer AJ. Inherited primary renal tubular hypokalemic alkalosis: A review of Gitelman and Bartter syndromes. *Am J Med Sci*. 2001;322:316-332.
4. Simon DB, Karet FE, Hamblan JM, et al. Bartter syndrome, hypokalemic alkalosis with hypercalciuria, is caused by mutations in the $Na^+K^+2Cl^-$ co-transporter NKCC2. *Nat Genet*. 1996;13:183-188.
5. International Collaborative Study Group for Bartter-like Syndromes. Mutations in the gene encoding the inwardly-rectifying renal potassium channel, ROMK, cause the antenatal variant of Bartter syndrome: Evidence for genetic heterogeneity. *Hum Mol Genet*. 1997;6:17-26.
6. Birkenhager R, Otto E, Schurmann MJ, et al. Mutations of BSND cause Bartter syndrome with sensorineural deafness and kidney failure. *Nat Genet*. 2001;29:310-314.
7. Zelikovic I, Szargel R, Hawash A, et al. A novel mutation in the chloride channel gene, ClCKB, as a cause of Gitelman and Bartter syndromes. *Kidney Int*. 2003;63:24-32.
8. Vargas-Poussou R, Huang C, Hulin P, et al. Functional characterization of a calcium-sensing receptor mutation in severe autosomal dominant hypocalcemia with a Bartter like syndrome. *J Am Soc Nephrol*. 2002;13:2259-2266.
9. Dillon MJ, Shah V, Mitchell MD. Bartter syndrome: 10 cases in childhood. Results of long term indomethacin therapy. *Q J Med*. 1979;48:429-446.
10. Simon DB, Nelson-Williams C, Bia MJ, et al. Gitelman variant of Bartter syndrome, inherited hypokalemic alkalosis, is caused by mutations in the thiazide-sensitive Na^+Cl^- co-transporter. *Nat Genet*. 1996;12:24-30.
11. Liddle GW, Bledsoe T, Coppage WS. A familial renal disorder simulating primary aldosteronism but with negligible aldosterone secretion. *Trans Assoc Am Physicians*. 1963;76:199-213.
12. Palmer BF, Alpern RJ. Liddle's syndrome. *Am J Med*. 1998;104:310-319.
13. Rossier BC, Pradervand S, Schild L, Hummler E. Epithelial sodium channel and the control of sodium balance: Interaction between genetic and environmental factors. *Annu Rev Physiol*. 2002;64:877-897.
14. Botero-Velez M, Curtis JJ, Warnock DG. Liddle's syndrome revisited: A disorder of sodium reabsorption in the distal tubule. *N Engl J Med*. 1994;330:178-181.
15. Geller DS, Farhi A, Pinkerton N, et al. Activating mineralocorticoid receptor mutation in hypertension exacerbated by pregnancy. *Science*. 2000;289:119-123.
16. White PC. Abnormalities of aldosterone synthesis and action in children. *Curr Opin Pediatr*. 1997;9:424-430.
17. Stewart PM, Krozowski Z, Gupta A, et al. Hypertension in the syndrome of apparent mineralocorticoid excess due to mutations of the 11β-hydroxysteroid dehydrogenase type 2 gene. *Lancet*. 1996;347:88-91.
18. White PC. 11β-hydroxysteroid dehydrogenase and its role in the syndrome of apparent mineralocorticoid excess. *Am J Med Sci*. 2001;322:308-315.
19. Palermo M, Delitala G, Mantero F, et al. Congenital deficiency of 11β-hydroxysteroid dehydrogenase (apparent mineralocorticoid excess syndrome): Diagnostic value of urinary free cortisol and cortisone. *J Endocrinol Invest*. 2001;24:17-23.
20. Li A, Tedde R, Krozowski ZS, et al. Molecular basis for hypertension in the "type II variant" of apparent mineralocorticoid excess. *Am J Hum Genet*. 1998;63:370-379.
21. Palermo M, Delitala G, Sorba G, et al. Does kidney transplantation normalise cortisol metabolism in apparent mineralocorticoid excess syndrome? *J Endocrinol Invest*. 2000;23:457-462.
22. McMahon GT, Dluhy RG. Glucocorticoid-remediable aldosteronism. *Cardiol Rev*. 2004;12:44-48.
23. Dillon MJ, Leonard JV, Buckler JM, et al. Pseudohypoaldosteronism. *Arch Dis Child*. 1980;55:427-434.
24. Geller DS, Rodriguez-Soriano J, Vallo Boado A, et al. Mutations in the mineralocorticoid receptor gene causes autosomal dominant pseudohypoaldosteronism type 1. *Nat Genet*. 1998;19:279-281.
25. Chang SS, Grunder S, Hanukoglu A, et al. Mutations in subunits of the epithelial sodium channel cause salt wasting with hyperkalemic acidosis, pseudohypoaldosteronism type 1. *Nat Genet*. 1996;12:248-253.
26. White PC. Aldosterone synthase deficiency and related disorders. *Mol Cell Endocrinol*. 2004;217:81-87.
27. Speiser PW. Congenital adrenal hyperplasia owing to 21-hydroxylase deficiency. *Endocrinol Metab Clin North Am*. 2001;30:31-59.
28. Mein CA, Caulfield MJ, Dobson RJ, et al. Genetics of essential hypertension. *Hum Mol Genet*. 2004;13:169-175.
29. Bichet DG. Vasopressin receptor mutations in nephrogenic diabetes insipidus. *Semin Nephrol*. 2008;28:245.
30. Sasaki S. Nephrogenic diabetes insipidus: Update of genetic and clinical aspects. *Nephrol Dial Transplant*. 2004;19:1351-1353.
31. Bichet DG, Oksche A, Rosenthal W. Congenital nephrogenic diabetes insipidus. *J Am Soc Nephrol*. 1997;8:1951-1958.
32. Heppner C, Kotzka J, Bullmann C, et al. Identification of mutations of the arginine vasopressin–neurophysin II gene in two kindreds with familial central diabetes insipidus. *J Clin Endocrinol Metab*. 1998;83:693-696.
33. Nguyen MK, Nielsen S, Kurtz I. Molecular pathogenesis of nephrogenic diabetes insipidus. *Clin Exp Nephrol*. 2003;7:9-17.

CHAPTER **48**

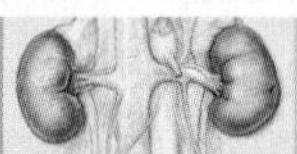

Fanconi Syndrome and Other Proximal Tubule Disorders

John W. Foreman

The proximal tubule is responsible for the reabsorption of the bulk of a number of solutes, including glucose, amino acids, bicarbonate, and phosphate. A number of disorders, mainly heritable, that affect proximal tubule reabsorption are described in this chapter, but renal tubular acidosis and familial forms of hyperphosphaturia are discussed in Chapters 12 and 10, respectively.

Most nonelectrolyte solutes are reabsorbed in the proximal tubule through specific transport proteins that cotransport them in conjunction with sodium (Fig. 48.1). The driving force for this solute transport is the electrochemical gradient for sodium entry maintained by the enzyme Na^+,K^+-ATPase. Most disorders of isolated solute reabsorption are related to defects in specific transport proteins, whereas disorders affecting multiple solutes, such as Fanconi syndrome, are probably secondary to defects in energy generation, Na^+,K^+-ATPase activity, or dysfunction of cellular organelles involved with membrane protein recycling.

FANCONI SYNDROME

Definition

In the 1930s, de Toni, Debré, and coworkers and Fanconi independently described several children with the combination of renal rickets, glycosuria, and hypophosphatemia. Fanconi syndrome nowadays refers to a global dysfunction of the proximal tubule leading to excessive urinary excretion of amino acids, glucose, phosphate, bicarbonate, and other solutes handled by this nephron segment. These losses lead to the clinical problems of acidosis, dehydration, electrolyte imbalance, rickets, osteomalacia, and growth failure. Numerous inherited or acquired disorders are associated with Fanconi syndrome (Fig. 48.2).

Etiology and Pathogenesis

The sequence of events leading to Fanconi syndrome is incompletely defined and probably varies with each cause. Possible mechanisms include widespread abnormality of most or all of the proximal tubule carriers, for example, a defect in sodium binding to the carrier or insertion of the carrier into the brush border membrane, "leaky" brush border membrane or tight junctions, inhibited or abnormal Na^+,K^+-ATPase pump, or impaired mitochondrial energy generation (see Fig. 48.1). An abnormality in energy generation has been implicated in a number of disorders, including hereditary fructose intolerance, galactosemia, mitochondrial cytopathies, and heavy metal poisoning as well as in a number of experimental models of Fanconi syndrome. Abnormal subcellular organelle function, such as the lysosome in cystinosis or the megalin-cubilin endocytic pathway in Dent disease, is also a cause of Fanconi syndrome (Fig. 48.3).

In adults, the most common causes of persistent Fanconi syndrome are an endogenous or exogenous toxin such as a heavy metal, a medication, and a dysproteinemia; in children, the most common persistent cause is an inborn error of metabolism, such as cystinosis. Specific causes of Fanconi syndrome are discussed after a general description of the clinical manifestations and treatment of the syndrome.

Clinical Manifestations of Fanconi Syndrome

Fanconi syndrome gives rise to a number of abnormalities (Fig. 48.4).

Aminoaciduria

Aminoaciduria is a cardinal feature of Fanconi syndrome. Virtually every amino acid is found in excess in the urine, hence the term *generalized aminoaciduria*. There are, however, no clinical consequences because the losses are trivial in relation to the dietary intake.

Glycosuria

Glycosuria secondary to proximal tubule dysfunction is another of the cardinal features of Fanconi syndrome and occurs because of impaired tubular reabsorption of glucose. It is often one of the first diagnostic clues. Like aminoaciduria, it rarely causes symptoms.

Hypophosphatemia

Hypophosphatemia, secondary to impairment in phosphate reabsorption, is a common finding in Fanconi syndrome. Assessment of tubular phosphate handling can be made by measuring the maximum phosphate reabsorption in relation to the glomerular filtration rate (TmP/GFR) on fasting urine and blood samples. Elevated parathyroid hormone (PTH) and low vitamin D levels also may play a role in the phosphaturia of Fanconi syndrome, although these hormonal abnormalities are not always present. A few patients have impaired conversion of 25-hydroxyvitamin D to 1,25-hydroxyvitamin D; metabolic acidosis, another feature of Fanconi syndrome, may also impair this conversion. Another mechanism for the hypophosphatemia is impairment of the megalin-dependent reabsorption and degradation of filtered PTH.[1] Unabsorbed PTH then binds to receptors in more distal portions of the proximal tubule, leading to increased endocytosis of apical phosphate transporters and increased phosphaturia. The hypophosphatemia, especially if it is accompanied by hyperparathyroidism and low

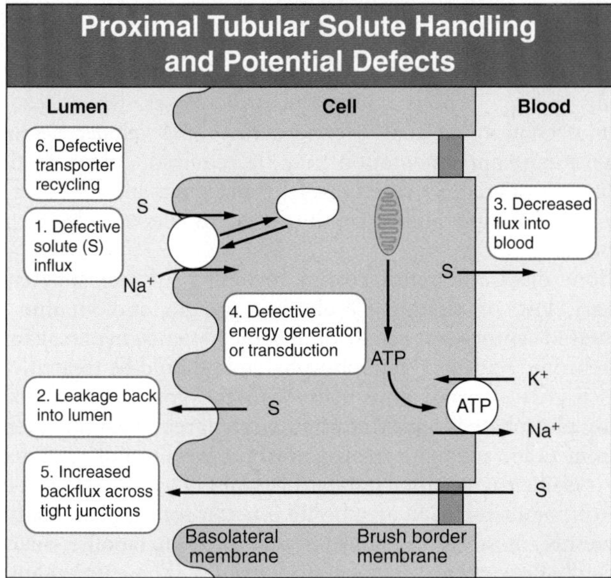

Figure 48.1 Defects and potential defects in proximal tubular solute handling. Solute uptake by the brush border membrane from the lumen is coupled to Na^+ influx. The favorable electrochemical driving force for luminal Na^+ is maintained by the Na^+,K^+-ATPase pump. Transported solute is then either used by the cell or returned to the blood across the basolateral membrane. Fanconi syndrome could arise because of a defect in one of six areas as shown. ATP, adenosine triphosphate.

Causes of Fanconi Syndrome

Inherited Causes
- Cystinosis
- Galactosemia
- Hereditary fructose intolerance
- Tyrosinemia
- Wilson's disease
- Lowe syndrome
- Dent disease
- Glycogenosis
- Mitochondrial cytopathies
- Idiopathic

Acquired Causes
- Drugs: *cisplatin, ifosfamide, tenofovir, cidofovir, adefovir,* didanosine, gentamicin, azathiopurine, valproic acid (sodium valproate), suramin, streptozocin (streptozotocin), ranitidine
- Dysproteinemias: *multiple myeloma, Sjögren's syndrome, light-chain proteinuria, amyloidosis*
- Heavy metal poisoning: lead, cadmium
- Other poisonings: Chinese herbal medicine, glue sniffing, diachrome
- Other: nephrotic syndrome, renal transplantation, acute tubular necrosis

Figure 48.2 Causes of Fanconi syndrome. More common causes are shown in italics.

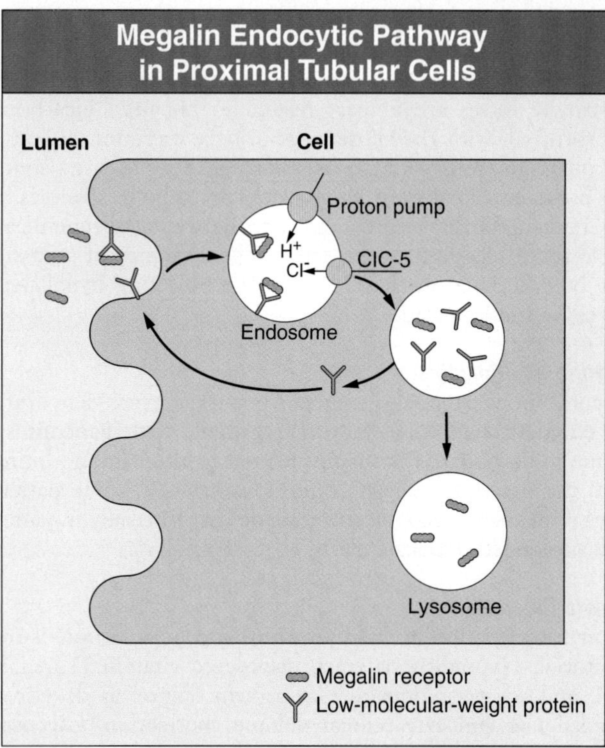

Figure 48.3 Megalin-cubilin endocytic pathway in proximal tubular cells. Low-molecular-weight proteins in the luminal fluid bind to the megalin-cubilin complex and are endocytosed. The recycling of megalin and further catabolism of these proteins are dependent on acidification of the vesicle by a proton pump. The ClC-5 chloride channel provides an electrical shunt for efficient functioning of the proton pump. This endocytosis pathway plays a role in membrane transporter recycling, and disruption of this pathway interferes with absorption of other luminal solutes.

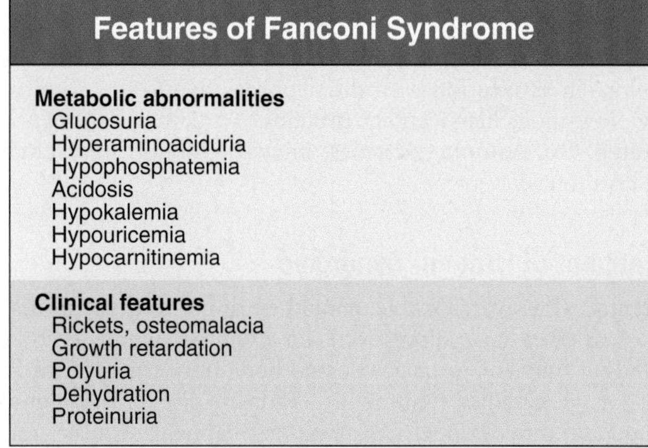
Features of Fanconi Syndrome

Metabolic abnormalities
- Glucosuria
- Hyperaminoaciduria
- Hypophosphatemia
- Acidosis
- Hypokalemia
- Hypouricemia
- Hypocarnitinemia

Clinical features
- Rickets, osteomalacia
- Growth retardation
- Polyuria
- Dehydration
- Proteinuria

Figure 48.4 Features of Fanconi syndrome.

1,25-hydroxyvitamin D levels, often leads to significant bone disease, presenting with pain, fractures, rickets, or growth failure.

Hyperchloremic Metabolic Acidosis

Hyperchloremic metabolic acidosis, another feature of Fanconi syndrome, is a result of impaired bicarbonate reabsorption by the proximal tubule (proximal or type 2 renal tubular acidosis; see Chapter 12). This impaired reabsorption can lead to the loss of more than 30% of the normal filtered load of bicarbonate. As the serum bicarbonate concentration falls, the filtered load falls, and excretion drops such that the serum bicarbonate concentration usually remains between 12 and 18 mmol/l. On occasion, there is an associated defect in distal acidification, usually in association with long-standing hypokalemia or nephrocalcinosis. Ammoniagenesis is usually normal or increased because of the hypokalemia and acidosis, unless there is an associated impairment in GFR.

Natriuresis and Kaliuresis

Natriuresis and kaliuresis are common in Fanconi syndrome and can give rise to significant, even life-threatening problems. These electrolyte losses are in part related to impaired bicarbonate reabsorption, with the subsequent urinary excretion of sodium and potassium ions with the bicarbonate. In some cases, sodium and potassium losses are so great that metabolic alkalosis and hyperaldosteronism result, simulating Bartter syndrome despite the lowered bicarbonate threshold. The clearance of potassium may be twice that of the GFR, and the resulting hypokalemia can cause sudden death.

Polyuria and Polydipsia

Polyuria, polydipsia, and frequent bouts of severe dehydration are common symptoms in young patients with Fanconi syndrome. The polyuria is mainly related to the osmotic diuresis from the excessive urinary solute losses; but in some patients, there is an associated concentrating defect, especially in patients with prolonged hypokalemia.

Growth Retardation

Growth retardation in children with Fanconi syndrome is multifactorial. Hypophosphatemia, disordered vitamin D metabolism, and acidosis contribute to growth failure, as do chronic hypokalemia and extracellular volume contraction. Glycosuria and aminoaciduria probably do not play a role. However, even with correction of all these metabolic abnormalities, most patients fail to grow, especially those with cystinosis.

Hypouricemia

Hypouricemia, caused by impairment in renal handling of uric acid, is often present in Fanconi syndrome, especially in adults. Urolithiasis from the uricosuria has only rarely been reported, probably because the urine flow and pH are increased, inhibiting uric acid crystallization.

Proteinuria

Proteinuria is usually minimal, except when Fanconi syndrome develops in association with the nephrotic syndrome. Typically, only low-molecular-weight proteins (<30,000 daltons) are excreted, for example, enzymes, immunoglobulin light chains, and hormones.

Treatment of Fanconi Syndrome

Therapy, whenever possible, should be directed at the underlying causes (see later discussion), for example, avoidance of the offending nutrient in galactosemia, hereditary fructose intolerance, or tyrosinemia; treatment of Wilson's disease with penicillamine and other copper chelators; or treatment of heavy metal intoxication by chelation therapy. In these cases, resolution of Fanconi syndrome usually is complete.

In other instances, therapy is directed at the biochemical abnormalities secondary to the renal solute losses and at the bone disease that is often present in these patients. The proximal renal tubular acidosis usually requires large doses of alkali for correction. Some patients benefit from hydrochlorothiazide to minimize the volume expansion associated with these large doses of alkali. Potassium supplementation is also commonly needed, especially if there is a significant renal tubular acidosis. The use of potassium citrate, lactate, or acetate will correct not only the hypokalemia but also the acidosis. A few patients will require sodium supplementation along with potassium. Again, the use of a metabolizable anion will aid in the correction of the acidosis. Rarely, patients may need sodium chloride supplementation. Usually, these patients have alkalosis when untreated as a result of large urinary sodium chloride losses, which lead to volume contraction that overrides the renal tubular acidosis. Magnesium supplementation may be required. Adequate fluid intake is essential. Correction of hypokalemia and its effect on the concentrating ability of the distal tubule may lessen the polyuria.

Bone disease is multifactorial, including hypophosphatemia, urinary loss of vitamin D–binding protein and vitamin D, decreased synthesis of calcitriol in some patients, hypercalciuria, and chronic acidosis. Hypophosphatemia should be treated with 1 to 3 g/day of oral phosphate with the goal of normalizing serum phosphate levels. Many patients will require supplemental vitamin D for adequate treatment of the rickets and osteomalacia. It is unclear whether standard vitamin D (calciferol [ergocalciferol]) or a vitamin D metabolite is better for supplementation. Currently, most clinicians use a vitamin D metabolite, such as 1,25-dihydroxycholecalciferol (calcitriol). These metabolites obviate the concern of inadequate vitamin D hydroxylation by the proximal tubule mitochondria and reduce the risk for prolonged hypercalcemia because of their shorter half-life. Vitamin D therapy will also improve the hypophosphatemia and lessen the risk for hyperparathyroidism. Supplemental calcium is indicated in those with hypocalcemia after supplemental vitamin D is started.

Hyperaminoaciduria, glycosuria, proteinuria, and hyperuricosuria usually do not lead to clinical difficulties and do not require specific treatment. Carnitine supplementation, to compensate for the urinary losses, may improve muscle function and lipid profiles, but the evidence is inconsistent.

INHERITED CAUSES OF FANCONI SYNDROME

Cystinosis

Definition

Cystinosis, or cystine storage disease, is characterized biochemically by excessive intracellular storage, particularly in lysosomes, of the amino acid cystine.[2] Three different types of cystinosis can be distinguished on the basis of the clinical course and the intracellular cystine content. Benign or adult cystinosis is associated with cystine crystals in the cornea and bone marrow only and the mildest elevation in intracellular cystine levels; there is no renal disease. Infantile or nephropathic cystinosis is the most common form and is associated with the highest intracellular levels of cystine and the earliest onset of renal disease. The intermediate or adolescent form has intracellular cystine levels in between those of the infantile and adult forms and later onset of renal disease.

Etiology and Pathogenesis

Nephropathic cystinosis is transmitted as an autosomal recessive trait localized to the short arm of chromosome 17, with an estimated incidence of 1 in 200,000 live births. The *CTNS* gene codes for a lysosomal membrane protein, cystinosin, that mediates the transport of cystine from the lysosome.[3] The benign and intermediate forms of cystinosis are also associated with mutations in this gene but still have some functional transport protein, leading to lower intracellular cystine levels and slower onset of renal disease in the intermediate form and no renal disease in the benign form.

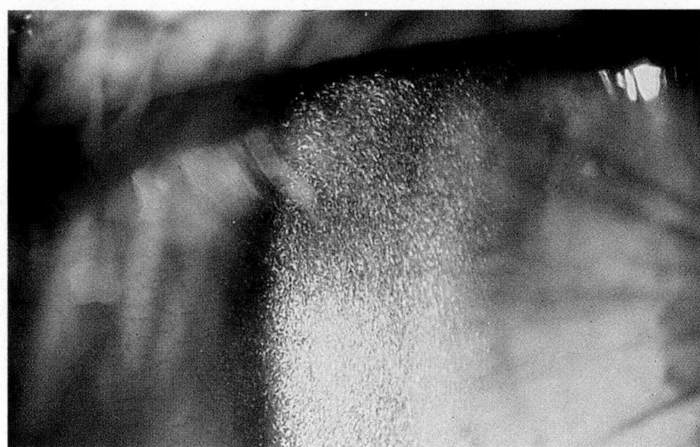

Figure 48.5 Corneal opacities in cystinosis. Tinsel-like refractile opacities in the cornea of a patient with cystinosis under slit-lamp examination. *(From reference 4.)*

Clinical Manifestations

The first clinical symptoms and signs in nephropathic cystinosis are those of Fanconi syndrome and usually appear in the second half of the first year of life. Subtle abnormalities of tubular function can be demonstrated earlier in families with index cases, but there always is a delay between birth and the first symptoms. Rickets is common after the first year of life, along with growth failure. The growth failure occurs before the GFR declines and despite correction of electrolyte and mineral deficiencies. The GFR invariably declines and end-stage renal disease (ESRD) occurs by late childhood. Nephrocalcinosis is relatively common, and a few patients have developed renal calculi. Photophobia is another common symptom that occurs by 3 years of age and is progressive. Older patients with cystinosis may develop visual impairment and blindness. Children with cystinosis usually have fair complexions and blond hair, but dark hair has been observed in some. Cystinosis has been observed in other ethnic groups but is less common than in Caucasians. The diagnosis is based on the demonstration of elevated intracellular levels of cystine, usually in white blood cells or skin fibroblasts. Patients with nephropathic and intermediate cystinosis have intracellular cystine levels that exceed 2 nmol half-cystine/mg protein. Normal patients have levels that are less than 0.2 nmol half-cystine/mg protein. Heterozygotes for cystinosis will have levels that range from 0.2 to 1 nmol half-cystine/mg protein. A slit-lamp demonstration of corneal crystals is strongly suggestive of the diagnosis (Fig. 48.5).[2] A prenatal diagnosis can be made with amniocytes or chorionic villi.

Common late complications of cystinosis include hypothyroidism, splenomegaly and hepatomegaly, decreased visual acuity, swallowing difficulties, pulmonary insufficiency, and corneal ulcerations.[5] Less commonly, older patients have developed insulin-dependent diabetes mellitus, myopathy, and progressive neurologic disorders. Decreased brain cortex has also been noted on imaging in some patients.

Pathology

The morphologic features of the kidney in cystinosis vary with the stage of the disease. Early in the disease, cystine crystals are present in tubular epithelial cells, interstitial cells, and rarely glomerular epithelial cells (Fig. 48.6A).[6,7] A swan-neck deformity or thinning of the first part of the proximal tubule is an early finding but is not unique to cystinosis. Later, there is pronounced tubular atrophy, interstitial fibrosis, and abundant crystal deposition with giant cell formation of the glomerular visceral epithelium, segmental sclerosis, and eventual glomerular obsolescence. Electron microscopy studies have demonstrated intracellular crystalline inclusions consistent with cystine (Fig. 48.6B). Peculiar "dark cells," unique to the cystinotic kidney, have also been observed.

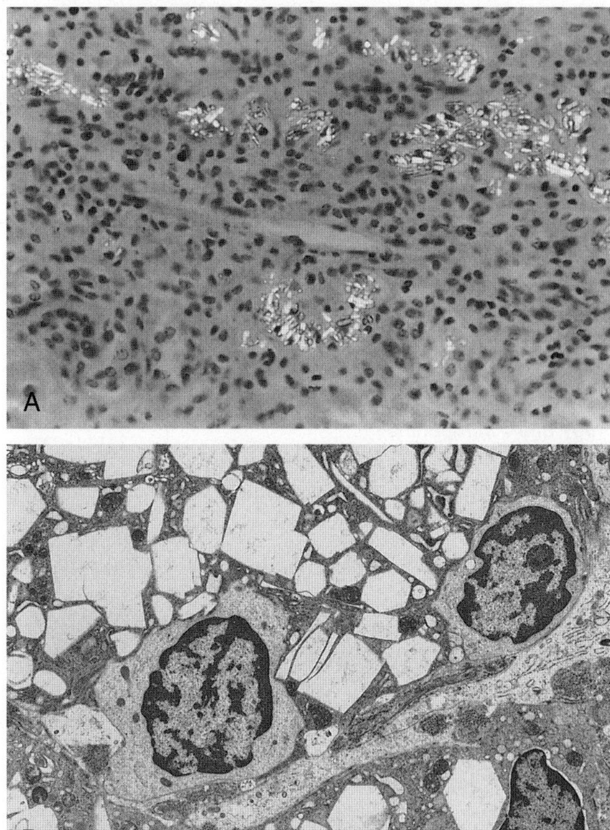

Figure 48.6 Cystine crystals in the kidney in cystinosis. A, Crystals are seen in a photomicrograph of an alcohol-fixed nephrectomy specimen, taken through incompletely crossed polarizing filters. Birefringent crystals are evident in tubular epithelial cells and free in the interstitium. **B,** Electron micrograph of a renal biopsy specimen showing hexagonal, rectangular, and needle-shaped crystals in macrophages within the interstitium. (Original magnification ×3000.) *(**A** from reference 6; **B** from reference 7.)*

Treatment

Nonspecific therapy for infantile cystinosis consists of vitamin D therapy and replacement of the urinary electrolyte losses, followed, in due course, by the management of the progressive renal failure (Fig. 48.7). Cysteamine has now been shown to lower tissue cystine and to slow the decline in GFR, especially in children with a normal serum creatinine concentration treated before 2 years of age (Fig. 48.8).[8] Cysteamine therapy also improves linear growth but not Fanconi syndrome. The most common problems associated with cysteamine therapy are nausea, vomiting, and a foul odor and taste. Treatment should begin with a low dose of cysteamine soon after the diagnosis is made, increased during 4 to 6 weeks to 60-90 mg/kg/day in four divided doses as close to every 6 hours as possible. Slowly increasing the dose minimizes the risk for a serum sickness–like reaction. Leukocyte cystine levels should be checked every 3 to 4 months to monitor effectiveness and compliance, with the goal of achieving and maintaining a cystine level of below 2.0 and preferably below 1.0 nmol half-cystine/mg protein. A 50-mM solution of cysteamine applied topically onto the eye has proved useful in depleting the cornea of cystine crystals but requires administration 6 to 12 times a day to be effective.

Treatment of ESRD in these children poses no greater problems than in other children. Successful renal transplantation reverses the renal failure and Fanconi syndrome but does not appear to improve the extrarenal manifestations of cystinosis. Cysteamine therapy should be continued after transplantation. Cystine does not accumulate in the transplanted kidney, except in infiltrating immunocytes.

Galactosemia

Etiology and Pathogenesis

Galactosemia is an autosomal recessively inherited disorder of galactose metabolism. It is most commonly the result of deficient activity of the enzyme galactose 1-phosphate uridyltransferase; this occurs with an incidence of 1 in 62,000 live births.[9] Deficiency of this enzyme leads to the intracellular accumulation of galactose 1-phosphate, with damage to the liver, proximal renal tubule, ovary, brain, and lens. A less frequent cause of galactosemia is a deficiency of galactose kinase, which forms galactose 1-phosphate from galactose. Cataracts are the only manifestation of this form of galactosemia. The pathogenesis of the symptoms of galactosemia is not clear. Accumulation of galactose 1-phosphate subsequent to the ingestion of galactose can inhibit a number of pathways for carbohydrate metabolism, and there is some correlation of its level with clinical symptoms. Defective galactosylation of proteins has also been postulated. Formation of galactitol from galactose by aldose reductase has been proposed as a pathogenetic mechanism, and this is probably responsible for the cataract formation.

Treatment of Cystinosis

Problem	Therapy
Removal of lysosomal cystine	Cysteamine, 0.325 g/m²q 6hr to maintain leukocyte cystine level <1 nmol half-cystine*/mg protein
Correction of Tubulopathy	
Dehydration	2–6 l/d fluid
Acidosis	2–15 mmol/kg/d K^+ citrate
Hypophosphatemia	1–4 g/d K^+ phosphate
Rickets	0.25–1 µg/d calcitriol
Adjunct therapies	NaCl, carnitine, indomethacin, hydrochlorothiazide
Later Therapies	
Growth failure	Growth hormone
Hypothyroidism	Thyroxine
Renal failure	Renal replacement therapy, ideally renal transplantation

Figure 48.7 Treatment of cystinosis. *By convention, units are half-cystine because the cystine originally was converted to two cysteine molecules, or "broken in half," before measurement.

Clinical Manifestations

Affected infants ingesting milk containing lactose, the most common source of galactose in the diet, rapidly develop vomiting, diarrhea, and failure to thrive. Jaundice from unconjugated hyperbilirubinemia is common, along with severe hemolysis. Continued intake of galactose leads to hepatomegaly and cirrhosis. Cataracts appear within days after birth, although at first they often are detectable only with a slit lamp. Mental retardation may develop within a few months. Fulminant *Escherichia coli* sepsis has been described in a number of infants; it may be a consequence of inhibited leukocyte bactericidal activity.

In addition to these clinical findings, galactose intake leads within days to hyperaminoaciduria and albuminuria. Raised urine sugar excretion is principally a result of galactosuria and not glycosuria. There seems to be little or no impairment in glucose handling by the renal tubule. Galactosemia should be suspected whenever there is a urinary reducing substance that does not react in a glucose oxidase test. The diagnosis can be confirmed by demonstration of deficient transferase activity in red blood cells, fibroblasts, leukocytes, or hepatocytes.

Treatment

Galactosemia is treated by elimination of galactose from the diet. Acute symptoms and signs resolve in a few days. Cataracts will also regress to some extent. However, even with early elimination of galactose, a common outcome in galactosemia is developmental delay, speech impairment, ovarian dysfunction, and growth retardation. Profound intellectual deficits are rare even in infants treated late.

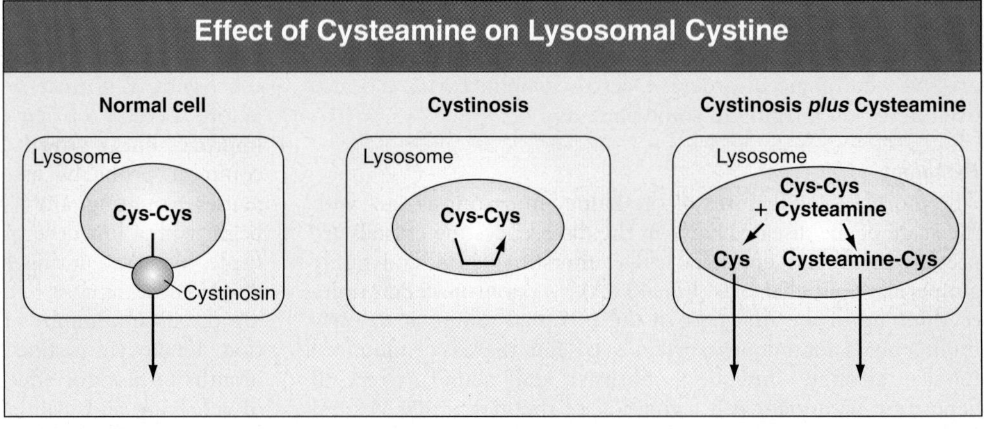

Figure 48.8 Effect of cysteamine on lysosomal cystine. In cystinosis, the transporter (cystinosin) for cystine (Cys-Cys) egress from the lysosome is defective. Cysteamine can easily enter the lysosome and combine with cystine, forming cysteine (Cys) and the mixed disulfide cysteamine-cysteine. Both of these compounds can exit the lysosome through a transporter other than the cystine carrier.

Hereditary Fructose Intolerance

Etiology and Pathogenesis

Hereditary fructose intolerance is another disorder of carbohydrate metabolism associated with Fanconi syndrome.[10] It is inherited as an autosomal recessive trait with an incidence estimated to be 1 in 20,000. It is caused by a deficiency of the B isoform of the enzyme fructose 1-phosphate aldolase, which cleaves fructose 1-phosphate into D-glyceraldehyde and dihydroxyacetone phosphate. Deficient activity of aldolase B leads to tissue accumulation of fructose 1-phosphate and reduced levels of ATP.

Clinical Manifestations

Symptoms of hereditary fructose intolerance appear at weaning when fruit, vegetables, and sweetened cereals that contain fructose or sucrose are introduced. Children with this disorder experience nausea, vomiting, and symptoms of hypoglycemia shortly after ingestion of fructose, sucrose, or sorbitol. These symptoms may progress to convulsions, coma, and even death, depending on the amount consumed. Young infants, when they are exposed to fructose, may have a catastrophic illness, with severe dehydration, shock, acute liver impairment, bleeding, and acute kidney injury. Concomitant serum biochemical findings after fructose ingestion are a fall in glucose, phosphate, and bicarbonate and a rise in uric acid and lactic acid. Chronic exposure to fructose leads to failure to thrive, hepatomegaly, jaundice, hepatic cirrhosis, and nephrocalcinosis. Children with hereditary fructose intolerance learn to avoid sweets and as a result have few dental caries.

Diagnosis

The diagnosis should be suspected when symptoms develop after the ingestion of fructose. Confirmation can be made either by a carefully applied fructose tolerance test or by assaying the activity of fructose 1-phosphate aldolase in a liver biopsy specimen.

Treatment

Treatment involves strict avoidance of foods containing fructose and sucrose, but because most patients develop a strong aversion to such foods, this is usually easy. The greatest risk occurs during infancy before affected individuals learn to avoid fructose.

Glycogenosis

Most patients with glycogen storage disease and Fanconi syndrome have an autosomal recessive disorder characterized by heavy glycosuria and increased glycogen storage in the liver and kidney, known as the Fanconi-Bickel syndrome, or glucose-losing syndrome, because the glucose losses can be massive.[11] The defect is deficient activity of the sugar transporter GLUT2 (see Fig. 48.10). GLUT2 facilitates sugar exit from the basolateral side of the proximal tubule and intestinal cell and sugar entry and exit from the hepatocyte and pancreatic ß-cell. A few patients with type I glycogen storage disease have mild Fanconi syndrome but not Fanconi-Bickel syndrome. The therapy for this disorder is directed at the renal solute losses, treatment of rickets (which can be severe), and frequent feeding to prevent ketosis. Uncooked corn starch has been shown to lessen the hypoglycemia and to improve growth.

Tyrosinemia

Definition

Hereditary tyrosinemia type I, also known as hepatorenal tyrosinemia, is a defect of tyrosine metabolism affecting the liver, kidneys, and peripheral nerves.[12]

Etiology and Pathogenesis

The cause of hereditary tyrosinemia type I is a deficiency of fumarylacetoacetate hydrolase (FAH) activity; it is an autosomal recessive disorder. Decreased or absent FAH activity leads to accumulation of maleylacetoacetate (MAA) and fumarylacetoacetate (FAA) in affected tissues. These compounds can react with free sulfydryl groups, reduce intracellular levels of glutathione, and act as alkylating agents. MAA and FAA are not detectable in plasma or urine but are converted to succinylacetoacetate and succinylacetone. Succinylacetone is structurally similar to maleic acid, a compound that causes Fanconi syndrome experimentally in rats and may be the cause of Fanconi syndrome in humans affected with tyrosinemia.

Clinical Manifestations

The liver is the major organ affected, and this may be evident as early as the first month of life. Such infants usually have severe disease and die in the first year of life. All children will eventually develop macronodular cirrhosis, and many develop hepatocellular carcinoma. Acute, painful peripheral neuropathy and autonomic dysfunction can also occur in tyrosinemia. Proximal renal tubular dysfunction is evident in all patients with tyrosinemia, especially those presenting after infancy. Nephromegaly is very common, and nephrocalcinosis may be seen. Glomerulosclerosis and impaired GFR may be seen with time.

Diagnosis

The diagnosis should be suspected with elevated plasma tyrosine and methionine levels together with their *p*-hydroxy metabolites. The presence of succinylacetone in blood or urine is diagnostic of hereditary tyrosinemia type I.

Treatment

The institution of a diet low in phenylalanine and tyrosine dramatically improves the renal tubular dysfunction. Nitisinone, which inhibits the formation of MAA and FAA, dramatically improves the renal and hepatic dysfunction.[12] Liver transplantation has been successfully used to treat patients with severe liver failure and to prevent the development of hepatocellular carcinoma. Liver transplantation leads to rapid correction of Fanconi syndrome.

Wilson's Disease

Definition

Wilson's disease is an inherited disorder of copper metabolism that affects numerous organ systems.[13,14] It has an overall incidence of 1 in 30,000. About 40% of patients present with liver disease, 40% with extrapyramidal symptoms, and 20% with psychiatric or behavioral abnormalities.

Etiology and Pathogenesis

Wilson's disease is a defect in the P-type copper-transporting ATPase ATP7B, which is highly expressed in the liver, kidney, and placenta. It impairs biliary copper excretion and the incorporation of copper into ceruloplasmin. These abnormalities cause excessive intracellular accumulation of copper in the liver, with subsequent overflow into other tissues such as brain, cornea, and renal proximal tubule.

Clinical Manifestations

Excessive storage of copper in the kidney leads to renal tubular dysfunction in most patients and full-blown Fanconi syndrome in some. Hematuria also has been noted. Renal plasma flow and GFR decrease as the disease progresses, but death from extrarenal causes occurs before the onset of renal failure. Fanconi syndrome usually appears before the onset of hepatic failure. Hypercalciuria with the development of renal stones and nephrocalcinosis also have been reported. Besides proximal tubular dysfunction, abnormalities in distal tubular function, decreased concentrating ability, and distal renal tubular acidosis have also been observed. Neurologic abnormalities, such as dysarthria and gait disturbances, may be the presenting symptom in young adults with Wilson's disease. Kayser-Fleischer rings, dense brown copper deposits around the iris, may be visible but typically can be seen only with a slit lamp.

Pathology

On histologic examination, the kidney in untreated Wilson's disease shows either no alteration on light microscopy or only some flattened proximal tubular cells without recognizable brush borders. Electron microscopy shows loss of the brush border, disruption of the apical tubular network, electron-dense bodies probably representing metalloproteins in the subapical region of tubule cell cytoplasm, and cavitation of the mitochondria with disruption of the normal cristae pattern. Rubeanic acid staining shows intracytoplasmic copper granules. The copper content of kidney tissue is markedly elevated.

Diagnosis

The diagnosis of Wilson's disease should be suspected in children and young adults with unexplained neurologic disease, chronic active hepatitis, acute hemolytic crisis, behavioral or psychiatric disturbances, or the appearance of Fanconi syndrome. In such patients, the presence of Kayser-Fleischer rings is an important clue in making the diagnosis. Serum ceruloplasmin levels are decreased in 96% of patients with Wilson's disease. A markedly increased urinary copper level is also useful in making the diagnosis, especially if it increases significantly with D-penicillamine. Liver copper levels are increased in untreated patients.

Treatment

Treatment with penicillamine, 1 to 1.5 g/day, reverses the renal dysfunction and may reverse the hepatic and neurologic disease, depending on the degree of damage before the onset of therapy. Recovery, however, is quite slow. Trientine can also chelate copper and is indicated in patients who cannot tolerate penicillamine. Tetrathiomolybdate is a potent agent in removing copper from the body and has been used in some patients with neurologic disease to prevent the immediate worsening of symptoms that can occur with penicillamine. Zinc salts, which induce intestinal metallothionein and blockade of intestinal absorption of copper, are useful in maintenance therapy. Liver transplantation has been successful in some patients but should be reserved for those with liver failure.

Lowe Syndrome

Lowe syndrome (oculocerebrorenal syndrome) is characterized by congenital cataracts and glaucoma, severe mental retardation, hypotonia with diminished to absent reflexes, and renal abnormalities.[15,16] Fanconi syndrome is followed by progressive renal impairment. ESRD usually does not occur until the third to fourth decade of life.

Lowe syndrome is transmitted as an X-linked recessive trait. Despite this inheritance pattern, Lowe syndrome has occurred in a few females. The defective gene codes for inositol polyphosphate 5-phosphatase, OCRL1, involved with cell trafficking and signaling.

Light microscopy of the kidney is normal early in the disorder, with endothelial cell swelling and thickening and splitting of the glomerular basement membrane seen by electron microscopy. In the proximal tubule cells, there is shortening of the brush border and enlargement of the mitochondria, with distortion and loss of the cristae. Only symptomatic treatment is available.

Dent Disease

Definition

Dent disease is an X-linked recessive disorder characterized by low-molecular-weight proteinuria, hypercalciuria, nephrolithiasis, nephrocalcinosis, and rickets.[17-19] In addition, affected males often have aminoaciduria, phosphaturia, and glycosuria. Renal failure is common and may occur by late childhood. Hemizygous females usually have only proteinuria and mild hypercalciuria. X-linked recessive nephrolithiasis and X-linked recessive hypophosphatemic rickets have similar features, and most have a defect in the renal ClC-5 chloride channel. Dent disease type 2 is a clinically similar disease affecting males, but there is a mutation in the same gene that causes Lowe syndrome, although they do not have the brain or eye involvement seen in Lowe syndrome.[17]

Etiology and Pathogenesis

Most of these disorders are caused by a mutation in the *CLCN5* gene leading to inactive ClC-5 chloride channel function (see Fig. 48.3). The ClC-5 chloride channel spans the membrane of pre-endocytic vesicles just below the brush border of the proximal tubule. There it facilitates the entry of Cl^- that is necessary for the active acidification of the vesicles by a proton pump. Lack of this Cl^- channel interferes with protein reabsorption from the tubule through the megalin-cubilin receptor system and cell surface receptor recycling, which may explain the phosphaturia, glycosuria, and aminoaciduria.

The defective OCRL1 in Dent disease type 2 patients interferes with normal cell protein trafficking. The renal disease is typical of Dent disease, without the eye and brain disease seen in Lowe syndrome.

Filtered PTH is also reabsorbed by the megalin-cubilin system for degradation in the lysosome. Decreased PTH reabsorption allows increased binding to luminal PTH receptors and increased endocytosis of luminal phosphate transporters, leading to increased phosphaturia.[1]

Mitochondrial Cytopathies

Definition

Mitochondrial cytopathies are a diverse group of diseases with abnormalities in mitochondrial DNA that lead to mitochondrial dysfunction in various tissues.[20]

Clinical Manifestations

Most of the mitochondrial cytopathies present with neurologic disorders such as myopathy, myoclonus, ataxia, seizures, external

Mitochondrial Cytopathies
MERRF: myoclonic epilepsy with ragged red fibers
NARP: neuropathy, ataxia, and retinitis pigmentosa
MELAS: mitochondrial encephalopathy, lactic acidosis, and strokelike episodes
LHON: Leber's hereditary optic neuropathy
Leigh disease: maternally inherited Leigh disease (somnolence, blindness, deafness, peripheral neuropathy, degeneration of brainstem)
Pearson's syndrome: pancytopenia, exocrine pancreatic deficiency, hepatic dysfunction
Kearns-Sayre syndrome: ophthalmoplegia, pigmentary retinopathy, heart block, ataxia
Alpers' disease: intractable epilepsy, liver disease, neuronal degeneration

Figure 48.9 Mitochondrial cytopathies.

ophthalmoplegia, stroke-like episodes, and optic neuropathy. Other manifestations include retinitis pigmentosa, diabetes mellitus, exocrine pancreatic insufficiency, sideroblastic anemia, sensorineural hearing loss, pseudo-obstruction of the colon, hepatic disease, cardiac conduction disorders, and cardiomyopathy. These various manifestations tend to group together in specific syndromes and reflect specific mutations in mitochondrial DNA (Fig. 48.9).

The most common renal manifestation associated with mitochondrial cytopathies is Fanconi syndrome, although a number of patients have been described with focal segmental glomerulosclerosis and corticosteroid-resistant nephrotic syndrome. All the patients with renal abnormalities have had extrarenal disorders, mainly neurologic disease. Most patients present in the first months of life and die soon afterward.

Diagnosis

A clue to these disorders is elevated serum or cerebrospinal fluid lactate levels, especially in association with an altered lactate to pyruvate ratio, suggesting a defect in mitochondrial respiration. The presence of "ragged red fibers," a manifestation of abnormal mitochondria, in a muscle biopsy specimen is another clue, especially with large abnormal mitochondria on electron microscopy of muscle tissue.

Treatment

There is little to offer these patients in terms of definitive therapy. Low mitochondrial enzyme complex III activity can be treated with menadione or ubidecarenone. Deficient mitochondrial enzyme complex I activity may be treated with riboflavin and ubidecarenone. Ascorbic acid has been used to minimize oxygen free radical injury. High-lipid, low-carbohydrate diet has been tried in cytochrome c oxidase deficiency.

Idiopathic Fanconi Syndrome

A number of patients develop the complete Fanconi syndrome in the absence of any known cause. Traditionally, these cases have been called adult Fanconi syndrome because it was thought that only adults were affected. However, it is clear that children may be affected, and a more proper designation is idiopathic Fanconi syndrome. Not all of the features of Fanconi syndrome may be present when the patients are first seen, but they do appear with time. Idiopathic Fanconi syndrome can be inherited in an autosomal dominant, autosomal recessive, or even X-linked pattern. However, most cases occur sporadically, without any evidence of genetic transmission. The prognosis is quite variable, and some develop chronic renal failure 10 to 30 years after the onset of symptoms. A few patients have undergone renal transplantation; in some of these, Fanconi syndrome has recurred in the allograft without evidence of rejection, suggesting an extrarenal cause of the idiopathic Fanconi syndrome. In one family, the gene defect was localized to chromosome 15.[21]

Renal morphologic descriptions of such cases are scanty. In some reports, no abnormalities were found, and in others, tubular atrophy with interstitial fibrosis was interspersed with areas of tubular dilation. Markedly dilated proximal tubules with swollen epithelium and grossly enlarged mitochondria with displaced cristae have also been noted.

ACQUIRED CAUSES OF FANCONI SYNDROME

Numerous substances can injure the proximal renal tubule (see Fig. 48.2), and this injury can range from an incomplete Fanconi syndrome to acute tubular necrosis or ESRD. The extent of the tubular damage is quite variable and is dependent on the type of toxin, the amount ingested, and the host. A careful history of possible toxin exposure and recent medications is important in patients with tubular dysfunction. The more common causes of acquired Fanconi syndrome are identified in Figure 48.2.

Heavy Metal Intoxication

A major cause of proximal tubular dysfunction is heavy metal intoxication, principally lead[22] and cadmium.[23] In lead poisoning, the renal tubular dysfunction, mainly aminoaciduria and mild glycosuria and phosphaturia, is usually overshadowed by the involvement of other organs, especially the central nervous system. Fanconi syndrome associated with cadmium poisoning is associated with severe bone pain, giving rise to the name itai-itai ("ouch-ouch") disease for its occurrence in Japanese patients affected by industrial contamination of the soil.

Tetracycline

Outdated tetracycline causes a reversible Fanconi syndrome even in therapeutic doses. Recovery is rapid when the degraded drug is stopped. The compound responsible for the tubule dysfunction is anhydro-4-tetracycline formed from tetracycline by heat, moisture, and low pH.

Cancer Chemotherapy Agents

A number of cancer chemotherapy agents have been associated with Fanconi syndrome and renal tubular dysfunction, especially cisplatin[24] and ifosfamide.[25] Carboplatin has been associated with reduced GFR and magnesium wasting but not Fanconi syndrome. The nephrotoxicity of both cisplatin and ifosfamide is dose dependent and often irreversible. Besides the usual manifestations of Fanconi syndrome, cisplatin toxicity is characterized by hypomagnesemia, caused by hypermagnesuria, which can be extremely severe, persistent, and difficult to treat. Ifosfamide is more commonly associated with hypophosphatemic rickets.

Chloroacetaldehyde, a metabolite of ifosfamide, appears experimentally to cause Fanconi syndrome. Both ifosfamide and cisplatin can cause an irreversible reduction in GFR.

Other Drugs and Toxins

Exposure to a wide range of toxins may give rise to Fanconi syndrome, often in association with a reduced GFR, including methyl-3-chromone (diachrome), 6-mercaptopurine, toluene (glue sniffing), and Chinese herbal medicines containing an *Aristolochia* species.[26] There have also been anecdotal reports associating Fanconi syndrome with valproic acid (valproate), suramin, Lysol (a cresol-based antiseptic), gentamicin, and ranitidine. Antiviral[27] medications, especially antiretroviral agents, are an increasingly common cause of Fanconi syndrome.

Dysproteinemias

Dysproteinemia[28] from multiple myeloma, light-chain proteinuria,[29] Sjögren's syndrome, and amyloidosis is sometimes associated with Fanconi syndrome, which appears to be correlated with urinary free light chains with specific physicochemical characteristics that crystallize within the tubular cells.

Glomerular Disease

Nephrotic syndrome has rarely been associated with Fanconi syndrome. Most of these patients have focal segmental glomerulosclerosis, and the occurrence of Fanconi syndrome heralds a poor prognosis.

After Acute Kidney Injury

Tubular dysfunction during recovery from acute kidney injury from any cause can occur, whether or not a known tubular toxin was originally implicated.

After Renal Transplantation

Fanconi syndrome has appeared rarely after renal transplantation. The pathogenesis probably is multifactorial, for example, sequelae of acute tubular necrosis, rejection, nephrotoxic drugs, ischemia from renal artery stenosis, and residual hyperparathyroidism.

FAMILIAL GLUCOSE-GALACTOSE MALABSORPTION AND HEREDITARY RENAL GLYCOSURIA

Definition

Renal glycosuria refers to the appearance of readily detectable glucose in the urine when the plasma glucose concentration is in a normal range. When the plasma glucose concentration is in a physiologic range, virtually all the filtered glucose is reabsorbed in the proximal tubule.[30] Filtered glucose enters the proximal tubule through two specific carriers (SGLT1 and SGLT2) coupled to sodium and exits the cell through the sugar transporters GLUT1 and GLUT2 (Fig. 48.10). However, when the plasma level exceeds the physiologic range, the filtered load exceeds the capacity of these carriers, and glucose begins to appear in the urine; this is termed the renal threshold.

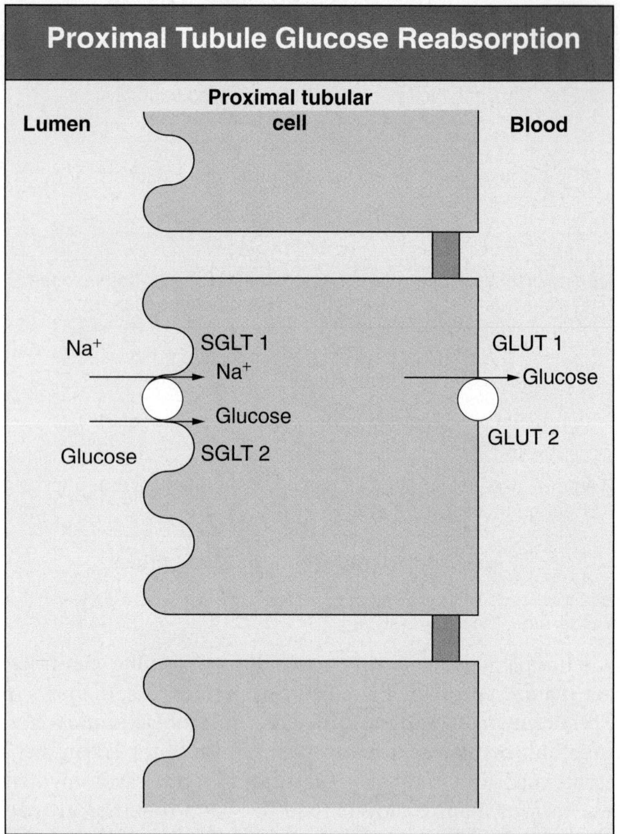

Figure 48.10 Proximal tubule glucose reabsorption. Glucose enters the proximal tubule cell coupled to Na^+ reabsorption from the lumen through a high-capacity, low-affinity transporter (SGLT2) in the early proximal tubule and a low-capacity, high-affinity transporter (SGLT1) in the late proximal tubule. Glucose exits the cell through the transporters GLUT1 and GLUT2 located in the late and early proximal tubule, respectively.

Etiology and Pathogenesis

Familial glucose-galactose malabsorption is a rare autosomal disorder that is due to mutations in the gene coding for the brush border sodium-glucose cotransporter SGLT1, which is found in the intestinal cell and the S_3 segment of the proximal renal tubule cell. The disorder is characterized by the neonatal onset of life-threatening diarrhea from the intestinal malabsorption of glucose and galactose that resolves rapidly with the removal of glucose and galactose and its dipeptide, lactose, from the diet. These patients frequently also have a mild renal glycosuria.

Hereditary renal glycosuria occurs with an incidence of 1 in 20,000 and appears to be inherited as a codominant trait with variable penetrance.[31] This disorder is due to mutations in SGLT2 glucose transporter found in the early portion of the proximal tubule. Renal glycosuria has been divided into three types based on the reabsorption patterns observed during glucose infusion studies (Fig. 48.11). In type A, there is lowering of both the threshold and the maximal rate of tubular reabsorption of glucose. In type B, the maximal rate of glucose reabsorption is normal, but the threshold is low, and there is exaggerated splay in the tubular reabsorption versus filtered load curve. In type 0, there is virtually no reabsorption of filtered glucose, with the clearance of glucose nearly the same as that of inulin.[32] This typing system has been called into question because clearance data suggest that patients with renal glycosuria have rates of glucose reabsorption that vary from virtually no reabsorption to

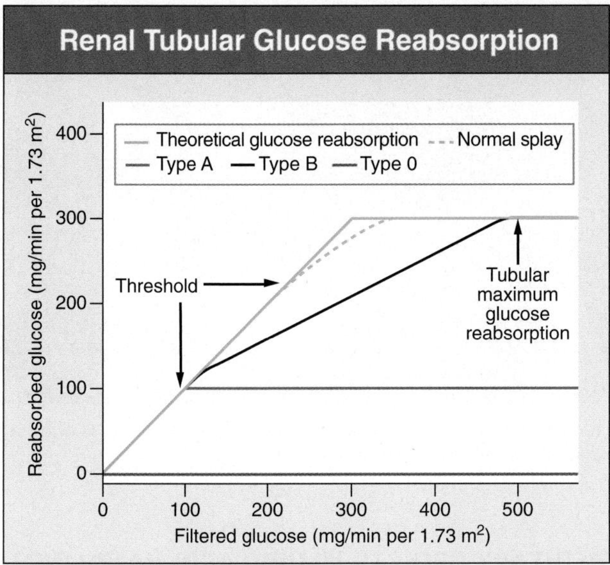

Figure 48.11 Renal glucose titration curves. The observed normal reabsorption curve follows the theoretical renal tubular glucose reabsorption until near the maximal reabsorption rate, when the observed rate deviates from the theoretical rate (splay). The point of deviation is the threshold. Stylized titration curves for types A, B, and 0 renal glycosuria are shown. *(Modified from reference 32.)*

nearly normal rates, rather than three distinct types, probably reflecting different mutations in the *SLC5A2* gene.[32]

Natural History

Patients with familial glucose-galactose malabsorption appear to grow and develop normally with removal of the offending sugars from the diet. The clinical course of hereditary renal glycosuria is benign, except for a few patients with polyuria, and it is not a precursor to diabetes mellitus. Patients need to be aware of the condition in order not to receive unnecessary diagnostic investigations or even treatment for presumed diabetes mellitus.

AMINOACIDURIAS

Like glucose, amino acids are nearly completely reabsorbed in the proximal tubule by a series of specific carriers. A number of inherited disorders resulting in the incomplete reabsorption of a specific amino acid or a group of amino acids have been described (Fig. 48.12).[33,34]

Inherited Aminoacidurias

Disease	Clinical Findings	Urine Amino Acids
Cystinuria	Urolithiasis	Cystine, lysine, ornithine, arginine
Hartnup disease	Rash, neurologic disease	Neutral amino acids
Iminoglycinuria	None	Proline, hydroxyproline glycine
Lysinuric protein intolerance	Hyperammonemia, vomiting, diarrhea	Dibasic amino acids

Figure 48.12 Inherited aminoacidurias.

Cystinuria

Definition

Cystinuria is characterized by the excessive urinary excretion of cystine and the dibasic amino acids ornithine, lysine, and arginine.[35]

Etiology and Pathogenesis

These four amino acids share a transport system on the brush border membrane of the proximal tubule. Because of the relative insolubility of cystine when its urine concentration exceeds 250 mg/l (1 mmol/l), patients with cystinuria have recurrent renal calculi.

Cystinuria is an autosomal recessive trait with a disease incidence of 1 in 15,000.[35] Initially, there appeared to be three genetic types on the basis of *in vitro* studies of intestinal transport and amino acid excretion in heterozygotes. More recently, two genes (*SLC3A1* and *SLC7A9*) have been identified that are defective in cystinuria. *SLC3A1* heterozygotes have normal excretion rates for cystine. *SLC7A9* heterozygotes have cystine excretion rates that range from normal to nearly that of homozygous patients. On the basis of these data, a new classification has been proposed. Type A involves mutations in both *SLC3A1* genes, and type B mutations in *SLC7A9*.[36] Type AB is compound heterozygote. Type A accounts for 38% of cystinuria patients, type B for 47%, and type AB for 14%.

Clinical Manifestations

Cystine stones are typically yellow-brown (Fig. 48.13A) and are radiopaque (Fig. 48.13B). Cystine crystals appear as microscopic, flat hexagons in the urine (Fig. 48.13C), and this is a clue to the diagnosis.

Diagnosis

Patients can be screened for cystinuria with the cyanide-nitroprusside test, but type B heterozygotes may also give a positive result. The definitive test is to quantify cystine and dibasic amino acid excretion in a 24-hour urine specimen. Homozygotes excrete more than 118 mmol cystine/mmol creatinine (250 mg/g).

Treatment

The aim of therapy in cystinuria is to lower the urine cystine concentration to below 300 mg/l (1.25 mmol/l). The first step is to increase fluid intake. However, because most patients with cystinuria excrete 0.5 to 1 g/day of cystine, a urine output of 2 to 4 l/day is needed to achieve this goal. Cystine solubility increases in alkaline urine, but the urine pH must be above 7.5 to be effective. In patients with recurrent stone disease, thiols, such as penicillamine, are extremely useful through the formation of a more soluble mixed disulfide of the thiol and cysteine from cystine. The thiols also reduce the overall excretion of cystine through an unknown mechanism. Penicillamine should be started at 250 mg/day and gradually increased (maximum, 2 g/day) during 3 months to achieve a urine cystine concentration below 300 mg/l in conjunction with a high fluid intake. Tiopronin is equally effective and is better tolerated than penicillamine. It should also be started at a low dose and slowly increased (maximum, 2 g/day). Captopril can be useful (an effect resulting

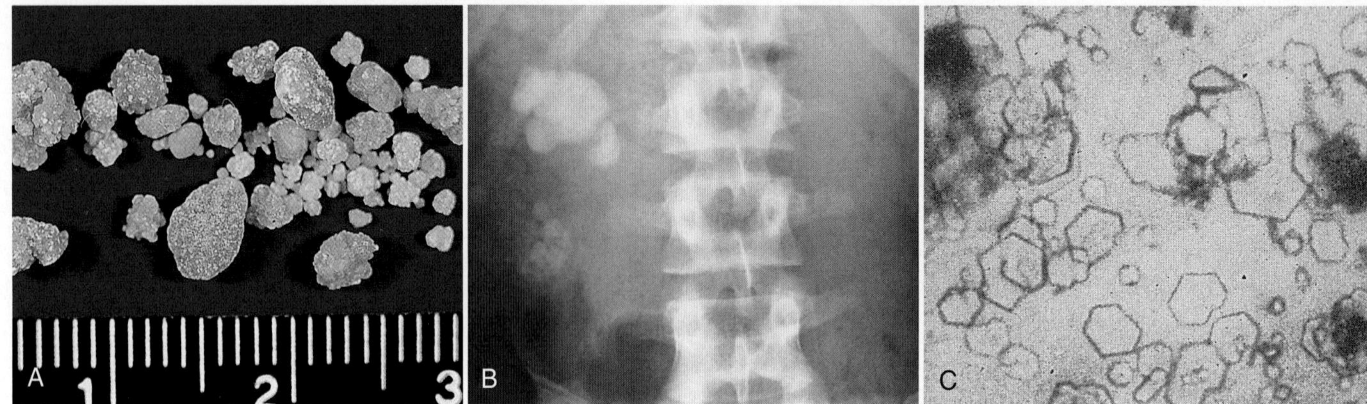

Figure 48.13 Cystinuria. A, Both rough and smooth cystine calculi. **B,** Plain radiograph of a cystine calculus in the right renal pelvis and further multiple parenchymal calculi. **C,** Urine microscopy showing characteristic flat hexagonal crystals (see also Fig. 4.7G).

from its thiol structure, not its angiotensin-converting enzyme inhibitor effect), but the dose range (75 to 150 mg/day) may be limited by its hypotensive effects.

Hartnup Disease

Hartnup disease is an autosomal recessive trait characterized by a neutral aminoaciduria that arises from a defect in a specific carrier for neutral amino acid transport present in both the intestine and the proximal renal tubule. The gene responsible for Hartnup disease is *SLC6A19*. It codes for the neutral amino acid transporter B^0AT1. From newborn screening programs, the genetic defect is more common than originally thought because most individuals with the aminoaciduria never manifest any symptoms. Individuals who become symptomatic with Hartnup disease have pellagra-like clinical features, including a photosensitive dermatitis, ataxia, and psychotic behavior. These symptoms appear to be secondary to niacin deficiency that is in part due to inadequate intestinal absorption of tryptophan, the precursor for niacin synthesis. However, most individuals who inherit the Hartnup transport defect do not have symptoms, so there must be other environmental or genetic factors that contribute to disease. Nicotinamide supplementation leads to clearing of the skin disease and, on occasion, some of the neurologic problems. The renal loss of neutral amino acids appears to have little clinical importance.

Iminoglycinuria

Iminoglycinuria is a benign heritable defect in the proximal tubule transporter PAT1, leading to incomplete reabsorption of proline, hydroxyproline, and glycine.

Lysinuric Protein Intolerance

Lysinuric protein intolerance is associated with recurrent bouts of hyperammonemia after a protein load, resulting from the decreased renal and intestinal dibasic amino acid transport.

Other Aminoacidurias

Rare individuals have been described with abnormalities in the excretion of other amino acids. These usually occur in association with mental retardation.

HEREDITARY DEFECTS IN URIC ACID HANDLING

Hereditary Renal Hypouricemia

Hereditary renal hypouricemia is a rare autosomal recessive disorder characterized by very low serum uric acid levels (<2.5 mg/dl [<150 μmol/l] in adult men and <2.1 mg/dl [<124 μmol/l] in adult women) and increased uric acid clearance, ranging from 30% to 150% of the filtered load.[37] In the normal kidney, uric acid is both reabsorbed and secreted in the proximal tubule by two different uric acid–anion exchange transporters and a voltage-sensitive pathway. In some patients, the defect is in the gene *SLC22A12* that codes for the protein URAT1; other patients have been found to have mutations in SLC2A9 (GLUT9). Most patients do not have symptoms and are found incidentally when a low serum uric acid concentration is noted during routine serum chemistry evaluation. About one fourth of patients with renal hypouricemia have had renal stones, but only one third of these were uric acid stones. There may also be hypercalciuria, and a few patients have had exercise-induced acute kidney injury, thought to be due to acute tubular injury by passage of urate "gravel" in association with volume depletion and reduced urine pH. Most patients require no treatment, but if they are forming uric acid stones, they should maintain a high fluid intake. Urine alkalinization and allopurinol can be used for patients with persistent uric acid stones.

Familial Juvenile Hyperuricemic Nephropathy and Medullary Cystic Kidney Disease Type 2

Familial juvenile hyperuricemic nephropathy (FJHN) is a rare autosomal dominant condition characterized by hyperuricemia associated with a tubular defect in uric acid excretion.[38] Children develop progressive renal impairment with interstitial fibrosis and glomerulosclerosis. The hyperuricemia is due to renal underexcretion of uric acid. Diagnosis is suggested by a fractional excretion of uric acid of less than 5% (normal, 10% to 15%). Controversy exists as to whether lowering of serum uric acid slows the progression of renal failure; the studies reporting benefit have usually involved starting of a xanthine oxidase inhibitor early in the course of the disease. Isosthenuria and hypertension are common, and some patients have renal salt wasting. Many of the features of FJHN are also seen in medullary cystic kidney disease type 2 (MCKD2).[39] Most of these patients have a defect in the gene *UMOD*, located on chromosome 16p12, coding for the Tamm-Horsfall/uromodulin protein. There is some evidence that this mutation may interfere with the function of the Na-K-2Cl transporter, leading to a secondary increase in proximal sodium and urate reabsorption. This mutation may also lead to deposition of abnormal protein in the endoplasmic reticulum and ultimately cell death.

REFERENCES

1. Saito A, Noriaki I, Takeda T, Gejyo F. Role of megalin, a proximal tubular endocytic receptor, in calcium and phosphate homeostasis. *Ther Apher Dial.* 2007;11(Suppl 1):S23-S26.
2. Gahl WA, Thoene JG, Schneider JA. Cystinosis. *N Engl J Med.* 2002;347:111-121.
3. Town M, Jean G, Cherqui S, et al. A novel gene encoding an integral membrane protein is mutated in nephropathic cystinosis. *Nat Genet.* 1998;18:319-324.
4. Foreman JW. Cystinosis and the Fanconi syndrome. In: Avner ED, Harmon WE, Niaudet P, eds. *Pediatric Nephrology*, 5th ed. Philadelphia: Lippincott Williams & Wilkins; 2004, p 789.
5. Gahl WA, Balog JZ, Kleta R. Nephropathic cystinosis in adults: Natural history and effects of oral cysteamine therapy. *Ann Intern Med.* 2007;147:241-250.
6. Schnaper HW, Cottel J, Merrill S, et al. Early occurrence of end-stage renal disease in a patient with infantile nephropathic cystinosis. *J Pediatr.* 1992;120:575-578.
7. van't Hoff WG, Ledermann SE, Waldron M, Trompter RS. Early-onset chronic renal failure as a presentation of infantile cystinosis. *Pediatr Nephrol.* 1995;9:483-484.
8. Kleta R, Gahl WA. Pharmacological treatment of nephropathic cystinosis with cysteamine. *Expert Opin Pharmacother.* 2004;5:2255-2262.
9. Bosch AM. Classical galactosemia revisited. *J Inherit Metab Dis.* 2006;29:516-525.
10. Wong D. Hereditary fructose intolerance. *Mol Genet Metab.* 2005; 85:165-167.
11. Santer S, Steinmenn B, Schaub J. Fanconi-Bickel syndrome: A congenital defect of facilitative glucose transport. *Curr Mol Med.* 2002;2: 213-227.
12. Santra S, Preece MA, Hulton SA, McKiernan PJ. Renal tubular function in children with tyrosinaemia type I treated with nitisinone. *J Inherit Metab Dis.* 2008;31:399-402.
13. Ala A, Walker AP, Ashkan K, et al. Wilson's disease. *Lancet.* 2007;369:397-408.
14. Riordan SM, Williams R. The Wilson's gene and phenotypic diversity. *J Hepatol.* 2001;34:165-171.
15. Charnas LR, Bernardini I, Rader D, et al. Clinical and laboratory findings in the oculocerebrorenal syndrome of Lowe, with special reference to growth and renal function. *N Engl J Med.* 1991;324:1318-1325.
16. Bockenhauer D, Bokencamp A, van't Hoff W, et al. Renal phenotype in Lowe syndrome: A selective proximal tubular dysfunction. *Clin J Am Soc Nephrol.* 2008;3:1430-1436.
17. Hoopes RR. Dent disease with mutations in OCRL1. *Am J Hum Genet.* 2005;76:260-267.
18. Cho HY, Lee NH, Choi HJ, et al. Renal manifestations of Dent disease and Lowe syndrome. *Pediatr Nephrol.* 2008;23:243-249.
19. Thakker RV. Pathogenesis of Dent's disease and related syndromes of X-linked nephrolithiasis. *Kidney Int.* 2000;57:787-793.
20. Niaudet P, Roetig A. Renal involvement in mitochondrial cytopathies. *Pediatr Nephrol.* 1996;10:368-373.
21. Lichter-Konecki U, Broman KW, Blau EB, Konecki DS. Genetic and physical mapping of the locus for autosomal dominant renal Fanconi syndrome, on chromosome 15q15.3. *Am J Hum Genet.* 2001;68: 264-268.
22. Loghman-Adham M. Aminoaciduria and glucosuria following severe childhood lead poisoning. *Pediatr Nephrol.* 1998;12:218-221.
23. Inaba T, Kobayashi E, Suwazono Y, et al. Estimation of the cumulative cadmium intake causing Itai-itai disease. *Toxicoloy Lett.* 2005;164: 189-190.
24. Cachat F, Nenadov-Beck M, Guignard JP. Occurrence of an acute Fanconi syndrome following cisplatin chemotherapy. *Med Pediatr Oncol.* 1998;31:40-41.
25. Rossi R, Pleyer J, Schafers P, et al. Development of ifosfamide-induced nephrotoxicity: Prospective follow-up in 75 patients. *Med Pediatr Oncol.* 1999;32:177-182.
26. Debelle FD, Vanherweghem JL, Nortier JL. Aristolochic acid nephropathy: A worldwide problem. *Kidney Int.* 2008;74:158-169.
27. Earle KE, Seneviratne T, Shaker J, Shoback D. Fanconi's syndrome in HIV+ adults: Report of three cases and literature review. *J Bone Miner Res.* 2004;19:714-721.
28. Merlini G, Pozzi C. Mechanisms of renal damage in plasma cell dyscrasias: An overview. *Contrib Nephrol.* 2007;153:66-86.
29. Rikitake O, Sakemi T, Yoshikawa Y, et al. Adult Fanconi syndrome in primary amyloidosis with lambda light-chain proteinuria. *Jpn J Med.* 1989;28:523-526.
30. Lee YJ, Lee YJ, Han HJ. Regulatory mechanisms of Na^+/glucose cotransporters in renal proximal tubule cells. *Kidney Int.* 2007;72: S27-S35.
31. Santer R, Kinner M, Lassen CL, et al. Molecular analysis of the SGLT2 gene in patients with renal glucosuria. *J Am Soc Nephrol.* 2003;14: 2873-2882.
32. Brodehl J, Oemer BS, Hoyer PF. Renal glucosuria. *Pediatr Nephrol.* 1987;1:502-508.
33. Camargo SM, Bockenhauer D, Kleta R. Aminoaciduria: Clinical and molecular aspects. *Kidney Int.* 2008;73:918-925.
34. Chillaron J, Roca R, Valencia A, et al. Heteromeric amino acid transporters: Biochemistry, genetics, and physiology. *Am J Physiol Renal Physiol.* 2001;281:F995-F1018.
35. Mattoo A, Goldfarb D. Cystinuria. *Semin Nephrol.* 2008;28:181-191.
36. Dello Strologo L, Pras E, Pontesilli C, et al. Comparison between SLC3A1 and SLC7A9 cystinuria patients and carriers: A need for a new classification. *J Am Soc Nephrol.* 2002;13:2547-2553.
37. Sperling O. Hereditary renal hypouricemia. *Mol Genet Metab.* 2006;89:14-18.
38. Wolf MT, Beck BB, Zaucke F, Kunze A. The uromodulin C744G mutation causes MCKD2 and FJHN in children and adults and may be due to a possible founder effect. *Kidney Int.* 2007;71:574-581.
39. Bleyer AJ, Hart TC, Willingham MC, Iskandar S. Clinicopathologic findings in medullary cystic kidney disease type 2. *Pediatr Nephrol.* 2005;20:824-827.

CHAPTER 49

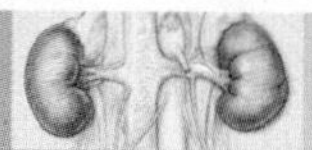

Sickle Cell Disease

Jan C. ter Maaten, Fatiu A. Arogundade

DEFINITIONS

Sickle cell disease is an autosomal recessive inherited disorder, predominantly of the African race. The gene for sickle hemoglobin (hemoglobin S, or HbS) results in the replacement of the normal glutamine by valine in the sixth position of the β-globin subunit, thereby changing the configuration of the hemoglobin molecule and enhancing the aggregation of hemoglobin molecules during cellular or tissue hypoxia, dehydration, or oxidative stress. This aggregation decreases the pliability of the erythrocytes and may distort their shape to a characteristic crescent or sickle, resulting in their premature destruction (hemolysis) and frequent, widespread vaso-occlusive episodes with subsequent acute and chronic organ damage. Sickle cell anemia occurs in those homozygous for HbS or in heterozygotes when HbS coexists with another abnormal hemoglobin (e.g., hemoglobin C, β-thal chains). *Sickle cell trait* occurs in those heterozygous for HbS when the other hemoglobin molecule is normal.

Sickle cell nephropathy describes the structural and functional abnormalities of the kidney in sickle cell disease.

SICKLE CELL DISEASE

Epidemiology

Sickle cell disease was first recognized in West Africa. The high prevalence of HbS in this region probably represents a survival benefit because the presence of sickle cell trait protects against malaria. Nowadays, sickle cell disease is a worldwide health problem because HbS has spread throughout Africa, around the Mediterranean, and to the Middle East and India as well as to the Caribbean, North America, and northern Europe. The prevalence of the sickle cell gene is about 8% in African Americans and about 25% in adult Nigerians and in some areas in equatorial Africa, Saudi Arabia, and India.

Restriction enzyme techniques have identified several hemoglobin S haplotypes, mutations of the HbS molecule, that have probably arisen independently of each other. There are four major types in Africa—the Benin, Senegal, Cameroon, and Bantu (or Central African Republic)—and one Asian haplotype. Variations in these haplotypes determine disease severity; for example, the Senegalese haplotype is associated with a higher hemoglobin F (HbF) concentration and has a better prognosis than others. In a sample population of Nigerians, Benin haplotype was detected in 92.3%.[1] Gender influences disease severity; female HbSS subjects with Benin haplotype have a higher HbF level than male subjects do.

Pathogenesis

Genetics

Sickle cell disease comprises a group of heterogenous disorders that share the presence of the gene for HbS, either homozygous (i.e., sickle cell anemia, HbSS) or double heterozygous (i.e., the combination of HbS with another abnormal hemoglobin).[2,3] Sickle cell anemia is the most common form. The most common double heterozygous disorders are the combinations of hemoglobin S with hemoglobin C (HbSC) and β-thalassemia (HbS-thal). Subjects with HbS-thal may produce reduced amounts of normal β chains (HbS–β^+-thal), but not always (HbS–β^0-thal). Subjects with a sickle cell trait or carrier state are heterozygous for HbS only.

Pathophysiology

The characteristic pathophysiologic feature in sickle cell disease is the episodic vaso-occlusive crisis, which can be triggered by several factors, including infection, hypoxia, hypovolemia, hypothermia, acidosis, and hyperosmolality. The common denominator is the occurrence of inflammation or cellular stress. The two key processes in the pathophysiology of vaso-occlusion are adhesive interactions between the sickle erythrocytes and the endothelium and the subsequent polymerization of HbS.

Sickle Cell Adherence Sickle cells have enhanced adherence to the endothelium compared with normal erythrocytes. This is increased by endothelial cell activation, from inflammation-associated proinflammatory cytokines such as tumor necrosis factor-α, interleukin-1β, and interferon-γ. Expression of leukocyte adhesion molecules on endothelial cells is induced, as is the release of procoagulant factors such as von Willebrand factor and thrombospondin (Fig. 49.1). The adhesion of sickle erythrocytes to the endothelium delays the capillary transit time, which allows polymerization of HbS and sickling to occur. Hypoxia distal to the occlusion further worsens the sickling process.

Polymerization of Hemoglobin S When HbS polymerizes, the hemoglobin molecules adhere to each other and aggregate into chain-like formations.[4] Polymerization changes the shape of the red cell, increases its rigidity, and causes sickling (Fig. 49.2). Polymerization is dynamic and depends on three independent variables: the degree of cellular hypoxia, the intracellular hemoglobin concentration, and the presence or absence of hemoglobin F (fetal hemoglobin, HbF).[4] Deoxygenation of HbS causes a change in the conformation of the β-globin subunits, which promotes the interaction of HbS molecules. The intracellular hemoglobin concentration can increase through cellular dehydration caused by membrane transport lesions, especially activated potassium-chloride cotransport and calcium-activated potassium efflux. The net efflux of potassium chloride leads to a decrease in intracellular volume, which increases the rate of HbS polymerization. Novel therapies minimizing the passive transport of cations may reduce cellular dehydration and consequent polymerization in experimental animals.[5] The presence of HbF decreases the polymerization tendency by reducing the concentration of HbS. Possible mechanisms of vaso-occlusion and ensuing vessel damage are shown in Figure 49.3.[6]

Clinical Manifestations

The clinical manifestations of sickle cell disease are individual and age dependent (Fig. 49.4). A chronic low-grade hemolytic anemia always occurs and predisposes to gallstones. The most prevalent clinical problem is periodic crises of bone pain. During the first years of life, it presents as the hand-foot syndrome, and in the course of life, it can result in avascular necrosis of the heads of the femur and humerus. Other disabling complications include stroke resulting from occlusion of major cerebral vessels, the acute chest syndrome, priapism, chronic leg ulceration, and chronic pulmonary disease with pulmonary hypertension.[7,8]

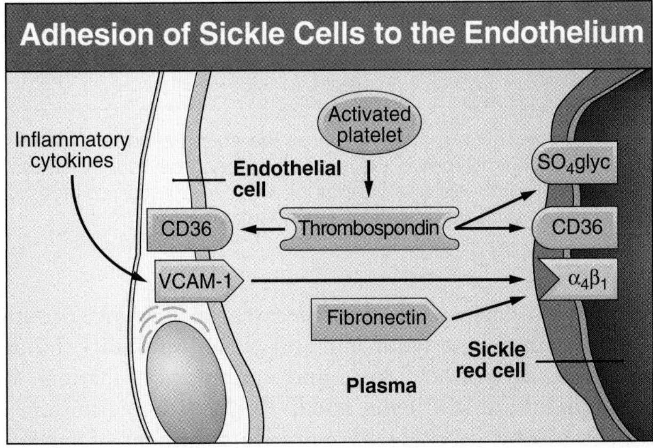

Figure 49.1 Principal interactions responsible for the adhesion of a sickle erythrocyte to the microvascular endothelium. Thrombospondin acts as a bridging molecule by binding to CD36 on the surface of an endothelial cell and to CD36 or sulfated glycans (SO$_4$glyc) on a sickle reticulocyte. Vascular cell adhesion molecule 1 (VCAM-1) on endothelial cells can bind directly to the $\alpha_4\beta_1$ integrin on the sickle reticulocyte. *(Modified with permission from reference 4.)*

Patients with sickle cell disease are prone to infections because of functional asplenia early in life as a result of splenic sequestration, recurrent splenic infarction, and consequent autosplenectomy. Ordinary bacterial infections, especially with encapsulated organisms, can be fatal in these patients. Bacterial isolates during invasive bacterial infections show *Streptococcus pneumoniae* (38%), *Salmonella* species (33%), *Haemophilus influenzae* (14%), *Escherichia coli* (11%), and *Klebsiella* species (4%).[9] *S. pneumoniae* and *H. influenzae* occur predominantly before 5 years of age, *Salmonella* increases almost linearly with age, and *Klebsiella* and *E. coli* predominate in patients older than 10 years. Pneumococcal infections carry high morbidity and mortality rates in the early years of life, necessitating vaccination or prophylaxis.[2]

Fever is common in patients with sickle cell disease. Common complications accompanying fever are painful crisis and acute chest syndrome. Bacteremia is not always confirmed, and in some cases, the fever may be viral in origin or related to infections due to atypical organisms. Nevertheless, early antibiotic treatment is recommended pending microbiologic information.

There are remarkable differences in clinical severity and outcome of disease. Sickle cell trait is a rather benign condition. Patients with HbSS tend to have more severe disease than do those with HbSC. Likewise, subjects with HbS–β^+-thal do better than those with HbS–β^0-thal. The Bantu haplotype is associated with the highest frequency of organ damage. However, the severity of disease may also differ among subjects with an identical genotype. In part, these differences can be explained by the amount of HbF present because it protects against clinical severity. In addition, endothelial factors probably play an important role. It has been shown that the degree of adherence between sickle erythrocytes and endothelial cells correlates with the clinical severity of disease. Also, a relation has been found between circulating activated endothelial cells of microvascular origin and the onset of painful sickle cell crises.[10]

Natural History

Life expectancy is reduced in sickle cell disease, especially in subjects with symptomatic disease. An increased risk for early death is associated with low levels of HbF, renal failure, the acute chest syndrome, and seizures.[8,11] Childhood survival to age 20 years has improved during the past decades. In the course of life, irreversible organ damage due to arterial and capillary microcirculation obstructive vasculopathy gradually becomes more prevalent. The diagnosis of a clinically evident form of organ damage, such as leg ulcer, osteonecrosis, or retinopathy, predicts the development of a more lethal form of organ damage, such as

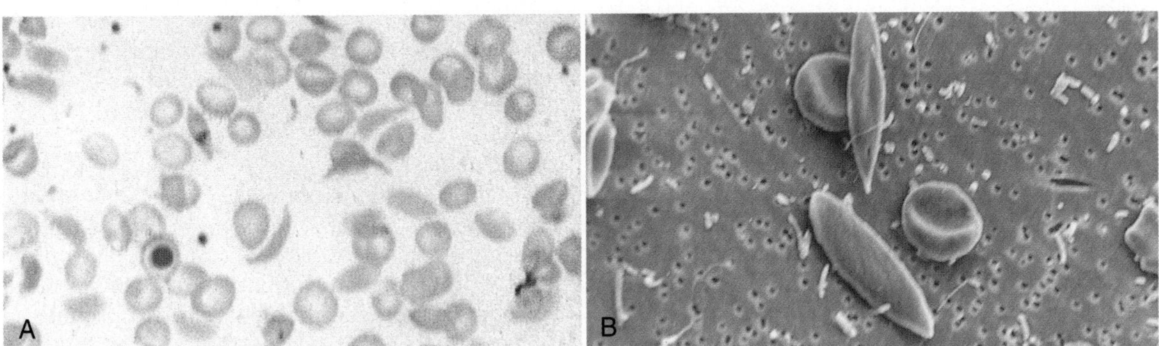

Figure 49.2 Sickle cells. A, Characteristic sickle cell erythrocytes in peripheral blood film of a patient with homozygous sickle cell anemia. **B,** Electron micrograph showing two normal and two sickle-shaped erythrocytes. *(Courtesy Professor Sally C. Davies.)*

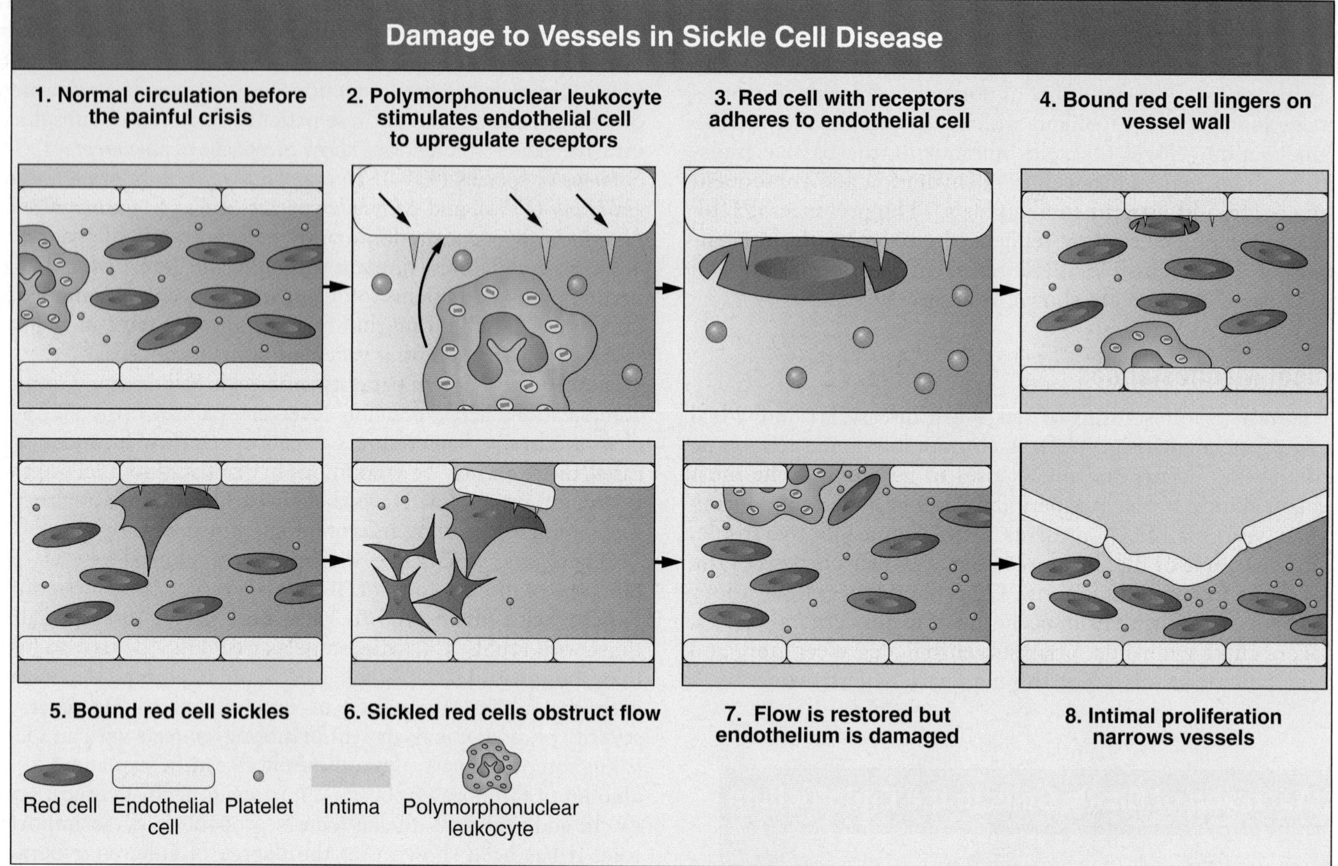
Damage to Vessels in Sickle Cell Disease
1. Normal circulation before the painful crisis
2. Polymorphonuclear leukocyte stimulates endothelial cell to upregulate receptors
3. Red cell with receptors adheres to endothelial cell
4. Bound red cell lingers on vessel wall
5. Bound red cell sickles
6. Sickled red cells obstruct flow
7. Flow is restored but endothelium is damaged
8. Intimal proliferation narrows vessels
Red cell
Endothelial cell
Platelet
Intima
Polymorphonuclear leukocyte

Figure 49.3 Pathophysiologic mechanisms of damage to vessels in sickle cell disease. Inflammation activates the endothelium and stimulates the upregulation of adhesion molecules and adherence of sickle cells to the endothelium. This promotes the sickling of erythrocytes, increases the blood viscosity, and causes sludging in the microcirculation (eventually with microvascular thrombosis and infarction). After restoration of blood flow, vascular remodeling may contribute to persistent impairment of tissue blood flow. *(Modified with permission from reference 6.)*

chronic lung disease, renal failure, or stroke.[12] Overall, the primary causes of death in patients with sickle cell anemia are chronic lung disease in 20%, renal failure in 14%, and stroke in 10%. In younger patients, the primary cause of death is infection; in older patients, the primary cause of death is irreversible organ damage (Fig. 49.5).

Treatment

Management of sickle cell disease is primarily directed at the relief of symptoms and prevention of complications, whereas newer treatments are being devised that target the pathophysiologic changes of the disease.[13] Daily oral penicillin for children 2 to 5 years of age is effective in reducing both the infection rate and the mortality related to pneumococcal infection.[14] Immunization against pneumococcus is recommended for children at 2 years of age, with booster doses at 5 years of age, although protection from current vaccines is imperfect. Immunization against influenza in children is also important.

Empiric broad-spectrum antibiotics effective against gram-positive and gram-negative organisms should be used in adults with fever pending microbiologic confirmation. A commonly prescribed antibiotic is amoxicillin.

Sickle cell crises are managed with oxygen therapy, rehydration with intravenous fluids, red cell transfusions, and analgesia. In severe cases, exchange red cell transfusions may be effective. Hydroxyurea treatment in subjects with sickle cell anemia and recurrent vaso-occlusive events decreases the incidence of painful crises and acute chest syndrome and overall mortality; butyrate compounds, deoxyazacytidine, and various combinations with erythropoietin are still being tried.[13,15] Hematopoietic stem cell transplantation is a potentially curative treatment of sickle cell disease; it is associated with an 80% to 85% disease-free survival rate in several series.[16] Young and presymptomatic patients with high-risk features of severe disease benefit the most from hematopoietic stem cell transplantation.

SICKLE CELL NEPHROPATHY

Pathogenesis

The hallmark of sickle cell nephropathy is the combination of impaired renal concentrating capacity and a normal diluting capacity.[17,18]

Concentrating Capacity

The defect in concentrating capacity results from loss of the countercurrent exchange mechanism in the inner renal medulla through loss of the vasa recta and long loops of Henle of the juxtamedullary nephrons (Fig. 49.6). The vasa recta of the juxtamedullary nephrons present an ideal setting for sickling. The renal medulla is relatively hypoxic and hyperosmotic, the blood viscosity is increased in the medullary circulation, and medullary blood flow is slow. Studies in transgenic sickle cell

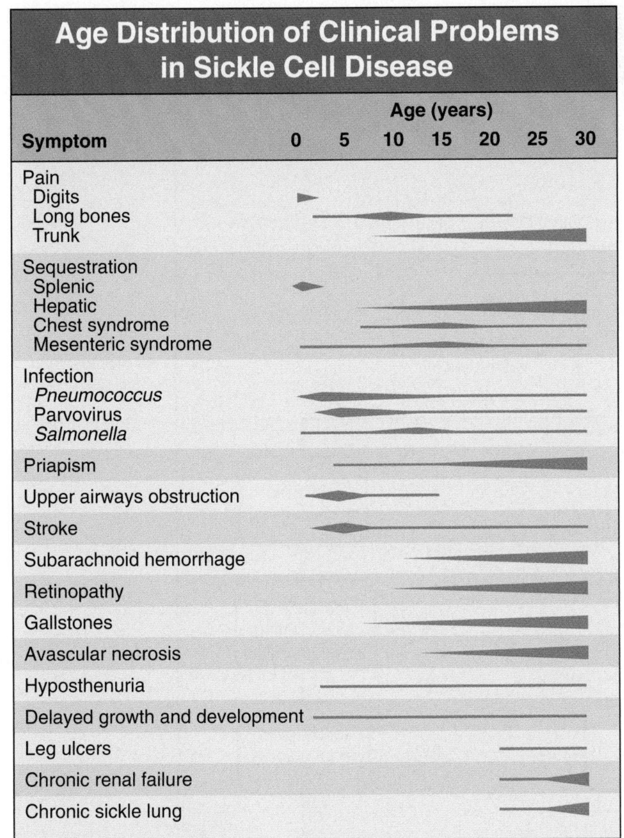

Figure 49.4 Age distribution of clinical problems in sickle cell disease. *(Modified with permission from reference 2.)*

mice have demonstrated distention and congestion of the vasa recta under hypoxic conditions. This environment facilitates the sickling of erythrocytes, formation of intravascular microthrombi, and obstruction of blood flow through the vasa recta. The loss of vasa recta has been confirmed by microradioangiographic studies (Fig. 49.7).[19] Histologic examination of the medulla shows edema, focal scarring, and interstitial fibrosis resulting in tubular atrophy. Ischemic infarction in the vasa recta sometimes causes papillary necrosis. The concentration defect is found to be reversible in young children when sickling is prevented after multiple transfusions of normal blood, but it becomes irreversible thereafter. Adults with sickle cell anemia cannot concentrate the urine above 450 mOsm/kg H_2O. This relates to the interstitial osmolality at the transition of the outer and inner medulla, at the tips of the short loops of Henle of the cortical nephrons. Subjects with sickle cell trait or hybrid sickling disorders show intermediate concentrating defects. Maximal osmolality varies from 400 to 900 mOsm/kg H_2O in sickle cell trait and from 400 to 700 mOsm/kg H_2O in HbSC and declines further with aging.

Diluting Capacity

The diluting capacity is normal as a result of the intact reabsorptive function of the superficial loops of Henle of the cortical nephrons. These are supplied by peritubular capillaries, which present a less ideal setting for sickling than the vasa recta. In contrast to the diluting capacity, the free water reabsorption, or capacity to generate negative free water balance, is impaired by defective trapping of solute in the inner medulla.

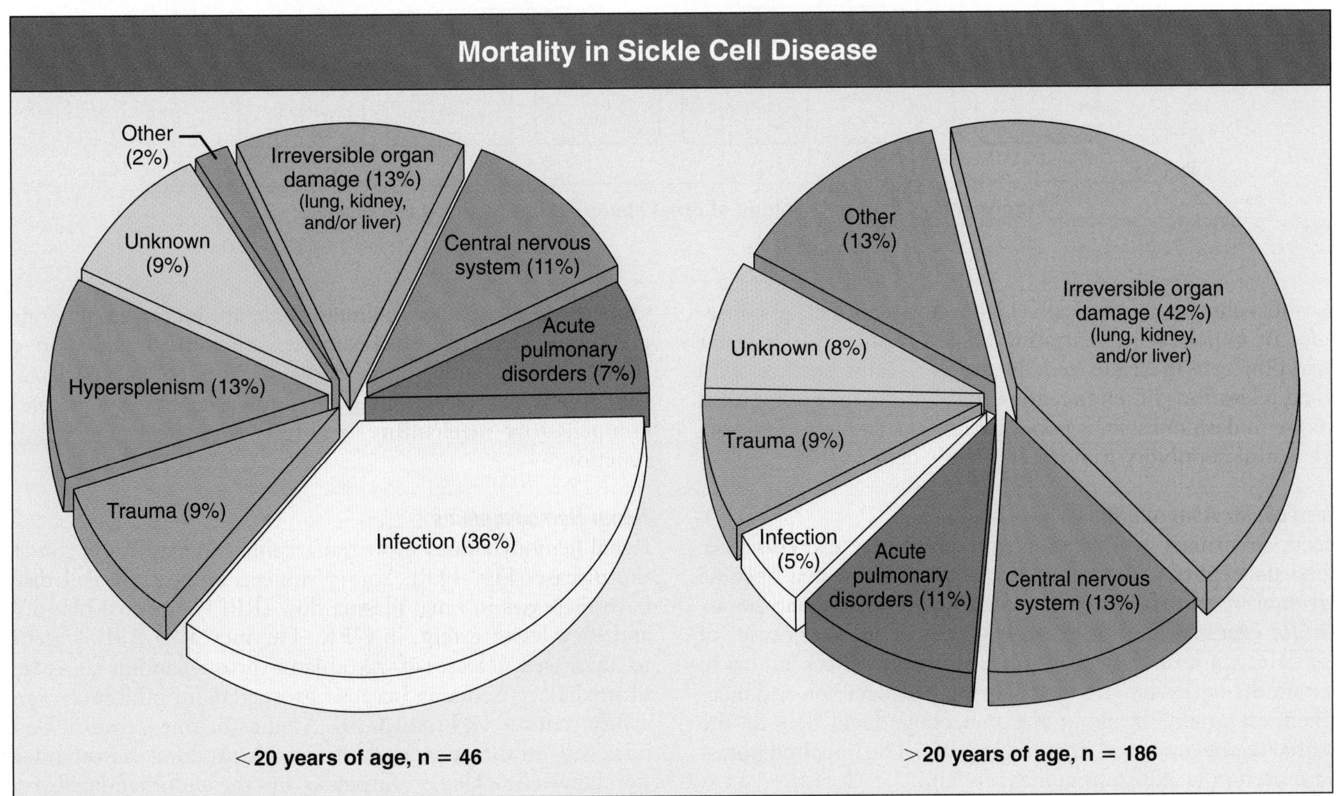

Figure 49.5 Mortality in sickle cell disease. Causes of death among 232 HbSS patients, comparing patients younger than 20 years (46 died) with patients older than 20 years (186 died). The infection category includes both bacterial and viral diseases. *(Modified with permission from reference 12.)*

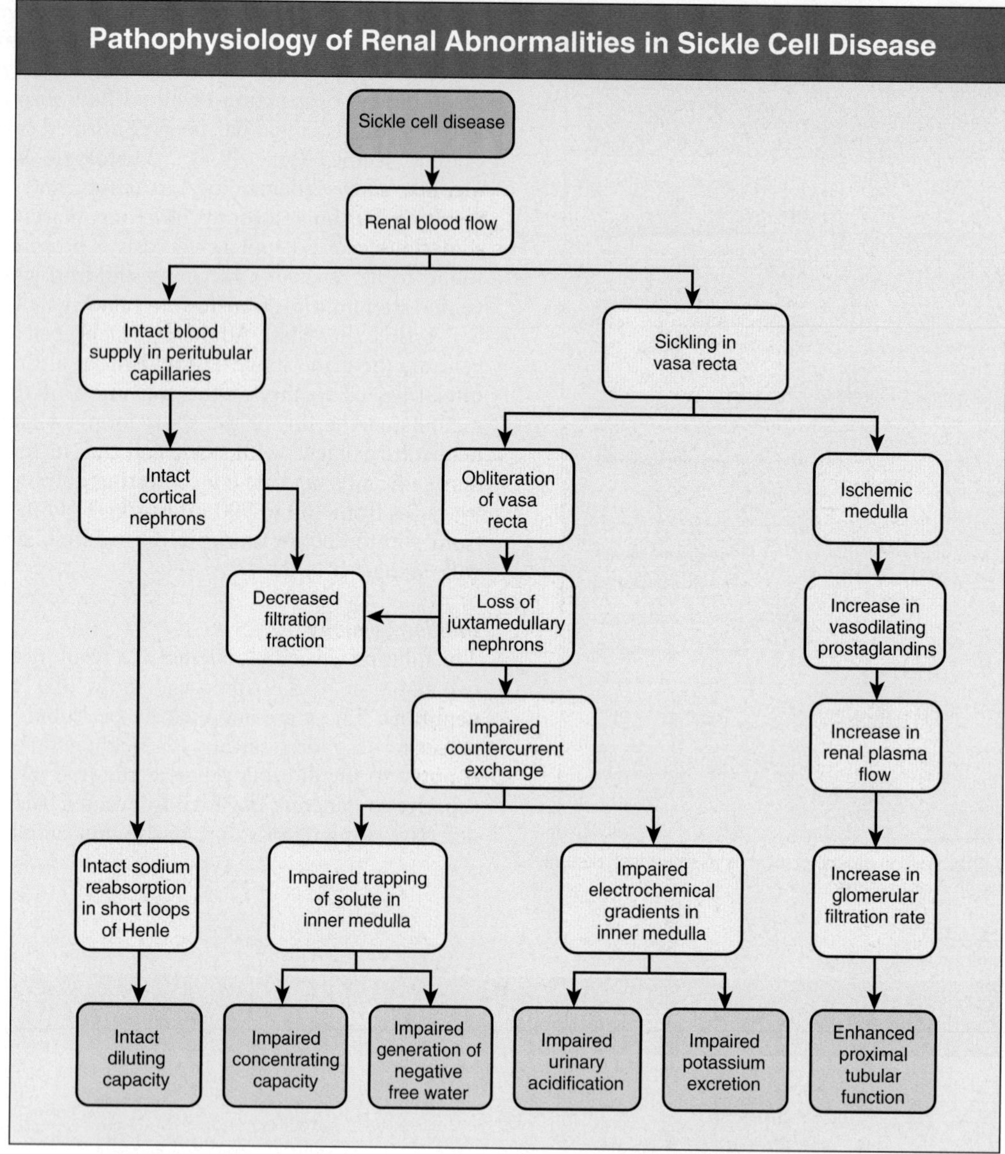

Figure 49.6 Pathophysiology of renal abnormalities in sickle cell disease.

Urine volumes are typically higher than normal, a consequence of impaired concentrating ability. Response to a water deprivation test in sickle cell disease is usually positive with marked elevation of endogenous antidiuretic hormone, and response to desmopressin is poor. Because isosthenuria is typical, there is a susceptibility to normonatremic dehydration.

Other Tubular Abnormalities

Defects in urinary acidification and potassium excretion are other distal nephron function abnormalities.[18] These may become overt only when there is an increased supply of acid and potassium, for example, during rhabdomyolysis. The exact causes of these defects are unknown, but they probably reflect failure to maintain the necessary energy-requiring hydrogen ion and electrochemical gradients along the collecting ducts due to the impaired medullary blood flow and hypoxia. The impaired potassium excretion is aldosterone independent.

In contrast to the functional abnormalities of the distal nephron, proximal tubular function is enhanced. Reabsorption of phosphate and β_2-microglobulin and secretion of uric acid and creatinine in the proximal tubule are increased. Therefore, creatinine clearance overestimates glomerular filtration rate (GFR) considerably. The cause of the enhanced proximal function is not clear, but it probably represents a secondary compensatory mechanism to correct for defects in medullary function.

Renal Hemodynamics

Renal hemodynamics show remarkable changes in the course of the disease (Fig. 49.8). Young subjects with sickle cell disease have increases in renal plasma flow (RPF) and renal blood flow and, to a lesser extent, in GFR. The increased RPF is ascribed to increased release of vasodilator prostaglandins as a result of medullary ischemia because prostaglandin inhibition significantly reduces RPF and GFR. Studies in transgenic sickle cell mice suggest that increased nitric oxide production from interaction between sickled erythrocytes and the endothelium also contributes to renal vasodilation. The decrease in filtration fraction may be caused by selective damage of juxtamedullary nephrons, which have the highest filtration fractions.

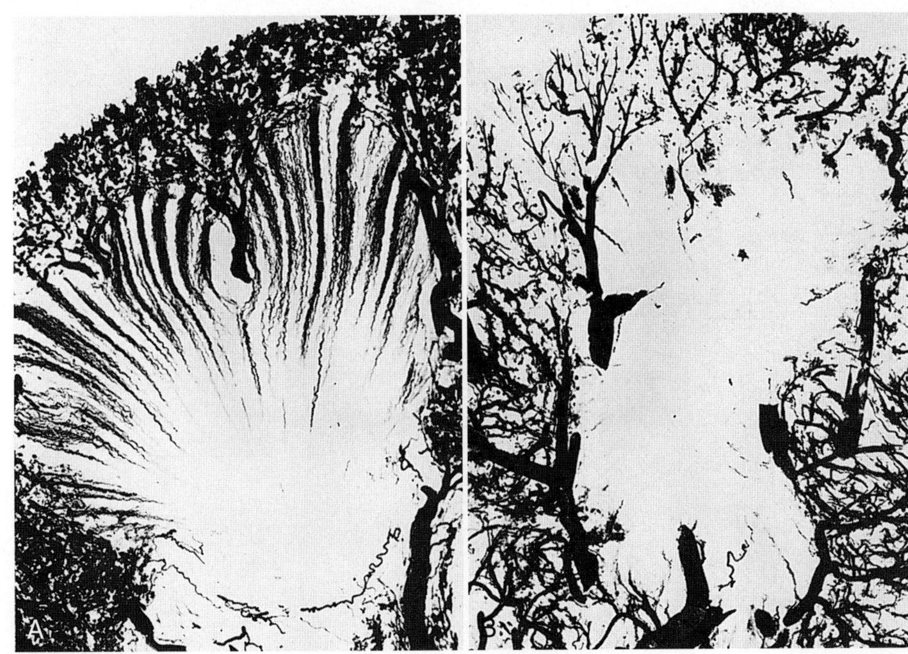

Figure 49.7 Microradioangiography showing loss of vasa recta in sickle cell nephropathy. A, Kidney from a control subject showing normal vasa recta. **B,** A patient with sickle cell anemia, with the absence of the vasa recta. *(Modified with permission from reference 19.)*

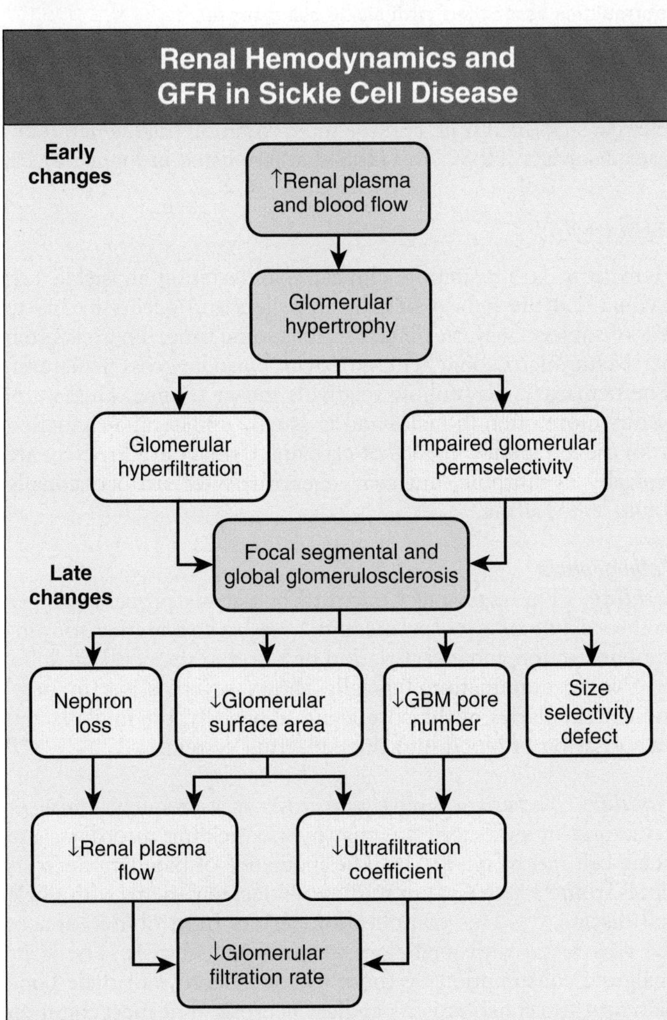

Figure 49.8 Renal hemodynamics and glomerular filtration in sickle cell nephropathy. GBM, glomerular basement membrane; GFR, glomerular filtration rate.

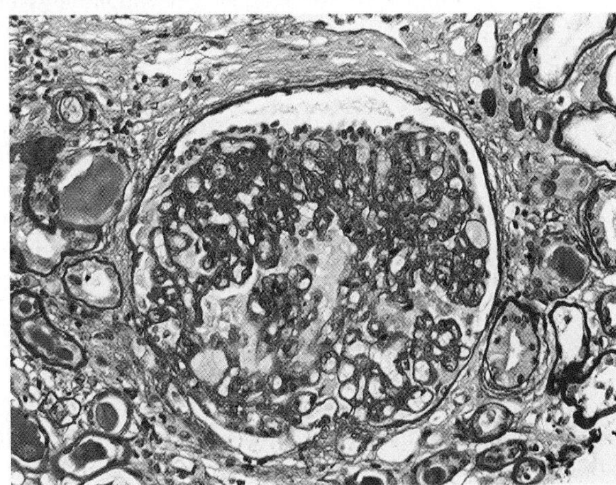

Figure 49.9 Focal segmental glomerulosclerosis in sickle cell nephropathy. Segmental sclerosis involving the upper half of the glomerulus. *(Courtesy Professor J. Weening.)*

Glomerular Injury

Glomerular hypertrophy is an early manifestation of sickle cell nephropathy. Histologic examination of the kidneys of young children shows glomerular enlargement and congestion, especially in the juxtamedullary glomeruli. Both afferent and efferent arterioles of these glomeruli may be dilated. In young adult patients with sickle cell anemia, there is a distinct pattern of glomerular dysfunction, with impaired glomerular permselectivity, increased ultrafiltration coefficient, glomerular hyperfiltration, and proteinuria.[20,21] Prolonged glomerular hyperfiltration may cause further glomerular injury. This is supported by the common histologic finding of focal segmental glomerulosclerosis (FSGS) in adult patients with sickle cell disease (Fig. 49.9).[22] Two patterns of FSGS have been described: a "collapsing" and an "expansive" pattern.[23] The initial collapsing pattern has been attributed to progressive obliteration of glomerular capillaries by red blood cell sickling in maximally hypertrophied glomeruli. The expansive pattern is characterized by an expansive sclerosis with increased mesangial matrix and further capillary obliteration; it is ascribed to sustained or increasing hyperfiltration.[23]

Frequencies and Etiology of Renal Abnormalities Associated with Sickle Cell Disease				
Type of Renal Disease	**Etiology**	**Sickle Cell Anemia**	**Sickle Cell Trait**	**HbSC and HbS-thal**
Impaired concentrating capacity	Loss of vasa recta of juxtamedullary nephrons	Irreversible defects in all adults	Intermediate defects in all adults' nephrons	Intermediate defects in all adults
Impaired urinary acidification	Incomplete form of distal renal tubular acidosis	Almost all, during acid loading	Rare	At least 30%, during acid loading
Impaired potassium excretion	Aldosterone independent	Almost all, during potassium loading	Rare	Unknown; probably at least 30%
Hematuria	Infarction, extravasation of blood in renal medulla	Common	3%–4%	Common
Proteinuria	Glomerular hyperfiltration plus impaired permselectivity	Up to 50%–60% with increasing age	Rare	20%–25%
Nephrotic syndrome	FSGS most common	About 4%	Rare	0%–4%
Chronic renal failure	See Figure 49.8	4.2%–4.6%	Rare	About 2.4%
Renal medullary carcinoma	Possible genetic predisposition	Rare	Absolutely rare, relatively frequent	Rare

Figure 49.10 Frequencies and etiology of renal abnormalities associated with sickle cell disease.

In older subjects, progressive ischemia and fibrosis with obliteration of glomeruli can be found. Glomerular function studies show a decrease in glomerular basement membrane pore number and a size selectivity defect in subjects with renal impairment.[24] Ultimately, a combined decrease in ultrafiltration capacity and RPF can result in end-stage renal disease (ESRD).[20]

Hormones in Sickle Cell Nephropathy

There is relative erythropoietin (EPO) deficiency in sickle cell disease; that is, EPO levels do not increase to the expected level for the degree of anemia, perhaps because of the right-shifted hemoglobin-oxygen dissociation curve. In addition, EPO levels fall with the decline in renal function, probably as a result of renal damage due to the sickling process.

Elevated serum renin and aldosterone have been reported in some studies, under standard and volume-depleted conditions, although in general normal values are found in sickle cell anemia.[17]

Hormone infusion studies have helped to localize sites of action in the kidney. Failure of low-dose infusion of atrial natriuretic peptide (ANP) to increase natriuresis in sickle cell anemia[25] suggests that ANP at this dosage exerts its natriuretic effect in the long loops of Henle of the juxtamedullary nephrons, whereas insulin induces a similar sodium retention in patients with sickle cell anemia and normal subjects,[25] suggesting that its antinatriuretic effect is probably localized at a distal tubular site other than the long loops of Henle. Urinary endothelin 1 is elevated in asymptomatic sickle cell disease patients. It correlates with a urine concentrating defect and microalbuminuria.[26]

CLINICAL MANIFESTATIONS OF SICKLE CELL NEPHROPATHY

The presentation of the clinical manifestations of sickle cell nephropathy shows an age-dependent pattern. The frequency and etiology of the renal abnormalities associated with sickle cell anemia, sickle cell trait, and the most common double heterozygous disorders (HbSC and HbS-thal) are listed in Figure 49.10.

Hematuria

Hematuria is a common clinical manifestation in sickle cell anemia and the hybrid sickling disorders and occurs in 3% to 4% of subjects with sickle cell trait at some time. There is often persistent microscopic hematuria with episodic gross hematuria. The hematuria may follow relatively minor trauma. Hematuria occurs more often in males and is usually unilateral, originating from the left kidney in 80% of patients. Urinary erythrocytes are typically isomorphic, but sickled erythrocytes are occasionally found in the urine.

Pathogenesis

Sickling The main mechanism of hematuria probably relates to the sickling of erythrocytes in the vasa recta and microthrombotic infarction and extravasation of blood in the renal medulla. Histologic examination typically shows severe stasis in peritubular capillaries of the cortex and, especially, the medulla and extravasation of blood into the collecting system.

Papillary Necrosis Papillary necrosis is a frequent cause of hematuria in sickle cell anemia, hybrid sickling disorders, and sickle cell trait (Fig. 49.11). The incidence of papillary necrosis varies from 23% to 67% in studies of selected patients with sickle cell disease.[18,27] This complication results from obliteration of the vasa recta, with medullary necrosis and fibrosis. The large analgesic consumption by these patients because of their bone pain may also contribute to papillary necrosis. The most common presenting symptom is painless macroscopic hematuria. Other presentations are renal colic caused by the passage of blood clots or necrotic papillae, microscopic hematuria, symptoms of urinary tract infection, and, rarely, acute renal failure. Papillary necrosis may also be asymptomatic and is frequently an incidental finding during imaging.

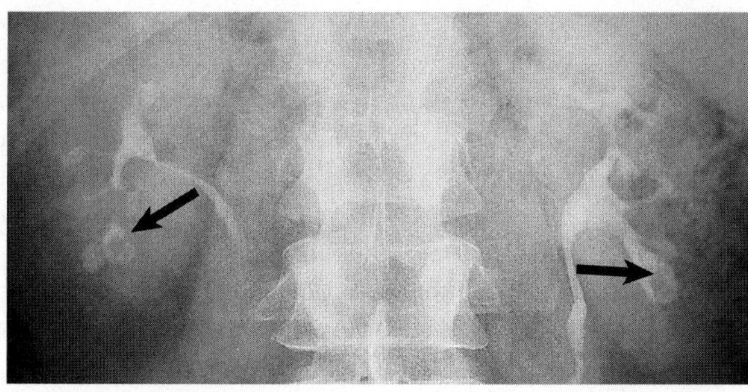

Figure 49.11 Papillary necrosis in sickle cell disease. Intravenous urography shows abnormal calyces with filling defects *(arrows).*

Nutcracker Phenomenon The left-sided predominance of hematuria has been attributed to the so-called nutcracker phenomenon, compression of the left renal vein between the aorta and the superior mesenteric artery, thereby increasing the pressure in the renal vein. This may especially contribute to the development of hematuria in sickle cell patients because the increased renal vein pressure could worsen anoxia in the renal medulla, thereby increasing the likelihood of sickling in the left kidney.

Clinical Manifestations

Painless macroscopic hematuria often presents after physical activity or minor renal trauma or is associated with hypoxic challenges, for example, airplane flights. It usually is accompanied by a substantial fall in hematocrit. Bleeding typically remits spontaneously within a few days.

Diagnosis and Differential Diagnosis

Urinalysis can exclude the presence of myoglobinuria and rhabdomyolysis, which can mimic hematuria. Rhabdomyolysis can be provoked during strenuous exercise and dehydration and may also occur during severe sickle cell crises. The coexistence of hematuria with leukocyturia is not unusual and does not necessarily indicate a urinary tract infection, even in combination with flank pain. Infection must be confirmed by examination of the urinary sediment and urine cultures.

Sickle cell trait has been reported in 50% of African Americans with ESRD caused by autosomal dominant polycystic kidney disease (ADPKD) but in only 7.5% of African American patients with other causes of ESRD. In addition, patients with ADPKD and sickle cell trait had an earlier onset of ESRD.[28] The prevalence of sickle cell disease in ADPKD has not been reported.

Recently, renal medullary carcinoma has been recognized as a specific entity in sickle cell nephropathy.[18,29] It is an aggressive form of renal cell carcinoma that appears uniquely to affect patients with sickle cell hemoglobinopathies, particularly sickle cell trait or HbSC, especially in teenagers and young adults. Chronic medullary hypoxia is thought to contribute to its pathogenesis.[9] The tumors are resistant to chemotherapy and tend to be metastatic at the time of diagnosis, with a reported mean survival from the time of surgery of only 15 weeks. It is not yet clear whether regular screening for renal medullary carcinoma in young patients with sickle cell disease or trait could result in an early diagnosis and a better survival.[29] Gross hematuria, flank pain, and weight loss are ominous signs of malignancy, particularly in young patients with sickle cell trait. The tumor is typically located deep in the parenchyma, unlike Wilms' tumor or renal cell carcinoma. Immunohistochemical analysis for epithelial cell markers (e.g., CAM 5.5), epithelial membrane antigen, and cytokeratin may assist in diagnosis.

von Willebrand disease has occasionally been described in subjects with sickle cell trait and gross hematuria.

Further evaluation is indicated for patients with severe or prolonged hematuria that is resistant to conservative therapeutic measures. Ultrasound examination will be normal unless there is papillary necrosis or a coincidental cause of hematuria, such as polycystic kidney disease, renal calculus, or tumor. Intravenous urography used to be the method of choice for diagnosis of papillary necrosis, but it does not distinguish reliably between papillary necrosis and other causes of filling defects in the pyelogram, including blood clots, neoplasm, calculus, and hemangioma. Ultrasound is therefore preferred, although it is suggested that contrast-enhanced computed tomography may better depict a full range of typical features.[30] The role of magnetic resonance imaging in this setting has not yet been sufficiently evaluated.

Cystoscopy is not routinely required but is indicated if the episode of hematuria is atypical, for example, a first episode of macroscopic hematuria in a patient older than 40 years or an episode that persists for more than 2 weeks. Cystoscopy may also be required to lateralize the source of the bleeding if surgical intervention is considered (see later).

Renal angiography only rarely identifies the bleeding source, but when it does so, it can be followed by embolization. However, the optimal approach in any institution depends on local experience with specific techniques.

Treatment

The therapeutic strategy for hematuria depends on the severity and duration of a specific bleeding episode. Bleeding will stop in most patients spontaneously or after a period of bed rest, although it may occasionally last for weeks or months. About half of patients will have recurrent episodes.

Initial therapeutic measures include bed rest and interventions aimed at retardation of the sickling process in the anoxic renal medulla. A high urine flow rate should be induced by intravenous fluid administration and diuretics to further reduce medullary tonicity and the urine alkalinized by administration of sodium bicarbonate by mouth or by vein, with a target urine pH of 8. Blood transfusion with normal HbA is indicated if anemia becomes severe; this may also decrease the sickling process. If necessary, bladder irrigation is performed for removal of blood clots.

Hyperbaric oxygen therapy may be helpful but has not been formally evaluated. Irrigation of the pelvicalyceal system with silver nitrate has also been described. The antifibrinolytic agent ε-aminocaproic acid, although effective, may be associated with adverse renal outcomes and is not recommended.

Unilateral nephrectomy has occasionally been necessary in patients with persistent, life-threatening hematuria refractory to conservative approaches. Full evaluation for another cause of hematuria, including cystoscopy to exclude a bladder lesion and to establish which kidney is the source of bleeding, is required before proceeding with nephrectomy.

Urinary Tract Infection

Subjects with sickle cell disease have an increased susceptibility to bacterial infections; even low-grade bacteremia with a common organism may be fatal. In addition to the impaired immunity that is a consequence of autosplenectomy, there is opsonic antibody deficiency, which predisposes to bacterial infections. The precise incidence of urinary tract infections is not well defined. However, the incidence of asymptomatic bacteriuria during pregnancy and the puerperium appears to be twice as high in women with sickle cell disease or trait as in women without sickle cell disease and requires appropriate therapy (see Chapter 42).

Pyelonephritis and urosepsis, like any other infection, may precipitate a sickle cell crisis. One should especially be aware of this possibility in young children, who often do not complain of urinary tract symptoms. Most common organisms isolated include *E. coli*, *Klebsiella* species, and other gram-negative Enterobacteriaceae. Invasive bacterial infections with *E. coli* occur especially in females after the age of 15 years, suggesting a greater chance of urinary tract infections in relation to sexual activity.

Acute Kidney Injury

People with sickle cell disease sometimes present with features of acute kidney injury (AKI). AKI, defined as a doubling of serum creatinine, is reported in 10% of hospitalized patients with sickle cell anemia.[31] A potentially reversible renal dysfunction with significant reduction in GFR could occur during vaso-occlusive crises.[32]

Etiology

A prerenal cause of AKI will be found in more than half of patients, especially volume depletion in the setting of sickle cell crisis. Patients with sickle cell disease are prone to AKI caused by volume depletion because of impaired urine concentrating capacity; it is therefore typically nonoliguric. A less frequent prerenal cause is congestive heart failure.

Typical intrinsic renal causes of AKI are rhabdomyolysis, sepsis, and drug nephrotoxicity. Less common are renal vein thrombosis and hepatorenal syndrome (caused by hemosiderosis-induced hepatic failure). Both exertional and nontraumatic rhabdomyolysis have been reported in patients with sickle cell disease; the latter especially occurs during a sickle cell crisis and has been ascribed to intravascular sickling and muscle ischemia. Rhabdomyolysis is a common finding in patients who develop multiorgan failure during severe sickle cell crises, in addition to the acute chest syndrome, which further contributes to AKI. The most typical postrenal cause of AKI is urinary tract obstruction by necrotic papillae or blood clots.

Treatment

Treatment and recovery of renal function depend on the specific underlying pathologic process. Metabolic acidosis may be prominent and should be actively corrected with sodium bicarbonate. Patients with volume depletion have a favorable outcome after fluid replacement.[31] Renal function may recover in patients with sepsis and rhabdomyolysis, although temporary renal replacement therapy may be necessary. AKI as a part of multiorgan failure during a severe sickle cell crisis may show a dramatic improvement with aggressive red cell transfusion therapy, although some renal function loss may persist.

Proteinuria and Nephrotic Syndrome

Microalbuminuria has been reported in 19% to 26% of children with sickle cell anemia.[33,34] The presence of microalbuminuria is directly related to age and inversely related to hemoglobin levels. Proteinuria has been reported in 17% to 33% of subjects with sickle cell disease by semiquantitative or dipstick measurement.[8] The prevalence of proteinuria is lower in subjects with coinheritance of sickle cell anemia and α-thalassemia than in those with sickle cell anemia and intact α-globin genes (13% versus 40%).[35] The "renoprotective" effect of α-globin gene microdeletions could be related to a lower mean corpuscular volume or lower erythrocyte hemoglobin concentration in sickle erythrocytes. The frequency of proteinuria increases with age (56% in subjects ≥40 years), and its presence is associated with renal impairment.

The nephrotic syndrome has been estimated to occur in 4% of patients with sickle cell anemia. The eventual development of renal failure appears virtually inevitable once the patient has nephrotic syndrome.

Pathology

The most common pathologic lesion is FSGS,[22,23] which is also the major lesion in patients who develop renal failure. Another specific pathologic lesion is a form of membranoproliferative glomerulonephritis (MPGN) with mesangial expansion and basement membrane duplication.[3] The general absence of immune complexes and electron-dense deposits discriminates this entity from idiopathic MPGN type I. It has been proposed that this form of MPGN is caused by intracapillary red cell fragmentation. Fragments of erythrocytes become lodged in isolated capillary loops and are continuously phagocytosed by mesangial cells. As a result, the mesangium expands and lays down new basement membrane material.

Patients may become hepatitis C positive from multiple blood transfusions, which may also be associated with MPGN, although it is rare with appropriate screening procedures before transfusion. In our series, hepatitis C positivity was observed in only 1 patient (0.26%), a reflection of the generally low seroprevalence rate in the environment.[8] On occasion, other causes have been reported, such as poststreptococcal glomerulonephritis, minimal change disease, and immune complex–mediated glomerulonephritis. Glomerulonephritis has also been described in association with aplastic crises in parvovirus infection. Renal vein thrombosis should be considered when nephrotic syndrome develops in sickle cell disease, but its incidence is not exactly known.

Treatment

Theoretically, dietary protein restriction may reduce hyperfiltration and retard the development of renal failure in those with FSGS, but this has not been evaluated specifically in sickle cell disease.

Short-term treatment with angiotensin-converting enzyme (ACE) inhibitors significantly reduces the degree of proteinuria without affecting blood pressure or renal hemodynamics. More prolonged ACE inhibition reduces proteinuria with a slight decrease in blood pressure. However, it remains to be established whether long-term treatment with ACE inhibitors or angiotensin receptor blockers (ARBs) delays the development of progressive renal failure. Combinations of ACE inhibitor and hydroxyurea have been found to be useful in retarding progression of microalbuminuria to overt proteinuria.[33,34,36]

Prevention of hyperfiltration can, theoretically, also be obtained with nonsteroidal anti-inflammatory drugs (NSAIDs), but these drugs reduce RPF and GFR in sickle cell anemia and are thus contraindicated.

Sodium and Acid-Base Disturbances

Distal Tubular Function

Impaired potassium excretion and impaired urinary acidification are caused by an incomplete form of distal tubular acidosis.

However, hyperkalemia and metabolic acidosis are not present under normal circumstances and may become manifested only during potassium or acid loading, with mild renal impairment or volume depletion, and during rhabdomyolysis.[17,18] Hyperkalemia may also develop more readily during treatment with NSAIDs, ACE inhibitors, β-blockers, potassium-sparing diuretics, or heparin.

Urine pH does not fall below 5 during acid loading tests unless maximal acidifying stimuli are used. The titratable acid and hydrogen ion excretion is reduced, whereas the ammonium excretion is either normal or decreased. Metabolic acidosis that develops during renal impairment or intercurrent diseases in sickle cell disease requires active treatment with sodium bicarbonate because acidosis stimulates the sickling process. Plasma bicarbonate should be monitored routinely and oral sodium bicarbonate supplements given to keep it within the reference range.

Proximal Tubular Function

Proximal tubular function abnormalities modify solute handling, producing increased reabsorption of phosphate and increased secretion of uric acid. Hyperphosphatemia may develop easily when renal function declines, necessitating dietary phosphate restriction and the use of phosphate binders early in renal impairment. The increased uric acid secretion protects patients with sickle cell disease against hyperuricemia, with elevated uric acid production resulting from hemolysis. However, the incidence of hyperuricemia and risk for gout increase with age as renal function declines.

Hypertension

Epidemiology

The prevalence of hypertension in patients with sickle cell anemia is about 2% to 6%, which is significantly lower than in age- and sex-matched control subjects.[8,17,37] However, blood pressure in patients with sickle cell anemia is higher than in matched subjects with β-thalassemia and similar degrees of anemia. Hypertension in sickle cell anemia especially occurs in the presence of advanced renal failure.

Pathogenesis

It is not yet clear whether the relative hypotension compared with control subjects relates to the pathologic renal medullary condition in sickle cell disease or to other mechanisms. The kidney in sickle cell disease has a normal overall capacity for sodium conservation, despite a tendency to lose sodium and water through the medullary defect.[17,37] This sodium conservation in sickle cell disease may follow stimulation of the renin-angiotensin system, which has been described in some but not all studies. The relative hypotension may be related to general vasodilation because skeletal vascular resistance is reduced in sickle cell patients. Increased production of vasodilatory prostaglandins or nitric oxide may be involved. Systemic vasodilation and increased flow is a compensatory mechanism for microcirculatory flow disturbances and intermittent microvascular occlusion.[38] Finally, reduced vascular reactivity has been demonstrated in sickle cell patients and may protect against blood pressure elevation.[37]

Treatment

The antihypertensive treatment of choice is an ACE inhibitor or ARB because of the potential beneficial effects on the progression of proteinuria and renal failure and because of the reported increments in plasma renin activity. However, the risk for hyperkalemia is increased. There are no specific recommendations on target blood pressure in sickle cell disease, and the targets for other nondiabetic nephropathies are appropriate.

An alternative therapeutic option is a calcium channel blocker, but those recognized to worsen proteinuria, like the short-acting dihydropyridines, should be avoided. Loop diuretics are less effective in patients with sickle cell disease because of the specific medullary defect.

Chronic Kidney Disease

Epidemiology

In a prospective, 25-year longitudinal study, chronic kidney disease (CKD) developed in 4.2% of 725 patients with sickle cell anemia and in 2.4% of 209 patients with HbSC.[39] The patients with sickle cell anemia were much younger at the time of the diagnosis of renal failure than those with HbSC (median age, 23.1 and 49.9 years, respectively). However, in another study of 368 patients with sickle cell anemia with an overall prevalence of CKD of 4.6%, the prevalence of CKD clearly increased with age.[40] The prevalence of CKD will probably increase even more in the future with further improved medical care and longer life expectancy. In our series, younger age at diagnosis and higher duration of sickle cell disease were found to strongly predict the development of nephropathy.[8]

Predictors of CKD are hypertension, proteinuria, hematuria, increasingly severe anemia, the nephrotic syndrome, and inheritance of the Bantu or Central African Republic β-globin gene cluster haplotype.[39] Apart from an apparent genetic predisposition, glomerular capillary hypertension and prolonged glomerular hyperfiltration seem to be important in the development of renal failure.

Natural History

Patients with sickle cell anemia and CKD have an increased mortality rate compared with patients without renal failure (Fig. 49.12). Patients with renal failure are also prone to

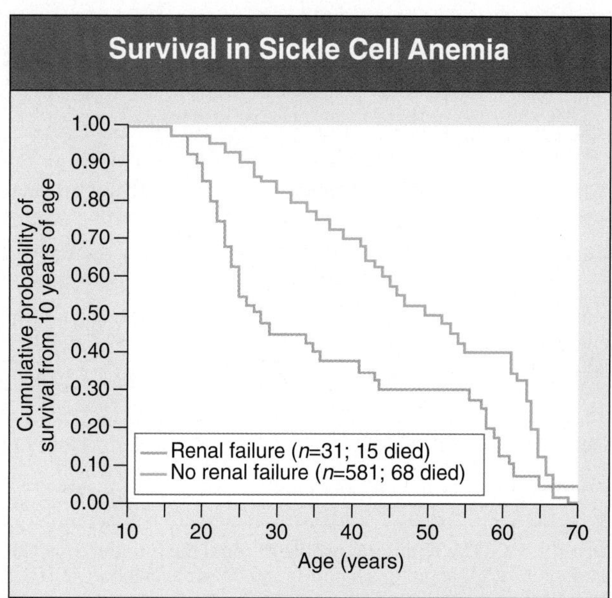

Figure 49.12 Survival in sickle cell anemia in the presence and absence of renal failure. *(Modified with permission from reference 40.)*

other manifestations of sickle-induced vasculopathy, such as cerebrovascular diseases, chronic restrictive lung disease, and leg ulcers, leading to frequent hospitalizations.[39] In the United States Renal Data System, patients with sickle cell nephropathy and ESRD had an increased mortality risk (hazard ratio, 1.52; 95% confidence interval, 1.27-1.82) compared with other patients with ESRD. However, patients with sickle cell nephropathy were less likely to receive renal transplantation, and the increased mortality risk did not persist after adjustment for transplantation.[41] As nephropathy progresses in sickle cell disease, strategies aimed at retarding progression and preparations for eventual renal replacement therapy should be initiated. The changing profile of renal dysfunction in sickle cell disease with age and available treatment options are summarized in Figure 49.13.[18]

Treatment

To delay the development of progressive renal failure, it is important to control hypertension and to avoid the use of nephrotoxic drugs, especially NSAIDs. Although plausible, it remains to be established whether the reduction of the degree of proteinuria with either ACE inhibitors or a low-protein diet retards the progression of renal failure.

The response to EPO therapy is poor, even when high doses are used during long treatment periods. EPO treatment predominantly results in the release of HbS-containing reticulocytes, with only a modest increase in the more stable HbF. A marked increase in hemoglobin levels, although unexpected, may precipitate sickle cell crisis. Routine use of EPO is therefore not recommended, but it can be tried on an individual basis with higher doses than needed in other forms of ESRD. As an

The Changing Profile of Renal Dysfunction in Sickle Cell Disease with Age and Available Treatment Options

Average Age (years)	Clinical Observations	Process	Modifiers + ameliorates – worsens	Treatment Options
1	Anemia, pain	Sickling	HbF Level (+)	Hypertransfusion, hydroxyurea, zinc supplements
			Level of aberrant β-globin (±)	β-globin gene therapy
			Increased HbA level (+)	Bone marrow transplantation
5–10	Hematuria	Medullary congestion	Increased WBC adhesion resultant RBC adhesion (–) High blood oxygen level (+)	Hydration
	Increased GFR, decreased serum creatinine	Hyperperfusion	High prostaglandin E production (+)	ACE inhibitor Avoid NSAIDs
		Hypertrophy	Hypoxia (–)	Somatostatin analogue
		Papillary necrosis	High NO synthesis (+) High caspase-3 level (+) High HSP70 level (+) Increased COX-2 production (+) High CRP level (–) High HO-1 level (+)	Hydration
		Hyperfiltration	Increased angiotensin II production (+)	ACE inhibitor or ARB
			High prostacyclin level (+)	Prostacyclin analogue
15	Microalbuminuria	Hyperperfusion	High prostaglandin E production (+)	ACE inhibitor
20	High urinary NAG and β_2-microglobulin	Tubular damage	Unknown	No specific treatment
30	Proteinuria	Glomerular hypertension, FSGS	Increased angiotensin II production (+)	ACE inhibitor or ARB
35	Low GFR	Loss of glomerular function	Unknown	Strategies to retard CKD progression
40	Falling GFR	Further loss of glomerular function	Unknown	Strategies to retard CKD progression, preparation for RRT

Figure 49.13 The changing profile of renal dysfunction in sickle cell disease with age and available treatment options. +, ameliorating factor; –, risk factor. ACEI, angiotensin-converting enzyme inhibitor; ARB, angiotensin receptor blocker; CKD, chronic kidney disease; COX-2, cyclooxygenase 2; CRP, C-reactive protein; FSGS, focal segmental glomerulosclerosis; GFR, glomerular filtration rate; HbA, hemoglobin A; HbF, fetal hemoglobin; HO-1, heme oxygenase 1; NAG, *N*-acetylglucosamine; NO, nitric oxide; NSAIDs, nonsteroidal anti-inflammatory drugs; RBC, red blood cell; RRT, renal replacement therapy; WBC, white blood cell. *(Modified with permission from reference 18.)*

alternative, supportive red cell transfusion may be necessary. Excessive iron accumulation should be prevented in patients undergoing regular transfusions, who are at risk for hemochromatosis, although organ dysfunction caused by tissue iron overload seems less predictable in sickle cell disease than in thalassemia major. Metabolic acidosis is also prominent and requires correction with sodium bicarbonate supplements.

ESRD in sickle cell disease has been treated successfully with hemodialysis, peritoneal dialysis, and transplantation. Hemodialysis has been used more frequently than peritoneal dialysis. Sickle cell crises are not common despite the potential for hypotension, hypoxemia, and cytokine release during hemodialysis. The 30-month survival rate of a group of 77 patients who were predominantly treated with hemodialysis was 59%, comparable to survival rates in other groups of patients with multisystem disorders receiving dialysis.

TRANSPLANTATION

Transplantation is an appropriate form of renal replacement therapy in sickle cell nephropathy. After kidney transplantation, 1- and 3-year patient survival rates are 90% and 75%, respectively; 1- and 3-year graft survival rates are 82% and 54%, respectively.[42] These outcomes compare unfavorably with kidney transplantation for most other groups of patients. The adjusted mortality risk in sickle cell patients undergoing transplantation is higher at 1 year (relative risk, 2.95) and at 3 years (relative risk, 2.82).[35] Nevertheless, there is a trend toward improved survival in transplant recipients compared with dialysis-treated patients with sickle cell disease on the transplant waiting list.[43]

In sickle cell disease, perioperative risks such as severe crisis and massive sickling can be reduced by preoperative transfusions of normal blood, thereby reducing the proportion of HbS. After transplantation, hematocrit increases and may even be higher than in patients with sickle cell disease and normal renal function. Sickle cell crisis may occur after transplantation, but it is not yet clear whether the increase in hematocrit enhances the risk for a crisis. Standard immunosuppressive therapy does not increase the risk for sickle cell crisis. However, caution is warranted with the use of antilymphocyte antibodies because the onset of a crisis has been related to this therapy in a few patients, perhaps as a consequence of increased cytokine release. The recurrence of hyposthenuria and sickle cell nephropathy after transplantation has occasionally been described.

REFERENCES

1. Adekile AD, Kitundu MN, Gu LH, et al. Haplotypes in SS patients from Nigeria; characterization of one atypical beta S haplotype no. 19 (Benin) associated with elevated Hb F and high G gamma levels. *Ann Hematol.* 1992;65:41-45.
2. Davies SC, Oni L. Management of patients with sickle cell disease. *BMJ.* 1997;315:656-660.
3. Serjeant GR. Sickle-cell disease. *Lancet.* 1997;350:725-730.
4. Bunn HF. Pathogenesis and treatment of sickle cell disease. *N Engl J Med.* 1997;337:762-769.
5. Bennekou P, Pedersen O, Møller A, Christophersen P. Volume control in sickle cells is facilitated by the novel anion conductance inhibitor NS1652. *Blood.* 2000;95:1842-1848.
6. Platt OS. Easing the suffering caused by sickle cell disease. *N Engl J Med.* 1994;330:783-784.
7. Stuart MJ, Nagel RL. Sickle-cell disease. *Lancet.* 2004;364:1343-1360.
8. Arogundade FA, Hassan MO, Sanusi AA, et al. Kidney dysfunction in patients with sickle cell disease: A retrospective review. Book of Abstracts, Joint meeting of 10th AFRAN and 21st NAN Congress; February. 2009; Abuja, Nigeria. Abstract T-PO 15, p 29.
9. Wierenga KJJ, Hambleton IR, Wilson RM, et al. Significance of fever in Jamaican patients with homozygous sickle cell disease. *Arch Dis Child.* 2001;84:156-159.
10. Solovey A, Lin Y, Browne P, et al. Circulating activated endothelial cells in sickle cell anemia. *N Engl J Med.* 1997;337:1584-1590.
11. Platt OS, Brambilla DJ, Rosse WF, et al. Mortality in sickle cell disease. Life expectancy and risk factors for early death. *N Engl J Med.* 1994;330:1639-1644.
12. Powars DR, Chan LS, Hiti A, et al. Outcome of sickle cell anemia: A 4-decade observational study of 1056 patients. *Medicine (Baltimore).* 2005;84:363-376.
13. Schechter AN. Hemoglobin research and the origins of molecular medicine. *Blood.* 2008;112:3927-3938.
14. Hord J, Byrd R, Stowe L, et al. *Streptococcus pneumoniae* sepsis and meningitis during penicillin prophylaxis era in children with sickle cell disease. *J Pediatr Hematol Oncol.* 2002;24:470-472.
15. Steinberg MH, Barton F, Castro O, et al. Effect of hydroxyurea on mortality and morbidity in sickle cell anemia: Risks and benefits up to 9 years of treatment. *JAMA.* 2003;289:1645-1651.
16. Vermylen C. Hematopoietic stem cell transplantation in sickle cell disease. *Blood Rev.* 2003;17:163-166.
17. de Jong PE, Statius van Eps LW. Sickle cell nephropathy: New insights into pathophysiology. *Kidney Int.* 1985;27:711-717.
18. Sheinman JI. Sickle cell disease and the kidney. *Nat Clin Pract Nephrol.* 2009;5:78-88.
19. Statius van Eps LW, Pinedo-Veels C, de Vries CH, de Koning J. Nature of concentrating defect in sickle-cell nephropathy. Microradioangiographic studies. *Lancet.* 1970;1:450-452.
20. Guasch A, Cua M, Mitch WE. Early detection and the course of glomerular injury in patients with sickle cell anemia. *Kidney Int.* 1996;49: 786-791.
21. Schmitt F, Martinez F, Brillet G, et al. Early glomerular dysfunction in patients with sickle cell anemia. *Am J Kidney Dis.* 1998;32:208-214.
22. Falk RJ, Scheinman J, Phillips G, et al. Prevalence and pathologic features of sickle cell nephropathy and response to inhibition of angiotensin-converting enzyme. *N Engl J Med.* 1992;326:910-915.
23. Bhathena DB, Sondheimer JH. The glomerulopathy of homozygous sickle hemoglobin (SS) disease: Morphology and pathogenesis. *J Am Soc Nephrol.* 1991;1:1241-1252.
24. Guasch A, Cua M, You W, Mitch WE. Sickle cell anemia causes a distinct pattern of glomerular dysfunction. *Kidney Int.* 1997;51: 826-833.
25. ter Maaten JC, Serné EH, Statius van Eps LW, et al. Effects of insulin and atrial natriuretic peptide on renal tubular sodium handling in sickle cell disease. *Am J Physiol.* 2000;278:F499-F505.
26. Tharaux PL, Hagege I, Placier S, et al. Urinary endothelin-1 as a marker of renal damage in sickle cell disease. *Nephrol Dial Transplant.* 2005;20: 2408-2413.
27. Osegbe DN. Haematuria in sickle cell disease. A report of 12 cases and review of literature. *Trop Geogr Med.* 1990;42:22-27.
28. Yium J, Gabow P, Johnson A, et al. Autosomal dominant polycystic kidney disease in blacks: Clinical course and effects of sickle-cell hemoglobin. *J Am Soc Nephrol.* 1994;4:1670-1674.
29. Watanabe IC, Billis A, Guimarães MS. Renal medullary carcinoma: Report of seven cases from Brazil. *Mod Pathol.* 2007;20:914-920.
30. Jung DC, Kim SH, Jung SI, et al. Renal papillary necrosis: Review and comparison of findings at multi-detector row CT and intravenous urography. *Radiographics.* 2006;26:1827-1836.
31. Sklar AH, Perez JC, Harp RJ, Caruana RJ. Acute renal failure in sickle cell anemia. *Int J Artif Organs.* 1990;13:347-351.
32. Aderibigbe A, Arije A, Akinkugbe OO. Glomerular function in sickle cell disease patients during crisis. *Afr J Med Med Sci.* 1994;23:153-160.
33. Marsenic O, Couloures KG, Wiley JM. Proteinuria in children with sickle cell disease. *Nephrol Dial Transplant.* 2008;23:715-720.
34. Thompson J, Reid M, Hambleton I, Serjeant GR. Albuminuria and renal function in homozygous sickle cell disease: Observations from a cohort study. *Arch Intern Med.* 2007;167:701-708.
35. Guasch A, Zayas CF, Eckman JR, et al. Evidence that microdeletions in the α globin gene protect against the development of sickle cell glomerulopathy in humans. *J Am Soc Nephrol.* 1999;10:1014-1019.
36. Kattamis A, Lagona E, Orfanou I, et al. Clinical response and adverse events in young patients with sickle cell disease treated with hydroxyurea. *Pediatr Hematol Oncol.* 2004;21:335-342.
37. Hatch FE, Crowe LR, Miles DE, et al. Altered vascular reactivity in sickle hemoglobinopathy. A possible protective factor from hypertension. *Am J Hypertens.* 1989;2:2-8.

38. ter Maaten JC, Serné EH, Bakker SJL, et al. Effects of insulin on glucose uptake and leg blood flow in patients with sickle cell disease and normal subjects. *Metabolism*. 2001;50:387-392.
39. Powars DR, Elliott-Mills DD, Chan L, et al. Chronic renal failure in sickle cell disease: Risk factors, clinical course, and mortality. *Ann Intern Med*. 1991;115:614-620.
40. Sklar AH, Campbell H, Caruana RJ, et al. Population study of renal function in sickle cell anemia. *Int J Artif Organs*. 1990;13:231-236.
41. Abbott KC, Hypolite IO, Agodoa LY. Sickle cell nephropathy at end-stage renal disease in the United States: Patient characteristics and survival. *Clin Nephrol*. 2002;58:9-15.
42. Bleyer AJ, Donaldson LA, McIntosch M, Adams PL. Relationship between underlying renal disease and renal transplantation outcome. *Am J Kidney Dis*. 2001;37:1152-1161.
43. Ojo AO, Govaerts TC, Schmouder RL, et al. Renal transplantation in end-stage sickle cell nephropathy. *Transplantation*. 1999;67:291-295.

CHAPTER 50

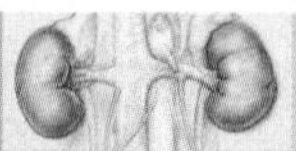

Congenital Anomalies of the Kidney and Urinary Tract

John O. Connolly, Guy H. Neild

This chapter discusses congenital anomalies of the kidney and urinary tract that can result in renal problems and renal failure. Nearly half of the children who develop end-stage renal disease (ESRD) have asymmetric, irregularly shaped kidneys.[1,2] This appearance, often referred to as bilateral renal scarring, is frequently associated with lower urinary tract anomalies including vesicoureteral reflux (VUR). The most serious conditions involve bladder outflow obstruction, and many can now be detected antenatally.

These cases were previously described as reflux nephropathy or chronic pyelonephritis; but with advances in genetics and developmental biology, it is becoming clear that many are due to primary renal malformations (renal dysplasia) often associated with congenital malformations of the ureter, bladder, and urethra. This is a change from the view that renal scarring and damage are secondary to the outflow problem and ureteral reflux. Although it is still a matter of some debate, the concept of acquired renal scarring is often wrong, and the British Association for Paediatric Nephrology now suggests that clinical distinction between reflux nephropathy and renal dysplasia is unnecessary.[1]

CLINICAL PRINCIPLES

Congenital renal tract abnormalities may present in one of five settings:

1. Antenatal diagnosis by fetal ultrasound screening.
2. Failure to thrive in an infant or young child.
3. Investigation of urinary tract infection (UTI).
4. An incidental finding in a child or adult.
5. An adult with abnormal urinalysis, stones, hypertension, or renal impairment.

The identification of these problems always poses the following questions:

- What is the cause?
- What is the natural history?
- Is surgical intervention required?

Such patients fall into two broad groups. First, there is a group of patients who appear to have normal bladders without outflow obstruction and normal-caliber ureters when not micturating, described as having either primary VUR or primary renal dysplasia. Second, there is a group with some form of bladder outflow dysfunction that causes secondary VUR and dilated upper urinary tracts, the most common cause of which is posterior urethral valves in males.

As predicted by the Brenner hypothesis,[3] small asymmetric kidneys with reduced glomerular filtration rate (GFR) develop all the features of glomerular hyperfiltration, with the onset of progressive renal failure signaled by increasing proteinuria. This can now be significantly modified by treatment with renin-angiotensin blockade.[4] The details of antenatal and pediatric management of these patients are beyond the scope of this chapter, which focuses on management in adolescence and adult life.

DEVELOPMENT OF THE URINARY TRACT

The urinary tract develops from the cloaca and intermediate mesoderm in parallel with the early differentiation of the metanephric blastema (future kidney) (Fig. 50.1).[5-7] At the fifth week of fetal life, the mesonephric (wolffian) duct connects to the allantois and the cloaca. By the sixth week, the urorectal fold appears and divides this cavity, which separates the urinary system (urogenital sinus) from the rectum. Growth of the anterior abdominal wall between the allantois and the urogenital membrane is accompanied by an increase in size and capacity of this bladder precursor. The allantois remains attached to the apex of the fetal bladder and extends into the umbilical root, although it loses its patency and persists as the urachal remnant, the median umbilical ligament, which connects the bladder to the umbilicus. By the seventh week, there is a separate opening of the mesonephric duct into the bladder at what will become the vesicoureteral opening and the area known as the trigone. The distal part of the primitive urogenital sinus will form the definitive urogenital sinus. In females, this gives rise to the entire urethra and the vestibule of the vagina. In males, it gives rise to the posterior urethra, whereas the anterior urethra is formed from the closure of the urethral folds.

In the 6-week embryo, the mesonephric and paramesonephric (müllerian) ducts run in parallel. By 7 weeks, in the male, the müllerian duct starts to regress, and the wolffian duct will eventually develop into the epididymis and the caudal part of the vas deferens. In the female, the müllerian ducts fuse to become the uterovaginal cord, which opens into the urogenital sinus and will develop into the vagina.

As the urogenital tract develops, there is simultaneous development of the fetal kidney (see Fig. 50.1). In the absence of the ureteral bud, the metanephric kidney does not form. Fetal urine makes a significant contribution to the amniotic fluid by 16 weeks.

Pathogenesis of Maldevelopment

Renal development is orchestrated by the expression of transcription factors, growth and survival factors, and adhesion molecules.[6,8,9] Mutations of genes encoding all classes of these

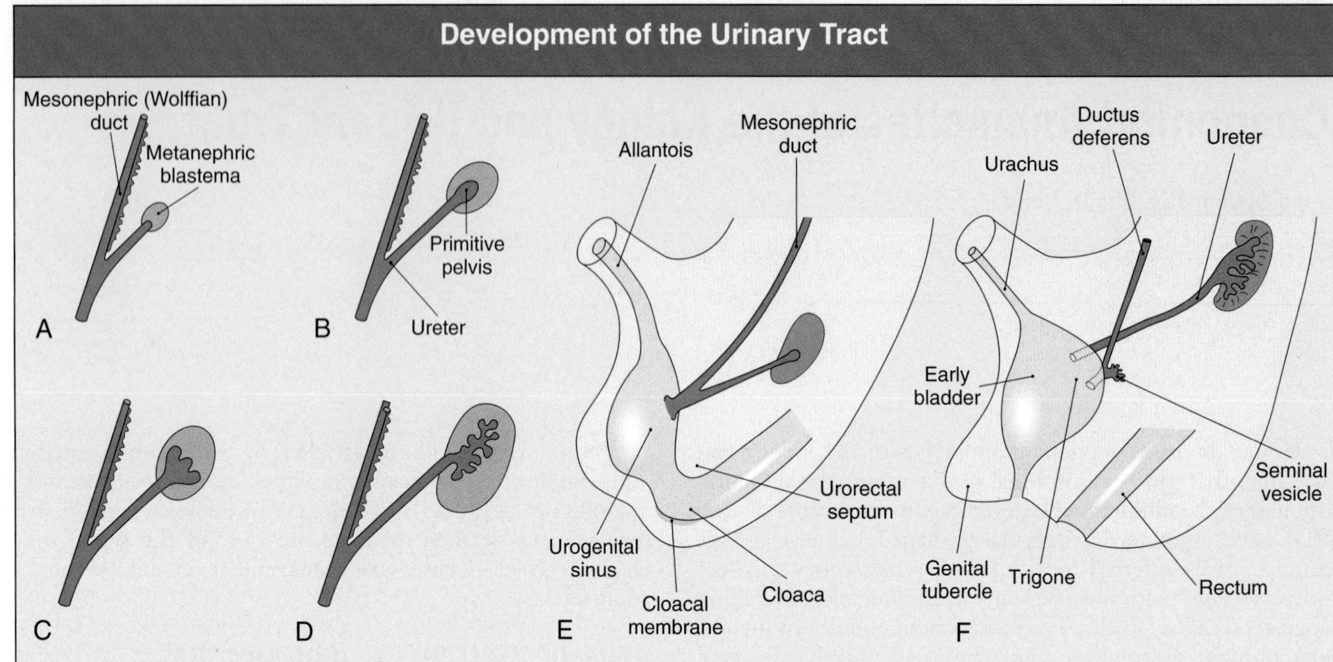

Figure 50.1 Development of the urinary tract. Growth and development of the ureter, pelvis, and calyces are shown in **A** to **D**. **A,** The metanephric kidneys first become detectable as small areas in the mesoderm close to the aorta. The primitive epithelial ureter buds off from the mesonephric duct and makes contact with the metanephric mesenchyme. **B,** Under the influence of signals from the ureter, the mesenchyme condenses and proliferates around the ureteral tip while there is simultaneous elongation and branching of the ureteral tip. **C** and **D,** A primitive pelvis appears, which then branches to form the divisions of the calyces. The branching process continues, with the epithelial system eventually differentiating into the nephrons of the renal parenchyma. As the fetus grows, there is ascent of the kidney due to the continuous rostral growth. **E,** Growth and development of the cloaca during weeks 5 to 6. **F,** Growth and development of the urogenital sinus into bladder and outflow tract during weeks 8 to 9.

molecules cause urinary tract malformations in mice.[8-10] One family of transcription factor proteins contains the paired DNA-binding domain and is encoded by the PAX genes. Studies in mice show that these PAX genes regulate the development of brain, eyes, lymphoid system, musculature, neural crest, and vertebrae.[11,12] PAX2 is expressed in the metanephros and in cell lineages that are forming nephrons and also in those that are destined to differentiate into the ureter, renal pelvis, and branching collecting duct system. The ablation of a single *PAX2* allele in knockout mice causes impaired metanephric growth and fewer nephrons than normal as well as megaureter, a finding consistent with gross VUR.[12] WT1, which is mutated in a proportion of Wilms' tumors, is another transcription factor whose mutation is associated with abnormal urinary tract development.

Normal development appears to depend on urine flow from the fetal kidney. This requires peristalsis and no anatomic obstruction to flow. A number of diverse defects can now be unified as it becomes clear they play some key role in peristalsis. This may be due to defects in smooth muscle development or innervations in the ureter. For example, mice lacking the transcription factor "teashirt 3" fail to develop normal smooth muscle in the ureter and have congenital hydronephrosis without anatomic obstruction.[13] Angiotensin plays a key role in initiating the peristalsis, and mice in whom the angiotensin type 1 receptor is knocked out fail to develop a renal pelvis and die of renal failure.[9]

Angiotensin type 2 receptor gene null mutant mice display congenital anomalies of the kidney and urinary tract. These include unilateral agenesis, unilateral megaureter and hydronephrosis, and pelviureteral junction (PUJ) obstruction and mimic a range of abnormalities found in humans.[9] Administration of angiotensin-converting enzyme (ACE) inhibitors throughout pregnancy in humans can cause hypotension and anuria in the baby with histologic features of renal tubular dysplasia. This phenotype is also caused by mutations in genes encoding renin, angiotensinogen, ACE, and angiotensin II receptor type 1.

Other syndromes associated with dysplasia and agenesis in which the mutation is now known include branchio-oto-renal syndrome (EYA1 mutation, transcription factor–like protein), Fraser syndrome (FRAS1 mutation, putative cell adhesion molecule), Kallmann syndrome (X-linked form, KAL1 mutation, cell adhesion molecule; autosomal form, FGFR1 mutation, growth factor receptor), and renal cysts and diabetes syndrome (HNF1 mutation, transcription factor).[14]

RENAL MALFORMATIONS

Congenitally abnormal kidneys may be large or small, cystic or irregular in outline, and absent or misplaced.

These conditions have traditionally been discussed on the basis of findings on intravenous urography (IVU), but the findings on computed tomography (CT) and magnetic resonance imaging (MRI) are now increasingly being emphasized.

Large Kidneys

Enlarged kidneys resulting from congenital problems are usually hydronephrotic or cystic. Wilms' tumor must also be considered. The differential diagnosis in adults of enlarged kidneys, both congenital and acquired, is shown in Chapter 5, Figure 5.4, and

Definitions of Renal Dysplasia and Malformation	
Term	**Characteristics**
Renal agenesis	Absence of the kidney or an identifiable metanephric structure
Renal aplasia	Severe dysplasia with an extremely small kidney, sometimes identifiable only by histologic examination
Renal dysplasia	Abnormal differentiation of the renal parenchyma with the development of abnormal structures, including primitive ducts surrounded by collars of connective tissue, metaplastic cartilage, a variety of nonspecific malformations such as preglomeruli of the fetal type, and reduced branching of the collecting ducts with cystic dilations and primitive tubules
Renal hypoplasia	Significantly reduced renal mass and nephron number without evidence of maldevelopment of the parenchyma
Renal multicystic dysplasia	Severe cystic dysplasia with extremely enlarged kidney full of cystic structures. It occurs as an isolated renal lesion in response to ureteral atresia and urethral obstruction. Ten percent of patients have a family history.

Figure 50.2 Definitions of renal dysplasia and malformation.

the differential diagnosis of cystic kidney disease is discussed further in Chapters 44 and 45.

Irregular Kidneys

Irregularity of the renal outline may result from fetal lobulation or a "dromedary hump," neither of which has any functional implications. Much more important is the diagnosis of renal dysplasia.

Renal Dysplasia

The range of dysplastic and other malformations of the kidney is presented in Figure 50.2. It is clear that abnormalities of the ureter, bladder, and urethra are often associated with renal dysplasia.[15,16] All types of renal dysplasia can also occur as isolated developmental anomalies. Renal dysplasia, although typically producing small, irregular kidneys, may sometimes be cystic or multicystic renal dysplasia.

Renal Hypoplasia (Oligomeganephronia)

Hypoplasia is defined as a congenitally small kidney (two standard deviations below the expected mean) that lacks evidence of parenchymal maldifferentiation (renal dysplasia) or of acquired disease sufficient to explain the reduced size. The term is often used loosely, however, and most patients with a small kidney and other malformations will have oligomeganephronia. This is a type of renal hypoplasia resulting from a congenital reduction in the number of nephrons. It results from arrested development of the metanephric blastema at 14 to 20 weeks of gestation with subsequent hypertrophy of glomeruli and tubules in the kidney. The hypertrophy and hyperfiltration result later in life in progressive nephron injury and sclerosis. Oligomeganephronia is recognized on renal biopsy by the large size of the glomeruli and tubules and the small number of glomeruli seen in a good core of renal cortex. It is reported in congenital syndromes caused by mutations in *PAX2* and hepatocyte nuclear factor 1β.

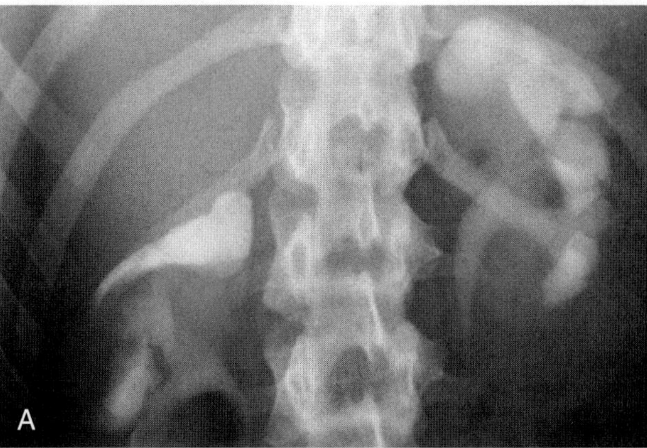

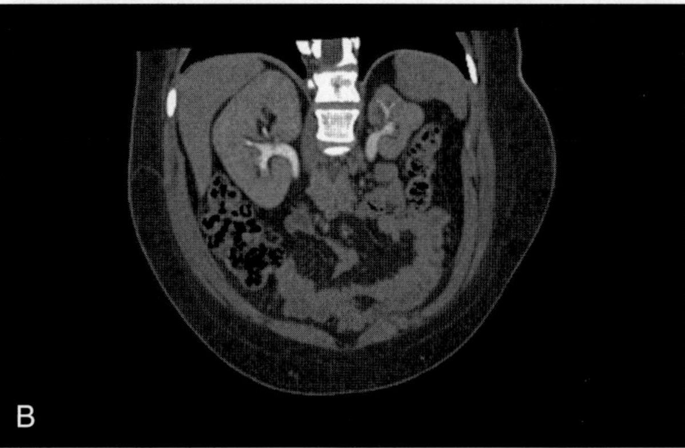

Figure 50.3 Renal dysplasia. A, Gross bilateral scarring in a 20-year-old woman who has been assessed since the age of 2 years. Progressive scarring has been observed in the absence of urinary tract infections and obstruction. This probably represents primary renal dysplasia. **B,** CT IVU showing gross scarring of right kidney. *(Courtesy Dr. A. Kirkham, University College Hospitals, London, UK.)*

Differential Diagnosis of Scarred Kidneys

Dysplasia Versus Reflux Progressive scarring and renal failure were once considered chronic parenchymal infection (so-called chronic pyelonephritis) and were regarded as a consequence of VUR. However, in the 1980s, there was a retreat from the paradigm of the primary role of infection, and emphasis was placed on scarring as a result of reflux and the progressive nature of the glomerular lesion associated with glomerular hypertension (or hyperfiltration), so-called reflux nephropathy.[3,17-19] The emphasis is changing again to the concept that scarring is often a consequence of renal dysplasia and that the reflux is a secondary feature (Fig. 50.3). Thus, irregular kidneys with normal-caliber ureters are more likely to be caused by primary dysplasia, and there may be no evidence of VUR.

Renal Scarring in Adults A practical clinical problem is the differential diagnosis of scarred, asymmetric kidneys. With older patients, the differential diagnosis of scarred or "lumpy bumpy" kidneys widens. Whereas this appearance was often attributed to analgesic nephropathy in the 1970s, today it is often designated reflux nephropathy. In older patients, multiple scarring from atheromatous arterial disease and embolization of the kidney is an increasingly important cause of renal failure. The diagnosis can be made by the radiologic features on IVU, but in practice, patients often have advanced renal impairment and are unable to excrete enough radiocontrast to delineate the anatomy of the calyces and pelvis and their relationship to the scarring. With

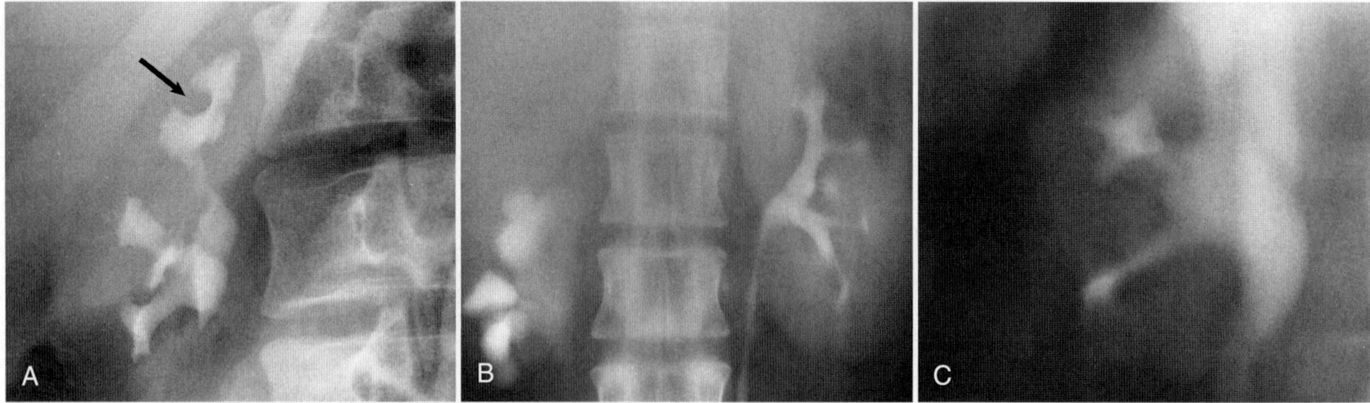

Figure 50.4 Differential diagnosis of "lumpy bumpy" kidneys from appearances on intravenous urography. A, Sickle cell disease: papillary necrosis. Missing papillae leave a round hole in the medulla *(arrow)* and give a clubbed appearance. Otherwise, the calyceal architecture is relatively well preserved. **B,** Reflux nephropathy. There is gross scarring and distortion of the calyceal pattern of the right kidney, giving rise to clubbed appearance of the dilated calyces. With reflux, there is a predilection for scarring of the upper and lower poles; with papillary necrosis or analgesic nephropathy, changes are less predictable. **C,** Analgesic nephropathy: the uniformly small shrunken kidney has relative preservation of the calyceal pattern. A plain film showed areas of calcification in both kidneys.

urologic conditions, there will be distortion and clubbing of calyces; with other conditions, the calyceal pattern should be normal, except for examples of papillary necrosis (Fig. 50.4). Scarring is best demonstrated by ^{99m}Tc-labeled dimercaptosuccinic acid (DMSA) scintigraphy.

Absent Kidneys

Unilateral Renal Agenesis

Complete absence of one kidney occurs in 1 in 500 to 1000 births. It can be familial, and the term *hereditary renal aplasia* is used by pediatricians. It is an autosomal dominant trait with incomplete penetrance and variable expression and can be associated with bilateral renal agenesis or severe dysplasia. In some families, mutations in uroplakin IIIa are found.[20]

Typically, there is no ureter, and the ipsilateral half of the bladder trigone is missing. The remaining kidney is usually hypertrophic, but it may be ectopic, malrotated, or hydronephrotic with a megaureter. The more severe the dysplasia of the remaining kidney, the earlier the presentation. The ipsilateral testis and seminal tract are usually absent, and in 10% of cases, the adrenal gland is also missing. Girls can have an absent fallopian tube or ovary or malformation of the vagina or uterus. Other associations include imperforate anus and malformations of the vertebrae and cardiovascular system. Agenesis could result from failure in formation of either the metanephros or the ureteral bud; however, in association with cloacal abnormalities, the latter is more likely.

Normality of the single kidney should be confirmed by ^{99m}Tc-DMSA scintigraphy, normal isotopic GFR, and absence of proteinuria. If the remaining kidney is not normal, lifelong follow-up is necessary. Ultrasound scanning of the kidneys is recommended in first-degree relatives in all families in which there is an individual with unilateral or bilateral renal agenesis.

Bilateral Renal Agenesis

Bilateral renal agenesis is lethal. It is associated with pulmonary hypoplasia and a characteristic facial appearance (Potter facies) caused by intrauterine compression, which is a consequence of oligohydramnios. The prevalence is about 1 in 10,000, with risk for occurrence in siblings of about 3%, unless there is a family history of agenesis, when risk rises to 15% to 20%.

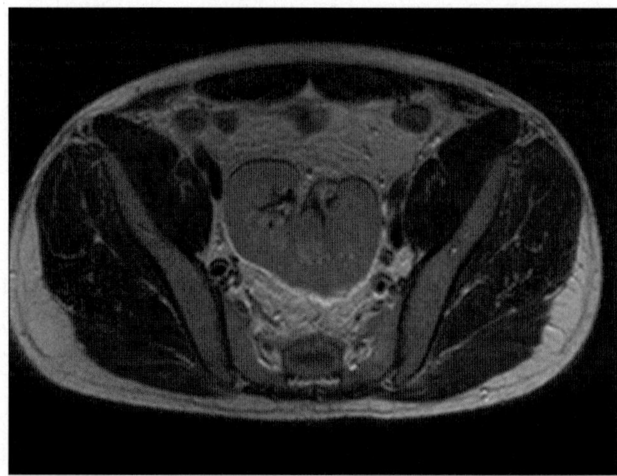

Figure 50.5 Single pelvic kidney. MRI scan, transverse section, showing single midline pelvic kidney. *(Courtesy Dr. A. Kirkham, University College Hospitals, London, UK.)*

Misplaced Kidneys

Renal Ectopia, Malrotation, and Crossed Fused Kidneys

The starting position of the fetal kidney is deep in the pelvis. Kidneys that fail to ascend properly and therefore remain lower than usual occur in 1 in 800 births (Fig. 50.5, see also Fig. 5.19). During development and ascent of the kidney, the renal pelvis comes to face more medially. The most common anomaly is for the pelvis to face forward. The more ectopic the kidney, the more severe the rotation and abnormal the appearance. In more than 90% of ectopia, there is fusion of both kidneys. This is now best visualized on CT or MR urography (Fig. 50.6). Symptoms and complications, if any, are caused by associated reflux or PUJ obstruction.

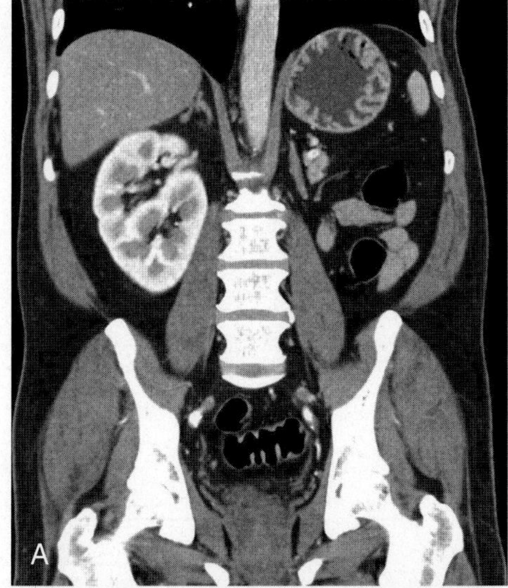

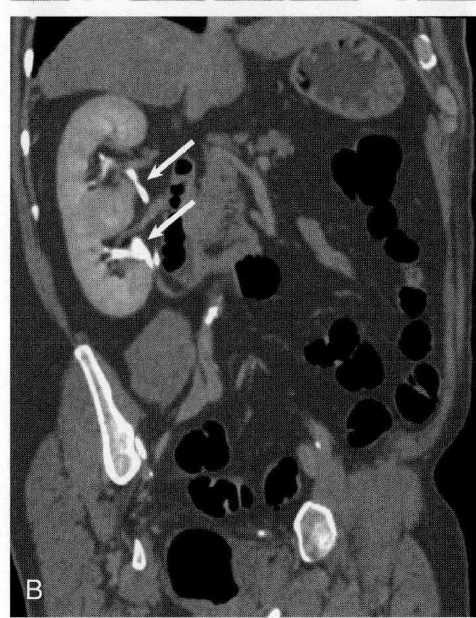

Figure 50.6 Crossed fused ectopia. A, MRI scan showing fused kidneys on right. **B,** There are two ureters *(arrows)*. *(Courtesy Dr. A. Kirkham, University College Hospitals, London, UK.)*

Horseshoe Kidney

If both kidneys are low, they may join at the lower pole and are usually drained by two ureters (Fig. 50.7). They lie lower than normal, and further ascent is prevented by the root of the inferior mesenteric artery. This occurs in 1 in 400 to 1800 births and is more common in males (2:1). Patients present, if at all, with complications of reflux, obstruction, or stone formation.

Calyceal Abnormalities

Hydrocalyx and Hydrocalycosis

Dilated calyces are usually caused by obstruction. Focal dilation can also be caused by congenital infundibular stenosis, extrinsic compression from vessel or tumor, stones, or tuberculosis. If obstruction is excluded, the appearance is likely to be a congenital abnormality and can be an incidental finding. Moreover, if the GFR is normal and the divided function of the kidneys is 50:50, surgery to "improve" the anatomy should not be attempted.

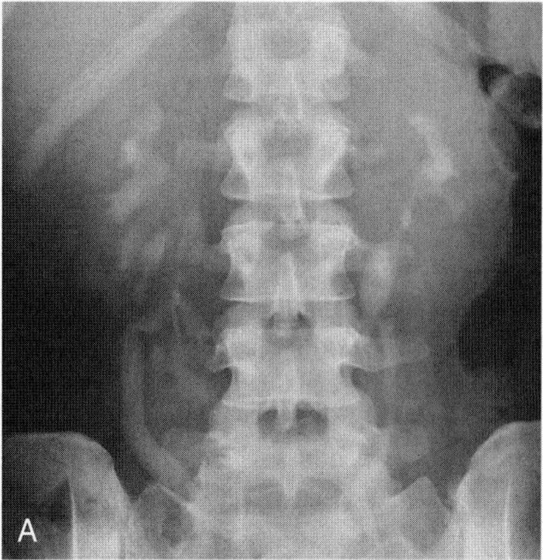

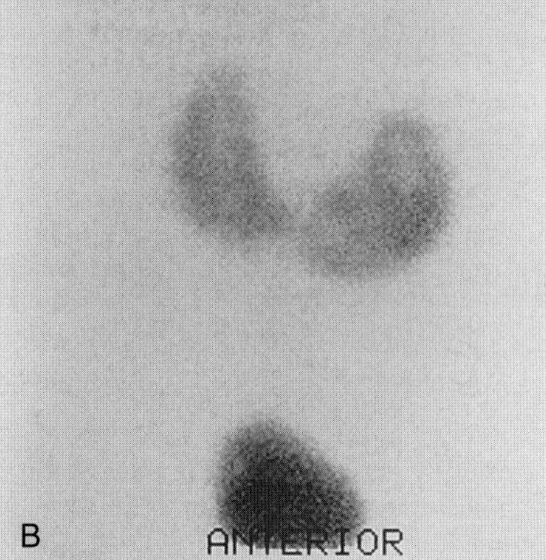

Figure 50.7 Horseshoe kidney. A, IVU soon after pregnancy in a 25-year-old woman shows not only the horseshoe kidney joining in the midline but also dilated ureters as a transient consequence of pregnancy. **B,** Dimercaptosuccinate scan showing a horseshoe kidney.

Megacalycosis

In megacalycosis, there is bizarre dysplasia of the calyceal system with an increase in the number of calyces. There is no obstruction, and it results from malformation of renal papillae. Megacalycosis is congenital, usually unilateral, and an incidental finding. It is much more common in males (6:1) and occurs only in Caucasians.

Bilateral disease is confined to males, and segmental, unilateral disease to females, which suggests an X-linked partially recessive gene with reduced penetrance in females. There may be an associated ipsilateral segmental megaureter, usually affecting the distal third.

Calyceal Diverticulum (Calyceal Cyst)

A calyceal diverticulum is a cavity peripheral to a minor calyx that is not a closed cyst but is connected to the calyx by a narrow channel. It is usually an incidental finding in 5 per 1000 IVUs and is best seen on a delayed film (Fig. 50.8). If it is present, symptoms relate to stones or infection within the cavity.

Bardet-Biedl Syndrome

Multiple calyceal clubbing and calyceal diverticula are the characteristic features of the renal dysplasia seen in Bardet-Biedl

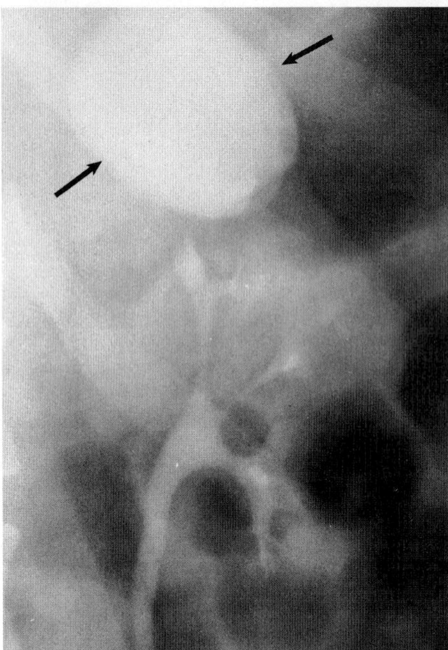

Figure 50.8 Calyceal cyst. IVU showing an upper pole calyceal cyst filled with contrast *(arrows)*. The plain abdominal film showed a group of stones in the floor of the cyst.

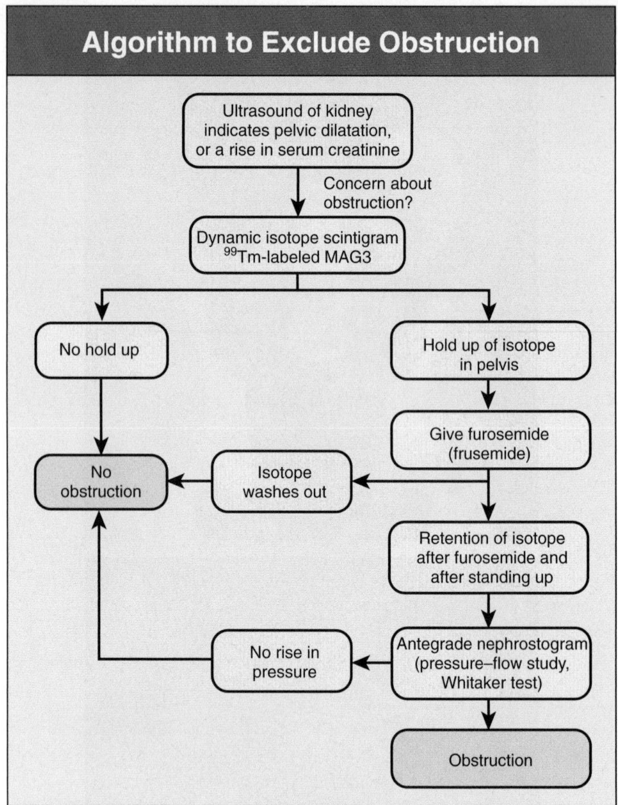

Figure 50.9 Algorithm to exclude obstruction.

syndrome (formerly known as Laurence-Moon-Biedl syndrome).[21] This autosomal recessive condition is characterized by retinitis pigmentosa, dysmorphic extremities (sometimes with polydactyly), obesity, and hypogonadism. Calyceal malformation is associated with parenchymal dysplasia; renal failure in early adult life is common.

Bardet-Biedl syndrome is probably the result of a lack of cilia formation or function caused by a defect of the basal body of ciliated cells. It is due to a mutation the *TTC8* gene which encodes a protein with a prokaryotic domain, pilF, involved in pilus formation and twitching mobility.[22]

Pelviureteral Junction Obstruction

PUJ obstruction is one of the most frequent causes of obstructive uropathy in children. The condition is usually congenital but can have an acquired mechanical basis caused by stenosis or external compression from adhesions, aberrant lower pole vessels, or kinking of the most proximal ureter. Associated abnormalities are common, and up to 50% of infants have another urologic abnormality, such as contralateral PUJ, contralateral renal dysplastic and multicystic kidney, minor degrees of VUR, and contralateral renal agenesis.

Older children can present with an abdominal mass or with pain in the flank, hematuria secondary to mild trauma, or UTI. Hypertension is unusual but can occur temporarily after surgical correction.

Diagnostic procedures have to differentiate between significant obstruction (Fig. 50.9) that requires surgical correction and congenital ectasia of the renal pelvis, in which case surgery is not indicated. Indications for surgical intervention include impairment of renal function, pyelonephritis, renal stones, and pain. Kidneys with good function can generally be left alone, and surgery is indicated only when function is clearly shown to deteriorate.[23]

Gonadal Dysgenesis

The problems of intersex, gender identity, and micropenis are beyond the scope of this chapter and rarely encountered in adult practice. Patients will be met, however, with ESRD who are phenotypically female but are genotype XY and have mutations of *WT1* (Denys-Drash and Frasier syndromes). They have gonadal dysgenesis and must have their streak ovaries removed; otherwise, gonadoblastomas will develop.

URETERAL ABNORMALITIES

Duplex Ureters

Duplication of the ureter and the renal pelvis is a common anomaly, with an incidence of about 1 in 150 births; unilateral duplication is six times more frequent than bilateral. It is more common in girls. If duplication has been detected in a patient, the likelihood of another sibling with duplication rises to 1 in 8.

Pathogenesis

If the ureteral bud bifurcates after its origin from the mesonephric duct but arises at a normal site, an incomplete ureteral duplication with a Y ureter will develop.[7] Complete ureteral duplication occurs if there are two ureteral buds, one in the normal location and the other in a low position. The normal bud ends in a correct site on the trigone in the bladder and is nonrefluxing. The lower bud, representing the ureter of the lower pole of the kidney, ends in the bladder as a lateral orifice with a short submucosal tunnel. The lower pole ureter is therefore often associated with VUR, and scarring of the lower pole can result.

If there are two ureteral buds, one with a normal location and one with a high position, the upper ureter is incorporated into the developing bladder, ending more distally and medial to the normal one. Thus, the upper pole ureter ends ectopically, and as a consequence of either obstruction or dysplasia, there is often severe scarring of the upper pole moiety.

Clinical Manifestations

In most adult patients, ureteral reduplication is asymptomatic and causes no long-term problems. Children with ureteral duplication often have VUR. The spontaneous disappearance of reflux is less common in duplex ureters than in patients with a single ureter.[24] Duplex ureters are best diagnosed by IVU and cystoscopy. PUJ obstruction of the ureter draining the lower pole of the kidney can occur.

Associated conditions, such as ectopic ureters and ureterocele (see later discussion), usually cause problems in early life and therefore have been dealt with by adolescence. Upper pole scarring is associated with an ectopic ureter, lower pole scarring with VUR (Fig. 50.10A).

Ectopic Ureters

Ectopic ureters are almost always associated with ureteral reduplication, and 10% are bilateral. There is a female to male ratio of 7:1. The ectopic ureter comes from the upper pole and inserts into the bladder more distally and toward the bladder neck, or it opens into the upper urethra. In females, the ureter may end in the urethra, vagina, or vulva, and patients present with incontinence, UTIs, or a persistent vaginal discharge, particularly if the external sphincter is damaged, for example, during labor.

Ectopic ureters are rare in males and present as UTI. Usually, there is a single ureter associated with a dysplastic kidney, which ends in the posterior urethra, ejaculatory duct, seminal vesicle, or vas. Males are usually continent because the ureter is proximal to the external sphincter.

Ectopic ureters are best visualized by IVU, although a small dysplastic kidney may be missed. A micturating cystourethrogram shows reflux into the lower pole of the kidney in 50% of patients.

Ureterocele

Ureteroceles are cystic dilations of the terminal segments of the ureter and are caused by maldevelopment of the caudal ureter. They occur more commonly in females (4:1) and almost exclusively in Caucasians, and 10% are bilateral.

Ectopic ureters and ureters with ureteroceles frequently (80%) drain the upper pole and are often associated with dysplastic or nonfunctional renal tissue. They usually present in childhood with infection; when large, they can obstruct the bladder neck or even the contralateral ureter. In adults, they commonly present with stones in the lower ureter. The treatment of simple ureteroceles is surgical excision with reimplantation of the ureter or simple incision if they subtend a well-functioning moiety. There are usually no medical sequelae.

Megaureter

Isolated dilation of the ureter does not necessarily imply obstruction. There are three broad groups of conditions with widely dilated ureters:

1. Obstruction of the ureter itself. This may be intrinsic (e.g., stone) or extrinsic (e.g., retroperitoneal fibrosis); it is not associated with reflux.

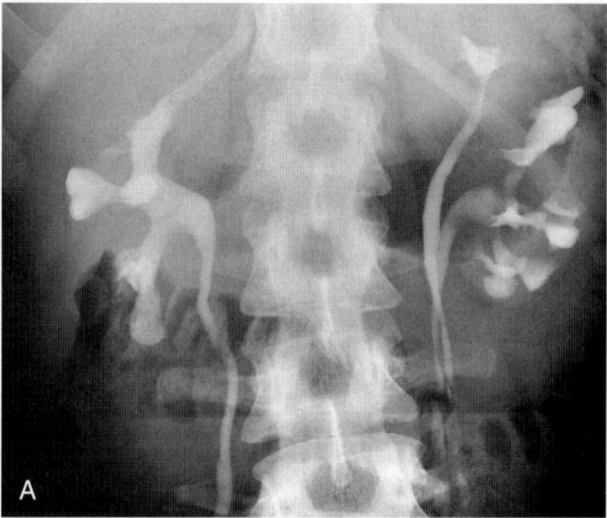

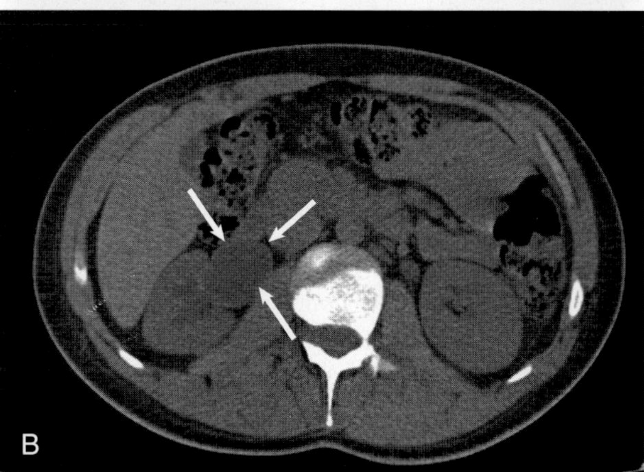

Figure 50.10 Duplex kidney. A, IVU shows a duplex left kidney. The lower pole is scarred and shows evidence of reflux damage. The two ureters entered the bladder separately, with the lower pole ureter in the abnormal location. The right kidney also shows features of reflux, with clubbing of the calyces and some scarring. **B,** CT scan showing an isolated right-sided megaureter *(arrows)*.

2. Bladder outflow obstruction, with secondary ureteral obstruction. Examples include a neuropathic bladder and posterior urethral valves; this may or may not be associated with reflux.
3. A dilated but nonobstructed ureter. This often occurs without reflux, and there can be normal renal function; sometimes, this is caused by an adynamic segment of the lower ureter (Fig. 50.10B).

Pathogenesis

In the normal ureter, there is a characteristic helical orientation of muscle fibers. When the megaureter is secondary to bladder outflow obstruction, there is muscle hyperplasia and hypertrophy of the ureteral wall. In megaureters for which there is no apparent cause, a variety of abnormalities of muscle orientation are described, or there may even be absence of muscle fibers at the proximal end of the undilated segment.

Electron microscopy shows an increase in collagen between the muscle bundles at the level of the obstructing segment.[25] Obstruction appears to be caused by a failure of peristalsis through the distal ureteral segment.

Clinical Manifestations

Most cases of megaureter associated with obstruction present in childhood with severe infections, often complicated by septicemia. In such cases, there is a high incidence of other congenital abnormalities. In less severe cases or when there is no obstruction, patients can present with abdominal pain, loin pain, hematuria, and UTI. Renal stones can form easily in the dilated systems. The exclusion of obstruction is often established only by an antegrade pressure-flow study (Whitaker test), in which a nephrostomy is placed in the renal pelvis and contrast material infused at 10 ml/min.[26]

Treatment

A definite diagnosis (is there obstruction or not?) must be made (see Fig. 50.9). The current view is that patients with nonobstructed asymptomatic disease should be managed conservatively, and most do very well with this approach.

BLADDER AND OUTFLOW DISORDERS

Prune-Belly Syndrome

The prune-belly syndrome occurs in males and consists of absence of the muscles of the anterior abdominal wall, bizarre malformations of the urinary tract with gross dilation of the bladder and ureters, and bilateral undescended testes.[27-29] When it is diagnosed early, renal outcome is related to the degree of renal dysplasia. There are incomplete forms of the syndrome (pseudo-prune). Rarely, a similar megacystis or megaureter may be seen in either sex.

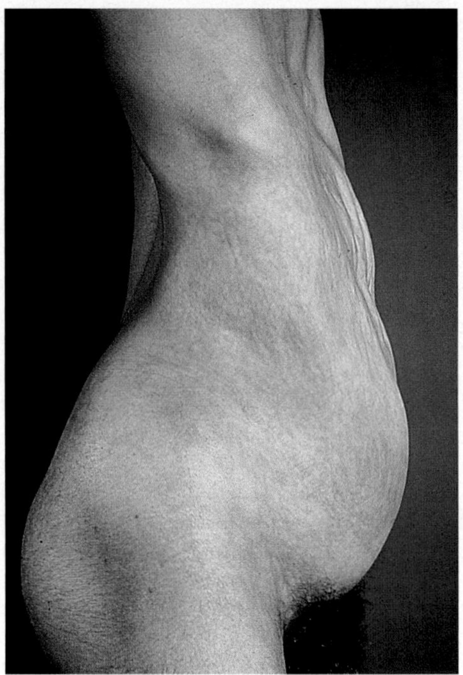

Figure 50.11 Prune-belly syndrome. Note the lax abdominal musculature leading to a pot-bellied appearance. There is also marked thoracic cage deformity. *(Courtesy Prof. C. R. J. Woodhouse, University College Hospital, London, UK.)*

Pathogenesis

No gene defect or unifying hypothesis has emerged to explain these features. The incidence varies from 1 in 30,000 to 50,000. There are a few familial cases, and the condition has been reported in twins, but there is 100% discordance reported in identical twins, which is a powerful argument against a genetic basis. There is evidence for a primary, localized arrest of mesenchymal development. This is supported by the lack of prostatic differentiation; the epithelial element in the prostate is absent or hypoplastic. Ultrastructure studies of the ureter show massive replacement of smooth muscle with fibrous and collagen tissue and the absence of nerve plexuses. A nearly identical syndrome can occur as a consequence of fetal urethral obstruction, including urethral atresia.

Clinical Manifestations

The prognosis is dependent on the degree of renal dysplasia and injury. Three groups can be distinguished. In group I, complete urethral obstruction causes stillbirth or neonatal death (20%); in group II, acute, early presentation requires diversion and reconstruction (20%); in group III, good health and renal function continue despite urologic appearances (60%).

There is complete absence or incomplete formation of the rectus abdominis and other muscles, which leads to the wrinkled abdominal wall of the prune infant (see Fig 50.12C). This gives way to a fairly smooth "pot belly" in later life (Fig. 50.11). Reconstructive surgery is not normally required. The patients grow up physically active and strong but cannot sit up directly from a supine position. Abnormalities of the thoracic cage, such as pectus excavatum, are common.

Although true outflow obstruction is sometimes present, the gross and irregular dilation of the urinary tract that is characteristic of this syndrome is primarily caused by a developmental defect with a variable degree of smooth muscle aplasia leading to aperistaltic ureters (Fig. 50.12). Urodynamic studies are often difficult to interpret because of gross VUR, but typically there is a low-pressure bladder. With late presentation, some patients have detrusor instability.

Differential Diagnosis

In severe cases of megacystis or megaureter with gross impairment of renal function (often with dysplastic kidneys), the differential diagnosis includes posterior urethral valves, renal dysplasia with or without multiple congenital defects, neuropathic bladder, and nephrogenic diabetes insipidus.

Natural History

Once any outflow obstruction is dealt with, usually in infancy, the renal function should remain stable despite the frightening radiologic appearances. In those patients observed in our unit for up to 40 years, renal deterioration and hypertension have been rare. In the small number who have progressed, recurrent infection, hypertension, and proteinuria have been warning signs of impending trouble.

Renal scarring should be assessed by isotopic DMSA scintigraphy and renal function followed by serial isotopic GFR measurements. Lifelong attention to blood pressure, UTIs, and stones is necessary.

Treatment

In all children, even with good renal function, there should be a careful search for obstruction, beginning with the urethra and working up to the PUJ, but often no obstruction is found and no surgery is required. In many others, the floppy bladder is not anatomically obstructed, but bladder emptying is improved by urethrotomy ("functional obstruction"). In infancy, there is debate about the need for reconstructive surgery. There is

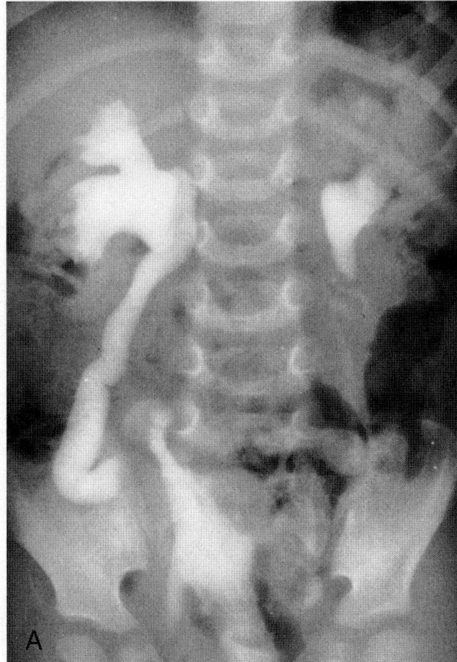

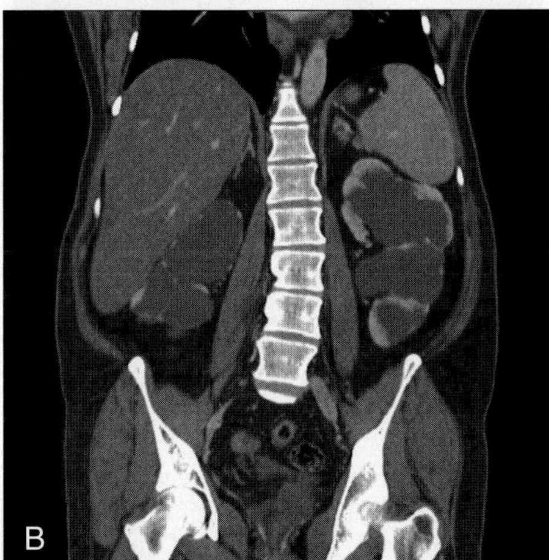

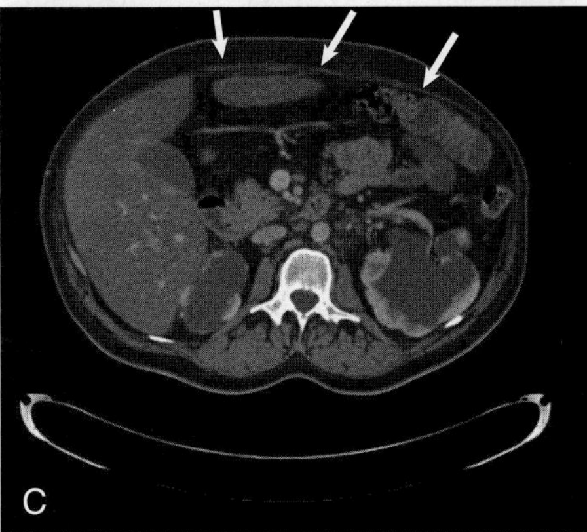

Figure 50.12 Prune-belly syndrome. A, Typical IVU appearance of a patient with prune-belly syndrome and good renal function. Often, the ureters are extremely dilated and tortuous. **B,** CT urogram showing gross bilateral hydronephrosis. **C,** Absence of anterior abdominal wall musculature *(arrows)*.

certainly a group of patients born with severely compromised renal function who do require reconstruction after stabilization by early diversion.[30]

The current view is that the testes should be brought down to the scrotum in infancy. It is hoped that earlier surgery will produce proper germ cell development and thus preserve fertility. So far, however, no prune-belly patient has been shown to be fertile.

Bladder Exstrophy (Ectopia Vesicae)

Classic exstrophy is the failure of the anterior abdominal wall and bladder to close, but there are a range of defects from epispadias of an otherwise normal penis to major cloacal abnormalities (Fig. 50.13).

Pathogenesis

Failure of growth of the lower abdominal wall between the allantois and the urogenital membrane coupled with breakdown of the urogenital membrane leaves a small, open bladder plate, a low-placed umbilical root, and diastasis of the pubic bones (Fig 50.14B). The genital tubercle is probably placed lower in these patients, and the cloacal membrane ruptures above it, leading to a penis with an open dorsal surface that is continuous with the bladder plate. A midline closure defect causes a failure of fusion of the lower anterior abdominal wall, including the symphysis pubis, lower urinary tract, and external genitalia. There are rare reports of a familial incidence. The condition occurs in 1 in 10,000 to 50,000 births. The male to female ratio is 2:1.

Clinical Manifestations

In severe cases, the bladder mucosa lies exposed on the lower abdominal wall, with the bladder neck and urethra laid open. The prostate and testes are normal. Most patients have normal kidneys at birth (although many reports do not record the state of the kidneys at birth). In one series, 33% had dilated ureters at presentation, but IVU was usually normal after diversion. However, in another series, one third of patients were said to have unilateral renal agenesis.[31] Renal function may be preserved after the diversion, although reflux is common (Fig. 50.14).

Other congenital abnormalities are only rarely present. More severe cloacal abnormalities are associated with imperforate anus and either high or low rectal atresia.

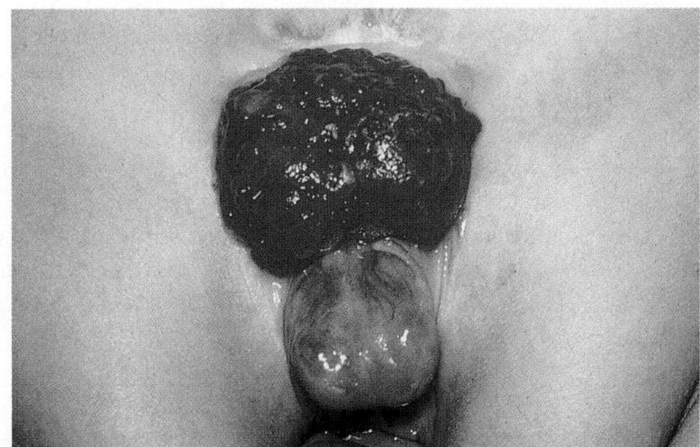

Figure 50.13 Bladder exstrophy. The entire length of the penis is also open (epispadias). *(Courtesy Prof. C. R. J. Woodhouse, University College Hospital, London.)*

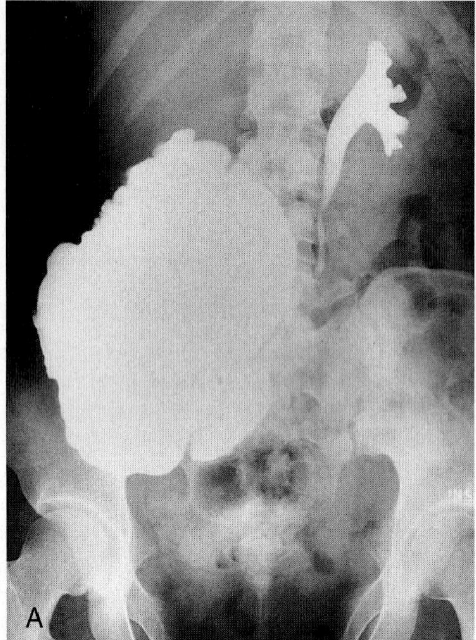

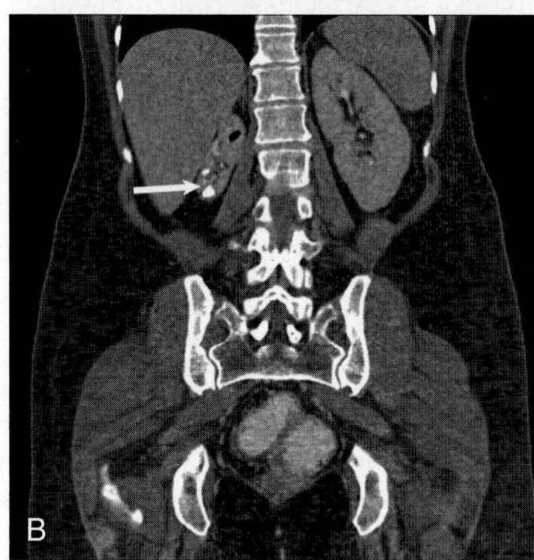

Figure 50.14 Cystography in bladder exstrophy. A, A 26-year-old woman with bladder exstrophy who has a continent Mitrofanoff system with use of the colon to create a reservoir. There is reflux into the left kidney. There is also reflux into the right kidney, but the kidney is obscured by the full reservoir. Her GFR is 130 ml/min. **B,** MRI scan of patient with bladder exstrophy showing small scarred left kidney with several renal calculi *(arrow)*. Note widely splayed symphysis pubis.

Natural History

Long-term renal outcome depends on the bladder. In the long term (up to 25 years), the kidneys survive much better with a well-functioning bladder; 13% of those with a good bladder had significant renal damage compared with 82% with ileal conduits, 22% with nonrefluxing colonic conduits, and 33% with ureterosigmoidostomy.[32] Today, the bladder is usually augmented (enterocystoplasty, ileocystoplasty, cecocystoplasty) or replaced by bowel (intestinal reservoir). In a study of 53 such patients who were observed for more than 10 years, renal function deteriorated (fall in GFR of 20% or more) in only 10 (20%).[33]

Treatment

When the infant is born, the three urologic treatment goals are to close the abdominal wall, to establish urinary continence and preserve renal function, and to reconstruct cosmetically acceptable genitalia.

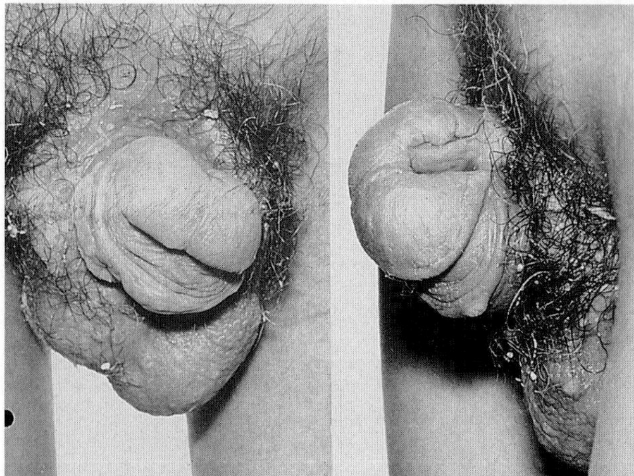

Figure 50.15 Epispadias. Result of multiple surgeries to close the epispadias and to lengthen the penis. *(Courtesy Prof. C. R. J. Woodhouse, University College Hospital, London, UK.)*

Causes of Neuropathic Bladder	
Site of Lesion	**Causes**
Cerebral	Cerebrovascular accident/cerebral palsy, encephalopathy, trauma, Parkinson's disease, dementia
Spinal	Isolated (no other neurologic features), trauma, multiple sclerosis, compression, spina bifida, spinal dysraphism, tethered cord, sacral agenesis, sacral teratoma
Peripheral nerve	Pelvic surgery, diabetes

Figure 50.16 Causes of neuropathic bladder.

The aim of initial surgery is to convert the defect to a complete epispadias (Fig. 50.15). At 4 years of age, reconstruction of the bladder neck and correction of the epispadias can be performed. If the bladder is small, intestinal augmentation is required. Patients may be able to void, but many have to use catheters. Incontinence may be a long-term problem.

Neuropathic Bladder

In childhood, the most common cause of a neuropathic bladder is myelomeningocele. A neuropathic bladder may also be seen without associated neurologic or other obvious causes (Fig. 50.16). The principal consequences are incontinence, infection, and reflux with upper tract dilation and subsequently renal failure. Early urodynamic assessment is essential (Fig. 50.17). Three different patterns of bladder behavior are seen: contractile, intermediate, and acontractile.

Contractile Behavior

An overactive detrusor (hyperreflexia) can produce some bladder emptying (incontinence). Unfortunately, 95% of patients have sphincter dyssynergia (inability to relax urethral sphincter), which results in no relaxation and incomplete emptying of the bladder. Patients with incomplete lesions may have some control of the distal sphincter and normal anal and sacral reflexes. Ironically, although this latter group has the least neurologic deficit, they have the worst bladder situation, generating high pressures

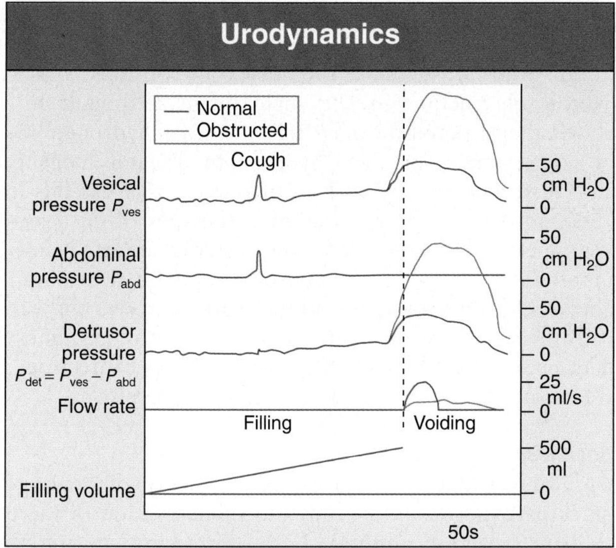

Figure 50.17 Urodynamic assessment by cystometrography. The vesical pressure is measured simultaneously with the abdominal pressure through the rectum; the detrusor pressure is the difference. A cough is used as a marker to show that the system is working. During filling, the first desire to void is normally at a detrusor pressure of less than 10 cm H_2O. This point is noted. The voiding pressure should normally be less than 40 cm H_2O (and is lower in women). Detrusor instability is an unstable (spontaneous) contraction occurring with a detrusor pressure above 15 cm H_2O. Higher pressure can cause incontinence. In combination with radiologic imaging (videocystometrography), the following are recorded: bladder neck, closed or open; bladder pressure, end filling; voiding detrusor pressure; bladder stability; compliance; flow rate, maximum; sensation, first; volume, voided and residual. *(Courtesy Prof. M. Craggs, University College London, UK.)*

and great risk for renal injury. The bladder becomes progressively hypertrophic, fibrotic, and poorly compliant.

Intermediate Behavior

These patients have some detrusor activity, but not sufficient to empty the bladder. Their bladders are poorly compliant, and they have no voluntary control of their sphincters, so any rise in bladder pressure tends to cause incontinence, or the high intravesical pressures lead to renal injury.

Acontractile Behavior

In about 25% of patients, there is no detrusor activity, and the bladder overflows when it is sufficiently full. This is not usually associated with renal failure.

Myelodysplasia

Myelodysplasia refers to a group of neural tube anomalies that primarily affect the lumbar and sacral segment of the spinal cord and are the most common cause of neurogenic bladder dysfunction in children. Spina bifida means the defective fusion of the posterior vertebral arches. Meningocele implies that the meninges extend beyond the confines of the vertebral canal with no neural elements contained inside. A myelomeningocele has neural tissue protruding with the meningocele. Spinal dysraphism (symptomatic spina bifida occulta) defines a group of structural anomalies of the caudal end of the spinal cord that do not result in an open vertebral canal but are associated with incomplete fusion of the posterior vertebral arches. Sacral agenesis is a rare anomaly in which part or all of two or more vertebral bodies is absent. It occurs early in fetal development when there is failure of ossification of the lowest vertebral segments. The only known teratogen is insulin. Sacral agenesis occurs in 1% of children born to insulin-dependent mothers. Partial sacral agenesis can be associated with an anterior meningocele.

Pathogenesis

The neural tube normally forms as the neural folds close over and fuse, starting in the cervical region and progressing caudally. It is believed that the embryologic defect is an incomplete tubularization of the neural tube, with inadequate mesodermal invagination and subsequent arrest of vertebral arch formation.

The incidence of myelodysplasia varies from 1 to 5 in 1000 live births, but there are wide geographic variations. Monozygotic twins are often discordant for spina bifida, but siblings are at increased risk (1:10-20), and children of affected parents have a 4% chance of having a similarly affected child. Myelomeningocele accounts for more than 90% of myelodysplastic infants. Folic acid supplements taken during the last trimester reduce the incidence of myelodysplasia by 50%.

Clinical Manifestations

All causes of tethered cord can produce a variable neurologic deficit. During development, some children develop progressive neurologic disturbance with bladder dysfunction, bowel dysfunction, scoliosis, and a syndrome of pes cavus and limb growth failure.

Bladder Dysfunction Neuropathic bladder can be an isolated problem with abnormal urodynamic studies but a normal neurologic examination.[34]

Bowel Dysfunction Bowel dysfunction is often present and needs to be treated accordingly. There may be severe constipation and overflow incontinence. The antegrade continent enterostomy procedure has been developed to improve the management. The appendix is brought out to the abdominal surface, and thus the colon can be irrigated antegradely with saline.

Intelligence Patients with myelomeningocele may have some intellectual impairment, especially those who have required ventriculoperitoneal shunting for associated hydrocephalus. Manual dexterity may also be affected. These are very important issues in long-term management.

Natural History

About 14% of patients have renal complications at birth and are at high risk in the next few years. Ultimately, about 50% will develop upper tract problems, although these can take up to 30 years to occur (Fig. 50.18). In one prospective study, renal outcome could be predicted by the urodynamic findings, with worst outcomes related to increased bladder wall thickness, degree of reflux, urethral pressures above 70 cm H_2O, and reduced bladder capacity. VUR occurs in 3% to 5% of newborns with detrusor hypertonicity or dyssynergia. Without treatment, this increases to 30% to 40% by the age of 5 years.[35]

Treatment

The management of the bladder depends on the urodynamic findings. In the 1970s, clean intermittent self-catheterization (CISC) was introduced,[36] but before that time, urinary diversion was the usual treatment. Today, when reflux and hydroureter are

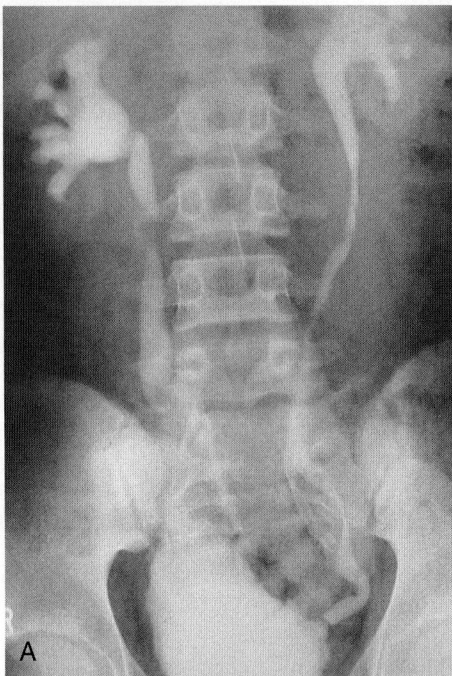

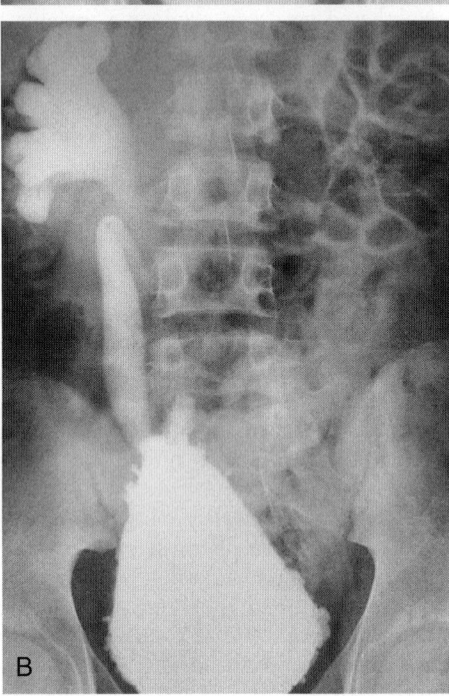

Figure 50.18 Sacral spina bifida with neuropathic bladder. A, IVU shows evidence of a previous hydronephrosis and subsequent scarring of the right kidney. The architecture of the left kidney is well preserved. **B,** Micturating cystogram. The typical tapering, hypertrophied, trabeculated bladder giving the characteristic fir cone appearance. Note the gross reflux on the right side. This is probably helping to protect the left kidney by acting as a pop-off mechanism. This is analogous to the protection that can occur in boys with posterior urethral valves.

present, the management is principally with CISC and anticholinergic drugs that increase bladder compliance.[37]

Bladder Neck Obstruction

Congenital bladder neck obstruction is rare and is usually caused by a neuropathic bladder, posterior urethral valves, or an ectopic ureterocele.

Posterior Urethral Valves

Posterior urethral valves are the most common cause of severe subvesical obstruction in the male infant (although in the newborn, they account for only 10% of cases of hydronephrosis). As a consequence, bilateral hydronephrosis and megaureter occur. Obstruction is caused by a diaphragm that extends from the floor to the roof of the urethra at the apex of the prostate. Valves appear as mucosal folds in the posterior urethra below the verumontanum. There is dilation of the proximal urethra and bladder wall hypertrophy and trabeculation. Above the valves, there is dilation of the prostatic urethra, which undermines the bladder neck. The valves obstruct flow only in one direction, and therefore a catheter can be passed without difficulty.

Pathogenesis

The urethra develops in two parts: differentiation of the urogenital sinus part (posterior urethra) and tubularization of the urethral plate (anterior urethra). Early obstruction during renal development can result in severe renal dysplasia.

Clinical Manifestations

Most cases of posterior urethral valves are now detected antenatally by ultrasound. Half of all patients present before the age of 1 year. Infants present with a palpably distended bladder and enlarged kidneys, abnormal urine stream, or failure to thrive due to renal failure. At diagnosis, 30% to 50% of children also have VUR. Children with less severe disease present with poor stream, hematuria, incontinence, acute UTI, or renal failure; however, late presentation is also associated with worse outcome.[38]

There are three abnormal features that can help protect the kidney; these all act to reduce the high pressures generated during voiding. They are massive unilateral reflux, usually with ipsilateral renal dysplasia (thereby protecting the other kidney); large bladder diverticulum; and urinary extravasation, often with urinary ascites. These protective mechanisms are referred to as "pop-off" mechanisms (see Fig. 50.18).[39] Ultrasound can show the bladder thickening, dilated system, and dilation of the posterior urethra. A specific diagnosis should be documented by videocystometrography (see later discussion).

Natural History

In the 1960s, 25% of children died within the first 12 months, and 25% died later in childhood, including "renal death" (i.e., ESRD). By the late 1990s, the early mortality rate was less than 5%, and after 15 years of follow-up, only 15% to 20% of patients had reached ESRD.[40]

The bladder may become stretched, resulting in poor emptying, or unstable, leading to poor compliance, unsuppressed detrusor contractions, and high storage pressure. Both these situations are exaggerated by progressive polyuria. It is not uncommon for such patients to have a daily urine volume of 5 liters. Urodynamic follow-up studies suggest that instability decreases with time; bladder capacity increases, but there are unsustained voiding contractions. The prognosis correlates with the nadir serum creatinine value once obstruction has been relieved. Despite adequate early treatment, chronic kidney disease (CKD) due to renal dysplasia develops in many children.[38,41]

Treatment

All children have had transurethral resection of their valves in infancy. Bladder diversion should be avoided. The question of "undiversion" of ileal conduits (created in earlier times) is discussed later. Bladder instability and poor bladder compliance must be treated, irrespective of whether they are causing symptoms. Boys with substantial residual volumes can be managed by CISC, but there is often poor compliance with this either because of urethral discomfort or because previous urethral surgery has made the passage of catheters difficult. Compliance is a particular problem with adolescents who are continent and for whom renal failure is too abstract a concept. Continence often improves spontaneously at puberty but can be helped by imipramine. Deterioration in renal function will require further examination of urine flow rate and exclusion of urethral stricture.

Urethral Diverticulum

Urethral diverticulum usually occurs in boys and is rare. It may present with UTI, obstruction, or stones. There are two types, anterior and posterior. The anterior type can be associated with anterior urethral valves and obstruction.

GENERAL MANAGEMENT OF CONGENITAL TRACT ABNORMALITIES

The principles of management of congenital tract abnormalities are shown in Figure 50.19. The most important part of the management is ensuring that the patient, family, and primary care physician know what can and must be done. The first thing to make clear is the necessity of long-term follow-up at no longer than annual intervals. ESRD commonly occurs when a patient is lost to follow-up, often presenting later with accelerated hypertension and rapid loss of renal function.

Clinical Evaluation

By the time the adolescent is passed on to an adult physician, it is assumed that the urinary tract is not obstructed and further surgery is not required. Nevertheless, it is the responsibility of the nephrologists and urologists who care for these children to review this aspect from time to time.

Symptomatic UTI is common and must be treated promptly. Increase in frequency or severity of infections must lead to investigations to find the cause.[42] The blood pressure must be monitored regularly and kept normal. Finally, renal function must be monitored, proteinuria assessed, and the cause of any deterioration identified. As in any other renal condition, the remnant kidney function may decline inexorably, and this is associated with increasing proteinuria and hypertension. As with other renal conditions, function is usually stable when there is little or no proteinuria. Deterioration in the absence of proteinuria must alert the physician to the likelihood of obstruction or the adverse effect of a nephrotoxic drug.

A number of routine investigations should be performed to document the current situation and to act as a reference point for the future (Fig. 50.20). If the bladder empties completely with an adequate flow rate (15 ml/s), no problems should arise. If there is any doubt about the condition of the bladder, urodynamic investigations are necessary. If the clinical situation changes, further investigations are required. An increase in UTIs might suggest a stone or increase in residual urine. With an unexpected decline in renal function, obstruction has to be excluded all over again.

It is helpful and important for the patient to keep a 24-hour urine volume diary every 6 to 12 months. Patients are asked to write down the time that they voided and to measure and record the volume passed. It is best to ask them to do this on 2 consecutive days, so that one can determine the maximum bladder capacity and the total 24-hour urine volume. This should be done before urodynamic investigations because results can be misleading if bladder is not filled to capacity.

Exclude Obstruction

Obstruction must always be excluded if there is a change in renal function. The possibility of obstruction may be raised by a routine ultrasound (see Fig. 50.9) and should be pursued with MAG3 scintigraphy to exclude obstruction (Fig. 50.21).

In patients with conduits, obstruction can be excluded by infusion of contrast material into the loop (loopogram) and demonstration of reflux up the ureter.

Rarely, in patients with large bladders or in transplant recipients, the kidney may become obstructed when the bladder reaches a certain volume. This can be investigated by filling the

Management of Congenital Renal Tract Abnormalities
Educate and explain to encourage compliance
Review urologic status
Find cause of urinary tract obstruction and treat
Control blood pressure
Monitor renal function and proteinuria
Treat acidosis
Prevent bone disease
Check for stones
Clean intermittent self-catheterization for chronic retention
Maintain bladder storage pressure below 40 cm H_2O
Maintain bladder volume below 400 ml

Figure 50.19 General principles of management of congenital renal tract abnormalities.

Monitoring Patients with Congenital Renal Tract Abnormalities

Baseline Measurements	Reason for Test
Radiology	
Abdominal x-ray	Exclude stones
Ultrasound of kidneys	Baseline
Ultrasound of bladder postmicturition	Assess residual volume
Urine flow rate	Ensure adequacy
Scintigraphy	
Glomerular filtration rate: ^{51}Cr-labeled EDTA	Baseline
Dynamic isotope scan with ^{99}Tc-labeled MAG3 or DTPA	Assess outflow obstruction/holdup
Static isotope scan with ^{99}Tc-labeled DMSA	Assess scarring and divided function
Biochemistry	
Urine-protein creatinine ratio	Baseline

Figure 50.20 Monitoring patients with congenital renal tract abnormalities. Routine investigations for assessment of clinical status.

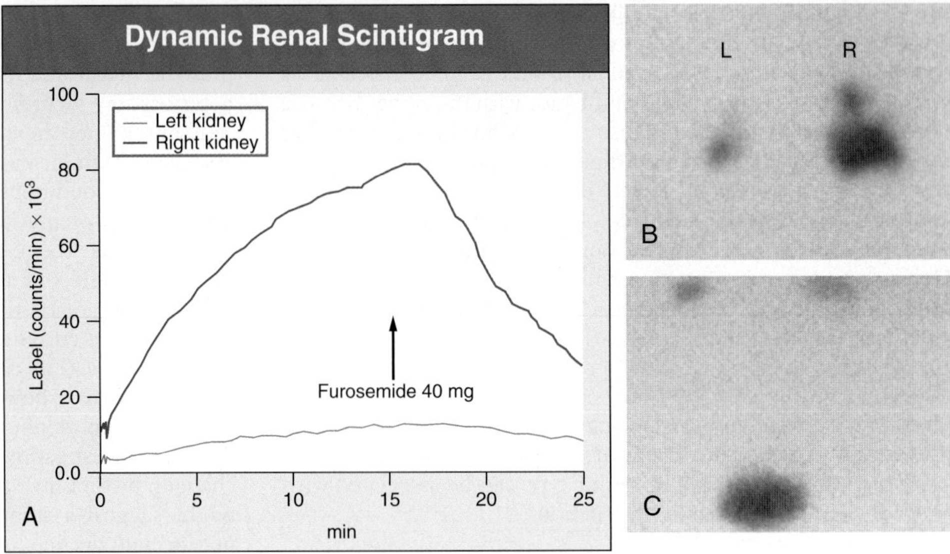

Figure 50.21 Dynamic ^{99m}Tc-labeled MAG3 renal scintigram. A, Time-activity curve showing accumulation of isotope in right kidney that washes out after furosemide, thus excluding significant obstruction. **B** and **C,** Images from the same study showing holdup of isotope in dilated right renal pelvis (**B**) that washes out into the bladder after furosemide (**C**), excluding significant obstruction.

bladder by a catheter and performing ^{99m}Tc-labeled MAG3 scintigraphy, initially with the bladder full. If there is no excretion, the bladder volume can be reduced in 100-ml increments until there is flow down the ureter (Fig. 50.22).

Urodynamics

Any urodynamic investigation should start with a free urine flow rate. Provided the flow rate is normal and the bladder empties completely (leaving no residual volume on postmicturition ultrasound), it can be assumed that there is no significant bladder outflow obstruction.

Complete investigation of abnormalities of bladder and urethral function requires synchronous recordings of intravesical and intrarectal pressures taken during bladder filling and emptying (see Fig. 50.17). Combined with radiologic imaging, the study is known as videocystometrography.

Surgical Correction of the Urinary Tract

A normal bladder acts as a low-pressure, good-volume urine reservoir that is continent, is sterile, and empties freely and completely. Any other form of urine reservoir aims to recreate such an environment. When this is not achieved in either a natural or a reconstructed bladder, complications such as sepsis and renal dysfunction can occur.

A variety of conduits and continent reservoirs have been developed to replace unusable bladders. Ileal conduit diversion has been most widely used for native kidneys, although deterioration in renal function commonly occurs secondary to long-term complications including urosepsis, renal calculi, and, most commonly, stenosis leading either to obstruction or to reflux with ureteral dilation. There is an overall complication rate of 45%, but with a high index of suspicion and an aggressive diagnostic and therapeutic approach, many of these problems can be detected and treated early, with resultant good long-term function of native kidneys. Similar results may be obtained when renal transplantation is performed in these patients.[43] Other forms of urinary diversion that are continent and therefore more socially acceptable to patients are now widely used in general urologic practice and are being encountered in renal transplantation (Fig. 50.23; see also Fig. 50.14). These forms include augmented bladders draining through the urethra and augmented or intestinal bladders draining through continent stomas.

Undiversion of Conduits

The only certain improvement with undiversion is cosmetic. Initially, undiversion was undertaken because of poor results or complications from conduits. Short-term results of undiversion are very promising, and the major indications today are convenience and cosmetic appearance (see Fig. 50.23). Long-term results, however, are not yet available.

Before undiversion is considered, four factors must be addressed:

1. Is there residual obstruction?
2. What is the function of the bladder?
3. What is the function of the sphincters?
4. What is the normal 24-hour urine volume?

In particular, the bladder storage pressure must be considered because a low-pressure reservoir must be achieved. This is a particular problem when patients are polyuric. The potential capacity of the bladder will often have to be reassessed after a period of bladder cycling, when the bladder is repeatedly filled through a suprapubic catheter and the volume, voiding capacity, and residual volume are determined. If the native bladder is not of sufficient volume and compliance, some form of augmentation will be required.

COMPLICATIONS

Urinary Tract Infections (To Treat or Not To Treat)

Symptomatic UTIs are common.[42] Risk factors include stagnation of urine, stones, foreign bodies (stents, catheters), previous infections, and renal scarring. UTIs must be treated promptly after a urine culture specimen (midstream or catheter specimen) has been taken. Recurrent UTIs, particularly after a period of stability, must lead to further investigations to exclude stones or obstruction, including abdominal radiography, renal ultrasound, and postmicturition bladder ultrasound.

Asymptomatic UTIs often do not require treatment (except during pregnancy). For patients with urinary diversions, it is

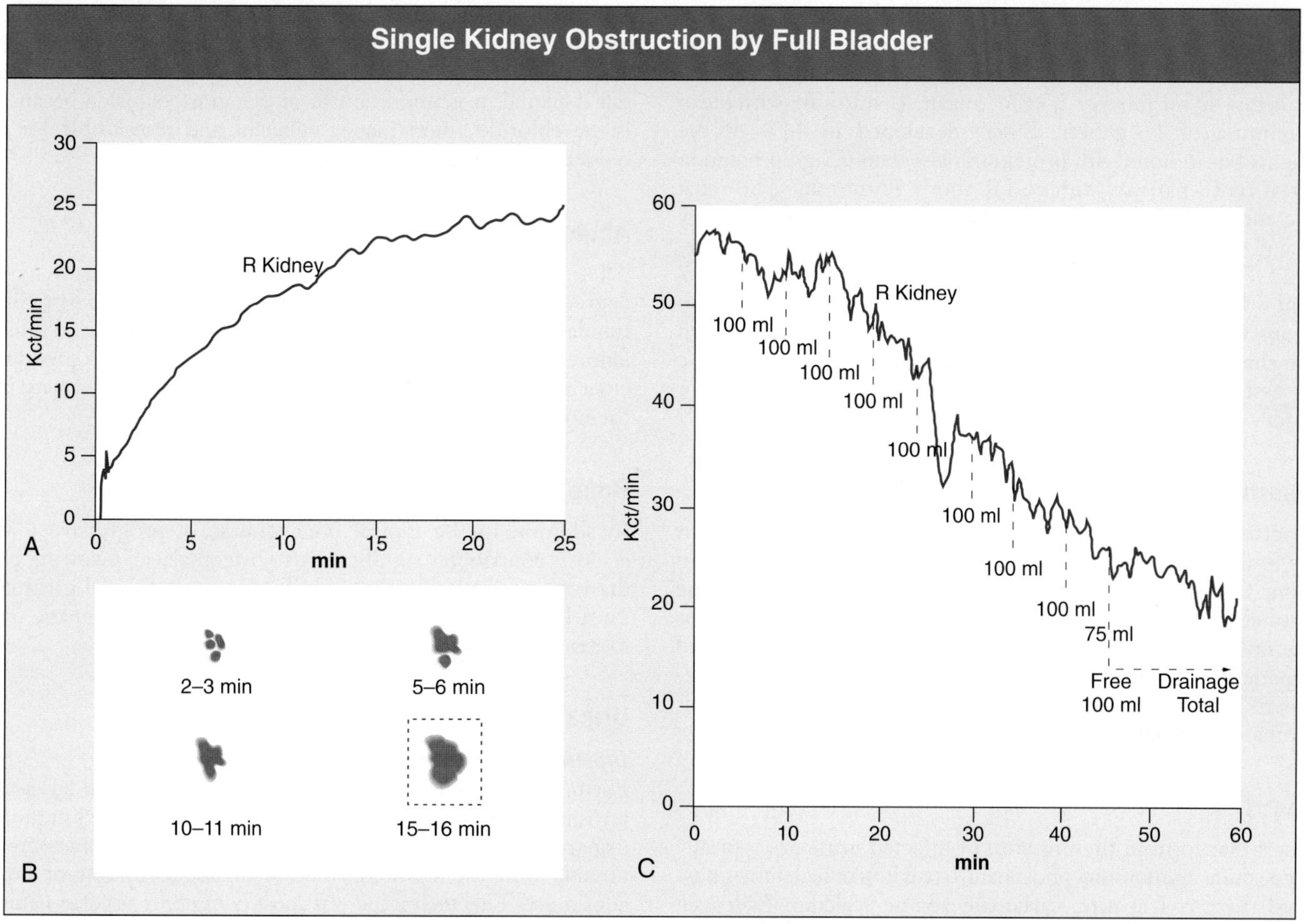

Figure 50.22 Dynamic isotope scan (MAG3) starting with bladder full in a patient with solitary right kidney. A, Rising curve of tracer accumulating in kidney and showing no excretion. **B,** Accumulation of isotope in hydronephrotic pelvis without excretion to bladder. **C,** The 100-ml increments of fluid removed from bladder result in eventual free drainage of the kidney.

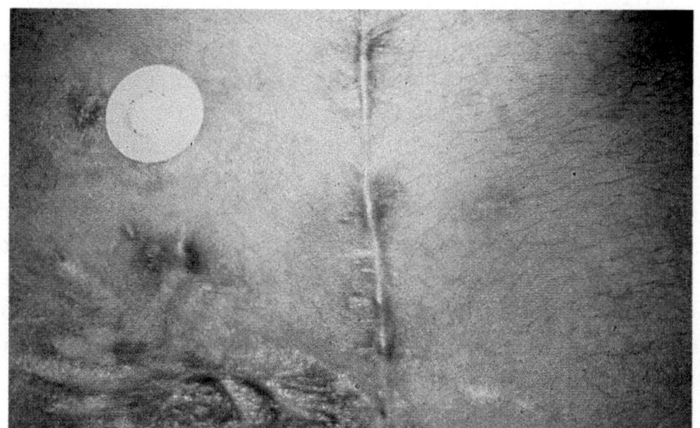

Figure 50.23 Mitrofanoff stoma. A patient born with bladder exstrophy who has had a successful renal transplant for the past 20 years. Her kidney is plumbed into a colonic reservoir, and she catheterizes herself through a continent Mitrofanoff stoma, which in the picture is covered by a small piece of bandage.

important to obtain a catheter specimen of urine because urine taken from a bag is invariably infected.

It is sometimes appropriate to give prophylactic antibiotics, such as trimethoprim or nitrofurantoin, to eradicate infection. Many patients believe that cranberry juice helps them; it reduces the incidence of *Escherichia coli* infection but will not treat a symptomatic infection. Tetracycline and oxytetracycline are contraindicated because they cause acute on chronic deterioration in renal function; doxycycline, however, can be used. Nitrofurantoin and nalidixic acid are avoided if GFR is reduced below 50 ml/min because they are both renally excreted and toxic in renal failure. Quinolones should not be used for prophylaxis, if possible, because of the risk for inducing resistance. Attempts to sterilize the urinary tract when foreign bodies such as stones remain are unlikely to be successful.

If prophylactic antibiotics are no longer effective at preventing infection, it is advisable to stop all antibiotics and to give the patient a supply of antibiotics to treat symptoms at home as they occur.

Hypertension and Glomerular Hyperfiltration

If renal function is declining with proteinuria and hypertension, glomerular hyperfiltration is likely, although all other causes of renal dysfunction must be excluded. Patients should be treated with renin-angiotensin blockade (ACE inhibitors and angiotensin receptor blockers [ARBs]).[4]

Proteinuria and Progressive Renal Failure

Can progression to ESRD be predicted, and does treatment with ACE inhibitors delay or prevent this?[4] We investigated this in a retrospective review of patients with scarred irregular kidneys as a consequence of either primary renal dysplasia or abnormal bladder function. All patients had at least 5 years of follow-up, and when ACE inhibitors were started, estimated GFR (eGFR) was below 60 ml/min per 1.73 m^2 (mean, 41 ml/min), with mean proteinuria of 1.7 g/24 h. ESRD developed in 46% of the patients but in none with proteinuria less than 0.5 g/24 h and in only 2 of 18 patients with eGFR above 50 ml/min. The renal outcome of the two groups was similar whether there was primary renal dysplasia or abnormal bladder function. There was a watershed GFR of 40 to 50 ml/min above which ACE inhibitor treatment improved renal outcome.[4] The similar outcome of the two groups indicates that progressive renal failure in young men born with abnormal bladders is due to intrinsic renal pathophysiologic processes, in contrast to the view that it is a consequence of poor bladder function.

Hypertension

Hypertension is common in the presence of scarred kidneys, but it is usually controlled easily with one or two drugs. Patients in whom CKD is secondary to obstruction tend to have volume contraction and therefore often have normal blood pressure or only mild hypertension. ACE inhibitors or ARBs are preferred for patients with proteinuria and progressive renal failure. Diuretics are likely to cause unacceptable side effects if the patient is volume contracted.

Stones

Stones that form in the presence of infected urine are typically magnesium ammonium phosphate (struvite) or calcium phosphate (hydroxyl apatite, carbonate apatite, calcium hydrogen phosphate [brushite], tricalcium phosphate [whitlockite]). These salts are poorly soluble in alkaline urine. In 90% of patients, the infecting organism is *Proteus* species,[44] but other urea-splitting organisms (including some staphylococci and *Pseudomonas* species) also generate ammonia.[42]

Stones, usually calcium phosphate, are common in conduits because of the alkaline environment and occur in 5% to 30% of ileal conduits. Stones must be suspected if UTIs recur or become more frequent, if renal function suddenly deteriorates, or if there is an unexplained sterile pyuria.

Tubular Dysfunction

In patients whose renal failure is secondary to obstruction, there is significant tubular injury. This may cause problems, in particular with urinary concentration, acidification, and sodium reabsorption.

Polyuria

Nocturia is one of the most significant symptoms in the assessment of patients in whom obstruction or tubular dysfunction is suspected. Overfilling of the bladder or reservoir is an important cause of intermittent upper tract obstruction and deteriorating function. The 24-hour urine volume diary is a simple way to assess this.

Salt Depletion

Patients with tubular damage may have a salt-losing tendency. Patients typically have a cool periphery and constricted hand veins with no peripheral edema. Increasing salt intake can relieve cramps, improve renal function, and reduce hyperuricemia, but at the cost of increasing blood pressure. With patients who are salt depleted, it is important to give sodium chloride because it is the chloride anion that is deficient and responsible for the reduction in circulating volume.

Acidosis

There is often a metabolic acidosis disproportionate to the degree of renal impairment. This is secondary both to a proximal tubular failure of bicarbonate reabsorption and to a distal tubular failure to secrete hydrogen ions. It is our practice to give sufficient sodium bicarbonate to correct the plasma bicarbonate into the normal range.

Bone Disease

In addition to the typical bone disease of progressive CKD, acidosis contributes significantly to osteomalacia. Growing children are particularly vulnerable to osteomalacia, and great care must be taken to correct acidosis and to actively manage bone disease.

Urinary Diversions

Ureterosigmoidostomy

Fortunately, it is now rare to meet a patient who still has a ureterosigmoidostomy, which was widely used as a technique for urinary diversion until the 1970s. The ureters were anastomosed directly into the sigmoid colon with no disruption of bowel continuity. This technique was most commonly used in patients with bladder exstrophy. Although patients start with normal renal function, there is frequently deterioration in function. In one series of 25 patients, significant renal damage occurred in 50%. Stones, infection, and ureteral strictures are common, and patients remain at risk for colonic carcinoma, with a 10% incidence of carcinoma at 20-year follow-up. However, this diversion is probably best known for the hyperchloremic, hypokalemic acidosis that occurs. Once the urine is in contact with the colonic mucosa, the urinary sodium exchanges for potassium and the chloride for bicarbonate, and large quantities of ammonium ions are produced by the action of the fecal bacteria on urinary ammonia. Ammonium ions are absorbed both with chloride and in exchange for sodium. The severe acidosis is a consequence of the ammonium ion retention and stool loss of bicarbonate. Patients are managed with large doses of oral sodium bicarbonate, which is titrated to keep the plasma bicarbonate in the normal range (>22 mmol/l).

Ileal Conduits

Unlike the sigmoidostomy, in which urine enters a reservoir, the ileal conduit is free flowing, with rapid urinary transit and no reservoir. Therefore, metabolic complications are much less common, although again the bowel can exchange sodium and chloride for potassium and bicarbonate.[45,46] There are a number of other complications of ileal and colonic conduits that can lead to progressive loss of renal function (Fig. 50.24).

Enterocystoplasty and Intestinal Urinary Reservoirs

In a study of 53 patients with bladder exstrophy who were observed for more than 10 years and had serial isotopic GFRs, renal function deteriorated (decrease in GFR of 20% or more)

Long-Term Complications of Urinary Diversion
Pyelonephritis and scarring
Calculi
Obstruction
Strictures
Bladder mucus causing obstruction
Cancer at intestinal–ureteral anastomosis
Hyperchloremic acidosis
Delayed linear growth in children
Effects of intestinal loss from gastrointestinal tract, e.g., vitamin B_{12} deficiency
Complications related to abnormal pelvic anatomy, e.g., in pregnancy
Psychological and body image problems

Figure 50.24 Long-term complications of urinary diversion.

in only 10 (20%).[33] Loss of function was caused principally by chronic retention with or without infection in poorly compliant patients who did not catheterize regularly. Patients must also be checked regularly to ensure that anastomotic stenoses and high-pressure reservoirs do not occur. Stones are very common and occur in up to 50% of patients.[47]

END-STAGE RENAL DISEASE AND TRANSPLANTATION

This group of patients presents two important problems at ESRD. First, because of multiple abdominal operations, continuous ambulatory peritoneal dialysis (CAPD) is often impossible, although if there is any doubt, CAPD should be attempted. Second, the bladder and urinary reservoir must be suitable for renal transplantation. If a bladder has just destroyed two perfectly good native kidneys, it is likely to do the same to a transplant kidney. Most patients will be maintained on hemodialysis, but it is frequently difficult to establish a good arteriovenous fistula because of chronic hypovolemia and venoconstriction. Patients on dialysis often continue to pass 1 liter or more of urine per 24 hours, and they also remain at risk for serious UTI and pyelonephritis.

Transplantation

Pretransplantation Assessment

Transplantation into the abnormal lower urinary tract requires careful evaluation and follow-up. Thorough preoperative assessment of bladder function is essential. Patients considered to have normal bladders require at least a postmicturition bladder ultrasound examination and urinary flow rate.

All patients with abnormal bladders or reservoir must have a full videocystometrogram to ensure that the bladder reservoir is large and adequately compliant. If the bladder is small or has not been used for some time, bladder cycling, which involves periodically filling and distending the bladder through a suprapubic catheter, may be required. A study of urodynamics before transplantation indicated that poor bladder function as shown by small bladder volumes is a predictor of graft loss even in patients with previously normal bladder function.[48]

Intermittent self-catheterization is safe and effective for a patient with a poor flow rate who fails to empty the bladder. This, however, is possible only with a normal urethra and a cooperative patient. When this is not practical, we attempt to establish suprapubic drainage through a continent stoma, for example, a Mitrofanoff stoma (see Fig. 50.23). If a conduit is to be used, then a loopogram and endoscopy must ensure that it is in good condition. We do not remove native kidneys unless they are causing recurrent UTI.

Transplant Outcome

In an 18-year experience, we transplanted 65 patients with abnormal bladders, with a total of 72 renal transplants.[49] In 52 cases, the ureters were transplanted into unaugmented bladder; in 20 cases, there was some form of augmentation or diversion. Results were compared with 59 transplants in 55 patients who had renal failure from renal dysplasia and whose bladder function was considered to be normal. There was no difference in actuarial graft survival in the two groups at 10 years (abnormal bladders, 66%; normal bladders, 61%), although longer follow-up showed an advantage for normal bladders, with a kidney half-life of 29 to 33 years compared with 15 years for the abnormal bladders.[49] UTIs were relatively common in all patients but produced problems only in patients with abnormal bladders.

Management

We routinely use double-J ureteral stents at the time of transplant surgery. Adequacy of urinary drainage must be assessed frequently, even when graft function seems to be good. Two months after transplantation, when the ureteral stent has been removed, we perform as a baseline the following tests:

- ^{51}Cr-EDTA GFR.
- Postmicturition ultrasound of kidney and bladder.
- Dynamic ^{99m}Tc-MAG3 scintigraphy.
- Static ^{99m}Tc-DMSA scintigraphy, as a baseline for renal scarring.

The GFR is repeated at 6 months and then annually. Ultrasound and ^{99m}Tc-MAG3 scintigraphy are repeated at 1 year and then when indicated. The protein-creatinine ratio is measured on a random urine sample at every outpatient visit. If there is renal dysfunction, imaging tests are repeated, and if there is a change from baseline, renal biopsy is performed to exclude an immunologic cause of graft dysfunction. If there is a documented deterioration in renal function in the absence of rejection or calcineurin inhibitor toxicity, the DMSA scan is repeated (to see whether there has been new scarring) and the bladder reassessed urodynamically.[50]

Complications

UTIs must be detected and treated early, and recurrent infections may require long courses of antibiotics or even removal of the native tracts.

In our experience, symptomatic UTIs are common in the first 3 months after transplantation (63%); fever and systemic symptoms occur in 39% with normal bladders and 59% with abnormal bladders. UTI directly contributes to graft loss in patients with abnormal bladders but causes no consequences in those with normal bladders.[43] In our practice, prophylactic administration of antibiotics for the first 6 months has halved the subsequent incidence of UTI.

When UTIs recur, a cause must be sought with ultrasound of kidney and bladder. A plain abdominal radiograph is essential to look for stones in native or transplant kidneys and the bladder or urinary diversion. If there is a residual volume after double micturition, the patient must be instructed to perform clean intermittent self-catheterization. With these measures, good results are obtained.

REFERENCES

1. Lewis MA. Demography of renal disease in childhood. *Semin Fetal Neonatal Med.* 2008;13:118-124.
2. Neild GH. What do we know about chronic renal failure in young adults? Adult outcome of pediatric renal disease. *Pediatr Nephrol.* 2009; 24:1921-1928.
3. Brenner BM, Meyer TW, Hostetter TH. Dietary protein intake and the progressive nature of kidney disease: The role of hemodynamically mediated glomerular injury in the pathogenesis of progressive glomerular sclerosis in aging, renal ablation, and intrinsic renal disease. *N Engl J Med.* 1982;307:652-659.
4. Neild GH, Thomson G, Nitsch D, et al. Renal outcome in adults with renal insufficiency and irregular asymmetric kidneys. *BMC Nephrol.* 2004;5:12-22.
5. Woolf AS, Winyard PJ, Hermanns MM, Welham SJM. Maldevelopment of the human kidney and lower urinary tract. In: Vize PD, Woolf AS, Bard JBL, eds. *The Kidney: From Normal Development to Congenital Disease*. London: Academic Press; 2003:377-394.
6. Woolf AS, Jenkins D. Development of the kidney. In: Jennette JC, Olson JL, Schwartz MM, Silva FG, eds. *Heptinstall's Pathology of the Kidney*, 6th ed. Philadelphia: Lippincott Williams & Wilkins; 2007:71-95.
7. Rascher W, Roesch WH. Congenital abnormalities of the urinary tract. In: Davison AM, Cameron JS, Grunfeld J-P, et al, eds. *Oxford Textbook of Clinical Nephrology*, 3rd ed. Oxford: Oxford University Press; 2005:2471-2494.
8. Woolf AS, Price KL, Scambler PJ, Winyard PJ. Evolving concepts in human renal dysplasia. *J Am Soc Nephrol.* 2004;15:998-1007.
9. Miyazaki Y, Ichikawa I. Ontogeny of congenital anomalies of the kidney and urinary tract, CAKUT. *Pediatr Int.* 2003;45:598-604.
10. Price KL, Woolf AS, Long DA. Unraveling the genetic landscape of bladder development in mice. *J Urol.* 2009;181:2366-2374.
11. Dressler GR, Wilkinson JE, Rothenpieler UW, et al. Deregulation of Pax-2 expression in transgenic mice generates severe kidney abnormalities. *Nature.* 1993;362:65-67.
12. Torres M, Gomez PE, Dressler GR, Gruss P. Pax-2 controls multiple steps of urogenital development. *Development.* 1995;121:4057-4065.
13. Caubit X, Lye CM, Martin E, et al. Teashirt 3 is necessary for ureteral smooth muscle differentiation downstream of SHH and BMP4. *Development.* 2008;135:3301-3310.
14. Schedl A. Renal abnormalities and their developmental origin. *Nat Rev Genet.* 2007;8:791-802.
15. Risdon RA, Yeung CK, Ransley PG. Reflux nephropathy in children submitted to unilateral nephrectomy: A clinicopathological study. *Clin Nephrol.* 1993;40:308-314.
16. Hiraoka M, Hori C, Tsukahara H, et al. Congenitally small kidneys with reflux as a common cause of nephropathy in boys. *Kidney Int.* 1997;52:811-816.
17. Cotran RS. Glomerulosclerosis in reflux nephropathy. *Kidney Int.* 1982;21:528-534.
18. Kincaid-Smith P, Becker G. Reflux nephropathy and chronic atrophic pyelonephritis: A review. *J Infect Dis.* 1978;138:774-780.
19. Bhathena DB, Weiss JH, Holland NH, et al. Focal and segmental glomerular sclerosis in reflux nephropathy. *Am J Med.* 1980;68:886-892.
20. Jenkins D, Bitner-Glindzicz M, Malcolm S, et al. De novo uroplakin IIIa heterozygous mutations cause human renal adysplasia leading to severe kidney failure. *J Am Soc Nephrol.* 2005;16:2141-2149.
21. O'Dea D, Parfrey PS, Harnett JD, et al. The importance of renal impairment in the natural history of Bardet-Biedl syndrome. *Am J Kidney Dis.* 1996;27:776-783.
22. Ansley SJ, Badano JL, Blacque OE, et al. Basal body dysfunction is a likely cause of pleiotropic Bardet-Biedl syndrome. *Nature.* 2003;425: 628-633.
23. Koff SA, Campbell KD. The nonoperative management of unilateral neonatal hydronephrosis: Natural history of poorly functioning kidneys. *J Urol.* 1994;152:593-595.
24. Lee PH, Diamond DA, Duffy PG, Ransley PG. Duplex reflux: A study of 105 children. *J Urol.* 1991;146:657-659.
25. Ehrlich RM, Brown WJ. Ultrastructural anatomic observations of the ureter in the prune belly syndrome. *Birth Defects Orig Artic Ser.* 1977;13:101-103.
26. Whitaker RH, Johnston JH. A simple classification of wide ureters. *Br J Urol.* 1975;47:781-787.
27. Woodhouse CRJ. *Long-Term Paediatric Urology*. Oxford: Blackwell Scientific Publications; 1991.
28. Woodhouse CR, Ransley PG, Innes WD. Prune belly syndrome: Report of 47 cases. *Arch Dis Child.* 1982;57:856-859.
29. Burbige KA, Amodio J, Berdon WE, et al. Prune belly syndrome: 35 years of experience. *J Urol.* 1987;137:86-90.
30. Woodard JR, Parrott TS. Reconstruction of the urinary tract in prune belly uropathy. *J Urol.* 1978;119:824-828.
31. Hurwitz RS, Manzoni GA, Ransley PG, Stephens FD. Cloacal exstrophy: A report of 34 cases. *J Urol.* 1987;138:1060-1064.
32. Husmann DA, McLorie GA, Churchill BM. A comparison of renal function in the exstrophy patient treated with staged reconstruction versus urinary diversion. *J Urol.* 1988;140:1204-1206.
33. Fontaine E, Leaver R, Woodhouse CR. The effect of intestinal urinary reservoirs on renal function: A 10-year follow-up. *BJU Int.* 2000;86: 195-198.
34. Johnston LB, Borzyskowski M. Bladder dysfunction and neurological disability at presentation in closed spina bifida. *Arch Dis Child.* 1998;79:33-38.
35. McLorie GA, Perez MR, Csima A, Churchill BM. Determinants of hydronephrosis and renal injury in patients with myelomeningocele. *J Urol.* 1988;140:1289-1292.
36. Lapides J, Diokno AC, Silber SJ, Lowe BS. Clean, intermittent self-catheterization in the treatment of urinary tract disease. *J Urol.* 1972;107:458-461.
37. Edelstein RA, Bauer SB, Kelly MD, et al. The long-term urological response of neonates with myelodysplasia treated proactively with intermittent catheterization and anticholinergic therapy. *J Urol.* 1995;154: 1500-1504.
38. Tejani A, Butt K, Glassberg K, et al. Predictors of eventual end stage renal disease in children with posterior urethral valves. *J Urol.* 1986; 136:857-860.
39. Rittenberg MH, Hulbert WC, Snyder HM, Duckett JW. Protective factors in posterior urethral valves. *J Urol.* 1988;140:993-996.
40. Smith GH, Canning DA, Schulman SL, et al. The long-term outcome of posterior urethral valves treated with primary valve ablation and observation. *J Urol.* 1996;155:1730-1734.
41. Parkhouse HF, Barratt TM, Dillon MJ, et al. Long-term outcome of boys with posterior urethral valves. *Br J Urol.* 1988;62:59-62.
42. Neild GH. Urinary tract infection. *Medicine (Baltimore).* 2003;31: 85-90.
43. Crowe A, Cairns HS, Wood S, et al. Renal transplantation following renal failure due to urological disorders. *Nephrol Dial Transplant.* 1998;13:2065-2069.
44. Dretler SP. The pathogenesis of urinary tract calculi occurring after ileal conduit diversion. I. Clinical study. II. Conduit study. 3. Prevention. *J Urol.* 1973;109:204-209.
45. McDougal WS. Metabolic complications of urinary intestinal diversion. *J Urol.* 1992;147:1199-1208.
46. Silverman SH, Woodhouse CR, Strachan JR, et al. Long-term management of patients who have had urinary diversions into colon. *Br J Urol.* 1986;58:634-639.
47. Woodhouse CR, Robertson WG. Urolithiasis in enterocystoplasties. *World J Urol.* 2004;22:215-221.
48. Kashi SH, Wynne KS, Sadek SA, Lodge JP. An evaluation of vesical urodynamics before renal transplantation and its effect on renal allograft function and survival. *Transplantation.* 1994;57: 1455-1457.
49. Neild GH, Dakmish A, Wood S, et al. Renal transplantation in adults with abnormal bladders. *Transplantation.* 2004;77:1123-1127.
50. Cairns HS, Spencer S, Hilson AJ, et al. ^{99m}Tc-DMSA imaging with tomography in renal transplant recipients with abnormal lower urinary tracts. *Nephrol Dial Transplant.* 1994;9:1157-1161.

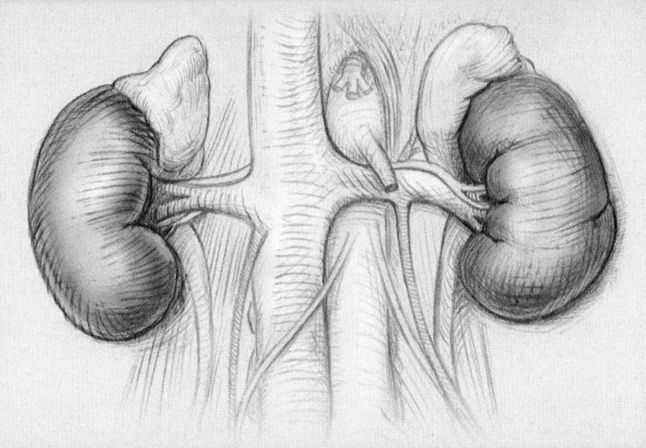

SECTION IX

Infectious Diseases and the Kidney

CHAPTER 51

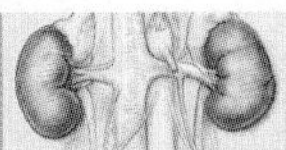

Urinary Tract Infections in Adults

Thomas Hooton

DEFINITION

Urinary tract infection (UTI) in adults can be categorized into six groups: young women with acute uncomplicated cystitis, young women with recurrent cystitis, young women with acute uncomplicated pyelonephritis, adults with acute cystitis and conditions that suggest occult renal or prostatic involvement, complicated UTI, and asymptomatic bacteriuria (Fig. 51.1).[1] A discussion of UTI in pregnancy is provided in Chapter 42 and of vesicoureteral reflux in children in Chapter 61.

Complicated UTI is defined as UTI that increases the risk for serious complications or treatment failure. Patients with various conditions, such as those presented in Figure 51.1, are at increased risk for complicated UTI. Complicated UTIs may require different pretreatment and post-treatment evaluation and type and duration of antimicrobial treatment than for uncomplicated UTI. On occasion, complicated UTIs are diagnosed only after a patient has a poor response to treatment. The physician often must decide, on the basis of limited clinical information, whether to embark on a more extensive evaluation and treatment course when confronted with a patient with UTI.

EPIDEMIOLOGY

Acute uncomplicated UTIs are extremely common, with several million episodes of acute cystitis and at least 250,000 episodes of acute pyelonephritis occurring annually in the United States. The incidence of cystitis in young sexually active women is about 0.5 per 1 person-year.[2] Acute uncomplicated cystitis may recur in 27% to 44% of healthy women, even though they have normal urinary tracts.[3] The incidence of pyelonephritis in young women is about 3 per 1000 person-years.[4] The self-reported incidence of symptomatic UTI in postmenopausal women is about 10% per year.[5] The incidence of symptomatic UTI in adult men younger than 50 years is much lower than in women, ranging from 5 to 8 per 10,000 men annually.

Complicated UTIs encompass an extraordinarily broad range of infectious entities (see Fig. 51.1). Nosocomial UTIs are a common type of complicated UTI and occur in 5% of admissions in the university tertiary care hospital setting; catheter-associated infections account for most of the infections. Catheter-associated bacteriuria is the most common source of gram-negative bacteremia in hospitalized patients.[6]

Asymptomatic bacteriuria is defined as two separate consecutive clean-voided urine specimens both with 10^5 or more colony-forming units (cfu)/ml of the same uropathogen in the absence of symptoms referable to the urinary tract.[7] Asymptomatic bacteriuria is found in about 5% of young adult women[8] but rarely in men younger than 50 years. The prevalence increases up to 16% of ambulatory women and 19% of ambulatory men older than 70 years and up to 50% of elderly women and 40% of elderly men who are institutionalized.[7] Asymptomatic bacteriuria may be persistent or transient and recurrent, and many patients have had previous symptomatic infection or develop symptomatic UTI soon after having asymptomatic bacteriuria. Asymptomatic bacteriuria is generally benign, although as discussed later, it may lead to serious complications in some clinical settings.

PATHOGENESIS

Uncomplicated Infection

Most uncomplicated UTIs in healthy women result when uropathogens (typically *Escherichia coli*) present in the rectal flora enter the bladder through the urethra after an interim phase of periurethral and distal urethral colonization. In the male, colonizing uropathogens may also come from a sex partner's vagina or rectum. Hematogenous seeding of the urinary tract by potential uropathogens such as *Staphylococcus aureus* is the source of some UTIs, but this is more likely to occur in the setting of persistent blood stream infection or urinary tract obstruction.

Many host behavioral, genetic, and biologic factors predispose young healthy women to uncomplicated UTI (Fig. 51.2).[9] Risk factors include sexual intercourse, use of spermicide products, and a history of previous recurrent UTI.[2,10] Nonsecretors of ABO blood group antigens have an increased risk for recurrent cystitis, the P_1 blood group phenotype is a risk factor for recurrent pyelonephritis in women, and mutations in the gene for CXCR1, the interleukin-8 receptor, are more frequent and expression of CXCR1 is lower in children prone to pyelonephritis compared with controls.[11] Factors protecting individuals from UTI include the host's immune response; maintenance of normal vaginal flora, which protects against colonization with uropathogens; and removal of bladder bacteriuria by micturition.

Certain strains of *E. coli* have a selective advantage for colonization and infection (see Fig. 51.2).[12] P-fimbriated strains of *E. coli* are associated with acute uncomplicated pyelonephritis, and their adherence properties may stimulate epithelial and other cells to produce proinflammatory factors that stimulate the inflammatory response. Other virulence determinants include adherence factors (types 1, S, and Dr fimbriae), toxins (hemolysin), aerobactin, and serum resistance. Bacterial virulence determinants associated with cystitis and asymptomatic bacteriuria have been less well characterized.

Categories of Urinary Tract Infection in Adults
Acute uncomplicated cystitis in young women
Recurrent acute uncomplicated cystitis in young women
Acute uncomplicated pyelonephritis in young women
Acute uncomplicated cystitis in adults with a following condition suggesting possible occult renal or prostatic involvement but without other known complicating factors: Male sex Elderly Pregnancy Diabetes mellitus Recent urinary tract instrumentation Childhood urinary tract infection Symptoms for more than 7 days at presentation
Complicated urinary tract infection* Obstruction or other structural factor: urolithiasis, malignancies, ureteral and urethral strictures, bladder diverticula, renal cysts, fistulas, ileal conduits, and other urinary diversions Functional abnormality: neurogenic bladder, vesicoureteral reflux Foreign bodies: indwelling catheter, ureteral stent, nephrostomy tube Other conditions: renal failure, renal transplantation, immunosuppression, multidrug-resistant uropathogens, health care associated (includes hospital-acquired [nosocomial]) infection, prostatitis-related infection, upper tract infection in an adult other than a young healthy woman, other functional or anatomic abnormality of the urinary tract
Asymptomatic bacteriuria

Figure 51.1 Categories of urinary tract infection in adults. *This is a selected list of complicating factors. Some factors complicate urinary tract infections through several mechanisms. *(Data for complicating factors from reference 1.)*

Factors Modulating Risk for Acute Uncomplicated Urinary Tract Infections in Women

Host Determinants	Uropathogen Determinants
Behavioral: sexual intercourse, use of spermicidal products, recent antimicrobial use, suboptimal voiding habits	***Escherichia coli*** virulence determinants: P, S, Dr, and type I fimbriae; hemolysin; aerobactin; serum resistance
Genetic: innate and adaptive immune response; enhanced epithelial cell adherence, antibacterial factors in urine and bladder mucosa, nonsecretor of ABO blood group antigens, P_1 blood group phenotype, reduced CXCR1 expression, previous history of recurrent cystitis	
Biologic: estrogen deficiency in postmenopausal women, micturition	

Figure 51.2 Factors modulating risk for acute uncomplicated urinary tract infections in women.

Factors affecting the large difference in UTI prevalence between men and women include the greater distance between the usual source of uropathogens (the anus and the urethral meatus), the drier environment surrounding the male urethra, and the greater length of the male urethra. Risk factors associated with UTIs in healthy men include intercourse with an infected female partner, anal intercourse, and lack of circumcision, although these factors are often not present in men with UTI. Most uropathogenic strains infecting young men are highly virulent, suggesting that the urinary tract in healthy men is relatively resistant to infection.

Complicated Infection

The initial steps leading to uncomplicated UTI discussed earlier probably also occur in most individuals who develop a complicated UTI. Factors that predispose individuals to complicated UTI generally do so by causing obstruction or stasis of urine flow, facilitating entry of uropathogens into the urinary tract by bypassing normal host defense mechanisms, providing a nidus for infection that is not readily treatable with antimicrobials, or compromising the host immune system (see Fig. 51.1).[1] UTIs are more likely to become complicated in the setting of impaired host defense, as occurs with indwelling catheter use, vesicoureteral reflux, obstruction, neutropenia, and immune deficiencies. Diabetes mellitus is associated with several syndromes of complicated UTI, including renal and perirenal abscess, emphysematous pyelonephritis and cystitis, papillary necrosis, and xanthogranulomatous pyelonephritis.[13] Uropathogen virulence determinants are less important in the pathogenesis of complicated UTIs compared with uncomplicated UTIs. However, infection with multidrug-resistant uropathogens is more likely with complicated UTI.

ETIOLOGIC AGENTS

Uncomplicated upper and lower UTI is most commonly due to *E. coli* (present in 70% to 95%) and *Staphylococcus saprophyticus* (present in 5% to more than 20%) (Fig. 51.3). *S. saprophyticus* only rarely causes acute pyelonephritis.[14] Less common causes of uncomplicated UTI include other Enterobacteriaceae, such as *Proteus mirabilis* or *Klebsiella* species; enterococci; group B streptococci; and rarely *Pseudomonas aeruginosa*, *Citrobacter* species, or other uropathogens.

A broader range of bacteria can cause complicated UTI, and many are resistant to broad-spectrum antimicrobial agents. Although *E. coli* is the most common, *Citrobacter* species, *Enterobacter* species, *P. aeruginosa*, enterococci, and *S. aureus* account for

Bacterial Etiology of Urinary Tract Infections		
	Urinary Tract Infection (%)	
Organisms	Uncomplicated	Complicated
Gram-negative organisms		
Escherichia coli	70–95	21–54
Proteus mirabilis	1–2	1–10
Klebsiella species	1–2	2–17
Citrobacter species	<1	5
Enterobacter species	<1	2–10
Pseudomonas aeruginosa	<1	2–19
Other	<1	6–20
Gram-positive organisms		
Coagulase-negative staphylococci (***S. saprophyticus***)	5–20 or more	1–4
Enterococci	1–2	1–23
Group B streptococci	<1	1–4
Staphylococcus aureus	<1	1–2
Other	<1	2

Figure 51.3 Bacterial etiology of urinary tract infections. *(Data for complicated infections from reference 1.)*

a relatively higher proportion of cases compared with uncomplicated UTIs (see Fig. 51.3).[1] The proportion of infections caused by fungi, especially *Candida* species, is increasing (see Chapter 53). Patients with chronic conditions, such as spinal cord injury and neurogenic bladder, are more likely to have polymicrobial (multiorganism) and multidrug-resistant infections.

CLINICAL SYNDROMES

Acute Uncomplicated Cystitis in Young Women

Women with acute uncomplicated cystitis generally present with acute onset of dysuria, frequency, urgency, or suprapubic pain. Acute dysuria in a young sexually active woman is usually caused by acute cystitis; acute urethritis from *Chlamydia trachomatis*, *Neisseria gonorrhoeae*, or herpes simplex virus infections; or vaginitis caused by *Candida* species or *Trichomonas vaginalis*.[6] These three entities can usually be distinguished by the history, physical examination, and simple laboratory tests. Pyuria is present in almost all women with acute cystitis as well as in most women with urethritis caused by *N. gonorrhoeae* or *C. trachomatis*, and its absence strongly suggests an alternative diagnosis. Hematuria (microscopic or gross) is common in women with UTI but not in women with urethritis or vaginitis.

Definitive diagnosis of UTI requires the presence of significant bacteriuria, the traditional standard for which is 10^5 or more uropathogens per milliliter of voided midstream urine. Studies have shown, however, that up to one third of patients with cystitis have lower colony counts, which are missed with use of the traditional definition. The Infectious Diseases Society of America consensus definition of cystitis is 10^3 cfu/ml or more (sensitivity, 80%; specificity, 90%).[15] Urine cultures are generally not in women with uncomplicated cystitis because the causative organisms are predictable and the culture results become available only after therapeutic decisions have been made.

E. coli in uncomplicated UTI is often resistant to sulfonamides and amoxicillin, and increasing resistance is also being observed for trimethoprim and trimethoprim-sulfamethoxazole (cotrimoxazole) among outpatient urinary strains in the United States and Europe.[16,17] Many drug-resistant *E. coli* are clonal and have been hypothesized to enter new environments by contaminated products ingested by community residents.[18] The prevalence of *E. coli* resistance to nitrofurantoin is generally less than 5%, although nitrofurantoin is inactive against *Proteus* species and some *Enterobacter* and *Klebsiella* strains. Fluoroquinolones remain active against most *E. coli* strains causing uncomplicated cystitis, although resistance is increasing in certain areas of the world.[16,17]

Three-day regimens are recommended for the treatment of acute uncomplicated cystitis because of comparable efficacy, better compliance, lower cost, and lower frequency of adverse reactions than with longer regimens. Single-dose regimens, although highly effective in most women (especially trimethoprim-sulfamethoxazole and fluoroquinolones), are less effective than longer regimens.[19] Higher cure rates have been observed with trimethoprim-sulfamethoxazole and fluoroquinolones than with β-lactams regardless of the site of infection and duration of treatment.

Optimal management of acute uncomplicated cystitis is summarized in Figures 51.4 and 51.5. Trimethoprim or trimethoprim-sulfamethoxazole in a 3-day oral regimen should be considered the first-line agents for uncomplicated cystitis in women who can tolerate them and in areas where resistance is infrequent.[20] Nitrofurantoin is equally effective in a 5-day regimen 20, and should also be considered a first-line agent for uncomplicated cystitis. Fluoroquinolones (3-day duration) are highly effective in the treatment of cystitis, but resistance is increasing worldwide, even among uropathogens causing uncomplicated cystitis, and many experts in UTI now recommend that they be considered as second-line therapy for uncomplicated cystitis to help preserve their usefulness in the treatment of other infections. In this regard, fosfomycin and pivmecillinam should be considered as fluoroquinolone-sparing antimicrobials in patients with uncomplicated cystitis, even though they may be less effective than other first-line agents.[21] Broad-spectrum oral cephalosporins (such as cefixime, cefpodoxime, cefprozil, and cefaclor) demonstrate in vitro activity against most uropathogens causing uncomplicated cystitis, but clinical data are sparse. A recent trial demonstrated that a 3-day regimen of amoxicillin-clavulanate is significantly inferior to a 3-day regimen of ciprofloxacin, even when the uropathogens were susceptible to the drugs with which they were treated.[22] β-Lactam antibiotics have generally been inferior to trimethoprim-sulfamethoxazole or fluoroquinolones in regimens of the same duration.[20]

Routine post-treatment cultures in women are not indicated unless the patient is symptomatic. If the patient remains symptomatic and has documented persistent infection, a longer course of therapy based on sensitivities, usually with a fluoroquinolone, should be used. The benefit of detecting and treating asymptomatic bacteriuria in healthy women has been demonstrated only in pregnancy and before urologic instrumentation or surgery.[7,23]

Recurrent Acute Uncomplicated Cystitis in Women

Most recurrent cystitis in healthy women is due to repeated infection, which in many cases is caused by persistence of the initially infecting strain in the fecal flora.[24] Experimental studies in mice also suggest that some same-strain recurrent UTIs may be caused by a latent reservoir of uropathogens in the bladder epithelium that persist after the initial UTI.[24,25]

Women with recurrent cystitis may benefit from behavioral modification (Fig. 51.6), such as increasing fluid intake and ensuring postcoital micturition, although the benefit of these practices has not been proved. Small studies suggest that ingestion of cranberry products has preventive properties, and *in vitro* studies have shown that cranberry juice blocks adherence of

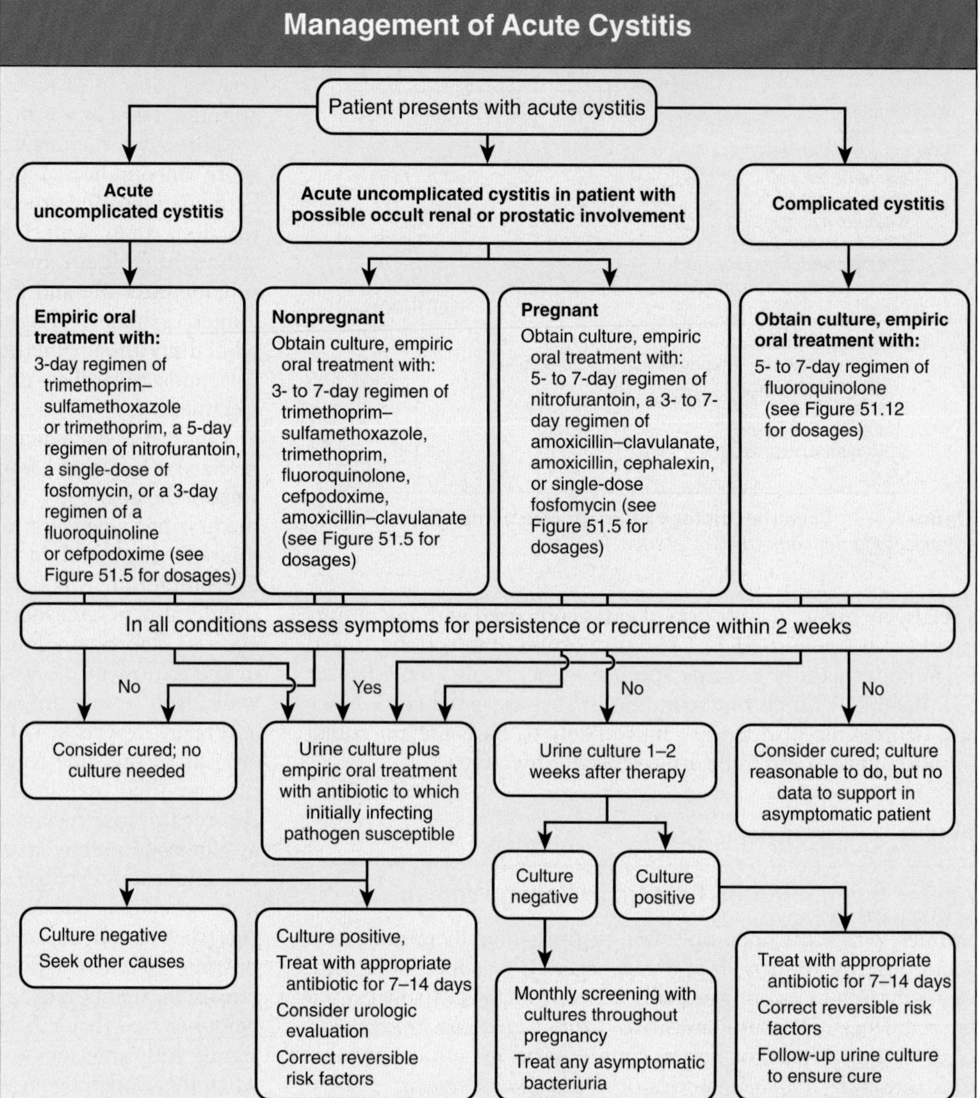

Figure 51.4 Algorithm for management of acute cystitis.

E. coli to epithelial cells. Clinical trials are currently in progress, but it is reasonable to recommend daily cranberry products to women with frequent recurrences of UTI. Women who do not wish to try or who obtain no benefit from the preceding approaches should be offered antimicrobial prophylaxis.

Antimicrobial prophylaxis is effective in preventing recurrent UTI in women (Fig. 51.7; see also Fig. 51.6). Prophylaxis should be considered for women who experience three or more infections during a 12-month period or whenever the woman thinks that her life is being adversely affected by frequent recurrences. Several approaches have been used, including continuous prophylaxis, postcoital prophylaxis, and intermittent self-treatment (which is really an early treatment method). In postmenopausal women with recurrent UTI, intravaginal estriol is effective, presumably by normalizing the vaginal flora, which reduces the risk for coliform colonization of the vagina.[24] This approach offers an alternative to antimicrobial strategies (see Fig. 51.6).

Acute Uncomplicated Pyelonephritis in Women

Acute pyelonephritis is suggested by fever (temperature ≥38.5°C), chills, flank pain, nausea and vomiting, and costovertebral angle tenderness. Cystitis symptoms are variably present. Symptoms may vary from a mild illness to a sepsis syndrome with or without shock and renal failure. Pyuria is almost always present, but leukocyte casts, specific for UTI, are infrequently seen. Gram stain of the urine sediment may aid in differentiating gram-positive and gram-negative infections, which can influence empiric therapy. A urine culture, which should be performed in all women with acute pyelonephritis, will have 10^4 cfu/ml or more uropathogens in up to 95% of patients.[15]

On pathologic examination, the kidney shows a focal inflammatory reaction with neutrophil and monocyte infiltrates, tubular damage, and interstitial edema (Fig. 51.8). Although imaging studies are generally not performed, the infected kidney is often enlarged, and contrast-enhanced computed tomography (CT) shows decreased opacification of the affected parenchyma, typically in patchy, wedge-shaped, or linear patterns (Fig. 51.9).

The availability of effective oral antimicrobials, especially the fluoroquinolones, allows initial oral therapy in appropriate patients or, in those requiring parenteral therapy, the timely conversion from intravenous to oral therapy and reduced need for hospitalization. Indications for admission to the hospital include inability to maintain oral hydration or to take

Oral Regimens for Acute Uncomplicated Cystitis			
Drug	**Dose (mg)**	**Interval**	**Comment**
Trimethoprim-sulfamethoxazole	160/800	q 12 h	If used in pregrancy (not approved use), avoid in first trimester.
Trimethoprim	100	q 12 h	If used in pregrancy (not approved use), avoid in first trimester.
Nitrofurantoin			Less active against ***Proteus*** species
Monohydrate/macrocrystals	100	q 12 h	
Macrocrystals	50	q 6 h	
Cefpodoxime proxetil	100	q 12 h	Comparable to Tmp-smx in efficacy, but data sparse
Fosfomycin	3000	Single dose	Less effective vs. fluoroquinolone or trimethoprim-sulfamethoxazole
Amoxicillin-clavulanate	500/125	q 12 h	Inferior to ciprofloxacin in 3-day regimen
Amoxicillin	500	q 12 h	Used only when causative pathogen is known to be susceptible or for empiric treatment of mild cystitis in pregnancy
Fluoroquinolones			Avoid fluoroquinolones if possible in pregnancy, nursing mothers, or persons <18 years old. Although highly effective, should be considered second line treatment to preserve its usefulness for other infections
Ciprofloxacin	100–250	q 12 h	
Ciprofloxacin extended release	500	q 24 h	
Levofloxacin	250	q 24 h	
Ofloxacin	200	q 12 h	

Figure 51.5 Oral antimicrobial agents for acute uncomplicated cystitis or cystitis in patients with possible occult renal or prostatic involvement. Duration of therapy depends on the clinical setting (see text and Fig. 51.4).

medications; uncertain social situation or concern about compliance; uncertainty about the diagnosis; and severe illness with high fevers, severe pain, and marked debility. Outpatient therapy is safe and effective for selected patients who can be stabilized with parenteral fluids and antibiotics in an urgent care facility and sent home with oral antibiotics under close supervision. In one population-based study of acute pyelonephritis in adult women, only 7% were hospitalized.[4]

The management strategy for acute uncomplicated pyelonephritis is shown in Figure 51.10. There are many effective parenteral (Fig. 51.11) and oral (Fig. 51.12) regimens for acute uncomplicated pyelonephritis. In the outpatient setting, an oral fluoroquinolone should be used for initial empiric treatment of infection caused by gram-negative bacilli.[20] Trimethoprim-sulfamethoxazole or other agents can be used if the infecting strain is known to be susceptible. If enterococci are suspected from the Gram stain, amoxicillin should be added to the treatment regimen until the causative organism is identified. Second- and third-generation cephalosporins also appear effective, although published data are sparse. Neither nitrofurantoin nor fosfomycin is approved or recommended for the treatment of pyelonephritis.

For hospitalized patients, ceftriaxone is an effective and inexpensive agent if the Gram stain is not suggestive of gram-positive bacterial infection. If enterococci are suspected on the basis of a stain showing gram-positive bacteria, ampicillin plus gentamicin, ampicillin-sulbactam, and piperacillin-tazobactam are reasonable broad-spectrum empiric choices. Trimethoprim-sulfamethoxazole should not be used alone for empiric therapy for pyelonephritis in areas with a high prevalence of resistance to this combination. Patients with acute uncomplicated pyelonephritis can often be switched to oral therapy after 24 to 48 hours, although longer intervals of parenteral therapy are occasionally indicated in patients whose symptoms and signs do not improve rapidly (such as those with continued high fever, severe flank pain, or persistent nausea and vomiting).

Treatment of acute uncomplicated pyelonephritis can be limited to 7 days for mildly to moderately ill patients who have a rapid response with resolution of fever and symptoms soon after initiation of treatment. However, β-lactam regimens shorter than 14 days have been associated with unacceptably high failure rates in some studies.[20] One study demonstrated superiority of a 7-day ciprofloxacin regimen over a 14-day trimethoprim-sulfamethoxazole regimen, with the difference accounted for entirely by the higher rate of resistance of the uropathogens to trimethoprim-sulfamethoxazole.[14]

Routine post-treatment urine cultures in asymptomatic patients are not cost-effective, but cultures should be performed if symptoms persist or recur. Recurrent infections are treated with a 7- to 14-day course of an antibiotic to which the organism is susceptible. Symptomatic patients who have persistent infection with the same strain as the initial infecting strain warrant 10 to 14 days of therapy, or even longer in some cases, and complicating factors should be looked for and corrected if found.

Acute Cystitis in Healthy Adults with Possible Occult Renal or Prostatic Involvement

Acute cystitis in healthy individuals other than young women are more likely to involve occult renal or prostatic infection (see Fig. 51.1) and may respond poorly to short-course therapy. We lack noninvasive tools to localize infections to the kidney or prostate, so our estimation of risk in a given patient is imprecise. Some patients, such as those with diabetes or pregnancy, warrant

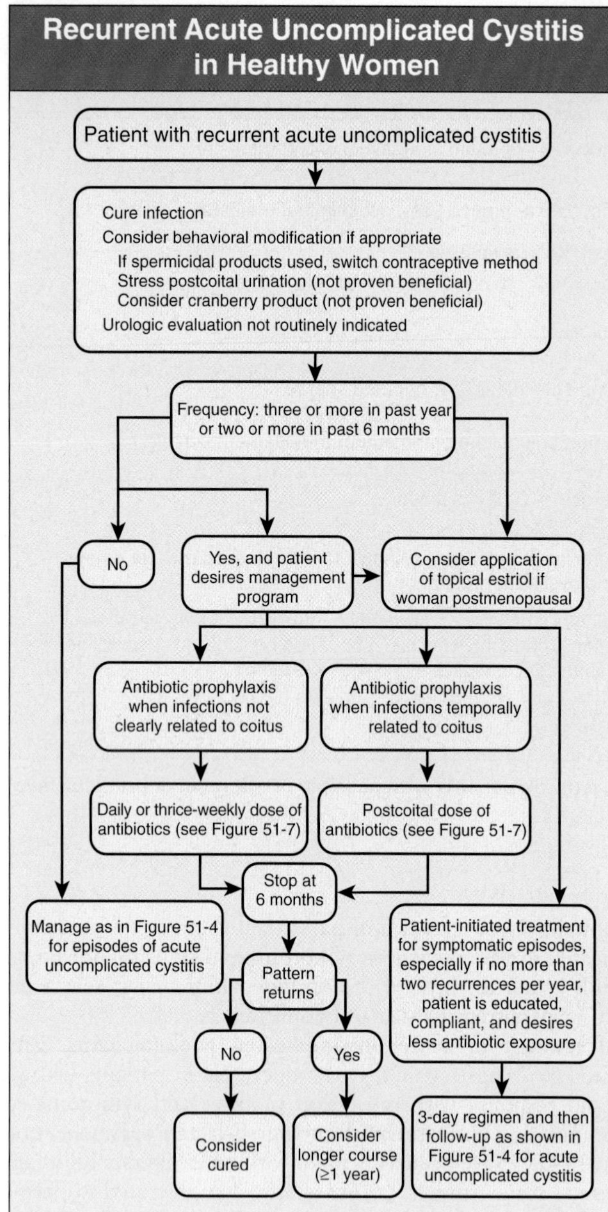

Recurrent Acute Uncomplicated Cystitis in Healthy Women
Patient with recurrent acute uncomplicated cystitis
Cure infection
Consider behavioral modification if appropriate
If spermicidal products used, switch contraceptive method
Stress postcoital urination (not proven beneficial)
Consider cranberry product (not proven beneficial)
Urologic evaluation not routinely indicated
Frequency: three or more in past year or two or more in past 6 months
No
Yes, and patient desires management program
Consider application of topical estriol if woman postmenopausal
Antibiotic prophylaxis when infections not clearly related to coitus
Antibiotic prophylaxis when infections temporally related to coitus
Daily or thrice-weekly dose of antibiotics (see Figure 51-7)
Postcoital dose of antibiotics (see Figure 51-7)
Stop at 6 months
Manage as in Figure 51-4 for episodes of acute uncomplicated cystitis
Pattern returns
Patient-initiated treatment for symptomatic episodes, especially if no more than two recurrences per year, patient is educated, compliant, and desires less antibiotic exposure
No
Yes
Consider cured
Consider longer course (≥1 year)
3-day regimen and then follow-up as shown in Figure 51-4 for acute uncomplicated cystitis

Figure 51.6 Management strategies for recurrent acute uncomplicated cystitis.

special attention because of the serious complications that can occur if treatment is inadequate. Symptoms, signs, and laboratory findings in this group are the same as those in uncomplicated cystitis. Urethritis must be excluded in dysuric sexually active men by a urethral Gram stain or a first-voided urine specimen wet mount evaluation for urethral leukocytosis.

A urine culture specimen should be obtained routinely in patients before treatment (see Fig. 51.4). Empiric treatment is similar to that used for uncomplicated cystitis in women. Nitrofurantoin treatment should be avoided except for cystitis in pregnancy, in which duration of treatment is 5 to 7 days, depending on the severity of symptoms.

The need for post-treatment culture is less certain, except in pregnant women (see Fig. 51.4). In men, early recurrence of UTI with the same species suggests a prostatic source of infection and warrants a 4- to 6-week regimen of either a fluoroquinolone (preferable) or trimethoprim-sulfamethoxazole.

Prophylaxis for Recurrent Acute Uncomplicated Cystitis

Drug	Dose (mg)	Frequency
Continuous prophylaxis		
Trimethoprim-sulfamethoxazole	40/200	Daily
Trimethoprim-sulfamethoxazole	40/200	Thrice weekly
Trimethoprim	100	Daily
Nitrofurantoin	50 or 100	Daily
Cefaclor	250	Daily
Cefalexin (cephalexin)	125 or 250	Daily
Norfloxacin*	200	Other fluoroquinolones are likely to be as effective*
Postcoital prophylaxis		
Trimethoprim-sulfamethoxazole	40/200	Single dose
Trimethoprim-sulfamethoxazole	80/400	Single dose
Nitrofurantoin	50 or 100	Single dose
Cefalexin	250	Single dose
Ciprofloxacin*	125	Single dose
Norfloxacin*	200	Single dose
Ofloxacin*	100	Single dose

Figure 51.7 Antimicrobial prophylaxis regimens for women with recurrent acute uncomplicated cystitis. See text and Figure 51.6 for management strategy. *Women should be cautioned about pregnancy when fluoroquinolones are being used.

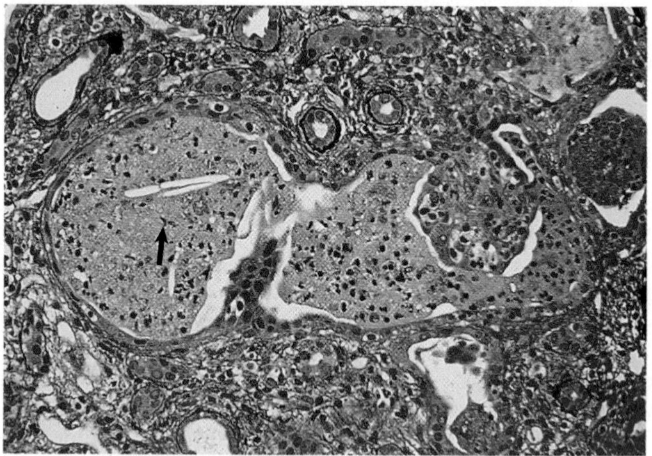

Figure 51.8 Acute pyelonephritis. Renal tissue shows a dilated tubule with neutrophils enmeshed in proteinaceous debris ("pus casts," *arrow*) with adjacent interstitial inflammation. *(Courtesy C. Alpers, University of Washington, Seattle, Washington, USA.)*

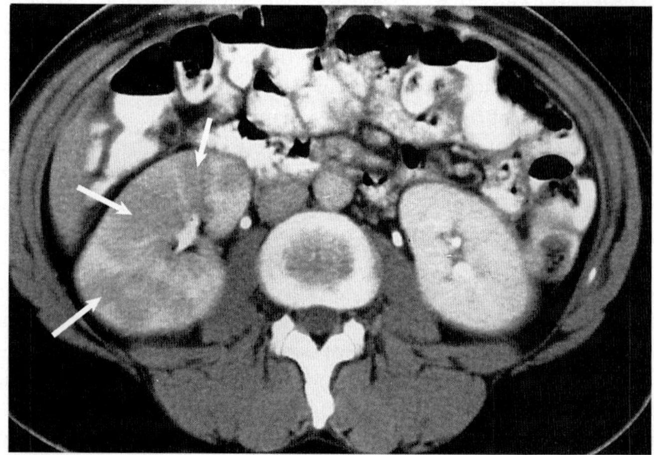

Figure 51.9 Acute pyelonephritis. Contrast-enhanced CT scan shows areas of lower density due to infection and edema *(arrows)*. *(Courtesy W. Bush, University of Washington, Seattle, Washington, USA.)*

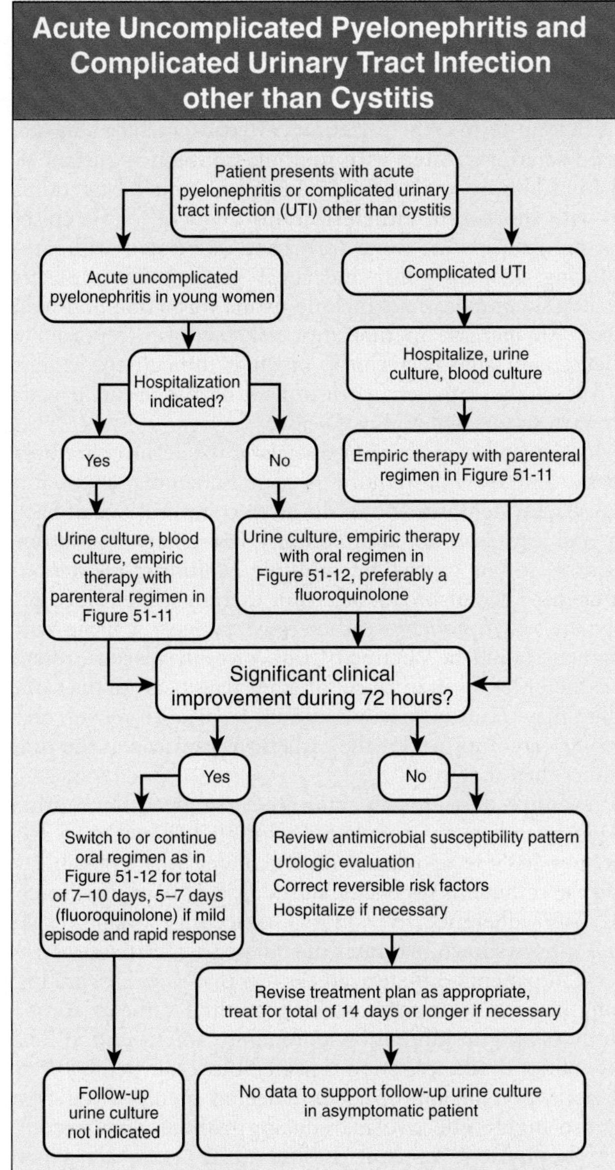

Figure 51.10 Management algorithm for acute uncomplicated pyelonephritis and complicated urinary tract infection other than cystitis.

Complicated Infections

Complicated UTI may present with classic signs of cystitis and pyelonephritis but may also be associated with vague or nonspecific symptoms, such as fatigue, irritability, nausea, headache, and abdominal or back pain. Signs and symptoms may exist for weeks to months before diagnosis. Complicated UTI, like uncomplicated UTI, is generally associated with pyuria and bacteriuria, although these may be absent if the infection does not communicate with the collecting system.

Urine culture should always be performed in patients with suspected complicated UTI. The Infectious Diseases Society of America consensus definition of complicated UTI is 10^5 cfu/ml or more in women and 10^4 cfu/ml or more in men,[15] but lower counts in symptomatic persons, as has been demonstrated in patients with uncomplicated UTI, may well represent significant bacteriuria. This is especially true when the specimen is collected from a urinary catheter. Thus, it is reasonable to use a colony count threshold of 10^3 cfu/ml or more to diagnose complicated UTI.

Parenteral Regimens for Acute Uncomplicated Pyelonephritis and Complicated Urinary Tract Infection

Drug	Dose (mg)	Interval
Ceftriaxone	1000–2000	q 24 h
Cefepime	1000–2000	q 12 h
Fluoroquinolones†		
Ciprofloxacin	200–400	q 12 h
Levofloxacin	250–750	q 24 h
Gentamicin (± ampicillin)	3–5 mg/kg body weight	q 24 h
	1 mg/kg body weight	q 8 h
Ampicillin (+ gentamicin)	1000	q 6 h
Trimethoprim-sulfamethoxazole†	160/800	q 12 h
Aztreonam	1000	q 8–12 h
Ampicillin-sulbactam	1500	q 6 h
Ticarcillin-clavulanate	3200	q 8 h
Piperacillin-tazobactam	3375	q 6–8 h
Imipenem-cilastatin	250–500	q 6–8 h
Ertapenem	1000	q 24 h
Vancomycin§	1000	q 12 h

Figure 51.11 Parenteral regimens for acute uncomplicated pyelonephritis and complicated urinary tract infection. Duration depends on clinical setting (see text and Fig. 51.10). †Avoid, if possible, in pregnancy. §Recommended if methicillin-resistant *S. aureus* (MRSA) is suspected or known.

The wide variety of underlying conditions (see Fig. 51.1), diverse bacterial agents (see Fig. 51.3), and paucity of controlled clinical trials make generalizations about antimicrobial therapy difficult. The management strategy for complicated cystitis is shown in Figure 51.4 and that for complicated infections other than cystitis in Figure 51.10.

Attempts to correct any underlying anatomic, functional, or metabolic defect must be made as antibiotics alone may not be successful.[1] For empiric therapy in patients with mild to moderate illness who can be treated with oral medication, the fluoroquinolones provide the broadest spectrum of antimicrobial activity, cover most expected pathogens, and achieve high levels in the urine and urinary tract tissue. Exceptions are trovafloxacin and moxifloxacin, which, in contrast to other fluoroquinolones such as ciprofloxacin and levofloxacin, may not achieve sufficient concentrations in urine to be effective for complicated UTI. If the infecting pathogen is known to be susceptible, trimethoprim-sulfamethoxazole or other agents are reasonable therapeutic choices.

For initial treatment in more seriously ill, hospitalized patients, several parenteral antimicrobial agents are available (see Fig. 51.11). The broader spectrum agents shown in Figure 51.11 are preferable for health care–associated infections. In contrast to uncomplicated UTI, *S. aureus* is more common in complicated UTIs, and if it is suspected, the therapeutic regimen should have activity against this pathogen. Studies show that a high proportion of *S. aureus* isolates, even in the community are methicillin-resistant (MRSA), so vancomycin should be included

Oral Regimens for Acute Uncomplicated Pyelonephritis and Complicated Urinary Tract Infection

Drug	Dose (mg)	Interval	Comment
Fluoroquinolones			Preferred for empiric treatment; avoid if possible in pregnancy, nursing mothers, or persons <18 years old
Ciprofloxacin	500	q 12 h	
Ciprofloxacin extended release	1000	q 24 h	
Levofloxacin	250–750	q 24 h	
Trimethoprim-sulfamethoxazole	160/800	q 12 h	Use only when the causative pathogen is known to be susceptible If used in pregnancy (not approved use), avoid in first trimester
Cefpodoxime proxetil	200	q 12 h	Data are sparse
Amoxicillin	500	q 8 h	Use only when the causative pathogen is known to be susceptible or in addition to a broad-spectrum agent when empiric coverage against enterococci is desirable

Figure 51.12 Oral regimens for acute uncomplicated pyelonephritis and complicated urinary tract infection. Duration depends on clinical setting (see text and Fig. 51.10).

in the empiric treatment regimen if *S. aureus* is suspected. Potential concerns that must be considered in the management of complicated UTI include the increasing prevalence of resistance to fluoroquinolones in institutional settings and the frequency of enterococcal infections.

The antimicrobial regimen can be modified when the infecting strain has been identified and antimicrobial susceptibilities are known. Patients who are given parenteral therapy can be switched to oral treatment after clinical improvement. Few studies have been performed that evaluate duration of treatment in populations with complicated UTIs. However, it is desirable to limit the duration of treatment, especially for milder infections, to reduce the selection pressure for drug-resistant flora. In one study, clinical and microbiologic success rates after treatment were almost identical in patients with acute pyelonephritis or complicated UTI treated with a 5-day course of levofloxacin or a 10-day course of ciprofloxacin.[27] These data suggest that a 7- to 10-day regimen is reasonable for most patients with complicated UTI, depending on their clinical response; shorter regimens, such as a 5-day regimen of a urinary fluoroquinolone, are likely to be sufficient in those patients who are less severely ill, are infected with uropathogens susceptible to the antibiotic used, and have a rapid response to treatment. At least 10 to 14 days of therapy is recommended in those patients who have a delayed response.

Catheter-Associated Infections

Approximately 15% to 25% of patients in general hospitals have a catheter inserted at some time during their stay, and approximately 5% to 10% of long-term care facility residents are managed with urethral catheterization, in some cases for years. The incidence of bacteriuria associated with indwelling catheterization is 3% to 10% per day of catheterization, and the duration of catheterization is the most important risk factor for the development of catheter-associated bacteriuria.

Catheter-associated bacteriuria is the most common source of gram-negative bacteremia in hospitalized patients. Complications of long-term catheterization (>30 days) include almost universal bacteriuria, often with multiple antibiotic-resistant flora, and (in addition to cystitis, pyelonephritis, and bacteremia as seen with short-term catheterization) frequent febrile episodes, catheter obstruction, stone formation associated with urease-producing uropathogens, and local genitourinary infections. Other rare complications include fistula formation and bladder cancer. An increase in mortality risk has been reported with catheter-associated bacteriuria, but it is difficult to distinguish the role of the catheter because most deaths occur in patients who have severe underlying disease.

Most episodes of catheter-associated bacteriuria are asymptomatic and do not require routine screening or treatment because treatment does not reduce the complications of bacteriuria and can lead to antimicrobial resistance.[7] Symptomatic infections, often caused by multiple multidrug-resistant uropathogens, warrant broad-spectrum therapy as described previously. In a symptomatic catheterized patient, a urine culture specimen should be obtained from a freshly placed catheter if the catheter has been in place for a few days because the catheter biofilm may result in spurious culture results. Moreover, clinical outcomes are improved if the catheter is replaced at the time of antimicrobial therapy.[28]

Preventive measures are indicated to reduce the morbidity, mortality, and costs of catheter-associated infection. Effective strategies include avoidance of a catheter when possible and, when the catheter is necessary, sterile insertion, prompt removal, and strict adherence to a closed collecting system.[6,29] Meta-analyses have shown that rates of catheter-associated bacteriuria, at least in patients catheterized for less than 2 weeks, are higher among patients with an indwelling urethral catheter compared with those on intermittent or suprapubic catheterization.[30] Likewise, condom catheterization is preferable to indwelling urethral catheterization in appropriately selected men.[31] Even though they are highly effective in reducing catheter-associated UTI rates, prophylactic systemic antimicrobial agents are generally not recommended for routine use because of concerns about selection for antimicrobial resistance. Antimicrobial-coated catheters appear to be effective in reducing catheter-associated bacteriuria in patients catheterized for less than 2 weeks, but they have not been shown to be effective in reducing symptomatic infection.

Spinal Cord Injury

Spinal cord injury alters the dynamics of voiding and often requires the use of bladder drainage with catheters. The diagnosis of UTI in patients with spinal cord injuries is often problematic and is based on the combination of symptoms and signs (which are often nonspecific), pyuria, and significant bacteriuria; uropathogens are often present in quantities of 10^5 cfu/ml or more. Fluoroquinolones are the empiric oral agents of choice in patients with mild to moderate infection, although many uropathogens, even in the outpatient setting, are resistant to this class of antibiotic, and parenteral antibiotics may be needed.

Treatment of asymptomatic bacteriuria in patients with spinal cord injuries is not of proven benefit and increases the risk for infection with antimicrobial-resistant uropathogens.[7,32] Likewise, antibiotic prophylaxis is generally not recommended, although it may be considered for selected outpatients with frequent symptomatic UTIs for whom there are no correctible risk factors.

Prostatitis

Prostatitis occurs in about 2% to 10% of men during their lifetime, but it is caused by acute or chronic bacterial infection in a minority.[33] The current National Institutes of Health classification system categorizes prostatitis within a complex series of syndromes that vary widely in clinical presentation and response to treatment. The most common organisms causing bacterial prostatitis are gram-negative bacilli, including *E. coli*, *Proteus* species, *Klebsiella* species, *P. aeruginosa*, and, less commonly, enterococci and *S. aureus*. The pathogenesis of prostatitis is believed to be related to reflux of infected urine from the urethra into the prostatic ducts. Prostatic calculi, commonly found in adult men, may provide a nidus for bacteria and protection from antibacterial agents.

Acute bacterial prostatitis is rare. Patients present with dysuria, frequency, urgency, obstructive voiding symptoms, fever, chills, and myalgias. The prostate is tender and swollen. Prostatic massage, as a diagnostic test, is contraindicated in men in whom the diagnosis of acute prostatitis is being considered because of the risk for precipitating bacteremia. The patient will usually have pyuria and a positive urine culture. Patients who are severely ill require hospitalization and parenteral antibiotics, but many patients can be treated in the outpatient setting with oral fluoroquinolones. The duration of treatment is recommended to be at least 30 days.[33] Abscess formation may rarely occur.

Chronic bacterial prostatitis is characterized by recurrent UTIs with the same uropathogen with intervening asymptomatic periods. The prostate typically is normal to palpation during asymptomatic periods. Chronic bacterial prostatitis is characterized microscopically by the presence of 10 or more leukocytes per high-power field in expressed prostatic secretions or postmassage voided urine in the absence of significant pyuria in first-voided and midstream urine specimens and a uropathogen colony count that is at least 10-fold higher in the expressed prostatic secretions or postmassage voided urine compared with the first-voided midstream urine. In addition, macrophage-laden fat droplets (oval fat bodies) are usually prominent in the prostatic secretions. These tests, however, are infrequently performed by urologists. Cure rates, which historically have been low, are 60% to 80% with the fluoroquinolones, which are the antibiotics of choice. The optimal duration of treatment is unknown, but most authorities recommend at least 1 to 3 months. Some patients require long-term, low-dose suppressive therapy to prevent symptomatic UTIs. Surgical intervention is only rarely considered and is associated with high morbidity.

Renal Abscess

Renal cortical and corticomedullary abscesses and perirenal abscesses occur in 1 to 10 per 10,000 hospital admissions.[34] Patients usually present with fever, chills, back or abdominal pain, and costovertebral angle tenderness but may have no urinary symptoms or findings if the abscess does not communicate with the collecting system, as is often the case with a cortical abscess. Bacteremia may be primary (cortical abscess) or secondary (corticomedullary or perirenal). The clinical presentation may be insidious and nonspecific, especially with perirenal abscess, and the diagnosis may not be made until admission to a hospital or at autopsy. CT is recommended to establish the diagnosis and location of a renal or perirenal abscess (Fig. 51.13). Empiric antibiotic therapy should be broad and cover *S. aureus* and other uropathogens causing complicated UTI (see Figs. 51.10 and 51.11) and modified once urine culture results are known.

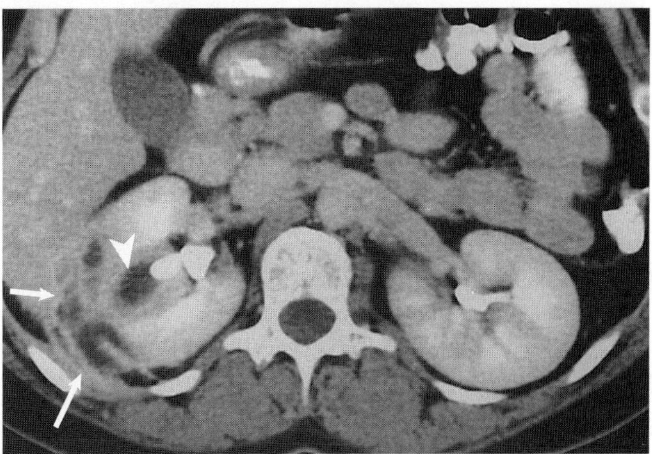

Figure 51.13 Renal abscess. Contrast-enhanced CT scan shows an abscess in the medulla of the kidney *(arrowhead)* with penetration and extension into the perinephric space *(arrows)*. *(Courtesy L. Towner.)*

A renal cortical abscess (renal carbuncle) is usually caused by *S. aureus*, which reaches the kidney by hematogenous spread. Treatment with antibiotics is usually effective, and drainage is not required unless the patient is slow to respond. A renal corticomedullary abscess, in contrast, usually results from ascending UTI in association with an underlying urinary tract abnormality, such as obstructive uropathy or vesicoureteral reflux, and is usually caused by common uropathogenic species such as *E. coli* and other coliforms. Such abscesses may extend deep into the renal parenchyma, perforate the renal capsule, and form a perirenal abscess. Treatment with antimicrobial agents without drainage may be effective if the abscess is small and if the underlying urinary tract abnormality can be corrected. Aspiration of the abscess may be necessary in some patients, and nephrectomy may occasionally be required in patients with diffuse renal involvement or with severe sepsis. Perirenal abscesses usually occur in the setting of obstruction or other complicating factors (see Fig. 51.1) and result from ruptured intrarenal abscesses, hematogenous spread, or spread from a contiguous infection. Causative uropathogens are those commonly found in complicated UTIs (see Fig. 51.3), including *S. aureus* and enterococci; polymicrobic infections are common. Anaerobes or *Mycobacterium tuberculosis* may be causative. A previously high mortality rate has been lowered with earlier diagnosis and therapy. In contrast to the other types of abscess, drainage of pus is the cornerstone of therapy, and nephrectomy is sometimes indicated.

Papillary Necrosis

More than half of those who develop papillary necrosis have diabetes, almost always in conjunction with a UTI, but the condition also complicates sickle cell disease, analgesic abuse, and obstruction. Renal papillae are vulnerable to ischemia because of the sluggish blood flow in the vasa recta, and relatively modest ischemic insults may cause papillary necrosis. The clinical features are those typical of pyelonephritis. In addition, passage of sloughed papillae into the ureter may cause renal colic, renal insufficiency or failure, or obstruction with severe urosepsis. Papillary necrosis in the setting of pyelonephritis is associated with pyuria and a positive urine culture. Causative uropathogens are those typical of complicated UTI. Spiral CT is the preferred diagnostic procedure. Radiologic findings include an irregular papillary tip; dilated calyceal fornix; extension of contrast material into the parenchyma; and a separated crescent-shaped papilla surrounded by contrast material, called the ring sign. Broad-spectrum antibiotics are indicated. Papillae obstructing the ureter may require removal with a cystoscopic ureteral basket or relief of obstruction by insertion of a ureteral stent.

Emphysematous Pyelonephritis

Emphysematous pyelonephritis is a fulminant, necrotizing, life-threatening variant of acute pyelonephritis caused by gas-forming organisms, including *E. coli*, *K. pneumoniae*, *P. aeruginosa*, and *Proteus mirabilis*.[35] Up to 90% of cases occur in diabetic patients, and obstruction may be present. Symptoms are suggestive of pyelonephritis, and there may be a flank mass. Dehydration and ketoacidosis are common. Pyuria and a positive urine culture are usually present. Gas is usually detected by a plain abdominal radiograph or ultrasound (Fig. 51.14). CT is the diagnostic modality of choice, however, because it can better localize the gas than ultrasound can. Accurate localization of gas is important because gas may also form in an infected obstructed collecting system or renal abscess; although serious, these conditions do not carry the same grave prognosis and are managed differently. Parenteral broad-spectrum antibiotics and percutaneous catheter drainage with relief of obstruction may be adequate for those less severely ill, but nephrectomy is warranted for those who are more severely ill and those less severely ill who do not respond to the preceding steps. Medical treatment is associated with a mortality rate of 60% to 80%, which is lowered to 20% or less with surgical intervention.

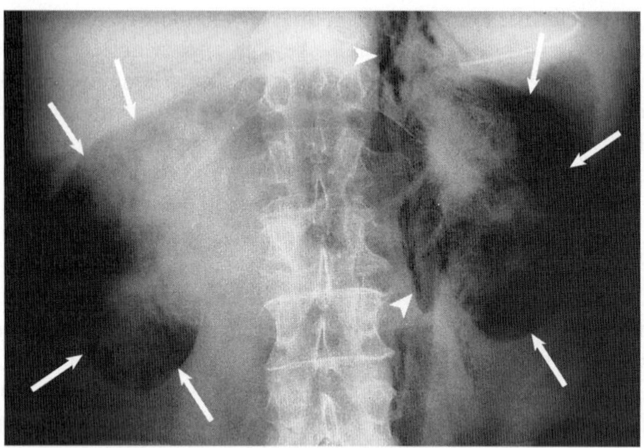

Figure 51.14 Emphysematous pyelonephritis. A plain radiograph in this febrile diabetic subject revealed diffuse gas formation throughout both kidneys *(outlined by arrows)* and gas dissecting in the left retroperitoneal space *(arrowheads)*. *(Courtesy W. Bush, University of Washington, Seattle, Washington, USA.)*

Renal Malacoplakia

Malacoplakia is a chronic granulomatous disorder of unknown etiology involving the genitourinary, gastrointestinal, skin, and pulmonary systems.[36] It is characterized by an unusual inflammatory reaction to a variety of infections and is manifested by the accumulation of macrophages containing calcified bacterial debris called Michaelis-Gutmann bodies (Fig. 51.15). The underlying disorder appears to be a monocyte-macrophage bactericidal defect. The diagnosis is made by histologic examination of involved tissue. Genitourinary malacoplakia, most commonly involving the bladder, is usually associated with gram-negative UTI. Patients with renal malacoplakia generally have fever, flank pain, pyuria and hematuria, bacteriuria, and, if both kidneys are involved, impaired renal function. CT scanning usually shows enlarged kidneys with areas of poor enhancement, and the condition may be indistinguishable from other infectious or neoplastic lesions. On occasion, the malacoplakia may extend through the renal capsule into the perinephric space, simulating a renal carcinoma (see Fig. 51.15). Treatment consists of therapy with a broad spectrum antimicrobial; correction of any underlying complicating conditions if possible, and improvement of renal function. Nephrectomy is recommended for advanced unilateral disease. When the disease is bilateral or occurs in a transplanted kidney, the prognosis is very poor.

Xanthogranulomatous Pyelonephritis

Xanthogranulomatous pyelonephritis is a poorly understood, uncommon, but severe chronic renal infection associated with obstruction of the urinary tract.[34] The renal parenchyma is replaced with a diffuse or segmental cellular infiltrate of foam cells, which are lipid-laden macrophages. The process may also extend beyond the renal capsule to the retroperitoneum. Its pathogenesis appears to be multifactorial, with infection

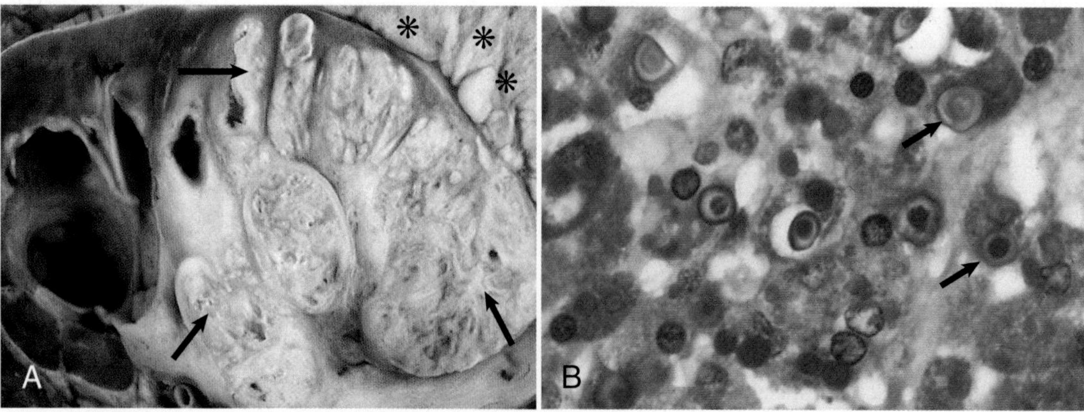

Figure 51.15 Renal malacoplakia. A, Malacoplakia involving most of the kidney *(arrows)* with extension through the capsule *(asterisks)*. A small portion of normal kidney is present that is associated with hydronephrosis secondary to obstruction by the malacoplakia. **B,** The kidney tissue shows many macrophages containing intracytoplasmic inclusions (*arrows* identify two particularly well demarcated macrophages with Michaelis-Gutmann bodies). *(Courtesy L. Truong, Baylor College of Medicine, Houston, Texas, USA and N. Sheerin, Guy's Hospital, London, United Kingdom.)*

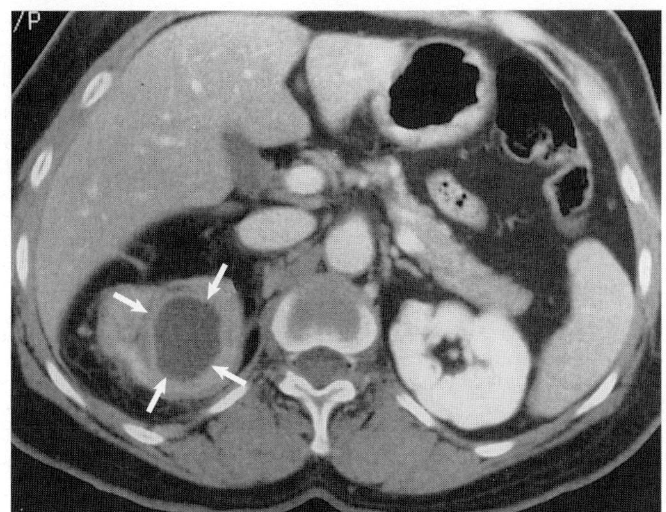

Figure 51.16 Xanthogranulomatous pyelonephritis. Contrast-enhanced CT scan with the inflammatory mass outlined by *arrows*. Pathologic diagnosis confirmed xanthogranulomatous pyelonephritis. *(Courtesy W. Bush, University of Washington, Seattle, Washington, USA.)*

complicating obstruction and leading to ischemia, tissue destruction, and accumulation of lipid deposits. Patients with xanthogranulomatous pyelonephritis are characteristically middle-aged women and have chronic symptoms such as flank pain, fever, chills, and malaise. Flank tenderness, a palpable mass, and irritative voiding symptoms are common. The urine culture is usually positive with *E. coli*, other gram-negative bacilli, or *S. aureus*. CT generally shows an enlarged nonfunctioning kidney, often the presence of calculi and low-density masses (xanthomatous tissue), and, in some cases, involvement of adjacent structures (Fig. 51.16). It may be difficult to distinguish from neoplastic disease. Broad-spectrum antimicrobials are indicated, but total or partial nephrectomy is usually necessary for cure.

Asymptomatic Bacteriuria

Asymptomatic bacteriuria, as noted previously, is a common and generally benign infection.[7,23] Pyuria is often present, especially in elderly people, and is a predictor for subsequent symptomatic UTI in some groups. Causative uropathogens are the same as those causing UTIs in the same population. Screening for and treatment of asymptomatic bacteriuria is generally not warranted.[7] However, patients at high risk for serious complications warrant a more aggressive approach to diagnosis and treatment, including pregnant women and patients undergoing urologic surgery. Current management strategies in patients with a renal transplant, including long-term antimicrobial prophylaxis, help prevent both asymptomatic bacteriuria and symptomatic urinary infection. It is not clear, however, whether screening for or treatment of asymptomatic bacteriuria in such patients is worthwhile.[7] Some authorities advise treatment of asymptomatic bacteriuria found in patients with anatomic or functional abnormalities of the urinary tract, diabetic patients, and patients with urea-splitting bacteria, such as *P. mirabilis*, *Klebsiella* species, and others.[23] Evidence-based guidelines for screening and treatment of asymptomatic bacteriuria in these populations are needed.

Asymptomatic bacteriuria in catheterized patients in hospitals and long-term care facilities, although thought to be generally benign, represents a large reservoir of antimicrobial-resistant urinary pathogens that increases the risk of cross-infection among catheterized patients and results in frequent inappropriate antimicrobial use.[29]

UROLOGIC EVALUATION

Urologic consultation and evaluation of the urinary tract should be considered in patients who present with symptoms or signs of obstruction, urolithiasis, flank mass, or urosepsis. Similarly, such an evaluation should be considered for those patients with presumptive uncomplicated or complicated UTI who have not had a satisfactory clinical response after 72 hours of treatment to exclude complicating factors. Contrast-enhanced CT scanning of the kidneys is the most effective imaging modality in adult patients with renal infection because of its superior resolution and sensitivity in detecting renal abnormalities and perirenal fluid collections.[37] Spiral (helical) CT may be superior to conventional CT.[38] Non–contrast-enhanced spiral CT is a rapid, safe, and sensitive method for evaluating patients with suspected renal stones. Renal ultrasound is useful for detection of stones and abscesses and is often more readily accessible than CT. However, it is less sensitive than CT for detection of many of the conditions present in patients with complicated UTI. The role of magnetic resonance imaging remains to be determined. Radionuclide imaging procedures have no role in the evaluation of adults with UTI, although they are very useful in children with pyelonephritis (see Chapter 61). A plain abdominal radiograph may be used to detect gas in the urinary tracts of diabetic patients with suspected pyelonephritis, but it is not as sensitive or specific as CT.

Excretory urography and cystoscopy in women with recurrent cystitis rarely demonstrate abnormalities or alter management[3] and are therefore not recommended. Likewise, routine urologic investigation of young women with acute pyelonephritis is generally not cost effective and has a low diagnostic yield, although it is reasonable to obtain such an evaluation after two episodes of pyelonephritis or if any complicating factor is present (see Fig. 51.1). A urologic evaluation is probably not necessary in a man who has had a single UTI with no obvious complicating factors and whose infection responds promptly to treatment.

REFERENCES

1. Nicolle LE. A practical guide to the management of complicated urinary tract infection. *Drugs*. 1997;53:583-592.
2. Hooton TM, Scholes D, Hughes JP, et al. A prospective study of risk factors for symptomatic urinary tract infection in young women. *N Engl J Med*. 1996;335:468-474.
3. Hooton TM, Stamm WE. Diagnosis and treatment of uncomplicated urinary tract infection. *Infect Dis Clin North Am*. 1997;11:551-581.
4. Scholes D, Hooton TM, Roberts PL, et al. Risk factors associated with acute pyelonephritis in healthy women. *Ann Intern Med*. 2005;142:20-27.
5. Foxman B, Barlow R, D'Arcy H, et al. Urinary tract infection: Self-reported incidence and associated costs. *Ann Epidemiol*. 2000;10:509-515.
6. Stamm WE, Hooton TM. Management of urinary tract infections in adults. *N Engl J Med*. 1993;329:1328-1334.
7. Nicolle LE, Bradley S, Colgan R, et al. Infectious Diseases Society of America guidelines for the diagnosis and treatment of asymptomatic bacteriuria in adults (IDSA GUIDELINES). *Clin Infect Dis*. 2005;40:643.
8. Hooton TM, Scholes D, Stapleton AE, et al. A prospective study of asymptomatic bacteriuria in young sexually active women. *N Engl J Med*. 2000;343:992-997.
9. Sobel JD. Pathogenesis of urinary tract infection: Role of host defenses. *Infect Dis Clin North Am*. 1997;11:531-549.

10. Scholes D, Hooton TM, Roberts PL, et al. Risk factors for recurrent urinary tract infection in young women. *J Infect Dis*. 2000;182: 1177-1182.
11. Lundstedt AC, McCarthy S, Gustafsson MC, et al. A genetic basis of susceptibility to acute pyelonephritis. *PLoS ONE*. 2007;2:e825.
12. Svanborg C, Godaly G. Bacterial virulence in urinary tract infection. *Infect Dis Clin North Am*. 1997;11:513-529.
13. Patterson JE, Andriole VT. Bacterial urinary tract infections in diabetes. *Infect Dis Clin North Am*. 1997;11:735-750.
14. Talan DA, Stamm WE, Hooton TM, et al. Comparison of ciprofloxacin (7 days) and trimethoprim-sulfamethoxazole (14 days) for acute uncomplicated pyelonephritis in women: A randomized trial. *JAMA*. 2000; 283:1583-1590.
15. Rubin RH, Shapiro ED, Andriole VT, et al. Evaluation of new anti-infective drugs for the treatment of urinary tract infection. *Clin Infect Dis*. 1992;15:S216-S227.
16. Zhanel GG, Hisanaga TL, Laing NM, et al. Antibiotic resistance in Escherichia coli outpatient urinary isolates: Final results from the North American Urinary Tract Infection Collaborative Alliance (NAUTICA). *Int J Antimicrob Agents*. 2006 Jun;27(6):468-475.
17. Naber KG, Schito G, Botto H, et al. Surveillance study in Europe and Brazil on clinical aspects and Antimicrobial Resistance Epidemiology in Females with Cystitis (ARESC): Implications for empiric therapy. *Eur Urol*. 2008 Nov;54(5):1164-1175.
18. Manges AR, Johnson JR, Foxman B, et al. Widespread distribution of urinary tract infection caused by a multi-drug-resistant *Escherichia coli* clonal group. *N Engl J Med*. 2001;345:1055-1057.
19. Norrby SR. Short-term treatment of uncomplicated lower urinary tract infections in women. *Rev Infect Dis*. 1990;12:458-467.
20. Warren JW, Abrutyn E, Hebel JR, et al. Guidelines for antimicrobial treatment of uncomplicated acute bacterial cystitis and acute pyelonephritis in women. *Clin Infect Dis*. 1999;29:745-758.
21. Gupta K, Hooton TM, Roberts PL, et al. Short-course nitrofurantoin for the treatment of acute uncomplicated cystitis in women. *Arch Intern Med*. 2007;167:2207-2212.
22. Hooton TM, Scholes D, Gupta K, et al. Amoxicillin-clavulanate vs ciprofloxacin for the treatment of uncomplicated cystitis in women: A randomized trial. *JAMA*. 2005;293:949-955.
23. Zhanel GG, Harding GKM, Guay DRP. Asymptomatic bacteriuria: Which patients should be treated? *Arch Intern Med*. 1990;150: 1389-1396.
24. Stapleton A, Stamm WE. Prevention of urinary tract infection. *Infect Dis Clin North Am*. 1997;11:719-733.
25. Anderson GG, Dodson KW, Hooton TM, et al. Intracellular bacterial communities of uropathogenic *Escherichia coli* in urinary tract pathogenesis. *Trends Microbiol*. 2004;12:424-430.
26. Rosen DA, Hooton TM, Stamm WE, et al. Detection of intracellular bacterial communities in human urinary tract infection. *PLoS Med*. 2007;4:e329.
27. Peterson J, Kaul S, Khashab M, et al. A double-blind, randomized comparison of levofloxacin 750 mg once-daily for five days with ciprofloxacin 400/500 mg twice-daily for 10 days for the treatment of complicated urinary tract infections and acute pyelonephritis. *Urology*. 2008;71: 17-22.
28. Raz R, Schiller D, Nicolle LE. Chronic indwelling catheter replacement before antimicrobial therapy for symptomatic urinary tract infection. *J Urol*. 2000;164:1254-1258.
29. Hooten TM, Bradley SF, Cardenas DD, et al. Diagnosis, prevention, and treatment of catheter-associated urinary tract infection in adults: 2009 International Clinical Practice Guidelines from the Infectious Diseases Society of America. *Clin Infect Dis*. 2010 Mar 1;50(5):625-663.
30. Niel-Weise BS, van den Broek PJ. Urinary catheter policies for short-term bladder drainage in adults. Cochrane Database Syst Rev. 2005;3:CD004203.
31. Saint S, Kaufman SR, Rogers MA, et al. Condom versus indwelling urinary catheters: A randomized trial. *J Am Geriatr Soc*. 2006;54: 1055-1061.
32. Cardenas DD, Hooton TM. Urinary tract infection in persons with spinal cord injury. *Arch Phys Med Rehabil*. 1995;76:272-280.
33. Habermacher GM, Chason JT, Schaeffer AJ. Prostatitis/chronic pelvic pain syndrome. *Annu Rev Med*. 2006;57:195-206.
34. Dembry LM, Andriole VT. Renal and perirenal abscesses. *Infect Dis Clin North Am*. 1997;11:663-680.
35. McHugh TP, Albanna SE, Stewart NJ. Bilateral emphysematous pyelonephritis. *Am J Emerg Med*. 1998;16:166-169.
36. Dobyan DC, Truong LD, Eknoyan G. Renal malacoplakia reappraised. *Am J Kidney Dis*. 1993;22:243-252.
37. Kaplan DM, Rosenfield AT, Smith RC. Advances in the imaging of renal infection. *Infect Dis Clin North Am*. 1997;11:681-705.
38. Wyatt SH, Urban BA, Fishman EK. Spiral CT of the kidneys: Role in characterization of renal disease. Part I: Nonneoplastic disease. *Crit Rev Diagn Imaging*. 1995;36:1-37.

CHAPTER 52

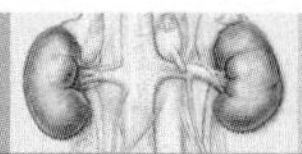

Tuberculosis of the Urinary Tract

R. Kasi Visweswaran, Suresh Bhat

DEFINITION

Tuberculosis (TB), caused mostly by *Mycobacterium tuberculosis*, affects 15 to 20 million people worldwide, half of whom are infectious. About 8 million people develop active disease annually from the stage of asymptomatic infection.[1] The World Health Organization estimates that between 1999 and 2020, nearly 1 billion more people will be newly infected if control measures are not improved. In developed countries, TB commonly affects older individuals and ethnic migrants. The incidence of TB is 100 times greater in human immunodeficiency virus (HIV)–infected subjects.[2] TB also is more common in patients with renal disease. In some endemic areas, TB has been reported to occur in up to 8.7% of subjects on hemodialysis, 9.3% of renal allograft recipients, and 12.3% of children with nephrotic syndrome.[3]

Genitourinary TB occurs in about 5% of active cases in the non–HIV-infected population.[4] It is almost always secondary to a symptomatic or asymptomatic primary lesion in the lung. Renal involvement may also occur as a complication of miliary (septicemic) TB.

ETIOLOGY

The tubercle bacillus is a nonmotile, nonsporing, strictly aerobic straight or slightly curved rod-like bacillus that is weakly gram positive and acid and alcohol fast. Mycobacteria have a lipid shell ("lipid barrier") containing mycolic acid that resists proteolysis and uptake into phagolysosomes; muramyl dipeptide, which stimulates a T-cell response that elicits the characteristic granuloma; and cell wall glycolipids that inhibit macrophage function. This surrounding coat of inert lipids and surface proteins allows mycobacteria to survive inside phagocytes, where they may remain dormant for years.[5]

Whereas most TB is due to *M. tuberculosis*, other mycobacteria may rarely cause clinical disease, especially in immunocompromised hosts. These include *M. avium-intracellulare*, *M. kansasii*, *M. bovis*, *M. fortuitum*, and *M. szulgai*. However, most cases of genitourinary TB are due to *M. tuberculosis*.[5]

PATHOGENESIS

The clinical and pathologic manifestations of TB depend on the virulence of the organism and the effectiveness of the host response. The host response may lead to complete containment of infection or result in an illness of varying severity. Strain differences may also determine whether an infected person develops primary TB, reactivation TB, or a chronic asymptomatic infection.

When an infected droplet with the size of 1 to 5 μm is deposited in the respiratory tract, tonsillar fossa, or gastrointestinal tract, a primary focus develops with the formation of a nonspecific asymptomatic granuloma. The organisms from the primary focus drain to the regional lymph gland, causing its enlargement, resulting in the *primary complex*. This is often asymptomatic and self-limited.

Bacilli from the regional lymph node may also enter through the thoracic duct into the blood, resulting in silent dissemination to various sites, including the cortex of the kidneys (Fig. 52.1). Here they elicit an inflammatory response resulting in granuloma formation that may heal and form a scar, remain dormant for many years, or rupture into the proximal tubule of the nephron. The bacilli in the nephron are trapped at the level of the loop of Henle, where they multiply. The relatively poor blood flow, hypertonicity, and high ammonia concentration in the renal medulla impair the immune responses and favor the formation of medullary granulomas. These granulomas (tuberculomas), which contain macrophages, may undergo coagulative necrosis, forming cheese-like caseous material (Fig. 52.2), and occasionally rupture into the calyx.[6]

The renal medulla is the most common site of involvement of clinical renal TB and is usually unilateral.[7] When this caseous focus ruptures into the collecting system, cavities and ulcers are formed, and involvement of renal papillae may lead to sloughing and papillary necrosis. Healing in the kidney occurs by fibrosis and scarring, resulting in strictures and obstruction. Calcification commences intracellularly by the accumulation of phosphate ions from the disintegration of nucleoproteins and calcium ions from cell membrane damage. These lesions may harbor live mycobacteria, and such dystrophic lesions should be considered active disease and not a sign of healing. Dystrophic calcification of damaged structures may result in a nonfunctioning kidney called "putty" or "cement" kidney. Spread of TB to contiguous structures may occur; ureteritis is common and may result in strictures and obstructive uropathy (Fig. 52.3).

The bladder may develop hyperemia near the ureteral orifice, followed by superficial ulcers and granulomatous changes involving all layers (pancystitis). Healing by fibrosis at the ureteral orifice results in a refluxing "golf-hole" ureter. Extensive fibrosis of the bladder wall results in a thick, small-capacity bladder ("thimble" bladder; Fig. 52.4). Bladder infection may also rarely result from instillation of bacille Calmette-Guérin (BCG) in the bladder as part of treatment of superficial bladder carcinomas.

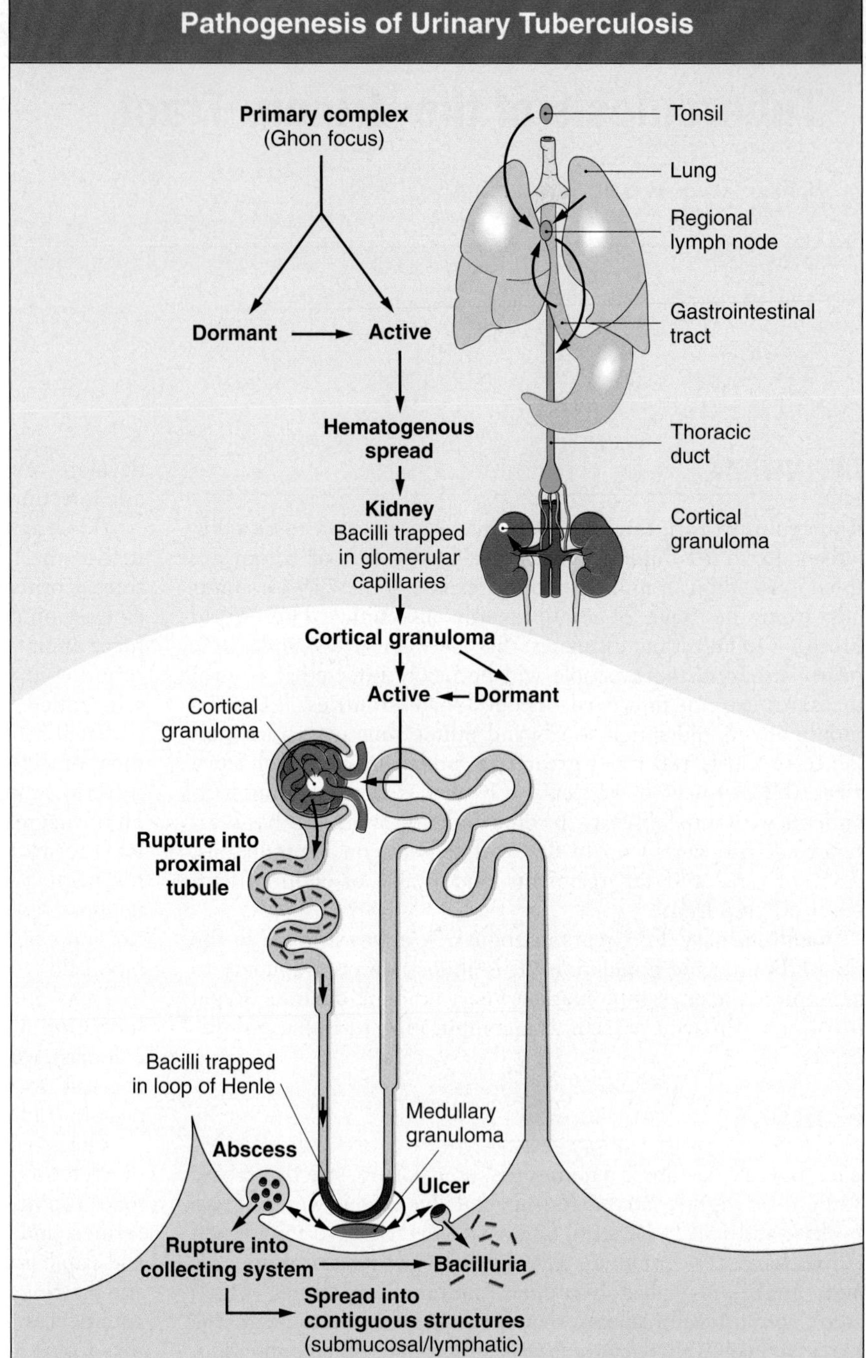

Figure 52.1 Pathogenesis of urinary tuberculosis.

Involvement of the genital tract is also common. As many as 70% to 80% of men with TB of the urinary tract have epididymitis, prostatitis, seminal vesiculitis, orchitis, or cold abscesses. In women, genital tract involvement is less common; but if it is present, it usually presents as salpingitis that is often diagnosed during investigation for infertility.

Transplanted kidneys may also transmit TB to their recipients.[8]

CLINICAL MANIFESTATIONS

Urinary tract TB may be asymptomatic or mimic other disorders. It may present with constitutional symptoms or symptoms related to the lower urinary tract, abdomen, or genitalia (Fig. 52.5). A high index of suspicion enables early diagnosis. Most patients are between 20 and 40 years of age, with a male to female ratio of 2:1. Because active genitourinary TB presents 5 to 15 years after primary infection, it is relatively rare in children. Increased risk factors for TB include close contact with sputum smear–positive individuals, vagrancy, social deprivation, neglect, immunosuppression, HIV infection or acquired immunodeficiency syndrome (AIDS), diabetes mellitus, renal failure, and other debilitating illness.

Nearly 25% of patients have no clinical or laboratory evidence of abnormality and the diagnosis is made on investigation for other diseases, during surgery, or at autopsy. Another 25%

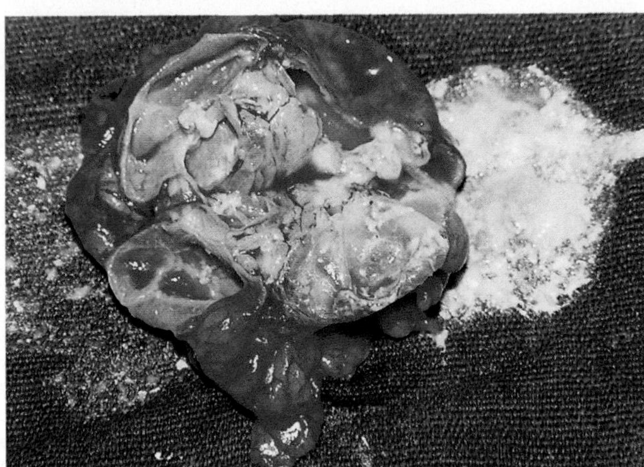

Figure 52.2 Renal tuberculosis. A cut section of kidney showing areas of cavitation and caseation necrosis (white chalky material).

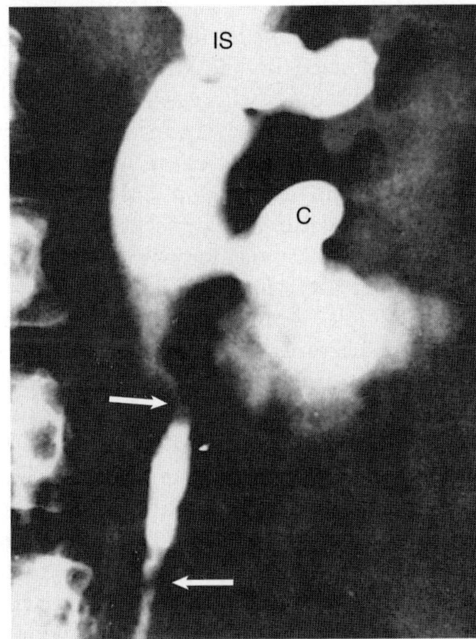

Figure 52.3 Multiple ureteral strictures. Strictures *(arrows)* associated with dilated ureter, infundibular stenosis (IS), and caliectasis (C) are seen in this intravenous urogram. *(Courtesy Professor K. Sasidharan, Kasthurba Medical College, Manipal, India.)*

have asymptomatic urinary abnormalities, usually persistent asymptomatic pyuria or hematuria. In patients with persistent pyuria, conventional urine cultures do not yield any growth, and the urine is usually acidic, hence the term *acid-sterile pyuria*. Of the patients who are symptomatic, lower urinary tract symptoms, such as frequency, urgency, dysuria, nocturia, frank pyuria, or hematuria, occur in more than 75%. Increased urinary frequency is one of the early symptoms and results from inflammation of the bladder. The defect in the urinary concentrating mechanism explains the nocturia.

Recurrent bouts of painless macroscopic hematuria should alert the clinician to the possible diagnosis of urinary TB, although glomerular diseases, for example, IgA nephropathy, should also be considered. Macroscopic hematuria in urinary TB is a result of bleeding from the ulcerating lesions, inflammation of the urothelium, or rupture of a blood vessel in the vicinity of a cavity. Colicky pain may occur as a presenting manifestation of urinary TB when it is associated with stone, clot, or acute obstruction.

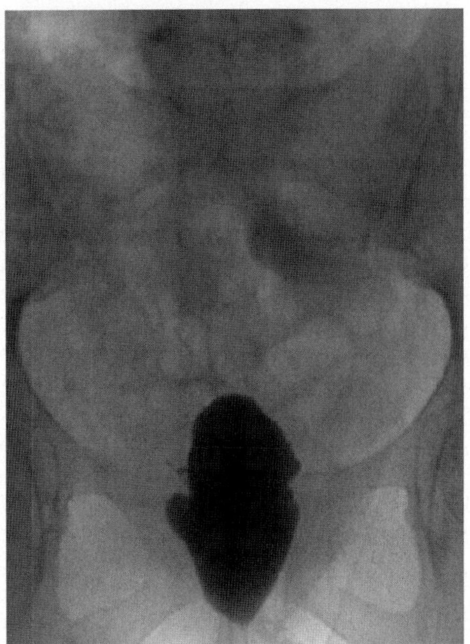

Figure 52.4 Cystogram showing thimble bladder.

Clinical Features of Urinary Tuberculosis

Features	Frequency (%)	Symptoms
Asymptomatic	25	Detected during autopsy, surgery, or investigations for other diseases
Asymptomatic urinary abnormalities	25	Persistent pyuria, microscopic abnormalities, hematuria
Lower urinary tract symptoms (most common)	40	Frequency, urgency, dysuria, incontinence, nocturia, suprapubic pain, perineal pain
Male genital tract involvement	75	Epididymitis, hemospermia, infertility, reduced semen volume
Female genital tract involvement	<5	Amenorrhea, infertility, vaginal bleeding, pelvic pain
Constitutional symptoms	<20	Fever, reduced appetite, anorexia, weight loss, night sweats
Miscellaneous	—	Urolithiasis, hypertension, acute kidney injury, chronic kidney disease, abdominal colic, abdominal mass

Figure 52.5 Clinical features of urinary tuberculosis.

In advanced disease, frequency and urgency related to reduced bladder capacity (thimble bladder) occur. Incomplete emptying, increased susceptibility to infection, and secondary vesicoureteral reflux may also occur. In chronic ureteral obstruction, enlargement of the kidney, infection, or perinephric collection leads to a dull aching loin pain. Severe suprapubic pain with backache and dysuria suggests acute tuberculous cystitis.

Episodes of pyuria, which may suggest secondary bacterial infection or drainage of a caseous focus into the collecting system, may also be a manifestation of renal TB. Persistence of pyuria after appropriate therapy should lead to an evaluation for urinary TB.

Long-standing renal TB may result in mild tubular proteinuria (<1 g/24 h) in up to 50% of patients. About 15% have proteinuria of more than 1 g/24 h, and nephrotic syndrome due to amyloidosis may develop in some patients. Rare cases of mesangial proliferative glomerulonephritis have also been reported.

Anemia is seen in less than 20% of patients with nonmiliary disease, but the frequency is higher in those with renal dysfunction.[9] A few patients have nephrogenic diabetes insipidus. Renal tubular acidosis may occur. Hyporeninemic hypoaldosteronism may result from the tubulointerstitial injury secondary to obstructive uropathy.[10] Renal function is usually normal, but chronic kidney disease may develop if both kidneys are extensively damaged.

Some patients may present with renal failure, pyuria, microscopic hematuria, and proteinuria, in whom the urine cultures for mycobacteria are repeatedly negative. These patients respond favorably to antituberculous chemotherapy combined with corticosteroids. The kidneys are of normal size and show diffuse interstitial nephritis, with caseating granulomas containing the bacilli in 75% of the biopsy samples.[11] Hypertension is unusual in renal TB, but intimal proliferation of vessels near inflamed areas may lead to segmental ischemia and renin release.[12] In association with a nonfunctioning kidney, nephrectomy may help improve the hypertension. Relief of any obstruction may also help lower the blood pressure. Nephrolithiasis may occur in 7% to 18% of patients. Secondary infection with *Escherichia coli* may be seen in 20% to 50% of patients.

As discussed earlier, genital involvement is common in men with urinary TB. Epididymitis may present with scrotal discomfort, mass, or a cold abscess that may rupture, leading to a nonhealing posterior scrotal sinus. Thickening of the vas deferens may result in the "beaded" vas. TB of the prostate may present with lower urinary symptoms and perineal pain. The prostate may be hard or boggy. Penile and urethral TB may present with strictures, fistulas, ulcers, or papillonecrotic skin lesions. Hemospermia, reduction of semen volume, and infertility are other manifestations of genital involvement. Direct spread of *M. tuberculosis* to the sexual partner is possible.

In women, the association between genital and renal TB is rare, occurring in 5% of cases. The major manifestation of genital involvement in women is infertility resulting from adherent salpingitis. Secondary amenorrhea, vaginal bleeding, and pelvic pain caused by inflammation may occur.

Constitutional symptoms, such as fever, weight loss, night sweats, fatigue, and anorexia, occur in less than 20% of patients and indicate active infection in other organs or secondary bacterial infection of the urinary tract. A careful examination to identify pulmonary, lymph node, or skeletal TB must be undertaken in all patients who present with constitutional symptoms. The chest radiograph may show evidence of active or healed tuberculous lesions in more than half of cases.

PATHOLOGY

Urinary TB may present as a miliary or ulcerocavernous pathologic process. The miliary form of TB is rare and is seen particularly in immunosuppressed individuals. The gross appearance of the kidney is characteristic; the cortex is studded with yellowish white, hard, pinhead-sized nodules that on microscopy show several coalescent granulomas with central caseation.

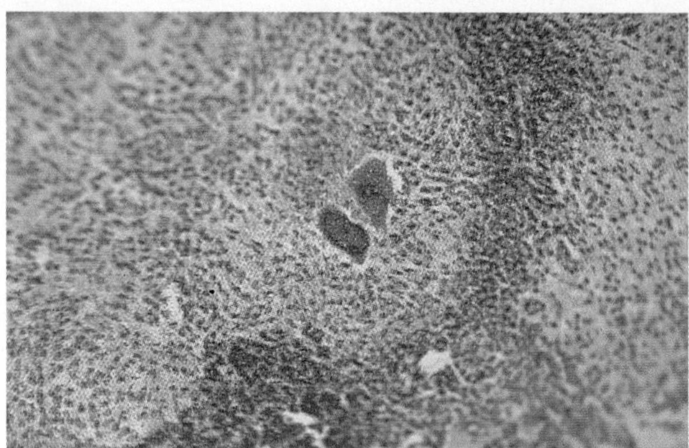

Figure 52.6 Tuberculous granuloma. The granuloma comprises Langhans giant cells (two large cells in the center), surrounding epithelioid cells, and a rim of lymphocytes. *(Courtesy Dr. Sathi Bai Panikker, Kottayam, India.)*

In the more common ulcerocavernous form, the kidneys will initially appear normal or show yellow nodules on the outer surface. On cut section, granulomas and ulcers in the renal pyramid or medullary cavities may be seen. Larger cavities filled with caseous material communicating with the collecting system may also occur. Other gross findings include multiple ulcers in the infundibular region of the calyces, calyceal stenosis with caliectasis, ulcers or strictures of the ureter with hydronephrosis, pyonephrosis, subcapsular collections, and perinephric abscesses. The bladder may show ulcers or be grossly fibrotic and contracted.

On microscopy, in early disease, neutrophilic infiltration with phagocytosis of the bacilli may be present. Subsequent histologic features depend on the virulence of the organism and the cell-mediated immunity. In those with an effective cell-mediated response, granulomas, characterized by the presence of macrophages with engulfed bacilli surrounded by epithelioid cells and Langhans giant cells, are seen (Fig. 52.6). There is often a cuff of lymphocytes and plasma cells surrounding the lesion. Healing occurs by fibrosis and scarring. In those with a less effective immune response, there is caseating necrosis, characterized by amorphous cheese-like eosinophilic material replacing the normal tissue architecture. The presence of caseous necrosis generally implies that the lesion is active. Later, this may calcify. Dystrophic calcification suggests activity rather than healing.

Kidneys may also be enlarged from amyloidosis or diffuse proliferative glomerulonephritis. In tuberculous interstitial nephritis, interstitial granuloma formation associated with normal-sized kidneys and negative urine cultures is seen.

DIAGNOSIS AND DIFFERENTIAL DIAGNOSIS

A high index of suspicion is necessary to diagnose genitourinary TB. Elderly subjects, those recently exposed to infection, immunocompromised individuals, and patients with TB elsewhere are at high risk. Suspicion may also occur if there is sterile pyuria, which is present in 50% of patients. The tuberculin test (Mantoux test) is useful for proving infection (or prior immunization with BCG), but not necessarily disease. A positive test response only suggests prior exposure to the antigen and does not indicate active infection. A negative test response in the absence of an immunosuppressed state rules out tuberculous infection. However, patients with uremia, particularly in the setting of malnutrition, may display anergy and have a false-negative test result.[13]

Isolation of *M. tuberculosis* by urine culture is the definitive diagnostic test. Fully voided early morning urine samples for 3 to 5 consecutive days are cultured on two standard solid mycobacterial culture media: the egg-based Lowenstein-Jensen medium and the agar-based Middlebrook 7H10 medium. These transparent media enable earlier visualization of microcolonies, which grow by 6 to 12 weeks. Sensitivity tests are performed to choose the optimum chemotherapeutic agents. However, this may take an additional 6 to 12 weeks. Any tissue specimen submitted for mycobacterial culture should be macerated with sterile sand by a mortar and pestle before inoculation. Direct demonstration of acid-fast bacilli in urine by Ziehl-Neelsen stain is not reliable for diagnosis because *Mycobacterium smegmatis*, a saprophyte, may be easily mistaken for *M. tuberculosis*.

Rapid methods for diagnosis of TB are increasingly available. With use of the radiometric broth method for acid-fast bacilli isolation, a positive growth can be obtained in about 9 days. Serologic tests with the soluble antigen fluorescent antibody test and the polymerase chain reaction can be used for early diagnosis of TB.[14] Enzyme linked immunospot assays are used as in-vitro diagnostic tests and they measure T cell specific *M tuberculosis* antigens. The test results are unaffected by prior tuberculin testing or low CD4 counts.[15] Another reliable and simple test using whole blood is based on quantifying the interferon-γ released from the white blood cells that have been exposed to some of the mycobacterial antigens. The availability of the result in 24 hours is the main advantage.[16] Sonographically guided fine-needle aspiration cytology is useful as a diagnostic tool in defining the granulomatous nature of the lesion in patients with positive urine culture. Histologic diagnosis is made by identifying the pathologic triad of caseating necrosis, loose aggregates of epithelioid histiocytes, and Langhans giant cells.

Imaging studies are essential to assess the extent and severity of involvement once a diagnosis of genitourinary TB is made. Extensive dystrophic calcification in advanced renal TB is described as "cumulus cloud" calcification (Fig. 52.7). Plain radiographs of chest and spine show active or healed tuberculous lesions in 60% to 70% of patients. Abnormalities in the excretory urogram may be seen in 70% to 90% of patients. Minimal erosion of the tip of the calyx with spasticity, incomplete filling, distortion, infundibular stenosis, hydrocalicosis, multiple ureteral strictures, hydronephrosis, hydroureter, or nonvisualization of the kidney may be present. The renal pelvis, which may be dilated initially, may eventually be obliterated, leading to a distorted appearance called hiked-up pelvis (Kerr kink sign). Irregularities or multiple strictures lead to a beaded or corkscrew appearance of the ureter or hydronephrosis. Later, thickening and straightening of the whole ureter may occur ("pipe-stem" ureter). The bladder may appear irregular and fibrosed, and vesicoureteral reflux may occur. Antegrade or retrograde pyelography can identify the number, length, or site of ureteral strictures and assist in placement of a ureteric stent across the stenotic segment.

High-resolution ultrasound is useful to rule out obstruction and to study the parenchyma closely to identify granulomas, small abscesses, bladder mucosal thickening, or calcification (Figs. 52.8 and 52.9).[17] The earliest finding is mucosal thickening and calyceal irregularity.

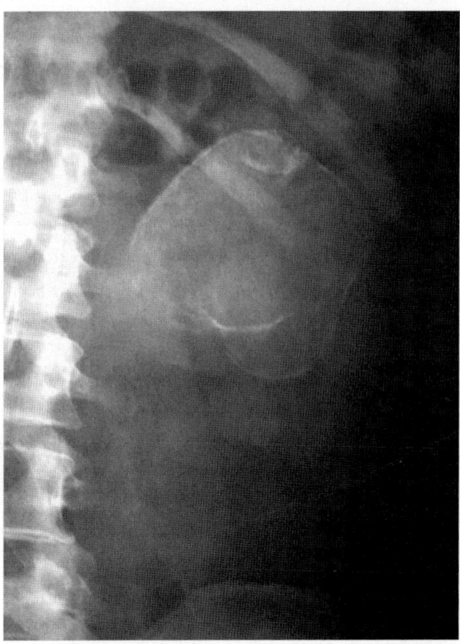

Figure 52.7 Plain radiograph showing calcified kidney.

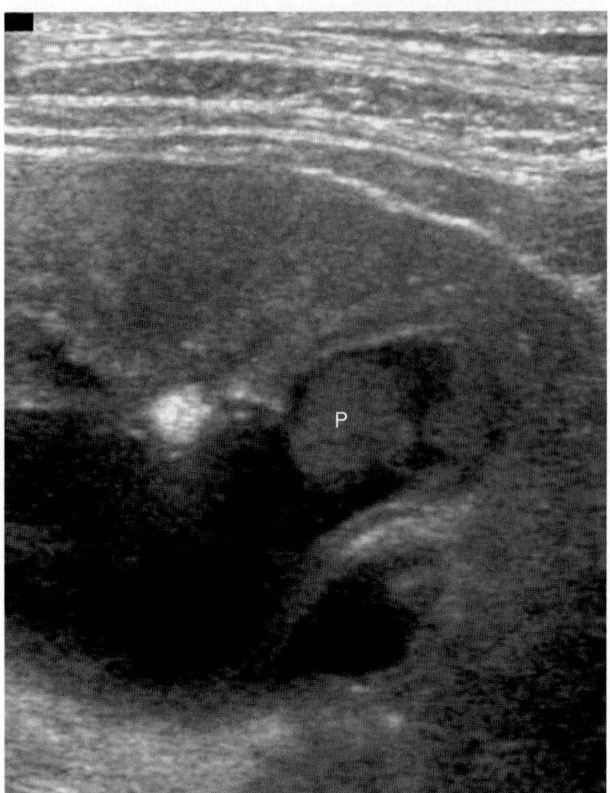

Figure 52.8 High-resolution ultrasound scan of the kidney showing a sloughed necrosed papilla (P) in the calyx. *(From reference 18, with permission of the American Institute of Ultrasound in Medicine.)*

Computed tomography (CT) is the most sensitive method for identifying renal parenchymal scarring, calcification, and cavitary lesions (Figs. 52.10 and 52.11). Cortical thinning is a common CT finding and may be either focal or global. These imaging modalities are helpful in the follow-up of patients with cavities or mass lesions in the kidney. Cystoscopy under general

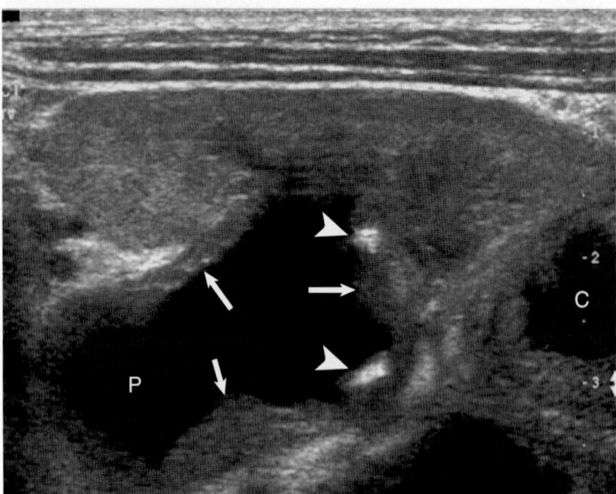

Figure 52.9 High-resolution transverse ultrasound scan of the kidney showing mucosal thickening *(arrows)* of calyces and the pelvis (P). There are calcifications of the wall of the calyx and pelvis *(arrowheads)*. A parenchymal cavity (C) is also shown. *(From reference 18, with permission of the American Institute of Ultrasound in Medicine.)*

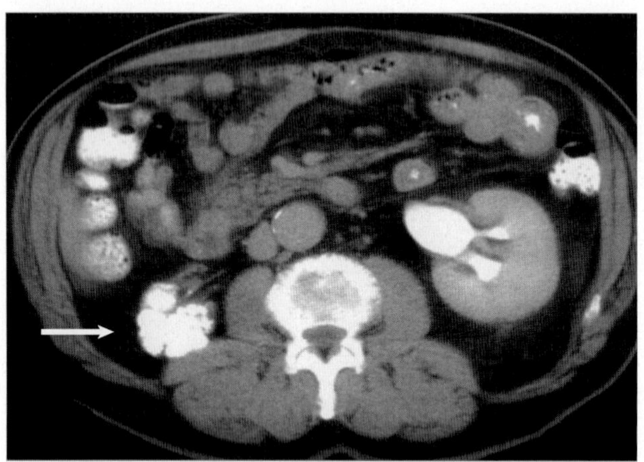

Figure 52.10 Contrast-enhanced CT image showing contracted calcified right kidney and normal opposite side.

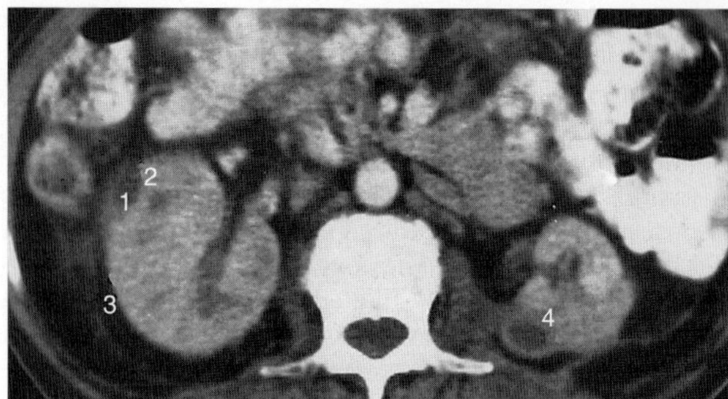

Figure 52.11 Renal tuberculosis. CT scan shows an enlarged left kidney with multiple cavities present bilaterally (marked 1, 2, 3, and 4). *(Courtesy Professor K. Sasidharan, Kasthurba Medical College, Manipal, India.)*

anesthesia helps visualize the mucosal lesions, the golf-hole ureteral orifice, or the efflux of toothpaste-like caseous material. Biopsy during the acute stage is avoided for fear of dissemination of TB.

TB mimics numerous diseases. Chronic nonspecific urinary infections may be confused with renal TB, and this is confounded by the fact that secondary bacterial infection may complicate 20% of cases of renal TB. Absence of response to usual antibiotics should arouse suspicion of urinary TB. Conditions causing recurrent painless hematuria, such as IgA nephropathy and schistosomiasis (see Chapter 54), are often misdiagnosed as TB in endemic areas. In interstitial cystitis, lower urinary symptoms similar to tuberculous cystitis may occur, but the urinalysis does not show gross pyuria, and cultures for acid-fast bacilli are negative. On radiologic examination, chronic pyelonephritis, renal papillary necrosis, medullary sponge kidney, calyceal diverticulum, renal carcinoma, xanthogranulomatous pyelonephritis, and multiple small renal calculi have to be differentiated from TB. Of late, a few cases of pseudotuberculous pyelonephritis have been reported in which caseating granulomas resembling TB were observed in the renal parenchyma but no mycobacteria or other microorganisms were detected in the renal tissue or urine culture.[18]

NATURAL HISTORY

The prognosis of genitourinary TB depends on the host resistance and the load and virulence of the organism. In many cases, foci in the urinary tract remain dormant indefinitely. Progression occurs through formation of tuberculous granuloma, caseation, ulceration, and dystrophic calcification. Most manifestations result from the complications, which can be prevented by timely chemotherapy and appropriate surgical intervention when indicated. With the advent of effective chemotherapeutic measures, the long-term complications and sequelae of TB have decreased significantly.

TREATMENT

Genitourinary TB is usually amenable to medical treatment. Many antituberculous drugs reach the kidneys, urinary tract, urine, and cavitary lesions in high concentration, and there are fewer organisms in the lesions compared with cavitary lung lesions. A wide variety of antituberculous agents are also available (Fig. 52.12).

A short-course regimen is recommended.[19] Treatment is started with daily rifampin (600 mg), isoniazid (300 mg), and pyrazinamide (1500 mg) in the morning. Unless the culture sensitivity indicates otherwise, pyrazinamide is discontinued after 2 months, and isoniazid and rifampin are continued for another 4 months. If the patient is very sick with irritative bladder symptoms, streptomycin in daily doses of 1 g may be added during the first 2 months. However, if the patient is older than 40 years, the daily dose of streptomycin is reduced to 0.75 g with periodic monitoring for ototoxicity and vestibular toxicity.

If the probability of drug resistance is high, ethambutol in daily doses of 800 to 1200 mg may also be used in the first 2 months. Longer courses of antituberculous treatment ranging from 9 months to 2 years are useful in patients who do not tolerate pyrazinamide, those responding slowly to a standard regimen, those with miliary or central nervous system disease, and children with multiple-site involvement.

Fixed-dose combinations of anti-TB drugs incorporating two or more drugs in the same tablet have advantages. These include increased compliance, administration of adequate dose, minimization of inadvertent medication errors, and avoidance of drug resistance.

Antituberculous Drugs

Drug	Dose Form	Dosage	Side Effects	Mode of Action	Remarks
Isoniazid	Tablet: 100 mg, 300 mg	5 mg/kg daily (oral) (maximum, 300 mg/day)	Peripheral neuritis, hepatitis, hypersensitivity reactions	Bactericidal for groups I and II	Pyridoxine (50 mg) prophylaxis necessary
Rifampin (Rifampicin)	Capsule or tablet: 150, 300, 450 mg	10 mg/kg daily (oral) (maximum, 600 mg/day)	Hepatitis, febrile reactions, acute interstitial nephritis	Bactericidal for groups I, II, and III	
Pyrazinamide	Tablet: 400, 500 mg	25 mg/kg daily (oral) (maximum, 2 g/day)	Hepatotoxicity, hyperuricemia	Bactericidal for group II	Combination with aminoglycoside useful
Streptomycin	Powder for injection: 1 g	15 mg/kg daily IM (maximum dose, 1 g; dose reduced in those >40 years of age)	Ototoxicity, nephrotoxicity	Bactericidal for group I	
Ethambutol	Tablet: 100, 400 mg	15–25 mg/kg daily (oral) (maximum, 2.5 g/day)	Optic neuritis (reversible), rash	Bacteriostatic for groups I and II	Used to inhibit development of resistant mutants; use with caution in renal failure
Thiacetazone	Tablet: 150 mg	150 mg (oral) (not for intermittent therapy)	Rashes, exfoliative dermatitis, hepatic failure	Bacteriostatic and inhibits emergence of isoniazid resistance	Not used in renal failure
Ciprofloxacin	Tablet: 250, 500 mg	500–1000 mg (oral)	Hypersensitivity, drug interaction		Not used in children
Ofloxacin	Tablet: 200, 400 mg	400–500 mg (oral)			Not approved by FDA for tuberculosis
Capreomycin Kanamycin		15–30 mg/kg daily IM	Ototoxicity, nephrotoxicity	Bactericidal for group I	Avoided in older patients and those with renal failure

Figure 52.12 Antituberculous drugs. The main drugs are listed with dosage form, dosage, side effects, and mode of action. *M tuberculosis* exists as 3 subpopulations. Group I is extracellular, occurs mainly in cavitating lesions, and respond to streptomycin, isoniazid and rifampin. Group II reside intracellularly in macrophages, replicate slowly, and respond to pyrazinamide, isoniazid or rifampin. Group III organisms exist within closed caseous lesions, survive better in neutral pH, replicate slowly, and respond best to rifampin.

During treatment, healing by fibrosis may lead to obstruction of one or both ureters, with hydronephrosis, parenchymal damage, and renal failure. Dehydration or salt depletion may occur from tubulointerstitial damage, resulting in altered tubular function. Adrenal involvement may contribute to salt wasting. Oliguric acute renal failure caused by allergic interstitial nephritis may occur in patients receiving intermittent rifampin therapy.

Surgical Treatment

The role of surgical treatment in urinary TB is limited. For ureteral strictures, timely introduction of stents across the narrow segment may avoid the need for major surgical procedures. Two broad types of surgical treatments are considered.

Reconstructive surgery involves the correction of obstruction to the ureter by pyeloplasty, ureteroureterostomy, correction of reflux by ureteral reimplantation, and increasing the bladder capacity by augmentation cystoplasty, which involves anastomosis of an isolated segment of bowel to the contracted bladder.

Ablative surgery involves removal of the diseased parts together with the infected material containing the dormant organisms. The need for removal of a unilateral nonfunctioning kidney is controversial. Because prolonged antituberculous treatment for 18 to 24 months effectively sterilizes caseous and calcified masses of the tuberculous cement kidney, nephrectomy is advocated only in cases of secondary sepsis, pain, bleeding, uncontrollable hypertension, or continued positive urinary cultures. Tuberculous abscesses can be aspirated under ultrasound or CT guidance and antituberculous drugs directly instilled into the cavity.

Treatment Regimens in Special Situations

Women During Pregnancy and Lactation

Most antituberculous drugs are safe for use during pregnancy. However, streptomycin is ototoxic to the fetus and must be avoided. If a four-drug schedule is indicated, streptomycin is replaced by ethambutol. There is no contraindication to the use of these drugs during breast-feeding, and it is not necessary to isolate the baby from the mother. The baby should receive BCG immunization and isoniazid prophylaxis. Because rifampin interacts with the efficacy of oral contraceptive pills, women taking these agents together should be advised to take a higher dose of estrogen or to use alternative methods of contraception.

Treatment of Patients with Liver Disease

The usual short-term (6-month) chemotherapy regimen can be used in patients with liver disorders if there is no evidence of chronic liver disease, hepatitis virus carrier state, past history of acute hepatitis, or excessive alcohol consumption. In chronic liver disease, isoniazid and two of the nonhepatotoxic drugs (streptomycin and ethambutol) can be used for 8 to 12 months. If rifampin is used, liver function should be closely monitored. Pyrazinamide is contraindicated. In those with acute hepatitis unrelated to TB or its therapy, it would be safer to defer the chemotherapy until the acute hepatitis has resolved. If immediate treatment of TB during acute hepatitis is mandatory, streptomycin plus ethambutol for a period of 3 months followed by isoniazid and rifampin for 6 months is advised.

Treatment of Patients with Renal Failure

In patients with renal failure, isoniazid, rifampin, and pyrazinamide, which are eliminated by the biliary route, can be given in normal dosages. Those receiving isoniazid should also be given pyridoxine (50 mg/day) to prevent peripheral neuropathy. Because streptomycin and ethambutol are excreted by the kidney, dosage modification of these drugs is necessary in renal failure. Streptomycin (15 mg/kg) is administered every 24 to 72 hours for a creatinine clearance between 10 and 50 ml/min and every 72 to 96 hours for a creatinine clearance of less than 10 ml/min to maintain a therapeutic peak level of 20 to 30 μg/ml. Monitoring for high-pitched tinnitus or sense of fullness in the ears and audiography may be useful. For ethambutol, the dose is administered every 24 to 36 hours if the creatinine clearance is between 10 and 50 ml/min and every 48 hours if the creatinine clearance is below 10 ml/min. Monthly questioning for symptoms of visual dysfunction (alterations in visual fields, acuity, and blue-green color vision) with early referral for ophthalmic examination may identify ethambutol toxicity early with potential reversibility.

Treatment in Renal Allograft Recipients

A modified treatment with adjusted doses of isoniazid and ethambutol for 18 months, combined with ofloxacin 200 mg twice daily for the first 9 months and pyrazinamide 750 mg twice daily for the first 3 months, has been recommended.[20] If rifampin is used in those who are receiving a non–cyclosporine-based immunosuppressive regimen, the maintenance dose of prednisolone may have to be doubled.

Treatment in AIDS

Short-term chemotherapy is sufficient. If the follow-up cultures are positive, prolonged therapy for up to 2 years may be needed on the basis of antibiotic sensitivity.

Patients Who Fail Treatment

Failure to show clinical or radiologic improvement with treatment may signify poor compliance, inadequate regimen and dosage, incorrect diagnosis, multidrug-resistant TB, delayed response, or the phenomenon of paradoxical reaction known as immune reconstitution inflammatory syndrome. This syndrome is characterized by unexpected worsening of symptoms or appearance of new lesions like lymphadenopathy, serosal effusions, and pleural infiltrates. This syndrome is more common in those prescribed antiretroviral treatment for coexisting HIV and TB infections.[21]

Monitoring of Patients

After 2 months of intensive chemotherapy, urine is cultured for *M. tuberculosis* for 3 consecutive days. If cultures remain positive, sensitivity is done and treatment modified accordingly. After completion of treatment, all patients should have three consecutive early morning samples of urine for *M. tuberculosis* culture, and this is repeated after 3 months and 1 year. Intravenous urography or ultrasound is repeated at the end of 2 months and at the completion of treatment to detect any evidence of obstruction. In cases of renal calcification, the patient should be evaluated yearly by three early morning samples of urine for culture of mycobacteria and by plain radiography of the abdomen for up to 10 years because calcification may harbor *M. tuberculosis* and may progress to destruction of the kidney.

REFERENCES

1. Raviglione MC, Srider DE, Kochi A. Global epidemiology of tuberculosis. *JAMA*. 1995;273:220-226.
2. Selwyn PA, Hartel D, Lewis VA, et al. A prospective study of the risk of tuberculosis among intravenous drug users with human immunodeficiency virus infection. *N Engl J Med*. 1989;370:546-547.
3. Gulati S, Kher V, Gulati K, Arora P. Tuberculosis in childhood nephrotic syndrome in India. *Pediatr Nephrol*. 1977;11:695-698.
4. Schafer M, Kim D, Weiss J, et al. Extrapulmonary tuberculosis in patients with HIV infection. *Medicine (Baltimore)*. 1991;70:384-396.
5. Ho JL, Rilay LW. Defenses against tuberculosis. In: Crystal RG, West JB, Weibel ER, Barnes PJ, eds. *The Lung: Scientific Foundations*. 2nd ed. Philadelphia: Lippincott-Raven; 1997:2381-2391.
6. Turk JL. Granulomatous diseases. In: McGee JOD, Isacson PG, Wright NA, eds. *Oxford Textbook of Pathology*. Oxford: Oxford University Press; 1992:394-404.
7. Simon HB, Weinstein AJ, Pasternak MS, et al. Genitourinary tuberculosis: Clinical features in a general hospital population. *Am J Med*. 1977;63:410-414.
8. Mourad G, Soullilon JP, Chong G, et al. Transmission of mycobacterium TB with renal allografts. *Nephron*. 1985;41:82-85.
9. Wisnia LG, Kukolj S, Lopez de Santa Maria J, Camuzzi F. Renal function damage in 131 cases of urogenital tuberculosis. *Urology*. 1978;11:457-461.
10. De Frongs RA. Hyperkalemia and hyporeninemic hypoaldosteronism. *Kidney Int*. 1980;17;118-134.
11. Mallinson WJW, Fuller RW, Levison DA, et al. Diffuse interstitial renal tuberculosis: An unusual cause of renal failure. *Q J Med*. 1981;50:137-148.
12. Marks LS, Poutasse EF. Hypertension from renal tuberculosis: Operative cure predicted by renal vein renin. *J Urol*. 1973;109:149-152.
13. Shankar MS, Aravindan AN, Sohal PM, et al. The prevalence of tuberculin sensitivity and anergy in chronic renal failure in an endemic area: Tuberculin test and the risk of post-transplant tuberculosis. *Nephrol Dial Transplant*. 2005;20:2720-2724.
14. Baniel J, Maunia A, Liamen G. Fine needle cytodiagnosis of renal tuberculosis. *J Urol*. 1999;146:689-691.
15. Richeldi L. An update on the diagnosis of tuberculosis infection. *Am J Respir Crit Care Med*. 2006;174:736-742.
16. Pai M, Gokhale K, Joshi R, et al. *Mycobacterium tuberculosis* infection in health workers in rural India: Comparison of whole blood interferon gamma assay with tuberculin skin testing. *JAMA*. 2005;293:2746-2755.
17. Vijayaraghavan SB, Kandasamy SV, Arul M, et al. Spectrum of high-resolution sonographic features of urinary tuberculosis. *J Ultrasound Med*. 2004;23:585-594.
18. Casasole SV, Muntaner LP, Alonso UJ. Pseudo tuberculous pyelonephritis. *Arch Esp Urol*. 1994;47:172-174.
19. Maher D, Chaulet P, Spinaci S, Harries A, eds. *Standardised treatment regimens. Treatment of Tuberculosis: Guidelines for National Programmes*. 2nd ed. Geneva: World Health Organization; 1997:25-31.
20. Sundaram M, Adhikary SD, John GT, Kekre NS. Tuberculosis in renal transplant recipients. *Indian J Urol*. 2008;24:396-400.
21. Manosuthi W, Kiertiburanakul S, Phoorisri T, Sungkanuparph S. Immune reconstitution inflammatory syndrome of tuberculosis among HIV infected patients receiving antituberculous and antiretroviral therapy. *J Infect*. 2006;53:357-363.

CHAPTER 53

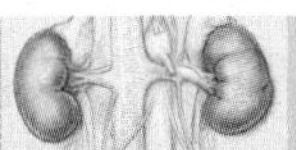

Fungal Infections of the Urinary Tract

Carol A. Kauffman

Funguria is a frequent finding in hospitalized patients. Almost always, the organisms found in urine are *Candida* species, although several other yeasts and less commonly molds and endemic fungi also can be found (Fig. 53.1). Candiduria is not a symptom, a sign, or a disease but frequently is a perplexing phenomenon for the physician to deal with. In reality, most patients with candiduria are asymptomatic and have colonization of the bladder or of an indwelling urinary catheter. The most difficult diagnostic problem that is encountered is determining when infection rather than colonization is present. Diagnostic tests to define whether candiduria is related to colonization or infection have not been standardized; similarly, diagnostic studies to localize the site of infection to either the bladder or the kidneys are not well established. In contrast to the situation with candiduria, growth in urine of organisms such as *Blastomyces dermatitidis*, *Aspergillus* species, and *Cryptococcus neoformans* almost always reflects disseminated infection. This chapter outlines an approach to the diagnosis and treatment of candiduria and other fungal urinary tract infections.

CANDIDA

Epidemiology

Candida species are common inhabitants of the perineum but are not found in urine in appreciable numbers in healthy hosts. However, a variety of predisposing factors allow these commensals to grow in the urine and in some instances to invade the bladder or the upper urinary tract and to cause infection. These factors are more commonly encountered in hospitalized patients, especially those in the intensive care unit and in patients in long-term care or rehabilitation units.[1] In a recent point prevalence survey of positive urine cultures obtained from hospitalized patients, *Candida* species were found in nearly 10% of specimens and were the third most common microorganism isolated from urine.[2]

The risk factors for candiduria, but not specifically for *Candida* urinary tract infection, have been established in several prospective surveillance studies and a few case-controlled studies.[3-5] Risk factors for candiduria are found to be similar in most of these studies and include increased age, female sex, antibiotic use, urinary drainage devices, prior surgical procedures, and diabetes mellitus (Fig. 53.2). In the largest surveillance study, urinary drainage devices, mostly indwelling urethral catheters, were present in 83% of patients who had candiduria; only 11% of patients with candiduria had no other risk factor.[3] In a multicenter study from Spain assessing candiduria in patients in an intensive care unit setting, independent risk factors associated with candiduria were age older than 65 years, female sex, diabetes mellitus, prior antibiotics, mechanical ventilation, parenteral nutrition, and length of hospital stay before admission to the intensive care unit.[4] A case-controlled study that compared candiduria due to *C. glabrata* with that due to *C. albicans* found that both species were associated with female sex, intensive care unit stay, and antibiotic use, whereas *C. glabrata* was more common in subjects with diabetes and in those who had received prior treatment with fluconazole (to which this species is typically resistant).[5] Most of the patients in these studies most likely had colonization and not infection with *Candida*.

Prospective controlled studies assessing risk factors for well-documented urinary tract infection due to *Candida* species have not been performed because firm diagnostic criteria for *Candida* urinary tract infection have not been established. However, clinical experience suggests that infection is more common in diabetic subjects and in those who have partial or complete urinary tract obstruction.

Pathogenesis

Candida has the propensity to cause disease by either the hematogenous or ascending route. This contrasts with urinary tract infections due to most bacteria, in which infection ascends from bladder to the collecting system of the kidney.

The pathogenesis of hematogenous seeding of *Candida* to the kidney was shown with animal models.[6] Multiple microabscesses develop throughout the cortex, with the yeasts penetrating through the glomeruli into the proximal tubules, where they are shed into the urine (Fig. 53.3). Healthy animals eventually clear the infection, but immunocompromised animals do not. Consistent with the experimental studies, renal microabscesses have been identified in 90% of patients with invasive candidiasis at autopsy.[7] The pathogenesis of ascending infection with *Candida* is not known. No animal model exists for this condition. Obstruction and stones are important factors in some patients, but specific mechanisms of adherence and subsequent growth in the collecting system have not been studied.

Microbiology

C. albicans accounts for 50% to 70% of all *Candida* urinary isolates; *C. glabrata*, present in approximately 20% of isolates, is the second most common,[3] *C. tropicalis* and *C. parapsilosis* are less common, and other species are rarely isolated. Certain populations of patients have a predominance of *C. glabrata*. For example, older adults frequently have *C. glabrata* isolated from urine, but urine cultures from neonates rarely yield *C. glabrata*. In a prospective survey of candiduria in renal transplant recipients, *C. glabrata* represented 53% and *C. albicans* only 35% of isolates.[8]

It is important to know the species causing candiduria for therapeutic reasons. Resistance to fluconazole, the primary agent

Fungal Genitourinary Tract Infections			
Fungal Infection	**Prostate**	**Bladder**	**Kidney**
Blastomycosis	+++	+	++
Histoplasmosis	+	+	++
Coccidioidomycosis	+	+	++
Aspergillosis	+	+	+++
Cryptococcosis	++	+	+++
Candidiasis	++	++++	++++

Figure 53.1 Fungal genitourinary tract infections.

Risk Factors for Different Types of *Candida* Urinary Tract Infections	
Type	**Risk Factors**
Renal (hematogenous)	Neutropenia, recent surgery, central venous catheter, parenteral nutrition, antibiotics, dialysis
Lower urinary tract	Indwelling bladder catheter, older age, female, diabetes, obstruction, antibiotics, urinary tract instrumentation
Upper urinary tract	Older age, diabetes, antibiotics, obstruction, urinary tract instrumentation (e.g., nephrostomy tube, ureteral sent)

Figure 53.2 Risk factors for candiduria.

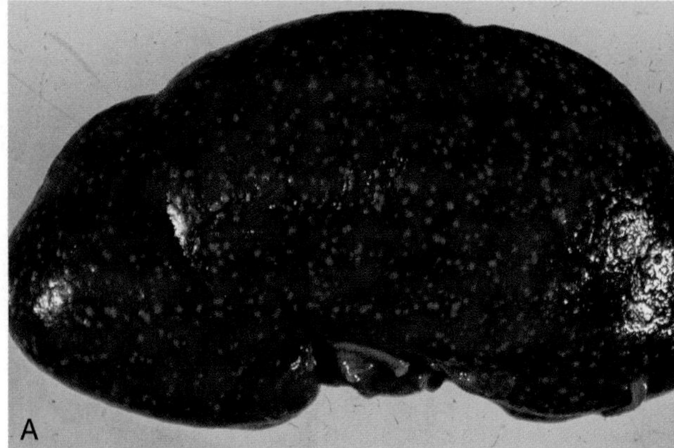

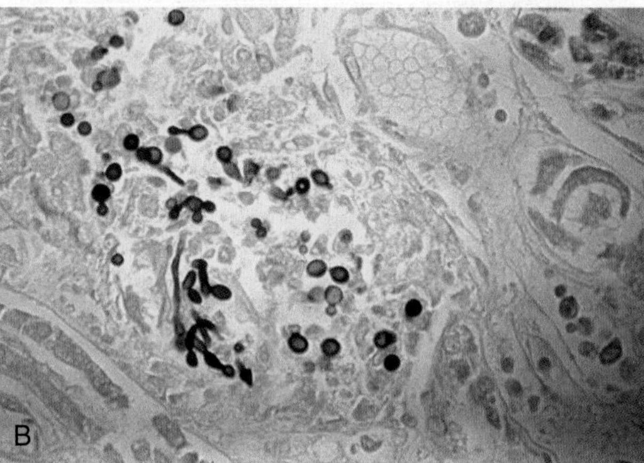

Figure 53.3 Hematogenous renal candidiasis. A, Multiple small abscesses are grossly obvious throughout the kidney. **B,** Histopathologic demonstration of a microabscess in the cortex of the kidney due to *Candida albicans* (Methenamine silver stain, yeast shown in grey-brown color).

used for the treatment of *Candida* urinary tract infections, occurs commonly among isolates of *C. glabrata* and occurs in all isolates of *C. krusei*. In contrast, almost all isolates of *C. albicans*, *C. tropicalis*, and *C. parapsilosis* are susceptible to fluconazole.

Clinical Manifestations

Most patients with candiduria are asymptomatic, and indeed, most do not have infection. A large prospective surveillance study of patients with candiduria noted that less than 5% of patients with candiduria had any symptoms suggesting urinary tract infection.[3] When patients have symptomatic cystitis or pyelonephritis, symptoms are indistinguishable from those noted with bacterial infections. Cystitis is manifested by dysuria, frequency, and urgency, and patients with upper tract infection can present with fever, chills, and flank pain. Uncommonly, urinary obstruction occurs from formation of a bezoar or fungal ball in the bladder or the collecting system. This may cause hydronephrosis, and uncommonly, acute kidney injury occurs.

Patients who have had seeding of the renal parenchyma during an episode of candidemia manifest the symptoms and signs associated with invasive candidiasis and not those of urinary tract infection. Chills, fever, hypotension, and other manifestations of sepsis are commonly noted in patients who are candidemic.

Diagnosis

Major diagnostic difficulties are encountered in trying to differentiate contamination of a urine specimen from colonization of the bladder or of an indwelling urethral catheter from invasive infection of the bladder or the kidney. Contamination is most easily differentiated by simply repeating the urine culture to determine if the candiduria persists. It may be necessary to obtain the second urine specimen by sterile bladder catheterization if the patient is unable to accomplish a clean-catch collection. In those patients who have an indwelling urethral catheter, the catheter should be replaced and a second urine specimen collected. For either of these circumstances, if the repeated culture yields no yeasts, no further diagnostic studies or therapeutic interventions are needed.

Distinguishing colonization from infection is not straightforward. In comparison with bacterial urinary tract infections, in which the diagnosis is based on appropriate symptoms combined with the findings of pyuria and quantitative bacterial counts, no studies have established the importance of quantitative urine cultures or pyuria for the diagnosis of *Candida* urinary tract infection.[1]

The techniques routinely used in most clinical laboratories for the detection of bacteria will also detect *Candida* in urine. However, *C. glabrata* grows more slowly than other species and more slowly than bacteria, and colonies may not appear for 48 hours, which is often after routine cultures of urine have been discarded in most laboratories.

The role of quantitative urine cultures to differentiate upper tract infection from bladder colonization was assessed by investigators in the 1970s and unfortunately showed broad ranges of

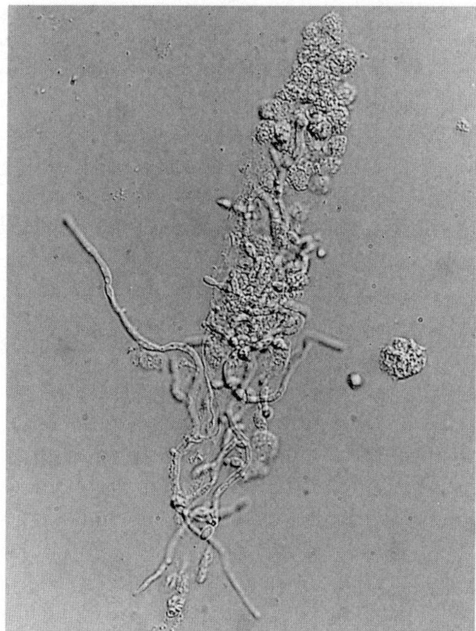

Figure 53.4 Photomicrograph of a renal tubular cast containing *Candida albicans,* showing both yeast forms and hyphae in a patient with fungal pyelonephritis.

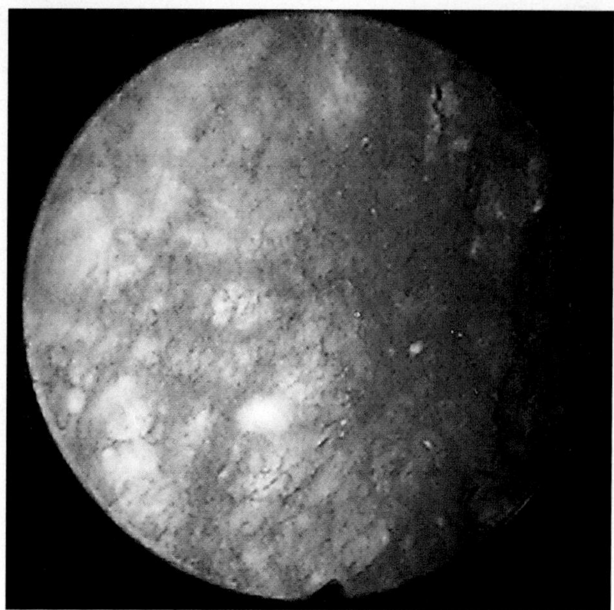

Figure 53.5 Cystoscopic appearance of extensive cystitis caused by *Candida krusei.*

colony counts for both colonization and infection.[9,10] In patients who did not have indwelling catheters, documented renal infection was found with colony counts as low as 10^4 yeasts/ml.[10] For patients who had indwelling catheters, colony counts between 2×10^4 and 10^5 cfu/ml or more were noted, and there was no correlation with biopsy-proven renal infection. A murine model of hematogenous renal candidiasis documented that renal involvement could be seen with any concentration of *Candida* in the urine.[11]

Pyuria is often not a helpful diagnostic criterion for infection in patients with candiduria. Concomitant bacteriuria is frequently noted in patients with candiduria and may be responsible for pyuria.[1] In patients who have an indwelling bladder catheter, pyuria is routinely noted, whether or not infection is present. In patients who do not have an indwelling bladder catheter or bacteriuria, the presence of pyuria is helpful.

Identification of casts containing yeasts in the urine appears to be specific for upper tract infection, but the technique is time-consuming, requires expert evaluation, and is not sensitive (Fig. 53.4). The finding of pseudohyphae in urine samples is no longer thought useful, especially because organisms such as *C. glabrata* cannot form pseudohyphae.

Imaging procedures, including abdominal ultrasound and computed tomography (CT), are essential to document obstruction at any level in the urinary tract and to determine the presence of fungus balls in bladder or kidneys.

In some patients, it is helpful to perform cystoscopy and biopsy of the bladder wall to determine whether inflammation is present and to evaluate the extent of invasion (Fig. 53.5). Retrograde studies can also be performed to establish whether obstruction is present.

Treatment with Systemic Antifungal Agents

Most patients who have candiduria do not need treatment with an antifungal agent. For patients who are asymptomatic, treatment should be given only to those who are at high risk for development of candidemia or in whom the presence of candiduria, regardless of symptoms, is likely to represent disseminated infection. The newly revised guidelines for the management of candidiasis published by the Infectious Diseases Society of America include the following in this category: patients undergoing urologic procedures, very low birth weight infants, and neutropenic patients (Fig. 53.6).[12] Patients who have candiduria and who are to undergo a urologic procedure are at increased risk for development of candidemia and should be treated with an antifungal agent a few days before and after the procedure. Candiduria in neutropenic patients and in very low birth weight infants has a high probability of representing disseminated candidiasis, and thus these groups also should be treated with an antifungal agent. Interestingly, asymptomatic candiduria in the renal transplant patient does not appear to warrant systemic antifungal treatment unless obstruction is present or symptoms suggestive of local or systemic infection develop.

In non–high-risk patients who have asymptomatic candiduria, removal of an indwelling urinary catheter will eradicate candiduria in many patients.[3] Follow-up urine culture can be performed a week later to determine if candiduria has cleared. If catheterization cannot be discontinued, the existing catheter should be removed and a new one inserted. This will often eradicate candiduria transiently, but it is highly likely that the organisms will return within a short time. Relief of obstruction, whether it is present in the upper or lower urinary tract, is essential for the long-term eradication of *Candida* from the urinary tract.

Patients who have symptoms suggestive of cystitis or pyelonephritis and in whom bacteria as well as *Candida* are found in the urine culture specimen should be treated initially with an antibacterial agent. If no bacteria are present, treatment with an antifungal agent is appropriate (see Fig. 53.6). Eradication of the organism with antifungal therapy is more likely if the indwelling catheter is also removed.[13] Oral fluconazole is the drug of choice. A loading dose of 400 mg should be given, followed by 200 mg daily for a total of 14 days.[12,13] Fluconazole is excreted as active

Treatment Recommendations for *Candida* Urinary Tract Infections

Asymptomatic candiduria	No treatment indicated except:	
	Urologic surgery	Treat a few days before and after the procedure with fluconazole 200–400 mg qd or Amphotericin 0.3–0.6 mg/kg/d
	Low birth weight infant or neutropenic patient	Treat as for disseminated candidiasis/candidemia
Cystitis	Preferred: oral fluconazole, 200 mg qd × 14 d	Alternatives include: Amphotericin 0.3–0.6 mg/kg/d × 1–7 d Flucytosine 25 mg/kg qid × 7–10 d
Pyelonephritis	Preferred: oral fluconazole, 200–400 mg qd × 14 d	Alternatives include: Amphotericin 0.5–0.7 mg/kg/d × 14 d Flucytosine 25 mg/kg qid × 14d
Renal (hematogenous)	Treat as for disseminated candidiasis/candidemia	
Fungus balls	Surgical removal and Fluconazole, 200–400 mg qd	Alternatives include: Amphotericin 0.5–0.7 mg/kg/d Flucytosine 25 mg/kg qid

Figure 53.6 Treatment recommendations for candiduria and *Candida* urinary tract infections.

drug in the urine and should effectively treat all *Candida* species, with the exception of those *C. glabrata* that are fluconazole resistant and *C. krusei.* The dosage of fluconazole should be reduced by 50% in patients with a creatinine clearance of 20 to 50 ml/min per 1.73 m^2 and by 75% when the creatinine clearance is below 20 ml/min per 1.73 m^2.

The possibility of drug-drug interactions should be evaluated before fluconazole is ordered. Phenytoin, warfarin, cyclosporine, tacrolimus, rifabutin, and sulfonylurea agents are some of the drugs for which serum concentrations will increase and may reach toxic levels after the addition of fluconazole to the therapeutic regimen.

The other available azole agents, itraconazole, voriconazole, and posaconazole, are not excreted into the urine as active drug. Whether tissue concentrations might be high enough to treat invasive kidney or bladder infections is not known, and there is no clinical experience to suggest that they will be effective.

Intravenous amphotericin B deoxycholate is effective in treating *Candida* urinary tract infections but should be reserved for those patients who have upper tract infection or for whom fluconazole therapy has failed. The toxicity, especially nephrotoxicity (see Chapter 66), associated with this agent precludes its use in many patients. The usual dosage is 0.3 to 0.6 mg/kg per day for 5 to 7 days, although this may be extended to 2 weeks for those with complicated upper tract infection.[12] Infusion-related side effects that are seen in some patients, even when they are treated with the lowest dosage, are rigors, fever, nausea, vomiting, and headache.

Lipid formulations of amphotericin are not recommended for treatment of fungal urinary tract infections. It is likely that the mechanism that leads to decreased nephrotoxicity with the addition of the lipid component precludes the drug's effectiveness by failing to achieve adequate levels in the urinary tract. Failures have been reported in a few patients.[14]

One of the few uses of flucytosine is for the treatment of *Candida* urinary tract infections. This agent, which is excreted into the urine as active drug in high concentrations, should be used only when fluconazole is not tolerated or the organism is fluconazole resistant. The usual dosage is 25 mg/kg orally every 6 hours for 7 to 10 days. Most species of *Candida*, with the exception of *C. krusei*, are susceptible to flucytosine, but resistance emerges quickly when this agent is used alone. Serious adverse effects of flucytosine include bone marrow suppression and hepatotoxicity. These effects are dose related, and the risk increases greatly with renal failure.

The echinocandins caspofungin, micafungin, and anidulafungin have minimal or no excretion into the urine as active drug. It is possible that the tissue concentrations achieved with these agents may be adequate to treat invasive *Candida* infections of the bladder or kidney. However, there are limited clinical data, and echinocandins currently cannot be recommended for the treatment of *Candida* urinary tract infections.

Local Antifungal Administration

Continuous bladder infusion of amphotericin, 50 mg in 1 liter of sterile water with a triple-lumen catheter, is sometimes used to treat *Candida* bladder infection. Bladder irrigation will clear candiduria more quickly than systemic antifungal agents will.[15] However, the effect is brief, and recolonization occurs within 1 to 2 weeks. It is likely that irrigation eliminates bladder colonization in the short term, but it is not evident that bladder infection can be treated with this maneuver. Recent literature suggests that amphotericin bladder irrigation is a strategy rarely needed given the need for catheter placement and the availability of more convenient treatment options, and this method of treatment is not recommended.[12,16] The one exception might be lower tract infection with *C. krusei* and *C. glabrata*, which are resistant to fluconazole and flucytosine.

In the setting of obstruction due to a fungus ball, irrigation through a percutaneous nephrostomy tube with amphotericin is recommended in addition to systemic antifungal therapy with fluconazole.[12] Absorption of amphotericin does not occur, and direct infusion is not nephrotoxic. Ultimately, surgical or endoscopic removal of the mass of fungal organisms is essential to eradicate the organism.

OTHER YEASTS

Cryptococcus neoformans infection in immunosuppressed hosts, especially patients with acquired immunodeficiency syndrome (AIDS), is a systemic illness with involvement of many organs, including the genitourinary tract. In autopsy series, kidney involvement has been noted in 25% to 50% of patients who died of cryptococcosis, but it is usually asymptomatic. The prostate is also frequently infected and can be a reservoir for *C. neoformans* infection. Viable *Cryptococcus* organisms have been shown to persist in the prostates of AIDS patients who had been successfully treated for cryptococcal meningitis.[17] Given the current use of fluconazole for treatment of cryptococcal meningitis and the high levels achieved by this agent in the prostate, this has become less of an issue.

Isolated prostatitis and epididymo-orchitis have been reported rarely in the absence of systemic cryptococcosis. The diagnosis is usually made at the time of biopsy of a mass or nodule; granulomatous inflammation is typically seen with highly encapsulated budding yeast shown by special stains. Treatment of local genitourinary tract cryptococcal infection is fluconazole, 400 mg daily for 6 to 12 months.

Saccharomyces cerevisiae rarely has been described as a cause of urinary tract infection. The presentation is the same as that noted with *Candida* species, and in those clinical microbiology laboratories that do not identify yeasts in urine to the species level, this organism will not be differentiated from *Candida*. *S. cerevisiae* is often resistant to fluconazole, and successful treatment may require amphotericin.

ASPERGILLUS AND OTHER MOLDS

The urinary tract is an uncommon site of infection with molds. However, individual case reports have noted genitourinary infections due to a variety of molds, including the Zygomycetes, *Aspergillus*, *Penicillium*, and *Paecilomyces*.[18] The most common mold infection is aspergillosis, as elsewhere in the body. Hematogenous spread to the kidney with invasive disease in immunosuppressed patients results in numerous renal microabscesses and infarcts. This may be an incidental finding in the face of massive dissemination at autopsy. Patients who have symptomatic urinary tract infection usually present with urinary tract obstruction due to masses of fungal elements causing fungal balls that can be visualized on CT scan or ultrasound examination. Treatment is surgical removal of the obstructing mass, often nephrectomy, and systemic antifungal therapy, usually with amphotericin. Mortality is extremely high.

ENDEMIC FUNGI

All of the major endemic mycoses have been reported to infect the genitourinary tract. For all of these organisms, infection is by hematogenous spread to the genitourinary tract. For upper tract infection, treatment is the same as that for disseminated infection. The treatment of focal infection, which is more likely to involve the lower genitourinary tract, is usually surgical removal of the infected tissue combined with antifungal therapy.

Blastomyces dermatitidis has the greatest propensity to cause symptomatic infection. In patients with disseminated blastomycosis, involvement of the genitourinary tract occurs in as many as a third of cases and usually is manifested by prostate or epididymal infection.[18] In most cases, this involvement is discovered incidentally when urine cultures yield the organism or when a biopsy is performed for a prostatic or epididymal mass.

Symptomatic genitourinary tract involvement with histoplasmosis is uncommon. However, at autopsy, kidney lesions are often found in patients who have disseminated histoplasmosis.[18] Patients are usually asymptomatic in regard to urinary symptoms. Rarely, individual cases of testicular abscesses, epididymitis, and prostate nodules have been reported.[19]

Coccidioidomycosis rarely causes symptomatic urinary tract infection. However, autopsy series of cases of disseminated coccidioidomycosis have noted kidney involvement in more than 50% of cases.[20] The finding of *Coccidioides* species in the urine in the absence of symptoms in such patients is not uncommon. Localized infection, presenting as abscesses or mass lesions of the epididymis or prostate, also occurs in patients with disseminated coccidioidomycosis.[18]

REFERENCES

1. Kauffman CA. Candiduria. *Clin Infect Dis*. 2005;41:S371-S376.
2. Bouza E, San Juan R, Munoz P, et al. A European perspective on nosocomial urinary tract infections. I. Report on the microbiology workload, etiology, and antimicrobial susceptibility (ESGNI-003 study). *Clin Microbiol Infect*. 2001;7:523-531.
3. Kauffman CA, Vazquez JA, Sobel JD, et al. Prospective multicenter surveillance study of funguria in hospitalized patients. *Clin Infect Dis*. 2000;30:14-18.
4. Alvarez-Lerma F, Nolla-Salas J, Leon C, et al. Candiduria in critically ill patients admitted to intensive care medical units. *Intensive Care Med*. 2003;29:1069-1076.
5. Harris AD, Castro J, Sheppard DC, et al. Risk factors for nosocomial candiduria due to *Candida glabrata* and *Candida albicans*. *Clin Infect Dis*. 1999;29:926-928.
6. Baghian A, Lee KW. Elimination of *Candida albicans* from kidneys of mice during short-term systemic infections. *Kidney Int*. 1991;40: 400-405.
7. Lehner T. Systemic candidiasis and renal involvement. *Lancet*. 1964;1:1414-1416.
8. Safdar N, Slattery WR, Knasinski V, et al. Predictors and outcomes of candiduria in renal transplant recipients. *Clin Infect Dis*. 2005;40: 1413-1421.
9. Goldberg PK, Kozinn PJ, Wise GJ, et al. Incidence and significance of candiduria. *JAMA*. 1979;241:582-584.
10. Wise GJ, Goldberg P, Kozinn PJ. Genitourinary candidiasis: Diagnosis and treatment. *J Urol*. 1976;116:778-780.
11. Navarro EE, Almario JS, Schaufele RL, et al. Quantitative urine cultures do not reliably detect renal candidiasis in rabbits. *J Clin Microbiol*. 1997;35:3292-3297.
12. Pappas PG, Kauffman CA, Andes D, et al. Clinical practice guidelines for the management of candidiasis: 2009 update by the Infectious Diseases Society of America. *Clin Infect Dis*. 2009;48:503-535.
13. Sobel JD, Kauffman CA, McKinsey D, et al. Candiduria: A randomized, double-blind study of treatment with fluconazole and placebo. *Clin Infect Dis*. 2000;30:19-24.
14. Augustin J, Raffalli J, Aguero-Rosenfeld M, Wormser GP. Failure of a lipid amphotericin B preparation to eradicate candiduria: Preliminary findings based on three cases. *Clin Infect Dis*. 1999;29:686-687.
15. Leu H-S, Huang C-T. Clearance of funguria with short-course antifungal regimens: A prospective, randomized, controlled study. *Clin Infect Dis*. 1995;20:1152-1157.
16. Drew RH, Arthur RR, Perfect JR. Is it time to abandon the use of amphotericin B bladder irrigation? *Clin Infect Dis*. 2005;40:1465-1470.
17. Larsen RA, Bozzette S, McCutchan JA, et al. Persistent *Cryptococcus neoformans* infection of the prostate after successful treatment of meningitis. *Ann Intern Med*. 1989;111:125-128.
18. Wise GJ, Talluri GS, Marella VK. Fungal infections of the genitourinary system: Manifestations, diagnosis, and treatment. *Urol Clin North Am*. 1999;26:701-718.
19. Schuster TG, Hollenbeck BK, Kauffman CA, Wei JT. Testicular histoplasmosis—a case report. *J Urol*. 2000;164:1652.
20. DeFelice R, Wieden MA, Galgiani JN. The incidence and implications of coccidioidouria. *Am Rev Respir Dis*. 1982;125:49-52.

CHAPTER 54

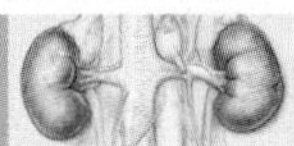

The Kidney in Schistosomiasis

Rashad S. Barsoum

Schistosomiasis is a parasitic disease usually acquired by teenagers, often leading to complications that may extend into the fourth and fifth decades of life. It was known to the ancient Egyptians as "the bloody urine disease"[1] and is also known as bilharziasis in honor of its discoverer, Theodor Bilharz, the German physician who practiced in Egypt in the 1850s.

The life cycle of the parasite is shown in Figure 54.1. Infection is acquired through contact with contaminated waters in the ponds and slow-flowing canals originating from certain rivers, such as the Nile. Cercariae enter through the skin or mucous membranes and migrate through the lymphatics and blood circulation into the portal or perivesical venous system, where they mature into sexually differentiated adult worms and live in almost continuous copulation. Females leave the males only to lay eggs, traveling against the blood flow, aiming at the rectal or bladder mucosa. The ova are driven out by visceral contraction during defecation or urination in the respective excreta. Contact with fresh water within a couple of days allows the eggs to hatch, releasing miracidia, which infect specific snails. In this "intermediate" host, they mature asexually into cercariae, which are eventually released, searching for their "definitive" host, usually humans and occasionally apes and cattle. The snail demography defines the endemicity and frequency of schistosomiasis in different geographic regions. Because this is largely influenced by climatic factors such as temperature and humidity, it is possible to accurately monitor the global epidemiology of schistosomiasis by satellite remote sensing.[2]

About 200 million inhabitants of 76 countries on five continents are infected, and an additional 400 million are at risk. Of the infected subjects, 60% are symptomatic, 10% have serious sequelae, and 1% die of the disease each year, mainly in China, the Philippines, Egypt, Brazil, northern Senegal, and Uganda.

Only three species are responsible for almost all the morbidity from the disease (Fig. 54.2): *Schistosoma haematobium*, throughout Africa and adjacent regions; *Schistosoma mansoni*, in Africa, South America, and the Caribbean islands; and *Schistosoma japonicum*, in the Far East. *S. haematobium* affects the urinary tract, whereas *S. mansoni* and *S. japonicum* affect the colon and rectum, ultimately reaching the liver and inducing periportal fibrosis. Sporadically, all three species cause "metastatic lesions" when ova are driven by the blood stream to the lungs, brain, spinal cord, heart muscle, eyes, and other sites.[3]

Morbidity from infection is variable and depends on the virulence of the infective strains, host resistance, environmental factors, and standards of primary medical care. For example, chronic lower urinary tract disease among infected subjects is reported to vary from 2% in Nigeria in the west of Africa to 52% in Tanzania in the east.[4]

PATHOGENESIS

Schistosomes cause morbidity through two major mechanisms (Fig. 54.3): (1) local reactions around the ova deposited in different tissues and (2) systemic effects attributed to the host's response to circulating antigens released from the worms or the ova.[4,5]

The local reaction is a cell-mediated immune response to soluble egg antigens diffusing out of trapped ova through micropores in the eggshell. The initial response is innate, being driven by tissue macrophages, and involves natural killer cells, neutrophils, and complement. This is followed by a specific immune response orchestrated by the helper $CD4^+$ T lymphocytes.

The schistosomal granuloma (Fig. 54.4) is composed of mononuclear cells, eosinophils, neutrophils, basophils, and fibroblasts, which are recruited and activated by a variety of T helper (Th) lymphokines as well as specific chemoattractants of parasitic origin. These cells are involved in the elimination of the parasite by direct phagocytosis (monocytes), lymphocytotoxicity (T lymphocytes), antibody-dependent cytotoxicity (eosinophils), and antibody- and complement-dependent cytotoxicity (neutrophils). Later, the granuloma is modulated by gradual switching from Th1 to Th2 activation, largely mediated by a change in the monokine profile that favors release of interleukin (IL)–4, which is associated with a phenotypic change of the committed tissue macrophages. At this stage, the intensity of the inflammatory reaction is reduced, and progressive fibrosis is induced largely through the release of IL-4, IL-5, IL-10, somatostatin, and transforming growth factor β. Finally, fibrotic granulomas in the bladder, lower ureters, and seminal vessels tend to become calcified.[6]

The systemic immune response is primarily a humoral reaction to circulating schistosomal antigens, which originate mainly from the worm's digestive enzymes (gut antigens), with a minor contribution from the tegument and ova. The gut antigens consist of a positively charged glycoprotein and a negatively charged proteoglycan (circulating cathodal antigens and circulating anodal antigens, respectively). These antigens are present in most of the schistosomal immune complex–mediated lesions, particularly in glomeruli.[7] The antibody response is biphasic, reflecting the successive Th1 and Th2 stages of lymphocyte activation. In the Th1 stage, B cells tend to synthesize IgM, IgG1, and IgG3 under the influence of IL-2. During the Th2 phase, IgG2, IgG4, and IgA predominate; these have a limited ability to fix complement and may even block its deposition, hence their importance in modulating the granulomas.[4,6]

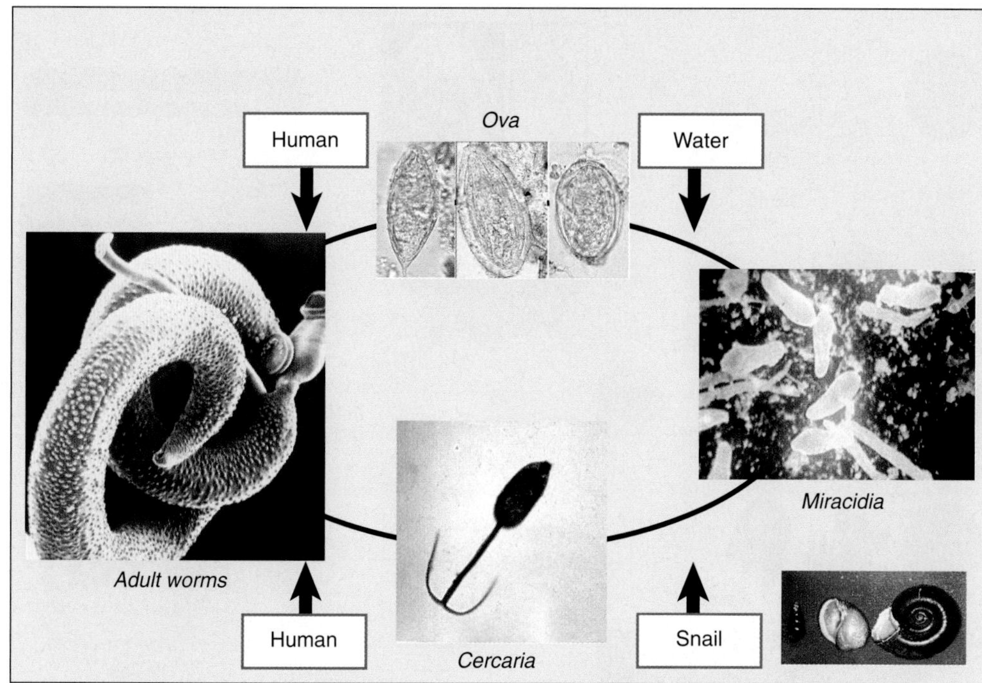

Figure 54.1 Life cycle of schistosomes.

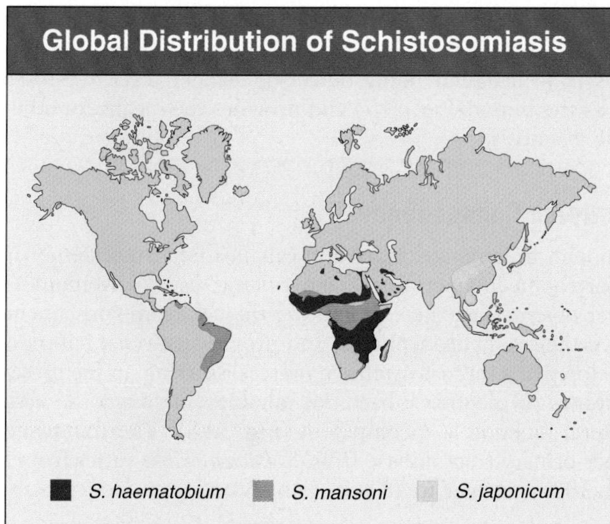

Figure 54.2 World map showing the geographic distribution of the main pathogenic schistosomes.

CLINICAL MANIFESTATIONS

Schistosomal lesions in the urinary system mirror the two major pathogenetic mechanisms. On one hand, there are local lesions, mostly affecting the lower urinary tract, caused by the local granulomatous response to *S. haematobium* ova.[8] On the other hand are those lesions caused by immune complex deposition in the glomeruli, usually associated with *S. mansoni* infections of the intestine and less commonly with *S. haematobium* infections.[9]

Lower Urinary Schistosomiasis

The lower urinary tract is the site of *S. haematobium* infection. Clinical disease starts by the coalescence of multiple granulomas that form small "pseudotubercles" in the bladder mucosa (Fig. 54.5). These may consolidate to form sessile, occasionally pedunculated masses or ulcerate, leading to painful terminal hematuria, the most typical presenting symptom. Ulcers eventually heal by fibrosis, with calcified granulomas under the atrophic and dirty mucosa, leading to the characteristic cystoscopic appearance of sandy patches and also the radiologic appearance of linear bladder calcifications. Similar lesions may occur in the lower ureters, bladder neck, seminal vesicles, and other organs in the vicinity (Fig. 54.6).

The bladder lesions predispose to secondary bacterial infection, particularly with *Pseudomonas* or *Proteus* species, after instrumentation. *Proteus* infection is notorious for favoring stone formation, which further complicates the scenario. The subsequent fibrotic process may involve the bladder neck, leading to outflow obstruction, or the vesicoureteral junction, leading to ureteral obstruction or vesicoureteral reflux. Involvement of the detrusor is a late event that may interfere with the motor function of the bladder, leading to an atonic or a hyperirritable viscus. Eventually, the bladder becomes a deformed, contracted, and calcified organ that accommodates a very small amount of urine that it can hardly void.

Bladder Cancer

Chronic bilharzial cystitis is precancerous. Up to 4.5% of patients with chronic urinary schistosomiasis develop bladder cancer, which is usually a squamous cell carcinoma (60%) or less commonly transitional cell carcinoma (20%) or adenocarcinoma (10%).[10] The tumor, particularly when it is of the squamous cell type, remains localized for a long time before spreading to the surrounding pelvic tissues or distant site, thanks to the occlusion of lymphatics by the preceding fibrotic process.

Associated infection with human papillomavirus is encountered in about one fourth of cases, which suggests an etiologic role in malignant transformation.[11] Specific p53 gene mutations were detected in one third of cases.[12] This may be attributed to neutrophil-generated reactive oxygen molecules, cleavage of

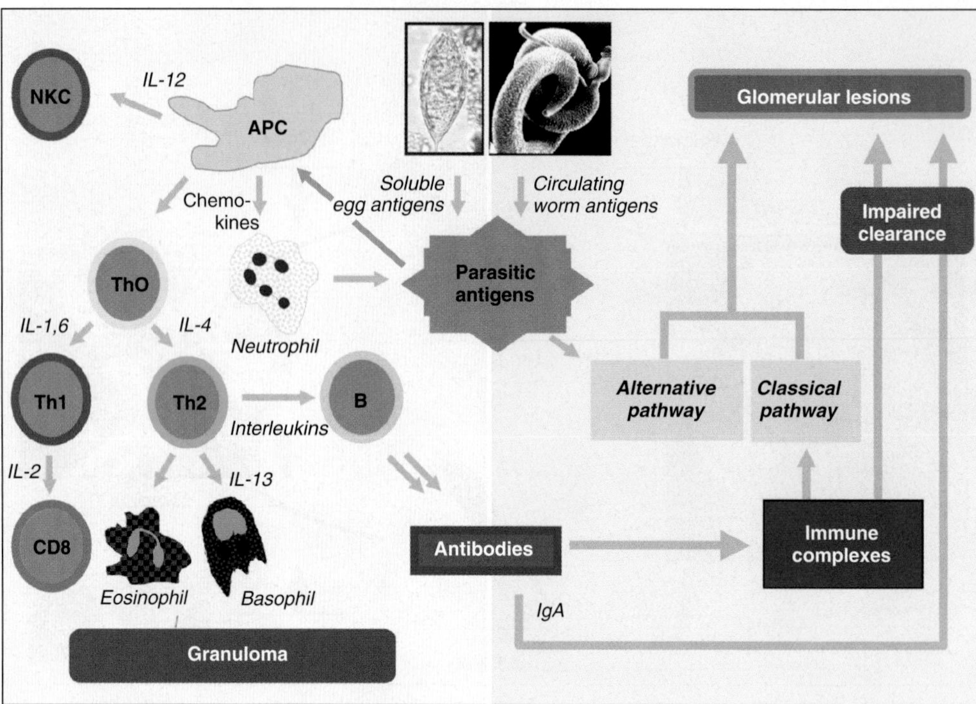

Figure 54.3 Immune response to schistosomal infection. The local immune response to deposited ova leading to granuloma formation is shown on the left; all cells shown in the diagram, in conjunction with antibodies or complement, participate in eventual parasite elimination (see text). The systemic immune response is shown on the right; note the important role of impaired clearance of schistosomal antigens and IgA in the development of glomerular lesions. APC, antigen-presenting cell; IL, interleukin; NKC, natural killer cell.

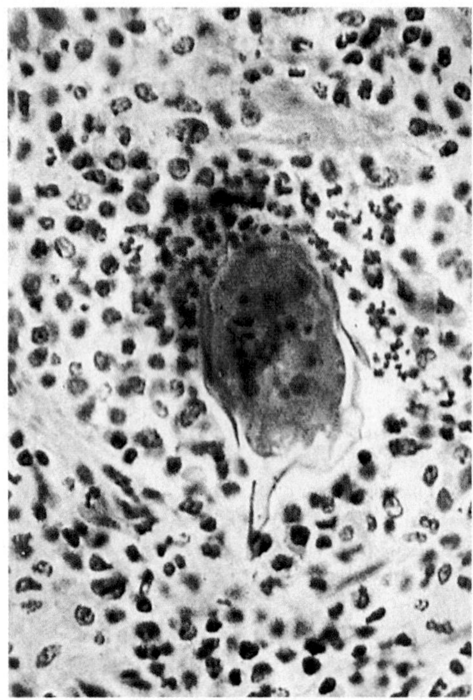

Figure 54.4 *Schistosoma haematobium* granuloma. Note the egg's terminal spike, which identifies *S. haematobium,* and the distortion of shell from proteases and oxidants released by the local neutrophil infiltration. (Hematoxylin and eosin; magnification ×500.)

conjugated urinary carcinogens, or production of nitrosamines by bacterial enzymes.[13]

Development of malignancy is suspected when the symptoms of chronic cystitis exacerbate, along with recurrence of hematuria many years after the initial presentation and the passage of small pieces of necrotic tissue with urine (necroturia). A characteristic radiologic sign is the irregular "eating up" of the bladder calcification on a plain radiograph. Cystography shows the tumor mass as an irregular filling defect or bladder ulcer. Cystoscopy shows the tumor (Fig. 54.7) and provides the means for a histologic diagnosis.

Upstream Consequences

Although ureteral strictures and calcifications are common, the hypertrophied upper ureteral musculature usually overcomes the lower obstruction, thereby limiting the upstream consequences. Nevertheless, hydronephrosis and progressive renal failure may develop when there is extensive ureteral scarring, in the presence of stones or secondary bacterial infection, or when the vesicoureteral junction is incompetent (Fig. 54.8). The frequency of upper urinary tract disease from *S. haematobium* varies from less than 10% in Niger to 48% in Cameroon.

Interstitial Nephritis

Chronic pyelonephritis is the eventual outcome of complicated *S. haematobium* infection, resulting from obstruction, reflux, and bacterial infection. Granulomas have occasionally been seen in the renal interstitium (Fig. 54.9) but tend to be discrete and of no functional significance. Immune-mediated tubulointerstitial nephritis has been described with *S. mansoni* in humans, but the role of immune mechanisms remains questionable in *S. haematobium* pyelonephritis.

The typical pathologic picture is that of a scarred kidney with calyceal dilation, distortion, and atrophic parenchyma. There is dense interstitial infiltration, fibrosis, and periglomerular scarring. The glomeruli may show ischemic collapse or other schistosomal lesions, such as proliferative glomerulonephritis or amyloidosis.

The clinical picture is that of chronic tubulointerstitial nephritis (see Chapter 62), often associated with residual manifestations of lower urinary involvement. Hypertension is a late feature, being checked by tubular salt wastage during the early

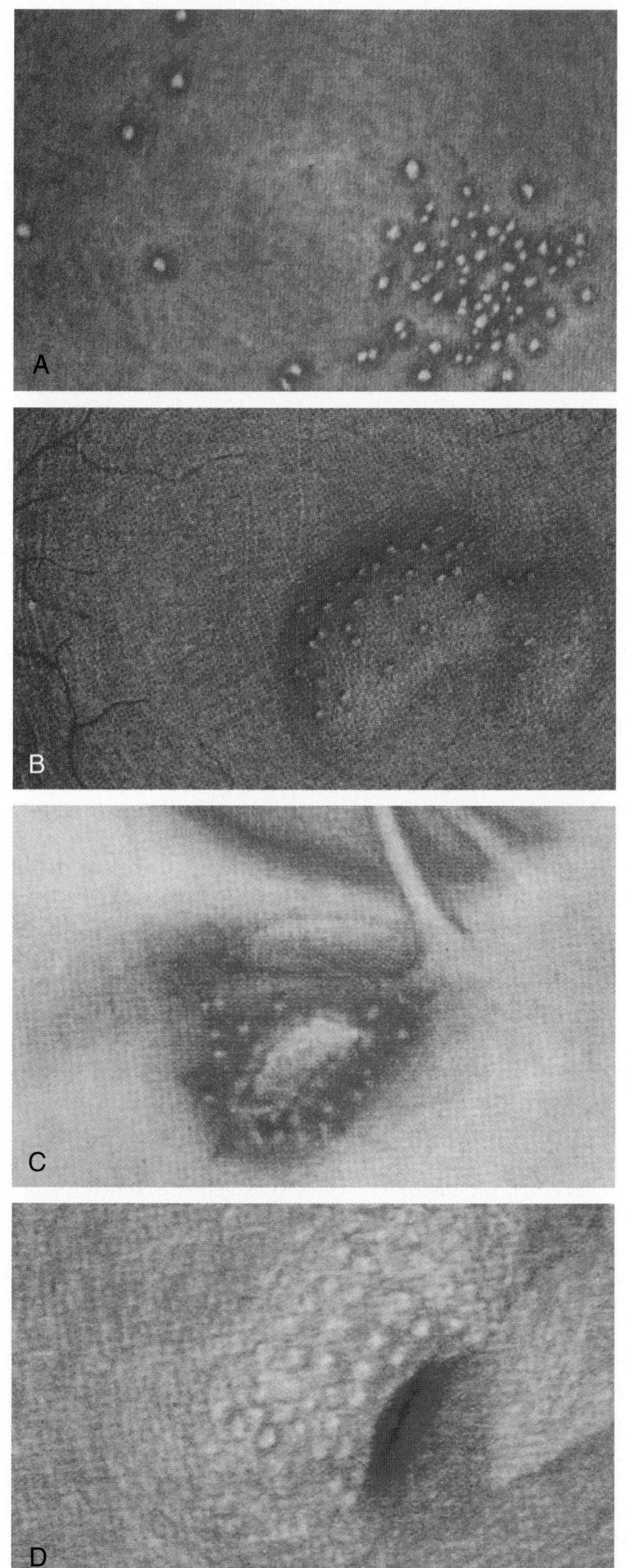

Figure 54.5 Cystoscopic appearances in urinary schistosomiasis. **A,** Pseudotubercles. **B,** Sessile mass covered by pseudotubercles. **C,** Ulcer surrounded by pseudotubercles. **D,** Sandy patches. *(Courtesy Professor Naguib Makar.)*

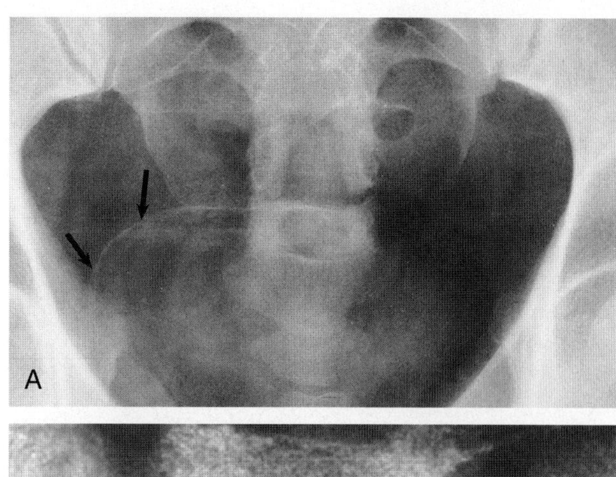

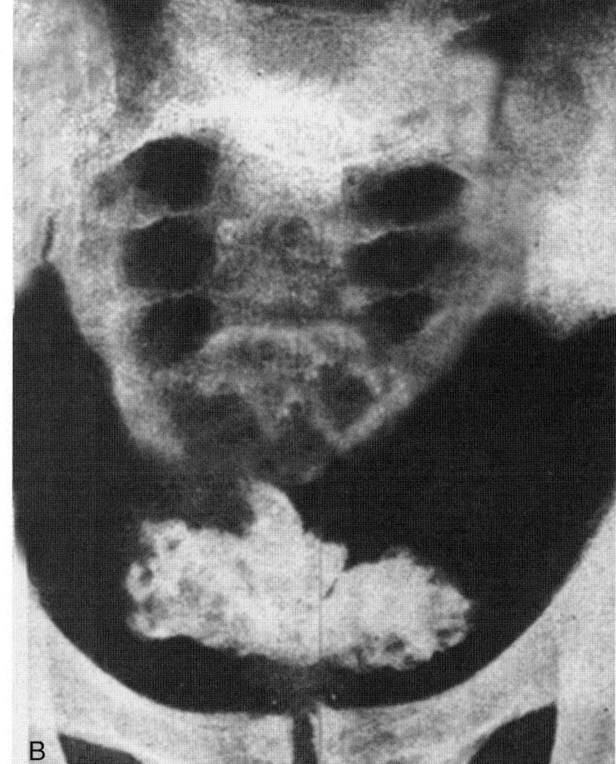

Figure 54.6 Plain radiographic appearances in *Schistosoma haematobium* infection. **A,** Faint linear calcification of the bladder wall *(arrows)*. **B,** Dense calcifications of contracted bladder and seminal vesicles.

phases of the disease. Anemia and osteodystrophy may be disproportionately severe because of the associated secondary distal tubular acidosis and nutritional deficiency in endemic areas.

Glomerulonephritis

Immune complex–mediated glomerulonephritis (GN) has been described in experimental[14] and human[9] infection, mainly with *S. japonicum* and *S. mansoni*, the latter accounting for most clinically significant disease in humans. *S. haematobium* GN is rare and usually subclinical, but a small epidemic of acute nephritis was reported in an Egyptian village where the infection had been recently introduced as a result of change in the agricultural irrigation system.[15]

Schistosomal gut antigens are present in circulating immune complexes as well as in the immune deposits in mesangial, subendothelial, and intramembranous locations. The presence of

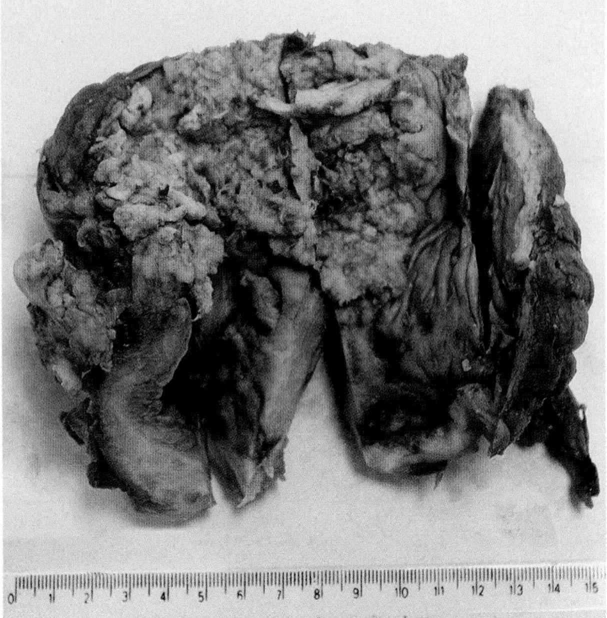

Figure 54.7 Bilharzial bladder cancer.

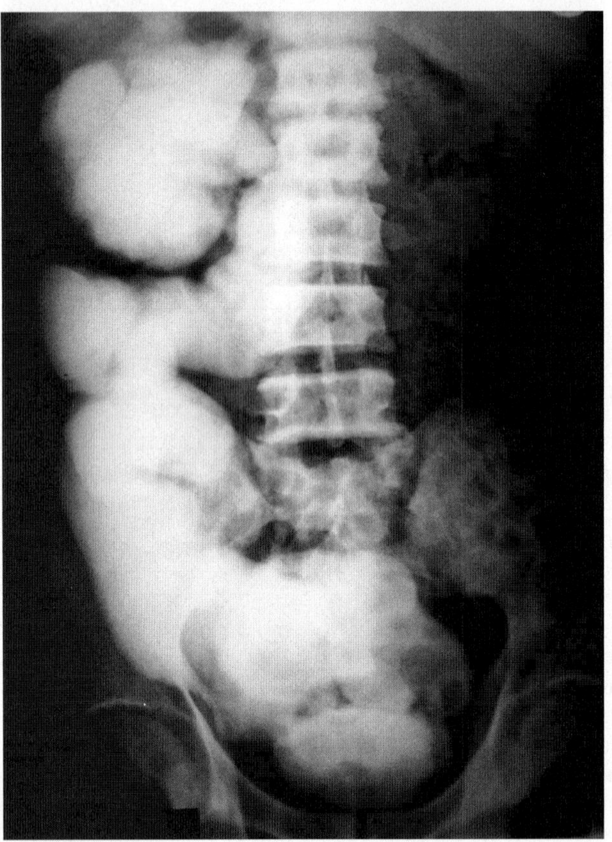

Figure 54.8 Ascending cystogram showing right megaureter due to vesicoureteral reflux.

liver fibrosis is critical because it results in impaired hepatic clearance of schistosomal antigens and immune complexes, which are mostly generated within the portal venous tributaries. Evidence of autoimmune reactivity has also been reported, but its potential pathogenetic role is undefined.

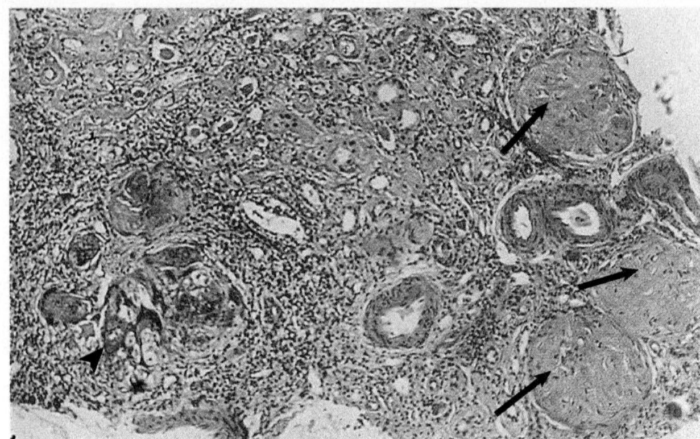

Figure 54.9 Schistosomal chronic interstitial nephritis. Note the dense cellular infiltration and fibrosis, atrophic dilated tubules, and thickened vessels. Three glomeruli heavily infiltrated with amyloid are seen on the right side *(arrows)*; a schistosomal granuloma is seen in the lower left corner *(arrowhead)*. (Hematoxylin and eosin stain; original magnification ×75.)

Most patients are 20- to 40-year-old men with evidence of hepatosplenic schistosomiasis. Renal involvement is asymptomatic in up to 40% of those, being identified by accidental or surveillance urinalysis, which may display microalbuminuria, various grades of proteinuria, or abnormal sediment. Some 15% of those with hepatosplenic schistosomiasis have overt GN, presenting with proteinuria and microhematuria, with or without the nephrotic syndrome, hypertension, and impaired renal function. Liver function test results are often normal. A polyclonal gammopathy is seen in most cases, whereas a monoclonal IgM response is seen in those with associated hepatitis C virus (HCV) and cryoglobulinemia. Rheumatoid factor activity and anti-DNA antibodies are detected in 5% to 10% of cases, particularly in association with *Salmonella* infection (see later discussion), but they do not correlate with clinical severity. Rheumatoid seropositivity is detected in much higher titers when HCV infection is associated.[13]

There are six histologic classes of schistosomal GN (Figs. 54.10 and 54.11).[4,6,9,16] Class I (mesangial proliferative), class III (membranoproliferative), and class IV (focal segmental glomerulosclerosis) result from the deposition of immune complexes representing different stages in the evolution of "pure schistosomal" hepatosplenic disease. The main deposits in class I are schistosomal antigens, IgM, and C3; and in class III and class IV, IgG and IgA, usually without schistosomal antigens. The IgA deposits parallel the severity of proteinuria and mesangial proliferation. Impaired hepatic clearance and increased mucosal synthesis of IgA have been documented in those patients.[17] Whereas class I lesions are seen in most asymptomatic cases, class III and class IV are usually symptomatic and progressive, even with eradication of the parasitic infection.

Class II (diffuse proliferative and exudative) is associated with coinfection with *Salmonella* strains, usually *Salmonella paratyphi* A in Africa and *Salmonella typhimurium* in Brazil, which are attached to specific receptors in the tissues of adult schistosomes. C3 and *Salmonella* antigens were detected in the glomerular capillary walls and the mesangium. In these patients, the clinical presentation is typical of acute postinfectious GN, associated with manifestations of *Salmonella*-related toxemia (fever, exanthema, and severe anemia).

Classification of Schistosomal Glomerulonephritis

Class	Histology	Immunofluorescence	Etiologic Agent	Prevalence	Clinical Findings	Treatment of Renal Disease
I	Mesangioproliferative GN	IgM, C3 Schistosomal gut antigens	*S. haematobium* *S. mansoni* *S. japonicum*	27%–60% of asymptomatic patients, 10%–40% of patients with renal disease	Microhematuria Proteinuria	May respond to antiparasitic treatment
II	Diffuse proliferative exudative GN	C3, Salmonella antigens	*S. haematobium* *S. mansoni* + *Salmonella* species	Salmonella infections Reduced serum C3	Acute nephritic syndrome, toxemia	May respond to treatment of Salmonella and Schistosomal infections
III	Membranoproliferative GN	IgG, IgA, C3, schistosomal antigens	*S. mansoni* *(S. haematobium?)*	7%–20% of asymptomatic patients and in 80% of patients with overt renal disease	Hepatosplenomegaly, nephrotic syndrome, hypertension, renal failure	No
IV	Focal segmental glomerulosclerosis	IgM, IgG (occasionally IgA)	*S. mansoni*	11%–38%	Hepatosplenomegaly, nephrotic syndrome, hypertension, renal failure	No
V	Amyloid	AA protein	*S. mansoni* *S. haematobium*	16%–39%	Hepatosplenomegaly, nephrotic syndrome, hypertension, renal failure	No
VI	Cryoglobulinemic GN	IgM, C3	*S. mansoni* + hepatitis C virus	Unknown	Hepatosplenomegaly, nephrotic syndrome, purpura, vasculitis, arthritis, hypertension, renal failure	Interferon + ribavirin, corticosteroids, immunosuppression, plasmapheresis

Figure 54.10 Classification of schistosomal glomerulonephritis.

Amyloid A protein deposits are detected by special stains or electron microscopy in up to 15% of biopsy samples from patients with class III and class IV, whereas amyloidosis may be the predominant lesion (class V) in less than 5% of patients with clinically overt schistosomal glomerulopathy. It occurs with heavy, often mixed infection regardless of the anatomic site. Minimal amyloid deposits do not seem to alter the clinical presentation or prognosis, but typical class V cases are grossly nephrotic and relentlessly progressive.

A class VI lesion was more recently described in patients with hepatosplenic schistosomiasis and HCV infection.[16] This association is common, particularly in Egypt, where it is believed that the virus was acquired many decades earlier, when intravenous injections were used for mass treatment of schistosomiasis. Some evidence also suggests that the virus may be transmitted with the infected cercariae. Regardless of the mode of infection, those patients appear to have created a critical pool in the community that became a reservoir for the spread of infection by other means. The lesion consists of a mixture of mesangial proliferation, amyloid deposition, fibrinoid necrosis, and cryoglobulinemic thrombi in the glomerular capillaries with tubular casts. Patients present with chronic hepatitis, cirrhosis, nephrotic syndrome, cryoglobulinemic skin vasculitis, polyarthritis, and rapidly progressive renal failure associated with severe protein-calorie malnutrition.

DIAGNOSIS

Schistosoma haematobium Urinary Tract Disease

The bedside diagnosis of lower urinary schistosomiasis is easily made, particularly if patients present with the typical pattern of painful terminal hematuria after exposure to fresh river waters in an endemic area. Diagnosis is more difficult when the history of exposure is less convincing (e.g., swimming pools) or when the clinical presentation is atypical (such as bacterial pyelonephritis, typhoid, or amyloidosis).

The diagnosis is made by finding ova in a fresh urine sample, which is easy because of their abundance, large size, and typical appearance. Live ova, containing mobile miracidia, indicate active infection, whereas dead, calcified ova may continue to be shed from fibrotic lesions for many months or even years.

Serologic diagnosis is based on finding circulating schistosomal antigens or antibodies by gel diffusion, precipitation, complement fixation, chromatography, immunoelectrophoresis, indirect hemagglutination, microfluorometry, radioimmunoassay, or various forms of enzyme-linked immunosorbent assay (ELISA) techniques. The circumoval precipitin is most frequently used in clinical laboratories. These techniques are useful in confirming the diagnosis in the absence of ova, which occurs with old infections when the worms are sterile but continue to

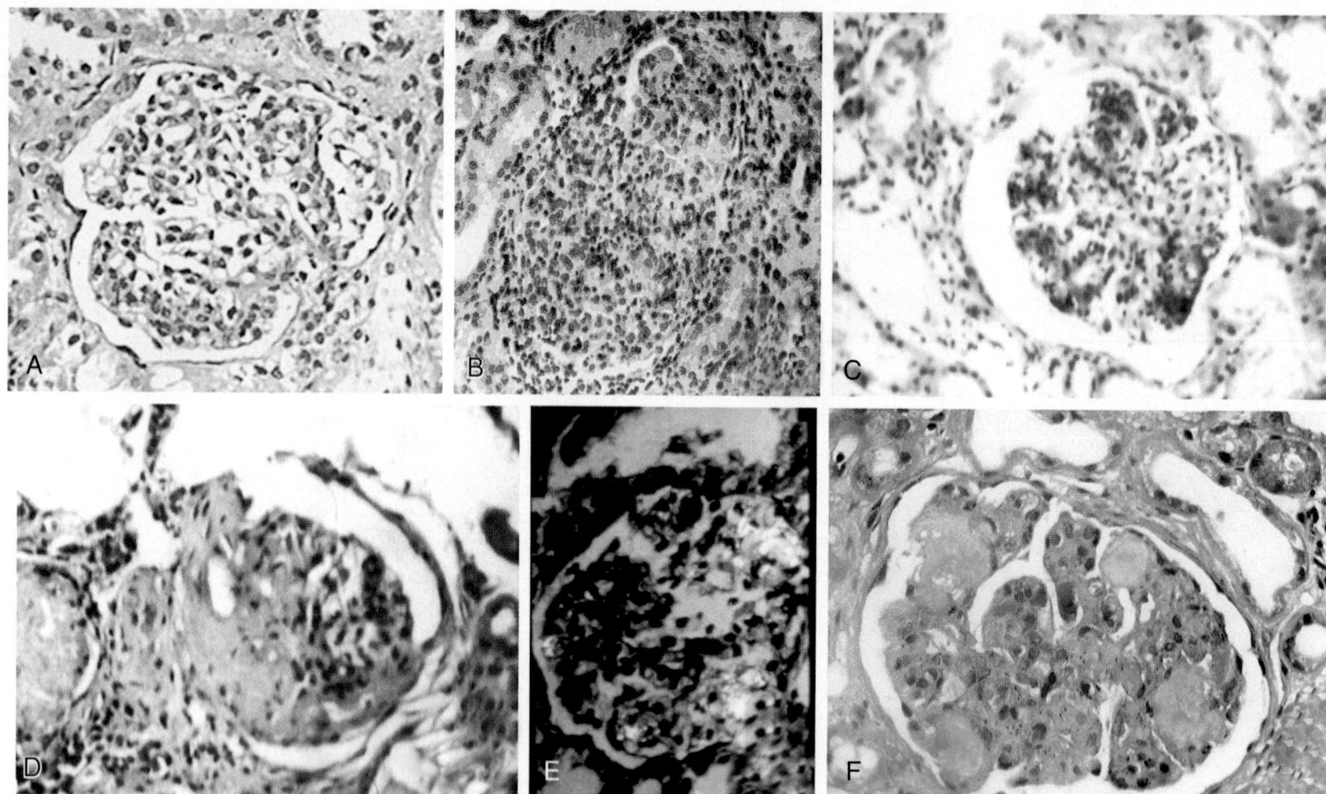

Figure 54.11 Schistosomal glomerulopathy. A, Mesangial proliferative glomerulonephritis, hematoxylin and eosin stain (class I). **B,** *Schistosoma*- and *Salmonella*-associated exudative glomerulonephritis, hematoxylin and eosin stain (class II). **C,** Membranoproliferative (mesangiocapillary) glomerulonephritis type I, hematoxylin and eosin stain (class III). **D,** Focal segmental glomerulosclerosis, Masson trichrome stain (class IV). **E,** Green birefringence under polarized light in a glomerulus with mesangial proliferation in a patient with mixed *S. haematobium* and *S. mansoni* infection, Congo red stain (class V). **F,** Amyloid deposits and cryoglobulin capillary thrombi (red stain) in a glomerulus displaying focal mesangial proliferation in a patient with schistosomal hepatic fibrosis and associated hepatitis C virus infection (class VI).

release their antigens. Serologic tests are also useful in assessing the response to treatment because titers usually become negative within 3 to 6 months of complete eradication of infection.

The radiologic appearances of bladder and seminal vesicle calcification are so typical that no further confirmatory tests are needed. Cystoscopic findings are equally pathognomonic although seldom required. Early pseudotubercles are easily distinguished from mycobacterial infection by their size and the surrounding mucosal pathologic changes. The presence of sandy patches with associated masses, polyps, and even neoplasms makes the diagnosis. Tissue biopsy confirms the parasitic nature of the lesions. Different imaging techniques (e.g., ultrasound, intravenous urography, voiding cystography) are useful in the diagnosis of upstream complications (see Chapter 58).

The main differential diagnosis for urinary schistosomiasis is tuberculosis, which also causes hematuria, strictures, back pressure, and chronic kidney disease. This differential can be resolved with appropriate parasitologic and bacteriologic techniques (see Chapter 52).

Schistosoma mansoni Glomerulonephritis

Overt glomerular disease in patients with hepatosplenic schistosomiasis is suspected in those who develop new hypertension, nephrotic or nephritic syndrome, or chronic kidney disease. Occult glomerular disease is detected by the presence of abnormal urinary sediment or renal function. Although renal biopsy is essential for the diagnosis and classification, none of the lesions

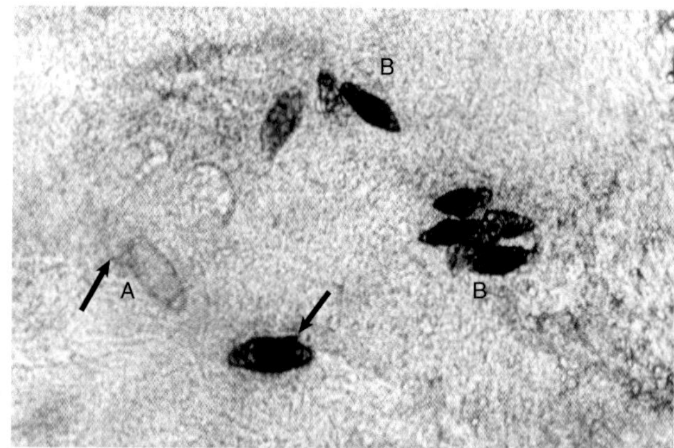

Figure 54.12 Stool smears showing living (A) and dead (B) *Schistosoma mansoni* ova. Species are identified by the lateral spike *(arrows)*.

is pathognomonic unless schistosomal antigens are detected by immunofluorescence, which is unusual in clinically overt cases. Identification of *S. mansoni* eggs in the stools (Fig. 54.12) or submucosal rectal snips supports the diagnosis. Concomitant *Salmonella* or HCV infection can be detected by appropriate microbiologic tests. The various serologic abnormalities described are of limited diagnostic value, except the high rheumatoid factor, monoclonal IgM expansion, and low C4 that are typical of class VI.

Other glomerular disorders associated with hepatic fibrosis, such as secondary IgA nephropathy and hepatic glomerulosclerosis, may be considered in the differential diagnosis. However, in both these conditions, the renal lesions are relatively mild, presenting mainly with microhematuria but rarely with significant proteinuria or impaired renal function. The glomerular deposits are mostly mesangial, in contrast to those seen in schistosomiasis, in which subendothelial and intramembranous deposits may also be present.

Treatment

Schistosoma haematobium Urinary Tract Disease

S. haematobium is susceptible to antimony compounds, organophosphates (metrifonate), and niridazole, but the current drug of choice is praziquantel, the most effective and least toxic. It is administered as a single oral dose of 40 mg/kg body weight. Antiparasitic treatment cures the early bladder disease, yet it has no effect on sandy patches or other fibrotic lesions. Interestingly, ureteral distention with radiologic evidence of hydronephrosis may be reversed a few weeks after successful treatment.

Antibacterial therapy usually controls acute episodes of cystitis and pyelonephritis. However, it must be combined with simultaneous eradication of parasitic infection if it is still active, especially if the urinary bacterial infection is due to typhoid (*Salmonella typhi*).

Chronic fibrotic lesions are difficult to treat. Surgery or the placement of stents may be necessary for the relief of an obstructive lesion. However, particular caution is required in dealing with the vesicoureteral junction to avoid induction of reflux. Several plastic procedures are available to restore the distorted ureteral, bladder, or urethral anatomy. Associated bacterial infections may require long-term low-dose antibiotics.

Regular dialysis in such patients can be difficult owing to the negative effects of chronic infection; the associated schistosomal lesions in the liver, lungs, and other organs; and the comorbid impact of undernutrition, viral infection, or malignant disease. The same factors reflect on the outcome of renal transplantation, with the additional risk for urinary leakage, which is many-fold higher than usual due to the presence of fibrotic granulomas and anatomic distortion in the bladder wall. Reinfection with *S. haematobium* has also been described in patients living in an endemic area.[18]

Schistosoma mansoni Glomerulonephritis

S. mansoni is more resistant to treatment but does respond to single-dose treatment with either praziquantel (40 to 60 mg/kg body weight) or oxamniquine (single dose of 15 mg/kg body weight in South America or two doses of 15 mg/kg body weight given 12 hours apart in Africa). However, eradication of the parasite can be curative only in classes I and II. In class II, it must be combined with antibiotics for the control of *Salmonella* infection (usually ampicillin and cotrimoxazole) Antischistosomal therapy (praziquantel or oxamniquine) and immunosuppressive therapy are ineffective in all other classes.[9]

Dialysis may be difficult in those who reach end-stage renal disease because of the frequent presence of esophageal or gastric varices that carry the risk for bleeding with anticoagulation for hemodialysis. Endoscopy is essential before starting of regular hemodialysis, with prophylactic sclerotherapy if necessary. Although peritoneal dialysis is a viable option in some cases, it is impossible in those with significant ascites because of the risk for excessive protein loss in the effluent.

The overall results of renal transplantation are not different from those with other renal disorders. Uncomplicated residual hepatic fibrosis in the recipient does not seem to significantly modify the pharmacokinetics of the immunosuppressive agents used in transplant recipients. However, variations in cyclosporine blood levels have been noted[15] and attributed to altered absorption of the drug. Associated viral hepatitis may have a considerable impact on the protocols of donor selection and prophylactic immunosuppression and on the eventual outcome (see Chapters 98 and 101).

Recurrence of schistosomal GN has been described in a few patients,[19] suggesting the persistent release of antigens from living worms. Prophylactic antischistosomal chemotherapy (i.e., praziquantel) is therefore recommended before renal transplantation for recipients known to have been previously infected with the parasite.

REFERENCES

1. Ghalioungui P. *Magic and Medical Science in Ancient Egypt*. London: Hodder and Stoughton; 1963.
2. Yang GJ, Vounatsou P, Zhou XN, et al. A review of geographic information system and remote sensing with applications to the epidemiology and control of schistosomiasis in China. *Acta Trop*. 2005;96:17-29.
3. Abdel-Wahab MF. *Schistosomiasis in Egypt*. Boca Raton, Fla: CRC Press; 1982.
4. Barsoum RS. Schistosomiasis. In Davison AM, Cameron JS, Grunfeld JP, et al, eds. *Oxford Textbook of Clinical Nephrology*. 3rd ed. Oxford: Oxford University Press; 2005:1173-1184.
5. Wahl SM, Frazier-Jessen M, Jin WW, et al. Cytokine regulation of schistosome-induced granuloma and fibrosis. *Kidney Int*. 1997;51:1370-1375.
6. Barsoum RS. Schistosomiasis and the kidney. *Semin Nephrol*. 2003;23:4-41.
7. deWater R, Van Marck EA, Fransen JA, Deelder AM. *Schistosoma mansoni:* Ultrastructural localization of the circulating anodic antigen and the circulating cathodic antigen in the mouse kidney glomerulus. *Am J Trop Med Hyg*. 1988;38:118-124.
8. Badr MM. Surgical management of urinary bilharziasis. In: Dudley H, Pories WJ, Carter DC, McDougal WS, eds. *Rob Smith's Operative Surgery*. London: Butterworth; 1986.
9. Barsoum RS. Schistosomal glomerulopathies. *Kidney Int*. 1993;44:1-12.
10. Ghoneim MA, El-Mekresh MM, El-Baz MA. Radical cystectomy for carcinoma of the bladder, critical evaluation of the results in 1026 cases. *J Urol*. 1997;158:393-399.
11. el-Mawla NG, el-Bolkainy MN, Khaled HM. Bladder cancer in Africa: Update. Semin Oncol. 2001;28:174-178.
12. Warren W, Biggs PJ, el-Baz M, et al. Mutations in p53 gene in schistosomal bladder cancer. Carcinogenesis. 1995;16:1181-1189.
13. Mostafa MH, Sheweita SA, O'Connor PJ. Relationship between schistosomiasis and bladder cancer. *Clin Microbiol Rev*. 1999;12:97-111.
14. Houba V. Experimental renal disease due to schistosomiasis. *Kidney Int*. 1979;16:30-43.
15. Ezzat E, Osman R, Ahmed KY, Soothill JF. The association between *Schistosoma haematobium* infection and heavy proteinuria. *Trans R Soc Trop Med Hyg*. 1974;68:315-317.
16. Barsoum R. The changing face of schistosomal glomerulopathy. *Kidney Int*. 2004;66:2472-2484.
17. Barsoum R, Nabil M, Saady G, et al. Immunoglobulin A and the pathogenesis of schistosomal glomerulopathy. *Kidney Int*. 1996;50:920-928.
18. Mahmoud KM, Sobh MA, El-Agroudy AE, et al. Impact of schistosomiasis on patient and graft outcome after renal transplantation: 10 years' follow-up. *Nephrol Dial Transplant*. 2001;16:2214-2221.
19. Azevedo LS, de Paula FJ, Ianhez LE, et al. Renal transplantation and schistosomiasis mansoni. *Transplantation*. 1987;44:795-798.

CHAPTER 55

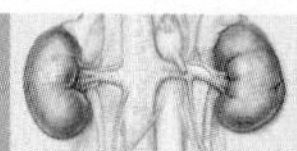

Glomerular Diseases Associated with Infection

Bernardo Rodríguez-Iturbe, Emmanuel A. Burdmann, Rashad S. Barsoum

GENERAL CHARACTERISTICS OF GLOMERULAR DISEASES ASSOCIATED WITH INFECTION

The observation of dark scanty urine in the convalescent period of scarlet fever is more than two centuries old. At the beginning of the last century, Clemens von Pirquet postulated that the disease resulted from antibodies that instead of having beneficial effects were pathogenic, an insight that constitutes a landmark that opened the field of immune-mediated renal disease.[1]

Today, infection-related glomerulonephritis (GN) is uncommon and usually associated with debilitating conditions such as diabetes, malignant neoplasia, acquired immunodeficiency syndrome (AIDS), and alcoholism. Most infection-associated GN is due to *Streptococcus* (27.7%) and *Staphylococcus* (24.4%), but a wide variety of pathogens have been reported (Fig 55.1). GN usually results from glomerular deposition of immune complexes containing bacterial antigens, but other mechanisms may also occur (see later discussion). The most common sites of infection are the upper respiratory tract (23%), skin (17%), lung (17%), and heart valves (11.6%).[2]

Histologic Patterns and Pathogenesis

The histologic patterns and the most typical infectious diseases associated with them are shown in Figure 55.2. Mesangial proliferative GN is usually acute and self-limited. Microscopic hematuria and non-nephrotic proteinuria are present in association with deposits of IgG, IgM, and C3. Serum complement may be transiently decreased. Diffuse proliferative GN is also acute and self-limited if the infection is eradicated. IgG, IgM, and C3 deposits are prominent in the mesangium and glomerular capillaries, and electron-dense deposits are present in mesangial, subendothelial, and subepithelial locations. The immune complexes deposited in the glomeruli may or may not contain bacterial antigens, and cryoglobulins may be present. Staphylococcal infections, particularly methicillin resistant, may induce diffuse proliferative GN, likely resulting from bacterial wall superantigens that induce a nonspecific polyclonal immunoglobulin response, with crescent formation and exclusive or predominant IgA deposition. The clinical presentation is the acute nephritic syndrome. Membranoproliferative GN (MPGN) is commonly observed with chronic infections. The clinical presentation is usually the nephrotic syndrome with microscopic hematuria and variable degrees of hypertension. Immunoglobulins and C3 deposits are present. In the setting of liver disease (as in *Schistosoma mansoni* infection), IgA may be a predominant component of the immune deposits. Membranous nephropathy (MN) is associated with chronic infections and presents as the nephrotic syndrome. Finally, vasculitis may develop in association with viral (especially hepatitis B virus and human immunodeficiency virus) or bacterial (rarely *Streptococcus*) infections.

Infection-related GN, especially when it is immune complex associated, occurs more frequently and has a worse prognosis in conditions in which there is difficulty clearing the infection or immune complexes. These conditions include human immunodeficiency virus infection, infections acquired in the neonatal period (when tolerance is often induced, such as is observed with hepatitis B virus infection), chronic liver disease, diabetes, and chronic alcoholism.

Infections may also be associated with renal disease by mechanisms that do not involve immune complexes. Focal segmental glomerulosclerosis (FSGS) with glomerular collapse (collapsing glomerulopathy) may occur with human immunodeficiency virus or parvovirus B19 infection. The hemolytic-uremic syndrome may result from verotoxin-producing *Escherichia coli* or *Shigella* species (see Chapter 28). Amyloidosis may result from chronic infections such as tuberculosis, leprosy, and schistosomiasis. Interstitial nephritis manifested as acute renal failure may result from several viral (especially Epstein-Barr virus) or bacterial (especially *Legionella*) infections. Hantavirus can also induce a hemorrhagic fever–renal failure syndrome in which infection of the interstitial capillaries and tubules leads to acute renal failure (see Chapter 66).

BACTERIAL INFECTIONS

Poststreptococcal Glomerulonephritis

Epidemiology

Poststreptococcal glomerulonephritis (PSGN) is more common in males (2:1) and usually affects children 2 to 14 years old. Traditionally, only certain nephritogenic strains of group A *Streptococcus pyogenes* result in GN. In the tropics and southern United States, PSGN usually follows streptococcal impetigo of M types 47, 49, 55, and 57. Throat infections with streptococcus types 1, 2, 4, and 12 are also nephritogenic.[3,4] More recently, ingestion of unpasteurized milk contaminated with group C streptococcus (*Streptococcus zooepidemicus*) has caused clusters of cases and at least one large epidemic.[5] The risk of nephritis in epidemics may range from 5% in throat infections to as high as 25% in M type 49 pyoderma. A genetic predisposition is suggested as there is an association of PSGN with HLA-DR4 and DR1 and higher attack rates in siblings than expected for the general population. The risk of PSGN is reduced by early antibiotic treatment.

Some Infectious Agents Associated with Renal Disease
Bacterial: *Streptococcus* (group A, *Streptococcus viridans*), *Staphylococcus (aureus, epidermidis), Salmonella (typhi, paratyphi), Escherichia coli, Leptospira, Treponema pallidum, Neisseria species, Mycobacterium leprae, Yersinia enterocolitica, Coxiella burnetii, Brucella abortus, Listeria monocytogenes*
Viral: Hepatitis A, B, and C; human immunodeficiency virus, varicella-zoster, parvovirus B19, cytomegalovirus, mumps, influenza, Epstein-Barr virus, coxsackievirus, and enteric cytopathic human orphan (ECHO) virus
Fungus: *Histoplasma capsulatum, Candida*
Protozoal: *Plasmodium* (*falciparum, malariae, vivax*, and *ovale*); *Trypanosoma*, *Toxoplasma*
Helminthic: *Schistosoma* (*mansoni, haematobium*), *Wuchereria bancrofti, Trichinella spiralis*, filaria (*Onchocerca volvulus, Loa loa*)

Figure 55.1 Some infectious agents associated with renal disease.

Renal Syndromes Associated with Infection

Clincical Presentation	Time Course	Pathologic Findings	Examples
Subclinical, microhematuria non-nephrotic proteinuria	Acute	Mesangioproliferative GN	Typhoid fever, *Pl. falciparum* PSGN
Acute nephritic syndrome	Acute	Diffuse proliferative GN	PSGN
Acute renal failure, nephrotic syndrome	Acute, chronic	Diffuse proliferative GN, cresents 1. IgM, IgG dominant 2. IgA dominant	1. Endocarditis, PSGN 2. Methicillin-resistant *S. Aureus*
Nephrotic syndrome reduced GFR	Chronic	1. MPGN type I ± cryoglobulins 2. Focal segmental glomerulosclerosis	1. Hepatitis C virus, infected AV shunts 2. HIV, parvovirus
Nephrotic syndrome	Chronic	1. Membranous nephropathy 2. Amyloid	1. Hepatitis B virus 2. Leprosy, *Schistosoma*, kala-azar
Acute renal failure, systematic symptoms, arthralgias, skin ulcers	Acute, chronic	Vasculitis, crescents, tubulointerstitial inflammation, atrophy and fibrosis	Hepatitis B virus, HIV
Hemplytic-uremic syndrome	Acute	Arteriolar thickening and occlusion, microthrombi, capillary wall thickening	*E. coli* O157-H7
Azotemia, non-nephrotic proteinuria, eosinophillia	Acute, chronic	Interstitial nephritis	Epstein-Barr virus, legionnaire's disease, Hantavirus, kala-azar

Figure 55.2 Renal syndromes associated with infection. AV, arteriovenous; GFR, glomerular filtration rate; GN, glomerulonephritis; HIV, human immunodeficiency virus; MPGN, membranoproliferative glomerulonephritis; PSGN, poststreptococcal glomerulonephritis.

PSGN is becoming less common in industrialized countries and is changing its epidemiologic pattern from one that primarily affects children to one that now occurs more commonly in debilitated elderly individuals, particularly alcoholics, diabetics, and intravenous drug users.[2] Nevertheless, PSGN remains common in developing countries, where it may affect 9.3 to 9.8 cases per 100,000 population,[4] especially in communities with poor socioeconomic conditions. The reduction in incidence of PSGN likely relates to more rapid and frequent use of antibiotics. The common practice of fluorination of water may also be protective as fluoride reduces the expression of virulence factors in cultures of *S. pyogenes*.

Pathogenesis

Two nephritogenic streptococcal antigens have been identified: nephritis-associated plasmin receptor (NAPLr), which was identified as glyceraldehyde-3-phosphate dehydrogenase (GAPDH)[6]; and streptococcal proteinase exotoxin B (SPEB) and its more immunogenic precursor, zymogen.[7] GAPDH and SPEB have been identified in renal biopsy specimens of acute PSGN, and antibody titers to both these antigens are elevated in most convalescent sera. GAPDH has been localized in areas of the glomeruli with plasmin-like activity, suggesting a local direct mechanism of glomerular inflammatory damage, but it is not co-localized with complement or immunoglobulin.[8] In contrast, SPEB is co-localized with both complement and IgG, suggesting a participation in the immune-mediated glomerular damage.[9] Furthermore, SPEB is the only putative streptococcal nephritogenic antigen that so far has been demonstrated in the subepithelial electron-dense deposits known as humps (Fig. 55.3), the most typical histologic lesion of acute PSGN. In studies from Latin America and central Europe, SPEB but not GAPDH is usually detectable in renal biopsy specimens of PSGN patients.[9] In contrast, GAPDH was present in PSGN in a study of Japanese patients.[6] These contrasting results raise the interesting possibility that different streptococcal antigens are capable of inducing acute nephritis in different ethnic groups. Indeed, a study of the group C *S. zooepidemicus* strain that caused the epidemic outbreak in Brazil revealed an absence of the gene related to SPEB, which documents that this antigen was not involved in that epidemic.[10]

PSGN is thought to occur when persistent streptococcal infection results in antigenemia and the development of circulating immune complexes that primarily deposit in the

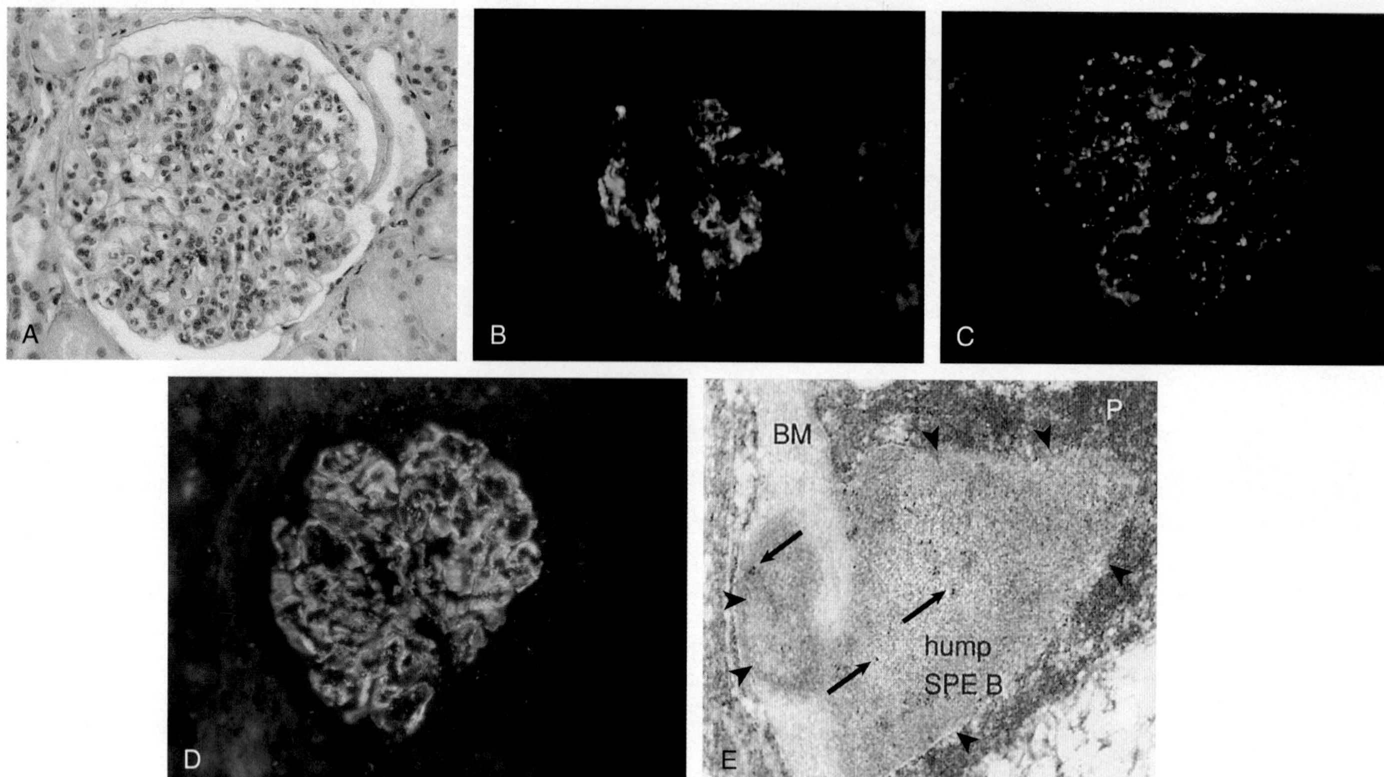

Figure 55.3 Poststreptococcal glomerulonephritis. A, A diffuse proliferative and exudative glomerulonephritis can be seen by light microscopy. **B-D,** Immunofluorescence showing the mesangial (**B**), starry sky (**C**), and garland (**D**) patterns. **E,** Immune electron microscopy showing the characteristic subepithelial electron-dense deposits (humps) *(arrowheads),* inside which streptococcal proteinase exotoxin B (SPEB) is demonstrated *(arrows)* (immunogold staining). BM, basement membrane; P, podocyte. *(Reprinted with permission from reference 9.)*

subendothelial and mesangial locations to initiate an inflammatory cascade with local complement activation and the recruitment of neutrophils and monocytes-macrophages. Subepithelial immune deposits (humps) develop because of the presence of cationic antigens (e.g., SPEB) or the dissociation of immune complexes in the subendothelial space with transit and re-formation on the outer aspect of the glomerular basement membrane. Cell-mediated immunity is supported by the presence of CD4 (helper) T lymphocytes. Cytokines also contribute to the local inflammation and injury. Urinary monocyte chemoattractant protein 1 correlates with the severity of proteinuria in the acute phase of PSGN.

Several issues remain unresolved. For example, immune complex disease generally results in activation of the classical complement pathway, yet in most cases, C4 levels are normal and only C3 is found in the deposits. This could be explained by the presence of antigens (such as GAPDH) that activate the alternative pathway. In some patients, C3Nef IgG antibodies have been demonstrated in sera that are capable of activating the alternative complement pathway. Activation of the lectin complement pathway by bacterial antigens has been postulated (see Chapter 16), but individuals genetically unable to activate this pathway may still develop PSGN.

Finally, the role of autoimmune mechanisms remains to be clarified. Rheumatoid factors (especially IgG rheumatoid factor) and cryoglobulins are found in the serum of one third of patients in the first week of the disease. Rheumatoid factors (antibody to IgG) have been shown in one third of the renal biopsy specimens and in the eluate from the kidney in a fatal case. Anti-IgG reactivity may result from the loss of sialic acid from autologous IgG due to streptococcal neuraminidase (sialidase) or from binding of the Fc fragment of IgG to type II Fc receptors in the streptococcal wall.[4] Additional manifestations of autoimmune reactivity include the anti-C1q antibodies, particularly in severe cases, and rarely anti-DNA reactivity, antineutrophil cytoplasmic antibody (ANCA), and autoimmune hemolytic anemia.[4]

Pathology

Renal biopsy shows a diffuse endocapillary GN with proliferation of mesangial and endothelial cells (see Fig. 55.3). There is glomerular and interstitial infiltration of monocytes and lymphocytes. Glomerular accumulation of neutrophils is common and is termed exudative GN. Glomerular immune deposits of C3 (100% of the cases), IgG (62%), IgM (76%), and properdin and the terminal membrane attack complex C5b-C9 (85% of the cases, usually codeposited with C3) are seen in glomerular capillary loops and in the mesangium. A seminal work by Sorger and colleagaues[11] described three patterns of immunofluorescence in the glomeruli and their clinical correlations: the mesangial pattern of irregular and heavy immune deposits, the starry sky pattern of deposits scattered in mesangium and in capillary walls, and the garland pattern formed by gross deposits in the capillary loops (see Fig. 55.3). The garland pattern is clinically relevant because it is associated with heavy proteinuria and a large number of electron-dense subepithelial immune deposits. Ultrastructural studies demonstrate the subepithelial humps, which are typical although not pathognomonic of PSGN as they may also be observed in postinfectious GN of other causes (classically endocarditis-associated GN secondary to *Staphylococcus* infection), cryoglobulinemia, and lupus nephritis.

GN resolves by apoptosis of the excess cells. Residual renal injury is common, and biopsy specimens years later show variable degrees of focal glomerulosclerosis and mesangial expansion even in the absence of clinical disease. The clinical significance of these changes is undetermined.

Clinical Manifestations

Most patients give a history of a previous streptococcal infection, although it has often resolved at presentation. The incubation period is longer after skin infections (several weeks) than after throat infections (2 weeks).

The classic presentation is acute nephritic syndrome. Hypertension is found in 80% of patients. Edema occurs in 80% to 90% of cases and is the chief complaint in 60%; yet ascites is distinctly unusual.[4] Primary sodium retention is the cause of expanded intravascular volume, hypertension, and edema. Plasma renin activity and aldosterone are reduced. Hematuria is universal and in 30% of cases is macroscopic.[4]

The nephrotic syndrome may occur at the onset in 2% of the children and 20% of adults. Rapidly progressive renal failure, resulting from extracapillary crescent formation, occurs in less than 1% of patients. Impaired renal function occurs in 25% to 40% of the children and in up to 83% of adults.

Positive cultures for *Streptococcus* are obtained in 10% to 70% of the cases during epidemics and in about 20% to 25% of sporadic cases. Antistreptolysin O (ASO) titers are increased in more than two thirds of patients with PSGN after throat infections, and anti-DNAse B titers are elevated in 73% of the post-impetigo cases. The streptozyme panel (which measures antibodies to four antigens, anti-DNAse B, antihyaluronidase, ASO, and antistreptokinase) is more sensitive, and the result is positive in more than 80% of subjects. Antibody titers to GAPDH and SPEB/zymogen, although more sensitive and specific,[10] are not clinically available.

Serum C3 levels are depressed in more than 90% of patients in the first week of disease and return to normal in less than 2 months. C4, a measure of classical complement pathway activation, may be normal. Serum IgG and IgM are elevated in 80% of the cases, and in contrast with another poststreptococcal disease, rheumatic fever, IgA is normal. Cryoglobulins, elevated rheumatoid factor, and anti-C1q antibodies are present in up to one third of patients, and rare patients may have low titers of anti-DNA and ANCA.

Subclinical disease, manifested by microscopic hematuria and fall in serum complement, occurs four to five times more frequently than clinically overt disease and often involves siblings of index cases.[7] On occasion, whole families have various manifestations of PSGN; it is thus important to inquire about a history of streptococcal infections and signs of nephritic syndrome among family members.

Management

Renal biopsy is not routinely indicated in PSGN but may be required to confirm the diagnosis when it presents with unusual clinical features, such as nephrotic proteinuria, decreased C3 levels lasting for more than a month (suggests lupus or hypocomplementemic MPGN), or increasing renal dysfunction (suggests crescentic GN).

Management includes culture and treatment of any remaining streptococcal infection. Early antibiotic treatment is likely to prevent PSGN. Treatment is with penicillin (1.2 million units of benzathine penicillin in adults or half this dose in small children, or alternatively, oral phenoxymethyl or phenoxyethyl penicillin G 250 mg [adults] or 125 mg [children], every 6 hours for 7 to 10 days) or, in persons allergic to penicillin, erythromycin (250 mg every 6 hours in adults and 40 mg/kg in children, for 7 to 10 days). Cephalosporins may be used with equal or even better results.[12] Preventive antibiotic treatment is justified in populations at risk during epidemics and in siblings of index cases.[13]

Treatment of the acute nephritic syndrome includes restriction of fluid and sodium intake and the use of loop diuretics to treat circulatory congestion. An oral long-acting calcium antagonist is usually sufficient to control hypertension. Nitroprusside is used in exceptional cases with hypertensive encephalopathy. Dialysis (either hemodialysis or peritoneal dialysis) is required in 25% to 30% of adults but seldom in children.

Rare complications of acute PSGN include cerebral vasculitis, cerebral vasogenic edema, and posterior reversible leukoencephalopathy. The last is manifested by mental disturbances, visual hallucinations, headache, and convulsions and may be confused with hypertensive encephalopathy. The diagnosis requires the use of magnetic resonance imaging studies.

Anecdotal reports suggest that the rare patients with crescentic GN associated with PSGN may benefit from pulse methylprednisolone therapy, and if spontaneous improvement is not observed in 2 weeks, this therapy may be tried. The prognosis of crescentic PSGN is significantly better than that of crescentic GN due to other causes, but a complete recovery may be expected in less than half of the cases.

Prognosis

Most children with PSGN recover. In older subjects, there are higher acute complication rates, including a higher prevalence of renal impairment (60% to 70%), congestive heart failure (40%), nephrotic proteinuria (20%), and mortality (25%).[3]

After recovery, mild proteinuria (<500 mg/day) and microscopic hematuria may persist for up to 1 year without worsening the long-term prognosis. Nevertheless, some subjects, especially adults, may have persistent impaired renal function, proteinuria, or hypertension. However, end-stage renal disease (ESRD) occurs in less than 1% of the children observed for 1 to 2 decades after the acute attack.[3]

Certain epidemics have reported a high incidence of chronicity, perhaps because of a predominantly adult population.[14] Risk factors for the development of chronic kidney disease include an onset with nephrotic-range proteinuria, older age, and coexistent diabetic nephropathy. Certain communities, such as Australian aborigines, also have a worse long-term prognosis.[15]

Endocarditis-Associated Glomerulonephritis

Community-acquired native valve endocarditis in the United States and western Europe has an incidence of 1.7 to 6.2 cases per 100,000 person-years, and as determined by population-based surveys, it is unchanged in the last 3 decades.[16] In the United States, 15,000 new cases of infective endocarditis occur each year. The most common infecting bacteria are *Staphylococcus aureus* and *Staphylococcus epidermidis; Streptococcus viridans* and *S. pyogenes; Enterococcus faecalis;* and less commonly, *E. coli, Proteus,* and microorganisms of the *Bartonella* and *Candida* species. The more significant changes observed in the epidemiology are the reduction in the proportion of cases associated with rheumatic heart disease and the increase in health care–associated cases.[16] Patients on chronic hemodialysis represent the most important subgroup, with 20 to 60 times the incidence in the general population. In this population, synthetic grafts and long-standing venous dialysis catheters are significant risk factors. One third of patients with bacterial endocarditis develop impaired renal function, and the risk increases with age, a history of hypertension, thrombocytopenia, and prosthetic valve infection.

In a recent survey of 62 patients with infective endocarditis in whom renal tissue was available for study, biopsy and autopsy material demonstrated GN in 26%, of which many cases were pauci-immune renal vasculitis. Other pathologic changes included localized infarcts in 31%, half of which were septic, and interstitial nephritis, mostly attributable to antibiotics, in 10%. Cortical necrosis was found in 10% of the cases.[16]

The most common glomerular pathologic change is diffuse proliferative GN. Less commonly, focal GN, MN, and MPGN type I may be found. Crescent formation is found in about half of the proliferative GN forms. Widespread deposition of IgM, IgG, and C3 and electron-dense subendothelial, mesangial, and subepithelial deposits (which resemble poststreptococcal humps) are usually evident. In subacute endocarditis, focal segmental proliferative lesions with fibrinoid necrosis or capillary thrombi and mesangial immune deposits may be present. Tubulointerstitial cellular infiltration and variable degrees of atrophy and fibrosis may be seen. Intense eosinophilic infiltration should suggest another diagnosis, such as acute interstitial nephritis secondary to antibiotics.[17]

The pathogenesis of endocarditis-associated GN involves the deposition of immune complexes containing bacterial antigens in glomeruli, a mechanism similar to that proposed for PSGN. Cryoglobulins (of the polyclonal or type III type) are present in 50% of subjects and may be found in glomeruli. Some bacteria (classically methicillin-resistant *S. aureus*) express superantigens that can also activate T cells directly and lead to a polyclonal gammopathy and immune complex GN (see later discussion).

Clinical Manifestations and Diagnosis

Patients often present with fever, arthralgias, anemia, and purpura. Infective endocarditis may rarely present as primary renal disease without characteristic systemic symptoms. Classic findings in endocarditis, such as Osler's nodes, Janeway lesions, and splinter hemorrhages, are seldom seen. The renal manifestations usually are microscopic hematuria and mild proteinuria (except in cases with membranous GN, which may have proteinuria in the nephrotic range), with or without mild impairment in renal function (except in cases with renal vasculitis, in which renal failure is common). A rapidly progressive clinical course or nephrotic syndrome is unusual. Abnormal serologic test results include decreased C3 and C4 levels (consistent with activation of the classical complement pathway), high titers of rheumatoid factor, circulating immune complexes, and type III cryoglobulins. These serologic findings are observed in 50% of subjects with subacute bacterial endocarditis and in a higher proportion of patients with endocarditis-associated GN, although complement levels may be normal in superantigen-mediated GN. Cytoplasmic ANCA has been reported in rare cases with subacute endocarditis and GN.[18]

The differential diagnosis includes antibiotic-associated nephrotoxicity, interstitial nephritis, and embolism. Embolism may originate from the left side of the heart or from the right if the foramen ovale is patent. Microscopic or large emboli may occlude small or large vessels, the latter observed with fungal or *Haemophilus* endocarditis. Large emboli may produce flank pain, hematuria, and pyuria; microemboli produce local infarcts and microabscesses that give the kidney the classic "flea-bitten" appearance. Interstitial nephritis is often associated with fever, eosinophilia, and eosinophiluria (see Chapter 60). Unfortunately, endocarditis-associated GN may also present with fever, and eosinophiluria can complicate crescentic nephritis of any etiology.

Antibiotic treatment for 4 to 6 weeks usually results in complete eradication of endocarditis with correction of serologic abnormalities, but microscopic hematuria, proteinuria, and elevation of serum creatinine may persist for months after eradication of the infection.[19] Normalization of C3 levels during therapy correlates with a good outcome. In cases with crescentic GN, pulse corticosteroid therapy and plasma exchange have been used in addition to effective antibiotic therapy, but the value of these treatments remains undefined. The overall mortality of bacterial endocarditis is 20% and increases to 36% in the patients who develop renal failure.[19]

Staphylococcal Infections with Glomerular IgA Deposition

In 1995, Koyama and coworkers[20] described a novel form of severe GN associated with methicillin-resistant staphylococcal infections that presented with renal impairment, nephrotic proteinuria, and variable degrees of crescent formation. There was IgA dominant or codominant deposition in association with other immunoglobulin and complement deposits, and the patients had increased serum IgA levels and specific T-cell receptor V_β^+ subsets during the course of the disease (Fig. 55.4). They postulated that staphylococcal superantigens were involved in the pathogenesis. The frequency of this condition is undefined, but it represents 1.6% of adult kidney biopsies in one institution.[21]

Clinical and Pathologic Characteristics

The initial cases all had severe GN with acute kidney injury, heavy proteinuria, and hematuria, but the condition may present with a milder clinical picture. Whereas most cases are associated with methicillin-resistant *Staphylococcus* infections, they may also occur in infection with methicillin-sensitive bacteria.[21] Diabetic glomerulosclerosis frequently coexists.[22] Complement levels may be low or normal.

Renal biopsy reveals variable degrees of mesangial and intracapillary hypercellularity with or without crescent formation. Interstitial fibrosis and tubular atrophy may be mild or severe. Electron microscopy shows electron-dense deposits in the mesangium in the glomerular basement membrane and in subendothelial areas. Large subepithelial electron-dense deposits are reported in some series. IgA deposition may be mild, moderate, or intense and is dominant or codominant with other Ig deposits. C3 deposits are usually present.

Pathogenesis

The pathogenesis of staphylococcal infection–related IgA GN is not entirely clear. Koyama and coworkers[20] have implicated staphylococcal superantigens that would bind directly to the major histocompatibility complex class II molecules on antigen-presenting cells, which then engage the V_β T-cell receptor region. The result is an intensive T-cell activation with cytokine production, which activates B cells that produce polyclonal IgG and IgA. They have identified a *S. aureus* cell envelope antigen that is co-localized with the glomerular IgA deposits.[23] Whether staphylococcus antigens are involved in the pathogenesis of IgA nephropathy (see Chapter 22) is a possibility that deserves further study.

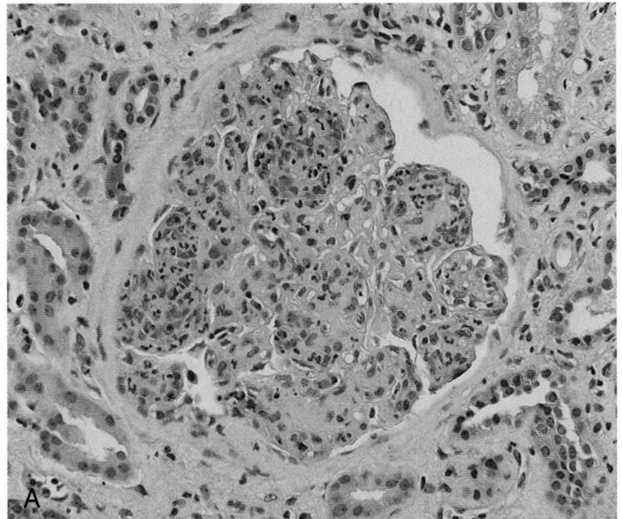

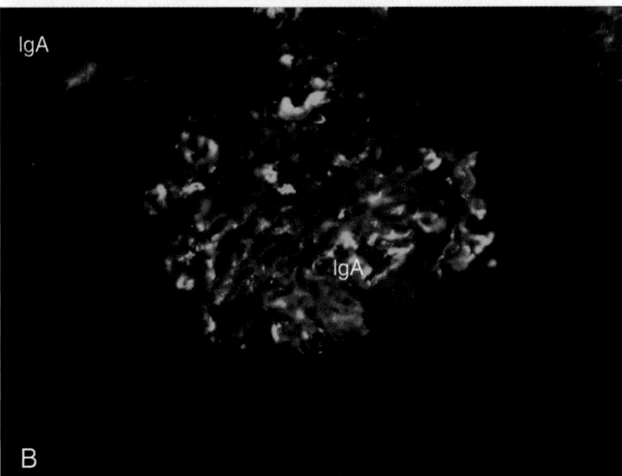

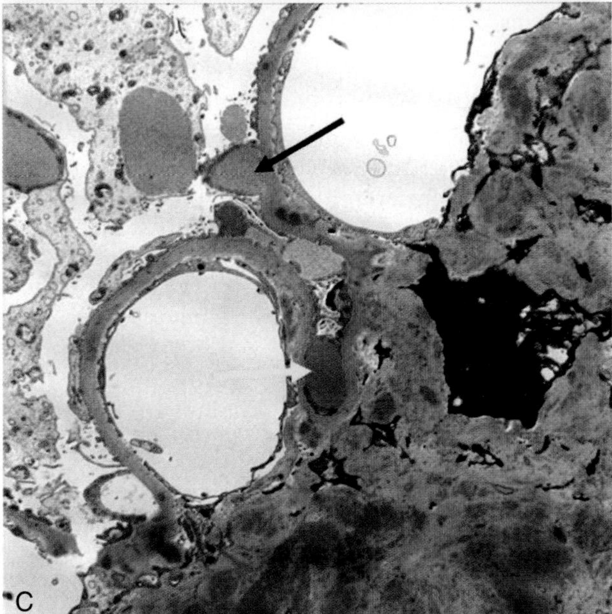

Figure 55.4 Glomerulonephritis in a diabetic subject with methicillin-sensitive *S. aureus* infection. A, A diffuse exudative GN is present with neutrophil infiltration. **B,** Immunofluorescence shows IgA-dominant mesangial deposits. **C,** Electron microscopy shows dome-shaped subepithelial deposits *(black arrow)* and mesangial deposits *(yellow arrow)*. *(Courtesy Surya Seshan.)*

Differential Diagnosis and Treatment

Antibiotic treatment of IgA-dominant staphylococcus-related GN is indicated because recovery of renal function may occur. Corticosteroid treatment is contraindicated, which makes it important to establish its differential diagnosis with IgA nephropathy, in which corticosteroids may be indicated in severe cases (see Chapter 22). Clinical characteristics that may be helpful in the differential diagnosis are the association with a staphylococcal infection (in contrast with upper respiratory infection in IgA nephropathy), the frequent occurrence of massive proteinuria (rare in IgA nephropathy), and the acute renal failure (uncommon in IgA nephropathy).

Shunt Nephritis

Atrioventricular shunts may become infected in about 30% of cases. GN may develop in 0.7% to 2% of those with infected atrioventricular shunts; this may occur 2 months to many years after insertion. The infective organisms are usually *S. epidermidis* and *S. aureus* and less frequently *Propionibacterium acnes*, diphtheroids, *Pseudomonas*, or *Serratia*. In contrast with atrioventricular shunts, ventriculoperitoneal shunts are rarely complicated with GN.

Patients present with insidious low-grade fever, arthralgias, weight loss, anemia, rash, hepatosplenomegaly, hypertension, and signs of increased intracranial pressure. Microscopic hematuria is present in 90% of subjects, and proteinuria is often in the nephrotic range. Serologic findings include positive rheumatoid factor titers, cryoglobulinemia, and decreased serum C3, C4, and CH50 levels. Raised c-ANCA titers may be found.[24]

Renal histology shows MPGN type I in nearly 60% of the cases and non-IgA mesangial proliferative GN in the remainder. IgM, IgG, and C3 deposits are present in the glomerular capillary and mesangium.

Treatment requires antibiotic therapy and the prompt removal of the infected atrioventricular shunt, which is usually replaced by a ventriculoperitoneal shunt. Delay in diagnosis and in removal of the shunt worsens the prognosis of the renal lesion. In the event that dialysis is required, hemodialysis is the preferred modality because peritonitis complicating chronic peritoneal dialysis carries the risk of meningitis in patients with a ventriculoperitoneal shunt. Complete recovery occurs in more than half of the patients; persistent urinary abnormalities have been found in 22% and ESRD in 6% of the patients.

Glomerulonephritis Associated with Other Bacterial Infections

Osteomyelitis and intra-abdominal, pelvic, pleural, and dental abscesses can be associated with GN. Infection is usually present for several months before it is diagnosed. Renal disease may vary from mild urinary abnormalities to rapidly progressive GN, but the most frequent presentation is nephrotic syndrome. Unlike with other infection-associated GN, complement levels are often normal. Renal histology reveals MPGN, diffuse proliferative GN, or mesangial proliferative GN. Crescents may be present. Antibiotic treatment may result in recovery of renal function if it is started early.

Congenital and secondary (or early latent) syphilis may be associated with GN. In congenital syphilis, patients present with anasarca 4 to 12 weeks after birth. Nephrotic syndrome occurs in 8% of the patients and may be the primary clinical manifestation (as opposed to the more classic triad of rhinitis,

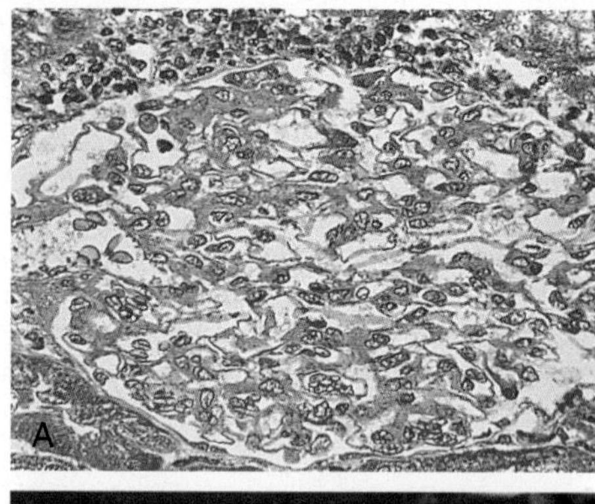

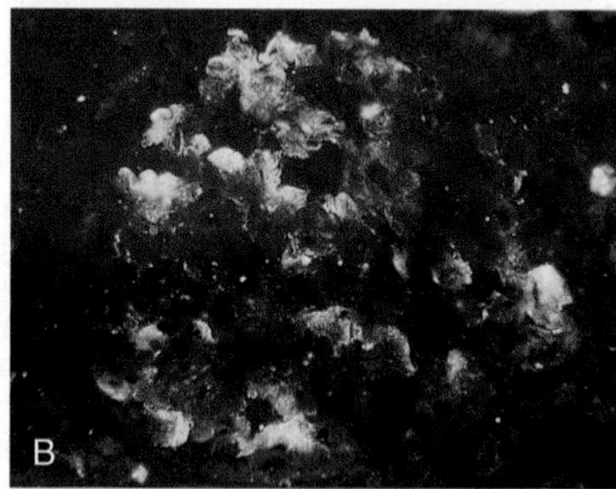

Figure 55.5 Glomerulonephritis in typhoid fever. A, Mesangial proliferative GN. **B,** Immunofluorescent staining demonstrates granular deposition of *Salmonella typhi* Vi antigens in the mesangium. *(Courtesy V. Boonpucknavig.)*

osteochondritis, and rash). In acquired syphilis, renal involvement occurs in 0.3% of all patients. Adults present with nephrotic syndrome or occasionally with an acute nephritic picture. Serologic test results for syphilis are positive (rapid plasmin reagin, VDRL, and fluorescent treponemal antibody absorption test). MN is the most common renal pathologic process, but diffuse proliferative GN with or without crescents, MPGN, and mesangial proliferative GN have also been observed. Treponemal antigens have been identified in the immune deposits. Syphilitic GN responds to antibiotic treatment, although remission may not occur for 4 to 18 months.

Acute typhoid fever from *Salmonella typhi* is characterized by fever, splenomegaly, and gastrointestinal symptoms. Severe cases may develop shock and acute renal failure as a part of disseminated intravascular coagulation or hemolytic-uremic syndrome, but these complications are rare. Overt mesangial proliferative GN occurs in 2% of the cases (Fig. 55.5), but microscopic hematuria and mild proteinuria may be present in 25% of the cases.[25] Diagnosis requires the culture of the organisms from blood or stools or rising antibody titers in the Widal test. GN may also occur in patients with schistosomiasis and coexisting *Salmonella* infection of the urinary tract (see Chapter 54).

Leprosy (*Mycobacterium leprae* infection) may be associated in autopsy studies with GN (5% to 14% of the cases), interstitial nephritis (4% to 54%), or amyloidosis (4% to 31%).[26] GN is manifested clinically in less than 2% of the patients. It remains controversial whether GN is more common in lepromatous leprosy than in tuberculoid leprosy. Urinary abnormalities consistent with GN often accompany episodes of erythema nodosum leprosum. Clinical manifestations are of nephrotic syndrome, less frequently of acute nephritic syndrome, and rarely of rapidly progressive GN. MPGN or diffuse proliferative GN with IgG, C3, IgM, IgA, and fibrin deposits is present on biopsy. Response of glomerular disease to treatment of leprosy is variable. Amyloidosis with nephritic syndrome may also rarely occur, especially in lepromatous leprosy. Other renal abnormalities associated with leprosy include interstitial nephritis. Prednisolone (40 to 50 mg/day) has been used in short courses to treat erythema nodosum leprosum associated with GN.

Pneumococcal pneumonia may rarely be associated with microhematuria and proteinuria, especially if treatment is delayed. Both diffuse proliferative GN and mesangial proliferative GN have been reported, and pneumococcal antigen is present in the immune deposits. Rarely, pneumococcal pneumonia can also be associated with hemolytic-uremic syndrome as a result of unmasking of the Thomsen-Friedenreich antigen in glomeruli by pneumococcal neuraminidase, which then allows preformed antibodies to bind and to elicit an immune response.

Gastroenteritis due to *Campylobacter jejuni* may be associated with mesangioproliferative or diffuse proliferative GN. GN may also occur with other bacterial infections, including those with *E. coli*, *Yersinia*, meningococcus, and *Mycoplasma pneumoniae*.

VIRAL INFECTIONS

Viral infections may cause acute GN (hepatitis A virus, parvovirus B19, measles, Epstein-Barr virus), chronic GN (hepatitis B virus [HBV], hepatitis C virus [HCV], human immunodeficiency virus [HIV], parvovirus B19), and interstitial nephritis (Hantavirus, influenza virus, dengue, BK virus, coronavirus, cytomegalovirus, hepatitis A virus). The most common infections are those associated with HBV, HCV, and HIV. Pathogenetic mechanisms include deposition or *in situ* formation of exogenous (viral) immune complexes; autoantibody formation directed to endogenous antigen modified by viral injury; virus-induced release of proinflammatory cytokines, chemokines, adhesion molecules, and growth factors; and direct cytopathic effects of viral proteins.[27]

Hepatitis A Virus–Associated Renal Disease

Renal failure associated with severe hepatitis A virus infection may be due to interstitial nephritis or acute tubular necrosis. Rarely, immune complex–related diffuse proliferative GN with immunoglobulin and C3 deposits and the clinical picture of nephritic or nephrotic syndrome may develop, at times with impaired renal function. Recovery from GN usually coincides with the improvement of hepatitis.

Hepatitis B Virus–Associated Renal Disease

HBV is a DNA virus of the Hepadnaviridae family; the human is its only known natural host. Hepatitis develops as a result of immune reactivity directed to infected hepatocytes.[28,29]

Acute HBV infection may present with nausea, vomiting, fever, hepatomegaly, and a short-lived serum sickness–like syndrome: urticaria or maculopapular rash, neuropathy, arthralgia or arthritis, microscopic hematuria, and non-nephrotic proteinuria.[28] Renal biopsy, if it is performed, shows a mesangial proliferative GN. The clinical picture resolves spontaneously as the hepatitis improves.

Whereas acute HBV infection may resolve uneventfully, more than 90% of infected infants, 25% to 50% of the children infected between the ages of 1 and 5 years, and 6% to 10% of older children and adults develop chronic infection (defined as persistence of HBsAg-positive serology but negative for IgM antibodies to HBV core antigen). Vertical (maternal-infant at birth) transmission is usually present in endemic areas, such as China and Southeast Asia. Horizontal transmission occurs through contamination with blood or direct contact with mucous membranes. In Europe and the United States, the prevalence is lower, and most carriers acquire the infection as adolescents or adults by horizontal transmission as a consequence of drug abuse, blood transfusions, or sexual relations.

HBV carriers may present with a variety of renal syndromes.

HBV-Associated Membranous Nephropathy

MN may occur in chronic HBV carriers. Children show a male predominance and often present with asymptomatic proteinuria or nephrotic syndrome, microscopic hematuria, and normal renal function, often with minimal evidence of liver disease. The prognosis is usually good, and spontaneous remission is common in association with the appearance of anti-HBe antibodies in circulation In contrast, adults are also nephrotic but often have impaired renal function and clinically apparent liver disease and are more at risk for progression to renal failure. C3 and C4 levels are decreased in 20% to 50%. Biopsy is consistent with MN, but mesangial immune deposits may also be present, in contrast with idiopathic MN. Virus-like particles have been identified in various areas of the glomeruli. HBeAg can often be demonstrated in the immune deposits by immunohistochemistry.[27,29]

HBV-Associated Membranoproliferative Glomerulonephritis

MPGN is the most common glomerular lesion in adult HBV carriers. Cryoglobulinemia may be present, especially if there is concurrent infection with HCV. Chronic liver disease is usually present but may be clinically asymptomatic. Nephrotic or non-nephrotic proteinuria, often associated with microhematuria, is common.[28] Biopsy shows typical type I MPGN, and HBsAg is occasionally shown in the immune deposits.

Mesangial Proliferative Glomerulonephritis with IgA Deposits

There are several reports of a renal lesion mimicking IgA nephropathy in HBV infection. It is possible that this is a consequence of chronic liver disease with impaired clearance of IgA circulating immune complexes, leading to hepatic IgA nephropathy (see Chapter 22).

Treatment of HBV-Associated Glomerulonephritis

Treatment is aimed at eradication of HBV virus. Interferon alfa (5 million units daily for 6 months) or pegylated interferon alfa may result in remission, especially in HBV-associated MN. Lamivudine (100 mg orally once daily for 52 weeks) has also been reported to clear HBV virus and to induce remission in HBV-associated MN. A reduction of the dose is necessary when the glomerular filtration rate (GFR) is reduced below 50 ml/min per 1.73 m^2. If the GFR is 30 to 49 ml/min per 1.73 m^2, the initial dose is 100 mg, and this is followed by 50 mg orally daily; if the GFR is 15 to 29 ml/min per 1.73 m^2, the initial dose is the same and subsequent does are reduced to 25 mg daily. In patients with ESRD, the initial dose is 35 mg followed by 10 mg daily.[30] Lamivudine-resistant strains may arise with prolonged use. Entecavir and adefovir dipivoxil may provide an alternative, but the nephrotoxicity of adefovir is a deterrent, although the risk is low at standard dosing if renal function is normal. Corticosteroid treatment is contraindicated because it is ineffective and may delay or prevent seroconversion and accelerate the progression of liver disease.

The prevailing view has been that treatment is not required for children with HBV-associated MN because the majority of children undergo spontaneous remission. However, clearance of HBV DNA and HBeAg has been achieved in about half of the children in controlled studies, with a higher incidence of resolution of the proteinuria in the treated group. Because HBV-associated MN may rarely progress to ESRD in children, it is reasonable to treat when proteinuria is severe or there is progression of renal disease.

Active immunization is the most effective prevention measure as shown by the 10-fold decline in the incidence in Taiwan and 67% reduction in the United States 10 years after universal vaccination was implemented in 1991.[27]

Polyarteritis Nodosa

HBV-related vasculitis (HBV-related polyarteritis nodosa [PAN]) has become progressively rare and is observed primarily in adult men who acquire HBV infection from drug use or transfusion, usually less than 12 months after a mild attack of hepatitis. It is almost never observed in children and is rare in areas of the world where HBV infection is acquired at birth or in childhood, such as in Asia. The typical patient with HBV-related PAN presents with signs of serum sickness preceding and during a mild or asymptomatic attack of hepatitis, unlike HBV-associated serum sickness, which resolves spontaneously with clearing of the HBsAg. In these patients, the disease progresses to involve numerous organs. It typically involves medium-sized arteries and may present with a variety of presentations, including myocardial ischemia, mesenteric angina, cerebral ischemia, and mononeuritis multiplex. Renal vasculitis is manifested by microhematuria, nephrotic or non-nephrotic proteinuria, and renin-dependent hypertension. Manifestations are in general similar to those observed in noninfectious PAN, but patients with HBV-associated PAN more frequently have orchitis and gastrointestinal and renal vessel involvement, whereas pulmonary and cutaneous manifestations are rare. Rapidly progressive GN, as seen in microscopic polyangiitis, is infrequent in HBV-related PAN.[31]

The pathogenesis of HBV-associated PAN is thought to be the deposition of HBsAg-antiHBs immune complexes in the arterial wall that results in a subsequent inflammatory reaction with the activation of complement. The vessels often show a predominance of IgM and HBsAg, suggesting that the injury is mediated by HBsAg-IgM complexes. Serologic tests reveal HBsAg and anti-HBc antibodies. Serum complement is usually normal, and ANCA are absent.

Diagnosis requires detection of circulating HBsAg in association with either biopsy or angiographic evidence of vasculitis. Biopsy studies demonstrate vascular lesions, which are typically panmural and in different stages of development. Variable degrees of fibrinoid necrosis, fibrin deposition, and leukocyte infiltration are present. HBsAg, IgM, and occasionally IgG are deposited in the vessel wall. Angiographic studies demonstrating narrow segments and saccular or fusiform aneurysms in celiac or renal arteries have higher diagnostic yield than biopsies do.

Liver biopsy demonstrates chronic active or persisting hepatitis or, rarely, acute hepatitis. The renal biopsy, in addition to the arteriolar lesions, may show relatively preserved glomeruli with variable degrees of collapse in the glomerular tuft likely resulting from ischemic changes. In contrast with idiopathic microscopic polyangiitis, necrotizing lesions with crescent formation are rare. Mesangial proliferative GN, diffuse proliferative GN, MPGN, and MN have all been reported.

Treatment consists of a short course of corticosteroids (prednisone 1 mg/kg per day for 2 weeks) and plasma exchange (9 to 12 exchanges during 3 weeks) followed by interferon alfa therapy or lamivudine.

Hepatitis C Virus–Associated Renal Disease

HCV is an RNA virus of the Flaviviridae family that is a common cause of chronic hepatitis, cirrhosis, and hepatoma. Chronic HCV infection can also be associated with the development of several types of glomerular disease.[32] The most common is MPGN with or without cryoglobulinemia, and this entity is discussed in Chapter 21. HCV may also be associated with MN, especially in renal transplant patients. The clinical and histologic findings are similar to those observed in idiopathic MN except that HCV RNA and anti-HCV antibodies are present in the blood. Other reported associations include fibrillary GN, focal glomerulosclerosis (especially in African Americans), and thrombotic microangiopathy with anticardiolipin antibodies (especially after renal transplantation).[33]

Human Immunodeficiency Virus–Associated Renal Disease

HIV infection may be associated with myriad renal complications, one of the most common of which is HIV-associated nephropathy. A discussion of HIV-associated nephropathy and other HIV-associated renal disorders is provided in Chapter 56.

Other Virus-Associated Renal Disease

Polyomavirus nephropathy due to BK virus is increasingly recognized in renal transplantation and can be a cause of decreased renal function. It is described in detail in Chapter 101.

Cytomegalovirus (CMV) infection commonly is manifested in renal transplant recipients, in whom it can infect tubular cells and macrophages in the interstitium, resulting in the characteristic intracytoplasmic "owl-like" inclusions. Whereas there is some evidence that this may be a cause of tubular dysfunction, there is no evidence that this results in glomerular injury. Rarely, however, CMV has been reported in nontransplant subjects to cause a diffuse proliferative GN with immune deposits containing CMV antigens. In addition, a rare report has linked CMV infection with collapsing glomerulopathy and ESRD in patients not infected with HIV.[34]

Parvovirus B19 is a single-stranded DNA virus with marked tropism for the erythroid precursor cells. In conditions in which there is increased destruction or decreased production of red cells, parvovirus infection may cause aplastic anemia as in renal transplantation and in sickle cell disease. In patients with sickle cell disease, parvovirus-induced aplastic crises are occasionally followed by nephritic or nephrotic syndrome, assumed to be the result of immune complex deposition. Diffuse proliferative GN, MPGN, and collapsing focal glomerulosclerosis (with similarities to heroin- and HIV-associated nephropathy) have been attributed to parvovirus B19 infection, and some studies but not others have detected viral DNA in kidney biopsy specimens. Granular deposition of C3 and IgG in capillary walls and subendothelial deposits have been found.[35] Studies have also suggested a relationship between renal parvovirus infection and chronic allograft nephropathy.[36]

Hantavirus causes hemorrhagic fever with acute interstitial nephritis (see Chapter 66). Severe cases, occurring more frequently in endemic areas, present with acute renal failure. Milder forms are manifested with fever, hepatitis, and mild renal functional impairment. Severe acute respiratory distress syndrome caused by coronavirus may cause tubulointerstitial nephritis; acute renal failure, when it is present, is probably associated with multiorgan failure.

Many viral infections, including varicella, mumps, adenovirus, coxsackievirus, and influenza, can be associated with transient microscopic hematuria, non-nephrotic proteinuria, and a mesangial proliferative GN or diffuse proliferative GN in which viral antigens can be identified in the mesangium. Measles may also cause a diffuse proliferative GN but is better known for its unique ability to induce remission in subjects with minimal change disease with nephrotic syndrome.

Dengue hemorrhagic fever may be caused by four serotypes of the family Flaviviridae. The clinical manifestations, reflecting increased vascular permeability, include muscle pains, gastrointestinal symptoms, and, in severe cases, bleeding manifestations and shock. Acute renal failure may accompany the severe cases; in some less severely ill patients, acute endocapillary GN with mesangial proliferation may develop and may be manifested by microhematuria and proteinuria. Intense granular deposits of IgG, IgM, and C3 in mesangial areas and to a lesser degree in capillary walls are usually present.

Mild renal abnormalities can also be observed with acute Epstein-Barr virus (EBV) infection, with microhematuria and proteinuria in 10% to 15% of cases. Acute interstitial nephritis is probably the most common renal complication, but diffuse proliferative GN and MPGN may also occur. Replicating EBV was localized not only to infiltrating macrophages but also to proximal tubular cells that were shown to express the CD21 receptor for EBV. It was posited that EBV might be a major cause of chronic interstitial nephritis.[27]

PARASITIC INFECTIONS

Kidney involvement is fairly common in different parasitic diseases. With the exception of schistosomiasis, malaria, and onchocercosis, such involvement is usually mild and transient and often masked by the manifestations of the primary disease (Fig. 55.6).

Schistosomiasis

See Chapter 54.

Malaria

Malaria, caused by the protozoan *Plasmodium*, is transmitted by *Anopheles* mosquitoes and is a major world health problem (Fig. 55.7). More than 90% of cases occur in Africa, India, Southeast Asia, and Latin America.[37] Malaria can also be acquired by blood transfusions,[38] transplantation of infected donor organs,[39] and bite by infected vectors introduced in aircraft ("airport malaria").

Four major species are responsible for malaria. *P. falciparum* is usually associated with heavy parasitemia because it invades red blood cells of any age. Because all red cells can be infected, *P. falciparum* can be associated with massive infection of the red cells, resulting in acute kidney injury and multiple organ failure. This entity is discussed in more detail in Chapter 66.

Acute glomerular injury may occur with *P. falciparum* infection. Transient urinary abnormalities, such as mild proteinuria

Renal Lesions in Parasitic Infection						
	Glomerular Lesions	**Tubulointerstitial Lesions**	**Amyloidosis**	**Local Tissue Infestation**	**Acute Kidney Injury**	**Post-transplant Disease**
Schistosomiasis						
*S. haematobium**	MesPGN	+++	++	Granulomas		+
*S. mansoni**	MesPGN, DPGN, MPGN, FSGS	+	++	Granulomas		+
S. japonicum	MesPGN	+				
S. mekongi		+++				
Malaria						
*P. malariae**	MPGN					
*P. falciparum**	DPGN, MPGN	+			++	+
Filariasis						
Onchocerciasis*	MCD, MesPGN, MPGN					+
Loiasis	MN, MesPGN					
Bancroftiasis	MesPGN, MPGN, DPGN			Chyluria		
Dirofilariasis	MPGN (dogs), MN (dogs, cats)					
Brugia malayi	MesPGN, MPGN, DPGN					
Kala-azar*	DPGN (human), MPGN (dogs)	++	++	Interstitial	+	+
Trichinosis	MesPGN					
Strongyloidiasis	MesPGN					
Echinococcosis	MPGN			Hydatid cysts		
Opisthorchiasis*	MesPGN	++	+		++	
Chagas' disease*	MesPGN (mice)					
Babesiosis	MesPGN				++	+
African trypanosomiasis	MesPGN (monkeys, mice)					
Toxoplasmosis*	MesPGN	+				

Figure 55.6 Renal lesions in parasitic infection. All conditions documented in humans unless otherwise indicated. *Parasitic antigens or specific antibodies detected in the glomeruli. DPGN, diffuse proliferative GN; FSGS, focal segmental glomerulosclerosis; MCD, minimal change disease; MPGN, membranoproliferative GN; MN, membranous nephropathy; MesPGN, Mesangial Proliferative GN.

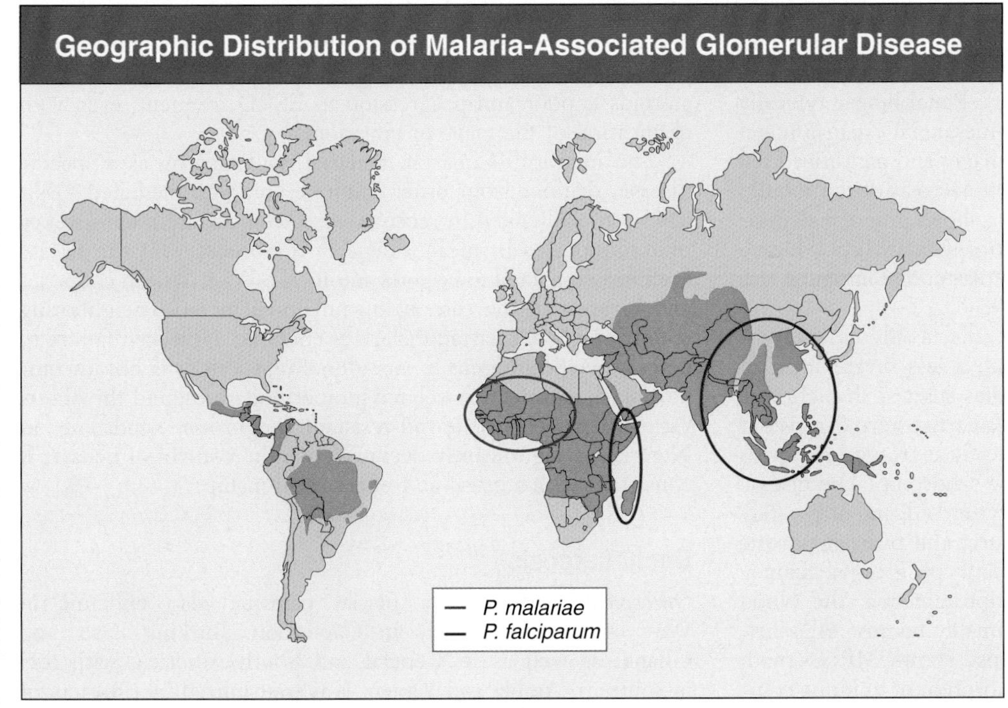

Figure 55.7 Geographic distribution of malaria-associated glomerular disease. Although malaria is endogenous to many areas of the world *(shaded orange),* the major areas where malaria-associated glomerular disease has been reported *(ringed)* and their respective species are shown.

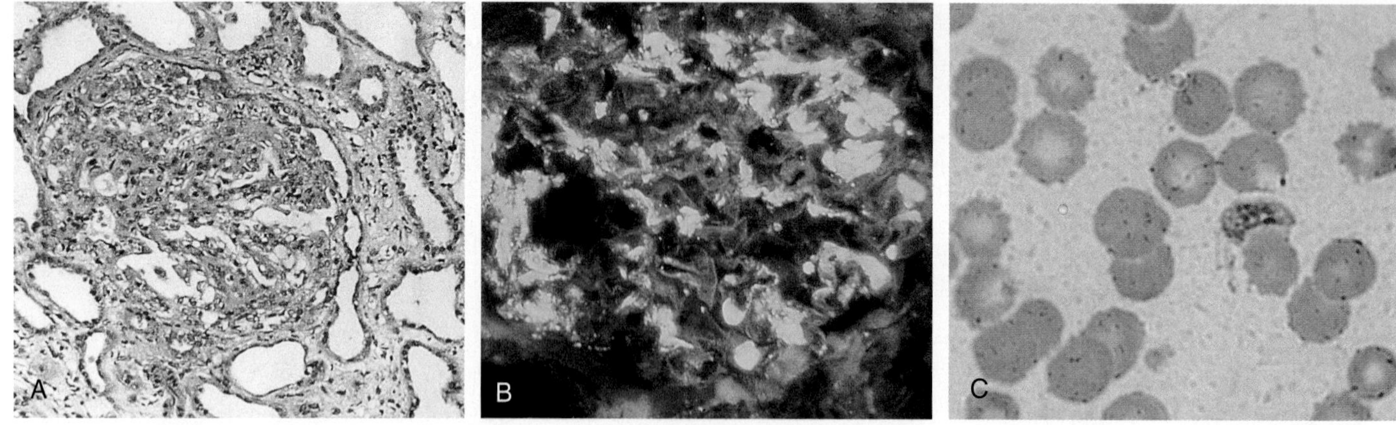

Figure 55.8 Glomerulonephritis associated with *Plasmodium falciparum* malaria. A, Light microscopy shows a mesangial proliferative GN. **B,** Immunofluorescence may reveal *P. falciparum* antigens in a mesangial pattern. **C,** Peripheral blood smear confirms acute *P. falciparum* infection, with banana-shaped gametocytes and multiple ring forms in erythrocytes. *(**A** reprinted with permission from reference 37; **B** and **C** courtesy of V. Boonpucknavig.)*

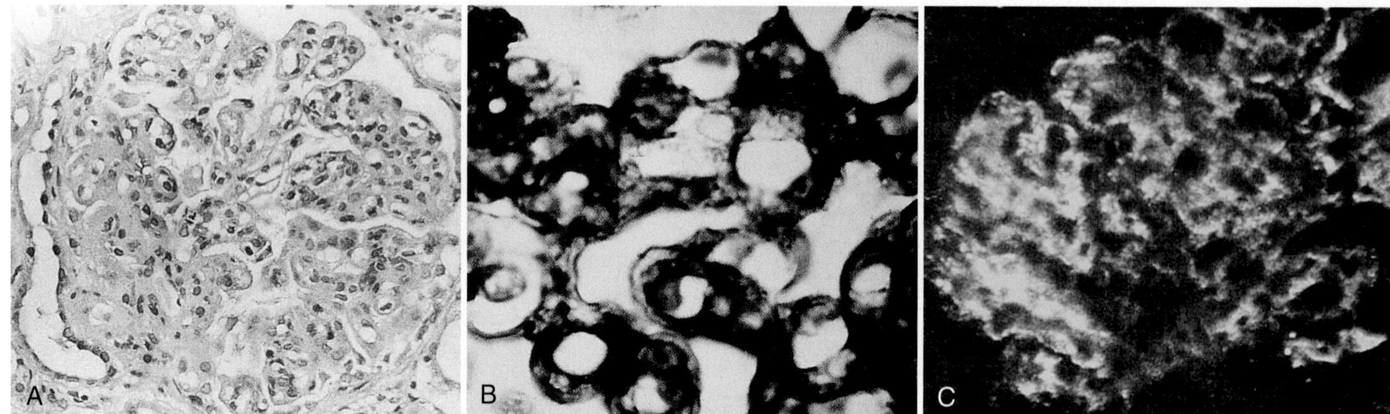

Figure 55.9 Quartan malarial nephropathy. A, Light microscopy shows a sclerosing membranoproliferative glomerulonephritis. **B,** Silver stain shows a double contour of the basement membrane. **C,** Malarial antigens are present by immunofluorescence. *(From reference 37.)*

and microhematuria, are encountered in 25% to 50% of patients; a full-blown nephritic syndrome with hypertension, edema, and impaired renal function is uncommon.[40] Serum complement C3 and C4 may be consumed in such cases. Renal biopsy typically shows endocapillary proliferation with mesangial expansion and infiltration with pigment-laden macrophages and parasitized red cells. Platelet-fibrin thrombi and patchy necrosis of the tubules may be associated. Immunofluorescence shows granular deposition of IgM, C3, malarial antigens, and occasionally IgG.[41] Dense immune complex deposits, containing plasmodial antigens, are seen by electron microscopy (Fig. 55.8).

Another malarial species, *P. malariae*, infects only aging erythrocytes and is therefore associated with a less severe form of malaria (quartan malaria). Several studies suggest that chronic quartan malaria may be associated with a corticosteroid-resistant nephrotic syndrome, referred to historically as tropical nephritis and more recently as tropical nephrotic syndrome. The disease typically affects children, usually 4 to 8 years old, and only rarely adults. It presents with heavy proteinuria and overt nephrotic syndrome, late-onset hypertension, and progressive kidney insufficiency. Despite the severe hypoproteinemia, the blood cholesterol level is often normal, presumably because of associated nutritional deficiency. Renal biopsy shows MPGN with intramembranous lacunae (due to reabsorption of immune complexes). Immunofluorescence shows coarsely granular IgG, IgM, and C3 deposits, and electron microscopy displays subendothelial electron-dense deposits (Fig. 55.9). The response to corticosteroids is poor and progression to ESRD frequent, even with eradication of the malarial infection.

The identity of quartan malarial nephropathy as a specific disease, distinct from other immune complex–mediated GNs, has been challenged in recent years owing to the inconsistency of immunohistochemical evidence.[42] It is unclear why the disease is almost restricted to Nigeria among the West African countries and Uganda in the east, being unknown in most neighboring countries where quartan malaria is endemic. However, failure to detect specific antigens in late glomerular lesions is not uncommon in most infection-related glomerulopathies, and the observation that corticosteroid-resistant nephrotic syndrome in Nigeria has significantly declined with the control of malaria is consistent with a cause-and-effect relationship.

Onchocercosis

Onchocerca volvulus is a filarial parasite, also endemic in West Africa, particularly in Cameroon, Burkina Faso, and Ghana, as well as in Central and South America, with foci in southern Arabia and Yemen. It is transmitted by a variety of black flies of the genus *Simulium*, usually found in the vicinity of rivers.

The mature parasite lives for many years in the affected host, usually protected from the immune response by hiding in subcutaneous nodules. However, migrating microfilariae are amenable to clearance by the innate immune system, releasing antigens that provoke production of antibodies and immune complexes.

The clinical syndrome of onchocerciasis includes (1) a variety of skin manifestations, such as papular and lichenified dermatitis, hyperpigmentation or depigmentation, and atrophy; (2) chronic lymphadenopathy, forming large masses, particularly in the inguinal region; (3) obstruction of the scrotal lymphatic drainage, leading to enlargement and progressive stretching under the effect of gravity (hanging scrotum syndrome); and (4) corneal opacities and anterior uveitis caused by microfilarial invasion, respective immune-mediated inflammation, and subsequent scarring (river blindness).

Corticosteroid-resistant nephrotic syndrome with progressive impairment of renal insufficiency is the most common renal presentation. Minimal change may occur, and also mesangial proliferative GN and MPGN, often with immune complexes containing onchocercal antigens. Antifilarial treatment does not halt the disease progression because of involvement of autoimmune mechanisms. Indeed, treatment with the antifilarial drug diethylcarbamazine may exacerbate proteinuria. Onchocercal GN may recur in transplanted kidneys.[43]

Other filarial infections, such as *Loa loa* and *Wuchereria bancrofti*, may induce mesangial proliferative GN, MN, or MPGN. Visceral leishmaniasis (kala-azar) frequently presents with microhematuria and interstitial nephritis or diffuse proliferative or membranous nephropathy. Trichinosis may also occasionally present with MPGN, manifested clinically with microhematuria and non-nephrotic proteinuria.

REFERENCES

1. Rodríguez-Iturbe B, Batsford S. Pathogenesis of poststreptococcal glomerulonephritis a century after Clemens von Pirquet. *Kidney Int.* 2007;71:1094-1104.
2. Nasr SH, Markowitz GS, Stokes MB, et al. Acute postinfectious glomerulonephritis in the modern era: Experience with 86 adults and review of the literature. *Medicine (Baltimore)*. 2008;87:21-32.
3. Rodríguez-Iturbe B, Musser JM. The current state of poststreptococcal nephritis. *J Am Soc Nephrol.* 2008;19:1855-1864.
4. Rodríguez-Iturbe B. Epidemic poststreptococcal glomerulonephritis. *Kidney Int.* 1984;25:129-136.
5. Balter S, Benin A, Pinto SW, et al. Epidemic nephritis in Nova Serrana, Brazil. *Lancet.* 2000;355:1776-1780.
6. Yoshizawa N, Yamakami K, Fujino M, et al. Nephritis-associated plasmin receptor and acute poststreptococcal glomerulonephritis: Characterization of the antigen and associated immune response. *J Am Soc Nephrol.* 2004;15:1785-1793.
7. Parra G, Rodríguez-Iturbe B, Batsford S, et al. Antibody to streptococcal zymogen in the serum of patients with acute glomerulonephritis: A multicentric study. *Kidney Int.* 1998;54:509-517.
8. Oda T, Yamakami K, Omasu F, et al. Glomerular plasmin-like activity in relation to nephritis-associated plasmin receptor in acute poststreptococcal glomerulonephritis. *J Am Soc Nephrol.* 2005;16:247-254.
9. Batsford SR, Mezzano S, Mihatsch M, et al. Is the nephritogenic antigen in poststreptococcal glomerulonephritis pyrogenic exotoxin B (SPE B) or GAPDH? *Kidney Int.* 2005;68:1120-1129.
10. Beres SB, Sesso R, Pinto SW, et al. Genome sequence of a Lancefield group C *Streptococcus zooepidemicus* strain causing epidemic nephritis: New information about an old disease. *PLoS ONE.* 2008;3:e3026. doi:10.1371/journal.pone.0003026.
11. Sorger K, Gessler M, Hübner FK, et al. Follow-up studies of three subtypes of acute postinfectious glomerulonephritis ascertained by renal biopsy. *Clin Nephrol.* 1987;27:111-124.
12. Casey JR, Pichichero ME. Meta-analysis of cephalosporin versus penicillin treatment of group A streptococcal tonsillopharyngitis in children. *Pediatrics.* 2004;113:866-882.
13. Johnston F, Carapetis J, Patel MS, et al. Evaluating the use of penicillin to control outbreaks of acute poststreptococcal glomerulonephritis. *Pediatr Infec Dis J.* 1999;18:327-332.
14. Sesso R, Pinto SWL. Five-year follow-up of patients with epidemic glomerulonephritis due to *Streptococcus zooepidemicus*. *Nephrol Dial Transplant.* 2005;20:1808-1813.
15. White AV, Hoy WE, McCredie DA. Childhood post-streptococcal glomerulonephritis as a risk for chronic renal disease in later life. *Med J Aust.* 2001;174:492-496.
16. Tlevjeh IM, Steckelberg JM, Murad HS, et al. Temporal trends in infective endocarditis: A population-based study in Olmsted County, Minnesota. *JAMA.* 2005;293:3022-3028.
17. Majumdar A, Chowdhary S, Ferreira MAAS, et al. Renal pathological findings in infective endocarditis. *Nephrol Dial Transplant.* 2000;15:1782-1787.
18. Fukuda M, Motokawa M, Usami T, et al. PR3-ANCA–positive crescentic necrotizing glomerulonephritis accompanied by isolated pulmonic valve infective endocarditis, with reference to previous reports of renal pathology. *Clin Nephrol.* 2006;66:202-209.
19. Badour LM, Wilson WR, Bayer AS, et al. Infective endocarditis. Diagnosis, antimicrobial therapy and management of complications. *Circulation.* 2005;111:3167-3184.
20. Koyama A, Kobayashi M, Yamaguchi N, et al. Glomerulonephritis associated with MRSA infection: A possible role of bacterial superantigen. *Kidney Int.* 1995;47:207-216.
21. Satoskar AA, Nadasdy G, Plaza JA, et al. *Staphylococcus* infection–associated glomerulonephritis mimicking IgA nephropathy. *Clin J Am Soc Nephrol.* 2006;1:1179-1186.
22. Nasr SH, Markowitz GS, Whelan JD, et al. IgA-dominant acute poststaphylococcal glomerulonephritis complicating diabetic nephropathy. *Hum Pathol.* 2003;34:1235-1241.
23. Koyama A, Sharmin S, Sakurai H, et al. *Staphylococcus aureus* cell envelope antigen is a new candidate for the induction of IgA nephropathy. *Kidney Int.* 2004;66:121-132.
24. Iwata Y, Ohta S, Kawai K, et al. Shunt nephritis with positive titers for ANCA specific for proteinase 3. *Am J Kidney Dis.* 2004;43:e11-e16.
25. Chugh KS, Sakhuja V. Glomerular disease in the tropics. *Am J Nephrol.* 1990;10:437-450.
26. Lomonte C, Chiarulli G, Cazzato F, et al. End-stage renal disease in leprosy. *J Nephrol.* 2004;17:302-305.
27. Lai ASH, Lai KN. Viral nephropathy. *Natur Clin Pract Nephrol.* 2006;2:254-262.
28. Johnson RJ, Couser WG. Hepatitis B infection and renal disease: Clinical, immunopathogenetic, and therapeutic considerations [editorial review]. *Kidney Int.* 1990;37:663-676.
29. Lai KN, Li PK, Lui SF, et al. Membranous nephropathy related to hepatitis B virus in adults. *N Engl J Med.* 1991;324:1457-1463.
30. Lau GK, Piratvisuth T, Luo KX, et al; Peginterferon Alfa-2a HBeAg-Positive Chronic Hepatitis B Study Group: Peginterferon alfa-2a, lamivudine, and the combination for HBeAg-positive chronic hepatitis B. *N Engl J Med.* 2005;352:2682-2695.
31. Pagnoux C, Cohen P, Guillevin L. Vaculitides secondary to infections. *Clin Exp Rheumatol.* 2006;24(Suppl 41):S71-S81.
32. Roccatello D, Fornasieri A, Giachino O, et al. Multicentric study on hepatitis C virus–related cryoglobulinemic glomerulonephritis. *Am J Kidney Dis.* 2007;49:69-82.
33. Alpers CE, Kowaleswska J. Emerging paradigms in renal pathology of viral diseases. *Clin J Am Soc Nephrol.* 2007;2:S6-S12.
34. Tomlinson L, Borskin Y, McPhee I, et al. Acute cytomegalovirus infection complicated by collapsing glomerulopathy. *Nephrol Dial Transplant.* 2003;18:187-189.
35. Waldman M, Kopp JB. Parvovirus B19 and the kidney. *Clin J Am Soc Nephrol.* 2007;2:S47-S56.
36. Barzon L, Murer L, Pacenti M, et al. Investigation of intrarenal viral infections in kidney transplant recipients unveils an association between parvovirus B19 and chronic allograft injury. *J Infect Dis.* 2009;199:372-380.
37. Barsoum RS. Malarial nephropathies. *Nephrol Dial Transplant.* 1998;13:1588-1597.
38. Okocha EC, Ibeh CC, Ele PU, Ibeh NC. The prevalence of malaria parasitaemia in blood donors in a Nigerian teaching hospital. *J Vector Borne Dis.* 2005;42:21-24.

39. Barsoum RS. Parasitic infections in transplant recipients. *Nat Clin Pract Nephrol*. 2006;2:490-503.
40. Rajapurkar MM. Renal involvement in malaria. *Trop Nephrol*. 1994; 40:132-134.
41. Ehrich JH, Eke FU. Malaria-induced renal damage: Facts and myths. *Pediatr Nephrol*. 2007;22:626-637.
42. Doe JY, Funk M, Mengel M, et al. Nephrotic syndrome in African children: Lack of evidence for "tropical nephrotic syndrome"? *Nephrol Dial Transplant*. 2006;21:672-676.
43. Ngu JL, Chatelanat F, Leke R. Nephropathy in Cameroon: Evidence for filarial derived immune complex pathogenesis in some cases. *Clin Nephrol*. 1985;24:128-132.

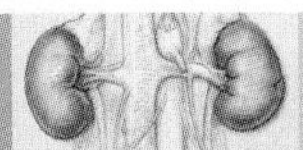

CHAPTER 56

Human Immunodeficiency Virus Infection and the Kidney

Jeffrey Kopp, June Fabian, Saraladevi Naicker

Human immunodeficiency virus (HIV) infection is the defining infectious disease of our era. In 2009, there were an estimated 33 million infected people and 2.5 million new infections; there have been 16 million deaths since the start of the epidemic, and there are 22 available antiretroviral medications. With regard to nephrologic issues, HIV-1 infection is associated with glomerular and tubulointerstitial disease, and patients with HIV infection are also at risk for nephrotoxicity from antiretroviral therapy (ART) as well as from other medications. Coinfections with other pathogens, in particular hepatitis B and hepatitis C viruses, can complicate the clinical picture. Acute kidney injury (AKI) and interstitial nephritis, due to medication and opportunistic infection, are not uncommon. As patients with HIV disease live longer with ART, patients are experiencing the complex, interacting effects of HIV infection itself, ART, and the worldwide diseases of development, including atherosclerosis, metabolic syndrome, type 2 diabetes, and end-stage renal disease (ESRD). Patients with HIV disease and chronic kidney disease (CKD) and ESRD, those receiving chronic dialysis therapy, and those undergoing kidney transplantation face particular issues and concerns.

In addition to HIV-1, HIV-2 can cause immunodeficiency but rarely causes kidney disease. In this chapter, we use HIV to stand for HIV-1.

HIV-ASSOCIATED KIDNEY DISEASE

General Approach

The evaluation of a patient with acute or chronic kidney disease in the setting of HIV infection resembles that in other settings: history, focused particularly on medication use and other infections; physical examination; examination of the urine sediment; serum and urine chemistries; and, in many cases, renal imaging studies. Urine chemistries may include 24-hour timed or spot urine measurement of protein and albumin (for suspected glomerular disease), glucose, phosphate, and uric acid (for suspected proximal tubular disease). Indications for kidney biopsy include AKI without clear associated cause, especially with a nephritic sediment; nephrotic proteinuria; clinical evidence of thrombotic microangiopathy; and unexplained CKD. In the past, some clinicians have argued that nephrotic proteinuria in an individual of African descent is likely to be HIV-associated collapsing glomerulopathy and that a biopsy is superfluous. Whether that once may have been true, the evolution of kidney diseases during the past decade with the widespread use of ART has rendered that judgment increasingly problematic, and it now appears more prudent to define the histologic features to guide prognosis and therapy.

GLOMERULAR DISORDERS

HIV-Associated Collapsing Glomerulopathy

HIV infection is associated with a number of glomerular disorders (Fig. 56.1). The classic glomerulopathy of HIV infection is collapsing glomerulopathy (CG). The pathologic changes were described in early reports as focal segmental glomerulosclerosis (FSGS) and more recently as HIV-associated nephropathy, but this latter term has also been used to describe other glomerular pathologic processes associated with HIV infection.

Etiology and Pathogenesis

There has been steady progress in deciphering how HIV infection results in injury to glomerular and tubular cells. HIV-associated CG occurs in both acute infection and chronic infection; in the latter case, it is associated with higher viral RNA levels and lower CD4 T-lymphocyte counts. It appears that HIV can infect glomerular and tubular cells, setting up a chronic and possibly latent infection.[1] There is also evidence that particular HIV accessory proteins damage renal cells, independent of direct infection. First, in transgenic mice, the expression of HIV-1 accessory protein Vpr or Nef in podocytes are associated with progressive CKD, leading to ESRD, loss of podocyte differentiation markers, and features suggestive of human CG and segmental glomerulosclerosis. Transgenic mouse experiments also suggest that HIV-1 gene products are toxic to tubular epithelial cells, resulting in apoptosis and a cytokinetic block. Second, Vpr and Nef proteins are toxic to cultured renal cells.

Host factors play a major role in determining susceptibility to HIV-associated CG. Individuals of African descent have a striking predilection for HIV-associated CG, with relative risk compared to individuals of European descent of approximately 20-fold. This predilection was originally identified as a consequence of variation in *MYH9*, encoding myosin heavy chain 9, a component of non-muscle myosin IIA. The *MYH9* risk haplotype contributes to risk for idiopathic FSGS (odds ratio 4) and HIV-associated CG (odds ratio 6). More recently, much of the risk attributed to MYH9 genetic variation has been shown to more closely associate with coding-region polymorphisms in APOL1 (encoding apolipoprotein L1), which is in close linkage disequilibrium with MYH9 polymorphisms. Apolipoprotein L1 is a constituent of high density lipoprotein. It remains unknown whether these APOL1 polymorphisms cause chronic kidney disease, and by what molecular mechanism. Nevertheless, homozygosity or dual heterozygosity for two risk alleles (labeled G1 and G2) are observed in 50% of African Americans with HIV-associated CG, compared to only 12% of African American control subjects. Interestingly, these variants appear to protect

Kidney Diseases Associated with HIV Infection

	Entity	Frequency	Associations
Glomerular	Collapsing glomerulopathy	Common	African descent; particularly advanced HIV disease
	Immune complex glomerulonephritis	Common	European, Asian descent, and black Africans in Africa
	Thrombotic microangiopathy	Uncommon	
	Membranoproliferative glomerulonephritis, with or without cryoglobulin-associated vasculitis	Rare*	Hepatitis C; enfuvirtide
	Membranous nephropathy	Rare*	Hepatitis B
	Fibrillary and immunotactoid glomerulopathies	Rare*	
	Amyloid nephropathy (AA type)	Rare*	
	Minimal change nephropathy	Rare*	Non-steroidal anti-inflammatory medication
Tubular	Acute kidney injury	Moderately common	Aminoglycosides, cidovofir, foscarnet
	Proximal tubule injury (Fanconi syndrome)	Moderately common	Tenofovir, adefovir, cidofovir, didanosine
	Diabetes insipidus	Uncommon	Amphotericin, tenofovir, didanosine, abacavir
	Chronic tubular injury	Moderately common	Amphotericin, cidofovir, adefovir, tenofovir
	Crystal nephropathy	Uncommon	Indinavir, atazanavir; sulfadiazine, ciprofloxacin, intravenous acyclovir
Interstitial	Interstitial nephritis	Uncommon	Allergy to beta-lactam, sulfa, ciprofloxacin rifampin, proton pump inhibitor, allopurinol, phenytoin; also causes of crystal nephropathy listed above BK virus; generally advanced disease Immune reconstitution inflammatory syndrome; generally advanced disease; following initiation of ART

Figure 56.1 Kidney diseases associated with HIV infection. Shown are diseases that are associated with HIV infection or its treatment. *Certain glomerular diseases are commonly associated with other viral infections or may occur on an idiopathic basis; a true association with HIV disease is uncertain or doubtful. Collapsing glomerulopathy is notable for glomerular, tubular, and interstitial disease but is classified under glomerular disease for simplicity. ART, antiretroviral therapy.

individuals from African sleeping sickness due to Trypanosoma brucei rhodesiense, and this may explain apparently rapid spread of these alleles in certain African populations that has occurred during the past 10,000 years.[2,3]

Clinical Manifestations

Patients with HIV-associated CG typically present with laboratory abnormalities, including proteinuria and renal insufficiency; some patients present with edema, although edema is less common than with other nephrotic conditions or with uremia. Imaging studies may reveal increased kidney size despite reduced glomerular filtration rate (GFR) and, in some cases, increased echogenicity; this unusual feature is shared with diabetic nephropathy and amyloid nephropathy. However, no radiologic features predict the renal histology, and renal biopsy is required for diagnosis.

Pathology

On histologic examination, HIV-associated CG is virtually indistinguishable from idiopathic CG and is a pan-nephropathy, with pathologic changes in the glomeruli (proliferation and dysregulation of podocytes or podocyte stem cells, together with glomerular collapse), tubules (acute and chronic injury, sometimes with microcystic tubular changes), and interstitium (chronic inflammation, fibrosis) (Fig. 56.2). Both HIV-associated CG and idiopathic CG may manifest tubuloreticular inclusions within dilated endosomal compartments within glomerular endothelial cells, which is believed to be a marker for cytokine (interferon) injury. Some pathologists make the diagnosis of classic FSGS in the setting of HIV infection, and others see this rarely; it is unclear whether these differences are due to population differences or to different diagnostic standards in distinguishing FSGS from CG. It may also be that in a patient with progressive loss of kidney function (e.g., from hypertensive nephrosclerosis or interstitial nephritis), the consequent glomerular hyperperfusion and hyperfiltration lead to glomerulomegaly and postadaptive FSGS.

Diagnosis and Differential Diagnosis

The diagnosis of glomerular disease is made by renal biopsy showing classic changes of HIV-associated CG. Among individuals of African descent, nephrotic proteinuria and low CD4 count suggest the diagnosis of HIV-associated CG; plasma HIV RNA of less than 400 copies/ml suggests that another disease is more likely. Potential diagnoses include hypertensive nephrosclerosis, diabetic nephropathy, and HIV-related immune

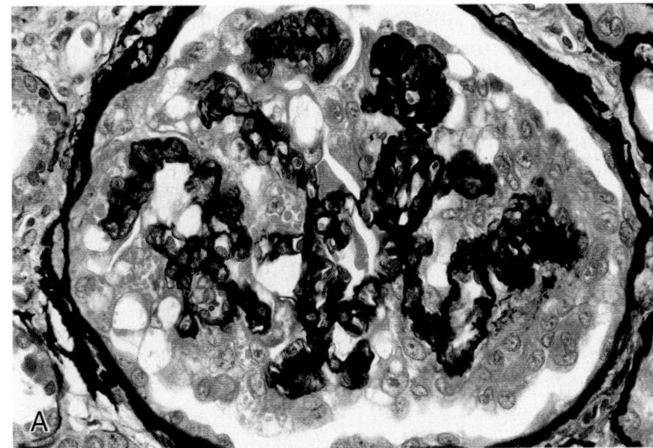

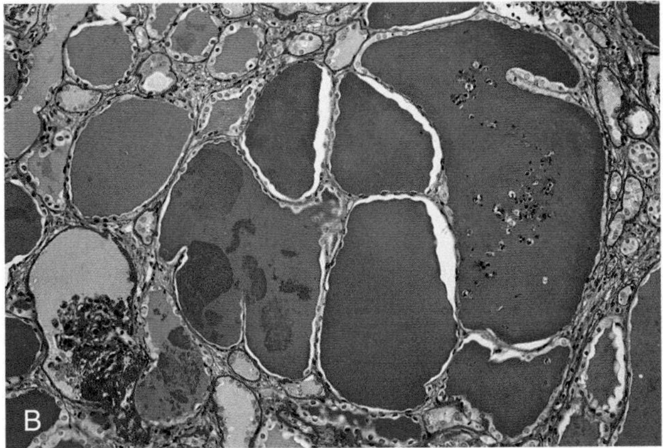

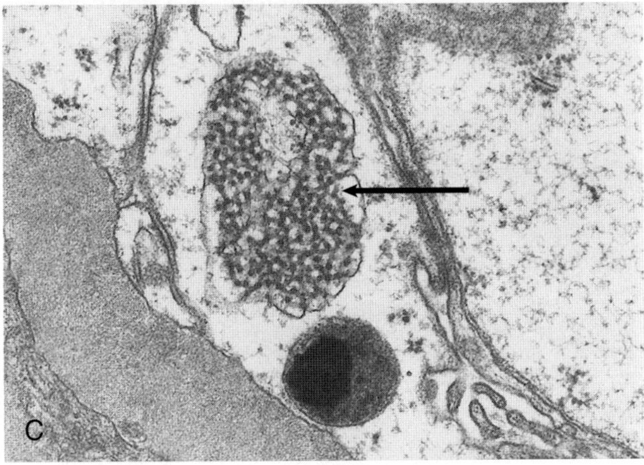

Figure 56.2 HIV-associated collapsing glomerulopathy. Typical histology in HIV-associated collapsing glomerulopathy (CG), often termed HIV-associated nephropathy. **A,** A globally collapsed glomerulus shows marked podocyte hypertrophy and hyperplasia (Jones methenamine silver). **B,** At low power, the renal parenchyma contains abundant tubular microcysts with proteinaceous casts. The glomerulus is collapsed with dilated urinary space (periodic acid–Schiff). **C,** The glomerular endothelial cell pictured here contains a large intracytoplasmic tubuloreticular inclusion ("interferon footprint"; arrow) composed of interanastomosing tubular structures within a dilated cisterna of endoplasmic reticulum (electron micrograph).

complex glomerulonephritis (ICGN) (see later discussion and Fig. 56.1).

Treatment

Current treatment guidelines suggest that the diagnosis of HIV-associated nephropathy is an indication for the initiation of ART in patients who are not currently receiving these medications and is not influenced by T-lymphocyte count.[4] It would seem reasonable to extend this recommendation to HIV-associated ICGN, but there are no systematic data that address this point.

There are several lines of evidence supporting a recommendation to use ART. In patients who are not receiving ART, the course of disease progression in HIV-associated CG may be fast, with patients reaching ESRD in months to a few years. By contrast, epidemiologic data (the decline in HIV-associated ESRD in the United States after the introduction of ART in 1995) suggest that effective control of viral replication with ART can prevent the appearance of HIV-associated CG. Retrospective studies suggest that the institution of ART after the diagnosis of HIV-associated CG may prolong renal survival.[5] A Ugandan study has demonstrated improvement of kidney function after 2 years of ART, but long-term outcomes are awaited.[6] Progression of CKD is more rapid in HIV-infected individuals of African descent, probably reflecting a racial predilection.[7] This is of particular relevance to the African population in sub-Saharan Africa that has the highest prevalence rates of HIV infection. Further support for screening has come from observations that ART improves renal outcome, preferably when it is initiated before the onset of severe renal disease[8-10]; the approach to CKD screening is discussed later. There are isolated case reports of improvement of renal function and, in some cases, regression of histologic lesions with ART.[10,11] For ethical reasons, a randomized control trial of this hypothesis has not and will not be undertaken.

Treatment of HIV-associated renal disease includes general and specific measures. Standard therapies for CKD are likely to be effective, including control of blood pressure to below 130/80 mm Hg and the use of angiotensin-converting enzyme (ACE) inhibitors or angiotensin receptor blockers (ARBs). Nonrandomized studies suggest benefit from these interventions, but randomized controlled studies have not been performed. Nonetheless, treatment guidelines prepared by the panel brought together by the National Institutes of Health suggest that one indication for initiation of ART is HIV-associated CG.[12] Several nonrandomized studies have suggested a benefit from corticosteroid therapy, but because the efficacy appears to be modest and often short-lived, this is not considered standard therapy.

HIV-Associated Immune Complex Glomerulonephritis

In populations of European and Asian ancestry, the most common glomerular disease associated with HIV disease is immune complex glomerulonephritis (ICGN); this is true among developed countries (e.g., European Union) and developing countries (e.g., Thailand). Importantly, HIV-associated ICGN is also seen in populations of African descent.[13] The pathogenesis of HIV-associated ICGN is not well understood. In some cases, immune complexes have been shown to include HIV antigen. It may be that other cases are due to the general polyclonal B-cell expansion that accompanies HIV disease. Clinically, these patients typically present with nephrotic proteinuria and hematuria and thus may be clinically indistinguishable from those with HIV-associated CG. On histologic examination, the glomeruli show diffuse or focal proliferative glomerulonephritis (GN) with endocapillary proliferation. In some cases, changes consistent with HIV-associated CG may also be present. Immune deposits are characterized by IgG and IgM or by IgG, IgM, and IgA (so-called full house deposits), often with C3. These forms resemble lupus nephritis, although lupus serologic test results are typically negative. Patients who have coinfection with hepatitis C virus (HCV) may manifest membranoproliferative glomerulonephritis (MPGN), with double glomerular capillary basement membrane contours. Other patients may have only IgA deposits, in the setting of microscopic hematuria and (typically) subnephrotic proteinuria, resembling idiopathic IgA nephropathy. The long-term outcome of HIV-associated ICGN has not been well defined but in general is believed to be relatively benign in most cases. There are few studies of therapy; presumably, control of HIV infection and conservative measures to control blood pressure and proteinuria are indicated.

TUBULAR DISORDERS

HIV infection is associated with a number of tubular disorders, many of which are secondary to various drugs commonly used in this disease (see Fig. 56.1).[14] AKI, as defined by the AIDS Clinical Trials Group, occurs with a creatinine concentration below 1.5 mg/dl or an increase of 1.3-fold that resolves within 3 months.[15] Most HIV-associated AKI occurs outside hospitals; major causes include prerenal impairment, postrenal impairment (including obstruction due to prostate disease, kidney stone, or crystalluria), medication toxicity (including interstitial nephritis due to antibiotics or indinavir, tubular injury due to tenofovir or other agents, and statin-associated rhabdomyolysis), and less commonly acute presentations of glomerular diseases. Risk factors reported in one or more cohorts have included male sex, black race, low CD4 count, high viral load, diabetes, CKD, and hepatic disease.[16]

Proximal tubular injury is moderately common, manifested as various combinations of glycosuria, phosphaturia (sometimes associated with clinically significant hypophosphatemia), uricosuria, proteinuria, and aminoaciduria. Diabetes insipidus may also be present, indicating that the distal nephron is also involved. The most common cause is tenofovir, which is taken up by proximal tubular cells by one or more organic anion transporters and is believed to impair mitochondrial function and also to inhibit DNA repair or replication. A mild decrease in GFR has also been associated with tenofovir use, but it was not severe enough for treatment to be discontinued.[17] Whereas three controlled studies have suggested minimal nephrotoxicity (perhaps 1%) when tenofovir is used for periods up to 48 weeks, a growing number of case series suggest that some patients manifest tubular injury that resolves during a period of months to years.[18] This apparent incongruity may be explained by the use of tenofovir in clinical practice in patients with other renal injury risk factors and by its frequent long-term use. Risk factors for tenofovir-induced renal toxicity include prior renal impairment and possibly combined therapy with didanosine.

Other protease inhibitors are also associated with variable risk for nephrotoxicity (Fig. 56.3). Nucleotide and nucleoside reverse transcriptase inhibitors (NRTIs) are associated with variable effects on tubular function. Besides the renal effects with tenofovir, the most common renal toxicities are seen with indinavir, which is associated with crystalluria, nephrolithiasis, or AKI (see Fig. 56.3). Although there have been cases of AKI, most of these case reports have been associated with multiple compounding factors (sepsis, concomitant nephrotoxic agents), and most are reversible.[17] Lopinavir and ritonavir may increase plasma

Renal Toxicity of Antiviral Therapy

Antiretroviral Class	Antiretroviral Therapy	Renal Effect	Clinical Recommendations
Protease Inhibitors	Indinavir	Nephrolithiasis, crystalluria, dysuria, papillary necrosis, acute kidney injury, interstitial nephritis Ritonavir and lopinavir may increase toxicity of indinavir	Daily fluid intake of >2 l/day
	Ritonavir	Reversible AKI (usually in combination with nephrotoxic drugs)	
	Saquinavir, nelfinavir	Renal calculi (rare)	Increased fluid intake
Reverse Transcriptase Inhibitors	Tenofovir, abacavir	Renal tubular damage: proximal tubular dysfunction, Fanconi syndrome, nephrogenic diabetes insipidus, acute tubular necrosis, AKI	Patients taking tenofovir should be monitored for signs of tubular dysfunction (elevated serum creatinine, hypophosphatemia, low serum uric acid, acidosis glycosuria, proteinuria)
	Didanosine, lamivudine, stavudine	Isolated case reports of tubular dysfunction	
Other	Cidofovir, adefovir	Renal tubular damage, proximal tubular dysfunction (cidofovir)	

Figure 56.3 Renal toxicity of antiviral therapy. The toxicity of these agents has been the subject of a recent review. *(From reference 17.)*

concentrations of tenofovir by 30%. NRTIs have a good renal safety profile.[17] Non-nucleoside reverse transcriptase inhibitors (NNRTIs) also have a good safety profile, with an isolated case report of AKI from interstitial nephritis due to a hypersensitivity reaction to efavirenz. The fusion inhibitor enfuvirtide has been associated with an isolated case report of MPGN in a diabetic patient.

CHRONIC KIDNEY DISEASE AND END-STAGE RENAL DISEASE IN THE PATIENT WITH HIV INFECTION

Epidemiology

The Developed World

Since the advent of highly active ART in 1996, increasing numbers of patients with HIV disease are receiving therapy, dramatically increasing the life span of patients and turning the disease into a chronic condition. This has been associated with an evolution in the pattern of renal disease. Early in the epidemic, the leading renal diagnoses included HIV-associated CG in individuals of African descent and ICGN associated with either IgA or all immunoglobulins in other individuals. In recent years, the range of common diagnoses has expanded to include diabetic nephropathy (DN) and hypertensive nephrosclerosis. In those with hepatitis, membranous nephropathy (MN) associated with hepatitis B and MPGN associated with hepatitis C should be considered. Uncommon but important diagnoses include MN (presumably idiopathic, but possibly related to the polyclonal B-cell expansion typical of HIV disease) and amyloid. Chronic tubular injury, especially associated with tenofovir therapy but possibly associated with other ART, is not uncommon; but when early diagnosis leads to cessation of the offending medication, CKD is usually averted. Despite the plethora of diagnoses, HIV-associated CG remains the leading cause of ESRD in patients with HIV disease.

The incidence of HIV-associated ESRD, typically not histologically examined by the United States Renal Data System, has remained relatively constant in the United States during the past decade, but the prevalence has risen because of increased survival of patients on dialysis. During the period 1995 to 2000, the number of *prevalent* ESRD cases in HIV-seropositive individuals rose by 159%, accounting for 1.2% of prevalent ESRD patients (this includes all individuals in the United States receiving dialysis or with a functioning renal allograft). In 2000, among *incident* ESRD cases, 851 (0.88%) were attributed to HIV-associated kidney disease, and another 320 cases (0.33%) were in HIV-seropositive individuals but attributed to other causes (the accuracy of the assessment of the cause of ESRD is unknown, as kidney biopsies may not be performed). In 2006, the annual incidence rate of ESRD attributed to HIV-associated renal disease for individuals of African descent, adjusted for age and sex, was 22 cases/million compared with 0.35 case/million among individuals of European descent, representing a relative risk of 63.[19] During the same period, first-year mortality for HIV-associated ESRD patients starting ESRD therapy, unadjusted for age, was 32%, which is higher than for ESRD patients as a group (24%). The prevalence rates are quite similar in France, where 0.6% of ESRD cases were HIV-positive during the period 2002 to 2004. Compared with the U.S. data, individuals had a more favorable 2-year patient survival rate of 89%, similar to that of other ESRD patients.[20]

The Developing World

More than two thirds of the total HIV-infected population in the world live in sub-Saharan Africa, and the majority infected are women (61%). Within the region, southern Africa is the worst affected, with the national adult HIV prevalence exceeding 15% in eight southern African countries from 2005. Transmission of HIV infection is largely heterosexual contact in most of the region. Only 30% of HIV-infected individuals have access to ART in Africa. Sub-Saharan Africa has a dearth of data describing the impact of HIV infection on the kidney, and renal histologic studies are scant. Access to renal replacement therapy (RRT) is also frequently limited. Reported prevalence of CKD has been assessed by the presence of albuminuria or (eGFR) (based on serum creatinine measurements) and ranges widely from 6% to 45%. This wide variation may be partly ascribed to differences in study design, populations studied, and definitions used for CKD based on dipstick proteinuria and quantitative measure of proteinuria or serum creatinine.

In terms of etiology, some studies have shown HIV-associated CG to be present in more than 80% of kidney biopsy specimens, which is consistent with findings in the United States, but others show a broader spectrum of disease, including ICGN due to postinfectious and other causes, MN and interstitial nephritis. There are nonspecific histologic changes, such as mesangial hyperplasia and chronic active interstitial nephritis, that do not necessarily fulfill the diagnostic criteria for HIV-associated CG but show regression on ART, which suggests that the histologic criteria for HIV-associated CKD may need to be revised.[21-23]

A significant response of HIV-associated CKD to ART has been shown, with the median eGFR improving by 21% after 2 years on ART.[6] The presence of kidney dysfunction, in the setting of HIV infection, acts as an independent predictor of poor outcome, with an increased mortality after 90 days.[24]

There are few data on the worldwide prevalence of CKD in HIV infection. In a cross-sectional study from 31 European countries, Israel, and Argentina, CKD (defined as an eGFR of ≤60 ml/min per 1.73 m^2) was present in 4.7% of HIV-infected subjects by use of the Modification of Diet in Renal Disease (MDRD) formula. A study from Hong Kong showed CKD (defined as eGFR ≤60 ml/min per 1.73 m^2 or proteinuria for more than 3 months) in 18% of HIV-infected Chinese patients, but this study excluded those with ESRD. Isolated screening studies with relatively small numbers using persistent proteinuria as a marker of CKD have been done in various countries with the following prevalence rates: 1.1% to 5.6% in Brazil, 18% in Switzerland, 27% in India, and 20% in Iran.

Dosing of Antiretroviral Therapy in Chronic Kidney Disease

Many antiretroviral medications are partially or completely eliminated by the kidney and require dose adjustment in CKD (Fig. 56.4). Certain drug classes, such as the protease inhibitors and the NNRTIs, are extensively metabolized by the liver and do not require dose adjustment.[25] Most of the NRTIs are excreted unchanged in the urine and require dose adjustment, with the exception of zidovudine and abacavir, which both have substantial extrarenal biotransformation that requires less or no dose adjustment. In uremia, drug dosing may be affected by altered gastric pH and variable volumes of distribution.[26] Factors that influence dialyzability of antiretroviral medications relate to the properties of the dialysis membrane and molecular weight,

Dose Adjustments for ART in CKD and ESRD			
Name	**CKD (adjusted according to creatinine clearance or by eGFR)**		**Dialysis**
Nucleoside or nucleotide analogues			
Abacavir	No adjustment		No adjustment HD: dosing independent of dialysis sessions
Azidothymidine (AZT), zidovudine[a]	CrCl ≥ 15 ml/min: no adjustment CrCl <15 ml/min: 100 mg PO q6-8h		HD:100 mg PO q6-8h[a] or 300 mg PO qd PD: no data
Didanosine (ddi)	Weight >60 kg CrCl 30-59 ml/min: 200 mg PO qd CrCl 10-29 ml/min: 150 mg PO qd CrCl <10 ml/min: 125 mg PO qd	Weight <60 kg 150 mg PO qd 100 mg PO qd 75 mg PO qd	Dose for CrCl <10 ml/min[b] HD, PD: same dose
Emtricitabine[d]	CrCl >50 ml/min: no adjustment CrCl 30-49 ml/min: 200 mg PO q48h CrCl 15-29 ml/min: 200 mg PO q72h CrCl <15 ml/min: 200 mg PO q96h		HD:200 mg PO q96h[b] PD: no data
Lamivudine[a] (3TC)	CrCl >50 ml/min: no adjustment CrCl 30-49 ml/min: 150 mg PO qd CrCl 15-29 ml/min: 150 mg first dose, then 100 mg PO qd CrCl 5-14 ml/min: 150 mg first dose, then 50 mg PO qd CrCl <5 ml/min: 50 mg first dose, then 25 mg PO qd		HD:50 mg first dose, then 25 mg PO qd[b]
Stavudine (d4T)	CrCl >50 ml/min: no adjustment CrCl 26-50 ml/min: 15-20 mg PO bid CrCl ≤25 ml/min: 15-20 mg PO qd		20 mg PO qd[b] PD: has been used safely
Tenofovir[d]	CrCl >50 ml/min: no adjustment CrCl 30-49 ml/min: 300 mg q48h CrCl 10-29 ml/min: 300 mg q72h		300 mg PO every 7 days[b]
Zalcitabine	CrCl ≥40 ml/min: no adjustment CrCl 10-40 ml/min: 0.75 mg q12h CrCl <10 ml/min: 0.75 mg q24h		HD: dose for CrCl <10 ml/min[b] PD: no data
Non-nucleoside reverse transcriptase inhibitors[c]	No adjustment		
Protease inhibitors[c]	No adjustment		No adjustment
Entry or fusion inhibitor	CrCl ≥35 ml/min: no adjustment		Unknown, use with caution
Enfuvirtide	CrCl <35 ml/min: unknown, use with caution		
CCR5 antagonist	No dosage recommendations		No data
Maraviroc	Patients with CrCl <50 ml/min should receive maraviroc and CYP3A inhibitor only if potential benefit outweighs the risk		
Integrase inhibitor[c]	No adjustment		No adjustment
Raltegravir			

[a] Combination AZT/lamivudine tablets (300mg/150mg) should be administered separately when eGFR<50ml/min
[b] Defer daily dose/s after hemodialysis (extraction of drug occurs on dialysis)
[c] No dose adjustment necessary for any drug from this class in patients with renal dysfunction, hemodialysis or pertoneal dialysis
[d] Combination emtricitabine/tenofovir tablets (200 mg/300 mg): if CrCl 30–49 ml/min: 1 tablet po q48h; if CrCl <30 ml/min the combination tablet should not be prescribed

Figure 56.4 Dose adjustments for ART in CKD and ESRD. FDA recommendations are based on CrCl or eGRF calculated as ml/min, but are likely valid for these expressed as ml/min per 1.73 m^2. Atripla (efavirenz, tenofovir, and emtricitabine is not recommended for CrCl < 5 ml/min. CrCl, creatinine clearance; HD, hemodialysis; PD, peritoneal dialysis.

degree of protein binding, molecular charge, and water solubility of the drug. If removal of the drug occurs during hemodialysis (HD), it should be taken after dialysis. If the drug is removed in peritoneal dialysis (PD) effluent, the dose may have to supplemented.[26] Dosing recommendations in both HD and PD are limited by the lack of reliable data. Fixed drug combinations should not be used in patients with eGFR below 30 to 50 ml/min.[25]

RENAL REPLACEMENT THERAPY IN THE PATIENT WITH HIV INFECTION

With the increasing survival of HIV-infected patients with treatment and the declining cost of ART, the magnitude of HIV-associated ESRD will likely increase worldwide, as it has in developed countries.[27] Life expectancy in HIV infection with ART has increased by 10 to 20 years in developed countries, and many of these patients are now dying of the complications of ESRD rather than of HIV infection. Currently, HIV-infected subjects requiring either HD or PD, who are stable on ART, are achieving survival rates comparable to those of dialysis patients without HIV infection, and choice of dialysis modality does not have an impact on survival.

Immunization schedules are the same as for non–HIV-infected dialysis patients and should include vaccinations for *Streptococcus pneumoniae*, influenza virus, hepatitis A, and hepatitis B.[15] In both CKD and HIV infection, the presence of anemia is independently associated with shorter survival. The response to recombinant erythropoietin (EPO) in HIV-infected patients with ESRD was similar to that in HIV-negative patients.[28] Measurements of iron indices are complicated in HIV-infected patients, especially as levels of ferritin are often elevated in patients with HIV infection.

Hemodialysis

Strict use of universal precautions is the best form of prevention of HIV transmission in dialysis units. HIV-infected patients do not have to be isolated from other patients or dialyzed on separate machines. Reprocessing of dialyzers from HIV-positive patients should not place staff members at increased risk for infection if necessary sterile precautions are undertaken. The risk of HIV seroconversion after a needle stick injury from an infected patient is estimated to be about 0.3%. Art may reduce the risk of transmission following a needle-stick injury and should be considered under certain circumstances, as recommended by the Centers for Disease Control and Prevention. Native arteriovenous fistulas are the preferred types of access because of excellent patency once established and lower complication rates compared with those associated with other access options.

Peritoneal Dialysis

HIV has been shown to survive in peritoneal effluents at room temperature for up to 7 days and in PD exchange tubing for up to 48 hours. Dialysate should therefore be handled as a contaminated body fluid.[29] Sodium hypochlorite (50% solution) and household bleach (10% solution), each further diluted 1:512, are effective at killing HIV in dialysate. PD patients should be instructed to pour dialysate into the home toilet and to dispose of dialysate bags and lines by tying them in plastic bags and disposing of the plastic bags in conventional home garbage.[15,30]

Kidney Transplantation

Kidney transplantation has been performed with success in HIV-infected patients. Preliminary short-term data in liver, kidney, and heart transplant recipients suggest that patient survival rates are similar to those of HIV-uninfected transplant recipients, and there has been no increase in the prevalence of opportunistic infection.[31] In spite of high rates of acute graft rejection, survival appears to be similar to that of HIV-uninfected recipients. In areas with high endemic rates of HIV infection, it has been proposed that HIV-infected cadaveric donor organs may be transplanted into HIV-infected recipients with ESRD.[32] Four such transplantations have been performed with good graft and recipient survival, but the data are preliminary.

SCREENING FOR CHRONIC KIDNEY DISEASE

As noted before, treatment of HIV-associated CG, and possibly HIV-associated ICGN, may slow progression of renal functional decline. Limited studies suggest that creatinine clearance and the eGFR equation provide suitable estimates of true GFR. Microalbuminuria may indicate early glomerular disease (diabetes, hypertensive nephrosclerosis, HIV-associated glomerular disease), tubular disease (drug toxicity), metabolic syndrome, or systemic inflammation. Its role in diagnosis and screening in the setting of HIV infection remains to be determined.

Patients with HIV disease are at increased risk for CKD and should receive regular screening. A committee of the Infectious Diseases Society of America has laid out a proposal for screening.[15] Support for screening has come from published data confirming that CKD in HIV infection is common, can occur at any stage of HIV infection (even before seroconversion), and can progress rapidly to ESRD if it is untreated.

The role of microalbuminuria in the natural history of HIV-associated CKD and screening is an area of active investigation. Microalbuminuria is associated with an increased risk of cardiovascular disease and mortality in certain well-defined high-risk settings, such as diabetes and hypertension. Han and colleagues[21] found that six of seven South African patients with persistent microalbuminuria had HIV-associated CG; these findings tell us that HIV-associated CG can present insidiously, at a stage when therapy may slow its progression. Nevertheless, these patients were ART naive, and this HIV-infected population may lack the high prevalence of diabetes, hypertension, and drug-induced renal toxicity that characterizes patients with HIV disease in developed countries. Szczech and colleagues[33] found microalbuminuria in 11% of patients with HIV disease compared with 2% of control subjects; the presence of microalbuminuria was associated with insulin resistance, systolic hypertension, and advanced HIV disease characterized by a low CD4 count. Whether this association predicts increased risk of cardiovascular disease and mortality in HIV disease needs to be investigated.

Screening, early detection, and treatment of HIV-associated CKD are strongly recommended (Fig. 56.5). In the algorithm, management of leukocyturia, in addition to proteinuria, has been included as it occurs commonly and the presence of sterile pyuria may be associated with comorbid disease. Urinary screening is inexpensive and easy to perform and to interpret, provided guidelines are given to staff at the primary health care level to initiate treatment, to investigate, and, if necessary, to refer. Effective screening programs are more realistic in resource-limited developing countries when the alternative is

Management Algorithm for Screening of HIV-Infected Antiretroviral Therapy-Naive Patients for Chronic Kidney Disease

Assessment for kidney disease in all HIV-infected individuals at presentation.
Risk factors: race, family history of CKD, use of nephrotoxic agents (including traditional medicines), diabetes mellitus, hepatitis C, HIV viral load >4000 copies/ml, CD4 count <200 cells mm^3.
Investigations: urine dipstick and serum creatinine, calculate eGFR (see Chapter 3).

↓

Urine dipstick for leukocytes.
If leukocytes or nitrites present: urine microscopy and culture.
UTI symptoms: treat empirically; adjust treatment according to culture results if indicated.
Sterile pyuria: exclude STI (including syphilis) and tuberculosis
Repeat urine dipstick at follow-up visit.

↓

Urine dipstick for proteinuria
If negative, test for microalbuminuria (see Chapters 29 and 76). If no proteinuria or microalbuminuria, repeat screen in 12 months in those at risk for development of CKD.

↓

Proteinuria or microalbuminuria: exclude potential causes of proteinuria: fever, infection (UTI, STI, tuberculosis), pregnancy, uncontrolled diabetes, uncontrolled hypertension, cardiac failure.
Treat comorbid conditions: repeat urine dipstick in 1 month.
If nephrotic, nephritic, or nephritic/nephrotic: refer for investigation and management.
Start ART.

↓

At follow-up: In patients with persistent proteinuria (random protein/creatinine ratio ≥2g/g) or MDRD eGFR <60 ml/min per 1.73 m^2, investigate with kidney ultrasound, serologic testing for hepatitis C and B, *Plasmodium malariae* (if appropriate, depending on infections endemic to the region), autoimmune screen. In patients with persistent microalbuminuria (random albumin/creatinine 17–250 mg/g in men, 25-355 mg/g in women), it is prudent to consider whether diabetic nephropathy might be present (an indication for ACE or ARB) and in other patients, to evaluate regulary for the appearance of macroproteinuria or reduced GFR.

Refer to a nephrologist, if available.

↓

If unable to refer: ART: adjust dose according to eGFR.
If still proteinuric after 3 months on ART: start antiproteinuric agents (see Chapter 76).
K^+ <5.0 mmol/l: ACE inhibitor or ARB and check K+ in 1 week.
K^+ >5.0 mmol/l: potassium-binding resin or use of nondihydropyridine calcium channel blocker: verapamil or diltiazem.
Manage stage of CKD appropriately (see Chapter 76).

Figure 56.5 Management algorithm for screening of HIV-infected antiretroviral therapy–naive patients for chronic kidney disease. Tuberculosis may be pulmonary or extrapulmonary. ACE, angiotensin-converting enzyme; ARB, angiotensin II receptor blocker; ART, antiretroviral therapy; CKD, chronic kidney disease; eGFR, estimated glomerular filtration rate, calculated by the Cockcroft-Gault formula or the modified MDRD formula; STI, sexually transmitted infection; UTI, urinary tract infection. Antiproteinuric agents may be used in normotensive individuals with gradual up-titration of dose, depending on tolerance and severity of proteinuria.

considered, which is that access to RRT is extremely limited and progression of CKD to ESRD is ultimately fatal for most patients.

REFERENCES

1. Bruggeman LA, Ross MD, Tanji N, et al. Renal epithelium is a previously unrecognized site of HIV-1 infection. *J Am Soc Nephrol.* 2000;11:2079-2087.
2. Genovese G, Friedman DJ, Ross MD, et al. Association of Trypanolytic ApoL1 Variants with Kidney Disease in African-Americans. *Science.* 2010 Jul 15. [Epub ahead of print]
3. Tzur S, Rosset S, Shemer R, et al. Missense mutations in the APOL1 gene are highly associated with end stage kidney disease risk previously attributed to the MYH9 gene. *Hum Genet.* 2010 Jul 16. [Epub ahead of print]
4. Hayabuchi Y, Inoue M, Watanabe N, et al. Assessment of systemic-pulmonary collateral arteries in children with cyanotic congenital heart disease using multidetector-row computed tomography: Comparison with conventional angiography. *Int J Cardiol.* 2008 Sep 12 [Epub ahead of print].
5. Atta MG, Gallant JE, Rahman MH, et al. Antiretroviral therapy in the treatment of HIV-associated nephropathy. *Nephrol Dial Transplant.* 2006;21:2809-2813.
6. Peters PJ, Moore DM, Mermin J, et al. Antiretroviral therapy improves renal function among HIV-infected Ugandans. *Kidney Int.* 2008;74:925-929.

7. Lucas GM, Lau B, Atta MG, et al. Chronic kidney disease incidence, and progression to end-stage renal disease, in HIV-infected individuals: a tale of two races. *J Infect Dis*. 2008;197:1548-1557.
8. Ifudu O, Rao TK, Tan CC, et al. Zidovudine is beneficial in human immunodeficiency virus associated nephropathy. *Am J Nephrol*. 1995; 15:217-221.
9. Michel C, Dosquet P, Ronco P, et al. Nephropathy associated with infection by human immunodeficiency virus: a report on 11 cases including 6 treated with zidovudine. *Nephron*. 1992;62:434-440.
10. Winston JA, Burns GC, Klotman PE. Treatment of HIV-associated nephropathy. *Semin Nephrol*. 2000;20:293-298.
11. Pope SD, Johnson MD, May DB. Pharmacotherapy for human immunodeficiency virus–associated nephropathy. *Pharmacotherapy*. 2005;25: 1761-1772.
12. Panel on Antiretroviral Guidelines for Adults and Adolescents Guidelines for the use of antiretroviral agents in HIV-1–infected adults and adolescents. Department of Health and Human Services. December 1, 2009.
13. Haas M, Kaul S, Eustace JA. HIV-associated immune complex glomerulonephritis with "lupus-like" features: a clinicopathologic study of 14 cases. *Kidney Int*. 2005;67:1381-1390.
14. Fine DM, Perazella MA, Lucas GM, Atta MG. Kidney biopsy in HIV: beyond HIV-associated nephropathy. *Am J Kidney Dis*. 2008;51: 504-514.
15. Gupta SK, Eustace JA, Winston JA, et al. Guidelines for the management of chronic kidney disease in HIV-infected patients: recommendations of the HIV Medicine Association of the Infectious Diseases Society of America. *Clin Infect Dis*. 2005;40:1559-1585.
16. Cohen SD, Chawla LS, Kimmel PL. Acute kidney injury in patients with human immunodeficiency virus infection. *Curr Opin Crit Care*. 2008;14:647-653.
17. Roling J, Schmid H, Fischereder M, et al. HIV-associated renal diseases and highly active antiretroviral therapy–induced nephropathy. *Clin Infect Dis*. 2006;42:1488-1495.
18. Szczech LA. Renal dysfunction and tenofovir toxicity in HIV-infected patients. *Top HIV Med*. 2008;16:122-126.
19. USRDS 2006 Annual Data Report. *Atlas of End-Stage Renal Disease in the United States*. Bethesda, Md: U.S. Renal Data System; 2006.
20. Tourret J, Tostivint I, du Montcel ST, et al. Outcome and prognosis factors in HIV-infected hemodialysis patients. *Clin J Am Soc Nephrol*. 2006;1:1241-1247.
21. Han TM, Naicker S, Ramdial PK, Assounga AG. A cross-sectional study of HIV-seropositive patients with varying degrees of proteinuria in South Africa. *Kidney Int*. 2006;69:2243-2250.
22. Fabian J. *Proteinuria in HIV seropositive individuals [Master of Medicine thesis]*. University of Witwatersrand, Johannesburg, 2008.
23. Gerntholtz TE, Goetsch SJ, Katz I. HIV-related nephropathy: a South African perspective. *Kidney Int*. 2006;69:1885-1891.
24. Mulenga LB, Kruse G, Lakhi S, et al. Baseline renal insufficiency and risk of death among HIV-infected adults on antiretroviral therapy in Lusaka, Zambia. *AIDS*. 2008;22:1821-1827.
25. Berns JS, Kasbekar JN. Highly active antiretrovial therapy and the kidney: an update on antiretroviral medications for nephrologists. *Clin J Am Soc Nephrol*. 2006;1:117-129.
26. Izzedine H, Launay-Vacher V, Baumelou A, Deray G. An appraisal of antiretroviral drugs in hemodialysis. *Kidney Int*. 2001;60:821-830.
27. Ahuja TS, Grady J, Khan S. Changing trends in the survival of dialysis patients with human immunodeficiency virus in the United States. *J Am Soc Nephrol*. 2002;13:1889-1893.
28. Shrivastava D, Rao TK, Sinert R, et al. The efficacy of erythropoietin in human immunodeficiency virus–infected end-stage renal disease patients treated by maintenance hemodialysis. *Am J Kidney Dis*. 1995;25: 904-909.
29. Farzadegan H, Ford D, Malan M, et al. HIV-1 survival kinetics in peritoneal dialysis effluent. *Kidney Int*. 1996;50:1659-1662.
30. Rao TK. Human immunodeficiency virus infection in end-stage renal disease patients. *Semin Dial*. 2003;16:233-244.
31. Roland ME, Stock PG. Review of solid-organ transplantation in HIV-infected patients. *Transplantation*. 2003;75:425-429.
32. Venter WD, Naicker S, Dhai A, et al. Uniquely South African: time to consider offering HIV-positive donor kidneys to HIV-infected renal failure patients? *S Afr Med J*. 2008;98:182-183.
33. Szczech LA, Grunfeld C, Scherzer R, et al. Microalbuminuria in HIV infection. *AIDS*. 2007;21:1003-1009.

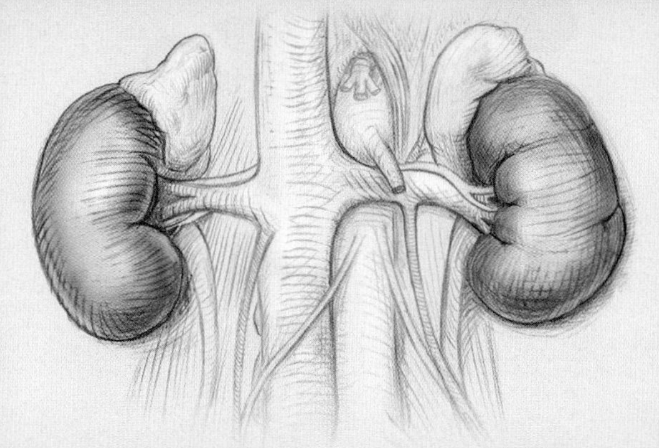

SECTION X

Urologic Disorders

CHAPTER 57

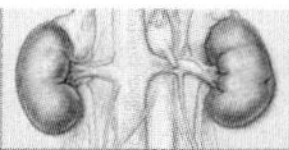

Nephrolithiasis and Nephrocalcinosis

Rebeca D. Monk, David A. Bushinsky

Kidney stones are common and are associated with significant morbidity. Nephrolithiasis refers to stone formation within the renal tubules or collecting system, although calculi are often found within the ureters or in the bladder. Most renal calculi are calcium oxalate, calcium phosphate, struvite, urate, and cystine. Clinical presentation varies from asymptomatic small stones to large, obstructing staghorn calculi that impair renal function and cause chronic kidney disease. The severity of stone disease depends on the pathogenesis as well as on the stone type, size, and location. Nephrolithiasis classically presents as ureteral colic but may also commonly present with hematuria or urinary tract infection (UTI). Diffuse renal parenchymal calcification is termed nephrocalcinosis. The calcifications are usually calcium phosphate or calcium oxalate and may be deposited in the renal cortex or medulla, depending on etiology.

NEPHROLITHIASIS

Epidemiology

Kidney stones are common in industrialized nations, with an annual incidence of more than 1 per 1000 persons and a lifetime risk of forming stones of 5% to 13%.[1-3] In the United States, the prevalence of nephrolithiasis has increased from 3.2% in the late 1970s to 5.2% in the 1990s,[4] in parallel with the rising incidence of obesity, insulin resistance, and type 2 diabetes mellitus.[5,6] Incidence peaks in the third and fourth decades and prevalence increases with age until approximately 70 years in men and 60 years in women.[7] Factors that determine renal stone prevalence include age, sex, race, and geographic distribution. In the United States, Caucasians are more likely to develop renal stones than are African Americans, Hispanics, or Asian Americans. Men are more prone to stone formation than are women, at a ratio of 2 to 4:1. In the United States, the tendency for the development of stones also depends on geographic location, with an increasing prevalence from north to south and, to a lesser degree, from west to east. The increase in nephrolithiasis rates in the American Southeast may be due to the greater sunlight exposure, leading to an increase in insensible losses through sweating and more concentrated urine.[2,8] The higher urine calcium excretion in a smaller urine volume will increase the risk for supersaturation for calcium, thereby promoting stone formation.

Stone type varies with worldwide geography and genetic predisposition. In the Mediterranean and Middle East, 75% of stones are composed of uric acid; whereas in the United States, the majority of stones are calcium oxalate or calcium phosphate (>70%), with less than 10% pure uric acid stones. Magnesium ammonium phosphate (struvite) stones account for 10% to 25% of stones formed (with a higher incidence in the United Kingdom), and cystine stones represent 2% of all stones formed (Fig. 57.1).[7,9,10]

Outbreaks of kidney stones can also be due to dietary supplements or medications. Recently, a large number of Chinese infants and toddlers developed kidney stones and, in some cases, renal failure due to obstructive stones. The outbreak was associated with melamine contamination in infant formulas and powdered milk as a means of raising the apparent concentration of protein in the products.[11-13]

Pathogenesis

Stones occur in urine that is supersaturated with respect to the ionic constituents of the specific stone. Supersaturation is dependent on the product of the free ion activities of stone components rather than on their molar concentrations. Whereas an increasing concentration of crystal components increases their free ion activity, other factors diminish it. When calcium and oxalate are dissolved in pure water, for example, the solution becomes saturated when the addition of any more calcium or oxalate does not result in further dissolution. However, urine, unlike pure water, contains numerous ions and molecules that can form soluble complexes with the ionic components of a stone. The interactions with these other solutes (e.g., citrate) may result in a decrease in free ion activity, which allows the stone constituents to increase in total concentration to levels that would normally cause stone formation in water. Urinary pH also influences free ion activity. The level of chemical free ion activity in which stones will neither grow nor dissolve is referred to as the equilibrium solubility product, or the upper limit of metastability. Above this level, the urine will be supersaturated, and any stone present will grow in size.

When the solution becomes supersaturated with respect to a solid phase, ions can join together to form the more stable, solid phase, a process termed nucleation. Homogeneous nucleation refers to the joining of similar ions into crystals. The more common and thermodynamically favored heterogeneous nucleation results when crystals grow around dissimilar crystals or other substances in the urine, such as sloughed epithelial cells. Calcium oxalate crystals, for example, can nucleate around uric acid crystals. For stones to grow sufficiently large in size to obstruct before being excreted in the urine, several small crystals generally bond together rapidly in a process termed aggregation.

Crystals then grow into a clinically significant calculus by anchoring to the renal epithelium. Calcium oxalate crystals anchor on areas of calcium phosphate deposits termed Randall's

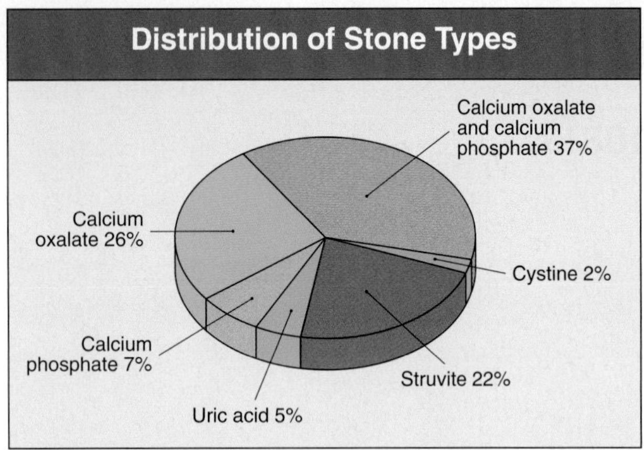

Figure 57.1 Proportion of stone types in a typical U.S. population.

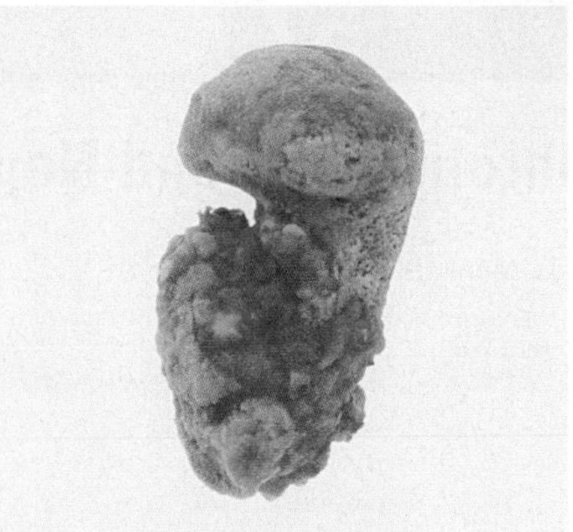

Figure 57.3 Ureteral calculus. A 1-cm-wide calcium oxalate stone that provoked ureteral colic and required surgical removal.

Clinical Presentations of Nephrolithiasis

Presentation	Characteristics
Pain	Ureteral colic, loin pain, dysuria
Hematuria	—
Urinary tract infection	Recurrent, chronic infection; pyelonephritis
Asymptomatic urine abnormality	Microscopic hematuria, proteinuria, sterile pyuria
Interruption of urinary stream	—
Calculus anuria	—

Figure 57.2 Clinical presentations of nephrolithiasis.

Causes of Hematuria

Nephrolithiasis
Infection: cystitis, prostatitis, urethritis, acute pyelonephritis, tuberculosis, schistosomiasis
Malignancy: renal cell carcinoma, transitional cell carcinoma, prostatic carcinoma, Wilms' tumor
Trauma
Glomerular disease
Interstitial nephritis
Polycystic kidney disease
Papillary necrosis
Medullary sponge kidney
Coagulopathy: bleeding disorders, anticoagulation therapy
Miscellaneous: loin pain hematuria syndrome, arteriovenous malformation, chemical cystitis, caruncle, factitious

Figure 57.4 Causes of hematuria.

plaques, which are located in the renal papillae and composed of apatite crystals. The apatite appears to originate around the thin loop of Henle, in the tubular basement membrane, and extends into the interstitium without filling the tubular lumen or damaging the tubular cells. Calcium oxalate crystals attach to these plaques, allowing significant stone growth.[14-16]

Clinical Manifestations

The two most characteristic symptoms of nephrolithiasis are pain and hematuria. Other presentations include UTI and acute kidney injury due to obstructive uropathy if stones cause bilateral renal tract obstruction or unilateral obstruction in a single functioning kidney (Fig. 57.2).

Pain

The classic presentation of pain in patients with nephrolithiasis is ureteral colic. Pain is of abrupt onset and intensifies over time into an excruciating, severe flank pain that resolves only with stone passage or removal. The pain may migrate anteriorly along the abdomen and inferiorly to the groin, testicles, or labia majora as the stone moves toward the ureterovesical junction. Gross hematuria, urinary urgency, frequency, nausea, and vomiting may occur. Stones smaller than 5 mm usually pass spontaneously with hydration, whereas larger stones often require urologic intervention (Fig. 57.3).[15,17] Ureteral colic may also occur with the passage of clots from hematuria of any cause ("clot colic") or with papillary necrosis. As well as colic, nephrolithiasis may provoke less specific loin pain that poorly localizes to the kidney and therefore has a wide differential diagnosis, particularly if it is not associated with other urinary symptoms. The finding of a stone on radiologic examination does not preclude a coincidental cause of pain from another etiology.

Hematuria

Stone disease is a common cause of hematuria. Macroscopic hematuria occurs more commonly with large calculi and during UTI and colic. Although it is typically associated with loin pain or ureteral colic, the hematuria of nephrolithiasis may also be painless. The clinical differential of hematuria is therefore wide (Fig. 57.4). Painless microscopic hematuria in children may occur with hypercalciuria in the absence of demonstrable stones.

Loin Pain–Hematuria Syndrome

Loin pain–hematuria syndrome is a poorly understood condition that must always be considered in the differential diagnosis of nephrolithiasis. It is diagnosed by exclusion when patients (most typically young and middle-aged women) present with loin pain and persistent microscopic or intermittent macroscopic hematuria.[18] Careful evaluation is required to exclude small stones, tumor, UTI, and glomerular disease. Angiographic abnormalities implying intrarenal vasospasm or occlusion have been reported, as have renal biopsy abnormalities typified by deposition of complement C3 in arteriolar walls. However, these findings are not consistent, nor do they provide a coherent framework to explain the pathogenesis of this condition.

In one study, 43 consecutive patients with clinical manifestations of loin pain–hematuria syndrome were evaluated by renal biopsy after other causes of their symptoms were excluded with at least two imaging studies.[19] Thirty-four subjects were considered to have idiopathic loin pain–hematuria syndrome after nine with histologic evidence of IgA nephropathy were excluded. Of these, 66% had glomerular basement membranes that were either unusually thick or thin on electron microscopy, and 47% had a history of kidney stones, although none had obstructing stones at the time of assessment. Evidence of glomerular hematuria was more common in biopsy specimens of patients with loin pain–hematuria syndrome compared with those of healthy living kidney donors who also underwent renal biopsy. The investigators postulated that the structurally abnormal glomerular basement membranes in the majority of these patients may lead to rupture of the glomerular capillary walls, with consequent hemorrhage into the renal tubules. Tubular obstruction by red blood cells or potentially by microcrystals ensues. Local and global renal parenchymal edema follows, ultimately resulting in stretching of the renal capsule and severe flank pain.

Loin pain–hematuria syndrome is a chronic condition requiring reassurance, careful management of analgesia, and ongoing psychological support. The condition usually remits after several years. Denervation of the kidney by autotransplantation is rarely successful.[20] The extreme measure of nephrectomy has been used, but pain often recurs promptly in the contralateral kidney. Bilateral nephrectomy with renal replacement therapy has been reported as an approach of very last resort. Referral to a pain clinic can assist in providing psychiatric counseling, analgesia, and exclusion of other disorders. In one retrospective study, patients who eventually came to accept a nonsurgical approach along with pain-coping strategies that did not involve narcotic analgesics had the most successful outcomes.[21]

Basic Evaluation of Nephrolithiasis
Stone history Number of stones formed Frequency of stone formation Age at first onset Size of stones passed or still present Kidney involved (left, right, or both) Stone type, if known Need for urologic intervention: ESWL, percutaneous nephrolithotomy, etc. Response to surgical procedure Are stones associated with urinary tract infections?
Medical history
Medications
Family history
Occupation, lifestyle
Fluid intake, diet
Physical examination Evidence of systemic causes of stones (e.g., tophi)
Laboratory data Urinalysis Urine culture Stone analysis
Blood chemistry Sodium, potassium, chloride, bicarbonate Creatinine, calcium, phosphorus, uric acid Intact parathyroid hormone level if calcium elevated
Radiologic evaluation KUB Helical CT IVU Ultrasound

Figure 57.5 Basic evaluation of nephrolithiasis. CT, computed tomography; ESWL, extracorporeal shock wave lithotripsy; IVU intravenous urography; KUB, kidneys, ureters, bladder.

Asymptomatic Stone Disease

Even large staghorn calculi may be asymptomatic and discovered during the investigation of unrelated abdominal or musculoskeletal symptoms. Obstructive uropathy caused by calculi may also be painless; therefore, nephrolithiasis should always be considered in the differential diagnosis of unexplained renal failure.

In the recent outbreak of melamine-associated nephrolithiasis in Chinese infants, the majority presenting to a screening clinic had no symptoms or signs of stones. The diagnosis of nephrolithiasis was made by ultrasound in at-risk infants and toddlers.[13]

Clinical Evaluation of Stone Formers

All patients with recurrent nephrolithiasis merit metabolic evaluation to determine the cause of their kidney stones. Complete evaluation of patients with a single stone is controversial because of the undetermined cost-benefit ratio. A National Institutes of Health Consensus Development Conference on the Prevention and Treatment of Kidney Stones determined that all patients, even those with a single stone, should undergo a basic evaluation, which need not include a 24-hour urine collection. Those with metabolically active stones (stones growing in size or number within 1 year), all children, non–calcium stone formers, and patients in demographic groups not typically prone to stone formation warrant a more complete evaluation that includes a 24-hour urine collection made with the patient taking the typical diet.[22]

Basic Evaluation

Clinic evaluation of stone formers includes a general history and physical examination. Specific data gathering on stone formation and the diet and specific laboratory studies are required, as shown in Figure 57.5.

History History serves to uncover a systemic etiology for nephrolithiasis. Any disease that can lead to hypercalcemia (including malignant neoplasm, hyperparathyroidism, and sarcoidosis) can result in hypercalciuria and increase the risk for calcium stone formation. A number of malabsorptive gastrointestinal disorders (including Crohn's disease and sprue [celiac disease]) can result in calcium oxalate stone formation as a result of volume depletion and hyperoxaluria. Uric acid stones often occur in patients with a history of gout and increasingly in patients with insulin resistance.[10]

Stone history (see Fig. 57.5) includes the number and frequency of stones formed, the age of the patient at occurrence of the first stone, the size of stones, the stone type (if known), and whether the patient required surgical removal of the calculi. This information indicates the severity of the stone disease and provides clues to the etiology of the stone formation. For example, large staghorn calculi that do not pass spontaneously and recur despite frequent surgical intervention are more consistent with struvite than with calcium oxalate stones. Stones that develop at a young age may be caused by cystinuria or primary hyperoxaluria. Stone response to intervention is also significant; cystine stones, for example, do not fragment well with lithotripsy. If stones recur frequently in a single kidney, a congenital abnormality in that kidney, such as megacalyx or medullary sponge kidney, should be explored.

Family history is important because a number of stone types have a genetic basis. Idiopathic hypercalciuria is most likely a polygenic disorder; cystinuria is usually autosomal recessive; and hyperuricosuria has been associated with rare inherited metabolic disorders. Nephrolithiasis and nephrocalcinosis can also result from a variety of monogenic disorders, such as Dent disease (X-linked recessive nephrolithiasis), McCune-Albright syndrome, osteogenesis imperfecta type I, and congenital lactate deficiency. The various genetic disorders can lead to hypercalciuria by their effect on increasing either bone resorption or intestinal absorption, by decreasing renal tubular reabsorption transport, or through other as yet unknown mechanisms.[2,15,16,23,24]

A number of medications are known to potentiate calcium stone formation (e.g., loop diuretics are calciuric) or may predispose to uric acid lithiasis (salicylates, probenecid) (Fig. 57.6). Certain drugs can precipitate into stones themselves, such as rapidly infused intravenous acyclovir, high-dose sulfadiazine, triamterene, and the antiretroviral agents indinavir and nelfinavir.[25]

Social history should include details about occupation and lifestyle. Cardiothoracic surgeons and real-estate agents, for example, may minimize fluid intake to avoid bathroom breaks during the workday. Those who engage in vigorous physical activities, such as running, may not rehydrate adequately to keep up with insensible losses, producing excessively concentrated urine and precipitation of stone crystals in those prone to nephrolithiasis.

Dietary history and review of fluid intake are essential in determining potential causes of or contributors to stone formation. The patient should be asked about commonly consumed foods, with attention paid to sodium-containing foods as well as quantities of calcium, animal protein, purine, and oxalate (Fig. 57.7). Dietary calcium intake should be reviewed as many patients with nephrolithiasis are erroneously instructed to eliminate all calcium from their diet, a suggestion that can result not only in bone demineralization, particularly in women and children, but also in an *increase* in stone formation.[3,26-29]

Physical Examination Most patients with idiopathic hypercalciuria are healthy and have normal physical examination

Medications Associated with Nephrolithiasis and Nephrocalcinosis
Calcium Stone Formation
Loop diuretics
Vitamin D
Corticosteroids
Calcium supplements
Antacids (calcium and noncalcium antacids)
Theophylline
Acetazolamide*
Amphotericin B*
Uric Acid Stone Formation
Salicylates
Probenecid
Allopurinol (usually associated with xanthine stones)
Melamine (in contaminated infant formula and milk products)
Medications That May Precipitate into Stones
Triamterene
Acyclovir (if infused rapidly intravenously)
Indinavir
Nelfinavir

Figure 57.6 Medications associated with nephrolithiasis and nephrocalcinosis. *Associated with nephrocalcinosis.

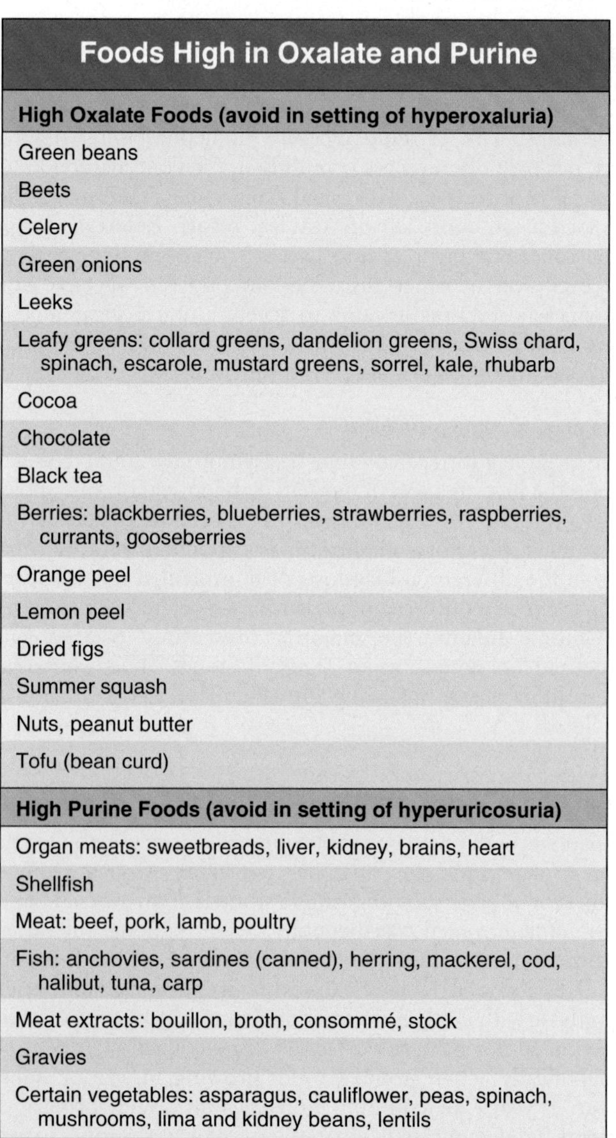

Foods High in Oxalate and Purine
High Oxalate Foods (avoid in setting of hyperoxaluria)
Green beans
Beets
Celery
Green onions
Leeks
Leafy greens: collard greens, dandelion greens, Swiss chard, spinach, escarole, mustard greens, sorrel, kale, rhubarb
Cocoa
Chocolate
Black tea
Berries: blackberries, blueberries, strawberries, raspberries, currants, gooseberries
Orange peel
Lemon peel
Dried figs
Summer squash
Nuts, peanut butter
Tofu (bean curd)
High Purine Foods (avoid in setting of hyperuricosuria)
Organ meats: sweetbreads, liver, kidney, brains, heart
Shellfish
Meat: beef, pork, lamb, poultry
Fish: anchovies, sardines (canned), herring, mackerel, cod, halibut, tuna, carp
Meat extracts: bouillon, broth, consommé, stock
Gravies
Certain vegetables: asparagus, cauliflower, peas, spinach, mushrooms, lima and kidney beans, lentils

Figure 57.7 Foods high in oxalate and purine.

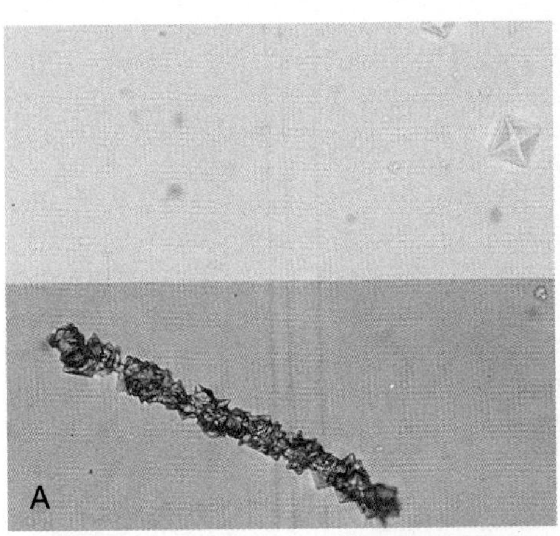

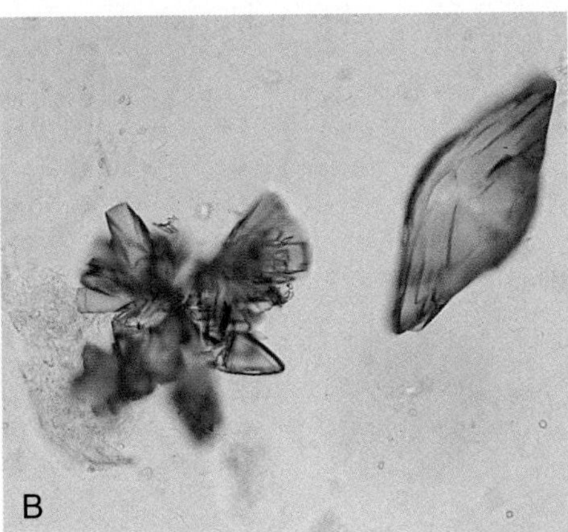

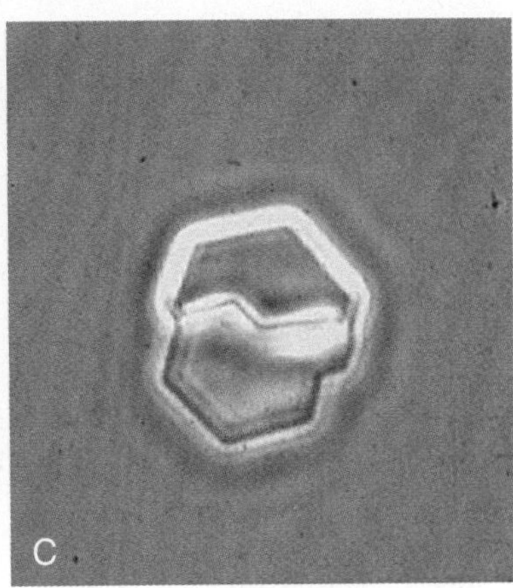

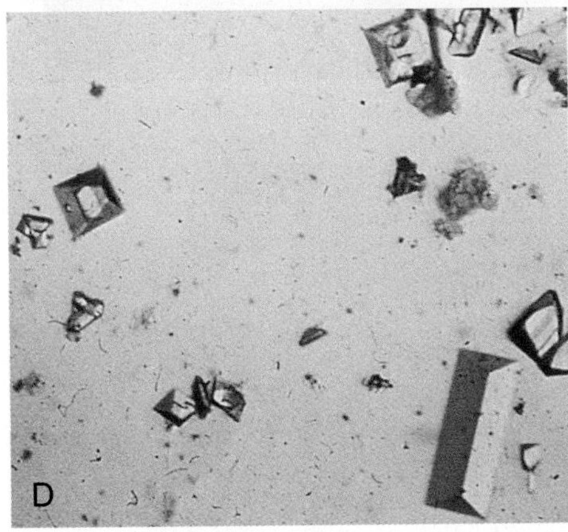

Figure 57.8 Urine crystals. A, Oxalate crystals: a pseudocast of calcium oxalate crystals accompanied by crystals of calcium oxalate dihydrate. **B,** Uric acid crystals: complex crystals suggestive of acute uric acid nephropathy or uric acid nephrolithiasis. **C,** A typical hexagonal cystine crystal; a single crystal provides a definitive diagnosis of cystinuria. **D,** Coffin lid crystals of magnesium ammonium phosphate (struvite). *(Courtesy Dr. Patrick Fleet, University of Washington, Seattle, Washington USA.)*

findings. In contrast, subjects with hyperuricosuria and uric acid stone formation may display tophi. Central obesity is associated with a predisposition to metabolic syndrome and uric acid stones. Similarly, paraplegic subjects with chronic indwelling bladder catheters may be predisposed to chronic UTI and struvite stones.

Laboratory Findings Urine pH is generally high in patients with struvite and calcium phosphate stones but low in patients with uric acid and calcium oxalate stones. The specific gravity, if it is high, will confirm inadequate fluid intake in many patients. Hematuria may imply active stone disease with crystal or stone passage. Examination of the urine may reveal red blood cells along with characteristic crystals (Fig. 57.8). Bacteriuria with urine pH above 6 to 6.5 suggests struvite stones. Urine should be cultured, and because many bacteria produce urease even when urine bacterial colony counts are low, the microbiology laboratory should be instructed to type the organism even if there are fewer than 100,000 colony-forming units/ml.

Blood tests required in the basic evaluation are serum electrolytes (sodium, potassium, chloride, and bicarbonate), creatinine, calcium, phosphorus, and uric acid. If the serum calcium concentration is elevated or at the upper limit of normal, especially if the serum phosphorus concentration is low, a serum parathyroid hormone level should be measured. A low potassium or bicarbonate level may indicate a cause of hypocitraturia, such as distal renal tubular acidosis.

Stone Analysis Patients should be encouraged to retrieve any stone they excrete for chemical analysis, which may define the underlying metabolic abnormality and guide therapy.

Imaging Patients should have a plain film of the abdomen performed with views of the kidneys, ureters, and bladder (KUB). This will reveal opacifications in the areas of the kidneys and ureters that could be due to calcium, cystine, or struvite stones (Fig. 57.9). Uric acid and xanthine calculi are radiolucent and will not be visible on plain films. The unenhanced helical computed tomography (CT) scan, also known as spiral CT or CT urography (Fig. 57.10), has replaced contrast-enhanced intravenous urography (IVU) as the diagnostic test of choice for acute ureteral colic; it has a higher sensitivity and specificity than IVU for detection of ureteral stones and ureteral obstruction[17] and avoids the need for administration of contrast material. CT urography is more likely to reveal causes of colic other than stones. It is more rapid, with results being available in minutes rather than hours, an advantage in the emergency department setting. However, an experienced radiologist, required for optimal interpretation of the images, may not be available at all times in urgent care facilities. Disadvantages of CT imaging include a radiation dose approximately three times that of conventional IVU and higher cost. Both tests should be avoided or limited in patients at risk for radiation exposure, such as children and pregnant women.[30-34]

Contrast material should generally be avoided in patients with renal impairment or other contraindications to the use of contrast agents. The IVU generally demonstrates urinary tract obstruction caused by calculi (Fig. 57.11) and can identify abnormalities of the genitourinary tract that may predispose to stone formation, such as medullary sponge kidney (see Chapter 45) and calyceal anomalies (see Chapter 50). During acute colic, the radiographic contrast material used in the IVU, by creating a strong osmotic diuresis, may assist in moving the stone along the ureter.

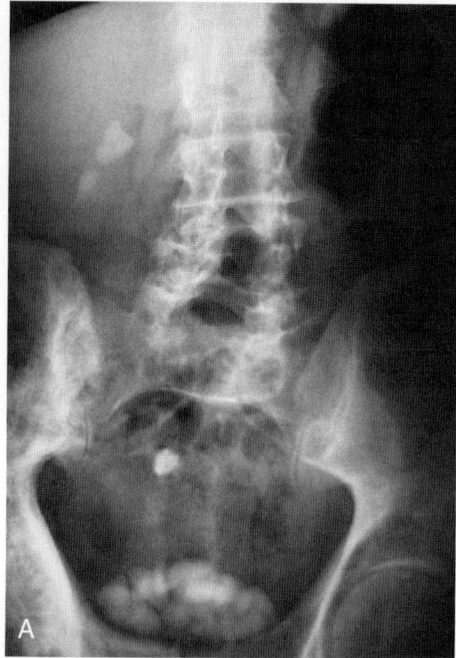

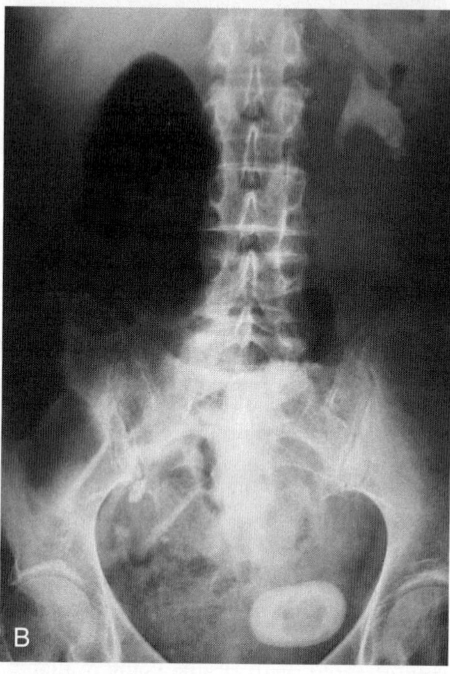

Figure 57.9 Radiopaque renal calculi. A, X-ray examination showing multiple cystine stones in the right kidney, right ureter, and bladder. **B,** Struvite stones: left staghorn calculus and a single bladder stone.

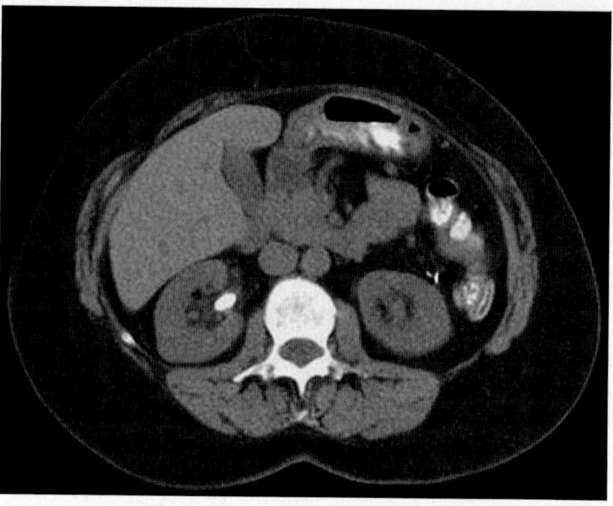

Figure 57.10 Stone in the right renal pelvis. Helical (spiral) CT scan showing a single stone in the right renal pelvis. There is no hydronephrosis. *(From www.gehealthcare.com/usen/ct/products/urologyimagegallery.html.)*

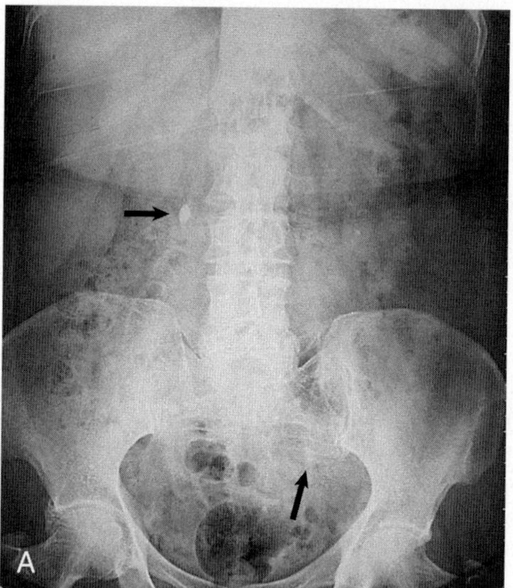

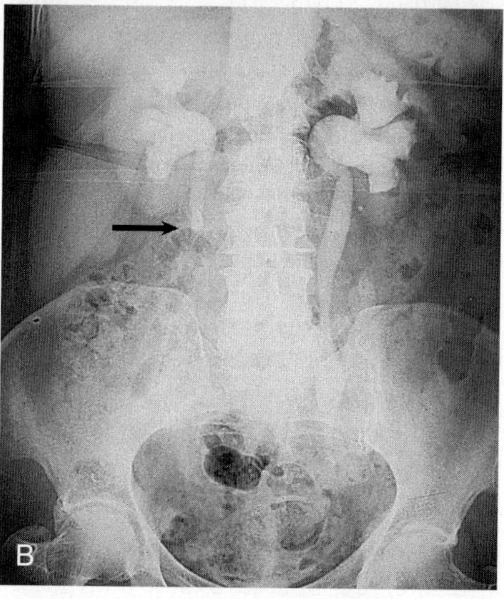

Figure 57.11 Obstructive uropathy resulting from nephrolithiasis in a patient with acute renal impairment. A, X-ray examination showing a stone in the right upper ureter and a very small stone in the lower left ureter *(arrows)*. **B,** Intravenous urography at the same time showing bilateral hydronephrosis caused by ureteral obstruction. Opacification of the right ureter ends at the site of the stone *(arrow)*.

Renal ultrasound provides great specificity in the evaluation of stones but is not a sensitive screening test. Both radiolucent and radiopaque stones within the kidneys should be detectable on ultrasound, but ureteral stones are often missed. Nonetheless, this is the test of choice for those patients who must avoid radiation exposure.

If stones are radiopaque, a KUB film can be obtained if a patient develops symptoms suggestive of recurrent stone disease. Periodic monitoring, if it is deemed necessary, should be obtained with a KUB film rather than with CT, whenever possible, to minimize radiation exposure.

Optimal 24-Hour Urine Values in Recurrent Nephrolithiasis		
Urine Values in 24 Hours		
Volume	>2–2.5 l	
Calcium	<4 mg/kg (0.1 mmol/kg), ~300 mg (7.5 mmol) in men, ~250 mg (6.3 mmol) in women	
Oxalate	<40 mg (0.36 mmol)	
Uric acid	<750 mg (4.5 mmol) in women, <800 mg (4.7 mmol) in men (can be pH dependent)	
Citrate	>320 mg (17 mmol)	
Sodium	<3000 mg (<130 mmol)	
Phosphorus	<1100 mg (35 mmol)	
Creatinine >10 mg/kg (88 µmol/kg) in women and >15 mg/kg (132 µmol/kg) in men, if specimen is a complete collection		
Urine Supersaturation Values*		
Calcium oxalate supersaturation	<5	
Calcium phosphate supersaturation	0.5–2	
Uric acid supersaturation	0–1	

Figure 57.12 Evaluation of nephrolithiasis: optimal 24-hour urine values. *The ratio between the actual ion activity product and its solubility product.

The Complete Evaluation

A complete evaluation should be undertaken in patients with multiple or metabolically active stones (i.e., stones that grow in size or increase in number within a year), in all children, in demographic groups not typically prone to stone formation, and in those with stones other than those containing calcium.

In addition to the basic evaluation, the complete evaluation includes a 24-hour urine collection for quantification of supersaturation for calcium oxalate, brushite (calcium phosphate), and uric acid (Fig. 57.12). Urine for supersaturation analysis has been shown to correlate well with stone composition.[35] Patients can bring their specimens to a local laboratory or may directly mail them to specialized laboratories that measure calcium, oxalate, citrate, uric acid, creatinine, sodium, potassium, magnesium, sulfate, phosphorus, chloride, urine urea nitrogen, and pH. Supersaturation is calculated for calcium oxalate, calcium phosphate, and uric acid by use of a software program such as EQUIL2.[36,37] Calculation of supersaturation from a 24-hour urine collection will provide values lower than the peak postprandial supersaturation that may initiate stone formation. Only an undersaturated urine ensures that stones will not recur; the risk of stone formation rises with increasing supersaturation.

JESS (Joint Expert Speciation System) is a different program that measures the concentration of the various complexes in solution under many different conditions. It may prove to be more accurate than supersaturation analysis but is currently used for research purposes only.[38,39] In the absence of supersaturation analysis, most laboratories assess urine volume and the quantity of calcium, oxalate, phosphorus, uric acid, sodium, citrate, and creatinine excreted in a 24-hour urine collection (see Fig. 57.12). Urine creatinine is useful in assessing adequacy of the collection; men should excrete more than 15 mg/kg (132 µmol/kg) and women should excrete more than 10 mg/kg (88 µmol/kg) daily. A disadvantage of the standard 24-hour urine collection is that laboratories vary in the preservatives required to process the various constituents. Many require more than one collection to measure all the urinary constituents, reducing compliance and therefore the accuracy of the results. Determination of supersaturation is far more informative than evaluation of the individual urinary constituents.

Patients should be encouraged to perform the urine collection on a typical day while eating a typical diet, although many patients prefer to collect the urine at weekends, when their diet and habits may differ from those on usual workdays. Specialized testing, such as the use of diets high or low in calcium, is not recommended.[22] Careful instructions should be given to avoid overcollection or undercollection.

General Treatment

Intervention for stone removal may be required when pain, obstruction, and infection due to nephrolithiasis do not respond to conservative management. Surgical management of stones includes extracorporeal shock wave lithotripsy and both endoscopic and percutaneous surgical removal of stones (see Chapter 59). The risk for development of renal impairment varies with types of stone, and this must be considered in planning management.[40]

Medical Management

Patients who are seen by stone "specialists" often have a decrease in stone recurrence even without pharmacologic intervention.[41] This phenomenon, termed the stone clinic effect, is probably due to modifications in diet and fluid intake. These nonpharmacologic measures include an increase in fluid intake, which increases urine volume; restriction of dietary sodium, which leads to a reduction of urine calcium excretion; restriction of animal protein, which also leads to a reduction of urine calcium excretion and an increase in excretion of the calcification inhibitor citrate; and ingestion of an age- and gender-appropriate amount of dietary calcium. Although dietary calcium restriction continues to be prescribed by many physicians, increasing evidence indicates that this is not beneficial and can actually increase the rate of stone formation (see later, Calcium Stones).[3,27,42]

Fluid Intake An increase in urine volume to more than 2 to 2.5 liters daily has been proven to reduce the incidence of stones.[41,43,44] Large urine volumes will reduce calcium oxalate supersaturation as well as precipitation of other crystals. Increased fluid intake to augment urine volume is also a mainstay of therapy for patients with uric acid and cystine stones. The period of maximum risk for stone formation is at night, when urine concentration is physiologically increased. Patients should be encouraged to drink enough fluid in the evening to provoke nocturia and then drink more fluid before returning to bed.

Salt Intake Urine sodium excretion augments urine calcium excretion.[45] Conversely, dietary salt restriction is associated with a decrease in calcium excretion. Patients should be instructed to limit daily sodium intake to 2 g (87 mmol sodium).

Dietary Protein Animal protein ingestion increases the frequency of renal stone formation by a number of mechanisms.

Metabolism of certain amino acids leads to generation of sulfate ions, which render urinary calcium ions less soluble.[46,47] The metabolic acidosis that results from protein ingestion causes calcium release from bone and a consequent increase in the filtered load of calcium.[46,47] Acidosis also decreases tubular calcium reabsorption, resulting in hypercalciuria. Urinary citrate excretion is also pH dependent, with acidosis leading to a decrease in citrate excretion. The result of increased animal protein intake is therefore an increase in urinary calcium ions that are rendered less soluble because of concomitant sulfate excretion and hypocitraturia. Low urine pH, coupled with increased uric acid excretion from the metabolism of animal protein, can result in uric acid lithiasis. For these reasons, stone formers should consume only a moderate-protein diet (0.8 to 1.0 g/kg daily).[7] Dietary fructose may also increase uric acid lithiasis.[48]

Dietary Calcium Despite conventional wisdom, studies have demonstrated a decrease in stone incidence when people consume diets adequate in calcium.[44,49-51] This beneficial effect has been attributed to the binding of ingested oxalate (which is highly lithogenic) by the additional dietary calcium. Whereas women have reduced stone formation on a higher calcium diet, an exception may be in those taking calcium supplements.[52] Some have postulated that this increased risk may be due to timing of the supplement calcium ingestion apart from meals, which would enhance calcium absorption without reducing oxalate absorption.

Previously, hypercalciuric patients were divided into those with excessive renal calcium excretion ("renal leak") and those who absorbed excessive amounts of calcium through the gastrointestinal tract ("absorptive hypercalciuria"). However, studies have shown that hypercalciuric patients generally do not have a transport defect limited to a single site. In both hypercalciuric rats and humans prescribed a low-calcium diet, there is a continuous, wide spectrum of calcium excretion, with many subjects excreting more calcium than they consume. This negative calcium balance must be derived from demineralization of bone, by far the largest repository of calcium in the body.[26,28,53] Support for the use of an age- and gender-appropriate amount of dietary calcium was provided by a randomized prospective study comparing the rate of stone formation in men assigned to a low-calcium diet with that in men assigned to a normal-calcium, low-sodium, and low–animal protein diet.[27] The men assigned to the low-calcium diet were twice as likely to have recurrent stones during 5 years compared with those on the normal-calcium, low-sodium, and low–animal protein diet. Urinary calcium oxalate supersaturation also diminished more rapidly in those on the higher calcium diet and remained lower than that of men on the low-calcium diet for most of the 5-year study. This reduction in supersaturation was due to a greater fall in urinary oxalate in the men eating the normal-calcium, low-sodium, and low–animal protein diet.[27,54]

Patients prescribed low-calcium diets can avoid excessive hyperoxaluria when they are adequately instructed to consume a low-oxalate diet.[55] Some experts contend that this approach may benefit patients with excessive intestinal absorption of calcium associated with severe hypercalciuria by allowing calcium restriction without risk of significant osteopenia.

We recommend, however, an age- and gender-appropriate calcium diet, although "excessive" dietary calcium intake and calcium supplements should be avoided in patients with calcium nephrolithiasis. Because stone formation can be reduced with normal calcium intake and there is a risk of bone demineralization with calcium restriction, we consider the low-calcium diet obsolete.[27,28,54]

SPECIFIC TYPES OF STONES

Calcium Stones

Calcium-containing kidney stones represent approximately 70% of all stones formed. Most calcium stones are composed of calcium oxalate, either alone or in combination with calcium phosphate or urate. A small percentage of stones are composed entirely of calcium phosphate.[7] Most calcium stones do not exceed 1 to 2 cm in width, although surgical intervention is often required for stones larger than 5 mm.

Calcium stones may develop as a result of excessive excretion of calcium (hypercalciuria), oxalate (hyperoxaluria), and uric acid (hyperuricosuria); insufficient citrate excretion (hypocitraturia); renal tubular acidosis; certain medications; and congenital abnormalities of the genitourinary tract (Fig. 57.13). Specific therapy for patients with calcium stones depends on the underlying metabolic abnormalities detected on evaluation. Nonspecific or general therapy as outlined before should always be instituted; however, more definitive treatment is often required.

Hypercalciuria

Etiology Hypercalciuria with no other demonstrable metabolic abnormality is termed idiopathic hypercalciuria. These patients typically have excessive intestinal calcium absorption and may also have decreased renal tubular calcium reabsorption and decreased bone mineralization. The etiology of this systemic disorder in calcium transport has, in hypercalciuric stone-forming rats and in humans, been linked to an excessive number of receptors for vitamin D.[56] Metabolic disorders leading to an elevation in serum calcium, parathyroid hormone, or $1,25(OH)_2D_3$ also may result in hypercalciuria.

Treatment For hypercalciuria, the usual first-line therapy is a thiazide diuretic, which acts to reduce urinary calcium. In the United States, chlorthalidone (25 to 50 mg) is the drug of choice as it requires only once-daily administration. Indapamide (1.25 to 2.5 mg daily) does not tend to raise serum lipids as much as other thiazides do and may be preferred for patients with cardiac risk factors or elevated serum lipids. On commencing these medications, patients should be instructed to increase their dietary potassium intake, and a serum potassium level should be checked 7 to 10 days later. If the level is low, oral potassium supplementation should be initiated. Potassium citrate is preferred to potassium chloride as citrate forms complexes with urinary calcium, further lowering supersaturation. However, most patients find potassium citrate liquid preparations unpalatable. A wax matrix tablet is well tolerated and is available in some countries. In general, patients are able to maintain a normal serum potassium level with 20 to 40 mmol of potassium citrate daily. The serum potassium and bicarbonate levels should be rechecked 7 to 10 days later for further dose adjustment. As citrate is a base, potassium citrate may excessively raise the serum bicarbonate level or urinary pH, and a change to potassium chloride may be required. The 24-hour urine calcium, sodium, and citrate excretion should be rechecked after several weeks. If the calcium excretion remains elevated, the thiazide dose should be increased. If the sodium excretion also remains high, patients should be encouraged to limit their sodium intake further as they will not have an adequate response to the diuretic on a

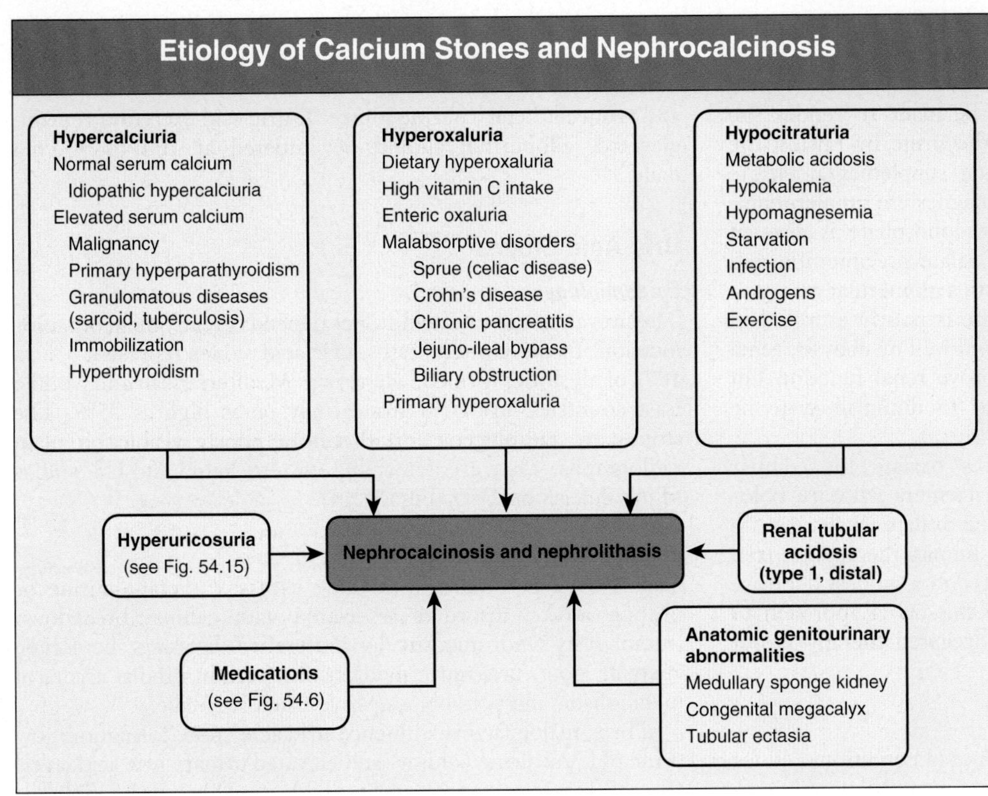

Figure 57.13 Etiology of calcium stones and nephrocalcinosis.

high-sodium diet. If the serum potassium remains low despite supplementation or the calcium excretion remains high despite increased thiazide dosing, addition of a potassium-sparing diuretic may be required to increase serum potassium. Triamterene itself can precipitate into stones; therefore, amiloride (starting dose, 5 mg daily) or a combination tablet that includes both a thiazide and amiloride should be added.[7,57,58]

Dietary Recommendations See General Treatment.

Hyperoxaluria

Etiology Elevated urinary oxalate results from excessive dietary intake (dietary oxaluria), gastrointestinal disorders that can lead to malabsorption (enteric oxaluria), or an inherited enzyme deficiency that results in excessive metabolism of oxalate (primary hyperoxaluria) (see Fig. 57.13).[59]

Dietary excess of oxalate generally does not raise urinary oxalate above 60 mg/24 h (0.54 mmol/24 h). Enteric oxaluria may occur when malabsorption results in excessive colonic absorption of oxalate due to sprue (celiac disease), Crohn's disease, chronic pancreatitis, or short bowel syndrome or after bariatric surgery. The anion exchange transporter Slc26a6 appears responsible for intestinal oxalate secretion, and mice with targeted inactivation of this transporter have hyperoxaluria.[60] It is not yet known whether patients with enteric hyperoxaluria have mutations in Slc26a6. Urinary oxalate is generally more than 60 mg/24 h and can exceed 100 mg/24 h (0.54 and 0.9 mmol/24 h).[61] In primary hyperoxaluria, the tremendous oxalate production results in widespread calcium oxalate deposition throughout the body at an early age. This infiltration of calcium oxalate into organs can result in cardiomyopathy, bone marrow suppression, and renal failure. Urinary oxalate values may range from 80 to 300 mg/24 h (0.72 to 2.70 mmol/24 h).

There are two types of primary hyperoxaluria with unique enzymatic defects in the liver glyoxylate pathway.[62] In type I, the defective enzyme is alanine–glyoxylate aminotransferase, encoded by the gene *AGXT* on chromosome 2. Type II tends to be a milder disorder and is caused by mutations in the *GRHPR* gene on chromosome 9, which results in failure of glyoxylate reduction to glycolate.[15,59,62]

Treatment of Dietary and Enteric Hyperoxaluria Treatment of dietary oxaluria consists of dietary oxalate restriction. Patients should be given a list of foods that have high oxalate content to be avoided or to be eaten in moderation (see Fig. 57.7). Calcium carbonate (1 to 1.5 g) may be added at each meal and snack to bind intestinal oxalate and to prevent its absorption.

Specific therapy for the malabsorptive disorder, such as a gluten-free diet for patients with sprue, is the first line of treatment of enteric hyperoxaluria. More generalized therapy for steatorrhea, such as a low-fat diet, cholestyramine, and administration of medium-chain triglycerides, may reduce fat malabsorption as well as oxalate absorption and subsequent excretion. The low-oxalate diet and mealtime calcium carbonate prescribed for patients with dietary oxaluria are also helpful for these patients. The diarrhea associated with these disorders may result in low urine volumes, hypokalemia, hypocitraturia, and hypomagnesuria. Patients should therefore be advised to increase their fluid intake and to take potassium citrate (in this case, the liquid, although unpalatable, is better absorbed than the tablets) as well as a magnesium supplement. Magnesium also serves as a urinary stone inhibitor and can be given as magnesium gluconate (0.5 to 1 g every 8 hours) or magnesium oxide (400 mg every 12 hours).

Treatment of Primary Hyperoxaluria Primary hyperoxaluria is a severe disorder that can be cured only with liver transplantation to replace the defective hepatic enzyme. Pyridoxine (vitamin B_6 in doses ranging from 2.5 to 15 mg/kg per 24 hours) may reduce oxalate production in patients with type I primary hyperoxaluria. Efforts should be made to render the calcium and oxalate more soluble in the urine by raising the urinary pH (to at least 6.5) and giving supplemental citrate and magnesium. Potassium citrate and magnesium supplementation can be prescribed as before. Orthophosphate is also an effective inhibitor of urinary calcium oxalate precipitation and can be safely administered in patients with a glomerular filtration rate (GFR) above 50 ml/min. As oxalate is poorly excreted in chronic kidney disease and is not removed well by dialysis, renal transplantation serves not only to improve renal function but also to improve oxalate excretion and to diminish systemic oxalosis.[15,63]

Oxalobacter formigenes primarily uses oxalate for cellular metabolism.[64,65] Calcium oxalate stone formers who are colonized with *O. formigenes* have lower urine oxalate levels than do those who are not colonized.[64] A small human therapeutic trial of administration of *O. formigenes* resulted in a modest decrease in urinary oxalate in some.[65] Whether this novel approach to reducing urinary oxalate will become accepted therapy is not yet clear.

Hypocitraturia

Citrate inhibits stone formation. A number of conditions reduce urinary citrate excretion, predisposing to stone formation. Excessive protein intake, hypokalemia, metabolic acidosis, exercise, hypomagnesemia, infections, androgens, starvation, and acetazolamide have all been implicated in decreased urinary citrate excretion. Therapy involves treatment of the underlying condition and potassium citrate supplementation. The potassium salt is preferred to sodium citrate as sodium promotes renal calcium excretion. Potassium citrate (15 to 25 mmol two or three times daily) is required, and tablets are considered by most patients to be more palatable than the liquid preparation. In patients with renal impairment, serum potassium concentration should be monitored, and dose reduction may be needed if hyperkalemia develops.[7,15,66]

Distal Renal Tubular Acidosis

Patients with distal (type 1) renal tubular acidosis have impaired distal tubular excretion of hydrogen ions with a non–anion gap metabolic acidosis and an alkaline urine (see Chapter 12). The acidosis causes calcium and phosphate to be released from bone with an ensuing increase in renal excretion of these ions. The acidosis also leads to an increase in citrate reabsorption by the proximal tubule. The end result is a high urinary pH, hypocitraturia (urinary citrate generally <100 mg/24 h [0.53 mmol/24 h]), and increased renal excretion of calcium and phosphate, all of which increase the propensity for calcium phosphate precipitation. Nephrocalcinosis in this setting is not uncommon. The metabolic acidosis and hypocitraturia should be treated with a combination of sodium citrate (or bicarbonate) and potassium citrate (or bicarbonate). Large amounts (1 to 2 mmol/kg daily in two or three divided doses) are often required to neutralize the acidosis.[7]

Hyperuricosuria

Calcium oxalate crystals often nucleate around other crystal types, such as uric acid. Hyperuricosuria contributes to nephrolithiasis in 10% to 15% of calcium stones. Patients with hyperuricosuric calcium oxalate nephrolithiasis have hyperuricosuria with normal urinary calcium and oxalate but often a higher urinary pH (>5.5) than that of patients with pure uric acid stones. Therapy for hyperuricosuria consists of increased fluid intake and reduced dietary purine intake. If uric acid excretion remains elevated, allopurinol should be initiated at 100 to 300 mg daily.[67,68]

Uric Acid Stones

Epidemiology

The prevalence of uric acid stones depends greatly on geographic location. In the United States, uric acid stones represent 5% to 10% of all stones formed, whereas in Mediterranean and Middle East countries, uric acid stones may be as high as 75%. The stones are radiolucent and therefore poorly visible on plain radiographs. They are detectable on ultrasound and CT and as filling defects on IVU (Fig. 57.14).

Etiology and Pathogenesis

Causes of hyperuricosuria include excessive dietary purine or protein intake, disorders associated with cellular breakdown (tumor lysis syndrome, myeloproliferative disorders, hemolytic anemia), gout, uricosuric medications, certain inborn errors of metabolism, and possibly excessive fructose intake.

Three major factors influence uric acid stone formation: low urine pH, low urine volume, and elevated urinary uric acid levels (Fig. 57.15). Uric acid is poorly soluble at pH below 5.5. Solubility increases with urine alkalinity, such that at urine pH 6.5, urine

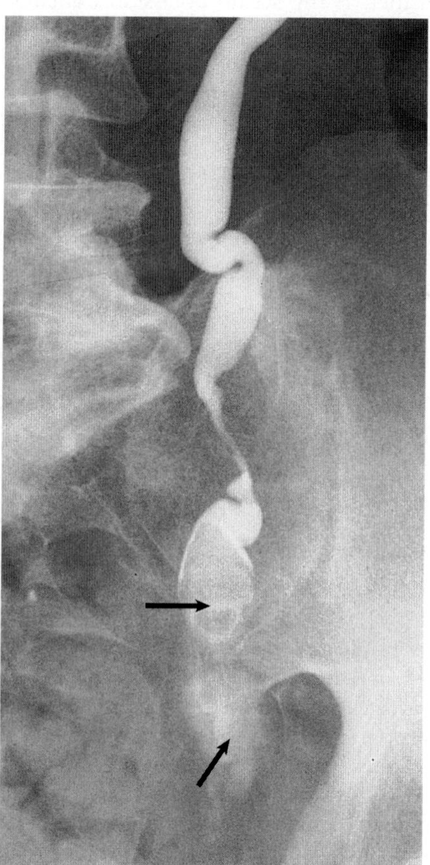

Figure 57.14 Radiolucent urate calculi. Antegrade pyelogram showing multiple radiolucent urate stones *(arrows)* obstructing the lower ureter.

Uric Acid Stones
Low Urine pH (≤5.5)
High animal protein diet
Diarrhea
Insulin resistance (high body mass index, metabolic syndrome, type 2 diabetes)
Low Urine Volume
Inadequate fluid intake
Excessive extrarenal fluid losses Diarrhea Insensible losses (e.g., perspiration)
Hyperuricosuria
Excessive dietary purine intake
Hyperuricemia Gout Intracellular-to-extracellular uric acid shift Myeloproliferative disorders Tumor lysis syndrome Inborn errors of metabolism Lesch-Nyhan syndrome Glucose-6-phosphatase deficiency
Medications (see Fig. 57.6)

Figure 57.15 Uric acid stones.

can contain more than six times the quantity of uric acid present at pH 5.3, without exceeding supersaturation. The rising incidence of obesity and insulin resistance in the United States has led to a parallel increase in uric acid lithiasis. The urinary acidosis is likely due to impaired ammoniagenesis, which results in excessive excretion of unbuffered acid and a very low urine pH.[6,10,69-71]

Treatment

Treatment of uric acid stones involves increasing urine volume and pH as well as decreasing uric acid excretion. Alkaline urine can prevent uric acid stone formation and may also result in stone dissolution. To raise urine pH, potassium citrate is recommended. Whereas sodium bicarbonate alkalinizes the urine and enhances uric acid solubility, the added sodium increases sodium urate formation, which serves as a nidus for calcium oxalate precipitation. Potassium citrate (40 to 50 mmol/day in divided doses) is given, increasing the dose as necessary to achieve a urine pH of 6.5 to 7. Patients should monitor pH with urine dipsticks at various times of the day and adjust dosing accordingly. If urine pH remains low despite potassium citrate above 100 mmol daily or if that dose results in hyperkalemia, acetazolamide is added. This carbonic anhydrase inhibitor produces an alkaline urine similar to that seen in renal tubular acidosis. Patients should be cautioned not to exceed a urine pH of 7 because this may result in calcium phosphate precipitation.

A low-purine and low–animal protein diet is also useful in raising urinary pH and decreasing uric acid excretion (see Fig. 57.7). If uric acid excretion remains high despite dietary intervention, as in patients with disorders of cellular catabolism, allopurinol should be prescribed, 100 mg increasing to 300 mg daily as needed to keep urinary uric acid excretion below 750 mg/24 h (4.5 mmol/24 h). See Figure 57.7 for high-purine foods to be avoided.[72]

Factors Associated with Struvite Stone Formation
Urease-producing bacteria* *Proteus* *Haemophilus* *Yersinia species* *Staphylococcus epidermidis* *Pseudomonas* *Klebsiella* *Serratia* *Citrobacter* *Ureaplasma*
Elevated urinary pH

Figure 57.16 Factors associated with struvite stone formation. **Escherichia coli* is not a urease producer.

Struvite Stones

Struvite stones are also referred to as infection stones or triple phosphate stones. The stones grow rapidly to a large size, can reduce renal function in the affected kidney, and are difficult to eradicate. Because of the significant morbidity in patients with struvite stones, they have also been termed stone cancer. Most staghorn calculi, large stones that penetrate more than one renal calyx, are composed of struvite. Their formation requires the presence of urease-producing bacteria in the urine (Fig. 57.16).[73]

Etiology and Pathogenesis

Struvite stones form when urease production by urinary bacteria results in the formation of ammonium ions as well as alkaline urine. In this setting, phosphate is present in its trivalent form and combines with three cations, ammonium, magnesium, and calcium, the last as a component of carbonate apatite. Women are more prone to struvite nephrolithiasis than men are because of an increased propensity to UTI. Others predisposed to development of struvite stones through infections or urinary stasis include patients with indwelling urinary catheters, neurogenic bladders, genitourinary tract anomalies, and spinal cord lesions. An alkaline urine (pH 7), urease-producing bacteria in the urine, and large stones suggest the diagnosis of struvite nephrolithiasis.[73]

A number of gram-negative and gram-positive bacteria have been implicated in urease production and consequent struvite formation; the most common are *Proteus* species (see Fig. 57.16). *Escherichia coli*, which is frequently present in urine cultures, is not a urease producer. If there is a strong suspicion of struvite stones but no organism is detected in the urine, a specific culture request for *Ureaplasma urealyticum* should be considered because it does not grow on routine culture media.

Treatment

Struvite stones require aggressive medical and surgical management. Antibiotic therapy is important to reduce further stone growth and for stone prevention. Bacteria will remain in the stone interstices, however, and stones will continue to grow unless chronic antibiotic suppression is maintained or the calculi are completely eradicated. Given the need for complete stone removal to effect a cure, early urologic intervention is advised. Stones smaller than 2 cm may respond well to extracorporeal shock wave lithotripsy; however, larger stones will likely require percutaneous nephrolithotomy often in combination with extracorporeal shock wave lithotripsy (see Chapter 59). Any stone fragments retrieved should be cultured and culture-specific antibiotics continued. Once the urine is sterile, usually around 2 weeks after initiation of therapy, the dose is halved. Monthly urine cultures should be obtained, and if they remain sterile for 3 consecutive months, antibiotics may be discontinued, although surveillance urine cultures should continue monthly for a full year.[74]

Adjunct medical therapies include urease inhibitors and chemolysis. The most commonly used urease inhibitor is acetohydroxamic acid. By inhibiting urease, these agents retard stone growth and prevent new stone formation. Unfortunately, they have numerous side effects that limit their use, although adverse effects resolve on discontinuation of the drug. In addition, they require adequate renal clearance to be effective and therefore are not useful in patients with renal impairment (estimated GFR <60 ml/min).[73,75] Chemolysis refers to irrigation of the kidney through a nephrostomy tube or the ureter with a solution designed to dissolve the stones. The most common solution is 10% hemiacidrin, which contains carbonic acid, citric acid, D-gluconic acid, and magnesium at pH 3.9. Lavage chemolysis is controversial as it has previously been associated with a high mortality rate, but it is now considered safe with appropriate monitoring for UTI, assessment of obstruction to flow by intrapelvic pressure measurement, and monitoring of serum magnesium levels. Although it is not a treatment of choice for large stones, it may be useful when surgical techniques have been effective but have left residual stone fragments.

Cystine Stones

Cystinuria is an autosomal disorder in which there is a tubular defect in dibasic amino acid transport, resulting in increased cystine, ornithine, lysine, and arginine excretion (see Chapter 48). The pattern of inheritance may be autosomal recessive or autosomal dominant with incomplete penetrance. The stone disease is usually clinically manifested by the second and third decades of life. Because of the high sulfur content of the cystine molecule, the stones are apparent on plain radiographs (see Fig. 57.9A) and will often present as staghorn calculi or multiple bilateral stones.

Cystine is poorly soluble, only approximately 300 mg/l (1.25 mmol/l) at a neutral pH. Normal cystine excretion of approximately 30 to 50 mg (0.12 to 0.21 mmol) per day is readily soluble in the usual daily urine output of approximately 1 liter. However, homozygote cystinurics often excrete 250 to 1000 mg (1.04 to 4.20 mmol) of cystine per day; heterozygotes excrete an intermediate amount. Treatment must be directed at decreasing the urinary cystine concentration below the limits of solubility. Because the dietary precursor of cystine, methionine, is an essential amino acid, it is impractical to reduce intake. Increasing urine volume so that cystine remains below the limits of solubility sometimes requires 4 liters of urine per day. A low-sodium diet has been reported to reduce urine cystine excretion.[76] Increasing urine pH above 7.5 will increase cystine solubility, but this is difficult to achieve on a long-term basis. D-Penicillamine (starting dose, 250 mg daily; maximum dose, 2 g daily) and tiopronin will bind cystine and reduce urinary supersaturation; however, side effects may limit their use. The angiotensin-converting enzyme inhibitor captopril may be effective by forming a thiol-cysteine disulfide bond that is more soluble than cystine.[77]

Stones Associated with Melamine Exposure

Since September 2008, more than 50,000 Chinese children younger than 3 years have been described with kidney stones associated with contaminated milk products. Powdered milk and infant formulas were noted to contain melamine, a nitrogenous substance synthesized from urea that increases the apparent protein content of the product.[11-13] Risk factors for nephrolithiasis after melamine exposure may include volume depletion, small body size, uricosuria, and low urine pH.

Whereas affected children often presented with dysuria and hematuria, many children who were subsequently screened were asymptomatic despite kidney stones identified by ultrasound.[13] On urinalysis, some children exhibited fan-shaped crystals. The kidney stones formed were radiolucent and fragile. Many were composed of a combination of uric acid with melamine and were amenable to dissolution by hydration and alkalinization. In animal studies of melamine exposure, the distal tubular crystal deposition may lead to tubulointerstitial inflammation and fibrosis. Whether a similar process may occur in humans is unknown.[11-13]

NEPHROCALCINOSIS

Nephrocalcinosis refers to augmented calcium content within the kidney.[16,78] This disorder may be symmetric or, in anatomic disorders such as medullary sponge kidney, involve only a single kidney.

Etiology and Pathogenesis

Medullary Nephrocalcinosis

Medullary nephrocalcinosis, in which the calcification tends to occur in the area of the renal pyramids, accounts for the majority of cases of nephrocalcinosis. It is typically associated with elevated urinary calcium, phosphate, and oxalate, or it can occur with alkaline urine (Fig. 57.17). Any disorder that can lead to hypercalcemia or hypercalciuria may be implicated. Instead of stone formation, smaller parenchymal calcifications are deposited in the medulla, which are usually bilateral and relatively symmetric (Fig. 57.18). Some metabolic disorders, particularly oxalosis due to primary hyperoxaluria, can result in both medullary and cortical nephrocalcinosis (Fig. 57.19).[78]

In adults, the most common causes of medullary nephrocalcinosis are primary hyperparathyroidism, distal renal tubular acidosis, and medullary sponge kidney (see Chapter 45) as well as medications including acetazolamide, amphotericin, and triamterene (see Fig. 57.6).

Whereas a similar range of disorders can be seen in children, the most common associations are with furosemide therapy and the hereditary disorders associated with hypercalciuria.[16,23] Furosemide, when it is used in premature neonates and older infants with congestive heart failure, can result in nephrocalcinosis with or without hypercalciuria. The lesions often resolve with discontinuation of therapy. A normal calcium to creatinine ratio at the time of diagnosis of nephrocalcinosis (approximately 0.40 [mg/mg] in premature infants) appears to be a good predictor of resolution.

Many uncommon hereditary disorders are associated with nephrocalcinosis. These include X-linked hypercalciuric nephrolithiasis, X-linked hypophosphatemic rickets, hypomagnesemia-hypercalciuria syndrome, and Bartter syndrome.

X-linked hypercalciuric nephrolithiasis is also termed Dent disease in the United Kingdom, low-molecular-weight protein-

Causes of Nephrocalcinosis
Medullary
Disturbed calcium metabolism Hyperparathyroidism Sarcoidosis Milk-alkali syndrome Rapidly progressive osteoporosis Idiopathic hypercalciuria
Other tubular disease Distal (type 1) renal tubular acidosis Oxalosis* Dent disease (X-linked hypercalciuric nephrolithiasis) X-linked hypophosphatemic rickets Bartter syndrome Hypomagnesemia-hypercalciuria syndrome
Anatomic disease Medullary sponge kidney Papillary necrosis
Medications Acetazolamide Amphotericin B Triamterene
Cortical
Cortical necrosis
Transplant rejection
Chronic glomerulonephritis
Trauma
Tuberculosis
Oxalosis*

Figure 57.17 Causes of nephrocalcinosis. *Oxalosis typically causes both cortical and medullary nephrocalcinosis.

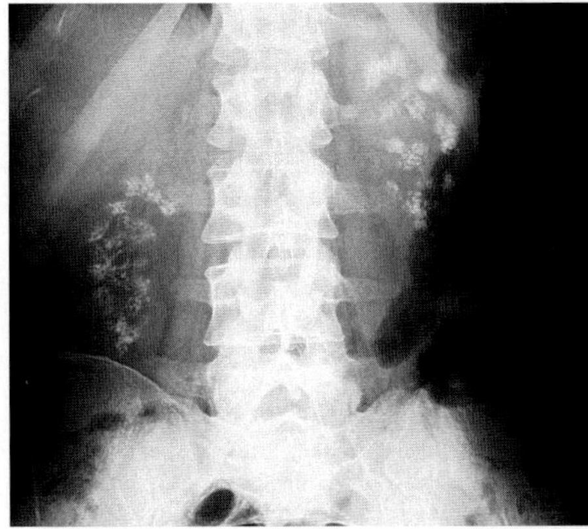

Figure 57.18 Medullary nephrocalcinosis. Plain radiograph showing bilateral metastatic medullary nephrocalcinosis in a patient with distal renal tubular acidosis.

uria with hypercalciuria and nephrocalcinosis in Japan, and X-linked recessive hypophosphatemic rickets in Italy.[79] A number of mutations affecting the *CLCN5* gene on the X chromosome have been identified that lead to inactivation of CLC-5 voltage-gated chloride channels. The result is a clinical syndrome typically affecting young boys and usually including hypercalciuria, nephrocalcinosis, nephrolithiasis, and hematuria as well as low-molecular-weight proteinuria, glycosuria, aminoaciduria, hypophosphatemia, renal failure, and rickets.[79,80]

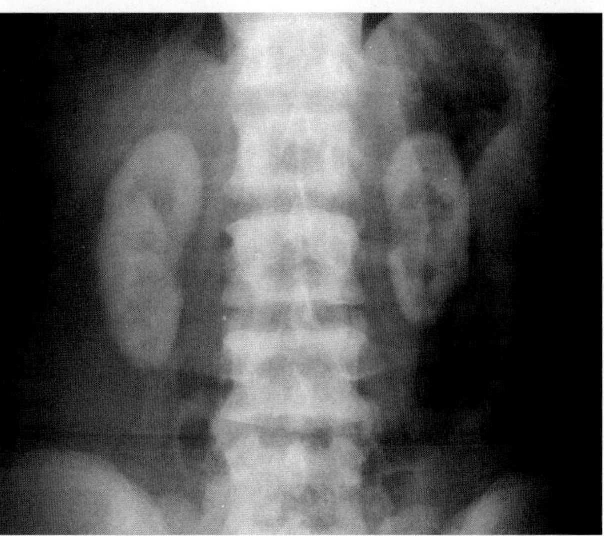

Figure 57.19 Nephrocalcinosis. Dense cortical and medullary calcification in the shrunken kidneys of a patient with oxalosis and long-standing renal failure.

In X-linked hypophosphatemic rickets, the recommended treatment, with phosphate repletion and vitamin D, may itself result in hypercalcemia, hypercalciuria, and nephrocalcinosis.

Another cause of medullary nephrocalcinosis in children is primary hypomagnesemia-hypercalciuria syndrome.[15,16,81] This rare autosomal recessive condition results from defective production of the cellular tight junction protein paracellin 1. This claudin family protein is necessary for adequate calcium and magnesium reabsorption in the thick ascending limb of the loop of Henle. Children typically present with symptoms of UTI (often with nephrolithiasis), polyuria, tetanic seizures (due to hypomagnesemia), and muscle cramps and weakness. Hypercalciuria, hypermagnesuria, and a urinary concentrating defect also occur. Patients often have renal impairment and may require renal replacement therapy by the third decade of life. Sensorineural hearing disorders and ocular impairment may accompany the renal manifestations in a subset of patients. These inherited tubular disorders are discussed further in Chapter 48.

Cortical Nephrocalcinosis

Cortical nephrocalcinosis is usually the result of dystrophic calcification, which follows parenchymal tissue destruction rather than the precipitation of excessive urinary constituents. It is secondary to infarction, neoplasm, and infection. It is typically asymmetric and is usually localized to the renal cortex (Fig. 57.20). Causes of cortical nephrocalcinosis include transplant rejection, cortical necrosis, tuberculosis, ethylene glycol toxicity, and chronic glomerulonephritis.

Clinical Manifestations

Patients who do not have nephrolithiasis associated with nephrocalcinosis are often asymptomatic. Ultrasound and CT scanning are sensitive diagnostic tests for both cortical and medullary nephrocalcinosis, demonstrating the parenchymal calcifications before they can be visualized on plain radiographs. The extent of calcification correlates poorly with renal function.

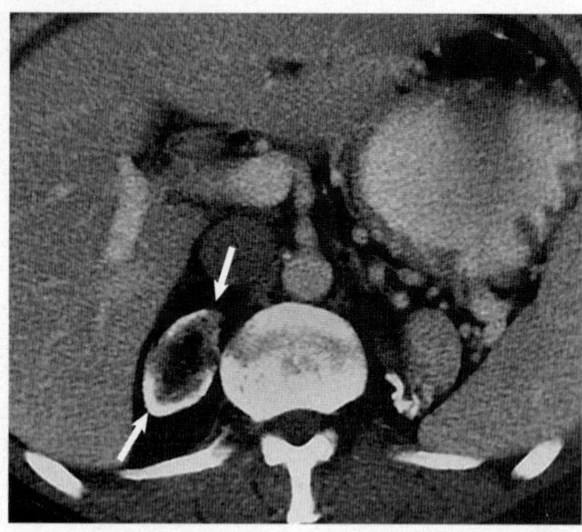

Figure 57.20 Cortical nephrocalcinosis. Non–contrast-enhanced CT scan showing cortical nephrocalcinosis *(arrows)* in the right kidney after cortical necrosis.

Treatment

Similar to treatment of nephrolithiasis, treatment of nephrocalcinosis relies on therapy for the underlying disease as well as measures to reduce hypercalcemia, hyperphosphatemia, and oxalosis, if possible.[82] The goal of treatment is usually to prevent further deposits as therapy cannot eradicate existing calcium deposits.

REFERENCES

1. Bushinsky DA, Coe FL, Moe OW. Nephrolithiasis. In: Brenner BM, ed. *The Kidney*. 8th ed. Philadelphia: WB Saunders; 2008:1299-1349.
2. Moe OW. Kidney stones: Pathophysiology and medical management. *Lancet*. 2006;367:333-344.
3. Monk RD, Bushinsky DA. Kidney stones. In: Kronenberg HM, Melmed S, Polonsky KS, Larsen PR, eds. *Williams Textbook of Endocrinology*. 11th ed. Philadelphia: Saunders Elsevier; 2008:1311-1326.
4. Stamatelou KK, Francis ME, Jones CA, et al. Time trends in reported prevalence of kidney stones in the United States: 1976-1994. *Kidney Int*. 2003;63:1817-1823.
5. Curhan GC, Willett WC, Rimm EB, et al. Body size and risk of kidney stones. *J Am Soc Nephrol*. 1998;9:1645-1652.
6. Sakhaee K, Maalouf NM. Metabolic syndrome and uric acid nephrolithiasis. *Semin Nephrol*. 2008;28:174-180.
7. Monk RD. Clinical approach to adults. *Semin Nephrol*. 1996;16: 375-388.
8. Soucie JM, Thun MJ, Coates RJ, et al. Demographic and geographic variability of kidney stones in the United States. *Kidney Int*. 1994; 46:893-899.
9. Mandel N. Mechanism of stone formation. *Semin Nephrol*. 1996;16: 364-374.
10. Maalouf NM, Cameron MA, Moe OW, Sakhaee K. Novel insights into the pathogenesis of uric acid nephrolithiasis. *Curr Opin Nephrol Hypertens*. 2004;13:181-189.
11. Hau AK, Kwan TH, Li PK. Melamine toxicity and the kidney. *J Am Soc Nephrol*. 2009;20:245-250.
12. Bhalla V, Grimm PC, Chertow GM, Pao AC. Melamine nephrotoxicity: An emerging epidemic in an era of globalization. *Kidney Int*. 2009; 75:774-779.
13. Guan N, Fan Q, Ding J, et al. Melamine-contaminated powdered formula and urolithiasis in young children. *N Engl J Med*. 2009; 360:1067-1074.
14. Evan AP, Lingeman JE, Coe FL, et al. Randall plaque of patients with nephrolithiasis begins in basement membranes of thin loops of Henle. *J Clin Invest*. 2003;111:607-616.
15. Coe FL, Evan A, Worcester E. Kidney stone disease. *J Clin Invest*. 2005;115:2598-2608.
16. Sayer JA, Carr G, Simmons NL. Nephrocalcinosis: Molecular insights into calcium precipitation within the kidney. *Clin Sci*. 2004;106: 549-561.
17. Teichman JMH. Acute renal colic from ureteral calculus. *N Engl J Med*. 2004;350:684-693.
18. Weisberg LS, Bloom PB, Simmons RL, Viner ED. Loin pain hematuria syndrome. *Am J Nephrol*. 1993;13:229-237.
19. Spetie DN, Nadasdy T, Nadasdy G, et al. Proposed pathogenesis of idiopathic loin pain–hematuria syndrome. *Am J Kidney Dis*. 2006;47: 419-427.
20. Sheil AG, Chui AK, Verran DJ, et al. Evaluation of the loin pain/hematuria syndrome treated by renal autotransplantation or radical renal neurectomy. *Am J Kidney Dis*. 1998;32:215-220.
21. Bass CM, Parrott H, Jack T, et al. Severe unexplained loin pain (loin pain haematuria syndrome): Management and long-term outcome. *QJM*. 2007;100:369-381.
22. Consensus Conference. Prevention and treatment of kidney stones. *JAMA*. 1988;260:977-981.
23. Moe OW, Bonny O. Genetic hypercalciuria. *J Am Soc Nephrol*. 2005; 16:729-745.
24. Gambaro G, Vezzoli G, Casari G, et al. Genetics of hypercalciuria and calcium nephrolithiasis: From the rare monogenic to the common polygenic forms. *Am J Kidney Dis*. 2004;44:963-986.
25. Daudon M, Jungers P. Drug-induced renal calculi: Epidemiology, prevention and management. *Drugs*. 2004;64:245-275.
26. Coe FL, Favus MJ, Crockett T, et al. Effects of low-calcium diet on urine calcium excretion, parathyroid function and serum $1,25(OH)_2D_3$ levels in patients with idiopathic hypercalciuria and in normal subjects. *Am J Med*. 1982;72:25-32.
27. Borghi L, Schianchi T, Meschi T, et al. Comparison of two diets for the prevention of recurrent stones in idiopathic hypercalciuria. *N Engl J Med*. 2002;346:77-84.
28. Asplin JR, Bauer KA, Kinder J, et al. Bone mineral density and urine calcium excretion among subjects with and without nephrolithiasis. *Kidney Int*. 2003;63:662-669.
29. Freundlich M, Alonzo E, Bellorin-Font E, Weisinger JR. Reduced bone mass in children with idiopathic hypercalciuria and in their asymptomatic mothers. *Nephrol Dial Transplant*. 2002;17:1396-1401.
30. Denton ER, Mackenzie A, Greenwell T, et al. Unenhanced helical CT for renal colic—is the radiation dose justifiable? *Clin Radiol*. 1999;54: 444-447.
31. Smith RC, Coll DM. Helical computed tomography in the diagnosis of ureteric colic. *BJU Int*. 2000;86:33-41.
32. Nakada SY, Hoff DG, Attai S, et al. Determination of stone composition by noncontrast spiral computed tomography in the clinical setting. *Urology*. 2000;55:816-819.
33. Smith RC, Verga M, McCarthy S, Rosenfield AT. Diagnosis of acute flank pain: Value of unenhanced helical CT. *AJR Am J Roentgenol*. 1996;166:97-101.
34. Smith RC, Rosenfield AT, Choe KA, et al. Acute flank pain: Comparison of non–contrast-enhanced CT and intravenous urography. *Radiology*. 1995;159:735-740.
35. Parks JH, Coward M, Coe FL. Correspondence between stone composition and urine supersaturation in nephrolithiasis. *Kidney Int*. 1997;51: 894-900.
36. Werness PG, Brown CM, Smith LH, Finlayson B. Equil2: A BASIC computer program for the calculation of urinary saturation. *J Urol*. 1985;134:1242-1244.
37. Asplin J, Parks J, Lingeman J, et al. Supersaturation and stone composition in a network of dispersed treatment sites. *J Urol*. 1998;159: 1821-1825.
38. Rodgers A, Allie-Hamdulay S, Jackson G. Therapeutic action of citrate in urolithiasis explained by chemical speciation: Increase in pH is the determinant factor. *Nephrol Dial Transplant*. 2006;21:361-369.
39. May PM, Muray K. Jess, a joint expert speciation system—II. The thermodynamic database. *Talanta*. 1991;38:1419-1426.
40. Gambaro G, Favaro S, D'Angelo A. Risk of renal failure in nephrolithiasis. *Am J Kidney Dis*. 2001;37:233-243.
41. Hosking DH, Erickson SB, Van Den Berg CJ, et al. The stone clinic effect in patients with idiopathic calcium urolithiasis. *J Urol*. 1983;130: 1115-1118.
42. Bushinsky DA. Renal lithiasis. In: Humes HD, ed. *Kelly's Textbook of Medicine*. New York: Lippincott Williams & Wilkins; 2000:1243-1248.
43. Borghi L, Meschi T, Amato F, et al. Urinary volume, water, and recurrences in idiopathic calcium nephrolithiasis: A 5-year randomized prospective study. *The Journal of Urology*. 1996;155:839-843.
44. Lemann J Jr, Pleuss JA, Worcester EM, et al. Urinary oxalate excretion increases with body size and decreases with increasing dietary calcium intake among healthy adults [erratum in Kidney Int 1996;50:341]. *Kidney Int*. 1996;49:200-208

45. Lemann J Jr, Worcester EM, Gray RW. Hypercalciuria and stones (Finlayson colloquium on urolithiasis). *Am J Kidney Dis.* 1991; 17:386.
46. Frassetto L, Morris RC Jr, Sebastian A. Long-term persistence of the urine calcium-lowering effect of potassium bicarbonate in postmenopausal women. *J Clin Endocrinol Metab.* 2005;90:831-834.
47. Lemann J Jr, Bushinsky DA, Hamm LL. Bone buffering of acid and base in humans. *Am J Physiol Renal Physiol.* 2003;285:F811-F832.
48. Taylor EN, Curhan GC. Fructose consumption and the risk of kidney stones. *Kidney Int.* 2007;73:207-212.
49. Curhan GC, Willett WC, Rimm EB, Stampfer MJ. A prospective study of dietary calcium and other nutrients and the risk of symptomatic kidney stones. *N Engl J Med.* 1993;328:833-838.
50. Stauffer JQ. Hyperoxaluria and intestinal disease: The role of steatorrhea and dietary calcium in regulating intestinal oxalate absorption. *Dig Dis.* 1977;22:921-928.
51. Curhan GC, Willett WC, Speizer FE, et al. Comparison of dietary calcium with supplemental calcium and other nutrients as factors affecting the risk for kidney stones in women. *Ann Intern Med.* 1997;126: 497-504.
52. Jackson RD, LaCroix AZ, Gass M, et al; the Women's Health Initiative Investigators. Calcium plus vitamin D supplementation and the risk of fractures. *N Engl J Med.* 2006;354:669-683.
53. Monk RD, Bushinsky DA. Pathogenesis of idiopathic hypercalciuria. In: Coe F, Favus M, Pak C, et al, eds. *Kidney Stones: Medical and Surgical Management.* Philadelphia: Lippincott-Raven; 1996;759-772.
54. Bushinsky DA. Recurrent hypercalciuric nephrolithiasis—does diet help? *N Engl J Med.* 2002;346:124-125.
55. Pak CYC, Odvina CV, Pearle MS, et al. Effect of dietary modification on urinary stone risk factors. *Kidney Int.* 2005;68:2264-2273.
56. Bushinsky DA, Frick KK, Nehrke K. Genetic hypercalciuric stone-forming rats. *Curr Opin Nephrol Hypertens.* 2006;15:403-418.
57. Coe FL, Parks JH, Asplin JR. The pathogenesis and treatment of kidney stones. *N Engl J Med.* 1992;327:1141-1152.
58. Coe FL, Parks JH, Bushinsky DA, et al. Chlorthalidone promotes mineral retention in patients with idiopathic hypercalciuria. *Kidney Int.* 1988;33:1140-1146.
59. Asplin JR. Hyperoxaluric calcium nephrolithiasis. *Endocrinol Metab Clin North Am.* 2002;31:927-949.
60. Sakhaee K. Recent advances in the pathophysiology of nephrolithiasis. *Kidney Int.* 2008;75:585-595.
61. Worcester EM. Stones from bowel disease. *Endocrinol Metab Clin North Am.* 2002;31:979-999.
62. Milliner DS. The primary hyperoxalurias: An algorithm for diagnosis. *Am J Nephrol.* 2005;25:154-160.
63. Smith LH. Hyperoxaluric states. In: Coe FL, Favus MJ, eds. *Disorders of Bone and Mineral Metabolism.* New York: Raven; 2000:707-727.
64. Kwak C, Kim HK, Kim EC, et al. Urinary oxalate levels and the enteric bacterium *Oxalobacter formigenes* in patients with calcium oxalate Urolithiasis. *Eur Urol.* 2003;44:475-481.
65. Hoppe B, Beck B, Gatter N, et al. *Oxalobacter formigenes:* A potential tool for the treatment of primary hyperoxaluria type 1. *Kidney Int.* 2006; 70:1305-1311.
66. Pak CYC, Fuller C. Idiopathic hypocitraturic calcium oxalate nephrolithiasis successfully treated with potassium citrate. *Ann Intern Med.* 1986;104:33-37.
67. Millman S, Strauss AL, Parks JH, et al. Pathogenesis and clinical course of mixed calcium oxalate and uric acid nephrolithiasis. *Kidney Int.* 1982;22:366-370.
68. Kwan TS, Padrines M, Theoleyre S, et al. IL-6, RANKL, TNF-α/IL-1: Interrelations in bone resorption pathophysiology. *Cytokine Growth Factor Rev.* 2004;15:49-60.
69. Daudon M, Traxer O, Conort P, et al. Type 2 diabetes increases the risk for uric acid stones. *J Am Soc Nephrol.* 2006;17:2026-2033.
70. Abate N, Chandalia M, Cabo-Chan AV, et al. The metabolic syndrome and uric acid nephrolithiasis: Novel features of renal manifestation of insulin resistance. *Kidney Int.* 2004;65:386-392.
71. Cameron MA, Maalouf NM, Adams-Huet B, et al. Urine composition in type 2 diabetes: Predisposition to uric acid nephrolithiasis. *J Am Soc Nephrol.* 2006;17:1422-1428.
72. Wainer L, Resnik BA, Resnick MI. *Nutritional Aspects of Stone Disease.* Boston: Martinus Nijhoff; 1987.
73. Rodman JS. Struvite stones. *Nephron.* 1999;81:50-59.
74. Wong HY, Riedl CR, Griffith DP. Medical management and prevention of struvite stones. In: Coe FL, Favus MJ, Pak CYC, eds. *Kidney Stones: Medical and Surgical Management.* Philadelphia: Lippincott-Raven; 1996:941-950.
75. Rodman JS. Struvite stones. In: Pak CYC, ed. *Renal Stone Disease: Pathogenesis, Prevention, and Treatment.* Boston: Martinus Nijhoff; 1987: 225-251.
76. Goldfarb DS, Coe FL, Asplin JR. Urinary cystine excretion and capacity in patients with cystinuria. *Kidney Int.* 2006;69:1041-1047.
77. Sakhaee K. Pathogenesis and medical management of cystinuria. *Semin Nephrol.* 1996;16:435-447.
78. Ramchandani P, Pollack HM. Radiologic evaluation of patients with urolithiasis. In: Coe FL, Favus MJ, Pak CYC, et al, eds. *Kidney Stones: Medical and Surgical Management.* Philadelphia: Lippincott-Raven; 1996:369-435.
79. Scheinman SJ. X-linked hypercalciuric nephrolithiasis: Clinical syndromes and chloride channel mutations. *Kidney Int.* 1998;53:3-17.
80. Scheinman SJ, Guay-Woodford LM, Thakker RV, Warnock DG. Genetic disorders of renal electrolyte transport. *N Engl J Med.* 1999;340:1177-1187.
81. Benigno V, Canonica CS, Bettinelli A, et al. Hypomagnesaemia-hypercalciuria-nephrocalcinosis: A report of nine cases and a review. *Nephrol Dial Transplant.* 2000;15:605-610.
82. Alon US. Nephrocalcinosis. *Curr Opin Pediatr.* 1997;9:160-165.

CHAPTER 58

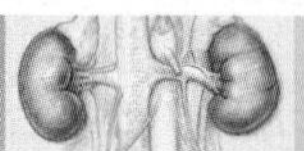

Urinary Tract Obstruction

Kevin P.G. Harris, Jeremy Hughes

DEFINITIONS

Obstructive uropathy refers to the structural or functional changes in the urinary tract that impede normal urine flow. Obstructive nephropathy refers to the renal disease caused by impaired flow of urine or tubular fluid. Hydronephrosis refers to dilation of the urinary tract. Importantly, hydronephrosis is not synonymous with obstructive uropathy as it can occur without functional obstruction to the urinary tract and can be absent in established obstruction. Obstructive uropathy and nephropathy frequently coexist, and their management requires close collaboration between nephrologists and urologists. Some surgical aspects of obstruction to the urinary tract are discussed in Chapter 59.

Obstructive uropathy is classified according to the site, degree, and duration of the obstruction. Acute or chronic obstruction can occur anywhere in the urinary tract and includes intrarenal causes (casts, crystals) and extrarenal causes. Acute or chronic obstruction is further subdivided into upper urinary tract obstruction (usually unilateral obstruction occurring above the vesicoureteral junction) and lower urinary tract obstruction (usually bilateral obstruction located below the vesicoureteral junction). Complete obstruction of the urinary tract is termed high grade, whereas partial or incomplete obstruction is termed low grade.

Unilateral obstruction in a patient with two normal kidneys will not result in significant renal impairment because the contralateral kidney compensates. However, bilateral obstruction or the obstruction of a single functioning kidney will result in renal failure. In acute urinary tract obstruction, changes are mainly functional, whereas structural damage to the kidney results from more chronic obstruction. The acute functional changes may recover after the effective release of the obstruction, but structural changes may be permanent and lead to chronic renal impairment. Urinary tract obstruction remains a major cause of renal impairment worldwide.

ETIOLOGY AND PATHOGENESIS

The causes of obstructive uropathy affecting the upper and lower urinary tracts are summarized in Figures 58.1 and 58.2.

Congenital Urinary Tract Obstruction

Congenital urinary tract obstruction occurs most frequently in males, most commonly as a result of either posterior urethral valves or pelviureteral junction obstruction. If obstruction occurs early during development, the kidney fails to develop and becomes dysplastic. If the obstruction is bilateral, there is a high mortality rate as a result of severe renal failure. If the obstruction occurs later in gestation and is low grade or unilateral, hydronephrosis and nephron loss will still occur, but renal function may be sufficient to allow survival, and such patients may not present until later in childhood. Pelviureteral junction obstruction, if it is mild, may not present until adulthood and in some patients may be an incidental finding (Fig. 58.3). However, with increased use and improved sensitivity of antenatal scanning, congenital abnormalities of the urinary tract are now frequently identified early, allowing prompt postnatal (and in some cases antenatal) intervention to relieve the obstruction and hence to preserve renal function. Congenital causes of obstruction are discussed further in Chapter 50.

Acquired Urinary Tract Obstruction

Acquired urinary tract obstruction may affect either the upper or lower urinary tract and can result from either intrinsic or extrinsic causes. Intrinsic causes of obstruction may be intraluminal or intramural.

Intrinsic Obstruction

Intraluminal Obstruction Intraluminal obstruction may result from tubular intrarenal obstruction, such as the deposition of uric acid crystals in the tubular lumen after treatment of hematologic malignant neoplasms (tumor lysis syndrome). It may also occur with the precipitation of Bence Jones protein in myeloma and with the precipitation or crystal formation of a number of drugs, including sulfonamides, acyclovir, methotrexate, and indinavir (see Chapter 66).

Extrarenal intraluminal obstruction in young adults is most commonly caused by renal calculi (see Chapter 57). Calcium oxalate stones are the most common and typically cause intermittent acute unilateral urinary tract obstruction but rarely result in marked chronic renal impairment. Less common causes of urinary lithiasis, such as struvite stones, uric acid stones, and cystinuria, are often bilateral and hence more likely to cause long-term renal impairment. Renal calculi lodge more commonly in the calyx, pelviureteral junction, or vesicoureteral junction and at the level of the pelvic brim. Surgical management of stones is discussed in Chapter 59. Intraluminal obstruction can also result from a sloughed papilla after papillary necrosis or blood clots after macroscopic hematuria (clot colic). Papillary necrosis may occur in diabetes mellitus, sickle cell trait or disease, analgesic nephropathy, renal amyloidosis, and acute pyelonephritis. Clot colic can occur with bleeding from renal tumors or

Causes of Upper Urinary Tract Obstruction	
Intrinsic Causes	**Extrinsic Causes**
Intraluminal Intratubular deposition of crystals (uric acid, drugs) *Stones* Papillary tissue Blood clots Fungal ball	Reproductive system Cervix: *carcinoma* Uterus: *pregnancy, tumors,* prolapse, endometriosis, pelvic inflammatory disease Ovary: abscess, tumor, cysts Prostate: *carcinoma*
Intramural Functional: pelvic-ureteral or vesicoureteral junction dysfunction Anatomic: tumors (benign or malignant) Infections, granulomas, strictures	Vascular system Aneurysms: aorta, iliac vessels Aberrant arteries: pelviureteral junction Venous: ovarian veins, retrocaval ureter
	Gastrointestinal tract Crohn's disease Pancreatitis Appendicitis Diverticulitis Tumors
	Retroperitoneal space Lymph nodes Fibrosis: idiopathic, drugs, or inflammatory Tumors: primary or metastatic Hematomas Radiation therapy
	Surgical disruption or ureteral ligation

Figure 58.1 Causes of upper urinary tract obstruction. The most common causes are in italics.

Causes of Lower Urinary Tract Obstruction
Urethral anatomic causes Urethal strictures: trauma, *postinstrumentation*, infections such as gonococcal urethritis, nongonococcal urethritis, tuberculosis *Posterior urethral valves* Stones Blood clots Periurethral abscess Phimosis Paraphimosis Meatal stenosis
Urethral functional causes Anticholinergic drugs, antidepressants, levodopa
Prostate *Benign prostatic hypertrophy* *Prostatic carcinoma* Prostatic calculi Prostatic infection
Bladder anatomic causes *Bladder cancer* *Schistosomiasis (Schistosoma haematobium* infection) Bladder calculi Bladder trauma, pelvic fracture
Bladder functional causes *Neurogenic bladder*: spinal cord defects or trauma, diabetes, multiple sclerosis, Parkinson's disease, cerebrovascular accidents

Figure 58.2 Causes of lower urinary tract obstruction. The most common causes are in italics.

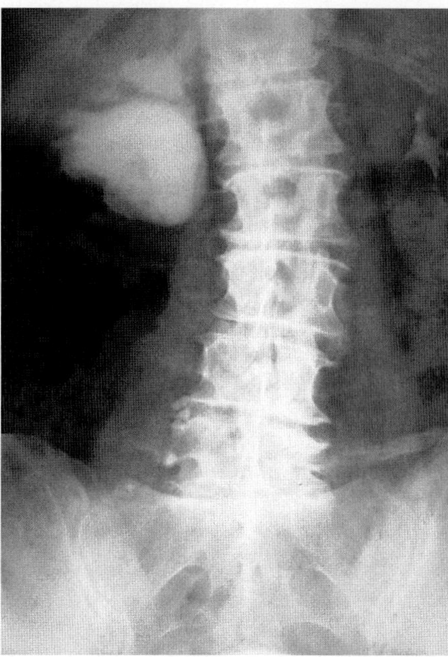

Figure 58.3 Intravenous urogram demonstrating pelviureteral junction obstruction. The study was performed in a previously asymptomatic adult to investigate nonspecific right loin pain. There is unilateral (right side) dilation of the pelvicalyceal system. The ureter has not been visualized.

arteriovenous malformations, after renal trauma, and in patients with polycystic kidney disease.

Intramural Obstruction Intramural obstruction can result from either functional or anatomic changes. Functional disorders include vesicoureteral reflux, adynamic ureteral segments (usually at the junction of the ureter with the pelvis or bladder), and neurologic disorders. The last may result in a contracted (hypertonic) bladder or a flaccid (atonic) bladder, depending on whether the lesion affects upper or lower motor neurons, and lead to impaired bladder emptying with vesicoureteral reflux. Bladder dysfunction is very common in patients with multiple sclerosis and after spinal cord injury and is also seen in diabetes mellitus, in Parkinson's disease, and after cerebrovascular accidents. Some drugs (anticholinergics, levodopa) can alter neuromuscular activity of the bladder and result in functional obstruction, especially if there is preexisting bladder outflow obstruction (e.g., prostatic hypertrophy).

Anatomic causes of intramural obstruction of the upper urinary tract include transitional cell carcinoma of the renal pelvis and ureter and ureteral strictures secondary to radiotherapy or retroperitoneal surgery. Rarely, obstruction may result from ureteral valve malfunction, polyps, or strictures after therapy for tuberculosis. Intramural obstruction of the lower urinary tract can result from urethral strictures, which are usually secondary to chronic instrumentation or previous urethritis, or malignant and benign tumors of the bladder. Infection with *Schistosoma haematobium*, when the ova lodge in the distal ureter and bladder, is a common cause of obstructive uropathy worldwide; up to 50% of chronically infected patients develop ureteral strictures and fibrosis, with contraction of the bladder.

Extrinsic Obstruction

The most common cause of extrinsic compression in women is pressure from a gravid uterus on the pelvic rim; the right ureter is more commonly affected. It is usually asymptomatic, and the changes resolve rapidly after delivery. Rarely, bilateral obstruction and acute kidney injury [AKI] may occur. Ureteral dilation may frequently be seen in pregnancy as a result of hormonal effects (especially progesterone) on smooth muscle, but this does not indicate functional obstruction (see Chapter 41, Fig. 41.1). Carcinoma of the cervix may also cause extrinsic obstruction because direct extension of the tumor to involve the urinary tract occurs in up to 30% of patients. Other pelvic pathologic processes that can cause ureteral compression include benign and malignant uterine and ovarian masses, abscesses, endometriosis, and pelvic inflammatory disease. Compression of the ureters outside the bladder may also occur with uterine prolapse. Although rare (<0.5%), inadvertent ureteric ligation may occur during surgical procedures, particularly those related to obstetrics and gynecology. Unilateral ligation may go undetected, but AKI will result from bilateral ligation.

In men, the most common cause of extrinsic obstruction of the lower urinary tract is benign prostatic hypertrophy. Carcinoma of the prostate can also result in obstruction either from direct tumor extension to the bladder outlet or ureters or from metastases to the ureter or lymph nodes.

Retroperitoneal disease may also result in extrinsic obstruction of the ureters, as can metastases or extension of tumors from the cervix, prostate, bladder, colon, ovary, and uterus. Primary tumors of the retroperitoneum, such as lymphomas and sarcomas, can commonly cause obstruction. Obstruction can also result from inflammatory conditions affecting the retroperitoneum, such as Crohn's disease and large bowel diverticulitis. In Crohn's disease, the obstruction is usually right sided as a result of ileocecal disease. Less common pathologic processes include retroperitoneal fibrosis, in which thick fibrous tissue extends out from the aorta to encase the ureters and draw them medially (Fig. 58.4). Retroperitoneal fibrosis may be idiopathic but can result from inflammatory aortic aneurysms, certain drugs (e.g., β-blockers, bromocriptine, and methysergide), previous irradiation, trauma or surgery, and granulomatous disease (e.g., tuberculosis, sarcoidosis). Ureteral compression may also be a result of vascular abnormalities, including aneurysmal dilation of the aorta or iliac vessels, aberrant vessels, and anatomic variations in the location of the ureter (retrocaval ureter).

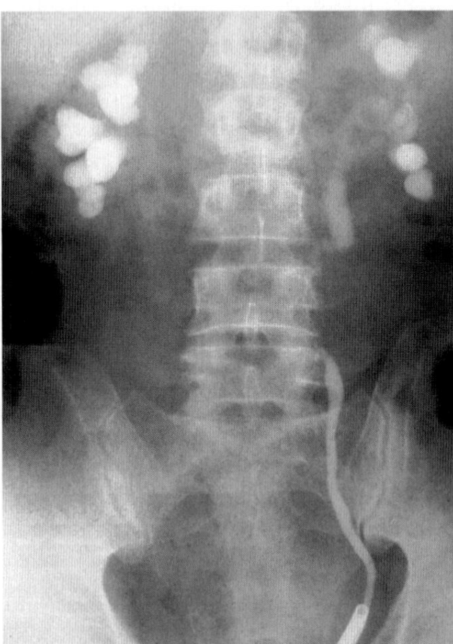

Figure 58.4 Retrograde pyelogram showing idiopathic retroperitoneal fibrosis. Dilation of the pelvicalyceal system is clearly demonstrated. The ureters, however, are not dilated, and the left ureter can be seen being pulled medially as a result of encasement in thick fibrous tissue.

PATHOPHYSIOLOGY

Obstruction to the renal tract causes profound functional and structural changes of the kidney.[1] Initially, changes are predominantly functional and potentially reversible, but with time, chronic and irreversible structural changes occur. Our understanding of the consequences of urinary tract obstruction stem mainly from the study of animal models.[2] Although many studies have focused on the effects of complete ureteral obstruction in rodents, investigators have also examined models of chronic complete, partial, or reversible obstruction in adult and neonatal animals.[3] Available experimental data show little species to species variation in the response to acute obstruction, suggesting that similar changes are likely to occur in humans. The complex effects of urinary tract obstruction on the kidney affect both glomerular hemodynamics and tubular function.[4]

Changes in Glomerular Function

Glomerular filtration rate (GFR) declines progressively after the onset of complete ureteral obstruction. Glomerular filtration is determined by the mean hydraulic pressure gradient between the glomerular capillary lumen and Bowman's space, the renal plasma flow, the ultrafiltration coefficient of the glomerular capillary wall, and the mean oncotic pressure difference across the glomerular wall. Obstruction can affect all of these, and the effects vary with the duration of the obstruction, the hydration state, and the presence or absence of a contralateral functioning kidney.

After complete ureteral obstruction, there is an initial rise in proximal tubular pressure. At the same time, afferent arteriolar dilation occurs as a result of the generation of vasodilatory prostaglandins (e.g., prostacyclin, prostaglandin E_2). Glomerular capillary hydraulic pressure increases, but this does not offset the rise in tubular pressure, and there is a net decrease in the hydraulic pressure gradient across glomerular capillaries, resulting in an 80% decline in GFR.

About 2 to 5 hours after obstruction, renal blood flow begins to decline, whereas intratubular pressure continues to increase. Within 5 hours, proximal tubular pressure begins to decline toward control values. From this time, the main determinant of the decrease in GFR is the fall in intraglomerular capillary pressure as a result of an increase in resistance of afferent arterioles. This results in a progressive fall in renal plasma flow, which reaches 30% to 50% of control values by 24 hours. Preferential constriction of the preglomerular blood vessels lowers both plasma flow and glomerular capillary pressure, resulting in a greater decrement in GFR than in plasma flow and a fall in filtration fraction. A falling filtration fraction also results from diversion of blood to nonfiltering areas of the kidney or a reduction in the ultrafiltration coefficient. The relative changes in ureteral pressure, renal plasma flow, and GFR are summarized in Figure 58.5.

The intrarenal vasoconstriction results from the generation of angiotensin II and thromboxane A_2, the release of vasopressin (antidiuretic hormone), and the decreased nitric oxide produc-

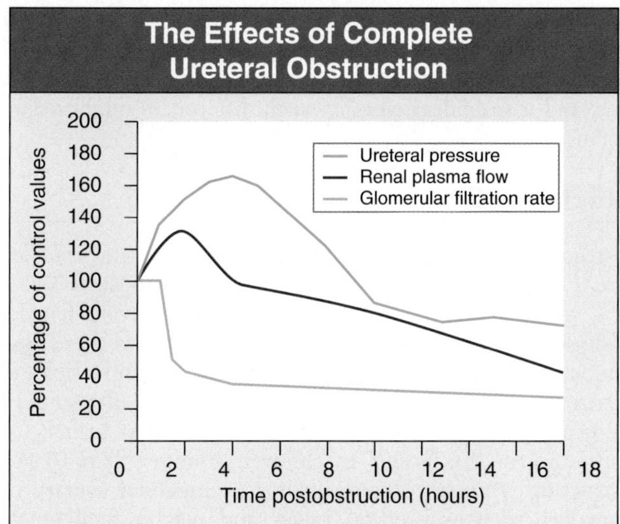

Figure 58.5 The effects of complete ureteral obstruction. The relative changes in ureteral pressure, renal plasma flow, and glomerular filtration rate are shown with data from experimental studies of unilateral ureteral obstruction in rats.

tion. Angiotensin II and thromboxane A_2 may also reduce the ultrafiltration coefficient.[4,5] The central role of these two vasoconstrictors has been demonstrated by studies in rats, in which pretreatment with angiotensin-converting enzyme inhibitors and thromboxane synthase inhibitors virtually normalized renal function after the relief of short-term ureteral obstruction.[6]

Intrarenal angiotensin II generation occurs secondary to an increase in renin release either through reduced delivery of sodium and chloride to the distal nephron (macula densa mechanism) or through a reduction in transmural pressure at the baroreceptor as a consequence of the prostaglandin-dependent dilation of the afferent arteriole. Generation of thromboxane A_2 occurs in both glomeruli and infiltrating interstitial cells.

An interstitial leukocyte infiltrate, predominantly macrophages, develops in response to chemoattractants such as monocyte chemoattractant protein 1 and osteopontin expressed by tubular cells. This infiltrate plays a key role in the acute functional changes after ureteral obstruction[7] and is implicated in the pathogenesis of the late structural changes that occur after obstruction as macrophage depletion limits interstitial fibrosis.[8]

The extent to which glomerular function recovers after the release of ureteral obstruction depends on the duration of the obstruction. Whole-kidney GFR may return to normal after short-term obstruction (days), whereas recovery may be incomplete after prolonged obstruction. Evidence from studies in rats now suggests that even with shorter periods of obstruction (72 hours), there may be a permanent loss of nephrons, and whole-kidney GFR returns to normal only at the expense of hyperfiltration (increase in single-nephron GFR) in the remaining functional nephrons.[9]

Changes in Tubular Function

Abnormalities in tubular function are common in urinary tract obstruction and are manifested as altered renal handling of electrolytes and changes in the regulation of water excretion.[4] The degree and nature of the tubular defects after obstruction depend in part on whether the obstruction is bilateral or unilateral. These differences could result from the dissimilar hemodynamic responses, different intrinsic changes within the nephron, differences in extrinsic factors (e.g., volume expansion and accumulation of natriuretic substances in bilateral obstruction) between the two states, or a combination of all three.

After ureteral obstruction, the ability to concentrate the urine is markedly impaired, with maximum values of 350 to 400 mOsm/kg reported in the rat. Causative factors include a loss of medullary tonicity, an overall decrease in GFR in deep nephrons, and a reduced expression of sodium transporters.[10] Also, the collecting duct is unresponsive to vasopressin because of a reduction in the expression of renal aquaporins that results from both cyclooxygenase 2 activity[11] and angiotensin II.[12]

Rats exhibit reduced expression of multiple acid-base transporters after ureteral obstruction,[13] and patients with urinary tract obstruction often exhibit urinary acidification defects. This may be detected only by exogenous acid loading, but hyperchloremic acidosis caused by impaired distal acid secretion, hyporeninemic hypoaldosteronism (type 4 renal tubular acidosis), and a combination of these findings have been described. This acidifying defect results from a marked increase in bicarbonate excretion or from a distal acidification defect, possibly as a result of abnormalities of the H^+-ATPase activity of intercalated cells of the collecting duct after ureteral obstruction.

Obstruction alters renal potassium handling. In the presence of a normal functioning contralateral kidney, potassium excretion is reduced after relief of obstruction, either in proportion to or perhaps even greater than the fall in GFR (i.e., fractional excretion of potassium is unaltered or slightly reduced). There is a defect in the distal potassium secretory mechanism after unilateral obstruction that may be secondary to reduced responsiveness of that nephron segment to aldosterone. By contrast, after release of bilateral ureteral obstruction, there is a marked increase in both net and fractional potassium excretion. The major mechanism by which potassium losses occur in this setting is an increased delivery of sodium to the distal tubule, resulting in an accelerated sodium-potassium exchange.

Recovery of tubular function after release of obstruction is slow and may remain abnormal even after whole-kidney GFR has returned to normal. In rats, acidification and potassium handling abnormalities persist for at least 14 days and urinary concentrating ability is abnormal for up to 60 days after the release of 24 hours of unilateral ureteral obstruction. These observations are consistent with persistent alterations in distal tubular and collecting duct function or a loss in functioning juxtaglomerular nephrons after the release of the obstruction.

Histopathologic Changes

The morphologic alterations in renal architecture are similar irrespective of the cause of the obstruction. Initially, there is renal enlargement and edema with pelvicalyceal dilation (Fig. 58.6). Tubular dilation that predominantly affects the collecting duct and distal tubular segments develops microscopically, although cellular flattening and atrophy of proximal tubular cells can also occur. Glomerular structures are usually preserved initially, although Bowman's space may be dilated and contain Tamm-Horsfall protein. Ultimately, some periglomerular fibrosis may develop.

Inadequately treated obstruction to the urinary tract eventually causes irreversible structural changes to the renal tract. The renal pelvis becomes widely dilated, with the renal papillae either flattened or hollowed out. The cortex and medulla become grossly thinned, such that the kidney becomes a thin rim of renal tissue surrounding a large saccular pelvis (Fig. 58.7). Histologic

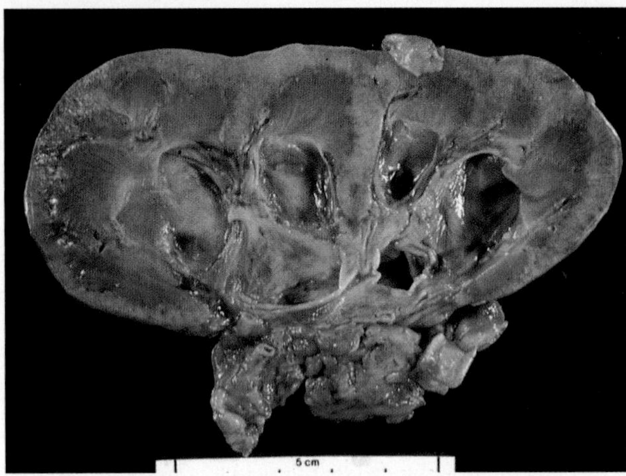

Figure 58.6 Autopsy specimen of a kidney showing the early effects of ureteral obstruction. The kidney is enlarged and edematous with pelvicalyceal dilation. There is good preservation of the renal parenchyma.

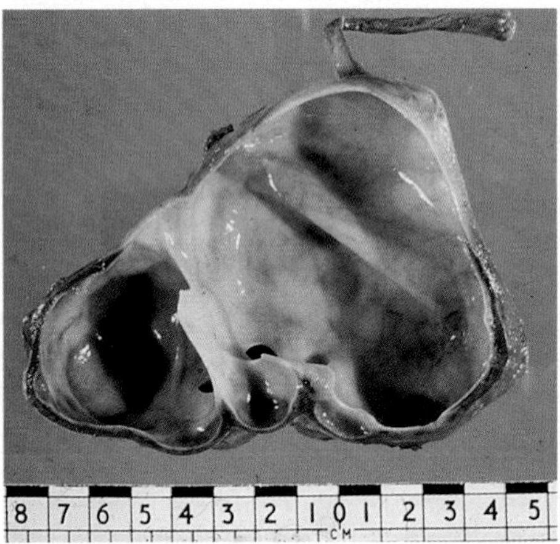

Figure 58.7 Chronic ureteral obstruction. Surgical specimen of a kidney showing gross dilation of the pelvicalyceal system and the reduction of the renal cortex to a thin fibrotic rim of tissue. There would have been no prospect for any significant functional recovery in this kidney after the relief of the obstruction.

examination demonstrates tubulointerstitial fibrosis and obliteration of nephrons. There is tubular proliferation and apoptosis, epithelial-mesenchymal transition, (myo)fibroblast accumulation, increased extracellular matrix deposition, and tubular atrophy. Ischemia as a result of the decreased renal blood flow contributes to the parenchymal damage after obstruction. In both genetic and interventional studies, an important pathologic role for angiotensin II and transforming growth factor β (TGF-β) has been established.[14,15]

Infiltrating macrophages play a pivotal role in the chronic tissue injury and fibrosis that result from prolonged ureteral obstruction (Fig. 58.8).[8,16] Interstitial macrophages release profibrogenic factors such as TGF-β and galectin-3, which promote progressive fibrosis. Local angiotensin II generation may also stimulate the production of TGF-β by tubular cells. Treatments shown to ameliorate chronic interstitial damage in experimental obstructive uropathy include angiotensin receptor blockers, pentoxifylline, simvastatin, and growth factors (such as bone morphogenetic protein 7, hepatocyte growth factor, and epidermal growth factor); beneficial effects include a reduction in tubulointerstitial inflammation and fibrosis, epithelial-mesenchymal transdifferentiation, and tubular cell apoptosis.[3] However, it is pertinent that differences have been noted in the response of adult and neonatal rodents to experimental therapeutic interventions, and it is unclear whether such differences might occur in humans.

EPIDEMIOLOGY

Obstructive uropathy is a common entity and can occur at all ages. The prevalence of hydronephrosis at autopsy is 3.5% to 3.8%, with about equal distribution between males and females,[17] although this underestimates the true incidence as these figures exclude transient obstruction. The frequency and etiology of obstruction vary in both sexes with age. Antenatal ultrasound has significantly increased the detection rate of lower urinary tract obstruction in the fetus.[18] In children younger than 10 years, obstruction is more common in boys; congenital urinary tract anomalies, such as urethral valves and pelviureteral junction obstruction, account for most cases. In North America, obstructive uropathy remains the most common cause of end-stage renal disease (ESRD) in pediatric patients registered for renal transplantation, accounting for 16% of cases. In addition, congenital obstructive uropathy accounts for 0.7% of all patients (median age, 31 years) maintained with renal replacement therapy, demonstrating the continued impact of this disease into adult life.[19] In young adults (<20 years of age), the frequency of urinary tract obstruction is similar in males and females. Beyond 20 years of age, obstruction becomes more common in women, mainly as a result of pregnancy and gynecologic malignant neoplasms. The peak incidence of renal calculi occurs in the second and third decades of life with a threefold increased incidence in men. After the age of 60 years, obstructive uropathy occurs more frequently in men secondary to benign prostatic hypertrophy and prostatic carcinoma. About 80% of men older than 60 years have some symptoms of bladder outflow obstruction, and up to 10% have hydronephrosis. In Europe, acquired urinary tract obstruction accounts for 3% to 5% of the cases of ESRD in patients older than 65 years, with most resulting from prostatic disease.[20] In the United States, the number of patients receiving renal replacement therapy as a result of acquired obstruction continues to increase, accounting for 1.4% of prevalent patients, although the rise is not as rapid as with other causes of ESRD.[19]

CLINICAL MANIFESTATIONS

Obstruction of the urinary tract can present with a wide range of clinical symptoms, depending on the site, degree, and duration of obstruction.[4] The clinical manifestations of upper and lower urinary tract obstruction differ. Symptoms can be caused by mechanical obstruction of the urinary tract (usually pain) or can result from the complex alterations in glomerular and tubular function that may occur in obstructive nephropathy. The latter commonly present as alterations in urine volume and as renal failure, which can be acute or chronic. For example, patients with complete obstruction present with anuria and AKI, whereas those with partial obstruction may present with polyuria and polydipsia as a result of acquired vasopressin resistance. Alternatively, there may be a fluctuating urine output, alternating from oliguria to polyuria. However, obstructive uropathy and hence obstructive nephropathy can occur without symptoms and with minimal clinical manifestations. Thus, obstruction of the urinary tract must be considered in the differential diagnosis of any patient with renal impairment.

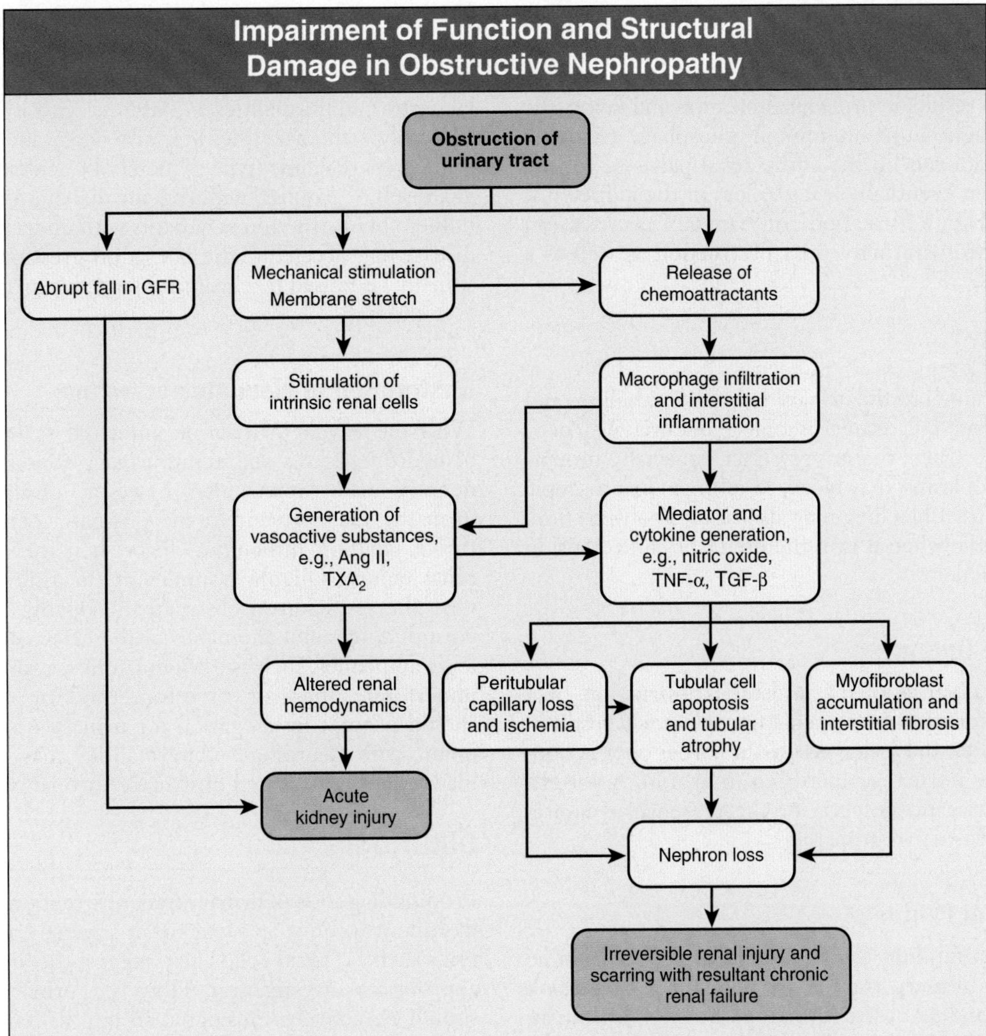

Figure 58.8 Events leading to acute impairment of renal function and chronic structural damage in obstructive nephropathy. Ang II, angiotensin II; GFR, glomerular filtration rate; TGF-β, transforming growth factor β; TNF-α, tumor necrosis factor α; TXA_2, thromboxane A_2.

Pain

Pain is a frequent complaint in patients with obstructive uropathy, particularly in those with ureteral calculi. The pain is believed to result from stretching of the collecting system or the renal capsule. Its severity correlates with the degree of distention and not with the degree of dilation of the urinary tract. On occasion, the location of the pain helps determine the site of obstruction. With upper ureteral or pelvic obstruction, flank pain and tenderness typically occur, whereas lower ureteral obstruction causes pain that radiates to the groin, the ipsilateral testicle, or the labia. Acute high-grade ureteral obstruction may be accompanied by a steady and severe crescendo flank pain radiating to the labia, the testicles, or the groin ("classic" renal colic). The acute attack may last less than half an hour or as long as a day. In contrast, pain radiating into the flank during micturition is said to be pathognomonic of vesicoureteral reflux. By comparison, patients with chronic, slowly progressive obstruction may have no pain or minimal pain during the course of their disease. In such patients, any pain that does occur is rarely colicky in nature. In pelviureteral junction obstruction, pain may occur only after fluid loading to promote a high urine flow rate.

Lower Urinary Tract Symptoms

Obstructive lesions of the bladder neck or bladder disease may cause a decrease in the force or caliber of the urine stream, intermittency, post-micturition dribbling, hesitancy, or nocturia. Urgency, frequency, and urinary incontinence can result from incomplete bladder emptying. Such symptoms commonly result from prostatic hypertrophy and are frequently referred to as prostatism, but they are not pathognomonic of this condition.

Urinary Tract Infections

Urinary stasis resulting from obstruction predisposes to urinary tract infections, and patients may develop cystitis with dysuria and frequency or pyelonephritis with loin pain and systemic symptoms. Infection occurs more often in patients with lower urinary tract obstruction than in those with upper urinary tract obstruction.

Urinary tract infection in men or young children of either sex, recurrent or persistent infections in women, infections with unusual organisms such as *Pseudomonas* species, and a single attack of acute pyelonephritis require further investigation to exclude obstruction. Also, the presence of obstruction makes effective eradication of the infection difficult. Infections of the urinary tract with a urease-producing organism such as *Proteus mirabilis* predispose to stone formation. These organisms generate ammonia, which results in urine alkalinization and favors the development of magnesium ammonium phosphate (struvite) stones. Struvite calculi can fill the entire renal pelvis to form a staghorn calculus that eventually leads to loss of the kidney if it is untreated. Thus, stone formation and papillary necrosis can also be a consequence of urinary tract obstruction as well as a cause of obstruction.

Hematuria

Calculi may cause trauma to the urinary tract uroepithelium and result in either macroscopic or microscopic hematuria. Any neoplastic lesion that obstructs the urinary tract, especially uroepithelial malignant neoplasms, may bleed, resulting in macroscopic hematuria. Urinary tract bleeding may also result in obstruction, giving rise to clot colic when it is in the ureter or clot retention when it is in the bladder.

Changes in Urine Output

Complete bilateral obstruction or unilateral obstruction of a single functioning kidney such as a renal transplant will result in anuria. However, when the lesion results in partial obstruction, urine output may be normal or increased (polyuria). A pattern of alternating oliguria and polyuria or the presence of anuria strongly suggests obstructive uropathy.

Abnormal Physical Findings

Physical examination findings can be completely normal. Some patients with upper urinary tract obstruction may have flank tenderness. Long-standing obstructive uropathy may result in an enlarged kidney that may be palpable. Hydronephrosis is a common cause of a palpable abdominal mass in children. Lower urinary tract obstruction causes a distended, palpable, and occasionally painful bladder. A rectal examination and, in women, a pelvic examination should be performed because they may reveal a local malignant neoplasm or prostatic enlargement.

Acute or chronic hydronephrosis, either unilateral or bilateral, may cause hypertension as a result of impaired sodium excretion with expansion of extracellular fluid volume or from the abnormal release of renin. On occasion, in patients with partial urinary tract obstruction, hypotension occurs as a result of polyuria and volume depletion.

Abnormal Laboratory Findings

Urinalysis may show hematuria, bacteriuria, pyuria, crystalluria, and low-grade proteinuria, depending on the cause of obstruction. However, urinalysis may be completely negative despite advanced obstructive nephropathy. In the acute phase of obstruction, urinary electrolyte values are similar to those seen in a "prerenal" state, with a low urinary sodium (<20 mmol/l), a low fractional excretion of sodium (<1%), and a high urinary osmolality (>500 mOsm/kg). However, with more prolonged obstruction, there is a decreased ability to concentrate the urine and an inability to reabsorb sodium and other solutes. These changes are particularly marked after the release of chronic obstruction and give rise to the syndrome commonly referred to as postobstructive diuresis. Obstructive nephropathy may cause secondary polycythemia as a result of increased erythropoietin production.

Increases in serum urea and creatinine are the most significant laboratory abnormalities in patients with obstructive uropathy. Electrolyte abnormalities may also occur, including a hyperchloremic hyperkalemic (type 4) metabolic acidosis or hypernatremia as a result of acquired nephrogenic diabetes insipidus. The development of obstruction in patients with underlying chronic kidney disease may accelerate the rate of progression. ESRD may occasionally be caused by chronic obstructive uropathy that had been asymptomatic.

Obstruction in Neonates or Infants

With the advent of routine antenatal scanning, the diagnosis of hydronephrosis and genitourinary abnormalities is now frequently made antenatally; however, unsuspected obstructive uropathy may present in the postnatal period with failure to thrive, voiding difficulties, fever, hematuria, or symptoms of renal failure. Oligohydramnios at the time of delivery should raise the suspicion of obstructive uropathy, as should the presence of congenital anomalies of the external genitalia. Nonurologic anomalies, such as ear deformities, a single umbilical artery, imperforate anus, or a rectourethral or rectovaginal fistula, should prompt investigation for urinary tract obstruction. Any infant with neurologic abnormalities may have a neurogenic bladder with associated obstructive uropathy.

DIAGNOSIS

Prompt diagnosis of urinary tract obstruction is essential to allow treatment to limit any long-term adverse consequences. Symptoms such as "renal colic" may suggest the diagnosis and prompt appropriate investigation. However, urinary tract obstruction should be actively considered in any patient with unexplained acute or chronic kidney impairment. The diagnostic approach has to be tailored to the clinical presentation (Fig. 58.9), but a careful history and thorough physical examination are mandatory in all patients.

Urinalysis may provide valuable diagnostic information. Hematuria suggests that the obstructing lesion is a calculus, sloughed papilla, or tumor. Bacteriuria suggests urinary stasis, especially in men or in pregnant women, but it may also be a complication of chronic obstruction. The presence of crystals in the urine sediment (cystine or uric acid) may be an indication of the type of stone causing the ureteral obstruction or the intrarenal obstruction resulting in AKI. Laboratory studies should include an assessment of renal function (serum creatinine and urea) and the measurement of serum electrolytes.

Imaging

Because the sites, causes, and consequences of obstruction to the renal tract are so variable, no single imaging investigation can diagnose renal tract obstruction with certainty. Thus, no single imaging investigation should be relied on to definitively exclude obstruction, especially if the clinical suspicion of obstruction is high. Therefore, the approach to the patient with suspected obstruction may require the complementary use of a number of different imaging techniques.

Ultrasound is the most widely used imaging modality, but the imaging approach to investigation of obstruction is changing. Computed tomography (CT) and magnetic resonance (MR)

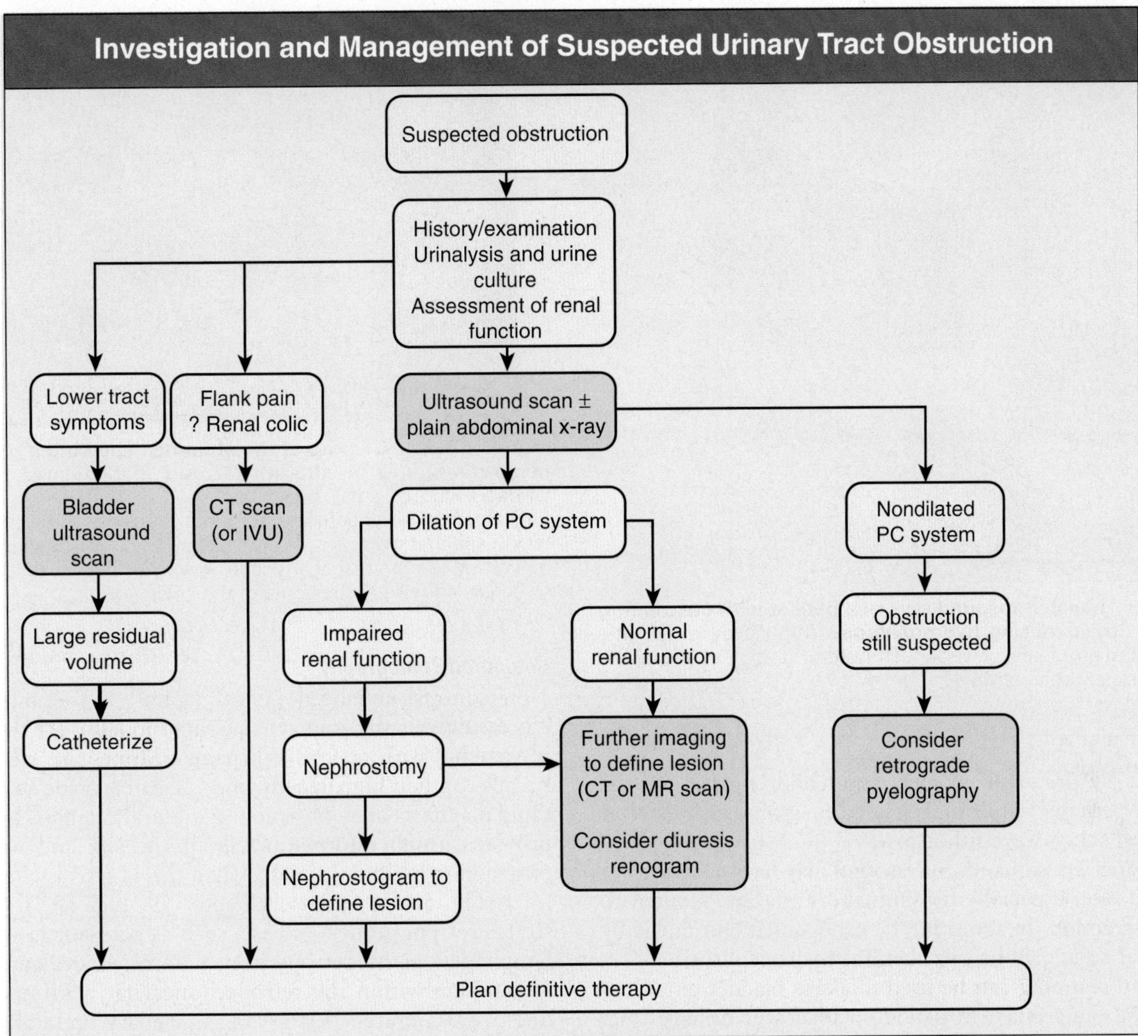

Figure 58.9 Investigation and management of suspected urinary tract obstruction. A full history and examination should be performed, together with urinalysis, urine microscopy and culture, and measurement of renal function and serum electrolytes. Ultrasound is a useful first-line investigation for any patient with suspected urinary tract obstruction. Helical (spiral) computed tomography (CT) is now the preferred imaging technique when renal calculi are suspected. Either CT or magnetic resonance (MR) urography can accurately diagnose both the site and the cause of obstruction in most cases. If there is renal impairment, insertion of a nephrostomy allows the effective relief of the obstruction and time for renal function to recover while definitive therapy is planned. IVU, intravenous urography; PC, pelvicalyceal.

urography are useful in accurately diagnosing both the site and the cause of obstruction, but the availability and expertise in the use of different imaging techniques vary from center to center, and older imaging techniques, such as intravenous urography (IVU), can still be used effectively to evaluate patients with obstructive uropathy. The role of imaging techniques is shown in Figure 58.9. Imaging is also discussed further in Chapter 5.

Ultrasound

Ultrasound can define renal size and demonstrate calyceal dilation[21] (Fig. 58.10) but depends on the expertise of the operator. Although it is sensitive for detection of hydronephrosis, ultrasound will often not detect its cause. Pathologic change within the ureter is difficult to demonstrate, and tiny stones will not generate acoustic shadows. However, unilateral hydronephrosis suggests obstruction of the upper urinary tract by stones, blood clots, or tumors. Bilateral hydronephrosis is more likely to result from a pelvic problem obstructing both ureters or obstruction of the bladder outlet, in which case the bladder will also be enlarged. Ultrasound is often combined with radiographic examination of the kidneys, ureters, and bladder (often known as KUB) to ensure that ureteral stones or small renal stones are not overlooked.

Ultrasound produces false-negative results in cases of nondilated obstructive uropathy.[21] Immediately after acute obstruction (<24 hours), the relatively noncompliant collecting system may not have dilated, such that an ultrasound examination may be normal. Furthermore, if urine flow is low, as in severe dehydration or renal failure, there may be little dilation of the urinary tract. Dilation may also be absent in slowly progressive obstruction when the ureters are encased by fibrous tissue (as in retroperitoneal fibrosis) or by tumor. The acoustic shadow of a staghorn calculus can also mask dilation of the upper urinary tract. The sensitivity of ultrasound for diagnosis of obstruction can be improved by measuring the resistive index with color Doppler ultrasound. A resistive index above 0.7 reflects the increased vascular resistance present in obstruction and effectively discriminates between obstructed and nonobstructed kidneys.[21] Such ultrasound techniques are particularly useful when it is especially important to minimize radiation exposure,

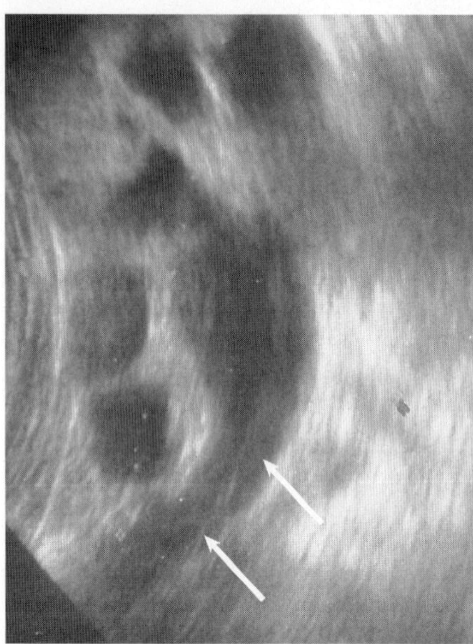

Figure 58.10 Renal ultrasound scan of a patient with obstruction of the urinary tract causing hydronephrosis. The kidney is hydronephrotic with dilation of the pelvicalyceal system; dilation of the upper ureter is also clearly seen *(arrows)*.

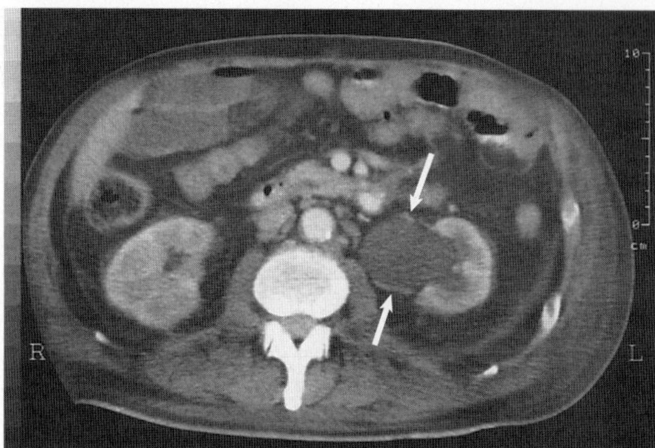

Figure 58.11 CT scan of the abdomen showing a grossly hydronephrotic kidney on the left (*arrows* mark dilated renal pelvis). Dilated loops of small bowel are seen in the right hypochondrium. Sequential sections demonstrated that the ureter was dilated along its length and that there was a pelvic mass, which was responsible for both bowel and left ureteral obstruction. The mass was subsequently shown to be arising from a carcinoma of the colon.

for example, in pregnant women and children, and in the follow-up of patients requiring repeated imaging, such as after extracorporeal shock wave lithotripsy.

Even in experienced hands, ultrasound may have a significant false-positive rate, especially if minimal criteria are adopted to diagnose obstruction. In addition, the echogenicity produced by multiple renal cysts may be mistaken for hydronephrosis.

Ultrasound scanning can be used to assess bladder emptying and should be undertaken in patients with lower urinary tract symptoms. A large post-micturition residual volume suggests bladder outflow obstruction, which should prompt further urologic investigation and treatment.

The investigation of neonates with hydronephrosis diagnosed antenatally depends on the grade of hydronephrosis identified. Neonates with grade 1 or 2 hydronephrosis (no calyceal dilation) undergo ultrasound scanning; neonates with grade 3 to 5 hydronephrosis (indicating increasingly severe pelvicalyceal dilation) require both ultrasound scanning and voiding cystourethrography. This combination can distinguish megaureter resulting from obstruction or reflux and diagnose posterior urethral valves and ureteropelvic junction obstruction.

Plain Abdominal Radiography

A plain abdominal radiograph (or KUB) allows an assessment of kidney size and contour and frequently demonstrates renal calculi because about 90% of calculi are radiopaque.

Intravenous Urography

IVU was formerly the first-choice investigation for suspected upper urinary tract obstruction. In patients with normal renal function, it can usually define both the site and the cause of the obstruction. However, the excretion of contrast material may be poor or delayed in patients with low GFR because of a decreased filtered load of the contrast agent, which is potentially nephrotoxic. IVU is no longer a first-line investigation to diagnose urinary tract obstruction, especially in patients with impaired renal function.

Computed Tomography

Non–contrast-enhanced helical (spiral) CT scanning is used increasingly as the primary imaging modality for the evaluation of patients with acute flank pain.[22] Stones are easily detected because of their high density, and CT can provide an accurate and rapid diagnosis of an obstructing ureteral calculus. In addition, it provides useful information about the site and nature of the obstructing lesion, especially when this is extrinsic to the urinary tract (Fig. 58.11; see also Chapter 59, Fig. 59.2). CT demonstrates retroperitoneal disease, such as para-aortic and paracaval lymphadenopathy; retroperitoneal fibrosis is evident as increased attenuation within the retroperitoneal fat, with encasement of one or both ureters. Hematomas, primary ureteral tumors, and polyps are also detectable. The diagnostic potential of CT is enhanced by the administration of contrast material, but this may limit its use in patients with renal impairment. In addition, it involves considerable exposure to ionizing radiation.

Magnetic Resonance Urography

MR urography (combined with KUB) can diagnose ureteral obstruction due to renal calculi with accuracy similar to that of spiral CT scanning but without exposure to contrast medium or ionizing radiation. The technique has less observer variability and is more accurate than CT in detecting indirect evidence of obstruction, such as perirenal fluid.[23] MR urography can rapidly and accurately depict the morphologic features of dilated urinary tracts and provide information about the degree and level of obstruction (Fig. 58.12).[24] MR urography is a particularly attractive imaging modality for the evaluation of hydronephrosis in children as it provides both anatomic and functional data and can indicate whether the hydronephrosis is compensated (symmetric changes of signal intensity of the nephrogram) or decompensated.[25] Signs of decompensation (acute on chronic obstruction) include edema of the renal parenchyma, a delayed and increasingly dense nephrogram, a delayed calyceal transit time, and a more than 4% difference in the calculated differential renal function. MR urography is likely to be increasingly used in the future.

Retrograde Pyelography

Retrograde pyelography (Fig. 58.13; see also Fig. 58.4) may be particularly useful to identify both the site and the cause of the

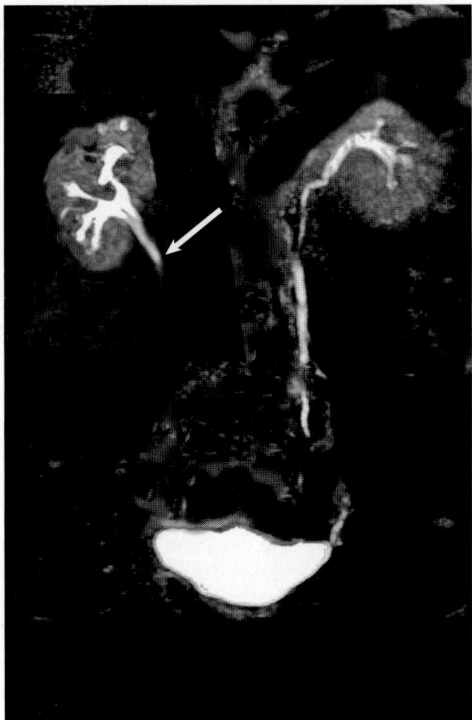

Figure 58.12 MR urography showing obstructive uropathy. T2-weighted MR image shows a proximal right-sided ureteral obstruction with an associated mild hydronephrosis. The obstruction was secondary to a ureteral calculus.

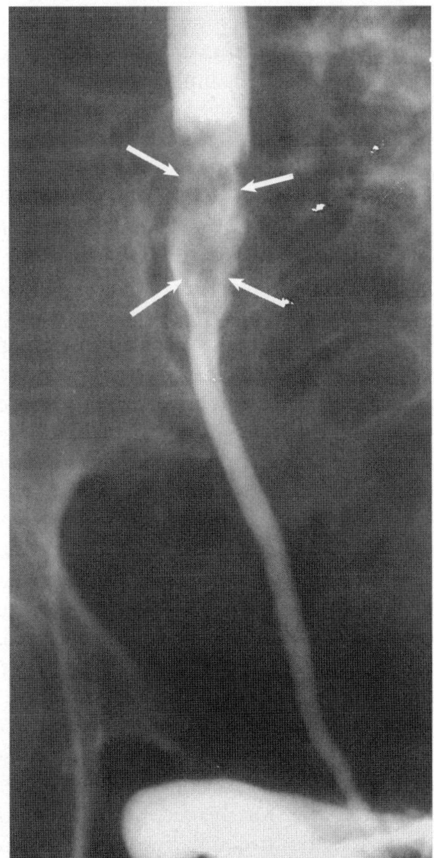

Figure 58.13 Ureteral obstruction by a tumor. A retrograde pyelogram shows that the tumor is within and obstructing the ureter *(arrows)*. Above the tumor, there is dilation of the ureter; but below it, the ureter is of a normal caliber.

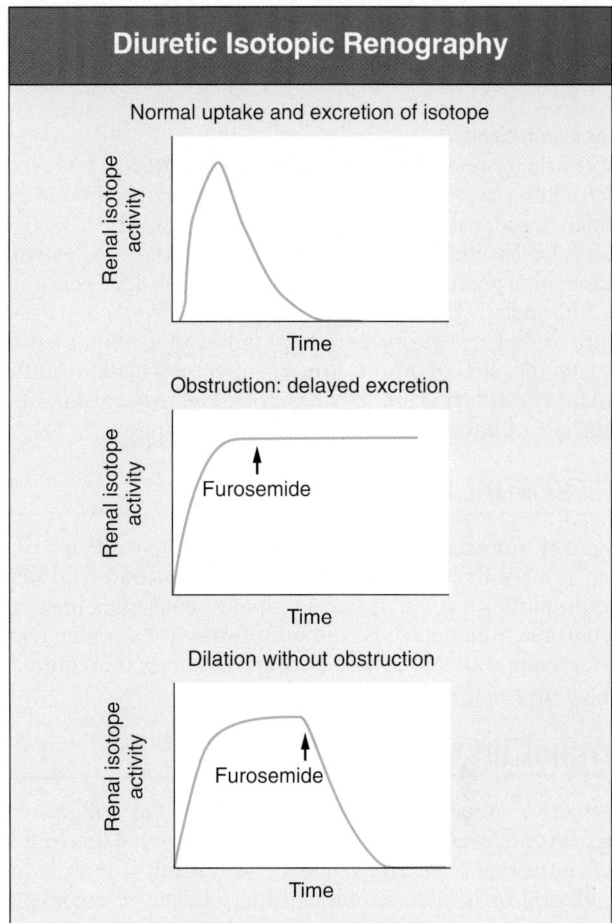

Figure 58.14 Diuretic isotopic renography. Idealized tracings for normal, obstructed, and dilated kidneys without obstruction of the upper urinary tract. In obstruction, there is delayed excretion of ^{99m}Tc-MAG3 despite administration of furosemide. When there is dilation of the upper urinary tract without obstruction, the isotope is retained but is rapidly excreted after the administration of furosemide.

obstruction. It is also helpful when nondilated urinary tract obstruction is suspected or when there is a history of allergic reactions to contrast material. Urinary tract infection that may become overwhelming if obstruction is present is a contraindication to retrograde pyelography.

Diuresis Renography

A diuresis renogram using technetium Tc 99m mercaptoacetyltriglycine (^{99m}Tc-MAG3), combined with intravenous furosemide administered 20 to 30 minutes after injection of the isotope (diuretic isotopic renography), can be used to distinguish between simple dilation of the collecting system and true obstruction.[26] Normally, there is a rapid washout of the isotope from the kidney, and persistence of the isotope suggests a degree of obstruction (Fig. 58.14). Poor renal function significantly limits the usefulness of renography as the diuretic response to furosemide may be absent. Diuresis renography may also be used for follow up of patients who have undergone surgical procedures to relieve obstruction, such as a pyeloplasty.

Pressure-Flow Studies

A pressure-flow study (Whitaker test[27]) involves puncture of the collecting system with a fine-gauge needle to perfuse fluid (at 10 ml/min) with concurrent measurement of the differential pressure between the bladder and the collecting system; a pressure above 20 cm H_2O indicates obstruction. This test is now rarely required.

Other Evaluations

Lower urinary tract obstruction may be evaluated by cystoscopy, which allows a visual inspection of the entire urethra and the bladder. Urodynamic studies (see Chapter 50, Fig. 50.17) can assess bladder outlet obstruction, measure the residual urine volume after voiding, and detect functional bladder abnormalities. Although IVU with oblique films of the bladder and urethra during voiding (excretory cystography) and after voiding can also evaluate the site of lower urinary tract obstruction and the amount of residual urine, this has now largely been superseded by the use of ultrasound, CT, and MR urography.

DIFFERENTIAL DIAGNOSIS

Diagnostic uncertainty arises with nonobstructive dilation of the upper urinary tract that may be seen with vesicoureteral reflux, diuretic administration, diabetes insipidus, congenital megacalyces, chronic pyelonephritis, and postobstructive atrophy. Diuresis renography or retrograde pyelography may be required to exclude obstruction.

NATURAL HISTORY

Obstructive uropathy is potentially curable but will result in progressive irreversible loss of nephrons and renal scarring if it is left untreated (Fig. 58.15). ESRD will result if both kidneys are affected or if there is only a solitary kidney. Outcome data for obstructive uropathy are limited, but the exact prognosis will depend on the pathologic process responsible for the obstruction, the duration of the obstruction, and the presence or absence of urosepsis. Relief of short-term obstruction (<1 to 2 weeks) usually results in an adequate return of renal function. With chronic progressive obstruction (>12 weeks), there is often irreversible and severe renal damage, and renal functional recovery may be limited even after relief of the obstruction. A single-center study identified 104 patients who presented with obstructive nephropathy.[28] The mean GFR at presentation and at 3, 12, and 36 months was 9 ml/min, 28 ml/min, 29 ml/min, and 30 ml/min (patients on dialysis excluded), demonstrating significant but nonprogressive renal impairment after relief of obstruction. It is likely that the prognosis for renal functional recovery is better the earlier the obstruction is diagnosed and relieved.

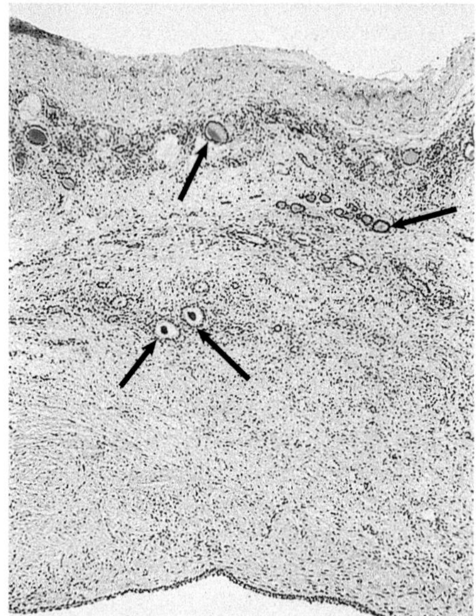

Figure 58.15 Pathology of chronic ureteral obstruction. This is a section of the rim of renal tissue from the kidney shown in Figure 58.7. The renal capsule is at the top, the urinary space at the bottom. The cortex is considerably thinned, and only a few atrophic tubules remain *(arrows)* within an interstitium comprising dense fibrous tissue and a mononuclear cell infiltrate (blue-staining nuclei). No glomeruli can be seen. This demonstrates why there would be no prospect for any significant functional recovery in this kidney even after the relief of the obstruction.

TREATMENT

General Considerations

Treatment is dictated by the location of the obstruction, the underlying cause, and the degree of any renal impairment. If renal impairment is present, the treatment of obstruction requires close collaboration between nephrologists and urologists to reduce the risks associated with the metabolic and electrolyte consequences of renal failure and to optimize the chances for long-term recovery of renal function. For example, complete bilateral ureteral obstruction presenting as AKI is a medical emergency and requires rapid intervention to salvage renal function. Prompt intervention to relieve the obstruction should result in a rapid improvement in renal function. Dialysis should rarely be required in patients with AKI secondary to obstruction except to make the patient fit for intervention, for example, by improving life-threatening hyperkalemia or severe fluid overload. The rapid relief of obstruction will limit permanent renal damage, but renal function may not recover immediately if acute tubular necrosis has resulted from obstruction or any accompanying sepsis.

Some surgical aspects of the management of obstructive uropathy are discussed in Chapter 59. The site of obstruction frequently determines the approach. If the obstruction is distal to the bladder, a urethral catheter or, if this cannot be passed, a suprapubic cystostomy will effectively decompress the kidneys. Placement of nephrostomy tubes or cystoscopy and passage of a retrograde ureteral catheter will relieve upper urinary tract obstruction. Percutaneous nephrostomy (PCN) is generally the appropriate emergency treatment of upper urinary tract obstruction, especially in the setting of AKI. PCN can be achieved with local anesthesia and should allow rapid recovery of renal function in most patients (>70%), avoiding the need for dialysis. After relief of the obstruction by PCN, the exact site and nature of the obstructing lesion can be determined by an antegrade study infusing radiographic contrast material into the nephrostomy tube (nephrostogram, Fig. 58.16), and time can be taken to plan definitive therapy. Major complications of nephrostomy insertion (abscess, infection, and hematoma) occur in less than 5% of patients. If both kidneys are obstructed, the nephrostomy should initially be placed in the kidney with the most preserved renal parenchyma, although bilateral nephrostomies may be required to maximize the potential for the recovery of renal function. If infection occurs above a ureteral obstruction (pyonephrosis), drainage of the kidney by PCN can play an important therapeutic role together with appropriate antibiotics.

A nephrostomy can be used to gauge the potential for functional recovery in patients with chronic obstruction. Failure of

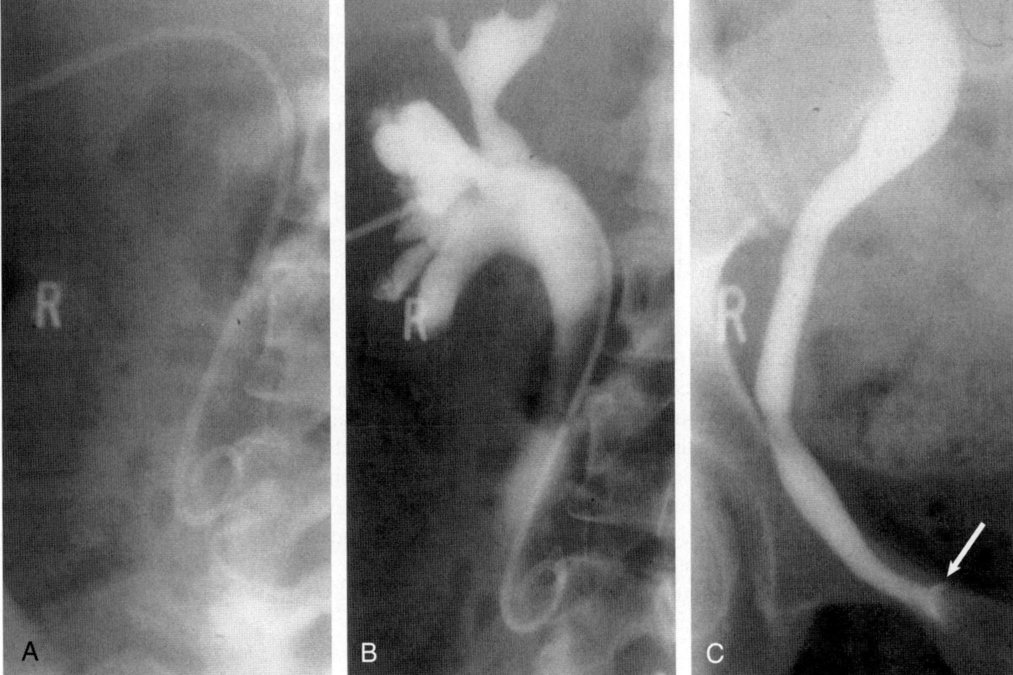

Figure 58.16 Nephrostogram. A nephrostomy has been placed percutaneously into the dilated collecting system of the kidney under ultrasound control (**A**). After infusion of contrast material down the nephrostomy, the dilated pelvicalyceal system and upper ureter (**B**) and the lower ureter (**C**) are outlined. The ureter is dilated along its length but tapers abruptly at the vesicoureteral junction *(arrow)*. In this case, the obstruction was caused by a radiolucent stone.

renal recovery after several weeks of nephrostomy drainage strongly suggests irreversible structural damage and thus no likely benefit from undertaking a more definitive surgical correction of the obstructing lesion. Long-term nephrostomy is increasingly used as a definitive therapy for patients who are unsuitable for major surgical intervention and those with incurable malignant disease (see Chapter 59 for further discussion).

Ureteral obstruction requiring intervention occurs in approximately 3% of renal transplant recipients.[29] It can be treated by nephrostomy and ureteric stenting, percutaneous incision or balloon dilation of the stricture, or open surgical repair (see Chapter 99).

Specific Therapies

Calculi are the most common cause of ureteral obstruction, and their treatment includes relief of pain, elimination of obstruction, and treatment of infection (see Chapter 59). Ureteral obstruction by papillary tissue, blood clots, or a fungus ball is treated by procedures similar to those used for calculi. When obstruction is caused by neoplastic, inflammatory, or neurologic disease, there is unlikely to be spontaneous remission of the obstruction, and some form of urinary diversion, such as an ileal conduit, should be considered. Some obstructing neoplastic lesions, such as lymphadenopathy from lymphoma, may respond to chemotherapy. Management of malignant urinary tract obstruction is discussed further in Chapter 59.

In idiopathic retroperitoneal fibrosis, ureterolysis (in which the ureters are surgically freed from their fibrous encasement) may be beneficial, especially in combination with corticosteroid therapy to prevent recurrence. A retrospective study demonstrated the effectiveness of ureteric stent insertion and corticosteroids in idiopathic retroperitoneal fibrosis.[30]

Functionally significant pelviureteral junction obstruction should be corrected surgically by either an open (Anderson-Hynes) pyeloplasty or a laparoscopic approach. The laparoscopic approach results in significantly less morbidity and has good long-term outcomes that are identical to those of the open procedure. Balloon dilation of the abnormal segment of ureter is also possible, but the recurrence rate is high.

Benign prostatic hypertrophy is the most common cause of lower urinary tract obstruction in men and may be mild and nonprogressive. A patient with minimal symptoms, no infection, and a normal upper urinary tract can continue with assessment until he and his physician agree that further treatment is desirable. Medical therapy with either α-adrenergic blockers (e.g., tamsulosin) or 5α-reductase inhibitors (e.g., finasteride) may be used in patients with moderate symptoms.[31] α-Blockers relax the smooth muscle of the bladder neck and prostate and decrease urethral pressure and outflow obstruction. 5α-Reductase inhibitors inhibit the conversion of testosterone to the active metabolite dihydrotestosterone and reduce prostatic hypertrophy. Combination therapy with these agents may be synergistic. Surgical intervention with transurethral resection of the prostate is generally required for failed medical treatment, debilitating symptoms, urinary retention, recurrent infection, or evidence of renal parenchymal damage. Holmium laser enucleation of the prostate is a less invasive alternative to transurethral resection of the prostate with good short-term and long-term outcomes.[32]

Urethral strictures in men can be treated by dilation or direct-vision internal urethrotomy. The incidence of bladder neck and urethral obstruction in women is low and treatment rarely required. Suprapubic cystostomy may be necessary for bladder drainage in patients unable to void after injury to the urethra or in those who have an impassable urethral stricture.

When obstruction results from neuropathic bladder function, urodynamic studies are essential to determine therapy. The goals of therapy are to establish the bladder as a urine storage organ without causing renal parenchymal injury and to provide a mechanism for bladder emptying that is acceptable to the patient. Patients may have either a flaccid atonic or an unstable hypertonic bladder. Ureteral reflux and parenchymal damage may develop in both cases, although it is more common in patients with a hypertonic bladder. Asking the patient to void at regular intervals may achieve satisfactory emptying of the bladder. Patients with an atonic bladder and significant residual urine retention associated with recurrent urosepsis need to undertake clean intermittent self-catheterization. The aim should be to catheterize four or five times per day to ensure that the amount of urine drained from the bladder on each occasion is less than 400 ml. External sphincterotomy has also been used in men with an atonic bladder and may relieve outlet obstruction and promote bladder emptying, but it may cause urinary incontinence and the need to wear an external collection device. In patients with a hypertonic bladder, improvement in the storage function of the bladder may be obtained with anticholinergic agents. On occasion, chronic clean intermittent self-catheterization is necessary.

Whenever possible, chronic indwelling catheters should be avoided in patients with a neurogenic bladder because they may lead to the formation of bladder stones, urosepsis, and urethral erosion, and they predispose to squamous cell carcinoma of the bladder. Patients who have chronic indwelling catheters for more than 5 years should have annual cystoscopic examinations. If deterioration in renal function occurs despite conservative measures or there is intractable incontinence or a small contracted bladder, an upper urinary tract diversion procedure such as an ileal conduit may be required.

Management of Postobstructive Diuresis

Marked polyuria (postobstructive diuresis) is frequently seen after the release of bilateral obstruction or obstruction of a single functioning kidney. Release of unilateral obstruction rarely results in a postobstructive diuresis[33] despite the presence of tubular dysfunction and a concentrating defect. This is due to intrinsic differences in the tubular response to unilateral and bilateral obstruction and, more important, the salt and water retention and renal impairment that occurred in bilateral obstruction (not evident in unilateral obstruction because of the contralateral normal kidney). The resultant increase in natriuretic factors (including atrial natriuretic peptide) and substances able to promote an osmotic diuresis, such as urea,[34] promote an appropriate postobstructive diuresis to excrete water and electrolytes that were retained during the period of obstruction. However, the postobstructive diuresis may also be inappropriate as a result of tubular dysfunction, and if it is not managed correctly, this may cause severe volume depletion and electrolyte imbalance with continued renal dysfunction. Intravenous and oral fluid replacement is usually required, with careful and regular clinical assessment of fluid balance and serum electrolytes to tailor the fluid replacement regimen appropriately. Once the patient is deemed euvolemic, urine losses plus an allowance for insensible losses should be replaced. Urine volume should be measured regularly (hourly) to facilitate fluid administration, and serum electrolytes should be measured at least daily and as frequently as every 6 hours when there is a massive diuresis. Daily weighing of the patient is also helpful. Replacement fluid regimens should include sodium chloride, a source of bicarbonate, and potassium. Calcium, phosphate, and magnesium replacement may also be necessary.

If fluid administration is overzealous, the kidney will not recover its concentrating ability, and a continued "driven" diuresis will result. It may then be necessary to decrease fluid replacement to levels below those of the urine output and to observe the patient carefully for signs of volume depletion.

Future Prospects

Understanding of the pathophysiologic changes that follow ureteral obstruction has allowed the development of rational interventional therapies to hasten the recovery of renal function and to limit permanent renal damage. Although the best treatment option in humans remains the prompt and effective relief of the obstruction, the development and implementation of improved imaging modalities that provide more sophisticated anatomic and functional information (including intrarenal oxygen content[35]) will undoubtedly refine management and increase the data available for making key clinical decisions, such as whether and when surgical intervention is required.

REFERENCES

1. Wen JG, Frøkiaer J, Jørgensen TM, et al. Obstructive nephropathy: An update of the experimental research. *Urol Res.* 1999;27:29-39.
2. Harris KPG. Models of obstructive nephropathy. In: Gretz N, Strauch M, eds. *Experimental and Genetic Rat Models of Chronic Renal Failure.* Basel: Switzerland; 1993:156-168.
3. Chevalier RL, Forbes MS, Thornhill BA. Ureteral obstruction as a model of renal interstitial fibrosis and obstructive nephropathy. *Kidney Int.* 2009;75:1145-1152.
4. Klahr S, Harris KPG. Obstructive uropathy. In: Seldin D, Giebisch G, eds. *The Kidney: Physiology and Pathophysiology.* 2nd ed. New York: Raven Press; 1992:3327-3369.
5. Klahr S, Harris K, Purkerson ML. Effects of obstruction on renal functions. *Pediatr Nephrol.* 1988;2:34-42.
6. Purkerson ML, Klahr S. Prior inhibition of vasoconstrictors normalizes GFR in postobstructed kidneys. *Kidney Int.* 1989;35:1305-1314.
7. Harris KP, Schreiner GF, Klahr S. Effect of leukocyte depletion on the function of the postobstructed kidney in the rat. *Kidney Int.* 1989;36:210-215.
8. Henderson NC, Mackinnon AC, Farnworth SL, et al. Galectin-3 expression and secretion links macrophages to the promotion of renal fibrosis. *Am J Pathol.* 2008;172:288-298.
9. Bander SJ, Buerkert JE, Martin D, et al. Long-term effects of 24-hr unilateral ureteral obstruction on renal function in the rat. *Kidney Int.* 1985;28:614-620.
10. Li C, Wang W, Kwon TH, et al. Altered expression of major renal Na transporters in rats with bilateral ureteral obstruction and release of obstruction. *Am J Physiol Renal Physiol.* 2003;285:F889-F901.
11. Nørregaard R, Jensen BL, Li C, et al. COX-2 inhibition prevents downregulation of key renal water and sodium transport proteins in response to bilateral ureteral obstruction. *Am J Physiol Renal Physiol.* 2005;289:F322-F333.
12. Jensen AM, Li C, Praetorius HA, et al. Angiotensin II mediates downregulation of aquaporin water channels and key renal sodium transporters in response to urinary tract obstruction. *Am J Physiol Renal Physiol.* 2006;291:F1021-F1032.
13. Wang G, Li C, Kim SW, et al. Ureter obstruction alters expression of renal acid-base transport proteins in rat kidney. *Am J Physiol Renal Physiol.* 2008;295:F497-F506.
14. Misseri R, Meldrum KK. Mediators of fibrosis and apoptosis in obstructive uropathies. *Curr Urol Rep.* 2005;6:140-145.
15. Bascands JL, Schanstra JP. Obstructive nephropathy: Insights from genetically engineered animals. *Kidney Int.* 2005;68:925-937.
16. Ricardo SD, Diamond JR. The role of macrophages and reactive oxygen species in experimental hydronephrosis. *Semin Nephrol.* 1998;18:612-621.
17. Bell ET. *Renal Diseases.* Philadelphia: Lea & Febiger; 1946.
18. Lissauer D, Morris RK, Kilby MD. Fetal lower urinary tract obstruction. *Semin Fetal Neonatal Med.* 2007;12:464-470.
19. U.S. Renal Data System, USRDS 2005. Annual Data Report: Atlas of End-Stage Renal Disease in the United States. Bethesda, Md: National

Institutes of Health, National Institute of Diabetes and Digestive and Kidney Diseases; 2005.
20. Sacks SH, Aparicio SA, Bevan A, et al. Late renal failure due to prostatic outflow obstruction: A preventable disease. *BMJ*. 1989;298:156-159.
21. Mostbeck GH, Zontsich T, Turetschek K. Ultrasound of the kidney: Obstruction and medical diseases. *Eur Radiol*. 2001;11:1878-1889.
22. Pfister SA, Deckart A, Laschke S, et al. Unenhanced helical computed tomography vs intravenous urography in patients with acute flank pain: Accuracy and economic impact in a randomized prospective trial. *Eur Radiol*. 2003;13:2513-2520.
23. Regan F, Kuszyk B, Bohlman ME, et al. Acute ureteric calculus obstruction: Unenhanced spiral CT versus HASTE MR urography and abdominal radiograph. *Br J Radiol*. 2005;78:506-511.
24. Blandino A, Gaeta M, Minutoli F, et al. MR pyelography in 115 patients with a dilated renal collecting system. *Acta Radiol*. 2001;42:532-536.
25. Grattan-Smith JD, Little SB, Jones RA. MR urography evaluation of obstructive uropathy. *Pediatr Radiol*. 2008;38(Suppl 1):S49-S69.
26. O'Reilly PH. Diuresis renography 8 years later: An update. *J Urol*. 1986;136:993-999.
27. Whitaker RH, Buxton-Thomas MS. A comparison of pressure flow studies and renography in equivocal upper urinary tract obstruction. *J Urol*. 1984;131:446-449.
28. Ravanan R, Tomson CR. Natural history of postobstructive nephropathy: A single-center retrospective study. *Nephron Clin Pract*. 2007;105:c165-c170.
29. Faenza A, Nardo B, Catena F, et al. Ureteral stenosis after kidney transplantation. A study on 869 consecutive transplants. *Transplant Int*. 1999;12:334-340.
30. Fry AC, Singh S, Gunda SS, et al. Successful use of steroids and ureteric stents in 24 patients with idiopathic retroperitoneal fibrosis: A retrospective study. *Nephron Clin Pract*. 2008;108:c213-c220.
31. Beckman TJ, Mynderse LA. Evaluation and medical management of benign prostatic hyperplasia. *Mayo Clin Proc*. 2005;80:1356-1362.
32. Suardi N, Gallina A, Salonia A, et al. Holmium laser enucleation of the prostate and holmium laser ablation of the prostate: Indications and outcome. *Curr Opin Urol*. 2009;19:38-43.
33. Gillenwater JY, Westervelt FBJ, Vaughan EDJ, et al. Renal function after release of chronic unilateral hydronephrosis in man. *Kidney Int*. 1975;7:179-186.
34. Harris RH, Yarger WE. The pathogenesis of post-obstructive diuresis. The role of circulating natriuretic and diuretic factors, including urea. *J Clin Invest*. 1975;56:880-887.
35. Thoeny HC, Kessler TM, Simon-Zoula S, et al. Renal oxygenation changes during acute unilateral ureteral obstruction: Assessment with blood oxygen level–dependent MR imaging—initial experience. *Radiology*. 2008;247:754-761.

CHAPTER 59

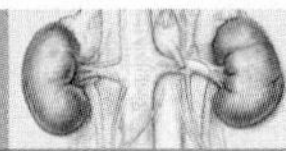

Urologic Issues for the Nephrologist

Evangelos G. Gkougkousis, Sunjay Jain, J. Kilian Mellon

Close interaction between nephrologists and urologists is crucial to the optimal management of a number of common clinical problems. A proper understanding of urologic strategies helps the nephrologist ensure that patients presenting with these problems are given clear information and are optimally managed. Areas in which such coordinated work is most important are discussed in this chapter. They include the management of stone disease, the surgical approach to urinary tract obstruction, the investigation of hematuria, and the management of urinary tract malignant neoplasms.

SURGICAL MANAGEMENT OF STONE DISEASE

The management of urinary tract stones has been irrevocably changed by the introduction of extracorporeal shock wave lithotripsy (ESWL), percutaneous nephrolithotomy (PCNL), and ureteroscopy. Because of the effectiveness of ESWL, many endoscopic procedures for stones are now more complex than previously. Open stone surgical techniques are a second- or third-line treatment in most cases. Figure 59.1 indicates the changing use of different modalities of stone treatment since the introduction of the newer techniques.[1]

Advances in Imaging for Urinary Tract Stones

In recent years, unenhanced computed tomography (CT) scanning of the abdomen and pelvis has replaced intravenous urography (IVU) as the standard imaging modality for stone diagnosis (Fig. 59.2). CT offers increased sensitivity compared with IVU (99% versus 70%) without the need for the intravenous administration of contrast material. An additional advantage is the ability of CT to demonstrate radiolucent stones (mainly uric acid and xanthine stones) and to detect concomitant lesions leading to alternative diagnoses. CT does require an increased radiation dose, but this is lessening with modern machines. Comparative doses are 0.42 mSv for plain radiography of the kidneys, ureters, and bladder (KUB); 2.5 mSv for IVU; and 4 mSv for non–contrast-enhanced CT.

Treatment of Urinary Tract Stones

Spontaneous stone passage can be expected in up to 80% of patients with a stone size smaller than 4 mm. Conversely, for stones with a diameter of more than 7 mm, the chance of spontaneous stone passage is very low. The location is also important; up to 70% of distal ureteral stones pass spontaneously, in contrast to only 45% of midureteral and 25% of proximal ureteral stones. Intervention is strongly recommended when there is persistent pain (>72 hours) despite adequate analgesia, persistent obstruction with risk of impaired renal function (e.g., with preexisting renal impairment or in a single kidney), bilateral obstruction, or associated urinary tract sepsis.

Another conservative treatment option is chemolysis, as several stone types are in principle amenable to dissolution by oral medications or by direct instillation of chemical solutions. However, in most cases, this form of treatment is either impractical or clinically ineffective. The major exception is uric acid stones, which can readily be dissolved by alkalization of the urine, usually with oral potassium citrate.

Acute Surgical Intervention

The main goal of acute surgical intervention is to relieve obstruction. If the patient is considered well enough for general anesthesia, ureteroscopic stone destruction can be attempted in most cases. Alternatively, a double-J stent (a ureteral stent with two coiled ends) can be inserted, which will relieve obstruction until definite treatment is performed (Fig. 59.3). However, in the setting of uncontrolled urinary tract infection, percutaneous nephrostomy (PCN) is the preferred option because it can be done under local anesthesia and is less likely than endoscopic surgery to cause septicemia (Fig. 59.4). Rarely, an open procedure to remove a stone or a grossly infected kidney may be necessary.

Elective Surgical Intervention

Extracorporeal Shock Wave Lithotripsy

During ESWL, acoustic shock wave energy is delivered to a stone under fluoroscopic or ultrasound guidance. Treatment sessions typically last about 30 minutes, during which 1500 to 2500 shock waves are delivered. Sessions are performed on an outpatient basis under analgesia or intravenous sedation and can be repeated at intervals of 10 to 14 days. Stones up to 20 mm in size can be treated effectively, and stone-free rates of 60% to 98% have been reported. However, ESWL is operator dependent, and outcome is influenced by the size, composition, and location of the stone and the type of lithotripter used. Cystine and calcium oxalate monohydrate stones are especially resistant. Targeting of the stone may be impossible in the presence of obesity and skeletal deformities, and ESWL is contraindicated in patients with aortic or renal artery aneurysm, uncontrolled urinary tract infection, coagulation disorders and in pregnant women.

Changing Use of Techniques for Stone Removal

	1984	1990	1999
Location (%)			
Calyceal stones	35	43	46
Pelvic stones	42	20	13
Staghorn stones	8	3	1
Ureteral stones	15	34	40
Treatment modality (%)			
ESWL	60	79	78
PCNL	20	5	2
Ureteroscopy	11	15	20
Open surgery	9	1	0.1

Figure 59.1 Changing use of techniques for stone removal. The changes in the application of surgical techniques for stone removal since the introduction of extracorporeal shock wave lithotripsy (ESWL) and percutaneous nephrolithotomy (PCNL). *(Data from reference 1.)*

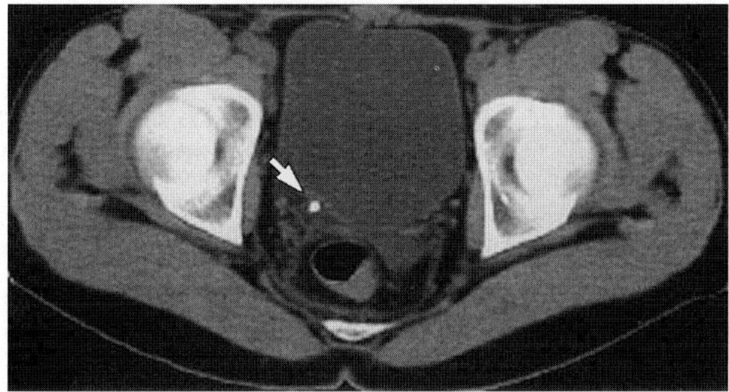

Figure 59.2 CT scan demonstrating a ureteral calculus. Non–contrast-enhanced CT scan showing a calculus *(arrow)* at the right vesicoureteral junction.

A double-J ureteral stent is sometimes placed endoscopically before ESWL treatment to prevent stone fragments from obstructing the distal ureter (Steinstrasse, literally "stone street"; Fig. 59.5). Other acute complications of ESWL include hemorrhage or hematoma, infection, and injury to adjacent organs. The risk for the later development of hypertension or renal impairment after ESWL remains controversial.

ESWL is the first-line treatment for more than 75% of stone patients. Figure 59.6 shows circumstances in which ESWL is less effective and PCNL becomes the preferred surgical approach or a combination of the two modalities is used. For lower pole stones in particular, ESWL may not provide optimal clearance because of problems with the drainage of residual fragments. A randomized controlled trial has shown that for lower pole stones larger than 10 mm, PCNL has much better clearance rates than ESWL (92% versus 23%).[2]

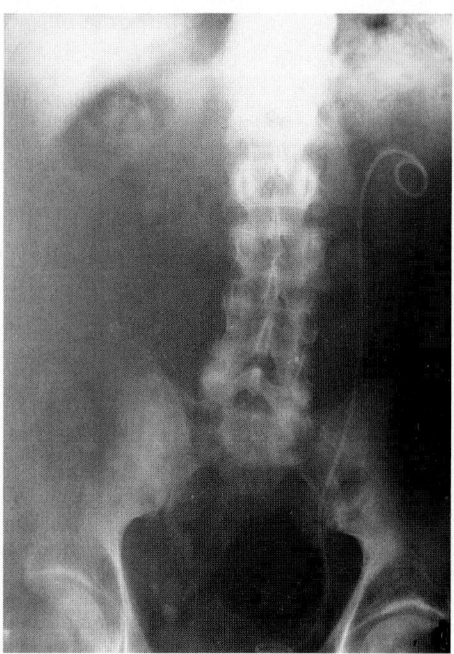

Figure 59.3 Ureteral stenting. Plain radiograph showing a double-J ureteral stent in the left ureter. Note that the curled ends of the stent remain in the pelvis and the bladder despite ureteral peristalsis.

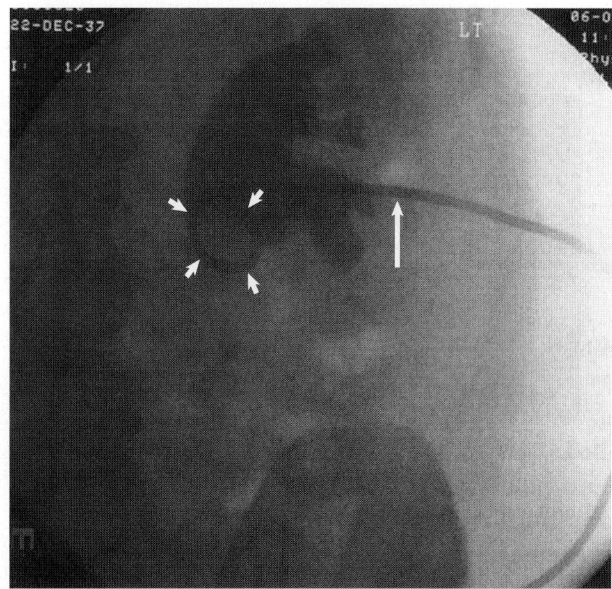

Figure 59.4 Nephrostogram in ureteral obstruction due to a stone. Contrast material is injected through a percutaneous nephrostomy tube placed in the lower pole calyx *(arrow)*. The contrast material outlines a single large calculus *(arrowheads)* producing complete obstruction at the pelviureteral junction.

Percutaneous Nephrolithotomy

During PCNL, a track is created between the skin and the collecting system of the kidney and used as a working channel to remove stones. Preoperatively, IVU or CT, sometimes with three-dimensional reconstruction, is used to accurately localize calculi and neighboring organs (e.g., spleen, liver, large bowel, pleura, or lungs) and to plan access. The most frequently used access site is the dorsal calyx of the lower pole, and stone fragmentation is undertaken by ultrasound, pneumatic, or laser devices. The PCNL technique is modified for special circumstances, usually by altering the site of puncture (e.g., directly into a calyceal diverticulum) or, if there are ureteral stones, by using a higher placed puncture to permit antegrade ureteroscopy. The percutaneous puncture may be facilitated by the preliminary placement of a retrograde ureteral catheter to dilate and to opacify the collecting system, which is then punctured under fluoroscopy. After completion of PCNL, a self-retaining balloon nephrostomy tube is used to tamponade the track and to provide

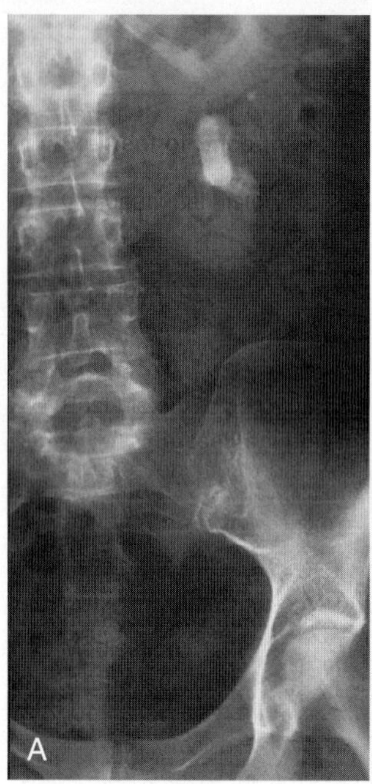

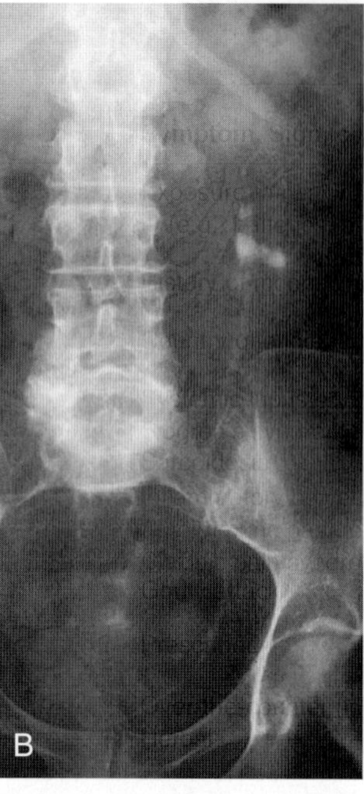

Figure 59.5 Extracorporeal shock wave lithotripsy complicated by Steinstrasse. A, Preoperative plain radiograph showing stones in the left renal pelvis. **B,** After ESWL, note the disappearance of the pelvic stone, the string of stone fragments throughout the length of the ureter, and the double-J ureteral stent placed to facilitate their passage.

Indications for Percutaneous Nephrolithotomy

Stone Size	Stone >3 cm or Staghorn	Treatment
Composition*	Struvite stones	Complete removal necessary to eliminate infection and minimize stone recurrence
	Calcium oxalate monohydrate stones	Difficult to pulverize by ESWL
	Cystine stones	Difficult to pulverize by ESWL
Stone position	Lower pole stones	Fragments less easily evacuated from dependent lower pole calyces, especially if collecting system dilated
Anatomic abnormalities	PUJ obstruction Calyceal diverticula	Prevent passage of fragments after ESWL
Patient characteristics	Morbid obesity Ureteral obstruction	Stone cannot be placed in focal point of ESWL machine

Figure 59.6 Indications for percutaneous nephrolithotomy. ESWL is the first choice for stone intervention, except in those circumstances that may favor PCNL. *Stone composition can be defined with certainty only by direct stone analysis, but advances in imaging may ultimately provide a means to accurately assess stone composition *in situ* before treatment, thus allowing the urologist to select the treatment most likely to be successful. PUJ, pelviureteral junction.

further access if needed. Hemorrhage can complicate PCNL (from renal or, rarely, intercostal arteries) and can usually be treated conservatively or by selective angioembolization. Other complications include sepsis; fluid overload ("transurethral resection syndrome"); injury to spleen, pleura, or colon; and extravasation. PCNL usually results in minimal parenchymal injury, averaging only 0.15% of the total renal cortex.[3]

Indications for PCNL are shown in Figure 59.6. These continue to evolve and are being challenged by developments in ureteroscopic techniques, which are allowing more upper ureteral and renal pelvis stones to be dealt with by a retrograde approach.

Open Stone Surgery

Although it is performed rarely, open surgery still has a place in the treatment of stone disease. It is reported that approximately 2% of stone cases are treated with open surgery, mainly when anatomic factors preclude the use of minimally invasive methods or when these techniques have failed. Other indications include complex stone burden and the presence of intrarenal anatomic abnormalities (e.g., pelviureteral junction obstruction). During surgery, the renal pelvis as well as the parenchyma can be opened along avascular planes, and clamping of the renal vessels and hypothermia of the kidney may be needed. In selected cases, a laparoscopic approach, can be employed for the treatment of stone disease.

Ureteroscopy

Recent advances in the design of endoscopes for ureteronephroscopy have rendered the entire urinary tract accessible to endoscopic examination and manipulation. Ureteroscopes may be semirigid or flexible, the latter allowing access to the renal pelvis and calyces. Stone fragmentation is achieved ideally by laser but also by ultrasound or pneumatic devices. Laser is equally effective for all types of stones and has additional advantages of a flexible fiber (allowing intrarenal stone fragmentation), low tissue penetration, and minimal stone displacement during use. Success rates for laser fragmentation of ureteral stones are high, in the region of 80%. Graspers and baskets can be used to manipulate stones or to remove fragments. However, because of the risk of ureteral avulsion, the use of baskets to remove intact stones is no longer recommended. Other complications of ureteroscopic techniques include perforation, extravasation, mucosal damage, hematuria, infection, and stricture.

Management of Staghorn Calculus

A staghorn calculus should usually be managed by intervention because reports of conservative therapy show a high rate of eventual nephrectomy (up to 50%) and an increase in associated morbidity (mainly renal failure) and mortality (up to 28%). Surgical options are ESWL monotherapy, complete endoscopic stone removal, and a combined approach using PCNL for debulking followed by ESWL. The advantage of the combined approach is the reduced need for additional renal access and secondary endourologic procedures. The choice of treatment depends on many factors, including the age and renal function of the patient. ESWL will not usually render the patient entirely stone free (the ideal goal of treatment), especially in the treatment of large staghorn stones; nevertheless, it can still be considered successful when less than 40% of a staghorn calculus persisting as fragments is achieved. Rarely, open surgical removal of the stone may be indicated.

Stones in Transplanted Kidneys

The management of stone disease in a transplanted kidney is challenging because of the solitary kidney, the anatomic location within the pelvis, and the difficulty with retrograde access to the ureter and kidney. Early active intervention is indicated; prophylactic stenting, ureteroscopy, and PCNL are preferred to ESWL because stone targeting may not be possible. Open surgery may be needed in selected cases.

MANAGEMENT OF URINARY TRACT OBSTRUCTION

The causes of upper tract obstruction are listed in Chapter 58, Figure 58.1, and a summary of the management of obstruction is given in Chapter 58, including Figure 58.9. Upper tract obstruction due to malignant disease can be a result of direct tumor invasion or external compression by metastatic lymph node involvement or, rarely, true metastasis to the ureter. Some 70% of tumors causing ureteral obstruction are genitourinary (cervical, bladder, prostate) in origin; breast and gastrointestinal carcinomas and lymphoma constitute the majority of the remainder.[4] The presentation of a patient with obstruction may vary significantly, and hydronephrosis may develop progressively and insidiously and remain unrecognized until the patient presents with anuria and uremia. Upper tract obstruction due to malignant disease rarely presents with classic acute ureteral colic, which is typically seen with a benign cause such as a stone. Bladder outflow obstruction may be acute and dramatic; or chronic, with few or no symptoms. To understand the immediate needs and longer term prognosis of these patients, the acute as well as the definitive management of the most common urologic diseases associated with obstruction and renal impairment is outlined.

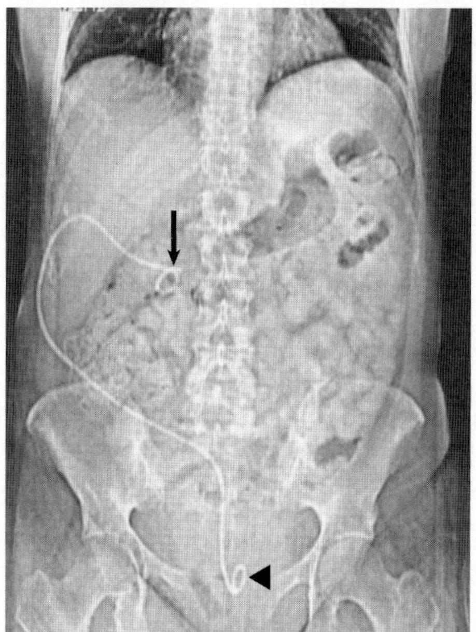

Figure 59.7 Extra-anatomic stenting for malignant ureteral obstruction. Plain radiograph showing placement of an extra-anatomic stent for malignant obstruction of the right ureter. The upper end of the double-J stent has been placed in the right renal pelvis *(arrow)*. The stent then runs through a subcutaneous tunnel before the lower end enters the bladder *(arrowhead)*.

Acute Management of Urinary Tract Obstruction

Relief of obstruction is crucial to reverse renal impairment and to preserve remaining renal function. In cases of bladder outflow obstruction, a urethral or suprapubic catheter is indicated; whereas in upper tract obstruction, a double-J ureteral stent is preferable, when possible. The most straightforward approach is endoscopic retrograde placement under fluoroscopy, with PCN reserved for cases in which the procedure fails. Bilateral stents should be placed if it is technically possible. However, tumor infiltration can distort trigonal anatomy, making identification of ureteral orifices for double-J stent insertion impossible at the time of cystoscopy. Furthermore, it has been suggested that stents fail to relieve obstruction in 40% to 50% of cases of external ureteral compression. Thus, these patients need to be closely monitored to ensure resolution of the obstruction. A new type of metallic, self-expanding stent, used alone or in conjunction with double-J stents, has good results in maintaining ureteral patency and avoiding PCN in malignant ureteral obstruction.

A stable patient with obstruction but without major signs of sepsis is a candidate for retrograde stent placement under general anesthesia. However, in a septic patient, endoscopic manipulation can lead to rapid deterioration. Furthermore, such patients may not be fit for general anesthesia, in which case the preferred initial approach is PCN, which can then be followed after an interval with antegrade ureteral stenting. The success rate of this combined approach is high (>90%).[5] In patients with bilateral ureteral obstruction, it is not always necessary to insert bilateral PCN tubes. Significant palliation and return to nearly normal renal function can be accomplished by drainage of a single kidney, preferably the unit with the better preserved parenchyma as determined by CT scan or ultrasound. Once they are placed, PCN tubes or double-J stents need to be replaced every 4 to 6 months. If they are left longer, they become increasingly brittle and encrusted and are liable to fracture or break when they are manipulated. Complications of ureteral stents include migration, obstruction with proteinaceous material, infection, fragmentation, and rarely erosion through the urinary tract.[6] As many as 70% of patients with stents report lower urinary tract symptoms, mainly urgency, frequency, and nocturia as well as pain along the urinary tract.

Morbidity after stenting or PCN is similar.[7] The main problem with indwelling stents is the increased risk of recurrent obstruction (11% for stents versus 1% for PCN). PCN may have an increased infection rate, and there may be psychological issues relating to the need for an external drainage bag.

Extra-anatomic stents are an alternative for patients in whom conventional stent insertion has failed or for whom permanent nephrostomy drainage is unacceptable. An extra-anatomic stent is placed by an initial percutaneous puncture and insertion of the upper end of a long (50-cm) double-J stent into the kidney. A subcutaneous tunnel is then created to bring the stent to the level of the iliac crest. Another tunnel is fashioned to bring the lower end of the stent out suprapubically, followed, finally, by suprapubic puncture of a full bladder and insertion of the lower end (Fig. 59.7).[8] Extra-anatomic stents are usually changed at 6-month intervals, and preliminary experience confirms their value in maintaining ureteral patency and avoiding PCN. Because of the effectiveness of minimally invasive methods, open surgery today is rarely indicated in the acute setting.

Pelviureteral Junction Obstruction

Until recently, the standard approach to pelviureteral junction obstruction was open surgical pyeloplasty. In recent years, laparoscopic pyeloplasty has emerged as the new gold standard, with success rates equal to those of open pyeloplasty (95%).[9] Alternatively, pelviureteral junction obstruction can be treated endoscopically, either antegrade (percutaneous endopyelotomy) or retrograde (ureteroscopic endopyelotomy).

Retroperitoneal Fibrosis

Retroperitoneal fibrosis can be treated medically or surgically. A causative factor should be excluded (see Chapter 58). There are reports of favorable outcome after immunosuppression with high doses of corticosteroids or azathioprine. Alternatively, surgery, consisting of ureterolysis and transposition of the ureters into the peritoneal cavity or omental flaps, can have good long-term results.

Malignant Obstruction

For upper tract transitional cell carcinoma, acute obstruction is best treated by internal stenting. PCN is avoided because of the risk of tumor seeding. Upper tract transitional cell carcinoma is an aggressive tumor and necessitates prompt extirpative surgery.

Bladder cancer can lead to hydronephrosis by invading the ureteral orifices and intramural ureter. Radical cystectomy is indicated, although temporary ureteral decompression may normalize renal function if neoadjuvant chemotherapy is planned. In selected cases, bladder preservation strategies combining systemic chemotherapy and radiotherapy can reverse the obstruction and offer long-term control of the disease.

Prostate cancer causes obstruction by occluding the urethra or invading the ureteral orifices. Hormonal treatment can shrink prostatic tissue and malignant deposits and offer long-term remission of symptoms. Limited resection of the prostate may sometimes be indicated.

The decision to offer ureteral decompression for upper tract obstruction due to cancer is not straightforward and requires input not only from the urologist but also from colleagues in radiation and medical oncology and the palliative care team. There must also be careful discussion of the options with the patient and family.

Ureteral decompression is justified when radiotherapy and systemic chemotherapy remain therapeutic options after improvement in renal function but may also be justified for palliation of pain or ongoing renal tract sepsis.

A review of patients undergoing PCN for obstructive uropathy secondary to pelvic malignant disease identified a group of patients with very poor survival in whom ureteral decompression is usually not justified (Fig. 59.8).[10] Patients with gastric or pancreatic cancer survive a median of only 1.4 months after ureteral decompression, calling into question the benefit of such a procedure in this setting.[11] In another report, the average survival of patients with advanced malignant neoplasms undergoing endourologic diversion was only 5 months, half of which time was spent in the hospital.[12]

Percutaneous Nephrostomy for Malignant Obstructive Uropathy

	Median Survival (wk)	5-yr Survival Rate (%)
Group I: primary untreated malignancy	27	10
Group II: recurrent malignancy with further treatment	20	20
Group III: recurrent malignancy with no further treatment	6.5	None survived >1 yr
Group IV: benign disease as a result of previous treatment	Not stated	64
Overall	26	22

Figure 59.8 Percutaneous nephrostomy for malignant obstructive uropathy. Outcome in 77 patients undergoing percutaneous nephrostomy for obstructive uropathy secondary to pelvic malignant disease. *(Data from reference 10.)*

Benign Ureteral Strictures

These can be secondary to stone disease, iatrogenic, or caused by various benign diseases. The treatment of choice is endoscopic balloon dilation or ureterotomy. Open surgical repair or major reconstructive surgery may be needed in cases of recurrent strictures.

Benign Prostatic Hyperplasia

Obstruction, upper tract dilation, and renal impairment due to benign prostatic hypertrophy are indications for surgical treatment. However, if long-term obstruction has severely weakened the detrusor muscle, prostatectomy will not restore voiding in up to 50% of cases. These patients will be treated best with intermittent clean self-catheterization or a permanent urethral or suprapubic catheter.

Neurologic Diseases of the Lower Urinary Tract

Diseases of the central or peripheral nervous system can present with bladder underactivity or detrusor-sphincter dyssynergia and lead to bilateral hydroureter and hydronephrosis. Diabetes mellitus can also produce a flaccid denervated bladder through destruction of the peripheral nerves and cause chronic retention and renal failure. Of diabetics who develop peripheral neuropathy, 75% to 100% will develop some neurogenic lower urinary tract dysfunction. The treatment of choice is generally intermittent clean self-catheterization, with a limited role for surgery.

INVESTIGATION OF HEMATURIA

Macroscopic (visible) hematuria is perhaps the most important symptom in urologic practice, and quite apart from being alarming to the patient, it can be the first presenting sign of an underlying malignant condition of the urinary tract (most often a transitional cell tumor of the bladder). Studies show that 15% to 22% of patients with visible hematuria have an underlying genitourinary tract malignant neoplasm.

Patients with macroscopic hematuria must be distinguished from those who have been found to have dipstick hematuria or microscopic hematuria, in whom the risk of malignant change is significantly lower (2% to 11%).

The outcome of full evaluation of a large group of patients (with both macroscopic and microscopic hematuria) attending a hematuria clinic is shown in Figure 59.9.[13] In addition to a small but important group of patients in whom malignant disease was identified, there was a significant pickup rate of parenchymal renal disease (about 10%), presenting with both macroscopic and microscopic hematuria. It is also important to note the sizable proportion of patients in whom a definitive diagnosis could not be reached.

Outcome of Evaluation in a Hematuria Clinic

Diagnoses Found	All (%)	Microscopic Hematuria (%)	Macroscopic Hematuria (%)
No diagnosis	1168 (60.5)	670 (68.2)	498 (52.5)
Renal cancer	12 (0.6)	3 (0.3)	9 (0.9)
Upper tract transitional cell carcinoma	2 (0.1)	1 (0.1)	1 (0.1)
Bladder cancer	230 (11.9)	47 (4.8)	183 (19.3)
Prostate cancer	8 (0.4)	2 (0.2)	6 (0.6)
Stone disease	69 (3.6)	39 (4.0)	30 (3.2)
Urinary tract infection	251 (13.0)	128 (13.0)	123 (13.0)
Renal parenchymal disease	190 (9.8)	92 (9.4)	98 (10.3)

Likelihood of Finding Malignancy*	Microscopic Hematuria	Macroscopic Hematuria
Male, age > 40 yr	8	24
Male, age < 40 yr	1.7 (1 case)	6.5
Female, age > 40 yr	5.2	19
Female, age < 40 yr	none	none

Figure 59.9 Outcome of evaluation in a hematuria clinic. *Percentage of cases investigated, according to age. *(Data from reference 13.)*

Evaluation of Macroscopic Hematuria

All adults with a single episode of macroscopic hematuria require full urologic evaluation, including renal imaging and cystoscopy. The only exception to this rule occurs when an adult younger than 40 years gives a history characteristic of glomerular hematuria, such as is typically seen in IgA nephropathy, in which dark brown hematuria lasting 24 to 48 hours coincides with intercurrent mucosal infection, usually of the upper respiratory tract. This hematuria may be painless, or there may be bilateral loin ache. These young adults should be referred first for nephrologic assessment.

Evaluation of Asymptomatic Microscopic Hematuria

The precise definition of microscopic hematuria remains contentious, and it has also been controversial whether these patients should be investigated by a urologist or nephrologist and how patients should be observed if investigation findings are normal.[14]

In 2001, the recommendations of the American Urological Association Best Practice Policy Panel on the management of asymptomatic microscopic hematuria in adults were published, providing an evidence-based set of guidelines for family physicians, urologists, and nephrologists in dealing with this condition.[15] Interpretation of the evidence continues to produce controversy about the likelihood of identifying a cause of hematuria.

Microscopic hematuria is common; the prevalence is at least 2% in the general population. It is more common in women and with increasing age (see Chapter 15, Fig. 15.7). There is no evidence to justify screening for microscopic hematuria except in specific high-risk groups, for example, those with occupational exposure to oncogenic chemicals or dyes (including benzidine and aromatic amines).

The typical definition of microscopic hematuria is three or more red blood cells per high-power field on microscopic evaluation of urinary sediment from two of three properly collected urinalysis specimens. Dipstick-positive hematuria may still herald significant disease in the absence of red cells on microscopy because red cells may lyse in alkaline or hypotonic urine before reaching the laboratory for analysis. Urine microscopy is discussed further in Chapter 4. If a careful history suggests a benign cause of the hematuria, the patient should undergo repeated urinalysis 48 hours after cessation of the implicated activity (i.e., menstruation, vigorous exercise, sexual activity, or trauma). No additional evaluation is warranted if the hematuria has resolved.

Two of three positive test results are sufficient to justify evaluation because intermittent hematuria still carries a significant risk for malignant disease. Full evaluation should still be considered if there is only a single positive test result or if there are only one or two red blood cells per high-power field when there are risk factors for significant disease (Fig. 59.10).

Complete evaluation of microscopic hematuria includes a history and physical examination, laboratory analysis, and radiologic imaging of the upper urinary tract, followed by cystoscopy (see Fig. 59.10). In women, urethral and vaginal examinations should be performed to exclude local causes of microscopic hematuria. In uncircumcised men, the foreskin should be retracted to expose the glans penis, if possible. If a phimosis is present, a catheter specimen of urine may be required. Patients with urinary tract infection should be treated appropriately, and urinalysis should be repeated 6 weeks after treatment. If the hematuria resolves with treatment, no additional evaluation is necessary. Serum creatinine should be measured. The remaining laboratory investigations are guided by specific findings of the history, physical examination, and urinalysis. In some instances, cytologic evaluation of exfoliated cells in the voided urine may also be performed. These American Urological Association guidelines are likely to undergo continuing review. Voided urine cytology is becoming controversial as part of the urologic evaluation of hematuria because most urothelial tumors are detected by other modalities. The role of cystoscopy in the evaluation of low-risk patients is also increasingly debated. There is now evidence to justify avoidance of cystoscopy in women younger than 40 years. However, many authorities still recommend cystoscopy in men younger than 40 years because the risk for bladder cancer, although very small, is higher than in young women. A number of urine tests are now available that claim to be more sensitive than urine cytology.[16] The ultimate aim is to avoid cystoscopy, but as yet none of the tests is sufficiently reliable. Virtual cystoscopy with three-dimensional reconstructions of cross-sectional imaging is also advancing to a level at which it may be an alternative to cystoscopy.

Significant proteinuria (>0.3 g/24 h), red cell casts, predominance of dysmorphic red blood cells in the urine (see Chapter 4), or renal impairment should prompt referral to a nephrologist and evaluation for parenchymal renal disease. When present, red cell casts are virtually pathognomonic of glomerular bleeding, but they are often absent in low-grade glomerular disease. Accurate determination of red blood cell morphology requires inverted phase contrast microscopy. In general, glomerular bleeding is associated with more than 80% dysmorphic red blood cells, and lower urinary tract bleeding is associated with more than 80% normal red blood cells.[17] This assessment is operator dependent. An alternative is to assess urinary red cell size by Coulter counter analysis because dysmorphic red cells are smaller

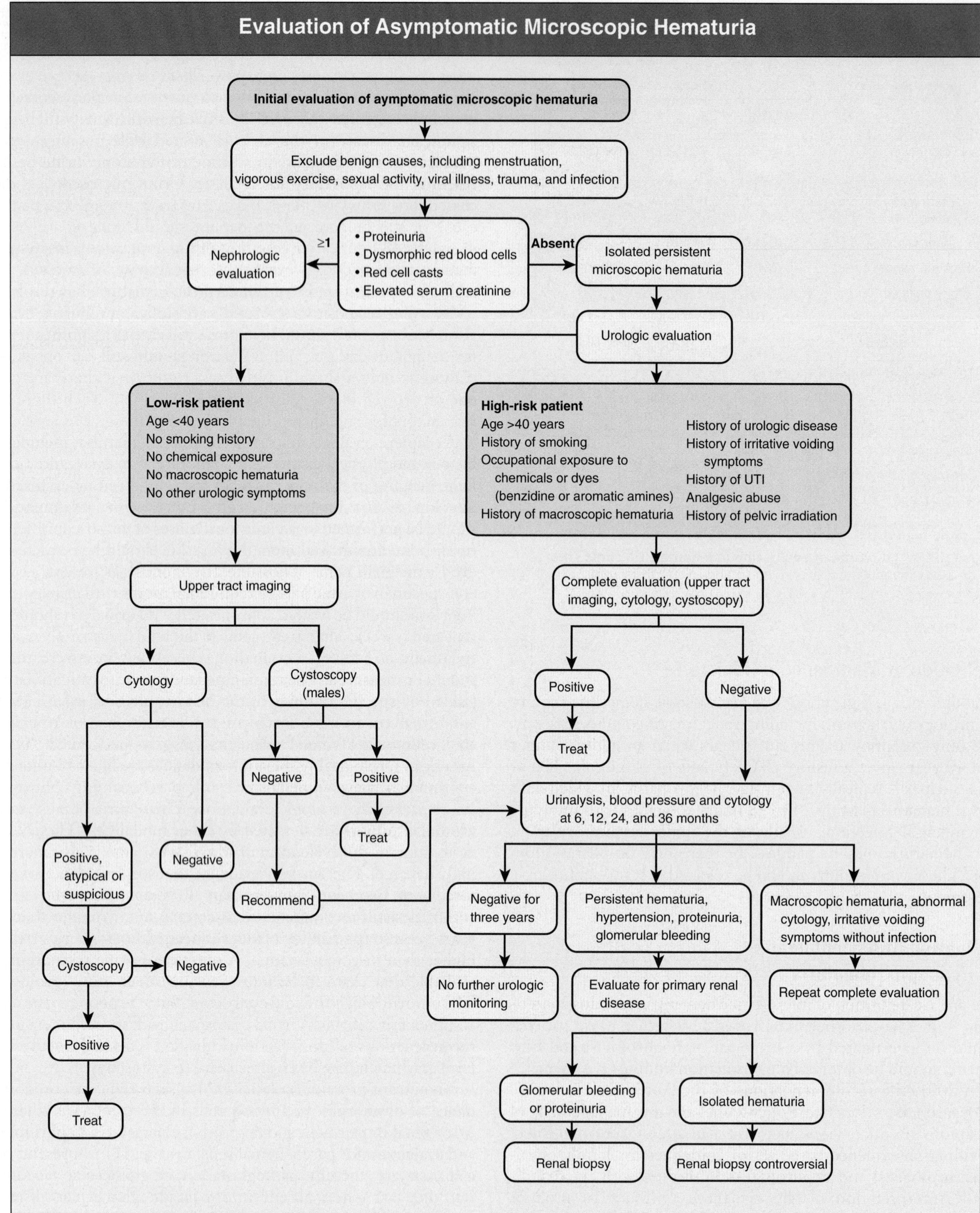

Figure 59.10 Evaluation of asymptomatic microscopic hematuria. UTI, urinary tract infection.

than normal red cells, but this method is not useful when red cell numbers in the urine are small. Even in the absence of features of glomerular bleeding, many patients with isolated microscopic hematuria have glomerular disease, most commonly IgA nephropathy or thin basement membrane nephropathy.[18] Because there is a low risk of progressive renal disease, renal biopsy in this setting is not usually recommended. Nevertheless, one study showed that microscopic hematuria unexplained by urologic evaluation carries a twofold risk for eventual development of ESRD,[19] so these patients should be observed for the development of hypertension, renal impairment, or proteinuria.

Cyclophosphamide

Past treatment with cyclophosphamide increases the risk of bladder cancer up to ninefold, probably in a dose- and duration-dependent manner. Tumors have been reported 6 to 13 years after cyclophosphamide exposure and are often high grade. Hematuria is also common after cyclophosphamide in the absence of cancer. If full evaluation does not identify a cause of hematuria, there is no agreed surveillance protocol; it is not clear whether routine follow-up by cystoscopy and urine cytology is valuable, although a high index of suspicion should be maintained.

INVESTIGATION AND MANAGEMENT OF A RENAL MASS

The incidence of renal cancer has more than doubled in the last 30 years and now accounts for 3% of all cancers. It is the third most common tumor of the urinary tract but is the most lethal. The apparent increased incidence is partly attributed to the widespread use of cross-sectional imaging; more than 50% of new cases are incidental findings on CT or magnetic resonance imaging (MRI).

The primary goal in investigating a renal mass is to exclude malignancy. Ultrasound has been reported to be 79% sensitive for the detection of renal parenchymal masses but does not detect lesions smaller than 5 mm. Until recently, the gold standard method of assessing renal masses was CT scanning with contrast enhancement, with use of no more than 5-mm slices. MRI, especially with T2-weighted images, may be superior to CT in the correct characterization of benign lesions.[20] Choice of imaging techniques and their interpretation are discussed further in Chapter 5.

Any solid mass larger than 3 cm should be regarded as malignant unless the radiologist can be confident that the mass is an angiomyolipoma by the presence of fat on CT images. A biopsy may be required if there is evidence suggestive of an alternative diagnosis (e.g., lymphoma or metastasis from another site) to guide appropriate management. Biopsy, however, has limited value in differentiating between malignant and benign primary renal lesions, mainly because of high false-negative rates.

The management of mixed cystic and solid masses is more of a problem. Figure 59.11 shows the Bosniak classification of cystic renal masses, which has recently been updated.[21] This classification, based on CT appearances, provides the basis for management according to risk of malignancy. The evaluation of multiple cystic lesions in the kidney is discussed further in Chapter 45.

Classification and Management of Cystic Renal Masses

Bosniak Class	Features on Imaging	Comment	Management
Class I: simple benign cyst	Round/oval Uniform density <20 H Unilocular No perceptible wall No contrast enhancement	Majority of asymptomatic cystic lesions	No further intervention required
Class II: benign cyst	One or two nonenhancing septa Calcifications in the wall or septum Hyperdense lesions (50-90HU, resulting from the presence of blood, protein, or colloid) < 3cm No contrast enhancement		No further intervention required
Class II F: probable benign cyst	Multiple hairline septa "Perceived" enhancement Nodular calcification Hyperdense lesions >3 cm	"Perceived" enhancement due to contrast within capillaries of septa	Surveillance with CT scans every 6–12 months
Class III: indeterminate cystic lesions	One or more of Thick, irregular borders Irregular calcifications Thickened or enhancing septa Multilocular form Uniform wall thickening Small nonenhancing nodules	About 40% are neoplastic Magnetic resonance imaging may improve characterization	Surgical exploration
Class IV: presumed malignant cystic masses	Appear malignant Heterogeneous cysts Shaggy, thickened walls or enhancing nodules	Appearances result from necrosis and liquefaction of a solid tumor or a tumor growing in the wall	Surgical exploration

Figure 59.11 Classification and management of cystic renal masses. Approach to renal mass found incidentally by ultrasound or CT scanning. All patients with symptomatic renal masses should be referred for urologic assessment. Classification after Bosniak. H, Hounsfield units. *(Data from reference 21.)*

Tumor size is important; in a large retrospective study of 2935 patients with surgically treated solid renal tumors, 46% of lesions smaller than 1 cm were benign compared with 22% and 10% of tumors 1 to 2 cm and 4 to 5 cm, respectively. Furthermore, only 2.3% of cancers smaller than 1 cm were of high grade, whereas for tumors larger than 7 cm, the percentage was 58%.[22] Surveillance studies of small renal tumors have shown a median growth rate of 0.28 cm per year; about 30% of these lesions will not increase in size. Biopsy of a renal mass is frequently nondiagnostic and may render radiographic follow-up more difficult.

The standard of care for localized kidney cancer is radical nephrectomy, open or laparoscopic; 5-year survival approaches 97% for tumors smaller than 4 cm. Partial nephrectomy can provide similarly good results and better preserve renal function. Usual indications for nephron-sparing surgery are an anatomic or functionally solitary kidney and a compromised contralateral kidney, but it can also be performed with a healthy contralateral kidney.

There is a growing trend for minimally invasive treatment of small renal tumors. Radiofrequency ablation and cryotherapy are the modalities most commonly used, and preliminary results show excellent short-term survival and metastasis-free rates, although concerns exist about local recurrence rates. The main disadvantages are that a tissue diagnosis is not always obtained and that radiologic follow-up can be difficult owing to the presence of necrosis and scar tissue. Interestingly, data from the United States show that the development of these newer technologies and the increased detection and treatment of renal tumors have not led to a corresponding decrease in age-specific renal cancer mortality rates.[23]

The Natural History of Renal Impairment After Surgical Treatment of Renal Cancer

It is well established that normal renal function can be preserved in the long term after donor transplant nephrectomy. However, donors are highly selected to minimize comorbidities and generally are younger than patients treated of renal tumors. After surgery for suspected renal cancer, when the residual renal mass is small, there is significant risk for late sequelae, including proteinuria, glomerulosclerosis, and progressive renal failure. These risks are greater when radical rather than partial nephrectomy is employed. A retrospective survey studied 662 patients who underwent surgery for a tumor 4 cm or less, with normal preoperative serum creatinine concentration and a normal contralateral kidney on imaging[24]; 26% of patients had postoperative glomerular filtration rate (GFR) lower than 60 ml/min, and mean GFR was 69 ml/min, significantly lower than reported after donor nephrectomy (92 to 103 ml/min). Postoperatively, the 3-year and 5-year probabilities of freedom from development of GFR below 60 ml/min were 80% and 67% after partial nephrectomy and 35% and 23% for radical nephrectomy. The probabilities of freedom from GFR below 45 ml/min were 95% and 93% after partial nephrectomy and only 64% and 57% for radical nephrectomy at 3 and 5 years postoperatively. Considering the excellent cancer-specific survival (>90%) of patients treated for renal tumors smaller than 4 cm, treatment-induced renal failure may have significant long-term consequences.

In another study, the effect of nephron-sparing surgery on solitary kidneys was assessed in a series of 400 patients.[25] Preoperatively, 56% of the patients had serum creatinine concentration above 1.5 mg/dl (136 μmol/l). Transient renal failure was observed in 21% of patients postoperatively; hemodialysis was necessary in 3.5%. At a mean follow-up of 44 months, 38% had more than 50% increase in serum creatinine, although only 5% of patients progressed to end-stage renal disease requiring renal replacement therapy. Overall, patients with a congenital single kidney tolerated partial nephrectomy better than did patients with acquired solitary kidneys. Other factors affecting long-term renal function were age and the percentage of parenchyma resected but not the use of hypothermia or the duration of renal ischemia during surgery.

Renal Cell Carcinoma in von Hippel–Lindau Disease

von Hippel–Lindau disease (VHL) is a rare autosomal dominant condition with a predisposition to the development of renal cell carcinoma. The genetics, clinical manifestations, and general management of VHL are discussed further in Chapter 45. The incidence of renal cell carcinoma in VHL is about 45%. On histologic examination, the tumors are of the clear cell type, often multifocal and bilateral, and can be solid or cystic. The mean age at diagnosis is 39 years, and there is a 30% to 35% risk for tumor progression, metastasis, and death.

A serial CT study[26] identified 228 renal lesions (on average, 8 per patient) in VHL patients, of which 74% were classified as cysts, 8% as cysts with solid components, and 18% as solid masses. The solid components of cysts and the solid lesions almost always contained renal cell carcinoma. During a mean 2.4-year follow-up (range, 1 to 12 years), most cysts remained the same size (71%) or enlarged (20%), and 9% became smaller. On the contrary, 95% of solid masses increased in size. Although it is generally thought that the cysts are premalignant, the transformation of a simple cyst to a solid lesion was observed in only two patients. VHL patients require multidisciplinary management. Surgical intervention is deferred for tumors smaller than 3 cm because metastasis is rare. In addition, bilateral nephrectomy should be avoided, if possible, because of the substantial morbidity associated with renal replacement therapy. The standard of care for these patients is partial nephrectomy, and 10-year survival rates of 81% have been reported.

The results of nephron-sparing surgery for VHL appear less satisfactory than for sporadic renal cell carcinoma because of a high risk of local tumor recurrence. Repeated surgery may be needed for new or growing lesions, and for this reason the use of minimally invasive methods is being investigated. Repeated ablation of tumors with radiofrequency and cryotherapy is possible with minimal morbidity; however, the long-term effectiveness of these methods has not yet been established.

REFERENCES

1. Rassweiler JJ, Renner C, Eisenberger F. The management of complex renal stones. *BJU Int.* 2000;86:919-928.
2. Albala DM, Assimos DG, Clayman RV, et al. Lower pole I: A prospective randomized trial of extracorporeal shock wave lithotripsy and percutaneous nephrostolithotomy for lower pole nephrolithiasis: Initial results. *J Urol.* 2001;166:72-80.
3. Webb DR, Fitzpatrick JM. Percutaneous nephrolithotripsy: A functional and morphological study. *J Urol.* 1985;134:587-591.
4. Zadra JA, Jewett MA, Keresteci AG, et al. Nonoperative urinary diversion for malignant ureteral obstruction. *Cancer.* 1987;60:1353-1357.
5. Chitale SV, Scott-Barrett S, Ho ET, Burgess NA. The management of ureteric obstruction secondary to malignant pelvic disease. *Clin Radiol.* 2002;57:118-121.

6. Saltzman B. Ureteral stents: Indications, variations, and complications. *Urol Clin North Am*. 1988;15:481-491.
7. Ku JH, Lee SW, Jeon HG, et al. Percutaneous nephrostomy versus indwelling ureteral stents in the management of extrinsic ureteral obstruction in advanced malignancies: Are there differences? *Urology*. 2004;64:95-99.
8. Minhas S, Irving HC, Lloyd SN, et al. Extra-anatomic stents in ureteric obstruction: Experience and complications. *BJU Int*. 1999;84:762-764.
9. Adeyoju AB, Hrouda D, Gill IS. Laparoscopic pyeloplasty: The first decade. *BJU Int*. 2004;94:64-67.
10. Lau MW, Temperley DE, Mehta S, et al. Urinary tract obstruction and nephrostomy drainage in pelvic malignant disease. *Br J Urol*. 1995;76:565-569.
11. Donat SM, Russo P. Ureteral decompression in advanced non-urologic malignancies. *Ann Surg Oncol*. 1996;3:393-399.
12. Shekarriz B, Shekarriz H, Upadhyay J, et al. Outcome of palliative urinary diversion in the treatment of advanced malignancies. *Cancer*. 1999;85:998-1003.
13. Khadra MH, Pickard RS, Charlton M, et al. A prospective analysis of 1,930 patients with hematuria to evaluate current diagnostic practice. *J Urol*. 2000;163:524-527.
14. Tomson C, Porter T. Asymptomatic microscopic or dipstick haematuria in adults: Which investigations for which patients? A review of the evidence. *BJU Int*. 2002;90:185-198.
15. Grossfeld GD, Wolf JS Jr, Litwin MS, et al. Asymptomatic microscopic hematuria in adults: Summary of the AUA best practice policy recommendations. *Am Fam Physician*. 2001;63:1145-1154.
16. van Rhijn BW, van der Poel HG, van der Kwast TH. Urine markers for bladder cancer surveillance: A systematic review. *Eur Urol*. 2005;47:36-48.
17. De Santo NG, Nuzzi F, Capodicasa G, et al. Phase contrast microscopy of the urine sediment for the diagnosis of glomerular and non-glomerular bleeding: Data in children and adults with normal creatinine clearance. *Nephron*. 1987;45:35-39.
18. Topham PS, Harper SJ, Harris KPG, et al. Glomerular disease as a cause of isolated microscopic haematuria. *Q J Med*. 1994;87:329-336.
19. Iseki K, Iseki C, Ikemiya Y, Fukiyama K. Risk of developing end-stage renal disease in a cohort of mass screening. *Kidney Int*. 1996;49:800-805.
20. Curry NS, Bissada NK. Radiologic evaluation of small and indeterminate renal masses. *Urol Clin North Am*. 1997;24:493-505.
21. Israel GM, Bosniak MA. An update of the Bosniak renal cyst classification system. *Urology*. 2005;66:84-88.
22. Frank I, Blute ML, Cheville JC, et al. Solid renal tumors: An analysis of pathological features related to tumor size. *J Urol*. 2003;170(pt 1):2217-2220.
23. Kunkle DA, Egleston BL, Uzzo RG. Excise, ablate or observe: The small renal mass dilemma—a meta-analysis and review. *J Urol*. 2008;179:1227-1233.
24. Huang WC, Levey AS, Serio AM, et al. Chronic kidney disease after nephrectomy in patients with renal cortical tumours: A retrospective cohort study. *Lancet Oncol*. 2006;7:735-740.
25. Fergany AF, Saad IR, Woo L, Novick AC. Open partial nephrectomy for tumor in a solitary kidney: Experience with 400 cases. *J Urol*. 2006;175:1630-1633.
26. Weld KJ, Landman J. Comparison of cryoablation, radiofrequency ablation and high-intensity focused ultrasound for treating small renal tumours. *BJU Int*. 2005;96:224-229.

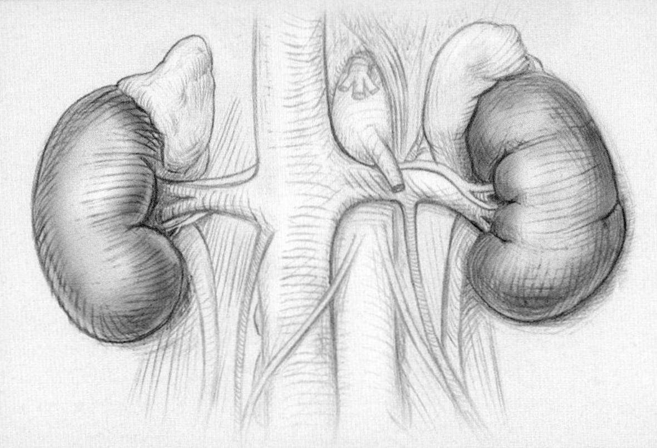

SECTION XI

Tubulointerstitial and Vascular Diseases

CHAPTER 60

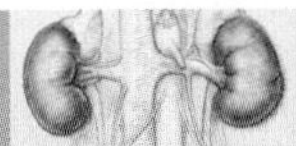

Acute Interstitial Nephritis

Jerome A. Rossert, Evelyne A. Fischer

DEFINITION

Acute interstitial nephritis (AIN) is an acute, often reversible disease characterized by inflammatory infiltrates within the interstitium. AIN is a rare cause of acute kidney injury (AKI), but it should not be overlooked because it usually requires specific therapeutic interventions.

PATHOGENESIS

Most studies suggest that AIN is an immunologically induced hypersensitivity reaction to an antigen that is classically a drug or an infectious agent. Evidence for a hypersensitivity reaction in drug-induced AIN includes the following: it occurs only in a small percentage of individuals; it is not dose dependent; it is often associated with extrarenal manifestations of hypersensitivity; it recurs after accidental reexposure to the same drug or to a closely related one; and it is sometimes associated with evidence of delayed-type hypersensitivity reaction (renal granulomas). Similarly, AIN secondary to infections can be differentiated from pyelonephritis by the relative absence of neutrophils in the interstitial infiltrates and the failure to isolate the infective agent from the renal parenchyma, again suggesting an immunologic basis to the disease.

Studies of experimental models of AIN have shown that three major categories of antigens can induce AIN.[1] Antigens may be tubular basement membrane (TBM) components (such as the glycoproteins 3M-1 and TIN-Ag/TIN1), secreted tubular proteins (such as Tamm-Horsfall protein), or nonrenal proteins (such as from immune complexes).

Although some types of human AIN may be secondary to an immune reaction directed against a renal antigen, the majority of cases of AIN are probably induced by extrarenal antigens, being produced in particular by drugs or infectious agents. These antigens may be able to induce AIN by a variety of mechanisms. These mechanisms include binding to kidney structures ("planted antigen"); acting as haptens that modify the immunogenicity of native renal proteins; mimicking renal antigens, resulting in a cross-reactive immune reaction; and precipitating within the interstitium as circulating immune complexes.

Studies of experimental models of AIN show that their pathogenesis involves either cell-mediated immunity or antibody-mediated immunity (Fig. 60.1). In humans, most forms of AIN are not associated with antibody deposition, which suggests that cell-mediated immunity plays a major role. This hypothesis is reinforced by the fact that interstitial infiltrates usually contain numerous T cells and that these infiltrates sometimes form granulomas. Nevertheless, deposition of anti-TBM antibodies or of immune complexes can be observed occasionally in renal biopsy specimens, and antibody-mediated immunity may play a role in the pathogenesis of the disease in these cases.

Formation of immune complexes within the interstitium, or interstitial infiltration with T cells, will result in an inflammatory reaction. This reaction is triggered by many events, including activation of the complement cascade by antibodies and release of inflammatory cytokines by T lymphocytes and phagocytes (see Fig. 60.1). Although the interstitial inflammatory reaction may resolve without sequelae, it sometimes induces interstitial fibroblast proliferation and extracellular matrix synthesis, leading to interstitial fibrosis and chronic renal failure. Cytokines such as transforming growth factor ß appear to play a key role in this latter process.

EPIDEMIOLOGY

AIN is an uncommon cause of AKI and is identified in only about 2% to 3% of all renal biopsy specimens.[2] However, it may account for up to 10% to 25% of patients undergoing renal biopsy for unexplained or drug-induced AKI, respectively.[2] Although AIN can occur at any age, it appears to be rare in children.

Before antibiotics were available, AIN was most commonly associated with infections, such as scarlet fever and diphtheria. Currently, AIN is most often induced by drugs, particularly antimicrobial agents, proton pump inhibitors, and nonsteroidal anti-inflammatory drugs (NSAIDs). Drug-induced AIN appears to account for about 75% to 90% of all cases.

DRUG-INDUCED ACUTE INTERSTITIAL NEPHRITIS

Clinical Manifestations

In the 1960s and 1970s, most cases of drug-induced AIN were caused by methicillin, and the clinical manifestations of methicillin-induced AIN were considered the prototypical presentation of AIN. Since then, many other drugs have been implicated in the induction of AIN (Fig. 60.2), of which antimicrobial agents (in particular, β-lactam antibiotics, sulfonamides, fluoroquinolones, and rifampin) and NSAIDs (especially fenoprofen) as well as cyclooxygenase 2 (COX-2) inhibitors have been most commonly involved. Antiulcer agents, diuretics, phenindione, phenytoin, and allopurinol have also been reported to cause AIN. There are increasing numbers of reports of AIN induced by proton pump inhibitors, with more than 70 reported biopsy-proven cases.[3] Recently, cases of drug-induced AIN have also been reported in human immunodeficiency virus (HIV)–infected patients treated with highly active antiretroviral therapy (HAART)[4] and in cancer patients treated with tyrosine kinase

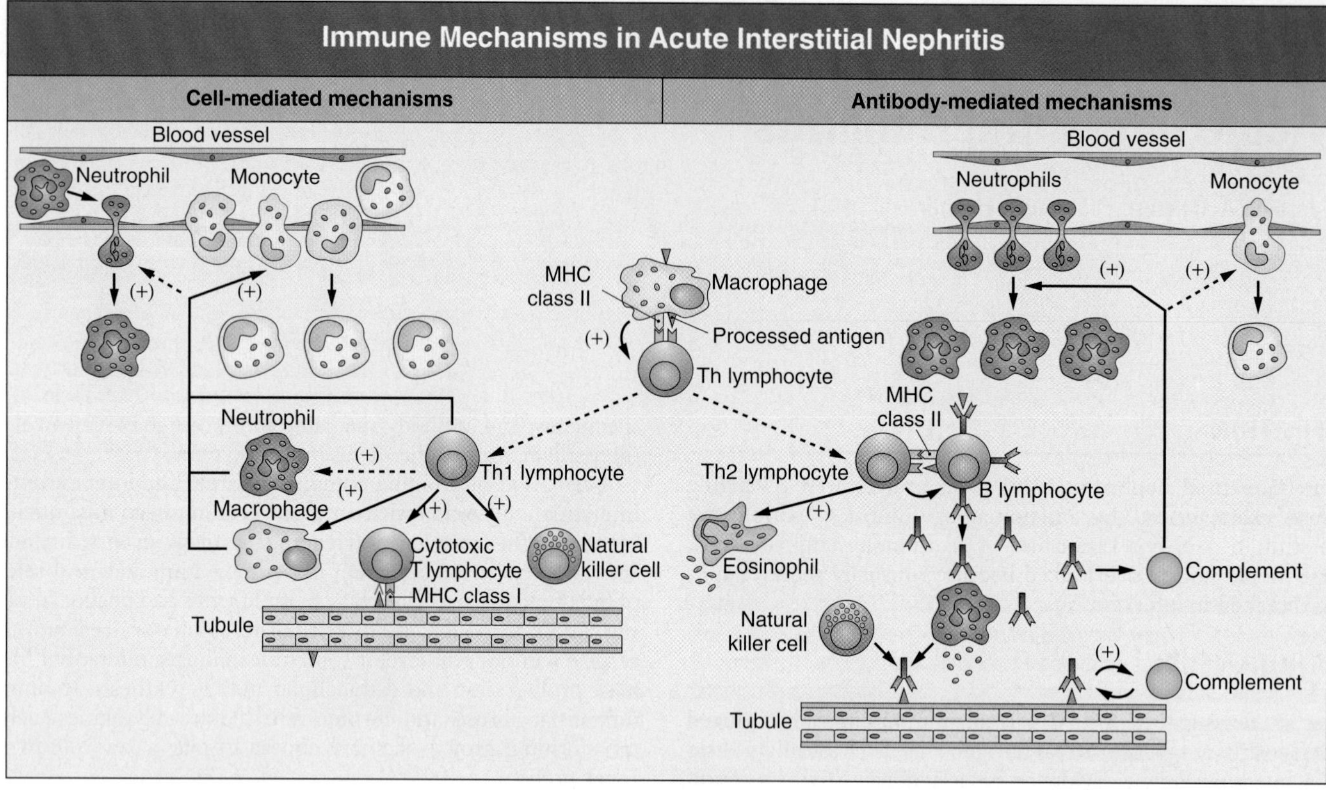

Figure 60.1 Immune mechanisms that can be involved in acute interstitial nephritis. Both cell-mediated and antibody-mediated mechanisms occur. The cell-mediated mechanism is primarily associated with macrophages and T cells. The antibody-mediated mechanism is frequently associated with neutrophil or eosinophil infiltration as well as with local complement activation. MHC, major histocompatibility complex.

inhibitors.[5] Most other drugs have only rarely been linked with AIN (see Fig. 60.2). The clinical characteristics of drug-induced AIN are now recognized as much more varied and nonspecific than the spectrum seen in classic methicillin-induced AIN (Fig. 60.3).[6,7]

Renal Manifestations

Symptoms of AIN usually develop a few days to a few weeks after the inciting drug is started, although cases have occurred months after initial exposure to the drug. The typical presentation is sudden impairment in renal function, associated with mild proteinuria (<1 g/day) and abnormal urinalysis, in a patient with flank pain, normal blood pressure, and no edema. In patients with AIN not caused by methicillin, the clinical presentation is often incomplete (see Fig. 60.3), and AIN should be considered in any patient with unexplained AKI.[6,7] The renal dysfunction may be mild or severe; dialysis is required in about one third of patients. Hematuria and pyuria are present in a little more than half of the patients, and although leukocyte casts are common, hematuria is almost never associated with red blood cell casts. Flank pain, reflecting distention of the renal capsule, is observed in about one third of the patients and can be the main complaint on hospital admission. On occasion, patients have a low fractional excretion of sodium.

Standard imaging procedures show kidneys normal in size or slightly enlarged. Ultrasound usually discloses an increased cortical echogenicity (comparable to or higher than that of the liver).

Extrarenal Manifestations

Extrarenal symptoms consistent with a hypersensitivity reaction are occasionally observed, including low-grade fever, maculopapular rash (Fig. 60.4), mild arthralgias, and eosinophilia. If patients with methicillin-induced AIN are not considered, each of these symptoms is present in less than half of the patients (see Fig. 60.3), and all these symptoms are present together in less than 10% of patients.[2,6,7] With some drugs, other manifestations of hypersensitivity, such as hemolysis or hepatitis, can be present. Serum IgE levels may also be elevated.

The association of AKI either with clinical signs suggestive of hypersensitivity or with eosinophilia should lead to consideration of a diagnosis of AIN. However, signs of hypersensitivity can also be observed in patients with AKI not related to AIN, including patients with drug-induced acute tubular necrosis.

Other Specific Drug Associations

The clinical and biologic manifestations of AIN may have some specificity, depending on the drug involved.

As outlined earlier, methicillin-induced AIN is characterized by a high frequency of abnormal urinalysis and extrarenal symptoms and by good preservation of renal function. Renal failure has been reported in only about 50% of patients (see Fig. 60.3).

More than 200 cases of rifampin-induced AKI have been reported. Most have been observed either after readministration of rifampin or several months after intermittent administration of the drug. Renal failure is usually associated with the sudden onset of fever, gastrointestinal symptoms (nausea, vomiting, diarrhea, abdominal pain), and myalgias. It may also be associated with hemolysis, thrombocytopenia, and less frequently hepatitis. Renal biopsy typically discloses tubular injury in addition to interstitial inflammatory infiltrates. Although circulating anti-rifampin antibodies are usually found in these patients, immunofluorescence staining of renal biopsy specimens has been

Drugs Responsible for Acute Interstitial Nephritis

ANTIMICROBIAL AGENTS

PENICILINS

Amoxicillin
Ampicillin*
Aztreonam
Carbenicillin
Cloxacillin
Methicillin*
Mezlocillin
Nafcillin
Oxacillin*
Penicillin G* (benzylpenicillin*)
Piperacillin

CEPHALOSPORINS

Cefaclor
Cefamandole
Cefazolin
Cefixim
Cefoperazone
Cefotaxime
Cefotetan
Cefoxitin
Ceftriaxone
Cephalexin
Cephaloridine
Cephalothin
Cephapirin
Cephradine
Latamoxef

QUINOLONES

Ciprofloxacin*
Levofloxacin*
Moxifloxacin
Norfloxacin

OTHERS

Abicavir
Acyclovir
Atazanavir
Azithromycin
Clarithromycin
Colistin
Cotrimoxazole*
Erythromycin*
Ethambutol
Flurithromycin
Foscarnet
Gentamicin
Indinavir
Interferon
Isoniazid
Lincomycin
Minocycline
Nitrofurantoin*
Piromidic acid
Polymixin B*
Quinine
Rifampin* (rifampicin*)
Spiramycine*
Sulfonamides*
Teicoplamin
Telithromycin
Tetracycline
Vancomycin*

NSAIDs INCLUDING SALICYLATES

SALICYLATES AND DERIVATIVES

Aspirin (acetyl salicylic acid)
Diflunisal*

PROPIONIC ACID DERIVATIVES

Benoxaprofen
Fenbufen
Fenoprofen*
Flurbiprofen
Ibuprofen*
Ketoprofen
Naproxen
Pirprofen
Suprofen

ACETIC ACID DERIVATIVES

Indomethacin* (indometacin)
Alclofenac
Diclofenac
Fenclofenac
Sulindac
Zomepirac

ENOLIC ACID DERIVATIVES

Meloxicam
Piroxicam*

FENAMIC ACID DERIVATIVES

Mefenamic acid
Niflumic acid

COXIBS

Celecoxib
Rofecoxib

OTHERS

Azapropazone
Mesalamine (mesalazine, 5-ASA)
Phenazone
Phenylbutazone
Sulfasalazine
Tolmetin

ANALGESICS

Aminopyrine
Antipyrine
Antrafenin
Clometacin* (clometazin*)
Dipyrone (noramidopyrine, metamizol)
Floctafenin*
Glafenin*

ANTICONVULSANTS

Carbamazepine*
Diazepam
Phenobarbital (phenobarbitone)
Phenytoin*
Valproic acid (valproate sodium)

DIURETICS

Chlortalidone
Ethacrynic acid
Furosemide* (frusemide*)
Hydrochlorothiazide*
Indapamide
Tienilic acid*
Triamterene*

ANTIULCER AGENTS

H2-RECEPTOR ANTAGONISTS

Cimetidine*
Famotidine
Ranitidine

PROTON PUMP INHIBITORS

Esomeprazole
Lansoprazole
Omeprazole
Pantoprazole
Rabeprazole

OTHERS

Allopurinol*
Alpha Methyl Dopa
Amlodipine
Azathioprine
Betanidine*
Bismuth salts
Captopril*
Carbimazole
Chlorpropamide*
Clofibrate
Clozapine
Cyamemazine*
Cyclosporine
Cytosine Arabinoside
Desferasirox
Diltiazem
D-penicillamine
Etanercept
Fenofibrate*
Fluindione
Gold salts
Griseofluvin
Interleukin 2
Lamotrigine*
Linezolid
Nicergolin
Phenindione*
Phenothiazine
Phentermine/ Phendimetrazine
Phenylpropanolamine
Probenecid
Propanolol
Propylthiouracil
Sorafenib
Streptokinase
Sulphinpyrazone
Sunitinib
Warfarin
Zopiclone

Figure 60.2 Drugs responsible for acute interstitial nephritis. Drugs most commonly involved are in bold. NSAIDs, nonsteroidal anti-inflammatory drugs. *Drugs that can cause granulomatous AIN.

negative in most cases, suggesting that cell-mediated immunity plays a key role in the induction of the nephritis. In a few cases, AIN developed after continuous treatment with rifampin for 1 to 10 weeks. It was almost never associated with extrarenal symptoms or with anti-rifampin antibodies, and renal biopsy specimens showed severe interstitial infiltrates but few tubular lesions.

Phenindione-induced AIN is generally associated with the development of hepatitis, which can be fatal.

Allopurinol-induced AIN appears to occur more often in patients with chronic kidney disease (CKD) and is usually seen in association with rash and liver dysfunction. It has been suggested that the decreased excretion of oxypurinol, a metabolite of allopurinol, might favor the occurrence of AIN. There is also

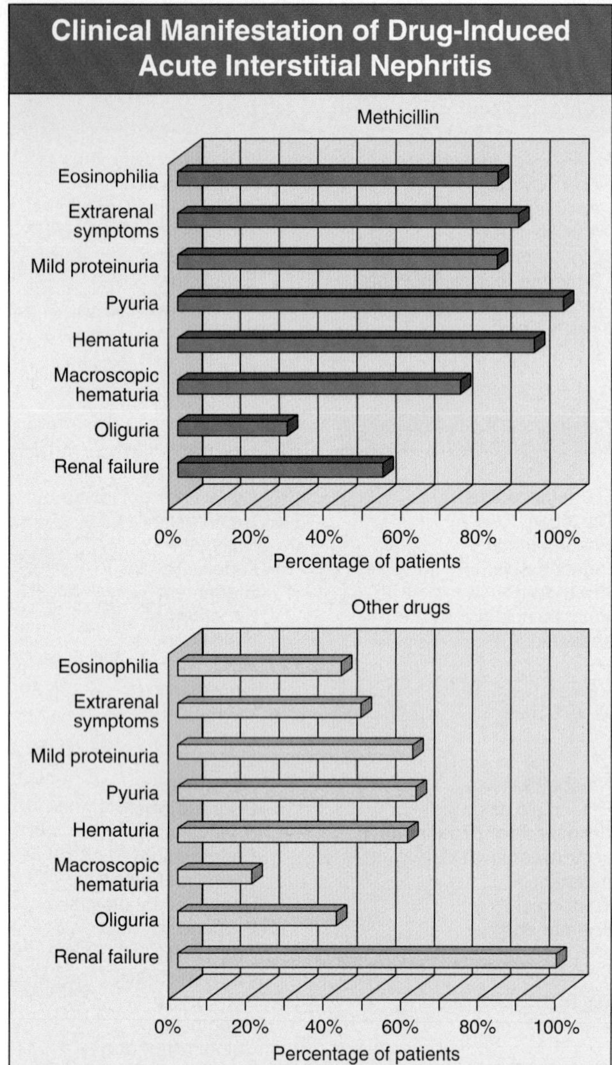

Figure 60.3 Clinical manifestations of drug-induced acute interstitial nephritis. Data were pooled from different case reports, including 95 patients with methicillin-induced AIN and more than 200 patients with other drug-induced AIN. Patients with AIN associated with a nephrotic syndrome are not included.

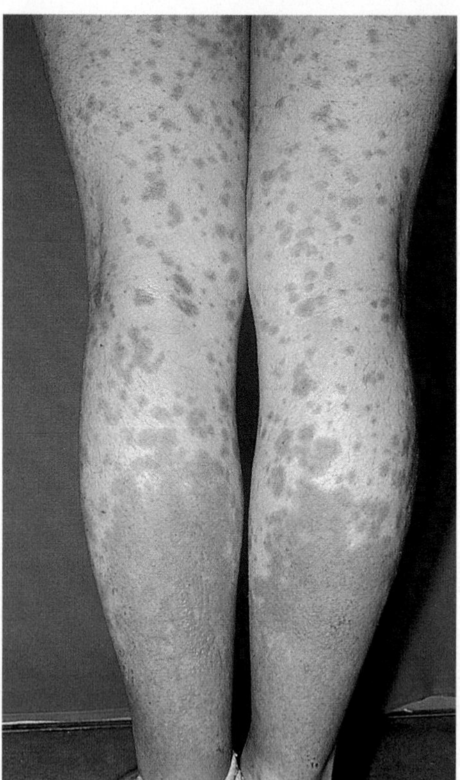

Figure 60.4 Maculopapular rash in a patient with drug-induced acute interstitial nephritis. Such cutaneous lesions occur in about 40% of patients with drug-induced AIN, but they can also be seen in patients with drug-induced acute tubular necrosis.

some experimental evidence that in the setting of renal impairment, allopurinol may precipitate as microcrystals or crystals and cause direct nephrotoxicity. Whether this can occur in humans is unknown, but it may provide an additional reason to reduce allopurinol doses in subjects with CKD.

AIN occurring secondary to NSAIDs is associated with nephrotic syndrome in about three fourths of cases. This usually occurs in patients older than 50 years, and although it has been observed with all NSAIDs, including COX-2–selective inhibitors, half of the incidents have been reported with fenoprofen. Most occurrences develop after the patient has taken NSAIDs for some months (mean, 6 months), but AIN can occur within days or after more than a year. With the exception of the heavy proteinuria and associated edema, the presentation of these patients is similar to that of patients with other drug-induced AIN (Fig. 60.5). The main difference is that extrarenal symptoms are present in only about 10% of patients. Renal disease caused by NSAIDs must be differentiated from other NSAID-induced nephropathies, including hemodynamically mediated AKI, papillary necrosis, and NSAID-induced membranous nephropathy. Drugs other than NSAIDs can rarely induce AIN associated with a nephrotic syndrome; a few cases have been reported after administration of ampicillin, rifampin, lithium, interferon, phenytoin, pamidronate, and D-penicillamine.

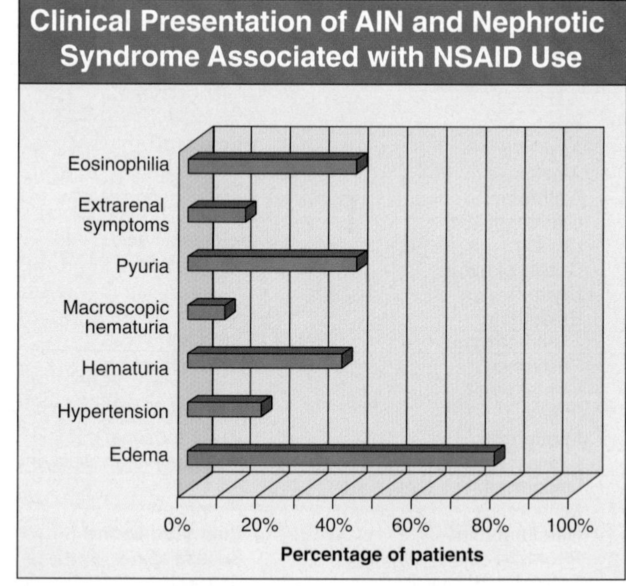

Figure 60.5 Clinical presentation of AIN and nephrotic syndrome associated with NSAID use. Data were pooled from different case reports from more than 60 patients.

Pathology

The hallmark of AIN is the presence of inflammatory infiltrates within the interstitium (Fig. 60.6). These infiltrative lesions are often patchy, predominating in the deep cortex and in the outer medulla, but they can be diffuse in severe cases. They are composed mostly of T cells and monocytes-macrophages, but plasma cells, eosinophils, and a few neutrophilic granulocytes may also be present. The relative number of $CD4^+$ T cells and $CD8^+$ T cells is variable from one patient to another. In some cases, T lymphocytes infiltrate across the TBM and between tubular cells, mainly in distal tubules, and the resulting lesion is referred to as tubulitis.

In some cases of drug-induced AIN, renal biopsy shows interstitial granulomas (Fig. 60.7). These granulomas are usually sparse and non-necrotic, with few giant cells, and are associated with nongranulomatous interstitial infiltrates. Granulomas are also found in AIN related to infection (see Fig 60.10), sarcoidosis, Sjögren's syndrome, and Wegener's granulomatosis.

Interstitial infiltrates are always associated with an interstitial edema, which is responsible for separating the tubules (see Fig. 60.6). They can also be associated with focal tubular lesions, which range from mild cellular alterations to extensive necrosis of epithelial cells and are sometimes associated with a disruption of the TBM. These tubular lesions usually predominate where the inflammatory infiltrates are most extensive.

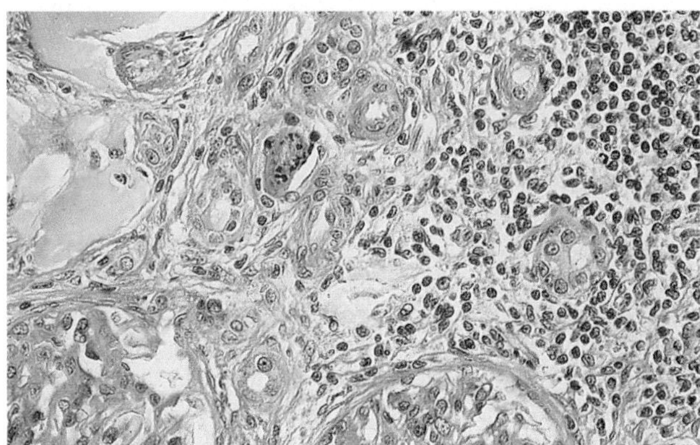

Figure 60.6 Drug-induced acute interstitial nephritis. On light microscopy, the characteristic feature is interstitial infiltration with mononuclear cells, with normal glomeruli. It is usually associated with interstitial edema and tubular lesions. *(Courtesy of Dr. B. Mougenot, Paris VI University, Paris France.)*

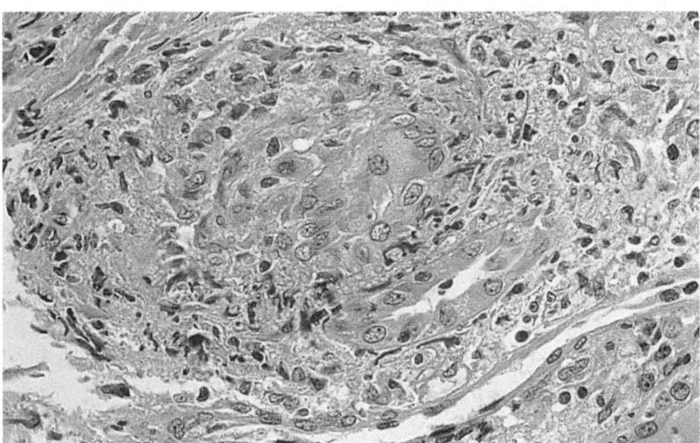

Figure 60.7 Drug-induced granulomatous acute interstitial nephritis. Some drugs can induce the formation of interstitial granulomas, which reflect a delayed-type hypersensitivity reaction. *(Courtesy of Dr. B. Mougenot, Paris VI University, Paris France)*

Tubulointerstitial lesions are not associated with vascular or glomerular lesions. Even in AIN associated with a nephrotic syndrome, glomeruli appear normal on light microscopy; glomerular lesions are similar to those seen in minimal change disease (see Chapter 17).

In most patients with AIN, renal biopsy specimens do not show immune deposits, and both immunofluorescence and electron microscopy are negative. Nevertheless, staining of the tubular or capsular basement membrane for IgG or complement may occasionally be seen by immunofluorescence; the staining pattern is either granular or linear (Fig. 60.8). Linear fixation of IgG along the TBM indicates the presence of antibodies directed against membrane antigens or against drug metabolites bound to the TBM, and circulating anti-TBM antibodies have been detected in some cases. These linear deposits are seen mostly in patients taking methicillin, NSAIDs, phenytoin, or allopurinol.

Diagnosis

The most accurate way to diagnose AIN is by renal biopsy. However, both eosinophiluria and gallium scanning have been suggested as helpful in making the diagnosis.

Eosinophils can be detected in urine with use of either the Wright stain or the Hansel stain, which both are eosin–methylene blue combinations, but the Hansel stain appears to be much more sensitive.[8,9] The result of this test is usually considered positive if more that 1% of urinary white blood cells are eosinophils. However, although eosinophiluria is frequently used to corroborate the diagnosis of drug-induced AIN, review of four large series shows that this test has rather poor sensitivity (67%) and a low positive predictive value, even when only patients with AKI are considered (50%) (Fig. 60.9).[8-11] In these series, the specificity of the test was 87%, and eosinophiluria was also observed in patients with acute tubular necrosis, postinfectious or crescentic glomerulonephritis, atheroembolic renal disease, urinary tract infection, urinary schistosomiasis, and even prerenal AKI. In particular, 28% of patients with urinary tract infection had eosinophiluria. Because of these limitations, eosinophiluria should no longer be used as a screening test.

An increased renal uptake of gallium 67 has been reported in AIN.[12] Analysis of available series shows that in 45 patients with AIN, 88% had an abnormal renal scan (maximum after 48 hours),

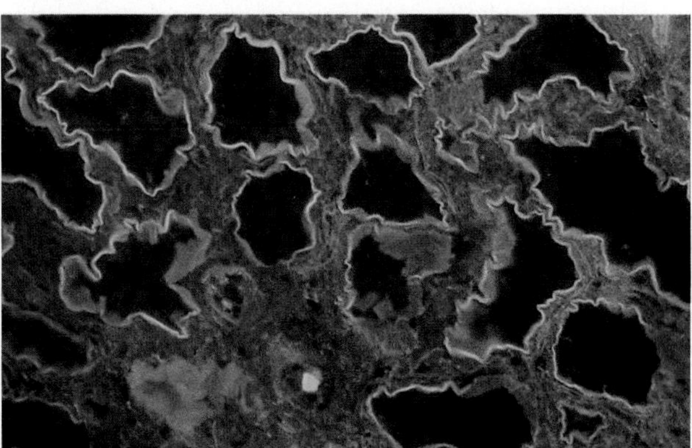

Figure 60.8 Linear deposits of IgG in methicillin-induced acute interstitial nephritis. Deposits along the TBM are shown on immunofluorescence microscopy. These antibodies recognize either a component of the TBM or a methicillin metabolite (dimethoxyphenylpenicilloyl) bound to the TBM. *(Courtesy of Dr. B. Mougenot, Paris VI University, Paris France.)*

Eosinophiluria and the Diagnosis of Acute Interstitial Nephritis					
	Corwin et al. [8]	Nolan et al. [9]	Corwin et al. [10]	Ruffin et al. [11]	All series n (%)
Patients with AIN (n)	**9**	**11**	**8**	**15**	**43**
Eosinophiluria	8	10	5	6	29 (67%)
No eosinophiluria	1	1	3	9	14 (33%)
Patients without AIN (n)	**56**	**81**	**175**	**184**	**496**
Eosinophiluria	27	12	15	10	64 (13%)
No eosinophiluria	29	69	160	174	432 (87%)
Patients with acute kidney injury					
	Corwin et al. [8]	Nolan et al. [9]	Corwin et al. [10]	Ruffin et al. [11]	All series
Patients with AIN (n)	9	11	8	15	43
Eosinophiluria	8	10	5	6	29 (67%)
No eosinophiluria	1	1	3	9	14 (33%)
Patients without AIN (n)	14	46	84	23	167
Eosinophiluria	6	5	2	6	19 (11%)
No eosinophiluria	8	41	82	17	148 (89%)

Figure 60.9 Eosinophiluria in the diagnosis of acute interstitial nephritis. The four large available series were analyzed to assess the value of eosinophiluria (defined by the presence of >1% of eosinophils in urine) for the diagnosis of drug-induced AIN. Only 67% of AIN was associated with eosinophiluria, whereas 13% of non-AIN was associated with eosinophiluria.

whereas it was normal in 17 of 18 patients with acute tubular necrosis. However, these studies were small and retrospective, and gallium 67 renal scanning is not specific for AIN and may be abnormal in patients with pyelonephritis, cancer, or glomerular diseases. Therefore, we also do not recommend use of gallium scanning as a diagnostic tool.

Because the clinical presentation of AIN may be polymorphic and because noninvasive diagnostic procedures have important limitations, renal biopsy is often essential for the diagnosis of AIN. Several studies have shown that prebiopsy diagnosis may be incorrect in a substantial number of patients.

Identification of the Causative Drug

Identification of the causative drug is relatively easy when AIN occurs in a patient taking only one drug. However, patients are often taking more than one drug capable of inducing AIN. Two biologic tests have been used, primarily in research laboratories, to help identify the causative drug: the lymphocyte stimulation test and the identification of circulating antidrug antibodies.

Identification of circulating antidrug antibodies has been used mostly for patients thought to have AIN induced by rifampin. Anti-rifampin antibodies are present in most patients with rifampin-induced AIN; but unfortunately, they have also been detected in patients taking rifampin and having no adverse reaction to the drug, so this test has a limited diagnostic value.

The lymphocyte stimulation test has been used since the 1960s to identify a sensitizing drug. It is based on the measurement of lymphocyte proliferation in the presence of different drugs; a high proliferative index reflects a sensitization of T lymphocytes against the drug. However, this test lacks specificity and we do not recommend using it.

Natural History

Drug-induced AIN was long considered benign, with complete recovery of renal function if the inciting agent was removed. For example, with methicillin-induced AIN, a complete normalization of serum creatinine has been observed in about 90% of uremic patients. Nevertheless, although hematuria, leukocyturia, and extrarenal symptoms usually disappeared within 2 weeks, complete recovery of renal function was often delayed, with an average recovery time of about 1.5 months.

More recent studies show that with drugs other than methicillin, the course of AIN is not always benign and that serum creatinine remains elevated in about 40% to 50% of patients.[6,13] Moreover, as for methicillin, recovery of renal function can be delayed, and an increase in serum creatinine can persist for several weeks. Unfortunately, few prognostic factors are available. The severity of renal failure does not appear to be linked with the prognosis.[6] It has been suggested that the presence on renal biopsy of diffuse neutrophil- or macrophage-rich infiltrates, interstitial granulomas, or tubular atrophy is associated with a poor prognosis, but this has not been consistently found in all series. The best prognostic factors may actually be the duration of AKI and the severity of interstitial fibrosis.

Treatment

In addition to removal of the inciting agent, corticosteroids have been used to treat AIN. Most commonly, patients received an initial daily dose of 1 mg/kg prednis(ol)one, which is then tapered during about 1 month; this oral therapy is sometimes associated with pulses of methylprednisolone. Analysis of series comparing patients who did or did not receive corticosteroids does not allow firm conclusion about the effect of corticosteroid therapy on long-term renal function, all the series being small, uncontrolled, and retrospective. However, some authors advocate an early and systematic use of a short course of corticosteroids.[7,13] In addition, it seems that a brief course of corticosteroids can hasten the recovery of renal function. In different series, corticosteroids rapidly induced a reduction in serum creatinine in patients whose renal function did not improve within about 1 week after discontinuation of the inciting agent. Interestingly, in patients with

NSAID-induced AIN, corticosteroids do not seem to modify the course of the nephrotic syndrome.

On the basis of anecdotal case reports, some authors have also advocated use of mycophenolate mofetil in patients resistant to corticosteroids.[14]

We recommend administration of a short course of prednis(ol) one in patients who are dialysis dependent or whose renal function fails to improve rapidly within 1 week after discontinuation of the inciting drug and return to baseline values, provided the diagnosis of AIN has been confirmed by renal biopsy. We initiate the treatment with 1 mg/kg per day of prednis(ol)one, and after 1 to 2 weeks, we progressively taper the dose so that the total duration of treatment is 4 to 6 weeks.

ACUTE INTERSTITIAL NEPHRITIS SECONDARY TO INFECTIOUS DISEASES

Infections were once the most common cause of AIN, but the frequency of AIN induced by an infection has dramatically decreased with the widespread use of antibiotics. Nevertheless, the diagnosis of infectious AIN should not be overlooked, and AIN occurring in patients treated with antibiotics should not always be attributed to the drug.

Infectious agents can cause renal parenchymal inflammation by direct infection, resulting in acute pyelonephritis (see Chapter 51). However, many infectious agents may also induce an immunologically mediated AIN in the absence of direct invasion (Fig. 60.10). In this case, the clinical presentation depends mostly on the underlying infection. On histologic examination, lesions are identical to those described for drug-induced AIN, and they can also occasionally result in granulomas (see Fig. 60.10). Infection-associated AIN usually resolves with the treatment of the underlying infection, and corticosteroid therapy is not recommended.

An important cause of infection-associated AIN is hantavirus.[15] Hantavirus infections occur worldwide and are responsible for a disease that has been known as hemorrhagic fever with renal syndrome, epidemic hemorrhagic fever, or nephropathia epidemica. Rodents are the main reservoir of the virus, and humans are most probably infected by the airborne route. Extrarenal symptoms usually include fever, headache, lightheadedness, abdominal pain, nausea and vomiting, and thrombocytopenia; the last can be responsible for hemorrhagic complications. AKI is almost always associated with proteinuria, sometimes in the nephrotic range, and with hematuria. When a kidney biopsy is performed, it discloses not only interstitial inflammatory infiltrates, which predominate in the medulla, but also vascular congestion and interstitial bleeding (Fig. 60.11). In about 50% of the patients, immunofluorescence studies show granular immune deposits along the TBM and within glomeruli. Serum creatinine concentration usually starts to decrease after a few days, and a complete recovery of renal function is the rule. Nevertheless, in the more severe cases, recovery can be complicated by the occurrence of hemorrhagic complications or severe shock. The diagnosis is based on serologic test results, which become positive early (within weeks) in the course of the disease.

Tubulointerstitial lesions are common in HIV-positive patients who undergo a renal biopsy for AKI. Interstitial infiltrates are often associated with glomerular lesions, but they can also be isolated. These forms of AIN have been observed in both white and black patients, and they might be related not only to drugs and opportunistic infections but also to the HIV infection itself.[16]

Infections that can be Associated with Acute Interstitial Nephritis

Bacteria	Viruses	Parasites	Others
Brucella species	Adenovirus	*Toxoplasma* species*	*Chlamydia* species
Campylobacter jejuni	Cytomegalovirus	*Leishmania donovani*	*Mycoplasma* species
Corynebacterium diphtheriae	Epstein-Barr virus*		
Escherichia coli	Hantaan virus		
Legionella species	Hepatitis A virus		
Leptospira species	Hepatitis B virus		
*Mycobacterium tuberculosis**	Herpes simplex virus		
Salmonella species*	Human immunodeficiency virus		
Staphylococcus species	Measles virus		
Streptococcus species	Polyomavirus		
Yersinia pseudotuberculosis	Rickettsia		

Figure 60.10 Infections that can be associated with acute interstitial nephritis. *Infections that can induce granulomatous AIN.

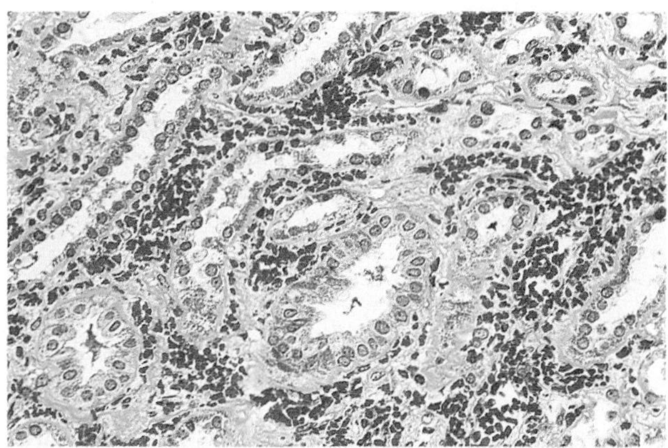

Figure 60.11 Acute interstitial nephritis secondary to hantavirus infection. Vascular congestion and foci of medullary hemorrhage are suggestive of the diagnosis. *(Courtesy Dr. B. Mougenot, Paris VI University, Paris France.)*

ACUTE INTERSTITIAL NEPHRITIS ASSOCIATED WITH SYSTEMIC DISEASES

Sarcoidosis

In sarcoidosis, renal impairment usually occurs as a complication of hypercalciuria and hypercalcemia, but granulomatous AIN associated with sarcoidosis has also been reported (Fig. 60.12).[17,18] The presentation is usually that of AKI, which can be isolated or associated with mild proteinuria and sterile leukocyturia. It is

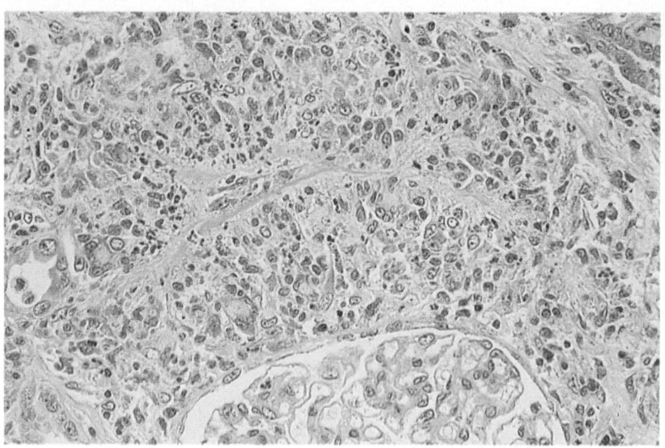

Figure 60.12 Granulomatous acute interstitial nephritis in a patient with sarcoidosis. *(Courtesy Dr. B. Mougenot, Paris VI University, Paris France.)*

associated with extrarenal symptoms of sarcoidosis in about 90% of patients, most frequently with lymphadenopathy and lung, eye, or liver involvement. Nevertheless, only slightly more than half of the patients have hilar lymphadenopathy or pulmonary interstitial fibrosis at the time of diagnosis.[19] Treatment with high-dose corticosteroids quickly improves renal function, but most patients do not recover completely. The starting dose should be 1 mg/kg prednis(ol)one daily, and corticosteroid therapy should be tapered slowly and not withdrawn before at least 1 year to prevent relapses. Whereas some authors advocate long-term maintenance therapy with low-dose corticosteroids, we usually stop corticosteroids after 2 to 3 years. Because of the risk of late relapse, these patients should be observed for a prolonged time.

Sjögren's Syndrome

Clinically significant interstitial nephritis is rare in Sjögren's syndrome and usually results in chronic tubular dysfunction.[20] Some patients may present with severe symptomatic hypokalemia with distal renal tubular acidosis. Rarely, Sjögren's syndrome presents with AKI due to AIN. In these patients, treatment with high-dose corticosteroids may dramatically improve renal function.

Systemic Lupus Erythematosus

About two thirds of renal biopsies performed in patients with systemic lupus show some tubulointerstitial involvement, but significant tubulointerstitial injury in the setting of minimal glomerular abnormalities is rare, with only about 10 cases reported in the literature.[21] In these cases, renal biopsy shows typical features of AIN on light microscopy, and immunofluorescence staining always discloses immune deposits along the TBM, usually with a granular pattern. Renal function improves after high-dose corticosteroids and does not usually require additional immunosuppressive drugs. However, azathioprine has been used as a corticosteroid-sparing agent.

Other Systemic Diseases

Among patients with cryoglobulinemia and AKI, a few exhibit significant interstitial inflammatory infiltrates associated with granular immune deposits in the interstitium and along the TBM. This AIN is usually associated with characteristic glomerular lesions and rarely lesions of the arterioles, and treatment is the same as for cryoglobulinemia-induced glomerulonephritis (see Chapter 21).

Most renal lesions associated with small-vessel vasculitis (such as Wegener's granulomatosis) consist of both an extracapillary glomerulonephritis and a tubulointerstitial nephritis. Nevertheless, a few patients with AIN and minimal glomerular lesions have been described.

ACUTE INTERSTITIAL NEPHRITIS ASSOCIATED WITH MALIGNANT NEOPLASMS

Infiltration of renal parenchyma by malignant cells is common in patients with leukemia or lymphoma. Most of the time, this infiltration is totally asymptomatic or only causes enlarged kidneys, but a few patients with AKI have been described.[22] Chemotherapy or radiotherapy may rapidly improve renal function in these patients, but before these treatments are started, it is important to exclude more common causes of AKI associated with neoplastic diseases (see Chapter 66).

IDIOPATHIC ACUTE INTERSTITIAL NEPHRITIS

More than 50 cases of idiopathic AIN with anterior uveitis have been reported (TINU syndrome).[23] This syndrome is found most commonly in girls of pubertal age but can also occur in pubertal boys and in adults. Initial symptoms may be ocular, with ocular pain and visual impairment, or pseudoviral, with fever, myalgia, and asthenia. AIN is responsible for AKI, ranging from mild to severe, that may or may not be associated with abnormal urinalysis. Renal biopsy shows diffuse interstitial inflammatory infiltrates, almost always without granulomas and without immune deposits. In children, renal prognosis is excellent, and serum creatinine usually returns to baseline values within a few weeks, with or without corticosteroid therapy. In adults, the renal prognosis seems to be less favorable, and corticosteroid therapy might be useful in preventing evolution to chronic renal failure. Uveitis, which can occur at any time in respect to AIN, is usually responsive to topical corticosteroids, but it may relapse without any recurrence of AIN.

A few cases of idiopathic AIN have been reported. Immunofluorescence studies of renal biopsy specimens can show linear deposits of IgG along the TBM, granular deposits of IgG along the TBM, or no immune deposits, suggesting that this entity is heterogeneous. The treatment of patients with idiopathic AIN is still controversial. Patients who receive corticosteroids usually show a dramatic improvement of renal function, but others have recovered normal renal function without any treatment.

ACUTE INTERSTITIAL NEPHRITIS IN RENAL TRANSPLANTS

Acute rejection is by far the most common cause of AIN in renal allograft recipients (see Chapter 100). Nevertheless, AIN can also be induced by drugs or infections. Cases of drug-induced AIN have been reported even in the first weeks after transplantation, when immunosuppression is maximal.[24] Among infectious AIN, the frequency of polyomavirus-induced AIN appears to be increasing, and it should be suspected in patients with acute deterioration of renal function and so-called decoy cells in urine (see Chapter 101).[25]

REFERENCES

1. Neilson EG. Pathogenesis and therapy of interstitial nephritis. *Kidney Int*. 1989;35:1257-1270.
2. Clarkson MR, Giblin L, O'Connell FP, et al. Acute interstitial nephritis: Clinical features and response to corticosteroid therapy. *Nephrol Dial Transplant*. 2004;19:2778-2783.
3. Brewster UC, Perazella MA. Acute kidney injury following proton pump inhibitor therapy. *Kidney Int*. 2007;71:589-593.
4. Schmid S, Opravil M, Moddel M, et al. Acute interstitial nephritis of HIV-positive patients under atazanavir and tenofovir therapy in a retrospective analysis of kidney biopsies. *Virchows Arch*. 2007;450:665-670.
5. Winn SK, Ellis S, Savage P, et al. Biopsy-proven acute interstitial nephritis associated with the tyrosine kinase inhibitor sunitinib: A class effect? *Nephrol Dial Transplant*. 2009;24:673-675.
6. Rossert J. Drug-induced acute interstitial nephritis. *Kidney Int*. 2001;60: 804-817.
7. Baker RJ, Pusey CD. The changing profile of acute tubulointerstitial nephritis. *Nephrol Dial Transplant*. 2004;19:8-11.
8. Corwin HL, Bray RA, Haber MH. The detection and interpretation of urinary eosinophils. *Arch Pathol Lab Med*. 1989;113:1256-1258.
9. Nolan CR 3rd, Anger MS, Kelleher SP. Eosinophiluria—a new method of detection and definition of the clinical spectrum. *N Engl J Med*. 1986;315:1516-1519.
10. Corwin HL, Korbet SM, Schwartz MM. Clinical correlates of eosinophiluria. *Arch Intern Med*. 1985;145:1097-1099.
11. Ruffing KA, Hoppes P, Blend D, et al. Eosinophils in urine revisited. *Clin Nephrol*. 1994;41:163-166.
12. Linton AL, Richmond JM, Clark WF, et al. Gallium 67 scintigraphy in the diagnosis of acute renal disease. *Clin Nephrol*. 1985;24:84-87.
13. Gonzalez E, Gutierrez E, Galeano C, et al. Early steroid treatment improves the recovery of renal function in patients with drug-induced acute interstitial nephritis. *Kidney Int*. 2008;73:940-946.
14. Preddie DC, Markowitz GS, Radhakrishnan J, et al. Mycophenolate mofetil for the treatment of interstitial nephritis. *Clin J Am Soc Nephrol*. 2006;1:718-722.
15. Ferluga D, Vizjak A. Hantavirus nephropathy. *J Am Soc Nephrol*. 2008;19:1653-1658.
16. Cohen SD, Chawla LS, Kimmel PL. Acute kidney injury in patients with human immunodeficiency virus infection. *Curr Opin Crit Care*. 2008;14:647-653.
17. Rajakariar R, Sharples EJ, Raftery MJ, et al. Sarcoid tubulo-interstitial nephritis: Long-term outcome and response to corticosteroid therapy. *Kidney Int*. 2006;70:165-169.
18. Mahevas M, Lescure FX, Boffa JJ, et al. Renal sarcoidosis: Clinical, laboratory, and histologic presentation and outcome in 47 patients. *Medicine (Baltimore)*. 2009;88:98-106.
19. Hannedouche T, Grateau G, Noel LH, et al. Renal granulomatous sarcoidosis: Report of six cases. *Nephrol Dial Transplant*. 1990;5:18-24.
20. Goules A, Masouridi S, Tzioufas AG, et al. Clinically significant and biopsy-documented renal involvement in primary Sjögren syndrome. *Medicine (Baltimore)*. 2000;79:241-249.
21. Mori Y, Kishimoto N, Yamahara H, et al. Predominant tubulointerstitial nephritis in a patient with systemic lupus nephritis. *Clin Exp Nephrol*. 2005;9:79-84.
22. Tornroth T, Heiro M, Marcussen N, et al. Lymphomas diagnosed by percutaneous kidney biopsy. *Am J Kidney Dis*. 2003;42:960-971.
23. Liakopoulos V, Ioannidis I, Zengos N, et al. Tubulointerstitial nephritis and uveitis (TINU) syndrome in a 52-year-old female: A case report and review of the literature. *Ren Fail*. 2006;28:355-359.
24. Josephson MA, Chiu MY, Woodle ES, et al. Drug-induced acute interstitial nephritis in renal allografts: Histopathologic features and clinical course in six patients. *Am J Kidney Dis*. 1999;34:540-548.
25. Hariharan S. BK virus nephritis after renal transplantation. *Kidney Int*. 2006;69:655-662.

CHAPTER 61

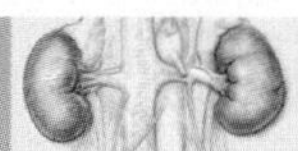

Primary Vesicoureteral Reflux and Reflux Nephropathy

Ranjiv Mathews, Tej K. Mattoo

DEFINITION

Vesicoureteral reflux (VUR) is a congenital or hereditary abnormality in which there is retrograde flow of urine from the bladder to the kidneys. This retrograde flow of urine, although normal in some animals, is not normal in humans. VUR may be an isolated abnormality (primary VUR) or may occur with other congenital anomalies of the kidney and urinary tract, including renal dysplasia, obstructive uropathy, and neurogenic bladder (secondary VUR).

VUR is usually identified by fetal ultrasound in pregnancy (in which renal pelvis dilation is observed) or after urinary tract infection (UTI) in childhood. It is commonly believed that the presence of VUR increases the risk of UTI, and the two together can cause renal injury leading to a contracted, scarred kidney termed reflux nephropathy. Reflux nephropathy may present as a UTI, hypertension, toxemia of pregnancy, chronic kidney disease (CKD), and even end-stage renal disease (ESRD). Whereas reflux nephropathy involves primary injury to the renal parenchyma, some subjects also have proteinuria due to secondary focal segmental glomerulosclerosis (FSGS).

Traditional management includes prompt treatment of UTI and long-term antimicrobial prophylaxis until the resolution of VUR. Surgical correction of the VUR may be recommended in those with high-grade VUR who have recurrent UTI in spite of antimicrobial prophylaxis or are noncompliant with medical management. Debate persists on the superiority of one intervention over the other; most studies have concluded that long-term outcomes are similar.

CLASSIFICATION

VUR is classified by radiologic evaluation on voiding cystourethrography (VCU) into five grades as defined by the International Reflux Study in Children (Figs. 61.1 and 61.2).[1] Grade I is reflux into the ureter; grade II is reflux into the renal pelvis, without any dilation of the calyces; grade III is reflux to the renal pelvis with mild dilation of the renal pelvis; grade IV is reflux to the renal pelvis with greater dilation of the renal pelvis; and grade V is reflux to the renal pelvis with ureteral and pelvic dilation. An example of grade V reflux is shown in Figure 61.3.

Grading of VUR is used to predict the outcomes of children with VUR. Because VUR may resolve spontaneously, grading is used to standardize management strategies as well as to compare clinical outcomes between institutions. Although it is widely used, the classification system is not perfect. Differences between grade III and grade IV are not always obvious. The degree of reflux may be modified by how aggressively the bladder is filled. Ureteral dilation may also be present without calyceal dilation, leading to difficulties with grading.

EPIDEMIOLOGY

VUR is often first suggested by dilation of the fetal kidney during ultrasound examination. VUR is suspected when the fetal renal pelvis is more than 5 mm in anteroposterior diameter; a diameter of more than 10 mm is associated with high-grade VUR. In neonates who had evidence of fetal dilation, as many as 13% to 22% will have VUR by VCU. Indeed, it is estimated that 1% to 2% of healthy children will have VUR, with a higher frequency in boys and premature infants.[2] The incidence of renal dysplasia is also greater in male infants with VUR.[3] Most cases associated with grades I to III VUR will spontaneously resolve within the first year of life, whereas grades IV and V are more likely to persist. Spontaneous resolution of VUR is greater in male infants.

VUR is also diagnosed in 30% to 40% of children presenting with UTI, predominantly girls. VUR is both less common and less severe in African American children.[4,5] Only about one third as many African American as Caucasian girls with UTI have VUR, and no significant differences in age or mode of presentation exist between the two races.

Reflux nephropathy may be responsible for up to 10% of ESRD and is one of the common causes of ESRD in children. In children, reflux nephropathy occurs equally in boys and girls; in adults, there is a slight female predominance.

ETIOLOGY AND PATHOGENESIS

Primary VUR is a congenital anomaly of the ureterovesical junction, probably due to a preexisting anatomic abnormality with shortening of the intravesical submucosal length of the ureter, leading to an incompetent valve (Fig. 61.4). The formation of the ureteral bud from the mesonephric duct signals the initial development of the metanephric kidney, the final stage of renal development. The ureteral bud interacts with the mesenchyme to give rise to the metanephric kidney. As the mesonephric duct is gradually absorbed into the enlarging urogenital sinus (the precursor of the developing bladder), the location of the ureteral bud plays a role in the eventual location of the ureteral meatus within the bladder. If the ureteral bud reaches the urogenital

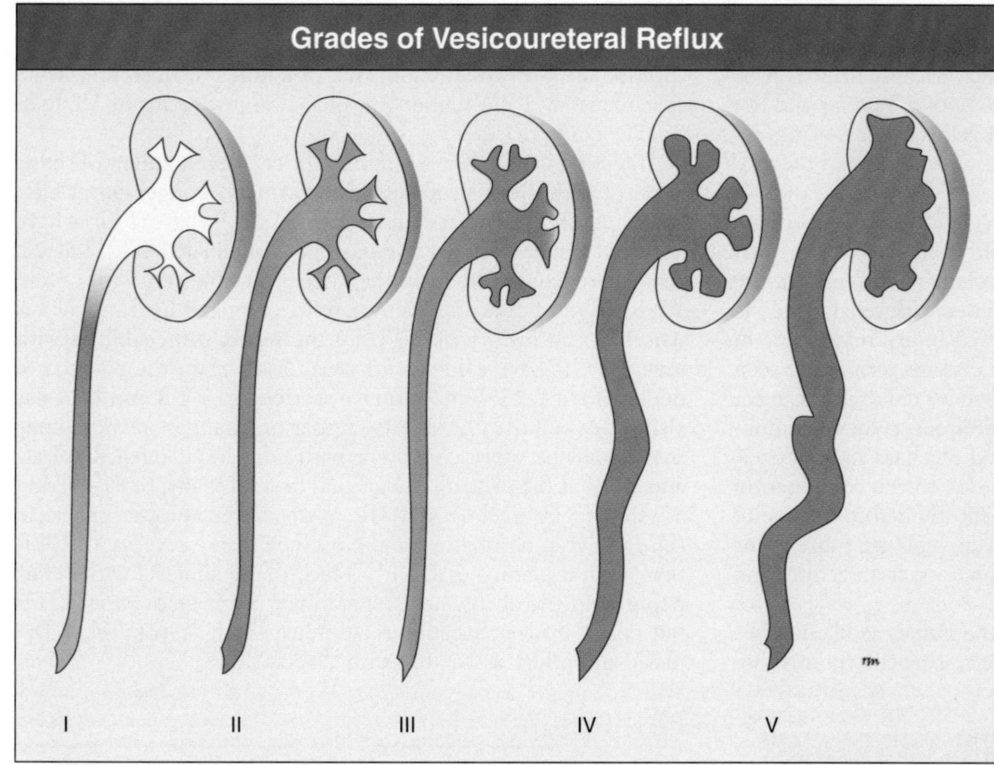

Figure 61.1 Grades of VUR.

International Reflux Study in Children Classification of VUR

Grade	Degree of VUR
I	Ureter only
II	Reflux into ureter, pelvis, and calyces with no dilation and with normal calyceal fornices
III	Mild or moderate dilation and/or tortuosity of the ureter and mild or moderate dilation of the pelvis; no or slight blunting of the fornices
IV	Moderate dilation and/or tortuosity of the ureter, and moderate dilation of the pelvis and calyces; complete obliteration of the pelvis and calyces; complete obliteration of the sharp angles of the fornices but maintenance of the papillary impressions in the majority of the calyces (see Fig. 61.12C)
V	Gross dilation and tortuosity of the ureter, pelvis, and calyces; the papillary impressions are no longer visible in the majority of calyces (see Fig. 61.3)

Figure 61.2 Classification of VUR. The International Reflux Study in Children classification.

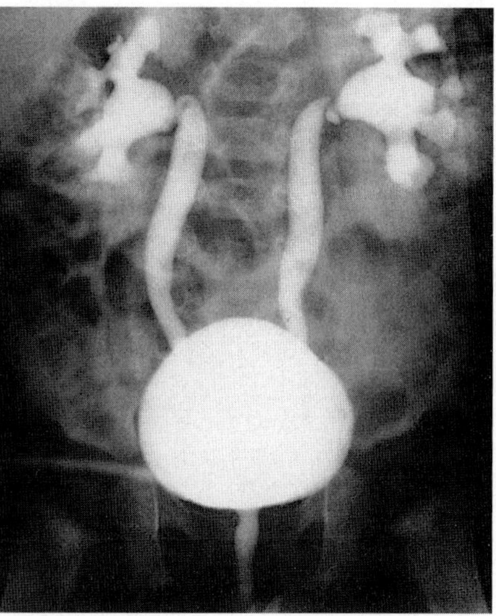

Figure 61.3 Gross VUR and intrarenal reflux. A voiding cystourethrogram shows grade V VUR with intrarenal reflux into several renal lobes in an infant.

sinus too early because of the absorption pattern of the mesonephric duct, it is eventually located more laterally and proximally in the bladder. This location is associated with the development of reflux as there is reduction in the intravesical submucosal length of the ureter.

Multiple genes are involved in the development of VUR. *PAX2* (necessary for ureteral budding in mice), glial-derived neurotrophic factor (*GDNF*), angiotensin II type 2 receptor, and uroplakin 3 (which is a component of tight junctions in uroepithelial cells) have been implicated in the development of VUR in mice; however, their role in human VUR remains controversial.[6,7] Neither autonomic innervation nor histology of the ureterovesical junction is different between subjects with VUR and controls.[8]

The ureterovesical junction is designed to prevent free reflux of urine from the bladder to the kidney. The ureters pass into the bladder through the detrusor in an oblique path. The distal end of the ureter is located submucosally within the bladder. The length of the submucosal ureter is critical in the prevention of VUR. The muscles of the ureter extend into the trigone of the bladder and mesh with the fibers from the opposite ureter. This intermingling of fibers helps anchor the ureters into the trigone of the bladder. The distal submucosal segment is compressed against the muscular bladder wall with bladder filling, acting as an additional mechanism to prevent reflux. Because urine is propulsed antegrade down the ureter, the tone of the ureter and the meatus in the bladder also help prevent reflux.

Reflux Nephropathy

Reflux nephropathy is thought to result from one of two processes (Fig. 61.5). In some subjects, especially males, renal injury may be due to severe VUR that is associated with renal dysplasia (congenital form). In these subjects, renal injury may occur in the absence of infection. These cases are more commonly seen in boys with grade IV or V VUR, and these children are most commonly identified with the antenatal discovery of renal dilation during fetal ultrasound. The second mechanism for development of reflux nephropathy is likely due to the combination of VUR and repeated UTI that occurs mostly before the age of 5 years (acquired form). In these children, who are more commonly female, the combination of upper tract infection and reflux causes permanent scarring.

In both conditions, the damage to the kidney is likely to be greatest in children younger than 2 years, particularly in those with severe VUR.[9] Renal injury is more common in this age group because of delay in diagnosis of UTI due to the nonspecific clinical presentation, the difficulties in obtaining urine specimens, and the higher prevalence and severity of VUR in smaller children.

Infection is not always required for the development of reflux nephropathy. Boys probably have primary, congenital, VUR-associated renal damage more commonly, whereas girls have acquired scarring related to recurrences of febrile UTI.[10] Indeed, renal parenchymal defects may occur in children with severe VUR diagnosed during follow-up for antenatal hydronephrosis who have no history of UTI. Furthermore, some siblings with severe VUR have evidence of renal scarring in the absence of documented UTI. Renal damage ascribed to VUR and UTI has also been found to be due to dysplastic changes in the kidney that would be more consistent with congenital renal dysplasia and VUR as the primary underlying cause. Finally, renal scarring as shown by technetium Tc 99m dimercaptosuccinic acid (DMSA) scan correlates more closely with the severity of VUR than with a history of UTI.[11] Thus, many subjects with reflux nephropathy probably have renal injury not from previous UTIs but rather from preexisting renal injury, such as from renal dysplasia and injury associated with severe VUR.

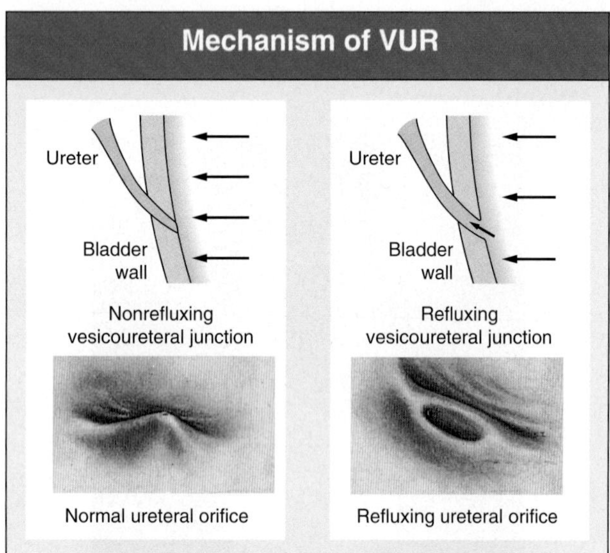

Figure 61.4 Pathogenesis of VUR. Competent *(left)* and incompetent *(right)* vesicoureteral junctions and ureteral orifices.

PATHOLOGY

The process of renal scarring may take several years; in one study, the mean time from discovery of VUR to the appearance of a renal scar was 6.1 years.[12] Grossly, the injury favors the renal poles and is associated with clubbed calyces with medullary and cortical damage. The injury results from the local inflammatory response that may persist with chronic inflammation, tubular injury, local fibroblast activation, and interstitial collagen deposition (Fig. 61.6).[13] The loss of nephrons is associated with hyperfiltration and hypertension that result in proteinuria and progressive loss of renal function. This can also lead to the development of FSGS (Fig. 61.7).

CLINICAL MANIFESTATIONS

Presentation with Vesicoureteral Reflux

Patients with primary VUR may present in a variety of ways (Fig. 61.8). The three most common presentations are after a diagnosis of UTI, during follow-up for antenatal hydronephrosis, and on screening of a sibling of a patient with VUR.

Types of Renal Damage Associated with VUR

	Congenital	Acquired
Time of occurrence	Often prenatal	Postnatally, sometimes in adulthood
Previous urinary infection	Not usually	Usually
Gender	Usually boys	Usually girls (particularly after infancy)
Grade of VUR	Usually grades IV and V	Grades IV and V less common
Renal scarring	Often present	Present in minority of cases*
Associated bladder dysfunction	Hypercontractile bladder common	Less commonly high capacity bladder with incomplete voiding

*depends on unilateral versus bilateral involvement, and the severity of renal involvement

Figure 61.5 Types of renal damage associated with VUR.

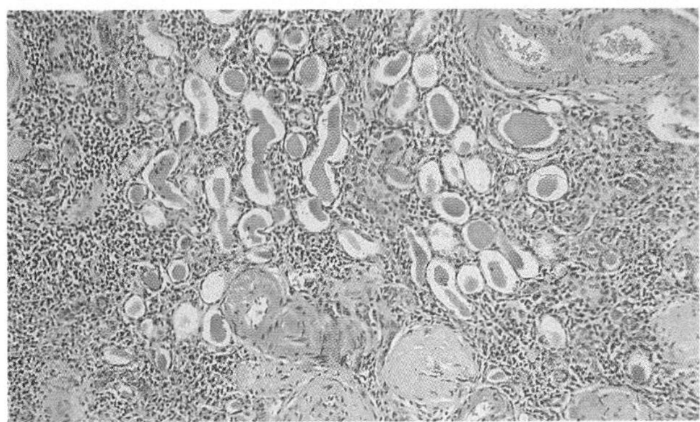

Figure 61.6 Histologic changes in reflux nephropathy. Sclerosed glomeruli, chronic inflammatory cell infiltration, and atrophic tubules with eosinophilic casts are present. (Hematoxylin and eosin; original magnification ×40.)

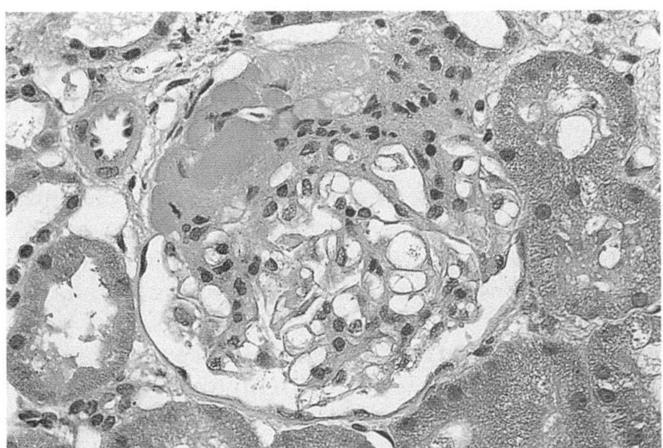

Figure 61.7 Focal segmental glomerulosclerosis in reflux nephropathy. Light microscopy of a glomerulus from a subject with reflux nephropathy shows FSGS. (Hematoxylin and eosin; original magnification ×400.)

Clinical Presentations of VUR

Complicated urinary infection – usually acute pyelonephritis in infants and children

Asymptomatic
- Detected by fetal ultrasound
- Detected in the workup of members of an affected family
- Detected in pregnant women with UTI
- Detected during workup of kidney stones in children
- Detected during assessment of other urologic congenital abnormalities

Figure 61.8 Clinical presentations of VUR.

Reflux Identified After a Urinary Tract Infection

VUR is most commonly found after UTI, particularly in a young child. The prevalence of VUR is higher in younger subjects and decreases with age (Fig. 61.9). In neonates and toddlers, UTI may be manifested as failure to thrive as opposed to typical symptoms of dysuria and frequency. VUR is more common in subjects with complicated or upper tract UTI. Because VUR may potentiate the effect of UTI in children, current recommendations for evaluation of UTI include ultrasound and VCU after resolution of the first UTI in both boys and girls (Fig. 61.10). If VUR is diagnosed, further testing involves a DMSA scan to determine whether renal scarring is present.

Prevalence of VUR in Patients with Urinary Tract Infection, According to Age

Age	Percentage with VUR
2–3 days	57
3–6 days	51
2–6 months	60
7–12 months	35
1–4 years	50
5–9 years	35
10–14 years	14
14 years	10
Adult	5

Figure 61.9 Prevalence of VUR in patients with urinary tract infection, according to age. *(From reference 14.)*

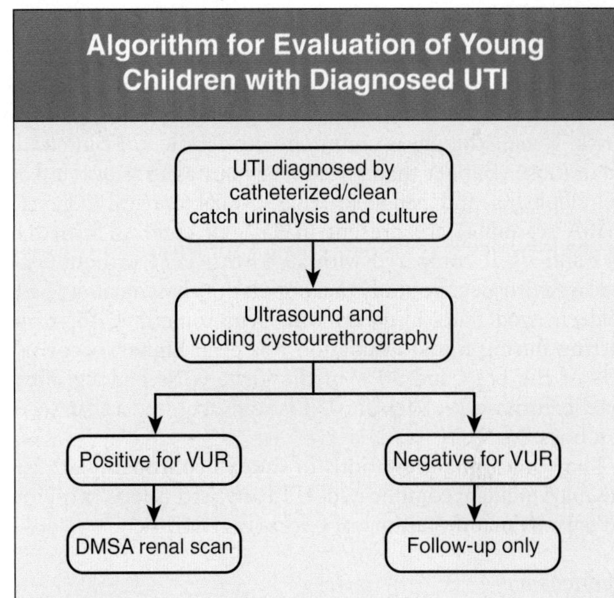

Figure 61.10 Current recommended algorithm for evaluation of young children with diagnosed UTI.

Most children diagnosed with VUR after a UTI are younger than 7 years. UTI in these subjects may be associated with modifiable host factors, such as voiding dysfunction and constipation. For example, toilet-trained children with VUR identified after a UTI, have a 43% incidence of dysfunctional voiding.[15]

Reflux Identified Secondary to Antenatal Hydronephrosis

Diagnosis of VUR may be suspected *in utero* with unilateral or bilateral hydronephrosis and confirmed at birth with VCU. There is a higher incidence of male infants diagnosed with VUR after identification of antenatal hydronephrosis.[16] Spontaneous resolution of the VUR occurs more commonly in boys with lower grades and unilateral reflux; infection rates are also lower in this cohort.[17] Female infants are more likely to have lower grades of VUR and are also less likely to develop renal damage compared with newborn boys. Reflux in newborn boys may be due to elevated bladder pressures secondary to dyssynergia of the urethral sphincter, which improves with time with secondary resolution of even higher grades of VUR.[18,19]

Sibling VUR

Approximately one third of siblings of an index patient with VUR also have VUR.[18] There is a slightly higher incidence of VUR in female siblings of female index patients; 75% of children with VUR identified by sibling screening are asymptomatic. The incidence of renal damage is also lower in the siblings diagnosed with reflux compared with the index patient with VUR.[20] For example, UTI with progression of scar was noted in only 5% of siblings with VUR observed for 3 to 7 years, and most of those with grades I and II VUR had resolution.[21] The more "benign" course of sibling reflux compared with reflux identified after a UTI has led many to suggest limitation of those being screened. At this time, most suggest screening of younger siblings (<5 years) of index children with VUR and reserve screening of older siblings for those who present with a UTI or other symptoms.

Reflux Nephropathy

VUR with or without UTI may cause renal scarring, which is known as reflux nephropathy.[22] Young children are particularly at risk. Renal scarring is common with febrile UTI in children, and in those younger than 5 years, as many as 75% develop acute pyelonephritis and renal scarring. Renal cortical defects (by DMSA scanning) are present in 45% of children with febrile UTI and VUR compared with 24% with UTI without VUR.[23] In a large prospective study of a population-based cohort of 1221 children aged 0 to 15 years with symptomatic UTI, primary scarring during initial evaluation was even higher, occurring in 86% of the boys and 30% of the girls. Girls had significantly more recurrences of febrile UTIs and acquired renal scarring than boys.[24]

The clinical manifestations of reflux nephropathy are varied and may include complicated UTI, hypertension, proteinuria, and various manifestations of CKD (Fig. 61.11).

Hypertension

Hypertension occurs in 10% to 30% of children and young adults with reflux nephropathy,[24,25] and according to one study, hypertension may take 8 years to develop.[12] The exact cause of hypertension due to renal scarring is not known, but it is believed to be due to impaired sodium excretion resulting from the renal injury. Hypertension is relatively uncommon in children with VUR, with an estimated probability of 2%, 6%, and 15% at 10, 15, and 21 years of age, respectively. However, hypertension increases in proportion to the degree of renal injury.[26] Renal scarring (noted by DMSA scans) was reported in 20% of newly diagnosed hypertension in children and adolescents.

Clinical Presentations of Reflux Nephropathy
Complicated urinary infection—usually acute pyelonephritis in infants and children
Hypertension: may be accelerated
During pregnancy: urinary infection, hypertension, preeclampsia
Proteinuria
Chronic renal impairment
Urinary calculi
Asymptomatic Detected in the workup of members of an affected family Detected by fetal ultrasound Detected during assessment of other urologic congenital abnormalities

Figure 61.11 Clinical presentations of reflux nephropathy.

Proteinuria

Patients may also present with microalbuminuria, persistent proteinuria, or rarely nephrotic-range proteinuria. The presence of proteinuria may suggest a histologic diagnosis of secondary FSGS, which can be confirmed by renal biopsy if kidney size is normal and diagnosis is uncertain (see Fig. 61.7).[27] Proteinuria is usually modest (0.5 to 4 g/day) and is commonly associated with hypertension and renal dysfunction. CKD progression often occurs gradually over 5 to 10 years.

End-Stage Renal Disease

According to the North American Pediatric Renal Transplant Cooperative Study (NAPRTCS) annual report of 2006, 8% of the 6405 children with ESRD had reflux nephropathy, which makes it the fourth most common cause of ESRD after obstructive uropathy, renal aplasia or hypoplasia or dysplasia, and FSGS.[28] Reflux nephropathy may also account for as much as 10% of ESRD in young to middle-aged adults.

Presentation of VUR in the Mother During Pregnancy

VUR may also first be manifested in the mother during pregnancy, when it can be associated with asymptomatic bacteriuria or symptomatic UTI, hypertension, preeclampsia, low-birth-weight babies, or miscarriage. VUR is present in approximately 5% of women with UTI in pregnancy and 4% to 5% of women with preeclampsia. VUR can be distinguished from the normal ureteral dilation that occurs in pregnancy, which preferentially affects the midportion of the ureter, and lack of involvement of the renal parenchyma.

Other Presentations

An increased risk of renal calculi has also been reported in children with VUR. Recurrent infections with urease-splitting organisms can lead to staghorn calculi. VUR or reflux nephropathy may also be discovered in adults after recurrent lower or upper UTI; indeed, about 5% of sexually active women with UTI have VUR.

DIAGNOSIS OF VESICOURETERAL REFLUX AND REFLUX NEPHROPATHY

An algorithm for diagnosis of VUR after the discovery of UTI is shown in Figure 61.10, and an example of the various tests in a child with UTI and VUR is shown in Figure 61.12. A similar approach should be performed in children after treatment of their first UTI.

Renal Ultrasound

Ultrasound is the initial modality for the evaluation of postnatal hydronephrosis and UTI in children. Ultrasound is also used as a screening tool in siblings of children with VUR to determine

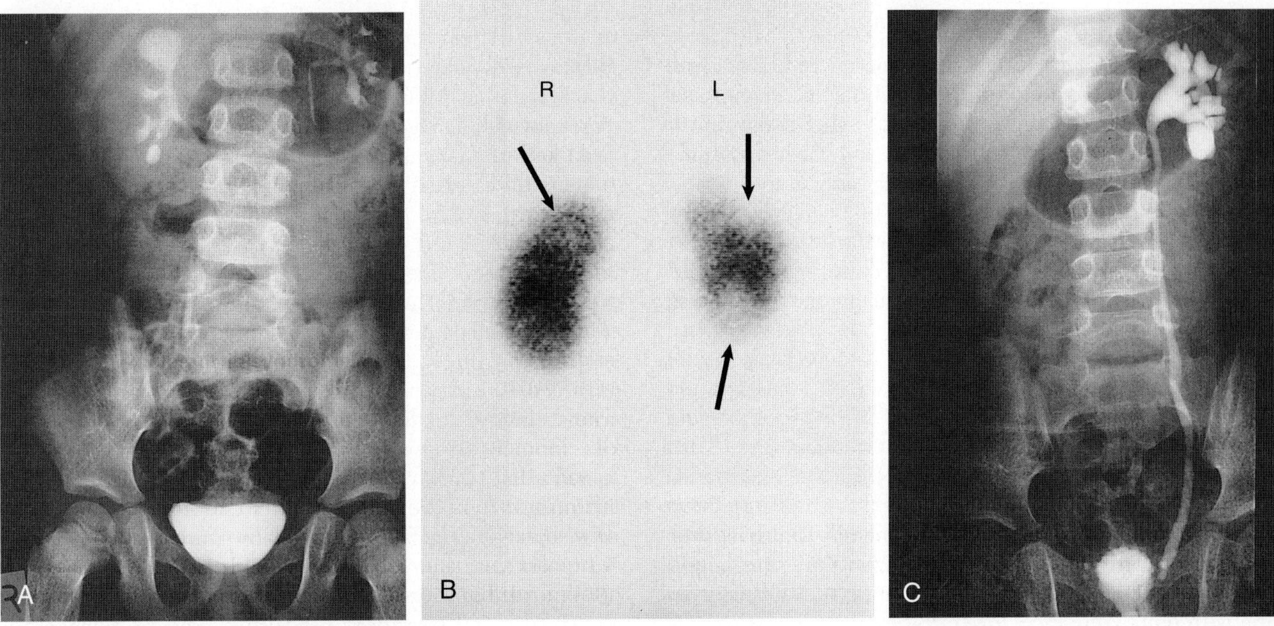

Figure 61.12 Investigation of reflux nephropathy. Investigation of a 3-year-old child with UTI. **A,** Intravenous urogram showing calyceal diverticulum in the upper pole of the right kidney and renal scarring in the upper pole and, probably, the lower pole of the left kidney. **B,** DMSA scintigraphy (posterior view) demonstrating upper and lower pole scarring *(arrows)* in the left kidney and scarring of the right upper kidney in association with the calyceal diverticulum *(arrowhead)*. **C,** Voiding cystourethrogram showing grade IV VUR on the left.

whether high-grade reflux is present. Whereas ultrasound can diagnose high-grade VUR, it has less sensitivity for diagnosis of acute pyelonephritis. In patients with acute pyelonephritis, abnormalities compatible with the diagnosis were reported in 20% to 69% by ultrasound compared with 40% to 92% by DMSA scintigraphy.[29] Nonetheless, ultrasound may be useful in detection of renal abscess and abnormalities of the perinephric space. Renal ultrasound is not a sensitive method for diagnosis of renal scars.

Voiding Cystourethrography

VCU is the primary diagnostic modality for identification of VUR. It requires catheterization, which can lead to significant distress among both children and parents. The grading of VUR is based on radiographic appearance by VCU (see Fig. 61.1). In children with UTI, VCU should be performed as soon as the child has completed the course of antibiotic therapy. Evaluation with VCU has been suggested after the first febrile infection in children younger than 5 years.

The results of VCU can be affected by size, type, and position of the catheter; rate of bladder filling; height of the column of contrast media; state of hydration of the patient; and volume, temperature, and concentration of the contrast medium.

Nuclear cystography has been used to reduce the radiation exposure for children during follow-up of VUR. Nuclear cystography, although it is more sensitive, does not permit specific grading of VUR or reveal anatomic defects, such as ureterocele and diverticulum. Nevertheless, it is useful in determining resolution of reflux during follow-up or after surgical correction.

DMSA Renal Scan

DMSA scintigraphy is currently the accepted gold standard for diagnosis of acute pyelonephritis and renal scarring. Single-photon emission computed tomography (SPECT) DMSA scintigraphy is superior to planar imaging for detection of renal cortical damage.[30,31] The sensitivity of DMSA scintigraphy in experimentally induced acute pyelonephritis in a pig model was reported to be 92% compared with histologic findings.[32] By use of standardized criteria for its interpretation, high levels of intraobserver and interobserver agreement were reported.[33]

An abnormal DMSA scan during a febrile UTI allows the identification of children at risk for development of renal scars. For acute pyelonephritis, DMSA scintigraphy can be performed within 2 to 4 weeks after the onset of UTI symptoms. For renal scarring, DMSA scintigraphy should ideally be performed 6 months after acute infection to allow acute reversible lesions to resolve.[34]

Dysplasia secondary to congenital reflux will appear similar to renal scarring after postnatal infections. In the context of a child presenting with VUR, obtaining a baseline DMSA renal scan allows identification of renal dysplasia and scarring, which can then be observed over time.

Magnetic Resonance Imaging

Magnetic resonance imaging (MRI) has recently been used for the diagnosis of renal scars because it discriminates swelling from scarring, both of which would be interpreted by DMSA scintigraphy as renal scarring. MRI may also diagnose other coexisting conditions, such as nephrolithiasis,[35,36] which is not diagnosed by DMSA scintigraphy. Newer imaging methods that show promise in diagnosis of renal scarring include dynamic contrast-enhanced MRI and MRI using a gadolinium-enhanced short-tau inversion-recovery (STIR) sequence. However, routine use of MRI is less practical because of limited availability, need for prolonged sedation, and high cost. Gadolinium is also contraindicated in the presence of significant renal impairment (glomerular filtration rate <30 ml/min per 1.73 m^2).

Proteinuria as a Marker for Reflux Nephropathy

Proteinuria predicts CKD progression due to reflux nephropathy.[37] Persistent microalbuminuria is helpful in diagnosis of glomerular damage at a very early stage.[38] Microalbuminuria increases with increasing severity of VUR and renal scarring.[39] In children with bilateral VUR with renal scarring and normal creatinine clearance, microalbuminuria was detected in 54% of the cases.[40] Microalbuminuria screening offers the possibility of early therapeutic intervention aimed at retarding CKD progress. Proteinuria, when it is severe, is usually associated with FSGS.

NATURAL HISTORY OF VESICOURETERAL REFLUX AND REFLUX NEPHROPATHY

Primary VUR, especially grades I to III, generally improves with time, and this is attributed to the lengthening of the submucosal segment of the ureter. Spontaneous resolution of VUR is more common with non–white race, lower grades of reflux, absence of renal damage, and lack of voiding dysfunction. Resolution of VUR occurs more slowly in children with bilateral VUR in most but not all studies. In one study of children younger than 5 years with grades I to III VUR, the resolution rate of left unilateral VUR was better than for right VUR.[41] In another study, the mean time until spontaneous resolution in black children was 15 months versus 21 months in white children.[42] Increasing age at presentation and bilateral VUR decrease the probability of resolution, and bilateral grade IV or grade V VUR has a particularly low chance of spontaneous resolution.[43]

The natural history of VUR in adults has been reported in few studies. In one study of adults (mean age of 24 years) with gross VUR diagnosed in infancy, proteinuria and CKD were present in 3 of the 13 patients with unilateral reflux nephropathy and 2 of the 4 patients with bilateral reflux nephropathy.[44] In another study of 127 adults (mean age of 41 years) with VUR diagnosed during childhood, 35% had unilateral renal scarring, 24% had bilateral renal scarring, 24% had albuminuria, and 11% had hypertension. Of the patients with bilateral renal scars, 83% had abnormal glomerular filtration rates.[45] An increased frequency of UTI and abnormal voiding patterns has also been noted in adults with VUR. UTIs may also be increased in frequency in adults who have had surgical management of VUR.

TREATMENT

For many decades, the management of VUR has been driven by the belief that VUR predisposes to recurrent UTI and renal parenchymal damage. Various treatment strategies have been used with the ultimate objective of preventing renal injury. The two main treatment modalities that have been practiced are long-term antimicrobial prophylaxis and surgical correction. Surgical correction of VUR was common until antimicrobial prophylaxis for childhood UTI was introduced in 1975.[46] Many subsequent studies have reported no significant differences in outcome with medical management of VUR versus surgical treatment. For example, in the International Reflux Study in Children, which involved 306 patients, no significant difference in outcome was found between medical and surgical management in terms of the development of new renal lesions or the progression of established renal scars.[47] In the International Reflux Study Group in Europe, 287 children with severe VUR were randomly allocated to medical or surgical groups. Follow-up with DMSA renal scans for a period of 5 years again revealed no difference in outcome.[9]

The 1997 American Urological Association guidelines reviewed seven treatment modalities used to manage VUR in children: intermittent antibiotic therapy; bladder training; continuous antibiotic prophylaxis; antibiotic prophylaxis and bladder training; antibiotic prophylaxis, anticholinergics, and bladder training; open surgical repair; and endoscopic repair. The key outcome measures were resolution of VUR, risk of pyelonephritis and scarring, and complications of medical versus surgical management. The study panel's recommendations are shown in Figure 61.13. Antibiotic prophylaxis is recommended for all grades of VUR in children younger than 1 year because of a very high rate of spontaneous resolution. For children 1 to 5 years old, the study panel recommended antibiotic prophylaxis for all grades of VUR, with surgical options in grades III to V if VUR is bilateral or renal scarring is present. For children older than 6 years, the study panel recommended antibiotic prophylaxis for grades I and II (unilateral or bilateral) and unilateral grades III and IV, with surgical options if renal scarring is present, and surgical repair for bilateral grades III and IV and unilateral or bilateral grade V with or without scarring as the VUR has the least possibility of spontaneous resolution.[48]

Medical Management

Medical management involves long-term antimicrobial prophylaxis, appropriate management of voiding dysfunction and

1997 AUA Panel Guidelines

Age		Grade 1	Grade II	Grade III	Grade IV	Grade V
<1 year of age	Unilateral VUR	Antibiotic prophylaxis	Antibiotic prophylaxis	Antibiotic prophylaxis	Antibiotic prophylaxis	Antibiotic prophylaxis
	Bilateral VUR	Antibiotic prophylaxis	Antibiotic prophylaxis	Antibiotic prophylaxis	Antibiotic prophylaxis	Antibiotic prophylaxis
	Scarring, dysplasia	Antibiotic prophylaxis	Antibiotic prophylaxis	Antibiotic prophylaxis	Antibiotic prophylaxis	Antibiotic prophylaxis
1-5 years of age	Unilateral VUR	Antibiotic prophylaxis	Antibiotic prophylaxis	Antibiotic prophylaxis	Antibiotic prophylaxis	Antibiotic prophylaxis
	Bilateral VUR	Antibiotic prophylaxis	antibiotic prophylaxis	Possible surgery	Possible surgery	Possible surgery
	Presence of scarring	Antibiotic prophylaxis	Antibiotic prophylaxis	Possible surgery	Possible surgery	Possible surgery
>6 years of age	Unilateral VUR	Antibiotic prophylaxis	Antibiotic prophylaxis	Antibiotic prophylaxis	Antibiotic prophylaxis	Surgery
	Bilateral VUR	Antibiotic prophylaxis	Antibiotic prophylaxis	Surgery	Surgery	Surgery
	Presence of scarring	Possible surgery	Possible surgery	Surgery	Surgery	Surgery

Figure 61.13 The 1997 American Urological Association (AUA) panel guidelines for management of VUR.

constipation, if present, and follow-up renal imaging to assess the resolution of VUR and the potential development of renal injury.

The antimicrobial agents most appropriate for prophylaxis include trimethoprim-sulfamethoxazole (TMP-SMZ), trimethoprim alone, nitrofurantoin, and cephalexin. Follow-up of patients with VUR and UTI requires rapid evaluation (within 72 hours of the onset of fever) to allow early detection and prompt treatment of UTI. The timing of follow-up VCU is not well defined, although most practitioners do it yearly.

The treatment of voiding dysfunction or dysfunctional elimination syndrome may include the use of laxatives and timed frequent voiding every 2 to 3 hours. Pelvic floor exercises, behavioral modification, or anticholinergic medication may be required. A combined conservative medical and computer game–assisted pelvic floor muscle retraining decreased the incidence of breakthrough UTI and facilitated VUR resolution in children with voiding dysfunction and VUR. Treatment of constipation by dietary measures, behavioral therapy, and laxatives helps reduce UTI recurrence and the resolution of enuresis and uninhibited bladder contractions.

Antibiotic Prophylaxis Versus Surveillance Only

Some studies challenge the benefit of long-term antimicrobial prophylaxis in the prevention of renal injury in patients with VUR. A randomized study involved 236 children aged 3 months to 18 years with acute pyelonephritis; 113 children had grades I to III VUR (age group 3 months to 12 years) and 115 patents none (age group 3 months to 17 years). Patients were randomly assigned to prophylactic antibiotic (TMP-SMZ) or no prophylaxis. At the end of 1 year, no difference was noted in the incidence of UTI, pyelonephritis, or renal scarring by DMSA scans between the two groups, suggesting that there is no role for prophylactic antibiotics in preventing the recurrence of infection and the development of renal scars in such children.[49] In another study, 225 children aged 1 month to 3 years with grades I to III VUR were randomized to daily antibiotic prophylaxis (TMP-SMZ) or no prophylaxis. After a follow-up period of 18 months, there was no significant difference in the occurrence of UTI. Antimicrobial prophylaxis did, however, reduce UTIs in boys ($P = .017$), particularly in those with grade III VUR.[50] In a third study, 100 babies 8 to 9 months old with grades II to IV VUR diagnosed after an upper tract UTI were randomized to TMP-SMZ prophylaxis for 2 years, then observed for another 2 years. There was no difference in recurrence of acute pyelonephritis during the 4 years of study. There was no difference in renal scarring at 2 years, and no patients were noted to have new renal scars after 4 years.[11] A fourth study of 338 children (aged 2 months to <7 years) with first febrile UTI included 128 children with grades I to III VUR. There was no effect of antimicrobial prophylaxis on the 12-month recurrence rate of febrile UTI in those with VUR.

These trials, although important, are not conclusive. Various study design limitations included small study size and short follow-up, lack of blinding, no use of placebo, urine collection by sterile bags in non–toilet-trained children, and exclusion of patients with high-grade VUR (who are normally associated with the highest risk of renal injury) as well as the issue of interobserver variability in the interpretation of DMSA renal scans.

Hypertension and Proteinuria

Appropriate management of hypertension and proteinuria includes the use of angiotensin-converting enzyme (ACE) inhibitors or angiotensin receptor blockers (ARBs) as in other renal diseases (see Chapter 76). ACE inhibitors reduce proteinuria in subjects with reflux nephropathy and also can reverse microalbuminuria. Combination of ACE inhibitor and ARB may provide additional lowering of proteinuria.[51] However, it is not known whether this antiproteinuric effect slows the progression of the renal disease. Historically, some patients also occasionally had their scarred kidney removed to help control hypertension, provided the contralateral kidney was healthy. However, this is

Surgical Techniques for Management VUR

Technique	Success Rates	Pros	Cons
Open reimplantation	95%	High success rates Limited requirement for follow-up VCU Reduction in hospital stays	Surgical incision Hospitalization required Catheters needed during postoperative management Pain control
Endoscopic injection Dextranomer/hyaluronidase (Deflux)	70%–80%	Reasonable success rates Outpatient management Minimal pain	Expensive Lower success rates Need for repeated procedures Need for follow-up VCU
Laparoscopic reimplantation	70%–90%	Reasonable success rates Small incisions Less discomfort	Lower success rates Requires hospitalization Need for follow-up VCU Long procedure Expensive equipment Significant surgical learning curve

Figure 61.14 Surgical techniques for VUR. VCU, voiding cystourethrography.

exceptionally rare these days because of the availability of many potent antihypertensive agents.

Surgical Management

Surgical management of VUR is now a second-line management strategy and is reserved for patients whose medical management with antimicrobial prophylaxis and follow-up has failed. Current indications for surgical management of VUR are recurrent infections despite compliance with a prophylactic antibiotic regimen, worsening of renal scars after a UTI, and repeated failure to comply with a prophylactic regimen. The recent introduction of minimally invasive modalities for the management of VUR has made some clinicians consider surgical correction a potential first-line therapy. Immediate correction could potentially offset the need for antibiotic prophylaxis in children. Although most surgical techniques have high success rates, most studies indicate that surgical correction of VUR does not prevent UTI or eventual renal scarring.[52] A review of surgical techniques is presented in Figure 61.14.

REFERENCES

1. Lebowitz RL, Olbing H, Parkkulainen KV, et al. International system of radiographic grading of vesicoureteric reflux. International Reflux Study in Children. *Pediatr Radiol.* 1985;15:105.
2. Gargollo PC, Diamond DA. Therapy insight: What nephrologists need to know about primary vesicoureteral reflux. *Nat Clin Pract Nephrol.* 2007;3:551.
3. Arena F, Romeo C, Cruccetti A, et al. Fetal vesicoureteral reflux: Neonatal findings and follow-up study. *Pediatr Med Chir.* 2001;23: 31.
4. Askari A, Belman AB. Vesicoureteral reflux in black girls. *J Urol.* 1982;127:747.
5. Kunin CM. A ten-year study of bacteriuria in schoolgirls: Final report of bacteriologic, urologic, and epidemiologic findings. *J Infect Dis.* 1970;122:382.
6. Shefelbine SE, Khorana S, Schultz PN, et al. Mutational analysis of the GDNF/RET-GDNFR alpha signaling complex in a kindred with vesicoureteral reflux. *Hum Genet.* 1998;102:474.
7. Cunliffe HE, McNoe LA, Ward TA, et al. The prevalence of PAX2 mutations in patients with isolated colobomas or colobomas associated with urogenital anomalies. *J Med Genet.* 1998;35:806.
8. Dixon JS, Jen PY, Yeung CK, et al. The structure and autonomic innervation of the vesico-ureteric junction in cases of primary ureteric reflux. *Br J Urol.* 1998;81:146.
9. Piepsz A, Tamminen-Mobius T, Reiners C, et al. Five-year study of medical or surgical treatment in children with severe vesico-ureteral reflux dimercaptosuccinic acid findings. International Reflux Study Group in Europe. *Eur J Pediatr.* 1998;157:753.
10. Wennerstrom M, Hansson S, Jodal U, et al. Primary and acquired renal scarring in boys and girls with urinary tract infection. *J Pediatr.* 2000;136:30.
11. Pennesi M, Travan L, Peratoner L, et al. North East Italy Prophylaxis in VUR study group: Is antibiotic prophylaxis in children with vesicoureteral reflux effective in preventing pyelonephritis and renal scars? A randomized, controlled trial. *Pediatrics.* 2008;121:e1489.
12. Shindo S, Bernstein J, Arant BS Jr. Evolution of renal segmental atrophy (Ask-Upmark kidney) in children with vesicoureteric reflux: Radiographic and morphologic studies. *J Pediatr.* 1983;102:847.
13. Eddy AA. Interstitial macrophages as mediators of renal fibrosis. *Exp Nephrol.* 1995;3:76.
14. Bailey RR. The relationship of vesicoureteral reflux to urinary tract infection and chronic pyelonephritis–reflux nephropathy. *Clin Nephrol.* 1973;11:132-141.
15. Koff SA, Wagner TT, Jayanthi VR. The relationship among dysfunctional elimination syndromes, primary vesicoureteral reflux and urinary tract infections in children. *J Urol.* 1998;160:1019.
16. Marra G, Barbieri G, Dell'Agnola CA, et al. Congenital renal damage associated with primary vesicoureteral reflux detected prenatally in male infants. *J Pediatr.* 1994;124:726.
17. Papachristou F, Printza N, Kavaki D, et al. The characteristics and outcome of primary vesicoureteric reflux diagnosed in the first year of life. *Int J Clin Pract.* 2006;60:829.
18. Yeung CK, Godley ML, Dhillon HK, et al. Urodynamic patterns in infants with normal lower urinary tracts or primary vesico-ureteric reflux. *Br J Urol.* 1998;81:461.
19. Godley ML, Desai D, Yeung CK, et al. The relationship between early renal status, and the resolution of vesico-ureteric reflux and bladder function at 16 months. *BJU Int.* 2001;87:457.
20. Noe HN. The long-term results of prospective sibling reflux screening. *J Urol.* 1992;148:1739.
21. Kenda RB, Zupancic Z, Fettich JJ, et al. A follow-up study of vesico-ureteric reflux and renal scars in asymptomatic siblings of children with reflux. *Nucl Med Commun.* 1997;18:827.
22. Bailey RR. The relationship of vesico-ureteric reflux to urinary tract infection and chronic pyelonephritis-reflux nephropathy. *Clin Nephrol.* 1973;1:132.
23. Ditchfield MR, de Campo JF, Nolan TM, et al. Risk factors in the development of early renal cortical defects in children with urinary tract infection. *AJR Am J Roentgenol.* 1994;162:1393.
24. Smellie JM, Prescod NP, Shaw PJ, et al. Childhood reflux and urinary infection: A follow-up of 10-41 years in 226 adults. *Pediatr Nephrol.* 1998;12:727.
25. Wallace DM, Rothwell DL, Williams DI. The long-term follow-up of surgically treated vesicoureteric reflux. *Br J Urol.* 1978;50:479.
26. Silva JM, Santos Diniz JS, Marino VS, et al. Clinical course of 735 children and adolescents with primary vesicoureteral reflux. *Pediatr Nephrol.* 2006;21:981.
27. Morita M, Yoshiara S, White RH, et al. The glomerular changes in children with reflux nephropathy. *J Pathol.* 1990;162:245.
28. 2006 annual report of the North American Pediatric Renal Trials and Collaborative Studies (NAPRTCS), pp 13-11 to 15-1.
29. Lavocat MP, Granjon D, Allard D, et al. Imaging of pyelonephritis. *Pediatr Radiol.* 1997;27:159.
30. Applegate KE, Connolly LP, Davis RT, et al. A prospective comparison of high-resolution planar, pinhole, and triple-detector SPECT for the detection of renal cortical defects. *Clin Nucl Med.* 1997;22:673.
31. Yen TC, Tzen KY, Lin WY, et al. Identification of new renal scarring in repeated episodes of acute pyelonephritis using Tc-99m DMSA renal SPECT. *Clin Nucl Med.* 1998;23:828.
32. Majd M, Nussbaum Blask AR, Markle BM, et al. Acute pyelonephritis: Comparison of diagnosis with ^{99m}Tc-DMSA, SPECT, spiral CT, MR imaging, and power Doppler US in an experimental pig model. *Radiology.* 2001;218:101.
33. Patel K, Charron M, Hoberman A, et al. Intra- and interobserver variability in interpretation of DMSA scans using a set of standardized criteria. *Pediatr Radiol.* 1993;23:506.
34. Stokland E, Hellstrom M, Jakobsson B, et al. Imaging of renal scarring. *Acta Paediatr Suppl.* 1999;88:13.
35. Kavanagh EC, Ryan S, Awan A, et al. Can MRI replace DMSA in the detection of renal parenchymal defects in children with urinary tract infections? *Pediatr Radiol.* 2005;35:275-281.
36. Chan YL, Chan KW, Yeung CK, et al. Potential utility of MRI in the evaluation of children at risk of renal scarring. *Pediatr Radiol.* 1999;29: 856.
37. Torres VE, Velosa JA, Holley KE, et al. The progression of vesicoureteral reflux nephropathy. *Ann Intern Med.* 1980;92:776.
38. Quattrin T, Waz WR, Duffy LC, et al. Microalbuminuria in an adolescent cohort with insulin-dependent diabetes mellitus. *Clin Pediatr (Phila).* 1995;34:12.
39. Bell FG, Wilkin TJ, Atwell JD. Microproteinuria in children with vesicoureteric reflux. *Br J Urol.* 1986;58:605.
40. Coppo R, Porcellini MG, Gianoglio B, et al. Glomerular permselectivity to macromolecules in reflux nephropathy: Microalbuminuria during acute hyperfiltration due to amino acid infusion. *Clin Nephrol.* 1993;40:299.
41. Arant BS Jr. Medical management of mild and moderate vesicoureteral reflux: Followup studies of infants and young children. A preliminary report of the Southwest Pediatric Nephrology Study Group. *J Urol.* 1992;148:1683.
42. Skoog SJ, Belman AB. Primary vesicoureteral reflux in the black child. *Pediatrics.* 1991;87:538.
43. Elder JS, Peters CA, Arant BS Jr, et al. Pediatric Vesicoureteral Reflux Guidelines Panel summary report on the management of primary vesicoureteral reflux in children. *J Urol.* 1997;157:1846.
44. Bailey RR, Lynn KL, Smith AH. Long-term followup of infants with gross vesicoureteral reflux. *J Urol.* 1992;148:1709.

45. Lahdes-Vasama T, Niskanen K, Ronnholm K. Outcome of kidneys in patients treated for vesicoureteral reflux (VUR) during childhood. *Nephrol Dial Transplant*. 2006;21:2491.
46. Gruneberg RN, Leakey A, Bendall MJ, et al. Bowel flora in urinary tract infection: Effect of chemotherapy with special reference to cotrimoxazole. *Kidney Int Suppl*. 1975;4:S122.
47. Smellie JM, Tamminen-Mobius T, Olbing H, et al. Five-year study of medical or surgical treatment in children with severe reflux: Radiological renal findings. The International Reflux Study in Children. *Pediatr Nephrol*. 1992;6:223.
48. Elder JS, Peters CA, Arant BS Jr, et al. Pediatric Vesicoureteral Reflux Guidelines Panel summary report on the management of primary vesicoureteral reflux in children. *J Urol*. 1997;157:1846.
49. Garin EH, Olavarria F, Garcia Nieto V, et al. Clinical significance of primary vesicoureteral reflux and urinary antibiotic prophylaxis after acute pyelonephritis: A multicenter, randomized, controlled study. *Pediatrics*. 2006;117:626.
50. Roussey-Kesler G, Gadjos V, Idres N, et al. Antibiotic prophylaxis for the prevention of recurrent urinary tract infection in children with low grade vesicoureteral reflux: Results from a prospective randomized study. *J Urol*. 2008;179:674.
51. Litwin M, Grenda R, Sladowska J, et al. Add-on therapy with angiotensin II receptor 1 blocker in children with chronic kidney disease already treated with angiotensin-converting enzyme inhibitors. *Pediatr Nephrol*. 2006;21:1716.
52. Yu TJ, Chen WF. Surgical management of grades III and IV primary vesicoureteral reflux in children with and without acute pyelonephritis as breakthrough infections: A comparative analysis. *J Urol*. 1997;157:1404.

CHAPTER 62

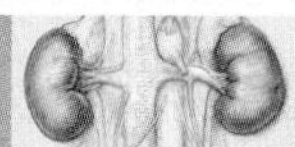

Chronic Interstitial Nephritis

Masaomi Nangaku, Toshiro Fujita

DEFINITION

Chronic interstitial nephritis is a histologic entity characterized by progressive scarring of the tubulointerstitium, with tubular atrophy, macrophage and lymphocytic infiltration, and interstitial fibrosis. Because the degree of tubular damage accompanying interstitial nephritis is variable, the term *tubulointerstitial nephritis* is used interchangeably with interstitial nephritis. *Tubulitis* refers to infiltration of the tubular epithelium by leukocytes, usually lymphocytes.

There are many primary as well as secondary causes of chronic interstitial nephritis (Fig. 62.1). Tubulointerstitial injury is clinically important because it is a better predictor than the degree of glomerular injury of present and future renal function. Although any glomerular disease can injure the tubulointerstitium secondarily through mechanisms involving the direct effects of proteinuria and ischemia, we restrict our discussion to primary chronic interstitial nephritis.

PATHOGENESIS

The tubulointerstitium can be injured by toxins (e.g., heavy metals), drugs (e.g., analgesics), crystals (e.g., calcium phosphate, uric acid), infections, obstruction, immunologic mechanisms, and ischemia. Regardless of the initiating mechanism, however, the tubulointerstitial response shows little variation. Tubular injury results in the release of chemotactic substances and the expression of leukocyte adhesion molecules that attract inflammatory cells into the interstitium. Tubular cells express human leukocyte antigens, serve as antigen-presenting cells, and secrete complement components and vasoactive mediators, all of which may further stimulate or attract macrophages and T cells. Growth factors released by tubular cells and macrophages, such as platelet-derived growth factor and transforming growth factor β, may stimulate fibroblast proliferation and activation, leading to matrix accumulation.[1] The source of fibroblasts in renal interstitial fibrosis remains controversial but may include an intrinsic fibroblast population, migration of circulating fibrocytes from perivascular areas, and transdifferentiation of tubular cells, pericytes, and endothelial cells into fibroblasts.[2] Over time, a loss of peritubular capillaries and decreased oxygen diffusion due to expansion of the interstitium render the kidney hypoxic, and progressive apoptosis leads to local hypocellularity and fibrosis.[3] Renal function becomes severely decreased, and renal replacement therapies are required.

EPIDEMIOLOGY

Whereas chronic interstitial nephritis occurs with progressive renal disease of all etiologies, primary chronic interstitial nephritis is not a common cause of end-stage renal disease (ESRD); reports range from 42% in Scotland to 3% to 4% in China and the United States.[4-6] This variability in incidence may relate to differences in how diagnoses are made, etiologies and toxin or drug exposure, and treatment modalities.

PATHOLOGY

The pathologic features of chronic interstitial nephritis are nonspecific. They include tubular cell atrophy or dilation; interstitial fibrosis that is composed of interstitial (types I and II) collagens; and mononuclear cell infiltration with macrophages, T cells, and occasionally other cell types (neutrophils, eosinophils, and plasma cells). Tubular lumina vary in diameter but may show marked dilation, with homogeneous casts producing a thyroid-like appearance, hence the term *thyroidization*.

Whereas a noncaseating granulomatous pattern is observed in sarcoidosis, interstitial granulomatous reactions also occur in response to infection of the kidney by mycobacteria (Fig. 62.2), fungi, or bacteria; drugs (rifampin, sulfonamides, and narcotics); and oxalate or urate crystal deposition. Interstitial granulomatous reactions also have been noted in renal malacoplakia, Wegener's granulomatosis, and heroin abuse and after jejunoileal bypass surgery.

CLINICAL MANIFESTATIONS

The impaired renal function is often insidious, and the early manifestations of the disease are those of tubular dysfunction, which may go undetected (Fig. 62.3).[7] Diagnosis is often made incidentally on routine laboratory screening or during evaluation of hypertension, in association with reduced glomerular filtration rate (GFR). Proteinuria is commonly less than 1 g/day. The urinalysis may show only occasional white blood cells and, rarely, white blood cell casts. Hematuria is uncommon. Anemia may occur relatively early because of loss of erythropoietin-producing interstitial cells.

The tubular dysfunction is often generalized, but some conditions may present with proximal tubular defects including aminoaciduria, phosphaturia, proximal renal tubular acidosis (RTA), or, rarely, a complete Fanconi syndrome. Distal tubular defects can be associated with type 4 RTA (see Chapter 12). Concentrating defects (increased urinary frequency and nocturia) can be a sign of medullary dysfunction and may be severe enough to result in nephrogenic diabetes insipidus. Some subjects will also have an inability to conserve salt on a low-salt diet with subsequent salt-wasting syndrome. Others, particularly with microvascular disease, may have a relative inability to excrete salt with resultant salt-sensitive hypertension.[8]

Major Etiologies of Chronic Interstitial Nephritis	
Diseases in which the Kidneys Are Macroscopically Normal	**Diseases in which the Kidneys Are Macroscopically Abnormal**
Drugs and toxins (e.g., aristolochic acid, lithium, cyclosporine, tacrolimus, indinavir, cisplatin)	Analgesic nephropathy
Metabolic (hyperuricemia, hypokalemia, hypercalcemia, hyperoxaluria, cystinosis)	Chronic obstruction (see Chapters 58 and 61)
Heavy metals (lead, cadmium, arsenic, mercury, gold, uranium)	Hereditary (nephronophtisis, medullary cystic kidney disease, familial juvenile hyperuricemic nephropathy, autosomal dominant polycystic kidney disease, autosomal recessive polycystic kidney disease)
Radiation	Infection (chronic pyelonephritis, malacoplakia, xanthogranulomatous pyelonephritis; see Chapter 51)
Balkan nephropathy	
Immune-mediated (systemic lupus erythematosus, Sjögren's syndrome, sarcoidosis, Wegener's granulomatosis, other vasculitides)	
Vascular diseases (atherosclerotic kidney disease) (see Chapter 64)	
Transplantation (chronic transplant rejection)	
Hematologic disturbances (multiple myeloma, light-chain deposition disease, lymphoma, sickle cell disease, paroxysmal nocturnal hemoglobinuria) (see Chapters 26, 49, and 63)	
Progressive glomerular disease of all etiologies (e.g., glomerulonephritides, diabetes, hypertension)	
Idiopathic	

Figure 62.1 Major etiologies of chronic interstitial nephritis. Note that kidneys of any clinical entity can be shrunken at end-stage. Some diseases categorized as macroscopically normal can show macroscopically abnormal kidneys. For example, kidneys of sickle cell nephropathy are macroscopically normal unless there is papillary necrosis.

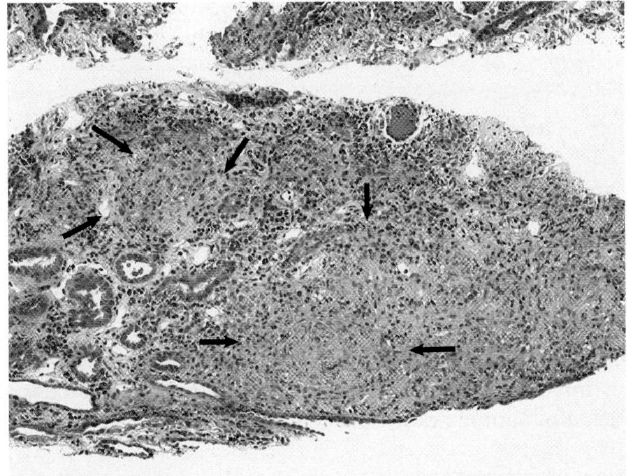

Figure 62.2 Renal tuberculosis. Noncaseating granulomas with epithelioid cells in miliary tuberculosis *(arrows)*. Although the typical pathologic change is granuloma with caseous necrosis with Langerhans-type giant cells, these nontypical granulomas can be observed in tuberculosis and should be differentiated from sarcoidosis. (Hematoxylin and eosin stain.) *(Courtesy Dr. Noriko Uesugi, Ibaraki, Japan.)*

Functional Manifestations of Chronic Interstitial Nephritis
Deterioration of glomerular filtration rate with insidious onset
Tubular proteinuria mainly composed of low-molecular-weight protein (generally <1 g/day)
Inactive urinary sediment
Renal anemia at a relatively early stage
Proximal tubular dysfunction (aminoaciduria, phosphaturia, proximal renal tubular acidosis, Fanconi syndrome)
Distal tubular dysfunction (type IV renal tubular acidosis)
Medullary dysfunction (concentrating defects)
Salt-wasting syndrome
Salt-sensitive hypertension

Figure 62.3 Functional manifestations of chronic interstitial nephritis.

Clues to tubulointerstitial nephritis by history and physical examination are shown in Figure 62.4.[9]

TREATMENT

Treatment includes identification and elimination of any exogenous agents (drugs, heavy metals), metabolic causes (hypercalcemia), or conditions (obstruction, infection) potentially causing the chronic interstitial lesion. Specific treatments may be required for a condition, such as corticosteroids for sarcoidosis. General measures include control of blood pressure. Most clinicians favor the use of angiotensin-converting enzyme (ACE) inhibitors or angiotensin receptor blockers (ARBs), which reduce glomerular and systemic pressures, decrease proteinuria, and increase renal blood flow. Specific therapies for each clinical entity are discussed later.

DRUG-INDUCED CHRONIC INTERSTITIAL NEPHRITIS

Several drugs and herbs can cause chronic interstitial nephritis. Cyclosporine- and tacrolimus-induced nephropathy is discussed in Chapter 100; aristolochic acid as a cause of aristolochic acid–associated nephropathy (Chinese herbs nephropathy) is discussed in Chapter 74.

Clues to Tubulointerstitial Nephritis by History and Physical Examination		
Element of Encounter	**Symptom, Sign, or Historical Clue**	**Potential Diagnosis**
Occupational history	Exposure to heavy metals (e.g., batteries, alloys)	Lead or cadmium nephropathy
Alcohol	History of moonshine ingestion	Lead nephropathy
Social history	Country of origin	Balkan nephropathy
Past history	Systemic lupus erythematosus Sjögren's syndrome, Sarcoidosis Inflammatory bowel disease Autoimmune pancreatitis	Disease-associated chronic interstitial nephritis
	Chronic pain syndrome	Analgesic nephropathy
	Gouty attack	Lead nephropathy
Medication	Prescribed	Drug-induced chronic interstitial nephritis
	Over-the-counter (NSAIDs)	Analgesic nephropathy
	Herbal	Aristolochic acid–associated nephropathy
	Indinavir	Cyrstal nephropathy
Physical examination	Dry eyes	Sjögren's syndrome
Laboratory examination	Hyperuricemia	Chronic urate nephropathy
	Hypokalemia	Hypokalemic nephropathy
	Hypercalcemia	Hypercalcemic nephropathy
	High serum IgG4 levels	IgG4-related sclerosing disease
Radiologic examination	Decreased volume, bumpy contours, and papillary calcification on CT	Analgesic nephropathy
	Microcysts on MRI or echography	Lithium nephropathy
	Nephrocalcinosis on CT	Hypercalcemic nephropathy

Figure 62.4 Clues to tubulointerstitial nephritis by history and physical examination. CT, computed tomography; MRI, magnetic resonance imaging; NSAIDs, nonsteroidal anti-inflammatory drugs. *(Modified from reference 9.)*

Lithium Nephropathy

Definition and Epidemiology

Lithium is commonly used in the treatment of bipolar disorder. Complications of lithium treatment include nephrogenic diabetes insipidus, acute lithium intoxication, and chronic lithium nephrotoxicity. A meta-analysis of the data of 14 studies involving 1172 patients receiving chronic lithium therapy showed that the prevalence of reduced GFR was 15%.[10]

Pathogenesis

Diabetes insipidus results from accumulation of lithium in the collecting tubular cells after entry into these cells through sodium channels in the luminal membrane. Lithium blocks vasopressin-induced reabsorption by inhibiting adenylate cyclase activity, and hence cyclic adenosine monophosphate production, and also by decreasing the apical membrane expression of aquaporin 2, the collecting tubule water channel. Chronic lithium-induced interstitial nephritis may also occur, possibly due to inositol depletion and inhibition of cell proliferation.

Pathology

Biopsies show focal chronic interstitial nephritis with interstitial fibrosis, tubular atrophy, and glomerular sclerosis. Whereas similar histologic changes have been reported in psychiatric subjects without a history of lithium therapy, subjects with lithium exposure often show microcystic changes in the distal tubule; interstitial inflammation and vascular changes are relatively minimal. The degree of interstitial fibrosis is related to the duration of administration and cumulative dose.

Clinical Manifestations

Lithium-Associated Diabetes Insipidus The most common presentation of lithium-induced nephrotoxicity is nephrogenic diabetes insipidus, characterized by resistance to vasopressin, polyuria, and polydipsia. Impaired renal concentrating ability is found in about 50% of patients, and polyuria due to nephrogenic diabetes insipidus occurs in about 20% of patients chronically treated with lithium.

Lithium is also rarely a cause of hypercalcemia, which could potentially exaggerate the tubular concentrating defect and contribute to the development of chronic interstitial nephritis in lithium-treated patients. Nephrogenic diabetes insipidus in lithium treatment may be associated with distal RTA, although this partial functional defect is virtually never of clinical importance.

Chronic Lithium Nephropathy Nephrogenic diabetes insipidus induced by lithium may persist despite the cessation of treatment, indicating irreversible renal damage.

In one study, the mean serum creatinine concentration of patients with biopsy-proven chronic lithium nephrotoxicity was 2.8 mg/dl (247 μmol/l) at the time of biopsy, and 42% of patients had proteinuria greater than 1 g/day.[11] After renal biopsy, all but one patient discontinued treatment with lithium, but seven patients nevertheless progressed to ESRD. A study of 74 lithium-treated patients in France showed that lithium-induced nephropathy developed slowly during several decades, with an average latency between the start of therapy and ESRD of 20 years.[12]

Magnetic resonance imaging or ultrasound may help in the detection of the microcysts in the kidney.[13]

Treatment

After other potential causes of polyuria and polydipsia have been excluded, particularly psychogenic polydipsia, the first step to consider is a reduction in lithium dosage. The potassium-sparing diuretic amiloride improves the polyuria and also blocks lithium uptake through sodium channels in the collecting duct. Thiazide diuretics should be avoided as they increase the risk for acute lithium intoxication because of the resultant volume contraction and an increase in sodium and lithium reabsorption in the proximal tubule.

Patients receiving long-term lithium treatment should have renal function (serum creatinine and estimated GFR) and 24-hour urine volume measured yearly. Lithium has a narrow therapeutic index, so levels should be monitored and maintained between 0.6 and 1.25 mmol/l. The severity of chronic lithium intoxication correlates directly with the serum lithium concentration and may be categorized as mild (1.5 to 2.0 mmol/l), moderate (2.0 to 2.5 mmol/l), or severe (>2.5 mmol/l). Once-daily regimens are less toxic than multiple daily dose schedules, perhaps because of the possibility of renal tubular regeneration with a once-daily dosing schedule.[14] Prevention of volume depletion is also important.

Because progressive renal injury with reduced GFR in patients without prior acute lithium intoxication is relatively unusual, raised serum creatinine concentration should initially be treated by a dose reduction. If there is persistently elevated serum creatinine, a renal biopsy should be considered, although the findings rarely mandate the complete cessation of lithium treatment. At all times, the risk for discontinuation in a patient with a severe unipolar or bipolar affective disorder needs to be balanced with the relatively low risk for progressive renal injury.

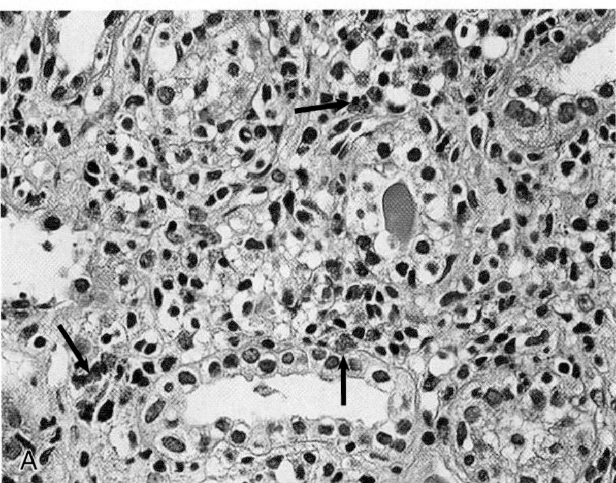

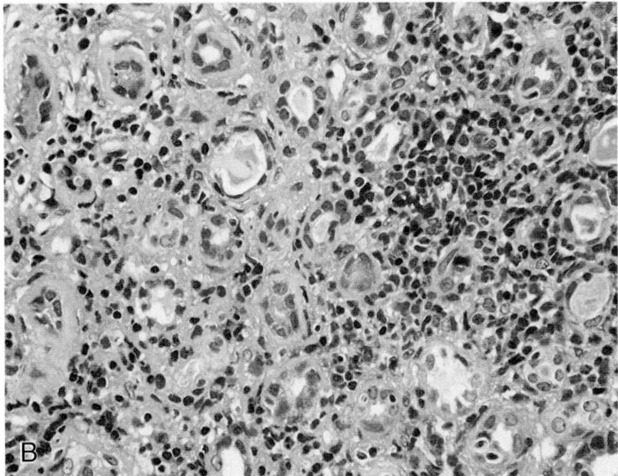

Figure 62.5 Histologic changes in analgesic nephropathy. A, Interstitial nephritis in a patient with analgesic nephropathy associated with marked mononuclear cellular infiltrate including eosinophils *(arrows)*. (Hematoxylin and eosin stain; original magnification ×600.) **B,** Analgesic nephropathy with interstitial fibrosis and inflammatory cell infiltration. (Masson trichrome stain; original magnification ×400.) *(Courtesy Drs. Akira Shimizu and Hideki Takano, Nippon Medical School, Tokyo, Japan.)*

Analgesic Nephropathy

Definition and Epidemiology

Analgesic nephropathy resulted from the abuse of analgesics, commonly mixtures containing phenacetin, aspirin, and caffeine that were available as over-the-counter preparations in Europe and Australia. It is now rare; indeed, some doubt that new cases are still presenting, following restrictions in compound analgesic sales.[15] Long-term use of aspirin alone is not associated with analgesic nephropathy, and although long-term nonsteroidal anti-inflammatory drug use has been associated with chronic interstitial nephritis in a small number of patients, a large-scale case-control study found no increased risk of ESRD in users of combined or single formulations of phenacetin-free analgesics.[16] A large study in the United States also showed no association between use of current analgesic preparations and increased risk of renal dysfunction.[17]

Pathogenesis and Pathology

The primary injury in analgesic nephropathy is medullary ischemia due to toxic concentrations of phenacetin metabolites combined with relative medullary hypoxia, aggravated by inhibition of vasodilatory prostaglandin synthesis. The main pathologic consequence is papillary necrosis, with secondary tubular atrophy, interstitial fibrosis, and a mononuclear cellular infiltrate (Fig. 62.5).

Clinical Manifestations

Analgesic nephropathy was five to seven times more common in women than in men. Renal manifestations are nonspecific and consist of slowly progressive chronic renal failure with impaired urine concentrating ability, urinary acidification defects, and impaired sodium conservation. Urinalysis showed sterile pyuria and mild proteinuria. Patients with analgesic nephropathy are at increased risk for transitional cell carcinoma of the uroepithelium.

Diagnosis

Papillary necrosis is present histologically in almost all patients, but it can be detected radiologically only if part or all of the

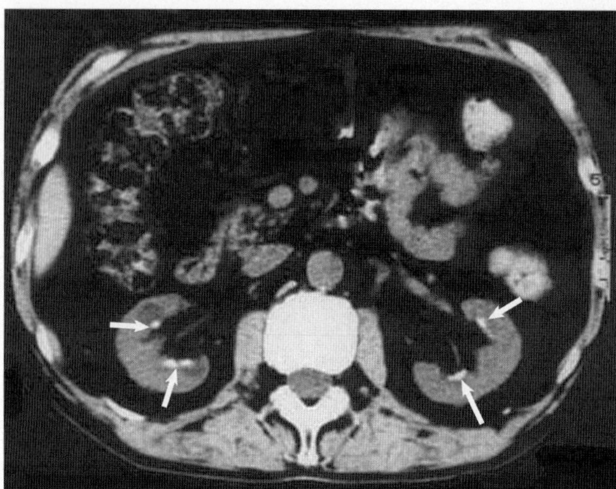

Figure 62.6 Papillary calcifications in analgesic nephropathy. Non–contrast-enhanced CT scan of a patient with long-time analgesic abuse showed thinning of the renal parenchyma and typical papillary calcifications *(arrows)*. *(Courtesy Dr. Yoshifumi Ubara, Toranomon Hospital, Tokyo, Japan.)*

papilla has sloughed. Papillary necrosis is not pathognomonic of analgesic nephropathy; it is also seen in diabetic nephropathy (particularly during an episode of acute pyelonephritis), sickle cell nephropathy, urinary tract obstruction, and renal tuberculosis. Non–contrast-enhanced computed tomography (CT) demonstrates a decrease in renal mass with either bumpy contours or papillary calcifications (Fig. 62.6).[18]

Treatment

Management consists of stopping or at least reducing the intake of analgesic medications. Because of the increased incidence of uroepithelial tumors, close follow-up is necessary. New hematuria requires early referral for urologic evaluation.

Analgesic nephropathy associated with over the counter medicines is also discussed in Chapter 74.

CHRONIC INTERSTITIAL NEPHRITIS DUE TO METABOLIC DISORDERS

Metabolic disorders causing interstitial nephritis are discussed here. Hyperoxaluria is described in Chapter 57 and cystinosis in Chapter 48.

Chronic Urate Nephropathy

Definition and Epidemiology

Historically, chronic interstitial nephritis associated with chronic hyperuricemia was called gouty nephropathy. Before drugs that lower uric acid levels became available, more than 50% of patients with gout had impaired renal function and nearly 100% had renal disease at autopsy. In the early 1980s, the concept of gouty nephropathy as a disease was challenged because the renal injury observed in subjects with gout was ascribed to coexistent hypertension, vascular disease, or aging-associated renal injury.[19] However, epidemiologic studies suggest that an elevated serum uric acid level may carry an independent and dose-dependent risk for kidney disease.[20] These increases in risk remained significant even after adjustment for estimated GFR, proteinuria, age, and components of the metabolic syndrome. These studies raise the interesting possibility that chronic hyperuricemia may be both a true risk factor for the development of chronic kidney disease (CKD) and a risk factor for progression of established CKD.

Pathogenesis

It has been suggested that chronic hyperuricemia and uricosuria result in intratubular sodium urate crystal deposition, with local obstruction, rupture into the interstitium, and subsequent granulomatous response and interstitial fibrosis. The determinants of uric acid solubility are its concentration and the pH of the tubular fluid, and the major sites of urate deposition are the renal medullae. If deposition occurs in an acid medium, as in the tubular fluid, birefringent uric acid crystals are formed; whereas in an alkaline medium, as in the interstitium, amorphous urate salts are deposited.

Crystalline deposits of urate may account for some degree of renal injury, but subjects with gouty nephropathy often have diffuse renal disease with arteriolosclerosis, focal and global glomerulosclerosis, and interstitial fibrosis. Although it is difficult to ascribe diffuse renal disease to the presence of focal crystalline deposits, experimental studies have suggested that hyperuricemia may induce chronic renal injury independent of crystal formation.[21] The mechanism appears to be the development of preglomerular arteriolar disease that impairs the renal autoregulatory response and thereby causes glomerular hypertension.

Pathology

Renal functional abnormalities are observed in 30% to 50% of patients who have had gout for many years, and histologic changes are observed in more than 90%.[22] On histologic examination, the lesion is characterized by tubulointerstitial fibrosis, often with arteriolosclerosis and glomerulosclerosis. Within the kidney, there are often precipitated uric acid crystals in the tubules and in the interstitium, particularly in the medulla (Fig. 62.7). On occasion, medullary renal tophi are found on gross anatomic dissection.

Clinical Manifestations

Patients present with hypertension with mildly impaired renal function, mild proteinuria, unremarkable urinary sediment, and minor tubular dysfunction (usually impairment of urine concentrating ability manifested as isosthenuria). Uric acid nephropathy should be particularly considered if there is a disproportionate elevation in serum uric acid in relation to the degree of renal impairment (Fig. 62.8).[23]

Diagnosis

The most important differential diagnosis for gouty nephropathy is chronic lead nephropathy. Familial juvenile hyperuricemic nephropathy is a rare autosomal dominant disease that mimics chronic gouty nephropathy but that presents in adolescence or during early childhood (see Chapter 48).

Treatment

Whether lowering of uric acid is renoprotective remains controversial. One prospective, randomized, controlled trial demonstrated that allopurinol therapy is associated with preservation of renal function in mild to moderate CKD.[24] Withdrawal of allopurinol from patients with stable CKD resulted in worsening of hypertension and acceleration of kidney dysfunction.[25] More studies are required before treatment of hyperuricemia should be routinely offered.

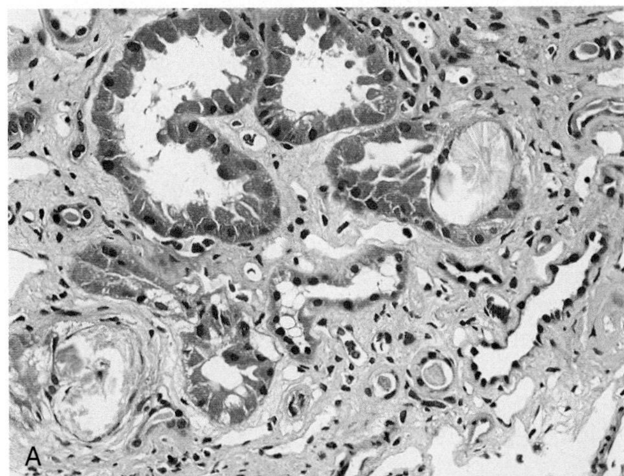

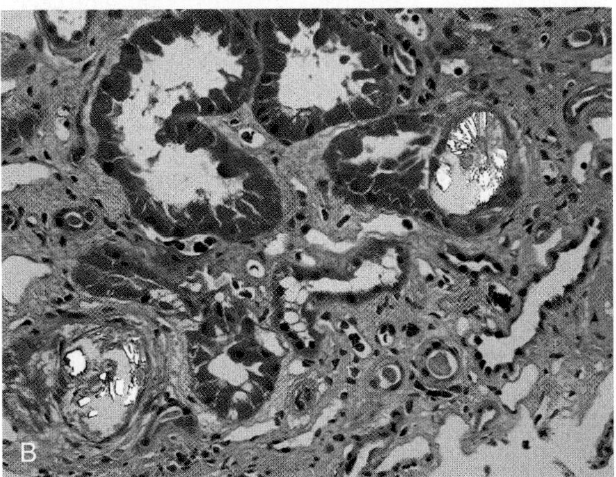

Figure 62.7 Chronic urate nephropathy. A, Large collections of elongated or fragmented urate crystals are present in association with atrophic tubules. (Hematoxylin and eosin stain; original magnification ×400.) **B,** The crystalline masses are refractile under polarized light. *(Courtesy Drs. Akira Shimizu and Hideki Takano, Nippon Medical School, Tokyo, Japan.)*

Expected Relationship of Serum Creatinine and Uric Acid Levels

Serum Creatinine		Corresponding Serum Uric Acid Level	
mg/dl	μmol/l	mg/dl	μmol/l
<1.5	132	9	536
1.5–2.0	132–176	10	595
>2.0	176	12	714

Figure 62.8 Expected relationship of serum creatinine and uric acid levels. Serum uric acid disproportionately elevated above the expected values for serum creatinine suggests a diagnosis of chronic uric acid nephropathy. *(Modified from reference 23.)*

One reason for caution is the accumulation of the xanthine oxidase inhibitor allopurinol in renal failure. It is prudent to initiate allopurinol at a dose of 50 to 100 mg/day, increasing to 200 or 300 mg/day if it is tolerated. A small minority of patients (0.1%) develop a hypersensitivity syndrome that can be fatal, and this risk is increased with renal dysfunction. Experimentally, allopurinol can also be associated with nephrotoxicity in the setting of significant renal dysfunction by formation of allopurinol microcrystals. The newer xanthine oxidase inhibitor febuxostat does not require modification of dose in renal failure, nor is it associated with hypersensitivity or nephrotoxicity, but more studies are required before its use can be recommended.

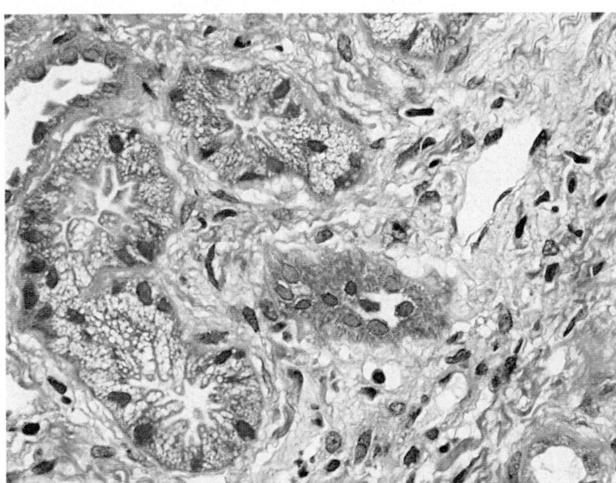

Figure 62.9 Hypokalemic nephropathy. Vacuolization of the renal tubules is observed in association with interstitial fibrosis in a patient with hypokalemic nephropathy. (Masson trichrome stain; original magnification ×400.) *(Courtesy Drs. Akira Shimizu and Hideki Takano, Nippon Medical School, Tokyo, Japan.)*

Hypokalemic Nephropathy

Definition and Epidemiology

Hypokalemia, if persistent for prolonged periods, can induce renal cysts, chronic interstitial nephritis, and progressive loss of renal function, so-called hypokalemic nephropathy, which can be inherited or acquired.

Pathology

The characteristic finding is vacuolation of the renal tubules due to dilation of cisternae of the endoplasmic reticulum and basal folding, which is generally limited to the proximal tubule segments (Fig. 62.9). This abnormality generally requires at least one month to develop and is reversible with potassium supplementation. More prolonged hypokalemia can lead to more severe changes, predominantly in the renal medulla, including interstitial fibrosis, tubular atrophy, and cyst formation. There is experimental evidence that hypokalemic injury may be due to hypokalemia-induced renal vasoconstriction with ischemia. Local ammonia production stimulated by hypokalemia may also lead to intrarenal complement activation that may contribute to the renal injury. Furthermore, the associated intracellular acidosis can stimulate cell proliferation, which may account for the occasional development of cysts in hypokalemic subjects.

Clinical Manifestations

Impaired urine concentration, presenting with nocturia, polyuria, and polydipsia, may occur, particularly when plasma potassium concentration is consistently below 3.0 mmol/l for months or years. The average duration of hypokalemia reported in patients with chronic hypokalemic nephropathy is between 3.5

and 9 years. The renal defect is associated with decreased collecting tubule responsiveness to vasopressin, possibly due to decreased expression of aquaporin 2.

Diagnosis

Although degenerative changes in proximal tubular cells are a consistent but nonspecific finding in hypokalemic nephropathy, a particularly characteristic finding is vacuolar changes in the proximal tubules. Similar vacuolization of the convoluted tubules is observed in ethylene glycol poisoning.

Treatment

Hypokalemia can usually be treated with oral potassium supplements. Details about treatment of hypokalemia are described in Chapter 9. Coarse cytoplasmic vacuoles may persist for some time after normalization of serum potassium values.

Hypercalcemic Nephropathy

Definition and Epidemiology

Hypercalcemia can cause both a transient and reversible renal vasoconstriction with a decrement in renal function and a chronic interstitial nephritis secondary to tubular cell necrosis and intratubular obstruction. In addition, hypoparathyroidism (especially surgically induced after treatment of hyperparathyroidism) can also result in marked hypercalciuria and a similar syndrome in the absence of hypercalcemia.

Pathology

Focal degeneration and necrosis of the tubular epithelium, primarily in the medulla where calcium is concentrated, develop soon with persistent hypercalcemia. Although focal degenerative and necrotic lesions of the tubular epithelium can be observed in acute hypercalcemic patients, the most distinctive histologic feature of long-standing hypercalcemia is calcific deposits in the interstitium (nephrocalcinosis; Fig. 62.10). Deposition begins in the medullary tubules, followed by deposition in the cortical proximal and distal tubules and within the interstitial space, and secondarily leads to mononuclear cell infiltration and tubular necrosis.

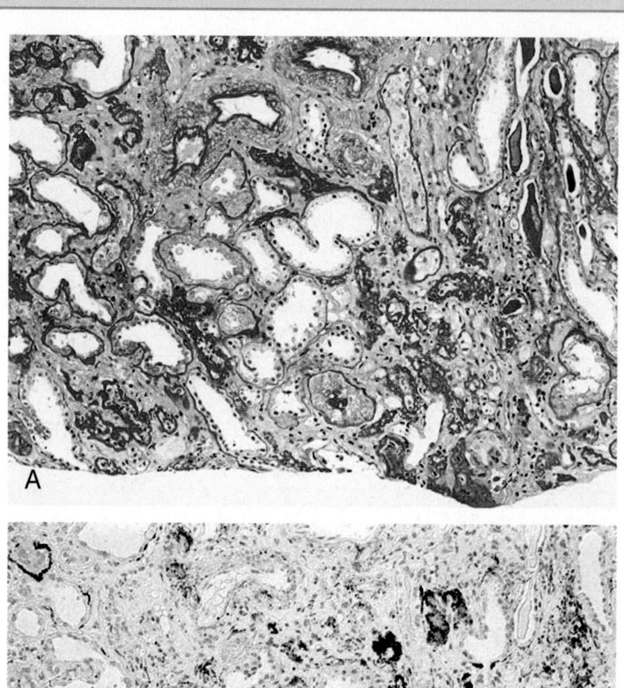

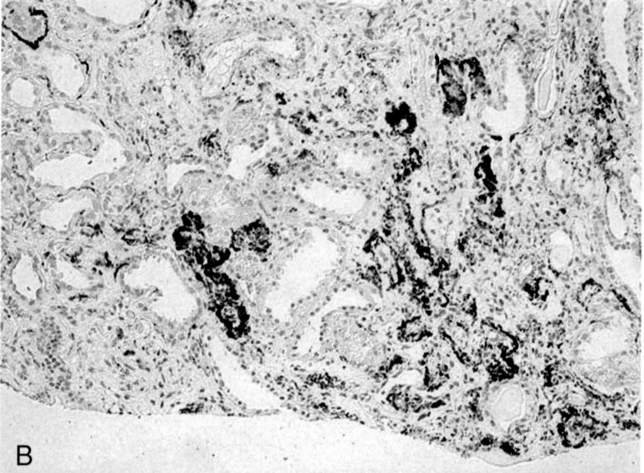

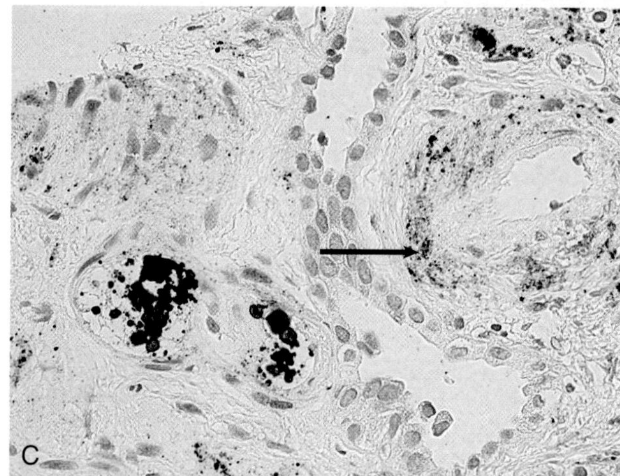

Figure 62.10 Hypercalcemic nephropathy due to sarcoidosis. A, Marked tubular atrophy and interstitial fibrosis with mild lymphocytic infiltrate. **B,** Dense calcium deposits are seen in the thickened basement membrane of the atrophic tubules and in the fibrotic area of interstitium (serial section of **A**). **C,** Intraluminal calcium plaque in the atrophic tubules. Granular calcium deposits are observed in the arterial wall *(arrow)*. (**A,** periodic acid–Schiff staining; **B** and **C,** von Kossa staining.) *(Courtesy Dr. Noriko Uesugi, Ibaraki, Japan.)*

Clinical Manifestations

Macroscopic nephrocalcinosis is often detected on radiography or ultrasound. A defect in urinary concentration is the most notable tubular dysfunction and is manifested as polyuria and polydipsia. The mechanism is incompletely understood, but the impairment relates both to a reduction in medullary solute content and to interference with the cellular response to vasopressin. Reversible impairment of renal function can result from either acute or chronic hypercalcemia by decreased renal blood flow and GFR. Irreversible renal failure is a rare consequence of long-standing hypercalcemia and is almost invariably associated with calcium crystal deposition in the interstitium of the kidney.

CHRONIC INTERSTITIAL NEPHRITIS DUE TO HEREDITARY DISEASES OF THE KIDNEY

Nephronophthisis (NPHP) and medullary cystic kidney disease (MCKD) (or the NPHP-MCKD complex) are hereditary diseases associated with renal cysts at the corticomedullary junction. These disorders are described in detail in Chapters 45 and 48.

CHRONIC INTERSTITIAL NEPHRITIS ASSOCIATED WITH HEAVY METAL EXPOSURE

Lead Nephropathy

Definition and Epidemiology

Acute lead intoxication is rare but may present with abdominal pain, encephalopathy, hemolytic anemia, peripheral neuropathy, and proximal tubular dysfunction (Fanconi syndrome). Because lead has a biologic half-life of several decades, both intermittent acute poisoning and low-level environmental exposure result in chronic cumulative lead poisoning. An epidemic of childhood lead poisoning in Queensland, Australia, established chronic lead nephropathy as a recognized clinical and pathologic entity.[26] The pathogenesis of the renal disease may be related to the accumulation of reabsorbed lead in the proximal tubule cells and effects of chronic lead exposure on the vasculature.

Epidemiologic studies have suggested that low-level exposure may be associated with CKD or hypertension in the general population.[27] Accelerated deterioration of renal function with low-level environmental lead exposure was confirmed in a prospective study of 121 patients with CKD.[28] Experimental studies showed that rats exposed to lead developed tubulointerstitial damage, peritubular capillary loss, and intrarenal arteriolar disease.[29]

Pathology

The kidneys are reduced in size. The characteristic morphology is relatively acellular interstitial nephritis. The earliest histologic finding is proximal tubular injury, with intranuclear inclusion bodies composed of a lead-protein complex. Glomeruli are normal, and arteries and arterioles demonstrate medial thickening and luminal narrowing, probably related to hypertension. Immunofluorescence studies are noncontributory.

Clinical Manifestations

Chronic lead nephropathy is usually identified when a source of high exposure is known (occupational hazard or consumption of illicitly distilled spirits [moonshine]). Hyperuricemia is common because of impaired uric acid excretion. Urine sediment is benign, and urinary protein excretion is less than 2 g/day. Hypertension is almost always present, and in the absence of appropriate testing or a careful exposure history, lead nephropathy is often misdiagnosed as hypertensive kidney disease. Gouty arthritis ("saturnine gout") affects about half of patients. Patients with chronic lead intoxication may occasionally manifest other signs, including peripheral motor neuropathies, anemia with "basophilic" stippling, and perivascular cerebellar calcifications.

Diagnosis

Lead nephropathy is underdiagnosed because no simple diagnostic blood test is available. Lead nephropathy is easily confused with chronic urate nephropathy, in which urate deposits (tophi) may form in the renal interstitium. All patients with hyperuricemia and renal insufficiency should have a history of occupational lead exposure excluded. The blood lead concentration is an insensitive measure of cumulative body stores. A clinical diagnosis of lead nephropathy is based on a history of exposure, evidence of renal dysfunction, and a positive result of a calcium disodium edetate ($CaNa_2$ EDTA) lead chelation test.[30] The association with gout and CKD is strong enough to merit lead chelation screening in patients with CKD who have gout and risk of lead exposure. $CaNa_2$ EDTA is administered (two doses of 0.5 g in 250 ml 5% dextrose given 12 hours apart), and urine is collected for 3 days because urinary excretion is slowed in the setting of renal failure. Normal urinary lead levels are less than 650 μg per 3 days. X-ray fluorescence, which provokes the emission of fluorescent photons from the target area, is an alternative method that detects increased bone lead levels, which are also a reflection of cumulative lead exposure.

Treatment

Treatment involves the infusions of $CaNa_2$ EDTA together with removal of the source of lead. The likelihood of a satisfactory response to $CaNa_2$ EDTA is influenced by the degree of interstitial fibrosis that has already occurred.

In industrial and occupational settings, such as in foundry workers and individuals working with lead-based paints and glazes, preventive measures to minimize exposure and low-level absorption are essential. The oral chelating agent succimer (Chemet) has proved highly successful in treating children. Chelation therapy may slow progressive CKD, even in patients with mild lead intoxication.[31] However, the chelation therapy has not been widely used in adults. It is generally not indicated for adults with blood lead concentrations of less than 45 μg/dl because of the potential risk of adverse drug events and concerns about remobilized lead.

Other Heavy Metal–Induced Nephropathies

Cadmium is a metal with a wide variety of industrial uses, including the manufacture of glass, metal alloys, and electrical equipment. Cadmium is preferentially concentrated in the kidney, principally in the proximal tubule, in the form of a cadmium-metallothionein complex that has a biologic half-life of about 10 years. A major outbreak of cadmium toxicity occurred in Japan as a result of industrial contamination. The disease was called *itai-itai*, or "ouch-ouch," because of the significant bone pain as the major clinical manifestation. Other manifestations included proximal tubular dysfunction, renal stones caused by hypercalciuria, anemia, and rarely progressive chronic interstitial nephritis. The mechanism by which cadmium elicits chronic inflammation and fibrosis in the kidney is relatively unstudied. The diagnosis is suggested by a history of occupational exposure, increased urinary β_2-microglobulin, and increased urinary cadmium levels (>7 μg/g creatinine). Once manifested, renal injury tends to be progressive, even if exposure is discontinued. Chelation has not been effective in humans, and prevention is the only effective treatment.

Arsenic, used as a poison gas in the First World War, is present in insecticides, weed killers, wallpaper, and paints. Chronic arsenic toxicity most commonly is manifested as sensory and motor neuropathies, distal extremity hyperkeratosis, palmar desquamation, diarrhea and nausea, Aldrich-Mees lines (white bands on the nails), and anemia. In rare cases, it may cause renal disease, manifested by both proximal RTA and chronic interstitial fibrosis. Diagnosis is made by demonstration of an elevated urinary arsenic level.

Mercury is found in alloy plants, mirror plants, and some batteries, and mercury intoxication usually occurs as a result of accidental exposure to mercury vapor. Although mercury has been shown to induce membranous nephropathy in experimental animals, the nephrotic syndrome is so uncommon in humans exposed to mercury that its etiologic role has been doubted. Neither elemental mercury nor the mercurous salt (Hg_2Cl_2) produces sustained renal tubular injury, but mercury dichloride

($HgCl_2$) may produce acute tubular necrosis and subsequent chronic interstitial nephritis. However, a report of endemic methyl mercury poisoning in Japan revealed a clinical picture dominated by neurologic sequelae; renal disease in these patients was surprisingly benign, consisting only of tubular proteinuria without changes in serum creatinine.

RADIATION NEPHRITIS

Definition and Epidemiology

Although radiation nephritis was relatively common decades ago, the incidence has decreased considerably because recognition of radiation-induced renal damage has altered protocols for the administration of therapeutic radiation. In general, direct exposure of the kidney to 20 to 30 Gy (1 Gy = 100 rad) during 5 weeks or less will produce radiation nephritis.

Pathology

The initial target of ionizing radiation within the kidney appears to be endothelial cells, leading to endothelial cell swelling. Subsequent vascular occlusion develops with resultant tubular atrophy. Electron microscopy reveals a split appearance of the capillary wall due to the mesangial interposition and widening of the subendothelial space by a nondescript fluffy material. These features are shared by hemolytic-uremic syndrome and thrombotic thrombocytopenic purpura, suggesting a common pathogenic mechanism originating from endothelial injury. Severe disease is characterized by progressive interstitial fibrosis and the presence of interstitial inflammatory cells.

Clinical Manifestations

In general, vascular and glomerular lesions of the thrombotic microangiopathy may predominate. However, tubulointerstitial changes of varying severity are also usually present. Hypertension is commonly observed. Progression to a "chronic" form of radiation nephritis may occur if resolution of acute radiation nephritis is incomplete. These patients present with proteinuria, progressive CKD, and eventual development of ESRD several years after irradiation in the absence of an acute phase.

Treatment

Prevention is the best approach. The risk for development of radiation nephritis can be minimized by shielding of the kidneys or fractioning the total-body irradiation into several small doses during several days. No specific treatment is available for established radiation nephritis; consequently, the general approach is control of hypertension and supportive treatment of CKD.

ENDEMIC DISEASES

Balkan Nephropathy

Definition and Epidemiology

This is an endemic kidney disease confined to discrete, well-defined settlements in the Balkans (i.e., Albania, Bosnia, Croatia, Serbia, Macedonia, Romania, Bulgaria; Fig. 62.11). The spatial distribution has remained unchanged with time, and the disease affects the same endemic clusters as 50 years ago. The disease occurs in indigenous or immigrant individuals who have resided in an endemic area for at least 15 to 20 years and does not occur among residents who move to nonendemic areas. The clinical features of Balkan nephropathy are essentially identical to those of aristolochic acid–associated nephropathy (see Chapter 74), and recent advances in the understanding of endemic nephropathy now favor the causative role of aristolochic acid over the ubiquitous mycotoxin (ochratoxin A), which had been previously implicated.[32]

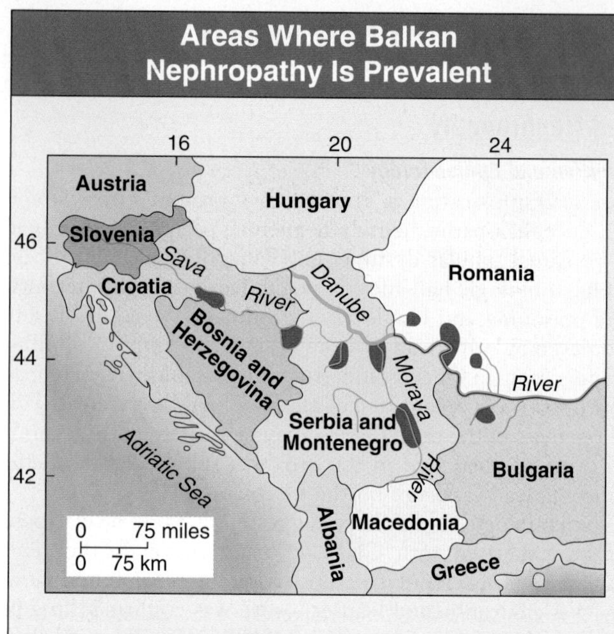

Figure 62.11 Balkan endemic nephropathy. Geographic regions where Balkan nephropathy is prevalent. The endemic areas are in *red*.

Pathogenesis

Most recent studies suggest that Balkan nephropathy results from contamination of wheat flour with aristolochic acids, which are derived from the seeds of *Aristolochia clematitis*. Analysis of the renal cortex of patients with Balkan nephropathy identified DNA adducts derived from aristolochic acid.[33] Thus, the disease most likely occurs in genetically predisposed individuals who are chronically exposed to a causative factor (aristolochic acid) in the environment within endemic areas.

Pathology

The kidneys are usually of normal size early in the course of the disease. A symmetric, smooth reduction in size is observed in late-stage disease. Renal biopsy findings are characterized by proximal tubular lesions in the early stage of disease, with predominantly focal tubular atrophy, interstitial edema and sclerosis, and sometimes mononuclear cell infiltrates. Disease progression is associated with marked tubular atrophy, peritubular capillary damage, and interstitial fibrosis. Early glomerular changes are mild and focal, whereas most glomeruli are hyalinized or sclerotic in advanced stages of the disease.

Clinical Manifestations

Balkan nephropathy typically is manifested clinically in the fourth or fifth decade of life and is only rarely seen in individuals younger than 20 years. One of the first signs, detected only when prospective monitoring is performed, is tubular proteinuria. Proteinuria is usually mild or intermittent but may increase in the advanced stages. An unremarkable urinary sediment is characteristic. Other manifestations of abnormal renal tubular dysfunction include impaired acidification, decreased ammonia and increased uric acid excretion, and urine concentrating defects with renal salt wasting, which may precede the decrease in GFR. The disease slowly progresses to ESRD.

An early feature is normochromic normocytic anemia disproportionate to the degree of renal impairment, whereas patients are usually without edema and are normotensive. Hypertension develops only with ESRD.

The increased incidence of uroepithelial carcinomas is similar to that observed in both analgesic nephropathy and aristolochic acid–associated nephropathy. Patients with macroscopic hematuria need attention and should be investigated for the presence of uroepithelial tumors.

Diagnosis

If screening by urinalysis and estimated GFR is negative, subjects should be followed up every 1 to 3 years, depending on risk factors. If abnormalities are found on screening, further evaluation is indicated; a diagnosis of Balkan nephropathy is currently made in inhabitants from endemic settlements by the criteria described in Figure 62.12.[34] Recent analysis of 182 patients in Serbia showed that proteinuria, urine α_1-microglobulin, and kidney length and volume are significant predictors of Balkan nephropathy, whereas variables related to kidney failure as well as several tubular disorders (urine specific gravity, fractional sodium excretion, and tubular phosphate reabsorption) had an insignificant predictive value.[35]

Treatment

Treatment is primarily supportive. For advancing disease with proteinuria or hypertension, ACE inhibitors or ARBs are recommended.

Diagnostic Procedures of Balkan Nephropathy

Diagnosis of Balkan nephropathy is made in inhabitants from endemic settlements using the following:

1. Epidemiologic criteria
2. Demonstration of
   - GFR decrease
   - Proteinuria generally below 1 g/24 hours
   - Microalbuminuria
   - Little urinary sediment
   - Tubular markers (renal glucosuria, increased urinary excretion of β2 microglobulin or alpha-1-microglobulin, and N-acetyl-β-D-glucosaminidase)
   - Typical renal histology showing hypocellular cortical interstitial fibrosis decreasing from the outer to the inner cortex (if renal biopsy feasible)
3. Exclusion of other known kidney disease (e.g., chronic pyelonephritis—obstructive and atrophic, adult dominant polycystic kidney disease, glomerulonephritis)

Figure 62.12 Diagnostic procedures of Balkan nephropathy. *(Modified from reference 34.)*

INTERSTITIAL NEPHRITIS MEDIATED BY IMMUNOLOGIC MECHANISMS

Sjögren's Syndrome

Definition and Epidemiology

Sjögren's syndrome may be associated with chronic interstitial nephritis. The reported prevalence of renal involvement in Sjögren's syndrome has varied widely, ranging from 2% to 67%, principally owing to different definitions of kidney involvement or disease. Recent analysis of 130 patients with primary Sjögren's syndrome in a Chinese hospital showed that the incidence of chronic interstitial nephritis was 80% among all the biopsy materials.[36]

Pathology

The lesion is characterized histologically by infiltration of lymphocytes and plasmacytes in the interstitium with tubular cell injury and, rarely, granuloma formation. This progresses to tubular atrophy and interstitial fibrosis over time. Immunofluorescence reveals granular deposits of IgG and C3 along the tubular basement membrane.

Clinical Manifestations

The clinical and biochemical manifestations of interstitial nephritis may be the presenting or only features of Sjögren's syndrome. Plasma creatinine concentration is generally only mildly elevated in association with a bland urine sediment and abnormalities in tubular function, including Fanconi syndrome, type 1 RTA, hypokalemia, and nephrogenic diabetes insipidus. Sjögren's syndrome is one of the most common causes of acquired distal (type 1) RTA in adults and the hypokalemia may be marked, resulting in a clinical presentation of severe weakness. Hypokalemia may occur in the absence of RTA, resulting from salt wasting and secondary hyperaldosteronism.

Treatment

Treatment with corticosteroids at the stage of cellular infiltration is frequently beneficial for protecting renal function. Although the renal disease has a slow and protracted course and CKD develops over time, progression to ESRD is rare.

Sarcoidosis

Definition and Epidemiology

Histologic evidence of interstitial nephritis with noncaseating granulomas is common in patients with sarcoidosis, but the frequency of clinically significant disease is low.[37] It may present as either an acute interstitial nephritis or a chronic interstitial nephritis.

Pathology

Renal biopsy reveals normal glomeruli; interstitial infiltration, mostly with mononuclear cells; tubular injury; and with more chronic disease, interstitial fibrosis. Whereas the classic finding is noncaseating granulomas in the interstitium, they are uncommon and nonspecific. Analysis of 18 cases with granulomatous interstitial nephritis in Glasgow showed that five cases were associated with sarcoidosis, two were associated with tubulointerstitial nephritis and uveitis, two were associated with medication, and nine were idiopathic.[38] Immunofluorescence and electron microscopic studies typically show no immune deposits.

Clinical Manifestations

Most affected patients have clear evidence of diffuse active sarcoidosis, although some present with an isolated elevation in plasma creatinine and only minimal extrarenal manifestations. The urinalysis, if not normal, shows only sterile pyuria or mild proteinuria.

In addition, hypercalcemia induced by increased production of calcitriol (1,25-dihydroxyvitamin D) by activated mononuclear cells (particularly macrophages) in the lung and lymph nodes occasionally results in renal problems (see the previous discussion of hypercalcemic nephropathy).

The serum ACE level is used best not as a primary diagnostic tool but as a marker of disease activity and response to therapy. A normal serum ACE level does not exclude renal disease.

Treatment

Corticosteroid therapy tends to improve renal function, although recovery is often incomplete. Rapid tapering of corticosteroid can result in relapse.

Systemic Lupus Erythematosus

Definition and Epidemiology

Interstitial nephritis with immune complexes is defined by granular deposits of immunoglobulins and complement in the tubular basement membrane, interstitium, or both. Systemic lupus erythematosus is the most common reason for this type of interstitial nephritis (Fig. 62.13), and interstitial involvement is present in half of kidney biopsy specimens in lupus. Rarely, tubulointerstitial immune complex disease may be the only manifestation of lupus nephritis.

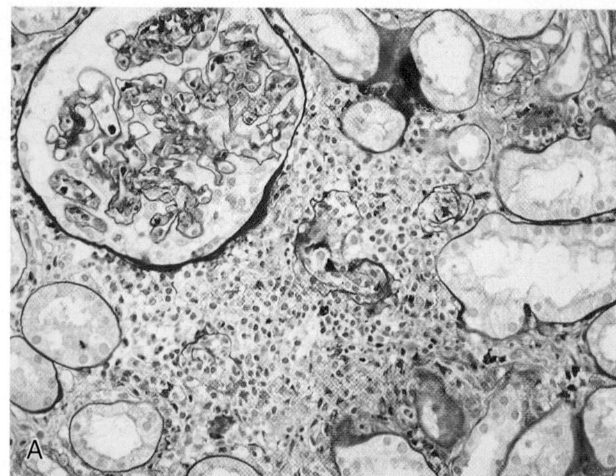

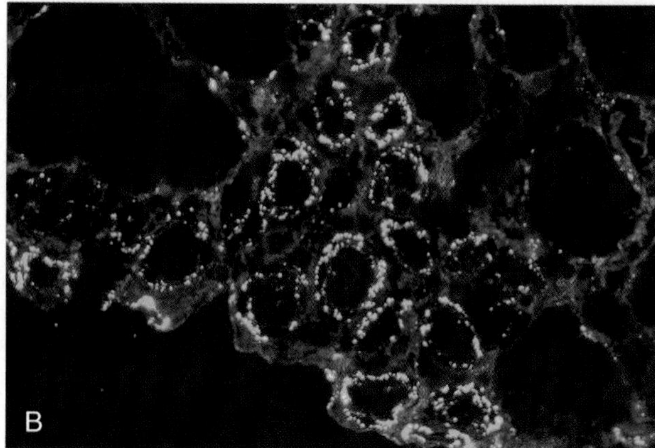

Figure 62.13 Chronic interstitial nephritis in lupus. A, Interstitial nephritis observed in patients with systemic lupus erythematosus. (Periodic acid–Schiff staining; original magnification ×400.) **B,** Immunofluorescence study of the same patient revealed deposition of IgG in the interstitium, in tubular cells, and along the tubular basement membrane. *(Courtesy Drs. Akira Shimizu and Hideki Takano, Nippon Medical School, Tokyo, Japan.)*

Clinical Manifestations

The presentation may be as an acute or chronic interstitial nephritis. The possibility of interstitial involvement (without glomerular disease) is suggested by a rising plasma creatinine concentration and a bland urine sediment. Interstitial involvement may be accompanied by signs of tubular dysfunction, such as type 1 or type 4 RTA; by isolated hyperkalemia resulting from impaired distal potassium secretion; or by hypokalemia resulting from salt wasting. The potentiating effects of sodium wasting on potassium secretion include an increase in sodium delivery to the potassium secretory site in the collecting tubules and associated volume depletion with subsequent stimulation of aldosterone secretion.

Treatment

Corticosteroid therapy is usually effective in subsiding tubular dysfunction and preserving renal function.

Inflammatory Bowel Disease

Although the most frequent renal complications of Crohn's disease are calcium oxalate stones and renal amyloidosis, several cases of interstitial nephritis were reported in patients treated for chronic inflammatory bowel disease. Whereas aminosalicylates (5-aminosalicylic acid, mesalazine, and sulfasalazine) are responsible for the development of chronic nephropathy in most cases, nephrotoxicity of these reagents is exceptional (mean rate of only 0.3% per patient-year).[39] Nephrotoxicity most often occurs in the first 12 months of treatment with aminosalicylate, but a delayed presentation after several years has also been reported. There is no clear relationship between aminosalicylate dose and the risk of nephrotoxicity, suggesting that this is an idiosyncratic response. Some patients were reported to have biopsy-proven interstitial nephritis before the diagnosis of Crohn's disease.

Aminosalicylates should be withdrawn when renal impairment is manifested in a patient with inflammatory bowel disease; if this does not result in a fall in plasma creatinine, renal biopsy should be considered. Corticosteroids may be recommended when renal function does not respond to drug withdrawal.

Interstitial Nephritis in IgG4-Related Sclerosing Disease

Definition and Epidemiology

On the basis of histologic and immunohistochemical examination of various organs of patients with autoimmune pancreatitis, a novel clinicopathologic entity of IgG4-related sclerosing disease has been proposed.[40] This is a systemic disease that is characterized by extensive IgG4-positive plasma cells and T-lymphocyte infiltration of various organs (Fig. 62.14). Most reports of IgG4-related sclerosing disease have come from Japan, but it has also been described in countries in Europe as well as in the United States and Korea, suggesting that it is a worldwide entity. The incidence may be increasing, perhaps because of increased recognition.

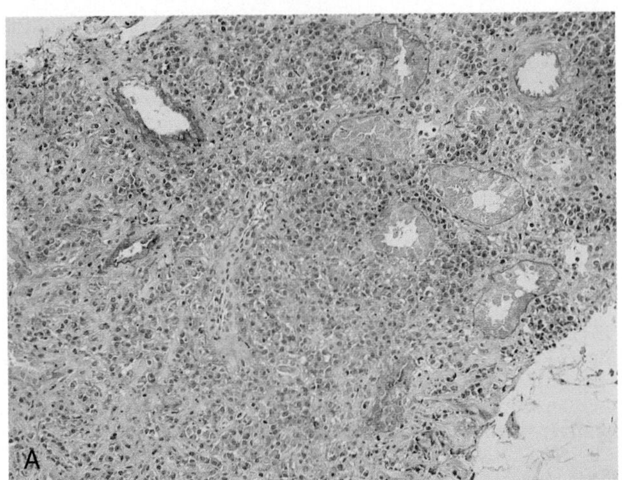

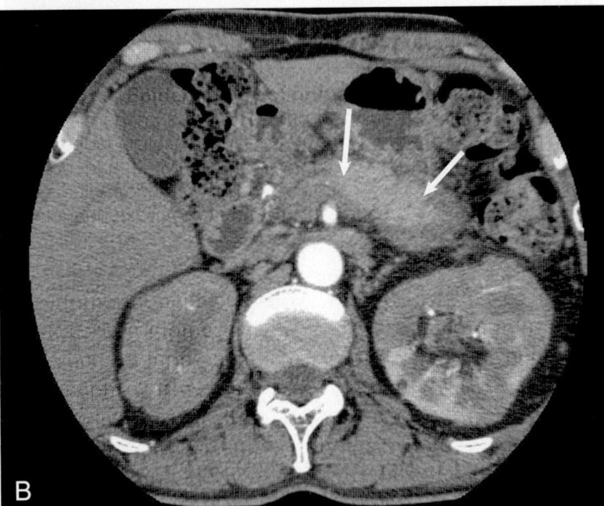

Figure 62.14 Chronic interstitial nephritis in IgG4-related sclerosing disease. A, Interstitial nephritis with numerous mononuclear cell infiltrates observed in patients with autoimmune pancreatitis. Many of these cells are positive for IgG4 in typical cases. (Periodic acid–Schiff staining; original magnification ×200.) **B,** CT scan of the patient revealed pancreatic swelling *(arrows). (Courtesy Dr. Hiroshi Nishi, University of Tokyo, Tokyo, Japan.)*

Pathology

There is tubulointerstitial nephritis with dense infiltrations of IgG4-positive mononuclear cells.

Clinical Manifestations

Clinical manifestations are observed in various organs, presenting as sclerosing cholangitis, cholecystitis, sialadenitis, retroperitoneal fibrosis, and so on. Whereas most IgG4-related sclerosing disease is most often associated with autoimmune pancreatitis, those without pancreatic involvement have also been described. The disease occurs predominantly in older men. Serum IgG4 levels are raised, and IgG4-positive cells are found in the interstitium.

Treatment

The response to corticosteroids is generally favorable.

Other Forms of Immune-Mediated Interstitial Nephritis

Primary anti–tubular basement membrane (TBM) nephritis is an extremely rare form of interstitial nephritis that usually is acute and characterized by linear deposits of immunoglobulins and complement in the TBM together with tubular interstitial inflammation and anti-TBM antibodies in the serum. Anti-TBM antibodies may also be found in 50% to 70% of patients with anti–glomerular basement membrane nephritis and occasionally in patients with membranous nephropathy, systemic lupus erythematosus, IgA nephropathy, minimal change disease, and malignant hypertension.

OBSTRUCTIVE UROPATHY

Complete or partial urinary tract obstruction is accompanied by pathologic changes in both the tubulointerstitium and glomeruli consisting of interstitial fibrosis, tubular atrophy, and occasionally focal glomerular sclerosis. Details are discussed in Chapters 58 and 61.

VASCULAR DISEASES

Kidney disease in this category is variably termed ischemic nephropathy, renovascular disease, and nephrosclerosis. Ischemia due to intrarenal vascular involvement causes tubular atrophy, interstitial fibrosis, and cellular infiltration. Of note, chronic ischemia in the tubulointerstitial compartment also plays a crucial role in the progression of a variety of glomerular and tubulointerstitial diseases.[3] For details, refer to Chapter 64.

VIRUS-ASSOCIATED CHRONIC INTERSTITIAL NEPHRITIS

Although a variety of bacterial and viral infections can be associated with acute interstitial nephritis (see Chapters 55 and 60), chronic interstitial nephritis secondary to infectious agents appears to be rare. Chronic bacterial infections can result in xanthogranulomatous pyelonephritis or renal malacoplakia (see Chapter 51).

REFERENCES

1. Boor P, Sebeková K, Ostendorf T, Floege J. Treatment targets in renal fibrosis. *Nephrol Dial Transplant*. 2007;22:3391-3407.
2. Zeisberg EM, Potenta SE, Sugimoto H, et al. Fibroblasts in kidney fibrosis emerge via endothelial-to-mesenchymal transition. *J Am Soc Nephrol*. 2008;19:2282-2287.
3. Nangaku M. Chronic hypoxia and tubulointerstitial injury: A final common pathway to end-stage renal failure. *J Am Soc Nephrol*. 2006; 17:17-25.
4. Rastegar A, Kashgarian M. The clinical spectrum of tubulointerstitial nephritis. *Kidney Int*. 1998;54:313-327.
5. Rychlík I, Jancová E, Tesar V, et al. The Czech registry of renal biopsies. Occurrence of renal diseases in the years 1994-2000. *Nephrol Dial Transplant*. 2004;19:3040-3049.
6. Chen H, Tang Z, Zeng C, et al. Pathological demography of native patients in a nephrology center in China. *Chin Med J*. 2003;116: 1377-1381.
7. Braden GL, O'Shea MH, Mulhern JG. Tubulointerstitial diseases. *Am J Kidney Dis*. 2005;3:560-572.
8. Johnson RJ, Herrera-Acosta J, Schreiner GF, Rodriguez-Iturbe B. Subtle acquired renal injury as a mechanism of salt-sensitive hypertension. *N Engl J Med*. 2002;346:913-923.
9. Beck LH Jr, Salant DJ. Glomerular and tubulointerstitial diseases. *Prim Care*. 2008;35:265-296.
10. Boton R, Gaviria M, Batlle DC. Prevalence, pathogenesis, and treatment of renal dysfunction associated with chronic lithium therapy. *Am J Kidney Dis*. 1987;10:329-345.

11. Markowitz GS, Radhakrishnan J, Kambham N, et al. Lithium nephrotoxicity: A progressive combined glomerular and tubulointerstitial nephropathy. *J Am Soc Nephrol.* 2000;11:1439-1448.
12. Presne C, Fakhouri F, Noel LH, et al. Lithium-induced nephropathy: Rate of progression and prognostic factors. *Kidney Int.* 2003;64: 585-592.
13. Farres MT, Ronco P, Saadoun D, et al. Chronic lithium nephropathy: MR imaging for diagnosis. *Radiology.* 2003;229:570-574.
14. Alexander MP, Farag YM, Mittal BV, et al. Lithium toxicity: A double-edged sword. *Kidney Int.* 2008;73:233-237.
15. Mihatsch MJ, Khanlari B, Brunner FP. Obituary to analgesic nephropathy—an autopsy study. *Nephrol Dial Transplant.* 2006;21: 3139-3145.
16. van der Woude FJ, Heinemann LA, Graf H, et al. Analgesics use and ESRD in younger age: A case-control study. *BMC Nephrol.* 2007;8:15.
17. Rexrode KM, Buring JE, Glynn RJ, et al. Analgesic use and renal function in men. *JAMA.* 2001;286:315-321.
18. Elseviers MM, De Schepper A, Corthouts R, et al. High diagnostic performance of CT scan for analgesic nephropathy in patients with incipient to severe renal failure. *Kidney Int.* 1995;48:1316-1323.
19. Yu TF, Berger L. Impaired renal function gout: Its association with hypertensive vascular disease and intrinsic renal disease. *Am J Med.* 1982;72:95-100.
20. Obermayr RP, Temml C, Gutjahr G, et al. Elevated uric acid increases the risk for kidney disease. *J Am Soc Nephrol.* 2008;19:2407-2413.
21. Feig DI, Kang DH., Johnson RJ. Uric acid and cardiovascular risk. *N Engl J Med.* 2008;359:1811-1821.
22. Johnson RJ, Kivlighn SD, Kim YG, et al. Reappraisal of the pathogenesis and consequences of hyperuricemia in hypertension, cardiovascular disease, and renal disease. *Am J Kidney Dis.* 1999;33:225-234.
23. Murray T, Goldgerg M. Chronic interstitial nephritis: Etiologic factors. *Ann Intern Med.* 1975;82:453-459.
24. Siu YP, Leung KT, Tong MK, Kwan TH. Use of allopurinol in slowing the progression of renal disease through its ability to lower serum uric acid level. *Am J Kidney Dis.* 2006;47:51-59.
25. Talaat KM, el-Sheikh AR. The effect of mild hyperuricemia on urinary transforming growth factor beta and the progression of chronic kidney disease. *Am J Nephrol.* 2007;27:435-440.
26. Inglis JA, Henderson DA, Emmerson BT. The pathology and pathogenesis of chronic lead nephropathy occurring in Queensland. *J Pathol.* 1978;124:65-76.
27. Muntner P, He J, Vupputuri S, et al. Blood lead and chronic kidney disease in the general United States population: Results from NHANES III. *Kidney Int.* 2003;63:1044-1050.
28. Yu CC, Lin JL, Lin-Tan DT. Environmental exposure to lead and progression of chronic renal diseases: A four-year prospective longitudinal study. *J Am Soc Nephrol.* 2004;15:1016-1022.
29. Roncal C, Mu W, Reunqjui S, et al. Lead, at low levels, accelerates arteriolopathy and tubulointerstitial injury in chronic kidney disease. *Am J Physiol Renal Phsyiol.* 2007;293:F1391-F1396.
30. Wedeen RP, Malik DK, Batuman V. Detection and treatment of occupational lead nephropathy. *Arch Intern Med.* 1979;139:53-57.
31. Lin JL, Lin-Tan DT, Hsu KH, Yu CC. Environmental lead exposure and progression of chronic renal diseases in patients without diabetes. *N Engl J Med.* 2003;348:277-286.
32. Bamias G, Boletis J. Balkan nephropathy: Evolution of our knowledge. *Am J Kidney Dis.* 2008;52:606-616.
33. Grollman AP, Shibutani S, Moriya M, et al. Aristolochic acid and the etiology of endemic (Balkan) nephropathy. *Proc Natl Acad Sci U S A.* 2007;104:12129-12134.
34. Stefanovic V, Jelakovic B, Cukuranovic R, et al. Diagnostic criteria for Balkan endemic nephropathy: Proposal by an international panel. *Ren Fail.* 2007;29:867-880.
35. Djukanovi L, Marinkovi J, Mari I, et al. Contribution to the definition of diagnostic criteria for Balkan endemic nephropathy. *Nephrol Dial Transplant.* 2008;23:3932-3938.
36. Ren H, Wang WM, Chen XN, et al. Renal involvement and followup of 130 patients with primary Sjogren's syndrome. *J Rheumatol.* 2008;35:278-284.
37. Berliner AR, Haas M, Choi MJ. Sarcoidosis: The nephrologist's perspective. *Am J Kidney Dis.* 2006;48:856-870.
38. Joss N, Morris S, Young B, Geddes C. Granulomatous interstitial nephritis. *Clin J Am Soc Nephrol.* 2007;2:222-230.
39. Gisbert JP, González-Lama Y, Mate J. 5-Aminosalicylates and renal function in inflammatory bowel disease: A systematic review. *Inflamm Bowel Dis.* 2007;13:629-638.
40. Kamisawa T, Okamoto A. IgG4-related sclerosing disease. *World J Gastroenterol.* 2008;14:3948-3955.

CHAPTER 63

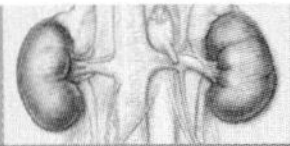

Myeloma and the Kidney

Ashley B. Irish

Myeloma is an uncommon hematologic malignant neoplasm, accounting for 1% of total and 10% of hematologic malignant neoplasms. Whereas all ethnic groups are affected, African Americans have twice the incidence of Caucasians, and males predominate over females. It is a disease of the elderly; the median age at diagnosis is older than 65 years. The characteristic feature of myeloma is the dysregulated overproduction of immunoglobulin and especially the light-chain component, which can be nephrotoxic. Various etiologies and manifestations of acute kidney injury (AKI) are possible in myeloma (Fig. 63.1), but the major risk is to due to myeloma cast nephropathy, which is a medical emergency that requires prompt diagnosis and intervention to avoid irreversible renal failure. This chapter primarily focuses on cast nephropathy; for other renal syndromes associated with myeloma, see Chapter 10 (hypercalcemia), Chapter 26 (amyloid and light-chain deposition disease), Chapter 48 (Fanconi syndrome), Chapter 57 (nephrolithiasis), and Chapter 66 (pathophysiology of AKI).

ETIOLOGY AND PATHOGENESIS OF MYELOMA

Myeloma is an incurable B cell–derived malignant neoplasm of incompletely differentiated plasma cells that have two prominent features, increased production of monoclonal immunoglobulin and bone destruction. Normally, plasma cells derive from mature uncommitted B cells and after antigen stimulation undergo heavy-chain class switching from μ (IgM) expression to α, δ, ε, or γ. Whole immunoglobulin production requires the intracellular assembly of two heavy chains and two light chains, κ or λ, to derive whole IgG, IgA, IgD, and IgE. Light chains are normally excreted in slight excess, with a κ:λ ratio of approximately 2:1. In myeloma, a clone of cells secretes excessive quantities of a specific immunoglobulin or light chain (the paraprotein or M protein). The genetic and somatic abnormalities underlying this malignant clone are complex and remain incompletely understood but have important implications for prognosis and treatment.[1] Both dysregulation of cell cycling and impaired apoptosis account for their progressive and dysfunctional accumulation within the bone marrow and occasionally other organs. Plasma cells express little surface immunoglobulin and are recognized by surface expression of CD38 and CD138; they normally reside only in the bone marrow. In myeloma, unrestrained plasma cell growth is supported by a complex milieu of autocrine and paracrine cytokines, especially interleukin (IL)–6. These cytokines are secreted from stromal cells, endothelial cells, or osteoclasts and maintain myeloma cell growth, survival, and migration; they also contribute to local organ dysfunction (e.g., bone resorption, fracture, and anemia).[2]

ETIOLOGY AND PATHOGENESIS OF RENAL DISEASE

Free light chains circulate as monomers (predominantly κ ≅ 25 kd) and dimers (predominantly λ ≅ 50 kd) with a very short half-life (2 to 6 hours) due to free glomerular filtration, whereas the much larger whole immunoglobulin circulates intact for several weeks. The filtered free light chain is reabsorbed in the proximal tubule cell (PTC) by receptor-mediated endocytosis after binding with the glycoprotein receptor cubilin (Fig. 63.2).[3] Light chains in excess can induce an inhibitory effect on endocytosis *in vitro* and are associated with lysosomal overload and rupture, releasing enzymatic contents into the cytosol, manifested histologically by evidence of crystallization, vacuolation, and desquamation of the PTC. Endocytosis of light chains induces the release of the proinflammatory cytokines IL-6 and IL-8 and monocyte chemoattractant protein 1 through the activation of nuclear factor κB in the PTC.[4] This mechanism suggests that light-chain overload induces factors promoting interstitial injury and fibrosis, as described in other proteinuric states. Light chains may also be cytotoxic to the PTC by direct DNA injury and the induction of apoptosis.[5] A less common manifestation of PTC injury is the Fanconi syndrome, which is invariably associated with specific variant κ light chains and often with pathologic evidence of crystalline inclusions.[6]

Injury to the PTC allows escape or overflow of the light chain to the distal nephron, where it can interact with the Tamm-Horsfall protein (THP) secreted by the cells of the thick ascending loop of Henle. Variations in the specificity of the binding region of different light chains modify the affinity of the light chain for binding with THP, which could in part explain the variable nephrotoxicity of light chains.[7] This specificity of the individual light chains for THP was illustrated by the finding that the intraperitoneal instillation of light chains isolated from humans with specific renal light chain–associated disease induces the same renal injury in animals.[8] Whereas renal injury occurs only in the presence of urinary light chains, not all light chains are associated with injury, and neither the amount nor type of urinary light chain correlates with the severity of cast formation. Nevertheless, in general, the higher the urinary excretion of light chains, the greater the risk for renal failure.[9,10] In addition to light chain–specific factors, tubular solute composition and tubular

Etiology of Renal Injury and Clinical Manifestations

	Cause	Manifestation
Prerenal		
Volume depletion	Hypercalcemia	Polyuria and polydipsia
	Gastrointestinal losses (nausea and vomiting)	Hypotension
	Sepsis	Fever
Hemodynamic	Hemodynamic from NSAIDs	Oliguria, hyperkalemia
Other	Hyperviscosity (IgA, IgG_3)	Mental state alterations
	Hyperuricemia	Tumor lysis
Renal	Proximal tubular injury from light chains, urate; distal tubular injury from casts	Fanconi syndrome
		Tubular proteinuria
		Crystalluria
	Glomerular disease (LCDD, amyloid)	Nephrotic proteinuria
		Hematuria, active sediment
Post Renal	Calculi	Colic

Figure 63.1 Etiology of renal injury and clinical manifestations. LCDD, light-chain deposition disease; NSAIDs, nonsteroidal anti-inflammatory drugs.

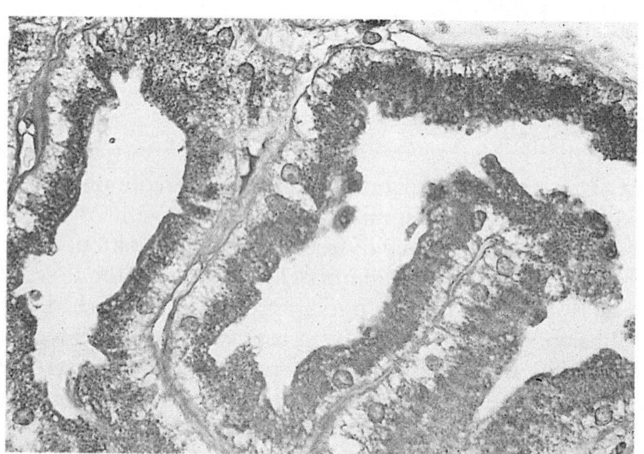

Figure 63.2 Uptake of light chains by proximal tubular cells. Renal biopsy specimen from a patient excreting κ light chains. Immunoperoxidase staining showing κ light chains along the brush border and in the cytoplasm of the PTC (brown stain).

flow rates modulate the risk for cast formation. In animals, urinary acidification, furosemide, and urinary sodium and calcium concentration may affect the tendency to increased binding or aggregation of light chains with THP; colchicine may reduce this tendency in animals but not in humans.[11,12] The formation and passage of casts distally can occlude the tubule and allow intratubular obstruction, with rupture and even backflow of contents (Fig. 63.3).

EPIDEMIOLOGY

Most myeloma presents *de novo*, although a small number evolve from patients with monoclonal gammopathy of undetermined significance (MGUS) each year. In Europe, approximately 50 cases per million occur annually. In patients with newly diagnosed myeloma, the prevalence of IgG, IgA, IgD, and free light chain–only myeloma was 52%, 21%, 2%, and 16%, respectively.[9] IgM and IgE myeloma are extremely uncommon. Approximately 70% of patients with myeloma also have a urinary M protein. At the time of diagnosis of myeloma, up to 50% of patients have evidence of impaired renal function judged by increased serum creatinine; around 25% present with serum creatinine concentration above 2 mg/dl (177 μmol/l).[9,10] In unselected series, 2% to 10% of patients present with severe renal failure requiring dialysis; this figure is higher in series reported from renal units. In contrast to the general distribution of M protein types in myeloma, light-chain and IgD myeloma are particularly associated with the risk of renal disease, being present in nearly 50% of patients with severe renal disease requiring dialysis.[13]

CLINICAL PRESENTATION

Most patients present with constitutional symptoms (fatigue, weight loss) and skeletal pain, especially back pain. Renal impairment is common and has a variety of causes (see Fig. 60.1). In a smaller proportion of patients, renal failure is the presenting manifestation of myeloma, and the diagnosis of myeloma is made or suggested by the renal biopsy findings. In general, these patients have more advanced disease with high morbidity and mortality.[13] Renal findings are nonspecific, usually with kidneys of normal size and bland urine. Urinary protein excretion may be marked because of the presence of light chains, whereas urinary dipstick may indicate only small amounts of protein because this measures albumin. Normal or elevated ionized calcium, decreased serum anion gap, lytic bone lesions on radiographic examination, hypogammaglobulinemia or reductions in levels of other immunoglobulin classes (immune paresis), abnormal serum free light chain ratio, significant cytopenias, and blood film changes (plasma cells or leukoerythroblastic film) are suggestive of myeloma. Clinical and laboratory findings that may distinguish myeloma cast nephropathy from other monoclonal immunoglobulin deposition diseases are listed in Figure 63.4 and discussed in Chapter 26.

PATHOLOGY

Histologic examination of the kidney in myeloma has diagnostic and prognostic utility, although it is not always required, and the risk of complications after biopsy may be increased. Biopsy is useful for the initial evaluation of AKI and to guide treatments designed to reverse AKI. Figure 63.5 lists the likely findings and prevalence of renal injury noted at histologic or autopsy sampling. Myeloma cast nephropathy, the most common histologic finding, occurs in 30% to 50% of patients (Figs. 63.6 and 63.7A). Myeloma cast nephropathy is characterized by many distal tubular casts that are strongly eosinophilic and consist of the monoclonal light chains and laminated THP, which often appear

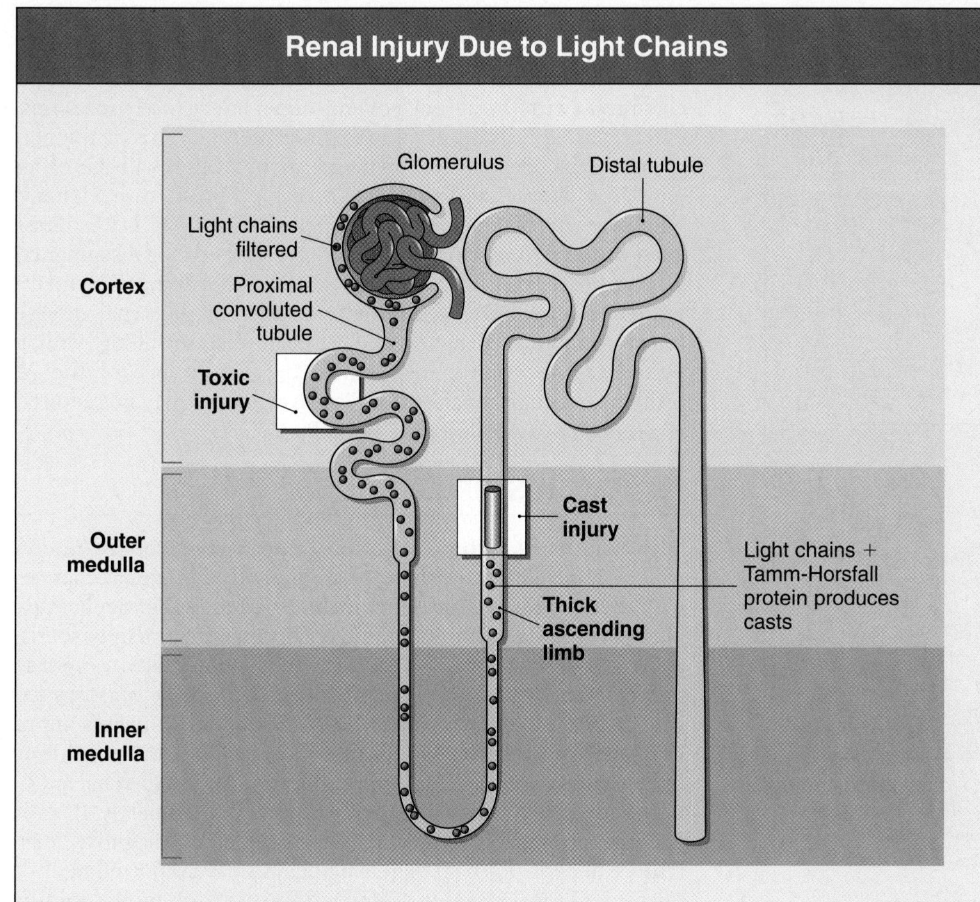

Figure 63.3 Renal injury caused by light chains. Sites *(shaded boxes)* where light chains injure the tubule. In the proximal tubule, there is direct tubular cytotoxicity. In the distal tubule, there is cast injury.

fractured after fixation. Casts promote local inflammation with giant cell formation.[14,15] In 30% of cases, cast formation may not be prominent despite extensive tubulointerstitial injury (Fig. 63.7B, C).[16] Glomeruli are usually spared unless there is associated light-chain deposition disease or amyloidosis (see Chapter 26).

DIAGNOSIS AND DIFFERENTIAL DIAGNOSIS

The International Myeloma Working Group (2003) diagnostic criteria for symptomatic myeloma require (1) detection and quantification of a monoclonal protein by serum electrophoresis (SEP) and characterization by immunofixation electrophoresis (IFE), (2) bone marrow (clonal) plasma cells or biopsy-proven plasmacytoma, and (3) demonstration of any end-organ damage not otherwise explained by other pathologic processes (including hypercalcemia, renal failure, anemia, and lytic bone disease).[17] The monoclonal M protein is the key abnormality required for diagnosis, and 97% of patients have an intact immunoglobulin or a free light chain by SEP and IFE. The quantity of the M protein is estimated from the SEP and may be used both for diagnosis and to monitor response to therapy. Urinary light chain (Bence Jones protein) concentration is determined from a concentrated sample, but despite this, light chains may still be below the level of detection by IFE. The new specific quantitative free light chain assay (which measures only light chains not bound to whole immunoglobulin) for both urine and serum is significantly more sensitive than SEP and IFE alone and is an automated assay that allows rapid diagnosis.[18-20] An abnormal monoclonal free light chain clone increases the specific light chain fraction and may suppress the other light chains, which alters the normal ratio of free light chains (0.26-1.65 κ:λ) to reflect the oversecretion of the abnormal light chain clone (e.g., <0.26 for λ free light chain clone, >1.65 for κ clone). The normal serum levels of free light chains are very low (7 to 13 mg/l), but in patients with impaired renal function, accumulation of both (κ and λ) free light chains is due to reduced excretion, and the ratio generally remains within the normal range. However, because λ free light chains tend to circulate as dimers, their clearance is reduced more than the monomeric κ free light chains, and this may alter the ratio such that the use of an extended reference range of 0.37 to 3.1 improves diagnostic sensitivity for myeloma to 99% with 100% specificity in the presence of renal failure.[20] The absolute value of the serum monoclonal light chains is of lesser importance in diagnosis. In general, patients with renal failure without myeloma have polyclonal increases in free light chains on the order of 10 to 20 times normal; but in biopsy-proven cast nephropathy, the ratios are highly abnormal, and the absolute increases in free light chains are on the order of 100 to 200 times normal and have values above 500 mg/l (usually >1000 mg/l) at presentation (Fig. 63.8).[20] Measurement of serum free light chains has significant advantages over SEP and IFE and is now incorporated into international clinical guidelines for the diagnosis and management of myeloma.[21]

Diagnostic difficulties can arise in elderly patients who are evaluated for newly diagnosed renal impairment and routine SEP reveals an M protein. Approximately 3% of the population older than 70 years will have a serum M protein, most consistent

Differentiating Features of Myeloma Kidney and Other Monoclonal Immune Deposition Diseases

	Myeloma Kidney	Other MIDDs
Proteinuria	<3 g/l	>3 g/l
Hematuria	Rare	LCDD, occasional Amyloidosis, rare
Hypercalcemia (or normal corrected calcium)	Common	Absent
Hypertension	Uncommon	LCDD common Amyloidosis uncommon
Cytopenias	Anemia very common Leukopenia and thrombocytopenia, occasional	Uncommon
Immunoparesis*	Very common	Uncommon
Lytic bone lesions	Very common	Absent
Renal impairment	Common	Common
Heavy chain	IgA, IgD, IgG	None
Type of light chain	Either	Amyloid λ > κ LCDD κ > λ
Urinary light-chain excretion	Higher	Lower

Figure 63.4 Clinical features of myeloma kidney versus monoclonal immunoglobulin deposition disease. LCDD, light-chain deposition disease; MIDDs, monoclonal immunoglobulin deposition diseases. *Defined as a reduction in the nonparaprotein globulin fractions.

Renal Pathology in Patients with Multiple Myeloma

Histological Finding	Prevalence
Myeloma kidney *(Myeloma cast nephropathy)*	30%-50%
Interstitial nephritis/fibrosis without cast nephropathy	20%-30%
Amyloidosis	10%
Light chain deposition disease	5%
Acute tubular necrosis	10%
Other (urate nephropathy, tubular crystals, hypercalcemia, FSGS)	5%

Figure 63.5 Renal pathology in patients with multiple myeloma. FSGS, focal segmental glomerulosclerosis. *(From references 25, 56-61.)*

Histologic Features of Myeloma Kidney

Histologic Features of Myeloma Kidney
Many eosinophilic, often fractured casts (medullary portion of the distal nephron predominantly)
Intratubular and interstitial macrophages and giant cells in response to casts
Interstitial inflammation, fibrosis, tubular atrophy, crystalline inclusions
Minimal glomerular abnormality
Minimal or no vascular changes

Figure 63.6 Histologic features of myeloma cast nephropathy.

with MGUS. A diagnosis of MGUS is more likely if the serum level of the M protein is low (<3 g/dl), urinary light chains are absent or very low (<1 g/24 h), and there is a normal free light chain ratio with the absence of end-organ injury (no lytic lesions, <10% plasma cells on bone marrow aspirate).[22] This distinction is important because most patients with MGUS will die of an unrelated disease, and only 1% a year progress to myeloma.[23] The majority of renal disease in patients with MGUS is unrelated to the M protein,[24] although rare cases of focal segmental glomerulosclerosis have been associated with a dysproteinemia.[25] Evidence supportive of alternative causes of the renal disease (most commonly diabetes and vascular disease) along with a period of observation may clarify the significance of the M protein, although renal or bone marrow biopsy may be required when diagnostic uncertainty persists.

NATURAL HISTORY

The majority of patients with renal impairment at presentation will show resolution of these predominantly functional changes with therapeutic measures that include withdrawal of nephrotoxins, rehydration, treatment of hypercalcemia, treatment of sepsis, and reduction in light-chain load with chemotherapy. Response to treatment with improvement in renal function is associated with improved clinical outcomes.[26] Reversibility occurs more frequently with lesser degrees of initial renal impairment, lower light-chain excretion, and hypercalcemia. Although renal function improves in the majority of patients, approximately 10% of patients presenting with renal impairment at diagnosis may require dialysis. Patients requiring dialysis have reported rates of recovery of renal function as low as 5% to 15% or, more recently, up to 30%.[27] This recovery sometimes occurs many months after presentation.

TREATMENT

There are three key issues in the management of myeloma cast nephropathy. The first is to suspect and to diagnose myeloma in the differential diagnosis of AKI, and the inclusion of serum free light chain measurement for routine evaluation of otherwise unexplained AKI in appropriate clinical circumstances is essential. This is because renal injury in myeloma is directly related to free light chain excess, and the increased sensitivity and specificity of free light chain measurement along with its rapid availability may implicate or refute myeloma as a likely diagnostic possibility days in advance of standard tests (SPE, IFE) or renal biopsy. Early diagnosis is crucial to allow implementation of the second strategy, which is to prevent or to reverse oliguria by rapid identification and management of possible contributing factors to renal impairment, which are present in around 50% of patients. Hypercalcemia, sepsis, and nonsteroidal anti-inflammatory agents are the most common precipitants. Intravenous volume expansion is helpful to increase glomerular filtration, to reduce single-nephron light-chain concentration, and to increase tubular flow. The use of furosemide to promote diuresis should be avoided as this may favor cast formation. There is no clinical evidence of the superiority of sodium bicarbonate over sodium chloride for volume expansion, although prevention of urinary acidification is in theory desirable and in severe renal failure may be necessary for management of metabolic acidosis. The maintenance of a high fluid intake (3 l/day) with water after initial volume correction and restoration of urine output with intravenous crystalloid is recommended

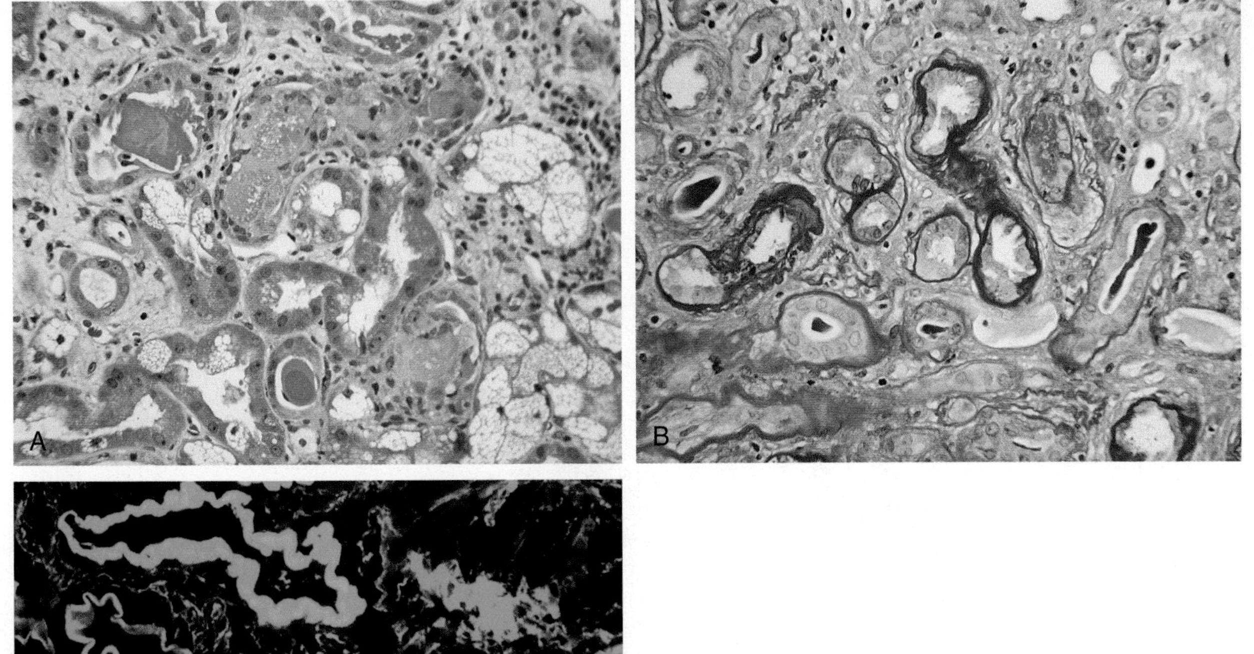

Figure 63.7 Myeloma cast nephropathy. A, Myeloma kidney. Many dilated tubules are obstructed by densely eosinophilic hard casts, with giant cell reaction and inflammatory cell infiltrates. There is also vacuolation and degeneration of tubules. (Hematoxylin and eosin stain; magnification ×160.) **B,** Light-chain deposition along tubular basement membrane in myeloma kidney without casts. There is marked thickening of the tubular basement membrane by deposits positive for periodic acid–Schiff, interstitial fibrosis, and mild chronic inflammation. (Periodic acid–Schiff stain; magnification ×160.) **C,** Light-chain deposition along tubular basement membrane: strong linear deposition of κ light chain in the thickened tubular basement membrane. (Direct immunofluorescence anti–κ light chain; magnification ×160.) *(Courtesy R. Sinniah, Perth, Australia.)*

to maintain high urine flow rates. Hydration before the use of contrast agents for radiologic or other procedures is essential.[28,29]

The third key requirement is the rapid reduction of free light chains in the serum by chemotherapy and, in patients with proven cast nephropathy, by enhanced dialysis (see later discussion) or in some cases plasma exchange. The immediate commencement of high-dose dexamethasone (40 mg daily) is recommended as plasma cells are highly responsive to corticosteroids, which induce rapid apoptosis and lowering of light-chain concentration. The addition of newer chemotherapy strategies (see later discussion) with high immediate light-chain lowering effects in combination with corticosteroids is also critical to rapid response.[30,31] The routine addition of plasma exchange to conventional treatment did not improve either recovery from renal failure or patient survival.[27] The large volume of distribution of light chains (which freely cross cell membranes) is not well suited to plasma exchange; however, in some circumstances, its use as an adjunct with chemotherapy may be considered beneficial.[32] The use of a new Polyflux dialysis membrane (HCO 1100, Gambro Scientific Research), with a high cutoff up to 50 kd, in conjunction with early chemotherapy has been shown to reverse renal failure in association with the rapid reduction in circulating free light chains in patients with cast nephropathy.[33] The optimal use of this membrane is under clinical trial and may differ according to the type of light chain, response to chemotherapy, use of convective therapies, and extended duration of dialysis.[34] A suggested algorithm for management of myeloma with AKI is shown in Figure 63.9.

Chemotherapy

Although myeloma is incurable, with a median survival of all patients around 3 years, chemotherapy will induce clinical improvement by control of the underlying disease. Until recently, no therapy had proved superior to cyclical melphalan and prednisone. The use of melphalan in patients with renal impairment (glomerular filtration rate <30 ml/min) requires dose adjustment to avoid the risk of significant hematologic toxicity.[35] Autologous stem cell transplantation (ASCT) significantly extends survival

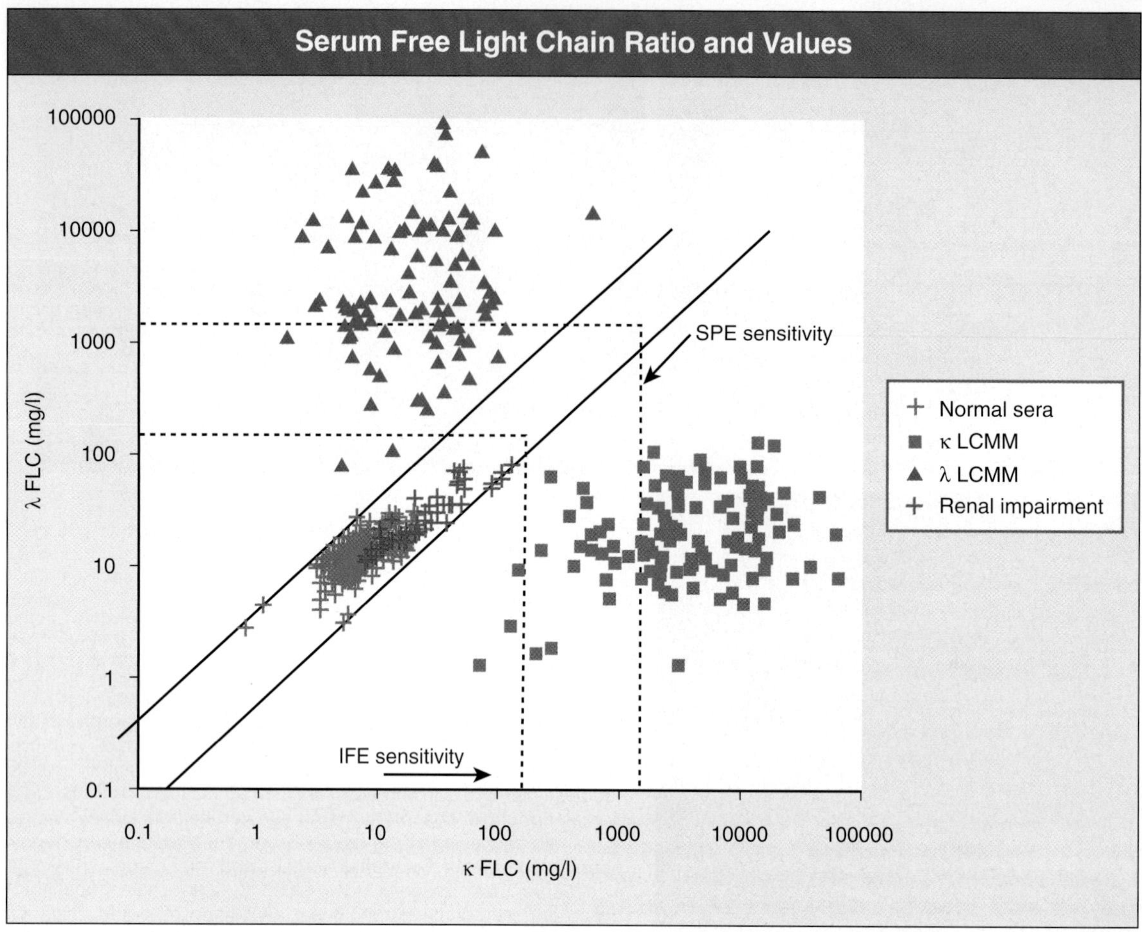

Figure 63.8 Serum free light chain ratio and values in normal individuals, patients with renal impairment, and light-chain myeloma. FLC, free light chain; IFE, immunofixation electrophoresis; SPE, serum protein electrophoresis; LCMM, light chain multiple myeloma. *(Reprinted with permission from reference 20.)*

and is now the treatment of choice for eligible patients.[36] Even patients with renal impairment and on dialysis may be suitable for ASCT, although increased morbidity and mortality are recognized.[37,38] For the very elderly, chemotherapy selection is dependent on comorbidity, and melphalan-prednisone or dexamethasone-thalidomide may be useful. Close multidisciplinary management and discussion with hematology and oncology services are required to individualize decision-making because of the rapid advances in this area.[39] Bortezomib, a reversible proteasome inhibitor whose clearance is independent of renal function, has been successfully and safely used in patients with severe degrees of renal failure and myeloma without significant toxicity and may be the agent of choice for rapid reduction of light chains in combination with dexamethasone and hemodialysis.[30] Thalidomide and lenalidomide are increasingly used first or as consolidation or maintenance therapy. Side effects of thalidomide include peripheral neuropathy, venous thrombosis, and teratogenicity. Preliminary data support use of thalidomide in patients with relapsed or refractory myeloma and renal failure, without need for dose alteration,[40] although concerns about hyperkalemia have been raised.[41] The newer and more potent agent lenalidomide may have reduced neurotoxicity; however, its use in renal failure is less well established, and myelosuppression may be more common in patients with reduced glomerular filtration rate.[42]

Infection and progression of disease remain the major impediments to survival, especially within the higher risk end-stage renal disease (ESRD) group. Median survival in recent ESRD series with conventional therapies before ASCT was only 4 to 8 months; however, survival of up to 5 years is reported in selected cases of ESRD managed with ASCT.[43]

Adjunctive Therapies

Patients with CKD or ESRD and myeloma respond to erythropoiesis-stimulating agents, and these should be used along with other hematopoietic agents including granulocyte colony-stimulating factor as required, although frequent transfusion may be necessary early in the disease.[44] Intravenous bisphosphonates rapidly correct hypercalcemia and are preferred to furosemide (which may aggravate tubular light-chain injury) and in the longer term reduce bone fracture.[45] However, there are several reports of toxicity (acute tubular necrosis, proteinuria) with high dose or rapid infusion of pamidronate and zoledronic acid; reduced doses (pamidronate, 30 to 60 mg; zoledronic acid, 2 to 4 mg) and slower infusion rates are recommended.[46,47] Replacement of profound immunoglobulin deficiency with regular intravenous immune globulin (IVIG) has been proven to reduce infectious complications in stable treated myeloma patients but is not widely adopted although recommended.[48] Caution is required to avoid further AKI due to the hyperosmolarity of IVIG because renal impairment and diabetes represent known risk factors for this complication.[49]

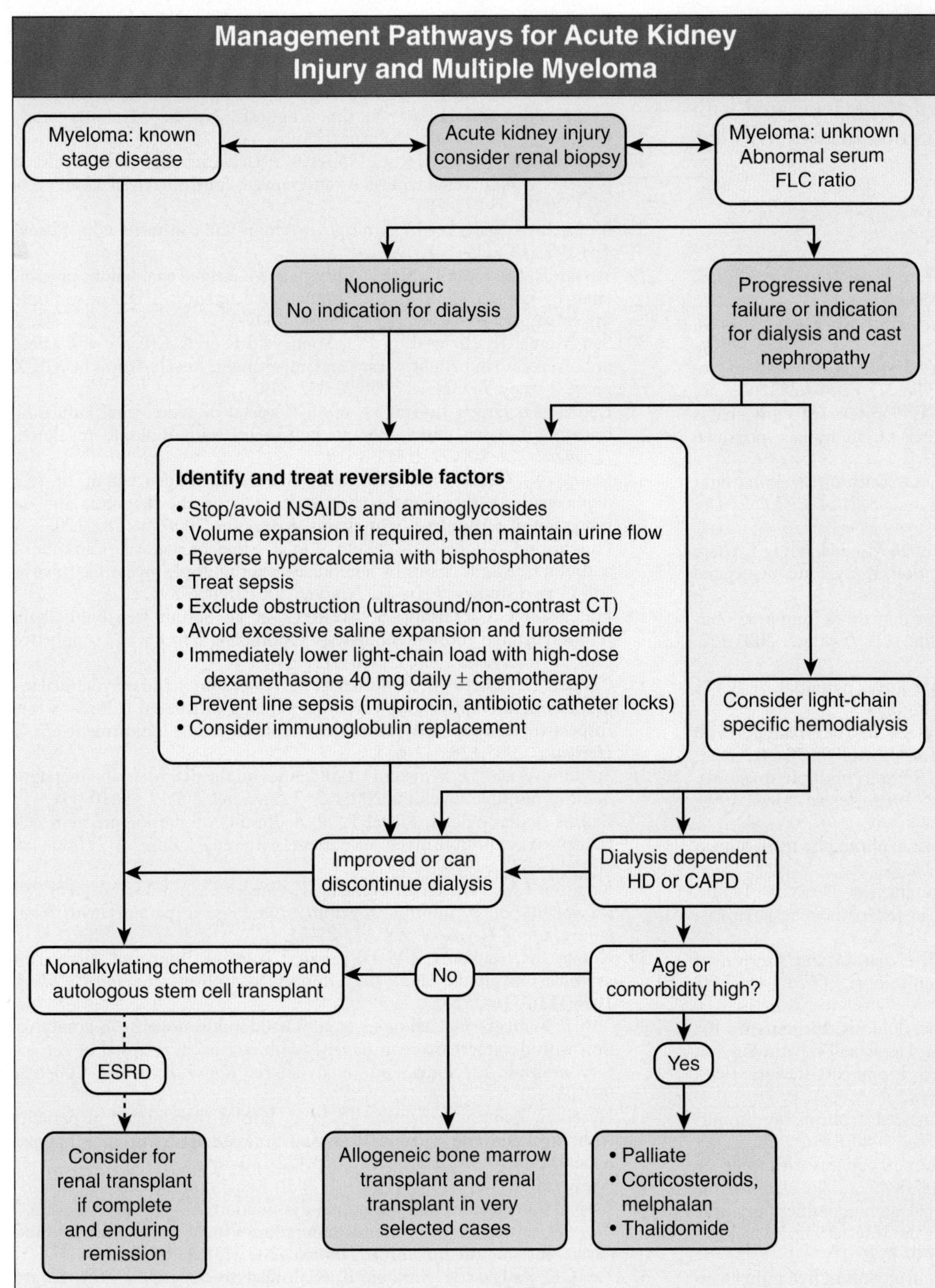

Management Pathways for Acute Kidney Injury and Multiple Myeloma
Myeloma: known stage disease
Acute kidney injury consider renal biopsy
Myeloma: unknown Abnormal serum FLC ratio
Nonoliguric No indication for dialysis
Progressive renal failure or indication for dialysis and cast nephropathy
Identify and treat reversible factors
• Stop/avoid NSAIDs and aminoglycosides
• Volume expansion if required, then maintain urine flow
• Reverse hypercalcemia with bisphosphonates
• Treat sepsis
• Exclude obstruction (ultrasound/non-contrast CT)
• Avoid excessive saline expansion and furosemide
• Immediately lower light-chain load with high-dose dexamethasone 40 mg daily ± chemotherapy
• Prevent line sepsis (mupirocin, antibiotic catheter locks)
• Consider immunoglobulin replacement
Consider light-chain specific hemodialysis
Improved or can discontinue dialysis
Dialysis dependent HD or CAPD
Nonalkylating chemotherapy and autologous stem cell transplant
No
Age or comorbidity high?
Yes
ESRD
Consider for renal transplant if complete and enduring remission
Allogeneic bone marrow transplant and renal transplant in very selected cases
• Palliate
• Corticosteroids, melphalan
• Thalidomide

Figure 63.9 Management of myeloma and AKI. CAPD, continuous ambulatory peritoneal dialysis; CT, computed tomography; ESRD, end-stage renal disease; FLC, free light chain; HD, hemodialysis; NSAIDs, nonsteroidal anti-inflammatory drugs.

Dialysis and Transplantation

Where renal replacement therapy is required long term, both hemodialysis and peritoneal dialysis have been successfully used, and there are no data to indicate that outcome is influenced by dialysis modality. Choice of long-term therapy requires individual assessment of patient circumstances. The majority of studies support the use of dialysis, although survival is substantially reduced and early mortality (30%) is high in this group due to the severity of tumor burden and the high rates of sepsis.[50-52] Aggressive measures to reduce risk of systemic infection by antibiotic line locking or mupirocin at exit sites and the use of IVIG replacement should be routinely considered because a dependency on central venous catheters for dialysis, plasma exchange, and chemotherapy is often required initially. The timing of placement of a permanent arteriovenous fistula requires an individualized risk assessment because it may be several months before irreversibility of renal failure and a response to chemotherapy are proven. Renal transplantation has a high risk of disease recurrence in the allograft and patient mortality, and given the incurability of the disease, it has rarely been appropriate.[53] Most recently, several cases of allogeneic bone marrow and renal allograft transplantation have been reported, demonstrating the ability to induce allograft tolerance in haploidentical pairs.[54] This treatment is limited in availability and suitability for the majority of patients. The use of renal transplantation after successful induction therapy and ASCT is unknown but may be suitable for younger patients when disease remission by standard criteria and normalization of the serum free light chain ratio are achieved. ASCT itself has been reported to be associated with recovery of renal function when the duration of dialysis is less than 6 months.[43,55]

REFERENCES

1. San Miguel JF, Garcia-Sanz R. Prognostic features of multiple myeloma. *Best Pract Res Clin Haematol.* 2005;18:569-583.
2. Chen-Kiang. Biology of plasma cells. *Best Pract Res Clin Haematol.* 2005;18:493-507.
3. Batuman V, Verroust PJ, Navar GL, et al. Myeloma light chains are ligands for cubilin (gp280). *Am J Physiol.* 1998;275:F246-F254.
4. Sengul S, Zwizinski C, Simon EE, et al. Endocytosis of light chains induces cytokines through activation of NF-κB in human proximal tubule cells. *Kidney Int.* 2002;62:1977-1988.
5. Pote A, Zwizinski C, Simon EE, et al. Cytotoxicity of myeloma light chains in cultured human kidney proximal tubule cells. *Am J Kidney Dis.* 2000;36:735-744.
6. Aucouturier P, Bauwens M, Khamlichi AA, et al. Monoclonal Ig L chain and L chain V domain fragment crystallization in myeloma-associated Fanconi's syndrome. *J Immunol.* 1993;150:3561-3568.
7. Ying WZ, Sanders PW. Mapping the binding domain of immunoglobulin light chains for Tamm-Horsfall protein. *Am J Pathol.* 2001;158:1859-1866.
8. Solomon A, Weiss DT, Kattine AA. Nephrotoxic potential of Bence Jones proteins. *N Engl J Med.* 1991;324:1845-1851.
9. Kyle RA, Gertz MA, Witzig TA, et al. Review of 1027 patients with newly diagnosed multiple myeloma. *Mayo Clin Proc.* 2003;78:21-33.
10. Alexanian R, Barlogie B, Dixon D. Renal failure in multiple myeloma. Pathogenesis and prognostic implications. *Arch Intern Med.* 1990;150:1693-1695.
11. Sanders PW, Booker BB. Pathobiology of cast nephropathy from human Bence Jones proteins. *J Clin Invest.* 1992;89:630-639.
12. Huang ZQ, Sanders PW. Biochemical interaction between Tamm-Horsfall glycoprotein and Ig light chains in the pathogenesis of cast nephropathy. *Lab Invest.* 1995;73:810-817.
13. Irish AB, Winearls CG, Littlewood T. Presentation and survival of patients with severe renal failure and myeloma. *QJM.* 1997;90:773-780.
14. Schwartz MM. The dysproteinemias and amyloidosis. In: Jennette JC, Olson JL, Schwartz MM, Silva FG, eds. Hepinstall's Pathology of the Kidney. vol 2. 5th ed. Philadelphia: Lippincott-Raven; 1998:1321-1369.
15. Start DA, Silva FG, Davis LD, et al. Myeloma cast nephropathy: Immunohistochemical and lectin studies. *Mod Pathol.* 1988;1:336-347.
16. Ivanyi B. Development of chronic renal failure in patients with multiple myeloma. *Arch Pathol Lab Med.* 1993;117:837-840.
17. Criteria for the classification of monoclonal gammopathies, multiple myeloma and related disorders: A report of the International Myeloma Working Group. *Br J Haematol.* 2003;121:749-757.
18. Nowrousian MR, Brandhorst D, Sammet C, et al. Serum free light chain analysis and urine immunofixation electrophoresis in patients with multiple myeloma. *Clin Cancer Res.* 2005;11:8706-8714.
19. Katzmann JA, Abraham RS, Dispenzieri A, et al. Diagnostic performance of quantitative kappa and lambda free light chain assays in clinical practice. *Clin Chem.* 2005;51:878-881.
20. Hutchison CA, Plant T, Drayson M, et al. Serum free light chain measurement aids the diagnosis of myeloma in patients with severe renal failure. *BMC Nephrol.* 2008;9:11.
21. Dispenzieri A, Kyle R, Merlini G, et al. International Myeloma Working Group guidelines for serum-free light chain analysis in multiple myeloma and related disorders. *Leukemia.* 2009;23:215-224.
22. Rajkumar SV, Kyle RA, Therneau TM, et al. Serum free light chain ratio is an independent risk factor for progression in monoclonal gammopathy of undetermined significance. *Blood.* 2005;106:812-817.
23. Kyle RA, Therneau TM, Rajkumar SV, et al. Long-term follow-up of 241 patients with monoclonal gammopathy of undetermined significance: The original Mayo Clinic series 25 years later. *Mayo Clin Proc.* 2004;79:859-866.
24. Paueksakon P, Revelo MP, Horn RG, et al. Monoclonal gammopathy: Significance and possible causality in renal disease. *Am J Kidney Dis.* 2003;42:87-95.
25. Dingli D, Larson DR, Plevak MF, et al. Focal and segmental glomerulosclerosis and plasma cell proliferative disorders. *Am J Kidney Dis.* 2005;46:278-282.
26. Knudsen LM, Hjorth M, Hippe E. Renal failure in multiple myeloma: Reversibility and impact on the prognosis. Nordic Myeloma Study Group. *Eur J Haematol.* 2000;65:175-181.
27. Clark WF, Stewart AK, Rock GA, et al. Plasma exchange when myeloma presents as acute renal failure: A randomized, controlled trial. *Ann Intern Med.* 2005;143:777-784.
28. McCarthy CS, Becker JA. Multiple myeloma and contrast media. *Radiology.* 1992;183:519-521.
29. Yussim E, Schwartz E, Sidi Y, Ehrenfeld M. Acute renal failure precipitated by non-steroidal anti-inflammatory drugs (NSAIDs) in multiple myeloma. *Am J Hematol.* 1998;58:142-144.
30. San-Miguel JF, Richardson PG, Sonneveld P, et al. Efficacy and safety of bortezomib in patients with renal impairment: Results from the APEX phase 3 study. *Leukemia.* 2008;22:842-849.
31. Ludwig H, Drach J, Graf H, et al. Reversal of acute renal failure by bortezomib-based chemotherapy in patients with multiple myeloma. *Haematologica.* 2007;92:1411-1414.
32. Leung N, Gertz MA, Zeldenrust SR, et al. Improvement of cast nephropathy with plasma exchange depends on the diagnosis and on reduction of serum free light chains. *Kidney Int.* 2008;73:1282-1288.
33. Hutchison CA, Cockwell P, Reid S, et al. Efficient removal of immunoglobulin free light chains by hemodialysis for multiple myeloma: In vitro and in vivo studies. *J Am Soc Nephrol.* 2007;18:886-895.
34. Hutchison CA, Harding S, Mead G, et al. Serum free–light chain removal by high cutoff hemodialysis: Optimizing removal and supportive care. *Artif Organs.* 2008;32:910-917.
35. Carlson K, Hjorth M, Knudsen LM. Toxicity in standard melphalan-prednisone therapy among myeloma patients with renal failure—a retrospective analysis and recommendations for dose adjustment. *Br J Haematol.* 2005;128:631-635.
36. Smith A, Wisloff F, Samson D. Guidelines on the diagnosis and management of multiple myeloma 2005. *Br J Haematol.* 2006;132:410-451.
37. Badros A, Barlogie B, Siegel E, et al. Results of autologous stem cell transplant in multiple myeloma patients with renal failure. *Br J Haematol.* 2001;114:822-829.
38. Knudsen LM, Nielsen B, Gimsing P, Geisler C. Autologous stem cell transplantation in multiple myeloma: Outcome in patients with renal failure. *Eur J Haematol.* 2005;75:27-33.
39. Kumar SK, Rajkumar SV, Dispenzieri A, et al. Improved survival in multiple myeloma and the impact of novel therapies. *Blood.* 2008;111:2516-2520.
40. Tosi P, Zamagni E, Cellini C, et al. Thalidomide alone or in combination with dexamethasone in patients with advanced, relapsed or refractory multiple myeloma and renal failure. *Eur J Haematol.* 2004;73:98-103.
41. Harris E, Behrens J, Samson D, et al. Use of thalidomide in patients with myeloma and renal failure may be associated with unexplained hyperkalaemia. *Br J Haematol.* 2003;122:160-161.
42. Niesvizky R, Naib T, Christos PJ, et al. Lenalidomide-induced myelosuppression is associated with renal dysfunction: Adverse events evaluation of treatment-naive patients undergoing front-line lenalidomide and dexamethasone therapy. *Br J Haematol.* 2007;138:640-643.
43. Lee CK, Zangari M, Barlogie B, et al. Dialysis-dependent renal failure in patients with myeloma can be reversed by high-dose myeloablative therapy and autotransplant. *Bone Marrow Transplant.* 2004;33:823-828.
44. Goldschmidt H, Lannert H, Bommer J, Ho AD. Multiple myeloma and renal failure. *Nephrol Dial Transplant.* 2000;15:301-304.
45. Ashcroft AJ, Davies FE, Morgan GJ. Aetiology of bone disease and the role of bisphosphonates in multiple myeloma. *Lancet Oncol.* 2003;4:284-292.
46. Desikan R, Veksler Y, Raza S, et al. Nephrotic proteinuria associated with high-dose pamidronate in multiple myeloma. *Br J Haematol.* 2002;119:496-499.
47. Munier A, Gras V, Andrejak M, et al. Zoledronic acid and renal toxicity: Data from French adverse effect reporting database. *Ann Pharmacother.* 2005;39:1194-1197.
48. Chapel HM, Lee M. The use of intravenous immune globulin in multiple myeloma. *Clin Exp Immunol.* 1994;97(Suppl 1):21-24.
49. Sati HIA, Ahya R, Watson HG. Incidence and associations of acute renal failure complicating high-dose intravenous immunoglobulin therapy. *Br J Haematol.* 2001;113:556-557.
50. Iggo N, Palmer AB, Severn A, et al. Chronic dialysis in patients with multiple myeloma and renal failure: A worthwhile treatment. *Q J Med.* 1989;73:903-910.

51. Korzets A, Tam F, Russell G, et al. The role of continuous ambulatory peritoneal dialysis in end-stage renal failure due to multiple myeloma. *Am J Kidney Dis*. 1990;16:216-223.
52. Sharland A, Snowdon L, Joshua DE, et al. Hemodialysis: An appropriate therapy in myeloma-induced renal failure. *Am J Kidney Dis*. 1997;30: 786-792.
53. Sammett D, Gagher F, Abbi R, et al. Renal transplantation in multiple myeloma. *Transplantation*. 1996;62:1577-1580.
54. Buhler LH, Spitzer TR, Sykes M, et al. Induction of kidney allograft tolerance after transient lymphohematopoietic chimerism in patients with multiple myeloma and end-stage renal disease. *Transplantation*. 2002;74:1405-1409.
55. Tauro S, Clark FJ, Duncan N, et al. Recovery of renal function after autologous stem cell transplantation in myeloma patients with end-stage renal failure. *Bone Marrow Transplant*. 2002;30:471-473.
56. Montseny JJ, Kleinknecht D, Meyrier A, et al. Long-term outcome according to renal histological lesions in 118 patients with monoclonal gammopathies. *Nephrol Dial Transplant*. 1998;13:1438-1445.
57. Touchard G. Renal biopsy in multiple myeloma and in other monoclonal immunoglobulin-producing diseases. *Ann Med Interne (Paris)*. 1992;143(Suppl 1):80-83.
58. Sanders PW, Herrera GA, Kirk KA, et al. Spectrum of glomerular and tubulointerstitial renal lesions associated with monotypical immunoglobulin light chain deposition. *Lab Invest*. 1991;64:527-537.
59. Ivanyi B. Frequency of light chain deposition nephropathy relative to renal amyloidosis and Bence Jones cast nephropathy in a necropsy study of patients with myeloma. *Arch Pathol Lab Med*. 1990;114:986-987.
60. Rota S, Mougenot B, Baudouin B, et al. Multiple myeloma and severe renal failure: A clinicopathologic study of outcome and prognosis in 34 patients. *Medicine (Baltimore)*. 1987;66:126-137.
61. Herrera GA, Joseph L, Gu X, et al. Renal pathologic spectrum in an autopsy series of patients with plasma cell dyscrasia. *Arch Pathol Lab Med*. 2004;128:875-879.

CHAPTER 64

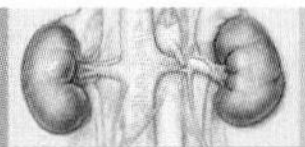

Thromboembolic Renovascular Disease

Barbara A. Greco, Jamie P. Dwyer, Julia B. Lewis

Renal arterial and venous thromboembolic disease presents as a wide variety of clinical syndromes, ranging from vascular catastrophe with acute renal infarction to progressive decline in renal function due to chronic renal ischemia. Appropriate imaging allows accurate and timely identification of renal infarction, renal artery or venous thrombosis, and other renovascular abnormalities.

Thrombotic microangiopathies are discussed in Chapter 28, and renovascular hypertension and atherosclerotic ischemic renal disease are discussed in Chapter 37.

NORMAL ANATOMY

Renal Artery

The anatomic considerations that affect the clinical outcome of renal arterial thromboembolic events include the size of the vessel involved, from the main renal artery and the branch vessels to the arterioles and glomerular capillaries, and the condition of the collateral blood supply. In most individuals, the kidney has a single artery ranging in diameter from 3 to 7 mm. The incidence of multiple renal arteries is about 30%.

Acute occlusion of the renal artery may result in sudden and irreversible renal infarction, particularly if there is a single vessel with inadequate collateral circulation. In the setting of chronic renal artery occlusive disease, such as might exist on a background of atheromatous renovascular disease, the collateral circulation may be more extensively developed.

The main collateral vessels to the kidney include the suprarenal, the lumbar, and the ureteral vessel complexes, which can maintain renal parenchymal viability in the face of main renal arterial occlusion. The collateral circulation to the kidney is depicted in Figure 64.1. In a study examining 301 aortograms, the adrenal arteries supplied collateral circulation to the kidney in 60% of cases, the lumbar in 55%, the ureteric in 15%, and the gonadal in 13%.[1] The factors determining the development and caliber of these vessels are poorly understood but are likely to relate to individual anatomy, state of the aorta, rate of progression of main renal artery narrowing, and condition of the intrarenal perforating arteries.

Renal Vein

Renal veins begin in the subcapsular region of the kidney. These stellate veins communicate with perirenal and cortical venous channels and empty into interlobular veins that drain into arcuate veins. The venae rectae drain the pyramids and join the arcuate veins. Arcuate veins leave the renal parenchyma through interlobar vessels, converging into four to six trunks near the hilum of the kidney (Fig. 64.2). The main renal veins empty into the inferior vena cava; the left renal vein is three times longer than the right (7.5 cm versus 2.5 cm). The left renal vein traverses behind the splenic vein and body of the pancreas before it crosses in front of the aorta near its termination in the inferior vena cava. The left renal vein collects the flow from the left ureteral, gonadal, adrenal, and inferior phrenic veins. In Gerota's fascia, the perirenal venous network communicates with the retroperitoneal collateral veins from the lumbar, azygos, and tributaries of the portal system.[2,3]

THROMBOEMBOLIC RENOVASCULAR DISEASE

Thromboembolic renovascular disease results in disruption of normal renal blood flow, leading to either renal ischemia or overt infarction. The caliber and type of vessels involved (artery, arteriole, vein) as well as whether one or both kidneys are affected determine the clinical presentation (Fig. 64.3).

THROMBOEMBOLIC ISCHEMIC RENAL DISEASE

Ischemic renal disease due to atherosclerotic renovascular disease is discussed in Chapter 37. On occasion, thrombosis of the renal artery or branch vessels occurs acutely and without overt renal infarction, providing a clinical opportunity for renal salvage. The clinical settings in which this might occur include spontaneous thrombosis of atherosclerotic renal artery occlusive disease, spontaneous dissection of the aorta involving the origin of the renal artery, dissection of the renal artery itself, and as a consequence of aortic or renal artery interventions including endovascular stenting.

The clinical presentation of renal artery or branch vessel thrombosis without infarction often involves acceleration of hypertension due to renin release, worsening renal function, and even anuria if all of the functioning renal mass is involved. Patients may develop volume overload, pulmonary edema, and symptoms of uremia.

The clinical evaluation of the patient includes ruling out overt renal infarction and defining renal parenchymal viability despite main renal or branch vessel thrombosis. This can be achieved by demonstrating a nephrogram on delayed venous-phase imaging by conventional renal arteriography, computed tomographic angiography (CTA) or contrast-enhanced computed tomography (CT), magnetic resonance angiography (MRA) with gadolinium enhancement, or nuclear isotope scintigraphy. The diagnostic approach is complicated in the setting of reduced renal function because of the concern of nephrotoxicity from radiocontrast dye. In addition, the use of gadolinium with MRA is contraindicated if glomerular filtration rate (GFR) is below

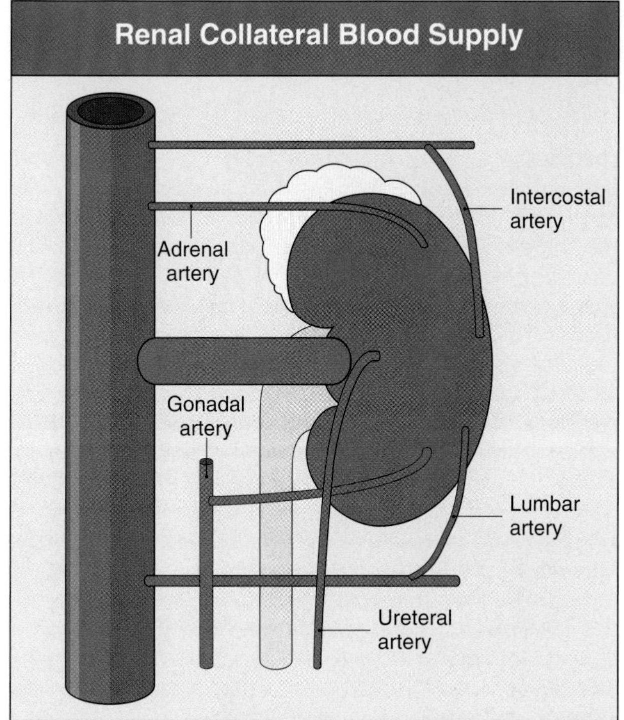

Figure 64.1 Renal collateral circulation. Diagrammatic representation of the potential collateral arterial vessels to the kidney.

30 ml/min because of the risk for nephrogenic systemic fibrosis.

Treatment involves assessment of the risks versus potential benefits of heroic revascularization procedures. The status of the contralateral kidney and overall residual renal function (RRF) should be weighed against the retrieval of the additional renal function from the ischemic kidney. The ischemic kidney's length and baseline function before thrombosis determine the potential benefits of renal revascularization. The cardiac and anesthesia risk from the intervention, such as surgical thrombectomy or bypass, has to be considered. Last, the intervention should be delayed until the clinical and renal status of the patient has recovered from any transient insults, such as acute kidney injury (AKI), decompensated pulmonary edema, congestive heart failure (CHF), myocardial infarction, and uremia.

Renal function can be salvaged by renal artery surgical revascularization and endovascular stenting in patients with dialysis-dependent renal failure due to occlusive renovascular disease.[4-6] Predictors of renal recovery are listed in Figure 64.4 and include preserved renal size, evidence of a renal "blush" or nephrogram by imaging, recent loss of GFR, and recent baseline creatinine concentration below 3 mg/dl.[7] Figure 64.5 shows thrombosis of a renal artery within a stent placed 1.5 years previously for atherosclerotic renal artery stenosis in a patient with a single functioning kidney. The patient presented with anuric AKI. Percutaneous thrombolytic therapy and renal artery angioplasty restored renal perfusion and renal function.

RENAL INFARCTION

When abrupt interruption of renal blood flow occurs without adequate collateral blood supply, renal infarction occurs. Renal infarction may involve the entire kidney or small areas of the cortex or medulla. Both arterial and venous thrombosis and renal

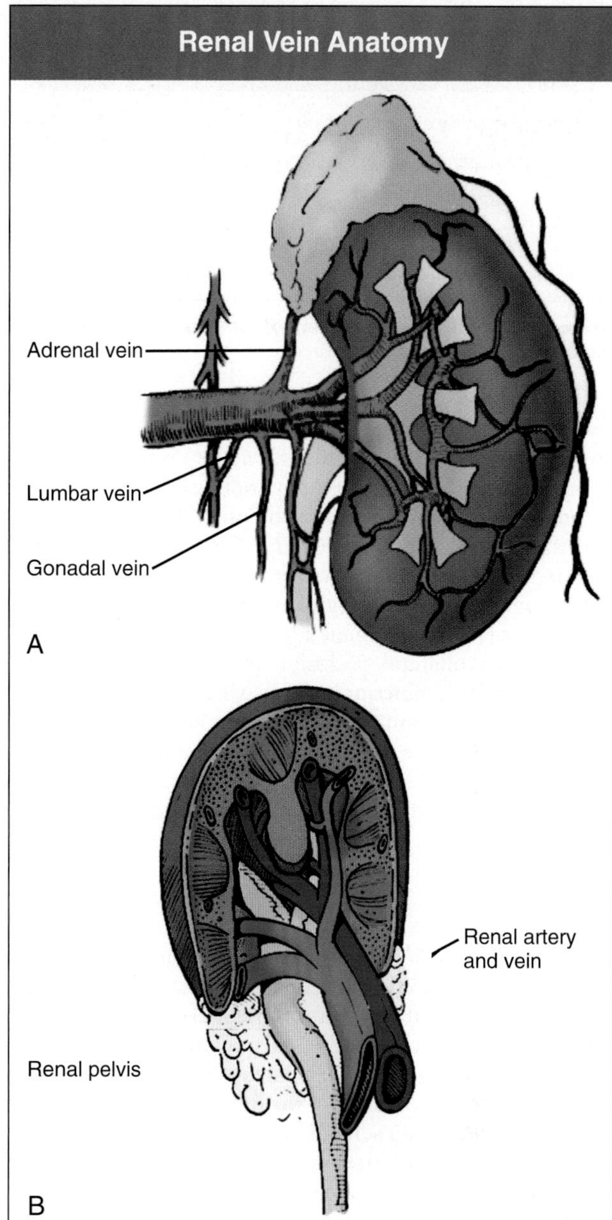

Figure 64.2 Renal vein anatomy. A, There is extensive communication between the renal venous plexus and lumbar, gonadal, and adrenal veins, which provide alternative outflow in the setting of renal vein thrombosis, particularly on the left. **B,** Transverse section of the kidney showing relative position of vascular structures in the renal pelvis. *(From reference 8.)*

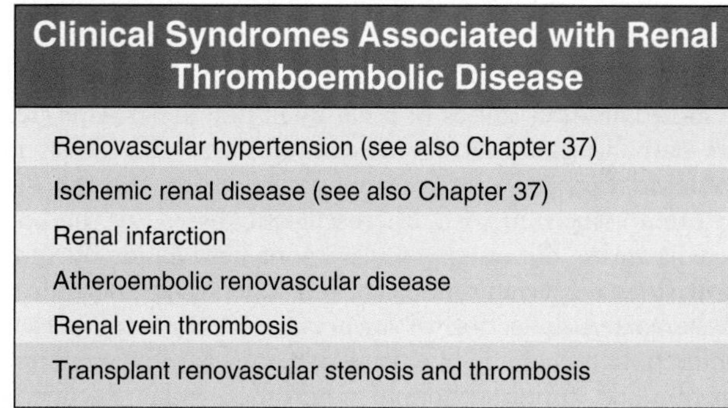

Clinical Syndromes Associated with Renal Thromboembolic Disease
Renovascular hypertension (see also Chapter 37)
Ischemic renal disease (see also Chapter 37)
Renal infarction
Atheroembolic renovascular disease
Renal vein thrombosis
Transplant renovascular stenosis and thrombosis

Figure 64.3 Clinical syndromes associated with renal thromboembolic disease.

Predictors of Recovery of Renal Function in Renal Artery Occlusion
Preserved renal size (>7–8 cm)
Recent baseline serum creatinine < 3 mg/dl (284 µmol/l)
Recent rapid loss of GFR
Nephrogram visible on delayed or venous phase imaging
Distal reconstitution of occluded renal artery

Figure 64.4 Predictors of recovery of renal function in renal artery occlusion. GFR, glomerular filtration rate.

artery embolism can cause renal infarction. Unlike thrombotic occlusion of a long-standing stenosis, acute vascular occlusion is often symptomatic. The most common presenting signs and symptoms include loin, flank, or abdominal pain; microscopic hematuria; and transient proteinuria (Fig. 64.6). Transient or accelerated hypertension may occur secondary to abrupt release of renin from the infarcted segment. Some cases may be asymptomatic but are noted as enhancing or functional defects on renal imaging. When bilateral occlusion of both kidney arteries or infarction of a single functioning kidney occurs, the patient presents with oliguric or anuric AKI. AKI is not uncommon, even when infarction is due to renal embolism rather than arterial thrombosis. Systemic signs of renal infarction include leukocytosis, fever, and elevations of lactate dehydrogenase, transaminases, creatine kinase, and alkaline phosphatase.[9]

Diagnosis

A high clinical suspicion is required for diagnosis. CT with the intravenous administration of contrast material is the imaging modality of choice and delineates those areas of the renal cortex that are not perfused. Other potential imaging techniques include MRA (with gadolinium if GFR remains above 30 ml/min or as time-of-flight or phase-contrast imaging) and nuclear renal scan with dimercaptosuccinic acid (DMSA). When the entire kidney is underperfused, it is often difficult to determine whether there may be salvageable renal parenchyma. Studies in experimental animals with acute renal artery occlusion have shown that the collateral circulation can maintain renal viability for up to 3 hours after occlusion.[10] In patients with underlying atherosclerotic renovascular disease, collateral vessels may be better developed and renal viability may be maintained for days to weeks. In these subjects, urgent arteriography to identify the location of the arterial thrombosis or embolus may allow percutaneous or surgical revascularization.

Etiology

The most common causes of renal infarction are trauma, renal artery embolism, and iatrogenic complications of endovascular procedures (Fig. 64.7). Spontaneous renal artery thrombosis is most often associated with atherosclerotic disease of the aortic or renal arteries, but other vascular anomalies include fibromuscular dysplasia, Marfan syndrome, and Ehlers-Danlos syndrome with associated dissection or aneurysms. Less common causes of infarction include hypercoagulable states, most commonly nephrotic and antiphospholipid syndromes; inflammatory diseases of the retroperitoneum or aortorenal vasculature; and thrombotic microangiopathies (TMAs).

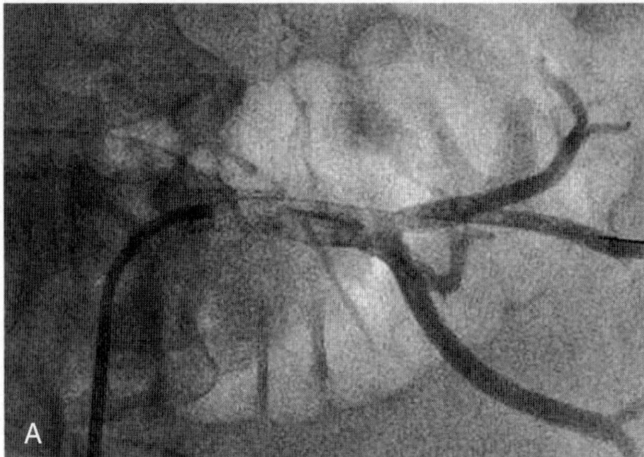

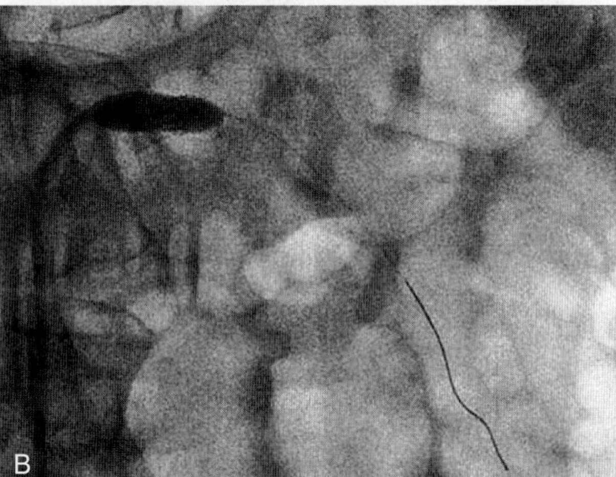

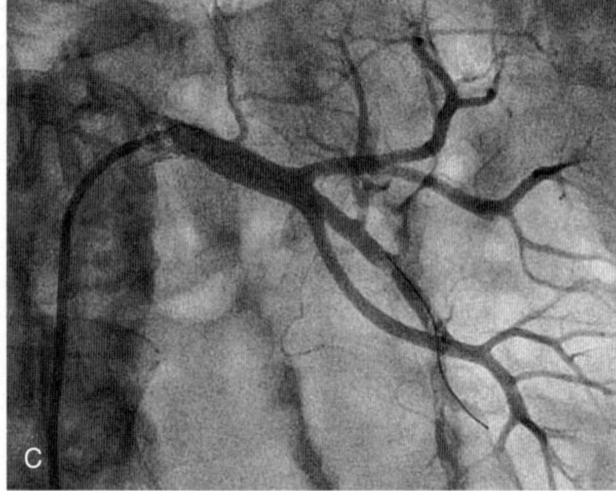

Figure 64.5 A, Thrombosis of renal artery within a previously placed stent. After tissue plasminogen activator thrombolytic infusion, recanalization allowed passage of a guide wire. **B,** Percutaneous renal artery balloon angioplasty of in-stent stenosis. **C,** Reperfusion of renal artery and kidney after percutaneous transluminal renal angioplasty.

Thrombosis due to Trauma

Traumatic injuries to the renal arteries make up 1% to 4% of all nonpenetrating abdominal trauma. Classically, kidney trauma results from a deceleration injury, such as a fall from a great height with an upright landing on impact. This results in stretching of the renal arteries as the kidneys continue downward after the rest of the body has stopped. The subsequent stretching and recoiling of the renal arteries can result in acute thrombosis,

Signs and Symptoms of Renal Infarction
Abdominal or flank pain
Leukocytosis
Fever
Hematuria
Elevations of serum LDH, transaminases, CK
Acceleration of preexisting hypertension or new onset hypertension
AKI
Incidental finding of perfusion defects on enhanced renal imaging

Figure 64.6 Signs and symptoms of renal infarction. AKI, acute kidney injury; CK, creatine kinase; LDH, lactate dehydrogenase.

which is typically bilateral. Direct blunt trauma to the loin or flank regions associated with motor vehicle crashes, street fights, and sports injuries can also result in renal artery thrombosis.

Evidence of lumbar vertebral injury should raise suspicion in the emergency department for renovascular trauma. Even when it is diagnosed early, the success rate for renal revascularization after trauma to the renal vessels remains low, between 0% and 29%.[11] Injuries to the renal pedicle that result in diminished perfusion to a single functioning kidney or to both kidneys require rapid intervention, and endovascular stabilization of renal blood flow may be helpful as a bridge to more definitive renal revascularization.

Thrombosis due to Hypercoagulable Disorders

Clotting disorders, such as protein C or protein S deficiency, antithrombin III deficiency, and rarely factor V Leiden mutations, can predispose to renal arterial thrombosis and infarction in addition to their association with renal vein thrombosis. Hypovolemia, polycythemia, and the use of oral contraceptive agents can increase the risk of thrombosis when these underlying disorders are present.

Antiphospholipid antibody syndrome is associated with both arterial and venous thrombotic events and can involve the renal circulation at any level. In patients younger than 50 years, the antiphospholipid syndrome can account for 15% to 20% of all deep venous thromboses and 30% of strokes. It is the most common cause of spontaneous arterial thrombosis. In one report of 16 cases of renal involvement with this syndrome, 15 of 16 subjects had either arterial or venous thrombosis, 10 had intrarenal microangiopathy, one had suprarenal aortic occlusion, and one had main renal artery thrombosis.[12] Concomitant thromboses in the mesenteric and cerebral circulation have been reported.[13]

Renal Artery Embolism

The kidneys are frequently the target for emboli from thrombus originating in the heart. In one series, 1.4% of the general population had renal artery embolism at autopsy, of which only 2 of 205 cases (1%) were diagnosed clinically.[14] The prevalences of left and right renal emboli are equal, and 12% of cases are bilateral.[15] Atrial fibrillation, cardiac thrombus after myocardial infarction, atrial myxoma or other cardiac tumors, endocarditis, paradoxical emboli, and aortic thrombus represent most of the conditions associated with renal embolism. Atrial fibrillation is the most common cause, with a rate of embolism four times higher than that of the general population; the highest risk is during the first year after the diagnosis of atrial fibrillation, when anticoagulation is subtherapeutic. When echocardiography is undertaken, cardiac thrombus is only rarely detected. Other causes of renal emboli include fiber or foam related to cardiac bypass procedures, calcium from valve annuli, and even "bullet emboli" in the setting of trauma. Aortic endovascular stenting has been associated with a 10% incidence of new renal infarcts, presumably of embolic etiology.[16]

Paradoxical renal artery embolism may occur in patients with right-to-left cardiac shunts. The most common cardiac shunt is

Causes of Renal Infarction

Thrombosis: spontaneous
- Atherosclerotic disease of aorta and renal artery
- Fibromuscular dysplasia of renal artery
- Aneurysms of aorta or renal artery
- Dissection of aorta or renal artery
  - Marfan syndrome
  - Ehlers-Danlos syndrome
- Vasculitis involving renal artery
  - Polyarteritis nodosa
  - Takayasu's arteritis
  - Kawasaki disease
  - Thromboangiitis obliterans
  - Other necrotizing vasculitides
- Inflammatory disease of the aorta or renal artery
  - Syphilis
  - Tuberculosis
  - Mycoses
- Hypercoagulable states
  - Nephrotic syndrome
  - Antiphospholipid syndrome
  - Antithrombin III deficiency
  - Homocystinuria
- Thrombotic microangiopathies
  - Hemolytic-uremic syndrome
  - Thrombotic thrombocytopenic purpura
  - Antiphospholipid syndrome
  - Malignant hypertension
  - Scleroderma
  - Sickle cell nephropathy
  - Polycythemia vera
  - Postpartum hemolytic-uremic syndrome
  - Hyperacute vascular allograft rejection

Thrombosis: induced
- Traumatic
- Following endovascular intervention
- Post renal transplantation

Embolism
- Cardiac source
  - Atrial fibrillation or other arrhythmias
  - Native and prosthetic valvular heart disease
  - Infective endocarditis
  - Marantic endocarditis
- Myocardial infarction with mural thrombi
  - Left atrial myxoma or other tumor
- Noncardiac sources
  - Atheromatous embolic disease
  - Paradoxical emboli
  - Fat emboli
  - Tumor emboli
- Therapeutic renal embolization
- Segmental renal infarction of childhood
- Cisplatinum and gemcitabine
- Sickle cell disease or sickle cell trait

Figure 64.7 Causes of renal infarction.

due to atrial septal defects, which are present in up to 9% to 35% of the general population. The diagnosis of paradoxical embolism requires clinical, angiographic, or pathologic evidence of systemic embolism and the presence of venous thrombus along with an abnormal communication between the right and left circulations and a favorable pressure gradient (typically diagnosed by "bubble" echocardiography) for the passage of clot from the right to the left side of the heart.

The clinical presentations of renal artery embolism mirror those of renal infarction (Fig. 64.8).[15] Pain is present in more than 90% of cases confirmed by radiologic imaging techniques. It is unclear from the literature how many go undiagnosed because of lack of clinical symptoms. There is a 30-day mortality rate of 10% to 13% among patients experiencing renal embolism in the setting of atrial fibrillation.[17] Up to 40% of cases have at least transient reduction in renal function.

Whereas angiography is the gold standard for diagnosis of renal artery embolism, nuclear isotope scanning is also very sensitive (97%). Contrast-enhanced CT detects 80% of renal embolic events.[15] In other reports, CT or CTA has a sensitivity nearly matching that of renal angiography.

Aortic and Renal Artery Dissection

Aortic dissection can involve the origin of either renal artery, with the false lumen occluding the vessel and impairing renal perfusion. In this setting, the predictors of renal salvage are the same as those for occlusion due to atherosclerotic renal artery stenosis and include preserved renal size, collateral circulation permitting renal viability, and blush on imaging studies. In one report, despite renal atrophy, aortic stent graft placement allowed renal reperfusion and restoration of renal size and function.[18] Aortic dissection occurs most commonly in association with atheromatous aneurysmal vascular disease of the thoracic aorta, but it can occur in collagen disorders, such as Ehlers-Danlos type IV or Marfan syndrome, and with arteritis, such as Takayasu disease.

Dissection of the renal artery can occur after percutaneous renal angioplasty or stenting (Fig. 64.9), spontaneously with atherosclerotic renovascular disease (ASRVD) or fibromuscular dysplasia of the renal artery, or as a complication of renal artery aneurysms. Risk factors for dissection include age, hypertension, connective tissue disorders, pregnancy, bicuspid aortic valve, and coarctation of the aorta. A high index of suspicion and rapid imaging are critical to improve chances of patient and renal survival. Although MRA is nearly 100% sensitive for diagnosis of aortic dissection, CTA has a sensitivity of 93% and is more readily available, has a more rapid turnaround time, is less dependent on patient factors, and is usually the imaging modality of choice.

Middle Aortic Syndrome

A rare entity, middle aortic syndrome is a diffuse narrowing of the aorta, considered a form of coarctation, causing renovascular hypertension (Fig. 64.10). The cause is unknown, but associations with fibromuscular dysplasia, congenital anomalies, neurofibromatosis, Williams syndrome, and Takayasu arteritis have been reported. It can present as aortic thrombosis involving the renal arteries. Repair of middle aortic syndrome before thrombosis is the goal, with angioplasty, surgical repair or autotransplantation of ischemic organs.

Thromboembolic Complication of Endovascular Interventions

Renal artery thrombosis, dissection, laceration, or embolism can occur secondary to vascular interventions, especially those involving placement of endovascular stents.[19] Occlusion of the vessel within the stent can occur many months to years after stent placement, particularly when in-stent restenosis is present. During the past decade, endovascular aortic stents have been used to treat infrarenal abdominal aortic aneurysms. When the stent crosses the orifice of the renal artery, renal perfusion is impaired, and there is a significant risk for renal artery thrombosis.[20] Renal artery stent placement may cause intimal

Clinical Presentation of Renal Embolism

Renal Embolism	Atheroembolic Renal Disease
Clinical Signs and Symptoms	
Flank/loin pain (91%)	Flank/abdominal/back pain NR
Fever (49%)	Fever (common)
Nausea or vomiting (40%)	Malaise/failure to thrive (common)
Oliguria (16%)	Nonoligruia (common)
Transient hypertension NR	Labile hypertension NR
	Skin manifestations 60%
	Livedo reticularis
	Blue toes
Laboratory Abormalities	
Elevated creatinine (53%)	Elevated creatinine (100%)
Elevated LDH (91%)	Elevated ESR (97%)
Elevated CPK NR	Elevated CPK or LDH 38–60%
Leukocytosis (85%)	Leukocytosis (57%)
Elevated transaminases NR	Elevated amylase (57%)
Hematuria (72%)	Eosinophilia (57%)
	Eosinophiluria (NR)
	Hematuria/transient proteinuria (NR)
	Bland sediment (common)
	Hypocomplementemia 25–70%
Diagnostic Testing	
Contrast enhanced CT or MR	Tissue biopsy: Skin, muscle kidney
Nuclear imaging/DMSA	
Renal angiogram	

Figure 64.8 Clinical presentation of renal embolic disease. CK, creatine kinase; CT, computed tomography; DMSA, dimercaptosuccinic acid; LDH, lactate dehydrogenase; MR, magnetic resonance. *(Modified with permission from reference 15.)*

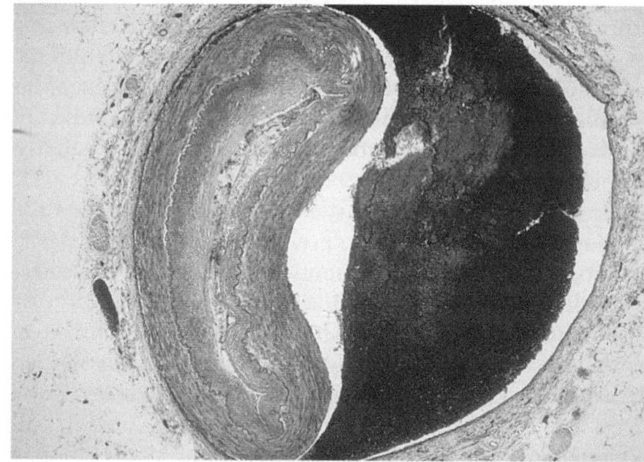

Figure 64.9 Cross section of a renal artery with dissection after renal angioplasty. Shown is the dissection with thrombus filling the false lumen. The kidney could not be salvaged.

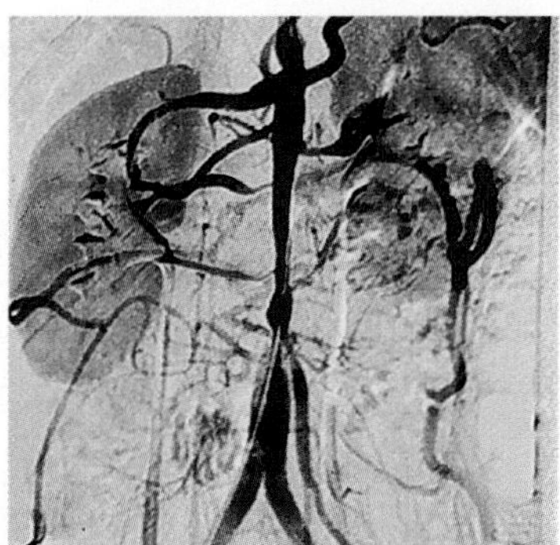

Figure 64.10 Middle aortic syndrome. Angiogram showing typical smooth narrowing of the aorta. There is bilateral stenosis of paired renal arteries. *(From reference 21.)*

dissection and thrombosis of the renal artery and even aortic dissection. Stent fracture or kinking can be associated with thrombosis of the lumen. Figure 64.11 demonstrates compression of a proximal renal artery stent with associated thrombotic occlusion of the vessel. Careful studies using filters to capture embolic material confirm that renal artery angioplasty with stenting of atherosclerotic renal arteries releases thousands of particles of various sizes in 70% to 100% of cases.[22] Preprocedure treatment with antiplatelet agents and intraprocedural use of embolic protection devices during renal stent implantation are under investigation as a means of reducing the frequency of this underdiagnosed cause of renal infarction.[23,24]

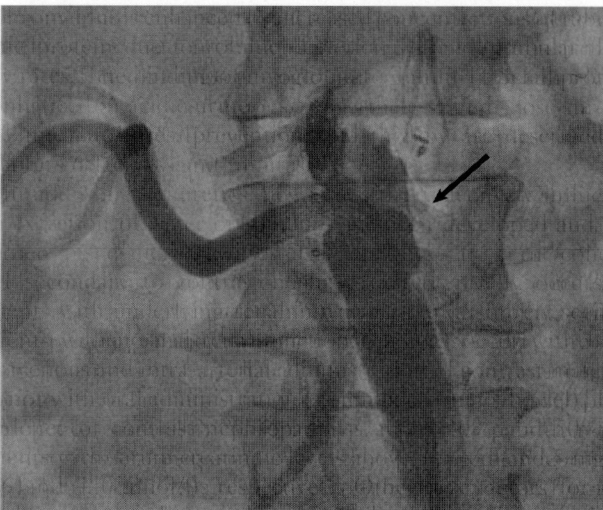

Figure 64.11 Thrombosis of renal artery complicating renal artery stenting. Right and left renal artery stents note the left renal stent *(arrow)* is triangular shaped indicating crimping of the proximal portion, which in this case, was associated with thrombosis of the renal artery seen here as no contrast entering the vessel. The right renal stent is patent.

Renal Artery Aneurysms

Renal artery aneurysms are rare and associated most commonly with atheromatous, fibromuscular, and vasculitic disease (Fig. 64.12). They are manifested clinically as renovascular hypertension, which is the presenting feature in 55% to 75% of cases. Thrombosis within an aneurysm can lead to distal thrombotic emboli and renal infarcts. Aneurysms with diameters of more than 1.5 cm have a higher risk of rupture. Elective repair of large renal aneurysms should be considered in women of childbearing age because of the risk of rupture during the third trimester of pregnancy and in patients with renovascular hypertension. Other complications of renal artery aneurysms include vessel dissection and arteriovenous fistula formation.

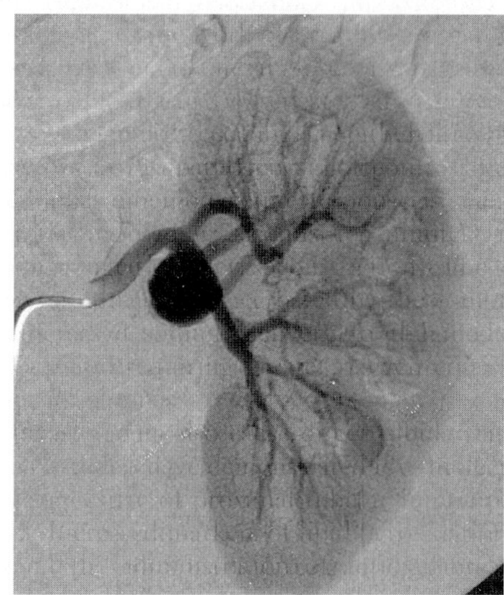

Figure 64.12 Renal artery aneurysm. Angiogram showing large renal artery aneurysm. The aneurysm is patent but is a risk factor for renal artery thrombosis.

Rare Causes of Renal Infarction

Rare causes of renal infarction include autoimmune diseases, such as Behçet's syndrome, systemic lupus, and other autoimmune diseases; Henoch-Schönlein purpura (HSP); chronic Chagas' disease; and drug abuse, such as intravenous injection or nasal insufflation of cocaine or even smoking marijuana. The exact mechanism involved in the pathogenesis of renal infarction in some of these conditions is unclear.

Treatment of Acute Renal Vascular Catastrophe

In the setting of renal infarction, a search for the cause of the renal vascular compromise should be undertaken to determine whether it is embolic or thrombotic. Treatment of the infarction itself is usually conservative and includes pain control and treatment of sometimes labile hypertension. If renal artery occlusion is due to thrombosis associated with hypercoagulable state or embolism from a central source, systemic anticoagulation is indicated. Salvage of the kidney by acute thrombolytic therapy has also been attempted with limited success. There is no evidence that thrombolytic therapy can limit infarct size if it is administered in the acute setting.

When embolism from a central source results in renal infarction or renal artery occlusion, a search for the source should include evaluation for atrial fibrillation, cardiac mural or atrial thrombus and mass, and valvular lesions. Except in the situation of septic emboli, anticoagulation is indicated to prevent recurrent embolic events.

Traumatic renal vascular occlusion leads to renal infarction within 3 to 6 hours. Attempts at renal salvage under these circumstances are often unsuccessful unless the diagnosis is made immediately on presentation of the patient and emergent renal revascularization surgery is feasible clinically.

Thrombosis of atherosclerotic renal arteries, because of prior collateral development in most cases, often results in marked ischemia but not infarction of the kidney and allows consideration of optimal surgical and sometimes percutaneous endovascular revascularization to restore renal function.

ATHEROEMBOLIC RENAL DISEASE

Atheroembolic renal disease is common and may account for up to 10% of unexplained renal failure in the elderly. It most commonly occurs after arterial manipulation in arteriography, vascular surgery, angioplasty, and stent placement. In patients with extensive atherosclerosis with unstable plaques, spontaneous atheroemboli may occur, especially after the administration of oral or intravenous anticoagulants or thrombolytic agents. The incidence of atheroembolic disease after vascular interventions is unclear, but recent data suggest that it is common.[25] A study evaluated the frequency of renal perfusion defects in patients after endovascular stent repair of abdominal aortic aneurysms; 18% of the cases had identifiable renal perfusion defects, and the occurrence of these infarcts was significantly associated with atherosclerotic burden.[26] Atheroembolism may therefore be expected to occur in up to 30% of patients with extensive aortic atherosclerosis after endovascular intervention. Ipsilateral renal artery stenosis may be present in up to 80% of patients with renal cholesterol embolization. Conversely, cholesterol emboli were found in the kidneys of 36% of the cases undergoing surgical revascularization.[27] Thus, cholesterol embolization may contribute to the loss of renal function in patients with atherosclerotic ischemic renal disease.

Most patients are older than 50 years with generalized atherosclerosis and have a history of recent endovascular procedures or signs or symptoms of atherosclerotic vascular disease, such as claudication, abdominal pain, angina, myocardial infarction, transient ischemic attacks, retinal artery emboli, amaurosis fugax, stroke, abdominal aortic aneurysm, renovascular hypertension, or ischemic renal disease. Many have a history of risk factors for atherosclerosis, including hypertension, hypercholesterolemia, diabetes, and smoking.

Clinical Presentation

Acute or subacute renal insufficiency due to renal microinfarctions developing as long as six months following the atheroembolic insult is the most common presentation leading to the diagnosis of cholesterol embolization. The clinical picture is multisystemic in nature and involves the kidneys in about 75% of patients. At autopsy, renal involvement is observed in 92% to 100%.

If a large shower of atheroemboli causes significant tubular damage, the AKI may have an oliguric phase characterized by a high fractional excretion of sodium. More often, the renal failure is nonoliguric and progressive because of ongoing embolization from a nidus of unstable ulcerative plaque. Some patients have only a moderate impairment in renal function, and others progress to end-stage renal disease (ESRD). Atheroembolic renal disease can also present as a more slowly progressive, often stair-stepping subacute renal insufficiency. Urinalysis findings are nonspecific but may include mild proteinuria, microhematuria, pyuria, and eosinophiluria. Renin release by ischemic zones in areas of embolization can lead to labile hypertension early in the course, sometimes associated with transient marked proteinuria. Fever, often low grade, is characteristic.

Although the kidneys are the organs most commonly involved, extrarenal cholesterol embolization will provide clues for

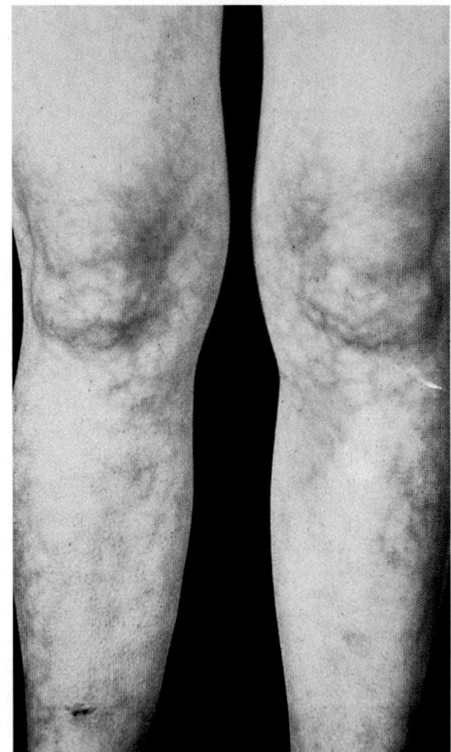

Figure 64.13 Livedo reticularis. The mottled skin changes associated with peripheral cholesterol embolization may be seen over the legs, buttocks, back, or flank and may be transient.

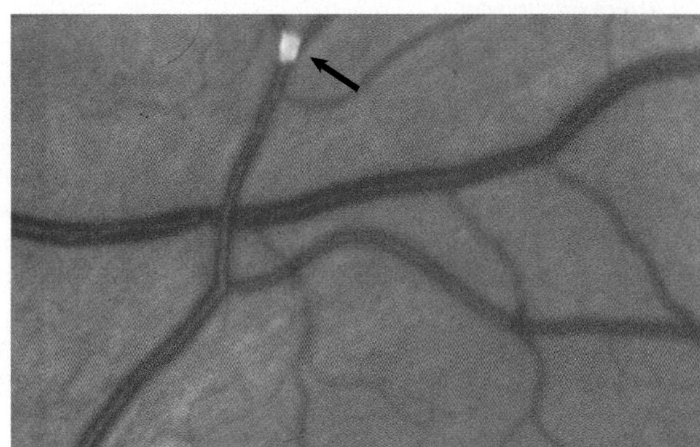

Figure 64.14 Hollenhorst bodies. Cholesterol embolus of a retinal arteriole *(arrow)*. *(Courtesy Richard Mills, University of Washington, Seattle, Washington, USA.)*

diagnosis. Cutaneous findings in up to 60% of patients at initial presentation include blue or purple toes, mottled skin or livedo reticularis, petechiae, and purpura or necrotic ulceration in areas of skin embolization, such as the lower back, buttocks, lower abdomen, legs, feet, or digits (Fig. 64.13).

Other organs often involved include spleen (in 55% of cases), pancreas (52%), gastrointestinal tract (31%), liver (17%), and brain (14%). This involvement can result in a number of clinical symptoms, including abdominal or muscle pain, nausea, vomiting, ileus, gastrointestinal bleeding, ischemic bowel, hepatitis, angina, and neurologic deficits. When retinal cholesterol embolization occurs, refractile yellow deposits known as Hollenhorst plaques may be seen at the bifurcation of retinal vessels on funduscopic examination (Fig. 64.14).

Diagnosis

The diagnosis of atheroembolic renal disease is suspected when subacute renal failure develops after a vascular intervention in the presence of livedo reticularis. Myriad laboratory abnormalities indicative of tissue injury are associated with cholesterol embolization, including elevated sedimentation rate (in 97% of cases), elevated serum amylase (60%), leukocytosis (57%), anemia (46%), hypocomplementemia (25% to 70%), and elevated lactate dehydrogenase and creatine kinase (38% to 60%). Eosinophilia, which may be transient, is seen in up to 57% of patients. The presence of eosinophilia should raise suspicion for atheroembolic renal disease in the appropriate clinical setting. Serum lactate is usually not elevated unless concomitant ischemic bowel is present. Definitive diagnosis is made by biopsy of an involved organ or system. A skin or muscle biopsy in an involved area may preclude the need for renal biopsy. In most circumstances, the diagnosis is made clinically.

Differential Diagnosis

Cholesterol embolization syndrome may mimic vasculitis, occult infection, neoplasm, or thrombotic microangiopathy. Contrast nephropathy with nonoliguric acute tubular necrosis (ATN) may also occur after angiography, angioplasty, or aortic vascular surgical procedures but is often more rapid as opposed to the subacute presentation of atheroemboli. Eosinophilia and eosinophiluria, rash, fever, and renal dysfunction may also be misdiagnosed as acute interstitial nephritis (AIN). Chronic cholesterol embolization syndrome may appear similar to hypertensive nephrosclerosis or ischemic renal disease. In the kidney transplant recipient, renal atheroembolism may mimic acute rejection or chronic allograft nephropathy (CAN).

Pathology and Pathophysiology

If clinical or other pathologic evidence has not secured the diagnosis, renal biopsy may be helpful. Diagnosis is based on the presence of birefringent, biconvex, elongated cholesterol crystals or biconcave clefts within the lumina of small vessels left behind in formalin-fixed tissue (Fig. 64.15). Because of the patchy nature of this disorder, open wedge renal biopsy guided by visualization of areas of ischemic infarction of the cortex has a higher likelihood of successful diagnosis than does percutaneous needle biopsy. The pathologist should be alerted by the clinician that cholesterol embolization is in the differential diagnosis before the biopsy specimen is processed. In frozen sections of tissue, the cholesterol material can be identified with polarized light microscopy. The pathologic findings may also include intimal thickening and concentric fibrosis of vessels, giant cell reaction to the cholesterol particles, vascular recanalization, endothelial proliferation, tubulointerstitial fibrosis with both eosinophil and mononuclear cell infiltrates, glomerular ischemia, and even focal segmental glomerulosclerosis (FSGS).[28] In the kidney, the most commonly affected vessels are the arcuate and interlobular arterioles, leading to patchy ischemic changes distal to these vessels.

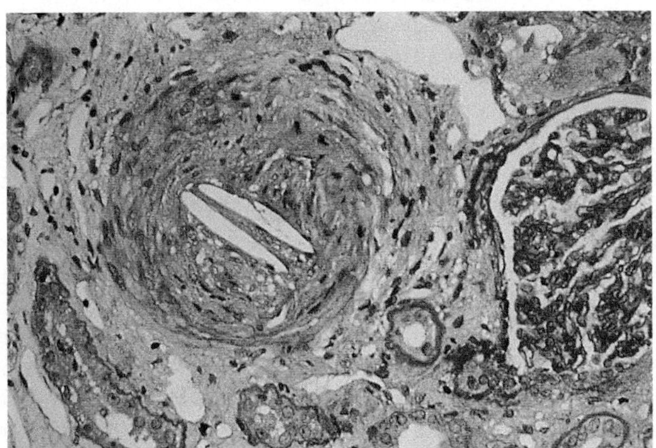

Figure 64.15 Cholesterol emboli in kidney biopsy specimen. Biconvex cholesterol clefts with giant cell reaction and recanalization of the lumen of a medium-sized renal vessel. (Periodic acid–Schiff stain.) *(Courtesy Dr. R. Horn, Vanderbilt University, Hashville, Tennessee, USA.)*

Natural History

The natural history is determined by the extent of organ involvement and the degree of the embolization. In one series of cases, renal function declined rapidly in 29%, with a more slowly progressive course seen in 79%.[29] Among the latter group, the decline in renal function was thought to result from a combination of cholesterol embolization and ischemic renal disease. In another series, the peak serum creatinine concentration occurred within 8 weeks after an angiographic procedure.[30] Patients may also manifest acute or subacute renal insufficiency followed by partial recovery of renal function. Conversely, the outcome can be dismal, particularly when cerebral embolization occurs or when there is a large unstable atheromatous burden. Some patients with cholesterol embolization may develop ESRD. These patients have a mortality rate of 35% to 40% during 5 years, even when dialysis is offered.[30]

Treatment

The risk for cholesterol embolization should be considered before angiographic and vascular surgical procedures are undertaken in patients with diffuse, extensive atherosclerotic disease. Because prevention is the most effective management strategy, patients with extensive aortic atherosclerosis should be considered for alternative approaches to cardiac catheterization, such as through the brachial artery. If vascular intervention is performed, signs of embolization should be sought both in the immediate postoperative period and for several months thereafter. When it is feasible, distal embolic protection devices should be used to trap embolic material for removal from the circulation to avoid end-organ damage by embolic debris.[31]

After the diagnosis of cholesterol embolization is established, further endovascular interventions should be avoided. Poor outcomes have been reported in patients with cholesterol emboli who subsequently undergo coronary artery bypass surgery. When clinical factors dictate the need for aortic, renal, or peripheral arterial surgery, optimal timing and surgical approach are critical. Conversely, there is a growing surgical experience with segmental aortic replacement to remove the source of emboli, particularly when atheroembolic disease occurs spontaneously. Transesophageal echocardiography is often used to identify mobile ulcerative plaque in the aorta to guide intervention.

Angiotensin-converting enzyme (ACE) inhibitors are effective in managing the labile hypertension seen early in the course of cholesterol embolization. Corticosteroids have been used with some success in patients with systemic cholesterol embolization and associated inflammatory symptoms.[32] There have also been several reports documenting improvement or stabilization of skin signs of cholesterol embolization after administration of statins,[33] which should be part of the treatment of the generalized atherosclerosis in these patients. Cholesterol embolization has also occurred after treatment with anticoagulants. Although direct causality between anticoagulants and cholesterol embolization has not been established, the proposed mechanism is that anticoagulants prevent thrombus organization over the ulcerative plaques. Therefore, anticoagulation should be avoided in the acute setting of cholesterol embolization unless a strong life-threatening indication for anticoagulation is present.

TRANSPLANT RENAL ARTERY STENOSIS AND THROMBOSIS

Epidemiology

Transplant renal artery stenosis is a common post-transplantation complication occurring most often in the period between 3 months and 2 years after transplantation. The highest reported incidence is 23% in a patient cohort screened angiographically, compared with reported incidences of between 1.3% and 12% when other screening tests are used.[34] In many cases, anastomotic stenoses are not hemodynamically significant.[34] The use of pediatric kidneys in adult recipients is associated with a higher rate of stenosis because of smaller donor vessel size, leading to greater turbulences and mismatch between donor and recipient vessels. As the transplant population ages, there has been increasing recognition of another subset of patients with pseudo–transplant renal artery stenosis, in which vascular disease proximal to the allograft artery, particularly involving the iliac vessel, results in renal ischemia.

Pathogenesis

The pathophysiologic basis for transplant renal artery stenosis is multifactorial and may include atheromatous disease in the donor artery, intimal scarring and hyperplasia in response to trauma to the vessel during harvesting, and anastomotic stenosis, which is most commonly associated with end-to-end anastomoses and may be related to suture technique. In end-to-side anastomoses, stenosis tends to develop in the postanastomotic site, suggesting that turbulence or other hemodynamic factors play a role. Immunologic causes of transplant renal artery stenosis have also been proposed on the basis of histologic similarities with chronic vascular rejection and association with prior acute rejection. Other proposed pathogenic mechanisms include calcineurin inhibitor (CNI) toxicity and cytomegalovirus (CMV) infection.

Clinical Presentation

Patients typically present with new-onset hypertension or difficult-to-control blood pressure (BP) with or without graft dysfunction occurring 3 to 24 months after transplantation. Patients may also present with AKI. When the stenosis occurs in the iliac artery above the anastomosis of the transplanted renal artery (pseudo–transplant renal artery stenosis), the patient often presents with ipsilateral lower extremity claudication associated with hypertension and worsening renal function in the allograft.[35] Systolic bruits over the transplant are not diagnostic because they may represent turbulent flow in the main vessels in the absence of stenosis or biopsy-related arteriovenous fistulas. Risk factors for the development of renal artery stenosis include male gender, hyperlipidemia, and elevated serum creatinine at discharge from transplantation.

Diagnosis

Renal duplex sonography is the screening test of choice for transplant renal artery stenosis because the vessel is superficial and easy to interrogate. The ratio of velocity in the renal and iliac vessels and the resistive index in the kidney have been shown to predict the hemodynamic response to percutaneous transluminal angioplasty. Phase-contrast MRA has an advantage over arteriography in viewing tortuous renal arteries and may provide information additional to Doppler ultrasound regarding the aorta and iliac vessels. However, with MRA, the surgical clip artifact may obscure the proximal renal artery, and it often cannot resolve peripheral renal vessels. High false-positive rates are associated with sharp anastomotic angles. CTA has the advantage over MRA from an imaging standpoint but requires a large amount of contrast material. The gold standard is selective renal angiography of the transplant and iliac artery. In situations in which the risk for contrast-induced nephrotoxicity is high, carbon dioxide angiography can be performed safely.

Treatment

Transplant renal artery stenosis often results in progressive loss of renal function.[36] Angioplasty is the preferred initial approach to transplant renal artery stenosis, with initial success rates of up to 75% and patency for follow-up periods of up to 30 months. The average complication rate for angioplasty of the allograft artery is 10%. It is often unsuccessful when there is arterial kinking and is associated with a high complication rate in this setting. The reported rates of late restenosis are between 10% and 33%, necessitating repeated procedures. Although stents are not usually required to treat stenoses within the transplant artery or at the anastomosis, they have been used successfully and are needed routinely to treat the pseudo–transplant renal artery stenosis due to iliac atherosclerotic occlusive disease proximal to the takeoff of the transplant artery.[37]

Surgical revascularization is reserved for patients in whom angioplasty or stenting has been unsuccessful or complicated. Surgical renal revascularization is difficult and is associated with significant mortality in the transplantation setting. Extensive fibrosis develops around the allograft and often involves the renal vessels, making surgical access risky. Complications include graft loss (in 15% to 30% of cases), ureteral injury (14%), and death (5%).

RENAL VEIN THROMBOSIS

Renal vein thrombosis (RVT) is rare and primarily observed in children with severe dehydration (with an incidence in neonates of 0.26% to 0.7%) or in adults with nephrotic syndrome, renal tumors, or hypercoagulable states and after surgery or trauma to the renal vessels.[38] When it occurs in adults, the diagnosis is often never considered. Thrombosis of the longer left (7.5 cm) renal vein may also involve the ureteric, gonadal, adrenal, and phrenic branches that drain into the left vein, whereas on the right side, the adrenal and gonadal veins drain directly into the inferior vena cava. The renal veins also communicate with perirenal veins outside of Gerota's fascia as part of the retroperitoneal collateral venous network: tributaries of the portal system, lumbar, azygos, and hemiazygos. Because of this network of venous complexes, occlusion of the left renal vein results in enlargement of the systemic collateral vessels and provides some protection against infarction.

Acute Versus Chronic Renal Vein Thrombosis

Experimentally, acute RVT is associated with immediate enlargement of the kidney with marked increase in renal vein pressure, leading to a marked decrease in renal arterial flow. Complications include hemorrhagic infarction, kidney rupture, and retroperitoneal hemorrhage. In the dog, the kidney enlarges during the course of 1 week, then proceeds to atrophy as a result of progressive fibrosis. In contrast, slow, progressive ("chronic") thrombosis may allow collateral formation, resulting in minimal symptoms.

Clinical Presentation

Acute RVT is usually symptomatic and associated with loin, testicular, or flank pain; low-grade fever; and in the setting of a single kidney or renal transplant, symptoms of renal failure. Nausea and vomiting often accompany acute RVT, and symptoms might be confused with acute pyelonephritis. Leukocytosis can accompany acute thrombosis. Clinical signs include renal enlargement, which in infants is manifested as a palpable abdominal mass. Hematuria is nearly universal and most often is microscopic. The high venous pressures result in a marked increase in proteinuria. Urinalysis sometimes reveals evidence of proximal tubule dysfunction, such as glycosuria. Oliguric renal failure occurs when RVT results in renal infarction of both kidneys or in subjects with a single kidney. In some cases, RVT is diagnosed only after the patient develops an acute pulmonary embolus and the source of the embolus is investigated or with worsening of renal function in the setting of proteinuric chronic kidney disease (CKD).

Chronic RVT may be asymptomatic and is associated with extensive venous collaterals and minimal impairment of renal function and structure. Often, however, microhematuria, increase in proteinuria, and evidence of either reduced GFR or tubular dysfunction are present, particularly when indices of differential renal function are sought, such as with nuclear studies.

When RVT causes renal infarction, the distribution of the hypoperfused region tends to be medullary or subcortical. The renal impairment tends to be patchy and subtotal. These patients can develop severe hypertension acutely. The swollen kidney can rupture the capsule and result in massive retroperitoneal hemorrhage.

Etiology

The causes of renal vein thrombosis are listed in Figure 64.16.

Neonatal Renal Vein Thrombosis

RVT occurs in neonates in situations of dehydration and thrombophilia. There is a greater predilection for development of RVT in male infants, with 67% of the reported cases occurring in boys.[39] Most cases are unilateral, with the left renal vein more commonly affected. Complications of neonatal RVT may include adrenal hemorrhage, renal atrophy, renal insufficiency, and hypertension. In neonates, the diagnosis is made by Doppler study of the renal veins. Fibrinolytic therapy may be associated with bleeding complications, including adrenal hemorrhage, and

Causes of Renal Vein Thrombosis
Malignant neoplasia Direct invasion of tumor into the renal vein Retroperitoneal adenopathy, fibrosis, or tumor compressing the renal vein Extension of inferior vena cava (IVC) obstruction by tumor invasion Hypercoagulable state associated with malignant disease
Complication of IVC filters
Complication of PICC lines
Nephrotic syndrome Membranous nephropathy Lupus nephritis
Acute pyelonephritis
Complicating inflammatory bowel disease
Acute pancreatitis
Inflammatory aortic aneurysm
Neonatal Congenital Dehydration Thrombophilia Complication of umbilical vein catheterization Transmission of maternal procoagulant factors
Hypercoagulable states Antiphospholipid antibody syndrome Factor V Leiden mutation Antithrombin III deficiency Protein S and C abnormalities Hyperhomocysteinemia Elevated levels of clotting factors VIII, IX, and XI Heparin-induced thrombocytopenia Birth control pill
Thrombophilia
Chuvash polycythemia
Post renal transplantation Acute rejection, OKT3 Vascular rejection Compression or kinking of renal vein Hypercoagulable disorders Sticky platelet syndrome Calcineurin inhibitors Viral infection of the allograft
Complication of surgical compression After aortic aneurysm surgery After pyeloplasty After partial nephrectomy
Traumatic renal vein thrombosis
Pregnancy Compression Preeclampsia, eclampsia
Complication of embolization of gastric varices
Budd-Chiari syndrome
Behçet's disease

Figure 64.16 Causes of renal vein thrombosis. PICC, peripherally inserted central catheter.

is usually not successful in restoring renal function unless it is undertaken within 24 hours of the thrombotic event.[40]

Nephrotic Syndrome

Patients with nephrotic syndrome have increased risk of venous thromboembolism; deep venous thrombosis is most commonly diagnosed (see Chapter 15).[41] The prevalence of RVT in nephrotic syndrome is unclear because it is largely undiagnosed; studies report frequencies between 5% and 62%.[38] Numerous abnormalities promoting a prothrombotic state occur secondary to heavy proteinuria. Interestingly, RVT appears more common in membranous nephropathy (MN) and lupus nephritis (LN), but RVT can complicate any cause of proteinuric renal disease. In this setting, RVT can lead to an increase in baseline proteinuria and present with AKI superimposed on chronic renal insufficiency.

After Renal Transplantation

RVT after transplantation is rare and occurs in less than 0.1% of transplants, usually within the first week after transplantation. It usually leads to graft infarction. Causes include compression of the renal vein, volume depletion, acute rejection, and hemostatic and hypercoagulable states. Factor V Leiden mutation, which occurs in 2% to 5% of the population, is a risk factor for transplant RVT and should be sought when it occurs. Another syndrome known as sticky platelet syndrome can result in post-transplant RVT. There are some data supporting the protective effects of low-dose aspirin in this population. Immunosuppression with cyclosporine and OKT3 may increase the risk of RVT. Unlike the native kidney, the transplant has only a single renal venous outflow, so the consequences of acute RVT are dire, often leading to loss or rupture of the allograft. Renal salvage is possible with early diagnosis and surgical exploration and thrombectomy.[42]

Pregnancy

Pregnancy and the postpartum state are hypercoagulable states. There have been reports of spontaneous RVT in the postpartum period associated with renal infarction. RVT complicating pregnancy should be suspected when clinical clues, such as flank pain and hematuria, are present.

Malignant Disease

Malignant disease accounts for the greatest number of cases of RVT.[43] RVT can result from invasion of tumor of renal origin into the renal vein. About half of renal cell carcinomas are associated with RVT at autopsy. In addition, neoplasia originating in the renal vein or inferior vena cava, such as leiomyosarcoma or cavernous hemangioma, can cause RVT. Extrinsic compression of the renal vein by a tumor or retroperitoneal fibrosis may also cause this syndrome.

Diagnosis

Diagnosis of RVT requires imaging. Conventional ultrasound may demonstrate alterations in size and echogenicity. Renal duplex sonography may show increases in resistive indices, and ultrasound can directly visualize the filling defect, but this may depend on the angle of the vein, the body habitus of the patient, and the operator's experience. In neonates, renal Doppler ultrasound is the diagnostic study of choice. In adults, both CT and magnetic resonance (MR) venography have much greater sensitivity than renal vein duplex studies. CT venography requires a significant contrast load, making MR venography preferable in patients with allergy to contrast agents or those at risk for contrast-associated nephrotoxicity. Figure 64.17 is a CT venogram demonstrating unilateral RVT.

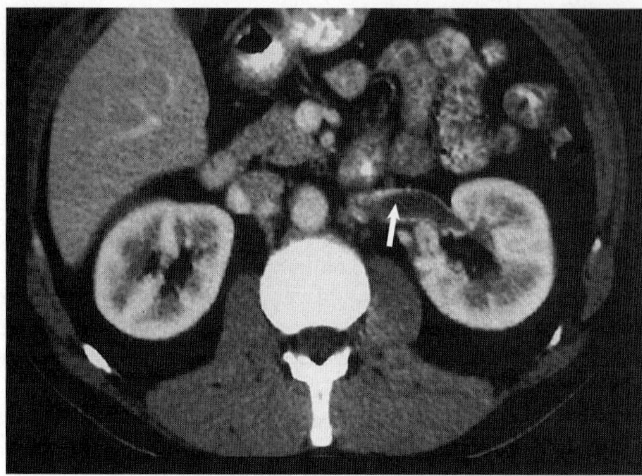

Figure 64.17 Computed tomography (CT) venogram demonstrating left renal vein thrombosis *(arrow)*. *(Courtesy Dr. S. Rankin, Guy's Hospital, London, United Kingdom.)*

Treatment

Treatment is controversial and depends on the setting, acuteness, and renal consequences. If there is no contraindication, most patients are treated with systemic anticoagulation acutely. In adults with acute RVT that is compromising renal function, catheter-directed thrombolytic therapy with urokinase or tissue plasminogen activator with or without percutaneous mechanical thrombectomy can be successful in regaining patency of the vessel and restoring renal function.[44] There are reports of successful thrombolytic therapy in pregnancy-associated RVT. The long-term benefit of this approach is unclear, and it is less successful when the thrombotic process begins in the small intrarenal venules rather than in the major veins, as is often the case when primary renal disease or a hypercoagulable state initiates the process. In neonatal RVT, which often results in renal nonfunction, thrombolytic therapy and anticoagulation have been used with variable results. In two recent reports of neonatal RVT, supportive care was recommended for unilateral RVT without extension into the inferior vena cava, whereas thrombolytics were used for bilateral cases with impending renal failure.

Surgical interventions include nephrectomy, thrombectomy, and retroperitoneal surgery for non–renal-associated abnormalities, such as tumor, retroperitoneal fibrosis, aortic aneurysm, and acute pancreatitis. Surgery tends to be reserved for situations in which the RVT results in hemorrhage from renal capsular rupture or for long-term consequences of RVT, such as hypertension or infection of a nonfunctioning kidney resulting from previous RVT.

A conservative approach may be favored when left RVT occurs because of the extensive collateral venous supply on that side, ultimately allowing venous drainage and improvement in renal function. Systemic anticoagulation is indicated acutely to prevent extension of thrombus into the inferior vena cava and for prevention of pulmonary emboli. Anticoagulation should be continued indefinitely in patients with persistent hypercoagulable state after RVT. In addition, eventual recanalization of the venous system can result in delayed improvement in renal function as measured by nuclear medicine studies.

REFERENCES

1. Yune Hy, Klatte EC. Collateral circulation to an ischemic kidney. *Radiology*. 1976;119:539-546.
2. Truty MJ, Bower TC. Congenital anomalies of the inferior vena cava and left renal vein: Implications during open abdominal aortic aneurysm reconstruction. *Ann Vasc Surg*. 2007;21:186-197.
3. Kaneko N, Kobayashi Y, Okada Y. Anatomic variations of the renal vessels pertinent to transperitoneal vascular control in the management of trauma. *Surgery*. 2008;143:616-622.
4. Hansen KJ, Cherr GS, Craven TE, et al. Management of ischemic nephropathy: Dialysis-free survival after surgical repair. *J Vasc Surg*. 2000;32:472-482.
5. Siddiqui S, Norbury M, Robertson S, et al. Recovery of renal function after 90 d on dialysis: Implications for transplantation in patients with potentially reversible causes of renal failure. *Clin Transplant*. 2008;22: 136-140.
6. Thatipelli M, Misra S, Johnson CM, et al. Renal artery stent placement for restoration of renal function in hemodialysis recipients with renal artery stenosis. *J Vasc Interv Radiol*. 2008;19:1563-1568.
7. Dean RH, Kieffer RW, Smith BM, et al. Renovascular hypertension: Anatomic and renal function changes during drug therapy. *Arch Surg*. 1981;116:1408-1415.
8. Graham SD, Keane TE, Glenn JF, eds. *Glenn's Urologic Surgery*. 7th ed. Philadelphia: Wolters Kluwer/Lippincott Williams & Wilkins Health; 2010.
9. Tsai SH, Chu SJ, Chen SJ, et al. Acute renal infarction: A ten-year experience. *Int J Clin Pract*. 2007;61:62-67.
10. Lohse JR, Shore RM, Belzer FO. Acute renal artery occlusion. *Arch Surg*. 1982;117:801-804.
11. van der Wal MA, Wisselink W, Rauwerda JA. Traumatic bilateral renal artery thrombosis: Case report and review of the literature. *Cardiovasc Surg*. 2003;11:27-29.
12. Nochy DE, Daugas E, Droz D, et al. The intrarenal vascular lesions associated with primary antiphospholipid syndrome. *J Am Soc Nephrol*. 1999;10:506-518.
13. Tektonidou MG. Renal involvement in the antiphospholipid syndrome (APS)—APS nephropathy. *Clin Rev Allergy Immunol*. 2009;36:131-140.
14. Hoxie HJ, Coggin CB. Renal infarction: Statistical study of two hundred and five cases and detailed report of an unusual case. *Arch Intern Med*. 1940;65:587-594.
15. Hazanov N, Somin M, Attali M, et al. Acute renal embolism: Forty-four cases of renal infarction in patients with atrial fibrillation. *Medicine (Baltimore)*. 2004;83:92-99.
16. Bockler D, Krauss, M, Mannsmann U, et al. Incidence of renal infarctions after endovascular AAA repair. *J Endovasc Ther*. 2003;10:1054.
17. Huang CC, Chen WL, Chen JH, et al. Clinical characteristics of renal infarction in an Asian population. *Ann Acad Med Singapore*. 2008;37: 416-420.
18. Verhoye J, De Latour B, Heautot J. Return of renal function after endovascular treatment of aortic dissection. *N Engl J Med*. 2005;352: 1824-1825.
19. Gorich J, Kramer S, Tomczak R, et al. Thromboembolic complications after endovascular aortic aneurysm repair. *J Endovasc Ther*. 2002;9:180.
20. Walsh SR, Boyle JR, Lynch AG, et al. Suprarenal endograft fixation and medium-term renal function: Systematic review and meta-analysis. *J Vasc Surg*. 2008;47:1364-1370.
21. Panayiotopoulos YP, Tyrrell MB, Koffman G, et al. Mid-aortic syndrome presenting in childhood. *Br J Surg*. 1996;83:235-240.
22. Edwards MS, Corriere MA, Craven TE, et al. Atheroembolism during percutaneous renal artery revascularization. *J Vasc Surg*. 2007;46: 55-61.
23. Urbano J, Manzarbetia F, Caramelo C. Cholesterol embolism evaluated by polarized light microscopy after primary renal artery stent placement with filter protection. *Vasc Interv Radiol*. 2008;19(Pt 1):189-194.
24. Henry M, Henry I, Polydorou A, Hugel MJ. Embolic protection for renal artery stenting. *Cardiovasc Surg (Torino)*. 2008;49:571-589.
25. Polu KR, Wolf M. Needle in a haystack. *N Engl J Med*. 2006;354: 68-73.
26. Harris JR, Fan CM, Geller SC, et al. Renal perfusion defects after endovascular repair of abdominal aortic aneurysms. *J Vasc Interv Radiol*. 2003;14:329-333.
27. Krishnamurthi V, Novick AC, Myles JL. Atheroembolic renal disease: Effect on morbidity and survival after revascularization for atherosclerotic renal artery stenosis. *J Urol*. 1999;161:93-96.
28. Greenberg A, Bastacky SI, Iqbal A, et al. Focal segmental glomerulosclerosis associated with nephrotic syndrome in cholesterol atheroembolism: Clinicopathologic correlations. *Am J Kidney Dis*. 1997;29: 334-344.
29. Blenfant X, Meyrier A, Jacquot C. Supportive treatment improves survival in multivisceral cholesterol crystal embolism. *Am J Kidney Dis*. 1999;33:840-850.
30. Scolari F, Ravani P, Pola A, et al. Predictors of renal and patient outcomes in atheroembolic renal disease: A prospective study. *J Am Soc Nephrol*. 2003;14:1584-1590.
31. Dubel GJ, Murphy TP. Distal embolic protection for renal arterial interventions. *Cardiovasc Intervent Radiol*. 2008;31:14-22.
32. Graziani G, Sanostasi S, Angelini C, et al. Corticosteroids in cholesterol emboli syndrome. *Nephron*. 2001;87:371-373.
33. Finch TM, Ryatt KS. Livedo reticularis caused by cholesterol embolization may improve with simvastatin. *Br J Dermatol*. 2000;143: 1319-1320.
34. Fervenza FC, Lafayette RA, Alfrey EJ, et al. Renal artery stenosis in kidney transplants. *Am J Kidney Dis*. 1998;31:142-148.
35. Becker BN, Odorico JS, Becker YT, et al. Peripheral vascular disease and renal transplant artery stenosis: A reappraisal of transplant renovascular disease. *Clin Transplant*. 1999;13:349-355.
36. Deglise-Favre A, Hiesse C, Lantz O, et al. Long-term follow-up of 40 untreated cadaveric kidney transplant renal artery stenoses. *Transplant Proc*. 1991;23:1342-1343.
37. Bertoni E, Zanazzi M, Rosat A, et al. Efficacy and safety of Palmaz stent insertion in the treatment of renal artery stenosis in kidney transplantation. *Transplant Int*. 2000;13:S425-S430.
38. Harris R, Ismail N. Extrarenal complications of nephrotic syndrome. *Am J Kidney Dis*. 1994;23:477-497.
39. Lau KK, Stoffman JM, Williams S, et al. Neonatal renal vein thrombosis: Review of the English language literature between 1992-2006. *Pediatrics*. 2007;120:e1276-e1284.
40. Messinger Y, Sheaffer JW, Mrozek J, et al. Renal outcomes of neonatal renal venous thrombosis: Review of 28 patients and effectiveness of fibrinolytics and heparin in 10 patients. *Pediatrics*. 2006;118: e1478-e1484.
41. Kayali F, Najjar R, Aswad F, et al. Venous thromboembolism in patients hospitalized with nephrotic syndrome. *Am J Med*. 2008;121:226-230.
42. Fathi T, Samhan M, Gawish A, et al. Renal allograft venous thrombosis is salvageable. *Transplant Proc*. 2007;39:1120-1121.
43. Wysokinski WE, Gosk-Bierska I, Greene EL, et al. Clinical characteristics and long-term follow-up of patients with renal vein thrombosis. *Am J Kidney Dis*. 2008;51:224-232.
44. Kim HS, Fine DM, Atta MG. Catheter-directed thrombectomy and thrombolysis for acute renal vein thrombosis. *J Vasc Interv Radiol*. 2006;17:815-822.

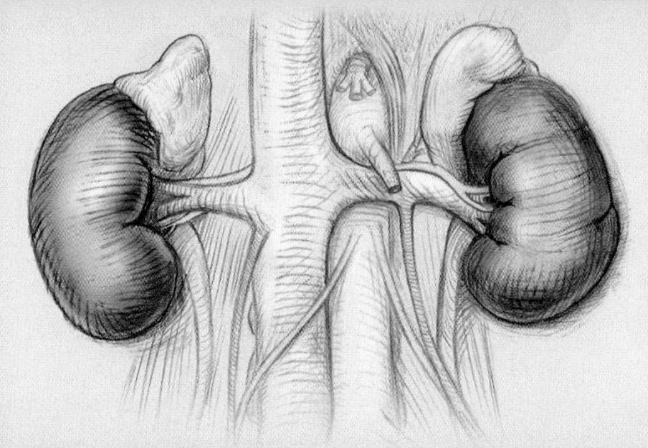

SECTION XII

Geriatric Nephrology

CHAPTER 65

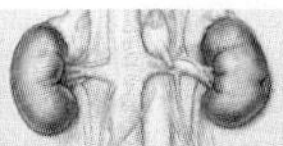

Geriatric Nephrology

Raimund Pichler, Christian Hugo, Richard J. Johnson

Aging is a slow, inflammatory biologic process that affects many organs, of which the kidney is one of the main targets. Aging is associated with a decline in renal function coincident with a progressive loss of nephrons, with glomerular and tubulointerstitial scarring. These changes begin in the fourth decade of life and accelerate between the fifth and sixth decades, resulting in alterations in glomerular and tubular function, systemic hemodynamics, and body homeostasis. Although aging-related changes begin in midlife, this chapter focuses on the management of the older population, defined as older than 65 years.

Aging-associated renal disease may not be inevitable. Some subjects do not show age-related decline in GFR. Hypertension does not increase with aging in non-westernized populations habitually on low-sodium diets. This has led some to hypothesize that aging-associated renal disease may be an active process that is potentially preventable.

AGING-ASSOCIATED DECLINE IN RENAL FUNCTION

Glomerular Filtration Rate

Inulin clearance studies document a progressive fall in glomerular filtration rate (GFR) after the age of 40 years, with a relatively greater decline in men (Fig. 65.1).[1] However, the fall in GFR is not inevitable; in as many as one third of subjects who remain normotensive, there is no decrease in creatinine clearance with age.[2]

In addition to the decrease in GFR with aging, there may be a reduction in renal "reserve." Whereas some studies suggest that aging humans show a normal increase in GFR after amino acid infusion, others have shown a marked reduction in increases in renal plasma flow and GFR in response to concurrent infusion of amino acids and dopamine in healthy elderly individuals.[3,4]

Renal Plasma Flow

Renal plasma flow (RPF) also decreases from a mean of 650 ml/min in the fourth decade to 290 ml/min by the ninth decade, with increasing renal vascular resistance (Fig. 65.2).[1] The fall in RPF with age is greater in men than in women and in those who are hypertensive.[5] Because RPF decreases relatively more than GFR, filtration fraction (defined as GFR/RPF) increases with age.

The decrease in RPF does not simply reflect a decrease in renal mass. Studies using a xenon washout technique demonstrated that there is a true reduction in renal blood flow when it is factored for renal mass.[6] The decrease in renal blood flow especially involves the cortex, and blood flow to the medulla is relatively preserved.

Proteinuria

The prevalence of both microalbuminuria (urinary albumin levels of 30 to 300 mg/day) and albuminuria increases progressively in the U.S. population after the age of 40 years. The increased prevalence is most marked in diabetic and hypertensive subjects but is also observed in patients lacking these risk factors (Fig. 65.3).[7] The prevalence of microalbuminuria and albuminuria is higher in African Americans, Mexican Americans, and those with elevated serum creatinine.[7] This is clinically relevant because microalbuminuria is an independent risk factor for cardiovascular disease (such as carotid disease and left ventricular hypertrophy) and cardiovascular mortality.

ASSESSMENT OF RENAL FUNCTION IN THE ELDERLY

Serum creatinine is a less reliable indicator of renal function in the aging population. This is because creatinine generation reflects muscle mass, and muscle mass decreases with aging. Men normally excrete 20 to 25 mg/kg body weight of creatinine in the urine each day, and women excrete 15 to 20 mg/kg body weight of creatinine. However, after the age of 60 years, there is a progressive decrease in urinary creatinine excretion, resulting in excretion rates lower than these ranges (Fig. 65.4).[8] For example, in one study, serum creatinine did not change between young subjects (mean age of 30 years) and older subjects (mean age of 80 years) despite a reduction in creatinine clearances from 140 ml/min per 1.73 m^2 at age 30 years to 97 ml/min per 1.73 m^2 at age 80 years.[9]

There is no consensus on the optimal approach to estimation of GFR in elderly people. Whereas the MDRD (Modification of Diet in Renal Disease) study equation and the Cockcroft-Gault formula for estimating GFR use age in their calculations (see Chapter 3), neither has been validated in a population older than 70 years, and both underestimate true GFR in those older than 65 years with standard techniques such as technetium Tc 99m. Although the MDRD equation may be more accurate than the Cockcroft-Gault formula,[10,11] serum cystatin C, which is independent of muscle mass, may be superior to both and is an independent risk factor for mortality in the elderly.[12] Renal function was assessed in a community-based survey of the elderly in Finland by

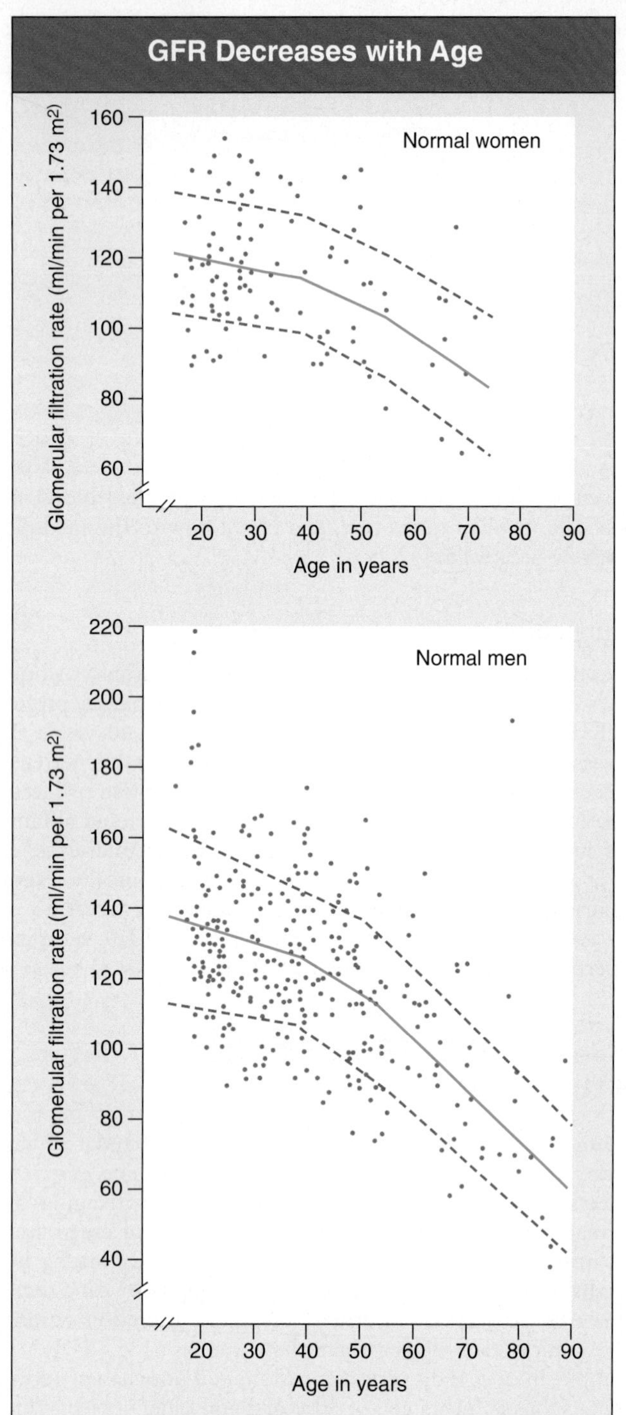

Figure 65.1 Glomerular filtration rate (GFR) decreases with age. GFR (inulin clearance) begins to fall at age 40 years, and the rate of decline is more rapid in men than in women. *(Modified from reference 1.)*

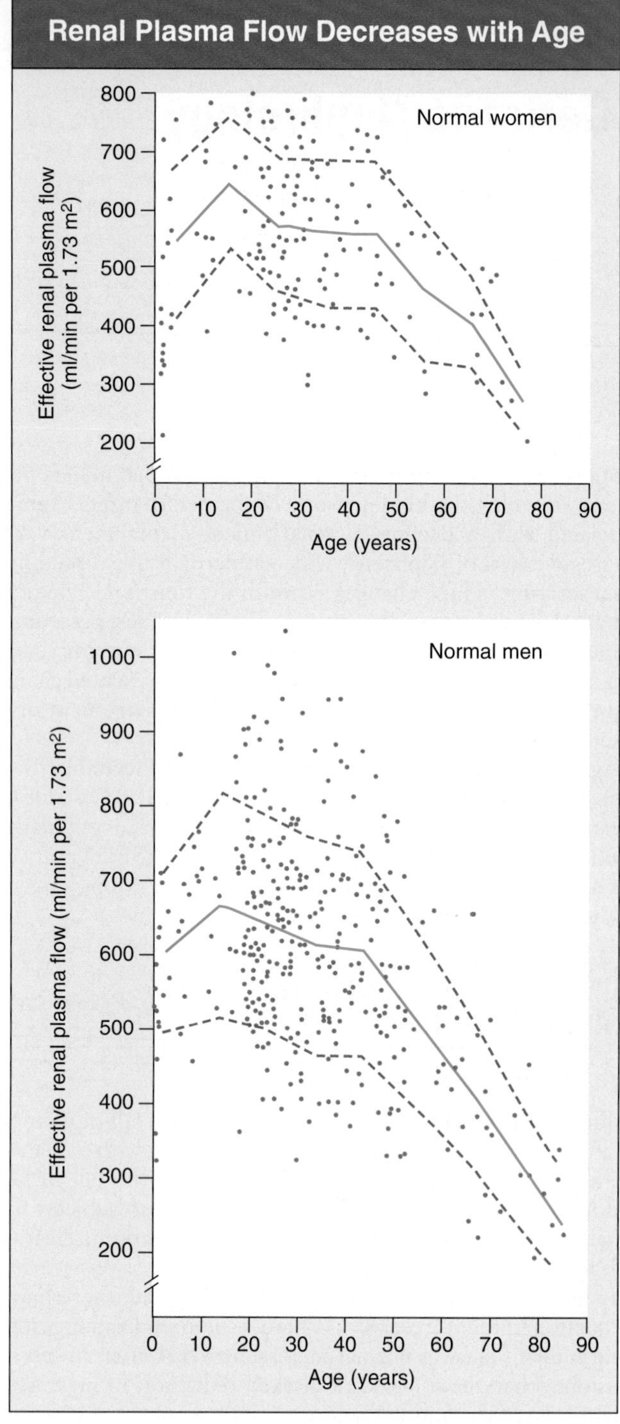

Figure 65.2 Renal plasma flow (RPF) decreases with age. RPF (*p*-aminohippurate clearance) begins to fall rapidly after the age of 50 years, and the rate of decline is more rapid in men than in women. *(Modified from reference 1.)*

use of the MDRD equation, Cockcroft-Gault formula, and serum cystatin C; only cystatin C correlated with albuminuria.[13]

PREVALENCE OF CHRONIC KIDNEY DISEASE IN THE ELDERLY

According to the National Health and Nutrition Examination Survey (NHANES; 1999-2004), nearly 45% of elderly subjects have chronic kidney disease (CKD, stages 1 to 4) in the United States compared with only 8% of the overall adult population (Fig. 65.5).[14] Elderly subjects older than 70 years account for half of people with CKD as defined by the KDOQI classification using the MDRD equation (see Fig. 65.5).[14] Furthermore, the prevalence of CKD in the elderly U.S. population appears to have increased by 10% compared with a decade ago.[14]

CKD is associated with an overall increase in all-cause cardiovascular mortality.[15] Nevertheless, reductions of eGFR to 50

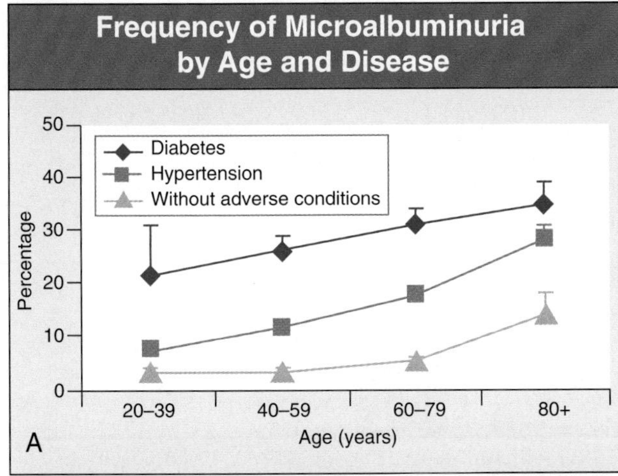

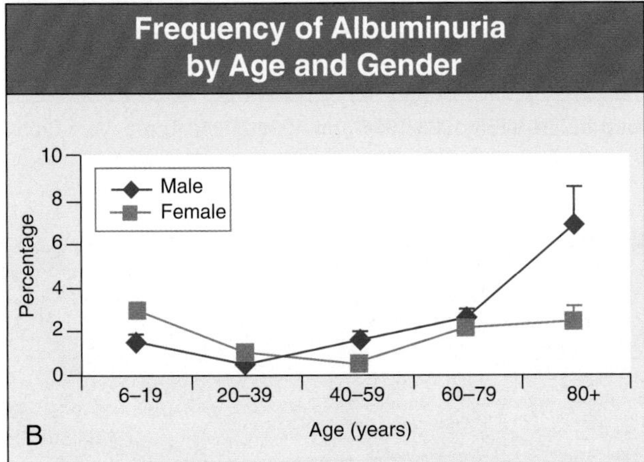

Figure 65.3 Increased proteinuria with aging. A, Microalbuminuria increases with age, with the greatest prevalence in diabetes, followed by hypertension and then the absence of either condition. **B,** Albuminuria increases with age, and the prevalence is greater in men than in women. *(Modified from reference 7.)*

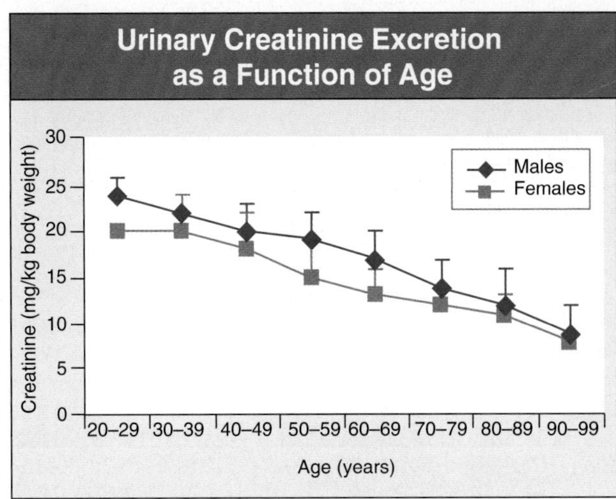

Figure 65.4 Urinary creatinine excretion (factored for body weight) decreases with age. *(Modified from reference 8.)*

to 59 ml/min per 1.73 m^2 do not increase mortality risk among patients age 65 years or older compared with patients with eGFR of more than 60 ml/min (Fig. 65.6).[16,17] These observations have led to the debate whether the decrease in GFR that occurs with aging should really be considered unhealthy and whether the term CKD should be applied to subjects with aging-associated decline in renal function.[18]

Risk Factors for Aging-Related Chronic Kidney Disease

The variability in the severity of aging-related renal disease in humans and experimental animals has suggested that there may be specific risk factors for its development. In experimental models, aging-related histologic changes vary according to the genetic strain, gender, body mass index, and diet. In general, aging-associated renal injury is worse in men, in obesity, or in the setting of endothelial dysfunction, and aging changes can be retarded with protein or calorie restriction or blockade of the renin-angiotensin system (RAS).[19]

Pathology

The human kidney reaches a maximum size of about 400 g (corresponding to 12 cm in length) in the fourth decade of life. After this, renal mass decreases at a rate of about 10% per decade, with a tendency for decrease to be greater in men than in women. Macroscopically, the kidneys develop an appearance of granularity and pitting of the external surface. There is progressive cortical thinning and loss in the number of functional nephrons (Fig. 65.7).

Glomerular number decreases from about 1 million per kidney to 600,000 or less by the eighth decade. Pathologic glomerular changes include glomerular hypertrophy, basement membrane thickening, and progressive development of focal segmental or, rarely, global glomerulosclerosis. At birth, less than 5% of glomeruli show glomerulosclerosis, but this increases to 10% to 30% of glomeruli by the eighth decade (Fig. 65.8).[20] It has been suggested that glomerulosclerosis should be considered "pathologic" if the percentage of globally sclerosed glomeruli exceeds (age/2) – 10.[21] The glomerulosclerosis is associated with mesangial matrix expansion and a progressive loss of capillary loops. Periglomerular fibrosis is often prominent, and there may be "atubular glomeruli," in which the exit from Bowman's capsule to the proximal tubular lumen is blocked by fibrosis.

Tubulointerstitial injury is greatest in the outer medulla and medullary rays, with tubular dilation and atrophy, mononuclear cell infiltration, and interstitial fibrosis. Distal tubules and collecting ducts may develop small diverticula; it has been suggested that these diverticula harbor bacteria predisposing to recurrent pyelonephritis.[2]

Arteriolar hyalinosis is common with aging but is observed almost exclusively in hypertensive individuals.[2] There is also increased tortuosity of the arcuate and interlobar vessels. Some afferent arterioles, particularly of juxtamedullary glomeruli, also develop vascular shunts to the efferent arterioles, thereby bypassing glomeruli, leading to "aglomerular arterioles."[22] Studies in rats have also demonstrated focal losses of glomerular capillary loops and peritubular capillaries consistent with a state of impaired angiogenesis.[23]

Pathogenesis of Aging-Associated Chronic Kidney Disease

A variety of mechanisms have been proposed for aging-related renal changes (Fig. 65.9).

One mechanism may involve *senescence*, in which there is telomere shortening of chromosomal DNA, loss of mitochondria,

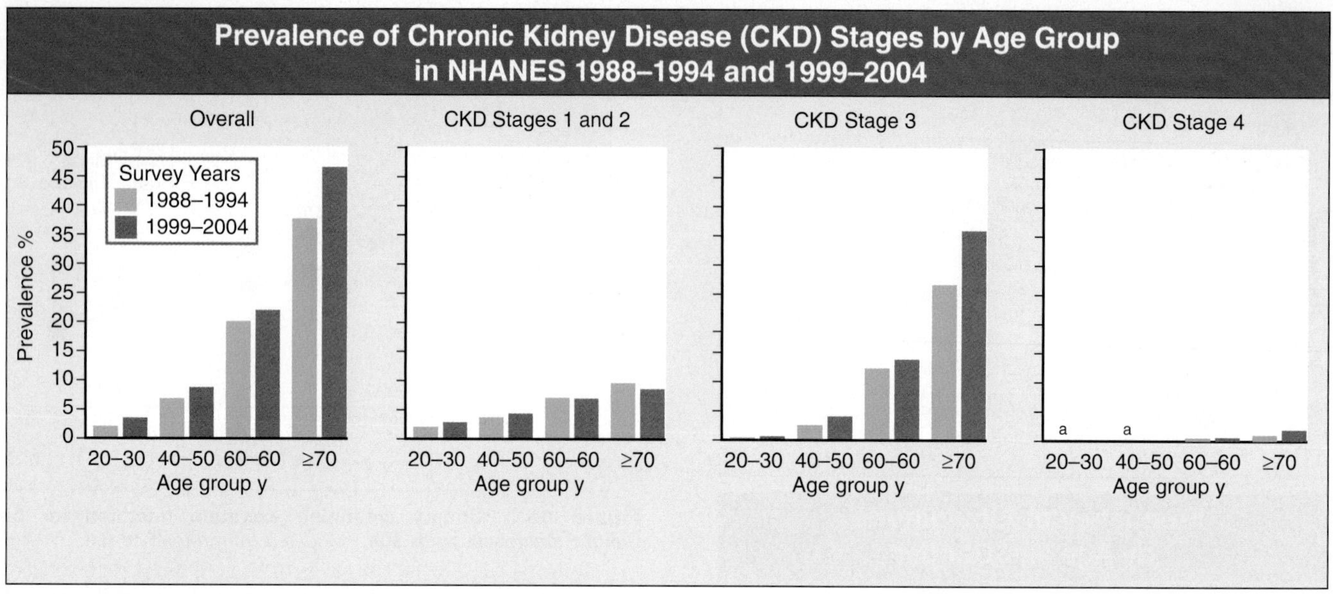

Figure 65.5 Prevalence of chronic kidney disease (CKD) stages by age group in NHANES 1988-1994 and 1999-2004. [a]There were no cases in 1988-1994. *(Modified from reference 14.)*

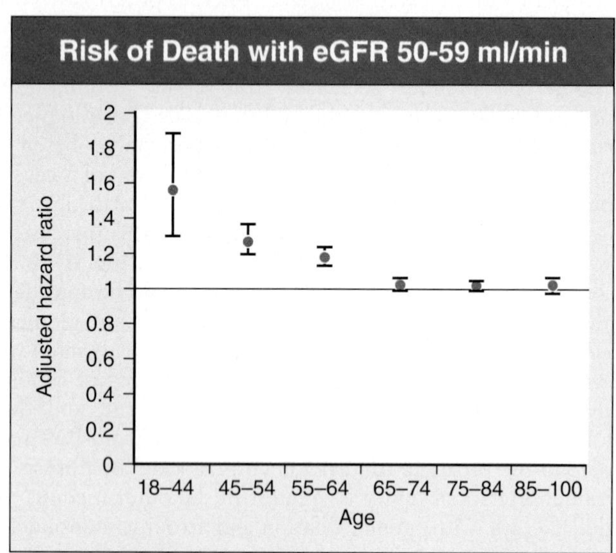

Figure 65.6 Adjusted hazard for death associated with an eGFR of 50 to 59 ml/min per 1.73 m². *(Modified from reference 16.)*

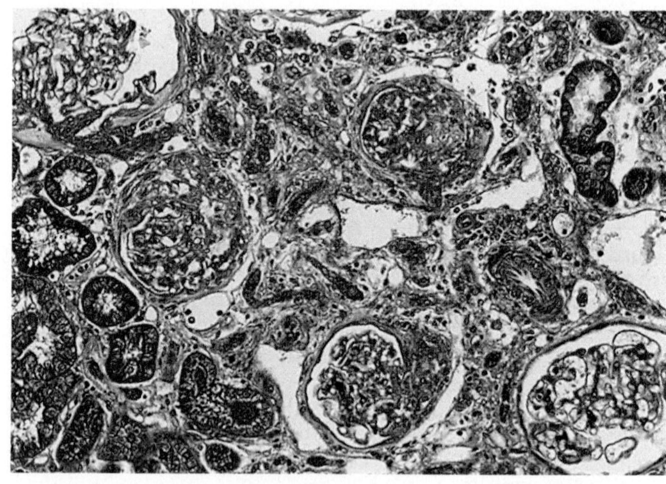

Figure 65.7 Glomerulosclerosis and tubulointerstitial fibrosis in an aging rat. Similar changes, consisting of focal segmental glomerulosclerosis, tubular atrophy, and interstitial fibrosis, occur in humans. (Trichrome stain; original magnification ×400.)

and accelerated apoptosis. Increased numbers of apoptotic tubular and interstitial cells have been shown in the aging rat.[24] This process may involve oxidative stress.[25]

Aging-associated renal disease may also be mediated by activation of the *renin-angiotensin system* (RAS). Although aging is associated with extracellular volume expansion and a reduction in plasma renin activity, there is evidence in aging rats that renal angiotensin II (Ang II) levels are elevated. Treatment of rats with angiotensin-converting enzyme (ACE) inhibitors reduces aging-associated oxidative stress and preserves mitochondria in renal proximal tubules in association with upregulation of cellular antioxidant enzymes.[26,27] Rats treated with ACE inhibitors shortly after birth also develop less glomerulosclerosis and tubulointerstitial fibrosis with aging.[28] The renoprotective mechanisms may be both hemodynamic (decreasing glomerular hydrostatic pressure and increasing renal blood flow) and nonhemodynamic

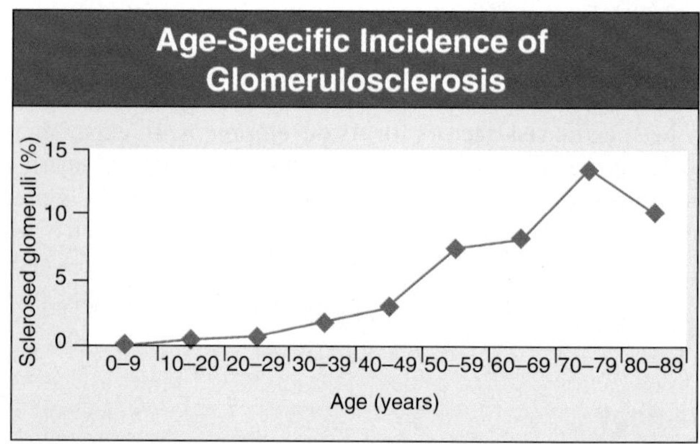

Figure 65.8 Glomerulosclerosis increases with aging. *(Modified from reference 20.)*

Proposed Mechanisms for Aging-Associated Renal Disease
Oxidative stress
Senescence (with telomere shortening and loss of mitochondria)
Glomerular hypertension and hyperfiltration
Intrarenal activation of the renin angiotensin system
Endothelial dysfunction (loss of nitric oxide)
Renal ischemia
Renal TGF-β expression
Accumulation of advanced glycation end products (AGEs)
Chronic effects of uric acid

Figure 65.9 Proposed mechanisms for aging-associated renal disease. TGF-β, transforming growth factor β.

(direct effect to block Ang II–mediated oxidative stress and cytokine [transforming growth factor β] production).[29] In addition, lifelong blockade of the RAS in rats results in less left ventricular hypertrophy and myocardial fibrosis, improvement in learning capacity, increased sexual activity, and decreased liver fibrosis.[26,29-31] Targeted disruption of the gene encoding for the AT_{1A} receptor also results in marked prolongation of life span in mice despite unchanged renal function or histology after 24 months.[31] The longevity in these mice was associated with a decrease of cardiac and vascular injury possibly through attenuation of oxidative stress and overexpression of prosurvival genes (also in the kidney).

A loss of nephrons results in *hyperfiltration* with increased glomerular hydrostatic pressure and glomerular hypertrophy, which are known risk factors for glomerular scarring.[32] However, studies in aging rats have shown that the initiation of renal damage with aging may occur independently of glomerular hypertension. Depending on the strain, glomerular hydrostatic pressures may be either elevated or normal with aging.[19] It is thus likely that glomerular hypertension, when it occurs with a decrease in nephron mass, is a contributor to rather than an initiator of the aging-associated decline in renal function.

With aging, there is dilation and stiffening of elastic arteries[33] that result in higher pulse wave velocity with increased pressure transmission to the microvasculature.[34] Measures of large artery stiffness are closely related to markers of renal microvascular injury, including albuminuria.[35] Aging-associated intimal hyperplasia of the interlobular arteries and disease of the afferent arteriole may also alter renal autoregulation, resulting in injury to the glomeruli.[36] Higher systemic pulse pressure, seen in aging individuals, has been associated with an accelerated decline in kidney function.[37]

Endothelial function also declines with aging, and this is greater in men than in women. The endothelial dysfunction is associated with a progressive reduction in nitric oxide production by endothelial cells and is reflected clinically by a reduction in brachial artery reactivity.[38] The loss of normal endothelial vasodilatory substances may account for the increased renal vasoconstrictive response observed in aging rats to agents such as Ang II and endothelin 1 and may also contribute to the development of renal microvascular disease. Endothelial dysfunction can also inhibit renal angiogenesis, resulting in progressive capillary loss and ischemia. Indeed, mice lacking endothelial nitric oxide synthase show a marked acceleration of aging-associated renal disease.

Aging is also associated with more pronounced *renal hypoxia*. Blood oxygenation level–dependent magnetic resonance imaging studies have shown that ambient Po_2 is about 20 mm Hg lower in both the renal cortex and the medulla in otherwise healthy aged individuals compared with young subjects.[39] The reduced ability of the aged kidney to generate nitric oxide and vasodilatory prostaglandins may also contribute to renal hypoxia.[40,41]

Advanced glycation end products (AGEs), although typically associated with diabetes, are also present in the diet and can accumulate in aging. The content of AGEs in the diet correlates with serum AGE levels, oxidant stress, organ dysfunction, and life span.[42] Calorie restriction may extend life span in animal models in part by reducing AGE levels.[42,43] Chronic administration of aminoguanidine (an inhibitor of AGE synthesis) also reduces glomerulosclerosis in the aging rat.

FLUID AND ELECTROLYTES IN AGING

Sodium Balance and Hypertension

Aging is associated with both impaired sodium excretion of a salt load[44] and defective conservation in the setting of sodium restriction.[45] Proximal sodium reabsorption (reflected by lithium clearance) is increased in aging, whereas distal sodium reabsorption may be reduced.[46] Studies in rats suggest that pressure natriuresis is impaired in aging.[19] Because the diet of most individuals in developed countries contains excess sodium (8 to 10 g salt/day), there is a tendency in the elderly population for total body sodium excess.

The relative defect in sodium excretion and increased total body sodium may be a predisposing factor for the development of hypertension. Blood pressure increases with age. After the age of 60 years, most of the population is hypertensive (Fig. 65.10).[47] Salt sensitivity occurs in more than 85% of the aging population, and sodium restriction will result in a significant fall (>10 mm Hg) in mean arterial pressure.[48] Populations that ingest low-sodium diets, such as the Yanomamo Indians of southern Venezuela, do not show an increase in blood pressure with age.[49] Loss of vascular compliance due to collagen deposition in the larger arterial vessels may also contribute to aging-associated hypertension, as may endothelial dysfunction, perhaps mediated by oxidative stress.

Aging-associated renal and vascular changes may explain why correction of secondary forms of hypertension (such as primary aldosteronism, Cushing's syndrome, renovascular hypertension, and hypothyroidism) is less effective at curing hypertension in older patients. In one study, diastolic blood pressure fell to below 90 mm Hg in 24 of 25 subjects younger than 40 years after treatment of the mechanism responsible for the secondary hypertension but in only 38 of 61 subjects older than 40 years.[50]

Osmoregulation and Water Handling

There is impaired water handling with aging. Both concentration and dilution are affected, and nocturia is common. There is a reduced maximal urinary osmolality and thirst response to hyperosmolality, which may predispose to dehydration and hypernatremia. The increase in urine osmolarity in response to antidiuretic hormone (vasopressin) is blunted compared with younger subjects. Total body water also decreases with age. Conversely, there is slower excretion of a water load, leading to an increased predisposition to hyponatremia.

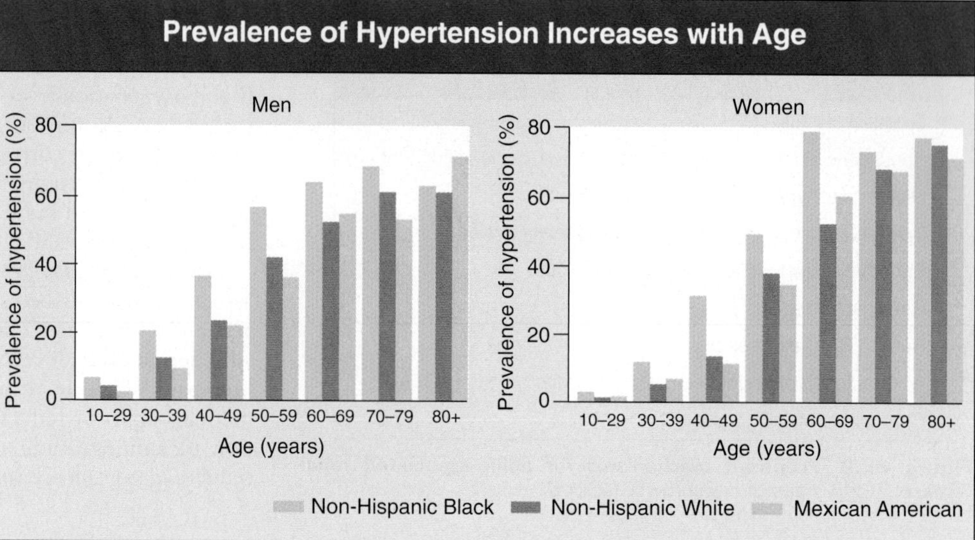

Figure 65.10 Prevalence of hypertension based on age, gender, and race. *(Modified from reference 47.)*

Other Tubular Defects and Electrolyte Problems

Potassium excretion is impaired, probably because of reduction in numbers of functioning tubules. Hyperkalemia occurs more frequently in elderly subjects treated with drugs that interfere with potassium excretion (such as potassium-sparing diuretics). Other factors contributing to the predisposition for hyperkalemia in the elderly include decreased GFR, lower basal levels of aldosterone, and tubulointerstitial scarring impairing the Na^+,K^+-ATPase transporters. Hypokalemia is also common because of renal or extrarenal losses.

Acid-base disturbances may result from the impaired distal tubular acidification that occurs with aging. Aging subjects do not excrete an acid load as effectively as younger subjects do.

Hypercalcemia occurs in 2% to 3% of institutionalized elderly patients. Causes include malignant tumors, hyperparathyroidism, immobilization, and use of thiazide diuretics. Hypocalcemia is less common and is observed mainly in patients with advanced CKD, chronic malabsorption, and severe malnutrition. Aging is associated with increased parathyroid hormone levels (which correlate inversely with GFR) and a decrease in serum calcitriol and phosphate.[46]

Hypomagnesemia is reported in 7% to 10% of elderly patients admitted to the hospital; most commonly, this is the result of malnutrition, laxatives, or diuretic use. Hypermagnesemia is less common and is found primarily in patients with CKD or who are taking large doses of magnesium-containing antacids. Gout (as well as an elevation in serum uric acid levels) is also more common in the aging population.

ENDOCRINE FUNCTION AND RENAL HORMONES

Erythropoietin (EPO) levels increase with age, probably related to a compensatory response to subclinical blood loss, increased erythrocyte turnover, and increased EPO resistance.[51] Nevertheless, EPO levels are significantly lower in the anemic elderly subject compared with the anemic younger individual, suggesting a blunted response to low hemoglobin.[52]

Elderly women with GFR below 60 ml/min have lower calcium absorption and lower 1,25-hydroxyvitamin D levels, probably due to diminished conversion of 25-hydroxyvitamin D to 1,25-dihydroxyvitamin D by the aging kidney.[53]

The kidney removes about 50% of insulin in the peripheral circulation by filtration and proximal tubular uptake and degradation. The decline of renal function in the elderly leads to a decrease in insulin clearance. This is in part offset by diminished glucose tolerance, which may relate to the increasing frequency of obesity observed in aging individuals.[54]

CLINICAL MANIFESTATIONS

General Considerations

Given the limitations of glomerular and tubular function in elderly people, fluid and electrolyte management needs constant vigilance to minimize morbidity. Fluid and electrolyte homeostasis is easily destabilized by intercurrent challenges that are well tolerated by younger patients. Moderate fluid loss (e.g., episode of diarrhea) and moderate fluid loading (e.g., inappropriate perioperative intravenous fluids) are both poorly tolerated and may lead to hypovolemia and fluid overload, respectively. Overzealous administration of water as 5% dextrose or 0.45% saline may result in hyponatremia. The acid load provoked by ischemic tissue injury or hypoxemia will be more severe in the elderly owing to inadequate renal compensation. Potassium homeostasis is easily altered by inaccurate estimation of intravenous or potassium requirements. The use of nonsteroidal anti-inflammatory drugs (NSAIDs) in the elderly is associated with increased risk for hyponatremia, hyperkalemia, hypertension, and impaired renal function.

Glomerular Diseases

Patterns of glomerular disease seen in elderly people are similar to those seen in the general population, although certain disorders may have an increased prevalence. Diabetic kidney disease is seen with increasing frequency in the aging population; however, older patients almost always have a mixture of different entities, most commonly of hypertensive nephrosclerosis and atherosclerosis. Also seen with increased frequency are membranous nephropathy, Wegener's granulomatosis, membranoprolif-

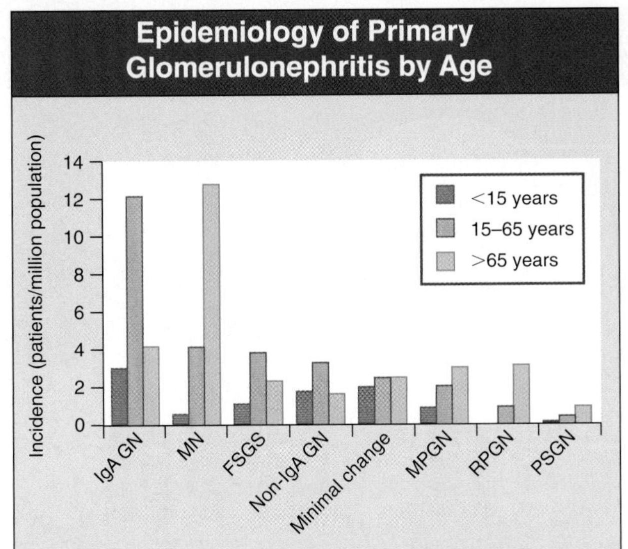

Figure 65.11 Epidemiology of primary glomerulonephritis by age. IgA GN, IgA nephropathy; MN, membranous nephropathy; FSGS, focal segmental glomerulosclerosis; non-IgA GN, other mesangial proliferative glomerulonephritis; MPGN, membranoproliferative glomerulonephritis; RPGN, rapidly progressive glomerulonephritis; PSGN, poststreptococcal glomerulonephritis. *(Modified from reference 55.)*

erative glomerulonephritis, and amyloidosis (Fig. 65.11).[18,55] In contrast, certain glomerular disorders are uncommon in elderly people, such as lupus nephritis, minimal change nephropathy, and IgA nephropathy. Only 2% of patients with systemic lupus erythematosus present after the age of 60 years.[18] As a consequence, most positive results of fluorescent antinuclear antibody tests performed in elderly patients are false-positive test results. Other diseases may be less typical in the elderly.

Renovascular and Atheroembolic Disease

There is also an increased frequency of renovascular and atheroembolic disease with aging. The observation of hypertension and elevated serum creatinine, especially in an individual with a history of vascular disease, should prompt a screening test for renovascular disease, such as by magnetic resonance angiography or by renal artery duplex scanning (see Chapter 37).

Acute Kidney Injury

Elderly subjects are at marked increased risk for acute kidney injury in many settings, including after surgery. Mechanisms involved include reduction in functional renal reserve, impaired renal autoregulation, defective fluid homeostasis, and increased susceptibility to drug nephrotoxicity.

Urinary Tract Infections

There is an increased risk for asymptomatic bacteriuria and symptomatic urinary tract infection with aging (see Chapter 51). In men, this may relate to the increased risk for prostatic hypertrophy and urinary calculi with age. Chronic use of indwelling catheters in elderly subjects is also associated with increased bacterial colonization rates; treatment of these urinary tract infections should generally be based on the presence of symptoms or signs (fever, elevated white blood cell count, or dysuria). Exceptions include high-risk subjects, such as those with frequent or recurrent urinary tract infections or structural defects of the urinary tract, patients scheduled to undergo urologic surgery, neutropenic patients, and renal transplant recipients. The treatment of catheter-associated infections is discussed in Chapter 51.

Transient Causes of Urinary Incontinence (DIAPPERS)

D	Delirium/confusional state
I	Infection—urinary (symptomatic)
A	Atrophic urethritis/vaginitis
P	Pharmaceuticals (diuretics, etc.)
P	Psychological, especially depression
E	Endocrine (hypercalcemia, hypokalemia, glycosuria)
R	Restricted mobility
S	Stool impaction

Figure 65.12 Transient causes of urinary incontinence in the elderly (DIAPPERS). *(Modified from reference 56.)*

Obstructive Uropathy

Obstructive uropathy (see Chapter 58) is common in elderly men, usually due to benign prostatic hypertrophy, prostate cancer, or urethral stricture. The incidence of obstructive uropathy in women is about one third to one half that in men and is primarily due to malignant neoplasms of the genitourinary tract. Lower urinary tract obstruction should be excluded by measuring the postvoid residual bladder volume, either by a bedside ultrasound bladder scan or by temporary placement of a urethral catheter. Ultrasound is the most appropriate imaging study for diagnosis of upper urinary tract obstruction (see Chapter 58).

Urinary Incontinence

The lower urinary tract also undergoes significant changes with aging. Decreased bladder contractility occurs secondary to weakening and thinning of the detrusor smooth muscle. This leads to a dysfunctional pattern, eventually culminating in involuntary detrusor contractions. Bladder capacity decreases, whereas postvoid residual bladder volume increases by about 50 to 100 ml. Elderly people also have a higher frequency of nocturia, due in part to the decrease in renal concentrating capacity and perhaps also associated with disordered sleep.

Transient urinary incontinence is very common in the elderly with multiple potentially treatable causes, which are best recalled by a mnemonic, DIAPPERS (Fig. 65.12).[56] In men, the most common cause is overflow incontinence from prostatic obstruction, whereas in women, a prolapsed uterus is frequently the cause. If a reversible cause is not promptly identified, referral to a neurologist (to rule out conditions such as normal-pressure hydrocephalus) or urologist is recommended.

In the absence of an easily reversible cause, nonsurgical therapeutic options for urinary incontinence include behavioral therapy and biofeedback, pelvic floor exercises, pharmacologic therapy (e.g., α-adrenergic antagonists to reduce prostatic hypertrophy), and, if it is unavoidable, long-term catheterization. Surgery may be required for large cystoceles, vaginal vault prolapse, and postprostatectomy stress incontinence.[56]

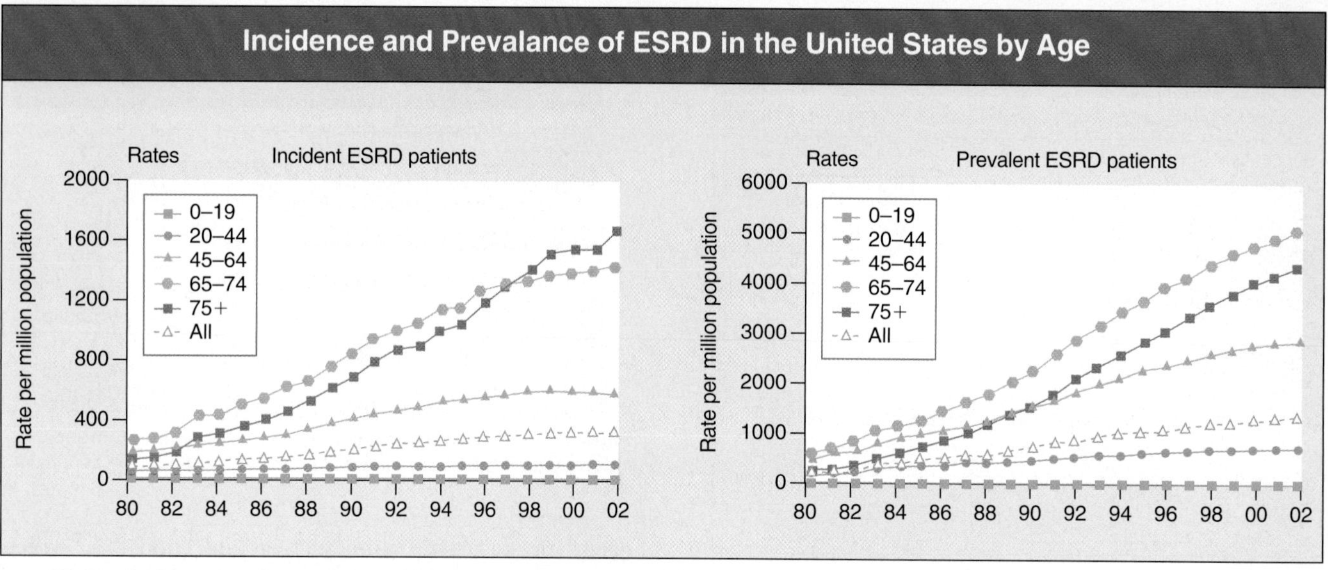

Figure 65.13 Incidence and prevalence of ESRD in the United States by age. Subjects older than 65 years have a higher incidence and prevalence of ESRD; factored for gender and race. *(Modified from U.S. Renal Data System [USRDS]: 2005 Annual Data Report. Am J Kidney Dis 2006;47[Suppl 1]:S65-S81.)*

Hematuria

Malignant neoplasms of the urinary tract are more common in older subjects. Bladder carcinoma is rarely observed before the age of 40 years in men and is even more uncommon in women younger than 40 years; it increases progressively after the fourth decade. Renal cell carcinomas are most commonly observed in the seventh decade. As a consequence, the development of microhematuria or macrohematuria requires thorough urologic evaluation. Other causes of hematuria may need to be considered, including glomerular disease and stone disease, as discussed in Chapter 59.

Nephrotoxicity and Drug Dosing

Elderly subjects are prone to increased nephrotoxicity both as a consequence of decreased renal mass and because they are often administered medicines on the assumption that a normal or nearly normal serum creatinine concentration is consistent with normal renal function. As a result, elderly subjects are commonly prone to nephrotoxicity from NSAIDs, cyclooxygenase 2 inhibitors, aminoglycosides, radiocontrast media, and chemotherapy (e.g., cisplatin).

Drug dosing needs to be carefully adjusted in the aging patient. Certain common drugs frequently need adjustment for renal function; these include aminoglycosides, digoxin, procainamide, tetracycline, and vancomycin. Certain drugs may be commonly associated with the development of hyponatremia; these include thiazides and chlorpropamide. Other drugs commonly prescribed in elderly subjects may rarely be associated with the development of nephrotic syndrome. These include NSAIDs and pamidronate.

End-Stage Renal Disease and Renal Replacement Therapy

Given the normal decrease in GFR with aging, it is not surprising that end-stage renal disease (ESRD) is common in the elderly. Both the incidence and prevalence of ESRD are higher in older subjects (Fig. 65.13). Indeed, the mean age for a patient to initiate renal replacement therapy is currently 63 years in the United States. Most cases of ESRD in older subjects are due to either diabetes or hypertension.

Despite the frequency of CKD among elderly patients, ESRD is far less common than cardiovascular morbidity or mortality.[57] Older patients with CKD stage 3 are more likely to die and less likely to reach ESRD than are their younger counterparts.[58]

The clinical presentation of ESRD in the elderly may also differ from that in younger patients. Patients may present with uremic symptoms (anorexia, nausea, and pruritus), with only modest elevations in serum creatinine, and such uremic manifestations may be attributed to the "aging process" or other comorbidities.

Occasional subjects may present with unexplained dementia or change in personality or behavior, unexplained exacerbation of congestive heart failure, or simply a change in sense of well-being. The decision to offer renal replacement therapy is no longer based on the age of the individual. Patients often do very well with either hemodialysis or peritoneal dialysis unless there are comorbid conditions such as cardiovascular disease. As with younger subjects, vascular access remains the Achilles heel of hemodialysis. Even in this population, the survival of arteriovenous fistulas is significantly greater than that of arteriovenous grafts. Some surgeons justify use of synthetic grafts in the elderly on the grounds that their blood vessels are fragile and significantly atherosclerotic. However, successful use of an arteriovenous fistula has results similar to those in younger people, with prolonged patencies and low incidence of infections and thromboses.

Transplantation should be considered in the management of elderly patients with ESRD because studies have clearly shown that the elderly recipient benefits from renal transplantation by a significant reduction in mortality (41%) compared with wait-listed ESRD patients.[59] This survival benefit is most striking for patients with ESRD caused by diabetes or hypertension,[59] but it becomes less apparent the longer the patient waits before transplantation.[60] The proportion of patients with ESRD who are older than 65 years and on the transplant waiting list has tripled in the past 10 years in the United States and currently exceeds 12%.[60]

Elderly subjects were thought to have a lower rate of graft rejection than younger patients. However, because they have a higher rate of death with functioning grafts, overall graft survival is similar to that in younger subjects.[60] On the basis of these studies, it has been argued that lower doses of immunosuppression are sufficient in elderly renal transplant recipients.[61] However, the Eurotransplant Senior Program allocating kidneys from donors 65 years or older to recipients 65 years or older regardless of HLA matching found 5% to 10% increased rejection rates in this "old to old" group compared with two better HLA-matched groups, the "old to any" and the "any to old," within the Eurotransplant Kidney Allocation System.[62] In a subanalysis of the ELITE-Symphony study, a large prospective, randomized trial comparing immunosuppressive regimens in renal transplant patients,[63] equal rates of rejection in elderly (≥60 years) versus younger (<60 years) recipients were demonstrated. Furthermore, this subanalysis suggested that older recipients who receive a marginal kidney from an older or expanded criteria donor may fare worse than younger recipients, with an increased likelihood of death, delayed graft function, graft loss, treatment failure, and reduced graft function. The use of a standard criteria donor kidney may therefore be especially important for elderly patient survival within the first year after renal transplantation. However, in the current dilemma of global organ shortage, in which expanded criteria donor kidneys represent about 17% of deceased donor kidney transplants in the United States,[64] this approach raises an ethical dilemma about fair kidney allocation.

REFERENCES

1. Wesson LG Jr. *Renal Hemodynamics in Physiological States*. New York: Grune & Stratton; 1969.
2. Lindeman RD, Goldman R. Anatomic and physiologic age changes in the kidney. *Exp Gerontol*. 1986;21:379-406.
3. Esposito C, Plati A, Mazzullo T, et al. Renal function and functional reserve in healthy elderly individuals. *J Nephrol*. 2007;20:617-625.
4. Fuiano G, Sund S, Mazza G, et al. Renal hemodynamic response to maximal vasodilating stimulus in healthy older subjects. *Kidney Int*. 2001;59:1052-1058.
5. Baylis C. Changes in renal hemodynamics and structure in the aging kidney; sexual dimorphism and the nitric oxide system. *Exp Gerontol*. 2005;40:271-278.
6. Hollenberg NK, Adams DF, Solomon HS, et al. Senescence and the renal vasculature in normal man. *Circ Res*. 1974;34:309-316.
7. Jones CA, Francis ME, Eberhardt MS, et al. Microalbuminuria in the US population: Third National Health and Nutrition Examination Survey. *Am J Kidney Dis*. 2002;39:445-459.
8. Epstein M. Aging and the kidney. *J Am Soc Nephrol*. 1996;7:1106-1122.
9. Rowe JW, Andres R, Tobin JD, et al. The effect of age on creatinine clearance in men: A cross-sectional and longitudinal study. *J Gerontol*. 1976;31:155-163.
10. Harmoinen A, Lehtimaki T, Korpela M, et al. Diagnostic accuracies of plasma creatinine, cystatin C, and glomerular filtration rate calculated by the Cockcroft-Gault and Levey (MDRD) formulas. *Clin Chem*. 2003;49:1223-1225.
11. Verhave JC, Fesler P, Ribstein J, et al. Estimation of renal function in subjects with normal serum creatinine levels: Influence of age and body mass index. *Am J Kidney Dis*. 2005;46:233-241.
12. Shlipak MG, Wassel Fyr CL, et al. Cystatin C and mortality risk in the elderly: The health, aging, and body composition study. *J Am Soc Nephrol*. 2006;17:254-261.
13. Wasen E, Isoaho R, Mattila K, et al. Renal impairment associated with diabetes in the elderly. *Diabetes Care*. 2004;27:2648-2653.
14. Coresh J, Selvin E, Stevens LA, et al. Prevalence of chronic kidney disease in the United States. *JAMA*. 2007;298:2038-2047.
15. Tonelli M, Wiebe N, Culleton B, et al. Chronic kidney disease and mortality risk: A systematic review. *J Am Soc Nephrol*. 2006;17:2034-2047.
16. O'Hare AM, Bertenthal D, Covinsky KE, et al. Mortality risk stratification in chronic kidney disease: One size for all ages? *J Am Soc Nephrol*. 2006;17:846-853.
17. Campbell KH, O'Hare AM. Kidney disease in the elderly: Update on recent literature. *Curr Opin Nephrol Hypertens*. 2008;17:298-303.
18. Glassock RJ. Glomerular disease in the elderly population. *Geriatr Nephrol Urol*. 1998;8:149-154.
19. Baylis C, Corman B. The aging kidney: Insights from experimental studies. *J Am Soc Nephrol*. 1998;9:699-709.
20. Kaplan C, Pasternack B, Shah H, Gallo G. Age-related incidence of sclerotic glomeruli in human kidneys. *Am J Pathol*. 1975;80:227-234.
21. Smith SM, Hoy WE, Cobb L. Low incidence of glomerulosclerosis in normal kidneys. *Arch Pathol Lab Med*. 1989;113:1253-1255.
22. Takazakura E, Sawabu N, Handa A, et al. Intrarenal vascular changes with age and disease. *Kidney Int*. 1972;2:224-230.
23. Kang DH, Anderson S, Kim YG, et al. Impaired angiogenesis in the aging kidney: Vascular endothelial growth factor and thrombospondin-1 in renal disease. *Am J Kidney Dis*. 2001;37:601-611.
24. Thomas SE, Anderson S, Gordon KL, et al. Tubulointerstitial disease in aging: Evidence for underlying peritubular capillary damage, a potential role for renal ischemia. *J Am Soc Nephrol*. 1998;9:231-242.
25. Beckman KB, Ames BN. The free radical theory of aging matures. *Physiol Rev*. 1998;78:547-581.
26. de Cavanagh EM, Piotrkowski B, Basso N, et al. Enalapril and losartan attenuate mitochondrial dysfunction in aged rats. *FASEB J*. 2003;17:1096-1098.
27. Ferder L, Inserra F, Romano L, et al. Effects of angiotensin-converting enzyme inhibition on mitochondrial number in the aging mouse. *Am J Physiol*. 1993;265:C15-C18.
28. Anderson S, Rennke HG, Zatz R. Glomerular adaptations with normal aging and with long-term converting enzyme inhibition in rats. *Am J Physiol*. 1994;267:F35-F43.
29. Basso N, Paglia N, Stella I, et al. Protective effect of the inhibition of the renin-angiotensin system on aging. *Regul Pept*. 2005;128:247-252.
30. Ferder LF, Inserra F, Basso N. Effects of renin-angiotensin system blockade in the aging kidney. *Exp Gerontol*. 2003;38:237-244.
31. Benigni A, Corna D, Zoja C, et al. Disruption of the Ang II type 1 receptor promotes longevity in mice. *J Clin Invest*. 2009;119:524-530.
32. Anderson S, Brenner BM. Progressive renal disease: A disorder of adaptation. *Q J Med*. 1989;70:185-189.
33. Laurent S, Cockcroft J, Van Bortel L, et al. Expert consensus document on arterial stiffness: Methodological issues and clinical applications. *Eur Heart J*. 2006;27:2588-2605.
34. Verhave JC, Fesler P, du Cailar G, et al. Elevated pulse pressure is associated with low renal function in elderly patients with isolated systolic hypertension. *Hypertension*. 2005;45:586-591.
35. Bakris G. Proteinuria: A link to understanding changes in vascular compliance? *Hypertension*. 2005;46:473-474.
36. Tracy RE, Newman WP 3rd, Wattigney WA, et al. Histologic features of atherosclerosis and hypertension from autopsies of young individuals in a defined geographic population: The Bogalusa Heart Study. *Atherosclerosis*. 1995;116:163-179.
37. Fesler P, Safar ME, du Cailar G, et al. Pulse pressure is an independent determinant of renal function decline during treatment of essential hypertension. *J Hypertens*. 2007;25:1915-1920.
38. Campo C, Lahera V, Garcia-Robles R, et al. Aging abolishes the renal response to L-arginine infusion in essential hypertension. *Kidney Int Suppl*. 1996;55:S126-S128.
39. Epstein FH, Prasad P. Effects of furosemide on medullary oxygenation in younger and older subjects. *Kidney Int*. 2000;57:2080-2083.
40. Baylis C. Nitric oxide deficiency in chronic kidney disease. *Am J Physiol Renal Physiol*. 2008;294:F1-F9.
41. Rathaus M, Greenfeld Z, Podjarny E, et al. Sodium loading and renal prostaglandins in old rats. *Prostaglandins Leukot Essent Fatty Acids*. 1993;49:815-819.
42. Cai W, He JC, Zhu L, et al. Reduced oxidant stress and extended lifespan in mice exposed to a low glycotoxin diet: Association with increased AGER1 expression. *Am J Pathol*. 2007;170:1893-1902.
43. Cai W, He JC, Zhu L, et al. Oral glycotoxins determine the effects of calorie restriction on oxidant stress, age-related diseases, and lifespan. *Am J Pathol*. 2008;173:327-336.
44. Luft FC, Grim CE, Fineberg N, Weinberger MC. Effects of volume expansion and contraction in normotensive whites, blacks, and subjects of different ages. *Circulation*. 1979;59:643-650.

45. Epstein M, Hollenberg NK. Age as a determinant of renal sodium conservation in normal man. *J Lab Clin Med.* 1976;87:411-417.
46. Fliser D, Franek E, Joest M, et al. Renal function in the elderly: Impact of hypertension and cardiac function. *Kidney Int.* 1997;51:1196-1204.
47. Burt VL, Whelton P, Roccella EJ, et al. Prevalence of hypertension in the US adult population. Results from the Third National Health and Nutrition Examination Survey, 1988-1991. *Hypertension.* 1995;25:305-313.
48. Weinberger MH, Fineberg NS. Sodium and volume sensitivity of blood pressure. Age and pressure change over time. *Hypertension.* 1991;18:67-71.
49. Oliver WJ, Cohen EL, Neel JV. Blood pressure, sodium intake, and sodium related hormones in the Yanomamo Indians, a "no-salt" culture. *Circulation.* 1975;52:146-151.
50. Streeten DH, Anderson GH Jr, Wagner S. Effect of age on response of secondary hypertension to specific treatment. *Am J Hypertens.* 1990;3:360-365.
51. Ershler WB, Sheng S, McKelvey J, et al. Serum erythropoietin and aging: A longitudinal analysis. *J Am Geriatr Soc.* 2005;53:1360-1365.
52. Carpenter MA, Kendall RG, O'Brien AE, et al. Reduced erythropoietin response to anaemia in elderly patients with normocytic anaemia. *Eur J Haematol.* 1992;49:119-121.
53. Gallagher JC, Rapuri P, Smith L. Falls are associated with decreased renal function and insufficient calcitriol production by the kidney. *J Steroid Biochem Mol Biol.* 2007;103:610-613.
54. Duckworth WC, Bennett RG, Hamel FG. Insulin degradation: Progress and potential. *Endocr Rev.* 1998;19:608-624.
55. Vendemia F, Gesualdo L, Schena FP, D'Amico G. Epidemiology of primary glomerulonephritis in the elderly. Report from the Italian Registry of Renal Biopsy. *J Nephrol.* 2001;14:340-352.
56. Sirls LT, Rashid T. Geriatric urinary incontinence. *Geriatr Nephrol Urol.* 1999;9:87-99.
57. Foley RN, Murray AM, Li S, et al. Chronic kidney disease and the risk for cardiovascular disease, renal replacement, and death in the United States Medicare population, 1998 to 1999. *J Am Soc Nephrol.* 2005;16:489-495.
58. Eriksen BO, Ingebretsen OC. The progression of chronic kidney disease: A 10-year population-based study of the effects of gender and age. *Kidney Int.* 2006;69:375-382.
59. Rao PS, Merion RM, Ashby VB, et al. Renal transplantation in elderly patients older than 70 years of age: Results from the Scientific Registry of Transplant Recipients. *Transplantation.* 2007;83:1069-1074.
60. Tesi RJ, Elkhammas EA, Davies EA, et al. Renal transplantation in older people. *Lancet.* 1994;343:461-464.
61. Meier-Kriesche HU, Ojo A, Hanson J, et al. Increased immunosuppressive vulnerability in elderly renal transplant recipients. *Transplantation.* 2000;69:885-889.
62. Frei U, Noeldeke J, Machold-Fabrizii V, et al. Prospective age-matching in elderly kidney transplant recipients—a 5-year analysis of the Eurotransplant Senior Program. *Am J Transplant.* 2008;8:50-57.
63. Ekberg H, Tedesco-Silva H, Demirbas A, et al. Reduced exposure to calcineurin inhibitors in renal transplantation. *N Engl J Med.* 2007;357:2562-2575.
64. Schold JD, Kaplan B, Baliga RS, Meier-Kriesche HU. The broad spectrum of quality in deceased donor kidneys. *Am J Transplant.* 2005;5:757-765.

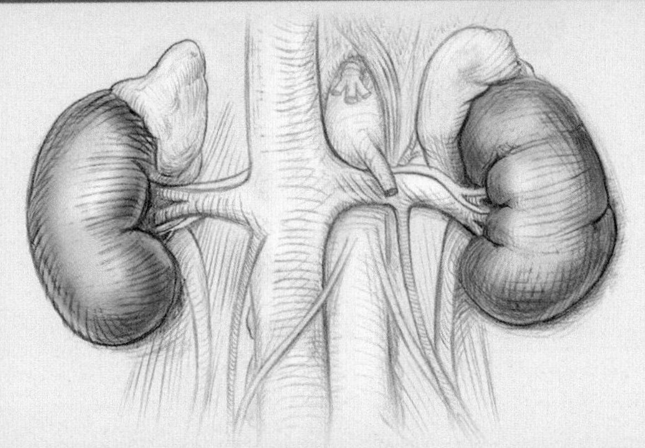

SECTION XIII

Acute Kidney Injury

CHAPTER 66

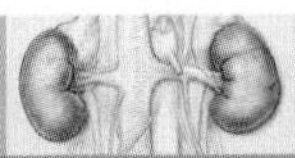

Pathophysiology and Etiology of Acute Kidney Injury

J. Ashley Jefferson, Joshua M. Thurman, Robert W. Schrier

DEFINITION

Acute kidney injury (AKI) is a clinical syndrome denoted by an abrupt decline in glomerular filtration rate (GFR) sufficient to decrease the elimination of nitrogenous waste products (urea and creatinine) and other uremic toxins. This has traditionally been referred to as acute renal failure (ARF), but in recent years, an effort has been made to implement the term AKI instead of ARF and to develop a standardized definition of AKI. One proposed definition of AKI, for example, is a decline in kidney function during 48 hours as demonstrated by an increase in serum creatinine of more than 0.3 mg/dl, an increase in serum creatinine of more than 50%, or the development of oliguria.[1] Staging criteria (see Chapter 68) have also been based on the magnitude of the rise in serum creatinine and changes in the volume of urine output during 1 week,[1] and studies have validated that these staging criteria are of prognostic value.

ETIOLOGY OVERVIEW

Although AKI is defined by a reduced GFR, the underlying etiology of the renal impairment is most frequently due to tubular and vascular factors. AKI can be due to a broad range of causes, and the differential diagnosis must be considered in a systematic fashion to avoid missing multiple factors that may be contributing to the condition. The traditional paradigm divides AKI into prerenal, renal, and postrenal causes. Prerenal AKI may be due to hypovolemia or a decreased effective arterial volume. Postrenal obstructive renal failure is usually diagnosed by urinary tract dilation on renal ultrasound or computed tomography scanning. Intrinsic renal causes of AKI should be considered under the different anatomic components of the kidney (vascular supply, glomerular, tubular, and interstitial disease; Fig. 66.1). Major extrarenal artery or venous occlusion must also be considered in the differential diagnosis (see Chapter 64). Similarly, disorders of the small intrarenal vasculature can result in AKI (e.g., vasculitis, thrombotic microangiopathy, malignant hypertension, eclampsia, postpartum states, disseminated intravascular coagulation, scleroderma; see Chapters 24, 28, 36, 42, and 62). All forms of acute glomerulonephritis can present as AKI, as can acute inflammation and space-occupying processes of the renal interstitium (e.g., drug-induced, infectious, and autoimmune disorders; leukemia; lymphoma; sarcoidosis).

In the hospital setting, prerenal uremia and acute tubular necrosis (ATN) account for the majority of AKI cases (Fig. 66.2).[2] The term *tubular necrosis* is a misnomer because the alterations are not limited to the tubular structures and true cellular necrosis in human ATN is often minimal. However, the term ATN is commonly employed in the clinical setting. To make things even more confusing, the terms ATN, ARF, and AKI are frequently used interchangeably in the literature. The term ATN should be reserved for cases of AKI in which a renal biopsy (if performed) would show the characteristic changes of tubular cell injury (Fig 66.3) or for patients with findings of tubular injury (such as renal tubular epithelial cells in the urine sediment) in an appropriate clinical setting.

There are also significant geographic differences in the causes of AKI; the spectrum of causes in tropical countries is described in Chapter 67. Obstetric AKI remains more common in emerging countries. There are also different patterns of accidental and deliberate self-poisoning. In Africa, herbal toxins are a common cause of AKI. Severe hemolysis may also occur in malaria; with drugs in association with glucose-6-phosphate dehydrogenase deficiency; and after spider, snake, and insect bites.

PATHOPHYSIOLOGY AND ETIOLOGY OF PRERENAL AZOTEMIA

Impaired renal perfusion with a resultant fall in glomerular capillary filtration pressure is a common cause of AKI. In this setting, tubular function is typically normal, renal reabsorption of sodium and water is increased, and consequently urine chemistries reveal a low urine sodium (<10 mmol/l) and a concentrated urine (urine osmolality >500 mOsm/kg).

A marked reduction in renal perfusion may overwhelm autoregulation and precipitate an acute fall in GFR. With lesser degrees of renal hypoperfusion, glomerular filtration pressures and GFR are maintained by afferent arteriolar vasodilation (mediated by vasodilatory eicosanoids) and efferent arteriolar vasoconstriction (mediated by angiotensin II). In this setting, AKI may be precipitated by agents that impair afferent arteriolar dilation (nonsteroidal anti-inflammatory drugs [NSAIDs]) or efferent vasoconstriction (angiotensin-converting enzyme [ACE] inhibitors and angiotensin receptor blockers [ARBs]).

Prerenal azotemia is commonly secondary to extracellular fluid volume depletion due to gastrointestinal losses (diarrhea, vomiting, prolonged nasogastric drainage), renal losses (diuretics, osmotic diuresis in hyperglycemia), dermal losses (burns, extensive sweating), or possibly sequestration of fluid, so-called third spacing (e.g., acute pancreatitis, muscle trauma). Renal perfusion may be impaired even in the setting of normal or even increased extracellular fluid. For example, renal perfusion may be reduced by a decreased cardiac output (heart failure) or by systemic arterial vasodilation with redistribution of cardiac output to extrarenal vascular beds (e.g., sepsis, liver cirrhosis).

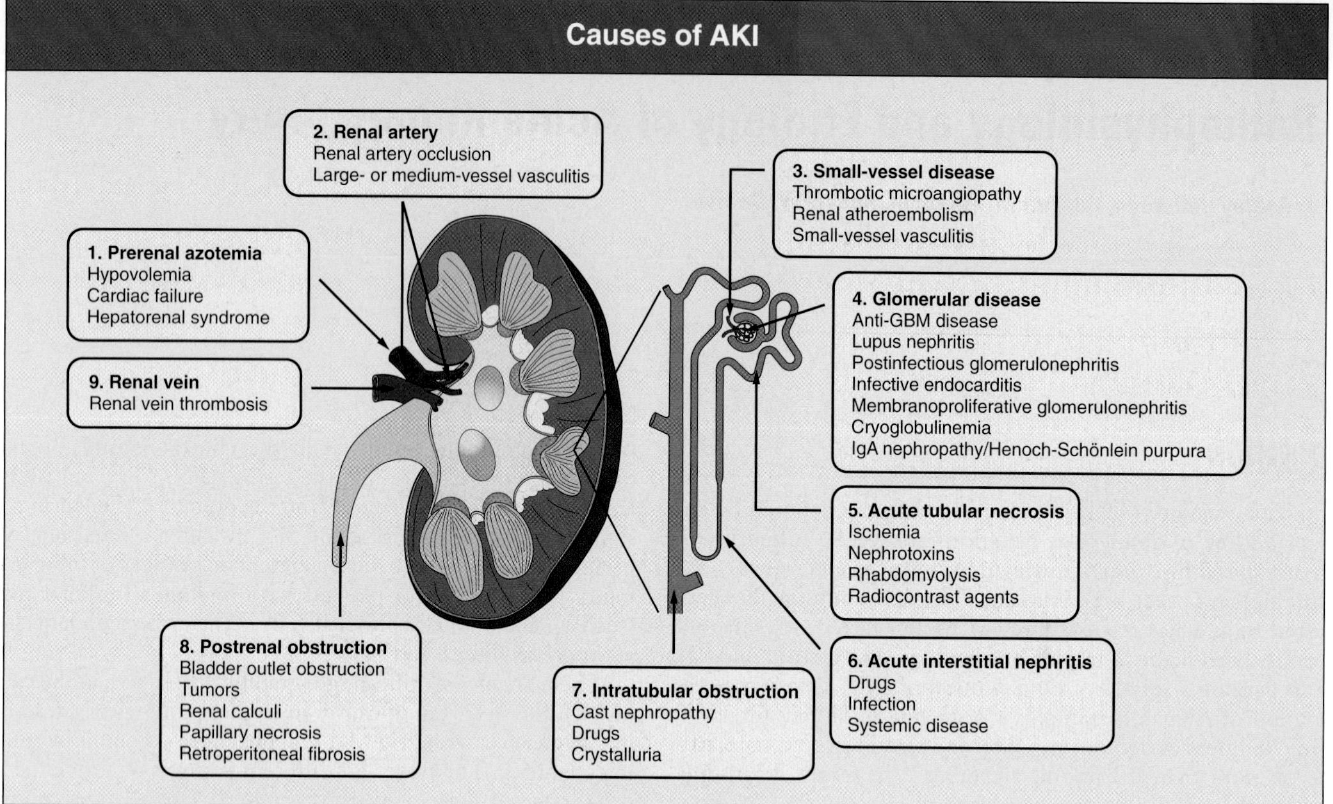

Figure 66.1 Causes of AKI. AKI is classified into prerenal, renal, and postrenal causes. Renal causes of AKI should be considered under the different anatomic components of the kidney (vascular supply, glomerular, tubular, and interstitial disease). GBM, glomerular basement membrane.

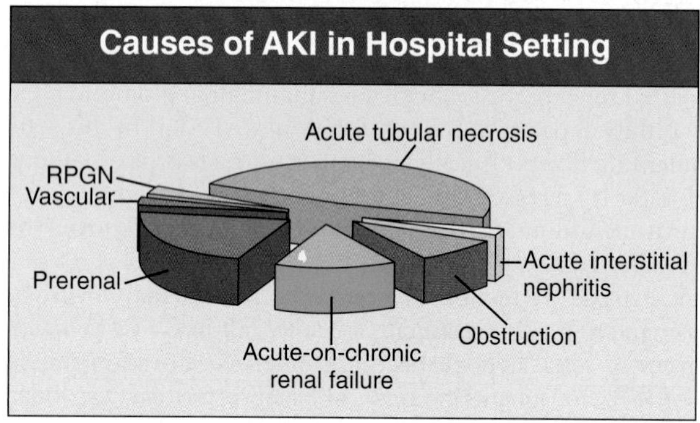

Figure 66.2 Causes of AKI in the hospital setting. RPGN, rapidly progressive glomerulonephritis.

The presence of AKI in the setting of severe heart failure has been termed the cardiorenal syndrome and is often exacerbated by the use of ACE inhibitors and diuretics.

An unusual cause of prerenal AKI is the hyperoncotic state. Infusion of large quantities of osmotically active substances, such as mannitol, dextran, and protein, can increase the glomerular oncotic pressure enough to exceed the glomerular capillary hydrostatic pressure, which stops glomerular filtration, leading to an anuric form of AKI.

Prerenal azotemia can be corrected if the extrarenal factors causing the renal hypoperfusion are rapidly reversed. Failure to restore renal blood flow during the functional prerenal stage will ultimately lead to ischemic ATN and tubular cell injury.

PATHOPHYSIOLOGY AND ETIOLOGY OF POSTRENAL ACUTE KIDNEY INJURY

In any patient presenting with AKI, an obstructive cause must be excluded because prompt intervention can result in improvement or complete recovery of renal function (see Chapter 58). Postrenal forms of AKI are divided into intrarenal (tubular) and extrarenal. Tubular precipitation of insoluble crystals (phosphate, methotrexate, acyclovir, sulfonamides, indinavir, uric acid, triamterene, oxalic acid) or protein (hemoglobin, myoglobin, paraprotein) can increase intratubular pressure. If it is sufficiently high, this opposes glomerular filtration pressure and can decrease GFR. Similarly, obstruction of the extrarenal collecting system at any level (renal pelvis, ureters, bladder, or urethra) can lead to postrenal AKI. Obstructive uropathy is common in older men with prostatic disease and in patients with a single kidney or intra-abdominal, particularly pelvic, cancer. Severe ureteral obstruction is also seen with small inflammatory aortic aneurysms. Most causes of obstructive uropathy are amenable to therapy, and the prognosis is generally good, depending on the underlying disease.

PATHOPHYSIOLOGY OF ACUTE TUBULAR NECROSIS

ATN commonly occurs in high-risk settings, which include after vascular and cardiac surgery, severe burns, pancreatitis, sepsis, and chronic liver disease. ATN is responsible for most cases of

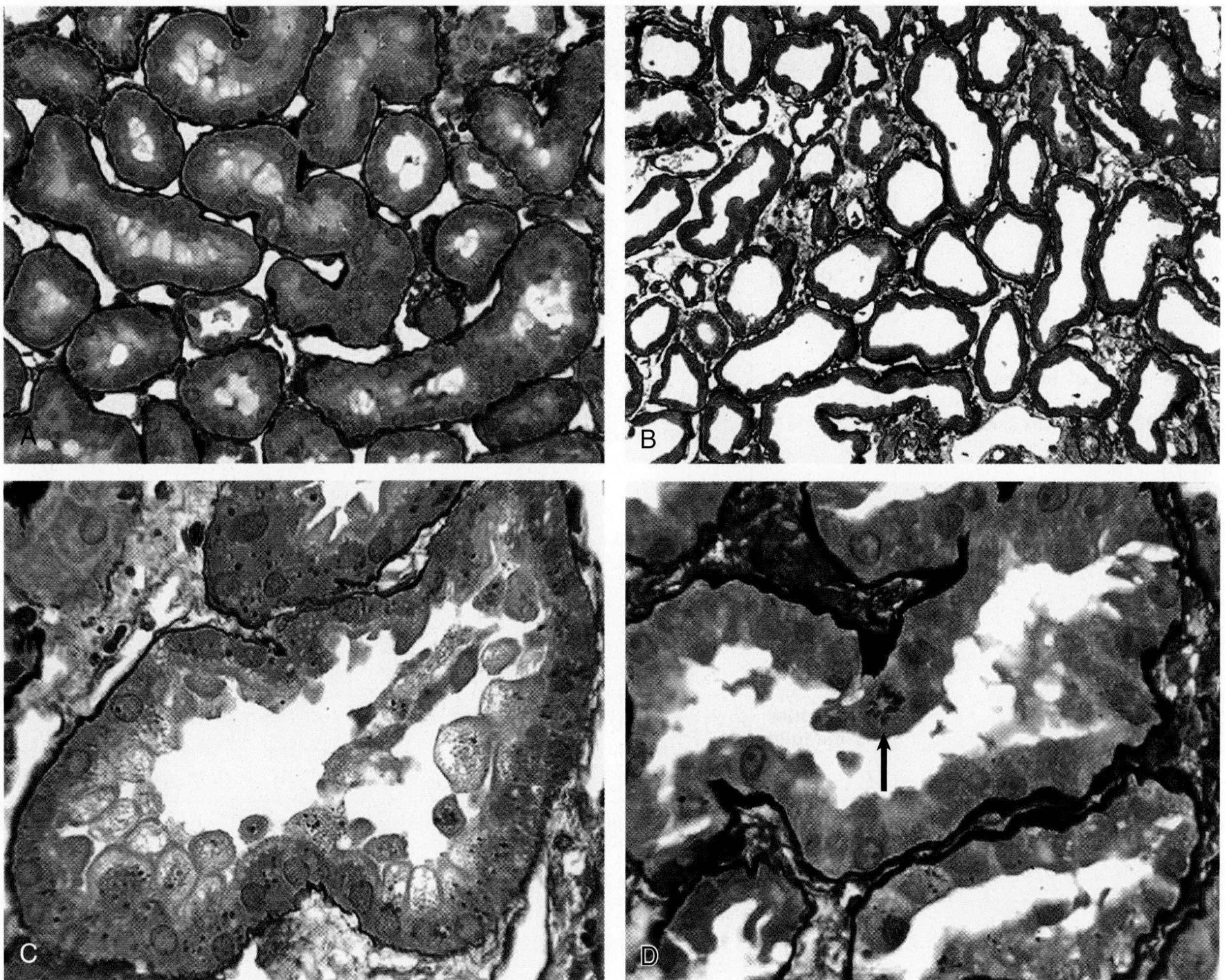

Figure 66.3 Renal pathology in acute tubular necrosis (ATN). A, Normal cortical renal tubules. **B** and **C,** ATN. Note the flattened epithelium, bare basement membranes, and intraluminal cellular debris. **D,** Recovering ATN showing a tubular epithelial cell mitotic figure *(arrow)*. *(Courtesy Erika Bracamonte, University of Washington, Seattle, USA.)*

hospital-acquired AKI and is usually due to ischemic or nephrotoxic injury.[3,4] In the intensive care unit, two thirds of cases of AKI are due to the combination of impaired renal perfusion, sepsis, and nephrotoxic agents.[5]

The importance of combined injurious mechanisms is also emphasized by experimental data. In animal studies, severe and prolonged hypotension (<50 mm Hg for 2 to 3 hours in the rat) does not cause ATN. Similarly, animal models require very high doses of single nephrotoxic agents to induce AKI. These features may reflect an inherent resistance to tubular injury in animal models but also illustrate the fact that a single insult alone is rarely sufficient to induce ATN. Fever may exacerbate ATN by increasing the renal tubular metabolic rate, thereby increasing adenosine triphosphate (ATP) consumption. In an experimental model (renal artery occlusion in the rat), renal ischemia for 40 minutes resulted in minimal renal injury at 32°C but marked renal injury at 39°C.

The typical course of uncomplicated ATN is recovery during 2 to 3 weeks. Superimposed renal insults often alter this pattern, however. For example, episodes of hypotension induced by hemodialysis may lead to additional ischemic lesions, potentially prolonging renal functional recovery, and patients with AKI often have multiple comorbidities.

Histology

The typical features of ATN on renal biopsy include vacuolization and loss of brush border in proximal tubular cells. Sloughing of tubular cells into the lumen leads to cast obstruction, manifested by tubular dilation. Interstitial edema can produce widely spaced tubules, and a mild leukocyte infiltration may be present (see Fig. 66.3).

Despite the term acute tubular "necrosis," frankly necrotic cells are not a common finding on renal biopsy, and histologic evidence of injury frequently involves only 10% to 15% of the tubules despite marked functional impairment. This implies that factors other than just tubular cell injury (such as vasoconstriction and tubular obstruction) are important in the loss of GFR.

Tubular Injury in Acute Tubular Necrosis

The tubular damage is usually due to a combination of ischemic injury resulting in depletion of cellular ATP and direct tubular epithelial cell injury by nephrotoxins. Most accept that the S_3 segment of the proximal tubule and the medullary thick ascending limb (mTAL) are particularly vulnerable to

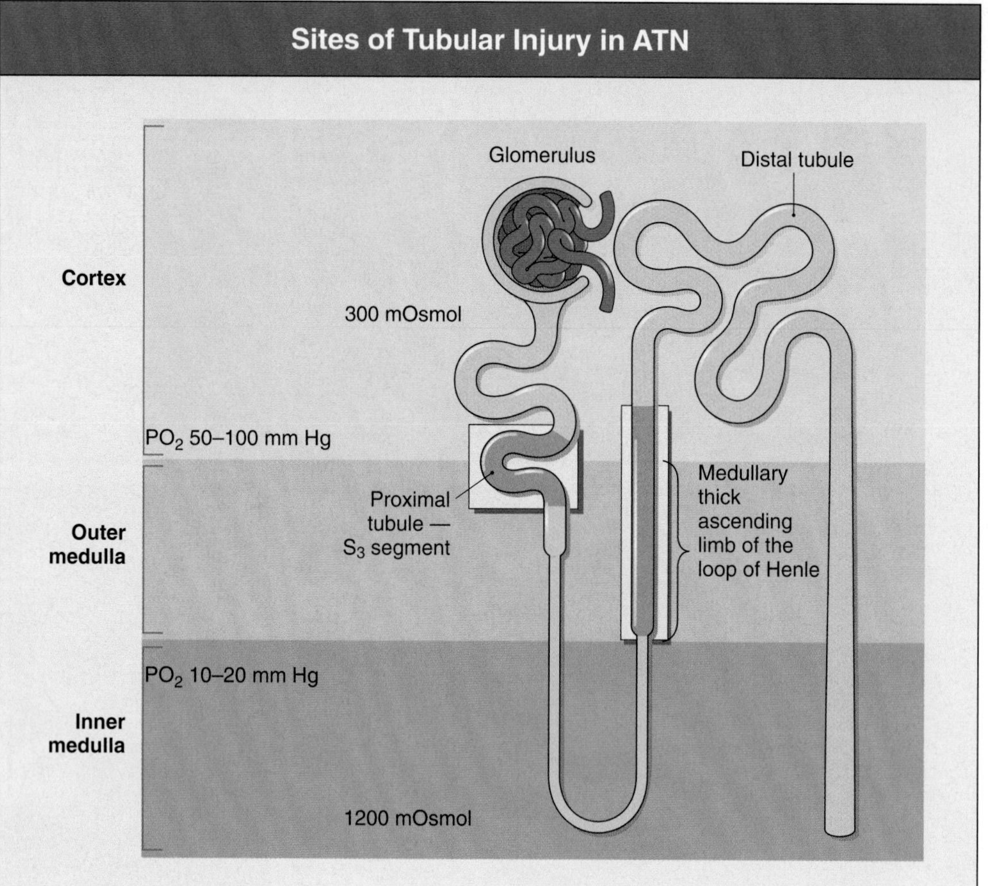

Figure 66.4 Sites of tubular injury in ATN. The S_3 segment of the proximal tubule and the medullary thick ascending limb are particularly vulnerable to ischemic injury because of the combination of borderline oxygen supply and high metabolic demands.

hypoxic injury (Fig. 66.4). There are several reasons for this vulnerability:

1. Blood supply. The blood flow to the kidney is not uniform, and most of it is directed to the renal cortex for glomerular filtration, where the cortical tissue Po_2 is 50 to 100 mm Hg. By contrast, the outer medulla and medullary rays are watershed areas receiving their blood supply from vasa recta. Countercurrent oxygen exchange occurs, leading to a progressive fall in Po_2 from cortex to medulla, which results in medullary cells living on the "brink of hypoxia" (medullary Po_2 as low as 10 to 15 mm Hg). The S_3 segments of proximal tubule cells and distal medullary thick ascending limbs are thus exposed to borderline chronic oxygen deprivation.
2. High tubular energy requirements. The cells of the S_3 region and mTAL have high metabolic activity, principally due to sodium reabsorption driven by basolateral membrane Na^+,K^+-ATPase. Indeed, blocking of sodium reabsorption in the mTAL with loop diuretics raises the medullary tissue Po_2 from about 15 to 35 mm Hg. Of note, the reduction of GFR in the setting of AKI may be renoprotective by diminishing sodium filtration and hence limiting ATP-dependent sodium reabsorption.
3. Glycolytic ability of tubular cells. Proximal tubular cells have minimal glycolytic machinery and rely almost solely on oxidative phosphorylation for the generation of ATP. In contrast, mTAL cells have a large glycolytic capacity and are more resistant to hypoxic or ischemic insults.

Hemodynamic Factors in the Development of Acute Tubular Necrosis

Impaired Renal Autoregulation

Autoregulation normally occurs between systolic blood pressures of 80 and 150 mm Hg, and between these ranges, renal blood flow, glomerular pressures, and GFR are maintained. Below 80 mm Hg, this autoregulation fails, and ischemic injury may result. In certain conditions, such as aging and chronic renal disease, autoregulation is abnormal, and ischemic injury may occur more easily with reductions in perfusion pressure. In addition, experimental studies demonstrate impaired autoregulation in ischemic ATN. In settings of low renal perfusion (e.g., volume depletion, left ventricular failure, edematous states, renal artery stenosis), GFR may be dependent on autoregulation mediated by vasodilatory prostaglandins acting on the afferent arteriole and angiotensin II–mediated efferent arteriolar vasoconstriction to maintain glomerular pressure. Any interference with these mechanisms (e.g., administration of ACE inhibitors or acute inhibition of cyclooxygenase 1 or 2 by NSAIDs) may produce a precipitous fall in GFR.

Intrarenal Vasoconstriction

In established ATN, renal blood flow is decreased by 30% to 50%. Indeed, in AKI, rather than the normal autoregulatory renal vasodilation that occurs in response to decreased perfusion pressure, there is evidence of renal vasoconstriction. A number of vasoconstrictors have been implicated in this vasoconstrictive

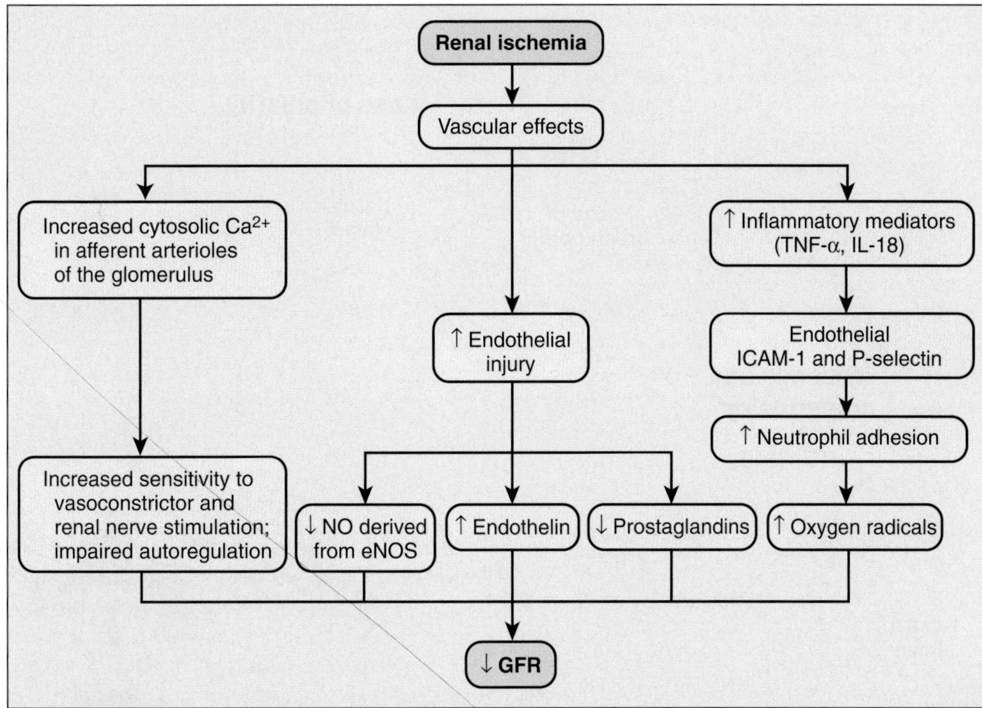

Figure 66.5 Vascular factors contributing to the development of acute tubular necrosis. ET, endothelin; ICAM-1, intercellular adhesion molecule 1; IL-18, interleukin-18; NO, nitric oxide; eNOS, endothelial nitric oxide synthase; PG, prostaglandin; TNF-α, tumor necrosis factor α. *(Modified with permission from reference 31.)*

response, including angiotensin II, endothelin 1, adenosine, thromboxane A_2, prostaglandin H_2, leukotrienes C_4 and D_4, and sympathetic nerve stimulation (Fig. 66.5). Tubuloglomerular feedback also contributes to this vasoconstriction. Some of these vascular abnormalities may be mediated by increased cytosolic calcium content in afferent arterioles as a result of ischemia, and disruption of the actin cytoskeleton in vascular smooth muscle cells may also impair autoregulation.

Tubuloglomerular Feedback

The role of tubuloglomerular feedback (see Chapter 2) in the setting of AKI may be partly beneficial because the resultant decrease in GFR limits sodium delivery to damaged tubules and decreases ATP-dependent tubular reabsorption, protecting against intracellular ATP depletion augmenting renal injury. In this respect, adenosine A_1 receptor knockout mice with absent tubuloglomerular feedback have augmented acute renal injury after ischemia-reperfusion.

Endothelial Cell Injury and the Development of Acute Tubular Necrosis

Renal cell injury is not limited to the tubular cell, and endothelial cell injury occurs partly as a result of acute renal ischemia and oxidant injury.[3] Endothelial injury is characterized by cell swelling, upregulation of adhesion molecules (with enhanced leukocyte–endothelial cell interactions), and impaired vasodilation (decreased endothelial nitric oxide synthase and vasodilatory prostaglandins) and may mediate some of the impaired autoregulation and intrarenal vasoconstriction described earlier. Endothelial injury within the peritubular capillaries (vasa recta) may produce congestion in the outer medulla, exacerbating hypoxic injury to the S_3 segment of the proximal tubule and the thick ascending loop of Henle.

Tubular Epithelial Cell Injury and the Development of Acute Tubular Necrosis

The tubular cell may be injured because of ischemia, with resulting depletion of cellular energy stores (ATP), or from direct cytotoxic injury. After acute renal ischemia, tubular cell injury may also result from the restoration of renal blood flow (reperfusion injury). Mediators of tubular cell injury include reactive oxygen species (ROS), intracellular calcium influx, nitric oxide, phospholipase A_2, complement, and cell-mediated cytotoxicity. ROS may be derived from local sources (including xanthine oxidase and cyclooxygenases and secondary to mitochondrial injury) or from infiltrating leukocytes. In models of ischemic ATN, a variety of methods that inhibit ROS protect against renal injury.[6]

Factors that affect the integrity and function of the renal tubular epithelial cells and contribute to the reduction in GFR include the following (Fig. 66.6):

1. Cell death. Despite the term acute tubular "necrosis," only a small percentage of tubular cells undergo cell death, and of these, many actually die by apoptosis rather than by necrosis. Indeed, studies in animal models have shown amelioration of renal injury with caspase inhibitors that inhibit apoptosis.
2. Disruption of actin cytoskeleton. A characteristic feature of sublethally injured cells is the disruption of the actin cytoskeleton. Activation of the cysteine protease calpain (partly due to increased intracellular calcium) can degrade actin-binding proteins such as spectrin and ankyrin. This leads to abnormal translocation of Na^+,K^+-ATPase and other proteins from the basolateral membrane to the cytoplasm or apical membranes. In the proximal tubular cell, this loss of polarity results in impaired proximal reabsorption of filtrate with increased distal NaCl delivery and activation of tubuloglomerular feedback.

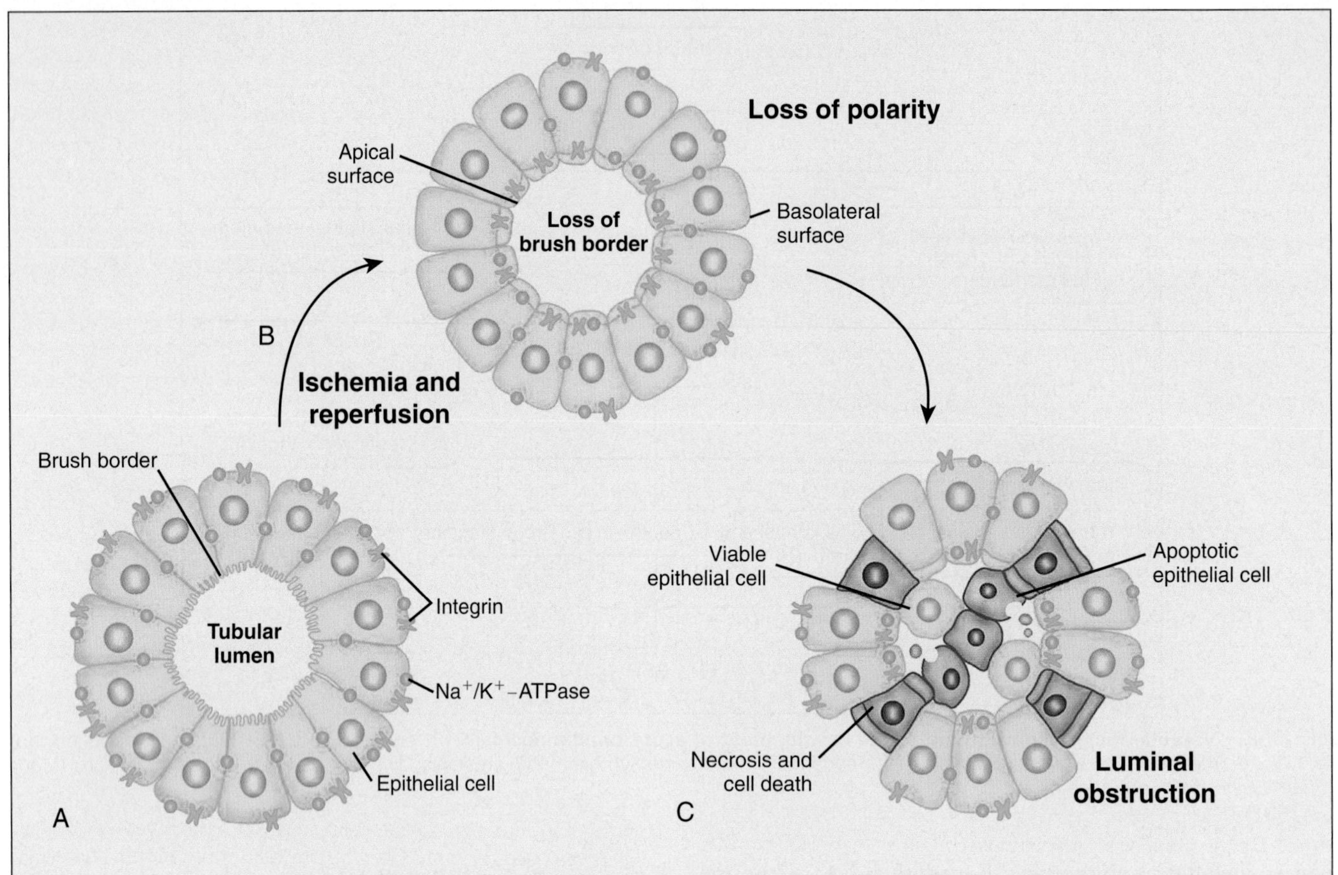

Figure 66.6 Tubular factors in the development of acute tubular necrosis. Loss of cell polarity weakens cell-cell and cell-matrix adhesion, resulting in cast obstruction and backleak of tubular fluid. *(Modified from reference 4.)*

3. Cast obstruction. Tubular cells are attached to the tubular basement membrane by $\alpha_3\beta_1$ integrins, which recognize RGD (arginine-glycine-aspartate) sequences in matrix proteins. Disruption of the actin cytoskeleton results in movement of integrins from basolateral positions to the apical membrane, leading to impaired cell matrix adhesion and cell detachment. Many of these detached cells are still viable and can be cultured from urine of patients with ATN. Sloughed proximal tubular cells can bind to RGD sequences in Tamm-Horsfall protein, resulting in cast formation and intratubular obstruction. In models of ischemic AKI, the elevation in tubular pressures may be inhibited by synthetic RGD peptides, mitigating the obstructive process.
4. Backleak. The loss of adhesion molecules (E-cadherin) and tight junction proteins (ZO-1, occludin) results in the weakening of junctions between cells, allowing filtrate to leak back into the renal interstitium. Although this does not alter the actual GFR at the level of the glomerulus, the net effect is a reduction in the measured GFR. Earlier dextran sieving experiments suggest only a modest effect of backleak on the decrement of GFR in AKI (about 10%); however, in the renal allograft with delayed graft function due to severe ATN, backleak has been calculated to account for up to 50% of the reduction in inulin clearance.

Inflammatory Factors in the Development of Acute Tubular Necrosis

The inflammatory response plays an important role in ATN.[7] Several proinflammatory cytokines (such as tumor necrosis factor α [TNF-α], interleukins IL-6 and IL-1β) and chemokines (such as MCP-1, IL-8, RANTES) are generated within the kidney and promote the infiltration of leukocytes. Renal hypoxia directly induces epithelial cells to produce some of these mediators. Ischemic injury also activates innate immune systems, including the complement system and Toll-like receptors 2 and 4 (TLR2 and TLR4). Activation of complement can cause direct injury of the renal tubular epithelial cells, and signaling through complement receptors and the Toll-like receptors induces the epithelial cells to produce chemokines.

Neutrophils and mononuclear cells may be seen in peritubular capillaries on renal biopsy. Experimental studies have helped to elucidate the role of the inflammatory cells in ATN. Neutrophil activation with the release of proteases and ROS can exacerbate injury. By contrast, neutrophil depletion with antibody, or inhibition of neutrophil adhesion molecules (ICAM-1) with antibody or antisense oligonucleotides, ameliorates injury in ischemic ATN. ICAM-1 knockout mice are similarly protected.

More recently, a role of T lymphocytes has emerged. Experimental ischemia-reperfusion injury may be ameliorated by T-cell depletion or blockade of T-cell costimulatory pathways. In addition, CD4-deficient mice (helper T cells) or mice that are unable to mount a Th1 response are protected against ischemia-reperfusion injury.

Recovery Phase

Recovery from ATN requires the restoration of tubular cell number and coverage of denuded tubular basement membrane. A marked increase in cell proliferation occurs in recovering human ATN, and mitotic figures may be seen by light microscopy (see Fig. 66.3). There has been some debate about the origin of the restored tubular cells. Some studies have suggested that mesenchymal stem cells may locate to areas of tubular injury and transform into proximal tubular cells. Indeed, experimental models of ischemia-reperfusion injury may be ameliorated by infusions of mesenchymal stem cells. More recent evidence, however, suggests that the restoration of tubular cell number is due to the dedifferentiation and proliferation of surviving tubular cells.[8] A number of growth factors have been implicated in the proliferative response, including insulin-like growth factor 1 (IGF-1) and hepatocyte growth factor; however, a therapeutic trial of subcutaneous recombinant IGF-1 in critically ill patients failed to show an acceleration in renal functional recovery.[9] After tubular epithelial cell proliferation, the dedifferentiated cells must migrate to areas of denuded tubular basement membrane, attach to the basement membrane, and differentiate into mature polar tubular epithelial cells.

SPECIFIC CAUSES OF ACUTE KIDNEY INJURY

Nephrotoxic Agents and Mechanisms of Toxicity

The avoidance of nephrotoxic agents in AKI is critical in the management of this condition because AKI may be rapidly reversible on removal of the offending agent. The mechanisms of nephrotoxicity are very broad and include alterations in renal hemodynamics, induction of direct tubular injury, generation of allergic reactions resulting in interstitial nephritis, and intratubular obstruction. The list is extensive, but the more common agents are presented in Figure 66.7.

Nonsteroidal Anti-inflammatory Drugs

NSAIDs are a common cause of AKI in the community because of the large amounts of these drugs either prescribed or bought over-the-counter.[10] The newer cyclooxygenase 2 (COX-2)–specific NSAIDs have effects on renal function similar to those of the nonselective NSAIDs.

This NSAID-related AKI may be due to a hemodynamically mediated reduction in GFR in particular clinical situations, such as atherosclerotic cardiovascular disease in elderly patients, preexisting chronic renal insufficiency, states of renal hypoperfusion (including sodium depletion, diuretic use, and hypotension), and sodium-avid states (such as cirrhosis, nephrotic syndrome, and congestive heart failure). There is little evidence that NSAIDs impair renal function in otherwise healthy individuals. This form of AKI is usually reversible in 2 to 7 days on discontinuation of the drug. Less frequently, NSAIDs induce ATN or, even more rarely, papillary necrosis.[10] NSAIDs, including the COX-2–specific NSAIDs, may also cause an acute interstitial nephritis (see Chapter 60). Other renal side effects of NSAIDs include fluid and electrolyte disturbances such as sodium retention exacerbating hypertension and congestive heart failure, hyponatremia, and hyperkalemia.

Angiotensin-Converting Enzyme Inhibitors and Angiotensin Receptor Blockers

ACE inhibitors and ARBs may also cause a hemodynamically induced AKI in the setting of reduced renal perfusion due to impaired vasoconstriction of the efferent arteriole. They may also directly impair renal perfusion by their antihypertensive effects. Patients in whom renal perfusion is compromised because of dehydration, renovascular disease, or functionally impaired autoregulation are at risk for development of AKI after initiation of therapy with ACE inhibitors or ARBs.

Patients chronically treated with ACE inhibitors have an increased risk for postoperative renal dysfunction,[11] probably as a consequence of intraoperative hypotensive episodes.

Gentamicin

Gentamicin is excreted by glomerular filtration, and toxicity may occur if the dose is not adjusted for underlying renal impairment. Cationic amino groups (NH_4^+) on the drug bind to anionic megalin on the brush border of proximal tubular epithelial cells, and the drug is then internalized by endocytosis. The drug accumulates in proximal tubular cell lysosomes and can reach 100 to 1000 times its serum concentration. The drug interferes with cellular energetics, impairs intracellular phospholipases, and induces oxidative stress; however, the exact pathways culminating in tubular necrosis remain unknown.[12]

Nonoliguric AKI usually occurs after 5 to 10 days of treatment with gentamicin. Involvement of distal tubular segments may produce polyuria and potassium and magnesium wasting. The risk for AKI correlates with the accumulation of gentamicin in proximal tubular cells and is related to the daily dose and duration of therapy. Prolonged accumulation in proximal tubular cells may allow development of AKI even after the drug has been discontinued. Additional risk factors for gentamicin toxicity include increasing age, preexisting renal disease, hypotension, concurrent liver disease, sepsis syndrome, and concurrent nephrotoxins.

Gentamicin serum levels should be followed to minimize nephrotoxicity. When possible, the drug may be administered in a single daily total dose, which leads to lower renal proximal tubular cell accumulation. Gentamicin, tobramycin, and netilmicin appear to have similar nephrotoxic effects. Amikacin, which has fewer amino groups per molecule, may be less nephrotoxic.

The macrolide antibiotic vancomycin has only rarely been associated with AKI when it is used as monotherapy, typically with toxic serum drug levels. However, when it is used with gentamicin, it may increase the risk for aminoglycoside-induced AKI.

Amphotericin

This polyene macrolide antibiotic binds to sterols in the cell membranes of fungal walls (ergosterol) and mammalian (cholesterol) cell membranes, resulting in the formation of aqueous pores, which increase membrane permeability. The increased sodium influx leads to increased Na^+,K^+-ATPase activity and depletion of cellular energy stores. In addition, the standard amphotericin formulation is suspended in the bile salt deoxycholate, which has a detergent effect on cell membranes.[13] Nephrotoxicity relates to cumulative dosage, usually occurring after administration of 2 to 3 g.

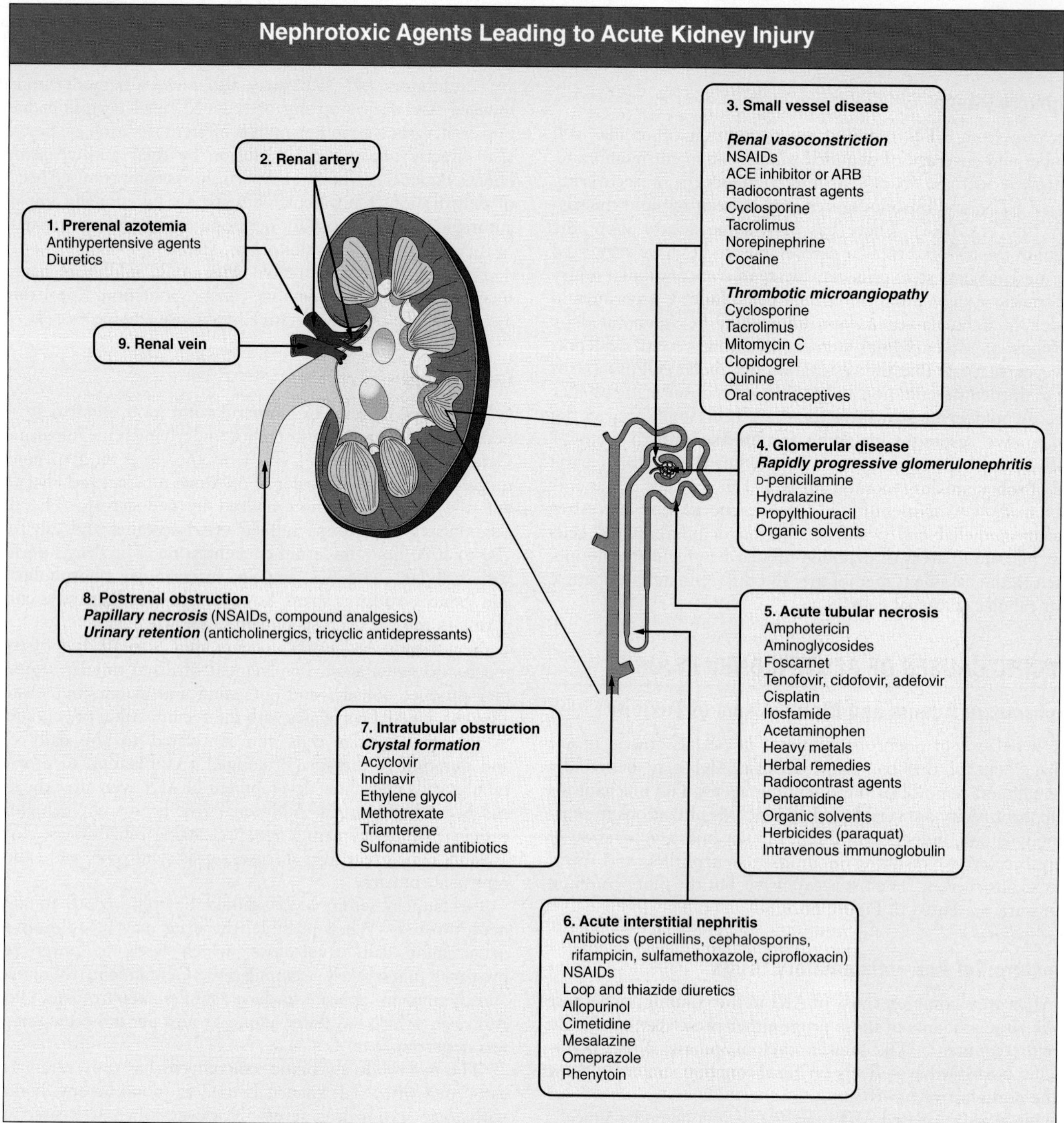

Figure 66.7 Common nephrotoxic agents leading to acute kidney injury. ACE, angiotensin-converting enzyme; ARB, angiotensin receptor blocker; NSAIDs, nonsteroidal anti-inflammatory drugs.

Early signs of nephrotoxicity include a loss of urine concentrating ability, followed by a decrease in GFR. Hypokalemia and hypomagnesemia due to distal tubular toxicity are common. A distal renal tubular acidosis may be due to proton backleak in the cortical collecting duct.

Prevention of nephrotoxicity requires the maintenance of high urine flow rates by saline loading during amphotericin administration. The more expensive liposomal amphotericin preparations reduce the incidence of AKI by 50%. The binding of amphotericin to ergosterol is more avid than to cholesterol, and by delivery of the drug as a cholesterol liposome, diminished binding to tubular epithelial cell membranes results without altering fungal binding. In addition, liposomal preparations do not contain deoxycholate. Amphotericin-induced AKI is usually reversible with discontinuation of treatment with the drug, although distal tubular injury as manifested by magnesium wasting may persist.

Antiviral Therapy

Acyclovir

Nephrotoxicity is typically seen after intravenous acyclovir administration and may be due to direct tubular cell toxicity and the formation of intratubular acyclovir crystals, which appear as birefringent needle-shaped crystals on urine microscopy. However, crystals may also be seen in non-AKI patients, and renal biopsy data suggest that acute interstitial nephritis may be the predominant mechanism of toxicity. Ceftriaxone appears to increase the risk for nephrotoxicity. By contrast, ganciclovir has little nephrotoxicity.

Oliguric AKI typically occurs within a few days of treatment and may be associated with abdominal or loin pain. High serum levels of acyclovir due to decreased renal clearance may produce neurologic toxicity. The AKI is usually mild and recovers on stopping of the drug.

Foscarnet

Foscarnet is a phosphate analogue used in the treatment of severe cytomegalovirus infection but also inhibits proximal tubule sodium-phosphate cotransport. AKI occurs in 10% to 20% of treated patients and may be due to ATN or intratubular crystal obstruction and acute interstitial nephritis. The AKI is usually nonoliguric and associated with mild proteinuria (<1 g) and a benign urine sediment. Hypocalcemia due to chelation of calcium may be present. The renal failure is usually reversible, although recovery may take several months. Prehydration markedly decreases the incidence of AKI.

Cidofovir and Adefovir

These nucleotide analogues have been associated with AKI secondary to proximal tubular injury in 12% to 24% of cases. They are transported into the proximal tubule by the human organic anion transporter (hOAT), and nephrotoxicity may be reduced by concurrent use of probenecid, which blocks hOAT and volume expansion.

Other Antiviral Agents

Most other antiviral agents are not nephrotoxic. In the treatment of hepatitis C, there have been rare reports of ATN secondary to interferon alfa.

Immunosuppressive Agents

See also Chapter 97.

Calcineurin Inhibitors

Cyclosporine and tacrolimus may cause acute renal impairment due to afferent arteriolar vasoconstriction partly mediated by endothelin. This is usually reversible on dose reduction. Persistent injury may lead to chronic interstitial fibrosis in a striped pattern along medullary rays, reflecting the ischemic nature of the insult as well as the development of arteriolar hyalinosis. Associated clinical features may include hypertension, hyperkalemia, hyperuricemia, and wasting of phosphate and magnesium from tubular injury. Calcineurin inhibitors may also cause endothelial injury, leading to thrombotic microangiopathy (see Chapter 28).

Other Immunosuppressive Agents

The monoclonal anti-CD3 antibody OKT3 or polyclonal antilymphocyte and antithymocyte preparations may cause a first-dose cytokine release syndrome and prerenal azotemia secondary to capillary leak. OKT3 has rarely been associated with a hemolytic-uremic syndrome. Intravenous immune globulin can cause AKI, which may be partly mediated by the high sucrose concentration in these products. Tubular uptake of sucrose may result in osmotic cell swelling and injury. Methotrexate is toxic to proximal tubular epithelial cells and rarely may cause intratubular crystal obstruction.

Acetaminophen (Paracetamol)

Isolated ATN with acetaminophen may occur in rare cases, but renal injury is more typically associated with acute hepatitis. Renal and liver toxic effects usually occur when more than 15 g has been taken, but in alcoholics, normal doses may be toxic. Acetaminophen is conjugated in the liver and undergoes renal excretion. Less than 5% undergoes metabolism by P-450 (CYP2E1) enzymes to form a toxic metabolite, *N*-acetylimidoquinone, which is inactivated by the thiol group of glutathione. With high levels of acetaminophen, glutathione becomes depleted, and *N*-acetylimidoquinone can bind to thiol groups on intracellular proteins, resulting in cell injury. Because glutathione is a major intracellular antioxidant, its loss may predispose to oxidative injury to the tubular cells.

Clinically, acute hepatitis and ATN only begin once glutathione levels are depleted, and clinical manifestations usually present 3 to 4 days after ingestion. *N*-Acetylcysteine can be protective, if it is administered early, because it provides a free thiol group, substituting for glutathione.

Ethylene Glycol

Ethylene glycol, found in antifreeze, remains a cause of both deliberate and accidental injury. It is rapidly metabolized by alcohol dehydrogenase to glycoaldehyde and glyoxylate, which are toxic to tubular cells. Further metabolism generates oxalic acid, which can precipitate in renal tubules, leading to intratubular obstruction.

The diagnosis is suggested by the presence of a severe anion gap metabolic acidosis and the presence of a serum osmolal gap. Oxalate crystals are typically but not always seen on urine microscopy (see Chapter 4, Fig. 4.7). Management includes inhibition of alcohol dehydrogenase with intravenous ethanol (aiming for blood levels of 100 to 200 mg/dl) or the specific alcohol dehydrogenase inhibitor fomepizole. Hemodialysis should be performed to remove the ethylene glycol and metabolites when the level is above 20 mg/dl and continued until it is below 5 mg/dl. Methanol intoxication may present with similar metabolic abnormalities but rarely causes AKI (see Chapter 12).

Illicit Drug Use

AKI is a common condition in those who abuse drugs. It may be due to nephrotoxicity of the drug, coexistent viral infection (human immunodeficiency virus [HIV] infection, hepatitis C virus [HCV] infection), sepsis, infective endocarditis, rhabdomyolysis, or alcohol abuse.

Cocaine induces intense vasoconstriction, which may lead to severe hypertension and rhabdomyolysis.[14] Mechanisms for rhabdomyolysis include coma and pressure necrosis, vasospasm leading to ischemic muscle injury, and adrenergic stimulation and hyperpyrexia leading to increased cellular metabolism. It typically occurs in those who inject cocaine, and the patient often presents with fever, hypertension, tachycardia, and a decreased mental state.

Other illicit drugs associated with AKI include opiates (coma-associated, pressure-induced rhabdomyolysis), phencyclidine (PCP; rhabdomyolysis secondary to hyperpyrexia and vasoconstriction), heroin (rhabdomyolysis), and amphetamines (AKI secondary to rhabdomyolysis, acute interstitial nephritis, or acute necrotizing angiitis).

Bisphosphonates

AKI due to tubular injury has been described with intravenous bisphosphonates (especially zoledronate and pamidronate), but not oral. This typically occurs after several months of treatment.

Bowel Preparations (Oral Sodium Phosphate and Polyethylene Glycol–Electrolyte Lavage Solution)

Bowel preparation for colonoscopic procedures is usually performed by the oral administration of high-osmolar agents such as oral sodium phosphate. These agents have been associated with the development of electrolyte disturbances, AKI, and chronic kidney disease (CKD).[15] AKI associated with oral sodium phosphate, also referred to as phosphate nephropathy, is believed to be caused by phosphaturia and calcium phosphate deposition within the renal tubules. This occurs most frequently in patients with CKD.

Occupational Toxins

Heavy Metals

Lead intoxication usually causes a chronic nephropathy (see Chapter 62). Rarely, acute tubular injury occurs that may be associated with Fanconi syndrome. ATN may also occur in cadmium and mercury poisoning.

Organic Solvents

Organic solvents may cause acute tubular injury by peroxidation of membrane lipids. A subacute renal failure due to anti–glomerular basement membrane (anti-GBM) antibody disease has also been reported with exposure to halogenated hydrocarbons.

Herbal Remedies

Specific herbs used in traditional African medicine (e.g., Cape aloes, *Callilepis laureola*) are common causes of AKI in parts of Africa. A subacute form of renal failure due to aristolochic acid found in certain herbs used in traditional Chinese medicine has also been described (see Chapter 62).

HEME PIGMENT NEPHROPATHY

Heme pigment nephropathy is a common cause of AKI and usually secondary to the breakdown of muscle fibers (rhabdomyolysis), which release potentially nephrotoxic intracellular contents (particularly myoglobin) into the systemic circulation. Less commonly, heme pigment nephropathy may be due to massive intravascular hemolysis. Prevention of and therapy for heme pigment nephropathy are discussed in Chapter 69.

Causes of Rhabdomyolysis

Muscle trauma is the most common cause of rhabdomyolysis. The initial description was by Bywaters and Beall during the bombing of London in World War II.[16] Other common causes of muscle injury include marked exercise, seizures, pressure necrosis secondary to coma, alcohol abuse, and limb ischemia (Fig. 66.8). In skeletal muscles confined to rigid compartments, cell swelling after injury may result in increased intracompartmental pressures impairing local microvascular circulation, leading to compartment syndrome (Fig. 66.9). In the patient with alcohol abuse, rhabdomyolysis is often multifactorial. Contributing causes include pressure necrosis from coma ("found down"), direct myotoxicity from ethanol, seizures, and electrolyte abnormalities (hypokalemia and hypophosphatemia). Therapy with statins may be associated with rhabdomyolysis. The risk is increased by concomitant therapy with fibrates, cyclosporine, or erythromycin. Familial myopathies such as McArdle's syndrome and carnitine palmityltransferase deficiency should be suspected in patients with a history of recurrent episodes of rhabdomyolysis associated with muscle pain, positive family history, onset in childhood, and absence of other identifiable causes.[17]

Causes of Rhabdomyolysis	
Muscle injury/ischemia	Trauma, pressure necrosis, electric shock, burns, acute vascular disease
Myofiber exhaustion	Seizures, excessive exercise, heat exhaustion
Toxins	Alcohol, cocaine, heroin, amphetamines, ecstasy, phencyclidine, snakebite
Drugs	Statins, fibrates, zidovudine, neuroleptic malignant syndrome, azathioprine, theophylline, lithium, diuretics
Electrolyte disorders	Hypophosphatemia, hypokalemia, excess water shifts (hyperosmolality)
Infections	Viral (influenza, HIV, Coxsackievirus, Epstein-Barr virus), bacterial (*Legionella, Francisella, Streptococcus pneumoniae, Salmonella, Staphylococcus aureus*)
Familial	McArdle's disease, carnitine palmitoyl transferase deficiency, malignant hyperthermia
Other	Hypothyroidism, polymyositis, dermatomyositis

Figure 66.8 Causes of rhabdomyolysis.

Causes of Hemoglobinuria

Intravascular hemolysis results in circulating free hemoglobin. If the hemolysis is mild, the released hemoglobin is bound by circulating haptoglobin. With massive hemolysis, however, haptoglobin becomes exhausted. Hemoglobin (69 kd) then dissociates into $\alpha\beta$ dimers (34 kd) that are small enough to be filtered, resulting in hemoglobinuria, hemoglobin cast formation, and heme uptake by proximal tubular cells. Like myoglobin, these processes can result in ATN and filtration failure. Causes of hemoglobinuric AKI include incompatible blood transfusion, autoimmune hemolytic anemia, malaria (blackwater fever), glucose-6-phosphate dehydrogenase deficiency, paroxysmal nocturnal hemoglobinuria, march hemoglobinuria, and toxins (dapsone, venoms).

Pathogenesis of Heme Pigment Nephropathy

The renal injury is due to a combination of factors, including volume depletion, renal vasoconstriction, direct heme protein–

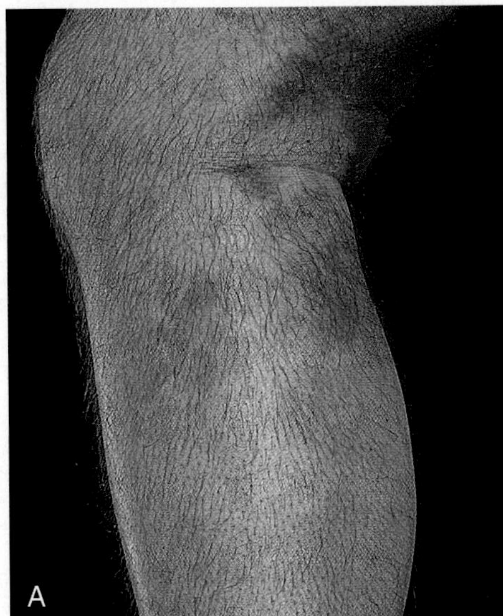

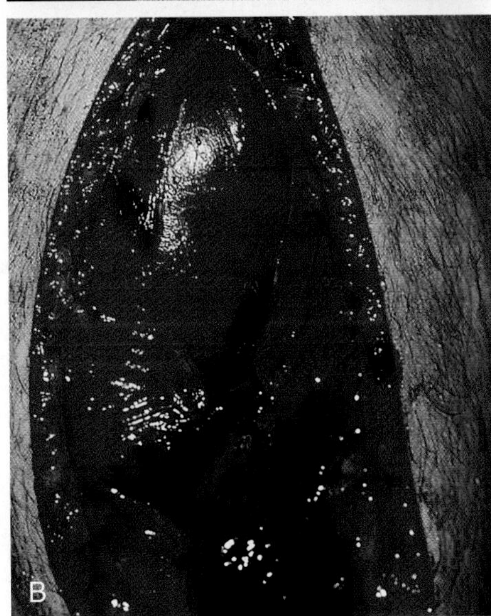

Figure 66.9 Compartment syndrome. A, Severe calf swelling due to anterior and posterior compartment syndromes after ischemia-reperfusion. **B,** Appearance after emergency fasciotomy. Note edematous muscle and hematoma. *(Courtesy Michael J Allen, FRCS, Leicester, UK.)*

mediated cytotoxicity, disseminated intravascular coagulation, and intraluminal cast formation (Fig. 66.10). Volume depletion is often prominent in patients with rhabdomyolysis owing to the sequestration of large amounts of fluid (up to 15 to 20 liters) in injured muscle. Volume depletion activates the sympathetic nervous system and renin-angiotensin system (RAS), resulting in renal vasoconstriction. This may be exacerbated by the scavenging of nitric oxide by circulating heme proteins. Myoglobin (17 kd) is freely filtered at the glomerulus and is toxic to tubular epithelial cells. The heme center of myoglobin may directly induce lipid peroxidation and renal injury,[18] and liberated free iron catalyzes the formation of hydroxyl radical through the Fenton reaction, inducing free radical–mediated injury. Renoprotection has been demonstrated in animal models with free iron scavengers and various antioxidants. Finally, the precipitation of myoglobin with Tamm-Horsfall protein and sloughed proximal tubular cells may result in obstructing casts in the distal nephron. This is enhanced by increased concentrations of tubular heme protein due to volume depletion with low tubular fluid flow rates. The binding of myoglobin to Tamm-Horsfall protein is enhanced in acidic urine.

Clinical features, prevention, and therapy are described in Chapters 68 to 70.

RADIOCONTRAST-INDUCED NEPHROPATHY

AKI secondary to contrast nephrotoxicity typically occurs in patients with underlying renal impairment and is rarely seen in patients with normal renal function.[19] It may occur with both intravenous and intra-arterial administration of contrast material but not with oral administration (assuming an intact bowel). The incidence of contrast nephropathy is about 20% and 50% in patients with serum creatinine levels above 2 mg/dl and 5 mg/dl (176 and 440 μmol/l), respectively. Other risk factors for the development of this condition include diabetic nephropathy, advanced age (>75 years), congestive heart failure, volume depletion, and high or repetitive doses of radiocontrast agent. A high-osmolar contrast agent is more nephrotoxic than low-osmolar or iso-osmolar contrast agents are. Concurrent use of potentially nephrotoxic agents, such as NSAIDs or ACE inhibitors, may increase the risk.

Pathogenesis

Medullary hypoxia and direct tubular epithelial cell toxicity are the main factors in the pathogenesis of contrast nephropathy. Typically, a biphasic hemodynamic response is seen. An initial vasodilation (lasting a few seconds to minutes) is followed by a more prolonged renal vasoconstriction. The consequent medullary hypoxia may be exacerbated by the osmotic diuresis, leading to increased sodium delivery to the medullary thick ascending loop and requiring greater oxygen consumption for reabsorption.

Radiocontrast agents also cause direct tubular epithelial cell injury. Human studies have demonstrated low-molecular-weight proteinuria, suggestive of proximal tubular injury, partly mediated by ROS. Increased markers of lipid peroxidation have been described, and the administration of antioxidants ameliorates contrast nephropathy in animals.

Clinical features, prevention, and therapy are described in Chapters 68 to 70.

ATHEROEMBOLIC RENAL DISEASE (SYNDROME OF MULTIPLE CHOLESTEROL EMBOLI)

This underrecognized condition occurs predominantly in older patients with atherosclerotic vascular disease, either spontaneously or, more frequently, precipitated by arteriography, vascular surgery, thrombolysis (streptokinase and tissue plasminogen activator), and anticoagulation. Destabilization of atherosclerotic plaques primarily in the aorta results in showers of cholesterol that lodge in small arteries in the kidneys (see Fig. 64.15) and the lower extremities (see Fig. 64.13). Characteristic needle-shaped clefts may be seen on renal or skin biopsy, denoting the localization of cholesterol plaques before dissolution with tissue fixation. The cholesterol emboli produce a marked and progressive inflammatory reaction, resulting in occlusion of the involved vasculature. Renal atheroembolism is discussed further in Chapter 64.

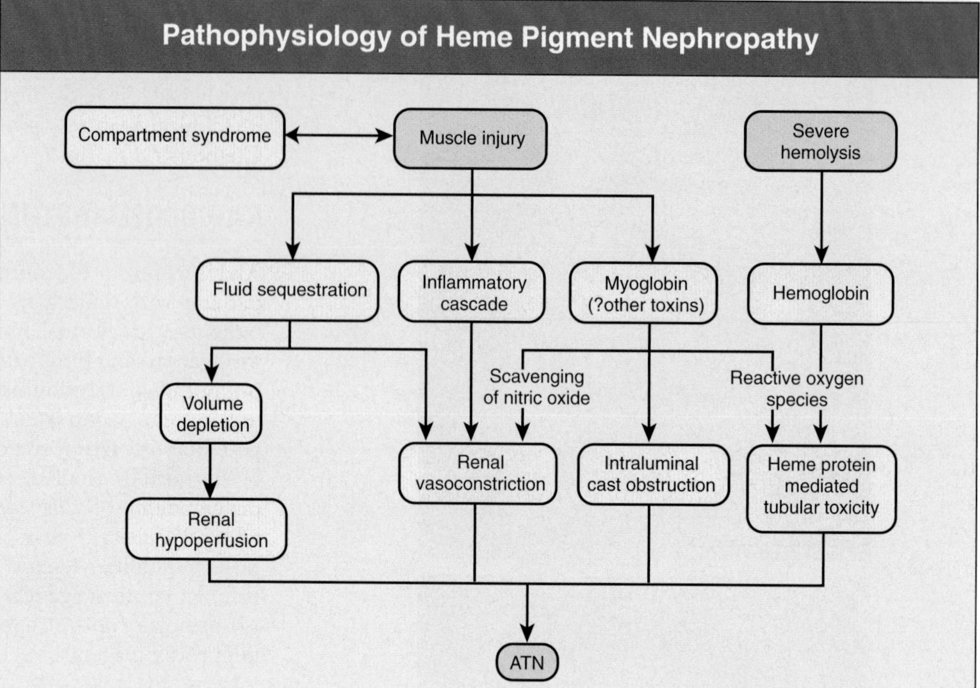

Figure 66.10 Pathophysiology of heme pigment nephropathy. ATN, acute tubular necrosis.

OTHER VASCULAR CAUSES OF ACUTE KIDNEY INJURY

AKI caused by complete renal artery thrombosis occurs when the occlusion is bilateral or, in the case of unilateral acute occlusion, with a single nonfunctioning kidney. Thrombosis of the renal artery or its intrarenal branches and noncholesterol emboli are more common in elderly patients. One important risk for intrarenal emboli is the presence of atrial fibrillation, in which the relative risk for peripheral embolization (aorta, renal and pelvic arteries, and arteries of the extremities) has been calculated to be 4.0 in men and 5.7 in women compared with the general population.

Renal vein thrombosis most commonly occurs in the setting of nephrotic syndrome and rarely may cause AKI if it is bilateral (see Chapter 64).

ACUTE INTERSTITIAL NEPHRITIS

This is most commonly a drug-induced phenomenon and is an important differential diagnosis in AKI because removal of the offending agent can result in reversal of the condition. Less commonly, it may be due to infection or immune-mediated diseases. Acute interstitial nephritis is discussed further in Chapter 60.

THROMBOTIC MICROANGIOPATHY

Thrombotic microangiopathy (TMA) constitutes a wide range of conditions that should be considered when a patient presents with AKI and thrombocytopenia, although the condition may occur in the absence of a low platelet count (see Figs. 28.10 and 28.12). Endothelial activation is followed by the formation of platelet thrombi, which occlude small vessels and lead to downstream ischemic injury. Endothelial injury may be triggered by infections, drugs, or immune complexes. Patients with reduced von Willebrand factor protease activity or impaired regulation of the complement system are at increased risk for development of TMA. Renal biopsy may be required to confirm the diagnosis, although histology is unable to differentiate among the different causes of TMA. TMA is discussed further in Chapter 28.

SPECIFIC CLINICAL SITUATIONS

Determination of the etiology of AKI is often aided by recognizing common patterns of presentation and determining the likely causes arising in each of these situations.

Acute Kidney Injury in the Patient with Multiorgan Failure

About 20% of patients with sepsis syndrome and 50% of those with septic shock develop AKI. This significantly worsens the prognosis, and when dialysis is required, intensive care unit mortality increases to 45% to 80%. Sepsis is classically associated with infection. A similar condition, termed the systemic inflammatory response syndrome (SIRS), may occur secondary to noninfectious insults such as acute pancreatitis, major trauma, and ischemia-reperfusion. Activation of the innate immune system may occur after the interaction of a number of bacterial products (lipopolysaccharide, flagellin, lipoteichoic acid, others) with pattern recognition receptors (such as Toll-like receptors) on immune cells. This leads to the activation of a wide range of cellular and humoral mediator systems, including the cytokine cascade (TNF-α, IL-1β, IL-6); the complement, coagulation, and fibrinolytic systems; and the release of mediators such as eicosanoids, platelet-activating factor, endothelin 1, and nitric oxide. Widespread endothelial injury results, leading to peripheral vasodilation, increased vascular permeability, and leukocyte infiltration. Peripheral vasodilation causes hypotension, with consequent activation of the RAS, increased vasopressin, and increased cardiac output to maintain organ perfusion. This neurohormonal activation may constrict the afferent arterioles of the kidney and further impair renal perfusion. The causes of the AKI in this setting are typically multifactorial, due to a combination of hypotension, impaired renal perfusion, inflammatory mediators, and nephrotoxic agents.[20-23]

Acute Kidney Injury in the Postoperative Patient

AKI in the postoperative period is commonly due to problems with fluid balance, perioperative hemodynamic instability, or nephrotoxic agents. The critically ill postoperative patient may develop SIRS. AKI may be particularly common after vascular, cardiac, and hepatobiliary surgery.

There is evidence that anesthetic agents may impair renal function. This may be partly due to their hypotensive effects, but the metabolism of fluorinated agents can lead to the production of potentially nephrotoxic fluoride ions. Modern inhaled agents (e.g., isoflurane, halothane, enflurane) all cause a transient decrease in GFR, and methoxyflurane had to be discontinued because of nephrotoxicity.

After Vascular Surgery

In patients with peripheral vascular disease, prior ischemic renal disease is often present, and preoperative diminished renal function is the strongest predictor of the risk for postoperative AKI. In aortic aneurysm surgery, most aneurysms are infrarenal; however, surgery that directly involves the renal arteries or aortic cross-clamping above the renal arteries can result in severe renal ischemia. Furthermore, aortic manipulation may dislodge atherosclerotic plaque, resulting in renal atheroembolism. Peripheral limb surgery may be complicated by rhabdomyolysis, and radiocontrast dye is frequently used for diagnostic purposes.

After Cardiac Surgery

Risk factors for postoperative AKI include duration of cardiac bypass, preoperative renal function, age, diabetes, valvular surgery, blood transfusions, and poor cardiac function.[24] Even a minor increase in serum creatinine after cardiac surgery is independently associated with an increased mortality and cost. The surgery is often performed with the patient cooled to less than 30°C to protect cells against ischemic injury; however, systemic hypothermia may cause intravascular coagulation. Aortic instrumentation and clamping may lead to renal atheroembolism. Cardiac bypass causes exposure of blood to a nonendothelialized surface, resulting in activation of neutrophils, platelets, complement, and fibrinolytic systems. Significant hemolysis may also occur, potentially resulting in hemoglobinuria. Perioperative myocardial infarction or left ventricular dysfunction may impair renal perfusion postoperatively, although the low cardiac output is often transient and recovers within 24 to 48 hours. Atrial fibrillation is a common complication and may be associated with peripheral embolization. Studies have suggested that off-pump coronary artery bypass operations have a lower risk of AKI than surgeries in which patients are put on cardiopulmonary bypass.

After Hepatobiliary Surgery

Surgery to relieve obstructive jaundice is more commonly associated with AKI than are other forms of abdominal surgery. This may be due to the absence of bile salts in the gut lumen, which normally break down lipopolysaccharide endotoxin, preventing absorption. One study suggested a decreased incidence of postoperative endotoxemia with treatment with oral bile salts. Other factors may include direct nephrotoxic effects of bilirubin or bile salts on renal tubular cells and an increased incidence of biliary sepsis.

Causes of Pulmonary-Renal Syndrome	
Systemic vasculitis	Anti-GBM disease (Goodpasture's) ANCA associated • Wegener's granulomatosis • Microscopic polyarteritis • Churg-Strauss syndrome • Drugs (penicillamine, hydralazine, propylthiouracil) Immune complex disease • Lupus erythematosus • Henoch-Schönlein purpura • Mixed cryoglobulinemia • Rheumatoid vasculitis
Infection	Severe bacterial pneumonia; postinfectious glomerulonephritis; *Legionella;* hantavirus; opportunistic infection in immunocompromised patients; infective endocarditis
Pulmonary edema and AKI	Volume overload; severe left ventricular failure
Multiorgan failure	Acute respiratory distress syndrome and AKI
Other	Paraquat poisoning; renal vein or IVC thrombosis with pulmonary emboli

Figure 66.11 Causes of pulmonary-renal syndrome. ANCA, anti-neutrophil cytoplasmic antibody; GBM, glomerular basement membrane; IVC, inferior vena cava.

Abdominal Compartment Syndrome

Markedly raised intra-abdominal pressures (>20 mm Hg) may occur after trauma, after abdominal surgery, or secondary to massive fluid resuscitation and can cause AKI.[25] The mechanism remains unclear but may be due to increased renal venous pressure and vascular resistance. Ureteral compression is not considered a factor. Efforts to reduce intra-abdominal pressures, including paracentesis, nasogastric suction, ultrafiltration, and surgical decompression, may occasionally improve renal function.

Pulmonary-Renal Syndromes

The term *pulmonary-renal syndrome* describes the presence of pulmonary hemorrhage in a patient with AKI and is most commonly due to anti-GBM disease (Goodpasture's syndrome), systemic vasculitis, or systemic lupus erythematosus (Fig. 66.11; see Chapters 23 to 25).

A similar clinical presentation may be due to pulmonary edema secondary to volume overload in AKI. Other conditions that may masquerade as a pulmonary-renal syndrome include upper respiratory infection triggering a flair of IgA nephropathy, severe bacterial pneumonia complicated by ATN or postinfectious glomerulonephritis, *Legionella* species infection causing a severe atypical pneumonia, and acute interstitial nephritis or rhabdomyolysis.

Acute Kidney Injury and Liver Disease

The patient with liver cirrhosis is predisposed to the development of AKI, and the differential diagnosis typically falls between prerenal azotemia, hepatorenal syndrome, and ATN. Assessment

Causes of Acute Kidney Injury and Liver Disease	
Prerenal uremia	Diuretic use, gastrointestinal loss, peritoneal aspiration, hypoalbuminemia
Hepatorenal syndrome	
Acute tubular necrosis	Hyperbilirubinemia, sepsis, toxic shock syndrome
Drugs	Acetaminophen (paracetamol), NSAIDs, tetracycline, rifampicin, isoniazid, anesthetic agents, sulfonamides, allopurinol, methotrexate
Infections	Hepatitis C and cryoglobulinemia, hepatitis B and polyarteritis nodosa, leptospirosis, hantavirus, Epstein-Barr virus, gram-negative sepsis, spontaneous bacterial peritonitis
Other	Papillary necrosis and obstruction, inhalation of chlorinated hydrocarbons, mushroom poisoning (*Amanita phalloides*)

Figure 66.12 Causes of acute kidney injury and liver disease. NSAIDs, nonsteroidal anti-inflammatory drugs.

Causes of Acute Kidney Injury in Patients with HIV infection	
Prerenal	Diarrhea, nausea and vomiting, cirrhosis and hepatorenal syndrome, sepsis
Vascular	Thrombotic microangiopathy
Glomerular	Immune complex glomerulonephritis (MPGN secondary to hepatitis C virus, postinfectious glomerulonephritis), HIVAN
Acute tubular necrosis	Sepsis, hypotension, nephrotoxins (aminoglycosides, amphotericin, acyclovir, cidofovir, tenofovir, pentamidine), rhabdomyolysis
Acute interstitial nephritis	Drug induced (cotrimoxazole, rifampicin, foscarnet, nevirapine), CMV infection, DILS
Drug-induced intratubular obstruction	Sulfadiazine, indinavir, foscarnet, acyclovir
Postrenal obstruction	Stones, tuberculosis, fungal ball, tumor
Associated with IV drug use	Sepsis, endocarditis, heroin-associated nephropathy (FSGS), rhabdomyolysis

Figure 66.13 Causes of acute kidney injury in patients with HIV infection. CMV, cytomegalovirus; DILS, diffuse infiltrative lymphocytosis syndrome; FSGS, focal segmental glomerulosclerosis; HIVAN, HIV-associated nephropathy; MPGN, membranoproliferative glomerulonephritis.

of intravascular volume status can be difficult, and a therapeutic trial of volume replacement is typically undertaken. Impaired renal perfusion and hyperbilirubinemia are predisposing risk factors. Alternatively, the same etiologic agent may be responsible for both the liver and renal injury. This occurs with certain infections (e.g., leptospirosis, hantavirus) and nephrotoxic agents (Fig. 66.12). Rarely, hyperbilirubinemia from hemolysis may cause jaundice in the absence of liver disease. AKI in patients with liver disease is discussed further in Chapter 72.

Acute Kidney Injury in Patients with HIV Infection

AKI is common in patients with HIV infection and may be related to the disease itself (e.g., HIV nephropathy; see Chapter 56), dehydration, therapeutic agents, opportunistic infections, or coexistent infections (HCV) and intravenous drug abuse (Fig. 66.13).[26] Prerenal azotemia is the most common cause of AKI in patients with HIV infection, and ATN caused by hypotension or nephrotoxic medications is also common. A hemolytic-uremic syndrome has also been described in HIV infection. In view of the wide differential diagnosis, renal biopsy should be considered when AKI does not respond to supportive measures. In the HIV-infected intravenous drug user, AKI may be due to concomitant HCV infection associated with membranoproliferative glomerulonephritis or to complications related to intravenous drug use (most notably endocarditis-associated renal disease or rhabdomyolysis).

Drug Therapy

Protease inhibitors may cause AKI in patients with HIV infection (see Chapter 56). This commonly occurs with indinavir, which can cause intratubular crystal obstruction or obstructing renal calculi, but it has also been reported with ritonavir. Reverse transcriptase inhibitors may also produce AKI. Tenofovir, a nucleoside reverse transcriptase inhibitor, is now commonly used in HAART regimens and is nephrotoxic.[27] Tenofovir toxicity initially is manifested as Fanconi syndrome and progresses to ATN. Several of the antiretroviral agents used to treat HIV infection can cause acute interstitial nephritis, including indinavir, atazanavir, and abacavir.

Treatment of opportunistic infections often requires the use of potentially nephrotoxic drugs, such as aminoglycosides and amphotericin. *Pneumocystis* species infection may be treated with high-dose cotrimoxazole (acute interstitial nephritis or intratubular crystal obstruction) or pentamidine (ATN in 25% of cases). Resistant cytomegalovirus infection may require foscarnet therapy (acute interstitial nephritis or intratubular crystal obstruction).

Acute Kidney Injury in the Cancer Patient

Patients with cancer are prone to AKI as a consequence of both their underlying disease and its treatment, and AKI may occur in up to 50% of critically ill cancer patients.[28] There is also a high incidence of prerenal azotemia in this group of patients due to the high frequency of nausea, vomiting, and diarrhea (Fig. 66.14). More specific causes of AKI are noted in the following sections.

Tumor Lysis Syndrome

Necrosis of large numbers of tumor cells, typically after chemotherapy, may release large amounts of nephrotoxic intracellular contents (uric acid, phosphate, xanthine) into the circulation.[29] It usually occurs after treatment of lymphomas (particularly Burkitt's) and leukemias, but it may occur spontaneously in patients with rapidly dividing tumor cells. It has also been seen with solid tumors. Rarely, a spontaneous form of tumor lysis syndrome occurs in rapidly growing tumors that outstrip their blood supply.

In earlier days, hyperuricemia resulted in acute urate nephropathy due to intratubular crystal obstruction and interstitial nephritis, but this is now less common because of the prophylactic use of allopurinol before chemotherapy. Other intracellular components are now more commonly involved, such as phosphate release with the precipitation of calcium phosphate in the tubules.

Causes of Acute Kidney Injury in Patients with Cancer

Prerenal	Nausea and vomiting, hypercalcemia, cardiomyopathy secondary to chemotherapy
Vascular	Thrombotic microangiopathy (adenocarcinoma of stomach, pancreas, prostate; radiation nephropathy), renal vein thrombosis secondary to hypercoagulability, disseminated intravascular coagulation (acute promyelocytic leukemia)
Glomerular	Rapidly progressive glomerulonephritis
Acute tubular necrosis	Sepsis and antibiotic nephrotoxicity, hypercalcemia
Malignant infiltration	Lymphoma, acute lymphoblastic leukemia
Intraluminal obstruction	Tumor lysis syndrome, cast nephropathy
Postrenal obstruction	Transitional cell carcinoma of the ureters/bladder, extrinsic ureteral compression (tumor, nodes, retroperitoneal fibrosis)
Chemotherapeutic agents	
Tubular toxicity	Cisplatin, ifosfamide, plicamycin (mithramycin); 5-fluorouracil, thioguanine (6-thioguanine), cytarabine
Thrombotic microangiopathy	Mitomycin C, bleomycin, cisplatin, calcineurin inhibitors
Other mechanisms	Capillary leak syndrome (IL-2 therapy), acute interstitial nephritis (interferon-α), intraluminal obstruction (methotrexate)

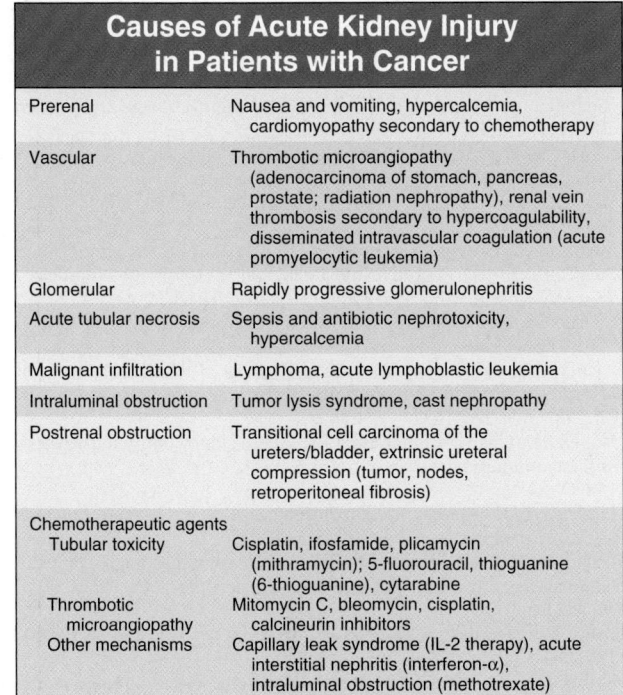

Figure 66.14 Causes of acute kidney injury in patients with cancer. IL-2, interleukin-2.

The AKI is typically oligoanuric, and the condition should be suspected in patients with high lactate dehydrogenase levels suggestive of massive cell lysis. Markedly elevated phosphate and urate levels may also be found. Hyperkalemia may be prominent and life-threatening.

Preventive measures include the use of high-dose allopurinol (600 to 900 mg/day) started 2 to 3 days before chemotherapy and either oral or intravenous fluid loading to ensure a urine output of more than 2.5 l/day. Urine alkalinization is of less benefit than merely maintaining a high urine flow with saline, and it may promote tubular calcium phosphate deposition. However, it should be considered when serum uric acid levels are elevated (>12 mg/dl [714 μmol/l]) or urinary uric acid crystals are present. Recombinant uricase (rasburicase) is effective in lowering serum uric acid levels (to <1 mg/dl in 24 hours) and should be considered for prophylaxis in high-risk patients.

Once the patient develops AKI with hyperuricemia, rasburicase, which lowers uric acid much more effectively than dialysis does, should be considered. It can lower uric acid levels within hours and also is effective in patients with impaired renal function. If this is not available or the patient is markedly hyperphosphatemic, early dialysis should be considered to remove these potential causes of further renal damage. Because phosphate is less well removed by dialysis than urate is, frequent (every 12 to 24 hours) or prolonged treatments should be considered.

Hypercalcemia

Volume depletion secondary to hypercalcemia-induced nausea and vomiting may cause AKI, which may be exacerbated by hypercalcemia-induced nephrogenic diabetes insipidus. Other hypercalcemia-associated factors that may contribute to AKI include direct intrarenal vasoconstriction, acute interstitial nephritis, and intratubular obstruction.

Renal Infiltration

Direct infiltration of the kidneys by tumor is not uncommon; however, this rarely results in renal failure. AKI may be seen with slow-growing lymphomas or leukemias, when the patient presents with nonoliguric AKI, a benign urine sediment, and enlarged kidneys on ultrasound scan. Renal function may improve, depending on the responsiveness of the tumor to treatment. Tumor-related urinary tract obstruction should also be considered.

Chemotherapeutic Agents

Cisplatin is commonly associated with a nonoliguric renal impairment.[30] Nephrotoxic injury affects both the proximal and distal nephron and clinically may be associated with magnesium wasting, impaired urinary concentration, and rarely salt wasting with volume depletion. Chloride ions in the *cis* position on the molecule may be replaced by water, releasing toxic hydroxyl radicals. Prophylaxis against nephrotoxicity includes volume loading, possibly with hypertonic saline, and the use of the antioxidant amifostine as a thiol donor. The alternative agent carboplatin appears to be less nephrotoxic. Once renal impairment is present, recovery may be poor, and magnesium wasting may persist.

Ifosfamide is a cyclophosphamide analogue with a nephrotoxic metabolite, chloroacetaldehyde. AKI is usually mild, although proximal tubular dysfunction (Fanconi syndrome) and hypokalemia may be prominent.

High-dose intravenous methotrexate is also nephrotoxic, possibly because of precipitation of the drug within the renal tubules and direct toxicity to the renal epithelial cells.

Cytosine arabinoside and 5-fluorouracil may increase the likelihood of AKI when they are included in multidrug regimens. Both agents, for example, are associated with AKI when they are given in combination with cisplatin.

Bone Marrow Transplant

AKI is common in patients undergoing hematopoietic cell transplantation (HCT), and some degree of renal dysfunction can be seen in more than 90% of the patients who undergo allogeneic HCT. These patients often have multiple risk factors for the development of AKI, including reactions to the infused hematopoietic cells, infections, nephrotoxic drugs, and dehydration. AKI is less common after autologous HCT, probably because the patients do not require chronic immunosuppression with nephrotoxic agents.

REFERENCES

1. Mehta RL, Kellum JA, Shah SV, et al. Acute Kidney Injury Network: Report of an initiative to improve outcomes in acute kidney injury. *Crit Care*. 2007;11:R31.
2. Liano F, Pascual J. Epidemiology of acute renal failure: A prospective, multicenter, community-based study. Madrid Acute Renal Failure Study Group. *Kidney Int*. 1996;50:811-818.
3. Bonventre JV, Weinberg JM. Recent advances in the pathophysiology of ischemic acute renal failure. *J Am Soc Nephrol*. 2003;14:2199-2210.
4. Schrier RW, Wang W, Poole B, Mitra A. Acute renal failure: Definitions, diagnosis, pathogenesis, and therapy. *J Clin Invest*. 2004;114:5-14.
5. Brivet FG, Kleinknecht DJ, Loirat P, Landais PJ. Acute renal failure in intensive care units—causes, outcome, and prognostic factors of hospital mortality; a prospective, multicenter study. French Study Group on Acute Renal Failure. *Crit Care Med*. 1996;24:192-198.
6. Nath KA, Norby SM. Reactive oxygen species and acute renal failure. *Am J Med*. 2000;109:665-678.

7. Kinsey GR, Li L, Okusa MD. Inflammation in acute kidney injury. *Nephron Exp Nephrol.* 2008;109:e102-e107.
8. Duffield JS, Park KM, Hsiao LL, et al. Restoration of tubular epithelial cells during repair of the postischemic kidney occurs independently of bone marrow–derived stem cells. *J Clin Invest.* 2005;115:1743-1755.
9. Hirschberg R, Kopple J, Lipsett P, et al. Multicenter clinical trial of recombinant human insulin-like growth factor I in patients with acute renal failure. *Kidney Int.* 1999;55:2423-2432.
10. Cheng HF, Harris RC. Renal effects of non-steroidal anti-inflammatory drugs and selective cyclooxygenase-2 inhibitors. *Curr Pharm Des.* 2005; 11:1795-1804.
11. Evenepoel P. Acute toxic renal failure. *Best Pract Res Clin Anaesthesiol.* 2004;18:37-52.
12. Rougier F, Claude D, Maurin M, Maire P. Aminoglycoside nephrotoxicity. *Curr Drug Targets Infect Disord.* 2004;4:153-162.
13. Deray G. Amphotericin B nephrotoxicity. *J Antimicrob Chemother.* 2002;49(Suppl 1):37-41.
14. Nzerue CM, Hewan-Lowe K, Riley LJ Jr. Cocaine and the kidney: A synthesis of pathophysiologic and clinical perspectives. *Am J Kidney Dis.* 2000;35:783-795.
15. Heher EC, Thier SO, Rennke H, Humphreys BD. Adverse renal and metabolic effects associated with oral sodium phosphate bowel preparation. *Clin J Am Soc Nephrol.* 2008;3:1494-1503.
16. Bywaters EG, Beall D. Crush injuries with impairment of renal function. *BMJ.* 1941;1:427-432.
17. Toledo Rojas R, Lopez Jimenez V, Martin Reyes G, et al. Rhabdomyolysis due to muscle enzyme deficiencies. *Nefrologia.* 2009;29:77-80.
18. Holt S, Moore K. Pathogenesis of renal failure in rhabdomyolysis: The role of myoglobin. *Exp Nephrol.* 2000;8:72-76.
19. Tumlin J, Stacul F, Adam A, et al. Pathophysiology of contrast-induced nephropathy. *Am J Cardiol.* 2006;98:14K-20K.
20. De Vriese AS. Prevention and treatment of acute renal failure in sepsis. *J Am Soc Nephrol.* 2003;14:792-805.
21. Riedemann NC, Guo RF, Ward PA. The enigma of sepsis. *J Clin Invest.* 2003;112:460-467.
22. Schrier RW, Wang W. Acute renal failure and sepsis. *N Engl J Med.* 2004;351:159-169.
23. Remick DG. Pathophysiology of sepsis. *Am J Pathol.* 2007;170: 1435-1444.
24. Shroyer AL, Coombs LP, Peterson ED, et al. The Society of Thoracic Surgeons: 30-day operative mortality and morbidity risk models. *Ann Thorac Surg.* 2003;75:1856-1864; discussion 64-65.
25. Sugrue M. Abdominal compartment syndrome. *Curr Opin Crit Care.* 2005;11:333-338.
26. Franceschini N, Napravnik S, Eron JJ Jr, et al. Incidence and etiology of acute renal failure among ambulatory HIV-infected patients. *Kidney Int.* 2005;67:1526-1531.
27. Cohen SD, Chawla LS, Kimmel PL. Acute kidney injury in patients with human immunodeficiency virus infection. *Curr Opin Crit Care.* 2008; 14:647-653.
28. Lameire NH, Flombaum CD, Moreau D, Ronco C. Acute renal failure in cancer patients. *Ann Med.* 2005;37:13-25.
29. Davidson MB, Thakkar S, Hix JK, et al. Pathophysiology, clinical consequences, and treatment of tumor lysis syndrome. *Am J Med.* 2004;116: 546-554.
30. Kintzel PE. Anticancer drug–induced kidney disorders. *Drug Saf.* 2001;24:19-38.
31. Kribben A, Edelstein CL, Schrier RW. Pathophysiology of acute renal failure. *J Nephrol.* 1999;12(Suppl 2):S142-S151.

CHAPTER 67

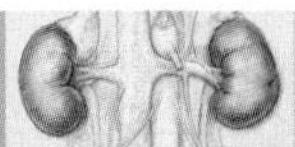

Acute Kidney Injury in the Tropics

Emmanuel A. Burdmann, Vivekanand Jha, Visith Sitprija

In tropical countries, the epidemiologic pattern of acute kidney injury (AKI) encountered in tertiary hospitals in densely inhabited cities will be similar to that in developed nontropical countries (see Chapter 66). In contrast, in the same cities and in the countryside, particular causes of AKI, such as malaria, yellow fever, hemorrhagic dengue, and leptospirosis, may be found, frequently affecting young and previously healthy individuals. Septic abortion is no longer a relevant cause of AKI in the developed world, but it remains a significant medical problem in some tropical countries. There are regions in Asia where venomous snakebite is the leading cause of community-acquired AKI. Rupture of the ecological balance by humans has induced particular causes of renal injury in the tropics, like accidents with the Africanized bee or *Lonomia* genus caterpillars. Natural medicines prescribed by traditional healers are an important cause of AKI in Africa and Asia.

In this chapter, specific causes of AKI, such as venomous snakebite, arthropod venom, and herbal and natural medicines, are discussed. Some of the most important infectious diseases causing AKI in the tropics (malaria, leptospirosis, and yellow fever) are reviewed.

SNAKEBITES

Snakebite is an occupational hazard in the rural tropics. Renal injury may develop after bites by several kinds of venomous snakes, such as Russell's viper, saw-scaled viper, puff adder, rattlesnake, tiger snake, green pit viper, *Bothrops*, *Lachesis*, *Crotalus*, boomslang, gwardar, dugite, *Hypnale*, *Cryptophis*, and sea snakes.[1-3] AKI is more frequent after Russell's viper (Fig. 67.1), *Bothrops*, or *Crotalus* bites, with incidences ranging from 10% to 32%.[1-3] The prevalence is higher in children, probably because of the higher venom dose in relation to the body size.[4]

Clinical Features

Manifestations depend on the nature of the venom and the injected dose. Pain, swelling, blister formation, ecchymosis of the bitten part, and tissue necrosis are frequent in Russell's viper and *Bothrops* bites (Figs. 67.2 and 67.3). The most common systemic manifestation in accidents by these snakes is coagulation abnormalities leading to bleeding diathesis (Fig. 67.3). Muscle paralysis may occur with *Crotalus* bites and rhabdomyolysis after bites by sea snakes and *Crotalus*. Renal injury develops within a few hours to as late as 96 hours after the bite. Cola-colored urine is noted in those with hemolysis or rhabdomyolysis. AKI is usually oliguric and catabolic, with rapidly rising levels of blood urea nitrogen, serum creatinine, and potassium. Oliguria generally lasts for 1 to 2 weeks, and its persistence suggests the likelihood of acute cortical necrosis.[1-4]

Investigations may show evidence of hemolysis (elevated free plasma hemoglobin, lactate dehydrogenase, and reduced haptoglobin) along with hypofibrinogenemia; reduced factors V, X, and XIIIa and protein C and antithrombin C; and elevated fibrin degradation products. Rhabdomyolysis may be indicated by raised creatine kinase. Other findings include leukocytosis and elevated hematocrit due to hemoconcentration.[1-4]

Pathology

In gross appearance, the kidneys may show petechial hemorrhages. Light microscopy usually discloses acute tubular cell injury ranging from mild changes to overt tubular necrosis, with hyaline or pigment casts, variable degrees of interstitial edema and cell infiltration, and scattered hemorrhages. Mesangiolysis is also common (especially with crotalid envenomation). Blood vessels may show fibrin thrombi. Electron microscopic findings include dense intracytoplasmic bodies representing degenerated organelles in the proximal tubules and electron-dense mesangial deposits. Less common findings are acute interstitial nephritis, necrotizing vasculitis, and proliferative and crescentic immune complex glomerulonephritis. Acute cortical necrosis is seen in about 20% to 25% of cases after Russell's viper and *Echis carinatus* bites and has been described after *Bothrops* accidents.[1-3]

Pathogenesis

Snake venom is a complex mixture of enzymes, toxins, and peptides. Renal injury may develop as a result of direct nephrotoxicity, renal vasoconstriction, hypovolemia, hemolysis, altered fibrinolysis, myoglobinuria, or disseminated intravascular coagulation.[1-4] Experimental studies have shown evidence of tubular injury manifested by increased excretion of tubular enzymes, altered fractional sodium excretion, and acute tubular necrosis.[1-5] Other changes including mesangiolysis, disrupted integrity of the cellular junctions, proteolysis of extracellular matrix, lysis of vessel wall (leading to mesangiolysis), and alterations in function of enzymes vital to cellular integrity have been noted.[1-3] Hypovolemia and hypotension secondary to bleeding, third spacing of fluids, and depression of the medullary vasomotor center or the myocardium may play a role.[2,3]

Management

The basic therapeutic approach is the same as that for AKI due to any cause. Key steps for reducing morbidity and mortality

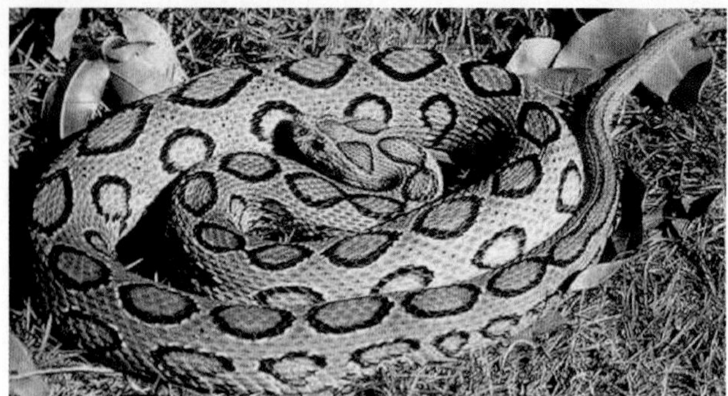

Figure 67.1 Russell's viper snake. This large snake is an important cause of venomous snakebite-induced AKI in Asia.

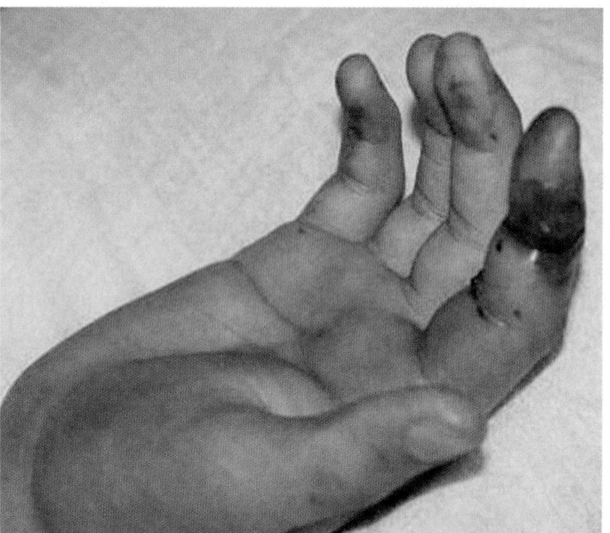

Figure 67.2 Necrotic finger injury after *Bothrops* snakebite. *(Courtesy Carlos A. C. Mendes, São José do Rio Preto, Brazil.)*

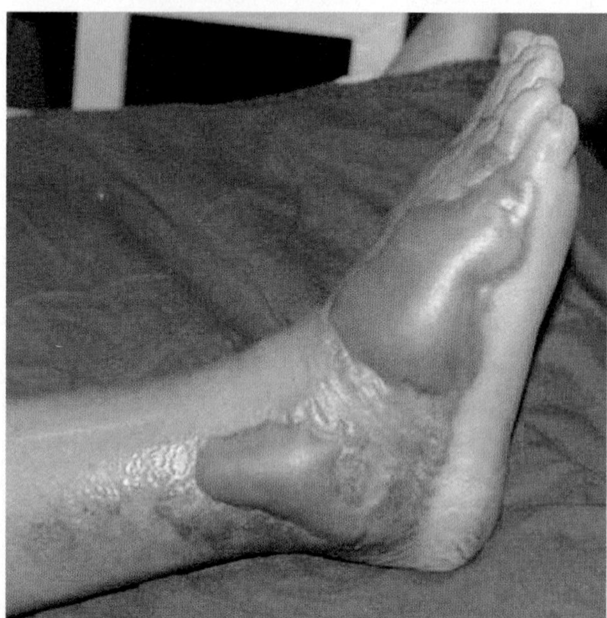

Figure 67.3 Hemorrhagic blister developing a few hours after *Bothrops* snakebite. *(Courtesy Carlos A. C. Mendes, São José do Rio Preto, Brazil.)*

include early administration of antivenom, appropriate volume replacement, maintenance of good urine flow, urinary alkalization in cases of rhabdomyolysis, correction of electrolyte imbalance, administration of tetanus immune globulin, and treatment of infections. Antivenom should be initiated in adequate amounts and by the appropriate route as soon as signs of local or systemic envenomation are noted.[1-5] Knowledge of the offending snake species allows administration of specific monovalent antivenom. Immunodiagnostic techniques can help in identification of venom antigen but are time-consuming. The overall mortality rate may reach 30%.[1-5] The prognosis is favorable in patients receiving early and adequate doses of antivenom. Renal functional recovery is usually complete except in those with acute cortical necrosis, who may be left with varying degrees of dysfunction, depending on the amount of viable parenchyma.

ARTHROPODS

Poisonous arthropods such as bees, wasps, caterpillars, and spiders may cause AKI. Patients receiving hundreds of simultaneous bee stings frequently have a multifaceted clinical picture, which may include intravascular hemolysis, rhabdomyolysis, low platelet count, coagulation disorders and bleeding, cardiovascular injury, hepatic injury, pulmonary injury, and AKI. In the same way, AKI can follow accidents with multiple wasp, yellow jacket, or hornet stings.[2,6] The mechanisms leading to renal injury are likely to be direct venom nephrotoxicity, intrarenal vasoconstriction, hemoglobinuria, myoglobinuria, and hypotension.[7] Renal histology usually shows acute tubular necrosis.[2,6,7]

Accidents with caterpillars of the genus *Lonomia* produce severe hemorrhagic disorders. The venom induces a complex hemorrhagic diathesis with both fibrinolytic and disseminated intravascular coagulation–like activity. Severe and prolonged AKI with renal histology suggesting ischemic injury has been reported after accidents with *Lonomia obliqua* (Fig. 67.4), and some patients did not recover renal function. Availability of *Lonomia* antivenom has led to an apparent decrease in the number of severe cases in Brazil.[6,8]

Spiders of the genus *Loxosceles* (Fig. 67.5) may induce late local necrosis at the bite site (Fig. 67.6), intravascular hemolysis, rhabdomyolysis, coagulation system changes, and acute renal injury. Even patients with mild cutaneous lesions may develop severe hemolysis and AKI, which is the main cause of death after theses accidents.[6,9]

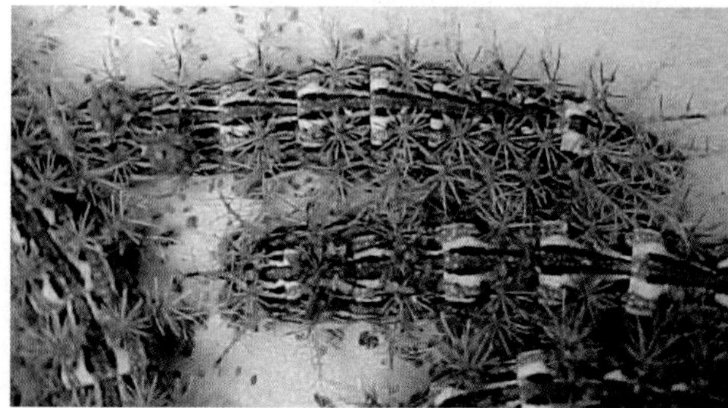

Figure 67.4 *Lonomia obliqua* caterpillars. Each hair works as a miniature hypodermic needle to inject the hemolymph, which contains powerful venom that is able to induce severe coagulation system changes. *(Courtesy Elvino J. G. Barros, Porto Alegre, Brazil.)*

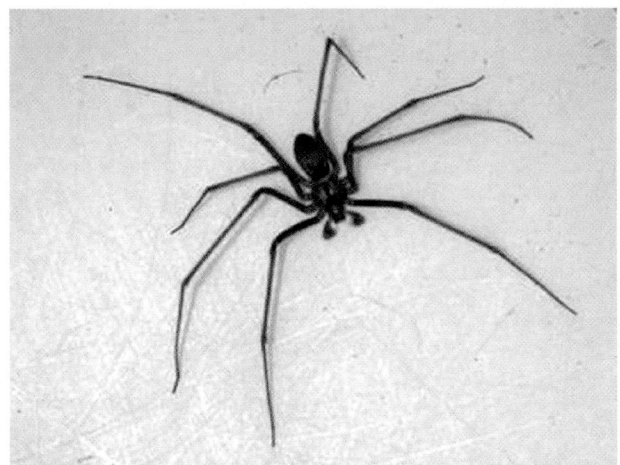

Figure 67.5 ***Loxosceles*** **sp. (brown recluse spider).** *(Courtesy Katia C. Barbaro, São Paulo, Brazil.)*

NATURAL MEDICINES

Herbs and indigenous remedies are used extensively in poor societies living in the tropics. About 50% to 80% of the population in Africa and China depends on traditional medicine for primary health care. Poisoning with traditional medicines is an important cause of mortality in sub-Saharan Africa. Herbalists and faith healers use unknown ingredients to prepare these medicines, which are not tested for efficacy and safety.[2,10,11]

AKI has been described in association with several of these natural remedies (see also Chapter 74). An accurate assessment of their contribution to AKI is rendered difficult by the failure of physicians to elicit a history because of ignorance or denial by the patients due to fear of stigmatization or social pressures. It is often difficult to discount the contribution of the original illness to the AKI.[10]

About 25% to 35% of all AKI due to medical causes in various African hospitals is related to herbal remedies. Accidental oral ingestion of the hair dye paraphenylenediamine is responsible for about 10% of all AKI cases in Morocco. The natural compounds more frequently associated with AKI are impila *(Callilepis laureola)*, djenkol beans *(Pithecolobium)*, mushrooms (genera *Amanita*, *Galerina*, *Cortinarius*, and *Inocybe*), cape aloe, and raw carp bile.[10,11] In addition, single case reports of other natural medicines inducing AKI can be found (Fig. 67.7).[10,11]

Kidney injury may be either the sole manifestation or part of a multisystem involvement that includes acid-base disturbances, liver failure, neurologic abnormalities, disseminated intravascular coagulation, or respiratory failure. Management of AKI is usually supportive (see Chapter 69) and includes volume replacement and correction of metabolic abnormalities. Dialytic support is given for usual indications (see Chapter 70). About 60% of all herbal remedy–related AKI cases need dialysis, with 25% to 75% mortality. Charcoal hemoperfusion is effective in clearing α-amanitin from the circulation in those with poisoning due to *Amanita* mushrooms.[10]

Pathogenesis of Natural Medicine–Induced Acute Kidney Injury

Several factors affect the toxicity and likelihood of kidney injury. Adulteration of indigenous medicines is common (see Chapter 74). Incorrect identification by inexperienced personnel may lead

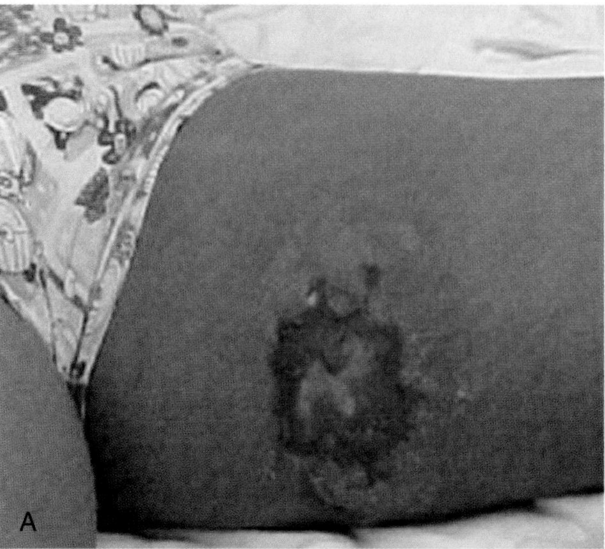

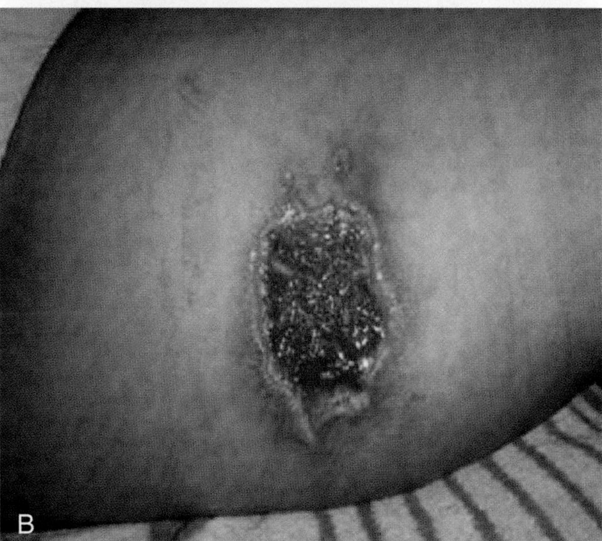

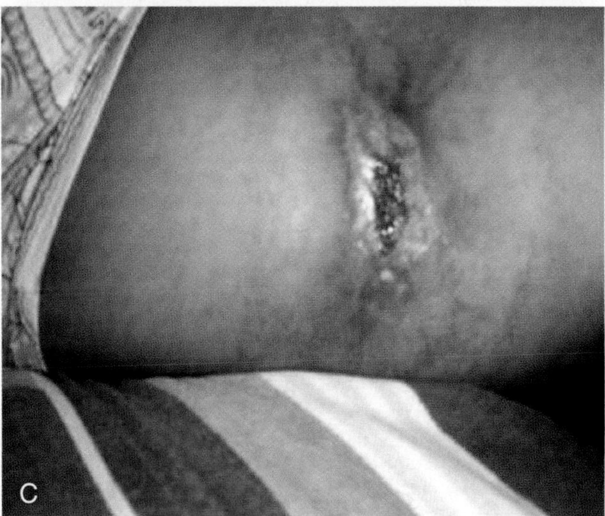

Figure 67.6 Local necrotic injury in the left leg of a female patient after ***Loxosceles*** **bite. A,** At 4 days after the bite. **B,** At 60 days after the bite. **C,** At 3 months after the bite. *(Courtesy Carlos A. C. Mendes, São José do Rio Preto, Brazil.)*

Traditional Remedies Associated with AKI in the Tropics

Plant	Reported from	Active molecule	Nature of kidney injury	Other manifestations
Averrhoa carambola (star fruit)	Hong Kong, Taiwan	Oxalate	Intratubular precipitation of oxalate crystals	Vomiting
Catha edulis (khat leaf)	East Africa, Arab peninsula	*S*-Cathinone, ephedrine	ATN	Hepatotoxicity
CKLS*	Atlanta, Georgia (USA)	Multiple toxins	AIN, hematuria	Diarrhea, abdominal pain
Cleistanthus collinus (Oduvan)	India	Cleistanthin A and B, collinusin, diphylline	AKI	Hypotension, hypokalemia, arrhythmia
Colchicum autumnale (meadow saffron)	Turkey	Colchicine	ATN	Hemorrhagic gastroenteritis, muscle paralysis, respiratory failure
Crotalaria laburnifolia (Bird flower)	Zimbabwe, Sri Lanka	Pyrrolizidine alkaloids	ATN, HRS	Hepatic veno-occlusive disease, pulmonary injury, thrombocytopenia
Cupressus funebris Endl (mourning cypress)	Taiwan	Flavonoid	ATN, AIN	AHF, hemolytic anemia, thrombocytopenia
Dioscorea quartiniana (yam)	Africa, Asia	Dioscorine, dioscin	ATN	Convulsions
Euphorbia metabelensis (spurge)	Zimbabwe	Irritant chemicals in plant latex	ATN	Thrombocytopenia
Glycyrrhiza glabrata (licorice)	Several countries	Glycyrrhizic acid	ATN	Rhabdomyolysis, hypokalemia, hypertension, cardiac arrhythmia
Larrea tridentate (chaparral)	Chile, South Africa	Nordihydroguaiaretic acid, S-quinone	Renal cysts, renal cell carcinoma	Hepatic failure
Lytta vesicatoria (Spanish fly)	South Africa, USA	Cantharidin	ATN, hematuria	GI symptoms, neuromuscular paralysis
Propolis	Brazil, Taiwan	Unknown	AIN	Contact dermatitis
Rhizoma rhei	Hong Kong	Anthraquinones (emodin, aloe emodin)	AIN	None
Securidacea longepedunculata (violet tree, wild wisteria)	Congo, Zambia, Zimbabwe	Methylsalicylate, securinine, saponins	ATN	Vomiting, diarrhea
Sutherlandia frufesces (cancer brush), *Dodonaea angustifolia*	South Africa	Unknown	AIN	Pulmonary embolism
Takaout roumia	Morocco, Sudan	Paraphenylenediamine	ATN	Rhabdomyolysis
Taxus celebia (Chinese yew)	Asia	Flavonoid	ATN, AIN	Hepatitis, hemolysis, DIC
Thevetia peruviana (yellow oleander)	India, Sri Lanka	Cardiac glycosides	ATN, mesangiolysis	Liver failure, cardiac arrhythmias
Tripterygium wilfordii Hook F (thunder god vine)	Taiwan	Triptolide	ATN	Diarrhea, shock
Uncaria tomentosa (cat's claw)	Peru	Alkaloids, flavonols	AIN	Diarrhea, hypotension, bruising, bleeding gums

*CKLS: Colon, Kidney, Liver, Spleen; mixture of ten plant products, exact toxic compound not known;
ATN: acute tubular necrosis; AIN: acute interstitial nephritis; AKI: acute kidney injury; HRS: hepatorenal syndrome, AHF: acute hepatic failure; GI: gastrointestinal; DIC: disseminated intravascular coagulation.

Figure 67.7 Traditional remedies associated with AKI in the tropics.

to substitution of a medicinal plant with a toxic one. An example is the substitution of Takaout el badia, a hair dye made from *Tamarix orientalis* seeds, with the toxic Takaout roumia (paraphenylenediamine). Finally, incorrect methods of preparation or consumption cause nephrotoxicity. Examples include consumption of improperly cooked djenkol beans, star fruit, or yam and failure to ingest impila in the prescribed way (with sufficient water, followed by regurgitation soon after consumption). Indirect mechanisms include interaction with metabolism of conventional drugs. St. John's wort *(Hypericum perforatum)* decreases plasma levels of drugs that are metabolized by the cytochrome P-450 enzyme system. In kidney transplant recipients, this interaction can lower levels of calcineurin inhibitors and precipitate AKI due to allograft rejection. Concomitant administration of other nephrotoxic medicines can also potentiate herbal nephrotoxicity.[10,11]

MALARIA

Malaria is caused by four species of malarial *Plasmodium* parasites: *falciparum*, *vivax*, *malariae*, and *ovale*. It has been estimated that globally, malaria afflicts nearly 250 million patients annually with one million deaths, mostly of children with *P. falciparum*.[12] The contribution of malaria as the cause of AKI among different geographic areas ranges from 2% to 39%. The incidence of AKI in *P. falciparum*–induced malaria can be as high as 60%. AKI is uncommon in the other forms of malaria but may be observed in complicated cases of *P. vivax* infection.[13] In this chapter, we focus on falciparum malaria–associated AKI. Glomerular disease associated with malaria infection is discussed in Chapter 55.

Pathophysiology

The inherent characteristics of each species of malarial parasite are important determinants in malaria pathogenesis. *P. vivax* and *P. ovale* infect young erythrocytes, and *P. malariae* infects aging cells. *P. falciparum* infects erythrocytes of all ages, producing a higher number of merozoites (Fig. 67.8). Heavy parasitemia is therefore commonly observed in falciparum malaria, creating adverse effects on microcirculation. The pathophysiologic process of malaria involves membrane changes, inflammation, and hemodynamic alterations.[14] *Plasmodium* parasites primarily infect erythrocytes with secondary effects on the microcirculation and immune system. Parasitized erythrocytes are integral to the pathophysiologic process of the disease through decreased erythrocyte deformability and sequestration, knobs and rosette formation, cytoadherence, and changes in membrane transport and permeability. Interestingly, nonparasitized erythrocytes also have decreased deformability. The presence of blebs on parasitized erythrocyte membranes and cytoadherence between parasitized erythrocytes and vascular endothelial cells are characteristic of falciparum malaria. Other forms of *Plasmodium* do not have this property. Similar to other infectious diseases, several proinflammatory cytokines and vasoactive mediators are released. Hemodynamic changes in malaria are similar to those of bacterial sepsis: decreased systemic vascular resistance, increased cardiac output, and increased renal vascular resistance. The initial hypervolemia is followed by hypovolemia and decreased cardiac output, with renal blood flow and glomerular filtration rate decrease. Increased blood viscosity, intravascular coagulation, hemolysis, rhabdomyolysis, jaundice, fever, lactic acidosis, complement activation, and reactive oxygen species further compromise renal blood flow. Activation of poly(ADP-ribose) polymerase by peroxynitrite and free radicals decreases oxygen utilization. AKI in malaria is therefore ischemic and hypoxic in origin and usually occurs in the patient with heavy parasitemia or intravascular hemolysis or rhabdomyolysis.[13,14]

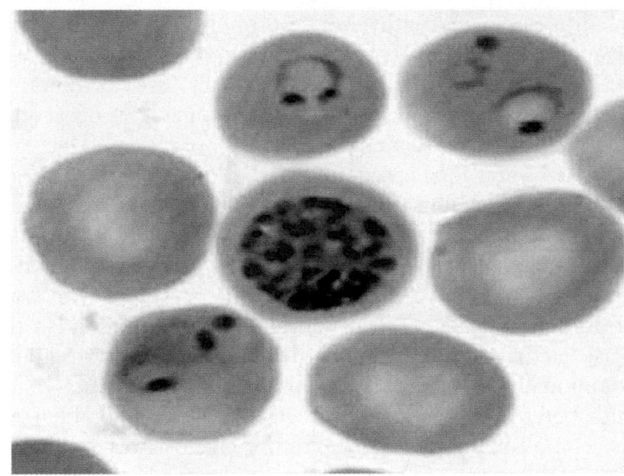

Figure 67.8 Ring form and merozoites of *Plasmodium falciparum* in infected erythrocytes.

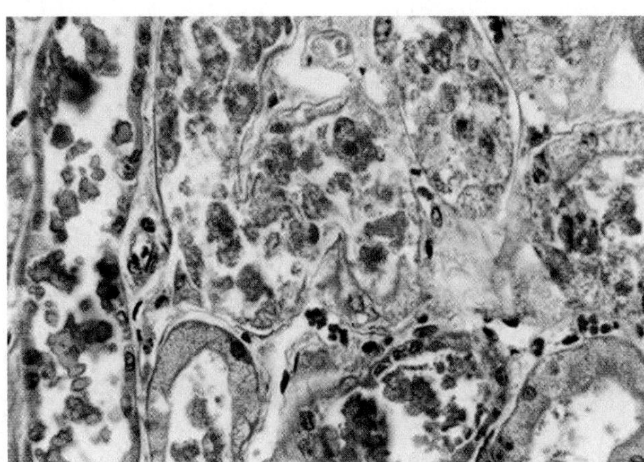

Figure 67.9 Acute tubular necrosis in falciparum malaria.

Immune responses in malaria involve both Th1 and Th2 activation. Immune complex glomerulonephritis is usually observed, with granular deposition of C3, IgM, and malarial antigen in the mesangial area and *in situ* immune complex deposition. Tubular changes vary from cloudy swelling to tubular degeneration with tubulorrhexis in the patient with AKI (Fig. 67.9). Bile and hemoglobin casts and Tamm-Horsfall protein are present in the tubular lumen. Interstitial mononuclear infiltration and edema can be observed. Malarial antigens are occasionally seen along the glomerular endothelium and medullary capillaries. Adhesion molecules and proinflammatory cytokines are overexpressed in the vascular endothelium and proximal tubules.[13,14]

Clinical Manifestations

Malarial AKI affects predominantly nonimmune adults, mostly infected by *P. falciparum*. Constitutional symptoms include fever, chills, headache, and prostration. Jaundice may be present. The urinalysis usually shows few erythrocytes, leukocytes, and granular casts and mild proteinuria (often less than 1 g/24 h). Hemoglobinuria is noted in the patient with intravascular hemolysis, frequently associated with glucose-6-phosphate dehydrogenase deficiency. Rhabdomyolysis with myoglobinuria has been observed. Fluid and electrolyte changes are common in malaria.[13-15] Hyponatremia, usually asymptomatic, is observed in 67% of patients and is related to the severity of malaria. Decreased response to water load is seen in 20% of hyponatremic patients. Fluid should be administered cautiously in hyponatremic patients to avoid fluid overload. Hyponatremia resolves within a few days after antimalarial treatment. The causes of hyponatremia are multiple, including increased antidiuretic hormone with water retention, intracellular shift of sodium due to decreased Na^+,K^+-ATPase activity, and sodium depletion. Hypernatremia is uncommon and when present indicates hypothalamic lesions with diabetes insipidus, being associated with unfavorable prognosis. Hypokalemia due to respiratory alkalosis occurs in 20% to 40% of the patients. Hyperkalemia is observed in patients with intravascular hemolysis, rhabdomyolysis, or AKI. Hypocalcemia with prolonged QTc interval occurs in 45% of severe malaria, is transient, and resolves when infection is controlled.[15] Decreased activities of Na^+,K^+-ATPase, Ca^{2+}-ATPase, and parathyroid hormone are considered the main causes. Hypophosphatemia secondary to respiratory alkalosis is observed in 6% to 30% of the patients. The clinical significance of both hypocalcemia and hypophosphatemia is unknown. Hypomagnesemia is seen in 30% of patients.[15]

AKI is characterized by a rapid increase in blood urea nitrogen and serum creatinine and is often associated with cholestatic jaundice. Hepatocellular jaundice may be observed with hypotension and secondary hepatic injury. Severe acidosis, hypoglycemia, and central nervous system symptoms can be observed. The duration of AKI ranges from one to several weeks and is oliguric in 60% of the patients. Quinine and artesunate are the antimalarial agents of choice. Early and frequent dialysis (hemodialysis or peritoneal dialysis) is lifesaving.[13] Continuous venovenous hemofiltration yields good results in patients with multiorgan involvement, especially those with pulmonary edema or acute respiratory distress syndrome.[13] Exchange blood transfusion and erythrocytapheresis are adjunctive for the patient with heavy parasitemia.[16] The mortality rate of malarial AKI ranges from 10% to 50%. Multiple organ involvement carries poor prognosis. The use of dopamine with furosemide in attenuating the progress of mild uncomplicated malarial renal injury has been successful.[14] This is in contrast to the experience in other causes of AKI (see Chapter 69) and requires larger randomized controlled studies to be validated.

LEPTOSPIROSIS

Leptospirosis, a worldwide zoonosis, is caused by *Leptospira* genus spirochetes. There are more than 200 pathogenic serovars of *Leptospira* occurring in tropical and subtropical areas, which makes this infection a major public health burden. In fact, the World Health Organization included leptospirosis as a reemerging infectious disease in both developed and developing areas. Wild and domestic mammals, such as rodents, dogs, pigs, cattle, and horses, are the typical vectors for leptospirosis. The infection is transmitted to humans through animal urine.[2,17,18]

Human leptospirosis is endemic in many tropical countries and usually reaches epidemic levels after either higher rainfall periods with flooding or natural disasters, such as hurricanes. Human cases range from 10 to 100 per 100,000/year in the humid tropics. This figure rises during outbreaks and in high-risk groups. Epidemic leptospirosis was recently reported in Nicaragua and Puerto Rico after hurricane strikes and in Brazil after summer floods. Some studies showed a high seroprevalence of anti-*Leptospira* antibodies in the general asymptomatic population, ranging from 18% to 33%. With use of polymerase chain reaction assay, 29% of wild small animals in the Peruvian Amazon were found to be infected by leptospiras.[2,17,18]

Leptospira interrogans, the only parasitic species, is mobile, aerobic, and unstained by the Gram method. Its endotoxins affect the tubulointerstitial cells. Glomerular changes are usually not relevant. The bacterial outer membrane contains lipopolysaccharide, cytotoxic glycolipoprotein, and lipoproteins (especially LipL 32, which is immunogenic and a new hope for a universal leptospiral human vaccine). As leptospiras have special tropism for kidneys, the effect of glycolipoprotein on tubular Na^+,K^+-ATPase activity is potentially involved in both the AKI cellular pathophysiologic process[19] and the paradoxical hypokalemia frequently seen in these patients.[2,17,18] High serum free fatty acids, mainly oleic acids (C18:1), are also potentially implicated in pulmonary hemorrhagic manifestations of the acute respiratory distress syndrome associated with this disease.[20]

Renal involvement is almost universal in leptospirosis but becomes relevant in Weil's disease, which represents the most severe form of the disease. Weil's syndrome is characterized by multiorgan involvement, with diffuse alveolar hemorrhage, pulmonary edema, acute respiratory distress syndrome, or a combination of these features, accompanied by AKI; it has a 50% mortality rate. The incidence of leptospirosis-associated AKI varies from less than 10% to more than 60% of these patients. AKI is typically nonoliguric and associated with hypokalemia.[2,17,18,21] Tubular changes characterized by high urinary fractional excretion of sodium and potassium precede glomerular filtration rate decrease, which could explain the high prevalence of hypokalemia. Antibiotic treatment is efficient in the early and late-severe phases.[17] Treatment recommendations include a high dialysis dose, conservative fluid intake, and approaches to minimize lung injury, such as low tidal volume and high positive end-expiratory pressure when artificial ventilation is required.[17,21]

HEMORRHAGIC FEVERS

Viral hemorrhagic fevers (VHF) are caused by RNA viruses of four different families (Flaviviridae, Arenaviridae, Bunyaviridae, and Filoviridae). They can be acquired by infected arthropod bite (dengue, Rift Valley, yellow fever, and the Crimean-Congo viruses) or by inhalation of infected rodent excreta particles (Lassa, Junin, Machupo, and Hantaan viruses). The clinical picture of VHF is characterized by fever, malaise, increased vascular permeability, and coagulation abnormalities that may lead to bleeding. AKI is an unusual complication of these diseases but has been reported in association with several forms of VHF.[2,18,22] Dengue and yellow fever are the most prevalent forms of VHF in the tropical regions.[22]

Dengue Fever

Dengue is an acute febrile disease caused by an arbovirus, transmitted primarily by mosquitoes, with a benign evolution in most cases. The main dengue vector is the *Aedes aegypti* female mosquito. It is currently the most important urban arboviral disease, affecting millions of people on all continents except Europe. It is more prevalent in tropical and subtropical areas where the environment is favorable for the mosquito's development. It is estimated that half the world's population lives in areas at risk for dengue disease, and about 50 to 100 million cases occur annually. Several factors account for the rising incidence and widespread distribution of dengue, such as climate changes (global warming, intensity and duration of rain season, hurricanes), ecosystem modifications, demographic increases, uncontrolled and unplanned urbanization, and migration of people.[22]

There are four serotypes of dengue flavivirus (DEN1 to DEN4). They are antigenically related, but one serotype does not confer enduring immunity to another. The introduction of a new serotype in a determinate area accounts for the occurrence of epidemics and the hemorrhagic fever dengue form, which is a more severe form of the disease that may be lethal.[22]

Dengue virus infection may be manifested as undifferentiated fever, dengue fever, dengue hemorrhagic fever (DHF), or dengue shock syndrome (DSS). Common clinical manifestations of dengue fever are high fever, myalgia, arthralgia, retro-ocular pain, headache, anorexia, nausea, vomiting, and a cutaneous rash similar to that of measles or rubella. DHF and DSS are severe forms of the disease characterized by fever, hemorrhagic phenomena, thrombocytopenia, evidence of plasma leakage (increased hematocrit, pleural effusion, ascites, and hypoalbuminemia), mental disorientation, breath shortness, tachycardia, shock, and death.

Renal involvement in dengue includes glomerulonephritis, AKI, and hemolytic-uremic syndrome. Dengue-induced AKI is usually associated with shock, hemolysis, or rhabdomyolysis,[22] but it may occur without any of these triggering factors.[23] There is no specific treatment of dengue fever. Therapy is mostly supportive, avoiding the use of aspirin and nonsteroidal anti-inflammatory drugs.

Yellow Fever

Yellow fever is a noncontagious infectious disease that is endemic in tropical Africa, South America, and Panama. The yellow fever virus is part of the *Flavivirus* genus (Flaviviridae family).[22]

Yellow fever is transmitted to humans by blood-eating insect bites, especially by the *Aedes* and *Haemagogus* genera. There are sylvatic and urban cycles. The sylvatic cycle affects sporadic individuals who come into contact with the vectors in performing economic or recreational activities in infested forests. The urban cycle is characterized by virus transmission through *A. aegypti* to individuals living in urban areas. The urban cycle was eliminated in the Americas from the 1940s to the 1950s, but its resurgence was recently documented in Bolivia. The movement of infected individuals when they are viremic to cities with high vector populations can potentially generate explosive urban epidemics affecting thousands of nonvaccinated people.[24] Interestingly, there is no evidence of yellow fever in Asia, despite an extensive presence of vectors. It is possible that the hyperendemicity of dengue in southwest Asia has afforded protection due to cross-reactive antibodies. This mechanism might also explain why urban yellow fever has not reemerged in Brazil after the reintroduction and spread of the *Aedes* vector and the occurrence of a large number of cases of dengue in the last 20 years.[22]

The diagnosis of yellow fever is made by measuring serum-specific IgM, by viral isolation in insect or mammal cells, and by molecular methods such as reverse transcription–polymerase chain reaction. The most specific pathologic finding of yellow fever is liver injury with formation of Councilman corpuscles. Both viral RNA and antigens are found in these cells, suggesting a direct viral cytopathy.[22,25]

Clinically, yellow fever infection might be asymptomatic, cause moderate febrile disease, or be severe, causing hemorrhagic fever, liver failure, AKI, and death. The majority of the patients (85%) fully recover after 3 to 4 days and become permanently immunized against the disease. About 20% develop the severe form, with mortality up to 50% of the cases.[22]

After 3 to 6 days of incubation, the clinical picture of yellow fever starts abruptly with high fever, chills, anorexia, myalgia, headache, vomiting, and bradycardia. Hemorrhagic manifestations may occur. There is then a remission period with symptom improvement, and mild cases do not have any further manifestations. In the severe forms, fever comes back, followed by vomiting, epigastric pain, and jaundice, the so-called intoxication phase. There are large increases in transaminases and bilirubin. Leukopenia and ST-segment abnormalities are also found. Hemorrhagic events, such as hematemesis, melena, petechiae, bruises, mucosal bleeding, and metrorrhagia in women, can occur in association with hepatic damage and consumptive coagulopathy. Microcirculatory thrombosis, disseminated intravascular coagulation, tissue anoxia, oliguria, and shock may follow.[22]

Yellow fever–associated renal injury is usually observed after 5 days of disease in the severe forms; it may evolve to anuria and acute tubular necrosis, with increased mortality. In Africa, AKI is observed earlier and in the absence of jaundice or liver abnormalities, with higher mortality. The mechanisms of kidney injury are poorly understood. In experimental studies performed in Rhesus monkeys in the 1980s, the renal disorder appeared to be prerenal until the last 24 hours of life of the animal. The final phase was characterized by marked oliguria, azotemia, and acidosis, with severe tubular necrosis seen at autopsy. In humans, an eosinophilic degeneration of the renal epithelial cells was described. Viral antigen identification in human renal tissue and after experimental infection in animals suggests a direct action of the virus on renal tissue.[22]

REFERENCES

1. Pinho FMO, Yu L, Burdmann EA. Snakebite-induced acute kidney injury in Latin America. *Semin Nephrol.* 2008;28:354-362.
2. Jha V, Chugh KS. Community-acquired acute kidney injury in Asia. *Semin Nephrol.* 2008;28:330-347.
3. Kanjanabuch T, Sitprija V. Snakebite nephrotoxicity in Asia. *Semin Nephrol.* 2008;28:363-372.
4. Pinho FMO, Zanetta DMT, Burdmann EA. Acute renal failure after *Crotalus durissus* snakebite. A prospective survey on 100 patients. *Kidney Int.* 2005;67:659-667.
5. Castro I, Burdmann EA, Seguro AC, et al. *Bothrops* venom induces direct renal tubular injury: Role for lipid peroxidation and prevention by antivenom. *Toxicon.* 2004;43:833-839.
6. Abdulkader RCRM, Barbaro KC, Barros EJG, et al. Nephrotoxicity of insect and spider venoms in Latin America. *Semin Nephrol.* 2008;28:373-382.
7. Grisotto LSD, Mendes GE, Castro I, et al. Mechanisms of bee venom–induced acute renal failure. *Toxicon.* 2006;48:44-54.
8. Gamborgi GP, Metcalf EB, Barros EJB. Acute renal failure provoked by toxin from caterpillars of the species *Lonomia obliqua. Toxicon.* 2006;47:68-74.
9. de Souza AL, Malaque CM, Sztajnbok J, et al. *Loxosceles* venom–induced cytokine activation, hemolysis, and acute kidney injury. *Toxicon.* 2008;51:151-156.
10. Jha V, Rathi M. Natural medicines causing acute kidney injury. *Semin Nephrol.* 2008;28:416-428.
11. Naicker S, Aboud O, Gharbi MB. Epidemiology of acute kidney injury in Africa. *Semin Nephrol.* 2008;28:348-353.
12. World Health Organization. *World Malaria Report.* Geneva: World Health Organization; 2008:10.
13. Mishra SK, Das BS. Malaria and acute kidney injury. *Semin Nephrol.* 2008;28:395-408.

14. Barsoum R, Sitprija V. Tropical nephrology. In: Schrier RW, ed. *Diseases of the Kidney and Urinary Tract*. 8th ed. Philadelphia: Lippincott Williams & Wilkins; 2007:2013-2055.
15. Sitprija V. Altered fluid, electrolyte and mineral status in tropical disease, with an emphasis on malaria and leptospirosis. *Nat Clin Pract Nephrol.* 2008;4:91-101.
16. Macallan DC, Pocock M, Robinson GT, et al. Red cell exchange, erythrocytapheresis, in the treatment of malaria with high parasitaemia in returning travelers. *Trans R Soc Trop Med Hyg*. 2003;94:353-356.
17. Andrade L, Daher EF, Seguro AC. Leptospiral nephropathy. *Semin Nephrol.* 2008;28:383-394.
18. Lombardi R, Yu L, Younes-Ibrahim M, et al. Epidemiology of acute kidney injury in Latin America. *Semin Nephrol.* 2008;28:320-329.
19. Younes-Ibrahim M, Burth P, Castro-Faria MV, et al. Inhibition of Na,K-ATPase by an endotoxin extracted from *Leptospira interrogans:* A possible mechanism for the physiopathology of leptospirosis. *C R Acad Sci (Paris).* 1995;318:619-625.
20. Burth P, Younes-Ibrahim M, Santos MCB, et al. Role of nonesterified unsaturated fatty acids in the pathophysiological processes of leptospiral infection. *J Infect Dis*. 2005;191:51-57.
21. Andrade L, Cleto S, Seguro AC. Door-to-dialysis time and daily hemodialysis in patients with leptospirosis: Impact on mortality. *Clin J Am Soc Nephrol.* 2007;2:739-744.
22. Lima EQ, Nogueira ML. Viral-hemorrhagic fever–induced acute kidney injury. *Semin Nephrol.* 2008;28:409-415.
23. Lima EQ, Gorayeb FS, Zanon JR, et al. Dengue haemorrhagic fever–induced acute kidney injury without hypotension, haemolysis or rhabdomyolisis. *Nephrol Dial Transplant.* 2007;22:3322-3326.
24. Massad E, Burattini MN, Coutinho FA, Lopez LF. Dengue and the risk of urban yellow fever reintroduction in São Paulo State, Brazil. *Rev Saude Publica*. 2003;37:477-484.
25. Quaresma JA, Barros VL, Pagliari C, et al. Hepatocyte lesions and cellular immune response in yellow fever infection. *Trans R Soc Trop Med Hyg*. 2007;101:161-168.

CHAPTER 68

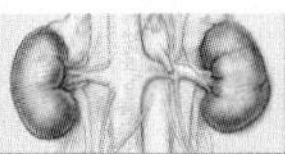

Diagnosis and Clinical Evaluation of Acute Kidney Injury

Li Yang, Joseph V. Bonventre

Acute kidney injury (AKI) occurs in response to a large number of pathophysiologic influences and is characterized by damage to one or more parts of the nephron with adverse functional consequences (see Chapters 66 and 68). Depending on the severity and duration of the kidney dysfunction, the clinical manifestations of AKI are accompanied by metabolic disturbances such as metabolic acidosis and hyperkalemia, abnormal body fluid balance, and effects on other organ systems. AKI can also be asymptomatic, which can result in the absence of a diagnosis or a significant delay in the diagnosis. In this case, asymptomatic AKI will be found on routine biochemical screening of hospitalized patients, revealing an increase in the concentration of blood urea nitrogen (BUN) and creatinine. It is increasingly recognized that AKI is much more common in the population of hospitalized patients and that even milder forms of dysfunction may have important consequences. Furthermore, there is emerging evidence that AKI episodes can lead to chronic kidney disease (CKD), accelerate the progression to end-stage renal disease (ESRD), and contribute to higher long-term mortality risk.[1,2]

AKI is a heterogeneous condition with a plethora of causes, which are generally categorized into prerenal, renal, and postrenal (see Chapter 66). Early detection and identification of the etiology of AKI are critical for designing and implementing prompt and efficient management and secondary prevention strategies. Despite significant improvements in management, the in-hospital mortality and morbidity associated with AKI remain high. A significant number of patients who survive the AKI have chronic sequelae with worsening of their underlying kidney disease and in some cases progression to ESRD requiring dialysis. Delay in the early detection of AKI due to insensitivity of serum creatinine as an early biomarker has been one of the important obstacles in evaluating and applying potentially effective early interventions.

DEFINITION AND CLASSIFICATION

Definition

There are many different published definitions of AKI based on changes of serum creatinine and urine output. Two recent and highly publicized consensus definitions and classification systems have been proposed. The Acute Dialysis Quality Initiative's RIFLE criteria stratified AKI into five groups: renal risk, renal injury, renal failure, renal loss, and ESRD (Fig. 68.1).[3] This classification has been proposed to allow consistency across studies for greater ability to compare clinical results.

With current data that even small changes in serum creatinine are associated with increased mortality,[4] the Acute Kidney Injury Network (AKIN) derived a consensus definition[5,6] that defines stage 1 of AKI as an absolute increase in creatinine concentration of 0.3 mg/dl (26 μmol/l) or greater or a 50% to 100% increase from baseline (see Fig. 68.1). Studies comparing the sensitivity of AKI detection between these two classification systems, however, showed contradictory results in different in-hospital populations.[7] Most attention has been focused on the first three categories of RIFLE (RIF) in comparisons with the three stages of AKIN. There remains some variation in how the criteria are interpreted and used in the literature, particularly with respect to the use of urine output criteria, the choice of baseline creatinine, and the use of the change in the estimated glomerular filtration rate (GFR) rather than the change in creatinine.

A recent analysis from the Program to Improve Care in Acute Renal Disease (PICARD) study group revealed that there is a changing spectrum of AKI in the critically ill, characterized by a large burden of comorbid disease and extensive extrarenal complications, resulting in the need for dialysis in the majority of patients. There is also wide variation across institutions in patient characteristics and practice patterns.[8] The general in-hospital incidence of AKI is at least 0.5% but may be as high as 13%, depending on the definitions used. In specialized settings (e.g., in intensive care units), the reported incidence of AKI varies from 25% to more than 45%; a study of 120,000 patients reported an incidence of AKI within 24 hours of admission to the intensive care unit of 36% with use of the RIFLE criteria.[9] We have recently reported that the time dependency of percentage changes in serum creatinine concentration after severe AKI are highly dependent on baseline kidney function, a feature that is not incorporated into the RIFLE criteria (Fig. 68.2).[10]

Classification

For the purpose of diagnosis and management, AKI can be broadly divided into prerenal, intrarenal, and postrenal (see Chapter 66 and Fig. 66.1). Most intrarenal AKI is related to tubular injury often associated with interstitial changes. Acute tubular injury is most often caused by ischemia or nephrotoxic injury to the kidney.

Although the term *acute tubular necrosis* has been generally applied to cases in which the AKI is due to tubular injury, it is a misnomer in many cases, especially when the insult is mild because necrosis may not dominate the pathologic picture. Rather, the cell death may be primarily apoptotic, and vasoconstriction may predominate in some cases; the cells may be injured but not so severely as to result in death. It is not appropriate to use the terms *acute kidney injury*, *acute renal failure*, and *acute tubular necrosis* interchangeably, as is often done.

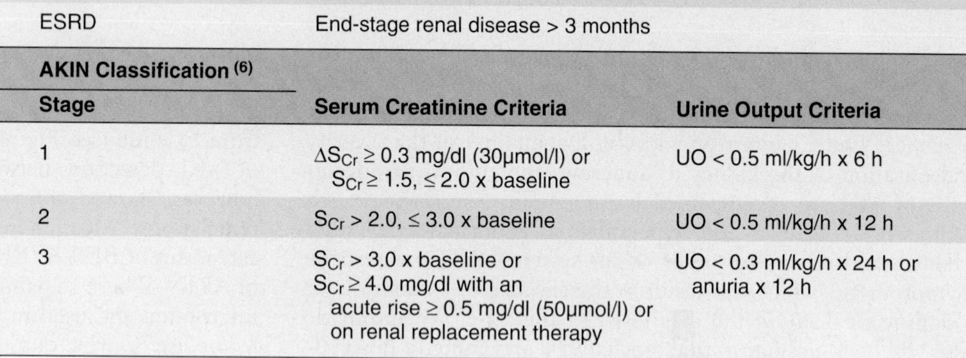

RIFLE and AKIN Criteria for Diagnosis of AKI

RIFLE Classification(3)	GFR Criteria	Urine Output Criteria
Risk	S_{Cr} >1.5 x baseline or ΔGFR >25% reduction	UO <0.5 ml/kg/h x 6 h
Injury	S_{Cr} >2.0 x baseline or ΔGFR >50% reduction	UO <0.5 ml/kg/h x 12 h
Failure	S_{Cr} >3.0 x baseline or ΔGFR >75% reduction or S_{Cr} >4.0 mg/dl	UO <0.3 ml/kg/h x 24 h or anuria x 12 h
Loss	Persistent acute renal failure = Complete loss of function for >4 wk	
ESRD	End-stage renal disease > 3 months	

AKIN Classification (6) Stage	Serum Creatinine Criteria	Urine Output Criteria
1	$\Delta S_{Cr} \geq$ 0.3 mg/dl (30µmol/l) or $S_{Cr} \geq$ 1.5, ≤ 2.0 x baseline	UO < 0.5 ml/kg/h x 6 h
2	S_{Cr} > 2.0, ≤ 3.0 x baseline	UO < 0.5 ml/kg/h x 12 h
3	S_{Cr} > 3.0 x baseline or $S_{Cr} \geq$ 4.0 mg/dl with an acute rise ≥ 0.5 mg/dl (50µmol/l) or on renal replacement therapy	UO < 0.3 ml/kg/h x 24 h or anuria x 12 h

Figure 68.1 RIFLE and AKIN criteria for diagnosis of AKI. RIFLE, risk, injury, failure, loss, ESRD; AKIN, Acute Kidney Injury Network; AKI, acute kidney injury; GFR, glomerular filtration rate; S_{Cr}, serum creatinine; UO, urinary output.

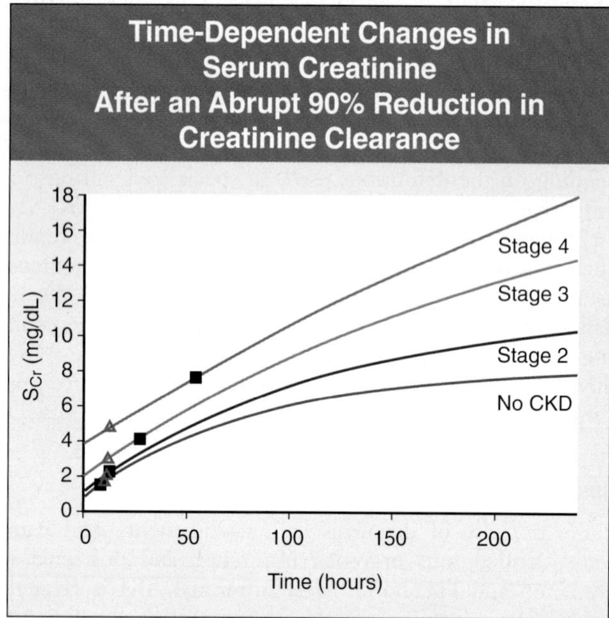

Figure 68.2 A model of time-dependent changes in S_{Cr} concentrations after an abrupt 90% reduction in CrCl, reflecting the pattern of increase at four different stages of baseline kidney function (no CKD and stages 2 to 4 CKD). *Solid squares* show the point at which a 100% increase in S_{Cr} has occurred; *open triangles* show the point at which an increase of 1.0 mg/dl in S_{Cr} has occurred. S_{Cr}, serum creatinine; CrCl, creatinine clearance; CKD, chronic kidney disease. *(Reprinted with permission from reference 10.)*

DIAGNOSIS AND CLINICAL EVALUATION OF ACUTE KIDNEY INJURY

Early Detection of Acute Kidney Injury

The delay in early diagnosis of AKI has been a major impediment to development of newer preventive strategies for AKI. The approaches to the early detection of AKI include identification and monitoring of at-risk populations and development of more sensitive biomarkers. Several risk stratification scoring systems for AKI after cardiac surgery, vascular surgery, general surgery, contrast-induced nephropathy, and trauma have been explored. These have included the Acute Physiology and Chronic Health Evaluation (APACHE) I or II score, which is not focused on the kidney but rather is a general severity of illness scoring system. The Cleveland Clinic Foundation (CCF) score is a preoperative AKI risk score consisting of 11 preoperative variables including gender, congestive heart failure, left ventricular ejection fraction, use of intra-aortic balloon counterpulsation, chronic lung disease, insulin-requiring diabetes mellitus, previous cardiac surgery, emergency surgery, valve surgery, procedures other than coronary bypass or valve, and serum creatinine. As an example of the use of the CCF scoring system, the factors found to be related to a higher incidence of AKI after cardiac surgery in a study of 34,562 surgeries were male gender, postoperative intra-aortic balloon pump, congestive heart failure, ejection fraction below 35%, coronary artery bypass grafting plus valve surgery, diabetes mellitus, chronic obstructive pulmonary disease, and peripheral vascular or cerebrovascular disease.[11] For contrast nephropathy, risk factors are age, CKD, diabetes mellitus, volume depletion, nephrotoxic drugs, hemodynamic instability, nonsteroidal anti-inflammatory agents, and other superimposed kidney injury such as atheroemboli or as occurs in sepsis.

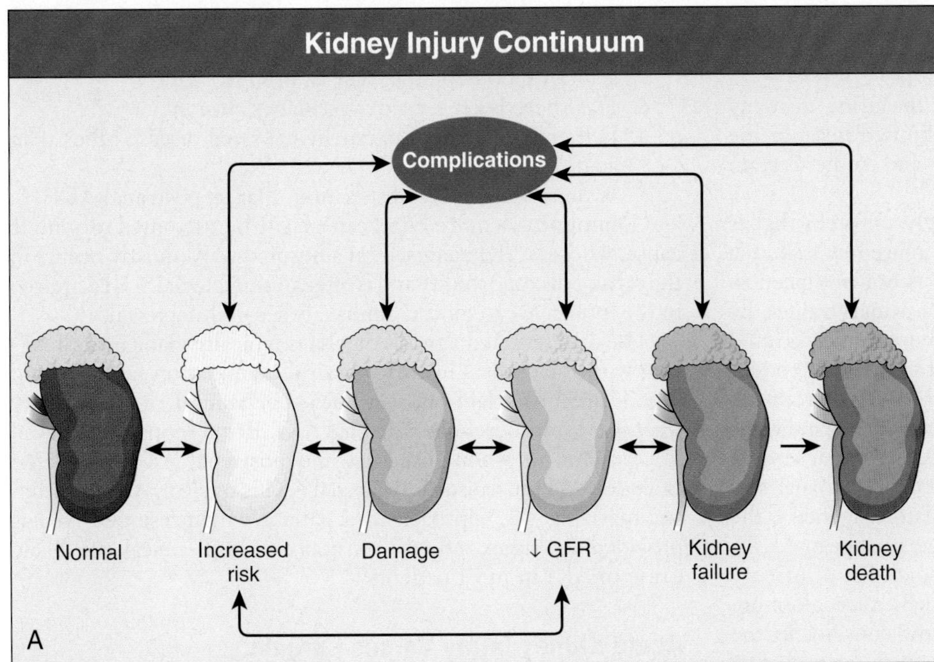

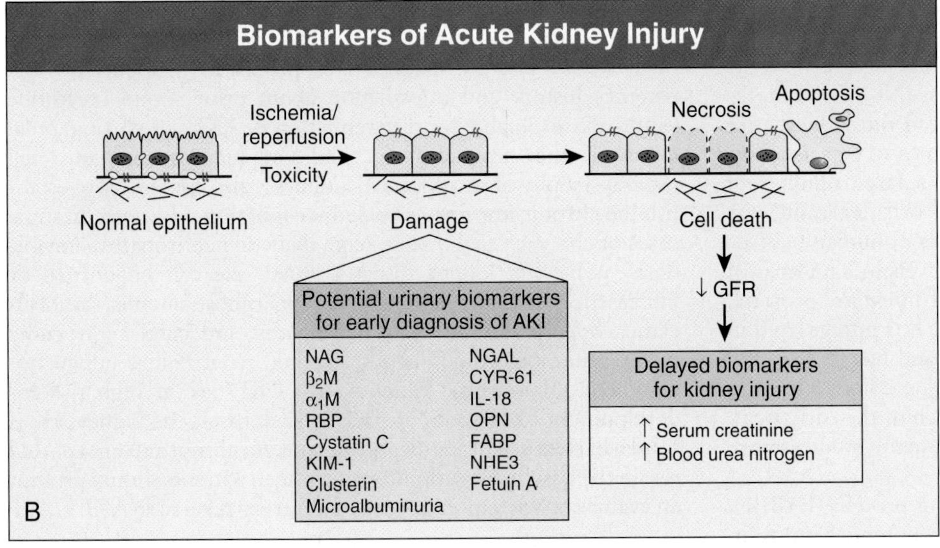

Figure 68.3 A, Kidney injury continuum. There are various reversible stages of AKI, depending on the severity of insult, ranging from increased risk to damage followed by decrease in GFR further progressing to kidney failure and death. **B,** Biomarkers of acute kidney injury. The traditional markers used to diagnose AKI, blood urea nitrogen and creatinine, are insensitive, are nonspecific, and do not adequately differentiate between the different stages of AKI. A group of urinary biomarkers of AKI are being evaluated, some of which will facilitate earlier diagnosis and specific preventive and therapeutic strategies, ultimately resulting in fewer complications and improved outcomes. GFR, glomerular filtration rate; NAG, *N*-acetylglucosaminidase; β_2M, β_2-microglobulin; α_1M, α_1-microglobulin; RBP, retinol-binding protein; KIM-1, kidney injury molecule 1; NGAL, neutrophil gelatinase-associated lipocalin; CYR-61, cysteine-rich protein 61; IL-18, interleukin-18; OPN, osteopontin; FABP, fatty acid–binding protein; NHE3, sodium-hydrogen exchanger isoform 3. *(Reprinted with permission from references 12 and 13.)*

There is a great deal of interest in the potential utility of various blood and urinary biomarkers, which can contribute either alone or in combination with the clinical markers described before to the diagnosis and prognosis of AKI. Figure 68.3 depicts the continuum of kidney injury severity and a number of biomarkers that have been proposed to be useful in early detection. Not all of these biomarkers are created equal, however, and a few are more likely than others to be useful because of stability of analytes, sensitivity and specificity, rapid assay availability, and cost-effectiveness. For a more complete overview of the potential urinary biomarkers, the reader is referred to recent reviews.[12,13]

Serum creatinine has limitations as a marker for the early detection of AKI. The serum creatinine concentration depends not only on urinary clearance of creatinine but also on the rate of production and the volume of distribution. Furthermore, serum creatinine concentration does not accurately reflect GFR in the non–steady-state condition of AKI. Substantial rises in serum creatinine are often not witnessed until 48 to 72 hours after the initial insult to the kidney. In addition, significant renal disease can exist with minimal or no change in creatinine; because a considerable "renal reserve" exists in the individual with normal renal function, the serum level of creatinine can be influenced by numerous nonrenal factors (see Chapter 3). Correct interpretation of serum creatinine concentrations across centers is also hampered by the variation in calibration of different creatinine assays.

Cystatin C has been receiving a great deal of attention as a better marker of kidney function compared with serum creatinine. Although it has not yet been well validated as a GFR indicator in AKI, studies have found cystatin C to be an early and reliable marker of AKI in patients in intensive care units.

β_2-Microglobulin and α_1-microglobulin have been reported as useful markers for proximal tubular damage. Limitations are associated with less specificity because diseases other than kidney injury can also affect their serum levels and thus affect the urinary concentrations.

N-Acetylglucosaminidase is increased in the urine in many AKI settings. Its value in AKI detection is limited because the enzyme activity is sensitive to urine pH and some certain nephrotoxins.

Kidney injury molecule 1 (KIM-1) is a glycoprotein that is highly upregulated in proximal tubular cells injured by ischemia or nephrotoxins in animals and humans and is not produced to any significant extent, at levels that will affect urinary values, by any other organ. The ectodomain of this membrane-associated mucin-rich molecule is shed into the urine of human and rodent kidneys with renal injury, but it is not found in urine produced by healthy kidneys. Recent evaluation in human disease indicates that it is much more highly upregulated in AKI compared with acute renal dysfunction not related to ischemia or toxins and chronic renal failure. Recently, the two regulatory agencies, the U.S. Food and Drug Administration and the European Medicines Agency, have included KIM-1 in the small list of urinary kidney tubular injury biomarkers (together with β_2-microglobulin, albumin, and total protein) that they will now consider in the evaluation of kidney tubular damage, as part of their respective drug review processes during animal studies of new drugs, and these regulatory agencies have encouraged its further use in clinical studies to amass more data on kidney biomarkers.[14,15] Importantly, KIM-1 is not elevated in prerenal disease.

Neutrophil gelatinase-associated lipocalin (NGAL) is markedly upregulated and abundantly expressed in the kidney after renal ischemia. Urinary NGAL has been shown to be a sensitive marker for the early detection of AKI in a large number of studies.[16] NGAL, also known as lipocalin 2 or siderocalin, was first discovered as a 25-kd protein in granules of human neutrophils. NGAL is normally expressed at low levels in a number of organs including kidney, breast, liver, small intestine, prostate, stomach, lymphoid cells, thymus, and lungs. It is upregulated in the distal tubule after injury to the kidney and has been found to be promising as an early diagnostic and predictive urinary marker of injury in many clinical states. Much of the early work on this molecule was done in children, but many studies more recently have been conducted in adults.

Urinary interleukin-18, fatty acid–binding protein (FABP1), and albuminuria also have shown important potential utility in the early diagnosis of AKI.

Given the urgent need for more timely diagnosis of AKI and the limitations of serum creatinine in the early detection of renal dysfunction, we believe that one or more of the new serum (cystatin C) and urine (such as KIM-1, *N*-acetylglucosaminidase, and NGAL) biomarkers will soon be monitored in high-risk patients. Additional regulatory approval, however, and more clinical studies in varying populations of patients will be necessary before physicians can be confident in the sensitivities and specificities of these markers either alone or in combination. In the future, we are likely to have point-of-care bedside technology including dipsticks to provide online noninvasive detection of the onset and severity of kidney injury.

DIFFERENTIAL DIAGNOSIS OF ACUTE KIDNEY INJURY

The differential diagnosis of AKI should aim to answer the following five questions:

1. Is the renal failure acute, acute on chronic, or chronic?
2. Is there evidence of true hypovolemia or reduced effective arterial blood volume, that is, prerenal AKI?
3. Has there been a major vascular occlusion?
4. Is there evidence of parenchymal renal disease other than acute tubular necrosis?
5. Is there renal tract obstruction, that is, postrenal AKI?

Community-acquired AKI can usually be attributed to a single cause, whereas AKI acquired on a hospital ward mostly occurs in the setting of comorbidity and is often multifactorial. AKI acquired in the intensive care unit is almost always multifactorial.

The differential diagnosis of AKI is typically made in conjunction with the clinical history, physical examination findings, and blood and urine laboratory values. Ultrasound of the urinary tract is useful to exclude postrenal AKI. Renal biopsy is reserved for patients in whom prerenal and postrenal AKI have been excluded and the cause of intrarenal AKI is unclear. An algorithm summarizing the approach to a patient with presumed AKI is provided in Figure 68.4. This approach will reveal the likely cause of AKI in most patients.

Acute Kidney Injury Versus Chronic Kidney Disease

It is extremely important to discriminate AKI from chronic renal failure because AKI can potentially resolve if the causal event can be removed and the patient is appropriately supported. The patient's history and information about prior serum creatinine values are invaluable for differentiation of AKI and chronic renal failure if they are available. Radiographic evidence of renal osteodystrophy or small scarred kidneys is also conclusive to establish the chronic impairment of kidney function. However, in some cases of chronic renal disease (e.g., diabetic nephropathy, amyloidosis, polycystic kidney disease), renal size can be normal or increased. The findings of anemia, hyperphosphatemia, hypocalcemia, hyperparathyroidism, neuropathy, and band keratopathy on presentation would suggest chronic renal failure (albeit not completely definitive). Patients with CKD are at high risk for development of episodes of AKI. In such cases, the kidney size is somewhat less useful as a diagnostic tool. An abrupt and unexpected rise in the baseline creatinine value in such patients should prompt an evaluation for superimposed, potentially reversible AKI.

Clinical Assessment

The assessment of patients with AKI requires a careful history and record review, a thorough physical examination, and the judicious interpretation of laboratory data. Careful recording of remote and recent serum creatinine levels over time, incorporating drug therapy and interventions, is invaluable for differential diagnosis and for the identification of the possible cause of AKI. Information obtainable by history should include type and duration of symptoms for urinary difficulty, estimates of volume of urine, history of urinary tract infection or stone disease, recent surgery and drugs used. Clinical, pharmacy, nursing, and radiology records should be reviewed for evidence of recent administration of nephrotoxic medications (e.g., nonsteroidal anti-inflammatory drugs, angiotensin-converting enzyme inhibitors, or angiotensin receptor blockers) or radiocontrast agents.

Physical examination will reveal signs important for the diagnosis of the etiology of AKI. Some of these include signs of sepsis or malignant disease, volume status, skin or pulmonary manifestations of systemic disease, cardiac rhythm abnormalities or

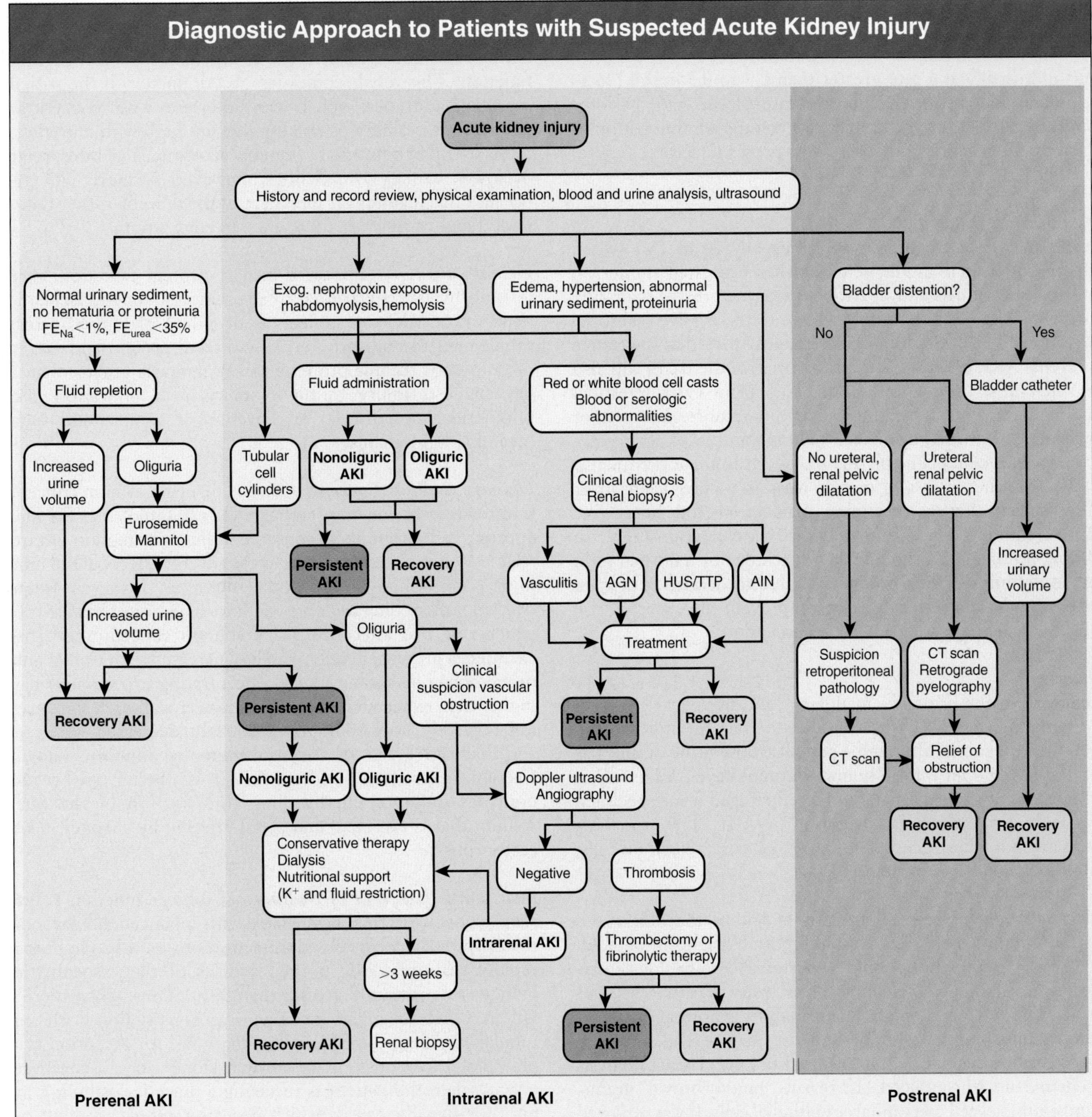

Figure 68.4 Diagnostic approach to patients with suspected AKI. AGN, acute glomerulonephritis; AIN, acute interstitial nephritis; CT, computed tomography; Exog., exogenous; HUS/TTP, hemolytic-uremic syndrome/thrombotic thrombocytopenic purpura.

congestive heart failure, manifestations of abnormal liver function, edema or ascites, and a hydronephrotic mass presenting as a mass in the flank or a distended bladder presenting as a suprapubic mass. A complete pelvic examination in women and a rectal examination for all patients are mandatory. Prerenal causes should be suspected especially in AKI patients with clinical symptoms of thirst or orthostatic hypotension or tachycardia, reduced jugular venous pressure, decreased skin turgor, and reduced axillary sweating. In critically ill patients, invasive hemodynamic monitoring (central venous or Swan-Ganz catheterization) is often necessary. Although most AKI is either prerenal or due to ischemia or nephrotoxins, patients should be assessed carefully for the evidence of other renal parenchymal diseases; many of these are treatable, and their diagnosis alters management and prognosis.

In any patients with AKI, an obstructive cause must be excluded because prompt intervention to relieve obstruction can result in improvement or complete recovery of renal function. If it is unnoticed, significant delays in the diagnosis can lead to adverse long-term sequelae.

Serum Creatinine Concentration

Although serum creatinine demonstrates poor sensitivity and specificity in early detection of AKI, in current clinical practice, renal function is still commonly monitored in patients with AKI by following the daily variations in serum creatinine concentration. The serum creatinine concentration tends to rise progressively and usually at a rate greater than 0.3 to 0.5 mg/dl (26 to 44 μmol/l) per day in AKI. A slow rate of rise with periodic downward fluctuations associated with volume administration or improvement in cardiac function favors prerenal factors as causes of the AKI.

Serum BUN/Creatinine Ratio

The plasma BUN/creatinine ratio is usually 10 to 15:1 (when both are expressed as mg/dl; 40 to 60 when expressed as mmol/l) in normal individuals and in AKI but may be greater than 20:1 in prerenal AKI because of the increase in the passive reabsorption of urea. Thus, a high ratio is frequently touted as suggestive of prerenal AKI, but this is unreliable because the BUN will also rise when urea production is increased from gastrointestinal bleeding, tissue breakdown, high catabolic status (e.g., sepsis), or impairment of protein anabolism (administration of corticosteroids or tetracycline). The plasma BUN/creatinine ratio can also exceed 20:1 when a loss of muscle mass in a chronically ill or elderly patient lowers creatinine production and hence the plasma creatinine concentration without a change in GFR. In addition, prerenal AKI should not be excluded by a normal ratio because diminished urea production (due to decreased protein intake or underlying liver disease) can prevent the expected rise in the BUN by increased tubular reabsorption.

Urinalysis

Assessment of the urine is a mandatory and inexpensive tool in the evaluation of AKI. Urine volume is of varying utility in the differential diagnosis, although a patient whose urine output has been less than 30 ml/h for 6 hours will often have AKI. Analysis of the sediment and supernatant of a centrifuged urine specimen is valuable for differential diagnosis of AKI. The urinalysis should involve a dipstick analysis for pH, glucose, red blood cells, white blood cells, and protein.

Urine Sediment Urine microscopy is one of the oldest and most commonly used tests for differential diagnosis of AKI. Microscopic examination should be performed on freshly centrifuged urine sediments, evaluating the presence of cells, casts, and crystals (Figs. 68.5 and 68.6). The urinalysis is normal or nearly normal in pure prerenal AKI; hyaline casts may be seen, but these are not an abnormal finding. In comparison, the classic urinalysis in ischemic or toxin-induced AKI reveals "muddy brown" granular and epithelial cell casts and free epithelial cells. It was reported recently that a simple urinary cast scoring system, based on grading the level of casts and epithelial cells, had potential value in diagnosis of tubular injury and might also be useful for predicting renal outcomes.[17] More data will be necessary to confirm the utility of this particular system. Casts may be absent, however, in approximately 20% to 30% of patients with ischemic or nephrotoxic AKI, and thus they are not a requisite for diagnosis. Patients with postrenal AKI may also present with benign sediment, although hematuria and pyuria are common in patients with intraluminal obstruction or prostatic disease.

Urine Osmolality Measurement of the urine osmolality can also be helpful in differential diagnosis. Loss of concentrating ability is an early and almost universal finding in AKI; the urine osmolality is below 450 mosmol/kg in almost all cases and often below 350 mosmol/kg. In contrast, a urine osmolality above 500 mosmol/kg is highly suggestive of prerenal AKI because it usually reflects both a hypovolemic stimulus to the secretion of antidiuretic hormone and the maintenance of normal tubular function. This test becomes less discriminatory if the patient is receiving diuretics, which can interfere with concentrating ability. If the urinary osmolality remains high with diuretics, the test is useful in pointing to prerenal azotemia. The interpretation of lower urinary osmolalities, however, is more ambiguous because this may reflect the effect of the diuretic rather than the underlying capacity of the kidney to concentrate.

Urinary Protein Increased urinary protein excretion, characteristically less than 1 g/day, is a common finding in ischemic or nephrotoxic AKI and reflects both failure of injured proximal tubule cells to reabsorb normally filtered protein and excretion of cell debris (tubule proteinuria). Proteinuria greater than 1 g/day suggests injury to the glomerular ultrafiltration barrier (glomerular proteinuria) or excretion of paraproteins such as myeloma light chains.

Urinary Sodium Concentration The urine sodium concentration tends to be low in prerenal AKI (<20 mmol/l) as the kidney appropriately attempts to conserve sodium and high in intrarenal AKI (>40 mmol/l) due in part to the adverse effects of the tubular injury on sodium reabsorption. There is, however, frequent overlap, often due to large variations in water reabsorption, which can also affect the urine sodium concentration. As an example, a prerenal patient who has increased secretion of antidiuretic hormone and an intact concentrating process may have a higher than expected urine sodium concentration despite excreting relatively little sodium. Conversely, decreased water reabsorption can lower the urine sodium by dilution. Thus, the fractional excretion of sodium (FE_{Na})* is a better test because it evaluates only sodium handling (the fraction of the filtered sodium that is excreted) and is not affected by changes in water reabsorption.

Fractional Excretion of Sodium If tubular function is intact, renal vasoconstriction is associated with enhanced tubular sodium reabsorption. Specifically, the fraction of filtered sodium that is rapidly reabsorbed by normal tubules of the vasoconstricted kidney is significantly greater than 99%. Thus, when there is a fall in GFR secondary to renal vasoconstriction with intact tubular function, the FE_{Na} is less than 1%. An exception to this physiologic response of the normal kidney to vasoconstriction occurs when the patient is receiving a diuretic, including mannitol, or has glucosuria, which decreases tubular sodium reabsorption and increases FE_{Na}. FE_{Na} is useful in many clinical scenarios but loses diagnostic value in patients receiving diuretics or with CKD because of intrinsic impairment of efficient sodium reabsorption associated with chronic tubulointerstitial disease and chronic adaptation of sodium excretion, leading to enhanced sodium excretion. The diagnostic specificity of FE_{Na} in distinguishing prerenal azotemia from intrarenal causes of AKI may also be affected by the fact that the patient may actually be progressing from a prerenal azotemic state to established AKI. The FE_{Na} has also been found to be less than 1% in some patients with a variety of conditions other than prerenal AKI (e.g., contrast media–induced or pigment-induced AKI, acute glomerulonephritis and vasculitis, and some cases of acute interstitial

*FE_{Na} = (urine sodium × plasma creatinine)/(plasma sodium × urine creatinine) = (urine sodium/plasma sodium)/(urine creatinine/plasma creatinine).

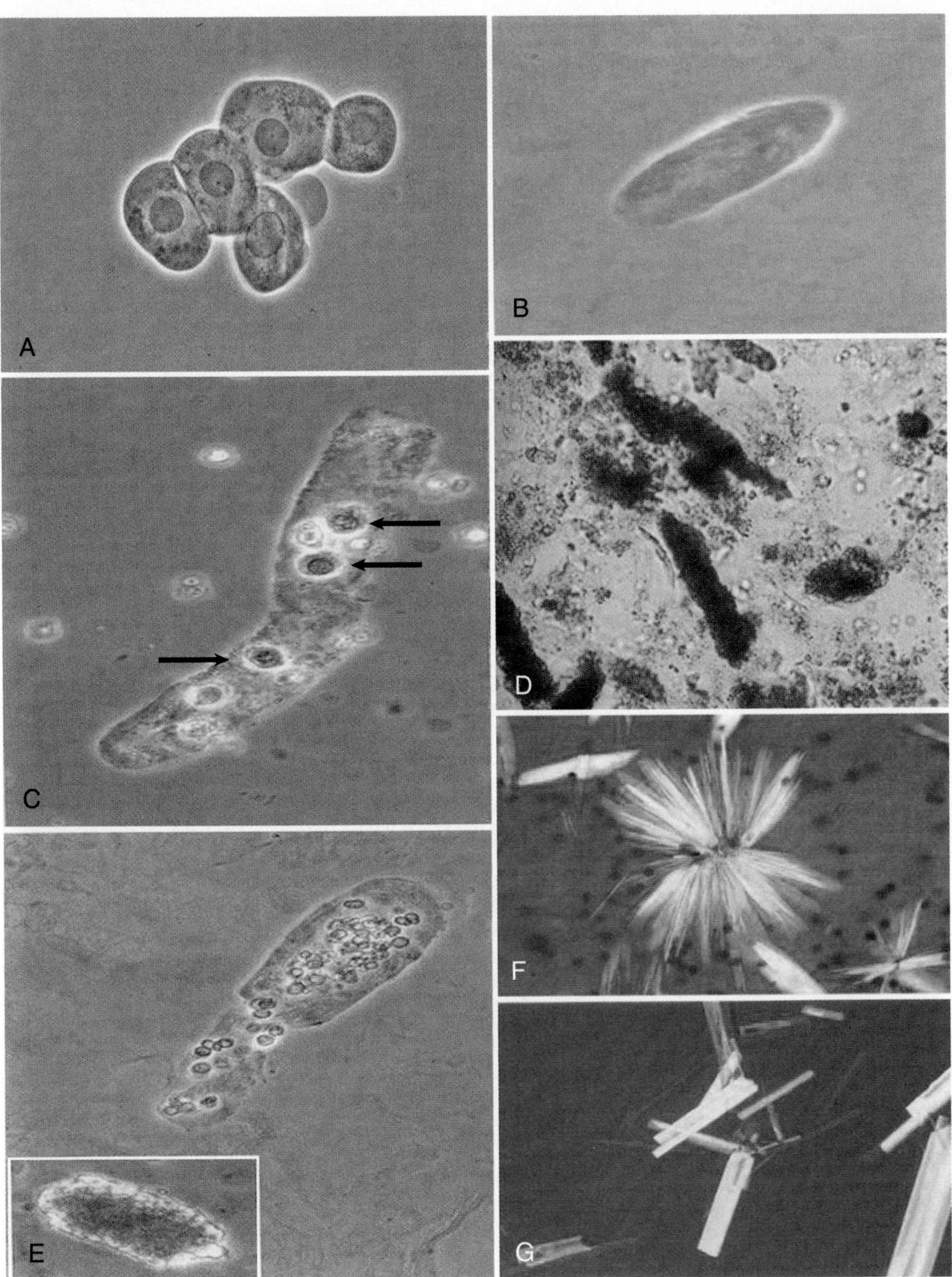

Figure 68.5 Examples of urinary sediments in common cases of AKI. **A,** Epithelial cell aggregate. **B,** Hyaline cast as can be seen in prerenal acute kidney injury. **C,** Epithelial cast as can be seen in early acute tubular necrosis (*arrows* indicate epithelial cells). **D,** Muddy brown cast, typical of established acute tubular necrosis. **E,** Erythrocyte cast as seen in glomerulonephritis and vasculitis. *Inset:* Hemoglobin cast. **F, G,** Two forms of indinavir crystals.

nephritis and obstruction). In patients who were not taking diuretics, FE_{Na} was reportedly able to distinguish transient from persistent AKI (determined by whether serum creatinine returned to baseline within 7 days). Despite these many caveats, FE_{Na} can be very useful when it is considered in the context of other clinical signs and laboratory studies. A fractional excretion of urea of less than 35% favors renal vasoconstriction rather than intrarenal AKI as a cause of the impaired kidney function in the presence of diuretics.[18]

Urine to Serum Creatinine Concentration The urine to plasma creatinine concentration (U_{Cr}/P_{Cr}) is a way to estimate tubular water reabsorption. The creatinine concentration in the glomerular filtrate is equal to that in the plasma and then rises progressively as water but not creatinine is reabsorbed; creatinine secretion will also make a modest contribution to the elevation in the ratio. Patients with prerenal AKI generally have a urine to plasma creatinine ratio above 40, indicating that more than 39/40 or 97.5% of the filtered water has been reabsorbed. Water reabsorption is less efficient in AKI, and the U_{Cr}/P_{Cr} is usually below 20. The most important clinical and laboratory variables in the differential diagnosis between prerenal and renal AKI are listed in Figure 68.7.

Imaging Studies

Imaging of the urinary tract by ultrasound (see Chapter 5) is useful to exclude postrenal AKI. Small kidneys are a clue to the diagnosis of chronic kidney diseases. A plain film of the abdomen, with tomography if necessary, is a valuable initial screening

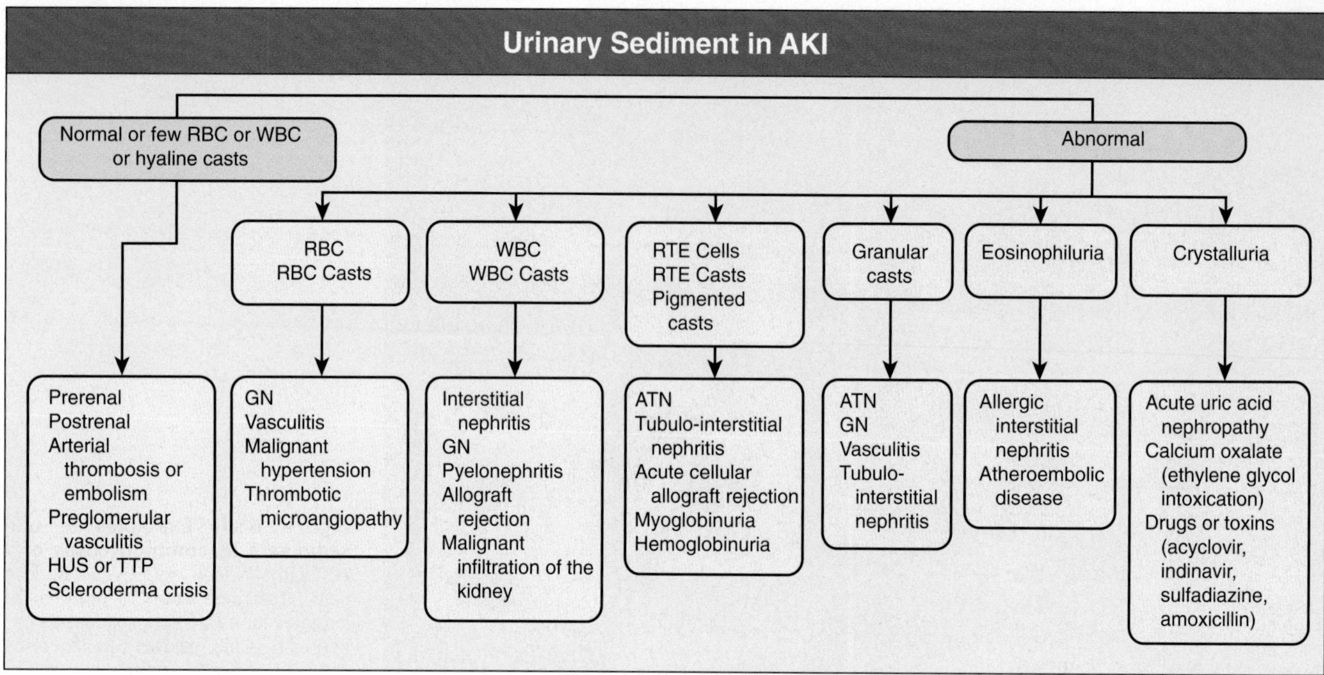

Figure 68.6 Urinary sediment in AKI. RBC, red blood cell; WBC, white blood cell; RTE, renal tubular epithelial; HUS, hemolytic-uremic syndrome; TTP, thrombotic thrombocytopenic purpura; GN, glomerulonephritis; ATN, acute tubular necrosis.

Clinical and Laboratory Variables in the Differential Diagnosis Between Prerenal and Renal AKI

	Prerenal	Renal
History	GI, urinary, skin volume loss, blood loss or third spacing	Drugs or toxin exposure, hemodynamic change
Clinical presentation	Hypotension or volume depletion	No specific symptoms or signs
Laboratory studies		
BUN/S_{Cr}	>20	<20
Sediment	Normal to few casts	"Muddy brown" casts
U_{osm} (mmol/kg)	>500	<350
Proteinuria	None to trace	Mild to moderate
U_{Na} (mmol/l)	<20	>40
FE_{Na} (%)	<1	>1
FE_{Urea} (%)	<35	>35
U_{Cr}/S_{Cr}	<20	>40
Novel biomarkers	None	KIM-1, cystatin C, NGAL, CYR61, others

Figure 68.7 Clinical and laboratory variables in the differential diagnosis between prerenal and renal AKI. GI, gastrointestinal; BUN, blood urea nitrogen; S_{Cr}, serum creatinine; U_{osm}, urinary osmolality; U_{Na}, urinary sodium; FE_{Na}, fractional excretion of sodium; FE_{Urea}, fractional excretion of urea; U_{Cr}, urinary creatinine; KIM-1, kidney injury molecule 1; NGAL, neutrophil gelatinase-associated lipocalin; CYR61, cysteine-rich protein 61.

technique in patients with suspected nephrolithiasis. Computed tomography and magnetic resonance imaging are also useful in detecting obstruction. Pelvicalyceal dilation is usual in patients with urinary tract obstruction (98% sensitivity); however, dilation may be absent immediately after obstruction or in patients with ureteral encasement (e.g., retroperitoneal fibrosis, neoplasia). Retrograde pyelography and anterograde pyelography are more definitive investigations in cases in which obstruction is highly suspected but imaging studies have not adequately defined the cause. These studies can provide precise localization of the site of obstruction. Doppler ultrasound and magnetic resonance angiography have proved useful for assessment of patency of renal arteries and veins in patients with suspected vascular compromise or obstruction as a prerenal cause of AKI; however, contrast angiography is usually required for definitive diagnosis, and the specific link of gadolinium as a causative agent in nephrogenic systemic fibrosis (see Chapter 84) makes it prudent to avoid this contrast agent.

Renal Biopsy

Renal biopsy is reserved for patients in whom prerenal and postrenal AKI have been excluded and the cause of intrinsic renal AKI remains unclear. Renal biopsy is particularly useful when clinical assessment and laboratory investigations suggest diagnoses other than ischemic or nephrotoxic injury that may respond to disease-specific therapy. Examples include rapidly progressive glomerulonephritis, vasculitis, systemic lupus erythematosus, and acute interstitial nephritis. Renal biopsy is also very useful when there is AKI in renal allograft recipients and the therapy will depend critically on whether this is due to immunologic rejection or another cause.

PATHOLOGY OF ACUTE KIDNEY INJURY

Tubular injury in ischemic AKI is usually most severe within the outer medulla of the kidney, involving both the pars recta (S_3 segments) of the proximal tubule and the medullary thick ascending limb of the distal nephron.[19] The typical histologic features of human proximal tubular injury include vacuolation, loss of brush border, and presence of intratubule casts (Fig. 66.3). Necrosis of tubular cells is patchy and is not usually dominant in the biopsy specimen, perhaps in part because most biopsy specimens are from the cortex and the outer medulla is not sampled adequately. Apoptosis of tubular cells is present in renal biopsy specimens from humans with AKI, and evidence of cellular regeneration is often seen, most commonly in those areas of greatest tubular cell loss. Furthermore, regenerative changes and signs of fresh epithelial injury are often observed in the same biopsy specimen, suggesting that recurrent episodes of tubular ischemia continue to occur during the maintenance phase of AKI. The morphologic appearance of the common forms of toxic AKI is similar to that of ischemic AKI. Correlations of morphologic findings to functional endpoints has been difficult, especially because the biopsy represents a limited view of the pathologic process at one point in time and usually samples only the cortex of the kidney.

REFERENCES

1. Macedo E, Bouchard J, Mehta RL. Renal recovery following acute kidney injury. *Curr Opin Crit Care*. 2008;14:660-665.
2. Ishani A, Xue JL, Himmelfarb J, et al. Acute kidney injury increases risk of ESRD among elderly. *J Am Soc Nephrol*. 2009;20:223-228.
3. Bellomo R, Ronco C, Kellum JA, et al. Acute renal failure—definition, outcome measures, animal models, fluid therapy and information technology needs: The Second International Consensus Conference of the Acute Dialysis Quality Initiative (ADQI) Group. *Crit Care*. 2004;8: R204-R212.
4. Chertow GM, Burdick E, Honour M, et al. Acute kidney injury, mortality, length of stay, and costs in hospitalized patients. *J Am Soc Nephrol*. 2005;16:3365-3370.
5. Molitoris BA, Levin A, Warnock DG, et al. Improving outcomes from acute kidney injury. *J Am Soc Nephrol*. 2007;18:1992-1994.
6. Mehta RL, Kellum JA, Shah SV, et al. Acute Kidney Injury Network: Report of an initiative to improve outcomes in acute kidney injury. *Crit Care*. 2007;11:R31.
7. Cruz DN, Ricci Z, Ronco C. Clinical review: RIFLE and AKIN—time for reappraisal. *Crit Care*. 2009;13:211.
8. Mehta RL, Pascual MT, Soroko S, et al. Spectrum of acute renal failure in the intensive care unit: The PICARD experience. *Kidney Int*. 2004;66: 1613-1621.
9. Bagshaw SM, George C, Gibney RT, Bellomo R. A multi-center evaluation of early acute kidney injury in critically ill trauma patients. *Ren Fail*. 2008;30:581-589.
10. Waikar SS, Bonventre JV. Creatinine kinetics and the definition of acute kidney injury. *J Am Soc Nephrol*. 2009;20:672-679.
11. Thakar CV, Arrigain S, Worley S, et al. A clinical score to predict acute renal failure after cardiac surgery. *J Am Soc Nephrol*. 2005;16:162-168.
12. Waikar SS, Bonventre JV. Biomarkers for the diagnosis of acute kidney injury. *Curr Opin Nephrol Hypertens*. 2007;16:557-564.
13. Vaidya VS, Ferguson MA, Bonventre JV. Biomarkers of acute kidney injury. *Annu Rev Pharmacol Toxicol*. 2008;48:463-493.
14. Vaidya VS, Ozer JS, Dieterle F, et al. Kidney injury molecule-1 outperforms traditional biomarkers of kidney injury in preclinical biomarker qualification studies. *Nat Biotechnol*. 2010;28:478-485.
15. Bonventre JV, Vaidya VS, Schmouder R, et al. Next-generation biomarkers for detecting kidney toxicity. *Nat Biotechnol*. 2010;28: 436-440.
16. Nguyen MT, Devarajan P. Biomarkers for the early detection of acute kidney injury. *Pediatr Nephrol*. 2008;23:2151-2157.
17. Perazella MA, Coca SG, Kanbay M, et al. Diagnostic value of urine microscopy for differential diagnosis of acute kidney injury in hospitalized patients. *Clin J Am Soc Nephrol*. 2008;3:1615-1619.
18. Carvounis CP, Nisar S, Guro-Razuman S. Significance of the fractional excretion of urea in the differential diagnosis of acute renal failure. *Kidney Int*. 2002;62:2223-2229.
19. Bonventre JV, Brezis M, Siegel N, et al. Acute renal failure. I. Relative importance of proximal vs. distal tubular injury. *Am J Physiol*. 1998;275: F623-F631.

CHAPTER 69

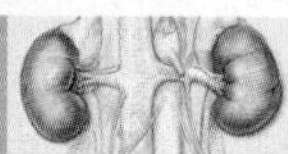

Prevention and Nondialytic Management of Acute Kidney Injury

Etienne Macedo, Josée Bouchard, Ravindra L. Mehta

Acute kidney injury (AKI) acquired in the hospital is often due to a combination of insults. The most common associated causes are failure of renal autoregulation, direct nephrotoxicity, ischemia-reperfusion, and inflammatory states. AKI severity predicts adverse outcomes, such as requirement for renal replacement therapy (RRT), length of hospital stay, and mortality. In addition, the widespread use of the RIFLE and AKI classification systems (see Chapter 68) has shown that even small changes in glomerular filtration rate (GFR) are associated with increased mortality.[1] Furthermore, AKI contributes to dysfunction of other organs, such as heart, lung, brain, and liver. Consequently, primary prevention and early diagnosis of AKI are of central clinical importance. Once a decline in GFR is detected, secondary prevention to attenuate the effects of injury and treatment of the consequences of injury are necessary.

RISK ASSESSMENT

Considering the conceptual model of AKI illustrated in Figure 69.1, the first step in preventing AKI is an adequate risk assessment. The initial care of patients at risk should be focused on identification and, if possible, reversal of the risk factors. Figures 69.2 and 69.3 summarize risk factors in different clinical settings. For a further discussion of risk factors and scoring systems, see Chapters 67 and 68.

PRIMARY PREVENTIVE MEASURES

Optimizing Volume Status and Hemodynamic Status

Regardless of the nature of an insult, hemodynamic stabilization with optimization of the cardiac output and blood pressure (BP) is a key factor in prevention of AKI. The general aim is to optimize volume status based on physiologic measurements, to maintain adequate hemodynamic status and cardiac output to ensure renal perfusion, and to avoid further insults (e.g., hypotension, hypovolemia). Therefore, fluid management is an important intervention for patients in the initiation or extension phase of AKI. Volume expansion can decrease the risk of AKI in the perioperative setting of major vascular surgeries, after renal transplantation and procedures to correct obstructive jaundice. In these clinical scenarios, fluid volume administration is most beneficial at the initiation phase. However, once the injury is initiated and the extension phase starts, the impact of volume expansion with intravenous fluids on clinical outcomes has not been well described and needs to be balanced with the unwanted consequence of fluid accumulation and overload.

Assessment of the volume status is challenging, particularly in patients in the intensive care unit.[2] In most cases, the effect of fluid expansion on the general hemodynamic status and renal function is retrospective and frequently evaluated by trial and error. In patients in the prerenal phase of AKI, fluid expansion will increase organ perfusion, and renal function can improve. In other circumstances, as in patients with severe congestive heart failure (CHF) or diastolic dysfunction, renal perfusion is inadequate despite normal volume status or volume overload. In these patients, fluid expansion can lead to worsening of cardiac function and pulmonary edema.

There are no specific guidelines for optimizing hemodynamic and fluid status for renal function preservation, but extrapolation of data from clinical settings associated with AKI can be instructive. To improve the evaluation of volume status, international guidelines for management of sepsis from the Surviving Sepsis Campaign recommend invasive monitoring with measurements of central venous pressure and venous oxygen saturation (superior vena cava or mixed) based on the early goal-directed therapy approach.[3] The Rivers study randomized patients with severe sepsis or septic shock to receive 6 hours of standard therapy or 6 hours of early goal-directed therapy before admission to the intensive care unit. The protocol ensured that all patients had a central venous pressure of between 8 and 12 mm Hg, a mean arterial pressure (MAP) above 65 mm Hg, and a urine output of more than 0.5 ml/kg per minute by the administration of 500-ml boluses of crystalloid or colloid and vasopressor agents as necessary. Early goal-directed therapy patients received a central venous catheter capable of measuring $Scvo_2$, and they also had to achieve $Scvo_2$ above 70%, pursued by red blood cell transfusion for anemic patients (hematocrit, <30%) and dobutamine therapy for patients above that threshold. This initial approach, applied for 6 hours, reduced the mortality rate, need of mechanical ventilation and therapy with vasopressors, and length of hospital stay.

A number of studies have since established the benefits of adequate fluid expansion and earlier vasopressor administration for rapid shock reversal,[4] and the concept of goal-directed therapy is an attempt to define resuscitation endpoints in early septic shock. However, fluid expansion should be stopped when patients are no longer fluid responsive; late and prolonged aggressive resuscitation in critically ill patients is associated with fluid overload and worse outcomes. Data from the Acute Respiratory Distress Syndrome (ARDS) Clinical Trials Network[5] indicate that after initial resuscitation, a conservative approach to fluid administration is associated with faster weaning from mechanical ventilation and decreased length of intensive care unit stay without any deterioration of kidney function or worse

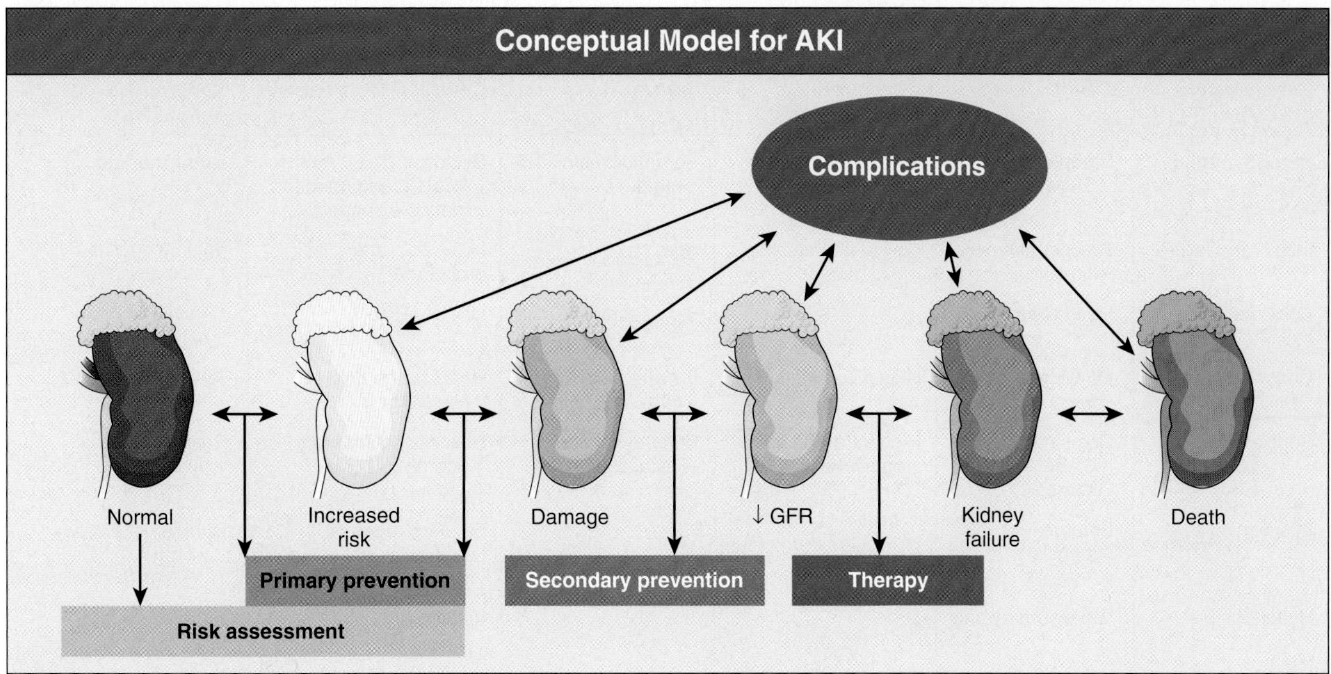

Figure 69.1 Conceptual model for acute kidney injury (AKI). GFR, glomerular filtration rate. *(Modified with permission from reference 2.)*

Major Risk Factors for Acute Kidney Injury

Patient Factors	Medications and Agents	Procedures
Pre-existing renal dysfunction	Nonsteroidal anti-inflammatory drugs	Cardiopulmonary bypass procedures
Sepsis		Surgery involving aortic clamp
Old age (>75)	Cyclooxgenase-2 inhibitors	Increased intra-abdominal pressure
Diabetes	Cyclosporine or tacrolimus	Large arterial catheter placement with risk for atheroembolization
Hepatic failure	Angiotensin-converting enzyme inhibitors	Liver transplantation
Atherosclerosis	Angiotensin receptor blockers	Kidney transplantation
Chronic hypertension		
Perioperative cardiac dysfunction	Use of venous or arterial radiocontrast agents	
Hypercalcemia		
Renal artery stenosis		

Figure 69.2 Major risk factors for acute kidney injury (AKI).

kidney outcomes.[5] In conclusion, a liberal fluid approach as part of early goal-directed therapy appears to be beneficial during the first 6 hours of shock, and a conservative approach should be followed after resolution of shock. Whether these same principles apply for patients with AKI in the absence of shock is unknown. The potential risks of fluid accumulations and overload in the setting of AKI need to be considered.[6]

There is controversy about the optimal fluid to use for resuscitation in critically ill patients. The recent Saline versus Albumin Fluid Evaluation (SAFE) trial of 6997 patients found that fluid resuscitation with saline or albumin resulted in similar relative risks of death in critically ill patients.[7] There were also no significant differences in the proportion of patients with new single-organ and multiple-organ failure, length of intensive care unit stay, length of hospital stay, days of mechanical ventilation, or days of RRT. However, a follow-up subgroup analysis showed that use of albumin may be deleterious in patients with traumatic brain injury.[8]

Specific Risk Factors for the Development of Acute Kidney Injury in Common Clinical Situations

Postoperative	Cardiac Surgery	Critically Ill	Sepsis	Contrast Nephropathy	Nephrotoxic Antibiotics
Hemodynamic	Preoperative S_{Cr}>2.1 mg/dl	Active cancer	Serum bilirubin >1.5 mg/dl	Systolic BP <80 mm Hg for >1 h and need for inotropic support	**Amphotericin**
Multiorgan failure	Preoperative IABP	Low serum albumin	Age	IABP 24 h after procedure	Volume depletion
Aortic cross-clamping	Heart failure		S_{Cr} >1.3 mg/dl	Use of IABP	Concurrent other nephropathy
Congestive heart failure	LV ejection fraction <35%	High A-a gradient*	Elevated CVP >8 cm	Heart failure (NYHA class 3 or 4)	**Aminoglycosides**
Sepsis	Combination of CABG + valve surgery	High intra-abdominal pressure	Hemodynamic instability	History of pulmonary edema	Preexisting renal dysfunction
Infection	Emergency surgery			S_{Cr} >1.5 mg/dl or eGFR <60 ml/min per m^2	Duration of therapy >7 days
Hypertension	Valve surgery only			Volume of contrast >100 ml	Sepsis
Cardiac instability	Previous cardiac surgery			Age >75 yr	Volume depletion
Major vascular surgery	Other cardiac surgery			DM	Divided-dose regimens
Gastrointestinal and endocrine	Insulin-requiring diabetes			Anemia, blood loss (Hct: <39% for men; <36% for women)	Liver disease
Liver cirrhosis	COPD			Intra-arterial injection	Old age
Biliary surgery	ACE inhibitor therapy				
Obstructive jaundice	Female gender				
DM					
Renal transplantation					
S_{Cr} >2 mg/dl					
Oliguria <400 ml/day					
Miscellaneous					
Massive blood transfusion					
Trauma					
Age >70 years					

Figure 69.3 Specific risk factors for the development of acute kidney injury (AKI) in common clinical situations. ACE, angiotensin-converting enzyme; BP, blood pressure; CABG, coronary arterial bypass graft; CVP, central venous pressure; IABP, intra-aortic balloon pump; COPD, chronic obstructive pulmonary disease; DM, diabetes mellitus; eGFR, estimated glomerular filtration rate; Hct, hematocrit; LV, left ventricular; NYHA, New York Heart Association. *A-a gradient, alveolar-arterial oxygen gradient calculated by the sea-level standard formula (713 × FIO_2) – (PCO_2/0.8) – PaO_2, where FIO_2 is fractional inspired oxygen concentration, PaO_2 is arterial partial oxygen pressure, and PCO_2 is partial carbon dioxide pressure. *(Modified with permission from reference 51.)*

Hydroxyethyl starch (HES) preparations are the most used nonprotein intravascular volume expanders. In addition to their efficiency in fluid management, they have anti-inflammatory properties and reduced cost compared with albumin. However, they potentially alter coagulation and platelet function as a result of their physicochemical characteristics and the electrolyte composition of the solvent. AKI is also a major concern with their use, and it is thought to be associated with the urine hyperviscosity leading to tubular lumen obstruction. This so-called osmotic nephrosis is characterized by tubular nephrosis–like lesions. The solutions exhibit different nephrotoxicity potential, as the pharmacokinetics of HES depends on the degree of substitution at carbons 2 and 6 in the glucose ring in combination with the molecular weight and molar substitution. They are identified by three numbers, indicating the concentration of the solution, the mean molecular weight, and, the most significant one, the molar substitution (e.g., 10% HES 200/0.5 or 6% HES 130/0.4). Current clinical data on the third-generation HES 130/0.4 have reported no adverse effects on renal function in patients who are considered to be at particular risk (mild to severe renal dysfunction, advanced age, and high-dose therapy). Therefore, older and newer generations of HES differ, and adverse effects reported with older generations of HES should not be extrapolated to newer compounds. In summary, in patients at risk for AKI, the newer generation iso-oncotic HES (130/0.4, 6%) should be preferred, the dose should be limited, and renal function should be closely monitored, preferably every 12 to 24 hours.

Prevention of Contrast Medium Nephropathy

Common among the various protocols is the need to establish and to maintain an adequate hydration status. To prevent contrast medium–induced nephropathy (CIN), low-risk patients should increase their oral fluid intake and high-risk patients should receive intravenous hydration (Fig. 69.4). Hydration with isotonic saline started the morning of the procedure or immediately before in cases of emergency interventions is superior to half-isotonic (0.45%) saline.[9] A randomized controlled trial (RCT) compared isotonic saline with isotonic sodium bicarbonate (154 mmol/l $NaHCO_3$ in 5% dextrose at 3 ml/kg per hour for 6 hours starting 1 hour before the procedure followed by 1 ml/kg per hour for the 6 hours after the procedure). CIN was significantly lower in the bicarbonate group, 2% versus 14% in the saline solution group.[10] The rationale for isotonic bicarbonate is based on animal studies showing that bicarbonate is capable of scavenging reactive oxygen species, and the increased pH in the proximal tubule and the renal medulla associated with bicarbonate administration could reduce generation of superoxide. In addition, isotonic saline contains high amounts of chloride, with a potential vasoconstrictor effect on renal vasculature. Considering that most hydration studies with isotonic bicarbonate use shorter infusion protocols (only 1 hour) than those with isotonic saline (usually 12 to 24 hours), hydration with bicarbonate is also an attractive alternative in the setting of emergency procedures.

Although the superiority of bicarbonate was confirmed by four additional randomized trials reported, four others did not show a difference and a large retrospective cohort study found that use of bicarbonate was associated with increased risk of CIN. Joannidis and colleagues[11] conducted a meta-analysis to address

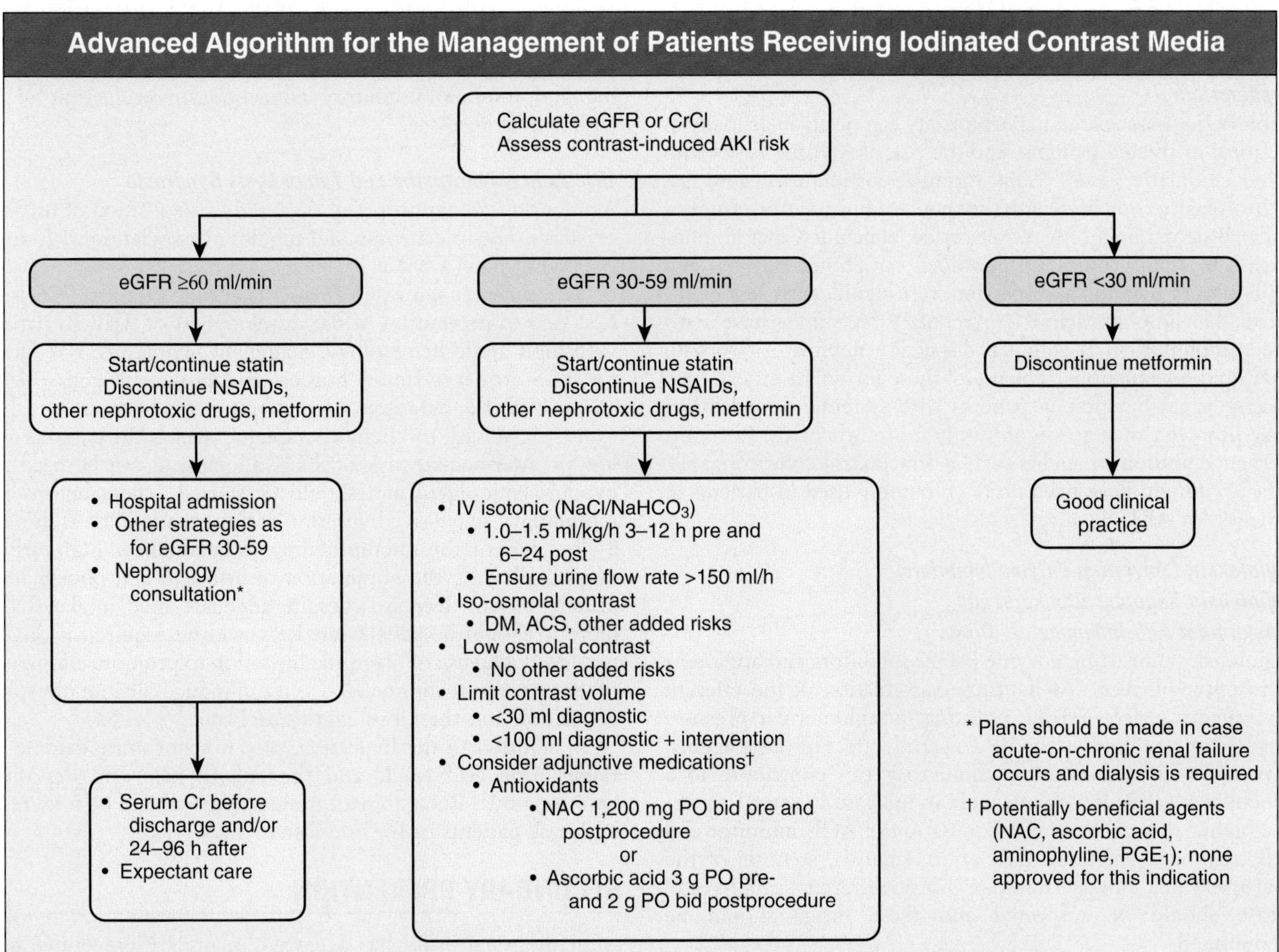

Figure 69.4 Advanced algorithm for the management of patients receiving iodinated contrast media. ACS, acute coronary syndromes; AKI, acute kidney injury; CrCl, creatinine clearance; DM, diabetes mellitus; eGFR, estimated glomerular filtration rate; NAC, *N*-acetylcysteine; NSAIDs, nonsteroidal anti-inflammatory drugs; PGE_1, prostaglandin E_1. *(Modified with permission from reference 52.)*

the discordant results of these trials. Although they confirmed that bicarbonate therapy is more effective in preventing CIN, the heterogeneity of the studies and publication bias were substantial, preventing clear and definitive conclusions.

Iodinated contrast medium can be categorized according to osmolality into high-osmolal contrast medium (~2000 mOsm/kg), low-osmolal contrast medium (600 to 800 mOsm/kg), and iso-osmolal contrast medium (290 mOsm/kg). The higher cost of the low-osmolality agents barred the complete replacement of high-osmolality iodinated contrast medium. The guidelines recommend the use of low-osmolality iodinated contrast medium for patients with increase risk of CIN. Evidence to date suggests that the iso-osmolal, nonionic contrast media are the least nephrotoxic, particularly after intraarterial administration, and should therefore be used in patients at high risk for CIN.

The volume of contrast material administered is also a crucial risk factor and an independent predictor of CIN. Based on the volume of contrast given (*V*) and the creatinine clearance (CrCl), a *V*/CrCl ratio above 3.7 was a significant and independent predictor of CIN in the general population. Administration of contrast material more than once in a short period is another risk factor, and contrast studies should be postponed at least 48 hours after the last infusion of contrast medium if possible.

The drugs used for CIN prevention are included in the section on pharmacologic approaches.

Prevention of Drug- and Nephrotoxin-Induced Acute Kidney Injury

Amphotericin

Amphotericin-associated nephrotoxicity can occur in as many as one third of treated patients, and the risk of AKI increases with higher cumulative doses. Lipid formulations seem to cause less nephrotoxicity compared with the standard formulation, amphotericin B deoxycholate. A recent review concluded that amphotericin B lipid complex, liposomal amphotericin B, and amphotericin B colloidal dispersion were significantly less nephrotoxic than amphotericin B deoxycholate. No studies have compared amphotericin B colloidal dispersion nephrotoxicity with other lipid formulations. The use of these formulations can help preserve renal function in patients with systemic fungal infections; however, they are significantly more expensive. Recently, alternative antifungal agents such as itraconazole, voriconazole, and caspofungin have been more commonly used in patients at high risk for AKI.

Angiotensin-Converting Enzyme Inhibitors, Angiotensin Receptor Blockers, and Nonsteroidal Anti-Inflammatory Drugs

Angiotensin-converting enzyme (ACE) inhibitors and angiotensin receptor blockers (ARBs) cause vasodilation of the efferent glomerular arteriole, further reducing intraglomerular pressure already compromised by the BP–lowering effect of these agents. In patients with renal dysfunction, they can contribute to a reduction in GFR. In patients with an increase in serum creatinine higher than 30% after the initiation of ACE inhibitor and ARB treatment, bilateral renal artery stenosis, stenosis of the renal artery in a solitary kidney, or diffuse intrarenal small-vessel disease should be suspected and these drugs should be discontinued.

Nonsteroidal anti-inflammatory drugs (NSAIDs) or cyclooxygenase 2 inhibitors should be used with caution in patients with atherosclerotic cardiovascular diseases (CVD), chronic kidney disease (CKD), and intravascular volume depletion. As NSAIDs cause acute inhibition of cyclooxygenase (type 1 or 2), they can reduce GFR and renal blood flow. In critically ill patients, renal hypoperfusion due to decreased effective circulating volume is relatively common, and inhibition of prostaglandin-induced vasodilation may further compromise renal blood flow and exacerbate ischemic injury.

Aminoglycosides

Clinical evidence of AKI due to aminoglycoside nephrotoxicity usually occurs 5 to 10 days after initiation of the treatment; it is typically nonoliguric and associated with decreased urine concentrating ability and urinary magnesium wasting. With multiple daily dosing schedules, elevated aminoglycoside peak levels appear to correlate with nephrotoxicity. Because aminoglycoside uptake by proximal tubular cells is a saturable process, once-daily dosing can decrease tubular cell toxicity by reducing drug taken up by proximal tubular cells. In the general population, extended intervals between doses maintains the target dose while decreasing the risk of nephrotoxicity compared with multiple daily dosing. However, intensive care patients have different volume of distribution and variable clearance, making it difficult to attain correct serum levels with longer intervals. As these drugs are entirely excreted by glomerular filtration, patients with compromised renal function are at increased risk for nephrotoxicity. In these patients, the administration of a large single dose can be associated with a decreased uptake and lower antimicrobial effect.[12] Therefore, for treatment of serious infections in critically ill patients, dosing with maximum concentration monitoring and minimal inhibitory concentration evaluation of the pathogen is necessary.[12]

Uric Acid Nephropathy and Tumor Lysis Syndrome

Acute uric acid nephropathy is caused by deposition of uric acid crystals in the interstitium and tubules in association with tumor lysis syndrome (TLS).

The early recognition of patients at high risk for TLS is the first step to prevention of the development of AKI. In patients with high-grade hematologic malignant neoplasms, risk factors for TLS are large tumor burden, lactate dehydrogenase levels above 1500 IU, extensive bone marrow involvement, and high tumor sensitivity to chemotherapeutic agents. In patients with low or intermediate risk of TLS, allopurinol can be used as a hypouricemic agent and should be started 2 days before chemotherapy. Aggressive hydration with isotonic saline is initiated 2 days before the chemotherapy to maintain a high urinary output, allowing the elimination of uric acid and phosphate. If urinary output decreases despite adequate fluid intake, a loop diuretic should be added, but RRT will be required if oliguria persists.[13] The use of urine alkalinization to promote elimination of urates is not recommended as it can induce calcium phosphate deposition and therefore aggravate TLS.

In addition to the hydration, recombinant urate oxidase can reduce uric acid levels and the risk of uric acid deposition nephropathy.[14] Recombinant urate oxidase should be initiated in high-risk patients or for established TLS.

SECONDARY PREVENTION

After the renal insult has occurred, secondary preventive measures should be directed to avoid further injury, to facilitate repair and recovery, and to prevent AKI complications. The timeliness of interventions is crucial to their effectiveness for secondary prevention. Various approaches have been applied but are best appreciated in the context of specific scenarios.

Traumatic and Nontraumatic Rhabdomyolysis

In the prevention of myoglobin-induced nephropathy after crush syndrome, intravenous hydration should be initiated with isotonic saline before the crushed limb is relieved to prevent precipitation of the pigment in the tubular lumen. A solution with 2.7% sodium bicarbonate (50 mmol/l) should be given every second or third liter to maintain urinary pH above 6.5 and to prevent intratubular deposition of myoglobin and uric acid. The urine output should be maintained around 300 ml/h, which may require an infusion of up to 12 liters of fluid per day. The volume administered is generally much greater than the urinary output; the accumulation of fluid in the damaged muscles may exceed 4 liters. This protocol should be continued until clinical or biochemical evidence of myoglobinuria disappears, usually by day 3. The addition of mannitol can help decompress the post-traumatic turgid edematous muscles, thus decreasing the development of compartmental syndromes.[15] If urinary flow is sustained above 20 ml/h, mannitol given at a rate of 5 g/h may be added to each liter of infusate not exceeding 1 to 2 g/kg per day.[16] Hypocalcemia can occur as a consequence of calcium sequestration in muscles and, as calcium is protein bound, the increased vascular permeability. Therefore, care must be taken to avoid a $NaHCO_3$-induced decrease in ionized calcium (due to metabolic alkalosis), which can trigger seizures and worsen existent muscle damage. An alkaline diuresis is ineffective if the patient has established AKI, and accumulation of mannitol in this setting may actually exacerbate renal injury.

In nontraumatic rhabdomyolysis, prevention of AKI involves vigorous fluid expansion to maintain renal perfusion pressure and to dilute myoglobin and other toxins. A urine output of 200 to 300 ml/h is desirable until myoglobinuria disappears. Urine alkalinization may help prevent tubular pigment cast formation; however, there is no clinical evidence that mannitol and bicarbonate are more effective than saline solution alone. Furthermore, there are potential risks to bicarbonate therapy, including precipitation of calcium phosphate and hypocalcemia.

In treating patients with rhabdomyolysis, one important consideration is when to stop aggressive fluid resuscitation. Although fluid expansion is the main therapeutic intervention to reduce the hemoglobin precipitation in the tubular lumen, the risk of fluid accumulation and compartmental expansion should always be part of the clinical judgment. Frequent assessment of renal functional parameters associated with uric acid and creatine kinase levels help the clinician decide how intense the volume expansion should be.

Hyperglycemia

After the first study showing a reduction in AKI incidence and mortality with strict control of blood glucose concentration, many studies presented conflicting results. A systematic review of intensive insulin therapy in critically ill patients found a 38% reduction in the incidence of AKI[17]; other negative trials showed no benefit and an increased risk of hypoglycemia. In a recent large, international, randomized trial in critically ill patients (NICE-SUGAR study), intensive glucose control increased the absolute risk of death at 90 days compared with conventional glucose control. Severe hypoglycemia was significantly more common with intensive glucose control. In a meta-analysis including 26 trials, a total of 13,567 patients, and data from the NICE-SUGAR study, the relative risk of death with intensive insulin therapy compared with conventional therapy was 0.93. Patients in surgical intensive care units had a benefit from intensive insulin therapy (RR 0.63), whereas patients in medical intensive care units did not (RR 1.0). On the basis of these studies, it appears that intensive insulin therapy significantly increased the risk of hypoglycemia and is not associated with a benefit in mortality among critically ill patients. Whether there is a benefit in preventing or ameliorating AKI is still unclear. We recommend maintaining appropriate control of blood glucose concentration in the range of 120 to 140 mg/dl.

Pharmacologic Approaches

A variety of drugs are effective in altering the course of experimental models of acute tubular necrosis (ATN). However, only a few have consistently shown benefits in established AKI (Fig. 69.5).

Acetylcysteine

N-Acetylcysteine (NAC) is a tripeptide analogous to glutathione able to cross cellular membranes. NAC may reduce vasoconstriction and oxygen free radical generation after the administration of contrast material. Because an increased production of free radicals by the kidneys is partly responsible for their cellular damage in postischemic and nephrotoxic AKI, several clinical studies have attempted to use NAC to prevent AKI, mainly in CIN and during cardiac surgery.

In the first study, NAC at a dose of 600 mg orally twice daily the day before and the day of the procedure prevented AKI after radiocontrast dye administration.[18] A large, single-center RCT[19] confirmed the preventive and dose-dependent effect of NAC in CIN prevention. Several meta-analyses have concluded that NAC, compared with periprocedural hydration alone, can lower the risk of CIN in high-risk patients. NAC use is recommended on the basis of its potential benefit, low cost, and excellent side effect profile. However, NAC should never replace intravenous fluids, which have a more substantial benefit. In practice, we combine both hydration and NAC in patients at risk for CIN.

Loop Diuretics and Natriuretics

Diuretic use is often associated with deterioration in kidney function and should be stopped when feasible if AKI is attributed to prerenal causes. One meta-analysis confirmed that the use of diuretics to prevent AKI did not reduce in-hospital mortality, the risk for requiring dialysis, the number of dialysis sessions required, or the proportion of oliguric patients.[20] No RCTs have been performed to assess the effect of natriuretics (ANP) on the prevention of AKI.

Vasoactive Agents

"Renal-dose" dopamine (0.5 to 3 µg/kg per minute), given as a specific vasodilator to increase renal blood flow and to prevent AKI, increases urine output but does not affect AKI outcome or mortality.[21] Dopexamine, a synthetic dopamine analogue, is a dopamine 1 and less potent dopamine 2 receptor agonist. Small studies performed in patients undergoing liver transplant surgery have not found a beneficial effect of dopexamine in preventing AKI.

No RCTs have assessed the effect of norepinephrine on prevention of AKI. In a meta-analysis, fenoldopam, a dopamine receptor 1 agonist increasing blood flow to the renal cortex and

Summary of Drugs Used in Prevention of Acute Kidney Injury

Drugs	Level of Evidence	Results	Administration
Dopamine	RCTs	No effect on kidney function	NA
Fenoldopam	Small RCTs	No effect on kidney function	Further studies required
	One meta-analysis	Beneficial effect on kidney function	
Loop diuretics	RCTs and meta-analysis	No effect on kidney function	NA
N-Acetylcysteine	RCTs and meta-analysis	Variable beneficial effect in CIN	N-Acetylcysteine 600 to 1200 mg PO bid before and the day of administration of the contrast agent along with saline or intravenous bicarbonate
Statins	Animal models	Beneficial effect on kidney function	Further studies required
	Prospective observational in CIN	Beneficial effect on kidney function	
Calcium channel blockers	RCT in peri-transplant period	No effect on kidney function	Further studies required
Adenosine antagonists	RCTs	Controversial effect on kidney function	Further studies required
Multipotent stem cells	Animal models	Beneficial effect on kidney function	Human studies required
Erythropoietin	Animal models	Beneficial effect on kidney function	Human studies required
Small interfering RNA targeting p53	Animal models	Beneficial effect on kidney function	Human studies required

Figure 69.5 Summary of drugs used in prevention of acute kidney injury (AKI). CIN, contrast-induced nephropathy; NA, not applicable; RCTs, randomized controlled trials.

outer medulla, was shown to reduce the risk of AKI in postoperative or critically ill patients (odds ratio, 0.43).[22] Intrarenal administration of fenoldopam allows the use of a substantial dose of fenoldopam mesylate while avoiding systemic adverse effects, such as hypotension. In a registry of 268 patients treated with intrarenal fenoldopam infused for at least 1 hour, the incidence of CIN was less than 1%, compared with 27% based in historic rates in that population. Although we are still waiting for additional studies to confirm these results, it may be a promising preventive measurement for patients at high risk for CIN.

Statins

Although the pathogenesis of CIN is not completely known, multiple mechanisms may be involved. Statins induce downregulation of angiotensin receptors, decrease endothelin synthesis, decrease inflammation and improve endothelial function by inhibiting nuclear factor (NF) κB, decrease expression of endothelial adhesion molecules, increase nitric oxide (NO) bioavailability, attenuate production of reactive oxygen species, and protect against complement-mediated injury. Those mechanisms may be involved in the protective effect against CIN. A number of publications support the potential for renal protection with statin administration.[23] A prospective study evaluated the effect of statins on decreasing the incidence of CIN during percutaneous coronary intervention. Patients receiving statins before the procedure had a significant decrease of CIN (3% versus 27%).[24] No benefit was observed in patients with a preexisting creatinine clearance below 40 ml/min. However, in a retrospective cohort study evaluating patients undergoing major vascular procedures,[25] perioperative statin administration did not improve renal function, reduce length of stay, or reduce mortality. Currently, there is no basis to recommend the initiation of statin therapy specifically for the pericontrast period to prevent CIN. Patients who are already receiving statin therapy or need it for other indications should be maintained on statins through the contrast procedures.

Calcium Channel Blockers

Calcium antagonists have been shown to reverse the afferent arteriolar vasoconstriction induced by a variety of stimuli and also have an independent natriuretic effect.[26] These drugs were exhaustively evaluated in the prevention of AKI, especially in the context of transplant-associated nephropathy. Administered prophylactically, calcium blockers protected against post-transplantation delayed graft failure in some studies. However, a large multicenter RCT evaluating the effect of isradipine on renal function, incidence and severity of delayed graft function, and acute rejection after kidney transplantation did not find any benefit.[27] A systematic review evaluated the benefits and harms of using calcium channel blockers (CCBs) in the peri-transplant period in patients at risk of ATN after cadaveric kidney transplantation[28] and did not find strong evidence for the routine use of CCBs to reduce the incidence of ATN after transplantation. Studies have shown improved long-term outcomes without any significant improvement in perioperative function. We believe the use of CCBs during renal transplant surgery may be of benefit in extended donor criteria transplants (e.g., donors older than 60 years, predonation serum creatinine level higher than 1.5 mg/dl, cerebrovascular disease as the cause of death) or those with prolonged ischemia times.

Adenosine Antagonists

Small clinical studies evaluating the role of theophylline, an adenosine antagonist, in the prevention of contrast nephropathy have shown discordant results. A meta-analysis including seven RCTs concluded that the prophylactic administration of theophylline or aminophylline appeared to protect against CIN.[29] However, this meta-analysis included studies that did not control for hydration status. A recent RCT adding theophylline to NAC showed reduced incidence of CIN. Additional selective blockers agents, such as rolofylline, have maintained renal function in patients with decompensated heart failure, although they have not been assessed for prevention of AKI. At the current moment, it remains unclear if theophylline as a solo agent might be useful in preventing CIN. Newer agents may be promising.

Emerging Agents

Multipotent mesenchymal stem cells were shown to prevent ischemia-reperfusion–induced AKI in rats. A phase 1 clinical trial is currently being performed in patients at high risk for AKI undergoing open heart surgery. In mice, erythropoietin (EPO) administered 30 minutes before the infusion of endotoxin significantly improved kidney function 16 hours after injury. EPO also seems to have a protective effect against ischemia-reperfusion injury in the rat kidney. There are ongoing RCTs looking at the effect of EPO or placebo on prevention of AKI in patients undergoing heart surgery or kidney transplantation. In the intensive care setting a recent study failed to show therapeutic renoprotective benefits of EPO. Although the timing to receive treatment was not ideal, more than 6 hours, this study using high-dose erythropoietin did not alter outcome in AKI patients.[30] Another RCT comparing the effect of EPO or placebo on prevention of AKI in patients receiving intravenous contrast material has just ended, but results are not currently available. In an animal model of AKI, those treated with small interfering ribonucleic acid targeting p53 presented a significant decrease in BUN and creatinine levels 24 hours after ischemic injury compared with animals treated with a placebo. Small interfering ribonucleic acids are currently being evaluated against placebo for prevention of AKI in a phase 1 clinical trial. Because p53 has, among other activities, a tumor suppression function, one of the major drawbacks to the use of an inhibitor of p53 is its potential carcinogenic effect.

TREATMENT OF ACUTE KIDNEY INJURY

Once measures to prevent AKI have failed, a key question is whether AKI can be managed with nondialytic therapy alone or if RRT is necessary (see Chapter 70). Management of AKI in the setting of cardiac failure and liver failure is discussed in Chapters 71 and 72, respectively.

General Management

Initial management of established AKI includes careful assessment of the etiology of renal dysfunction and the patient's volume status. The main goal includes maintenance of adequate hemodynamic status to ensure renal perfusion and avoidance of further kidney injury. Appropriate therapeutic interventions to reduce kidney function loss and for prevention and treatment of the associated complications of AKI need to be instituted concurrently. Any potentially nephrotoxic agents should be avoided, including intravascular radiocontrast dye. Antimicrobial agents such as aminoglycosides, amphotericin, acyclovir, and pentamidine should be avoided or their dose adjusted to prevent further insult. Any other medications associated with AKI (hemodynamic, nephrotoxic, immune mediated) should also be avoided if possible.

Fluid and Electrolyte Management

Whereas early and vigorous resuscitation with crystalloid solutions and aggressive infection control can reduce the incidence of AKI (see earlier discussion), the role of fluid resuscitation in established AKI is less clear. Volume status is one of the most difficult parameters to assess, and fluid resuscitation should target a predefined preload, stroke volume, or cardiac output rather than a set MAP. Nevertheless, many clinical studies have emphasized the poor value of right atrial pressure and pulmonary artery occlusion pressure in predicting volume expansion efficacy. Other bedside indicators of preload, such as the right ventricular end-diastolic volume (evaluated by thermodilution) and the left ventricular end-diastolic area (measured by echocardiography), have also been shown to be ineffective in differentiating volume responder from nonresponder patients.[31]

In critically ill patients receiving mechanical ventilation, respiratory changes in left ventricular stroke volume can predict fluid responsiveness. In hypovolemic patients, positive-pressure ventilation may induce a fall in the venous return and consequently in cardiac output. Based on the positive relationship between ventricular end-diastolic volume and stroke volume, the expected hemodynamic response to volume expansion is an increase in right ventricular end-diastolic volume, left ventricular end-diastolic volume, stroke volume, and cardiac output. Because a decrease in ventricular contractility decreases the slope of the relationship between end-diastolic volume and stroke volume, the increase in stroke volume as a result of end-diastolic volume increase depends on ventricular function.

Volume expansion in critically ill patients can frequently result in a relative increase in body weight of 10% to 15% or more, sometimes doubling the total body water in a short time. Some studies have demonstrated an association between fluid accumulation and mortality and the benefits of restrictive fluid management strategies in acute respiratory distress syndrome. A prospective multicenter observational study (PICARD) found that patients with fluid overload, defined as an increase in body weight relative to baseline of more than 10%, had significantly higher mortality at 60 days (46% versus 32%).[6] In addition, increases in the total body water alter the volume of distribution of creatinine, resulting in underestimation of serum values. The resulting underestimation of the severity of renal dysfunction may delay recognition and adequate treatment of AKI. In AKI patients presenting with fluid overload, the evaluation of renal function should consider the effect of fluid balance to prevent underestimation of AKI severity, to modify drug dosing correctly, and to avoid use of nephrotoxic agents.

Summary of Drugs Used in Treatment of Acute Kidney Injury

Drug	Level of Evidence	Results	Comment
Loop diuretics	RCTs and meta-analyses	No effect	Further studies required; use for short periods of time if needed
Atrial natriuretic peptide	RCTs	Possible beneficial effect on survival and kidney function	Further studies required
Dopamine	RCTs	No effect on mortality or kidney function	
Norepinephrine	Prospective observational studies	Possible beneficial effect on kidney function	Further studies required
Fenoldopam	RCTs	No effect on mortality or kidney function	Further larger studies required
	One meta-analysis	Beneficial effect on mortality and need for dialysis	
Insulin	Meta-analyses	Controversial effect	NA
Mesenchymal stem cells	Animal models	Beneficial effect on kidney function	Further studies required
Erythropoietin	Animal models	Beneficial effect on kidney function	Further studies required
Alkaline phosphatase	Small RCT	Beneficial effect on kidney function	Further studies required

Figure 69.6 Summary of drugs used in treatment of acute kidney injury (AKI). NA, not applicable; RCTs, randomized controlled trials.

Drugs to Promote Recovery from Acute Kidney Injury

See Fig. 69.6 for a summary of drugs used in treatment of acute kidney injury.

Loop Diuretic Therapy

Although loop diuretics are often prescribed in established AKI,[32] a meta-analysis confirmed that their use is not associated with reduced mortality or better kidney recovery.[33] However, in this meta-analysis, there was an association between diuretic use and a shorter duration of dialysis (mean 1.4 days). Two other meta-analyses have shown that loop diuretics do not affect mortality, need for dialysis, or number of dialysis sessions required.[20,34] Two prospective cohort studies evaluating diuretic use in AKI and mortality yielded controversial results; one study showed an increase,[35] and the other study showed no effect.[36] In regard to morbidity, diuretics are associated with an increased risk of ototoxicity.[20] Concomitant prescription of aminoglycosides and diuretics should be avoided because of an increased risk of ototoxicity. Well-designed trials of diuretics are required to assess their benefits and potential side effects in AKI. In the meantime, we suggest that a trial of diuretics may be used to enhance urine output; however, if it is not successful, escalating doses of diuretics should be avoided.

Natriuretics

Atrial natriuretic peptide (ANP) has been studied as a treatment of AKI in four RCTs.[37-40] ANP was shown to reduce need for dialysis but not mortality.[37] In the largest study published so far, ANP improved overall dialysis-free survival in the subgroup of oliguric patients only.[38] Unfortunately, a subsequent trial including 222 oliguric patients did not confirm that ANP reduces mortality or dialysis-free survival.[40] Both trials delivered ANP for 24 hours and at high doses, which could have influenced the results. The most recent study included 61 patients who underwent cardiac surgery and were treated with ANP for a mean of 5.3 ± 0.8 days. In this small study, the use of ANP decreased the probability of dialysis and improved dialysis-free survival.[39] Larger studies are required to confirm the benefits of ANP in AKI.

Nesiritide, a B-type natriuretic peptide, is currently approved by the Food and Drug Administration for the treatment of heart failure. Nesiritide induces vasodilation and an indirect increase in cardiac output but has no inotropic effects and neutral effect on heart rate. In addition, it inhibits adverse neurohormonal activation and can result in natriuresis and diuresis in some individuals. In adults with acute decompensated heart failure, nesiritide reduces pulmonary capillary wedge pressure, right atrial pressure, and systemic vascular resistance; decreases symptoms of heart failure; and enhances clinical status. However, questions about the risks of nesiritide therapy have been raised. The most frequently reported adverse effect is dose-related hypotension and an acute increase in serum creatinine concentration. This effect on renal function has not been shown to negatively affect mortality, and reviews of large, observational registry databases do not suggest an adverse inpatient mortality effect compared with other vasodilator therapies.

Vasoactive Agents

As in the case of prevention, dopamine use for the treatment of established AKI is no longer recommended (see earlier discussion).

Vasopressors are often considered to be detrimental for organ perfusion. In septic shock, a small prospective study including 14 patients showed that norepinephrine improved serum creatinine and creatinine clearance when MAP was raised above 70 mm Hg.[41] However, in a small RCT including 28 patients, increasing MAP from 65 to 85 mm Hg with norepinephrine did not improve renal function.[42]

In a meta-analysis, fenoldopam decreased the need for dialysis (7% versus 10%) and in-hospital mortality (15% versus 19%) in postoperative or critically ill patients.[22] Several limitations were present in this meta-analysis, such as no standardized criteria for initiation of dialysis, heterogeneity of populations and AKI definitions, dosage and duration of treatments, and absence of an independent measure of GFR. In addition, fenoldopam has hypotensive properties and may be more dangerous in the "real world" outside of RCTs.[22,43] No single prospective study has shown that fenoldopam can reduce the need for dialysis. Therefore, before the use of fenoldopam is widely promoted, these results need to be confirmed with an adequately powered trial.

Specific therapy for patients presenting with the hepatorenal syndrome includes the use of terlipressin in combination with octreotide (see Chapter 72). In the United States, terlipressin has not been available, and most centers use a combination of midodrine, octreotide, and albumin infusions. Norepinephrine has also been used in these settings with good response, equivalent to terlipressin (see Chapter 72).

Other Agents

Other agents have been studied to treat established AKI. Mesenchymal stem cells were used to treat AKI in rats suffering from ischemia-reperfusion–induced AKI. In this study, the administration of mesenchymal stem cells significantly reduced creatinine levels on days 2 and 3. Human clinical trials are required to confirm these findings. EPO might also be beneficial in the treatment of AKI, as shown in two animal models. However, in a retrospective study including 187 patients with AKI, the use of EPO was not associated with renal recovery. In severe sepsis and septic shock, a study including 36 patients has shown that the infusion of alkaline phosphatase improves kidney function, possibly through reduced NO metabolite production and attenuated tubular enzymuria.[44]

Treatment of Acute Kidney Injury Complications

Fluid Overload

When fluid overload occurs in a patient with AKI, all intakes should be minimized and medical treatment should be attempted before dialysis initiation. In patients with positive fluid balance with large fluid intakes and inadequate urine output and in those presenting with symptomatic volume overload, loop diuretic therapy can be initiated in conjunction with measures to optimize systemic and renal perfusion. Intravenous bolus doses of diuretics may be necessary to optimize the response, especially in patients with CHF and nephrotic syndrome, but there is no other benefit from continuous infusions over bolus therapy.

Although administration of loop diuretics facilitates fluid management in critically ill patients with AKI, concerns of possible harm from loop diuretics in AKI arose after studies associated diuretic use with an increased adjusted risk of death and nonrecovery of renal function. A systematic review of furosemide including nine randomized studies of furosemide found no significant effect on in-hospital mortality, risk for requiring RRT, or number of dialysis sessions. Nevertheless, high-dose furosemide (1 to 3.4 g daily) was associated with an increased risk of temporary deafness and tinnitus.

In addition to diuretics, new drugs that selectively influence the excretion of water or sodium have been developed and can be used in specific clinical settings. Aquaretics act in the collecting duct of the kidney in the vasopressin 2 receptors, contributing to free water excretion. Natriuretic peptides inhibit sodium reabsorption in the nephron, resulting in net sodium excretion. There is currently no evidence to support the use of natriuretic peptides as an adjunctive treatment in AKI. Nesiritide (brain natriuretic peptide, BNP) is the latest natriuretic peptide introduced for clinical use, only for the therapy of acute decompensated heart failure, and data suggest that kidney function deteriorates under therapy with nesiritide (see earlier discussion). Vasopressin receptor antagonists are an alternative for volume management of patients with heart failure; further studies are under way to establish their role in the treatment of AKI with volume overload and hyponatremia.

Morphine and nitrates can be used to alleviate the respiratory symptoms in urgent situations. Morphine reduces the patient's anxiety and decreases the work of breathing; it can be administered intravenously at an initial dose of 2 to 4 mg during a 3-minute period and can be repeated if necessary at 5- to 15-minute intervals. Nitrates are the most commonly used vasodilators in pulmonary edema. Nitroglycerin reduces left ventricular filling pressure through venodilation; an initial dose of 5 μg/min of intravenous nitroglycerin can be used, commonly in addition to diuretic therapy. When fluid overload cannot be quickly treated with medical management, positive-pressure ventilation may need to be initiated with or without endotracheal intubation and dialysis, depending on the clinical situation (see Chapter 70).

Potassium Disorders

Hyperkalemia, covered in detail in Chapter 9, is a frequent complication of AKI. Its primary risk is on cardiac conduction, and it may cause bradycardia or asystole. If electrocardiographic changes are present, the intravenous administration of calcium is urgent. Concomitantly, sources of oral or intravenous potassium should be identified and removed, including drugs with effect on potassium handling, such as β-adrenergic antagonists, potassium-sparing diuretics, ACE inhibitors, ARBs, and other drugs that inhibit renal potassium excretion.

The next step is to enhance the shift of potassium to the intracellular space by parenteral glucose and insulin infusions. The onset of action is within 20 to 30 minutes, and their effect lasts 2 to 6 hours. Continuous infusions of insulin and glucose-containing intravenous fluids can be used to prolong their effect. Sodium bicarbonate also promotes shift of K^+ into the intracellular space; the effect occurs in less than 15 minutes and has 1 to 2 hours of duration. This therapy can be started if there is no concern of fluid overload (44.6 mEq intravenously during 5 minutes), although the potassium-lowering effect of sodium bicarbonate is most prominent in patients with metabolic acidosis. β-Adrenergic agonists given as aerosols are effective but more likely to produce side effects and therefore not often prescribed to treat hyperkalemia.

Potassium excretion should be increased by the administration of saline, loop diuretics, and cation exchange resins such as

Kayexalate or calcium resins. The resins can be administered orally or rectally as a retention enema. In case of hyperkalemic emergencies, rectal administration is preferred, as the colon is the major site of action of this drug. If hyperkalemia is unresponsive to conservative measures or occurs in patients with end-stage renal disease (ESRD), emergency hemodialysis (HD) is the treatment of choice. Continuous renal replacement therapy (CRRT) techniques can also be used for hyperkalemia with higher volumes of replacement solution or dialysate with low or no potassium levels. As it may take some time to initiate RRT, medical management should always be used while waiting for dialysis to be initiated. Monitoring of potassium levels should continue after conservative or dialytic management to prevent and to treat rebound hyperkalemia from the underlying process.

Sodium Disorders

Hyponatremia is not common in AKI unless heart failure, liver failure, or diuretics are present. In these settings, water restriction to below the level of output is mandatory. Sodium restriction is usually necessary to treat fluid overload and edema. In cases of true volume depletion with associated prerenal AKI, isotonic saline will need to be administered to correct both disorders (see Chapters 7 and 8).

Intensive care patients with hypernatremia are more prone to AKI. In most cases, treatment of the underlying cause will be necessary and water deficit will need to be estimated. Water should be administered orally or intravenously as dextrose in water to correct serum sodium concentration at a maximum rate of 10 mmol/l per day. Dialysis and CRRT in particular may be required to optimally correct sodium disorders in AKI.

Calcium, Phosphorus, and Magnesium Disorders

Hyperphosphatemia and hypocalcemia are common in AKI. Hyperphosphatemia is usually due to a reduced excretion by the kidneys, although it can also be caused by a continuous release from rhabdomyolysis or TLS (see Chapters 66 and 68). As phosphorus levels increase, calcium levels decrease, resulting in hypocalcemia. The levels of reduction are usually mild to moderate, with total calcium levels dropping to 7 to 8 mg/dl (1.75 to 2.0 mmol/l). Other causes of hypocalcemia in AKI are skeletal resistance to parathyroid hormone (PTH) and low calcitriol production from the dysfunctional kidney. Hypocalcemia can also occur during rhabdomyolysis and pancreatitis, two conditions often associated with AKI. Hypocalcemia is also aggravated when bicarbonate is administered to correct acidosis. A high calcium-phosphorus product (>60 mg^2/dl^2; >4.64 $mmol^2/l^2$) could theoretically trigger tissue calcium deposition, which can cause cardiac arrhythmia. No randomized study has evaluated the benefits of treating these disorders. However, because hyperphosphatemia due to oral phosphorus-containing medications and TLS can cause AKI,[45] severe hyperphosphatemia should be avoided to prevent further damage. Calcium-base phosphate binders and other phosphate binders can be used in this setting.[46] If there are symptoms of hypocalcemia or hemodynamic instability, a calcium gluconate infusion should be administered.

Hypercalcemia is rare in AKI and is usually seen in the recovery phase of rhabdomyolysis when calcium is released from calcium-containing complexes in muscle (see Chapters 66 and 68). In addition, when production of calcitriol is reestablished by the recovering kidney, an enhanced responsiveness to PTH can be seen. Hypercalcemia in this setting is rarely problematic and can be easily treated with medical management. Mild hypermagnesemia is frequent in AKI and usually does not have clinical consequences.

Acid-Base Disorders

In AKI, metabolic acidosis is the most common acid-base abnormality (see Chapter 12) and is due to reduced regeneration of bicarbonate and failure to excrete ammonium ions. Accumulation of phosphate and unexcreted unmeasured anions, such as sulfate, urate, hippurate, hydroxypropionate, furanpropionate, and oxalate, is contributory. Hypoalbuminemia can attenuate this acidification process, and it is exacerbated by lactic acidosis. Despite retention of unmeasured anions, the anion gap remains within normal limits in 50% of patients. Whereas metabolic acidosis is frequent, triple acid-base disturbances can also occur.

The approach to acid-base disturbances in AKI needs to be adjusted to the underlying causes.

There is controversy surrounding the optimal treatment of acute metabolic acidosis. When metabolic acidosis is simply a complication of AKI, sodium bicarbonate can be administered if the serum bicarbonate concentrations fall below 15 to 18 mmol/l. Volume overload can occur after the administration of bicarbonate. Bicarbonate administration in lactic acidosis due to an underlying shock is controversial given the possibility of an increase in carbon dioxide generation, worsening of the intracellular acidosis, and volume overload. Rapid improvement in the metabolic status may also enhance hypocalcemia, which may lower cardiac output. Therefore, because the benefit of bicarbonate in patients with lactic acidosis due to an underlying shock seems limited, most physicians would restrict the administration of sodium bicarbonate to patients with severe metabolic acidosis (arterial pH below 7.10 to 7.15) to maintain the pH above 7.15 to 7.20 until the primary process can be reversed. Alternative forms of base treatment have not been studied extensively in patients with AKI. Tris(hydroxymethyl)aminomethane (THAM) is excreted in the urine, and its clinical efficacy compared with sodium bicarbonate remains unproven.[47] We do not recommend its use in patients with AKI, especially in patients with hyperkalemia, because THAM does not decrease potassium levels in contrast to bicarbonate and can even cause hyperkalemia. Restriction of protein intake has also been suggested as a method of acidosis control because protein breakdown has been associated with worsening acidosis, such as in CKD.[48] However, no studies have clearly demonstrated the benefit of protein restriction on acid-base status in AKI.

Nutritional Considerations

AKI patients have an increased risk of protein-energy malnutrition due to poor nutrient intakes and high catabolic rates. Nutritional support should be directed to ensure adequate nutrition, to prevent protein-energy wasting with its concomitant metabolic complications, to promote wound healing and tissue repair, to support immune system function, to accelerate recovery, and to reduce mortality.

Nutritional assessment is difficult, especially in AKI patients presenting higher metabolic demands. Subjective global assessment evaluates nutritional status, requires no additional laboratory testing, and is highly predictive of outcome.[49]

Patients with AKI should receive a basic intake of at least 1.5 g/kg per day of protein and an energy intake of no more than 30 kcal nonprotein calories or 1.3 times the basal energy expenditure, calculated by the Harris-Benedict equation. Thirty percent to 35% of calories should come from lipid, as lipid emulsions.

Monitoring of nitrogen balance to assess the effectiveness of supplemental nutritional therapy is determined by measuring protein intake during 12 or 24 hours and urinary excretion of urea nitrogen during the same time interval. A positive or negative protein balance is used to determine the adequacy of protein intake of the patient. It is calculated as follows:

$$\text{Nitrogen balance} = (\text{protein intake}/6.25) - (\text{UUN} + 4)$$

Protein intake and urinary urea nitrogen (UUN) are each expressed in grams.

The enteral route should be the first choice for nutritional support if the gastrointestinal tract is functioning; parenteral nutrition should be reserved for when the gastrointestinal tract cannot be used or when the enteral route appears inadequate to reach nutrient intake goals.[50] AKI itself and other factors commonly present in critically ill patients, such as medications, hyperglycemia, and electrolyte disorders, can impair gastrointestinal motility.

REFERENCES

1. Ricci Z, Cruz D, Ronco C. The RIFLE criteria and mortality in acute kidney injury: A systematic review. *Kidney Int*. 2008;73:538-546.
2. Mehta RL, Kellum JA, Shah SV, et al. Acute Kidney Injury Network: Report of an initiative to improve outcomes in acute kidney injury. *Crit Care*. 2007;11:R31.
3. Rivers E, Nguyen B, Havstad S, et al. Early goal-directed therapy in the treatment of severe sepsis and septic shock. *N Engl J Med*. 2001; 345:1368-1377.
4. Durairaj L, Schmidt GA. Fluid therapy in resuscitated sepsis: Less is more. *Chest*. 2008;133:252-263.
5. Wiedemann HP, Wheeler AP, Bernard GR, et al. Comparison of two fluid-management strategies in acute lung injury. *N Engl J Med*. 2006; 354:2564-2575.
6. Bouchard J, Soroko S, Chertow G, et al. Fluid accumulation, survival and recovery of kidney function in critically ill patients with acute kidney injury. *Kidney Int*. 2009;76:422-427.
7. Finfer S, Norton R, Bellomo R, et al. The SAFE study: Saline vs. albumin for fluid resuscitation in the critically ill. *Vox Sang*. 2004;87(Suppl 2):123-131.
8. Finfer S, Bellomo R, Boyce N, et al. A comparison of albumin and saline for fluid resuscitation in the intensive care unit. *N Engl J Med*. 2004; 350:2247-2256.
9. Mueller C, Buerkle G, Buettner HJ, et al. Prevention of contrast media–associated nephropathy: Randomized comparison of 2 hydration regimens in 1620 patients undergoing coronary angioplasty. *Arch Intern Med*. 2002;162:329-336.
10. Merten GJ, Burgess WP, Gray LV, et al. Prevention of contrast-induced nephropathy with sodium bicarbonate: A randomized controlled trial. *JAMA*. 2004;291:2328-2334.
11. Joannidis M, Schmid M, Wiedermann CJ. Prevention of contrast media–induced nephropathy by isotonic sodium bicarbonate: A meta-analysis. *Wien Klin Wochenschr*. 2008;120:742-748.
12. Rea RS, Capitano B. Optimizing use of aminoglycosides in the critically ill. *Semin Respir Crit Care Med*. 2007;28:596-603.
13. Cairo MS, Bishop M. Tumour lysis syndrome: New therapeutic strategies and classification. *Br J Haematol*. 2004;127:3-11.
14. Coiffier B, Mounier N, Bologna S, et al. Efficacy and safety of rasburicase (recombinant urate oxidase) for the prevention and treatment of hyperuricemia during induction chemotherapy of aggressive non-Hodgkin's lymphoma: Results of the GRAAL1 (Groupe d'Etude des Lymphomes de l'Adulte Trial on Rasburicase Activity in Adult Lymphoma) study. *J Clin Oncol*. 2003;21:4402-4406.
15. Better OS, Rubinstein I, Winaver JM, Knochel JP. Mannitol therapy revisited (1940-1997). *Kidney Int*. 1997;52:886-894.
16. Sever MS, Vanholder R, Lameire N. Management of crush-related injuries after disasters. *N Engl J Med*. 2006;354:1052-1063.
17. Thomas G, Rojas MC, Epstein SK, et al. Insulin therapy and acute kidney injury in critically ill patients a systematic review. *Nephrol Dial Transplant*. 2007;22:2849-2855.
18. Tepel M, van der Giet M, Schwarzfeld C, et al. Prevention of radiographic-contrast-agent-induced reductions in renal function by acetylcysteine. *N Engl J Med*. 2000;343:180-184.
19. Marenzi G, Assanelli E, Marana I, et al. *N*-Acetylcysteine and contrast-induced nephropathy in primary angioplasty. *N Engl J Med*. 2006;354: 2773-2782.
20. Ho KM, Sheridan DJ. Meta-analysis of frusemide to prevent or treat acute renal failure. *BMJ*. 2006;333:420.
21. Friedrich JO, Adhikari N, Herridge MS, Beyene J. Meta-analysis: Low-dose dopamine increases urine output but does not prevent renal dysfunction or death. *Ann Intern Med*. 2005;142:510-524.
22. Landoni G, Biondi-Zoccai GG, Tumlin JA, et al. Beneficial impact of fenoldopam in critically ill patients with or at risk for acute renal failure: A meta-analysis of randomized clinical trials. *Am J Kidney Dis*. 2007; 49:56-68.
23. Yasuda H, Yuen PS, Hu X, et al. Simvastatin improves sepsis-induced mortality and acute kidney injury via renal vascular effects. *Kidney Int*. 2006;69:1535-1542.
24. Patti G, Nusca A, Chello M, et al. Usefulness of statin pretreatment to prevent contrast-induced nephropathy and to improve long-term outcome in patients undergoing percutaneous coronary intervention. *Am J Cardiol*. 2008;101:279-285.
25. Kor DJ, Brown MJ, Iscimen R, et al. Perioperative statin therapy and renal outcomes after major vascular surgery: A propensity-based analysis. *J Cardiothorac Vasc Anesth*. 2008;22:210-216.
26. Epstein M. Calcium antagonists and the kidney. Implications for renal protection. *Am J Hypertens*. 1993;6:251S-259S.
27. van Riemsdijk IC, Mulder PG, de Fijter JW, et al. Addition of isradipine (Lomir) results in a better renal function after kidney transplantation: A double-blind, randomized, placebo-controlled, multi-center study. *Transplantation*. 2000;70:122-126.
28. Shilliday IR, Sherif M. Calcium channel blockers for preventing acute tubular necrosis in kidney transplant recipients. Cochrane Database Syst Rev. 2004;1:CD003421.
29. Ix JH, McCulloch CE, Chertow GM. Theophylline for the prevention of radiocontrast nephropathy: A meta-analysis. *Nephrol Dial Transplant*. 2004;19:2747-2753.
30. Endre ZH, Walker RJ, Pickering JW, et al. Early intervention with erythropoietin does not affect the outcome of acute kidney injury (the EARLYARF trial). *Kidney Int*. 2010;77:1020-1030.
31. Tousignant CP, Walsh F, Mazer CD. The use of transesophageal echocardiography for preload assessment in critically ill patients. *Anesth Analg*. 2000;90:351-355.
32. Bagshaw SM, Delaney A, Jones D, et al. Diuretics in the management of acute kidney injury: A multinational survey. *Contrib Nephrol*. 2007;156: 236-249.
33. Bagshaw SM, Delaney A, Haase M, et al. Loop diuretics in the management of acute renal failure: A systematic review and meta-analysis. *Crit Care Resusc*. 2007;9:60-68.
34. Sampath S, Moran JL, Graham PL, et al. The efficacy of loop diuretics in acute renal failure: Assessment using Bayesian evidence synthesis techniques. *Crit Care Med*. 2007;35:2516-2524.
35. Mehta RL, Pascual MT, Soroko S, Chertow GM. Diuretics, mortality, and nonrecovery of renal function in acute renal failure. *JAMA*. 2002;288:2547-2553.
36. Uchino S, Doig GS, Bellomo R, et al. Diuretics and mortality in acute renal failure. *Crit Care Med*. 2004;32:1669-1677.
37. Rahman SN, Kim GE, Mathew AS, et al. Effects of atrial natriuretic peptide in clinical acute renal failure. *Kidney Int*. 1994;45:1731-1738.
38. Allgren RL, Marbury TC, Rahman SN, et al. Anaritide in acute tubular necrosis. Auriculin Anaritide Acute Renal Failure Study Group. *N Engl J Med*. 1997;336:828-834.
39. Sward K, Valsson F, Odencrants P, et al. Recombinant human atrial natriuretic peptide in ischemic acute renal failure: A randomized placebo-controlled trial. *Crit Care Med*. 2004;32:1310-1315.
40. Lewis J, Salem MM, Chertow GM, et al. Atrial natriuretic factor in oliguric acute renal failure. Anaritide Acute Renal Failure Study Group. *Am J Kidney Dis*. 2000;36:767-774.
41. Albanese J, Leone M, Garnier F, et al. Renal effects of norepinephrine in septic and nonseptic patients. *Chest*. 2004;126:534-539.
42. Bourgoin A, Leone M, Delmas A, et al. Increasing mean arterial pressure in patients with septic shock: Effects on oxygen variables and renal function. *Crit Care Med*. 2005;33:780-786.

43. Kellum JA. Prophylactic fenoldopam for renal protection? No, thank you, not for me—not yet at least. *Crit Care Med*. 2005;33:2681-2683.
44. Heemskerk S, Masereeuw R, Moesker O, et al. Alkaline phosphatase treatment improves renal function in severe sepsis or septic shock patients. *Crit Care Med*. 2009;37:417-423, e1.
45. Tsokos GC, Balow JE, Spiegel RJ, Magrath IT. Renal and metabolic complications of undifferentiated and lymphoblastic lymphomas. *Medicine (Baltimore)*. 1981;60:218-229.
46. Lameire N, Van Biesen W, Vanholder R. Acute renal failure. *Lancet*. 2005;365:417-430.
47. Hoste EA, Damen J, Vanholder RC, et al. Assessment of renal function in recently admitted critically ill patients with normal serum creatinine. *Nephrol Dial Transplant*. 2005;20:747-753.
48. Clinical practice guidelines for nutrition in chronic renal failure. K/DOQI, National Kidney Foundation. *Am J Kidney Dis*. 2000;35:S1-S140.
49. Jeejeebhoy KN, Detsky AS, Baker JP. Assessment of nutritional status. *JPEN J Parenter Enteral Nutr*. 1990;14:193S-196S.
50. Fiaccadori E, Maggiore U, Giacosa R, et al. Enteral nutrition in patients with acute renal failure. *Kidney Int*. 2004;65:999-1008.
51. Lameire N, Van Biesen W, Vanholder R. Epidemiology, clinical evaluation, and prevention of acute renal failure. In: Feehally J, Floege J, Johnson RJ, eds. *Comprehensive Clinical Nephrology*. Philadelphia: Mosby-Elsevier; 2007:771-785.
52. McCullough PA. Radiocontrast-induced acute kidney injury. *Nephron Physiol*. 2008;109:61-72.

CHAPTER 70

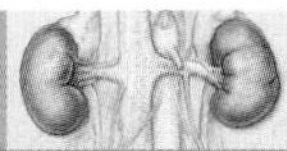

Dialytic Management of Acute Kidney Injury and Intensive Care Unit Nephrology

Mark R. Marshall

Intensive care unit nephrology can be defined as a subspecialty that focuses on abnormalities of fluid, electrolyte, and pH homeostasis in intensive care unit (ICU) patients and the prevention and management of acute kidney injury (AKI).

By use of the RIFLE (risk, injury, failure, loss, and end stage) criteria (see Fig. 68.1), up to 65% of ICU patients have evidence of AKI, an independent risk factor for death. The nondialytic therapy for AKI is discussed in Chapter 69. Approximately 5% of ICU patients receive acute renal replacement therapy (ARRT). Mortality in this population appears to be gradually improving over time despite a higher degree of illness severity, although it remains high in absolute terms.[1] Death attributable to AKI appears to be due to nonresolving infection, hemorrhage, or nonresolving shock, despite optimal care. Such conditions may therefore comprise an acute uremic syndrome that is specific to AKI and a possible target for modulation with ARRT as opposed to the traditional uremic syndrome of end-stage renal disease (ESRD).

ORGANIZATIONAL ASPECTS OF ACUTE RENAL REPLACEMENT THERAPY PROGRAMS

ICUs can be referred to as open (patient care remains under the attending physician of record), closed (patient care is transferred to an intensivist), or co-managed (an open ICU in which patients receive mandatory consultation from an intensivist). Most ICUs in the United States are open, whereas most in Australia and New Zealand are closed. Those in Europe are approximately equally split. In considering AKI and ARRT, advantages of intensivist-based management include immediate availability of service, cost containment, and decreased fragmentation of care. This model of care is supported by ecological studies suggesting improved patient outcomes in health care systems with closed ICUs, although these studies often lack internal validity because of important residual confounding. Alternatively, advantages of nephrology-based management include greater understanding of dialysis dosing and membrane design and of the processes underlying AKI and their implications. This model of care is supported by studies showing improved outcomes in ICU patients with AKI associated with earlier consultation to nephrology, although these studies often lack external validity in health care systems with closed ICUs where expertise is "in-house." Clinical governance over ARRT is therefore likely to remain a point of contention between intensivists and nephrologists in the future, although the individual expertise of staff providing care probably influences patient outcomes more than the specialty to which they belong. Specific training in ICU nephrology with exposure to ARRT is inadequate in many critical care and nephrology training fellowships, and it should be a component of both core curriculums.

In many parts of the world, all modalities of ARRT are now delivered by ICU nursing staff; in other countries, support from nephrology staff is still sought. As machinery platforms are becoming universal for continuous renal replacement therapy and intermittent hemodialysis, it is likely that ICU expertise in all modalities of renal replacement therapy will grow, provided in-service education and support are sufficient to develop and to maintain the skill base.

OVERVIEW OF ACUTE RENAL REPLACEMENT THERAPIES

The four main modalities of ARRT are acute intermittent hemodialysis (iHD); continuous renal replacement therapy (CRRT); prolonged intermittent renal replacement therapy (PIRRT), otherwise known as sustained low-efficiency dialysis (SLED); and acute peritoneal dialysis. Globally, CRRT is the most popular modality, although practice patterns vary regionally because of cost, availability of technology, and reimbursement policies. PIRRT is becoming more popular, and for reasons of cost and convenience, it may become the dominant ARRT in the future. Acute peritoneal dialysis is only occasionally used in adults and is not considered further in this chapter.

Therapeutic goals for ARRT are not well defined. The usual minimum recommendation is to correct acidosis or hyperkalemia, refractory hypervolemia, and traditional uremic features such as pericarditis and coma. Serum electrolyte and bicarbonate concentrations should be maintained in the normal range. Targets for uremic solute control are discussed later in this chapter. Importantly, the process of ARRT itself should not jeopardize the patient by exacerbating hemodynamic instability, increasing end-organ damage, or delaying renal recovery.

Determination of therapeutic goals with respect to the patient's fluid status is not straightforward. Assessment itself is difficult; physical signs such as jugular venous distention are not often informative, especially for mechanically ventilated patients. Moreover, baseline values of central venous pressure, pulmonary capillary wedge pressure, and echocardiographic left ventricular diastolic dimensions may be inaccurate surrogates for intravascular volume status, especially for septic patients. More reliable approaches use the effect of therapeutic maneuvers such as fluid challenge on blood pressure, stroke volume, or vena cava collapsibility obtained by bedside echocardiography. Even once fluid status is adequately assessed, determination of the therapeutic goal is also difficult; patients with extracellular fluid excess in the absence of intravascular hypervolemia may benefit from fluid removal if they develop abdominal compartment syndrome, impairment of lung compliance and oxygenation, or poor wound healing. Patients with acute respiratory distress syndrome (ARDS, defined as low Pao_2 relative to inspired oxygen, diffuse pulmonary infiltrates, and no left atrial hypertension) require a shorter period of ventilation with less fluid loading (guided by central filling pressures). However, the benefit of fluid removal in ARDS by means of ARRT has not been established.

Increasingly, ARRT is being used to facilitate adsorption or clearance of unconventional uremic markers and mediators such as proinflammatory cytokines, which might contribute to the purported acute uremic syndrome by their cardiodepressant, vasodilatory, and immunomodulatory properties. Because ARRT will remove both proinflammatory and anti-inflammatory cytokines, there is the potential to inadvertently exacerbate the inflammatory milieu.[2] The evolving technique of high-volume hemofiltration (HVHF) in septic shock is an area of intense study, supported by observations in septic ICU patients with AKI of improved outcomes with higher doses of hemofiltration (≥45 ml/kg per hour) and improved hemodynamic stability with HVHF (60 to 100 ml/kg per hour) applied either as a "pulse" or continuous maneuver. Presently, there are insufficient outcome data to justify routine clinical use of HVHF. Clinical trials of this approach, such as the IVOIRE (hIgh VOlume in Intensive Care) study, are under way.[3]

Timing of ARRT initiation remains controversial and current practices vary widely. A large multinational cohort study showed that ARRT was initiated when the median (IQR) serum creatinine and urea levels were 309 (202 to 442) µmol/l and 24 (15 to 35) µmol/l, respectively, and when urine output was 576 (192 to 1272) ml/day.[4] Observational studies suggest that earlier rather than later initiation might achieve better outcomes, and none suggests that it is harmful. There is no high-quality evidence to guide practice, and the single clinical trial designed to answer the question was insufficiently powered.[5] Proponents of early initiation argue that it is in the patient's interest to prevent rather than to treat the acute uremic syndrome and recommend initiation to prevent or to minimize fluid overload and biochemical abnormalities once kidney injury or failure is present. Timing of ARRT initiation is currently the leading priority for research in AKI.[6]

An important determinant of modality choice is cost. More complex extracorporeal circuits and replacement fluids make CRRT generally more expensive than iHD or PIRRT. Pharmacoeconomic studies comparing ARRT modalities are all limited by wide variation in ICU cost and reimbursement structures.

ACUTE INTERMITTENT HEMODIALYSIS

Acute intermittent hemodialysis (iHD) is still a widely used modality for the management of AKI when the patient has sufficient hemodynamic stability. Hemodialysis techniques and adequacy are discussed in the context of maintenance treatment of ESRD in Chapters 89 and 90.

Techniques for Acute Intermittent Hemodialysis

Acute iHD is categorized according to hemodialyzer membrane and mechanism of solute removal. High-flux membranes allow greater convective removal of middle and larger solutes, but there are only limited clinical data on high-flux dialysis in the critically ill with AKI, and these do not show obvious advantages.[7] Biocompatibility defines a membrane with a low capacity for activating complement and leukocytes. After complement activation, there is stasis of leukocytes in the lungs, renal parenchyma, and other organs, and the release of products of leukocyte activation. By minimizing these processes, use of biocompatible membranes should in principle favorably affect mortality and recovery of renal function in ICU patients with AKI. Unfortunately, studies to resolve this issue have often been confounded by poor design, and meta-analyses have not clarified this issue. A reasonable recommendation can be made against the use of less biocompatible unsubstituted cuprophane membranes.

Hemodiafiltration (HDF) is usually performed in the ICU as a continuous modality. However, acute intermittent HDF can be performed in this setting with standard machinery, using sterile online replacement fluid generated from ultrapure dialysate, which is then diverted by a separate pump to be infused directly into the extracorporeal blood circuit. As with high-flux dialysis, limited clinical data do not show obvious advantages.

Dialysate for the single-pass machines is generated online with a proportioning system from concentrate using reverse osmosis–treated tap water. There is concern about the possibility of backfiltration of bacterial contaminants, specifically endotoxin, which could perpetuate microcirculatory insult and cytokine-mediated injury. As a minimum, dialysate for iHD should be of the same purity as that accepted for ESRD settings. Online replacement fluid for intermittent HDF is produced by cold sterilization using ultrafilters in the dialysate pathway fluid and does not differ from commercial hemofiltration (HF) solutions in terms of microbial counts, endotoxin concentration, and cytokine-inducing activity. Dialysate cold sterilization is also suggested by some for acute iHD, although there are insufficient data to support a strong recommendation.

Strategies to Reduce Intradialytic Hemodynamic Instability

Hypotension is detrimental for end-organ function and recovery. Fresh ischemic lesions in kidney biopsy specimens can be found in patients with RIFLE failure stage of more than 3 weeks in duration. The relatively high ultrafiltration rate (UFR) with iHD often leads to intradialytic hypotension, which reduces residual renal function. A frequent schedule of iHD and prolonged treatment time will minimize ultrafiltration goals and rates and is the most effective measure to minimize hypotension.

Bicarbonate-buffered dialysate should be used routinely in critically ill AKI patients. It is associated with less hypotension than acetate dialysate, which has a peripheral vasodilating and myocardial depressant effect.

The rapid reduction in serum osmolality with iHD promotes water movement into cells, thus reducing effective circulating volume. Sodium profiling mitigates this process by promoting water flux into the vascular compartment, although the simpler approach of a high-sodium dialysate without profiling also may achieve this and needs to be tested in the ICU setting. A randomized study showed that iHD with sodium profiling (160 mmol/l initially, reducing to 140 mmol/l) combined with ultrafiltration profiling (50% of ultrafiltration volume removed in first third of treatment) improved hemodynamic stability.[8] Profiling therefore seems to be safe and effective, although it should be used judiciously in the patients with dysnatremias, in which serum sodium concentrations should be corrected slowly to minimize the risk of neurologic complications (see Chapter 7).

Relative blood volume monitoring with a biofeedback system automatically adjusts UFR and dialysate sodium content in response to a decrease in circulating blood volume. Although it is effective for ESRD patients, relative blood volume monitoring does not correlate with volumetric and hemodynamic parameters measured with transpulmonary thermodilution and does not appear useful for preventing hypotension in ICU patients.[9]

High dialysate calcium (1.75 mmol/l) has been used to improve hemodynamic stability during iHD in ESRD patients with cardiomyopathy. This technique is limited by the development of hypercalcemia, however, and has not been studied in ICU patients with AKI.

Vasoconstriction due to lower body temperatures has been used to increase vascular resistance and to improve hemodynamic stability during iHD in ESRD. Hypothermia, however, may be undesirable in ICU patients because of adverse effects on myocardial function, end-organ perfusion, blood clotting, and probably renal recovery. With blood temperature monitoring, the patient's blood temperature is precisely maintained at target value by a series of feedback loops controlling thermal transfer to and from the dialysate. Blood temperature monitoring is effective in ameliorating hemodynamic instability for ESRD patients. Blood temperature monitoring might conceivably allow controlled cooling in ICU patients without the risk of hypothermic damage, but it has not been evaluated in this setting.

In the ESRD setting, hemodynamic stability may be better during intermittent HDF compared with conventional iHD, although prospective controlled studies are contradictory. This could theoretically be related to heat loss in the circuit, lower sodium removal, higher calcium flux, and enhanced removal of endogenous vasoactive substances leading to increased peripheral vasoconstriction. There are insufficient data in ICU patients with AKI to support a strong recommendation.

Measures to reduce hemodynamic instability during iHD are summarized in Figure 70.1.[10] Should these measures fail, modality change to PIRRT or CRRT is recommended.

Dosing of Acute Intermittent Hemodialysis

The relationship between acute iHD dose and mortality has been clarified in several studies. A retrospective observational study showed that delivered single-pool *Kt/V* (*spKt/V*; see Chapter 90) above 1.0 per treatment was associated with improved survival in patients with intermediate illness severity.[11] This study did not relate outcomes to frequency of treatments. A prospective, controlled trial demonstrated that delivered *spKt/V* of 0.9 to 1.0 per treatment six or seven times per week improved survival compared with this dose three or four times per week. In this study, the time-averaged blood urea nitrogen (BUN) in the lower dose group (104 mg/dl) indicates underdialysis by current standards.[12] Most recently, a prospective, randomized controlled trial showed that delivered *spKt/V* of 1.2 to 1.4 per treatment five or six times per week did not improve survival compared with this dose thrice weekly.[13]

Optimal iHD dose therefore appears to be related to small rather than to larger solute clearance, and there appears to be a dose above which survival becomes dose independent. This "breakpoint" in the iHD dose-response curve suggests a recommended iHD dose: delivered *spKt/V* of 1.2 or more per treatment at least thrice weekly. This mandates routine measurement of *spKt/V* for iHD treatments in ICU patients with AKI to guide appropriate adjustment of operating parameters. Delivered dose tends to be low in this population and is optimized by measures summarized in Figure 70.2.[10] If delivered *spKt/V* of 1.2 or more per treatment cannot be achieved, dose should be maintained as high as possible and treatment frequency increased. The required number of treatments per week and dosing interval can be established from the nomogram in Figure 70.3 expressing combinations of iHD dose and treatment frequency as a continuous small-solute clearance (expressed as the corrected equivalent

Measures to Improve Hemodynamic Stability During Intermittent HD
Minimize ultrafiltration rate requirements by Increased frequency of treatments (up to daily) Increased duration of treatments (up to 6 hours), then consider PIRRT (SLED) or CRRT
Bicarbonate-buffered dialysate
Sodium/ultrafiltration profiling
? Increase dialysate [Ca^{2+}]
? Change modality from hemodialysis to hemodiafiltration
? Blood temperature monitoring

Figure 70.1 Measures to improve hemodynamic stability during intermittent HD. CRRT, continuous renal replacement therapy; PIRRT, prolonged intermittent renal replacement therapy; SLED, sustained low-efficiency dialysis. *(Modified from reference 10.)*

Measures to Increase Intermittent Hemodialysis Dose
Maximize hemodialyzer surface area (up to 2–2.2 m^2)
Maximize hemodialyzer porosity (high flux)
Maximize blood flow rate by Maximizing internal lumen diameter of catheter (up to 2.0–2.2 mm) Titrating blood flow to maximum arterial and venous pressure (up to – and + 300–350 mm Hg, respectively) Correcting position of catheter tip in SVC and IVC as appropriate Use right-sided IJ and SC in preference to left-sided IJ and SC
Minimize access recirculation by correcting position of catheter tip in superior or inferior vena cava as appropriate using internal jugular and subclavian, rather than femoral, catheters
Maximize dialysate flow (up to 800–1000 ml/min)
Add postdilution HDF
Optimize anticoagulation to reduce hemodialyzer fiber bundle clotting
Optimize circulation to reduce compartmental urea sequestration
Increased treatment frequency (up to daily)
Increased treatment duration (up to 6–8 hours, then consider PIRRT (SLED) or CRRT)

Figure 70.2 Measures to increase intermittent hemodialysis dose. CRRT, continuous renal replacement therapy; HDF, hemodiafiltration; IJ, internal jugular; IVC, inferior vena cava; PIRRT, prolonged intermittent renal replacement therapy; SC, subclavian; SLED, sustained low-efficiency dialysis; SVC, superior vena cava. *(Modified from reference 10.)*

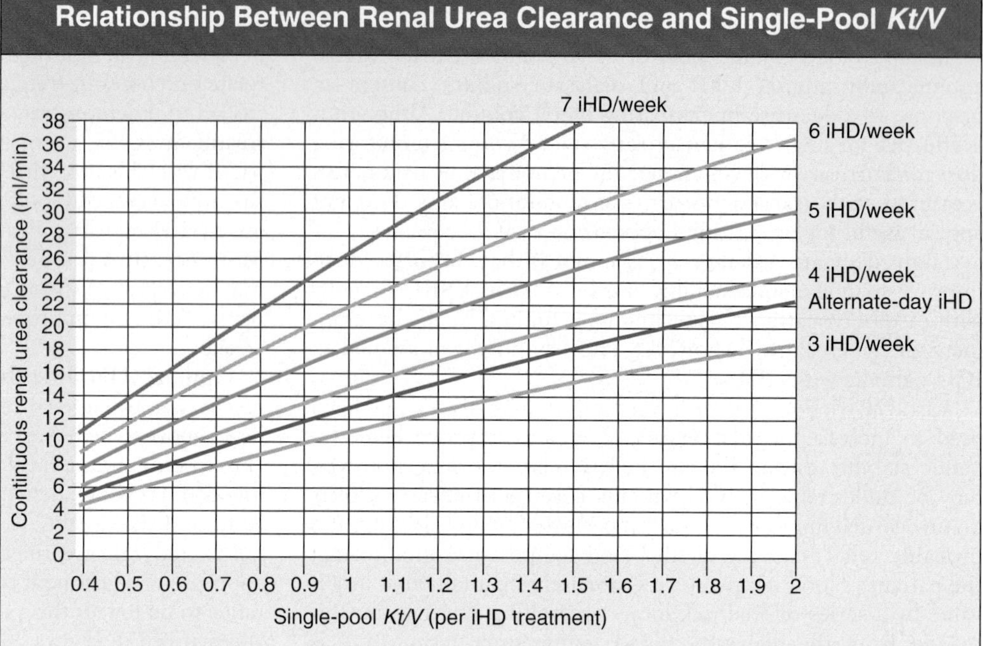

Figure 70.3 Relationship between corrected continuous renal urea clearance (weekly urea clearance/volume of distribution of urea) and single-pool *Kt/V*) per treatment for a frequency of three to seven treatments per week. iHD, intermittent hemodialysis. *(From reference 14.)*

renal urea clearance), aiming for a value of 12.6 ml/min or more.[14]

CONTINUOUS RENAL REPLACEMENT THERAPY

CRRT involves the application of lower UFR and solute clearances for substantial periods every day. Solute removal is achieved by diffusion, convection, or a combination. CRRT is used to complement or to supplant iHD. The lower UFR provides comparatively better hemodynamic stability than with iHD, especially during ultrafiltration of large obligatory fluid loads, and the lower solute clearances result in single-pool solute kinetics despite discrepancies in regional blood flow due to pressor use. The longer treatment duration results in better and more consistent control of uremic solutes, especially for severely catabolic patients.

Interruptions to CRRT because of circuit clotting or out-of-unit procedures lead to a reduction in dose from downtime as well as expense related to blood circuitry changes. Mean operating time for CRRT has been reported at 21.9 h/day.[15]

Techniques of Continuous Renal Replacement Therapy

The Acute Dialysis Quality Initiative group (*www.adqi.net*) has proposed standardized classification, with nomenclature based on the type of vascular access and the method of solute removal.

Arteriovenous (AV) denotes an extracorporeal blood circuit in which an arterial catheter allows blood to circulate by systemic blood pressure. A venous catheter is placed for return. AV circuits are simple but involve arterial puncture, which can lead to distal embolization, hemorrhage, and vessel damage. A blood flow (*Qb*) of 90 to 150 ml/min is typical in patients with mean arterial pressure above 80 mm Hg, although flow can be erratic, predisposing to clotting. Venovenous (VV) denotes a circuit with a central venous catheter, achieving more reliable and rapid *Qb* of ~250 ml/min by a mechanical pump. Pumped VV circuits have the disadvantage of potential inadvertent disconnection of lines, resulting in hemorrhage or air embolism with continued pump operation; this risk is minimized but not eliminated by monitors and alarms.

Mechanisms of Solute Removal

Hemodialysis

Continuous hemodialysis (HD) provides diffusive small-solute transport that can be quantified according to the degree to which dialysate is saturated with urea (expressed as the ratio of dialysate to blood urea nitrogen or DUN/BUN). *Qb* and dialysate flow (*Qd*) during CRRT are usually relatively low (100 to 200 ml/min and 1 to 2 l/h, respectively). Under these conditions, the dialysate to blood urea nitrogen ratio (DUN/BUN) is 1.0, indicating complete saturation. Urea clearance therefore equals *Qd* and is unaffected by *Qb* until it decreases to less than 50 ml/min.

With increasing *Qd*, there are proportionally decreasing gains in small-solute clearance as the DUN/BUN progressively decreases. Figure 70.4 illustrates this principle.[16] The flattening of the curves describes the conditions in which increasing *Qb* does not enhance clearance. At *Qb* of 200 ml/min, urea clearance will correspond to *Qd* at a rate of 2 l/h (or less) and will not increase with increased *Qb*. If *Qd* is increased to 4 l/h, this will correspond to a urea clearance of ~3 l/h that will progressively increase with increased *Qb*.

Hemofiltration

Continuous HF provides convective transport of small and medium-sized solutes that can be similarly quantified by use of filtrate saturation with urea (FUN/BUN). An important determinant of clearance is the site of fluid replacement, which can be infused either into the arterial blood line leading to the hemofilter (predilution) or into the venous blood line leaving the hemofilter (postdilution). The standard method is postdilution.

However, higher UFR can lead to hemoconcentration in the hemofilter, increased resistance in the blood flow pathway, reductions in *Qb*, and ultimately hemofilter clotting. In practice, UFR should not exceed 30% of the plasma water flow rate (i.e., filtration fraction should be <0.30). The problem can be resolved by increasing *Qb* to ≥200 to 250 ml/min or by diluting the blood and clotting factors with replacement fluid before it reaches the hemofilter (predilution), thereby improving filter patency and decreasing anticoagulant requirements.

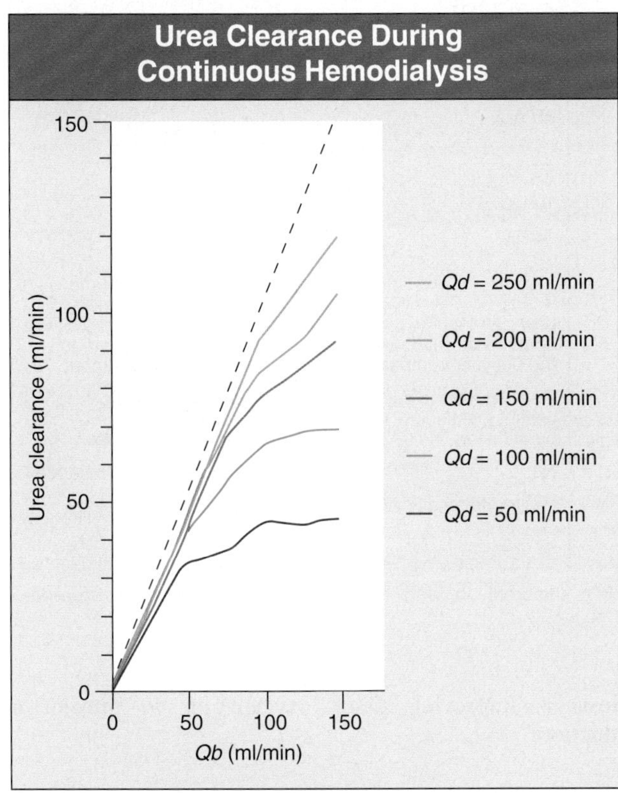

Figure 70.4 Determinants of urea clearance during continuous hemodialysis. Relationship between urea clearance, *Qb* (blood flow), and *Qd* (dialysate flow) during continuous hemodialysis. The flattening of the urea clearance curves describes the conditions in which increases in *Qb* do not enhance clearance. *(From reference 16.)*

The disadvantage of predilution is that filtrate is generated from blood diluted with replacement fluid and therefore contains a lower concentration of uremic solutes. Small-solute clearance is reduced by ~15% at low UFR, although this figure increases to ~40% with a higher UFR.[17,18] Clearance of any given solute during continuous HF is

$$K\ (\text{postdilution}) = \text{UFR} \times S$$

$$K\ (\text{predilution}) = \text{UFR} \times S \times [Qbw/(Qbw + Qr)]$$

where *K* is clearance (ml/min), *S* is the sieving coefficient of the solute, *Qbw* is blood water flow rate equal to the product of *Qb* and (1 – hematocrit), and *Qr* is the replacement fluid rate.

Hemodiafiltration

Continuous HDF refers to a combination of the preceding techniques. With large enough membranes, the small-solute clearances obtained approach the sum of the individual techniques.[17]

Specific Techniques

CRRT techniques are shown in Figures 70.5 and 70.6. The choice of technique is dependent on equipment availability, clinician expertise, prospects for vascular access, and whether the primary need is for fluid or solute removal. This last factor is often the most important because each technique provides different rates of fluid and solute removal. Most clinicians avoid AV circuits because of higher vascular complication rates. The potential complications of the techniques are listed in Figure 70.7.[19]

For isolated fluid removal, slow continuous ultrafiltration (SCUF) can be used. Given its minimal solute clearance (equal to the UFR at generally 4 to 5 ml/min), SCUF has primarily proved useful for treatment of the cardiorenal syndrome (see Chapter 71).

Most ICU patients require removal of solute in addition to that of fluid. For this, most clinicians prefer pumped VV rather than AV circuits because of higher and more reliable *Qb*, allowing greater solute clearance. The substantially enhanced clearance capabilities of continuous HDF combine diffusion and convection for removal of both small and medium-sized solutes

Comparison of Continuous Renal Replacement Modalities

Modality	Blood Pump	Dialysate (D) Replacement Fluid (RF)	Urea Clearance (l/day)	Urea Clearance (ml/min)	Middle Molecular Clearance	Complexity
Slow continuous ultrafiltration	Yes/no	No	1–4	1–3	+	+
Continuous arteriovenous hemofiltration	No	RF	10–15	7–10	++	+
Continuous venovenous hemofiltration	Yes	RF	22–24	15–17	+++	++
Continuous arteriovenous hemodialysis	No	D	24–30	17–21	–	+
Continuous venovenous hemodialysis	Yes	D	24–30	17–21	–	++
Continuous arteriovenous hemodiafiltration	No	RF+D	36–38	25–26	+++	+++
Continuous venovenous hemodiafiltration	Yes	RF+D	36–38	25–26	+++	+++

Figure 70.5 Comparison of different continuous renal replacement modalities. +, simplest; +++, most complex. *(Modified from reference 20.)*

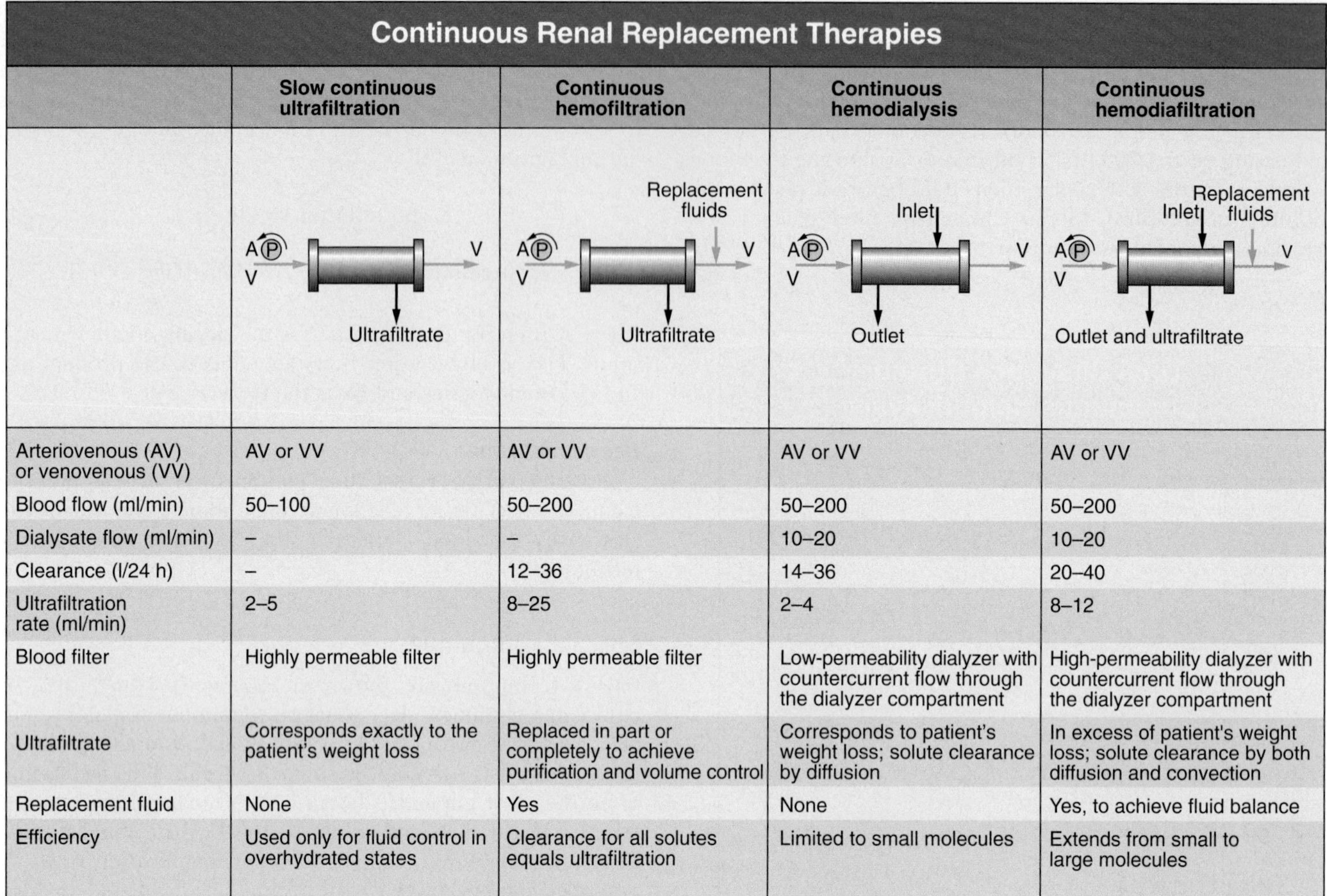

Continuous Renal Replacement Therapies

	Slow continuous ultrafiltration	Continuous hemofiltration	Continuous hemodialysis	Continuous hemodiafiltration
	A (P) V → V; Ultrafiltrate	A (P) V → V; Replacement fluids; Ultrafiltrate	A (P) V → V; Inlet; Outlet	A (P) V → V; Inlet; Replacement fluids; Outlet and ultrafiltrate
Arteriovenous (AV) or venovenous (VV)	AV or VV	AV or VV	AV or VV	AV or VV
Blood flow (ml/min)	50–100	50–200	50–200	50–200
Dialysate flow (ml/min)	–	–	10–20	10–20
Clearance (l/24 h)	–	12–36	14–36	20–40
Ultrafiltration rate (ml/min)	2–5	8–25	2–4	8–12
Blood filter	Highly permeable filter	Highly permeable filter	Low-permeability dialyzer with countercurrent flow through the dialyzer compartment	High-permeability dialyzer with countercurrent flow through the dialyzer compartment
Ultrafiltrate	Corresponds exactly to the patient's weight loss	Replaced in part or completely to achieve purification and volume control	Corresponds to patient's weight loss; solute clearance by diffusion	In excess of patient's weight loss; solute clearance by both diffusion and convection
Replacement fluid	None	Yes	None	Yes, to achieve fluid balance
Efficiency	Used only for fluid control in overhydrated states	Clearance for all solutes equals ultrafiltration	Limited to small molecules	Extends from small to large molecules

Figure 70.6 Continuous renal replacement therapy modalities. The pump (P) is used only in venovenous modes. *(Modified from reference 21.)*

Complications of Continuous Renal Replacement Therapy

Technical	Clinical
Vascular access malfunction	Hemorrhage
Circuit clotting	Hematomas
Catheter and circuit kinking	Thrombosis
Line disconnections	Hypothermia
Insufficient blood flow	Allergic reactions
Air embolism	Nutrient losses
Fluid balance errors	Insufficient clearance
Loss of efficiency	Hypotension
	Arrhythmias

Figure 70.7 Complications of continuous renal replacement therapy. *(Reproduced from reference 19.)*

and can be applied to hypercatabolic and intoxicated patients. The benefit of larger solute clearance is uncertain in this population, whereas the benefits of small-solute clearance are more evident (see later discussion). The long cherished practice of treating lactic acidosis with CRRT should be discarded. Extracorporeal lactate clearance is between 10- and 100-fold lower than plasma clearance, and the only effective treatment of lactic acidosis is improving tissue oxygenation to prevent acid production.

Dosing of Continuous Renal Replacement Therapy

The relationship between CRRT dose and mortality has been established in several prospective, randomized controlled trials. The first demonstrated that an effluent volume flow rate above 35 ml/kg per hour (based on premorbid or pre-ICU weight) of postdilution continuous HF was associated with highest survival. The external validity of this study, however, is limited by the small patient size and the predominantly postsurgical causes of AKI.[22] Another demonstrated that the addition of 18 ml/kg per hour of continuous HD to ~25 ml/kg per hour of predilution continuous HF resulted in improved survival.[23] Most recently, two more trials demonstrated that more than 35 ml/kg per hour of predilution continuous HDF did not improve survival compared with 20 ml/kg per hour, and another demonstrated that 40 ml/kg per hour of postdilution continuous HDF did not improve survival compared with 20 ml/kg per hour.[13,24,25]

Optimal CRRT dose therefore appears to be related to small as much as to larger solute clearance, and as with iHD, there appears to be a dose above which survival becomes dose independent. This breakpoint in the CRRT dose-response curve varies by study but suggests a minimum recommendation for CRRT dose: an effluent volume flow rate of 20 ml/kg per hour. As for iHD, this mandates routine measurement of dose on a regular basis.

Technical Aspects of Continuous Renal Replacement Therapy

Equipment

VV CRRT requires a blood pump, a hemofilter or hemodialyzer, arterial and venous pressure monitors, an air detection system, a method for removal of air bubbles, and a system to balance dialysate inflow/replacement fluid with dialysate outflow/filtrate. Integrated machinery dedicated to CRRT is commercially available with computerized volumetric or gravimetric balancing, allowing accurate and reliable treatment delivery.

Hemofilters

Specific devices for CRRT are usually referred to as hemofilters. However, conventional inexpensive hemodialyzers can serve as hemofilters by occlusion of one of the dialysate ports and connection of the other to a drainage system. To achieve adequate UFR, the surface area must be large (~2 m^2) for low-flux or, alternatively, more modest (~0.5 m^2) for high-flux hemodialyzers. Some CRRT machines use a specific hemofilter because of a unique cartridge system. Sieving coefficients of small solutes are usually preserved throughout the life of all such hemofilters.

A promising innovation has been the recent use of so-called superflux hemofilters with a cutoff of 100 to 150 kd. When they are used with CRRT and iHD *ex vivo* or in healthy volunteers, significant convective removal of cytokines can be achieved, and studies are under way to determine effects on clinical outcomes. Albumin losses may prevent prolonged use of such filters.

Replacement Fluids and Dialysate

CRRT requires sterile replacement fluid or dialysate for blood purification, with composition that is determined by the clinical requirements for acid-base control and electrolyte management. Fluids are available commercially or can be prepared aseptically in hospital pharmacies. A commonly used regimen consists of a blended mixture of 1 liter of each of four different solutions, which are kept separate until allowed to mix through a multiprong adapter just before entering the blood pathway:

1. Isotonic saline (0.9% NaCl) plus 7.5 ml 10% calcium chloride (5.2 mmol calcium).
2. Isotonic saline plus 1.6 ml 50% magnesium sulfate (3.2 mmol magnesium).
3. Half-isotonic saline.
4. Half-isotonic saline plus 150 mmol sodium bicarbonate.

Options for replacement fluids are summarized in Figure 70.8.

Buffer choice is between bicarbonate and lactate, which metabolizes in the liver to bicarbonate in a 1:1 ratio. Although many patients tolerate lactate solutions, bicarbonate solutions are superior in terms of acid-base control, hemodynamic stability, urea generation, cerebral dysfunction, and possibly survival in patients with a history of cardiovascular disease. Overall, bicarbonate has become the buffer of choice and is preferred in patients with lactic acidosis or liver failure. If lactate-buffered fluids are used, the development of lactate intolerance (>5 mmol/l increase in serum lactate during CRRT) may require a switch to bicarbonate-based fluid. Bicarbonate concentrations in fluid are typically 25 to 35 mmol/l; concentrations in the lower part of this range are indicated during high-dose or prolonged CRRT and during regional citrate anticoagulation therapy to prevent metabolic alkalosis.

Glucose concentrations in fluids range from 0.1% in commercially prepared fluids to 1.5% to 4.25% in peritoneal dialysis fluids adapted for use with CRRT. Up to 3600 kcal/day may be derived from these latter solutions, although hyperglycemia may supervene to the detriment of patient outcomes. It is recommended that glucose intake be less than 5 g/kg per day and that glucose concentration in fluid be ~100 to 180 mg/dl (~5.5 to 10 mmol/l) to maintain zero glucose balance.

Replacement Fluids for CRRT

Component (mmol/l)	Dialysis Machine Generated*	Peritoneal Dialysis Fluid†	Lactated Ringer's Solution	Accusol† (2.5-liter bag)	Prismasate (5-liter bag)	NxStage§ (5-liter bag)	Normocarb¶
Sodium	140	132	130	140	140	140	140
Potassium	Variable	—	4	0 or 2 or 4	0 or 2 or 4	0 or 2 or 4	0
Chloride	Variable	96	109	109.5 to 116.3	108 to 120.5	109 to 113	106
Bicarbonate	Variable	—	—	30 or 35	22 or 32	35	35
Calcium	Variable	3.5	2.7	2.8 or 3.5	0 or 2.5 or 3.5	3	0
Magnesium	1.5	0.5	—	1 or 1.5	1.0 or 1.5	1	1.5
Lactate	2	40	28	0	3	0	0
Glucose (mg/dl)	100	1360	—	0 or 110	0 or 110	100	—
Preparation method	6-liter bag via membrane filtration	Premix	Premix	Two-compartment bag	Two-compartment bag or Premix	Two-compartment bag or Premix	Vial mix added to 3-liter sterile water bag
Sterility	No	Yes	Yes	Yes	Yes	Yes	Yes

Figure 70.8 Replacement fluids for CRRT. Examples of replacement fluids that are suitable for CRRT. Dialysis machine–generated ultrapure dialysate and peritoneal dialysis fluid are used for continuous hemodialysis only. Lactated Ringer's solution and commercial hemodiafiltration fluids are used for continuous hemodialysis, hemofiltration, and hemodiafiltration. *Leblanc et al.[26] †Dianeal 1.5%, Baxter Healthcare Corp. ‡Gambro Renal Products. §Nxstage Medical Inc. ¶B. Braun Medical Inc.

Intravenous phosphate supplementation is often required during CRRT and is usually administered separately because of the potential for precipitation with calcium and magnesium in dialysate or replacement fluid. This concern may have been overstated in the past, and phosphate has been safely supplemented by injection of phosphate into these solutions.

PROLONGED INTERMITTENT RENAL REPLACEMENT THERAPY

PIRRT should replace alternative names such as sustained low efficiency dialysis (SLED), slow low efficiency dialysis, go slow dialysis, extended dialysis, extended daily dialysis, accelerated venovenous filtration. PIRRT uses standard iHD equipment and accessories, but with lower solute clearances and UFR maintained for prolonged periods.[27] Typical operating parameters would be *Qb* of 200 to 300 mL/min and *Qd* of 300 ml/min for regimens of 8 hours or less, and *Qb* of 100 to 200 ml/min and *Qd* of 100 to 200 mL/min for regimens longer than 8 hours. The systems are fully monitored with computerized ultrafiltration control. *Qd* and urea clearances are higher than in conventional CRRT, which allows scheduled downtime without compromise in dialysis dose.

PIRRT provides a high dose of dialysis with minimal urea disequilibrium, online bicarbonate dialysate, excellent control of electrolytes, and good tolerance to ultrafiltration. PIRRT is usually delivered as a diffusive therapy (a subgroup of PIRRT referred to as extended dialysis), although there is increasing experience with combined diffusive and convective clearance using online replacement fluid (extended diafiltration). Survival in the reported observational series has not differed from that predicted by a variety of illness severity scores. ARRT that is easiest to administer will be the most popular if all such outcomes are equivalent, and PIRRT may become the therapy of choice in this setting as it is safe, convenient, inexpensive, and effective in achieving goals for solute and fluid removal.

VASCULAR ACCESS

A prerequisite for all ARRT modalities is reliable vascular access. This is usually through uncuffed, untunneled (temporary) double-lumen polyurethane or silicone catheters in the internal jugular (IJ), subclavian (SC), or femoral (FE) veins. SC catheters are associated with a higher incidence of procedural complications, venous stenosis, and thrombosis.

For CRRT and PIRRT, *Qb* below 250 ml/min is usually sufficient. For acute iHD, higher *Qb* is required to provide sufficient solute clearance, and it can be safely increased until venous and arterial pressures are plus and minus 350 mm Hg, respectively, after which hemolysis can occur. Left-sided IJ and SC catheters provide flows that are more erratic and up to 100 ml/min lower than elsewhere because their tips abut the vein walls. FE and right-sided IJ or SC catheters provide the best *Qb*.[25] Catheters with larger bore lines are preferred.

Access recirculation for all sites is approximately 10% at *Qb* of 250 to 350 ml/min and may increase to as much as 35% at *Qb* above 500 ml/min. It is least in IJ catheters and highest in FE catheters shorter than 20 cm. Up to half of acute iHD treatments will require catheters to be used in reversed configuration, such that the original venous line is used as for blood inflow (relative to dialyzer), and the original arterial line for outflow. Access recirculation in this situation doubles to ~20% at 250 to 350 ml/min.[28] Access recirculation also affects dialysis dose; in one study, the urea reduction ratio was significantly higher with SC (63%) versus FE (55%) catheters despite identical iHD operating parameters.[29]

Infection of temporary catheters is common. Blood stream, exit site, and distant infections occurred in one series at 6.2, 3.6, and 1.1 episodes per 1000 catheter-days.[28] The risk of bacteremia is highest with FE catheters and lowest with SC catheters. Although there are generally fewer data than for tunneled catheters, both povidone and mupirocin ointments with dry gauze exit site dressings and antimicrobial locks using taurolidine or 30% trisodium citrate have been shown to reduce the risk of blood stream infection from temporary catheters.

The Centers for Disease Control and Prevention recommend that temporary catheters in the ICU setting be changed when it is clinically indicated rather than routinely because the risks of the catheterization outweigh the supposed benefit of reduced infection risk.[30] KDOQI (Kidney Disease Outcomes Quality Initiative) recommends that SC and IJ catheters be changed after 3 weeks and FE catheters after 5 days in the non-ICU setting because of increased infection risk.[31]

ANTICOAGULATION IN ACUTE RENAL REPLACEMENT THERAPY

Anticoagulation during ARRT ideally should prevent clotting in the extracorporeal circuit without producing significant systemic anticoagulation. Most commonly, unfractionated heparin is infused into the most proximal part of the extracorporeal circuit, keeping the activated partial thromboplastin time in the venous blood line 1.5 to 2 times the control value and the systemic activated partial thromboplastin time below 50 seconds. This typically requires an initial bolus dose of ~2000 U and maintenance infusion of ~500 U/h. Low-molecular-weight heparin is theoretically advantageous because of increased antithrombotic activity and decreased hemorrhagic risk. However, disadvantages include a prolonged half-life (approximately doubled in RIFLE failure stage), incomplete reversal with protamine, and limited availability of appropriate monitoring by serial anti–factor Xa determinations. Most experience is with dalteparin, and the optimal dose appears to be an initial bolus of ~20 to 30 U/kg (all ARRT modalities), followed by an infusion of ~10 U/kg per hour (CRRT and PIRRT). Other systemic anticoagulants include lepirudin (recombinant hirudin, notable for its very long half-life in those with reduced renal function) and argatroban, which are direct thrombin inhibitors, and fondaparinux, which is a synthetic pentasaccharide that inhibits factor Xa by binding to antithrombin. Experience with these anticoagulants is limited, although they are the anticoagulants of choice in patients with heparin-induced thrombocytopenia who also require ARRT.

For those receiving systemic anticoagulation with heparin, the incidence of significant bleeding complications is 25% to 30%, and 4% of such patients die as a result of hemorrhage. Most patients can successfully avoid any anticoagulation during iHD, but only a minority can during PIRRT or CRRT. Alternatives to systemic anticoagulation include regional citrate anticoagulation, regional heparin anticoagulation, and prostacyclin (epoprostenol), which is a potent inhibitor of platelet aggregation that essentially acts as a regional anticoagulant. The lowest rates of hemorrhage and greatest prolongation of filter life are associated with regional citrate anticoagulation, and it is the preferred regional technique.

Regional citrate anticoagulation involves calcium chelation in the extracorporeal blood circuit with calcium reversal. For iHD and PIRRT, this most commonly involves an infusion of 4% trisodium citrate into the proximal circuit, with zero calcium dialysate and an infusion of calcium chloride into the venous blood line. A simpler approach has been described in which the trisodium citrate infusion is combined with normal calcium dialysate and no calcium infusion. The positive calcium flux through the hemodialyzer maintains calcium balance without the need for a separate infusion and provides partial chelation of the undialyzed citrate.

For CRRT, regional citrate anticoagulation may be performed with 4% trisodium citrate or with ACD-A solution (anticoagulant citrate dextrose A). ACD-A is preferred to trisodium citrate as it is less hypertonic, potentially reducing complications from overinfusion and mixing errors. For continuous HD, a prefilter infusion of 3% to 7% of *Qb* with a postfilter infusion of calcium chloride is used. This requires dialysate that is hyponatremic and devoid of alkali because citrate metabolizes to bicarbonate in the liver in a 1:3 ratio. For continuous HF, a prefilter infusion of substitution fluid that contains no calcium but citrate as buffer can be used (Fig. 70.9). Frequent monitoring and titration of citrate dose are needed to keep the ionized calcium within a therapeutic range. The major complications of regional citrate anticoagulation are systemic hypocalcemia and metabolic alkalosis from citrate toxicity, particularly in patients with liver dysfunction.

Regional heparin anticoagulation involves neutralization of heparin by infusion of protamine into the venous blood line. It may be complicated by rebound bleeding, occurring when neutralization with protamine wears out faster than the anticoagulation from heparin. Furthermore, protamine may cause sudden hypotension, bradycardia, or anaphylactoid reactions.

Prostacyclin is an effective alternative anticoagulant. However, it is a vasodilator, causing a variable but occasionally marked decrease in blood pressure.

MODALITY CHOICE AND OUTCOMES IN ACUTE RENAL REPLACEMENT THERAPY

The prime advantage of CRRT appears to be the increased hemodynamic stability and solute control; patient survival does not appear to differ between AV and VV CRRT when dose is the same. Observational reports have previously suggested improved survival with CRRT compared with iHD, but numerous confounding variables have made definitive comparison with iHD difficult. Small randomized clinical trials and subsequent meta-analyses comparing iHD and CRRT have shown no difference in patient survival.[32]

The relationship between modality choice and outcomes is currently under study in specific clinical situations, such as acute lung injury, sepsis, and acute cardiac decompensation. Such studies may yet yield definitive data, but in the interim, modality choice depends on the patient's condition and the clinical objectives. In most cases, iHD can provide safe and effective renal replacement therapy, with recourse to other therapies as the individual situation dictates. For example, CRRT will be more

Comparison of Regional Citrate Anticoagulation Protocols

	Modality	Blood Flow (ml/min)	Replacement Fluid Composition (mmol/l)	Dialysis Fluid Composition (mmol/l)	Citrate Source
Mehta et al.[33] (1990)	CAV-HD	52–125	Normal saline	Na 117, Cl 122.5, Mg 0.75, K 4, dextrose 2.5%	4% Trisodium citrate
Hoffmann et al.[34] (1995)	CVV-HD	125	Prefilter: normal saline + KCl 4, alternate with 0.45% saline + KCl 4 Postfilter: 0.45% saline $+MgSO_4 + CaCl_2$	—	4% Trisodium citrate
Palsson and Niles[35] (1999)	CVV-HD	180	Citrate 13.3, Na 140, Cl 101.5, Mg 0.75, dextrose 0.2%	—	Customized citrate solution
Tolwani et al.[36] (2001)	CVV-HD	125–150	—	Normal saline + $MgSO_4$ 1.0, KCl 3	4% Trisodium citrate
Tobe et al.[37] (2003)	CVV-HDF	100	Normal saline	Normocarb	ACD-A
Mitchell et al.[38] (2003)	CVV-HD	75	—	Variable Ca 1.75–1.78	ACD-A
Swartz et al.[39] (2004)	CVV-HD	200	—	Na 135, HCO_3 28, Cl 105, $MgSO_4$ 1.3, glucose 1g/l	ACD-A
Gupta et al.[40] (2004)	CVV-HDF	150	Normal saline ± $MgSO_4$ and KCl	PD fluid: Na 132, Ca 1.25, Cl 95, Mg 0.5, lactate 360 mg/dl, 1.5% dextrose	ACD-A

Figure 70.9 Comparison of regional citrate anticoagulation protocols. ACD-A, anticoagulant citrate dextrose form A; CAV-HD, continuous arteriovenous hemodialysis; CVV-HD, continuous venovenous hemodialysis; CVV-HDF, continuous venovenous hemodiafiltration; PD, peritoneal dialysis.

appropriate for a patient unable to achieve ultrafiltration goals with iHD because of hemodynamic instability, and HVHF may be more appropriate than iHD for a highly catabolic septic patient.

Ultimately, the skill and experience of the staff providing renal replacement therapy probably influence patient outcomes as much as the choice of modality does.

DRUG DOSING IN ACUTE RENAL REPLACEMENT THERAPY

For patients undergoing CRRT, 20 liters of daily filtrate correspond to a glomerular filtration rate of ~14 ml/min, and the dose of drugs should be calculated accordingly. Any drug with a low therapeutic index that can be readily measured should be measured frequently early in the course of ARRT, until a stable pattern appears. One day of CRRT is in general comparable to one iHD treatment with regard to drug removal.

REFERENCES

1. Bagshaw SM, George C, Bellomo R. Changes in the incidence and outcome for early acute kidney injury in a cohort of Australian intensive care units. *Crit Care*. 2007;11:R68.
2. De Vriese AS, Colardyn FA, Philippé JJ, et al. Cytokine removal during continuous hemofiltration in septic patients. *J Am Soc Nephrol*. 1999; 10:846-853.
3. Joannes-Boyau O, Honore PM, Boer W, Collin V. Are the synergistic effects of high-volume haemofiltration and enhanced adsorption the missing key in sepsis modulation? *Nephrol Dial Transplant*. 2009;24: 354-357.
4. Bagshaw SM, Uchino S, Bellomo R, et al. Timing of renal replacement therapy and clinical outcomes in critically ill patients with severe acute kidney injury. *J Crit Care*. 2009;24:129-140.
5. Bouman C, Oudemans-Van Straaten HM, Tijssen JG, et al. Effects of early high-volume continuous venovenous hemofiltration on survival and recovery of renal function in intensive care patients with acute renal failure: A prospective, randomized trial. *Crit Care Med*. 2002;30: 2205-2211.
6. Kellum JA, Mehta RL, Levin A, et al. Development of a clinical research agenda for acute kidney injury using an international, interdisciplinary, three-step modified Delphi process. *Clin J Am Soc Nephrol*. 2008;3: 887-894.
7. Ponikvar JB, Rus RR, Kenda RB, et al. Low-flux versus high-flux synthetic dialysis membrane in acute renal failure: Prospective randomized study. *Artif Organs*. 2001;25:946-950.
8. Paganini E, Sandy D, Moreno L, et al. The effect of sodium and ultrafiltration modelling on plasma volume and haemodynamic stability in intensive care patients receiving haemodialysis for acute renal failure: A prospective, stratified, randomized, cross-over study. *Nephrol Dial Transplant*. 1996;11(Suppl):32-37.
9. Tonelli M, Astephen P, Andreou P, et al. Blood volume monitoring in intermittent hemodialysis for acute renal failure. *Kidney Int*. 2002;62: 1075-1080.
10. Marshall M, Golper T. Intermittent hemodialysis. In: Murray P, Brady H, Hall J, eds. *Intensive Care In Nephrology*. Oxon, UK: Taylor & Francis; 2006:181-198.
11. Paganini EP, Tapolyai M, Goormastic M, et al. Establishing a dialysis therapy/patient outcome link in intensive care unit acute dialysis for patients with acute renal failure. *Am J Kidney Dis*. 1996; 28(Suppl):S81-S89.
12. Schiffl H, Lang S, Fischer R. Daily hemodialysis and the outcomes of acute renal failure. *N Eng J Med*. 2002;346:305-310.
13. Palevsky PM, Zhang JH, O'Connor TZ, et al. Intensity of renal support in critically ill patients with acute kidney injury. *N Engl J Med*. 2008; 359:7-20.
14. Casino F, Lopez T. The equivalent renal urea clearance: A new parameter to assess dialysis. *Nephrol Dial Transplant*. 1996;11:1574-1581.
15. Frankenfield D, Reynolds HN, Wiles CE 3rd, et al. Urea removal during continuous hemodiafiltration. *Crit Care Med*. 1993;22:407-412.
16. Kudoh Y, Iimura O. Slow continuous hemodialysis—new therapy for acute renal failure in critically ill patients—Part 1. Theoretical considerations and new technique. *Jpn Circ J*. 1988;52:1171-1182.
17. Brunet S, Leblanc M, Geadah D, et al. Diffusive and convective solute clearances during continuous renal replacement therapy at various dialysate and ultrafiltration flow rates. *Am J Kidney Dis*. 1999;34:486-492.
18. Troyanov S, Cardinal J, Geadah D, et al. Solute clearances during continuous venovenous haemofiltration at various ultrafiltration flow rates using Multiflow-100 and HF1000 filters. *Nephrol Dial Transplant*. 2003;18:961-966.
19. Ronco C, Bellomo R. Complications with renal replacement therapy. *Am J Kidney Dis*. 1996;28(Suppl 3):S100-S104.
20. Manns M, Sigler MH, Teehan BP. Continuous renal replacement therapies: An update. *Am J Kidney Dis*. 1998;32:185-207.
21. Ronco C. Continuous renal replacement therapies for the treatment of acute renal failure in intensive care patients. *Clin Nephrol*. 1993;40:187-198.
22. Ronco C, Bellomo R, Homel P, et al. Effects of different doses in continuous veno-venous haemofiltration on outcomes of acute renal failure: A prospective randomised trial. *Lancet*. 2000;356:26-30.
23. Saudan P, Niederberger M, De Seigneux S, et al. Adding a dialysis dose to continuous hemofiltration increases survival in patients with acute renal failure. *Kidney Int*. 2006;70:1312-1317.
24. Tolwani AJ, Campbell RC, Stofan BS, et al. Standard versus high-dose CVVHDF for ICU-related acute renal failure. *J Am Soc Nephrol*. 2008;19:1233-1238.
25. Bellomo R, Cass A, Cole L, et al. Intensity of continuous renal-replacement therapy in critically ill patients. *N Engl J Med*. 2009;361: 1627-1638.
26. Leblanc M, Moreno L, Robinson OP, et al. Bicarbonate dialysate for continuous renal replacement therapy in intensive care unit patients with acute renal failure. *Am J Kidney Dis*. 1995;26:910-917.
27. Marshall MR, Golper TA, Shaver MJ, et al. Sustained low-efficiency dialysis for critically ill patients requiring renal replacement therapy. *Kidney Int*. 2001;60:777-785.
28. Oliver M. Acute dialysis catheters. *Semin Dial*. 2001;14:432-435.
29. Leblanc M, Fedak S, Mokris G, Paganini E. Blood recirculation in temporary central catheters for acute hemodialysis. *Clin Nephrol*. 1996;45:315-319.
30. Centers for Disease Control and Prevention. Guidelines for the prevention of intravascular catheter-related infections. *MMWR*. 2002; 51(RR-10).
31. National Kidney Foundation. K/DOQI Clinical Practice Guidelines for Vascular Access, 2000. *Am J Kidney Dis*. 2001;37(Suppl 1): S137-S181.
32. Pannu N, Klarenbach S, Wiebe N, et al. Renal replacement therapy in patients with acute renal failure: A systematic review. *JAMA*. 2008; 299:793-805.
33. Mehta RL, McDonald BR, Aguilar MM, Ward DM. Regional citrate anticoagulation for continuous arteriovenous hemodialysis in critically ill patients. *Kidney Int*. 1990;38:976-981.
34. Hoffmann JN, Hartl WH, Deppisch R, et al. Hemofiltration in human sepsis: Evidence for elimination of immunomodulatory substances. *Kidney Int*. 1995;48:1563-1570.
35. Palsson R, Niles JL. Regional citrate anticoagulation in continuous venovenous hemofiltration in critically ill patients with a high risk of bleeding. *Kidney Int*. 1999;55:1991-1997.
36. Tolwani AJ, Campbell RC, Schenk MB, et al. Simplified citrate anticoagulation for continuous renal replacement therapy. *Kidney Int*. 2001;60:370-374.
37. Tobe SW, Aujla P, Walele AA, et al. A novel regional citrate anticoagulation protocol for CRRT using only commercially available solutions. *J Crit Care*. 2003;18:121-129.
38. Mitchell A, Daul AE, Beiderlinden M, et al. A new system for regional citrate anticoagulation in continuous venovenous hemodialysis (CVVHD). *Clin Nephrol*. 2003;59:106-114.
39. Swartz R, Pasko D, O'Toole J, Starmann B. Improving the delivery of continuous renal replacement therapy using regional citrate anticoagulation. *Clin Nephrol*. 2004;61:134-143.
40. Gupta M, Wadhwa NK, Bukovsky R. Regional citrate anticoagulation for continuous venovenous hemodiafiltration using calcium-containing dialysate. *Am J Kidney Dis*. 2004;43:67-73.

CHAPTER 71

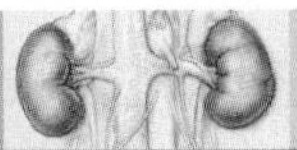

Ultrafiltration Therapy for Refractory Heart Failure

Edward A. Ross, Claudio Ronco

Nephrologists are being increasingly consulted for fluid management in patients with refractory congestive heart failure (CHF), a condition in part due to poorly controlled hypertension and the growing prevalence of obesity and the metabolic syndrome. Renal expertise extends beyond diuretics and electrolyte homeostasis and now includes recent advances in extracorporeal fluid removal by dialysis machines or isolated ultrafiltration modalities. In this chapter, we review the treatment options for severe CHF and develop clinical recommendations from the perspective of the cardiorenal syndrome.

DEFINITION AND SCOPE OF THE PROBLEM

CHF and renal dysfunction may coexist, but each disease can also cause or exacerbate the other. Poor cardiac output may result in kidney ischemia and progressive chronic kidney disease (CKD). Conversely, CKD may result in salt and water retention, hypertension, activation of the renin-angiotensin-aldosterone system (RAS), and vascular calcification that causes cardiac dysfunction, accelerated atherosclerosis, and left ventricular hypertrophy and remodeling.

In the Acute Decompensated Heart Failure National Registry (ADHERE), an analysis of more than 100,000 patients with CHF, 57% had stage 3 or stage 4 CKD, 7% were at stage 5 (68% receiving dialysis), and only 9% had normal kidney function. In subjects with CHF who presented with CKD at the time of admission, there was greater use of diuretics and inotropes, less angiotensin-converting enzyme (ACE) inhibitor and angiotensin receptor blocker (ARB) administration, and 5% higher in-hospital mortality.[1]

The cardiorenal syndrome has undergone a classification into several categories (Fig. 71.1),[2] including cardiorenal (heart causing kidney disease), renocardiac (CKD leading to CHF), and syndromes with both being primary disorders or secondary to systemic conditions.

PATHOGENESIS

In cardiorenal syndrome, low cardiac output worsens renal perfusion and function, activating the RAS and other systems, leading to salt and water retention (see also Chapter 7), then a paradoxical worsening of cardiac function. Central to this vicious circle is tubuloglomerular feedback (described in Chapter 2), which is maladaptive in heart failure and in the case of some drugs that alter tubular sodium delivery. Secondary aldosteronism (resulting in increased sodium retention), increased systemic vascular resistance (thereby putting more strain on the heart), and higher cardiac filling pressures lead to a reduction in cardiac output as described by the Starling curve. Low stroke volume further activates the sympathetic nervous system (SNS), which in turn worsens vasoconstriction, cardiac function, and renal perfusion. Excessive activation of both the RAS and SNS pathways has long been considered the hallmark of worsened CHF. However, other pathophysiologic mechanisms that could have important therapeutic implications have now been elucidated.

Adenosine Mediators Adenosine receptors are involved with tubuloglomerular feedback signaling and maintain intrarenal vascular tone through a number of complex pathways, which include A_1 receptors (A_1R), causing afferent arteriolar vasoconstriction, and A_2 receptors, inducing efferent vessel dilation. Actions of adenosine at the macula densa and mesangium depend on angiotensin, renin, nitric oxide, and prostaglandin levels. Mechanisms by which adenosine may also directly influence distal and collecting tubule transporters and vasopressin function are still under investigation. A_1R antagonists could thereby not only restore diuretic sensitivity but also allow appropriate aquaresis in severe CHF.

Venous Congestion Apart from low cardiac output, CHF frequently causes high right-sided pressures and venous congestion. High renal vein pressures combined with arterial hypoperfusion will narrow the arterial to venous pressure gradient and hydraulic forces and are thought to lower renal plasma flow and glomerular filtration rate (GFR).

Inflammatory Cytokines Chronic and acute exacerbations of CHF are associated with widespread inflammation and high levels of proinflammatory cytokines, such as tumor necrosis factor and interleukins 6 and 10. These are thought to contribute to the vicious circle that further boosts cardiac, renal, and other tissue dysfunction.

Anemia Anemia may be due to "chronic disease" or coexistent CKD. The importance of both recognizing and treating anemia has led to the term *cardiorenal anemia syndrome*, emphasizing this pharmacologically remediable aspect of CHF.

Diuretic Tolerance and Adverse Effects Many patients with CHF develop tolerance to chronic diuretic therapy, fail to have appropriate natriuresis despite escalating doses, and have worsening of neurohumoral mediator levels.[3] Thus, some of the cardiac benefits of ACE inhibitors might be from blocking of diuretic-induced RAS activation. Consistent with this paradigm,

Classification of the Cardiorenal Syndrome

General definition: a pathophysiologic disorder of the heart and kidneys in which acute or chronic dysfunction in one organ may induce acute or chronic dysfunction in the other organ

Type I, Acute Cardiorenal Syndrome
Abrupt worsening of cardiac function leading to acute kidney injury
Examples: acute cardiogenic shock, acutely decompensated congestive heart failure

Type II, Chronic Cardiorenal Syndrome
Chronic abnormalities in cardiac function leading to acute kidney injury
Example: chronic congestive heart failure

Type III, Acute Renocardiac Syndrome
Abrupt worsening of renal function causing acute cardiac disorder
Examples: acute kidney ischemia, glomerulonephritis

Type IV, Chronic Renocardiac Syndrome
Chronic kidney disease contributing to decreased cardiac function, cardiac hypertrophy, or increased risk of adverse cardiovascular events
Example: chronic glomerular or interstitial disease

Type V, Secondary Cardiorenal Syndrome
Systemic condition causing both cardiac and renal dysfunction
Examples: diabetes mellitus, sepsis

Figure 71.1 Classification of the cardiorenal syndrome. *(Modified with permission from reference 2.)*

morbidity and mortality in advanced CHF increased up to fourfold with higher doses of diuretics despite the fact that there were no clinical or echocardiographic parameters to suggest that the high-dose group had any worse cardiac function.[4] Similar conclusions were reached in the Management to Improve Survival in Congestive Heart Failure (MISCHF) study and the large ADHERE database. Finally, in a multicenter analysis, patients receiving high-dose diuretics had worsening of GFR compared with the control group on alternative medications, despite equivalent fluid losses.[5]

TREATMENT

General Approach and Limitations

A pragmatic approach for this challenging disorder (Fig. 71.2) is first to address potentially treatable problems, such as valvular disease, conduction disorders and arrhythmias, pericardial effusion, and coronary ischemia (e.g., by angioplasty and stenting). The clinician can then approximate the volume of excess fluid and craft a daily therapeutic goal concurrent with efforts to ensure compliance with salt restriction. Medication-naive patients can then be cautiously treated as described in the following sections, with serial monitoring because hypotension or renal dysfunction commonly limits the use of pharmaceuticals. Determination of the degree to which a particular patient may be able to tolerate drug-induced hypotension (e.g., from afterload-reducing agents) is clinically challenging. Indeed, marked sensitivity of the blood pressure or renal function to low doses of RAS blockade should lead to a consideration of bilateral renal artery stenosis, a potentially remediable problem that can exacerbate the cardiorenal syndrome and also be a cause of flash pulmonary edema.

Stepwise Treatment Approach for Decompensated CHF and the Cardiorenal Syndrome

Step 1: Initial Evaluation
1. Compliance: Optimize adherence for medication regimen and salt restriction.
2. Electromechanical: Evaluate and treat arrhythmias and dyssynchrony
3. Anatomic, with imaging (cardiac catheterizaton, echocardiography) as appropriate for:
   a. Ischemia: angioplasty, stents, or surgery when appropriate for coronary artery stenoses
   b. Other remediable disorders, such as valvular heart disease, pericardial effusions, constrictive pericarditis
4. Anemia control: iron repletion, erythropoiesis-stimulating agents, or transfusions for Hb < 10 g/dl
5. Pharmacologic, with dose reductions for hypotension:
   Diuretics
   ACE inhibitors and ARBs
   Other agents: after load-reducing medications (i.e., hydralazine), digoxin

Step 2: For worsening renal function, ineffective diuresis, persistent CHF
1. Further pharmaceutical dose reductions to avoid hypotension
2. Re-evaluate for concurrent renal disease (i.e., renocardiac syndrome)
   a. Consider primary nephrologic disorders (i.e., parenchymal, obstruction)
   b. Consider evaluation for unilateral or bilateral renal artery stenosis

Step 3: For persistent hypotension, renal dysfunction, and CHF
1. Begin vasopressor (i.e., dobutamine) or consider ultrafiltration
2. Begin extracorporeal ultrafiltration, especially if patient is refractory to pressor:
   a. Intermittent slow ultrafiltration, when hypotension does not preclude adequate fluid removal during typically 4 to 6 hour sessions
   b. Continuous ultrafiltration, when equipment is available and patient becomes hypotensive or has worsening renal function with intermittent treatment sessions

Figure 71.2 Stepwise treatment approach for decompensated CHF and the cardiorenal syndrome. ACE-I, angiotensin-converting enzyme inhibitors; ARBs, angiotensin receptor blockers; Hb, hemoglobin.

Treatment Modalities for the Cardiorenal Syndrome

Traditional
- Diuretics: loop diuretics, long-acting thiazides
- Digoxin
- ACE-I and ARBs
- Vasodilators
- Blood transfusions

Recent Pharmaceuticals
- Inotropes: milrinone, dobutamine
- Atrial natriuretic peptides
- Aquaretics: vasopressin antagonists
- Erythropoiesis-stimulating agents
- Adenosine receptor blockade

Mechanical
- Biventricular pacing
- Ventricular assist devices

Ultrafiltration
- Peritoneal dialysis
  - Manual (CAPD) and automated using a cycler (APD)
- Extracorporeal therapies
  - Intermittent short-duration ultrafiltration
  - Slow continuous ultrafiltration

Figure 71.3 Treatment modalities for the cardiorenal syndrome. ACE-I, angiotensin-converting enzyme inhibitors; ARBs, angiotensin receptor blockers; CAPD, continuous ambulatory peritoneal dialysis; APD, automated peritoneal dialysis.

Pharmacologic Therapeutic Strategies

The pharmacologic management of CHF is summarized in Figure 71.3 and includes traditional cardiology approaches for arrhythmias (e.g., for atrial fibrillation) and afterload reduction. Use of inotropes is challenging in that there is limited efficacy from digoxin (other than rate control), and the intravenous agents (i.e., dobutamine and milrinone) are typically reserved for inpatients. An adequate diuresis by use of traditional medications in patients admitted with acute heart failure is not easily achieved; the ADHERE registry indicated that approximately 16% were discharged at a higher body weight. Specific pharmacologic strategies include the following.

Diuretics Despite the preceding concerns, some initially respond to escalating doses of diuretics. Loop diuretics need to be administered at frequent intervals in a high enough dose to achieve adequate drug levels within the glomerular filtrate. Coadministration of a long-acting thiazide diuretic can help maintain a natriuresis. In severe CHF, continuous low-dose infusion of a loop diuretic may be required.

RAS Antagonists ACE inhibitors and ARBs may worsen GFR in patients undergoing diuresis or those with advanced CKD, requiring temporary decrease in dose or withdrawal. Alternatively, diuretic dosage may need to be reduced before adjusting that of the ACE inhibitor. Hyperkalemia may also limit the use of RAS antagonists, including aldosterone antagonists.

Adenosine Antagonists It is hoped that by affecting tubuloglomerular feedback, A_1R antagonists could increase GFR, a benefit that theoretically could be partially offset by increased distal nephron workload and ischemia. In a pilot study, 300 patients with acute heart failure and renal dysfunction received the selective A_1R antagonist rolofylline intravenously for 3 days.[6] At days 14 and 60, some treatment benefits in dyspnea, smaller rises in serum creatinine levels, mortality, and readmission rates were noted. On the basis of these results, the 2000-patient PROTECT trial is ongoing.

Erythropoiesis-Stimulating Agents In a large registry, 25% of CHF individuals were moderately to severely anemic (hemoglobin 5 to 10.7 g/dl), and anemia (hemoglobin <12.1 g/dl) was associated with higher in-hospital mortality, longer length of stay, and more readmissions at 90 days.[7] Improvements in anemia and cardiac function may also benefit GFR. In small patient series, correction of severe anemia (hemoglobin <10 g/dl) improved CHF and clinical outcomes. Prospective multicenter trials to test whether further benefit can be achieved from normalization of hemoglobin values in CHF are ongoing. Until such data are available, we believe the most prudent course is to follow renal disease targets (see Chapter 79).

Antidiuretic Hormone Antagonists Release of vasopressin by (nonosmotic) low cardiac output results in water retention and hyponatremia. In clinical trials, V_2-selective antagonists such as tolvaptan and lixivaptan or a nonselective oral V_{1A}/V_2 antagonist indeed increased urine output and serum sodium, but it has not yet been proved that this results in clinically relevant improvement in CHF. Treatment of 537 patients for a minimum of 60 days had no effect at 10 months on all-cause mortality or heart failure–related morbidity.[8]

Natriuretic Peptides Early clinical trials were encouraging for a cardiac benefit, but there was no improvement in renal function. These agents should no longer be used for CHF because of subsequent data demonstrating increased short-term mortality in such patients.[9]

Nonrenal Salt and Water Removal

Nonrenal methods of salt and water removal are advantageous because they avoid tubuloglomerular feedback–mediated neurohumoral pathway activation and are effective in patients refractory to pharmaceutical treatment.

Paracentesis

In a small study of five patients, removal of approximately 3 liters of ascites resulted in a decrease in intra-abdominal pressure and improved renal function.[10] Repeated intermittent paracentesis, however, causes significant protein losses, often the need for albumin repletion, and the possibility of subsequent fluid leakage or infection. Nevertheless, the role for this approach in select patients needs to be better defined, especially in those settings in which the more elaborate and costly nonpharmacologic methodologies are not available.

Ultrafiltration: Peritoneal Dialysis

The techniques and potential complications of peritoneal dialysis (PD) are described in Chapters 92 and 93, but there are specific issues in regard to its use for CHF. The rapid use of PD catheters for acute CHF patients increases the risk of early fluid leaks and peritoneal infection. PD-induced electrolyte disturbances may worsen rhythm control. Large peritoneal fluid volumes can potentially compromise respiration that might already be tenuous in CHF, which could be avoided by frequent lower volume exchanges through automated cyclers.

Early small case series highlighted the safety of catheter placement and efficacy of outpatient PD for fluid removal in CHF patients. Intermittent PD accomplished ultrafiltration (UF) and also restored diuretic sensitivity. In one of the larger uncontrolled investigations,[11] 20 patients with severe CHF were treated with automated PD for 8 hours thrice weekly, achieving UF of 2.1 ± 0.5 l/session. At 1-year follow-up, there were improvements in echocardiographic measures of cardiac contractility, NYHA class, and hospitalization days; but some of the benefit may have been from resolving salt and fluid excesses due to concurrent CKD. Improvements in cardiac parameters were similarly described in 15 CHF patients.[12] This study, however, noted a high rate of complications, and 16% of the patients had peritoneal or abdominal wall infections, difficulty with dialysate effluent drainage, or displaced catheters requiring replacement.

A number of review articles have attempted to reconcile the diverse published dialysis protocols.[13] These support the efficacy of PD in cardiorenal (apart from renocardiac) patients for fluid removal, better NYHA class,[12] bridging to cardiac transplantation, decrease in hospitalization days, and improved quality of life.

Ultrafiltration: Conventional Hemodialysis or Hemofiltration

There is extensive experience with intermittent hemodialysis techniques for fluid removal in CHF. Traditionally, acute temporary or tunneled dual-lumen catheters are inserted (see Chapter 87). Permanent access is often precluded from a cardiac standpoint because these arteriovenous fistulas or grafts may shunt a liter or more of blood per minute. When the intention is to provide UF only, no dialysate is used ("isolated UF"; see Chapter 89); however, when electrolyte disorders are already present, they can be slowly corrected by temporary use of traditional dialysis techniques. The major risk from UF is hemodynamic instability due to excess fluid removal. Even with careful setting of the UF rate, many unstable CHF patients will not tolerate removal of 2 liters or more during typical 2- to 4-hour treatment times. Importantly, episodes of hypotension not only will prevent further fluid removal but also can induce acute kidney injury and potentially make the patient dialysis dependent.

It is believed that the key to hemodynamic stability is to dramatically slow the UF rate to allow adequate refill of the vascular space (see later), and this approach led to longer and then continuous treatment modalities: slow extended-duration isolated UF and continuous venovenous hemofiltration. There are multiple case reports and small series of patients treated with such techniques, but most had heterogeneous patient populations and lacked appropriate control groups, well-defined outcome measures, or strict treatment protocols.

Ultrafiltration: Recent Advances in Extracorporeal Techniques

Widespread use of these modalities so far has been limited by the logistic hurdles of performing them outside of an ICU setting. The barriers of extended treatment times and the need for 1:1 supervision by nurses have been overcome with commercially available modern devices dedicated to isolated UF. These now have small extracorporeal blood volumes (<100 ml) and allow blood flows low enough (<50 ml/min) to permit use of temporary peripheral vein catheters; they have pre-prepared tubing for one-step loading, computerized simple user interfaces with embedded help screens, remote monitoring capabilities, and miniaturization for portability. Treatment times range from 6 hours a day to continuous during multiple days. One such compact UF-dedicated device for use outside of the ICU setting has been extensively tested.

The first feasibility study[14] demonstrated that 16- to 18-gauge catheters could deliver blood at up to 40 ml/min and resulted in 2611 ± 1002 ml (up to 3725 ml) of UF during approximately 7 hours. In another study[15] of 20 patients with decompensated CHF and serum creatinine levels of at least 1.5 mg/dl or diuretic resistance, the UF rate was as high as 500 ml/h (decreased to 200 ml/h if hypotension occurred), and the therapy was continued until the CHF symptoms resolved. With more than 8 liters of fluid removal, patients were discharged in just 3.7 days without changes in their serum urea or creatinine values and had improved heart failure scores; seven had resolution of hyponatremia, and subjects appeared to have a decreased rate of readmission. Finally, in the prospective UNLOAD trial, 200 CHF patients were randomized to early UF or intravenous diuretics and observed for 90 days.[16] The UF achieved by the study was 241 ml/h for 12.3 ± 12 hours, which led to a weight reduction of 5.0 ± 3.1 kg during the 2 days. This was approximately 2 kg more than for those in the control diuretic group. Although dyspnea was improved in those undergoing UF at 8 hours, that score was no different at 48 hours. The groups were statistically similar for rises in serum creatinine of more than 0.3 mg/dl, blood urea nitrogen and sodium levels, heart failure scores, episodes of hypotension, and hospitalization length of stay. At 90 days, the UF group exhibited fewer total rehospitalizations (18% versus 32%), rehospitalization days (1.4 versus 3.8 days), and unscheduled office and emergency department visits (21% versus 44%). Potential weaknesses of the study design included sponsorship by the manufacturer, submaximal medical therapy in the diuretic group, and uncertainties as to post-hospitalization care and readmission. Last, there are small case series of patients who underwent long-term UF treatments for up to approximately a year and reportedly had sustained CHF benefits.

The Effect of Ultrafiltration on the Pathophysiology of Congestive Heart Failure

In 24 patients with refractory CHF, removal of up to 4 liters of fluid in a few hours[17] did not affect plasma volume, thereby confirming the matching of UF and plasma refill rate. Even at 24 hours after the procedure, the patients had reduced right atrial, pulmonary artery, and wedge pressures; increased stroke volume; stable heart rates and systemic vascular resistance; and improved responsiveness to diuretics.

UF in CHF patients decreases levels of norepinephrine, aldosterone, and renin.[18] UF also reduced systemic levels of inflammatory cytokines, a phenomenon that was not observed in patients treated with just diuretics. Some patients reportedly also have improved exercise capacity and pulmonary function. Last, in comparing UF with diuretics, it is important to appreciate that salt losses vary between these therapies. Part of the benefit from UF may be due to the convection of isotonic fluid, compared with less removal of sodium in the diuretic-induced hypotonic urine.

The Effect of Ultrafiltration on Renal Function

Benefits of UF for renal function appear to occur predominantly in patients with low baseline urine output (<1 l/day); UF reverses the RAS and SNS activation, thereby improving renal perfusion and GFR and restoring sensitivity to diuretics.[19] In contrast, in

CHF patients with a mean baseline GFR of 48 ml/min and preserved diuretic sensitivity, there were no significant differences in the kidney parameters before or after 2 days of either UF or intravenous diuretic therapy.[20]

There are thus encouraging but not unanimous reports of improving renal function with UF compared with diuretics, but it is important that cautious fluid removal can be accomplished without harming the kidney. Multiple studies have demonstrated that patients can undergo extracorporeal UF without a significant rise in serum creatinine or detriment to renal hemodynamics.[15,16] Determination of a safe rate of UF can be difficult, however, and excessive fluid removal can unquestionably lead to kidney injury. In a 25-patient retrospective study[21] of relatively high volume UF compared with usual care, the fluid removal rate was 325 ± 117 ml/h for 37 ± 25 hours. This resulted in greater weight reduction than in the historical control group but was associated with more patients having a rise in serum creatinine of more than 0.5 mg/dl (44% versus ≤24%). This led the investigators to alter their treatment protocol so that the rate of UF would be reduced to 100 to 200 ml/h.

Ultrafiltration: Setting the Rate of Fluid Removal

The key concept is to avoid intravascular fluid depletion by ensuring that the UF rate does not exceed the rate at which the vascular plasma compartment is being refilled from interstitial spaces. The plasma refill rate can vary during the course of fluid removal, as it is dependent on Starling forces (generated by the plasma oncotic pressure and the gradient between interstitial and vascular hydrostatic pressures) and the permeability of vascular basement membranes. If the UF rate exceeds the plasma refill rate, hemoconcentration, hypovolemia, hypotension, and decreased renal function develop. Equipment has been developed for hemodialysis machines that optically monitors hemoconcentration, and this approach can also be used as a guide for UF in patients with refractory CHF. So far, body fluid determination by bioimpedance vector analysis (see Chapter 90) has had little application in cardiology, despite being a validated important tool in nephrology.

Safety and Risks of Extracorporeal Therapies

Whereas newer simplified devices for isolated UF have improved the ease of patient care, these modalities are not risk free. In a small outpatient 1-year study, two deaths of 14 patients were attributed to complications of the UF.[22] In the larger UNLOAD trial,[16] however, the UF therapy proved very safe, without increased mortality or hemorrhage compared with those undergoing standard care. It is hoped that newer machines dedicated to isolated UF will have an added margin of safety conferred by low rates of filtration and blood flow as well as more robust automated monitoring software. Nevertheless, all complications that can occur in hemodialysis therapies are of course also relevant for CHF patients receiving isolated UF (see Chapter 91).

REFERENCES

1. Heywood JT, Fonarow GC, Costanzo MR, et al. High prevalence of renal dysfunction and its impact on outcome in 118,465 patients hospitalized with acute decompensated heart failure: A report from the ADHERE database. *J Card Fail*. 2007;13:422-430.
2. Ronco C, House AA, Haapio M. Cardiorenal syndrome: Refining the definition of a complex symbiosis gone wrong. *Intensive Care Med*. 2008;34:957-962.
3. Bayliss J, Norell M, Canepa-Anson R, et al. Untreated heart failure: Clinical and neuroendocrine effects of introducing diuretics. *Br Heart J*. 1987;57:17-22.
4. Eshaghian S, Horwich TB, Fonarow GC. Relation of loop diuretic dose to mortality in advanced heart failure. *Am J Cardiol*. 2006;97:1759-1764.
5. Butler J, Forman DE, Abraham WT, et al. Relationship between heart failure treatment and development of worsening renal function among hospitalized patients. *Am Heart J*. 2004;147:331-338.
6. Cotter G, Dittrich HC, Weatherley BD, et al. The PROTECT pilot study: A randomized, placebo-controlled, dose-finding study of the adenosine A_1 receptor antagonist rolofylline in patients with acute heart failure and renal impairment. *J Card Fail*. 2008;14:631-640.
7. Young JB, Abraham WT, Albert NM, et al. Relation of low hemoglobin and anemia to morbidity and mortality in patients hospitalized with heart failure (insight from the OPTIMIZE-HF registry). *Am J Cardiol*. 2008;101:223-230.
8. Konstam MA, Gheorghiade M, Burnett JC Jr, et al. Effects of oral tolvaptan in patients hospitalized for worsening heart failure: The EVEREST Outcome Trial. *JAMA*. 2007;297:1319-1331.
9. Sackner-Bernstein JD, Kowalski M, Fox M, Aaronson K. Short-term risk of death after treatment with nesiritide for decompensated heart failure: A pooled analysis of randomized controlled trials. *JAMA*. 2005;293:1900-1905.
10. Mullens W, Abrahams Z, Francis GS, et al. Prompt reduction in intra-abdominal pressure following large-volume mechanical fluid removal improves renal insufficiency in refractory decompensated heart failure. *J Card Fail*. 2008;14:508-514.
11. Gotloib L, Fudin R, Yakubovich M, Vienken J. Peritoneal dialysis in refractory end-stage congestive heart failure: A challenge facing a no-win situation. *Nephrol Dial Transplant*. 2005;20(Suppl 7):vii32-36.
12. Ryckelynck JP, Lobbedez T, Valette B, et al. Peritoneal ultrafiltration and treatment-resistant heart failure. *Nephrol Dial Transplant*. 1998;13(Suppl 4):56-59.
13. Mehrotra R, Kathuria P. Place of peritoneal dialysis in the management of treatment-resistant congestive heart failure. *Kidney Int Suppl*. 2006;103:S67-S71.
14. Jaski BE, Ha J, Denys BG, et al. Peripherally inserted veno-venous UF for rapid treatment of volume overloaded patients. *J Card Fail*. 2003;9:227-231.
15. Costanzo MR, Saltzberg M, O'Sullivan J, Sobotka P. Early ultrafiltration in patients with decompensated heart failure and diuretic resistance. *J Am Coll Cardiol*. 2005;46:2047-2051.
16. Costanzo MR, Guglin ME, Saltzberg MT, et al. Ultrafiltration versus intravenous diuretics for patients hospitalized for acute decompensated heart failure. *J Am Coll Cardiol*. 2007;49:675-683.
17. Marenz G, Lauri G, Grazi M, et al. Circulatory response to fluid overload removal by extracorporeal ultrafiltration in refractory congestive heart failure. *J Am Coll Cardiol*. 2001;38:963-968.
18. Cipolla CM, Grazi S, Rimondini A, et al. Changes in circulating norepinephrine with hemofiltration in advanced congestive heart failure. *Am J Cardiol*. 1990;66:987-994.
19. Marenzi G, Grazi S, Giraldi F, et al. Interrelation of humoral factors, hemodynamics, and fluid and salt metabolism in congestive heart failure: Effects of extracorporeal ultrafiltration. *Am J Med*. 1993;94:49-56.
20. Rogers HL, Marshall J, Bock J, et al. A randomized, controlled trial of the renal effects of ultrafiltration as compared to furosemide in patients with acute decompensated heart failure. *J Card Fail*. 2008;14:1-5.
21. Bartone C, Saghir S, Menon SG, et al. Comparison of ultrafiltration, nesiritide, and usual care in acute decompensated heart failure. *Congest Heart Fail*. 2008;14:298-301.
22. Sheppard R, Panyon J, Pohwani AL, et al. Intermittent outpatient ultrafiltration for the treatment of severe refractory congestive heart failure. *J Card Fail*. 2004;10:380-383.

CHAPTER 72 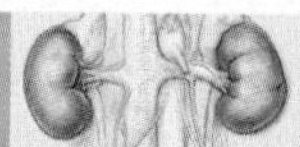

Hepatorenal Syndrome

Ignatius K.P. Cheng, Felix F.K. Li

DEFINITION

Hepatorenal syndrome (HRS) is a reversible and functional renal failure that occurs in patients with acute or chronic liver disease, advanced hepatic failure, and portal hypertension. It is characterized by impaired renal function and marked abnormalities in the arterial circulation and endogenous vasoactive systems. In the kidney, there is pronounced vasoconstriction resulting in low glomerular filtration rate (GFR). In the splanchnic circulation, there is a predominance of arteriolar vasodilation resulting in reduction of systemic vascular resistance and arterial hypotension.[1,2] Two forms of HRS can be identified on the basis of the progression of the disease (Fig. 72.1). An acute form (type 1) is characterized by a rapid deterioration in renal function, whereas a chronic form (type 2) is marked by an insidious onset and a slowly progressive course.

Pseudohepatorenal Syndrome

Pseudohepatorenal syndrome describes concurrent hepatic and renal dysfunction secondary to a wide variety of infectious, systemic, circulatory, genetic, and other diseases and after exposure to a variety of drugs and toxins. In these conditions, the liver does not play an etiologic role in the pathogenesis of renal failure, and they must be excluded before the diagnosis of HRS can be established.

PATHOPHYSIOLOGY AND PATHOGENESIS

Renal and Systemic Hemodynamic Changes

In HRS, reduction in GFR occurs mainly as a result of renal cortical hypoperfusion after intense cortical renal vasoconstriction, which can be demonstrated angiographically as marked beading and tortuosity of the interlobular and proximal arcuate arteries and the absence of a distinct cortical nephrogram and vascular filling of the cortical vessels (Fig. 72.2).[3] Intense renal vasoconstriction occurs in the presence of splanchnic vasodilation, which gives rise to a low peripheral vascular resistance and a low systemic mean arterial blood pressure (MAP). This further compromises renal perfusion because intense renal vasoconstriction results in blunting of the autoregulation of renal blood flow, so that renal perfusion becomes more pressure dependent. In HRS, filtration fraction is also reduced, reflecting a dominant increase in afferent arteriolar tone and a decrease in the ultrafiltration coefficient. Serial systemic hemodynamic studies showed that HRS occurs in the setting of reduced MAP, cardiac output, and wedge pulmonary pressure without change of systemic vascular resistance. These findings suggest that the inability of the heart to increase its output to compensate for a decrease in cardiac preload also significantly contributes to the pathogenesis of HRS.[4] Vasoconstriction is not confined to the renal vascular bed, and in type 1 HRS in particular, it is also observed in the vasculature of other organs, including the liver, brain, muscle, and skin.[2]

Neurohumoral Abnormalities

The renal and systemic hemodynamic changes that characterize HRS are a direct consequence of neurohumoral disturbances.[2] The sympathetic nervous system is activated, and the sympathetic discharges through the renal nerves are markedly increased. Increases in the plasma and urinary levels of vasoconstrictors and in the plasma level of vasodilators are observed in patients suffering from HRS. The vasoconstrictors include plasma renin activity, norepinephrine, neuropeptide Y, arginine vasopressin, endothelin and F_2 isoprostanes, and urinary cysteinyl leukotrienes; the vasodilators include plasma endotoxin, nitrite and nitrate (end product of nitric oxide metabolism), and glucagon. Activation of the vasoconstrictor systems is thought to be the cause of renal vasoconstriction; activation of the vasodilator systems is thought to occur mainly in the splanchnic circulation and to lead to splanchnic vasodilation.

Most of these neurohumoral abnormalities found in HRS are also detected, albeit to a lesser extent, in decompensated cirrhosis (with ascites) with normal renal function and in compensated cirrhosis (without ascites). These findings support the hypothesis that HRS most likely represents one end of the spectrum of homeostatic abnormalities that occur in liver failure and portal hypertension.

In contrast to increased plasma and urinary levels of vasoconstrictors and plasma level of vasodilators, decreased levels of urinary vasodilators have been observed in HRS. These include prostaglandin E_2, 6-keto-prostaglandin F_1 (a stable metabolite of renal prostacyclin), and kallikrein. As the level of these urinary vasodilators is normal in compensated cirrhosis and higher than normal in decompensated cirrhosis with ascites and normal renal function, it is postulated that a reduction of renal vasodilators is the final event that leads to the development of HRS.

Summary of Pathogenetic Events

Figure 72.3 is a simplified diagram of the pathogenetic events that lead to HRS. Liver failure and portal hypertension through

Definition of Hepatorenal Syndrome Type 1 and Type 2
Type 1 Hepatorenal Syndrome
Doubling of serum creatinine >2.5 mg/dl (220 μmol/l) or a 50% reduction in 24-hr creatinine clearance to <20 ml/min <2 weeks
Frequently follows a precipitating event (e.g. infection)
Median survival without treatment: 2 weeks
Type 2 Hepatorenal Syndrome
Less rapid renal functional deterioration than type 1
Mainly presents with refractory ascites
Median survival without treatment: 4–6 months

Figure 72.1 Definition of hepatorenal syndrome type 1 and type 2.

endotoxemia and increased shear stress increase vascular production of vasodilators, including nitric oxide and glucagon in the splanchnic circulation, leading to the initiating event of splanchnic arteriolar vasodilation (the peripheral arterial vasodilation hypothesis). Splanchnic vasodilation leads to a decrease in systemic vascular resistance, but MAP is initially maintained by an increase in cardiac output, resulting in a hyperdynamic circulation. Splanchnic vasodilation also decreases arterial filling and reduces the effective arterial blood volume. The subsequent stimulation of the central volume receptors leads to compensatory activation of the vasoconstrictor systems, in particular the arginine vasopressin system, renin-angiotensin-aldosterone system (RAAS), and sympathetic nervous system (including its hormones norepinephrine and neuropeptide Y), which help restore effective arterial blood volume. This restoration is achieved in patients with compensated cirrhosis but not in patients with decompensated cirrhosis, in whom progressive splanchnic arteriolar vasodilation leads to increased splanchnic capillary pressure, resulting in an increase in lymph formation that exceeds reabsorption capacity. In parallel, further contraction of the effective arterial blood volume leads to reduction of systemic MAP and further stimulation of the vasoconstrictor systems, resulting in sodium and water retention. The net result of these combined effects is continuous ascites formation (the forward theory of ascites formation).

As the splanchnic circulation is resistant to the effects of vasoconstrictors because of local release of vasodilators, progressive splanchnic vasodilation continues to occur as liver failure and portal hypertension progress. This leads to continued contraction of effective arterial blood volume, which, in combination with the progressive inability of the cirrhotic heart to respond to reduced preload consequent to splanchnic vasodilation, results in further reduction of MAP and more intense stimulation of the vasoconstrictor systems. Normally, the effect of vasoconstrictors on the renal circulation is counterbalanced by the reactive production of intrarenal vasodilators. It is postulated that HRS develops when the balance of activities between the renal vasoconstrictors and intrarenal vasodilators finally breaks down. The likelihood that this will occur increases with progressive or acute deterioration in liver function or increasing severity of portal hypertension (e.g., after acute alcoholic hepatitis) and is precipitated by events that lead to further volume contraction and reduction of the effective arterial blood volume (see later discussion).

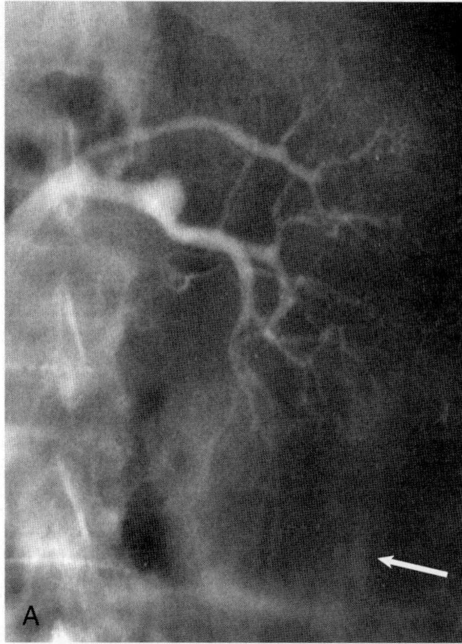

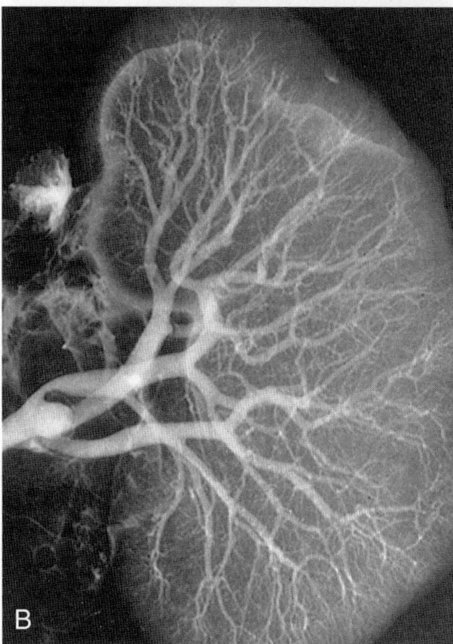

Figure 72.2 Hepatorenal syndrome (HRS). A, Renal angiogram (the *arrow* marks the edge of the kidney). **B,** The angiogram carried out in the same kidney at autopsy. Note complete filling of the renal arterial system throughout the vascular bed to the periphery of the cortex. The vascular attenuation and tortuosity seen previously (**A**) are no longer present. The vessels are also histologically normal. This indicates the functional nature of the vascular abnormality in HRS.[3]

EPIDEMIOLOGY

The possibility for development of HRS in the cirrhotic patient is estimated at 18% at 1 year and 39% at 5 years.[5] Neither the etiology nor the Child-Pugh score (*http://homepage.mac.com/sholland/contrivances/childpugh.html*) predicts the incidence of HRS. Rather, independent predictors of HRS include low serum sodium concentration, high serum renin activity,[4,5] absence of hepatomegaly,[5] abnormal renal duplex Doppler ultrasound study (resistive index >0.7),[6] and low cardiac output.[4]

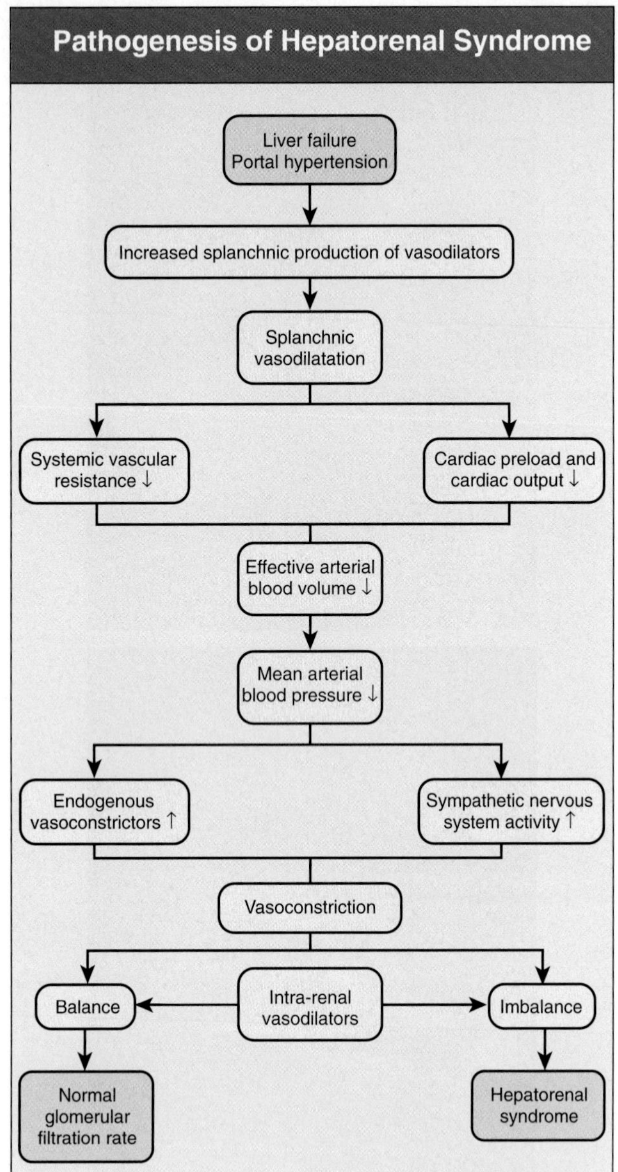

Figure 72.3 The pathogenesis of hepatorenal syndrome.

CLINICAL MANIFESTATIONS

Type 1 and type 2 HRS are considered to be different syndromes rather than different expressions of a common underlying disorder.[2] Type 1 HRS is characterized by a rapid decline in renal function and is most often observed in patients suffering from acute liver failure, acute alcoholic hepatitis, or acute decompensation on a background of cirrhosis (see Fig. 72.1). This group of patients, apart from suffering from rapidly progressive renal failure, also suffers from multiorgan dysfunction including severe hepatic failure (severe hyperbilirubinemia, prolongation of prothrombin time), hepatic encephalopathy, and relative adrenal insufficiency. Hyponatremia is almost always present, and arterial blood pressure is usually low. Acute decompensation in type 1 HRS may be precipitated by bacterial infections (especially spontaneous bacterial peritonitis), gastrointestinal bleeding, vigorous diuretic therapy, abdominal paracentesis, or the administration of substances such as nonsteroidal anti-inflammatory drugs (NSAIDs) that further suppress intrarenal generation of vasodilators (e.g., prostaglandins). Left untreated, it tends to run a rapid and progressive downhill course, resulting in death of the patient within weeks.[5]

Type 2 HRS is characterized by insidious onset and slowly progressive deterioration of renal function. This is most often observed in patients with decompensated cirrhosis and portal hypertension. This group of patients tends to be less severely jaundiced and mainly presents with refractory ascites. Low-normal arterial blood pressure, modest prolongation of prothrombin time, and hyponatremia are usually present. It tends to run a slowly progressive downhill course during months and most likely reflects the natural course of the disease because additional precipitating factors are not usually identified.[2,5]

PATHOLOGY

HRS is, by definition, a functional renal disorder, and the presence of significant glomerular and tubular disease excludes the diagnosis. However, glomerular abnormalities, including mesangial expansion, capillary wall thickening, mesangial and capillary wall electron-dense deposits, and immune deposits of C3 and the immunoglobulins IgA, IgM, and IgG, are frequently found in cirrhotic patients with normal renal function and minimal urinary abnormalities. The presence of such glomerular abnormalities in a cirrhotic patient, therefore, does not exclude the diagnosis of HRS. Protrusion of the proximal tubular epithelium into Bowman's space (glomerulotubular reflux) is not specific for HRS and is found in other conditions associated with profound renal ischemia and terminal hypotension. Although early autopsy studies demonstrated normal tubular morphology in patients dying of HRS, detailed light and electron microscopic studies have documented proximal tubular lesions consistent with ischemic injury.

DIAGNOSIS AND DIFFERENTIAL DIAGNOSIS

The diagnostic criteria for HRS were established by the International Ascites Club[1] in 1996 (Fig. 72.4) and have recently been revised (Fig. 72.5).[7] The main differences between the new and old criteria include the exclusion of creatinine clearance as a measure of renal function because of the difficulty in obtaining an accurate urine collection, the removal of ongoing bacterial infection as an exclusion criterion so that treatment of HRS is not delayed in these patients, the substitution of albumin for saline as the preferred fluid for plasma volume expansion, and the removal of the minor criteria as they are not thought to be essential.

The diagnosis of HRS is mainly one of exclusion and should be suspected in any patient with acute or chronic liver disease with advanced liver failure and portal hypertension who develops progressive renal impairment. There may be significant renal impairment despite a normal serum creatinine or blood urea nitrogen concentration because these patients are frequently malnourished, with reduced lean body mass, and often have a low urea generation rate because of liver failure and low protein intake. Severe hyperbilirubinemia, which is often present in patients with HRS, interferes with the Jaffe reaction for creatinine quantification and may cause falsely low results. Enzymatic creatinine assays are less susceptible to high bilirubin levels. In cases of uncertainty, GFR may be assessed with use of serum cystatin C, ^{125}I-iothalamate, ^{51}Cr-labeled EDTA, or inulin clearance.[8]

Pseudohepatorenal syndrome (Fig. 72.6)[9] is usually easy to exclude because the etiologic agent is frequently known and both

Diagnostic Criteria for Hepatorenal Syndrome
Major Criteria
Chronic or acute liver disease with advanced hepatic failure and portal hypertension
Low glomerular filtration rate, as indicated by serum creatinine >1.5 mg/dl (135 μmol/l) or 24-hr creatinine clearance <40 ml/min
Absence of shock, ongoing bacterial infection, and current or recent treatment with nephrotoxic drugs
Absence of gastrointestinal fluid losses (repeated vomiting or intense diarrhea)
Absence of renal fluid losses (weight loss >500 g/day for several days in patients with ascites without peripheral edema or 1000 g/day in patients with peripheral edema)
No sustained improvement in renal function (decrease in serum creatinine to 1.5 mg/dl [135 μmol/l] or less or increase in creatinine clearance to 40 ml/min or more) following diuretic withdrawal and expansion of plasma volume with 1.5 liters of isotonic saline
Proteinuria <500 mg/day and no ultrasonographic evidence of obstructive uropathy or parenchymal renal disease
Additional Criteria
Urine volume <500 ml/day
Urine sodium <10 mmol/l
Urine osmolality greater than plasma osmolality
Urine red blood cells <50 per high-power field
Serum sodium concentration <130 mmol/l

Figure 72.4 Diagnostic criteria for hepatorenal syndrome. *(Modified from reference 1.)*

Revised Diagnostic Criteria for Hepatorenal Syndrome
Cirrhosis with ascites
Serum creatinine > 1.5 mg/dl (133 μmol/l)
No improvement in serum creatinine (decrease to a level of 1.5 mg/dl) after at least 2 days with diuretic withdrawal and volume expansion with albumin. The recommended dose of albumin is 1 gm/kg of body weight per day up to a maximum of 100 gm/day.
Absence of shock
No current or recent treatment with nephrotoxic drugs
Absence of parenchymal kidney disease as indicated by proteinuria >500 mg/day, microhaematuria (>50 red blood cells per high power field) and/or abnormal renal ultrasound

Figure 72.5 Revised diagnostic criteria for hepatorenal syndrome. *(Modified from reference 7.)*

renal and liver functional abnormalities are often found at first clinical presentation, when there is no evidence of advanced liver failure and portal hypertension. In contrast, HRS invariably occurs after liver failure and portal hypertension are fully established and frequently develops when the patient is undergoing treatment of these conditions or their complications.

In patients with preexisting liver failure and portal hypertension, nephrotoxic agents (e.g., NSAIDs and aminoglycosides) must be stopped, and conditions leading to renal failure must be excluded by careful history, physical examination, urine examination, and ultrasound study before the diagnosis of HRS can be considered. The absence of shock, gastrointestinal bleeding, and

Causes of Pseudohepatorenal Syndrome

Potential Causes	Predominantly Tubulointerstitial Involvement	Predominantly Glomerular Involvement
Infections	Sepsis, leptospirosis, brucellosis, tuberculosis, Epstein-Barr virus, hepatitis A virus	Hepatitis B and C viruses, HIV infection, *Schistosoma mansoni*, liver abscess
Drugs	Tetracycline, rifampin (rifampicin), sulfonamide, phenytoin, allopurinol, fluroxene, methotrexate (high dose), acetaminophen (overdose)	
Toxins	Carbon tetrachloride, trichloroethylene, chloroform, elemental phosphorus, arsenic, copper, chromium, barium, amatoxins,* raw carp bile toxins†	
Systemic disease	Sarcoidosis, Sjögren's syndrome	Systemic lupus erythematosus, vasculitis, cryoglobulinemia, amyloidosis
Circulatory failure	Hypovolemic or cardiogenic shock	
Malignancy	Lymphoma, leukemia	
Congenital and genetic disorders	Polycystic liver and kidney disease, nephronophthisis and congenital hepatic fibrosis	
Miscellaneous	Fatty liver of pregnancy, Reye's syndrome	Eclampsia, HELLP syndrome, cirrhotic glomerulopathy

Figure 72.6 Causes of pseudohepatorenal syndrome. *Accidental poisoning after ingestion of mushrooms of the *Amanita* genus. †Accidental poisoning after ingestion of the raw gallbladder or bile of the grass carp (a common practice in rural East Asia). *(Modified from reference 9.)*

excess gastrointestinal, peritoneal, or renal fluid loss must also be documented. Prerenal acute renal failure must be excluded by withdrawal of diuretics and fluid challenge either with 1.5 liters of normal saline or preferably with albumin, 1 g/kg of body weight per day up to the maximum of 100 g/day for 2 days. Fewer than 50 urinary red blood cells per high-power field and urinary protein of less than 500 mg/l help exclude significant coexisting glomerular or tubulointerstitial disease leading to renal failure and support the diagnosis of HRS.

NATURAL HISTORY

The prognosis of HRS is poor. Without treatment, the median survival rate for type 1 HRS is about 2 weeks; that of type 2 HRS is about 4 to 6 months.[5] Recovery of renal function coincides with recovery of liver function and liver regeneration and follows therapeutic intervention. Renal failure is infrequently an immediate cause of death, and most patients succumb to the other complications of liver failure and portal hypertension, such as hepatic encephalopathy, gastrointestinal bleeding, and sepsis. Despite this, renal failure refractory to therapy is an important determinant of outcome.

TREATMENT

Preventive Measures

Accepting the hypothesis that HRS represents one end of the spectrum of the homeostatic abnormalities in liver failure and portal hypertension and is precipitated by such events as volume contraction, sepsis, and the administration of potential nephrotoxic agents, it follows that a major focus of treatment must be to avoid the occurrence of such events and to treat them promptly when they occur. In patients with decompensated liver disease, the common events that lead to volume contraction include gastrointestinal bleeding, injudicious use of lactulose (for treatment of hepatic encephalopathy) resulting in profuse diarrhea, and excessive diuretic therapy or paracentesis for the treatment of ascites. To avoid the last, a stepwise approach to the treatment of ascites is recommended. All patients are advised to have bed rest and to follow a low-sodium diet (60 to 90 mmol/day, equivalent to about 1.5 to 2 g of salt per day). After this, spironolactone is prescribed at increasing doses (100 mg/day as initial dosages; if there is no response within 4 days, 200 mg/day; if no further response, 400 mg/day). When there is no response to the highest dose of spironolactone, furosemide is added at increasing dosages every 2 days (40 to 160 mg/day). In cases of diuretic resistance, therapeutic paracentesis, when it is combined with plasma volume expansion using albumin (8 g per liter of ascites removed), is helpful and is associated with a low incidence of circulatory dysfunction after treatment. The use of potentially nephrotoxic agents, including angiotensin-converting enzyme inhibitors, angiotensin receptor blockers, NSAIDs, aminoglycosides, and radiocontrast media, should be avoided as far as possible. Therapeutic agents (e.g., β-blockers and somatostatin) that are employed for the treatment of bleeding esophageal and gastric varices reduce GFR, and their use must be monitored carefully. There should be a low threshold for antibiotic therapy for suspected sepsis. Spontaneous bacterial peritonitis must be excluded by regular examination of ascites fluid and treated not only with broad-spectrum antibiotics but also with albumin infusion (1.5 g/kg initially and 1 g/kg 2 days later) because the latter has been shown to prevent the subsequent development of HRS.[10] Primary prophylaxis of spontaneous bacterial peritonitis with norfloxacin has recently been shown not only to prevent its development but also to delay the development of HRS and to improve patient survival in cirrhotic patients at high risk for complications (low ascitic protein level <15 g/l, advanced liver failure with Child-Pugh score ≥9 and serum bilirubin ≥3 mg/dl, or impaired renal function with serum creatinine ≥1.2 mg/dl or serum sodium ≤130 mmol/l).[11] Norfloxacin is thought to exert its renoprotective effect by reducing bacterial translocation from the intestine, endotoxemia, and nitric oxide generation, which in turn leads to improved hemodynamics. Prophylactic use of pentoxifylline (400 mg orally three times per day) also prevents the development of HRS in patients suffering from acute alcoholic hepatitis, probably by inhibiting the synthesis of tumor necrosis factor α.[12]

General Approach to Treatment

Once the diagnosis of HRS is made, patients should be assessed for orthotopic liver transplantation (OLT). Suitable candidates, especially those suffering from type 1 HRS, should be placed on the urgent waiting list for cadaveric or living donor liver transplantation. In patients who are transplantation candidates but do not yet have a donor, bridge treatments to OLT include pharmacotherapy, mechanical shunt, extracorporeal liver support therapy, and, in patients with advanced uremia, renal replacement therapy. In some patients who are not transplantation candidates, prolonged survival in terms of months may still be achievable with some of these therapies.

Pharmacotherapies for Hepatorenal Syndrome
*Terlipressin, IV 0.5-1 mg q4–6 h to start, doubling every 2 days up to a maximum of 12 mg/day if serum creatinine decreases < 25% after 2 days. Maximum duration of treatment 14 days
Vasopressin, 0.01 U/min to start and titrating the dose upwards to a maximum of 0.8 U/min to achieve an increase of MAP of at least 10 mmHg. Maximum duration of treatment 11 days
Norepinephrine, IV 0.5 mg/h to start, increasing dose by 0.25 to 0.5 mg/h every 4 hours up to maximum of 3 mg/h to achieve an increase of MAP of at least 10 mmHg. Maximum duration of treatment 15 days
Midodrine, oral 7.5 mg tid + Octreotide SC 100 μg tid to start, increasing midodrine dose to maximum of 12.5–15 mg tid and octreotide dose to maximum of 200 μg tid to achieve an increase of MAP of at least 15 mmHg. Maximum duration of treatment not defined

Figure 72.7 Pharmacotherapies for hepatorenal syndrome. All patients should also receive albumin, 1 g/kg up to 100 g in the first day and 20 to 40 g/day afterward. Central venous pressure monitoring to achieve a reading of 10 to 15 mm Hg is desirable but not mandatory. *Terlipressin is the preferred treatment. MAP, mean arterial blood pressure. *(Modified from references 7 and 24.)*

Pharmacotherapy

At present, the most promising pharmacotherapy appears to be vasoconstrictor therapy targeted at reversal of splanchnic arteriolar vasodilation and restoration of the effective arterial blood volume with use of albumin (Fig. 72.7). Vasodilator therapy, which aims at reversal of renal vasoconstriction, is limited by profound hypotension because activation of the vasoconstrictor systems of the extrasplanchnic circulation is essential for maintaining the systemic MAP.

Vasopressin analogues have attracted the most attention, given their preferential vasoconstrictor action on the splanchnic versus the renal vascular bed. Terlipressin (triglycyllysine vasopressin) is a synthetic analogue of vasopressin that apart from having a greater effect on the vascular vasopressin receptors (V_1) than the renal vasopressin receptors (V_2) is a prodrug requiring transformation to the active form, lysine vasopressin. Because of this, terlipressin has a prolonged half-life and can be given as an intravenous bolus instead of a continuous intravenous infusion. This significantly reduces the incidence of systemic ischemic complications. Long-term prospective studies[13-17] and a large retrospective study[18] in patients with type 1 and type 2 HRS have shown that terlipressin combined with daily albumin infusion improved renal function in 60% of the treated patients, with 37% surviving beyond 1 month, 60% without OLT. Reversal of HRS was associated with improved survival.[16,18] The efficacy of terlipressin in the treatment of HRS has recently been confirmed in four randomized trials (Fig. 72.8).[19-22] Terlipressin was given at a starting dose of 2 to 6 mg/day, and in two studies, the dose was titrated upward on the basis of response to a maximum dose of 12 mg daily. Both treated patients and controls were given

Randomized Studies of Terlipression or Norepinephrine in Patients with HRS

Investigators	Treatment	No. of patients*	Dose of treatment	Duration of treatment (days)	Reversal of HRS† complete/partial	Patients surviving 1/3/6 months	Patients surviving with OLT at 1/3/6 months
Solanki et al., 2003[19]	T	12 (0)	1mg/12 hr	<15	5‡	NA	NA
	P	12 (0)	-	<15	0	0	0
Sanyal et al, 2008[20]	T	56 (0)	1-2 mg/6 hr	6.3	19/NA‡	NA/NA/24	NA/NA/17
	P	56 (0)	-	5.8	7/NA	NA/NA/21	NA/NA/16
Neri et al., 2008[21]	T	26 (0)	1-0.5 mg/8 hr	<19	21/4‡	19/14/11‡	NA
	C	26 (0)	-	<19	5/11	11/5/4	NA
Martin-Llahl et al., 2008[22]	T	23 (6)	1-2 mg/4 hr	7 ± 5	9/1‡	NA/6/NA	NA
	C	23 (5)	-	8 ± 5	1/1	NA/4/NA	NA
Alessandria et al., 2007[26]	T	12 (7)	1-2 mg/4 hr	6 (2-11)	10/0	11/8/8	3/7/8
	N	10 (6)	0.1-0.7 μg/kg/min	5 (2-10)	7/0	8/7/7	7/7/7
Sharma et al., 2008[27]	T	20 (0)	0.5-2 mg/6 hr	7 (4-15)	10/4	11/NA/NA	NA
	N	20 (0)	0.5-3 mg/hr	6.5 (4-15)	10/3	11/NA/NA	NA

Figure 72.8 Randomized studies of terlipressin or norepinephrine in HRS. T, terlipressin; P, placebo; C, control; N, norepinephrine. All patients received albumin infusion. *Number of patients with type 2 hepatorenal syndrome in parentheses. †Complete reversal: serum creatinine ≤1.5 mg/dl; partial reversal: serum creatinine <30% to 50% baseline level but >1.5 mg/dl. ‡$P < .05$ versus placebo or control. OLT, orthotopic liver transplantation; NA, information not available.

daily albumin infusion of 20 to 40 g/day. Reversal of HRS was associated with improved survival, but a significant improvement in survival compared with controls was observed in only one study.[21] The inclusion of patients with more severe renal failure in the treated group[20] and the unexpected high response and survival rate in controls[22] may explain the inability of some of these studies to show a survival benefit of treatment despite success in reversing HRS. The latter is likely to be due to the more aggressive use of albumin infusion in these studies as such an approach has been shown to reverse HRS in a high proportion of patients.[23]

Recurrence rates of HRS after successful treatment are variable and tend to be more common in type 2 than in type 1 HRS.[13,14,16,17,20,22] Re-treatment with terlipressin is successful in most patients.[14,16,20] Younger age,[18,21] lower baseline serum creatinine level,[22] Child-Pugh score of 12 or lower,[18,21] and administration of albumin[16] are independent predictors for a successful response to treatment; Child-Pugh score (≤12)[16,18,20,21] and model for end-stage liver disease (MELD) score[22] were independent predictors for patient survival. Transient abdominal pain and diarrhea after the first dose of terlipressin treatment are common. Significant ischemic side effects attributed to terlipressin occurred in an average of 4% of cases.[13-17,19-22] Deterioration of liver function or hepatic encephalopathy during treatment was not observed in most studies.[13,14,18,20,22]

Intravenous vasopressin has been used as an alternative to terlipressin in the treatment of HRS in countries where this drug is not available and was successful in reversing type 1 and type 2 HRS in 42% of patients in a retrospective study.[24] Responders had significantly lower mortality and higher liver transplantation rate than nonresponders did. No adverse effect related to therapy was observed.

Intravenous norepinephrine combined with intravenous albumin and furosemide reversed type 1 HRS in 10 of 12 patients; three survived with OLT, and four survived for a median of 332 days without OLT.[25] With use of a similar dosing regimen, two randomized comparative studies showed that norepinephrine is as effective as terlipressin in the treatment of type 1 and type 2 HRS (see Fig. 72.8).[26,27] All recurrences were successfully re-treated with the original regimen. Significant treatment-related side effects were low, and the cost of treatment with norepinephrine was 3 and 15 times lower, respectively, than with terlipressin.

Administration of midodrine (an orally active α-mimetic drug), subcutaneous octreotide, and albumin infusion was successful in reverting type 1 HRS in all of five treated patients, compared with only one of eight patients treated with subpressor dose of dopamine and albumin.[28] Four of five treated patients survived longer than 1 month, two with OLT and two without OLT. Treatment could be maintained for up to 2 months, with three patients receiving treatment at home. Side effects were self-limited, including tingling, goose bumps, and diarrhea. These findings were confirmed in a retrospective study that used a similar drug dosing regimen but without daily albumin infusion.[29] Significant side effects of treatment were observed in only one treated patient. In another study, oral midodrine given in a lower dose in combination with intravenous octreotide (25-μg bolus followed by 25 μg/h) and albumin for 14 ± 3 days (range, 5 to 47 days) reversed type 1 HRS in 10 of 14 patients.[30] Octreotide may contribute to normalizing the response of the vasodilated splanchnic arterial vessels to midodrine, thereby avoiding the extrasplanchnic side effects of vasoconstrictor therapy. Thus, midodrine in combination with octreotide is an effective alternative treatment of type 1 HRS and allows treatment on an outpatient basis. In contrast, monotherapy with octreotide was ineffective in a randomized prospective double-blind placebo crossover trial[31] and in a retrospective study in HRS.[24]

Transjugular Intrahepatic Portosystemic Stent-Shunt

Portal hypertension is central in the pathogenesis of the homeostatic abnormalities in HRS. The high operative mortality precludes side-to-side portacaval shunts in HRS patients. Transjugular intrahepatic portosystemic stent-shunting (TIPS) creates a parenchymal track between branches of the hepatic and portal vein (Fig. 72.9). In experienced hands, operative mortality rates are 1% to 2%, and the morbidity rate is 10%. Procedure-related complications include intra-abdominal bleeding, cardiac arrhythmia, shunt migration and thrombosis, hemolytic anemia, fever, infection, and reactions to radiocontrast media (including nephrotoxicity). The resultant diversion of portal blood flow from the liver to the systemic circulation may result in transient deterioration of liver function and development of encephalopathy. In an earlier study, TIPS improved renal function in six of seven HRS patients (all with Child-Pugh score <12) and achieved a mean survival of 4.7 (0.3 to 17) months.[32] A long-term study of 31 nontransplantable cirrhotic patients with HRS (14 type 1 and 17 type 2) without severe liver failure confirmed that TIPS improved renal function and survival compared with controls.[33] Shunt stenosis and occlusion occurred in seven patients and could be treated in six by balloon dilation or stent prolongation, and 11 developed hepatic encephalopathy during follow-up.

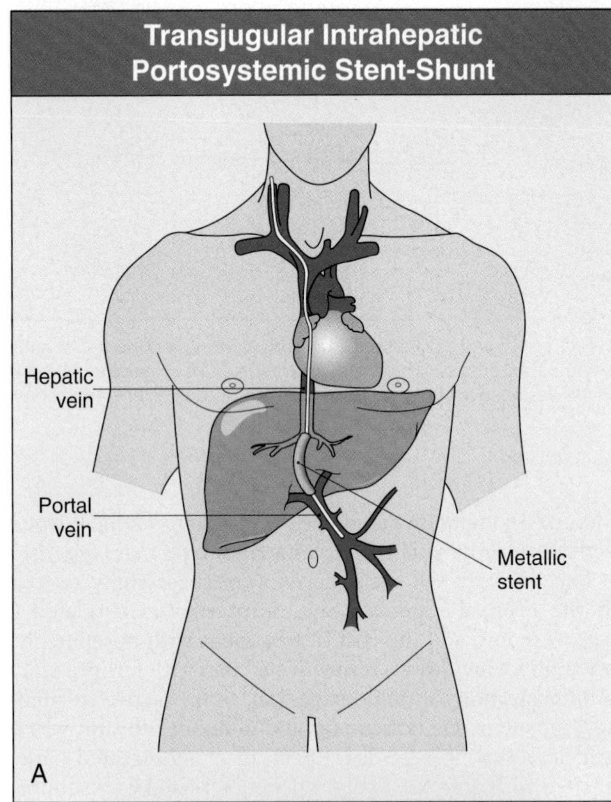

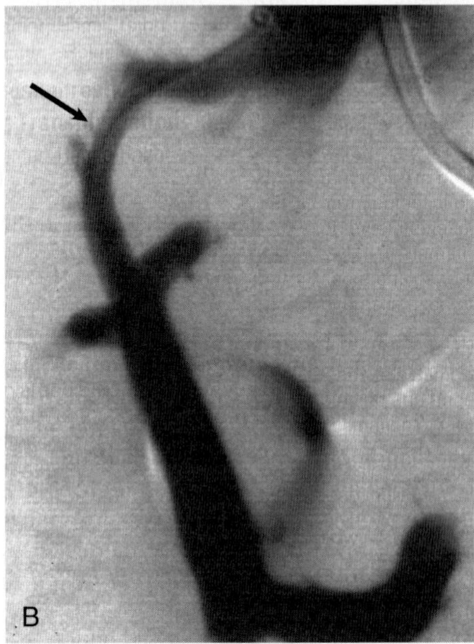

Figure 72.9 Transjugular intrahepatic portosystemic stent-shunt. **A,** An intrahepatic track has been created between the right hepatic vein and the right portal vein. **B,** The track is dilated *(arrow)* and stented, creating a shunt as demonstrated on shuntogram. *(Courtesy Dr. W. K. Tso, Queen Mary Hospital, Hong Kong.)*

Combined TIPS and intravenous terlipressin therapy was performed in nine patients with type 2 HRS.[17] All seven patients who responded to terlipressin and relapsed after treatment cessation responded to TIPS. In another study, TIPS was performed in five patients with type 1 HRS after successful treatment with midodrine, octreotide, and albumin.[30] Complete normalization of renal function was observed in all patients 12 months after TIPS. In both studies, improvement or elimination of ascites was an added benefit.

Extracorporeal Liver Support Therapy

Extracorporeal liver support therapy, as a bridge to OLT, relies on biologic (hepatocytes or whole liver organ from human or animal source in an *ex vivo* perfusion system) or nonbiologic methods, including hemodialysis, hemofiltration, plasma exchange, and hemoperfusion through charcoal or other adsorbent. In a small prospective randomized controlled trial, a mean of five treatments with the molecular adsorbents recirculating system (MARS) effectively removed albumin-bound toxic metabolites (i.e., bilirubin and bile acids), improved renal function, and prolonged survival in eight patients (mean survival, 25 ± 5 days) with type 1 HRS and severe liver failure compared with five control patients treated only with hemodiafiltration (mean survival, 5 ± 2 days).[34] In another study of eight encephalopathic patients (five with type 1 and two with type 2 HRS), MARS improved renal function, bilirubin, prothrombin time, grade of encephalopathy, MAP, systemic vascular resistance, and cardiac output, with four patients still alive without OLT at 3 months.[35] In both studies, therapy was well tolerated. Thrombocytopenia was the only MARS-related adverse event observed.

Renal Replacement Therapy

Hemodialysis and peritoneal dialysis in HRS patients with advancing uremia are both difficult. Conventional hemodialysis is hampered by the invariable systemic hypotension, and the efficacy of peritoneal dialysis is reduced by the presence of large amounts of ascites creating huge "dead spaces." The latter could be overcome by complete drainage of the abdominal fluid between cycle exchanges, but this would result in substantial derangement of body fluid distribution, with resultant hypotension. Continuous venovenous hemofiltration (CVVH) has been advocated for the treatment of advancing uremia in HRS.[36] CVVH allows the administration of nutritional support, which is often vital to the survival of these patients and would optimize their condition before OLT. Furthermore, CVVH is associated with a fall in intracranial pressure in patients with HRS, an important consideration, especially in patients suffering from hepatic encephalopathy, whereas an increase is observed with intermittent hemofiltration or hemodialysis. It is therefore also safer to use in patients who suffer from severe hepatic encephalopathy. Anticoagulation should be minimized or may be avoided totally, especially in patients with preexisting coagulopathy, by giving the replacement fluid in the predilutional mode. When anticoagulation is needed, conventional or low-molecular-weight heparin is generally recommended. Because the liver plays a significant role in citrate metabolism, dose adaptation and close metabolic monitoring would be required for regional citrate anticoagulation, especially after prolonged use. Bicarbonate should be used instead of lactate as the buffer for the replacement solution to minimize metabolic acidosis. MARS may be combined with either CVVH or hemodialysis for the treatment of HRS. This approach may be most desirable in patients who also suffer from severe hepatic encephalopathy. For both MARS and CVVH, the site of dialysis catheter placement should be carefully chosen in a potential liver transplant recipient so that the right jugular and right femoral vein may be preserved for cannulation when going into bypass at the time of liver transplantation.

Orthotopic Liver Transplantation

OLT is the only definitive treatment of patients suffering from HRS. After OLT, the 5-year patient and graft survival rates are about 10% lower for those who had HRS before OLT compared with those who did not.[37] Although renal function improves after transplantation in HRS patients, it never reaches that observed in non-HRS patients.[37] Pretransplantation or post-transplantation dialysis did not affect the clinical outcome. The incidence of end-stage renal disease in the HRS group was 7%, compared with 2% in the non-HRS group. Retransplantation rates and long-term liver function were similar in the two groups.[37] Thus, OLT is associated with comparable liver outcome but inferior renal outcome in patients with HRS compared with those without HRS. This problem cannot be overcome by performing combined kidney and liver transplantation in HRS, which overall produces outcomes no better than with OLT alone.[38] However, in the subgroup of patients with HRS who required prolonged pretransplant dialysis for more than 2 months, combined kidney and liver transplantation did confer an advantage in patient survival and use of hospital resources.[39] In addition, the liver appeared to be immunoprotective for the kidney. The reason for the inferior outcome of HRS patients after OLT is most likely related to the enhanced nephrotoxic effect of calcineurin inhibitors in ischemic kidneys. As the hemodynamic and neurohumoral abnormalities associated with HRS take time to resolve, these drugs should be withheld in the first few days after OLT to give the kidney a chance to recover. A study showed that pretransplantation reversal of HRS allows HRS patients to achieve renal and liver outcomes comparable to those of patients without HRS after OLT.[40] These results suggest that HRS should be treated before OLT, and this strategy may improve the renal outcome in these patients.

THERAPEUTIC STRATEGY AND CHOICE OF TREATMENT MODALITIES

Figure 72.10 is an algorithm for the management of HRS. Recent recommendations for therapy have also been

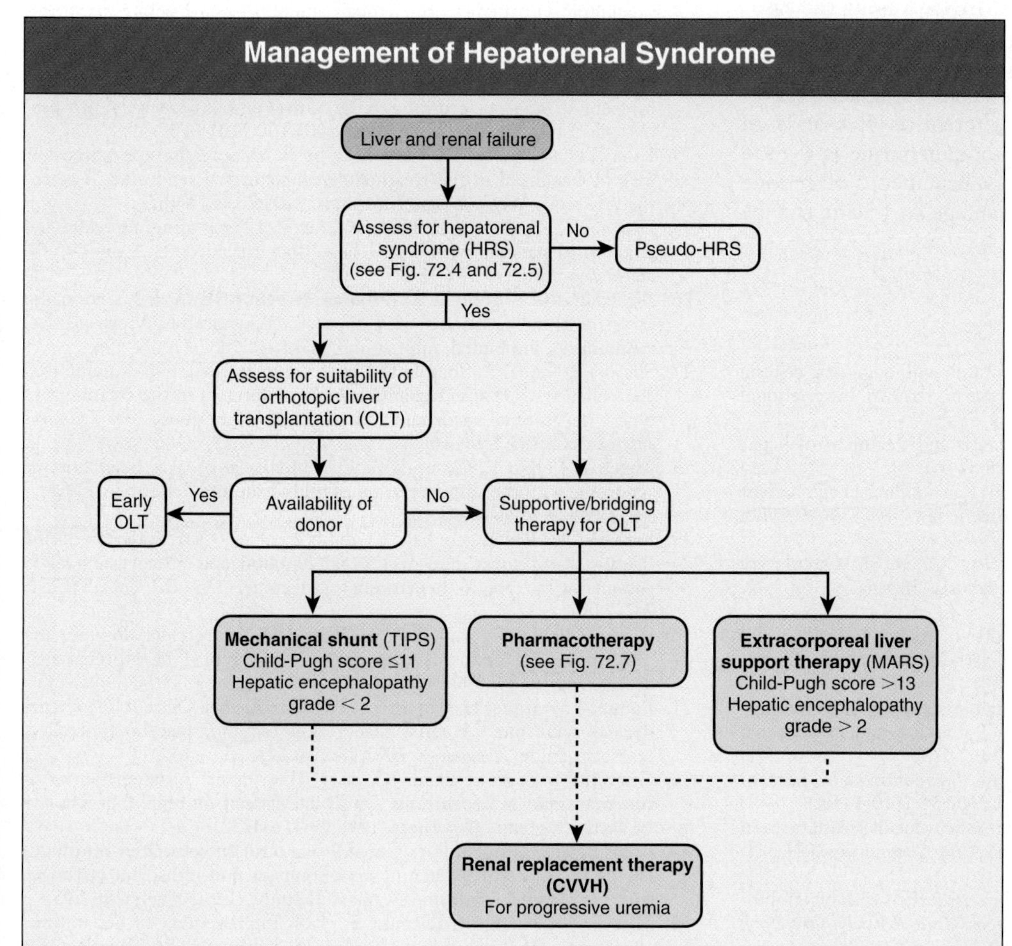

Figure 72.10 Algorithm for the management of hepatorenal syndrome. CVVH, continuous venovenous hemofiltration; MARS, molecular adsorbents recirculating system; TIPS, transjugular intrahepatic portosystemic stent-shunt.

published by the Consensus Workshop of the International Ascites Club.[7]

OLT is undoubtedly the treatment of choice for patients suffering from HRS, but other treatments described earlier may be used as a bridge to OLT, and they may improve the renal outcome after successful OLT. In patients who are not transplantation candidates, these treatments are their only chance for increased survival and, in some cases, may improve their condition to an extent that may allow them to be reconsidered for transplantation. The choice of therapeutic modalities depends on the availability of resources and expertise on the one hand and the severity of underlying renal and liver failure and the general condition of the patient on the other. All patients without clinical evidence of significant atherosclerotic or cardiovascular disease should be considered for vasoconstrictor therapy combined with albumin infusion. In patients with relatively well preserved liver function (bilirubin <5 mg/dl and Child-Pugh score ≤11) without severe hepatic encephalopathy (grade <2) or history of recurrent encephalopathy, concurrent severe bacterial infection, and serious cardiovascular or pulmonary disease, TIPS should be considered, especially in patients with recurrence after vasoconstrictor therapy, a situation more commonly observed in HRS type 2 patients. In these patients, TIPS may have the added benefit of relieving refractory ascites. TIPS also appears to achieve complete normalization of renal function in selected patients after an initial successful response to vasoconstrictor therapy. In patients with severe liver failure (Child-Pugh score >13) and severe hepatic encephalopathy (grade >2), MARS should be considered. In patients with advancing renal failure, CVVH is the treatment of choice and may be combined with other therapeutic modalities, especially MARS. Among the vasoconstrictor therapies, intravenous terlipressin, combined with daily albumin infusion, is most established and is the preferred therapy. In countries where terlipressin is not available, intravenous vasopressin may be used as an alternative. If cost is an important consideration, intravenous norepinephrine is a good choice. Oral midodrine combined with subcutaneous octreotide is another alternative and has the advantage in that it can be administered on an outpatient basis.

REFERENCES

1. Arroyo V, Gines P, Gerbes AL, et al. Definition and diagnostic criteria of refractory ascites and hepatorenal syndrome in cirrhosis. International Ascites Club. *Hepatology*. 1996;23:164-176.
2. Arroyo V, Fernandez J, Gines P. Pathogenesis and treatment of hepatorenal syndrome. *Semin Liver Dis*. 2008;28:81-95.
3. Epstein M, Berk DP, Hollenberg NK, et al. Renal failure in the patient with cirrhosis. The role of active vasoconstriction. *Am J Med*. 1970; 49:175-185.
4. Ruiz-Del-Arbol L, Monescillo A, Arocena C, et al. Circulatory function and hepatorenal syndrome in cirrhosis. *Hepatology*. 2005;42: 439-447.
5. Gines A, Escorsell A, Gines P, et al. Incidence, predictive factors, and prognosis of the hepatorenal syndrome in cirrhosis with ascites. *Gastroenterology*. 1993;105:229-236.
6. Platt JF, Ellis JH, Rubin JM, et al. Renal duplex Doppler ultrasonography: A noninvasive predictor of kidney dysfunction and hepatorenal failure in liver disease. *Hepatology*. 1994;20:362-369.
7. Salerno F, Gerbes A, Gines P, et al. Diagnosis, prevention and treatment of hepatorenal syndrome in cirrhosis. *Gut*. 2007;56:1310-1318.
8. Demirtas S, Bozbas A, Akbay A, et al. Diagnostic value of serum cystatin C for evaluation of hepatorenal syndrome. *Clin Chim Acta*. 2001;311: 81-89.
9. Levenson D, Korecki KL. Acute renal failure associated with hepatobiliary disease. In: Brenner BM, Lazarus JM, eds. *Acute Renal Failure*. New York: Churchill Livingstone; 1988:535-580.
10. Sort P, Navasa M, Arroyo V, et al. Effect of intravenous albumin on renal impairment and mortality in patients with cirrhosis and spontaneous bacterial peritonitis. *N Engl J Med*. 1999;341:403-409.
11. Fernandez J, Navasa M, Planas R, et al. Primary prophylaxis of spontaneous bacterial peritonitis delays hepatorenal syndrome and improves survival in cirrhosis. *Gastroenterology*. 2007;133:818-824.
12. Akriviadis E, Botla R, Briggs W, et al. Pentoxifylline improves short-term survival in severe acute alcoholic hepatitis: A double-blind, placebo-controlled trial. *Gastroenterology*. 2000;119:1637-1648.
13. Uriz J, Gines P, Cardenas A, et al. Terlipressin plus albumin infusion: An effective and safe therapy of hepatorenal syndrome. *J Hepatol*. 2000;33:43-48.
14. Mulkay JP, Louis H, Donckier V, et al. Long-term terlipressin administration improves renal function in cirrhotic patients with type 1 hepatorenal syndrome: A pilot study. *Acta Gastroenterol Belg*. 2001;64:15-19.
15. Halimi C, Bonnard P, Bernard B, et al. Effect of terlipressin (Glypressin) on hepatorenal syndrome in cirrhotic patients: Results of a multicentre pilot study. *Eur J Gastroenterol Hepatol*. 2002;14:153-158.
16. Ortega R, Gines P, Uriz J, et al. Terlipressin therapy with and without albumin for patients with hepatorenal syndrome: Results of a prospective, nonrandomized study. *Hepatology*. 2002;36:941-948.
17. Alessandria C, Venon WD, Marzano A, et al. Renal failure in cirrhotic patients: Role of terlipressin in clinical approach to hepatorenal syndrome type 2. *Eur J Gastroenterol Hepatol*. 2002;14:1363-1368.
18. Moreau R, Durand F, Poynard T, et al. Terlipressin in patients with cirrhosis and type 1 hepatorenal syndrome: A retrospective multicenter study. *Gastroenterology*. 2002;122:923-930.
19. Solanki P, Chawla A, Garg R, et al. Beneficial effects of terlipressin in hepatorenal syndrome: A prospective, randomized placebo-controlled clinical trial. *J Gastroenterol Hepatol*. 2003;18:152-156.
20. Sanyal AJ, Boyer T, Garcia-Tsao G, et al. A randomized, prospective, double-blind, placebo-controlled trial of terlipressin for type 1 hepatorenal syndrome. *Gastroenterology*. 2008;134:1360-1368.
21. Neri S, Pulvirenti D, Malaguarnera M, et al. Terlipressin and albumin in patients with cirrhosis and type I hepatorenal syndrome. *Dig Dis Sci*. 2008;53:830-835.
22. Martin-Llahl M, Pepin MN, Guevara M, et al. Terlipressin and albumin vs albumin in patients with cirrhosis and hepatorenal syndrome: A randomized study. *Gastroenterology*. 2008;134:1352-1359.
23. Peron JM, Bureau C, Gonzalez L, et al. Treatment of hepatorenal syndrome as defined by the International Ascites Club by albumin and furosemide infusion according to the central venous pressure: A prospective pilot study. *Am J Gastroenterol*. 2005;100:2702-2707.
24. Kiser TH, Fish DN, Obritsch MD, et al. Vasopressin, not octreotide, may be beneficial in the treatment of hepatorenal syndrome: A retrospective study. *Nephrol Dial Transplant*. 2005;20:1813-1820.
25. Duvoux C, Zanditenas D, Hezode C, et al. Effects of noradrenalin and albumin in patients with type I hepatorenal syndrome: A pilot study. *Hepatology*. 2002;36:374-380.
26. Alessandria C, Ottobrelli A, Debernardi-Venon W, et al. Noradrenalin vs terlipressin in patients with hepatorenal syndrome: A prospective, randomized, unblinded, pilot study. *J Hepatol*. 2007;47:499-505.
27. Sharma P, Kumar A, Shrama BC, et al. An open label, pilot, randomized controlled trial of noradrenaline versus terlipressin in the treatment of type 1 hepatorenal syndrome and predictors of response. *Am J Gastroenterol*. 2008;103:1689-1697.
28. Angeli P, Volpin R, Gerunda G, et al. Reversal of type 1 hepatorenal syndrome with the administration of midodrine and octreotide. *Hepatology*. 1999;29:1690-1697.
29. Esrailian E, Pantangco ER, Kyulo NL, et al. Octreotide/midodrine therapy significantly improves renal function and 30-day survival in patients with type 1 hepatorenal syndrome. *Dig Dis Sci*. 2007;52: 742-748.
30. Wong F, Pantea L, Sniderman K. Midodrine, octreotide, albumin, and TIPS in selected patients with cirrhosis and type 1 hepatorenal syndrome. *Hepatology*. 2004;40:55-64.
31. Pomier-Layrargues G, Paquin SC, Hassoun Z, et al. Octreotide in hepatorenal syndrome: A randomized, double-blind, placebo-controlled, crossover study. *Hepatology*. 2003;38:238-243.
32. Guevara M, Gines P, Bandi JC, et al. Transjugular intrahepatic portosystemic shunt in hepatorenal syndrome: Effects on renal function and vasoactive systems. *Hepatology*. 1998;28:416-422.
33. Brensing KA, Textor J, Perz J, et al. Long term outcome after transjugular intrahepatic portosystemic stent-shunt in non-transplant cirrhotics with hepatorenal syndrome: A phase II study. *Gut*. 2000;47:288-295.
34. Mitzner SR, Stange J, Klammt S, et al. Improvement of hepatorenal syndrome with extracorporeal albumin dialysis MARS: Results of a

prospective, randomized, controlled clinical trial. *Liver Transplant*. 2000;6:277-286.

35. Jalan R, Sen S, Steiner C, et al. Extracorporeal liver support with molecular adsorbents recirculating system in patients with severe acute alcoholic hepatitis. *J Hepatol*. 2003;38:24-31.
36. Epstein M, Perez GO. Continuous arterio-venous ultrafiltration in the management of the renal complications of liver disease. *Int J Artif Organs*. 1986;9:217-218.
37. Gonwa TA, Klintmalm GB, Levy M, et al. Impact of pretransplant renal function on survival after liver transplantation. *Transplantation*. 1995;59: 361-365.
38. Jeyarajah DR, Gonwa TA, McBride M, et al. Hepatorenal syndrome: Combined liver kidney transplants versus isolated liver transplant. *Transplantation*. 1997;64:1760-1765.
39. Ruiz R, Kunitake H, Wilkinson AH, et al. Long-term analysis of combined liver and kidney transplantation at a single center. *Arch Surg*. 2006;141:735-741.
40. Restuccia T, Ortega R, Guevara M, et al. Effects of treatment of hepatorenal syndrome before transplantation on posttransplantation outcome. A case-control study. *J Hepatol*. 2004;40:140-146.

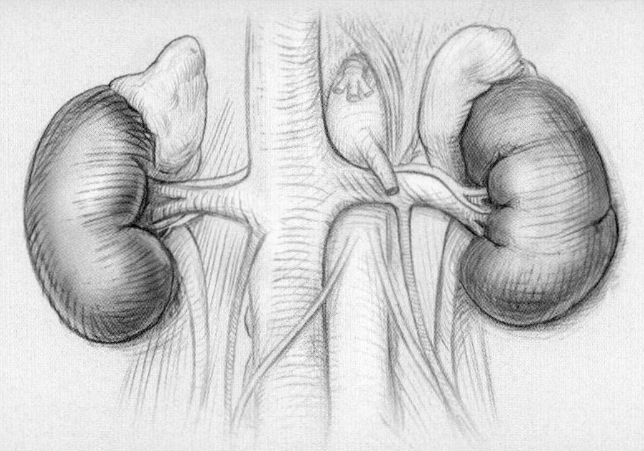

SECTION **XIV**

Drug Therapy in Kidney Disease

CHAPTER 73

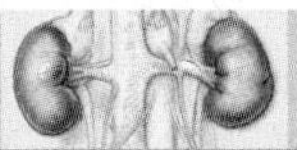

Principles of Drug Therapy, Dosing, and Prescribing in Chronic Kidney Disease and Renal Replacement Therapy

Matthew J. Cervelli, Graeme R. Russ

Renal impairment can alter drug pharmacokinetics and pharmacodynamics, and consequently patients with renal impairment are at risk for adverse effects. In addition, these patients take multiple drugs and are at high risk for drug interactions and drug-related problems.[1] To prescribe safely and effectively in these patients, clinicians should be familiar with the pharmacokinetic behavior of drugs in varying stages of renal impairment and renal replacement therapy (RRT) and ideally rely on data from these populations. Unfortunately, such information is not always readily available. Exclusion of these patients from clinical studies can lead to restrictive licensed recommendations. Although newer drugs are usually studied in small numbers of renally impaired patients, the applicability of this information to individual patients is difficult. This chapter describes pharmacokinetic principles and highlights common prescribing issues in renal impairment, dialysis, and transplantation. Specific dose recommendations and pharmacokinetic data are not included but can be obtained from references developed specifically to provide concise, reliable, and practical information to assist decision-making for prescribing in renal impairment, dialysis, and transplantation.[2-5]

PHARMACOKINETIC PRINCIPLES

Pharmacokinetics describes the behavior of a drug (or metabolite) with regard to absorption, distribution, metabolism, and elimination (Figs. 73.1 and 73.2).[6,7]

Absorption

Bioavailability

Absolute bioavailability (F) is the portion of a drug dose that appears in the systemic circulation after administration by an alternative route compared with the intravenous route. Drugs given intravenously have 100% bioavailability, reach the central compartment directly, and usually have a rapid onset of action. Drugs given by alternative routes pass through a series of biologic membranes before entering the systemic circulation so that only a fraction may reach the circulation.

After oral administration, the liver can metabolize a drug during "first pass" when it is absorbed or later when it is delivered through systemic blood flow. First-pass metabolism can significantly reduce absorption. The gastrointestinal mucosa also acts as a barrier to absorption by metabolizing drugs or retarding absorption.[8] Renal impairment can influence absorption, although the effect is difficult to quantify and the number of drugs for which this is clinically significant is limited. Gastrointestinal edema can limit oral absorption of furosemide. Nausea and vomiting from uremia can impair absorption and contact time between the drug and gastrointestinal mucosa. In advanced uremia, the alkalinizing effect of salivary urea may decrease absorption of drugs optimally absorbed in an acid milieu. Oral iron requires acidic conversion from the ferrous to ferric state for absorption, and acid suppression can impair absorption. Commonly prescribed metallic phosphate binders can decrease drug absorption by forming nonabsorbable complexes with drugs (Fig. 73.3).[9] Changes in cardiac output in renal failure can reduce the rate and extent of absorption for drugs with significant first-pass metabolism. Increased absorption in renal impairment from reduced first-pass metabolism is seen with some β-blockers, dextropropoxyphene, and dihydrocodeine. Comorbidities in renal patients also have an effect; for example, absorption can be erratic in patients with diabetic nephropathy as coexisting gastrointestinal neuropathy slows gastric emptying and the rate of drug absorption.

Distribution

Volume of Distribution

After absorption, drugs may distribute from plasma to an extravascular compartment. Each drug has a characteristic volume of distribution (V_D), which is really an apparent V_D because it does not correspond to an anatomic space but instead relates the amount of drug in the body to its plasma concentration. For drugs with low plasma concentration relative to dose, V_D may exceed total body water. Drugs that are restricted to the circulation have a low V_D. V_D is used to calculate the loading dose to achieve a desired plasma concentration (V_D = dose/[plasma]). Water-soluble drugs tend to be restricted to the extracellular fluid space and have a relatively small V_D. Lipid-soluble drugs penetrate body tissues and have a large V_D. Increased V_D can occur in edema, ascites, or infection, particularly for water-soluble drugs. If usual doses are given, low concentrations result. Conversely, muscle wasting or volume depletion can decrease the V_D of water-soluble drugs, and usual doses produce high concentrations.

Plasma Protein Binding

Drugs can bind extensively to plasma proteins.[10] The free (or unbound) fraction of a drug is usually the portion that exerts a pharmacologic effect. If protein binding is reduced, a greater free fraction is available for any given total drug concentration, which may increase drug activity. Organic acids usually have a single binding site on albumin, whereas organic bases have multiple binding sites on glycoproteins. Protein binding can be altered in renal impairment, especially when serum albumin is low (e.g., nephrotic syndrome) or when uremic toxins displace drugs from binding sites (Fig. 73.4). Predicting the effect of changes in protein binding is difficult because even though more free drug is available at the site of action, more is available for metabolism or renal excretion. Hence, lower plasma concentrations can occur and drug half-life may decrease rather than increase. Phenytoin, for example, has marked decreases in protein binding in renal impairment, and toxicity can occur despite normal or low total plasma concentrations because of an increase in the active free fraction. With albuminuria, bound drug may also be lost, which may partially explain the refractoriness of nephrotic patients to diuretics. In chronic kidney disease (CKD), high plasma levels of α_1-acid glycoprotein are induced in acute and chronic inflammation, which can increase drug binding.

Metabolism

Drug metabolism is primarily a hepatic function converting drugs to more water-soluble entities to promote elimination by the kidneys and bile. Despite the assumption that nonrenal

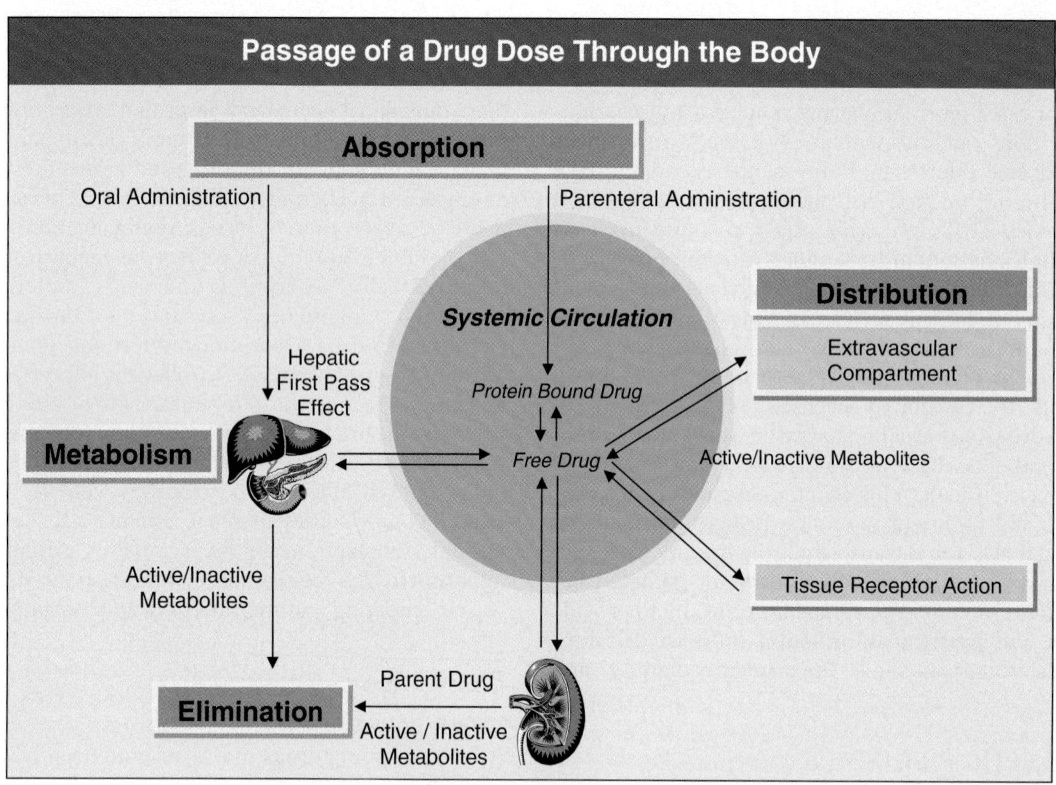

Figure 73.1 Passage of a drug dose through the body.

Figure 73.2 Pharmacokinetic parameters.

Pharmacokinetic Parameters

Parameter	Definition	Application
Bioavailability (*F*)	% of a dose that appears in the systemic circulation after administration by an alternative route compared with intravenously	Determines the amount of drug reaching the systemic circulation
Volume of distribution (V_D)	Proportionality constant relating the amount of drug in the body at a given time to a simultaneously occurring drug concentration in plasma, blood, or other reference fluid at an identical time	Determines the size of loading doses
Clearance (Cl)	Proportionality constant between rate of drug elimination from the body (units = mass/unit time) and the concentration of the drug in plasma or blood at the same point in time	Determines the maintenance dose
Half-life ($t_{1/2}$)	Time taken for the drug concentration in plasma to fall to half its current value	Determines frequency of administration and time to steady state

Effect of Food and Phosphate Binders on Oral Drug Absorption

Drug	Effect of Food
Captopril	Decrease in serum drug levels
Bisphosphonates (oral)	Significantly reduces drug absorption
Cinacalcet	Significantly increases drug absorption
Iron (oral)	Decreases absorption
Ketoconazole/Itraconazole	Increases absorption with reduced pH
Sirolimus	High fat meals increase absorption
Tacrolimus	Reduces drug absorption
Drug	**Effect of Metallic Phosphate Binders**
Bisphosphonates (oral)	Ca^{2+} based binders significantly reduce absorption
Fluoroquinolones	Reduction in absorption
Tetracycline	Reduction in absorption
Thyroid hormones	Reduction in absorption

Figure 73.3 Effect of food and phosphate binders on oral drug absorption.

Protein Binding of Drugs in Renal Disease

Albumin: Binding Sites for Acidic Compounds	
Major Effects	**Minor Effects**
Barbiturates (↓)	Ascorbic acid
Benzodiazepine	Valproate (↓)
Carbamazepine	Fatty acids
Fibrates	Nafcillin
Furosemide (↓)	Phenylbutazone (↓)
Mycophenolate mofetil	Probenecid
Penicillins	Thiopental (↓)
Phenytoin (↓)	Warfarin (↓)
Sulfonamides (↓)	Thyroxine (↓)
Globulins: Binding Site for Basic Compounds	
Major Effects	**Minor Effects**
Digoxin (↓)	Adenosine
Methadone	Amitriptyline
Propranolol	Chloramphenicol

Figure 73.4 Protein binding of drugs in renal disease. (↓) indicates reduced protein binding in renal impairment. For all other drugs listed there is increased protein binding. The therapeutic effect is however not easily predicted (see text).

clearance is unchanged in renal impairment, renal impairment can alter and slow drug metabolism.[11] For high hepatic extraction drugs, this may increase bioavailability. Importantly, some drugs have renally cleared active or toxic metabolites that, although insignificant in normal renal function, can accumulate in renal impairment.

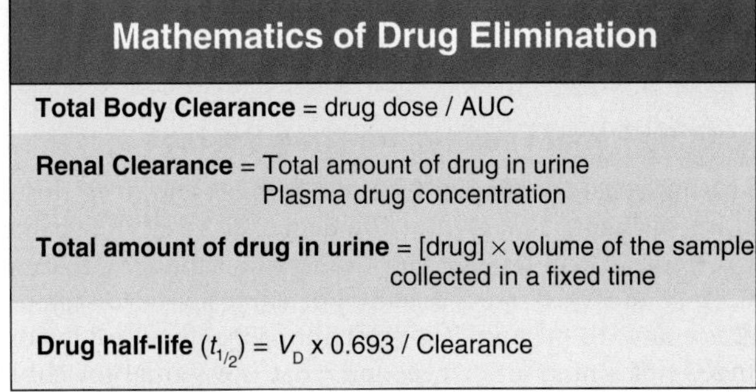

Mathematics of Drug Elimination

Total Body Clearance = drug dose / AUC

Renal Clearance = $\frac{\text{Total amount of drug in urine}}{\text{Plasma drug concentration}}$

Total amount of drug in urine = [drug] × volume of the sample collected in a fixed time

Drug half-life ($t_{1/2}$) = V_D x 0.693 / Clearance

Figure 73.5 Mathematics of drug elimination. AUC = area under the concentration-time curve; V_D = volume of distribution (dose/blood concentration).

Elimination

The kidney is the most important organ for drug and metabolite elimination. Terms to describe drug clearance are shown in Figure 73.5. Total drug clearance equals the apparent volume of blood or plasma from which the drug is cleared per unit of time and is expressed as the dose divided by the area under the drug concentration curve (AUC). Half-life describes the time taken for plasma concentrations to halve and is related to V_D and clearance. Quantitation of drug elimination by the kidney is expressed as renal clearance, which depends on renal blood flow and the ability of the kidney to remove the drug. Renal drug clearance is the balance of its glomerular filtration rate (GFR), renal tubular secretion, and tubular reabsorption. Glomerular filtration depends on molecular size (<10 kd), charge, and protein binding (increased when binding decreases). Secretion of drugs eliminated by tubular transport may change in renal disease, but measurement of tubular function is difficult. Practically, as GFR decreases, drugs dependent on tubular secretion are also excreted more slowly. Assuming no change in nonrenal clearance, as GFR falls, clearance of drugs (and metabolites) eliminated by the kidney decreases, and their half-life is prolonged.

PRESCRIBING PRINCIPLES IN CHRONIC KIDNEY DISEASE AND RENAL REPLACEMENT THERAPY

Ideally, the pharmacokinetics of a drug at varying stages of renal impairment should be compared with that at normal function. This approach underpins many dose modification recommendations. However, lack of reliable data and individual patient factors limit such generalities, and clinical judgment about a particular patient's ability to handle a drug is vital.[12] Dose nomograms, tables, and computer recommendations are helpful but not necessarily associated with better outcomes. Any fixed approach to dosing will probably fail because of the clinical complexity of renal failure. Physicians should use clinical judgment to evaluate every situation individually, choose a dose regimen based on factors in that patient, and continually re-evaluate the response to therapy.

Initial Assessment and Laboratory Data

A targeted history is important in assessing dose in renal impairment. Previous drug efficacy or toxicity should be determined. The current drug list should be reviewed for potential interactions or nephrotoxins. Physical and laboratory parameters indicate volume status, height, weight, and the presence of extrarenal disease (e.g., liver).

Estimating Renal Function for Drug Dosing

Estimating renal function is essential in assessing drug dose in renal impairment. The greater the degree of renal impairment, the greater the potential need for dose modification. With exceptions, dose modification is usually not clinically necessary until GFR is below 30 ml/min. Assessment of renal function for drug dosing is not a precise science, and what is essential for clinical decision-making is awareness that a patient's renal function is impaired, and approximately to what extent, rather than knowing the precise GFR.[13] For drug prescribing, renal impairment is usually graded as mild (30 to 60 ml/min), moderate (10 to 30 ml/min), or severe (dialysis). For drug dosing, methods of estimating GFR are sufficient (see Chapter 3). The Cockcroft-Gault equation has been the most widely used and accepted method for assessing renal drug dosing. The Modification of Diet in Renal Disease (MDRD) formula is not routinely recommended and, if not corrected for body surface area, can lead to recommendations different from those obtained by the Cockcroft-Gault equation. An important limitation of many renal function estimates is the inaccuracy of single-point estimates when renal function is rapidly changing. This may lead to overestimation or underestimation of renal function and underdosing or overdosing of drugs. In severe acute kidney injury (AKI), the decline in GFR is so rapid that patients should be dosed as if the GFR is below 10 ml/min. The opposite is true in patients with rapidly improving renal function after AKI or in the early post-transplantation phase.

Activity and Toxicity of Metabolites

It is essential to consider the activity (and toxicity) of drug metabolites in addition to that of the parent drug itself. Renally cleared metabolites can accumulate, leading to enhanced drug action or toxicity (Fig. 73.6).

Fraction of Active Drug (and Active or Toxic Metabolite) Excreted Unchanged in Urine

The greater the fraction of active drug or metabolite excreted unchanged by the kidneys (fe), the greater the need for dose modification. However, it is usually clinically necessary to modify doses only if the fe of the active component is more than 25% to 50%. The reported fe is often determined from studies that do not distinguish between parent drug and metabolites. The contribution of inactive nontoxic metabolites to overall renal drug elimination may exaggerate the potential for harm. Active or toxic metabolites should be assessed separately for their dependence on renal excretion in the same way as the parent drug (Fig. 73.7).

Therapeutic Index of the Drug or Metabolites

The decision to dose modify in renal impairment is influenced by the therapeutic index or therapeutic window of the drug. The therapeutic window is the range of plasma drug concentrations

Drugs with Active/Toxic Metabolites Requiring Dose Modification

Drug	Active Metabolite	Consequence
Allopurinol	Oxypurinol	
Cefotaxime	Desacetylcefotaxime	
Glyburide	4-*trans*-Hydroxyglibenclamide 3-*cis*-Hydroxyglibenclamide	Hypoglycemia
Morphine	Morphine-6-glucuronide	CNS side effects
Tramadol	*O*-Desmethyltramadol	CNS side effects
Venlafaxine	*O*-Desmethylvenlafaxine	CNS/ cardiovascular side effects
Drug	**Toxic Metabolite**	**Consequence**
Dapsone	Monoacetylated metabolite	
Mepiridine (pethidine)	Normeperidine (norpethidine)	CNS (seizures)
Nitroprusside	Thiocyanate	Cyanide toxicity
Procainamide	*N*-Acetylprocainamide (NAPA)	Arrhythmia
Propoxyphene	Norpropoxyphene	Cardiac toxicity

Figure 73.6 Drugs with renally cleared active or toxic metabolites. CNS, central nervous system.

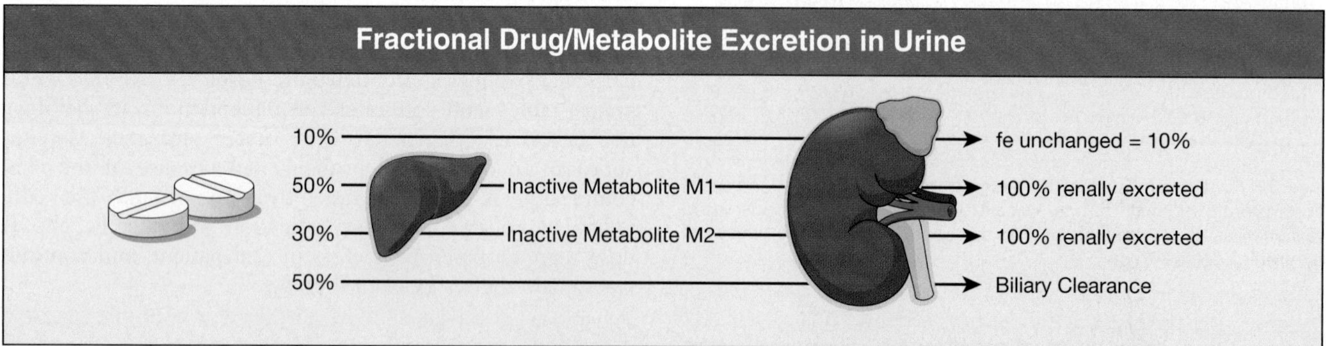

Figure 73.7 Fraction of drug/metabolite excreted in urine. In this hypothetical example, 10% of the dose is excreted unchanged in urine (fe = 10%); 50% of the dose is metabolized to inactive metabolite M1, which is then 100% excreted renally; 30% of the dose is metabolized to inactive metabolite M2, which is 100% renally excreted; and the remaining 10% is excreted unchanged in bile. For this drug, the total excretion of drug dose in urine is 90%. However, this 90% comprises 10% as parent drug and 80% as inactive metabolites, and dose modification is probably not essential even in severe renal impairment. Total renal excretion of the dose is 90%; however, the clinically significant fraction of active drug excreted in urine is 10%.

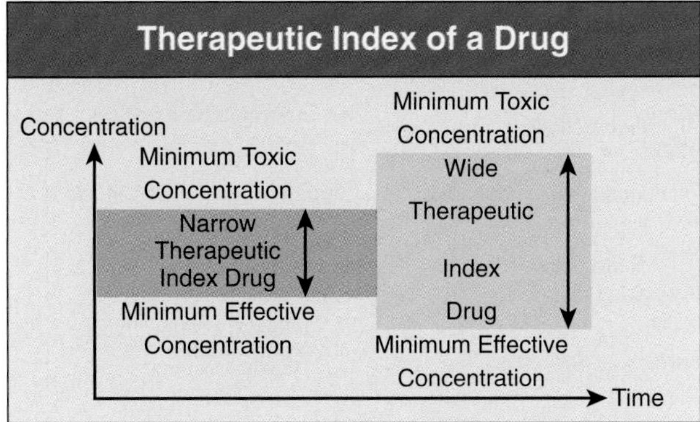

Figure 73.8 Therapeutic index of a drug.

spanning the minimum concentration for clinical efficacy and toxicity. The therapeutic index is the ratio of these concentrations (Fig. 73.8). If the therapeutic window is wide (e.g., many penicillins), there may be no clinical need for dose modification despite significant renal elimination. If the therapeutic window is narrow (e.g., digoxin), dose modification is more critical. The clinician should judge the clinical relevance of increased exposure to drug or metabolites.

Avoid Nephrotoxic Drugs

A wide range of drugs can cause nephrotoxicity (Fig. 73.9; see also Fig. 66.7). Idiosyncratic nephrotoxicity (e.g., interstitial nephritis) is unpredictable and independent of dose. Predictable hemodynamic-related nephrotoxicity can occur with angiotensin-converting enzyme (ACE) inhibitors, angiotensin receptor blockers (ARBs), nonsteroidal anti-inflammatory drugs (NSAIDs), diuretics, antihypertensives, and laxatives. Direct tubular nephrotoxins include aminoglycosides, vancomycin, amphotericin, cisplatin, calcineurin inhibitors, and radiographic contrast media. Obstructive uropathy can occur with tubular crystallization of acyclovir, statin-induced rhabdomyolysis, or tricyclic antidepressants. In dialysis patients who do not have potential for further significant loss of renal function, use of nephrotoxic drugs may be acceptable.

Drugs That Aggravate the Metabolic Effects of Renal Impairment

A number of drugs have no direct adverse effect on renal function but when used in renal impairment can aggravate the metabolic consequences of renal failure. Hyperkalemia is worsened with potassium supplements, potassium-sparing diuretics, eplerenone, ACE inhibitors, ARBs, and the catabolic effects of tetracycline (also exacerbates uremia). Many renal patients are intolerant of sodium loading, which may provoke fluid overload and hypertension. Sodium-containing drugs and those that promote sodium and water retention should be used cautiously.

Effect of Renal Impairment on Pharmacodynamic or Physiologic Mechanisms

Renal disease may alter a pharmacodynamic response or physiologic process that in turn affects clinical response. For example, the inability of impaired kidneys to activate vitamin D precursors means that vitamin D_2 and D_3 therapy may be less effective in renal impairment. Patients with renal impairment often have a coagulopathy due to the effects of uremia on platelet function and may be more prone to the bleeding complications of anticoagulant and antiplatelet therapy.

Effect of Renal Impairment on the Concentration of Drug at the Site of Action

Renal impairment can significantly alter drug concentration at the site of action. Some diuretics and antibiotics are clinically ineffective in renal impairment because they do not achieve adequate concentrations at their site of action in the renal tubules or bladder. This may preclude the use of particular drugs (e.g., thiazide diuretics, nitrofurantoin, and hexamine hippurate) or require increased doses of others (e.g., loop diuretics).

Location of Drug Action

Drugs that have negligible bioavailability and that are used for a local or topical effect may be used safely at normal dose despite toxicity with systemically administered doses. These include topical NSAIDs, nebulized gentamicin, and oral vancomycin.

Method of Administration

In fluid-restricted renal patients, administration of intravenous drug infusions with approved fluid volumes may be undesirable. When administration will exceed daily fluid restrictions, consider alternatives or more concentrated solutions if physiochemical parameters allow. Similarly, oral drug administration with large fluid volumes (e.g., bisphosphonates) may not be advisable. In severe nausea and vomiting, essential immunosuppressants should be administered intravenously.

Drug Interactions

Pharmacokinetic drug interactions are frequently problematic, and awareness of clinically significant interactions is essential, especially for those receiving transplant immunosuppressants. The most important of these are cyclosporine, tacrolimus, everolimus, and sirolimus, which are substrates of both the CYP3A4 enzyme system and P-glycoprotein that are expressed in gastrointestinal mucosa and liver.[14] Co-prescription of drugs that inhibit these systems (e.g., some azole antifungals, calcium channel blockers, macrolides, and grapefruit juice) can increase absorption and reduce metabolism of the immunosuppressant, causing toxicity. Conversely, drugs that induce these systems (e.g., barbiturates, phenytoin, carbamazepine, rifampin, and St. John's wort [*Hypericum*]) can reduce absorption and increase metabolism and therefore increase the risk of rejection (Figs. 73.10 and 73.11). All drug changes in patients receiving transplant immunosuppressants should be considered for their potential to interact and appropriate dose modifications or alternatives used.

Clinical Condition of the Patient

The patient's welfare should override theoretical concerns. Higher than recommended doses may be appropriate when there is a strong clinical indication. For example, excessive reduction in initial antibiotic doses based on renal function may be inappropriate in the setting of life-threatening infection when the consequences of failed therapy are greater than potential toxicity.

Nephrotoxic Drugs

Examples	Mechanism	Prevention/Management
ACE inhibitors/ARBs	Impairment of angiotensin II–mediated afferent arteriole dilation during renal hypoperfusion	Withdraw in renal hypoperfusion
Aminoglycosides Amikacin Gentamicin Tobramycin	In proximal tubules, aminoglycosides bind to anionic phospholipid, are delivered to megalin, are taken up into the cell, accumulate, and cause direct toxicity	Alternative if possible Monitor drug concentrations Avoid multiple daily dosing Withdraw if creatinine rises
Antifungals Amphotericin	Afferent vasoconstriction and direct action to reduce GFR Distal tubular injury via creation of pores that increase membrane permeability leading to hypokalemia, hypomagnesemia, metabolic acidosis due to tubular acidosis, polyuria due to nephrogenic diabetes insipidus	Avoid use Administer slowly with hydration Use liposomal preparation
Antivirals Acyclovir	Deposition of drug crystals → intratubular obstruction and foci of interstitial inflammation	Avoid bolus dose Reduce dose in renal impairment Hydrate during therapy
Cidofovir	Induces apoptosis in proximal tubule → tubular dysfunction, diabetes insipidus, renal failure	Oral probenecid and hydration
Foscarnet	Direct tubular toxicity → acute tubular necrosis, nephrogenic diabetes insipidus Crystals in glomerular capillary lumen and proximal tubular lumen	Hydration
Indinavir	Crystal neuropathy, nephrolithiasis → obstructive AKI	Hydration
Calcineurin Inhibitors Cyclosporine Tacrolimus	↓ PG and ↑20-HETE acid production → vasoconstriction, generation of H_2O_2 resulting in depleted glutathione → decreased GFR, ischemic collapse or scarring of the glomeruli, vacuolization of the tubules, and focal areas of tubular atrophy and interstitial fibrosis	Measure plasma concentrations Avoid interacting drugs Withdraw drug (switch to mTOR inhibitor)
Chemotherapeutics Cisplatin	Cis chloride replaced by H_2O → highly reactive OH radical → DNA injury, tubular cell death Nephrogenic diabetes insipidus, hypomagnesemia (may be persistent)	Forced diuresis and hydration
Ifosfamide	Direct tubular injury and mitochondrial damage→renal tubular acidosis, Fanconi-like syndrome, nephrogenic diabetes insipidus hypokalemia	
Intravenous immunoglobulin (sucrose-containing products)	Accumulation of sucrose in proximal convoluted tubules forms vesicle, ↑osmolarity → cell swelling, vacuolization, and tubular luminal occlusion	Infusion rate <3 mg sucrose/kg/min Avoid radiocontrast Avoid sucrose-containing product Hydration
Lithium	Impairment of collecting duct concentrating ability → diabetes insipidus Chronic tubulointerstitial nephropathy (tubular atrophy and interstitial fibrosis)	Measure plasma concentrations Prevent dehydration Avoid thiazides
NSAIDs	Hemodynamically induced AKI due to vasoconstriction via reduced prostaglandin production	Avoid use Withdraw during hypoperfusion
	Recruitment and activation of lymphocytes → acute and chronic tubulointerstitial nephritis, with or without nephrotic syndrome	Withdraw (add corticosteroids)
Proton pump inhibitors	Interstitial nephritis	Withdraw (add corticosteroids)
Radiocontrast media	High osmolarity, medullary vasoconstricition, ↑active transport in thick ascending loop of Henle → ↑O_2 demand	Hydration pre- and post-procedure Acetylcysteine
Sulphonamides	Intrarenal precipitation → Kidney stone formation	Fluid intake >3 l/day and monitor urine for crystals. Alkalinize urine to >7.15 if crystal seen

Figure 73.9 Some examples of nephrotoxic drugs. ACE, angiotensin-converting enzyme; ARBs, angiotensin receptor blockers; AKI, acute kidney injury; GFR, glomerular filtration rate; NSAIDs, nonsteroidal anti-inflammatory drugs; PG, prostaglandin.

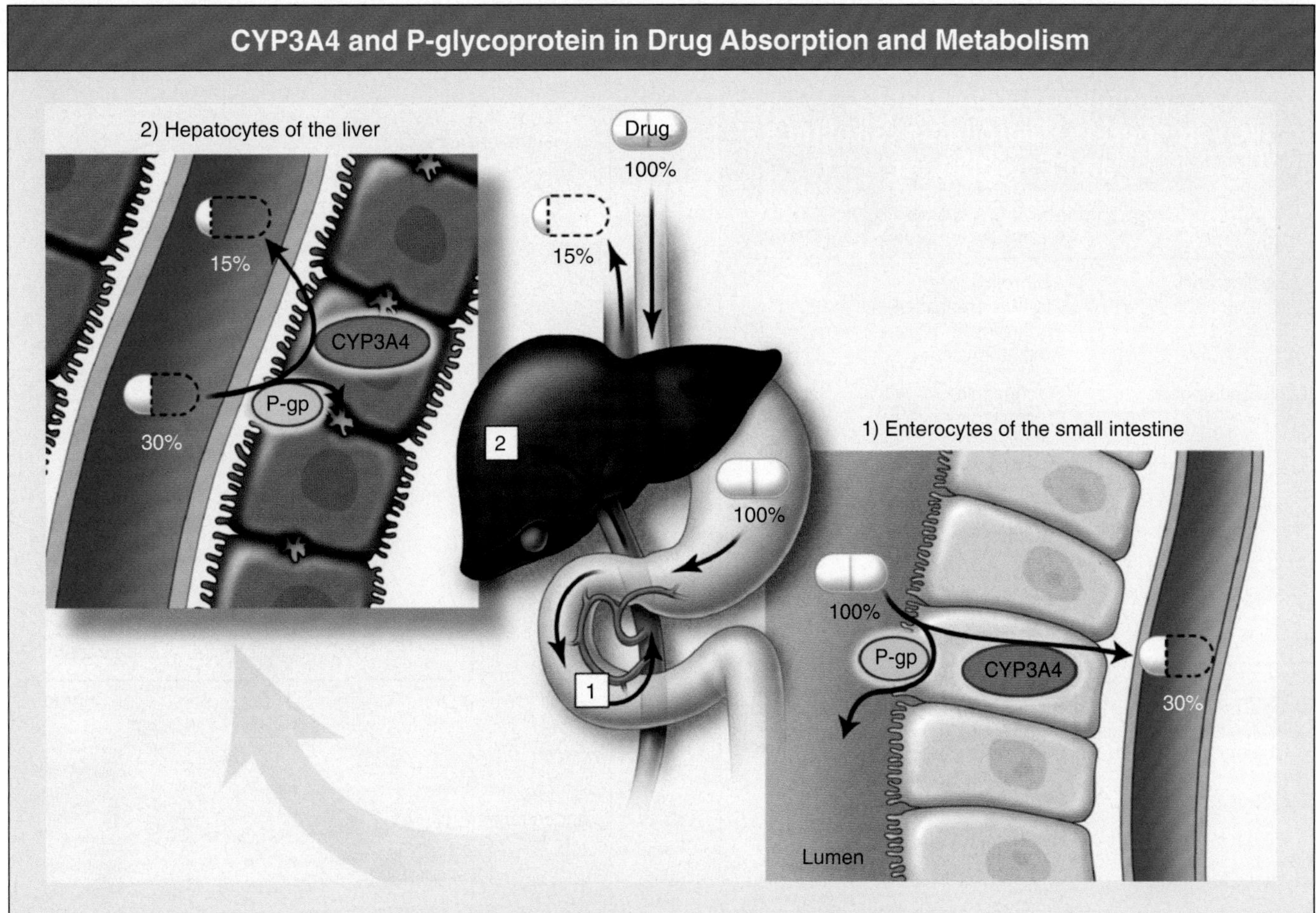

Figure 73.10 CYP3A4 and P-glycoprotein in drug absorption/metabolism. Schema for absorption and metabolism of drugs which are substrates for CYP3A4 and p-glycoprotein. Overall ~15% of ingested drug reaches the systemic circulation. 1) Enterocyte: p-glycoprotein on the apical surface of enterocytes prevents drug absorption, maintaining drug in the gastrointestinal lumen; CYP3A4 in enterocytes metabolizes drug. The net effect is ~30% of ingested drug reaches the portal circulation. 2) Hepatocyte: p-glucoprotein on the cell surface prevents drug entry into hepatocytes; CYP3A4 in hepatocytes metabolizes drug. The net effect is that drug entry to the systemic circulation is further reduced.

Methods of Dose Reduction

Loading Doses

For most drugs, steady-state concentrations are achieved after five drug half-lives. Hence, for some drugs, a loading dose is given to reduce the time to steady state. Because renal impairment may prolong the half-life, simply reducing drug doses could be a therapeutic error because this would further delay achievement of steady state. The loading dose (mg/kg) is equal to the product of the desired plasma concentration (mg/ml) and V_D (ml/kg) and is independent of clearance. Provided the desired concentration and V_D are unchanged, loading doses do not require modification in renal impairment. In some instances, V_D is altered, especially with hypoproteinemia or fluid overload. Hence, some clinicians alter the loading dose of drugs with a narrow therapeutic index, such as digoxin, in renal impairment. Aminoglycoside doses may need to be increased in fluid-overloaded or septic patients who have an increased V_D.

Maintenance Dosing

When specific pharmacokinetic information is not available, and assuming no change in nonrenal clearance, maintenance doses should be reduced in proportion to the extent of renal impairment and renal drug elimination. For example, if renal function is 50% of normal and the drug is 100% renally excreted, a maintenance dose of 50% is required. If the drug is 50% renally cleared and the patient has 20% renal function, the dose should be 60% of normal. The dose reduction factor is usually estimated from first principles or the following formula:

$$\text{dose rate}_{(\text{in renal impairment})}/\text{dose rate}_{(\text{in normal renal function})} = (1 - \text{fe}) \times (1 - \text{fraction remaining renal function})$$

(fe = fraction of active drug excreted unchanged in urine)

Once a dose reduction factor is determined, the clinician must decide on a dose reduction method. Two methods are used either alone or in combination (Fig. 73.12).

Interval Method Because drug clearance is reduced, a reduction to the total delivered dose is achieved by administration of the same dose less frequently. This method is particularly useful when the size of the dose and peak blood concentrations are important for efficacy (e.g., aminoglycosides). If this method is used, practical dose intervals should be recommended (e.g., once daily or alternate daily) rather than inconvenient or complex intervals.

Dose Method An alternative method is to administer a smaller dose at the usual interval. This method is common especially when the size of a dose and peak concentrations are less critical

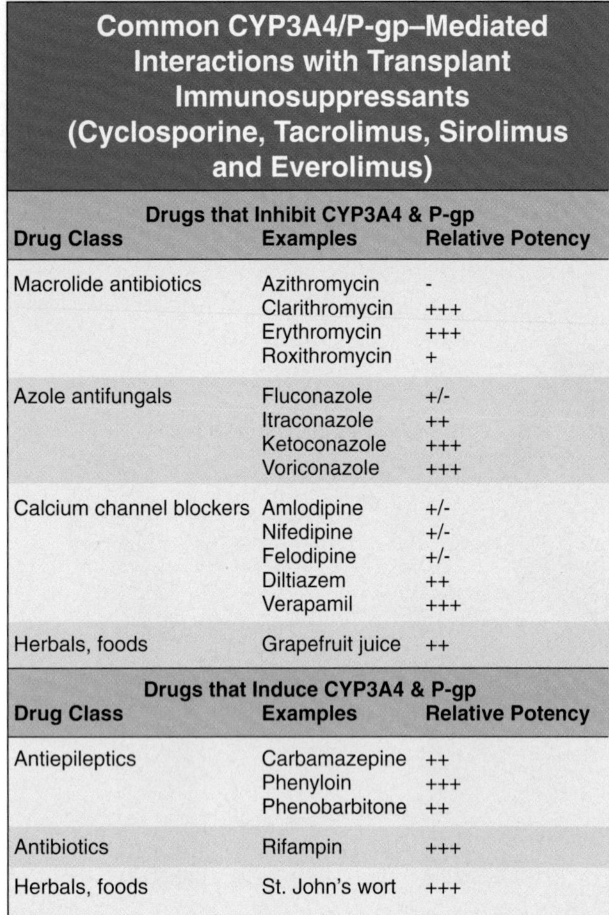

Common CYP3A4/P-gp–Mediated Interactions with Transplant Immunosuppressants (Cyclosporine, Tacrolimus, Sirolimus and Everolimus)

Drug Class	Examples	Relative Potency
Drugs that Inhibit CYP3A4 & P-gp		
Macrolide antibiotics	Azithromycin	-
	Clarithromycin	+++
	Erythromycin	+++
	Roxithromycin	+
Azole antifungals	Fluconazole	+/-
	Itraconazole	++
	Ketoconazole	+++
	Voriconazole	+++
Calcium channel blockers	Amlodipine	+/-
	Nifedipine	+/-
	Felodipine	+/-
	Diltiazem	++
	Verapamil	+++
Herbals, foods	Grapefruit juice	++
Drugs that Induce CYP3A4 & P-gp		
Drug Class	**Examples**	**Relative Potency**
Antiepileptics	Carbamazepine	++
	Phenyloin	+++
	Phenobarbitone	++
Antibiotics	Rifampin	+++
Herbals, foods	St. John's wort	+++

Figure 73.11 Common CYP3A4/P-gp–mediated drug interactions with transplant immunosuppressants (cyclosporine, tacrolimus, sirolimus, everolimus). P-gp, P-glycoprotein.

for efficacy. If this method is used, clinicians should consider the availability of smaller dose formulations and the ability of the patient to accurately and safely divide available dosage forms.

Combination Method In some instances, especially for drugs with a narrow therapeutic index, for which tight control of concentrations is required (e.g., digoxin), a combination of the dose and interval methods is used.

Ongoing Assessment

Even with appropriate consideration and dose modification in renal impairment, clinicians should always remain vigilant and closely monitor the response to therapy to guide dose titration.

Therapeutic Drug Monitoring

Therapeutic drug monitoring can provide objective information to guide dosing strategies and is valuable in monitoring drugs such as aminoglycosides, glycopeptides, digoxin, lithium, antiepileptics, and immunosuppressants (Fig. 73.13). Assays usually measure total blood concentrations and may significantly underestimate plasma levels of the active or free form of the drug.

Clinical Response

Ultimately, clinical response should influence the need to modify doses. Doses should be carefully titrated according to the desired response and adverse effects. For example, blood pressure offers

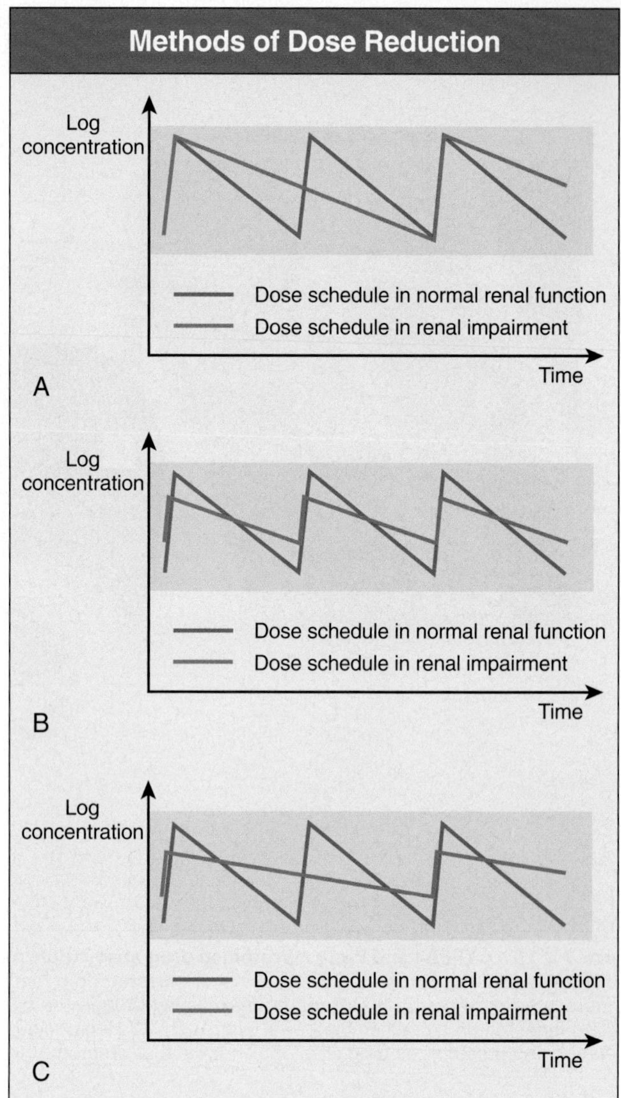

Figure 73.12 Methods of dose reduction. A, Interval method. **B,** Dose method. **C,** Combination method.

the best guide for dosing of antihypertensives; blood glucose concentration and HbA_{1c} for monitoring of oral hypoglycemics; and renal function for toxicity from calcineurin inhibitors, ACE inhibitors, or ARBs.

Extracorporeal Drug Losses

Dialysis drug clearance may significantly reduce drug efficacy if it is not accounted for.[5,7] Alternatively, it may be used in overdose to assist drug removal (see Chapter 94). Studies of drug clearance with different RRT modalities have often used variations in dialysis technique that alter drug clearance and make it difficult to compare results. In particular, many older studies before the 1990s reported data by standard hemodialysis with low-flux membranes, which are less efficient at drug removal than the high-flux membranes now widely used. Many recommendations report the effect of dialysis on the clearance of specific drugs and the need for supplemental doses. Clinically, supplemental doses are rarely used, especially if less than 30% of the drug is cleared or the drug has a wide therapeutic index. Rather, drugs known to be significantly cleared by dialysis should be dosed after dialysis (Fig. 73.14). When drugs are given in multiple daily doses, at

Therapeutic Drug Monitoring in Renal Impairment

Drug	Therapeutic Range When to draw sample
Aminoglycosides (24-h dosing)	Peak (30 min after a 30-min infusion) Trough (6–12-h after dose)
Gentamicin	Peak: >10 mg/l
Tobramycin	Trough: depends on time post dose 0.5–2 mg/l
Amikacin	Peak: >30 mg/l Trough: depends on time post dose 1.5–6 mg/l
Immunosuppressants Cyclosporine	C_0 (trough): 150–400 μg/ml C_2 (2-h post dose): 1200–1500 μg/ml $AUC_{0\text{-}4}$ >4400 μg/ml/h
Tacrolimus	C_0 (trough): 4–12 μg/ml
Sirolimus	C_0 (trough): 5–15 μg/ml
Antiarrhythmics Digoxin	0.8–2.0 μg/ml (trough at least 6-h after dose)
Lidocaine	1–5 μg/ml 8-h after IV infusion starts or changed
Antipsychotics Lithium	Acute: 0.8–1.2 mmol/l (trough) Chronic: 0.6–0.8 mmol/l (trough)
Antiepileptics Carbamazepine Phenytoin Free phenytoin Phenobarbital Valproic acid	 4–12 μg/ml (trough prior to dosing) 10–20 μg/ml (trough prior to dosing) 1–2 μg/ml (trough prior to dosing) 15–40 μg/ml (trough prior to dosing) 40–100 μg/ml (trough prior to dosing)
Vancomycin	Trough: 10-20 mg/l

Figure 73.13 Therapeutic drug monitoring in renal impairment. Target levels are dependent on assay methodology and clinical context.

least one of the daily doses should be administered soon after the completion of dialysis. For some drugs for which the relative time of administration is important (e.g., sleeping tablets, SSRIs, and bisphosphonates), this will take precedence over dialysis-related issues.

Hemodialysis

Hemodialysis drug clearance occurs mainly by passive diffusion along a concentration gradient but also by convectional movement of soluble drug with ultrafiltrated plasma water.[7,15] The efficiency of drug removal depends on physiochemical drug properties. As molecular size decreases (<500 daltons) and water solubility increases, drug removal increases. Conversely, as protein binding and V_D increase, dialysis clearance decreases. Hemodialysis factors influencing drug removal include membrane type and surface area, blood flow rates, and dialysis frequency and duration. High-flux membranes have larger pore sizes and allow removal of molecules of 500 to 1500 daltons. Hemodialysis can remove drug from plasma faster than it can redistribute from tissue, so drug concentrations determined from samples drawn soon after beginning or completion of

Dialysis Clearance of Commonly Prescribed Drugs

Drugs significantly cleared by hemodialysis that require administration after dialysis or a supplement post dialysis	Drugs not significantly cleared by hemodialysis and that do not require administration after dialysis or a supplement post dialysis or that must be administered at specific times independent of hemodialysis
Analgesics Morphine 6-glucuronide (in toxicity) Normeperidine (in toxicity) Aspirin, high dose (contraindicated) **Antibiotics** Aminoglycosides Amikacin Gentamicin Tobramycin Cephalosporins Cefotaxime Cefazolin Ceftazidime Carbapenems Imipenem Meropenem Metronidazole Penicillins Amoxicillin Ticarcillin Piperacillin Fluoroquinolones Ciprofloxacin Glycopeptides Vancomycin (high-flux dialysers) Teicoplanin Miscellaneous antibiotics Ethambutol Cotrimoxazole **Antifungals** Fluconazole **Antivirals** Acyclovir Cidofovir Famciclovir Foscarnet Gancicolovir Ribavirin Valganciclovir Zidovudine **Antineoplastics** Cyclophosphamide Methotrexate **Anticoagulants** Lepirudin **Antiepileptics** Gabapentin Pregabalin Levetiracetam **Cardiovascular** Sotalol **Antidiabetic** Metformin (in overdose) **Vitamins** Water-soluble B, C, and folate **Psychotropics** Lithium	**Anemia** Erythropoietins Iron **Analgesics** Morphine Paracetamol Fentanyl Oxycodone NSAIDs **Antibiotics** Penicillins Amoxicillin Flucloxacillin Fluoroquinolones Moxifloxacin Rifamycins Rifampin Rifabutin Glycopeptides Vancomycin (oral or "low flux") Tetracyclines Tetracycline Doxycycline Minocycline **Antifungals** Amphotericin Voriconazole Ketoconazole Itraconazole **Antivirals** Amphotericin **Antiepileptics** Carbamazepine **Cardiovascular** Amiodarone Perhexiline Nitrates **Anticoagulants** Heparin Warfarin LMWHs **Antiplatelets** Low-dose aspirin Clopidogrel Dipyridamole **Immunosuppressants** Azathioprine Cyclosporine/tacrolimus Mycophenolate Prednisolone Sirolimus/everolimus T Cell–depleting antibodies Rituximab Anti-CD25 antibodies **Antidabetic** Sulfonylureas **Musculoskeletal** Bisphosphonates **Antiepileptics** Sodium valproate Carbamazepine **Antidepressants** SSRIs (dose in morning) **Vitamins** Fat-soluble vitamins ADEK

Figure 73.14 Dialysis clearance of drugs. NSAIDs, nonsteroidal anti-inflammatory drugs; LMWHs, low-molecular-weight heparins; SSRIs, serotonin-specific reuptake inhibitors.

hemodialysis may be low. Samples should preferably be drawn before dialysis or about 1 to 2 hours after to allow drug redistribution.

Peritoneal Dialysis

Many drug properties that affect removal by hemodialysis also apply to peritoneal dialysis, but peritoneal dialysis is usually less efficient.[16] For significant removal by peritoneal dialysis, the drug must have a very low V_D and low protein binding. For most drugs, there is little evidence of significant removal during chronic peritoneal dialysis. A few studies have examined drug clearance from automated peritoneal dialysis that uses large volumes of short dwells at night, often accompanied by one or more longer daytime dwells. Clearance of some drugs on automated peritoneal dialysis is increased because of the increased drug concentration gradient between blood and dialysate. Increased drug dialyzability may occur with increased peritoneal dialysate flow rates or during peritonitis.

Continuous Renal Replacement Therapy

Drug clearance by continuous RRT (CRRT) with arteriovenous or venovenous hemofiltration, hemodialysis, or hemodiafiltration differs from intermittent hemodialysis.[17] Relying on continuous ultrafiltration of plasma water, CRRT can remove large quantities of ultrafilterable drug. CRRT generally uses membranes with larger pore sizes and involves convective transport of solute. Hence, these methods allow the passage of larger molecules (up to 5000 daltons). A large V_D and protein binding still prevent removal by CRRT. Protein binding and the device filtration rate determine the rate of removal. A series of sieving coefficients is available that allows calculation of the amount of drug actually lost if the ultrafiltration flow rate is known.[5] The sieving coefficient is the ratio of drug concentration in the ultrafiltrate to the pre-filter plasma water drug concentration. The closer the sieving coefficient is to 1.0, the more it passes across the filter. Again, there are few detailed studies of drug clearance with use of these methods, and clinicians must rely on estimates from hemodialysis, known physiochemical properties, and clinical response.

COMMON PRESCRIBING ISSUES IN CHRONIC KIDNEY DISEASE AND RENAL REPLACEMENT THERAPY

Anemia

Erythropoiesis-Stimulating Proteins

The pharmacokinetics of erythropoiesis-stimulating agents is not affected by renal function *per se*. However, as renal function decreases, their dose may need to be increased to account for reduced production of endogenous erythropoietin (EPO). Because of the absorption rate–limited increase in half-life of subcutaneous compared with intravenous EPO, epoetin alfa and beta are approximately 30% more efficient given subcutaneously than intravenously[18] compared with no difference between subcutaneous and intravenous darbepoetin.[19]

Iron Therapy

Oral supplements may be sufficient in mild anemia in the early stages of CKD or in continuous ambulatory peritoneal dialysis patients who do not have the same degree of regular blood loss as hemodialysis patients do. Maximum absorption of oral iron occurs with frequent administration of small doses away from food. Gastrointestinal intolerance is a limiting complication, and although this is reduced by administration with food, absorption is reduced. It is important to avoid interactions with drugs whose absorption is affected by oral iron. Patients with severe iron deficiency and those on hemodialysis often require regular intravenous rather than oral supplementation to maintain iron stores (see Chapter 79 for further discussion of anemia management).

Analgesics

Various analgesics (or their metabolites) undergo significant renal excretion or are nephrotoxic, and dose modification or avoidance is required.[20,21] Fear of adverse effects often prevents the use of sufficient doses to manage pain appropriately. Adequate initial doses should be followed by careful assessment and titration to the minimal effective dose for the shortest period.

Acetaminophen (Paracetamol)

Despite suggestions that acetaminophen may be nephrotoxic, lack of platelet inhibition and gastrointestinal irritation makes it a safer base analgesic in CKD and RRT compared with NSAIDs and opioids. Acetaminophen is hepatically metabolized and does not require dose adjustment in renal impairment.

Opioid Analgesics

Opioids have primary metabolites with variable activity and dependence on renal excretion.[22,23] Metabolite accumulation in renal impairment prolongs drug action and predisposes to central nervous system (CNS) toxicity (sedation, respiratory depression, confusion, hallucinations, and seizures), which is often difficult to distinguish from the symptoms of uremia. Regular opioid use in fluid-restricted patients can exacerbate constipation, particularly in peritoneal dialysis. Opioids should be used cautiously in renal impairment, giving adequate doses to establish control and titrating to the smallest effective dose for the shortest period.[24]

There is wide variation in opioid pharmacokinetics and response even in those with normal renal function. Morphine is metabolized to two renally cleared active metabolites (morphine 3-glucuronide and morphine 6-glucuronide). Their accumulation in renal impairment may be responsible for CNS toxicity and respiratory depression or sedation.[25] Morphine is best avoided in renal impairment, but if it is essential, significant dose reduction is recommended. Meperidine (pethidine) is metabolized to a renally cleared metabolite (normeperidine) that can cause CNS toxicity (seizures, myoclonus, mental state changes, respiratory depression, and psychosis).[26] It too should be avoided in moderate to severe renal impairment. Dextropropoxyphene should also be avoided as it is metabolized to the renally cleared metabolite norpropoxyphene, which can accumulate and cause cardiac toxicity. Hydromorphone is metabolized to hydromorphone 3-glucuronide, which has minor activity and does not accumulate substantially. Buprenorphine is metabolized to relatively inactive metabolites, which are excreted in bile, and is relatively safe in renal impairment. Weaker opioids (codeine, dihydrocodeine, and hydrocodone) can still cause CNS and respiratory depression. They should be avoided or used cautiously in severe renal impairment. With appropriate titration, alfentanil, fentanyl, sufentanil, methadone, and oxycodone are relatively safer choices as they do not have significantly active metabolites. The partial opioid tramadol is metabolized to a renally cleared active metabolite, *O*-desmethyltramadol, whose half-life doubles in renal impairment and predispose to seizures, respiratory depression, and other CNS adverse effects. The maximum dose should be lower in renal impairment. In opioid intoxication, naloxone may be used at normal dose to reverse the effect.

Nonsteroidal Anti-inflammatory Drugs

The most frequent nephrotoxic effect of NSAIDs is to cause acute renal impairment by preventing renal prostaglandin-mediated afferent arteriolar vasodilation (see Chapter 66). In healthy individuals, cyclooxygenase (COX) inhibition has little effect on renal function. Nephrotoxicity is more likely in those with a high renin state or renal hypoperfusion, in which renal prostaglandins are upregulated and play a supportive role in maintaining glomerular filtration through afferent arteriole dilation. Use of NSAIDs with ACE inhibitors, ARBs, diuretics, or antihypertensives significantly increases the potential for nephrotoxicity, and these combinations should be prescribed cautiously. When they are required, NSAIDs should be used at the lowest effective dose for the shortest period with monitoring of response and renal function. Increases in potassium, sodium, and fluid retention may also occur in renally impaired patients treated with NSAIDs.

Various NSAIDs cause a rare idiosyncratic nephritis that may present with acute interstitial nephritis or nephrotic syndrome with minimal change disease.[27] This form of renal failure typically has a protracted course. NSAIDs have also been associated with renal papillary necrosis and other pathologic changes during long-term administration. Selective COX-2 inhibition was initially thought to have less renal toxicity. However, because COX-2 is expressed in the kidney, COX-2–selective agents offer no advantage in renal toxicity over nonselective inhibitors.[28] The potential for cardiovascular complications of COX-2 inhibitors is also undesirable in renal patients at high risk for cardiovascular disease.

Drugs for Neuropathic Pain

Low-dose tricyclic antidepressants are used at normal doses in renal impairment, although patients may be more sensitive to anticholinergic side effects. Low-dose valproate and carbamazepine are used at normal doses. Extreme caution is required with gabapentin[29] and pregabalin[30] as they are extensively renally cleared and can cause significant CNS adverse effects (somnolence, lethargy, dizziness, and ataxia).

Antihistamines

Normal doses of sedating antihistamines can be used initially with titration based on response and typical cholinergic side effects to which renal patients may be more susceptible. Sedating antihistamines should be used cautiously in bladder outflow obstruction as they may cause or aggravate urinary frequency or retention. Newer, less sedating antihistamines are better tolerated. They have a wide therapeutic index, and accumulation rarely causes significant complications during short-term treatment. Cetirizine relies more on renal clearance, and dose reduction is suggested. Loratadine and desloratadine have active metabolites but are safe. Fexofenadine is safe; however, terfenadine should be avoided because of the risk of arrhythmias.

Anti-infective Agents

The kidneys excrete many anti-infectives in whole or in part, and dose reduction is often required in severe impairment or extended therapy. However, many others have a wide therapeutic index, and dose adjustment is clinically unnecessary despite their reliance on renal excretion. An important principle of anti-infective dosing in renal impairment is to initiate effective drugs at sufficient doses. Excessive dose reductions may fail to achieve effective drug concentrations. Normal doses or doses larger than expected on the basis of renal function may be appropriate in treating less susceptible organisms and when drug distribution to the site of infection is reduced (e.g., meningitis). Loading doses equivalent to the dose in normal renal function may be appropriate to achieve therapeutic concentrations. More severe infection, particularly in severely immunocompromised patients, may require extended therapy. In urinary tract infection, if GFR is below 30 ml/min and the drug does not undergo tubular secretion, inadequate renal tract concentrations may result and systemic accumulation could lead to toxicity. Nitrofurantoin becomes ineffective in advanced renal impairment,[31] and accumulation causes peripheral neuropathy. Anti-infective prescribing in urinary tract infection is discussed further in Chapter 51.

Antibacterials

Variations in pharmacokinetics of antibiotics with impaired renal function have significant impacts on clinical care.[32]

Aminoglycosides

Aminoglycosides are extensively excreted unchanged by the kidneys and can cause nephrotoxicity and ototoxicity (see Chapter 66).[33] When use is essential, the total daily dose should be reduced, treatment courses kept to a minimum, and serum concentrations and renal function monitored closely. Because aminoglycosides undergo tubular secretion, high urine concentrations are achieved even in advanced renal impairment, and lower doses may be appropriate in uncomplicated urinary tract infections.

Aminoglycoside Dosing Schedules Despite short half-life (2 to 3 hours with normal renal function), aminoglycosides are usually given once daily rather than in divided daily doses for most indications other than endocarditis and in pregnancy. This is based on data showing that their action is dependent on "peak" concentration and that once-daily regimens have reduced toxicity. The required dose regimen depends on V_D and renal clearance. Dosing in renal impairment first involves reducing the "normal daily dose" (5 to 7 mg/kg for gentamicin and tobramycin or 15 mg/kg for amikacin) according to renal function (e.g., with 25% remaining renal function, reduce the total daily dose to 25% of normal). Because of their peak concentration–dependent activity, aminoglycosides should be administered at a minimum effective dose (≥2.5 mg/kg for gentamicin and tobramycin; ≥7.5 mg/kg for amikacin) to achieve target peak serum concentrations (>10 μg/ml for gentamicin and tobramycin; >30 μg/ml for amikacin). The reduced normal daily dose calculated might be lower than the minimum individual dose required to achieve target peak concentrations. If this is true (e.g., moderate to severe renal impairment), it may be necessary to administer the minimally effective dose at an extended interval (i.e., every 36 or 48 hours) rather than to reduce the size of the individual dose. Although commonly practiced, efficacy with longer dosing intervals (>48 hours) relies on a post-antibiotic effect, and it is uncertain whether this effect lasts for extended dosing schedules.

Aminoglycoside Concentration Monitoring Because of pharmacokinetic variability in infection and renal impairment as well as toxicity, monitoring is essential to guide aminoglycoside dosing. It is particularly important at the initiation of therapy or when significant changes occur in renal function or clinical condition. Routine monitoring is not required for short treatment of less than 48 hours. Graphical methods that use a single-point concentration 6 to 14 hours after dosing are valid only with relatively normal renal function. They do not provide information on attainment of peak concentrations and are not recommended in renal impairment.

Trough concentrations can be measured to determine drug accumulation and to reduce the risk of toxicity. Trough samples must be interpreted in the context of the time after the dose when the sample was drawn. Trough monitoring does not provide information on the attainment of peak concentrations and may be below the limit of quantification of some assays. Some patients, especially those with severe sepsis and renal impairment, may have altered (usually higher) V_D, which results in lower peak concentrations. Measurement of peak concentrations (30 minutes after dosing) is the only certain way to determine if adequate peak concentrations are achieved and to assist in determining the size of subsequent doses. Combining peak and trough monitoring provides information on both V_D and clearance and can therefore be used to determine both the size of individual doses and the dosage interval. Provided the relationship between the time of dosing and blood sampling is known, simple dose modifications are made on first principle estimates (see earlier, Methods of Dose Reduction).

Carbapenems

Ertapenem, doripenem, imipenem,[34] and meropenem[35] are significantly excreted in urine but with appropriate dose modification can be used safely in CKD and transplantation. Imipenem can cause significant neurotoxicity (myoclonic activity, seizures, and confusion), especially when it is given in high dose to those with underlying CNS disorders or renal impairment. Meropenem and doripenem may be preferable as they appear less neurotoxic. Imipenem is inactivated by renal dehydropeptidase 1 and is combined with cilastatin to prevent this.

Cephalosporins

Despite being predominantly renally cleared, the relative safety of many cephalosporins means that normal doses of many agents can be used for most short-course therapies even in dialysis patients (e.g., ceftriaxone, cefaclor, and cephalexin). High-dose parenteral therapy and prolonged courses of some agents require dose reduction in severe impairment to prevent electrolyte disturbances and neurotoxicity. Reduction is suggested in severe impairment for cefepime,[36] cefotaxime,[37] ceftazidime,[38] cefoxitin, and cefazolin.[39] Therapeutic concentrations of cefazolin are maintained after doses of 20 mg/kg (~2 g) post dialysis three times per week.[40] Some cephalosporins give a creatinine-like reaction in assays based on the picrate method. This can falsely elevate serum creatinine and be mistaken for nephrotoxicity.[41]

Fluoroquinolones

Renal excretion is significant with ciprofloxacin, norfloxacin, and gatifloxacin, and doses of these agents should be halved if GFR is below 30 ml/min.[42,43] Moxifloxacin is only 20% renally excreted, and dose reduction is not required. Norfloxacin is well secreted by the kidney and thus useful in urinary tract infections. Quinolones are generally well tolerated but have been known to cause CNS effects (headache, dizziness, insomnia, depression, restlessness, and tremors), interstitial nephritis, and crystalluria. Fluids should be encouraged (if tolerated) and excessively alkaline urine avoided to prevent crystalluria. Quinolones show reduced absorption when they are coadministered with compounds containing metals such as magnesium, calcium, aluminum, and iron. As the timing of phosphate binders with meals is vital, quinolones should be administered away from meals and metallic phosphate binders.[9]

Glycopeptides

Glycopeptides (vancomycin and teicoplanin) are extensively renally excreted. Because of potential nephrotoxicity and ototoxicity, dose modification is essential even in mild to moderate renal impairment. Nephrotoxicity is greater in those with renal impairment, prolonged therapy, high doses, and concomitant nephrotoxins. Nephrotoxicity may be less common with teicoplanin. Ototoxicity may involve sensorineural deafness and tinnitus. Permanent deafness is more likely with previous auditory compromise or impaired renal function. If glycopeptides are essential, duration of therapy should be minimized with regular monitoring of serum concentrations and renal function. Glycopeptides demonstrate time-dependent antibacterial activity, so dosing should be repeated once serum concentrations fall below minimum inhibitory concentrations. In dialysis patients, single doses of vancomycin maintain therapeutic concentrations (>15 μg/ml) for 3 to 5 days.[44] Vancomycin is removed more extensively with high-flux than with low-flux dialysis membranes.

Lincosamides

Lincosamides (e.g., clindamycin and lincomycin) are relatively safe in renal impairment and transplantation and are not significantly excreted by the kidneys. A significant adverse effect is pseudomembranous colitis. If this occurs, the drug should be stopped. Fluid management and treatment with oral metronidazole or vancomycin are required to prevent hypovolemia and electrolyte disturbances.

Macrolides

Macrolides are mostly hepatically cleared, and dose modifications are usually not required even in end-stage renal disease (ESRD). However, dose reduction is required with high-dose or intravenous erythromycin,[45] which may prolong the QT interval and cause ototoxicity. Various macrolides are potent inhibitors of CYP3A4 and P-glycoprotein, so there may be significant interactions with and increased exposure to coadministered drugs that rely on CYP3A4- or P-glycoprotein–mediated absorption and metabolism (cyclosporine, tacrolimus, sirolimus, everolimus, and statins). Erythromycin and clarithromycin are the most significant inhibitors, and dose modification of the concomitant drug is required. Roxithromycin is a much weaker inhibitor and usually causes little or no clinically significant interactions. Azithromycin does not interact.

Penicillins

Most penicillins have a short half-life and are rapidly eliminated by filtration and secretion into urine. Many have a relatively wide therapeutic window, and so despite their significant renal clearance, many are used at normal dose for short courses of oral therapy. High-dose parenteral therapy or prolonged high-dose oral therapy may require dose reduction to prevent electrolyte disturbances and neurotoxicity in advanced renal failure. Because most penicillins exert little or no post-antibiotic effect, the amount of time above the minimum inhibitory concentration is more important than their maximum concentration. Severe reductions in frequency of administration are not advised. Dose reduction of ticarcillin-clavulanate[46] and piperacillin is advised in severe renal impairment.

Rifamycins

Rifamycins are mainly hepatically metabolized and used at normal dose even in severe renal impairment. Orange-red coloration of body fluids (e.g., urine and peritoneal dialysis fluid) is common. Infrequently, they cause hepatotoxicity and blood dyscrasias. Rifampin is a potent enzyme inducer and significantly increases metabolism of drugs, including immunosuppressants. Although it is structurally similar, rifabutin does not induce CYP450 enzymes to the same extent. If rifampin use is essential, the impact on the dose of concomitant drugs should be considered.

Tetracyclines

Tetracycline depends more on renal excretion than doxycycline and minocycline do. In renal impairment, tetracycline is anti-anabolic and can cause uremia, hyperphosphatemia, and metabolic acidosis; it may also aggravate preexisting renal failure.[47] Tetracycline should be avoided in renal impairment; however, doxycycline, minocycline, and tigecycline are not anti-anabolic and may be used as usual. Nephrotoxicity has occurred in association with "acute fatty liver" with high-dose tetracyclines. Degraded tetracycline (anhydro-4-epitetracycline) may result in renal tubular damage and a Fanconi-like syndrome.

Sulfonamides and Trimethoprim

Most sulfonamide use is accounted for by cotrimoxazole (sulfamethoxazole in a 5:1 combination with trimethoprim). This ratio was chosen to provide the optimal synergistic ratio of 20:1 in blood; however, the ratio in urine is closer to 1:1. Sulfonamides are eliminated by acetylation followed by renal excretion. Acetylated metabolites may cause crystalluria and tubular damage. Sulfamethoxazole and trimethoprim display similar renal excretion except at extremes of urine pH. Alkaline urine promotes sulfamethoxazole excretion, whereas acidic urine promotes trimethoprim excretion. Accumulation of both occurs in renal impairment,[48] and dose reduction is advisable except perhaps in the initial treatment of *Pneumocystis jiroveci* infection, in which the risk of toxicity is balanced against the seriousness of infection. Trimethoprim inhibits tubular secretion of creatinine, resulting in a reversible increase in serum creatinine[49] that can be misinterpreted as trimethoprim nephrotoxicity.

Other Antibiotics

Linezolid is used at normal dose. Metronidazole has a partially active, renally cleared metabolite, although only 15% of parent drug is renally cleared. It is usually given in usual doses or reduced to twice daily in dialysis.[50]

Antimycobacterials

Antimycobacterial treatment (see also Chapter 52) in renal impairment and RRT requires dose modification according to renal function and avoidance of drug interactions.[51] Of the first-line drugs, ethambutol is significantly renally cleared (80%) and has a prolonged half-life in renal impairment. Dose reduction is essential to avoid visual toxicity. Isoniazid, pyrazinamide, and rifampin-rifabutin can be given in usual doses. Rifampin can cause induction of hepatic enzymes and severe drug interactions with transplant immunosuppressants. Of the second-line agents, amikacin, kanamycin, streptomycin, capreomycin, and gatifloxacin are extensively renally cleared, are nephrotoxic, and require significant dose reduction.

Antifungals

Amphotericin

Amphotericin use is limited by nephrotoxicity (see Chapters 53 and 66). Nephrotoxicity with crystalline amphotericin may be minimized with pre-hydration and administration by continuous infusion. Newer liposomal formulations have fewer infusion-related problems and are less nephrotoxic[52] but significantly more expensive. In maintenance dialysis patients who do not have potential for further clinically significant loss of renal function, liposomal or lipid preparations offer no major advantage except a lower incidence of infusion reactions. Oral amphotericin is not absorbed and does not contribute to nephrotoxicity.

Azole Antifungals

Most azole antifungals (ketoconazole, itraconazole, and voriconazole) are extensively metabolized and do not require dose reduction in renal impairment. Fluconazole,[53] however, is renally excreted; after an adequate loading dose, maintenance doses should be reduced in moderate to severe renal impairment, and it should be given after dialysis. Fluconazole is significantly excreted in urine and therefore the first choice in fungal urinary tract infections. The manufacturer recommends avoiding the intravenous formulation of voriconazole because of possible accumulation of the intravenous vehicle (sulfobutyl betadex sodium). Ketoconazole and itraconazole require an acidic environment for absorption. Given the widespread use of acid suppressants in renal impairment, this is a clinically important interaction. Voriconazole, ketoconazole, and itraconazole are potent inhibitors of CYP3A4 and P-glycoprotein, which are involved in the metabolism and absorption of a variety of drugs, including cyclosporine, tacrolimus, sirolimus, everolimus, and statins. A 2- to 10-fold reduction of the concomitant drug may be required with drug monitoring; however, the magnitude of interaction may restrict the ability to use the concomitant drug. Interactions between ketoconazole and calcineurin inhibitors or mTOR inhibitors have been exploited as a cost-reducing, "immunosuppressant-sparing" strategy. Increased exposure to statins (except pravastatin) increases the risk of rhabdomyolysis-induced renal impairment. Fluconazole is a weak enzyme inhibitor, and although caution should be exercised, the need for preemptive dose reduction of concomitant drugs is less certain. Topical azole antifungals including bifonazole, clotrimazole, econazole, ketoconazole (topical), tinidazole, and miconazole are minimally absorbed and do not cause interactions.

Other Antifungals

Absorption of nystatin from topical and oral preparations is minimal and safe in renal impairment. Terbinafine is hepatotoxic, and dose reduction of 50% is suggested in moderate to severe renal impairment. Griseofulvin and caspofungin can be given in usual doses. Flucytosine[54] is extensively renally cleared and requires dose reduction. All these agents do not interfere with CYP450 enzymes or P-glycoprotein.

Antivirals

Many antivirals (or their active metabolites) are extensively renally excreted and can cause nephrotoxicity (see Chapter 66).

Guanine Analogues

Acyclovir, its prodrug valacyclovir, and famciclovir[55] are extensively renally cleared and can crystallize in tubules, causing obstructive uropathy. High concentrations also cause severe CNS toxicity (cerebral irritation, ataxia, and myoclonus). Strict dose reduction based on renal function is essential. Ganciclovir and its prodrug valganciclovir are extensively renally cleared,[56] and accumulation can lead to severe bone marrow toxicity. Dose reduction is essential even in mild renal impairment. All these agents are freely dialyzed and should be given after hemodialysis.

Hepatitis B and C

Pegylated interferon alfa-2a has a larger metabolic clearance than pegylated interferon alfa-2b,[57] which has higher renal clearance requiring dose reduction in renal impairment. Interferons can upregulate cell surface expression of class II histocompatibility antigens, which increases the potential for transplant rejection. Many oral antivirals used in hepatitis are extensively renally cleared, requiring avoidance or significant dose reduction. Ribavirin and its metabolites rely on renal excretion, and accumulation causes severe anemia; therefore, it is contraindicated if GFR is below 50 ml/min. Some have reported the use of ribavirin in dialysis with dose reduction and drug and blood count monitoring. Adefovir,[58] entecavir, lamivudine,[59] and telbivudine[60] are extensively renally excreted, and significant dose reduction is essential.

Neuraminidase Inhibitors

Oseltamivir is converted by hepatic esterases to its active metabolite, oseltamivir carboxylate, which is extensively (99%) renally cleared through filtration and secretion.[61] The AUC is increased 10-fold in severe renal impairment (GFR <30 ml/min). Although it is well tolerated, a doubling of the dose interval is recommended with GFR below 30 ml/min. Despite intravenous doses showing significant reliance of zanamivir on renal clearance, dose modification is not clinically necessary because its absolute bioavailability from inhaled doses is approximately 2% and high intravenous doses are well tolerated.[61]

Other Antivirals

Cidofovir[62] and foscarnet[63] are extensively renally cleared and require dose reduction in renal impairment. Both are nephrotoxic and require close monitoring of renal function and should be administered with hydration. Cidofovir is often administered with probenecid to slow renal secretion and to minimize nephrotoxicity.

Anticoagulants, Antiplatelet Agents, Thrombolytics, and Hemostatics

The risk of bleeding complications with these agents is increased in CKD and ESRD.[64,65]

Unfractionated Heparin

Unfractionated heparin (UFH) clearance occurs by a rapid saturable mechanism of the endothelium and reticuloendothelial system and a slower nonsaturable mechanism through the kidneys.[64,66] Half-life is slightly prolonged (1.5-fold) in renal impairment, especially at higher doses, when renal elimination is more significant. However, UFH is initially used at normal dose in renal impairment with titration based on activated partial thromboplastin time monitoring and response. In some centers, UFH is preferred in severe renal impairment because its effect is shorter and more easily measured and reversed.

Low-Molecular-Weight Heparin

Low-molecular-weight heparin (LMWH) relies more on renal clearance than UFH does. In moderate to severe renal impairment, LMWHs can accumulate, increasing the risk of serious bleeding.[67] Strong consideration should be given to use of UFH in this setting. Some studies suggest that enoxaparin dose does not need reduction in the first 48 hours of therapy and that tinzaparin is less likely to accumulate. If prolonged treatment doses of LMWHs are used, the dose should be reduced in severe renal impairment and, if possible, anti-Xa activity measured to guide therapy.

Other Parenteral Anticoagulants

Other anticoagulants that accumulate in renal impairment and that should be avoided or used with significant dose reduction include bivalirudin,[68] danaparoid,[69] fondaparinux,[70] lepirudin,[71] ximelagatran,[72] and melagatran.[72] Argatroban may be used at normal dose.[73] Prostacyclin used to prevent platelet aggregation in hemodialysis circuits is rapidly hydrolyzed and not affected by renal impairment.

Oral Anticoagulants

The liver extensively metabolizes warfarin. In renal impairment, it is usually commenced at normal dose and titrated according to the international normalized ratio. Warfarin is highly protein bound, and in renal patients with hypoalbuminemia, there may be increased sensitivity to warfarin.[74] Similarly, hepatic metabolism may be altered in renal impairment, increasing sensitivity.[75]

Antiplatelet Drugs

Commonly prescribed doses of oral antiplatelets (aspirin, clopidogrel, and dipyridamole) do not require initial adjustment for renal function. In acute coronary syndromes or percutaneous coronary intervention, moderate or severe renal dysfunction may influence the choice of intravenous glycoprotein IIb/IIIa inhibitors. Despite their efficacy in reduced renal function, eptifibatide[76] and tirofiban are renally excreted and have been associated with bleeding in this setting. Abciximab is cleared by platelet binding and is not associated with increased bleeding risk in renal impairment.

Thrombolytics

Streptokinase, anistreplase, and alteplase are used as normal in renal impairment, but the high risk of hemorrhage should be considered. Urokinase is also used to unclot dialysis catheters.

Hemostatics

Tranexamic acid requires dose reduction in moderate to severe renal impairment. Protamine and vitamin K are used as normal, as are fresh frozen plasma and whole blood in critical bleeding.

Diuretics

Most diuretics must reach the renal tubule lumen unbound to exert an effect.[77] Pharmacokinetic and pharmacodynamic properties of diuretics can change in proteinuria or renal impairment, usually causing a resistance to their effect. In excessive proteinuria, binding of diuretics to tubular protein can reduce their effectiveness.[77] Tubular secretion of various organic acid diuretics is reduced because of competition from uremic organic acids. The effects and use of diuretics are also discussed in Chapter 7. Diuretics must be used cautiously in AKI or renal hypoperfusion to avoid nephrotoxicity. Diuretic use in the immediate post-transplantation setting may increase urine flow in the native kidneys, giving a false appearance of transplant function. In addition to fluid status, diuretics can significantly alter serum electrolytes.

Thiazide Diuretics

Thiazide diuretics generally become ineffective as diuretics when GFR is below 30 ml/min, although they may augment the effectiveness of a loop diuretic and retain their antihypertensive effects. Metolazone can maintain efficacy at a lower GFR.

Loop Diuretics

Loop diuretics (furosemide, bumetanide, torsemide, and ethacrynic acid) remain effective at low GFR and are generally the preferred diuretics in renal impairment, although higher doses are usually required.

Potassium-Sparing Diuretics

Potassium-sparing diuretics are the least effective diuretics and are often contraindicated in moderate to severe renal impairment because of the risk of life-threatening hyperkalemia.

Antihypertensives

Hypertension is both a cause and consequence of renal disease and may be severe, requiring aggressive treatment with multiple drugs. Antihypertensives should be used cautiously according to clinical response to avoid renal hypoperfusion.[78] Hypotension from hemodialysis may require antihypertensives to be withheld or delayed on dialysis days.

Angiotensin-Converting Enzyme Inhibitors and Angiotensin Receptor Blockers

Although various ARBs and the active metabolites of ACE inhibitors are renally excreted, they can be used effectively in CKD but should be initiated at low to moderate doses and titrated cautiously to clinical response, renal function, and serum potassium concentration. An increase in serum creatinine (up to 20% in the first 2 months in closely monitored patients) may be associated with blood pressure response. All ACE inhibitors and ARBs can cause acute renal impairment by inhibiting the angiotensin II–mediated homeostatic vasoconstriction of the efferent renal arteriole during renal hypoperfusion (e.g., dehydration, hypotension, blood loss, and infection) or preexisting renal impairment (see also Chapter 66). Nephrotoxicity is more likely with coadministration of drugs that reduce renal perfusion, including diuretics, antihypertensives, and NSAIDs.[79] Hyperkalemia is more likely to be provoked by ACE inhibitors and ARBs in those with renal impairment and those taking potassium-sparing diuretics or supplements, which should be used cautiously in this setting. Rarely, ACE inhibitors or ARBs can worsen anemia and increase the requirement for erythropoiesis-stimulating agents.

β-Blockers

Most β-blockers (carvedilol, labetalol, metoprolol, pindolol, and propranolol) are hepatically metabolized and used at conventional doses in CKD according to response. However, sotalol[80] and atenolol[81] rely more on renal clearance. Sotalol dose reduction and titration are essential in renal impairment, although atenolol can be titrated up to normal doses even in dialysis patients. β-Blockers may slightly elevate serum potassium.

Calcium Channel Blockers

Pharmacokinetic parameters of calcium channel blockers are essentially unaltered in renal impairment. They are generally well tolerated and used in normal doses according to response. Dihydropyridine calcium channel blockers can cause significant edema, which can aggravate the edema of renal impairment. To varying extents, calcium channel blockers inhibit CYP3A4 and P-glycoprotein, causing increased absorption and reduced elimination of various substrate drugs, including cyclosporine, tacrolimus, sirolimus, and everolimus. Verapamil and diltiazem are moderately potent inhibitors, and dose modification and monitoring of the concomitant drug are required. This interaction has been exploited so that the calcium channel blocker is used as an immunosuppressant-sparing agent.[82] Other calcium channel blockers do not usually cause clinically significant changes in concomitant drug concentrations, and dose modification is usually not required.

Other Antihypertensives

Methyldopa, clonidine, prazosin, terazosin, doxazosin, and minoxidil are renally cleared but can be initiated and titrated at conventional dosage. However, they are often associated with a higher incidence of adverse effects in renal impairment. α-Blockers cause profound orthostatic hypotension. Nitroprusside must be used cautiously because the toxic metabolite thiocyanate may accumulate in renal impairment but is hemodialyzable.[83]

Antianginal Agents

Most antianginals (β-blockers, nitrates, calcium channel blockers, nicorandil, and perhexiline) can be used as normal, although atenolol may require initial dose reduction.

Antiarrhythmics

Various antiarrhythmics (digoxin, disopyramide, procainamide,[84] and sotalol[80]) rely on renal excretion and require dose modification in renal impairment. Digoxin is most commonly used, and because of its significant reliance on renal excretion and narrow therapeutic window, dose reduction is essential even in mild impairment. Because of reduced tissue protein binding and V_D, some physicians use a smaller loading dose of digoxin than in normal renal function. Cautious monitoring and titration should be exercised to prevent accumulation and further toxicity, which may present as the arrhythmia the drug was intended to correct. When it is possible, monitoring of antiarrhythmic drug concentrations and the electrocardiogram is recommended. Other agents (amiodarone, flecainide, metoprolol, mexiletine, and verapamil) are used at normal doses.

Lipid-Lowering Agents

Bile Acid–Binding Resins

Bile acid–binding resins are now rarely used. The large fluid volumes required to administer them can limit their use in renal impairment. They can interfere with absorption and enterohepatic recirculation of various drugs, including mycophenolate.

Statins

Statins (HMG-CoA reductase inhibitors) can be used effectively in renal impairment and transplantation.[85] Most are extensively metabolized to products with varying activity; however, normal doses may be used in the first instance and then titrated to target cholesterol values. Rhabdomyolysis with acute renal impairment can occur with statins, although the risk does not appear to be greatly increased with renal impairment. The risk increases with use of fibrates and drugs that inhibit the CYP3A4 metabolism of statins. Patients commencing therapy should have lipids, renal function, and creatine kinase monitored regularly.

Fibrates

Fenofibrate but not gemfibrozil is extensively renally excreted, and dose reduction is required in moderate to severe impairment. Combination of statins and fibrates significantly increases the risk of rhabdomyolysis and should be used only when benefits outweigh risks and with monitoring for muscle symptoms, creatine kinase, and alanine aminotransferase.

Diabetes

The kidney plays an important role in insulin metabolism,[86] and thus renal impairment influences glycemic control. Diabetes is also common after renal transplantation due to resumption of insulin metabolism by the functioning transplant and the effect of drugs (tacrolimus and corticosteroids). Various antidiabetic drugs (or their metabolites) depend on renal excretion, and accumulation in renal impairment can cause adverse effects.[87] Patients with renal impairment are therefore at increased risk for hypoglycemia, and drugs should be initiated and titrated cautiously.[88] Management of diabetes in CKD is discussed in Chapter 31.

Diabetes Management in Peritoneal Dialysis

Peritoneal dialysis patients may have higher antihyperglycemic requirements because of the glucose load in peritoneal dialysis fluid. If intraperitoneal insulin is used, dosing may vary from intravenous requirements. Icodextrin solutions can significantly interfere with blood glucose monitoring as a result of metabolites (maltose, maltotriose, or maltotetraose), which falsely elevate blood glucose readings from monitors that use the enzyme glucose dehydrogenase pyrroloquinoline quinone. A glucose-specific test strip is required to avoid interference.

Biguanides

Metformin is almost entirely excreted unchanged in urine, and accumulation in renal impairment can contribute to severe or fatal lactic acidosis (see Chapter 31).[89] Metformin should be temporarily discontinued in situations known to increase the risk of lactic acidosis or to reduce renal function (e.g., acute tissue hypoxia, dehydration, serious infection or trauma, and 24 to 48 hours before anticipated surgery or use of iodinated radiocontrast media). Although metformin is not usually recommended if GFR is below 60 ml/min and certainly below 30 ml/min, low-dose protocols may be considered in a specialized setting. Nevertheless, stability of a patient with renal impairment receiving low-dose metformin does not abolish the risk of lactic acidosis. Lactic acidosis has occurred with doses as low as 500 mg/day, and any acute deterioration in renal function can result in reduced drug clearance at any time. Patients on this regimen should be advised to seek early medical advice in any cases of acute deterioration in health.

Insulin

As renal function decreases, insulin clearance decreases (see Chapter 31). Uremia, however, can cause peripheral resistance to insulin, requiring increased doses. Most insulin regimens can be used in CKD or transplantation with cautious titration and monitoring. Theoretically, insulin glargine is preferable to insulin detemir in renal impairment because the latter is highly bound to serum albumin, and in patients with decreased or unstable serum albumin, a higher free fraction may occur.

Meglitinides

The non-sulfonylurea insulin secretagogues repaglinide and nateglinide can be used in renal failure without dose adjustment.

Sulfonylureas

Sulfonylureas are metabolized and some (glibenclamide and glimepiride) have active, renally excreted metabolites. In moderate to severe renal impairment, hypoglycemic risk is increased.[90] These agents should be initiated at low dose and titrated to response. Gliclazide and glipizide are preferable in renal impairment as they do not have active metabolites. Regardless of which agent is used, the effect of sulfonylureas may still be increased because the insulin released by the drug will itself have a prolonged duration of action in renal impairment.

Thiazolidinediones

Thiazolidinediones are extensively metabolized and excreted in bile. Their pharmacokinetics are not significantly altered by renal impairment and in fact show reduced exposure, possibly due to reduced protein binding.[91,92] However, they can cause fluid retention and edema, exacerbating the difficulties of fluid management and heart failure.[87] Thiazolidinediones have been associated with dilutional anemia due to an increase in plasma volume, which may complicate management of renal anemia.

Drugs for Thyroid Disorders

Thyroid hormones generally do not require dose alteration in CKD.[93] Doses should be initiated and titrated to thyroid-stimulating hormone levels and clinical effect. In circulation, thyroxine (T_4) is 99.98% protein bound (0.02% free) and triiodothyronine (T_3) is 99.8% bound (0.2% free). T_3 and T_4 bind partially, in slightly different proportions, to three different plasma proteins: thyroid-binding globulin, thyroid-binding prealbumin, and albumin. In protein-deficient states (e.g., nephrotic syndrome), there is the possibility of transient or permanent changes in thyroid hormone protein binding that may alter the free fraction of T_3 and T_4, leading to transient toxicity. Uremic toxins can also inhibit enzymes associated with conversion of T_4 to T_3. Oral absorption of thyroid hormones is affected by coadministration with metallic phosphate binders and iron, so thyroid hormone supplements should be dosed away from binders. Hyperthyroid or hypothyroid states may alter the metabolism of drugs, including immunosuppressants. Achieving a euthyroid state helps avoid complications of altered drug metabolism. Euthyroid patients with CKD may have abnormal thyroid function test results, possibly due to decreased peripheral conversion of T_4 to T_3, decreased clearance of reverse T_3 generated from T_4, or decreased binding of thyroid hormones to proteins. Antithyroid drugs can be used at usual doses.

Mineral and Bone Disorders

Phosphate Binders

Phosphate binders should be taken with meals for maximal efficacy. Patients can be instructed to tailor phosphate binder intake to the phosphate content and frequency of meals. Dosing is not affected by renal function except that reducing function increases the need for phosphate binders. Dosing is based on phosphate levels and the need to avoid biochemical abnormalities (see Chapter 81). Acid suppression may reduce the effectiveness of phosphate binders by inhibiting hydrolysis of metallic ions in the gut. Phosphate binders may reduce gastrointestinal absorption of drugs, including thyroid hormones, fluoroquinolones, tetracyclines, digoxin, and immunosuppressants.

Vitamin D

In renal impairment, inability of the kidneys to activate 25-hydroxycholecalciferol to calcitriol may produce relative vitamin D deficiency and hypocalcemia. In combination with hyperphosphatemia, this may trigger secondary hyperparathyroidism (see Chapter 81). For this reason, active 1,25 vitamin D is often preferred to the less active precursors D_2 and D_3, or a combination is sometimes given. Hypercalcemia is the most common and dose-limiting toxicity of vitamin D (see Chapter 10). Patients treated with ergocalciferol (D_2) and cholecalciferol (D_3) at physiologic doses (e.g., ≤2,000 IU/day) are not usually at risk for hypercalcemia. The risk for and magnitude of hypercalcemia are significantly higher with active forms of vitamin D, calcitriol or alfacalcidol; however, hypercalcemic episodes may be shorter and easier to treat than with longer acting substances. Hypercalcemia is exacerbated by concurrent use of high-dose calcium salts (e.g., used as phosphate binders). Calcitriol also stimulates gastrointestinal absorption of phosphate, thus worsening the hyperphosphatemia of CKD.

Calcimimetics

Cinacalcet (see Chapter 81) dosing is independent of renal function except that progressive renal impairment exacerbates secondary hyperparathyroidism. When it is possible, cinacalcet should be dosed with the evening meal to increase absorption and ensure that morning parathyroid hormone blood samples are drawn at least 12 hours after dosing.

Dyspepsia, Gastroesophageal Reflux Disease, and Peptic Ulcers

Proton pump inhibitors and H_2 receptor blockers are commonly used in CKD (see Chapter 83). Acid suppression may reduce the effectiveness of phosphate binders by inhibiting the release of free metallic ions in the gastrointestinal tract.

Antacids

Alginates, magnesium trisilicate, and sodium bicarbonate are useful for symptom control but have high sodium content, which exacerbates hypertension and fluid status. Magnesium and aluminum salts can reduce the absorption of mycophenolate.

H_2 Antagonists

Most H_2 antagonists are renally cleared but relatively safe; in practice, most clinicians do not reduce their dose.[94] Protein binding and V_D are unaltered; however, the bioavailability of nizatidine is reduced in renal impairment. Accumulation of cimetidine[95] produces CNS effects, and it also causes significant interactions through the CYP450 system and falsely elevates serum creatinine.[96] It should be avoided in renal impairment.

Proton Pump Inhibitors

Proton pump inhibitors are generally safe and well tolerated in renal impairment and have a wide therapeutic index. Proton pump inhibitors have rarely been associated with interstitial nephritis.[97]

Antiemetics

Dopamine Antagonists

Domperidone, metoclopramide, and prochlorperazine are not significantly renally cleared and can be used in CKD; however, extrapyramidal and CNS effects may be more prevalent, especially in high dose. Dosing should be cautiously titrated to effect. Domperidone does not cross the blood-brain barrier and may be preferable for long-term management. Metoclopramide and domperidone increase gastric emptying, which may alter drug pharmacokinetics.

5-HT_3 Antagonists

Most 5-HT_3 antagonists are minimally excreted in urine with a wide therapeutic window. Dolasetron, granisetron, ondansetron, and tropisetron are safe, and dose modification is not required.

Aperients and Laxatives

Common low-potency agents including docusate, bisacodyl, glycerin, lactulose, liquid paraffin, senna, and sorbitol may be used for acute or chronic constipation in renal impairment. Normal doses should be titrated to effect while avoiding significant dehydration, fluid shifts, or electrolyte disturbances. High-potency laxatives and bowel preparations should be used cautiously. They can cause significant fluid and electrolyte disturbances, especially in susceptible renal patients. Preparations containing high amounts of phosphate should be avoided. Despite the large fluid volumes required for administration, iso-osmotic laxatives may be used for bowel preparation in renal impairment and dialysis.

Antidiarrheals

Opioids or their derivatives should be used with the same caution as when they are used as analgesics. Loperamide and diphenoxylate-atropine can be given in usual dose.

Antiobesity Drugs

Drug therapy for obesity can prevent absorption of intestinal material or suppress appetite, which may cause nutrient deficiency. Sibutramine is used without modification, although it can increase heart rate and blood pressure. Sympathomimetics can cause CNS stimulation. Laxative and diuretic use is discouraged as they predispose to fluid and electrolyte disorders and renal hypoperfusion.

Drugs for Erectile Dysfunction

Phosphodiesterase-5 Inhibitors

The AUCs of sildenafil (twofold), tadalafil (fourfold), and vardenafil (20% to 30%) are increased in severe renal impairment despite minimal dependence on renal excretion.[98] However, provided relevant cardiovascular and drug contraindications are excluded, phosphodiesterase-5 inhibitors can be used in renal impairment and transplantation. They should be initiated at low dose and titrated to response. In renal impairment, shorter acting agents (sildenafil and vardenafil) may be preferable. Vardenafil can prolong the QT interval.

Intracavernosal Therapy

Drugs given directly by intracavernosal injection do not achieve significant concentrations in the systemic circulation and can be used in renal impairment.

Immunosuppressants

Immunosuppression in renal transplantation as well as its adverse effects is discussed in Chapters 97 and 103. In organ transplantation, immunosuppressants from different classes are combined to increase efficacy and to minimize adverse effects. Initial and maintenance doses in any individual are highly variable and depend on local protocol, concomitant therapy, risk of rejection, serum drug concentrations, and response. Immunosuppression is required for the life of the transplant and should never be withheld except in exceptional circumstance (life-threatening infection or malignant disease). Regimens should preferably be limited to twice daily, spread at convenient times about 12 hours apart. In practice, the precise timing of doses or intake relative to time and food is not as important as consistency in relation to time and food. Patients should take their medications consistently, and doses can be titrated to levels and response. Most immunosuppressants are cleared by hepatic metabolism and require little or no dose modification based on altered drug excretion in renal impairment.

Immunosuppressants are prone to a range of significant drug interactions. As the consequences of altered drug action are so great, all changes to drug regimens in transplant patients should be considered for their potential to interact. Significant interactions can also occur with "natural" or "herbal" medicines (e.g., St. John's Wort; see also Chapter 74). If these products are deemed essential, it is advisable to monitor response, renal function, blood counts, and serum drug concentrations regularly. Therapeutic monitoring is recommended for several immunosuppressants[99] (tacrolimus, cyclosporine, everolimus, sirolimus, and mycophenolate). Target levels should be interpreted in the context of the patient's response, immunosuppressive regimen, time after transplantation, and assay methodology.[100] Pharmacokinetics may vary in relation to food (e.g., tacrolimus) or concomitant drugs (e.g., sirolimus with or without cyclosporine), so blood sampling should aim to reflect the patient's usual routine.

Calcineurin Inhibitors

Calcineurin inhibitors are extensively metabolized to numerous inactive metabolites, and initial dosing is not adjusted on the basis of altered exposure in renal impairment. The major toxicity of calcineurin inhibitors is nephrotoxicity (acute and chronic),[101] and regular assessment of renal function is essential. Nephrotoxicity may increase with concurrent use of mTOR inhibitors (sirolimus and everolimus). Early detection of calcineurin inhibitor nephrotoxicity on biopsy assists in planning maintenance therapy (see Chapters 97 and 103). Because of nephrotoxicity, lower doses or temporary withdrawal may be used when calcineurin inhibitors have caused or are likely to cause nephrotoxicity (e.g., delayed graft function).

Calcineurin inhibitors are substrates of P-glycoprotein and CYP3A4. Drugs that inhibit or compete as substrates for these enzymes can increase absorption and reduce metabolism of calcineurin inhibitors, causing increased serum concentrations and adverse effects. Drugs that induce these enzymes can reduce absorption and increase metabolism of calcineurin inhibitors, causing reduced serum concentrations, and increase the risk of rejection (see Fig. 73.11). Cyclosporine but not tacrolimus interferes with the enterohepatic recirculation of mycophenolate, and so the mycophenolate dose may need to be higher if it is coadministered with cyclosporine compared with the use of mycophenolate alone or with other immunosuppressants. Tacrolimus trough concentrations (C_0) show good correlation with drug exposure (AUC) and are used to monitor therapy. Debate remains about the optimal method of monitoring cyclosporine. Clinically, a combination of C_0 (trough), C_2 (concentration 2 hours post dose), and $AUC_{0\text{-}4}$ (multipoint area under curve, 0 to 4 hours) are used. Different assay methodologies (high-performance liquid chromatography [HPLC], immunoassays) have differing ability to detect parent compound from metabolites. Specific HPLC methods are recommended, and results from different laboratories may not be interchangeable.[100]

Corticosteroids

Corticosteroids are predominantly cleared by hepatic metabolism to inactive metabolites. Dose modification based on impaired renal function is not required.

Antiproliferative and Cytotoxic Agents

Various antiproliferatives and cytotoxics are used to prevent rejection (azathioprine and mycophenolate) and in autoimmune and inflammatory disorders (azathioprine, cyclophosphamide, chlorambucil, methotrexate, and mycophenolate). Their primary dose-limiting toxicity is bone marrow suppression, which is exacerbated by combined use with other bone marrow suppressants (e.g., ganciclovir, cotrimoxazole, and mTOR inhibitors). Regular blood monitoring is needed to guide dosing in renal impairment and transplantation.

Methotrexate relies significantly on renal clearance and should be avoided or used cautiously at a significantly reduced dose. It can also cause obstructive uropathy. Renal clearance is significant with cyclophosphamide[102] (which also causes hemorrhagic cystitis) and chlorambucil, and dose modification is required. Accumulation of mycophenolate metabolites in severe renal impairment predisposes to adverse effects. Allopurinol significantly interferes with the metabolism of the active metabolite of azathioprine (6-mercaptopurine), and co-prescription can lead to life-threatening bone marrow suppression. The combination should be avoided by exchanging azathioprine with mycophenolate or by significant (75%) dose reduction of azathioprine or mercaptopurine.

mTOR Inhibitors

Although not nephrotoxic when they are used alone, mTOR inhibitors (sirolimus, everolimus) can potentiate the nephrotoxicity of calcineurin inhibitors, particularly in ongoing maintenance therapy. mTOR inhibitors are almost entirely hepatically metabolized to essentially inactive metabolites. Dosing is independent of renal function and based on clinical situation, serum drug levels, and specific toxicities (especially hematologic and lipids). mTOR inhibitors are substrates of CYP3A4 and P-glycoprotein. Drugs that inhibit or compete as substrates for these enzymes can increase absorption and reduce metabolism of mTOR inhibitors, causing increased blood concentrations and adverse effects. Drugs that induce these enzymes can reduce absorption and increase metabolism of mTORs and consequently reduce serum concentrations and increase the risk of rejection (see Fig. 73.11). Bone marrow toxicity (neutropenia, anemia, and thrombocytopenia) is increased when they are used in combination with other myelosuppressants (azathioprine, mycophenolate, ganciclovir, and cotrimoxazole). Trough levels show good correlation with drug exposure (AUC) and are used to monitor mTOR inhibitor therapy. Different assay methodologies (HPLC versus immunoassays) vary in their ability to detect parent drug from metabolites. Specific HPLC methods are recommended, and results from different laboratories or methods may not be interchangeable.

Immunosuppressant Antibodies

Biologic agents used for immunosuppression include T cell–depleting antibodies (antithymocyte globulin, anti-CD3 antibodies [OKT3]), anti–interleukin-2 receptor (CD25) antibodies (basiliximab and daclizumab), and B cell–depleting antibodies (rituximab). Their use and adverse effects are discussed in Chapter 97. Dosing of these agents is independent of renal function, and they should be administered after concurrent plasma exchange[103] to avoid drug removal. They are not removed by hemodialysis.

Musculoskeletal Drugs

Nonsteroidal Anti-Inflammatory Drugs

NSAIDs can cause significant nephrotoxicity (see Chapter 66) and should be avoided or used with extreme caution in patients with renal impairment and in transplantation.

Miscellaneous Arthritis Drugs

Gold salts and penicillamine[104] are now rarely used for rheumatoid arthritis; both were associated with nephrotic syndrome due to membranous nephropathy. Glucosamine and fish oil have been used without apparent increase in toxicity in renal impairment or transplantation.

Gout and Hyperuricemia

Gout is highly prevalent in renal impairment, and treatment is complicated by several factors. In acute therapy, short courses of oral corticosteroids are safe and often preferable in renal impairment and transplantation and avoid the need for NSAIDs. Colchicine[105] accumulation in renal impairment may cause diarrhea and hypoperfusion-induced renal impairment as well as myelosuppression. It is best avoided or used at lower doses with careful attention to avoid gastrointestinal and hematologic toxicity. In maintenance therapy, allopurinol is effective but should initially be dose reduced in moderate to severe renal impairment because of formation of a renally cleared active metabolite (oxypurinol).[106] Despite this, some ESRD patients tolerate normal doses. Allopurinol significantly interacts with azathioprine, with a risk of severe myelosuppression. If the combination is unavoidable, the dose of azathioprine should be reduced to 75% and blood counts monitored carefully. Uricosuric agents (e.g., probenecid) inhibit secretion of acids in the proximal tubule and prevent reabsorption of uric acid from the tubular lumen. They often become ineffective with diminishing renal function and are best avoided if the GFR is below 40 ml/min unless clear benefit is demonstrated.[107] Probenecid also interferes with the tubular secretion of many drugs, causing interactions.

Bisphosphonates

Bisphosphonates are extensively excreted in urine. The fraction not excreted is incorporated into bone, from which it slowly dissociates. In renal impairment, impaired clearance of absorbed drug may increase the fraction available for incorporation into bone and thus the risk of adynamic bone disease. Their long terminal elimination half-life reflects rate-limiting dissociation from bone and may not significantly be altered in renal impairment. Oral bisphosphonates appear to be safe in stage 2 to stage 3 CKD.[108] Their safety in CKD stages 4 and 5 is less well established; they may worsen low bone turnover in adynamic bone disease. Rapid administration of intravenous bisphosphonates (pamidronate and zoledronic acid[109]) without hydration has been associated with acute nephrotoxicity. Intravenous preparations should be administered slowly with hydration, and renal function should be assessed regularly. Oral bisphosphonate dosing may be complicated by the volumes of fluid recommended for administration. In addition, many patients with renal impairment are taking calcium-based phosphate binders or supplements that impair the absorption of oral bisphosphonates. Once-weekly dosing given at least 30 minutes before food and any calcium-based medications or supplements is preferable to daily doses. This reduces the total weekly fluid load required to administer the tablets and helps ensure absorption.

Antiepileptics

Renally impaired patients may be more prone to seizures (e.g., uremic encephalopathy and dialysis disequilibrium syndrome) and to the CNS effects of antiepileptics. Some antiepileptics rely on renal excretion, and dose modification is essential. Some antiepileptics (barbiturates, phenytoin, and carbamazepine) are strong inducers of drug-metabolizing enzymes. Coadministration with drugs reliant on hepatic metabolism (e.g., immunosuppressants) can reduce exposure and efficacy of the concomitant drug. Therapeutic drug monitoring is available for many antiepileptics and should be used to guide dosing.

Barbiturates

Phenobarbitone and primidone are now rarely used. Significant amounts of active drug and metabolites are excreted in urine, necessitating lower initial doses. Patients with renal impairment may be more prone to CNS adverse effects, such as sedation. Barbiturates are potent enzyme inducers, and care must be taken to account for drug interactions, particularly in transplantation. In renal impairment, barbiturates should be titrated cautiously to response, adverse effects, and drug concentrations.

Benzodiazepines

See later, Psychotropic Drugs.

Carbamazepine

Carbamazepine is initially dosed as normal in renal impairment and titrated to response and blood concentrations. It is a potent enzyme inducer, and care must be taken to account for important drug interactions, particularly in the transplant setting.

Gabapentin and Pregabalin

Extreme caution is advised with pregabalin[30] and gabapentin[29] as they are almost completely renally cleared. Accumulation in renal impairment causes significant CNS adverse effects (somnolence, lethargy, dizziness, and ataxia). They should be avoided or used extremely cautiously at significantly lower doses even in mild to moderate renal impairment. Both are freely dialyzable, which can be beneficial in overdose.

Phenytoin

Caution should be exercised with phenytoin in renal impairment because of its erratic absorption, saturable metabolism, nonlinear pharmacokinetics, reduced protein binding, and increased V_D. The concentration of free drug may be higher than in those with normal renal function; because most laboratories measure total drug concentration, a low serum total phenytoin level in renal impairment should not be mistaken as subtherapeutic. Nystagmus, cerebellar ataxia, and seizures can occur in overdose, and small dose increases may result in disproportionate increases in serum concentrations. Physical findings such as nystagmus are helpful in deciding not to increase the dose. Cautious titration based on effect and monitoring of free plasma concentration is advised. Phenytoin is a potent enzyme-inducing agent, and care must be taken to account for drug interactions, especially in the transplant setting.

Other Antiepileptics

Levetiracetam, topiramate, and vigabatrin undergo significant renal excretion, and dose modification is required in renal impairment. Valproate and lamotrigine are not significantly renally excreted and do not cause enzyme induction or inhibition. They are initiated as normal in renal impairment and transplantation with titration according to concentration and effect. Protein binding changes can increase the free fraction of valproic acid, predisposing to increased responsiveness.

Antiparkinsonian Drugs

In addition to their use in Parkinson's disease and hyperprolactinemia disorders, dopaminergic drugs are used to treat restless legs and other limb movement disorders in renal impairment. Most are hepatically cleared and safe in renal impairment and transplantation, although dopaminergic agents may exacerbate postural hypotension. Amantadine[110] is highly dependent on renal excretion, and dose modification is essential.

Antimigraine Drugs

Simple analgesics (acetaminophen) are used as normal, although aspirin should be avoided at therapeutic doses and opioids used cautiously (see Analgesics). NSAIDs are best avoided because of potential nephrotoxicity. 5-HT_1 agonists are effective in renal impairment and transplantation. Naratriptan relies the most on renal excretion (50%), and a lower maximum dose is recommended. Sumatriptan and zolmitriptan are preferred as they are less dependent on renal excretion.

Psychotropic Drugs

Most psychotropics are fat soluble, are nondialyzable, undergo significant hepatic metabolism, and are excreted as inactive compounds. Even so, patients with renal impairment are often more susceptible to common adverse effects (especially CNS effects).[111,112] Consequently, slow titration and dose modifications are required. Adverse effects are not easily distinguished from symptoms of uremia. Despite being metabolized extensively by CYP450 enzymes, very few psychotropics cause clinically significant inhibition or induction of CYP3A4.

Monoamine Oxidase Inhibitors

Monoamine oxidase inhibitors are extensively metabolized by the liver. Although they are less commonly used in current practice, normal doses of reversible monoamine oxidase inhibitors (moclobemide) are preferred, and these can be titrated cautiously up to full doses in renal impairment. Monoamine oxidase inhibitors can cause peripheral edema, which is not usually associated with fluid retention and is unresponsive to diuretics. Prostatic hypertrophy and urinary retention may also occur.

Serotonin-Specific Reuptake Inhibitors

Serotonin-specific reuptake inhibitors (SSRIs) have become the most common drugs for treating depression in renal impairment and transplantation. Most are extensively metabolized to compounds without significant SSRI activity.[113] Normal doses of most SSRIs (citalopram, fluvoxamine, paroxetine, and sertraline) can be used with cautious dose titration. Fluoxetine is metabolized to an active metabolite (norfluoxetine), but single- and multiple-dose studies have shown little change in pharmacokinetics even in dialysis patients.[114] Patients with renal impairment may be more prone to the CNS toxicity of SSRIs and serotonin syndrome. SSRIs can cause the syndrome of inappropriate antidiuretic hormone secretion and platelet aggregation or hemorrhagic complications, which theoretically increases the risk of bleeding in uremic patients who are already prone to bleeding complications. SSRIs vary in their potential to inhibit CYP450 enzymes, with citalopram having the lowest capacity. Although most SSRIs have some inhibitory effect on CYP3A4, this is usually not significant. Fluoxetine and fluvoxamine are more likely to interact than citalopram and sertraline, but all can be used in patients taking immunosuppressants. Cinacalcet can cause significant inhibition of CYP2D6-mediated metabolism of SSRIs and perhexiline. This may increase the possibility of serotonin syndrome or perhexiline toxicity.

Tricyclic Antidepressants

Tricyclic antidepressants are now infrequently used for depression but more for neuropathic pain and their anticholinergic properties in urinary tract disorders. They are predominantly metabolized in the liver to metabolites with varying activity. Patients with renal impairment may be more prone to the common anticholinergic adverse effects, particularly urinary retention, orthostatic hypotension, confusion, and sedation.[115] Obstructive uropathy can occur from the anticholinergic properties. Cautious initial dosing and titration of tricyclic antidepressants are recommended. Depending on response, many agents can be used at up to normal or maximal doses in renal impairment.

Other Antidepressants

Venlafaxine dose should be initially reduced in severe renal impairment because of reduced clearance of the active metabolite, *O*-desmethylvenlafaxine.[116] Nefazodone is used at normal dose.

Antipsychotics

Conventional antipsychotics cause a variety of side effects to which patients with renal impairment may be susceptible (sedation, confusion, and postural hypotension). Caution is advised for atypical antipsychotics that prolong the QT interval (e.g., pimozide, thioridazine, mesoridazine, droperidol, and ziprasidone). Newer atypical agents are more commonly used and better tolerated. Clozapine, olanzapine, quetiapine, and aripiprazole are commenced at normal doses in renal impairment and titrated to response. Risperidone[117] and its active metabolite, 9-hydroxyrisperidone, are renally excreted, and clearance is reduced by 60% in severe renal impairment. Lithium is filtered and reabsorbed mainly in the proximal tubules. It is extensively renally excreted and accumulates even in mild renal impairment, causing toxicity, and it should be avoided if possible. If use is essential, the dose must be reduced with monitoring of plasma concentrations.

In hyponatremic patients, tubular reabsorption of lithium is increased, leading to increased plasma concentrations and toxicity. NSAID co-prescription may also increase toxicity. Hemodialysis is efficient in removal of lithium and can be used in overdose; however, multiple dialysis treatments are usually required as plasma concentrations rebound soon after hemodialysis. Chronic lithium nephrotoxicity is discussed further in Chapter 62.

Benzodiazepines

Benzodiazepines are extensively metabolized by the liver to a range of active and inactive metabolites. Enhanced CNS toxicity, especially sedation, is the main concern in renal patients.[118,119] Because of the potential for accumulation, chronic use should be discouraged when possible. Short-acting benzodiazepines are preferred, and dosing should be titrated cautiously according to response. The dose of midazolam should be reduced because of changes in plasma protein binding. Hemoperfusion and dialysis are not useful in benzodiazepine intoxication. Flumazenil may be used as normal in cases of benzodiazepine overdose.

Vaccines

Live vaccines (Bacille Calmette-Guérin, oral poliovirus, rubella, typhoid, yellow fever, and varicella) in immunosuppressed transplant patients are contraindicated because of the potential for causing disease. Attenuated vaccines (diphtheria-tetanus, hepatitis B, influenza, meningococcal, and pneumococcal) may be used; however, the immune reaction required for vaccine response may be diminished in immunocompromised individuals, and appropriate protection may not occur. Hepatitis B may need more doses for seroconversion to be achieved in hemodialysis patients. Immunization should preferably occur at least 1 month before initiation of immunosuppression. After transplantation, the immune response may be inadequate for at least 6 to 8 months, meaning that vaccination should be withheld until then.[120] Immunization in renal impairment is discussed further in Chapter 80.

Vitamin Supplementation

Patients with renal impairment may become vitamin deficient as a result of poor dietary intake and the effect of dialysis on removal of water-soluble vitamins. Administration of vitamin supplements (B, C, and folic acid) is recommended after dialysis.

REFERENCES

1. Manley HJ, McClaran ML, Overbay DK, et al. Factors associated with medication related problems in ambulatory hemodialysis patients. *Am J Kidney Dis*. 2003;41:386-393.
2. Cervelli MJ, ed. *The Renal Drug Reference Guide*. Adelaide: MJC Pharma; 2007. Available at: www.renaldrugreference.com.au.
3. Ashley C, Currie A, eds. *The Renal Drug Handbook*, 2nd ed. Oxford: Radcliffe Medical Press; 2004.
4. Aronoff GR, Berns JS, Brier ME, et al, eds. *Drug Prescribing in Renal Failure (Dosing Guidelines for Adults)*. 4th ed. Philadelphia: American College of Physicians; 1999. Available at: www.kdp-baptist.lousville.edu/renalbook.
5. Johnson CA. *Dialysis of Drugs*. Verona, Wisconsin: CKD Insights; 2009.
6. Meibohm B, Evans WE. Clinical pharmacokinetics and pharmacodynamics. In: Helms R, Quan D, Herfindal ET, eds. *Textbook of Therapeutics: Drug and Disease Management*. Philadelphia: Lippincott Williams & Wilkins; 2006:1-30.
7. Matzke GR, Comstock TJ. Influence of renal function and dialysis on drug disposition. In: Burton ME, Shaw LM, Schentag JJ, et al, eds. *Principles of Therapeutic Drug Monitoring*. 4th ed. Philadelphia: Lippincott Williams & Wilkins; 2006.
8. Zhang Y, Benet LZ. The gut as a barrier to drug absorption: Combined role of cytochrome P450 3A and P-glycoprotein. *Clin Pharmacokinet*. 2001;40:159-168.
9. Frost RW, Lasseter KC, Noe AJ, et al. Effects of aluminum hydroxide and calcium carbonate antacids on the bioavailability of ciprofloxacin. *Antimicrob Agents Chemother*. 1992;36:830-832.
10. Reidenberg MM, Drayer DE. Alteration of drug-protein binding in renal disease. *Clin Pharmacokinet*. 1984;9(Suppl 1):18-26.
11. Dreisbach AW, Lertora JJL. The effect of chronic renal failure on hepatic drug metabolism and drug disposition. *Semin Dial*. 2003;16:45-50.
12. Lam YWF, Banergi S, Hatfield C, et al. Principles of drug administration in renal insufficiency. *Clin Pharmacokinet*. 1997;32:30-57.
13. Reidenberg M. Kidney function and drug action. *N Engl J Med*. 1985;313:816-817.
14. Elbarbry FA, Marfleet T, Shoker AS. Drug-drug interactions with immunosuppressive agents: Review of the in vitro functional assays and role of cytochrome P450 enzymes. *Transplantation*. 2008;85:1222-1229.
15. Lee C-S, Marbury TC. Drug therapy in patients undergoing haemodialysis (clinical pharmacokinetic considerations). *Clin Pharmacokinet*. 1984;9:42-66.
16. Paton TW, Cornish WR, Manuel A, et al. Drug therapy in patients undergoing peritoneal dialysis: Clinical pharmacokinetic considerations. *Clin Pharmacokinet*. 1985;10:404-426.
17. Bohler J, Donauer J, Keller F. Pharmacokinetic principles during continuous renal replacement therapy: Drugs and dosage. *Kidney Int*. 1999;56(Suppl 72):S24-S28.
18. Besarab A, Reyes CM, Hornberger J. Meta-analysis of subcutaneous versus intravenous epoetin in maintenance treatment of anemia in hemodialysis patients. *Am J Kidney Dis*. 2002;40:439-446.
19. Cervelli MJ, Gray N, McDonald S, et al. Randomized cross-over comparison of intravenous and subcutaneous darbepoetin dosing efficiency in hemodialysis patients. *Nephrology*. 2005;10:129-135.
20. Kurella M, Bennett WM, Chertow GM. Analgesia in patients with ESRD: A review of the available evidence. *Am J Kidney Dis*. 2003;42:217-228.
21. Davison SN. Pain in hemodialysis patients: Prevalence, cause, severity, and management. *Am J Kidney Dis*. 2003;42:1239-1247.
22. Davies G, Kingswood C, Street M. Pharmacokinetics of opioids in renal dysfunction. *Clin Pharmacokinet*. 1996;31:410-422.
23. Dean M. Opioids in renal failure and dialysis patients. *J Pain Symptom Manage*. 2004;28:497-504.
24. Murtagh FEM, Chai M-O, Donohoe P, et al. The use of opioid analgesia in end-stage renal disease patients managed without dialysis. *J Pain Palliat Care Pharmacother*. 2007;21:5-16.
25. Peterson GM, Randall CT, Paterson J. Plasma levels of morphine and morphine glucuronides in the treatment of cancer pain: Relationship to renal function and route of administration. *Eur J Clin Pharmacol*. 1990;38:121-124.
26. Clark RF, Wei EM, Anderson PO. Meperidine: Therapeutic use and toxicity. *J Emerg Med*. 1995;13:797-802.
27. Rose BD, Post TW. NSAIDs: Acute kidney injury (acute renal failure) and nephrotic syndrome. UpToDate. Online 2009;version 17.1.
28. Perazella M, Tray K. Selective cyclooxygenase-2 inhibitors: A pattern of nephrotoxicity similar to traditional nonsteroidal anti-inflammatory drugs. *Am J Med*. 2001;111:64-67.
29. Blum RA, Comstock TJ, Sica DA, et al. Pharmacokinetics of gabapentin in subjects with various degrees of renal function. *Clin Pharmacol Ther*. 1994;56:154-159.
30. Randinitis EJ, Posvar EL, Alvey CW, et al. Pharmacokinetics of pregabalin in subjects with various degrees of renal function. *J Clin Pharmacol*. 2003;43:277-283.
31. Sullivan JM, Bueschen AJ, Schlegel JU. Nitrofurantoin, sulfamethizole and cephalexin urinary concentrations in unequally functioning pyelonephritic kidneys. *J Urol*. 1975;114:343-347.
32. St. Peter WL, Redic-Kill KA, Halstenson CE. Clinical pharmacokinetics of antibiotics in patients with impaired renal function. *Clin Pharmacokinet*. 1992;22:169-210.
33. Decker BS, Molitoris BA. Manifestations of and risk factors for aminoglycoside nephrotoxicity. UpToDate. Online 2009;version 17.1.
34. Gibson TP, Demetriades JL, Bland JA. Imipenem/cilastatin: Pharmacokinetic profile in renal insufficiency. *Am J Med*. 1985;78:54-61.
35. Christensson BA, Nilsson-Ehle I, Hutchison M, et al. Pharmacokinetics of meropenem in subjects with various degrees of renal impairment. *Antimicrob Agents Chemother*. 1992;36:1532-1537.

36. Barbhaiya RH, Knupp CA, Forgue ST, et al. Pharmacokinetics of cefepime in subjects with renal insufficiency. *Clin Pharmacol Ther.* 1990;48:268-276.
37. Doluisio JT. Clinical pharmacokinetics of cefotaxime in patients with normal and reduced renal function. *Rev Infect Dis.* 1982;4(Suppl): S333-S345.
38. Lin M-S, Wang L-S, Huang J-D. Single- and multiple-dose pharmacokinetics of ceftazidime in infected patients with varying degrees of renal function. *J Clin Pharmacol.* 1989;29:331-337.
39. Brogard JM, Pinget M, Brandt C, et al. Pharmacokinetics of cefazolin in patients with renal failure; special reference to hemodialysis. *J Clin Pharmacol.* 1977;17:225-230.
40. Ahern JW, Possidente CJ, Hood V, et al. Cefazolin dosing protocol for patients receiving long-term hemodialysis. *Am J Health Syst Pharm.* 2003;60:178-181.
41. Kroll MH, Hagengruber C, Elin RJ. Reaction of picrate with creatinine and cepha antibiotics. *Clin Chem.* 1984;30:1664-1666.
42. Fillastre JP, Leroy A, Moulin B, et al. Pharmacokinetics of quinolones in renal insufficiency. *J Antimicrob Chemother.* 1990;26(Suppl B): 51-60.
43. Shah A, Lettieri J, Blum R, et al. Pharmacokinetics of intravenous ciprofloxacin in normal and renally impaired subjects. *J Antimicrob Chemother.* 1996;38:103-116.
44. Decker BS, Molitoris BA. Vancomycin dosing and serum concentration monitoring in adults. UpToDate. Online 2009;version 17.1.
45. Kanfer A, Stamatakis G, Torlotin JC, et al. Changes in erythromycin pharmacokinetics induced by renal failure. *Clin Nephrol.* 1987;27: 147-150.
46. Parry MF, Neu HC. Pharmacokinetics of ticarcillin in patients with abnormal renal function. *J Infect Dis.* 1976;133:46-49.
47. Phillips ME, Eastwood JB, Curtis JR, et al. tetracycline poisoning in renal failure. *Br Med J.* 1974;5:149-151.
48. Siber GR, Gorham CC, Ericson JF, et al. Pharmacokinetics of intravenous trimethoprim-sulfamethoxazole in children and adults with normal and impaired renal function. *Rev Infect Dis.* 1982;4:566-578.
49. Dijkmans BAC, Van Hooff JP, de Wolff FA, et al. The effect of co-trimoxazole on serum creatinine. *Br J Clin Pharmacol.* 1981;12: 701-703.
50. Houghton GW, Dennis MJ, Gabriel R. Pharmacokinetics of metronidazole in patients with varying degrees of renal failure. *Br J Clin Pharmacol.* 1985;19:203-209.
51. Launay-Vacher V, Izzedine H, Deray G. Pharmacokinetic considerations in the treatment of tuberculosis in patients with renal failure. *Clin Pharmacokinet.* 2005;44:221-235.
52. Saliba F, Dupont B. Renal impairment and amphotericin B formulations in patients with invasive fungal infections. *Med Mycol.* 2008;46: 97-112.
53. Berl T, Wilner KD, Gardner M, et al. Pharmacokinetics of fluconazole in renal failure. *J Am Soc Nephrol.* 1995;6:242-247.
54. Cutler RE, Blair AD, Kelly MR. Flucytosine kinetics in subjects with normal and impaired renal function. *Clin Pharmacol Ther.* 1978;24: 333-342.
55. Boike SC, Pue MA, Freed MI, et al. Pharmacokinetics of famciclovir in subjects with varying degrees of renal impairment. *Clin Pharmacol Ther.* 1994;55:418-426.
56. Czock D, Scholle C, Rasche FM, et al. Pharmacokinetics of valganciclovir and ganciclovir in renal impairment. *Clin Pharmacol Ther.* 2002;72:142-150.
57. Gupta SK, Swan SK, Marbury T, et al. Multiple-dose pharmacokinetics of peginterferon alfa-2b in patients with renal insufficiency. *Br J Clin Pharmacol.* 2007;64:726-732.
58. Fontaine H, Vallet-Pichard A, Chaix M-LL, et al. Efficacy and safety of adefovir dipivoxil in kidney recipients, hemodialysis patients, and patients with renal insufficiency. *Transplantation.* 2005;80:1086-1092.
59. Heald AE, Hsyu PH, Yuen GJ, et al. Pharmacokinetics of lamivudine in human immunodeficiency virus–infected patients with renal dysfunction. *Antimicrob Agents Chemother.* 1996;40:1514-1519.
60. Zhou X-J, Swan S, Smith WB, et al. Pharmacokinetics of telbivudine in subjects with various degrees of renal impairment. *Antimicrob Agents Chemother.* 2007;51:4231-4235.
61. Karie S, Launay-Vacher V, Janus N, et al. Pharmacokinetics and dosage adjustment of oseltamivir and zanamivir in patients with renal failure. *Nephrol Dial Transplant.* 2006;21:3606-3608.
62. Brody SR, Humphreys MH, Gambertoglio JG, et al. Pharmacokinetics of cidofovir in renal insufficiency and in continuous ambulatory peritoneal dialysis or high-flux hemodialysis. *Clin Pharmacol Ther.* 1999;65: 21-28.
63. Aweeka FT, Jacobson MA, Martin-Munley S, et al. Effect of renal disease and hemodialysis on foscarnet pharmacokinetics and dosing recommendations. *J Acquir Immune Defic Syndr Hum Retrovirol.* 1999;20:350-357.
64. Grand'Maison A, Charest AF, Geerts WH. Anticoagulant use in patients with chronic renal impairment. *Am J Cardiovasc Drugs.* 2005;5:291-305.
65. Lobo BL. Use of newer anticoagulants in patients with chronic kidney disease. *Am J Health Syst Pharm.* 2007;64:2017-2026.
66. Follea G, Laville M, Pozet N, et al. Pharmacokinetic studies of standard heparin and low molecular weight heparin in patients with chronic renal failure. *Haemostasis.* 1986;16:147-151.
67. Crowther M, Lim W. Low molecular weight heparin and bleeding in patients with chronic renal failure. *Curr Opin Pulm Med.* 2007;13: 409-413.
68. Robson R, White H, Aylward P, et al. Bivalirudin pharmacokinetics and pharmacodynamics: Effect of renal function, dose, and gender. *Clin Pharmacol Ther.* 2002;71:433-439.
69. Danhof M, de Boer A, Magnani HN, et al. Pharmacokinetic considerations on Orgaran (Org 10172) therapy. *Haemostasis.* 1992;22: 73-84.
70. Donat F, Duret JP, Santoni A, et al. The pharmacokinetics of fondaparinux sodium in healthy volunteers. *Clin Pharmacokinet.* 2002;41(Suppl 2):1-9.
71. Tschudi M, Lämmle B, Alberio L. Dosing lepirudin in patients with heparin-induced thrombocytopenia and normal or impaired renal function: A single-center experience with 68 patients. *Blood.* 2009;113: 2402-2409.
72. Eriksson UG, Johansson S, Attman P-O, et al. Influence of severe renal impairment on the pharmacokinetics and pharmacodynamics of oral ximelagatran and subcutaneous melagatran. *Clin Pharmacokinet.* 2003;42:743-753.
73. Swan SK, Hursting MJ. The pharmacokinetics and pharmacodynamics of argatroban: Effects of age, gender, and hepatic or renal dysfunction. *Pharmacotherapy.* 2000;20:318-329.
74. Bachmann K, Shapiro R, Maciewicz J. Warfarin elimination and responsiveness in patients with renal dysfunction. *J Clin Pharmacol.* 1977;17:292-299.
75. Dreisbach AW, Japa S, Gebrekal AB, et al. Cytochrome P4502C9 activity in endstage renal disease [letter]. *Clin Pharmacol Ther.* 2003;73:475-477.
76. Gretler DD, Gueriolini R, Williams PJ. Pharmacokinetic and pharmacodynamic properties of eptifibatide in subjects with normal or impaired renal function. *Clin Ther.* 2004;26:390-398.
77. Wilcox CS. New insights into diuretic use in patients with chronic renal disease. *J Am Soc Nephrol.* 2002;13:798-805.
78. Carter BL. Dosing of antihypertensive medications in patients with renal insufficiency. *J Clin Pharmacol.* 1995;35:81-86.
79. Thomas MC. Diuretics, ACE inhibitors and NSAIDs—the triple whammy. *Med J Aust.* 2000;172:184-185.
80. Berglund G, Descamps R, Thomis JA. Pharmacokinetics of sotalol after chronic administration to patients with renal insufficiency. *Eur J Clin Pharmacol.* 1980;18:321-326.
81. Flouvat B, Decourt S, Aubert P, et al. Pharmacokinetics of atenolol in patients with terminal renal failure and influence of hemodialysis. *Br J Clin Pharmacol.* 1980;9:379-385.
82. McDonald SP, Russ GR. Associations between use of cyclosporin-sparing agents and outcome in kidney transplant recipients. *Kidney Int.* 2002;61:2259-2265.
83. Schulz V. Clinical pharmacokinetics of nitroprusside, cyanide, thiosulphate and thiocyanate. *Clin Pharmacokinet.* 1984;9:239-251.
84. Vlasses PH, Ferguson RK, Rocci MLJ, et al. Lethal accumulation of procainamide metabolite in severe renal insufficiency. *Am J Nephrol.* 1986;6:112-116.
85. Strippoli GFM, Navaneethan SD, Johnson DW, et al. Effects of statins in patients with chronic kidney disease: Meta-analysis and meta-regression of randomised controlled trials. *Br Med J.* 2008;336: 645-651.
86. Duckworth WC. Insulin degradation: Mechanisms, products and significance. *Endocr Rev.* 1988;9:319-345.
87. Yale J-F. Oral antihyperglycemic agents and renal disease: New agents, new concepts. *J Am Soc Nephrol.* 2005;16:S7-S10.
88. Management of diabetes in chronic renal failure. *Indian J Nephrol.* 2005;15(Suppl 1):S23-S31.
89. Salpeter S, Greyber E, Pasternak G, et al. Risk of fatal and nonfatal lactic acidosis with metformin use in type 2 diabetes mellitus. Cochrane Database Syst Rev. 2006;25:CD002967.

90. Krepinsky J, Ingram AJ, Clase CM. Prolonged sulfonylurea induced hypoglycemia in diabetic patients with end stage renal disease. *Am J Kidney Dis*. 2000;35:500-505.
91. Chapelsky MC, Thompson-Culkin K, Miller AK, et al. Pharmacokinetics of rosiglitazone in patients with varying degrees of renal insufficiency. *J Clin Pharmacol*. 2003;43:252-259.
92. Budde K, Neumayer H-H, Fritsche L, et al. The pharmacokinetics of pioglitazone in patients with impaired renal function. *Br J Clin Pharmacol*. 2003;55:368-374.
93. Iglesias P, Díez JJ. Thyroid dysfunction and kidney disease. *Eur J Endocrinol*. 2009;160:503-515.
94. Manluca J, Tonelli M, Ray JG, et al. Dose-reducing H_2 receptor antagonists in the presence of low glomerular filtration rate: A systematic review of the evidence. *Nephrol Dial Transplant*. 2005;20:2376-2384.
95. Larsson R, Norlander B, Bodemar G, et al. Steady-state kinetics and dosage requirements of cimetidine in renal failure. *Clin Pharmacokinet*. 1981;6:316-325.
96. Dubb JW, Stote RM, Familiar RG, et al. Effect of cimetidine on renal function in normal man. *Clin Pharmacol Ther*. 1978;24:76-83.
97. Geevasinga N, Coleman P, Roger S. *Proton pump inhibitors: The most common iatrogenic cause of acute interstitial nephritis?* Singapore: Third World Congress of Nephrology; 2005.
98. Mehrotra N, Gupta M, Kovar A, et al. The role of pharmacokinetics and pharmacodynamics in phosphodiesterase-5 inhibitor therapy. *Int J Impot Res*. 2007;19:253-264.
99. Kahan BD, Keown P, Levy GA, et al. Therapeutic drug monitoring of immunosuppressant drugs in clinical practice. *Clin Ther*. 2002;24:330-350.
100. Morris RG: Immunosuppressant drug monitoring: Is the laboratory meeting clinical expectations? *Ann Pharmacother*. 2005;39:119-127.
101. Naesens M, Kuypers DRJ, Sarwal M. Calcineurin inhibitor nephrotoxicity. *Clin J Am Soc Nephrol*. 2009;4:481-508.
102. Haubitz M, Bohnenstengel F, Brunkhorst R, et al. Cyclophosphamide pharmacokinetics and dose requirements in patients with renal insufficiency. *Kidney Int*. 2002;61:1495-1501.
103. Ibrahim RB, Liu C, Cronin SM, et al. Drug removal by plasmapheresis: An evidence-based review. *Pharmacotherapy*. 2007;27:1529-1549.
104. Lange K. Nephropathy induced by D-penicillamine. *Contrib Nephrol*. 1978;10:63-74.
105. Wallace SL, Singer JZ, Duncan GJ, et al. Renal function predicts colchicine toxicity: Guidelines for the prophylactic use of colchicine in gout. *J Rheumatol*. 1991;18:264-269.
106. Day RO, Graham GG, Hicks M, et al. Clinical pharmacokinetics and pharmacodynamics of allopurinol and oxypurinol. *Clin Pharmacokinet*. 2007;46:623-644.
107. Cunningham RF, Israili ZH, Dayton PG. Clinical pharmacokinetics of probenecid. *Clin Pharmacokinet*. 1981;6:135-151.
108. Jamal SA, Bauer DC, Ensrud KE, et al. Alendronate treatment in women with normal to severely impaired renal function: An analysis of the fracture intervention trial. *J Bone Miner Res*. 2007;22:503-508.
109. Chang JT, Green L, Beitz J. Renal failure with the use of zoledronic acid. *N Engl J Med*. 2003;349:1676-1679.
110. Horadam VW, Sharp JG, Smilack JD, et al. Pharmacokinetics of amantadine hydrochloride in subjects with normal and impaired renal function. *Ann Intern Med*. 1981;94:454-458.
111. Cohen LM, Tessier EG, Germain MJ, et al. Update on psychotropic medication use in renal disease. *Psychosomatics*. 2004;45:34-48.
112. Levey NB. Psychopharmacology in patients with renal failure. *Int J Psychiatry Med*. 1990;20:325-334.
113. Preskorn SH. What are the clinically relevant pharmacokinetic differences among SSRIs? In *Clinical Pharmacology of SSRIs*. Caddo, Oklahoma: Professional Communications, Inc.; 1996.
114. Blumenfield M, Levy NB, Spinowitz B, et al. Fluoxetine in depressed patients on dialysis. *Int J Psychiatry Med*. 1997;27:71-80.
115. Lieberman JA, Cooper TB, Suckow RF, et al. Tricyclic antidepressant and metabolite levels in chronic renal failure. *Clin Pharmacol Ther*. 1990;37:301-307.
116. Troy SM, Schultz RW, Parker VD, et al. The effect of renal disease on the disposition of venlafaxine. *Clin Pharmacol Ther*. 1994;56:14-21.
117. Heykants J, Haung ML, Mannens G. The pharmacokinetics of risperidone in humans: A summary. *J Clin Psychiatry*. 1994;55(Suppl 5):13-17.
118. Schmith VD, Piraino B, Smith RB, et al. Alprazolam in end-stage renal disease: I. Pharmacokinetics. *J Clin Pharmacol*. 1991;31:571-579.
119. Ochs HR, Greenblatt DJ, Kaschell HJ, et al. Diazepam kinetics in patients with renal insufficiency or hyperthyroidism. *Br J Clin Pharmacol*. 1981;12:829-832.
120. Cohn J, Blumberg EA. Immunizations for renal transplant candidates and recipients. *Nat Clin Pract Nephrol*. 2009;5:46-53.

CHAPTER 74 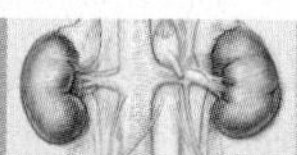

Herbal and Over-the-Counter Medicines and the Kidney

Mark S. Segal, Xueqing Yu

In recent years, the use of herbal medicines and dietary supplements to promote health and to treat various chronic diseases has increased globally. An estimated one third of adults in developed countries and more than 80% of the population in many developing countries are using herbal and folk medicines to promote health and to manage common maladies such as cold, hay fever, inflammation, heart disease, indigestion, constipation, liver cirrhosis, cancer, acquired immunodeficiency syndrome, diabetes, and central nervous system diseases.[1] In Africa, up to 80% of the population depends on traditional medicine for primary health care; in China, herbal preparations account for up to 50% of the total consumption of pharmaceutical agents. There has been a surge in the popularity of herbal medicine in the West. For instance, the size of the U.S. herbal medicine market has increased from U.S. $1.6 billion in 1994 to U.S. $3.9 billion in 1998, and the proportion of U.S. citizens who consulted a provider of herbal medicine in a 1-year period increased from 10.2% in 1993 to 15.1% in 1998.[2] In addition, European countries spent almost $5 billion (at manufacturers' prices to wholesalers) on over-the-counter herbal medicines in 2003. Germany and France are the indisputable leaders in over-the-counter sales (Fig. 74.1) and also have large markets for prescription herbal preparations.[3] Complementary and alternative medicines including Chinese herbal medicines and herbal plants have been used by about 50% of Australians.[1]

Herbal medicine use has been recorded in all of the ancient literature. To date, there are at least 11,000 species of plants for medicinal use, and about 500 of them are commonly used by various ethnic groups.[1,4] These herbal plants may be used either in their primary forms or as mixtures. However, the source and composition of botanical medicines vary by prevalent local practices. Notably, these herbal remedies have not been tested for efficacy and safety, their ingredients are unknown, and the dosage and route of administration are not standardized. Although the prevalence of toxicity of organs caused by traditional medicines is directly related to a combination of ignorance, poverty, lack of medical facilities, lack of legislation, and widespread belief in indigenous systems of medicine in rural areas, it has been realized recently that the problems and concerns of herbal medicines arise from intrinsic toxicity, adulteration, contamination, substitution, misidentification, mistaken labeling, unfavorable herb-drug interactions, lack of standardization, or poor quality control.[1,4] Increasing evidence for both adverse drug reactions and poisoning events associated with the use of herbal medicines has been reported worldwide. Adulteration of synthetic drugs and other potentially toxic compounds to herbal medicines has been identified. On the other hand, coadministration of herbal medicines with conventional drugs raises the potential of herb-drug interactions, which may cause altered drug elimination, undertreatment, or toxicity.[1,4,5]

HERBAL MEDICATIONS AND THE KIDNEY

Kidneys are particularly vulnerable to toxic injury because of their high blood flow rate, large endothelial surface area, high metabolic activity, active uptake by tubular cells, medullary interstitial concentration, and low urine pH. Renal tubules are involved in active transport and urinary concentration, and therefore the local concentration of toxins is potentially high, leading to direct injury to tubular cells. Herbal medicines may be toxic through one or more common pathogenic mechanisms. These include alteration of intraglomerular hemodynamics, tubular cell toxicity, inflammation, crystal nephropathy, rhabdomyolysis, and thrombotic microangiopathy. Compared with 30 years ago, patients today are usually taking multiple medications because of more underlying disease and have been exposed to more diagnostic and therapeutic procedures with the potential to harm kidney function. Thus, drug-related nephrotoxicity tends to be more common clinically. The patient-related risk factors for drug-induced nephrotoxicity include age older than 60 years, underlying renal insufficiency, glomerular filtration rate of less than 60 ml/min per 1.73 m^2, volume depletion, diabetes, heart failure, and sepsis.[6] These risk factors may also make individuals susceptible to the renal toxicity of herbal medicines. An overview of the potential renal side effects of herbal medicines is shown in Figure 74.2. This chapter reviews current knowledge of the hazards related to herbal medicines for the kidneys.

Herbs That Lead to Kidney Injury

Tubulointerstitial Nephritis: Aristolochic Acid Nephropathy

Aristolochic acids (AAs) are a family of structurally related nitrophenanthrene carboxylic acids that are primarily derived from herbs of the genus *Aristolochia*, including *Aristolochia fangchi*, *Aristolochia clematitis*, and *Aristolochia manshuriensis* (Fig. 74.3). The predominant AAs are AAI (8-methoxy-6-nitro-phenanthro-(3,4-*d*)-1,3-dioxolo-5-carboxylic acid) and AAII (6-nitro-phenanthro-(3,4-*d*)-1,3-dioxolo-5-carboxylic acid). Long-term consumption of *A. fangchi* for slimming purposes was reported in Belgium. More than 100 young women suffered kidney damage, and several patients developed renal and urinary tract cancer (Fig. 74.4).[7] Increasing evidence shows that AAs present in the herb are the compounds responsible for this renal toxicity.[8,9] The nephrotoxic and carcinogenic effects of AAs in animals have been reported, and similar toxicities have been observed in

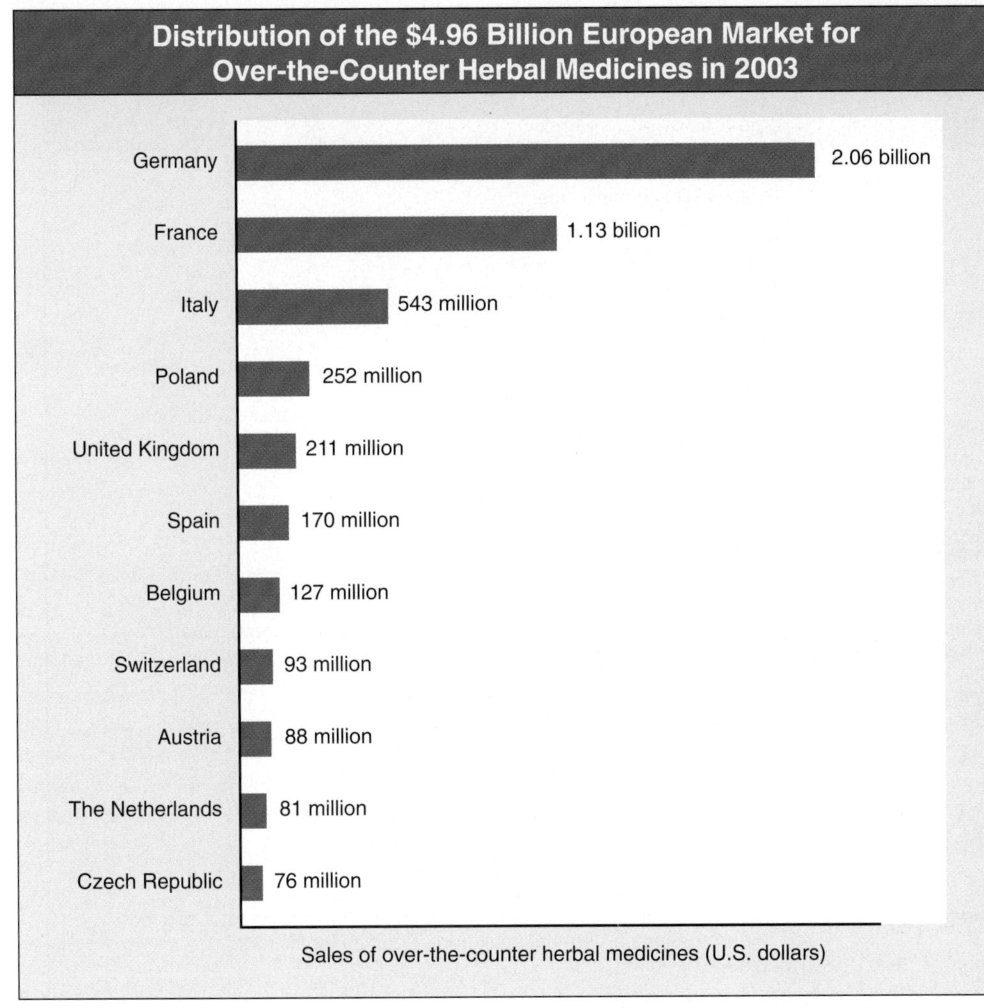

Figure 74.1 Distribution of the U.S. $4.96 billion European market for over-the-counter herbal medicines in 2003. *(From reference 3.)*

Kidney Syndromes Induced by Herbal Medicines

Syndrome	Herbal medicines
Hypertension	• *Glycyrrhiza* species (Chinese herbal teas, gancao, boui-ougi-tou) • *Ephedra* species (ma huang)
Acute tubular necrosis	• Traditional African medicine: toxic plants (*Securidaca longepedunculata, Euphoria matabelensis, Callilepsis laureola,* Cape aloes, or adulteration by dichromate) • Chinese medicine: *Taxus celebica* • Morocco: Takaout roumia (paraphenylenediamine)
Acute interstitial nephritis	• Peruvian medicine (*Uno degatta*) • Tung Shueh pills (adulterated by mefenamic acid)
Fanconi syndrome	• Chinese herbs containing AAs (*Akebia* species, Boui, Mokutsu) • Chinese herbs adulterated by cadmium
Papillary necrosis	• Chinese herbs adulterated by phenylbutazone
Chronic interstitial renal fibrosis	• Chinese herbs or Kampo containing AAs (*Aristolochia* species, *Akebia* species, Mutong, Boui, Mokutsu)
Urinary retention	• *Datura* species, *Rhododendron molle* (atropine, scopolamine)
Kidney stones	• Ma huang (ephedrine) • Cranberry juice (oxalate)
Urinary tract carcinoma	• Chinese herbs containing AAs

Figure 74.2 Kidney syndromes induced by herbal medicines. AAs, aristolochic acids. *(From reference 6.)*

Botanicals Known to Contain or Suspected of Containing Aristolochic Acid

Botanical Name	Common or other names
Aristolochia spp.	Aristolochia, Guan Mu tong, Guang Mu tong
Aristolochia acuminota (Syn. *Aristolochia tagala*)	Oval leaf Dutchman's pipe
Aristolochia bracteata	Ukulwe
Aristolachia clematitis	Birthwort
Aristolochia contorta	Ma Dou Ling (fruit), Bei Ma Dou Ling (root), Tian Xian Teng (herb)
Aristolochia cymbifera	Mil homens
Aristolochia debilis (Syn. *Aristolochia Janga, A. recurvilabra, A. sinarum*)	Ma Dou Ling *(fruit),* Tian Xian Teng *(herb),* Qing Mu Xiang (root), Sei-Mokkou (Japanese), Birthwort, Long birthwort, Slender Dutchman's pipe
Aristolochia fanachi	Guang Fank ji (root), Fang ji, Fang chi, Makuboi (Japanese), Kou-boui (Japanese), Kwangbanggi (Korean)
Aristolochia heterophylla	Han Fang Ji
Aristolochia indica	Indian birthwort (root), Yin Du Ma Dou Ling
Aristolochia kaempferi (Syn. *Aristolochia chrysaps, A. feddei, A. heterophylla, A. mollis, A. setchuenensis, A. shimadoi, A. thibetica isotrema chrysops, I heterophylla, I lasiops)*	Yellowmouth Dutchman's pipe, Zhu Sha Lian
Aristolochia macrophylla (Syn. *Aristolochia sipho*)	Dutchman's pipe
Aristolochia manschuriensis (Syn. *Hacquartia manchuriensis*, Syn. *Isotrema manchuriensis*)	Manchurian birthwort, Manchurian Dutchmans's pipe (stem), Guan Mutong (stem), Kan-Mokutsu (Japanese), Mokubai (Japanese), Kwangbanggi (Korean)
Aristolochia maxima (Syn. *Howardia hoffmanü*)	Maxima Dutchman's pipe, Da Ma Dou Ling
Aristolochia mollissima	Wooly Dutchman's pipe, Mian Mao Ma Dou Ling
Aristolochia moupinensis	Moupin Dutchman's pipe, Huai Tong
Aristolochia sarpentaria (Syn. *Aristolochia serpentaria*)	Virginia snakeroot, Serpentaria, Virginia serpentary
Aristolochia triangularis	Triangular Dutchman's pipe, San Jiao Ma Dou Ling
Aristolochia tuberosa	Tuberous Dutchman's pipe, Kuai Jing Ma Dou Ling
Aristolochia tubifluru	Tubeflower, Dutchman's pipe, Guan Hua Ma Dou Ling
Aristolochia versicolar	Versicoloraus Dutchman's pipe, Bian Se Ma Dou Ling
Asarum canodense (Syn. *Asarum acuminarum, A. ambiguum, A. canadense, A. furcarum, A. medium, A. parvifolium, A. reflexurn, A. rubracincrum)*	Wild ginger, Indian ginger, Canada snakeroot, False coltsfoot, Colic root, Heart snakeroot, Vermont snakeroot, Southern snakeroot, Jia Na Da Xi Xin
Asarum himala(y)cum	Tanyou-satshin (Japanese)
Asarum splendens	Do-satshin (Japanese)

Figure 74.3 Botanicals known to contain or suspected of containing aristolochic acid and their vernacular names. *(From reference 9.)*

humans. The renal syndrome was initially referred to as Chinese herb nephropathy (CHN) and later as AA nephropathy (AAN), a name more specific and mechanistic than CHN. AAN was soon recognized as a global health problem.[7,8,10] Since the publication of the index cases, new cases of AAN have been reported, not only in Belgium but also worldwide (Fig. 74.4A). The true incidence of AAN is largely unknown and probably underestimated as numerous ingredients known to contain or suspected of containing AA are used in traditional medicine in China, Japan, and India (Fig. 74.5).[11]

AAN is characterized by tubulointerstitial nephritis that rapidly progresses to fibrosis with deterioration of renal function, ultimately leading to end-stage renal failure in several months. The renal toxicity of AAI is dependent on the dosage and the duration of administration.[12] After multiple dosages or even a single dose, AAI is detectable in the kidneys for a long time. Human AAN is reproducible in rodents, in which AA intoxication results in tubular atrophy and interstitial fibrosis, leading to renal failure.[13] The progressive tubular atrophy is related to impaired regeneration and apoptosis of proximal tubular epithelial cells, which is considered a possible mechanism of tubular epithelial cell deletion. The resident fibroblast activation plays a critical role in the process of renal fibrosis during AA toxicity.[14]

Clinically, the initial presentation of AAN is usually silent and the renal failure is discovered by routine blood testing. However, a few cases reported in the literature have presented with Fanconi's syndrome or acute kidney injury due to acute tubular necrosis.[15] Anemia is present and is often unusually severe in patients with severe renal impairment. In most of the cases, the urinary sediment is unremarkable, and dipstick analysis for albuminuria is negative. However, urinary excretion of low-molecular-weight proteins (e.g., β_2-microglobulin, cystatin C) is markedly increased, and the urinary low-molecular-weight protein/albumin ratio is higher than in control patients with glomerular diseases.[16]

On pathologic examination, AAN is characterized by extensive renal interstitial fibrosis and tubular atrophy, which generally decreases in severity from the outer to the inner cortex (see Fig. 74.4C). The glomeruli are relatively spared, although, in the later stage of the disease, they also display a mild collapse of the capillaries and a wrinkling of the basement membrane.

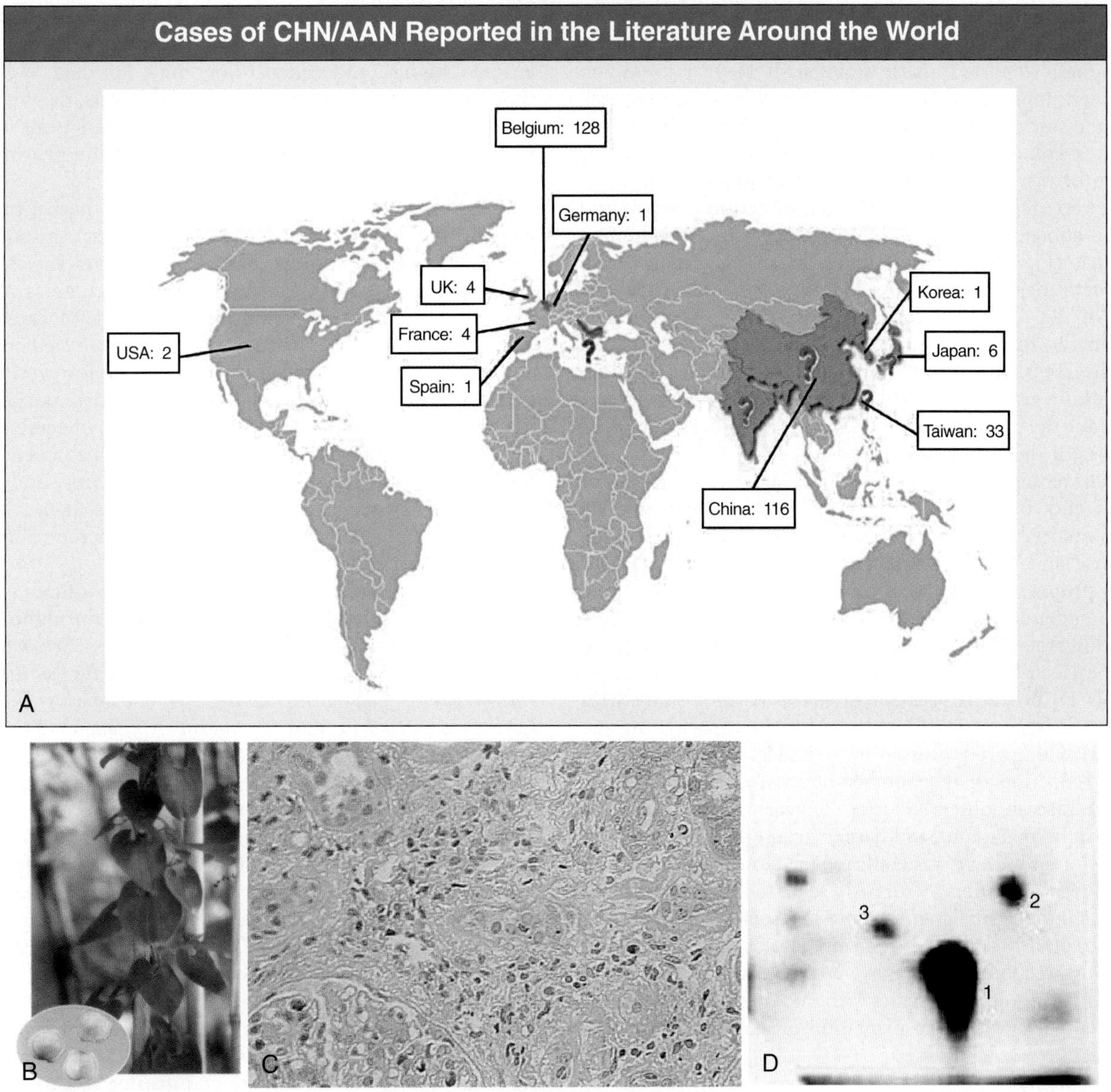

Cases of CHN/AAN Reported in the Literature Around the World

Belgium: 128
Germany: 1
UK: 4
France: 4
Spain: 1
USA: 2
Korea: 1
Japan: 6
Taiwan: 33
China: 116
A

B C D

Figure 74.4 Chinese herb nephropathy/aristolochic acid nephropathy (CHN/AAN). A, Cases of CHN/AAN reported around the world. **B,** Guang Mu Tong, a Chinese herb which contains AAs. **C,** Extensive paucicellular interstitial fibrosis and tubular atrophy typically found in CHN/AAN. **D,** Autoradiographic pattern of specific AA DNA adducts detected in human renal tissue. *(Modified in part from reference 9.)*

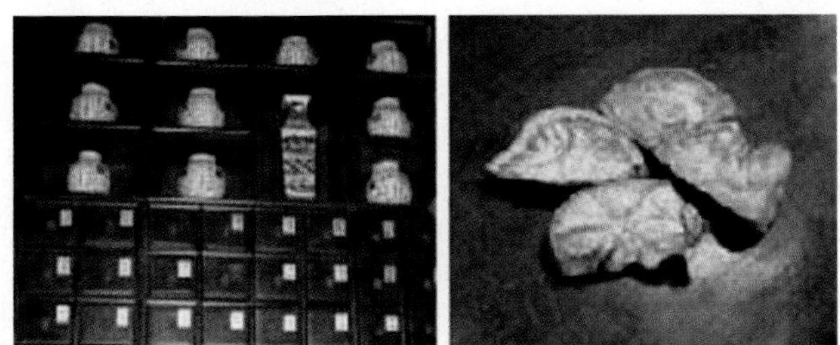

Figure 74.5 A pharmacy selling traditional herbal remedies (left) including fang chi and mu tong (right). The true incidence of AAN is largely unknown and probably underestimated as numerous ingredients known to contain or suspected of containing aristolochic acid are used in traditional medicine in India and eastern Asia. *(From reference 9.)*

Immune deposits are not found, but endothelial cell swelling is often apparent with consequent thickening of interlobular and afferent arterioles.[11,17] An early and massive interstitial inflammation characterized by activated monocytes-macrophages and cytotoxic $CD8^+/CD103^+$ T lymphocytes has been demonstrated during the progression of experimental AAN,[18] suggesting an immunologic process as a possible pathophysiologic mechanism.

The striking association between AA exposure and urothelial abnormalities was described for the first time by Cosyns and associates,[19] who observed moderate atypia and atypical hyperplasia of the urothelium in four pieces of nephroureterectomies removed from three patients with AAN before or at the time of transplantation. The persistence of AA-DNA adducts in renal tissues of the cohort of Belgian women is consistent with the postulated role of AA in urothelial cancer. It accounts for 40%

to 45% of AAN patients who display multifocal high-grade transitional cell carcinomas, mainly in the upper urinary tract.[9] Lemy and colleagues[20] reported a case series with 15-year follow-up and identified upper tract urothelial carcinoma as a potent risk factor for the subsequent development of bladder urothelial carcinoma after kidney transplantation for AAN. The molecular mechanism of AA-induced carcinogenesis shows a strong association between DNA adduct formation, mutation pattern, and tumor development. Analysis of DNA adducts formed in human target tissues (Fig. 74.4D) and studies in animal models have pointed out a major role of AAs in carcinogenesis. After oral ingestion of AA, extensive formation of AA-DNA adducts is observed in the forestomach, accompanied by development of tumors.[1] In 2002, the International Agency for Research on Cancer working group concluded that there is sufficient evidence in humans for the carcinogenicity of herbal remedies containing plant species of the genus *Aristolochia*.[21]

Studies have demonstrated that AA is a significant risk factor for Balkan endemic nephropathy,[22] which is characterized by chronic interstitial fibrosis with slow progression to end-stage renal disease and urothelial malignant neoplasia (see Chapter 62). AA is proposed as one of the environmental causal factors for Balkan endemic nephropathy affecting thousands of people living in Bulgaria, Bosnia, Croatia, Romania, and Serbia along the Danube River basin.[23]

There is no proven treatment of AAN. A pilot study with corticosteroids was performed in 35 AAN patients with chronic renal failure. Compared with an untreated group, there was a significant reduction of the number of patients reaching end-stage renal disease observed after 1 year of corticosteroid therapy.[24] Eight years later, in a larger group of AAN patients, the corticosteroid therapy was confirmed to slow the progression of renal failure.[25] As patients with AAN seem to be at an increased risk for uroepithelial malignant neoplasms, such patients should at least be regularly screened by urine cytologic examinations. Some authors recommend prophylactic removal of the native kidneys and ureters in all patients with end-stage AAN who are being treated with either transplantation or dialysis.[26]

Acute Kidney Injury

The nephrotoxicity of medicinal herbs most frequently reported in the literature is from countries in southern Africa and Asia. The use of traditional herbal remedies has been implicated in 37.5% of all cases of acute kidney injury in Nigeria.[27] Herbal plants reported as the cause of renal damage include *Securidaca longepedunculata* (or violet tree), which contains methylsalicylate and saponin; *Euphorbia matabelensis*, which contains latex; *Crotalaria laburnifolia*, which contains hepatonephrotoxic alkaloids; *Uncaria tomentosa* (cat's claw); *Lepidium meyenii* (common name: maca); *Tripterygium wilfordii* (lei gong teng); licorice *(Glycyrrhiza glabra)* root; and *Callilepsis laureola* (impila). This section describes some of the important examples of nephrotoxicity caused by herbal remedies.

Tripterygium wilfordii Hook F (TWHF) is a kind of Chinese herbal medicine used for 2000 years. It was applied externally for treatment of arthritis and inflammatory tissue swelling for many years. This drug has been found to have immunosuppressive effects that could successfully induce remission of some autoimmune disorders. Its side-effects include gastrointestinal upset, infertility, and suppression of lymphocyte proliferation. A case was reported of a previously healthy young man who developed profuse vomiting and diarrhea, leukopenia, renal failure, profound hypotension, and shock after ingestion of an extract of TWHF. In addition to his hypovolemic shock, he had evidence of cardiac injury by electrocardiography, cardiac enzyme studies, and echocardiography. He died of intractable shock 3 days after the abuse of TWHF. In rats, daily intragastric ingestion of an effective compound extracted from *T. wilfordii* Hook F for 16 days led to dysfunction of the proximal tubule of the kidney.[28]

Cat's claw, or uno de gato, is a Peruvian herbal preparation made from *Uncaria*, a woody vine found in the Amazon basin. It has been used for various diseases, such as cirrhosis, gastritis, gonorrhea, cancers of the female genital tract, and rheumatism. The oxindole alkaloids from the root bark of cat's claw are thought to invoke its most widely sought-after medicinal effects as an herbal remedy against inflammation. However, it appears that additional unknown substances have an important role in the overall effect of cat's claw extracts. A case of acute interstitial nephritis after the use of this preparation has been reported; renal biopsy showed acute interstitial nephritis, and the renal failure was reversed after withdrawal of the agent. The acute interstitial nephritis is likely to be an idiosyncratic allergic reaction to the remedy.[29]

A variety of nephrotoxic mushrooms are confused with edible mushrooms, resulting in acute kidney injury throughout Europe and North America. The *Cortinarius* species (*Cortinarius callisteus*, *Cortinarius cinnamomeus* group, *Cortinarius gentilis*, *Cortinarius orellanus*, *Cortinarius rainierensis*, *Cortinarius speciosissimus*, *Cortinarius splendens*, and *Cortinarius semisanguineus* group) are the most notorious. In North America, the most common mushroom is probably *C. gentilis*. In 2004, mushroom exposures accounted for 8601 cases and five fatalities, but only three exposures were attributed to the *Cortinarius* group.[30] However, because more than 80% of mushroom exposures fell into the unknown mushroom category, *Cortinarius* exposures certainly are higher.[30] Clinically, the history of mushroom ingestion may be remote, particularly with *Cortinarius*. Although early gastrointestinal symptoms are usually noted at the time of intake, they may not be severe enough for patients to seek medical attention, and symptoms of renal failure may not be manifested until 1 to 3 weeks after exposure. Presentation with a shorter latent period suggests a more severe toxicity and greater risk of severe renal failure than with delayed presentation. Improvement in renal injury may occur within several weeks to months; however, renal injury may last months to years, and patients may require chronic hemodialysis or renal transplantation.

A more recently described mushroom syndrome involves *Amanita smithiana/proxima*. It is thought that the toxin is 2-amino-4,5-hexadienoic acid.[31] Although it causes acute tubular necrosis within hours of ingestion, the clinical outcome is usually good.

Herbal Remedies and Renal Complications

Hypertension

Ma huang, an ephedra-containing herbal preparation, is used in the treatment of bronchial asthma, cold and influenza symptoms, fever and chills, headaches and other aches, edema, and lack of perspiration. In Western countries, ephedrine and herbal ephedra preparations have been used to promote weight loss and to enhance athletic performance. Dietary supplements that contain ephedra alkaloids have been reported to possibly induce hypertension, palpitations, tachycardia, and stroke. A report showed that prescribed ephedrine is not associated with a substantially increased risk of adverse cardiovascular outcomes in a registry-based case-crossover study.[32] However, ephedra may pose a serious health risk to some users, such as renal patients who are particularly prone to hypertension.

The dried roots of the licorice plant *(Glycyrrhiza glabra)* have been consumed for the past 6000 years and are used as flavoring and sweating agents, as demulcents and expectorants in the Western world, and as antiallergic and anti-inflammatory agents in Asian countries, including China, Japan, and Korea. Licorice contains glycyrrhizin. After oral administration of licorice preparations, glycyrrhizinic acid is hydrolyzed by intestinal bacteria into glycyrrhetic acid. Glycyrrhetic acid can inhibit the enzyme 11β-hydroxysteroid dehydrogenase 2, which in the distal kidney tubules converts the steroid hormone cortisol to cortisone. A decreased activity of 11β-hydroxysteroid dehydrogenase 2 leads to an excess of cortisol and an overstimulation of this mineralocorticoid receptor, leading to water and sodium retention and an increased excretion of potassium. With exposure to large doses of glycyrrhizinic acid for a prolonged period, it can cause hypokalemia, hypernatremia, arrhythmia, edema, pseudoaldosteronism, hypertension, and cardiac disorders.[1] To minimize the adverse effects, it is recommended that licorice not be ingested for longer than 4 to 6 weeks.[33]

Crystalluria and Nephrocalcinosis

Many health drinks that are well tolerated by individuals with normal renal function can cause serious problems in patients with limited renal function. One example of this is oxalate crystalluria. Star fruit carambola juice can contain as much as 800 mg of oxalate in 4 ounces (120 ml). Sour carambola juice is a popular beverage in Taiwan, and although commercial carambola juice prepared by pickling and dilution has markedly reduced oxalate content, fresh juice or only mildly diluted post-pickled juice may contain high quantities of oxalate. Cranberry concentrate tablets also can lead to an increase in urinary excretion of oxalate. Ma huang ingestion also has been reported to lead to kidney stones, and the use of ephedrine and guaifenesin individually or in combination has been shown to cause more than 35% of urinary stones that are related to pharmaceutical metabolites and 0.1% of all urinary stones.[34]

Hyperkalemia

One of the most common recommendations made for people with renal impairment is tight control of potassium intake. This is especially true in light of the side effects with regard to increased potassium for many of the medications we prescribe to slow the progression of renal disease. The normal food sources for increased intake are oranges, bananas, tomatoes, and potatoes. However, some health drinks are also very high in potassium. Noni juice is often taken to increase energy, but it contains more potassium than any other fruit juice. The legume alfalfa *(Medicago sativa)* and the plants dandelion *(Taraxacum officinale)*, stinging nettle *(Urtica dioica)*, and horsetail *(Equisetum arvense)* all contain significant amounts of potassium as well[35] and may induce hyperkalemia, especially in patients with chronic kidney injury.

Urinary Obstruction

Djenkol beans or jering *(Pithecellobium jeringa)* are broad, round, reddish beans that grow during monsoon season in Myanmar, Indonesia, and Malaysia and are considered a delicacy. The jering seeds are extolled for their supposed ability to prevent diabetes and high blood pressure. In addition, the seeds do have bladder spasmodic properties and are also used as a remedy to eliminate stones from the bladder. The jering poisoning or djenkolism is characterized by spasmodic pain, urinary obstruction, and acute kidney injury.[36] The underlying pathologic process is an obstructive uropathy. On a more chronic basis, djenkol bean consumption is associated with a fourfold higher risk of nonglomerular hematuria.[37]

Renal Toxicity from Contaminants in Herbal Medicines

Herbal medicines may be contaminated with excessive or banned pesticides, microbial contaminants, heavy metals, and chemical toxins or adulterated with orthodox drugs. These contaminants are related to the source of these herbal materials, if they are grown in a contaminated environment, or to collection of the plant materials. The herbal materials may be contaminated with chemical toxins unintentionally or intentionally during the storage of the herbs. The presence of orthodox drugs is often due to the intentional alteration of the herbal remedy by the manufacturers.[38] A federal government report found undeclared pharmaceuticals or heavy metals in 32% of Asian medicines sold in the state of California. These include ephedrine, chlorpheniramine, methyltestosterone and phenacetin, sildenafil, steroids, and fenfluramine; 10% to 15% have lead, mercury, or arsenic. Of more than 500 Chinese drugs, approximately 10% contain undeclared drugs or heavy metals.[4]

A number of case reports have demonstrated adulterations leading to renal injury. One described a 73-year-old Malaysian woman who presented with renal failure and bilateral papillary necrosis. She had osteoarthritis and had been consuming two tablets of a traditional herbal preparation, freely available from Chinese medical halls, daily for the past 10 years. She denied the consumption of other analgesics. The product inserts of these preparations stipulated that their only active ingredients were Chinese herbs. However, analysis of the herbal preparation demonstrated the presence of 120 mg of phenylbutazone per tablet. The second report described a 34-year-old housewife who had been taking a mixture of Chinese herbs to strengthen her health. She presented with Fanconi's syndrome and a nephrogenic diabetes insipidus and was found to have a urinary excretion of cadmium 50 times greater than normal. Another report described a patient who presented with a rapid onset of dialysis-requiring acute kidney injury, with marked albuminuria, microscopic pyuria, and hematuria after a 4-week treatment with Tung Shueh pills for arthralgias. A renal biopsy demonstrated acute interstitial nephritis with an inflammatory infiltrate consisting of lymphocytes and eosinophils. The Tung Shueh pills were analyzed and found to contain both diazepam and mefenamic acid as additives. In Morocco, the traditional el badia, a powder made of the seeds of *Tamarix orientalis*, is used by women for hair dye; however, when the *T. orientalis* seeds are scarce, they are replaced with roumia, which contains paraphenylenediamine. This substitution is responsible for about 10% of all cases of acute kidney injury, 50% of all cases of rhabdomyolysis, 25% of intensive care unit admissions for poisonings, and two thirds of poisoning-related deaths in Morocco.[4,6]

In Thailand and other parts of Southeast Asia and India, herbal remedies have been shown to be contaminated with lead, cadmium, and mercury. In South Africa, about 15% of herbs have been found to be contaminated with uranium. In the United States, ginseng dietary supplements have been shown to contain the pesticides quintozene and hexachlorobenzene or to have exceeded the standard for lead content.

Herb-Drug Interactions Resulting in Adverse Renal Effects

Herbs are often administered in combination with therapeutic drugs, raising the potential of pharmacokinetic or pharmacodynamic herb-drug interactions. A number of herb-drug interactions have been noted to alter efficacy and adverse events. Pharmacokinetic herb-drug interactions are due to altered absorption, metabolism, distribution, and excretion of drugs. Frequently, one of the underlying mechanisms of altered drug concentrations by concomitant herbal medicines is the induction or inhibition of hepatic and intestinal cytochrome P-450. By searching the literature, it has been found that a total of 32 drugs interact with herbal medicines in humans. These drugs mainly include anticoagulants (warfarin, aspirin, and phenprocoumon), sedatives and antidepressants (midazolam, alprazolam, and amitriptyline), oral contraceptives, anti-HIV agents (indinavir, ritonavir, and saquinavir), cardiovascular drugs (digoxin), immunosuppressants (cyclosporine and tacrolimus), and anticancer drugs (imatinib and irinotecan). Most of them are substrates for cytochromes or P-glycoprotein, and many have narrow therapeutic indices. Toxicity arising from drug-herb interactions may be minor, moderate, or even fatal, depending on a number of factors associated with the patients, herbs, and drugs.[1]

St. John's wort, derived from the plant *Hypericum perforatum*, has been used since ancient times for depression and anxiety. It is the most common antidepressant used in Germany. St. John's wort induces a hepatic enzyme through activation of the cytochrome P-450 system. Through these mechanisms, St. John's wort can decrease plasma levels of a wide range of prescribed drugs, with possible serious clinical consequences. For example, St. John's wort ingested for 10 days by a group of healthy volunteers reduced the bioavailability of digoxin by an average of 25%. St. John's wort ingested for 2 weeks reduced total absorption of indinavir by 50%, which is large enough to cause treatment failure. Case reports indicated significant increases in the metabolism of other drugs, including warfarin, theophylline, oral contraceptives, and cyclosporine. In transplant recipients, toxicity and underdosage of calcineurin inhibitor–based immunosuppression have been linked to phytochemically triggered activity changes of cytochrome P-450 isoenzyme CYP3A4 metabolism and drug transport proteins. Concomitant use of St. John's wort in renal transplant recipients treated with cyclosporine or tacrolimus could favor graft rejection.[39,40]

Gingko biloba, one of the most popular plant extracts in Europe, recently received approval in Germany for treatment of dementia. *G. biloba* is composed of several flavonoids, terpenoids (e.g., gingkolides), and organic acids believed to act synergistically as free radical scavengers. It has been suggested that *G. biloba* should not be administered with concomitant anticoagulation or in patients with bleeding disorders. Hence, concomitant use of aspirin or any of the nonsteroidal anti-inflammatory drugs (NSAIDs), as well as of anticoagulants such as warfarin and heparin, is ill-advised. Spontaneous hyphema and spontaneous bilateral subdural hematomas have been observed in patients taking *G. biloba* and attributed to ginkgolide B, a potent inhibitor of platelet-activating factor needed to induce arachidonate-independent platelet aggregation. Hemorrhagic complications were observed often in patients administered concomitant antiaggregant or anticoagulant therapy. The exact mechanism of the interaction of *G. biloba* with aspirin, warfarin, and NSAIDs remains unclear. Experimental data from rats suggest that a *G. biloba* diet markedly increased the content of cytochrome P-450 and activity of glutathione *S*-transferase and markedly induced the level of CYP2B1/2, CYP3A1, and CYP3A2 messenger RNA in the liver.[41]

In summary, herbal medicines may exert renal toxicity through their inherent properties, occasionally dose-related or idiosyncratic toxicity, herb-drug interactions, and misidentification and adulteration of the preparation. Various renal syndromes have been reported after the use of herbal medicines. They include acute tubular necrosis, acute interstitial nephritis, Fanconi's syndrome, hypokalemia, hypertension, papillary necrosis, chronic interstitial nephritis, nephrolithiasis, urinary retention, and cancer of the urinary tract. Conversely, herbal medicine may also be hazardous for renal patients because it may interact with such drugs as cyclosporine or carry significant amounts of potassium. Until now, most published data about the toxicity of herbal medicines are case reports. Precise identities of the culprit substances, the toxicologic characteristics, and the pathogenic mechanisms in herbal medicines remain largely unknown. Whereas many herbs have been used for centuries without incidence of acute kidney injury, insidious damage caused by long-term use is a concern because many herbs have not been rigorously tested for toxicity. Some Web sites provide data on herbal therapy hazards (Fig. 74.6),[6] which may be helpful for nephrologists to obtain specific information about specific herbs that their patients may use.

OVER-THE-COUNTER MEDICINES AND THE KIDNEY: ANALGESIC NEPHROPATHY

In recent years, we have witnessed the increasing popularity of over-the-counter (OTC) health foods, nutraceuticals, and medicinal products from plants or other natural sources in the developed countries. However, OTC analgesics are one of the most widely used classes of drugs in the United States. The primary indications for use of OTC analgesics include fever and minor aches and pains. NSAIDs, such as aspirin, ibuprofen, and naproxen sodium, are also used to treat inflammatory conditions, and aspirin is used prophylactically as an anticoagulant in thrombosis-related disorders. Acetaminophen, aspirin, ibuprofen, and naproxen sodium are available over the counter. Population studies and World Health Organization statistics indicate that 10% to 50% of individuals have a history of musculoskeletal disorders. Easy access to some of these OTC analgesics and combinations by the general public runs the risk of unwarranted and unsupervised chronic intake. Although studies on the association between the long-term use of aspirin, NSAIDs, and other analgesics and end-stage renal disease have given conflicting results, many studies have suggested an association between chronic ingestion of analgesics and kidney disease. A retrospective cohort study using data from the Australia and New Zealand Dialysis and Transplant registry showed that of 31,654 patients with incident renal replacement therapy, 10.2% had analgesic nephropathy. Patients with analgesic nephropathy have more comorbidities and poorer survival on renal replacement therapy, especially among younger patients.[42] Because of the widespread use of analgesics, even a small increased risk of kidney disease will have major public health implications.

A National Kidney Foundation position paper defines analgesic nephropathy as a disease resulting from the habitual consumption during several years of a mixture containing at least two antipyretic analgesics and usually codeine or caffeine. It is characterized by kidney papillary necrosis and chronic interstitial

Websites Providing Data on Herbal Therapy Hazards

Web Address	Website
http://www.fda.gov or http://www.vmcfsan.fda.gov/~dms/aems/html.	On the Food and Drug Administration Website under the title Medwatch, some herb warnings can be found ("special adverse event monitoring system" link)
http://www.faseb.org/aspet/H&MIG3.htm#top.	ASPET Herbal and Medicinal Plant Interest Group: a site for an herb discussion group with pharmacologists
http://www.nnlm.nlm.nih.gov/pnr/uwmhg/.	University of Washington Medicinal Herb Garden
http://www.nim.nih.gov/medlineplus/herbalmedicine.html	Provides an update on ongoing clinical studies involving herbal products, news, and many links
http://www.update-software.com/abstracts/mainindex.html	The Cochrane Collaboration maintains an updated international database of clinical trials involving complementary and alternative medicine
http://www.amfoundation.org/	Providing consumers and professionals with responsible evidence-based information on the integration of alternative and conventional medicine
http://www.herbmed.org/	An interactive electronic herbal database provides hyperlinked access to scientific data underlying the use of herbs for health; an evidence-based information resource for professionals, researchers, and general public
http://nccam.nih.gov/	The National Center for Complementary and Alternative Medicine is 1 of 27 institutes and centers that make up the U.S. National Institutes of Health; their mission is to support rigorous research on complementary and alternative medicine, train researchers, and disseminate information to the public and professionals
http://toxnet.nlm.nih.gov/	A cluster of databases on toxicology, hazardous chemicals, and related areas

Figure 74.6 Websites providing data on herbal therapy hazards. *(From reference 6.)*

nephritis that leads to insidious onset of progressive kidney failure. NSAIDs, such as aspirin, ibuprofen, and naproxen sodium, inhibit cyclooxygenase and may inhibit lipoxygenase, decreasing the production of prostaglandins and leukotrienes, which accounts for many NSAID-induced renal effects. In patients with volume depletion, renal perfusion depends on circulating prostaglandins to vasodilate the afferent arterioles, allowing more blood flow through the glomerulus. The contribution of prostaglandins to renal homeostasis is most critical in elderly patients and those with circulatory disturbances, such as renal or liver dysfunction, congestive heart failure, or volume depletion.[43]

The early-phase changes of analgesic nephropathy in humans were first demonstrated in patients with normal kidney function with a history of phenacetin and acetylsalicylic acid consumption (ingestion of a minimum of five tablets a day for 5 years). Histologic lesions seen in experimentally induced analgesic nephropathy are similar to those seen in humans. Medullary ischemia seems to be the initiating event. Light microscopy and electron microscopy reveal irreversible damage to medullary interstitium, characterized by interstitial cell nuclear degeneration, abnormal interstitial matrix, loss of medullary interstitial cells, and increased collagen. The earliest changes involve sclerosis of vasa recta capillaries and patchy tubular necrosis. Later changes include areas of papillary necrosis and secondary focal segmental glomerulosclerosis, cortical scarring, and interstitial fibrosis. Papillary necrosis may also be the result of reactive metabolic products of the drug or the accumulation of phospholipids in the papilla.

The clinical symptoms of analgesic nephropathy include polyuria, sterile leukocyturia, and microscopic hematuria. Progression is insidious, and clinical findings in later stages are related to advanced renal failure. Diagnosis can be made by ultrasound or intravenous urography (see Fig. 50.4C), but a computed tomography (CT) scan finding of irregular kidneys with papillary necrosis and calcification is the most sensitive and specific method of diagnosis of analgesic nephropathy (Fig. 74.7).[44] A staging system for analgesic nephropathy based on CT scan appearances has been proposed by Elseviers and coworkers.[44]

It is important to highlight the potential adverse effects of analgesic agents on the kidney. Patients who warrant chronic therapy with these agents should be closely monitored for any early signs of kidney injury. Early detection and removal of the offending agent could halt or even reverse analgesic-induced kidney injury. There is a pressing need for multicenter trials to assess the true incidence of this problem and to study the effects of various analgesic agents (alone and in combination) in at-risk populations. Analgesic nephropathy is also discussed in Chapter 62.

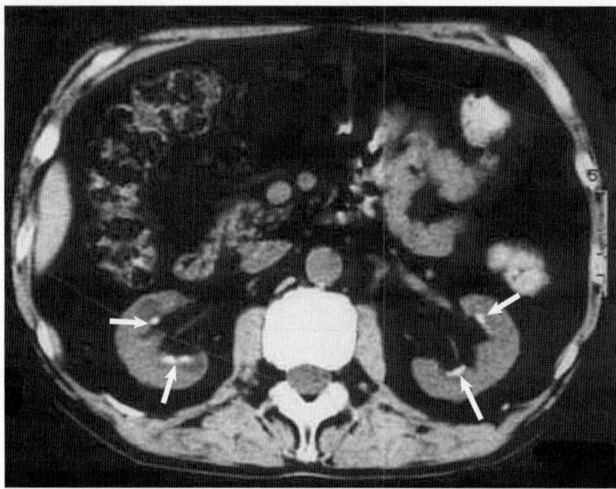

Figure 74.7 Papillary calcifications in analgesic nephropathy. Non–contrast-enhanced CT scan of a patient with long-time analgesic abuse showed thinning of the renal parenchyma and typical papillary calcifications *(arrows)*. *(Courtesy Dr. Yoshifumi Ubara, Toranomon Hospital, Tokyo, Japan.)*

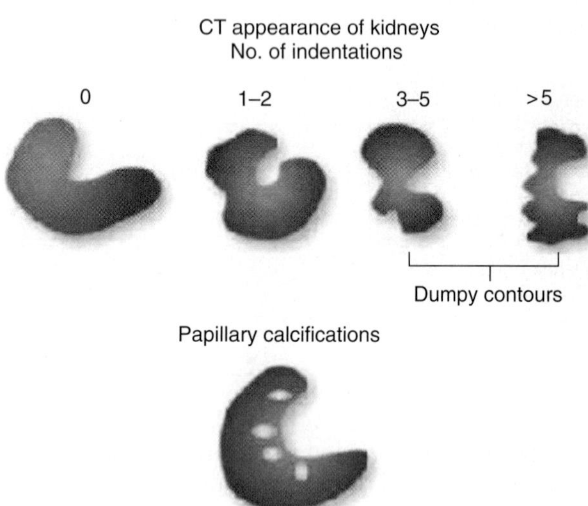

Figure 74.8 CT imaging criteria of analgesic nephropathy. *(Modified from reference 44.)*

REFERENCES

1. Zhou SF, Xue CC, Yu XQ, et al. Metabolic activation of herbal and dietary constituents and its clinical and toxicological implications: An update. *Curr Drug Metab*. 2007;8:526-553.
2. De Smet PA. Herbal remedies. *N Engl J Med*. 2002;347:2046-2056.
3. De Smet PA. Herbal medicine in Europe—relaxing regulatory standards. *N Engl J Med*. 2005;352:1176-1178.
4. Jha V, Rathi M. Natural medicines causing acute kidney injury. *Semin Nephrol*. 2008;28:416-428.
5. Naughton CA. Drug-induced nephrotoxicity. *Am Fam Physician*. 2008; 78:743-750.
6. Isnard Bagnis C, Deray G, Baumelou A, et al. Herbs and the kidney. *Am J Kidney Dis*. 2004;44:1-11.
7. Vanherweghem JL, Depierreux M, Tielemans C, et al. Rapidly progressive interstitial renal fibrosis in young women: Association with slimming regimen including Chinese herbs. *Lancet*. 1993;341:387-391.
8. Lord GM, Cook T, Arlt VM, et al. Urothelial malignant disease and Chinese herbal nephropathy. *Lancet*. 2001;358:1515-1516.
9. Nortier JL, Vanherweghem JL. Renal interstitial fibrosis and urothelial carcinoma associated with the use of a Chinese herb *(Aristolochia fangchi)*. *Toxicology*. 2002;181-182:577-580.
10. Gillerot G, Jadoul M, Arlt VM, et al. Aristolochic acid nephropathy in a Chinese patient: Time to abandon the term "Chinese herbs nephropathy"? [comment]. *Am J Kidney Dis*. 2001;38:E26.
11. Debelle FD, Vanherweghem JL, Nortier JL. Aristolochic acid nephropathy: A worldwide problem. *Kidney Int*. 2008;74:158-169.
12. Lai MN, Lai JN, Chen PC, et al. Increased risks of chronic kidney disease associated with prescribed Chinese herbal products suspected to contain aristolochic acid. *Nephrology (Carlton)*. 2008 Dec 4 [Epub ahead of print].
13. Debelle F, Nortier J, De Prez E, et al. Aristolochic acids induce chronic renal failure with interstitial fibrosis in salt-depleted rats. *J Am Soc Nephrol*. 2002;13:431-436.
14. Pozdzik AA, Salmon IJ, Debelle FD, et al. Aristolochic acid induces proximal tubule apoptosis and epithelial to mesenchymal transformation. *Kidney Int*. 2008;73:595-607.
15. Kong PI, Chiu YW, Kuo MC, et al. Aristolochic acid nephropathy due to herbal drug intake manifested differently as Fanconi's syndrome and end-stage renal failure—a 7-year follow-up. *Clin Nephrol*. 2008;70: 537-541.
16. Kabanda A, Jadoul M, Lauwerys R, et al. Low molecular weight proteinuria in Chinese herbs nephropathy. *Kidney Int*. 1995;48:1571-1576.
17. Depierreux M, Van Damme B, Vanden Houte K, et al. Pathologic aspects of a newly described nephropathy related to the prolonged use of Chinese herbs. *Am J Kidney Dis*. 1994;24:172-180.
18. Pozdzik AA, Salmon IJ, Husson CP, et al. Patterns of interstitial inflammation during the evolution of renal injury in experimental aristolochic acid nephropathy. *Nephrol Dial Transplant*. 2008;23:2480-2491.
19. Cosyns JP, Jadoul M, Squifflet JP, et al. Chinese herbs nephropathy: A clue to Balkan endemic nephropathy? *Kidney Int*. 1994;45:1680-1688.
20. Lemy A, Wissing KM, Rorive S, et al. Late onset of bladder urothelial carcinoma after kidney transplantation for end-stage aristolochic acid nephropathy: A case series with 15-year follow-up. *Am J Kidney Dis*. 2008;51:471-477.
21. IARC Working Group on the Evaluation of Carcinogenic Risks to Humans. Some traditional herbal medicines, some mycotoxins, naphthalene and styrene. *IARC Monogr Eval Carcinog Risks Hum*. 2002;82:118.
22. de Jonge H, Vanrenterghem Y. Aristolochic acid: The common culprit of Chinese herbs nephropathy and Balkan endemic nephropathy. *Nephrol Dial Transplant*. 2008;23:39-41.
23. Lincoln T. Toxicology: Danger in the diet. *Nature*. 2007;448:148.
24. Vanherweghem JL, Abramowicz D, Tielemans C, et al. Effects of steroids on the progression of renal failure in chronic interstitial renal fibrosis: A pilot study in Chinese herbs nephropathy. *Am J Kidney Dis*. 1996;27:209-215.
25. Muniz Martinez MC, Nortier J, Vereerstraeten P, et al. Steroid therapy in chronic interstitial renal fibrosis: The case of Chinese-herb nephropathy. *Nephrol Dial Transplant*. 2002;17:2033-2034.
26. Nortier JL, Martinez MC, Schmeiser HH, et al. Urothelial carcinoma associated with the use of a Chinese herb *(Aristolochia fangchi)* [comment]. *N Engl J Med*. 2000;342:1686-1692.
27. Kadiri S, Ogunlesi A, Osinfade K, et al. The causes and course of acute tubular necrosis in Nigerians. *Afr J Med Med Sci*. 1992;21:91-96.
28. Dan H, Peng RX, Ao Y, et al. Segment-specific proximal tubule injury in tripterygium glycosides intoxicated rats. *J Biochem Mol Toxicol*. 2008;22:422-428.
29. Hilepo JN, Bellucci AG, Mossey RT. Acute renal failure caused by "cat's claw" herbal remedy in a patient with systemic lupus erythematosus. *Nephron*. 1997;77:361.
30. Watson WA, Litovitz TL, Rodgers GC Jr, et al. 2004 Annual report of the American Association of Poison Control Centers Toxic Exposure Surveillance System. *Am J Emerg Med*. 2005;23:589-666.
31. Saviuc P, Danel V. New syndromes in mushroom poisoning. *Toxicol Rev*. 2006;25:199-209.
32. Hallas J, Bjerrum L, Støvring H, et al. Use of a prescribed ephedrine/caffeine combination and the risk of serious cardiovascular events: A registry-based case-crossover study. *Am J Epidemiol*. 2008;168:966-973.
33. de Klerk GJ, Nieuwenhuis MG, Beutler JJ. Hypokalaemia and hypertension associated with use of liquorice flavoured chewing gum. *BMJ*. 1997;314:731-732.
34. Bennett S, Hoffman N, Monga M. Ephedrine- and guaifenesin-induced nephrolithiasis. *J Altern Complement Med*. 2004;10:967-969.
35. Leung AY, Foster S. *Encyclopedia of Common Natural Ingredients Used in Food, Drugs, and Cosmetics*. New York: Wiley; 1996.

36. Segasothy M, Swaminathan M, Kong NC, Bennett WM. Djenkol bean poisoning (djenkolism): An unusual cause of acute renal failure. *Am J Kidney Dis*. 1995;25:63-66.
37. Vachvanichsanong P, Lebel L. Djenkol beans as a cause of hematuria in children. *Nephron*. 1997;76:39-42.
38. Chan K. Some aspects of toxic contaminants in herbal medicines. *Chemosphere*. 2003;52:1361-1371.
39. Ernst E. The risk-benefit profile of commonly used herbal therapies: Ginkgo, St. John's Wort, Ginseng, Echinacea, Saw Palmetto, and Kava. *Ann Intern Med*. 2002;136:42-53.
40. Yang XX, Hu ZP, Duan W, et al. Drug-herb interactions: Eliminating toxicity with hard drug design. *Curr Pharm Des*. 2006;12: 4649-4664.
41. Shinozuka K, Umegaki K, Kubota Y, et al. Feeding of Ginkgo biloba extract (GBE) enhances gene expression of hepatic cytochrome P-450 and attenuates the hypotensive effect of nicardipine in rats. *Life Sci*. 2002;70:2783-2792.
42. Chang SH, Mathew TH, McDonald SP. Analgesic nephropathy and renal replacement therapy in Australia: Trends, comorbidities and outcomes. *Clin J Am Soc Nephrol*. 2008;3:768-776.
43. Schlondorff D. Renal prostaglandin synthesis. Sites of production and specific actions of prostaglandins. *Am J Med*. 1986;81:1-11.
44. Elseviers MM, De Schepper A, Corthouts R, et al. High diagnostic performance of CT scan for analgesic nephropathy in patients with incipient to severe renal failure. *Kidney Int*. 1995;48:1316-1323.
45. Vadivel N, Trikudanathan S, Singh AK. Analgesic nephropathy. *Kidney Int*. 2007;72:517-520.

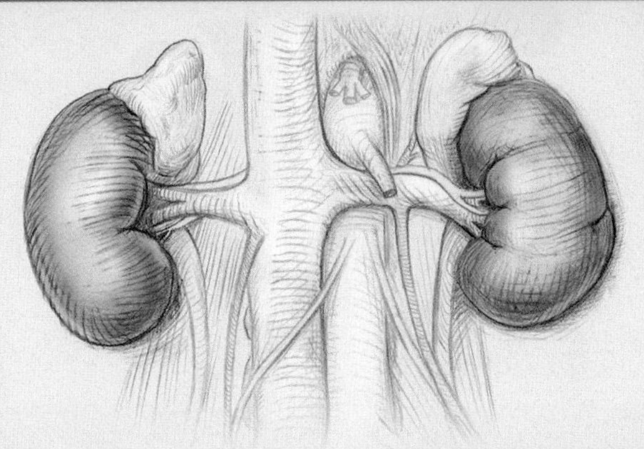

SECTION XV

Chronic Kidney Disease and the Uremic Syndrome

CHAPTER 75

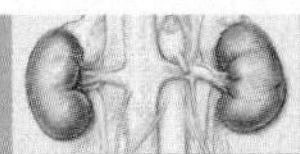

Epidemiology and Pathophysiology of Chronic Kidney Disease

Aminu Bello, Bisher Kawar, Mohsen El Kossi, Meguid El Nahas

DEFINITION

Chronic kidney disease (CKD) is defined as kidney damage or glomerular filtration rate (GFR) below 60 ml/min per 1.73 m^2 for 3 months or more irrespective of the cause. The Kidney Disease Outcomes Quality Initiative (KDOQI) guidelines have classified CKD into five stages.[1] This classification, although useful in simplifying the categorization of CKD, has its limitations, which include classifying people with isolated microalbuminuria as suffering from CKD, labeling mild and stable kidney damage as CKD, and not differentiating between age-related impaired kidney function and progressive disease-induced CKD.[2]

In 2005, the Kidney Disease: Improving Global Outcomes (KDIGO) group suggested clarifications including the addition of the suffix T for patients with renal allografts and D to identify CKD stage 5 patients on dialysis.[3]

The U.K. National Institute of Health and Clinical Excellence (NICE) has modified, in 2008, the KDOQI CKD classification by subdividing CKD stage 3 into 3A and 3B, estimated GFR of 45 to 59 ml/min per 1.73 m^2 and 30 to 44 ml/min per 1.73 m^2, respectively.[4] The NICE CKD guidelines also stipulated that the suffix *p* be added to the stages in proteinuric patients (Fig. 75.1). This refinement of the initial CKD classification by NICE assumes that there is a distinction between patients with GFR below 60 ml/min per 1.73 m^2 and those with GFR below 45 ml/min per 1.73 m^2 in terms of prognosis and that the presence of significant proteinuria has to be acknowledged in the classification.[4]

EPIDEMIOLOGY OF CHRONIC KIDNEY DISEASE

The true incidence and prevalence of CKD within a community are difficult to ascertain as early to moderate CKD is usually asymptomatic. However, various epidemiologic studies attempted to clarify that issue and have made relatively similar observations suggesting a prevalence of CKD of around 10%, albuminuria (mostly microalbuminuria) of around 7%, and GFR below 60 ml/min per 1.73 m^2 of around 3% (Fig. 75.2).

Of note, most of these studies are limited by the fact that individuals were tested only once, thus precluding a clear assumption of chronicity. The high prevalence of CKD is confounded by a number of facts:

1. Microalbuminuria is considered a marker of CKD when it may merely reflect underlying vascular disease, endothelial dysfunction, or atherosclerosis or chronic inflammatory conditions such as hepatitis, dermatitis, and colitis. Also, microalbuminuria is associated with aging, obesity, and smoking. Finally, it is often transient and reversible.
2. The majority of those screened within the community and found to have reduced GFR are elderly individuals. Age is known to be associated with a decline in kidney function that some consider physiologic, whereas others attribute it to underlying vascular aging and pathologic processes, mostly atherosclerosis and progressive renal ischemia.
3. Formulae such as the Modification of Diet in Renal Disease (MDRD) and Cockcroft-Gault are used to estimate GFR in spite of their known limitations and underestimation of normal kidney function (bias and imprecision) (see Chapter 3).

All these limitations of current CKD screening strategies may tend to overinflate the overall prevalence of significant CKD.

EPIDEMIOLOGY OF END-STAGE RENAL DISEASE

Incidence of end-stage renal disease (ESRD) refers to the number of patients with ESRD beginning renal replacement therapy (RRT) during a given time (usually a year) in relation to the general population; it is usually expressed as number of patients per million population per year. Of note, the incidence of ESRD according to most national registries does not take into account patients not treated by RRT; therefore, it underestimates the overall true incidence of ESRD (CKD stage 5).

The prevalence of ESRD is the proportion in a specific population who have ESRD at a given time; it encompasses both new and continuing patients on RRT; it is expressed as patients per million population. Prevalence is a function of the incidence (new cases) and outcomes (transplantation or death) rates of ESRD in a given population.

The global epidemiology of ESRD is heterogeneous and influenced by several factors. Consequently, the incidence and prevalence of ESRD vary widely from country to country (Fig. 75.3).

Disparities in the incidence and prevalence of ESRD within and between developed countries reflect racial and ethnic diversities as well as their impact on the prevalence of diabetes and hypertension in respective countries and communities. Recently, different progression rates of CKD in the population, referral patterns, and quality of pre-ESRD care have been linked to the heterogeneity of ESRD rates in different parts of the world. Disparities with developing countries are likely to reflect availability of and access to RRT in low and middle economies.

The cost of treating patients with ESRD is substantial and has an impact on provision of care. In this context, it has been proposed that there is a clear and direct relationship between nations' gross national product and the availability of RRT in most countries.[5] It was pointed out that during the next decade, even the industrialized nations will struggle to meet the demands of expanding ESRD programs; in the United States, it has been estimated that the annual expenditure on ESRD will reach more than U.S. $52 billion by 2030.[6] In the United Kingdom, renal services currently consume about 2% of the National Health Service budget, and this is set to rise with increasing numbers of individuals requiring RRT.[7] Globally, it has been estimated that by 2010, more than 2 million individuals will be treated by RRT at a cost of $1 trillion during the decade.[8] The great majority (90%) of those treated live in high economies. More than 100 of 212 countries worldwide with low and middle economies do not have any provision for RRT.[9] Consequently, in many low and middle economy countries, ESRD is a death sentence.

Classification of CKD Based on GFR

CKD Stage	Definition
1	Normal or increased GFR; some evidence of kidney damage reflected by microalbuminuria, proteinuria, and hematuria as well as radiologic or histologic changes
2	Mild decrease in GFR (89–60 ml/min per 1.73 m^2) with some evidence of kidney damage reflected by microalbuminuria, proteinuria and hematuria as well as radiologic or histologic changes
3	GFR 59-30 ml/min per 1.73 m^2
3A	GFR 59 to 45 ml/min per 1.73 m^2
3B	GFR 44 to 30 ml/min per 1.73 m^2
4	GFR 29-15 ml/min per 1.73 m^2
5	GFR <15 ml/min per 1.73 m^2; when renal replacement therapy in the form of dialysis or transplantation has to be considered to sustain life

The suffix p to be added to the stage in proteinuric patients (proteinuria >0.5 g/24h)

Figure 75.1 Classification of CKD based on GFR as proposed by the Kidney Disease Outcomes Quality Initiative (KDOQI) guidelines and modified by NICE in 2008. *(From references 1 and 4.)*

SCREENING FOR CHRONIC KIDNEY DISEASE

Current Screening Guidelines

In view of the rising number of those suffering from ESRD and the perceived high prevalence of CKD in communities, interest has focused on the early detection of CKD and those at risk. Several guidelines for screening, mostly targeted to high-risk individuals, have been issued and implemented worldwide. Those include the U.S. KDOQI, the U.K. CKD NICE, and the Australian Caring for Australasians with Renal Impairment (CARI) guidelines, to name a few.[1,4,10] There are few differences as to the recommended targeted populations, but they invariably include individuals with hypertension and diabetes mellitus. Other groups include those with a family history of CKD; obese individuals; those with cardiovascular diseases, especially congestive heart failure; people with multisystem diseases; ethnic groups with high prevalence of CKD; and those with urologic conditions, such as nephrolithiasis. The KDOQI guidelines additionally recommend screening those older than 65 years. Screening should consist of a urine albumin/protein estimation as well as measurement of serum creatinine and estimation of GFR (see Chapter 3). General population CKD screening is unlikely to be realistic or cost-effective. Targeted screening is the most cost-effective approach (Fig. 75.4).

Overall, CKD screening would best be associated with broader national strategies and programs to minimize cardiovascular disease (CVD). This is the essence of the U.K. national vascular campaign/strategy launched in 2009 and aiming to screen those older than 40 years for CVD risk, including, when appropriate, CKD. Similar strategies have been initiated by the Centers for Disease Control and Prevention in the United States and in Australia.

NATURAL HISTORY OF CHRONIC KIDNEY DISEASE

The natural history of CKD stages 1 and 2 remains to be fully defined. It has generally been assumed that the majority of patients with CKD stages 3B to 5 progress relentlessly to ESRD.

Representative Population-based Studies on CKD Epidemiology

Study	Country	Design	N	Outcome (%) MA	Outcome (%) CKD
NHANES III	United Sates	CS/L	15,626	12	11
PREVEND	Netherlands	CS/L	40,000	7	
NEOERICA	United Kingdom	CS/ service based	130,226		11 (F), 6 (M)
HUNT II	Norway	CS	65,181	6	10
EPIC-Norfolk	United Kingdom	CS	23,964	12	
MONICA Augsburg	Germany	CS	2,136	8	
AusDiab	Australia	CS	11,247	6	10
Taiwan	Taiwan	CS/L	462,293		12
Beijing	China	CS	13,925		13
Takahata	Japan	CS	2,321	14	

Figure 75.2 Representative population-based studies on CKD epidemiology. Outcome = subjects with chronic kidney disease (CKD) or microalbuminuria (MA). NHANES, National Health and Nutrition Evaluation Survey; PREVEND, Prevention of Renal and Vascular Endstage Disease; NEOERICA, New Opportunities for Early Renal Intervention by Computerised Assessment; HUNT, Nord-Trøndelag health study; EPIC, European Prospective Investigation into Cancer Study; AusDiab, Australian Diabetes, Obesity and Lifestyle study; CS, cross-sectional; F, female; L, longitudinal; M, male; N, number of participants; service based, collecting patients' data from general practitioner computer records.

Global Incidence and Prevalence of RRT (Per Million Population) in 2006		
Country	**Incidence**	**Prevalence**
United States	360	1,626
Caucasians	279	1,194
African Americans	1,010	5,004
Native Americans	489	2,691
Asians	388	1,831
Hispanics	481	1,991
Australia	115	778
Aboriginal/Torres Strait	441	2,070
Japan	275	1,956
Europe	129	770
United Kingdom	113	725
France	140	957
Germany	213	1,114
Italy	133	1,010
Spain	132	991

Figure 75.3 Global incidence and prevalence of RRT (per million population) in 2006. *(Source: USRDS, ANZDATA, ERA-EDTA, and U.K. renal registries.)*

International Recommendations for Targeted Screening for CKD				
Targeted group	**Guidelines**			
	KDOQI	**UK NICE**	**CARI**	**CSN**
Elderly	•			
Hypertension	•	•	•	•
Diabetes mellitus	•	•	•	•
Atherosclerotic		•	•	•
Cardiovascular disease heart failure		•		•
Urologic disease, stone disease, recurrent urinary infections	•	•		
Systemic autoimmune conditions	•	•		•
Nephrotoxic drugs	•	•		•
High-risk ethnic groups	•		•	•
Family history of CKD	•	•		
Other high-risk groups may include smokers, metabolic syndrome, obesity, low birth weight, systemic infections, reduced renal mass, and previous acute kidney injury				

Figure 75.4 International recommendations for targeted screening for CKD. KDOQI, Kidney Disease Outcomes Quality Initiative; U.K. NICE, U.K. National Institute of Health and Clinical Excellence; CARI, Australian Caring for Australasians with Renal Impairment; CSN, Canadian Society of Nephrology.

This has recently been challenged as progression is variable, and a sizable percentage of these patients have stable kidney function or die prematurely of CVD.[11] A Canadian study showed the natural history of CKD stages 3 and 4 to be variable and reflecting the patient's risk factor profile.[12] Many CKD patients with GFR below 60 ml/min per 1.73 m^2 die from cardiovascular or other causes before reasing reaching ESRD.

A straight-line relationship is often found between the reciprocal of serum creatinine ($1/S_{Cr}$) values or the estimated GFR and time (for methodologic aspects, refer to Chapter 76). However, a significant percentage of patients do not progress in a predictable linear fashion and have breakpoints in their progression slopes, suggesting acceleration or slowing down of the rate of progression of CKD. These breakpoints could be either spontaneous or secondary to events such as infections, dehydration, changes in the adequacy of systemic blood pressure control, and exposure to nephrotoxins, in particular nonsteroidal anti-inflammatory drugs (NSAIDs) or radiocontrast agents. Attention has also been drawn recently to the impact of intercurrent acute kidney injury (AKI) events on the rate of progression of CKD. It is also important to appreciate that some patients with mild to moderate CKD have stable renal function for sustained periods.[11,12]

The rate of progression of CKD also varies according to the underlying nephropathy and between individual patients. Historically, the rate of decline in GFR of patients with diabetic nephropathy has been among the fastest, averaging around −10 ml/min per year. Control of systemic hypertension slows the rate of GFR decline to −5 ml/min per year, with further improvement (−1 to −2 ml/min per year) expected in patients whose glycemia and hypertension are optimally controlled and in those treated with inhibitors of the renin-angiotensin-aldosterone system (RAS). In nondiabetic nephropathy, the rate of progression of CKD was 2.5 times faster in patients with chronic glomerulonephritis than in those with chronic interstitial nephritis and 1.5 times faster than in those with hypertensive nephrosclerosis. The association of proteinuria and faster progression of CKD was highlighted in a number of studies (reviewed in reference 13). Relief of obstruction, discontinuation of nephrotoxic agents, and control of hypertension often stabilize renal function in a large percentage of patients. Patients with polycystic kidney disease and impaired renal function, CKD stage 3B and beyond, may also have a faster rate of progression compared with other nephropathies. The rate of progression of CKD in the elderly has been associated with incident and progressive underlying cardiovascular disease. This is of interest as an increasing number of elderly patients reach ESRD, and renovascular disease has become one of the most common causes of ESRD in some countries.[14]

FACTORS AFFECTING INITIATION AND PROGRESSION OF CHRONIC KIDNEY DISEASE

CKD is likely to be a multi-hit process. Risk factors for CKD include susceptibility, initiation, and progression factors. Susceptibility factors predispose to CKD, whereas initiation factors directly trigger kidney damage. Progression factors are associated with worsening of already established kidney damage. The aim of identifying susceptibility and initiation factors for CKD is to define individuals at high risk for development of CKD; with progression factors, the aim is to define individuals at high risk for worsening (CKD) kidney damage and subsequent loss of kidney function (Fig. 75.5).

Summary of Risk Factors Associated with the Initiation and Progression of CKD

Initiation Factors	Progression Factors
Systemic hypertension	Older age
Diabetes mellitus	Gender (male)
Cardiovascular disease	Race/ethnicity
Dyslipidemia	Genetic predisposition
Obesity/metabolic syndrome	Poor blood pressure control
Hyperuricemia	Poor glycemia control
Smoking	Proteinuria
Low socioeconomic status	Cardiovascular disease
Nephrotoxins exposure: NSAIDs, analgesics, traditional herbal use, heavy metals exposure (such as lead)	Dyslipidemia Smoking Obesity/metabolic syndrome Hyperuricemia Low socioeconomic status Alcohol consumption Nephrotoxins; NSAIDs, RCM, herbal remedies Acute kidney injury

Figure 75.5 Summary of risk factors associated with the initiation and progression of CKD. NSAIDs, nonsteroidal anti-inflammatory drugs; RCM, radiocontrast material.

These risk factors are further classified according to feasibility for intervention as modifiable and nonmodifiable (see Fig. 75.5). The classification can also be clinical (diabetes, hypertension, autoimmune diseases, systemic infections, drugs, or toxins) and sociodemographic (age, race, poverty/low income). A number of these risk factors have been identified in longitudinal community-based studies (see Fig. 75.5).

Known CKD susceptibility factors include genetic and familial predisposition, race (Afro-Caribbeans, Indo-Asians), maternal-fetal factors (low birth weight, malnutrition *in utero*), age (elderly), and gender (male) (reviewed in references 1 and 15). Beyond the susceptibility to CKD, additional initiation factors are likely to trigger disease. These are listed in Figure 75.5.

CHRONIC KIDNEY DISEASE PROGRESSION FACTORS

Once it is established, CKD (eGFR <60 ml/min) progression is influenced by a number of modifiable and nonmodifiable risk factors.[16]

Nonmodifiable Progression Risk Factors

Age

The rate of progression of CKD is influenced by age; elderly patients affected by glomerulonephritis seemingly have a faster rate of GFR decline. However, longitudinal studies of subjects without CKD have observed a decline in GFR with increasing age in some subjects, implying that nephron loss may be part of normal aging. This is corroborated by recently published longitudinal data from Norway.[17] However, in one such study, the Baltimore Longitudinal Study, more than a third of individuals did not have a decline in kidney function with aging. Age-related progression may be affected by underlying CVD and atherosclerosis.[18]

Gender

This is an important demographic factor associated with development and progression of CKD. It has been reported that ESRD due to all causes occurs more frequently in men than in women. According to the USRDS Annual Data Report,[6] there is preponderance in the prevalence of all-cause ESRD in favor of men, but this has not been reported to be so marked in Europe. In most CKD studies and meta-analyses, women have a slower rate of progression compared with men.[6]

Race

In the United States, for all causes of ESRD, African Americans have a faster rate of progression than their Caucasian cohorts do. The incidence and prevalence of diabetic and hypertensive CKD are higher in African and Hispanic Americans compared with Caucasians.[19] Their rate of CKD progression also seems faster, although few studies confirmed this by multivariate analysis. The mechanisms underlying these associations remain to be elucidated, but possible explanations include racial and genetic factors, lower nephron endowment, and increased susceptibility to salt-sensitive hypertension as well as environmental, lifestyle, and socioeconomic differences. The last may have an impact on access to health care and compliance with treatment.

Genetics

Studies have demonstrated that genetic factors play a crucial role in CKD and ESRD, mostly through linkage and association analyses with candidate gene approaches. Recent technologic advancements in genome-wide association studies are likely to uncover new CKD susceptibility genes.

Associations have been described between certain major histocompatibility complex loci and the rate of CKD progression. Patients with polycystic kidney disease carrying the genotype *PKD1* are thought to have a worse prognosis than others. Progression of CKD may also be influenced by polymorphisms of genes coding for putative mediators of renal scarring, including those coding for the renin-angiotensin-aldosterone system (RAAS) (reviewed in reference 20). The human homologue of the rat renal failure (*Rf*) gene has been localized to the long arm of chromosome 10. In African Americans with ESRD due a variety of nephropathies, an association between two markers (D10S1435 and D10S249) spanning 21 polymorphic regions of chromosome 10 approached significance in nondiabetic patients. It was also reported that genetic variation at the *MYH9* locus or sequence variants in the APOL1 gene could explain the increased burden of focal segmental glomerulosclerosis and hypertensive ESRD among African Americans (see Chapter 19). Recent observations showed that single-nucleotide polymorphisms in the genes *TCF7L2*[21] and *MTHFS*[22] are associated with CKD progression in population-based cohorts.

Phenotypically, diabetic and nondiabetic nephropathies cluster in families, particularly in African Americans. In diabetes mellitus, a family history of CVD or hypertension is associated, respectively, with a twofold or fourfold increase in the risk for development of diabetic nephropathy.

Loss of Renal Mass

The threshold to natural progression after nephron loss is likely to be lowered by the presence of hypertension, obesity, hyperlipidemia, hyperglycemia, and black race. Recent evidence

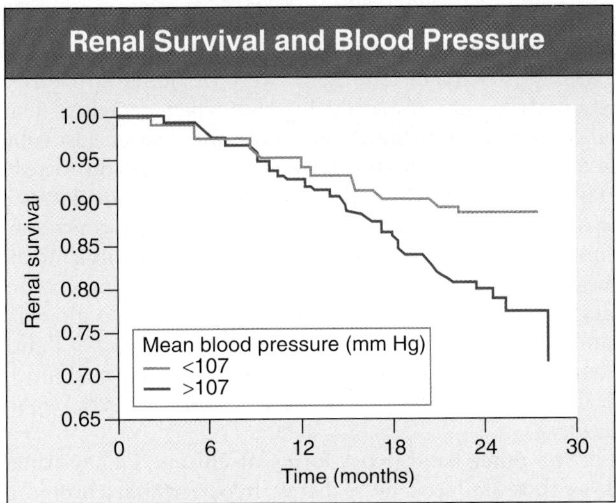

Figure 75.6 Actuarial renal survival in relation to blood pressure. *(Modified from reference 23.)*

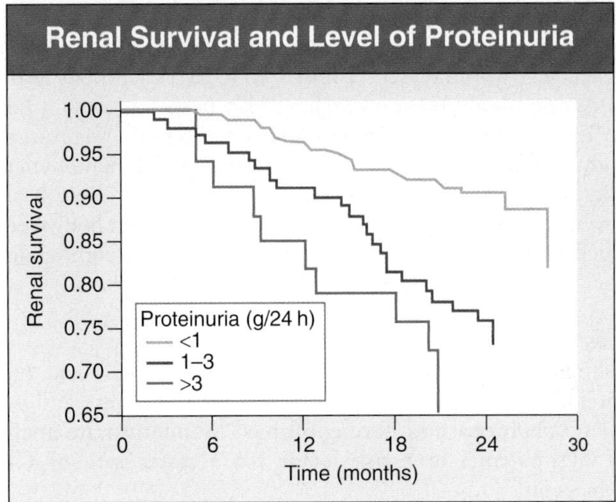

Figure 75.7 Actuarial renal survival in relation to proteinuria. *(Modified from reference 23.)*

also points to the impact of episodes of AKI on the decline in kidney function, with the elderly being more susceptible.[24]

Modifiable Progression Risk Factors

These include systemic hypertension, proteinuria, and metabolic factors. In addition, interest has focused on the contribution of cigarette smoking, alcohol consumption, and recreational drug use to the risk for development of ESRD (see also Chapter 76).

Hypertension

Systemic hypertension is an important cause, consequence, and presenting feature of CKD. It is one of the leading causes of ESRD worldwide,[6] the second leading cause in the United States after diabetes. Some experimental and epidemiologic studies have shown that sustained hypertension is indeed a significant contributor to the progression of CKD. Strong evidence links the progression of CKD to systemic hypertension in diabetic and nondiabetic nephropathies (reviewed in reference 1). It is believed that the transmission of systemic hypertension into the glomerular capillary beds and the resulting glomerular hypertension contribute to the progression of glomerulosclerosis (Fig. 75.6).

Proteinuria

A large number of studies in patients with diabetic and nondiabetic glomerular disease and nonglomerular diseases confirmed, by multivariate analysis, that heavy proteinuria is associated with a faster rate of CKD progression (Fig. 75.7).[1,25] Furthermore, reduction of proteinuria by diet, angiotensin-converting enzyme inhibition, or angiotensin receptor blockade predicts a better outcome[26] (see also Chapter 76); the extent of reduction in proteinuria is often proportional to the benefit accrued by such intervention on CKD progression. Experimental data suggest that proteinuria may contribute directly to the progression of CKD (see later discussion). The threshold for natural progression attributed to proteinuria appears to be crossed when proteinuria exceeds 1 g/day.

Albuminuria, Chronic Kidney Disease, and Cardiovascular Disease

Urinary albumin excretion rate is independently associated with the presence and severity of CVD in the general population.[27] Even low-grade albuminuria (below the current microalbuminuria threshold [albumin to creatinine ratio <3 mg/mmol]) in middle-aged nondiabetic and nonhypertensive individuals is associated with increased CVD risk. The risk associated with albuminuria in the general population matches, and sometimes exceeds, that attributed to better known risk factors of CVD, such as hypertension and hyperlipidemia. Diffuse endothelial and vascular dysfunction may be the common pathway linking albuminuria to the manifestations and prognosis of CKD and CVD (see also Chapter 78). Albuminuria has been linked in a number of studies to underlying systemic atherosclerosis, diffuse vascular stiffness, and maladaptive vascular remodeling.[28,29]

CKD is now defined as a CVD risk equivalent, and patients with moderate to severe CKD are taken to be in the "highest risk group" for development of CVD.[1,30] Patients with CVD are also at a higher risk for development of CKD. Overall, these observations may, in part, be explained by the fact that CVD and CKD share many risk factors, including obesity, metabolic syndrome, hypertension, diabetes mellitus, dyslipidemia, and smoking. In addition, CVD may have direct hemodynamic effects on the kidneys that may promote initiation and progression of CKD, including decreased kidney perfusion in heart failure and atherosclerosis of the renal arteries, with subsequent ischemic nephropathy. Evidence is linking faster rate of CKD progression to severe atherosclerotic disease.[18]

Renin-Angiotensin System

The links between systemic hypertension, proteinuria/albuminuria, and CVD may be mediated by changes in the RAS in CKD. A number of experimental and clinical data have implicated the RAS in the pathogenesis of hypertension, proteinuria, and renal fibrosis throughout the course of CKD (reviewed in reference 31). Consequently, interventions aimed at inhibition of the RAS have proved extremely effective in slowing the progression of CKD (discussed in Chapter 76).

Glycemia

A number of observations as well as randomized clinical trials have demonstrated during the last 25 years that tight diabetes control can potentially slow the rate of progression of diabetic microvascular complications, including diabetic nephropathy in both type 1 and type 2 diabetes mellitus.[32,33]

Obesity

Several studies have linked obesity, and the associated metabolic syndrome, with increased risk of CKD. Excessive body weight and a raised body mass index have also been linked to a faster rate of progression of CKD. Anecdotal reports suggest that weight reduction reduces obesity-related renal hemodynamic changes as well as CKD-associated proteinuria. Recent data derived from general population studies suggest that body weight reduction reduces albuminuria, and increased weight gain is associated with its progression.[34]

Lipids

Dyslipidemia may contribute to glomerulosclerosis and tubulointerstitial fibrosis. A number of studies of diabetic and nondiabetic nephropathies have confirmed by multivariate analysis that dyslipidemia is a risk factor for a faster rate of CKD progression.[1]

Smoking

Smoking has been shown to increase the risk of albuminuria as well as that of progression of CKD (reviewed in reference 35). Possible mechanisms whereby cigarette smoking may contribute to kidney damage include sympathetic nervous system activation, hypertension, endothelial injury, and potential direct tubulotoxicity.

Uric Acid

Hyperuricemia has been associated with systemic hypertension, CVD, and CKD[36] (see also Chapter 33). Hyperuricemia may cause hypertension and renal injury through crystal-independent pathways, notably a stimulation of the RAAS. In a small Japanese study, hyperuricemic patients with IgA nephropathy had a worse prognosis compared with those with normal serum uric acid levels, and a serum uric acid of 6.0 mg/dl or higher was an independent predictor of ESRD in women. However, a more recent observation from the United States suggested that in patients with CKD, hyperuricemia appears to be an independent risk factor for all-cause and CVD mortality but not for kidney failure.[37]

Additional Factors Implicated in Progression of Chronic Kidney Disease

- Alcohol and recreational drugs
- Analgesics and NSAIDs
- Lead and heavy metals exposure

MECHANISMS OF PROGRESSION OF CHRONIC KIDNEY DISEASE

The progression of CKD is associated with changes in kidney structure characterized by scarring associated with glomerulosclerosis, tubulointerstitial fibrosis, and vascular sclerosis. Whereas injury to the glomeruli, tubules, interstitium, or vessels may predominate initially, CKD progression is often associated with damage and scarring affecting all structural components of the kidney.

The kidney responds to injury by adaptive changes that lead to remodeling evolving toward either healing and functional recovery or scarring with loss of kidney function and progressive CKD.[38] During the last 25 years, considerable progress has been made in the understanding of the pathways leading to healing and recovery and those favoring the progression to scarring and fibrosis. However, little is known about what determines the kidney's predilection for one or the other pathway.

Healing is characterized by recovery of kidney structure and function. It occurs primarily in AKI when acutely damaged tubules recover from the initial insult and replace lost tubular cells to reconstitute the integrity of the tubules and to restore kidney function. Healing also takes place in acute interstitial nephritis when treatment is instituted early in the course of the inflammatory process, leading to resolution of the inflammatory process and tubule recovery. Healing is also the hallmark of acute postinfectious glomerulonephritis, when the acute glomerular inflammation resolves through the death (apoptosis) of infiltrating leukocytes or their efflux from the glomeruli. Renal function typically recovers within a few weeks from the acute nephritic process.

On the other hand, most forms of chronic kidney damage, such as those induced by diabetes, hypertension, chronic glomerulonephritis, or chronic exposure to infections or nephrotoxins, evolve to progressive scarring with loss of function and CKD. Scarring is characterized by the progressive loss of intrinsic renal cells and their replacement by fibrous tissue made of collagenous extracellular matrix (ECM; Fig. 75.8). This affects the glomeruli (glomerulosclerosis; Fig. 75.9), tubules and interstitium (tubulointerstitial fibrosis; Fig. 75.10), and vessels (vascular sclerosis). In this section, we describe the generic elements of renal scarring and fibrosis in an attempt to identify stages potentially amenable to future therapies.[39]

Renal Cell Loss, Activation, and Transformation

Loss of intrinsic renal cells is one of the hallmarks of progressive renal scarring. Experimental and clinical models of glomerulo-

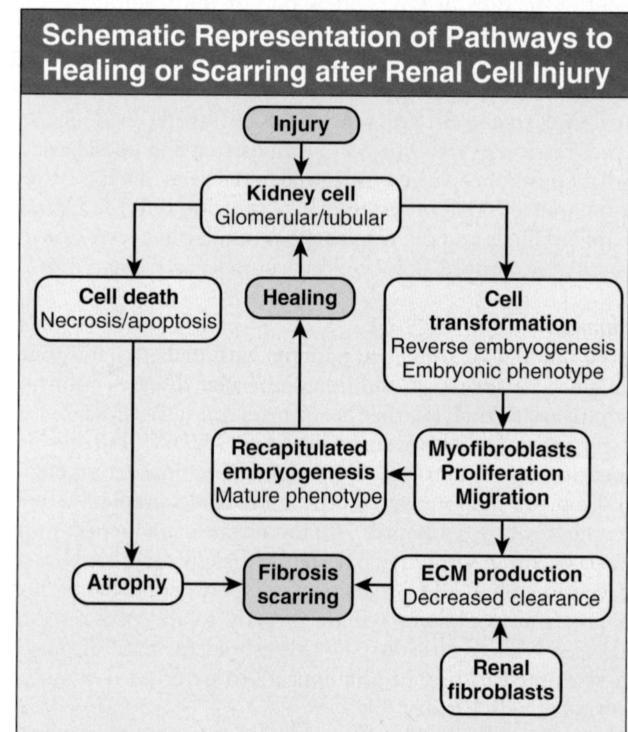

Figure 75.8 Schematic representation of pathways to healing or scarring after renal cell injury. Cell death through necrosis or apoptosis would ultimately lead to renal atrophy and favors replacement by fibrous tissue. Cell injury may lead to dedifferentiation as a step toward recovery and healing.

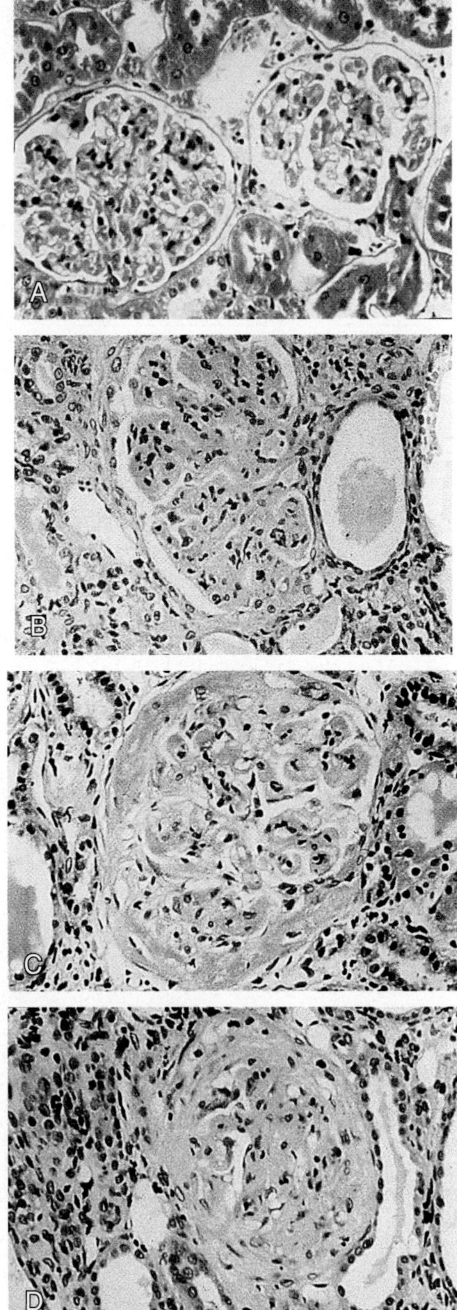

Figure 75.9 Histologic development of glomerulosclerosis. **A,** Normal glomerulus. **B,** Mesangial hypercellularity. **C** and **D,** Glomerulosclerosis of increasing severity. Note the tubular atrophy and dilation in **B** to **D**, indicating the parallel development of tubulointerstitial scarring.

nephritis display a progressive loss of the fine glomerular capillary structure and the disappearance of the glomerular cellular elements with their replacement by an expanding ECM and fibrous tissue. Loss of glomerular cells through necrosis or apoptosis has been described and can be triggered by a severe glomerular inflammatory process, as in glomerulonephritis with glomerular endothelial and capillary damage, or by continuing damage to glomerular cells, as in subacute and chronic glomerulonephritis affecting the mesangium or the podocytes (Fig. 75.11). Similarly, progressive renal scarring is associated with progressive tubular cell loss and atrophy.

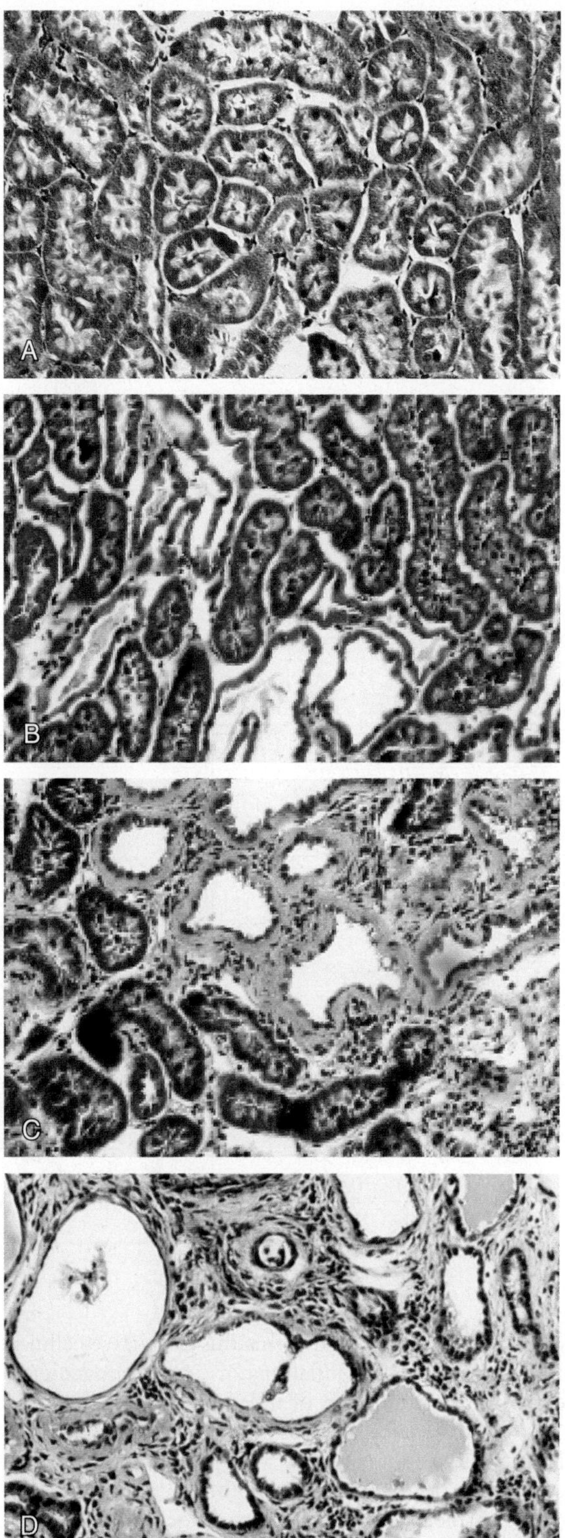

Figure 75.10 Histologic development of tubulointerstitial fibrosis. **A,** Normal tubulointerstitium. **B,** Mild tubulointerstitial scarring with tubular atrophy and interstitial edema. **C,** Segmental interstitial fibrosis. **D,** Diffuse interstitial fibrosis with tubular atrophy and dilation.

Endothelial Cells

In acute and severe glomerulonephritis, damage to the glomerular endothelial lining triggers further injury. The endothelial capillary lining normally displays protective anticoagulant, anti-inflammatory, and antiproliferative functions.[40] Damage to the

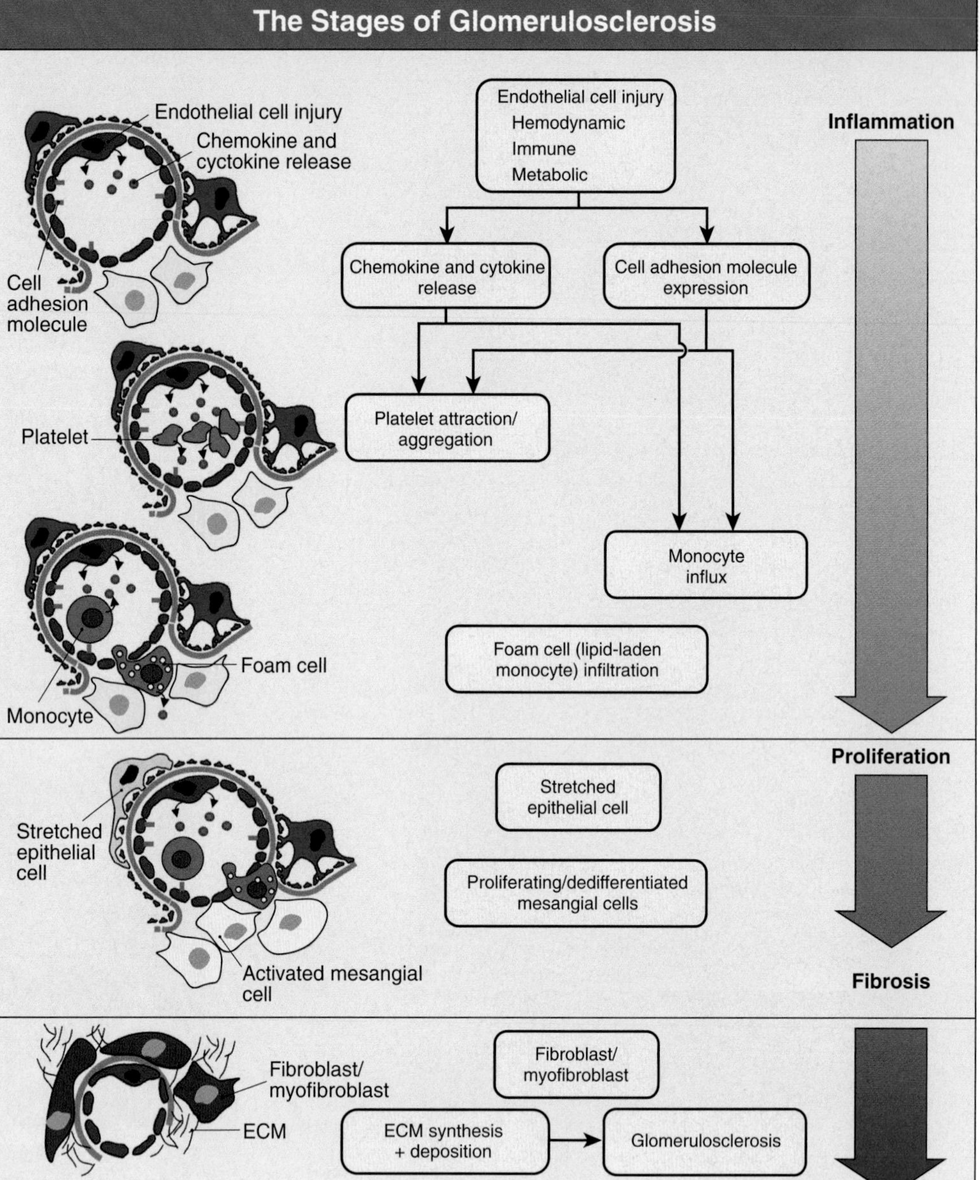

Figure 75.11 The stages of glomerulosclerosis. ECM, extracellular matrix.

glomerular endothelium transforms this protective cellular layer to a proaggregatory, pro-inflammatory, and mitogenic surface, leading to the accumulation of inflammatory cells and platelets within glomerular capillaries as well as the stimulation of the proliferation of the mesangium. This process bears strong similarities to atherosclerosis with microthrombi formation, infiltration of the glomerular tufts by macrophages and foam cells, and proliferation of the smooth muscle cell equivalent, the mesangial cell. Glomerular endothelial damage can be clearly triggered by an acute inflammatory process but also by a metabolic insult, as in diabetes, or hemodynamic shear stress, as in hypertension.

Mesangial Cells

Mesangial cells are the glomerular capillary equivalent to the smooth muscle cell and in that capacity respond to injury in a similar fashion: death, transformation, proliferation, and migration as well as synthesis and deposition of ECM. Mesangial death through necrosis, lysis, and apoptosis has been well documented in response to injury. Injury is also followed by the engagement of the mesangial cells in the repair, healing, or scarring process. Dedifferentiation of mesangial cells into an embryonic phenotype with the acquisition of stress fibers and α-smooth muscle actin allows these cells to proliferate, to migrate, and to restore the glomerular structural integrity.[38] They also lay down collagenous ECM to seal the wound and to repair structural damage. However, scarring is often characterized by uncontrolled mesangial proliferation and excessive deposition of mesangial matrix. These are the forebears of glomerulosclerosis. Mesangial activation, transformation, proliferation, migration, and ECM synthesis seem to be driven by a number of cytokines and growth factors, including transforming growth factor β1 (TGF-β1), platelet-derived growth factor (PDGF), and fibroblast growth factor.[41] These growth factors activate, through their respective mesangial cell surface receptors, a number of intracellular signal transduction pathways. These in turn mediate mesangial events and scarring (see Fig. 75.11).

Podocytes

The relative inability of podocytes to replicate in response to injury may lead to their stretching along the glomerular basement membrane, exposing areas of denuded glomerular basement membrane that would attract and interact with parietal epithelial cells, leading to the formation of capsular adhesions and subsequent segmental glomerulosclerosis.[42] However, inability of podocytes to replicate was challenged by the hypothesis that glomerular parietal epithelial cells could differentiate into podocytes. It has also been suggested that changes in podocytes' derived growth factors, including vascular endothelial growth factor (VEGF) and PDGF, may also be instrumental in contributing to intraglomerular injury. Capsular adhesions formed by contact between the glomerular basement membrane and the parietal epithelial lining of Bowman's capsule may lead to misdirected filtration with the accumulation of amorphous material in the paraglomerular space and the subsequent disruption of glomerular-tubular junction, resulting in atubular glomeruli. Misdirected filtration may also contribute to tubular atrophy and interstitial fibrosis. Tuft-capsule adhesions may allow the influx of periglomerular fibroblasts into the glomerular tuft, thus contributing to glomerulosclerosis. Podocytopathy and ECM deposition in diabetic nephropathy are believed to be mediated by increased proinflammatory cytokines and growth factor production by podocytes, including VEGF, TGF-β1, macrophage migration inhibitory factor, and monocyte chemoattractant protein 1.[43]

Tubular Cells

As with glomerular cells, injury to tubule cells is followed by an attempt at regeneration and repair.[44] After an acute insult, some tubular cells die through necrosis or apoptosis. Apoptosis has been well documented during the course of experimental and clinical models of CKD. Surviving cells attempt to restore tubule integrity by dedifferentiation into an embryonic phenotype that allows them, through the acquisition of cytoplasmic α-smooth muscle actin and stress fibers, to proliferate, to migrate, and to repopulate acellular tubules. Healing and recovery of renal function ensue. On the other hand, repeated or sustained insult is likely to stimulate sustained epithelial mesenchymal transformation (EMT) of tubule cells into a myofibroblastic phenotype with excessive production and deposition of ECM, contributing to fibrosis. Thus, tubular injury with subsequent activation and transformation can directly contribute to renal fibrogenesis. A number of stimuli have been shown to induce tubular EMT, including cytokines (interleukins) and growth factors (TGF-β1, epidermal growth factor) as well as advanced glycation products. Also, recent evidence suggests that excessive exposure of tubule cells in culture to albumin, simulating albuminuria, has the capacity to induce EMT. It has been postulated that proteinuria/albuminuria itself is capable of activating the proximal tubules to release proinflammatory mediators and to initiate interstitial inflammation (reviewed in reference 45). Inflammatory cells would lead to more damage and also stimulate resident renal fibroblasts to produce and deposit ECM (Fig. 75.12).

Vascular Cells

Vascular sclerosis is an integral feature of the renal scarring process. Renal arteriolar hyalinosis is present in CKD at an early stage, even in the absence of severe hypertension. Furthermore, these vascular changes are often out of proportion to the severity of systemic hypertension. Vascular sclerosis is associated with progressive kidney failure in glomerulonephritis. Hyalinosis of afferent arterioles has been implicated in the pathogenesis of diabetic glomerulosclerosis. Changes in postglomerular arterioles and damage to peritubular capillaries may further exacerbate interstitial ischemia and fibrosis. Ischemia and the ensuing hypoxia are fibrogenic influences that stimulate tubular cells and kidney fibroblasts to produce ECM components and to reduce their collagenolytic activity.[46]

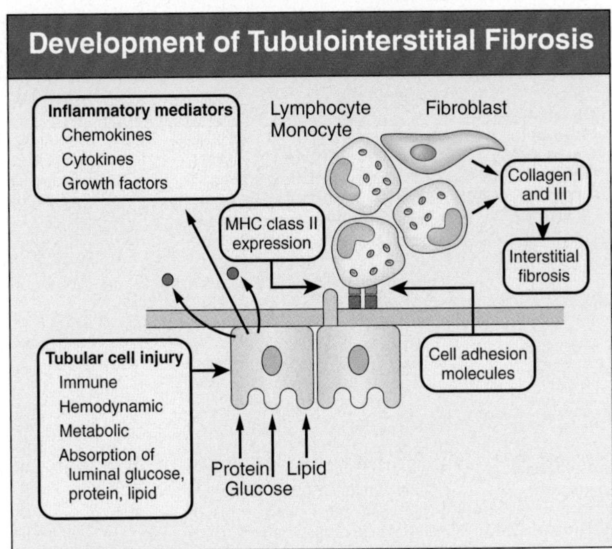

Figure 75.12 Development of tubulointerstitial fibrosis. MHC, major histocompatibility complex.

Loss of peritubular capillaries with the associated impaired angiogenesis has been linked in experimental models of renal scarring to a fall in the renal expression of the proangiogenic VEGF. Together with an overexpression by scarred kidneys of thrombospondin, an antiangiogenic factor, this would perpetuate microvascular deletion and ischemia.[47] The administration of VEGF preserves peritubular capillaries and improves scarring and functional outcome. Finally, the vascular endothelium, adventitia, and pericytes may be a source of interstitial myofibroblasts, contributing to the development of interstitial renal fibrosis.[48]

Recent evidence also points to lymphatic neoangiogenesis in association with interstitial inflammation and progressive renal fibrosis.[49] Such a process appears to be driven by macrophages that express the lymphangiotropic growth factor VEGF-C. It may play a role in interstitial remodeling as it provides an exit route for inflammatory cells involved in interstitial inflammation.

Inflammation and Infiltration by Extrinsic Cells

Infiltration of the glomeruli and renal interstitium by inflammatory cells is an early and common pathway in the pathogenesis of glomerulosclerosis (see Fig. 75.11) and tubulointerstitial fibrosis (see Fig. 75.12).

Platelets

Platelets and their release products have been detected within glomeruli in experimental and clinical nephropathies. The stimulation of the coagulation cascade is likely to activate mesangial cells and to induce sclerosis. Thrombin stimulates glomerular TGF-β1 production, leading to production of mesangial ECM as well as that of inhibitors of metalloproteinases. The upregulation within damaged glomeruli of plasminogen activator

Experimental Interventions to Slow CKD with Potential for Clinical Translation

Target	Intervention	Mechanism of Action	Evidence Level
Growth factors			
Fibrosis-modulating growth factors (TBF–β1, HGF, BMP-7)	Neutralizing anti–TGF–β1 antibodies	Neutralization of the growth factor (TGF–β1)	Experimental models of CKD
	ALK1 (TGF–β1 receptor) inhibitors	Inhibition of receptor-mediated signal transduction	Experimental models of CKD
	Administration of bone morphogenic protein 7 (BMP-7)	Inhibitor of the TGF–β1–Smad signaling pathway	Experimental models of CKD
	Administration of hepatocyte growth factor (HGF)	Inhibits nuclear translocation of receptor-regulated Smads and upregulates the expression of Smad corepressors	Experimental models of CKD Clinical trials in promoting angiogenesis
	Inhibition of connective tissue growth factor (CTGF)	Mediator of TGF-β1– induced fibrosis	Experimental models of CKD Phase II clinical trial completed in diabetic nephropathy
	Tranilast	Inhibits TGF-β1–induced ECM synthesis	Experimental models of CKD Used in the treatment of hypertrophic scars and scleroderma Preliminary clinical data in diabetic nephropathy
	Decorin	Sequesters TGF-β1 in the extracellular matrix	Experimental models of CKD
Proliferative growth factors (PDGF, EGF)	Neutralizing anti–platelet-derived growth factor CR002 (PDGF) antibodies including CR002	CR002 monoclonal antibody targeting PDGF-D	Experimental data indicate potential of CR002 in mesangioproliferative disease
	PDGF antagonists; aptamers, imatinib mesylate, trapidil	Direct inhibition of PDGF; imatinib mesylate: tyrosine kinase inhibitor of PDGF transduction	Phase I clinical trial completed in MPGN Clinical use limited by cardiotoxicity
	Anti–epidermal growth factor (EGF) antibody	Neutralize EGF action	Inhibition of renal fibroblast proliferation and collagen expression
	Inhibition of epidermal growth factor receptor (EGF-R)	Inhibition of EGF-R by ascofuranone, an isoprenoid antibiotic, that inhibits phosphorylation of EGFR and downstream kinases	
Angiogenic growth factors (VEGF)	Administration of vascular endothelial growth factor	To stimulate/restore glomerular and peritubular capillary angiogenesis However, may also stimulate glomerular hypertrophy and albuminuria in models of diabetic nephropathy	Experimental models of CKD Experimental mesangioproliferative GN and diabetic nephropathy
Intracellular transduction pathways	Ras-Raf-Mek-Erk pathway inhibition by: 1: Ras: prenylation inhibitors (statins), prenyltransferase inhibitors farnesylthiosalicylic acid (FTS) 2:Raf and Mek kinase inhibitors	Inhibition of cellular proliferation, differentiation, and apoptosis	Experimental models of CKD Role of statins in progressive clinical CKD not yet defined
	Rho kinase inhibition: fasudil	Interference with cell proliferation, tubulointerstitial fibrosis, and glomerular hemodynamics	Experimental models of CKD Phase II studies in ischemic heart disease Fasudil in clinical use in Japan for cerebral vasospasm
	p38 mitogen–activated protein kinase inhibitors	Inhibition of proinflammatory and profibrotic mediators	Experimental models of CKD Clinical trials in rheumatoid arthritis and type 1 diabetes mellitus
	Protein kinase C inhibitors, such as ruboxistaurin	Inhibition of cell growth most evident in diabetic nephropathy	Experimental models of CKD Phase II clinical trials in diabetic nephropathy, reduce albuminuria
Cell cycle inhibitors	Cyclin-dependent kinase inhibitors, such as roscovitine	Inhibition of cell cycle progression	Experimental models of CKD
Immuno suppressive agents	Mycophenolate mofetil (MMF)	Inhibitor of inosine monophosphate dehydrogenase; inhibiting cell proliferation	Experimental models of CKD Used in clinical CKD associated with vasculitis
	Sirolimus (rapamycin)	mTOR inhibitor; interference with cell proliferation by regulating ribosomal biogenesis and protein translation	Variable data in experimental models of CKD but can induce/increase proteinuria Promising in experimental PDKD Clinical trials completed in PKD
Other agents	Endothelin antagonists	Reduce cellular proliferation and intraglomerular hypertension; antiproteinuric effect	Experimental models of CKD Clinical trials in diabetic nephropathy Reduce albuminuria in diabetic nephropathy Risk of increased CVD mortality
	Pirfenidone	Inhibits ECM accumulation	Experimental models of CKD Phase II trials in diabetic nephropathy
	Peroxisome proliferator-activated receptor γ agonists	Reduce cell growth, inflammation; antiproteinuric effect	Experimental models of CKD Reduces proteinuria in clinical diabetic nephropathy Risk of increased CVD mortality
	Prolyl hydroxylase domain (PHD) inhibitors, e.g., cobalt chloride, FG-2216	Upregulation of HIF-regulated genes, such as VEGF and EPO	Experimental models of CKD Phase II clinical trials of FG-2216 for treatment of anemia
	Pentoxifylline	Antioxidant	Experimental models of CKD Phase II clinical trials assessing role in proteinuric CKD
	N–Acetylcysteine (NAC)	Antioxidant	Experimental models of CKD Used for AKI prophylaxis in CKD
	Tocopherols	Antioxidant	Experimental models of CKD Tocopherols and α–lipoic acid in clinical trials in CKD

Figure 75.13 Experimental interventions to slow CKD with potential for clinical translation. AKI, acute kidney injury; CVD, cardiovascular disease; ECM, extracellular matrix; EPO, erythropoietin; GN, glomerulonephritis; HIF, hypoxia-inducible transcription factor; MPGN, membranoproliferative glomerulonephritis; PKD, polycystic kidney disease.

inhibitor 1 is also likely to affect outcome as its inhibition of the proteolytic enzyme plasmin may lead to ECM accumulation and glomerulosclerosis.[50] Glomerulosclerosis may depend on the balance between thrombotic/antiproteolytic and anticoagulant/proteolytic activities, with a key role played by the plasminogen regulatory system.

Lymphocytes, Monocytes-Macrophages, and Dendritic Cells

Lymphocytes, including helper and cytotoxic T cells, as well as monocytes-macrophages are often identified within damaged glomeruli.[51] It has been postulated that the balance between proinflammatory Th1 and anti-inflammatory Th2 lymphocytes may be a key factor in the resolution or progression of glomerulosclerosis.

The relevance of monocytes-macrophages to the initiation and progression of glomerulosclerosis has been supported by experiments in which depletion of these cells had a protective effect. The release by these cells of cytokines, growth factors, and procoagulant factors is likely to contribute to the pathogenesis of glomerulosclerosis. However, these cells may also contribute to the termination and resolution of the glomerular inflammatory response. Phenotypic and functional macrophage changes may determine the outcome of glomerular inflammation and sclerosis.

Interstitial inflammation is a common precursor of tubulointerstitial fibrosis. The severity of the interstitial inflammatory infiltrate correlates closely with the severity of renal dysfunction and predicts progressive CKD. Interstitial lymphocytes and monocytes have been implicated in the pathogenesis of renal fibrosis with variable degree of involvement. Limited evidence also implicates mast cells, but this area is more controversial.[52]

Dendritic cells, a subset of cells that play an essential role in immunopathology of the kidney and the crosstalk with other proinflammatory cells including T lymphocytes, also have a central role in the pathogenesis of kidney inflammation in different disease processes.[53] In the interstitium, inflammatory infiltrates of B cells, T cells, and dendritic cells form nodular aggregates surrounded by neolymphatic vessels.

Bone Marrow–Derived Cells

Glomerular remodeling (repair-healing or scarring) may depend on the influx of hematopoietic stem cells with the potential for repair or scarring (reviewed in references 54 and 55). The detection of cells displaying embryonic mesenchymal characteristics in glomeruli has led to the hypothesis that hematopoietic stem cells may be involved in normal glomerular cell turnover as well as in the response of glomeruli to injury. Experiments based on bone marrow transplantation have demonstrated the potential involvement of bone marrow–derived cells in normal mesangium turnover and in glomerular repair-repopulation after experimental mesangial injury.

It has also been postulated that bone marrow–derived mesenchymal stem cells may be involved in fibrogenesis by migrating into scarred kidneys and contributing to the pool of fibroblasts.

Extracellular Matrix Processing

Loss of intrinsic renal cells and their transformation into fibroblastic phenotypes are likely to be key events in the pathogenesis of renal fibrosis.[48] In addition to transformed tubular cells, there is growing evidence that other renal cells, including vascular endothelial and pericytic cells, have the capacity to transform into mesenchymal myofibroblasts, thus contributing to the renal fibroblastic pool. The other main source of renal fibroblasts is likely to be derived from quiescent renal fibroblasts activated by tubules and inflammatory cells through the release of a range of cytokines and growth factors. Finally, bone marrow–derived stem cells are also thought to participate in renal fibrogenesis.[48]

One of the most potent inducers of EMT and fibroblast activation is thought to be TGF-ß1. This growth factor is thought to be a key factor in wound healing and scarring. It acts through its type 1 and 2 receptors and activates a number of intracellular signal transduction pathways including STATs and Smads. Connective tissue growth factor is one of the TGF-β1 effectors that enhances TGF-β1 intracellular signaling pathways. Two growth factors, hepatocyte growth factor and bone morphogenic protein 7 (BMP-7), have so far been shown *in vitro* and *in vivo* to inhibit and even to reverse EMT and to counteract the fibrogenic influences of TGF-β1. Of interest, uterine sensitization–associated gene 1, the natural antagonist of BMP-7, is abundant in renal tissue and modulates many of the effects of BMP-7 on the kidney.

Fibroblast activation, proliferation, migration, and synthesis of ECM constitute a major step in fibrogenesis and renal scarring. Deposited ECM undergoes quantitative and qualitative changes. For instance, within scarred glomeruli, interstitial type III collagen is deposited. Interstitial fibrosis is associated with excessive deposition of collagens I, III, and IV. The normal homeostasis of ECM turnover is likely to be compromised in the course of renal scarring through excessive synthesis, decreased breakdown, or resistance to breakdown.

Renal ECM breakdown is regulated by a number of collagenolytic enzymes including the matrix metalloproteinases and the plasmin system. These are in turn regulated by a number of inhibitors, such as the tissue inhibitors of matrix metalloproteinases (TIMPs) and the plasminogen activator inhibitors. Decreased matrix metalloproteinase activities or increased TIMPs and plasminogen activator inhibitor 1 activity have been implicated in the deposition of ECM in CKD.

Recent evidence points to another putative pathway to excessive deposition of ECM, namely, resistance to breakdown through structural modification and cross-link of deposited ECM by an enzyme called tissue transglutaminase. This enzyme is upregulated during the course of experimental and clinical nephropathies.[56] Mice lacking this enzyme have reduced propensity to renal scarring. Synthetic inhibitors of this enzyme have been shown to considerably attenuate experimental renal fibrosis.

A number of potential interventions affecting and modulating different pathways of renal fibrosis are under investigation with variable degrees of promise and success (Fig. 75.13).[39]

REFERENCES

1. National Kidney Foundation. K/DOQI kidney disease outcome quality initiative. *Am J Kidney Dis*. 2002;39(Suppl 1):S1-S266.
2. Glassock RJ, Winearls C. An epidemic of chronic kidney disease: Fact or fiction? *Nephrol Dial Transplant*. 2008;23:1117-1121.
3. Levey AS, Atkins R, Coresh J, et al. Chronic kidney disease as a global public health problem: Approaches and initiatives—a position statement from Kidney Disease Improving Global Outcomes. *Kidney Int*. 2007;72: 247-259.
4. National Collaborating Centre for Chronic Conditions. *Chronic kidney disease: National clinical guideline for early identification and management in*

adults in primary and secondary care. London: National Institute for Health and Clinical Excellence; September 2008. Clinical guideline 73.
5. Schena FP. Epidemiology of end-stage renal disease; international comparisons. *Kidney Int*. 2000;57:S39-S45.
6. U.S. Renal Data System. *USRDS 2007 Annual Data Report: Atlas of End Stage Renal Disease in the United States*. Bethesda, Md: National Institutes of Health, National Institutes of Diabetes and Digestive and Kidney Diseases; 2007. Available at: www.usrds.org.
7. Ansell D, Feehally J, Feest TG, et al. *UK Renal Registry Report 2007*. Bristol, UK: UK Renal Registry; 2007.
8. Lysaght MJ. Maintenance dialysis population dynamics: Current trends and long-term implications. *J Am Soc Nephrol*. 2002;13(Suppl 1): S37-S40.
9. Lacson E, Kuhlmann MK, Shah K. Outcomes and economics of ESRF. In: El Nahas AM, ed. *Kidney Disease in Developing Countries and Ethnic Minorities*. New York: Taylor & Francis; 2005:15-38.
10. Caring for Australasians with renal impairment. Available at: http://www.cari.org.au/. Updated February 2009.
11. Keith DS, Nichols GA, Gullion CM, et al. Longitudinal follow-up and outcomes among a population with chronic kidney disease in a large managed care organization. *Arch Intern Med*. 2004;164:659-663.
12. Levin A, Djurdjev O, Beaulieu M, Er L. Variability and risk factors for kidney disease progression and death following attainment of stage 4 CKD in a referred cohort. *Am J Kidney Dis*. 2008;52:661-671.
13. Locatelli F, Del Vecchio L. Natural history and factors affecting the progression of chronic renal failure. In: El Nahas AM, Anderson S, Harris KPG, eds. *Mechanisms and Management of Progressive Renal Failure*. London: Oxford University Press; 2000:20-79.
14. Gansevoort RT, van der Heij B, Stegeman CA, et al. Trends in the incidence of treated end-stage renal failure in The Netherlands: Hope for the future? *Kidney Int Suppl*. 2004;92:S7-S10.
15. Meguid El Nahas A, Bello AK. Chronic kidney disease: The global challenge. *Lancet*. 2005;365:331-340.
16. Taal MW, Brenner BM. Renal risk scores: Progress and prospects. *Kidney Int*. 2008;73:1216-1219.
17. Eriksen BO, Ingebretsen OC. The progression of chronic kidney disease: A 10-year population-based study of the effects of gender and age. *Kidney Int*. 2006;69:375-382.
18. Shlipak MG, Katz R, Kestenbaum B, et al. Clinical and subclinical cardiovascular disease and kidney function decline in the elderly. *Atherosclerosis*. 2009;204:298-303.
19. Traver-Carr ME, Powe NR, Eberhardt MS, et al. Excess risk of chronic kidney disease among African-American versus white subjects in the United States: A population-based study of potential explanatory factors. *J Am Soc Nephrol*. 2002;13:2363-2370.
20. El Nahas AM. Mechanisms of experimental and clinical renal scarring. In: Davison AM, Cameron JS, Grunfeld J-P, et al, eds. *Oxford Textbook of Clinical Nephrology*. 3rd ed. London: Oxford University Press; 2005:1647-1686.
21. Köttgen A, Hwang SJ, Rampersaud E, et al. TCF7L2 variants associate with CKD progression and renal function in population-based cohorts. *J Am Soc Nephrol*. 2008;19:1989-1999.
22. Köttgen A, Kao WH, Hwang SJ, et al. Genome-wide association study for renal traits in the Framingham Heart and Atherosclerosis Risk in Communities Studies. *BMC Med Genet*. 2008;9:49.
23. Locatelli F, Marcelli D, Comelli M, et al. Northern Italian Cooperative Study Group: Proteinuria and blood pressure as causal components of progression to end-stage renal failure. *Nephrol Dial Transplant*. 1996;11:461-467.
24. Ishani A, Xue JL, Himmelfarb J, et al. Acute kidney injury increases risk of ESRD among elderly. *J Am Soc Nephrol*. 2009;20:223-228.
25. Jafar TH, Stark PC, Schmid CH, et al. Proteinuria as a modifiable risk factor for the progression of non-diabetic renal disease. *Kidney Int*. 2001;60:1131-1140.
26. Jafar TH, Stark PC, Schmid CH, et al. Progression of chronic kidney disease: The role of blood pressure control, proteinuria, and angiotensin-converting enzyme inhibition: A patient-level meta-analysis. *Ann Intern Med*. 2003;139:244-252.
27. Arnlov J, Evans JC, Meigs JB, et al. Low-grade albuminuria and incidence of cardiovascular disease events in nonhypertensive and nondiabetic individuals: The Framingham Heart Study. *Circulation*. 2005;112: 969-975.
28. Hermans MM, Henry R, Dekker JM, et al. Estimated glomerular filtration rate and urinary albumin excretion are independently associated with greater arterial stiffness: The Hoorn Study. *J Am Soc Nephrol*. 2007;18:1942-1952.
29. Hermans MM, Henry RM, Dekker JM, et al. Albuminuria, but not estimated glomerular filtration rate, is associated with maladaptive arterial remodeling: The Hoorn Study. *J Hypertens*. 2008;26:791-797.
30. Menon V, Sarnak MJ. The epidemiology of chronic kidney disease stages 1 to 4 and cardiovascular disease: A high-risk combination. *Am J Kidney Dis*. 2005;45:223-232.
31. Remuzzi G, Perico N, Macia M, Ruggenenti P. The role of renin-angiotensin-aldosterone system in the progression of chronic kidney disease. *Kidney Int Suppl*. 2005;99:S57-S65.
32. Retinopathy and nephropathy in patients with type 1 diabetes four years after a trial of intensive therapy. The Diabetes Control and Complications Trial/Epidemiology of Diabetes Interventions and Complications Research Group. *N Engl J Med*. 2000;342:381-389.
33. Effect of intensive blood-glucose control with metformin on complications in overweight patients with type 2 diabetes (UKPDS 34). UK Prospective Diabetes Study (UKPDS) Group. *Lancet*. 1998;352: 854-865.
34. Bello AK, de Zeeuw D, El Nahas M, et al. Impact of weight change on albuminuria in the general population. *Nephrol Dial Transplant*. 2007;22:1619-1627.
35. Orth SR, Hallan SI. Smoking: A risk factor for progression of chronic kidney disease and for cardiovascular morbidity and mortality in renal patients—absence of evidence or evidence of absence? *Clin J Am Soc Nephrol*. 2008;3:226-236.
36. Johnson RJ, Kivlighn SD, Kim YG, et al. Reappraisal of the pathogenesis and consequence of hyperuricemia in hypertension, cardiovascular disease and renal disease. *Am J Kidney Dis*. 1999;33:225-234.
37. Madero M, Sarnak MJ, Wang X, et al. Uric acid and long-term outcomes in CKD. *Am J Kidney Dis*. 2009;53:796-803.
38. El-Nahas AM. Plasticity of kidney cells: Role in kidney remodeling and scarring. *Kidney Int*. 2003;64:1553-1563.
39. Khwaja A, El Kossi M, Floege J, El Nahas M. The management of CKD: A look into the future. *Kidney Int*. 2007;72:1316-1323.
40. Savage CO. The biology of the glomerulus: Endothelial cells. *Kidney Int*. 1994;45:314-319.
41. Wynn TA. Cellular and molecular mechanisms of fibrosis. *J Pathol*. 2008;214:199-210.
42. Endlich K, Kriz W, Witzgall R. Update in podocyte biology. *Curr Opin Nephrol Hypertens*. 2001;10:331-340.
43. Boor P, Sebeková K, Ostendorf T, Floege J. Treatment targets in renal fibrosis. *Nephrol Dial Transplant*. 2007;22:3391-3407.
44. Christensen EI, Verroust PJ. Interstitial fibrosis: Tubular hypothesis versus glomerular hypothesis. *Kidney Int*. 2008;74:1233-1236.
45. Bruzzi I, Benigni A, Remuzzi G. Role of increased glomerular protein traffic in the progression of renal failure. *Kidney Int Suppl*. 1997;62: S231.
46. Fine LG, Orphanides C, Norman JT. Progressive renal disease: The chronic hypoxia hypothesis. *Kidney Int*. 1998;53(Suppl 65):S74-S78.
47. Kang DH, Kanellis J, Hugo C, et al. Role of the microvascular endothelium in progressive renal disease. *J Am Soc Nephrol*. 2002;13: 806-816.
48. Strutz F. How many different roads may a cell walk down in order to become a fibroblast? *J Am Soc Nephrol*. 2008;19:2246-2248.
49. Sakamoto I, Ito Y, Mizuno M, et al. Lymphatic vessels develop during tubulointerstitial fibrosis. *Kidney Int*. 2009;75:828-838.
50. Ma LJ, Fogo AB. PAI-1 and kidney fibrosis. *Front Biosci*. 2009; 14:2028-2041.
51. Nikolic-Paterson DJ, Lan HY, Hill PA, Atkins RC. Macrophages in renal injury. *Kidney Int Suppl*. 1994;45:S79-S82.
52. Eddy AA. Mast cells find their way to the kidney [erratum in Kidney Int. 2001;60:1216-1127]. *Kidney Int*. 2001;60:375-377.
53. Heymann F, Meyer-Schwesinger C, Hamilton-Williams EE, et al. Kidney dendritic cell activation is required for progression of renal disease in a mouse model of glomerular injury. *J Clin Invest*. 2009;119: 1286-1297.
54. Bussolati B, Hauser PV, Carvalhosa R, Camussi G. Contribution of stem cells to kidney repair. *Curr Stem Cell Res Ther*. 2009;4:2-8.
55. Hewitson TD. Renal tubulointerstitial fibrosis: Common but never simple. *Am J Physiol Renal Physiol*. 2009;296:F1239-F1244.
56. Johnson TS, Griffin M, Thomas GL, et al. The role of transglutaminase in the rat subtotal nephrectomy model of renal fibrosis. *J Clin Invest*. 1997;99:2950-2960.

CHAPTER 76

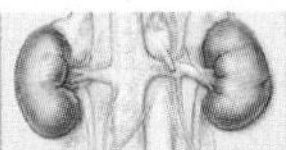

Retarding Progression of Kidney Disease

Christopher Brown, Nabil Haddad, Lee A. Hebert

Progression to end-stage renal disease (ESRD) usually occurs through the mechanisms of the primary kidney disease or by natural progression (see Chapter 75). This chapter focuses on therapies to slow natural progression.[1,2] The goal is to preserve enough nephron function to avoid the vicious circle of natural progression.

GLOMERULAR FILTRATION RATE LOSS AND THE RISK OF NATURAL PROGRESSION

The tendency for kidney disease to progress independently of underlying etiology does not occur until a certain degree of renal function has been lost, which typically is when the loss of nephron function exceeds 50%. For example, unilateral nephrectomy in living kidney donors does not usually lead to natural progression. However, a normal solitary kidney can be vulnerable to natural progression if it is congenital or acquired early in life or if it is accompanied by hypertension, obesity, hyperlipidemia, or hyperglycemia.[1,2] Increased risk of natural progression, even though nephron loss is less than 50%, can also occur in persons of African ancestry with hypertensive nephrosclerosis.[2] Low birth weight, particularly in men, may also cause chronic kidney disease (CKD) and its natural progression, presumably because of inadequate nephron development.[3]

PROTEINURIA MAGNITUDE AND THE RISK OF NATURAL PROGRESSION

The threshold for natural progression attributable to proteinuria appears to be crossed when proteinuria exceeds 500 mg/day. In most CKD, proteinuria is the single strongest risk factor for progression. An exception is highly selective proteinuria (the urine protein is almost entirely albumin), which can persist in the nephrotic range for more than 10 years without causing renal structural damage.[1]

MONITORING KIDNEY DISEASE PROGRESSION

In contrast to natural progression, in which the first sign is increasing proteinuria, the first sign of progression is declining glomerular filtration rate (GFR) in many forms of CKD (Fig. 76.1). Total proteinuria may remain in the normal range, but microalbuminuria is generally present and is the most useful test for the early detection of progression due to the primary CKD, natural progression, or both.[4]

Monitoring Proteinuria Trends

Proteinuria is the strongest single predictor of GFR decline (Fig. 76.2). Furthermore, therapies that reduce proteinuria slow GFR decline, probably through multiple mechanisms (see also Chapter 75). The Modification of Diet in Renal Disease (MDRD) and Ramipril Efficacy in Nephropathy (REIN) trials reported that for each 1g reduction in proteinuria achieved by 4 to 6 months of antiproteinuric intervention, GFR decline was slowed by about 1 to 2 ml/min per year. GFR loss in CKD is typically 4 to 10 ml/min per year.[1,2] Thus, each reduction of 1 g/day should result in important slowing of GFR decline and delay of ESRD (Fig. 76.3). Figure 76.3 may be an optimistic projection because there is now evidence that as CKD progresses, the rate of decline of GFR accelerates. Nevertheless, the available evidence suggests that substantial benefit can be achieved by measures that reduce proteinuria.

The recommended method for assessing proteinuria is the serial measurement of urine protein-creatinine (PC) ratio (mg/mg) of intended 24-hour urine collections that are at least 50% complete on the basis of their creatinine content. The PC ratios of such collections are generally within ±10% of the PC ratio of complete 24-hour collections.[5] This recommendation differs from the current National Kidney Foundation Kidney Disease Outcomes Quality Initiative (KDOQI) guidelines, which recommend random spot urine PC ratios. This is because within a given patient, the concordance between random spot PC ratio and 24-hour urine PC ratio is poor, particularly over the moderate proteinuria range (Fig. 76.4).[5] Also, the random spot urine PC ratio is not a suitable screening test because overestimates and underestimates occur with about equal frequency.[6] Another advantage of 24-hour urine testing is measurement of dietary sodium and protein intake (see later discussion).

Measurements of total proteinuria and albuminuria are highly correlated in glomerular diseases, and measurement of urine total protein is less expensive than measurement of urine albumin.[4,5] Proteinuria testing is recommended every 2 to 3 months for those with nephrotic-range proteinuria and every 6 months for those with subnephrotic proteinuria.

Monitoring Glomerular Filtration Rate Trends

In individual patients, it is usually sufficient to monitor GFR trends by serial measurements of serum creatinine. However, one must keep in mind circumstances that can increase serum creatinine by increasing creatinine production (eating cooked meat, creatine ingestion, increased exercise, or increased muscle mass) or decrease creatinine production (vegetarian diet, muscle wasting, decreased exercise).[1,2] Serum creatinine can also be spuriously increased by serum ketones (from fasting or poor diabetes control) or by drugs that interfere with tubular secretion of creatinine (cimetidine, trimethoprim). If a chronic progressive change in creatinine production is occurring (e.g., muscle wasting), GFR trends can be monitored by measuring serial 24-hour urine creatinine clearance, which is not affected by change in creatinine production. If creatinine clearance is used, an accurate 24-hour collection is essential.[2]

The Cockcroft-Gault and MDRD-4 equations provide similar estimates of GFR, especially in the mid range of estimated glomerular filtration rate (eGFR) values (see Chapter 3). The MDRD-4 equation is more easily implemented in clinical laboratories because it does not require knowledge of body weight, it is accurate in many CKD patients, and it takes into account the influence of age. The last is important in assessing a patient's GFR trend during 10 years or more.[7,8] MDRD-4 is inaccurate in CKD stages 1 and 2 and in those with high-normal creatinine production (GFR is underestimated) or low-normal creatinine production (GFR is overestimated). During longitudinal testing, MDRD-4 also underestimates GFR decline assessed by iothalamate clearance by about 28%. For those with slowly progressive renal disease, this underestimate can mean a difference of several years between the actual and predicted onset of ESRD.[7] A newer version of the MDRD equation (CKD-EPI) has been developed but is not yet validated (see Chapter 3).

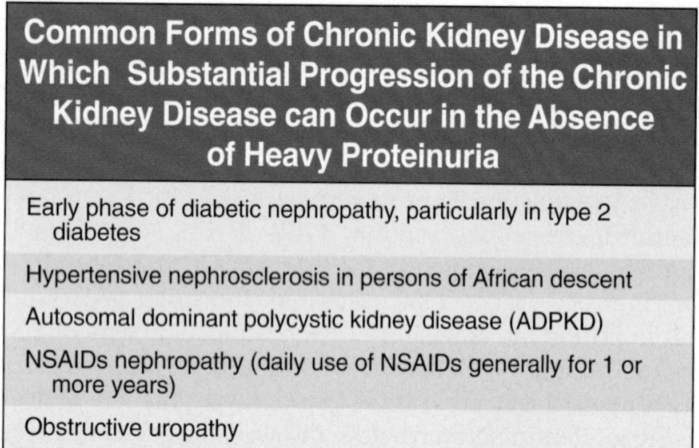

Common Forms of Chronic Kidney Disease in Which Substantial Progression of the Chronic Kidney Disease can Occur in the Absence of Heavy Proteinuria
Early phase of diabetic nephropathy, particularly in type 2 diabetes
Hypertensive nephrosclerosis in persons of African descent
Autosomal dominant polycystic kidney disease (ADPKD)
NSAIDs nephropathy (daily use of NSAIDs generally for 1 or more years)
Obstructive uropathy

Figure 76.1 Common forms of chronic kidney disease (CKD) in which substantial progression of the CKD can occur. NSAIDS, nonsteroidal anti-inflammatory drugs (e.g., serum creatinine increases to >2.0 mg/dl) but proteinuria remains low (e.g., 24-hour urine protein/creatinine ratio <0.3).

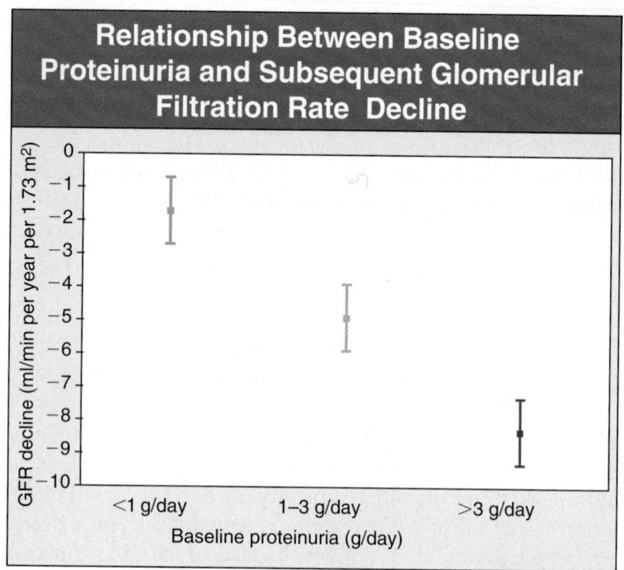

Figure 76.2 Relationship between baseline proteinuria and subsequent glomerular filtration rate (GFR) decline. Data from study A of the Modification of Diet in Renal Disease study. *(Modified from reference 9.)*

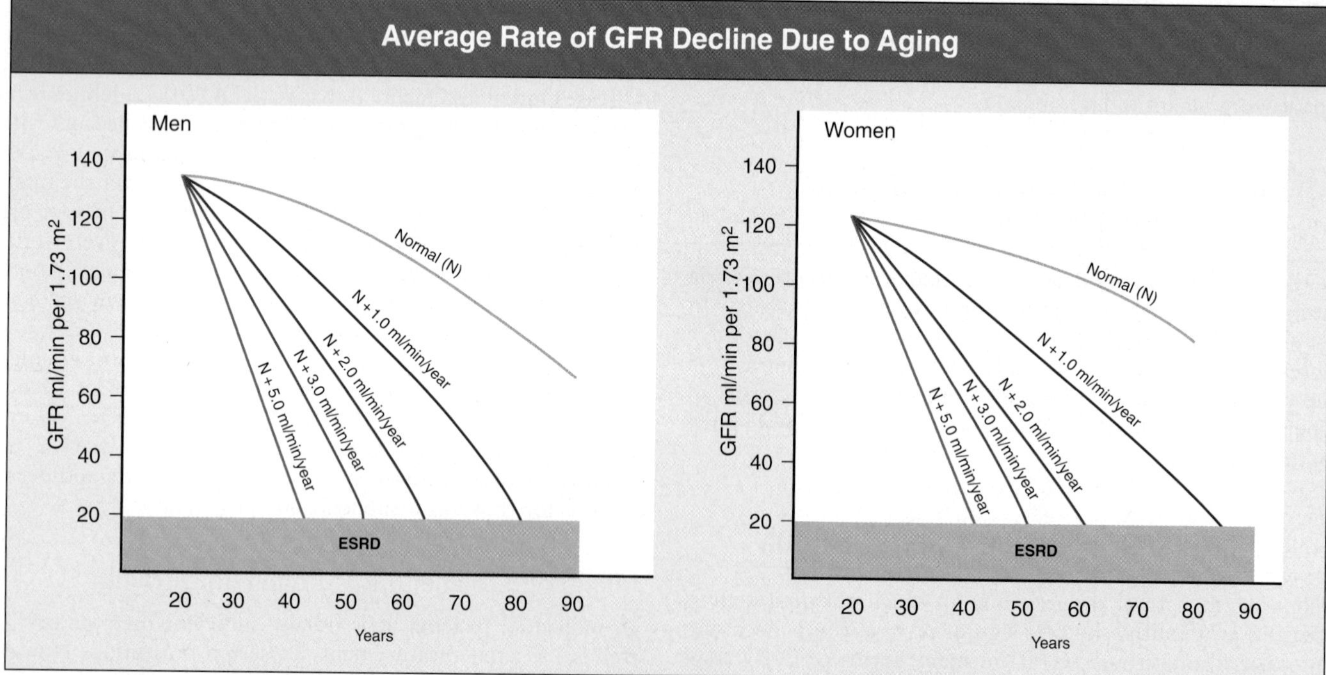

Figure 76.3 Average rate of GFR decline due to aging *(top curve)* in comparison to hypothetical patients each with the onset of a progressive kidney disease at age 25 years but with different rates of GFR decline superimposed on the GFR decline of aging (*left panel,* men; *right panel,* women). Note that small differences in GFR decline rate can result in large differences in time to onset of end-stage renal disease (ESRD). GFR, glomerular filtration rate. *(Modified with permission from reference 2.)*

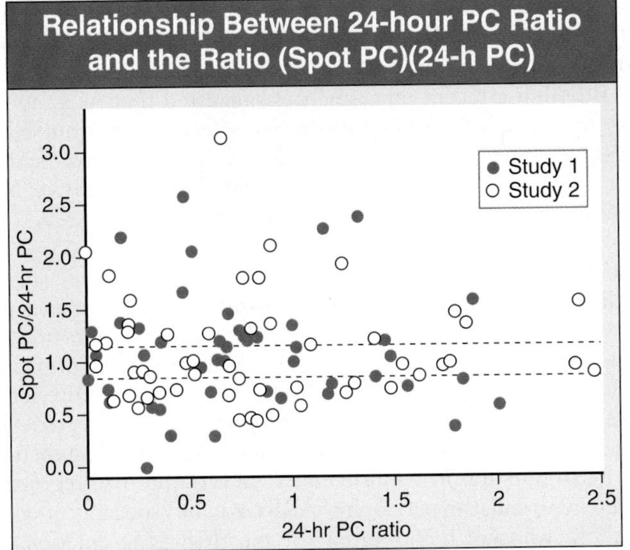

Figure 76.4 Relationship between 24-hour PC ratio and the ratio (spot PC)/(24-h PC) for the cohorts of study 1 *(closed circles)* and study 2 *(open circles)* with PC ratios 0.5 to 3.0. These data are shown in relationship to the expected limits of agreement *(dashed horizontal lines)* between random spot urine PC ratio and 24-hour urine PC ratio, if they were equally precise in estimating 24-hour proteinuria. These data show that random spot urine PC ratio is an unreliable estimate of 24-hour urine PC ratio.[6]

Recommended Kidney Protective Therapies According to Level of Recommendation*

Level 1 Recommendations

1. Control blood pressure (BP)
2. ACE inhibitor therapy
3. ARB therapy
4. Combination ACE inhibitor and ARB therapy
5. Renin inhibitor therapy
6. Avoid DHP-CCBs unless needed for BP control
7. Control protein intake

Level 2 Recommendations

1. Restrict NaCl intake/diuretic therapy
2. Control fluid intake
3. NDHP-CCB therapy
4. Control each component of the metabolic syndrome
5. Aldosterone antagonist therapy
6. β-blocker therapy
7. Smoking cessation
8. Allopurinol therapy

Figure 76.5 Recommended kidney protective therapies according to level of recommendation.* *The goal for the chronic kidney disease (CKD) patient is to implement all level 1 recommendations and as many level 2 recommendations as feasible. ACE, angiotensin-converting enzyme; ARB, angiotensin receptor blocker; DH-CCB, dihydropyridine calcium channel blocker; NDHP-CCB, nondihydropyridine calcium channel blocker.

Measurement of serum cystatin C may provide a better estimate of the GFR than serum creatinine–based measures (see also Chapter 3) but is more expensive. Diabetes, obesity, inflammation and thyroid hormone status can alter cystatin C levels independently of kidney function.[10] The role of cystatin C in CKD management remains to be defined.

THERAPY FOR NATURAL PROGRESSION

Because of the gravity of ESRD and the benefit of even small decreases in CKD progression rate (see Fig. 76.3), a strong argument can be made for an aggressive, multiple risk factor intervention to slow GFR decline.[1,2] This, however, does not apply for patients with low ESRD risk. This includes corticosteroid-responsive minimal change disease (MCD), a solitary kidney that is normal and acquired in adulthood and not accompanied by other CKD risk factors, hereditary nephritis or thin glomerular basement membrane disease in a normotensive adult whose only renal manifestation is microscopic hematuria, and the elderly with idiopathic and moderately elevated serum creatinine (1.30 to 2.00 mg/dl) and minor proteinuria (24-hour urine PC ratio <1.0) and whose renal parameters have been stable for at least 1 year. The last group is much more likely to die of cardiovascular disease (CVD) than to progress to ESRD.[1,2]

Recommended therapies in this chapter are listed in Figure 76.5. The recommendations categorized as level 1 (highest) are based on one or more large randomized clinical trials (RCTs) that have documented effects on GFR decline. Level 2 recommendations are based on secondary analysis of the level 1 RCTs, or RCTs that have documented effects on proteinuria but not GFR decline, or RCTs that appear to be of high quality but may not be definitive because of study size.

The goals of progression therapy are (1) to reduce proteinuria as much as possible, ideally to less than 500 mg/day,[1,2] and (2) to slow GFR decline as much as possible, ideally to about 1 ml/min per year, which is the rate of GFR decline attributable to aging (see Fig. 76.3).

Level 1 Recommendations to Slow Natural Progression

Control Blood Pressure

The low blood pressure goal is recommended for all CKD patients.[1,2] On the basis of the relevant RCTs, we suggest a sitting systolic blood pressure in the 120s or lower, if it is tolerated. "Optimal" blood pressure (systolic blood pressure <120 mm Hg) is associated with significantly lower CVD risk than "normal" blood pressure (systolic blood pressure of 120 to 129 mm Hg),[2] and there is no convincing evidence that systolic blood pressure below 120 mm Hg is harmful if it is well tolerated (not associated with fatigue, lightheadedness, tachycardia, or decline in kidney function).[1,2] Sitting blood pressure is recommended because it is the position used in the relevant RCTs. Systolic blood pressure is the recommended goal because in the relevant RCTs, achieved systolic blood pressure strongly correlated with GFR decline, but achieved diastolic blood pressure did not. Specifying a goal with both a systolic and diastolic blood pressure component is not recommended. It can be confusing to the physician and the patient and can lead to overtreatment.[2] Isolated diastolic hypertension probably represents an artifact, particularly in white hypertensives.[2]

The greater the proteinuria, the greater is the benefit of the low blood pressure goal in slowing GFR decline. Current guidelines do not recommend the low blood pressure goal for those with low-level proteinuria, although the low blood pressure goal does prevent progressive increase in proteinuria compared with the usual blood pressure goal (135/85 mm Hg) and probably further reduces CV risk.[1,2] Home blood pressure monitoring is recommended to assess whether the patient is achieving the blood pressure goal.[1,2] Treatment of nocturnal hypertension, assessed by ambulatory blood pressure monitoring, may also provide benefit.[2]

Antihypertensive drug selection can play an important role in maximizing the CV benefits of hypertension control (see also Chapter 78). For example, in the Antihypertensive and Lipid-Lowering Treatment to Prevent Heart Attack Trial (ALLHAT), diuretic therapy in nonblack hypertensives lowered blood pressure significantly better than angiotensin-converting enzyme (ACE) inhibitors but did not lower cardiovascular (CV) risk more than ACE inhibitors.[11] In the Ongoing Telmisartan Alone and in Combination with Ramipril Global Endpoint Trial (ONTARGET), ACE inhibitors plus angiotensin receptor blockers (ARBs) lowered blood pressure significantly better than ACE inhibitors or ARBs alone but did not lower CV risk better than either drug alone.[12] In the Avoiding Cardiovascular Events Through Combination Therapy in Patients Living with Systolic Hypertension (ACCOMPLISH) trial, ACE inhibitor plus CCB lowered systolic blood pressure comparable to ACE inhibitor plus thiazide diuretic, but the cohort receiving ACE inhibitor and CCB experienced significantly fewer CV events.[13]

The classes of drugs used to lower blood pressure also importantly influence CKD progression.[1,2] An evidence- and experience-based algorithm for blood pressure control in CKD is shown in Figures 76.6 and 76.7. Delay in achieving the low blood pressure goal increases the risk for progression to ESRD.[2] If systolic blood pressure is 20 mm Hg or more above goal, two or more antihypertensive agents will usually be needed to achieve blood pressure goal.[2]

ACE Inhibitor Therapy

This drug class is recommended as first-line therapy in all CKD patients. Although the ALLHAT study suggested that diuretics should be first-line therapy in CKD with low-level proteinuria,[2] the study protocol did not use ACE inhibitors optimally (with diuretic, if needed), which confounds its interpretation. Also, the benefits of diuretics were seen mainly in black patients. Diuretics as monotherapy may induce metabolic dysfunctions that include hypokalemia, hyperglycemia, hyperuricemia, and stimulation of the renin-angiotensin-aldosterone system (RAS),[1,2] each of which increases CV risk. However, if the diuretic is used with an ACE inhibitor (or ARB), most of the metabolic dysfunctions associated with diuretic use should be mitigated.[1,2,14]

Although both ACE inhibitors and ARBs are kidney protective, ACE inhibitors are the first choice because it is not yet clear if ARBs give equivalent cardioprotection.[2] ACE inhibitors should be used even if the patient is not hypertensive.[1,2] Measures that may increase ACE inhibitor–associated kidney protection include a low-sodium and reduced-protein diet, diuretic therapy, lower blood pressure goal, and statin therapy.[1,2] ACE inhibitors are antiproteinuric even in inflammatory glomerulonephritis (GN). ACE inhibitors should be continued even though GFR declines to stage 4 CKD (15 to 29 ml/min per 1.73 m^2). To prevent hyperkalemia, dietary potassium restriction and the concomitant use of furosemide and sodium bicarbonate may be indicated.[2]

CV and renal benefits of ACE inhibitors appear to be a class effect. There is no firm evidence of additional benefits for any particular ACE inhibitor. A plausible argument can be made for the preferential use of ramipril and benazepril, which have relatively long half-lives and strong are inhibitors of tissue ACE, the most important component of the RAS.

Advancing the ACE inhibitor dose to tolerance increases its antiproteinuric effect and decreases the likelihood of aldosterone escape (increasing plasma aldosterone levels during stable ACE inhibitor therapy), which could diminish ACE inhibitor–associated renoprotection.[2] ACE inhibitors may be particularly effective in those who are homozygous for the *ACE* gene insertion (I) polymorphism.[15]

Although a recent meta-analysis suggested that ACE inhibitors may not have kidney protective effects apart from blood pressure control, that analysis included heterogeneous studies that did not all use ACE inhibitor treatment optimally or have ideal methodologic rigor.[2]

ARB Therapy

ARBs are protective in the nephropathy of type 2 diabetes and probably in other nephropathies.[2] ARBs are recommended as first-line therapy in those who are ACE inhibitor intolerant (cough, angioedema, or allergy). In CKD, ARBs may raise serum potassium less than ACE inhibitors.[2] The highest tolerated ARB dose, up to the maximum recommended dose, is recommended for maximum antiproteinuric effect[2] and to optimize regression of left ventricular hypertrophy.[2] ARBs may be especially effective in those who are homozygous for the *ACE* gene deletion (D) polymorphism.[15] There is recent evidence that the ARBs that became available after losartan may have better CV and renal protective effects.

Combination ACE Inhibitor and ARB Therapy

Combined ACE inhibitor and ARB therapy may be more antiproteinuric than ACE therapy inhibitor or ARB alone.[16] However, there is uncertainty about the scientific validity of the COOPERATE study, the only long-term study of combination ACE inhibitor and ARB therapy in CKD.[16]

Furthermore, there are puzzling data from the ONTARGET study suggesting that combination ACE inhibitor and ARB therapy increased the risk of renal endpoints, despite achieving lower blood pressure than either ACE inhibitor or ARB therapy alone. One possible explanation is unfavorable outcome when blood pressure is reduced too far in patients with severe atheromatous renovascular disease. Combination ACE inhibitor and ARB therapy should therefore be used with caution in those with evidence of advanced atherosclerotic CV disease, but it may still be warranted, especially if there is heavy proteinuria.

Renin Inhibitor Therapy

Aliskiren, a direct renin inhibitor, has been combined with losartan in the Aliskiren in the Evaluation of Proteinuria in Diabetes (AVOID) study in patients with hypertension and diabetic nephropathy, resulting in greater reduction in proteinuria compared with losartan alone; the antiproteinuric effect was independent of its effect on blood pressure. Aliskiren is well tolerated and is a promising agent, although more data are required before its role in CKD with proteinuria can be defined.

Avoidance of Dihydropyridine CCBs

Avoid therapy with dihydropyridine calcium channel blockers (DHP-CBBs) unless they are needed for blood pressure control. DHP-CBBs lowered blood pressure better than ACE inhibitors or β-blockers did; however, in those with hypertensive nephrosclerosis, it led to accelerated GFR decline and increased the risk of a composite endpoint of doubling of serum creatinine, ESRD, or death.[1,2] The clearest evidence that DHP-CBBs are not kidney protective is the REIN-2 trial, in which nondiabetic proteinuric renal disease patients receiving ramipril were randomized to the usual or a low blood pressure goal. DHP-CBBs (felodipine) was used to achieve the low blood pressure goal. Despite achieving the low blood pressure goal, the DHP-CBBs group did not

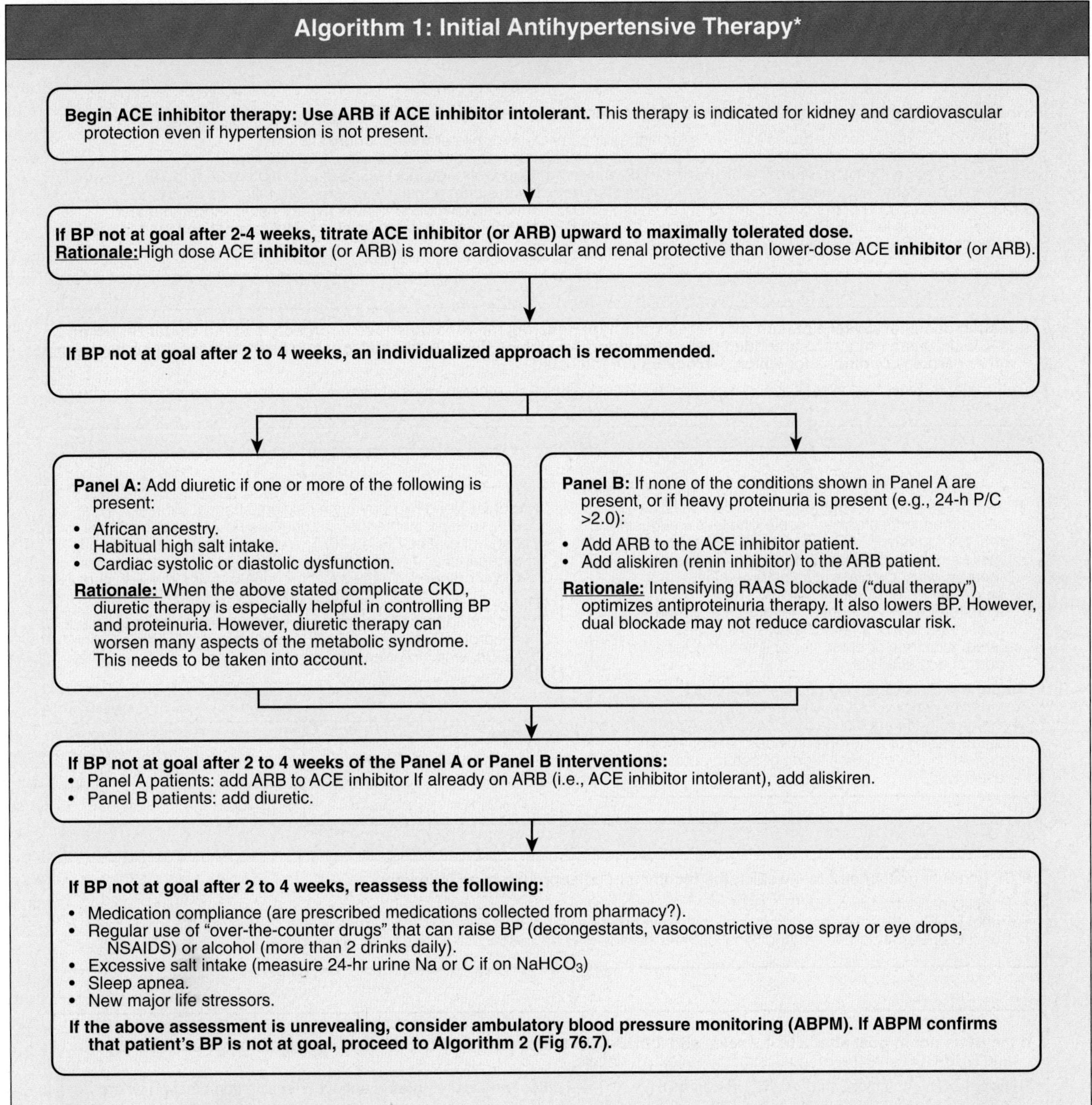

Algorithm 1: Initial Antihypertensive Therapy*
Begin ACE inhibitor therapy: Use ARB if ACE inhibitor intolerant. This therapy is indicated for kidney and cardiovascular protection even if hypertension is not present.
If BP not at goal after 2-4 weeks, titrate ACE inhibitor (or ARB) upward to maximally tolerated dose.
Rationale: High dose ACE inhibitor (or ARB) is more cardiovascular and renal protective than lower-dose ACE inhibitor (or ARB).
If BP not at goal after 2 to 4 weeks, an individualized approach is recommended.
Panel A: Add diuretic if one or more of the following is present:
• African ancestry.
• Habitual high salt intake.
• Cardiac systolic or diastolic dysfunction.
Rationale: When the above stated complicate CKD, diuretic therapy is especially helpful in controlling BP and proteinuria. However, diuretic therapy can worsen many aspects of the metabolic syndrome. This needs to be taken into account.
Panel B: If none of the conditions shown in Panel A are present, or if heavy proteinuria is present (e.g., 24-h P/C >2.0):
• Add ARB to the ACE inhibitor patient.
• Add aliskiren (renin inhibitor) to the ARB patient.
Rationale: Intensifying RAAS blockade ("dual therapy") optimizes antiproteinuria therapy. It also lowers BP. However, dual blockade may not reduce cardiovascular risk.
If BP not at goal after 2 to 4 weeks of the Panel A or Panel B interventions:
• Panel A patients: add ARB to ACE inhibitor If already on ARB (i.e., ACE inhibitor intolerant), add aliskiren.
• Panel B patients: add diuretic.
If BP not at goal after 2 to 4 weeks, reassess the following:
• Medication compliance (are prescribed medications collected from pharmacy?).
• Regular use of "over-the-counter drugs" that can raise BP (decongestants, vasoconstrictive nose spray or eye drops, NSAIDS) or alcohol (more than 2 drinks daily).
• Excessive salt intake (measure 24-hr urine Na or C if on NaHCO3)
• Sleep apnea.
• New major life stressors.
If the above assessment is unrevealing, consider ambulatory blood pressure monitoring (ABPM). If ABPM confirms that patient's BP is not at goal, proceed to Algorithm 2 (Fig 76.7).

Figure 76.6 Algorithm 1: initial antihypertensive therapy.* *Assumes nonpharmacologic therapy to control blood pressure is in place (see text) and that the patient does not have renovascular hypertension, congestive heart failure, ischemic heart disease, or hypertensive urgency. This approach focuses on blood pressure control in proteinuric nephropathies but is also appropriate for nephrosclerosis, polycystic kidney disease (PKD), and interstitial nephropathies. ACEI, angiotensin-converting enzyme inhibitor; ARB, angiotensin receptor blocker; BP, blood pressure; CKD, chronic kidney disease; NSAIDs, nonsteroidal anti-inflammatory drugs; RAAS, renin-angiotensin-aldosterone system.

experience slower GFR decline or proteinuria reduction compared with those maintained at the usual blood pressure goal, despite concomitant ramipril therapy. The mechanism may be that the DHP-CBBs, by causing afferent arteriolar vasodilation, do not reduce glomerular hypertension.[1,2] Although DHP-CBBs should generally be avoided in CKD management, DHP-CBBs clearly are important in blood pressure management to reduce CV risk; for example, in the ACCOMPLISH trial, ACE inhibitor and DHP-CBBs reduced CV risk more than ACE inhibitor and diuretic did. However, for kidney protection, if a CCB is needed, the first choice should be a nondihydropyridine CCB (see Fig. 76.6 and later discussion).

Control Protein Intake

Reducing dietary protein intake from the usual level (about 1 to 1.5 g/kg ideal body weight per day) to about 0.7 g/kg ideal body weight per day (low-protein diet) slows GFR decline in those with proteinuria of more than 1 g/day.[1] Another benefit of the lower protein intake is that it slows proteinuria progression in CKD, even in those who at baseline have low-level proteinuria

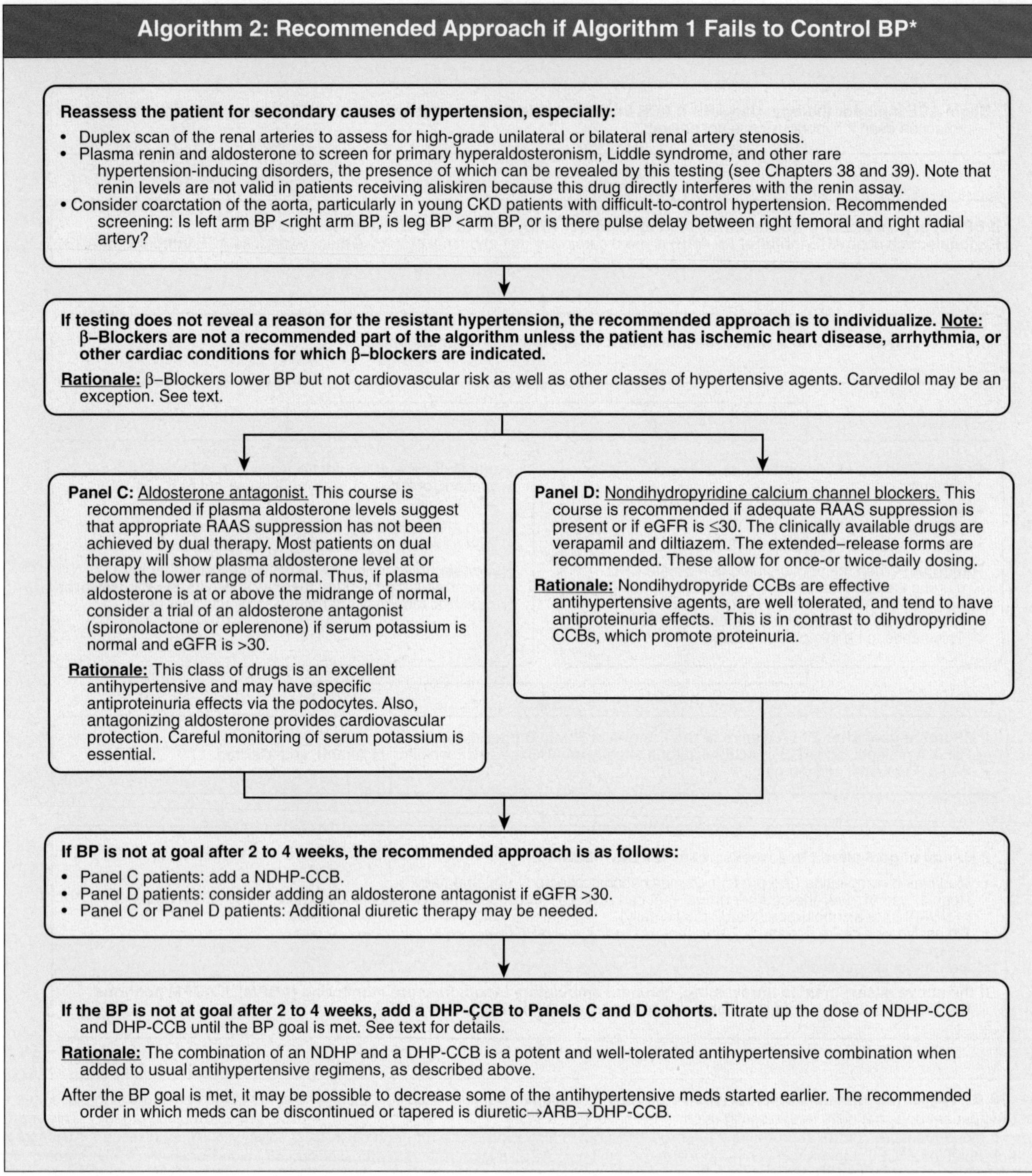

Algorithm 2: Recommended Approach if Algorithm 1 Fails to Control BP*

Reassess the patient for secondary causes of hypertension, especially:

- Duplex scan of the renal arteries to assess for high-grade unilateral or bilateral renal artery stenosis.
- Plasma renin and aldosterone to screen for primary hyperaldosteronism, Liddle syndrome, and other rare hypertension-inducing disorders, the presence of which can be revealed by this testing (see Chapters 38 and 39). Note that renin levels are not valid in patients receiving aliskiren because this drug directly interferes with the renin assay.
- Consider coarctation of the aorta, particularly in young CKD patients with difficult-to-control hypertension. Recommended screening: Is left arm BP <right arm BP, is leg BP <arm BP, or is there pulse delay between right femoral and right radial artery?

↓

If testing does not reveal a reason for the resistant hypertension, the recommended approach is to individualize. Note: β–Blockers are not a recommended part of the algorithm unless the patient has ischemic heart disease, arrhythmia, or other cardiac conditions for which β–blockers are indicated.

Rationale: β–Blockers lower BP but not cardiovascular risk as well as other classes of hypertensive agents. Carvedilol may be an exception. See text.

↓

Panel C: Aldosterone antagonist. This course is recommended if plasma aldosterone levels suggest that appropriate RAAS suppression has not been achieved by dual therapy. Most patients on dual therapy will show plasma aldosterone level at or below the lower range of normal. Thus, if plasma aldosterone is at or above the midrange of normal, consider a trial of an aldosterone antagonist (spironolactone or eplerenone) if serum potassium is normal and eGFR is >30.

Rationale: This class of drugs is an excellent antihypertensive and may have specific antiproteinuria effects via the podocytes. Also, antagonizing aldosterone provides cardiovascular protection. Careful monitoring of serum potassium is essential.

Panel D: Nondihydropyridine calcium channel blockers. This course is recommended if adequate RAAS suppression is present or if eGFR is ≤30. The clinically available drugs are verapamil and diltiazem. The extended–release forms are recommended. These allow for once-or twice-daily dosing.

Rationale: Nondihydropyride CCBs are effective antihypertensive agents, are well tolerated, and tend to have antiproteinuria effects. This is in contrast to dihydropyridine CCBs, which promote proteinuria.

↓

If BP is not at goal after 2 to 4 weeks, the recommended approach is as follows:

- Panel C patients: add a NDHP-CCB.
- Panel D patients: consider adding an aldosterone antagonist if eGFR >30.
- Panel C or Panel D patients: Additional diuretic therapy may be needed.

↓

If the BP is not at goal after 2 to 4 weeks, add a DHP-ÇCB to Panels C and D cohorts. Titrate up the dose of NDHP-CCB and DHP-CCB until the BP goal is met. See text for details.

Rationale: The combination of an NDHP and a DHP-CCB is a potent and well-tolerated antihypertensive combination when added to usual antihypertensive regimens, as described above.

After the BP goal is met, it may be possible to decrease some of the antihypertensive meds started earlier. The recommended order in which meds can be discontinued or tapered is diuretic→ARB→DHP-CCB.

Figure 76.7 Algorithm 2: recommended approach if algorithm 1 fails to control blood pressure.* *If patient is intolerant of or allergic to the drugs recommended in the algorithms, suggested alternatives include ethacrynic acid for thiazide diuretics, aliskiren for ACE inhibitor or ARB, and minoxidil for calcium channel blocker. Carvedilol or doxazosin may be appropriate in algorithm 2 at any point in patients in whom stress may play an important role in their hypertension or in whom BP is particularly labile, in the absence of correctable factors to account for the lability (pseudopheochromocytoma). ACE, angiotensin-converting enzyme; ARB, angiotensin receptor blocker; BP, blood pressure; CCBs, calcium channel blockers; CKD, chronic kidney disease; DHP-CCB, dihydropyridine calcium channel blocker; eGFR, estimated glomerular filtration rate; NDHP-CCB, nondihydropyridine calcium channel blocker; RAAS, renin-angiotensin-aldosterone system.

(e.g., <250 mg/day).[1,2] Diets incorporating soy proteins may induce less proteinuria than those composed of only animal proteins.[2] Dietary protein intake should be monitored periodically, for example, each 4 to 6 months, by measuring urine urea excretion in 24-hour urine collections. For a 70-kg person, ingestion of about 50 g of protein daily would achieve the dietary goal of 0.7 g/kg ideal body weight per day. In such a patient, the 24-hour urine collection would contain about 8 g of urea nitrogen. Monitoring protein intake is particularly important in those who are not achieving their proteinuria goal. Men and those with glomerular disease may particularly benefit from the low-protein diet.[2] Severe protein restriction should be avoided; in the MDRD study, long-term follow-up of those on a very low protein intake (<0.6 g/kg per day) showed no further reduction in GFR decline but appeared to have an increased risk of death.[17]

Level 2 Recommendations to Slow Natural Progression

Restrict NaCl Intake and Diuretic Therapy

A high salt intake (e.g., 200 mmol NaCl/day, 4.6 g sodium, 11.6 g NaCl) can completely override the antiproteinuric effects of ACE inhibitor, ARB, or NDHP-CCB therapy.[1,2] The recommended NaCl intake in CKD (assuming that renal salt wasting is not present) is about 80 to 120 mmol/day (2 to 3 g Na). The NaCl intake in the average North American adult is about 170 mmol/day (3.9 g Na, 9.9 g NaCl). Salt intake should be monitored periodically (e.g., each 4 to 6 months) by 24-hour urine collection.[2] With achievement of the goal for salt intake, a complete 24-hour urine collection would have about 80 to 120 mEq of sodium. The monitoring of 24-hour urine sodium content is particularly important in those not achieving the blood pressure or proteinuria goal. In patients receiving $NaHCO_3$ therapy, urine chloride rather than sodium should be monitored, taking account of concomitant KCl.[2] High fructose intake (in the form of table sugar or high-fructose corn syrup) should be avoided because it increases renal sodium reabsorption and can worsen blood pressure control.[18]

Diuretic therapy improves blood pressure control and reduces proteinuria in those receiving ACE inhibitor or ARB.[2] Nevertheless, the ideal is to avoid diuretics because of the multiple metabolic dysfunctions, which include hypokalemia, hyperglycemia, hyperlipidemia, and stimulation of the RAAS, all of which are known to increase the CV risk. Furosemide may be more effective than thiazide diuretics with serum creatinine concentration of more than 2.0 mg/dl.

Control Fluid Intake

A retrospective analysis of MDRD study A showed that urine volumes exceeding 2 l/day were associated with faster GFR decline, especially in patients with polycystic kidney disease (PKD).[1,2] The patients with the higher urine volumes showed higher blood pressure, lower serum sodium, and frankly hypotonic urine, suggesting that they were intentionally taking in excess fluid ("pushing fluids"). Also, in the African American Study of Kidney Disease (AASK) trial, urine volume measured at baseline was the seventh strongest predictor of GFR decline of the 35 baseline predictors tested, predicting GFR decline to the same degree as baseline systolic blood pressure.[19] Excessive fluid intake in a CKD subject may be difficult to excrete and can lead to volume overload. CKD is associated with both impaired concentration and dilution. Thus, one should neither restrict nor push fluids in CKD.

Nondihydropyridine Calcium Channel Blocker Therapy

This class of agents, which includes diltiazem and verapamil, is antiproteinuric and may be renoprotective. NDHP-CCB together with a DHP-CCB is a potent antihypertensive combination when it is used along with other antihypertensive therapies (see Fig. 76.6).[1,2]

Control Each Component of the Metabolic Syndrome

The metabolic syndrome is defined as any three of the following:

- Blood pressure ≥130/85 mm Hg or requiring antihypertensive therapy.
- Fasting blood glucose concentration >100 mg/dl (5.6 mmol/l) or treatment for hyperglycemia.
- Fasting serum high-density lipoprotein cholesterol level <40 mg/dl for men, <50 mg/dl for women.
- Fasting serum triglycerides ≥150 mg/dl or drug therapy needed to control hypertriglyceridemia.
- Waist circumference >40 inches (102 cm) in men or >35 inches (88 cm) in women.

Each component of the metabolic syndrome is a risk factor for CKD progression. Also, the prevalence of microalbuminuria and CKD increases proportionately with the number of components of the metabolic syndrome.

Obesity increases the risk for CKD and is associated with glomerulomegaly, focal and segmental glomerulosclerosis, and proteinuria, which can be progressive. Reducing even moderate obesity can reduce proteinuria. In moderately obese CKD patients (mean body mass index, 32; mean proteinuria, 2.8 g/day), a 4% decrease in body weight during 5 months reduced proteinuria by 31%.[2]

Management of lipids in CKD is discussed in Chapters 77 and 78. Although definitive evidence of benefit is lacking, we recommend statin therapy to control lipids in CKD patients not on dialysis, in view of their increased CV risk of CKD.

Aldosterone Antagonist Therapy

Spironolactone and the more selective aldosterone antagonist eplerenone have substantial antihypertensive, cardioprotective, and antiproteinuric effects even in low doses (e.g., spironolactone, 25 mg daily) and in the presence of combined ACE inhibitor and ARBs.[20] The mechanism may involve benefits of aldosterone blockade on endothelium and the profibrotic effects of aldosterone. If these drugs are used in combination with ACE inhibitor or ARBs, monitoring for hyperkalemia is necessary. Although there are no strong trial data with hard endpoints such as ESRD, the available evidence supports the use of aldosterone antagonists in high-risk CKD patients who have not reached their blood pressure or proteinuria goals despite other therapy (see Fig. 76.7). However, the use of aldosterone antagonists should be restricted to those with an eGFR above 30 ml/min per 1.73 m^2.[20]

β-Blocker Therapy

The AASK study showed that β-blocker therapy is more antiproteinuric and slows GFR decline more than DHP-CCB. However, β-blockers increase the likelihood of diabetes and, as monotherapy or combined with diuretic, increase the mortality rate of hypertension management compared with ACE inhibitors plus diuretic.[14] β-Blockers should be used in CKD to manage heart disease but should not be first-line therapy for blood pressure and proteinuria. Carvedilol, which possesses both β-blocker and α_1-blocker effects, may be better tolerated than metoprolol when it is used in combination with an ACE inhibitor.[2]

Smoking Cessation

There is strong epidemiologic evidence that cigarette smoking promotes progression of all forms of kidney disease and that this effect may be of greater magnitude in African Americans.[2]

Allopurinol Therapy

In a placebo-controlled, randomized trial, allopurinol therapy resulted in a 40% lesser increase in serum creatinine during 1 year of follow-up and improved blood pressure control (~13 mm Hg lower systolic blood pressure).[2] In another trial allopurinol or placebo was administered to 113 subjects with CKD stage 3 for 2 years. There was a slight improvement in the allopurinol group (+1.3 mL vs −4 ml per min per 1.73 m^2) and a substantial (70%) reduction in cardiovascular events.[21] These findings are consistent with an abundance of evidence that serum uric acid elevation is a strong risk factor for the development of CV and renal disease.[22] Allopurinol therapy mitigates these risk factors, perhaps by mechanisms beyond lowering of serum uric acid. However, allopurinol can be associated with a severe allergic reaction (Stevens-Johnson–like syndrome). If allopurinol is administered to CKD subjects, the dose needs to be reduced.

Although there is substantial evidence supporting the use of allopurinol in hyperuricemic CKD patients, some experts recommend that allopurinol not be used for asymptomatic hyperuricemia in CKD until better information becomes available because of the risk of severe toxicity.[22] A new xanthine oxidase inhibitor, febuxostat, is now available. It is safe in patients allergic to allopurinol and does not need dose adjustment in CKD. To date, severe reactions have not been reported; however, experience in the use of this drug in CKD is limited.

Other Measures to Retard Progression of Chronic Kidney Disease

- Avoid multiple daily doses of acetaminophen, particularly in women, because of the evidence that it is significantly associated with rising serum creatinine during prolonged follow-up.[2]
- Avoid nonsteroidal anti-inflammatory drugs (NSAIDs) altogether (or, at most, take no more than once or twice weekly) because of their known nephrotoxicity. Daily low-dose aspirin, however, appears to provide net benefit in CKD.[2]
- Avoid herbal therapy unless the safety of the herb has been proved. Many herbals appear to be nephrotoxic (see Chapter 74).[2]
- Avoid prolonged severe hypokalemia because it can cause progressive renal interstitial fibrosis.[2]
- Avoid phosphate cathartics. These can cause acute kidney injury (AKI) and CKD by causing intratubular calcium phosphate deposits.
- Avoid intravenous bisphosphonates in CKD. Some may exacerbate renal failure.
- Avoid oral estrogen in elderly women with CKD. It may promote progression.
- $NaHCO_3$ to correct metabolic acidosis should be considered because of its anticatabolic effects. Also, the nephrotoxicity of nonselective proteinuria appears to be strongly related to activation of the alternative complement pathway in the renal tubular compartment. $NaHCO_3$ inhibits this process by raising tubular fluid pH.[2]
- Control hyperphosphatemia and hyperparathyroidism. In animal models and in human studies, control of hyperphosphatemia slows CKD progression. Also, active 1,25-dihydroxyvitamin D therapy has been found to be potentially antiproteinuric (dipstick protein) in CKD in one *post hoc* analysis of an RCT and by this mechanism might be kidney protective.[2]

REFERENCES

1. Haddad N, Brown C, Hebert LA. Retarding progression of kidney disease. In: Johnson R, Fehally J, eds. *Comprehensive Clinical Nephrology*. 3rd ed. Philadelphia: Elsevier; 2007:823-830.
2. Agarwal A, Haddad N, Hebert LA. Progression of kidney disease: Diagnosis and management. In: Molony D, Craig J, eds. *Evidence-Based Nephrology*. Hoboken, NJ: Wiley; 2008:311-322.
3. Li S, Chen SC, Shlipak M, et al. Low birth weight is associated with chronic kidney disease only in men. *Kidney Int*. 2008;73:637-642.
4. Birmingham DJ, Rovin BH, Shidham G, et al. Relationship between albuminuria and total proteinuria in systemic lupus erythematosus nephritis: Diagnostic and therapeutic implications. *Clin J Am Soc Nephrol*. 2008;3:1028-1033.
5. Birmingham DJ, Rovin BH, Shidham G, et al. Spot urine protein/creatinine ratios are unreliable estimates of 24 h proteinuria in most systemic lupus erythematosus nephritis flares. *Kidney Int*. 2007;72:865-870.
6. Hebert LA, Birmingham DJ, Shidham G, et al. Random spot urine protein/creatinine ratio is unreliable for estimating 24-hour proteinuria in individual systemic lupus erythematosus nephritis patients. *Nephron Clin Pract*. 2009;113:c177-c182.
7. Xie D, Joffe MM, Brunelli SM, et al. A comparison of change in measured and estimated glomerular filtration rate in patients with nondiabetic kidney disease. *Clin J Am Soc Nephrol*. 2008;3:1332-1338.
8. Stevens LA, Coresh J, Greene T, et al. Assessing kidney function—measured and estimated glomerular filtration rate. *N Engl J Med*. 2006;354:2473-2483.
9. Wilmer WA, Rovin BH, Hebert CJ, et al. Management of glomerular proteinuria: a commentary. *J Am Soc Nephrol*. 2003;14:3217-3232.
10. Stevens LA, Schmid CH, Greene T, et al. Factors other than glomerular filtration rate affect serum cystatin C levels. *Kidney Int*. 2009;75:652-660.
11. Hebert LA, Rovin BH, Hebert CJ. The design of ALLHAT may have biased the study's outcome in favor of the diuretic cohort. *Nature Clin Pract Nephrol*. 2007;3:60-61.
12. ONTARGET Investigators. Telmisartan, ramipril, or both in patients at high risk for vascular events. *N Engl J Med*. 2008;358:1547-1559.
13. Jamerson K, Weber MA, Bakris GL, et al. Benazepril plus amlodipine or hydrochlorothiazide for hypertension in high-risk patients. *N Engl J Med*. 2008;359:2417-2428.
14. Messerli FH, Bangalore S, Julius S. Risk/benefit assessment of β-blockers and diuretics precludes their use for first-line therapy in hypertension. *Circulation*. 2008;117:2706-2715; discussion 2715.
15. Ruggenenti P, Bettinaglio P, Pinares F, et al. Angiotensin converting enzyme insertion/deletion polymorphism and renoprotection in diabetic and nondiabetic nephropathies. *Clin J Am Soc Nephrol*. 2008;3:1511-1525.
16. Arici M, Erdem Y. Dual blockade of the renin-angiotensin system for cardiorenal protection: An update. *Am J Kidney Dis*. 2009;53:332-345.
17. Menon V, Kopple JD, Wang X, et al. Effect of a very low-protein diet on outcomes: Long-term follow-up of the Modification of Diet in Renal Disease (MDRD) Study. *Am J Kidney Dis*. 2009;53:208-217.
18. Choi ME. The not-so-sweet side of fructose. *J Am Soc Nephrol*. 2009;20:457-459.
19. Wang X, Lewis J, Appel L, et al. Validation of creatinine-based estimates of GFR when evaluating risk factors in longitudinal studies of kidney disease. *J Am Soc Nephrol*. 2006;17:2900-2909.
20. Navaneethan SD, Nigwekar SU, Sehgal AR, et al. Aldosterone antagonists for preventing the progression of chronic kidney disease: A systematic review and meta-analysis. *Clin J Am Soc Nephrol*. 2009;4:542-551.
21. Goicoechea M, de Vinuesa SG, Verdalles U, et al. Effect of allopurinol in chronic kidney disease progression and cardiovascular risk. *Clin J Am Soc Nephrol*. 2010;5:1388-139.
22. Feig DI, Kang DH, Johnson RJ. Uric acid and cardiovascular risk. *N Engl J Med*. 2008;359:1811-1821.

CHAPTER 77

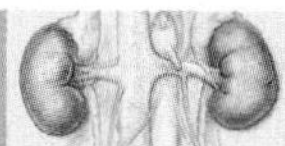

Clinical Evaluation and Management of Chronic Kidney Disease

David C. Wheeler

Although many patients with chronic kidney disease (CKD) progress to end-stage renal disease (ESRD) and require renal replacement therapy, the majority die of nonrenal causes, particularly premature cardiovascular events.[1] Early diagnosis of CKD is therefore important because it provides opportunities to delay progression of CKD (see Chapter 76) and to prevent cardiovascular complications (see Chapter 78).

DEFINITIONS

The U.S. Kidney Disease Outcomes Quality Initiative (KDOQI) guidelines[2] classify CKD (Fig. 77.1) into five stages (Fig. 75.1). This system, which is based on disease severity rather than cause, was endorsed in modified format by the international Kidney Disease: Improving Global Outcomes (KDIGO) organization.[3] Because of the impracticalities of using radioisotopes and 24-hour urine collections, the KDOQI classification system recommends that kidney function be assessed by estimating the glomerular filtration rate (GFR) with an appropriate equation. Two formulae are in common use, one developed by Cockcroft and Gault, the other derived from the Modification of Diet in Renal Disease (MDRD) study (see Chapter 3).[4] Although standardization of creatinine assays remains an issue, the KDOQI staging system provides a useful framework for the management of CKD.

CLINICAL PRESENTATION

Early diagnosis of CKD with the introduction of an algorithm-based disease management plan may slow the rate of decline of kidney function and reduce cardiovascular risk.[5] Many patients with CKD are known to health care professionals because they are receiving treatment for hypertension, cardiovascular disease, or diabetes. They may be identified because an elevated serum creatinine level or urinary abnormality is detected at routine follow-up. Unfortunately, others remain undiagnosed until they present with symptomatic acute or chronic kidney disease or with a cardiovascular event.

Evaluation of the Patient with Suspected Chronic Kidney Disease

The detection of an estimated GFR (eGFR) of less than 60 ml/min in a patient in whom renal function was previously unknown or normal requires a history and examination with attention to the blood pressure and urinalysis (for protein and blood) to assess whether the disease is acute or chronic. Imaging of the kidneys by ultrasound is useful as small kidneys suggest chronic disease.

Proteinuria is an important diagnostic and prognostic marker, and its presence indicates a higher risk for both progression of kidney disease and cardiovascular complications.[6] Measurement of proteinuria in a 24-hour urine collection has been largely abandoned in favor of the "spot" urine albumin/creatinine ratio, although an argument can be made for timed urine collections (see Chapter 76). Dipstick urinalysis and urine culture are also recommended.[7] Workup of hematuria is discussed in Chapters 4 and 59.

Blood pressure should be checked in all patients. Those with stage 3 to stage 5 CKD need to be assessed for other complications, such as dyslipidemia, anemia, and the biochemical abnormalities that characterize the CKD–mineral bone disorder.

When to Refer to the Nephrologist

Although management of patients with early nonprogressive CKD is increasingly becoming the responsibility of primary care physicians, nephrologists need to assess those individuals likely to progress to ESRD and to require renal replacement therapy. Criteria for referral are included in management algorithms, such as those developed by the U.K. National Institute for Clinical Excellence (NICE; Fig 77.2). Such criteria are not absolute but should provide a guide to the primary care physician as to which patients are likely to benefit from secondary care. Unfortunately, because CKD is not associated with symptoms in the early stages, a substantial proportion of such patients are referred late, often when they need dialysis. Late referral is often avoidable,[8] particularly among patients with known CKD, and may be due to the lack of recognition by physicians of the nonlinear relation between serum creatinine and GFR. In other cases, late referral is unavoidable because the patient may have had a truly silent illness or an acute presentation of a disease that causes a rapid decline in kidney function.

Late presentation is disadvantageous as it limits the time for patients to select the mode of dialysis or to be listed for "preemptive" kidney transplantation. Furthermore, because an arteriovenous fistula takes weeks to mature, patients presenting late are required to start hemodialysis using central venous catheters. Catheters are prone to infectious complications and inevitably damage central veins, leading to thromboses and stenoses, which may be manifested at a later stage when venous return from one or the other arm is increased by the subsequent construction of an arteriovenous fistula (see Chapter 87).[9] Late presentation of CKD precludes treatment of uremic complications, such as hypertension and anemia,[10] both of which contribute to cardiovascular damage, which may ultimately limit life span.[11] These factors compound psychological stress, making it difficult for the patient to come to terms with the illness. Importantly, late presentation is associated with a worse prognosis,[12] and the cost of initiating dialysis in ESRD patients presenting late is higher than for those in whom dialysis is initiated electively.[13]

CLINICAL MANIFESTATIONS

A detailed discussion of the complications of CKD is provided in Chapters 78 to 85. With the exception of hypertension, there are usually few clinical manifestations during CKD stages 1 and 2 (GFR >60 ml/min per 1.73 m^2), the presence of proteinuria or hematuria being largely dependent on the underlying cause of kidney disease. Other complications (discussed in the following sections) tend to develop progressively as GFR declines below 60 and in particular below 30 ml/min per 1.73 m^2 (i.e., during stages 4 and 5 CKD).

Hypertension

Between 50% and 75% of individuals with CKD stages 3 to 5 have hypertension (if it is defined as a systolic blood pressure ≥140 mm Hg or diastolic blood pressure ≥80 mm Hg).[14] Casual clinic blood pressure is useful, but ambulatory monitoring correlates better with cardiovascular outcomes and is particularly informative if there is suspicion that readings taken in the hospital are not representative. In patients with atherosclerotic vascular disease and CKD, the presence of renal artery stenosis should be considered (see Chapter 37).

Control of blood pressure both slows the rate of decline of renal function (see Chapter 76) and reduces cardiovascular complications. All classes of antihypertensive agent can be used in CKD patients, although agents blocking the renin-angiotensin system (RAS) may provide better renoprotection (see Chapter 76). Multidrug regimens are usually necessary to achieve blood pressure control, and most recommendations suggest targeting lower blood pressures (125/75 mm Hg), especially in those with diabetes or proteinuria.[14] Lifestyle modifications should be encouraged (see Chapter 34). Fluid retention occurs in CKD stages 3 to 5, and a diuretic can be included in the antihypertensive regimen. In general, thiazides are recommended in patients with CKD stages 1 to 3 and loop diuretics in those with more severely impaired kidney function.[14] Potassium-sparing diuretics can be associated with hyperkalemia in CKD stages 4 and 5 as well as in subjects receiving angiotensin-converting enzyme (ACE) inhibitors or angiotensin receptor blockers (ARBs). The available evidence supports a target blood pressure below 130/80 mm Hg for most CKD patients not receiving dialysis but below 125/75 mm Hg for those with a urinary protein excretion of more than 1 g/24 hours.[14]

Dyslipidemia

Patients with CKD stage 3 frequently develop dyslipidemia with elevated plasma triglycerides and low high-density lipoprotein cholesterol due to the accumulation of very low density lipoprotein particles and a disturbance in the maturation of high-density lipoprotein.[16] Total and low-density lipoprotein cholesterol levels are generally normal but may be low in patients with concomitant inflammation and malnutrition.[17]

Current guidelines for the treatment of dyslipidemia in CKD patients recommend extrapolation of treatment thresholds and targets from non-CKD populations.[16] Nevertheless, whereas *post hoc* analysis of large randomized controlled trials suggests that statin therapy may benefit patients with CKD stage 3 with vascular disease,[18] to date there is no robust evidence to suggest that these drugs benefit CKD patients without overt vascular disease or those with more advanced stages of CKD. Furthermore, the risks for myopathy with the use of fibrates and statins is increased

Criteria for Definition of Chronic Kidney Disease

Kidney damage for ≥3 months, as defined by structural or functional abnormalities of the kidney, with or without decreased GFR, that can lead to decreased GFR, manifest by either:
- Pathologic abnormalities
- Markers of kidney damage, including abnormalities in the composition of blood or urine, or abnormalities in imaging tests
- GFR <60 ml/min/1.73 m^2 for ≥3 months, with or without kidney damage

Figure 77.1 Criteria for definition of chronic kidney disease. GFR, glomerular filtration rate. *(Modified from reference 15.)*

Suggested Criteria for Referral of Patients with Chronic Kidney Disease to a Nephrologist

New Diagnosis	Stage 3	Stage 4
eGFR <30 ml/min/per 1.73 m^2	eGFR falling by >4 ml/min per year	eGFR <20 ml/min per 1.73 m^2
Hemoglobin <11g/dl	eGFR < 50 ml/min in patient younger than 50 years	eGFR falling by >4 ml/min per year
K^+ >6 mmol/l	Hemoglobin < 11 g/dl	Hemoglobin <11 g/dl
Ca <2.1 mmol/l	K^+ >6 mmol/l	K^+ >6 mmol/l
Pi >1.5 mmol/l	Ca <2.1 mmol/l	Ca <2.1 mmol/l
PTH >3× upper limit normal	Pi >1.5 mmol/l	Pi >1.5 mmol/l
Hematuria		PTH >3× upper limit normal
Urine ACR >30 mg/mmol		
Suspected renovascular disease		

Figure 77.2 Suggested criteria for referral of patients with chronic kidney disease (CKD) to a nephrologist. ACR, albumin to creatinine ratio; eGFR, estimated glomerular filtration rate; PTH, parathyroid hormone. *(Modified from NICE CKD guideline.)*

in CKD. Fibrate dosage should therefore be reduced in patients with CKD stages 3 and 4 and fibrates should be avoided in CKD stage 5. Statins should be initiated with low starting doses because of drug accumulation.[16]

Anemia

Anemia is common in CKD stages 3 to 5 and is caused by a relative deficiency of erythropoietin (EPO), although reduced availability of iron and chronic inflammation are frequent contributory factors.[19] Anemia may contribute to cardiac dysfunction by increasing cardiac output and may thereby exacerbate left ventricular hypertrophy. Although reversal of anemia with erythropoietin has been associated with regression of left ventricular hypertrophy,[20] there is currently no evidence that treatment is associated with an improved longer term cardiac prognosis, although its use may be associated with better quality of life.[21] Debate remains as to the optimal target range of hemoglobin concentrations, with most guidelines recommending a level of 11 to 13 g/dl (see Chapter 79).[22] Partial correction of anemia does not accelerate the decline of renal function but may necessitate increases in antihypertensive therapy.[23]

Bone and Mineral Metabolism

Hyperphosphatemia together with a deficiency of 1,25-dihydroxyvitamin D_3 contribute to secondary hyperparathyroidism and ultimately to the development of renal bone disease. These biochemical and endocrine changes, in association with the closely related histologic abnormalities of bone and soft tissue calcification, are collectively termed the CKD–mineral bone disorder.[24] Bone disease may already be manifested in CKD stage 3 and is well established in ESRD, even though the subject is often asymptomatic (see Chapter 81). Prevention of secondary hyperparathyroidism requires dietary phosphate restriction and administration of phosphate binders.[25] Patients are also prescribed biologically active vitamin D (e.g., calcitriol) or vitamin D prohormones that are converted to active dihydroxy compounds in the liver (e.g., 1α-hydroxyvitamin D_3).[26] Many patients with CKD stages 3 and 4 are also deficient in 25-hydroxyvitamin D_3,[27] and oral replacement with parent vitamin D_3 (cholecalciferol) may increase plasma levels of the 1,25-dihydroxy derivative.[28]

Metabolic Acidosis

The metabolic acidosis associated with CKD is caused by failure of hydrogen ion excretion and may be compounded by bicarbonate loss, particularly in interstitial kidney diseases and the accumulation of organic acids. Clinical symptoms from acidosis are rare until patients reach CKD stage 5, when dyspnea may occur. Other causes of dyspnea in advanced CKD, including anemia and pulmonary edema, should always be considered. Acidosis aggravates hyperkalemia, inhibits protein anabolism, and accelerates calcium loss from bone where the hydrogen ions are buffered.[29] There is also emerging evidence that correction of metabolic acidosis slows progression of renal disease.[30] Severe metabolic acidosis (e.g., serum bicarbonate <20 mmol/l) associated with symptoms in a patient with CKD stage 5 is an indication to start dialysis. If dialysis is not immediately available, oral sodium bicarbonate in a dose up to 1.2 g four times daily may be considered, but sodium loading may aggravate hypertension.

Malnutrition

Malnutrition is common among patients on dialysis but also occurs in CKD stages 4 and 5 (see Chapter 83) and is associated with an increased risk for death.[17] The causes are multifactorial and include anorexia, acidosis, insulin resistance, inflammation, oxidative stress, and urinary protein loss. Biochemical indicators include a decrease in serum albumin, transferrin, and cholesterol. Weight should be monitored in patients who progress to CKD stages 4 and 5. Serum creatinine concentrations, which in part reflect muscle mass, may stop rising despite a progressive loss of kidney function because of compromised nutritional status. If patients do not readily respond to dietary supplementation, initiation of dialysis should be considered.

Sodium and Water Retention

Sodium handling by the kidney is altered in CKD (see Chapter 8), although plasma sodium concentrations are generally within the normal range. As GFR falls, sodium homeostasis is initially maintained because a greater proportion of sodium and water filtered by the glomerulus is excreted as a result of reduced tubular reabsorption (glomerulotubular balance). One of the earliest effects of CKD is to limit the ability of the kidney to compensate for large changes in sodium and water intake. Although water excretion in healthy individuals can vary from about 20 to 1500 ml/h, depending on hydration status, this range becomes restricted in CKD. Excessive oral water intake may lead to dilutional hyponatremia, and in those whose daily fluid intake exceeds 2 liters, it may accelerate progression of CKD (see Chapter 76). As kidney function declines, most patients develop sodium retention and extracellular volume expansion. They may complain of ankle swelling or shortness of breath as a result of pulmonary edema. Restriction of dietary sodium intake to 2.4 g (100 mmol) per day may help alleviate such symptoms and control the associated increase in blood pressure. Salt substitutes containing potassium should be avoided because of the risk for hyperkalemia.

Potassium

Hyperkalemia may develop in CKD stages 4 and 5 and can be managed by dietary restriction to less than 60 mmol potassium daily. Patients with CKD may tolerate higher serum potassium concentrations without electrocardiographic changes or arrhythmias than those with acute kidney injury (AKI), but this is not a consistent feature, and hyperkalemia should always be actively managed (see Chapter 9). Acute reductions in serum potassium are best achieved by glucose and insulin infusion; sodium bicarbonate is less effective in the setting of impaired renal function. Oral resins (such as Kayexalate with sorbitol) are widely used in some countries but may cause gastrointestinal upset and can raise blood pressure because of sodium retention. Dialysis may be required acutely if the serum potassium concentration is markedly elevated (levels >6.5 mmol/l). For chronic management of hyperkalemia, dietary potassium restriction and loop diuretics may be required.

Endocrine Abnormalities

Thyroid Hormones

Total plasma thyroxine (T_4) levels may be low, with an associated increase in triiodothyronine (T_3) as a result of impaired conversion of T_3 to T_4. Loss of thyroid-binding globulin in urine may further lower total circulating T_4 concentrations.[31] However, patients do not become clinically hypothyroid, and measurement of thyroid-stimulating hormone remains a reliable diagnostic test for hypothyroidism in CKD.

Growth Hormone

Plasma growth hormone levels may be elevated in patients with CKD stage 5 because of delayed clearance and alterations in hypothalamic-pituitary control.[32] In children, growth retardation may result and can be corrected by treatment with exogenous recombinant growth hormone given in supraphysiologic doses.[33]

Insulin

Decreased clearance of insulin is balanced by increased peripheral resistance to the effects of the hormone. As a result, there are usually no clinical manifestations, and patients are not particularly prone to hypoglycemia. However, in patients with diabetes, these effects may lead to a falling requirement for insulin as kidney function declines (see Chapter 31), a trend that may be reversed by the initiation of dialysis.[34]

Sex Hormones

Males Prolactin levels are elevated in CKD stage 5 and may contribute to gynecomastia and sexual dysfunction. Testosterone levels are often low-normal, and gonadotropins may be raised, implying testicular failure.[35] This is accompanied by poor spermatogenesis, leading to low sperm counts and reduced fertility. It may be appropriate to prescribe androgen replacement treatment if testosterone is unequivocally low, not least because this may help prevent osteoporosis or erectile dysfunction.[36] Erectile dysfunction is also common in the absence of testosterone deficiency and may result from neurological, psychological, and vascular abnormalities. Treatment with phosphodiesterase type 5 inhibitors, such as sildenafil citrate, may be appropriate if there is no evident cardiovascular disease.

Females The pituitary-ovary axis may be disturbed in CKD stages 4 and 5.[37] Although luteinizing hormone levels are raised, the normal pulsatile release and the preovulation surge are absent. Cycles may be irregular or anovulatory and associated with amenorrhea. Raised prolactin levels may also contribute to infertility. Nevertheless, conception can occur, and increasingly there are successful pregnancy outcomes (see Chapter 43).

Immunity

Infection is the second most common cause of death after cardiovascular disease in the patient with ESRD, which is due to CKD being a state of chronic immunosuppression[38] with defects in both cellular and humoral immunity (see Chapter 80).

T-cell responses to *de novo* antigens are deficient, partly because of impaired antigen presentation by monocytes. Neutrophil activation is defective, and although serum immunoglobulin levels are normal, antibody responses to immunization are poor. In practical terms, this is a problem in immunizing the CKD patient against hepatitis B and other T cell–dependent antigens, such as pneumococcus species and *Haemophilus influenzae* type b (see Chapter 80).

Patients with CKD have an increased susceptibility to bacterial infection (particularly staphylococcal), increased risk of reactivation of tuberculosis (typically with a negative tuberculin skin test response), and failure to eliminate hepatitis B and C viruses after infections. CKD patients should be immunized against hepatitis B as early as is feasible in an effort to maximize the chances of seroconversion.[39]

Immunization is still worthwhile in patients presenting with CKD stage 5, but an intensified regimen is recommended (see Chapter 80).

Psychological Manifestations

Anxiety and depression are common in patients with severe CKD and are due to the loss of health and lifestyle changes. Management consists of education and counseling. Short-term antidepressant therapy may help, and some patients benefit from night sedation, particularly during hospital admissions.

Other Complications of Chronic Kidney Disease

CKD patients, particularly those with stage 5 disease, may develop a bleeding diathesis (see Chapter 80), neurologic problems including uremic encephalopathy (see Chapter 82), and dermatologic manifestations (see Chapter 84). Uremic pericarditis may occur in CKD stage 5 and can usually be detected clinically by the presence of a pericardial rub. Administration of anticoagulants to such patients may lead to hemorrhage into the pericardial cavity, causing life-threatening tamponade.

MANAGEMENT OF CHRONIC KIDNEY DISEASE STAGES 4 AND 5

The management of a CKD patient according to the stage of disease is shown in Figure 77.3. For subjects with CKD stage 5 who have symptoms consistent with advanced uremia, dialysis treatment should be initiated. Earlier presentation to a nephrologist increases opportunities to treat complications and to prepare patients for renal replacement therapy. To optimize the management of such individuals, many centers observe patients with CKD stages 4 and 5 in clinics where care is delivered by a multidisciplinary team, including the nephrologist, surgeon, nurse, social worker, dietitian, and psychologist.

Treating the Uremic Emergency

For patients presenting with symptomatic uremia, the priority is to deal with life-threatening complications, such as hyperkalemia, pulmonary edema, metabolic acidosis, encephalopathy, and pericarditis. The uremic emergency can be the initial presentation of either AKI or ESRD resulting from CKD, but the immediate management is the same. Patients presenting with uremic emergencies should be admitted to an intensive care unit or to a high-dependency area. Here, the nephrologist determines treatment priorities, optimizes composition and timing of dialysis, monitors complications, and oversees the medications.

Acute Kidney Injury Versus Chronic Kidney Disease

An important issue is to distinguish acute from chronic kidney disease. There may be hints of a past history of kidney problems (e.g., hypertension, proteinuria, microscopic hematuria) or symptoms suggestive of prostatic disease. The physical examination is not usually helpful, although skin pigmentation (Fig.

Management Plan for Patients with Chronic Kidney Disease, According to Stage

KDOQI Classification	GFR (ml/min)	Typical Serum Creatinine in 65-kg Subject	Consequences	Actions to Consider
3	30–59	2mg/dl (170 μmol/l)	Hypertension, secondary hyperparathyroidism	6-monthly eGFR initially 12-monthly eGFR if stable Annual Hb, K, Ca, P Treat hypertension Immunize against hepatitis B
4	15–29	4 mg/dl (350 μmol/l)	*Plus* anemia, hyperphosphatemia	3-monthly eGFR initially 6-monthly eGFR is stable 6-monthly Hb, K, Ca, P, and PTH Start phosphate-restricted diet and phosphate binders Correct vitamin D deficiency Start vitamin D analogue Plan renal replacement therapy, including vascular access
5	<15	8 mg/dl (700 μmol/l)	*Plus* sodium and water retention, anorexia, vomiting, reduced higher mental function	Plan elective start of dialysis or preemptive renal transplant
5	<5	17 mg/dl (1500 μmol/l)	*Plus* pulmonary edema, coma, fits, metabolic acidosis, hyperkalemia, death	Start dialysis *or* provide palliative care

Figure 77.3 Management plan for patients with chronic kidney disease (CKD), according to stage. The table gives a rough guide to the level of serum creatinine corresponding to each stage of CKD in a typical 65-kg subject and shows the approximate timing of the anticipated clinical problems and interventions required as CKD progresses. At each stage, the action plan for the previous CKD stage should be followed if it has not already been initiated. eGFR, estimated glomerular filtration rate; PTH, parathyroid hormone.

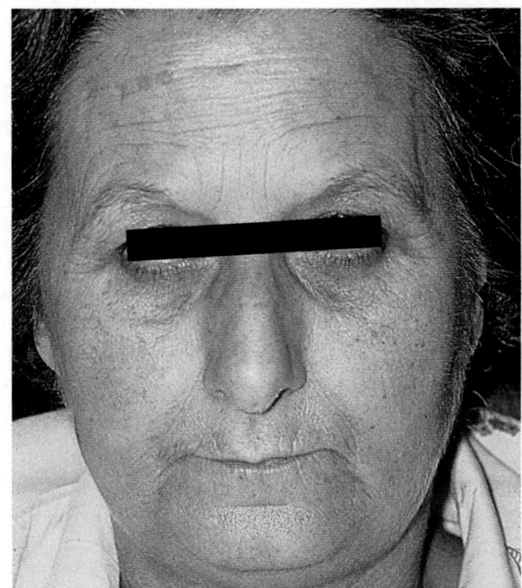

Figure 77.4 Uremic pigmentation. Diffuse brown pigmentation as seen here suggests chronic kidney disease rather than acute kidney injury.

77.4), scratch marks, left ventricular hypertrophy, and hypertensive fundal changes favor a chronic presentation.

The renal ultrasound examination is the most useful distinguishing test. Small kidneys with reduced cortical thickness, showing increased echogenicity, scarring, or multiple cysts, suggest a chronic process. Blood tests are less helpful unless they indicate evidence of an acute illness that may be the cause of kidney failure, such as systemic vasculitis or multiple myeloma. A normochromic normocytic anemia is usual in CKD but may also be a feature of acute systemic illnesses, so it is not discriminatory. Low serum calcium and raised phosphate levels also have little discriminatory value, but normal levels of parathyroid hormone are more in keeping with AKI. Patients with grossly abnormal biochemical values (e.g., blood urea nitrogen >140 mg/dl, serum creatinine 13.5 mg/dl (>1200 μmol/l), blood urea >300 mg/dl (>50 mmol/l) who appear relatively well and are still passing normal volumes of urine are much more likely to have chronic than acute kidney disease.

Establishing the Cause of Chronic Kidney Disease

Establishing the cause of CKD is important as there may be a treatable condition, and those with genetic causes, such as adult polycystic kidney disease (PKD), may require appropriate counseling. Some kidney diseases may also recur after transplantation, and an accurate diagnosis may therefore influence later management. However, the cause of CKD is often unclear, with an unhelpful past medical history, minimal abnormalities of urinalysis, and small kidneys on ultrasound, in which case investigation should not be pursued relentlessly because the implications for treatment are often minimal. Attempting to obtain biopsy material from small kidneys is also risky, and if biopsy is performed, it may show only nonspecific chronic scarring.

Minimizing Progression of Chronic Kidney Disease

Delay or prevention of the progression of kidney failure is a management priority in CKD. In some cases, the underlying cause can be modified or arrested. In all patients, there will be modifiable factors, most notably hypertension (see Chapter 76).

Unexpected Deterioration of Kidney Function

CKD patients may require reassessment if kidney function suddenly declines faster than predicted during follow-up (Fig. 77.5); the possible causes are listed in Figure 77.6. Because subjects with CKD frequently have impaired urinary concentrating ability, the most common cause is volume depletion due to the overzealous use of diuretics, insufficient fluid intake in hot weather, diarrhea, or vomiting. Dehydration substantial enough to cause a rise in serum creatinine may not cause symptoms, although there may be a fall in body weight of at least 3 kg and a postural drop in blood pressure. Kidney perfusion can also be compromised by heart failure, myocardial infarction, and tachyarrhythmias and may be affected by drugs, including nonsteroidal anti-inflammatory drugs (NSAIDs), ACE inhibitors, and ARBs. Other common causes include acute interstitial nephritis (see Chapter 60), obstructive nephropathy (see Chapter 58), and intercurrent infection.

Additional causes include hypercalcemia, which may be caused by the coadministration of high doses of vitamin D compounds and calcium-containing phosphate binders; accelerated-phase hypertension; and renal vein thrombosis. The clinician should also be alert to the possibility of relapse of a treated underlying disease.

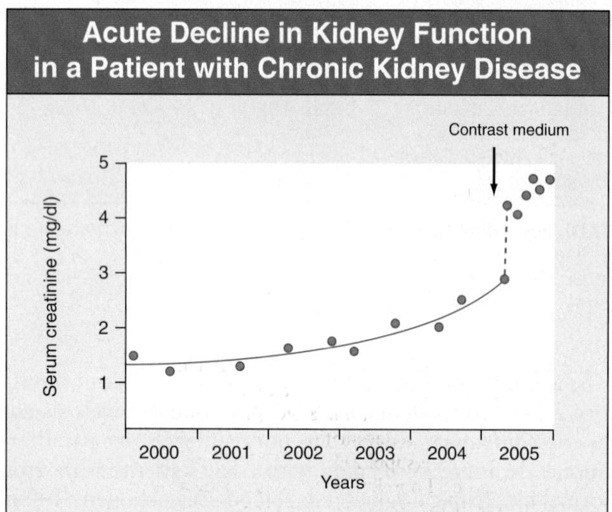

Figure 77.5 Acute decline in kidney function in a patient with chronic kidney disease (CKD). Serum creatinine plot for a 58-year-old man with CKD secondary to diabetic nephropathy. An exponential increase over time is seen between 2000 and 2004. However, an abrupt rise occurs in April 2005, when the patient receives contrast medium for coronary angiography without prior hydration. The patient's kidney function never recovered to the previous baseline, and he began hemodialysis in December 2005.

Causes of Acute-on-Chronic Kidney Failure
Dehydration
Drugs
Disease relapse
Disease acceleration
Infection
Obstruction
Hypercalcemia
Hypertension
Heart failure
Interstitial nephritis

Figure 77.6 Causes of acute-on-chronic kidney failure.

Assessing Stage of Chronic Kidney Disease and Preparation for Renal Replacement Therapy

Despite all attempts to optimize the management of CKD, many patients will progress to ESRD. The KDOQI staging system (see Fig. 75.1) provides management guidelines according to CKD stage (see Fig. 77.3). In CKD stage 3, prophylaxis against secondary hyperparathyroidism should be started by restricting dietary phosphate; if this fails to control phosphate levels, prescription of oral phosphate binders is appropriate (see Chapter 81). Patients should be checked for deficiency of 25-hydroxyvitamin D_3, and ergocalciferol or cholecalciferol should be commenced if deficiency is shown. Immunization against hepatitis B should be performed. Anemia and iron status should be evaluated and treated or corrected, if necessary (see Chapter 79).

At a GFR of 15 to 20 ml/min (late stage 4 or stage 5), patients should receive education and counseling to aid their selection of the most appropriate renal replacement modality. If hemodialysis is the preferred option, an arteriovenous fistula should be constructed, remembering that it may take 8 to 12 weeks for veins to become adequately arterialized before needling can be attempted (see Chapter 87). Because early kidney transplantation improves long-term outcome,[40] patients should be assessed for their suitability and, when feasible, activated on the waiting list before dialysis is commenced. This maximizes the chances of the potential recipient remaining in reasonably good health. The availability of a live donor should be explored to increase the chances of preemptive transplantation before the patient begins dialysis.

The decision to start dialysis is generally considered in any patient with CKD stage 5 who develops uremic symptoms, shows evidence of malnutrition, or develops life-threatening complications of CKD, such as pericarditis, hyperkalemia, acidosis, or fluid overload (see Chapter 86). The case for starting dialysis earlier than stage 5 is not strong,[41] but all patients with CKD stages 4 and 5 are best monitored in a multidisciplinary specialist clinic. A plan for assessment of such patients is provided in Figure 77.7.

CONSERVATIVE MANAGEMENT OF TERMINAL UREMIA

There will be patients for whom dialysis is considered inappropriate and others who decide to discontinue treatment. The decision not to initiate dialysis should be made, if possible, in consultation with the patient and family long before the need arises, preferably in the context of a multidisciplinary clinic (see Chapter 86). The patient should be educated about the expected benefits of dialysis as well as its complications and cost (in terms of inpatient stays, travel time, and lifestyle restrictions). One compelling argument not to offer dialysis to elderly patients with high levels of associated comorbidity is that such individuals are unlikely to benefit in terms of life expectancy.[42] It may also be

Continuing Assessment of the Chronic Kidney Disease Patient
Kidney Function
Has kidney function declined?
Has kidney function declined at the predicted rate?
If not, are there exacerbating factors?
Should dialysis be started?
Are there life-threatening complications? Pericarditis Fluid overload Resistant hypertension Hyperkalemia Uncompensated metabolic acidosis
Should access be created or transplantation planned?
Supportive Treatment
Can salt, potassium, and fluid balance be improved by diet or diuretics?
Is the phosphate controlled?
Is the dose of vitamin D compound appropriate?
Should erythropoietin (EPO) be prescribed?
Are nutritional supplements needed?
Does the patient need counseling?

Figure 77.7 Continuing assessment of the patient with chronic kidney disease (CKD). Questions to be posed in evaluation of the patient.

inappropriate to offer dialysis to patients with other comorbid conditions that lead to major limitations or limit life span, such as malignant disease.

In the context of a uremic emergency, when the background history may not be readily available and the patient's premorbid state is unknown, dialysis treatment should not be withheld, particularly when dialysis may provide symptomatic relief. However, subsequently, withdrawal of dialysis or death while on dialysis treatment may be traumatic for both the patient's family and staff. The legal issues are complex and may vary in some respects from country to country, but it is always a requirement for patients to make the decision not to receive or to discontinue dialysis when they are fully informed and able to do so.

Properly managed, death from uremia should be free of suffering. One must ensure that the patient is comfortable with the decision and that family members are understanding and supportive. Symptoms such as dyspnea from pulmonary edema and acidosis are best controlled with an opiate infusion and nausea with regular chlorpromazine or ondansetron. Pain is often underestimated as a symptom of terminal uremia and should be actively managed, usually with opiates. The mouth can become dry and crusted from mouth breathing, and regular mouth washes and gum care should be offered. Pruritus can be managed by cooling the skin and by application of emollients. Myoclonic jerks are distressing and may be reduced by prescription of benzodiazepines.

REFERENCES

1. Keith DS, Nichols GA, Gullion CM, et al. Longitudinal follow-up and outcomes among a population with chronic kidney disease in a large managed care organization. *Arch Intern Med.* 2004;164:659-663.
2. National Kidney Foundation. KDOQI clinical practice guidelines for chronic kidney disease: evaluation, classification and stratification. *Am J Kidney Dis.* 2002;39(suppl 1):S1-S266.
3. Levey AS, Eckardt KU, Tsukamoto Y, et al. Definition and classification of chronic kidney disease: a position statement from Kidney Disease: Improving Global Outcomes (KDIGO). *Kidney Int.* 2005;67: 2089-2100.
4. Froissart M, Rossert J, Jacquot C, et al. Predictive performance of the Modification of Diet in Renal Disease and Cockcroft-Gault equations for estimating renal function. *J Am Soc Nephrol.* 2005;16:763-773.
5. Richards N, Harris K, Whitfield M, et al. Primary care–based disease management of chronic kidney disease (CKD), based on estimated glomerular filtration rate (eGFR) reporting, improves patient outcomes. *Nephrol Dial Transplant.* 2008;23:549-555.
6. Brantsma AH, Bakker SJ, Hillege HL, et al. PREVEND study group. Cardiovascular and renal outcome in subjects with K/DOQI stage 1-3 chronic kidney disease: the importance of urinary albumin excretion. *Nephrol Dial Transplant.* 2008;23:3851-3858.
7. Arm JP, Peile EB, Rainford DJ, et al. Significance of dipstick haematuria. 1. Correlation with microscopy of the urine. *Br J Urol.* 1986;58: 211-217.
8. Roderick P, Jones C, Drey N, et al. Late referral for end-stage renal disease: a region-wide survey in the south west of England. *Nephrol Dial Transplant.* 2002;17:1252-1259.
9. Roy-Chaudhury P, Kelly BS, Melhem M, et al. Vascular access in hemodialysis: issues, management, and emerging concepts. *Cardiol Clin.* 2005;23:249-273.
10. Landray MJ, Thambyrajah J, McGlynn FJ, et al. Epidemiological evaluation of known and suspected cardiovascular risk factors in chronic renal impairment. *Am J Kidney Dis.* 2001;38:537-546.
11. Go AS, Chertow GM, Fan D, et al. Chronic kidney disease and risk of death, cardiovascular events, and hospitalization. *N Engl J Med.* 2004;351:1296-1305.
12. Winkelmayer WC, Owen WF, Levin R, Avorn J. A propensity analysis of late versus early nephrologist referral and mortality on dialysis. *J Am Soc Nephol.* 2003;14:486-492.
13. Lameire N, Wauters JP, Teruel JL, et al. An update on the referral pattern of patients with end-stage renal disease. *Kidney Int Suppl.* 2002;80:27-34.
14. National Kidney Foundation. K/DOQI clinical practice guidelines on hypertension and antihypertensive agents in chronic kidney disease. *Am J Kidney Dis.* 2004;43(Suppl 1):S1-S290.
15. National Kidney Foundation. KDOQI clinical practice guidelines for chronic kidney disease: evaluation, classification and stratification. *Am J Kidney Dis.* 2002;39(suppl 2):S1-S266.
16. National Kidney Foundation. KDOQI clinical practice guidelines for management of dyslipidemias in patients with chronic kidney disease. *Am J Kidney Dis.* 2003;41(suppl 3):S1-S91.
17. Kalantar-Zadeh K. Recent advances in understanding the malnutrition-inflammation-cachexia syndrome in chronic kidney disease patients: what is next? *Semin Dial.* 2005;18;365-369.
18. Tonelli M, Isles C, Curhan GC, et al. Effect of pravastatin on cardiovascular events in people with chronic kidney disease. *Circulation.* 2004;110:1557-1663.
19. Obrador GT, Pereira BJ. Anaemia of chronic kidney disease: an under-recognized and under-treated problem. *Nephrol Dial Transplant.* 2002; 17(Suppl 11):44-46.
20. Locatelli F, Pozzoni P, Del Vecchio L. Anemia and heart failure in chronic kidney disease. *Semin Nephrol.* 2005;25:392-396.
21. Weisbord SD, Kimmel PL. Health-related quality of life in the era of erythropoietin. *Hemodial Int.* 2008;12:6-15.
22. Locatelli F, Aljama P, Barany P, et al; European Best Practice Guidelines Working Group. Revised European best practice guidelines for the management of anaemia in patients with chronic renal failure. *Nephrol Dial Transplant.* 2004;19(suppl 2):ii1-ii47.
23. Jungers P, Choukroun G, Oualim Z, et al. Beneficial influence of recombinant human erythropoietin therapy on the rate of progression of chronic renal failure in predialysis patients. *Nephrol Dial Transplant.* 2001;16:307-312.
24. Moe S, Drüeke T, Cunningham J, et al. Definition, evaluation, and classification of renal osteodystrophy; a position statement from Kidney Disease: Improving Global Outcomes (KDIGO). *Kidney Int.* 2006;69: 1945-1953.
25. Locatelli F, Cannata-Andia JB, Drueke TB, et al. Management of disturbances of calcium and phosphate metabolism in chronic renal insufficiency, with emphasis on the control of hyperphosphataemia. *Nephrol Dial Transplant.* 2002;17:723-731.
26. Martin KJ, Gonzalez EA. Vitamin D analogues for the management of secondary hyperparathyroidism. *Am J Kidney Dis.* 2001;38(suppl 5):S34-S40.

27. Levin A, Bakris GL, Molitch M, et al. Prevalence of abnormal serum vitamin D, PTH, calcium, and phosphorus in patients with chronic kidney disease: results of the study to evaluate early kidney disease. *Kidney Int*. 2007;71:31-38.
28. National Kidney Foundation. K/DOQI clinical practice guidelines for bone metabolism and disease in chronic kidney disease. *Am J Kidney Dis*. 2003;42(suppl 3):S1-S201.
29. Alpern RJ, Sakhaee K. The clinical spectrum of chronic metabolic acidosis: homeostatic mechanisms produce significant morbidity. *Am J Kidney Dis*. 1997;29:291-302.
30. de Brito-Ashurst I, Varagunam M, Raftery MJ, Yaqoob MM. Bicarbonate supplementation slows progression of CKD and improves nutritional status. *J Am Soc Nephrol*. 2009;20:2075-2084.
31. Lim VS. Thyroid function in patients with chronic renal failure. *Am J Kidney Dis*. 2001;38(suppl 1):S80-S84.
32. Johannasson G, Ahlmen J. End-stage renal disease: endocrine aspects of treatment. *Growth Horm IGF Res*. 2003;13(suppl A):S94-S101.
33. Vimalachandra D, Hodson EM, Willis NS, et al. Growth hormone for children with chronic kidney disease. Cochrane Database Syst Rev. 2006;3:CD003264.
34. Snyder RW, Berns JS. Use of insulin and oral hypoglycaemic medications in patients with diabetes mellitus and advanced kidney disease. *Semin Dial*. 2004;17:365-370.
35. Schmidt A, Luger A, Horl WH. Sexual hormone abnormalities in male patients with renal failure. *Nephrol Dial Transplant*. 2002;17:368-371.
36. Johansen KL. Treatment of hypogonadism in men with chronic kidney disease. *Adv Chronic Kidney Dis*. 2004;11:348-356.
37. Holley JL. The hypothalamic-pituitary axis in men and women with chronic kidney disease. *Adv Chronic Kidney Dis*. 2004;11:337-341.
38. Descamps-Latscha B, Herbelin A, Nguyen AT, et al. Immune system dysregulation in uraemia. *Semin Nephrol*. 1994;14:253-260.
39. Da Roza G, Loewen A, Djurdjev O, et al. Stage of chronic kidney disease predicts seroconversion after hepatitis B immunization: earlier is better. *Am J Kidney Dis*. 2003;42:1184-1192.
40. Wolfe RA, Ashby VB, Milford EL, et al. Comparison of mortality in all patients on dialysis, patients on dialysis awaiting transplantation, and recipients of a first cadaveric transplant. *N Engl J Med*. 1999;341:1725-1730.
41. Korevaar JC, Jansen MA, Dekker FW, et al; Netherlands Co-operative Study on the Adequacy of Dialysis Study Group. When to initiate dialysis: effect of proposed US guidelines on survival. *Lancet*. 2001;358:1046-1050.
42. Smith C, Da Silva-Gane M, Chandna S, et al. Choosing not to dialyse: evaluation of planned non-dialytic management in a cohort of patients with end-stage renal failure. *Nephron Clin Pract*. 2003;95:c40-c46.

CHAPTER 78

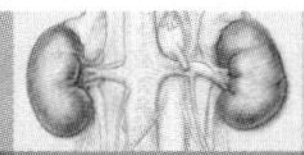

Cardiovascular Disease in Chronic Kidney Disease

Peter Stenvinkel, Charles A. Herzog

The life span of patients with chronic kidney disease (CKD), particularly those with end-stage renal disease (ESRD), is reduced. In the United States, the all-cause mortality rate of prevalent dialysis patients in 2006 was 221 deaths per 1000 patient-years, 41% attributable to cardiac causes.[1] Diminished estimated glomerular filtration rate (eGFR) is a powerful graded, independent predictor of cardiovascular morbidity and mortality[2] (Fig. 78.1) and all-cause mortality.[3] Even subtle kidney dysfunction, as suggested by albuminuria, increases cardiovascular risk,[4] as it may reflect microvasculature health, including endothelial function. There is a strong association between urinary albumin excretion and other cardiovascular risk factors (Fig. 78.2).[1] ESRD patients face an extraordinary risk for premature death, due largely to cardiovascular complications. However, the numbers of patients with non–dialysis-dependent CKD are much larger, and those with eGFR below 60 ml/min per 1.73 m^2 are much more likely to die than to develop ESRD,[5] reflecting the burden of cardiovascular disease (CVD) in this high-risk population. The most effective strategy for reducing cardiovascular morbidity and mortality would be to target patients with mild renal impairment for prevention and treatment before severe CKD develops.

Unfortunately, CKD patients were often excluded from randomized controlled trials targeting CVD, or renal function was poorly described,[6] possibly reducing acceptance of evidence-based therapies (validated in nonrenal patients) and fostering "therapeutic nihilism" in clinicians who treat CKD patients.

Like conventional atheromatous occlusive vascular disease, CKD is characterized by generalized vasculopathy with other characteristics, including left ventricular hypertrophy (LVH), vascular calcification, and vascular noncompliance. Numerous CVD risk factors are specific for CKD and operate in addition to conventional risk factors found in the general population.

EPIDEMIOLOGY

Prevalence of Cardiovascular Complications in Chronic Kidney Disease

Interpretation of epidemiologic studies of CVD in CKD is problematic because of the difficulty defining cause of death, but this difficulty is not limited to renal disease patients. Unexpected sudden death is most likely due to arrhythmia, but a subarachnoid hemorrhage, massive embolic stroke, or aortic dissection might be indistinguishable from a primary arrhythmic event without an autopsy. The real conundrum, however, is defining "coronary heart disease." In the general population, sudden cardiac death is rightly considered a primary complication of coronary artery disease (CAD); evidence-based interventions (e.g., statins) aimed at quelling the progression of atherosclerotic disease reduce the incidence of sudden death. However, in dialysis patients, sudden cardiac death is likely *not* to be a surrogate for coronary heart disease. Even using a history of angina to classify a patient as having coronary heart disease is problematic, as angina (due to supply-demand mismatch) can occur in patients with LVH and angiographically pristine coronary arteries. This probably relates to the increased myocardial fibrosis, diminished relative capillary density, and increased thickening of the intramyocardial vessel walls in uremia.

Of incident ESRD patients, 75% have LVH. Hypertension prevalence increases progressively with falling GFR; 75% to 85% of dialysis patients have hypertension (Fig. 78.3). With hypertension, anemia, vascular noncompliance, and volume overload contribute to LVH. Published data are sparse regarding left ventricular systolic function in incident ESRD patients after erythropoiesis-stimulating agents (ESAs) were introduced. Based on echocardiography, 85% to 90% of patients have preserved left ventricular systolic function, despite frequent congestive heart failure (CHF). As CHF is diagnosed in about 40% of incident ESRD patients within the first year,[7] many volume overload episodes may be attributable to "diastolic dysfunction" or "circulatory congestion." Whatever the mechanism, these hospitalizations are associated with high long-term mortality.[8] Although occlusive CAD is common in CKD patients, acute myocardial infarction (AMI) accounts for only 15% of cardiac deaths; 66% of deaths in the United States Renal Data System (USRDS) database are attributable to arrhythmic mechanisms.[1]

Cardiovascular Disease Is Present Before the Start of Renal Replacement Therapy

In elderly CKD patients at stage 2 or 3, traditional risk factors seem to be the major contributors to cardiovascular mortality. Atherosclerosis Risk in Communities (ARIC) data suggest that both traditional and novel risk factors are relevant at CKD stage 4,[9] and studies of dialysis patients suggest that novel risk factors are far more prevalent than in the general population (Fig. 78.4). The Framingham predictive instrument does not accurately predict coronary events in CKD,[10] another reflection of the necessary consideration of novel risk factors in predictive models for these patients.

Racial and International Differences in Cardiovascular Disease Prevalence

In the United States, after adjustment for demography and comorbid conditions, African American dialysis patients have better survival than do Caucasian patients. Differences in

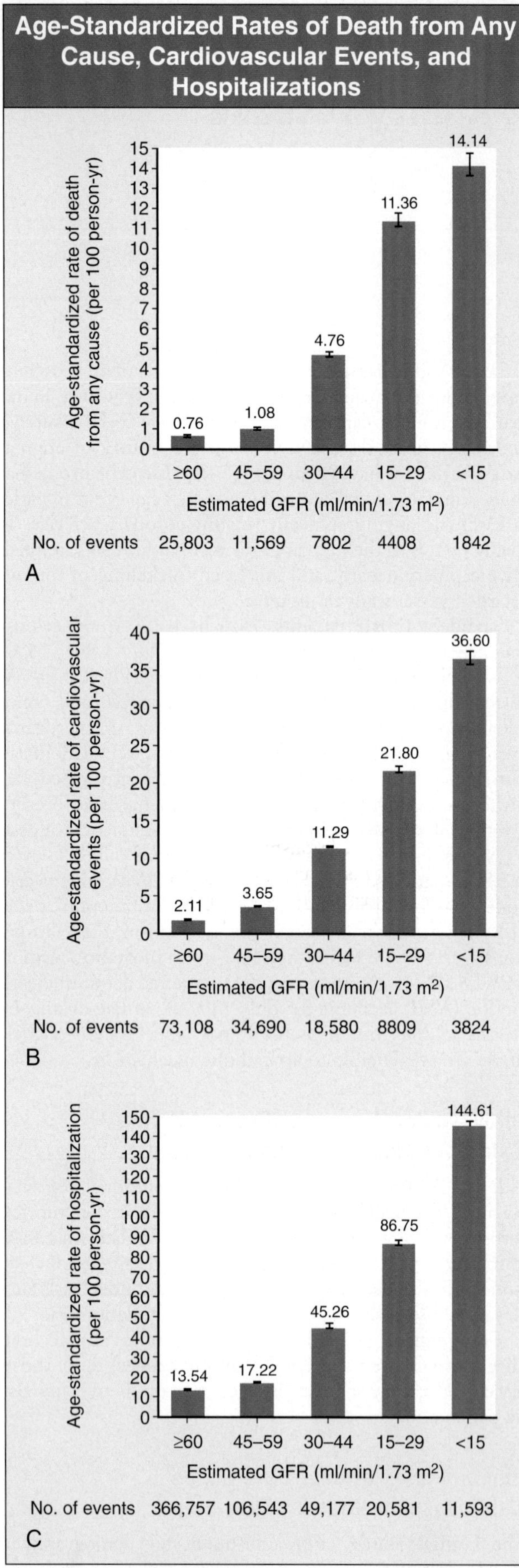

cardiovascular mortality among dialysis patients from the United States, Japan, and Europe are striking,[11] even after adjustment for standard risk factors and dialysis dose. Higher mortality rates in U.S. dialysis patients may be related to higher prevalence of sicker or diabetic patients or to differences in dialysis practice patterns; however, cultural habits, differences in diet, or genetic variations may also contribute.

Reverse Epidemiology

"Reverse epidemiology" is the seemingly paradoxical observation that the association between hypercholesterolemia, hypertension, obesity, and poor outcomes, including cardiovascular death, in the general population does not exist and may be reversed in the CKD population.[12] This concept is needlessly confusing and should be replaced by "confounded epidemiology." Causality must not be confused with association. It is assumed (but open for debate) that wasted, inflamed patients account for poor survival and confounded epidemiology.

ETIOLOGY AND RISK FACTORS

Traditional Risk Factors

Age, Gender, and Smoking

The U.S. National Health and Nutrition Examination Survey (NHANES) shows the prevalence of cardiovascular risk factors and CVD prevalence in relation to age and CKD stage (Figs. 78.5 and 78.6). In the United States, the average age at initiation of renal replacement therapy is 63 years, when CVD is common. Female gender is associated with a 4% independent increased risk of mortality in incident dialysis patients.[1] Smoking is associated with an independent 52% increased risk of mortality in dialysis patients.[13]

Diabetes Mellitus

Diabetes accounted for 44% of incident U.S. ESRD patients in 2006[7] and is the most common cause of ESRD in many countries. Diabetic patients starting renal replacement therapy exhibit a multifactor CVD risk factor profile, including dyslipidemia, hypertension, signs of inflammation, increased oxidative stress, and protein-energy wasting. Not surprisingly, diabetes at dialysis initiation is an independent risk factor for all-cause and CVD-related deaths, including after coronary revascularization or AMI; diabetic ESRD confers a 34% mortality risk after AMI compared with nondiabetic ESRD.

Hypertension

Hypertension is common and not always well treated in CKD patients. Of NHANES[1] participants with CKD stages 3 and 4, 80% were hypertensive (defined as blood pressure ≥130/≥80 mm Hg for CKD patients); 25% of these were unaware of being hypertensive, 7% were aware but untreated, 48% were treated but inadequately controlled (defined as blood pressure <130/<80 mm Hg), and only 20% were treated and adequately

Figure 78.1 Age-standardized rates of death from any cause (A), cardiovascular events (B), and hospitalization (C) according to estimated GFR among 1,120,295 ambulatory adults. A cardiovascular event was defined as hospitalization for coronary heart disease, heart failure, ischemic stroke, and peripheral arterial disease. Error bars represent 95% confidence intervals. The rate of events is listed above each bar. *(Reprinted with permission from reference 2.)*

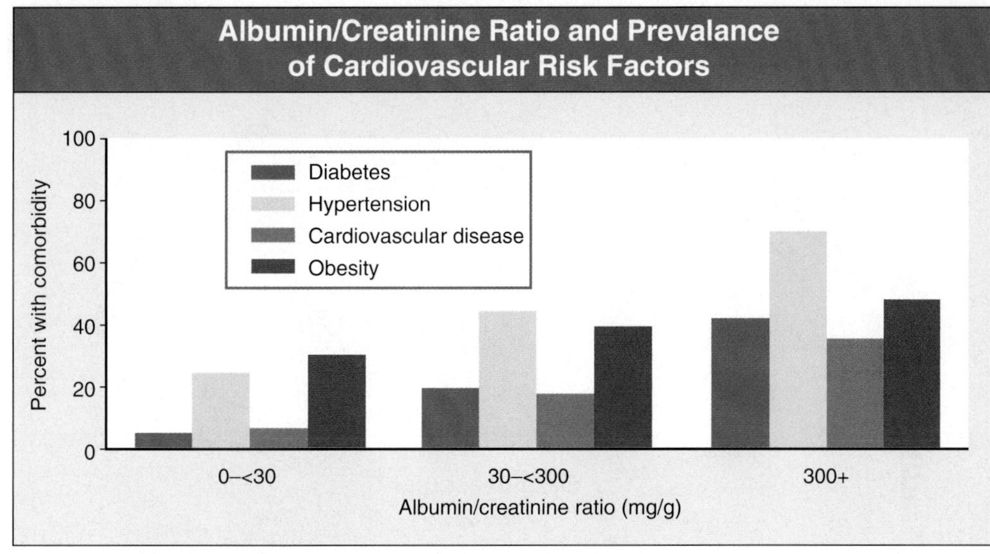

Figure 78.2 Albumin/creatinine ratio and prevalence of cardiovascular risk factors. *(U.S. Renal Data System. USRDS 2008 Annual Data Report: Atlas of Chronic Kidney Disease and End-Stage Renal Disease in the United States. Bethesda, Md, National Institutes of Health, National Institute of Diabetes and Digestive and Kidney Diseases, 2008.)*

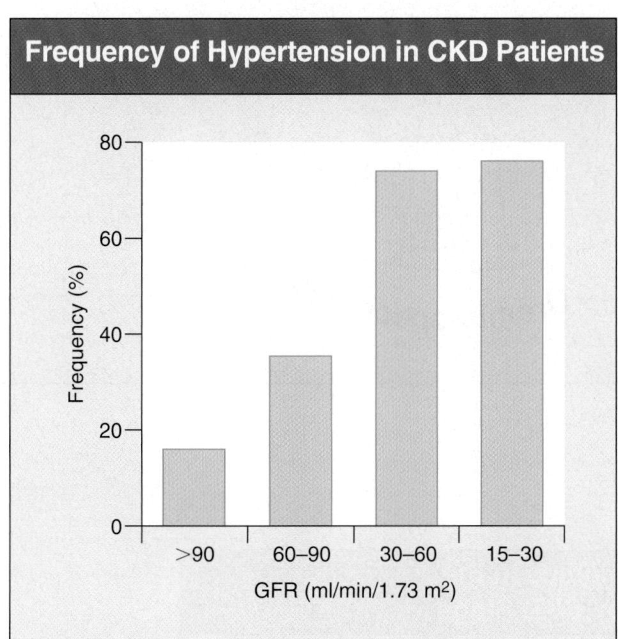

Figure 78.3 Frequency of hypertension in CKD patients according to glomerular filtration rate (GFR). *(Data from NHANES III.)*

controlled. Of participants with CKD stages 1 and 2, 63% were hypertensive; 40% of these were unaware, 13% were aware but untreated, 36% were treated but inadequately controlled, and only 11% were treated and adequately controlled. Low blood pressure is correlated with mortality in some dialysis patients (see Reverse Epidemiology). However, as in the general population, hypertension predicts mortality in CKD patients before or at dialysis initiation. Isolated systolic hypertension with increased pulse pressure is by far the most prevalent blood pressure anomaly in dialysis patients due to arterial medial sclerosis with secondary stiffening. Stiff vessels cause increased pulse wave velocity, resulting in increased systolic peak pressure by a prematurely reflected pulse wave, progressive left ventricular dysfunction, and finally CHF. This may subsequently result in decreased mean arterial and diastolic pressure and increased risk for cardiovascular death. The relationship between blood pressure and mortality is U shaped; isolated systolic hypertension and increased pulse pressure probably indicate high long-term risk in dialysis patients, whereas low mean and diastolic blood pressures predict early mortality. The "invisible" hypertension danger relates to numerous CKD patients being "nondippers" (see Chapter 32). CKD patients frequently also experience sleep apnea, associated with nondipping, sympathetic nervous system activation, and cardiovascular risk.

Dyslipidemia

In CKD patients, the relationship between hypercholesterolemia, CVD, and mortality is weak because some major cardiovascular abnormalities, such as cardiomyopathy and arteriosclerosis, may be less dependent on dyslipidemia than on other factors. Paradoxically, low rather than high serum cholesterol level is associated with poor survival in hemodialysis patients,[12] confounded epidemiology related to protein energy wasting and inflammation. After adjustment for C-reactive protein levels, high cholesterol level predicted risk in relatively healthy ESRD patients without inflammation.[14]

Progressive CKD leads to changes in blood lipids associated with vascular disease, including decreased levels of apoA-containing lipoproteins and increased levels of apoB-containing lipoproteins (Fig. 78.7). Plasma triglyceride levels are elevated in most ESRD patients, whereas total serum cholesterol levels may be elevated, normal, or low, depending on nutritional status and presence of inflammation. High-density lipoprotein (HDL) cholesterol is typically reduced, and low-density lipoprotein (LDL), intermediate-density lipoprotein, and very low density lipoprotein cholesterol as well as lipoprotein(a) levels tend to be increased. Compared with long-term hemodialysis patients, peritoneal dialysis patients more often exhibit both hypercholesterolemia and hypertriglyceridemia. Both groups are characterized by low HDL and elevated oxidized LDL cholesterol levels; elevated lipoprotein(a) levels are associated with increased CVD mortality.

Insulin Resistance and Atherosclerosis

In the general population, impaired insulin-stimulated glucose disposal in muscle is often part of a metabolic syndrome that

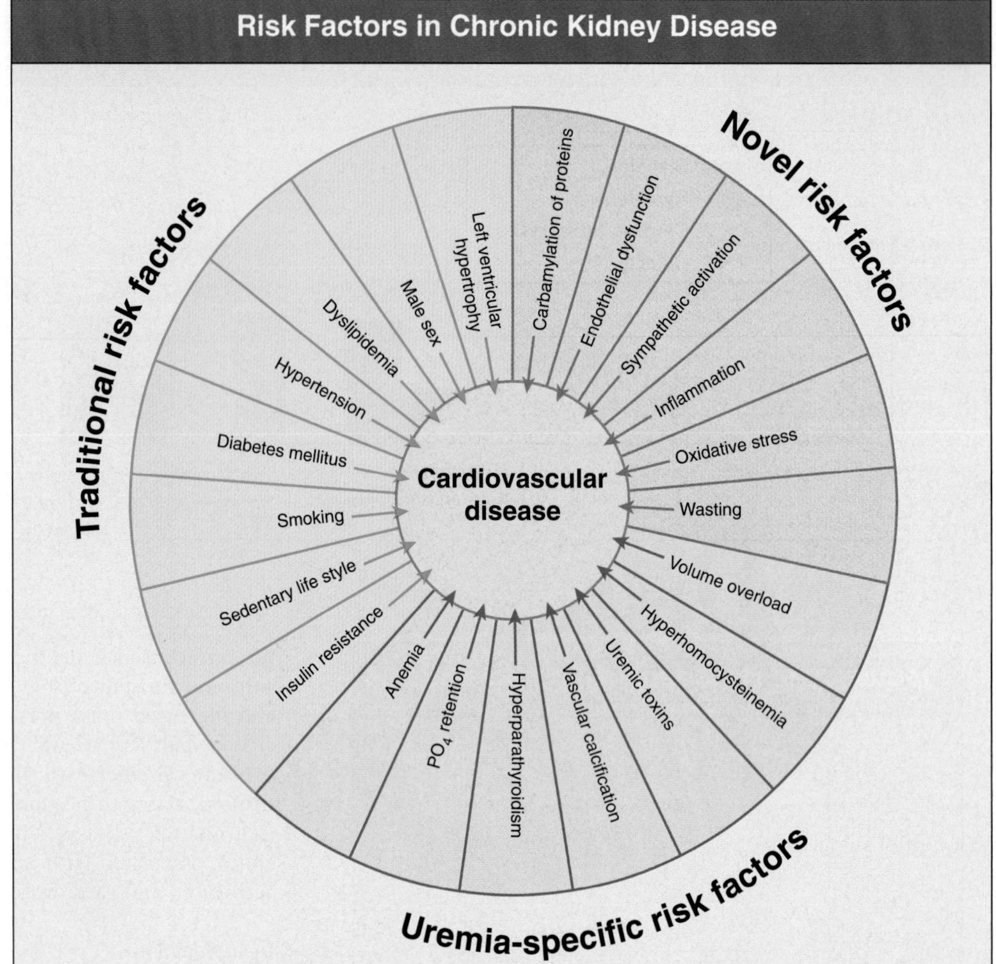

Figure 78.4 Risk factors. Schematic overview of traditional (i.e., Framingham) risk factors *(green)*, "novel" risk factors *(orange)*, and more or less "uremia-specific" risk factors *(blue)*.

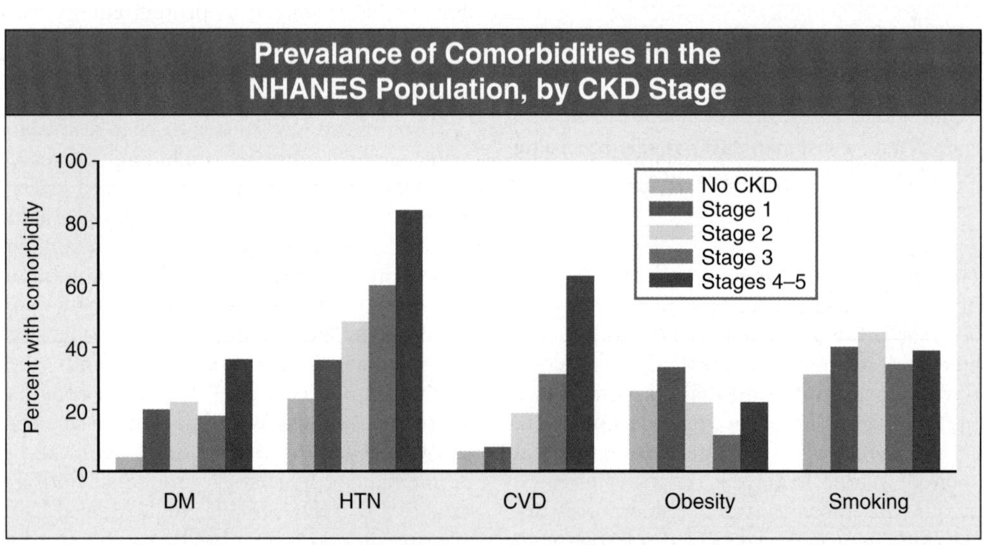

Figure 78.5 Prevalence of comorbidities in the NHANES population, by CKD stage. DM, diabetes mellitus; HTN, hypertension; CVD, cardiovascular disease. *(U.S. Renal Data System. USRDS 2008 Annual Data Report: Atlas of Chronic Kidney Disease and End-Stage Renal Disease in the United States. Bethesda, Md, National Institutes of Health, National Institute of Diabetes and Digestive and Kidney Diseases, 2008.)*

includes dyslipidemia, hypertension, endothelial dysfunction, and sympathetic overactivity. Many of these abnormalities are present in CKD. Although insulin resistance was found to be an independent predictor of cardiovascular mortality in dialysis patients,[15] its contribution to CKD patient mortality is uncertain.

Nontraditional and Uremia-Specific Risk Factors

Several large prospective population studies have shown that even mild CKD is an independent risk factor for CVD, independent of hypertension, diabetes, and albuminuria (Fig. 78.8). Because about 10% of low-risk and 30% of high-risk CVD populations have mild CKD, it is now regarded as an independent cardiovascular risk factor similar in magnitude to diabetes and hypertension. The uremic milieu may affect both quality and quantity of the atherosclerotic plaques. Coronary lesions in uremic patients, compared with nonrenal controls, are characterized by increased media thickness, infiltration, and activation of macrophages and marked calcification.[16] The mechanism by which a uremic milieu may accelerate atherosclerosis is not well established, but prevalence and magnitude of several nontraditional risk factors, such as oxidative stress, inflammation, vascular calcification, and advanced glycation end products (AGEs), increase as renal function deteriorates. Other uremic retention solutes, such as asymmetric dimethylarginine (ADMA), homocysteine, guanidine, indoxyl sulfate, and *p*-cresol, which accumulate in CKD, may have proatherogenic properties.[17] Finally, the kidneys produce substances that may inhibit CVD and atherogenesis, for example, renalase, a soluble monoamine oxidase that regulates cardiac function and blood pressure.[18]

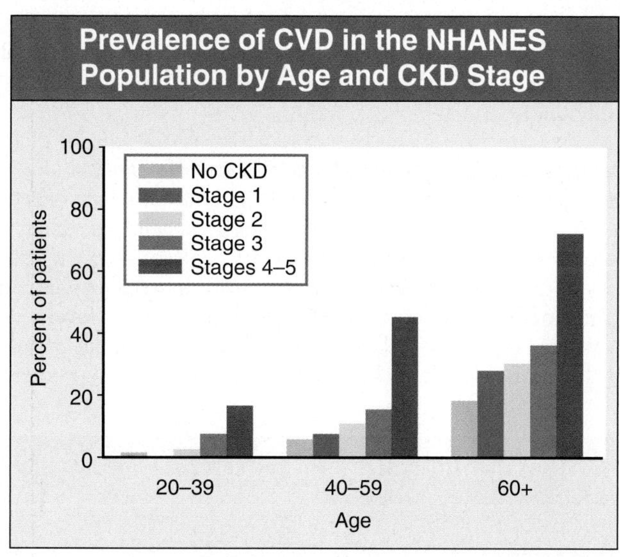

Figure 78.6 Prevalence of CVD in the NHANES population, by age and CKD stage. *(U.S. Renal Data System. USRDS 2008 Annual Data Report: Atlas of Chronic Kidney Disease and End-Stage Renal Disease in the United States. Bethesda, Md, National Institutes of Health, National Institute of Diabetes and Digestive and Kidney Diseases, 2008.)*

Oxidative Stress

Oxidative stress may be implicated in the pathogenesis of atherosclerosis and the increased risk of atherosclerotic cardiovascular events and in other CKD complications, such as protein-energy wasting and anemia.[19] Increased production of reactive oxygen species in the vascular wall is a characteristic feature of atherosclerosis.[19] Early CKD (stage 3), and in particular uremia, is a pro-oxidant state resulting from reduced antioxidant systems (vitamin C and selenium deficiency, reduced intracellular vitamin E levels, reduced glutathione system activity) and increased pro-oxidant activity associated with advanced age, diabetes, chronic inflammation, retained uremic solutes, and bioincompatibility of dialysis membranes and solutions.[19] Four oxidative stress pathways can be hypothesized in CKD: carbonyl stress, nitrosative stress, chlorinated stress, and classical oxidative stress (Fig. 78.9).

Inflammation

Most dialysis patients are in a state of chronic inflammation; inflammatory biomarkers such as C-reactive protein, interleukin-6, fibrinogen, and white blood cell count are robust and independent predictors of mortality in CKD patients. Hypoalbuminemia, a biochemical factor strongly associated with systemic inflammation, is another strong outcome predictor in CKD. Whereas both dialysis-related (dialysis system bioincompatibility) and non–dialysis-related (infection, comorbidity, genetic factors, diet, renal function loss) factors may contribute to chronic inflammation, its primary causes are not always evident. As in the general population, it is unclear in CKD whether the acute-phase response only reflects established atherosclerotic disease or is involved in the initiation and progression of atherosclerosis. Some inflammatory biomarkers, such as interleukin-6, pentraxin 3, and tumor necrosis factor α, may have

Lipid Abnormalities in Renal Disease

	Cholesterol Levels			
Stage of Renal Disease	Total	High-Density Lipoproteins	Low-Density Lipoproteins	Triglycerides
Nephrotic syndrome	↑↑↑	↓	↑↑	↑
Chronic kidney disease	→	↓	→*	↑↑
Hemodialysis	→	↓	→*	↑↑
Peritoneal dialysis	↑	↓	↑	↑
Transplantation	↑↑	→	↑	↑

Figure 78.7 Lipid abnormalities in renal disease. Common patterns of hyperlipidemia in different stages of renal disease. *Composition altered.

proatherogenic properties, such as promoting vascular calcification, oxidative stress, and endothelial dysfunction (Fig. 78.10). Evidence also suggests associations between inflammation and development of albuminuria. The link between septicemia and subsequent increased risk of death and cardiovascular events, including AMI, in observational studies further supports inflammation as a trigger for cardiovascular events.[20]

Endothelial Dysfunction

As in other clinical disorders characterized by a high burden of vascular disease, endothelial dysfunction (as evaluated by impaired endothelium-dependent vasodilation) is a prominent feature of CKD. Reasons include inflammation, ADMA retention, oxidative stress, hyperhomocysteinemia, dyslipidemia, hyperglycemia, and hypertension. Surrogate markers of endothelial dysfunction, such as ADMA, pentraxin 3, and adhesion molecules, independently predict death.[21] Detached circulating endothelial cells serve as potential markers of endothelial damage in renal and nonrenal patients and have prognostic value in hemodialysis patients.[21] Normally, in response to ischemic insult and cytokine stimulation, endothelial progenitor cells are mobilized from the bone marrow to act as "repair" cells for the endothelial injury. As CKD patients seem to have reduced numbers or functional impairment of endothelial progenitor cells due to inflammation or uremic toxins, they seem predisposed to endothelial dysfunction. Recent data support an independent association between circulating fibroblast growth factor 23 (FGF-23) and endothelial dysfunction,[22] and future studies are required to validate whether FGF-23 is a modifiable cardiovascular risk factor.

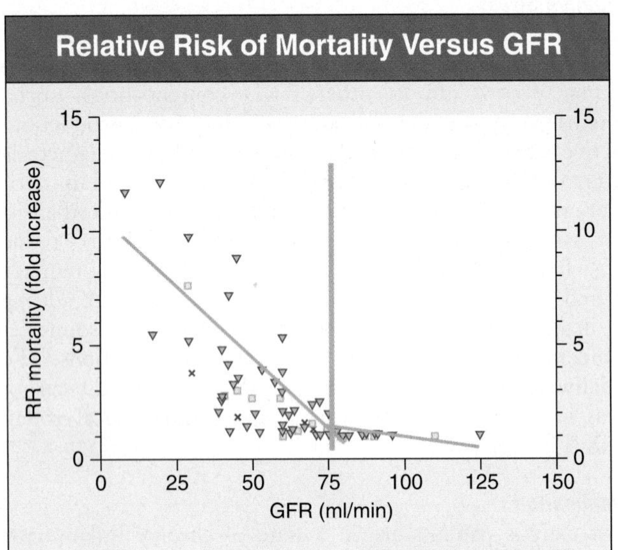

Figure 78.8 Relative risk for mortality (RR mortality) versus GFR. The majority of studies used the Cockroft and Gault formulae to estimate clearance (triangles). Studies using the MDRD formula are indicated by the squares and unadjusted studies by the crosses.

Anemia

Anemia is a major cause of LVH and left ventricular dilation in CKD. Although partial correction of anemia with ESAs results in LVH regression, current information does not suggest any cardiovascular outcome benefit of normalized hemoglobin (see Chapter 79).

Secondary Hyperparathyroidism and Mineral Metabolism

Disturbances of calcium and phosphate metabolism starting as early as CKD stages 3 and 4 might accelerate calcifying atherosclerosis and arteriosclerosis. In registry data, a strong independent mortality risk is predicted by hyperphosphatemia, an intermediate risk by elevated serum calcium levels, and a weak but significant risk by high or low serum intact parathyroid hormone levels. The overall mortality risk prediction

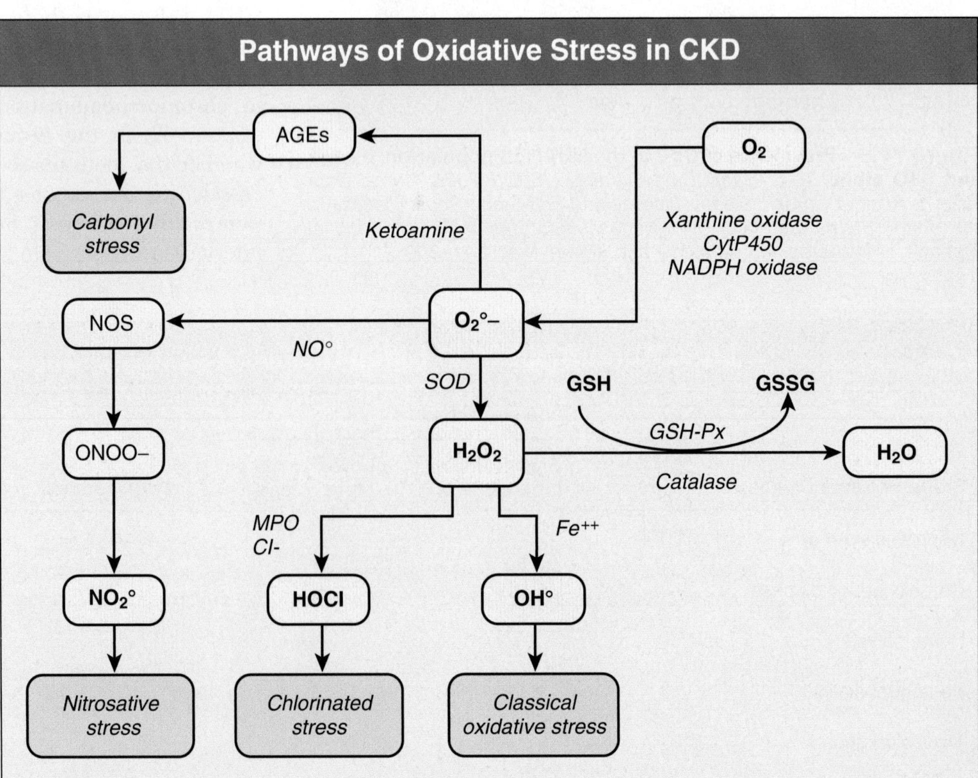

Figure 78.9 Pathways of oxidative stress in CKD. MPO, myeloperoxidase; SOD, superoxide dismutase; AGEs, advanced glycation end products; GSH, gluthathione; GSH-Px, glutathione peroxidase; GSSG, glutathione disulfide; NOS, nitric oxide synthase, NO, nitric oxide, HOCL, hypochlorous acid, OH, hydroxyl radical

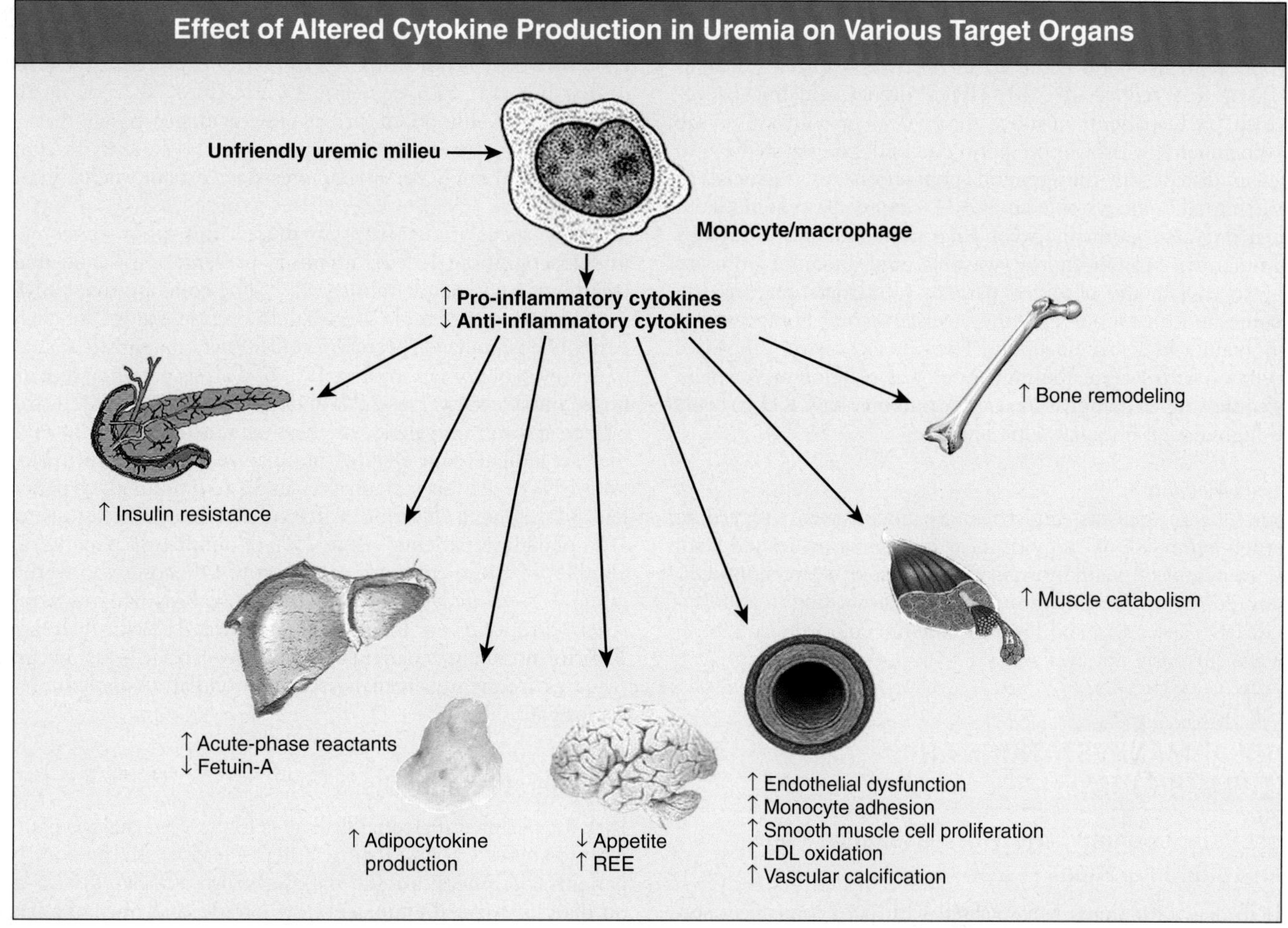

Figure 78.10 Potential mechanisms by which elevated circulating levels of proinflammatory and anti-inflammatory cytokines may promote accelerated atherosclerosis, other uremic complications, and wasting. LDL, low-density lipoprotein; REE, resting energy expenditure. *(From reference 17).*

attributable to mineral metabolism disorders is estimated to be about 17% in hemodialysis patients.[23]

Cardiovascular Calcification

Cardiovascular calcification may affect the arterial media, atherosclerotic plaques, myocardium, and heart valves. Medial calcification causes arterial stiffness and, consequently, increased pulse pressure. The pathophysiologic role of plaque calcification is less clear because soft plaques are assumed to rupture and to cause AMI; atherosclerotic calcification is a potent risk marker of cardiovascular events, but its utility as a risk marker for clinical management of CKD patients remains controversial. Valvular calcification mostly affects the aortic and mitral (annulus) valves in dialysis patients and contributes to progressive stenosis and associated morbidity; mitral annular calcification is associated with increased mortality.[24] In dialysis patients, extensive vascular, especially coronary artery, calcification can be observed at young ages. Calcium and phosphate metabolism disturbance is an important factor in cardiovascular calcification in ESRD. Serum phosphate level of 5.0 mg/dl or higher (≥1.62 mmol/l) is associated with increased risk for valvular heart surgery in hemodialysis patients.[25] Calciphylaxis (calcific uremic arteriolopathy), characterized by severe calcifications of cutaneous arterioles and tissue necrosis, is discussed in Chapter 84.

Vascular calcification is not derived only from passive calcium and phosphate precipitation. Rather, it is a highly regulated active process involving differentiation of vascular smooth muscle cells toward osteoblasts induced by phosphate, calcium, and other factors, such as calcitriol and pro-inflammatory. One way by which chronic inflammation promotes vascular calcification may involve downregulation of fetuin-A, the most potent circulating inhibitor of extraosseous calcification. In cross-sectional studies, dialysis patients with low serum fetuin-A levels showed significantly poorer survival than did those with normal values.[26] Apart from fetuin-A, other inhibitors probably counteract unwanted calcification. Leptin, matrix GLA protein, pyrophosphates, bone morphogenic proteins (e.g., BMP-2 and BMP-7), and osteoprotegerin may be related to accelerated vascular calcification in ESRD.

Advanced Glycation End Products

AGEs accumulate in CKD patients as a result of nonenzymatic glycation, oxidative stress, and diminished clearance of AGE precursors. Stable AGE residues of long-lived proteins are biomarkers of cumulative metabolic, inflammatory, and oxidative stress; carbonyl stress is speculated to contribute to tissue aging and long-term CKD complications. Whether AGE inhibition may be a useful intervention to reduce cardiovascular events and mortality is unknown.

Hyperhomocysteinemia

Homocysteine is a nonprotein sulfur-containing amino acid that may be protein bound (70% to 80%), free oxidized (20% to 30%), or free reduced (~1%). Hyperhomocysteinemia prevalence in CKD patients is more than 90%. In contrast to the well-documented association between total homocysteine and vascular disease in the general population, the association between total homocysteine and CVD is not consistent in CKD. The strong associations between total homocysteine and hypoalbuminemia, protein-energy wasting, and inflammation are likely to explain the observed paradoxical association between outcome and total homocysteine levels. As total homocysteine exists mainly in a protein-bound form, it has a strong positive correlation with serum albumin, and this association may explain why some studies demonstrate better outcome in CKD patients with higher total homocysteine levels.

Dialysis Modality

Reports from dialysis registries are inconsistent regarding whether hemodialysis or peritoneal dialysis is associated with better outcomes.[27] Valid mortality comparisons between modalities would require stratification of patients according to underlying ESRD cause, age, and level of baseline comorbidity.[27] Such data are currently not available.

CLINICAL MANIFESTATIONS AND NATURAL HISTORY

Chest Pain, Coronary Artery Disease, and Acute Myocardial Infarction

AMI in dialysis patients is associated with poor long-term survival. The unadjusted 73% 2-year mortality rate (Fig. 78.11) has changed minimally during 25 years, despite dramatic improvements in AMI outcomes in the general population. This heightened mortality is not restricted to ESRD patients, as in-hospital deaths increase with decreasing GFR (Fig. 78.12).[29] Furthermore, the likelihood of prescribing evidence-based therapies including aspirin and β-blockers in CKD patients is diminished,[29,30] although these therapies decrease mortality in such patients.

Prior speculations have attributed this poor outcome to underrecognition due to "atypical" presentations[30] and undertreatment (therapeutic nihilism).[30,31] The collaborative USRDS/National Registry of Myocardial Infarction study[31] of dialysis patients hospitalized for AMI found a lower diagnostic suspicion of acute coronary syndromes; 45% of dialysis patients were diagnosed incorrectly versus 21% of nondialysis patients. This partly reflects a lower prevalence of chest pain, experienced by 44% of dialysis patients and 68% of nondialysis patients. Surprisingly, only 19% of dialysis patients (versus 36% of nondialysis patients) had ST-segment elevation. After other clinical exclusions, only 10% of dialysis patients, versus 25% of nondialysis patients, were eligible for acute coronary reperfusion. Of those who were eligible, 47% of dialysis and 75% of nondialysis patients actually received reperfusion. In-hospital death was 21% for dialysis and 12% for nondialysis patients. In-hospital cardiac arrest occurred twice as frequently in dialysis as in nondialysis patients (11% versus 5%).

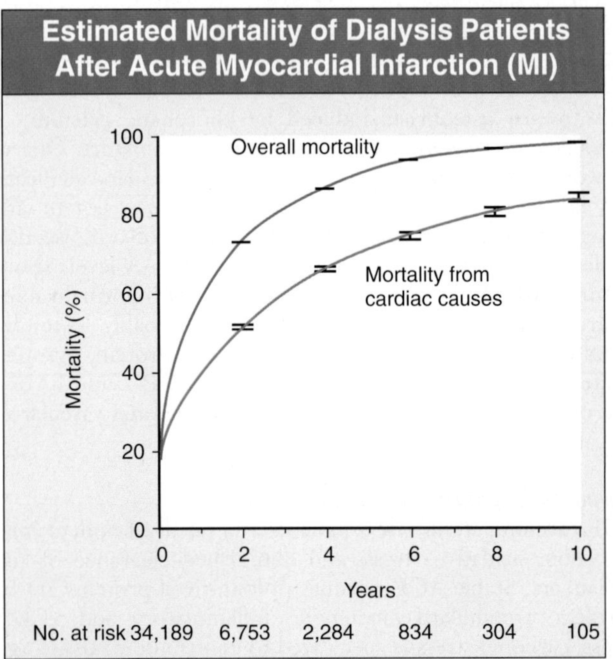

Figure 78.11 Estimated mortality of dialysis patients after acute myocardial infarction. *(Reprinted with permission from reference 28. © 2003 American Society of Nephrology.)*

Peripheral Arterial Disease

Risk for peripheral arterial disease is highest for dialysis patients with diabetes or preexisting atherosclerosis. In hemodialysis patients, peripheral arterial disease is also associated with time on dialysis, hypoalbuminemia, low parathyroid hormone levels, and low predialysis diastolic blood pressure. Vascular medial calcification of large peripheral arteries may not indicate presence of occlusive disease, and peripheral gangrene is often caused by diabetic or other small-vessel disease or rarely by calcific uremic arteriolopathy (see Chapter 84). Peripheral arterial disease is associated with increased mortality; outcomes after revascularization are worse than for the general population,[32] in part reflecting advanced vasculopathy.

Cerebrovascular Disease

Cognitive impairment is underrecognized in dialysis patients; in one study, more than a third of patients showed severe cognitive impairment and only 15% normal cognition.[33] Cognitive impairment prevalence increases approximately 10% per 10 ml/min per 1.73 m^2 of eGFR less than 60 ml/min per 1.73 m^2.[34] Microalbuminuria and stage 3 CKD increased stroke risk 1.5- to 2-fold in a multivariate model.[35,36] Incident dialysis patients have a sixfold age-adjusted relative risk of stroke compared with the general population; the unadjusted rate for stroke hospitalization for dialysis patients was 48 per 1000 patient-years, and 10.6% were attributed to hemorrhagic stroke.[37] Stroke accounts for 4% of ESRD deaths in the USRDS registry (see Chapter 82 for more details).[1]

Left Ventricular Remodeling and Hypertrophy

LVH is a potent predictor of mortality in ESRD patients. LVH is associated with a 60% increased risk of sudden death and a more than twofold increased risk of stroke.[38] LVH occurs early

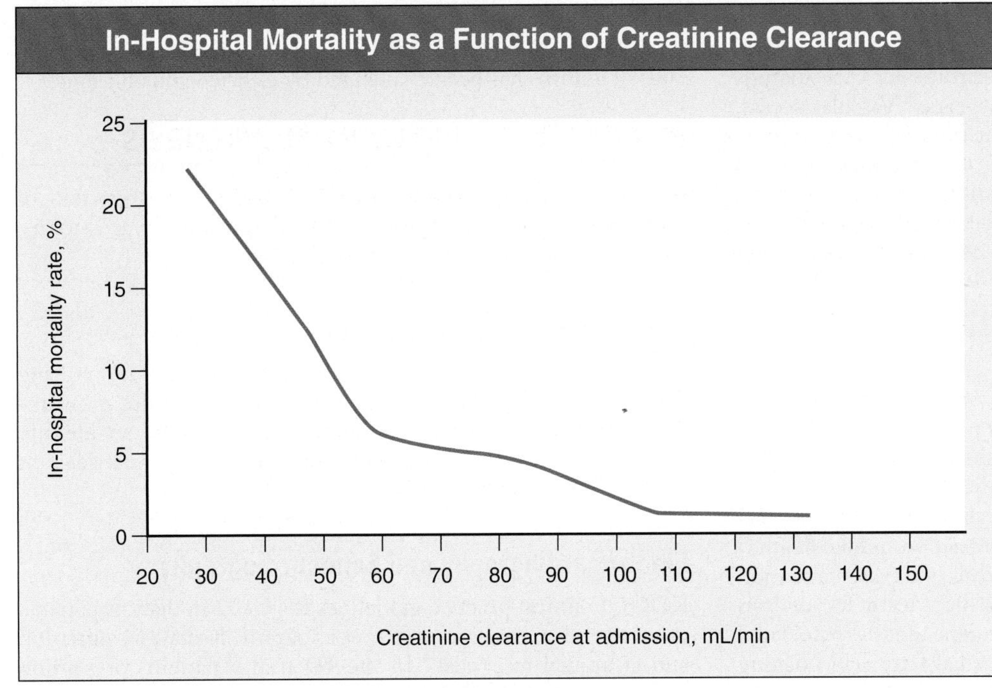

Figure 78.12 In-hospital mortality as a function of creatinine clearance. *(Reprinted with permission from reference 29. © 2003 American Society of Nephrology.)*

in progressive CKD, probably because of high hypertension prevalence, including frequent nocturnal hypertension. Pressure overload, caused by hypertension and arterial stiffness, results in concentric hypertrophy. Volume overload is manifested as "eccentric" hypertrophy. Left ventricular dilation strongly predicts poor outcome. It may be an end result of severe LVH, diffuse ischemic damage, or recurrent volume overload; high-output arteriovenous fistula may contribute. Diastolic dysfunction is strongly associated with LVH and with increased risk for intradialytic hypotension because relatively small reductions in left atrial filling have significant effects on cardiac output in these stiff, hypertrophied preload-sensitive hearts, together with Bezold-Jarisch reflex activation through stimulation of left ventricular posterior wall stretch receptors in "underfilled," hypercontractile, hypertrophied ventricles.

Extracellular Volume Overload

Extracellular volume overload resulting from loss of sodium excretory capacity is the major cause of hypertension in dialysis patients. Whether prevention of recurrent hypervolemia reduces cardiovascular morbidity and mortality remains unproved. If adjusted for comorbidity and advanced age, a strong, incremental risk of all-cause and cardiovascular mortality is associated with interdialytic weight gains.[39] Recurrent hypervolemia may result in LVH and left ventricular dilation, peripheral or pulmonary edema, raised jugular vein pulse, or a third heart sound, or it may be largely asymptomatic. Tolerance of large ultrafiltration volumes may indicate that the dry weight target (see Chapter 90) has not been reached. Reaching an optimal dry weight, however, does not necessarily lead to immediate blood pressure correction; a lag phase of some weeks can precede improvement.

Pericarditis

Pericarditis from untreated uremia is rare today. The more common dialysis-associated pericarditis may be related to intercurrent illnesses (including viral infections), fistula recirculation, or underlying diseases such as systemic lupus erythematosus, but the exact pathogenesis remains obscure. Fever with pericardial pain or a rub on heart auscultation, unexplained cardiomegaly on chest films, or hemodynamic instability should prompt echocardiography. An effusion causing overt hemodynamic compromise (i.e., pericardial tamponade) or large pericardial effusions judged unlikely to resolve with conservative measures require echocardiographically or computed tomography (CT)–guided pericardiocentesis or surgical drainage. Intensive dialysis is indicated for "true" uremic pericarditis; the optimal treatment of "dialysis-associated" pericarditis is much less clear in patients without hemodynamic compromise.[40] Aggressive anticoagulation should be avoided because of increased (but not well defined) risk for development of hemorrhagic pericarditis and pericardial tamponade.

Autonomic Dysfunction

CKD involves decreased baroreflex sensitivity, which has been linked to increased risk of sudden death.[41] Increased sympathetic nerve activity, including secondary to sleep apnea, is a common alteration in CKD patients and associated with adverse outcome.[42]

Valvular Disease

The calcific aortic stenosis progression rate is approximately three times faster in dialysis patients than in the general population (0.23 versus 0.05 to 0.1 cm^2 per year).[43] Annual Doppler echocardiographic follow-up is recommended for asymptomatic dialysis patients who are suitable candidates for cardiac surgery with aortic valve area of 1.0 cm^2 or less.[44] A USRDS study of 5825 dialysis patients undergoing valvular replacement surgery found no difference in survival for patients receiving tissue versus nontissue valves.[45] The overall mortality is high, with in-hospital mortality about 20% and 2-year survival 40%.

Infective Endocarditis

Estimated incidence of infective endocarditis in U.S. dialysis patients is 267 cases per 100,000 patient-years.[46] Vascular access, including temporary and semipermanent catheters, is an important source of infection; heightened risk of bacteremia related to hemodialysis therapy is likely an important aspect of endocarditis risk. Dialysis patients with bacterial endocarditis have poor long-term survival. In-hospital mortality was 24% and 1-year survival only 38% for patients hospitalized in 1997-2000.[47]

Sudden Cardiac Arrest

In the USRDS database, 60% to 65% of cardiac deaths (25% to 27% of all-cause mortality) in dialysis patients are attributable to arrhythmic mechanisms.[1] Although obstructive CAD is likely to be an important cause of sudden cardiac death, it is probably not the major one (unlike in the general population). The 4D study found that statin therapy had no impact on sudden death,[48] and a USRDS study found that coronary revascularization does not nullify the risk of sudden cardiac death for dialysis patients.[49] Sudden cardiac death is independently associated with inflammatory biomarkers.[50] Myocardial fatty acid imaging might identify patients at risk for sudden death.[51] Factors probably contributing to the special vulnerability of ESRD patients to sudden cardiac arrest include LVH; rapid electrolyte shifts and hyperkalemia in hemodialysis; autonomic dysfunction and sympathetic overactivity, including sleep apnea; and abnormalities in myocardial ultrastructure and function, including endothelial dysfunction, interstitial fibrosis, decreased perfusion reserve, and diminished ischemia tolerance.[30,52] Sudden death may be attributable to the rapid electrolyte shifts that occur in hemodialysis, particularly because risk of death increases by 50% on the day after dialysis[53]; however, although the rate of cardiac arrest is 50% higher for hemodialysis than for peritoneal dialysis patients 3 months after initiation of renal replacement therapy, it is higher for peritoneal dialysis patients at 3 years.[54] One study of cardiac arrests occurring in hemodialysis centers found that the predominant rhythm was ventricular fibrillation (66%), followed by pulseless electrical activity (23%) and asystole (10%).[55]

Non–dialysis-dependent CKD is also associated with increased risk of sudden cardiac death. In women with coronary heart disease in the Heart and Estrogen Replacement Study, eGFR below 40 ml/min per 1.73 m^2 was associated with a 2.3-fold increased risk of sudden cardiac death. Despite a graded, incremental risk of arrhythmic death and impaired renal function, the overall magnitude of risk in stage 3 CKD patients is small compared with dialysis patients.

The role that implantable cardioverter-defibrillators (ICDs) may play in reducing mortality in CKD patients is controversial, particularly regarding "primary prevention" of sudden death in patients with left ventricular ejection fraction of 35% or lower (comparable general population patients receive ICDs under current U.S. implant guidelines). CKD may attenuate the survival advantage of ICDs for primary prevention of sudden cardiac death,[56,57] but older age and medical comorbidity should not routinely exclude patients from receiving ICDs. Nevertheless, ICDs were underused in dialysis patients who survived cardiac arrest in 1996-2001, and ICD implantation was associated with a 42% reduction in long-term mortality.[58]

The reported rate of cardiac arrest in hemodialysis centers is 3.8 to 7.1 events per 100,000 dialysis sessions.[55,59,60] On-site defibrillation capability (preferably with automatic external defibrillators) was recommended as a U.S. practice guideline in 2005,[44] but this has been challenged by Lehrich and colleagues.[59]

DIAGNOSIS AND DIFFERENTIAL DIAGNOSIS

Key issues in the diagnosis of CVD are underrecognition of symptoms, underuse of appropriate diagnostic investigations, and interpretation of those investigations.

Blood Pressure Measurements

Outcome prediction by ambulatory blood pressure monitoring is not necessarily better than by office blood pressure measurements. However, ambulatory monitoring is useful to identify high-risk nondippers and inverted dippers, allowing consequent treatment adjustments.

Electrocardiography and Echocardiography

KDOQI clinical practice guidelines for CVD in dialysis patients recommend a baseline electrocardiogram at dialysis initiation and at annual intervals.[44] In the 4D trial,[38] patients presenting without sinus rhythm (11% of the cohort) were 89% more likely to die (based on multivariate analysis) and 164% more likely to sustain a stroke. In the Cardiovascular Health Study, CKD patients (eGFR <60 ml/min per 1.73 m^2) with increased QRS duration had 15% greater risk of incident CHF, 13% greater risk of incident coronary heart disease, and 17% greater risk of mortality per 10-millisecond increase; prolongation of the QT interval was also independently associated with adverse outcome.[61]

KDOQI guidelines recommend routine echocardiograms in all dialysis patients after they achieve "dry weight" targets, preferably 1 to 3 months after dialysis initiation on an interdialytic day for hemodialysis patients and at 3-year intervals thereafter.[44] The rationale for this guideline is that diminished left ventricular systolic function is independently associated with incident CHF, recurrent CHF, incident ischemic heart disease, and increased mortality,[44] and it is not accurately diagnosed by history, physical examination, or chest radiography. Detection of unsuspected cardiomyopathy is also important, given that carvedilol therapy in such patients improved left ventricular systolic function, decreased hospitalization, and reduced mortality.[62] As in the general population, CKD patients with a left ventricular ejection fraction below 40% should be evaluated for CAD (exceptions are pediatric or young adult patients with nondiabetic renal failure and other patients known to be at low risk for CAD).

Stress Tests and Screening Renal Transplant Candidates

ESRD patients are poorly suited for conventional exercise stress electrocardiography because of limited exercise tolerance and frequent resting electrocardiographic abnormalities. Accuracies of pharmacologic stress echocardiographic and nuclear scintigraphic techniques are remarkably variable over the world; they clearly are operator dependent, and the approach of individual sites to cardiac screening should rely on institutional expertise. Moreover, prediction of the likelihood of future events may differ considerably from prediction of coronary anatomy. In severe CKD, dobutamine stress echocardiography is an independent predictor of long-term mortality.[63] Sensitivities and

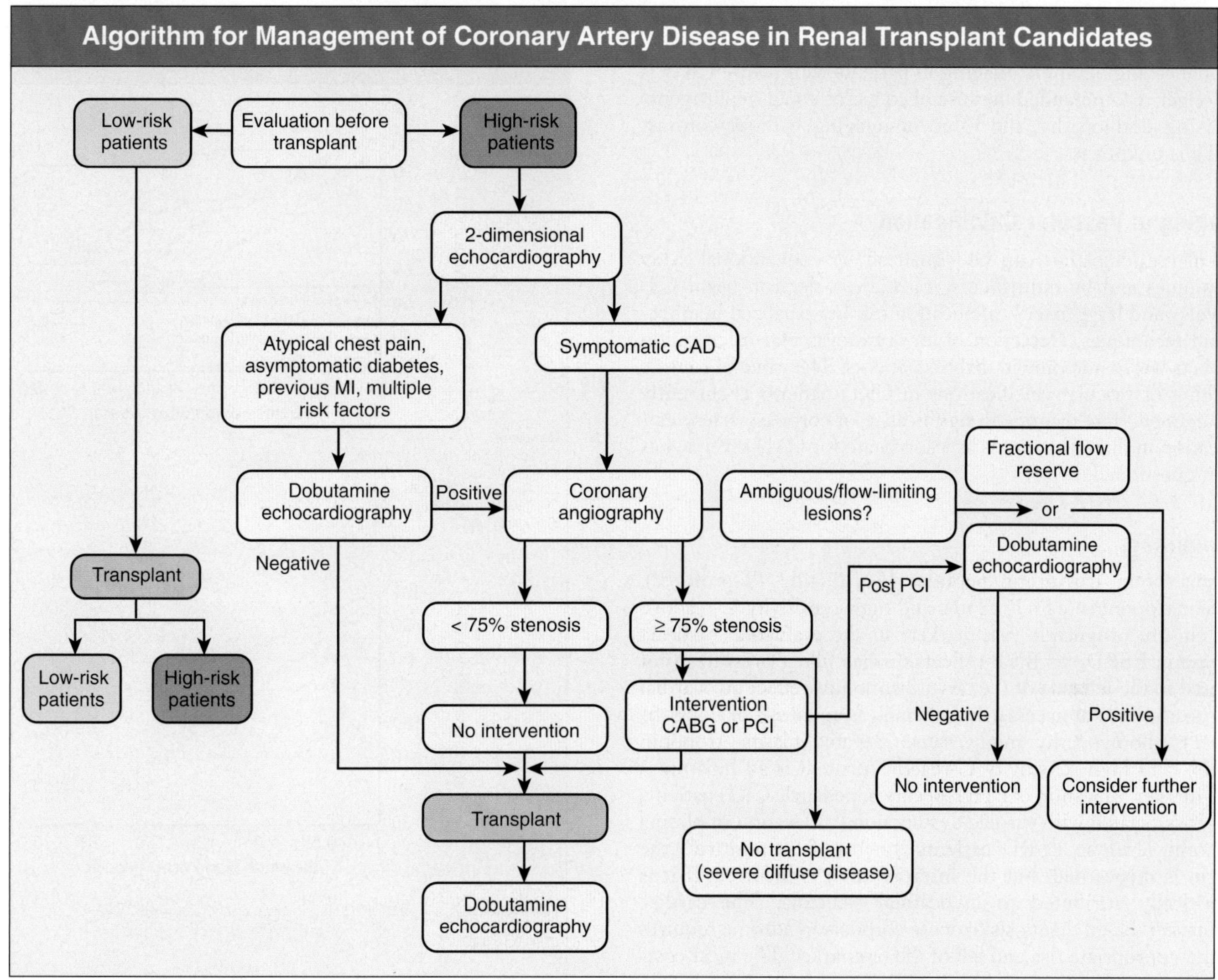

Figure 78.13 Algorithm for management of coronary artery disease in renal transplant candidates. CABG, coronary artery bypass graft surgery; CAD, coronary artery disease; MI, myocardial infarction; PCI, percutaneous coronary intervention. *(Modified from reference 64.)*

specificities for detection of CAD in renal transplant candidates have been reported to range from 44%[65] to 75%[66] and up to 90%.[67] A meta-analysis[68] concluded that presence of inducible myocardial ischemia by any stress imaging test is independently predictive of increased AMI risk and cardiac death, whereas a fixed or resting defect or abnormality is predictive of cardiac death but not AMI.

The major problem with "screening" is use of test results for clinical management. The evidence base for "prophylactic" revascularization of asymptomatic renal transplant candidates (or any other patient group) is weak[30]; optimal medical therapy (which should constitute the treatment strategy for all patients) may potentially attenuate the putative benefit of prophylactic coronary revascularization. In our institution, we use the algorithm presented in Figure 78.13 for screening and management of CAD in renal transplant candidates. All patients undergo resting echocardiography, and high-risk patients (most of our ESRD patients) undergo stress echocardiography. For patients subsequently found to have angiographically indeterminate lesions, measurement of fractional flow reserve is used to make decisions about revascularization.[69]

Coronary Angiography

Coronary angiography, the gold standard in evaluating CAD in CKD, should be considered in stable ESRD patients with evidence for inducible myocardial ischemia, unstable patients with acute coronary syndrome (performed urgently for ST-segment elevation myocardial infarction), and patients with a left ventricular ejection fraction below 40%. Some reports suggest a predilection for more proximal CAD in CKD patients, which may predict worse outcome.[70,71]

In CKD and ESRD with residual renal function, fear of contrast nephropathy may restrain use of coronary angiography (see Chapter 69 for preventive measures). Echocardiography should be performed before any nonemergent coronary angiography in CKD patients to diagnose clinically unsuspected valvular disease or cardiomyopathy, to gauge preprocedure volume status, and to assess left ventricular function (to avoid excessive exposure to radiocontrast media through unwarranted ventriculography).

Noninvasive coronary CT angiography may be problematic in dialysis patients because of medial calcification interfering with angiographic interpretation. Another problem may be the requirement for a large-bore intravenous line for rapid injection of radiocontrast media. Noninvasive gadolinium-based magnetic resonance angiographic imaging in patients with severe CKD is no longer recommended because of concerns about nephrogenic fibrosing dermopathy; the value of imaging without contrast media is unknown.

Imaging of Vascular Calcification

Vascular calcification can be visualized by conventional x-ray techniques and by multislice spiral CT or electron-beam CT. Valvular and large artery calcification can be visualized by ultrasound techniques. Detection of any cardiovascular calcification predicts worse outcome in dialysis patients. The value of routine imaging of vascular calcifications in CKD patients is currently not defined. The diagnostic significance of coronary artery calcification in dialysis patients as a surrogate for CAD severity has been questioned.[72]

Biomarkers

Plasma brain natriuretic peptides (BNP and NT-proBNP), cardiac troponins (cTnT, cTnI), and high-sensitivity C-reactive protein are prognostic risk markers in the evaluation of heart disease in ESRD.[73-75] BNP reflects cardiac filling pressures (not limited to the left side of the heart), troponins reflect myocardial cell death (but not necessarily ischemia, as apoptosis or nonischemic cardiomyopathy might cause elevated plasma troponin levels), and high-sensitivity C-reactive protein is an inflammatory marker. Elevation of cTnT occurs in pediatric CKD patients and is associated with cardiac dysfunction.[76] Elevation of plasma troponin levels in ESRD patients is *not* a "false positive"; the origin is myocardial, but the interpretation is incorrect if it is uncritically attributed to myocardial ischemia. The cardiac biomarker–based diagnosis of acute coronary syndrome requires a time-appropriate rise and fall of the biomarker. The most cost-effective combination of biomarkers for risk stratification in dialysis patients might be cTnT and high-sensitivity C-reactive protein, but this is controversial. In asymptomatic non–dialysis-dependent CKD patients, plasma cTnT and cTnI were elevated in at least a third of patients, but only cTnT was predictive of death.[77] In CKD, NT-proBNP and BNP are equivalent predictors of decompensated heart failure, but NT-proBNP is a better predictor of survival.[78] Figure 78.14 graphically displays the relationship of cTnT and cTnI levels in asymptomatic dialysis patients and long-term survival. On the basis of these data, the U.S. Food and Drug Administration approved the measurement of cTnT in dialysis patients for the indication of risk stratification (mortality prediction) in 2004[44]; however, utility of the information in clinical practice remains unclear.

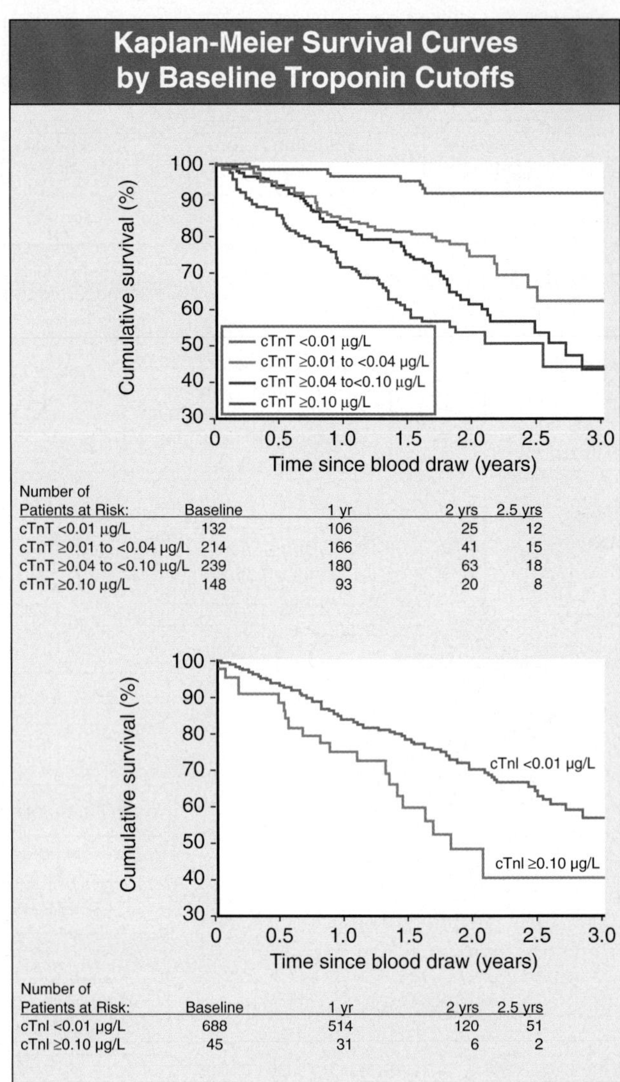

Figure 78.14 Kaplan-Meier survival curves by baseline troponin cutoffs. cTnT, cardiac troponin T; cTnI, cardiac troponin I. *(From reference 73.)*

TREATMENT AND PREVENTION OF CARDIOVASCULAR DISEASE

Risk Factor Reduction

Smoking

It is clearly imperative to strongly encourage smoking cessation at any CKD stage.

Weight and Diet

Lifestyle changes, including balanced diets with regard to saturated fat and carbohydrates (in diabetic patients), probably reduce cardiovascular morbidity and should be encouraged. However, in all CKD stages, protein energy wasting must be avoided; especially in dialysis patients, increased body mass index has been associated with improved outcomes in the United States,[79] possibly reflecting confounded epidemiology. Correction of obesity should be encouraged. Low-salt diet and phosphate restriction are discussed in Chapter 83.

Hypertension and Coronary Artery Disease

Arterial hypertension is undertreated in many CKD and ESRD patients, and despite controversial data about the risk prediction by diastolic and systolic blood pressure in dialysis patients, antihypertensive treatment is associated with improved survival. Blood pressure targets for CKD patients, in particular those with diabetes or proteinuria exceeding 1 g/day, are discussed in Chapter 76. Hallmarks of therapy are volume control (see Chapter 90) and prevention of salt overload, particularly through dietary sodium restriction. Longer or more frequent hemodialysis sessions may be beneficial in controlling hypertension. Because of their parallel cardioprotective effects, angiotensin-converting enzyme (ACE) inhibitors, angiotensin receptor blockers (ARBs), and vasodilating ß-blockers (e.g., carvedilol) are the first-line drugs to treat CKD- and ESRD-related hypertension. Calcium channel blockers and most other antihypertensive drugs, including centrally acting sympathetic inhibitors, are useful when administered complementarily. Pure vasodilators (e.g., minoxidil) must be used with caution because they may increase volume overload or occasionally cause pericardial effusions.

CAD and CAD-related events should be treated with the same medications and active interventions indicated in the nonrenal population in the absence of convincing CKD-specific data to the contrary. Medical treatment includes use of antiplatelet agents, ACE inhibitors, ARBs, β-blockers, nitroglycerin, and statins. There is no rationale for a less aggressive therapeutic approach for CKD and ESRD patients than for the nonrenal population.

Diabetes Mellitus

Optimal glycemic control, reaching blood pressure target levels, and lipid monitoring (with subsequent dyslipidemia treatment) are all crucial in managing diabetic CKD patients. CAD and other CVD should be treated aggressively in this high-risk group.

Dyslipidemia

If CKD (like diabetes) is considered a "CHD equivalent," CKD patients should be treated to secondary prevention LDL cholesterol target guidelines (<100 mg/dl or 2.6 mmol/l). However, this contention is currently unsupported by clinical trials targeting CKD patients, notably the 4D trial of atorvastatin in type 2 diabetic dialysis patients.[48] The AURORA study[80] found that rosuvastatin failed to reduce time to cardiovascular death, nonfatal AMI, or stroke in hemodialysis patients. *Post hoc* subgroup analyses in the Heart Protection Study,[81] Cholesterol and Recurring Events study,[82] and Treating to New Targets study,[83] together with a meta-analysis,[84] provide inferential support for the role of statins in improving outcomes in CKD stage 1 or 2 patients. The Study of Heart and Renal Protection (SHARP) testing the effect of lipid lowering in CKD stage 3 and stage 4 patients is ongoing. Statin treatment is recommended in CKD patients older than 20 years with goals of LDL cholesterol levels above 130 mg/dl (3.4 mmol/l) or above 100 mg/dl (2.6 mmol/l) for secondary prevention; however, the negative 4D and AURORA results do not support this guideline in dialysis patients.

Volume

In predialysis CKD, sodium restriction and diuretics are important to counteract fluid retention. In ESRD, longer and more frequent hemodialysis sessions may permit more effective volume control. In the hemodialysis center in Tassin, France, more than 90% of patients were normotensive with 8 hours of dialysis three times per week, with dietary salt restriction and no antihypertensive drugs. Episodes of dialysis-related hypotension should prompt re-evaluation of dry weight, antihypertensive treatment, and exclusion of pericardial effusions, valvular disease, cardiomyopathy, or silent myocardial ischemia (see Chapter 91).

Anemia

Partial correction of severe anemia with ESAs results in regression of LVH. Treatment of severe anemia is also associated with fewer ischemic symptoms in CAD patients. However, evidence for reduction of cardiovascular mortality by ESAs is based on observational data only. To date, a randomized controlled trial in hemodialysis patients,[85] and the CHOIR[86] and CREATE[87] studies in CKD patients, have shown no benefit of normalized anemia (>13.5 g/dl) on mortality as a primary endpoint (see Chapter 79). Until results from the ongoing TREAT study on the effects of darbepoetin on outcome are available, anemia correction in CKD patients to a hemoglobin interval between 11 and 12 g/dl appears logical.

Inflammation

Anti-inflammatory treatment strategies, such as statins and aspirin, have beneficial effects on cardiovascular mortality in the general population, but few data are available to support that such therapies decrease inflammation in CKD patients. Recent data from the 4D study[48] show that whereas C-reactive protein baseline levels were not significantly different between treated and placebo groups and remained stable at 6 months with atorvastatin, they increased significantly in the placebo group.[88] Until data are available from such trials, careful search for infectious processes and use of biocompatible dialysis membranes and ultrapure water are recommended. Restriction of catheter use is also important; short daily dialysis with better fluid status was associated with decreasing C-reactive protein levels compared with conventional hemodialysis.[89] Volume status should be carefully monitored.

Oxidative Stress

Oxidative stress probably plays a role in mediating CVD in CKD. Two placebo-controlled interventional studies showed that vitamin E[90] and *N*-acetylcysteine[91] decreased the number of cardiovascular events in hemodialysis patients. Unfortunately, both studies were small and of limited duration. As *N*-acetylcysteine administration led to reduced atheromatous lesions in an apoE knockout model of CKD-enhanced atherosclerosis, adequately powered randomized trials with antioxidative treatment strategies are warranted.

Vascular Calcification

In the prospective Treat-to-Goal study, 200 hemodialysis patients were randomized to receive calcium-containing phosphate binders (calcium acetate or carbonate) or the calcium-free binder sevelamer.[92] For calcium binder patients, coronary and aortic calcification progressed during the year but was halted for sevelamer-treated patients. In the subsequent Dialysis Clinical Outcomes Revisited trial, sevelamer versus calcium-based phosphate binder therapy did not reduce mortality.[93] As vitamin D treatment is associated with improved survival in dialysis patients,[94] vitamin D insufficiency should also be considered. KDOQI and KDIGO targets for parathyroid hormone, calcium, and phosphate are discussed in Chapter 81.

Hyperhomocysteinemia

Despite suggestive epidemiologic data linking hyperhomocysteinemia to adverse outcomes, to date, all randomized clinical trials on homocysteine lowering with use of folic acid or multivitamin supplementation have shown no benefit in the general population or in CKD patients.[95]

Revascularization

There is a strong inverse relationship between renal function and survival after percutaneous coronary intervention (PCI)[96] and coronary artery bypass graft surgery (CABG).[97] Coronary revascularization complicated by acute kidney injury is associated with excess mortality; operative mortality for non-ESRD patients who require acute dialysis after cardiac surgery is 44%.[98]

Data comparing coronary revascularization with medical therapy in CKD are limited by their retrospective, observational nature; studies have not always compared revascularization with optimal medical therapy, including β-blockers. Observational studies suggest lower mortality in CKD (including dialysis) patients undergoing coronary revascularization compared with no revascularization.[99,100] A *post hoc* analysis of CKD patients in the FRISC II (Fast Revascularization During InStability in Coronary Artery Disease) trial indicated a superior outcome with an early invasive strategy in acute coronary syndrome compared with conservative management.[101]

The optimal coronary revascularization method for CKD patients remains controversial because of absence of adequate clinical trial data; the largest studies are derived from observational data, particularly the USRDS database. A *post hoc* analysis of CKD patients enrolled in the ARTS (Arterial Revascularization Therapies Study)[102] trial found similar outcomes for CABG or multivessel PCI with non–drug-eluting stents for death, myocardial infarction, or stroke; unsurprisingly, CABG was associated with less repeated revascularization. Dialysis patient survival after CABG was better than after PCI with non–drug-eluting stents,[103] but 2-year mortality was still very high at 44% (versus 52% for PCI). Preliminary data from USRDS studies indicate that drug-eluting stents provide the best 1-year survival for dialysis patients, but unadjusted long-term survival is best after CABG and increases with number of arteries bypassed and use of the internal mammary artery as a graft conduit. Because of higher periprocedural surgical mortality, short-term dialysis patient survival after PCI is better. However, for dialysis patients with four or more vessels bypassed, including use of internal mammary artery grafting, survival outcome more than 6 months after CABG is superior to drug-eluting stents. The best outcome thus depends on the length of postprocedure follow-up, and the optimal revascularization strategy may depend on particular clinical circumstance (a patient with a limited life expectancy might choose a treatment associated with less morbidity and only a short-term survival advantage). In elderly non–dialysis-dependent CKD patients, preliminary USRDS data indicate better 2-year survival with drug-eluting stents (with an 18% reduction in mortality compared with CABG).[104] In the general population, one proven advantage of drug-eluting stents (compared with non–drug-eluting stents) is lower incidence of in-stent restenosis. In dialysis patients, reliance on clinical surrogates (e.g., chest pain) for detection of restenosis can be problematic and lead to underestimation of the true incidence. The most complete angiographic follow-up of drug-eluting stents (performed in Japanese dialysis patients) noted 22% to 31% angiographically detected incidence of restenosis with drug-eluting stents and 24% to 37% with non–drug-eluting stents.[105,106] Clinically inapparent restenosis is a rationale for surveillance stress imaging to detect occult restenosis as part of our management strategy for dialysis patients undergoing PCI (see Fig. 78.13).

REFERENCES

1. U.S. Renal Data System. *USRDS 2008 Annual Data Report: Atlas of Chronic Kidney Disease and End-Stage Renal Disease in the United States.* Bethesda, Md: National Institutes of Health, National Institute of Diabetes and Digestive and Kidney Diseases; 2008.
2. Go AS, Chertow GM, Fan D, et al. Chronic kidney disease and the risks of death, cardiovascular events, and hospitalization. *N Engl J Med.* 2004;351:1296-1305.
3. Tonelli M, Wiebe N, Culleton B, et al. Chronic kidney disease and mortality risk: A systematic review. *J Am Soc Nephrol.* 2006;17:2034-2047.
4. Gerstein HC, Mann JF, Yi Q, et al. Albuminuria and risk of cardiovascular events, death, and heart failure in diabetic and nondiabetic individuals. *JAMA.* 2001;286:421-426.
5. Foley RN, Murray AM, Li S, et al. Chronic kidney disease and the risk for cardiovascular disease, renal replacement, and death in the United States Medicare population, 1998 to 1999. *J Am Soc Nephrol.* 2005;16:489-495.
6. Coca SG, Krumholz HM, Garg AX, Parikh CR. Underrepresentation of renal disease in randomized controlled trials of cardiovascular disease. *JAMA.* 2006;296:1377-1384.
7. U.S. Renal Data System. *USRDS 2007 Annual Data Report: Atlas of Chronic Kidney Disease and End-Stage Renal Disease in the United States.* Volume II. Bethesda, Md: National Institutes of Health, National Institute of Diabetes and Digestive and Kidney Diseases; 2007.
8. Banerjee D, Ma JZ, Collins AJ, Herzog CA. Long-term survival of incident hemodialysis patients who are hospitalized for congestive heart failure, pulmonary edema, or fluid overload. *Clin J Am Soc Nephrol.* 2007;2:1186-1190.
9. Muntner P, He J, Astor BC, et al. Traditional and nontraditional risk factors predict coronary heart disease in chronic kidney disease: Results from the atherosclerosis risk in communities study. *J Am Soc Nephrol.* 2005;16:529-538.
10. Weiner DE, Tighiouart H, Elsayed EF, et al. The Framingham predictive instrument in chronic kidney disease. *J Am Coll Cardiol.* 2007;50:217-224.
11. Yoshino M, Kuhlmann MK, Kotanko P, et al. International differences in dialysis mortality reflect background general population atherosclerotic cardiovascular mortality. *J Am Soc Nephrol.* 2006;17:3510-3519.
12. Kalantar-Zadeh K, Block G, Humphreys MH, Kopple JD. Reverse epidemiology of cardiovascular risk factors in maintenance dialysis patients. *Kidney Int.* 2003;63:793-808.
13. Foley RN, Herzog CA, Collins AJ. Smoking and cardiovascular outcomes in dialysis patients: The United States Renal Data System Wave 2 study. *Kidney Int.* 2003;63:1462-1467.
14. Liu Y, Coresh J, Eustace JA, et al. Association between cholesterol level and mortality in dialysis patients: Role of inflammation and malnutrition. *JAMA.* 2004;291:451-459.
15. Shinohara K, Shoji T, Emoto M, et al. Insulin resistance as an independent predictor of cardiovascular mortality in patients with end-stage renal disease. *J Am Soc Nephrol.* 2002;13:1894-1900.
16. Schwarz U, Buzello M, Ritz E, et al. Morphology of coronary atherosclerotic lesions in patients with end-stage renal failure. *Nephrol Dial Transplant.* 2000;15:218-223.
17. Vanholder R, Massy Z, Argiles A, et al. Chronic kidney disease as cause of cardiovascular morbidity and mortality. *Nephrol Dial Transplant.* 2005;20:1048-1056.
18. Xu J, Li G, Wang P, et al. Renalase is a novel, soluble monoamine oxidase that regulates cardiac function and blood pressure. *J Clin Invest.* 2005;115:1275-1280.
19. Himmelfarb J, Stenvinkel P, Ikizler TA, Hakim RM. The elephant in uremia: Oxidant stress as a unifying concept of cardiovascular disease in uremia. *Kidney Int.* 2002;62:1524-1538.
20. Ishani A, Collins AJ, Herzog CA, Foley RN. Septicemia, access and cardiovascular disease in dialysis patients: the USRDS Wave 2 study. *Kidney Int.* 2005;68:311-318.
21. Stenvinkel P, Carrero JJ, Axelsson J, et al. Emerging biomarkers for evaluating cardiovascular risk in the chronic kidney disease patient: How do new pieces fit into the uremic puzzle? *Clin J Am Soc Nephrol.* 2008;3:505-521.
22. Mirza MA, Larsson A, Lind L, Larsson TE. Circulating fibroblast growth factor-23 is associated with vascular dysfunction in the community. *Atherosclerosis.* 2009;205:385-390.
23. Block GA, Hulbert-Shearon TE, Levin NW, Port FK. Association of serum phosphorus and calcium × phosphate product with mortality risk in chronic hemodialysis patients: A national study. *Am J Kidney Dis.* 1998;31:607-617.
24. Sharma R, Pellerin D, Gaze DC, et al. Mitral annular calcification predicts mortality and coronary artery disease in end stage renal disease. *Atherosclerosis.* 2007;191:348-354.
25. Rubel JR, Milford EL. The relationship between serum calcium and phosphate levels and cardiac valvular procedures in the hemodialysis population. *Am J Kidney Dis.* 2003;41:411-421.
26. Ketteler M, Bongartz P, Westenfeld R, et al. Association of low fetuin-A (AHSG) concentrations in serum with cardiovascular mortality

in patients on dialysis: A cross-sectional study. *Lancet*. 2003;361: 827-833.
27. Vonesh EF, Snyder JJ, Foley RN, Collins AJ. The differential impact of risk factors on mortality in hemodialysis and peritoneal dialysis. *Kidney Int*. 2004;66:2389-2401.
28. Herzog CA, Ma JZ, Collins AJ. Poor long-term survival after acute myocardial infarction among patients on long-term dialysis. *N Engl J Med*. 1998;339:799-805.
29. Wright RS, Reeder GS, Herzog CA, et al. Acute myocardial infarction and renal dysfunction: A high-risk combination. *Ann Intern Med*. 2002;137:563-570.
30. Herzog CA. How to manage the renal patient with coronary heart disease: The agony and the ecstasy of opinion-based medicine. *J Am Soc Nephrol*. 2003;14:2556-2572.
31. Herzog CA, Littrell K, Arko C, et al. Clinical characteristics of dialysis patients with acute myocardial infarction in the United States: A collaborative project of the United States Renal Data System and the National Registry of Myocardial Infarction. *Circulation*. 2007;116: 1465-1472.
32. Reddan DN, Marcus RJ, Owen WF Jr, et al. Long-term outcomes of revascularization for peripheral vascular disease in end-stage renal disease patients. *Am J Kidney Dis*. 2001;38:57-63.
33. Murray AM, Tupper DE, Knopman DS, et al. Cognitive impairment in hemodialysis patients is common. *Neurology*. 2006;67:216-223.
34. Kurella Tamura M, Wadley V, Yaffe K, et al. Kidney function and cognitive impairment in US adults: The Reasons for Geographic and Racial Differences in Stroke (REGARDS) Study. *Am J Kidney Dis*. 2008;52:227-234.
35. Ovbiagele B. Impairment in glomerular filtration rate or glomerular filtration barrier and occurrence of stroke. *Arch Neurol*. 2008;65: 934-938.
36. Koren-Morag N, Goldbourt U, Tanne D. Renal dysfunction and risk of ischemic stroke or TIA in patients with cardiovascular disease. *Neurology*. 2006;67:224-228.
37. Seliger SL, Gillen DL, Longstreth WT Jr, et al. Elevated risk of stroke among patients with end-stage renal disease. *Kidney Int*. 2003;64: 603-609.
38. Krane V, Heinrich F, Meesmann M, et al. Electrocardiography and outcome in patients with diabetes mellitus on maintenance hemodialysis. *Clin J Am Soc Nephrol*. 2009;4:394-400.
39. Kalantar-Zadeh K, Regidor DL, Kovesdy CP, et al. Fluid retention is associated with cardiovascular mortality in patients undergoing long-term hemodialysis. *Circulation*. 2009;119:671-679.
40. Alpert MA, Ravenscraft MD. Pericardial involvement in end-stage renal disease. *Am J Med Sci*. 2003;325:228-236.
41. Johansson M, Gao SA, Friberg P, et al. Baroreflex effectiveness index and baroreflex sensitivity predict all-cause mortality and sudden death in hypertensive patients with chronic renal failure. *J Hypertens*. 2007;25:163-168.
42. Zoccali C, Mallamaci F, Parlongo S, et al. Plasma norepinephrine predicts survival and incident cardiovascular events in patients with end-stage renal disease. *Circulation*. 2002;105:1354-1359.
43. Ureña P, Malergue MC, Goldfarb B, et al. Evolutive aortic stenosis in hemodialysis patients: Analysis of risk factors. *Nephrologie*. 1999;20: 217-225.
44. K/DOQI clinical practice guidelines for cardiovascular disease in dialysis patients. *Am J Kidney Dis*. 2005;45(Suppl 3):S1-153.
45. Herzog CA, Ma JZ, Collins AJ. Long-term survival of dialysis patients in the United States with prosthetic heart valves: Should ACC/AHA practice guidelines on valve selection be modified? *Circulation*. 2002;105: 1336-1341.
46. Abbott KC, Agodoa LY. Hospitalizations for bacterial endocarditis after initiation of chronic dialysis in the United States. *Nephron*. 2002;91:203-209.
47. Shroff GR, Herzog CA, Ma JZ, Collins AJ. Long-term survival of dialysis patients with bacterial endocarditis in the United States. *Am J Kidney Dis*. 2004;44:1077-1082.
48. Wanner C, Krane V, Marz W, et al. Atorvastatin in patients with type 2 diabetes mellitus undergoing hemodialysis. *N Engl J Med*. 2005;353: 238-248.
49. Herzog CA, Strief JW, Collins AJ, Gilbertson DT. Cause-specific mortality of dialysis patients after coronary revascularization: Why don't dialysis patients have better survival after coronary intervention? *Nephrol Dial Transplant*. 2008;23:2629-2633.
50. Parekh RS, Plantinga LC, Kao WH, et al. The association of sudden cardiac death with inflammation and other traditional risk factors. *Kidney Int*. 2008;74:1335-1342.
51. Nishimura M, Tsukamoto K, Hasebe N, et al. Prediction of cardiac death in hemodialysis patients by myocardial fatty acid imaging. *J Am Coll Cardiol*. 2008;51:139-145.
52. Herzog CA, Mangrum JM, Passman R. Sudden cardiac death and dialysis patients. *Semin Dial*. 2008;21:300-307.
53. Bleyer AJ, Russell GB, Satko SG. Sudden and cardiac death rates in hemodialysis patients. *Kidney Int*. 1999;55:1553-1559.
54. U.S. Renal Data System. *USRDS 2006 Annual Data Report: Atlas of Chronic Kidney Disease and End-Stage Renal Disease in the United States*. Bethesda, Md: National Institutes of Health, National Institute of Diabetes and Digestive and Kidney Diseases; 2006.
55. Davis TR, Young BA, Eisenberg MS, et al. Outcome of cardiac arrests attended by emergency medical services staff at community outpatient dialysis centers. *Kidney Int*. 2008;73:933-939.
56. Cuculich PS, Sanchez JM, Kerzner R, et al. Poor prognosis for patients with chronic kidney disease despite ICD therapy for the primary prevention of sudden death. *Pacing Clin Electrophysiol*. 2007;30:207-213.
57. Amin MS, Fox AD, Kalahasty G, et al. Benefit of primary prevention implantable cardioverter-defibrillators in the setting of chronic kidney disease: A decision model analysis. *J Cardiovasc Electrophysiol*. 2008;19: 1275-1280.
58. Herzog CA, Li S, Weinhandl ED, et al. Survival of dialysis patients after cardiac arrest and the impact of implantable cardioverter defibrillators. *Kidney Int*. 2005;68:818-825.
59. Lehrich RW, Pun PH, Tanenbaum ND, et al. Automated external defibrillators and survival from cardiac arrest in the outpatient hemodialysis clinic. *J Am Soc Nephrol*. 2007;18:312-320.
60. Karnik JA, Young BS, Lew NL, et al. Cardiac arrest and sudden death in dialysis units. *Kidney Int*. 2001;60:350-357.
61. Kestenbaum B, Rudser KD, Shlipak MG, et al. Kidney function, electrocardiographic findings, and cardiovascular events among older adults. *Clin J Am Soc Nephrol*. 2007;2:501-508.
62. Cice G, Ferrara L, D'Andrea A, et al. Carvedilol increases two-year survival in dialysis patients with dilated cardiomyopathy. A prospective, placebo-controlled trial. *J Am Coll Cardiol*. 2003;41:1438-1444.
63. Bergeron S, Hillis GS, Haugen EN, et al. Prognostic value of dobutamine stress echocardiography in patients with chronic kidney disease. *Am Heart J*. 2007;153:385-391.
64. Herzog C. Acute MI in dialysis patients: How can we improve the outlook? *J Crit Illn*. 1999;14:613-621.
65. De Lima JJ, Sabbaga E, Vieira ML, et al. Coronary angiography is the best predictor of events in renal transplant candidates compared with noninvasive testing. *Hypertension*. 2003;42:263-268.
66. Herzog CA, Marwick TH, Pheley AM, et al. Dobutamine stress echocardiography for the detection of significant coronary artery disease in renal transplant candidates. *Am J Kidney Dis*. 1999;33: 1080-1090.
67. Sharma R, Pellerin D, Gaze DC, et al. Dobutamine stress echocardiography and cardiac troponin T for the detection of significant coronary artery disease and predicting outcome in renal transplant candidates. *Eur J Echocardiogr*. 2005;6:327-335.
68. Rabbat CG, Treleaven DJ, Russell JD, et al. Prognostic value of myocardial perfusion studies in patients with end-stage renal disease assessed for kidney or kidney-pancreas transplantation: A meta-analysis. *J Am Soc Nephrol*. 2003;14:431-439.
69. Tonino PA, De BB, Pijls NH, et al. Fractional flow reserve versus angiography for guiding percutaneous coronary intervention. *N Engl J Med*. 2009;360:213-224.
70. Charytan D, Kuntz RE, Mauri L, deFilippi C. Distribution of coronary artery disease and relation to mortality in asymptomatic hemodialysis patients. *Am J Kidney Dis*. 2007;49:409-416.
71. Charytan DM, Kuntz RE, Garshick M, et al. Location of acute coronary artery thromboses in patients with and without chronic kidney disease. *Kidney Int*. 2009;75:80-87.
72. Fujimoto N, Iseki K, Tokuyama K, et al. Significance of coronary artery calcification score (CACS) for the detection of coronary artery disease (CAD) in chronic dialysis patients. *Clin Chim Acta*. 2006;367: 98-102.
73. Apple FS, Murakami MM, Pearce LA, Herzog CA. Predictive value of cardiac troponin I and T for subsequent death in end-stage renal disease. *Circulation*. 2002;106:2941-2945.
74. Apple FS, Murakami MM, Pearce LA, Herzog CA. Multi-biomarker risk stratification of N-terminal pro-B-type natriuretic peptide, high-sensitivity C-reactive protein, and cardiac troponin T and I in end-stage renal disease for all-cause death. *Clin Chem*. 2004;50:2279-2285.
75. Wang AY, Lai KN. Use of cardiac biomarkers in end-stage renal disease. *J Am Soc Nephrol*. 2008;19:1643-1652.

76. Lipshultz SE, Somers MJ, Lipsitz SR, et al. Serum cardiac troponin and subclinical cardiac status in pediatric chronic renal failure. *Pediatrics*. 2003;112:79-86.
77. Lamb EJ, Kenny C, Abbas NA, et al. Cardiac troponin I concentration is commonly increased in nondialysis patients with CKD: Experience with a sensitive assay. *Am J Kidney Dis*. 2007;49:507-516.
78. deFilippi CR, Seliger SL, Maynard S, Christenson RH. Impact of renal disease on natriuretic peptide testing for diagnosing decompensated heart failure and predicting mortality. *Clin Chem*. 2007;53:1511-1519.
79. Kalantar-Zadeh K, Abbott KC, Salahudeen AK, et al. Survival advantages of obesity in dialysis patients. *Am J Clin Nutr*. 2005;81:543-554.
80. Fellström B, Jardine AG, Schmieder R, et al. Rosuvastatin and cardiovascular events in patients undergoing hemodialysis. *N Engl J Med*. 2009;360:1395-1407.
81. MRC/BHF Heart Protection Study of cholesterol lowering with simvastatin in 20,536 high-risk individuals: A randomised placebo-controlled trial. *Lancet*. 2002;360:7-22.
82. Tonelli M, Moye L, Sacks FM, et al. Pravastatin for secondary prevention of cardiovascular events in persons with mild chronic renal insufficiency. *Ann Intern Med*. 2003;138:98-104.
83. Shepherd J, Kastelein JJ, Bittner V, et al. Intensive lipid lowering with atorvastatin in patients with coronary heart disease and chronic kidney disease: the TNT (Treating to New Targets) study. *J Am Coll Cardiol*. 2008;51:1448-1454.
84. Strippoli GF, Navaneethan SD, Johnson DW, et al. Effects of statins in patients with chronic kidney disease: Meta-analysis and meta-regression of randomised controlled trials. *BMJ*. 2008;336:645-651.
85. Besarab A, Bolton WK, Browne JK, et al. The effects of normal as compared with low hematocrit values in patients with cardiac disease who are receiving hemodialysis and epoetin. *N Engl J Med*. 1998;339:584-590.
86. Singh AK, Szczech L, Tang KL, et al. Correction of anemia with epoetin alfa in chronic kidney disease. *N Engl J Med*. 2006;355:2085-2098.
87. Drueke TB, Locatelli F, Clyne N, et al. Normalization of hemoglobin level in patients with chronic kidney disease and anemia. *N Engl J Med*. 2006;355:2071-2084.
88. Krane V, Winkler K, Drechsler C, et al. Effect of atorvastatin on inflammation and outcome in patients with type 2 diabetes mellitus on hemodialysis. *Kidney Int*. 2008;74:1461-1467.
89. Ayus JC, Mizani MR, Achinger SG, et al. Effects of short daily versus conventional hemodialysis on left ventricular hypertrophy and inflammatory markers: A prospective, controlled study. *J Am Soc Nephrol*. 2005;16:2778-2788.
90. Boaz M, Smetana S, Weinstein T, et al. Secondary prevention with antioxidants of cardiovascular disease in endstage renal disease (SPACE): Randomised placebo-controlled trial. *Lancet*. 2000;356:1213-1218.
91. Tepel M, van der Giet M, Statz M, et al. The antioxidant acetylcysteine reduces cardiovascular events in patients with end-stage renal failure: A randomized, controlled trial. *Circulation*. 2003;107:992-995.
92. Chertow GM, Burke SK, Raggi P. Sevelamer attenuates the progression of coronary and aortic calcification in hemodialysis patients. *Kidney Int*. 2002;62:245-252.
93. Suki WN, Zabaneh R, Cangiano JL, et al. Effects of sevelamer and calcium-based phosphate binders on mortality in hemodialysis patients. *Kidney Int*. 2007;72:1130-1137.
94. Naves-Diaz M, Alvarez-Hernández D, Passlick-Deetjen J, et al. Oral active vitamin D is associated with improved survival in hemodialysis patients. *Kidney Int*. 2008;74:1070-1078.
95. Jamison RL, Hartigan P, Kaufman JS, et al. Effect of homocysteine lowering on mortality and vascular disease in advanced chronic kidney disease and end-stage renal disease: A randomized controlled trial. *JAMA*. 2007;298:1163-1170.
96. Best PJM, Lennon R, Ting HH, et al. The impact of renal insufficiency on clinical outcomes in patients undergoing percutaneous coronary interventions. *J Am Coll Cardiol*. 2002;39:1113-1119.
97. Cooper WA, O'Brien SM, Thourani VH, et al. Impact of renal dysfunction on outcomes of coronary artery bypass surgery: Results from the Society of Thoracic Surgeons National Adult Cardiac Database. *Circulation*. 2006;113:1063-1070.
98. Mehta RH, Grab JD, O'Brien SM, et al. Bedside tool for predicting the risk of postoperative dialysis in patients undergoing cardiac surgery. *Circulation*. 2006;114:2208-2216.
99. Hemmelgarn BR, Southern D, Culleton BF, et al. Survival after coronary revascularization among patients with kidney disease. *Circulation*. 2004;110:1890-1895.
100. Yasuda K, Kasuga H, Aoyama T, et al. Comparison of percutaneous coronary intervention with medication in the treatment of coronary artery disease in hemodialysis patients. *J Am Soc Nephrol*. 2006;17:2322-2332.
101. Johnston N, Jernberg T, Lagerqvist B, Wallentin L. Early invasive treatment benefits patients with renal dysfunction in unstable coronary artery disease. *Am Heart J*. 2006;152:1052-1058.
102. Aoki J, Ong AT, Hoye A, et al. Five year clinical effect of coronary stenting and coronary artery bypass grafting in renal insufficient patients with multivessel coronary artery disease: Insights from ARTS trial. *Eur Heart J*. 2005;26:1488-1493.
103. Herzog CA, Ma JZ, Collins AJ. Comparative survival of dialysis patients in the United States after coronary angioplasty, coronary artery stenting, and coronary artery bypass surgery and impact of diabetes. *Circulation*. 2002;106:2207-2211.
104. Herzog CA, Gilbertson D. Comparative long-term survival of general Medicare patients with surgical versus percutaneous coronary intervention in the era of drug-eluting stents, and the impact of chronic kidney disease. *Circulation*. 2008;118:S741.
105. Aoyama T, Ishii H, Toriyama T, et al. Sirolimus-eluting stents vs bare metal stents for coronary intervention in Japanese patients with renal failure on hemodialysis. *Circ J*. 2008;72:56-60.
106. Ishio N, Kobayashi Y, Takebayashi H, et al. Impact of drug-eluting stents on clinical and angiographic outcomes in dialysis patients. *Circ J*. 2007;71:1525-1529.

CHAPTER 79

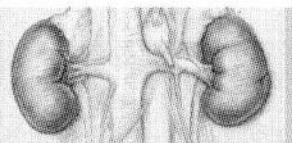

Anemia in Chronic Kidney Disease

Iain C. Macdougall, Kai-Uwe Eckardt

Anemia is an almost universal complication of chronic kidney disease (CKD). It contributes considerably to reduced quality of life of patients with CKD and has been associated with a number of adverse clinical outcomes. Before the availability of recombinant human erythropoietin (rHuEPO, or epoetin), patients on dialysis frequently required blood transfusions, exposing them to the risks of iron overload, transmission of viral hepatitis, and sensitization, which reduced the chances of successful transplantation. The advent of rHuEPO in the late 1980s changed this situation completely. The ability to correct anemia has shown that its consequences go beyond general fatigue and reduced physical capacity to affect a broad spectrum of physiologic functions. Thus, there is a strong rationale for managing anemia in CKD patients, and yet the optimal treatment strategies are still incompletely defined. Apart from therapy with erythropoiesis-stimulating agents (ESAs), iron replacement is essential for anemia management. Importantly, CKD patients require target thresholds of iron parameters different from those for normal individuals to ensure optimal rates of red cell production. The costs of anemia management are considerable; therefore, a rational and careful consideration of the risks and benefits is mandatory.

PATHOGENESIS

Renal anemia is typically an isolated normochromic, normocytic anemia with no leukopenia or thrombocytopenia. Both red cell life span and the rate of red cell production are reduced, but the latter is more important. The normal bone marrow has considerable capacity to increase the rate of erythropoiesis, and the reduction in erythrocyte life observed in association with CKD would normally be easily compensated. However, this EPO-induced compensatory increase in erythrocyte production is impaired in CKD. Serum EPO levels remain within the normal range and fail to show the inverse exponential relationship with blood oxygen content characteristic of other types of anemia. EPO is normally produced by interstitial fibroblasts in the renal cortex, in close proximity to tubular epithelial cells and peritubular capillaries.[1,2] In addition, hepatocytes and perisinusoidal Ito cells in the liver can produce EPO (Fig. 79.1). Hepatic EPO production dominates during fetal and early postnatal life but cannot compensate for the loss of renal production in adult organisms. Subtle changes in blood oxygen content induced by anemia reduce environmental oxygen concentrations, and high altitude stimulate the secretion of EPO through a widespread system of oxygen-dependent gene expression.[2-4] Central to this process is a family of hypoxia-inducible transcription factors (HIFs). The two most important members of this family, HIF-1 and HIF-2, are composed of an oxygen-regulated α subunit (HIF-1α or HIF-2α) and a constitutive β subunit. The production of HIF-1α and HIF-2α is largely independent of oxygen, but their degradation is related to cellular oxygen concentrations. Hydroxylation of specific prolyl and asparagyl residues of HIF-α, for which molecular oxygen is required as a substrate, determines HIF proteasomal destruction and inhibits its transcriptional activity. Apart from EPO, more than 100 HIF target genes have been identified. HIF-2, rather than HIF-1, is the transcription factor primarily responsible for the regulation of EPO production.[5,6]

The role of renal EPO production in the pathogenesis of renal anemia is supported by the observation that anemia is particularly severe in anephric individuals. However, the mechanisms impairing renal EPO production in diseased kidneys remain poorly understood. The production capacity for EPO remains significant, even in end-stage renal disease. Thus, patients with anemia and CKD can respond with a significant increase in EPO production to an additional hypoxic stimulus.[1] The main problem therefore appears to be a failure of EPO production in response to chronically reduced hemoglobin (Hb) concentrations. In line with this view, endogenous EPO production can be induced in CKD patients by pharmacologic inhibition of HIF degradation (see later discussion).

EPO is a glycoprotein hormone consisting of a 165–amino acid protein backbone and four complex, heavily sialylated carbohydrate chains.[1,2] The latter are essential for the biologic activity of EPO *in vivo* because partially or completely deglycosylated EPO is rapidly cleared from the circulation. This is also why rHuEPO has to be manufactured in mammalian cell lines because bacteria lack the capacity to glycosylate recombinant proteins.

EPO stimulates red cell production through binding to homodimeric EPO receptors, which are primarily located on early erythroid progenitor cells, the burst-forming units erythroid (BFU-e) and the colony-forming units erythroid (CFU-e). Binding of EPO to its receptors salvages these progenitor cells and the subsequent earliest erythroblast generation from apoptosis, thereby permitting cell division and maturation into red blood cells.[7] Inhibition of red cell production by uremic inhibitors of erythropoiesis may also contribute to the pathogenesis of renal anemia, although they have so far not been identified. Nevertheless, dialysis *per se* can improve renal anemia and the efficacy of ESAs. Moreover, the interindividual dose requirements for ESAs vary significantly among CKD patients, and the average weekly dose is much higher than estimated production rates of endogenous EPO in healthy individuals. An alternative view to the accumulation of inhibitors of erythropoiesis in CKD is that in

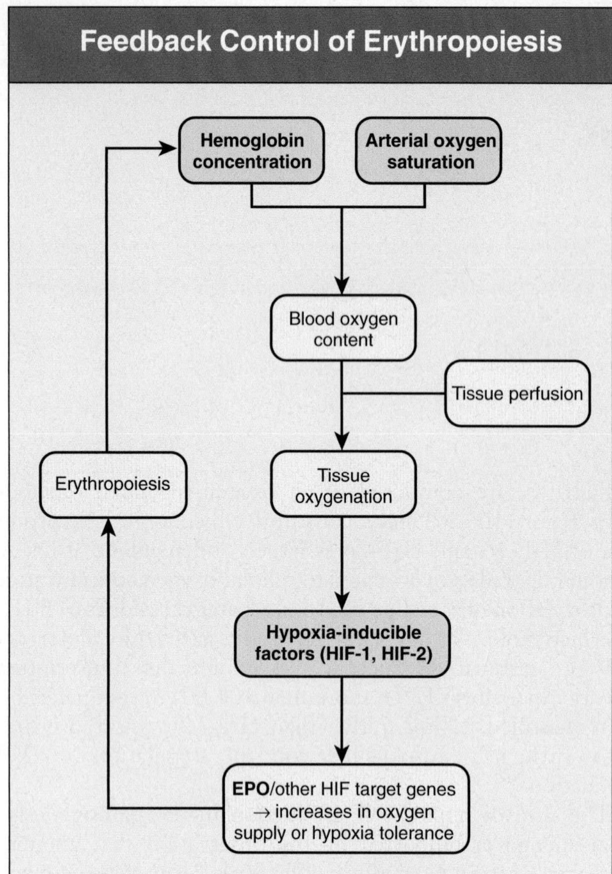

Figure 79.1 Feedback control of erythropoiesis.

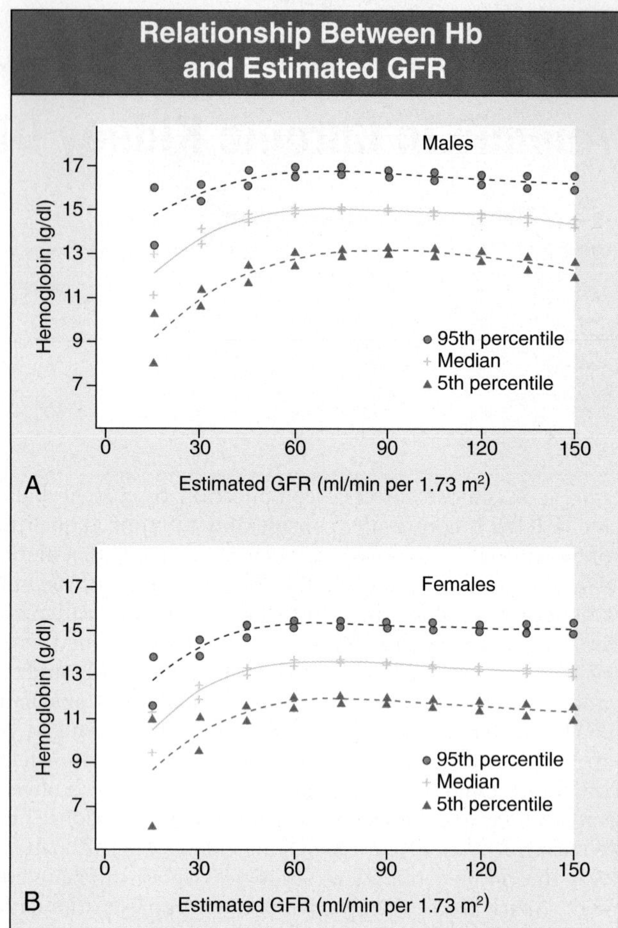

Figure 79.2 Relationship between hemoglobin (Hb) concentration and estimated glomerular filtration rate (GFR). Data are from a cross-sectional survey of individuals randomly selected from the general U.S. population (NHANES III). Results and 95% confidence interval are shown for males **(A)** and females **(B)** at each estimated GFR interval. *(From reference 11.)*

many patients, there is overlap between renal anemia and the anemia of chronic disease, which is characterized by inhibition of EPO production and EPO efficacy as well as by reduced iron availability, mediated through the effects of inflammatory cytokines.[8] Recently, hepcidin was discovered as a key mediator of iron metabolism. Its hepatic release is upregulated in states of inflammation; it simultaneously blocks iron absorption from the gut and promotes iron sequestration in macrophages.[9]

EPIDEMIOLOGY AND NATURAL HISTORY

In general, there is a progressive increase in the incidence and severity of anemia with declining renal function. The reported prevalence of anemia by CKD stage varies significantly and depends to a large extent on the definition of anemia and whether study participants are selected from the general population, are at high risk for CKD, are diabetic, or are already under the care of a physician. Data from the National Health and Nutrition Examination Survey (NHANES) showed that the distribution of Hb levels starts to fall at an estimated glomerular filtration rate (eGFR) of less than 75 ml/min per 1.73 m^2 in men and 45 ml/min per 1.73 m^2 in women (Fig. 79.2).[10] The prevalence of Hb values below 13 g/dl increases below a threshold eGFR of 60 ml/min per 1.73 m^2 in men and 45 ml/min per 1.73 m^2 in women in the general population. Among patients under regular care and known to have CKD, the prevalence of anemia was found to be much greater, with mean Hb levels of 12.8 ± 1.5 (CKD stages 1 and 2), 12.4 ± 1.6 (CKD stage 3), 12.0 ± 1.6 (CKD stage 4), and 10.9 ± 1.6 (CKD stage 5).[11] Although anemia develops largely independently of the etiology of kidney disease, there are two important exceptions. Diabetic patients develop anemia more frequently, at earlier stages of CKD, and more severely at a given level of renal impairment.[12,13] Conversely, in patients with polycystic kidney disease, Hb is on average higher than in other patients with similar degrees of renal failure, and polycythemia may occasionally develop.[1]

Many patients not yet on dialysis still receive no specific treatment for their anemia. In patients on dialysis, in contrast, average Hb values have steadily increased during the past 15 years, following the advent of EPO and the development of clinical practice guidelines for anemia management.[12,13] The average Hb value, however, varies considerably between countries, reflecting considerable variability in practice patterns (Fig. 79.3).[14] Moreover, Hb values vary considerably between patients in the same treatment setting as well as within patients, and at each time a large proportion of patients continues to have Hb values below recommended target levels (see later discussion).

DIAGNOSIS AND DIFFERENTIAL DIAGNOSIS

The diagnosis of anemia and the assessment of its severity are best made by measuring the Hb concentration rather than the hematocrit. Hb is a stable analyte that is measured directly in a standardized fashion, whereas the hematocrit is relatively

Hemoglobin Levels in Patients on Dialysis						
	Among Patients on Dialysis >180 Days			Among Patients New to ESRD, at Start of Dialysis		
Country	n	Mean Hb (g/dl)	Hb <11 g/dl (% of patients)	n	Mean Hb (g/dl)	Hb <11 g/dl (% of patients)
Sweden	466	12.0	23	168	10.7	55
United States	1690	11.7	27	458	10.4	65
Spain	513	11.7	31	170	10.6	61
Belgium	442	11.6	29	213	10.3	66
Canada	479	11.6	29	150	10.1	70
Australia and New Zealand	423	11.5	36	108	10.1	70
Germany	459	11.4	35	142	10.5	61
Italy	447	11.3	38	167	10.2	68
United Kingdom	436	11.2	40	93	10.2	67
France	341	11.1	45	86	10.1	65
Japan	1210	10.1	77	131	8.3	95

Figure 79.3 Mean hemoglobin (Hb) levels and percentage of patients with Hb levels below 11 g/dl who have been on dialysis therapy for more than 180 days and at the time of starting dialysis, by country. Data are from the Dialysis Outcomes and Practice Patterns Study, phase II (DOPPS 2), and are derived from 308 randomly selected, representative dialysis facilities. Note that there are marked differences between countries, but at least one fourth and up to three fourths of dialysis patients and, in most countries, more than two thirds of patients starting chronic dialysis have Hb values below the recommended lower target of 11 g/dl. ESRD, end-stage renal disease. *(Modified from reference 14.)*

unstable, indirectly derived by automatic analyzers, and lacking in standardization. Within-run and between-run coefficients of variation in automated analyzer measurements of Hb are one half and one third those for hematocrit, respectively.[12]

There is considerable variability in the Hb threshold used to define anemia. According to the most recent definition in the Kidney Disease Outcomes Quality Initiative (KDOQI) guidelines, anemia should be diagnosed at Hb concentrations of less than 13.5 g/dl in adult men and less than 12.0 g/dl in adult women.[12] These values represent the mean Hb concentration of the lowest 5th percentile of the sex-specific general adult population. In children, age-dependent differences in the normal values have to be taken into account. Normal Hb values are increased in high-altitude residents.[12] Adjustment is not recommended for age in adults.

In addition to the Hb value, the evaluation of anemia in CKD patients should include a complete blood count with red blood cell indices (mean corpuscular Hb concentration [MCHC], mean corpuscular volume [MCV]), white blood cell count (including differential), and platelet count. Although renal anemia is typically normochromic and normocytic, deficiency of vitamin B_{12} or folate may lead to macrocytosis, whereas iron deficiency or inherited disorders of Hb formation (such as thalassemia) may produce microcytosis. Macrocytosis with leukopenia or thrombocytopenia suggests a generalized disorder of hematopoiesis caused by toxins, nutritional deficit, or myelodysplasia. Hypochromia probably reflects iron-deficient erythropoiesis. An absolute reticulocyte count, which normally ranges between 40,000 and 50,000 cells/μl of blood, is a useful marker of erythropoietic activity.

Iron status tests should be performed to assess the level of iron in tissue stores or the adequacy of iron supply for erythropoiesis. Although serum ferritin is so far the only available marker of storage iron, several tests reflect the adequacy of iron for erythropoiesis, including transferrin saturation, MCV, and MCHC; the percentage of hypochromic red blood cells (PHRC); and the content of Hb in reticulocytes (CHr). Storage time of the blood sample may elevate PHRC, and MCV and MCHC are below the normal range only after long-standing iron deficiency.

It is important to identify anemia in CKD patients because it may signify nutritional deficits, systemic illness, or other conditions that warrant attention, and even at modest degrees, anemia reflects an independent risk factor for hospitalizations, cardiovascular disease, and mortality.[12] The diagnosis of renal anemia, that is, an anemia caused by CKD, requires careful judgment of the degree of anemia in relation to the degree of renal impairment and exclusion of other or additional causes. Because there is significant variability in the degree of anemia in relation to the impairment in renal function, no simple diagnostic criteria can be applied. Causes of anemia other than EPO deficiency should be considered when (1) the severity of anemia is disproportionate to the impairment of renal function, (2) there is evidence of iron deficiency, or (3) there is evidence of leukopenia or thrombocytopenia. Concomitant conditions such as sickle cell disease may exacerbate the anemia, as can drug therapy. For example, inhibitors of the renin-angiotensin system may reduce Hb levels by (1) direct effects of angiotensin II on erythroid progenitor cells,[15] (2) accumulation of *N*-acetyl-seryl-lysyl-proline (Ac-SDKP), an endogenous inhibitor of erythropoiesis in patients treated with angiotensin-converting enzyme (ACE) inhibitors,[16] and (3) reduction of endogenous EPO production, potentially due to the hemodynamic effects of angiotensin II inhibition. Myelosuppressive effects of immunosuppressants may further contribute to anemia.[17] The measurement of serum EPO concentrations is usually not helpful in the diagnosis of renal anemia because there is relative rather than absolute deficiency, with a wide range of EPO concentrations for a given Hb concentration that extends far beyond the normal range of EPO levels in healthy, nonanemic individuals. Abnormalities of other laboratory parameters should be looked for, such as a low MCV or MCHC (may indicate an underlying hemoglobinopathy), a high MCV (may

Secondary Effects of Anemia Correction on the Cardiovascular System
Reduction in high cardiac output
Reduced stroke volume
Reduced heart rate
Increase in peripheral vascular resistance
Reduction in anginal episodes
Reduction in myocardial ischemia
Regression of left ventricular hypertrophy
Stabilization of left ventricular dilation
Increase in whole blood viscosity

Figure 79.4 Secondary effects of anemia correction on the cardiovascular system.

Other Secondary Effects of Anemia Correction
Reduced blood transfusions
Increased quality of life
Increased exercise capacity
Improved cognitive function
Improved sleep patterns
Improved immune function
Improved muscle function
Improved depression
Improved nutrition
Improved platelet function
(Hypertension)
(Vascular access thrombosis)

Figure 79.5 Other secondary effects of anemia correction. Parentheses indicate negative and adverse effects.

indicate vitamin B_{12} or folate deficiency), or an abnormal leukocyte or platelet count (may suggest a primary bone marrow problem, such as myeloma or myelodysplastic syndrome), and further tests should be performed as indicated to explore these potential conditions. However, when there are no such pointers to other confounding causes of anemia and iron deficiency has been excluded, a trial with rHuEPO or its derivatives is warranted, even when the eGFR is only moderately reduced.

CLINICAL MANIFESTATIONS

In the early clinical trials of EPO performed in the late 1980s, the mean baseline Hb concentration was about 6 to 7 g/dl, and this progressively increased to about 11 or 12 g/dl after treatment. Patients subjectively felt much better, with reduced fatigue, increased energy levels, and enhanced physical capacity, and there were also objective improvements in cardiorespiratory function.[18] Thus, it is now clear that many of the symptoms previously attributed to the "uremic syndrome" are indeed due to the anemia associated with CKD (Figs. 79.4 and 79.5). Although the avoidance of blood transfusions and improvement in quality of life are obvious early changes, there are also possible effects on the cardiovascular system (see Fig. 79.4). The physiologic consequences of long-standing anemia are an increase in cardiac output and a reduction in peripheral vascular resistance. Anemia is a risk factor for the development of left ventricular hypertrophy in CKD patients and thought to exacerbate left ventricular dilation. Sustained correction of anemia in CKD patients results in a reversal of most of these cardiovascular abnormalities, with the notable exception of left ventricular dilation. Once the left ventricle is stretched beyond the limits of its elasticity, correction of anemia cannot reverse this.[19] It may, however, prevent further progression in some patients. Other effects of anemia correction reported in clinical trials include improvements in quality of life, cognitive function, sleep patterns, nutrition, sexual function, menstrual regularity, immune responsiveness, and platelet function.

There has been considerable debate in recent times about the optimal target range of Hb in CKD patients. The improvement in quality of life with increasing Hb concentrations supports a level above 10 to 11 g/dl in all CKD patients,[12,13] but some studies have indicated increased risks associated with attempts to completely correct anemia. No survival benefit is evident at a higher level of anemia correction,[20-22] although quality of life and exercise capacity may be greater. Thus, there is a possible tradeoff between improved quality of life and increased cost and risk for harm, so that a target level of Hb above 13 g/dl should be avoided.[12]

TREATMENT

Erythropoiesis-Stimulating Agents

Epoetin Therapy

Manufacture of rHuEPO is achieved by gene transfer into a suitable mammalian cell line such as Chinese hamster ovary cells or induction of the human gene in a hepatoma cell line. The early clinical trials of rHuEPO were conducted with both EPO alfa and EPO beta. Like the endogenous hormone, rHuEPO consists of a 165–amino acid backbone with one *O*-linked and three *N*-linked glycosylation chains. Invariably, however, there are some differences in the glycosylation pattern between different preparations of rHuEPO and the endogenous hormone. Several formulations of EPO are now available, including "biosimilar" EPO preparations, which have been developed after patent expiry of the innovator compounds. Other "copy" EPOs are available elsewhere in the world (e.g., China, India, Peru, Argentina, Russia, and Cuba), which are not necessarily produced to the same regulatory standards as the EPO preparations marketed in the United States and Europe. Another EPO that was initially developed for the European market was EPO delta, which differed from other EPOs in its glycosylation pattern because it was produced in a human fibrosarcoma cell line.

Before 1998, EPO alfa in Europe was formulated with human serum albumin, but because of a change in European regulations, this was replaced with polysorbate 80. EPO beta is formulated with polysorbate 20, along with urea, calcium chloride, and five amino acids as excipients. The importance of the formulation of the EPO products was highlighted in 2002 with an upsurge in cases of antibody-mediated pure red cell aplasia in association with the subcutaneous use of EPO alfa after its change of formulation. Patients affected by this complication develop neutralizing antibodies against both rHuEPO and the endogenous hormone, which result in severe anemia and transfusion dependence.[23] The cause of this serious complication in which there is a break in B-cell tolerance remains obscure, although it seems likely that factors such as a breach of the cold storage chain were relevant, and the subcutaneous application route was a prerequisite; circumstantial evidence also suggested that rubber stoppers of prefilled syringes used in one of the albumin-free EPO alfa formulations may have released organic compounds that acted as immunologic adjuvants.[24] Although this unfortunate combination of adverse factors was specific for one compound, a low baseline rate of pure red cell aplasia also occurs with EPO beta and darbepoetin alfa.

The EPOs are administered either intravenously or subcutaneously. The bioavailability after intraperitoneal administration (in peritoneal dialysis patients) is too low. The earliest clinical trials of EPO used intravenous injections two or three times per week. This was partly due to the short half-life of EPO (6 to 8 hours after intravenous administration)[25] and partly due to the convenience for the patient on dialysis. With use of this regimen, 90% of patients show a significant increase in Hb concentration. Good iron management is pivotal for the success of EPO therapy (see later discussion). Adverse effects of EPO therapy are uncommon, apart from a moderate increase in blood pressure and an increased rate of vascular access thrombosis. Whereas these effects are probably dependent to a large degree on the increase in Hb concentrations, there are some concerns that ESA therapy may enhance thrombogenicity and tumor growth in patients with malignant disease as well as exacerbate vascular events in CKD independently of Hb concentrations.

Although the bioavailability of subcutaneous EPO is between 20% and 30%, the prolonged half-life after subcutaneous compared with intravenous administration allows less frequent injections. Furthermore, the dose required to achieve the same Hb response is about 30% lower with subcutaneous compared with intravenous administration.[26] There appears to be little difference between the thigh, arm, or abdomen as injection sites.

Darbepoetin Alfa

Darbepoetin alfa is a second-generation ESA that is a supersialylated analogue of EPO, possessing two extra *N*-linked glycosylation chains. This property confers greater metabolic stability and a lower clearance rate *in vivo*, and the elimination half-life of this compound in humans after a single intravenous administration is three times greater than that of epoetin alfa (25.3 hours versus 8.5 hours). Thus, this agent can generally be given less frequently than the standard epoetins, with dosing intervals of once weekly and once every alternate week.[27] In contrast to the epoetins, dosage requirements for darbepoetin alfa for the correction of anemia and maintenance of Hb concentration in CKD patients are the same for intravenous and subcutaneous administration. The conversion factor for switching patients from epoetin alfa or beta to darbepoetin alfa is usually quoted as 200:1, but there may be considerable variability in this, depending on the patient population, the dose, and the route of administration.[25]

C.E.R.A. (Methoxypolyethylene Glycol–Epoetin Beta)

Alternative bioengineering techniques to prolong the half-life of EPO further resulted in the development of C.E.R.A., which is a pegylated derivative of epoetin beta with an elimination half-life of around 130 hours when it is administered either intravenously or subcutaneously. Phase III studies suggested that many patients are able to be maintained with once-monthly administration of C.E.R.A., and a superiority study (PATRONUS) suggested greater efficacy with this frequency of administration compared with once-monthly dosing of darbepoetin alfa when it is administered intravenously to hemodialysis patients.[28]

Other Erythropoiesis-Stimulating Agents

Several other ESAs are currently in clinical development,[29] including Hematide and the "HIF stabilizers."

Hematide is an erythropoietin mimetic peptide, the amino acid sequence of which is completely unrelated to native or recombinant erythropoietin,[29] although it shares the same functional and biologic properties of EPO. Hematide is currently in phase III of its clinical development program. The potential advantages of this compound include a greater *ex vivo* stability, allowing storage at room temperature; a prolonged pharmacodynamic action, allowing once-monthly administration; a different immunogenicity profile with no cross-reactivity between Hematide and anti-EPO antibodies, allowing effective treatment of anti-EPO antibody–mediated pure red cell aplasia[30]; and a simple manufacturing process involving synthetic peptide chemistry.

The HIF stabilizers are competitive inhibitors of HIF prolyl hydroxylases[29] and asparagyl hydroxylase, enzymes involved in the metabolism of HIF and its transcriptional activity. The HIF stabilizers therefore cause an increase in endogenous EPO production.[29] The first of the prolyl hydroxylase inhibitors is currently being tested in phase II studies, and these drugs are orally active.[29] There is much discussion about whether these agents will upregulate not only EPO gene expression but also other HIF target genes, such as those involved in iron metabolism and neoangiogenesis. Whereas some of these effects may facilitate an increase in Hb concentrations, the long-term consequences of these potential additional effects have not been established.[29,31]

Initiation of and Maintenance Therapy with Erythropoiesis-Stimulating Agents

According to current guidelines, all CKD patients should be investigated and treated if their Hb concentration decreases to less than 11 g/dl.[12,13] Before ESA therapy is started, it is essential to exclude and to correct causes of anemia other than EPO deficiency, such as hematinic deficiencies (Fig. 79.6). If the ferritin concentration is below 100 μg/l, iron supplementation may be administered either first or concurrently. Iron is best given by intravenous administration, although oral iron can be considered in patients not yet on dialysis. Some patients may respond to intravenous iron alone (see later discussion). If the ferritin level is above 100 μg/l (in the absence of systemic inflammation) or there is a suboptimal response to iron, ESA therapy should be commenced. The usual starting dose of epoetin is about 25 to 50 IU/kg (e.g., 2000 IU) two or three times weekly, either by intravenous or subcutaneous administration. Within 3 to 4 days, an increase in the reticulocyte count is seen, and within 1 to 2 weeks, there is a significant rise in the Hb concentration, usually on the order of 0.25 to 0.5 g/dl per week. Thus, during the course of 1 month, a significant increase of 1 to 2 g/dl in the Hb concentration is usually achieved. If a patient fails to respond satisfactorily to ESAs, the dose is increased in stepwise upward titrations of 25% to 50%, and if there is still an inadequate response, causes of resistance to EPO therapy should be investigated (see later discussion). The optimal target range of Hb

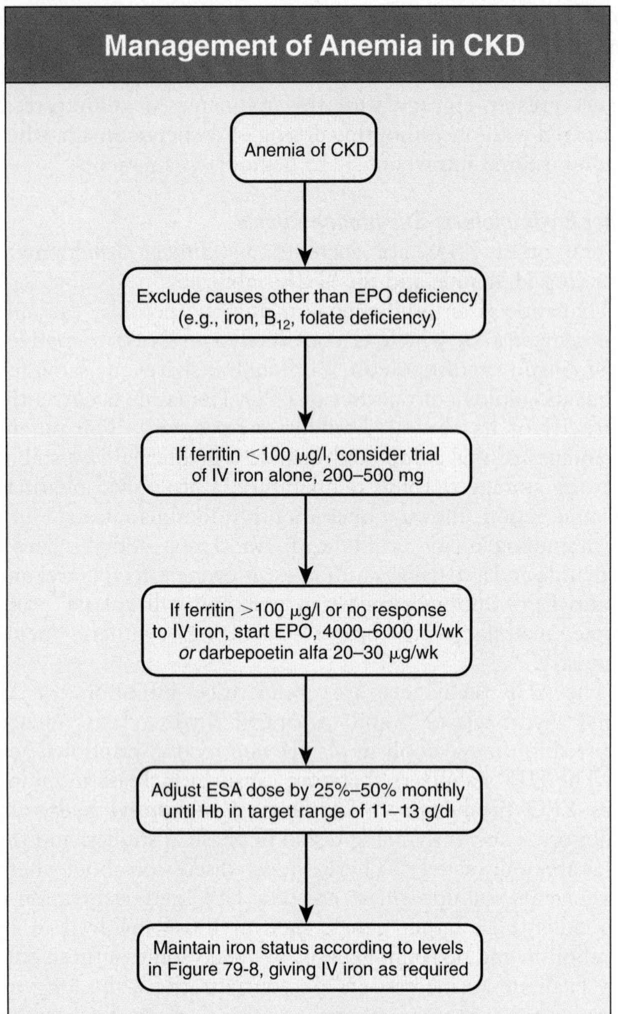

Figure 79.6 Management of anemia in patients with chronic kidney disease (CKD). EPO, erythropoietin; ESA, erythropoiesis-stimulating agent.

Causes of a Poor Response to ESA Therapy

Major (Frequent)	Minor (Less Common)
Iron deficiency	Poor compliance, poor adherence to ESA therapy
Infection, inflammation Underdialysis	Blood loss Hyperparathyroidism Aluminum toxicity (rare nowadays) Vitamin B_{12} or folate deficiency Hemolysis Primary bone marrow disorders (e.g., myelodysplastic syndrome) Hemoglobinopathies (e.g., sickle cell disease) ACE inhibitors, angiotensin receptor blockers Carnitine deficiency Anti-EPO antibodies causing PRCA

Figure 79.7 Causes of a poor response to erythropoiesis-stimulating agent (ESA) therapy. ACE, angiotensin-converting enzyme; EPO, erythropoietin; PRCA, pure red cell aplasia.

concentration for CKD patients is considered to be 11 to 13 g/dl[12] (see earlier discussion), and iron supplementation should be administered to maximize the response to ESA therapy (see later discussion). A possible starting dose of darbepoetin alfa is 20 to 30 μg once weekly intravenously or subcutaneously; an appropriate starting dose of C.E.R.A. is 30 to 60 μg once every 2 weeks intravenously or subcutaneously.

Hyporesponsiveness to Erythropoiesis-Stimulating Agents

There is no absolute definition of hyporesponsiveness to ESA therapy, but it is usually identified when the Hb concentration remains below 11 g/dl despite increasing doses of ESA. The causes of resistance to ESA therapy are listed in Figure 79.7, and it is important to correct them when possible. The major causes include iron deficiency (see later discussion), infection or inflammation,[32] and underdialysis.[33] If the patient is self-administering (e.g., for peritoneal dialysis patients), poor adherence to or compliance with therapy must be excluded. If there is any doubt about the possibility of iron deficiency, a trial of intravenous iron may be useful. Vitamin B_{12}, folate, and thyroxine deficiency may be excluded easily by the appropriate laboratory tests, as may severe hyperparathyroidism. Aluminum toxicity is no longer a significant cause of ESA resistance. Depending on the ethnic origin of the patient, a hemoglobinopathy should be excluded by performing Hb electrophoresis. Some patients taking ACE inhibitors or angiotensin receptor blockers may require higher doses of ESA therapy, although it is rarely necessary or indeed advisable to stop these drugs. Primary bone marrow disorders, such as myelodysplastic syndrome, should be investigated by a bone marrow examination (aspirate and trephine) if all other causes have been excluded. A bone marrow test may also be necessary in the diagnosis of antibody-mediated pure red cell aplasia, although measurement of the reticulocyte count and anti-erythropoietin antibodies may provide an earlier clue.[23] If a patient receiving ESA therapy has a high reticulocyte count, the bone marrow is generating more than adequate quantities of new red cells, and bleeding or hemolysis should be investigated by means of upper gastrointestinal endoscopy, colonoscopy, or hemolysis screen (Coombs test, bilirubin measurement, lactate dehydrogenase levels, haptoglobin levels).

There is no defined upper dose limit of ESA, and doses of 60,000 IU per week of EPO are not uncommon in the United States, but there is recent concern that high doses of ESA may increase side effects independently of Hb concentrations by presumed pleiotropic effects and may enhance cardiovascular and other thrombotic events. However, because the requirement of high doses usually reflects a high degree of comorbidity and inflammation, it is difficult to establish the cause and effect of the association between high ESA doses and adverse outcomes; consequently, no "safe" upper dose level has been determined. Studies in cancer patients have found that targeting a normal Hb concentration with high ESA doses may also be associated with adverse outcomes compared with targeting a subnormal Hb target,[34,35] but whether this is due to vascular complications or effects on tumor growth is still controversial. Although no study has investigated anemia management in patients with CKD and cancer, it appears reasonable to apply the subnormal Hb target recommendation for CKD patients also to this special group and to avoid high ESA doses. In patients with acute illness requiring hospitalization, Hb frequently falls despite continued ESA therapy, indicating increased blood loss and temporary hyporesponsiveness. The optimal management of anemia under these conditions remains unclear. Whereas cost considerations may speak for withholding of ESA therapy until responsiveness is reestablished, it has also been proposed that doses should be increased in an attempt to overcome hyporesponsiveness. Very high doses have been demonstrated to be effective even in critically ill patients on intensive care units, but a pivotal trial[36] failed to demonstrate a reduction in transfusion requirements. From a practical point of view, and pending evidence to the contrary, it seems sensible to continue the same dose of ESA or to attempt one dose increase (e.g. doubling), but further dose escalations are probably not advisable or cost-effective.

Iron Management

Iron is an essential ingredient for heme synthesis, and adequate amounts of this mineral are required for the manufacture of new red cells. Thus, under enhanced erythropoietic stimulation, greater amounts of iron are used, and many CKD patients (particularly those on hemodialysis) have inadequate amounts of available iron to satisfy the increased demands of the bone marrow.[37] Even before the introduction of ESA therapy, many CKD patients were in negative iron balance as a result of poor dietary intake, poor appetite, and increased iron losses due to occult and overt blood losses (see Chapter 83). Losses in hemodialysis patients are up to 5 or 6 mg a day, compared with 1 mg in healthy individuals, and this may exceed the absorption capacity of the gastrointestinal tract, particularly when there is any underlying inflammation. Iron absorption capacity in patients with CKD is considerably lower than in nonuremic individuals, particularly in the presence of systemic inflammatory activity, and this is probably mediated by hepcidin upregulation (see earlier discussion).[9] For this reason also, oral iron is ineffective in many CKD patients, and parenteral iron administration is required, particularly in those receiving hemodialysis.[37] However, even with these limitations of oral iron absorption, the cheap costs of using this route, along with convenience for the patient, often persuade physicians to try oral iron supplementation first in nondialysis patients; if, however, there is insufficient response after 2 to 3 months, intravenous iron should be administered.

Inadequate supply of iron to the bone marrow may be due to an absolute or a functional iron deficiency.[37] *Absolute* iron deficiency occurs when there are low whole-body iron stores, as indicated by a serum ferritin level less than 30 μg/l. *Functional* iron deficiency occurs when there is ample or even increased storage iron but the iron stores fail to release iron rapidly enough to satisfy the demands of the bone marrow. Several markers of iron status are available, but none of them is ideal (Fig. 79.8). The serum ferritin is a marker of storage iron but is spuriously raised in inflammatory conditions and liver disease. The transferrin saturation is a function of the circulating plasma iron in relation to the total iron-binding capacity and is often regarded as a better measure of available iron; however, levels can be highly fluctuant owing to significant diurnal variation in the measurement of plasma iron.[37] The percentage of hypochromic red cells and the CHr are red cell and reticulocyte parameters, respectively, that are indirect measures of how much iron is being incorporated into the newly developing or mature red cell.[33] No one measure of iron status is usually adequate to exclude iron deficiency, and the recommended levels for these measures are based on limited scientific evidence. Functional iron deficiency is usually diagnosed when there is a normal or increased ferritin level and a reduced transferrin saturation (<20%) or increased hypochromic red cells (>10%). The U.S.[12] and European[13] guidelines on renal anemia management suggest

Markers of Iron Status in CKD Patients

Test	Recommended Range
Serum ferritin	100–500 μg/L (CKD) 200–500 μg/L (HD)
Transferrin saturation	20%–40%
Hypochromic red cells	<10%
Reticulocyte hemoglobin content (CHr)	>29 pg/cell
Serum transferrin receptor	Not established
Erythrocyte zinc protoporphyrin	Not established

Figure 79.8 Markers of iron status and the recommended target ranges in chronic kidney disease (CKD).

that the ferritin level be maintained in the range of 200 to 500 μg/l, with an upper limit of 800 μg/l (see Fig. 79.8). Levels of ferritin above this threshold usually do not confer any clinical advantage and may exacerbate iron toxicity. The optimal transferrin saturation is above 20% to 30% to ensure a readily available supply of iron to the bone marrow. Several studies support the maintenance of the percentage of hypochromic red cells at levels of less than 6% and the CHr at levels greater than 29 pg/cell. Other measures of iron status, such as serum transferrin receptor levels and erythrocyte zinc protoporphyrin levels, are mainly research tools and have not been established in routine clinical practice.

Iron supplementation is often required in CKD patients. Oral iron is poorly absorbed in uremic individuals, and there is a high incidence of gastrointestinal side effects. Intramuscular administration of iron is not recommended in CKD, given the enhanced bleeding tendency, the pain of the injection, and the potential for brownish discoloration of the skin. Thus, intravenous administration of iron has become the standard of care for many CKD patients, particularly those receiving hemodialysis.[37] There are several intravenous iron preparations available worldwide, including iron dextran, iron sucrose, and iron gluconate. All of these preparations contain elemental iron surrounded by a carbohydrate shell, which allows them to be injected intravenously. The lability of iron release from these preparations varies, with iron dextran being the most stable, followed by iron sucrose and then iron gluconate. Iron is released from these compounds to plasma transferrin and other iron-binding proteins and is eventually taken up by the reticuloendothelial system.

In hemodialysis patients, it is easy and practical to give low doses of intravenous iron (e.g., 10 to 20 mg every dialysis session) or, alternatively, 100 mg weekly. In peritoneal dialysis and nondialysis CKD patients, however, such low-dose regimens are impractical, and larger doses may be administered. The more stable the iron preparation, the larger the dose administration rate that can be used. For example, 1 g of iron dextran may be given by intravenous infusion, whereas the maximum recommended dose of iron sucrose at any one time is 500 mg. For iron gluconate, doses in excess of 125 to 250 mg are best avoided. All intravenous iron preparations carry a risk for immediate reactions, which may be characterized by hypotension, dizziness, and nausea. These reactions are usually short-lived and caused by too large a dose given during too short a time. Iron dextran also carries the risk for acute anaphylactic reactions due to preformed dextran antibodies, and although this risk may be less with the lower molecular weight iron dextrans, the potential for anaphylaxis still remains. Other, longer term concerns about intravenous administration of iron include the potential for increased susceptibility to infections and oxidative stress. Much of the scientific evidence for this has been generated in *in vitro* experiments, the clinical significance of which is unclear. Recently, two new iron preparations have become available for intravenous use (ferumoxytol in the United States and ferric carboxymaltose in Europe). Both of these compounds allow higher doses of intravenous iron to be administered rapidly as a bolus injection, without the need for a test dose.

There is emerging evidence that intravenous iron may improve the anemia of CKD in up to 30% of patients not receiving ESA therapy who have a low ferritin level.[38] In such patients, a response to intravenous iron alone may occur within 2 to 3 weeks of iron administration. In those already receiving ESAs, there is considerable evidence that concomitant intravenous iron may enhance the response to the ESAs and result in lower dose requirements.[13,14,37]

REFERENCES

1. Eckardt KU. Erythropoietin: Oxygen-dependent control of erythropoiesis and its failure in renal disease. *Nephron*. 1994;67:7-23.
2. Jelkmann W. Molecular biology of erythropoietin. *Intern Med*. 2004;43:649-659.
3. Schofield CJ, Ratcliffe PJ. Oxygen sensing by HIF hydroxylases. *Nat Rev Mol Cell Biol*. 2004;5:43-54.
4. Maxwell P. HIF-1: An oxygen response system with special relevance to the kidney. *J Am Soc Nephrol*. 2003;14:712-722.
5. Warnecke C, Zaborowska Z, Kurreck J, et al. Differentiating the functional role of hypoxia-inducible factor (HIF)-1α and HIF-2α (EPAS-1) by the use of RNA interference: Erythropoietin is a HIF-2α target gene in Hep3B and Kelly cells. *FASEB J*. 2004;18:462-464.
6. Scortegagna M, Morris MA, Oktay Y, et al. The HIF family member EPAS1/HIF-2α is required for normal hematopoiesis in mice. *Blood*. 2003;102:634-640.
7. Chen C, Sytkowski AJ. The erythropoietin receptor and its signalling cascade. In: Jelkmann WFP, ed. *Erythropoietin: Molecular Biology and Clinical Use*. Johnson City, Tenn: Graham Publishing; 2003:165-194.
8. Weiss G, Goodnough LT. Anemia of chronic disease. *N Engl J Med*. 2005;352:11-23.
9. Verga Falzacappa MV, Muckenthaler MU. Hepcidin: Iron-hormone and anti-microbial peptide. *Gene*. 2005;364:37-44.
10. Astor BC, Muntner P, Levin A, et al. Association of kidney function with anemia: The Third National Health and Nutrition Examination Survey, 1988-1994. *Arch Intern Med*. 2002;162:1401-1408.
11. McClellan W, Aronoff SL, Bolton WK, et al. The prevalence of anemia in patients with chronic kidney disease. *Curr Med Res Opin*. 2004;20:501-510.
12. K/DOQI. Anemia guidelines in CKD patients. *Am J Kidney Dis*. 2006;47(Suppl 3):S1-S146.
13. European Best Practice Guidelines Working Group. Revised European best practice guidelines for the management of anaemia in patients with chronic renal failure. *Nephrol Dial Transplant*. 2004;19(Suppl 2):1-47.
14. Pisoni RL, Bragg-Gresham JL, Young EW, et al. Anemia management and outcomes from 12 countries in the Dialysis Outcomes and Practice Patterns Study (DOPPS). *Am J Kidney Dis*. 2004;44:94-111.
15. Cole J, Ertoy D, Lin H, et al. Lack of angiotensin II–facilitated erythropoiesis causes anemia in angiotensin-converting enzyme–deficient mice. *J Clin Invest*. 2000;106:391-398.
16. Le Meur Y, Lorgeot V, Comte L, et al. Plasma levels and metabolism of AcSDKP in patients with chronic renal failure: Relationship with erythropoietin requirements. *Am J Kidney Dis*. 2001;38:10-17.
17. Winkelmayer WC, Kewalramani R, Rutstein M, et al. Pharmacoepidemiology of anemia in kidney transplant recipients. *J Am Soc Nephrol*. 2004;15:347-352.
18. Macdougall IC, Lewis NP, Saunders MJ, et al. Long-term cardiorespiratory effects of amelioration of renal anaemia by erythropoietin. *Lancet*. 1990;335:489-493.
19. Parfrey PS, Foley RN, Wittreich BH, et al. Double-blind comparison of full and partial anemia correction in incident hemodialysis patients without symptomatic heart disease. *J Am Soc Nephrol*. 2005;16:2180-2189.
20. Besarab A, Bolton WK, Browne JK, et al. The effects of normal as compared with low hematocrit values in patients with cardiac disease who are receiving hemodialysis and epoetin. *N Engl J Med*. 1998;339:584-590.
21. Drueke TB, Locelli F, Clyne N, et al. Normalization of hemoglobin level in patients with chronic kidney disease and anemia. *N Engl J Med*. 2006;355:2071-2084.
22. Singh AK, Szczech L, Tang KL, et al. Correction of anemia with epoetin alfa in chronic kidney disease. *N Engl J Med*. 2006;355:2085-2098.
23. Rossert J, Casadevall N, Eckardt KU. Anti-erythropoietin antibodies and pure red cell aplasia. *J Am Soc Nephrol*. 2004;15:398-406.
24. Boven K, Stryker S, Knight J, et al. The increased incidence of pure red cell aplasia with an Eprex formulation in uncoated rubber stopper syringes. *Kidney Int*. 2005;67:346-353.
25. Macdougall IC, Padhi D, Jang G. Pharmacology of darbepoetin alfa. *Nephrol Dial Transplant*. 2007;22(Suppl 4):iv2-iv9.
26. Kaufman JS, Reda DJ, Fye CL, et al. Subcutaneous compared with intravenous epoetin in patients receiving hemodialysis. Department of Veterans Affairs Cooperative Study Group on Erythropoietin in Hemodialysis Patients. *N Engl J Med*. 1998;339:578-583.
27. Vanrenterghem Y, Barany P, Mann JF, et al, for the European/Australian NESP 970200 Study Group. Randomized trial of darbepoetin alfa for treatment of renal anemia at a reduced dose frequency compared with rHuEPO in dialysis patients. *Kidney Int*. 2002;62:2167-2175.
28. Carrera F, Lok CE, de Francisco A, et al. Maintenance treatment of renal anaemia in haemodialysis patients with methoxy polyethylene glycol-epoetin beta versus darbepoetin alfa administered monthly: a randomized comparative trial. *Nephrol Dial Transplant*. 2010 Jun 3.
29. Macdougall IC, Eckardt KU. Novel strategies for stimulating erythropoiesis and potential new treatments for anaemia. *Lancet*. 2006;368:947-953.
30. Macdougall IC, Rossert J, Casadevall N, et al. A peptide-based erythropoietin-receptor agonist for pure red-cell aplasia. *N Engl J Med*. 2009;361:1848-1855.
31. Bunn HF. New agents that stimulate erythropoiesis. *Blood*. 2007;109:868-873.
32. Macdougall IC, Cooper AC. Hyporesponsiveness to erythropoietic therapy due to chronic inflammation. *Eur J Clin Invest*. 2005;35(Suppl 3):32-35.
33. Locatelli F, Del Vecchio L. Dialysis adequacy and response to erythropoietic agents: What is the evidence base? *Nephrol Dial Transplant*. 2003;18(Suppl 8):29-35.
34. Glaspy JA. Erythropoietin in cancer patients. *Annu Rev Med*. 2009;60:181-192.
35. Bennett CL, Silver SM, Djulbegovic B, et al. Venous thromboembolism and mortality associated with recombinant erythropoietin and darbepoetin administration for the treatment of cancer-associated anemia. *JAMA*. 2008;299:914-924.
36. Corwin HL, Gettinger A, Fabian TC, et al, EPO Critical Care Trials Group. Efficacy and safety of epoetin alfa in critically ill patients. *N Engl J Med*. 2007;357:965-976.
37. Macdougall IC. Monitoring of iron status and iron supplementation in patients treated with erythropoietin. *Curr Opin Nephrol Hypertens*. 1994;3:620-625.
38. Mircescu G, Garneata L, Capusa C, Ursea N. Intravenous iron supplementation for the treatment of anaemia in pre-dialyzed chronic renal failure patients. *Nephrol Dial Transplant*. 2006;1:120-124.

CHAPTER 80

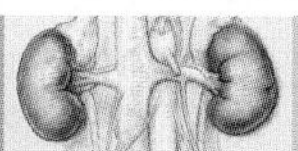

Other Blood and Immune Disorders in Chronic Kidney Disease

Walter H. Hörl

Whereas anemia (see Chapter 79) is the clinically most prominent hematologic alteration in patients with chronic kidney disease (CKD), a variety of other changes also occur. These include altered platelet function, which together with abnormal coagulation may result in a uremic bleeding tendency but can also result in a prothrombogenic state. In addition, leukocyte function is altered, resulting in increased susceptibility to infections and abnormal immune responses (e.g., after vaccinations).

PLATELET DYSFUNCTION AND COAGULATION DEFECTS

Normal hemostasis (Figs. 80.1 and 80.2) begins with platelet adhesion to vascular endothelium and requires a relatively vasoconstricted vessel wall, the integrity of platelet glycoproteins, and a normal quantity of large-molecular-weight, multimeric von Willebrand factor (vWF). Main platelet glycoproteins are GpIb, the platelet receptor for vWF, involved in platelet adhesion, and GpIIb/IIIa, the platelet receptor for fibrinogen, involved in platelet aggregation. Under static conditions, GpIb and vWF have no affinity for each other. However, these molecules develop a specific affinity for one another at high shear stress, resulting in arterial platelet adhesion. Aggregated fibrinogen-platelet mesh acts as a trap for binding and activation of other plasma clotting factors. The exposure of preceding clotting factors to tissue factors, present on damaged endothelial cells, catalyzes the conversion of prothrombin to thrombin, which converts fibrinogen to fibrin. Subsequent cross-linking of insoluble fibrin results in a stable hemostatic plug.

BLEEDING DIATHESIS IN UREMIA

Uremic bleeding caused by acquired platelet dysfunction is a major cause of morbidity and mortality in end-stage renal disease (ESRD) patients. The bleeding problems are characterized by abnormal prolongation of bleeding time and hemorrhagic symptoms, manifested usually as ecchymoses or petechiae in the skin, epistaxis, gastrointestinal or gingival oozing, or prolonged hemorrhage from needle puncture or postoperative sites. Hemorrhagic complications in ESRD patients may also be manifested as hemorrhagic pericarditis or hemorrhagic pleural effusion as well as intracranial, retroperitoneal, ocular, or uterine bleeding. The pathogenesis of platelet dysfunction in uremia is multifactorial (Fig. 80.3) and includes diminished adherence of platelets to vascular endothelium. In uremic patients, total platelet GpIb content is reduced, whereas the total content of GpIIb and GpIIIa is normal. Platelet membrane GpIb levels and GpIIb/IIIa expression have been described as normal, decreased, or increased in uremic platelets. Plasma vWF level is normal or elevated in uremia. However, the observation that the administration of agents that increase plasma vWF or the factor VIII:vWF complex results in a shortening of prolonged bleeding time and a transient reversal of bleeding tendency in uremia suggests abnormalities in vWF metabolism, structure, or function. Mean platelet vWF antigen is reduced in uremia. Some ESRD patients display a decrease in all components, especially those with high molecular weight in their platelet vWF multimer pattern.

A variety of circulating plasma proteases, such as plasmin, cleave α chain of platelet GpIb. The resulting proteolytic degradation product glycocalicin contains binding sites for thrombin and vWF. Elevated plasma glycocalicin levels in uremic patients may contribute to diminished binding of uremic platelets to subendothelium due to the vWF binding site of glycocalicin. Furthermore, glycocalicin contains the thrombin binding site of GpIb, which may also contribute to diminished platelet function in uremia.

Low GpIb expression on resting platelets obtained from patients with CKD correlates with the severity of impaired kidney function. However, GpIb expression in uremic platelets increases after stimulation. In contrast, GpIIb/IIIa expression on resting uremic platelets is normal but reduced after stimulation, indicating hyporesponsiveness of the uremic platelets.

The ability to bind both vWF and fibrinogen to glycoproteins is reduced in uremia because of a conformational change in the GpIIb/IIIa receptor. Improvement of fibrinogen binding to GpIIb/IIIa by hemodialysis (HD) treatment suggests that uremic toxins, such as methylguanidine, guanidinosuccinic acid, phenolic acid, and hydroxyphenylacetic acid, also contribute to platelet dysfunction. HD and peritoneal dialysis (PD) correct platelet abnormalities at least partly, because conventional dialysis therapy does not remove all uremic toxins effectively. Interactions between platelets and HD membranes may alter platelet membrane receptors for vWF and fibrinogen, thus preventing normal platelet–vessel wall and platelet-platelet interactions. This can be demonstrated by a more prolonged bleeding time, a more decreased platelet responsiveness to thrombin, and a decreased platelet agglutination in response to ristocetin immediately after the HD procedure. Thus, heparin administered during HD treatment is not alone responsible for the prolonged bleeding time immediately after HD. Platelet contact with the artificial surfaces may result in GpIb internalization, which may also occur during platelet activation.

Prostacyclin and nitric oxide (NO) inhibit platelet function, modulate vascular tone, and affect platelet–vessel wall interaction as well as platelet-platelet interaction. Uremic platelets generate

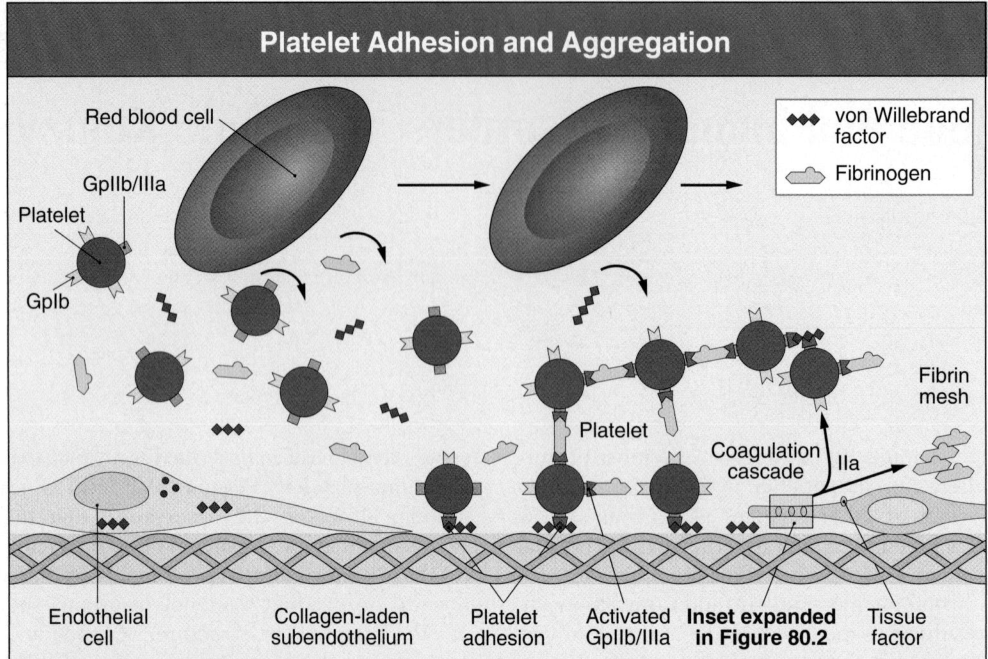

Figure 80.1 Platelet adhesion and aggregation. Platelets are pushed peripherally toward the vascular wall by red blood cells traversing centrally through the blood stream. Damage to the vessel wall results in a disruption of the nonthrombogenic endothelial cell lining and exposure of subendothelial structures. Whereas collagen supports initial platelet adhesion (and subsequent aggregation), von Willebrand factor (vWF) deposition on the subendothelium serves as the main anchor for platelet adhesion through platelet GpIb receptor. Postadhesion conformational change in platelet GpIIb/IIIa receptor (fibrinogen/vWF receptor) results in interlinking platelet aggregation.

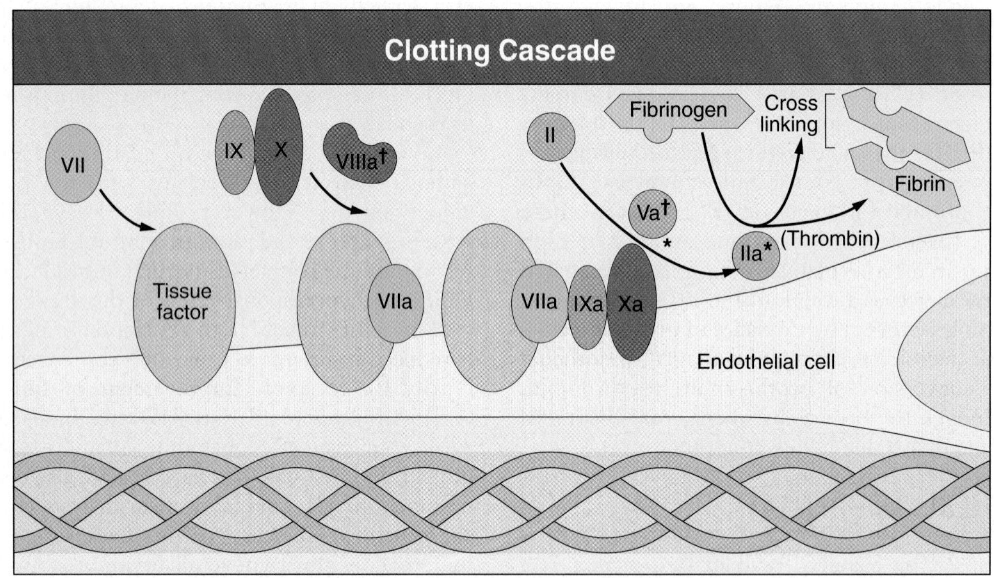

Figure 80.2 Clotting cascade. Expansion of the inset in Figure 80.1 shows the clotting cascade that takes place at the damaged vessel wall. Exposure of subendothelial tissue factor, present on pericytes and fibroblasts, allows eventual activation of prothrombin (factor II) to thrombin. Thrombin converts fibrinogen to fibrin, activates fibrin cross-linking, stimulates further platelet aggregation, and activates anticoagulant protein C. Naturally occurring anticoagulants antithrombin III, protein C, and protein S help maintain control and counterbalance on coagulation. *Site of anticoagulant effect for antithrombin III. †Site of anticoagulant effect for protein C–protein S complex.

more NO than platelets obtained from healthy subjects do. Uremic plasma induces NO synthesis in endothelial cells. Bleeding tendency in uremic patients is related to the increased platelet nitric oxide synthase (NOS) activity. The NOS substrate L-arginine inhibits platelet aggregation, whereas the NOS inhibitors N^G-monomethyl-L-arginine (L-NMMA) and N^G-nitro-L-arginine methyl ester (L-NAME) restore platelet adhesion and aggregation. Inhibition of NOS by L-NMMA restores the increased bleeding time in experimental uremia to normal.

Renal anemia is another determinant of the prolonged bleeding time in ESRD patients. Within the normal circulation, red blood cells increase platelet–vessel wall contact by displacing platelets away from the axial flow and toward the vessel wall. Red blood cells improve platelet function by releasing adenosine

Pathogenesis of Platelet Dysfunction in Uremia

Platelet abnormalities
- Alterations in membrane fluidity
- Reduction in intracellular ADP and serotonin
- Enhanced intracellular cAMP
- Impaired release of β-thromboglobulin and ATP
- Increased NO production
- Increased intracellular Ca^{2+} (due to secondary hyperparathyroidism)
- Abnormal mobilization of platelet Ca^{2+}
- Defective cyclooxygenase activity
- Reduced thromboxane A_2 generation
- Decreased platelet factor 3 availability
- Reduced total GPIb content (with increased glycocalixin formation)
- Reduced GPIIb/IIIa after stimulation
- Diminished responsiveness to platelet agonists
- Decreased clott retraction
- Aggregation abnormalities (mostly hyperaggregation)
- Abnormal platelet adherence

Uremic toxins

Anemia

vWf abnormalities

Vessel abnormalities

Drugs (β-lactam antibiotics, nonsteroidal anti-inflammatory drugs, antiplatelet agents)

Figure 80.3 Pathogenesis of platelet dysfunction in uremia. ADP, adenosine diphosphate; ATP, adenosine triphosphate; cAMP, cyclic adenosine monophosphate; NO, nitric oxide; vWF, von Willebrand factor.

diphosphate (ADP) and inactivating prostacyclin. Vasodilating effects of prostacyclin and NO increase vessel luminal diameter and decrease peripheral dispersion of platelets and their contact with the vessel wall. Erythropoiesis-stimulating agents (ESAs) improve platelet function mainly through increasing hematocrit.

However, ESAs can also enhance the risk for thrombotic events through an increase in blood viscosity. Platelet aggregation in uremia is increased by ESAs even at a dose that does not influence hematocrit by the release of young platelets to the blood. Low-dose ESA therapy also improves impaired platelet aggregation in uremia stimulated by ADP and ristocetin (for review, see reference 1).

The hemorrhage risk of ESRD patients is evaluated by the determination of the bleeding time. It is the most sensitive indicator of the extent of platelet dysfunction and measures primary platelet adhesion to the vessel wall and correlates with the abnormal platelet–vessel wall interaction that characterizes uremic bleeding. Bleeding times of more than 10 to 15 minutes have been associated with high risk of hemorrhage.

PLATELET NUMBER IN UREMIA

Thrombocytopenia is a common finding in ESRD patients. The platelet number is reduced in 16% to 55% of the uremic patients. However, the platelet count is rarely less than 80×10^9/l, a platelet number generally considered adequate for normal hemostasis. In HD patients, the interaction of blood with the HD membrane material may lead to complement activation and transient thrombocytopenia during the dialysis procedure. In contrast, thrombocytopenia does not occur with biocompatible non–complement-activating dialyzers. Heparin may induce antibody-mediated thrombocytopenia (see later discussion).

Reduced platelet half-life and low-normal platelet number in uremia suggest increased platelet turnover, which is reflected by an increased percentage of reticulated platelets. Healthy subjects have a mean of 2.77% ± 0.17% reticulated platelets; PD and HD patients have a significantly higher mean percentage of reticulated platelets of 6.92% ± 0.68% and 8.21% ± 0.36%, respectively. Shortened platelet survival in uremia may be the result of increased exposure of negatively charged phosphatidylserine. This signal is recognized by macrophages and promotes phagocytosis (for review, see reference 1).

CORRECTION OF UREMIC BLEEDING

The bleeding disorder of uremic patients has been classically defined as an acquired defect of primary hemostasis, characterized by prolongation of bleeding time. Several options are available to prevent or to treat uremic bleeding (Fig. 80.4).

Correction by Dialysis

Adequate dialysis (*Kt/V* >1.2 in HD and *Kt/V* >1.7 in PD patients) (see Chapters 90 and 92) and the use of biocompatible high-flux dialyzers in HD patients ameliorate prolonged bleeding times in ESRD patients and the risk of hemorrhagic complications, probably by removal of uremic plasma factors. Hemorrhagic problems are fewer with PD compared with HD. Deep tissue biopsies or invasive surgical procedures that require improved hemostasis should ideally be scheduled 12 to 24 hours after dialysis in HD patients. Residual anticoagulant effects last as long as 2½ hours with use of unfractionated heparin (UFH) during HD or even longer with low-molecular-weight heparin (LMWH). In case of clinical urgency or high risk of postoperative bleeding, heparin use should be minimized, eliminated (using predilutional saline), or replaced by regional anticoagulation with citrate during HD. Protamine sulfate administration (1 mg per 100 U of heparin infused during 10 minutes) should be considered if there is marked HD-induced prolongation of the partial thromboplastin time and severe bleeding.

Correction of Anemia

The use of ESAs has diminished hemorrhagic problems in uremic patients. Increased intraoperative bleeding complications have been reported in ESRD patients with low preoperative hematocrit levels (see Fig. 80.4). In ESRD patients, intraoperative transfusion of packed red blood cells may cause or aggravate hyperkalemia. If surgery is elective, ESAs (in combination with intravenous iron therapy) may be administered preoperatively to raise the hemoglobin to the upper acceptable values (12 g/dl). The maintenance dose of ESAs and the average time to reach target hemoglobin levels are highly variable from patient to patient. International guidelines recommend partial correction of renal anemia in CKD patients, targeting hemoglobin levels between 10 and 12 g/dl (hematocrit 30% to 36%; see Chapter 79). It remains to be clarified whether a patient prepared for surgery may have a benefit or risk in pushing hemoglobin levels even higher preoperatively.

ESA therapy improves uremic bleeding tendency by several mechanisms:

- Displacement of platelets closer to the vascular endothelium with the increase in circulating red blood cells

Treatment and Prevention of Uremic Bleeding

Treatment	Mechanism	Prescription	Dose	Onset of Action	Maximum Effect	Duration of Effect after Cessation
Dialysis	Removes uremic platelet receptor Allows re-expression of platelet vWF and fibrinogen receptors		Per *Kt/V*	Bleeding time may not improve immediately	Unknown	> 48 h
HD		Avoid surgery or biopsy immediately after HD	*Kt/V* > 1.2	Progressive improvement in bleeding time > 4 h after HD	Bleeding time returns to baseline > 16 h after HD	Until next HD
CAPD	Avoids platelet-dialyzer membrane interactions		*Kt/V* > 1.7	24 h	4–7 days	Unknown
Correct anemia (to a hematocrit 30%–36%)	Enhances platelet-vessel interaction	Transfusion of packed red blood cells Intravenous or subcutaneous epoetin	See Chapter 79	Immediate	To hematocrit 30%–36%	NA
Estrogen	Vasoconstriction: enhances platelet-vessel and platelet-platelet interaction	Intravenous, conjugated	0.6 mg/kg per day (3 mg total)	6 h	6 days	14 days
		Oral conjugated Topical (patch) estradiol	50 mg per day 50–100 mg patch q3.5/day	3-5 days 24–48 h	7 days 5–7 days	4 days unknown
DDAVP (arginine vasopressin; desmopressin)	Enhanced platelet adhesion by increasing vWF serum levels and vWF platelet receptors (GpIb).	Intravenous	0.3-0.4 μ/kg in 50 ml normal saline during 30 min	1 h		4-6 h
		Intranasal Subcutaneous	2–3 μg/kg 0.3 μg/kg	2 h	Unknown	Unknown
Cryoprecipitate	Enhances platelet adhesion by increasing vWF levels	Intravenous	10 U/30 min	1 h	4–8 h	24 h

Figure 80.4 Treatment and prevention of uremic bleeding. CAPD, continuous ambulatory peritoneal dialysis; HD, hemodialysis; vWF, von Willebrand factor.

- Increase in reticulated (metabolically active) platelets
- Increase in platelet aggregation
- Improvement of platelet signaling (and thereby better response to stimuli)
- Scavenging of NO by hemoglobin, resulting in increased platelet adhesion.[2]

Cryoprecipitate

Cryoprecipitate is a blood product rich in factor VII, vWF, and fibrinogen. In uremic patients at high risk of bleeding or with active bleeding, a beneficial effect of cryoprecipitate on bleeding time should occur within 4 to 12 hours. Disadvantages include the risk of exposure to various blood-borne pathogens and allergic reactions.[2]

Desmopressin

Desmopressin acetate (1-deamino-8-D-arginine-vasopressin, DDAVP) is a synthetic derivative of the antidiuretic hormone vasopressin. The compound has been shown to be useful in a variety of inherited and acquired hemorrhagic conditions, such as uremia, and in patients with hemostatic defects induced by therapeutic use of antiplatelet drugs, such as aspirin, dipyridamole, clopidogrel, or ticlopidine. Moreover, DDAVP shortens bleeding time and activated partial thromboplastin time (APTT) of patients receiving heparin. It is therefore helpful for the management of hemorrhagic complications during treatment with heparin. Desmopressin shortens the prolonged APTT and bleeding time by an increase in plasma levels of factor VIII and vWF. The increase in larger vWF–factor VIII multimers after infusion of DDAVP is associated with shortening of bleeding time. It also increases platelet GpIb expression.

Desmopressin is the most common agent used in uremic patients for bleeding disorders. The recommended doses range from 0.3 to 0.4 μg/kg administered intravenously in 50 ml normal saline during 20 to 30 minutes as a single infusion. Subcutaneous (0.3 μg/kg) or intranasal (2 to 3 μg/kg) routes of administration are also effective. One important advantage of DDAVP is its rapid onset of action in the setting of acute bleeding. Desmopressin decreases bleeding time within approximately 1 hour after administration. This advantage is important for CKD patients with prolonged bleeding time needing biopsies or major surgery. Disadvantages of DDAVP include tachyphylaxis caused by depletion of vWF from endothelial stores even after one single dose, headache, facial flushing, and rare thrombotic events. Because of the short duration of DDAVP activity (4 to 6 hours), bleeding time tends to return to baseline within

24 hours, indicating that patients are once again at risk of bleeding.[2]

Estrogens

Estrogens are still used for the treatment of uremic bleeding. The hormones decrease production of L-arginine, which is a precursor of NO, resulting in less production of cyclic guanosine monophosphate as well as in an increased production of thromboxane A_2, and ADP is crucial for the formation of platelet plugs. Estrogens may also decrease antithrombin III and protein S and increase factor VII concentrations, indicating that estrogens also display effects on coagulation factors.[2] The recommended dose of conjugated estrogens needed to improve bleeding time and clinical bleeding in uremia is 0.6 mg/kg intravenously during 30 to 40 minutes once daily for 5 consecutive days. The time to onset of action is about 6 hours; the maximum effect is evident at 5 to 7 days. Conjugated estrogens are effective for 14 to 21 days. Oral and transdermal estrogen therapy has also been shown to be beneficial.[2] Side effects include flushes, hypertension, and abnormal liver function test results.

Tranexamic Acid

Tranexamic acid is an antifibrinolytic drug. In the majority of patients with ESRD, bleeding time improves or normalizes within 6 days of treatment with tranexamic acid (20 to 25 mg/kg per day) administered intravenously or orally. Improvement of bleeding time was observed as soon as 24 to 48 hours after intake of tranexamic acid. If other treatment options do not elicit the desired response, tranexamic acid may be added to the regimen. For example, DDAVP and tranexamic acid have concomitantly been used to prevent or to treat bleeding in patients with CKD.

HEPARIN-INDUCED THROMBOCYTOPENIA

Heparin-induced thrombocytopenia (HIT) type II is a serious immune-mediated complication of heparin therapy. Thrombocytopenia (mean platelet number, 60,000/mm^3) due to platelet consumption usually occurs between 4 and 14 days after the administration of heparin and is associated with arterial ("white clot syndrome") and particularly venous thromboembolism in 20% to 50% of the cases. HIT type II should be considered whenever the platelet count falls by 50% in a patient receiving heparin. Even though these patients develop thrombocytopenia, the threat is not bleeding but thrombosis. Antibodies against the complex of heparin with platelet factor 4 are the cause of this devastating disease. These antibodies activate platelets in the presence of heparin.[3] A negative HIT antibody test result does not exclude the diagnosis of HIT type II syndrome; a positive antibody test result does not prove it.

In contrast, HIT type I presents with nonimmune mild transient decrease in the platelet count (rarely <100,000/mm^3) 1 to 4 days after initiation of heparin therapy. It occurs in 10% to 20% of patients without appreciable clinical consequences and usually resolves spontaneously even though heparin therapy is continued.

The diagnosis of HIT type II requires immediate substitution of heparin with an alternative anticoagulation for HD to prevent possible life-threatening complications. In addition, heparin skin ointments and heparin-coated catheters have to be avoided. The use of LMWH is also contraindicated because of a high rate of cross-reactivity once UFH has induced HIT antibody formation.

In a summary of six trials performed in HD patients,[4] a total of 21 patients were found to have a positive test result for the HIT antibody (2.6%); the percentage was lower with use of LMWH compared with UFH. Very few of the HD patients were noted to be thrombocytopenic (n = 6), and none had severe thrombotic complications. A recent survey reported a prevalence of 0.26 per 100 patients and an incidence of 0.32 per 100 patients of HIT type II syndrome in the U.K. HD population. Only 17% of the patients have had complications of HIT type II syndrome. Thirty-six percent of renal units used danaparoid as anticoagulant of choice for these patients.[5] In HIT type II patients, warfarin should not be used until the platelet count has recovered.[3]

Alternative Anticoagulation for Hemodialysis Patients with Heparin-Induced Thrombocytopenia Type II

Danaparoid

Danaparoid, a heparinoid of 5.5 kd, consists of heparan sulfate (83%), dermatan sulfate, and chondroitin sulfate. It is used as an alternative anticoagulant in HD patients with HIT type II in Canada and the European community. Danaparoid binds to antithrombin and heparin cofactor II. It inhibits factor Xa more selectively than LMWH does.[6] In 6.5% of patients with HIT, cross-reactivity against HIT antibodies may result in thrombocytopenia. For monitoring of danaparoid therapy, anti-Xa activity has to be measured. The half-life of the anti-Xa activity of danaparoid is 25 hours in patients with normal kidney function and is further prolonged in uremia. An antidote is not available.[6]

Lepirudin

Lepirudin is a recombinant hirudin preparation. It is mainly eliminated by the kidney. Thus, its half-life is markedly prolonged in patients with ESRD. After a single loading dose (0.1 mg/kg), therapeutic anticoagulation may persist for 1 week or even longer. Hirudin does not cross-react with HIT antibodies, but 44% to 74% of patients treated with hirudin for more than 5 days develop antihirudin antibodies. Antilepirudin antibodies are not necessarily associated with a decrease in efficacy. Only in 2% to 3% of patients with antilepirudin antibodies is an inhibitory effect seen, and dose adjustments are required. Target APTT is 1.5 to 2.5 times the normal value.[6,7]

Argatroban

Argatroban is a potent arginine-derived synthetic thrombin inhibitor. It is metabolized primarily by the liver. Its half-life is only moderately extended in patients with impaired kidney function. Argatroban does not cross-react with HIT antibodies. A loading dose of 250 μg/kg before HD and a maintenance dose of 1.7 to 3.3 μg/kg per minute are recommended. Target APTT of argatroban-treated HD patients is 1.5 to 3.0 times mean of normal range.[6]

In critically ill patients with HIT type II and necessity for continuous renal replacement therapy (CRRT) due to acute renal failure, critical illness scores such as the Acute Physiology and Chronic Health Evaluation (APACHE) II, the Simplified Acute Physiology Score (SAPS) II, and the indocyanine green plasma disappearance rate (ICG-PDR) can help predict the required argatroban maintenance dose for anticoagulation.[8] Argatroban dosing during CRRT in those patients is recommended as follows: the loading argatroban dose is 100 μg/kg followed by a maintenance infusion rate (μg/kg per minute), which is

- 2.15–0.06 × APACHE II (for APACHE II)
- 2.06–0.03 × SAPS II (for SAPS II)
- −0.35 + 0.08 × ICG-PDR (for ICG-PDR)

Fondaparinux

Fondaparinux, a fully synthetic pentasaccharide, is a selective factor Xa inhibitor. Its half-life is prolonged in patients with impaired kidney function, but it is safe. Subgroup analysis of the Fifth Organization to Assess Strategies in Acute Ischemic Syndromes (OASIS 5) showed that benefits of fondaparinux over enoxaparin (when it is administered for non–ST-segment elevation acute coronary syndrome) are most marked among patients with renal dysfunction (GFR <58 ml/min per 1.73 m^2) and are largely explained by lower rates of major bleeding with fondaparinux.[9] In addition, fondaparinux had significant benefit in decreasing the composite outcome of death, myocardial infarction, and refractory ischemia at day 30 in this population of patients. It is, however, not yet recommended for use in patients with HIT type II.

Regional Anticoagulation with Citrate

Citrate infused into the arterial line during HD inhibits the coagulation cascade in the extracorporeal circulation by the chelation of calcium and magnesium. The local deficit in ionized calcium is corrected by calcium substitution into the venous line before the blood is reinfused to the patient. In HD patients, regional citrate anticoagulation reduces bleeding complications and improves biocompatibility of dialysis membranes compared with systemic anticoagulation with UFH or LMWH (see also Chapter 89).

THROMBOTIC EVENTS IN UREMIA

Apart from a bleeding tendency, uremic patients also have a thrombophilic tendency and an increased incidence of thrombotic events. In dialysis patients, this frequently is manifested as thrombosis at the site of vascular access as well as in the coronary, cerebral, and retinal arteries. Thrombophilia is due to both platelet hyperaggregability and hypercoagulability.

Platelet Hyperaggregability

Binding of activated factor V to platelet surface–exposed phosphatidylserine induces coagulation. In uremic patients receiving murine monoclonal antibody to CD3 as prophylaxis for graft rejection, platelet procoagulant activity increases by binding of anti–factor V/Va as a result of increased exposure of anionic phospholipids in platelets.

Platelet activation also results in shape change, activation of surface receptors for fibrinogen and other adhesion proteins, and secretion of platelet factor 4, β-thromboglobin, thromboxane B_2, and serotonin as well as induction of procoagulant activity. In HD patients, a relationship between recurrent vascular access failure and increase in CD62P-positive platelets and an increase in fibrinogen receptor (PAC-1)–positive platelets has been demonstrated.

Chronically activated circulating platelets seen in ESRD patients interact with leukocytes and erythrocytes, resulting in platelet-erythrocyte aggregates and platelet-leukocyte aggregates. Platelet-erythrocyte aggregates enhance platelet reactivity, as detected by their thromboxane B_2 formation and release of β-thromboglobulin. Low levels of platelet-erythrocyte aggregates are found in healthy subjects (1.2% ± 0.1%). This percentage increases approximately 6-fold in ESRD patients but approximately 8- or 10-fold during HD. Platelet-leukocyte aggregates trigger neutrophil oxidative burst.

Platelets release small particles, so-called platelet microparticles (PMPs), after they are activated. PMPs expose procoagulant proteins such as tissue factor and contain a membrane receptor for coagulation factor V. In addition, PMPs provide a highly catalytic surface for the prothrombinase reaction due to high amounts of negatively charged phospholipids at the outer membrane. Significantly higher PMP counts were detected in predialysis patients and in patients undergoing regular PD or HD compared with healthy subjects.[3] The HD procedure does not affect PMP counts. However, rHuEPO therapy increases PMP release. Some studies suggest higher PMP counts in uremic patients with thrombotic events, but not all studies confirmed these findings (for review, see reference 1).

Hypercoagulability

Apart from enhanced platelet aggregability (see earlier discussion), hypercoagulability in uremic patients results from diminished protein C anticoagulant activity, deficient release of tissue plasminogen activator, and elevated plasma levels of antiphospholipid and anticardiolipin antibodies, anti–protein C and anti–protein S antibodies, factor VIII levels, prothrombin fragments 1 and 2, fibrinogen, homocysteine, and lipoprotein(a). ESRD patients suffer from thrombocytic complications as the result of changes in the secondary hemostasis and impaired fibrinolytic system activity. Antiphospholipid antibodies can trigger activation of the coagulation cascade at the endothelial surface. These antibodies cross-react with protein C and protein S, rendering them functionally deficient (see also Antiphospholipid Antibody Syndrome in Chapter 27). Reduced antithrombin III activity in uremia results in increased thrombin formation. Activated factor V (factor Va) serves as a cofactor for the conversion of prothrombin to thrombin. Its inactivation occurs by activated protein C. Heterozygosity for factor V Leiden mutation occurs in 2% to 5% of the Western population. Its prevalence is not increased in CKD patients, but factor V Leiden deficiency increases the risk of thrombotic complications.

Antiplatelet Agents in Patients with End-Stage Renal Disease

Antiplatelet agents may prevent vascular access thrombosis often seen in ESRD patients (see also Chapter 87). Small studies of aspirin and sulfinpyrazone, dipyridamole, or ticlopidine suggest effectiveness of these drugs in the prevention of vascular access thrombosis. However, antiplatelet agents may increase bleeding complications in ESRD patients with the well-known bleeding diathesis discussed before. In a prior randomized controlled trial of clopidogrel (75 mg/day) plus aspirin (375 mg/day) versus placebo in HD patients during a period of at least 2 years, there was no significant benefit of active treatment in the prevention of access thrombosis, but the cumulative incidence of bleeding events was significantly greater in the patients treated with clopidogrel plus aspirin.[10] Early failure of fistulas due to thrombosis or inadequate maturation is a common problem among patients treated with HD. Clopidogrel (loading dose of 300 mg followed by daily dose of 75 mg for 6 weeks starting within 1 day after fistula creation) has been shown to reduce the frequency of early thrombosis of new arteriovenous fistulas compared with placebo (12% versus 20%; RR, 0.6; $P = .02$).[11]

In patients with non–ST elevation acute coronary syndrome, clopidogrel treatment (loading dose of 300 mg followed by 75 mg daily) was beneficial in all patients, but impairment of kidney function increased the risk of major or life-threatening bleeding.[12] In patients undergoing an elective percutaneous coronary intervention of a single vessel or multiple vessels, clopidogrel treatment for 1 year markedly reduced death, myocardial infarction, and stroke compared with placebo in patients with normal kidney function (10% versus 4%; $P < .001$) but not in those with CKD stage 2 or above.[13] A *post hoc* analysis of the Clopidogrel for High Atherothrombotic Risk and Ischemic Stabilization, Management and Avoidance (CHARISMA) trial revealed that asymptomatic patients with diabetic nephropathy assigned to aspirin plus clopidogrel had significantly increased overall and cardiovascular mortality compared with those treated with aspirin and placebo. It was thus suggested that clopidogrel may be harmful in patients with diabetic nephropathy.[14]

Because antiplatelet agents such as aspirin, dipyridamole, clopidogrel, and ticlopidine increase bleeding time, these drugs should not be given within at least 72 hours before biopsies and major surgery. Other drugs that may increase the risk of intraoperative bleeding in uremic patients include β-lactam antibiotics, nonsteroidal anti-inflammatory drugs, and diphenhydramine.

Anticoagulant Therapy in Patients with End-Stage Renal Disease

Approximately 6% of ESRD patients at risk of thrombosis or thromboembolic events may have an indication for oral anticoagulants. However, these indications are usually by extrapolation from patients without CKD or mild CKD at best. Vitamin K antagonism (e.g., by warfarin or other coumarins) in dialysis patients is associated with a marked increase in the frequency of hemorrhages. Moreover, vitamin K antagonists in the dialysis population contribute to vascular and valvular calcifications.[15] Thus, the value of long-term vitamin K antagonism, for example, in dialysis patients with atrial fibrillation, is currently not well established. Management of warfarin is challenging in patients with CKD because warfarin dose, anticoagulation control, and risk for hemorrhagic complications are influenced not only by genetic factors (such as the genes for cytochrome P-450 2C9 and vitamin K epoxide reductase complex 1) as in each patient population but also by the kidney function. Patients with stage 4 or stage 5 CKD require significantly lower warfarin dosages, spend less time with their international normalized ratio (INR) within the target range of 2 to 3, and are at a higher risk for overanticoagulation (INR >4) compared with patients with no, mild, or moderate CKD.[16] These problems may even be aggravated in ESRD patients and particularly in those undergoing regular dialysis treatment.

With regard to the high risk of stroke in ESRD patients with atrial fibrillation and the conflicting data about oral anticoagulation, an individualized approach based on the Cardiac Failure, Hypertension, Age, Diabetes, and Stroke ($CHADS_2$) score, on the one hand, and the Outcome Bleeding Risk Index has been recommended.[17] In other words, ESRD patients with atrial fibrillation and a high risk of ischemic stroke but low risk for bleeding events should receive oral anticoagulants, whereas ESRD patients with atrial fibrillation and a low or moderate risk for stroke but high risk for bleeding complications should probably not be treated with oral anticoagulants.[18]

Standard oral anticoagulation with an INR between 2 and 3 is not sufficient to prevent clotting during HD. Additional low-dose LMWH or UFH is needed to facilitate adequate extracorporeal treatment.

IMMUNE DYSFUNCTION IN UREMIA

Uremia-related immune dysfunction is a complex interaction between alterations in both the innate and adaptive immune systems. In uremic patients, immune activation, characterized by elevated cytokine levels and acute-phase response, and immunosuppression, characterized by impaired responses to infections and poor development of adaptive immunity, coexist.

Pathogenesis

Immunosuppression

Altered Function of Polymorphonuclear Leukocytes ESRD is characterized by deranged functions of polymorphonuclear leukocytes. Polymorphonuclear leukocytes are cells of the first-line nonspecific immune defense and migrate to the site of infection along a chemotactic gradient. Polymorphonuclear leukocytes ingest the invading microorganisms by phagocytosis and kill them with proteolytic enzymes and toxic radicals produced during the oxidative burst. Disturbances of any essential polymorphonuclear leukocyte function increase the risk for infectious complications.[19]

Uremic toxins have been isolated from the ultrafiltrate of HD patients or the dialysis effluent of PD patients that inhibit specific neutrophil responses *in vitro*. Among these are soluble low- and high-molecular-weight molecules, including granulocyte inhibitory proteins with homology to immunoglobulin light chains and β_2-microglobulin, monomers and dimers of free immunoglobulin light chains, angiogenin, complement factor D, ubiquitin, advanced glycation end products, retinol-binding protein, leptin, and resistin. These molecules have been found to interfere with polymorphonuclear leukocyte and lymphocyte functions, including reduced chemotaxis, adherence, oxidative burst activity in response to phagocytosis, and intracellular killing of bacteria.[19] Advanced glycation end products are formed by the reaction of aldehyde or ketone groups of carbohydrates with amino acids. Accumulation of advanced glycation end products in uremia promotes inflammation but also immune dysfunction by the modulation of polymorphonuclear leukocyte apoptosis. Polyclonal free immunoglobulin light chains are usually excreted in the urine and thus accumulate in the serum of patients with progressive CKD. Monomers and dimers of free immunoglobulin light chains isolated from uremic patients inhibit stimulated glucose uptake (a measurement of the state of activation of phagocytic cells) and polymorphonuclear leukocyte chemotaxis. Free immunoglobulin light chains attenuate polymorphonuclear leukocyte apoptosis, contributing to preactivation of polymorphonuclear leukocytes and interfering with normal resolution of inflammation. By these mechanisms, polyclonal free immunoglobulin light chains contribute to the chronic inflammatory state seen in uremia. HD with newer, high cutoff dialyzers allows removal of large amounts of free immunoglobulin light chains, but the effect on polymorphonuclear leukocyte function and infections in HD patients remains unknown at present.

Immunologic functions in uremic patients are compromised by three different mechanisms targeting polymorphonuclear leukocytes[20]: inhibition, pre-activation, and priming. Inhibition of immune cells on stimulation reflects diminished immune responses leading to infections or impairing the resolution of infectious complications. Priming of immune cells is an important physiologic mechanism controlling host defense responses. During priming of leukocytes by a primary agent such as oxidants, the functional response to a stimulus is amplified. Pre-activation of leukocytes in uremia reflects enhanced polymorphonuclear leukocyte activity under basal conditions but does not allow adequate response to a stimulus.

Dendritic Cell Function Uremia impairs blood dendritic cell function,[21] a factor likely to contribute to the higher rates of infectious complications observed in these patients. Dendritic cells are antigen-presenting cells that coordinate both innate and adaptive immunity. The subsets of circulating dendritic cell precursors derived from CD34$^+$ bone marrow hematopoietic progenitor cells in the peripheral blood include precursor myeloid dendritic cells and precursor plasmacytoid dendritic cells. Precursor myeloid dendritic cells are immunosurveillant cells, and precursor plasmacytoid dendritic cells are critical in antiviral and possibly antitumor immunity. Isolated myeloid dendritic cells and plasmacytoid dendritic cells from HD patients are functionally impaired *in vitro* with reduced cell surface costimulatory molecule expression and interferon-α production after appropriate stimulation. Myeloid dendritic cells incubated with uremic sera demonstrate impaired maturation and decreased allostimulatory capacity. Similarly, herpes virus–stimulated plasmacytoid dendritic cells incubated with uremic sera produced significantly less interferon-α compared with dendritic cells incubated in the control media. Improving clearance of small-molecular-weight uremic toxins by use of a more efficient dialysis membrane improved myeloid dendritic cell function but not plasmacytoid dendritic cell function. Thus, the immunodeficiency of HD patients is at least partially due to dialyzable uremic toxins.[21] These data are in agreement with previous observations that HD patients exhibit significantly lower polymorphonuclear leukocyte killing than healthy subjects do and that HD treatment can partially improve this.

Immune Stimulation

Chronic Stimulation of the Inflammatory Response Chronic stimulation of the inflammatory response in uremia results from uremic toxins plus dialysis-related factors (such as interaction between blood and the dialyzer membrane, presence of endotoxins in the dialysate), access-related infection, periodontal disease, other chronic infections (e.g., nasal sinuses), and peritoneal dialysis solution (high glucose concentration, low pH, and presence of glucose degradation products). Vitamin D and calcitriol deficiency is a common finding in patients with CKD stages 3 to 5 (see Chapter 81). Pleiotropic effects of activated vitamin D and its analogues include a role of this hormone as a potent immunomodulator. The link between Toll-like receptors (TLRs) and vitamin D–mediated innate immunity suggests that differences in the ability of human populations to produce vitamin D may contribute to susceptibility to microbial infection. TLR activation in human macrophages upregulates expression of the vitamin D receptor and the vitamin D 1-hydroxylase genes, leading to induction of the antimicrobial peptide cathelicidin. Patients with low 25-hydroxyvitamin D are inefficient in supporting cathelicidin messenger RNA induction.[22] However, controlled randomized studies are needed to clarify the role of vitamin D deficiency and its correction for impaired host deficiency in uremia.

Infections in Patients with Chronic Kidney Disease

Infections are the main reason for hospitalization and the second common cause of death in ESRD patients. In addition, dialysis patients exhibit a higher annual mortality rate caused by sepsis compared with the general population. An increased risk of blood stream infection is also observed in older adults with non–dialysis-dependent CKD stages 4 and 5.[23] Infections develop primarily as a consequence of deranged functions of polymorphonuclear leukocytes (see earlier discussion). Other factors predisposing to infections include an inadequate response to vaccinations as a consequence of a deficient T lymphocyte–dependent immune response[20] and an impairment of blood dendritic cell function.[21] A variety of additional factors, such as the accumulation of uremic toxins, iron overload, renal anemia, dialyzer bioincompatibility, vascular access–related infections, or vitamin D deficiency of ESRD patients, may also contribute to infections.[19]

VACCINATION IN PATIENTS WITH CHRONIC KIDNEY DISEASE

Hepatitis B Virus

Blood is a major vehicle for the transmission of the hepatitis B virus (HBV). Therefore, patients undergoing regular HD are at particularly high risk of exposure to HBV infection, with a wide variation in endemicity between the countries. In addition, immunodeficiency renders patients with ESRD susceptible to infection and subsequent disease. Uremia impairs not only the clearance of the virus but also antigen presentation, T-cell activation, and subsequent antibody production. Thus, responses to HBV vaccination range from 50% to 90% in this population of patients. HBV vaccination (Fig. 80.5) is recommended for all predialysis and dialysis patients, but the seroconversion rate (anti-HBs>10 IU/l) and adequate responses (anti-HBs>100 IU/l) are markedly lower, quite variable, and shorter lasting than in healthy immunocompetent subjects. Therefore, patients with CKD should undergo vaccination in the early stages of the disease when the primary immune response is still intact. Reasons for poor response to HBV vaccination in ESRD patients include cellular immunodeficiency, dialysis inadequacy, inflammation, malnutrition, diabetes mellitus, and older age.

Careful monitoring of antibody titers and booster doses are necessary to maintain protection against HBV. A cutoff of 100 IU/l is considered a necessary threshold for maintaining protection in immunocompromised patients. A study confirmed that seroprotection rates decrease rapidly over time in HD patients. It also documented, however, better persistence of circulating anti-HBs antibodies up to 42 months after primary vaccination with HBV-AS04 (HBV vaccine formulated with a new adjuvant system) compared with standard HBV vaccine (78% versus 51%). No difference in seroprotection rates was observed in the two groups 1 month after completion of the immunization course (92% versus 87%) or at month 12 and month 24, whereas it became significant at month 30 (85% versus 63%).[24]

Different approaches have been used to overcome the nonresponsiveness of chronically uremic patients, such as the intra-

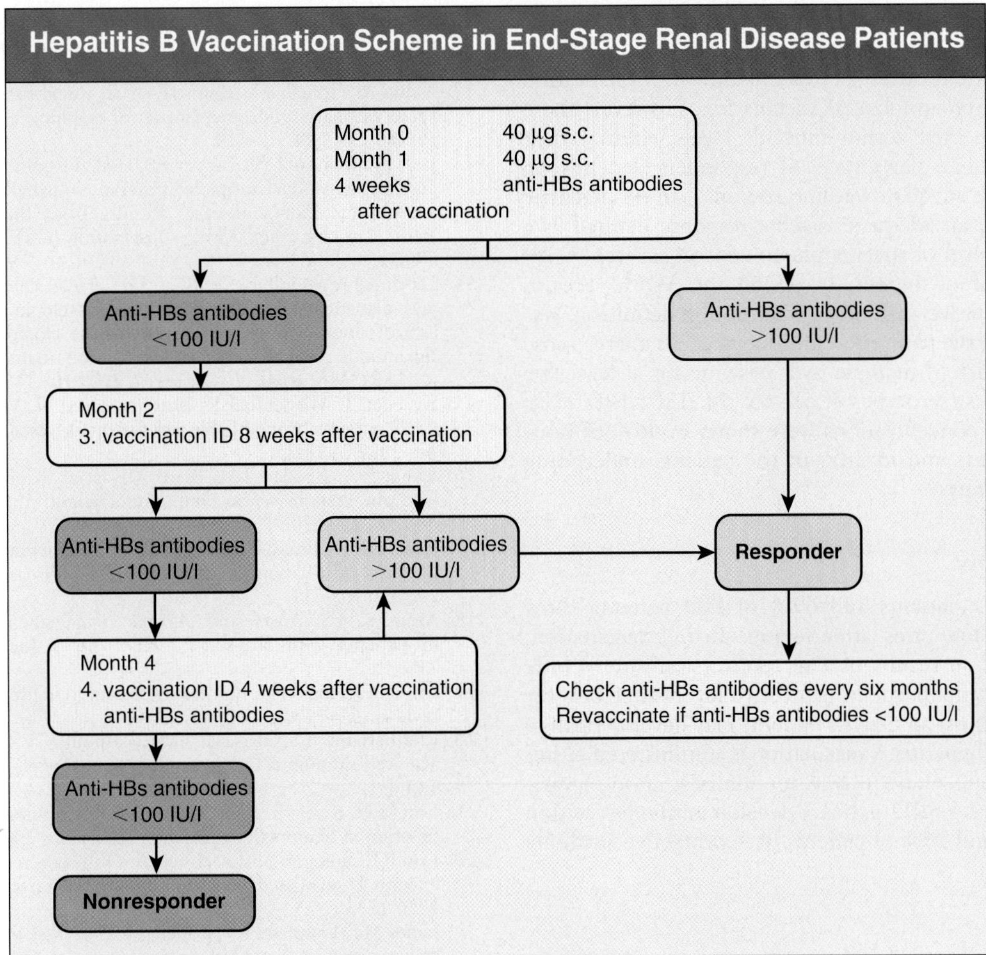

Figure 80.5 Hepatitis B vaccination scheme in end-stage renal disease patients. All patients receive three doses of hepatitis B vaccine, 40 µg subcutaneously. An additional dose is given if anti-HBs antibody response is less than 100 IU/l.

muscular administration of multiple doses or double doses, the coadministration of immunomodulators, and the intradermal administration of HBV vaccine. In a prospective open-label randomized controlled trial, HD patients nonresponsive to primary HBV vaccination were revaccinated with either intradermal (5 µg of vaccine every week for 8 weeks) or intramuscular (40 µg of vaccine at weeks 1 and 8) HBV vaccine. Seroconversion rates were 79% intradermally but only 40% intramuscularly (P = .002). There was also a trend toward longer duration of seroprotection with intradermal vaccination. It was concluded that intradermal vaccination should become the standard of care in this setting. However, it remains unclear whether the greater efficacy of intradermal vaccination is the cumulative effect of multiple injections or route of administration.[25]

A variety of studies have demonstrated that granulocyte-macrophage colony-stimulating factor (GM-CSF) may be an effective adjuvant to HBV vaccine response in HD patients. GM-CSF induced a significant effect in terms of response rate and achievement of an earlier seroconversion to the vaccine in the overall populations examined, in renal failure patients, and in healthy subjects.[26] Because GM-CSF primarily acts on monocytes and dendritic cells, it may be reasonable to assume a direct effect of GM-CSF on antigen-presenting cells including dendritic cells to overcome dysfunctional antigen presentation/costimulation and overall cellular function[21] that leads to impaired antibody responses after HBV vaccination.

Influenza Virus

Chronic dialysis patients benefit from influenza vaccination in reducing mortality and hospitalization rate. Response to such a vaccination has been reported to be suboptimal or normal. A first vaccination of HD patients with the influenza vaccine was followed by protective hemagglutination antibody titers (≥1:40) in 95% of the vaccinees 1 month after vaccination. A booster dose of influenza vaccine did not improve the humoral response in this population of patients.[27] In 201 long-term HD patients and 41 healthy volunteers, the immunogenicity of a standard trivalent inactivated influenza vaccine was evaluated.[28] More than 80% of HD patients showed seroprotection 1 month after vaccination. Their immune response was not different from that of healthy volunteers. High serum ferritin level was the only parameter independently associated with a better vaccination-induced antibody response in HD patients, whereas nutrition, inflammation, and dialysis adequacy did not have a significant impact. Therefore, the clinical relevance of disturbances in acquired immunity in contemporary HD patients was questioned.[28]

Pneumococcus

HD patients and patients after successful kidney transplantation respond well to antipneumococcal vaccination. However, these patients rapidly lose their serum antibody levels within 1 year after vaccination.[29] The percentage of responders depends on the definition of the adequate vaccine response. In 48 pediatric patients with CKD, an adequate vaccine response defined as a postimmunization level of specific pneumococcal serotype antibody of 0.35 μg/ml or higher, based on the World Health Organization's protective antibody concentration definition, was obtained in 100% of the patients. If an adequate vaccine response was defined as a fourfold increase over baseline for at least five of the seven antigens (serotypes 4, 6B, 9V, 14, 18C, 19F, 23F), protective antibody concentrations were found in 46% of nondialysis CKD patients and in 38% of the patients undergoing regular dialysis therapy.[30]

Other Vaccinations

Only 55% of CKD patients and 69% of HD patients show normal seroconversion rates after tetanus toxoid vaccination. Diphtheria vaccination results in a seroconversion rate of only 37%, and 33% of patients retain protective levels after booster administration.[31] Almost all dialysis patients may develop protective antibodies after hepatitis A vaccination is administered either intramuscularly or subcutaneously. After administration of varicella vaccine, 85% of ESRD patients develop antibodies within the first 6 months, and 76% of patients have protective antibody titer at 1 year.

REFERENCES

1. Hörl WH. Thrombozytopathie und Blutungskomplikationen bei Urämie [Thrombocytopathy and blood complications in uremia]. *Wien Klin Wochenschr*. 2006;118:134-150.
2. Hedges SJ, Dehoney SB, Hooper JS, et al. Evidence-based treatment recommendations for uremic bleeding. *Nat Clin Pract Nephrol*. 2007;3: 138-153.
3. Ahmed I, Majeed A, Powell R. Heparin induced thrombocytopenia: Diagnosis and management update. *Postgrad Med J*. 2007;83:575-582.
4. Reilly RF. The pathophysiology of immune-mediated heparin-induced thrombocytopenia. *Semin Dial*. 2003;16:54-60.
5. Hutchinson CA, Dasgupta I. National survey of hepatic-induced thrombocytopenia in the haemodialysis population of the UK population. *Nephrol Dial Transplant*. 2007;22:1680-1684.
6. Fischer KG. Essentials of anticoagulation in hemodialysis. *Hemodial Int*. 2007;11:178-189.
7. Greinacher A, Warkentin TE. The direct thrombin inhibitor hirudin. *Thromb Haemost*. 2008;99:819-829.
8. Link A, Girndt M, Selejan S, et al. Argatroban for anticoagulation in continuous renal replacement therapy. *Crit Care Med*. 2009;37: 105-110.
9. Fox KA, Bassand JP, Mehta SR, et al. Influence of renal function on the efficacy and safety of fondaparinux relative to enoxaparin in non ST-segment elevation acute coronary syndromes. *Ann Intern Med*. 2007;147:304-310.
10. Kaufman JS, O'Connor TZ, Zhang JH, et al. Randomized controlled trial of clopidogrel plus aspirin to prevent hemodialysis access graft thrombosis. *J Am Soc Nephrol*. 2003;14:2313-2321.
11. Dember LM, Beck GJ, Allon M, et al. Effect of clopidogrel on early failure of arteriovenous fistulas for hemodialysis: A randomized controlled trial. *JAMA*. 2008;299:2164-2171.
12. Keltai M, Tonelli M, Mann JF, et al. Renal function and outcomes in acute coronary syndrome: Impact of clopidogrel. *Eur J Cardiovasc Prev Rehabil*. 2007;14:312-318.
13. Best PJ, Steinhubl SR, Berger PB, et al. The efficacy and safety of short- and long-term dual antiplatelet therapy in patients with mild or moderate chronic kidney disease: Results from the Clopidogrel for the Reduction of Events During Observation (CREDO) trial. *Am Heart J*. 2008;155:687-693.
14. Dasgupta A, Steinhubl SR, Bhatt DL, et al. Clinical outcomes of patients with diabetic nephropathy randomized to clopidogrel plus aspirin versus aspirin alone (a post hoc analysis of the clopidogrel for high atherothrombotic risk and ischemic stabilization, management, and avoidance [CHARISMA] trial). *Am J Cardiol*. 2009;103:1359-1363.
15. Krueger T, Westenfeld R, Ketteler M, et al. Vitamin K deficiency in CKD patients: A modifiable risk factor for vascular calcification? *Kidney Int*. 2009;76:18-22.
16. Limdi NA, Beasley TM, Baird MF, et al. Kidney function influences warfarin responsiveness and hemorrhagic complications. *J Am Soc Nephrol*. 2009;20:912-921.
17. Reinecke H, Brand E, Mesters R, et al. Dilemmas in the management of atrial fibrillation in chronic kidney disease. *J Am Soc Nephrol*. 2009;20:705-711.
18. Aronow WS. Acute and chronic management of atrial fibrillation in patients with late-stage CKD. *Am J Kidney Dis*. 2009;53:701-710.
19. Cohen G, Hörl WH. Immune dysfunction in uremia: An update [invited review]. *Blood Purif*. in press.
20. Eleftheriadis T, Antoniadi G, Liakopoulos V, et al. Disturbances of acquired immunity in hemodialysis patients. *Semin Dial*. 2007;20: 440-451.
21. Lim WH, Kireta S, Russ GR, et al. Uremia impairs blood dendritic cell function in hemodialysis patients. *Kidney Int*. 2007;71:1122-1131.
22. Liu PT, Stenger S, Li H, et al. Toll-like receptor triggering of a vitamin D–mediated human antimicrobial response. *Science*. 2006;311: 1770-1773.
23. James MT, Laupland KB, Tonelli M, et al. Risk of bloodstream infection in patients with chronic kidney disease not treated with dialysis. *Arch Intern Med*. 2008;168:2333-2339.
24. Kong NC, Beran J, Kee SA, et al. A new adjuvant improves the immune response to hepatitis B vaccine in hemodialysis patients. *Kidney Int*. 2008;73:856-862.
25. Barraclough KA, Wiggins KJ, Hawley CM, et al. Intradermal versus intramuscular hepatitis B vaccination in hemodialysis patients: A prospective open-label randomized controlled trial in nonresponders to primary vaccination. *Am J Kidney Dis*. 2009;54:95-103.
26. Cruciani M, Mengoli C, Serpelloni G, et al. Granulocyte macrophage colony-stimulating factor as an adjuvant for hepatitis B vaccination: A meta-analysis. *Vaccine*. 2007;25:709-718.
27. Tanzi E, Amendola A, Pariani E, et al. Lack of effect of a booster dose of influenza vaccine in hemodialysis patients. *J Med Virol*. 2007;79: 1176-1179.
28. Scharpé J, Peetermans WE, Vanwalleghem J, et al. Immunogenicity of a standard trivalent influenza vaccine in patients on long-term hemodialysis: An open-label trial. *Am J Kidney Dis*. 2009;54:77-85.
29. Pourfarziani V, Ramezani MB, Taheri S, et al. Immunogenicity of pneumococcal vaccination in renal transplant recipients and hemodialysis patients: A comparative controlled trial. *Ann Transplant*. 2008;13: 43-47.
30. Vieira S, Baldacci ER, Carneiro-Sampaio M, et al. Evaluation of antibody response to the heptavalent pneumococcal conjugate vaccine in pediatric chronic kidney disease. *Pediatr Nephrol*. 2009;24:83-89.
31. Dinits-Pensy M, Forrest GN, Cross AS, et al. The use of vaccines in adult patients with renal disease. *Am J Kidney Dis*. 2005;46:997-1011.

CHAPTER 81

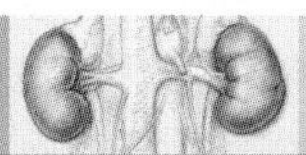

Bone and Mineral Metabolism in Chronic Kidney Disease

Kevin J. Martin, Jürgen Floege, Markus Ketteler

DEFINITION

Disturbances of mineral metabolism are common if not ubiquitous during the course of chronic kidney disease (CKD) and lead to serious and debilitating complications unless these abnormalities are addressed and treated. The spectrum of disorders includes abnormal concentrations of serum calcium, phosphate, and magnesium and disorders of parathyroid hormone (PTH) and vitamin D metabolism. These abnormalities as well as other factors related to the uremic state affect the skeleton and result in the complex disorders of bone known as renal osteodystrophy; it is now recommended that this term be used exclusively to define the bone disease associated with CKD. The clinical, biochemical, and imaging abnormalities heretofore identified as correlates of renal osteodystrophy should be defined more broadly as a clinical entity or syndrome called chronic kidney disease–mineral and bone disorder (CKD-MBD).[1] The spectrum of skeletal abnormalities seen in renal osteodystrophy (Fig. 81.1) includes the following:

- Osteitis fibrosa, a manifestation of hyperparathyroidism characterized by increased osteoclast and osteoblast activity, peritrabecular fibrosis, and increased bone turnover.
- Osteomalacia, a manifestation of defective mineralization of newly formed osteoid most often caused by aluminum deposition; bone turnover is decreased.
- Adynamic bone disease, a condition characterized by abnormally low bone turnover.
- Osteopenia or osteoporosis.
- Combinations of these abnormalities termed mixed renal osteodystrophy.
- Other abnormalities with skeletal manifestations (e.g., chronic acidosis, β_2-microglobulin amyloidosis).

EPIDEMIOLOGY

The prevalence of the various types of renal bone disease in patients with end-stage renal disease (ESRD) is illustrated in Figure 81.2.[2] In patients on hemodialysis, osteitis fibrosa and adynamic bone disease now occur with almost equal frequency. In contrast, in patients on peritoneal dialysis, the adynamic bone lesion predominates. Osteomalacia represents only a small fraction of cases in either group but is more common in certain ethnic groups, particularly Indo-Asians. The abnormalities of the skeleton start relatively early in the course of CKD.

PATHOGENESIS

Several biochemical and hormonal abnormalities that are encountered during the course of CKD contribute to renal bone disease and can be affected by efforts at prevention and therapy. The major factors that are operative in early CKD may vary as CKD progresses. Similarly, the predominance of one particular pathogenetic mechanism over another may contribute to the heterogeneity of bone disorders. We therefore discuss separately the two major entities, namely, high- and low-turnover osteodystrophy.

Osteitis Fibrosa: Hyperparathyroidism: High-Turnover Renal Bone Disease

Elevated levels of PTH in blood and hyperplasia of the parathyroid glands are seen early in CKD. Whereas the level of free (i.e., non–protein bound) calcium in blood is normally the principal determinant of PTH secretion, during the course of CKD, several metabolic disturbances also alter the regulation of the secretion of PTH.

Abnormalities of Calcium Metabolism

There are three main body pools of calcium: the bony skeleton (mineral component), the intracellular pool (mostly protein bound), and the extracellular pool (see Chapter 10). The calcium in the extracellular pool is in continuous exchange with that of bone and cells and is altered by diet and excretion. Calcium metabolism depends on the close interaction of two hormonal systems: PTH and vitamin D. Perturbations of both of these systems occur during the course of CKD, with adverse consequences on the skeleton. Total serum calcium tends to decrease during the course of CKD as a result of phosphate retention and decreased production of 1,25-dihydroxyvitamin D (calcitriol) from the kidney, decreased intestinal calcium absorption, and skeletal resistance to the calcemic action of PTH, but the levels of free calcium remain within the normal range in most patients (Fig. 81.3)[3] as a result of compensatory hyperparathyroidism. Because calcium is a major regulator of PTH secretion, persistent hypocalcemia is a powerful stimulus for the development of hyperparathyroidism and also contributes to parathyroid growth.

Abnormalities of Phosphate Metabolism

With progressive CKD, phosphate is retained by the kidney. However, hyperphosphatemia usually does not become evident before CKD stage 4. Until then, compensatory hyperparathyroidism and increases in circulating fibroblast growth factor 23 (FGF-23) result in increased phosphaturia, maintaining serum phosphate levels in the normal range.[4]

One mechanism by which phosphate retention may lead to hyperparathyroidism (Fig. 81.4) is by a decrease in serum free calcium, which in turn stimulates the secretion of PTH. Thus, a new steady state is achieved in which serum phosphate is restored to normal at the expense of a sustained high level of PTH. This cycle is repeated as renal function declines until

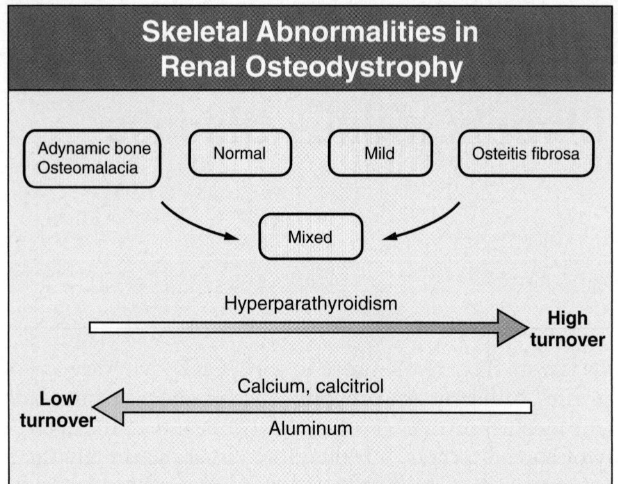

Figure 81.1 The spectrum of renal osteodystrophy. The range of skeletal abnormalities in renal bone disease encompasses syndromes with both high and low bone turnover.

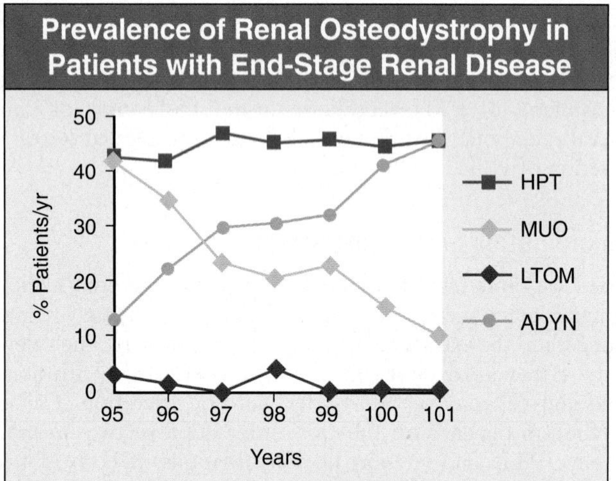

Figure 81.2 Prevalence of renal osteodystrophy in patients with end-stage renal disease. HPT, high-turnover renal osteodystrophy; MUO, mixed uremic osteodystrophy; LTOM, low-turnover osteomalacia; ADYN, adynamic bone disease. *(From reference 37.)*

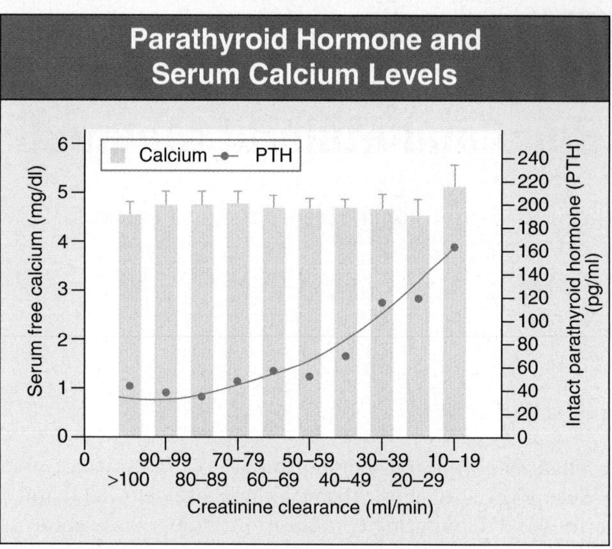

Figure 81.3 Ionized calcium and parathyroid hormone (PTH) levels in chronic renal failure. Levels of ionized calcium are maintained in advancing renal failure by progressive increases in PTH.

sustained and severe hyperparathyroidism is present. Second, phosphate retention leads to decreased production of calcitriol by the kidney, either directly or by increasing the levels of FGF-23 (which decreases the activity of 1α-hydroxylase). The decrease in calcitriol allows increases in PTH gene transcription by direct action and also decreases intestinal calcium absorption, leading to hypocalcemia, which in turn stimulates PTH secretion. Third, hyperphosphatemia is associated with resistance to the actions of calcitriol in the parathyroid glands, which also favors the development of hyperparathyroidism and also induces resistance to the actions of PTH in bone. Finally, phosphate *per se* appears to affect PTH secretion independently of changes in serum calcium or serum calcitriol.[5,6] Phosphate may also have an effect on parathyroid growth independent of serum calcium.[7,8] Regardless of the mechanism by which phosphate retention causes hyperparathyroidism, restriction of dietary phosphate in proportion to the decrease in glomerular filtration rate (GFR) can prevent the development of hyperparathyroidism. Current evidence suggests that FGF-23 also acts directly on the parathyroid gland and has inhibitory effects on PTH secretion and parathyroid growth.[9,10] This would suggest that the main effects of FGF-23 on the pathogenesis of hyperparathyroidism appear to be indirect as a result of the potent effect of FGF-23 to decrease calcitriol production. These various actions may explain the association of the levels of FGF-23 with patient outcome.[11]

Abnormalities of Vitamin D Metabolism

The conversion of 25-hydroxyvitamin D to its active metabolite 1,25-dihydroxyvitamin D occurs mainly in the kidney by the enzyme 1α-hydroxylase. Extrarenal production of calcitriol also occurs and contributes to the circulating levels of calcitriol. Renal calcitriol production progressively declines during the course of CKD as a result of several mechanisms (Fig. 81.5).

Calcitriol production is compromised in the setting of CKD by a reduction in 25-hydroxyvitamin D levels[12] and the decrease in GFR, which further limits the delivery of 25-hydroxyvitamin D to the site of the 1α-hydroxylase in the proximal tubule. Phosphate retention either directly or by inducing an increase in FGF-23 also decreases the activity of 1α-hydroxylase. Finally, it appears that circulating PTH fragments may also directly decrease calcitriol production. The resultant decreased levels of calcitriol contribute to the pathogenesis of hyperparathyroidism by several direct and indirect mechanisms (Fig. 81.6). Low levels of calcitriol directly release the gene for PTH from suppression by the vitamin D receptor and allow increased PTH secretion. In many tissues, vitamin D regulates its own receptor by positive feedback; the vitamin D receptor content is decreased in parathyroid tissue in CKD. Administration of calcitriol has been shown to increase the vitamin D receptor content in the parathyroid glands coincident with the suppression of PTH secretion. Studies *in vitro* have shown that calcitriol is a negative growth regulator of parathyroid cells; therefore, calcitriol deficiency in CKD may facilitate parathyroid cell proliferation. Other direct consequences of low levels of calcitriol that contribute to the pathogenesis of secondary hyperparathyroidism include increasing the parathyroid set point for calcium-regulated PTH secretion and, possibly, decreasing the expression of calcium receptors.

Low levels of calcitriol may also promote the development of hyperparathyroidism indirectly. First, decreased calcitriol

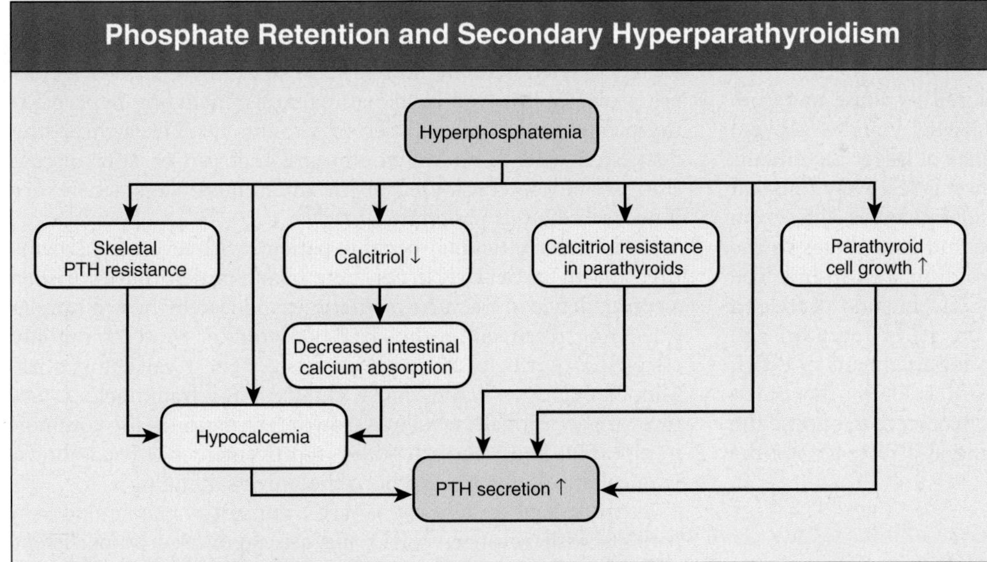

Figure 81.4 Role of phosphate retention in the pathogenesis of secondary hyperparathyroidism. Hyperphosphatemia stimulates parathyroid hormone (PTH) secretion indirectly by inducing hypocalcemia, skeletal resistance to PTH, low levels of calcitriol, and calcitriol resistance. Hyperphosphatemia also has direct effects on the parathyroid gland to increase PTH secretion and parathyroid cell growth.

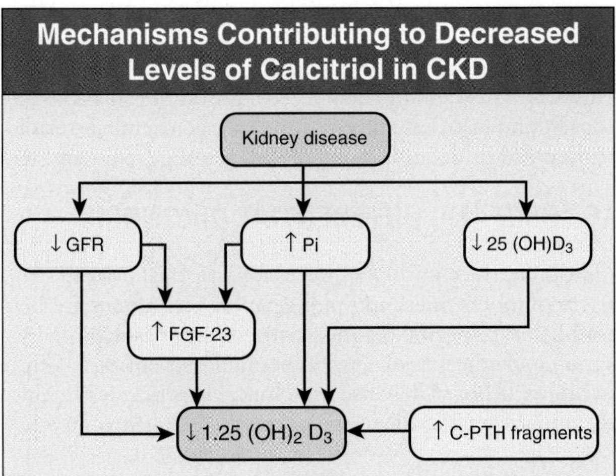

Figure 81.5 Mechanisms contributing to decreased levels of calcitriol in CKD.

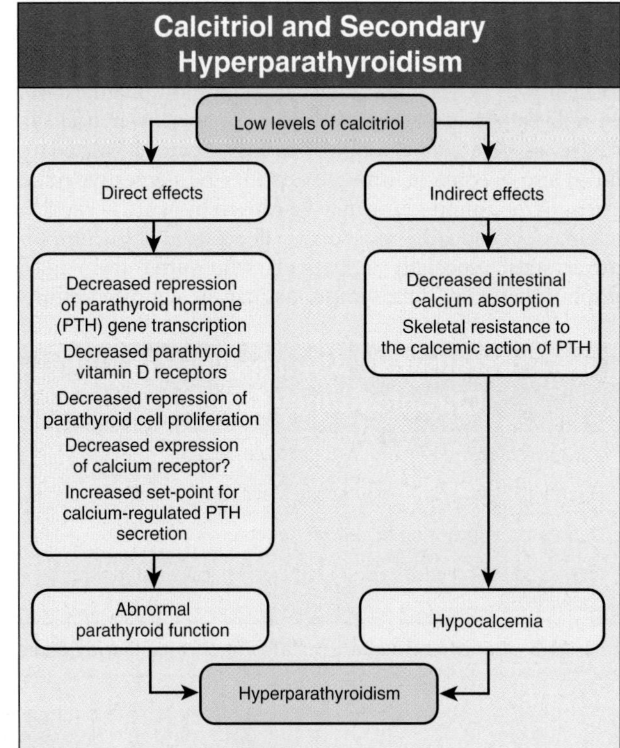

Figure 81.6 Role of low levels of calcitriol in the pathogenesis of secondary hyperparathyroidism.

production as renal function decreases can lead to progressive reductions in intestinal absorption of calcium, leading to hypocalcemia and stimulation of PTH release. Second, low levels of calcitriol have been implicated in skeletal resistance to the calcemic actions of PTH, which may also contribute to the development of hyperparathyroidism.

Abnormalities of Parathyroid Gland Function

There are intrinsic abnormalities in parathyroid gland function in the course of CKD in addition to those caused by hypocalcemia, low levels of calcitriol, and skeletal resistance to the actions of PTH (Fig. 81.7).

Parathyroid hyperplasia is an early finding in CKD. In experimental models, hyperplasia begins within a few days after the induction of CKD and can be prevented by dietary phosphate restriction or by the use of calcimimetic agents.[7,13] Resected parathyroids from patients with severe hyperparathyroidism have nodular areas throughout the gland, which represent monoclonal expansions of parathyroid cells.[14] Within these nodules, there is decreased expression of vitamin D receptors as well as of calcium receptors.[15,16] The decreased expression of calcium receptors renders efforts to therapeutically affect these enlarged hyperplastic glands difficult.

The parathyroid calcium receptor is centrally involved in the regulation of PTH secretion by calcium.[17] Its expression and synthesis are decreased in parathyroid glands from hyperparathyroid subjects,[16] leading to altered calcium-regulated PTH secretion. Increased concentrations of calcium are required *in vitro* to suppress PTH release from the parathyroid cells of uremic patients compared with those of normal controls. Thus, the set point for the concentration of calcium required to decrease PTH release by 50% appears to be increased.

Abnormal Skeletal Response to Parathyroid Hormone

In patients with CKD, there is an impaired response of serum calcium to the administration of PTH and a delay in the recovery from induced hypocalcemia in the presence of larger increments in PTH levels. Thus, in CKD, the skeleton is relatively resistant to the calcemic actions of PTH. The resultant decrease in serum calcium levels stimulates PTH secretion and contributes to the pathogenesis of secondary hyperparathyroidism. Factors involved in the skeletal resistance to PTH in CKD include decreased levels of calcitriol, downregulation of the PTH receptor, and phosphate retention. In addition, circulating fragments of PTH, truncated at the N-terminus, which still react in the older, second-generation two-site PTH assays, may serve to oppose the calcemic actions of PTH, probably acting at a receptor for the C-terminal region of PTH.[18,19]

CLINICAL MANIFESTATIONS OF HIGH-TURNOVER RENAL OSTEODYSTROPHY

Clinical manifestations of hyperparathyroidism are usually nonspecific and are often preceded by biochemical or imaging abnormalities. Aches and pains are common manifestations, often nonspecific in nature, and occur in the lower back, hips, and legs, aggravated by weight bearing. Acute, localized bone pain can also become manifested and may be suggestive of acute arthritis. Pain around joints may be caused by acute periarthritis, which is associated with periarticular deposition of calcium phosphate crystals, especially in patients who suffer from marked hyperphosphatemia. The symptoms may be confused clinically with gout or pseudogout and often respond to nonsteroidal anti-inflammatory drugs (NSAIDs). The gradual onset of muscle weakness is also common in patients with ESRD. Many factors are probably involved in its pathogenesis, including hyperparathyroidism and abnormalities of vitamin D. The arthropathy associated with β_2-microglobulin amyloidosis (see later discussion) should be considered in the differential diagnosis in very long term dialysis patients.

Bone deformities may occur in patients with severe hyperparathyroidism, particularly in children. In adults, deformities arise as a consequence of fractures, sometimes induced by brown tumors (see later discussion); the axial skeleton is most commonly affected. This can lead to kyphoscoliosis or chest wall deformities. Slipped epiphysis may occur in children, and frank rachitic features are occasionally evident. Growth retardation is also common in children, and although some improvement has been shown with calcitriol, this has not been the universal finding.

Extraskeletal calcifications are frequently encountered in patients with advanced CKD and are aggravated by persistent elevation of the calcium-phosphate product. Most commonly, vascular calcifications are seen, but calcifications may also occur in other sites, such as the lung, myocardium, and periarticular areas (Fig. 81.8).

In the skin, hyperparathyroidism can be manifested as pruritus (discussed in detail in Chapter 84). Rarely, it can also underlie the development of calciphylaxis, or calcific uremic arteriolopathy (discussed in detail in Chapter 84; see Figs. 84.6 and 84.7).

Parathyroid Abnormalities in Chronic Kidney Disease
Parathyroid gland hyperplasia: diffuse, nodular
Decreased expression of vitamin D receptors
Decreased expression of calcium receptors
Increased set-point of calcium-regulated parathyroid hormone secretion

Figure 81.7 Parathyroid abnormalities in chronic kidney disease.

DIAGNOSIS AND DIFFERENTIAL DIAGNOSIS

In addition to the clinical manifestations of renal osteodystrophy, a variety of biochemical and radiographic techniques are helpful to establish the specific diagnosis and to serve as a guide for the initiation and adjustment of therapeutic interventions. Although bone biopsy is not widely used in clinical practice, it remains the gold standard for the diagnosis of renal osteodystrophy.

Serum Biochemistry

The levels of free calcium and phosphate in serum are usually normal in patients with mild to moderate CKD. Usually in stage 4 CKD, the levels of serum calcium tend to fall, and hyperphosphatemia is manifested. Hypercalcemia may result from the administration of large doses of calcium-containing antacids or

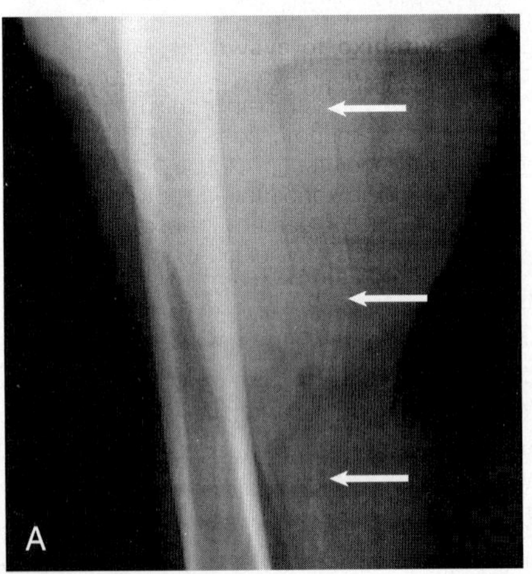

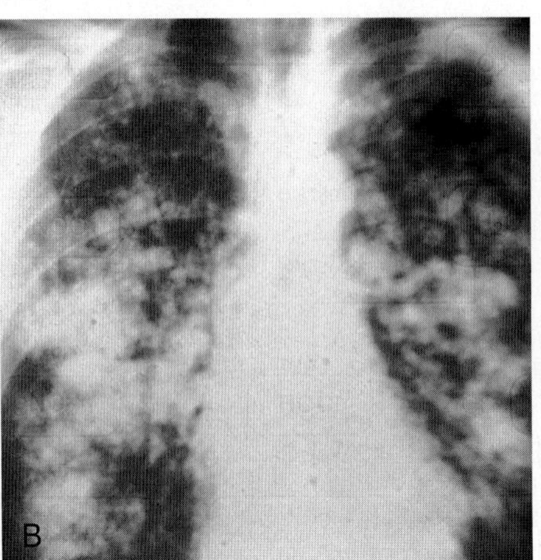

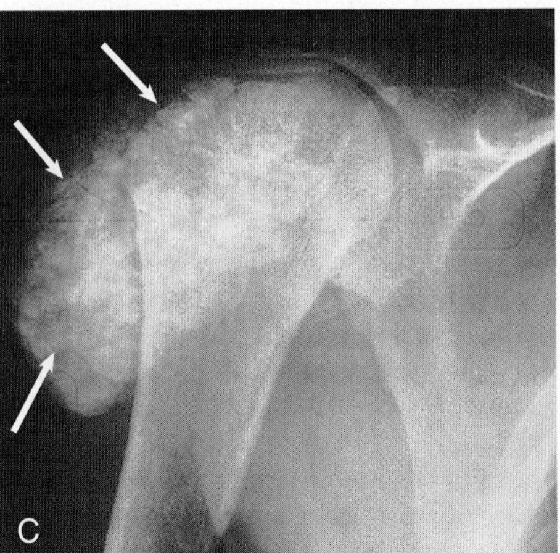

Figure 81.8 Extraskeletal calcification in chronic renal failure. A, Arterial calcification *(arrows).* **B,** Pulmonary calcification. **C,** Periarticular calcification *(arrows).*

the administration of vitamin D metabolites. Patients with severe hyperparathyroid bone disease may develop hypercalcemia. It is important to differentiate between the different causes of hypercalcemia in the setting of CKD (see Chapter 10) because the management will vary greatly according to the cause. Also, the levels of serum calcium and phosphate, when used alone, are not useful in predicting the specific type of bone disease.

Parathyroid Hormone

Measurements of PTH are important for diagnostic purposes and for therapeutic guidance in the management of renal osteodystrophy. With renal impairment, there is accumulation of circulating PTH fragments, which complicates the interpretation of PTH assays, including the two-site immunometric assays, which measure intact PTH (iPTH). Refinements in PTH assays have demonstrated that these "intact" PTH assays also measure some large fragments of PTH, which are truncated at the N-terminus and may have important biologic activity. Although more specific assays for so-called biointact PTH have been developed that exclude these fragments from measurement, work continues to define the clinical utility of such more specific assays.[20-22] It is hoped that continued efforts will lead to improved standardization between different PTH assays from various laboratories and various manufacturers of assay reagents.[18] With existing intact PTH assays (upper limit of the reference range, approximately 60 pg/ml), only values at the extremes are useful in the noninvasive diagnosis of renal osteodystrophy. In dialysis patients, iPTH levels above approximately 600 pg/ml are characteristic of patients with osteitis fibrosa. It is well accepted that there is an element of skeletal resistance to PTH in patients with CKD; therefore, supranormal levels of PTH appear to be required to maintain normal bone turnover. Serial measurements of PTH are useful in the initial evaluation of patients with renal bone disease and are essential during the management of these disorders to assess response to therapy and to avoid overtreatment and undertreatment because either can have detrimental effects on bone histology. There are marked differences between commercial PTH assay results so that precise recommendations of desired ranges cannot reliably be provided.[23]

Vitamin D Metabolites

The levels of calcitriol in patients with CKD are not helpful in differentiating the histologic lesions of renal osteodystrophy. Measurements of calcitriol are not used routinely for diagnostic purposes unless extrarenal production of this metabolite is suspected, as in granulomatous disorders (see Chapter 10).

Vitamin D deficiency in CKD rarely results in osteomalacia in the United States and Europe but may contribute to hyperparathyroidism. In patients with CKD with proteinuria, there is loss of vitamin D–binding protein in the urine, which may result in decreased levels of 25-hydroxyvitamin D. Vitamin D deficiency may be encountered in patients with limited sun exposure, in those with intestinal malabsorption or malnutrition, and in susceptible racial groups, particularly Indo-Asians. Assessment of vitamin D nutrition is by measurement of serum 25-hydroxyvitamin D_3.

Markers of Bone Formation and Bone Resorption

Levels of circulating alkaline phosphatase offer an approximate index of osteoblast activity in patients with CKD. High levels are commonly present in hyperparathyroid bone disease. The discriminatory power of alkaline phosphatase measurements is enhanced by measurement of bone-specific alkaline phosphatase isoenzyme and in particular in conjunction with PTH values. Serial measurements of alkaline phosphatase may be useful in assessing the progression of bone disease. Osteocalcin is another marker of osteoblastic activity, but it is not superior to alkaline phosphatase. Tartrate-resistant acid phosphatase and collagen degradation products are both markers of osteoclastic activity but are considered investigational at present.

Radiology of the Skeleton

Routine x-ray examination of the skeleton is relatively insensitive for the diagnosis of renal osteodystrophy, and radiographs can appear virtually normal in patients with severe histologic evidence of renal bone disease. However, subperiosteal erosions are often present in severe secondary hyperparathyroidism, detected in the hands (Fig. 81.9), clavicles, and pelvis. Skull radiographs may show focal radiolucencies and a ground-glass appearance, known as "pepper pot" skull. Osteosclerosis of the vertebrae is responsible for the "rugger-jersey" appearance of the spine (Fig. 81.10). Very rarely, brown tumors, focal collections of giant cells and typical of severe hyperparathyroidism, are seen as well-demarcated radiolucent zones in long bones, clavicles, and digits. They may be confused with osteolytic metastases. Looser zones or pseudofractures are characteristic of osteomalacia. Routine skeletal radiographs are not indicated unless there are symptoms.

Measurements of Bone Density

Dual-energy x-ray absorptiometry is widely used to assess bone density. However, there is no clear utility for this technique in the assessment of renal bone disease (see later discussion) because bone density measurements do not correlate with bone histology in renal bone disease. Vascular and soft tissue calcifications may contribute to errors in bone density measurements.

Bone Biopsy

Biopsy of bone and the microscopic analysis of undercalcified sections after double tetracycline labeling provide definitive and

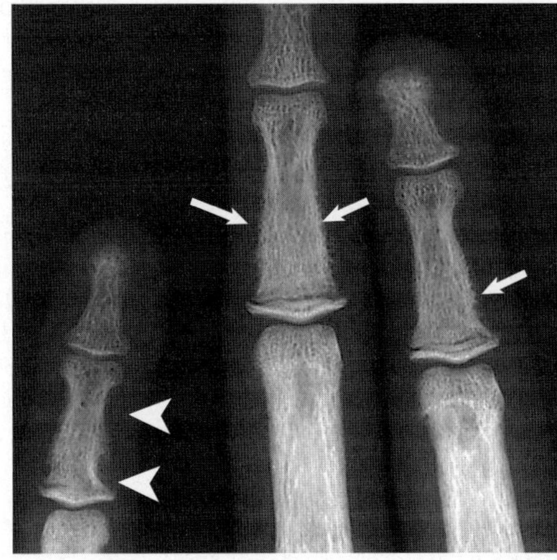

Figure 81.9 Subperiosteal erosions in hyperparathyroidism. Severe subperiosteal erosions as a manifestation of hyperparathyroidism *(arrows)*. The extensive scalloped appearance of the middle phalanx on the left *(arrowheads)* represents a small brown tumor.

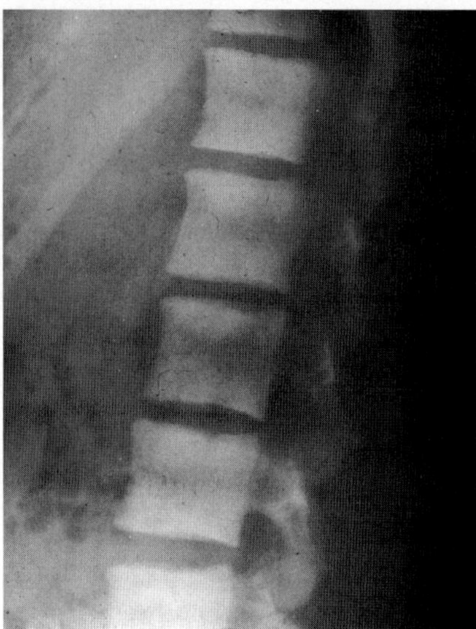

Figure 81.10 "Rugger-jersey spine" in hyperparathyroidism. Vertebral bodies show the increased density of the ground plates and central radiolucency, which gives the appearance of a rugger jersey.

quantitative diagnosis of renal bone disease.[24] To standardize reports on bone histology, the Kidney Disease: Improving Global Outcomes (KDIGO) CKD-MBD work group initialized the TMV classification, an assessment of turnover (T), mineralization (M), and bone volume (V).[1] Bone mineralization is assessed by the administration of two different tetracyclines spaced apart (e.g., tetracycline 500 mg three times daily for 2 days followed by a 10-day interval, then demeclocycline 300 mg three times daily for 3 days) and biopsy 4 days later; the quantitation of bone mineralization rate is achieved by measuring the distance between the two fluorescent tetracycline bands.

Bone biopsy is not routinely performed in clinical practice because of the invasive nature of the procedure. Although noninvasive testing is useful to distinguish normal from high bone turnover, there is considerable overlap, and therefore biopsy might be required for definitive diagnosis when biochemistry is not conclusive (e.g., PTH in recommended range but bone alkaline phosphatase elevated, hypercalcemia with PTH only modestly elevated, or bone pain).

Osteitis fibrosa (hyperparathyroid bone disease) is characterized by increased bone turnover, increased number and activity of osteoblasts and osteoclasts, and variable amounts of peritrabecular fibrosis (Fig. 81.11A). Osteoid may be increased but usually has a woven pattern distinct from the normal lamellar appearance. Osteomalacia is characterized by increased osteoid seam width, increase in the trabecular surface covered with osteoid, and decreased bone mineralization as assessed by tetracycline labeling (Fig. 81.11B). The presence of aluminum can be detected on the mineralization front by specific staining (Fig. 81.11C). Aluminum-related bone disease is defined by aluminum staining exceeding 15% of the trabecular surface and a bone formation rate of less than 220 mm^2 per day. Features of osteitis fibrosa may occur together with features of osteomalacia; the combination is termed mixed renal osteodystrophy.

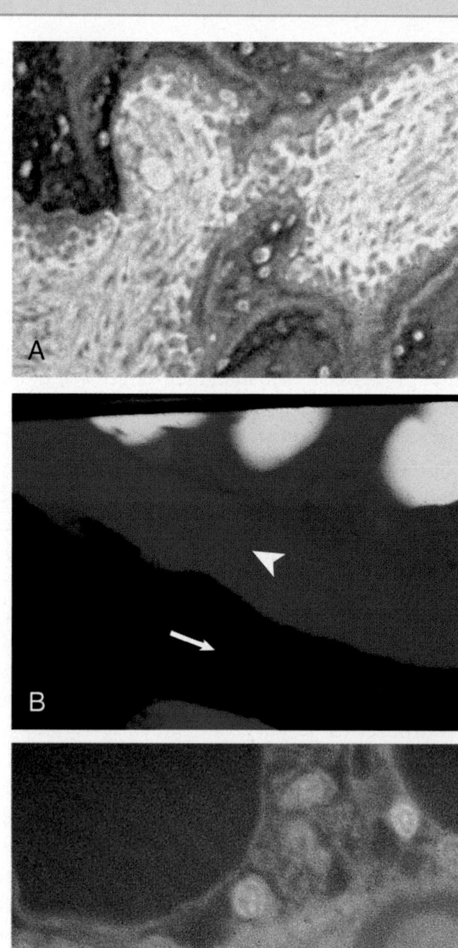

Figure 81.11 Bone histology in renal osteodystrophy. A, Osteitis fibrosa: characteristic manifestations of severe hyperparathyroidism with increased osteoclast and osteoblast activity and peritrabecular fibrosis. **B,** Osteomalacia: marked excess of unmineralized osteoid stained red *(arrowhead)* surrounding the mineralized bone stained black *(arrow)*. **C,** Aluminum bone disease: specific red staining shows the deposition of aluminum at the mineralization front *(arrow)*.

TREATMENT OF HIGH-TURNOVER BONE DISEASE

Prevention is the primary goal in the management of renal osteodystrophy. Therapy for hyperparathyroidism should ideally be initiated in CKD stage 3 so that parathyroid gland hyperplasia can be prevented. Because renal osteodystrophy is usually asymptomatic early in the course of CKD, attention is often not paid to secondary hyperparathyroidism. By the time CKD is advanced, patients may have already developed significant skeletal abnormalities or nodular parathyroid hyperplasia, and more aggressive therapy is required to prevent the long-term consequences of renal bone disease. The successful approach to the prevention and management of this disorder involves the integration of a variety of measures directed toward the suppression of PTH secretion and the prevention of parathyroid hyperplasia.

Prevention of Hypocalcemia

Hypocalcemia, if present, should be corrected because it is a potent stimulus for PTH secretion. In patients with hypoalbuminemia, free calcium should be measured. The initial approach to therapy for hypocalcemia in mild to moderate CKD is the administration of calcium supplements such as calcium carbonate, taken between meals with increasing doses as required.

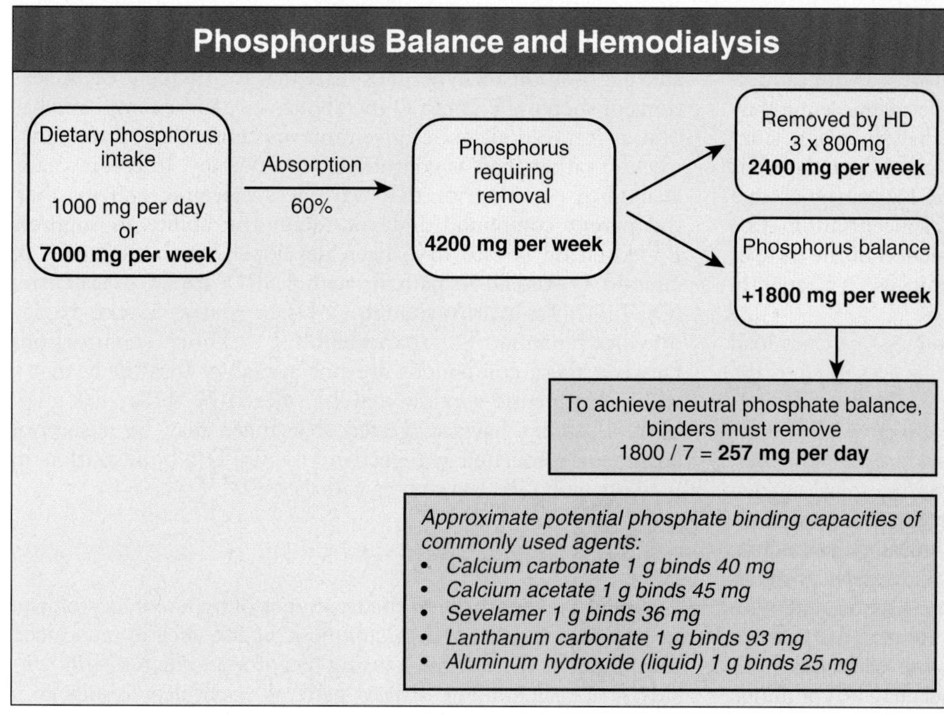

Figure 81.12 Phosphate balance and phosphate binders used in hemodialysis patients.

Assessment of vitamin D status should be undertaken by measurement of 25-hydroxyvitamin D, and this should be corrected if it is below 30 ng/ml. Assessment of efficacy of therapy is by follow-up determinations of serum calcium and PTH. Adjunctive therapy with active vitamin D sterols should be considered if hyperparathyroidism or hypocalcemia persists. In patients with ESRD, active vitamin D sterols are often required. In dialysis patients, the goal is to achieve levels of iPTH that are approximately two to nine times above the upper limit of the assay used.[25] Also, iPTH trends over time should be closely monitored. In CKD stages 3 to 5, progressive rises of iPTH above the normal range should be abrogated by correction of hypocalcemia, vitamin D deficiency, and hyperphosphatemia.

Control of Phosphate

Control of phosphate is the cornerstone of effective management of secondary hyperparathyroidism. In mild to moderate CKD, a normal serum phosphate concentration does not necessarily indicate normal parathyroid status, and except for the late stages of CKD, normophosphatemia may be maintained at the expense of elevated serum PTH. Therefore, efforts to control phosphate, including dietary phosphate restriction and the use of phosphate binders, should not be delayed until frank hyperphosphatemia develops.

Dietary Phosphate Restriction

Dietary phosphate intake should already be restricted in CKD stage 2 or 3. In experimental animals with mild CKD, dietary phosphate restriction can prevent excessive PTH synthesis and secretion, as well as parathyroid cell proliferation, independently of changes in serum calcium and calcitriol concentrations. The input of a dietitian is essential. Protein restriction and avoidance of dairy products are the mainstays of the regimen. In addition to reducing CKD progression, phosphate-protein restriction has been shown to increase the serum levels of calcitriol in patients with mild to moderate CKD. Restriction of phosphate by severe dietary protein restriction should be avoided because it may lead to protein-calorie malnutrition. Restriction of the daily dietary protein intake to 0.8 g/kg should be sufficient to provide phosphate restriction without the risk for malnutrition.

Phosphate Binders

Whereas dietary phosphate restriction is usually sufficient in early CKD, the control of phosphate becomes more difficult as renal function deteriorates. It then becomes necessary to also use agents that bind ingested phosphate in the intestinal lumen to limit its absorption. Compounds used for this purpose include aluminum hydroxide, calcium-containing antacids, magnesium salts, and, in recent years, non–calcium-containing, non–aluminum-containing phosphate binders (Fig. 81.12).

Aluminum-containing antacids are effective phosphate binders, but in patients with CKD, their use can no longer be recommended because of the risk for aluminum toxicity. There are certain circumstances that limit the use of calcium-containing phosphate binders, such as hypercalcemia, extensive vascular calcification, and calciphylaxis. In such cases, aluminum-containing antacids may be used for a short period, but the dose should be restricted to no more than 40 to 45 mg/kg per day, and frequent reassessments should be made to institute alternative therapy as soon as possible. Ingestion of aluminum-containing antacids together with foods containing citric acid (such as fruit juices and foods with sodium, calcium, or potassium citrate) may significantly increase aluminum absorption and therefore should be avoided.

Calcium carbonate or calcium acetate taken with meals effectively binds phosphates and limits their absorption. They are effective phosphate binders in 60% to 70% of patients on hemodialysis. The doses required to prevent hyperphosphatemia may vary according to the patient's compliance with dietary phosphate restriction as well as the CKD stage. Hypercalcemia is the major potentially serious side effect. Calcium citrate potentiates aluminum uptake and should be avoided in CKD. Current recommendations are to limit the ingestion of elementary calcium to 1500 mg/day.

Magnesium salts are also effective phosphate binders for patients who become hypercalcemic with calcium-containing phosphate binders, but they should be administered with caution in CKD patients not on dialysis because hypermagnesemia may have serious adverse effects. In patients on dialysis, magnesium carbonate (200 to 500 mg elemental magnesium per day) has been used successfully, with prevention of hypermagnesemia through a reduction in dialysate magnesium concentration. The use of magnesium carbonate also allows reduction of the dose of calcium carbonate required by about half, but its use is frequently complicated by diarrhea.

The risks for hypercalcemia because of the high calcium load of calcium-containing phosphate binders can be prevented by the use of nonabsorbable polymers. Sevelamer hydrochloride in a dose range of 2.4 to 4.8 g daily provides effective phosphate control without hypercalcemia[26] and also produces a significant reduction in total and low-density lipoprotein cholesterol. Agents such as sevelamer may offer great advantage over calcium-containing phosphate binders in terms of limiting the calcium load, although they are significantly more expensive. Studies have suggested that the use of sevelamer is associated with decreased progression of vascular calcification.[27] At present, sevelamer hydrochloride is being replaced by sevelamer carbonate, which has similar properties.[28] Sevelamer may be combined with both calcium- and magnesium-containing phosphate binders if necessary. Lanthanum carbonate also is an effective phosphate binder[29] but is expensive. No significant toxicity has been observed, although some lanthanum appears to accumulate in bone and liver.[30]

Use of Vitamin D Metabolites

Calcitriol and other 1α-hydroxylated vitamin D sterols, such as 1α-hydroxyvitamin D_3 (alfacalcidol), 1α-hydroxyvitamin D_2 (doxercalciferol), and 19-nor-1α,25-dihydroxyvitamin D_2 (paricalcitol), are effective in the control of secondary hyperparathyroidism. Calcitriol lowers PTH levels and improves bone histology. In patients with very high levels of PTH and markedly enlarged glands with severe nodular hyperplasia, the effectiveness of vitamin D metabolites may be limited because the levels of vitamin D receptor are low in such tissue. Accordingly, it would appear rational to initiate treatment of secondary hyperparathyroidism with vitamin D metabolites early in CKD when the parathyroid glands are more sensitive to such therapy and thereby prevent the progression to a refractory stage. A beneficial effect of vitamin D metabolite therapy in the treatment of secondary hyperparathyroidism in patients with mild to moderate CKD has been shown, but the concern with initiation of vitamin D therapy at this stage of CKD is acceleration of the progression of renal disease should hypercalcemia occur. Because of the effect of calcitriol to increase intestinal phosphate absorption, hyperphosphatemia and elevations in calcium-phosphate product may predispose patients to the development of metastatic calcification; however, it appears that doses of 1α-hydroxyvitamin D_3 or calcitriol up to 0.5 μg/day are not commonly associated with hypercalcemia, hyperphosphatemia, or worsening renal insufficiency. Another concern with the use of vitamin D metabolites before dialysis is that oversuppression of hyperparathyroidism may increase the risk for adynamic bone. Accordingly, vitamin D therapy should be monitored carefully and should not be instituted without documentation of hyperparathyroidism, correction of 25-hydroxyvitamin D deficiency, and prior control of serum phosphate.

In patients with ESRD, indications for therapy with vitamin D metabolites are better defined; however, hypercalcemia and aggravation of hyperphosphatemia are frequent complications of therapy. Vitamin D metabolites are increasingly used as oral or intravenous pulses given intermittently (e.g., three times weekly) rather than as continuous oral therapy. In recent years, analogues of calcitriol that have less calcemic activity than the parent compound and yet retain the ability to suppress PTH release *in vivo* have been developed. Such analogues of vitamin D studied in patients with ESRD are 22-oxacalcitriol (OCT), 1α-hydroxyvitamin D_2, and 19-nor-1α,25-dihydroxyvitamin D_2 (paricalcitol).[31-33] Direct comparisons between these compounds are not available. It is likely that a wider therapeutic window may be offered by these analogues. Several studies have suggested that there may be a survival advantage associated with active vitamin D administration in patients with CKD as well as with ESRD.[34,35]

Role of Calcimimetics

An additional approach to the treatment of hyperparathyroidism in ESRD is the use of a calcimimetic agent, such as cinacalcet, which targets the calcium-sensing receptor and increases its sensitivity to calcium. In dialysis patients, cinacalcet results in a significant fall in PTH levels and when administered daily can facilitate the control of hyperparathyroidism. As illustrated in Figure 81.13, the addition of cinacalcet to standard therapy in patients with iPTH serum levels exceeding 300 pg/ml while receiving standard therapy allowed significantly more dialysis patients to achieve Kidney Disease Outcomes Quality Initiative (KDOQI) practice guideline targets for calcium, phosphate, and iPTH.[36] Cinacalcet is especially useful in patients with marginal or frank hypercalcemia or with hyperphosphatemia and can be used in conjunction with other therapies. Studies investigating the effect of cinacalcet on progression of vascular calcification and survival in dialysis patients with hyperparathyroidism are ongoing. In CKD patients not on dialysis, the use of calcimimetics is accompanied by significant phosphate retention and is currently not recommended.

Role of Parathyroidectomy

Although the strategies discussed previously are effective for the control of hyperparathyroidism in many patients, there are occasions when these steps fail or are contraindicated and surgical removal of the parathyroids should be considered (Fig. 81.14). Parathyroidectomy is indicated for patients with severe hyperparathyroidism that cannot be controlled medically (phosphate binders, vitamin D sterols, or calcimimetic). Severe hyperphosphatemia in these patients precludes the use of vitamin D metabolites because of the risk for metastatic calcification. Some control of iPTH levels may be obtained with calcimimetics, but even these compounds may fail in severe hyperparathyroidism because of downregulated calcium-sensing receptors in the parathyroid glands. Some patients with severe hyperparathyroidism may become hypercalcemic in the absence of calcitriol therapy; consequently, calcitriol and calcium-containing phosphate binders cannot be administered. In this circumstance, calcimimetic and non–calcium-containing phosphate binders should be administered. It is important to be certain that hypercalcemia represents severe hyperparathyroidism and is not caused by adynamic bone or other disease. For hypercalcemia to occur because of hyperparathyroidism in CKD, the levels of iPTH generally

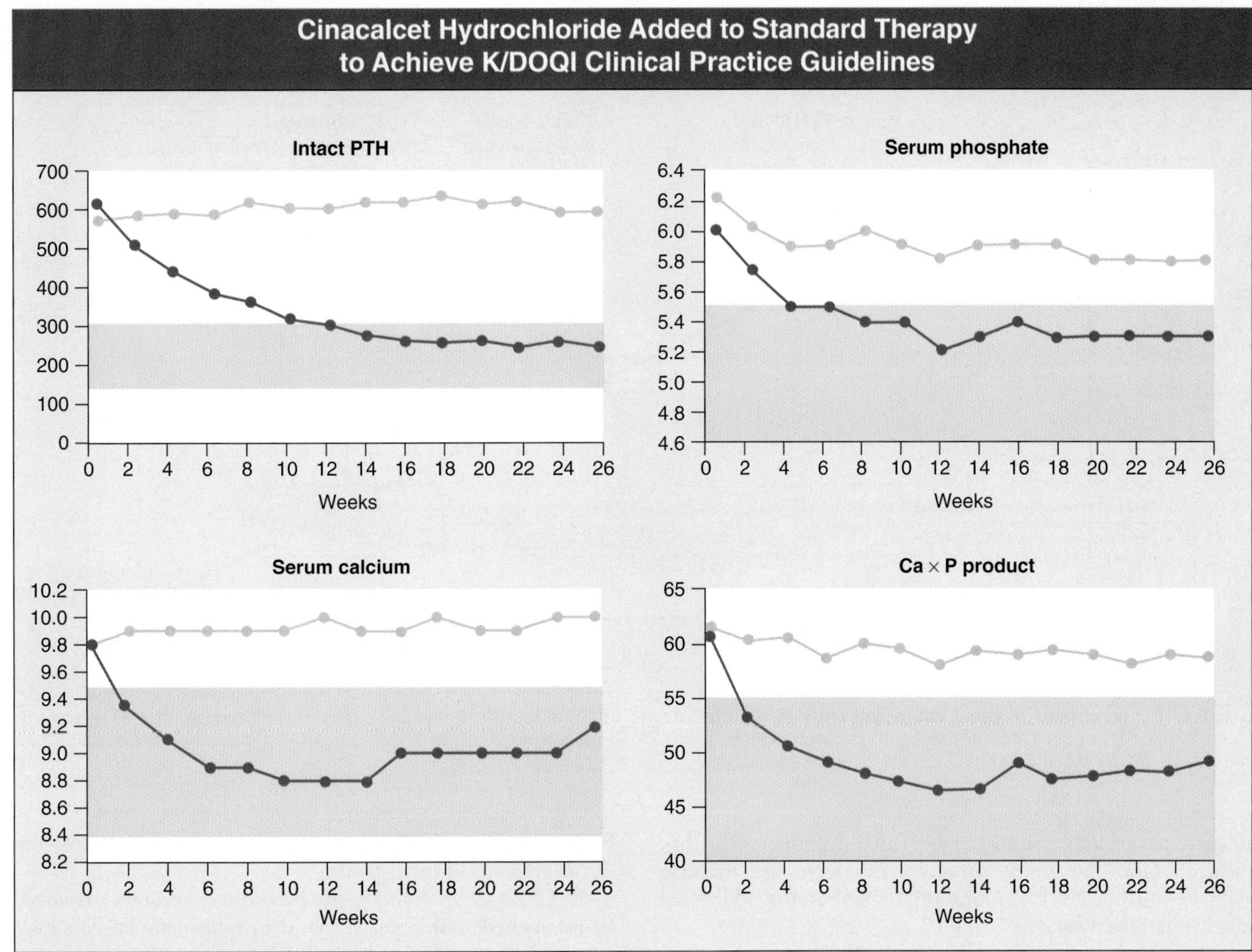

Figure 81.13 Cinacalcet hydrochloride *(dark blue line)* added to standard therapy *(light blue line)* facilitates the achievement of the Kidney Disease Outcomes Quality Initiative (KDOQI) clinical practice guidelines. KDOQI target ranges are indicated by the *shaded green* areas. PTH, parathyroid hormone. *(Modified from reference 36.)*

Indications for Parathyroidectomy
Severe hyperparathyroidism With persistent hyperphosphatemia Unresponsive to calcitriol and calcium With hypercalcemia In renal transplantation candidate With evidence of metastatic calcification
Calciphylaxis with evidence of hyperparathyroidism
Severe pruritus, only if additional evidence of hyperparathyroidism

Figure 81.14 Indications for parathyroidectomy.

exceed 1000 pg/ml, and bone-specific alkaline phosphatase is usually elevated. Surgical parathyroidectomy might also be considered in patients with very severe hyperparathyroidism who may receive a renal transplant in the near future, particularly if they are female and have significant osteopenia. Parathyroidectomy in these cases can help avoid post-transplantation hypercalcemia and hypophosphatemia (due to PTH-induced phosphaturia) as well as osteopenia. By avoiding hypercalcemia, this may lead to improved graft function and possibly to less intragraft calcification. Parathyroidectomy might also be considered in patients with severe hyperparathyroidism who have evidence of metastatic calcification. The development of calciphylaxis is an urgent indication for parathyroidectomy if PTH levels are elevated (see Chapter 84). Before parathyroidectomy, consideration should also be given to the possibility of coexisting aluminum accumulation, using deferoxamine testing and bone biopsy if necessary, because this might predispose to osteomalacia after parathyroidectomy.

The choice of surgical procedure for parathyroidectomy has been controversial. The most commonly used procedures are subtotal removal of the parathyroids and total removal of the parathyroids with reimplantation of parathyroid tissue in the forearm. Recurrence of hyperparathyroidism occurs in about 10% of patients. Total parathyroidectomy alone is less commonly performed; although this is an appropriate procedure for patients remaining on dialysis, there is concern that hypoparathyroidism after a renal transplantation may be a disadvantage of this approach if there is no residual parathyroid tissue. Unregulated tumor-like growth of parathyroid tissue implants has been described and may be related to the monoclonal nature of the nodular hyperplasia of severe hyperparathyroidism. Total parathyroidectomy with forearm implantation (our preference) or subtotal parathyroidectomy in the neck, marking remaining tissue with clips, may be performed.

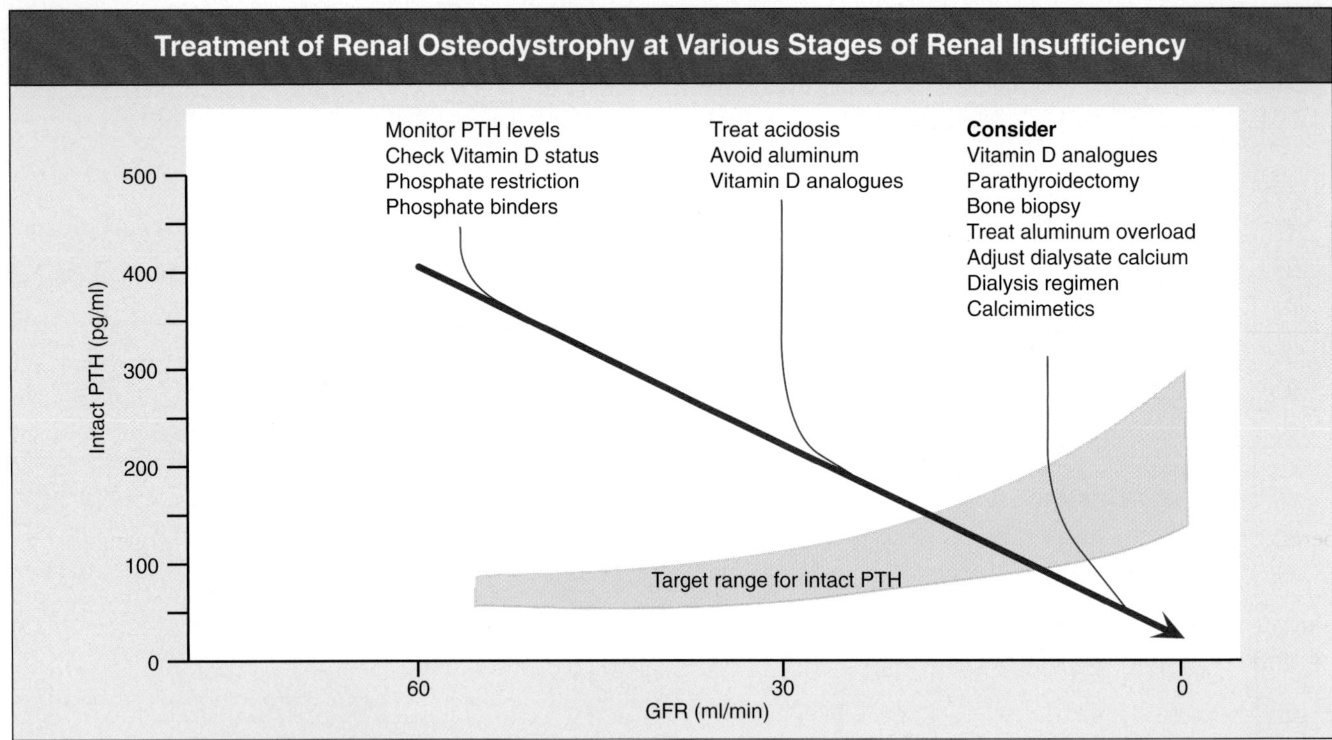

Figure 81.15 Treatment of renal osteodystrophy at various stages of renal insufficiency. GFR, glomerular filtration rate; PTH, parathyroid hormone. Note: PTH target range in this figure is based on the older KDOQI recommendation of 150-300 pg/ml, whereas the newer KDIGO target range is about 120 to about 540 pg/ml.

Recurrence of hyperparathyroidism may respond to further medical therapy, but more surgery to remove the forearm implant or further neck exploration to search for additional glands is often necessary.

Synthesis of Therapeutic Strategies

The general recommendations for the prevention and therapy of renal osteodystrophy are summarized in Figure 81.15, in which therapeutic maneuvers are stratified according to the degree of CKD.

Therapy should be initiated if possible in stage 2 or 3 CKD (GFR, 30 to 90 ml/min), and dietary phosphate intake should be restricted once patients enter CKD stage 3. Levels of iPTH should be measured; if elevated above the normal range, the levels of 25-hydroxyvitamin D should be measured and corrected if less than 30 ng/ml. If hyperparathyroidism persists, calcium-based phosphate binders, 1 to 3 g/day administered with meals, should be initiated and the dose adjusted as required to achieve control of hyperparathyroidism.

As CKD progresses within stage 3, dietary phosphate restriction should be continued or intensified, and the doses of calcium-containing phosphate binders should be adjusted on the basis of serial measurements of iPTH, with careful attention to avoid hypercalcemia or excessive calcium load. Acidosis, if present, should be treated with oral sodium bicarbonate because persistent acidosis has deleterious effects on the skeleton. The additional sodium load may require further salt restriction or increases in diuretics. Aluminum-based phosphate binders should be avoided. If hyperparathyroidism (iPTH >100 pg/ml) persists despite these measures, consideration should be given to the addition of calcitriol (0.25 to 0.5 μg/day), vitamin D analogues, or vitamin D prohormones to the regimen. Such therapy should be monitored carefully to avoid hypercalcemia and acceleration of progression of renal failure.

In CKD stages 4 and 5, the preceding therapies may need to be intensified, and larger amounts of phosphate binders may be required to avoid hyperphosphatemia. The use of aluminum-containing phosphate binders is particularly undesirable at this stage in view of the increased risk for aluminum accumulation with worsening renal function. In patients on dialysis, calcitriol therapy can be intensified, with attention to the serum levels of calcium and phosphate and monitoring of iPTH levels. In CKD stage 5, iPTH levels should be maintained approximately two to nine times above the upper limit of the assay used to maintain normal bone turnover. Calcitriol may be administered orally either daily or intermittently (pulse therapy) or administered intravenously to patients on hemodialysis. During therapy with calcitriol, it is imperative to ensure that serum phosphate remains controlled and that elevations of serum calcium do not occur to prevent metastatic calcification. Vitamin D analogues, which are less calcemic and phosphatemic than calcitriol and yet retain the ability to suppress the levels of PTH, may be useful. The calcimimetic cinacalcet provides additional effective control of hyperparathyroidism in patients with ESRD and may be used alone or in combination with the other strategies if iPTH levels do not fall into the target range. Parathyroidectomy needs to be considered in selected circumstances. Bone biopsy may be indicated in selected patients, particularly if aluminum overload is suspected. Aluminum overload may require chelation therapy with deferoxamine in selected circumstances, especially if it is symptomatic, but in most cases, the prevention of further aluminum exposure is sufficient to allow a gradual reduction in the serum levels of aluminum. During therapy with potent vitamin D metabolites, attention should be given to the dialysate calcium concentrations because high concentrations may aggravate

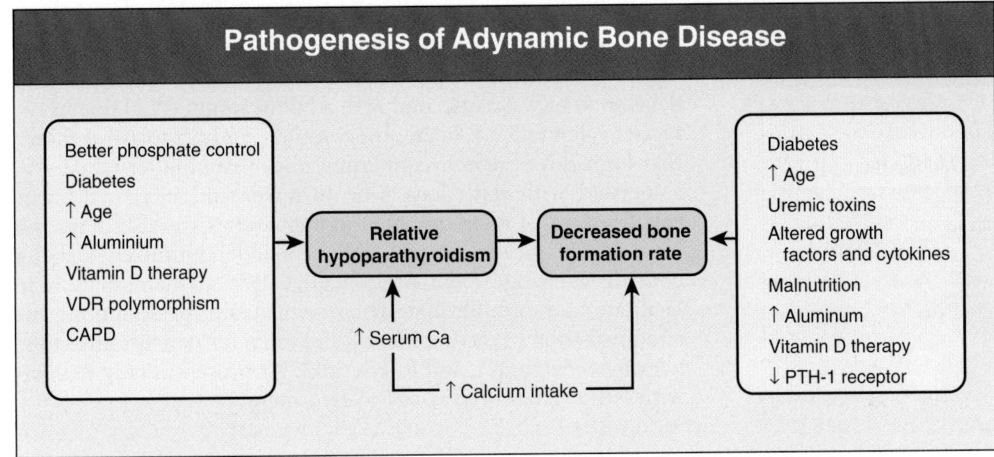

Figure 81.16 Pathogenesis of adynamic bone disease. CAPD, continuous ambulatory peritoneal dialysis; PTH, parathyroid hormone; VDR, vitamin D receptor. *(Modified from reference 59.)*

hypercalcemia. However, the increasingly frequent use of lower dialysate calcium levels, such as 1.25 mmol/l, requires careful monitoring of the patient to ensure compliance with calcium-containing phosphate binders and vitamin D metabolites to avoid progressive negative calcium balance. Dialysate calcium should not be taken outside the range of 1.25 to 1.75 mmol/l and, when possible, should be individually prescribed.

LOW-TURNOVER RENAL OSTEOPATHY

Adynamic bone disease (ABD) describes the morphologic consequences of low-turnover osteopathy in CKD. As CKD progresses, high-turnover renal osteodystrophy initially develops as an adaptive response to counteract the increasing skeletal PTH resistance and phosphate overload. ABD probably results from too rigorous suppression of this adaptive response. ABD is increasingly important in CKD-MBD because of the high percentage of affected individuals (>40% in CKD stage 5) and because of its association with cardiovascular calcification and mortality.[37,38] Furthermore, fracture incidence is estimated to be twice as high in individuals with low than in those with high bone turnover. The ABD prevalence is markedly increasing in bone biopsy registries of dialysis patients, which may relate to the increasing prevalence of its central risk factors, namely, advanced age and diabetes mellitus. Peritoneal dialysis also represents a risk factor, possibly because of a continuous exposure of the patient to high dialysate calcium as opposed to hemodialysis, in which calcium exposure is cyclic.

Pathogenesis of Adynamic Bone Disease

As pointed out earlier, the bone develops a relative resistance of the PTH-1 receptor to its ligand PTH as CKD progresses. Therefore, PTH levels above the normal range are required to maintain adequate bone turnover. Unfortunately, there are no definite ranges of elevated PTH levels that can reliably differentiate an adaptive response (normal bone turnover) from a maladaptive response (increased bone turnover) because PTH resistance individually varies and because it depends on the stage of CKD. Accordingly, ABD is a consequence of inadequately low PTH levels, which cause suppression or cessation of both osteoblast and osteoclast activities, resulting in a reduced bone formation rate and low bone mass. Iatrogenic oversuppression of PTH in CKD mostly results from high-dose active vitamin D metabolite treatment, from calcium loading (high doses of calcium-containing phosphate binders, high dialysate calcium concentration), or after parathyroidectomy. The effects of intensified calcimimetic treatment on bone turnover have not yet been systematically evaluated. Finally, diabetes, uremic toxins, malnutrition, and a disproportionate appearance of C-terminal PTH fragments may be additional factors favoring a state of low bone turnover (Fig. 81.16).

Diagnosis and Differential Diagnosis

Serum Biochemistry

Low iPTH levels (<100 pg/ml) are almost always indicative of low bone turnover in CKD stage 5. However, histologically proven ABD may occur in many dialysis patients with iPTH levels of up to 300 pg/ml and, in exceptions, of up to 600 pg/ml.[39,40] Therefore, PTH levels alone are not a sensitive biomarker of ABD. Serum levels or activities of alkaline phosphatase or bone-specific alkaline phosphatase are usually normal or low; downward trends may indicate the development of ABD. Serum calcium and phosphate can be normal or elevated, dependent on the choices of co-treatment (phosphate binders, vitamin D metabolites) and on the nutritional status. Particularly in instances of calcium and phosphate loading, hypercalcemia and hyperphosphatemia may be pronounced because adynamic bone is no more able to buffer calcium and phosphate loads by osseous deposition (Fig. 81.17).

In CKD stages 3 and 4, there are uncertainties with regard to the diagnosis of ABD and its clinical consequences. It is unclear which PTH levels are required to maintain adequate bone turnover in these stages. It seems reasonable to correct vitamin D deficiency, hyperphosphatemia, and hypocalcemia when PTH levels start to rise, but beyond that, no firm recommendations can be given at this time.

Bone Biopsy

The gold standard for diagnosis of ABD is bone biopsy. According to the TMV classification (see earlier discussion), ABD is characterized by low turnover, normal (or high secondary) mineralization, and low bone (osteoid) volume. The individual indication to perform bone biopsy should be considered in symptomatic subjects on the basis of inconsistencies of biochemical parameters associated with unexplained fractures, bone pain, progressive extraosseous calcifications, or hypercalcemia. The KDIGO initiative currently investigates 800 or more bone biopsy and concomitant serum samples to identify biomarker

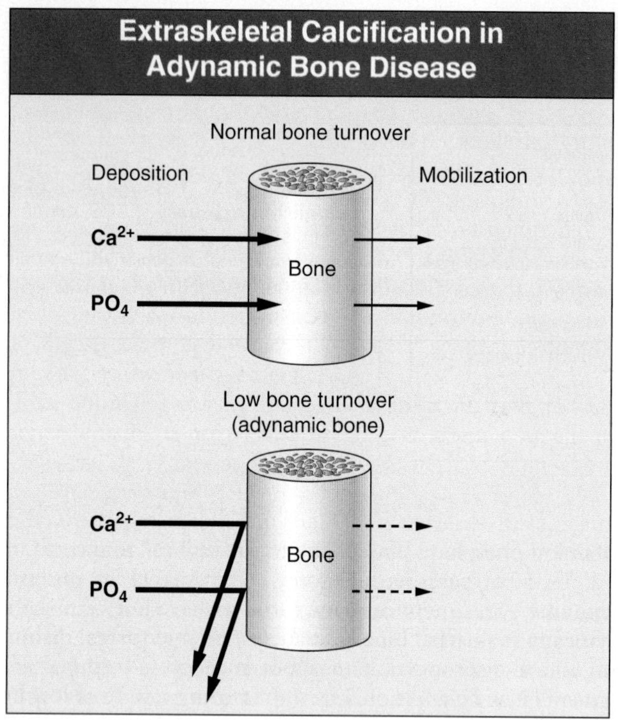

Figure 81.17 Bone turnover in adynamic bone disease. Reduced bone turnover leads to increased extraskeletal calcification.

patterns that may allow noninvasive testing of bone turnover status. Aluminum toxicity is a relevant differential diagnosis versus ABD. Thus, if the patient's history suggests significant aluminum exposure, aluminum bone deposition should be excluded by specific staining.

Radiology and Measurements of Bone Density

There are no typical features of ABD in conventional bone radiographs and in dual-energy x-ray absorptiometry. In the latter, bone density may be low, normal, or high, depending on the primary or secondary mineralization state, but it never reflects the actual turnover and is therefore not a helpful diagnostic test (Fig. 81.18). A very high cardiovascular calcification burden on conventional radiographs may raise the suspicion of a low bone turnover state if accompanying biochemical parameters are compatible with this diagnosis. Biopsy-proven ABD is associated with the highest magnitude of vascular calcification in dialysis patients.[38]

Treatment of Adynamic Bone Disease

The key therapeutic approaches in the treatment of ABD are to avoid PTH overexpression and to restore adequate PTH levels, without triggering the progressive development of secondary hyperparathyroidism. Such a stepwise treatment approach may include reduction or withdrawal of active vitamin D metabolites, reduction or withdrawal of calcium-containing phosphate binders, and reduction of the dialysate calcium concentration (usually to 1.25 mmol/l). Any aluminum should be withdrawn. After these interventions, biochemical parameters (PTH, calcium, phosphate, perhaps alkaline phosphatases) should be monitored more frequently than usual.

The best study data on this issue are available from studies comparing calcium-containing versus non–calcium-containing phosphate binders in dialysis patients.[39,41] In comparing baseline with follow-up bone biopsies in such cohorts, the administration of calcium-containing phosphate binders was associated with a higher percentage of individuals who developed ABD. This development was associated with a fall in serum PTH due to the higher calcium load. In an observational study, it was also shown that high-dose calcium-containing phosphate binder intake was associated with both low bone turnover and increased aortic calcification.[42] Other therapeutic approaches to ABD have not been systematically studied. They include optimized diabetes control, a change from peritoneal dialysis to hemodialysis to facilitate a more flexible dialysate calcium prescription, the administration of recombinant PTH (e.g., for patients after total parathyroidectomy), and calcilytics.[43] At present, many patients with ABD remain refractory to treatment.

OSTEOPOROSIS IN CHRONIC KIDNEY DISEASE

Whereas abnormal bone is common and fracture risk is increased in CKD patients, the relative contribution of classic osteoporosis (as defined by World Health Organization criteria) to the CKD-MBD complex is not well defined. Data from studies of antiosteoporosis agents are available only for patients in CKD stages 1 to 3. Nevertheless, postmenopausal women and elderly men nowadays are highly prevalent in late-stage CKD populations, and it is thus likely that classic osteoporosis also contributes to their bone disease.

Pathogenesis of Osteoporosis in Chronic Kidney Disease

Osteoporosis may be associated with low, normal, or high bone turnover and is characterized by thin and disconnected trabeculae and the loss of the plate-like bone structure. Many patients with CKD have abnormal mineralization and increased osteoid, which is quite untypical for osteoporosis. Typical pathogenetic factors of osteoporosis including hypoestrogenemia, immobilization, and corticosteroid use are frequent in CKD patients, although some postmenopausal women in late-stage CKD may have relatively normal estrogen levels. However, the sum of CKD-MBD–related biochemical disturbances probably represents the decisive factors as to which bone phenotype predominates. Secondary hyperparathyroidism, relative hypoparathyroidism (as in ABD), and 25-hydroxyvitamin D as well as 1,25-dihydroxyvitamin D deficiencies may dominate and "overrule" the bone phenotype of osteoporosis even if classic risk factors are present.

Diagnosis and Differential Diagnosis

In patients with advanced CKD, bone turnover biomarkers and measurements of bone mineral density by dual-energy x-ray absorptiometry are useless tools (Fig. 81.18) in the differential diagnosis of classic osteoporosis from other CKD-MBD–related bone disease. Assays for biomarkers such as β-crosslaps (C-terminal cross-linked, CTX; marker of bone collagen degradation), procollagen type I N-terminal propeptide (PINP; marker of bone collagen synthesis), and tartrate-resistant alkaline phosphatase 5b (TRAP5b; marker of osteoclast activity) are insufficiently validated in CKD patients, and low bone mineral density can be found in CKD-MBD–induced high-turnover bone disease, ABD, and osteomalacia (Fig. 81.18). Further, bone mineral density does not predict fracture risk in CKD patients

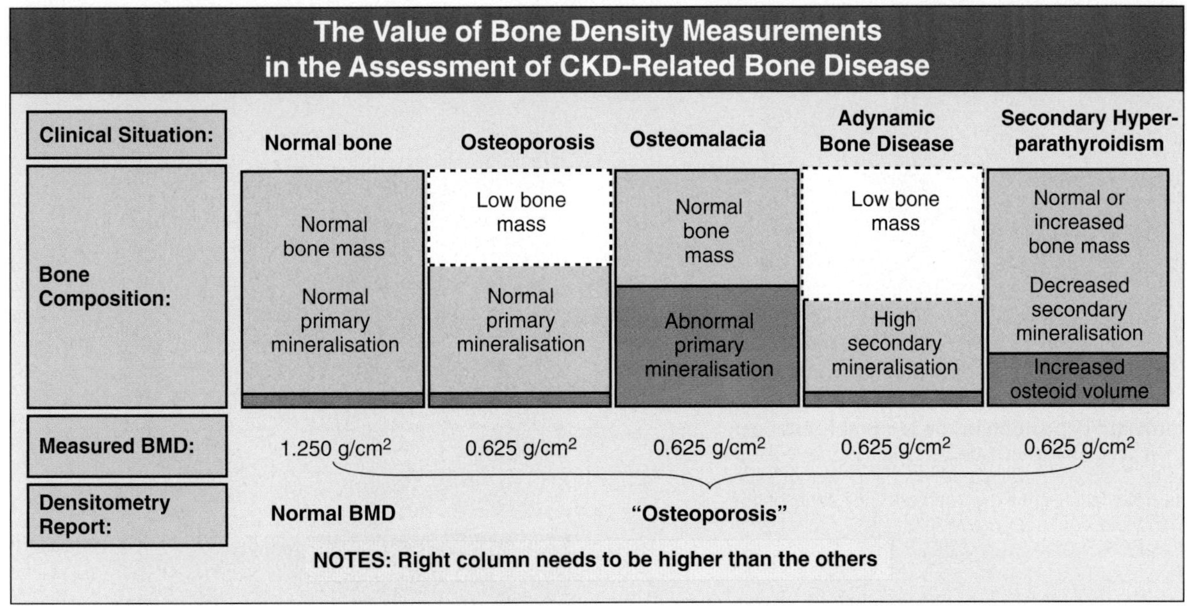

Figure 81.18 The value of bone density measurements in the assessment of CKD-related bone disease. Pink boxes indicate mineralized bone; red boxes indicate osteoid; BMD, bone mineral density. *(Courtesy Prof. M. H. Lafage-Proust, St. Etienne, France.)*

as it does in the general population, implying that abnormal bone quality rather than density is the major disturbance in such patients. The only reliable methodology to diagnose osteoporosis and to discriminate it from other bone manifestations in CKD patients is bone biopsy. In a large bone biopsy study including 1429 samples from dialysis patients, osteoporosis was diagnosed in 52% of individuals, and 49% of them also had ABD.[44] These percentages may be quite different in patients in earlier CKD stages, but there are no systematic data available on such cohorts.

Treatment of Osteoporosis in Chronic Kidney Disease

Post hoc analyses of large prospective treatment studies using antiosteoporotic medications demonstrated that it seems safe and efficacious to treat postmenopausal women in stages CKD 1 to 3 if they have a high risk of fractures (according to World Health Organization criteria) and no features of CKD-MBD.[45-48] In such populations, bisphosphonates, raloxifene, and teriparatide appear to be feasible therapeutic options. In contrast, for patients in CKD stages 3 to 5 with features of CKD-MBD, there are no data available on the safety and efficacy of any of these antiosteoporotic medications. In CKD patients with ABD, bisphosphonates may aggravate osteoclast paralysis. In CKD patients with secondary hyperparathyroidism, bisphosphonates may upregulate PTH secretion. None of these antiosteoporotic compounds can thus be recommended in patients with CKD-MBD to date, unless bone biopsy proves the exclusive presence of osteoporosis.

β_2-MICROGLOBULIN–DERIVED AMYLOID

β_2-Microglobulin–derived (Aβ_2M) amyloidosis, also termed dialysis-associated amyloidosis, exclusively affects patients with stage 5 CKD. It is a systemic amyloidosis. Clinical manifestations are largely confined to the musculoskeletal system. In recent years, the disease has become notably infrequent.

Pathogenesis

Fibrils of Aβ_2M amyloid are derived from the circulating precursor protein β_2-microglobulin, the nonvariable light chain of the HLA class I complex. The pathogenesis appears to involve three events: (1) pronounced renal retention of β_2-microglobulin (11.8 kd), leading to plasma levels that can be elevated up to 60-fold in dialysis patients[49]; (2) modifications of the β_2-microglobulin molecule that render it more amyloidogenic, such as limited proteolysis or the formation of different sugar-protein cross-links[50,51]; and (3) local factors that contribute to and determine the particular spatial localization of the amyloidosis.

Epidemiology

Histologic studies from the 1990s observed amyloid deposits in 100% of dialysis patients treated for more than 13 years.[52] Most amyloid deposits never cause clinical problems. Main risk factors for Aβ_2M amyloid deposition are age at onset of renal replacement therapy and the duration of (nontransplant) renal replacement therapy.[49,50] Aβ_2M amyloid–related symptoms nowadays are largely confined to patients who have been dialyzed for more than 15 years.

Clinical Manifestations and Diagnosis

Aβ_2M amyloidosis mainly is manifested at osteoarticular sites, particularly synovial membranes; visceral manifestations are rare.[49,50] Carpal tunnel syndrome typically worsens at night and during hemodialysis. It is often bilateral and usually requires surgery. Osteoarthropathy of peripheral joints, resulting from amyloid deposition in periarticular bone and the synovial capsule (Fig. 81.19), is characterized by recurrent or persistent arthralgias, stiffness of large and medium-sized joints, and swelling of capsules and adjacent tendons. Recurrent joint effusions and synovitis, often in the shoulders and knees, may occur. The clinical presentation may vary from frank, acute arthritis to slow, progressive destruction of the affected joints. Destructive spondylarthropathy (Fig. 81.20) resulting from Aβ_2M amyloidosis can be manifested as asymptomatic deposits, radiculopathy, stiffness, "mechanical

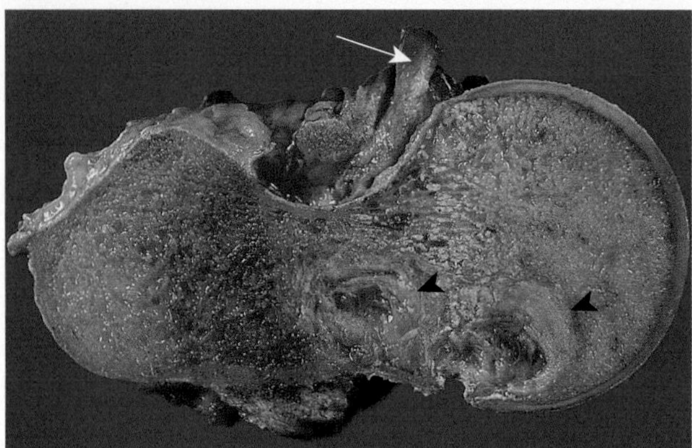

Figure 81.19 Aβ_2M amyloid deposition in the femoral head. Postmortem specimen from a long-term hemodialysis patient. Two large lesions *(arrowheads),* partly filled with grayish amyloid and partly cystic, are noted in the femoral head. Also note the marked thickening of the synovial capsule due to amyloid deposition *(arrow).*

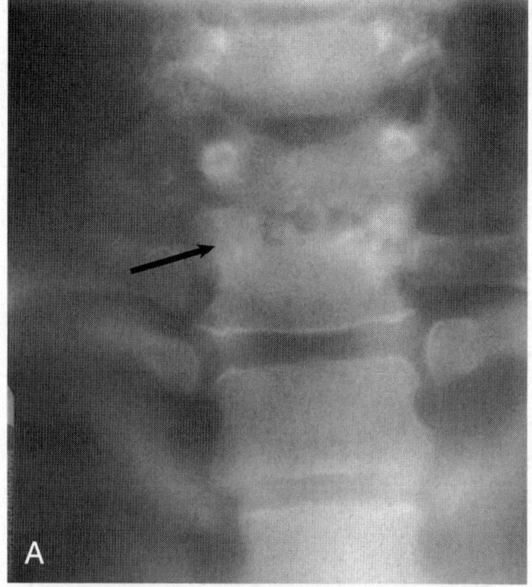

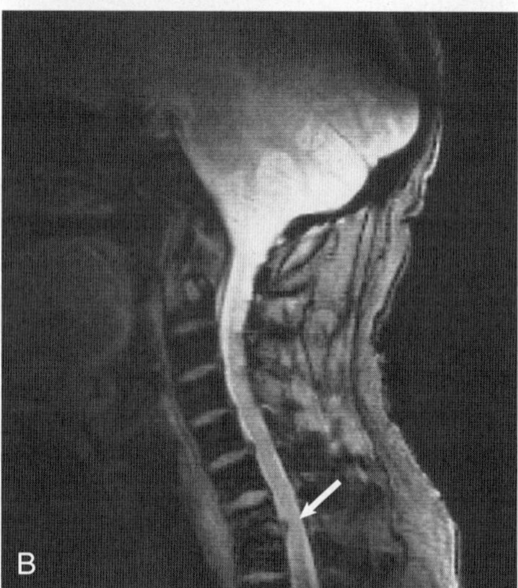

Figure 81.20 Aβ_2M amyloidosis–associated spondylarthropathy. A, Destruction of an intervertebral disk *(arrow)* in the neck vertebrae of a long-term hemodialysis patient. **B,** Magnetic resonance image of the same patient as in **A**. Note destruction of the intervertebral space and protrusion of material into the spinal canal *(arrow).*

ache," and, finally, medullary compression with resulting paraplegia or cauda equina syndrome.[49,50] Other manifestations include camptodactyly (a flexion deformity resulting in bent fingers that cannot completely extend or straighten) resulting from amyloid deposits along the flexor tendons of the hands (Fig. 81.21). Patients undergoing dialysis can also have subcutaneous tumorous deposits of Aβ_2M amyloid; however, diffuse infiltration of the subcutaneous fat or skin has not been observed.

Case reports of clinically relevant organ manifestations are usually in patients treated with hemodialysis for more than 15 years and have described heart failure, odynophagia, intestinal perforation of both small and large bowel, gastrointestinal bleeding and pseudo-obstruction, gastric dilation, paralytic ileus, persistent diarrhea, macroglossia or functional tongue disturbances (abnormal taste, mobility, articulation), ureteral stenosis, and renal calculi.[49,50]

Diagnosis

Plasma levels of β_2m do not distinguish between patients with the amyloidosis and those without. Ultrasound can detect synovial Aβ_2M amyloidosis as thickening of the joint capsules of the hip and knee, biceps tendons, and rotator cuffs as well as the presence of echogenic structures between muscle groups and joint effusions.[50] On radiologic examination, affected joints may present with single or multiple juxta-articular, "cystic" (i.e., amyloid-filled) bone radiolucencies (Fig. 81.22; see also Fig. 81.19). Such bone defects are prone to pathologic fractures. Diagnostic criteria for Aβ_2M amyloid–induced cystic bone radiolucencies have been published.[53] They include (1) diameter of lesions more than 5 mm in wrists and more than 10 mm in shoulders and hips, (2) normal joint space adjacent to the bone defect, (3) exclusion of small subchondral cysts in the immediate weight-bearing area of the joint and of defects of the "synovial inclusion" type, (4) increase of defect diameter of more than 30% per year, and (5) presence of defects in at least two joints. Scintigraphy, employing either radiolabeled serum amyloid P component or β_2-microglobulin,[54] offers more specific detection of amyloid deposits but is not widely available. The definitive diagnosis of Aβ_2M amyloidosis relies on histology. Fat aspiration and rectal biopsy are not helpful in Aβ_2M amyloidosis, but diagnostic material can be obtained from synovial membranes, synovial fluid, or bone lesions.[49]

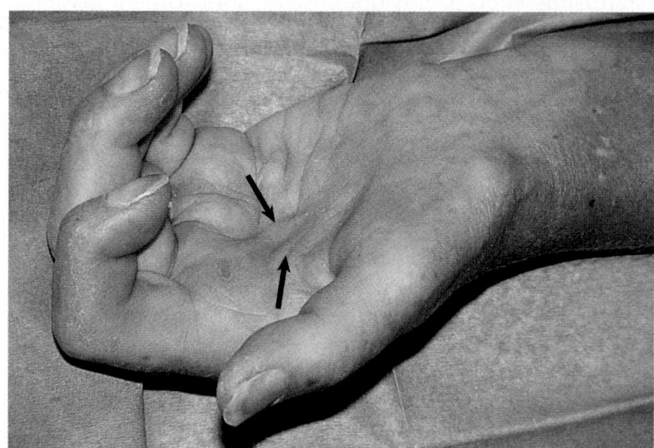

Figure 81.21 Hand involvement in Aβ_2M amyloidosis. Hand of a long-term hemodialysis patient showing maximal extension. Note the prominence of shrunken flexor tendons *(arrows).* This is also known as the "guitar string" sign.

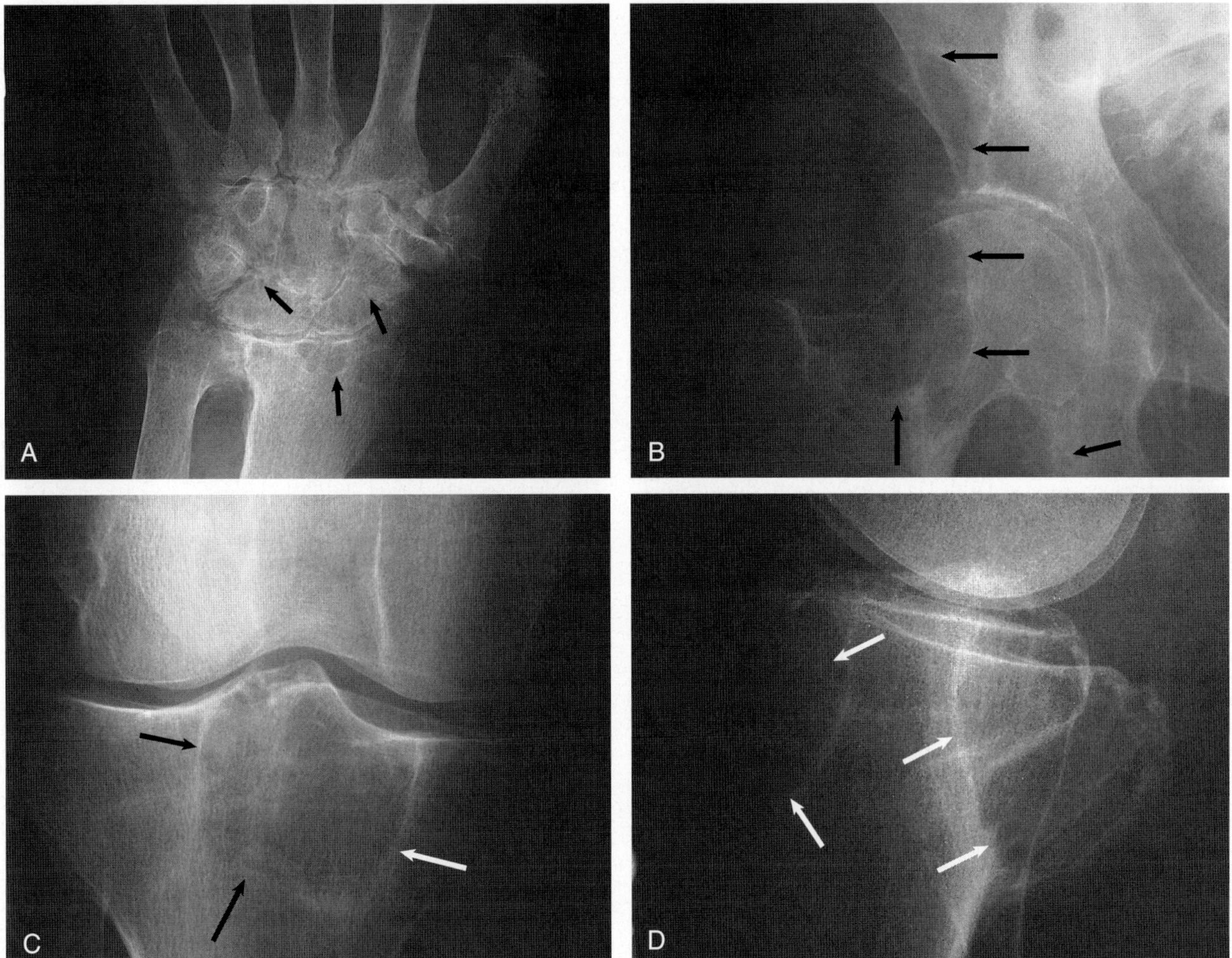

Figure 81.22 Peripheral bone cystic radiolucencies in Aβ_2M amyloidosis. Radiographic findings in a long-term hemodialysis patient. **A,** Multiple cystic lesions *(arrows)* are present in the hand bones. **B,** Large cysts *(arrows)* in the neck of the femur and adjacent pelvic bones. **C** and **D,** Anterior and lateral views of the head of the tibia with two very large, cystic lesions *(arrows)* resulting in posterior bulging of the tibial plateau.

Treatment and Prevention

Therapy for established Aβ_2M amyloidosis is symptomatic. NSAIDs and physical and surgical measures such as carpal tunnel decompression, endoscopic coracoacromial ligament release, and bone stabilization in areas of cystic destruction are all used.[49] Although some dialysis modalities allow significant removal of β_2-microglobulin, there is at present no convincing evidence that this is of therapeutic value in an established Aβ_2M amyloidosis. Renal transplantation is the preferred treatment because it leads to rapid symptomatic improvement and halts further progress of the disease, but it is controversial whether this can actually lead to regression of established Aβ2M amyloid deposits.

A number of strategies exist for prevention of the clinical manifestations of Aβ_2M amyloidosis.[49,50] The risk of carpal tunnel syndrome is reduced by 40% to 50% in patients treated with high-flux hemo(dia)filtration[55] and minimal in patients receiving online hemodiafiltration.[56] A dramatic reduction in the prevalence of carpal tunnel syndrome occurred in patients dialyzed with ultrapure dialysate.[57] In another study, an 80% reduction of amyloid signs in a chronic hemodialysis population appeared to relate to dialysate factors such as microbiologic purity and the use of bicarbonate buffer.[58]

REFERENCES

1. Moe S, Drueke T, Cunningham J, et al. Definition, evaluation, and classification of renal osteodystrophy: A position statement from Kidney Disease: Improving Global Outcomes (KDIGO). *Kidney Int.* 2006;69:1945-1953.
2. Sherrard DJ, Hercz G, Pei Y, et al. The spectrum of bone disease in end-stage renal failure—an evolving disorder. *Kidney Int.* 1993;43:436-442.
3. Martinez I, Saracho R, Montenegro J, Llach F. The importance of dietary calcium and phosphorous in the secondary hyperparathyroidism of patients with early renal failure. *Am J Kidney Dis.* 1997;29:496-502.
4. Gutierrez O, Isakova T, Rhee E, et al. Fibroblast growth factor-23 mitigates hyperphosphatemia but accentuates calcitriol deficiency in chronic kidney disease. *J Am Soc Nephrol.* 2005;16:2205-2215.
5. Almaden Y, Canalejo A, Hernandez A, et al. Direct effect of phosphorus on PTH secretion from whole rat parathyroid glands in vitro. *J Bone Miner Res.* 1996;11:970-976.
6. Slatopolsky E, Finch J, Denda M, et al. Phosphorus restriction prevents parathyroid gland growth. High phosphorus directly stimulates PTH secretion in vitro. *J Clin Invest.* 1996;97:2534-2540.
7. Naveh-Many T, Rahamimov R, Livni N, Silver J. Parathyroid cell proliferation in normal and chronic renal failure rats. The effects of calcium, phosphate, and vitamin D. *J Clin Invest.* 1995;96:1786-1793.
8. Denda M, Finch J, Slatopolsky E. Phosphorus accelerates the development of parathyroid hyperplasia and secondary hyperparathyroidism in rats with renal failure. *Am J Kidney Dis.* 1996;28:596-602.

9. Ben-Dov IZ, Galitzer H, Lavi-Moshayoff V, et al. The parathyroid is a target organ for FGF23 in rats. *J Clin Invest.* 2007;117:4003-4008.
10. Krajisnik T, Bjorklund P, Marsell R, et al. Fibroblast growth factor-23 regulates parathyroid hormone and 1α-hydroxylase expression in cultured bovine parathyroid cells. *J Endocrinol.* 2007;195:125-131.
11. Gutierrez OM, Mannstadt M, Isakova T, et al. Fibroblast growth factor 23 and mortality among patients undergoing hemodialysis. *N Engl J Med.* 2008;359:584-592.
12. Gonzalez EA, Sachdeva A, Oliver DA, Martin KJ. Vitamin D insufficiency and deficiency in chronic kidney disease. A single center observational study. *Am J Nephrol.* 2004;24:503-510.
13. Wada M, Furuya Y, Sakiyama J, et al. The calcimimetic compound NPS R-568 suppresses parathyroid cell proliferation in rats with renal insufficiency. Control of parathyroid cell growth via a calcium receptor. *J Clin Invest.* 1997;100:2977-2983.
14. Arnold A, Brown MF, Urena P, et al. Monoclonality of parathyroid tumors in chronic renal failure and in primary parathyroid hyperplasia. *J Clin Invest.* 1995;95:2047-2053.
15. Fukuda N, Tanaka H, Tominaga Y, et al. Decreased 1,25-dihydroxyvitamin D_3 receptor density is associated with a more severe form of parathyroid hyperplasia in chronic uremic patients. *J Clin Invest.* 1993;92:1436-1443.
16. Gogusev J, Duchambon P, Hory B, et al. Depressed expression of calcium receptor in parathyroid gland tissue of patients with hyperparathyroidism. *Kidney Int.* 1997;51:328-336.
17. Brown EM, Gamba G, Riccardi D, et al. Cloning and characterization of an extracellular Ca^{2+}-sensing receptor from bovine parathyroid. *Nature.* 1993;366:575-580.
18. Slatopolsky E, Finch J, Clay P, et al. A novel mechanism for skeletal resistance in uremia. *Kidney Int.* 2000;58:753-761.
19. Murray TM, Rao LG, Divieti P, Bringhurst FR. Parathyroid hormone secretion and action: Evidence for discrete receptors for the carboxyl-terminal region and related biological actions of carboxyl-terminal ligands. *Endocr Rev.* 2005;26:78-113.
20. Monier-Faugere MC, Geng Z, Mawad H, et al. Improved assessment of bone turnover by the PTH-(1-84)/large C-PTH fragments ratio in ESRD patients. *Kidney Int.* 2001;60:1460-1468.
21. Martin KJ, Akhtar I, Gonzalez EA. Parathyroid hormone: New assays, new receptors. *Semin Nephrol.* 2004;24:3-9.
22. Coen G, Bonucci E, Ballanti P, et al. PTH 1-84 and PTH "7-84" in the noninvasive diagnosis of renal bone disease. *Am J Kidney Dis.* 2002;40:348-354.
23. Souberbielle JC, Boutten A, Carlier MC, et al. Inter-method variability in PTH measurement: Implication for the care of CKD patients. *Kidney Int.* 2006;70:345-350.
24. Malluche HH, Monier-Faugere MC. The role of bone biopsy in the management of patients with renal osteodystrophy. *J Am Soc Nephrol.* 1994;4:1631-1642.
25. KDIGO Guidelines, 2009.
26. Chertow GM, Burke SK, Lazarus JM, et al. Poly[allylamine hydrochloride] (RenaGel): A noncalcemic phosphate binder for the treatment of hyperphosphatemia in chronic renal failure. *Am J Kidney Dis.* 1997;29:66-71.
27. Chertow GM, Burke SK, Raggi P. Sevelamer attenuates the progression of coronary and aortic calcification in hemodialysis patients. *Kidney Int.* 2002;62:245-252.
28. Delmez J, Block G, Robertson J, et al. A randomized, double-blind, crossover design study of sevelamer hydrochloride and sevelamer carbonate in patients on hemodialysis. *Clin Nephrol.* 2007;68:386-391.
29. Hutchison AJ. Oral phosphate binders. *Kidney Int.* 2009;75:906-914.
30. Hutchison AJ, Barnett ME, Krause R, Siami GA. Lanthanum carbonate treatment, for up to 6 years, is not associated with adverse effects on the liver in patients with chronic kidney disease stage 5 receiving hemodialysis. *Clin Nephrol.* 2009;71:286-295.
31. Martin KJ, Gonzalez EA, Gellens M, et al. 19-Nor-1-α-25-dihydroxyvitamin D_2 (Paricalcitol) safely and effectively reduces the levels of intact parathyroid hormone in patients on hemodialysis. *J Am Soc Nephrol.* 1998;9:1427-1432.
32. Kurokawa K, Akizawa T, Suzuki M, et al. Effect of 22-oxacalcitriol on hyperparathyroidism of dialysis patients: Results of a preliminary study. *Nephrol Dial Transplant.* 1996;11(Suppl 3):121-124.
33. Tan AU Jr, Levine BS, Mazess RB, et al. Effective suppression of parathyroid hormone by 1α-hydroxy-vitamin D_2 in hemodialysis patients with moderate to severe secondary hyperparathyroidism. *Kidney Int.* 1997;51:317-323.
34. Kovesdy CP, Ahmadzadeh S, Anderson JE, Kalantar-Zadeh K. Association of activated vitamin D treatment and mortality in chronic kidney disease. *Arch Intern Med.* 2008;168:397-403.
35. Shoben AB, Rudser KD, de Boer IH, et al. Association of oral calcitriol with improved survival in nondialyzed CKD. *J Am Soc Nephrol.* 2008;19:1613-1619.
36. Moe SM, Chertow GM, Coburn JW, et al. Achieving NKF-K/DOQI bone metabolism and disease treatment goals with cinacalcet HCl. *Kidney Int.* 2005;67:760-771.
37. Malluche HH, Mawad H, Monier-Faugere MC. The importance of bone health in end-stage renal disease: Out of the frying pan, into the fire? *Nephrol Dial Transplant.* 2004;19(Suppl 1):i9-i13.
38. London GM, Marty C, Marchais SJ, et al. Arterial calcifications and bone histomorphometry in end-stage renal disease. *J Am Soc Nephrol.* 2004;15:1943-1951.
39. Ferreira A, Frazao JM, Monier-Faugere MC, et al. Effects of sevelamer hydrochloride and calcium carbonate on renal osteodystrophy in hemodialysis patients. *J Am Soc Nephrol.* 2008;19:405-412.
40. Barreto FC, Barreto DV, Moyses RM, et al. K/DOQI-recommended intact PTH levels do not prevent low-turnover bone disease in hemodialysis patients. *Kidney Int.* 2008;73:771-777.
41. D'Haese PC, Spasovski GB, Sikole A, et al. A multicenter study on the effects of lanthanum carbonate (Fosrenol) and calcium carbonate on renal bone disease in dialysis patients. *Kidney Int Suppl.* 2003;85:S73-S78.
42. London GM, Marchais SJ, Guerin AP, et al. Association of bone activity, calcium load, aortic stiffness, and calcifications in ESRD. *J Am Soc Nephrol.* 2008;19:1827-1835.
43. Brandenburg VM, Floege J. Adynamic bone disease. *Nephrol Dial Transplant Plus.* 2008;1:135-147.
44. Ballanti P, Wedard BM, Bonucci E. Frequency of adynamic bone disease and aluminum storage in Italian uraemic patients—retrospective analysis of 1429 iliac crest biopsies. *Nephrol Dial Transplant.* 1996;11:663-667.
45. Miller PD, Roux C, Boonen S, et al. Safety and efficacy of risedronate in patients with age-related reduced renal function as estimated by the Cockcroft and Gault method: A pooled analysis of nine clinical trials. *J Bone Miner Res.* 2005;20:2105-2115.
46. Jamal SA, Bauer DC, Ensrud KE, et al. Alendronate treatment in women with normal to severely impaired renal function: An analysis of the fracture intervention trial. *J Bone Miner Res.* 2007;22:503-508.
47. Neer RM, Arnaud CD, Zanchetta JR, et al. Effect of parathyroid hormone (1-34) on fractures and bone mineral density in postmenopausal women with osteoporosis. *N Engl J Med.* 2001;344:1434-1441.
48. Ishani A, Blackwell T, Jamal SA, et al. The effect of raloxifene treatment in postmenopausal women with CKD. *J Am Soc Nephrol.* 2008;19:1430-1438.
49. Floege J, Ketteler M: β_2-Microglobulin–derived amyloidosis: An update. *Kidney Int Suppl.* 2001;78:S164-S171.
50. Miyata T, Jadoul M, Kurokawa K, et al. β_2-Microglobulin in renal disease. *J Am Soc Nephrol.* 1998;9:1723-1735.
51. Nangaku M, Miyata T, Kurokawa K. Pathogenesis and management of dialysis-related amyloid bone disease. *Am J Med Sci.* 1999;317:410-415.
52. Jadoul M, Garbar C, Noel H, et al. Histological prevalence of β_2-microglobulin amyloidosis in hemodialysis: A prospective post-mortem study. *Kidney Int.* 1997;51:1928-1932.
53. van Ypersele de Strihou C, Jadoul M, Malghem J, et al. Effect of dialysis membrane and patient's age on signs of dialysis-related amyloidosis. The Working Party on Dialysis Amyloidosis. *Kidney Int.* 1991;39:1012-1019.
54. Ketteler M, Koch KM, Floege J. Imaging techniques in the diagnosis of dialysis-related amyloidosis. *Semin Dial.* 2001;14:90-93.
55. Locatelli F, Marcelli D, Conte F, et al. Comparison of mortality in ESRD patients on convective and diffusive extracorporeal treatments. The Registro Lombardo Dialisi e Trapianto. *Kidney Int.* 1999;55:286-293.
56. Nakai S, Iseki K, Tabei K, et al. Outcomes of hemodiafiltration based on Japanese dialysis patient registry. *Am J Kidney Dis.* 2001;38:S212-S216.
57. Baz M, Durand C, Ragon A, et al. Using ultrapure water in hemodialysis delays carpal tunnel syndrome. *Int J Artif Organs.* 1991;14:681-685.
58. Schwalbe S, Holzhauer M, Schaeffer J, et al. β_2-Microglobulin associated amyloidosis: A vanishing complication of long-term hemodialysis? *Kidney Int.* 1997;52:1077-1083.
59. Couttenye MM, D'Haese PC, Verschoren WJ, et al. Low bone turnover in patients with renal failure. *Kidney Int Suppl.* 1999;73:S70-S76.

CHAPTER 82

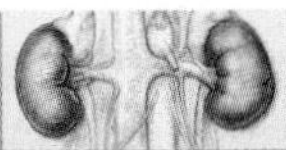

Neurologic Complications of Chronic Kidney Disease

Julian Lawrence Seifter, Martin A. Samuels

Disorders of the nervous system are associated with renal disease in patients with systemic disorders (e.g., hypertensive encephalopathy, thrombotic microangiopathies, atheroembolic and atherosclerotic disease, vasculitides), fluid and electrolyte abnormalities, and multisystem disease in the intensive care unit setting and with chronic kidney disease (CKD). Furthermore, patients with CKD are at increased risk of toxin- and pharmacologic agent–induced neurotoxicity. This chapter focuses on the direct neurologic consequences of CKD.

UREMIC ENCEPHALOPATHY

The syndrome of uremic encephalopathy (UE) involves a spectrum of brain abnormalities that may clinically range from nearly imperceptible changes to coma.

Pathogenesis

The brain in CKD has decreased metabolic activity and oxygen consumption.[1,2] As long as the underlying renal disease has not affected cerebral hemodynamics and responsiveness to carbon dioxide, these functions appear intact, but subtle disturbances have been detected after dialysis.

Many theories support the role of uremic toxins that accumulate in CKD. The balance of excitatory and inhibitory neurotransmitters may be disrupted by organic substances,[3] in particular guanidino compounds, which are increased in the cerebrospinal fluid.[4,5] These compounds antagonize γ-aminobutyric acid ($GABA_A$) receptors and at the same time have agonistic effects on *N*-methyl-D-aspartate glutamate receptors, leading to enhanced cortical excitability. Asymmetric dimethylarginine,[6] which is increased in CKD, inhibits endothelial nitric oxide synthase, and levels correlate with cerebrovascular complications in uremia. Disturbances in monoamine metabolism include a depletion of norepinephrine and suppression of central dopamine, which has been linked to the impairment of motor activity in uremic rats. Myoinositol, carnitine, indoxyl sulfate, polyamines, and decreased transport functions and increased permeability of the central nervous system have also been implicated in the neuronal dysfunction of uremia. Metabolites of drugs, including cimetidine and acyclovir, may be increased in uremia because of inhibition of the organic anion transporter (OAT3), and neurotoxic syndromes may result.[7] Levels of opiates and in particular metabolites of meperidine increase in plasma because of decreased excretion through cation secretory transport, with subsequent neurotoxicity.

Secondary hyperparathyroidism may also play a role in UE[8,9] as brain calcium is increased in CKD and calcium transporters within neurons are parathyroid hormone sensitive. Increased cellular calcium may play a role in neuroexcitation.

Appetite regulation is abnormal in uremia (see Chapter 83). A high rate of tryptophan entry across the blood-brain barrier may increase the synthesis of serotonin, a major appetite inhibitor.[10] High levels of cholecystokinin, a powerful anorectic, and low levels of neuropeptide Y, an appetite stimulant, have been observed. Cachexia may result from anorexia, acidosis, and inflammation. Inflammatory cytokines such as leptin, tumor necrosis factor α, and interleukin-1 may signal anorexigenic neuropeptides such as pro-opiomelanocortin and α-melanocyte–stimulating hormone in the arcuate nucleus of the hypothalamus.

Clinical Manifestations

Whereas 20% of patients with acute kidney injury in an intensive care unit setting developed neurologic impairment,[11] the syndrome in CKD is more subtle, not correlating closely to the level of uremia.[1,12] Cross-sectional studies in hemodialysis (HD) patients found cognitive impairment in 30%, with about 10% exhibiting severe impairment. Neurocognitive deficits may have special implications for CKD in early childhood, adversely affecting development of the brain.[13]

UE can be manifested as complex mental changes or motor disturbances (Fig. 82.1). The full-blown syndrome is a risk factor for morbidity and mortality.[1,2] Mental changes include emotional changes, depression, disturbing and disabling cognitive and memory deficits, and, in the most severe form, a generalized disorder characterized by delirium, psychosis, seizures, coma, and ultimately death. Such advanced UE is usually seen only in patients in whom a decision has been made not to initiate renal replacement therapy (see also Chapter 75). Severe motor symptoms or signs are rare. Depression, anxiety, and even suicide are important underdiagnosed and undertreated aspects of uremia and may be related to metabolic or poor nutritional state and fear of dialysis or death. Other known causes of depression should always be sought.

Stable UE is manifested by fine action tremor, asterixis, and hyperreflexia. Asterixis is characterized by intermittent loss of

Clinical Manifestations of Uremic Encephalopathy	
Early Encephalopathy	**Late Encephalopathy**
Mental Changes	
Mood swings	Altered cognition and perception
Impaired concentration, loss of recent memory	Illusions, visual hallucinations, agitation, delirium
Insomnia, fatigue, apathy	Stupor, coma
Motor Changes	
Hyper-reflexia	Myoclonus, tetany
Tremor, asterixis	Hemiparesis
Dysarthria, altered gait, clumsiness, unsteadiness	Convulsions

Figure 82.1 Clinical manifestations of uremic encephalopathy (UE).

muscle tone in antigravity muscles. It is distinguished from tremor by the fact that it is not an oscillation but rather an intermittent loss of tone. Myoclonus is also seen in patients with UE. It is similar in timing to asterixis (10 to 100 milliseconds) but is due to activation of antigravity muscles. For this reason, some consider asterixis to be a form of negative myoclonus. The distinction between asterixis and myoclonus is less important than once thought as both or either may be present in many metabolic encephalopathies and some structural brain diseases as well. Asterixis and myoclonus may be elicited with the hands outstretched but may be more sensitively assessed by looking at the protruded tongue or the index finger raised with the hand resting on a firm surface. Asterixis and myoclonus may be seen in patients with renal impairment who have received various drugs (e.g., metoclopramide, phenothiazines, antiepileptic drugs including gabapentin, and opioids, especially meperidine). Metabolic acidosis may also produce an indistinguishable encephalopathy, as can aluminum toxicity. Therefore, before it is considered a clinical feature of advanced uremia requiring renal replacement therapy, a careful search for other causes should be initiated.

Advanced UE is usually characterized by a reduced level of consciousness, anorexia, asterixis, myoclonus, and upper motor neuron signs that result in disturbances of gait and speech.

Diagnosis and Differential Diagnosis

The diagnosis of UE is based on clinical findings and their improvement after adequate therapy (see next section). Lumbar puncture, electroencephalography, and imaging procedures largely serve to exclude other causes in patients in whom the clinical diagnosis is doubtful. In UE, the cerebrospinal fluid is often abnormal, sometimes demonstrating a modest pleocytosis (usually <25 cells/mm^3) and increased protein (usually <100 mg/dl). The electroencephalogram is usually abnormal but nonspecific. Generalized slowing with an excess of delta and theta waves is found.[14] Brain imaging (Fig. 82.2) usually shows cerebral atrophy and enlargement of the ventricles.

The differential diagnosis of UE is shown in Figure 82.3. Seizure activity may be secondary to UE, hypertensive encephalopathy, cerebral embolism, cerebral venous thrombosis, or electrolyte and acid-base abnormalities. Tetany can develop when treatment involves alkalinization of an acidemic patient with renal disease and hypocalcemia.

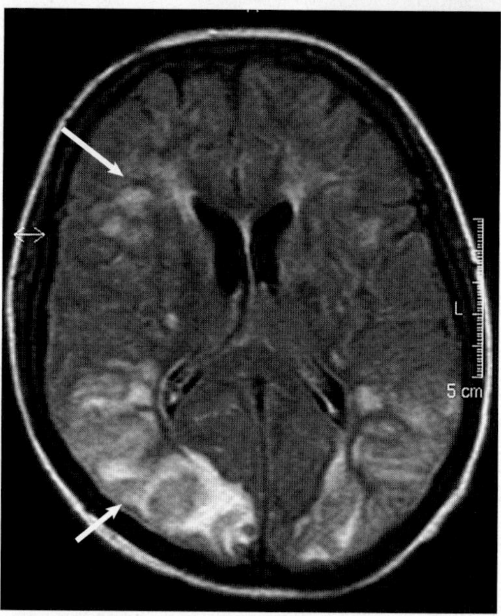

Figure 82.2 Magnetic resonance imaging (MRI) findings in uremic encephalopathy. Axial T2-weighted MRI (fluid-attenuated inversion recovery) in a 40-year-old woman. The extensive hyperintense lesion involves the cortical and subcortical areas of both occipital lobes and, in a more focal distribution, the basal ganglia and the frontal white matter (arrows). The volume of the affected brain parenchyma is increased. Reversibility of the MRI changes was noted 2 weeks later after the initiation of regular dialysis. *(Courtesy A. Thron, Aachen, Germany.)*

Treatment

Most nephrologists consider advanced cognitive or memory impairment an indication for initiation of renal replacement therapy. Most of the manifestations of central nervous system involvement are reversible with dialysis within days or weeks, but mild signs of UE may persist. In dialyzed patients with persistent or recurrent symptoms, increasing the delivered dialysis dose may improve clinical findings. Successful renal transplantation usually results in resolution of the UE syndrome within days.

Correction of anemia with recombinant erythropoietin in the dialysis patient to a target hemoglobin level of 11 to 12 g/dl (see Chapter 79) may be associated with improved cognitive function and decreased slowing on the electroencephalogram.[15] Too rapid overcorrection of anemia may be associated with seizures. Similarly, parathyroid hormone suppression with vitamin D analogues and cinacalcet is important given the potential role of parathyroid hormone as neurotoxin (see Chapter 81). Treatment of psychosis in kidney disease must take into account the pharmacokinetics of the specific agent. For example, risperidone may have utility, but dose reduction is necessary because of a prolonged half-life with CKD.

PERIPHERAL NEUROPATHY

Patients with CKD are susceptible to both polyneuropathies and mononeuropathies. The pathophysiologic process of polyneuropathy involves axonal degeneration in a length-dependent fashion. Primary demyelinating neuropathies are rare in the context of CKD except when the renal disease is the result of an illness that also causes demyelination (e.g., multiple myeloma). Mononeuropathies may be due to entrapment with compression of metabolically weakened nerves, particularly in wheelchair-bound or bed-bound patients. Mononeuritis multiplex should

Differential Diagnosis of Uremic Encephalopathy

Differential Diagnosis	Comment
Hypertensive encephalopathy	
Systemic inflammatory response syndrome (SIRS)	Observed in septic patients
Systemic vasculitis	Vasculitis or lupus with cerebral involvement
Drug-induced neurotoxicity	
Analgesics	Meperidine, codeine, morphine, gabapentin
Antibiotics	High-dose penicillins (may cause seizures), acyclovir, ethambutol (optic nerve damage), erythromycin and aminoglycosides (may cause ototoxicity), nitrofurantoin and isoniazid (peripheral neuropathy)
Psychotropics	Lithium, haloperidol, clonazepam, diazepam, chlorpromazine
Immunosuppressants	Cyclosporine, tacrolimus
Chemotherapeutics	Cisplatinum, ifosfamide
Others	High doses loop diuretics (ototoxic), ephedrine, methyldopa, aluminum
Cerebral atheroembolic disease	Follows recent aortic or cardiac angiography; associated with peripheral manifestations, including lower extremity cyanosis, livedo reticularis, and eosinophilia
Subdural hematoma	
Posterior leukoencephalopathy	Observed particularly following renal transplantation due to reversible, abnormal permeability of the blood-brain barrier Often manifests as headache followed by mental depression, visual loss, and seizures in the context of volume expansion, acute hypertension, and often treatment with corticosteroids or calcineurin inhibitors Lesions in the parietal, temporal, and occipital lobes may be seen on imaging studies.

Figure 82.3 Differential diagnosis of uremic encephalopathy.

raise the question of vasculitic neuropathy, especially when systemic vasculitis (e.g., ANCA-positive small-vessel vasculitis or polyarteritis nodosa) is causing the CKD. Functional sparing of small-diameter axons in uremia is suggested by relatively intact thermal thresholds (hot and cold thermal threshold testing is a surrogate for pain threshold). The modestly slowed nerve conduction velocities in the polyneuropathies of uremia may be related to the reversible inhibition of the sodium-potassium adenosine triphosphatase by a uremic toxin. According to the middle molecule hypothesis, accumulated toxins in the range of 300 to 12,000 d, including peptide hormones and polyamines, may lead to progression of neuropathy in HD patients.[4,8,9] Lower limb motor axons in uremic patients are depolarized before but not after dialysis, consistent with a role of hyperkalemia in the development of altered nerve excitability.[16] Elevated magnesium levels will also slow nerve conduction velocity. *In vitro*, extracellular acidosis contributes to decreased sodium conductance in large sensory neurons. Very slow nerve conduction velocities (i.e., less than half normal) suggest a demyelinating neuropathy, a finding that should lead the physician to seek a specific cause (e.g., a paraprotein).

Polyneuropathies occur in about two thirds of uremic patients and may progress rapidly in advanced CKD.[1,16,17] Characteristic symptoms and signs are sensory loss, pain, paresthesias, and insensitivity to temperature, particularly cold. These findings can advance to include motor findings, such as footdrop. Phrenic neuropathy may cause dyspnea, whereas hiccups are more likely due to the central nervous system effects of uremia. The distal lower extremities are usually affected first because axonal polyneuropathies are length dependent. Decrease in vibratory sensation and position sense and Romberg sign (i.e., greater instability of stance with eyes closed than with eyes open) are common signs. Muscle stretch reflexes are reduced or absent. In the diabetic dialysis patient who has progressive neuropathy, it is important to establish adequacy of the dialysis as well as glucose control. Uremic polyneuropathy is aggravated by malnutrition, inadequately controlled hypertension, and a number of comorbid conditions, including diabetes mellitus, alcohol abuse, atherosclerotic vascular disease, and medications (e.g., nitrofurantoin, isoniazid, hydralazine).

The diagnosis of uremic polyneuropathy can usually be made on clinical findings. Nerve conduction velocity is modestly reduced, and needle electromyography shows evidence of chronic denervation and sometimes reinnervation. If electromyography and nerve conduction tests are performed, they should not be done in an extremity bearing an arteriovenous fistula as the surgery may cause local nerve injury, which can complicate the interpretation of the clinical neurophysiologic studies.[16]

Lead polyneuropathy should be considered, particularly when there is a known exposure history. Lead accumulates in the dialysis patient but could also be the cause of CKD. A lower motor neuron syndrome due to lead toxicity may be mistaken for amyotrophic lateral sclerosis. A bone lead scan using K-line x-ray fluorescence spectroscopy of the tibia is a promising new noninvasive test that may become useful. Serum lead values and red cell protoporphyrin levels may be normal if exposure is remote. There may be associated depression, the so-called saturnine temperament, so named because the ancients believed that Saturn was made of lead and was associated with a melancholy disposition. Gout, hypertension, renal glycosuria, and microcytic anemia also may be caused by lead toxicity.

Other conditions in the differential diagnosis of mixed polyneuropathy include other heavy metals (such as arsenic and mercury), nutritional deficiencies (such as pyridoxine, thiamine, and niacin), human immunodeficiency virus–related neuropathy, amyloid, vasculitis, sarcoid, lupus, and a paraneoplastic syndrome.

Progressive polyneuropathy may be an indication for initiation of dialysis or for renal transplantation. Symptoms usually will not deteriorate further or may even show a slow improvement thereafter. If polyneuropathic symptoms worsen in a dialysis patient, the dialysis dose should be increased. Physical therapy is an important component of the management. Patients experiencing neuropathic pain may be treated with tricyclic antidepressants (e.g., amitriptyline, 10 to 25 mg, increasing to 75 to 150 mg at bedtime) or antiepileptic drugs (e.g., carbamazepine, 200 to 400 mg initially, increasing to 1200 mg maximally; phenytoin, 100 to 200 mg initially, maximally 600 mg).[1,2] Gabapentin is an antiepileptic drug that is sometimes used to treat neuropathy but is quite toxic in renal disease and is rarely necessary. When it is used, it should be monitored closely at reduced doses. Deficiencies of cobalamin (vitamin B_{12}), folate, and pyridoxine may be reflected in an elevated serum homocysteine level. Thiamine deficiency, often associated with malnutrition, can also aggravate neuropathy, but whether replacement of any of these vitamins is effective in preventing or curing polyneuropathy in uremic patients is not well established. Thiamine deficiency is the cause of Wernicke's encephalopathy in dialysis or malnourished patients. This syndrome is suspected when the triad of mental change (often amnesia), ataxia, and oculomotor disturbances (most often abducens palsies with gaze-evoked nystagmus) is seen in any patient whose diet is deficient in B vitamins. When amnesia is combined with a polyneuropathy, the term *Korsakoff psychosis* applies. In malnourished patients, the cause of Korsakoff psychosis is usually multiple subclinical attacks of Wernicke's encephalopathy, hence the term *Wernicke-Korsakoff disease*.

Specific mononeuropathic syndromes include ulnar nerve entrapment, associated with uremic humoral calcinosis and subsequent ischemia, and carpal tunnel syndrome, for example, due to β_2-microglobulin–derived amyloidosis (see Chapter 81) or to an arteriovenous fistula.[1,17] These syndromes may be treated with anti-inflammatory agents, anticonvulsants, and surgical decompression. It is important to ensure adequacy of dialytic treatment.

AUTONOMIC NEUROPATHY

Autonomic neuropathy is also very common in patients with advanced CKD, probably because diabetes is a common cause of CKD. Hyperglycemia may be more difficult to control in CKD as glucose filtration is decreased. Amyloidosis, a less common cause of CKD, also is associated with autonomic neuropathy. A typical manifestation is orthostatic hypotension, which is most severe in patients with diabetes mellitus or amyloidosis as a cause of CKD. The low blood pressure may preclude antiproteinuric treatment with angiotensin antagonists in the predialysis patient and may complicate fluid removal during dialysis. CKD patients were thought to have decreased baroreceptor function, but normal baroreceptor responses to graded decrements in mean arterial blood pressure have been described.[18] Instead, CKD patients have sympathetic hyperactivity, which contributes to hypertension, more rapid progression to renal failure in the predialysis patient, and greater cardiovascular risk. Accordingly, α- and β-adrenergic blockade has been advocated in CKD.[18] Autonomic neuropathy is due to axonal disease and thus is length dependent. For that reason, the longest autonomic nerve, the vagus, is usually the first affected, resulting in the loss of the normal sinus arrhythmia, significant reductions of day-night blood pressure variation, and possibly sudden cardiac death related to the loss of the balance between the sympathetic and parasympathetic limbs of the autonomic nervous system. Gastrointestinal complaints include gastroparesis, particularly problematic for the diabetic patient. In the predialysis patient, nausea and early satiety associated with gastroparesis may be confused with uremia. Nocturnal diarrhea is another consequence of vagal neuropathy. Erectile dysfunction and incontinence (urinary more common than fecal) may also be related to autonomic neuropathy.

CRANIAL NEUROPATHIES

Cranial nerve involvement is most often vestibulocochlear. Hearing loss needs to be distinguished from drug-induced ototoxicity or the neurosensory deafness of hereditary nephropathy.[1,2] Bilateral vestibular failure leads to inability to stand or to walk normally without vertigo or nystagmus. It is often related to the use of aminoglycoside antibiotics in the patient with CKD, unless the dose is properly adjusted. *N*-Acetylcysteine given with aminoglycosides may reduce the risk of cochlear toxicity. Sulfa-based loop diuretics often used at high dose in CKD may cause vestibular or cochlear damage. Decreased olfactory function, especially a reduced ability to discriminate among and to identify odors, and dysgeusia are commonly seen in patients with CKD.

SLEEP DISORDERS

Many HD and peritoneal dialysis patients exhibit obstructive sleep apnea that is independent of obesity.[19] The associated sleep deprivation contributes to fatigue and cognitive impairment and increases the risk of cardiovascular complications.[19] Both obstructive and central sleep apnea are seen in patients with CKD. Treatment of obstructive sleep apnea, with use of continuous positive airway pressure in a fashion similar to the treatment of nonuremic individuals, is effective. Nocturnal HD significantly reduced the occurrence of sleep apnea.[19]

Daytime sleepiness is common and underdiagnosed in patients with CKD and contributes not only to worsened hypertension and increased cardiovascular risk but also to social dysfunction. Whether obstructive sleep apnea and its associated excessive daytime sleepiness is an independent risk factor for the progression of renal failure is not yet settled. It is assessed by a multiple sleep latency test, that is, the duration of time from "lights out" to the onset of sleep. If it is less than 5 minutes, it is consistent with sleep deprivation. There was also a reduced proportion of rapid eye movement sleep. An increased arousal frequency is related to periodic limb movements during sleep and the presence of sleep apnea.

Sleep-wake complaints are common in patients on dialysis, with an incidence of up to 80%. Contributors include peripheral neuropathy, pain, and pruritus.

RESTLESS LEGS SYNDROME (THE EKBOM SYNDROME)

Restless legs syndrome (RLS), described by K. A. Ekbom in 1944,[20] is frequent in CKD, particularly in women. It may result from a decrease in dopaminergic modulation of intracortical excitability, with reduced supraspinal inhibition and increased spinal cord excitability. RLS is characterized by unpleasant "creeping" sensations in the extremities and a compulsive need to move the limbs, usually the legs.[21-23] The movement is worsened by periods of rest or inactivity and is relieved by walking or stretching. Symptoms are worse at night and may lead to insomnia and consequent daytime sleepiness and reduced quality of life. Nocturnal muscle cramps are also common in CKD and should be distinguished from the RLS. The Ekbom syndrome consists of restless legs plus other obsessive-compulsive–like disorders including various pica behaviors, such as pagophagia (ice eating), geophagia (clay eating), and amylophagia (starch eating).

Periodic limb movements is a disorder characterized by episodes of involuntary repetitive extension of the big toe and dorsiflexion of the ankle as well as flexion of the knee and hip.[22,23] This disorder is more likely to occur in those with RLS.

Iron deficiency or iron transport into the central nervous system plays a central role in RLS. Iron is a cofactor for the enzyme tyrosine hydroxylase, the rate-limiting step in the biosynthesis of dopamine, possibly explaining the link between iron deficiency and dopamine deficiency in RLS. Overt iron deficiency is easily diagnosed and should be treated.[22,23] In patients with normal red blood cell indices and serum iron and total iron-binding capacity, serum ferritin should be tested. Transferrin saturation ratio may be an even more sensitive indicator of iron deficiency. If these are both normal, a spinal fluid ferritin analysis may reveal a subtle central nervous system iron deficiency syndrome. RLS often persists after initiation of dialysis but may improve after transplantation and has been linked to abnormalities in calcium and phosphorus metabolism as well as to anemia. Iron replacement should be initiated if there is any indication of iron deficiency. Oral replacement is the safest method. Although intravenous iron may be effective, this has not been demonstrated in carefully controlled clinical trials in this setting. Dopaminergic treatment is often helpful, usually starting with the dopamine receptor agonists pramipexole and ropinirole. Levodopa combined with decarboxylase inhibitors (e.g., Sinemet) may be used as well as gabapentin, opioids, and benzodiazepines.[21-23] Care should be taken with gabapentin because of toxicity with accumulation, the symptoms of which are sedation, cognitive slowing, and various movement disorders including tremor and asterixis (see previous discussion). Older dopamine receptor agonists, such as bromocriptine and pergolide, are rarely used now for RLS.

NEUROLOGIC SYNDROMES ASSOCIATED WITH RENAL REPLACEMENT THERAPY

Renal replacement therapy is associated with an increased incidence of subdural hematoma and intracranial hemorrhage, presumably connected to hypertension and anticoagulation with HD as well as Wernicke's encephalopathy (see earlier discussion).[1,2] A syndrome of muscle weakness has been attributed to L-carnitine depletion from dialysis, leading to decreased mitochondrial fatty acid utilization.

Dialysis disequilibrium syndrome is a rare complication of rapid metabolic changes occurring with HD, usually affecting patients in whom HD is being initiated (see also Chapter 91).[24] It is most common in those patients with severe uremia of long duration and with severe hypertension. Characterized by acute onset of headache, nausea, vomiting, disorientation, a confusional state, and seizures, it is a diagnosis of exclusion. It usually results from acute changes in osmolality during HD, in which the rapid decrease in urea in the extracellular fluid favors water movement into brain cells, resulting in cerebral edema. Alternatively, other intracellular osmolytes within brain cells may draw water from the extracellular fluid. The syndrome normally reverses spontaneously after a period of regular HD. If no improvement is seen after a month of HD, one should investigate for other possible causes of the clinical syndrome by imaging the brain, obtaining an electroencephalogram, and examining the spinal fluid. Dialysis disequilibrium syndrome may be prevented by decreasing HD length to 2 to 3 hours, dialyzing daily, and reducing HD efficacy during the first sessions.

Dialysis encephalopathy (formerly called dialysis dementia) is probably a multifactorial syndrome occurring in sporadic-endemic and epidemic types. In particular, in the epidemic type, aluminum-based phosphate binders and exposure to a dialysate containing more than 20 μg/l aluminum are considered to be major causes.[25,26] Aluminum transferred to the nervous system by transferrin results in a characteristic clinical condition with prominent stuttering that usually worsens toward the end of a dialysis session and encephalopathy, initially responding well to intravenous benzodiazepines but then becoming unresponsive, leading to a severe encephalopathy and death. With the almost universal preparation of dialysate water by reverse osmosis and the marked reduction in aluminum-containing phosphate binder use, aluminum-induced encephalopathy has virtually disappeared. If it is present, aluminum toxicity is treated with deferoxamine (see Chapter 81). Renal transplantation is an effective treatment of dialysis dementia.

REFERENCES

1. Brouns R, De Deyn PP. Neurologic complications in renal failure: A review. *Clin Neurol Neurosurg*. 2004;107:1-16.
2. Burn DJ, Bates D. Neurology and the kidney. *J Neurol Neurosurg Psychiatry*. 1998;65:810-821.
3. Smogorzewski MJ. Central nervous dysfunction in uremia. *Am J Kidney Dis*. 2001;38:S122-S128.
4. Vanholder R, Glorieux G, DeSmet R, Lameire N. New insights in uremia toxins. *Kidney Int*. 2003;63:S6-S10.
5. De Deyn PP, D'Hooge R, Van Bogaert PP, Mareskau B. Endogenous guanidine compounds as uremic neurotoxins. *Kidney Int*. 2001;59: S77-S83.
6. De Deyn PP, Vanholder R, D'Hooge R. Nitric oxide in uremia: Effects of several potentially toxic guanidine compounds. *Kidney Int*. 2003;63: S25-S28.
7. Ohtsuki S, Asaba H, Takanaga H, et al. Role of blood-brain barrier organic anion transporter 3 (OAT3) in the efflux of indoxyl sulfate, a uremic toxin: Its involvement in neurotransmitter metabolite clearance from the brain. *J Neurol Chem*. 2002;83:57-66.
8. Fraser CL, Arieff AI. Nervous system complications in uremia. *Ann Intern Med*. 1988;109:143-153.
9. Lockwood AH. Neurologic complications of renal disease. *Neurol Clin*. 1989;7:617-627.
10. Aguilera A, Codoceo R, Bajo MA, et al. Eating behavior disorders in uremia: A question of balance in appetite regulation. *Semin Dial*. 2004;17:44-52.
11. Mehta RL, Pascual MT, Soroko S, et al. Spectrum of acute renal failure in the intensive care unit: The PICARD experience. *Kidney Int*. 2004; 66:1613-1621.
12. Tyler HR. Neurologic disorders seen in the uremic patient. *Arch Intern Med*. 1970;126:781-786.
13. Gipson DS, Wetherington CE, Duquette PJ, Hooper SR. The nervous system and chronic kidney disease in children. *Pediatr Nephrol*. 2004; 19:832-839.
14. Balzar E, Saletu B, Khoss A, Wagner U. Quantitative EEG: Investigation in children with end stage renal disease before and after haemodialysis. *Clin EEG*. 1986;17:195-202.
15. Stivelman JC. Benefits of anaemia treatment on cognitive function. *Nephrol Dial Transplant*. 2000;15:29-35.
16. Krishnan AV, Phoon RKS, Pussell BA, et al. Altered motor nerve excitability in end-stage kidney disease. *Brain*. 2005;128:2164-2174.
17. Krishnan AV, Phoon RKS, Pussell BA, et al. Sensory nerve excitability and neuropathy in end stage kidney disease. *J Neurol Neurosurg Psychiatry*. 2006;77:548-551.
18. Koomans HA, Blankestijn PJ, Joles JA. Sympathetic hyperactivity in chronic renal failure: A wake-up call. *J Am Soc Nephrol*. 2004;15: 524-537.
19. Hanly P. Sleep apnea and daytime sleepiness in end-stage renal disease. *Semin Dial*. 2004;17:109-114.
20. Ekbom KA. Asthenia crurum paraesthetica (irritable legs). *Acta Med Scand*. 1944;118:197-209.
21. Earley CJ. Restless legs syndrome. *N Engl J Med*. 2003;348:2103-2109.
22. Collado-Seidel V, Winkelmann J, Trenkwalder C. Aetiology and treatment of restless legs syndrome. *CNS Drugs*. 1999;12:8-20.
23. Barriere G, Cazalets JR, Bioulac B, et al. The restless legs syndrome. *Prog Neurobiol*. 2005;77:139-165.
24. Arieff AI. Dialysis disequilibrium syndrome: Current concepts on pathogenesis and prevention. *Kidney Int*. 1994;45:629-635.
25. Alfrey AC. Dialysis encephalopathy. *Kidney Int*. 1986;29(Suppl 18):S53-S57.
26. Nayak P. Aluminum: Impacts and disease. *Environ Res A*. 2002;89: 101-115.

CHAPTER 83

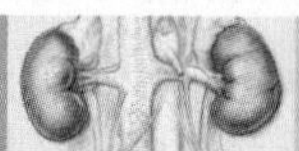

Gastroenterology and Nutrition in Chronic Kidney Disease

Gemma Bircher, Graham Woodrow

GASTROINTESTINAL PROBLEMS IN CHRONIC KIDNEY DISEASE

Gastrointestinal (GI) symptoms and disease are common in patients with chronic kidney disease (CKD), including those receiving renal replacement therapy (Fig. 83.1). Anorexia, nausea, and vomiting can arise from uremic toxicity. These may indicate the need to start dialysis or may be a manifestation of inadequate dialysis clearances. GI disturbances contribute to the development of malnutrition and wasting. These common complications of advanced CKD carry an adverse prognosis for survival. Some GI conditions are a result of uremia or the effects of renal replacement therapy. Other GI symptoms are manifestations of conditions also responsible for the renal disease. Medications used in patients with CKD may result in a range of GI complications.

GASTROINTESTINAL DISEASE IN CHRONIC KIDNEY DISEASE

Oral Disease in Chronic Kidney Disease

Glossitis can result from iron, vitamin B_{12}, or folic acid deficiency anemia. Halitosis is a feature of uremia, and reduced taste sensation or abnormal or unpleasant taste can impair dietary intake. Dental disease may prevent adequate nutrition. Gingival hyperplasia is a frequent complication of treatment with calcium channel blockers or cyclosporine. Oral candidiasis occurs in patients receiving immunosuppressive drugs including corticosteroids, with antibiotic therapy, in patients with diabetes, and in older malnourished individuals. If extensive, particularly with esophageal involvement, it may lead to dysphagia (Fig. 83.2).

Gastroesophageal Reflux Disease and Esophagitis

This common complaint is defined by symptoms of heartburn or mucosal changes arising from reflux of caustic gastric contents into the esophagus. It occurs more frequently in CKD because of GI dysmotility or delayed gastric emptying and may be more prevalent in peritoneal dialysis (PD) because of increased intra-abdominal pressure.[1] It is more common in patients with scleroderma because of reduced esophageal peristalsis. Esophagitis also results from the irritant effects of drugs, including slow-release potassium preparations, tetracyclines, iron preparations, aspirin, nonsteroidal anti-inflammatory drugs, and bisphosphonates. The diagnosis is made from the patient's symptoms. Typical features occur on endoscopy but may be absent in symptomatic patients. Other investigations include 24-hour ambulatory esophageal pH monitoring and demonstration of reflux on barium swallow examination. It is important to consider ischemic cardiac disease in CKD as an alternative cause of atypical symptoms. Management includes weight loss if the patient is obese; avoidance of bedtime snacks, fatty foods, cigarettes, and alcohol; and raising the head of the patient's bed. Proton pump inhibitors are the most effective medical treatment, and maintenance therapy may be required. Other drugs include H_2 receptor antagonists and antacid preparations. Sucralfate should be avoided in CKD because of the risk of aluminum accumulation.

Peptic Ulcer Disease, Gastritis, and Duodenitis

In the early days of dialysis, peptic ulceration and GI hemorrhage were major complications of renal failure. However, with effective drug therapies and improvement in dialysis therapy, peptic ulcer disease is not more common in CKD than in the general population, although it remains an important cause of GI hemorrhage. Peptic ulcers in CKD are more often multiple than in the general population and situated in a post-bulbar position.[2] Hemorrhage occurs more often, but pain is less frequent.[2]

Gastritis and duodenitis are common in patients with CKD and abdominal symptoms. Hypergastrinemia occurs in CKD but is not important in causation of gastritis, duodenitis, or peptic ulcers. Despite high urea concentrations in patients with CKD, *Helicobacter pylori* infection is not increased. Increased susceptibility of gastric and duodenal mucosa to damage in CKD may be an underlying mechanism. The presence of *H. pylori* infection in PD has been suggested as a possible cause of anorexia, inflammation, and malnutrition.[3]

Dyspepsia without other warning features (weight loss, vomiting, hemorrhage) may be managed by testing for *H. pylori* with a breath test or stool antigen test (which are valid in CKD) and an empirical course of acid-suppressing therapy. Persistent symptoms of new onset in patients older than 55 years warrant upper GI endoscopy to exclude malignant disease. The frequent coexistence of other symptoms in CKD, such as nausea, vomiting, and weight loss, may lead to a lower threshold for performing endoscopy. Management includes use of proton pump inhibitors and H_2 receptor antagonists. There is a risk of excess calcium and magnesium absorption with some antacids in CKD, and aluminum- or bismuth-containing preparations should be avoided.

Important Causes of Common GI Symptoms in Patients with CKD

Clinical Feature	Important Causes in CKD
Anorexia	Uremic toxicity Inadequate dialysis clearances Delayed gastric emptying
Nausea and vomiting	Uremic toxicity Delayed gastric emptying Gastritis/duodenitis Peptic ulcer disease
Constipation	Drugs – including opioid analgesia GI pseudo-obstruction Diverticular disease
Diarrhea	Diabetic enteropathy Dialysis-related amyloidosis Diverticular disease Clostridium difficile infection
GI hemorrhage	Gastritis/duodenitis Esophagitis Peptic ulcer disease Angiodysplasia Intestinal ischemia Dialysis-related amyloidosis Vasculitis
Acute abdominal pain	Gastritis/duodenitis Complications of peptic ulcer disease Acute pancreatitis Intestinal ischemia Diverticulitis GI pseudo-obstruction Colonic perforation due to fecal impaction Complications of peritoneal dialysis (peritonitis, dialysis catheter malposition, dialysate infusion pain) Complications of autosomal dominant polycystic kidney disease Retroperitoneal hemorrhage

Figure 83.1 Important causes of common GI symptoms in patients with CKD.

Delayed Gastric Emptying and Gastroparesis

Gastric emptying is impaired in uremia (possibly to a greater degree in PD)[4,5] and is affected by some conditions leading to renal disease, particularly diabetes and amyloidosis. This results in reduced appetite, early satiety, nausea, vomiting, and malnutrition. Mechanisms in uremia may include autonomic neuropathy and retained GI peptides. The diagnosis is confirmed by scintigraphic measurement of gastric emptying. It may be suspected when endoscopy demonstrates residual gastric contents despite fasting. Endoscopy is important to exclude gastric outlet obstruction. Reversible causes should be addressed, including optimization of diabetic control, correction of electrolyte abnormalities, and discontinuation of drugs that impair gastric emptying (e.g., those with anticholinergic and opioid effects). Dietary measures, with frequent smaller low-fat meals and avoidance of nondigestible solids, are often disappointing. Antiemetic agents are also often ineffective. The mainstay of treatment is prokinetic drug therapy, including metoclopramide, domperidone, and erythromycin. Prokinetic drugs improve nutritional state in patients with delayed gastric emptying.[6] Nutritional support through feeding nasoenteric or jejunostomy tubes may be required.

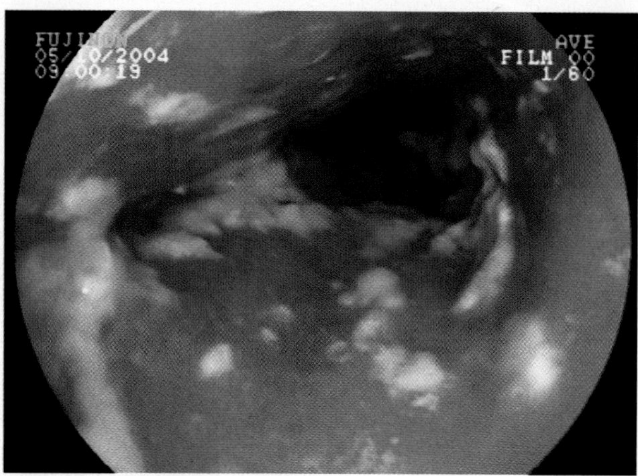

Figure 83.2 Endoscopic appearance of esophageal candidiasis. *(Courtesy Dr. B. Rembacken, Leeds, UK.)*

Large Bowel Disorders

Diverticular disease has an incidence in CKD similar to that in the general population, except in patients with autosomal dominant polycystic kidney disease (ADPKD), in whom it is increased.[7] It presents as acute diverticulitis or colonic perforation and is associated with PD peritonitis due to enteric organisms. There is a greater risk of bleeding in CKD (due to uremic bleeding tendency) and perforation with high-dose corticosteroids (e.g., after renal transplantation).

Constipation is common in CKD. Predisposing factors include drugs, dietary restrictions, low oral fluid intake, and electrolyte abnormalities, including hypercalcemia. In PD, constipation results in impaired dialysate drainage and catheter malposition. Severe constipation is a risk factor for large bowel perforation. Management includes stool-softening agents, stimulant laxatives, and fiber preparations. Drugs predisposing to constipation include calcium-based phosphate binders, sevelamer, oral iron, opioid analgesics, and calcium resonium.

Colonic perforation may occur in CKD from a number of causes. These include diverticulitis, fecal impaction, and dialysis-related amyloidosis. This condition has a higher mortality in CKD patients.

Gastrointestinal Pseudo-obstruction

Pseudo-obstruction presents with acute or more chronic clinical features of abdominal pain, vomiting, constipation, or diarrhea. It arises from disordered gut motility and is more common in dysmotility states, such as diabetes, amyloidosis, and scleroderma. Drugs reducing bowel motility and electrolyte disturbance such as hypokalemia predispose to pseudo-obstruction, and it may be acutely precipitated by surgery, constipation, and retroperitoneal hemorrhage. Investigations include plain abdominal radiography, computed tomographic scanning, and bowel

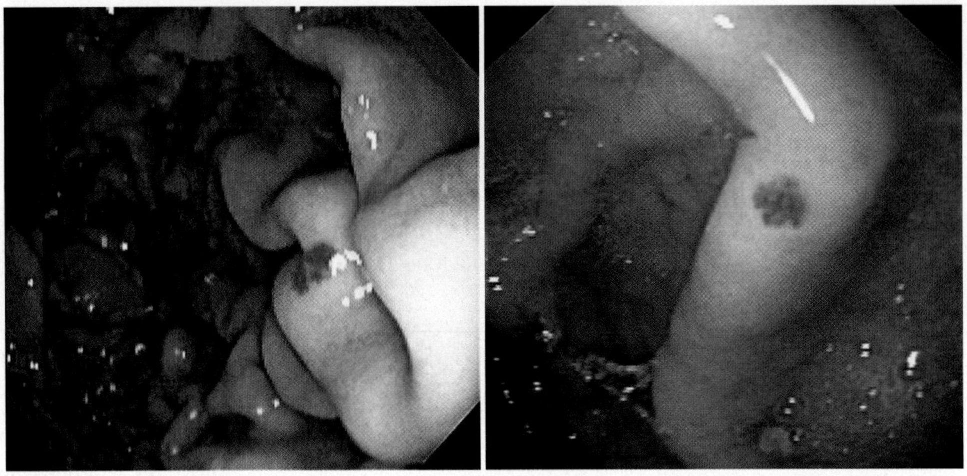

Figure 83.3 Two examples of gastric angiodysplasia in a dialysis patient. *(Courtesy Drs. R. Winograd and C. Trautwein, Aachen, Germany.)*

contrast studies. Management includes nutritional support (which may require parenteral feeding) and prokinetic agents. Nasogastric tube insertion and aspiration may be required for symptomatic control. Complications include intestinal perforation[8] and bacterial overgrowth.

Vascular Disease of the Gastrointestinal Tract

Intestinal ischemia is an important cause of an acute abdomen in older CKD patients. A proportion of cases result from nonocclusive mesenteric ischemia, in which there is no critical vascular occlusion.[9] It may be precipitated by excess fluid removal by hemodialysis (HD). Predisposing factors include hypotension, cardiac failure, hypoxia, increased plasma viscosity, and constipation (which increases intraluminal pressure, impairing vascular perfusion). Presentation is with abdominal pain, diarrhea, or lower GI bleeding. Abdominal signs such as peritonism can be misleadingly modest at presentation, but there is often peripheral neutrophil leukocytosis and progressive lactic acidosis. Milder cases may settle with hemodynamic resuscitation. More severe cases with features of peritonism and intestinal infarction require laparotomy and have a high mortality.

Gastrointestinal Hemorrhage

GI hemorrhage is an important complication of CKD, with increased incidence compared with the general population. Causes include a greater incidence of lesions such as gastritis and duodenitis,[10] angiodysplasia (Fig. 83.3), and, more rarely, dialysis-related amyloidosis and systemic vasculitis. Uremic hemostatic defects and anticoagulation during HD are also important. Upper GI endoscopy is the major diagnostic investigation in upper GI bleeding and also allows therapeutic procedures to stop bleeding. Flexible sigmoidoscopy and colonoscopy are performed in lower GI bleeding. Investigations where the cause remains unclear include angiography, small bowel enteroscopy or capsule study, and radiolabeled red cell scanning.

Resuscitation requires careful monitoring in CKD. Adequate fluid replacement to maintain renal perfusion in subjects not on dialysis or residual renal function in patients on dialysis, but avoiding fluid overload, is crucial. Monitoring of serum potassium with avoidance of hyperkalemia complicating blood transfusion is also important. Correction of coagulation defects in

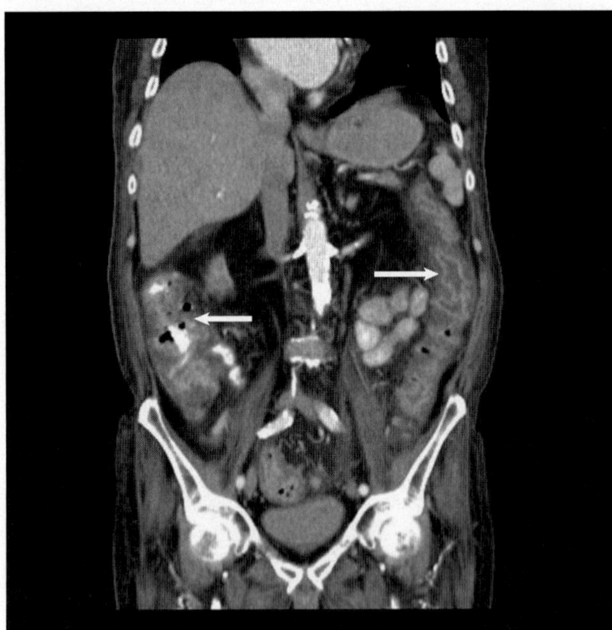

Figure 83.4 Computed tomographic appearance of *Clostridium difficile* colitis in a hemodialysis patient, demonstrating pancolitis with markedly edematous haustra *(arrows)* after treatment with broad-spectrum antibiotics. *(Courtesy Dr. M. Weston, Leeds, UK.)*

CKD includes optimization of dialysis clearance, correction of anemia, and use of DDAVP or cryoprecipitate. Drugs increasing bleeding risk should be discontinued when possible. HD, when it is required, should be performed without heparin for anticoagulation. Specific treatment is directed against the cause of hemorrhage. Bleeding from angiodysplasia in HD may improve on transfer to PD.[11] The presence of CKD increases the risk of mortality in GI hemorrhage.[10]

Clostridium difficile Infection

Clostridium difficile is a major cause of nosocomial diarrheal illness. Clinical manifestations vary from mild diarrheal illness to severe pseudomembranous colitis (Fig. 83.4). Patients with CKD are at risk of more frequent or severe infection and have a higher resulting mortality.[12] Reasons include the older age of CKD patients, frequent use of acid-suppressing drugs, and antibiotics. Diagnosis is made by identifying *C. difficile* toxin in diarrheal stools. In severe cases, there are radiologic appearances of acute colitis with mucosal edema, but these are not specific for *C. difficile*. A pseudomembrane may be visualized on sigmoidoscopy, but diarrhea can occur in its absence. The precipitating antibiotic should be stopped if possible. Oral metronidazole is first-line therapy; oral vancomycin is used if there is intolerance of or failure to respond to metronidazole. Drugs to reduce diarrhea or impairing gut motility must be avoided as they may precipitate toxic megacolon. Colectomy may be required in life-threatening disease. *C. difficile* infection is a major problem in the hospital setting, including renal units. Preventive measures, including hand washing, cleanliness of physical environment, and isolation of affected inpatients with barrier nursing, are essential. Antibiotic policies should minimize use of broad-spectrum antibiotics, which induce *C. difficile* infection.

Acute Pancreatitis

There is some evidence suggesting that acute pancreatitis is more common in CKD, and incidence may be greater in PD than in other CKD patients.[13] Most cases are secondary to biliary tract disease or alcohol or are idiopathic. Rarer causes, in CKD patients, are hypercalcemia, vasculitis, and drugs including corticosteroids, azathioprine, angiotensin-converting enzyme (ACE) inhibitors, and diuretics. Serum amylase is the usual diagnostic measure, although concentrations are normally elevated up to threefold in renal failure and are lowered in PD patients receiving icodextrin dialysate. Serum lipase is an alternative diagnostic marker (although it is also elevated in uremia). Amylase and lipase concentrations may be measured in dialysate in PD patients with suspected pancreatitis. Radiology, including ultrasound, computed tomography, and magnetic resonance imaging, is useful to confirm the diagnosis and to detect underlying biliary disease and complications such as pancreatic necrosis and pseudocyst formation. In PD patients with acute pancreatitis, dialysate may become cloudy with increased leukocytes, hemorrhagic, or dark brown (cola colored).

Acute Abdomen

Some causes of acute abdominal pain occur more commonly in or are specific to CKD patients. A high index of suspicion for ischemic bowel is important because of the frequency of vascular disease in CKD. Pain may result from complications of autosomal polycystic kidney disease. Retroperitoneal hemorrhage can arise from anticoagulation, including during HD. In PD, abdominal pain arises from peritonitis, dialysate infusion pain due to acidity of the fluid, catheter malposition, constipation, and encapsulating peritoneal sclerosis. Other surgical conditions need to be distinguished from dialysis-specific causes. Although air uncommonly enters the peritoneal cavity during PD, in the setting of acute abdominal symptoms, the finding of free gas on radiologic imaging of the abdomen suggests visceral perforation.

GASTROINTESTINAL-RENAL SYNDROMES

A number of conditions result in both renal and GI manifestations (Fig. 83.5).

Diabetes

Diabetes is commonly complicated by disordered gut motility. Gastroparesis needs to be distinguished from uremic upper GI symptoms. Diarrhea due to diabetic enteropathy is also common, classically is nocturnal, and usually is neurogenic in origin. Bacterial overgrowth is uncommon and is diagnosed by the hydrogen breath test. GI symptoms may be exacerbated by drug treatments for diabetes, including metformin and α-glucosidase inhibitors. Gastroparesis results in difficulties with glycemic control, fluid and electrolyte imbalance, drug malabsorption, and malnutrition. Colonic transport time is increased in diabetes, resulting in constipation.

Gastrointestinal-Renal Syndromes: Conditions Typically Resulting in Both Renal and GI Disease

Disorder	Renal involvement	GI involvement
Diabetes	Proteinuria, CKD	Gastroparesis, diabetic enteropathy, constipation
Systemic vasculitis	Proliferative glomerulonephritis, CKD	Intestinal ischemia, GI hemorrhage, bowel perforation, hepatobiliary involvement, acute pancreatitis
Systemic amyloidosis	Nephrotic syndrome, CKD	Diarrhea, malabsorption, splenic rupture
Autosomal dominant polycystic kidney disease	CKD, cyst hemorrhage and infection	Abdominal pain (from renal or hepatic cysts), diverticular disease, hernia
Inflammatory bowel disease	AA amyloidosis, drug-induced interstitial nephritis, IgA nephropathy, oxalate renal calculi (with terminal ileal Crohn's disease)	Abdominal pain, diarrhea, GI hemorrhage, malabsorption
Scleroderma	CKD, acute scleroderma renal crisis	Dysphagia, constipation, malabsorption and bacterial overgrowth
Fabry's disease	Hematuria, proteinuria, CKD	Abdominal pain, episodes of diarrhea or constipation
Coeliac disease	IgA nephropathy	Malabsorption, iron-deficiency anemia

Figure 83.5 Gastrointestinal-renal syndromes: conditions typically resulting in both renal and GI disease.

GI Side Effects of Drugs Commonly Used in Patients with CKD	
Drug	**GI Side Effects**
Calcium-based phosphate binders	Constipation, abdominal discomfort
Sevelamer	Constipation, dyspepsia, bowel obstruction (very rare)
Lanthanum carbonate	Dyspepsia, nausea, diarrhea
Cinacalcet	Anorexia, nausea, vomiting
Statins	Abdominal discomfort, diarrhea, constipation
ACE inhibitors	Nausea, constipation, diarrhea, acute pancreatitis
Iron supplements	Nausea, epigastric pain, constipation, diarrhea
Bisphosphonates	Esophagitis, esophageal ulcers and strictures
Polystyrene sulphonate (calcium resonium/kayexalate)	Severe constipation, colonic necrosis
Calcium channel blockers	Constipation, intestinal pseudo-obstruction
Metformin	Anorexia, nausea, vomiting, diarrhea
Proton pump inhibitors	Nausea, vomiting, abdominal pain, constipation, diarrhea
Mycophenolate mofetil	Diarrhea, abdominal pain, vomiting
Azathioprine	Dyspepsia, acute pancreatitis, hepatitis

Figure 83.6 GI side effects of drugs commonly used in patients with CKD. ACE inhibitors, angiotensin-converting enzyme inhibitors.

Systemic Vasculitis

GI manifestations of vasculitis include intestinal ischemia or infarction, hemorrhage, and perforation with peritonitis. Abnormal liver function test results arise from hepatitis, and cholecystitis and pancreatitis have been described. Serositis with abdominal pain is a feature of systemic lupus erythematosus. Abdominal pain, vomiting, and GI hemorrhage are typical of Henoch-Schönlein purpura.

Systemic Amyloidosis

Primary AL amyloidosis may result in both renal and GI involvement. Conversely, inflammatory bowel disease is an important cause of secondary AA amyloidosis, which may result in renal involvement. Thus, in a patient with renal amyloidosis who has GI symptoms, it is important to characterize the type of amyloid and the underlying cause of GI disturbance.

Autosomal Dominant Polycystic Kidney Disease

Abdominal hernias are more common in ADPKD[14] and are a particular problem in PD patients. Colonic diverticular disease occurs more frequently. The enlarged kidneys can result in abdominal pain, hemorrhage, abdominal fullness, and anorexia. Hepatic cysts and occasionally massive hepatomegaly may cause chronic abdominal pain and fullness. Common bile duct dilation, of uncertain significance, occurs more frequently in ADPKD.

Inflammatory Bowel Disease

Inflammatory bowel disease may be complicated by AA amyloidosis and IgA nephropathy. Drug therapy, such as aminosalicylates, can lead to renal disease, including chronic interstitial nephritis. Terminal ileal disease in Crohn's disease can lead to hyperoxaluria and oxalate calculi.

Celiac Disease

Celiac disease is a relatively common condition and occurs with increased frequency in association with other autoimmune conditions, such as diabetes mellitus. There is also a reported association with IgA nephropathy.[15]

DRUGS AND GASTROINTESTINAL DISEASE IN CHRONIC KIDNEY DISEASE

Drugs commonly used in CKD can lead to GI problems (Fig. 83.6). Phosphate-binding drugs commonly result in abdominal symptoms. Nausea and vomiting are important complications of cinacalcet. Other drugs important in CKD that may cause GI problems include statins, ACE inhibitors, iron supplements, sodium bicarbonate, bisphosphonates, and metformin. Acid-suppressing drugs including proton pump inhibitors and H_2 receptor blockers are commonly prescribed in CKD. They are often inappropriately continued for long periods[16] and have their own associated side effects. They increase the risk of *C. difficile* infection. Proton pump inhibitors can result in symptoms including nausea, vomiting, abdominal pain, diarrhea, and constipation.

SPECIFIC GASTROINTESTINAL COMPLICATIONS OF RENAL REPLACEMENT THERAPY

Idiopathic Dialysis-Related Ascites

Idiopathic ascites occurs in HD patients and may be due to suboptimal dialysis clearances. Diagnosis is by exclusion of other causes of ascites. Aspirated fluid usually has an elevated protein content. Management includes fluid and sodium intake restriction and ultrafiltration by dialysis. Small solute clearance must be optimized, and paracentesis may be required for symptom

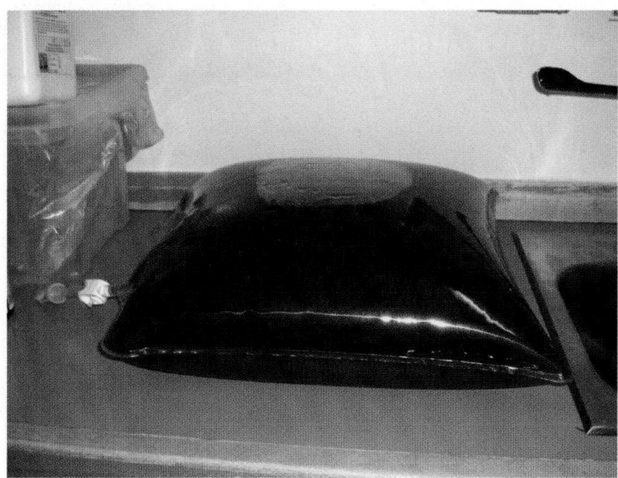

Figure 83.7 Hemoperitoneum: blood-stained peritoneal dialysate in a peritoneal dialysis patient who has developed acute pancreatitis.

control. It may resolve after renal transplantation, and switching to PD can be tried.

Peritoneal Dialysis–Related Gastrointestinal Conditions

A number of complications relating to PD may affect the abdomen, including infectious peritonitis, pain on dialysate infusion and drainage, and encapsulating peritoneal sclerosis (see Chapter 93). Hemoperitoneum in PD is typically related to the menstrual cycle, occurring during menstruation or ovulation, or may be self-limited, probably resulting from minor peritoneal membrane trauma from the PD catheter (Fig. 83.7). Rarely, underlying pathologic causes are present, including encapsulating peritoneal sclerosis, malignant disease, pancreatitis, hepatobiliary disease, and hemorrhage from polycystic kidneys.

Dialysis-Related Amyloidosis

Amyloidosis due to deposition of β_2-microglobulin in very rare patients on long-term dialysis can result in GI manifestations. These include GI hemorrhage, diarrhea, pseudo-obstruction, ischemia, and perforation (see Chapter 81).

Transplantation and Gastrointestinal Disturbance

A variety of GI problems occur after renal transplantation (see Chapters 100 and 101). Gastritis or duodenitis results from corticosteroid therapy, and mycophenolate mofetil commonly leads to diarrhea, abdominal pain, or vomiting. Infectious complications of the GI tract include oral and esophageal candidiasis, cytomegalovirus disease, and diarrhea from *C. difficile*. Posttransplantation lymphoproliferative disease may also involve the GI tract.

NUTRITION IN CHRONIC RENAL FAILURE

Nutrition plays an important role in the management of hypertension, obesity, hyperlipidemia, and diabetes, all of which affect CKD progress. As the glomerular filtration rate (GFR) deteriorates, retention of nitrogenous metabolites, decreased ability to regulate levels of electrolytes and water, and certain vitamin deficiencies can be affected by dietary changes. In addition, protein-energy depletion predicts a poor outcome.

Malnutrition: Protein-Energy Wasting

In kidney disease, there are often conditions that lead to wasting that are not related to reduced intake alone. Many terms exist to indicate malnutrition in CKD, including uremic malnutrition, protein-energy malnutrition, and malnutrition–inflammation complex syndrome. In 2008, the International Society of Renal Nutrition and Metabolism recommended that the term *protein-energy wasting* be used for loss of body protein and fuel reserves.[17]

The prevalence of protein-energy wasting in dialysis patients ranges from 10% to 70%, depending on the choice of nutritional marker and the population studied.[18,19] There is also diminished nutritional status before initiation of dialysis, which strongly predicts mortality on dialysis. Paradoxically, several investigators have found a significant inverse relationship between mortality risk and body size in HD populations, a phenomenon termed reverse epidemiology (see Chapter 78).

Several factors related to the uremic state may contribute to the high incidence of protein-energy wasting:

- Inadequate protein and calorie intake: nutrient intake parallels the decrease of GFR and is largely driven by CKD-associated anorexia.[20] This anorexia is due to impaired taste acuity and diminished olfactory function, medications, autonomic gastroparesis, psychological and socioeconomic factors, and inadequate dialysis. Elevated serum leptin, a long-term regulator of appetite, has also been linked to the anorexia seen in CKD.[21]
- Nutritional losses occur during treatment: 8 to 12 g of amino acids is lost per HD treatment, and 5 to 10 g of protein is lost daily during PD, depending on the peritoneal membrane transport type. This may be significantly higher during episodes of PD peritonitis.
- Metabolic acidosis, periods of acute or chronic illnesses, and the use of bioincompatible dialysis membranes, such as cuprophane, may induce protein catabolism. This is mediated in large part through the ubiquitin-proteasome pathway of protein degradation.[22]
- Protein catabolic effects that can further compromise patients early after transplantation include large doses of corticosteroids, the stress response to surgery, and delayed graft function.
- Inflammatory state of uremia (see also Chapter 78).[23]
- Endocrine disorders, such as insulin resistance, increased parathyroid hormone concentrations (which may promote amino acid catabolism and gluconeogenesis), and vitamin D deficiency (which can contribute to proximal myopathy), may have an adverse effect on nutritional status.

Assessment of Nutritional Status

The measurement of nutritional status does not lend itself to one simple test, and a panel of measures is required for optimal screening of nutritional status. Figure 83.8 summarizes some of the methods used for assessment of nutritional status.

Estimation of Intake

Diet history, recall, and food diaries are the mainstays for estimation of dietary intake. In addition, a gradual decrease in blood urea nitrogen and reduced phosphate and potassium levels may indicate a decrease in protein intake in dialysis-dependent

Assessment of Nutritional Status

Area	Assessments
Physical examination	
Assessment of dietary intake	Diet history, food diaries, appetite assessment questionnaires
Anthropometric measurements	Body weight, height, body mass index Percentage weight change Skinfold thickness Midarm muscle circumference
Body composition	Neutron activation Near-infrared resistance Bioelectrical impedance Dual-energy x-ray absorptiometry (DEXA) Total body potassium
Biochemical determinations	Serum electrolytes Serum proteins PNA, PCR Serum cholesterol Creatinine index
Nutritional scoring systems	Subjective global assessment
Immunologic assays	Blood lymphocytes Delayed cutaneous hypersensitivity tests
Functional tests	Grip strength

Figure 83.8 Assessment of nutritional status. Methods used to assess nutritional status are shown. PNA, protein equivalent of total nitrogen appearance; PCR, protein catabolic rate (mathematically identical to PNA). The creatinine index is measured as the sum of creatinine removed from the body (measured from the creatinine removed in dialysate, ultrafiltrate and/or urine), any increase in the body creatinine pool, and the creatinine degradation rate. See also http://www.kidney.org/professionals/kdoqi

patients, and low serum cholesterol level may indicate a poor calorie intake.

The excretion of the protein end-product urea is easily measured and is often used to estimate adequacy of dialysis. The protein equivalent of total nitrogen appearance (PNA) can be estimated on HD from interdialytic changes in urea nitrogen concentration in serum and the urea nitrogen content of urine and dialysate. nPNA is the term for PNA related to body weight. On the basis of the assumption that nitrogen excretion equals nitrogen intake in steady state, nPNA has been used to approximate dietary protein intake in the short term. Results, however, need to be interpreted with caution (urea kinetic modeling and adequacy of dialysis are further discussed in Chapters 89 and 90). Equations for estimation of nPNA have been recommended by the Kidney Disease Outcomes Quality Initiative (KDOQI).[24]

Body Composition

A range of techniques are available that can distinguish body compartments on the basis of physical characteristics, which can provide information about nutritional state (body lean tissue and fat content) and hydration.

Skinfold thickness can be used to assess body fat, and muscle mass can be assessed by measurement of mid–upper arm muscle circumference (MAMC; Fig. 83.9). The midpoint of the upper dominant arm is used, as this is the arm less likely to have an arteriovenous fistula.

$$\text{MAMC (cm)} = \text{midarm circumference (cm)} - [3.14 \times \text{triceps skinfold (cm)}]$$

The measurement is taken after dialysis for patients on HD. Although they are inexpensive and relatively easy to learn and quick to carry out, these anthropometric measurements are limited by intervariability and intravariability. Nevertheless, serial measures over time can be useful to track changes in the same patient when they are used in conjunction with other nutritional indices.

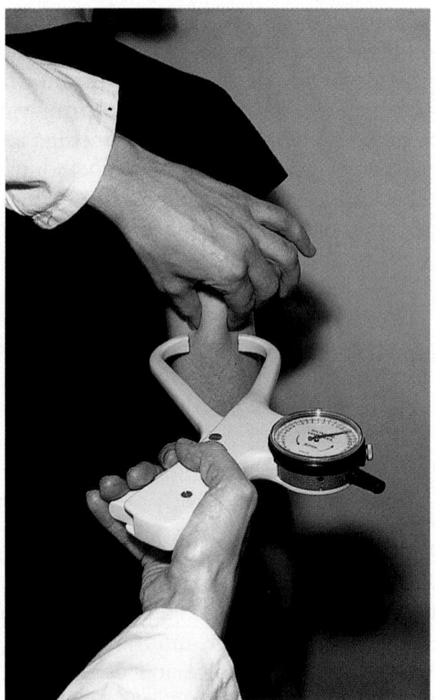

Figure 83.9 Routine measurement of skinfold thickness. The dominant arm that does not have an arteriovenous fistula or graft is used in patients with renal failure.

Subjective global assessment (SGA) is a reliable nutritional assessment tool for patients on dialysis.[25] A series of questions

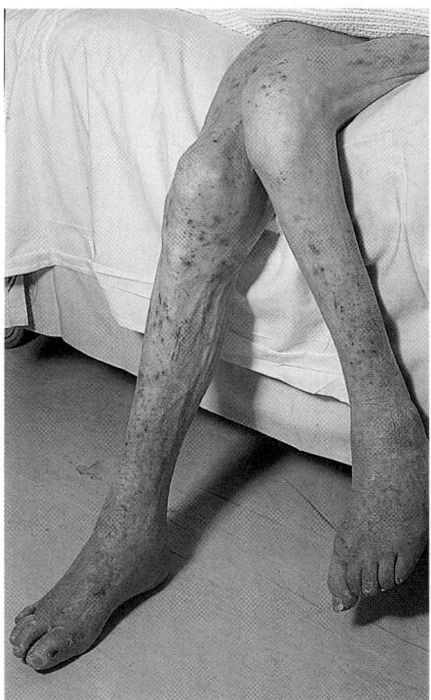

Figure 83.10 A severely malnourished hemodialysis patient. There is marked wasting of the quadriceps and calf muscles.

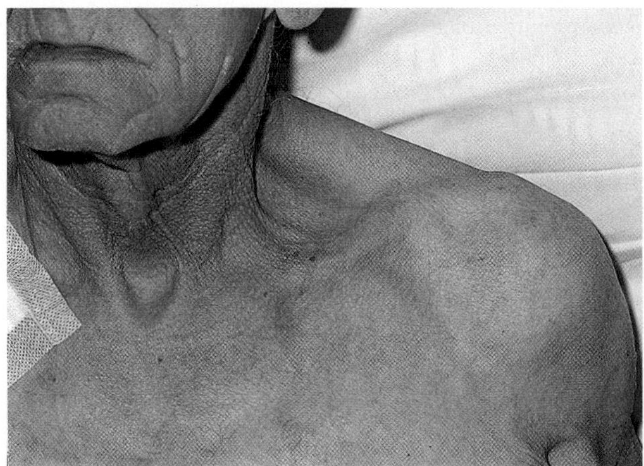

Figure 83.11 A severely malnourished hemodialysis patient. Muscle wasting around clavicle and shoulder.

about recent changes in nutrient intake are used with simple observations of the patient's body weight and muscle mass to determine subjectively the nutritional status of the individual; patients are classified as well nourished, mildly malnourished/suspected malnutrition, or severely malnourished. Figures 83.10 and 83.11 show muscle wasting in a patient on HD classified by SGA as severely malnourished. SGA is by definition subjective and has been criticized for being insufficiently sensitive to define the degree of malnutrition. Other scoring systems using components of the conventional SGA are presently being evaluated.

Visceral Protein

Fluid status, impaired liver function, age, and acute inflammatory conditions can all affect albumin levels. However, despite its relatively long half-life (20 days), albumin still remains an important measure of nutritional status and health of the patient.

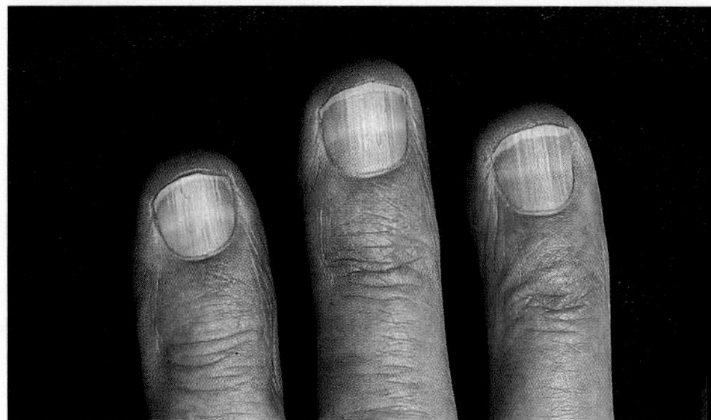

Figure 83.12 White nails in hypoalbuminemia. The white band grew during a transient period of hypoalbuminemia caused by nephrotic syndrome.

Some Indices of Malnutrition

Assessment	Indices
Biochemical parameters	Serum albumin below the normal range Serum prealbumin <300 mg/l (30 mg/dl) (for maintenance dialysis patients only as levels may vary according to GFR level for CKD 2-5) Low serum creatinine, phosphate, potassium, urea in patients on dialysis Serum cholesterol <150 mg/dl (3.8 mmol/l) Low creatinine index Low PNA, PCR
Anthropometric parameters	Continuous decline in weight, skinfold thickness, midarm muscle circumference Body mass index <20 Body weight <90% of ideal Abnormal muscle strength

Figure 83.13 Some indices of malnutrition. GFR, glomerular filtration rate; PNA, protein equivalent of total nitrogen appearance; PCR, protein catabolic rate.

Clinically, it may be possible to observe the growth of white nails when there has been a transient period of hypoalbuminemia (Fig. 83.12). Other serum protein markers of nutritional status are also difficult to interpret because of the influence of factors other than nutrition. Serum transferrin is linked to body iron stores and may be altered with changes in iron status. Prealbumin levels can be increased by CKD because of impaired metabolism in the kidney. Levels of prealbumin also decline rapidly during episodes of acute inflammation.

With the low specificity and sensitivity of many of the anthropometric and biochemical markers, it becomes clear that integration of a range of measurements along with evaluation of the subjective well-being of the patient is needed to assess nutritional status (Fig. 83.13).

Nutritional Guidelines

Guidelines are useful, but it is important that dietary restrictions are not unnecessarily imposed and that advice is tailored to the individual and altered as circumstances dictate. Figure 83.14 summarizes the nutritional recommendations for CKD.

Hyperlipidemia

Although disturbances of lipid metabolism are commonly seen in CKD, there is a paucity of data on the effect of diet therapy in this group. A diet low in fat, particularly saturated fat, with an increased intake of soluble fiber may be helpful in reducing cholesterol level, although the role of cholesterol lowering in CKD patients is controversial (see Chapter 78). Losing weight if overweight and consuming a diet lower in sugar may improve hypertriglyceridemia, but a balance needs to be struck between healthy eating concepts and nutritional adequacy. Additional fiber, within the confines of the diet, has the benefit of helping to regulate bowel function, particularly important in PD patients.

Bone and Mineral Disorders

Guidelines for phosphorus and calcium intake as well as vitamin D type and dose in CKD have been provided by KDOQI and recently updated by the Kidney Disease: Improving Global Outcomes (KDIGO) organization (see also Chapter 81).

Vitamins, Minerals, and Trace Elements

Vitamin, mineral, and trace element abnormalities in CKD relate to dietary restriction, dialysate losses, and the necessity of intact kidney function for normal metabolism of certain vitamins. However, the dietary requirements for patients with CKD are not clear-cut.

Protein and potassium restrictions can lead to inadequate intakes of pyridoxine, vitamin B_{12}, folic acid, vitamin C, iron, and zinc. The use of recombinant human erythropoietin may increase the requirement for iron and folic acid (see Chapter 79).

Increased serum homocysteine is a known risk factor for cardiovascular morbidity in CKD (see Chapter 78). However, lowering of serum homocysteine concentration with folic acid, vitamin B_{12}, and pyridoxine supplements has had no effect on cardiovascular outcomes in patients with advanced CKD.[26] A variety of multivitamin preparations are available that contain a recommended vitamin profile for dialysis patients (vitamin C, 60 mg; biotin, 300 µg; calcium pantothenate, 10 mg; cyanocobalamin, 6 µg; folic acid, 800 µg; niacinamide, 20 mg; pyridoxine, 10 mg; riboflavin, 1.7 mg; and thiamine, 1.5 mg).[27] In the absence of firm guidance, it is prudent to have a low threshold for commencing such a vitamin preparation. The European Best Practice Guidelines (EBPG) on nutrition give opinion-based recommendations for intakes of vitamins, minerals, and some trace elements in patients on HD.[28]

High-dose vitamin C supplements, popular in the general population, should not be taken as they may lead to oxalosis and extensive soft tissue calcification, including blood vessels, heart, and retina. Supplementation with fat-soluble vitamins is generally not recommended (with the exception of vitamin E, which the EBPG recommend can be supplemented in HD patients for secondary prevention of cardiovascular events and prevention of recurrent muscle cramps)[28] because diets do not tend to be deficient, dialysis losses are minimal, and accumulation can occur.

Recommendations for mineral intakes are shown in Figure 83.14.

Nutritional Recommendations in Renal Disease

Daily Intake	Predialysis CRF	Hemodialysis	Peritoneal Dialysis
Protein (g/kg ideal BW) (see KDOQI[24] for estimation of adjusted edema-free body weight)	0.6–1.0 Level depends on the view of the nephrologist 1.0 for nephrotic syndrome	1.1–1.2 [24, 28] This is a broad recommendation as protein intake would be individualized for the patient's nutritional status, serum phosphate levels, and dialysis adequacy	1.0–1.3 [24,32]
Energy (kcal/kg BW)	35 [24] (<60 yr) 30–35 [24] (>60yr)	35 [24] (<60 yr) 30–35 [24] (>60 yr)	35 [24] including dialysate calories (<60 yr) 30–35 [24] including dialysate calories (>60 yr)
Sodium (mmol)	<100 (more if salt wasting)	<100	<100
Potassium	Reduce if hyperkalemic If hyperkalemic, advice will take the form of decreasing certain foods (e.g. some fruits and vegetables) and giving information about cooking methods	Reduce if hyperkalemic	Reduce if hyperkalemic; potassium restriction is generally not required
Phosphorous	Reduce; level dependent on protein intake Advice will take the form of reducing certain foods (e.g. dairy, offal, some shellfish) and giving information about the timing of binders with high phosphorus meals and snacks		
Calcium	In CKD stages 3–5, total intake of elemental calcium (including dietary calcium) should not exceed 2000 mg/day	Total intake of elemental calcium (including dietary calcium) should not exceed 2000 mg/day	Total intake of elemental calcium (including dietary calcium) should not exceed 2000 mg/day

Figure 83.14 Nutritional recommendations in chronic kidney disease. Recommendations are for typical patients but should always be individualized on the basis of clinical, biochemical, and anthropometric indices. BW, body weight; CKD, chronic kidney disease; CRF, chronic renal failure; KDOQI, Kidney Disease Outcomes Quality Initiative.

Monitoring and Treatment

Monitoring of patients with CKD involves a combination of nutritional assessment, noting relevant biochemistry (potassium, phosphate, lipids), and observation of fluid status. The challenge comes in giving advice that carefully balances control of electrolytes while not compromising nutritional status. When anorexia is present, strategies to treat this should be considered and nutrient intake maximized by use of one or more of the methods discussed in the following sections.

Enteral Supplementation

If food fortification advice is insufficient, supplements, in the form of high-protein, high-calorie drinks, powders, and puddings, should be administered. Enteral tube feeding is also an option if nutrient intake cannot be increased sufficiently by use of oral supplements. Renal-specific tube feeds and supplements are available that have lower fluid and electrolyte contents. A systematic review suggested that enteral multinutrient support increases serum albumin concentration and improves total dietary intake in patients receiving maintenance dialysis.[29]

Supplementation of Dialysate Fluids

Intradialytic parenteral nutrition (IDPN) can be used to provide intensive parenteral nutrient therapy with use of concentrated hypertonic solutions three times weekly during HD treatments without the need for establishing a central venous line. The nutrients, usually a mixture of amino acids, glucose, and lipid, are infused into the venous blood line, and only about 10% of infused amino acids are lost into the dialysate. In 2007, a prospective, randomized trial of oral supplements with and without a year of IDPN failed to show any advantage of adding IDPN to oral supplements. However, the study did show that nutrition supplementation improved prealbumin levels, which was associated with a decrease in morbidity and mortality in malnourished HD patients.[30]

Intraperitoneal amino acids (IPAA) are sometimes used in PD. A 1.1% amino acid solution is substituted for glucose in PD fluid, and about 80% of the amino acids are absorbed in a 4-hour period.[31] The long-term effects of IPAA on nutritional status and clinical outcomes are not known.

KDOQI has suggested that IPAA (for PD) or IDPN (for HD) should be considered for patients who have evidence of protein or energy malnutrition and inadequate protein or energy intake and are unable to tolerate adequate oral supplements or tube feeding.[24]

Appetite Stimulants

Megestrol acetate, a progesterone derivative, moderately improved appetite in HD patients in small studies. However, as megestrol acetate is not without its side effects, larger trials are required before recommendations can be made for CKD patients. More studies are also required for ghrelin, an orexigenic hormone, and melanocortin-receptor antagonists.

Metabolic Acidosis

Although some trials have shown no detrimental effect of mild metabolic acidosis, many others have reported that normalization of the predialysis serum bicarbonate concentration is beneficial for protein nutritional status and bone metabolism. Medical management of metabolic acidosis is discussed further in Chapter 12. Current guidelines recommend the correction of acidosis in dialysis-dependent patients.[28,32]

REFERENCES

1. Kim MJ, Kwon KH, Lee SW. Gastroesophageal reflux in CAPD patients. *Adv Perit Dial.* 1998;14:98-101.
2. Kang JY, Ho KY, Yeoh KG, et al. Peptic ulcer and gastritis in uremia, with particular reference to the effect of *Helicobacter pylori* infection. *J Gastroenterol Hepatol.* 1999;14:771-778.
3. Aguilera A, Codoceo R, Bajo MA, et al. *Helicobacter pylori* infection: A new cause of anorexia in peritoneal dialysis patients. *Perit Dial Int.* 2001;21(Suppl 3):S152-S156.
4. DeSchoenmakere G, Vanholder R, Rottey S, et al. Relationship between gastric emptying and clinical and biochemical factors in chronic HD patients. *Nephrol Dial Transplant.* 2001;16:1850-1855.
5. Strid H, Simrén M, Stotzer PO, et al. Delay in gastric emptying in patients with chronic renal failure. *Scand J Gastroenterol.* 2004; 39:516-520.
6. Silang R, Regaldo M, Cheng TH, et al. Prokinetic agents increase plasma albumin in hypoalbuminemic chronic dialysis patients with delayed gastric emptying. *Am J Kidney Disease.* 2001;37:287-293.
7. Scheff RT, Zuckerman G, Harter HR, et al. Diverticular disease in patients with chronic renal failure due to polycystic kidney disease. *Ann Intern Med.* 1980;92:202-204.
8. Adams DL, Rutsky EA, Ostand SG, et al. Lower gastrointestinal tract dysfunction in patients receiving long-term hemodialysis. *Arch Intern Med.* 1982;142:303-306.
9. Zeier M, Weisel M, Ritz E. Non-occlusive mesenteric infarction (NOMI) in dialysis patients: Risk factors, diagnosis, intervention and outcome. *Int J Artif Organs.* 1992;15:387-389.
10. Tsai C-J, Hwang J-C. Investigation of upper gastrointestinal hemorrhage in chronic renal failure. *J Clin Gastroenterol.* 1996;22:2-5.
11. Yorioka K, Hamaguchi N, Taniguchi Y, et al. Gastric antral vascular ectasia in a patient on hemodialysis improved with CAPD. *Perit Dial Int.* 1996;16:177-178.
12. Cunney RJ, Magee C, McNamara E, et al. *Clostridium difficile* colitis associated with chronic renal failure. *Nephrol Dial Transplant.* 1998; 13:2842-2846.
13. Lankisch PG, Weber-Dany B, Maisonneuve P, et al. Frequency and severity of acute pancreatitis in chronic dialysis patients. *Nephrol Dial Transplant.* 2008;23:1401-1405.
14. Morris-Stiff G, Coles G, Moore R, et al. Abdominal wall hernia in autosomal dominant polycystic kidney disease. *Br J Surg.* 1997;84:615.
15. Woodrow G, Innes A, Boyd SM, et al. A case of IgA nephropathy and coeliac disease responding to a gluten free diet. *Nephrol Dial Transplant.* 1993;8:1382-1383.
16. Strid H, Simrén M, Björnsson ES. Overuse of acid suppressant drugs in patients with chronic renal failure. *Nephrol Dial Transplant.* 2003;18: 570-575.
17. Fouque D, Kalantar-Zadeh K, Kopple J, et al. A proposed nomenclature and diagnostic criteria for protein-energy wasting in acute and chronic kidney disease. *Kidney Int.* 2008;73:391-398.
18. Bergstom J. Nutrition and mortality in hemodialysis. *J Am Soc Nephrol.* 1995;6:1329-1341.
19. Churchill DN, Taylor DW, Keshaviah PR. The CANUSA Peritoneal Dialysis Study Group: Adequacy of dialysis and nutrition in continuous peritoneal dialysis: Association with clinical outcomes. *J Am Soc Nephrol.* 1996;7:198-207.
20. Kopple JD, Greene T, Chumlea W. Relationship between nutritional status and the glomerular filtration rate: Results from the MDRD Study. *Int Soc Nephrol.* 2000;57:1688-1703.
21. Cheung W, Yu P, Little B, et al. Role of leptin and melanocortin signaling in uremia-associated cachexia. *J Clin Invest.* 2005;115: 1659-1665.
22. Mitch W. Mechanisms causing loss of lean body mass in kidney disease. *Am J Clin Nutr.* 1998;67:359-366.
23. Stenvinkel P, Heimburger O, Paultre F, et al. Strong association between malnutrition, inflammation and atherosclerosis in chronic renal failure. *Kidney Int.* 1999;55:1899-1911.
24. K/DOQI Clinical Practice Guidelines for Nutrition in Chronic Renal Failure. National Kidney Foundation. *Am J Kidney Dis.* 2000;35(Suppl 2):S1-S140.
25. Enia G, Sicuso C, Alati G, Zoccali C. Subjective global assessment of nutrition in dialysis patients. *Nephrol Dial Transplant.* 1993;8: 1094-1098.
26. Jamison RL, Hartigan P, Kaufman JS, et al. Effect of homocysteine lowering on mortality and vascular disease in advanced chronic kidney disease and end-stage renal disease: A randomized controlled trial. *JAMA.* 2007;298:1163-1170.

27. Makoff R. Vitamin replacement therapy in renal failure patients. *Miner Electrolyte Metab*. 1999;25:349-351.
28. Fouque D, Vennegoor M, ter Wee P, et al. EBPG guideline on nutrition. *Nephrol Dial Transplant*. 2007;22(Suppl 2):ii45-ii87.
29. Stratton RJ, Bircher G, Fouque D, et al. Multinutrient oral supplements and tube feeding in maintenance dialysis: A systematic review and meta-analysis. *Am J Kidney Dis*. 2005;46:387-405.
30. Cano NJ, Fouque D, Roth H, et al. Intradialytic parenteral nutrition does not improve survival in malnourished hemodialysis patients: A 2-year multicenter, prospective, randomized study. *J Am Soc Nephrol*. 2007;18:2583-2591.
31. Bruno M, Gabella P, Ramello A. Use of amino acids in peritoneal dialysis solutions. *Perit Dial Int*. 2000;20(Suppl 2):s166-s171.
32. Dombros N, Dratwa M, Feriani M, et al. European best practice guidelines for peritoneal dialysis. 8. Nutrition in peritoneal dialysis. *Nephrol Dial Transplant*. 2005;20(Suppl 9):ix28-ix33.

CHAPTER **84**

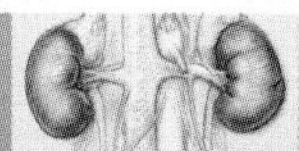

Dermatologic Manifestations of Chronic Kidney Disease

Pieter Evenepoel, Dirk R. Kuypers

Cutaneous disorders are common in patients with end-stage renal disease (ESRD), with the most prevalent disorder being hyperpigmentation. Many of these cutaneous disorders are due to the underlying renal disease, whereas others relate to the severity and duration of uremia.

Skin lesions associated with cutaneous aging have a high incidence in ESRD patients, including wrinkling, senile purpura, actinic keratoses, and diffuse hair loss. The prevalence of skin cancers does not appear to be increased unless the patient had received or is receiving immunosuppression.

Improved treatments in dialysis patients have resulted in changes in the frequency and types of skin disorders observed in conjunction with ESRD. Dermatologic conditions such as uremic frost, erythema papulatum uremicum, uremic roseola, and uremic erysipeloid now rarely occur. Pigmentary alterations, xerosis, ichthyosis, half-and-half nails, acquired perforating dermatosis (Fig. 84.1), bullous dermatoses, pruritus, and calcific uremic arteriolopathy are prevalent, whereas nephrogenic systemic fibrosis remains a rare entity.[1] The last four skin disorders are the focus of this chapter because they are associated with significant morbidity or mortality and represent an ongoing diagnostic or therapeutic challenge.

UREMIC PRURITUS

Clinical Manifestations

Uremic pruritus (UP) is a frequent symptom of ESRD with a reported prevalence ranging from 22% to 48%. Although its incidence in adult dialysis patients has declined as a result of improved dialysis efficacy and the introduction of so-called biocompatible dialysis membranes, pruritus remains a frustrating problem for patients, causing serious discomfort and skin damage, often in association with disturbance of day and night rhythm, sleeping disorders, depression, anxiety, and diminished quality of life.[2,3] The intensity and spatial distribution of UP vary significantly between patients and over time throughout the course of renal disease. Excoriations, induced by uncontrollable scratching with or without superimposed infection, are frequently encountered in severely affected patients and rarely lead to prurigo nodularis, that is, a treatment-resistant lichenified or excoriated papulonodular chronic skin eruption (Fig. 84.2). The most frequently involved body areas are the back, limbs, chest, and face; 20% to 50% of patients complain of generalized pruritus.[4]

Pathogenesis

Many uremic factors are thought to contribute to UP. Parathyroid hormone (PTH) and divalent ions (calcium, phosphate, and magnesium) have been implicated as itching is a frequent symptom accompanying severe secondary hyperparathyroidism and elevated calcium-phosphate product. However, the lack of consistent correlations between serum and skin levels of PTH, calcium, phosphorus, and magnesium with the severity of UP indicates that other factors contribute to its development. Histamine released by mast cells has been implicated in UP. The number of dermal mast cells is increased in uremic patients, and higher tryptase and histamine plasma concentrations are reported in severe cases. Histamine release is triggered by substance P, a neurotransmitter involved in itch sensation. The role of elevated serotonin (5-hydroxytryptamine [5-HT_3]) levels in dialysis patients with UP is debated as clinical trials using a selective inhibitor of 5-HT_3 have yielded conflicting results (see later discussion). Xerosis is a common skin problem (60% to 90%) in dialysis patients that predisposes to UP. Skin dryness is caused by primary dermal changes associated with uremia, such as atrophy of sweat glands with impaired sweat secretion, disturbed stratum corneum hydration, sebaceous gland atrophy, and abnormal arborization of free cutaneous nerve fiber endings.

There are two major hypotheses of the mechanisms of UP. The opioid hypothesis proposes that UP is caused by overexpression of opioid μ receptors in dermal cells and lymphocytes. Consistent with this hypothesis, activation of the κ opioid system using a κ-receptor agonist was efficient in reducing pruritus in a mouse model. In contrast, the immune hypothesis considers UP an inflammatory systemic disease rather than a local skin disorder. Studies examining the beneficial effects of ultraviolet B (UVB) exposure on pruritus showed that UVB attenuates the development of Th1-type lymphocytes in favor of the Th2 type. Indeed, the number of CXCR3-expressing and interferon-γ–secreting $CD4^+$ cells (indicating Th1 differentiation) is significantly increased in the circulation of dialysis patients with pruritus compared with those without. Serum markers of inflammation, such as C-reactive protein and interleukin-6, are also higher in subjects with UP.

Treatment

Common causes of UP in chronic kidney disease (CKD) and dialysis patients like primary skin disorders (e.g., urticaria, psoriasis, atopic dermatitis), liver disease (e.g., hepatitis), and endocrine diseases (e.g., hypothyroidism, diabetes mellitus) should be ruled out and adequately treated. The treatment approach to UP is shown in Figure 84.3.

Optimizing Dialysis Therapy

Improving both dialysis efficacy and the nutritional status of the dialysis patient will result in a reduced prevalence and severity of UP. The use of so-called biocompatible hemodialysis (HD) membranes also has a beneficial effect. Adequate control of

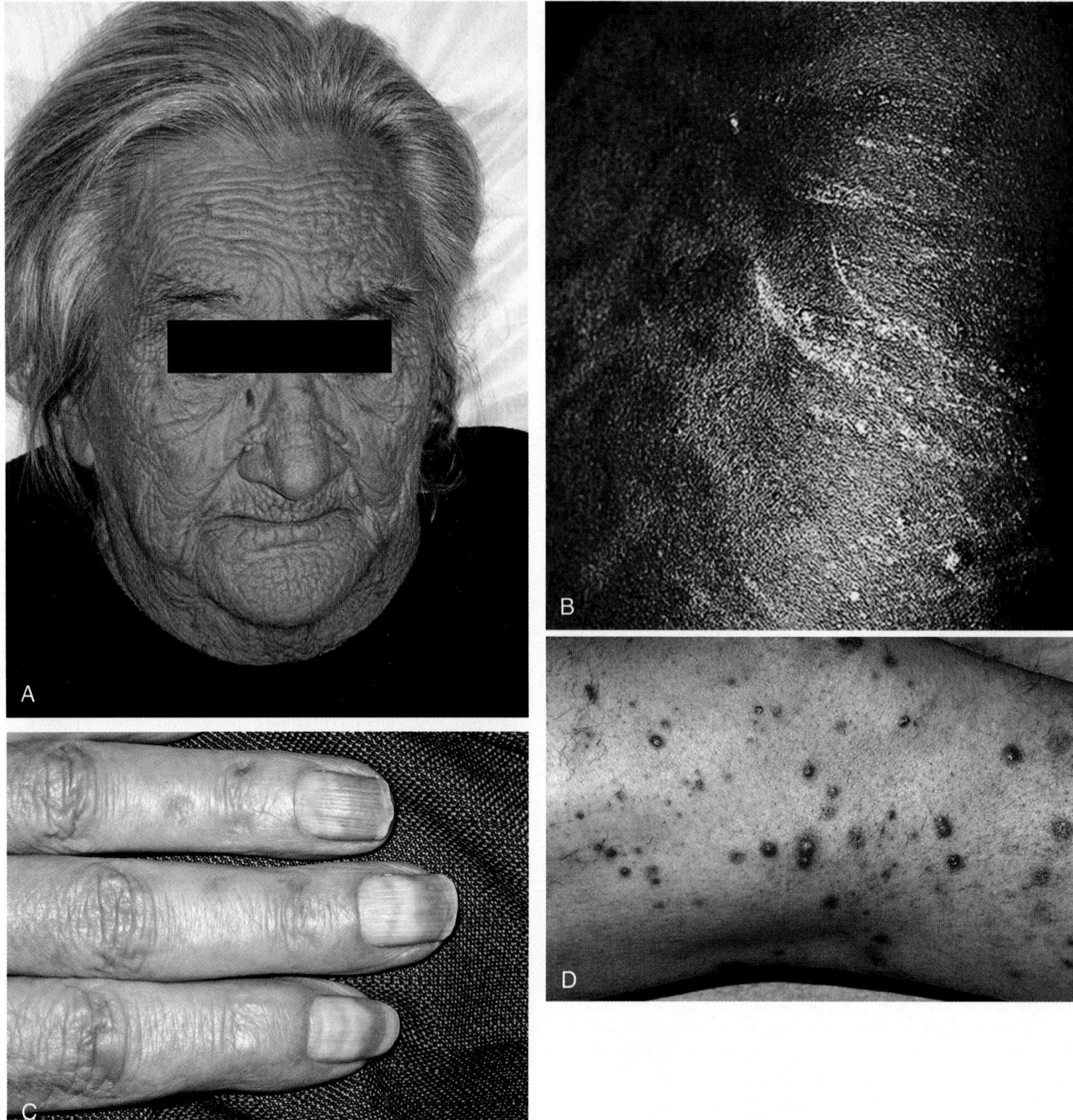

Figure 84.1 Cutaneous disorders in patients with end-stage renal disease. A, A spectrum of pigmentary alterations occurs in dialysis patients, brownish hyperpigmentation in sun-exposed areas being the most prevalent. **B,** Xerosis, a dry or roughened skin texture, is seen in up to 75% of dialysis patients. **C,** Half-and-half nails (also termed red and white nails) occur in as many as 40% of patients on dialysis. The nails exhibit a whitish or normal proximal portion and an abnormal brown distal portion. **D,** Acquired perforating dermatosis affects approximately 10% of the dialysis population. The lesion is usually asymptomatic and consists of grouped dome-shaped papules and nodules, 1 to 10 mm in diameter. The trunk and the extremities are most commonly involved.

calcium and phosphorus plasma concentrations by short-term use of dialysate with low calcium and magnesium concentrations ameliorated pruritus symptoms in only a few small studies and may lead to worsening of renal osteodystrophy in cases of prolonged use. Parathyroidectomy is not advocated for relief of UP because no consistent beneficial effects have been demonstrated.

Skin Emollients

The application of emollients is probably still the primary therapeutic action undertaken by many nephrologists despite contradictory results in the literature. The use of simple emollients without perfumes or other additives is preferred. Continuous bath oil therapy containing polidocanol, a mixture of monoether compounds of lauryl alcohol and macrogol, seems to be of value for some patients.

Antihistaminic Drugs

Classic antihistamines have limited efficacy and do not differ in efficacy compared with emollients; newer, second-generation antihistamines might have some effect but have not been formally tested in UP. Ketotifen (2 to 4 mg/day), a putative mast cell stabilizer, was beneficial in one small study.

Phototherapy

UV light, especially UVB (wavelength, 280 to 315 nm), is effective for treatment of UP and is well tolerated except for occasional sunburn. The duration of the antipruritic effect of thrice-weekly total body UVB therapy (total, 8 to 10 sessions) is variable but may last for several months. Potential carcinogenic effects of UV radiation require serious consideration, and its prolonged use is contraindicated in patients with a fair complexion (skin phototypes I and II).

5-Hydroxytryptamine Antagonist

Ondansetron, a selective 5-HT_3 antagonist, was used successfully in a small study in peritoneal dialysis patients. However, a subsequent larger randomized, placebo-controlled study failed to show superiority over placebo in HD patients.

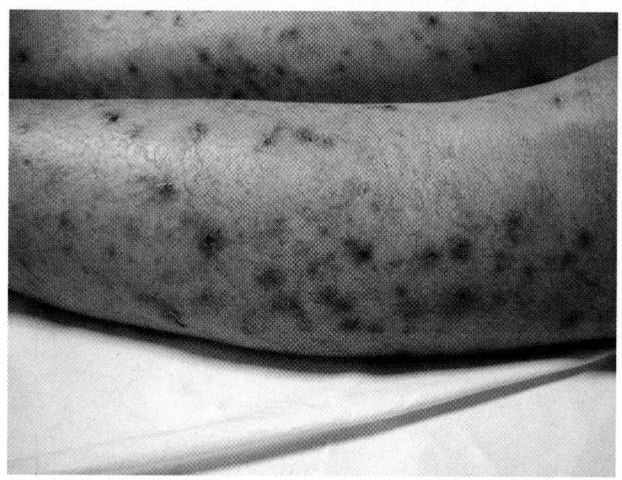

Figure 84.2 Prurigo nodularis. *(Courtesy I. Macdougall, London, UK.)*

Opioid Receptor Antagonists and Agonists

The oral μ opiate receptor antagonist naltrexone seemed effective for the treatment of UP in a small randomized, crossover trial in 15 dialysis patients. In a subsequent larger trial, a significant difference in efficacy could not be demonstrated between 4 weeks of treatment with naltrexone (50 mg/day) or placebo. More recently, a κ-receptor agonist, nalfurafine, given intravenously after HD, was tested in two randomized, double-blind, placebo-controlled trials comprising 144 patients. Itching intensity, excoriations, and sleep disturbances were significantly reduced in patients receiving the active compound without an excess of drug-related side effects compared with placebo.[5] In some patients, symptom relief between dialysis sessions was incomplete, and central nervous system side effects such as drowsiness, dizziness, and somnolence occurred.

Gabapentin

Gabapentin, an anticonvulsant drug, administered after dialysis (300 mg) was effective in reducing pruritus. A reduced dose is required if it is given chronically to subjects with ESRD as it has a narrow therapeutic window, and it can accumulate and cause neurotoxic side effects.[6]

Immunomodulators and Immunosuppressive Agents

A 7-day course of thalidomide reduced the intensity of UP by up to 80% in a placebo-controlled crossover study of 29 HD patients. Because of its strong teratogenic properties, thalidomide should probably be reserved for therapy-resistant severe UP in individuals outside the reproductive-age category. Adverse effects of thalidomide, such as peripheral neuropathy and cardiovascular side effects, limit its continuous longer use. A prospective, single-center study of 25 chronic dialysis patients with UP demonstrated that 6 weeks of treatment with tacrolimus ointment (0.1%) significantly reduced the severity of UP. Tacroli-

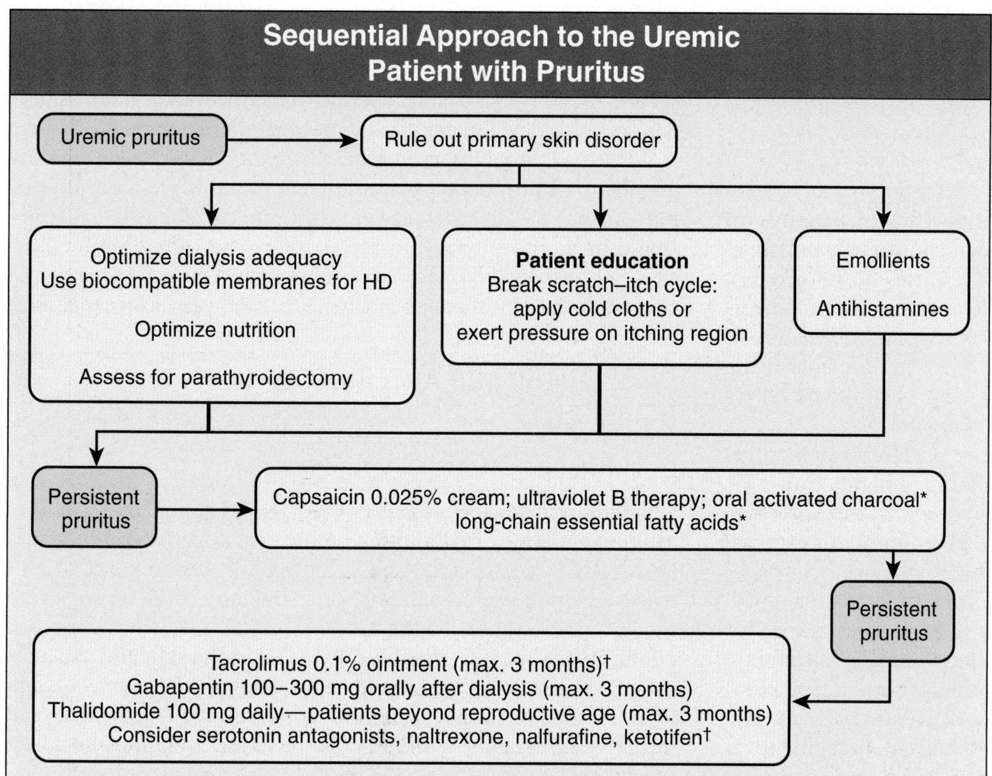

Figure 84.3 Sequential approach to the uremic patient with pruritus. *See text for details. †Therapeutic benefit in studies has been described variably; see text for details. HD, hemodialysis.

mus was well tolerated in this trial and caused no detectable systemic exposure or side effects.[7] However, a subsequent smaller vehicle-controlled trial showed equal relief of UP with vehicle and tacrolimus. The risks of long-term topical use of these agents are currently unknown, and their prolonged use is not recommended until more data are available.

Long-Chain Essential Fatty Acids

Oral administration of γ-linoleic acid (GLA)–rich primrose oil resulted in significant improvement of UP in chronic dialysis patients. Supplementation of GLA-rich primrose oil is thought to augment synthesis of anti-inflammatory eicosanoids. Similar effects could be obtained by use of fish oil, olive oil, and safflower oil.

Capsaicin

Capsaicin (*trans*-8-methyl-*N*-vanillyl-6-nonenamide) is a natural alkaloid found in the pepper plant that depletes the cutaneous type C sensory nerve endings of substance P. Two clinical studies showed that application of a 0.025% capsaicin cream significantly alleviated UP in dialysis patients while exhibiting no side effects.

Oral Activated Charcoal

Pruritus symptoms completely disappeared or were significantly reduced in chronic dialysis patients treated with activated charcoal (6 g/day) for 8 weeks. In two different clinical studies, comparable results were obtained with this inexpensive and well-tolerated compound, rendering it a valuable alternative for patients with UP.

Miscellaneous

Various other types of therapies have been examined in the treatment of pruritus but are, despite the effectiveness of some, not considered first choice in chronic HD patients because of undesirable side effects, cumbersome use, or incompatibility with renal replacement therapy (sauna, cholestyramine, nicergoline). Others that have not reduced UP in a controlled setting and are therefore not advocated include acupuncture, low-protein diet, intravenous lidocaine, and mexiletine.

BULLOUS DERMATOSES

Bullous dermatoses are reported in up to 16% of patients on maintenance dialysis. They can be subdivided into true porphyrias (e.g., porphyria cutanea tarda [PCT], variegate porphyria), pseudoporphyrias (e.g., secondary to nonporphyrinogenic drugs and chemicals, dialysis-porphyria), and other photodermatoses.[8] They are clinically and histologically similar and are characterized by a blistering photosensitive skin rash. The dorsal hands and the face are the most affected areas (Fig. 84.4).

PCT is caused by abnormalities in the porphyrin-heme biosynthetic pathway leading to an accumulation of highly carboxylated uroporphyrins in the plasma and skin. Phenotypic expression of the disease also requires one or more of a number of external contributory factors, including alcohol, estrogens, iron, and infection with hepatitis B and C. It is important to distinguish PCT from other porphyrias in which patients are at risk for development of potentially fatal neurologic attacks if they are exposed to porphyrinogenic drugs and other precipitants. Therapeutic options include avoidance of environmental triggers, HD with high-flux membranes, repeated small-volume phlebotomies, and iron chelators.

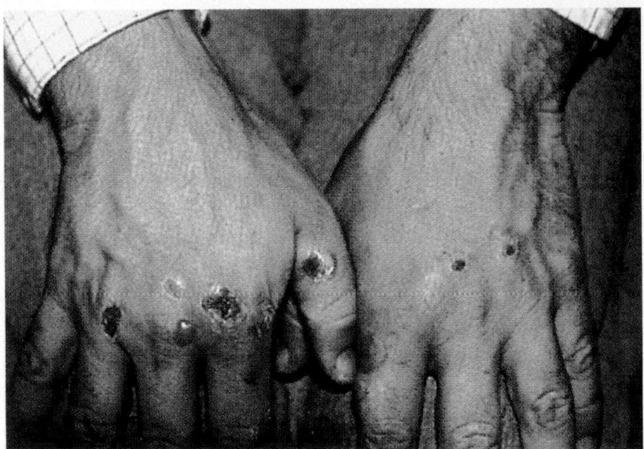

Figure 84.4 Porphyria cutanea tarda. Tense bullae, erosions, and crusts of the dorsal hands. *(From reference 9.)*

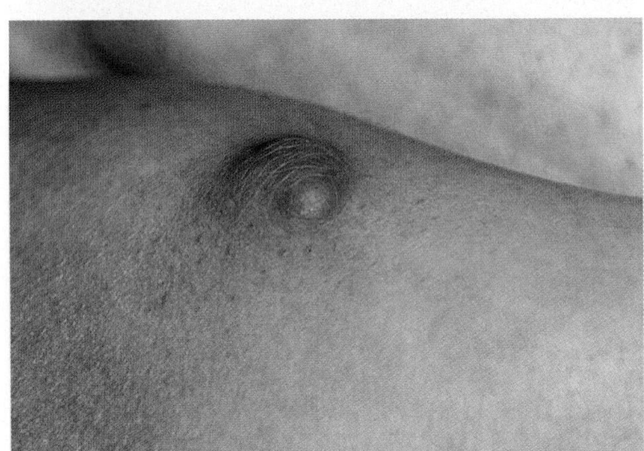

Figure 84.5 Benign nodular calcification (calcinosis cutis). Firm subcutaneous nodule adjacent to the elbow.

The term *pseudoporphyria* was originally used for patients with normal plasma porphyrins who exhibited PCT-like skin lesions secondary to drugs and chemicals. However, some dialysis patients also develop similar skin lesions that spontaneously heal and leave a hypopigmented area; this entity is known as dialysis-porphyria; a proportion of these have raised plasma porphyrins but without the disturbances in porphyrin metabolism classically found in the porphyrias. In rare patients, an offending medication can be identified. However, in most dialysis patients, protection from sun exposure appears to be the only preventive measure.

CALCIFIC UREMIC ARTERIOLOPATHY (CALCIPHYLAXIS)

Definition

Calcific uremic arteriolopathy (CUA), or calciphylaxis, is a devastating and life-threatening ischemic vasculopathy confined primarily to patients with CKD. There are also reports of this disease in nonuremic patients. The ischemia may be so severe that frank infarction of downstream tissue develops. The most common and most noticeable damage is in the skin and subcutaneous tissues.[10] CUA should be distinguished from benign nodular calcification (calcinosis cutis; Fig. 84.5), which can develop in patients with very high serum calcium-phosphate product.

Pathogenesis

The pathogenesis of CUA involves abnormalities in mineral metabolism in uremia that predispose to vascular and soft tissue calcification, but no single abnormality is sufficient to predict the development of this disorder. Elevated levels of PTH and therapy with vitamin D analogues have been associated with an increased risk of CUA, although the evidence is not always striking. A perturbation of the calcium and phosphate homeostasis most probably underlies the positive association. Insufficient activation or expression of inhibitors of calcification should also be considered in the pathogenesis. Inhibitors of vascular calcification include matrix GLA protein (MGP), osteoprotegerin, pyrophosphate, and fetuin-A. MGP requires vitamin-K mediated γ-carboxylation for its functional activity. As a consequence, coumarin anticoagulants and vitamin K deficiency may antagonize MGP function and stimulate vascular calcification. Levels of both osteoprotegerin and fetuin-A decline with inflammation. Finally, several lines of evidence indicate that a hypercoagulable state secondary to an absolute or functional protein C or protein S deficiency may be involved in the pathogenesis of CUA.[10]

Epidemiology and Risk Factors

Although hard epidemiologic data are lacking, the incidence of CUA may be increasing. This might be due in part to increased physician awareness and possibly the practice of treating severe hyperparathyroidism with calcium-based phosphate binders plus vitamin D analogues. The estimated incidence ranges between 1 and 4 per 100 patient-years.

Female gender, Caucasian race, obesity, diabetes, use of coumarin anticoagulants, and dialysis vintage are established risk factors. Probable risk factors include low serum albumin concentrations, the use of calcium salts and vitamin D analogues, and exposure to high doses of iron salts. There is no correlation between the severity of any of these factors and the development of CUA.[10]

Clinical Manifestations

CUA is frequently precipitated by a specific event, such as local skin trauma or a hypotensive episode. CUA is typically characterized by areas of ischemic necrosis of the dermis, subcutaneous fat, and, less often, muscle. These ischemic changes lead to livedo reticularis or violaceous, painful, plaque-like subcutaneous nodules on the trunk, buttocks, or proximal extremity, that is, in areas of greatest adiposity (proximal CUA; Fig. 84.6A). The early purpuric plaques and nodules progress to ischemic or necrotic ulcers with eschars that often become infected. CUA can also affect the hands, fingers, and lower extremities, thereby mimicking atherosclerotic peripheral vascular disease (distal CUA; Fig. 84.6B). Peripheral pulses are preserved distal to the area of necrosis. Myopathy, hypotension, fever, dementia, and infarction of the central nervous system, bowel, or myocardium have been described in association with cutaneous necrosis. This condition is termed systemic CUA.[10,11]

Pathology

The histologic features of CUA are suggestive but not pathognomonic. Specimens from incisional biopsies of early lesions show subtle histologic changes. Late lesions characteristically show epidermal ulceration, dermal necrosis, and mural calcification with intimal hyperplasia of small and medium-sized blood vessels in the dermis and subcutaneous tissue (Fig. 84.7).

Diagnosis and Differential Diagnosis

Many clinicians base the diagnosis of CUA on physical examination findings only. Although ulceration is an obvious presentation of CUA, increasing awareness of the condition should allow diagnosis at an earlier, nonulcerative stage.[11] Biopsies are discouraged because of potential ulceration in the region of the incision and the risk of sample error. Other potentially useful diagnostic procedures include measurements of transcutaneous oxygen saturation, bone scintigraphy (Fig. 84.8), and xeroradiography.[11]

The following conditions should be considered in the differential diagnosis: systemic vasculitis, peripheral vascular disease, pyoderma gangrenosum, atheroemboli, cryoglobulinemia, warfarin-induced skin necrosis, and systemic oxalosis. Considering these risks, a skin biopsy should be performed only when clinical circumstances do not suggest CUA or when detailed clinical and technical examinations, including the assessment of coagulation and immunologic parameters, point to an alternative diagnosis.

Natural History

Despite intensive combined treatments, the prognosis of CUA remains poor; the overall 1-year survival is 45% and the 5-year survival is 35%, with a relative risk of death of 8.5 compared with other dialysis patients. Patients with ulcerative or proximal CUA have the worst prognosis. Infection accounts for up to 60% of the mortality.[11]

Prevention and Treatment

Preventive approaches include attention to calcium, phosphorus, PTH homeostasis, and nutritional state. Specific therapeutic regimens have been limited to uncontrolled case series (Fig. 84.9). A reasonable plan of intervention should include an aggressive program of wound care and prevention of superinfection, adequate pain control, and correction of underlying abnormalities in plasma calcium and phosphorus concentrations. This includes cessation of vitamin D supplementation, intensification of the dialysis treatment, and use of a low-calcium dialysate and non–calcium-containing phosphate binders (e.g., sevelamer, lanthanum carbonate). Furthermore, local tissue trauma, including subcutaneous injections, should be avoided. Parathyroidectomy is effective in the control of CUA in some series but not in others and should be reserved for patients with severe hyperparathyroidism.[10] In such patients, calcimimetic agents may be a suitable noninvasive alternative. Vitamin K supplementation is advised in patients with coumarin-associated CUA. Novel and experimental therapies include hyperbaric oxygen therapy and bisphosphonates. Sodium thiosulfate has repeatedly been used to enhance the solubility of calcium deposits[12] because exchange of calcium for sodium results in extremely soluble calcium thiosulfate. Besides being a chelator of calcium, sodium thiosulfate is also a potent antioxidant. Sodium thiosulfate is given intravenously at the end of every HD session (12.5 to 25 g during 30 to 60 minutes). Apart from nausea and vomiting, the therapy is well tolerated. The major side effect of sodium thiosulfate infusion is the development of metabolic acidosis. The optimal duration of treatment and potential effects of long-term treatment on bone are unknown.

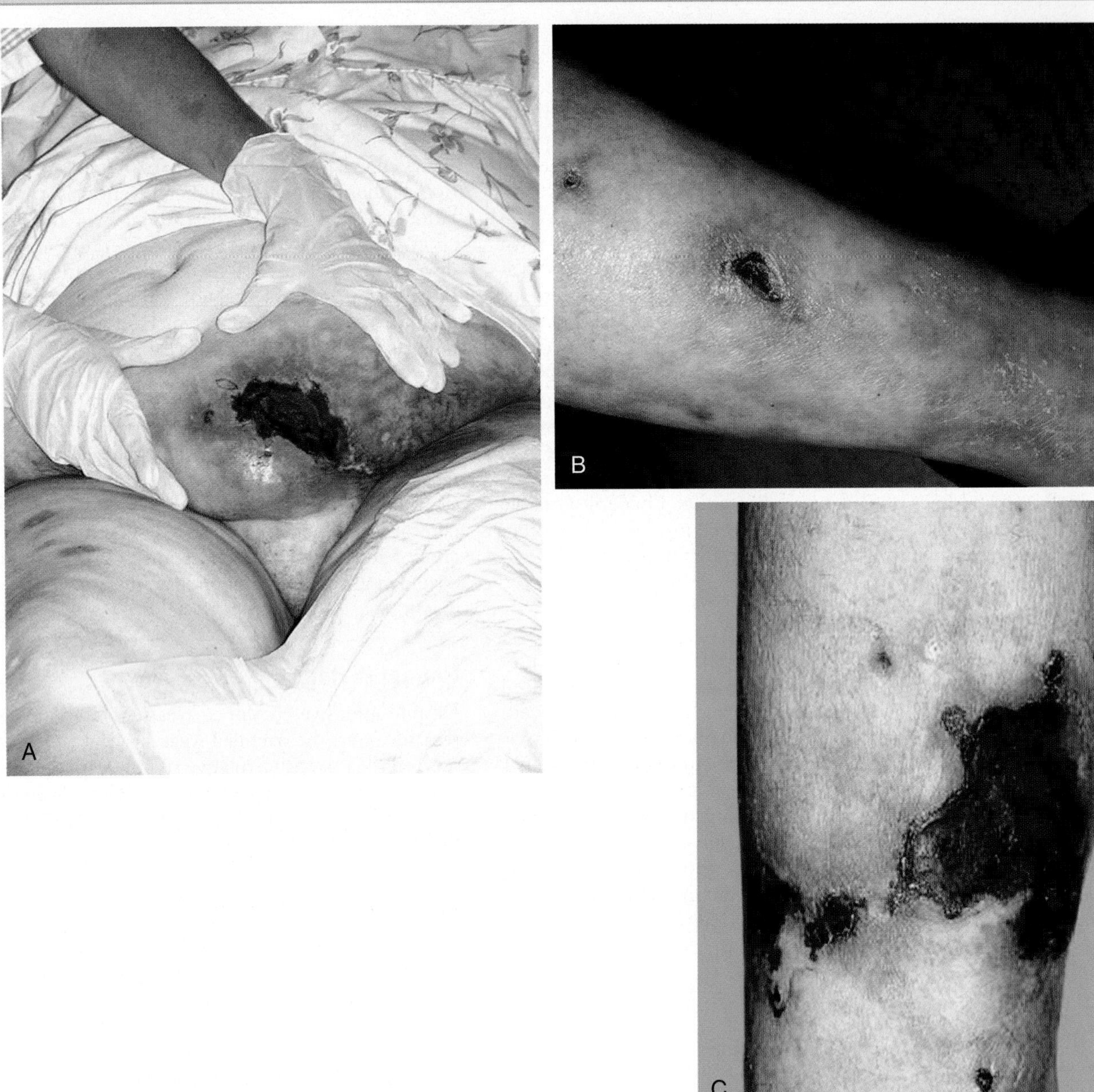

Figure 84.6 Proximal **A,** and distal **B, C,** calcific uremic arteriolopathy.

NEPHROGENIC SYSTEMIC FIBROSIS

Definition

Nephrogenic systemic fibrosis (NSF), formerly known as nephrogenic fibrosing dermopathy, is a scleroderma-like fibrosing disorder that develops in the setting of renal failure. The fibrotic process affects the dermis, subcutaneous tissues, fascia, and other organs, including striated muscles, heart, and lungs.[13,14]

Pathogenesis

The role of gadolinium-based contrast (GBC) agents in the development of NSF is increasingly recognized; exposure to gadolinium before the onset of disease was confirmed in more than 95% of reported cases. Free gadolinium ions are highly toxic to tissues. The toxic effects of gadolinium are circumvented by sequestration of the metal by chelates, large organic molecules that form a stable complex with gadolinium and make the ion biochemically inert and nontoxic. Under normal circumstances, GBC agents are eliminated by the kidney through glomerular filtration. Evidence points toward aberrant activation of circulating fibrocytes as a central event in the genesis of NSF. Other investigators have suspected that the strongly profibrotic mediator transforming growth factor ß may be involved in the pathogenesis of NSF.

Epidemiology

NSF is a rare disorder. Since the identification of the first cases of NSF in 1997, the NSF registry has confirmed more than 215 cases from medical centers worldwide. NSF equally affects men and women. The risk for development of NSF after GBC agent exposure is related to the degree of renal failure and stability of the chelate. Gadodiamide (marketed as Omniscan in the United States), the linear nonionic chelate–based formulation, maintains

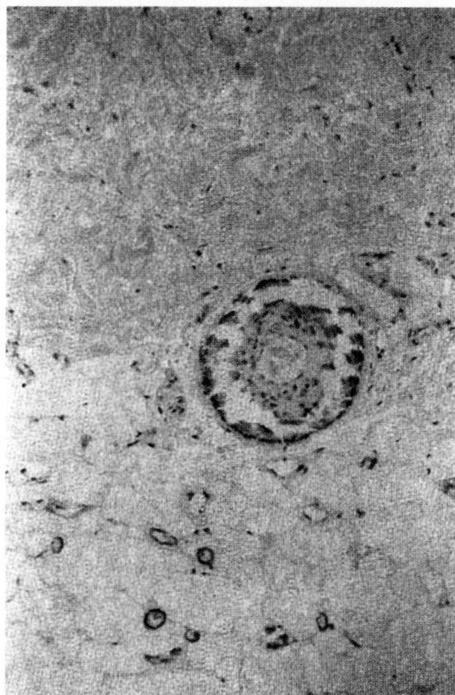

Figure 84.7 Histopathologic features of calcific uremic arteriolopathy. Medial calcification and intimal hyperplasia of an arteriole at the dermal-subcutaneous junction. Note calcification of interlobular capillaries in the subcutaneous tissue *(arrows)*. Van Kossa staining. *(From reference 9.)*

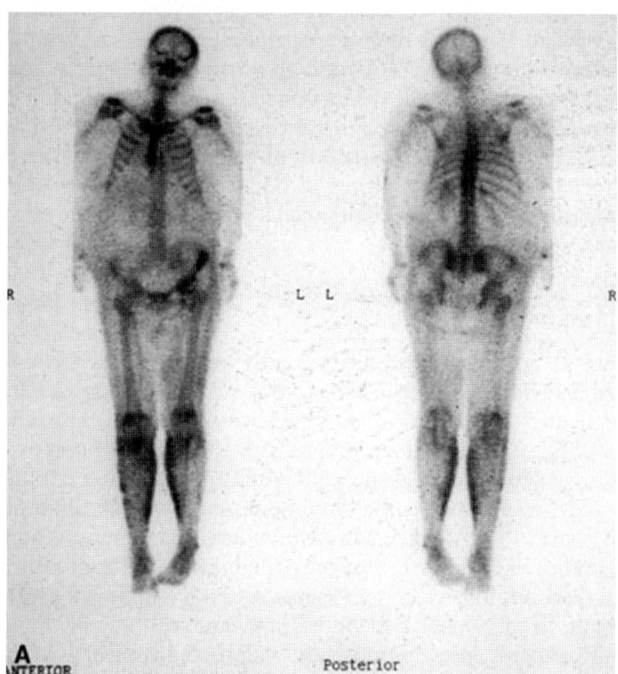

Figure 84.8 Bone scintigraphic abnormalities in calcific uremic arteriolopathy. Calf calcification in a patient with gross ulcerations in both legs from the popliteal fossae to the ankles *(arrows)*. *(From reference 15.)*

Treatment Options in Patients with CUA

1. Reduction of pro-calcifying factors
- Intensified (e.g., daily, hemodialysis; switch from peritoneal dialysis to hemodialysis; low-calcium dialysate)
- Avoidance of vitamin D and calcium supplements; administration of calcium-free phosphate binders; bisphosphonate administration (caution if adynamic bone disease is suspected)
- Parathyroidectomy (in case of hyperparathyroidism) or administration of cinacalcet

2. Improving the status of calcification inhibitors
- Halt vitamin K antagonists (warfarin)
- Aggressive treatment of infections or other proinflammatory stimuli to increase fetuin-A levels (a negative acute-phase protein)
- Experimental:
  Administration of high-dose vitamin K_2?
  Administration of fetuin-A (e.g., by fresh frozen plasma or plasma exchange?)

3. Prevention or reversal of calcium-phosphate precipitation
- Administration of sodium thiosulfate

4. Supportive measures
- Avoidance of additional local tissue trauma by atraumatic wound care with gentle debridement of necrotic tissue and avoidance of subcutaneous injections
- Improving oxygen supply by hyperbaric oxygen therapy
- Anticoagulation (heparin and low-molecular-weight heparins)
- Adequate pain management
- Adequate infection control

Figure 84.9 Treatment options in patients with CUA (calciphylaxis). Theoretical options, based on pathophysiologic considerations, which have not been tested in clinical practice, are printed in italics. *(Modified from reference 12.)*

the highest risk on the basis of epidemiologic data and animal studies. Gadopentetate, the linear ionic chelate–based product, probably has a medium risk, less than linear nonionic chelates but more than macrocyclic chelates. Other factors reported to be associated with NSF (without definitive proof) include coagulation abnormalities and deep venous thrombosis, recent surgery (particularly vascular surgery), hyperphosphatemia, and the use of high doses of recombinant erythropoietin. Angiotensin-converting enzyme (ACE) inhibitors might protect against NSF.

Clinical Manifestations and Natural History

The lesions of NSF are typically symmetric and develop on limbs and trunk. A common location is between the ankles and midthighs and between the wrists and mid–upper arms bilaterally. On occasion, swelling of the hands and feet, sometimes associated with bullae, is noted. The primary lesions are skin-colored to erythematous papules that coalesce into erythematous to brawny plaques with a peau d'orange appearance (Fig. 84.10A). These plaques have been described as having an ameboid advancing edge. Nodules are sometimes also described. Involved skin becomes markedly thickened and woody in texture. Joint contractures may develop rapidly, with patients becoming wheelchair dependent within days to weeks of onset (Fig. 84.10B). Patients often complain of pruritus, causalgia,

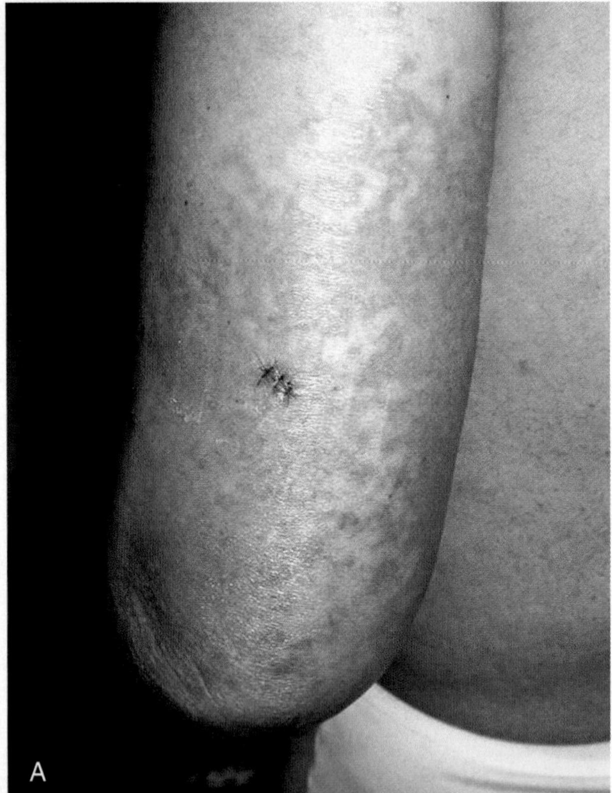

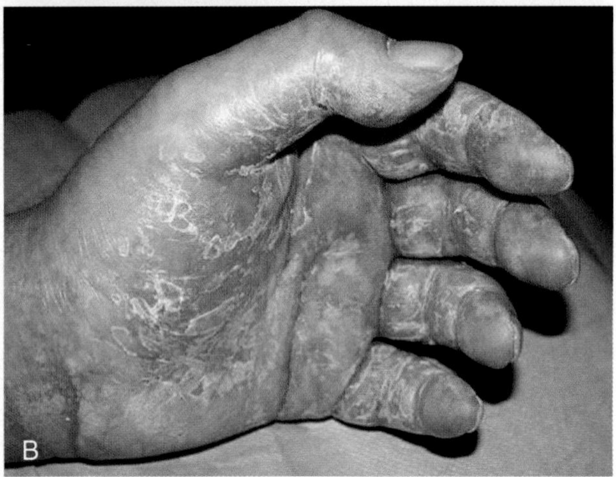

Figure 84.10 Nephrogenic systemic fibrosis. A, Peau d'orange appearance. **B,** Swelling of the hands, accompanied by palmar erythema, blisters, and contracture of the fingers.

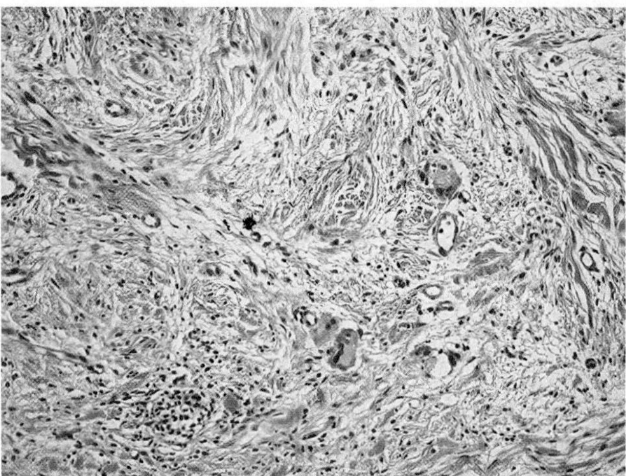

Figure 84.11 Histopathologic features of nephrogenic systemic fibrosis. Haphazardly arranged dermal collagen bundles with surrounding clefts and a strikingly increased number of similarly arranged spindled and plump fibroblast-like cells.

and sharp pains in the affected areas.[13] In almost all cases of NSF, the disease course parallels the course of the underlying renal dysfunction. Although NSF has not been reported as a cause of death, the impairment of mobility seen in this disorder has led to fractures that ultimately resulted in a protracted hospital course and death.

Pathology

The histopathologic changes in affected skin include marked proliferation of spindle cells, the presence of numerous dendritic cells, and accumulation of mucinous material and thick collagen bundles (Fig. 84.11). Most dermal spindle cells in NSF have the immunophenotype of a circulating fibrocyte, a recently characterized circulating cell that expresses markers of both connective tissue cells and circulating leukocytes. Metastatic calcification and NSF may be found in the same lesion.

Diagnosis and Differential Diagnosis

The gold standard of diagnosis is histopathologic examination of skin biopsy specimens from an involved site. Skin lesions can also be visualized by [^{18}F]-fluorodeoxyglucose whole-body positron emission tomography. NSF resembles other fibrosing skin disorders including scleromyxedema, scleroderma, eosinophilic fasciitis, eosinophilia-myalgia syndrome, and Spanish toxic oil syndrome. The specific distribution of cutaneous involvement, the occurrence in the setting of renal failure, and the unique histopathologic features distinguish NSF from the other fibrotic disorders.

Treatment and Prevention

There is no consistently effective therapy for NSF. There is variable evidence for the efficacy of plasma exchange. Other therapeutic modalities that have been used (or are under investigation) include imatinib, oral and topical corticosteroids, selective histamine blockade, calcipotriene ointment, cyclophosphamide, cyclosporine, thalidomide, interferon alfa, photophoresis, and PUVA (psoralen ultraviolet A) therapy. Intense physiotherapy is advised in every patient to prevent or to reverse limb disability related to contractures of the joints.[13] At present, prevention of NSF seems more important than any of the currently available interventions, and widespread clinical awareness of this condition is required. Avoidance of GBC agents in high-risk patients (acute kidney injury [AKI] and subjects with CKD with an estimated glomerular filtration rate <30 ml/min per 1.73 m^2) is the best measure to prevent this catastrophic complication. If GBC agent exposure is required, use of the smallest dosage of a macrolytic chelate is strongly advised. HD (three sessions within 48 hours) should be considered after GBC agent exposure in patients who are already on this modality.

REFERENCES

1. Abdelbaqi-Salhab M, Shalhub S, Morgan MB. A current review of the cutaneous manifestations of renal disease. *J Cutan Pathol.* 2003;30: 527-538.
2. Zucker I, Yosipovitch G, David M, et al. Prevalence and characterization of uremic pruritus in patients undergoing hemodialysis: Uremic pruritus is still a major problem for patients with end-stage renal disease. *J Am Acad Dermatol.* 2003;49:842-846.
3. Mathur vs Lindberg J, Germain M, et al. A longitudinal study at uremic pruitus in nemodialysis patients. *Clin J Am Soc Nephrol.* 2010;5:1410-1419.
4. Mettang T, Pauli-Magnus C, Alscher DM. Uremic pruritus—new perspectives and insights from recent trials. *Nephrol Dial Transplant.* 2002;17:1558-1563.
5. Wikstrom B, Gellert R, Soren D, et al. Kappa opioid system in uremic pruritus: Multicenter, randomized, double-blind, placebo-controlled clinical studies. *J Am Soc Nephrol.* 2005;16:3742-3747.
6. Gunal AI, Ozalp G, Kurtulus Yoldas T, et al. Gabapentin therapy for pruritus in hemodialysis patients: A randomized, placebo-controlled, double-blind trial. *Nephrol Dial Transplant.* 2004;19:3137-3139.
7. Kuypers DK, Claes K, Evenepoel P, et al. A prospective proof of concept study of the efficacy of tacrolimus ointment on uremic pruritus (UP) in patients on chronic dialysis therapy. *Nephrol Dial Transplant.* 2004;19: 1895-1901.
8. Robinson-Bostom L, DiGiovanna JJ. Cutaneous manifestations of end-stage renal disease. *J Am Acad Dermatol.* 2000;43:975-986.
9. Robinson-Bostom L, DiGiovanna JJ. Cutaneous manifestations of end-stage renal disease. *J Am Acad Dermatol.* 2000;43:975-986.
10. Wilmer WA, Magro CM. Calciphylaxis: Emerging concepts in prevention, diagnosis, and treatment. *Semin Dial.* 2002;15:172-186.
11. Fine A, Zacharias J. Calciphylaxis is usually non-ulcerating: Risk factors, outcome and therapy. *Kidney Int.* 2002;61:2210-2217.
12. Schlieper G, Brandenburg V, Ketteler M, Floege J. Sodium thiosulfate in the treatment of calcific uremic arteriolopathy. *Nat Rev Nephrol.* 2009;5:539-543.
13. Cowper SE. Nephrogenic fibrosing dermopathy: The first 6 years. *Curr Opin Rheumatol.* 2003;15:785-790.
14. Kuypers DR. Skin problems in chronic kidney disease. *Nat Clin Pract Nephrol.* 2009;5:157-170.
15. Fine A, Zacharias J. Calciphylaxis is usually non-ulcerating: risk factors, outcome and therapy. *Kidney Int.* 2002;61:2210-2217.

CHAPTER 85

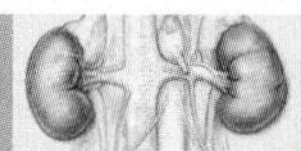

Acquired Cystic Kidney Disease and Malignant Neoplasms

Frank Eitner

DEFINITION

Acquired cystic kidney disease (ACKD) was first recognized in 1847 by John Simon in patients with chronic Bright's disease. He described the development of cystic renal changes with cysts ranging from "mustard seed to as large as cocoa nuts" and also noted that they "run a slow and insidious progress during life, and often leave in the dead body no such obvious traces as would strike the superficial observer." ACKD was "rediscovered" by Dunnill and colleagues[1] in 1977 in kidneys from dialysis patients.

ACKD is a disease of chronic renal failure of any etiology and has to be differentiated from other types of cystic kidney disease (see Chapters 44 and 45). It is usually defined as more than three to five macroscopic cysts in each kidney of a patient who does not have a hereditary cause of cystic disease. ACKD is associated with renal neoplasms with such high frequency that some authors consider ACKD preneoplastic.[2]

PATHOGENESIS

Most cysts are lined by a single layer of epithelium composed of flat nondescript cells, cells with abundant cytoplasm and hyaline droplets, or small cuboidal cells resembling those from distal tubules or collecting ducts.[2] Others have argued that the presence of a brush border on the luminal membrane suggests that the cysts arise primarily from proliferation of proximal tubular epithelial cells. Although the mechanisms of tubule transformation into cysts are not entirely clear, tubular epithelial cell hyperplasia is currently viewed as a central early event in ACKD pathogenesis (Fig. 85.1).[3] Various factors have been implicated in the development of tubular hyperplasia, including plasticizer, ischemia, and uremic metabolites. However, the most important factor appears to be slow, progressive parenchymal loss, which could explain why the development or progression of ACKD does not appear to be influenced by the type of underlying renal disease or the choice of dialysis modality. The loss of intact nephrons is a strong stimulus for compensatory growth of the remaining, still intact nephrons, which is achieved by initial hypertrophy and later by hyperplasia. In these hyperplastic tubules, a cyst will develop if transepithelial fluid secretion continues, and if it is due to anatomic distortion or obstruction, the distal outflow is impaired.

With the continuing presence of mitogenic stimuli, the epithelial layer of the cyst becomes multilayered and atypical cells form intracystic papillary structures or mural adenomas. Activation of proto-oncogenes, chromosomal abnormalities, and additional factors such as genetic background, environmental chemicals, and sex hormones thereafter probably account for the transition of the proliferative process into malignant growth (see Fig. 85.1).[3]

EPIDEMIOLOGY

Among patients entering dialysis treatment, prevalences of ACKD ranging from 5% to 20% have been described. ACKD can occur in some patients even before dialysis is initiated. In both chronic hemodialysis and peritoneal dialysis patients, prevalence then increases at a similar rate and reaches 80% to 100% after 10 years of treatment (Fig. 85.2).[3-5] Children are also prone to the development of ACKD. Several but not all studies have reported an increased frequency or faster progression in men than in women. The rate of progression appears to slow after 10 to 15 years of dialysis.

The frequency of ACKD as well as of renal tumors in dialysis patients may be underestimated on the basis of imaging methods alone. Renal cysts are detectable by ultrasound with a minimum size of 0.5 cm. Data obtained in 260 native nephrectomy specimens at the time of transplantation with a median dialysis duration of 1.0 year identified ACKD in 33%, renal adenomas in 14%, and renal cell carcinomas (RCCs) in 4% of the cases.[6]

CLINICAL MANIFESTATIONS

ACKD can be manifested as unilateral or bilateral cysts, which are mostly cortical and variable in size and number. Rarely, severe ACKD can become macroscopically indistinguishable from adult polycystic kidney disease (PKD). In contrast to hereditary cystic diseases, the cysts of ACKD are strictly confined to the kidneys. The disease is usually asymptomatic and discovered accidentally during abdominal imaging procedures. Alternatively, it may be manifested by potential complications or consequences of ACKD:

- Cystic hemorrhage with or without hematuria; bleeding may occur with cyst rupture with subsequent perinephric hemorrhage or retroperitoneal hemorrhage, which may in rare cases be severe enough to lead to hypovolemic shock.
- Calcifications in or around cysts and in rare cases stone formation (calcium-containing stones or β_2-microglobulin stones).
- Cyst infection, abscess formation, or sepsis.
- Erythrocytosis in advanced cases, similar to erythrocytosis observed in polycystic kidney disease.
- Malignant transformation.[7]

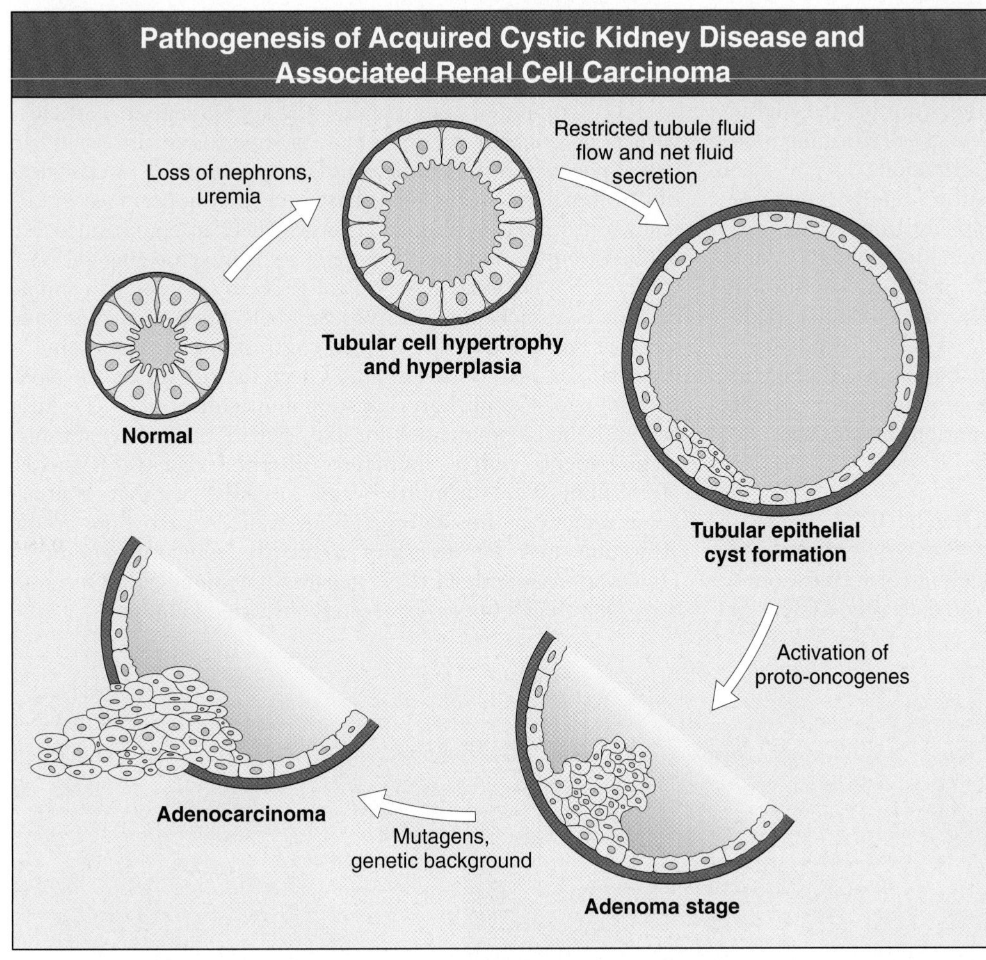

Figure 85.1 Pathogenesis of acquired cystic kidney disease (ACKD) and associated renal cell carcinoma. Diagram of events leading to the development of ACKD and subsequent malignant transformation. *(Modified from reference 3.)*

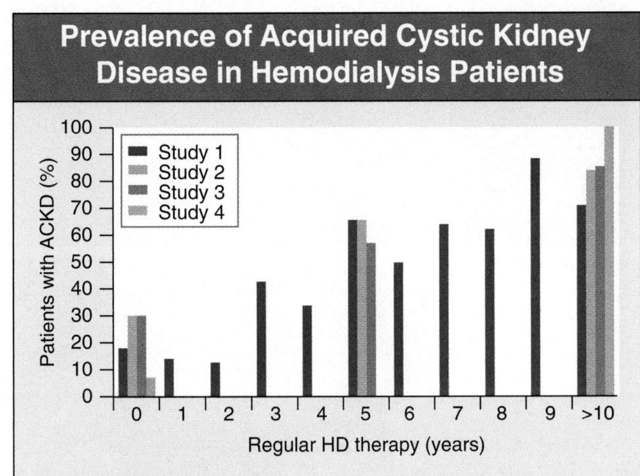

Figure 85.2 Prevalence of acquired cystic kidney disease (ACKD) in hemodialysis patients. Summary of reported ACKD prevalences in chronic hemodialysis patients in relation to the length of hemodialysis treatment. Four separate studies are shown.

Acquired Cystic Kidney Disease–Associated Renal Cell Carcinoma

Malignant transformation, the most feared complication of ACKD, accounts for about 80% of the renal cell neoplasms observed in uremic patients. In an unselected series of chronic dialysis or transplant patients, the cumulative incidence of RCC complicating ACKD is probably below 1%, although rates up to 7% have been reported in some small studies. These data indicate an up to 40-fold increased risk for RCC in ACKD patients compared with RCC in the general population. Risk factors include male gender (male-to-female ratio, 7 : 1), African American ethnicity, long duration of dialysis, and severe ACKD with marked organ enlargement. It is unknown whether the risk of malignant transformation differs between hemodialysis and peritoneal dialysis patients. However, cases of malignant transformation in patients treated exclusively with peritoneal dialysis have been described.

About 85% of ACKD-associated RCCs are asymptomatic. The remaining cases mostly are manifested with bleeding, usually gross hematuria, from the tumor. In cases in which nephrectomy had to be performed in dialysis patients for intractable hematuria, RCCs, not visualized before surgery, were diagnosed in about one third of the patients.

Compared with sporadic RCCs, ACKD-associated RCCs are characterized by younger age of the patient, male predominance, more frequent multicentric and bilateral manifestation, and less frequent metastases.[2]

PATHOLOGY

Cystic changes in ACKD are typically bilateral but may vary between kidneys. Most ACKD kidneys are smaller than normal. An increase in size above normal can be observed in cases of cyst hematoma formation or malignant transformation. The cysts are usually restricted to the renal cortex. The size of the cysts ranges from microscopic to about 2 cm; about 60% of the cysts are smaller than 0.2 cm.[2] Preneoplastic changes can be detected in ACKD kidneys, including atypical cyst-lining cells forming multiple cell layers and intracystic nodular formations.

Up to 25% of kidneys with ACKD harbor tumors, about one third of which are carcinomas. RCCs arising from ACKD are multicentric in about 50% of cases, bilateral in about 10%, and papillary as well as clear cell carcinoma by histology. Transitional cell carcinoma has been reported in ACKD, occasionally in addition to the presence of RCC. However, ACKD does not seem to increase the risk for transitional cell carcinoma. Rather, its development may be related to analgesic nephropathy as the underlying renal disease, although this notion remains speculative so far.

DIAGNOSIS AND DIFFERENTIAL DIAGNOSIS

The diagnostic approach to ACKD usually involves ultrasound (Fig. 85.3), which is a sensitive means of detecting ACKD or large RCCs.[4,8] However, the differentiation between simple cysts and renal carcinomas can be difficult given the echogenicity of end-stage kidney parenchyma and the complexity of cysts in ACKD. Computed tomography (CT) scanning, in particular with early contrast enhancement, is superior to ultrasound in detecting small malignant lesions (see Fig. 86.3).[4,8,9] A classification of renal cysts (Fig. 85.4) based on their appearance in CT scans, introduced by Bosniak, is now widely accepted and is also applied to ultrasound and magnetic resonance imaging (MRI).[10] Criteria that favor the diagnosis of RCC as opposed to a simple cyst include thickened and irregular walls, the presence of septa or renal tissue within the lesions, contrast enhancement, multilocularity, and large size (>4 cm). Given the risk for the development of nephrogenic fibrosis, gadolinium-enhanced MRI cannot currently be recommended for dialysis patients and renal transplant patients with a glomerular filtration rate (GFR) below 60 ml/min. The diagnostic value of MRI without contrast enhancement in this setting is not well defined. Fine-needle aspiration may be necessary to clarify equivocal findings.[11] However, even with all these imaging techniques, RCCs (up to 8 cm) have been missed in severely distorted kidneys.

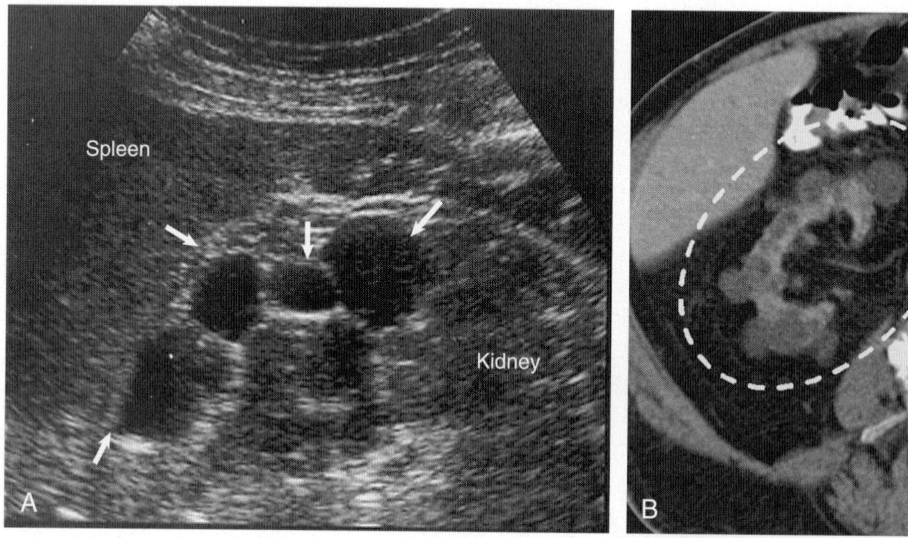

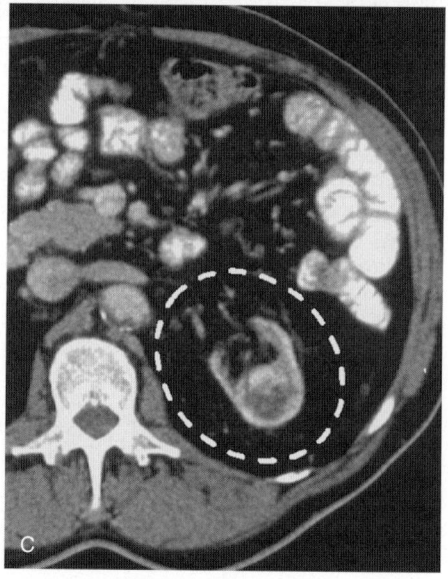

Figure 85.3 Imaging studies in acquired cystic kidney disease (ACKD). A, Ultrasound image of the left native kidney of a patient after 16 years of chronic hemodialysis (HD). Multiple cysts are present in the renal cortex *(arrows).* **B,** CT image of a patient after 5 years of chronic HD demonstrating multiple cysts within the right kidney *(dashed circle).* **C,** Contrast-enhanced CT image of a renal transplant patient who developed a renal cell carcinoma *(arrow)* originating from the left native kidney with ACKD *(dashed circle).*

Renal Cyst Classification System		
Category	**Synonymous**	**Description**
I	Benign simple cyst	Hairline thin cyst wall; no septa; no calcifications; no solid components; no contrast enhancement
II	Benign cyst	Minimal regular thickening of the cyst wall; few, hairline thin septa; smooth, hairline thin calcifications in wall or septa; no contrast enhancement
IIF	Moderately complex cyst	Minimal regular thickening of the cyst wall; multiple, minimal smooth thickening septa; thick, nodular calcifications in wall or septa; no contrast enhancement
III	Indeterminate cystic mass	Irregular thickening of cyst wall; multiple, measurably thick, irregular septa; thick, nodular, irregular calcifications in wall or septa; contrast enhancement present
IV	Clearly malignant cystic mass	Gross irregular thickening of cyst wall; irregular gross thickening of septa; thick, nodular irregular calcifications in wall or septa; contrast enhancement present in tissue and cysts

Figure 85.4 Renal cyst classification system. *(Modified from reference 12.)*

Because of the risk of malignant transformation, screening for ACKD on a regular basis, as well as regular follow-up imaging in cases of established ACKD, has been advocated. A proposal for ACKD and tumor screening is outlined in Figure 85.5. However, there is at present no consensus on screening strategies. This is because of the cost of screening as well as the risk-benefit ratio of nephrectomy in dialysis patients. A decision analysis[5] concluded that screening for ACKD (by either ultrasound or CT scanning) in young patients with a life expectancy of 25 years offers as much as a 1.6-year gain in life expectancy. This is similar to the gain obtained in young healthy people who stop smoking. In contrast, in ACKD patients older than 60 years, no significant gain in life expectancy is achieved by regular screening.[5] In a different analysis of 797 dialysis patients who had developed RCCs (90% identified by screening, 10% by clinical symptoms), screening provided a mean survival benefit of 3.3 years after adjustment for age and dialysis vintage.[13] Screening during transplant evaluation by ultrasound followed by CT in the case of suspicious lesions is recommended on the basis of recent data showing a prevalence of renal cancer in up to 4% of the patients and concerns about the role of immunosuppression in accelerating tumor growth.[14]

NATURAL HISTORY

Cystic dilations of renal tubules develop microscopically once the creatinine clearance falls below 70 ml/min.[15] Macroscopic cysts start to develop when serum creatinine rises above 3 mg/dl (264 µmol/l). As discussed before, ACKD thereafter progresses and reaches a prevalence of nearly 100% after more than 10 years of dialysis (see Fig. 85.2). In malignant transformation, tumor growth rates are highly variable. The incidence of metastases at diagnosis (15% to 30% of cases) and 5-year survival rates (35%) are comparable to those observed in RCC in the general population. Death is usually associated with widespread metastases and accounts for about 2% of the deaths in renal transplant patients.

After renal transplantation, the course of ACKD is variable. There may be retardation of the progressive course of the disease or regression of the cysts, particularly if good long-term graft function is maintained. However, especially in grafts with impaired or failing renal function, there may be further progression in the native kidneys as well as the development of *de novo* ACKD in the graft. It is not established whether renal transplantation affects the natural history of RCC complicating ACKD, although immunosuppression has been suggested as a risk factor for RCC in transplant patients with ACKD.[7] A prospective, single-center ultrasound screening of the native kidneys in 561 renal transplant recipients identified ACKD in 23%.[16] The mean duration of dialysis was 4 to 5 years, and the mean time after transplantation was 9 years. In this cohort, ACKD was slightly less frequent than had been reported in dialysis patients, possibly indicating that renal transplantation might inhibit the development of ACKD.[16] The prevalence of RCCs among all 561 patients was 4.8%. However, among the patients with ACKD, RCCs were detected in almost 20%, whereas among the patients without ACKD, RCCs were detected in only 0.5%.[16]

TREATMENT

Treatment of ACKD is warranted only when complications such as hemorrhage, cyst infection, or malignant transformation develop. Whereas the first two complications may be handled conservatively and only rarely require surgery, malignant transformation should raise the question of nephrectomy. Given the perioperative morbidity and mortality of nephrectomy, in particular in multimorbid dialysis or transplant patients, it is not surprising that the threshold for surgical intervention in cases of RCC is still controversial.

Most authors agree that tumors larger than 3 cm in diameter justify nephrectomy because above this size, RCCs in the general population frequently metastasize (see Fig. 85.5).[7] However, this strategy is based on an extrapolation from otherwise healthy persons, and a more aggressive approach may be required under certain circumstances. This is particularly true because tumor size in ACKD is often difficult to establish by imaging studies (given its frequent multilocular development) and because metastases have been described in ACKD even when renal tumors were not detected by imaging studies.

In the case of tumors of less than 3 cm in diameter with no complications, the slow tumor growth may justify observation with repeated imaging studies (see Fig. 85.5). Patients with high life expectancy or patients listed for transplantation might be

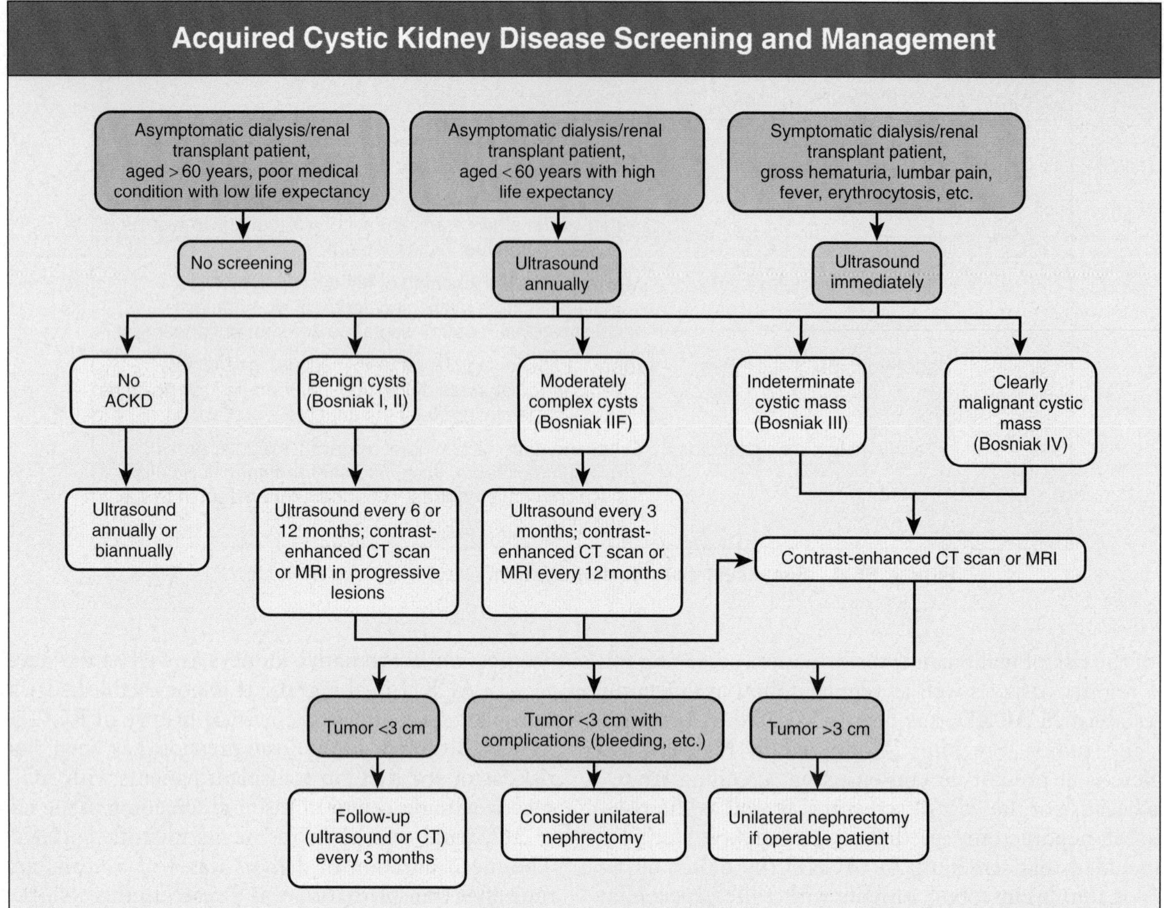

Figure 85.5 Proposed approach to acquired cystic kidney disease (ACKD) screening and management of suspected renal cell carcinoma. ACKD, acquired cystic kidney disease; CT, computed tomography; MRI, magnetic resonance imaging. *(Modified from references 5, 7, and 16.)*

considered for nephrectomy also in case of tumors with diameters less than 3 cm. In general, tumor enlargement should be used as an indication for nephrectomy if it is permitted by the patient's status. When complications such as back pain and persistent hematuria are present, nephrectomy has been recommended by some but not all authors.[7]

A prophylactic contralateral nephrectomy, in the case of unilateral tumors, is not routinely recommended because of the morbidity associated with the procedure, the worsening of anemia, and the loss of residual renal function in those who are not considered transplant candidates. A delay of transplantation is generally not suggested in patients who have had an asymptomatic RCC associated with ACKD in their nephrectomy. In such a setting, a contralateral nephrectomy can be recommended to decrease the potential risk of neoplastic growth and to avoid a delay of transplantation.

MALIGNANT NEOPLASMS IN DIALYSIS PATIENTS

Even if the risk of malignant transformation of ACKD is disregarded, dialysis patients have a slightly higher cancer risk compared with the general population. Analysis of more than 800,000 dialysis patients in three registries from the United States, Europe, and Australia/New Zealand revealed that most of the increased risk was due to cancers of the kidney, bladder, and endocrine organs (Fig. 85.6).[17] Besides the specific risk associated with malignant transformation of ACKD, some of the increased risk is directly related to the underlying renal disease or to the immunosuppression that may have been administered to patients with immune-mediated renal disease. Cyclophosphamide therapy, for example, may predispose to bladder and ureteral cancer that presents after patients have been initiated on dialysis. Renal disease or immunosuppressive therapy may underlie the apparent risk of dialysis patients for development of multiple myeloma (see Fig. 85.6). In addition, patients with analgesic nephropathy or Chinese herbs/aristolochic acid nephropathy are at high risk for development of transitional cell carcinoma of the upper urinary tract.[18] Particularly after renal transplantation, these tumors tend to be less differentiated and in an advanced stage, and therefore the patients have a relatively poor outcome. For this reason, patients with analgesic nephropathy and aristolochic acid nephropathy should be screened for the presence of transitional cell carcinoma before transplantation and annually after transplantation. It has been advocated that screening should include cystoscopy, retrograde ureteral catheterization with washings and brushings, and sonography imaging.[19] Other malignant neoplasms that have been observed at increased frequencies in dialysis patients include carcinoma of the cervix, thyroid and other endocrine neoplasias (see Fig. 85.6), and, at least in the USRDS database, a 1.5- to 2-fold increase in the risk for non-Hodgkin's lymphoma, Hodgkin's disease, and leukemias.[17] This suggests that female dialysis patients should undergo gynecologic screening including cervical smear in the same intervals as suggested for the general population. Regular

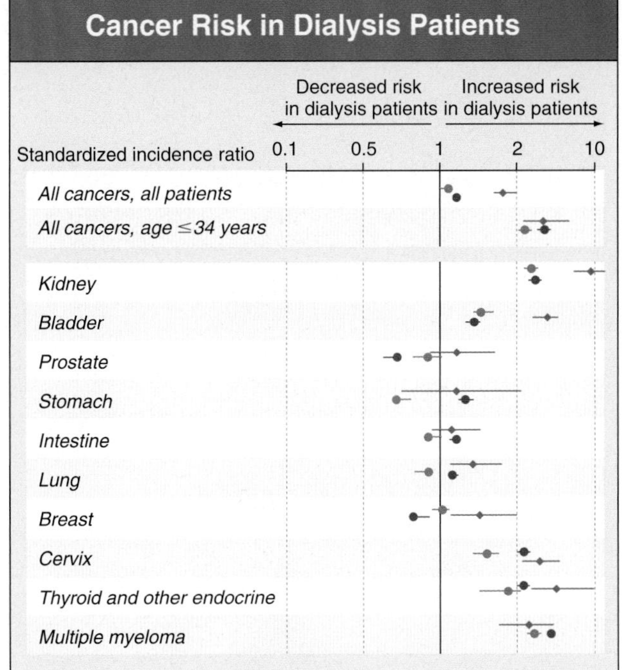

Figure 85.6 Cancer risk in dialysis patients. Relative risk of cancer (plus 95% confidence interval) compared with the general populations in 831,804 dialysis patients from Australia/New Zealand *(blue diamonds)*, Europe *(orange circles)*, and the United States *(purple circles)*. *(Modified from reference 17.)*

thyroid ultrasound is probably also justified, although no formal decision analysis is available to support this recommendation; lymphoma and leukemia screening will be difficult to impose, and clinical vigilance is advocated.

REFERENCES

1. Dunnill MS, Millard PR, Oliver D. Acquired cystic disease of the kidneys: A hazard of long-term intermittent maintenance haemodialysis. *J Clin Pathol.* 1977;30:868-877.
2. Truong LD, Choi YJ, Shen SS, et al. Renal cystic neoplasms and renal neoplasms associated with cystic renal diseases: Pathogenetic and molecular links. *Adv Anat Pathol.* 2003;10:135-159.
3. Grantham JJ. Acquired cystic kidney disease. *Kidney Int.* 1991;40:143-152.
4. Levine E. Acquired cystic kidney disease. *Radiol Clin North Am.* 1996;34:947-964.
5. Sarasin FP, Wong JB, Levey AS, Meyer KB. Screening for acquired cystic kidney disease: A decision analytic perspective. *Kidney Int.* 1995;48:207-219.
6. Denton MD, Magee CC, Ovuworie C, et al. Prevalence of renal cell carcinoma in patients with ESRD pre-transplantation: A pathologic analysis. *Kidney Int.* 2002;61:2201-2209.
7. Truong LD, Krishnan B, Cao JT, et al. Renal neoplasm in acquired cystic kidney disease. *Am J Kidney Dis.* 1995;26:1-12.
8. Choyke PL. Acquired cystic kidney disease. *Eur Radiol.* 2000;10:1716-1721.
9. Takebayashi S, Hidai H, Chiba T, et al. Using helical CT to evaluate renal cell carcinoma in patients undergoing hemodialysis: Value of early enhanced images. *AJR Am J Roentgenol.* 1999;172:429-433.
10. Israel GM, Bosniak MA. An update of the Bosniak renal cyst classification system. *Urology.* 2005;66:484-488.
11. Todd TD, Dhurandhar B, Mody D, et al. Fine-needle aspiration of cystic lesions of the kidney. Morphologic spectrum and diagnostic problems in 41 cases. *Am J Clin Pathol.* 1999;111:317-328.
12. Israel GM, Bosniak MA. An update of the Bosniak renal cyst classification system. *Urology.* 2005;66:484-488; and modified according to Eknoyan G. A clinical view of simple and complex renal cysts. *J Am Soc Nephrol.* 2009;20:1874-1876.
13. Ishikawa I, Honda R, Yamada Y, Kakuma T. Renal cell carcinoma detected by screening shows better patient survival than that detected following symptoms in dialysis patients. *Ther Apher Dial.* 2004;8:468-473.
14. Gulanikar AC, Daily PP, Kilambi NK, et al. Prospective pretransplant ultrasound screening in 206 patients for acquired renal cysts and renal cell carcinoma. *Transplantation.* 1998;66:1669-1672.
15. Liu JS, Ishikawa I, Horiguchi T. Incidence of acquired renal cysts in biopsy specimens. *Nephron.* 2000;84:142-147.
16. Schwarz A, Vatandaslar S, Merkel S, Haller H. Renal cell carcinoma in transplant recipients with acquired cystic kidney disease. *Clin J Am Soc Nephrol.* 2007;2:750-756.
17. Maisonneuve P, Agodoa L, Gellert R, et al. Cancer in patients on dialysis for end-stage renal disease: An international collaborative study. *Lancet.* 1999;354:93-99.
18. Stewart JH, Buccianti G, Agodoa L, et al. Cancers of the kidney and urinary tract in patients on dialysis for end-stage renal disease: Analysis of data from the United States, Europe, and Australia and New Zealand. *J Am Soc Nephrol.* 2003;14:197-207.
19. Swindle P, Falk M, Rigby R, et al. Transitional cell carcinoma in renal transplant recipients: The influence of compound analgesics. *Br J Urol.* 1998;81:229-233.

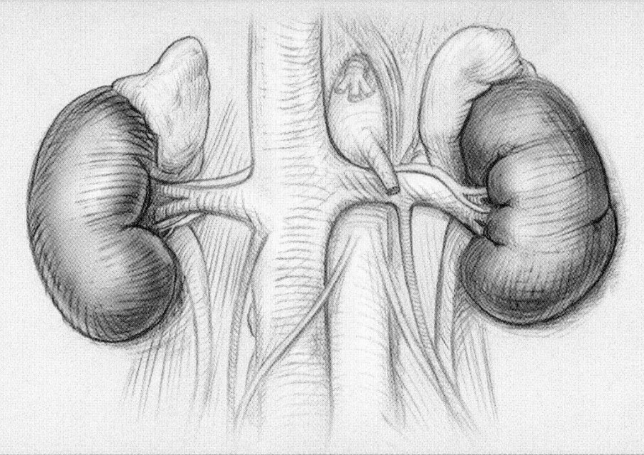

SECTION XVI

Dialytic Therapies

CHAPTER **86**

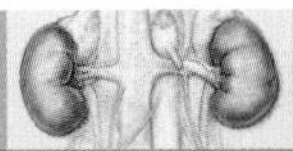

Approach to Renal Replacement Therapy

Hugh C. Rayner, Enyu Imai

TREATMENT OPTIONS FOR RENAL REPLACEMENT THERAPY

Resources available for renal replacement therapy (RRT) vary substantially between countries. If effective chronic kidney disease (CKD) management minimized progression to end-stage renal disease (ESRD) and RRT were universally available for everyone who could benefit from it and wished to have it, the incidence rates of new dialysis patients would reflect the epidemiology of irremediably progressive kidney disease. In reality, incidence rates of ESRD treatment show huge variation, far larger than can be explained by disease incidence alone (Fig. 86.1). Clearly, there are other factors involved in the transition from CKD to RRT.

Each modality of RRT needs particular preparation, has substantial costs, and once started may continue for years. Education about RRT should be given to all patients and their families as they approach ESRD and should include the rationale, efficacy, and prognosis of each RRT modality as well as information about any relevant limitations of medical resources.

PREDICTION OF THE START OF DIALYSIS

Predicting the start of dialysis is important for preparation for RRT and is made easier if renal function is routinely measured by an estimate of the glomerular filtration rate (eGFR) derived by the Modification of Diet in Renal Disease (MDRD) formula (see Chapter 3). It is very easy to underestimate the severity of renal impairment from serum creatinine values, especially in elderly patients. Graphs of eGFR against time make it easy to identify those patients whose renal function is deteriorating at a rate that predicts they will require dialysis in the next 1 to 2 years and who therefore should be referred to the multidisciplinary team (Fig. 86.2). This is preferable to adopting an arbitrary threshold eGFR.[1]

MULTIDISCIPLINARY PREDIALYSIS CARE

Multidisciplinary care should begin at CKD stage 4 (eGFR <30 ml/min per 1.73 m^2). One aim of a predialysis program is to ensure that patients and their families know as much as they wish to know about renal failure and its treatment before dialysis needs to be started. To achieve this aim, sufficient time is needed to allow the large amount of information to be absorbed and its implications for that individual to be understood. This may take months rather than days in patients who have difficulty accepting information about their illness but who may gain particular benefit from the program.[2] It is our practice to transfer patients to the care of a multidisciplinary team at least 12 months before the predicted date of dialysis.

Predialysis care should address a number of issues: preserving residual renal function; preventing or treating complications of CKD; ensuring that patients have sufficient understanding of their condition to decide whether they wish to have dialysis or not and to choose between PD and HD; arranging appropriate access; and in appropriate patients, preparing for kidney transplantation.

Predialysis care is best delivered by a multidisciplinary team.[3,4] Such teams commonly include a dietitian, a nurse educator, a pharmacist, a social worker, and sometimes a trained peer-support volunteer. Patients receiving this additional care have better biochemical results, are more likely to start dialysis in a planned way with less hospitalization, and may even have improved survival rates once they have started dialysis.[5] As well as being good practice, these programs make good financial sense as the savings in inpatient costs from such programs outweigh those required to run the clinics. Lack of access to effective predialysis care is a significant issue in the United States. Only one third of patients older than 67 years who started RRT in the United States between 1996 and 1999 had seen a nephrologist at least 4 months before starting dialysis,[6] and this may partly explain the higher incidence rate of RRT in the United States compared with Europe.[7]

Predialysis Education Programs

Patients with advanced CKD may not gain sufficient knowledge and understanding of their condition from conventional office consultations, even when they have been seen on multiple occasions by a nephrologist. This education gap is greater among African Americans than among Asians and Caucasians.[8]

To be effective, education of the patient should follow the principles of adult learning: assess the patient's existing level of knowledge and understanding; build on this knowledge by the delivery of appropriate information in an appropriate form; and establish that the patient has understood and accepted the information given. Education can be delivered individually or in groups.[9] In a group session, the wide range of patients' pre-existing understanding may make it difficult for the organizer to achieve the right level of detail and complexity. On the other hand, patients probably learn as much from fellow patients within a support group as they do from the group's facilitator. Furthermore, a group will help patients and their relatives appreciate that they are not alone in facing the demands of ESRD. The educational value of individual patient

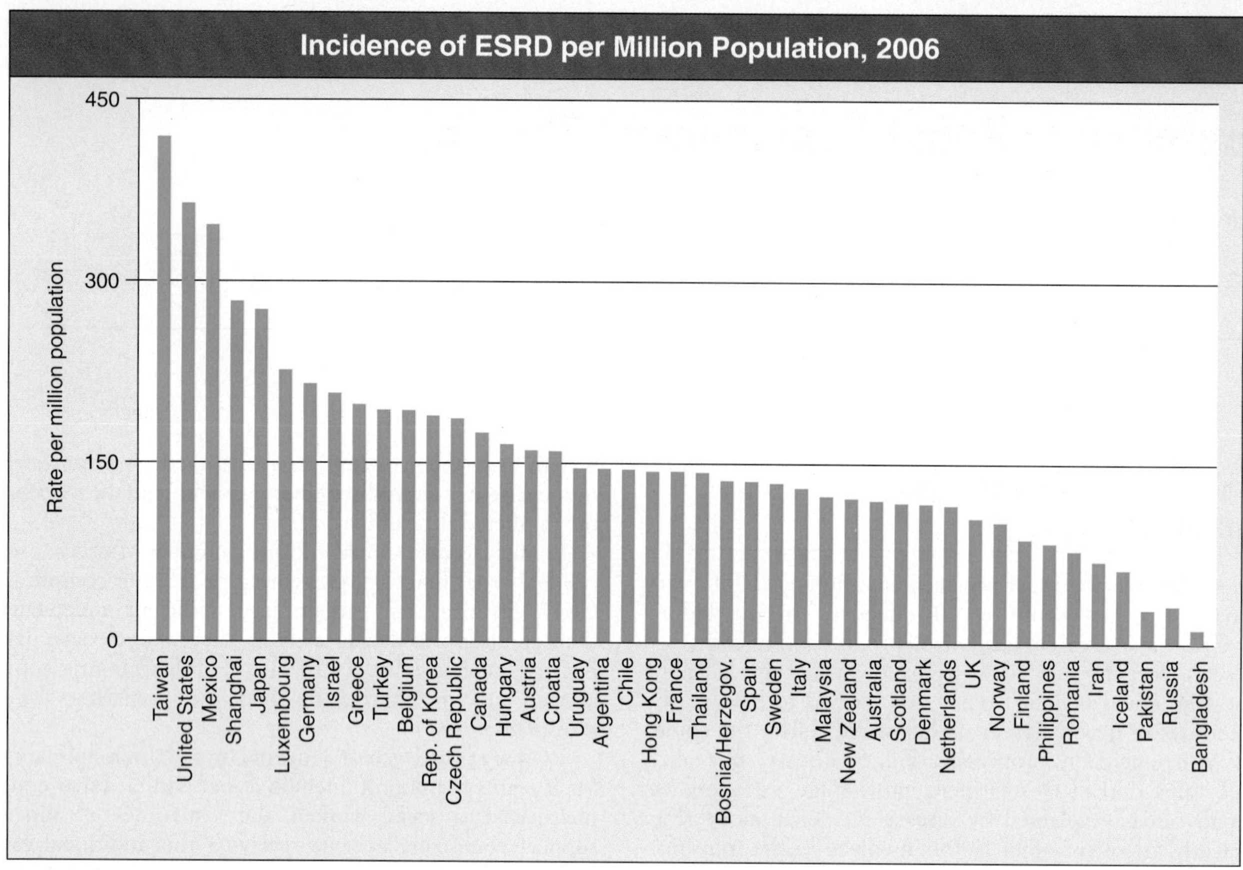

Figure 86.1 Incidence of end-stage renal disease (ESRD) per million population, 2006. Data are presented only for those countries from which relevant information was available.

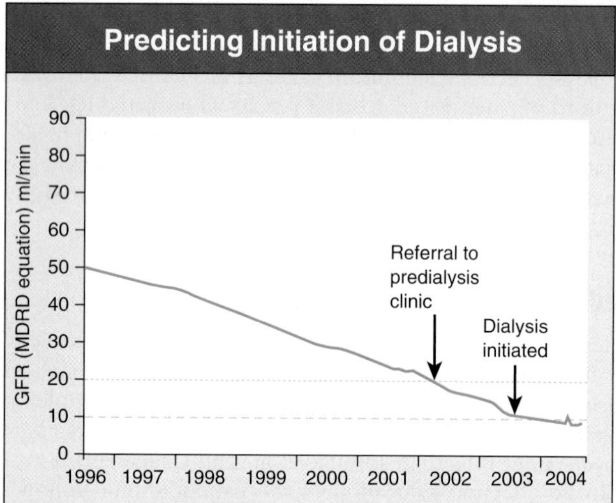

Figure 86.2 Predicting initiation of dialysis. Use of graph of estimated GFR (by MDRD equation) against time to schedule preparation for dialysis. Symptoms of renal failure increase as GFR falls below 20 ml/min per 1.73 m^2 and usually become sufficiently severe to justify dialysis below 10 ml/min per 1.73 m^2. The patient is referred to the predialysis multidisciplinary clinic when GFR falls below 20 ml/min per 1.73 m^2 or at least 12 months before the predicted need for dialysis.

consultations can be increased by the physician writing a letter to the patient summarizing the patient's medical details and the discussion about his or her treatment. This can be in addition to or in place of the conventional letter to the patient's general practitioner.

The predialysis program should be delivered by representatives of all members of the multidisciplinary team, both medical and nonmedical. For example, a controlled trial from California has studied the value of social worker input to the predialysis program in reducing unemployment.[10] In the intervention group, patients and their relatives met regularly with a licensed social worker both before and after starting dialysis to explore strategies for continuing the patient's current employment. The aim of the education and counseling was to change the perception among patients, relatives, and employers that dialysis patients are unable to continue working. Blue-collar workers in the intervention group were 2.8 times more likely to continue working. Patients in work had a better quality of life, greater self-esteem, and a more positive attitude to work. As it is difficult for dialysis patients to regain jobs once they are lost, this result is particularly valuable for the long-term rehabilitation of patients.

In addition to formal sessions, patients should be made aware of the wide range of educational materials available. A number of books have been written specifically for dialysis patients. Many national organizations provide information on the Internet and produce patient information leaflets and audio-visual material, for example, the National Kidney Foundation *(www.kidney.org)*.

Education About Transplantation

The possibility of kidney transplantation should be considered for each new patient with ESRD. For those who are suitable, transplantation offers the prospect of improved survival and quality of life. In a U.S. study, although the risk of death was 2.8 times higher in the first 2 weeks after transplantation compared with remaining on dialysis, the long-term mortality rate was 48% to 82% lower among transplant recipients than among patients remaining on the waiting list, with relatively larger benefits among patients who were 20 to 39 years old, Caucasian patients, and younger patients with diabetes.[11]

The options of deceased donor and live donor kidney transplants, as well as combined kidney and pancreas transplants for people with diabetes, should be discussed. Whereas outcome data from the local transplanting centers should be made available, published data can be used to inform patients.

The ideal time for the transplant to be performed is before dialysis is ever begun, so-called preemptive transplantation. A U.S. study showed that preemptive transplantation was associated with a 52% reduction in the risk of graft failure during the first year after transplantation, an 82% reduction during the second year, and an 86% reduction during subsequent years compared with transplantation after dialysis. Increasing duration of dialysis was associated with increasing odds of rejection within 6 months of transplantation, possibly due to immunologic stimulation during long-term dialysis.[12]

WHEN SHOULD DIALYSIS BE STARTED?

Patients with eGFR below 15 ml/min per 1.73 m^2 should be monitored regularly and dialysis started when symptoms of uremia develop. The serum levels of urea and creatinine will vary according to the patient's protein intake and muscle mass, respectively, and there is no single value of either that can be used as a threshold for starting dialysis.

The mean eGFR at the start of dialysis varies between countries and has steadily increased during recent years. The mean eGFR at start of RRT in the United Kingdom has increased from 6 ml/min per 1.73 m^2 in 1997 to 8.5 ml/min per 1.73 m^2 in 2006 (*www.renalreg.com*, U.K. Renal Registry 2007 Report), which compares with 11 ml/min per 1.73 m^2 in the same year in the United States (*www.USRDS.org*, 2008 Report).

A higher threshold may be used in diabetics, as they tend to tolerate uremia poorly and are frequently troubled by sodium retention and fluid overload. Other measurements to be taken into consideration include rising serum phosphate, falling serum bicarbonate, and protein-energy malnutrition, which develops and persists despite vigorous attempts to optimize intake. A fall in serum albumin is a late sign of reduced protein intake and debility. National Kidney Foundation Disease Outcomes Quality Initiative guidelines for initiation of dialysis are shown in Figure 86.3.

Arbitrary guidelines have been established to gain Medicare approval for dialysis reimbursement in the United States. These include eGFR below 15 ml/min per 1.73 m^2 for patients older than 18 years and below 20 ml/min per 1.73 m^2 (Schwartz formula) for those younger than 18 years. Alternatively, adults should have a serum creatinine concentration of more than 8 mg/dl (700 µmol/l; >6 mg/dl [530 µmol/l] in diabetes). Patients may also qualify for Medicare if they do not meet these criteria but have uremic symptoms (nausea, vomiting, pericardial pain, acidosis, or hyperkalemia) or pulmonary edema refractory to diuretics.

Limitations of a Purely Clinical Approach to the Initiation of Dialysis

Waiting for patients to develop uremic symptoms, such as anorexia, nausea, vomiting, and loss of lean body weight, carries the risk that the patient will start dialysis in a malnourished state with an increased risk of mortality. Renal failure itself is a catabolic state, and it is commonly difficult for patients on dialysis to regain lost weight.

When to Initiate Dialysis

Indications for early start on dialysis
- Intractable fluid overload
- Intractable hyperkalemia
- Malnutrition due to uremia
- Uremic neurologic dysfunction
- Uremic serositis
- Functional deterioration otherwise unexplained

Uremic cognitive dysfunction can affect learning
Therefore, home-based self-dialysis may need to start earlier than center-assisted dialysis.

Start of dialysis may be delayed if patient is
asymptomatic, awaiting imminent kidney transplant, awaiting imminent placement of permanent HD or PD access, or, after appropriate education, has chosen conservative therapy.

If start of dialysis is delayed,
patient should be re-evaluated regularly to see if dialysis has become necessary.

Patients who choose PD
should not be required to have HD access placed, but venous sites for possible future HD access in arms should be preserved since HD may be required in the future.
Incremental start on PD may be considered if there is significant residual renal function.

Nephrologists should consider conservative (nondialysis) treatment of kidney failure an integral part of their clinical practice.

Figure 86.3 When to initiate dialysis. HD, hemodialysis; PD, peritoneal dialysis. *(Modified from NKF KDOQI Clinical Practice Guideline for initiation of dialysis. http://www.kidney.org/professionals/Kdoqi/guideline_upHD_PD_VA/pd_rec1.htm.)*

Given the chronic nature of renal disease, patients frequently remain unaware of the severity of their illness. Protein intake may fall spontaneously with the result that symptoms of uremia do not develop, but this is at the expense of a loss of lean body mass. Similarly, patients may gradually reduce their activities as their exercise tolerance declines. It is only when dialysis is started that many patients appreciate how ill they have become.

Lack of awareness is a trap that can be avoided by carefully questioning the patient for insidious symptoms of uremia. For example, the patient should be asked to compare his or her current eating habits and lifestyle with those 6 to 12 months previously. Close friends and relatives provide a useful third-party view of the patient's well-being.

Limitations of a Purely "Laboratory Result–Based" Approach to the Initiation of Dialysis

Routine early initiation of dialysis would need to confer significant benefits to justify the added inconvenience to the patient, the additional risk of dialysis-related complications, and the additional cost. As dialysis treatment has a finite life, from loss of peritoneal function or failure of hemodialysis (HD) access, starting treatment earlier will bring forward the time when more procedures or a change of modality is necessary.

Moreover, there is likely to be resistance from many patients to the suggestion that they should start dialysis when they have no symptoms of uremia. The nephrologist would need complete confidence in the laboratory values as well as in the evidence supporting early commencement of dialysis to persuade a reluctant, asymptomatic patient.

Starting dialysis is the first step in a lifelong commitment to RRT. Patients will be asked to comply with a wide variety of inconvenient and sometimes unpleasant treatments. A high level of compliance is required for a successful outcome, and particularly in the United States, there is concern about the level of noncompliance, which is associated with increased mortality.[13] It seems reasonable to presume that the commitment to dialysis is likely to be greater if the patient feels better after it has started.

A prospective study in Holland provides useful data to help the patient and nephrologist agree when to commence treatment.[14] Those patients who started dialysis with less residual renal function (5 ml/min per 1.73 m^2 versus 7 ml/min per 1.73 m^2) had a poorer quality of life in the early period after starting dialysis. However, this difference was no longer present by the end of the first 12 months of treatment. The study was too small to demonstrate a difference in mortality.

Starting dialysis earlier will lead to an apparent increase in survival if survival is measured from the time dialysis begins, so-called lead-time bias. A randomized controlled trial of early (GFR 10-14 ml/min) or late (GFR 5-7 ml/min) or when symptoms supervened initiation of HD showed no difference in mortality or other clinical outcomes.[15]

THE CHOICE BETWEEN PERITONEAL DIALYSIS AND HEMODIALYSIS

The majority of patients with ESRD are suitable for treatment with either peritoneal dialysis (PD) or HD. It is difficult to envisage an ethically acceptable trial in which patients are allocated randomly to PD or HD, and the various possible modifications within each modality make a simple comparative trial impractical. Retrospective comparative studies have failed to indicate a consistent survival advantage for either modality.[16,17] A prospective cohort study from 81 U.S. dialysis clinics attempted to overcome the limitations of these studies, although it was still not a randomized study.[18] No significant difference in outcomes was found between HD and PD during the first year of treatment; but in the second year, the risk of death was significantly greater in those on PD. The increased risk was mainly in patients with cardiovascular comorbidity and is consistent with two other U.S. studies that showed patients with coronary artery disease and congestive heart failure have a shorter survival on PD than on HD. This contradicts a commonly expressed opinion that PD is more "gentle" for such patients as it avoids rapid fluid shifts and causes less "stress" on the heart.[19,20]

When making their choice, patients should be aware that the chances of a change in treatment modality may be up to fivefold greater for PD (to HD) than for HD (to PD) and that change in treatment from PD to HD is associated with an increased risk of hospitalization and mortality.[21] A planned change from PD to HD may not be associated with this increased risk, although this has not been studied systematically in a large population.

Contraindications to Peritoneal Dialysis

There are a few situations in which PD is contraindicated (Fig. 86.4). These have been agreed to by the consensus panel of the National Kidney Foundation Dialysis Outcomes Quality Initiative.[22] Relative contraindications to PD include the following.

Contraindications to Dialysis Modalities

Peritoneal Dialysis	
Absolute	**Relative**
Loss of peritoneal function	Recent abdominal aortic graft
Producing inadequate clearance	Ventriculoperitoneal shunt
Adhesions blocking dialysate flow	Intolerance of intra-abdominal fluid
Surgically uncorrectable abdominal hernia	Large muscle mass
Abdominal wall stoma	Morbid obesity
Diaphragmatic fluid leak	Severe malnutrition
Inability to perform exchanges in absence of suitable assistant	Skin infection
	Bowel disease
Hemodialysis	
Absolute	**Relative**
No vascular access possible	Difficult vascular access
	Needle phobia
	Cardiac failure
	Coagulopathy

Figure 86.4 Contraindications to dialysis. Absolute and relative contraindications to hemodialysis and peritoneal dialysis. *(Modified with permission from reference 22.)*

Fresh Intra-abdominal Foreign Body

Patients with prosthetic aortic grafts have been successfully treated with PD. HD is usually used initially for up to 16 weeks to allow the graft to be covered with epithelium and so avoid the risk of graft infection through peritoneal dialysate. However, this risk must be balanced against that of bacterial seeding from the patient's HD access.

Body Size Limitations and Intolerance of Intra-abdominal Fluid Volume

Body size can be a problem at both ends of the spectrum. Small patients may be intolerant of the volume of dialysate needed to achieve adequate dialysis, particularly if they have negligible residual renal function. Alternative methods of fluid exchange, such as nocturnal automated PD, can be used to overcome this limitation. It may also be difficult to achieve adequate clearances in patients with a body mass index above 35 kg/m^2. Discomfort due to increased intra-abdominal volume can be significant in patients with chronic respiratory disease, low back pain, or large polycystic kidneys. In general, it is difficult to predict a patient's tolerance of intra-abdominal fluid, and so these limitations usually appear after a patient has started PD.

Bowel Disease and Other Sources of Infection

The presence of ischemic bowel disease, inflammatory bowel disease, or diverticulitis is likely to increase the incidence of peritonitis due to organisms passing through the bowel wall into the peritoneum. Abdominal wall infection may lead to peritonitis through the exit site and catheter tunnel.

Screening for methicillin-resistant *Staphylococcus aureus* (MRSA) before all elective surgical procedures is National Health Service policy in the United Kingdom. Nasal carriage of *S. aureus* increases the risk of subsequent staphylococcal exit site infection and peritonitis, and clearance of nasal *S. aureus* with topical mupirocin cream has been shown to reduce significantly the risk of staphylococcal infection at the exit site.[23]

Severe Malnutrition or Morbid Obesity

Patients should ideally commence PD in an adequate nutritional state. Severe malnutrition may lead to poor wound healing and to leakage from the catheter tunnel. In addition, peritoneal protein losses during dialysis may exacerbate hypoalbuminemia and be particularly severe with continuous ambulatory PD (CAPD) peritonitis. At the other end of the spectrum, it may prove difficult to place a peritoneal catheter satisfactorily through the abdominal wall in patients with morbid obesity. Thereafter, absorption of glucose from the dialysate, which may average as much as 800 calories per day, may contribute to further weight gain.

Contraindications to Hemodialysis

Contraindications to HD are few (see Fig. 86.4). As discussed in Chapter 87, access to the circulation can usually be obtained, even in patients with extensive vascular disease or previous surgery. An aversion to needle puncture of the arteriovenous (AV) fistula is common in the early stages but can usually be overcome by careful use of local anesthetic and nursing encouragement. Severe coagulopathy may make management of anticoagulation for the extracorporeal circuit difficult.

HOME HEMODIALYSIS

In the last two decades, the use of home HD has declined. For example, in the United Kingdom, the percentage of the dialysis population on home HD fell from 35% in 1984 to 2% in 2006. France, Australia, and New Zealand are the only countries with a significant proportion of patients on home HD (Fig. 86.5). This has occurred for a variety of reasons. First, HD usually requires the presence of an assistant throughout the period of dialysis in case the patient becomes hypotensive or unconscious. As an increasing proportion of new dialysis patients are elderly, there may be no one available who is able or willing to take on this considerable responsibility. Second, there is the added cost of installing a dialysis machine and its associated water treatment, which is not required for PD. However, the subsequent running costs are less for home than in-center HD.

Home HD can provide significant benefits for appropriate patients. It removes the inconvenience of traveling to and from the dialysis facility and gives patients the freedom to dialyze at a time to suit themselves. As a result, they are able to perform more hours of treatment per week with less disruption to their lives. Although there is no randomized, controlled trial comparing hospital and home HD, comparative studies, in which correction has been made for differences in comorbidity, do suggest that patients on home HD have a better outcome in terms of morbidity and mortality.[24] Selected patients are able to dialyze every night at home. This gives much greater clearance than is possible with thrice-weekly dialysis, and major improvements in anemia, blood pressure, and phosphate control have been demonstrated. The inconvenience of nightly treatment is balanced by the removal of dietary restrictions and antihypertensive medications and an improved quality of life.[25] In 2002, the U.K. National Institute for Health and Clinical Excellence recommended that "all patients who are suitable . . . should be offered the option of

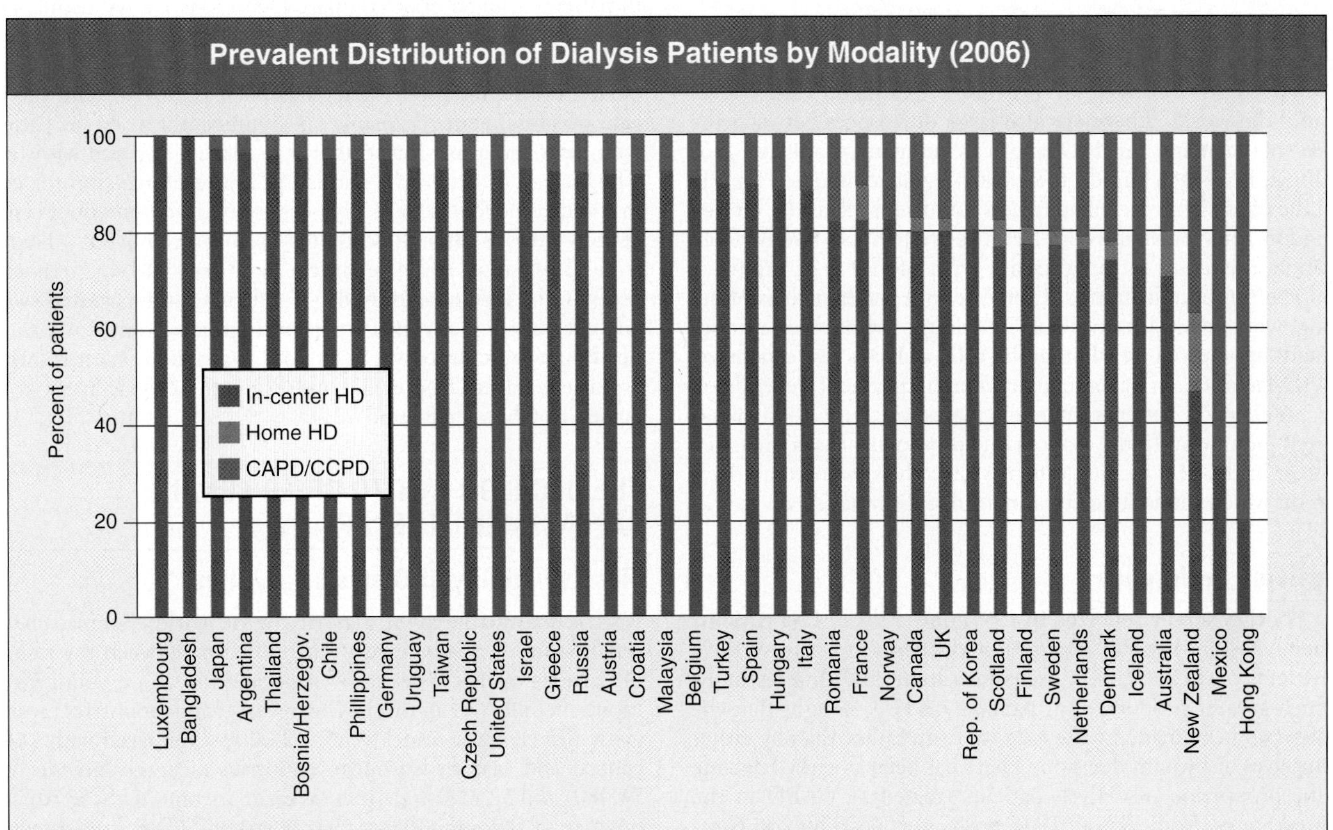

Figure 86.5 Prevalent distribution of dialysis patients by modality, 2006. Data are presented only for those countries from which relevant information was available. All rates are unadjusted. CAPD, continuous ambulatory PD; CCPD, continuous cycling PD; HD, hemodialysis.

having HD in the home" (*www.nice.org.uk/Guidance/TA48*), and with improvements in dialysis machine technology, this form of treatment is becoming more widespread.

PATIENT'S CHOICE OF HEMODIALYSIS OR PERITONEAL DIALYSIS

In the facility of one of the authors (HCR) in Birmingham, U.K., all patients entering the ESRD program are given "modality-neutral" counseling and allowed to select their preferred mode of treatment.[26] Between 1992 and 1998, the patient's choice was restricted for medical reasons by the physician in 54 of 333 patients (16%), PD being contraindicated in 51 of the 54. Of the remainder, 55% chose HD and 45% PD. These relative proportions are the same as those found in a study of 5466 U.S. patients who received a program of predialysis education.[27] Independent predictors for choosing HD in our study were increasing age and male sex. Independent predictors for choosing CAPD in the United Kingdom and the United States include being married, being counseled before the start of dialysis, and increasing distance from home to the base unit.[28]

Of those able to choose, almost all patients can be started on their preferred modality of dialysis.[24] However, in the United States, whereas 45% of patients chose PD, only 33% actually started dialysis on this modality.[27] Furthermore, the major differences in dialysis modality between countries (see Fig. 86.5) suggest that the type of dialysis is more often decided by physicians rather than by patients. Possible factors affecting these decisions are discussed next.[29,30]

Arrangements for the Reimbursement of Physicians and Funding of Dialysis Facilities

The arrangements by which physicians and dialysis facilities are reimbursed for the cost of providing treatment vary widely around the world. There are also large differences between the levels of payment for HD and PD in many countries. For example, in French clinics, the facility is not reimbursed for PD and the physicians receive no fee. In countries such as the United Kingdom and Canada, where facilities are publicly funded from taxation, the use of more expensive types of HD (e.g., high-flux hemodiafiltration) is limited. Conversely, in places such as Hong Kong, where dialysis is available only in the private sector, more patients are treated by PD than by HD, as PD is less expensive. In HD facilities, an arrangement whereby payment depends on the number of patients treated creates pressure to increase patient numbers. If the patient's nephrologist has a financial interest in the HD facility, this may directly influence the decision on which modality of treatment to recommend.

Physician Preference

In a USRDS survey reported in 1997, only 25% of HD patients remembered having PD discussed with them. In contrast, 68% of patients on PD reported discussions about HD. Interestingly, a much greater proportion of patients on HD thought that the choice had been made by the medical team rather than by either themselves or by joint decision. There has been a marked decline in the proportion of dialysis patients treated by CAPD in the United States, from 14% in 1995 to 8% in 2006. This compares with 20% in the United Kingdom in 2006. In Japan, approximately 50% of ESRD patients will survive on dialysis for more than 10 years; the physician therefore needs to consider the suitability of a dialysis modality for 10 years or more of treatment. Most Japanese physicians prefer HD because of better long-term outcome; alternatively, they start with PD and change to HD after 5 to 7 years of treatment.

THE IMPORTANCE OF DIALYSIS ACCESS

Ideally, every patient would make an informed choice between PD and HD after a period of in-depth counseling and preparation, and dialysis access would be established in advance of starting dialysis. Sadly, dialysis is frequently started in less than ideal circumstances. Late presentation is a worldwide phenomenon, indicating that no system of health care has overcome the problems of identifying patients with CKD and bringing them to the attention of nephrologists in time (Fig. 86.6).[31,32]

Reports from both Europe and the United States document the excess morbidity and mortality for patients presenting late in ESRD and requiring dialysis as an emergency procedure.[33] Patients starting dialysis as an emergency usually receive HD through a catheter and tend to remain on HD rather than converting to PD. Compared with nonemergency patients, their length of hospital stay is significantly greater, and during this time, there is a higher incidence of major complications and death. A significant part of the increased mortality is related to the use of a catheter rather than a permanent AV fistula. In the United States, many incident patients receive an AV graft rather than a fistula as it is believed that grafts can be cannulated more easily and earlier than fistulas (Fig. 86.7).[34]

International data from the Dialysis Outcomes and Practice Patterns Study showed a 37% increase in the relative risk of death in patients dialyzing through a catheter and a 19% increase in patients using a graft compared with a native AV fistula, after adjustment for a wider range of demographic and comorbid factors.[34] The detrimental effects of central venous catheters persist even after the catheter has been removed. The survival rate of subsequent AV fistulas is significantly worse in patients who have had a previous catheter in place compared with those who started directly on a fistula, even after correction for casemix and comorbidity, possibly because of development of central venous stenosis after the catheter has been removed.[31] There is wide variation in countries in the time required for permanent access to be created and used.[31] If a fistula can be created swiftly and used as soon as it is mature, perhaps after only 2 weeks, the need for a catheter may be avoided. Details of HD access surgery are discussed in Chapter 87, and PD catheter placement is discussed in Chapters 88 and 92.

THE DECISION NOT TO OFFER RENAL REPLACEMENT THERAPY

The Availability of Dialysis Facilities

RRT is unavailable to the majority of the world's population with renal failure.[35] A strong relationship exists between the number of patients on RRT per million population and a country's per capita income: 644 in the 15 European Union countries (average gross per capita income, >U.S. $22,000) compared with 166 in central and eastern European countries (average income, U.S. $4,480) and 52 in Bangladesh (average income, U.S. $370). The practice of rationing dialysis has been candidly documented in a report from a South African center[36] in which more than half the patients with ESRD assessed between 1988 and 2003 were not

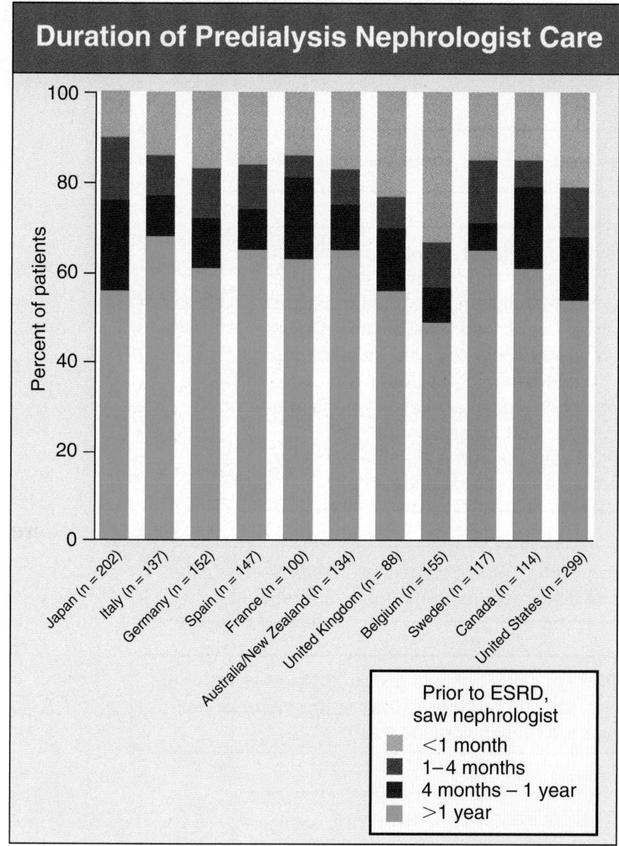

Figure 86.6 Variations in predialysis care. Percentage of patients starting hemodialysis having seen a nephrologist more than 1 month or 4 months previously by country. *(Data from the Dialysis Outcomes and Practice Patterns Study.* www.dopps.org.*)*

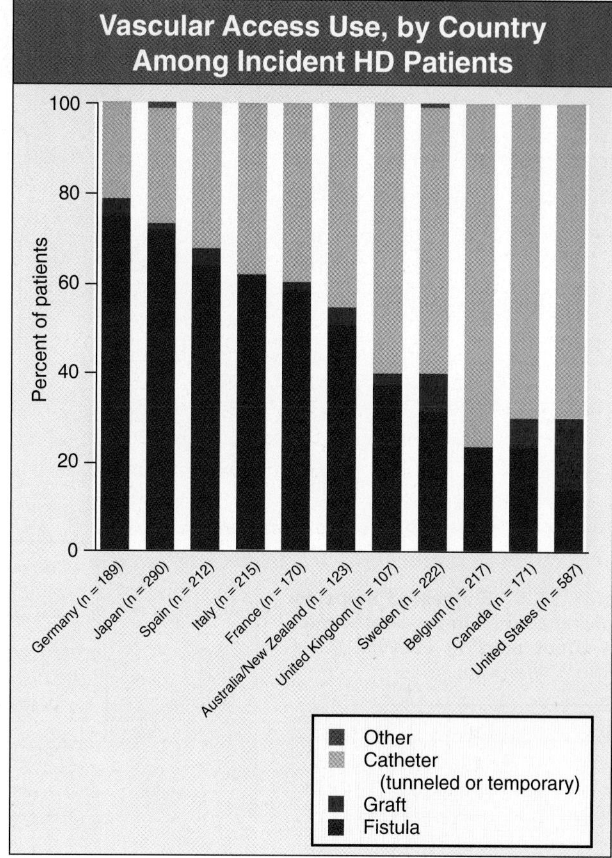

Figure 86.7 Country differences in vascular access use at start of hemodialysis. Percentage of patients starting hemodialysis with an arteriovenous fistula, an arteriovenous graft, or an intravenous catheter, by country. *(Data from the Dialysis Outcomes and Practice Patterns Study.* www.dopps.org.*)*

offered dialysis; socioeconomic factors such as age, race, employment, and marital status outweighed medical factors in the decision to begin treatment.

Selection of Patients by Physicians and Nephrologists

Incidence rates of RRT have steadily increased during recent decades. Some but not all of this is due to the increasing prevalence of ESRD. A long-term study from California has shown a steady increase in the likelihood of going on to receive RRT without there being an increase in risk factors for ESRD, such as age, diabetes, high blood pressure, proteinuria, and reduced eGFR, or a fall in premature deaths from other causes.[37] This indicates a greater enthusiasm to start RRT in recent years.

In the developed world, the practice of starting dialysis in patients who are very elderly or dependent on others for their care or who have multiple comorbid conditions varies significantly between countries and between nephrologists within those countries.[38,39] For example, the percentage of patients who were living in a nursing home or who were unable to eat independently within 90 days of starting dialysis is much higher in the United States (11.6%) and Japan (19.2%) than in France (1.3%), Germany (6.4%), Italy (4.7%), Spain (2.0%), and the United Kingdom (1.5%).[38] The average age at start of dialysis in Japan is 66.8 years. In 2008, 6065 patients in Japan were older than 80 years at the initiation of dialysis, and 422 patients were older than 90 years.[40] The odds of new patients being older than 80 years are significantly lower in units whose medical directors agree that they do not start dialysis in the very elderly.[38]

Severe intellectual impairment in a patient would much more strongly influence a nephrologist in the United Kingdom not to start dialysis than in the United States.[38,39] Furthermore, nephrologists in the United States were much more likely than those in the United Kingdom and Canada to start dialysis in patients with dementia or in a persistent vegetative state, if pressured to do so by family members. In a recent report from the Japanese Society for Dialysis Therapy, 1326 of 15,239 new dialysis patients (8.7%) had some intellectual impairment.[40] Fear of litigation was particularly influential in persuading Japanese, U.S., and Canadian nephrologists to offer treatment.[39]

The Renal Physicians Association and American Society of Nephrology (RPA/ASN) guidelines for the initiation of dialysis in the United States provide a systematic approach to conflict resolution if there is disagreement about the benefits of dialysis (Fig. 86.8).[41]

RATIONING OF DIALYSIS TREATMENT

On the grounds that the greatest good should be derived from the limited resources available, it has been argued that patients who are expected to survive for only a few months should not be offered dialysis. This is supported by the view that it is preferable to avoid suffering by not starting dialysis than to withdraw treatment when

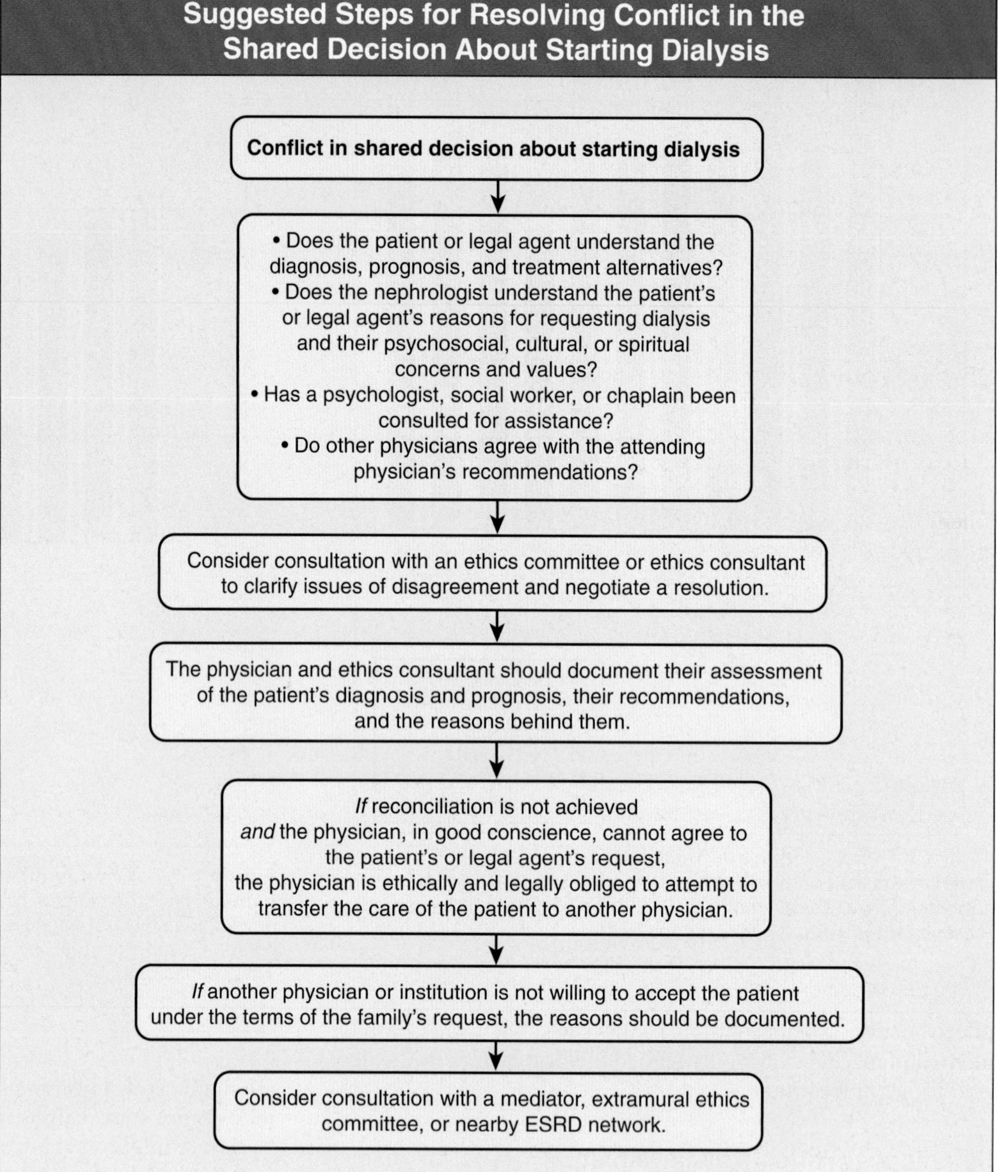

Suggested Steps for Resolving Conflict in the Shared Decision About Starting Dialysis
Conflict in shared decision about starting dialysis
• Does the patient or legal agent understand the diagnosis, prognosis, and treatment alternatives?
• Does the nephrologist understand the patient's or legal agent's reasons for requesting dialysis and their psychosocial, cultural, or spiritual concerns and values?
• Has a psychologist, social worker, or chaplain been consulted for assistance?
• Do other physicians agree with the attending physician's recommendations?
Consider consultation with an ethics committee or ethics consultant to clarify issues of disagreement and negotiate a resolution.
The physician and ethics consultant should document their assessment of the patient's diagnosis and prognosis, their recommendations, and the reasons behind them.
If reconciliation is not achieved and the physician, in good conscience, cannot agree to the patient's or legal agent's request, the physician is ethically and legally obliged to attempt to transfer the care of the patient to another physician.
If another physician or institution is not willing to accept the patient under the terms of the family's request, the reasons should be documented.
Consider consultation with a mediator, extramural ethics committee, or nearby ESRD network.

Figure 86.8 Suggested steps for resolving conflict in the shared decision about starting dialysis. *(Modified from reference 41.)*

the patient's condition becomes distressing.[42] Withdrawal of dialysis seems more like actively causing death than withholding of dialysis, where death is allowed to occur "naturally."

This utilitarian approach to the allocation of resources is contrary to the instincts of most physicians to act in the patient's best interest and may be unacceptable to many physicians. Furthermore, it does not take into account the value of even a short extension of life that allows the patient and his or her family to prepare for death. It also makes only a small contribution to minimizing the use of resources as the costs of a HD program are in proportion to the length of time that the patient continues to receive treatment.

Against this ethical background, are there any objective criteria that can be applied to identify patients who are unsuitable for dialysis? One criterion to be dismissed is age. Although advanced age was used as a simple exclusion criterion in the early days of dialysis, the elderly are now the most rapidly growing section of the dialysis population.

Predictive Factors

Two studies have attempted to identify other predictive factors. In a prospective Canadian study of patients starting dialysis,[43] a comorbidity scoring system was used to quantify factors likely to predict early death. The predictive value of this scoring system was compared with the value of an estimate made by the patient's nephrologist of the probability that the patient would die within 6 months. It was not possible to predict early death accurately by either the comorbidity scoring system or the clinician's opinion. Indeed, it was impossible even to identify the small proportion of patients with a very poor prognosis. Clinicians were more accurate than the scoring system in identifying patients with less than a 50% risk of death by 6 months, but they tended to overestimate the risk of death in the worst prognostic groups. For example, 30% of patients whose predicted probability of death was considered to be 80% or higher survived for more than 6 months.

In a U.K. study,[44] a high-risk group of 26 patients was identified by factors associated with poor survival in a statistical model, which included poor functional status at presentation, comorbidity, and underlying disease. Although these patients had a 1-year survival of only 19.2%, four patients survived at least 2 years. Furthermore, the cost incurred by this high-risk group was only 3.2% of the total cost of the chronic dialysis program.

ADVISING PATIENTS ABOUT PROGNOSIS ON DIALYSIS

Despite these uncertainties, an individual patient should be given an estimate of his or her likely future on dialysis. Factors associated with a poorer prognosis in a large number of studies include advanced age, male gender, decreased serum albumin, malnutrition, impaired functional status, diabetes mellitus, and coronary heart disease. Quality of life is strongly predictive of mortality, even after statistical correction for these comorbid factors.[45]

For patients whose prognosis is particularly uncertain, or when there is disagreement between the views of the patient and the dialysis team, a time-limited trial of dialysis may be offered.[41] This will give the patient and his or her family a better understanding of what life on dialysis entails and allow time for further discussion between all parties. The duration of the trial should be judged for each individual and clinical and biochemical parameters reviewed regularly. In our experience of 31 patients older than 79 years on HD, 10 patients who were hypoalbuminemic at the start of dialysis and whose serum albumin had fallen by more than 3 g/l to 30 g/l or less after 4 weeks on dialysis had all died by 6 months. The median survival of the other 21 patients was 1.3 years.

Most people would agree that patients who are certain to have an unacceptable quality of life should not be subjected to the discomfort of dialysis. Elderly patients with multiple comorbidities, particularly ischemic heart disease, have been shown to have survival rates with conservative therapy without dialysis that are equivalent to those of patients receiving dialysis.[46] Sparing such patients the inconvenience and discomfort of hospital attendances, surgical access procedures, and dialysis treatments is a major benefit.

Many of the symptoms and complications of ESRD (e.g., anemia, acidosis, pruritus, insomnia, depression, fluid overload, and hypertension) can be treated with medication and low-protein diet,[47] and so a decision not to start dialysis is not the same as a decision to withhold active treatment. Such "conservative" therapy is best delivered by the specialist multidisciplinary team that delivers care to all patients with ESRD not yet on dialysis, which should include a dietitian, social worker, and psychological support. The team should have close links with palliative care specialists so that there is a smooth transition from active medical therapy to terminal care.

THE PATIENT WHO DOES NOT WANT DIALYSIS

Nephrologists may be presented with the dilemma of a mentally competent patient whom they would normally treat but who does not wish to have dialysis.[41] From an ethical viewpoint, decisions not to start dialysis and to withdraw dialysis are justified on the principle of individual autonomy. Legally, they are based on the individual's common-law right to self-determination in the United Kingdom and on the constitutional right of liberty in the United States. Where the patient is able to express a clear wish, the physician is obliged to respect this because to treat a patient against his or her will would constitute an assault. The physician must nonetheless ensure that all reversible factors have been addressed, such as unfounded fears about what dialysis will entail or a depressive illness affecting the patient's judgment, and ideally request a psychiatric evaluation. It is not uncommon for patients to express a strong desire not to have dialysis, particularly if they are relatively asymptomatic, only to change their mind when they become more symptomatic. At this late stage, the basic "will to survive" comes to the fore. An advance directive written by the patient should never be held as a reason against a change of mind.

DISAGREEMENT ABOUT A DECISION TO DIALYZE A PATIENT

There will inevitably be differences of opinion about the benefits of dialysis for individual patients. Dialysis nurses may disagree with the nephrologist's decision to treat a patient. If the dialysis nurses and physicians are functioning well as a team, they should be able to express these reservations and have the issue adequately discussed. It is very demoralizing for individual staff and the team as a whole if they feel pressured into giving treatment that they think is inappropriate.

The nephrologist may remain unwilling to offer dialysis despite the insistence of either the patient or, more often, the patient's care providers, the legal agent, or another physician (see Fig. 86.8). Dialysis must never be given at the insistence of others if it is against the patient's clearly expressed wishes. However, if the patient insists on treatment against the nephrologist's advice, dialysis should usually be given while a resolution is reached. Extensive discussions and explanations of the treatment options and prognosis may be needed to gain a better understanding of the reasons behind the differing views. Helpful advice may be obtained from another physician, particularly the patient's family physician, who will have a broader understanding of the patient's circumstances. It may be appropriate to involve a psychologist, social worker, or religious counselor. If the conflict persists, it may be necessary to refer the case to a formal ethics committee, if one exists locally, to clarify the issues of disagreement and to enable a resolution. A physician cannot be compelled to offer treatment against his or her considered professional judgment, but the physician is ethically and legally obliged to attempt to transfer the care of the patient to another physician. Only as a last resort, if no alternative dialysis unit can be found and after adequate advance notice has been given, should dialysis be withdrawn.[41]

MANAGEMENT OF DISRUPTIVE PATIENTS ON DIALYSIS

Most nephrologists have had experience of treating a small number of patients who, for one reason or another, will not comply with the discipline required for maintenance dialysis and who become disruptive to the staff and other patients. This behavior can range from noncompliance with treatment, which harms the patient but is merely inconvenient to the staff, to verbal or even physical aggression toward the staff and other patients in the unit. The impact of this small number of patients can be very great.

The strategy for dealing with such patients must be tailored to the individual. However, useful suggestions for resolving conflict have been provided in the RPA/ASN Clinical Practice Guideline[41] (Fig. 86.9); they are available at *www.esrdnetworks.org/networks/net6/policies/po-recom.html* and have been reviewed

Suggested Steps for Dealing with Disruptive Patients
Identify and document problem behaviors and discuss them with the patient.
Seek to understand the patient's perspective.
Identify the patient's goals for treatment.
Share control and responsibility for treatment with the patient: Educate the patient so that he or she can make informed decisions. Involve the patient in the treatment as much as possible. Negotiate a behavioral contract with the patient.
Consult a psychiatrist, psychologist, or social worker for assistance in patient management or determination of decision-making capacity.
Be patient and persistent; try not to be adversarial.
Allow the patient to air concerns but do not tolerate verbal abuse or threats to staff or patients (see www.nhs.uk/zerotolerance/intro.htm).
Contact law enforcement officials if physical abuse is threatened or occurs.
If satisfactory resolution has not occured with the above strategies, contact the local end-stage renal disease network to discuss the situation and ensure due process.
Consider transferring the patient to another facility or discharging the patient.
Consult with legal counsel before proceeding with plans for discharge and do not discharge without advance notice and a full explanation of future treatment options.

Figure 86.9 Suggested steps for dealing with disruptive patients. *(Modified from reference 41.)*

recently.[48] They emphasize the importance of understanding, information, patience, and persistence. However, the bottom line for patients who are aggressive toward staff while on dialysis must be that they are taken off treatment and sent home.

RESUSCITATION AND WITHDRAWAL OF DIALYSIS

Cardiopulmonary Resuscitation

If patients are to be fully involved in decision-making about their treatment, two sensitive issues need to be discussed: cardiopulmonary resuscitation (CPR) and the possibility of withdrawal of dialysis.[49] The two are not necessarily linked; patients may wish to continue with dialysis but express a desire that resuscitation not be attempted should they suffer a cardiac arrest. Such a decision would be supported by evidence on the outcome of CPR in dialysis patients: only 6 of 74 dialysis patients who received CPR survived to hospital discharge, and at 6 months after CPR, only two were still alive, significantly less than 23 of 247 "control" patients not on dialysis still alive at 6 months; this difference was not explained by age or comorbid conditions.[50] Successful CPR often resulted in a "poor-quality" death, 20 of the 27 successfully resuscitated dialysis patients dying a few days later on mechanical ventilation in an intensive care unit.

A decision not to attempt CPR must be carefully documented in the patient's medical and nursing records, and all nursing staff must be made aware of it. It is important to be clear about what is meant by "cardiac arrest" and for there to be agreement on how the nursing staff are to respond should the patient suffer a hypotensive "crash" while on dialysis. These notes may form part of a complete advance directive, as discussed next.

Withdrawal of Dialysis

As discussed earlier, it is not possible to predict accurately which patients will gain prolonged benefit from dialysis. Many nephrologists therefore maintain a liberal policy of offering dialysis to all patients with ESRD who wish to have it. This policy ensures that no patients are denied dialysis but has the inevitable consequence that a number of patients will be started on dialysis who subsequently do not enjoy an acceptable quality of life. The possibility of withdrawing dialysis needs to be addressed if these patients are not to suffer unreasonably.

Rates of withdrawal vary widely between countries and cultures. Withdrawal rates in Italy and France are much lower than in the United Kingdom and the United States.[49] In the United States, African Americans have about one-third the withdrawal rate of Caucasians. Rates of withdrawal vary between dialysis units and are significantly associated with the medical director's opinion about whether withdrawal is allowed or facilitated in that unit.[38] This suggests that patients' wishes are not always fully included in these decisions. Patients may be very reticent to express a wish to withdraw from dialysis. Many see it as their duty as a patient to go along with the treatment recommended by the physician and do not wish to appear ungrateful for the efforts that are being made to keep them alive. The physician may be the last member of the team to learn about the patient's views, and it is very important that good communication exist within the multidisciplinary team so that any clues that the patient gives are passed on and acted on.

Staff should adopt a proactive approach and raise the issue of withdrawal of dialysis with patients who are not thriving. There is good evidence that early discussion of these issues can lead to a more satisfactory outcome for patients, relatives, and staff when the patient eventually dies.[51] In the United States, formal advance directives play an important part in these discussions, and helpful guidance on how to conduct sensitive interviews has been published.[52] In the United Kingdom, there has been less enthusiasm for formalizing this process. This may stem from a fear that raising the subject of death with patients may destroy their hope for the future. Qualitative research suggests that the opposite may be the case.[53] Advance directives do not obviate the need for staff to continue to communicate closely with the patient and his or her family in case the decision changes as death comes closer.

When a patient is no longer competent to make a decision, an advance directive can provide a clear legal basis for the decision to stop dialysis. Indeed, in the absence of clear and convincing written evidence, some American states (e.g., Missouri, New York) insist that dialysis must be continued. In other American states and the United Kingdom, the physician is given the task of deciding on the patient's behalf. Helpful advice for dialysis staff and patients wishing to complete an advance directive is available in the RPA/ASN Clinical Practice Guideline[41] and at the website *www.ageingwithdignity.org*.

Once a patient has expressed a wish for dialysis to be withdrawn or the issue has been raised by his or her relatives, the first priority must be to identify any reversible factors that may improve the patient's health sufficiently for the decision to be reversed. In particular, any depression must be identified and treated.[54] Once all these factors have been ruled out, the process of withdrawing dialysis should be managed according to some key principles (Fig. 86.10).

Withdrawal of dialysis should be seen not as an admission of failure but as a final stage in the process of RRT. The

Principles Underlying Withdrawal of Dialysis
The ultimate responsibility for the decision rests with the physician, not the relative.
The patient's interests and dignity should be protected at all times.
The process should not be rushed. If there is any doubt about the correctness of the decision, treatment should continue.
There should be an open discussion among the multidisciplinary team to avoid any damaging disagreements.
The psychological needs of the health care team should not be overlooked.
Palliative care must be given in the most appropriate environment, e.g., a hospice or, ideally, the patient's own home.

Figure 86.10 Key principles underlying the process of withdrawal of dialysis.

opportunity for patients to complete unfinished emotional and financial business can make the subsequent bereavement period much less traumatic. Managing this terminal phase can be uniquely rewarding, particularly if it allows a patient and his or her family and care givers to prepare themselves for the patient's death.[55]

REFERENCES

1. O'Hare AM, Bertenthal D, Walter LC, et al. When to refer patients with chronic kidney disease for vascular access surgery: Should age be a consideration? *Kidney Int*. 2007;71:555-561.
2. Devins GM, Mendelssohn DC, Barré PE, Binik YM. Predialysis psychoeducational intervention and coping styles influence time to dialysis in chronic kidney disease. *Am J Kidney Dis*. 2003;42:693-703.
3. Curtis BM, Ravani P, Malberti F, et al. The short- and long-term impact of multi-disciplinary clinics in addition to standard nephrology care on patient outcomes. *Nephrol Dial Transplant*. 2005;20:47-154.
4. Goldstein M, Yassa T, Dacouris N, McFarlane P. Multidisciplinary predialysis care and morbidity and mortality of patients on dialysis. *Am J Kidney Dis*. 2004;44:706-714.
5. Hemmelgarn BR, Manns BJ, Zhang J, et al. Association between multidisciplinary care and survival for elderly patients with chronic kidney disease. *J Am Soc Nephrol*. 2007;18:993-999.
6. Zhao Y, Brooks JM, Flanigan MJ, et al. Physician access and early nephrology care in elderly patients with end-stage renal disease. *Kidney Int*. 2008;74:1596-1602.
7. Hallan SI, Coresh J, Astor BC, et al. International comparison of the relationship of chronic kidney disease prevalence and ESRD risk. *J Am Soc Nephrol*. 2006;17:2275-2284.
8. Finkelstein FO, Story K, Firanek C, et al. Perceived knowledge among patients cared for by nephrologists about chronic kidney disease and end-stage renal disease therapies. *Kidney Int*. 2008;74:1178-1184.
9. Trento M, Passera P, Borgo E, et al. A 5-year randomized controlled study of learning, problem solving ability and quality of life modifications in people with type 2 diabetes managed by group care. *Diabetes Care*. 2004;27:670-675.
10. Razgone S, Schwankovsky L, James-Rogers A, et al. An intervention for employment maintenance among blue-collar workers with end stage renal disease. *Am J Kidney Dis*. 1993;22:403-412.
11. Wolfe RA, Ashby VB, Milford EL, et al. Comparison of mortality in all patients on dialysis, patients on dialysis awaiting transplantation, and recipients of a first cadaveric transplant. *N Engl J Med*. 1999;341:1725-1730.
12. Mange KC, Joffe MM, Feldman HI. Effect of the use or nonuse of long-term dialysis on the subsequent survival of renal transplants from living donors. *N Engl J Med*. 2001;344:726-731.
13. Saran R, Bragg-Gresham JL, Rayner HC, et al. Nonadherence in hemodialysis: Associations with mortality, hospitalization, and practice patterns in the DOPPS. *Kidney Int*. 2003;64:254-262.
14. Korevaar JC, Jansen MA, Dekker FW, et al. Evaluation of DOQI guidelines: Early start of dialysis treatment is not associated with better health-related quality of life. National Kidney Foundation–Dialysis Outcomes Quality Initiative. *Am J Kidney Dis*. 2002;39:108-115.
15. Cooper BA, Branley P, Bulfone L, et al. A randomized, controlled trial of early versus late initiation of dialysis. *N Engl J Med*. 2010;363:609-619.
16. Fenton SS, Schaubel DE, Desmeules M, et al. Hemodialysis versus peritoneal dialysis: A comparison of adjusted mortality rates. *Am J Kidney Dis*. 1997;30:334-342.
17. Held PJ, Port FK, Turenne MN, et al. Continuous ambulatory peritoneal dialysis and hemodialysis: Comparison of patient mortality with adjustment for comorbid conditions. *Kidney Int*. 1994;45:1163-1169.
18. Jaar BG, Coresh J, Plantinga LC, et al. Comparing the risk for death with peritoneal dialysis and hemodialysis in a national cohort of patients with chronic kidney disease. *Ann Intern Med* 2005;2(143):174-183.
19. Ganesh SK, Hulbert-Shearon T, Port FK, et al. Mortality differences by dialysis modality among incident ESRD patients with and without coronary artery disease. *J Am Soc Nephrol*. 2003;14:415-424.
20. Stack AG, Molony DA, Rahman NS, et al. Impact of dialysis modality on survival of new ESRD patients with congestive heart failure in the United States. *Kidney Int*. 2003;64:1071-1079.
21. Rayner HC, Pisoni RL, Bommer J, et al. Mortality and hospitalization in haemodialysis patients in five European countries: Results from the Dialysis Outcomes and Practice Patterns Study (DOPPS). *Nephrol Dial Transplant*. 2004;19:108-120.
22. NKF-K/DOQI Clinical Practice Guidelines for Peritoneal Dialysis Adequacy 2000. *Am J Kidney Dis*. 2001;37(Suppl 1):S65-S136. Available at: www.kidney.org/professionals/doqi/index.cfm.
23. Mupirocin Study Group. Nasal mupirocin prevents *Staphylococcus aureus* exit site infection during peritoneal dialysis. *J Am Soc Nephrol*. 1996;7:2403-2408.
24. Woods JD, Port FK, Stannard D, et al. Comparison of mortality with home hemodialysis and center hemodialysis: A national study. *Kidney Int*. 1996;49:1464-1470.
25. Pierratos A. Daily nocturnal home hemodialysis. *Kidney Int*. 2004;65:1975-1986.
26. Little J, Irwin A, Marshall T, et al. Predicting a patient's choice of dialysis modality: Experience in a United Kingdom renal department. *Am J Kidney Dis*. 2001;37:981-986.
27. Golper TA, Vonesh EF, Wolfson M, et al. The impact of pre-ESRD education on dialysis modality selection. *J Am Soc Nephrol*. 2000;11:231A.
28. Stack AG. Determinants of modality selection among incident US dialysis patients: Results from a national study. *J Am Soc Nephrol*. 2002;13:1279-1287.
29. Nissenson AR, Prichard SS, Cheng IKP, et al. Non-medical factors that impact on ESRD modality selection. *Kidney Int*. 1993;43(Suppl 40):S120-S127.
30. Mendelssohn DC, Mullaney SR, Jung B, et al. What do American nephrologists think about dialysis modality selection? *Am J Kidney Dis*. 2001;37:22-29.
31. Rayner HC, Pisoni RL, Young EW, et al. Creation, cannulation and survival of arteriovenous fistulae—data from the DOPPS. *Kidney Int*. 2003;63:323-330.
32. Jungers P. Late referral: Loss of chance for the patient, loss of money for society. *Nephrol Dial Transplant*. 2002;17:371-375.
33. Dhingra RK, Young EW, Hulbert-Shearon TE, et al. Type of vascular access and mortality in US hemodialysis patients. *Kidney Int*. 2001;60:1443-1451.
34. Pisoni RL, Albert JM, Elder SE, et al. Lower mortality risk associated with native arteriovenous fistula (AVF) vs graft (AVG) use in patient and facility-level analyses: Results from the DOPPS. *J Am Soc Nephrol*. 2005;16:259A.
35. Schieppati A, Remuzzi G. Chronic renal diseases as a public health problem: Epidemiology, social, and economic implications. *Kidney Int Suppl*. 2005;98:S7-S10.
36. Moosa MR, Kidd M. The dangers of rationing dialysis treatment: The dilemma facing a developing country. *Kidney Int*. 2006;70:1107-1114.
37. Hsu C, Go AS, McCulloch CE, et al. Exploring secular trends in the likelihood of receiving treatment for end-stage renal disease. *Clin J Am Soc Nephrol*. 2007;2:81-88.
38. Lambie M, Rayner HC, Bragg-Gresham JL, et al. Starting and withdrawing haemodialysis—associations between nephrologists' opinions, patient characteristics and practice patterns (data from the Dialysis Outcomes and Practice Patterns Study). *Nephrol Dial Transplant*. 2006;10:2814-2820.
39. McKenzie JK, Moss AH, Feest TG, et al. Dialysis decision making in Canada, the United Kingdom, and the United States. *Am J Kidney Dis*. 1998;31:12-18.

40. Japanese Society for Dialysis Therapy. Available at: http://docs.jsdt.or.jp/overview/index.html.
41. Renal Physicians Association and American Society of Nephrology. *Shared Decision-Making in the Appropriate Initiation of and Withdrawal from Dialysis. Clinical Practice Guideline, Number 2.* Washington, DC: Renal Physicians Association; 2000.
42. Singer PA. Nephrologists' experience with and attitudes towards decisions to forego dialysis. *J Am Soc Nephrol.* 1992;2:1235-1240.
43. Barrett BJ, Parfrey PS, Morgan J, et al. Prediction of early death in end-stage renal disease patients starting dialysis. *Am J Kidney Dis.* 1997;29:214-222.
44. Chadna SM, Schulz J, Lawrence C, et al. Is there a rationale for rationing chronic dialysis? A hospital based cohort study of factors affecting survival and morbidity. *BMJ.* 1999;318:217-222.
45. Mapes DL, Lopes AA, Satayathum S, et al. Health-related quality of life as a predictor of mortality and hospitalization: The Dialysis Outcomes and Practice Patterns Study (DOPPS). *Kidney Int.* 2003;64:339-349.
46. Murtagh FEM, Marsh JE, Donohoe P, et al. Dialysis or not? A comparative survival study of patients over 75 years with chronic kidney disease stage 5. *Nephrol Dial Transplant.* 2007;22:1955-1962.
47. Brunori G, Viola BF, Parrinello G, et al. Efficacy and safety of a very-low-protein diet when postponing dialysis in the elderly: A prospective randomized multicenter controlled study. *Am J Kidney Dis.* 2007;49:569-580.
48. Hashmi A, Moss AH. Treating difficult or disruptive dialysis patients: Practical strategies based on ethical principles. *Nat Clin Pract Nephrol.* 2008;4:515-520.
49. Fissell RB, Bragg-Gresham JL, Lopes AA, et al. Factors associated with "do not resuscitate" orders and rates of withdrawal from hemodialysis in the international DOPPS. *Kidney Int.* 2005;68:1282-1288.
50. Moss AH, Holley JL, Upton MB. Outcomes of cardiopulmonary resuscitation in dialysis patients. *J Am Soc Nephrol.* 1992;3:1238-1243.
51. Swartz RD, Penny E. Advance directives are associated with good deaths in chronic dialysis patients. *J Am Soc Nephrol.* 1993;3:1623-1630.
52. Davison SN, Torgunrud C. The creation of an advance care planning process for patients with ESRD. *Am J Kidney Dis.* 2007;49:27-36.
53. Davison SN, Simpson C. Hope and advance care planning in patients with end stage renal disease: Qualitative interview study. *BMJ.* 2006;333:886. doi:10.1136/bmj.38965.626250.55.
54. Lopes AA, Albert JM, Young EW, et al. Screening for depression in hemodialysis patients: Associations with diagnosis, treatment, and outcomes in the DOPPS [erratum in Kidney Int. 2004;66:2486]. *Kidney Int.* 2004;66:2047-2053.
55. Moss A, Holley J, Davison S, et al. Palliative care. *Am J Kidney Dis.* 2004;43:172-185.

CHAPTER 87

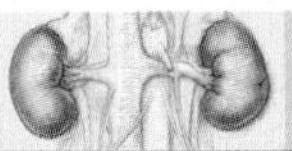

Vascular Access for Dialytic Therapies

Jan H. M. Tordoir

Functional vascular access is needed for all extracorporeal dialytic therapies and remains the lifeline for patients with end-stage renal disease who need chronic intermittent hemodialysis (HD) therapy. The ideal HD access should have a long length of a suitable superficial vein for cannulation in two places more than 5 cm apart with a sufficient blood flow for effective dialysis, usually in excess of 400 ml/min. A vascular access should have good primary patency, have a low risk of complications and side effects, and leave opportunities for further procedures in the event of failure. Ideally, a first access should be an arteriovenous (AV) fistula placed peripherally at the wrist. However, upper arm and lower limb access sites are increasingly used because the aging dialysis population, with multiple comorbidities, has poor and diseased arm vessels that may be unsuitable for the creation of a simple wrist fistula.

Vascular access should be performed with minimal delay by a surgeon experienced in vascular access creation and, wherever possible, in advance so that dialysis may start with permanent access rather than with use of a central venous catheter. Central venous catheter use should be minimized because of the increased risk of sepsis, the increased mortality, and the development of central venous stenosis or thrombosis, which compromises further access in the upper limbs. Unfortunately, many patients require a central venous catheter either to start dialysis or as a bridge between the failure of a permanent access and the creation of a new AV fistula.[1]

The need for revisional procedures because of access-related complications, including thrombosis, central venous obstruction, and ischemia, is increasing. A multidisciplinary approach to access creation and maintenance, involving nephrologists, interventional radiologists, access surgeons, and dialysis nurses, is mandatory to meet the burden of HD vascular access on health care facilities and costs.

EVALUATION OF THE PATIENT FOR VASCULAR ACCESS

The earlier a patient with chronic kidney disease (CKD) is seen by a vascular access surgeon, the better the chance for the patient to have a well-functioning access at the initiation of HD. An early decision on the type, side, and site of the first vascular access will be based on the following:

- *Clinical examination* with careful palpation of arterial pulses and venous vasculature. Particular attention is paid to the venous filling capacity, with use of a blood pressure cuff and variable pressures, and to the presence of venous collaterals and swelling. The dominant arm is not necessarily the preferred side, and the decision should be based on the quality of the vessels.
- *Vascular mapping by Doppler ultrasound.* This provides information about the venous vasculature, particularly in obese patients and in the upper arm, and about the diameter of the brachial, radial, and ulnar arteries; detects vascular calcifications; and reveals the blood flow volume in the brachial artery. The resistance index, a measure of arterial compliance, can be calculated from the differences between the high-resistance triphasic Doppler signal with clenched fist and the low-resistance biphasic waveform after the fist is released. A preoperative resistance index of 0.7 or higher in the feeding artery indicates insufficient arterial compliance (often associated with arterial calcification) so that the chance of successful creation of an AV fistula is reduced. Current guidelines recommend ultrasound mapping in all patients. Additional angiography is needed only in very difficult cases; the use of radiocontrast media should be minimized.

Preservation of veins during the earlier stages of CKD is crucial for the success of vascular access. Patients should be instructed to protect their veins, restricting blood sampling to the dorsum of the hand whenever possible.

PRIMARY AUTOGENOUS VASCULAR ACCESS

Radiocephalic AV Fistula

A well-functioning distal radiocephalic AV fistula in the non-dominant arm is the ideal permanent access for HD. This usually gives an adequate blood flow and a long length of superficial vein for needling. It also leaves proximal sites for further procedures in the event of failure. A distal radiocephalic AV fistula should be possible in a majority of incident patients but may be compromised if the cephalic and antecubital fossa veins are unusable because of thrombophlebitis from previous intravenous cannulae or venipunctures. For this reason, it is essential that these veins be avoided for intravenous cannulae, which should be restricted to the dorsum of the hand in all patients with CKD, except in the emergency situation when rapid access to the circulation is required.

A radiocephalic AV fistula is usually created at the wrist (Fig. 87.1) but can be performed more proximally in the forearm if distal vessels are inadequate. On occasion, three or four radiocephalic AV fistulas can be created at progressively more proximal sites in the forearm before resorting to a brachiocephalic AV fistula. The radiocephalic AV fistula at the wrist was initially described by Brescia and Cimino in 1966 as a side-to-side anastomosis, but an end-to-side configuration is preferred by most to reduce the risk of venous hypertension in the radial aspect of the hand. An end-to-end anastomosis is advocated by some surgeons to eliminate the small risk of steal.

The primary patency of radiocephalic fistulas varies from center to center, but recent publications report high primary failure rates varying from of 5% to 41% and 1-year primary patencies from 52% to 71% (Fig. 87.2).[2-7] Early thrombosis and nonmaturation of an AV fistula in the older comorbid population, who have poor upper limb vessels, are the major causes of these high primary failure and low patency rates. The patency of radiocephalic AV fistulas is poorer in women, so a proximal AV fistula might be preferable if the cephalic vein or radial artery is small.

Nonmaturation of Radiocephalic AV Fistula

The autogenous radiocephalic AV fistula needs time to mature and for the vein to enlarge to a size at which it can be needled for dialysis. Usually 6 weeks for maturation is advised. Earlier cannulation can damage the thin veins. Nonmaturation rates vary from 25% to 33%. The essential components of a successful AV fistula are a sufficient vein diameter of 4 to 5 mm for needling and a high blood flow so that blood can be drawn from the fistula at between 300 and 400 ml/min. In reality, this requires a fistula flow of about 600 ml/min to prevent excessive recirculation and to permit adequate dialysis within the usual 4-hour time frame of a HD treatment. Fistulas that fail immediately are the consequence of poor selection of vessels or poor technique. Regular duplex ultrasound investigation early after AV fistula formation, especially in fistulas that are not maturing, can detect poor flow, stenosis, and accessory branches, guiding the interventional radiologist and surgeon to the appropriate treatment.

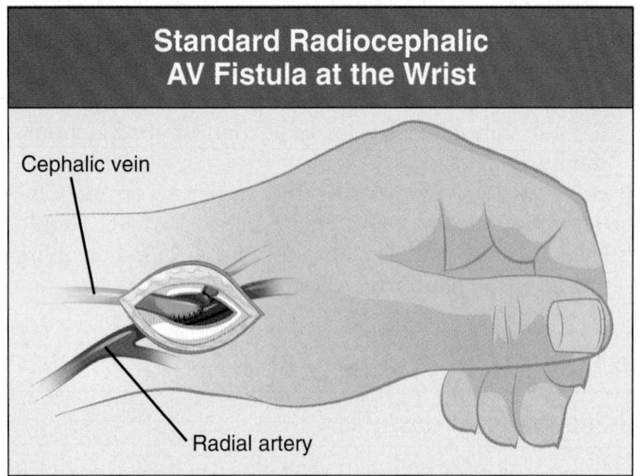

Figure 87.1 Standard radiocephalic AV fistula at the wrist. Anastomosis of end of vein to side of artery.

SECONDARY AUTOGENOUS VASCULAR ACCESS

Although a primary radiocephalic AV fistula is preferable, the first-choice procedure is increasingly an upper arm AV fistula with use of an autogenous deeply located arm vein, especially in the dialysis population with associated comorbidities such as diabetes mellitus, coronary artery disease, and peripheral arterial occlusive disease.[1]

The upper limb is preferred to the lower limb for vascular access because of the ease of cannulation, comfort for the patient, and considerably lower incidence of complications. Similarly, autogenous conduits are preferable to the use of prosthetic grafts because of improved patency and lower risk of infection.

Forearm Cephalic and Basilic Vein Transposition and Elevation

Superficial vein transposition or elevation increases the possibilities of creating a forearm fistula. The cephalic vein is preferred, but if it is unsuitable, the basilic vein can be transposed from the ulnar to the radial side along a straight subcutaneous course from the elbow to the radial artery. Alternatively, a basilic vein to ulnar artery anastomosis can be performed with additional volar transposition to facilitate needling for dialysis.

Different surgical techniques, with or without transposition, have been advocated according to the forearm artery and vein location. In one study,[8] 91% fistula maturation was achieved with a range of techniques; 15% were suitable for a straightforward AV fistula, 33% required vein transposition from dorsal to volar for anastomosis to the appropriate artery, and the remaining 52% required superficial transposition of a vein on the volar aspect of the forearm before arterial anastomosis. Primary patency rates were 84% at 1 year and 69% at 2 years.

Needle cannulation may be difficult, particularly in obese patients. A forearm cephalic vein that is too deeply located may be made accessible for cannulation by transposition or elevation. In one study, the elevation technique was applied in obese patients with radiocephalic AV fistulas and cannulation difficulties; primary failure rate was 15%, with a 1-year patency rate of 84%. After operation, all patients could be successfully cannulated for dialysis.[9]

Early Failure and 1-Year Patency Rates of Radiocephalic AVF

Author	Year	No. Fistulae	Early Failure (%)	1-Year Patency (%)
Wolowczyk et. al.	2000	208	20	65
Gibson et. al.	2001	130	23	56
Allon et. al.	2001	139	46	42
Ravani et. al.	2002	197	5	71
Roijens et. al.	2005	86	41	52
Biuckians et. al.	2008	80	37	63

Figure 87.2 Early failure and 1-year patency rates of radiocephalic AV fistulas.

Elbow and Upper Arm Cephalic Vein AV Fistula

The brachiocephalic and antecubital fistulas are two possible AV anastomoses in the elbow region. In addition, anastomosis between the transposed cephalic vein and brachial artery 2 cm proximal to the elbow may be executed, which provides an optimal situation for cannulation along the cephalic vein (Fig. 87.3). The outcome of the brachiocephalic AV fistula is usually good, with a high primary function rate and good long-term patency; studies showed a 10% early failure rate due to nonmaturation and an 80% 1-year patency rate.[10,11] Two-year primary, assisted primary, and secondary patency rates were 40%, 59%, and 67%, respectively. (Primary patency is functioning access without any intervention; assisted primary patency is functioning access after preemptive intervention for flow decline; secondary patency is functioning access after intervention for thrombosis.) Predictors of failure include diabetes mellitus and a history of contralateral forearm AV graft (indicating poor vessels). Therefore, the primary patency of brachiocephalic fistulas is comparable to that of radiocephalic fistulas. The early failure and 1-year patency rates of brachiocephalic AV fistulas are shown in Figure 87.4.[10-14]

Upper Arm Basilic Vein AV Fistula

The upper arm basilic vein is usually inaccessible for dialysis cannulation because of its medial and deep position. Therefore, the basilic vein needs to be superficialized and transposed to an anterolateral position. The original technique of brachiobasilic AV fistula construction is a two-step approach. First, a brachiobasilic anastomosis is constructed, and in the second operation, usually after 6 weeks, the arterialized vein is mobilized into a subcutaneous position, becoming accessible for needling (Fig. 87.5); nowadays, the brachiobasilic AV fistula may be performed as a one-stage surgical procedure, with elevation or transposition of the vein to a subcutaneous and anterolateral position at the time of creation of the AV anastomosis. A nonrandomized study comparing the different techniques of brachiobasilic AV fistula

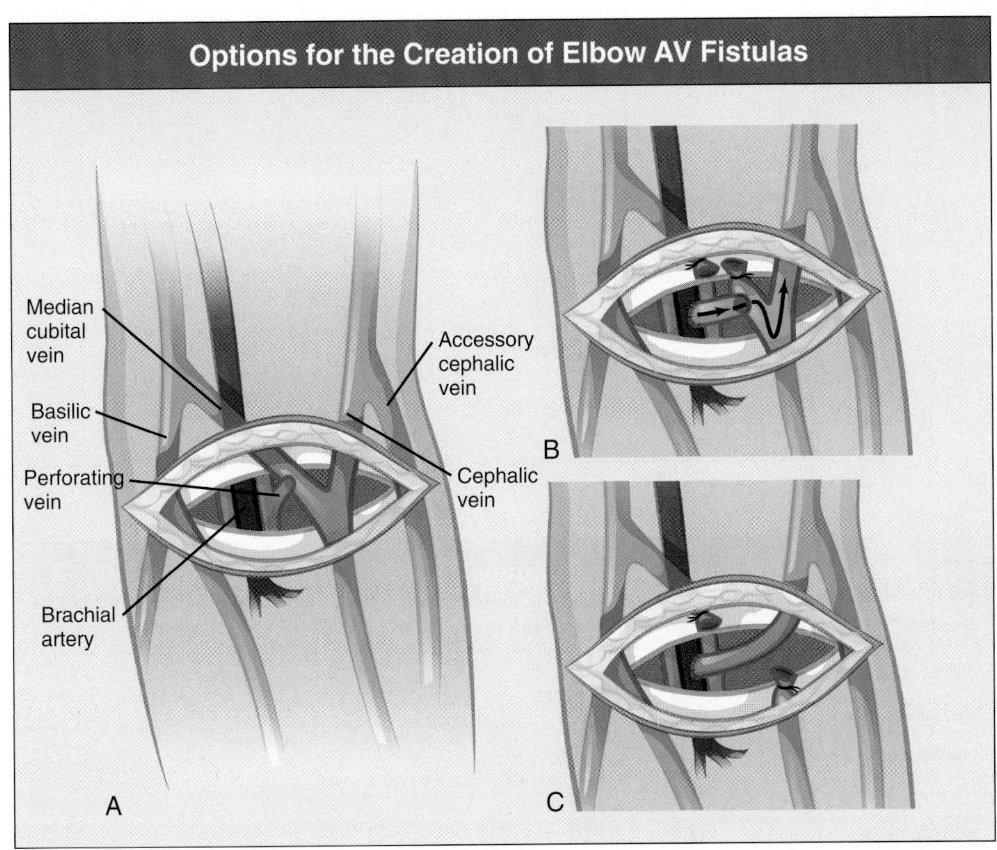

Figure 87.3 Options for the creation of elbow AV fistulas. A, Brachiocubital AV fistula. **B,** Brachiocubital AV fistula with ligation of proximal cubital vein. **C,** Brachiocephalic AV fistula.

Early Failure and 1-Year Patency Rates of Brachiocephalic AVF

Author	Year	No. Fistulae	Early Failure (%)	1-Year Patency (%)
Murphy et. al.	2002	208	16	75
Zeebregts et. al.	2005	100	11	79
Lok et. al.	2005	186	9	78
Woo et. al.	2007	71	12	66
Koksoy et. al.	2009	50	10	87

Figure 87.4 Early failure and 1-year patency rates of brachiocephalic AV fistulas.

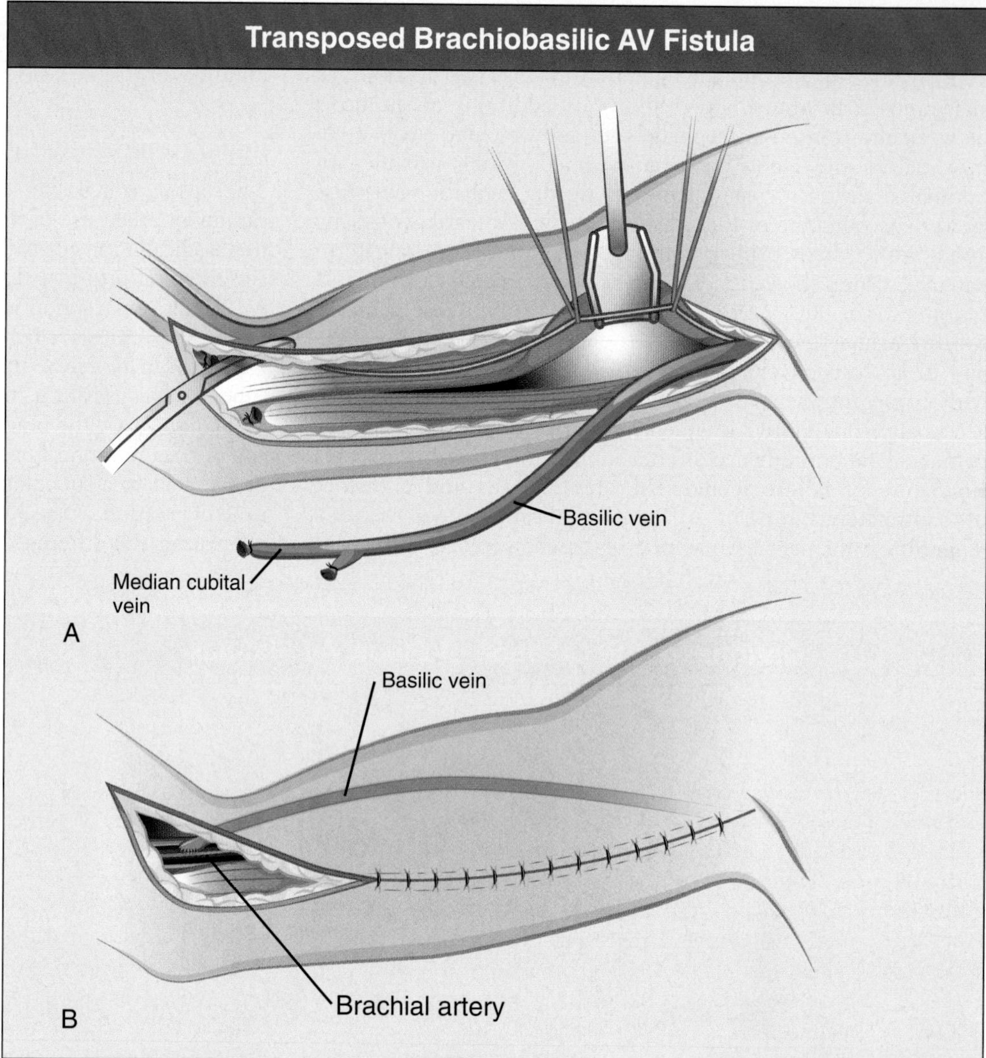

Figure 87.5 Transposed brachiobasilic AV fistula. A, Dissection of the basilic vein. **B,** Anterolateral transposition and brachial artery anastomosis.

Figure 87.6 Early failure and 1-year patency rates of brachiobasilic AV fistulas.

Early Failure and 1-Year Patency Rates of Brachiobasilic AVF

Author	Year	No. Fistulae	Early Failure (%)	1-Year Patency (%)
Segal et. al.	2003	99	23	64
Wolford et. al.	2005	100	20	47
Harper et. al.	2008	168	23	66
Keuter et. al.	2008	52	2	89
Koksoy et. al.	2009	50	4	86

creation reported 86% to 90% 1-year patencies in all groups, with only 5% to 7% nonmaturation rates.[15] Primary failure rates of 2% to 23% with 1-year patencies varying from 55% to 89% have been reported (Fig. 87.6).[12,16-19] In comparison with brachiocephalic fistulas, brachiobasilic AV fistulas are more likely to mature, although they are more susceptible to late thrombosis. However, a randomized study showed similar patencies of brachiocephalic and brachiobasilic AV fistulas.[12]

The technique of subcutaneous placement of the basilic vein has several advantages over forearm or upper arm graft implantation, with less infection and thrombosis. A meta-analysis comparing brachiobasilic AV fistulas with prosthetic grafts has shown superiority of the brachiobasilic AV fistula in primary and secondary patency rates, and it should therefore be used early in difficult access cases before the use of prosthetic grafts.[20]

NONAUTOGENOUS PROSTHETIC VASCULAR ACCESS

When autogenous AV fistula creation is impossible or the fistulas have failed, graft implantation should be considered as a vascular

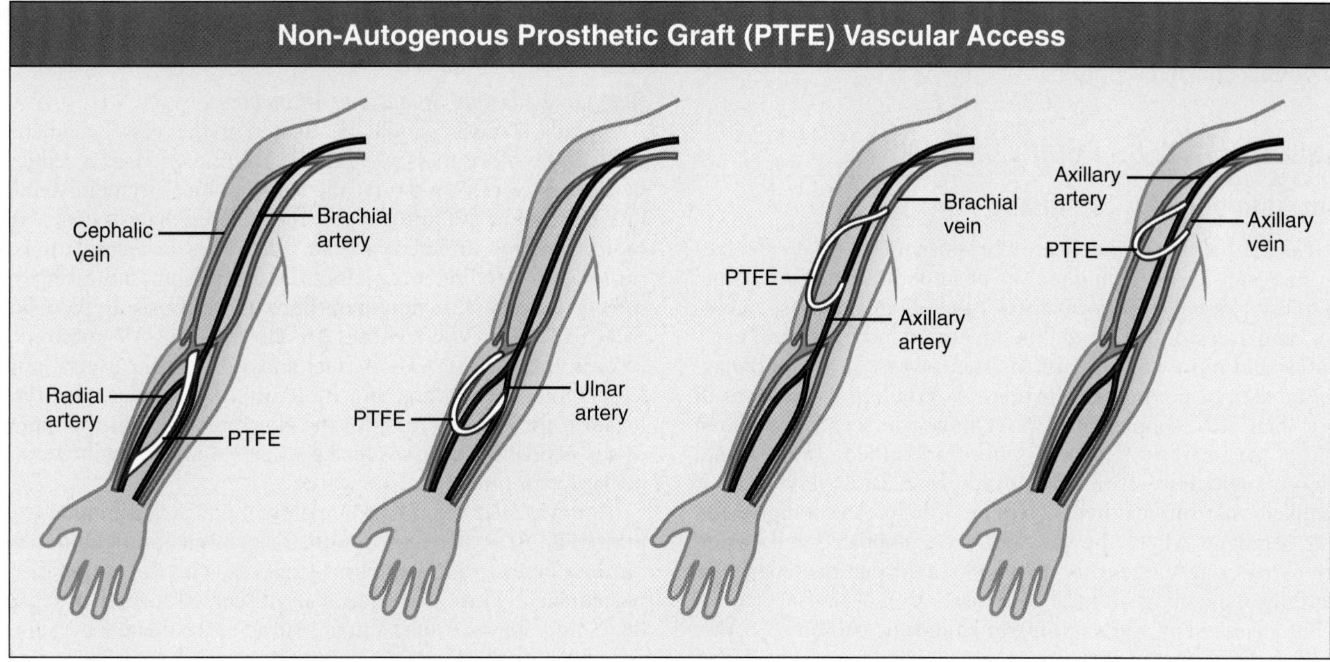

Figure 87.7 Nonautogenous prosthetic graft (PTFE) vascular access. Straight and loop configuration in upper limb.

access conduit. Xenografts such as the ovine sheep (Omniflow) and bovine cow ureter graft (SynerGraft) are popular materials as an alternative access conduit, with acceptable patency and low infection rates. The most frequently used implants are prosthetic grafts made of either polyurethane (Vectra) or polytetrafluoroethylene (PTFE). These prosthetic grafts can be implanted in a wide variety of locations and configurations in the upper limb (Fig. 87.7). Short-term functional patency is usually good, but stenosis (mostly at the graft-vein anastomosis) may lead to thrombotic occlusion within 12 to 24 months. The primary patency rates of prosthetic AV grafts vary from 60% to 80% at 1 year and from 30% to 40% at 2 years of follow-up. Secondary patency ranges from 70% to 90% and from 50% to 70% at 1 and 2 years, respectively.[21-24] Intimal hyperplasia, with smooth muscle cell migration and proliferation and matrix deposition, is the major cause of stenosis formation and thrombosis. The etiology of the intimal hyperplasia is uncertain, although the high wall shear stress, caused by the access flow, may denude the endothelial cell layer, resulting in platelet adhesion and initiation of a cascade of proteins that stimulate the smooth muscle cells to proliferate and to migrate.

Measures to Improve Graft Patency

Numerous experimental and clinical studies have defined the influence of graft material and graft design on AV graft patency. Modulating the geometry of the arterial inlet or venous outlet of the graft may have a beneficial effect on intimal hyperplasia. Clinical studies using tapered (at the arterial side of the graft) grafts did not improve patency rates, nor did cuff implantation at the venous anastomosis.[25,26] However, primary patency did improve with the use of a cuff-shaped prosthesis (Venaflo).[27] Grafts such as polyurethane, which are more distensible, could in principle influence intimal hyperplasia by the better matching of the stiff prosthesis with the compliant vein at the anastomotic site; however, in clinical studies, this feature was not of proven benefit.[28]

PHARMACOLOGIC APPROACHES FOR ACCESS PATENCY

Aspirin, ticlopidine, and dipyridamole have some beneficial effect in maintaining patency of AV fistulas and grafts but increase the risk of hemorrhage.[29] Clopidogrel may also be effective in reducing thrombosis of AV grafts and fistulas. Warfarin reduces AV graft thrombosis but increases the risk of hemorrhage.[30] A recent large trial showed that dipyridamole plus aspirin had a significant but modest effect in reducing the risk of stenosis and improving the duration of primary unassisted patency of newly created AV grafts.[31] In a large randomized study, clopidogrel improved primary radiocephalic fistula function but not maturation.[32] On the available evidence, antiplatelet agents should be used routinely in patients with AV grafts but not fistula. Warfarin should be considered only when there is recurrent thrombosis in the absence of anatomic stenosis.

There have been suggestions that other drugs, such as calcium channel blockers and angiotensin-converting enzyme inhibitors, might be associated with improved AV fistula patency, but this requires confirmation with randomized studies.[33] Fish oil reduced AV graft thrombosis in one randomized trial.[34]

Efforts have been made to inhibit the development of intimal hyperplasia pharmacologically with the cytotoxic agent paclitaxel. Paclitaxel wraps have been shown to reduce prosthetic graft intimal hyperplasia in animal models but have yet to be clinically evaluated.

LOWER LIMB VASCULAR ACCESS

Probably the only indication for lower limb vascular access is bilateral central venous or caval obstruction, which endangers the outflow of upper limb AV fistulas. Saphenous and superficial femoral vein transposition is a primary option for thigh AV fistulas, although this carries a relatively high risk of distal ischemia. If clinical evaluation indicates incipient ischemia, primary flow reduction by tapering of the anastomosis is indicated to prevent ischemia.[35] Prosthetic graft implantation in the thigh bears a high risk of infection and septicemia.

VASCULAR ACCESS COMPLICATIONS

Nonmaturation of AV Fistulas

Fistulas that fail immediately are the consequence of poor selection of vessels, poor technique, or postoperative hemodynamic instability. Vascular abnormalities, including stenoses, occlusions, and accessory veins, will be identified in virtually all early failures, and more than half of the stenoses are in the perianastomotic area of nonmatured fistulas. Arterial inflow stenoses of more than 50% coupled with poor flows are seen in less than 10% of nonmaturing fistulas, but if identified, they should undergo angioplasty. If this fails to improve fistula flow rates, it is unlikely that surgical bypass will be of help. Anastomotic and swing segment (where the vein has been mobilized and swung over to the artery) stenosis may be treated percutaneously or surgically, depending on local expertise.

The diameter of the angioplasty balloon is chosen to correspond to the diameter of the vessel next to the stenotic or occlusive lesion and is usually not smaller than 5 mm for venous stenoses and not smaller than 4 mm for arterial or anastomotic stenoses. Ultrahigh-pressure balloons inflatable up to 30 atm are used when necessary to abolish the waist of the stenosis on the balloon. Apart from local infection, contraindications to balloon angioplasty are anastomotic stenoses in fistulas less than 4 to 6 weeks after surgical construction, which increases the risk of anastomotic disruption at angioplasty. Percutaneous balloon angioplasty is further discussed in Chapter 88.

The surgical approach is to reconstruct the AV fistula, usually under local anesthesia. The anastomosis is exposed and ligated; the vein can then be divided, mobilized proximally, and reanastomosed to the proximal radial artery.

A prospective nonrandomized study of 64 patients showed that outcomes were similar with angioplasty or surgery.[36] Restenosis rates were significantly higher after angioplasty, but overall costs of treatment were similar.

Nonmatured fistulas are rescued by angioplasty of stenoses or occlusions, ligation of accessory veins, or both. Accessory veins can be obliterated through coil embolization, percutaneous ligation, or surgical ligation. The use of coils with a diameter of 1 mm in excess of the target vessel diameter will prevent coil dislocation. Although ligation of accessory veins is usually performed in a single surgical intervention, three variants of vein ligation in a stepped approach have also been described.[37] By use of this approach, surgery is limited to ligation of the accessory veins if the AV fistula appears to be of adequate size to allow cannulation. If the fistula is still considered to be too small, the median cubital vein is ligated. If the AV fistula is still believed inadequate, temporary banding of the main venous channel is performed. Apart from surgical ligation, accessory veins can also be ligated percutaneously.

Stenosis and Thrombosis

The development of vessel stenosis in both autogenous AV fistulas and prosthetic AV grafts is usually initiated by intimal hyperplasia due to migrating and proliferating vessel smooth muscle cells, which form extracellular matrix. Progressive stenosis leads to access flow deterioration and subsequently thrombotic occlusion. Prophylactic repair of access stenoses may prevent thrombosis and prolong access patency.

Autogenous Fistula Stenosis or Thrombosis

AV fistula stenosis should be treated if the vessel diameter is reduced by more than 50% and is accompanied by a reduction in access flow (25% flow decline between measurements or absolute flow below 500 ml/min) or in measured dialysis dose. Other indications for intervention are difficulties in cannulation and prolonged bleeding time after decannulation, indicating high intra-access pressure due to outflow vein stenosis. In AV fistulas, 55% to 75% of the stenoses are close to the AV anastomosis, 25% in the venous outflow tract and 15% in the arterial inflow. In brachiocephalic and brachiobasilic AV fistulas, the typical location for stenosis (besides the anastomosis) is at the junction of the cephalic with the subclavian vein and the basilic with the axillary vein (junctional stenosis).

Endovascular treatment by percutaneous transluminal angioplasty (PTA) is the first option for arterial inflow and venous outflow stenoses and junctional stenoses, with the option of stent placement.[38] These techniques are discussed further in Chapter 88. Some stenoses may not be sufficiently dilated by conventional balloons (12 to 16 atm), and in these patients, cutting balloons or ultrahigh-pressure balloons (up to 32 atm) may be applied. Anastomotic stenoses in forearm and upper arm fistulas are primarily treated with PTA; however, surgical revision with a more proximal reanastomosis for swing segment stenosis is indicated in failed PTA of radiocephalic AV fistula.

Fistula thrombosis should be treated as soon as possible because timely declotting allows immediate use of the access without the need for a central venous catheter; fistula salvage usually requires intervention within 6 hours (grafts may be salvaged up to 24 hours). The duration and site of AV fistula thrombosis as well as the type of access are important determinants of treatment outcome. Thrombi become progressively fixed to the vein wall, which makes surgical removal more difficult. When the clot is localized at the anastomosis in radiocephalic and brachiocephalic fistulas, the outflow vein may remain patent because of continuing flow in its tributaries, making it possible to create a new proximal anastomosis.[39]

Thrombolysis can be performed mechanically or pharmacomechanically.[40-42] Whereas the immediate success rate is higher in AV grafts than in autogenous AV fistulas (99% versus 93% in forearm fistulas), the primary patency rate of the forearm AV fistula at 1 year is much higher (49% versus 14%). One-year secondary patency rates are 80% in forearm and 50% in upper arm AV fistulas.

In AV fistulas, the combination of a thrombolytic agent (urokinase or tissue plasminogen activator [tPA]) with balloon angioplasty resulted in an immediate success rate of 94%.[41]

AV Graft Stenosis or Thrombosis

The most common cause of graft dysfunction and thrombosis is venous anastomotic stenosis. Because grafts should be implanted only in patients with exhausted peripheral veins, vein-saving procedures like PTA or patch angioplasty are preferred to graft extensions to more central venous segments. When a stent or a patch fails, graft extension is still possible. Graft monitoring by access flow measurement is recommended; with preemptive endovascular treatment, this may diminish graft thrombosis but does not extend graft patency.

Intra-graft (or mid-graft) stenoses are found in the cannulation segment of grafts. They result from excessive ingrowth of fibrous tissue through puncture holes. These stenoses can be treated by PTA, graft curettage, or segmental graft replacement. When only a part of the cannulation segment is replaced, the access can be used for HD without the need of a central venous catheter. When restenosis occurs in a nonexchanged part of the graft, this can be replaced after healing of the new segment.

Prosthetic graft thrombosis can be treated with various percutaneous techniques and tools, including combinations of thromboaspiration, thrombolytic agents such as tPA, and mechanical thrombectomy. An initial success rate of 73% and primary patency rates of 32% and 26% at 1 and 3 months, respectively, are reported.[43-46] It is important to perform thrombolysis as soon as possible to avoid the need for a central venous catheter and as an outpatient procedure to decrease costs, whenever possible. Postprocedural angiography to detect and to correct inflow, intra-access, or venous outflow stenosis is mandatory.

When endovascular treatment fails or is not possible, surgical thrombectomy may be performed with a Fogarty catheter after venotomy, with correction of the underlying obstruction. On-table angiography should be performed after completion of thrombectomy of both the arterial and venous limbs of the graft.

Central Venous Obstruction

In the majority of patients, central vein obstruction is due to previously inserted central venous catheters or pacemaker wires. In 40% of patients with subclavian vein and 10% with jugular vein catheters, venous stenosis or occlusion will develop. Chronic swelling of the access arm is the most important sign, usually with prominent superficial collateral veins around the shoulder. The indications for intervention, by PTA and stent placement, are severe and disabling arm swelling, finger ulceration, and pain or inadequate HD. Contrast angiography of the access and complete venous outflow tract must be performed because the central veins can be difficult to examine with ultrasound in their retroclavicular position.

Endovascular Intervention

Endovascular intervention is the first option for central venous obstruction treatment. PTA alone results in low primary patency rates of 10% or less at 1 year, and numerous restenoses may develop. Primary or additional stent implantation gives much better outcome, with 1-year patency rates up to 56% or more.[47,48] Reinterventions are usually required to maintain patency and to achieve long-term clinical success.

Stent placement should avoid overlapping the ostium of the internal jugular vein because this vein is essential for future placement of central venous catheters. Similarly, a stent placed in the innominate vein should not overlap the ostium of the contralateral vein; otherwise, contralateral stenosis may occur and preclude future use of the contralateral limb for access creation.

Surgical Intervention

When interventional treatment of central venous obstruction fails, surgical revision with bypass grafting is indicated. Surgical bypass to the ipsilateral jugular vein or contralateral subclavian or jugular vein is the first option in these patients. Alternative surgical approaches for upper limb vascular accesses with compromised venous outflow are axillary vein to femoral, saphenous, or popliteal vein and right atrial bypasses.[49] In case of bilateral obstruction of the mediastinal veins, including the superior vena cava, it will not be possible to sustain upper limb access, and lower limb access will be required.

Ultimately, ligation of the upper limb access can be considered, which will relieve local symptoms but loses a valuable dialysis access.

Vascular Access–Induced Ischemia

Vascular access–induced upper limb ischemia is a serious complication that without prompt intervention may lead to amputation. The incidence of symptomatic ischemia varies from 2% to 8% of the HD population.[50] Elderly patients, diabetics, and patients with peripheral or coronary arterial occlusive disease are most at risk of ischemia. In addition, previous ipsilateral vascular access increases the risk. Access-induced ischemia occurs more often with proximally located fistulas. These high-flow AV fistulas induce a steal phenomenon with lowering of distal perfusion pressures, and when collateral circulation is inadequate, symptoms may occur. Pain during HD is a characteristic early symptom. A grade 1 to 4 classification for access-induced ischemia can be used to outline the severity of the disease; this ranges from minor symptoms to finger necrosis.

Grade 1: pale/blue or cold hand without pain
Grade 2: pain during exercise or HD
Grade 3: ischemic pain at rest
Grade 4: ulceration, necrosis, and gangrene

For grades 1 and 2, ischemia conservative treatment is advocated. With grades 3 and 4, interventional treatment is mandatory.

Diagnosis of Ischemia

Physical examination, including observation and palpation of peripheral vessels, may be inadequate and misleading for the diagnosis of symptomatic ischemia. Additional noninvasive testing with measurement of digital pressures and calculation of the digit to brachial index, transcutaneous oximetry, ultrasound of forearm arteries, and access blood flow measurement are important steps in the diagnosis and decision-making process. Finally, contrast angiography with visualization of the upper extremity arterial tree from the proximal subclavian artery to the distal palmar arches with and without AV fistula compression to enhance distal flow is obligatory to outline the strategy for treatment and to determine whether interventional or surgical options are preferred.

Endovascular and Surgical Management of Ischemia

The treatment strategy depends on the etiology of the ischemia. Inflow arterial obstruction and distal arterial lesions are recanalized with small-caliber balloons or stent placement[51]; high-flow AV fistulas are suitable for flow-reducing procedures like access banding (Fig. 87.8) and arterial inflow reduction by an interposition graft to a smaller forearm artery (revision using distal inflow).[52,53] Steal in itself may be cured by ligation of the artery distal to the arteriovenous anastomosis (distal radial artery ligation). In most patients, it is necessary to add a saphenous vein or prosthetic graft bypass to the forearm arteries to augment distal hand perfusion (distal revascularization and interval ligation; Fig. 87.9). The results of these procedures are usually good, with relief of symptoms and preservation of the access site (Fig. 87.10).[54-58] A simpler alternative to the distal revascularization–interval ligation procedure is the proximal arteriovenous anastomosis technique, in which the AV anastomosis at the elbow is disconnected and moved to the axilla, with

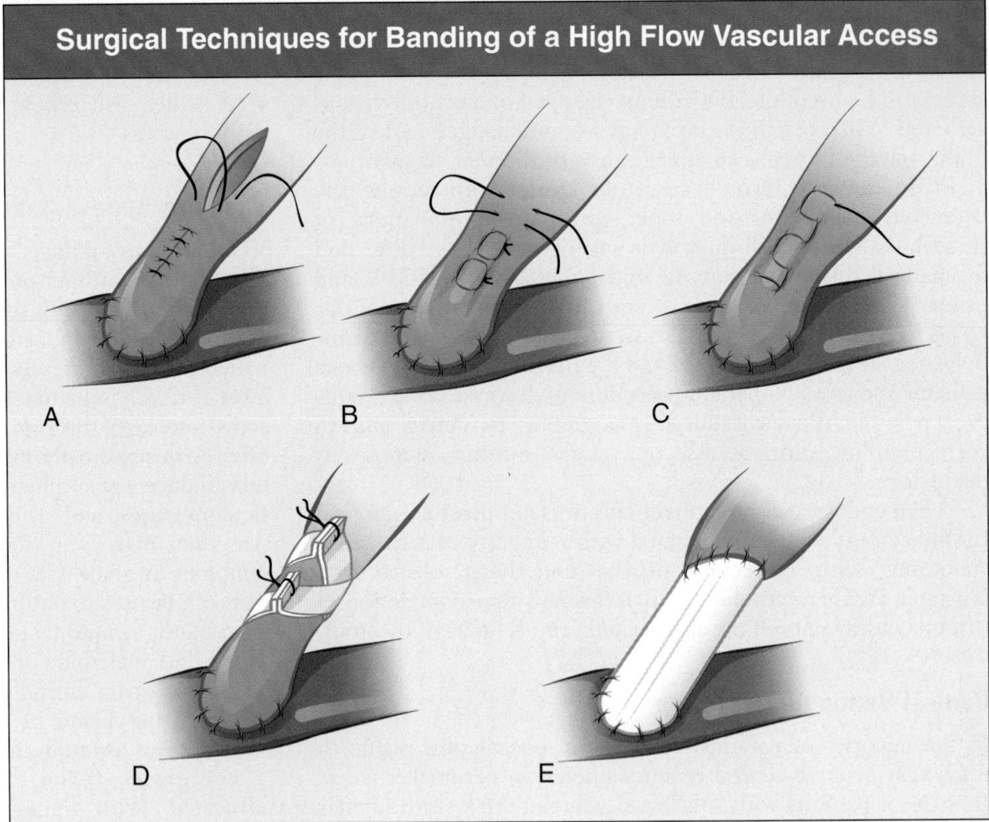

Figure 87.8 Surgical techniques for banding of a high-flow vascular access. A, Open venoplasty; **B,** Interrupted mattress suturing; **C,** Continuous mattress suturing; **D,** PTFE banding; **E,** PTFE interposition graft. The choice of technique is made by the surgeon on a case by case basis.

anastomosis to the axillary artery by means of a graft interposition.[59] Recently, the minimally invasive limited ligation endoluminal-assisted revision procedure was described, using a minimally invasive percutaneous technique with banding of the access over a 4-mm balloon.[60]

Intraoperative digital pressure measurement or transcutaneous oximetry ($TcPo_2$) is mandatory to guarantee an adequate surgical intervention with acceptable outcome. A digital-brachial pressure index above 0.60 or $TcPO_2$ above 40 mm Hg is indicative of sufficient distal hand perfusion. In some patients, AV fistula ligation and transition to chronic catheter dialysis access or a change in renal replacement modality to peritoneal dialysis may be the only solution.

CENTRAL VENOUS CATHETER ACCESS

Central venous catheters are still widely used as vascular access for HD. Data from the DOPPS study[61] indicate that 25% of HD patients in the United States are dialyzed with catheters; in other countries, the use of catheters is even more common (Belgium, 41%; United Kingdom, 28%). Central venous catheters are the preferred vascular access for patients presenting with acute kidney injury and for chronic patients without permanent AV access or with failed vascular access. Two types of catheters are used in practice: nontunneled catheters for short-term dialysis, with a limited use and high morbidity; and tunneled cuffed catheters, which can be used up to several months or years with low morbidity. The physical characteristics (i.e., design and geometry) not only influence the performance (blood flow rate, recirculation, and resistance) but also affect the overall efficiency of the HD therapy and the morbidity risk (infection, thrombosis).

Nontunneled Catheters

Single- or double-lumen catheters are usually made of polymers (polyethylene, polyurethane), enabling a simple and direct implant possibility. The length of the catheter must be chosen in accordance with the insertion site. The femoral route requires catheters of 30 to 35 cm in length for the distal tip to be located in the inferior vena cava. The internal jugular vein route needs shorter catheters of 20 to 25 cm in length, with tip location at the inferior vena cava–right atrium junction. The subclavian vein should not be used because of the very high risk of subsequent venous stenosis. For sufficient blood flow rates to be achieved, the diameter of these catheters must be ideally between 12 and 14 French. It is recommended that the use of nontunneled catheters not exceed 7 days.

Tunneled Catheters

Tunneled central venous catheters have two lumens, each having a length of 40 cm, 10 cm of which is tunneled under the skin; the cannulae are made of synthetic polymer with a large internal lumen and a Dacron cuff to ensure subcutaneous anchoring. The catheter characteristics rely on the type of polymer, design, and geometry (double-lumen catheters, dual catheters, split catheters). The use of a tunneled central venous catheter is associated with reduced morbidity as well as better and constant performance compared with uncuffed catheters.[62]

Both tunneled and nontunneled catheters are inserted percutaneously by the Seldinger technique and ultrasound guidance. These techniques are described in Chapter 88. The internal jugular vein (Fig. 87.11) and femoral vein routes are preferred because of ease of implantation and low risk of complications, such as central vein stenosis.

Catheter Infection

Catheter-related blood stream infections are a significant cause of mortality in HD patients. Results of the HEMO study indicate that patients with central venous catheters have an increased relative mortality risk of 3.4 compared with patients with AV fistulas. Switching from central venous catheters to AV fistulas decreases the relative mortality risk to 1.4.[63] The most likely explanation for this increased mortality risk is infection and sepsis related to the central venous catheter, including exit site infection. Typical infection rates are 3 episodes of infection per 1000 tunneled catheter–days and higher with nontunneled catheters.[64] These localized infections can progress to metastatic complications of osteomyelitis, septic arthritis, epidural abscess, and endocarditis. Various societies have issued recommendations for the management of catheter infections.[65] A recommended treatment algorithm is shown in Figure 87.12.

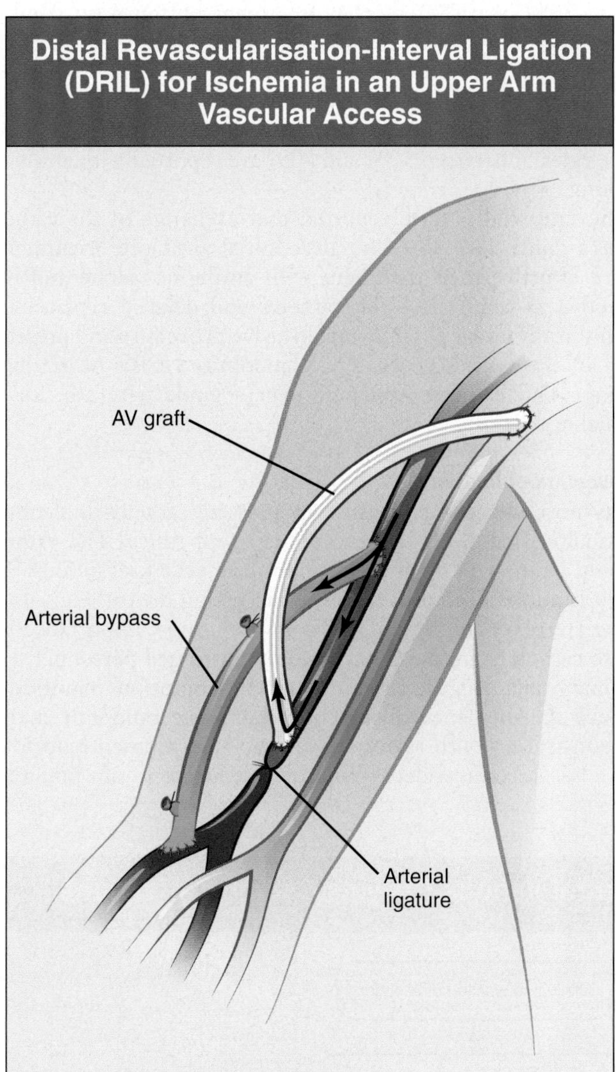

Figure 87.9 Distal revascularization–interval ligation for ischemia in an upper arm vascular access.

Infections Involving Temporary Catheters

When a temporary dialysis catheter becomes infected, it should always be removed. There is no role for trying to salvage temporary catheters.[65]

Exit Site Versus Tunnel Track Infections

An exit site infection is a localized cellulitis confined to the 1 to 2 cm where the catheter exits the skin. The majority of these cases respond well to systemic antibiotics and meticulous exit site care, and the removal of the catheter is generally not required.[65] However, exit site infections can progress to tunnel track infections, which involve the potential space surrounding the catheter more than 2 cm from the exit site (Fig. 87.13). Patients with a tunnel track infection sometimes but not always have an associated exit site infection; untreated, they can rapidly develop bacteremia. Patients with a tunnel track infection present with fever as well as local signs of pain, swelling, fluctuance, and erythema along the track of the catheter. Because tunnel track infections involve a potential space, in an area with limited vascular supply, and an implanted synthetic material, they respond poorly to antibiotics alone and require catheter removal.[65]

Catheter-Associated Bacteremia

When a patient with a dialysis catheter has a fever, catheter infection must always be considered. If the patient does not have a clear and convincing alternative explanation for the fever, blood culture specimens should be obtained peripherally as well as through the catheter, and the patient should be started on antibiotic therapy, which is subsequently adjusted on the basis of culture results.[65] The most common organism is *Staphylococcus*, although a wide range of gram-positive and gram-negative organisms have been reported (Fig. 87.14). The percentage of patients with methicillin-resistant *Staphylococcus aureus* (MRSA) varies greatly between centers, with higher rates associated with

Results of the DRIL Procedure for Angio-Access Related Ischemia

Author	Year	No. fistulae	Ischemia cured (%)	Ischemia improved (%)	Ischemia not improved (%)	Access patency (%)
Haimov et. al.	1996	23	86	14	–	95
Knox et. al.	2002	55	55	25	11	86
Waltz et. al.	2007	36	100	–	–	54
Yu et. al.	2008	24	96	–	4	88
Huber et. al.	2008	64	78	–	NS	68

Figure 87.10 Results of the distal revascularization–interval ligation (DRIL) procedure for vascular access–related ischemia. NS, not stated.

greater antibiotic use. An aminoglycoside or a cephalosporin is a good choice for gram-negative coverage; however, local microbiologic epidemiology must be taken into consideration, especially concerning antibiotic resistance.

Catheter Removal

The decision to remove a tunneled cuffed dialysis catheter for an episode of catheter-associated bacteremia is not straightforward. The clinical condition of the patient and response to initial therapy, the presence of metastatic complications, the infecting organism, and the availability of other vascular access sites must all be taken into consideration before deciding on a treatment plan (see Fig. 87.12).

The conventional approach is to remove the catheter with interval replacement at a different site after the infection has resolved. Although this is effective, it leads to an additional temporary catheter if dialysis is needed before the catheter can be replaced. Attempts to "salvage" an infected catheter with systemic antibiotic therapy lead to resolution of infection in only about 30% of cases. Another treatment option is to combine systemic antibiotics with antibiotic "lock" solutions. Many different cocktails of antibiotics mixed with either heparin or citrate have been tested; a popular regimen is vancomycin 2.5 mg/ml, gentamicin 1 mg/ml, and heparin 2500 U/ml. Infection clearance rates of between 50% and 70% are reported with antibiotic locking.

Several studies have reported that exchange of the catheter over a guide wire 48 hours after initial antibiotic treatment is more effective then treatment with antibiotics alone and is as effective as removal of the catheter and delayed replacement, with the advantages of only one invasive procedure and preservation of the venous access site. Randomized trials of antibiotic locking and catheter exchange over a guide wire are not yet available.

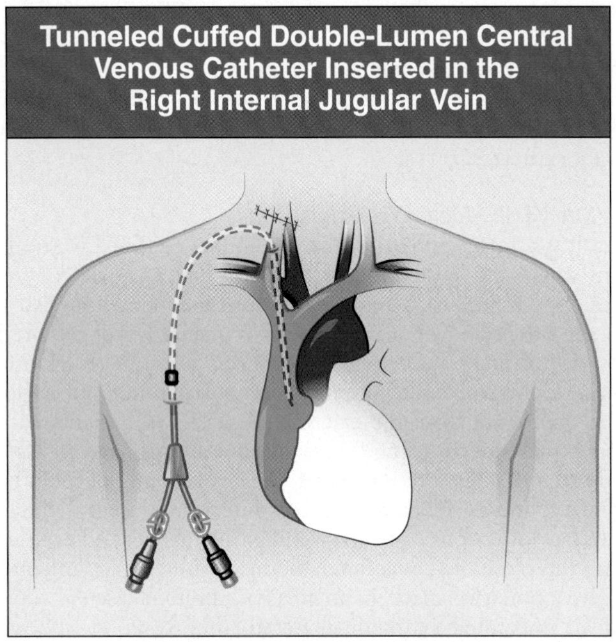

Figure 87.11 Tunneled cuffed double-lumen central venous catheter inserted in the right internal jugular vein.

Prevention of Infection

The most important measure to prevent catheter infection is meticulous handling of the catheter at all times. The catheter should be inserted with use of maximal sterile precautions. The dialysis nurses need procedures for accessing the catheters under strict sterile conditions, and it is of the utmost importance that these catheters are never accessed by untrained personnel. Preliminary data suggest that antibiotic lock solutions significantly reduce the incidence of infection, but large randomized trials demonstrating both safety and efficacy are awaited before this can be recommended. Topical application of mupirocin

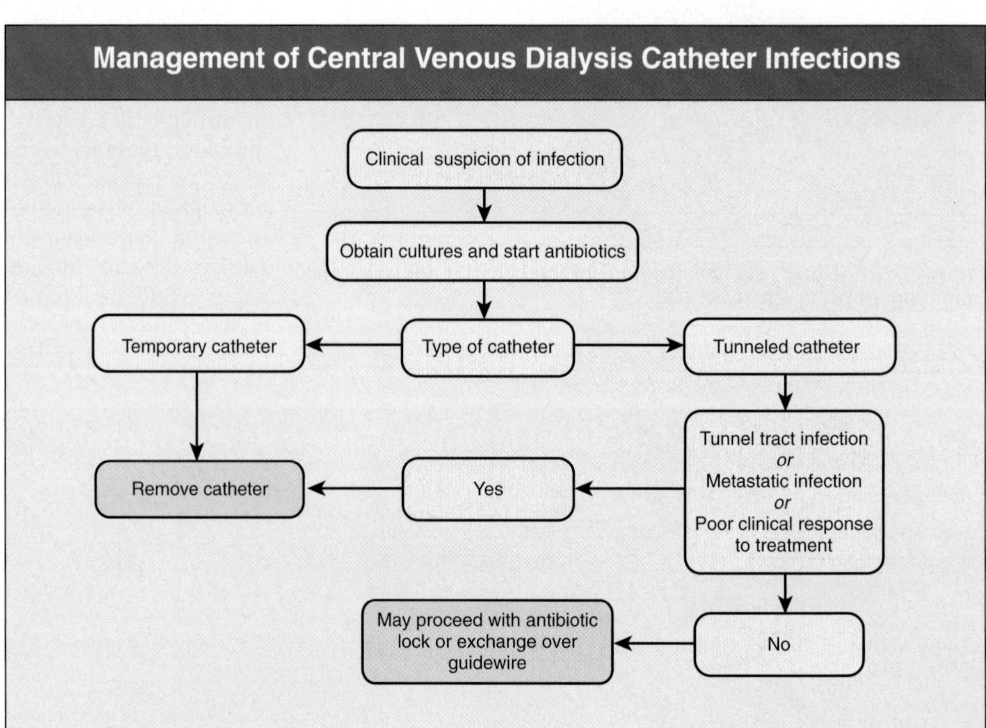

Figure 87.12 Algorithm for the management of central venous dialysis catheter infections. *(Modified with permission from reference 65.)*

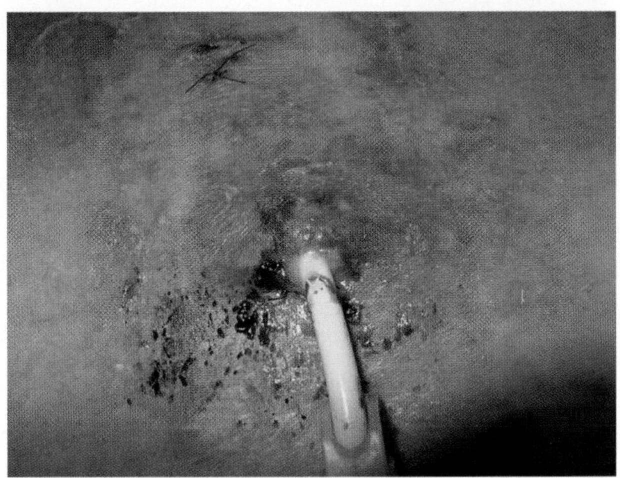

Figure 87.13 Dialysis catheter tunnel infection. *(Courtesy Dr. I. M. Leidig, University Hospital Erlangen, Germany.)*

Causative Organisms in Dialysis Catheter Infections		
Polymicrobial		16%
Gram positive		89%
	Staphylococcus aureus	30%
	Staphylococcus epidermidis	37%
	Enterococcus	17%
	Corynebacterium	49%
Gram negative		33%
	Enterobacter	11%
	Pseudomonas	7%
	Acinetobacter	4%
	Citrobacter	4%
	Serratia	2%
	Klebsiella	3%
	Other Gram negative	3%
Mycobacteria		2%

Figure 87.14 Causative organisms in dialysis catheter infections. Numbers do not add up to 100% because 16% of infections were polymicrobial. *(Modified with permission from reference 66.)*

ointment to tunneled exit sites has been reported to reduce the incidence of catheter-associated bacteremia.

Catheter Obstruction

Catheter obstruction may be due to endoluminal fibrin deposits, restricting the catheter lumen or obstructing catheter side holes at the tip, or external fibrin sleeves surrounding the catheter, resulting in inadequate flow and excessive extracorporeal blood pressure alarms during the dialysis session. Depending on the location of the fibrin clot (arterial or venous line), there may be high negative arterial pressure (obstruction at the arterial catheter line) or high positive venous pressure (obstruction at the venous catheter line).

Prevention of clot formation in the catheter tip during the interdialytic period is crucial. This is achieved by installing an antithrombotic lock solution (sodium citrate is superior to standard heparin or low-molecular-weight heparin). A certain amount of the antithrombotic lock solution may leak into the circulation through side and central catheter holes, facilitating catheter clot formation while increasing risk of hemorrhage. Regular use of low-dose warfarin or antiplatelet agents has failed to improve catheter function in dialysis patients in randomized trials.

To prevent or to correct catheter dysfunction, it is recommended that the catheter lumen be cleaned periodically by applying a fibrinolytic agent (urokinase or tPA) as a lock solution or by continuous infusion on both arterial and venous lines. Occluded catheters are reopened either by means of a mechanical method (brush) or pharmacologically (urokinase or tPA). Removal of the fibrin sleeve may be achieved by lasso wire stripping or by infusion of a fibrinolytic solution (urokinase, tPA) during 3 to 6 hours. Alternatively, the catheter may be exchanged over a guide wire.

REFERENCES

1. Pisoni RL, Young EW, Dykstra DM, et al. Vascular access use in Europe and the United States: Results from the DOPPS. *Kidney Int.* 2002;61: 305-316.
2. Wolowczyk L, Williams AJ, Donovan KL, et al. The snuffbox arteriovenous fistula for vascular access. *Eur J Vasc Endovasc Surg.* 2000;19: 70-76.
3. Gibson KD, Caps MT, Kohler TR, et al. Assessment of a policy to reduce placement of prosthetic hemodialysis access. *Kidney Int.* 2001;59:2335-2345.
4. Allon M, Lockhart ME, Lilly RZ, et al. Effect of preoperative sonographic mapping on vascular access outcomes in hemodialysis patients. *Kidney Int.* 2001;60:2013-2020.
5. Ravani P, Marcelli D, Malberti F. Vascular access surgery managed by renal physicians: The choice of native arteriovenous fistulas for hemodialysis. *Am J Kidney Dis.* 2002;40:1264-1276.
6. Rooijens PP, Burgmans JP, Yo TI, et al. Autogenous radial-cephalic or prosthetic brachial-antecubital forearm loop AVF in patients with compromised vessels? A randomized, multicenter study of the patency of primary hemodialysis access. *J Vasc Surg.* 2005;42:481-486.
7. Biuckians A, Scott EC, Meier GH, et al. The natural history of autologous fistulas as first-time dialysis access in the KDOQI era. *J Vasc Surg.* 2008;47:415-421.
8. Silva MB, Hobson RW, Pappas PJ, et al. Vein transposition in the forearm for autogenous hemodialysis access. *J Vasc Surg.* 1997;26: 981-986.
9. Weyde W, Krajewska M, Letachowicz W, et al. Obesity is not an obstacle for successful autogenous arteriovenous fistula creation in haemodialysis. *Nephrol Dial Transplant.* 2008;23:1318-1323.
10. Lok CE, Oliver MJ, Su J, et al. Arteriovenous fistula outcomes in the era of the elderly dialysis population. *Kidney Int.* 2005;67:2462-2469.
11. Zeebregts CJ, Tielliu IF, Hulsebos RG, et al. Determinants of failure of brachiocephalic elbow fistulas for haemodialysis. *Eur J Vasc Endovasc Surg.* 2005;30:209-214.
12. Koksoy C, Demirci RK, Balci D, et al. Brachiobasilic versus brachiocephalic arteriovenous fistula: A prospective randomized study. *J Vasc Surg.* 2009;49:171-177.
13. Murphy GJ, Saunders R, Metcalfe M, et al. Elbow fistulas using autogenous vein: Patency rates and results of revision. *Postgrad Med J.* 2002;78:483-486.
14. Woo K, Farber A, Doros G, et al. Evaluation of the efficacy of the transposed upper arm arteriovenous fistula: A single institutional review of 190 basilic and cephalic vein transposition procedures. *J Vasc Surg.* 2007;46:94-99.
15. Hossny A. Brachiobasilic arteriovenous fistula: Different surgical techniques and their effects on fistula patency and dialysis-related complications. *J Vasc Surg.* 2003;37:821-826.
16. Segal JH, Kayler LK, Henke P, et al. Vascular access outcomes using the transposed basilic vein arteriovenous fistula. *Am J Kidney Dis.* 2003;42:151-157.
17. Wolford HY, Hsu J, Rhodes JM, et al. Outcome after autogenous brachial-basilic upper arm transpositions in the post–National Kidney Foundation Dialysis Outcomes Quality Initiative era. *J Vasc Surg.* 2005;42:951-956.
18. Harper SJ, Goncalves I, Doughman T, et al. Arteriovenous fistula formation using transposed basilic vein: Extensive single centre experience. *Eur J Vasc Endovasc Surg.* 2008;36:237-241.

19. Keuter XH, De Smet AA, Kessels AG, et al. A randomized multicenter study of the outcome of brachial-basilic arteriovenous fistula and prosthetic brachial-antecubital forearm loop as vascular access for hemodialysis. *J Vasc Surg*. 2008;47:395-401.
20. Lazarides MK, Georgiadis GS, Papasideris CP, et al. Transposed brachial-basilic arteriovenous fistulas versus prosthetic upper limb grafts: A meta-analysis. *Eur J Vasc Endovasc Surg*. 2008;36:597-601.
21. Glickman MH, Stokes GK, Ross JR, et al. Multicenter evaluation of a polyurethane vascular access graft as compared with the expanded polytetrafluoroethylene vascular access graft in hemodialysis applications. *J Vasc Surg*. 2001;34:465-472.
22. Kaufman JL, Garb JL, Berman JA, et al. A prospective comparison of two expanded polytetrafluoroethylene grafts for linear forearm hemodialysis access: Does the manufacturer matter? *J Am Coll Surg*. 1997;185:74-79.
23. Lenz BJ, Veldenz HC, Dennis JW, et al. A three-year follow-up on standard versus thin wall ePTFE grafts for hemodialysis. *J Vasc Surg*. 1998;28:464-470.
24. Garcia-Pajares R, Polo JR, Flores A, et al. Upper arm polytetrafluoroethylene grafts for dialysis access. Analysis of two different graft sizes: 6 mm and 6-8 mm. *Vasc Endovasc Surg*. 2003;37:335-343.
25. Dammers R, Planken RN, Pouls KP, et al. Evaluation of 4-mm to 7-mm versus 6-mm prosthetic brachial-antecubital forearm loop access for hemodialysis: Results of a randomized multicenter clinical trial. *J Vasc Surg*. 2003;37:143-148.
26. Lemson MS, Tordoir JH, van Det RJ, et al. Effects of a venous cuff at the venous anastomosis of polytetrafluoroethylene grafts for hemodialysis vascular access. *J Vasc Surg*. 2000;32:1155-1163.
27. Sorom AJ, Hughes CB, McCarthy JT, et al. Prospective, randomized evaluation of a cuffed expanded polytetrafluoroethylene graft for hemodialysis vascular access. *Surgery*. 2002;132:135-140.
28. Hofstra L, Bergmans DC, Hoeks AP, et al. Mismatch in elastic properties around anastomoses of interposition grafts for hemodialysis access. *J Am Soc Nephrol*. 1994;5:1243-1250.
29. DaSilva AF, Escofet X, Rutherford PA. Medical adjuvant treatment to increase patency of arteriovenous fistulas and grafts. Cochrane Database Syst Rev. 2003;2:CD002786.
30. Crowther MA, Clase CM, Margetts PJ, et al. Low-intensity warfarin is ineffective for the prevention of PTFE graft failure in patients on hemodialysis: A randomized controlled trial. *J Am Soc Nephrol*. 2002;13:2331-2337.
31. Dixon BS, Beck GJ, Vazquez MA, et al. Effect of dipyridamole plus aspirin on hemodialysis graft patency. *N Engl J Med*. 2009;360:2191-2201.
32. Dember LM, Besk GJ, Allon M, et al. Effect of clopidogrel on early failure of arteriovenous fistulas for hemodialysis: A randomized controlled trial. *JAMA*. 2008;299:2205-2207.
33. Saran R, Dykstra DM, Wolfe RA, et al. Association between vascular access failure and the use of specific drugs: The Dialysis Outcomes and Practice Patterns Study (DOPPS). *Am J Kidney Dis*. 2002;40:1255-1263.
34. Schmitz PG, McCloud LK, Reikes ST, et al. Prophylaxis of hemodialysis graft thrombosis with fish oil: Double-blind, randomized, prospective trial. *J Am Soc Nephrol*. 2002;13:184-190.
35. Gradman WS, Laub J, Cohen W. Femoral vein transposition for arteriovenous hemodialysis access: Improved patient selection and intraoperative measures reduce postoperative ischemia. *J Vasc Surg*. 2005;41:279-284.
36. Tessitore N, Mansueto G, Lipari G, et al. Endovascular versus surgical preemptive repair of forearm arteriovenous fistula juxta-anastomotic stenosis: Analysis of data collected prospectively from 1999 to 2004. *Clin J Am Soc Nephrol*. 2006;1:448-454.
37. Beathard GA, Arnold P, Jackson J, et al. Aggressive treatment of early fistula failure. *Kidney Int*. 2003;64:1487-1494
38. Turmel-Rodrigues L, Pengloan J, Rodrigue H, et al. Treatment of failed native arteriovenous fistulas for hemodialysis by interventional radiology. *Kidney Int*. 2000;57:1124-1140.
39. Oakes DD, Sherck JP, Cobb LF. Surgical salvage of failed radiocephalic arteriovenous fistulas: Techniques and results in 29 patients. *Kidney Int*. 1998;53:480-487.
40. Patel AA, Tuite CM, Trerotola SO. Mechanical thrombectomy of hemodialysis fistulas and grafts. *Cardiovasc Intervent Radiol*. 2005;28:704-713.
41. Schon D, Mishler R. Salvage of occluded autologous arteriovenous fistulas. *Am J Kidney Dis*. 2000;36:804-810.
42. Haage P, Vorwerk D, Wildberger JE, et al. Percutaneous treatment of thrombosed primary arteriovenous hemodialysis access fistulas. *Kidney Int*. 2000;57:1169-1175.
43. Marston WA, Criado E, Jaques PF, et al. Prospective randomized comparison of surgical versus endovascular management of thrombosed dialysis access grafts. *J Vasc Surg*. 1997;26:373-380.
44. Beathard GA. Thrombolysis versus surgery for the treatment of thrombosed dialysis access grafts. *J Am Soc Nephrol*. 1995;6:1619-1624.
45. Beathard GA, Welch BR, Maidment HJ. Mechanical thrombolysis for the treatment of thrombosed hemodialysis access grafts. *Radiology*. 1996;200:711-716.
46. Falk A, Mitty H, Guller J, et al. Thrombolysis of clotted hemodialysis grafts with tissue-type plasminogen activator. *J Vasc Interv Radiol*. 2001;12:305-311.
47. Mansour M, Kamper L, Altenburg A, et al. Radiological central vein treatment in vascular access. *J Vasc Access*. 2008;9:85-101.
48. Mickley V, Görich J, Rilinger N, et al. Stenting of central venous stenoses in hemodialysis patients: Long-term results. *Kidney Int*. 1997;51:277-280.
49. Mickley V. Central vein obstruction in vascular access. *Eur J Vasc Endovasc Surg*. 2006;32:439-444.
50. Morsy AH, Kulbaski M, Chen C, et al. Incidence and characteristics of patients with hand ischemia after a hemodialysis access procedure. *J Surg Res*. 1998;74:8-10.
51. Guerra A, Raynaud A, Beyssen B, et al. Arterial percutaneous angioplasty in upper limbs with vascular access devices for haemodialysis. *Nephrol Dial Transplant*. 2002;17:843-851.
52. van Hoek F, Scheltinga MR, Luirink M, et al. Access flow, venous saturation, and digital pressures in hemodialysis. *J Vasc Surg*. 2007;45:968-973.
53. Minion D, Moore E, Endean E, et al. Revision using distal inflow: A novel approach o dialysis-associated steal syndrome. *Ann Vasc Surg*. 2005;19:625-628.
54. Haimov M, Schanzer H, Skladani M. Pathogenesis and management of upper-extremity ischemia following angioaccess surgery. *Blood Purif*. 1996;14:350-354.
55. Knox RC, Berman SS, Hughes JD, et al. Distal revascularization–interval ligation: A durable and effective treatment for ischemic steal syndrome after hemodialysis access. *J Vasc Surg*. 2002;36:250-256.
56. Walz P, Ladowski JS, Hines A. Distal revascularization and interval ligation (DRIL) procedure for the treatment of ischemic steal syndrome after arm arteriovenous fistula. *Ann Vasc Surg*. 2007;21:468-473.
57. Yu SH, Cook PR, Canty TG, et al. Hemodialysis-related steal syndrome: Predictive factors and response to treatment with the distal revascularization–interval ligation procedure. *Ann Vasc Surg*. 2008;22:210-214.
58. Huber TS, Brown MP, Seeger JM, Lee WA. Midterm outcome after the distal revascularization and interval ligation (DRIL) procedure. *J Vasc Surg*. 2008;48:926-932.
59. Zanow J, Kruger Ulf, Scholz H. Proximalization of the arterial inflow: A new technique to treat access-related ischemia. *J Vasc Surg*. 2006;43:1216-1221.
60. Goel N, Miller GA, Jotwani MC, et al. Minimally invasive limited ligation endoluminal-assisted revision (MILLER) for treatment of dialysis access–associated steal syndrome. *Kidney Int*. 2006;70:765-770.
61. Ethier J, Mendelssohn DC, Elder SJ, et al. Vascular access use and outcomes: An international perspective from the dialysis outcomes and practice patterns study. *Nephrol Dial Transplant*. 2008;23:3219-3226.
62. Weijmer MC, Vervloet MG, ter Wee PM. Compared to tunnelled cuffed haemodialysis catheters, temporary untunnelled catheters are associated with more complications already within 2 weeks of use. *Nephrol Dial Transplant*. 2004;19:670-677.
63. Allon M, Daugirdas J, Depner TA, et al. Effect of change in vascular access on patient mortality in hemodialysis patients. *Am J Kidney Dis*. 2006;47:469-477.
64. Gersch MS. Treatment of dialysis catheter infections in 2004. *J Vasc Access*. 2004;5:99-108.
65. NKF-K/DOQI Clinical Practice Guidelines for Vascular Access: update 2000. *Am J Kidney Dis*. 2001;37:S137-S181.
66. Weijmer MC, van den Dorpel MA, van de Ven PJ, et al; CITRATE Study Group. Randomized controlled trial comparison of trisodium citrate 30% and heparin as catheter-locking solution in hemodialysis patients. *J Am Soc Nephrol*. 2005;16:2769-2777.

CHAPTER 88

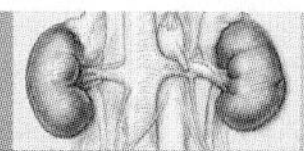

Diagnostic and Interventional Nephrology

W. Charles O'Neill, Haimanot Wasse, Arif Asif, Stephen R. Ash

A variety of procedures are essential to the care of nephrology patients and include ultrasound, renal biopsy, insertion of hemodialysis and peritoneal dialysis (PD) catheters, creation of arteriovenous (AV) fistulas, and diagnostic and interventional procedures on hemodialysis accesses. These procedures have traditionally been performed by other specialists, and this may lead to fragmented care. The desire to provide more continuity of care has led an increasing number of nephrologists to perform these procedures, the field of diagnostic and interventional nephrology. It is most developed in the United States, where the American Society of Diagnostic and Interventional Nephrology *(www.asdin.org)* has established training standards and certification procedures. This chapter covers ultrasound, insertion of dialysis catheters, and interventions on vascular access, focusing on their applications and their performance by nephrologists. Renal biopsy is covered in Chapter 6, placement of AV fistulas and AV grafts in Chapter 87.

ULTRASOUND

An important reason for nephrologists to be involved in this procedure is that many of the findings on ultrasound are not specific and require clinical correlation. The role and interpretation of ultrasound are further covered in Chapter 5.

Applications and Limitations of Ultrasound

Ultrasound is an excellent tool for examination of the kidneys and urinary tract. Under optimal conditions, both kidneys, the renal artery and vein, the proximal and distal ureter (when enlarged), and the bladder can be visualized. The ureter is usually apparent only when it is dilated. The middle portion of the ureter is usually obscured by overlying bowel but still may be visible when it is very dilated. In transplants, the entire ureter can be visualized, even when it is not markedly dilated, because of the proximity to the probe and the lack of overlying bowel. In very ill patients who cannot be optimally positioned or cannot control their breathing or have abdominal wounds or distention, views of the kidneys may be limited, but it is still possible in most of these patients to determine whether hydronephrosis is present.

Chronic Kidney Disease

Ultrasound is indicated in any patient presenting with chronic kidney disease (CKD) to establish renal size and to rule out polycystic kidney disease or urinary tract obstruction. Small, echogenic kidneys indicate severe irreversible disease, eliminating the need for a biopsy.[1]

Acute Kidney Injury

Although the diagnostic yield is very low in patients in whom the basis for renal failure is likely to be acute tubular necrosis or prerenal causes, ultrasound is still indicated in certain patients to rule out obstruction and to identify preexisting CKD.[2]

Renal Transplant

Ultrasound is indicated when there is an acute decline in renal transplant function because urinary obstruction is common in this setting.[3] In the immediate post-transplantation period, Doppler evaluation of renal blood flow should also be performed to rule out thrombosis. Additional indications in transplant patients are pain, swelling, ipsilateral leg edema, and infection. Another important indication in both native and transplanted kidneys is guidance for percutaneous biopsy, nephrostomy, or drainage of fluid collections.

Renal Biopsy

Ultrasound is the method of choice to guide percutaneous renal biopsy.[4] Except in rare cases, computed tomography offers no advantages over ultrasound[5] and results in unnecessary irradiation. This is discussed further in Chapter 6.

Urinary Bladder

Ultrasound is the procedure of choice for measurement of postvoid residual volume because it is painless and sufficiently accurate[6] and, when a scanner is readily available, a simple task. Additional indications include checking the location and patency of Foley catheters and examination of the distal ureters. Placement of the catheter in the proximal urethra is uncommon but not rare, and obstruction of catheters is frequent, so examination of the bladder should always be considered when urine output decreases. Prostatic hypertrophy, prostatitis, bladder carcinoma, mucosal edema, blood clots, stones, stents, and other foreign bodies can be recognized by ultrasound, but transabdominal ultrasound is not the appropriate test to rule out bladder cancer (which requires cystoscopy) or prostatic cancer (which requires transrectal ultrasound and biopsy).

Hemodialysis Access

Ultrasound is essential in the management of vascular access, including guidance of catheter insertion, evaluation of fistula dysfunction, preoperative vein mapping, and monitoring of access flow. Of these, the first two can be readily performed by nephrologists. Guidance of catheterization is best performed with a dedicated scanner but can be done with any scanner that has a vascular probe and does not require Doppler imaging.

Examination of dysfunctional fistulas is also straightforward and does not necessarily require Doppler analysis. Vein mapping and monitoring of access flow are both best performed by an experienced vascular technician.

Renovascular Ultrasound

Doppler ultrasound of renal arteries and veins is a difficult study requiring an experienced operator and is not usually practical for nephrologists. Tracings from segmental arteries are more easily obtained and can be useful in diagnosis of renal vein thrombosis. However, measurement of resistive index can be unreliable (it can be influenced by external factors such as systemic blood pressure and heart rate) and is of questionable clinical utility. Doppler ultrasound is also useful in distinguishing between cystic and vascular lesions and between renal vein and ureter.

Equipment

Important considerations in the choice of equipment are image quality, probe type and frequency, cost, size, portability, and output. Image quality is difficult to quantitate and is related to the number of elements (crystals) in the probe and the number of channels that can be processed. Probes should be electronic and in the frequency range of 2.0 to 5.0 MHz (up to 7.5 MHz for pediatric use) for abdominal imaging. Preferably, these should be variable frequency, curvilinear probes. Probes for vascular imaging are usually linear probes with a frequency between 7.5 and 12 MHz. For gray-scale renal ultrasound, portable, lightweight scanners with good image quality are available; Doppler capability can add to the cost but is increasingly being offered as a standard feature. Larger and more expensive scanners are difficult to maneuver and have additional features that are of little use to the nephrologist. Controls on the scanner allow adjustment of scanning depth, focal length, time-gain compensation, sound intensity, and gray scale. Although this seems a daunting number of variables, adjustment is usually straightforward and mostly empirical. Images can be printed directly or digitally stored.

Procedure

Description of the scanning procedures cannot substitute for hands-on training because scanning is an acquired skill that requires practice. Ideally, the patient should be fasting for abdominal scanning to minimize interference from intestinal gas, but this is not essential for examination of kidneys and of no consequence for examination of the bladder or transplanted kidneys. There must be an airtight connection between the probe and the skin, which is accomplished by placing gel on the probe or skin and applying firm pressure against the skin. To avoid compression of the vessels, minimal pressure should be applied for vascular examinations, with the use of more gel. Gel specifically designed for ultrasound should be used because other gels, such as lubricating gel, give poorer image quality. Ambient light should be dimmed to optimize viewing of the monitor.

The patient should be flat in the supine or lateral decubitus position with imaging through the abdomen for examination of native kidneys. Initial attempts should be made in the supine position before resorting to the lateral decubitus position. Imaging through the back is not recommended for diagnostic imaging because of sound attenuation by muscle and fascia and limitations on angling of the probe. Placement of the ipsilateral arm over the head, removal of pillows from under the head, and deep inspiration aid in moving overlying ribs superiorly. Transplanted kidneys and the urinary bladder are examined in the supine position, but the patient need not be completely flat.

Initially, longitudinal images should be obtained to determine maximal kidney length. On the right side, this view should be obtained through the liver if possible (Fig. 88.1A). The probe should be oriented so that the upper pole is toward the left-hand side of the image. The probe should then be rotated 90 degrees to obtain transverse views (Fig. 88.1B), and the kidney is scanned from pole to pole to ensure visualization of the entire kidney. Examination of each kidney should include longitudinal images with adjacent liver or spleen if possible as well as transverse images through the mid kidney and each pole.[7] Measurements other than length are of no clinical utility, and measurements of kidney volume are inaccurate and no better than length in judging kidney size.[8] Sagittal and transverse views of the urinary bladder are obtained with the probe just superior to the symphysis pubis and angled inferiorly (Fig. 88.1C, D). Volume is obtained by multiplying the two transverse dimensions and the sagittal length by 0.523.[6] The technique for renal biopsy is discussed in Chapter 6.

Training and Certification

There are no data on what constitutes adequate training for renal ultrasound. Training is required for both performance and interpretation and should include didactic, hands-on, and supervised components. The last can vary considerably, depending on case volume and particularly type because any quantity of studies will be inadequate if they are all normal. Thus, the number of studies required for competence is inversely related to the frequency of pathology. Minimal qualifications for physician-sonographers have been established by the American Institute of Ultrasound in Medicine[9] and the American College of Radiology,[6] but neither organization has developed guidelines for limited abdominal ultrasound. The American Society of Diagnostic and Interventional Nephrology *(www.asdin.org)* has established training standards for ultrasound limited to kidneys and bladder that specify 50 hours of training and 125 studies (at least 80 being supervised and the remaining having confirmatory follow-up).[10] Because renal ultrasound is not usually a formal component of nephrology training, a course for nephrologists has been established in the United States *(www.medicine.emory.edu/divisions/renal/ultrasound)*.[7] Training and certification are available in vascular ultrasound but are not limited to applications specific to nephrology. Such training is important for vascular studies of kidneys but not necessary for examination of dysfunctional AV fistulas and grafts (unless flow is measured) because this does not require Doppler analysis. There are currently no guidelines or training established for vascular ultrasound related to nephrology.

PERITONEAL DIALYSIS CATHETERS

Successful PD is dependent on proper catheter insertion and management. The feasibility, safety, and success of these procedures when they are performed by nephrologists have been well documented,[11-13] and this leads to greater use of PD. Chronic PD catheters are constructed of silicone rubber with a 5-mm external diameter and internal diameters of 2.6 to 3.5 mm. Some commonly used designs of PD catheters are shown in Figure 92.6. The intraperitoneal portion can be straight, straight with perpendicular silicone disks, or curled with side holes or T shaped with linear grooves or slots rather than side holes. These

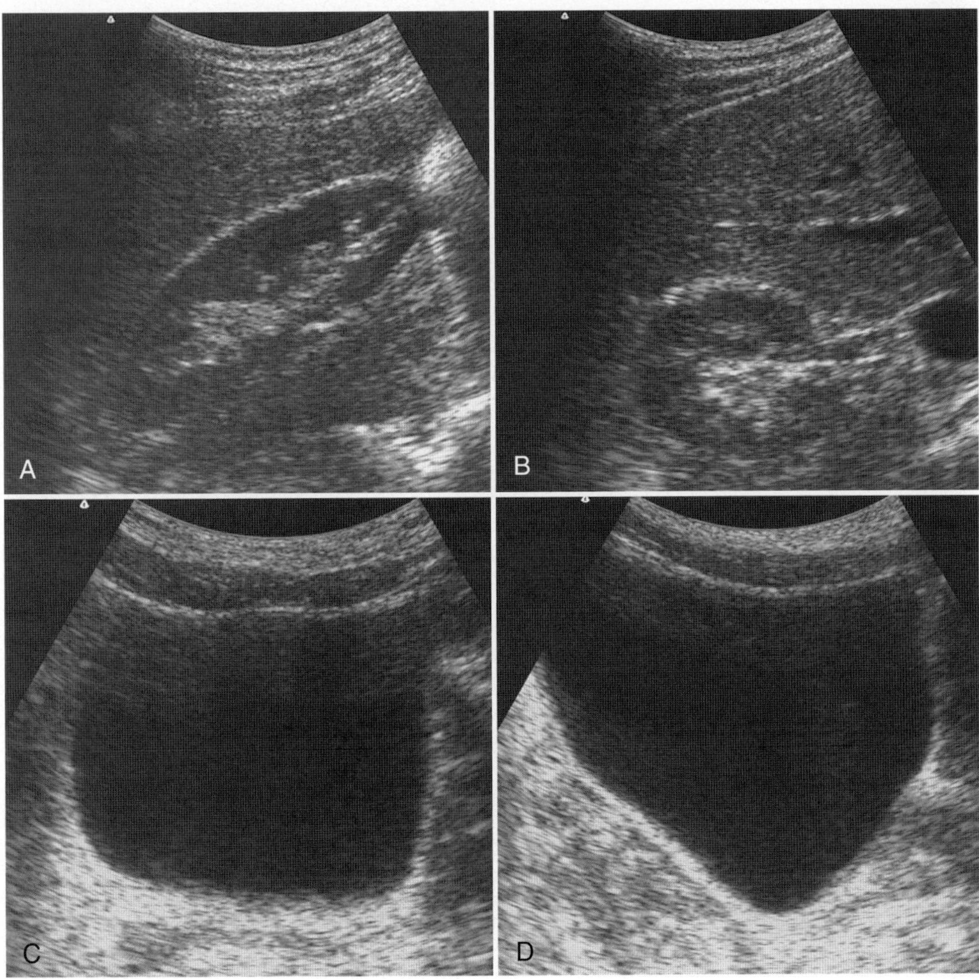

Figure 88.1 Imaging planes for renal and bladder sonography. A, Longitudinal image of right kidney. Upper pole should be on left side of the image. **B,** Transverse image of right kidney through the renal hilum. **C,** Transverse image of urinary bladder. Anteroposterior and mediolateral dimensions are obtained in this plane. **D,** Sagittal image of the urinary bladder. Superior portion of the bladder is to the left. Superoinferior dimension is obtained in this plane.

designs are created to diminish outflow obstruction. The subcutaneous portion is either straight or bent and has one or two extraperitoneal Dacron cuffs that prevent fluid leaks and bacterial migration around the catheter. The subcutaneous catheter shapes all provide a lateral or downward direction of the exit site. An upwardly directed exit site collects debris and fluid, increasing the risk of exit site infection. Currently, the method of placement of the catheter has more effect on the outcome than catheter choice does.

Catheter Insertion

The four techniques for PD catheter insertion are dissection (surgical), the Seldinger technique (blind or with fluoroscopy), peritoneoscopic, and laparoscopic.[14] The Seldinger and peritoneoscopic techniques are most frequently used by nephrologists. Peritoneoscopic insertion is a single-puncture technique using a small (2.2-mm diameter) optical peritoneoscope for direct inspection of the peritoneal cavity and identification of a suitable site for the optimal intraperitoneal portion of the catheter. Peritoneoscopic placement is usually performed with local anesthesia (sometimes with conscious sedation) and manual infusion of about 1 liter of air. Laparoscopic techniques are performed under general anesthesia, with larger scopes, multiple insertion sites, and automated gas infusion. Both peritoneoscopic and laparoscopic techniques allow direct visualization of intraperitoneal structures.

The choice of technique must take into account the local experience with complications (pericatheter leakage, outflow failure, exit site and tunnel infection) and long-term catheter function associated with each technique, costs, ease and timely insertion of the catheter, and factors contributing to mortality risk (local versus general anesthesia). Both randomized and nonrandomized studies have documented that the peritoneoscopic and fluoroscopic Seldinger techniques result in fewer catheter complications (infection, outflow failure, pericatheter leak) and improved catheter survival compared with surgical placement.[12,15] The superior results with peritoneoscopic placement may relate to direct visualization of the abdominal cavity, less tissue dissection, and avoidance of general anesthesia. Because tissue dissection is minimal, the catheter can be used immediately (after 36 hours), although a 2- to 3-week delay is recommended.[16]

For peritoneoscopic insertion (Fig. 88.2), a small skin incision (2 to 3 cm) is made and dissection is carried down only to the subcutaneous tissue. The anterior rectus sheath is identified but not incised. A preassembled cannula with trocar and a spiral sheath is then inserted at a 40°-50° angle into the abdominal cavity through the rectus muscle (Figs. 88.2A and 88.3). The trocar is then removed and replaced by the peritoneoscope to confirm the intra-abdominal position of the cannula (Figs. 88.2B and 88.4). Air is then infused (600 to 1000 ml) to separate visceral and parietal peritoneum. Alternatively, a Veress needle can be used.[17] Bowel loops, the dome of the bladder, and any intra-abdominal adhesions are identified. The cannula and spiral

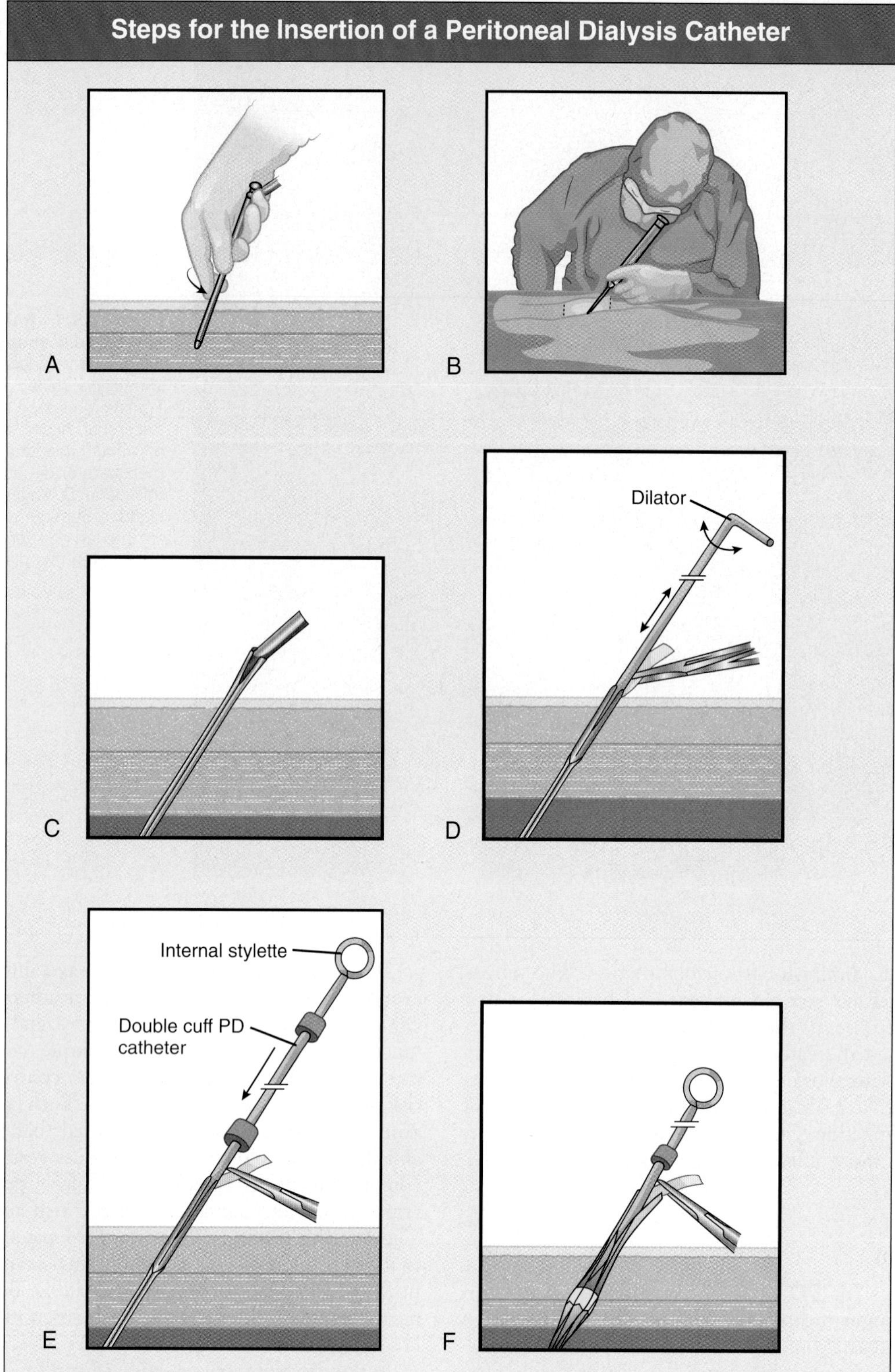

Figure 88.2 Steps for the insertion of a peritoneal dialysis catheter. A, A trocar and cannula with a sheath are inserted into the abdominal cavity. **B,** A peritoneoscope is passed through and locked into the cannula. **C,** The sheath has been passed into the abdominal cavity and the peritoneoscope and cannula removed sequentially. **D,** The sheath is secured with a forceps while it is being dilated. **E,** A PD catheter (with double cuff) is passed through the dilated sheath by use of an internal stylet. **F,** The deep cuff is implanted into the rectus muscle. *(Redrawn from Y-Tec Instructions: Laparoscopic and Peritoneoscopic Placement of Peritoneal Dialysis Catheters. Medigroup Inc. [division of Janin Group, Inc.], Oswego, Ill, 2004, pp 1-5.)*

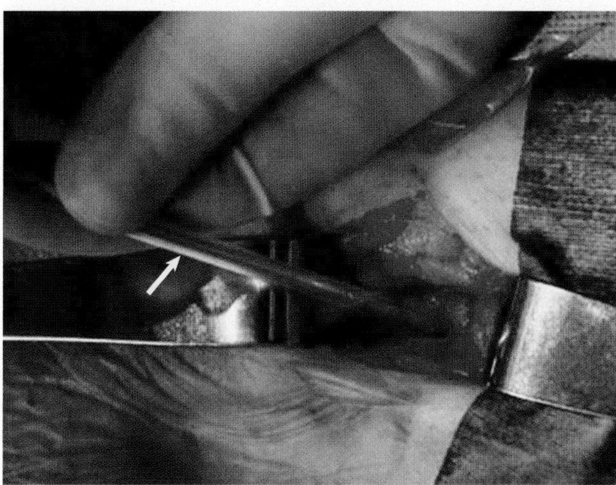

Figure 88.3 Peritoneoscopic insertion of a peritoneal dialysis catheter. During peritoneoscopic insertion of a peritoneal dialysis catheter, a Quill guide trocar and cannula *(arrow)*, with its wrapped spiral sheath, is being inserted through the rectus muscle under local anesthesia.

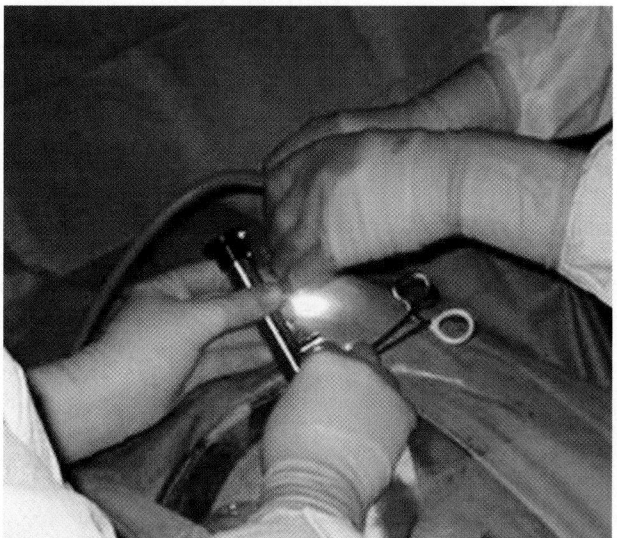

Figure 88.4 Peritoneoscopic insertion of a peritoneal dialysis catheter. A peritoneoscope has been introduced into the abdominal cavity through the cannula, and the fiberoptic light source is being connected to the scope.

sheath are advanced into the pelvis (Fig. 88.2C). The cannula and the peritoneoscope are then removed, the spiral sheath is dilated to 6-mm diameter (Fig. 88.2D), and the catheter is inserted through the sheath by a stylet (Fig. 88.2E). The deep cuff is implanted into the rectus muscle with use of an implanter tool without dissection of the anterior rectus sheath or the muscle (Fig. 88.2F). A tunnel and an exit site are created (Fig. 88.5), and the superficial cuff is implanted into the subcutaneous tissue. The subcutaneous tissue is sutured with absorbable material; the skin is closed with nylon. No sutures are placed on the external rectus sheath or at the skin exit site.

The Seldinger technique using fluoroscopy begins with blunt dissection down to the level of the lateral border of the rectus sheath. A 22-gauge needle from a 5-French micropuncture set is inserted at an angle of 45 degrees, directed toward the lower

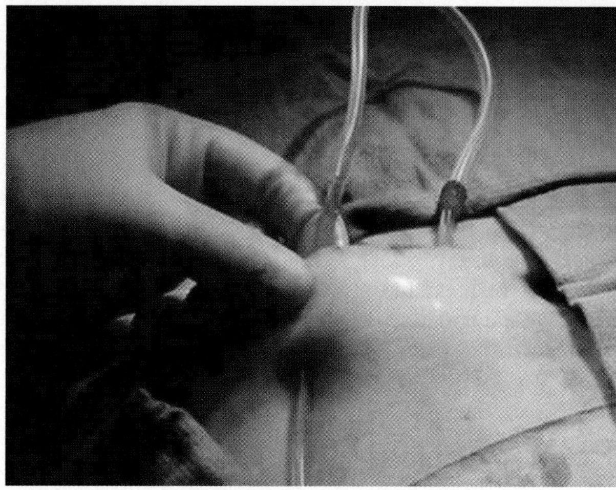

Figure 88.5 Peritoneoscopic insertion of a peritoneal dialysis catheter. With use of a disposable tool, a subcutaneous tunnel is created for the catheter. The superficial cuff shown will be implanted in the subcutaneous tunnel.

pelvis into the peritoneum (ultrasound can be helpful). The location of the needle within the peritoneal cavity is confirmed by injecting 3 to 5 ml of contrast material, which is seen surrounding bowel loops. A micropuncture 0.018-inch wire is then inserted through the needle under fluoroscopy. Once it is in the lower pelvis, a 5-French catheter is placed over the wire. Contrast material can again be injected to confirm the position. A 0.035-inch guide wire is then passed through the catheter, and dilators are advanced sequentially up to the final 18-French dilator and peel-away sheath. The guide wire is removed and the PD catheter is inserted over a metal stylet through the sheath, splitting the sheath as the deep Dacron cuff advances. This cuff is pushed into the rectus muscle while the sheath is in place, and the sheath is then removed around the cuff and catheter. The catheter is tunneled laterally with a tunneling tool.[18,19]

Burying the Peritoneal Dialysis Catheter

If the catheter will not be used immediately, it can be implanted (buried) under the skin for weeks to months before it is tunneled to the outside and used. The placed in the usual manner, then blocked with a plug and tunneled in a straight line under the skin. Some centers tie off the catheter with silk suture and coil it into a pouch under the exit site. This allows ingrowth of tissue into the cuffs of the catheter without an opportunity for bacterial colonization and diminishes the incidence of early pericatheter infections.[20,21] Catheters buried in this fashion have been successfully used more than 1 year after insertion.[22] We recommend burial when the catheter will not be used for at least a month.

Complications of Peritoneal Dialysis Catheter Insertion

Bowel perforation is the most feared complication of catheter insertion. The incidence is 1% to 1.4% with surgical insertion[12,13] but 0% to 0.8% with the peritoneoscopic insertion.[11,13] The diagnosis is established by direct peritoneoscopic visualization of bowel mucosa, bowel contents or hard stool, return of fecal material, or emanation of foul-smelling gas through the cannula. Whereas some investigators suggest that this complication should be treated with surgical intervention,[24] successful conservative management of bowel perforation with bowel rest and intravenous antibiotics has also been reported.[19,25] To minimize the risk of perforation, a needle (such as a Veress needle) that is smaller and has a blunt, self-retracting end can be used instead of a trocar to gain access to the abdominal cavity.[17] Previous abdominal surgery is mentioned as a relative contraindication to PD because of intraperitoneal adhesions.[26,27] However, with peritoneoscopy, which can identify intraperitoneal adhesions, assess their extent, and locate a suitable site for catheter placement, the incidence of bowel perforation is no higher than in patients without prior abdominal surgery, and the success rate exceeds 95%.[11,13]

Catheter Repositioning

Migration of the PD catheter to the upper abdomen is a frequent cause of catheter failure. A variety of techniques have been used for repositioning, including guide wire or stylet insertion, Fogarty catheters, and laparoscopy, and are feasible for nephrologists. The long-term success rate is only 27% to 48%,[28,29] probably because the migration of the catheter is the result of encasement by the omentum. Thus, insertion of a new catheter is required in many cases. Fogarty catheter manipulation is perhaps the most cost-effective, safe, and simple method. A Fogarty catheter is advanced into the PD catheter, and the balloon is inflated. Manipulation is performed by tugging movements to reposition the catheter into the pelvic area. Infusion and drainage of dialysate as well as radiography are performed to determine patency and position of the PD catheter, respectively.

Removal of Peritoneal Dialysis Catheters

A Tenckhoff curled or straight PD catheter can be safely removed without need for an operating room or general anesthesia.[16] Local anesthetic is infiltrated at the site of the primary incision, and dissection is carried down to the subcutaneous portion of the catheter by longitudinal incisions with scissors while the catheter is held with toothed forceps. The catheter is clamped with a hemostat, a nylon suture is placed in the catheter beyond the hemostat as a tag, and the catheter is cut between the two. Dissection is continued toward the deep cuff (Fig. 88.6), and additional anesthetic is infiltrated around the deep cuff. For catheters that have been in place for less than a month, blunt dissection is usually sufficient to free the deep cuff. Older catheters require sharp dissection. Exposure of the deep cuff and the anterior rectus sheath is required. Once the deep cuff is separated from the surrounding tissue, the intraperitoneal portion of the catheter is gently withdrawn from the peritoneal cavity, and the defect in the rectus sheath is closed with an absorbable purse-string suture. The nylon tag is then pulled to expose the remaining subcutaneous portion of catheter segment, and dissection is performed in the direction of the superficial cuff. Once the superficial cuff is free, this portion of the catheter is removed through the primary incision site or the exit site. Absorbable suture material is used to close the subcutaneous tissue; nylon is used to close the skin. The exit site is not sutured.

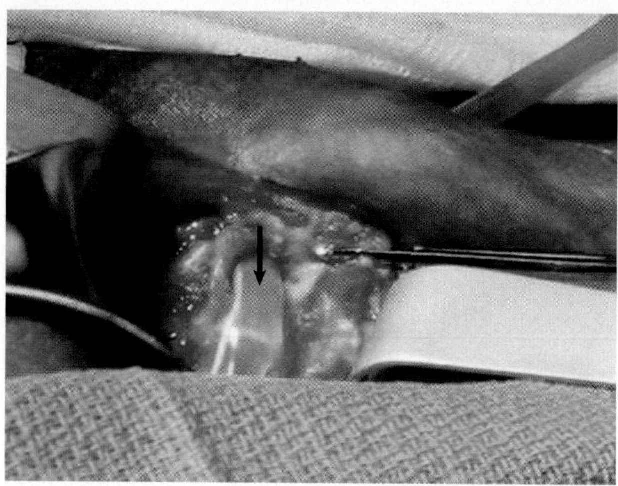

Figure 88.6 Peritoneal dialysis catheter removal. The catheter (*arrow*) has been exposed by dissection of the subcutaneous tunnel.

Training and Certification

The American Society of Diagnostic and Interventional Nephrology has established training guidelines and criteria for certification of physicians in the insertion of PD catheters (*www.asdin.org*).[10] In addition to appropriate didactic training, there should be two practice insertions (into models, animals, or human cadavers), observation of two insertions into patients, and then six successful insertions into patients as primary operator.

TUNNELED HEMODIALYSIS CATHETERS

Central venous catheters are used as a temporary hemodialysis access, as a bridge to AV fistula or graft use, and when all other permanent access sites have been exhausted. Nontunneled catheters are used when a limited number of dialysis sessions are anticipated or there are contraindications to tunneled catheters (systemic infection, risk of bleeding) and are appropriate for use only in the inpatient setting. Tunneled catheters can be placed in both inpatient and outpatient settings, can be inserted at multiple vein locations, are relatively low in cost, and provide immediate access. However, there are significant disadvantages, including morbidity due to infection and thrombosis and risk of central vein stenosis or occlusion.[30,31] The role of the tunneled dialysis catheter in the provision of vascular access for hemodialysis is discussed further in Chapter 87.

Catheter Insertion

The right internal jugular vein is the preferred catheter location compared with the left internal jugular and subclavian vein sites; it provides a straight route to the right atrium, thereby reducing the risk of central vein stenosis. Catheters may also be placed in the femoral veins.

Catheter insertion is performed in a sterile setting, ideally in an operating room environment with fluoroscopy available or at a minimum in a dedicated procedure room with cardiac monitoring. Before cannulation, the vein should be located by ultrasound to detect anatomic variation or venous thrombosis. The patient's neck is then prepared and draped in sterile fashion; under ultrasound guidance, the vein is cannulated with a micropuncture needle (18- to 22-gauge), and a micropuncture guide wire is inserted and positioned in the superior vena cava. The needle is then removed, and the micropuncture dilator is inserted over the guide wire so that it can be replaced with a standard guide wire. The use of the smaller needle rather than the standard 15-gauge

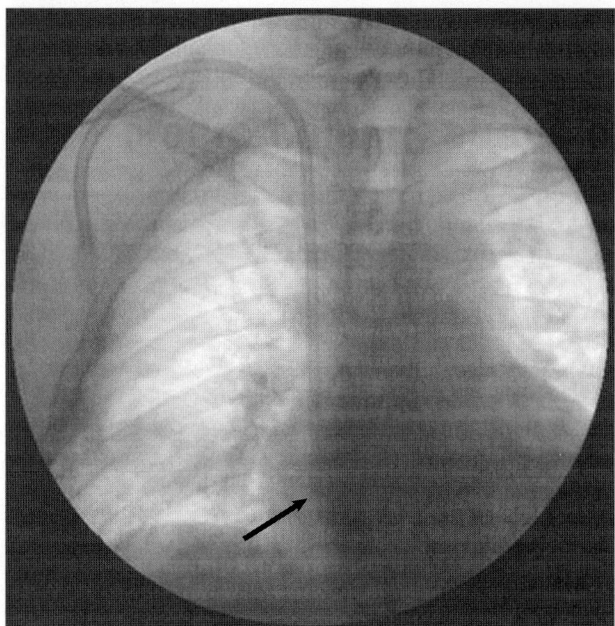

Figure 88.7 Insertion of a venous catheter for hemodialysis. Chest radiograph confirming that the tip of the catheter *(arrow)* is at the junction of the superior vena cava and the right atrium.

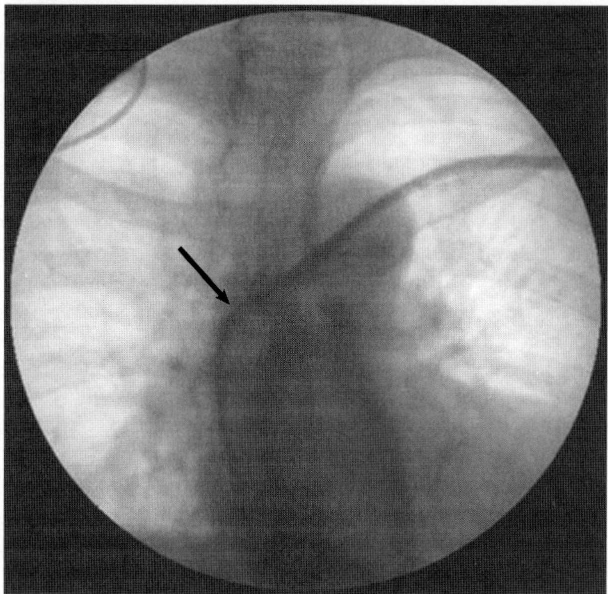

Figure 88.8 Fibrin sheath on a tunneled venous catheter. Contrast material has been injected into a tunneled catheter after the tip *(arrow)* has been pulled back into the innominate vein. The contrast material fills a sheath that extends from the catheter tip.

needle minimizes trauma to the vein. A small subcutaneous incision is made adjacent to the dilator or guide wire, additional dilation is performed, and the catheter is placed over the guide wire with care taken to hold the guide wire in place. If a tunneled catheter is to be placed, a catheter exit site is selected inferior to the clavicle and sufficiently lateral to the venotomy to avoid a kink in the catheter. A 1-cm superficial incision is made at this point, and a subcutaneous track adjacent to the venotomy is infiltrated with lidocaine. A double-lumen catheter, generally 28 or 32 cm in length, is attached to the tunneling device and pulled through the subcutaneous tunnel in a curved path. A guide wire is passed through the dilator and into the inferior vena cava. The venotomy site is then serially dilated over the guide wire. The catheter can then be inserted over the guide wire through the venous port. When a split-tip catheter is used, the guide wire is passed in and out of the two venous ports and through an arterial port or through a hollow intracatheter stiffener. Alternatively, a peel-away sheath is placed over the guide wire and the catheter inserted through the sheath after the removal of the guide wire; however, this method has greater potential for blood loss and air embolism. Fluoroscopy is used to confirm tip placement at the level of the right atrium, with the arterial port facing away from the atrial wall, and to ensure that there are no kinks in the catheter (Fig. 88.7). Each port of the catheter is then flushed with saline and locked with the appropriate amount of heparin based on catheter length and priming volume designation, followed by placement of the catheter hub caps.

Catheter Dysfunction

Catheter dysfunction is defined as the failure to maintain a blood flow sufficient to perform hemodialysis without significantly extending treatment time; this is usually 300 ml/min.[39] Causes of immediate dysfunction include a kink in the catheter, incorrect position or orientation (arterial port against the vessel wall), and errant venous cannulation. These problems should be ascertained and corrected at the time of catheter placement. Catheter thrombosis is the most common cause of late dysfunction. Extrinsic thrombosis is less common than intrinsic thrombosis and is caused by central vein, mural, or right atrial thrombosis. Intrinsic obstruction results from thrombus within the catheter lumen or tip or most commonly from a fibrin sheath. Fibrin sheaths typically develop weeks to months after catheter insertion and result when a sleeve of connective tissue forms at the venotomy site and extends and encases the catheter tip, creating a flap-valve. First-line treatment of catheter thrombosis includes forceful flush of the catheter with saline. If flow is not restored, a fibrinolytic agent should be instilled. Tissue plasminogen activator (tPA) is commonly used and appears more effective than urokinase in restoring patency and adequate flow.[32,33] Typically, 2 mg of tPA is instilled into the occluded catheter lumen and allowed to dwell 30 minutes. If this fails, the catheter should be exchanged. Strategies to minimize dialysis catheter thrombosis are discussed in Chapter 87.

Catheter Exchange and Fibrin Sheath Removal

Catheter exchange over a guide wire is useful in the setting of catheter thrombosis or bacteremia and allows the preservation of the venotomy, tunnel, and exit sites. The tunnel and exit sites must appear free of infection if the same sites are to be used. Catheter exchange should take place within 72 hours of the initiation of antibiotic therapy.[39] Under sterile conditions, the exit site is anesthetized and the cuff is freed. Once the catheter is pulled back 8 to 10 cm, contrast material is injected through the catheter under fluoroscopy to check for a fibrin sheath (Fig. 88.8). To obliterate a sheath, a guide wire is passed down the venous port of the catheter and into the inferior vena cava. The catheter is then removed, and a balloon catheter is inserted over the guide wire to the sheath location and inflated to disrupt the sheath. The guide wire is then wiped with povidone-iodine (Betadine), and a new catheter is inserted over the guide wire.

When the catheter tip is beyond the venotomy site, near the superior vena cava, contrast material can be injected again to check for sheath removal before proceeding with catheter insertion.

Training and Certification

The American Society of Diagnostic and Interventional Nephrology guidelines for hemodialysis vascular access procedure certification specify formal didactic training in central venous anatomy, sonographic examination of central veins, fluoroscopy, and catheter design and complications. In addition, practical training for certification includes satisfactory insertion of 25 tunneled long-term catheters. More information may be obtained at *www.asdin.org*.

PROCEDURES ON ARTERIOVENOUS FISTULAS AND GRAFTS

The most common indications for intervention are inadequate flow during dialysis, thrombosis, and failure of AV fistulas to mature. Specific interventions include angiography, thrombectomy, angioplasty, and stenting. All of these procedures require a dedicated facility, either inpatient or outpatient, with fluoroscopy, monitoring equipment, and staff to assist with the procedures and to deliver conscious sedation. There are many different techniques for AV access procedures and few data to indicate superiority of one method over the other, so the choice is generally one of personal preference and cost. However, the first step should always include a careful physical and ultrasound examination of the access. An examination will generally identify the problem and allow detection of access infection, an absolute contraindication to intervention. Appropriate intervention can then be planned. Monitoring and management of vascular access to minimize stenosis, thrombosis, and failure are discussed further in Chapter 87.

Percutaneous Balloon Angioplasty

Stenosis in AV grafts and fistulas is routinely managed by percutaneous balloon angioplasty, which can be safely performed on an outpatient basis, causes minimal discomfort, and allows immediate use of the access. Not all stenotic lesions are responsive, however, and some require repeated treatment. In fistulas, the stenosis is most commonly located at the "swing point," the portion of the native vein mobilized during creation of the AV anastomosis (Fig. 88.9); in grafts, the venous anastomosis is the most common site of stenosis.[34-38] Angioplasty is indicated if the stenosis is 50% or more and is associated with clinical or physiologic abnormalities.[39] Treatment of stenosis increases access blood flow and longevity, reduces access thrombosis, and reduces vascular access–related hospitalization.[38,40,41] A relative contraindication to angioplasty is a newly created access (<4 to 6 weeks old).

The access is cannulated with an introducer needle, a sheath is inserted, and initial angiography is performed. This should include views of the access, draining veins (peripheral and central), and arterial anastomosis and is used to confirm the location and degree of stenosis. Unless it is contraindicated, sedation and analgesia are then given with short-acting agents once a lesion has been identified on initial angiography, as angioplasty is painful.

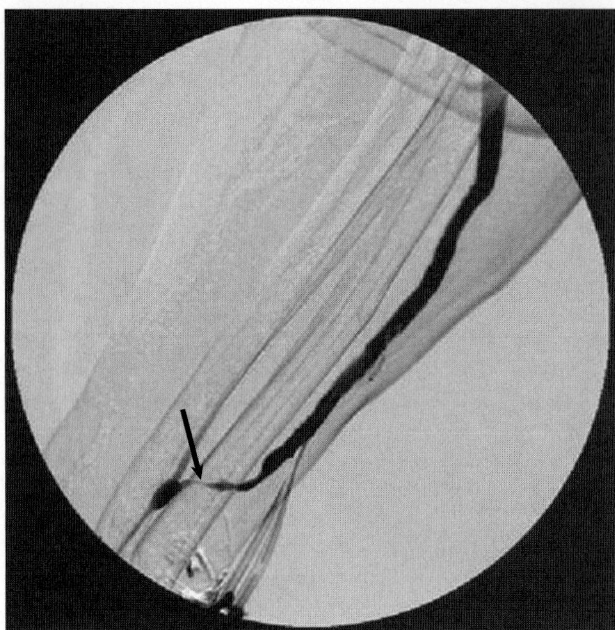

Figure 88.9 Juxta-anastomotic stenosis in a radiocephalic arteriovenous fistula. Contrast material was injected at the arterial anastomosis *(bottom left of image)* and demonstrates a narrowing in the initial portion of the fistula *(arrow)*.

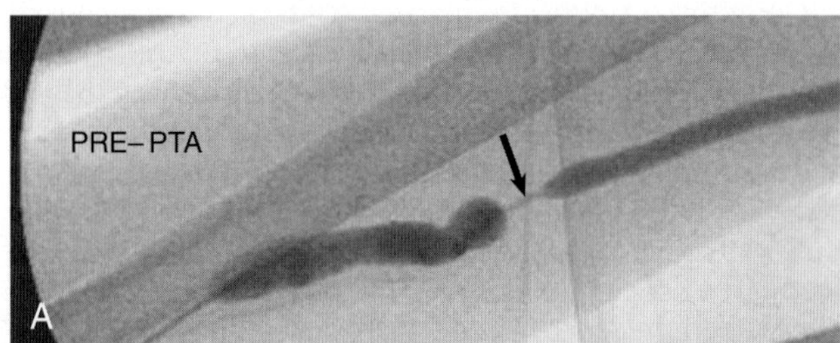

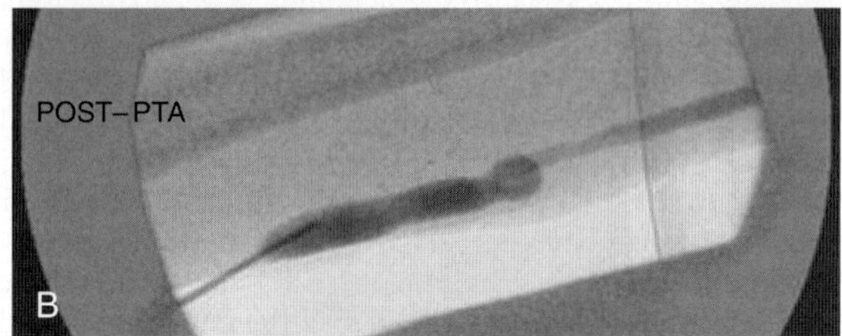

Figure 88.10 Arteriovenous graft stenosis. A, Stenosis in the outflow vein of an upper arm AV graft *(arrow)*. **B,** Angiogram performed immediately after percutaneous angioplasty.

A guide wire is passed through the sheath and across the stenosis. An angioplasty balloon catheter is passed over the guide wire, positioned at the stenotic site, and inflated with a syringe to 18 to 20 atm (Fig. 88.10). A variety of sheaths, guide wires, balloon sizes, and maximum pressures are available. The guide wire is left in place, and angiography is repeated to identify residual stenosis or any complications. Angioplasty is repeated for residual stenosis or when multiple lesions are present and may require a second cannulation of the access in the opposite direction for inflow stenoses. After removal of all devices, hemostasis at the cannulation site is achieved by manual pressure or suture placement. There is no evidence to support the use of antiplatelet agents or anticoagulation after intervention.

According to Kidney Disease Outcomes Quality Initiative (KDOQI) guidelines, a successful angioplasty is achieved when there is no more than 30% residual stenosis and physical indicators of stenosis have resolved.[39]

Percutaneous Thrombectomy

There are a variety of techniques for thrombus removal. Thromboaspiration is the least costly and is as effective and efficient as mechanical and pharmacomechanical thrombolysis, in which low-dose tPA is instilled into the thrombosed access, the clot is manually macerated, flow returns, and angioplasty is used to dilate access stenoses.[42] Thrombectomy by thromboaspiration combines angiography with balloon angioplasty and thrombectomy by clot aspiration. Absolute contraindications to thromboaspiration include access infection and known right-to-left cardiac shunt; relative contraindications include a large clot burden and long-standing access occlusion.

The access is cannulated in an antegrade direction, and a guide wire is passed to the level of the central veins. A straight catheter is inserted over the wire to the central veins, and angiography is performed to confirm central venous patency. Anticoagulation and short-acting sedative and analgesic medications are administered in the central circulation. An angiogram is then obtained as the catheter is pulled back to identify the location of stenosis. The guide wire is then inserted beyond the stenotic lesion, followed by an angioplasty balloon catheter. The balloon catheter is insufflated by hand with a syringe, and the stenotic lesion is dilated. The access is then cannulated in the retrograde direction, a sheath is inserted, and a Fogarty catheter is passed across the arterial anastomosis, inflated, and pulled back through the entire length of the access while clot fragments are aspirated. On return of flow through the access, angiography is performed to evaluate the inflow and the arterial anastomosis, and angioplasty is repeated if necessary. Hemostasis is achieved by manual pressure or a suture at the cannulation sites.

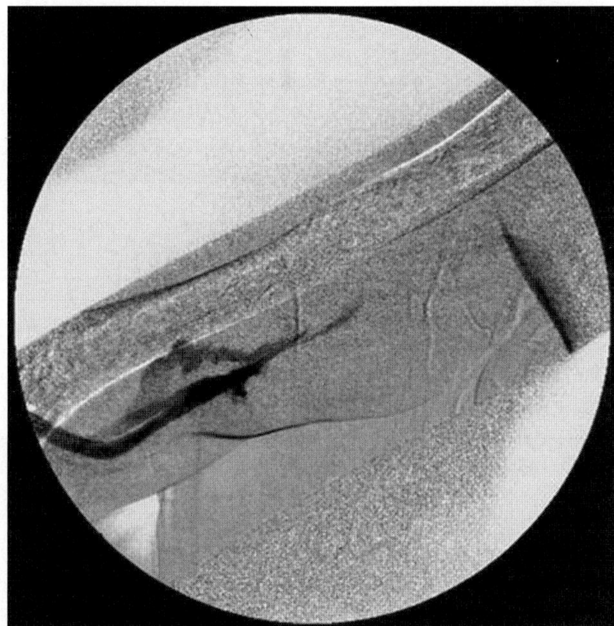

Figure 88.11 Vein rupture. A postangioplasty angiogram of an AV fistula showing extravasation of dye indicative of a vein rupture. *(Courtesy Dr. G. Beathard, Austin, Texas, USA.)*

Stents

The precise role of the endovascular stent in AV fistulas and grafts has not been defined. Results from nonrandomized studies differ as to the patency benefit of primary stent use versus angioplasty alone within a stenotic access or central vein.[43-46] Stents are expensive and have often been used in situations in which their use will not extend the life of the access. Stents should be considered in the setting of failed balloon angioplasty (an elastic lesion), when there are few remaining access sites, if the patient is not a surgical candidate for a new access, or when an outflow vein ruptures after balloon angioplasty (Figs. 88.11 and 88.12).[47,48] Finally, a stent may be useful in the setting of an expanding pseudoaneurysm.[49,50]

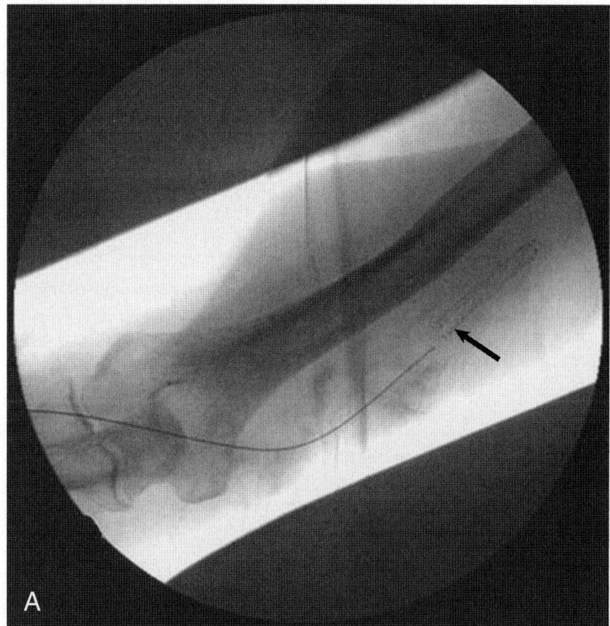

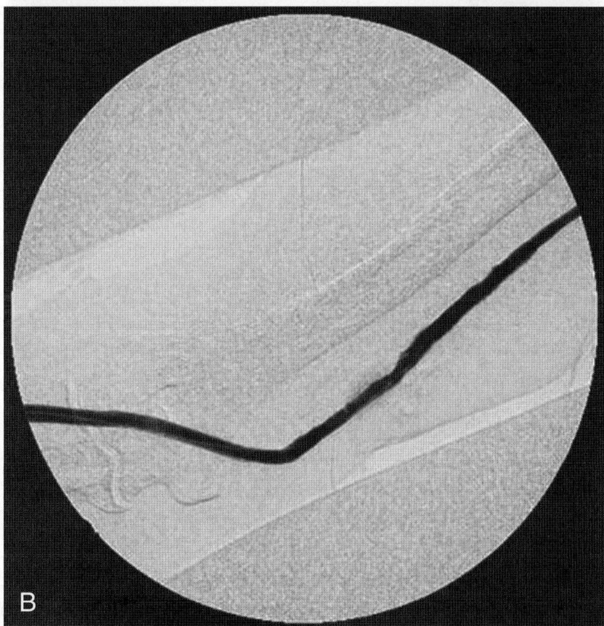

Figure 88.12 Treatment of vein rupture with an intraluminal stent. A, Placement of the stent *(arrow)*. **B,** An angiogram obtained after stent placement showing that venous outflow has been re-established. *(Courtesy Dr. G. Beathard, Austin, Texas, USA.)*

Training and Certification

The American Society of Diagnostic and Interventional Nephrology guidelines for hemodialysis vascular access procedure certification specify didactic training in venous anatomy, fluoroscopy, procedural equipment, and sedation and analgesia. Requirements for practical training include 25 cases in both fistulas and grafts of each of the following: angiography, angioplasty, and thrombectomy as primary operator (refer to *www.asdin.org* for more information). In general, several times that number as secondary operator will be required to become a primary operator.

REFERENCES

1. Moghazi S, Jones E, Schroepple J, et al. Correlation of renal histopathology with sonographic findings. *Kidney Int.* 2005;67:1515-1520.
2. Gottlieb RH, Weinberg EP, Rubens DJ, et al. Renal sonography: Can it be used more selectively in the setting of an elevated serum creatinine level? *Am J Kidney Dis.* 1997;29:362-367.
3. O'Neill WC, Baumgarten DA. Ultrasonography in renal transplantation. *Am J Kidney Dis.* 2002;39:663-678.
4. Korbet SM. Percutaneous renal biopsy. *Semin Nephrol.* 2002;22:254-267.
5. Nass K, O'Neill WC. Bedside renal biopsy: Ultrasound guidance by the nephrologist. *Am J Kidney Dis.* 1999;34:955-959.
6. Riccabona M, Nelson TR, Pretorius DH, Davidson TE. In vivo three-dimensional sonographic measurement of organ volume: Validation in the urinary bladder. *J Ultrasound Med.* 1996;5:627-632.
7. O'Neill WC. Renal ultrasonography: A procedure for nephrologists. *Am J Kidney Dis.* 1997;30:579-585.
8. Emamian SA, Nielsen MB, Pedersen JF. Intraobserver and interobserver variations in sonographic measurements of kidney size in adult volunteers. A comparison of linear measurements and volumetric estimates. *Acta Radiol.* 1995;36:399-401.
9. Training Guidelines for Physicians Who Evaluate and Interpret Diagnostic Ultrasound Examinations. Laurel, Md, American Institute of Ultrasound in Medicine, 1997.
10. Guidelines for training, certification, and accreditation in placement of permanent tunneled and cuffed peritoneal dialysis catheters. *Semin Dial.* 2002;15:440-442.
11. Asif A, Byers P, Vieira CF, et al. Peritoneoscopic placement of peritoneal dialysis catheter and bowel perforation: Experience of an interventional nephrology program. *Am J Kidney Dis.* 2003;42:1270-1274.
12. Pastan S, Gassensmith C, Manatunga AK, et al. Prospective comparison of peritoneoscopic and surgical implantation of CAPD catheters. *ASAIO Trans.* 1991;37:M154-M156.
13. Gadallah MF, Pervez A, el-Shahawy MA, et al. Peritoneoscopic versus surgical placement of peritoneal dialysis catheters: A prospective randomized study on outcome. *Am J Kidney Dis.* 1999;33:118-122.
14. Ash SR. Chronic peritoneal dialysis catheters: Procedures for placement, maintenance, and removal. *Semin Nephrol.* 2002;22:221-236.
15. Scalamogna A, De Vecchi A, Castelnovo C, Ponticelli C. Peritoneal catheter outcome effect of mode of placement. *Perit Dial Int.* 1994;14:S81.
16. Asif A, Byers P, Gadalean F, Roth D. Peritoneal dialysis underutilization: The impact of an interventional nephrology peritoneal dialysis access program. *Semin Dial.* 2003;16:266-271.
17. Asif A, Tawakol J, Khan T, et al. Modification of the peritoneoscopic technique of peritoneal dialysis catheter insertion: Experience of an interventional nephrology program. *Semin Dial.* 2004;17:171-173.
18. Zaman F, Pervez A, Atray NK, et al. Fluoroscopy-assisted placement of peritoneal dialysis catheters by nephrologists. *Semin Dial.* 2005;18:247-251.
19. Maya ID. Ultrasound/fluoroscopy-assisted placement of peritoneal dialysis catheters. *Semin Dial.* 2007;20:611-615.
20. Moncrief JW, Popovich RP, Broadrick LJ, et al. The Moncrief-Popovich catheter. A new peritoneal access technique for patients on peritoneal dialysis. *ASAIO J.* 1993;39:62-65.
21. Prischl FC, Wallner M, Kalchmair H, et al. Initial subcutaneous embedding of the peritoneal dialysis catheter—a critical appraisal of this new implantation technique. *Nephrol Dial Transplant.* 1997;12:1661-1667.
22. Ash SR. Chronic peritoneal dialysis catheters: Overview of design, placement, and removal procedures. *Semin Dial.* 2003;16:323-334.
23. Ash SR. Bedside peritoneoscopic peritoneal catheter placement of Tenckhoff and newer peritoneal catheters. *Adv Perit Dial.* 1998;14:75-79.
24. Simkin EP, Wright FK. Perforating injuries of the bowel complicating peritoneal catheter insertion. *Lancet.* 1968;1:64-66.
25. Rubin J, Oreopoulos DG, Lio TT, et al. Management of peritonitis and bowel perforation during chronic peritoneal dialysis. *Nephron.* 1976;16:220-225.
26. Nkere UU. Postoperative adhesion formation and the use of adhesion preventing techniques in cardiac and general surgery. *ASAIO J.* 2000;46:654-656.
27. Brandt CP, Franceschi D. Laparoscopic placement of peritoneal dialysis catheters in patients who have undergone prior abdominal operations. *J Am Coll Surg.* 1994;178:515-516.
28. Gadallah MF, Arora N, Arumugam R, Moles K. Role of Fogarty catheter manipulation in management of migrated, nonfunctional peritoneal dialysis catheters. *Am J Kidney Dis.* 2000;35:301-305.
29. Siegel RL, Nosher JL, Gesner LR. Peritoneal dialysis catheters: Repositioning with new fluoroscopic technique. *Radiology.* 1994;190:899-901.
30. Schwab SJ, Beathard G. The hemodialysis catheter conundrum: Hate living with them, but can't live without them. *Kidney Int.* 1999;56:1-17.
31. Vanherweghem JL, Yassine T, Goldman M, et al. Subclavian vein thrombosis: A frequent complication of subclavian vein cannulation for hemodialysis. *Clin Nephrol.* 1986;26:235-238.
32. Haire WD, Atkinson JB, Stephens LC, Kotulak GD. Urokinase versus recombinant tissue plasminogen activator in thrombosed central venous catheters: A double-blinded, randomized trial. *Thromb Haemost.* 1994;72:543-547.
33. Zacharias JM, Weatherston CP, Spewak CR, Vercaigne LM. Alteplase versus urokinase for occluded hemodialysis catheters. *Ann Pharmacother.* 2003;37:27-33.
34. Falk A, Teodorescu V, Lou WY, et al. Treatment of "swing point stenoses" in hemodialysis arteriovenous fistulae. *Clin Nephrol.* 2003;60:35-41.
35. Beathard GA, Arnold P, Jackson J, Litchfield T. Aggressive treatment of early fistula failure. *Kidney Int.* 2003;64:1487-1494.
36. Maya ID, Oser R, Saddekni S, et al. Vascular access stenosis: Comparison of arteriovenous grafts and fistulas. *Am J Kidney Dis.* 2004;44:859-865.
37. Sivanesan S, How TV, Bakran A. Sites of stenosis in AV fistulae for haemodialysis access. *Nephrol Dial Transplant.* 1999;14:118-120.
38. Badero OJ, Salifu MO, Wasse H, Work J. Frequency of swing-segment stenosis in referred dialysis patients with angiographically documented lesions. *Am J Kidney Dis.* 2008;51:93-98.
39. III. NKF-K/DOQI Clinical Practice Guidelines for Vascular Access: update 2000. *Am J Kidney Dis.* 2001;37:S137-S181.
40. Schwab SJ, Oliver MJ, Suhocki P, McCann R. Hemodialysis arteriovenous access: Detection of stenosis and response to treatment by vascular access blood flow. *Kidney Int.* 2001;59:358-362.
41. Beathard GA. Angioplasty for arteriovenous grafts and fistulae. *Semin Nephrol.* 2002;22:202-210.
42. Schon D, Mishler R. Pharmacomechanical thrombolysis of natural vein fistulas: Reduced dose of TPA and long-term follow-up. *Semin Dial.* 2003;16:272-275.
43. Chan MR, Bedi S, Sanchez RJ, et al. Stent placement versus angioplasty improves patency of arteriovenous grafts and blood flow of arteriovenous fistulae. *Clin J Am Soc Nephrol.* 2008;3:699-705.
44. Vesely TM, Amin MZ, Pilgram T. Use of stents and stent grafts to salvage angioplasty failures in patients with hemodialysis grafts. *Semin Dial.* 2008;21:100-104.
45. Bakken AM, Protack CD, Saad WE, et al. Long-term outcomes of primary angioplasty and primary stenting of central venous stenosis in hemodialysis patients. *J Vasc Surg.* 2007;45:776-783.
46. Vogel PM, Parise C. Comparison of SMART stent placement for arteriovenous graft salvage versus successful graft PTA. *J Vasc Interv Radiol.* 2005;16:1619-1626.
47. Vesely TM, Hovsepian DM, Pilgram TK, et al. Upper extremity central venous obstruction in hemodialysis patients: Treatment with Wallstents. *Radiology.* 1997;204:343-348.
48. Funaki B, Szymski GX, Leef JA, et al. Wallstent deployment to salvage dialysis graft thrombolysis complicated by venous rupture: Early and intermediate results. *AJR Am J Roentgenol.* 1997;169:1435-1437.
49. Vesely TM. Use of stent grafts to repair hemodialysis graft-related pseudoaneurysms. *J Vasc Interv Radiol.* 2005;16:1301-1307.
50. Barshes NR, Annambhotla S, Bechara C, et al. Endovascular repair of hemodialysis graft-related pseudoaneurysm: An alternative treatment strategy in salvaging failing dialysis access. *Vasc Endovasc Surg.* 2008;42:228-234.

CHAPTER 89

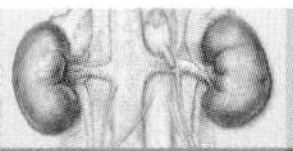

Hemodialysis: Principles and Techniques

Peter Kotanko, Martin K. Kuhlmann, Nathan W. Levin

Despite the widespread use of peritoneal dialysis and renal transplantation, hemodialysis (HD) remains the main renal replacement therapy in most countries worldwide. More than 1.7 million patients are currently treated with HD in about 28,500 dialysis units worldwide. The HD population is projected to grow to 2.0 million in 2010. Despite significant advances in our understanding of the biology of chronic kidney disease and the risk factors for poor outcome on HD and improved dialysis technology, the annual mortality in HD patients varies from 10% to 25% internationally, depending on demographic and possibly genetic factors.

DIALYSIS SYSTEM

The aim of the HD system is to deliver blood in a fail-safe manner from the patient to the dialyzer, to enable an efficient removal of uremic toxins and fluid, and to deliver the cleared blood back to the patient. The main components of the dialysis system are the extracorporeal blood circuit, the dialyzer, the dialysis machine, and the water purification system.[1] The dialysis machine delivers dialysis fluid with the intended flow rate, temperature, and chemical composition. The dialysis machine has monitoring and safety systems for air, blood, conductivity, and pressure; blood and dialysate pumps; a heating system; a dialysate mixing and degassing unit; and an ultrafiltrate balancing system. The role of the water purification system is to produce water for dialysis that complies with set chemical and microbiologic standards.

DIALYZER DESIGNS

The dialyzer provides controllable transfer of solutes and water across the semipermeable membrane. The flows of dialysate and blood are separated and countercurrent. The dialyzer has four ports, one inlet and one outlet port each for blood and dialysate. The semipermeable dialysis membrane separates the blood compartment and the dialysate compartment. The transport processes across the membrane are diffusion (dialysis) and convection (ultrafiltration). The removal of small solutes occurs primarily by diffusion; larger components, such as β_2-microglobulin, are more effectively removed by convection. The hollow-fiber dialyzer is currently the most effective design; it delivers high dialysis efficiency with low resistance to flow in a small device.

DIALYSIS MEMBRANES

Membranes vary with respect to chemical structure, biophysical properties such as transport characteristics, and biocompatibility (Fig. 89.1).

Materials

The original widely used membrane material was cellulose, which is made up of repetitive polysaccharide units containing hydroxyl groups. In cellulose acetate, 80% of the hydroxyl groups are replaced by acetate radicals. Synthetic tertiary amino compounds are added during cellulose membrane synthesis to form cellulosynthetic membranes. More recent membranes are not cellulose based but instead are built of entirely synthetic materials, such as polyacrylonitrile, polysulfone, polycarbonate, polyamide, and polymethylmethacrylate. These synthetic membranes provide superior biocompatibility and are widely used.

Transport Properties

Transport of molecules across the dialysis membrane is due to (1) the concentration gradient (diffusive transport) and (2) the hydrostatic pressure gradient across the membrane (convective transport) and is dependent on membrane pore size. Dialyzer efficiency in terms of urea removal depends on the surface area (usually 0.8 to 2.1 m^2). High-efficiency dialyzers have a high surface area irrespective of pore size and possess a superior clearance for small molecules but may have small pores and thus a low ability to remove large molecules such as β_2-microglobulin. The dialyzer mass transfer area coefficient (K_oA) for urea is a measure of the theoretically maximal possible urea clearance (ml/min) at infinite blood and dialysate flow rates. Dialyzer efficiency can be categorized according to K_oA for urea as low (<500 ml/min), moderate (500 to 700 ml/min), and high (>700 ml/min). In contrast to the dialyzer clearance of a substance, its K_oA is independent of the flows in the blood and in the dialysate compartment. High-flux dialyzers have pores large enough to allow the passage of larger molecules such as β_2-microglobulin (M_r 11,800 d). Water permeability is described by the ultrafiltration coefficient (K_{uf}, in ml transmembrane ultrafiltration/h/mm Hg transmembrane pressure). K_{uf} is high in high-flux dialyzers, with ultrafiltration coefficients up to 80 ml/h/mm Hg. During high-flux HD, backfiltration (the flow of dialysate into the blood due to higher hydrostatic pressure on the dialysate side) may result in a transfer of 5 to 10 liters of dialysate into the blood. Therefore, water quality is of paramount importance when high-flux dialyzers are used.

In the recent prospective, randomized Membrane Permeability Outcome (MPO) study, a survival benefit of high-flux membranes was seen among patients with serum albumin levels of 4 g/dl or lower.[2] This finding contrasts with the HEMO study, which did not show any effect in patients with hypoalbuminemia but did show survival benefit in patients on dialysis for more than 3.7 years before the trial.[3] These differences may be related in

Dialysis Membrane Properties

Membrane	Membrane Name (example)	High or Low Flux	Biocompatibility
Cellulose	Cuprophane	Low	Low
Semisynthetic cellulose			
Cellulose diacetate	Cellulose acetate	High and low	Intermediate
Cellulose triacetate	Cellulose triacetate	High	Good
Diethylaminoethyl-substituted cellulose	Hemophane	High	Intermediate
Synthetic polymers			
Polymethylmethacrylate	PMMA	High	Good
Polyacrylonitrile methacrylate coplymer	PAN	High	Good
Polyacrylonitrile methallyl sulfonate copolymer	PAN/AN-69	High	Good
Polyamide	Polyflux	High and low	Good
Polycarbonate/polyether	Gambrane	High	Good
Polyethylene/vinyl alcohol	EVAL	High	Good
Polysulfone	Polysulfone	High and low	Good

Figure 89.1 Dialysis membrane properties.

part to population characteristics (race, recruitment of incident or prevalent patients) and fluxes achieved.

SAFETY MONITORS

Safety monitors are important integral parts of the dialysis machine. Pressure monitors are in most machines integrated to monitor the system pressure in critical positions[1] (Fig. 89.2):

- Between the arterial side and the blood pump (pre-pump arterial pressure) to assess the suction pressure. Overly negative values may signal reduced arterial inflow and access problems.
- Between the blood pump and the dialyzer inlet (post-pump or dialyzer inflow pressure) to assess the dialyzer inflow pressure. A high pressure may signal dialyzer clotting.
- Between the dialyzer outlet and the air trap (venous pressure) to control the return pressure. A high pressure may point to an obstruction in the venous limb; it is important to consider that in the event of venous needle displacement, the venous pressure will remain positive because of the needle's flow resistance, and no pressure alarm may occur.

A venous air detector and air trap are located downstream of the venous pressure monitor. A positive signal at the air detector automatically clamps the venous line and stops the blood pump. A blood leak detector is placed in the dialysate outflow line. Dialysate temperature is constantly monitored. Dialysate is produced by a proportioning system that mixes acid and bicarbonate concentrates with water. The osmolarity of the dialysate translates into conductivity, which is measured by the dialysis conductivity monitor. The ultrafiltration rate has to be controlled precisely, nowadays in most machines by a volumetric control system.

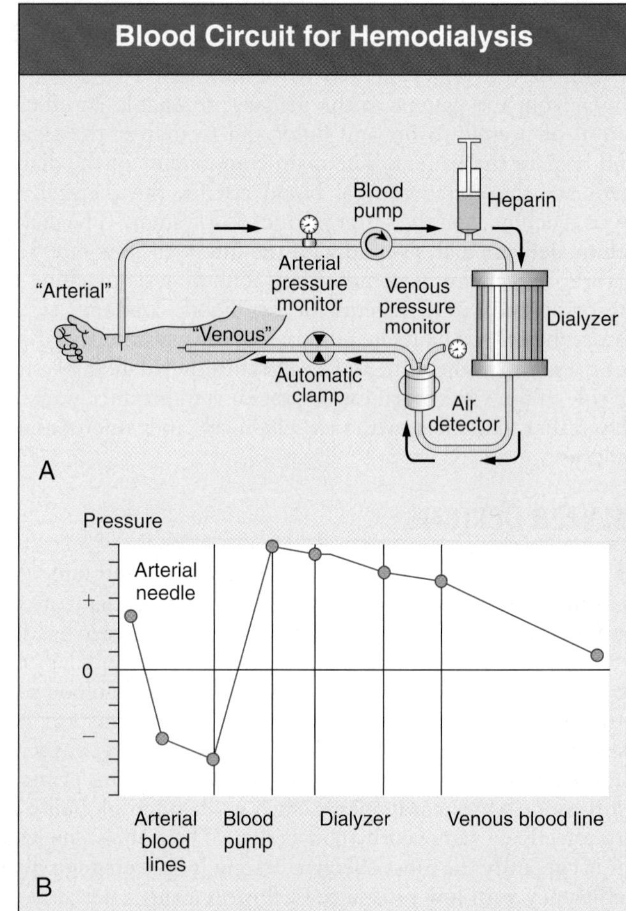

Figure 89.2 Blood circuit for hemodialysis. A, The blood circuit. **B,** The pressure profile in the blood circuit with an arteriovenous fistula as the vascular access.

ANTICOAGULATION

Usually unfractionated or, in some countries, low-molecular-weight (LMW) heparin is used to prevent blood clotting in the extracorporal circuit. Constant infusion of heparin, repeated bolus of heparin, or single bolus of LMW heparin is used. A number of alternative modalities are available for patients at high risk for bleeding or who have contraindications to heparin, such as saline flushes, regional citrate anticoagulation, prostacyclin, danaparoid, argatroban (direct thrombin inhibitor), and lepirudin (recombinant hirudin). Lepirudin has the disadvantage of very long half-life in dialysis patients. In some institutions, regional citrate anticoagulation is used routinely, especially in patients with recent surgery, coagulopathies, thrombocytopenia, active bleeding, pericarditis, and heparin-associated side effects (such as heparin-induced thrombocytopenia type II, pruritus, rapidly progressive osteoporosis, alopecia). Neutrophil activation may be reduced with regional citrate anticoagulation compared with heparin anticoagulation.

A typical routine prescription of constant infusion heparin is to administer an initial bolus of 2000 IU followed by a heparin infusion (800 to 1200 IU/h) ending 30 to 60 minutes before the end of the session. Applying the repeated bolus method, an initial heparin bolus of, for example, 4000 IU is followed by, for example, 1000 to 2000 IU after 2 hours Although the half-life of LMW heparin may be prolonged with renal failure, it has proved safe with fewer bleeding episodes, if appropriate dose reductions are made. LMW heparin has become the anticoagulant of choice in many centers in Europe for routine outpatient HD sessions. LMW heparin is given as a bolus at the beginning of the session. Routine monitoring of whole-blood partial thromboplastin time, activated clotting time, or factor Xa (with LMW heparin) is usually not necessary.

DIALYSATE FLUID

Water and Water Treatment

A standard 4-hour HD session exposes the patient to 120 to 160 liters of water. Therefore, water quality is of paramount importance to the patient's well-being. Water for the dialysate may be subjected to filtration, softening, and deionization, but it is ultimately purified in most centers by reverse osmosis. Reverse osmosis entails forcing water through a semipermeable membrane at very high pressure to remove microbiologic contaminants and more than 90% of dissolved ions.

Standards for chemical quality of water are widely accepted, but there is less consensus as to acceptable levels of bacterial and endotoxin contamination.[4] Municipal water supplies may contain a variety of contaminants that are toxic to HD patients. Substances added to the water, such as aluminum and chloramines, cause significant morbidity. Aluminum accumulation may result in a severe neurologic disorder (speech abnormalities, muscle spasms, seizures, and dementia), bone disease, and erythropoietin-resistant anemia. Plasma aluminum concentration should be monitored regularly; levels should be less than 1 μmol/l, and levels above 2 μmol/l should prompt the search for excessive exposure (aluminum-based phosphate binders may be an important source). Chloramines have been associated with hemolysis and methemoglobinemia. Copper and zinc may leach from plumbing components and may cause hemolysis. Lead has been associated with abdominal pain and muscle weakness. Nitrate and nitrite may cause nausea and seizures. High concentrations of calcium may cause the hard water syndrome, characterized by acute hypercalcemia and hypomagnesemia, hemodynamic instability, nausea, vomiting, muscle weakness, and somnolence.

Gram-negative bacteria produce endotoxins (pyrogenic lipopolysaccharides from the outer bacterial cell wall), and fragments of these endotoxins may be responsible for some dialysis-related symptoms. Exposure to bacteria and endotoxin is associated with rigors, hypotension, and fever; even low levels of microbiologic contaminants may contribute to chronic inflammation in HD patients. Bacteria may proliferate in the biofilm, a coating on surfaces consisting of microcolonies of bacteria embedded in an extracellular matrix secreted by the cells, protecting the bacteria from antibiotics and disinfectants. The microbiologic standards for HD water, acid and basic concentrates, dialysis fluid, and online substitution fluid vary between regions (Fig. 89.3).[4] The harm done by the passage of endotoxin through the dialysis membrane by backfiltration includes stimulation of inflammation, decreased response to erythropoiesis-stimulating agents, and possible aggravation of atherosclerosis. Use of a polysulfone or polyamide filter in the dialysate line may be adequate to remove endotoxins, but smaller molecules including bacterial DNA fragments may pass through the dialyzer and stimulate immune cells. In the absence of routine hot-water disinfection of the machine and the connections to the water loop, the only way that endotoxin concentration can be kept low is by frequent measurement and disinfection when concentration exceeds accepted standards.

Ultrapure water is defined as bacterial count below 0.1 colony-forming unit/ml and endotoxin below 0.03 endotoxin unit/ml and is recommended by both European and American guidelines for use with high-flux dialyzers. Ultrapure water represents a basic prerequisite for dialysis modalities using online production of substitution fluid (online hemofiltration or hemodiafiltration).

Liquid bicarbonate dialysis fluid concentrate distributed in a central system with piping may be a source of bacterial growth. Acid concentrates in canisters and bicarbonate powder represent no bacterial growth risk.

Dialysis Solution

Dialysis fluid can be considered a drug to be adjusted to the individual patient's needs. In modern machines, dialysate is made by mixing two concentrate components, which may be provided as liquid or dry (powder) concentrates. The bicarbonate component contains sodium bicarbonate and sodium chloride; the acid component contains chloride salts of sodium, potassium (if needed), calcium, magnesium, acetate (or citrate), and glucose (optional). These two components are mixed simultaneously with purified water to make the dialysate. Dialysate proportioning pumps ensure proper mixing. The relative amounts of water, bicarbonate, and acid components define the final dialysate composition. Bicarbonate has replaced acetate as the dialysate buffer in most countries. Typical concentrations of dialysate components are given in Figure 89.4. Dialysate containing citrate (0.8 mmol/l) has recently been introduced, which may allow a reduction in heparin dose. Dialysate composition can be further modified by changing the mixing fraction and by adding salt solutions; potential advantages and disadvantages of dialysate modifications are shown in Figure 89.5. Modern machines allow an alteration of the bicarbonate concentration by changing the mixing ratio of water to bicarbonate. A variable sodium option allows the adaptation of the dialysate sodium concentration to the patient's needs. Glucose is usually added to prevent intradialytic hypoglycemia, but glucose concentrations of 200 mg/dl (11 mmol/l) may result in hyperglycemia and hyperinsulinemia.

Microbiologic Standards for Water, Concentrates, and Dialysis Fluids[4]

National and International Standards	Year Issued	Microorganisms, CFU/mL	Endotoxins, EU/mL
Water			
EDTA	2001	<100	<0.25
USA (AAMI RD 52)	2004	200 (alert 50)	2 (alert 1)
ISO/DIS 13959 (draft)	2009	100	0.25
Concentrates (acid and basic)			
USA (AAMI RD 52)	2004	200 (alert 50)	2 (alert 1)
Ph Eur, 5th ed.	2005	—	<0.5*
Dialysis fluid			
EDTA	2001	<100	<0.25
USA (AAMI RD 52)	2004	200 (alert 50)	2 (alert 1)
ISO/DIS 11663 (draft)	2009	100 (alert 50)	0.5
Ultrapure dialysis fluid prior to last filter for hemodiafiltration on-line			
EDTA	2001	<0.1	<0.03
USA (AAMI RD 52)	2004	0.1	0.03
ISO/DIS 11663	2009	<0.1	<0.03
Substitution fluid on-line			
EDTA	2001	$<10^{-6}$	<0.25
USA (AAMI RD 52)	2004	$<10^{-6}$	<0.03
ISO/DIS 11663	2009	Sterile	Non-pyrogenic

EDTA = European Dialysis and Transplant Association; Ph Eur = European Pharmacopoeia: AAMI = Association for the Advancement of Medical Instrumentation; ISO/DIS = International Organization for Standardization/Draft International Standard.

Figure 89.3 Microbiologic standards for water, concentrates, and dialysis fluids.[4] EDTA, European Dialysis and Transplant Association; Ph Eur, European Pharmacopoeia; AAMI, Association for the Advancement of Medical Instrumentation; ISO/DIS, International Organization for Standardization/Draft International Standard. *Diluted to user concentration.

Composition of Dialysates for Bicarbonate Dialysis

Component	Concentration: Range	Concentration: Typical
Electrolytes (mmol/l)		
Sodium	135–145	140
Potassium	0–4.0	2.0
Calcium	0–2.0	1.25
Magnesium	0.5–1.0	0.75
Chloride	87–124	105
Buffers (mmol/l)		
Acetate	2–4	3
Bicarbonate	20–40	35
pH	7.1–7.3	7.2
PCO_2 (mmHg)	40–100	
Glucose	0–11 (0–200 mg/dl)	5.5 (100 mg/dl)

Figure 89.4 Composition of dialysates for bicarbonate dialysis.

To avoid the need for large volumes of water, spent dialysate can be regenerated by sorbents. These systems may need as little as 6 liters of tap water for a regular dialysis treatment, which makes them particularly attractive for home HD or arid areas.

BIOCOMPATIBILITY

The contact of blood with lines and some types of membranes triggers an inflammatory response akin to that seen in infection. Biocompatibility indicates a membrane that does not produce a toxic, injurious, or immunologic response on contact with blood. Although many components of the dialysis procedure contribute to the degree of biocompatibility, it is the membrane itself that is most important. Biocompatibility is of particular importance with the use of cellulose membranes, whereas synthetic membranes and reused membranes activate complement to a much lesser extent (see Fig. 89.1). Blood contact with the dialysis membrane activates the complement cascade (most prominent in cellulose membranes), the coagulation cascade, and cellular mechanisms (Fig. 89.6). Activation of complement peaks at 15 minutes after the start of dialysis and lasts up to 90 minutes. Regional citrate anticoagulation may improve biocompatibility by reduced granulocyte degranulation.[5] Dialyzer reuse with appropriate antibacterial substances is also associated with improved biocompatibility.

HEMOFILTRATION

Hemofiltration (HF; Fig. 89.7) differs markedly from HD in the mechanisms by which the composition of the blood is modified. In the simplest form of HF, blood under pressure passes down one side of a highly permeable membrane, allowing both water and substances up to about 20 kd to pass across the membrane by convective flow, depending on the membrane and its permeability. During HF, the filtrate is discarded and the patient receives a substitution fluid either before (predilution) or after (postdilution) the dialyzer. The substitution fluid contains the major crystalloid components of the plasma at physiologic levels. Both bicarbonate and lactate are used as buffers. The rate of fluid removal and substitution fluid infusion can be adapted to the patient's need. HF is particularly useful as a continuous renal replacement therapy in an intensive care setting.[6]

Advantages and Disadvantages of Modifications of Dialysate Composition

Component	Advantage	Disadvantage
Sodium		
Increased	Hemodynamic stability	Thirst; intradialytic weight gain; high blood pressure; sodium toxicity?
Decreased	Reduced osmotic stress in the presence of predialytic hyponatremia	Intradialytic hemodynamic instability
Potassium		
Increased	Fewer arrhythmias in digoxin intoxication with hypokalemia; may improve hemodynamic stability	Hyperkalemia
Decreased	Increased dietary potassium intake	Arrhythmias; risk of sudden death
Calcium		
Increased	Suppresses PTH, increased hemodynamic stability	Hypercalcemia, vascular calcification, adynamic bone disease due to PTH suppression
Decreased	Permits more liberal use of calcium containing phosphate binders	Stimulation of PTH, reduced hemodynamic stability
Bicarbonate		
Increased	Acidosis control improved	Postdialytic alkalosis; increased mortality
Decreased	No postdialytic alkalosis	Promotes acidosis; increased mortality
Magnesium		
Increased	Hemodynamic stability, less arrhythmias, suppresses PTH	Altered nerve conduction, pruritus, renal bone disease
Decreased	Permits use of magnesium containing phosphate binders; improved bone mineralization; less bone pain	Arrhythmias, muscle weakness and cramps, elevated PTH
Glucose		
Decreased	Avoidance of intradialytic hyperglycemia and hyperinsulinemia	Increased risk of disequilibrium (rare), hypoglycemia
Increased	Lower risk of disequilibrium	Intradialytic hyperglycemia and hyperinsulinism
Citrate	Heparin-sparing effect	High blood citrate levels in liver failure

Figure 89.5 Advantages and disadvantages of modifications in the dialysate composition. PTH, parathyroid hormone. *(Modified from http://www.kidneyatlas.org/book5/adk5-02.ccc.QXD.pdf.)*

HEMODIAFILTRATION

Hemodiafiltration (HDF; Fig. 89.8) combines the benefits of HD (high transport rate of low-molecular-weight solutes by diffusion) and HF (high convective transport of substances). HDF is used as both a continuous and an intermittent renal replacement therapy. HDF offers potential benefits regarding anemia correction, inflammation, oxidative stress, lipid profiles, and calcium-phosphate product.[7] Higher costs and, in some countries, the decisions of regulatory boards concerning fluid infusion prevent the widespread use of HDF, despite its likely benefits over conventional HD. Randomized controlled trials of HD and HDF will determine its true value.

DIALYSIS TIMES

HD has conventionally been delivered in three treatment sessions per week. This developed as a practical compromise between the physiologic benefits of replacing renal function by HD ("the more the better") and the practicalities of delivering HD in terms of both the patient's tolerability and the facility's organization. There is good evidence that twice-weekly HD provides inferior outcomes to three times weekly, except in occasional patients with substantial residual renal function. Treatment times of 3 to 4 hours per session are now typical, but a few centers have maintained the longer hours (up to 8 hours per session) that were originally necessary because of the relative inefficiency of the available HD techniques. It remains controversial whether the excellent long-term outcomes of patients receiving prolonged HD are related to selection bias rather than real advantages. If longer hours of HD were of proven benefit, this would provide major planning challenges to HD units organized around three times weekly shorter HD and might renew interest in nocturnal HD either in the home or in treatment facilities.

Two large trials organized by the Frequent Hemodialysis Network (FHN) are currently under way to investigate the effect of increased HD frequency on outcomes.[8] Primary endpoints are changes in left ventricular mass as measured by magnetic resonance imaging and quality of life, including cognitive measures. One FHN randomized trial is comparing in-center six times per week short daily HD versus conventional three times per week in-center HD. The other is comparing nocturnal home HD with conventional in-center HD. The results of these trials may become available in 2010.

ADDITIONAL DEVICES AND TECHNOLOGIES

Blood Volume Monitoring

A decrease in blood volume due to ultrafiltration is one of the main causes of intradialytic hypotension. Blood volume monitors provide continuous noninvasive monitoring of relative changes in blood volume by continuous measurement of plasma protein concentration by ultrasound or of hematocrit by optical scattering. Too rapid changes in blood volume from baseline indicate decreased plasma refilling rates and may precede intradialytic hypotension. Blood volume monitoring can be particularly useful for monitoring of hemodynamically unstable dialysis patients. Because blood volume is only loosely related to the volume of the extracellular fluid, monitoring of relative blood volume is of no help in determining dry weight.[9] In some dialysis machines,

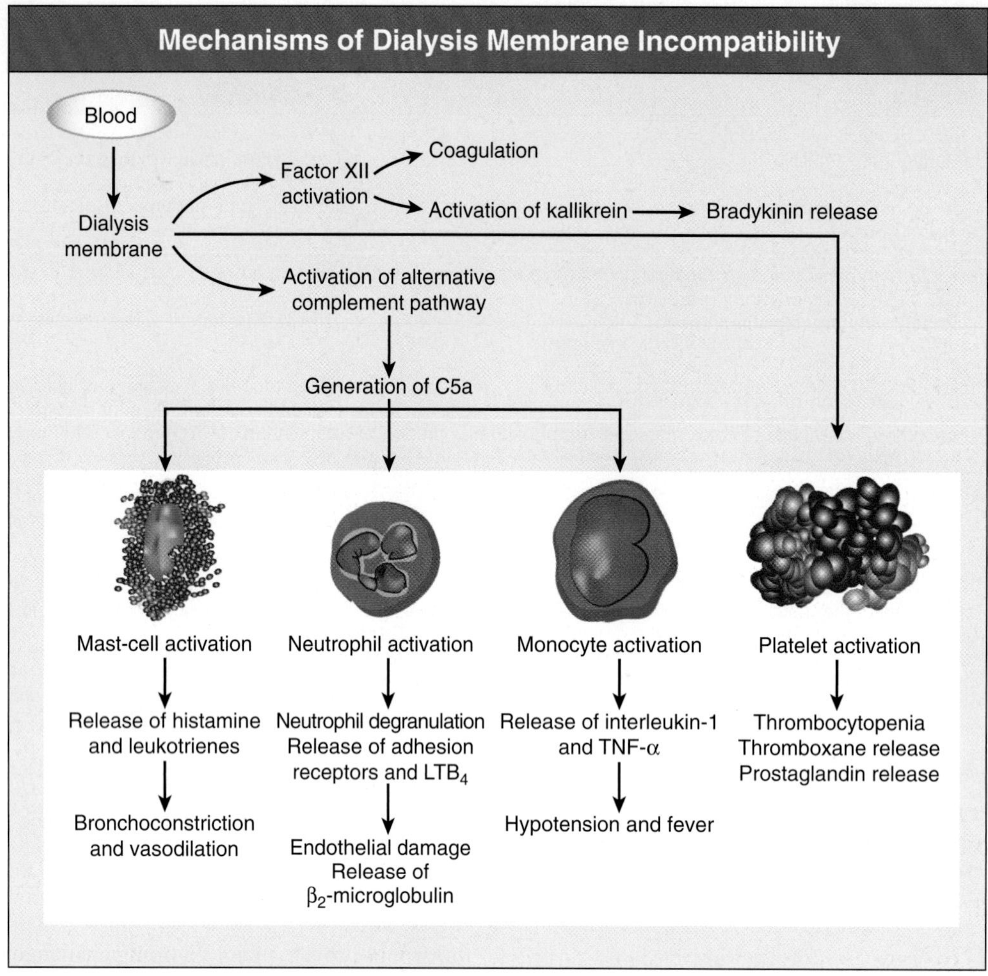

Figure 89.6 Mechanisms of dialysis membrane incompatibility. Pathways involved in the body's response to dialysis membranes. LTB_4, leukotriene B_4; TNF-α, tumor necrosis factor α.

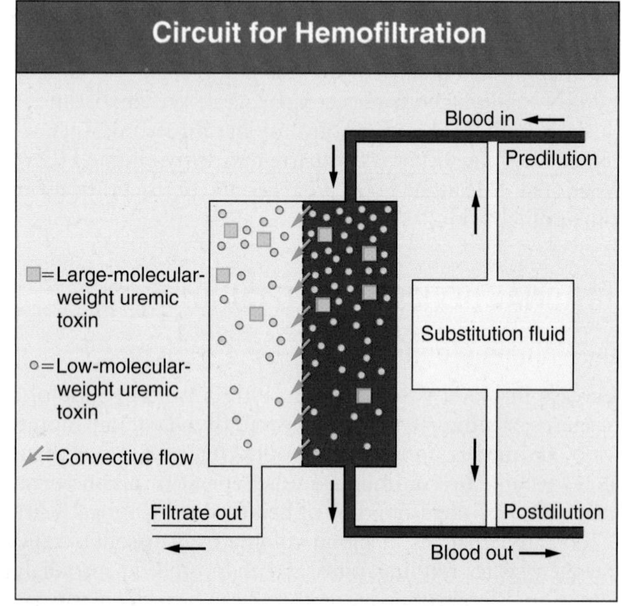

Figure 89.7 The principle of hemofiltration. Substitution fluid is usually given either pre- or postdilution, but not both.

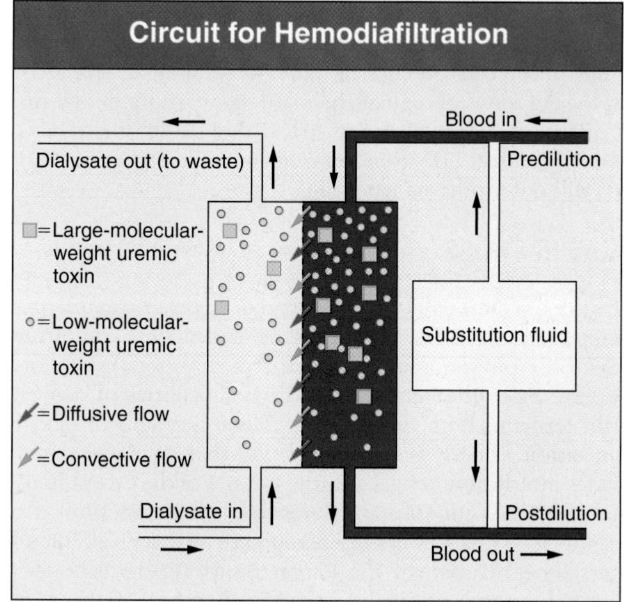

Figure 89.8 The principle of hemodiafiltration. Substitution fluid is usually given either pre- or postdilution, but not both.

blood volume monitor signals are used to automatically adjust ultrafiltration rates. This approach has been shown to reduce the frequency of symptomatic intradialytic hypotension.[10]

Ultrafiltration Profiling

The ultrafiltration rate is usually kept constant but can be changed during the dialysis session in a preprogrammed manner (ultrafiltration profiling). It may be advantageous to remove a large proportion (e.g., two thirds) of the ultrafiltration volume in the first half of the HD session. Because of a high initial plasma refilling rate, severely overhydrated patients may tolerate a higher ultrafiltration rate in the early stages, and dry weight may be reached more easily. In some machines, predefined ultrafiltration profiles are incorporated, for example, triangular ultrafiltration ramps and exponential profiles; in most instances, the ultrafiltration rate is initially high and then turned down. The clinical benefits of ultrafiltration profiling are under debate; in the absence of clear evidence-based recommendations, we suggest that ultrafiltration profiling be considered in patients prone to intradialytic complications, such as hypotensive episodes.

Sodium Profiling

The dialysate sodium concentration is normally kept constant throughout the dialysis treatment. The variable sodium option allows dynamic changes of the dialysate sodium concentration during the treatment (sodium profiling). Although high-grade evidence is lacking, patients with hemodynamic instability may benefit from sodium profiling in which the initial sodium concentration is kept high and then slowly reduced by a degree similar to the initial sodium rise. Otherwise, sodium profiling usually results in a sodium load to the patient in the absence of equivalent reductions in dialysate sodium concentrations that may result in thirst and consequent increased interdialytic weight gain.

Online Clearance Monitoring

Sodium and urea clearances are identical for practical purposes. Because the conductivity of the dialysate is largely a function of the dialysate sodium concentration, online clearance monitors can use this feature to compute the urea clearance (*K*) of a dialyzer. Changes in inflow dialysate sodium concentration are related to the respective changes of conductivity in the dialysate outflow. The conductivity clearance is equivalent to urea clearance, and *Kt* is easily calculated. Together with estimates of *V* (total body water), *Kt/V* can be determined with each treatment.

Blood Temperature Monitoring

During standard HD, the core temperature usually increases. Because the thermoregulatory response to rising core temperature (dilation of thermoregulatory vessels) may offset the vascular response to hypovolemia (vasoconstriction), this increase in internal heat production might be in part responsible for the intradialytic hemodynamic instability. Reducing dialysate temperature to a level of 0.5°C below core temperature is in general safe. "Cool" dialysate has been shown to improve vascular stability during dialysis. The core temperature can be controlled by the blood temperature monitor, which adapts the dialysate temperature according to the desired core temperature. A meta-analysis of 22 studies concluded that intradialytic hypotension occurred 7.1 times less frequently with cool dialysis[11] without reduction in urea clearance. When no blood temperature monitor is available, the dialysate temperature can be set initially to the patient's core temperature. If this is well tolerated and intradialytic hypotension still occurs, the dialysate temperature may be reduced up to 0.5°C below the patient's core temperature, unless cold discomfort occurs.

Hemodiafiltration

High-volume HDF (removal and replacement of up to 50 liters per treatment) is in common use in parts of Europe and Asia. The beneficial effects are controversial, but a study suggests favorable short-term outcomes. A large trial of 800 chronic HD patients randomized between online HDF and low-flux HD observed for 3 years is under way with all-cause mortality as the primary endpoint.[12]

Sorbents, Nanotechnology, Wearable Artificial Kidney

Use of sorbents to absorb nondialyzable molecules will test the relevance as uremic toxins of the many protein-derived substances that accumulate in the plasma of uremic patients. Nanotechnological approaches to dialysis therapy are under intensive investigation.[13] A study has reported the successful short-term use of a wearable artificial kidney.[14]

REFERENCES

1. Misra M. The basics of hemodialysis equipment. *Hemodial Int.* 2005;9:30-36.
2. Locatelli F, Martin-Malo A, Hannedouche T, et al. Effect of membrane permeability on survival of hemodialysis patients. *J Am Soc Nephrol.* 2009;20:645-654.
3. Eknoyan G, Beck GJ, Cheung AK, et al. Effect of dialysis dose and membrane flux in maintenance hemodialysis. *N Engl J Med.* 2002; 347:2010-2019.
4. Nystrand R. Microbiology of water and fluids for hemodialysis. *J Chin Med Assoc.* 2008;71:223-229.
5. Bohler J, Schollmeyer P, Dressel B, et al. Reduction of granulocyte activation during hemodialysis with regional citrate anticoagulation: Dissociation of complement activation and neutropenia from neutrophil degranulation. *J Am Soc Nephrol.* 1996;7:234-241.
6. Forni LG, Hilton PJ. Continuous hemofiltration in the treatment of acute renal failure. *N Engl J Med.* 1997;336:1303-1309.
7. Vaslaki L, Major L, Berta K, et al. On-line haemodiafiltration versus haemodialysis: Stable haematocrit with less erythropoietin and improvement of other relevant blood parameters. *Blood Purif.* 2006;24:163-173.
8. Suri RS, Garg AX, Chertow GM, et al. Frequent Hemodialysis Network (FHN) randomized trials: Study design. *Kidney Int.* 2007;71:349-359.
9. Raimann J, Liu L, Tyagi S, et al. A fresh look at dry weight. *Hemodial Int.* 2008;12:395-405.
10. Santoro A, Mancini E, Basile C, et al. Blood volume controlled hemodialysis in hypotension-prone patients: A randomized, multicenter controlled trial. *Kidney Int.* 2002;62:1034-1045.
11. Selby NM, McIntyre CW. A systematic review of the clinical effects of reducing dialysate fluid temperature. *Nephrol Dial Transplant.* 2006;21:1883-1898.
12. Penne EL, Blankestijn PJ, Bots ML, et al. Resolving controversies regarding hemodiafiltration versus hemodialysis: The Dutch Convective Transport Study. *Semin Dial.* 2005;18:47-51.
13. Cruz D, Bellomo R, Kellum JA, de Cal M, Ronco. The future of extracorporeal support. *Crit Care Med.* 2008;(Suppl 4):S243-S252.
14. Davenport A, Gura V, Ronco C, et al. A wearable haemodialysis device for patients with end-stage renal failure: A pilot study. *Lancet.* 2007; 370:2005-2010.

CHAPTER 90

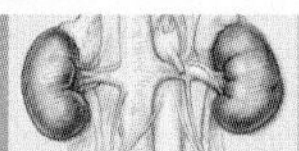

Hemodialysis: Outcomes and Adequacy

Martin K. Kuhlmann, Peter Kotanko, Nathan W. Levin

From an idealistic clinical perspective, an adequately treated hemodialysis (HD) patient is physically active, well nourished, nonanemic, and nonhypertensive with a maintained quality of life and a life expectancy that is not inferior to that of healthy subjects. Despite these idealistic goals, outcomes for dialysis patients expressed in terms of mortality, hospitalization, and quality of life regrettably remain comparable to those observed in patients with solid organ cancer. The mean life expectancy of an average 60-year-old HD patient currently can be estimated between 5 and 7 years, with an annual mortality rate between 13% and 20% (*www.usrds.org*). Mortality in HD patients differs by gender and race; in the United States, there is lower mortality in African Americans compared with Caucasians, in Hispanics compared with non-Hispanics, and in Asians compared with any other racial group. Data from the Dialysis Outcomes and Practice Pattern Study (DOPPS) suggest that variations in practice patterns, such as prescribed dialysis treatment time, average epoetin dose, preferred vascular access type, and number of patients with central venous catheters, may account for some of these differences. Outcomes are also directly related to comorbid factors occurring during evolution of chronic kidney disease (CKD), such as atherosclerotic vascular disease, diabetes, and arterial hypertension, and to background cardiovascular mortality of the respective general population.[1] Indeed, the majority of CKD patients die mainly of cardiovascular causes before reaching end-stage renal disease (ESRD). Besides cardiovascular disease (discussed further in Chapter 78), other major factors influencing outcome that are common to all patients with ESRD include anemia (see Chapter 79) and control of bone and mineral metabolism (see Chapter 81).

In this chapter, we discuss dialysis-related factors influencing outcome in patients receiving maintenance HD (see summary in Fig. 90.1). A key factor influencing outcome is "adequacy" of dialysis, a term originally used exclusively to describe dialysis dosing measured by small solute removal. However, dialysis adequacy now has a broader meaning encompassing all aspects of the replacement of excretory and endocrine functions of the kidney that affect outcome.

Unfortunately, randomized, controlled trials are few in HD, and lower grades of evidence support the published clinical practice guidelines, which are listed in Figure 90.2.

ADEQUACY OF DIALYSIS DOSE

Uremic Toxins

The retention in the body of compounds that normally are metabolized or secreted into the urine by healthy kidneys results in the uremic syndrome. These compounds are called uremic retention solutes or uremic toxins when they interact negatively with biologic functions. Uremic toxins include a small group of inorganic compounds, such as water, potassium, phosphate, and trace elements, and a much larger group of organic compounds that are further subdivided into small water-soluble solutes (<500 d), middle molecules (>500 d), and protein-bound solutes (Fig. 90.3). A continuously updated list of uremic toxins is provided at *http://www.uremic-toxins.org/*. The catalogue of uremic toxins is long, but only a few compounds have been associated with outcomes. Mortality has repeatedly been shown to be associated with the clearance of urea. Of commonly measured protein-derived substances, only the serum concentration of β_2-microglobulin correlates with mortality. Recently, a higher free concentration of the protein-bound solute *p*-cresol has also been reported to be associated with mortality.[2] Uremic toxicity is more than the retention of urea or water-soluble compounds alone, but current dialysis and dialysis-related treatments do not remove any significant quantity of substances larger than 10 to 15 kd. Future means of removing higher molecular weight toxins or protein-bound substances may include the use of sorbents in addition to traditional diffusive and convective dialysis strategies.

Urea as a Surrogate Marker of Uremic Toxicity

Among all potential uremic toxins, only urea, a 60-dalton small water-soluble compound, is established as a classic marker of uremic solute retention and removal. Urea, which itself shows little toxicity, is a metabolite of amino acid metabolism; urea generation therefore depends on protein intake and the balance between protein anabolism and catabolism. The removal of urea was originally considered to be representative for the removal of other water-soluble solutes with a higher pathogenic impact, although it is now clear that urea removal does not closely parallel that of other small water-soluble compounds, protein-bound solutes, or middle molecules.[3] Nevertheless, adequacy of HD dosing remains conventionally evaluated by removal of urea.

Assessment of Dialysis Dose

Adequacy in terms of dialysis dose refers to delivery of a treatment dose that is considered sufficient to promote an optimal long-term outcome. The delivered dose of dialysis is assessed by the removal of urea and expressed either by the urea reduction ratio or by the treatment index *Kt/V*. Simply following predialysis blood urea nitrogen (BUN) or serum urea is insufficient; low serum urea may much more reflect malnutrition due to inadequate protein intake rather than adequate dialysis urea removal.

Factors Related to Dialysis Outcomes			
Factor	**Effects of Dialysis**	**Effect on Dialysis**	**Effect on Outcome**
Patient Characteristics			
Age		Hemodynamic instability	Profound increase in CV disease
Gender		Intensified therapy in case of pregnancy	Possible interaction with increased dialysis dose
Race/Ethnicity			Definite effects on cardiac outcomes esp. atherosclerosis
Body size (BMI)		Requires longer Tx-time	Small people worse outcomes
Comorbidities			
Diabetes mellitus	Worse metabolic control; falsely low Hb_{A1C}	Autonomic dysfunction→ ↑ IDWG	Increased mortality due to CVD; increased risk of calciphylaxis
Arterial hypertension	Increase or decrease	low BP→ ↑ dialysis time; high BP→↓ dry weight	Both low and high blood pressure associated with ↑mortality
Cardiomyopathy	May be worsened	Makes UF difficult	Associated with poorer survival
Depression	Dialysis dose; organizational issues	Missed treatments Incompliance	Increased morbidity, reduced QoL
Transplant eligibility	May be improved by dialysis adequacy	Use of HDF in non-eligible patients	Lower mortality in patients on waiting list
Anemia			
Hemoglobin (Hb)	Rises during ultrafiltration	High Hb may limit phosphate elimination	Low Hb associated with LVH High Hb associated with access thrombosis and mortality
Epo resistance	May be improved by adequate dialysis dose	Switch from catheter to fistula	Association with poor survival
Epo variability			Possibly associated with poor outcomes
Mineral and Bone Disease			
PTH	↑ with low dialysate Ca^{++} ↓ with high dialysate Ca^{++}	Hypocalcemia→vascular instability	↑PTH possibly related to morbidity and mortality
Vitamin D		Hypocalcemia→vascular instability	Associated with osteomalacia Vit D use associated with increased survival
Hyperphosphatemia	Affected by dialysis time and frequency		Increased morbidity and mortality,
Nutrition/Inflammation			
Inflammation	Induced by dialysate impurities and bioincompatibility	Choice of access	Increased morbidity and mortality induces Epo resistance
Protein-energy malnutrition	Affected by dialysis dose, membrane flux	Volume control poorer	Increased morbidity and mortality
Low serum albumin	Induced by dialysate impurities	May limit refilling of plasma volume	Risk of IDH, increased morbidity and mortality
Overhydration	Increased with positive sodium balance	Easier dialysis due to rapid plasma refilling	Increased morbidity and mortality Increased BP and LVH
Central venous catheter		Reduced dialysis dose due to low QB, thrombosis and infection	Increased mortality, Epo resistance, inflammation
Beta-2 microglobulin	↓ with high flux dialyzers		High plasma concentration associated with mortality

Figure 90.1 Factors related to dialysis outcome. BMI, body mass index; BP, blood pressure; CVD, cardiovascular disease; EPO, erythropoietin; HDF, hemodiafiltration; IDH, intradialytic hypotension; IDWG, interdialytic weight gain; LVH, left ventricular hypertrophy; PTH, parathyroid hormone; *Qb*, blood flow rate; QoL, quality of life; Tx, treatment; UF, ultrafiltration.

If urea removal is inadequate, then dialysis is inadequate, regardless of the serum urea level.

Intradialytic Urea Kinetics

Dialyzers are highly efficient in removal of urea from the blood, reducing the urea concentration during one passage by 80% to 90%. Intradialytic serum urea kinetics were originally described by single-compartment (single-pool) models, assuming that full equilibration between blood and tissue compartments occurs immediately and without time delay. In such models, the change in BUN follows first-order kinetics, with a linear decline and no urea rebound (Fig. 90.4, *dashed line*). *In vivo,* however, intercompartmental urea redistribution is delayed, and the intradialytic urea concentration in the blood compartment is always lower than in the tissue compartments. Full equilibration between blood and tissue compartments is only completed by 30 to 60 minutes after dialysis. These features of urea kinetics are more accurately described by double-pool models that take into account delayed intercompartmental urea redistribution and postdialysis urea rebound (Fig. 90.4, *solid line*).

Current methods for assessment of dialysis dose are based on the predialysis and postdialysis difference in BUN and include the urea reduction ratio (URR), the single-pool *Kt/V* (*spKt/V*), the equilibrated *Kt/V* (*eKt/V*), and the weekly standard *Kt/V* (*std-Kt/V*).

Web-Based Resources
Guidelines
NKF-KDOQI (National Kidney Foundation–Kidney Disease Outcomes Quality Initiative); http://www.kidney.org/professionals/kdoqi/guidelines.cfm
European Best Practice Guidelines for Haemodialysis (Part 1)–European Renal Association–European Dialysis and Transplant Association http://www.ndt-educational.org/guidelinesvanbiesen.asp
CARI (Caring for Australians with Renal Impairment)–Australian and New Zealand Society of Nephrology (ANZSN) and Kidney Health Australia (KHA) http://www.cari.org.au/guidelines.php
KDIGO (Kidney Disease Improving Global Outcomes); international cooperation in the development and implementation of clinical practice guidelines in nephrology; http://www.kdigo.org
The Renal Association (UK) guidelines provide a template for the management of patients with kidney disease in the UK http://www.renal.org/Clinical/GuidelinesSection/Guidelines.aspx
Canadian Society of Nephrology Clinical Practice Guidelines, 1999; http://csnscn.ca/local/files/guidelines/CSN-Guidelines-1999.pdf
National Guideline Clearinghouse lists an index of clinical practice guidelines of various organizations; http://www.guideline.gov/index.aspx
Foundations, Associations and Initiatives
USRDS (United States Renal Data System); comprehensive analyses of renal disease epidemiology in United States; http://www.usrds.org
NKF (National Kidney Foundation); committed to education of healthcare professionals and public, research support, expanding healthcare resources, and shaping health policies in the field of nephrology; http://www.kidney.org
Kidney and Urology Foundation of America; promoting renal research and accessibility of new therapies to renal disease patients; http://www.kidneyurology.org/
HDCN (Hypertension, Dialysis and Clinical Nephrology); an official educational program of Renal Physicians Association and American Society of Nephrology; http://www.hdcn.com

Figure 90.2 Web-based resources for hemodialysis.

Urea Reduction Ratio

URR refers to the treatment-related reduction of serum urea concentration and is computed as follows:

$$\text{URR}(\%) = (1 - C_t/C_0) \times 100\%$$

where C_t is postdialysis and C_0 is predialysis serum urea concentration.

URR is a simple but rather imprecise way to quantify dialysis dose because it does not take into account intradialytic urea generation and convective urea removal by ultrafiltration. Despite these limitations, URR correlates well with dialysis outcome and is an accepted method for assessment of dialysis adequacy. A minimum URR of 65% to 70% is recommended for adequate HD.

Treatment Index *Kt/V*

The treatment index *Kt/V* is the most widely used parameter to assess dialysis dose. *Kt/V* is a dimensionless number representing volume cleared ($K \times t$, in liters) divided by volume of distribution (V, in liters). The concept of *Kt/V* may be applied to any substance but in clinical practice is almost exclusively used for urea, where K is the dialyzer blood water urea clearance (liters per hour), t is dialysis session length (hours), and V is the distribution volume of urea (liters), which equates closely to total body water. A delivered *Kt/V* of 1.0 implies that the volume of plasma cleared of urea ($K \times t$) during a dialysis session is equal to urea distribution volume (V). *Kt/V* and URR are mathematically linked by the following equation:

$$Kt/V = -\ln(1 - \text{URR})$$

where ln represents the natural logarithm.

Accordingly, *Kt/V* equals 1.0 when URR equals 0.63, or 63% of whole-body urea has been removed. The equation is formally based on a single-pool model and does not take into account intradialytic urea generation and convective urea removal by ultrafiltration. This formula, however, has built the basis for further development of *spKt/V* and *eKt/V* equations.

Single-Pool *Kt/V* (*spKt/V*)

Daugirdas[4] has adjusted the equation for intradialytic urea generation and for ultrafiltration volume. His second-generation formula is validated for a *Kt/V* range between 0.8 and 2.0 and is widely used because of its simplicity and accuracy.

$$spKt/V = -\ln(R - 0.008 \times t) + (4 - 3.5 \times R) \times UF/W$$

where ln is the natural logarithm, R is the postdialysis/predialysis serum urea ratio, t is the treatment time (hours), UF is ultrafiltration volume (liters), and W is the patient's postdialysis body weight (kilograms).

Accurate computation of *spKt/V* requires a nonequilibrated post-HD serum urea concentration and accurate timing of blood collections. Pre-HD blood samples must be collected right at the start of the treatment and post-HD samples immediately after termination of dialysis, at the beginning of urea rebound. The nonequilibrated post-HD serum urea concentration is always lower than the equilibrated value, and thus nonequilibrated URR and *Kt/V* values are always higher than the respective equilibrated values.

Equilibrated *Kt/V* (*eKt/V*)

Dialysis dose is more accurately estimated by *eKt/V* based on the equilibrated postdialysis serum urea concentration. The amount of urea rebound depends on the intensity of dialysis: the shorter and more intense a treatment, the higher the urea rebound. Rebound can be predicted from nonequilibrated postdialysis serum urea concentration and the intensity of the dialysis treatment expressed as the number of *Kt/V* units per hour (*Kt/V* per time unit = *K/V*):

$$eKt/V = spKt/V - (0.6 \times spK/V) - 0.03 \text{ (arterial access)}$$

The *arterial* access equation is valid only for dialysis treatments using arterial access, such as arteriovenous fistulas or grafts. For treatments using central venous catheters, in which cardiopulmonary recirculation is less and rebound therefore lower, the following *venous* access equation should be applied:

$$eKt/V = spKt/V - (0.47 \times spK/V) - 0.02 \text{ (venous access)}$$

Organic Uremic Solutes

Free Water-Soluble Low-Molecular-Weight Solutes	MW	Protein-Bound Solutes	MW	Middle Molecules	MW
Guanidines		**AGE**		**Cytokines**	
ADMA	202	3-Deoxyglucosone	162	Interleukin-1β	32000
Argininic acid	175	Fructoselysine	308	Interleukin-6	24500
Creatinine	113	Glyoxal	58	Tumor necrosis factor-α	26000
Guanidine	59	Pentosidine	342	**Peptides**	
Methylguanidine	73	**Hippurates**		Adrenomedulin	5729
Peptides		Hippuric acid	179	ANP	3080
β-Lipotropin	461	**Indoles**		β-2-Microglobulin	11818
Polyols		Indoxyl sulfate	251	β-Endorphin	3465
Erythritol	122	Melatonin	126	Cholecystokinin	3866
Myoinositol	180	Quinolinic acid	167	Cystatin C	13300
Sorbitol	182	**Phenols**		Delta sleep-inducing peptide	848
Threitol	122	Hydroquinone	110	Hyaldronic acid	25000
Purines		P-Cresol	108	Leptin	16000
Cytidine	234	Phenol	94	Neuropeptide Y	4272
Hypoxanthine	136	**Polyamines**		PTH	9225
Uracil	112	Putrescine	88	Retinol-binding protein	21200
Uric acid	168	Spermidine	145	**Others**	
Xanthine	152	Spermine	202	Complement factor D	23750
Pyrimidines		**Others**			
Orotic acid	174	Homocysteine	135		
Thymine	126				
Uridine	244				
Ribonucleosides					
1-Methyladenosin	281				
Pseudouridine	244				
Xanthosine	284				
Others					
Malondialdehyde	71				
Oxalate	90				
Urea	60				

Figure 90.3 Organic uremic solutes. ADMA, asymmetric dimethylarginine; AGE, advanced glycation end product; ANP, atrial natriuretic peptide; PTH, parathyroid hormone.

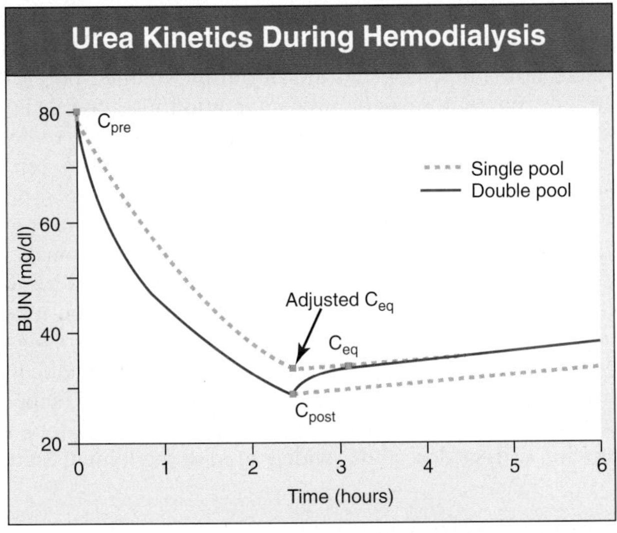

Figure 90.4 Urea kinetics during hemodialysis. BUN, blood urea nitrogen; C_{pre}, predialysis BUN; C_{post}, postdialysis BUN; C_{eq}, postdialysis equilibrated BUN.

From these equations, it is clear that *eKt/V* is always lower than *spKt/V*. With a conventional 4-hour HD treatment, *eKt/V* is about 0.2 *Kt/V* units lower than *spKt/V*. The difference is even larger with short, high-efficiency HD or hemodiafiltration, in which urea rebound is higher. Typical results of *spKt/V* and *eKt/V* for identical treatment characteristics are shown in Figure 90.5.

Single-pool *Kt/V* or, even better, *eKt/V* should be assessed monthly, and dialysis prescription should be adapted accordingly. In large cross-sectional studies, mortality increases when *spKt/V* falls below 1.2, and international guidelines (e.g., KDOQI) recommend a target *spKt/V* of 1.3 for a conventional dialysis schedule of three times per week.

Weekly Standard *Kt/V* (*std-Kt/V*)

The weekly dialysis dose is not equivalent to the product of session *Kt/V* and the number of treatments per week because the total urea mass removed per time unit decreases with increasing dialysis treatment time and dose as a result of lowering of serum urea concentration over time. This is exemplified by looking at a doubling of *Kt/V* from 1.0 to 2.0, when the total mass of urea removed is not doubled but only increased by about 24% (Fig. 90.6). With the weekly *std-Kt/V* concept, the *intermittently* provided dialysis urea clearance during 1 week is converted to an equivalent *continuous* "extracorporeal" urea clearance (ml/min), then multiplied by 10,080 (minutes per week) and divided by

Computation of Dialysis Dose: Results Derived from Different Model Equations

Formula	Result	Comment
$URR = (1 - C_t / C_0) \times 100\%$	67%	Urea rebound, urea generation, and ultrafiltration not taken into account
$Kt/V = \ln (C_0 / C_t)$	1.10	Urea rebound, urea generation, and ultrafiltration not taken into account
$spKt/V = -\ln (R - 0.008 \times t) + (4 - 3.5\ R) \times UF/W$	1.33	Single-pool model; urea rebound not taken into account
$eKt/V = spKt/V - 0.6 \times spKt/V/t + 0.03$	1.16	Double-pool model for arteriovenous access including urea rebound
$eKt/V = spKt/V - 0.47 \times spKt/V/t + 0.02$	1.20	Double-pool model for central venous access including urea rebound

Figure 90.5 Computation of dialysis dose: results derived from different model equations. Calculations based on dialysis duration (t) = 4 hours; predialysis BUN (C_0) = 90 mg/dl; nonequilibrated postdialysis BUN (C_t) = 30 mg/dl; ultrafiltration volume (UF) = 3 liters; postdialysis body weight (W) = 72 kg; $R = C_t/C_0$; URR, urea reduction ratio.

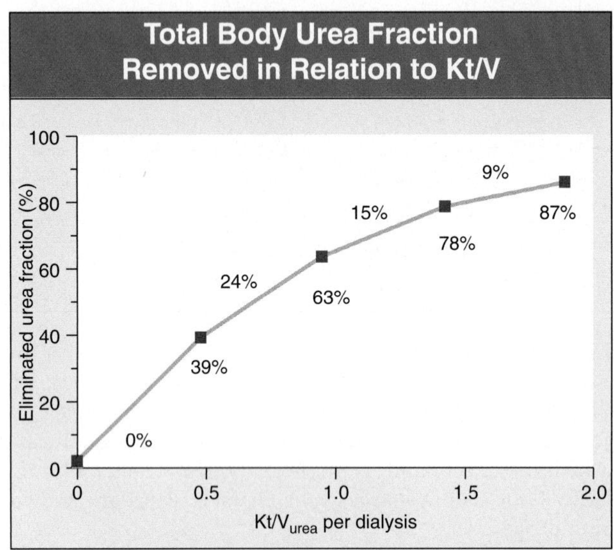

Figure 90.6 Total body urea fraction removed in relation to *Kt/V*. In this example, 63% of total body urea fraction is removed with *Kt/V* of 1; doubling of *Kt/V* to 2 increases the removed urea fraction by an additional 24%.

urea distribution volume V (ml).[5] The resulting dimensionless *std-Kt/V* value is directly compatible with peritoneal dialysis weekly *Kt/V* and with native residual renal *Kt/V*. Weekly *std-Kt/V* can be derived graphically by plotting *eKt/V* of a representative dialysis session onto the respective frequency curve (Fig. 90.7). A maximum *std-Kt/V* of 2.8/week can be achieved with a conventional thrice-weekly dialysis schedule. To deliver higher *std-Kt/V*, dialysis frequency needs to be increased. Residual renal function expressed as weekly renal *Kt/V* can simply be added to dialysis *std-Kt/V*.

Independent of the treatment schedule, a minimum target *std-Kt/V* of 2.0/week including renal *Kt/V* is recommended for all patients. This is exactly the value that is achieved with a *spKt/V* of 1.2 given three times per week in an anuric patient.

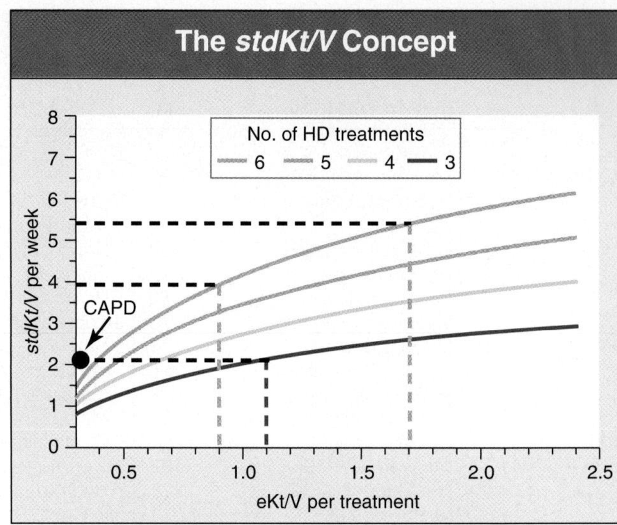

Figure 90.7 The *std-Kt/V* concept. The *std-Kt/V* for any hemodialysis (HD) frequency is derived by plotting *eKt/V* of a representative dialysis session onto the respective frequency curve. CAPD, continuous ambulatory peritoneal dialysis; CHD, conventional hemodialysis regimen (3×/week); SHD, short daily hemodialysis (6×/week); NHD, nocturnal home hemodialysis (6×/week).

Formal Urea Kinetic Modeling

Formal urea kinetic modeling (UKM) is the most accurate method for assessment of delivered dialysis dose. Besides this, it is the only kinetics-based method for prescription of *Kt/V* and for measurement of urea distribution volume. UKM has formed the basis for retrospective interpretation of the National Cooperative Dialysis Study and for prescription and control of the HEMO and the Frequent Hemodialysis Network studies. Single-pool *Kt/V* is modeled from the prescribed dialyzer clearance (K), derived from the intrinsic dialyzer overall transport coefficient K_oA (for details, see Chapter 89), and from prescribed blood and dialysate flow rates, targeted ultrafiltration volume, prescribed treatment time, interdialytic urea generation rate, and assumed urea distribution volume. By comparing modeled *Kt/V* to delivered *Kt/V*, the accuracy of delivery of dialysis dose can be assessed.

UKM also accounts for ultrafiltration, intradialytic urea generation, and unconventional dialysis frequencies. Additional benefits of formal UKM in addition to *spKt/V*, *eKt/V*, and *std-Kt/V* include the estimation of the normalized protein nitrogen appearance, a marker of spontaneous dietary protein intake, and regular assessment of urea distribution volume. Because of its mathematical complexity, UKM requires advanced computer support. UKM is the most rigorous available method for prescribing and evaluating dialysis dose and is widely used in the United States.

Prescription of Dialysis Dose

Delivered dialysis dose depends on dialysate and blood flow rates, dialyzer efficiency (K_oA), session length (t), and the distribution volume (V) of the uremic toxin studied. For urea, this is total body water volume; but for other small-molecular-weight compounds, V may be substantially different. A standard dialysis prescription should include a minimum treatment time of 4 hours, a blood flow rate of at least 250 ml/min, and a dialysate flow rate of 500 to 800 ml/min. In a new dialysis patient, V is unknown and has to be estimated (men, 58% of body weight; women, 55% of body weight).

Example

Male, body weight: 76 kg; V = 58% of body weight = 44 liters

Target blood flow rate: 300 ml/min; dialyzer efficiency: 80%; effective dialyzer urea clearance (K_d) = 240 ml/min; target *spKt/V* = 1.3

Required treatment time (min): 1.3 × V (ml)/K_d (ml/min) = 238 min

Once dialysis is delivered and *Kt/V* has been measured, the prescription is adjusted to meet the *Kt/V* target. In severe and long-standing uremia, the target dose is approached slowly during the course of several sessions to avoid the dialysis disequilibrium syndrome.

Is *V* the Adequate Denominator for $K \times t$?

Several studies have suggested that patients with small urea V, typically women, tend to do poorly relative to larger people. Because total body water is much more closely related to muscle mass than to body weight, small urea V is a good indicator for low muscle mass. Interestingly, in the HEMO study, a beneficial effect of higher *Kt/V* was reported for women but not for men.[4] This implies that individuals with low muscle mass may require a higher clearance in relation to V and therefore raises the question of whether V is the appropriate denominator for dialysis dose. Native renal clearances, in contrast, are commonly related to body surface area (BSA), not to total body water. By analogy, it has been proposed to relate dialysis clearances to BSA. The ratio of BSA to urea V is generally higher in women than in men and decreases with an increment in V. Prescribing dialysis dose in relation to BSA ($K \times t$/BSA) would result in more dialysis for smaller patients of either gender and for women of any size. A nomogram approach for a BSA-adjusted target *spKt/V* has been published recently.[6] Although this new approach has not yet been fully validated, it may be recommended for subpopulations with low muscle mass and associated high mortality risk.

Factors Affecting Delivered *Kt/V*

The effective dialyzer urea clearance *Kd* depends on blood and dialysate flow rates, dialyzer K_oA, effective dialyzer surface area, hematocrit, anticoagulation, and recirculation. Treatment time t is important for reaching the *Kt/V* target. Effective treatment time can be substantially shorter than prescribed treatment time because of intermittent pump stops or patient demand. V does not substantially change during a single HD session but may change over time. Dialysis dose needs to be adjusted for an increase in V. On the contrary, if there is a loss in body mass, which is associated with a decrease in V, *Kt/V* should not be reduced but rather adjusted to the higher, ideal patient V or, as pointed out before, to BSA.

Confronted with an inadequate delivered *Kt/V*, it is sensible to check whether the studied session was representative of an average session because unusual problems may have occurred (e.g., shortened time, single-needle HD). A frequent cause of low *Kt/V* is a vascular access problem leading to recirculation. Blood sampling errors should be considered because delayed post-HD sampling will reduce *Kt/V*. Blood sampling procedures should be standardized in each center (for recommendations, see KDOQI guidelines). If, despite these checks, a low *Kt/V* remains unexplained, treatment time should be increased to 4.5 or 5 hours.

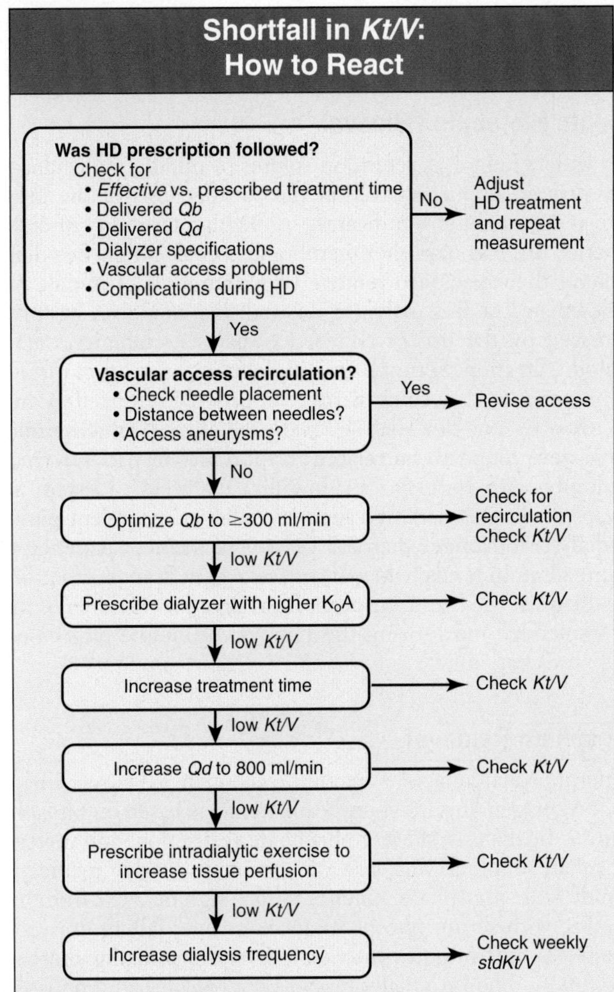

Figure 90.8 Management of low *Kt/V*. HD, hemodialysis; K_oA, the dialyzer urea mass transfer area coefficient; *Qb*, blood flow rate; *Qd*, dialysate flow rate.

Prescription of a more efficient dialyzer and higher blood and dialysate flow rates should also be considered (Fig. 90.8). Muscle exercise before or during dialysis improves *Kt/V* by increasing blood supply to poorly perfused urea rich muscle tissue and thus facilitates urea equilibration. Delivered *Kt/V* should be checked whenever the dialysis prescription has been modified substantially. Online clearance monitoring allows assessment of *Kt/V* during each single session without blood sampling.

Recommendations for Dialysis Dose Adequacy

Current recommendations in the United States are as follows:

- A minimum *spKt/V* of at least 1.2 for both adult and pediatric HD patients. When URR is used, the delivered dose should be equivalent to a *Kt/V* of 1.2, that is, an average URR of 65%.
- To prevent the delivered dose of HD from falling below the recommended minimum dose, the prescribed dose of HD should be *spKt/V* 1.3, which corresponds to an average URR of 70%.
- The delivered dose of HD should be measured at least once per month in all adult and pediatric HD patients.

Details on these and other recommendations can be found at the various Web sites listed in Figure 90.2.[7]

OTHER DIALYSIS FACTORS RELATED TO OUTCOMES

Middle Molecule Removal

It is widely held that retention solutes of middle molecular size may play an important role in the pathogenesis of the uremic state and contribute significantly to the high mortality of dialysis patients. Because of higher membrane porosity, high-flux dialyzers have the capacity to remove larger amounts of middle molecules than low-flux dialyzers do, and this may even be further increased by the use of convective dialysis strategies, such as hemodiafiltration. Serum β_2-microglobulin, a surrogate for other uremic middle molecules, is more effectively removed by high-flux than by low-flux dialysis, and predialysis β_2-microglobulin levels were found to be related to mortality in patients treated randomly with high-flux or low-flux dialyzers.[8] Certain subgroups of dialysis patients, such as diabetics, prevalent patients on dialysis for longer than 3.7 years, and incident patients with serum albumin levels below 40 g/l, may benefit most from high-flux dialysis.[9,10] The European Best Practice Guidelines have recommended maximizing the removal of middle molecules in all dialysis patients.[11]

Phosphate Removal

Hyperphosphatemia is a major problem in HD (see Chapter 81).[12] Management of hyperphosphatemia is based on phosphate removal by dialysis, dietary phosphate restriction, and intestinal phosphate binding with use of phosphate binder medication. Intradialytic phosphate kinetics differ significantly from urea kinetics, with serum phosphate levels steeply falling during the first 90 to 120 minutes into dialysis and stabilizing thereafter (Fig. 90.9). The intradialytic plateau is explained by phosphate mobilization from various compartments at a rate similar to that of dialyzer phosphate removal. Phosphate removal can be improved by high-flux HD and hemodiafiltration, by the use of larger dialyzer surface area, and, most dramatically, by higher frequency dialysis schedules, such as short daily or daily nocturnal HD. Long frequent dialysis schedules may result in hypophosphatemia so that phosphate has to be added to the dialysate. Target predialysis phosphate levels should be in the normal range.

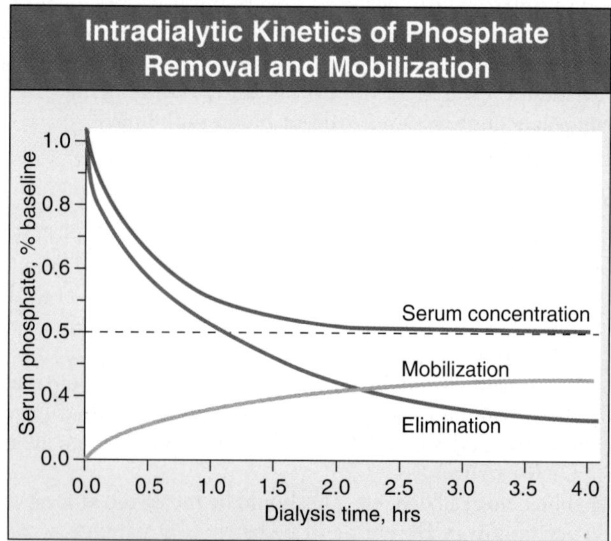

Figure 90.9 Intradialytic kinetics of phosphate removal and mobilization.

Preservation of Residual Renal Function

Most patients starting dialysis still have considerable residual renal function (RRF); but by the end of the first year, the majority have lost RRF completely. Only 10% to 20% of patients still have RRF after more than 3 years of dialysis. RRF of 2 to 3 ml/min urea clearance contributes significantly to the elimination of uremic toxins.[13] This translates into lower serum β_2-microglobulin, phosphate, potassium, urea, creatinine, and uric acid levels; higher hemoglobin concentration; enhanced nutritional status; better quality of life scores; and a reduced need for dietary and fluid restrictions. Loss of RRF, in contrast, is associated with left ventricular hypertrophy. To assess the relative contribution of RRF to total delivered dialysis dose, weekly dialysis dose should be expressed as *std-Kt/V*. For a patient with an estimated total body water of 40 liters, a residual urea clearance of 2 to 3 ml/min is equivalent to a *std-Kt/V* of 0.5 to 0.75/week. Risk factors for the loss of RRF include activation of the immune system by bioincompatible membranes and dialysate water impurities; intradialytic hypotension; use of angiotensin-converting enzyme inhibitors or nephrotoxic agents, such as radiocontrast media, aminoglycosides, and nonsteroidal anti-inflammatory drugs; and hypercalcemia. Loss of RRF may be delayed by the use of calcium antagonists and adequate target post-HD weight prescription.

Dialysate Composition

Dialysate composition may have a strong long-term impact on outcome. During a standard treatment session, a patient's blood is exposed to 120 to 200 liters of dialysate. The several ingredients of dialysate should therefore be prescribed with great care.

Sodium

Sodium retention is a typical feature of ESRD and an important factor in the pathogenesis of hypertension in HD patients. Judicious control of sodium balance is effective in normalizing blood pressure, and dietary sodium intake should be restricted to 6 g salt or 100 mmol sodium per day. Sodium is mainly removed through ultrafiltration; but depending on the ratio of dialysate to plasma water sodium concentration, it will be additionally removed or delivered to the patient by diffusion. To avoid a positive sodium balance, dialysate sodium should not exceed the patient's average predialysis serum sodium concentration by more than 2 or 3 mmol/l.

Potassium

Potassium removal during dialysis should ideally be equal to the amount accumulated during the interdialytic period. The dialysate potassium concentration has to be set at a level that avoids pre-HD hyperkalemia as well as intradialytic hypokalemia, which may provoke dialysis-induced arrhythmia. The typical dialysate potassium concentration is set between 2.0 and 4.0 mmol/l.

Calcium

In light of the interdialytic positive calcium balance and accelerated vascular calcification as a major cardiovascular risk factor in ESRD, intradialytic calcium delivery to the patient should be avoided. In patients using calcium salts as phosphate binders, a negative intradialytic calcium mass balance is desirable.[14] A standard dialysate calcium concentration of 1.25 to 1.50 mmol/l is recommended by KDIGO. These and higher dialysate calcium concentrations may be associated with tissue calcium accumulation, whereas lower dialysate calcium will stimulate PTH secretion.

Bicarbonate

Chronic metabolic acidosis is associated with decreased protein synthesis and increased protein catabolism and contributes to mineral and bone disorders. Normalized pre-HD bicarbonate levels in the range of 20 to 23 mmol/l are associated with improved survival. Dialysate bicarbonate concentration is typically set between 35 and 40 mmol/l to generate a transmembrane concentration gradient favoring bicarbonate delivery to the patient. Overalkalinization may result in reduced cerebral perfusion.

Treatment Time

Conventional three times a week dialysis remains the standard of care in most countries, where treatment time is typically governed by dialysis dose (*Kt/V*), with the consequence of longer dialysis in patients with higher urea distribution volumes.

In some countries, such as Germany, a minimum treatment time of 4 hours per HD session is mandatory for demonstration of adequacy. Great care should be given to prescribing and delivering *effective* treatment times, which exclude periods of pump stops or any other interruptions of the treatment session. Even with similar *Kt/V*, longer treatment times are associated with higher mass removal of urea, creatinine, phosphate, and β_2-microglobulin compared with shorter treatment times.[15]

Weekly treatment time is the one factor with the highest impact on dialysis dosing. More frequent in-center dialysis and longer dialysis hours delivered by in-center or home nocturnal dialysis are increasingly used alternatives to three times weekly treatment. Both modalities offer the opportunity for improved solute clearance and complete removal of interdialytic weight gain with fewer problems because ultrafiltration rates are lower and hypotension is less likely. However, scientific evidence for the extension of weekly treatment time is currently based on only a few small-scale randomized or nonrandomized studies.[16] The results of a larger randomized, controlled study, the Frequent Hemodialysis Network study, are awaited in 2011.

Hydration Status

Overhydration, which is found in the majority of HD patients, is an established risk factor for the development of arterial hypertension, left ventricular hypertrophy, and cardiovascular mortality. It is the goal of an adequate HD treatment to normalize body water homeostasis and extracellular volume to a level comparable with that of subjects of similar age and normal renal function. In clinical practice, this idealized postdialysis body weight is termed dry weight, which may differ substantially from the target weight prescribed by the physician. Because of the difficulties in detecting overhydration of 2 to 3 liters clinically from the presence of edema, high blood pressure, dyspnea, and distended jugular veins, technical methods such as ultrasound (diameter of inferior vena cava), chest radiography, and whole-body bioimpedance should be applied regularly.[17] The prescribed post-HD target weight is achieved by ultrafiltration. High ultrafiltration rates above 1000 ml/h are associated with an increased risk of intradialytic hypotension, which in turn is associated with an increased long-term mortality risk. Intradialytic hemodynamics are stabilized by isothermic HD, in which the physiologic intradialytic rise in body core temperature, a key factor in the pathogenesis of intradialytic hypotension, is prevented through cooling of the dialysate.[18] In hemodynamically unstable patients, only low ultrafiltration rates and therefore longer dialysis treatment times can accomplish the goal of adequate fluid removal.

Dialysis patients are advised to limit daily fluid intake to 0.5 to 0.75 liter in excess of their average daily diuresis. A positive interdialytic and intradialytic sodium balance is a major factor governing thirst and interdialytic water intake. Dietary salt restriction to 6 g salt per day is recommended to prevent high interdialytic weight gain and the development of arterial hypertension and congestive heart failure.

Dietary Protein and Calorie Intake

HD patients are at risk of malnutrition due to protein-energy wasting, decreased appetite, infection, intercurrent illnesses, hospital admissions, and missed meals after dialysis. The recommended daily intake of 1.0 to 1.2 g protein per kilogram of ideal body weight and 35 kcal per kilogram of ideal body weight is often not met. The nutritional status of dialysis patients should be assessed regularly by clinical and biochemical means, including measurement of protein nitrogen appearance (see Chapter 83).

Vascular Access

The choice of vascular access strongly affects outcome in dialysis patients. A functioning vascular access is a major precondition for adequate dialysis treatment. Native fistulas should always be the first-line vascular access. In cases in which a native fistula cannot be created, a vascular graft may be an alternative. Central venous catheters may be used for bridging until a vascular access can be used for dialysis. Only when a native fistula or a graft is not available may subcutaneous tunneled central venous catheters be used as permanent access. Worldwide, there are large differences in the fraction of patients with central venous catheters used as permanent access. Long-term catheter use is associated with a higher rate of chronic inflammation and acute infection, lower serum albumin levels, impaired response to erythropoietin, and higher hospitalization and mortality rates, mainly due to infection (see Chapter 87). The quality of the vascular access should be assessed regularly by clinical means, such as inspection, palpation, and auscultation, as well as by technical means, including intradialytic measurement of recirculation or access flow rate and Doppler ultrasound technology.

Quality of Life

Quality of life measures may be among the most sensitive indicators of the efficacy of dialysis therapies.[19] Measures of physical and mental aspects of quality of life are recognized to assess the physical and psychological disturbances that can accompany the uremic state and can be modified by renal replacement therapy. Various standardized quality of life tests are now routinely used in clinical trials involving HD patients. Besides dialysis adequacy, quality of life may also be significantly affected by factors related to organizational issues, for example, travel delays, waiting time at the dialysis facility for treatment to start, time of dialysis in relationship to work or educational needs, and lack of exercise.

Depression is one of the major mental aspects affecting quality of life and may be assessed separately by validated standardized questionnaires, such as the Beck Depression Index.[20] Depression is frequently associated with biochemical evidence of inflammation or infection and may improve with appropriate treatment. One potential way to make some impact on some of these issues is to modify the "assembly line" character of many dialysis centers with variations including physical exercise and occupational therapy programs and opportunities for the patients to have regular meetings with staff to discuss their questions.

REFERENCES

1. Yoshino M, Kuhlmann MK, Kotanko P, et al. International differences in dialysis mortality reflect background general population atherosclerotic cardiovascular mortality. *J Am Soc Nephrol.* 2006;17:3510-3519.
2. Vanholder R, De Smet R, Glorieux G, et al. Review on uremic toxins: Classification, concentration, and interindividual variability. *Kidney Int.* 2003;63:1934-1943.
3. Vanholder R, Van Laecke S, Glorieux G. What is new in uremic toxicity? *Pediatr Nephrol.* 2008;23:1211-1221.
4. Daugirdas JT. Second generation logarithmic estimates of single-pool variable volume Kt/V: an analysis of error. *J Am Soc Nephrol.* 1993;4:1205-1213.
5. Gotch FA. The current place of urea kinetic modelling with respect to different dialysis modalities. *Nephrol Dial Transplant.* 1998;13(Suppl 6):10-14.
6. Daugirdas JT, Depner TA, Greene T, et al. Surface-area-normalized Kt/V: A method of rescaling dialysis dose to body surface area—implications for different-size patients by gender. *Semin Dial.* 2008;21:415-421.
7. National Kidney Foundation. KDOQI Clinical Practice Guidelines and Clinical Practice Recommendations for 2006 Updates: Hemodialysis Adequacy, Peritoneal Dialysis Adequacy and Vascular Access. *Am J Kidney Dis.* 2006;48(Suppl 1):S1-S322.
8. Cheung AK, Rocco MV, Yan G, et al. Serum β_2-microglobulin levels predict mortality in dialysis patients: Results of the HEMO study. *J Am Soc Nephrol.* 2006;17:546-555.
9. Eknoyan G, Beck GJ, Cheung AK, et al. Effect of dialysis dose and membrane flux in maintenance hemodialysis. *N Engl J Med.* 2002;347:2010-2019.
10. Locatelli F, Martin-Malo A, Hannedouche T, et al. Effect of membrane permeability on survival of hemodialysis patients. *J Am Soc Nephrol.* 2009;20:645-654.
11. European Best Practice Guidelines Expert Group on Hemodialysis, European Renal Association. *Nephrol Dial Transplant.* 2002;17(Suppl 7):16-31.
12. Levin NW, Gotch FA, Kuhlmann MK. Factors for increased morbidity and mortality in uremia: Hyperphosphatemia. *Semin Nephrol.* 2004;24:396-400.
13. Bargman JM, Golper TA. The importance of residual renal function for patients on dialysis. *Nephrol Dial Transplant.* 2005;20:671-673.
14. Gotch FA. Calcium and phosphorus kinetics in hemodialysis therapy. *Contrib Nephrol.* 2008;161:210-214.
15. Eloot S, Van Biesen W, Dhondt A, et al. Impact of hemodialysis duration on the removal of uremic retention solutes. *Kidney Int.* 2008;73:765-770.
16. Lindsay RM, Leitch R, Heidenheim AP, et al. The London daily/nocturnal hemodialysis study—study design, morbidity and mortality results. *Am J Kidney Dis.* 2003;42(Suppl 1):5-12.
17. Kuhlmann MK, Zhu F, Seibert E, Levin NW. Bioimpedance, dry weight and blood pressure control: New methods and consequences. *Curr Opin Nephrol Hypertens.* 2005;14:543-549.
18. Selby NM, McIntyre CW. A systematic review of the clinical effects of reducing dialysate fluid temperature. *Nephrol Dial Transplant.* 2006;21:1883-1898.
19. Unruh ML, Weisbord SD, Kimmel PL. Health-related quality of life in nephrology research and clinical practice. *Semin Dial.* 2005;18:82-90.
20. Kimmel PL, Peterson RA. Depression in patients with end-stage renal disease treated with dialysis: Has the time to treat arrived? *Clin J Am Soc Nephrol.* 2006;1:349-352.

CHAPTER 91

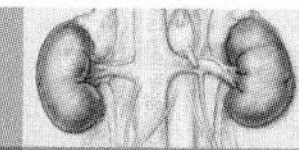

Acute Complications During Hemodialysis

Victor F. Seabra, Bertrand L. Jaber

CARDIOVASCULAR COMPLICATIONS

Intradialytic Hypotension

Intradialytic hypotension, which occurs in 10% to 30% of treatments, ranges from asymptomatic episodes to marked compromise of organ perfusion resulting in myocardial ischemia, cardiac arrhythmias, vascular thrombosis, loss of consciousness, seizures, or death. Further, in patients with acute kidney injury, intradialytic hypotension may induce more renal ischemia and retard recovery of renal function. Intradialytic hypotension and postdialysis orthostatic hypotension have been shown to be independent risk factors for mortality.[1] The pathogenesis of intradialytic hypotension is complex[2] and is summarized in Figure 91.1.

The immediate treatment is to restore the circulating blood volume by placing the patient in the Trendelenburg position, reducing or stopping ultrafiltration, and infusing boluses of 0.9% isotonic saline (100 ml or more, as necessary). Salt-poor albumin offers no advantage over isotonic saline and costs more. Blood flow rate should not be routinely reduced to manage hypotension as it has not been shown to be beneficial. If the blood pump rate is reduced transiently, particular attention should be paid to minimizing underdialysis from such a practice. Because cardiac factors can precipitate intradialytic hypotension, if hypotension is accompanied by chest pain or dyspnea, an electrocardiogram should be obtained to rule out ischemia. Similarly, recurrent and unexplained episodes of hypotension might warrant echocardiography to rule out pericarditis.

Preventive strategies include correction of anemia and hypoalbuminemia and treatment of congestive heart failure or arrhythmias, avoidance of antihypertensive drugs before dialysis, and avoidance of food before and during dialysis. Patients should be counseled to avoid excessive interdialytic weight gain, and accurate assessment of the patient's dry weight is required. Midodrine, an oral selective α_1-agonist, is a useful preventive therapy.[3]

Preventive strategies through modification of the dialysis procedure include the use of bicarbonate dialysate, volumetric control of ultrafiltration, sodium modeling, and short daily dialysis.[4] Online blood volume monitoring and biofeedback techniques have also been used to improve intradialytic cardiovascular stability.[5] Dialysate cooling to 35.5°C to 36°C, a measure that induces release of catecholamines, resulting in vasoconstriction, may lessen hypotension. This can be achieved through a new device with thermal sensors able to measure blood temperature at the arterial and venous sides of the extracorporeal circuit and accordingly modify the dialysate temperature. This technique allows isothermic dialysis and has been shown to reduce symptomatic intradialytic hypotension.[6]

Intradialytic Hypertension

Intradialytic hypertension occurs in 8% to 30% of treatments.[7] Hypertension during or immediately after dialysis constitutes an important risk factor for cardiovascular mortality. Moreover, intradialytic increase in systolic blood pressure is associated with an increased risk of hospitalization or death.[8]

Its mechanism is primarily volume dependent. However, in a number of patients, blood pressure remains elevated despite fluid removal, a syndrome called dialysis-refractory hypertension. These patients are usually young with preexisting hypertension and have excessive interdialytic weight gain and a hyperactive renin-angiotensin system in response to fluid removal.[9] There may be a lag time of several weeks between achieving dry weight and becoming normotensive.

Erythropoietin and other erythropoiesis-stimulating agents have been associated with a 20% to 30% incidence of new onset or exacerbation of hypertension. Further, among patients receiving intravenous (not subcutaneous) erythropoietin, elevated levels of endothelin-1 (a potent vasoconstrictor) have been shown to correlate with increased blood pressure. Intradialytic hypertension can be precipitated by the use of hypernatric dialysate, which is intended to mitigate the intradialytic decrease in serum osmolality that occurs with the diffusive removal of urea and sodium.[10] Although this approach stabilizes blood pressure during dialysis, hypernatric dialysate results in a positive intradialytic sodium balance and is associated with increased postdialysis thirst, resulting in significant weight gain in the interdialytic period. To circumvent these problems, sodium modeling has been adopted as an approach that uses variable sodium concentrations in the dialysate, generally with sodium reduced in a continuous or stepwise manner from an initial level of 150 to 154 mmol/l to 138 to 142 mmol/l. Other hypothesized mechanisms of intradialytic hypertension include hyperactivity of the sympathetic nervous system[11] and increased cardiac output due to fluid removal, particularly among patients with cardiomyopathy.[12] Clinicians should also be aware of possible dialytic removal of certain antihypertensive drugs, such as angiotensin-converting enzyme (ACE) inhibitors and β-blockers.

Increasing hypertension during a dialysis session requires intervention if systolic blood pressure is greater than 180 mm Hg. This is best treated with a centrally acting agent such as clonidine

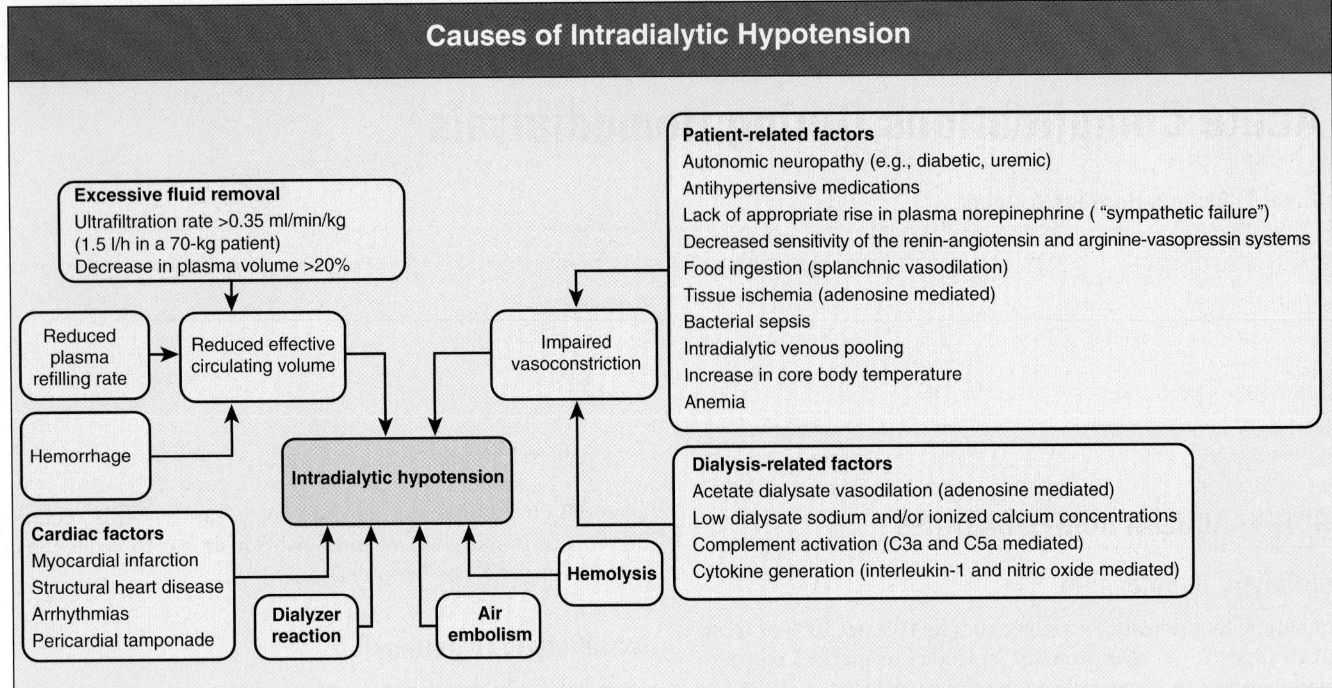

Figure 91.1 Pathogenesis and causes of intradialytic hypotension.

or a short-acting ACE inhibitor such as captopril. Successful treatment of hypertension for a longer period requires an accurate determination of the patient's dry weight and its achievement by gradual ultrafiltration during several weeks of dialysis. Sodium modeling can be instituted, targeting serum sodium concentrations of 135 mmol/l at the end of dialysis; reduce the dry weight in 0.5-kg increments, observe the clinical response, and reevaluate periodically. Once dry weight is achieved, optimization of antihypertensive drug therapy is warranted, including the use of minimally dialyzable or nondialyzable medications such as angiotensin receptor blockers, calcium channel blockers, clonidine, and carvedilol.

Cardiac Arrhythmias

Intradialytic arrhythmias are common and are often multifactorial in origin.[13,14] Left ventricular hypertrophy, congestive cardiomyopathy, uremic pericarditis, silent myocardial ischemia, and conduction system calcification are frequently encountered in adult dialysis patients. In addition, polypharmacy coupled with the constant alterations in fluid, electrolyte, and acid-base homeostasis may precipitate intradialytic arrhythmias. The range of electrocardiographic abnormalities that may be encountered in renal failure is shown in Figure 91.2. QTc dispersion, the difference between maximum and minimum QTc interval on a standard 12-lead electrocardiogram, is prolonged after hemodialysis (HD) and has been proposed as a prognostic indicator of cardiac complications in dialysis patients.[15]

Preventive measures include the use of bicarbonate dialysate and careful attention to dialysate potassium and calcium levels. Use of zero potassium dialysate should be discouraged because of its arrhythmogenic potential, particularly in patients receiving digoxin, should serum potassium concentration decrease to less than 3.5 mmol/l. Serum digoxin levels should be regularly monitored and the need for the drug regularly reassessed.

Electrocardiographic Abnormalities in Renal Failure

Function	Abnormality Seen in Renal Failure
PR interval	Usually normal; prolongation in long-term hemodialysis Calcification of mitral valve annulus may involve His-bundle giving complete heart block
QRS interval	
Amplitude	Increases during ultrafiltration (correlates with reduction in left ventricular [LV] dimensions) LV hypertrophy (LVH) on voltage criteria found in up to 50%
Duration	Prolonged (within normal range) by hemodialysis Late potentials increased only in patients with preexisting ischemic heart disease Prolonged in hyperkalemia
ST segment	Depression during hemodialysis does not predict coronary artery disease Depression or elevation may occur in hyperkalemia Depression during ambulatory monitoring poorly predictive of coronary artery disease
QTc interval	Increases during hemodialysis (correlates with reduction in [K^+] and [Mg^{2+}]) Increased QT dispersion reported in patients on dialysis
T wave	Peaking or inversion may occur in hyperkalemia Inversion in anterolateral leads in LVH with strain pattern
Rhythm	High incidence of atrial and ventricular arrhythmias during hemodialysis

Figure 91.2 Electrocardiographic abnormalities in renal failure. Risk factors include left ventricular dysfunction, wall motion abnormalities, known coronary artery disease, abnormal thallium redistribution tests (even without coronary artery disease), use of cardiac glycosides, and low dialysate potassium concentration.

Sudden Death

Cardiac arrest occurs at a rate of 7 per 100,000 HD sessions and is more common in the elderly, patients with diabetes, and patients using central venous catheters.[16] Some 80% of sudden deaths during dialysis are due to ventricular fibrillation and are more frequently observed after the long interdialytic interval on thrice-weekly dialysis.[17,18] Although ischemic heart disease increases the risk of sudden death, other catastrophic intradialytic events need to be ruled out. The prompt recognition and treatment of life-threatening hyperkalemia, often encountered in young, noncompliant patients, is imperative. Profound generalized muscle weakness may be a warning sign of imminent life-threatening hyperkalemia.

When cardiopulmonary arrest occurs during dialysis, an immediate decision must be made as to whether the collapse is due to an intrinsic disease or technical errors, such as air embolism, unsafe dialysate composition, overheated dialysate, line disconnection, or sterilant in the dialyzer. Air in the dialysate, grossly hemolyzed blood, and hemorrhage due to line disconnection can be easily detected. However, if no obvious cause is identifiable, blood should not be returned to the patient, particularly if the arrest occurred immediately on initiation of dialysis. A patient exposed to formaldehyde may have complained earlier of burning at the access site. If the possibility of a problem with dialysate composition is remote, blood may be returned to the patient. However, blood and dialysate samples should be immediately sent for electrolyte analysis, the dialyzer and blood lines saved for later analysis, and the dialysis machine replaced until all its safety features have been thoroughly evaluated for possible malfunction. It should be a standard practice to have defibrillators in dialysis units. The management of cardiopulmonary arrest during dialysis should follow the standard principles of cardiopulmonary resuscitation; the diagnosis and management of technical errors are discussed later.

Prevention of sudden cardiac death in HD patients, including the role of implantable defibrillators, is further discussed in Chapter 78.

Pericarditis

The management of pericarditis in dialysis patients is discussed in Chapter 78.

Dialysis-Associated Steal Syndrome

The construction of an arteriovenous fistula or graft frequently results in reduction of blood flow to the hand. Although clinically significant ischemia does not usually result, symptoms are by no means rare, particularly in diabetics or elderly patients with peripheral vascular disease. Dialysis-associated steal syndrome has been reported in 6.4% and 1% of patients with radiocephalic fistulas and grafts, respectively. The clinical presentation, differential diagnosis, and evaluation of dialysis-associated steal syndrome are summarized in Figure 91.3 and are discussed further in Chapter 87.[19,20]

Treatment depends on the clinical severity of ischemia and vascular access anatomy.[20] Severe ischemia can cause irreparable injury to nerves within hours and must be considered a surgical emergency. Mild ischemia, manifested by mild pain during HD, subjective coldness and paresthesias, and objective reduction in skin temperature but with no loss of sensation or motion, is common and generally improves with time.[21] Patients with mild

Dialysis-Associated Vascular Steal Syndrome

Clinical presentations (symptoms often aggravated on dialysis)
- Hand numbness, pain, or weakness
- Coolness of distal arm
- Diminished pulses
- Acrocyanosis, gangrene

Differential diagnosis
- Dialysis-associated cramp
- Polyneuropathy—diabetes, uremia
- Entrapment neuropathy—Aβ_2M amyloid
- Reflex sympathetic dystrophy
- Calciphylaxis

Evaluation of steal severity
- Pulse oximetry
- Plethysmography
- Doppler flow
- Angiography

Treatment options (depending on severity)
- Symptomatic (e.g., gloves)
- Surgical, with preservation of vascular access: banding to reduce flow, DRIL procedure (see Figure 87-9)
- With loss of vascular access; ligation

Figure 91.3 Dialysis-associated vascular steal syndrome. DRIL, distal revascularization and interval ligation.

ischemia should undergo symptom-specific therapy (e.g., wearing a glove) and frequent physical examination, with special attention to subtle neurologic changes and muscle wasting.[22] Failure to improve may require surgical intervention with banding or access correction or ligation. More serious manifestations, such as fingertip necrosis, require ligation of the fistula,[21] which provides immediate improvement in perfusion but results in the elimination of a site for vascular access and the immediate need to construct another one. Other techniques that do not sacrifice the access and yet improve distal perfusion include ligation of the artery distal to the origin of the fistula or graft with or without establishment of an arterial bypass (see Chapter 87) and narrowing of the fistula or graft to reduce flow, thereby improving distal perfusion. Percutaneous luminal angioplasty or laser recanalization is reserved for patients with inflow or outflow arterial disease. A modified brachiocephalic fistula extension technique, in which the median vein is anastomosed to the radial or ulnar artery just below the brachial bifurcation, is thought to preserve part of the blood supply to the hand and to prevent the arterial steal syndrome.[23] Persistence of symptoms after an apparently successful correction of the vascular access flow should alert the clinician to other unrelated causes.

NEUROMUSCULAR COMPLICATIONS

Muscle Cramps

Muscle cramps occur in 5% to 20% of patients late during dialysis and frequently involve the legs. They account for 15% of premature discontinuations of dialysis.[24] Electromyography shows increased tonic muscle electrical activity throughout dialysis, and serum creatine kinase may be elevated.

Although the pathogenesis is unknown, dialysis-induced volume contraction and hypo-osmolality are common predisposing factors. Indeed, the onset of muscle cramps often gives an indication that the target weight has been reached. However, hypomagnesemia and carnitine deficiency may also play a role.

The acute management is directed at increasing plasma osmolality. Cessation of ultrafiltration is not useful. Parenteral infusion of 23.5% hypertonic saline (15 to 20 ml), 25% mannitol (50 to 100 ml), or 50% dextrose in water (25 to 50 ml) is equally effective. However, hypertonic saline may result in postdialytic thirst, and both hypertonic saline and mannitol cause transient warmth and flushing during the infusion. Furthermore, large and repetitive infusions of mannitol may lead to increased thirst, interdialytic weight gain, and fluid overload. Overall, dextrose in water is preferred, particularly in nondiabetics.

Preventive measures include dietary counseling about excessive interdialytic weight gain. In patients without clinical signs of fluid overload, it is reasonable to increase the dry weight by 0.5 kg and to observe the clinical response. Quinine sulfate (250-300 mg) or oxazepam (5 to 10 mg) given 2 hours before dialysis may also be effective. Although the U.S. Food and Drug Administration regards quinine sulfate as both unsafe and ineffective for the prevention of cramps, this drug works well in some patients, and it is used freely in most parts of the world. The use of sodium gradient during dialysis is effective as well. Proposed strategies include starting with a dialysate sodium concentration of 145 to 155 mmol/l and a linear decrease to 135 to 140 mmol/l by the completion of the treatment. A comparison of sodium modeling with an exponential, linear, or step program has yielded similar results.[25] In anecdotal reports, 5 mg of enalapril twice weekly may be effective, presumably by inhibiting angiotensin II–mediated thirst. Stretching exercises, creatine monohydrate (12 mg before dialysis),[26] and L-carnitine supplementation (20 mg/kg per dialysis session) may also be beneficial.[27] An intradialytic blood volume biofeedback control system has been shown to effectively reduce the incidence of muscle cramps.[28]

Restless Legs Syndrome

Restless legs syndrome is common in dialysis patients. The typical complaint is of crawling sensations in the legs that occur with inactivity, and symptoms may worsen during dialysis. The etiology, prevention, and management of restless legs syndrome are discussed in Chapter 82.

Dialysis Disequilibrium Syndrome

Despite a decline in its incidence, dialysis disequilibrium syndrome (DDS) is still observed sporadically in patients who are initiated on HD on high-flux dialyzers with large surface areas and short dialysis time. Risk factors include young age, severe azotemia, low dialysate sodium concentration, and preexisting neurologic disorders (see Chapter 82).

DDS commonly presents with restlessness, headache, nausea, vomiting, blurred vision, muscle twitching, disorientation, tremor, and hypertension. More severe manifestations include obtundation, seizures, and coma. DDS usually develops toward the end of dialysis but may be delayed for up to 24 hours. Although cerebral edema is a consistent finding on computed tomographic scanning, DDS remains a clinical diagnosis because laboratory tests, including electroencephalography, are nonspecific. It is usually self-limited, but full recovery may take several days.

The pathogenesis of DDS is still a subject of debate. The reverse urea effect theory, which proposes that a transient osmotic disequilibrium occurs during dialysis as a result of a more rapid removal of urea from blood than from cerebrospinal fluid, has been disputed.[29] In animals undergoing rapid dialysis, despite the correction of systemic acidosis, a paradoxical cerebrospinal fluid acidosis develops that is aborted by slower dialysis. An additional mechanism is the intracerebral accumulation of idiogenic osmoles, such as inositol, glutamine, and glutamate.

In high-risk patients, preventive measures include the use of volumetric-controlled machines, bicarbonate dialysate, sodium modeling, earlier recognition of uremic states, and earlier initiation of dialysis. In addition, short and more frequent dialysis treatments are recommended with use of small surface area dialyzers and reduced blood flow rates. The target reduction in blood urea should initially be limited to 30%. The prophylactic use of mannitol or anticonvulsants is not recommended.

Seizures

Intradialytic seizures occur in less than 10% of patients and tend to be generalized but easily controlled. However, focal or refractory seizures warrant evaluation for focal neurologic disease, particularly intracranial hemorrhage. Causes of seizures are summarized in Figure 91.4 and are discussed further in Chapter 82.

Treatment of established seizures requires cessation of dialysis, maintenance of airway patency, and investigation for metabolic abnormalities. Intravenous diazepam, alprazolam or clonazepam, and phenytoin may be required. Intravenous 50% dextrose in water should be administered promptly if hypoglycemia is suspected.

Headache

Dialysis headache is common and consists of a bifrontal discomfort that develops during dialysis and may become intense and throbbing, accompanied by nausea and vomiting. It is usually aggravated by the supine position, but there are no visual disturbances.

Although its etiology has not been elucidated, dialysis headache may be a subtle manifestation of DDS or may be related to the use of acetate dialysate. Furthermore, it may be a manifestation of caffeine withdrawal due to dialytic removal of caffeine.

Management consists of oral analgesics (e.g., acetaminophen [paracetamol]). Preventive measures include slow dialysis with reduced blood flow rates, change to bicarbonate dialysate, sodium and ultrafiltration modeling, coffee ingestion during dialysis, and use of reprocessed dialyzers.

HEMATOLOGIC COMPLICATIONS

Complement Activation and Dialysis-Associated Neutropenia

During dialysis with unsubstituted cellulose dialyzers, which are infrequently used nowadays, the free hydroxyl groups present on the membrane cause activation of the alternative pathway of complement.[30] This results in activation and increased adherence of circulating neutrophils to the endothelial capillary pulmonary vasculature, leading to transient neutropenia that reaches a nadir after 15 minutes of dialysis, followed by a rebound leukocytosis 1 hour later. Neutropenia has also been detected with other more widely used dialyzer membranes, including cellulose acetate and polysulfone, but to a lesser degree. Although the long-term clinical relevance of this phenomenon remains speculative, its contribution to acute intradialytic morbidity is discussed later.

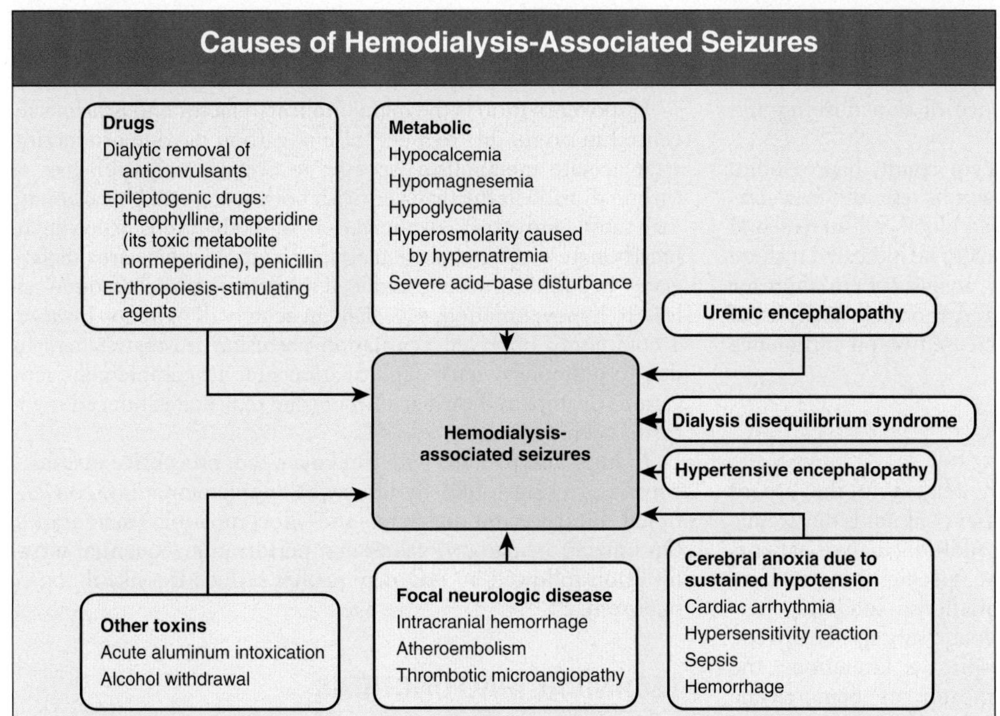

Figure 91.4 Causes of hemodialysis-associated seizures.

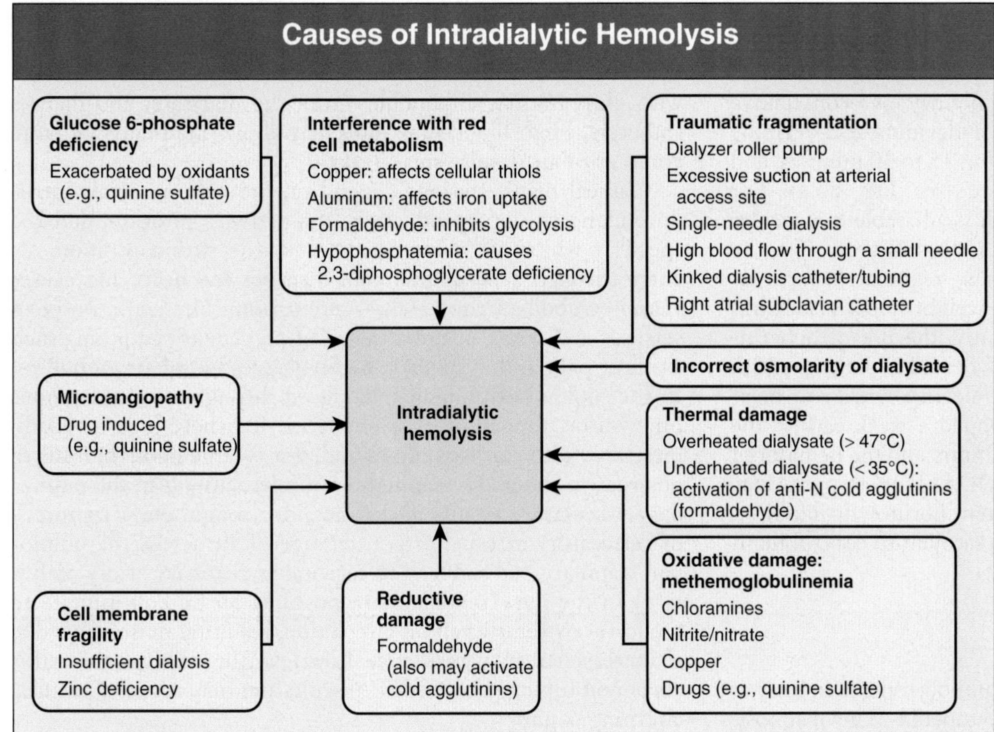

Figure 91.5 Causes of intradialytic hemolysis.

Intradialytic Hemolysis

Acute hemolysis can be due to faulty dialysis equipment, chemicals, drugs, toxins, or patient-related factors (Fig. 91.5).[31] With the advent of better dialysis equipment and the widespread use of deionization systems, traumatic red blood cell fragmentation caused by poorly designed blood pumps and methemoglobinemia caused by water contamination with chloramine or copper are never seen today. However, nitrate/nitrite intoxication causing methemoglobinemia still occurs sporadically in patients on home HD who use well water that is contaminated with urine from domesticated animals. Further, during dialyzer reprocessing, formaldehyde retention can result in hemolysis by inducing formation of cold agglutinins or inhibiting red cell metabolism.

The diagnosis of acute hemolysis is evident when grossly translucent hemolyzed blood is observed in the tubing. Patients with methemoglobinemia have nausea, vomiting, hypotension, and cyanosis, and oxygen therapy does not improve the black blood present in the extracorporeal circuit. Copper contamination should be suspected in the presence of skin flushing and abdominal pain or diarrhea.

Evaluation should include reticulocyte count, haptoglobin, lactate dehydrogenase, blood smear, Coombs test, and measurement of methemoglobin. ^{51}Cr-labeled red blood cell survival and bone marrow examination may occasionally be indicated if there is recurrent hemolysis. More important, analysis of tap water for chloramines and metal contaminants and thorough analysis of the dialysis equipment for clues of increased blood turbulence are recommended.

Hemorrhage

Bleeding complications are commonly related to the use of intradialytic anticoagulation, which further confounds the uremic bleeding diathesis (see Chapter 80).[32] In addition, dialysis patients are prone to spontaneous bleeding at specific sites, such as gastrointestinal arteriovenous malformations; subdural, pericardial, pleural, retroperitoneal, and hepatic subcapsular spaces; and the ocular anterior chamber. Despite its limitations, the bleeding time remains the best indicator of hemorrhagic tendency.

In addition to specific measures directed to the site of hemorrhage, reversal of uremic platelet dysfunction is imperative. Strategies include the use of erythropoiesis-stimulating agents or red blood cell transfusions to achieve a hematocrit above 30% to improve rheologic platelet–vessel wall interactions, intravenous conjugated estrogens at 0.6 mg/kg per day for 5 consecutive days, intravenous or subcutaneous 1-deamino-8-D-arginine vasopressin (DDAVP) at 0.3 μg/kg during 15 to 30 minutes, and intravenous infusion of cryoprecipitate (see Fig. 80.4). For patients experiencing severe bleeding, it is advisable to consider heparin-free dialysis, using normal saline flushes every 15 to 30 minutes with ultrafiltration adjustments, regional heparin or citrate anticoagulation, low-molecular-weight heparin, heparin modeling, or prostacyclin. More recently, the use of heparin-bound Hemophan dialyzers has been advocated in patients at risk of bleeding.[33] In patients scheduled for elective surgery or invasive procedures, aspirin should be stopped a week earlier, the dose of anticoagulant reduced to a minimum, and the hematocrit maintained above 30%. In some cases, DDAVP or estrogens may also be required. Tranexamic acid, a potent fibrinolytic inhibitor, has recently been used as an adjuvant treatment to control hemorrhage in dialysis patients.[34]

Thrombocytopenia

An increasingly important cause of thrombocytopenia in dialysis patients is heparin-induced thrombocytopenia. The diagnosis and management, including alternative strategies for anticoagulation strategies for HD, are discussed in Chapter 80.

PULMONARY COMPLICATIONS

Dialysis-Associated Hypoxemia

In most patients, the arterial P_{AO_2} decreases by 5 to 20 mm Hg (0.6 to 4 kPa) during dialysis, reaching a nadir at 30 to 60 minutes, and resolves within 60 to 120 minutes after discontinuation of dialysis. This decrease is usually of no clinical significance to patients unless there is preexisting chronic cardiopulmonary disease.

Hypoventilation is the main implicated factor and is primarily central in origin due to a decrease in carbon dioxide production after acetate metabolism (specific to acetate dialysate), loss of carbon dioxide in the dialyzer (with both acetate and bicarbonate dialysate), and rapid alkalinization of body fluids (specific to bicarbonate dialysate, particularly with large surface area dialyzers).[35] In addition, acetate-induced respiratory muscle fatigue can lead to hypoventilation, especially in acutely ill patients. Further, a commonly observed ventilation-perfusion mismatch may be due to pulmonary leukoagglutination (due to complement activation) or impaired cardiac output (due to acetate-induced myocardial depression).

In high-risk patients with fluid overload, preventive measures consist of using intradialytic oxygen supplementation, conventional bicarbonate dialysate, and biocompatible membranes. Optimizing hematocrit values and performing sequential ultrafiltration followed by HD may further reduce the likelihood of hypoxemia.

TECHNICAL MALFUNCTIONS

Air Embolism

The most vulnerable source of air entry into the extracorporeal circuit is the pre-pump tubing segment, where significant subatmospheric pressures prevail. However, other sources need to be considered, including intravenous infusion circuits especially with glass bottles, air bubbles from the dialysate, and dialysis catheters. High blood flow rates may allow rapid entry of large volumes of air despite small leaks.

Clinical manifestations depend on the volume of air introduced, the site of introduction, the patient's position, and the speed at which air is introduced.[36] In the sitting position, air entry through a peripheral vein bypasses the heart and causes venous emboli in the cerebral circulation. The acute onset of seizures and coma in the absence of precedent symptoms such as chest pain and dyspnea is highly suggestive of air embolism. In the supine position, air introduced through a central venous line will be trapped in the right ventricle, where it forms foam, interferes with cardiac output, and, if it is large enough, leads to obstructive shock. Dissemination of microemboli to the pulmonary vasculature results in dyspnea, dry cough, chest tightness, or respiratory arrest. Further, passage of air across the pulmonary capillary bed can lead to cerebral or coronary artery embolism. In the left Trendelenburg position, air emboli migrate to the lower extremity venous circulation, resulting in ischemia due to increased outflow resistance. Foam may be visible in the extracorporeal tubing, and cardiac auscultation may reveal a peculiar churning sound.

The immediate management of clinically suspected air embolism is summarized in Figure 91.6. Prevention depends primarily on dialysis machines that are equipped with venous air bubble traps and foam detectors located just distal to the dialyzer and a venous pressure monitor at the venous end. The detector is attached to a relay switch that simultaneously activates an alarm, shuts off the blood pump, and clamps the venous blood line if air is detected. Therefore, dialysis should never be performed in the presence of an inoperative air detection alarm system. Glass bottles should be avoided because they create vacuum effects that

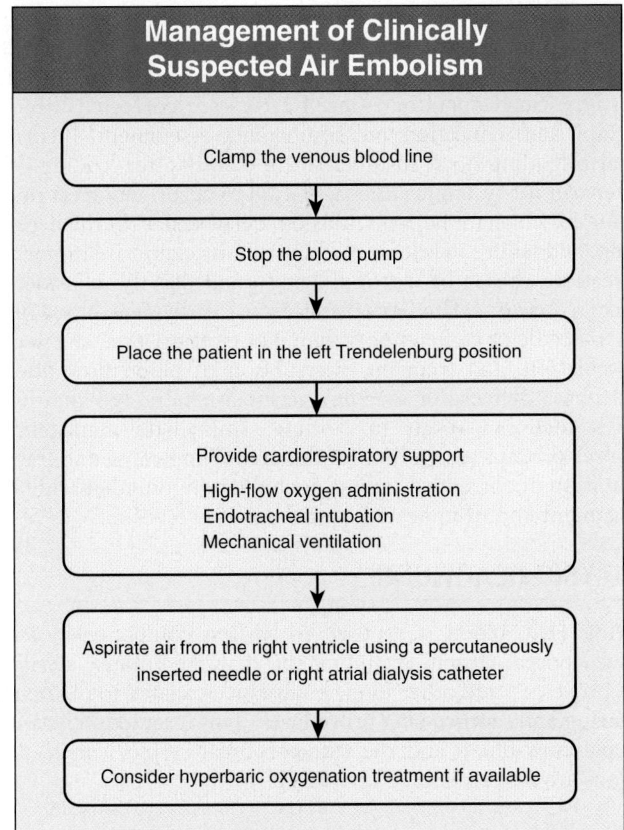

Management of Clinically Suspected Air Embolism
Clamp the venous blood line
Stop the blood pump
Place the patient in the left Trendelenburg position
Provide cardiorespiratory support
High-flow oxygen administration
Endotracheal intubation
Mechanical ventilation
Aspirate air from the right ventricle using a percutaneously inserted needle or right atrial dialysis catheter
Consider hyperbaric oxygenation treatment if available

Figure 91.6 Management of clinically suspected air embolism.

can permit air entry into the extracorporeal system. Dialysis catheters should be aspirated and flushed with saline before connection. Dialyzer rinsing, before use, should expand all compartments to remove residual air bubbles.

Incorrect Dialysate Composition

Incorrect dialysate composition results from technical or human errors. Because the primary solutes constituting the dialysate are electrolytes, the dialysate concentration will be reflected by its electrical conductivity. Therefore, proper proportioning of concentrate to water can be achieved by the use of a meter that continuously measures the conductivity of the dialysate solution as it is being fed to the dialyzer. Life-threatening electrolyte and acid-base abnormalities are avoidable if the conductivity alarm is functioning properly and the alarm limits are set correctly. However, in dialysis machines that are equipped with conductivity-controlled mixing systems, the system automatically changes the mixing ratio of the concentrates until the dialysate solution conductivity falls within the set limits. This may inadvertently lead to dialysate without any bicarbonate, with apparently acceptable conductivity. Therefore, if conductivity-controlled systems are used, it is safer to also check the dialysate pH before dialysis. Conductivity monitors can fail or can be improperly adjusted by human error. Therefore, it is important to add human monitoring of dialysate composition before every treatment, whenever a machine has been sterilized or moved about, or whenever a new concentrate is used. Furthermore, many nonstandardized solutions are available, some of which may be used with an inappropriate proportioning system. Therefore, it is also essential that the supplies match the machine-proportioning ratio for which they were prepared for the appropriate final dialysate composition to be obtained.

Hypernatremia

Hypernatremia occurs when concentrate or the ratio of concentrate to water is incorrect and the conductivity monitors or the alarms are not functioning properly. Hyperosmolality results in intracellular water depletion. Clinical manifestations include thirst, headache, nausea, vomiting, seizures, coma, and death. Aggressive treatment is mandatory and includes cessation of dialysis, hospitalization, and infusion of 5% dextrose in water. Dialysis should be resumed with a different machine; the dialysate sodium level should be 2 mmol/l lower than the plasma level, and isotonic saline should be concurrently infused. Dialysis against a sodium level 3 to 5 mmol/l lower than the serum level may increase the risk of disequilibrium. Ultrafiltration with equal volume replacement with normal saline is another option.

Hyponatremia

Failure to add concentrate, inadequate concentrate to water ratio, or conductivity monitor or alarm malfunction can cause hyponatremia. Hyponatremia can also occur during the course of dialysis with a proportioning system if the concentrate container runs dry and the conductivity set limits are inappropriate. Acute hypo-osmolality causes hemolysis with hyperkalemia and hemodilution of all plasma constituents. Symptoms include restlessness, anxiety, pain in the vein injected with the hypotonic hemolyzed blood, chest pain, headache, nausea, and occasional severe abdominal or lumbar cramps. Pallor, vomiting, and seizures may be observed. Treatment consists of clamping the blood lines and discarding the hemolyzed blood in the extracorporeal circuit. High-flow oxygen and cardiac monitoring are imperative because of hyperkalemia and potential myocardial injury. Dialysis should be restarted with a new dialysate batch containing low potassium, and high transmembrane pressure should be applied to remove excess water. Correction of serum sodium concentration should be achieved by no more than 1 to 2 mmol/l per hour. Anticonvulsants are indicated for seizures and blood transfusions for severe anemia. Successful correction of severe hyponatremia has been reported in a single 3-hour HD session with a dialysate sodium concentration of 135 mmol/l without any adverse neurologic consequences despite a serum sodium correction rate of 3 mmol/l per hour.[37] This suggests that elevated blood urea levels might protect uremic patients from the development of demyelinating syndromes when hyponatremia is rapidly corrected.

Metabolic Acidosis

Although acute intradialytic metabolic acidosis can be a manifestation of improper mixing of concentrates or failure of pH monitors, other causes need to be ruled out, including diabetic or alcoholic ketoacidosis, lactic acidosis, toxic ingestions, and dilutional acidosis.[38] The diagnosis is usually suggested by the acute onset of hyperventilation during HD and confirmed by laboratory evaluation. In most circumstances, correction of the underlying cause and use of bicarbonate dialysate at the appropriate concentration (35 mmol/l) are adequate measures.

Metabolic Alkalosis

Severe intradialytic metabolic alkalosis is rare and may be due to error in dialysate concentrates, reversed connection of bicarbonate and acid concentrate containers to the entry ports of the dialysis machine, pH monitor malfunction, or use of regional citrate anticoagulation. The most common cause, however, is hydrochloric acid loss as a result of vomiting or nasogastric suction. Attention should also be directed to identification of sources of added alkali.[39] Furthermore, the combination of sodium polystyrene sulfonate and aluminum hydroxide can lead to absorption of alkali that is normally neutralized in the small intestine.

Acute treatment is rarely necessary unless a technical error has occurred. Removal of the alkali source is usually sufficient, and H_2 antagonists or proton pump inhibitors may be successful if there is gastric acid loss. The administration of sodium chloride to anephric patients with chloride-sensitive alkalosis will not repair the alkalosis. If a more rapid reduction in serum bicarbonate is desired, modification of the dialysate bath by replacement of alkali with chloride, substitution of bicarbonate with acetate dialysate, use of acid dialysate, and infusion of hydrochloric acid are effective but cumbersome measures. The use of conventional or low-bicarbonate (25 to 30 mmol/l) dialysate is probably as effective.

Temperature Monitor Malfunction

Malfunction of the thermostat in the dialysis machine can result in the production of excessively cool or hot dialysate. Whereas cool dialysate is not dangerous and may have beneficial hemodynamic effects, overheated dialysate can cause immediate hemolysis and life-threatening hyperkalemia, particularly if the dialysate temperature increases to more than 51°C. In such an event, dialysis must be stopped immediately and blood in the system discarded. The patient should be monitored for hemolysis and hyperkalemia. Dialysis should be resumed to cool the patient by use of a dialysate temperature of 34°C to treat hyperkalemia and to allow blood transfusions if necessary. Visual and audible alarms are mandatory to prevent this complication.

Blood Loss

Intradialytic blood loss can result from arterial or venous needle disengagement from the access, separation of the venous or arterial line connections, femoral or central line dialysis catheter perforation or dislodgment, or rupture of a dialysis membrane with or without malfunction of the blood leak detector. Clinical findings include hypotension, loss of consciousness, and cardiac arrest. In addition, after traumatic insertion of a dialysis catheter, blood loss can result in pain or mass from a rapidly expanding hematoma; chest, shoulder, or neck pain from intrapericardial blood loss; back, flank, groin, or lower abdominal pain or distention from retroperitoneal bleeding; or hemoptysis from pulmonary bleeding. Acute management includes the discontinuation of HD, pressure application for local hemostasis, hemodynamic support, oxygen administration, and surgical intervention if needed.

Clotting of Dialysis Circuit

Clotting of the extracorporeal circuit during dialysis is a common practical problem, has many underlying causes, and warrants a thorough investigation. Technical factors include an inadequate or poor priming technique, resulting in retention of air in the dialyzer, and lack of or inadequate priming of the heparin infusion line. Such operator-induced errors are corrected through ongoing staff education and competency assessment. Incorrect heparin loading dose, insufficient time lapse after loading dose of heparin for systemic anticoagulation to occur, incorrect pump setting for constant heparin infusion, delayed start of the heparin pump, and failure to release the heparin line clamp are important correctible causes of clotting that should also be considered. Vascular access–related problems from inadequate blood flow due to needle or catheter positioning or clotting, excessive access recirculation, and frequent interruption of blood flow due to inadequate delivery or machine alarm situations are additional causes that can result in clotting. Immediate management requires prompt recognition of the underlying cause and implementation of corrective actions, including ongoing heparin dose adjustment and, if indicated, vascular access revision.

DIALYSIS REACTIONS

During HD, blood is exposed to surface components of the extracorporeal circuit, including the dialyzer, tubing, sterilization processes, and other foreign substances related to the manufacturing and reprocessing procedures. This interaction between the patient's blood and the extracorporeal system can lead to various adverse reactions (Fig. 91.7).[40]

Anaphylactic and Anaphylactoid Reactions

Clinical Presentation

Anaphylaxis is the result of an IgE-mediated acute allergic reaction in a sensitized patient, whereas anaphylactoid reactions result from the direct release of mediators by host cells. The onset of symptoms usually occurs within the first 5 minutes of initiation of dialysis, although a delay of up to 20 minutes is possible. Symptoms vary from subtle to severe and include burning or heat throughout the body or at the access site; dyspnea, chest tightness, and angioedema or laryngeal edema; paresthesias involving the fingers, toes, lips, or tongue; rhinorrhea, lacrimation, sneezing, or coughing; skin flushing; pruritus; nausea or vomiting; abdominal cramps; and diarrhea. Predisposing factors include a history of atopy, elevated total serum IgE, eosinophilia, and the use of ACE inhibitors. The etiology of dialysis reactions is diverse and requires a thorough investigation.

First-Use Reactions

The majority of these reactions are ascribed to the manufacturer's dialyzer sterilant ethylene oxide (ETO), which is now rarely used. The potting compound that anchors the hollow fibers in the dialyzer housing acts as a reservoir for ETO and may impede its washout from the dialyzer, leading to sensitization. When it is conjugated to human serum albumin (HSA), ETO acts as an allergen. By use of a radioallergosorbent test (RAST), specific IgE antibodies against ETO-HSA are detected in two thirds of patients with such reactions. However, 10% of patients with no history of dialysis reactions have a positive RAST result.

Reuse Reactions

As most residual ETO is washed out of the dialyzer during first use, reuse reactions are likely to be due to the disinfectants used for dialyzer reprocessing. These agents include formaldehyde,

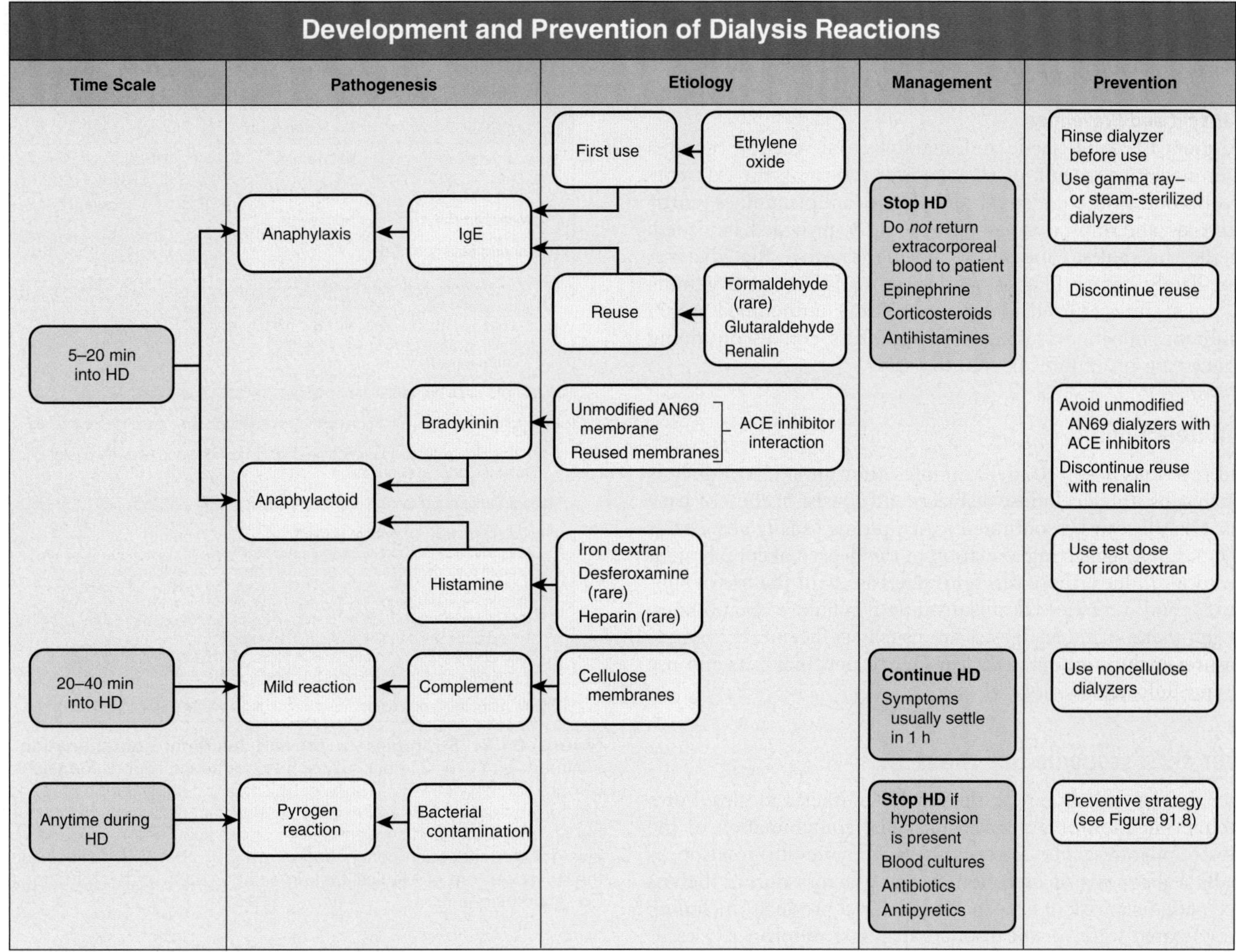

Figure 91.7 Development and prevention of dialysis reactions. ACE, angiotensin-converting enzyme; HD, hemodialysis.

glutaraldehyde, and peracetic acid–hydrogen peroxide (renalin); in allergic patients, specific IgE antibodies against formaldehyde are occasionally detectable.

Bradykinin-Mediated Reactions

In the early 1990s, anaphylactoid reactions appeared in Europe among patients dialyzed with AN69 dialyzers who were also taking ACE inhibitors. Investigation of these incidents revealed that binding of factor XII to this sulfonate-containing, negatively charged membrane resulted in the formation of kallikrein and release of bradykinin, which in turn led to the production of prostaglandin and histamine, with subsequent vasodilation and increased vascular permeability. ACE inactivates bradykinin, and therefore ACE inhibitors can prolong the biologic activities of bradykinin.[41] These membranes have since been chemically modified, thereby reducing this risk.

Anaphylactoid reactions have also been observed in patients taking ACE inhibitors who were dialyzed with membranes that had been reprocessed. Renalin was the sterilant used, and the reactions abated once reprocessing was discontinued, despite continued use of ACE inhibitors. It has been speculated that renalin may oxidize cysteine-containing proteins that are adsorbed on the dialyzer membrane, leading to the formation of cysteine sulfonate and contact activation of factor XII.

Drug-Induced Reactions

Anaphylactoid reactions to parenteral iron dextran occur in 0.6% to 1% of HD patients. Significantly higher rates of anaphylactoid reactions have been observed among users of higher molecular weight compared with lower molecular weight iron dextran.[42] *In vitro*, dextran produces a dose-dependent basophil histamine release. In light of hypersensitivity reactions, the National Kidney Foundation's Clinical Practice Guidelines recommend that resuscitative medication and personnel trained to evaluate and to resuscitate anaphylaxis should be available whenever a dose of iron dextran is administered.[43] Intravenous iron gluconate and sucrose are alternative preparations that have rapidly replaced iron dextran for patients requiring intravenous iron supplementation because of fewer anaphylactoid reactions than with high-molecular-weight dextran. Life-threatening adverse drug events, defined as reactions requiring resuscitative measures, appear to be more frequent among recipients of iron dextran than among recipients of sodium ferric gluconate complex and iron sucrose.[43-45] Ferumoxytol, a new iron formulation that might be as safe as iron gluconate and sucrose with a better dosing regimen, was recently approved for use in patients with chronic kidney disease.[46]

Hypersensitivity to heparin formulations is rare and usually responds by substitution of beef with pork heparin, or vice versa.

A recent nationwide outbreak in the United States of severe adverse reactions in HD patients was attributed to vials of heparin contaminated with oversulfated chondroitin sulfate.[47]

Treatment and Prevention

Treatment of anaphylactic and anaphylactoid reaction requires the immediate cessation of HD without returning the extracorporeal blood to the patient. Epinephrine, antihistamines, corticosteroids, and respiratory support should be provided, if needed. Specific preventive measures include rinsing the dialyzer immediately before first use, substituting ETO- with gamma ray– or steam-sterilized dialyzers, avoiding unmodified AN69 membranes in patients taking ACE inhibitors, and discontinuing reprocessing procedures in selected cases.

Mild Reactions

Mild reactions occur 20 to 40 minutes after initiation of dialysis with unsubstituted cellulose dialyzers and consist of chest or back pain. Dialysis can be continued as symptoms usually abate after the first hour, suggesting a relation to the degree of complement activation. Indeed, these reactions decrease with the use of substituted and reprocessed unsubstituted cellulose membranes. Oxygen therapy and analgesics are usually sufficient. Preventive measures include automated cleansing of new dialyzers and use of noncellulose dialyzers.

Fever and Pyrogenic Reactions

Fever during dialysis can be the result of either a localized or a systemic infection or excessive microbial contamination of the dialysis apparatus. The latter, known as pyrogenic reaction, is usually a diagnosis of exclusion. Several factors during dialysis place patients at risk of exposure to bacterial products, including contaminated water or bicarbonate dialysate, improperly sterilized dialyzers, use of central venous dialysis catheters, and cannulation of infected arteriovenous grafts or fistulas.[40] Soluble bacterial products can diffuse across the dialyzer into the blood, resulting in cytokine production and, consequently, pyrogenic reactions. Strategies for the prevention of pyrogenic reactions are summarized in Figure 91.8.[48]

When fever develops during HD, the first step is to address hemodynamic stability. If the patient is hypotensive, administration of fluids, cessation of ultrafiltration, and discontinuation of dialysis are often required, and refractory hypotension suggesting severe sepsis should trigger hospitalization.

The next step is to identify a potential source of infection. Careful examination of the dialysis vascular access is warranted. If a non–vascular access–related infectious source is identified, specific therapy should be instituted on the basis of the working diagnosis. Nontunneled and tunneled central venous dialysis catheters should always be suspected as a likely cause of infection, even in the absence of local signs of infection such as erythema and exit site drainage. Nontunneled catheters with evident signs of infection at the insertion site should be removed and the tip cultured.

Antipyretics should be administered and blood culture specimens should be obtained before initiation of antibiotic therapy. The initial choice of antibiotics should include vancomycin plus empiric gram-negative bacterial coverage (e.g., cefepime), and the regimen should be adjusted according to the culture results.[49]

In the presence of a dialysis catheter, paired blood culture specimens should be obtained from both a peripheral vein and the catheter lumen, and the aforementioned broad-spectrum antibiotic regimen should be initiated. Although the use of antibiotic lock solutions has recently emerged as an adjunct therapy aimed at preservation of the dialysis catheter, this approach warrants further investigation.[49,50] In the case of a catheter-related *Staphylococcus aureus* infection, the use of an antibiotic lock has been associated with a cure rate of less than 55%,[51] arguing for the removal of the dialysis catheter in this setting, performance of transesophageal echocardiography to rule out endocarditis, and completion of at least 14 days of antibiotic therapy.[49]

An outbreak of bacteremia among several dialysis patients involving a similar organism should prompt a thorough search for bacterial contaminants in the dialysis equipment.[40] Attention should also be paid to single-use vials that are punctured several times, such as erythropoietin, which has been linked to an outbreak of blood stream infection.[52]

Strategies to Prevent Bacterial Contamination

Strict adherence to the AAMI standards		
Type of Fluid	**Microbial Count**	**Endotoxin**
Water products	<200 cfu/ml	<2 EU
Dialysate	<2000 cfu/ml	No standard
Reprocessed dialyzers	No growth	—
Use appropriate germicide 4% formaldehyde* 1% formaldehyde heated to 40°C*† Glutaraldehyde† Hydrogen peroxide–peracetic acid mixture (renalin)*† Heat sterilization (105°C for 20 hours) for reprocessing of polysulfone membranes†		
Wash and rinse the vascular access arm with soap and water		
Prior to cannulation, inspect vascular access for local signs of inflammation		
Scrub the skin with povidone-iodine or chlorhexidine and allow to dry for 5 minutes prior to cannulation		
Record temperature before and after dialysis		
When central delivery system is used Clean and disinfect connecting pipes regularly Remove residual bacteria or endotoxin by additional filtration		
When single-patient proportioning dialysis machine is used Freshly prepare bicarbonate dialysate on a daily basis Discard unused solutions at the end of each day Rinse and disinfect containers with fluids that meet AAMI standards Air-dry containers prior to dialysate preparation		
Follow manufacturer's guidelines for use of preservative-free medications		

Figure 91.8 Strategies to prevent bacterial contamination. *A minimum of 11- or 24-hour exposure to peracetic acid or formaldehyde is required, respectively. †These germicides are equivalent or superior to 4% formaldehyde. The action level for the total viable microbial count in the product water and conventional dialysate is 50 cfu/ml, and the action level for the endotoxin concentration is 1 EU/ml. AAMI, Association for the Advancement of Medical Instrumentation; cfu, colony-forming units; EU, endotoxin units.

Investigation of a Dialysis Outbreak

Although causes of dialysis outbreaks are usually easily identifiable, many times the reason for the outbreak is less clear, such as water contamination with bacterial toxins,[53] medication chemical impurities,[47] bacterial contaminants,[52] systemic embolization of degraded dialyzer membrane polymer due to prolonged or improper storage,[54] and hemolysis due to faulty blood tube sets.[55] Investigation of a dialysis outbreak requires a methodical

Investigation of Dialysis Outbreak
Review of Medical Records
Demographics Underlying diseases Dialysis schedule Dialysis machine Dialyzer used • Membrane • Type • Manufacturer's sterilization method • Reuse germicide (if applicable) Medication history Signs and symptoms of illness Laboratory tests Interview of medical staff caring for patient during incident
Procedural Review
Water treatment systems and practices • Disinfection • Distribution • Storage procedures Disinfection and maintenance of reprocessed dialyzers Disinfection and maintenance of dialysis machines Review of patient's dialysis sessions

Figure 91.9 Investigation of a dialysis outbreak.

approach including a critical review of the medical records and the various steps of the dialysis procedure (Fig. 91.9).

MISCELLANEOUS COMPLICATIONS

Postdialysis Fatigue

An ill-defined "washed out" feeling or malaise during or after HD is a common nonspecific symptom that is observed in about one third of patients[56] and has multifactorial origins. Reduced cardiac output, peripheral vascular disease, depression, poor conditioning, postdialysis hypotension, hypokalemia or hypoglycemia, mild uremic encephalopathy, myopathy due to carnitine deficiency, and membrane bioincompatibility through cytokine production have all been incriminated. The use of glucose or bicarbonate dialysate and L-carnitine supplementation (20 mg/kg per day) has been shown to improve postdialysis well-being. A recent trial of thrice-weekly L-carnitine at 20 mg/kg for 6 months resulted in a marked decrease in C-reactive protein level, which was paralleled by an increase in body mass index.[57] To date, however, there are insufficient data to support the use of L-carnitine to improve quality of life in unselected dialysis patients.[43]

Compared with thrice-weekly HD, more frequent dialysis, including short daily and nocturnal HD, has been associated with a marked shortening in the time it takes for patients to recover from a dialysis session and to resume their daily activities, which is a surrogate for postdialysis fatigue.[58]

Pruritus

Pruritus is common. The etiology is often multifactorial, including xerosis, hyperparathyroidism, neuropathy, derangements in the immune system, and inadequate dialysis. In many cases, pruritus is more severe during or after dialysis and may be an allergic manifestation to heparin, ETO, formaldehyde, or acetate. In this subgroup of patients, use of gamma ray–sterilized dialyzers, discontinuation of formaldehyde use, switching to bicarbonate dialysate, and use of low dialysate calcium and magnesium might result in cessation of itching. Eczematous reactions to antiseptic solutions, rubber glove or puncture needle components, puncture needles, or cellophane used to secure dialysis needles should also be considered.[59]

Therapies include the use of emollients and antihistamines, activated charcoal, ultraviolet therapy, sunbathing, ketotifen (a mast cell stabilizer), erythropoietin therapy, topical capsaicin, and topical tacrolimus ointment. Dialysis adequacy should always be assessed. The management of uremic pruritus is discussed further in Chapter 84 (see Fig. 84.3).

Priapism

Priapism occurs in less than 0.5% of male HD patients. It is not related to sexual activity and occurs while the patient is on dialysis. The patient is usually awakened from sleep by a painful erection. Although the majority of cases are idiopathic, secondary causes include heparin-induced hyperviscosity; high hematocrit due to androgen or epoetin therapy; dialysis-induced hypoxemia and hypovolemia due to excessive ultrafiltration, particularly in African American men with sickle cell disease; and use of α-blockers, such as prazosin, or an antidepressant, such as trazodone.

Urologic referral is mandatory. Acute treatment consists of corporal aspiration and irrigation. Although surgical bypass provides venous egress from the corpora cavernosa, secondary impotence commonly develops but may be effectively treated by a penile prosthesis.

Hearing and Visual Loss

Intradialytic hearing loss may be due to bleeding in the inner ear as a consequence of anticoagulation or cochlear hair cell injury from edema.

Intradialytic visual loss is rare but can be caused by central retinal vein occlusion, precipitation of acute glaucoma, ischemic optic neuropathy secondary to hypotension, or Purtscher-like retinopathy secondary to leukoembolization.

Concomitant ocular and hearing impairment can occur after the use of outdated cellulose acetate dialyzer membranes.[54]

REFERENCES

1. Shoji T, Tsubakihara Y, Fujii M, et al. Hemodialysis-associated hypotension as an independent risk factor for two-year mortality in hemodialysis patients. *Kidney Int.* 2004;66:1212-1220.
2. Daugirdas JT. Dialysis hypotension: A hemodynamic analysis. *Kidney Int.* 1991;39:233-246.
3. Cruz DN, Mahnensmith RL, Brickel HM, et al. Midodrine and cool dialysate are effective therapies for symptomatic intradialytic hypotension. *Am J Kidney Dis.* 1999;33:920-926.
4. Okada K, Abe M, Hagi C, et al. Prolonged protective effect of short daily hemodialysis against dialysis-induced hypotension. *Kidney Blood Press Res.* 2005;28:68-76.
5. Locatelli F, Buoncristiani U, Canaud B, et al. Haemodialysis with on-line monitoring equipment: Tools or toys? *Nephrol Dial Transplant.* 2005;20:22-33.
6. Cogliati P. Thermal sensor and on-line hemodiafiltration [in Italian]. *G Ital Nefrol.* 2005;22(Suppl 31):S111-S116.
7. Chen J, Gul A, Sarnak MJ. Management of intradialytic hypertension: The ongoing challenge. *Semin Dial.* 2006;19:141-145.
8. Inrig JK, Oddone EZ, Hasselblad V, et al. Association of intradialytic blood pressure changes with hospitalization and mortality rates in prevalent ESRD patients. *Kidney Int.* 2007;71:454-461.

9. Rahman M, Dixit A, Donley V, et al. Factors associated with inadequate blood pressure control in hypertensive hemodialysis patients. *Am J Kidney Dis.* 1999;33:498-506.
10. Sang GL, Kovithavongs C, Ulan R, et al. Sodium ramping in hemodialysis: A study of beneficial and adverse effects. *Am J Kidney Dis.* 1997;29:669-677.
11. Ligtenberg G, Blankestijn PJ, Oey PL, et al. Reduction of sympathetic hyperactivity by enalapril in patients with chronic renal failure. *N Engl J Med.* 1999;340:1321-1328.
12. Gunal AI, Karaca I, Celiker H, et al. Paradoxical rise in blood pressure during ultrafiltration is caused by increased cardiac output. *J Nephrol.* 2002;15:42-47.
13. Bailey RA, Kaplan AA. Intradialytic cardiac arrhythmias: I. *Semin Dial.* 1994;7:57-58.
14. Kant KS. Intradialytic cardiac arrhythmias: II. *Semin Dial.* 1994;7:58-60.
15. Nakamura S, Ogata C, Aihara N, et al. QTc dispersion in haemodialysis patients with cardiac complications. *Nephrology (Carlton).* 2005;10:113-118.
16. Karnik JA, Young BS, Lew NL, et al. Cardiac arrest and sudden death in dialysis units. *Kidney Int.* 2001;60:350-357.
17. Chazan J. Sudden deaths in patients with chronic renal failure on hemodialysis. *Dial Transplant.* 1987;16:447-448.
18. Bleyer AJ, Russell GB, Satko SG. Sudden and cardiac death rates in hemodialysis patients. *Kidney Int.* 1999;55:1553-1559.
19. Kwun KB, Schanzer H, Finkler N, et al. Hemodynamic evaluation of angioaccess procedures for hemodialysis. *Vasc Surg.* 1979;13:170-177.
20. Schanzer H, Skladany M, Haimov M. Treatment of angioaccess-induced ischemia by revascularization. *J Vasc Surg.* 1992;16:861-864; discussion 864-866.
21. Clinical practice guidelines for vascular access. *Am J Kidney Dis.* 2006;48(Suppl 1):S176-S247.
22. Mattson WJ. Recognition and treatment of vascular steal secondary to hemodialysis prostheses. *Am J Surg.* 1987;154:198-201.
23. Ehsan O, Bhattacharya D, Darwish A, et al. "Extension technique": A modified technique for brachio-cephalic fistula to prevent dialysis access–associated steal syndrome. *Eur J Vasc Endovasc Surg.* 2005;29:324-327.
24. Canzanello VJ, Burkart JM. Hemodialysis-associated muscle cramps. *Semin Dial.* 1992;5:299-304.
25. Sadowski RH, Allred EN, Jabs K. Sodium modeling ameliorates intradialytic and interdialytic symptoms in young hemodialysis patients. *J Am Soc Nephrol.* 1993;4:1192-1198.
26. Chang CT, Wu CH, Yang CW, et al. Creatine monohydrate treatment alleviates muscle cramps associated with haemodialysis. *Nephrol Dial Transplant.* 2002;17:1978-1981.
27. Eknoyan G, Latos DL, Lindberg J, et al. Practice recommendations for the use of L-carnitine in dialysis-related carnitine disorder. National Kidney Foundation Carnitine Consensus Conference. *Am J Kidney Dis.* 2003;41:868-876.
28. Basile C, Giordano R, Vernaglione L, et al. Efficacy and safety of haemodialysis treatment with the Hemocontrol biofeedback system: A prospective medium-term study. *Nephrol Dial Transplant.* 2001;16:328-334.
29. Arieff AI. Dialysis disequilibrium syndrome: Current concepts on pathogenesis and prevention. *Kidney Int.* 1994;45:629-635.
30. Cheung AK. Biocompatibility of hemodialysis membranes. *J Am Soc Nephrol.* 1990;1:150-161.
31. Eaton JW, Leida MN. Hemolysis in chronic renal failure. *Semin Nephrol.* 1985;5:133-139.
32. Remuzzi G. Bleeding in renal failure. *Lancet.* 1988;1:1205-1208.
33. Lee KB, Kim B, Lee YH, et al. Hemodialysis using heparin-bound Hemophan in patients at risk of bleeding. *Nephron Clin Pract.* 2004;97:c5-c10.
34. Sabovic M, Lavre J, Vujkovac B. Tranexamic acid is beneficial as adjunctive therapy in treating major upper gastrointestinal bleeding in dialysis patients. *Nephrol Dial Transplant.* 2003;18:1388-1391.
35. Cardoso M, Vinay P, Vinet B, et al. Hypoxemia during hemodialysis: A critical review of the facts. *Am J Kidney Dis.* 1988;11:281-297.
36. O'Quin RJ, Lakshminarayan S. Venous air embolism. *Arch Intern Med.* 1982;142:2173-2176.
37. Oo TN, Smith CL, Swan SK. Does uremia protect against the demyelination associated with correction of hyponatremia during hemodialysis? A case report and literature review. *Semin Dial.* 2003;16:68-71.
38. Gennari FJ. Acid-base balance in dialysis patients. *Semin Dial.* 2000;13:235-239.
39. Gennari FJ, Rimmer JM. Acid-base disorders in end-stage renal disease: Part II. *Semin Dial.* 1990;3:161-165.
40. Jaber BL, Pereira BJG. Dialysis reactions. *Semin Dial.* 1997;10:158-165.
41. Coppo R, Amore A, Cirina P, et al. Bradykinin and nitric oxide generation by dialysis membranes can be blunted by alkaline rinsing solutions. *Kidney Int.* 2000;58:881-888.
42. Chertow GM, Mason PD, Vaage-Nilsen O, et al. On the relative safety of parenteral iron formulations. *Nephrol Dial Transplant.* 2004;19:1571-1575.
43. KDOQI Clinical Practice Guidelines and Clinical Practice Recommendations for Anemia in Chronic Kidney Disease. *Am J Kidney Dis.* 2006;47:S11-S145.
44. Aronoff GR, Bennett WM, Blumenthal S, et al. Iron sucrose in hemodialysis patients: Safety of replacement and maintenance regimens. *Kidney Int.* 2004;66:1193-1198.
45. Michael B, Coyne DW, Fishbane S, et al. Sodium ferric gluconate complex in hemodialysis patients: Adverse reactions compared to placebo and iron dextran. *Kidney Int.* 2002;61:1830-1839.
46. Singh A, Patel T, Hertel J, et al. Safety of ferumoxytol in patients with anemia and CKD. *Am J Kidney Dis.* 2008;52:907-915.
47. Blossom DB, Kallen AJ, Patel PR, et al. Outbreak of adverse reactions associated with contaminated heparin. *N Engl J Med.* 2008;359:2674-2684.
48. Dialysate for Hemodialysis. Arlington: American National Standards, Association for the Advancement of Medical Instrumentation; 2009:1-66.
49. Mermel LA, Allon M, Bouza E, et al. Clinical practice guidelines for the diagnosis and management of intravascular catheter-related infection: 2009 Update by the Infectious Diseases Society of America. *Clin Infect Dis.* 2009;49:1-45.
50. Jaffer Y, Selby NM, Taal MW, et al. A meta-analysis of hemodialysis catheter locking solutions in the prevention of catheter-related infection. *Am J Kidney Dis.* 2008;51:233-241.
51. Allon M. Treatment guidelines for dialysis catheter-related bacteremia: An update. *Am J Kidney Dis.* 2009;54:13-17.
52. Grohskopf LA, Roth VR, Feikin DR, et al. *Serratia liquefaciens* bloodstream infections from contamination of epoetin alfa at a hemodialysis center. *N Engl J Med.* 2001;344:1491-1497.
53. Carmichael WW, Azevedo SM, An JS, et al. Human fatalities from cyanobacteria: Chemical and biological evidence for cyanotoxins. *Environ Health Perspect.* 2001;109:663-668.
54. Hutter JC, Kuehnert MJ, Wallis RR, et al. Acute onset of decreased vision and hearing traced to hemodialysis treatment with aged dialyzers. *JAMA.* 2000;283:2128-2134.
55. Duffy R, Tomashek K, Spangenberg M, et al. Multistate outbreak of hemolysis in hemodialysis patients traced to faulty blood tubing sets. *Kidney Int.* 2000;57:1668-1674.
56. Parfrey PS, Vavasour HM, Henry S, et al. Clinical features and severity of nonspecific symptoms in dialysis patients. *Nephron.* 1988;50:121-128.
57. Savica V, Santoro D, Mazzaglia G, et al. L-Carnitine infusions may suppress serum C-reactive protein and improve nutritional status in maintenance hemodialysis patients. *J Ren Nutr.* 2005;15:225-230.
58. Lindsay RM, Heidenheim PA, Nesrallah G, et al. Minutes to recovery after a hemodialysis session: A simple health-related quality of life question that is reliable, valid, and sensitive to change. *Clin J Am Soc Nephrol.* 2006;1:952-959.
59. Weber M, Schmutz JL. Hemodialysis and the skin. *Contrib Nephrol.* 1988;62:75-85.

CHAPTER 92

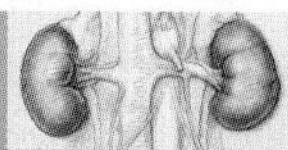

Peritoneal Dialysis: Principles, Techniques, and Adequacy

Bengt Rippe

Peritoneal dialysis (PD) is presently used by ~170,000 end-stage renal disease (ESRD) patients worldwide, representing approximately 8% of the total dialysis population.[1] In PD, the peritoneal cavity, which is the largest serosal space in the body, is used as a container for 2 to 2.5 liters of sterile, usually glucose-containing dialysis fluid, which is exchanged four or five times daily through a permanently indwelling catheter. The dialysis fluid is provided in plastic bags. The peritoneal membrane, by the peritoneal capillaries, acts as an endogenous dialyzing membrane. Across this membrane, waste products diffuse to the dialysate; excess body fluid is removed by osmosis induced by the glucose or another osmotic agent in the dialysis fluid, usually denoted ultrafiltration (UF). PD is usually provided 24 hours a day and 7 days a week in the form of continuous ambulatory peritoneal dialysis (CAPD). Approximately one third of the patients in most centers are on automated peritoneal dialysis (APD, sometimes also referred to as continuous cycler-supported peritoneal dialysis), in which nightly exchanges are delivered through an automatic PD cycler. The use of PD as a modality for ESRD treatment varies widely among countries, mostly because of nonmedical factors, such as the reimbursement policy. In one study, 81% of all dialysis patients in Hong Kong were treated with CAPD or APD in 2006, followed by Mexico (71%) and New Zealand (39%), whereas PD was used by only 7.5% in the United States and by 4.8% in Germany.[1]

ADVANTAGES AND LIMITATIONS OF PERITONEAL DIALYSIS

Assuming that the patients or their care givers are competent to undertake PD, the only absolute contraindications are large diaphragmatic defects, excessive peritoneal adhesions, surgically uncorrectable abdominal hernias, and acute ischemic or infectious bowel disease. These and other relative contraindications are discussed further in Chapter 93. PD is best used for patients with some residual renal function, although anuric patients may also do well. Most patients who start PD will eventually, after several years, transfer to other modalities of renal replacement therapy, such as hemodialysis (HD), if adequacy cannot be maintained or because of other complications, such as recurrent peritonitis or exit site or catheter problems. Only rarely do HD patients transfer to PD.

PD offers a number of advantages over HD, at least during the first 2 or 3 years of treatment. First, PD represents a "slow," continuous, "physiologic" mode of removal of small solutes and excess body water, associated with relatively stable blood chemistry and body hydration status. Second, there is no need for vascular access. The absence of vascular access and the absence of the blood-membrane contact of HD make catabolic stimuli less prominent in PD than in HD. This, and the continuous nature of PD, may be the major reason that the small solute clearance needed to yield an adequate dialysis is only ~50% of that in HD. Thus, for the same protein intake in PD compared with HD, the need for clearance of uremic waste products is reduced. Furthermore, residual renal function is better preserved in PD patients than in HD patients.

PD is a home-based therapy, and most patients are trained to do the bag exchanges themselves. In general, home dialysis patients have a better quality of life than those on other types of dialysis. The number of hospital visits is reduced and the ability to travel is increased. There is also some evidence that PD patients may be better candidates than HD patients for transplantation; several studies have shown a lower incidence and severity of delayed graft function in PD patients after transplantation.[2] In children, PD (usually APD) is the preferred dialysis modality because it is noninvasive and socially acceptable, reducing hospital visits and allowing the child to attend school. Advocates of PD often recommend that renal replacement therapy begin with PD according to the patient's choice and then proceed, as required when residual renal function declines, to HD or transplantation. PD should thus be regarded as part of an "integrated" renal replacement therapy together with HD and transplantation.[3] Factors influencing the choice of dialysis modality between PD and HD as well as global variations in the use of PD are discussed further in Chapter 86.

PRINCIPLES OF PERITONEAL DIALYSIS

The Three-Pore Model

The major principles governing solute and fluid transport across the peritoneal membrane are *diffusion*, driven by concentration gradients, and *convection* (filtration or UF), driven by osmotic or hydrostatic pressure gradients. The barrier separating the plasma in the peritoneal capillaries from the fluid in the peritoneal cavity is represented by the capillary wall and the interstitium. The interstitium can be regarded as a barrier coupled in series with that of the capillary wall; the mesothelium lining the peritoneal cavity is of much lesser significance as a transport hindrance.

For the transport of fluid (UF) and of large solutes, the capillary wall is by far the dominating transport barrier. However, for small solute diffusion, the interstitium accounts for approximately one third of the transport (diffusion) resistance. The

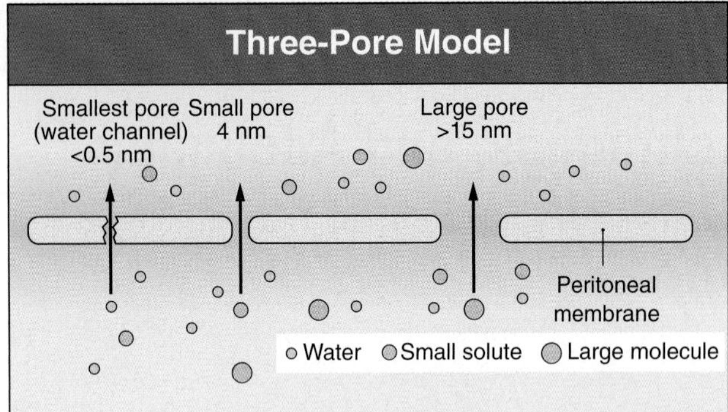

Figure 92.1 Three-pore model. The small pores in the middle represent the major pathway across the peritoneum through which small solutes move by diffusion and water moves by convection driven by hydrostatic, colloid osmotic, and crystalloid osmotic pressure differences. Across large pores *(to the right),* macromolecules move out slowly by convection from plasma to the peritoneal cavity. The smallest pores *(to the left)* are represented by aquaporins permeable to water but impermeable to solutes. Water moves here exclusively by crystalloid osmotic pressure.

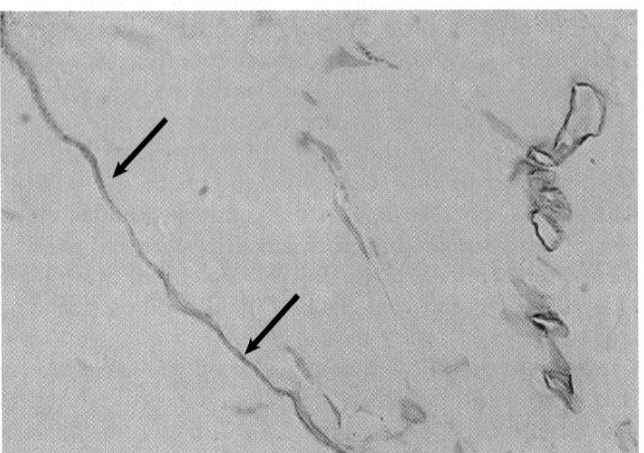

Figure 92.2 Light microscopic section of a peritoneal membrane with capillaries and venules *(to the right)* in an "amorphous" interstitium. The peritoneum is lined by a thin layer of mesothelium *(arrows).* Capillaries and venules as well as the mesothelium are immunocytochemically stained for aquaporin-1 (brownish). *(From reference 45.)*

permeability of the capillary wall can be described by a three-pore model of membrane transport (Fig. 92.1).[4,5] In the capillary wall, the major route for small solute and fluid exchange between the plasma and the peritoneal cavity is the space between individual endothelial cells, the so-called interendothelial clefts. The functional radius of the permeable pathways in these clefts, denoted sma ll pores, is 40 to 50 Å, slightly larger than the radius of albumin (36 Å). The size of these pores markedly impedes the transit of albumin and completely prevents the passage of larger molecules (e.g., immunoglobulins and α_2-macroglobulin). However, larger proteins can transit through very rare large pores (radius ~250 Å) in capillaries and postcapillary venules. The large pores constitute only 0.01% of the total number of capillary pores, and the transport across them occurs by hydrostatic pressure–driven unidirectional filtration from the plasma to the peritoneal cavity. In addition, the capillary wall has a high permeability to osmotic water transport through "water-only pores" of radius ~2 Å, present in the endothelial cell membranes. These pores have been identified as aquaporin 1 (AQP1) channels (Fig. 92.2).[6]

Fluid Kinetics

Under normal (non-PD) conditions, most transport occurs through the small pores. Only 2% of peritoneal water transport occurs by AQP1. In PD, fluid removal is markedly enhanced by infusion of a hyperosmolar dialysate into the peritoneal cavity. The type of osmotic agent used markedly affects the mechanism of osmosis. Very small osmotic agents (e.g., glycerol) will exert a rather low osmotic effect on the small pores and thereby act primarily on AQP1 channels. In contrast, glucose will induce fluid flow through both AQP1 (~40%) and small pores (~60%), whereas large molecules, such as polyglucose (icodextrin), will remove fluid mainly through small pores (~90%). Thus, glucose osmosis will result in a rapid dilution of the peritoneal dialysate, as reflected by a fall in sodium concentration (sodium sieving) during the first 2 hours of the dialysate dwell, because of relatively large transport through the water-only AQP1 channel; this tends to be corrected later as diffusion across the small pores eventually increases the sodium concentration to that in the plasma.

Glucose, the commonly used osmotic agent, is usually available at three concentrations: 1.36%, 2.27%, and 3.86%. Figure 92.3A demonstrates the intraperitoneal fluid kinetics, computer simulated by use of the three-pore model, during 12 hours of dwell time with these three solutions. Glucose is an intermediate-size osmolyte with a low osmotic efficiency (osmotic reflection coefficient $\sigma = 0.03$) across small pores, whereas glucose is 100% efficient as an osmotic agent across AQP1 (σ = 1). For that reason, glucose will markedly (30-fold) boost the transport of fluid through aquaporins and thus redistribute fluid transport away from the small pores toward AQP1, resulting in significant sodium sieving. For example, for 3.86% glucose in the PD solution, the dialysate sodium concentration will drop from 132 to 123 mmol/l in 60 to 100 minutes, which later increases toward plasma sodium concentration (Fig. 92.3B). On the other hand, icodextrin, with an average molecular weight of 17 kd, has a high osmotic efficiency (σ ~0.5) across small pores and in relative terms is rather inefficient across aquaporins. Hence, during icodextrin-induced osmosis, only a very minor fraction of the UF will occur through AQP1, producing insignificant sodium sieving (see Fig. 92.7B).

In addition to the size of the osmotic agent, the degree of sodium sieving is dependent on the presence and quantity of AQP1 and also on the total rate of net UF (which is mainly determined by the glucose concentration) and the diffusion capacity of sodium. A high rate of small solute transport, and thereby of sodium diffusion, in so-called fast transporters will show up as rapid equilibration of small solutes (creatinine and glucose) in the peritoneal equilibration test (see later discussion) and will also reduce sodium sieving.

In the absence of an osmotic agent in the PD fluid, the dialysate would be reabsorbed to the plasma within a few hours, mainly driven by the difference in colloid osmotic pressure between plasma and the peritoneum. This absorption will, to a major extent, occur through small pores, whereas ~30% of the peritoneal fluid will be removed by lymphatic absorption. The partial fluid flows in the peritoneal membrane modeled across different fluid conductive pathways in the three-pore model (for 3.86% glucose) are shown in Figure 92.4. It is the presence of relatively high concentrations of glucose in the peritoneal fluid that prevents the reabsorption of fluid to the plasma during the first few hours of the dwell.

Patients who have a high rate of sodium diffusion (fast transporters) will have more difficulty in achieving effective fluid

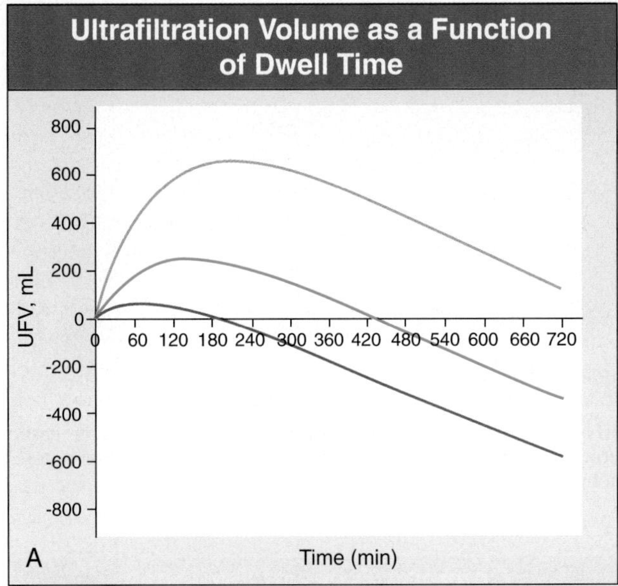

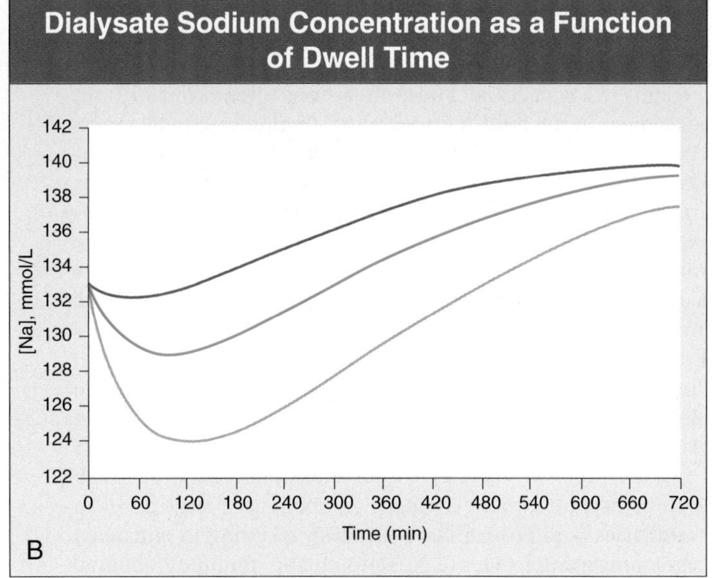

Figure 92.3 A, Ultrafiltration as a function of dwell time. Net ultrafiltration volume (UFV) as a function of dwell time for 3.86% *(yellow line),* 2.27% *(green line),* and 1.36% *(blue line)* glucose, computer simulated by the three-pore model of peritoneal transport. **B, Dialysate sodium concentration as a function of dwell time.** Dialysate sodium concentration as a function of dwell time for 3.86% *(yellow line),* 2.27% *(green line),* and 1.36% *(blue line)* glucose, computer simulated according to the three-pore model of peritoneal transport.

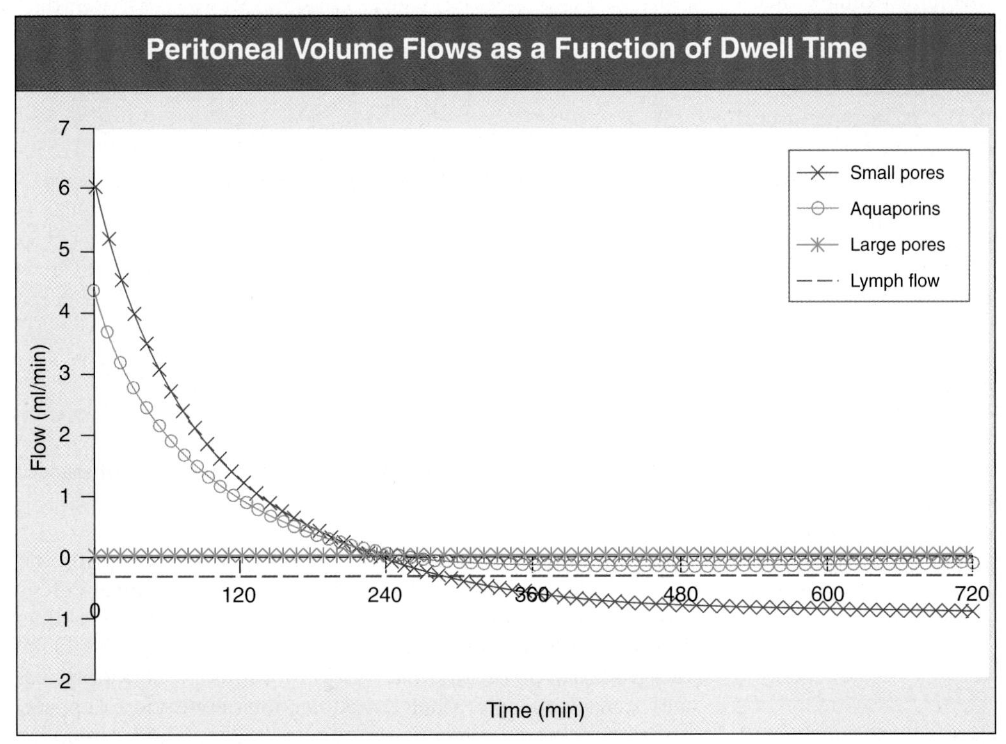

Figure 92.4 Peritoneal volume flows as a function of dwell time. Peritoneal volume flows as a function of dwell time for 3.86% glucose partitioned among aquaporins, small pores, large pores, and lymphatic absorption. The small-pore volume flow is initially approximately 60% of total volume flow and becomes negative after peak time (220 minutes). The aquaporin-mediated water flow becomes slightly negative after approximately 250 minutes. The large-pore volume flow is negligible and remains constant throughout the dwell, as does lymphatic absorption (0.3 ml/min).[33]

removal compared with slow transporters. In fast transporters, the maximum UF volume is reduced and the peak of the UF versus time curve occurs earlier. There is usually also a more rapid reabsorption of fluid in the late phase of the dwell. The issue of fluid loss from the peritoneum is controversial, however, because some authors claim that the peritoneal fluid loss occurring in the late phase of the PD dwell is dominated by lymphatic absorption.[7]

Effective Peritoneal (Vascular) Surface Area

The functional surface area of the peritoneum reflects the "effective" surface area of the peritoneal capillaries.[8] The transport of small solutes, such as urea, creatinine, and glucose, is partly limited by the degree of perfusion of these capillaries, the "effective" peritoneal membrane blood flow. Furthermore, as mentioned before, some of the diffusion resistance for the smallest solutes (urea and creatinine) is located in the interstitium. Vasodilation of arterioles results in an increase in the number of effectively perfused capillaries, whereas vasoconstriction results in a reduction. These alterations often occur without large changes in the fluid "permeability" (hydraulic conductance, L_pS) of the peritoneum. Thus, during vasodilation or vasoconstriction, there is usually a dissociation between changes in the permeability–surface area product (PS or mass transfer area coefficient [MTAC]) for small solutes and changes in L_pS of the membrane. Vasodilation, with recruitment of capillary surface area, occurs early in the dwell when glucose is used as the osmotic agent, causing early, transient increases in PS.[9]

Peritonitis is also associated with marked vasodilation, again leading to increases in small solute PS, in the absence of large changes in L_pS, during the first 60 to 100 minutes of the dwell. However, in some subjects with peritonitis, an increase in L_pS will result in relative increased fluid transport across the small pores. Furthermore, there is usually an opening of large pores in the capillaries (and postcapillary venules), resulting in enhanced leakage of macromolecules (e.g., albumin and immunoglobulins) from plasma to peritoneum. Peritonitis may thus result in a relative difficulty in removal of fluid (due to rapid dissipation of intraperitoneal glucose), a reduced sodium sieving (due to the reduced UF and increased sodium diffusion), and a markedly increased leakage of proteins to the dialysate.

The contact area between the dialysate and the peritoneal tissue varies according to posture and fill volume. Adult subjects usually tolerate 2 to 2.5 liters of instilled volume. An intraperitoneal hydrostatic pressure of less than 18 cm H_2O (supine position) is usually tolerated.[10] At higher pressures (>18 cm H_2O), the patient usually feels some discomfort. At intraperitoneal volumes of less than 2 liters, there is a reduction in small solute PS, whereas PS is only moderately increased at high fill volumes. Overall, an increased fill volume implies a more efficient exchange with regard to both small solute exchange and UF, the latter being much more pronounced for hypertonic solutions.[11] For a long time, it was thought that increased fill volumes would directly affect peritoneal fluid reabsorption by the hydrostatic pressure effect (increases in intraperitoneal hydrostatic pressure). However, because 80% of any increase in intraperitoneal hydrostatic pressure is transmitted by vein compression back to the capillaries, the actual changes in the transcapillary hydrostatic pressure gradient, which governs UF, will be rather small.[12] On the other hand, because an elevated intraperitoneal hydrostatic pressure will cause some peritoneal tissue edema and hence a lower tissue oncotic pressure, an elevated intraperitoneal hydrostatic pressure may actually (moderately) increase fluid reabsorption across the peritoneal capillaries.[13]

PERITONEAL ACCESS

The key to successful chronic PD is a safe and permanent access to the peritoneal cavity (Fig. 92.5). Despite improvements in catheter survival during the past few years, catheter-related complications still occur, causing significant morbidity and sometimes forcing the removal of the catheter. Catheter-related problems are a cause of permanent transfer to HD in up to 20% of all patients. Most catheters nowadays are derived from that originally devised by Tenckhoff and Schechter.[14] The Tenckhoff catheter is a Silastic tube with side holes along its intraperitoneal portion. There are usually one or two Dacron cuffs, allowing tissue ingrowth, which secures the catheter in place and prevents pericatheter leakage and infection. The Tenckhoff catheter is straight, having one cuff lying on the peritoneum, with the catheter tip pointing in the caudal direction; the outer cuff is close to the skin exit. Several centimeters of the catheter is thus located transcutaneously. There have been a variety of catheter designs based on the original Tenckhoff catheter. Intraperitoneal and transcutaneous catheter modifications continue to appear, indicating that no single design is perfect (Fig. 92.6). A number of studies report less frequent catheter drainage failures with use of the arcuate "swan neck" catheter (see Fig. 92.6) compared with straight catheters. The swan neck catheter appears superior to a straight catheter when it is not tunneled through an arcuate pathway with a downwardly directed exit site. A cranially directed exit site may result in an increased risk of exit site infection. However, previous catheter studies have not taken into account confounding factors such as nasal carriage of *Staphylococcus aureus* and comorbid conditions such as diabetes mellitus, both known as risk factors for exit site infection, which may put these results into doubt. Thus, there is no hard evidence that any of the

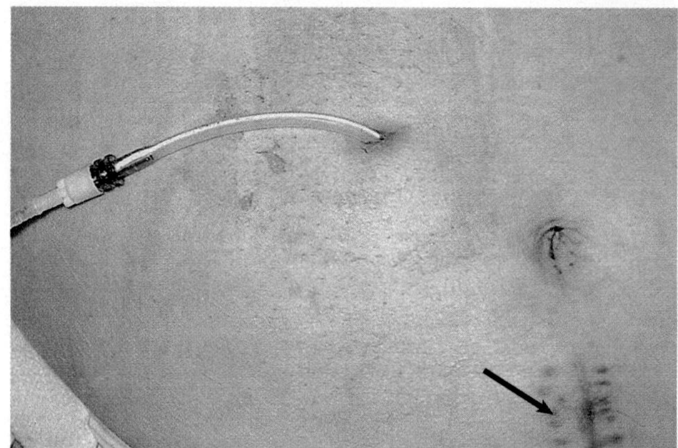

Figure 92.5 A recently implanted peritoneal dialysis catheter *in situ*. Note the subumbilical midline scar where the catheter enters the peritoneal cavity *(arrow)*.

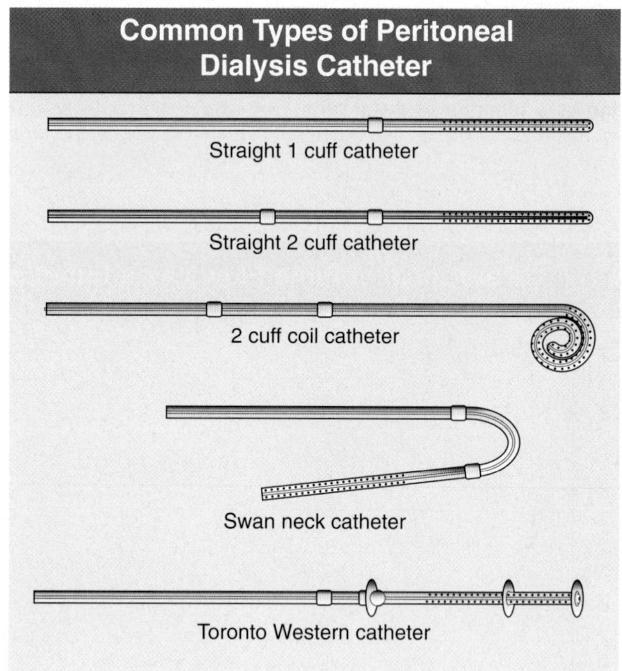

Figure 92.6 Common types of peritoneal dialysis catheter.

modified catheters on the market is actually superior to the original (one- or two-cuff) Tenckhoff catheter.[15]

Ideally, catheter insertion should be undertaken by an experienced operator, under operating room sterile conditions. In various centers, that operator may be a surgeon or a nephrologist trained in interventional nephrology techniques. Presurgical assessment for herniation or any weakness of the abdominal wall is essential; if present, it may be possible to correct this at the time of catheter insertion. Before the operation, eradication of nasal carriage of *S. aureus* with locally applied antibacterials (such as mupirocin) significantly reduces exit site infection rates. A single preoperative intravenous dose of a first- or second-generation cephalosporin is also recommended. To avoid development of vancomycin-resistant enterococcus, vancomycin should not be used as a prophylactic agent. Several placement techniques have been described and practiced: surgical minilaparotomy and dissection, blind placement using the Tenckhoff trocar, blind placement using a guide wire (Seldinger technique), mini-trocar peritoneoscopy placement, and laparoscopy. These techniques are discussed further in Chapter 88.

TECHNIQUES OF PERITONEAL DIALYSIS

In CAPD, 2 to 2.5 liters of dialysis fluid is exchanged with the peritoneal cavity four or five times daily. In 4 to 5 hours, there is nearly full (95%) equilibration of urea and approximately 65% equilibration of creatinine; the glucose gradient has dissipated to approximately 40% of the initial value. For glucose as an osmotic agent, 4 to 5 hours is a suitable dwell time, although for night dwell exchanges, longer dwell times can be accepted (8 to 10 hours). Furthermore, there is room for individual exchange schedules that can be adjusted to suit the individual patient's convenience. Dwell times shorter than 4 to 5 hours can be performed with a machine (cycler) and can be used when the patient needs to reduce intraperitoneal volume, for example, to minimize leakage. This is often the case in conjunction with catheter insertion, hernia repair, or abdominal operations. Rapid exchanges may also be required during treatment of peritonitis or in patients with fluid overload when the patient's hydration status needs to be corrected rapidly.

Nowadays, double-bag systems (so-called Y systems) are in general use according to the principle "flush before fill." The double-bag system contains the unused dialysis fluid connected to an empty sterile drain bag by a Y-set tubing system. After the patient has connected the system and flushed the connection (for 2 or 3 seconds), a frangible (breakable) pin to the drain bag is opened, and the peritoneal cavity is drained during 10 to 15 minutes to fill the drain bag. This bag is then clamped, and the "fresh" bag is opened to fill the peritoneal cavity during another 10 to 15 minutes. The time for exchange (instillation and drainage), if the catheter is in good order, should not exceed a total of 30 minutes. The first 1.6 to 1.8 liters will usually drain rapidly (at ≥200 ml/min), whereas the last 200 to 300 ml will drain much more slowly. The "breakpoint" between the rapid and the slow phases may vary markedly from individual to individual.

APD is usually performed with a cycler overnight (8 to 10 hours), during which large volumes (10 to 20 liters) can be exchanged. During daytime, the APD patient usually has a so-called wet day, that is, a long dwell, usually with icodextrin as the osmotic agent in the dialysis fluid. Some patients with nightly APD perform one daily exchange so that there are two long (6 to 8 hours) daily dwells. Most cyclers can be programmed to vary inflow volume, inflow time, dwell time, and drain time. Cyclers usually warm the fluid before inflow, and they also monitor outflow volume and the excess drainage (UF volume). Current APD machines have alarms for inflow failure, overheating, and poor drainage. Some cyclers interrupt drainage at the breakpoint between the fast and slow phases to make the exchange more efficient. Another way to accelerate exchanges is to allow a considerable "sump volume" in the peritoneal cavity by not letting all the fluid drain; subsequent inflow volumes are proportionally reduced, and after a number of cycles, complete drainage occurs. This technique is called tidal PD.

The exchange volume should be adjusted according to the patient's size. Adult patients weighing less than 60 kg should start with 1.5-liter bags. The average patient (60 to 80 kg) should receive 2-liter exchanges; and if the patient weighs more than 80 kg, 2.5 liters should be used. If pressure monitoring systems are available, the intraperitoneal hydrostatic pressure may inform the choice of exchange volume. In the supine position, most patients have an intraperitoneal hydrostatic pressure of 12 cm H_2O. If the intraperitoneal hydrostatic pressure is higher than 18 cm H_2O, the patient usually feels some discomfort.

PERITONEAL DIALYSIS FLUIDS

The majority of PD fluids used today have the composition of a lactate-buffered, "balanced" salt solution devoid of potassium, with glucose (1.36%, 2.27%, and 3.86%) as the osmotic agent. The potassium concentration in current PD fluids is zero to aid control of potassium balance.

Lactate is used as a buffer instead of bicarbonate because bicarbonate and calcium may precipitate (to form calcium carbonate) during storage. With the advent of newer multichambered PD delivery systems, it is possible to replace lactate with bicarbonate and to make a number of other solution modifications that previously were not feasible. However, the high cost of a number of the newer, more physiologic fluid formulations should be borne in mind.

Electrolyte Concentration

In current PD fluids, the concentrations of sodium, chloride, calcium, and magnesium are selected to be close to the plasma (equilibrium) concentration. The removal of these ions across the peritoneum is therefore due to the low diffusion gradient, more or less completely dependent on convection. For every deciliter of fluid removed in a 4-hour dwell, approximately 10 mmol/l of sodium[16] and 0.1 mmol/l of calcium are removed, provided plasma sodium and calcium concentrations are within the reference ranges.[12]

The frequent use of calcium-containing phosphate binders requires an understanding of calcium kinetics for various types of dialysis fluids to avoid hypercalcemia. The calcium concentration of current PD solutions is usually 1.25 to 1.75 mmol/l. However, because calcium, like sodium and magnesium, has a UF-dominated transport, 1.25 mmol/l may be considered appropriate only for 1.36% glucose to achieve a zero ("neutral") peritoneal calcium removal. To reach the same objective for 4% glucose, the dialysis fluid calcium would have to be increased to 2.3 mmol/l to prevent UF-driven calcium loss during a 4-hour dwell. With use of a three-compartment system for the PD bags, it would be possible to adapt the dialysis fluid calcium concentration either to obtain net zero peritoneal calcium transport across the peritoneum or to reach a preset calcium removal target for each PD fluid glucose concentration used.[17] However, in currently available PD solutions, calcium concentration is not variable as a function of glucose concentration; therefore, 1.25 mmol/l of calcium is recommended when patients use calcium-containing phosphate binders. However, net peritoneal calcium removal with a calcium level of 1.25 mmol/l can be achieved only by PD fluids containing 2.27% or 3.86% glucose.

The magnesium concentration commonly used in current PD solutions is 0.25 to 0.75 mmol/l. For 1.36% glucose, 0.25 mmol/l would be appropriate for zero magnesium transport during the dwell, whereas for higher dialysis fluid glucose concentrations, there will be net magnesium loss with this concentration.

Osmotic Agents

Glucose is the principal osmotic agent used for fluid removal (UF) in PD. Alternative commercially available osmotic agents are amino acids and icodextrin. Icodextrin is a polydispersed glucose polymer with an average molecular weight of 17 kd.[18] However, because of the polydispersity of icodextrin, ~70% of the molecules have a molecular weight of 3 kd or less.[11] Icodextrin is available as a 7.5% solution with essentially the same electrolyte composition as glucose-based dialysates. The osmolality of the glucose polymer solution, unlike that of 1.36% glucose (osmolality = 350 mosmol/kg) dialysis fluid, is within the same range as or actually slightly lower than that of normal plasma. The presence of larger molecules in the icodextrin solution, compared with those in glucose-based solutions, improves the osmotic efficiency markedly across the small pores ($\sigma = 0.5$) and also reduces the dissipation of the osmotic gradient over time. This yields a sustained UF during 8 to 12 hours (Fig. 92.7A). Therefore, icodextrin is preferably used for long dwell exchanges, for example, overnight, and particularly for patients who tend to absorb glucose rapidly (fast transporters, see later).

Another alternative osmotic agent, which is commercially available, is a 1.1% amino acid mixture having the same osmolality as 1.36% glucose.[19] According to some studies, regular use of this dialysate may increase certain nutritional indices, although there is also some evidence that amino acid solutions increase acidosis and raise plasma urea concentration. Both icodextrin-based and amino acid–based solutions may be used to reduce the glucose exposure of the peritoneal membrane and the total glucose load to the patient.

Until recently, conventional PD solutions have had a low pH and a high concentration of glucose degradation products (GDPs). GDPs are reactive carbonyl compounds that form during heat sterilization or storage of glucose-based solutions. GDPs are toxic to a variety of cells *in vitro* and also potentially toxic *in vivo*.[20] By the use of multicompartment systems, it has been possible to compose new solutions with much lower concentrations of GDPs and a neutral pH and also to use bicarbonate or bicarbonate-lactate mixtures as buffer.[21-23] Solutions using bicarbonate or bicarbonate-lactate mixtures result in significantly less infusion pain and are as effective as lactate at correction of acidosis when they are used at the same total buffer ion concentration.[24] In prospective, randomized studies, these fluids have been associated with improvement in dialysate effluent markers of peritoneal membrane integrity, particularly cancer antigen 125 (CA-125), a measure of peritoneal mesothelial cell mass.[21-23] There have also been some indications of improved residual renal function in patients with PD solutions low in GDPs,[23] although this was not confirmed in a prospective randomized study.[25]

Pyruvate is an alternative buffer to lactate (or bicarbonate) but is not yet clinically available. Finally, certain additives may help preserve the peritoneal membrane, such as *N*-acetylglucosamine, hyaluronic acid, citrate, and low-molecular-weight heparin. Low-molecular-weight heparin, 4500 IU in every morning bag daily for 3 months, increased UF by reduced glucose reabsorption during the dwell.[26] This may be due to reduction of the initial vasodilation that regularly occurs with intraperitoneal instillation of glucose-based PD solutions.[26] Hyaluronic acid seems to reduce the reabsorption of fluid that occurs in the late

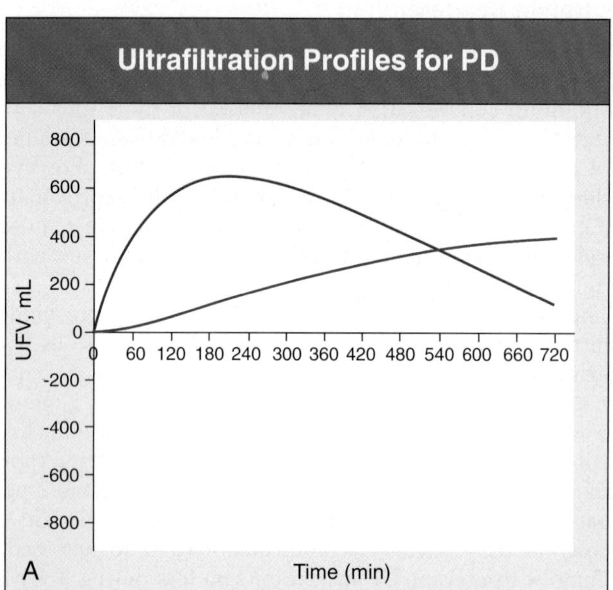

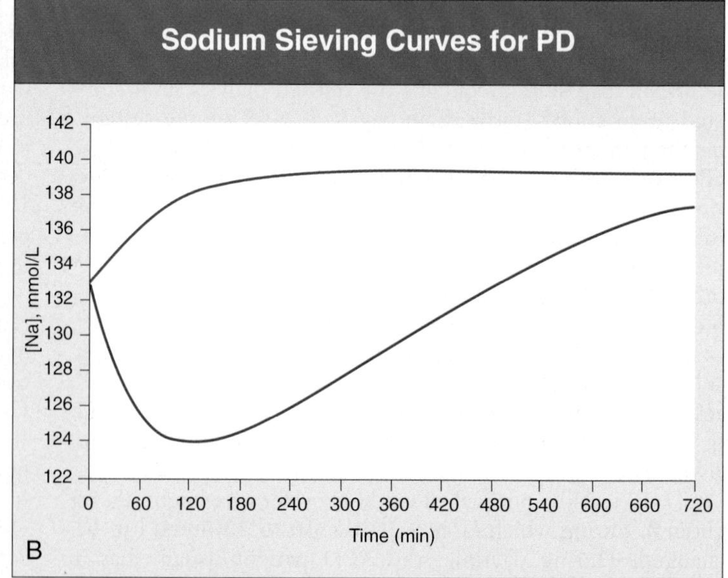

Figure 92.7 A, Ultrafiltration profiles for PD. UF profile for 7.5% icodextrin *(blue line)*, computer simulated according to the three-pore model in an average patient who is not naive to icodextrin, in comparison with the computer-simulated UF curve for 3.86% *(red line)* glucose (see Fig. 92.3). **B, Sodium sieving curves for PD.** Sodium sieving curves for 7.5% icodextrin *(blue line)* and 3.86% glucose *(red line)* (see Fig. 92.3). *(**A** from reference 11.)*

phase of the dwell, possibly by producing a "filter cake" at the peritoneal surface.[27] None of the additives (*N*-acetylglucosamine, hyaluronic acid, or low-molecular-weight heparin) or buffers (pyruvate, citrate) can yet be recommended in routine clinical practice, and further trial data are awaited.

ASSESSMENTS OF PERITONEAL SOLUTE TRANSPORT AND ULTRAFILTRATION

Small Solute Removal

The net removal of solutes and fluid during PD, in excess of residual renal excretion, can be measured by evaluating the drained dialysate. For this purpose, the concentrations of urea and creatinine are measured in dialysate and plasma. The dialysate to plasma concentration ratios (D/P) of either of these solutes multiplied by the daily drain volume gives the 24-hour clearance. Weekly creatinine and urea clearances are obtained by multiplying these figures by 7. For comparison between patients, creatinine clearances are conventionally related to body standard surface area (1.73 m^2); urea clearance (mostly for comparison with HD) is expressed as *Kt/V* (where *Kt* is the weekly clearance and *V* the volume of distribution of urea). In PD, routine assessment of *V* is imprecise, in contrast to the situation in HD, in which *V* can be mathematically derived directly from urea kinetics. *V* should preferably be determined by direct techniques, such as from the dilution of isotopic water (total body water); in practice, however, *V* is usually approximated from standard tables using body weight and height as anthropometric parameters together with gender.[28] The *Kt/V* concept in conjunction with PD is open to criticism, mostly because of the uncertainty of determining a correct value for *V*.

Large Solute Removal

To gain more insight into peritoneal transport, the clearance of larger solutes, such as β_2-microglobulin, as well as of markers for transport across the large pores, such as albumin, immunoglobulins, and α_2-macroglobulin, can be measured. Whereas many centers assess the daily peritoneal removal of total protein or albumin, measurements of most other solutes are not made in routine clinical practice.

Ultrafiltration

UF can be assessed with a 24-hour collection. Even if it is done accurately, there is a considerable dwell-to-dwell and day-to-day variability in UF, depending on drainage conditions, posture, and varying levels of residual (sump) intraperitoneal volume. Reasonably accurate estimations of daily UF volume can be obtained by averaging collections of all fluid during a period of several days. In clinical practice, the patient's own daily dialysis records should also be examined with respect to dwell-to-dwell UF volumes and the number of hypertonic bags used per day. UF volume can also be determined by the so-called peritoneal equilibration test as described later. For a 3.86% glucose dwell, a UF volume of less than 400 ml will indicate insufficient UF, that is, UF failure. In a routine 2.27% glucose peritoneal equilibration test (see later), less than 200 ml of UF in 4 hours signals UF failure. More accurate determination of intraperitoneal volume can be achieved as a function of time with use of an intraperitoneal volume marker, such as ^{125}I-labeled human serum albumin or dextran 70 (while correcting for marker clearance from the peritoneal fluid). With such marker techniques, more precise UF volume estimations can be made, which is a prerequisite for accurate estimations of true membrane parameters in terms of permeability–surface area products (PS or MTAC) for small solutes or clearance for macromolecules.

Peritoneal Membrane Function

Peritoneal Equilibration Test

The peritoneal equilibration test (PET) yields approximate estimations of the rate of peritoneal transport of small solutes and of UF capacity.[29] The rate of small solute transport is dependent on the effective peritoneal surface area, which is essentially dependent on the number of effectively perfused capillaries available for exchange (and the blood flow). The volume ultrafiltrated in 4 hours is a function of the so-called osmotic conductance to glucose (the peritoneal UF coefficient times the reflection coefficient for glucose) as well as the rate of dissipation of the glucose osmotic gradient (= rate of small solute transport). In general, when the rate of glucose disappearance is high (for fast transporters, see later), UF volume is low. The PET procedure is summarized in Figure 92.8. After an overnight dwell (8 to 12 hours), the dialysate fluid is drained, and a 2-liter 2.27% glucose bag is infused during 10 minutes with the patient in the supine position (rolling from side to side every 2 minutes). At 10 minutes (after start), that is, at completion of the infusion, 200 ml is drained into the drainage bag and mixed, and a zero time dialysate sample is taken. At the end of the 4-hour dwell period, dialysate is drained out and measured. The net volume is noted. Concentrations of glucose and creatinine in the outflow and plasma are measured, as is the concentration of glucose in the zero sample. The results are expressed as the ratio of dialysate to plasma (D/P) solute concentration and as the ratio of glucose concentration at 4 hours to dialysate glucose concentration at time zero (D/D_0). The higher the D/P ratio is for creatinine, the faster the rate of transport for small solutes. According to D/P ratios for creatinine or D/D_0 for glucose, patients can be described as slow, slow average, fast average, and fast transporters (Fig. 92.9). However, D/P measurements give only an approximate estimation of small solute transport rate. An increased D/P-creatinine is usually accompanied by a lower UF volume, but a lower UF volume will *per se* automatically (due to less dilution) tend to increase the D/P.

Peritoneal Equilibration Test
1. The night bag (8–12 hours) must be 1.36% or 2.27% glucose, drained for 20 minutes with patient sitting.
2. 2 liters (warm) 2.27% fluid instilled for 10 minutes with the patient supine and rolling from side to side every 2 minutes.
3. Exactly at 10 minutes after start of the infusion, 200 ml is drained into the bag. Draw 5 ml (discard); 5 ml taken for creatinine and glucose determination.
4. After 2 hours, new samples collected as under 3.
5. After 4 hours (exactly) drainage during 20 minutes. Note total bag weight. Subtract empty bag weight. Take samples (after mixing) for creatinine and glucose.
6. The glucose at 4 hours to dialysate glucose at time zero for glucose and dialysate to plasma ratio for creatinine are D/D_0 plotted versus time in a graph demonstrated in Figure 92.9. The drained volume is noted (D/P-creatine)

Figure 92.8 Peritoneal equilibration test.

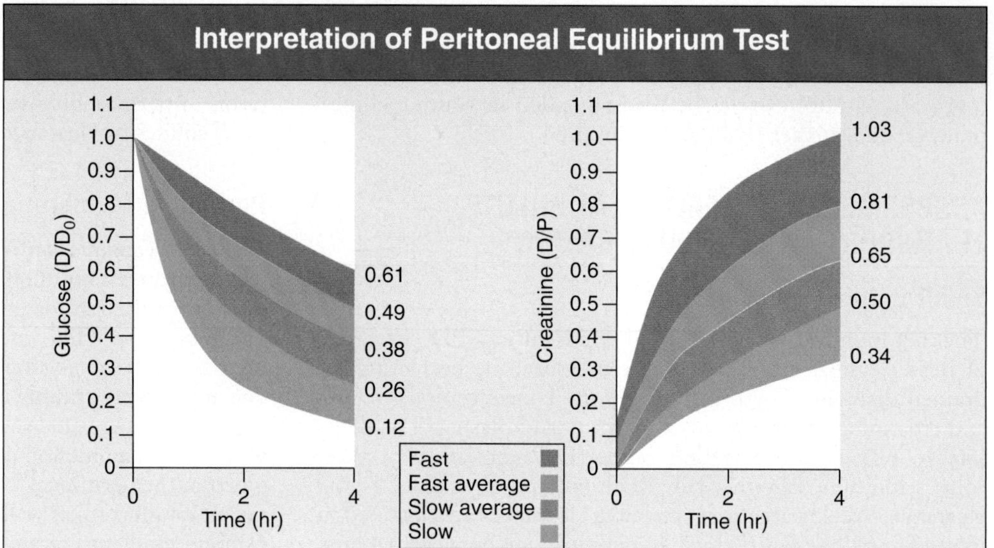

Figure 92.9 Interpretation of the peritoneal equilibration test. Changes in solute concentration allow classification into different transport types. *(Modified from reference 29.)*

Standard Permeability Analysis and the Fast-Fast Peritoneal Equilibration Test

In the standard permeability analysis (SPA), a 3.86% glucose bag is instilled, but the test is otherwise performed like the PET.[30] After a dwell time of 1 hour, a dialysate sample is taken and the sodium concentration is compared with that of the zero (time) value. This is done to assess the degree of sodium sieving and hence to obtain a measure of aquaporin-mediated water flow.[31] In SPA, UF volume below 400 ml at 4 hours suggests UF failure. A variant of SPA has been suggested with complete drainage of a 3.86% glucose bag at 1 hour and measurement of the total drained volume.[32] By such a technique, it is theoretically possible to assess the fraction of "free" water transport (across AQP1) in the early phase of the dwell when sodium diffusion is negligible from the 1-hour drained volume. First, the peritoneal clearance of sodium during 1 hour (i.e., the mass of sodium drained minus that instilled divided by the average sodium concentration in plasma) is calculated. The peritoneal clearance of sodium approximately equals the peritoneal small solute clearance of fluid (water) during the first hour of the dwell. This value is then subtracted from total UF volume. Thereby, a surprisingly accurate estimate of the free (aquaporin-mediated) water transport during the first 60 minutes is obtained, even without the application of a correction algorithm.[33] The apparent fraction of free water transport and the osmotic conductance may decline in long-term patients with UF failure, usually combined with increases in D/P-creatinine and a decline in D/D_0-glucose.[34]

Residual Renal Function

In PD, residual renal function is of considerable importance for patient and technique survival. Residual renal function is better preserved over treatment time in PD than in HD.[35] Residual renal function can be assessed by collecting all urine during a day and by assessing the urine concentrations of urea and creatinine and total urine volume. Because renal creatinine clearance, due to tubular secretion, yields an overestimate of the glomerular filtration rate (GFR) by 1 to 2 ml/min when GFR is 10 ml/min or less, and renal urea clearance yields an underestimate of GFR by 1 to 2 ml/min in the same interval of reduced GFR, a good estimate of actual GFR can be calculated as the average of renal creatinine clearance and urea clearance. However, if the daily urine volume is less than 200 ml, residual renal function will be too small to be measured accurately.

Criteria for Peritoneal Dialysis Adequacy

Clinical	The patient feels well and has a stable lean body mass No symptoms of anorexia, asthenia, nausea, emesis, insomnia Stable nerve conductance velocity
Small solute clearance	Weekly Kt/V urea >1.7 (renal + peritoneal) Weekly creatinine clearance >50 l/1.73 m^2
Large solute clearance	Albumin clearance <0.15 ml/min
Fluid balance	No edema No hypertension No postural hypotension
Electrolyte balance	Serum potassium <5 mmol/l
Acid-base balance	Serum bicarbonate >24 mmol/l
Nutrition	Daily protein intake ≥1.2 g/kg Caloric intake >35 kcal/kg/day Serum albumin >35 g/l Body mass index 20–30 kg/m^2 Stable midarm muscle circumference

Figure 92.10 Criteria for peritoneal dialysis adequacy.

ADEQUACY

An important measure of dialysis adequacy is the general clinical state of the patient, as manifested by a good nutritional status (maintained muscle mass) and the absence of anemia, edema, hypertension, electrolyte and acid-based disturbances, neurologic symptoms, pruritus, and insomnia. Management of anemia and bone disease in ESRD patients is discussed in Chapters 79 and 81, respectively. Some criteria for PD adequacy are given in Figure 92.10.

Small Solute Clearance

There are few prospective randomized studies that define adequate PD. From a clinical point of view, it has been suggested

Typical PD Regimens Required to Achieve Adequate Solute Clearances

Patient Body Surface Area (m^2)	Peritoneal Solute Transport Characteristics—D/P Creatinine at 4 Hours			
	Slow (<0.5)	Slow Average (0.5 to <0.65)	Fast Average (0.65–0.82)	Fast (>0.83)
<1.7	CAPD/APD	CAPD/APD+	APD+*	APD*
	10–12.5 liters	10–12.5 liters	10–12.5 liters	10–12.5 liters
1.7–2.0	CAPD+/APD	APD+	APD+*	APD+*
	12.5–15 liters	12.5–15 liters	12.5–15 liters	12.5–15 liters
>2.0	CAPD+, HD	APD+	APD+*	APD+*
		15–20 liters	15–20 liters	15–20 liters

Figure 92.11 Peritoneal dialysis regimens. Typical peritoneal dialysis regimens required to achieve adequate solute clearance according to patient size and membrane characteristics in anuric patients. The total volume of dialysate fluid required increases with body size, using 2.5- or even 3.0-liter exchanges. As solute transport increases, the use of automated peritoneal dialysis (APD) with shorter overnight exchanges is favored over continuous ambulatory peritoneal dialysis (CAPD). Both CAPD and APD may have to be augmented with an additional exchange (denoted by +); this is given by way of an additional afternoon exchange in CAPD patients or by employing an exchange device that delivers a single additional exchange at night. HD, hemodialysis. *The use of glucose polymer (icodextrin) solution for the long exchange will enhance both solute clearance and ultrafiltration.

that a weekly *Kt/V* above 1.7 and a weekly creatinine clearance above 50 l/1.73 m^2 would be minimally adequate for patients on CAPD. This represents only approximately 50% to 60% of the urea and creatinine clearance considered adequate in HD patients. In a large prospective study in the United States and Canada, the CANUSA study, the outcome for a cohort of 680 patients starting CAPD was studied with an average follow-up of 2 years.[36] In the CANUSA study, patients who maintained a high *Kt/V* or creatinine clearance over time did better than those who did not. An increase of 0.1 unit of *Kt/V* (peritoneal and renal) per week was associated with a 5% decrease in relative risk of death, and an increase of 5 l/1.73 m^2 of creatinine clearance per week (peritoneal and renal) was associated with a 7% decrease in the relative risk of death. Further analysis of the CANUSA study indicated that the survival advantage of patients with higher total small solute clearance was entirely attributed to the residual renal function. For each increase of 250 ml of urine output per day, there was a 36% decrease in the relative risk of death. In the ADEMEX study,[37] a large randomized controlled clinical trial designed to test the value of increasing peritoneal small solute clearance in a Mexican PD cohort, there was no obvious survival advantage of increasing the peritoneal clearance to obtain a total creatinine clearance above 60 l/1.73 m^2 compared with less than 50 l/1.73 m^2.

From these studies, it seems that renal clearance and peritoneal clearance are not mutually comparable. High residual renal function is of greater survival advantage than high peritoneal solute transport capacity. The mere fact that the survival of PD patients is equal to or supersedes that of HD patients during the first 2 to 3 years of dialysis (see later), despite the fact that PD provides ~50% of the total *Kt/V* of HD, indicates that the benefit of PD goes beyond the clearance of small solutes. In a European multicenter study of APD, the EAPOS study, small solute clearance did not correlate with survival in anuric patients.[38] On the contrary, total volume removal and hydration state were important factors. Still, there is reasonably good evidence that a weekly *Kt/V* above 1.7 and a weekly creatinine clearance above 50 l/1.73 m^2 are adequacy targets that should be reached and maintained in a majority of patients. As residual renal function declines, attempts should be made to increase the dose of dialysis, either by increasing the exchange volumes or by prescribing more frequent exchanges.

The concept of *Kt/V*, a kinetic parameter obtained from HD practice, is somewhat questionable in PD. Theoretically, body surface area would be superior to urea distribution volume to normalize urea clearance. Furthermore, the long-term PD patient is often overhydrated or has an increased fat mass, which makes the estimation of *V* cumbersome.[39] A patient with a high solute transport will achieve peritoneal creatinine clearance targets rather easily, whereas obese individuals may have difficulties in reaching an adequate Kt/V_{urea}.

Commercially available computer programs* can predict urea and creatinine clearances and peritoneal UF performance and provide suggestions for treatment options based on drained volumes and on plasma and dialysate creatinine and urea values. These parameters are often obtained by PET or standardized schedules for specified dwell exchanges. Some of the programs yield an estimate of peritoneal albumin clearance, which to a great extent is dependent on the filtration occurring across large pores, being increased in "inflammation." Recommended dialysis schedules based on the categorization of the PET are given in Figure 92.11.

Fluid Balance

As in all types of renal replacement therapy, long-term maintenance of adequate fluid and electrolyte balance is of crucial importance for the survival of patients on PD. As already mentioned, the outcome of PD is directly related to residual renal function, particularly a high urine output. Furthermore, patients with fast transport in the PET (a more rapid absorption of glucose and a more rapid loss of the osmotic gradient) have a reduced technique survival. It seems evident that after 2 or 3 years of PD, when residual renal function is low, most patients on PD are fluid overloaded. It is likely that volume overload not only

*www.baxter.com/products/renal/software/pdadequest/index.html
www.gambro.com/int/2713/Peritoneal-Dialysis/Products/Synergy/.
www.fmc-ag.com/internet/fmc/fmcag/neu/fmcpub.nsf/Content/
Software_%28Peritoneal_Dialysis%29.

aggravates hypertension but also leads to progression of left ventricular hypertrophy, often already present at the start of PD. However, during the first year of PD, there is often a fall in blood pressure and a reduced need for antihypertensive agents. Unfortunately, with time on PD, blood pressure usually rises and the number of antihypertensive drugs needed usually again increases.[40] Therefore, it is advisable to regularly assess fluid removal in the patients over time, at least every 6 months, either separately (using SPA) or in conjunction with PET measurements.

Management of Fluid Overload

As total urinary water (and sodium) excretion and peritoneal UF volume decline, it is advisable to instruct patients to restrict salt and water intake. In view of the difficulty in compliance with salt restriction, the use of PD solutions with lower sodium concentration has been advocated. Preliminary studies of low-sodium PD solutions have been very promising, reducing the need for blood pressure–lowering drugs to control hypertension[41]; however, low-sodium solutions are not yet commercially available. Loop diuretics such as furosemide (250 to 500 mg daily) can be used to maintain urine volumes but do not maintain renal clearance. If salt and water restriction and diuretics are not effective in maintaining UF, it can be enhanced by increasing the dialysis glucose concentration to 2.27% (or 3.86%). Patients with alterations in peritoneal membrane function appearing in the first few years of PD usually have an increased small solute transport combined with only a moderate increase in peritoneal UF capacity,[34] and there is an increased reabsorption of fluid in the late phase of the dwell. These patients can benefit from switching to APD and to the use of icodextrin for one of the daily exchanges. Randomized controlled trials using icodextrin for the long daytime dwell in APD have demonstrated an improved UF and a reduced extracellular fluid volume.[42] Patients who have been on PD for several years may have a reduced UF capacity (reduced osmotic conductance to glucose).[34] These patients would theoretically benefit less from switching to icodextrin because of the reduced UF capacity.

Nutrition

During their first year of treatment, CAPD patients typically have evidence of net anabolism; the average weight gain may exceed 5 kg without any clinical signs of fluid overload. Contributing to this weight gain is the peritoneal glucose reabsorption (on average, 100 to 150 g daily), which adds 400 to 600 kcal of energy intake daily. As residual renal function declines, the nutritional and metabolic abnormalities in CAPD become increasingly manifested, with reductions in lean body mass. The main cause of protein-energy malnutrition and wasting, apart from poor food intake, is the impaired metabolism of protein and energy in uremia. Despite glucose absorption, many patients on long-term CAPD have signs of energy malnutrition, a major component of the uremic wasting syndrome. Contributing factors are low-grade inflammation associated with carbonyl and oxidative stress and accelerated atherosclerosis, the so-called malnutrition-inflammation-atherosclerosis syndrome.[43] It is important for CAPD patients to be prescribed an adequate amount of protein (>1.2 g of protein per kilogram per day) and energy (total energy intake >35 kcal per kilogram per day) and a sufficient dose of dialysis, enabling the patient to ingest this diet. The daily losses of protein to the dialysate are not negligible but approximate 5 to 7 g daily, of which ~4 to 5 g is albumin. This actually compares to the losses occurring in nephrotic-range proteinuria. The nutritional management of PD patients should include frequent assessments of their nutritional status, and if it is inadequate, referral for HD (or transplantation) should be considered. Nutrition in PD patients is discussed further in Chapter 83.

OUTCOME OF PERITONEAL DIALYSIS

Registry data[1] have indicated a lower risk of death in patients treated with PD during the first 2 years of treatment compared with those treated with HD, although overall, the mortality in PD compared with HD is not significantly different. Survival differences seem to vary substantially according to the underlying cause of ESRD, age, and baseline comorbidity. In a study based on U.S. Medicare registry data,[44] HD was associated with a higher risk of death among diabetic patients with no comorbidity and among younger patients (18 to 44 years), whereas PD was associated with a higher risk of death among older patients (45 to 64 years). In patients with mortality rates adjusted for comorbidity at start of dialysis, there were no differences between HD and PD among nondiabetic patients and among younger diabetic patients (18 to 44 years), but mortality was higher on PD for older diabetic patients with baseline comorbidity.

REFERENCES

1. Collins AJ, Foley RN, Herzog C, et al. United States Renal Data System 2008 Annual Data Report Abstract. *Am J Kidney Dis*. 2009;53:vi-vii, S8-374.
2. Bleyer AJ, Burkart JM, Russell GB, Adams PL. Dialysis modality and delayed graft function after cadaveric renal transplantation. *J Am Soc Nephrol*. 1999;10:154-159.
3. Coles GA, Williams JD. What is the place of peritoneal dialysis in the integrated treatment of renal failure? *Kidney Int*. 1998;54:2234-2240.
4. Rippe B, Stelin G. Simulations of peritoneal solute transport during continuous ambulatory peritoneal dialysis (CAPD). Application of two-pore formalism. *Kidney Int*. 1989;35:1234-1244.
5. Rippe B, Stelin G, Haraldsson B. Computer simulations of peritoneal fluid transport in CAPD. *Kidney Int*. 1991;40:315-325.
6. Ni J, Verbavatz JM, Rippe A, et al. Aquaporin-1 plays an essential role in water permeability and ultrafiltration during peritoneal dialysis. *Kidney Int*. 2006;69:1518-1525.
7. Krediet RT. The effective lymphatic absorption rate is an accurate and useful concept in the physiology of peritoneal dialysis. *Perit Dial Int*. 2004;24:309-313; discussion 316-307.
8. Flessner MF. Peritoneal transport physiology: Insights from basic research. *J Am Soc Nephrol*. 1991;2:122-135.
9. Waniewski J, Heimbürger O, Werynski A, Lindholm B. Diffusive mass transport coefficients are not constant during a single exchange in continuous ambulatory peritoneal dialysis. *ASAIO J*. 1996;42:M518-M523.
10. Fischbach M, Dheu C. Hydrostatic intraperitoneal pressure: An objective tool for analyzing individual tolerance of intraperitoneal volume. *Perit Dial Int*. 2005;25:338-339.
11. Rippe B, Levin L. Computer simulations of ultrafiltration profiles for an icodextrin-based peritoneal fluid in CAPD. *Kidney Int*. 2000;57:2546-2556.
12. Rippe B, Venturoli D, Simonsen O, de Arteaga J. Fluid and electrolyte transport across the peritoneal membrane during CAPD. *Perit Dial Int*. 2004;1:10-27.
13. Rippe B. Is intraperitoneal pressure important? *Perit Dial Int*. 2006;26:317-319; discussion 411.
14. Tenckhoff H, Schechter H. A bacteriologically safe peritoneal access device. *Trans Am Soc Artif Intern Organs*. 1973;10:363-370.
15. Flanigan M, Gokal R. Peritoneal catheters and exit-site practices toward optimum peritoneal access: A review of current developments. *Perit Dial Int*. 2005;25:132-139.
16. Heimbürger O, Waniewski J, Werynski A, Lindholm B. A quantitative description of solute and fluid transport during peritoneal dialysis. *Kidney Int*. 1992;41:1320-1332.

17. Simonsen O, Wieslander A, Venturoli D, et al. Mass transfer of calcium across the peritoneum at three different peritoneal dialysis fluid Ca and glucose concentrations. *Kidney Int*. 2003;64:208-215.
18. Mistry CD, Gokal R, Peers E. A randomized multicenter clinical trial comparing isosmolar icodextrin with hyperosmolar glucose solutions in CAPD. MIDAS Study Group. Multicenter Investigation of Icodextrin in Ambulatory Peritoneal Dialysis. *Kidney Int*. 1994;46:496-503.
19. Kopple JD, Bernard D, Messana J, et al. Treatment of malnourished CAPD patients with an amino acid based dialysate. *Kidney Int*. 1995;47:1148-1157.
20. Wieslander AP, Nordin MK, Kjellstrand PT, Boberg UC. Toxicity of peritoneal dialysis fluids on cultured fibroblasts, L-929. *Kidney Int*. 1991;40:77-79.
21. Rippe B, Simonsen O, Heimbürger O, et al. Long-term clinical effects of a peritoneal dialysis fluid with less glucose degradation products. *Kidney Int*. 2001;59:348-357.
22. Jones S, Holmes CJ, Krediet RT, et al. Bicarbonate/lactate-based peritoneal dialysis solution increases cancer antigen 125 and decreases hyaluronic acid levels. *Kidney Int*. 2001;59:1529-1538.
23. Williams JD, Topley N, Craig KJ, et al. The Euro-Balance Trial: The effect of a new biocompatible peritoneal dialysis fluid (balance) on the peritoneal membrane. *Kidney Int*. 2004;66:408-418.
24. Mactier RA, Sprosen TS, Gokal R. Bicarbonate and bicarbonate/lactate peritoneal dialysis solutions for the treatment of infusion pain. *Kidney Int*. 1998;53:1061-1067.
25. Fan SL, Pile T, Punzalan S, et al. Randomized controlled study of biocompatible peritoneal dialysis solutions: Effect on residual renal function. *Kidney Int*. 2008;73:200-206.
26. Sjøland JA, Smith Pedersen R, Jespersen J, Gram J. Intraperitoneal heparin reduces peritoneal permeability and increases ultrafiltration in peritoneal dialysis patients. *Nephrol Dial Transplant*. 2004;19:1264-1268.
27. Rosengren B-I, Carlsson O, Rippe B. Hyaluronan and peritoneal ultrafiltration: A test of the "filter-cake" hypothesis. *Am J Kidney Dis*. 2001;37:1277-1285.
28. Watson PE, Watson ID, Batt RD. Total body water volumes for adult males and females estimated from simple anthropometric measurements. *Am J Clin Nutr*. 1980;33:27-39.
29. Twardowski ZJ, Nolph DK, Khanna R, et al. Peritoneal equilibration test. *Perit Dial Bull*. 1987;7:138-147.
30. Pannekeet MM, Imholz AL, Struijk DG, et al. The standard peritoneal permeability analysis: A tool for the assessment of peritoneal permeability characteristics in CAPD patients. *Kidney Int*. 1995;48:866-875.
31. Smit W, Struijk DG, Ho-Dac-Pannekeet MM, Krediet RT. Quantification of free water transport in peritoneal dialysis. *Kidney Int*. 2004;66:849-854.
32. La Milia V, Di Filippo S, Crepaldi M, et al. Mini–peritoneal equilibration test: A simple and fast method to assess free water and small solute transport across the peritoneal membrane. *Kidney Int*. 2005;68:840-846.
33. Venturoli D, Rippe B. Validation by computer simulation of two indirect methods for quantification of free water transport in peritoneal dialysis. *Perit Dial Int*. 2005;25:77-84.
34. Davies SJ. Longitudinal relationship between solute transport and ultrafiltration capacity in peritoneal dialysis patients. *Kidney Int*. 2004;66:2437-2445.
35. Rottembourg J, Issad B, Gallego JL, et al. Evolution of residual renal function in patients undergoing maintenance haemodialysis or continuous ambulatory peritoneal dialysis. *Proc Eur Dial Transplant Assoc*. 1983;19:397-403.
36. Adequacy of dialysis and nutrition in continuous peritoneal dialysis: Association with clinical outcomes. Canada-USA (CANUSA) Peritoneal Dialysis Study Group. *J Am Soc Nephrol*. 1996;7:198-207.
37. Paniagua R, Amato D, Vonesh E, et al. Effects of increased peritoneal clearances on mortality rates in peritoneal dialysis: ADEMEX, a prospective, randomized, controlled trial. *J Am Soc Nephrol*. 2002;13:1307-1320.
38. Brown EA, Davies SJ, Rutherford P, et al. Survival of functionally anuric patients on automated peritoneal dialysis: The European APD Outcome Study. *J Am Soc Nephrol*. 2003;14:2948-2957.
39. Johansson AC, Samuelsson O, Attman PO, et al. Limitations in anthropometric calculations of total body water in patients on peritoneal dialysis. *J Am Soc Nephrol*. 2001;12:568-573.
40. Faller B, Lameire N. Evolution of clinical parameters and peritoneal function in a cohort of CAPD patients followed over 7 years. *Nephrol Dial Transplant*. 1994;9:280-286.
41. Davies S, Carlsson O, Simonsen O, et al. The effects of low-sodium peritoneal dialysis fluids on blood pressure, thirst and volume status. *Nephrol Dial Transplant*. 2009;24:1609-1617. Epub 2009 Jan 14.
42. Davies SJ, Woodrow G, Donovan K, et al. Icodextrin improves the fluid status of peritoneal dialysis patients: Results of a double-blind randomized controlled trial. *J Am Soc Nephrol*. 2003;14:2338-2344.
43. Stenvinkel P, Heimburger O, Paultre F, et al. Strong association between malnutrition, inflammation, and atherosclerosis in chronic renal failure. *Kidney Int*. 1999;55:1899-1911.
44. Vonesh EF, Snyder JJ, Foley RN, Collins AJ. The differential impact of risk factors on mortality in hemodialysis and peritoneal dialysis. *Kidney Int*. 2004;66:2389-2401.
45. Carlsson O, Nielsen S, Zakaria el R, Rippe B. In vivo inhibition of transcellular water channels (aquaporin-1) during acute peritoneal dialysis in rats. *Am J Physiol*. 1996;271:H2254-H2262.

CHAPTER 93

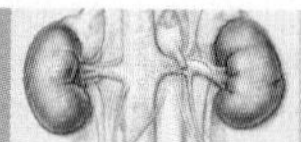

Complications of Peritoneal Dialysis

Simon J. Davies, John D. Williams

CHANGES IN PERITONEAL STRUCTURE AND FUNCTION

Loss of peritoneal function is a major factor leading to late treatment failure in peritoneal dialysis (PD).[1] Although the precise biologic mechanisms responsible for these changes are not fully understood, it is widely assumed that alterations in peritoneal function, a combination of an increased rate of small solute transport and loss of ultrafiltration (UF) capacity, are related to structural changes in the peritoneal membrane.[2] There is accumulating evidence that continuous exposure to dialysis solution components and repeated episodes of bacterial peritonitis (Fig. 93.1) are the main drivers of this process. Whereas the relationship between structure and function has not been fully defined, increased solute transport is likely to reflect a greater vascular surface area, which in turn causes reduced UF due to early loss of the osmotic gradient and enhanced fluid reabsorption (type 1 UF failure). There is also evidence of an additional mechanism by which membranes exhibit a reduced UF capacity for a given osmotic gradient (type 2 failure, reduced osmotic conductance) that might be explained by progressive fibrosis.

Studies that have quantified these changes within the submesothelial collagenous zone suggest a progressive increase in thickness with time on PD (Figs. 93.2 and 93.3). Changes within the peritoneal vascular bed have also been identified. These include progressive changes to the structure of small venules ranging from subtle thickening of the subendothelial matrix to complete obliteration of vessels (Fig. 93.4).[3] In one study, the extent of these changes in a small group of patients correlated with the loss of ultrafiltration.[4] Thus there is accumulating evidence that changes occur in both the interstitial and vascular compartments of the dialyzed peritoneal membrane.

Given that one of the likely drivers of membrane damage is the toxic profile of conventional dialysis solutions (low pH, lactate buffers, high concentration of glucose degradation products), new, more biocompatible solutions have been developed that variably correct these factors. Initial studies using these fluids indicated that dialysate effluent biomarkers thought to represent membrane integrity improve, with a reduction in circulating glucose degradation products.[5-7] There is still little evidence that this translates into clinically relevant endpoints, in part because of the inherent difficulties in undertaking sufficiently powered randomized trials. There is suggestive evidence from some studies that residual renal function might be better preserved, but these data are confounded by a concomitant reduction in peritoneal UF. Whereas these solutions are more biocompatible, to achieve adequate UF, it remains necessary to use high glucose concentrations that are unphysiologic and may still damage the membrane. When possible, excessive glucose exposure should be avoided to preserve the membrane.

REDUCED ULTRAFILTRATION AND ULTRAFILTRATION FAILURE

Recognizing the Problem

There is increasing evidence that reduced UF is associated with poor survival in PD.[8-10] The cause and effect in this relationship are not clear because the studies are observational, but in the only study with a preset UF target (>750 ml/day), mortality was significantly worse in those patients who were identified as having reduced peritoneal UF capacity, resulting in daily UF consistently below this level.[9] UF failure, often defined as less than 400 ml at 4 hours after a 3.86% exchange, is also associated with technique failure. This occurs in up to 31% of patients by 6 years of treatment.

Problems with UF should be suspected if patients have signs of fluid overload or are using excessive numbers of hypertonic exchanges and when the total fluid removal per day (urine plus dialysate) is less than 1 liter. It is important to check the actual drainage volumes by asking the patient to bring the bags to the unit and to remember to include the overfill flush volume in the calculation of net UF. In these circumstances, peritoneal membrane function tests should be performed to establish the solute transport rate and UF capacity of the membrane. If membrane function is normal and ultrafiltration adequate, it is likely that fluid or salt intake is excessive, and educational measures must be undertaken to correct this. Diabetics may require improved blood glucose control, which will be helped by reducing the glucose prescription and using icodextrin and amino acid solutions.[11] If the UF capacity is less than 200 ml (including overfill, otherwise zero net UF) by a routine peritoneal equilibration test (PET)[12] with 2.27% glucose or less than 400 ml by a modified standard permeability analysis (SPA)[13] with 3.86% glucose, then treatment strategy is determined by transport status (4-hour dialysate to plasma creatinine ratio). It is recommended that patients undergo routine membrane function tests (PET or SPA) at 6 weeks after starting PD and then at least on an annual basis or when clinical problems with fluid management are manifested.

Management of Fast Solute Transport Ultrafiltration Failure (Dialysate to Creatinine Ratio >0.64 at 4 hours)

In observational studies, increased solute transport is consistently associated with increased mortality and technique failure, independent of age, gender, and comorbidity. In patients with fast transport, there is a more rapid absorption of glucose from the peritoneal cavity, which results in the early loss of the osmotic gradient, leading to reduced net UF and more rapid fluid reabsorption once the osmotic gradient has dissipated. Short dwell periods reduce the degree of fluid reabsorption, and a change to automated PD (APD) using several (typically four or five) short overnight cycles may improve the situation. If there is a significant urine output, a loop diuretic in high dose should be tried. Furosemide, 250 mg/day, has been shown in a randomized study to maintain urine volume and sodium excretion without affecting clearances.[14]

For the long dwells, icodextrin, a glucose polymer that is iso-osmotic with plasma, can generate prolonged UF due to a sustained oncotic pressure gradient that also avoids fluid reabsorption. A number of randomized trials have shown that this prevents fluid reabsorption in the long dwell, resulting in a significant benefit compared with glucose 2.27% in fast transporters.[15] It also improves the fluid status of these patients by reducing the extracellular fluid (EF) volume, usually by ~15%.[16] When patients are started on icodextrin, care needs to be taken to avoid a rapid change in fluid status, typically seen in individuals in whom excessive fluid reabsorption was occurring, as this might result in a loss of residual renal function (RRF). When icodextrin has been used in long-term studies (e.g., in anuric patients using APD), fast peritoneal transport is no longer a risk factor for mortality and technique failure, and there is stable membrane function. Some patients, usually long term, will fail to achieve adequate UF despite these measures. These patients have usually acquired both fast solute transport and low osmotic conductance and have combined type 1 and type 2 UF failure (see later discussion).

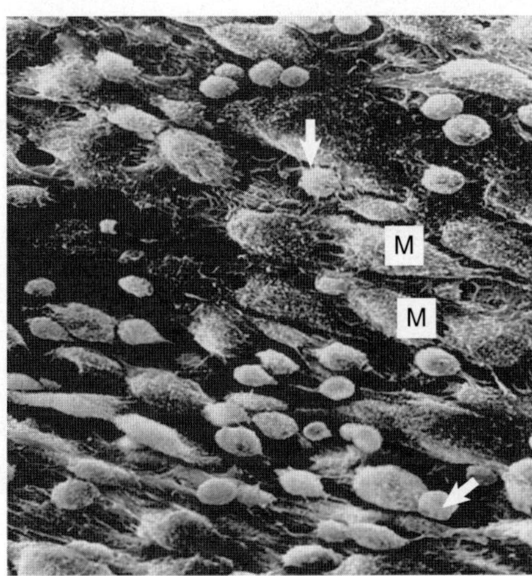

Figure 93.1 Peritonitis. Scanning electron micrograph of the peritoneum from a patient receiving peritoneal dialysis (PD) who has peritonitis. The small round cells *(arrows)* are phagocytes, which are widely distributed among the mesothelial cells (M). (Magnification ×1800.)

Management of Slow Transport Ultrafiltration Failure (Dialysate to Plasma Creatinine Ratio <0.64)

Although slow transport ultrafiltration failure is less common, its management is more difficult. It is essential to exclude any form of mechanical failure, such as an occult peritoneal cuff leak or an inguinal hernia, by contrast-enhanced computed tomography (CT). Once mechanical problems have been excluded, it is possible to determine whether the poor UF is due to a failure of UF or of excessive fluid reabsorption by determining whether sodium sieving is present. Typically, slow transport patients will have a sustained glucose gradient and will therefore exhibit sodium sieving (a decrease in the dialysate sodium concentration)

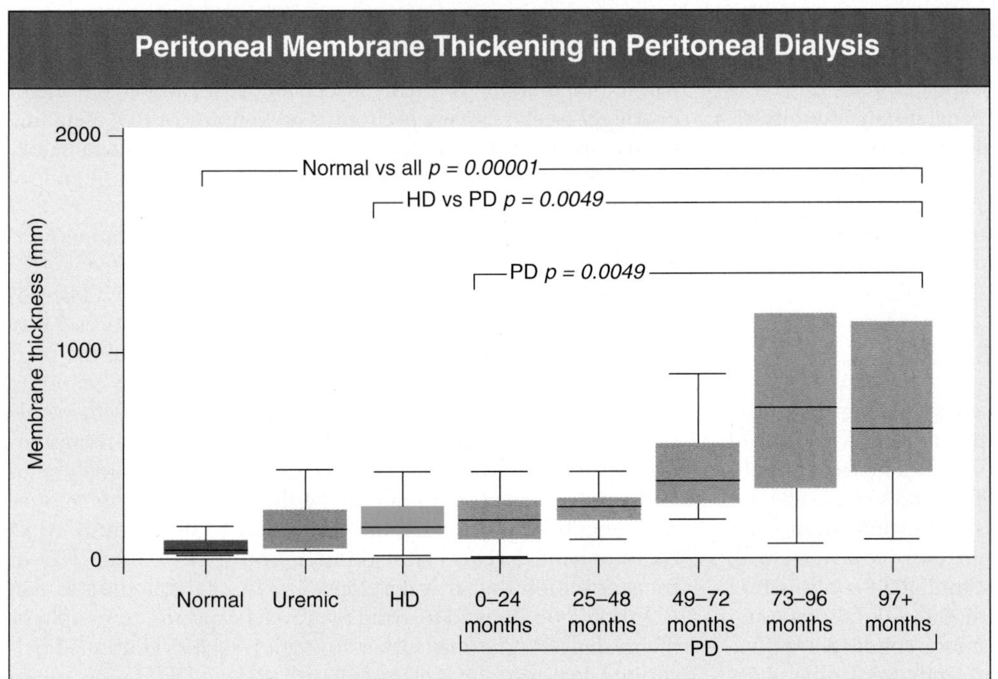

Figure 93.2 Peritoneal membrane thickening in peritoneal dialysis (PD). The thickness of the submesothelial collagenous zone of the peritoneal membrane in normal individuals, in undialyzed uremics, in hemodialysis (HD), and in those who have received PD for different periods. Membrane thickness is significantly increased in all uremic and dialysis patients compared with normal. Membrane thickness increases significantly with duration of PD and is increased in PD patients as a group compared with HD patients.

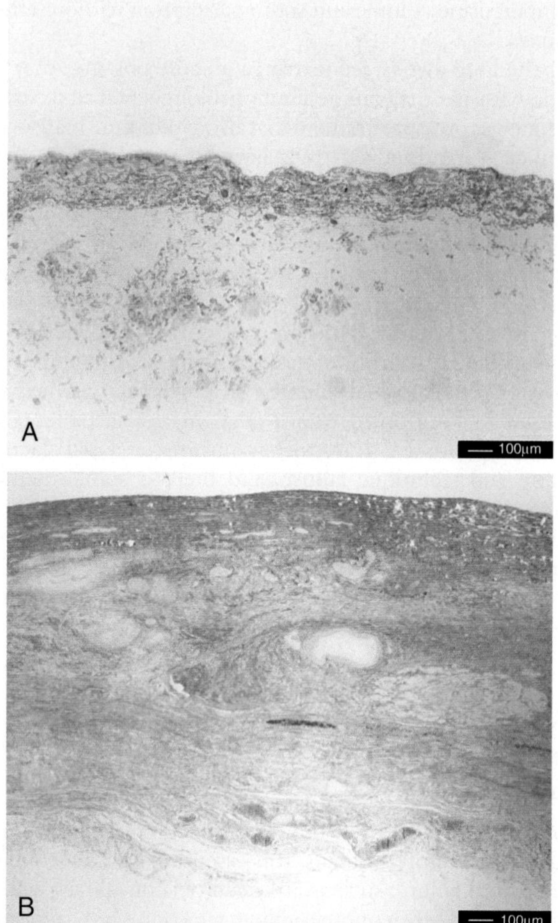

Figure 93.3 Morphologic changes in the parietal peritoneal membrane. A, Normal. **B,** A patient who has been on peritoneal dialysis (PD) for 10 years. Note the marked thickening of the submesothelial compact zone (toluidine blue).

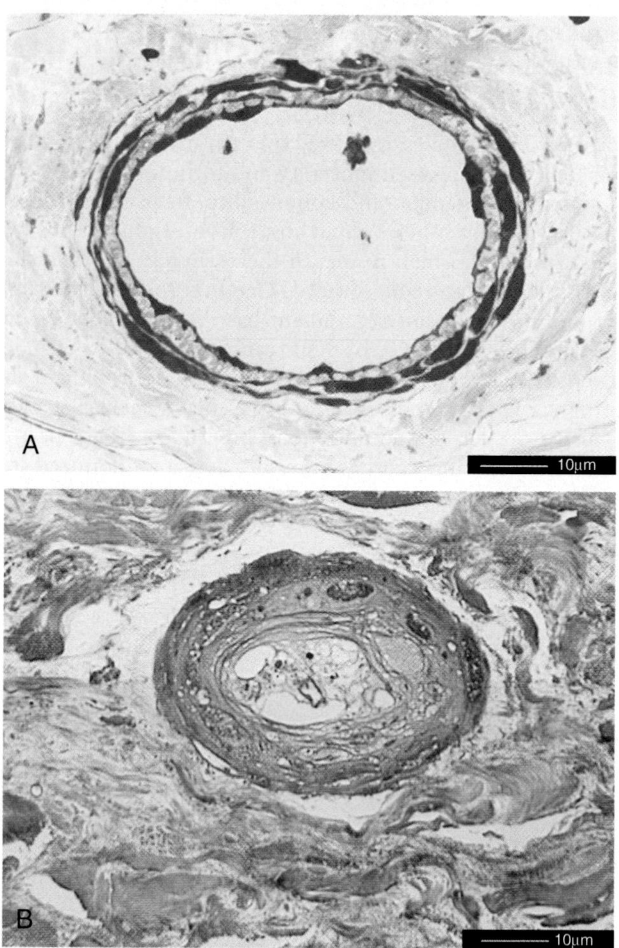

Figure 93.4 Blood vessels in the parietal peritoneum: transverse sections of peritoneal arterioles. A, Normal. **B,** Vasculopathy in a patient on peritoneal dialysis; the vascular lumen is occluded by connective tissue containing fine calcific stippling.

during the first 60 minutes of a 3.86% dwell. This occurs because of the convective transport of water through water exclusive pathways, now known to be capillary aquaporins. Lack of sieving indicates failure of the membrane to generate an ultrafiltrate. Patients with loss of sodium sieving will require regular hypertonic exchanges as well as strategies to preserve urine volume, such as use of diuretics[14] or angiotensin-converting enzyme (ACE) inhibitors.[17] For many of these patients, a planned transfer to hemodialysis (HD) once RRF is lost is the only practical outcome.

ENCAPSULATING PERITONEAL SCLEROSIS

A minority of patients on PD develop encapsulating peritoneal sclerosis, in which the bowel is enveloped in a thick cocoon of fibrous tissue, causing obstruction (Fig. 93.5). The current definition of this syndrome requires clinical features of obstructive bowel symptoms leading to weight loss and malnutrition (with or without features of systemic inflammation) combined with either typical features on imaging (CT scanning) or confirmation of fibrous cocooning at laparotomy. Although UF failure, especially when it is associated with loss of osmotic conductance (type 2), appears to be a risk factor, there are important differences suggesting that this is at least in part a different pathologic process. It is predominantly a disease of visceral as opposed to parietal membrane, is usually associated with another risk factor or trigger (such as severe peritonitis or stopping of PD, including for transplantation), and frequently has a systemic inflammatory phase; biopsy material more often shows inflammation and, of note, fibrinous exudates.

The single most important risk factor for encapsulating peritoneal sclerosis is time on PD; at 5 years, the incidence is ~2% to 3%, whereas by 10 years, this rises to 6% to 20%.[18] There is increasing evidence that the most successful treatment is surgery in the form of extensive adhesion lysis and excision of the peritoneum while avoiding enterotomy, especially when there are obstructive symptoms.[19] Parenteral nutrition can be used, mainly as a preparation for surgery but occasionally as a long-term solution. In about 50% of cases, symptoms are less severe and gradually resolve. There appears to be little role for preemptive screening by CT scanning, but this is helpful in diagnosis. Most commonly, it develops after transfer from PD to either HD or transplantation; but if it develops on PD, the consensus is that PD should be stopped to avoid continued exposure to nonphysiologic dialysis solutions. Other strategies, such as continued irrigation, dual-modality treatment with PD and HD, and use of

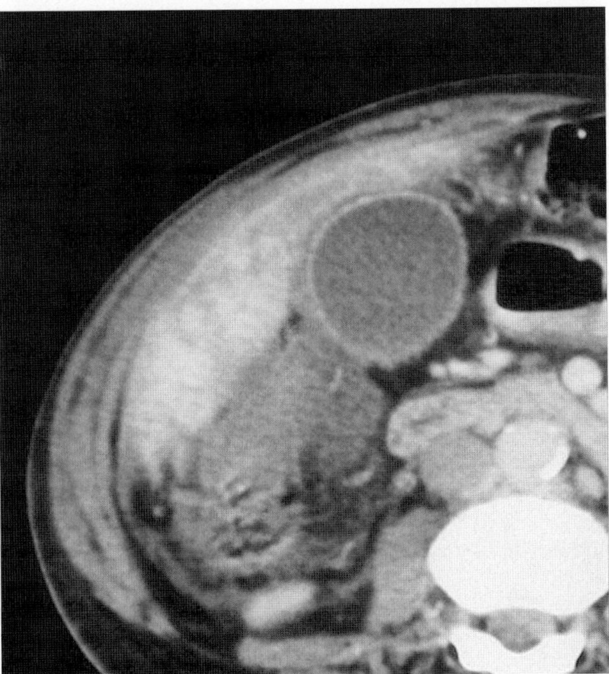

Figure 93.5 Encapsulating peritoneal sclerosis. Abdominal CT scan of a patient with encapsulating peritoneal sclerosis showing extensive peritoneal thickening.

antifibrotic drugs such as tamoxifen, are practiced, but an evidence base is lacking.

CATHETER MALFUNCTION

Inflow Failure

A 2-liter bag of dialysate should take 15 minutes or less to run into the peritoneal cavity. If inflow is significantly slowed or even stopped completely, mechanical causes should be suspected. After it is checked that the tubing and catheter are not kinked, that all clamps or rollers are open to the inflow position, and that any frangible seal is fully broken, the catheter should be flushed vigorously with 20 ml of heparinized saline. If the catheter is cleared, then heparin should be added (500 U/l) to the next few cycles because the cause of the blockage is often a fibrin plug. Should the catheter remain blocked, a plain abdominal radiograph is required. If this shows that the catheter is in a satisfactory position in the pelvis, an attempt to restore patency should be made with urokinase. Urokinase (25,000 U in 2 ml of saline) is infused into the lumen of the catheter and left *in situ* for 2 to 4 hours. The catheter is then flushed. If inflow is restored, heparin should be added to the dialysate for the next few cycles. Should this procedure not be successful but fibrin is still thought to be the cause, an endoscopy brush may sometimes prove successful in unblocking the catheter.

If the radiograph shows the catheter to be malpositioned (Fig. 93.6), an attempt should be made to reposition the catheter tip into the pelvis. This can be done by use of a sterile semirigid rod, shaped into a curve and slid down the lumen of the catheter under radiographic screening control. This technique is not practical when the catheter has a swan neck configuration. Alternatively, the catheter can be repositioned at laparotomy or peritoneoscopy. Sometimes the catheter becomes wrapped in

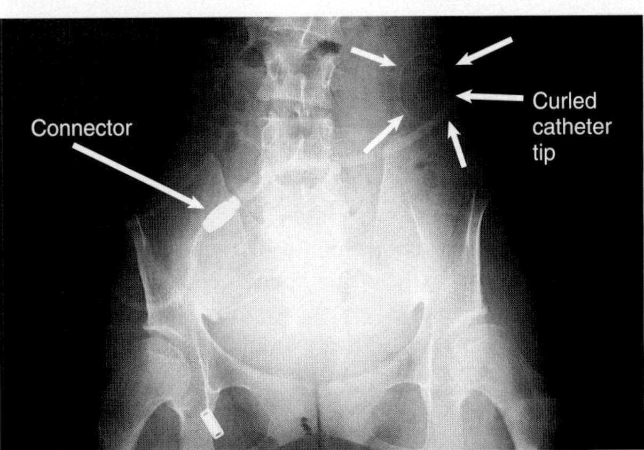

Figure 93.6 Catheter malposition. Plain radiograph of the abdomen with curled catheter *(arrows)* misplaced in the upper left abdomen.

omentum, suggested usually by complete inflow and outflow failure. This requires a partial omentectomy or an omental hitch, a surgical procedure in which the omentum is temporarily held away from the catheter by a dissolvable suture.

Outflow Failure

The most common reason for outflow failure is constipation, although causes of inflow failure discussed previously should also be considered. Loading of the bowel with fecal material is often obvious on a plain radiograph, but treatment for constipation should be initiated without recourse to this investigation as it is so common. Constipation should be treated with oral laxatives or an enema. Subsequently, bowel action should be kept regular by increasing the fiber in the diet and, if necessary, the addition of a mild laxative such as lactulose or senna. Slow outflow can be a problem in APD patients, resulting in excessive machine alarms. This is best dealt with by switching to tidal APD and using a relatively large residual volume (>50% of the fill volume).

Fibrin in the Dialysate

During peritonitis, fibrin in the dialysate is common. If fibrin causes restriction to dialysate flow, heparin (500 U/l) should be added to each bag. A small number of patients have fibrin formation in the absence of peritonitis. Immediately on drainage, the bag may appear cloudy, but on standing, the fibrin will aggregate. The first time this happens, a sample must be sent to the microbiology laboratory to exclude infection. If this proves negative, the patient can be reassured. If catheter plugging occurs subsequently, regular use of heparin is recommended.

FLUID LEAKS

External Leaks

On occasion, fluid may leak from the exit site or even the incision used to insert the catheter into the peritoneal cavity. This is usually a problem that occurs early, particularly if dialysis is started soon after catheter insertion. Whenever possible, elective insertion of the catheter should be performed at least 10 days before dialysis is required to avoid early leaks. Catheters can be used immediately in the case of acute PD start by using APD, low fill volumes, and bed rest. In addition, the use of the paramedian approach for the peritoneal entry site is thought to minimize the chances of this complication. If a leak occurs, PD should be withheld for as long as possible. If dialysis is necessary, APD can be used overnight with a dry day for at least 10 days.

Internal Leaks

Isolated edema of the abdominal wall suggests an internal leak from the peritoneal cavity, either spontaneously or in association with a surgical hernia. In contrast, genital edema suggests an inguinal hernia or patent processus vaginalis. On occasion, both can be present. The site of the leak can be visualized by CT scanning after intraperitoneal instillation of contrast material. It may be necessary for the patient to stand or to perform other maneuvers to increase intra-abdominal pressure before the leak is demonstrated (Fig. 93.7A). An alternative diagnostic test is to perform scintigraphy after injection of a compound such as technetium Tc 99m diethylenetriaminepentaacetic acid (^{99m}Tc-DTPA; Fig. 93.7B). A surgical repair will be required if a major leak is visualized and should always be considered in association with a hernia. Most leaks, however, will heal after resting or with APD, using dry days, or temporary HD.

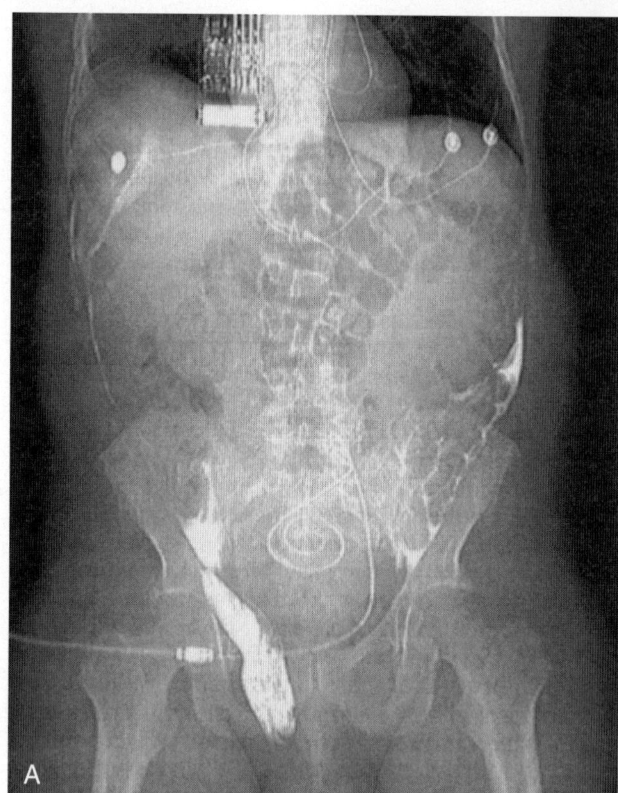

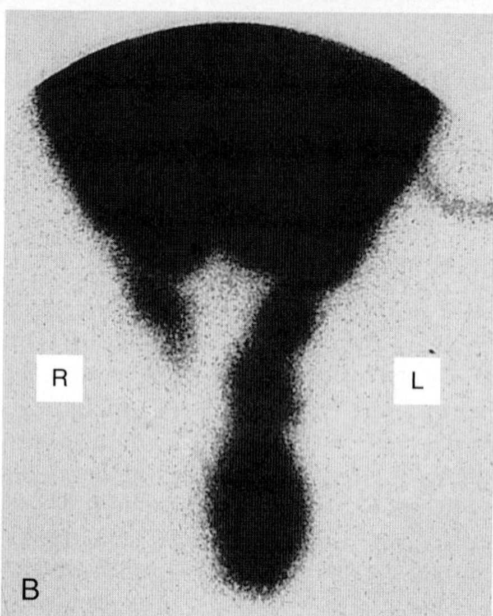

Figure 93.7 Inguinal hernia during peritoneal dialysis. A, CT scan after intraperitoneal injection of contrast material in a male patient showing dialysate flowing into a right inguinal hernia. **B,** Peritoneal scintigram of a male patient on peritoneal dialysis showing bilateral inguinal hernias. The left hernia extends into the scrotum; the right hernia is less extensive. *(**A** from reference 21.)*

Hydrothorax

A pleural effusion can occur with generalized fluid overload or local lung disease, but it is occasionally caused by a leakage of dialysate through the diaphragm (Fig. 93.8). This more commonly occurs on the right side. A leak is most simply confirmed by aspirating a sample of the effusion and demonstrating that its glucose concentration is higher than the patient's blood glucose concentration. Initially, conservative measures should be tried. These include stopping PD, aspirating the effusion to dryness, and leaving the abdomen dry for 2 weeks (using HD, if necessary). This regimen is effective in a number of patients. If the condition recurs, pleurodesis can be tried; various agents have been advocated, but introduction of tetracycline or talc under direct vision with video-thoracoscopy is the best described.

PAIN RELATED TO PERITONEAL DIALYSIS

Inflow Pain

Soon after starting PD, patients may experience pain during fluid inflow. This is particularly likely to occur if dialysis begins immediately or within a few days of catheter insertion. Slowing the rate of fluid inflow will often reduce the symptoms, and peritonitis should be excluded and treated. A small number of individuals have persistent inflow pain. Randomized controlled trials have demonstrated that bicarbonate/lactate–buffered dialysis fluids at physiologic pH are associated with a dramatic improvement in infusion pain in such individuals.[20]

Backache

Backache occurs in a minority of PD patients; the presence of a large volume of fluid in the abdomen distorts the normal posture, exacerbating any tendency to lordosis of the spine. Patients with preexisting back problems are most likely to have an exacerbation of their backache, although not all will be affected. It is important to investigate the symptom to exclude treatable or serious disease. Adjusting the dialysis regimen to reduce the daytime volume or leaving the abdomen empty of fluid during the day can help symptoms, provided dialysis treatment is not compromised.

Outflow Pain

Some patients have discomfort or even pain when the fluid runs out. This emptying sensation is abolished when the next cycle

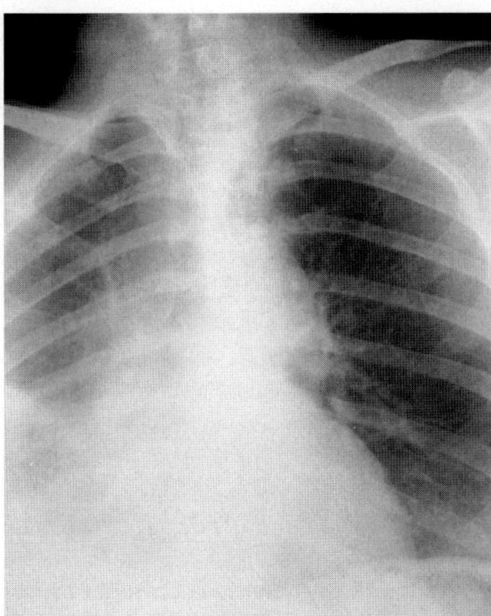

Figure 93.8 Hydrothorax in peritoneal dialysis. Chest radiograph showing a right-sided pleural effusion with partial collapse of the right lung caused by a diaphragmatic leak.

runs in. This commonly occurs during peritonitis but may be experienced in the absence of infection during the first few weeks of PD. Switching to tidal APD will often solve this problem. Tidal therapy enables a prescribed amount of fluid to remain in the peritoneal cavity throughout treatment. If this is set to between 50% and 80% of the inflow volume, pain and drainage alarms are often prevented.

BLEEDING

Exit Site

The exit site can be a source of blood loss at any time while a peritoneal catheter is in place. A common cause is the removal of a crust before natural separation has occurred. The bleeding almost invariably stops with local pressure, but a new raw area that is liable to become infected remains. Regular cleansing of the exit site with povidone-iodine will reduce the chances of this complication. Patients must be instructed not to pull off the crust but to await its natural separation. Severe infection of the exit site may, on occasion, be accompanied by secondary hemorrhage. This will usually respond to firm pressure. The subsequent management is the same as for any exit site infection.

Blood-Stained Dialysate

Blood-stained dialysate is uncommon. It is rarely serious but causes considerable alarm to the patient. There is sometimes a clear history of trauma to the abdomen or of unexpected strain. A few female patients relate the episode to their time of ovulation or menstruation. The treatment is to flush the abdomen with a few cycles of dialysate containing heparin (500 U/l) to minimize the chances of clotting in the catheter. The problem usually resolves spontaneously and often is visible only in one outflow. It is unusual for the blood-stained dialysate to be associated with infection, although it is wise to have the fluid cultured. Routine use of antibiotics is not necessary. Blood-stained dialysate can be a presenting feature of encapsulating peritoneal sclerosis, so if this is suspected clinically, a CT scan or laparoscopy and biopsy should be performed.

NUTRITIONAL PROBLEMS

Malnutrition

Cross-sectional surveys of patients receiving PD show that about 40% have malnutrition and 8% have severe protein-calorie depletion. Malnutrition is an adverse risk factor for morbidity and mortality of patients on PD; this poor nutrition is multifactorial. The assessment and management of malnutrition are discussed further in Chapter 83. It has been suggested that ideally, patients should consume daily at least 1.2 to 1.3 g of protein per kilogram of body weight. In practice, many subjects take only about 0.8 g/kg per day and seem to be nutritionally stable. It is likely that they have achieved a steady state but with a lower total body nitrogen or lean body mass.

Patients on continuous ambulatory peritoneal dialysis (CAPD) have abnormal eating behavior with smaller meals, slow eating, and impaired gastric emptying compared with normal subjects. The full peritoneal cavity may produce easy satiety, and some patients complain of feeling bloated. However, studies have shown that there is no actual difference in food consumption with or without dialysate in the abdomen.

One obvious contributing factor is protein loss through the peritoneum, which averages 8 g/day but can be as high as 20 g/day. It increases considerably during peritonitis. Patients with fast solute transport also have high peritoneal protein losses, in particular albumin. In both cases, the protein loss is a reflection of a larger effective peritoneal surface area. The ensuing hypoalbuminemia complicates poor UF and exacerbates the extracellular fluid (ECF) expansion in these patients.

Acid-Base Status

Another important influence on nutrition is the acid-base status of the patient. Correction of acidosis reduces protein catabolism. One study compared the use of 35 mmol/l lactate dialysate with fluid containing 40 mmol/l lactate.[25] After 1 year, the group receiving the higher lactate concentration had increased serum bicarbonate levels and, more important, had gained more weight with a greater increase in midarm muscle circumference. This implies that protein anabolism had taken place as the result of better acid-base correction. Correction of malnutrition is not easy. Clearly, patients should be encouraged to increase protein and calorie intake. Food supplements are of particular value during intercurrent illness. One report suggested that the regular use of a calorie supplement was associated with increased total body nitrogen after several months, but this remains to be confirmed. Correction of acidosis is best achieved by use of dialysate with higher levels of potential buffer,[22] but if necessary, oral bicarbonate may be added.

Amino acid–based dialysate improves nitrogen balance in malnourished patients, but the long-term benefits are still unclear.[23] One bag per day is usually recommended during the daytime when calories are being consumed to promote anabolism and to avoid the risk of the absorbed amino acids being used for energy production. Earlier reports noted a tendency to acidosis with this type of dialysate, which would negate any beneficial effect. Close observation of the serum bicarbonate is necessary, with supplementation as required.

Lipids and Obesity

The use of glucose-based hyperosmolar solutions for PD results in a significant increase in the glucose load experienced by the patient. A number of reports have measured the daily glucose absorption, which is estimated to be 100 and 200 g/day, producing 400 to 800 kcal. The resultant metabolic effect is a tendency for patients on CAPD to develop central obesity, hyperglycemia, and hyperinsulinemia; they may even develop frank diabetes. These problems can be reduced by use of icodextrin in place of glucose.[22] Serum triglycerides and cholesterol increase during the first year on CAPD, with increases in very-low-density and low-density lipoproteins. The greater the degree of hyperlipidemia at the start of therapy, the worse will be the changes with time on CAPD. In addition, there is some evidence that lipoprotein(a) levels may increase with time on CAPD (although this has not been consistently confirmed). Proatherogenic lipid levels are more common in patients on CAPD than in patients on HD. A number of studies have demonstrated the effectiveness of cholesterol-lowering agents in patients on CAPD. Statins are of proven efficacy in reducing total cholesterol and low-density lipoprotein cholesterol while increasing high-density lipoprotein cholesterol. However, the long-term effects of such intervention on cardiovascular (CV) morbidity and mortality in CAPD patients have yet to be established.

There is no evidence to suggest that PD should be avoided in obese patients despite these concerns. The survival advantage seen in HD associated with a higher body mass index is not seen.[24]

INFECTIOUS COMPLICATIONS

Peritonitis

Although the introduction of disconnect delivery systems has reduced the incidence of peritonitis, it remains one of the most important complications of PD and is a major cause of treatment failure. Guidelines for the diagnosis and management of PD peritonitis are published by the International Society for Peritoneal Dialysis (ISPD; *www.ispd.org*).[25] The spectrum of peritonitis and its management in children have also recently been described in detail.[26]

Diagnosis of Peritonitis

The diagnosis of peritonitis should be suspected in any patient who develops a cloudy bag when PD fluid is drained or abdominal pain. Fever may also be present but is not a universal feature. Patients should be advised to contact their dialysis unit immediately if they observe a cloudy bag or develop persistent abdominal pain. Samples of the dialysate should be taken for cell count and microbiologic examination. The diagnosis is confirmed by finding more than 100 white blood cells/mm^3 (1×10^7 cells/l). A Gram stain of the spun deposit should also be performed to help identify the type of causative organism, although initial treatment will usually be empiric pending culture and sensitivity results. Various culture techniques have been proposed, but white cell lysis and inoculation into blood culture media is often helpful in increasing the yield of a positive growth.

The dialysate leukocyte count will be affected by dwell length, and this needs to be taken into account in APD patients. In short dwells, the count will be lower, and under these circumstances, if the proportion of cells that are neutrophils exceeds 50%, empiric treatment of peritonitis should be commenced.

Antibiotic Regimens for Bacterial Peritoneal Dialysis Peritonitis

Culture	Antibiotic
Enterococci (including vancomycin-resistant enterococci)	Ampicillin
*Staphylococcus aureus** Methicillin resistant*	Cephalosporin/floxacillin (flucloxacillin) Vancomycin
Other gram-positive organism†	Cephalosporin/floxacillin
Gram-negative organisms (including *Pseudomonas* species)*	Cefazolin, quinolone, or aminoglycoside‡, depending on sensitivities and residual renal function
Multiple/anaerobic organisms*	Metronidazole ± laparotomy
Culture negative	Continue empirical treatment

Figure 93.9 Antibiotic regimens for bacterial peritoneal dialysis (PD) peritonitis. Suggested antibiotic regimens when dialysate fluid culture is available. Except for culture-negative episodes, empiric treatment is stopped once the sensitivities are known. All antibiotic regimens should be developed in consultation with local microbiology practices. *Three-week treatment. †Two-week treatment. ‡Avoid unnecessary use if there is residual function.

Conversely, if the patient has had a dry abdomen during the day, the initial drain on connection may be cloudy. This will clear within one or two cycles, however, and the majority of the cells found will be mononuclear leukocytes.

Treatment of Peritonitis

The empiric treatment of peritonitis will vary according to center and should be developed in close collaboration with the local microbiology service, taking into account sensitivity patterns and infection control policy. Initial regimens must cover both gram-positive and gram-negative organisms; in the latest ISPD guidelines, examples of appropriate antibiotics include vancomycin, cephalosporins, and aminoglycosides.[25] Dosing regimens will depend on whether the patient is on CAPD or APD. For CAPD, the antibiotic is administered as a loading dose in the first bag and then as a maintenance dose in subsequent bags. Although it was customary to transfer APD patients to CAPD for the purpose of treating peritonitis, this is no longer necessary. APD patients are now given large loading doses into dialysis fluid with a minimum 6-hour dwell (e.g., vancomycin 30 mg/kg) and then are given further doses every 3 to 5 days according to checked blood levels. Once the culture result is available, the regimen should be modified accordingly (Fig. 93.9). If the organism is methicillin-resistant *Staphylococcus aureus* (MRSA), vancomycin will continue as part of the regimen.

If the culture is negative, empiric therapy should be continued for 2 weeks, assuming there is a clinical response. If a gram-negative organism is identified, the subsequent management will depend on the sensitivity (Fig. 93.10). The isolation of multiple organisms including anaerobes strongly suggests major bowel disease. Metronidazole should be added to the regimen and consideration given to surgical intervention.

A wide variety of antibiotics other than those cited have been used with success. In particular, a commonly used strategy is to include an oral quinolone, such as ciprofloxacin, instead of an aminoglycoside because ototoxicity and loss of residual renal function may occur with aminoglycosides. Current recommendations are that for gram-positive organisms, therapy should be

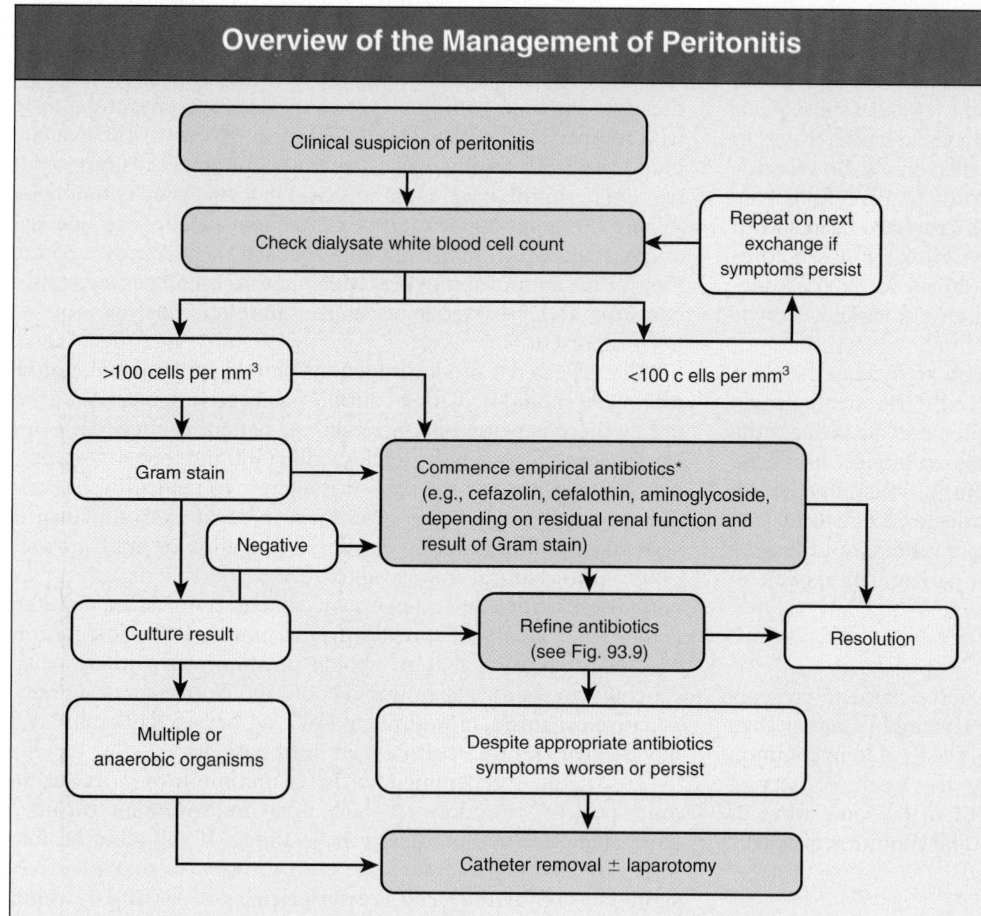

Figure 93.10 Overview of the management of peritonitis.

for 14 days except in the case of *S. aureus,* for which 21 days is suggested. For culture-negative episodes, 14 days of therapy should suffice. The same is true in the case of single-organism gram-negative peritonitis. For *Pseudomonas, Xanthomonas* species, or multiple organisms, 21 days is recommended.

Many patients can be treated successfully as outpatients. It is extremely important, however, that they are followed up either in the clinic or by telephone. In most cases, clinical resolution, as judged by the clearing of the bags, starts within 48 hours. If there is no improvement within 96 hours despite use of the correct antibiotic, as judged by sensitivity tests, the fluid must be retested by cell count, Gram stain, and culture. In the case of a persistent *S. aureus* infection, an underlying tunnel infection should be excluded. In all other situations in which there is a failure to improve, serious consideration should be given to removal of the catheter. In addition, the possibility of intra-abdominal or gynecologic disease or the presence of unusual organisms such as mycobacteria should be considered. Under these circumstances, a mini-laparotomy should be performed to exclude intra-abdominal disease, and if mycobacterial infection is suspected, a peritoneal biopsy specimen should be obtained for culture.

Fungal Peritonitis

If peritonitis is caused by yeasts or fungi, the peritoneal catheter should always be removed. This should be combined with antifungal treatment using fluconazole, with flucytosine initially intraperitoneally until sensitivities are known. Oral antifungals should be continued for at least 10 days and up to 4 weeks after catheter removal, at which point catheter replacement can be considered.[25]

Relapsing Peritonitis

Relapsing or recurrent peritonitis is defined as a separate infective episode caused by the same organism within 4 weeks of completion of an appropriate course of antibiotics. In the case of a relapsing gram-positive infection, a 4-week course of intraperitoneal cephalosporin together with oral rifampin should be tried. Recurrence of *S. aureus* infection should trigger the search for pericatheter infection. Relapsing MRSA peritonitis will require a prolonged course (4 weeks) of intraperitoneal vancomycin or clindamycin. If enterococci or gram-negative organisms are the cause of a relapse, the possibility of intra-abdominal disease or an abscess should be considered (although these organisms are frequently water-borne). If a patient has other gastrointestinal symptoms, such as change in bowel habit, colonoscopy should be performed, but this is essential only if multiple organisms have been isolated. Again, a repeated course of antibiotics chosen by sensitivity testing should last 4 weeks. Removal of the catheter should be considered if there is no improvement within 4 days of commencing treatment or earlier if it is clinically indicated. Current practice in most units is to allow a period of up to 3 weeks before a new catheter is inserted. Simultaneous removal and replacement of the catheter, under antibiotic cover, can be achieved successfully when the causative organism is a skin commensal.

Prevention of Peritonitis

The latest ISPD guidelines place increased emphasis on prevention of peritonitis. Antibiotic cover with vancomycin (1 g) at the time of catheter insertion is recommended to prevent subsequent exit site infection and peritonitis.[25] No particular catheter design has been shown to reduce infection rates, but a downward-pointing exit site of the catheter assists in catheter care. Enhanced training schedules and improved exit site care have been shown in a randomized study to reduce infection rates.[27] Flush-before-fill dialysate delivery systems have been shown to reduce infections associated with touch contamination and should now be standard.[28]

S. aureus nasal carriage is associated with an increased chance of peritonitis caused by this organism. Daily use of mupirocin either intranasally or applied to the catheter exit site reduces the rate of *S. aureus* peritonitis; occasional resistance has been reported, but this has not been a significant problem to date. Of greater concern is a relative increase in infections due to *Pseudomonas*.[26] One randomized trial has shown a reduction in *Pseudomonas* peritonitis associated with topical gentamicin applied to the exit site (see later discussion).[29]

Eosinophilic Peritonitis

Eosinophilic peritonitis is diagnosed when a patient presents with a cloudy bag of effluent containing eosinophils rather than neutrophils. The fluid is also culture negative. It is an uncommon event but tends to occur within the first few weeks of starting PD. The cause is unknown but assumed to be some form of reaction to the catheter or the dialysate. The condition is usually self-limited, and no treatment is required.

Exit Site Infection

Exit site infection is an important complication of long-term PD, occurring on average at a rate of 0.48 episode per patient-year. The diagnosis is suspected on clinical grounds, usually by the presence of marked erythema or discharge from the exit site (Fig. 93.11). A scoring system for exit sites has been developed to determine the likelihood of infection and to grade its severity, with 1 or 2 points awarded for crusting, swelling, pain, and discharge according to severity (score >4 indicates infection), although if the discharge is purulent, this mandates treatment.[25] Extension of the infection into the tunnel may be assessed either clinically or by ultrasound, enabling measurement of any abscess formation. The most common infecting organism is *S. aureus*.

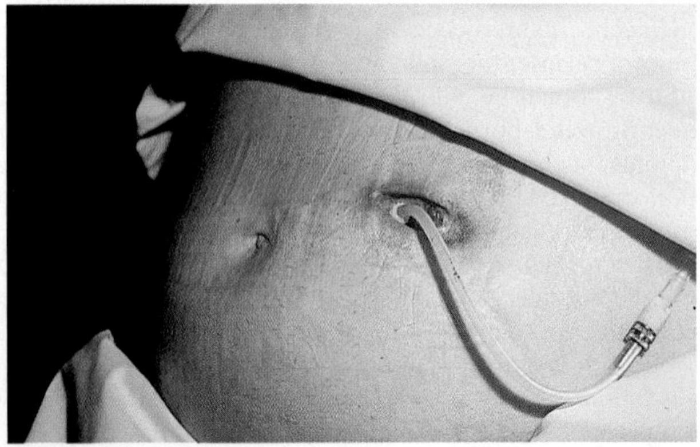

Figure 93.11 Exit site infection. A severe exit site infection that has exposed the outer cuff of the catheter.

Regular use of topical mupirocin can reduce the frequency of infection episodes substantially with the additional benefit of reducing the risk of peritonitis due to this organism. Otherwise, the most common pathogen is *Pseudomonas*. A recent randomized trial comparing mupirocin and gentamicin cream at the exit site found that both staphylococcal and pseudomonal infections (exit site and peritonitis) were less common in those using gentamicin. Whereas regular application of gentamicin to exit sites infected at any stage with gram-negative organisms is currently advised, the routine application of gentamicin cream for all patients raises concerns about bacterial resistance, although this has not yet been reported.[29]

All suspected exit site infections should be swabbed. Initial treatment should be with an antibiotic effective against *S. aureus* unless there is prior evidence that the patient carries MRSA or *Pseudomonas*, for example, flucloxacillin (500 mg four times a day) or a cephalosporin if the patient is allergic to penicillin. In most patients, the drug can be given orally; but if the individual is systemically ill, the antibiotics should be administered intravenously until clinical improvement occurs. Hospitalization, parenteral antibiotics, and often urgent catheter removal are required if there is evidence of spread into the tunnel. If the infection is MRSA, eradication therapy should be attempted with systemic vancomycin, as for peritonitis. Should the culture grow a gram-negative organism, ciprofloxacin (500 mg twice a day orally) will be effective empiric treatment in most patients.

Treatment is recommended for a minimum of 2 weeks. In gram-positive infections, if there is no improvement within 7 days, rifampin (600 mg/day) can be added. If complete healing does not take place after 4 weeks of therapy, further measures should be considered, such as exteriorizing and shaving the outer cuff. Should this cuff be visible or even close to the exit site, it is likely to be involved in the infection. There is often temporary resolution of infection after this procedure. If, despite this step, the infection persists or relapses, catheter removal must be considered because there is a high risk that the exit site infection will lead to peritonitis. It is important that the new exit site be formed in a different part of the anterior abdominal wall. If the infection is controlled and there is no evidence of sepsis along the tunnel, it is possible to insert a new catheter under antibiotic cover at the same time as the old one is removed.

REFERENCES

1. Davies SJ, Phillips L, Griffiths AM, et al. What really happens to people on long-term peritoneal dialysis? *Kidney Int*. 1998;54:2207-2217.
2. Davies SJ. Longitudinal relationship between solute transport and ultrafiltration capacity in peritoneal dialysis patients. *Kidney Int*. 2004;66:2437-2445.
3. Williams JD, Craig KJ, Topley N, et al. Morphologic changes in the peritoneal membrane of patients with renal disease. *J Am Soc Nephrol*. 2002;13:470-479.
4. Honda K, Nitta K, Horita S, et al. Morphological changes in the peritoneal vasculature of patients on CAPD with ultrafiltration failure. *Nephron*. 1996;72:171-176.
5. Jones S, Holmes CJ, Krediet RT, et al. Bicarbonate/lactate-based peritoneal dialysis solution increases cancer antigen 125 and decreases hyaluronic acid levels. *Kidney Int*. 2001;59:1529-1538.
6. Rippe B, Simonsen O, Heimburger O, et al. Long-term clinical effects of a peritoneal dialysis fluid with less glucose degradation products. *Kidney Int*. 2001;59:348-357.
7. Williams JD, Topley N, Craig KJ, et al. The Euro-Balance Trial: The effect of a new biocompatible peritoneal dialysis fluid (balance) on the peritoneal membrane. *Kidney Int*. 2004;66:408-418.
8. Jansen MA, Termorshuizen F, Korevaar JC, et al. Predictors of survival in anuric peritoneal dialysis patients. *Kidney Int*. 2005;68:1199-1205.

9. Brown EA, Davies SJ, Rutherford P, et al. Survival of functionally anuric patients on automated peritoneal dialysis: The European APD Outcome Study. *J Am Soc Nephrol.* 2003;14:2948-2957.
10. Paniagua R, Amato D, Mujais S, et al. Predictive value of brain natriuretic peptides in patients on peritoneal dialysis: Results from the ADEMEX trial. *Clin J Am Soc Nephrol.* 2008;3:407-415. Epub 2008 Jan 16.
11. Marshall J, Jennings P, Scott A, et al. Glycemic control in diabetic CAPD patients assessed by continuous glucose monitoring system (CGMS). *Kidney Int.* 2003;64:1480-1486.
12. Davies SJ, Brown B, Bryan J, Russell GI. Clinical evaluation of the peritoneal equilibration test: A population-based study. *Nephrol Dial Transplant.* 1993;8:64-70.
13. Smit W, van Dijk P, Langedijk MJ, et al. Peritoneal function and assessment of reference values using a 3.86% glucose solution. *Perit Dial Int.* 2003;23:440-449.
14. Medcalf JF, Harris KP, Walls J. Role of diuretics in the preservation of residual renal function in patients on continuous ambulatory peritoneal dialysis. *Kidney Int.* 2001;59:1128-1133.
15. Wolfson M, Piraino B, Hamburger RJ, Morton AR. A randomized controlled trial to evaluate the efficacy and safety of icodextrin in peritoneal dialysis. *Am J Kidney Dis.* 2002;40:1055-1065.
16. Davies SJ, Woodrow G, Donovan K, et al. Icodextrin improves the fluid status of peritoneal dialysis patients: Results of a double-blind randomized controlled trial. *J Am Soc Nephrol.* 2003;14:2338-2344.
17. Li PK, Chow KM, Wong TY, et al. Effects of an angiotensin-converting enzyme inhibitor on residual renal function in patients receiving peritoneal dialysis. A randomized, controlled study. *Ann Intern Med.* 2003; 139:105-112.
18. Augustine T, Brown PW, Davies SD, et al. Encapsulating peritoneal sclerosis: Clinical significance and implications. *Nephron Clin Pract.* 2009;111:c149-c154; discussion c154. Epub 2009 Jan 16.
19. Kawanishi H, Watanabe H, Moriishi M, Tsuchiya S. Successful surgical management of encapsulating peritoneal sclerosis. *Perit Dial Int.* 2005;25(Suppl 4):S39-S47.
20. Mactier RA, Sprosen TS, Gokal R, et al. Bicarbonate and bicarbonate/lactate peritoneal dialysis solutions for the treatment of infusion pain. *Kidney Int.* 1998;53:1061-1067.
21. Tintillier M, Coche E, Malaise J, Goffin E. Peritoneal dialysis and an inguinal hernia. *Lancet.* 2003;362:1893.
22. Mujais S. Acid-base profile in patients on PD. *Kidney Int Suppl.* 2003; 88:S26-S36.
23. Li FK, Chan LY, Woo JC, et al. A 3-year, prospective, randomized, controlled study on amino acid dialysate in patients on CAPD. *Am J Kidney Dis.* 2003;42:173-183.
24. Abbott KC, Glanton CW, Trespalacios FC, et al. Body mass index, dialysis modality, and survival: Analysis of the United States Renal Data System Dialysis Morbidity and Mortality Wave II Study. *Kidney Int.* 2004;65:597-605.
25. Piraino B, Bailie GR, Bernardini J, et al. Peritoneal dialysis–related infections recommendations: 2005 update. *Perit Dial Int.* 2005;25: 107-131.
26. Schaefer F, Feneberg R, Aksu N, et al. Worldwide variation of dialysis-associated peritonitis in children. *Kidney Int.* 2007;72:1374-1379. Epub 2007 Sep 19.
27. Hall G, Bogan A, Dreis S, et al. New directions in peritoneal dialysis patient training. *Nephrol Nurs J.* 2004;31:149-154, 159-163.
28. MacLeod A, Grant A, Donaldson C, et al. Effectiveness and efficiency of methods of dialysis therapy for end-stage renal disease: Systematic reviews. *Health Technol Assess.* 1998;2:1-166.
29. Bernardini J, Bender F, Florio T, et al. Randomized, double-blind trial of antibiotic exit site cream for prevention of exit site infection in peritoneal dialysis patients. *J Am Soc Nephrol.* 2005;16:539-545.

CHAPTER 94

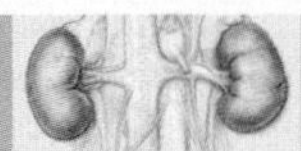

Dialytic Therapies for Drug Overdose and Poisoning

Nigel S. Kanagasundaram, Andrew Lewington

Poisoning and drug overdose, whether intentional or accidental, remain common medical emergencies, accounting for more than 100,000 hospital admissions per year in the United Kingdom (around 1% of all admissions).[1] Most human exposures, however, do not require hospital admission; 73% of the nearly 2.5 million cases in the United States in 2007 were managed at the site of the incident, in a non–health care facility.[2] The spectrum of agents ingested is wide, ranging from overdose of prescription or proprietary drugs to poisoning with nonpharmacologic substances and recreational drugs.

The pattern of toxin ingestion has changed over the years but also varies according to geographic location. Frequently implicated agents in industrialized societies include analgesics (acetaminophen, opioids, salicylates), antidepressants, sedatives, and antipsychotics. Barbiturate poisoning is now less common but was in the past a major contributor. Pesticides remain a frequent cause of poisoning in areas of the developing world.[3] Changes in legislation have been instituted to try to affect availability of potential toxins; in the United Kingdom, for instance, paraquat was withdrawn from sale in July 2008, although this has yet to be reflected in the incidence of poisoning because stored product is still available.[1]

U.S. data indicate a low mortality rate, 1239 attributable fatalities in 2007 of 2.5 million episodes.[2] However, poisoning remains a major cause of death in young people.[3]

The mainstays of management include hemodynamic, respiratory, and other supportive care; prevention of further drug absorption (oral activated charcoal in specific cases); neutralization of drug toxicity (e.g., intravenous *N*-acetylcysteine after significant acetaminophen overdose or Digibind for digitoxicity); and enhancement of drug elimination.

Extracorporeal therapy is one method of achieving poison removal, either by dialysis or by a nondialytic technique, such as hemoperfusion. These enhanced elimination techniques are only occasionally needed. Just more than 2100 patients have been recorded as requiring extracorporeal therapy in the United States in 2007.[2] In that report, the treatment was predominantly hemodialysis, with only 16 cases recorded as receiving hemoperfusion, a decline in use of hemoperfusion perhaps due to the rarity of theophylline and barbiturate overdose in the modern era, as historically these two agents were the main indications for hemoperfusion.

Aspects of the management of poisoning beyond those related to extracorporeal therapies are well covered through resources such as TOXBASE in the United Kingdom *(www.toxbase.org)* and those of the American Association of Poison Control Centers *(www.aapcc.org)*. Other local and regional poisons information services are linked through the Web site of the European Association of Poisons Centres and Clinical Toxicologists *(www.eapcct.org)*.

TREATMENT MODALITIES

Intermittent Hemodialysis and Hemofiltration

Diffusion against a steep concentration gradient, the physical process employed in intermittent hemodialysis, encourages the rapid removal of the smaller solutes that are the usual agents of overdose. Clearances can be enhanced by increasing dialyzer efficiency (indicated by the K_oA, the urea mass transfer area coefficient) or membrane surface area. Larger solute removal can be enhanced by increasing dialyzer flux when intermittent hemodialysis is used (for toxins >500 d and up to 10,000 d, e.g., deferoxamine, aminoglycosides) or by switching to hemofiltration (usually applied continuously; see later), in which the physical process of higher volume convection and larger membrane pore size can allow removal of toxins up to ~40,000 d.

A range of physical and biologic factors determine whether a given toxin can be eliminated by hemodialysis and whether that elimination is actually therapeutic (Fig. 94.1). In addition to molecular weight, other important physical characteristics relevant to dialyzability are water solubility and the degree of protein binding.

In each individual case, it should be determined whether hemodialysis is expected to contribute significantly to total toxin removal. Dialysis will have a limited impact if the rate of drug removal is significantly faster by endogenous routes. The risks of therapy (acute transfer to a specialist center, vascular access, anticoagulation) also have to be balanced against the clinical relevance of any gain in drug elimination. If endogenous elimination is minimal, either because these routes are naturally limited or because of toxin-associated attenuation of elimination (liver or renal failure, for instance), hemodialysis can be effective. It is generally accepted that if at least 30% can be added to total body clearance by extracorporeal treatment, its use is justified. This is not a threshold that is readily derived at the bedside without knowledge of endogenous clearance rates and the expected contribution from exogenous therapy. The summary of product characteristics may help determine the endogenous clearance rate (at least for pharmaceuticals; available from, for instance, *www.emc.medicines.org.uk*) but may not account for the impact of disease on specific endogenous routes of elimination. An estimate of dialyzer clearances of a variety of solutes of different molecular weights can be obtained from its product insert. For

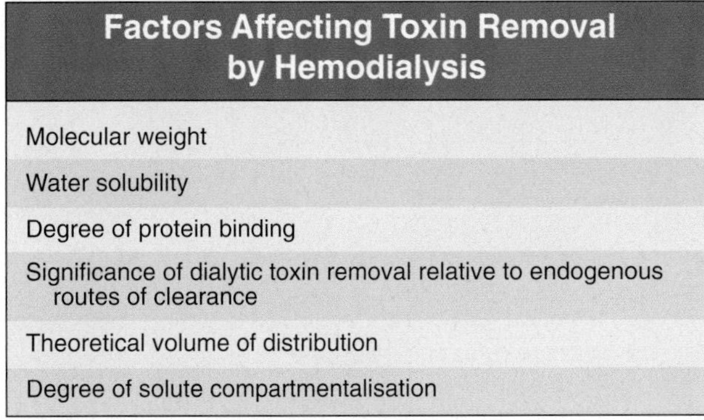

Factors Affecting Toxin Removal by Hemodialysis
Molecular weight
Water solubility
Degree of protein binding
Significance of dialytic toxin removal relative to endogenous routes of clearance
Theoretical volume of distribution
Degree of solute compartmentalisation

Figure 94.1 Factors affecting toxin removal by hemodialysis. See text for explanation.

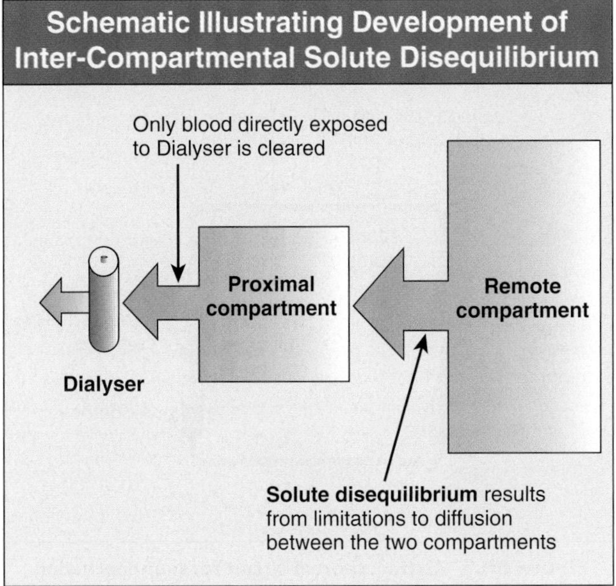

Figure 94.2 Intercompartmental solute disequilibrium. Access of dialyzer to toxin is limited by disequilibrium, which retains toxin in remote compartment.

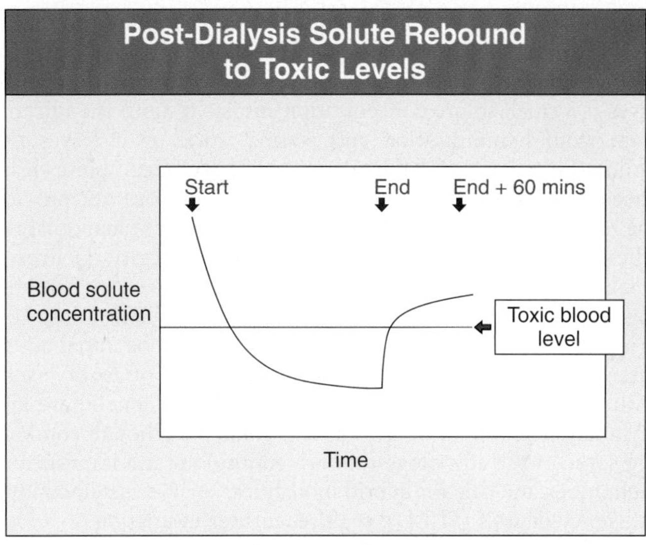

Figure 94.3 Post-dialysis solute rebound. Falling solute concentration during dialysis with rapid postdialysis rebound to toxic levels.

hemofiltration (see later, Continuous Renal Replacement Therapy), an estimate of clearance can be provided by the ultrafiltration rate.

The efficacy of toxin removal is also influenced by its theoretical volume of distribution (V_D). Substances confined to the blood stream will have a low V_D (~ 0.07 l/kg body weight); those distributed in the extracellular space, a V_D of ~0.2 l/kg; and those confined to total body water, ~0.6 l/kg. Higher distribution volumes are, however, not uncommonly found in those substances with avid tissue binding or sequestration. As V_D increases, more solute must be removed to achieve a particular blood level. The ideal solute would therefore have a low distribution volume, which would also be a single, well-mixed compartment that is directly accessible by the dialysis process. However, as shown in Figure 94.2, solute is often distributed across at least one remote body compartment that is not directly accessible during hemodialysis. If there is any resistance to solute movement between the accessible proximal and remote compartments, disequilibrium will develop during the course of the dialysis session, reducing the overall efficiency of toxin removal. This may be significant, as in the case of lithium, and will be manifested as a large, postdialysis rebound in blood levels as solute re-equilibrates from the remote compartment. A significant solute rebound to a potentially toxic level may be missed if the immediate postdialysis blood level is relied on as a measure of elimination (Fig. 94.3).

Extending the hemodialysis session beyond 4 hours can to some extent ameliorate rebound, but intermittent hemodialysis is an inherently inefficient process that depends on the solute concentration presented to the dialyzer. Most solute removal occurs at the start of dialysis. Any gains in solute removal will be disproportionately low in comparison to the increases in dialysis time. An alternative or adjunctive solution is to increase dialysis session frequency.

Compartmentalization need not preclude hemodialysis-related toxin removal, but the closer that its distribution is to a single compartment, the easier that removal becomes.

In summary, intermittent hemodialysis is usually the first-choice extracorporeal modality because of its common availability, the rapidity of toxin removal, and the low molecular weight of the common agents of poisoning. The role of other renal replacement modalities is less clear because of a lack of published data.

Peritoneal Dialysis

Peritoneal dialysis is rarely used in the treatment of poisoning because of the comparatively slow rate of clearance, the risks associated with acute peritoneal dialysis catheter insertion, and the widespread availability of extracorporeal techniques (at least in the industrialized world). It may have a role in the treatment of poisoning in children as the lower clearance may be sufficient for their smaller solute distribution volumes. There may, in addition, be technical challenges making hemodialysis less satisfactory, especially in very young children.

Continuous Renal Replacement Therapy

Continuous renal replacement therapy (CRRT) may be used when intermittent hemodialysis is not immediately available or when more rapid solute removal will be compromised by significant intercompartmental disequilibrium. For small solute clearances, continuous hemofiltration and continuous hemodialysis have nearly kinetic equivalence; full saturation of dialysate effluent in continuous hemodialysis, due to its slow flow rates, gives it a small solute concentration similar to both the ultrafiltrate from hemofiltration and plasma water as it leaves the hollow-fiber device. CRRT gives better longer term solute clearances (during the course of several days) but does not provide the rapidity of elimination afforded by intermittent hemodialysis when minimizing toxin exposure is a high priority. Delivered small solute clearances of CRRT can be maximized by combining techniques in the form of continuous hemodiafiltration. If it is logistically possible, an ideal combination may be initial use of intermittent hemodialysis for rapid reduction of toxin levels, with continuous therapy then being applied to ameliorate any postdialysis rebound, where this is predicted. Although combining some of the advantages of both continuous and intermittent techniques, the role for hybrid modalities, such as sustained low-efficiency dialysis (SLED), requires further evaluation.

Although small solute clearances are similar in continuous hemofiltration and continuous hemodialysis, continuous hemofiltration should be used in preference if larger toxins (as described earlier for intermittent hemodialysis) require removal.

Renal replacement therapy is also indicated for acute kidney injury (AKI), which can result from ingestion of a variety of different agents (e.g., acetaminophen), and for other complications of poisoning, such as pulmonary edema, electrolyte and acid-base disturbances, and hypothermia and hyperthermia.

Because renal replacement therapy modalities are often applied for drug elimination in the absence of any actual renal dysfunction or serious electrolyte disturbance, careful monitoring for evolving biochemical abnormalities is required. Hypokalemia can be corrected by adjusting the dialysate or replacement fluid composition and by supplementation. Hypophosphatemia can be addressed with standard supplements. At least for intermittent hemodialysis, the risk for development of a metabolic alkalosis can be attenuated by dialing in a dialysate bicarbonate concentration at the lower end of the physiologic range, provided there is no coexistent renal impairment and no metabolic acidosis or the risk of it. Manipulation of the bicarbonate concentration of premanufactured replacement or dialysate fluid in CRRT is not practical; this is another advantage of intermittent hemodialysis in this setting because it affords flexibility of bicarbonate dialysate concentration if a severe metabolic alkalosis is present.

Hemoperfusion

The technique involves the extracorporeal circulation of blood through a hemoperfusion cartridge (Fig. 94.4) containing an adsorbent material such as activated charcoal or a resin. The charcoal sorbent particles are coated with a polymer to increase biocompatibility and to reduce the risk of thrombocytopenia. Hemoperfusion removes those substances that can bind to the adsorbent material. It is effective at removal of uncharged molecules through competitive binding, especially those that are significantly plasma protein bound and lipophilic. As with hemodialysis and hemofiltration, the likely proportional contribution to total toxin elimination should be considered before embarking on hemoperfusion.

Other than the cartridge itself and the lack of dialysate and other replacement fluid circuits, the disposables and hardware are those used for standard intermittent hemodialysis (Fig. 94.5). It is much less widely available than hemodialysis or hemofiltration but may have its principal utility in the removal of protein-bound drugs that are not eliminated effectively by those modalities.[4]

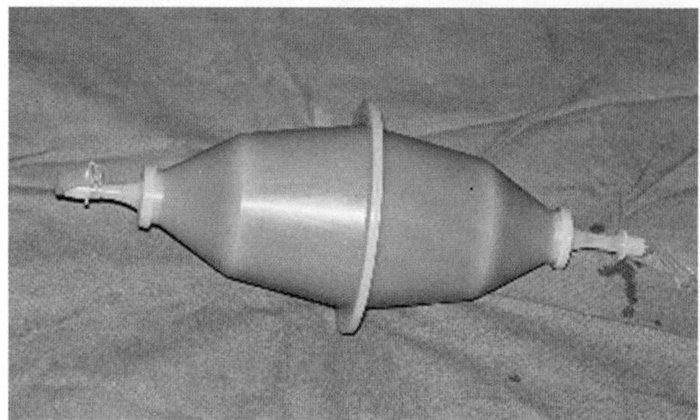

Figure 94.4 A charcoal hemoperfusion cartridge.

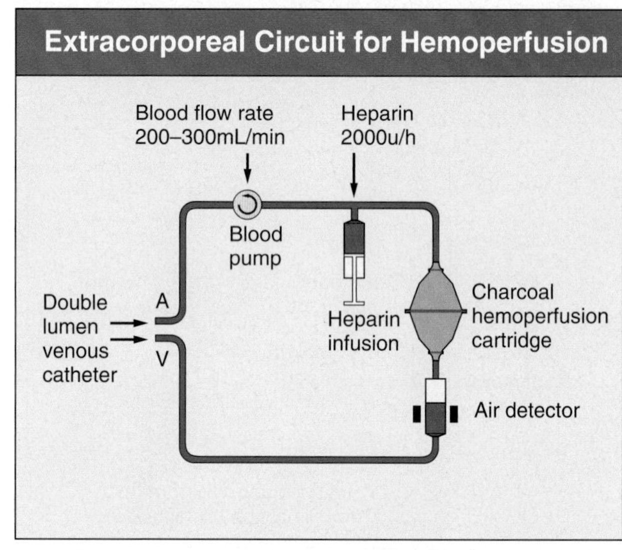

Figure 94.5 Extracorporeal circuit for hemoperfusion.

Standard anticoagulation protocols may be insufficient for hemoperfusion as heparin is also adsorbed. A larger unfractionated heparin initial bolus and maintenance dose (e.g., ≥2000 U/h) is usually required, with subsequent adjustments guided by regular monitoring of clotting times during the procedure. The cartridge manufacturer's instructions should be reviewed carefully, as some require specific priming with dextrose solution to prevent hypoglycemia. Other complications include hypocalcemia, charcoal embolization, leukopenia, thrombocytopenia, and adsorption of coagulation factors.

Saturation of the adsorbent material limits the duration of treatment with any individual hemoperfusion cartridge to around 3 hours, although this is usually adequate for a significant lowering of blood levels. Continuous hemoperfusion can help attenuate the post-session rebound that can occur with intermittent treatment, with cartridges being changed every 4 hours.

If a toxin is equally removed by intermittent hemodialysis and hemoperfusion, intermittent hemodialysis should be used preferentially as it also allows fluid, electrolyte, and other metabolic control. Combined hemoperfusion-hemodialysis has also been used but only rarely, and its role is not defined.

Some Poisonings for which Extracorporeal Removal May be Indicated		
Hemodialysis	**Hemofiltration**	**Hemoperfusion**
Alcohols Ethanol Methanol Ethylene glycol Isopropanol	Aminoglycosides Desferoxamine Sodium edetate Theophylline	*Amanita* mushroom Barbiturates Carbamazepine Meprobamate Theophylline
Betablockers Atenolol Sotalol		
Lithium		
Meprobamate		
Metformin		
Salicylates		
Theophylline		

Figure 94.6 Some poisonings for which extracorporeal removal may be indicated.

Criteria for Considering Extracorporeal Therapy for a Removable Substance
Toxic blood levels (if a threshold of toxicity can be defined)
Serious clinical manifestations despite optimal support
Delayed action possible (e.g. ethylene glycol, methanol, paraquat)
Metabolic effects (e.g. acidosis)
Endogenous routes of clearance, impaired (e.g. liver or renal failure)

Figure 94.7 Criteria for considering extracorporeal therapy for poisoning.

Other Modalities

There are a few reports of the use of plasma exchange and the molecular adsorbent recirculating system (MARS) in poisoning. In principle, both should be useful for those toxins that are strongly protein bound. Plasma exchange can also clear the red cell fragments and free hemoglobin that result from poisoning with sodium chlorate or other agents that can cause hemolysis.

WHEN SHOULD EXTRACORPOREAL REMOVAL BE CONSIDERED?

A wide range of drugs and other toxins can be removed by extracorporeal therapy, but those for which such treatment may actually be indicated is much more limited as supportive measures and orally administered activated charcoal may be equally effective. More common indications for extracorporeal drug removal are shown in Figure 94.6.

Principles guiding the decision to deploy extracorporeal therapy are shown in Figure 94.7.

EXTRACORPOREAL THERAPY FOR SPECIFIC DRUGS AND POISONS

Alcohols

Ethylene glycol and methanol poisoning may present with nausea, vomiting, abdominal pain, impaired consciousness that may progress to severe metabolic acidosis, AKI, optic nerve damage, convulsions, coma, and ultimately death. The presence of needle-shaped crystals of calcium oxalate monohydrate in the urine is pathognomonic for ethylene glycol toxicity. Ingestion of relatively small amounts of ethylene glycol and methanol may result in significant toxicity (see Chapter 12). This toxicity results from metabolism of ethylene glycol and methanol by alcohol dehydrogenase to the toxic metabolites formic acid and glycolic acid, respectively.

Early recognition is essential, allowing institution of treatment to inhibit alcohol dehydrogenase with ethanol or fomepizole. Fomepizole has now replaced ethanol as first-line therapy[5,6]; it is safe with minimal side effects, and although it is expensive, this can be offset compared with the increased cost of hemodialysis and intensive care unit admission if fomepizole is not used.

Fomepizole should be prescribed if there is a clear history of ethylene glycol or methanol ingestion with an osmolal gap above 10 (indicating significant toxicity) or the ethylene glycol or methanol blood level is more than 200 mg/l. Fomepizole is administered as a loading dose of 15 mg/kg intravenously. This is then followed by 10 mg/kg every 12 hours for four doses and then 15 mg/kg every 12 hours until the metabolic acidosis has resolved and the serum concentration of ethylene glycol and methanol is less than 200 mg/l or less than 100 mg/l in the presence of end-organ damage. Patients who have ingested methanol should also receive folinic acid, 50 mg intravenously every 6 hours, to enhance the metabolism of formic acid. If fomepizole is not available, intravenous 10% ethanol should be administered as a loading dose of 10 ml/kg followed by an infusion of 0.15 ml/kg per hour to achieve a serum ethanol concentration of about 1 to 1.5 g/l. Ethanol should be administered until no ethylene glycol or methanol is detectable in the blood.

Immediate hemodialysis is recommended if ingestion of ethylene glycol or methanol is confirmed with serum concentration of more than 500 mg/l in the setting of severe metabolic acidosis or the presence of end-organ damage such as AKI or visual disturbance. It is important to recognize that fomepizole is removed by hemodialysis. Therefore, if a loading dose of fomepizole has already been administered, a continuous infusion of 1 to 1.5 mg/kg per hour should be prescribed for the duration of the hemodialysis. Similarly, if ethanol has been used as a competitive inhibitor of alcohol dehydrogenase, its dose will have to be doubled because of its removal by hemodialysis.

To achieve optimal clearance, the dialyzer should have a large surface area (>1.5 m^2) and the blood flow rate should be more than 300 ml/min. Bicarbonate buffer should be used, and serum concentrations of ethylene glycol and methanol should be measured 2 hours after cessation of treatment to take account of rebound. Patients who have ingested large quantities of ethylene glycol and methanol may require further hemodialysis. Continuous extracorporeal treatment is less effective in removal of ethylene glycol and methanol but may be used if intermittent hemodialysis is not available.

β-Blockers

Symptomatic β-blocker overdose will be manifested within 4 hours of ingestion in the majority of patients with bradycardia and hypotension. Clinical presentation may also include changes in mental status, seizures, bronchospasm, and hypoglycemia. An increased risk of severe toxicity occurs in patients who have co-ingested other drugs that act on the cardiovascular system. The principles of medical management involve implementation of immediate life support. Bradycardia can be treated with intravenous atropine at 0.5 to 1 mg, and bronchospasm can be treated initially with high-dose nebulized salbutamol. Intravenous fluids (crystalloid) should be administered to treat hypotension. Symptomatic hypoglycemia requires intravenous dextrose. Activated charcoal should be administered orally to all patients presenting within 1 to 2 hours of β-blocker overdose.

Extracorporeal removal of β-blockers is rarely required and only in those patients who have not improved despite maximal medical therapy. Extracorporeal removal is effective only for hydrophilic, minimally protein bound drugs such as atenolol, sotalol, nadolol, and acebutolol. Intermittent hemodialysis is recommended in hemodynamically stable patients. Continuous venovenous hemodialysis or continuous venovenous hemodiafiltration may be considered in patients who are hemodynamically unstable. There are few data regarding the effectiveness of β-blocker removal by continuous venovenous hemofiltration.

Lithium

In cases of severe lithium poisoning, patients may present with arrhythmias, hypotension, confusion, coma, or seizures. Hemodialysis is recommended if the serum lithium concentration is above 4 mmol/l or above 2.5 mmol/l in a patient with central nervous system manifestations. Lithium (M_r 74 d) is removed easily by hemodialysis because of its low molecular weight and negligible protein binding. The clearance of lithium by hemodialysis is superior to that achieved by the kidneys, which is limited by significant proximal tubule reabsorption of lithium. Because lithium equilibrates relatively slowly between the extracellular and intracellular compartments, a rebound increase in serum levels of lithium follows hemodialysis.[7] Therefore, extended[8] or frequent hemodialysis treatment may be needed to minimize the impact of disequilibrium. Serum lithium levels should be checked 6 hours after completion of treatment to guide further therapy. Continuous modalities, including continuous venovenous hemodialysis and continuous venovenous hemofiltration, may be advantageous and have been used successfully.[9]

Metformin

Metformin (M_r 166 d) overdose can present with a severe lactic acidosis. Medical management will involve immediate life support and the intravenous administration of sodium bicarbonate. In patients who are unresponsive to medical management or who also present with AKI, extracorporeal therapy will be necessary to correct the acidosis. Intermittent hemodialysis is effective, and more recently there have been reports of successful continuous extracorporeal therapy, including continuous venovenous hemofiltration.[10]

Salicylates

The clinical manifestations of salicylate overdose include fever, sweating, tinnitus, epigastric pain, nausea, vomiting, diarrhea, vertigo, and blurring of vision. In severe overdoses, clinical presentation may progress to depression of mental status, noncardiogenic pulmonary edema, and death. Salicylate intoxication initially results in activation of the respiratory center with hyperventilation and a respiratory alkalosis. This is then followed by a metabolic acidosis due to the accumulation of lactic acid and keto acids. Therefore, the patient may present with either a respiratory alkalosis or a mixed respiratory alkalosis–metabolic acidosis. Diagnosis is based on the presenting history and clinical examination and confirmed with plasma salicylate levels. Moderate toxicity occurs with salicylate levels above 500 mg/l. Ingestion of enteric-coated salicylate preparations may delay detection of peak levels for up to 36 hours.

General management includes immediate life support and stabilization of the patient. Gastric lavage should be attempted up to 12 hours after ingestion if the airway is protected, and activated charcoal should be administered orally. Hypoglycemia should be treated with intravenous dextrose.

Increased salicylate tissue penetration and toxicity can occur with only small decreases in the pH because of increased concentration of nonionized salicylate. Intravenous sodium bicarbonate should be given to decrease tissue penetration and to facilitate the excretion of salicylate through the kidneys. Sodium bicarbonate can be administered as an initial bolus of 1 to 2 mmol/kg of 8.4% sodium bicarbonate and then as an infusion of 150 mmol of sodium bicarbonate in 1 liter of 5% dextrose during 2 hours. Blood pH should be measured every 2 hours and the pH kept between 7.5 and 7.55 (not rising above a pH of 7.6). Urinary volume should be monitored, and urinary pH should be kept above 7.5 to optimize salicylate excretion. Urinary alkalinization is contraindicated if the patient has AKI, pulmonary edema, or cerebral edema.

Extracorporeal therapy is indicated in patients who do not respond to this medical management. It is also indicated in patients who have AKI (preventing salicylate excretion), pulmonary edema, or altered mental status or in whom the serum salicylate concentration is more than 800 mg/l. Intermittent hemodialysis has the advantage over hemoperfusion because of its more rapid correction of associated electrolyte abnormalities and acidemia. There are few data on use of continuous venovenous hemofiltration.

Theophylline

The clinical presentation of theophylline overdose includes nausea, vomiting, diarrhea, gastrointestinal hemorrhage, hypokalemia, seizures, arrhythmias, and hypotension. Indications for extracorporeal removal of theophylline include acute intoxication with a serum level above 100 mg/l, chronic intoxication in a patient older than 60 years with a serum level above 40 mg/l, and recurrent seizure activity. Theophylline is readily cleared by either hemodialysis or hemoperfusion because of its low volume of distribution.[11] Hemoperfusion is preferred to hemodialysis because of higher removal rates unless there are severe electrolyte abnormalities, when hemodialysis is the preferred modality. Continuous venovenous hemofiltration can be used but requires a more sustained period of treatment.

Valproate

Valproate (M_r 144 d) overdose may present with clinical features that include mild confusion, lethargy, nausea, vomiting, tachycardia, hypotension, metabolic acidosis, and electrolyte disturbances (hyponatremia and hypocalcemia). Extracorporeal therapy is rarely indicated for the removal of valproate except in cases of refractory metabolic acidosis or hemodynamic instability. Valproate is poorly cleared despite a low molecular weight and a low volume of distribution because of its high degree of protein binding. However, at higher serum levels (>1000 mg/l), the valproate protein-binding sites become saturated, resulting in unbound free drug. Hemodialysis and hemoperfusion readily clear the unbound drug and reverse associated metabolic abnormalities.[12] Despite a number of case reports detailing the use of extracorporeal removal of valproate, there is no clear-cut evidence that it improves clinical outcomes.

REFERENCES

1. Good AM, Bateman DN. *National Poisons Information Service Annual Report 2007/2008*. London: Health Protection Agency; September 2008.
2. Bronstein AC, Spyker DA, Cantilena LR Jr, et al. 2007 Annual Report of the American Association of Poison Control Centers' National Poison Data System (NPDS): 25th Annual Report. *Clin Toxicol (Phila)*. 2008;46: 927-1057.
3. Bradberry S, Vale A. Epidemiology and clinical presentation. *Clin Med*. 2008;8:86-88.
4. Shalkham AS, Kirrane BM, Hoffman RS, et al. The availability and use of charcoal hemoperfusion in the treatment of poisoned patients. *Am J Kidney Dis*. 2006;48:239-241.
5. Brent J, McMartin K, Phillips S, et al. Fomepizole for the treatment of ethylene glycol poisoning. Methylpyrazole for Toxic Alcohols Study Group. *N Engl J Med*. 1999;340:832-838.
6. Brent J, McMartin K, Phillips S, et al. Fomepizole for the treatment of methanol poisoning. *N Engl J Med*. 2001;344:424-429.
7. Clendeninn NJ, Pond SM, Kaysen G, et al. Potential pitfalls in the evaluation of the usefulness of hemodialysis for the removal of lithium. *J Toxicol Clin Toxicol*. 1982;19:341-352.
8. Jacobsen D, Aasen G, Fredricksen P, Eisenga B. Lithium intoxication: Pharmacokinetics during and after terminated hemodialysis in acute intoxications. *J Toxicol Clin Toxicol*. 1987;25:81-94.
9. Goodman JW, Goldfarb DS. The role of continuous renal replacement therapy in the treatment of poisoning. *Semin Dial*. 2006;19:402-407.
10. Lalau JD, Andrejak M, Moriniere P, et al. Hemodialysis in the treatment of lactic acidosis in diabetics treated by metformin: A study of metformin elimination. *Int J Clin Pharmacol Ther Toxicol*. 1989;27:285-288.
11. Benowitz NL, Toffelmire EB. The use of hemodialysis and hemoperfusion in the treatment of theophylline intoxication. *Semin Dial*. 1993;6:243.
12. Bowdle TA, Patel IH, Levy RH, Wilensky AJ. Valproic acid dosage and plasma protein binding and clearance. *Clin Pharmacol Ther*. 1980;28:486.

CHAPTER 95

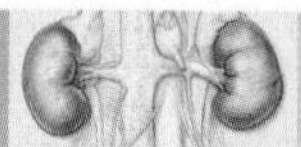

Plasma Exchange

Jeremy Levy, Charles D. Pusey

The place of plasma exchange (plasmapheresis) in the management of renal disease has become clearer in the past 5 years, with increasing numbers of controlled studies comparing therapeutic plasma exchange with other treatments. Despite this, in many renal diseases, the quality of published data still remains poor and the precise role for plasma exchange unclear. Plasma exchange came into widespread clinical use after early reports of beneficial effects in Goodpasture's disease in the mid-1970s. It is used to remove many large-molecular-weight substances from plasma, including pathogenic antibodies, cryoglobulins, and lipoproteins. Newer techniques have also been developed to allow more selective removal of plasma components, such as double filtration plasmapheresis, cryofiltration, and immunoadsorption.

TECHNIQUES

Plasma exchange can be carried out either by centrifugal cell separators or, more commonly in renal units, with hollow-fiber plasma filters and standard hemodialysis equipment (Figs. 95.1 and 95.2). Centrifugal devices allow withdrawal of plasma from a bowl with either synchronous or intermittent return of blood cells to the patient. There is no upper limit to the molecular weight of proteins removed by this method. The bowls and circuits are single use and disposable, and blood flow rates are generally relatively low (90 to 150 ml/min). Platelet loss is a particular problem with centrifugal devices, and platelet counts can decrease by as much as 50%. Membrane plasma filtration uses highly permeable hollow fibers with membrane pores of 0.2 to 0.5 μm. Plasma readily passes through the membrane while the cells are simultaneously returned to the patient. All immunoglobulins will cross the membrane (IgG more efficiently than IgM); however, some large immune complexes and cryoglobulins may not be adequately cleared, although many membranes allow clearance of molecules up to 3 million daltons. There is no loss of platelets, but hemolysis can occur if transmembrane pressures are too high (a rare complication). Blood flow rates required are 90 to 200 ml/min; there is no increase in rate of plasma filtration at higher blood flows, but there is an increased risk of hemolysis. Membranes used in plasma filters are polysulfone, polypropylene, cellulose diacetate, polymethylmethacrylate, or polyacrylonitrile. It has been suggested that the adsorptive properties of the membrane for cytokines and other biomolecules may account for some of the beneficial effects of plasma filtration. There have been occasional reports of mild adverse reactions in patients taking angiotensin-converting enzyme inhibitors when plasma is filtered with ethylene vinyl alcohol or acrylic copolymer membranes. Reuse of plasma filters is not advised, but performance data do not indicate a major loss of function during routine plasma exchange.

Vascular access is usually achieved with use of standard central venous catheters; but if a patient already has an arteriovenous (AV) fistula, then of course this can be used. However, it is also sometimes possible to perform plasma exchange by peripheral access through large-bore, short, intravenous cannulae, placed in the antecubital fossa, because the blood flow rates required are low. Single-needle access with an AV fistula is also relatively easy to accommodate, especially for centrifugal plasma exchange, in which the blood removal and return can be asynchronous, but also for membrane filtration. Anticoagulation is almost always needed and must be carefully managed in patients with a bleeding risk, for example, those with hemolytic-uremic syndrome, recent or ongoing pulmonary hemorrhage, or recent renal biopsy. In general, citrate is used for centrifugal plasma exchange and heparin for membrane plasma filtration; however, citrate has particular advantages in patients at higher bleeding risk in view of its lack of systemic anticoagulant actions. When heparin is used, higher doses may be needed than in hemodialysis as a result of increased losses during the procedure (heparin is protein bound). Bolus doses of unfractionated heparin 2000 to 5000 U are given initially, and then 500 to 2000 U/h. Anticoagulant is administered prefilter.

Both methods of plasma exchange require large volumes of colloid replacement. A single plasma volume exchange will lower plasma macromolecule levels by approximately 60%, and five exchanges during 5 to 10 days will clear 90% of the total body immunoglobulin (Fig. 95.3).[1] For most patients, this is achieved by removal of 50 ml of plasma per kilogram of body weight at each procedure (~4 liters for a 75-kg person). Daily plasma exchange is likely to be most effective in rapidly depleting total body load in view of redistribution of immunoglobulins from the extravascular compartments, but there is no good evidence that intensity of exchanges has a major effect on outcomes except in patients with hemolytic-uremic syndrome with poor prognostic markers (see later discussion). Indeed, alternate-day exchanges are of proven efficacy in antineutrophil cytoplasmic antibody (ANCA)–associated diseases. Replacement with crystalloid is untenable because of the need to maintain colloid oncotic pressure. Synthetic gelatin-based plasma expanders can be used as part of a replacement regimen but have a shorter half-life than human albumin, which is the mainstay replacement fluid. The major disadvantage of albumin solutions is the lack of clotting factors, with the potential development of depletion coagulopathy after plasma exchange. Fresh frozen plasma (FFP) should be given, usually in addition to human albumin solution, in patients at particular risk of bleeding. However, almost all the serious

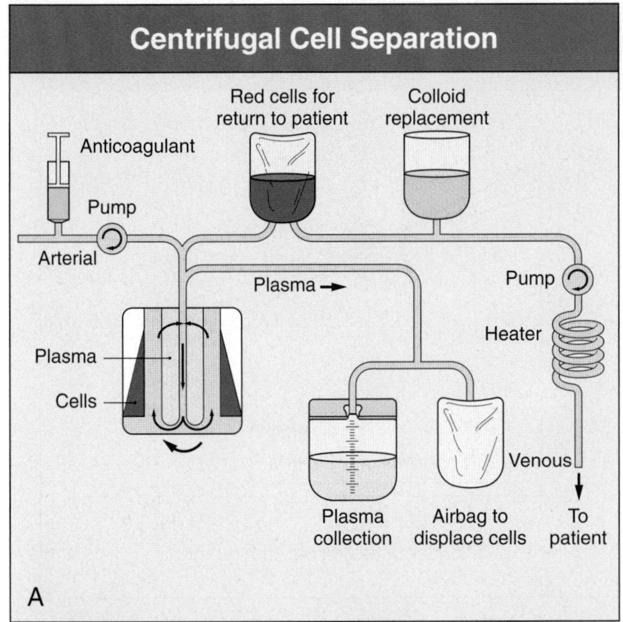

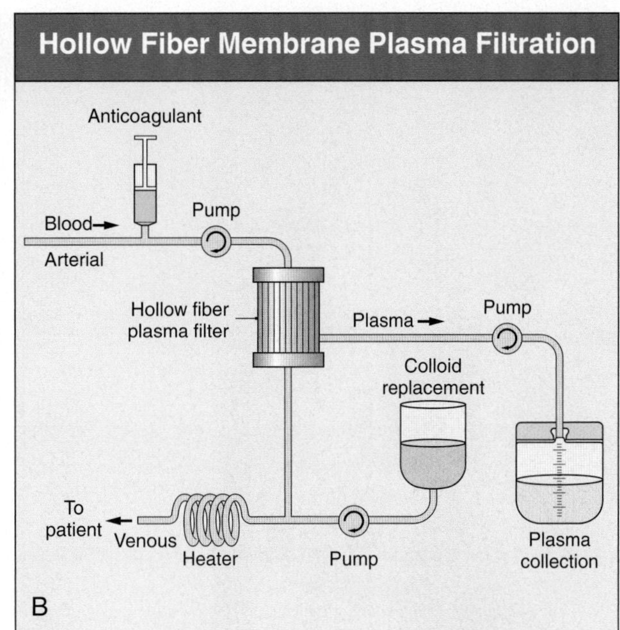

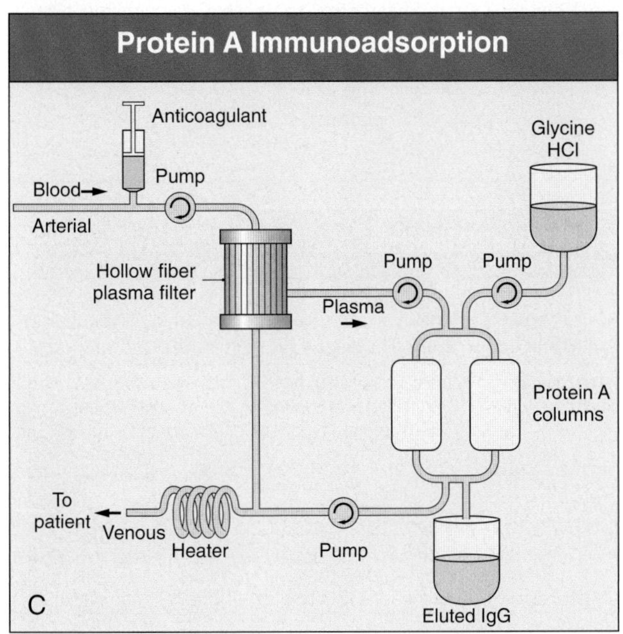

Figure 95.1 Plasma exchange and immunoadsorption techniques. Techniques include centrifugal cell separation **A,** hollow-fiber membrane plasma filtration **B,** and protein A immunoadsorption **C.**

complications of plasma exchange (hypotension, anaphylaxis, citrate-induced paresthesia, urticaria) have been reported in patients receiving FFP rather than albumin (see later discussion).[2,3] Both human products carry a tiny risk of transmission of infectious diseases, especially viral. Standard regimens for plasma exchange are summarized in Figure 95.4. Human albumin solution should be used for all exchanges except in thrombotic microangiopathies (in which plasma should provide the total exchange; see Chapter 28), and FFP should form part of the exchange when bleeding risk is high (ongoing pulmonary hemorrhage or within 48 hours of biopsy or surgery). If fibrinogen levels decrease to less than 1.25 to 1.5 g/l or prothrombin time is increased 2 to 3 seconds above normal, FFP should also be administered.

Double filtration plasmapheresis (or cascade filtration) uses membrane filtration to separate cells from plasma and then a secondary plasma filtration (pore size, 0.01 to 0.03 μm) to remove plasma solutes based on molecular size. Most albumin is therefore returned to the patient together with lower molecular weight proteins, reducing the need for replacement fluids. Cryofiltration uses a similar principle but exposes the filtrate to 4°C during the procedure, with the aim of precipitating cryoproteins. These techniques are not widely available.

Selective and specific immunoadsorption techniques are increasingly available. Protein A immunoadsorption has been used to remove immunoglobulin alone from plasma, without the need for replacement fluids and without depletion of clotting factors and complement (see Fig. 95.1C). Protein A selectively binds the Fc domains of immunoglobulin molecules, and the immunoadsorption columns can be repeatedly regenerated. Columns have been used for 1 year for a single patient on up to 30 occasions; however, the repeated acid stripping during

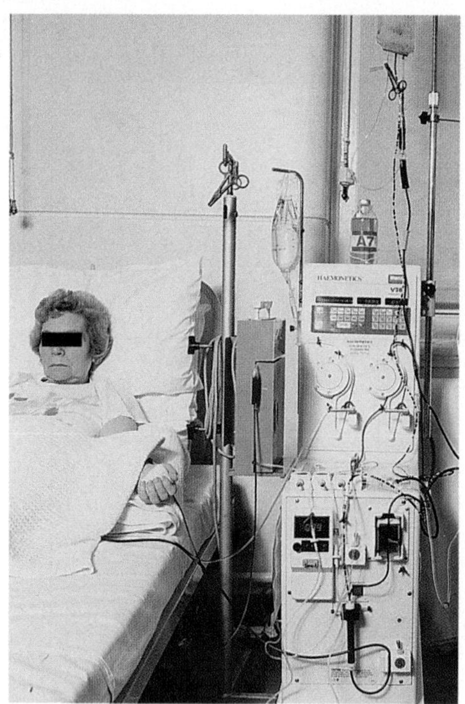

Figure 95.2 **A centrifugal cell separator used for plasma exchange.**

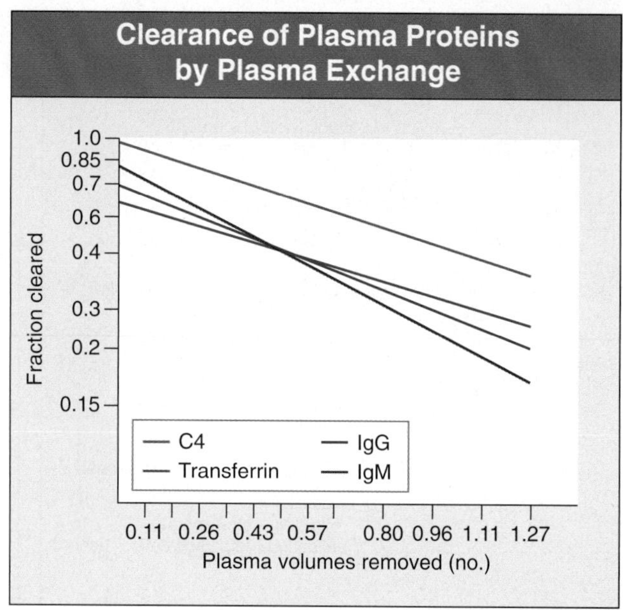

Figure 95.3 **Clearance of plasma proteins by plasma exchange.** Clearance from the intravascular compartment varies with the plasma volume exchanged and between individual proteins. *(Modified from reference 1.)*

Regimens for Plasma Exchange in Renal Disease

Indication	Antiglomerular Basement Membrane Antibody (anti-GBM) Disease	Small Vessel Vasculitis	Cryoglobulinemia	Recurrent FSGS After Transplantation	HUS/TTP
Duration of treatment	Daily, at least 14 days until anti-GBM antibodies 20%	Daily, 7–10 days depending on clinical response	At least 7–10 days or until clinical response	Daily, at least 10 days initially, then continuing less frequently, often for months	Daily for 7–10 days or until platelet count 80–100 × 10^9/l (sometimes needed twice daily)
Exchange volume	50 ml/kg each treatment	As for anti-GBM disease	As for anti-GBM disease	As for anti-GBM disease	As for anti-GBM disease
Replacement fluid	Human albumin 5% (unless bleeding risk)	As for anti-GBM disease	As for anti-GBM disease	As for anti-GBM disease	Fresh-frozen plasma (FFP) or cryo-poor FFP
Additions to replacement fluid	20 ml 10% calcium gluconate (occasionally more), 3 ml 15% KCl if not dialysis dependent, heparin 5000–10,000 U (unless citrate anticoagulation)	As for anti-GBM disease	As for anti-GBM disease	As for anti-GBM disease	As for anti-GBM disease (may need more calcium because of increased volume of FFP-containing citrate)
Immunosuppression	Prednisolone and cyclophosphamide	As for anti-GBM disease	Prednisolone and cyclophosphamide in type II (caution if HCV positive)	None	None
Variations	FFP 5–8 ml/kg as part of exchange volume if hemorrhage risk (renal biopsy in last 48 hr, lung hemorrhage, platelets <40 ×10^9/l, fibrinogen <1.5 g/l); immunoadsorption may be as effective	As for anti-GBM disease Immunoadsorption may be as effective	As for anti-GBM disease	As for anti-GBM disease; may need to include replacement immunoglobulins if continuing long term; immunoadsorption may be as effective	

Figure 95.4 **Practical regimens for plasma exchange in renal disease.** FSGS, focal segmental glomerulosclerosis; FFP, fresh frozen plasma; HUS/TTP, hemolytic-uremic syndrome/thrombotic thrombocytopenic purpura.

regeneration does reduce the efficacy of antibody binding. This technique has been used to treat conditions in which autoantibodies are thought to play a key pathogenic role and usually in place of plasma exchange, such as in Goodpasture's disease, rheumatoid arthritis, and systemic lupus vasculitis, and to remove anti-ABO or anti-HLA antibodies in highly sensitized transplant recipients. In general, the reported efficacy has been equal to that of plasma exchange. Specific ligands have also been immobilized onto columns for more specific removal of potentially pathogenic serum factors; ligands used include anti-human IgG, C1q, phenylalanine, hydrophobic amino acids, acetylcholine receptor and β-adrenoreceptor peptides, and blood group–related oligosaccharides.

COMPLICATIONS

Plasma exchange is expensive (mostly the cost of replacement fluids) and time-consuming and requires trained staff and large-bore vascular access. However, the complication rate is not high. The Swedish registry reported no fatalities during 20,485 procedures and an overall adverse incidence rate of only 4.3% of all exchanges (0.9% for severe adverse events), of which 27% were paresthesias, 19% transient hypotension, 13% urticaria, and 8% nausea.[3] The Canadian apheresis registry has collected data on 144,432 apheresis procedures since 1981 and reported adverse events occurring in 12% of procedures (mostly minor) and overall in 40% of patients. Severe events occurred in only 0.4% of procedures. Three deaths were probably related directly to the procedure, one from a transfusion-related acute lung injury and two from complications from central venous catheters.[4] An overall complication rate of 1.4% has been reported in more than 15,000 treatments in patients receiving albumin and 20% in patients receiving FFP.[2,3] Plasma exchange by centrifugation had a lower risk for adverse events than by filtration.

Other complications directly attributable to plasma exchange include citrate-induced hypocalcemia (presenting with perioral tingling and paresthesias) and citrate-induced metabolic alkalosis. Citrate is usually present in FFP (up to 14% by volume) or is administered in the extracorporeal circuit as an anticoagulant; it binds free calcium in plasma. Symptomatic hypocalcemia can be averted by infusion of 10 to 20 ml of 10% calcium gluconate during each plasma exchange. Alkalosis is rare and is caused by metabolism of citrate to bicarbonate and failure to excrete bicarbonate in patients with renal impairment.

Plasma exchange predictably increases the risk of bleeding as a result of depletion of coagulation factors in patients receiving albumin as sole replacement colloid. Prothrombin time is increased by 30% and partial thromboplastin time by 100% after a single plasma volume exchange. Patients at risk of bleeding (pulmonary hemorrhage, after biopsy, postoperative) should receive FFP (300 to 600 ml) with replacement fluids. Dilutional hypokalemia is avoided by adding potassium to the replacement albumin. An increased incidence of infection secondary to hypogammaglobulinemia has not been confirmed in recent series.[4] Sepsis related to intravenous access is the most common infectious complication of plasma exchange. Cascade filtration can lead to hemolysis (in up to 20% patients) but rarely necessitates transfusion.

MECHANISMS OF ACTION

Plasma exchange removes large-molecular-weight substances from the plasma, including antibodies, complement components, immune complexes, endotoxin, lipoproteins, and von Willebrand factor (vWF) multimers. The pathogenicity of autoantibodies in anti–glomerular basement membrane (anti-GBM) disease provided the impetus for development of plasma exchange therapy, but it is now clear that antibodies, although necessary, are not alone sufficient to cause the necrotizing glomerulonephritis in Goodpasture's disease. Therefore, plasma exchange may well have benefits in addition to simply clearance of autoantibodies. The clearance of antibodies from patients is variable and depends on a number of factors, including the rate of equilibration of macromolecules between the intravascular and extravascular compartments. IgM antibodies are cleared more effectively by centrifugal plasma exchange than are other classes of immunoglobulin as they are retained in the vascular compartment almost wholly. Rebound increase in antibody production will occur unless there is concomitant immunosuppression to prevent resynthesis.

Plasma exchange has also been shown to remove immune complexes, which may have clinical significance in cryoglobulinemia and systemic lupus, and fibrinogen and complement components. There is no good evidence that removal of cytokines has any clinical significance. Plasma exchange reduces plasma viscosity, with consequent improved blood flow in the microvasculature.

INDICATIONS FOR PLASMA EXCHANGE

Evidence to support specific indications for plasma exchange is variable in quality. Direct comparison between randomized controlled trials can be unsatisfactory because of variations in dose and frequency of plasma exchange and in immunosuppressive and other adjunctive therapy. The American Society for Apheresis reviewed all indications for plasma exchange in 2007 and summarized available trial data.[7,8] In this chapter, evidence from available randomized trials is discussed alongside observational data. The indications are summarized in Figures 95.5 and 95.6.

Anti–Glomerular Basement Membrane Antibody Disease (Goodpasture's Disease)

Plasma exchange removes anti-GBM antibodies effectively. Most patients can be depleted of pathogenic antibodies after 7 to 10 plasma volume exchanges if further antibody synthesis is inhibited by the concurrent use of cyclophosphamide and corticosteroids. Before the introduction of this therapy, the mortality from Goodpasture's disease was more than 90%, and only 11% of patients who were not dialysis dependent at presentation survived with preserved renal function. The use of plasma exchange improved the outcome considerably; 70% to 90% of patients now survive. However, only 50% of survivors and no more than 10% of those who are dialysis dependent at presentation retain independent renal function. There has been only one small controlled trial of plasma exchange in the treatment of Goodpasture's disease that used a low intensity of plasma exchange.[7,9] A total of 17 patients were randomized to receive corticosteroids and cyclophosphamide, with or without plasma exchange. Only two of the eight receiving plasma exchange developed end-stage renal disease compared with six of the nine receiving drugs alone.

Long-term data from 71 patients with Goodpasture's disease confirmed the benefit of a treatment regimen including plasma exchange because most patients with mild to moderate renal failure retained independent renal function during 10 to 25

Conditions for Which There is Strong Evidence for the Benefit of Plasma Exchange					
Indication	**Randomized Controlled Trial (no. of Patients)**	**Controlled Trial (no. of Patients)**	**Case Series (no. of Patients)**	**Replacement Fluid**	**Comments**
ANCA-associated systemic vasculitis	8 (300)	1 (26)	21 (294)	Albumin unless pulmonary hemorrhage or need to prevent coagulopathy	Only proven benefit in dialysis-dependent patients Should consider daily exchanges in fulminant cases or with pulmonary hemorrhage
Anti-GBM antibody disease	1 (17)	0	17 (430)	Albumin unless pulmonary hemorrhage or need to prevent coagulopathy	Minimum course 14 days to remove antibodies effectively Especially beneficial in nonoliguric patients before dialysis Patients with creatinine >5.5 mg/dl (500 μmol/l) unlikely to benefit
Cryoglobulinemia	0	0	18 (195)	Albumin	Long-term maintenance treatment needed in some patients Ensure blood warmer on return lines or warm replacement fluids
Thrombotic thrombpcytopenic purpura	3 (237)	2 (133)	17 (915)	Plasma or cryo-poor plasma	Daily; often with corticosteroids The only treatment that has improved mortality
ABO incompatible kidney transplantation	0	0	22 (>500)	Albumin +/– plasma (compatible with donor and recipient or AB)	Used before transplantation to reduce titers of antibodies and often continued for a few days after surgery Allows successful transplantation
HLA desensitization for transplantation (in highly sensitized patients)	0	1 (61)	18 (219)	Albumin	Always in combination with immunosuppression and continued until crossmatch negative Usually needs 5 plasma exchanges to reduce Ab levels sufficiently
Antibody-mediated kidney transplant rejection	3 (61)	5 (240)	24 (396)	Albumin	Daily or alternate day Significantly better evidence has emerged in the last 15 years for benefit

Figure 95.5 Conditions for which there is strong evidence for the benefit of plasma exchange. ANCA, antineutrophil cytoplasmic antibody.

years,[10] and renal recovery was possible even in some of those with the most severe renal disease. Combining all the available published data for patients with Goodpasture's disease, 76% of patients presenting with serum creatinine concentration below 5.5 to 6.8 mg/dl (500 to 600 μmol/l) will retain renal function, in contrast to 8% of those presenting dependent on dialysis.

Recommendation

All patients presenting before dialysis should receive intensive plasma exchange with daily 4-liter exchanges initially for 14 days (regimen shown in Fig. 95.5). For dialysis-dependent patients, we recommend plasma exchange with immunosuppression only for those who have biopsy or clinical evidence of recent-onset disease. Pulmonary hemorrhage is an independent indication for plasma exchange. Treatment of Goodpasture's disease is discussed further in Chapter 23.

Small-Vessel Vasculitis

The majority of patients with rapidly progressive glomerulonephritis (RPGN), other than anti-GBM disease, have small-vessel vasculitis with ANCA detectable in their serum, and there is increasing evidence that these autoantibodies are pathogenic (see Chapter 24). Plasma exchange was initially introduced in such patients because of the similarity of the histologic changes to those seen in Goodpasture's disease and the supposition that immune complexes may be instrumental in disease pathogenesis. Several trials of plasma exchange in non–anti-GBM RPGN have been reported.[7,11] Most of the early trials included patients with a variety of diseases, used a low intensity of plasma exchange, and often excluded those with oligoanuria. These trials showed no overall benefit of plasma exchange in addition to conventional immunosuppression; however, those patients with the most

Conditions for Which There is Some Evidence for the Benefit of Plasma exchange

Indication	Randomized Controlled Trial (no. of patients)	Controlled Trial (no. of patients)	Case Series (no. of patients)	Replacement Fluid	Comments
Catastrophic antiphospholipid antibody syndrome	0	0	(280)	Plasma	Should be done daily Combination of plasma exchange or IVIG, heparin, and corticosteroids (from registry data) gives best outcomes
Primary or recurrent FSGS	0	0	40 (98)	Albumin	Sometimes in combination with cyclophosphamide May be more effective in recurrent disease after transplantation May need long-term maintenance treatment
Atypical hemolytic-uremic syndrome (aHUS) or thrombotic microangiopathy	1 (35)	1 (37)	49 (>1000)	Plasma or cryo-poor plasma	Conflicting reports on benefit in aHUS but prognosis without very poor Daily plasma exchange intitially but duration variable
Myeloma	5 (182)	0	6 (105)	Albumin	Daily or alternate daily for 7–10 exchanges Despite negative randomized trial in 2005, plasma exchange should be considered if high light-chain load, severe renal failure, and oliguria despite aggressive hydration and conservative management
Rapidly progressive glomerulonephritis (may include patients with ANCA-associated disease in older literature	7 (196)	0	20 (273)	Albumin	No good evidence for benefit in immune complex disease of any cause
Scleroderma	0	3 (75)	6 (60)	Albumin	No good evidence for benefit, but some patients have reported improvement with therapeutic trial of plasma exchange
SLE (not nephritis)	1 (20)	1 (4)	13 (124)	Albumin	For cerebritis, lupus-associated TTP, or pulmonary hemorrhage

Figure 95.6 Conditions for which there is some evidence for the benefit of plasma exchange. ANCA, antineutrophil cytoplasmic antibody; FSGS, focal segmental glomerulosclerosis; IVIG, intravenous immune globulin; SLE, systemic lupus erythematosus; TTP, thrombotic thrombocytopenic purpura.

severe disease did seem to benefit. Combining the results of the controlled trials, 31 of 42 (74%) dialysis-dependent patients treated with plasma exchange recovered renal function compared with only 8 of 25 (32%) treated with drugs alone. The most recent randomized, controlled trial (MEPEX: methylprednisolone or plasma exchange in severe ANCA-associated vasculitis) randomized 137 patients with ANCA-associated systemic vasculitis and serum creatinine concentration above 5.5 mg/dl (500 μmol/l) to plasma exchange or intravenous methylprednisolone in addition to oral corticosteroids and cyclophosphamide[11]; 69% of patients recovered renal function when treated with plasma exchange compared with 49% of those receiving intravenous methylprednisolone. Patients with both ANCA and anti-GBM antibodies (so-called double-positive patients) and RPGN do not seem to respond so well to plasma exchange and rarely if ever recover renal function.[12]

Recommendation

We perform plasma exchange in patients with small-vessel vasculitis who present with severe renal failure (serum creatinine concentration above 5.5 mg/dl [~500 μmol/l] or dialysis dependent) or pulmonary hemorrhage. The regimen is shown in Figure 95.5.

Other Crescentic Glomerulonephritis

Crescent formation is a common histologic finding in a number of other patterns of glomerulonephritis (GN), including postinfectious GN, GN associated with infective endocarditis, IgA nephropathy, membranoproliferative glomerulonephritis (MPGN), and membranous nephropathy. Patients historically were often included in studies of treatment of RPGN, and plasma exchange has been used in the treatment of a number of these conditions. More than 400 patients with such diseases have been treated with plasma exchange with no good evidence for any benefit in RPGN not due to anti-GBM disease or vasculitis.[7,8] In crescentic IgA nephropathy, there are anecdotal reports of short-term benefit in patients with severe renal impairment, but longer term follow-up has proved disappointing.

Recommendation

We reserve plasma exchange in IgA nephropathy and other GN for patients with rapidly deteriorating renal function and extensive fresh crescents in the biopsy specimen.

Focal Segmental Glomerulosclerosis

Plasma exchange and protein A immunoadsorption have been used to treat patients with primary focal segmental glomerulosclerosis (FSGS) or recurrent disease after transplantation. The results have been less good in primary disease; less than 40% of patients achieve either partial or complete remission,[7,8,13] and we do not recommend plasma exchange in this setting. Plasma exchange for recurrent disease is discussed later and in Chapter 104.

Hemolytic-Uremic Syndrome/Thrombotic Thrombocytopenic Purpura

In both hemolytic-uremic syndrome (HUS) and thrombotic thrombocytopenic purpura (TTP), endothelial activation leads to thrombotic microangiopathy, but through independent mechanisms (see Chapter 28).

Diarrhea-Associated Hemolytic-Uremic Syndrome

Childhood diarrhea-associated HUS (D^+ HUS) is usually caused by bacterial verotoxins and has a good prognosis. Most children will recover fully with supportive care and management of fluid and electrolyte imbalance and hypertension. Two controlled trials of plasma infusion (at least 10 ml/kg daily) in childhood HUS complicated by dialysis-dependent renal failure showed no clinical benefit (as determined by hypertension, renal dysfunction, and proteinuria) in either short- or medium-term follow-up.[14] There has been no study of plasma exchange in childhood D^+ HUS. Plasma exchange and infusion have not been subjected to any controlled trials in adult D^+ HUS, but uncontrolled observations suggest possible benefit.[7,15]

Thrombotic Thrombocytopenic Purpura

Patients with TTP have a defective vWF-cleaving protease (ADAMTS13), an enzyme that normally degrades large vWF multimers, because of either inherited deficiency or autoantibodies directed against the protease. Accumulation of vWF multimers leads to systemic platelet activation under conditions of high shear stress (the microcirculation) and thrombosis. The rationale for plasma infusion and plasma exchange in TTP is therefore to replenish vWF-cleaving protease, to remove antibodies against it, and to remove the large vWF multimers from circulation.

The first prospective, controlled trial compared plasma infusion with plasma exchange (1 to 1.5 plasma volumes at least seven times in the first 9 days).[16] All patients received aspirin and dipyridamole. Of patients receiving plasma exchange, 47% had a platelet count above 150×10^9 cells/l and no new neurologic features, compared with only 25% of those receiving plasma infusion during the first 2 weeks. At 6 months, survival was substantially better in the plasma exchange group (50% versus 78%). More recent series using plasma exchange have reported mortality rates as low as 15%,[7] and there may be an association of reduced early mortality with more intensive plasma exchange. Renal impairment is not an independent predictor of poor outcome in TTP and does not in itself warrant more intensive therapy. Fever, age older than 40 years, and hemoglobin level below 9 g/dl have been associated with a worse outcome. Whether FFP or its cryosupernatant fraction is better as replacement fluid remains unclear.

D^- Hemolytic-Uremic Syndrome

The cause of adult HUS remains unclear in most cases in which there is no clear diarrheal prodrome (D^- HUS; atypical HUS). Some patients have defective regulation of the complement pathway (e.g., factor H deficiency), leading to uninhibited activation of complement; in others, infections or drugs cause platelet or leukocyte activation and complement activation and consumption. Direct activation of endothelial cells may also be a cause. Plasma exchange and infusion have not been subjected to any controlled trials in adult D^- HUS, but uncontrolled series suggest benefit (see Chapter 28).[7] HUS/TTP occurring after renal transplantation has also responded to plasma exchange.

Recommendation

We use plasma exchange in all adults with TTP or D^- HUS and perform all exchanges against FFP or cryo-poor FFP.

Systemic Lupus

Plasma exchange has been used extensively in patients with lupus. Most studies have included patients with diverse patterns of disease and often only mild renal involvement. A randomized, prospective trial could show no benefit of plasma exchange over conventional immunosuppression for renal, serologic, or clinical outcomes, in both the short and long term.[17] However, patients with crescentic lupus nephritis and those with the most severe renal dysfunction (dialysis dependency) were excluded. Anecdotal evidence suggests that plasma exchange may benefit patients with crescentic glomerulonephritis, pulmonary hemorrhage, cerebral lupus, catastrophic antiphospholipid syndrome, lupus-associated TTP, or severe lupus unresponsive to conventional drugs and patients for whom cytotoxic therapy has been withdrawn because of bone marrow suppression or other toxicity. Immunoadsorption may be more successful in the severe forms of lupus nephritis. A variety of techniques have been used, including standard protein A and anti-Ig absorption, and also phenylalanine, tryptophan, and dextran sulfate ligands, all of which bind immunoglobulin, rheumatoid factors, and immune complexes to varying degrees and all of which have been reported to induce remission in patients with severe disease after failure of conventional therapy.

Recommendation

We reserve plasma exchange for lupus patients with rapidly progressive renal failure and class IV renal histology with crescents, for severe neurologic involvement and hemolysis, for those likely to suffer bone marrow suppression from cyclophosphamide, and for those with catastrophic antiphospholipid syndrome. The treatment of lupus is further discussed in Chapter 25.

Cryoglobulinemia

In type I cryoglobulinemia, usually associated with myeloma or lymphoma, a monoclonal immunoglobulin causes hyperviscosity and cryoprecipitation. Such antibodies are easily removed by plasma exchange, often with immediate clinical benefit. Cytotoxic agents are used simultaneously to inhibit further paraprotein production. There are no controlled trials of the use of plasma exchange, but symptoms are closely related to the presence of the cryoimmunoglobulin, and hence treatment with plasma exchange appears effective.[7]

Patients with type II (mixed essential) cryoglobulinemia develop a monoclonal antibody (usually IgM) with specificity for a second, usually polyclonal, immunoglobulin. Type II cryoglobulins occur most commonly in association with lymphoma and hepatitis C virus infection. The resulting immune complexes can be deposited in the microcirculation and are particularly associated with MPGN (see Chapter 21). Plasma exchange is effective at clearing the immune complexes, although in long-term follow-up, the cryoglobulins often recur, and sustained benefit has not been clearly demonstrated. However, many of the acute features of cryoglobulinemia do resolve with plasma exchange, particularly arthralgia, skin lesions, and digital necrosis, and patients with RPGN can recover renal function. Concomitant immunosuppression with cytotoxic agents or rituximab may prevent resynthesis of the cryoproteins, although some patients require long-term intermittent plasma exchange to control symptoms. Immunosuppressive treatment should be used with caution in patients with hepatitis C virus–associated cryoglobulinemia who may respond to antiviral therapies, such as interferon and ribavirin. Cryofiltration apheresis (in which a normal plasma filter is used to separate plasma, which is then cooled to precipitate the cryoglobulin before return to the patient) selectively removes cryoglobulins, avoids large volumes of replacement fluids, and avoids deficiency of clotting factors, but it needs to be combined with immunosuppression to prevent synthesis of further cryoglobulin. Few centers currently perform this technique.

Myeloma

Plasma exchange has benefit in myeloma with either cast nephropathy or light-chain renal toxicity. Two small controlled trials performed more than 15 years ago provided conflicting results. Recently, a large prospective, controlled trial was reported in which 97 patients with myeloma and progressive acute kidney injury (creatinine >200 μmol/l [2.3 mg/dl] with an increase >50 μmol/l during the previous 2 weeks despite conventional management) were randomized to receive plasma exchange (five to seven sessions of 50 ml/kg during 10 days) in addition to chemotherapy (vincristine-doxorubicin-dexamethasone [VAD] or melphalan and prednisolone).[18] This study showed no benefit of plasma exchange on mortality or recovery of renal function. However, patients had a wide degree of renal dysfunction, and relatively few had a renal biopsy performed to confirm cast nephropathy. A retrospective review from the Mayo Clinic suggested that those with myeloma and high light-chain loads or severe renal failure may benefit if plasma exchange reduced light chains rapidly.[19] Promising early data suggest that hemodialysis with novel membranes allowing the removal of large-molecular-weight molecules and lengthy dialysis sessions (6 to 8 hours) may prove superior to plasma exchange in removing light chains and improving renal function (see Chapter 63).

Recommendation

We reserve plasma exchange in myeloma for patients with high light-chain loads and cast nephropathy on biopsy.

Transplantation

Antibody-Mediated Rejection

Studies in the 1980s suggested that combining plasma exchange with cyclophosphamide could deplete circulating antibodies in patients with vascular or antibody-mediated rejection, but a review of 157 patients included in five trials could not demonstrate any significant difference in the outcome of acute vascular rejection in patients treated with or without plasma exchange.[7,8] More recently, at least eight trials including more than 300 patients with more clearly defined antibody-mediated rejection and case series of more than 400 patients have suggested that plasma exchange, usually combined with intravenous immune globulin but sometimes antithymocyte globulin, may effectively reverse such rejection episodes in 55% to 100% of episodes.[7]

There is no convincing evidence that plasma exchange has any role in the treatment of chronic rejection.

Anti-HLA Antibodies

Highly sensitized patients with preformed anti-HLA antibodies have been treated both before and after transplantation with plasma exchange or immunoadsorption to reduce cytotoxic antibody levels.[7] Patients usually received intensive immunoadsorption or plasma exchange before transplantation to ensure a current negative crossmatch immediately before transplantation; some received longer term immunoadsorption or plasma exchange in combination with corticosteroids and cyclophosphamide in the months preceding transplantation. Treatment of 100 patients with high-titer cytotoxic antibodies with plasma exchange or immunoadsorption in addition to cyclophosphamide and prednisolone led to graft survival rates at 1 and 4 years of 77% and 64%, respectively, in living donor recipients, and 70% and 57%, respectively, in first deceased donor graft recipients.

ABO-Incompatible Renal Transplantation

Plasma exchange is widely used to remove natural anti-A or anti-B blood group antibodies from the recipient before living related transplantation from an ABO-incompatible donor. Various protocols are in use, but all rely on depleting specific antibody during 4 to 6 days before transplantation by exchanging a single plasma volume for human albumin solution (in addition to routine immunosuppression, sometimes including rituximab and intravenous immune globulin). Plasma exchange is sometimes continued for one or two sessions after transplantation or if antibody-mediated rejection occurs.[20] One-year graft survival rates of up to 85% have been reported with such protocols, although rejection episodes are more common than in ABO-compatible transplants. Patients with increasingly high antibody titers are being treated in this way. More recently, immunoadsorption using synthetic A- or B-oligosaccharide epitopes linked to Sepharose has been developed. Such columns specifically remove anti-A or anti-B antibodies, but any clinical benefit remains uncertain.

Recurrent Focal Segmental Glomerulosclerosis

Plasma exchange, double filtration plasmapheresis, and protein A immunoadsorption have all been used to treat recurrence of nephrotic syndrome after transplantation in patients with recurrent FSGS.[7,21] An incompletely defined circulating factor causing increased permeability of glomerular capillaries can be found in most patients with recurrent FSGS. There are no controlled trials of plasma treatments in recurrent FSGS, and most series are small. One study demonstrated an 82% reduction in urinary protein excretion in eight patients with recurrent nephrosis during plasma protein adsorption; however, the effect was transient and persisted for less than 2 months in seven of the eight patients.[21] Other investigators have obtained remissions in approximately 50% of patients and a significant reduction in graft loss due to recurrent disease compared with historic controls. More intensive treatment regimens have led to more persistent remissions. All three apheresis modalities have also been used prophylactically in patients deemed to be at high risk of recurrence, with variable success. Management of recurrent FSGS is discussed further in Chapter 104.

REFERENCES

1. Derksen RH, Schuurman HJ, Meyling FH, et al. The efficacy of plasma exchange in the removal of plasma components. *J Lab Clin Med.* 1984;104:346-354.
2. Reutter JC, Sanders KF, Brecher ME, et al. Incidence of allergic reactions to FFP or cryo-supernatant in the treatment of thrombotic thrombocytopenic purpura. *J Clin Apher.* 2001;16:134-138.
3. Norda R, Stegmayr B. Therapeutic apheresis in Sweden. *Transfus Apher Sci.* 2003;9:159-166.
4. Rock G, Clark B, Sutton D, et al. The Canadian apheresis registry. *Transfus Apher Sci.* 2003;29:167-177.
5. Stegmayr B, Ptak J, Wikstrom B, et al. World apheresis registry 2003-2007 data. *Tansfus Apher Sci.* 2008;39:247-254.
6. Malchesky PS, Koo AP, Roberson GA, et al. Apheresis technologies and clinical applications: The 2005 international apheresis registry. *Ther Apher Dial.* 2007;11:341-362.
7. Szczepiorkowski ZM, Bandarenko N, Kim HC, et al. Guidelines on the use of therapeutic apheresis in clinical practice—evidence based approach from the Apheresis Applications Committee of the American Society for Apheresis. *J Clin Apher.* 2007;22:106-175.
8. Shaz BW, Linenberger ML, Bandarenko N, et al. Category IV indications for therapeutic apheresis—ASFA fourth special issue. *J Clin Apher.* 2007;22:176-180.
9. Johnson JP, Whitman W, Briggs WA, Wilson CB. Plasmapheresis and immunosuppressive agents in antibasement membrane antibody–induced Goodpasture's syndrome. *Am J Med.* 1978;64:354-359.
10. Levy JB, Turner AN, Rees AJ, Pusey CD. Long term outcome of anti–glomerular basement membrane antibody disease treated with plasma exchange and immunosuppression. *Ann Intern Med.* 2001;134:1033-1042.
11. Jayne DR, Gaskin G, Rasmussen N, et al. Randomized trial of plasma exchange or high dose methylprednisolone as adjunctive therapy for severe renal vasculitis. *J Am Soc Nephrol.* 2007;18:2180-2188.
12. Levy JB, Hammad T, Coulthart A, et al. Clinical features and outcome of patients with both ANCA and anti-GBM antibodies. *Kidney Int.* 2004;66:1535-1540.
13. Bosch T, Wendler T. Extracorporeal plasma exchange in primary and recurrent focal segmental glomerulosclerosis. A review. *Ther Apher.* 2001;5:155-160.
14. Rizzoni G, Claris-Appiani A, Edefonti A, et al. Plasma infusion for hemolytic uremic syndrome in children. *J Pediatr.* 1988;112:284-290.
15. Nguyen TC, Stegmayr B, Busund R, et al. Plasma therapies in thrombotic syndromes. *Int J Artif Organs.* 2005;28:459-465.
16. Rock GA, Shumak KH, Buskard NA, et al. Comparison of plasma exchange with plasma infusion in the treatment of thrombotic thrombocytopenic purpura. Canadian Apheresis Study Group. *N Engl J Med.* 1991;325:393-397.
17. Korbet SM, Lewis EJ, Schwartz MM, et al. Factors predictive of outcome in severe lupus nephritis. Lupus Nephritis Collaboration Group. *Am J Kidney Dis.* 2000;35:904-914.
18. Clark WF, Stewart AK, Rock GA, et al. Plasma exchange when myeloma presents as acute renal failure. *Ann Intern Med.* 2005;143:777-784.
19. Leung N, Gertz MA, Zeidenrust SR, et al. Improvement of cast nephropathy with plasma exchange depends on the diagnosis and on reduction of serum light chains. *Kidney Int.* 2008;73:1282-1288.
20. Winters JL, Gloor JM, Pineda AA, et al. Plasma exchange conditioning for ABO-incompatible renal transplantation. *J Clin Apher.* 2004;19:79-85.
21. Dantal J, Bigot E, Bogers W, et al. Effect of plasma protein adsorption on protein excretion in kidney-transplant recipients with recurrent nephrotic syndrome. *N Engl J Med.* 1994;330:7-14.

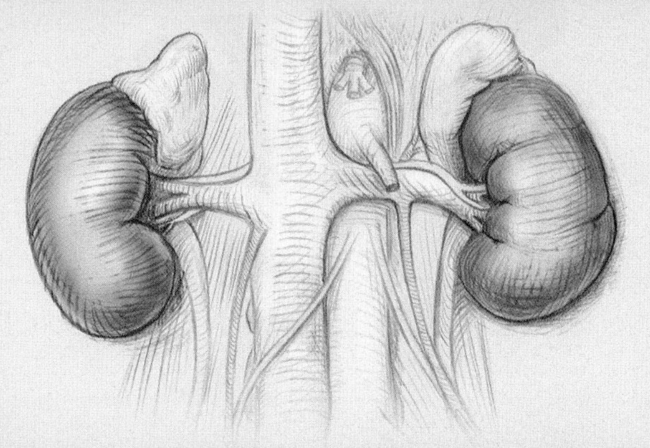

SECTION XVII

Transplantation

CHAPTER 96

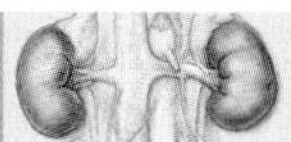

Immunologic Principles in Kidney Transplantation

Karl Womer, Hamid Rabb

The human immune system has evolved into a complex and highly sophisticated defense mechanism against the invasion of foreign pathogens and the growth of tumor cells. Important to an effective immune response is the ability of T cells to recognize a wide variety of non-self antigens, which allows restrained immune activation and subsequent antigen-specific killing. This task is accomplished through the generation of a diverse repertoire of T cells in a single individual with specificity for an enormous number of potential foreign antigens presented as peptides on the surface of major histocompatibility complex (MHC) molecules. Variations in MHC structure from individual to individual increase the variety of peptides that can be presented to T cells, which protects the species as a group by ensuring adequate T-cell responses to a given foreign organism in at least one member of the population. Although slight, these MHC polymorphisms are recognized as foreign after kidney transplantation between nongenetically identical humans and induce alloresponses that in the absence of immunosuppression result in rejection of the allograft (see Fig. 96.1 for graft terminology). In this chapter, we review basic immunologic principles important to the field of kidney transplantation.

ISCHEMIA-REPERFUSION INJURY

The immunologic responses that occur after kidney transplantation are a series of relatively well defined stages, as depicted in Figure 96.2. Initial insults to the graft occur during donor organ procurement and subsequent transplantation into the recipient and are referred to as ischemia-reperfusion injury (IRI). The pathogenesis of IRI represents a complex interplay between biochemical, cellular, vascular endothelial, and tissue-specific factors, with inflammation as a common feature.[1] Acute ischemia leads to tissue damage and endothelial cell activation, with production of oxygen free radicals, secretion of inflammatory cytokines and chemokines, and upregulation of adhesion molecules that are important initiators of the innate or antigen-nonspecific immune response. Toll-like receptors (TLRs) are primarily expressed on resident antigen-presenting cells (APCs), mostly dendritic cells (DCs), but also on endothelial and stromal cells. Activation of TLRs by noninfectious stimuli during IRI leads to release of cytokines, including tumor necrosis factor α (TNF-α) and interleukin-6 (IL-6). These proinflammatory mediators induce tubular epithelial cell production of the chemokine CXCL8 (IL-8), which attracts neutrophils by activation of their surface chemokine receptor, CXCR2. Neutrophil accumulation is the prime cellular mediator of microvascular plugging and local tissue destruction in IRI. However, monocyte-macrophage infiltration also occurs during IRI and probably contributes to extension of early injury as well as repair.[2] TLR activation induces the maturation of DCs, which leads to the adaptive or antigen-specific phase of transplantation immunity. Natural killer (NK) cells probably also function as a bridge between innate and adaptive immunity in IRI, in part through bidirectional crosstalk between NK cells and DCs, which plays a relevant role in the mechanisms leading to maturation of DCs.[3] Likewise, although activation of the alternative pathway of complement plays an important role in IRI as a manifestation of the innate immune system, complement may also regulate adaptive immune responses. Whereas both T and B cells constitute the primary arms of the adaptive immune response, they also play an important role in the acute and possibly healing phases of IRI.[1] The immunologic events described are not specific to allografts, as they also occur in syngeneic grafts.

ANTIGEN PRESENTATION

Antigen-Presenting Cells

APCs are specialized cells capable of activating T cells. Antigen is endocytosed by APCs and then displayed by MHC molecules on their surface. T cells recognize and interact with the antigen:MHC complex to become activated. DCs, macrophages, and B cells are all considered "professional APCs," although DCs are the most potent at antigen presentation. Alloimmune responses are initiated by activation of APCs (mostly DCs) through innate immune recognition systems, as described previously. DCs are highly versatile cells, determining whether the environment indicates that antigen should lead to an immune response or, alternatively, tolerance.[4] In the graft and surrounding tissues after transplantation, DCs of either donor or host origin become activated and move to T-cell areas of secondary lymphoid organs (SLOs). The trafficking pattern of naive T cells is restricted to SLOs, such as the lymph node and spleen, but also possibly tertiary lymphoid structures formed in tissues after inflammation.[5] They traverse from blood to lymphoid organs, where they pass through the T-cell areas and become activated on encounter of donor antigen (alloantigen) presented by activated DCs in the context of MHC molecules. Thus, the movement of DCs and naive T cells is coordinated to bring them into contact in the T-cell areas of SLOs, which appears essential for effective priming.[6] Once activated, T cells are able to leave SLOs through lymph vessels to enter the blood and ultimately peripheral tissues, particularly into sites of inflammation. B cells are activated when antigen engages their antigen receptors, initially in the border of T-cell and B-cell areas of SLOs, where helper T-cell function is provided.[7]

Antigen-experienced memory cells may be activated by other APCs, such as graft endothelium.[8] Patients normally have no

Figure 96.1 **Graft terminology.**

Graft Terminology
Autograft (autologous graft): A graft from one part of the body to another. Examples include skin and vascular grafts. No rejection occurs.
Isograft (isogenic or syngeneic graft): A graft from one member of a species to a genetically identical member of the same species. Examples include grafts between identical twins; or members of the same inbred rodent strain. No rejection typically occurs.
Allograft (allogeneic graft): A graft between nonidentical members of the same species. Examples include grafts between unrelated or related nonidentical humans; or members of different inbred rodent strains. Rejection occurs by lymphocytes reactive to alloantigens on the graft (i.e., alloresponse).
Xenografts (xenogeneic graft): A graft between members of different species. Examples include pig or baboon to human; or rat to mouse. Rejection occurs by lymphocytes reactive to xenoantigen on the graft (i.e., xenoresponse).

preexisting immunoreactivity to alloantigen unless they have been exposed to alloantigen through pregnancy, blood transfusion, or prior transplantation. However, viral antigens that cross-react with alloantigens can lead to the generation of alloantigen-specific memory cells through a process termed heterologous immunity.[9]

T-Cell Ontogeny and MHC Specificity

Allografts induce alloimmune responses due to the recognition of non-self antigens (e.g., MHC) from the graft by recipient T cells. During T-cell ontogeny, multilineage bone marrow precursors migrate to the thymus, where ultimate rearrangement of the T-cell receptor (TCR) gene occurs, resulting in irrevocable T-cell commitment. TCR gene rearrangement is random and ensures that a diverse repertoire of T cells exists to be able to respond to the enormous number of potential foreign antigens.[10] The mature T-cell repertoire is determined in the thymus by two processes, positive and negative selection. Positive selection is dependent on a certain degree of antigen-specific T-cell affinity to self MHC molecules on thymic cortical epithelial cells. This process ensures that mature T cells will interact effectively with MHC to allow recognition of foreign antigen in the context of self MHC. Negative selection occurs by deletion of T cells with high affinity for self peptide and MHC, thereby preventing release of high-affinity T cells with autoimmune potential.

Mature T cells expressing their clone-specific TCRs then exit the thymus as either CD4 or CD8 T cells. The TCRs of CD4 T cells (also called helper T cells) are selected to interact with class II MHC molecules; the TCRs of CD8 T cells (precursors of cytotoxic T lymphocytes or CTLs) interact with class I MHC molecules. A fundamental principle of immunology is that T cells do not recognize intact foreign proteins directly but instead as peptides presented by self MHC on APCs. However, allelic variation among MHC molecules from individual to individual is quite small, resulting in similarities between donor and recipient MHC structure. Thus, unique to the transplant setting, recipient TCRs have a strong affinity for intact donor MHC molecules and can recognize them directly, which explains in large part the high proportion of T cells responding to alloantigen.[11] In fact, roughly $1/10^5$ to $1/10^6$ T cells will respond to any given nominal antigen (e.g., peptide derived from tetanus toxin or influenza hemagglutinin). However, the frequency of T cells that respond to foreign MHC molecules (alloantigens) is much higher (up to 5% to 10% of all T cells).

Pathways of Allorecognition

Recipient T cells may encounter alloantigen by either the direct or indirect pathway of allorecognition (Fig. 96.3). As previously alluded to, direct antigen presentation involves recipient T-cell recognition of donor MHC peptides in the context of intact donor MHC molecules on the surface of donor APCs. By this mechanism, *donor* APCs migrate from the graft to recipient lymphoid organs and activate alloreactive recipient T cells to initiate the alloimmune response. It has been suggested that the direct pathway may be particularly active early after transplantation, when a large number of donor APCs are present in the allograft. However, direct antigen presentation may also occur when recipient T cells recognize intact donor MHC molecules on cells of the graft (e.g., endothelium). B cells also recognize intact donor MHC antigen through their B-cell receptors. The best evidence of direct allorecognition is the strong *in vitro* response generated in the mixed lymphocyte reaction, in which lymphocytes are cultured with allogeneic APCs.

Indirect antigen recognition is the physiologic mechanism of foreign antigen presentation. Foreign antigen is taken up by APCs, processed intracellularly, and then presented as peptides on MHC molecules. During indirect allorecognition, donor MHC molecules are shed from the graft and processed by *recipient* APCs, where they are presented as peptides to recipient T cells in the context of recipient MHC molecules.[12] As donor MHC molecules are continually shed from the graft and presented by recipient APCs, indirect allorecognition may play a larger role in the late alloresponse, including chronic rejection. Indirect allorecognition may also be necessary for effective alloantibody production and isotype switching after transplantation.[13] Although the true relative contribution of direct versus indirect allorecognition to the alloresponse and transplant rejection remains open to question, recent work using transgenic T cells recognizing allo-MHC either directly or indirectly indicates that the direct alloresponse is short-lived, whereas the indirect alloresponse eventually becomes the driving force behind the rejection process, at least for CD4 T cells.[14]

Major Histocompatibility Complex

Class I and class II MHC molecules are designed for presentation of antigen from different sources for different purposes. The class I system is designed to sample cytosolic proteins to detect tumors or intracellular pathogens, such as virus and intracellular

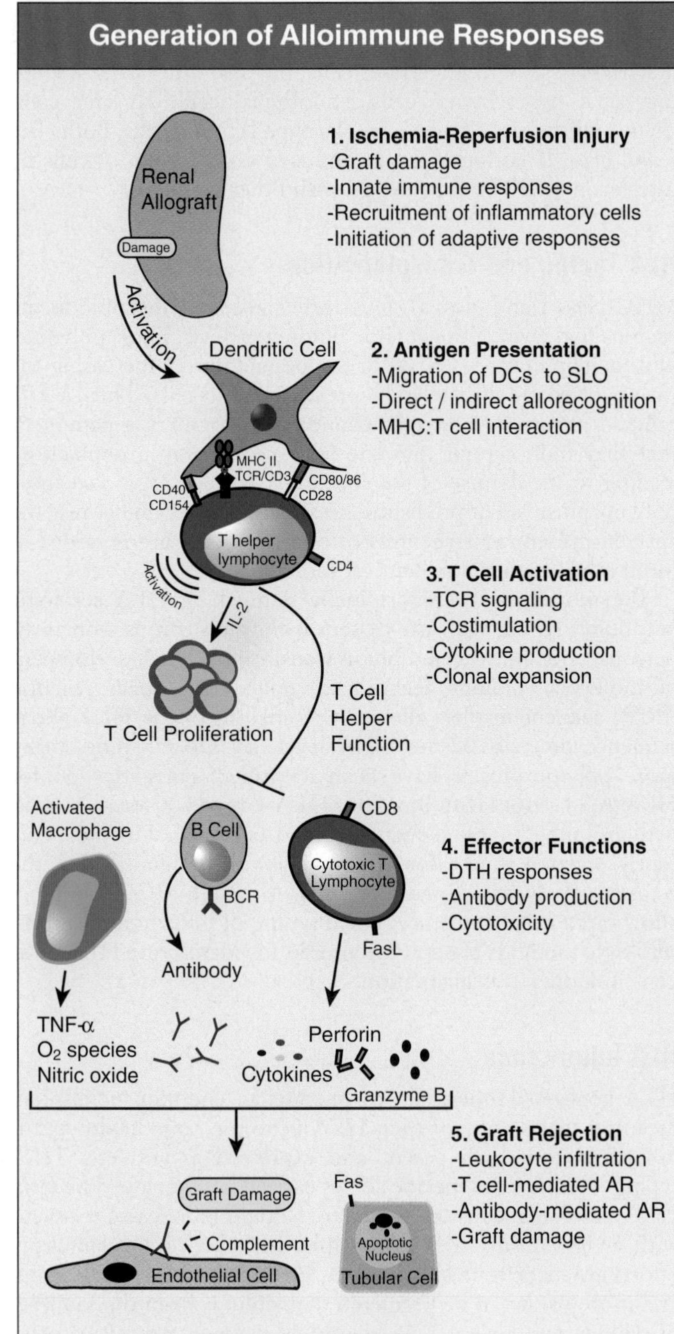

Figure 96.2 Generation of alloimmune responses. Immunologic responses after renal transplantation represent a series of well-defined stages that result in rejection of the allograft in the absence of exogenous immunosuppression. Graft damage that follows ischemia-reperfusion injury during procurement and transplantation activates innate (antigen-nonspecific) immune responses, which recruit inflammatory cells and initiate adaptive (antigen-specific) immune responses. After activation, dendritic cells (DCs) of donor (direct pathway) or recipient (indirect pathway) origin migrate to secondary lymphoid organs (SLO), where they present alloantigen to T cells through MHC structures on their cell surface. After T-cell receptor (TCR) signaling and appropriate costimulation, T cells become activated to produce large amounts of cytokine and undergo clonal expansion. CD4 T cells provide help to B cells, CD8 T cells, and macrophages for the production of alloantibody, cellular cytotoxicity, and delayed-type hypersensitivity (DTH) responses, respectively. These effector functions result in destruction of the graft by acute rejection (AR), which may be T cell or antibody mediated.

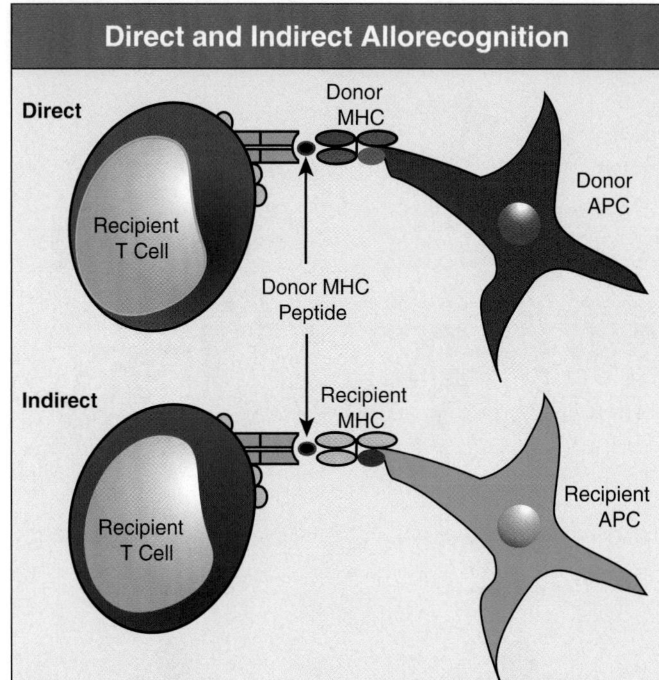

Figure 96.3 Direct and indirect antigen presentation. In direct allorecognition, donor antigen *(shown in red)* is presented to recipient T cells as a peptide in the context of intact *donor* major histocompatibility complex (MHC) molecules on the surface of donor antigen-presenting cells (APCs). In indirect allorecognition, the donor antigen is processed by recipient APCs and presented as a peptide in the context of *recipient* MHC molecules.

bacteria. Class I proteins are recognized by CD8 T cells and thus provide a surveillance mechanism to target infected or malignant cells for destruction by CTLs. The class II system is designed to sample extracellular proteins that have been taken up and processed by APCs. Class II proteins are recognized by CD4 T helper cells and allow the generation of immune responses to invading pathogens that are phagocytosed by APCs. Cross-presentation is a process by which certain APCs take up, process, and present extracellular antigen on class I molecules to CD8 T cells.[15] This mechanism is necessary for immunity against tumors and viruses that do not infect APCs. MHC products also play other important roles, including the positive and negative selection of developing T cells, stimulation of naive T cells that is necessary for their survival (homeostatic proliferation), induction of T-cell tolerance and anergy, tumor surveillance, and interaction with NK cells and other inhibitory or activating receptors.

The MHC gene locus (in humans, HLA) maps to a 3.5-million base pair region on the short arm of chromosome 6 and is divided into three regions: the class II region, the class III region, and the class I region. Only the class I and class II regions encode proteins involved in antigen presentation. The key MHC genes are the class I genes (HLA-A, HLA-B, and HLA-C) and the class II genes (HLA-DP, HLA-DQ, and HLA-DR). The class I and class II proteins share overall structural homology but are functionally different.[16]

MHC class I molecules are single polypeptide chains of 45-kd noncovalently associated with a smaller 12-kd protein, β_2-microglobulin (Fig. 96.4). The class I heavy chain consists of three α domains (α1, α2, and α3) and a short cytoplasmic tail. The membrane proximal α3 domain and β_2-microglobulin are immunoglobulin domains and serve as a membrane anchor. The

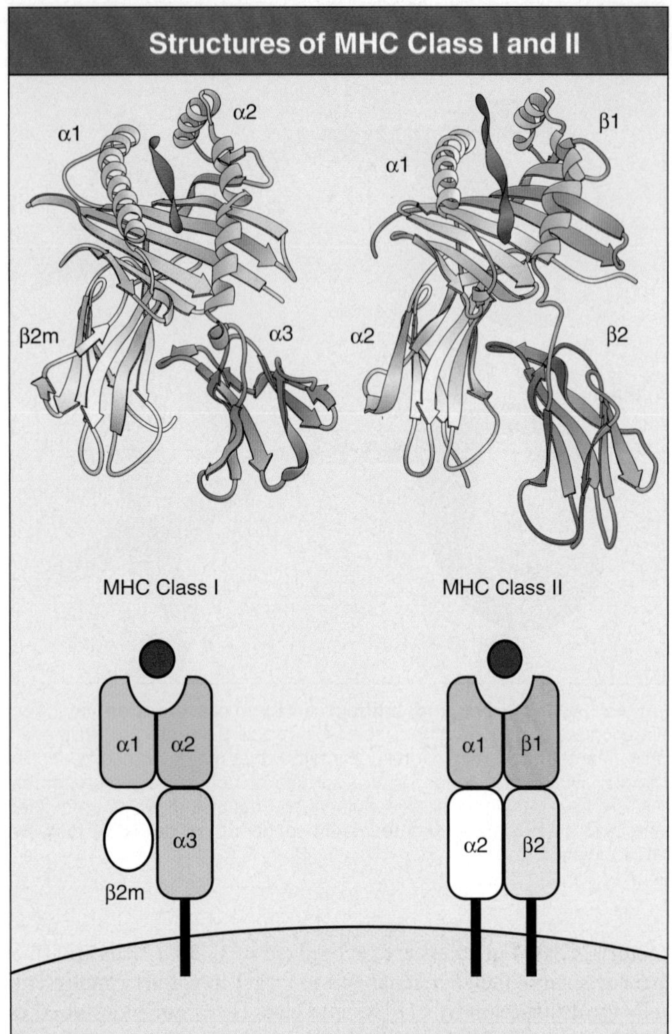

Figure 96.4 Structures of MHC class I and II. MHC class I is composed of a heavy chain divided into α1, α2, and α3 domains noncovalently associated with β_2-microglobulin (β2m). The α1 and α2 domains each form a long α helix and β sheet to make up the floor and walls of the peptide binding groove (peptide indicated by *red ribbon*). MHC class II is a dimer composed of α and β chains. Each chain is divided into two domains, with α1 and β1 domains forming the two α helices and β pleated sheet that surround the peptide binding groove.

α1 and α2 domains are sheet-and-helix domains, each constructed to form a long α helix and an antiparallel β sheet. The two sheet-and-helix domains assemble face to face to form a long β sheet bounded by two α helices, making up the peptide binding groove. This groove can hold peptides of 8 to 10 amino acids.[17]

Class II proteins are heterodimers of α and β chains, each spanning the membrane.[18] The α2 and β2 domains are adjacent to the cell membranes and are immunoglobulin domains; the peptide binding groove is composed of the α1 and β1 domains (see Fig. 96.4). The structural elements of class II are two α helices, a β pleated sheet, and two membrane proximal immunoglobulin domains, with two membrane anchors. The class II peptide binding groove is open on both ends, which accommodates larger peptides of 10 to 30 amino acids, although longer peptides are likely trimmed by peptidases to a length of 13 to 17 amino acids in most cases.

Class I proteins are expressed on virtually all nucleated cells, although the amount expressed varies. Class II proteins have a more restricted cell distribution, generally limited to bone marrow–derived "professional" APCs, including DCs, B cells, macrophages, and Langerhans cells, but also other cells, including renal parenchymal cells, endothelial cells, Kupffer cells, thymic epithelial cells, and alveolar type II lining cells. Both class I and class II antigens can be induced on a variety of cells by interferon-γ (IFN-γ) in synergy with other cytokines.

HLA Typing and Transplantation

MHC class I and class II genes are highly polymorphic in the regions that encode the peptide binding groove. These polymorphisms help ensure survival of the population by increasing the variety of peptides that can be presented to T cells. Thus, MHC polymorphisms decrease the chance of encountering pathogens that may induce poor immune responses within a population, leading to the demise of the species.[19] However, it is also these polymorphisms that predispose to allograft rejection because the antigen-presenting structures of one individual are regarded as foreign by another nonidentical individual.

Polymorphisms were originally defined by HLA serologic (antibody) typing with use of sera from multiparous women or persons who had received blood transfusions. The development of molecular biology techniques (polymerase chain reaction [PCR] sequencing) has allowed the analysis of the HLA allelic sequence diversity at the DNA level. By DNA typing, many more polymorphisms have been identified: currently 733 for HLA-A, 1115 for HLA-B, 392 for HLA-C, and 700 for HLA-DR, with around 450 new sequences added each year. The most currently updated source for HLA alleles can be identified at the website *http://www.ebi.ac.uk/imgt/hla*. Although PCR techniques allow rapid DNA sequence–based typing of human populations, serologic methods are still often used for identifying HLA antigens in kidney transplantation.

HLA Inheritance

HLA genes are inherited in a mendelian codominant fashion, meaning that a copy of each HLA gene (i.e., one haplotype) is inherited from each parent and expressed as antigens. HLA typing identifies the specific alleles carried by a person. The term HLA *matching* means assignment of a donor kidney to a recipient with as few mismatches as possible. In kidney transplantation, efforts are made to match HLA-A, HLA-B, and HLA-DR genes and proteins. It can be predicted that siblings from the same set of parents will have a 25% chance of having zero mismatches, 50% chance of having one mismatch, and 25% chance of having two mismatches (Fig. 96.5).

Non-MHC Antigens

Minor histocompatibility antigens are normal proteins that are themselves polymorphic in a given population. Even when a transplant donor and recipient are identical with regard to MHC genes, amino acid differences in these minor proteins can lead to rejection. Minor antigens are encoded by a large number of chromosomes and are presented only as peptides in the context of recipient MHC (indirect allorecognition). Minor antigens are responsible for the need for immunosuppression after donation between HLA-matched nonidentical twin siblings. The prototypic minor histocompatibility antigen, the male or H-Y antigen, is derived from a group of proteins encoded on the Y chromosome. Alloresponses to this antigen may explain reduced

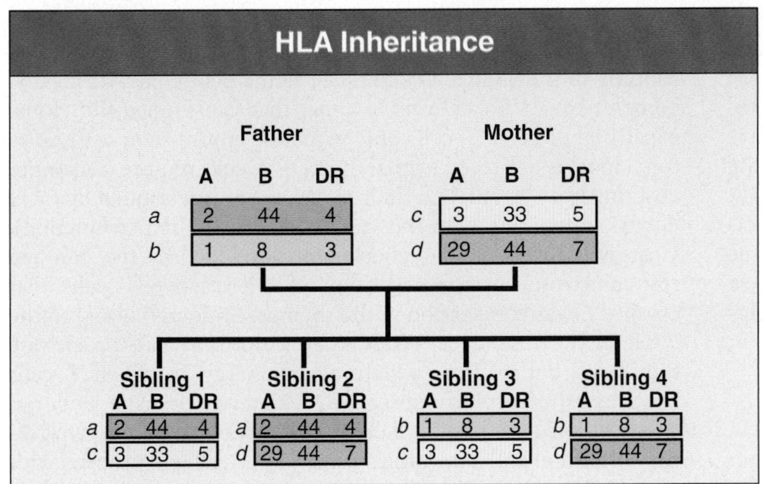

Figure 96.5 HLA inheritance. HLA antigens are inherited and expressed in a mendelian codominant fashion, whereby one copy of each HLA gene, called a haplotype (e.g., *a, b, c, d*), is inherited from each parent. Efforts are made to match both class I (HLA-A and HLA-B) and class II (HLA-DR) antigens.

long-term graft survival observed in male-to-female donations. MHC I–related chain A (MICA) antigens are surface glycoproteins with functions related to innate immunity. Exposure to allogeneic MICA during transplantation can elicit antibody formation.[20] ABO blood group glycolipids expressed on endothelial and red blood cells are other notable non-MHC antigens. Finally, immune responses to autoantigens have been associated with allograft damage.[21]

T-CELL ACTIVATION

T cells are required for rejection because animals experimentally deprived of T cells through mutation or genetic manipulation are unable to reject allografts. Alloreactive T cells can be found in the naive and memory T-cell populations, but both require recognition of non-self MHC molecules to become activated. Reactions mediated by naive T cells take longer to develop than those mediated by memory T cells, which can be generated more quickly and with higher numbers of cells (secondary response). During allograft rejection, both populations are activated simultaneously.

T-Cell Receptor

Each T cell bears about 30,000 identical antigen receptor molecules. Each receptor consists of two different polypeptide chains, termed the TCR α and β chains, which are linked by a disulfide bond. The genes encoding the TCR chains are members of the immunoglobulin supergene family, which are found on B, T, and NK cells. The α:β heterodimers are very similar in structure to the Fab fragment of an immunoglobulin molecule and account for antigen recognition by most T cells (Fig. 96.6). In contrast to the immunoglobulin receptors of B cells, TCRs do not recognize antigen in its native state but instead recognize a composite ligand of a peptide bound to an MHC molecule. A minority of T cells bears an alternative but structurally similar receptor composed of a different polypeptide heterodimer (γ:δ). These γ:δ TCRs seem to have different antigen recognition properties, although their function during alloimmune responses is not known.

Both chains of the TCR have an amino-terminal (V) domain with homology to an immunoglobulin V domain, a constant (C) domain with homology to an immunoglobulin C domain, and a

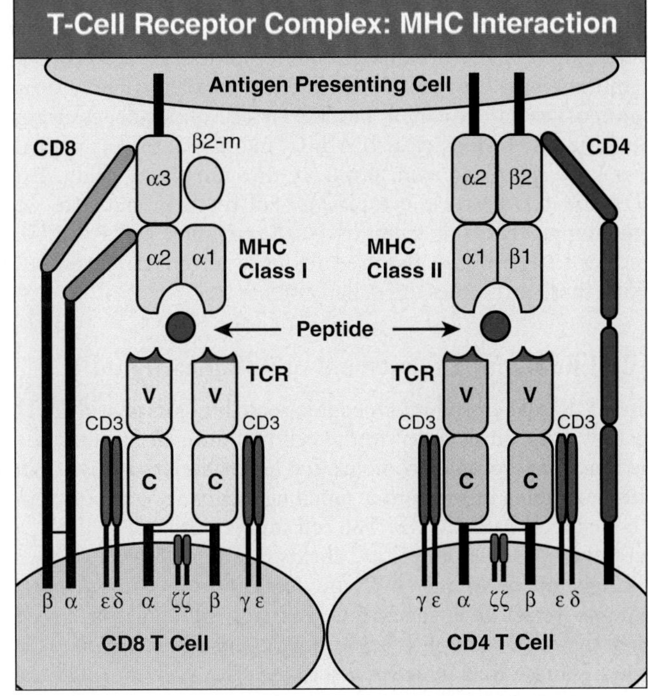

Figure 96.6 T-cell receptor complex:MHC interaction. Each T-cell receptor (TCR) consists of an α and β chain linked by a disulfide bond. The α:β heterodimers are similar in structure to the Fab fragment of an immunoglobulin molecule (see Fig. 96.9), including variable (V) and constant (C) regions. Diversity in the T-cell repertoire is encoded in the V domains of the α and β chains in three complementarity-determining regions that form the antigen binding site at the end of the TCR *(highlighted in red)*. CD8 is a disulfide-linked α:β heterodimer or α:α homodimer, with each chain containing a single immunoglobulin-like domain linked to the membrane by a polypeptide chain. CD8 binds to the conserved region of the α3 domain of the class I MHC molecule on antigen-presenting cells (APCs) but also interacts with the class I MHC α2 domain, probably through the α chain.CD4 is composed of four immunoglobulin-like domains and binds to a conserved site on the β2 domain of the class II MHC molecule on APCs. Triggering of the TCR by antigen initiates a signaling cascade started by the signaling complex made up of CD3 γ, ε, and δ chains as well as the ζ chain homodimer.

short hinge region containing a cysteine residue that forms the interchain disulfide bond. Each chain spans the cell membrane by a hydrophobic transmembrane domain and ends in a short cytoplasmic tail. The diversity in the TCR repertoire is encoded in the V domains of the α and β chains. These V domains have three hypervariable loops or complementarity-determining regions that form the antigen binding site at the end of the TCR, interacting with the sheet-and-helix domains of the MHC molecule and the presented peptide. This interaction enhances the specificity of antigen recognition by T cells because the most variable of the complementarity-determining regions interacts with the diverse peptides presented in the MHC complex.

CD4 and CD8 Coreceptors

T cells fall into two major classes with different effector functions, distinguished by the expression of the cell surface proteins CD4 and CD8. CD4 is a single-chain molecule composed of four immunoglobulin-like domains and binds to a conserved site on the β2 domain of the class II MHC molecule well away from the site where the TCR binds (see Fig. 96.6). CD8 is a disulfide-linked α:β heterodimer or α:α homodimer, with each chain containing a single immunoglobulin like domain linked to the membrane by a polypeptide chain. CD8 binds to the conserved region of the α3 domain of the class I MHC molecule, equivalent to where CD4 binds class II MHC, but also interacts with the class I MHC α2 domain, probably through the α chain. Both CD4 and CD8 have a cytoplasmic tail that can associate with signaling proteins important in T-cell activation. CD4 and CD8 binding to MHC are required to make an effective response. Thus, these molecules are called coreceptors.

T-Cell Receptor Engagement of Antigen: Signal 1

The TCR α:β heterodimer recognizes and binds its peptide:MHC ligand[22] but cannot signal to the cell that antigen has bound. In the functional receptor complex, α:β heterodimers are associated with a complex of four other signaling chains (two ε, one δ, one γ) collectively called CD3. The cell surface receptor is also associated with a homodimer of ζ chains (see Fig. 96.6).

Engagement of the TCR by MHC, along with the other required receptor engagements, initiates the signaling process from the CD3 complex.[23] The first event is activation of the protein kinase Lck, which is associated with CD4 or CD8 molecules. Activated Lck phosphorylates tyrosine residues on the CD3 molecules that then serve as anchoring sites for the protein tyrosine kinase ZAP-70. ZAP-70 phosphorylates several downstream substrates, including adaptor and linker molecules, which leads to activation of phospholipase C (PLC-γ) and the Ras-MAP kinase pathway. PLC-γ cleaves phosphatidylinositol bisphosphate to yield diacylglycerol (DAG) and inositol triphosphate (IP_3). DAG activates protein kinase C, leading to activation of the nuclear factor κB (NF-κB) pathway. IP_3 acts on the endoplasmic reticulum to induce the release of intracellular Ca^{2+}, which leads to activation of the protein-serine phosphatase calcineurin. Calcineurin dephosphorylates the transcription factor nuclear factor of activated T cells (NF-AT), allowing it to translocate into the nucleus. Translocation of NF-AT and NF-κB, along with activator protein 1 (AP-1) activated by the Ras-induced kinase cascade, allows the transcription of the genes for IL-2 and other cytokines as well as the genes for the high-affinity subunit of the IL-2 receptor (CD25), leading to cell proliferation and differentiation.

T-Cell Costimulation: Signal 2

Binding of the TCR:CD3 complex to the peptide:MHC class II complex on APCs delivers a signal that can induce the clonal expansion of naive T cells only when the appropriate costimulatory signal is delivered (signal 2). CD8 T cells require a stronger costimulatory signal, and their clonal expansion is aided by CD4 T cells interacting with the same APC (i.e., T helper function). Costimulation is likely a checkpoint developed by the immune system to prevent the activation of self-reactive T cells that escaped negative selection in the thymus. Antigen binding to the TCR in the absence of costimulation not only fails to activate the T cell but leads to a state called anergy, in which T cells become refractory to subsequent activation or even undergo apoptosis (programmed cell death). Thus, costimulation removes this inhibition and determines whether a T cell will proceed with clonal expansion and the development of effector functions. It is now clear that costimulatory molecules can provide positive or negative signals to T cells (Fig. 96.7). Thus, it is the integration of both positive and negative costimulatory signals during and after initial T-cell activation, dictated by their temporal and spatial expression patterns, that ultimately determines the fate and functional status of the T-cell response.[24] In transplant models, rejection can occur when costimulatory molecules are absent from the donor APCs and MHC class II is absent from the recipient APCs, suggesting that bystander APCs can provide trans-costimulation.[25]

CD28 and its ligands B7.1 (CD80) and B7.2 (CD86) are the best characterized costimulatory molecules and are members of the immunoglobulin superfamily.[26] CD28 is constitutively expressed on all naive CD4 and CD8 T cells. However, a significant proportion of memory T cells, especially memory CD8 T cells, are CD28 negative. Ligation of CD28 by B7 molecules is required for clonal expansion of naive CD4 T helper cells. Once activated, T cells express increased levels of CTLA-4 (CD152). CTLA-4 has a higher affinity than CD28 for B7 molecules and thus binds most or all of the B7 molecules, effectively shutting down the proliferative phase of the response. This effect can also be achieved by the administration of CTLA-4Ig, a fusion protein with high affinity for B7 molecules. B and T lymphocyte attenuator (BTLA) and programmed death 1 (PD-1) are two other costimulatory molecules of the immunoglobulin superfamily that, when engaged by their ligands (HVEM and PD-L1/PD-L2, respectively), provide inhibitory signals to T cells.

Activated T cells express a number of proteins that contribute to sustainment or modification of the costimulatory signal to drive clonal expansion and differentiation. The inducible costimulatory molecule (ICOS) is a CD28 homologue, but unlike CD28, it is not constitutively expressed on naive T cells. Rather, ICOS is induced only after T-cell activation. The ligand for ICOS is B7H (also called ICOS-L, B7RP-1, B7H-2, and GL-50), and although it is structurally related to B7 molecules, it does not bind to either CD28 or CTLA-4. Engagement of ICOS by B7H enhances T-cell proliferation, cytokine production, and survival. ICOS is also expressed on B cells and provides help for antibody production by activated B cells. Finally, ICOS is expressed on memory T cells and $FOXP3^+$ T regulatory cells (Tregs).

Costimulatory molecules of the TNF and TNF-R superfamily include CD40 ligand (CD40L, CD154) on T cells and its receptor CD40 on APCs, such as B cells, DCs, macrophages, and endothelial cells. Binding of CD40 by CD40L transmits

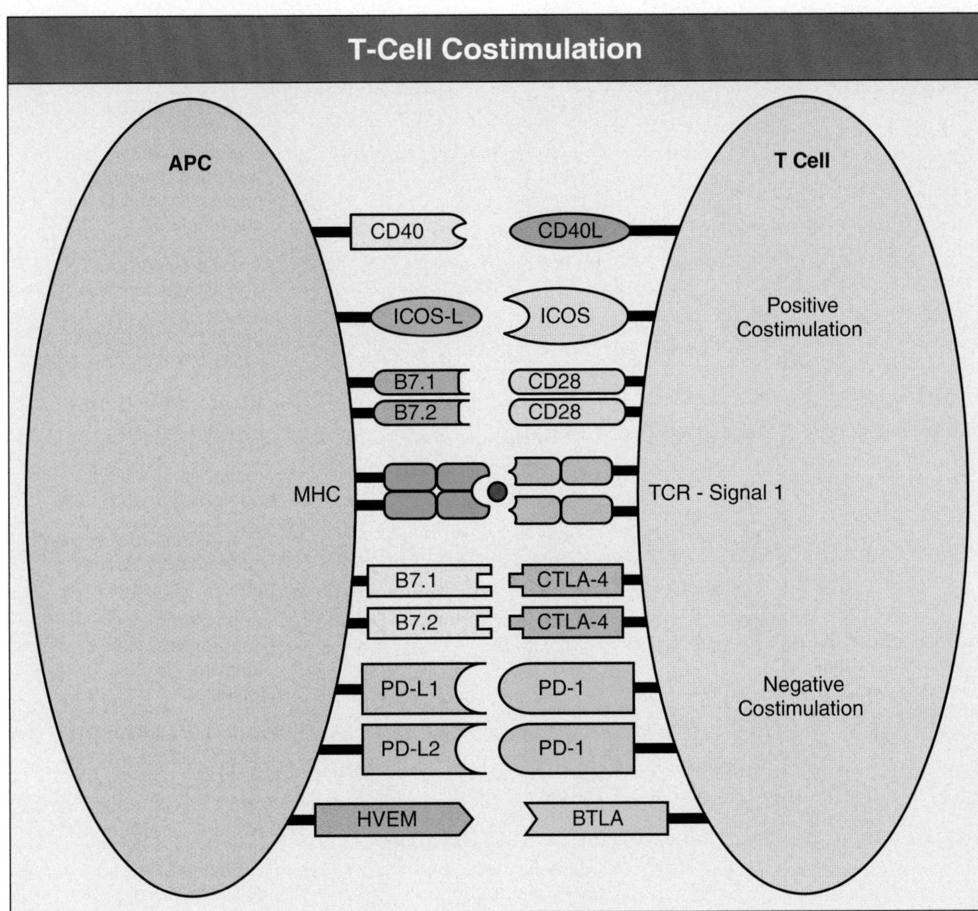

Figure 96.7 T-cell costimulation.

activating signals to the T cell but also activates the APCs to secrete proinflammatory molecules and to express B7 molecules, thus stimulating further T-cell proliferation. Engagement of CD40 on DCs by T helper cells allows proper priming of precursor CTLs. CD40 ligation on B cells promotes their survival and proliferation and induces class switching, allowing the production and secretion of specialized, higher affinity antibodies. Costimulatory molecules of the TNF:TNF-R superfamily include many other receptor-ligand pairs and, with the exception of CD27, are expressed only on T-cell activation.[26] This finding has given rise to the general view that costimulatory molecules in this family are more important for the effector and memory phases of the immune response rather than for the initial phase of T-cell priming.

TIM (T-cell immunoglobulin and mucin domain) molecules are type I transmembrane glycoproteins that like other molecules in this family consist of an extracellular domain, a transmembrane domain, and a cytoplasmic domain. The extracellular domain of all TIM molecules contains an immunoglobulin V motif and a heavily glycosylated mucin motif, a structural feature that distinguishes this family member from other costimulatory molecules. Similar to other costimulatory molecules, however, the cytoplasmic domain contains a tyrosine phosphorylation motif that is involved in signal transduction on ligand binding. The human TIM gene family has three members (TIM-1, TIM-3, and TIM-4) and is involved in regulating a wide array of immune-related responses that are not yet fully understood.

T-Cell Clonal Expansion and Differentiation

In most instances, the number of T cells that react to a given antigen is quite small. Therefore, effective immune responses generally require clonal expansion and differentiation of T cells. These processes are largely driven by cytokines, including IL-2, which acts on the T cell in an autocrine fashion or by paracrine secretion to neighboring T cells. Activated T cells produce the α subunit of the IL-2 receptor (IL-2R or CD25), enabling a fully functional signaling receptor composed of α, β, and γ subunits that can bind IL-2 with high affinity, which in turn activates T-cell proliferation pathways. The list of cytokines is large and continues to grow. Figure 96.8 lists selected cytokines involved in allograft rejection, their sources, and their effects.

CD4 and CD8 T cells have different roles during immune responses. CD4 T cells are both effectors and regulators and are notable for heavy cytokine secretion. After prolonged stimulation, CD4 T cells sometimes tend to express groups of several cytokines, probably depending on the local environment, the nature of the antigen, and the type and activation status of the APC. The so-called Th1 (for T helper 1) clones produce IL-2, IFN-γ, and lymphotoxin; Th2 clones produce IL-4, IL-5, and IL-10. As the effects of these cytokines became known, it was apparent that the subdivision of production correlated with a categorization of function. Th1-derived cytokines are growth and maturation factors for CTLs (especially IL-2) and macrophages (particularly IFN-γ); Th2-derived cytokines act similarly on B cells. Rejecting allografts typically express high levels of

Cytokines Involved in Allograft Rejection

Cytokine	Source	Biologic activity
IL-1	Macrophages, DC, EC, NK cells	Proinflammatory, adhesion molecule expression on EC, NK cell function
IL-2	Activated T cells	T cell proliferation, CTL and NK cell function, Treg maintenance, Ig production by B cells, AICD of activated T cells
IL-4	Activated T cells	Activated T and B cell proliferation, Th2 differentiation, allergic responses, MHC II upregulation on B cells
IL-6	T cells, macrophages, EC	Proinflammatory and anti-inflammatory, acute-phase responses
IL-10	T cells, macrophages, DC	Anti-inflammatory, suppression of APC function, NK cell inhibition
IL-12	Macrophages, DC	Proinflammatory, Th1 differentiation, NK cell and CTL activity, IFN-γ and TNF-α production by NK and T cells
IL-15	Epithelial cells, stromal cells, macrophages	NK cell proliferation, T cell proliferation, memory T cell survival
IL-17	T cells	Proinflammatory and allergic responses, Th17 function, cytokine production from many cell types
IFN-γ	Activated Th1 cells, CTL, DC, NK cells	MHC expression by EC, macrophage function, Th1 differentiation, Th2 suppression, adhesion and binding of T cells to EC, NK cell activity
TGF-β	T and B cells, macrophages, platelets	Anti-inflammatory, wound healing, fibrosis
TNF-α	Macrophages, T and B cells, EC, NK cells	Proinflammatory, acute phase responses, cytotoxicity

Figure 96.8 Cytokines involved in allograft rejection. IL, interleukin; DC, dendritic cells; EC, endothelial cells; NK, natural killer; CTL, cytotoxic T lymphocytes; Treg, regulatory T cells; Ig, immunoglobulin; AICD, activation-induced cell death; Th, T helper (cell); IFN-γ, interferon-γ; TNF-α, tumor necrosis factor α; TGF-β, transforming growth factor β.

mRNA for both subsets of cytokines and cannot be considered a pure Th1 response. T helper 17 (Th17) cells are a subset of T helper cells distinct from Th1 and Th2 clones[27] that produce IL-17, IL-21, and IL-22.[28] Th17 cells are thought to play a key role in autoimmune disease, and their role in transplantation is currently under intense investigation.

Memory Cells

Although there is limited knowledge of how memory T cells are generated or maintained, these cells are an important component of the immune response after transplantation. The principle of immunologic memory is that the immune response to a previously encountered antigen is swifter and more effective than the response to a new antigen. Memory cells seem to be more easily activated than naive T cells and in addition produce more cytokines. Furthermore, there is an increase in antigen-specific T-cell frequency after exposure to a given antigen. Finally, exposure to antigen leads to a refinement of the antibody repertoire, resulting in a more effective memory response. Effector memory T cells are specialized to quickly enter inflamed tissues, as they can rapidly mature into effector T cells and secrete larger amounts of cytokines after restimulation. Central memory T cells probably remain in the SLOs and do not produce as much cytokine.[29] Memory cells are believed to persist after an initial immune response through expression of the antiapoptotic genes Bcl-2 and Bcl-xL, which are induced primarily by IL-2 and

CD28 stimulation. IL-15 may also provide survival signals. Long-term memory cell survival is likely to be a function of periodic interactions with self MHC–peptide complexes (i.e., homeostatic proliferation).

EFFECTOR FUNCTIONS

Once activated and expanded, T cells exert effector functions that result in destruction of graft tissue. Although T cells are essential for acute organ allograft rejection, the precise mechanisms by which they mediate graft injury are uncertain. CD4 T helper cells may release numerous cytokines that affect the alloimmune response. For example, they may promote delayed-type hypersensitivity (DTH) responses that involve stimulating production of nitric oxide, reactive oxygen species, and TNF-α by macrophages. T-cell cytokines may also act directly on parenchymal cells or indirectly through effects on the endothelium and vascular supply. TNF-α and TNF-β exert local cytotoxic effects on receptors on the graft, including endothelial cells (TNF-R1) and tubular cells (TNF-R2). IFN-γ, the prototypical Th1 cytokine, is released by both CD4 and CD8 T cells during rejection. IFN-γ induces MHC class II expression on endothelium and MHC class I expression on vascular endothelial cells, epithelial cells, and parenchymal cells in the graft. The precise role of class II expression by donor cells in the graft remains controversial because mouse kidney grafts lacking class II are rejected more vigorously. Although IFN-γ is strongly associated with rejection, it probably has other signaling roles that actually help to stabilize the graft. As cytokine production by CD8 T cells is generally lower than that of CD4 T cells, production of cytokines such as IL-2 by CD4 T cells provides help for the generation of CTLs from their CD8 T-cell precursors. CD4 T cells may themselves become cytolytic T cells, by mechanisms similar to those used by CD8 CTLs (described later). CD4 T cells also provide help to B cells to enhance their production of alloantibodies. Finally, Tregs may have important roles in suppressing immune responses and maintaining tolerance.

CTL Differentiation and Function

With rare exceptions, virtually all CTLs are MHC class I–restricted CD8 T cells. Activated CTLs possess two mechanisms to kill target cells that require cell-cell contact.[30] The first mechanism is by the release of specialized lytic granules. Perforin and granzyme B are two proteins found in granules of most CTLs and NK cells. Perforin, like complement components, has the ability to induce transmembrane pores. The granzyme B–perforin complex enters the cell through the mannose 6-phosphate receptor, and after internalization, perforin allows granzyme B to enter the cell through the vesicle surface to induce programmed cell death through apoptosis.[31] A third cytotoxic protein, granulysin, is also able to induce apoptosis in target cells. The second mechanism is by Fas/Fas ligand (FasL) interactions. Fas (CD95) is a member of the TNF-R family and is the surface mediator of a pathway that, when activated by FasL on activated CTLs, induces the target cell to undergo apoptosis. Both pathways induce apoptosis through activation of the caspase cascade in target cells. As previously alluded to, CD8 CTLs also release several cytokines that exert direct cytotoxic effects, including IFN-γ, TNF-α, and TNF-β.[32] Effector CD4 T cells that can mediate class II–restricted cytotoxicity to minor antigens have also been detected.

Macrophage Activation

The activated macrophage is an important mediator of DTH responses, which lead to localized tissue destruction. Resting macrophages must be activated to exert full inflammatory and cytopathic effects. Th1 cells provide help for this activation by interaction of CD40L with CD40 on the macrophage and by production of IFN-γ, which sensitizes the macrophage to respond to IFN-γ. It is possible that T-cell membrane–associated TNF-α and TNF-β can substitute for CD40L. CD8 T cells also produce IFN-γ and can activate macrophages. Production of TNF-α, oxygen radicals, and nitric oxide by activated macrophages is important for their cytopathic effects. Activated macrophages can also produce IL-12, which directs the differentiation of activated naive CD4 T cells into Th1 effector cells. Macrophage activation is inhibited by cytokines such as transforming growth factor β (TGF-β) and IL-10, many of which are produced by Th2 cells.

Humoral Immune Response

The extracellular spaces of the body are protected by humoral immune responses, in which antibodies produced by B cells cause the destruction of extracellular microorganisms and prevent the spread of intracellular infections. Membrane-bound immunoglobulin on the B-cell surface serves as the antigen receptor and is known as the B-cell receptor (BCR; Fig. 96.9). It is associated with antigen-nonspecific signaling molecules, Igα and Igβ.

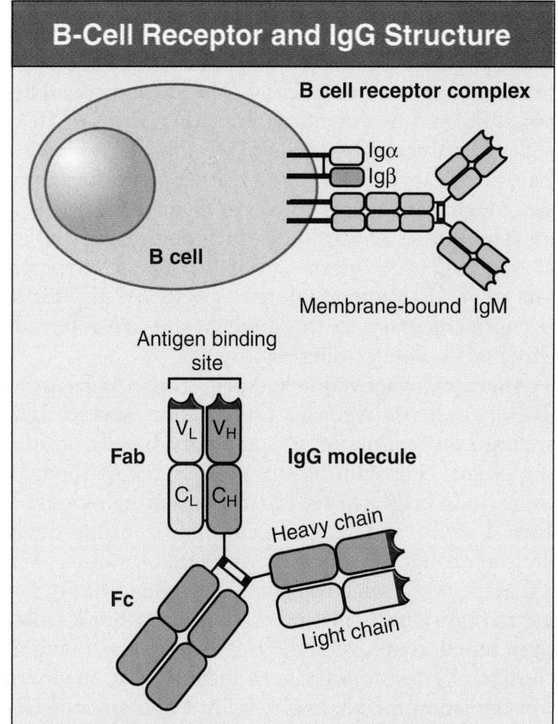

Figure 96.9 B-cell receptor and IgG structure. B-cell surface membrane–bound immunoglobulin M (IgM) associated with antigen-nonspecific signaling molecules, Igα and Igβ, forms the B-cell receptor complex. The IgG molecule is made up of four polypeptide chains, comprising two identical light (L) chains *(yellow)* and two identical heavy (H) chains *(green)*. Each of the four chains has a variable (V) region at its amino terminus (Fab portion), which contributes to the antigen binding site, and a constant (C) region (Fc portion), which determines the isotype. The V domains contain hypervariable regions that determine antigen specificity called complementarity-determining regions *(highlighted in red)*.

Immunoglobulin of the same specificity is then secreted as antibody by terminally differentiated B cells (i.e., plasma cells). B cells develop in the bone marrow and undergo sequential rearrangement of immunoglobulin gene segments to generate a diverse repertoire of antigen receptors that can interact with antigen in their environment. In a process similar to that for developing T cells in the thymus, immature B cells that are strongly self-reactive at this stage are inactivated by negative selection. In contrast to T cells, new B cells are continually produced in adulthood.

B-cell activation requires binding of antigen to the BCR. Although some polysaccharides and polymeric proteins can activate B cells directly, antibody responses to most proteins require both binding of the antigen to the BCR and interaction of the B cell with antigen-specific helper T cells. Helper T cells recognize peptide fragments derived from the antigen that are internalized and presented as peptide:MHC class II complexes on the B-cell surface. Helper T cells stimulate B cells through the binding of CD40L with CD40 on B cells, through interaction of other TNF:TNF-R family ligands, as well as by the directed release of cytokines. Although these helper T cells are generally of the Th2 subset, Th1 cells can also assist with B-cell activation. Activated B cells also provide signals to T cells through B7 family molecules that promote their continued activation.

Secretion of antibodies, which bind pathogens or their toxic products, is the main effector function of B cells in adaptive immunity. The antibody molecule has two separate functions: one is to bind specifically to molecules from the pathogen that elicited the immune response; the other is to recruit other cells and molecules to destroy the pathogen bound by the antibody. The five major classes of antibodies are IgM, IgD, IgG, IgA, and IgE. IgG is by far the most abundant immunoglobulin and has several subclasses (IgG1, 2, 3, and 4). The IgG molecule is made up of four polypeptide chains, comprising two identical light (L) chains of 25-kd and two identical heavy (H) chains of 50-kd that form a flexible Y-shaped structure (see Fig. 96.9). Each of the four chains has a variable (V) region at its amino terminus (Fab portion), which contributes to the antigen binding site, and a constant (C) region (Fc portion), which determines the isotype. The V regions of a given antibody contain hypervariable segments that determine antigen specificity by forming a surface complementary to the antigen and are referred to as complementarity-determining regions.

After appropriate activation and help from T cells, previously naive B cells undergo vigorous proliferation, secrete IgM, and then undergo differentiation into memory B cells or antibody-secreting plasma cells. During this process, the antibody isotype can change (to IgA, IgG, or IgE) in response to cytokines released by helper T cells, and the antigen-binding properties of the antibody can change by somatic hypermutation of the V region genes. T helper cells selectively activate higher affinity mutants, resulting in high-affinity plasma cells and memory B cells. Antibodies can function in several different ways once bound to their target antigen. These mechanisms include fixation of complement, opsonization for phagocytosis by Fc receptor (FcR)–positive cells, opsonization for cell lysis by cells capable of antibody-dependent cellular cytotoxicity (ADCC), and induction of eosinophil degranulation.

Natural Killer Lymphocytes

NK cells, a subset of peripheral lymphocytes, share certain developmental and functional features with the more numerous CD8 T lymphocytes.[33] Unlike T or B cells, NK cells do not possess a clonotypically distributed, antigen-specific cell surface receptor that is generated by gene recombination. Instead, NK cells use an array of receptors that recognize the loss of HLA class I molecules on susceptible targets. Peripheral NK cells are mature, do not require costimulation and differentiation as with T cells, and immediately release cytotoxic granules and inflammatory cytokines such as TNF-α and IFN-γ on detection of relevant targets. Given the strong cytolytic function and potential for autoreactivity, NK cell activity is tightly regulated. Mechanisms of activation include cytokines, binding of antibody to Fc receptors, and binding of ligands to activating and inhibitory receptors. NKG2D is an activating receptor expressed on all NK cells and NKT lymphocytes.[3] The presence of NKG2D ligands, including MHC class I–related antigen, has been reported on human transplant samples undergoing acute allograft rejection and acute tubular necrosis. Thus, NKG2D ligands in the graft may stimulate a cytolytic cellular immune response after transplantation by interacting with cells bearing NKG2D, including NK cells. Recent animal models, however, have questioned whether NK cells play a significant role during rejection.[34]

Termination of the Immune Response

To avoid massive continued expansion of the lymphoid pool, it is important to have mechanisms in place to terminate the immune response. Once the source of antigen is destroyed, there is no longer an inciting stimulus to induce further activation and proliferation of lymphocytes. However, preexisting effector cells can cause antigen-specific tissue damage and must be deactivated. Several mechanisms accomplish this task. Once they are terminally mature, DCs switch cytokine production from IL-12 to IL-10, favoring the generation of regulatory phenomena that suppress the function of effector T cells. As mentioned previously, induction of CTLA-4 after T-cell activation provides regulatory feedback to provide inhibitory signals to T cells that induce anergy. In the absence of continued cytokine production, T cells lack the necessary growth factors and undergo passive cell death. Finally, activated T cells undergo activation-induced cell death (AICD) by the expression of Fas and FasL on their surface. Engagement of Fas by its ligand triggers a death signal, leading to apoptosis of the cell. Because both molecules are expressed on the same cell, elimination of T cells can be through "suicide" as well as by "fratricide." Although IL-2 is important for the clonal expansion of T cells, it is also essential for AICD. Finally, Tregs are important in maintaining self-tolerance after removal of effector T cells.

ALLOGRAFT REJECTION

Allograft rejection is defined as tissue injury produced by the effector mechanisms of the alloimmune response, leading to deterioration of graft function. There are two types of rejection: T cell–mediated rejection (TCMR) and antibody-mediated rejection (AMR). Both types of rejection can be early or late, fulminant or indolent, and isolated or concomitant. For the purposes of this chapter, the two types are described separately.

Recruitment of Cells into the Interstitium of Kidney Allografts

Allograft rejection is caused by several cellular elements of the immune system, including T cells, macrophages, B cells, plasma cells, eosinophils, and neutrophils. Although there are a variety

Proteins Involved in the Recruitment of Leukocytes into Allografts

Protein type	Name	Ligand	Function
Selectins	CD62L/L-selectin CD62P/P-selectin CD62E/E-selectin	Sialated glycoproteins	Initial rolling of leukocytes on endothelium
Chemokines	MCP-1/CCL2	CCR2	Recruitment of monocytes, immature DC, T cells, and NK cells
	MIP-1α/CCL3	CCR1	Recruitment of monocytes, immature DC, T cells, and neutrophils
	RANTES/CCL5	CCR1,CCR4, CCR5	Recruitment of monocytes, DC, T cells, NK cells, and neutrophils
	IL-8/CXCL8	CXCR1, CXCR2	Recruitment of neutrophils
	MIG/CXCL9	CXCR3	Recruitment of activated memory T cells
	IP-10/CXCl10	CXCR3	Recruitment of activated memory T cells
	Lymphotactin/XCL1	XCL1	Recruitment of T cells
Immunoglobulin superfamily	CD54/ICAM-1	LFA-1	Tight adhesion of leukocytes to endothelium
	CD102/ICAM-2 CD50/ICAM-3	LFA-1	Tight adhesion of leukocytes to endothelium (not as strong as ICAM-1)
	CD106/VCAM-1	VLA-4	Rolling and tight adhesion of leukocytes to endothelium
	CD31/PECAM-1	CD31	Extravasation of leukocytes across endothelium

Figure 96.10 Proteins involved in the recruitment of leukocytes into allografts. DC, dendritic cells; ICAM, intercellular adhesion molecule; NK, natural killer; PECAM, platelet–endothelial cell adhesion molecule; VCAM, vascular adhesion molecule.

of target cells in the graft, endothelial and tubular cells are particularly affected by these mediators. T cells serve as the main effectors and regulators of the alloimmune response; macrophages serve as possible effectors but also aid in the removal of apoptotic cells. B cells and plasma cells serve in the production of alloantibodies, and neutrophils probably cause significant damage during AMR.

A three-step model has been proposed to explain the entry of cellular infiltrates into the allograft: tethering, adhesion, and transmigration. Figure 96.10 lists several of the proteins involved in this process. The endothelium of postcapillary venules in the graft serves as the entry point of recipient leukocytes from the blood stream. Selectins are constitutive and inducible lectin-like molecules on the endothelium that cause leukocytes to roll along the vessel wall, a process called tethering. Leukocytes slowed down by selectins come into more prolonged contact with the endothelium. As a result, leukocytes are stimulated by chemokines, a group of small proinflammatory molecules produced by inflamed tissue that are fundamentally important in attraction of cells into an inflammatory infiltrate. Once they are secreted, chemokines bind locally to cell surface proteoglycans on endothelial cells, allowing them to activate leukocytes as they roll by. As chemokines bind to receptors on leukocytes, they activate the adhesion function of integrins.

Integrins are αβ heterodimers formed by noncovalent association. The best characterized integrin, LFA-1, is expressed on most leukocytes. The ligands for LFA-1, including ICAM-1, ICAM-2, and ICAM-3 (immunoglobulin superfamily gene

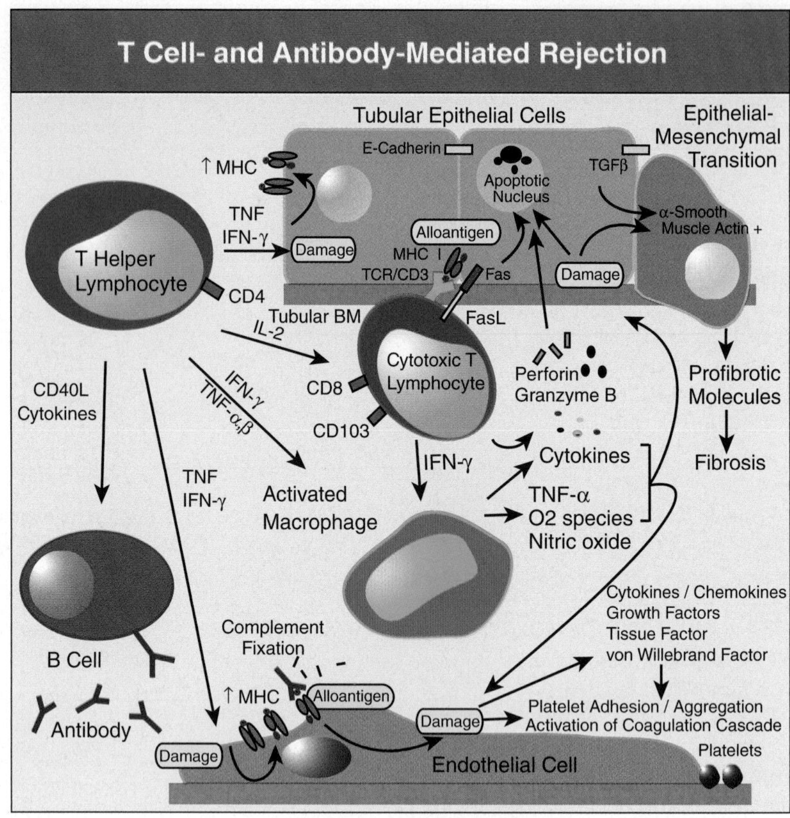

Figure 96.11 T cell– and antibody-mediated rejection. CD4 T cells induce epithelial and endothelial cell damage directly by secretion of cytokines but also indirectly by activation of cytotoxic T lymphocytes (CTLs) and macrophages. CTLs may cause apoptosis by releasing cytolytic granules containing granzymes and perforin or by exposure of Fas ligand (FasL) on the T-cell surface. The integrin component CD103 is postulated to help retain T cells in epithelial layers by binding to E-cadherin, expressed most strongly in the distal nephron. Macrophages induce local tissue damage through secretion of cytokines, oxygen species, and nitric oxide (delayed-type hypersensitivity response). CD4 T cells secrete cytokines, which induce upregulation of major histocompatibility complex (MHC) molecules on epithelial and endothelial cells. CD4 T cells also provide help to B cells for production of alloantibody by engagement of CD40L and production of cytokines. Antigraft antibody is usually directed at MHC molecules, followed by activation of complement. Damaged endothelial cells secrete factors that activate coagulation systems and result in formation of microthrombi. Tubular cells chronically exposed to transforming growth factor β (TGF-β) may undergo epithelial-mesenchymal transition, an aberrant phenotype evidenced by epithelial cell expression of α-smooth muscle actin and loss of E-cadherin expression. These cells then may infiltrate the interstitium and contribute to fibrosis.

members), are expressed weakly on resting endothelium but are induced by activation with cytokines, such as IL-1 and TNF-α. Likewise, activation of leukocytes by chemokines triggers the transition of their surface LFA-1 to a high-affinity state for ICAM, resulting in tight adhesion of the leukocyte to the endothelium. This adhesion contributes to antigen recognition, and through a process called haptotaxis, leukocytes are induced to move along the vessel wall by an adhesion gradient.

Transmigration is the final step in the process of cellular entry into the allograft. Rapidly after integrin engagement of their ligands, leukocytes flatten and then undergo diapedesis through gaps between endothelial cells. Leukocyte secretion of proteases degrades the basement membrane, allowing the escape of leukocytes from the vessel. Once they are in the interstitium, secretion of metalloproteinases allows leukocytes to digest extracellular matrix to move through the tissue on a chemokine gradient by a process called chemotaxis. Confronted with foreign antigen in the allograft, previously activated T cells are capable of releasing proinflammatory cytokines (helper T cells) or of directly killing foreign cells (cytotoxic T cells). Recent work in mouse models of renal allograft rejection indicates that allorecognition by T cells occurs in perivascular sites by day 1 after allotransplantation; alloimmune parenchymal damage begins at day 3, coinciding with the emergence of T-cell and monocyte-macrophage and DC (MMDC) infiltrates; and finally tubulitis and arteritis develop by day 7.[34]

Acute T Cell–Mediated Rejection

Tubulitis, invasion of the tubular epithelium by infiltrating T cells and myeloid cells of the MMDC series, is a characteristic feature of acute TCMR (Fig. 96.11). In fact, deterioration of renal function during TCMR correlates with tubulitis and arterial inflammation (endothelialitis), which is much less common. Although it is generally agreed that T cells orchestrate the process that results in damage to the allograft, the precise mechanisms are not clear. As described earlier, CTLs can kill target cells by release of cytotoxic molecules (perforin, granzyme B, and granulysin) or by engagement of Fas on target cells by FasL, with both mechanisms resulting in apoptotic death of the target cell. Human gene expression studies show an increase in mRNA for CTL-associated transcripts, including granzyme B, perforin, and FasL, as well as T-bet, a master transcription factor for effector Th1 lymphocytes. Moreover, lymphocytes expressing mRNA and perforin protein are closely associated with tubular epithelial cells. Some studies suggest that tubulitis may involve a specific subset of CTLs expressing the integrin CD103, which binds to its ligand E-cadherin on epithelial cells, resulting in retention of T cells in the tubules.

Proof of mechanisms in organ transplantation, however, relies on *in vivo* models in animals. Although class I MHC–mismatched heart allografts show prolonged survival in perforin knockout mice, most available evidence with perforin/granzyme, Fas/FasL, and CD103 knockouts indicates that any one of these individual cytolytic pathways is dispensable because acute rejection still occurs with these deficiencies in fully mismatched combinations.[35] These studies argue against cytotoxicity as a primary mechanism to explain graft epithelial cell deterioration. Likewise, CD103:E-cadherin interactions may not be responsible for creating the lesions of tubulitis but rather may reflect damaged cells that lose the ability to exclude inflammatory cells. Thus, tubulitis may not be the cause of tubular cell deterioration but instead a sign that is has already occurred.

T cells may mediate rejection instead through the secretion of cytokines, either through direct effects of soluble products or through the ability to activate macrophages to organize a DTH response. DTH responses involve the release of reactive oxygen species, proteolytic enzymes, icosanoids, and other products. These products may act directly on tubular epithelium and interstitial matrix or indirectly by effects on endothelium and the vascular supply.

Endarteritis is detected in a minority of biopsy specimens taken for acute TCMR and often responds only to anti–T cell therapies, arguing for a pathogenic role for T cells. Endarteritis is not always associated with interstitial inflammation, arguing for a T-cell pathway distinct from that of tubulointerstitial rejection. Glomerulitis is an occasional feature of acute TCMR, and cells are typically a mixture of T cells and macrophages. Why the glomerulus becomes the target in only a minority of cases is not currently known. FOXP3$^+$ CD4 Tregs are concentrated in tubules during rejection, although their role during TCMR continues to be debated.

Acute Antibody-Mediated Rejection

Acute AMR is recognized as a distinct clinicopathologic entity and may occur with or without a component of TCMR (see Fig. 96.11). Although it is typically a response to donor HLA antigens expressed on endothelial cells, AMR can occur to non-HLA antigens. Examples include ABO blood group antigens and the putative endothelial alloantigens, as suggested by the rare occurrence of AMR in HLA-identical sibling grafts. Even autoantibodies have been implicated, such as those to angiotensin II type 1 receptors. The kidney typically shows an accumulation of neutrophils and monocytes in peritubular and glomerular capillaries, although the infiltrate can be quite sparse.[36] Tubulitis and endarteritis are generally minimal, unless a component of TCMR is present. FOXP3$^+$ Tregs are more rare in the AMR infiltrate than that of TCMR,[37] perhaps indicating a factor in the poorer prognosis. A subset of acute AMR that can result in immediate graft failure is hyperacute rejection, which is due to the presence of preformed anti–donor HLA antibody in sensitized recipients or of antibodies to mismatched ABO blood group loci. This type of AMR is rare now that crossmatching practices and desensitization protocols are routinely employed by transplant centers.

Alloantibodies are cytotoxic through their ability to activate complement. The classical pathway appears most relevant, as other pathways have not been shown to participate in acute or chronic AMR. C4d is an inactive fragment of C4b, an activation product of the classical pathway. C4b and C4d contain an occult sulfhydryl group that forms a covalent thioester bond with nearby proteins bound in the tissue after activation by immunoglobulin and C1. No functional role for C4d has been reported, but it remains in the tissue for several days after immunoglobulin and C1 have been released. C4d deposition is strongly associated with circulating antibody to donor HLA class I or class II antigens and is currently the best single marker of complement-fixing circulating antibodies to the endothelium.

The acute effects of complement are well described and include chemoattraction of neutrophils and macrophages through C3a and C5a, vasospasm through the release of prostaglandin E_2 from macrophages, and edema through the release of histamine from mast cells. C3a and C5a increase endothelial adhesion molecules and various cytokines and chemokines.[38] The membrane attack complex, C5b-9, causes lysis of endothelial cells. Alloantibodies may also induce cell damage through complement-independent pathways by recruitment of leukocytes with FcγIIRs (CD16), including NK cells and macrophages (antibody-dependent cellular cytotoxicity). Finally, antibodies without leukocyte or complement participation can activate endothelial cells to produce chemokines and to promote rejection in some animal models.[39]

A common feature of all types of AMR is the presence of microthrombi. As a result of antibody-mediated damage, von Willebrand factor is released from the endothelium, leading to platelet aggregation.[40] Animal models indicate that clotting activation is a direct consequence of complement fixation. Activation of endothelial protease-activated receptors by coagulation proteases, including thrombin, leads to the secretion of many proinflammatory cytokines.[41]

Chronic Rejection

Late allograft dysfunction is due to a combination of alloimmune mechanisms (i.e., chronic rejection) and alloimmune-independent mechanisms, including hypertension, calcineurin inhibitor toxicity, and recurrent disease.[42] Chronic rejection may occur by either cellular or humoral mechanisms, or both. Histologic features characteristic of chronic rejection are transplant glomerulopathy, peritubular capillaropathy (see later), transplant arteriopathy, and, less specifically, tubular atrophy and interstitial fibrosis.

Transplant glomerulopathy is defined by the widespread duplication or multilamination of the glomerular basement membrane (GBM), sometimes accompanied by mesangial expansion and accumulation of mononuclear cells in glomerular capillaries. GBM duplication may be caused by a number of insults to the allograft glomerulus, including recurrent or *de novo* immune complex glomerular disease and thrombotic microangiopathy. However, it is believed that chronic antibody-mediated injury predominates, as the majority of cases of transplant glomerulopathy are associated with circulating antibody to donor class II MHC antigens (sometimes class I antigens), and approximately 30% to 50% of these cases have C4d deposition in the peritubular capillaries.[43] It is believed that the absence of C4d deposition in the remainder of cases represents intermittent antibody involvement.

Similar to findings in transplant glomerulopathy, multilamination of peritubular capillaries can be demonstrated by electron microscopy (peritubular capillaropathy). It is believed that repeated episodes of antibody-mediated injury to the endothelium result in repair mechanisms that are characterized by duplication of the basement membrane. What leads to episodic antibody injury is unknown but may represent the fluctuating donor-specific antibody levels observed in some patients followed up longitudinally. Neointimal thickening can be observed in either C4d positive or negative chronic rejection. Known as transplant arteriopathy, this lesion is characterized histologically by thickening of the arterial intima without duplication of the elastica (in contrast to fibroelastic thickening seen in hypertension). Macrophages and T cells may sometimes be demonstrated within the thickened intima, providing evidence of cell-mediated immunologic activity.

Although it is not specific for rejection, interstitial fibrosis with tubular atrophy is another important histologic feature of chronically rejected allografts. One putative mechanism of fibrosis is by epithelial-mesenchymal transition of tubular cells to an activated myofibroblast that migrates into the interstitium.[44] Steps in this conversion include loss of cell-cell adhesion, loss of

E-cadherin, acquisition of α-smooth muscle actin, actin reorganization, tubular basement membrane disruption, cell migration, and profibrotic molecules. TGF-β may play an important role in the pathogenesis of fibrosis and epithelial-mesenchymal transition (see Fig. 96.11).

The current criteria for chronic active AMR are histologic evidence of chronic injury (in the absence of other possible causes), immunopathologic evidence of antibody action (i.e., C4d staining), and evidence of circulating antibody reactive to the donor. Chronic AMR appears to arise through a series of stages.[36] The first common event is alloantibody production (stage I), followed by antibody interaction with alloantigens, resulting in the deposition of C4d in the peritubular capillaries and possibly glomeruli (stage II), followed by pathologic changes (stage III) and finally graft dysfunction (stage IV). Whereas the factors promoting progression from stage I to stage IV are not currently understood, the hypothesized stages provide a useful organizing structure for ongoing clinical trials to intervene in the earlier stages (I or II).

TRANSPLANTATION TOLERANCE

Transplantation tolerance is a state characterized by the absence of a destructive immune response in the recipient toward a well-functioning donor allograft, with a fully intact immune system and no exogenous immunosuppression.[45] Like self-tolerance, transplantation tolerance is achieved through control of T-cell reactivity by both central and peripheral mechanisms. Central tolerance involves thymic deletional mechanisms that eliminate T cells with reactivity against self antigens (or donor antigens in the case of transplantation tolerance) and positive selection of T cells without such reactivity. In experimental transplant models, central tolerance is achieved by elimination of the preexisting mature T-cell population by irradiation or cytotoxic agents, followed by infusion of donor hematopoietic progenitor cells. Reconstituted donor antigen "re-educates" the thymus to delete developing T cells with antidonor reactivity, leading to a state of chimerism, in which both donor and recipient cells coexist. Translating this approach to the clinical setting, however, requires a functional thymus, which may not be present in the adult human. Peripheral tolerance mechanisms include deletion, anergy, and regulation. With self-tolerance, these mechanisms serve to prevent deleterious autoimmune responses from T cells that escape central deletion. Various approaches to induce peripheral transplant tolerance are currently under investigation, including costimulatory blockade, pharmacologic manipulation of DCs, and induction of donor antigen–specific Tregs. One of the most significant hurdles to the development of clinical tolerance strategies is the lack of reproducible immune monitoring assays to detect the presence or absence of tolerance, which would determine when immunosuppressive medications could be safely withdrawn. Although transplantation tolerance is not yet a clinical reality, progress in the field is being made.[46,47]

REFERENCES

1. Huang Y, Rabb H, Womer KL. Ischemia-reperfusion and immediate T cell responses. *Cell Immunol.* 2007;248:4-11.
2. Swaminathan S, Griffin MD. First responders: Understanding monocyte-lineage traffic in the acutely injured kidney. *Kidney Int.* 2008;74:1509-1511.
3. Suarez-Alvarez B, Lopez-Vazquez A, Baltar JM, et al. Potential role of NKG2D and its ligands in organ transplantation: New target for immunointervention. *Am J Transplant.* 2009;9:251-257.
4. Morelli AE, Thomson AW. Tolerogenic dendritic cells and the quest for transplant tolerance. *Nat Rev Immunol.* 2007;7:610-621.
5. Chalasani G, Dai Z, Konieczny BT, et al. Recall and propagation of allospecific memory T cells independent of secondary lymphoid organs. *Proc Natl Acad Sci U S A.* 2002;99:6175-6180.
6. Lakkis FG, Arakelov A, Konieczny BT, et al. Immunologic "ignorance" of vascularized organ transplants in the absence of secondary lymphoid tissue. *Nat Med.* 2000;6:686-688.
7. Pape KA, Kouskoff V, Nemazee D, et al. Visualization of the genesis and fate of isotype-switched B cells during a primary immune response. *J Exp Med.* 2003;197:1677-1687.
8. Valujskikh A, Lakkis FG. In remembrance of things past: Memory T cells and transplant rejection. *Immunol Rev.* 2003;196:65-74.
9. Adams AB, Williams MA, Jones TR, et al. Heterologous immunity provides a potent barrier to transplantation tolerance. *J Clin Invest.* 2003;111:1887-1895.
10. Schwartz RS. Shattuck lecture: Diversity of the immune repertoire and immunoregulation. *N Engl J Med.* 2003;348:1017-1026.
11. Hennecke J, Wiley DC. Structure of a complex of the human alpha/beta T cell receptor (TCR) HA1.7, influenza hemagglutinin peptide, and major histocompatibility complex class II molecule, HLA-DR4 (DRA*0101 and DRB1*0401): Insight into TCR cross-restriction and alloreactivity. *J Exp Med.* 2002;195:571-581.
12. Gokmen MR, Lombardi G, Lechler RI. The importance of the indirect pathway of allorecognition in clinical transplantation. *Curr Opin Immunol.* 2008;20:568-574.
13. Steele DJ, Laufer TM, Smiley ST, et al. Two levels of help for B cell alloantibody production. *J Exp Med.* 1996;183:699-703.
14. Brennan TV, Jaigirdar A, Hoang V, et al. Preferential priming of alloreactive T cells with indirect reactivity. *Am J Transplant.* 2009;9:709-718.
15. Bevan MJ. Cross-priming. *Nat Immunol.* 2006;7:363-365.
16. Jones EY. MHC class I and class II structures. *Curr Opin Immunol.* 1997;9:75-79.
17. Bouvier M, Wiley DC. Importance of peptide amino and carboxyl termini to the stability of MHC class I molecules. *Science.* 1994;265:398-402.
18. Dessen A, Lawrence CM, Cupo S, et al. X-ray crystal structure of HLA-DR4 (DRA*0101, DRB1*0401) complexed with a peptide from human collagen II. *Immunity.* 1997;7:473-481.
19. Gao X, Nelson GW, Karacki P, et al. Effect of a single amino acid change in MHC class I molecules on the rate of progression to AIDS. *N Engl J Med.* 2001;344:1668-1675.
20. Zou Y, Stastny P, Susal C, et al. Antibodies against MICA antigens and kidney-transplant rejection. *N Engl J Med.* 2007;357:1293-1300.
21. Bates RL, Frampton G, Rose ML, et al. High diversity of non-human leukocyte antigens in transplant-associated coronary artery disease. *Transplantation.* 2003;75:1347-1350.
22. Reiser JB, Darnault C, Guimezanes A, et al. Crystal structure of a T cell receptor bound to an allogeneic MHC molecule. *Nat Immunol.* 2000;1:291-297.
23. Wange RL, Samelson LE. Complex complexes: Signaling at the TCR. *Immunity.* 1996;5:197-205.
24. Li XC, Rothstein DM, Sayegh MH. Costimulatory pathways in transplantation: Challenges and new developments. *Immunol Rev.* 2009;229:271-293.
25. Mandelbrot DA, Kishimoto K, Auchincloss H Jr, et al. Rejection of mouse cardiac allografts by costimulation in trans. *J Immunol.* 2001;167:1174-1178.
26. Li XC, Rothstein DM, Sayegh MH. Costimulatory pathways in transplantation: Challenges and new developments. *Immunol Rev.* 2009;229:271-293.
27. Wynn TA. T_H-17: a giant step from T_H1 and T_H2. *Nat Immunol.* 2005;6:1069-1070.
28. Ouyang W, Kolls JK, Zheng Y. The biological functions of T helper 17 cell effector cytokines in inflammation. *Immunity.* 2008;28:454-467.
29. Willinger T, Freeman T, Hasegawa H, et al. Molecular signatures distinguish human central memory from effector memory CD8 T cell subsets. *J Immunol.* 2005;175:5895-5903.
30. Barry M, Bleackley RC. Cytotoxic T lymphocytes: All roads lead to death. *Nat Rev Immunol.* 2002;2:401-409.
31. Buzza MS, Bird PI. Extracellular granzymes: Current perspectives. *Biol Chem.* 2006;387:827-837.
32. Al-Lamki RS, Wang J, Skepper JN, et al. Expression of tumor necrosis factor receptors in normal kidney and rejecting renal transplants. *Lab Invest.* 2001;81:1503-1515.

33. Young NT. Immunobiology of natural killer lymphocytes in transplantation. *Transplantation*. 2004;78:1-6.
34. Einecke G, Mengel M, Hidalgo L, et al. The early course of kidney allograft rejection: Defining the time when rejection begins. *Am J Transplant*. 2009;9:483-493.
35. Einecke G, Fairhead T, Hidalgo LG, et al. Tubulitis and epithelial cell alterations in mouse kidney transplant rejection are independent of CD103, perforin or granzymes A/B. *Am J Transplant*. 2006;6:2109-2120.
36. Colvin RB. Antibody-mediated renal allograft rejection: Diagnosis and pathogenesis. *J Am Soc Nephrol*. 2007;18:1046-1056.
37. Veronese F, Rotman S, Smith RN, et al. Pathological and clinical correlates of FOXP3[+] cells in renal allografts during acute rejection. *Am J Transplant*. 2007;7:914-922.
38. Colvin RB, Smith RN. Antibody-mediated organ-allograft rejection. *Nat Rev Immunol*. 2005;5:807-817.
39. Rahimi S, Qian Z, Layton J, et al. Non-complement- and complement-activating antibodies synergize to cause rejection of cardiac allografts. *Am J Transplant*. 2004;4:326-334.
40. Ota H, Fox-Talbot K, Hu W et al. Terminal complement components mediate release of von Willebrand factor and adhesion of platelets in arteries of allografts. *Transplantation*. 2005;79:276-281.
41. Camerer E, Huang W, Coughlin SR. Tissue factor- and factor X–dependent activation of protease-activated receptor 2 by factor VIIa. *Proc Natl Acad Sci U S A*. 2000;97:5255-5260.
42. Womer KL, Vella JP, Sayegh MH. Chronic allograft dysfunction: Mechanisms and new approaches to therapy. *Semin Nephrol*. 2000;20:126-147.
43. Sis B, Campbell PM, Mueller T, et al. Transplant glomerulopathy, late antibody-mediated rejection and the ABCD tetrad in kidney allograft biopsies for cause. *Am J Transplant*. 2007;7:1743-1752.
44. Robertson H, Ali S, McDonnell BJ, et al. Chronic renal allograft dysfunction: The role of T cell–mediated tubular epithelial to mesenchymal cell transition. *J Am Soc Nephrol*. 2004;15:390-397.
45. Salama AD, Womer KL, Sayegh MH. Clinical transplantation tolerance: Many rivers to cross. *J Immunol*. 2007;178:5419-5423.
46. Fudaba Y, Spitzer TR, Shaffer J, et al. Myeloma responses and tolerance following combined kidney and nonmyeloablative marrow transplantation: In vivo and in vitro analyses. *Am J Transplant*. 2006;6:2121-2133.
47. Kawai T, Cosimi AB, Spitzer TR, et al. HLA-mismatched renal transplantation without maintenance immunosuppression. *N Engl J Med*. 2008;358:353-361.

CHAPTER 97

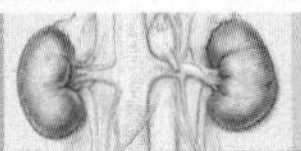

Immunosuppressive Medications in Kidney Transplantation

Karl Womer, Hamid Rabb

Much of the success of kidney transplantation is a result of advancements in immunosuppressive medications that are used during the induction and maintenance phases and for treatment of acute rejection.[1] The term *maintenance immunosuppression* is usually used to describe drug regimens consisting historically of small molecule agents that are administered to stable kidney transplant recipients, particularly after the first year. Increasingly, community nephrologists and primary care physicians are becoming involved in the care of stable kidney transplant recipients during the maintenance phase. In contrast, biologic agents that are used as induction protocols before the maintenance stage or for the treatment of early or late acute rejection episodes are commonly managed by transplant surgeons and nephrologists in inpatient settings. This chapter discusses the immunosuppressive agents that either are approved for prevention of rejection in renal transplantation or are commonly used as such by most transplant centers, with specific emphasis on their biologic mechanisms of action, pharmacokinetics, and side effect profile. These agents are divided into small molecule drugs and biologic agents for the purposes of this discussion.

SMALL MOLECULE DRUGS

Corticosteroids

Corticosteroids have been a cornerstone of transplant immunosuppression for the past 50 years, both as maintenance immunosuppression and for treatment of acute rejection.

Mechanism of Action

Corticosteroids suppress production of numerous cytokines and vasoactive substances, including interleukin (IL)–1, tumor necrosis factor α (TNF-α), IL-2, major histocompatibility complex class II, chemokines, prostaglandins (by inhibition of phospholipase A_2), and proteases. Corticosteroids also cause neutrophilia (often with a left shift), but neutrophil chemotaxis and adhesion are inhibited. They also affect nonhematopoietic cells.

Corticosteroids act as agonists of glucocorticoid receptors but at higher doses have receptor-independent effects. Corticosteroid receptors (CRs) belong to a family of ligand-regulated transcription factors called nuclear receptors. CRs are normally present in the cytoplasm in an inactive complex with heat shock proteins (HSP90, HSP70, and HSP56). The binding of corticosteroids to the CRs dissociates HSP from the CR and forms the active corticosteroid-CR complex, which migrates to the nucleus and dimerizes on palindromic DNA sequences in many genes, called the corticosteroid response element. The binding of CR in the promoter region of the target genes can lead to either induction or suppression of gene transcripts (e.g., of cytokines). CRs also exert effects by interacting directly with other transcription factors independent of DNA binding.

A key way by which corticosteroids regulate immune responses is by regulation of the transcription factors activator protein 1 (AP-1) and nuclear factor κB (NF-κB). Normally, NF-κB is present as an inactive complex with inhibitor of nuclear factor κB (IκB), but it can be released by IκB kinase. Corticosteroids stimulate IκB, which then competes with the IκB:NF-κB complex for degradation by the IκB kinase. Corticosteroids also stimulate lipocortin, which inhibits phospholipase A_2, thereby inhibiting the production of leukotrienes and prostaglandins. The total immunosuppressive effect of corticosteroids is complex, reflecting effects on cytokines, adhesion molecules, apoptosis, and activation of inflammatory cells.

Pharmacokinetics

The major corticosteroids used are oral prednisone (or prednisolone) and intravenous methylprednisolone. The oral agents have good oral bioavailability (60% to 100%) and have short half-lives (60 to 180 minutes) but long biologic half-lives (18 to 36 hours). Corticosteroids are eliminated by hepatic conjugation and are excreted by the kidneys as inactive metabolites. Coadministration of inducers of enzymes that metabolize corticosteroids (e.g., phenytoin, rifampin) decreases their half-life, whereas concomitant use of P-450 3A4 inhibitors (e.g., ketoconazole) has the opposite effect. As corticosteroid levels are not routinely monitored, dosage adjustment during concurrent therapy with these medications becomes problematic. For treatment of acute rejection, pulse doses of 250 to 1000 mg of methylprednisolone are typically used, with no evidence that the higher dosage is more efficacious.

Side Effects

Side effects of corticosteroid therapy are common and associated with significant morbidity, particularly cataracts, osteoporosis, and avascular necrosis of the femoral heads (Fig. 97.1). Other side effects include hypertension, hyperglycemia, hyperlipidemia, cushingoid features, psychiatric disturbances, sleep disorders, peptic ulcer disease, pancreatitis, colonic perforation, increased appetite with weight gain, growth retardation, and myopathy. Infection risk is also increased and is excessive if high-dose pulse therapy is prolonged. Interestingly, corticosteroids are not associated with increased incidence of malignant disease.

Common Side Effects of Small Molecule Immunosuppressive Medications							
	Cyclosporine	Tacrolimus	Mycophenolate	Azathioprine	Corticosteroids	mTOR Inhibitors	Leflunomide
Renal	Nephrotoxicity, type IV RTA, HTN, diuretic resistance, hyperkalemia, hypomagnesemia, hypophosphatemia	Nephrotoxicity, type IV RTA, HTN, diuretic resistance, hyperkalemia, hypomagnesemia, hypophosphatemia			HTN, hypokalemia, diuretic resistance	Synergistic nephrotoxicity with CNIs, delayed recovery from ATN, proteinuria, hypokalemia, HTN	
Gastrointestinal		Diarrhea, abdominal pain	Diarrhea, nausea and vomiting, gastritis, esophagitis, oral and colonic ulcers	Nausea and vomiting, hepatotoxicity, pancreatitis	Peptic ulcers, gastritis, esophagitis, diarrhea, colonic perforation	Diarrhea	Nausea, diarrhea, hepatitis
Hematologic	Thrombotic microangiopathy	Thrombotic microangiopathy	Anemia, leukopenia, thrombocytopenia	Anemia, leukopenia, thrombocytopenia	Leukocytosis, polycythemia	Thrombotic microangiopathy, anemia, thrombocytopenia	Anemia, leukopenia
Metabolic	Hyperlipidemia, hyperuricemia, gout, glucose intolerance	New onset diabetes			Hyperlipidemia, hyperuricemia, hyperglycemia, osteoporosis, vascular necrosis, increased appetite and weight gain	Hyperlipidemia	
Cosmetic	Gingival hyperplasia, coarsened facial features	Alopecia			Hirsutism, acne, cushingoid facies, buffalo hump	Impaired wound healing, oral ulcers	Alopecia
Neuromuscular	Encephalopathy, insomnia, myopathy, tremors	Encephalopathy, insomnia, myopathy, tremors			Psychosis, insomnia, myopathy	Reflex sympathetic dystrophy	
Other	Edema	Myocardial hypertrophy	Viral infections, pulmonary edema in elderly, progressive multifocal leukoencephalopathy		Cataracts	Lymphocele, interstitial pneumonitis, rash, edema	Rash

Figure 97.1 Common side effects of small molecule immunosuppressive medications. ATN, acute tubular necrosis; CNIs, calcineurin inhibitors; HTN, hypertension; mTOR, mammalian target of rapamycin; RTA, renal tubular acidosis.

Although corticosteroids are generally considered safe in pregnancy, orofacial clefts and fetal adrenal suppression have been reported.

Calcineurin Inhibitors

Calcineurin inhibitors (CNIs), including cyclosporine and tacrolimus, are fungus-derived small molecules that are the mainstays of current maintenance immunosuppressive regimens. Considerable variability exists in their pharmacokinetics, interactions, and side effect profiles, which raises the question of which agent to use in the individual patient. Cyclosporine is a cyclic, lipophilic peptide endecapeptide with several *N*-methylated amino acids, which may explain its resistance to inactivation in the gastrointestinal tract. Tacrolimus is a macrolide lactone antibiotic. Both drugs are highly soluble in lipids and other organic solvents.

Mechanism of Action

Both CNIs exert their effect by binding to cytoplasmic proteins called immunophilins (Fig. 97.2). Cyclosporine binds to cyclophilin, and tacrolimus binds to FK-binding protein 12 (FKBP12).[2] Such binding enhances the immunophilin's affinity to and subsequent inhibition of calcineurin, which is a calmodulin-activated serine phosphatase important for dephosphorylation of inactive nuclear factor of activated T cells (NF-AT). Nuclear translocation of dephosphorylated (active) NF-AT, in association with other transcription factors, initiates downstream events leading to T-cell activation (see section on T-cell activation in Chapter 96). The tacrolimus:FKBP12 active complex inhibits calcineurin with greater molar potency than the corresponding cyclosporine complex. Cyclosporine and tacrolimus can interfere with activation of calcineurin on substrates other than NF-AT, which likely explains many of the side effects of calcineurin inhibition. Treatment with CNIs also causes upregulation of the cytokine transforming growth factor β (TGF-β), which has significant immunosuppressive properties but also promotes the deposition of matrix proteins and tissue fibrosis. Finally, these two agents can suppress the immune response by calcineurin-independent pathways as well. This mechanism generally involves blockade of intracellular signaling pathways specific for T cells.

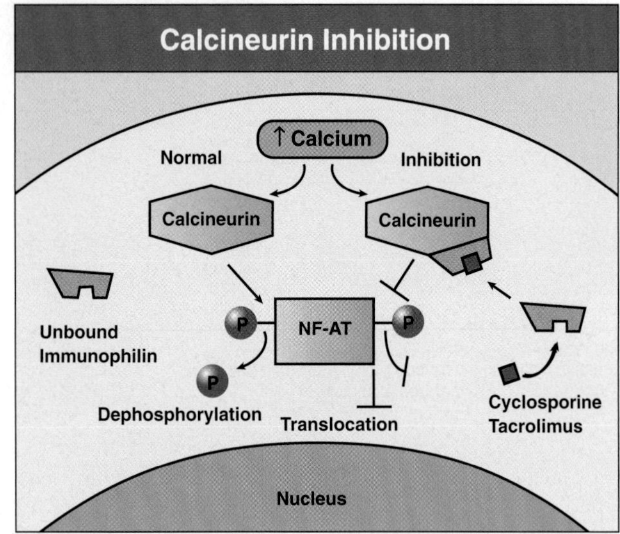

Figure 97.2 Calcineurin inhibition. During normal T-cell activation, calcium release activates calcineurin's phosphatase activity, causing dephosphorylation of the transcription factor nuclear factor of activated T cells (NF-AT) and subsequent translocation to the nucleus. Cyclosporine and tacrolimus form a complex with immunophilins (cyclophilin or FK-binding protein 12, respectively), which bind calcineurin and sterically inhibit the phosphatase activity, preventing dephosphorylation and nuclear translocation of NF-AT.

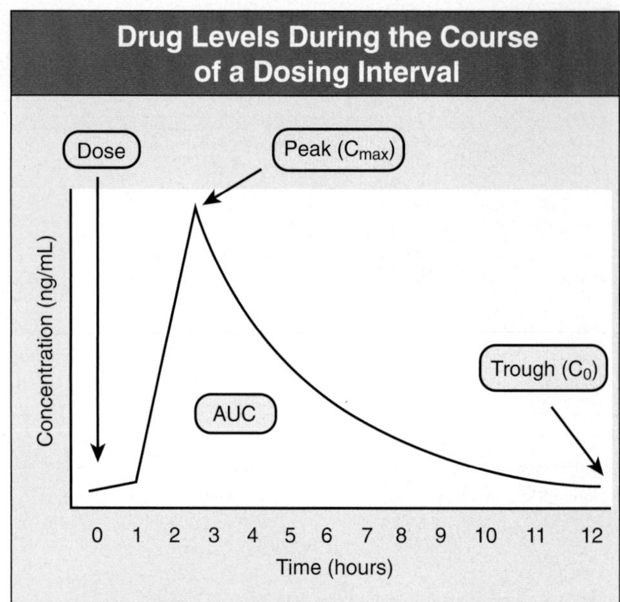

Figure 97.3 Drug levels during the course of a dosing interval. The drug concentration is lowest just before the dose is taken (C_0), then rises to a peak concentration at a certain time after the dose (C_{max}). The area under the concentration-time curve (AUC) describes total drug exposure during the entire dosing interval.

The ability of these agents to interfere with two distinct mechanisms of T-cell activation contributes to their highly specific immunosuppressive properties.

Pharmacokinetics, Monitoring, and Drug Interactions

After a dose of CNI, there is an initial absorptive phase, during which blood concentrations reach a peak level (C_{max}).[3] Typically, C_{max} occurs during the first 2 to 3 hours after the dose and corresponds to the time of maximum calcineurin inhibition. Drug levels then fall as a result of metabolism (also known as elimination phase) until they are at the lowest, or trough, level (C_0) immediately before the next dose. The total drug exposure throughout the period from one dose until the next is the area under the concentration-time curve (AUC; Fig. 97.3). For both CNIs, most of the interpatient and intrapatient variability occurs in the absorption rather than in the elimination phase.

The oil-based formulation of cyclosporine requires solubilization in bile and is plagued by highly variable and unpredictable bioavailability (up to 60% AUC), which is influenced by age, ethnicity, variability of gastric milieu (bile flow, concomitant ingestion of certain foods and medications), and comorbidities such as diabetes and cystic fibrosis. The microemulsion preparation of cyclosporine (modified) has enhanced bioavailability and less dependence on bile secretion, with 70% to 135% higher blood concentrations. In blood, cyclosporine resides primarily in erythrocytes (60% to 70%) and leukocytes (9%), with some binding to lipoproteins and, to lesser extent, other plasma proteins. Cyclosporine is metabolized primarily by CYP3A4, a member of the cytochrome P-450 superfamily. Metabolism occurs mostly in the liver, although other organs, including the kidneys and gut mucosa, contain this enzyme. Interindividual differences in CYP3A4 activity and the large number of exogenous and endogenous substances capable of altering its function and expression explain the wide variation in clearance rates. One factor is the multidrug resistance 1 gene product, P-glycoprotein, which is variably expressed in the intestine and reduces the absorption of several xenobiotics, including CNIs, by transport out of intestinal epithelial cells. The average half-life of cyclosporine is about 19 hours, with excretion primarily in bile. Generic formulations of cyclosporine modified exist, although they may not have identical pharmacokinetics and therefore may not be readily interchangeable.

The absorption of tacrolimus, like that of cyclosporine, is highly variable; bioavailability ranges from 5% to 67%. Absorption is not bile dependent but does depend on gastrointestinal transit time and is affected by the presence or absence of food as well as the lipid content of food. Clearance appears to be faster in the pediatric population, requiring administration of higher or more frequent doses. Ethnic differences exist as well, with African Americans requiring higher doses than Caucasians to achieve equivalent therapeutic levels. These differences may in part be due to expression of alternative subtypes of CYP3A (e.g., CYP3A5). In blood, tacrolimus distributes primarily to erythrocytes, with whole-blood concentrations 10 to 30 times higher than in plasma. In contrast to cyclosporine, no lipoprotein binding occurs. Tacrolimus has 20- to 30-fold higher potency than cyclosporine on a molecular weight basis. Similar to cyclosporine, metabolism occurs through the CYP3A4 system, with pharmacokinetics also affected by intestinal P-glycoprotein. Both CNIs are generally administered twice daily.

Because of their narrow therapeutic index, the variability of concentrations between patients after a dose, and the potential for drug interactions, monitoring of CNIs is required to ensure both safety and adequacy. Both cyclosporine and tacrolimus bind to cells and to plasma components (primarily lipoproteins for cyclosporine and albumin for tacrolimus) in the blood and therefore must be assayed in the whole blood. Four assays are currently used to monitor levels of CNIs in the blood: high-performance liquid chromatography (HPLC), monoclonal radioimmunoassay (RIA), monoclonal and polyclonal fluorescent polarization immunoassays, and the specific enzyme-multiplied immunoassay. Cyclosporine trough levels measured by HPLC

Drugs and Other Substances that Interact with Calcineurin Inhibitors	
Increase Blood Levels (P450-3A4 and/or p-glycoprotein inhibitors)	**Decrease Blood Levels (P450-3A4 and/or p-glycoprotein inducers)**
Ketoconazole	Rifampin
Fluconazole	Rifabutin
Itraconazole	Phenytoin
Voriconazole	Carbamazepine
Erythromycin	Phenobarbital
Clarithromycin	St John's Wort
Diltiazem	Caspofungin
Verapamil	
Nicardipine	
Cimetidine	
Methylprednisolone	
Metronidazole	
Ezetimibe	
Metoclopramide	
Fluvoxamine	
HIV protease inhibitors	
Grapefruit juice	
Chamomile	
Wild cherry	
Lovastatin	
Atorvastatin	
Simvastatin	

Figure 97.4 Drugs and other substances that interact with calcineurin inhibitors.

or RIA are comparable, as both techniques measure levels of the parent compound only. However, these concentrations are one-third lower compared with concentrations measured by techniques that detect the parent compound plus its metabolites. See Chapter 100 for standard dosing and target blood levels.

Given the complementary influence of both CYP3A4 and P-glycoprotein on their pharmacokinetic profiles, it is assumed that CNI-drug interactions are similar. Interestingly, drugs that competitively inhibit CYP3A4 activity, such as ketoconazole, usually also inhibit P-glycoprotein, thereby increasing the bioavailability of CNIs and potential for toxicity. In contrast, drugs like phenobarbital that increase CYP3A4 levels tend to upregulate P-glycoprotein, decreasing overall bioavailability. In this case, the likelihood of rejection increases. Despite similar drug interactions, the age and ethnic differences in pharmacokinetics between the two CNIs are likely to influence the degree and importance of such interactions. See Figure 97.4 for common interactions.

Side Effects

Cyclosporine and tacrolimus have similarities and differences in their toxicity profiles (see Fig. 97.1). Both can cause nephrotoxicity, hyperkalemia, hypomagnesemia and hypophosphatemia (secondary to urinary loss), renal tubular acidosis (type 4), hypertension, diabetes, and neurotoxicity. Certain side effects, such as gingival hyperplasia, hirsutism, hypertension, hyperuricemia, and hyperlipidemia, are more common with cyclosporine, whereas tremor and glucose intolerance are more common with tacrolimus. Cyclosporine may also be associated with coarsening of facial features, especially in children, and bone pain responsive to calcium channel blockers. Tacrolimus, especially in combination with mycophenolate mofetil, has been suspected of inducing more BK virus nephropathy.

The most common and vexing problem with CNIs is nephrotoxicity, with the importance evident from cardiac and liver transplant recipients, in whom large doses of CNIs are associated with progression to end-stage renal disease. Both reversible hemodynamic and irreversible structural components underlie the nephrotoxicity of CNIs. Reversible vasoconstriction is caused by direct vascular effects but is also due to activation of the renin-angiotensin system (RAS), endothelin, thromboxane, and the sympathetic nervous system. Over time, chronic renal injury occurs, which is notable for afferent arterial hyalinosis and tubulointerstitial fibrosis. It is presumed that these lesions are the result of prolonged renal vasoconstriction with ischemia. Experimentally, chronic cyclosporine nephropathy is exacerbated by the presence of sodium restriction and volume depletion, which stimulates the RAS, and can be ameliorated by angiotensin-converting enzyme inhibitors or angiotensin receptor blockers. Cyclosporine toxicity and to a lesser extent tacrolimus toxicity are potentiated in combination with sirolimus and everolimus. Finally, CNIs in high doses can cause thrombotic microangiopathy, probably by direct endothelial cell injury and dysfunction.

Mycophenolate

Mycophenolate mofetil (MMF) and enteric-coated mycophenolate sodium (EC-MPS) are important components of immunosuppressive regimens that are associated with some of the most successful outcomes in kidney transplantation.[4] Because of its well-documented efficacy and acceptable side effect profile, MMF has become by far the most frequently used antiproliferative agent.

Mechanism of Action

The immunosuppressive effects of both these agents are likely to be mediated through the active metabolite mycophenolic acid (MPA). MMF is a morpholinoethyl ester of MPA, a potent reversible inhibitor of inosine monophosphate dehydrogenase (IMPDH), isoform 2. EC-MPS is a salt that combines an acid-MPA with a base-sodium. The enteric coating delays MPS release so that the MPA is absorbed in the small intestine rather than in the stomach. MPA noncompetitively inhibits IMPDH, which is the rate-limiting enzyme in the *de novo* synthesis of guanosine monophosphate (GMP). Inhibition of IMPDH creates a relative deficiency of GMP and a relative excess of adenosine monophosphate (AMP). GMP and AMP levels act as a control on *de novo* purine biosynthesis; therefore, MPA, by inhibiting IMPDH, creates a block in *de novo* purine synthesis that selectively interferes with proliferative responses of T and B cells. Some other cell types, including gastrointestinal epithelial cells, use the *de novo* pathway. Thus, MPA may act directly to inhibit replication of gastrointestinal epithelial cells, leading to disruption of fluid absorption and diarrhea. However, most other cell types, including neurons, depend primarily on the alternative pathway for DNA synthesis and cell division and thus are relatively spared from toxicity.

Pharmacokinetics

MMF, being a prodrug of MPA, is absorbed rapidly and completely from the gastrointestinal tract and undergoes extensive presystemic de-esterification to become MPA, the active moiety. Food intake can delay the rate of MMF absorption but does not affect the extent. However, coadministration of antacids or cholestyramine decreases absorption by approximately 20% and 40%, respectively. EC-MPS has shown bioavailability equivalent to that of MMF. MPA undergoes enterohepatic circulation, and its plasma concentration shows a secondary peak at 6 to 12 hours after intravenous or oral dosing. The mean contribution of enterohepatic circulation to the overall AUC of MPA is 37% (range, 10% to 61%). The majority of MPA is metabolized in the liver (and possibly other sites, including intestine and kidney) through a phase II glucuronidation process. The major metabolite of MPA is the pharmacologically inactive 7-0-glucuronide metabolite (MPAG), although two other metabolites, MPA-acyl-glucuronide (AcMPAG) and MPA-phenyl-glucoside (glucoside-MPA), are isolated from the plasma of renal transplant patients. AcMPAG has shown *in vitro* pharmacologic activity (inhibition of IMPDH) as well as proinflammatory effects and potentially is responsible for the gastrointestinal toxicity of MPA.

The glucuronide metabolites are excreted into the bile, a process that is mediated by the multidrug resistance–related protein 2 (MRPR2), then undergo de-glucuronidation back to MPA by enzymes that are produced by colonic bacteria. Blockade of MRPR2 by an inhibitor, such as cyclosporine but not tacrolimus, decreases the biliary excretion of MPAG and increases plasma MPAG levels. This eventually leads to lower plasma levels of MPA because the glucuronide metabolites no longer can be reabsorbed as MPA by enterohepatic cycling. Thus, tacrolimus-treated patients have higher exposure to MPA than cyclosporine-treated patients do, and it is possible that tacrolimus results in greater intestinal exposure to the metabolites of MPA because of greater enterohepatic circulation.[5] The ultimate elimination pathway for the glucuronide metabolites is through the kidney, and more than 95% of an administered dose eventually is found in the urine as glucuronide metabolites.

For the most part, MMF and EC-MPS have been used exclusively in a fixed-dose regimen. However, studies have established a strong association of MPA AUC and its pharmacologic effects, specifically prevention of acute rejection. Furthermore, considerable interindividual variability is found in MPA AUC and trough concentrations in patients who receive a fixed dose of MMF. These data lend support to recent efforts to evaluate the role of therapeutic drug monitoring in increasing the therapeutic potential of MMF and EC-MPS.

Side Effects

MMF and EC-MPS have similar side effect profiles, including gastrointestinal toxicity, bone marrow suppression, and increased infections, especially those of viral etiology (see Fig. 97.1). Gastrointestinal disturbances include oral ulcerations, esophagitis, gastritis, nausea and vomiting, diarrhea, and colonic ulcers. Diarrhea and leukopenia frequently necessitate dose reduction, which can precipitate rejection. As the metabolites of MPA appear to play a major role in the gastrointestinal disturbances associated with MMF, there is little rationale for enteric coating of the prodrug to reduce these symptoms. In fact, randomized controlled trials have found no significant difference in gastrointestinal adverse events between MMF and EC-MPS.[6,7] MMF is not routinely used during pregnancy because of its teratogenicity in experimental animal models and clinical reports of major fetal malformations.

Azathioprine

The use of azathioprine has decreased dramatically in kidney transplantation with the introduction of MMF. Azathioprine is metabolized in the liver to 6-mercaptopurine and further converted to the active metabolite thio-inosinic acid by hypoxanthine-guanine phosphoribosyltransferase. Because allopurinol (a xanthine oxidase inhibitor) will increase the levels of thio-inosinic acid, doses of azathioprine must be reduced by two thirds in patients taking allopurinol. More often, MMF is substituted for azathioprine.

Azathioprine suppresses the proliferation of activated T and B cells and reduces the number of circulating monocytes by arresting the cell cycle of promyelocytes in the bone marrow. The antiproliferative effect is mediated by the metabolites of azathioprine, including 6-mercaptopurine, 6-thiouric acid, 6-methylmercaptopurine, and 6-thioguanine. These compounds are incorporated into replicating DNA and halt replication. They also block the *de novo* pathway of purine synthesis by formation of thio-inosinic acid; this effect confers specificity of action on lymphocytes that lack a salvage pathway for purine synthesis.

The major side effect of azathioprine is bone marrow suppression, leading to leukopenia, thrombocytopenia, and anemia (see Fig. 97.1). The mean cell volume is commonly increased in patients taking azathioprine, and red cell aplasia can occasionally occur. The hematologic side effects are dose related and usually reversible on dose reduction or temporary discontinuation of the drug. Other common side effects are increased risk of malignant disease (especially of skin cancers), hepatotoxicity, pancreatitis, and hair loss. Azathioprine is generally considered safe in pregnancy, although some fetal immunosuppression may occur.

mTor Inhibitors

The mTOR inhibitors are proliferation signal inhibitors with potent immunosuppressive activity. Sirolimus, also called rapamycin, was the first agent used in transplantation and is a macrolide product of a soil fungus found in Easter Island.[8] Everolimus is a rapamycin analogue with similar mechanism of action, immunosuppressive properties, and side effect profile. Although initially used in regimens with the intent of minimizing exposure to CNIs, the mTOR inhibitors have been associated with their own set of toxicities that have prevented their widespread use.

Mechanism of Action

Sirolimus has structural similarity to tacrolimus and binds the immunophilin FKBP12. The affinity of sirolimus for FKBP12 is higher than that of everolimus. mTOR inhibitors do not inhibit calcineurin or the calcium-dependent activation of cytokine genes but instead inhibit cytokine receptor–mediated signal transduction and cell proliferation and block lymphocyte responses to cytokines and growth factors. The sirolimus:FKBP12 or everolimus:FKBP12 complex binds with high affinity a kinase enzyme called mammalian target of rapamycin or mTOR, which is a serine-threonine kinase of the phosphatidylinositol 3-kinase pathway that acts during costimulatory and cytokine-driven pathways. mTOR inhibits an inhibitor (4E-BP1) and activates a ribosomal enzyme (p70 S6 kinase), both of which are important for translation of the mRNAs for certain proteins needed for progression from the G_1 phase to the S phase of DNA synthesis. mTOR has been identified as the principal controller of cell growth and proliferation. The sirolimus:FKBP12 complex inhibits mTOR-mediated signal transduction pathways by blocking postreceptor immune responses to costimulatory signal 2 during G_0 to G_1 transition and to cytokine signaling during G_1 progression. It also inhibits IL-2– and IL-4–dependent proliferation of T and B cells, leading to suppression of new ribosomal protein synthesis and arrest of the G_1-S phase of the cell cycle. Proliferation of nonimmune cells, such as fibroblasts, endothelial cells, hepatocytes, and smooth muscle cells, is also impaired by inhibition of the growth factor–mediated responses (e.g., basic fibroblast growth factor, platelet-derived growth factor, vascular endothelial cell growth factor, and TGF-β). In addition, it has been shown that mTOR contributes to several protein synthesis pathways that could be involved in oncogenesis.

Pharmacokinetics

The oral bioavailability of sirolimus is poor (10% to 16%), with significant interindividual and intraindividual variability. Peak concentrations occur approximately 1 to 2 hours after an oral dose, and sirolimus distributes extensively into tissues, including blood cells. The oral bioavailability of everolimus is higher than that of sirolimus. High-fat meals increase sirolimus levels while decreasing everolimus levels. Because sirolimus has a relatively long half-life (approximately 62 hours), it is reasonable to wait 1 week (approximately three half-lives to achieve steady state) before monitoring sirolimus blood levels after initiation or dose adjustment. Sirolimus is metabolized by the P-450 3A4 isoenzyme and P-glycoprotein system and thus has interactions similar to those described for the CNIs (see Fig. 97.4). When sirolimus or everolimus is administered simultaneously with cyclosporine, C_{max} and AUC for both the compounds are increased. Thus, it is recommended that cyclosporine and mTOR inhibitors be administered 4 hours apart. Cyclosporine clearance may be reduced during concurrent therapy.

Side Effects

The mTOR inhibitors have a wide variety of toxicities (see Fig. 97.1). The most common adverse effects associated with sirolimus are dose-dependent hyperlipidemia (particularly hypertriglyceridemia), thrombocytopenia, and leukopenia. Other adverse effects include anemia (especially in combination with MMF), hypokalemia, impaired wound healing and dehiscence, formation of lymphoceles, rashes, oral ulcers, reduced testosterone levels, pneumonitis, and diarrhea. Although not inherently nephrotoxic, the mTOR inhibitors result in renal graft damage through several mechanisms. When it is used in combination with full-dose cyclosporine (and probably also tacrolimus), sirolimus potentiates CNI-induced toxicity, perhaps by increasing TGF-β expression. In patients with renal insufficiency, sirolimus is associated with marked yet potentially reversible proteinuria and worsening of established proteinuria. Sirolimus can also cause delayed recovery from acute tubular necrosis. Finally, cases of thrombotic microangiopathy have been reported, and there is concern that higher doses of sirolimus may inhibit endothelial cell growth. Sirolimus-based regimens have been associated with a reduced incidence of post-transplantation malignant neoplasms. Some physicians regard sirolimus as the preferred immunosuppressive agent in transplant patients who develop malignant neoplasms. Sirolimus is not routinely used during pregnancy because of its teratogenicity in experimental animal models, although successful pregnancies have been reported.

Dihydro-orotate Dehydrogenase Inhibitors

Leflunomide and its derivative, FK778, are pyrimidine synthesis inhibitors with immunosuppressive as well as antiproliferative effects. These agents inhibit dihydro-orotate dehydrogenase, which is a key rate-limiting enzyme in *de novo* pyrimidine synthesis. Unlike other cell types, activated lymphocytes expand their pyrimidine pool by nearly eightfold during proliferation, whereas purine pools increase only twofold. Thus, inhibition of dihydro-orotate dehydrogenase prevents lymphocytes from accumulating sufficient pyrimidines to support DNA synthesis.

Leflunomide tablets are 80% bioavailable. After oral administration, leflunomide is metabolized to teriflunomide (previously A77 1726), which is responsible for essentially all of the activity *in vivo* and is monitored during therapy. Metabolism occurs in the liver, with excretion in the urine and bile. Because of its very long half-life (approximately 2 weeks), a loading dose of 100 mg for 3 to 5 days is generally used to reach steady-state levels quickly. Side effects include gastrointestinal adverse events, alopecia, bone marrow suppression, severe hepatitis, interstitial lung disease, and life-threatening skin reactions. Leflunomide use is not safe during pregnancy, and unless female leflunomide users receive cholestyramine therapy to eliminate the drug from the body, pregnancy must be avoided for 2 years after discontinuation. Although it is not approved by the Food and Drug Administration (FDA) for use in kidney transplantation, leflunomide has recently been assigned orphan drug status for the prevention of rejection in solid organ transplantation, largely on the basis of modest antiviral activity *in vitro* against BK virus and cytomegalovirus. However, the efficacy and safety of leflunomide have not been completely assessed in well-controlled and adequate studies. Furthermore, the manufacturers of FK778 discontinued development owing to a lack of benefit over current options with regard to prevention of rejection and treatment of BK virus nephropathy.

BIOLOGIC AGENTS

Biologic agents in the form of polyclonal antibodies and monoclonal antibodies (mAbs) are frequently used in kidney transplantation either as induction therapy or for the treatment of rejection. Polyclonal antibodies are derived from horses or rabbits; historically, mAbs have been murine in origin. However, because foreign proteins can elicit an immune response, there has been an attempt to replace murine monoclonal products with humanized or chimeric mAbs (Fig. 97.5). Humanized antibodies are produced by merging the DNA that encodes the antigen-binding portion of a monoclonal mouse antibody with human antibody–producing DNA. Mouse hybridomas are then used to express this DNA to produce hybrid antibodies that are not as immunogenic as the murine variety. Chimeric antibodies use the same strategy but for the entire variable region and thus are more immunogenic than humanized antibodies. Polyclonal antibodies and mAbs can be divided further into two groups: depleting agents and immune modulators.

Polyclonal Antilymphocyte Sera

Polyclonal antilymphocyte agents are produced by immunizing animals with human thymus-derived lymphoid cells. Although rabbit antithymocyte globulin (ATG) is currently the preferred preparation, equine preparations have historically been used. Most regimens involve daily intravenous administration of ATG for 5 to 7 days either as induction therapy or for treatment of corticosteroid-resistant rejection. ATG contains antibodies that react against a variety of targets, including red blood cells, neutrophils, dendritic cells, and platelets. ATG binds to multiple epitopes on the surface of T cells and induces a rapid lymphocytopenia by several mechanisms, including complement-dependent cytolysis, cell-dependent phagocytosis, and apoptosis. ATG is a potent immunosuppressive, and T- and B-lymphocyte

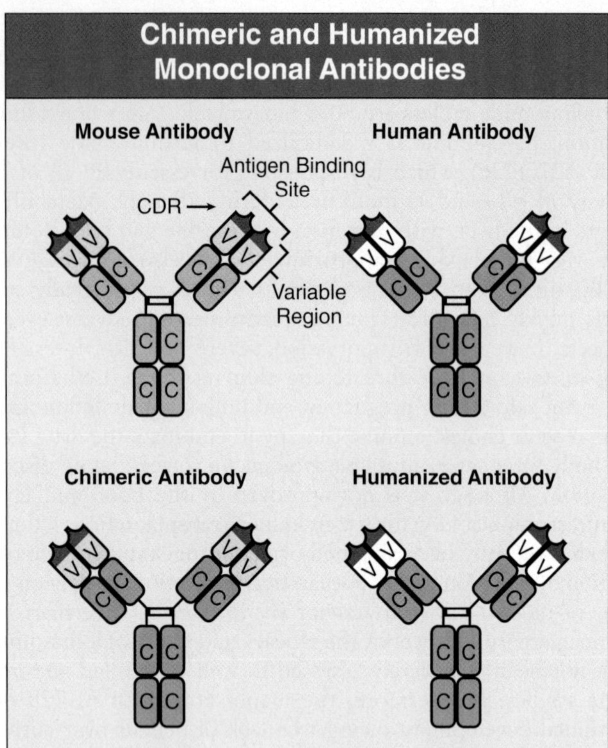

Figure 97.5 Chimeric and humanized antibodies. Chimeric antibodies consist of human constant (C) regions and mouse variable (V) regions. A chimeric antibody therefore retains the antigen binding site of the mouse antibody but fewer amino acid sequences foreign to the human immune system than a standard mouse antibody. Humanized monoclonal antibodies retain only the minimum necessary parts of the mouse antibody for antigen binding, the complementarity-determining region (CDR, *highlighted in red*), and therefore are even less immunogenic in the human host.

counts can remain depressed up to 24 hours after administration. The lack of specificity coupled with marked immunosuppression increases the risk of infection and malignant neoplasms. As polyclonal agents are xenogeneic proteins, they may elicit a number of side effects, including fever and chills. The initial lysis and activation of T cells that follow ATG administration may generate significant first-dose effects, with release of TNF-α, interferon-γ (IFN-γ), and other cytokines. Less commonly, ATG can induce a serum sickness–like syndrome and rarely acute respiratory distress syndrome (ARDS).

Murine Monoclonal Anti-CD3 Antibody

OKT3 is a murine IgG2a mAb targeting the ε chain of the CD3:T-cell receptor complex and was first approved for the treatment of rejection. Soon after OKT3 administration, T cells disappear from circulation as a result of opsonization and subsequent removal from circulation by mononuclear cells in the liver and spleen. Initially, OKT3 can activate T cells and result in release of several cytokines, including IL-2, IFN-γ, IL-6, and TNF-α. These cytokines cause a syndrome referred to as the cytokine release syndrome, which consists of fever, chills, headache, gastrointestinal complaints, and, less commonly, ARDS, aseptic meningitis, and encephalopathy. The availability of other agents and the severity of side effects associated with the cytokine release syndrome have resulted in a marked reduction in the use of OKT3. Furthermore, OKT3 is immunogenic in humans, and approximately 50% of patients will make antibodies to it after a course of treatment, decreasing the efficacy of subsequent courses. Although several humanized anti-CD3 mAbs (huOKT3g1, HuM291) have been generated, they have not been developed for use in renal transplantation.

Humanized Monoclonal Anti-CD52 Antibody

Alemtuzumab is a humanized IgG1 mAb directed against CD52, a glycoprotein present on circulating T and B cells, monocytes-macrophages, NK cells, and granulocytes. Although it is currently approved only for the treatment of B-cell chronic lymphocytic leukemia, alemtuzumab has been used as an induction agent in renal transplantation, given its powerful depletional properties and favorable cost profile compared with other induction agents. Treatment results in a rapid and effective depletion of peripheral and central lymphoid cells that may take months to return to pretransplantation levels. Side effects of alemtuzumab include first-dose reactions, neutropenia, anemia, and, rarely, pancytopenia and autoimmunity (e.g., hemolytic anemia, thrombocytopenia, and hyperthyroidism). The risks of immunodeficiency complications such as infection and malignant neoplasia with alemtuzumab are still not clear, and further controlled trials are necessary to establish dosing, safety, and efficacy.

Monoclonal Anti-CD25 Antibody

The α subunit of the IL-2R (CD25) is upregulated on activated T cells and leads to the expression of the high-affinity IL-2R that on engagement by IL-2 triggers the activated T cell to undergo proliferation. Two mAbs, daclizumab (humanized) and basiliximab (chimeric), have been developed with specificity for CD25. These antibodies induce relatively mild immunosuppression and are used as induction agents to prevent rejection[9,10] but not to treat established rejection. Although the exact mechanism of action is not fully understood, it is clear that significant depletion of T cells does not play a major role. Saturation of the IL-2R α subunit persists for up to 120 days after daclizumab induction and 25 to 35 days after treatment with basiliximab. Although saturation is important as a determinant of minimal blood concentrations, it is not predictive of rejection. No major side effects have been associated with anti-CD25 therapy.

B Cell–Depleting Monoclonal Anti-CD20 Antibody

Rituximab is an engineered chimeric mAb that contains murine heavy- and light-chain variable regions directed against CD20 plus a human IgG1 constant region.[11] The CD20 antigen, a transmembrane protein, is found on immature and mature B cells as well as on malignant B cells. CD20 mediates proliferation and differentiation of B cells. Rituximab directly inhibits B-cell proliferation and induces apoptosis and lysis by complement-dependent cytotoxicity, antibody-dependent cell cytotoxicity, and activation of tyrosine kinases as a direct effect of the antibody's binding to its CD20 ligand. Rapid and sustained depletion of circulating and tissue-based B cells occurs after intravenous administration, and recovery does not begin until approximately 6 months after completion of treatment. Although plasma cells are usually CD20 negative, many are short-lived and require replacement from CD20-positive precursors. In addition, CD20-positive B cells can act as secondary antigen-presenting cells, thereby enhancing T-cell responses. Thus, by targeting CD20 on precursor B cells, rituximab decreases the production of activated B cells and limits their antibody production as well as antigen presentation capability.

Most adverse events are first-infusion effects, such as fevers and chills, and are generally of mild severity. Moreover, these adverse effects occur less frequently during subsequent infusions. Viral infections, including reactivation of hepatitis B virus and JC virus (progressive multifocal leukoencephalopathy), have been reported, although it is not known whether these events are specific to the agent or instead reflect the overall state of immunosuppression. Antichimeric antibodies develop in some cases, but their true incidence and therapeutic significance are uncertain.

Rituximab is currently approved by the FDA only for treatment of B-cell non-Hodgkin's lymphoma and rheumatoid arthritis. However, given the effects on B-cell depletion, this agent has been used in kidney transplantation to treat antibody-mediated rejection as well as in combination with intravenous immune globulin to reduce high-titer anti-HLA antibodies in highly sensitized patients awaiting renal transplantation.[12] Rituximab is also used as induction therapy after desensitization therapy for ABO blood group–incompatible and high-risk positive-crossmatch kidney transplantation. Finally, rituximab is often used to treat post-transplantation lymphoproliferative disease.

Intravenous Immune Globulin

Intravenous immune globulin (IVIG) products are known to have powerful immunomodulatory effects on inflammatory and autoimmune conditions. The mode of action of IVIG is not understood. In renal transplantation, the most important effect appears to be a reduction of alloantibodies through inhibition of antibody production and increased catabolism of circulating antibodies. Additional potential mechanisms include inhibition of complement-mediated injury, inhibition of inflammatory cytokine generation, and neutralization of circulating antibodies by anti-idiotypes.

Side effects related to IVIG administration include minor self-limited reactions, such as flushing, chills, headache, myalgia, and arthralgia. Rarely, anaphylactic reactions may occur. Delayed reactions include severe headache and aseptic meningitis, which respond to analgesics. More recently, severe thrombotic events have been linked to the administration of IVIG products. Of concern to renal transplant recipients is the development of acute renal failure due to osmotic injury of the proximal tubular epithelium after administration of sucrose-containing IVIG preparations. This tubular injury is self-limited and can be minimized or avoided by use of sucrose-free preparations.

In combination with plasmapheresis, IVIG appears to offer significant benefits in the desensitization of positive-crossmatch and ABO-incompatible patients to allow successful transplantation as well as in the treatment of antibody-mediated rejection. Alone or in combination with rituximab, IVIG has been successful in the desensitization of highly sensitized wait-listed patients to increase the chances of finding a compatible donor.

REFERENCES

1. Samaniego M, Becker BN, Djamali A. Drug insight: Maintenance immunosuppression in kidney transplant recipients. *Nat Clin Pract Nephrol.* 2006;2:688-699.
2. Ho S, Clipstone N, Timmermann L, et al. The mechanism of action of cyclosporin A and FK506. *Clin Immunol Immunopathol.* 1996;80(pt 2):S40-S45.
3. Schiff J, Cole E, Cantarovich M. Therapeutic monitoring of calcineurin inhibitors for the nephrologist. *Clin J Am Soc Nephrol.* 2007;2:374-384.
4. Jeong H, Kaplan B. Therapeutic monitoring of mycophenolate mofetil. *Clin J Am Soc Nephrol.* 2007;2:184-191.
5. Heller T, van Gelder T, Budde K, et al. Plasma concentrations of mycophenolic acid acyl glucuronide are not associated with diarrhea in renal transplant recipients. *Am J Transplant.* 2007;7:1822-1831.
6. Budde K, Curtis J, Knoll G, et al. Enteric-coated mycophenolate sodium can be safely administered in maintenance renal transplant patients: Results of a 1-year study. *Am J Transplant.* 2004;4:237-243.
7. Salvadori M, Holzer H, de Mattos A, et al. Enteric-coated mycophenolate sodium is therapeutically equivalent to mycophenolate mofetil in de novo renal transplant patients. *Am J Transplant.* 2004;4:231-236.
8. Morath C, Arns W, Schwenger V, et al. Sirolimus in renal transplantation. *Nephrol Dial Transplant.* 2007;22(Suppl 8):viii61-viii65.
9. Nashan B, Moore R, Amlot P, et al. Randomised trial of basiliximab versus placebo for control of acute cellular rejection in renal allograft recipients. CHIB 201 International Study Group. *Lancet.* 1997;350:1193-1198.
10. Vincenti F, Kirkman R, Light S, et al. Interleukin-2-receptor blockade with daclizumab to prevent acute rejection in renal transplantation. Daclizumab Triple Therapy Study Group. *N Engl J Med.* 1998;338:161-165.
11. Salama AD, Pusey CD. Drug insight: Rituximab in renal disease and transplantation. *Nat Clin Pract Nephrol.* 2006;2:221-230.
12. Vo AA, Lukovsky M, Toyoda M, et al. Rituximab and intravenous immune globulin for desensitization during renal transplantation. *N Engl J Med.* 2008;359:242-251.

CHAPTER 98

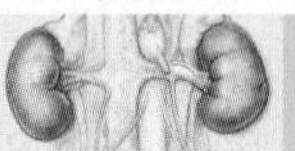

Evaluation and Preoperative Management of Kidney Transplant Recipient and Donor

William R. Mulley, John Kanellis

Renal transplantation provides superior long-term outcomes compared with dialysis, in both quantity and quality of life, although the benefit gained varies between individuals.[1] The improvement in outcomes coupled with the shortage of available organs has led to an expansion of donor criteria and an increasing tendency for centers to accept marginal donor kidneys.[2] In this chapter, we review current recommendations for the evaluation and preoperative management of both the kidney transplant donor and recipient.

RECIPIENT EVALUATION

Many units now accept patients who were previously excluded from transplantation, such as those with human immunodeficiency virus (HIV) infection, obesity, and diabetes. This is due to the availability of newer treatment options for some conditions and a greater understanding of the impact of these conditions on patient and graft survival along with changing societal attitudes on equality of access to transplantation. Some absolute contraindications to transplantation remain (Fig. 98.1), including significant current infection or malignant disease, noncompliance or substance abuse, and any condition likely to severely limit life expectancy (<1 to 2 years).[3-5]

Whereas the application of guidelines for transplant suitability may be relatively straightforward for patients with a single comorbidity, it is not as simple for those with multiple medical conditions who represent a growing group of transplant recipients. Determination of suitability in such patients often requires input from specialists in a variety of medical and surgical disciplines along with allied health professionals. The final decision needs to be a joint one between clinician and patient after full and open discussion of the likely risks and benefits followed by regular reassessment of suitability while the patient awaits transplantation.

A summary of guidelines published by national and international transplantation associations[3-5] is presented in Figure 98.2. Some of the important areas to consider in evaluating the transplant recipient are discussed here.

Cardiovascular Disease

Cardiovascular disease is the major cause of death in renal transplant recipients. Hence, cardiovascular evaluation is critical in the evaluation of the transplant recipient.

Coronary Heart Disease and Left Ventricular Dysfunction

Renal failure itself is a major risk factor for coronary artery disease. However, the vascular lesion, clinical features, and response to treatment may be quite different in patients with renal failure compared with the normal population. Because of a lack of conclusive evidence, the role of pretransplantation screening and intervention for coronary artery disease is controversial, making definite recommendations difficult. However, given the high incidence of cardiac events in the peritransplantation period and its major contribution to post-transplantation mortality, we favor aggressive screening and intervention in at-risk patients while avoiding unnecessary tests and procedures in low-risk candidates. Patients may be stratified into risk groups on the basis of history and examination, resting electrocardiography, and chest radiography. Further screening is unnecessary in asymptomatic patients without risk factors because of a very low incidence of coronary events.[6] Further investigation is recommended, however, in patients with abnormal test results or significant risk factors, such as previous ischemic events, diabetes, smoking, age older than 50 years, hypertension, dyslipidemia, prolonged renal failure (>2 years), or a family history of ischemic heart disease.[3-5]

Symptomatic patients should proceed directly to coronary angiography; noninvasive functional testing should be used to screen the need for angiography in asymptomatic patients.[7] Exercise echocardiography or thallium imaging is preferred; however, pharmacologically driven testing may be necessary if exercise is not possible. Whereas a normal result does not exclude coronary artery disease, it has a negative predictive value for myocardial infarction or cardiac death in excess of 96% in patients with renal failure.[8] If significant coronary artery disease is identified, treatment before transplantation should be instituted. Treatment consists of medical management including aggressive risk factor modification and angioplasty and stenting or coronary artery bypass grafting in patients with significant stenoses.[7] A suggested approach is presented in Figure 98.3.

In patients with clinical or radiologic evidence of left ventricular dysfunction, transthoracic echocardiography should be performed to assess the severity and nature of the dysfunction. If it is significant, a cause should be sought and treated when possible. Whereas mild to moderate left ventricular dysfunction may improve after transplantation, severe dysfunction in a patient with a short life expectancy is considered a contraindication to transplantation unless, in rare instances, combined heart and kidney transplantation is appropriate.[3-5]

Cerebrovascular Disease

Patients with a history of recent transient ischemic attack or stroke are at greatest risk of recurrence early after the primary event; and because stroke after transplantation is associated with a high rate of mortality,[9] a waiting time of 6 months is

Contraindications to Renal Transplantation

Current Absolute Contraindications to Transplantation	Previous Contraindications to Transplantation (now acceptable under certain circumstances – see text)
• Active Sepsis • Current uncontrolled malignant disease • Uncontrolled psychosis • Active drug dependence • Any medical condition with a severely shortened life expectancy (<1–2 years) • Positive T-cell CDC cross match	• HIV Infection • Hepatitis B and C • Obesity • Mood disorders • Age > 60 years • Previous malignant disease • Blood group incompatibility

Figure 98.1 Contraindications to renal transplantation. CDC, complement-dependent cytotoxicity; HIV, human immunodeficiency virus.

Recipient Evaluation Checklist

History and Examination
Cause of renal failure and risk of recurrence Sensitization (transfusion, pregnancy, previous transplant) Past and current infections (TB, hepatitis, HIV) Immunization (especially hepatitis B) Malignancy Cardiovascular risks (smoking, hypertension, diabetes) Pulmonary, gastrointestinal disease Genitourinary tract Psychiatric, psychological history Surgical issues (weight, iliac vessels, abdomen, previous surgery)
Laboratory and Radiologic Investigations
Viral serology (HIV, CMV, EBV, hepatitis B and C) Liver function tests Bone-related issues (PTH, calcium, phosphate) Chest radiograph Electrocardiogram Prostate-specific antigen (for men >50-60 years old) Mammogram or breast ultrasound (women >50 years old or with family history of breast cancer) Pap smear (sexually active women)
Immunologic Investigations
ABO blood group and HLA typing Screening for HLA antibodies and autoreactive antibodies Crossmatching

Figure 98.2 Recipient evaluation. CMV, cytomegalovirus; EBV, Epstein-Barr virus; HIV, human immunodeficiency virus; PTH, parathyroid hormone; TB, tuberculosis.

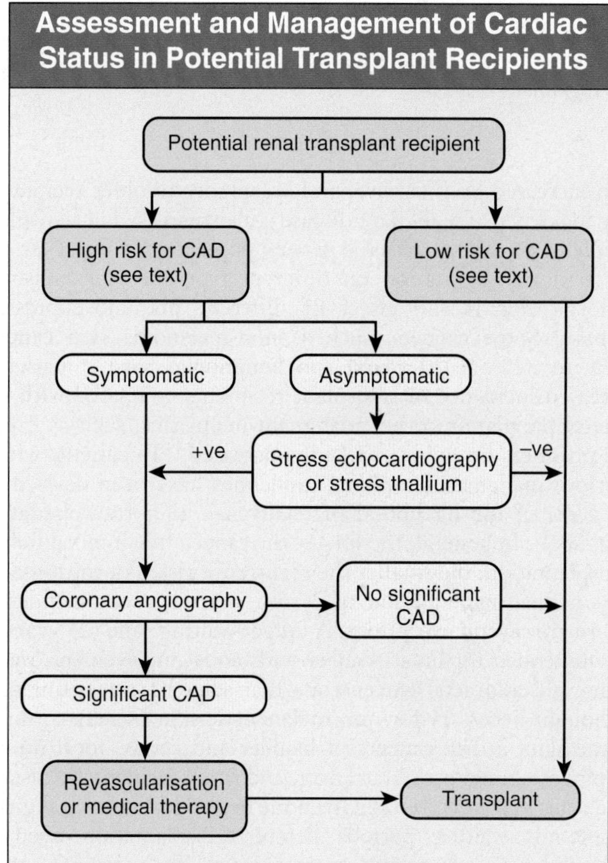

Figure 98.3 Assessment and management of cardiovascular disease in potential transplant recipients. CAD, coronary artery disease; +ve, positive; –ve, negative.

recommended. Meanwhile, aggressive risk factor modification should be undertaken to limit the likelihood of further stroke. Routine screening for cerebrovascular disease is not advocated in asymptomatic patients. Recent evidence suggests a benefit in further investigation of patients with a carotid bruit and treatment with carotid endarterectomy if a significant stenosis is found.[10] Evidence on the merits of screening for and treatment of asymptomatic cerebral artery aneurysms in patients with polycystic kidney disease is inconclusive, making definite recommendations difficult at this time.

Peripheral Vascular Disease

Asymptomatic patients with strong femoral and peripheral pulses generally require no further investigation. Patients with diabetes, history of claudication, or reduced pulses require vascular imaging beginning with Doppler ultrasound. Significant disease involving the iliac vessels may make transplantation difficult or impossible and may worsen ischemia in the distal leg. Although it is not an absolute contraindication to transplantation, peripheral vascular disease is associated with increased mortality[11] and should be considered in conjunction with the patient's other comorbidities.

Cancer

Cancer is a major cause of death in renal transplant recipients. Further increases in the incidence of malignant disease are likely

Guidelines for Transplantation in Patients with Previous Malignancies
Usual Waiting Time of 2 Years
Most cancers
No Waiting Time Necessary
Incidental renal carcinoma
In situ carcinoma
Focal neoplasm (defined as a localized tumor without metastases)
Low-grade bladder cancer
Basal cell skin cancer
Waiting Time of >2 Years May Be Necessary
Melanoma
Breast cancer
Colorectal cancer
Uterine cancer

Figure 98.4 Guidelines for transplantation in patients with previous malignant disease.[63]

with increased graft survival and acceptance of older recipients. The incidence of malignant disease is also increased in transplant recipients compared with the general population.[12] However, the effect of transplantation on different types of cancers is not uniform, nor is the effect of different immunosuppressive agents.[13] Some cancers, such as non-melanoma skin cancers (61% to 82% at 20 years) and lymphoma, have a markedly increased incidence in transplant recipients compared with the general population; other malignant neoplasms, such as breast and prostate, are not as markedly increased.[14] In patients with a previous malignant neoplasm, guidelines have been devised on the basis of the likelihood of recurrence after transplantation (Fig. 98.4). In general, the longer the cancer-free interval before transplantation, the smaller the recurrence risk. For most malignant neoplasms, a period of 2 to 5 years is recommended.[3-5] There are several exceptions. A longer waiting time (≥5 years) is recommended for breast cancer with nodal involvement, melanoma, and colorectal cancer worse than stage B1; no waiting time is thought necessary for non-melanocytic skin cancers confined to the skin, *in situ* cancers of bladder and cervix, focal microscopic low-grade prostate cancer, and small incidentally discovered renal cell carcinomas. Given the heterogeneity of malignant neoplasms, waiting periods before transplantation need to be individualized, taking into account the patient's other comorbidities.

Although extensive screening of all potential recipients is not warranted, guidelines appropriate for the general population should be adopted in screening for breast, cervical, prostate, and colorectal cancer. Chest radiography is performed as part of the routine assessment. More comprehensive and targeted evaluation is recommended in patients with a strong family history or suggestive clinical features of malignant disease or conditions associated with an increased risk of malignant disease, such as renal imaging in patients with acquired cystic disease of the kidney for possible renal cell carcinoma.[3,4]

Infectious Complications

All patients are screened for previous exposure to Epstein-Barr virus and cytomegalovirus (CMV) to assess the risk of infection,

Routine Serology	Where Indicated, Tests for	Other Routine Investigations
Hepatitis B virus	Human herpesvirus 8	Urine culture
Hepatitis C virus	HTLV	Chest radiograph
HIV	*Strongyloides stercoralis*	
Cytomegalovirus	Malaria	
Epstein-Barr virus	*Trypanosoma cruzi*	
	Schistosomiasis	

Figure 98.5 Screening tests for occult infection. Routine screening tests for occult infection. HIV, human immunodeficiency virus; HTLV, human T-cell lymphotropic virus.

either primary or reactivation. This guides the appropriate use of prophylactic antiviral agents. For example, patients who are negative for CMV IgG who receive a kidney from a CMV-positive donor are at the highest risk of infection and may benefit from prolonged prophylaxis compared with the lower risk CMV-negative donor to CMV-negative recipient (see Chapter 101). Screening for other infections should be tailored to geographic location; a guide for screening is presented in Figure 98.5. Immunization against hepatitis B should be undertaken in all potential recipients. Immunization against encapsulated organisms (pneumococcus, *Haemophilus influenzae*, and meningococcus) should also be considered in patients at high risk of antibody-mediated rejection in case splenectomy is required.

Before highly active antiretroviral therapies (HAART), HIV infection was considered an absolute contraindication to transplantation because of very poor patient survival.[15] In the HAART era, HIV infection is seen as a manageable chronic disease, and transplantation is offered to HIV-positive patients at many major centers. Short- to medium-term results in the small studies reported suggest excellent patient and graft survival.[16] Larger studies are under way to further explore these outcomes. Patients with sustained CD4 counts above 200/ml and undetectable HIV viral loads, without an AIDS-defining illness, could be considered for transplantation at a center experienced in managing HIV infection and transplantation.

Patients with hepatitis B may be considered for renal transplantation if there is no evidence of active viral replication (hepatitis B virus [HBV] DNA or hepatitis B early [HBe] antigen positive), advanced liver disease or cirrhosis (as determined by liver biopsy), or hepatocellular carcinoma.[3-5] Immunosuppression can increase HBV replication; hence, treatment before transplantation is indicated in patients with active disease, and although data to support prophylactic antiviral therapy after transplantation are scarce, it is commonly practiced while immunosuppression is at its highest (initial 12 to 24 months). Early reports suggest that mortality may be increased in HBV-positive patients after transplantation compared with HBV-negative recipients.[17] The significance of these findings is unclear in the current era with more effective treatment options and if only patients with inactive disease are transplanted. Frank disclosure of possible risks involved is recommended.[3-5]

Patients with hepatitis C should be assessed by measurement of hepatitis C viral (HCV) load and a liver biopsy. Treatment should be instituted before transplantation; however, candidates who do not clear the virus may still proceed with transplantation as mortality in this group is improved compared with those remaining on dialysis.[18] HCV-positive patients may in some units, with informed consent, receive a kidney from an HCV-positive donor. Any possible increased risk may be offset by a significantly reduced waiting time. Patients with hepatitis B and C should be screened every 12 months for hepatocellular carcinoma by liver ultrasound and serum alpha-fetoprotein. Those with cirrhosis may be considered for combined kidney-liver transplantation.

The risk of tuberculosis reactivation after transplantation should be assessed by chest radiography and a tuberculin skin test. Whereas a positive test response correlates with past infection, false-negatives in uremic patients are common.[19] Patients at high risk (previous tuberculosis, abnormal chest radiograph or positive skin test response, or resident in an endemic area) who have not been previously treated should receive prophylactic isoniazid after transplantation (see Chapter 101).

Previous graft loss due to polyoma (BK) viral nephropathy is not a contraindication to repeated transplantation. Limited data currently prevent specific recommendations on the benefit of waiting for serum and urine BK polymerase chain reaction test results to become negative or on the value of graft nephrectomy before repeated transplantation. Vigilant screening for recurrence is recommended.[5]

Obesity

Transplantation in obese patients (body mass index [BMI] >30 kg/m^2) generally improves survival compared with matched waiting list controls, but inferior outcomes for patient and graft survival, delayed graft function and wound healing, and infective complications have been reported in obese compared with non-obese patients, particularly those with a BMI above 36 kg/m^2.[20] There are several reports to the contrary, however, including a recent multivariate analysis of registry data suggesting that obesity is not associated with worse graft and patient survival when comorbidities are controlled for.[21]

However, the overweight or obese are more likely to develop new-onset diabetes after transplantation, which can adversely affect graft and patient survival. Potential transplant recipients with obesity should be advised to lose weight as a means to decrease this risk before transplantation.

Recurrent Disease

The risk of disease recurrence needs to be discussed as part of the informed consent process, particularly in certain primary renal diseases (e.g., focal segmental glomerulosclerosis). Graft loss attributed to recurrent disease has increased in recent years but still accounts for only 5% of graft loss.[22] The risks and management of recurrent disease are discussed in Chapter 104.

Gastrointestinal Disease

Screening for gastrointestinal disease is not warranted in the asymptomatic patient.[4,5] Patients with active acute or chronic pancreatitis should not undergo transplantation until they have been clear of symptoms for 12 months. Patients with active peptic ulcer disease should be treated before transplantation with proton pump inhibitors, and this should be continued to prevent ulceration after transplantation. Patients with symptomatic diverticular disease require colonoscopy and potential colonic resection in severe cases before transplantation as they are at increased risk of perforation on immunosuppressive medications.[4] Whereas symptomatic cholecystitis should be treated surgically before transplantation, asymptomatic cholelithiasis does not require surgery before transplantation because cholecystectomy after transplantation is required in less than 10% of these patients and results in no increased mortality or morbidity compared with pretransplantation cholecystectomy and no deleterious effects on graft function.[23]

Genitourinary Disorders

Screening for genitourinary disorders before transplantation is indicated in those with a history or renal ultrasound suggestive of urinary obstruction, especially in children, in whom urologic problems are a major cause of end-stage renal disease. If obstruction is found, urologic assessment, which may include voiding cystourethrography and urodynamic studies, is indicated to determine the best course of action to limit bladder pressures after transplantation; this may involve bladder augmentation, urinary diversion, or self-catheterization.

Native nephrectomy before transplantation should be considered for recurrent or persistent renal sepsis, particularly in the setting of nephrolithiasis. Very large polycystic kidneys may need to be removed to accommodate the transplant kidney. Whether previous grafts should be removed before repeated transplantation is controversial. Nephrectomy of a failed graft is commonly performed on withdrawal of immunosuppression in patients with early graft failure (<12 months)[24] to alleviate symptoms such as pain over the graft, fever, and weight loss.[25] Other indications include graft sepsis and to allow room for the new graft. However, unless there is a convincing reason to remove the graft, it is generally left *in situ*. In these circumstances, the patient may need to stay on a minimal amount of immunosuppression (e.g., prednisolone, 5 mg/day) to minimize graft tenderness and inflammation. Graft nephrectomy may be associated with an increased risk of HLA sensitization,[24] perhaps relating to loss of antigen-dependent tolerogenic mechanisms[26]; this, however, is not a universal finding. Another advantage of leaving the previous transplant *in situ* is preservation of any residual renal function and urine output.

Pulmonary Disease

Initial assessment by physical examination and chest radiography is indicated for all potential recipients; further testing, such as pulmonary function tests or computed tomographic scanning, is performed if it is clinically indicated. Recent guidelines suggest that patients with a short life expectancy associated with pulmonary disease, such as cor pulmonale, uncontrolled asthma, and severe obstructive lung disease (FEV_1 <25% of predicted or Po_2 <60 mm Hg on room air), or those needing home oxygen be excluded from transplantation.[5] Many units require patients to cease smoking before acceptance as smokers have an increased risk of death and graft loss. Cessation of smoking demonstrates positive lifestyle behavior and good compliance, suggesting these factors will be optimized in the post-transplantation period.

Psychosocial Issues

Psychosocial issues can have a major impact on transplant outcomes. Patients should be evaluated by a social worker or other health professional experienced in judging capacity to consent and assessing likely compliance with a transplant medication regimen. Compliance with the post-transplantation treatment regimen is vital to minimize premature graft loss. Predicting

Re-Evaluation of Suitability for Transplantation		
Cardiac re-evaluation every 1–2 years depending on risk factors (e.g. diabetes)	**Cancer surveillance relevant to age, sex, and risk Factors**	**Comorbidity re-assessment**
Stress echo or thallium scan Angiography if indicated (see Figure 2)	Prostate specific antigen Mammography Pap smear Colonoscopy if indicated Skin cancer check	Viral hepatitis Liver function tests Alpha-fetoprotein Liver ultrasound HIV CD4 count ? AIDS defining illness Other (see discussion of individual organ systems)

Figure 98.6 Re-evaluation of suitability for transplantation.

compliance can be challenging and may be based on pretransplantation compliance, such as adherence to dialysis management regimens. If compliance is unlikely, as judged by medical, psychiatric, psychological, and social work assessment, transplantation should not proceed.[3-5]

Cognitive impairment is not an absolute contraindication to transplantation as long as appropriate supports and proxy arrangements are in place. Patients with psychiatric illnesses including depression, bipolar affective disorder, and psychosis require assessment by a psychiatrist to determine transplant suitability and to devise a management plan to cope with possible consequences of immunosuppressive medications such as corticosteroids.[3-5] Drug and alcohol addiction should be addressed with rehabilitation and demonstrated abstinence before listing for transplantation.

Re-evaluation of Patients on the Waiting List

Patients may wait several years on the transplant list before receiving an opportunity to be transplanted. It is vital that when their opportunity comes, they are still suitable. A targeted reassessment of waiting list patients therefore should be conducted at regular intervals (Fig. 98.6). General measures, such as sun avoidance and cancer screening (e.g., prostate, breast, and cervical), should be continued on a regular basis as indicated. Reassessment of cardiac status is advocated on the basis of risk. Diabetic and other high-risk patients should be reassessed every 1 to 2 years.[7] The value of reassessing low-risk patients is more questionable, but given that renal failure is a strong risk factor for cardiac disease, repeated stress testing by exercise or pharmacologically driven echocardiography or thallium scanning at least every 3 years seems appropriate. Patients with preexisting medical conditions (e.g., HIV infection and viral hepatitis) require regular specialist reviews, with any issues arising brought to the attention of the transplant team. Surgical reassessment may be needed in patients with peripheral vascular disease, with weight gain, or if a complication such as peritonitis occurs while awaiting transplantation. Patients should be temporarily removed from the waiting list if they develop a serious infection or other illness until it is resolved.

DONOR EVALUATION

Donor kidneys can be obtained from both deceased and living donors.

Deceased Donors

Classification of the Deceased Donor

Deceased donors can be classified as either heart-beating donors with loss of brainstem function (donation after brain death or DBD) or non–heart-beating donors (donation after cardiac death or DCD). In recent years, the proportion of DCD donors is increasing in many countries as a result of policies aiming to maximize the opportunities for donation.

DBD donors can be further divided into standard criteria donors and extended criteria donors. Whereas the definition of extended criteria donor varies, in the United States it refers to heart-beating donors older than 60 years or 50 to 59 years old with two or three of the following criteria: a history of hypertension; elevated serum creatinine at donation (>1.5 mg/dl or 130 μmol/l); death from a cerebrovascular accident. In some jurisdictions, the term *marginal donor* is loosely used to describe donors who are less than optimal for some reason. This is usually due to the presence of significant underlying disease (hypertension, diabetes, vascular disease, renal impairment) or advanced age (>65 years).

Donation after cardiac death can occur by several mechanisms. The Maastricht classification separates these types of donors into controlled and uncontrolled categories (Fig. 98.7).[27] Controlled donors are those who suffer cardiac arrest after withdrawal of support or after brain death. Uncontrolled donors are those who are deceased on arrival to the hospital or who have a failed cardiopulmonary resuscitation. From a practical point of view, a system that uses controlled donors is easier to implement than one using uncontrolled donors. This is largely related to factors surrounding ethical considerations and the consent process involving relatives of the donor.

The survival of kidneys from extended criteria donors and from some categories of DCD donors is generally inferior to that of kidneys retrieved from standard criteria donors.[28,29] Many matching schemes attempt to allocate these less ideal grafts to recipients who are predicted to have a lower than average overall survival, but practice varies considerably between countries with regard to these issues.

Evaluation of the Deceased Donor

In most circumstances, organ donor coordinators screen potential deceased donors after referral from hospital intensive care units or emergency departments. Patient records are assessed and relatives are interviewed about important aspects of the

Classification of Donation after Cardiac Death Donors
As per Maastricht classification (Kootstra, 2007) (also known as non–heart–beating donors)
Uncontrolled
Category I: Dead on arrival to hospital Cause of death is usually obvious (e.g. severe head injury) and no resuscitation is given
Category II: Unsuccessful resuscitation The subject is brought to the emergency department while being resuscitated, but this is not effective. Alternatively, arrest occurs in hospital and subject is unable to be resuscitated
Controlled
Category III: Awaiting cardiac arrest Severe brain injury without brain death. Subjects are usually ventilator dependent. Arrest occurs once support is withdrawn
Category IV: Cardiac arrest while brain dead Subject suffers cardiac arrest after being declared brain dead. Alternatively, this occurs during brain death testing and the subject is not or cannot be successfully resuscitated
Category V (see Ch. 99)

Figure 98.7 Classification of donation after cardiac death (DCD) donors.[27]

clinical history. The assessment focuses on general health (including history of infections and cancer), social history (especially drug use and sexual history), and laboratory evidence of renal impairment or other diseases (Fig. 98.8). Patients with sepsis, acute hepatitis, or HIV infection are excluded from donation, as are those with a history of malignant disease. Nonmelanomatous skin cancers do not lead to exclusion, nor do primary brain tumors unless they are of a high grade or the donor has received chemotherapy or had a craniotomy or cerebral shunt inserted.[30] In some centers, donors potentially carrying hepatitis B or hepatitis C virus are accepted only for those positive for these viruses. The risk of an unknown donor malignant neoplasm is approximately 1.3%; however, the risk of transmitting a donor malignant neoplasm is lower at approximately 0.2%.[31]

Evaluation of renal function is determined by history, urinalysis, and serum creatinine concentration. In some cases, a biopsy (often performed at retrieval) may provide useful information, particularly with extended criteria donors.[32] Serum creatinine concentration at admission should be in the near-normal range (estimated glomerular filtration rate [GFR] >60 ml/min), but a temporary decline in renal function is acceptable if the function is expected to recover. Proteinuria (>0.5 g/24 h) indicates structural renal damage and is a valid reason for nonacceptance.

The use of kidneys from very small donors varies between centers. Donors younger than 5 or 6 years are generally associated with high risk of failure, especially from vascular thrombosis.[33] For this reason, some centers occasionally transplant two kidneys—transplanted en bloc, using the aorta and inferior vena cava as conduits.[34]

Deceased Donor Management Before Transplantation

In the brain-dead donor, maintenance of an adequate blood pressure and oxygenation are important to avoid warm ischemic renal injury. The use of pressor agents, volume resuscitation, and other conditioning strategies is complex and has been the subject of several guideline documents (see the Intensive Care Society website, *www.ics.ac.uk*). In this category of donor, the kidneys are generally not subject to significant warm ischemia at the time of organ retrieval unless the donor suffers prolonged hemodynamic compromise.

Deceased Donor Evaluation Checklist
Medical History
Hypertension, diabetes
Malignant disease
Infections: past and current (TB, hepatitis, HIV)
Transfusions
Trauma
Surgical history
Hospitalizations
Social History
Intravenous drug use
Alcohol, smoking
Sexual behavior
Tattoos, acupuncture
Overseas Travel
Incarceration
Examination
Blood pressure
Cardiac, vascular
Lymphadenopathy
Abdominal
Laboratory/Technical
Serum creatinine
Urinalysis, urine culture
Liver function tests
Coagulation profile, complete blood count
Blood culture
Virology: antibodies to CMV, EBV, HSV-1 and -2; HHV-6, -7, -8; HCV, HBV (include HBsAG, anti-HBc IgG and IgM), HIV, West Nilevirus, rabies, HTLV-1
Parasites, depending on geographic region: malaria, babesiosis, toxoplasmosis, Chagas, syphilis
Fungi in appropriate regions: Coccidioides, Histoplasma
Tuberculosis (depending on geographic region)
Chest radiograph
Electrocardiogram
Biopsy if there is concern for chronic kidney disease
Operating Room Evaluation
Intra-abdominal examination to detect occult malignant diseases
Macroscopic appearance of kidneys

Figure 98.8 Deceased donor evaluation checklist. CMV, cytomegalovirus; EBV, Epstein-Barr virus; HBc, hepatitis B core antigen; HBsAg, hepatitis B surface antigen; HBV, hepatitis B virus; HCV, hepatitis C virus; HHV, human herpesvirus; HIV, human immunodeficiency virus; HSV, herpes simplex virus; HTLV-1, human T-cell lymphotropic virus 1; TB, tuberculosis.

In donation after cardiac death, once death is certified and deemed irreversible, either rapid surgical exposure of the great vessels with cooling of the organs followed by prompt retrieval is required or, alternatively, the kidneys are cooled *in situ* by insertion of perfusion catheters through the femoral vessels. Surgical retrieval can then take place after a period of delay to variably allow one or more of the following: family counseling, donor assessment, or relocation from one hospital area to another (e.g., from the intensive care unit or emergency department to the operating theater). Donation after cardiac death is inevitably associated with warm ischemic renal injury. This is responsible for the higher rate of delayed graft function that is seen in this group. The need for dialysis support after transplantation is on average 50% but varies from 30% to 90%, depending on the category of donor.[27]

Living Donors

Live kidney donation is currently justifiable in most countries on the basis of the demand for deceased donor organs—which far outweighs the supply—as well as the apparent very low level of risk to the majority of healthy donors.[35] Added to this are the detrimental effects for the recipient of waiting on dialysis and the excellent, generally superior results obtained through use of live donors.

Living donors may be related, unrelated, altruistic, or part of a donor exchange or list-exchange program. In many countries with well-established transplant programs, half or more of all transplants are now performed with living donors. In Japan, Brazil, and the Middle East, more than 80% of transplants use living donors. The superior success of transplantation from live donors compared with that from deceased donors has supported the development of live donor paired exchange and live donor–deceased donor exchange.[36] In the first instance, live donors who are incompatible with their intended recipients are exchanged between recipients. In the other instance, the donor donates to the wait list in exchange for the intended recipient's receiving priority on the list.[37]

In some countries, either a state-organized or free-market system results in the purchase of live donor kidneys; this is a highly controversial area and under active international policy development.[38] The Declaration of Istanbul on organ trafficking and transplant tourism and the World Health Organization both condemn the exploitation of living donors who are thought to be vulnerable (illiterate, impoverished, undocumented immigrants, prisoners, and political or economic refugees).[39]

In recent times, many units have extended their selection of donors to include subjects who are mildly hypertensive, overweight, or hyperlipidemic or have other abnormalities (such as isolated hematuria or previous stone disease).[40] Whereas donation appears to be safe in the short to medium term for most of these subjects, adequate studies have not been performed to assess the longer term medical or psychological effects.

Mortality and Morbidity

Mortality related to living donation is a catastrophic and unexpected event. Registry data and institutional surveys suggest the perioperative risk of donor death is approximately 3 in 10,000.[41] Donor mortality and major complications appear equivalent with laparoscopic and open donor nephrectomy. In open surgery, the risks are related to perioperative complications, including pulmonary emboli, pneumonia, and ischemic events. With laparoscopic surgery, complications are largely due to catastrophic intraoperative events or postoperative bleeding related to securing of the vascular pedicle.[41,42]

In the longer term, survival of donors appears to be similar to that of control subjects in the general population (Fig. 98.9).

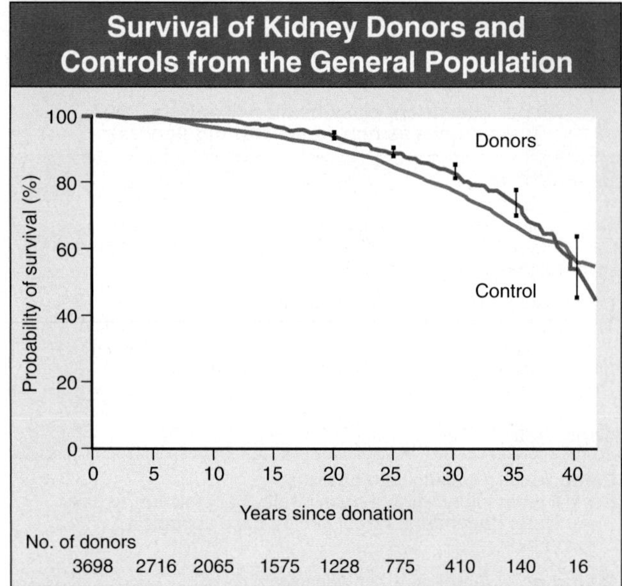

Figure 98.9 Survival of living kidney donors. The survival of living related donors is similar to the expected survival derived from the general population. Error bars at 5-year intervals indicate 95% confidence intervals for the probability of survival among kidney donors. *(Modified with permission from reference 35.)*

Numerous series report early operative complications after laparoscopic and open donor nephrectomy with rates of between 3% and 38%.[41] These reports variably include events such as bleeding, wound infection, urinary retention, pneumonia, asymptomatic and symptomatic pneumothorax, ileus, and need for transfusion, among other things. This enormous variability relates to both definition of complication and accuracy of reporting.

Case series report that physical and psychological function in living donors is higher than the community norm. Physical issues reported by donors after donation frequently include a temporary decrease from baseline in energy; some note a longer time to full recovery than anticipated and incision pain that lasts longer than expected. Psychological factors usually include an improved relationship with the recipient, an improved self-image, and frequently a positive effect on the donor's life. Longer term psychological morbidity appears minimal; however, some series have reported an association with anxiety, depression, or other psychological issues in a small proportion of the subjects.[43,44] Even though most donors have a positive experience, a small number for a variety of reasons do regret the decision to donate (0% to 5%). Psychological evaluation before donation is therefore extremely important, as is the need to provide support and counseling after donation. This issue is particularly important when the transplant does not go as well as anticipated.

Evaluation of the Live Donor

Several groups have developed guidelines for the evaluation of the living donor, including the Amsterdam forum[45] and consensus guidelines published by several U.S. transplant centers.[46] An outline of the usual donor evaluation is shown in Figures 98.10 and 98.11. It includes a thorough history and examination, blood and urine screening tests, chest radiography, electrocardiography, age- and family history–appropriate cardiac stress test, and radiographic assessment of the kidneys and vessels. An assessment of the anatomy may be achieved by computed tomographic

Live Donor Evaluation Checklist: History and Examination
History
Hypertension
Diabetes (including gestational)
Infections
Cancer (including skin lesions)
Vascular disease
Renal calculi
Gout
Urinary tract
Family history
Medications (including NSAIDs, herbs)
Smoking
Elicit and intravenous drug use
Sexual history
Vocation, sport interests
Level of physical activity/exercise
Psychiatric history/psychological factors
Willingness to donate
Relationship with recipient
Examination
Blood pressure
Weight and height, BMI
Joints, skin
Cancer (including skin lesions, breast)
Lymph nodes
Vascular disease
Heart and lungs
Abdomen

Figure 98.10 Live donor evaluation checklist: history and examination. NSAIDs, nonsteroidal anti-inflammatory drugs; BMI, body mass index.

Live Donor Evaluation Checklist: Investigations
Laboratory and Radiologic Investigations
Urinalysis (blood, protein)
Urine microscopy and culture (blood, organisms)
Serum electrolytes, urea and creatinine
Liver function tests
Full blood examination
Fasting blood glucose and/or oral glucose tolerance test
Fasting lipids
24-hour urine, creatinine clearance, protein excretion (or GFR measurement by other methods, [e.g., iothalamate clearance, nuclear GFR by Cr-EDTA, DTPA; protein excretion by other methods], [e.g., protein-creatinine ratio])
Serum uric acid, calcium, phosphate
Viral screening: HBV, HCV, HIV, CMV, EBV serology
Syphilis screening (RPR)
TB screening (PPD)
Electrocardiogram
Chest radiograph
Females: Pap smear, mammography (according to age/family history)
Males: prostate-specific antigen (according to age/family history)
Additional cardiac investigations (where indicated by age/history/risk factors)
Stress test
Echocardiography
Ambulatory blood pressure
Renal Anatomy (as per local expertise)
Computed tomographic angiography
Magnetic resonance imaging angiography
Catheter angiography

Figure 98.11 Live donor evaluation checklist: investigations. CMV, cytomegalovirus; Cr-EDTA, chromium-labeled ethylenediaminetetraacetic acid; DTPA, diethylenetriaminepentaacetic acid; EBV, Epstein-Barr virus; GFR, glomerular filtration rate; HBV, hepatitis B virus; HCV, hepatitis C virus; HIV, human immunodeficiency virus; PPD, purified protein derivative test; RPR, rapid plasmin reagent; TB, tuberculosis.

angiography or magnetic resonance angiography, depending on the particular center. Formal renal arteriography, although informative, is no longer necessary given the anatomic detail obtainable noninvasively with modern radiologic techniques.

Assessment of Renal Function

Most centers use a GFR of 80 ml/min per 1.73 m^2 as the lower limit for donors. It is accepted that this is an overgeneralization, potentially representing too low a limit for the younger donor (e.g., <40 years) and too high a limit for the older donor (e.g., >60 to 65 years). For this reason, an alternative approach is to consider the age-specific GFR and to accept donors only if they fall within the average for this figure. This method has been recommended by the British Transplantation Society (guidelines available at *www.bts.org.uk*) and is presented in Figure 98.12. An alternative approach uses the life expectancy of the donor.[47] By use of these calculations, a 30-year-old donor would require a GFR of 123 ml/min per 1.73 m^2; the level for a 70-year-old would be approximately 68 ml/min per 1.73 m^2.

Hypertension in the Live Donor

Donation may be acceptable for some hypertensive individuals if blood pressure is well controlled, GFR is as expected for donation and age, and there are no features of end-organ involvement from hypertension.[45,46] The evaluation for hypertension should include blood pressure measurements on three separate occasions. Borderline elevated levels should be further evaluated with ambulatory blood pressure monitoring. If elevated blood pressure is detected and the prospective donor is still under consideration, echocardiography (looking for left ventricular hypertrophy), ophthalmologic evaluation (looking for hypertensive retinal changes), and assessment for microalbuminuria (suggesting hypertensive renal damage) should be undertaken. The prospective donor should be excluded if any of these features are present.

Obesity and Abnormal Glucose Tolerance in the Live Donor

Although many centers accept obese living donors, several issues need to be addressed. This includes the impact of obesity on perioperative complications, future renal function, and cardio-

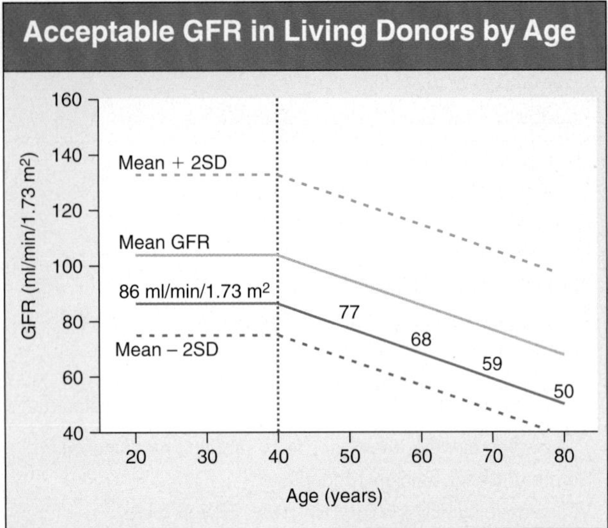

Figure 98.12 Acceptable glomerular filtration rate (GFR) in living donors by age. Diagram explaining the minimum acceptable age-associated GFR in living donor candidates. The *solid orange line* shows the variation with age of mean GFR. The *outer dashed lines* show the +2 and −2 population standard deviation (SD) limits. GFR is constant up to the age of 40 years and then declines at the rate of 9 ml/min per 1.73 m^2 per decade. The reference plot is based on an analysis of data for 428 live renal transplant donors who had ^{51}Cr-ETDA GFR measurements. The *solid blue line* shows the safety limit of 86 ml/min per 1.73 m^2 for young adults, declining to 50 ml/min per 1.73 m^2 at age 80 years. For transplant donors with preoperative GFR values above the solid blue line, the GFR of the remaining kidney will still be above 37.5 ml/min per 1.73 m^2 at age 80 years. *(Modified with permission from the revised British Transplantation Society/Renal Association U.K. guidelines for living donor kidney transplantation available at* www.bts.org.uk/.*)*

vascular health. In one study, obese (BMI >30 kg/m^2) subjects had an increased rate of proteinuria and renal impairment 10 to 20 years after nephrectomy.[48] Obese individuals may therefore be more prone to development of renal disease after donation, but this issue has not been carefully studied.

Future risk of diabetes is another important consideration. As well as close assessment of those who are overweight, prospective donors with an abnormal fasting glucose concentration, a history of gestational diabetes, or a first-degree relative with diabetes should be evaluated with an oral glucose tolerance test. An abnormal glucose tolerance test result is a contraindication to donation. Subjects often lose weight and otherwise change their lifestyle (exercise, diet), leading to an improvement in their results and eventual acceptance as donors. It is important that these lifestyle and risk modifications be sustained after donation occurs.

Renal Abnormalities in the Live Donor

As well as factors identified in the history (e.g., previous calculi, urinary tract infections, prostatic disease), a variety of previously unidentified renal abnormalities can be encountered in prospective donors during their assessment. These include microscopic hematuria, evidence of reflux disease, renovascular abnormalities, and renal masses and cysts.

Isolated hematuria in a prospective donor necessitates consideration of thin basement membrane nephropathy, Alport's syndrome (carrier status in women may have minor or moderate abnormalities), and IgA nephropathy as well as urinary tract infection, malignant disease, and nephrolithiasis. Microscopic hematuria is a relatively common problem, with persistent microscopic hematuria evident in approximately 3% of the general population.[49] Among the possible disorders, IgA nephropathy is generally a contraindication to live donation, whereas thin basement membrane disease may not necessarily be so.[50] The implications of isolated mesangial IgA without other manifestations of nephropathy require further study, and donation should be decided in the context of family history, absolute renal function, presence of interstitial disease, and age. If persistent isolated asymptomatic hematuria is detected during live donor evaluation, a workup should include cystoscopy and urinary cytology if the hematuria is not clearly glomerular in origin. A renal biopsy should be considered when there is glomerular hematuria or the possibility of familial disease (e.g., Alport's syndrome, IgA nephropathy) because this aids the decision-making process by clarifying the prospective donor's future risk of progressive renal disease.[51]

Those with a history of bilateral or recurrent stones and those with systemic conditions associated with recurrent stone disease should not donate. An asymptomatic potential donor with a current single stone is suitable if the donor does not have a high risk of recurrence, if the stone is smaller than 1.5 cm, and especially if the stone is potentially removable during transplantation.[45] The evaluation of an asymptomatic donor with a single prior episode of nephrolithiasis should include evaluation of serum calcium, creatinine, albumin, and parathyroid hormone levels; spot urine for cystine; urinalysis and urine culture; spiral computed tomographic scan; chemical analysis of the stone, if available; and 24-hour urine measurement of oxalate, urate, and creatinine.

Atherosclerotic renal vascular disease is a relative contraindication to living donation. If it is discovered, the donor should be normotensive, have normal renal function, and have only unilateral disease.[52] Careful evaluation for coronary disease and peripheral vascular disease should be undertaken, given the significant association of renovascular disease with atherosclerosis elsewhere. Fibromuscular dysplasia is found in 2% to 4% of prospective donors. Donors with severe and diffuse disease should not be accepted for donation. The age of the prospective donor should also be considered, with the outcome in donors older than 50 years more predictable and benign than in younger donors.[53]

Malignant Disease

A past history of certain malignant neoplasms is considered a contraindication to live kidney donation. These include melanoma, testicular cancer, renal cell carcinoma, bronchial and breast cancer, choriocarcinoma, hematologic malignant neoplasm, and multiple myeloma.[45] A history of malignant disease may be acceptable for donation if prior treatment of the malignant neoplasm does not decrease renal reserve or place the donor at increased risk of renal disease and prior treatment of malignant disease does not increase the operative risk of nephrectomy. A history of malignant disease may be acceptable if the specific cancer is curable and transmission of the cancer can reasonably be excluded; consultation with an oncologist may be required. Consent to receive a renal transplant must include a discussion with the donor and the recipient that risk of transmission of malignant disease cannot be completely excluded.

Cardiovascular and Pulmonary Disease

In prospective donors, the cardiac assessment should be based on the history, risk factors, examination, and electrocardiographic findings. An exercise or pharmacologic stress test and echocardiography may be warranted in certain circumstances.

Individuals with myocardial dysfunction or coronary ischemia are at increased anesthetic risk and should generally not donate. Pulmonary contraindications to donation include chronic lung diseases that significantly increase the anesthetic risk. If it is indicated by history and examination, pulmonary function testing, echocardiography, or sleep studies should be performed. In all cases, donors should cease smoking for at least 8 to 12 weeks before surgery to minimize the risk of postoperative pneumonia.

COMPATIBILITY AND IMMUNOLOGIC CONSIDERATIONS

Blood Group Compatibility

Traditionally, transplantation across incompatible blood groups has been avoided owing to the risk of hyperacute rejection mediated by preformed anti-A or anti-B antibodies to the carbohydrate blood group antigens, expressed by endothelial cells as well as by red blood cells. In recent years, ABO-incompatible transplantation has become more widespread, largely on the basis of excellent outcomes described initially by Japanese units.[54] "Desensitizing" the recipient can avert hyperacute rejection. This involves removal of blood group antibodies by plasma exchange or immunoadsorption to achieve target titers. Preemptive splenectomy or rituximab administration (anti-CD20 monoclonal antibody) is often also employed; however, the need for these measures is not clear.[55] Rejection is predicted by high initial antibody titers and high rebound titers early after transplantation.[56] Further plasma exchange or immunoadsorption is generally required after transplantation for at least 2 weeks to reduce the chances of rejection. With use of this protocol, patient and graft survival appears to be equivalent to that of blood group–compatible transplantation for the short to medium term (up to 9 years).[54] Longer term results are awaited. A comprehensive overview and summary of current approaches relating to antibody-incompatible transplants is available at the British Transplantation Society website, *www.bts.org.uk*.

HLA Compatibility

"Tissue typing" of recipient and donor determines their human leukocyte antigen (HLA) match. HLA antigens are coded on chromosome 6, with half (one haplotype) inherited from each parent. The major histocompatibility class I HLA-A and HLA-B and class II HLA-DR antigens are routinely determined as rejection responses are thought to most commonly stem from mismatches at these alleles. There is an increasing awareness of the importance of immune responses to other HLA antigens, and many centers now look for the presence of antibodies to HLA-C, HLA-DQ, and HLA-DP. A six-antigen (HLA-A, HLA-B, and HLA-DR) match confers a graft survival advantage compared with 0 antigen matches for both cadaveric and live donor transplantation of 10% at 10 years.[57,58] In addition to determination of the HLA compatibility, crossmatching and screening for anti-HLA antibodies are performed to assess the risk of rejection.

Assessing HLA Sensitization

The principle of screening for antibodies against HLA antigens using panel reactivity is shown in Figure 98.13. IgG antibodies against class I (HLA-A and HLA-B) antigens are highly associated with acute rejection and are a contraindication to transplantation. IgM antibodies against HLA antigens may also predict rejection if they are present in current but not past sera; however, they may also be falsely positive. Prior treatment of sera with dithiothreitol can remove IgM antibodies and aid in the interpretation of the test (Fig. 98.14). Autoantibodies (such as may occur in lupus) may also give false-positive results and can be determined by prior absorption with autologous lymphocytes.

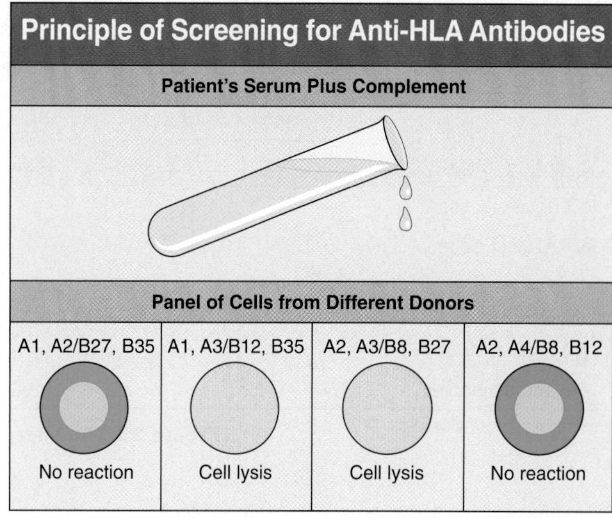

Figure 98.13 Principle of screening for anti-HLA antibodies. The patient's serum is tested with a panel of cells of known HLA types. The most common HLA antigens are represented in such panels. In this example, the A3 antigen is the only antigen present in the two lysed cell populations and absent from the nonlysed samples. Therefore, the patient's serum contains anti-HLA A3 antibodies.

Sensitization to HLA antigens generally occurs through blood transfusion, pregnancy, or prior transplantation. Presence in the recipient of antibodies to donor-specific HLA antigens can result in hyperacute rejection. Crossmatching of donor lymphocytes with recipient serum allows screening for this possibility. Terasaki and coworkers pioneered the complement-dependent cytotoxicity (CDC) crossmatch.[59] This assay determines the presence of antibodies thought to be of clinical significance by mixing donor T or B lymphocytes with recipient serum in the presence of complement. The sensitivity of the assay can be augmented by the addition of anti–human globulin. Presence of a positive T-cell CDC crossmatch to the donor is highly predictive of hyperacute rejection,[59,60] whereas a B-cell CDC crossmatch is more subject to false-positives but should prompt a search for donor-specific antibodies.[61] A positive T-cell crossmatch is an absolute contraindication to transplantation.

The flow crossmatch is more sensitive than the CDC in detecting antibody capable of binding to donor T or B lymphocytes. Binding of antibody from donor serum is detected by flow cytometry after probing with a fluorescein-labeled anti-immunoglobulin antibody. The predictive value of a positive flow crossmatch for rejection is less than that of a CDC crossmatch because of its increased sensitivity, and it does not assess the ability of the antibody to fix complement. In most centers, it is not routinely performed before cadaveric donor transplants, but it is commonly performed in a live donor transplant workup. A positive flow crossmatch (with a negative CDC crossmatch) is not an absolute contraindication to proceeding; however, it may lead the team to alter the immunosuppressive regimen (e.g., desensitization protocol) to decrease the risk or severity of antibody-mediated rejection.

Interpretation of the Crossmatch Test					
	Crossmatch (normal procedure)		Crossmatch (dithiothreitol)		Risk of Antibody-Mediated Graft Damage
Antibody to MHC Class	T Cells	B Cells	T Cells	B Cells	
IgG against class I	+	+	+	+	Yes
IgM against class I	+	+	–	–	Yes, IgM class I antibodies may be harmless if present in old sera only but not in the current serum
IgG against class II	–	+	–	+	Yes
IgM against class II	–	+	–	–	Unknown
IgM autoantibodies	+	+	–	–	No

Figure 98.14 Interpretation of the crossmatch test.

Determination of the presence of anti-HLA antibodies in the recipient's serum is increasingly used as a means of predicting rejection. This virtual crossmatch compares the specificity of the antibodies identified with the prospective donor's HLA typing. Donor-specific anti-HLA antibodies are correlated with worse graft survival even in the setting of a negative crossmatch.[62] As well as through panel reactive antibody testing, antibodies can be detected by enzyme-linked immunosorbent assay or more sensitive antigen-coated bead technology (Luminex). Beads are coated with a single HLA antigen and are mixed with recipient serum and probed with a fluorescein-labeled anti-immunoglobulin antibody. Beads that bind antibody are therefore identified by fluorescence. The decision on whether to proceed with transplantation in the context of this information is complex. Current recommendations for detection and characterization of clinically relevant antibodies in solid organ transplantation are summarized by the British Society of Histocompatibility and British Transplantation Society and are available at *www.bts.org.uk*.

REFERENCES

1. Wolfe RA, Ashby VB, Milford EL, et al. Comparison of mortality in all patients on dialysis, patients on dialysis awaiting transplantation, and recipients of a first cadaveric transplant. *N Engl J Med.* 1999;341:1725-1730.
2. Fritsche L, Vanrenterghem Y, Nordal KP, et al. Practice variations in the evaluation of adult candidates for cadaveric kidney transplantation: A survey of the European Transplant Centers. *Transplantation.* 2000;70:1492-1497.
3. European Best Practice Guidelines for Renal Transplantation (part 1). *Nephrol Dial Transplant.* 2000;15(Suppl 7):1-85.
4. Kasiske BL, Cangro CB, Hariharan S, et al. The evaluation of renal transplantation candidates: Clinical practice guidelines. *Am J Transplant.* 2001;1(Suppl 2):3-95.
5. Knoll G, Cockfield S, Blydt-Hansen T, et al. Canadian Society of Transplantation: Consensus guidelines on eligibility for kidney transplantation. *CMAJ.* 2005;173:S1-S25.
6. Kasiske BL, Malik MA, Herzog CA. Risk-stratified screening for ischemic heart disease in kidney transplant candidates. *Transplantation.* 2005;80:815-820.
7. Pilmore H. Cardiac assessment for renal transplantation. *Am J Transplant.* 2006;6:659-665.
8. Rabbat CG, Treleaven DJ, Russell JD, et al. Prognostic value of myocardial perfusion studies in patients with end-stage renal disease assessed for kidney or kidney-pancreas transplantation: A meta-analysis. *J Am Soc Nephrol.* 2003;14:431-439.
9. Oliveras A, Roquer J, Puig JM, et al. Stroke in renal transplant recipients: Epidemiology, predictive risk factors and outcome. *Clin Transplant.* 2003;17:1-8.
10. Chambers BR, Donnan GA. Carotid endarterectomy for asymptomatic carotid stenosis. Cochrane Database Syst Rev. 2005;4:CD001923.
11. Makisalo H, Lepantalo M, Halme L, et al. Peripheral arterial disease as a predictor of outcome after renal transplantation. *Transpl Int.* 1998;11(Suppl 1):S140-S143.
12. Webster AC, Craig JC, Simpson JM, et al. Identifying high risk groups and quantifying absolute risk of cancer after kidney transplantation: A cohort study of 15,183 recipients. *Am J Transplant.* 2007;7:2140-2151.
13. Buell JF, Gross TG, Woodle ES. Malignancy after transplantation. *Transplantation.* 2005;80:S254-S264.
14. Vajdic CM, McDonald SP, McCredie MR, et al. Cancer incidence before and after kidney transplantation. *JAMA.* 2006;296:2823-2831.
15. Spital A. Should all human immunodeficiency virus–infected patients with end-stage renal disease be excluded from transplantation? The views of U.S. transplant centers. *Transplantation.* 1998;65:1187-1191.
16. Roland ME, Barin B, Carlson L, et al. HIV-infected liver and kidney transplant recipients: 1- and 3-year outcomes. *Am J Transplant.* 2008;8:355-365.
17. Fabrizi F, Martin P, Dixit V, et al. HBsAg seropositive status and survival after renal transplantation: Meta-analysis of observational studies. *Am J Transplant.* 2005;5:2913-2921.
18. Pereira BJ, Natov SN, Bouthot BA, et al. Effects of hepatitis C infection and renal transplantation on survival in end-stage renal disease. The New England Organ Bank Hepatitis C Study Group. *Kidney Int.* 1998;53:1374-1381.
19. Abbott KC, Klote MM. Update on guidelines for prevention and management of *Mycobacterium tuberculosis* infections after transplant. *Am J Transplant.* 2005;5:1163.
20. Meier-Kriesche HU, Arndorfer JA, Kaplan B. The impact of body mass index on renal transplant outcomes: A significant independent risk factor for graft failure and patient death. *Transplantation.* 2002;73:70-74.
21. Chang SH, Coates PT, McDonald SP. Effects of body mass index at transplant on outcomes of kidney transplantation. *Transplantation.* 2007;84:981-987.
22. Chadban S. Glomerulonephritis recurrence in the renal graft. *J Am Soc Nephrol.* 2001;12:394-402.
23. Kao LS, Flowers C, Flum DR. Prophylactic cholecystectomy in transplant patients: A decision analysis. *J Gastrointest Surg.* 2005;9:965-972.
24. Johnston O, Rose C, Landsberg D, et al. Nephrectomy after transplant failure: Current practice and outcomes. *Am J Transplant.* 2007;7:1961-1967.
25. Ayus JC, Achinger SG. At the peril of dialysis patients: Ignoring the failed transplant. *Semin Dial.* 2005;18:180-184.
26. Nishinaka H, Nakafusa Y, Hirano T, et al. Graft persistence effectively induces and maintains donor-specific unresponsiveness. *J Surg Res.* 1997;68:145-152.
27. Kootstra G, van Heurn E. Non-heartbeating donation of kidneys for transplantation. *Nat Clin Pract Nephrol.* 2007;3:154-163.
28. Chapman J, Bock A, Dussol B, et al. Follow-up after renal transplantation with organs from donors after cardiac death. *Transpl Int.* 2006;19:715-719.
29. Pascual J, Zamora J, Pirsch JD. A systematic review of kidney transplantation from expanded criteria donors. *Am J Kidney Dis.* 2008;52:553-586.

30. Buell JF, Trofe J, Sethuraman G, et al. Donors with central nervous system malignancies: Are they truly safe? *Transplantation*. 2003;76: 340-343.
31. Morath C, Schwenger V, Schmidt J, Zeier M. Transmission of malignancy with solid organ transplants. *Transplantation*. 2005;80: S164-S166.
32. Remuzzi G, Cravedi P, Perna A, et al. Long-term outcome of renal transplantation from older donors. *N Engl J Med*. 2006; 354:343-352.
33. Singh A, Stablein D, Tejani A. Risk factors for vascular thrombosis in pediatric renal transplantation: A special report of the North American Pediatric Renal Transplant Cooperative Study. *Transplantation*. 1997;63: 1263-1267.
34. Foss A, Gunther A, Line PD, et al. Long-term clinical outcome of paediatric kidneys transplanted to adults. *Nephrol Dial Transplant*. 2008;23:726-729.
35. Ibrahim HN, Foley R, Tan L, et al. Long-term consequences of kidney donation. *N Engl J Med*. 2009;360:459-469.
36. Segev DL, Kucirka LM, Gentry SE, Montgomery RA. Utilization and outcomes of kidney paired donation in the United States. *Transplantation*. 2008;86:502-510.
37. Roth AE, Sonmez T, Unver MU, et al. Utilizing list exchange and nondirected donation through "chain" paired kidney donations. *Am J Transplant*. 2006;6:2694-2705.
38. Friedman EA, Friedman AL. Payment for donor kidneys: Pros and cons. *Kidney Int*. 2006;69:960-962.
39. The Declaration of Istanbul on organ trafficking and transplant tourism. *Transplantation*. 2008;86:1013-1018.
40. Davis CL, Delmonico FL. Living-donor kidney transplantation: A review of the current practices for the live donor. *J Am Soc Nephrol*. 2005;16:2098-2110.
41. Matas AJ, Bartlett ST, Leichtman AB, Delmonico FL. Morbidity and mortality after living kidney donation, 1999-2001: Survey of United States transplant centers. *Am J Transplant*. 2003;3:830-834.
42. Friedman AL, Peters TG, Jones KW, et al. Fatal and nonfatal hemorrhagic complications of living kidney donation. *Ann Surg*. 2006;243:126-130.
43. Johnson EM, Anderson JK, Jacobs C, et al. Long-term follow-up of living kidney donors: Quality of life after donation. *Transplantation*. 1999;67:717-721.
44. Minz M, Udgiri N, Sharma A, et al. Prospective psychosocial evaluation of related kidney donors: Indian perspective. *Transplant Proc*. 2005;37:2001-2003.
45. Delmonico F. A Report of the Amsterdam Forum On the Care of the Live Kidney Donor: Data and Medical Guidelines. *Transplantation*. 2005;79:S53-S66.
46. Bia MJ, Ramos EL, Danovitch GM, et al. Evaluation of living renal donors. The current practice of US transplant centers. *Transplantation*. 1995;60:322-327.
47. Thiel GT, Nolte C, Tsinalis D. Living kidney donors with isolated medical abnormalities: The SOL-DHR experience. In: Gaston RS, Wadström J, eds. *Living Donor Kidney Transplantation*. London: Taylor & Francis; 2005:55-74.
48. Praga M, Hernandez E, Herrero JC, et al. Influence of obesity on the appearance of proteinuria and renal insufficiency after unilateral nephrectomy. *Kidney Int*. 2000;58:2111-2118.
49. Jaffe JS, Ginsberg PC, Gill R, Harkaway RC. A new diagnostic algorithm for the evaluation of microscopic hematuria. *Urology*. 2001;57:889-894.
50. Ierino FL, Kanellis J. Thin basement membrane nephropathy and renal transplantation. *Semin Nephrol*. 2005;25:184-187.
51. Koushik R, Garvey C, Manivel JC, et al. Persistent, asymptomatic, microscopic hematuria in prospective kidney donors. *Transplantation*. 2005;80:1425-1429.
52. Zierler RE, Bergelin RO, Davidson RC, et al. A prospective study of disease progression in patients with atherosclerotic renal artery stenosis. *Am J Hypertens*. 1996;9:1055-1061.
53. Indudhara R, Kenney, Bueschen AJ, Burns JR. Live donor nephrectomy in patients with fibromuscular dysplasia of the renal arteries. *J Urol*. 1999;162:678-681.
54. Takahashi K, Saito K, Takahara S, et al. Excellent long-term outcome of ABO-incompatible living donor kidney transplantation in Japan. *Am J Transplant*. 2004;4:1089-1096.
55. Tobian AA, Shirey RS, Montgomery RA, et al. The critical role of plasmapheresis in ABO-incompatible renal transplantation. *Transfusion*. 2008;48:2453-2460.
56. Shimmura H, Tanabe K, Ishikawa N, et al. Role of anti-A/B antibody titers in results of ABO-incompatible kidney transplantation. *Transplantation*. 2000;70:1331-1335.
57. Opelz G, Wujciak T, Dohler B, et al. HLA compatibility and organ transplant survival. Collaborative Transplant Study. *Rev Immunogenet*. 1999;1:334-342.
58. Opelz G. Impact of HLA compatibility on survival of kidney transplants from unrelated live donors. *Transplantation*. 1997;64:1473-1475.
59. Patel R, Mickey MR, Terasaki PI. Serotyping for homotransplantation. XVI. Analysis of kidney transplants from unrelated donors. *N Engl J Med*. 1968;279:501-506.
60. Stegall MD, Gloor J, Winters JL, et al. A comparison of plasmapheresis versus high-dose IVIG desensitization in renal allograft recipients with high levels of donor specific alloantibody. *Am J Transplant*. 2006;6: 346-351.
61. Pollinger HS, Stegall MD, Gloor JM, et al. Kidney transplantation in patients with antibodies against donor HLA class II. *Am J Transplant*. 2007;7:857-863.
62. Lefaucheur C, Suberbielle-Boissel C, Hill GS, et al. Clinical relevance of preformed HLA donor-specific antibodies in kidney transplantation. *Am J Transplant*. 2008;8:324-331.
63. Penn I. The effect of immunosuppression on pre-existing cancers. *Transplantation*. 1993;55:742-747.

CHAPTER 99

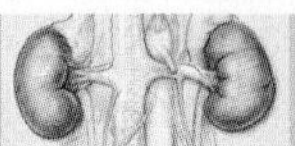

Kidney Transplantation Surgery

Adam D. Barlow, Nicholas R. Brook, Michael L. Nicholson

SOURCES OF KIDNEYS FOR TRANSPLANTATION

The usual and most frequent source of kidneys for transplantation has been donation before cardiac death (DBD), formerly known as the heart-beating cadaveric donor. The increasing worldwide discrepancy between the availability of and need for renal allografts[1] has led to the increasing use of alternative sources of organs, including donation after cardiac death (DCD) cadaveric donors (previously known as non–heart-beating donors) and live donors. The evaluation and selection of donors are discussed in Chapter 98. Here we discuss surgical aspects of retrieval and transplantation of kidneys.

DONATION BEFORE CARDIAC DEATH DONORS

The potential DBD donor is maintained by artificial ventilation in a critical care setting until death has been diagnosed by brainstem death criteria,[2] the consent of the next of kin for donation has been given, and the necessary legal and institutional approvals have been obtained.

In the operating room, the initial step is cannulation of the aorta and inferior vena cava while the heart is still beating. This allows perfusion of the organs with cold preservative solution immediately before cardiac arrest, minimizing warm ischemia. The priorities of the organ retrieval team are influenced by the range of organs being donated. Heart, lung, and liver retrieval take priority over kidney retrieval, which may significantly lengthen the ischemic time. The kidneys are removed *en bloc*, and the artery is typically retrieved with a cuff of aorta (Carrel patch), with the maximum achievable length of renal vein and 10 to 15 cm of ureter. The length of the right renal vein may be maximized by including a portion of inferior vena cava in continuity. Care is taken to avoid damage to polar and other accessory arteries, especially the lower pole artery, which may supply the ureter; stripping of adventitial tissue from the ureter must also be avoided, which may also compromise its blood supply.

The kidneys are flushed with ice-cold preservation fluid until the effluent is clear and then are stored for transport in crushed ice or on a perfusion machine (see Renal Preservation).

DONATION AFTER CARDIAC DEATH DONORS

Before consensus on the definition of brainstem death, DCD donors were the main source of transplant organs. These donors were intensive care unit based and had suffered head injuries or cerebrovascular accidents deemed irrecoverable, but organ retrieval could proceed only after cardiorespiratory death. This changed with the introduction of brainstem death legislation, but the use of DCD kidneys has recently increased again in response to the shortage of suitable organs for transplantation. An international consensus has defined categories of DCD donors[3] to facilitate legal and ethical discussion and to highlight possible differences in organ viability (see Fig. 98.7). DCD kidneys suffer a period of warm ischemia (the period between cardiac death and the time that *in situ* cold perfusion is started). The duration of ischemia correlates with rates of primary nonfunction, delayed graft function, acute rejection, and allograft and patient survival. The main requirement of organ procurement from DCD donors is therefore to achieve rapid *in situ* perfusion of the kidneys to limit warm ischemia. This requires an emergency response team of surgeons and transplant coordinators, with considerable on-call and logistic commitments.

DCD donors may be either uncontrolled (Maastricht categories I and II) or controlled (Maastricht categories III to V) (Fig. 98.7). In controlled donors, cardiac arrest is expected, and it is therefore possible to reduce the warm ischemia time to only a few minutes, as the surgical retrieval team will be on standby. Unexpected donor cardiac arrest may result in prolonged warm ischemia times. The duration of reversible warm ischemia time that the human kidney can sustain is unknown, but DCD kidneys with warm ischemia exceeding 60 minutes are considered by many to be of marginal suitability.

Donation After Cardiac Death Protocol

Centers involved with DCD donation should adhere to the Maastricht protocol,[4] which includes the following principles:

- Approval by the local medical ethics committee.
- Diagnosis of death by physicians who are independent of the transplantation team.
- 10-minute rule (after declaration of cardiac death, the body is left untouched for a period of 10 minutes before intervention).
- Rapid *in situ* cooling by a catheter inserted into the aorta.
- Organ retrieval by standard surgical techniques.

Uncontrolled DCD Donors

After a period of unsuccessful resuscitation and confirmation of cardiac death and observation of the 10-minute rule, cardiac massage and ventilation with 100% oxygen are recommenced in an attempt to deliver oxygenated blood to the kidneys. A mechanical resuscitation device may be used. *In situ* renal cooling is effected by placing a double-balloon, triple-lumen perfusion catheter into the aorta through a femoral artery cutdown (Fig. 99.1), with instillation of preservation solution.

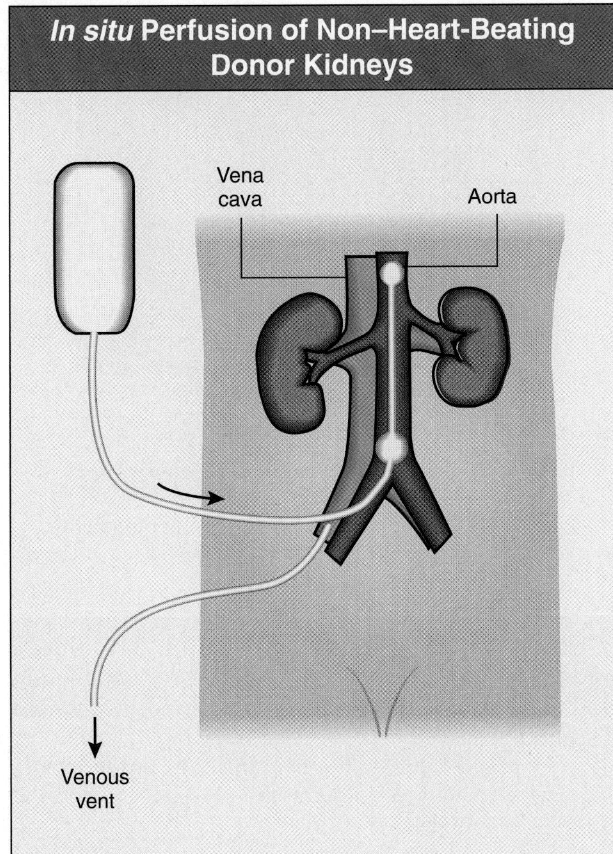

Figure 99.1 Technique for *in situ* perfusion of donation after cardiac death kidneys. A double-lumen, double-balloon arterial catheter is introduced through the femoral artery; the lower balloon is inflated at the aortic bifurcation and the upper balloon above the renal arteries. Ice-cold perfusion fluid is introduced and vented through the femoral vein until the effluent becomes clear.

Alternatively, the donor can be moved to an operating room as soon as death has occurred, and the aortic perfusion catheter is placed directly at laparotomy rather than through a femoral artery cutdown.

Controlled DCD Donors

Here the transplantation team awaits cardiac arrest; after confirmation of death, the 10-minute rule is observed, and then the perfusion catheter is inserted through the femoral artery. Alternatively, the patient can be taken to the operating room before cardiac death if the next of kin gives consent.

LIVE KIDNEY DONORS

In the United States in 2008, 45% of renal transplants were from live donors,[5] compared with 25% in the United Kingdom.[6] After a rapid increase in live donor transplantation at the beginning of this decade, rates have become more static. The superior recipient post-transplantation outcome compared with kidneys from deceased donors,[7] the potential for preemptive transplantation before dialysis, and the ability to plan the procedure (allowing optimization of the recipient's condition) are major advantages and justify continued efforts to expand live donation. The medical evaluation of the live donor is discussed in Chapter 98 (see Figs. 98.10 and 98.11).

Preoperative Imaging

Preoperative imaging of live donors confirms the presence of two functioning kidneys, indicates disease that would preclude donation, and provides anatomic information necessary for planning of the procedure. Imaging assumes paramount importance before minimal access donor nephrectomy because of the reduced operative exposure and particular difficulties in the identification of complex renal vein tributaries. The location, size, and number of renal veins and tributaries need to be accurately described preoperatively. Angiography combined with excretion urography is now obsolete. For preoperative description of the main renal artery and vein anatomy, magnetic resonance angiography and computed tomographic angiography are comparable,[8] but computed tomographic angiography is more sensitive and specific for complex vascular anatomy and provides excellent correlation between imaging and surgical findings (Fig. 99.2).[9]

Minimal Access Donor Nephrectomy

Live donor nephrectomy has traditionally been performed through an open incision, necessitating a prolonged period of recovery. This and the cosmetic implications of a large flank wound may discourage potential donors (Fig. 99.3). To reduce such disincentives, there has been a move toward minimally invasive donor nephrectomy, first performed as a transperitoneal laparoscopic procedure (laparoscopic donor nephrectomy [LapDN]).[10] LapDN is associated with decreased severity and duration of postoperative pain, shorter inpatient stay, quicker return to work and normal activities, and improved cosmetic result compared with open donor nephrectomy (Fig. 99.4).[11] Furthermore, the overall societal cost of LapDN is lower, and the recipient's quality of life scores are higher.[12] The procedure is technically demanding, however, and there is potential for damage to the renal parenchyma, vessels, and ureter during dissection. It takes longer than open nephrectomy and exposes the allograft to a longer period of warm ischemia.[11]

Nevertheless, retrospective data suggest that minimal access donor nephrectomy not only offers postoperative advantages to the donor but also increases the number of transplants performed by reducing donor disincentives; estimates range from a 25% to a 100%[13] increase in transplantation activity. The widespread introduction of LapDN at the beginning of this decade saw an initial dramatic increase in the number of live kidney donors. However, rates have been static in both the United States and the United Kingdom during the last 5 years, suggesting that we may have seen the maximum benefits of this effect. Three minimal access approaches have been described: transperitoneal, extraperitoneal, and hand-assisted live donor nephrectomy.

Transperitoneal Laparoscopic Donor Nephrectomy

Pneumoperitoneum is established, and four laparoscopic ports are usually required (Fig. 99.5). After laparoscopic dissection, a Pfannenstiel incision is made through which the kidney is brought out within an endoscopy retrieval bag after control and division of the artery, vein, and ureter.

Hand-Assisted Laparoscopic Donor Nephrectomy

The hand-assisted technique allows tactile sense to facilitate dissection, retraction, and exposure. It is said to be easier to learn and can be safely and efficiently performed by surgeons with less laparoscopic experience. The hand-assisted device allows the

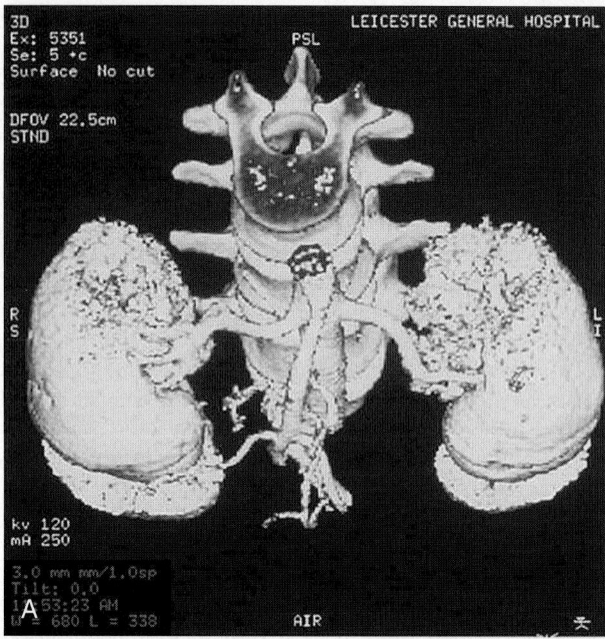

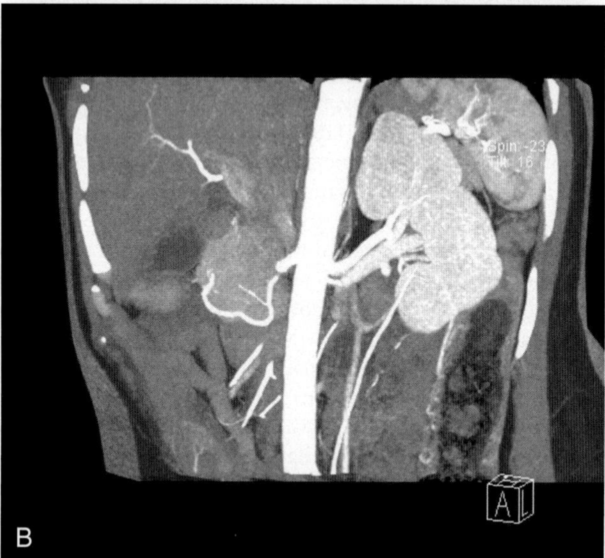

Figure 99.2 Live donor preoperative computed tomographic angiography. A, Three-dimensional reconstruction of arterial supply. Note the lower pole artery to the right kidney *(arrow)*, which may supply the ureter as well as the lower pole parenchyma. **B,** Conventional image showing single artery and vein to the left kidney.

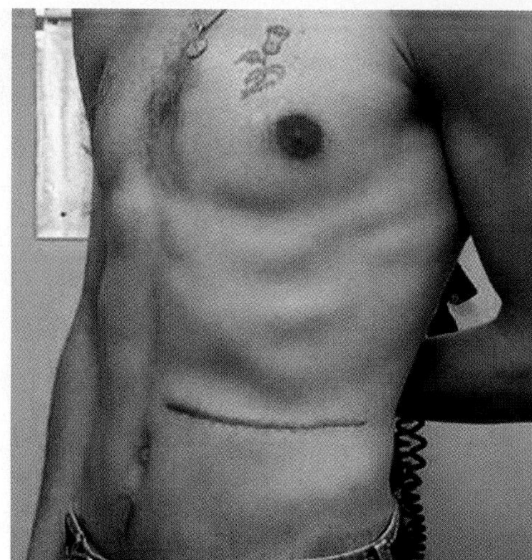

Figure 99.3 Flank wound from open nephrectomy.

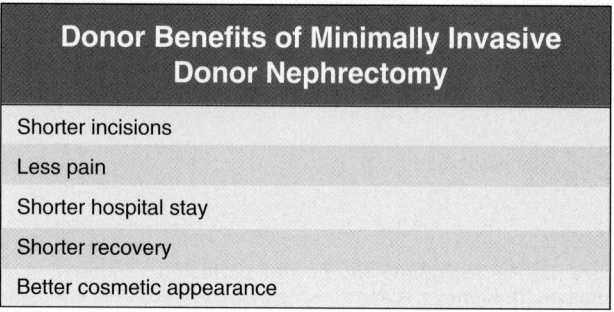

Donor Benefits of Minimally Invasive Donor Nephrectomy
Shorter incisions
Less pain
Shorter hospital stay
Shorter recovery
Better cosmetic appearance

Figure 99.4 Donor benefits of minimally invasive donor nephrectomy.

operator's nondominant hand to enter the abdomen through an airtight system.

Retroperitoneoscopic Operative Technique

The retroperitoneal approach avoids breaching the peritoneum, displays the renal anatomy in a very different manner, and may be easier for retrieval of the full length of the vessels, especially on the right side. The disadvantage is that a more limited operating space is available than with the transperitoneal or hand-assisted laparoscopic techniques.

Contraindications to Minimal Access Donor Nephrectomy

There are no absolute contraindications other than those applying to the open operation. The relative contraindications are dictated by donor factors and the experience of the surgeon. The donor must be fit for anesthesia, including the physiologic stress of pneumoperitoneum. Obesity is a relative contraindication to both open and laparoscopic surgery, and the hand-assisted approach may be better suited in such patients. Previous abdominal surgery is another relative contraindication because of the potential for adhesions. Multiplicity of renal vessels should not hinder LapDN.

Effect of Pneumoperitoneum

Transient intraoperative oliguria secondary to decreased renal blood flow is a frequent occurrence during laparoscopic procedures. Proposed mechanisms include decreased cardiac output, renal vein compression, ureteral obstruction, renal parenchymal compression, and systemic hormonal effects. Intracranial pressure increases during pneumoperitoneum, with release of vasoconstrictor agents that decrease renal blood flow. Use of a lower pressure reduces the adverse effects of pneumoperitoneum on renal perfusion. In donor nephrectomy, impaired renal blood flow may compromise early allograft function and compound the damaging effects of warm and cold ischemia and operative manipulation of the kidney. Laparoscopically derived donor kidneys have higher serum creatinine up to 1 month after transplantation compared with open surgery, but thereafter graft function is equivalent.[14] The pioneers of LapDN report using high volumes of crystalloid preoperatively and intraoperatively to maintain renal perfusion in the presence of pneumoperitoneum. The authors have seen two episodes of unilateral

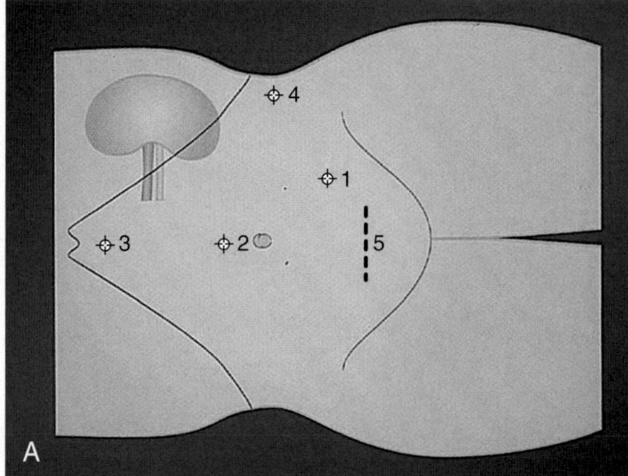

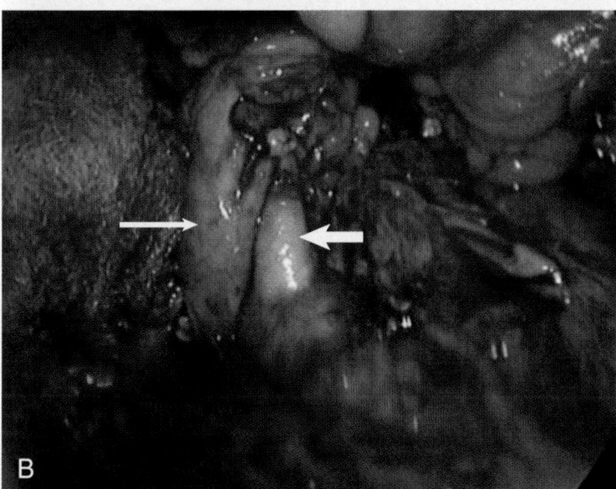

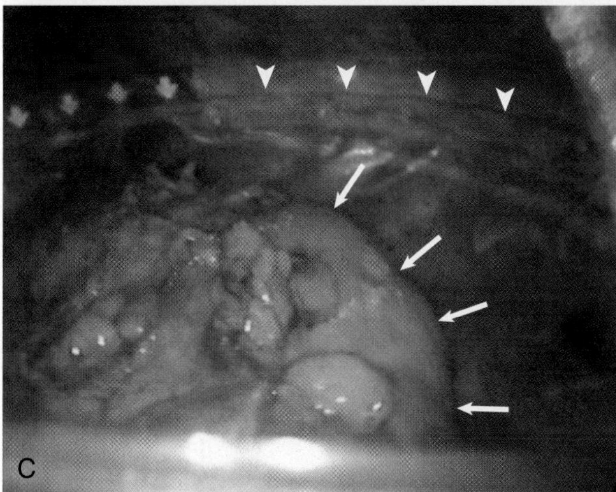

Figure 99.5 Technique for laparoscopic donor nephrectomy. A, Positions for four laparoscopic ports (1 to 4) and Pfannenstiel incision (5) through which the kidney is removed. **B,** Intraoperative view showing left renal artery *(short arrow)* and vein *(long arrow)* prepared for control and division. **C,** Intraoperative view showing the kidney *(arrows)* in the endoscopic retrieval bag *(arrowheads mark edge of bag)*.

pulmonary edema in the dependent lung, and we now recommend volume loading of the donor with 2 liters of crystalloid the night before surgery and use of replacement fluid only during surgery. This protocol has led to no apparent detriment to graft function.

Graft Function and Acute Rejection

There is no consistent evidence that graft function differs between kidneys retrieved by open, laparoscopic, or hand-assisted donor nephrectomy. The exception is that rates of delayed graft function and acute rejection may be higher in pediatric recipients, especially the 0- to 5-year age group.

Pretransplantation ischemia could, in theory, render the donor kidney more immunogenic by inducing major histocompatibility complex class II expression. However, despite the longer warm ischemia time, acute rejection rates and severity of rejection are not higher in laparoscopic than in open live donor kidneys.

Technical Issues

Ureteral ischemia was more common in early experience of LapDN, but it can be avoided if care is taken to ensure that sufficient periureteral tissue is taken and that the dissection does not occur too close to the renal pelvis.

Multiple arteries need not be a barrier to successful use of grafts from laparoscopic donors. In open donor nephrectomy, the right kidney is retrieved in 20% to 30% of cases, whereas LapDN uses the right kidney in less than 10%,[15] reflecting concern about the operative safety of the right-sided laparoscopic operation, principally the difficulties involved in obtaining an adequate length of renal vein. It has been argued that this practice has led to compromise of the principle that the better kidney should remain with the donor.

Postoperative Recovery

After uneventful open nephrectomy, the donor can expect to be discharged from the hospital in 5 or 6 days and can return to work in 8 to 12 weeks. After LapDN, the donor usually leaves the hospital in 2 to 4 days and can return to work in 4 to 6 weeks.

Choice of Donor Operative Technique

The choice of operative procedure depends on the local expertise of the surgeons. There is accumulating evidence that the laparoscopic operation removes some of the disincentives to donation, and this approach is likely to be adopted widely in the future.

RENAL PRESERVATION

Preservation of deceased donor organs is crucial to allow time for matching, sharing of organs, and preparation of the recipient. Damage from hypothermia and reperfusion must be minimized. There is little standardization of the type of preservation solution used. Marshall's hyperosmolar citrate solution and histidine-tryptophan-ketoglutarate are popular choices in Europe, but the University of Wisconsin solution is more commonly used in the United States as extended preservation times are more commonly required.

Organs can be preserved by cold storage (kept in crushed ice after flushing with preservation solution) or by machine-driven pulsatile perfusion. The proposed benefits of machine perfusion come from allowance of aerobic function through provision of oxygen and substrate and removal of metabolic end products. Although machine perfusion has been used for many years, there is still no consensus about its superiority to cold storage or about the best perfusion parameters.

Decisions on the use of a kidney from a marginal donor can be supported by data from machine perfusion. High perfusion pressures are associated with primary nonfunction and delayed graft function.

RENAL TRANSPLANTATION PROCEDURE

The transplanted kidney is placed heterotopically in one or other iliac fossa. The inferior epigastric vessels are ligated, as is the round ligament of the uterus in female patients. On occasion, the inferior epigastric artery may be preserved and used for revascularization of small polar arteries. In male patients, the spermatic cord is mobilized and preserved. The peritoneum should not be breached but instead swept superiorly to reveal the extraperitoneal bed into which the transplanted kidney will be placed. The iliac blood vessels are then mobilized, with care taken to meticulously ligate all the associated lymphatic channels to reduce the risk of post-transplantation lymphatic leak.

Vascular Anastomosis

The renal vein is anastomosed end to side to the external iliac vein. The arterial anastomosis can be performed either end to side to the external iliac artery or end to end to the divided internal iliac artery (Fig. 99.6). The end-to-side anastomosis is technically easier and is the usual method employed in cadaveric transplantation, in which it is possible to include a Carrel aortic patch with the renal artery.

With live donor kidneys, it is not possible to include a Carrel patch, and it is preferable to anastomose the renal artery end to end to the divided internal iliac artery. If there is no Carrel patch and the internal iliac artery is not available for anastomosis because of severe atheroma, it is possible to anastomose the renal artery directly to the external iliac artery without a patch. However, the external iliac artery has a much thicker wall than the renal vessel, increasing the likelihood of technical errors, in particular, narrowing of the anastomosis.

After completion of the vascular anastomoses, the kidney must sit in such a position that the renal vessels are not kinked. The transplanted kidney can be placed laterally in the iliac fossa, or it may be placed in a subrectus pouch fashioned specifically for the purpose.[16] In the latter case, the renal vessels run laterally from the kidney, and this needs to be noted in performing a post-transplantation biopsy. An operative diagram of the position of the kidney and vessels is therefore a vital component of the clinical notes.

If there are multiple renal vessels, the number of anastomoses should be minimized. This can usually be achieved by careful bench surgery before implantation. If there are two or more renal arteries, their aortic patches are joined in such a way that a single arterial anastomosis is required. If necessary, recipient iliac artery or saphenous vein is used to facilitate reconstruction. Small polar arteries will occasionally be recognized only after a kidney has been retrieved, and it is particularly important to reanastomose lower polar arteries accurately as these may provide all the ureteral blood supply. In the case of double renal veins, the most common course of action is simply to ligate the smaller vein; the larger one is usually sufficient to drain the whole kidney. If there are two equally sized veins, both may need to be anastomosed separately to the external iliac vein.

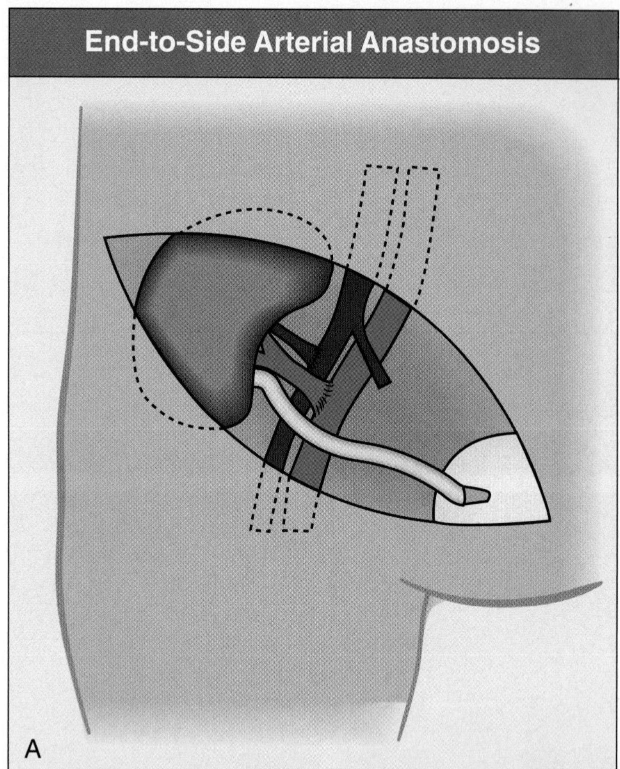

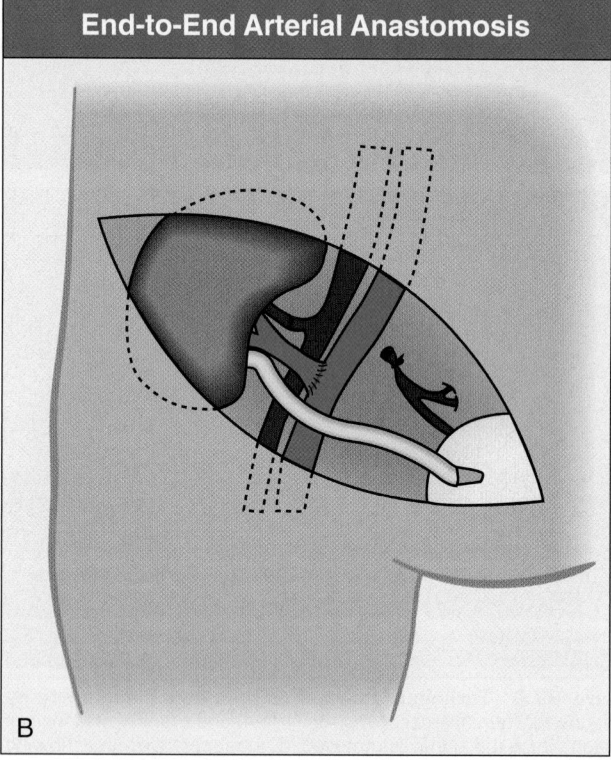

Figure 99.6 Vascular anastomosis techniques for renal transplantation. A, End-to-side anastomosis to the external iliac artery. **B,** End-to-end anastomosis to the divided internal iliac artery, suitable for live donor transplantation in which no aortic patch is available.

Urinary Drainage

The traditional method of ureteral anastomosis is the Politano-Leadbetter technique, involving a transvesical ureteroneocystostomy with creation of a submucosal antireflux tunnel. The end of the transplanted ureter is drawn through a submucosal tunnel from outside to inside and sutured to the bladder mucosa. Many surgeons now prefer the technically simpler extravesical ureteroneocystostomy onlay, in which the spatulated end of the ureter is anastomosed to the cystostomy and the divided muscle layer is then resutured over the ureter to create a short antireflux muscle tunnel. The onlay method has the advantage of being possible with only a short length of ureter. The shorter the ureter, the less likely it is that there will be an inadequate blood supply to the distal end, thereby reducing the risks of ischemic ureteral leaks or stenosis. A temporary double-J ureteral stent is usually placed. Stents reduce the impact of small technical errors while the ureter is leaking and reduce major urologic complications to an incidence of 1.5%.[17] However, they are a potential source of urinary infection, can become encrusted or blocked by debris, and can migrate or fragment. Nevertheless, antibiotic prophylaxis is not justified as it increases the risk of infection with multiresistant organisms. Another danger is the forgotten stent that has not been removed, which should always be considered in patients with unexplained and persistent lower urinary tract symptoms after transplantation. Stents are usually removed 4 to 6 weeks after transplantation, and this can be performed without general anesthesia by use of a flexible cystoscope.

Alternative Techniques of Urinary Reconstruction

Renal transplantation is commonly performed in patients who have abnormal bladders. In many cases, it is possible to anastomose the transplanted ureter to the bladder in the hope that the bladder can be rehabilitated, if necessary, by post-transplantation intermittent self-catheterization. Nonetheless, some patients require urinary diversion with an ileal conduit. The conduit should be fashioned at least 6 weeks before transplantation, but it may have been present for many years. If so, a CT conduitogram should be performed before transplant to exclude conduit stenosis (rare) and to delineate conduit anatomy and position. The transplanted kidney is best placed in the ipsilateral iliac fossa to avoid tension in the ureter, and it may be preferable to deliberately place the transplanted kidney upside down so that the ureter runs cranially and has a more direct route to the conduit. After revascularization, the peritoneum is opened and the ureter is anastomosed to the conduit over a double-J stent. Excellent long-term results have been achieved with this technique.[18]

Drainage and Wound Closure

Both the transplant bed and the subcutaneous tissues are drained to prevent the accumulation of serosanguineous fluid or lymph around the transplanted kidney. The skin is best closed with a subcuticular absorbable suture and then dressed with a clear adhesive dressing so that ultrasound scanning can be performed early without disturbing the wound. Metal skin clips make ultrasound more difficult, and some units avoid using them for this reason.

Postoperative Course

The recipient is nursed in a general ward with standard precautions and no need for reverse barrier nursing. If recovery is straightforward, the bladder catheter and wound drains are usually removed by day 5, and the recipient is fit for discharge after 7 to 10 days to be kept under close outpatient monitoring.

SURGICAL COMPLICATIONS OF RENAL TRANSPLANTATION

There is a small but significant incidence of technical complications, which can be minimized by avoiding damage to the kidneys at the time of the retrieval. Nonetheless, the presence of multiple renal vessels and donor atherosclerotic disease do increase the likelihood of technical problems in the recipient, as do recipient obesity, atherosclerosis, and previous transplantation.

The two most common clinical presentations requiring evaluation in the early postoperative period are sudden oliguria or anuria and pain or swelling over the graft. Algorithms to aid in the management of these problems can be found in Figures 99.7 and 99.8. A discussion of common surgical complications follows.

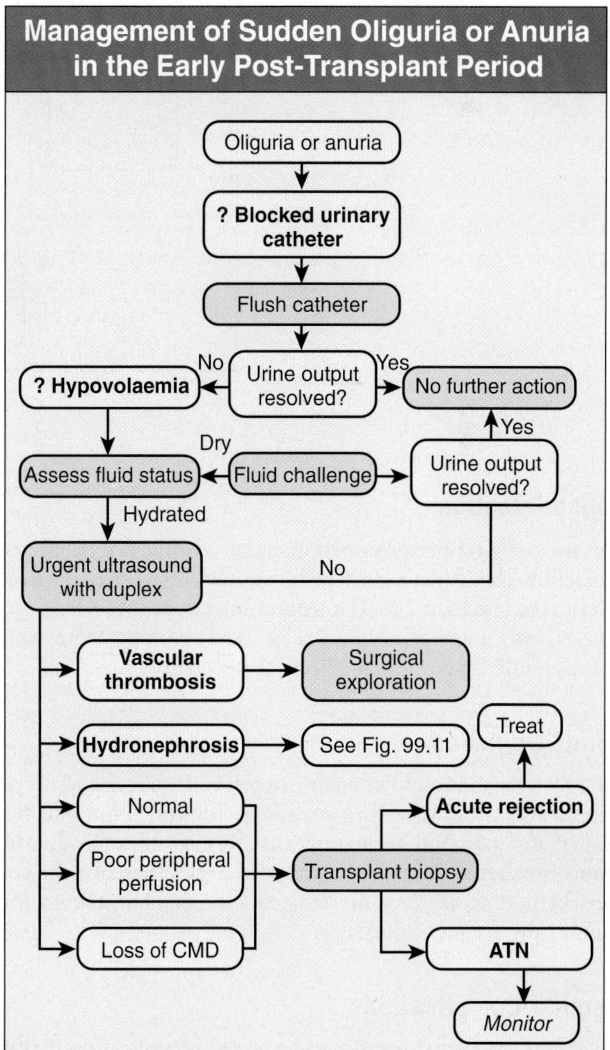

Figure 99.7 Management of sudden oliguria or anuria in the early post-transplantation period. ATN, acute tubular necrosis; CMD, corticomedullary differentiation.

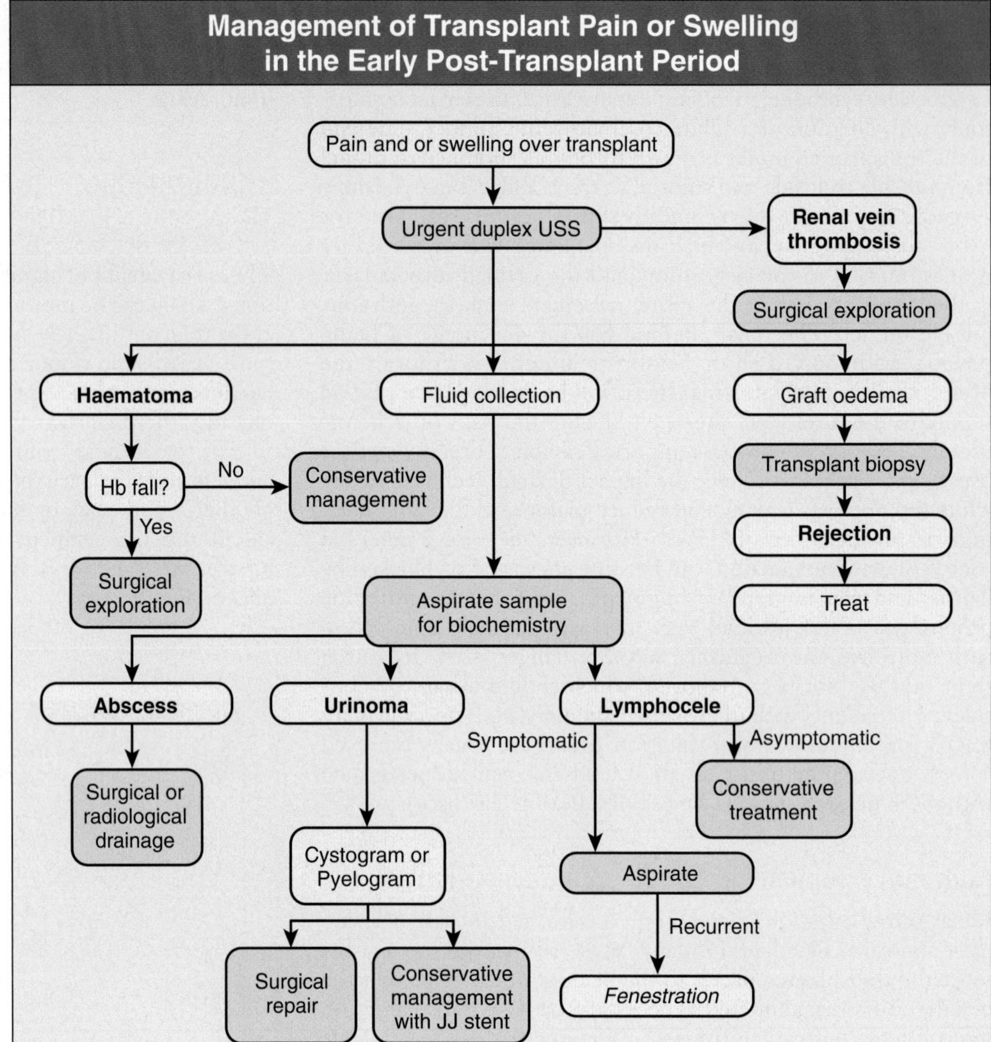

Figure 99.8 Management of transplant pain or swelling in the early post-transplantation period. Hb, hemoglobin; USS, ultrasound scan.

Wound Infection

The use of preoperative prophylactic antibiotics, commonly amoxicillin-clavulanate, has reduced the incidence of wound infection to less than 1%. If a wound infection does occur, treatment is with antibiotics, guided by microbiology from wound swabs, and drainage of collections as necessary.

Wound Dehiscence

The risk of wound dehiscence is increased in obese and diabetic patients and those receiving sirolimus. Identification and treatment of any infection are mandatory. Resuturing of a superficial wound breakdown is rarely justified. Large areas of dehiscence often benefit from vacuum-assisted closure, but the majority require only frequent dressing.

Vascular Complications

Transplant vascular thrombosis is a feared complication that may cause early and irreversible graft failure. Although there are also significant hemorrhagic risks, routine perioperative prophylaxis may be given with subcutaneous low-molecular-weight heparin, and some units prescribe aspirin for the first few postoperative months.

Bleeding from Vessels in the Renal Hilum

Careful postoperative observations, with regular hemoglobin and hematocrit measurements, are crucial for the early detection of bleeding. Output from the transplant drains may give an early indication of heavy blood loss. Unsecured small vessels in the renal hilum may not be obvious during surgery, but they may start bleeding postoperatively. This form of blood loss can be slow, persistent, and serious. If the patient's condition allows, urgent imaging may be performed to secure a diagnosis, but the best course of action is usually emergency exploration of the transplant under general anesthesia.

Anastomotic Hemorrhage

This is a rare occurrence, usually due to a technical surgical error, and is more common with multiple arteries and use of antiplatelet agents.[19,20] Early after transplantation, the patient may complain of pain over the graft. This symptom should always be taken seriously. There may also be pain in the back or the rectum caused by a tension hematoma in the retroperitoneum or pelvis. Significant hemorrhage will be attended by circulatory collapse, with tachycardia and hypotension. There will be a decrease in the hemoglobin and hematocrit, sometimes to alarmingly low levels. The patient must be returned to the operating theater immediately and the transplant re-explored.

Hemorrhage can also occur some weeks after transplantation because of the development of a mycotic aneurysm of the renal artery. In the rare case of a ruptured mycotic aneurysm, an immediate graft nephrectomy is required, but the mortality is high.

Renal Artery Thrombosis

This is a rare event, occurring in less than 1% of transplants. The usual outcome is loss of the kidney. Acute arterial thrombosis may occur intraoperatively or during the first days or weeks after transplantation. Potential causes include hyperacute rejection and a procoagulant state, but most cases are due to a technical error during the anastomosis of small or atheromatous vessels.[20] Successful vascular anastomosis requires that the vessels are not under tension and that there is a smooth transition between the two intimal surfaces; sutures must be placed through all layers of the vessel walls so that an intimal flap is avoided. Vascular adventitia is thrombogenic and must be excluded from the lumen of the anastomosis.

Renal artery thrombosis presents with sudden anuria; the differential diagnoses are a blocked urinary catheter, dehydration, acute tubular necrosis, and a urologic complication. A high index of suspicion is required to make this diagnosis, particularly in the immediate postoperative period. The only worthwhile investigation is an urgent duplex ultrasound scan, but if the diagnosis is seriously entertained, then the only hope of saving the transplant is to re-explore it immediately in the hope that a correctable cause can be found. The reality is that unless the acute arterial thrombosis occurs on-table, there is little chance of saving the transplanted kidney. Acutely thrombosed grafts must nevertheless be explored and removed to avoid the development of sepsis in a necrotic graft, a potentially fatal complication.

Renal Vein Thrombosis

Renal vein thrombosis is more common than arterial thrombosis and occurs in 1% to 6% of renal transplants.[20,21] It may result from a technical error at the time of surgery, but its cause is usually less certain. The renal vein can certainly be twisted or kinked if it is not correctly placed after completion of the vascular and ureteral anastomoses. The peak incidence of renal vein thrombosis is 3 to 9 days after transplantation[22]; a transplant with good initial graft function will have a sudden loss of urine output, which is often markedly blood stained, associated with severe pain arising from swelling and (very rarely) rupture of the allograft. The ipsilateral leg may also swell if there is involvement of the iliac venous system. Renal vein thrombosis may also be occult and is one differential diagnosis of delayed graft function. Duplex ultrasound scanning is the best investigation. In an established renal vein thrombosis, this may show an obviously swollen allograft with surrounding hematoma and an absence of renal perfusion. Lesser degrees of thrombosis, or indeed incipient thrombosis, may be highlighted by an absence of arterial flow in diastole. An even later development is a reversal of flow in diastole.

As with arterial thrombosis, if this diagnosis is entertained, the best course of action is to re-explore the transplant as an emergency. The renal vein anastomosis can be opened to allow clot to be extracted, and the venotomy is then closed and the kidney observed for improvement. A more radical alternative is to immediately explant the kidney by taking down the arterial, venous, and ureteral anastomoses. The kidney can then be reflushed with cold perfusion fluid on the back table and held in preservation fluid at 4°C. This allows much more time to assess the cause of the venous thrombosis, and if the kidney remains viable, the transplant operation can then be repeated. If the transplant is already infarcted or cannot be adequately flushed with preservation fluid, the organ will need to be discarded anyway and nothing is lost by immediate explantation. Successful emergency surgical exploration with subsequent long-term function is rare. Interventional radiographic techniques offer an alternative to surgery. The renal vein can be selectively catheterized through the ipsilateral femoral vein, and graft thrombolysis may then be attempted. This technique is particularly useful when renal vein thrombosis occurs late after transplantation and the risk of systemic anticoagulation is low. The use of various thrombolytic agents has been reported, including heparin, urokinase, streptokinase, and tissue plasminogen activator, with no consensus as to which is the most appropriate.

Transplant Renal Artery Stenosis

Transplant renal artery stenosis is a later complication occurring 3 to 48 months after transplantation. Not all stenoses are of functional or clinical significance, as shown by studies in which all functioning transplants have undergone angiography.[23] Causal factors include donor and recipient atherosclerosis, factors associated with surgical technique, and severe acute rejection.[24] The presentation and management of transplanted renal artery stenosis are discussed in Chapter 64.

Lymphocele

Small, clinically insignificant lymphatic collections can be demonstrated by ultrasound scan in up to 50% of renal transplants.[25] Larger lymphoceles that cause complications or require treatment occur in 2% to 10% of cases.[26] The source of peritransplant lymph leaks is the lymphatic channels around the iliac arterial system rather than the lymphatics of the transplanted kidney itself.[27] Therefore, during the dissection of the iliac arterial system, all the surrounding lymphatic channels must be meticulously secured with nonabsorbable ligatures or metals clips. Wound suction drains should not be removed postoperatively until less than 30 ml of fluid is produced on 2 consecutive days. It is safe to leave drains in place for several weeks after transplantation to allow a low-volume lymphatic leak to seal by gradual fibrosis. Despite the theoretical risk of infection, this does not seem to be a problem in practice. If necessary, the patient can be discharged from the hospital with the drain *in situ*.

Compression of the transplanted ureter leading to renal dysfunction is produced only by very large lymphoceles (volume >300 ml). The peak incidence is at 6 weeks, but a lymphatic collection may present between 2 weeks and 6 months after transplantation.[25] Most lymphatic collections are found anterior to the iliac vessels and lying between the transplant and the bladder (Fig. 99.9). Presenting features may include wound or ipsilateral thigh swelling in association with suprapubic discomfort and urinary frequency due to bladder compression. Other presentations include pain over the transplanted kidney sometimes associated with fever, ureteral obstruction with graft dysfunction, and ipsilateral thrombophlebitis. However, most are asymptomatic and present as an incidental finding during an ultrasound scan being performed for another reason. It is important to aspirate all peritransplant fluid collections under ultrasound control to aid diagnosis. Macroscopic findings are usually sufficient to

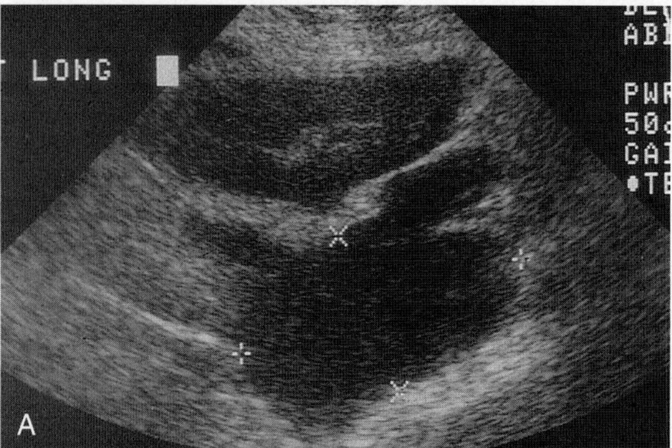

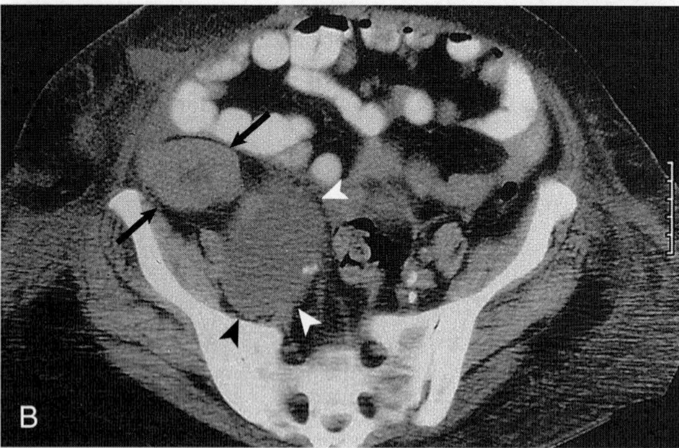

Figure 99.9 Post-transplantation lymphocele. A, Ultrasound appearance. A large echolucent lymphocele can be seen inferior to the transplanted kidney. **B,** Computed tomographic appearance. A 5- × 5-cm lymphocele *(arrowheads)* is present under the transplanted kidney *(arrows)*.

differentiate infected from noninfected lymph, and biochemical analysis of the fluid allows a urine leak to be excluded. Computed tomography or magnetic resonance imaging is an essential investigation if surgery is being contemplated, particularly if a laparoscopic procedure is planned. This allows accurate definition of the relationship between the lymphocele and the transplanted ureter. If the ureter is bow-strung across the superior surface of the lymphocele, it could be damaged during a laparoscopic fenestration procedure.

Many small lymphoceles are asymptomatic and will resolve spontaneously given enough time. If action is deemed necessary, first-line treatment is aspiration under ultrasound control. If there is a recurrence, further aspirations can be performed or an external drain can be placed with ultrasound guidance. If these simple measures fail, open or laparoscopic surgical drainage may be required. A 5-cm-diameter disk of the lymphocele wall is removed to create a large opening into the peritoneal cavity, allowing reabsorption of the lymph through the abdominal lymphatic drainage system. These peritoneal fenestrations have a tendency to heal before the lymphocele is completely reabsorbed, leading to early recurrence; this can be minimized by use of a metal or omental plug.

Urologic Complications

Urinary tract complications are relatively common after renal transplantation, with an incidence of between 5% and 14%.[28] Although they can be difficult to manage, they only rarely cause graft loss or mortality. The relatively high incidence of urologic problems is a consequence of the tenuous blood supply of the transplanted ureter. After kidney retrieval, the only ureteral blood supply that is preserved is derived from the renal artery near the hilum of the kidney, and this can be easily damaged during retrieval.

Urinary Leaks

These most commonly occur because of ischemic necrosis in any part of the transplanted urinary collecting system. The distal ureter has the poorest blood supply and is therefore the most common site. Less commonly, leaks occur from the renal pelvis or the midportion of the ureter, which may be due to unrecognized direct damage to the ureter during organ retrieval. Urinary leaks tend to occur in the first few days after transplantation but can present much later. The usual presentation is with straw-colored fluid leaking directly from the transplant wound or accumulating in the drains in association with oliguria. Alternatively, extravasating urine may accumulate as a peritransplant fluid collection. This presents as a painful swelling of the wound, and the patient may have a fever. In either case, the extravasated fluid must be differentiated from lymph by biochemical analysis of the fluid and a simultaneous serum sample. Urine will have markedly elevated urea and creatinine levels compared with the patient's serum, whereas lymph will have a similar biochemical profile.

The presence of a urinary fistula should be confirmed by antegrade or retrograde pyelography. Both of these techniques present challenges. Antegrade puncture of a nondilated pelvicalyceal system is technically difficult but usually possible. Retrograde cannulation of the transplanted ureteral orifice can be attempted with a flexible cystoscope. This is also a difficult maneuver because the transplanted ureter is implanted into the dome of the bladder rather than at its base. If the urine leak is contained as a urinoma, ultrasound will demonstrate a fluid collection between the transplanted kidney and the bladder that can be sampled by needling or drained by the placement of a suitable percutaneous catheter.

The management of urinary leaks has changed significantly in recent years. The former practice of early re-exploration and surgical reconstruction[29] is no longer always necessary. Interventional radiographic techniques offer an alternative, at least for initial treatment. The aim is to place a double-J ureteral stent across the region of damage through an antegrade nephrostomy; this may allow time for the urinary fistula to heal.[30] This technique, however, is unlikely to be successful if there is significant ischemic necrosis of the ureter, in which case surgery still has a role. Re-exploration of kidney transplants is straightforward in the early postoperative period but may be a considerable challenge later because of the development of an intense peritransplant fibrotic reaction. The choice of operative procedure for a necrotic distal ureter depends on the length of remaining viable ureter. If there is sufficient length after excision of the necrotic distal portion, the transplanted ureter may be simply reimplanted into the bladder. If this is not possible, the urinary tract should be reconstructed with use of the patient's native ureter (Fig. 99.10). Depending on length of viable transplanted ureter, there is a choice of anastomosis of the native ureter to the transplanted ureter proximal to the ischemic segment (ureteroureterostomy) or to the transplanted renal pelvis (ureteropyelostomy). Whichever technique is chosen, the anastomosis should be protected with a double-J stent. Although these techniques require the native ureter to be ligated proximally, there is usually no need to perform an ipsilateral nephrectomy.[31] Postoperatively, the

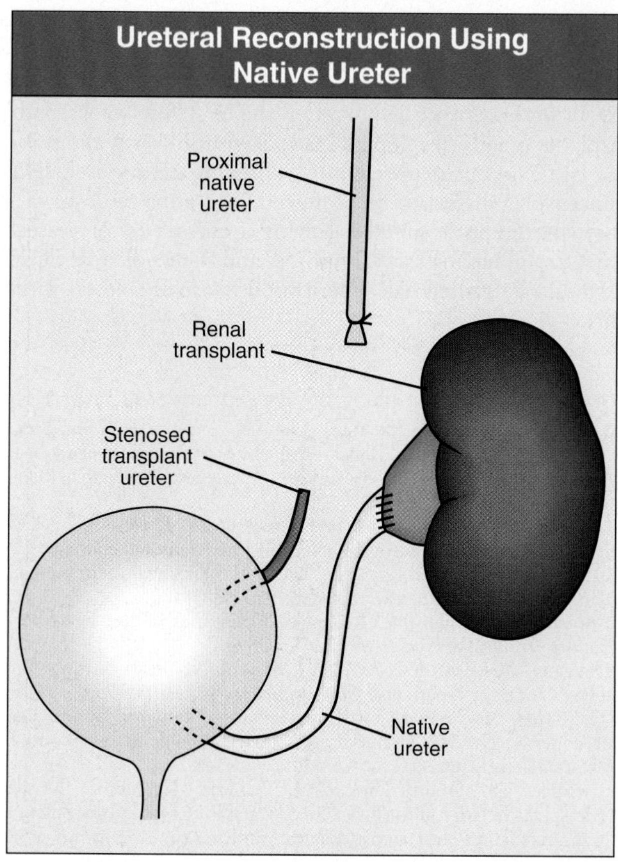

Figure 99.10 Ureteral reconstruction using native ureter.

antegrade nephrostomy can be left *in situ* so that a contrast study can be performed after 7 to 10 days to confirm healing of the new anastomosis. If the transplanted recipient has undergone an ipsilateral nephrectomy in the past or the native ureter is too diseased to be used for reconstruction, a Boari bladder flap can be used to reconstruct the urinary tract.

Ureteral Obstruction

Obstruction of the transplanted ureter may occur at any time after transplantation. It should always be considered in the differential diagnosis of acute transplant dysfunction and excluded by ultrasound examination. The management of transplant ureteral obstruction is summarized in Figure 99.11. Early obstruction is uncommon and suggestive of a technical error, such as creation of a submucosal bladder tunnel that is too tight, kinking of a redundant length of ureter, and incorrect suture placement during anastomosis. Early obstruction may also be caused by blood clot in the ureter, bladder, or catheter. Bleeding may occur from the ureterovesical anastomosis or cystostomy or after a transplant biopsy. It is common practice to drain the urinary bladder with a three-way irrigating catheter as small-diameter two-way Foley catheters are easily blocked by blood clot.

Late ureteral obstruction may occur at the vesicoureteral or pelviureteral junctions. Ischemia that is not severe enough to cause necrosis is presumed to be the cause of most vesicoureteral obstructions. Renal transplants invariably excite a pronounced perigraft fibrotic response, and this is more likely to be the cause of an obstruction at the level of the pelviureteral junction. It is possible that acute rejection episodes contribute to ureteric stenosis, but this has never been unequivocally demonstrated.[32]

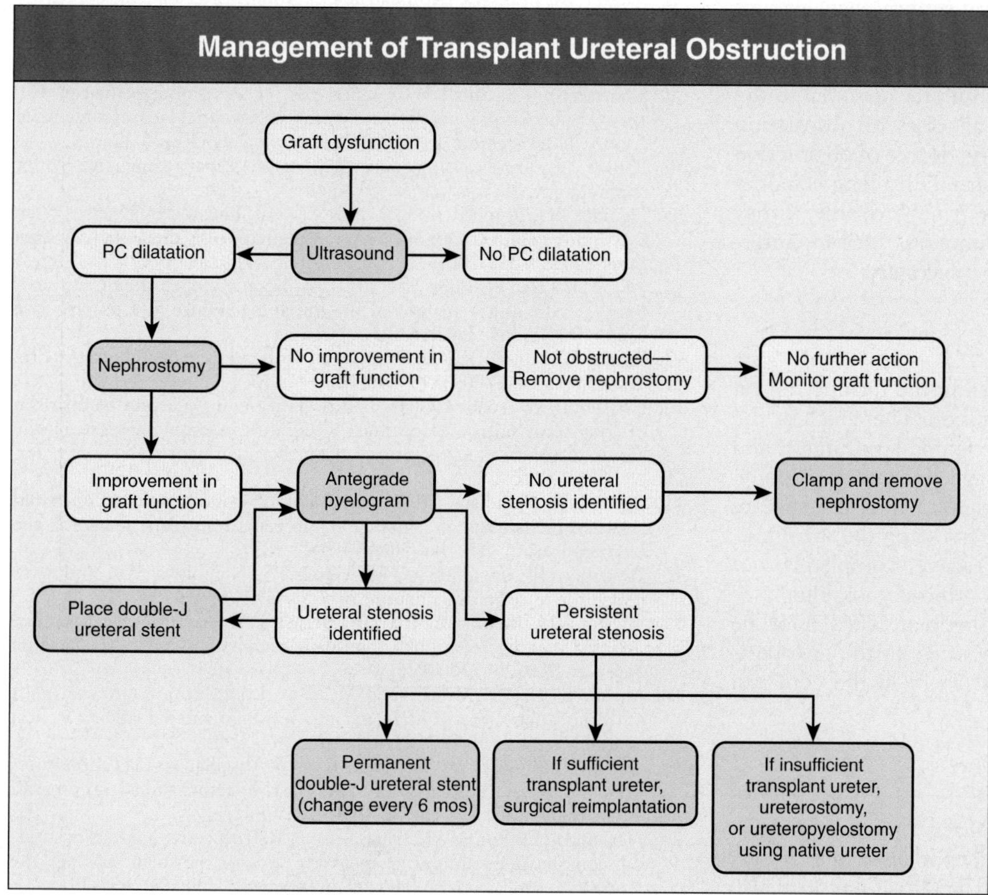

Figure 99.11 Management of transplant ureteral obstruction. PC, pelvicalyceal.

An ultrasound scan will demonstrate a dilated pelvicalyceal system. However, long-standing kidney transplants may have marked pelvicalyceal dilation without being obstructed. This most commonly causes uncertainty in assessing whether obstruction may be contributing to chronic allograft dysfunction in a patient with biopsy-proven chronic allograft nephropathy. Further investigation is needed to confirm or to refute the presence of obstruction and to define its anatomy. Retrograde pyelography has a low success rate because of the difficulty of catheterizing the transplanted ureteral orifice at cystoscopy. Therefore, percutaneous nephrostomy followed by antegrade pyelography is the investigation of choice in suspected transplant ureteral obstruction. The nephrostomy is performed under antibiotic cover using ultrasound control, and the nephrostomy tube should be left in place for a few days. If serum creatinine decreases during this period, obstruction is confirmed. If there is no improvement in renal function, significant obstruction can be confidently excluded. This simple observation avoids the need for an antegrade pressure study (Whittaker test), which may be difficult to interpret in transplanted kidneys. After external decompression of the transplanted kidney for a few days, an antegrade pyelogram is obtained to accurately define the anatomy of the obstructing lesion.

Nonoperative approaches to the treatment of transplant ureteral stricture are often preferred.[33] The simplest approach is to place a double-J stent across the stricture through a percutaneous nephrostomy. This may require initial balloon dilation.[34] The stent can be removed after 6 weeks, but the restenosis rate is high. An alternative is long-term stenting, changing the stent every 6 months. The disadvantage of this method is a high incidence of urinary tract infection, with potential severe consequences for immunosuppressed patients, and long-term antibiotic prophylaxis is a sensible precaution. Open surgical management still has a place in the management of ureteral obstruction. The operation performed depends on the site of obstruction and the remaining length of healthy transplanted ureter proximal to the obstruction (see Urinary Leaks). Not all cases of obstruction require intervention. When there is a mild degree of obstruction not associated with urinary tract infection and in a long-standing kidney that is affected by chronic allograft nephropathy, it may be better to simply monitor transplant function, reserving intervention for a later date should it become necessary.

Complications in the Transplant Bed

A number of nerves may be encountered in the retroperitoneal dissection required for kidney transplantation. These include the lateral femoral cutaneous nerve and the femoral, obturator, and sacral nerves. Each of these may be damaged by a traction injury, particularly when modern fixed wound retraction systems are used as these can exert a great deal of pressure on the surrounding tissues. Such neurapraxias should recover completely, but this may take some months, and they can be very disabling.

In male transplant recipients, the spermatic cord must be mobilized during the dissection to gain access to the retroperitoneal space. Damage to the testicular artery in the cord can result in testicular atrophy.

TRANSPLANT NEPHRECTOMY

An early graft nephrectomy may be required for arterial thrombosis, capsular rupture (due to severe rejection or venous thrombosis), or other technical reasons. Graft nephrectomy may also be required after graft failure for persisting pain, malaise, fever, and thrombocytopenia, although a nonfunctioning graft left *in situ* will usually shrink and become fibrotic. Early graft nephrectomy is straightforward, but after the first few weeks, kidney transplants usually develop intense perigraft fibrosis, and this can make late allograft nephrectomy a difficult technical challenge. A subcapsular dissection is preferred, and after removal of the kidney, the hilum is sutured, leaving a cuff of donor vessels in place. Careful hemostasis is required, and the whole raw capsular bed should be cauterized. The wound is usually closed without drains.

REFERENCES

1. Koffman G, Gambaro G. Renal transplantation from non–heart-beating donors: A review of the European experience. *J Nephrol*. 2003;16: 334-341.
2. Criteria for the diagnosis of brain stem death. Review by a working group convened by the Royal College of Physicians and endorsed by the Conference of Medical Royal Colleges and their Faculties in the United Kingdom. *J R Coll Physicians Lond*. 1995;29:381-382.
3. Kootstra G, Daemen JH, Oomen AP. Categories of non–heart-beating donors. *Transplant Proc*. 1995;27:2893-2894.
4. Daemen JW, Kootstra G, Wijnen RM, et al. Nonheart-beating donors: The Maastricht experience. *Clin Transplant*. 1994;303-316.
5. The Organ Procurement and Transplantation Network. Donors Recovered in the U.S. by Donor Type, 2005. Available at: www.optn.org/latestData/rptData.asp.
6. Statistics and Audit Directorate. United Kingdom Transplant. Transplant Activity in the UK 2008. Available at: www.uktransplant.org.uk/ukt/statistics/latest_statistics/latest_statistics.jsp current_activity_reports.jsp/ukt/tx_activity_report_2005_uk_complete-v2.pdf.
7. Ratner LE, Montgomery RA, Kavoussi LR. Laparoscopic live donor nephrectomy: The four year Johns Hopkins University experience. *Nephrol Dial Transplant*. 1999;14:2090-2093.
8. Rankin SC, Jan W, Koffman CG. Noninvasive imaging of living related kidney donors: Evaluation with CT angiography and gadolinium-enhanced MR angiography. *AJR Am J Roentgenol*. 2001;177:349-355.
9. Namasivayam S, Small WC, Kalra MK, et al. Multidetector-row CT angiography for preoperative evaluation of potential laparoscopic renal donors: How accurate are we? *Clin Imaging*. 2006;30:120-126.
10. Ratner LE, Ciseck LJ, Moore RG, et al. Laparoscopic live donor nephrectomy. *Transplantation*. 1995;60:1047-1049.
11. Nanidis TG, Antcliffe D, Kokkinos C, et al. Laparoscopic versus open live donor nephrectomy in renal transplantation: A meta-analysis. *Ann Surg*. 2008;247:58-70.
12. Pace KT, Dyer SJ, Phan V, et al. Laparoscopic v open donor nephrectomy: A cost-utility analysis of the initial experience at a tertiary-care center. *J Endourol*. 2002;16:495-508.
13. Ratner LE, Buell JF, Kuo PC. Laparoscopic donor nephrectomy: Pro. *Transplantation*. 2000;70:1544-1546.
14. Nogueira JM, Jacobs CJ, Harinan A, et al. A single center comparison of long-term outcomes of renal allografts procured laparoscopically versus historical controls procured by the open approach. *Transpl Int*. 2008;21:2908-2915.
15. Brook NR, Nicholson ML. An audit over 2 years' practice of open and laparoscopic live-donor nephrectomy at renal transplant centres in the UK and Ireland. *BJU Int*. 2004;93:1027-1031.
16. Wheatley TJ, Doughman TM, Veitch PS, Nicholson ML. Subrectus pouch for renal transplantation. *Br J Surg*. 1996;83:419.
17. Wilson CH, Bhatti AA, Rix DA, Manas DM. Routine intraoperative ureteric stenting for kidney transplant recipients. Cochrane Database Syst Rev. 2005;4:CD004925.
18. Abusin K, Rix D, Mohammed M, et al. Long-term adult renal graft outcome after ureteric drainage into an augmented bladder or ileal conduit. *Transpl Int*. 1998;11(Suppl 1):S147-S149.
19. Osman Y, Shokeir A, Ali-el-Dein B, et al. Vascular complications after live donor renal transplantation: Study of risk factors and effects on graft and patient survival. *J Urol*. 2003;169:859-862.
20. Hernandez D, Rufino M, Armas S, et al. Retrospective analysis of surgical complications following cadaveric kidney transplantation in the modern transplant era. *Nephrol Dial Transplant*. 2006;21:2908-2915.

21. Reuther G, Wanjura D, Bauer H. Acute renal vein thrombosis in renal allografts: Detection with duplex Doppler US. *Radiology*. 1989;170:557-558.
22. Beyga ZT, Kahan BD. Surgical complications of kidney transplantation. *J Nephrol*. 1998;11:137-145.
23. Lacombe M. Arterial stenosis complicating renal allotransplantation in man: A study of 38 cases. *Ann Surg*. 1975;181:283-288.
24. Bruno S, Remuzzi G, Ruggenenti P. Transplant renal artery stenosis. *Am Soc Nephrol*. 2004;15:134-141.
25. Pollak R, Veremis SA, Maddux MS, Mozes MF. The natural history of and therapy for perirenal fluid collections following renal transplantation. *J Urol*. 1988;140:716-720.
26. Zincke H, Woods JE, Leary FJ, et al. Experience with lymphoceles after renal transplantation. *Surgery*. 1975;77:444-450.
27. Ward K, Klingensmith WC 3rd, Sterioff S, Wagner HN Jr. The origin of lymphoceles following renal transplantation. *Transplantation*. 1978;25:346-347.
28. Mundy AR, Podesta ML, Bewick M, et al. The urological complications of 1000 renal transplants. *Br J Urol*. 1981;53:397-402.
29. Palmer JM, Chatterjee SN. Urologic complications in renal transplantation. *Surg Clin North Am*. 1978;58:305-319.
30. Nicholson ML, Veitch PS, Donnelly PK, Bell PR. Urological complications of renal transplantation: The impact of double J ureteric stents. *Ann R Coll Surg Engl*. 1991;73:316-321.
31. Lord RH, Pepera T, Williams G. Ureteroureterostomy and pyeloureterostomy without native nephrectomy in renal transplantation. *Br J Urol*. 1991;67:349-351.
32. Brook NR, Waller JR, Pattenden CJ, Nicholson ML. Ureteric stenosis after renal transplantation: No effect of acute rejection or immunosuppression. *Transplant Proc*. 2002;34:3007-3008.
33. Goldstein I, Cho SI, Olsson CA. Nephrostomy drainage for renal transplant complications. *J Urol*. 1981;126:159-163.
34. Streem SB, Novick AC, Steinmuller DR, et al. Long-term efficacy of ureteral dilation for transplant ureteral stenosis. *J Urol*. 1988;140:32-35.

CHAPTER 100

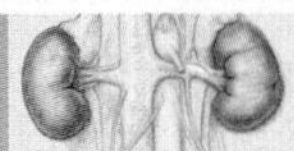

Prophylaxis and Treatment of Kidney Transplant Rejection

Alexander C. Wiseman

The clinical presentation of the immune response to transplanted tissue, referred to as rejection, became apparent in 1960 when, after successful proof-of-principle kidney transplants were performed in identical twins, kidney transplantation was attempted between immunologically dissimilar individuals.[1] Eleven patients underwent lymphoid irradiation to prevent rejection after kidney transplantation from nonidentical donors. Whereas 10 of 11 died of overwhelming infection, illustrating the potential consequences of immunosuppression, the lone surviving patient from this series subsequently underwent two episodes of acute rejection, both of which were successfully treated with cortisone with successful graft function. Thus began the development of immunosuppressive agents that could prevent and treat rejection while not inducing severe life-threatening side effects and the characterization of the histologic patterns of injury that quantify the type and severity of rejection.

The occurrence of acute rejection in the first year after transplantation has significantly diminished from a nearly universal occurrence of rejection in the earlier era to present-day rates of 10% to 15%,[2] primarily due to the development of newer immunosuppression medications. Although the incidence of acute rejection has diminished (Fig. 100.1), the management of chronic rejection has remained a challenge, with continued attempts to better define the nature of injury and methods to prevent or to reverse this process. However, as attention shifts to limiting the toxicity of immunosuppression medications in corticosteroid withdrawal and calcineurin inhibitor (CNI) withdrawal protocols and attempts are made to increase access to transplantation by performing transplants across human leukocyte antigen (HLA) and blood type barriers, management of acute rejection will continue to be an important clinical issue. The purpose of this chapter is to summarize our current understanding of rejection from a histologic standpoint and to describe methods for prevention and treatment of this entity.

DEFINITION

Rejection (both acute and chronic) is defined by histologic findings after kidney transplant biopsy. A biopsy considered adequate for analysis involves sampling of at least 10 glomeruli and two small arteries, stained by hematoxylin and eosin, periodic acid–Schiff or silver, and trichrome stains; a biopsy specimen with seven to nine glomeruli and one artery is considered of marginal adequacy. When biopsy is performed for clinical indications (renal dysfunction), two separates cores should be obtained because the findings of rejection are often patchy in distribution (Fig. 100.2).[3] There is not a consensus for the number of cores required when biopsies are performed for nonclinical indications (e.g., in protocol-driven practice), although adequate tissue sampling defined by the preceding criteria is recommended.

The Banff Working Classification of Renal Allograft Pathology forms the basis of the histologic definition of rejection and is reviewed and updated biannually. First developed in 1993 with a primary focus on T cell–mediated acute inflammatory infiltrates to classify the degree of rejection, the most recent (2007) classification (Fig. 100.3) now differentiates a humoral (antibody-mediated) response from the T-cell response and further distinguishes a chronic humoral form of injury previously included within the term *chronic allograft nephropathy* (see Chapter 103).[4] This has been possible because of the identification of antibody-mediated injury indirectly through evidence of complement deposition. C4d is a fragment of C4b that is generated on IgG and IgM deposition and activation of the classical complement pathway. C4b/C4d forms a covalent bond with proteins on tissue such as capillary endothelial cells through a sulfhydryl group and persists bound to tissue after immunoglobulin and other complement products have been released.[5] Staining for C4d is currently the most sensitive marker for antibody-mediated injury and should be routinely performed on renal transplant biopsy specimens.

Antibody-Mediated Rejection

Acute antibody-mediated (humoral) rejection is estimated to occur in 3% to 10% of all transplants and is present in 20% to 30% of episodes of acute rejection,[6] occurring typically within the first few weeks of transplantation or in association with a change in immunosuppression. Whereas patients who have preexisting donor-specific HLA alloantibodies (donor-specific antibodies) are at higher risk for the development of acute humoral rejection, the identification of *de novo* donor-specific antibodies at the time of graft dysfunction is common. The diagnosis of acute humoral rejection requires (1) evidence of donor-specific antibodies, (2) C4d deposition in peritubular capillaries, and (3) evidence of tissue injury (Fig. 100.4). Patterns of injury associated with acute humoral rejection range from acute tubular cell injury suggestive of acute tubular necrosis (ATN) to thrombotic microangiopathy but typically will be associated with neutrophils or macrophages in peritubular capillaries.

Chronic active antibody-mediated rejection is likely due to an indolent alloimmune response that results in transplant glomerulopathy and arteriolopathy. Although transplant glomerulopathy is often associated with circulating donor-specific antibodies and with C4d deposition, 30% to 50% of cases will be identified in the absence of these diagnostic markers.[7] This suggests that these lesions are not solely due to a humoral response or that the lack

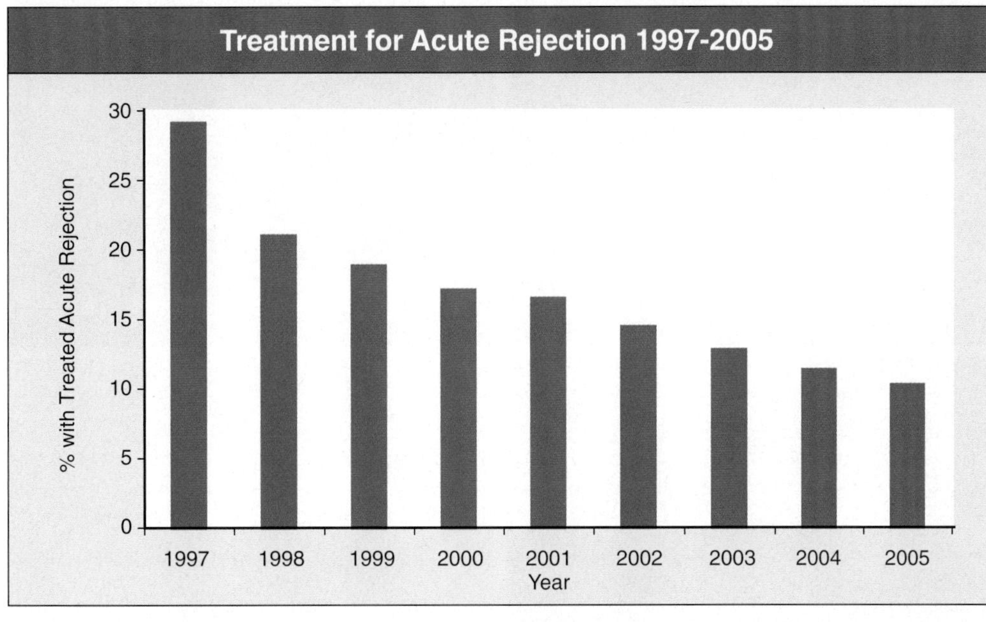

Figure 100.1 Treatment for acute rejection 1997-2005. *(As reported to the Scientific Registry of Transplant Recipients, SRTR Report 2007.)*

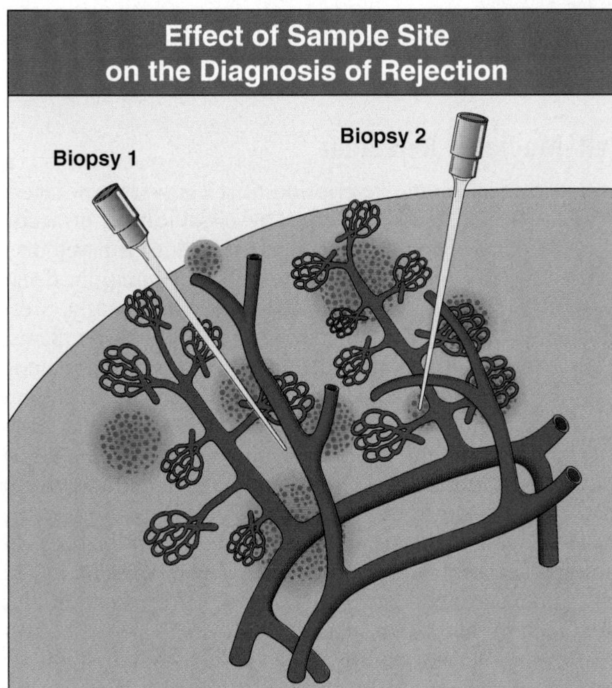

Figure 100.2 Effect of sample site on the diagnosis of rejection. Acute rejection begins as patchy, focal infiltrates and becomes homogeneous only in advanced stages. The intensity of mononuclear infiltrate seen on biopsy would differ between core 1 and core 2. Routinely taking two core biopsy samples can help decrease the sampling errors, which can affect the histologic interpretation of rejection.

Classification of Rejection

Antibody Mediated

Acute

C4d+, presence of circulating antidonor antibodies and acute tissue injury

I. ATN-like (minimal inflammation)

II. Capillary and/or glomerular inflammation and/or thromboses

III. Arterial inflammation

Chronic

C4d+, presence of circulating antidonor antibodies and chronic tissue injury

(1) Glomerular double contours, (2) peritubular capillary basement membrane multilayering, (3) tubular atrophy/interstitial fibrosis, and/or (4) fibrous intimal thickening in arteries

T Cell Mediated

Acute

Mononuclear cell interstitial inflammation and tubulitis and/or arteritis

IA: >25% Interstitial infiltration, 4–10 mononuclear cells/tubular cross section

IB: >25% Interstitial infiltration, >10 mononuclear cells/tubular cross section

IIA: Intimal arteritis, mild to moderate (0%–25% of luminal area)

IIB: Intimal arteritis, severe (>25% of luminal area)

III: Transmural arteritis and/or fibrinoid change and necrosis of medial smooth muscle cells with accompanying lymphocyte inflammation

Chronic

Arterial intimal fibrosis with mononuclear cell infiltration in fibrosis, formation of neointima

Borderline

10%–25% Interstitial infiltration, <4 mononuclear cells/tubular cross section

Figure 100.3 Classification of rejection. ATN, acute tubular necrosis. *(Modified from reference 8.)*

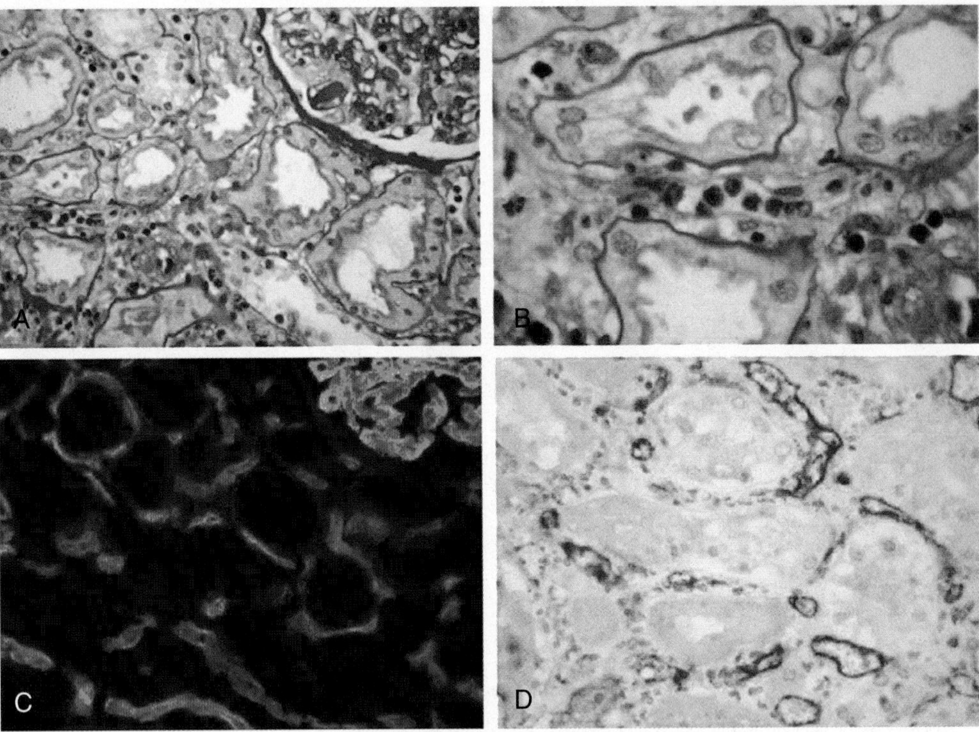

Figure 100.4 Acute antibody-mediated rejection. A, Peritubular and glomerular capillaries contain numerous polymorphonuclear leukocytes and mononuclear cells. **B,** Numerous polymorphonuclear leukocytes are observed in a peritubular capillary. Interstitial edema is noted. (Periodic acid–Schiff; magnification ×200.) **C,** Immunofluorescence staining of peritubular capillaries with C4d. (Fresh frozen tissue sample; magnification ×250.) **D,** Immunohistochemistry demonstrating peritubular capillary staining of C4d. (Paraffin-embedded tissue; magnification ×480.) *(From reference 9.)*

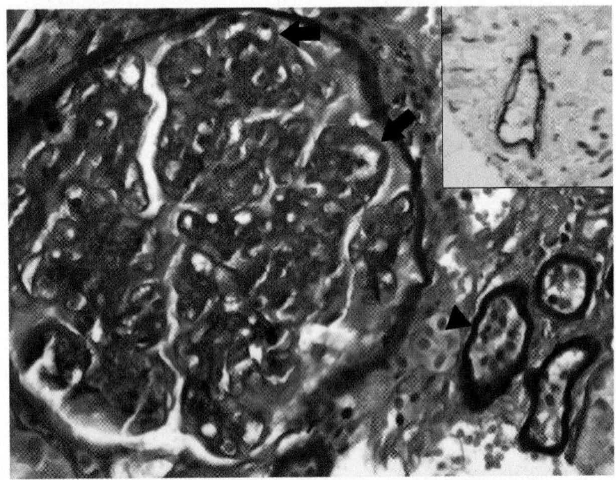

Figure 100.5 Chronic antibody-mediated rejection. Glomerular double contours *(arrows)* and tubular atrophy *(arrowhead).* (Periodic acid–Schiff; magnification ×400.) *Inset:* Diffuse C4d deposition in peritubular capillaries by immunohistochemistry. *(Photomicrographs courtesy Dr. Maxwell Smith, University of Colorado, Denver, Colorado, USA.)*

of a temporal relationship of donor-specific antibodies or C4d deposition to biopsy findings is related to the waxing and waning nature of the humoral response. The diagnosis of chronic humoral rejection requires (1) evidence of donor-specific antibodies, (2) C4d deposition in peritubular capillaries, and (3) evidence of chronic tissue injury. The forms of chronic tissue injury may include duplication of the glomerular basement membrane (GBM), multilamination of the peritubular capillary basement membrane, arterial intimal fibrosis without elastosis, and interstitial fibrosis with tubular atrophy (Fig. 100.5). It has been recommended that if only two of these are present, the diagnosis should be considered "suspicious" for chronic humoral rejection.

T Cell–Mediated Rejection

The classical pathologic description of rejection is now referred to as T cell–mediated rejection. The classification of acute T cell–mediated rejection (acute cellular rejection) is based on the degree and location of mononuclear cell inflammation. Because interstitial inflammation and tubulitis are frequently present immediately beneath the renal capsule (subcapsular inflammation) in stable allografts, this histologic feature is not taken into account in interpreting an allograft biopsy sample for the presence of rejection. When it is severe, interstitial inflammation may extend into tubules by injury to the tubular basement membrane (TBM) (tubulitis). The predominant phenotype of these infiltrates is a mixture of $CD4^+$ and $CD8^+$ T cells; however, B cells, eosinophils, and macrophages may also be present. Less commonly, endarteritis (endothelialitis) may be present, in which T cells and macrophages extend under the arterial endothelium, a phenomenon that may or may not be accompanied by interstitial inflammation or tubulitis. The finding of interstitial infiltrates and tubulitis in a kidney transplant biopsy specimen is not specific to acute cellular rejection, and other causes, such as viral nephropathy (BK virus, less commonly cytomegalovirus [CMV]), pyelonephritis, and post-transplantation lymphoproliferative disease, should be considered on the basis of the clinical presentation. In contrast, the histologic finding of endothelialitis is pathognomonic of acute cellular rejection.

Acute T cell–mediated rejection is histologically classified in the Banff criteria on the basis of the presence or absence of endothelialitis, the degree of interstitial inflammation, and the quantity of infiltrating cells into tubules. Type I acute cellular rejection (Fig. 100.6) is characterized by the absence of endothelialitis, with interstitial inflammation of at least 25% of the parenchyma and tubulitis (type IA requires 4 to 10 mononuclear cells/tubular cross section; type IB requires >10 mononuclear cells/tubular cross section). Type II acute cellular rejection (Fig. 100.7) is characterized by vascular involvement/endothelialitis

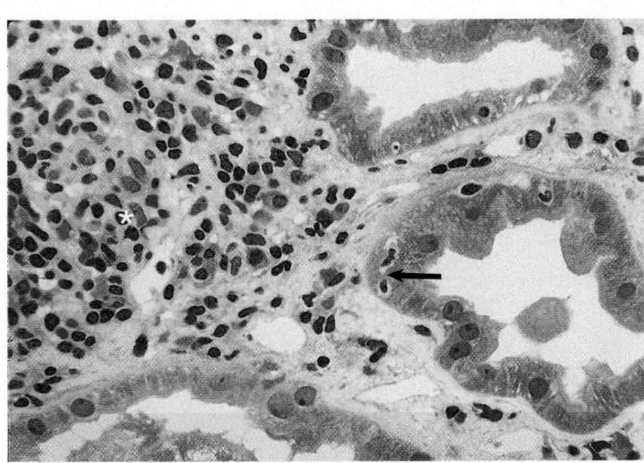

Figure 100.6 Type I acute cellular rejection. Type I acute rejection is manifested by interstitial mononuclear cell infiltration *(asterisk)* with invasion of the tubules *(arrow)*. (Periodic acid–Schiff; magnification ×200.)

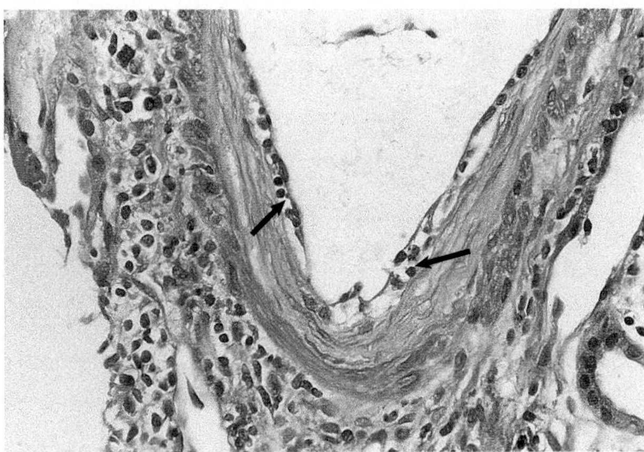

Figure 100.7 Type II acute cellular rejection. Type II rejection, called acute vascular rejection, is manifested by endothelialitis with mononuclear cell infiltration *(arrows)* beneath the arterial endothelium. (Periodic acid–Schiff; magnification ×200.) *(Courtesy Dr. Agnes Fogo, Vanderbilt University, Nashville, Tennessee, USA.)*

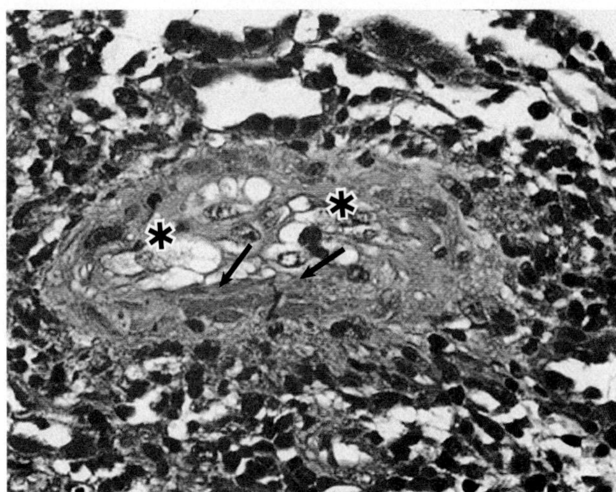

Figure 100.8 Type III acute cellular rejection. Severe small-vessel vasculitis with transmural mononuclear cell infiltration, fibrinoid necrosis *(arrows)*, and very swollen endothelial cells *(asterisks)*. (Periodic acid–Schiff; magnification ×400.) *(From reference 10.)*

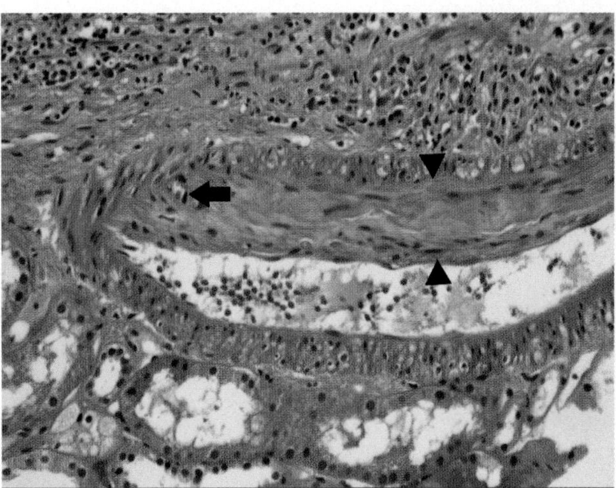

Figure 100.9 Chronic active T cell–mediated rejection. Chronic allograft arteriopathy with the formation of a fibrous neointima *(between arrowheads)* and embedded mononuclear cell infiltration *(arrow)*. (Hematoxylin and eosin; magnification ×200.) *(Photomicrographs courtesy Dr. Maxwell Smith, University of Colorado, Denver, Colorado, USA.)*

(type IIA requires mild to moderate intimal arteritis; type IIB requires arteritis with at least 25% of the luminal area lost in at least one arterial cross section). Type III acute cellular rejection (Fig. 100.8) is characterized by vascular inflammation that extends to the media (transmural) and may be accompanied by fibrinoid change and necrosis of the smooth muscle cells. Type II and type III acute cellular rejection may or may not be associated with elements of type I acute cellular rejection; thus, the pathologic description of rejection should not be viewed as a pathogenic continuum. However, type II and type III acute cellular rejection appear to require different therapeutic interventions and carry prognostic implications different from those of type I acute cellular rejection (see later sections).

Chronic active T cell–mediated rejection is a histologic diagnosis that refers to arterial intimal fibrosis specifically with evidence of mononuclear cell infiltration and formation of neointima (Fig. 100.9). This is distinguished from chronic humoral rejection by the location of vascular injury and lack of evidence of pathogenic antibody, and it is distinguished from other nonimmunologic processes that may lead to vascular and interstitial fibrosis by the presence of persistent infiltrating cells within vessels. This is covered in greater detail in Chapter 103.

Borderline Rejection

The finding of inflammation in 10% to 25% of the interstitium with tubulitis of fewer than four cells per tubular cross section is classified as borderline rejection. This currently remains a pathologic definition without clear clinical significance. When it is identified in the setting of graft dysfunction or with other findings such as glomerulitis, the risk of progression to clinical rejection on subsequent biopsies is increased, and thus treatment may be considered.[11]

CLINICAL MANIFESTATIONS

The clinical presentation of acute rejection is common to both T cell– and antibody-mediated rejection. Patients typically present with a rapid rise in serum creatinine and in severe cases

Differential Diagnosis of Renal Allograft Dysfunction
Week 1 Post-Transplantation
Acute tubular necrosis
Hyperacute/accelerated rejection
Urologic Obstruction Urine leak
Vascular thrombosis Renal artery Renal vein
<12 Weeks Post-Transplantation
Acute rejection
Calcineurin inhibitor toxicity
Volume contraction
Urologic Obstruction
Infection Bacterial pyelonephritis Viral infections
Interstitial nephritis
Recurrent disease
>12 Weeks Post-Transplantation
Acute rejection
Volume contraction
Calcineurin inhibitor toxicity
Urologic Obstruction
Infection Bacterial pyelonephritis Viral infections
Chronic allograft nephropathy
Recurrent disease
Renal artery stenosis
Post-transplantation lymphoproliferative disorder

Figure 100.10 Differential diagnosis of renal allograft dysfunction.

Risk Factors for Acute Rejection
High Risk
Sensitization (high panel reactive antibody percentage) Previous transplantation Pregnancy Transfusion
Delayed graft function Deceased donor source Increased donor age Prolonged ischemic time Donor brain death Donor acute renal dysfunction
HLA mismatching
Positive pretransplantation B-cell crossmatch
ABO incompatibility
Corticosteroid minimization
Infection Bacterial pyelonephritis Cytomegalovirus
Adolescent recipient
African American recipient
Previous rejection episode
Low Risk
Zero HLA mismatch
Elderly recipient of young donor kidney
Pre-emptive transplantation
Living donor source
First transplant

Figure 100.11 Risk factors for acute rejection.

may have a decreasing diuresis, weight gain, fever, or graft tenderness. The clinical findings are commonly nonspecific, and other causes of graft dysfunction are often considered at the time of presentation (Fig. 100.10) in the context of an individual's risk for the development of acute rejection (Fig. 100.11). Because of the increase in transplantation of presensitized patients, patients with known donor-specific antibody in desensitization protocols, and ABO-incompatible transplants, approximately 25% of acute rejection episodes now have a humoral component. In acute humoral rejection, there may be features of thrombotic microangiopathy with microangiopathic anemia and thrombocytopenia. If there is immediate cyanosis of the graft on revascularization (hyperacute rejection) or an abrupt decline in urine output and graft tenderness 3 to 14 days after transplantation (delayed hyperacute or accelerated rejection), donor-specific antibody is implicated. Typically, there is type III acute cellular rejection and interstitial hemorrhage on biopsy.

PROPHYLAXIS AND PREVENTION

Prophylaxis

The primary goal of transplant management is prevention of immunologic graft loss in the early period after transplantation. Over time, the risk for acute rejection diminishes and goals of immunosuppression therapy shift toward considerations of side effects of medications and risks for other events, such as cardiovascular disease (CVD) and malignancy. Therefore, current clinical practice follows a general strategy of intensive immunosuppression and monitoring in the first months after transplantation with a reduction or alteration of treatment after the initial period of risk.

Prevention of Acute T Cell–Mediated Rejection: Induction Therapy

The use of a brief course of potent immunosuppression at the time of transplantation, referred to as induction therapy, has become a common strategy for the prevention of acute rejection in all transplant recipients, including those at both higher and lower immunologic risk. According to the Scientific Registry of Transplant Recipients (SRTR) Annual Report in 2007, the use of induction therapy overall in the United States has increased from 52% to 80% during the period 2000-2006. For higher risk patients, such as those with prior sensitization (the presence of HLA antibodies quantified by percentage reactivity against a panel of common HLA types, referred to as percent panel reactive antibodies), prior transplantation, or African American ethnicity, induction therapy is usually combined with standard doses of immunosuppression to prevent rejection. For those with lower risk (living donor kidney recipients, primary kidney transplants), induction therapy is often employed in an effort to minimize exposure to maintenance immunosuppression. The use of race as a risk factor for rejection has recently been questioned with a study demonstrating similar acute rejection rates in African Europeans compared with European Caucasians in France.[12] However, most studies still report a higher risk of rejection for African Americans than for American Caucasians; thus, induction therapy is commonly used in this population.[13]

Induction agents can be classified as T-cell depleting or nondepleting. Nondepleting agents include the monoclonal humanized interleukin (IL)–2 receptor antibodies (IL-2Ra) daclizumab (Zenapax) and basiliximab (Simulect). The IL-2 receptor was identified as a potential immunosuppressive target as it is present on T cells and inhibition of IL-2/IL-2R signaling inhibits T-cell proliferation (see Chapter 96). The IL-2Ra have shown a reduction in acute rejection rates with minimal side effects in combination with cyclosporine-based immunosuppression in the absence of mycophenolate.[14] Importantly, these agents have not been studied in a prospective randomized fashion in combination with a tacrolimus/mycophenolate-based maintenance regimen; thus, questions still remain about the relative benefits of the addition of IL-2Ra with more potent, commonly used maintenance agents.

Depleting agents include antithymocyte globulin, OKT3, and anti-CD52. Unlike the IL-2Ra agents, none of these agents has been compared with placebo for the prevention of rejection, and thus their use as induction agents is considered "off label" in the United States. Antithymocyte globulin is a polyclonal preparation of antibodies directed at T cells prepared by immunizing animals with human lymphoid cells derived from the thymus. Earlier preparations were created from equine sources (Atgam), but this preparation is inferior to other depleting agents in the treatment of rejection, and its use has diminished.[15] Currently, the most common antilymphocyte preparation in use is rabbit antithymocyte globulin (rATG, Thymoglobulin). Anti-CD3 (OKT3, muromonab-CD3), a mouse monoclonal antibody directed to the CD3 subunit of the T-cell receptor, also results in depletion of T cells but has fallen out of favor as an induction agent because of a significant innate immune response to foreign antibody that results in a cytokine release syndrome presenting with fevers, hemodynamic changes, pulmonary edema, and, less commonly, seizures.

Recently, use of anti-CD52 (alemtuzumab, Campath-1H) has increased in kidney transplantation. This agent binds to CD52, an antigen of unclear physiologic significance that is present on both B and T cells, and results in depletion of both lymphoid cell lines. Its ability to induce prolonged, significant lymphopenia for up to 6 to 12 months after dosing led to its use in refractory chronic lymphocytic leukemia. Unlike other depleting agents, it is a humanized antibody and therefore has fewer infusion-related side effects than either antithymocyte globulin or OKT3. Initial trials suggest equivalence to other depleting agents in the prevention of rejection, but the long-term impact of prolonged lymphopenia on the risk for infection or post-transplantation lymphoproliferative disorder has yet to be determined, and comparative trials of induction agents are lacking (see later discussion).

Although effective in the inhibition of the T-cell response, all depleting agents carry concerns for long-term safety. Registry analyses suggest that there is an increased risk of future development of lymphoma with depleting agents compared with nondepleting agents or no induction therapy,[16,17] an association that appears to be dose dependent. For this reason, repeated or prolonged courses of depleting antibody therapy must be considered with this risk balanced by the potential for graft recovery or prolongation.

Few trials have compared the efficacy of induction agents in the prevention of acute rejection. Recently, a multicenter trial in patients at high risk for acute rejection (patients with an elevated risk of delayed graft function, elevated panel reactive antibodies, repeated transplants, or HLA mismatches) compared the IL-2Ra basiliximab to antithymocyte globulin with maintenance immunosuppression of cyclosporine, mycophenolate mofetil (MMF), and prednisone.[18] At 12 months, the rate of acute rejection in the basiliximab cohort was 26% versus 16% ($P = .02$) in the antithymocyte globulin arm. Whereas the number of infections overall was higher in the antithymocyte globulin arm (86% versus 75%; $P = .03$), the rate of CMV disease was lower with antithymocyte globulin (8%) than with basiliximab (18%; $P = .02$). Thus, for patients at increased risk for rejection, antithymocyte globulin provided greater prevention from acute rejection, supporting its use in higher risk populations. An ongoing clinical trial comparing anti-CD52 to antithymocyte globulin in high-risk patients and IL2-Ra versus antithymocyte globulin in low-risk patients followed by early corticosteroid withdrawal may help clarify the relative benefits of each induction agent. In general, the issues of the need for induction therapy in low-risk patients and the optimal induction agent for high-risk patients are not fully resolved and require further prospective head-to-head trials. Common dosing regimens of induction agents are listed in Figure 100.12.

Prevention of Acute Antibody-Mediated Rejection: Desensitization

The patient who has donor-specific antibodies or is blood type incompatible to the donor before transplantation has a nearly universal risk for development of acute antibody-mediated rejection after transplantation without pretransplantation therapeutic intervention. Experimental protocols have recently emerged that incorporate interventions, referred to as desensitization, that may permit transplantation of these donor-recipient combinations. Desensitization protocols typically involve removal of preformed antibody with plasma exchange and suppression of antibody production and action with intravenous immune globulin (IVIG). These may be coupled with other experimental agents such as rituximab, a humanized anti-CD20 monoclonal antibody that depletes B cells, or splenectomy to reduce B-cell development and thus antibody production.[19-21] Coupled with depleting antibody induction therapy and standard immunosuppression, acute antibody-mediated rejection rates of 39% have been reported.[22]

Agents Used for Induction/Desensitization Therapy and Treatment of Rejection			
Agent	**Target**	**Dose (induction)**	**Dose (rejection)**
Methylprednisolone	B cells, T cells, macrophages	500 mg IV intraoperatively, followed by taper during 1–5 days	3-5 mg/kg (250-500 mg) IV × 3–5 days
Basiliximab	IL-2 receptors on T cells	20 mg IV x 2 on days 0, 4	N/A
Dacilizumab	IL-2 receptors on T cells	1–2 mg/kg IV every 2 weeks for 5 doses post-transplantation	N/A
OKT3	CD3 on T cells	5 mg IV x 7–14 days	5 mg IV x 7-14 days
rATG	T-cell surface antigens	1–1.5 mg/kg IV × 4–14 days	1–1.5 mg/kg IV × 7–14 days
Anti-CD52	CD52 on T and B cells	30–60 mg x 1–2 on days 0 and 2	Same as induction
IVIG	B cell inhibition?	1–2 g/kg total dose during 1–5 IV infusions	Same as desensitization
Rituximab	CD20 on B cells	375 mg/m^2	Same as desensitization

Figure 100.12 Agents used for induction/desensitization therapy and treatment of rejection. NA, not applicable.

Common Immunosuppression Regimens in the United States, 2005		
Regimen	**At Time of Hospital Discharge**	**At One Year Post-Transplantation**
Standard Regimens		
TAC/MMF-MPA/Pred	50%	44%
CSA/MMF-MPA/Pred	10%	9%
Avoidance Regimens		
CNI-free (any)	5%	4%
Steroid-free (any)	23%	26%
TAC/MMF-MPA	20%	21%
CSA/MMF-MPA	1%	3%

Figure 100.13 Common immunosuppression regimens in the United States, 2005. CNI, calcineurin inhibitor; CSA, cyclosporine; MMF, mycophenolate mofetil; MPA, mycophenolate sodium; Pred, prednisone; TAC, tacrolimus. *(Modified from OPTN/SRTR Annual Report 2007.)*

Maintenance Therapy for the Prevention of Acute Rejection

Current maintenance immunosuppression most commonly includes a CNI, an antiproliferative agent, and corticosteroids. This combination of agents forms the standard against which novel strategies are compared, such as corticosteroid withdrawal/avoidance and CNI withdrawal/avoidance. Cyclosporine has been replaced by tacrolimus as the preferred CNI in the United States and together with the antiproliferative agent MMF forms the most common immunosuppressive regimen in current practice in the United States and most Western countries (Fig. 100.13).

Calcineurin Inhibitors in the Prevention of Acute Rejection

Since the early 1980s, when the introduction of cyclosporine resulted in a reduction in the incidence of acute rejection and improvements in projected graft survival,[23] calcineurin inhibition has been a cornerstone of maintenance immunosuppression. Tacrolimus, first introduced in the 1990s and compared head-to-head with cyclosporine in a number of trials, appears to provide greater protection from acute rejection but with a different side effect profile. A recent meta-analysis of trials that compared tacrolimus- and cyclosporine-based immunosuppression demonstrated a reduction in risk of acute rejection of 31% but an increase in risk for development of diabetes of 86%. Tacrolimus was also associated with a better death-censored graft survival (HR, 0.56), particularly at target trough doses of less than 10 ng/ml, a finding that was not shown in individual studies.[24]

Antiproliferative Agents in the Prevention of Acute Rejection

The first antiproliferative agent used in kidney transplantation, azathioprine, was introduced in the early 1960s and was used initially in conjunction with corticosteroids and later with cyclosporine. Whereas its development was critical in the advancement of allotransplantation, acute rejection was common, with acute rejection rates of 35% to 40% in a number of clinical trials using cyclosporine/azathioprine/prednisone. Newer antiproliferative agents emerged in the 1990s with MMF and later with sirolimus that significantly reduced the incidence of acute rejection.

MMF, a purine antagonist that interferes with DNA synthesis in rapidly dividing cells such as activated lymphocytes, gained popularity after a number of multicenter prospective clinical trials demonstrated an approximately 50% reduction in the incidence of acute rejection compared with azathioprine.[25,26] A large registry analysis suggests that there is a beneficial effect of MMF on graft survival, independent of acute rejection.[27] One drawback of MMF has been its gastrointestinal tolerability, which often results in reduction of therapy with attendant risks of acute rejection[28] and graft loss.[29] A mycophenolate analogue, enteric-coated mycophenolate sodium (EC-MPS), has been developed and appears to be "noninferior" in efficacy to MMF,[30] with less gastrointestinal side effects reported in one open-label study.[31]

Like MMF, sirolimus was initially tested in clinical trials as a substitute for azathioprine and demonstrated reductions in acute rejection rates similar to MMF.[32] An antiproliferative agent that inhibits the progression from G_1 to S phase of the cell cycle, sirolimus appears to have additional antiproliferative effects on nonimmune cells that may contribute to an increase in side effects (impaired wound healing, lymphocele formation, proteinuria, and slower recovery from delayed graft function) but also may reduce the incidence of viral infection and malignant disease.[33]

Acute Rejection Rates in Calcineurin Inhibitor– and Corticosteroid-Sparing Immunosuppression Regimens

Given the advances in immunosuppression during the last decade, attempts to eliminate undesirable side effects of immunosuppression have assumed a greater importance in the management of patients. Avoidance of CNIs offers the hope of prolonged graft survival, given the inherent nephrotoxicity of this medication class, whereas avoidance of corticosteroids offers the hope of reducing a number of cosmetic, metabolic, and cardiovascular (CV) side effects attributable to prednisone.

Early corticosteroid cessation (within 7 days after transplantation) has become increasingly popular in the United States. In 2006, more than 30% of all patients were discharged after transplantation without maintenance prednisone therapy. In general, patients at lower immunologic risk (low panel reactive antibodies, first transplants) are selected,[34,35] and immunosuppression includes induction therapy, a CNI, and an antiproliferative agent. Acute rejection rates in single-center studies range from 10% to 15%. In the largest prospective, multicenter study of corticosteroid cessation to date,[36] a standard corticosteroid taper or a rapid elimination of corticosteroids at 7 days after transplantation was compared on the background of induction therapy plus a tacrolimus/MMF-based immunosuppression. Corticosteroid withdrawal was associated with less bone disease, less weight gain, and lower triglyceride levels with similar graft function at 5 years. However, rejection rates were higher in the corticosteroid withdrawal arm (18% versus 11%; $P = .04$), and a *post hoc* analysis suggested a higher rate of chronic allograft nephropathy in the corticosteroid withdrawal arm.

CNI avoidance has been studied with both dual therapy (MMF/prednisone) and triple therapy (sirolimus/MMF/prednisone) with two antiproliferative agents in combination with induction therapy. In general, MMF/prednisone maintenance immunosuppression does not appear to be effective in the prevention of rejection (70% incidence in a pilot study[37]), and although single-center studies report acute rejection rates of 6% to 13% with sirolimus/MMF/prednisone therapy,[38,39] a large multicenter trial using this combination and target trough concentrations of sirolimus of 4 to 8 ng/ml also revealed an excessively high acute rejection rate (38%).[40] Whereas newer agents such as the costimulation blocker belatacept may permit CNI avoidance in the future,[41] and CNI withdrawal with sirolimus 2 to 6 months after transplantation may be more feasible than *de novo* avoidance,[42,43] CNI-based initial immunosuppression is appropriately considered the standard of care at present.

Acute rejection rates by treatment regimen reported in recent multicenter clinical trials are shown in Figure 100.14. These rates are often higher than rates reported to registries (see Fig. 100.1) because of the more rigorous follow-up and mandatory reporting within the context of clinical trials.

TREATMENT

Acute T Cell–Mediated Rejection

Treatment of T cell–mediated acute rejection is often directed by the findings on biopsy and the clinical response to pulse corticosteroids. For the patient with graft dysfunction and biopsy-proven rejection, treatment with intravenous methylprednisolone, 3 to 5 mg/kg (250 to 500 mg/day), for 3 to5 days is often effective if the histologic injury is tubulointerstitial (Banff class IA or IB). Remarkably few studies of the clinical response to corticosteroids in the treatment of acute rejection have been performed under modern immunosuppression, but prior data suggest that 60% to 70% of patients will respond with improved urine output and decreasing serum creatinine within 5 days. If there is inadequate response after corticosteroid pulse therapy or if there is vascular involvement (Banff class IIA, IIB), corticosteroids often must be supplemented with T cell–depleting antibody therapies in a similar dosing strategy but longer treatment course compared with their use for induction (see Fig. 100.12). Most studies have used these agents in 7- to 14-day treatment courses, with no clinical trials investigating the efficacy of shorter courses versus longer courses. For patients who are on a maintenance regimen that is not tacrolimus based, tacrolimus conversion may also be considered in the setting of rejection with an inadequate response to corticosteroids[44]; for patients on a corticosteroid-free regimen, reinstitution of maintenance prednisone may be warranted.[45]

The question of the most effective depleting agent for treatment of acute rejection remains a matter of debate. In general, the number and quality of trials comparing agents do not permit firm conclusions. In a meta-analysis of randomized trials comparing monoclonal (OKT3) versus polyclonal (antilymphocyte globulin, antithymocyte globulin) antibody therapy, no differences were noted in reversing rejection, preventing subsequent rejection, or preventing graft loss, whereas OKT3 was three times more likely to induce reactions of fever, chills, and malaise.[46] Given a more favorable side effect profile, antithymocyte globulin has become the most common antibody agent used in the treatment of refractory rejection. According to the SRTR Annual Report 2007, in 2005 75% of patients with acute rejection were treated with corticosteroids with or without additional agents, whereas 28%, 5%, and 2% of patients were treated with antithymocyte globulin, OKT3, and alemtuzumab, respectively.

Acute Antibody-Mediated Rejection

Treatment of acute humoral rejection is indicated when the triad of graft injury, $C4d^+$ staining in peritubular capillaries on biopsy, and circulating donor-specific antibody is present, but it should also be considered in high-risk circumstances (prior desensitization or known donor-specific antibody) even if all three criteria are not met. Treatment entails removal of the pathogenic immunoglobulins with plasma exchange and inhibition/suppression of antibody production with IVIG. In general, at least five plasma exchange treatments should be administered with 1 to 2 g/kg total dose of IVIG. As IVIG is removed by plasma exchange, a common strategy employed is to administer IVIG 100 to 200 mg/kg after each exchange. For refractory acute humoral rejection, rituximab may be considered despite targeting of B cells at an earlier phase of maturation than the antibody-producing plasma cell line.[47] Finally, there are case reports of splenectomy for refractory acute humoral rejection.[48] These therapies are typically coupled with targeted T-cell therapy, such as high-dose

Maintenance Immunosuppression and Reported Rejection Rates in Randomized Multi-Center Trials				
Regimen	**Induction**	**CNI Dose or Trough Goal**	**Antiproliferative Dosing**	**Acute Rejection at 6 Months**
Low Immunologic Risk				
CSA/AZA/Pred		4.0 mg/kg/d	1.5–2 mg/kg/d	36%[26]
CSA/AZA/Pred	IL-2Ra	Not stated	Not stated	22%[14]
CSA/MMF/Pred		150–300 ng/ml × 3 mo, 100–200 ng/ml	1 g bid	24%[40]
CSA/MMF/Pred	IL-2Ra	125–400 ng/ml × 3 mo, 100–300 ng/ml	1 g bid	12%[54]
TAC/AZA/Pred	OKT3 or Atgam	5–13.9 ng/ml	1.5 mg/kg/d	32%[55]
TAC/MMF/Pred	OKT3 or Atgam	5–13.9 ng/ml	1 g bid	7%[55]
TAC/MMF/Pred	IL-2Ra	7–16 ng/ml × 3 mo, 5–15 ng/ml	1 g bid	4%[54]
CSA/SRL/Pred		200–350 ng/ml × 1 mo, 200–300 ng/ml × 1 mo, 150–250 ng/ml	2 mg daily	17%[32]
TAC/SRL/Pred		8–16 ng/ml × 3 mo, 5–15 ng/ml	4–12 ng/ml	13%[56]
High Immunologic Risk				
CSA/SRL/Pred	IL-2Ra or rATG	200–300 ng/ml 0-14 d 150–200 ng/ml	10–15 ng/ml	14%[57]
TAC/SRL/Pred	IL-2Ra or rATG	10–15 ng/ml 0-14 d 5–10 ng/ml	10–15 ng/ml	17%[57]
Drug Minimization/Avoidance				
CSA (low)/MMF/Pred	IL-2Ra	50–100 ng/ml	1 g bid	23%[40]
TAC (low)/MMF/Pred	IL-2Ra	3–7 ng/ml	1 g bid	12%[40]
TAC/MMF	IL-2Ra or rATG	10–20 ng/ml × 3 mo, 5–15 ng/ml	1.5 g bid x 14 d 1 g bid	9%[36]
SRL/MMF/Pred	IL-2Ra	N/A	SRL 4–8 ng/ml MMF 1 g bid	38%[40]

Figure 100.14 Maintenance immunosuppression and reported rejection rates in randomized multicenter trials. Anti-proliferative dosing is shown as SRL trough level goals and for MMF as dose. Mycophenolate trough levels are of limited value. *A higher percentage of living donor kidney transplant recipients were enrolled in this clinical trial. For general comparison only. In comparing acute rejection rates from various clinical trials, the study population and treatment algorithms may be different between trials. AZA, azathioprine; CSA, cyclosporine; IL-2Ra, interleukin-2 receptor antibodies; MMF, mycophenolate mofetil; Pred, prednisone; rATG, rabbit antithymocyte globulin; SRL, sirolimus; TAC, tacrolimus.

corticosteroids or depleting antibody therapy, because helper T-cell function may contribute to an enhanced B-cell response.

Chronic Rejection (T Cell or Antibody Mediated)

T cell– or antibody-mediated injury in a graft without features of acute tissue injury remains a therapeutic dilemma in kidney transplantation. No specific intervention has been proven to be effective in reversing the chronic tissue injury; however, consideration should be given to optimizing or enhancing the maintenance immunosuppression by transitioning to tacrolimus/MMF therapy or increasing the dose of these agents if CNI nephrotoxicity is not identified.[49] Any intervention should be weighed against the potential for risk of enhanced immunosuppression and the lack of any long-term data describing the impact of enhancing immunosuppression. This topic is discussed in greater detail in Chapter 103.

PROGNOSIS

Episodes of acute rejection may predispose to chronic graft dysfunction, with increased histologic findings of chronic rejection or interstitial fibrosis and tubular atrophy and clinical findings of reduced graft survival. The clinical response to antirejection therapy appears to be critical in this regard, as the change in renal function from 6 and 12 months after transplantation is more predictive of long-term graft survival than the occurrence of prior episodes of acute rejection.[50] Two analyses (one examining the United States experience[51] and another examining the Australia/New Zealand experience[52]) have shed light on risk factors for graft loss after episodes of acute rejection. In general, acute T cell–mediated rejection that responds to therapy with return to near-baseline renal function does not portend worse graft survival. However, vascular rejection, late rejection (after 3 months), and rejection that does not respond to within 75% of baseline serum creatinine level is associated with worse graft outcomes. Although acute rejection rates have fallen significantly during the past decade, graft survival rates have not improved in similar fashion; one explanation for this finding is that the rejection now identified tends to be less responsive to therapy, with fewer cases achieving near-baseline serum creatinine levels. The long-term prognosis after episodes of acute antibody-mediated rejection has not been fully defined in prospective analyses; however, from single-center and retrospective studies, it appears that episodes of acute humoral rejection are likely to have an impact on long-term graft survival. Similarly, the emergence of *de novo* HLA antibodies at any time after transplantation has been shown to be associated with a 5% worse graft survival *per year* compared with those who do not form anti-HLA antibodies.[53] For this reason, patients who have suffered episodes of acute rejection must be rigorously monitored with optimization of baseline maintenance immunosuppression. Remaining questions include the value of escalated immunosuppression, such as longer term scheduled antibody therapy, and additional IVIG treatment for those without adequate clinical response or with persistently elevated titers of HLA antibodies.

REFERENCES

1. Hamburger J, Vaysse J, Crosnier J, et al. Renal homotransplantation in man after radiation of the recipient. Experience with six patients since 1959. *Am J Med.* 1962;32:854-871.
2. Meier-Kriesche HU, Li S, Gruessner RW, et al. Immunosuppression: Evolution in practice and trends, 1994-2004. *Am J Transplant.* 2006;6(Pt 2):1111-1131.
3. Racusen LC, Solez K, Colvin RB, et al. The Banff 97 working classification of renal allograft pathology. *Kidney Int.* 1999;55:713-723.
4. Solez K, Colvin RB, Racusen LC, et al. Banff 07 classification of renal allograft pathology: Updates and future directions. *Am J Transplant.* 2008;8:753-760.
5. Colvin RB. Antibody-mediated renal allograft rejection: Diagnosis and pathogenesis. *J Am Soc Nephrol.* 2007;18:1046-1056.
6. Watschinger B, Pascual M. Capillary C4d deposition as a marker of humoral immunity in renal allograft rejection. *J Am Soc Nephrol.* 2002; 13:2420-2423.
7. Cosio FG, Gloor JM, Sethi S, Stegall MD. Transplant glomerulopathy. *Am J Transplant.* 2008;8:492-496.
8. Banff 07 classification of renal allograft pathology: updates and future directions. *Am J Transplant.* 2008;8:753-760.
9. Moll S, Pascual M. Humoral rejection of organ allografts. *Am J Transplant.* 2005;5:2611-2618.
10. Racusen LC, Colvin RB, Solez K, et al. Antibody-mediated rejection criteria—an addition to the Banff 97 classification of renal allograft rejection. *Am J Transplant.* 2003;3:708-714.
11. Meehan SM, Siegel CT, Aronson AJ, et al. The relationship of untreated borderline infiltrates by the Banff criteria to acute rejection in renal allograft biopsies. *J Am Soc Nephrol.* 1999;10:1806-1814.
12. Pallet N, Thervet E, Alberti C, et al. Kidney transplant in black recipients: Are African Europeans different from African Americans? *Am J Transplant.* 2005;5:2682-2687.
13. Young CJ, Gaston RS. Renal transplantation in black Americans. *N Engl J Med.* 2000;343:1545-1552.
14. Vincenti F, Kirkman R, Light S, et al. Interleukin-2-receptor blockade with daclizumab to prevent acute rejection in renal transplantation. Daclizumab Triple Therapy Study Group. *N Engl J Med.* 1998;338: 161-165.
15. Gaber AO, First MR, Tesi RJ, et al. Results of the double-blind, randomized, multicenter, phase III clinical trial of Thymoglobulin versus Atgam in the treatment of acute graft rejection episodes after renal transplantation. *Transplantation.* 1998;66:29-37.
16. Caillard S, Dharnidharka V, Agodoa L, et al. Posttransplant lymphoproliferative disorders after renal transplantation in the United States in era of modern immunosuppression. *Transplantation.* 2005;80:1233-1243.
17. Kirk AD, Cherikh WS, Ring M, et al. Dissociation of depletional induction and posttransplant lymphoproliferative disease in kidney recipients treated with alemtuzumab. *Am J Transplant.* 2007;7: 2619-2625.
18. Brennan DC, Daller JA, Lake KD, et al. Rabbit antithymocyte globulin versus basiliximab in renal transplantation. *N Engl J Med.* 2006;355: 1967-1977.
19. Gloor JM, Lager DJ, Fidler ME, et al. A comparison of splenectomy versus intensive posttransplant antidonor blood group antibody monitoring without splenectomy in ABO-incompatible kidney transplantation. *Transplantation.* 2005;80:1572-1577.
20. Ishida H, Miyamoto N, Shirakawa H, et al. Evaluation of immunosuppressive regimens in ABO-incompatible living kidney transplantation—single center analysis. *Am J Transplant.* 2007;7:825-831.
21. Montgomery RA, Locke JE, King KE, et al. ABO incompatible renal transplantation: A paradigm ready for broad implementation. *Transplantation.* 2009;87:1246-1255.
22. Burns JM, Cornell LD, Perry DK, et al. Alloantibody levels and acute humoral rejection early after positive crossmatch kidney transplantation. *Am J Transplant.* 2008;8:2684-2694.
23. Hariharan S, Johnson CP, Bresnahan BA, et al. Improved graft survival after renal transplantation in the United States, 1988 to 1996. *N Engl J Med.* 2000;342:605-612.
24. Webster AC, Woodroffe RC, Taylor RS, et al. Tacrolimus versus ciclosporin as primary immunosuppression for kidney transplant recipients: Meta-analysis and meta-regression of randomised trial data. *BMJ.* 2005;331:810.
25. Sollinger HW. Mycophenolate mofetil for the prevention of acute rejection in primary cadaveric renal allograft recipients. U.S. Renal Transplant Mycophenolate Mofetil Study Group. *Transplantation.* 1995;60: 225-232.
26. A blinded, randomized clinical trial of mycophenolate mofetil for the prevention of acute rejection in cadaveric renal transplantation. The Tricontinental Mycophenolate Mofetil Renal Transplantation Study Group. *Transplantation.* 1996;61:1029-1037.
27. Ojo AO, Meier-Kriesche HU, Hanson JA, et al. Mycophenolate mofetil reduces late renal allograft loss independent of acute rejection. *Transplantation.* 2000;69:2405-2409.
28. Knoll GA, MacDonald I, Khan A, Van Walraven C. Mycophenolate mofetil dose reduction and the risk of acute rejection after renal transplantation. *J Am Soc Nephrol.* 2003;14:2381-2386.
29. Bunnapradist S, Lentine KL, Burroughs TE, et al. Mycophenolate mofetil dose reductions and discontinuations after gastrointestinal complications are associated with renal transplant graft failure. *Transplantation.* 2006;82:102-107.
30. Salvadori M, Holzer H, de Mattos A, et al. Enteric-coated mycophenolate sodium is therapeutically equivalent to mycophenolate mofetil in de novo renal transplant patients. *Am J Transplant.* 2004;4:231-236.
31. Bolin P, Tanriover B, Zibari GB, et al. Improvement in 3-month patient-reported gastrointestinal symptoms after conversion from mycophenolate mofetil to enteric-coated mycophenolate sodium in renal transplant patients. *Transplantation.* 2007;84:1443-1451.
32. Kahan BD. Efficacy of sirolimus compared with azathioprine for reduction of acute renal allograft rejection: A randomised multicentre study. The Rapamune US Study Group. *Lancet.* 2000;356:194-202.
33. Campistol JM, Eris J, Oberbauer R, et al. Sirolimus therapy after early cyclosporine withdrawal reduces the risk for cancer in adult renal transplantation. *J Am Soc Nephrol.* 2006;17:581-589.
34. Matas AJ, Kandaswamy R, Gillingham KJ, et al. Prednisone-free maintenance immunosuppression—a 5-year experience. *Am J Transplant.* 2005;5:2473-2478.
35. Kaufman DB, Leventhal JR, Axelrod D, et al. Alemtuzumab induction and prednisone-free maintenance immunotherapy in kidney transplantation: Comparison with basiliximab induction—long-term results. *Am J Transplant.* 2005;5:2539-2548.
36. Woodle ES, First MR, Pirsch J, et al. A prospective, randomized, double-blind, placebo-controlled multicenter trial comparing early (7 day) corticosteroid cessation versus long-term, low-dose corticosteroid therapy. *Ann Surg.* 2008;248:564-577.
37. Asberg A, Midtvedt K, Line PD, et al. Calcineurin inhibitor avoidance with daclizumab, mycophenolate mofetil, and prednisolone in DR-matched de novo kidney transplant recipients. *Transplantation.* 2006;82:62-68.
38. Larson TS, Dean PG, Stegall MD, et al. Complete avoidance of calcineurin inhibitors in renal transplantation: A randomized trial comparing sirolimus and tacrolimus. *Am J Transplant.* 2006;6:514-522.
39. Flechner SM, Goldfarb D, Modlin C, et al. Kidney transplantation without calcineurin inhibitor drugs: A prospective, randomized trial of sirolimus versus cyclosporine. *Transplantation.* 2002;74:1070-1076.

40. Ekberg H, Tedesco-Silva H, Demirbas A, et al. Reduced exposure to calcineurin inhibitors in renal transplantation. *N Engl J Med*. 2007; 357:2562-2575.
41. Vincenti F, Larsen C, Durrbach A, et al. Costimulation blockade with belatacept in renal transplantation. *N Engl J Med*. 2005;353:770-781.
42. Mota A, Arias M, Taskinen EI, et al. Sirolimus-based therapy following early cyclosporine withdrawal provides significantly improved renal histology and function at 3 years. *Am J Transplant*. 2004;4:953-961.
43. Mulay AV, Hussain N, Fergusson D, Knoll GA. Calcineurin inhibitor withdrawal from sirolimus-based therapy in kidney transplantation: A systematic review of randomized trials. *Am J Transplant*. 2005;5: 1748-1756.
44. Jordan ML, Shapiro R, Vivas CA, et al. FK506 "rescue" for resistant rejection of renal allografts under primary cyclosporine immunosuppression. *Transplantation*. 1994;57:860-865.
45. Humar A, Gillingham K, Kandaswamy R, et al. Steroid avoidance regimens: A comparison of outcomes with maintenance steroids versus continued steroid avoidance in recipients having an acute rejection episode. *Am J Transplant*. 2007;7:1948-1953.
46. Webster AC, Pankhurst T, Rinaldi F, et al. Monoclonal and polyclonal antibody therapy for treating acute rejection in kidney transplant recipients: A systematic review of randomized trial data. *Transplantation*. 2006;81:953-965.
47. Faguer S, Kamar N, Guilbeaud-Frugier C, et al. Rituximab therapy for acute humoral rejection after kidney transplantation. *Transplantation*. 2007;83:1277-1280.
48. Locke JE, Zachary AA, Haas M, et al. The utility of splenectomy as rescue treatment for severe acute antibody mediated rejection. *Am J Transplant*. 2007;7:842-846.
49. Theruvath TP, Saidman SL, Mauiyyedi S, et al. Control of antidonor antibody production with tacrolimus and mycophenolate mofetil in renal allograft recipients with chronic rejection. *Transplantation*. 2001;72: 77-83.
50. Hariharan S, McBride MA, Cherikh WS, et al. Post-transplant renal function in the first year predicts long-term kidney transplant survival. *Kidney Int*. 2002;62:311-318.
51. Meier-Kriesche HU, Schold JD, Srinivas TR, Kaplan B. Lack of improvement in renal allograft survival despite a marked decrease in acute rejection rates over the most recent era. *Am J Transplant*. 2004;4:378-383.
52. McDonald S, Russ G, Campbell S, Chadban S. Kidney transplant rejection in Australia and New Zealand: Relationships between rejection and graft outcome. *Am J Transplant*. 2007;7:1201-1208.
53. Terasaki PI, Ozawa M, Castro R. Four-year follow-up of a prospective trial of HLA and MICA antibodies on kidney graft survival. *Am J Transplant*. 2007;7:408-415.
54. Silva HT Jr, Yang HC, Abouljoud M, et al. One-year results with extended-release tacrolimus/MMF, tacrolimus/MMF and cyclosporine/ MMF in de novo kidney transplant recipients. *Am J Transplant*. Mar 2007;7(3):595-608.
55. Miller J, Mendez R, Pirsch JD, Jensik SC. Safety and efficacy of tacrolimus in combination with mycophenolate mofetil (MMF) in cadaveric renal transplant recipients. FK506/MMF Dose-Ranging Kidney Transplant Study Group. *Transplantation*. Mar 15 2000;69(5):875-880.
56. Gonwa T, Mendez R, Yang HC, et al. Randomized trial of tacrolimus in combination with sirolimus of mycophenolate mofetil in kidney transplantation: results at 6 months. *Transplantation*. Apr 27 2003;75(8): 1213-1220.
57. Gaber AO, Kahan BD, Van Buren C, et al. Comparison of sirolimus plus tacrolimus versus sirolimus plus cyclosporine in high-risk renal aliograft recipients: results from an open-label, randomized trial. *Transplantation*. Nov 15 2008;86(9):1187-1195.

CHAPTER 101

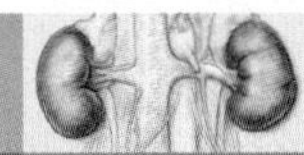

Medical Management of the Kidney Transplant Recipient: Infections and Malignant Neoplasms

Phuong-Thu T. Pham, Gabriel M. Danovitch, Phuong-Chi T. Pham

Patient and graft survival rates in recipients of solid organ transplants have improved significantly because of refinement in surgical techniques and the advent of potent immunosuppressive agents. Nonetheless, malignant neoplasms and infectious complications continue to adversely affect post-transplantation morbidity and mortality. Although rare, donor-derived infections or malignant disease can arise by delayed donor seroconversion after a recent acute infection, unidentified pathogens in the organ donor, occult neoplastic disease at the time of organ procurement, or malignant transformation of donor cells. This chapter discusses infections and post-transplantation–related malignant neoplasms in recipients of renal transplants. Post-transplantation infectious and drug-related gastrointestinal complications are also discussed.

INFECTIOUS DISEASES

Despite prophylactic therapy against common bacterial, viral, and opportunistic pathogens in the perioperative and postoperative period, infections are the second most common cause of death after cardiovascular disease (CVD) in renal transplant recipients. According to the U.S. Renal Data System (USRDS), infections occurred at a rate of 45 per 100 patient-years during the first 3 years after transplantation.[1] The most common infections are bacterial, followed by viral and fungal. Parasitic infections are rare. Notably, cytomegalovirus (CMV) and herpes simplex virus (HSV) infection rates have decreased since the mid-1990s as a result of effective antiviral prophylaxis; hepatitis B virus (HBV) and hepatitis C virus (HCV) infection rates increased during the same period for unclear reasons.

Infectious Etiologies

Both the type and occurrence of infections in the immunocompromised transplant recipient follow a "timetable pattern" (Fig. 101.1).[2]

Infection with Transplantation

Although rare, both blood-borne and kidney infections have been transmitted during donation. These include viral infections (e.g., HCV, HBV, human immunodeficiency virus (HIV), CMV, and BK, among others), parasitic infections (malaria, *Babesia*), and bacterial infections (from undiagnosed bacteremia or renal infections).

Month 1 After Transplantation

Most infections in the first month are due to common bacteria and *Candida* acquired in the hospital setting. Except for HSV, other viral infections are uncommon during this period. Similar to those that follow any major surgical procedure, most bacterial infections during this period involve wounds, catheters, and drainage sites. Aspiration pneumonia and urinary tract infections (UTIs) are common. Infections specific to renal transplant recipients include perinephric fluid collections due to lymphoceles, wound hematomas, or urine leaks; indwelling urinary stents; and UTIs secondary to urinary tract abnormalities, such as ureteral stricture, vesicoureteral reflux, or neurogenic bladder. Most UTIs are caused by common gram-negative bacteria (*Escherichia coli*, Enterobacteriaceae, and *Pseudomonas)* and gram-positive bacteria (enterococcus). Preventive measures for UTIs include early urethral catheter removal and antibiotic prophylaxis. Trimethoprim-sulfamethoxazole or ciprofloxacin prophylaxis during the first 3 months after transplantation effectively reduces the frequency of UTIs to less than 10% and essentially eliminates urosepsis unless anatomic or functional derangement of the urinary tract is present.

Infections with multidrug-resistant microorganisms have recently emerged as an important cause of morbidity and mortality in organ transplantation. Hence, in some centers, the routine use of antibiotic prophylaxis is no longer recommended. Although strict aseptic surgical techniques and perioperative use of first-generation cephalosporins reduce the incidence of wound infections, infections are still observed, especially in subjects with comorbid conditions such as diabetes mellitus (DM) and obesity. Antibiotic-associated *Clostridium difficile* infection (particularly cephalosporins, ciprofloxacin, and amoxicillin-clavulanate) has become a serious epidemiologic problem worldwide. Judicious use of antibiotic prophylactic therapy may decrease the incidence of iatrogenic *C. difficile* infections. Whereas most infections during the first month are due to routine bacterial infections, nosocomial outbreaks have also been reported for rarer infections, such as *Legionella* from contaminated hospital water supplies.

Months 1 to 6

During months 1 to 6, opportunistic infections secondary to immunosuppression are most common. Viral infections, such as CMV, HSV, varicella-zoster virus (VZV), Epstein-Barr virus (EBV), HBV, and HCV, may occur from exogenous infection or reactivation of latent disease due to the immunosuppressed state. Repeated courses of antibiotics and corticosteroid therapy increase the risk of fungal infections, whereas viral infections may not only result from the immunosuppression but may themselves further impair immunity to increase the risk for additional opportunistic infections. Opportunistic infections may occur with *Pneumocystis jiroveci* (previously *Pneumocystis carinii*), *Aspergillus* species, *Listeria monocytogenes*, *Nocardia* species, and *Toxoplasma gondii*. Trimethoprim-sulfamethoxazole prophylaxis (see

Figure 101.1 Timetable of infections.* *Geographically focused infections will need to be considered in certain cases, such as malaria, leishmaniasis, trypanosomiasis, and strongyloidiasis. [1]Sources of infections specific to recipients of renal transplant: perinephric fluid collections (e.g., lymphoceles, wound hematomas, urine leaks), indwelling urinary stents, or anatomic or functional genitourinary tract abnormalities (e.g., ureteral stricture, vesicoureteric reflux, neurogenic bladder). CMV, cytomegalovirus; EBV, Epstein-Barr virus; HBV, hepatitis B virus; HCV, hepatitis C virus; HHV, human herpesvirus; HIV, human immunodeficiency virus; HSV, herpes simplex virus; RSV, respiratory syncytial virus; VZV, varicella-zoster virus. *(Modified from reference 2.)*

Timetable of Infections*

Month 1 After Transplantation	Months 1–6	After 6 Months
Postoperative bacterial infections Urinary tract Respiratory Vascular access related Wound Intra-abdominal infections[1] Bacteremia **Nosocomial**, including *Legionella* species **Viral:** HSV, HBV, HCV, HIV **Fungal:** *Candida* **Organisms transmitted with donor organ** Untreated infection in recipient	**Opportunistic** or **unconventional infections** **Viral:** CMV, HHV-6, HHV-7, EBV, VZV, influenza, RSV, adenovirus **Fungal:** *Aspergillus* species, *Cryptococcus, Mucor* **Bacterial:** *Nocardia, Listeria, Mycobacterium* species *Legionella*, tuberculosis **Parasitic:** Pneumocystis, jiroveci, *Toxoplasma* and *Strongyloides* species, leishmaniasis	**Late opportunistic infections** *Cryptococcus*, CMV retinitis or colitis, VZV, parovirus-B-19, polyomavirus BK, *Listeria*, tuberculosis **Persistent infections:** HBV, HCV **Associated with malignancy** EBV, papillomavirus, HSV, HHV-8 **Community acquired** **Unusual sites** (e.g., paravertebral abscess)

Fig. 101.2 for trimethoprim-sulfamethoxazole allergy) eliminates or reduces the incidence of *Pneumocystis* pneumonia, *L. monocytogenes* meningitis, *Nocardia* species infection, and *T. gondii* infection.

After 6 Months

After 6 months, the infection risk can be categorized on the basis of the patient's status.

The first category consists of the majority of transplant recipients (70% to 80%), who have satisfactory or good allograft function, relatively low doses of immunosuppression medication, and no history of chronic viral infection. The risk of infection in these patients is similar to that of the general population, with community-acquired respiratory viruses constituting the major infective agents. Opportunistic infections are unusual unless environmental exposure has occurred.

The second group (approximately 10% of patients) consists of those with chronic viral infection that may include HBV, HCV, CMV, EBV, BK virus, or papillomavirus. In the setting of immunosuppression, such viral infections may lead to the development of progressive liver disease or cirrhosis (HBV, HCV), BK nephropathy, post-transplantation lymphoproliferative disease (EBV), or squamous cell carcinoma (papillomavirus).

The third group (approximately 10% of patients) consists of those who experience multiple episodes of rejection requiring repeated exposure to heavy immunosuppression. These patients are the most likely to develop chronic viral infections and superinfection with opportunistic organisms. Causative opportunistic pathogens include *P. jiroveci*, *L. monocytogenes*, *Nocardia asteroides*, and *Cryptococcus neoformans* and geographically restricted mycoses (coccidioidomycosis, histoplasmosis, blastomycosis, and paracoccidioidomycosis). In these high-risk candidates, lifelong prophylactic therapy with trimethoprim-sulfamethoxazole (80 mg/400 mg daily) has been advocated. Lifelong antifungal prophylaxis should also be considered and environmental exposure minimized (primarily avoidance of pigeons and areas of active building construction).

Newly Recognized Viral Infections

Several uncommon viral infections have recently been reported in both the early and late post-transplantation periods.[3] In the early post-transplantation period, outbreaks of donor-transmitted viral infections, such as lymphocytic choriomeningitis and West Nile virus, have been reported. Lymphocytic choriomeningitis occurs within the first 4 weeks after transplantation and is associated with a greater than 90% mortality rate.[3] In the late post-transplantation period, infections with community-acquired viral pathogens, including vaccine-preventable diseases such as mumps and measles, have reemerged. There is currently no effective antiviral therapy against either infection, and adherence to current guidelines for vaccinations in solid organ transplantation is recommended (discussed later). Other emerging or reemerging viral infections include adenovirus, human herpesvirus 6, metapneumovirus, parainfluenza, and respiratory syncytial virus. Interestingly, only rare cases due to severe acute respiratory syndrome (SARS) coronavirus have been reported.

The following sections discuss selected infections in renal transplant recipients. Suggested prophylactic therapy is shown in Figure 101.2.

Cytomegalovirus Infection

CMV infection may be a primary infection in a seronegative recipient (donor seropositive, recipient seronegative), reactivation of endogenous latent virus (donor seropositive or seronegative, recipient seropositive), or superinfection with a new virus strain in a seropositive recipient (donor seropositive, recipient seropositive). Primary CMV infection is usually more severe than reactive infection or superinfection.

CMV infection occurs primarily after the first month of transplantation and continues to be a significant cause of morbidity in the first 6 months after organ transplantation through both direct and indirect effects.

Clinical Manifestations

CMV infection may be asymptomatic, presenting as a mononucleosis-like syndrome or influenza-like illness with fever and leukopenia or thrombocytopenia, or a severe systemic disease. Hepatitis, esophagitis, gastroenteritis with colonic ulceration, pneumonia, chorioretinitis (associated with retinal hemorrhage), and even otitis[4] may occur. In enterically drained pancreas transplantation, CMV has been reported to cause bleeding ulcer from the duodenal segment. Clinical manifestations usually

Suggested Prophylactic Therapy for Recipients of Renal Transplants

	Comments
Trimethoprim-sulfamethoxazole (TMP–SMZ)* (80/400 mg) one tablet daily × 3 months	Its routine use reduces or eliminates the incidence of *Pneumocystis jiroveci, Listeria monocytogenes, Nocardia asteroides,* and *Toxoplasma gondii* In renal transplant recipients, TMP–SMZ reduces the incidence of urinary tract infection from 30%–80% to <5%–10%
Monthly intravenous or aerosolized pentamidine > dapsone† > or atovaquone‡	Replaces TMP–SMZ for patients with sulfa allergies
Nystatin 100,000 units/ml, 4 ml after meals and before bedtime *or* Fluconazole§ 200 mg one tablet daily × 2 months	For fungal prophylaxis Close monitoring of cyclosporine or tacrolimus levels when starting and stopping antifungal agents
Acyclovir/valganciclovir/ganciclovir	For CMV prophylaxis, see Figure 101.3

Figure 101.2 Suggested prophylactic therapy for recipients of renal transplants. *Prophylactic therapy for the first 3 months after transplantation is generally recommended. For patients receiving sirolimus immunosuppression, 1 year of therapy is recommended. †Check glucose-6-phosphate dehydrogenase deficiency before initiation of therapy. ‡In order of efficacy. §Fluconazole is recommended for recipients of combined kidney-pancreas or combined kidney-liver transplants.

Consider reinstitution of prophylactic therapy for 3 months after acute rejection episodes requiring intensification of immunosuppression. CMV, cytomegalovirus.

occur 1 to 4 months after transplantation except for chorioretinitis, which occurs later in the transplant course.[5] Quantitative CMV assays of serum in patients with invasive colitis and gastritis or neurologic disease including chorioretinitis are often negative. Diagnosis in such cases may require invasive testing and biopsies.

Immunomodulating Effects of CMV Infection

CMV infection is associated with immune modulation and dysregulation of helper/suppressor T cells and may be a risk factor for chronic allograft rejection, secondary infection with opportunistic agents (such as *P. jiroveci, Candida,* and *Aspergillus*), reactivation of human herpesvirus HHV-6 and HHV-7, and the development of post-transplantation lymphoproliferative disease. CMV infection is also associated with acceleration of HCV infection and the development of new-onset DM after transplantation.[6]

Risk Factors for CMV Infection

Donor and recipient seropositive status and the use of blood products from a CMV-seropositive donor are well-established risk factors for CMV infection. Other factors associated with an increased risk of CMV infection include the use of antilymphocyte antibodies, prolonged or repeated course of antilymphocyte preparations, comorbid illnesses, neutropenia, and acute rejection episodes. Mycophenolate mofetil (MMF) has been reported to increase the risk for CMV viremia and CMV disease in some studies, especially in patients receiving more than 3 g/day. Although the cause-effect of allograft rejection and CMV infection remains conjectural, several studies suggest that one may increase the risk for the other, possibly owing to the release of inflammatory cytokines. Prevention of CMV infection, for example, results in a lower incidence of graft rejection.[7]

Prevention and Treatment

Prophylactic therapy begins in the immediate postoperative period. Preemptive therapy involves treatment of those who are found to seroconvert by quantitative laboratory assays of the blood, such as CMV DNA polymerase chain reaction (PCR) or pp65 antigenemia during surveillance studies. The former assay is highly specific and sensitive for the detection of CMV viremia. The latter is a semiquantitative fluorescent assay in which circulating neutrophils are stained for nonspecific uptake of CMV early antigen (pp65).

Various prophylactic and preemptive protocols have been developed. Oral acyclovir provides effective CMV prophylaxis solely in recipients of seronegative donor organs. Oral or intravenous ganciclovir or oral valganciclovir provides superior prophylactic or preemptive therapy against primary CMV infection or CMV reactivation. Prophylactic or preemptive therapy should be based on the intensity of immunosuppression (i.e., during antilymphocyte antibody therapy) and the seropositive status of the donor, the recipient, or both. Seronegative individuals who receive organs from latently infected seropositive donors are at greatest risk for primary infection and severe CMV disease. A suggested CMV prophylaxis protocol is shown in Figure 101.3.

Clinical CMV disease is treated with intravenous ganciclovir (5 mg/kg twice daily for 3 weeks, dose adjusted for renal dysfunction) with reduction of immunosuppression, such as withholding of MMF. Treatment is continued until clearance of viremia as assessed by PCR or antigenemia. Anecdotal reports have suggested that calcineurin inhibitor (CNI) to sirolimus switch in conjunction with ganciclovir therapy may be beneficial in patients with apparent ganciclovir-resistant CMV.[8]

In patients with gastrointestinal CMV infection, the use of these assays is unreliable, and repeated endoscopy should be considered to assess response to therapy. In patients who have primary infection and respond slowly to therapy, the addition of CMV hyperimmune globulin (150 mg/kg per dose given intravenously every 3 to 4 weeks for 3 months) may be of benefit.[5] In patients with tissue invasive disease, intravenous ganciclovir is recommended with conversion to oral therapy when there is evidence of a good response, followed by a 3-month course of oral ganciclovir or valganciclovir prophylaxis.[5] Whereas oral valganciclovir provides good bioavailability and may be effective in mild CMV disease, it is not recommended for the treatment of

Suggested Cytomegalovirus Prophylaxis Protocol[1]

For CMV– recipients of a CMV– organ
Acyclovir 400 mg daily (or valganciclovir 450 mg daily) × 3 months
CMV DNA every 2 weeks × 3 months

For CMV– recipients of a CMV+ organ
During antibody treatment, DHPG[2] 5.0 mg/kg IV everyday, then following antibody treatment/valganciclovir 900 mg PO everyday × 6 months
If no antibody treatment: valganciclovir 900 mg everyday for 6 months
CMV DNA every 2 weeks x 3 months

For CMV+ recipients of a CMV– organ
During antibody treatment, DHPG 5.0 mg/kg IV everyday, then following antibody treatment, valganciclovir 900 mg PO everyday × 6 months
If no antibody treatment: acyclovir 400 mg daily (or valganciclovir 450 mg daily) × 3 months
CMV DNA every 2 weeks × 3 months

For CMV+ recipients of a CMV+ organ
During antibody treatment, DHPG 5.0 mg/kg IV everyday, then following antibody treatment, valganciclovir 900 mg PO everyday × 6 months
If no antibody treatment: acyclovir 400 mg daily (or valganciclovir 450 mg daily)[3] × 3 months
CMV DNA every 2 weeks × 3 months

Figure 101.3 Suggested cytomegalovirus prophylaxis protocol. [1]If CMV status is unknown, give intravenous DHPG until CMV status is determined. [2]Dose adjustment for renal function is necessary. DHPG, 9-(1,3-dihydroxy-2-propoxymethyl) guanine. [3]Although low-dose valganciclovir, 450 mg daily, has been shown to be effective, the Canadian Society of Transplantation Consensus Workshop on CMV management recommends dosing valganciclovir at 900 mg daily for CMV+ recipients of a CMV+ organ (kidney, liver, pancreas, heart). *(From reference 9.)*

established CMV disease, and intravenous ganciclovir is required. Cidofovir and foscarnet are alternative therapeutic agents, but in view of their nephrotoxicity and potential synergistic nephrotoxicity with CNIs, they are reserved for use when ganciclovir-resistant strains are clinically suspected.

Candida Infections

Candida infections are common in transplant recipients; *Candida albicans* and *Candida tropicalis* account for 90% of the infections. DM, high-dose corticosteroids, and broad-spectrum antibacterial therapy predispose patients to mucocutaneous candidal infections such as oral candidiasis, intertriginous candidal infections, esophagitis, vaginitis, and UTI. Skin infections are treated with nystatin and topical clotrimazole; candidal UTIs are treated with fluconazole or voriconazole or more rarely with liposomal amphotericin or caspofungin for fluconazole-resistant species (see Chapter 53). Whenever possible, foreign objects such as bladder catheters, surgical drains (e.g., percutaneous nephrostomy tube), and urinary stents should be promptly removed. The ideal management of asymptomatic candiduria in immunocompromised patients remains uncertain (see Chapter 53), but a short course (7 to 10 days) of fluconazole is generally recommended. Systemic antifungal therapy is indicated in the presence of any positive blood culture for *Candida* species.

BK Infection

BK virus is a ubiquitous human virus with a peak incidence of primary infection in children 2 to 5 years of age and a seroprevalence rate of more than 60% to 90% among the adult population worldwide. After primary infection, BK virus preferentially establishes latency within the genitourinary tract and frequently is reactivated in the setting of immunosuppression. In renal transplant recipients, BK virus is associated with a range of clinical syndromes including asymptomatic viruria with or without viremia, ureteral stenosis and obstruction, interstitial nephritis, and BK allograft nephropathy. During the last decade, BK nephropathy has emerged as an important cause of allograft dysfunction after renal transplantation. Most series report that 30% to 40% of renal transplant recipients develop BK viruria, 10% to 20% develop BK viremia, and 2% to 5% develop BK nephropathy. The highest prevalence of BK viruria and viremia occurs at 2 to 3 months and 3 to 6 months, respectively. The risk for development of BK viremia increases when urine viral load is greater than 10^4 copies/ml, whereas BK nephropathy is unusual in the absence of BK viremia. BK nephropathy commonly presents with an asymptomatic rise in serum creatinine during the first post-transplantation year. However, BK nephropathy may occur as early as the first week to as late as 6 years after transplantation. Diagnosis is made by allograft biopsy, which demonstrates BK viral inclusions in renal tubular cell nuclei and occasionally in glomerular parietal epithelium (Fig. 101.4A). There are variable degrees of interstitial mononuclear inflammation (Fig. 101.4B), often with plasma cells, degenerative changes in tubules, and focal tubulitis, which may mimic acute rejection. BK nephropathy often is associated with very focal and sharply demarcated areas of tubulointerstitial inflammation, corresponding to foci of viral infection. Immunohistochemistry (Fig. 101.4C), *in situ* hybridization, or electron microscopy is required to confirm the diagnosis. BK infection and acute rejection may occur simultaneously, and distinguishing between BK nephropathy and acute rejection or the presence of both can be a diagnostic challenge. In late BK nephropathy, few characteristic intranuclear inclusions are seen, and the histologic changes may be indistinguishable from chronic rejection. A histologic classification system for BK nephropathy based on the degree of active inflammation, acute tubular injury, and tubulointerstitial scarring may have prognostic significance.[10] Urine cytology for decoy cells and quantitative determinations of viruria and of viral load in blood have been proposed as surrogate markers for the diagnosis of BK nephropathy.

Treatment strategies include reduction in immunosuppression that involves reduction or discontinuation of MMF and azathioprine with judicious reduction in CNI therapy or other immunosuppressive regimen. Switching from tacrolimus to cyclosporine or to sirolimus (rapamycin) has resulted in resolution of BK nephropathy and viremia or viruria in anecdotal case reports. Switching from CNI to sirolimus may have the added benefit of avoiding the long-term nephrotoxic effect of CNI therapy. Although no approved antiviral drug is available, adjunctive therapy with leflunomide, cidofovir, quinolones, or intravenous immune globulin (IVIG) may be beneficial, especially in patients with progressive allograft dysfunction. Quinolones are preferred by some centers because of low cost and ease of administration; leflunomide is used by others because of its potential simultaneous antiviral and immunosuppressive properties. Cidofovir is highly concentrated in urine and renal tissue, and the use of low-dose cidofovir in BK nephropathy has been reported to be devoid of nephrotoxicity or serious adverse events. Anecdotal

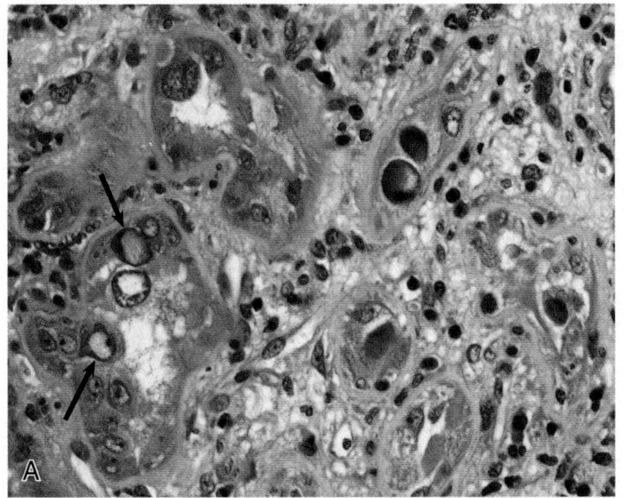

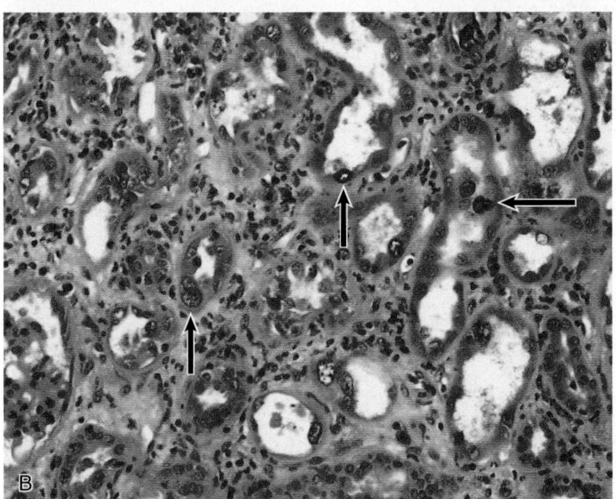

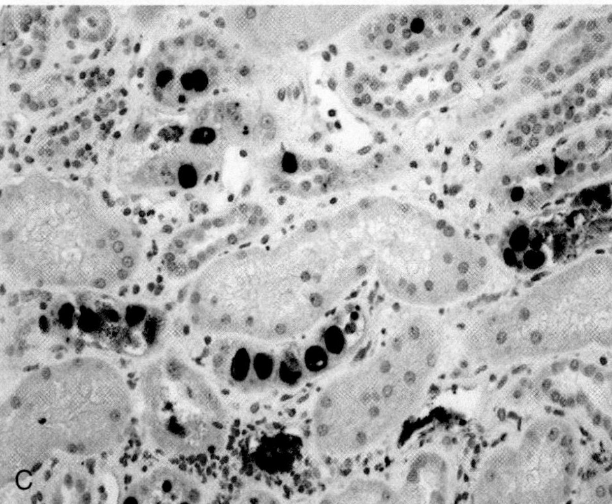

Figure 101.4 BK virus nephropathy. A, Prominent intranuclear viral inclusions are present within tubular epithelial cells *(arrows)*. (Hematoxylin and eosin; original magnification ×400.) **B,** Tubulointerstitial nephritis with diffuse intranuclear *Polyomavirus* inclusions *(arrows)*. (Hematoxylin and eosin; original magnification ×200). **C,** Immunohistochemistry staining highlights intranuclear *Polyomavirus* inclusions. (SV40 immunoperoxidase stain; original magnification ×200.) *(Courtesy Charles Lassman and William Dean Wallace, David Geffen School of Medicine at UCLA, Los Angeles, California, USA.)*

reports have suggested that IVIG may be effective in treating corticosteroid-resistant rejection,[11] and its use may be beneficial in patients with concomitant rejection and BK nephropathy or in those with histopathologic changes that are indistinguishable from those of rejection.

Despite treatment, 30% to more than 60% of patients with established BK nephropathy developed progressive decline in renal function with graft loss. Early diagnosis and intervention may improve prognosis. Intensive monitoring of urine and serum for BK by PCR during the first year with preemptive reduction of immunosuppressive therapy may lead to the resolution of viremia and prevent BK nephropathy. In the absence of active viral replication, patients with graft loss due to BK nephropathy can safely undergo retransplantation. Active surveillance for BK virus reactivation after transplantation is recommended. Suggested guidelines for post-transplantation screening and monitoring for BK replication are shown in Figure 101.5.

Other Infections

Tuberculosis (TB) infection in the renal transplant recipient varies according to the prevalence in the general population (e.g., the incidence of TB in transplant recipients has been reported to occur in 0% to 1.3% in the United States, compared with 11% in South Africa and 11% to 14% in India and Pakistan).[12] Most TB infection in the transplant recipient results from reactivation of dormant lesions in the setting of immunosuppressive therapy. Hence, all renal transplant candidates should have a PPD skin test (tuberculin skin test) placed before transplantation. A positive skin test response or a prior history of TB mandates further evaluation to rule out active disease. Isoniazid prophylaxis for a total of 9 months is recommended for those who have a positive skin test response. Of interest, most of the patients who develop TB after transplantation had negative PPD skin test results before transplantation.[13] Some centers recommend isoniazid prophylactic therapy in selected PPD-negative patients with (1) a history of inadequately treated TB, (2) radiographic evidence of granulomatous disease and no history of adequate treatment, (3) an organ from a PPD-positive donor, or (4) close and prolonged contact with a case of active TB.[13] In patients with a known history of adequately treated TB infection, we advocate the use of isoniazid prophylaxis for the first 9 months after transplantation and during intensification of immunosuppression. Others, however, have suggested that isoniazid prophylaxis is not indicated for those patients whose TB had been properly treated.[12] Clinical, radiologic, or culture evidence of active TB infection is a contraindication to transplantation. Enzyme-linked immunospot (ELISPOT), which detects T cells specific for *Mycobacterium tuberculosis* antigens, is unaffected by bacille Calmette-Guérin (BCG) vaccination and has become a major advance in TB screening. In some centers, the tuberculin skin test has been replaced by the ELISPOT assays (T-SPOT.TB assay).

A rare but important cause of infection in transplant patients, particularly those from endemic areas such as Southeast Asia, is *Strongyloides*. In the presence of immunosuppression, a "hyperinfection" syndrome may be observed with parasitic pneumonia (Fig. 101.6) and gastrointestinal involvement.

GASTROINTESTINAL DISEASE

Post-transplantation gastrointestinal complications are common and can arise from a variety of causes. Only selected complications are discussed; for a comprehensive review of

Suggested Guidelines for Screening and Monitoring for BK Nephropathy

Screening assays for BK virus replication
Plasma and/or urine* DNA load by PCR
Month 1, 2, 3, 6, 12, 24 post-transplantation, *or* when allograft dysfunction occurs, *or* when allograft biopsy (including surveillance biopsy) is performed

Positive Screening
NB: Plasma DNA load >10^4 copies/ml and/or urine DNA load >10^7 copies/ml
→ Possible BKN

Negative Screening
Continue to monitor

Decrease immunosuppression at the discretion of the clinician†

Repeat plasma and/or urine assay q 2-4 weeks until clear

BK load increase

NO (or improving)

YES

?

Intervention

Discontinue antimetabolites if not already done
Consider antiviral‡/ biopsy if ↑creatinine
Consider IVIG for biopsy-documented severe BKN (or BK + superimposed AR)‡

Monitor plasma and/or urine BK q 2-4 weeks

Figure 101.5 Guidelines for screening and monitoring for BK nephropathy. *Institution dependent. †Preemptive immunosuppression reduction may be associated with resolution of viruria or viremia and ↓ incidence of BK nephropathy. ‡See text. AR, acute rejection; BKN, BK nephropathy; IVIG, intravenous immune globulin; NB: note well; PCR, polymerase chain reaction.

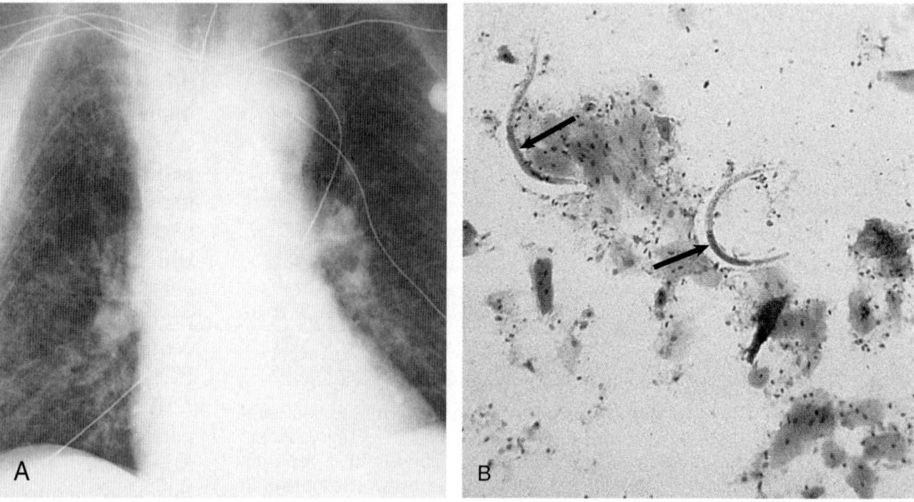

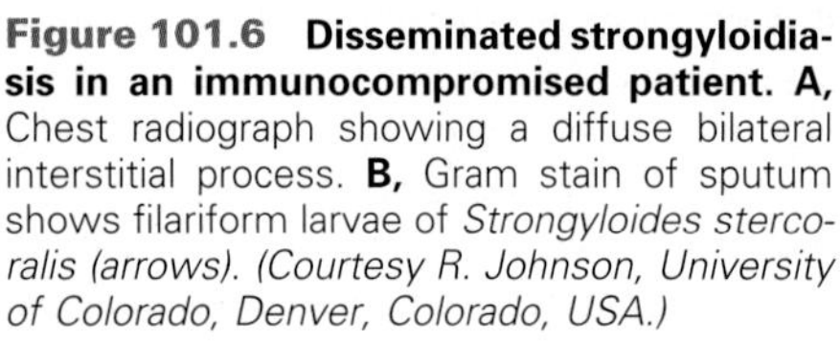

Figure 101.6 Disseminated strongyloidiasis in an immunocompromised patient. A, Chest radiograph showing a diffuse bilateral interstitial process. **B,** Gram stain of sputum shows filariform larvae of *Strongyloides stercoralis (arrows). (Courtesy R. Johnson, University of Colorado, Denver, Colorado, USA.)*

post-transplantation gastrointestinal complications, readers are referred to Chapter 83 and references 13 and 14.

Drug-Related Gastrointestinal Complications

MMF commonly causes gastrointestinal side effects, including nausea, vomiting, dyspepsia, anorexia, flatulence, and diarrhea. Dose reduction, transient discontinuation of the drug, or dividing the dose into three or four times a day often ameliorates or resolves the symptoms. Switching to the enteric-coated formulation of MMF may improve gastrointestinal tolerability in some patients but has not been consistently shown to be better than the original formulation. A large randomized double-blind study using patient-reported outcomes to assess the impact of gastrointestinal symptoms on patients' health-related quality of life and symptom burden is currently under way. Sirolimus may cause oral mucocutaneous lesions that can be confused with HSV or CMV infection but are culture negative. Drug-related oral ulcers usually resolve after discontinuation of the offending agent. Sirolimus, tacrolimus, and cyclosporine have also been suggested to cause diarrhea in some patients.

Infections

Post-transplantation infections of the gastrointestinal tract may be viral, fungal, or bacterial in etiology. Viral infections are most commonly caused by CMV and HSV; *C. albicans* and *C. tropicalis* are common opportunistic fungal infections. Leukoplakia and post-transplantation lymphoproliferative disorder (PTLD) may develop in patients with EBV infection (PTLD is discussed in a later section). Commonly encountered bacterial pathogens include *Clostridium difficile* and *Helicobacter pylori.*

Cytomegalovirus Infection

CMV can affect any segment of the gastrointestinal tract. Patients may present with dysphagia, odynophagia, nausea, vomiting, gastroparesis, abdominal pain, diarrhea, or gastrointestinal bleeding. Leukopenia and elevated transaminases are common. Persistent or unexplained symptoms of nausea, vomiting, or diarrhea, particularly in the early post-transplantation period or during intensification of immunosuppression, warrant further investigation with upper or lower endoscopies and biopsies.

Herpes Simplex Virus Infection

HSV infection results primarily from reactivation of endogenous latent virus, causing clinical infection within the first 1 to 2 months after transplantation. Patients commonly present with oral mucocutaneous lesions or gingivostomatitis with or without odynophagia and dysphagia. HSV esophagitis has been noted to occur in patients receiving high-dose corticosteroids and antilymphocyte preparations for acute rejection. Limited oral mucocutaneous lesions are treated with oral acyclovir; extensive infections require intravenous acyclovir or ganciclovir. Rare cases of HSV hepatitis have been reported.[14] The routine use of acyclovir prophylaxis in the early post-transplantation period is recommended.

Fungal Infections

Candida stomatitis and esophagitis are common during the first 6 months after transplantation and are increased in subjects with leukopenia or with severe immunosuppression, diabetes, or concomitant infections. Bleeding or perforation with formation of tracheoesophageal fistulas has been reported. Prophylactic oral nystatin "swish and swallow" during the first month after transplantation is recommended. In high-risk candidates, including liver or pancreas transplant recipients and those receiving antilymphocyte antibody therapy, fluconazole prophylactic therapy (3 to 6 months) is warranted.

Clostridium Infection

Clostridium difficile infection may be asymptomatic or present with diarrhea, intestinal obstruction, or even fulminant pseudomembranous colitis with toxic megacolon and perforation. *C. difficile* colitis is reported in 3.5% to 16% of transplant recipients.[15] Risk factors include young (<5 years) or advanced age, female gender, use of monoclonal antibodies to treat acute rejection episodes, and intra-abdominal graft placement. Among transplant recipients receiving antimicrobial therapy, *C. difficile*–associated diarrhea develops in approximately 50% of patients.[15] In mild cases of *C. difficile* infection, oral metronidazole is as effective as oral vancomycin and is the preferred first-line treatment. Treatment failure, however, requires treatment with oral vancomycin. In severely ill patients with gastrointestinal dysmotility or ileus, in which oral agents may not reach the colonic mucosa, metronidazole should be administered intravenously. Severe colonic disease refractory to medical treatment may necessitate colectomy.

Helicobacter Infection

Helicobacter pylori infection is associated with a wide range of gastrointestinal complications including chronic gastritis, duodenal and gastric ulcers, mucosa-associated lymphoid tissue (MALT) lymphoma, and gastric carcinoma, both in the general population and in recipients of solid organ transplants. Treatment includes a triple-drug regimen consisting of two antibiotics and an acid-suppressive agent such as an H_2 blocker or a proton pump inhibitor. The first-line *H. pylori* regimen as recommended by the American College of Gastroenterology is shown in Figure 101.7. In recipients of orthotopic heart transplants, triple-drug therapy resulted in a lower eradication rate compared with the general population, suggesting that immunosuppression may hinder the clearance of *H. pylori*. Unexplained dyspeptic or reflux symptoms should be investigated further with endoscopy and biopsy to exclude malignant transformation. *H. pylori* is now recognized as a risk factor for MALT lymphoma, which may occur in kidney, liver, and heart transplant recipients. In renal transplant recipients infected with *H. pylori*, MALT lymphoma may be less aggressive than other lymphomas, and the disorder may be cured by eradication of *H. pylori*.

Colon Disorders

Post-transplantation colonic complications, such as diverticulitis and colonic perforation, may be life-threatening and difficult to diagnose because symptoms may be masked by immunosuppressive therapy, particularly in the early postoperative period. Diverticulitis complicated by perforation, abscess formation, phlegmon, or fistula has been reported to occur in 1.1% of renal transplant recipients[16] and may be increased in patients with polycystic kidney disease (PKD).

Early post-transplantation colonic perforations are largely due to high-dose corticosteroids, diverticulitis, CMV colitis, and intestinal ischemia; perforations occurring late or years after transplantation are commonly due to diverticulosis or malignant disease. Abdominal symptoms may be absent because of the effects of immunosuppression and may only be suggested by the

First-Line Treatment Regimens for *Helicobacter pylori* as Recommended by the American College of Gastroenterology

Penicillin allergies	
No*	Standard-dose PPI twice daily (or esomeprazole once daily) + clarithromycin 500 mg twice daily + amoxicillin 1000 mg twice daily for 10–14 days
Yes†	Standard–dose PPI twice daily + clarithromycin 500 mg twice daily + metronidazole 500 mg twice daily for 10–14 days
Yes	Bismuth subsalicylate 525 mg orally 4 times daily + metronidazole 250 mg orally 4 times daily + tetracycline 500 mg orally four times daily + ranitidine 150 mg orally twice daily (or standard-dose PPI once daily to twice daily) for 10–14 days

Figure 101.7 First-line treatment regimens for *Helicobacter pylori* as recommended by the American College of Gastroenterology. *For patients who have not previously received a macrolide antibiotic. †For patients who have not previously received a macrolide antibiotic or who are intolerant of bismuth quadruple therapy. PPI, proton pump inhibitor.

presence of tachypnea and tachycardia. Mortality after colonic perforation is high. Management includes prompt exterioration of the perforated colon, early and broad-spectrum antimicrobial therapy, and minimization of immunosuppressive therapy. Although uncommon, the presence of abdominal pain and gastrointestinal bleeding with unexplained fevers or weight loss should raise the suspicion for gastrointestinal TB. The characteristic endoscopic findings include circular ulcers, small diverticula, and sessile polyps. The presence of caseating granulomas or acid-fast bacilli, or both, confirms the diagnosis.

Immunizations Before and After Transplantation

All potential renal transplant candidates should receive immunization for hepatitis B, pneumococcus, and other standard immunizations appropriate for age. Up-to-date recommendations for routine adult immunizations are available through the Centers for Disease Control and Prevention website (*www.cdc.gov/nip/rec/adult-schedule.pdf*). Immunizations should ideally be administered at least 4 to 6 weeks before transplantation to achieve optimal immune response and to minimize the possibility of live vaccine–derived infection in the post-transplantation period. Household members, close contacts, and health care workers should also be fully immunized.

Live virus or live organism vaccines should be avoided after transplantation. These include measles-mumps-rubella (MMR), live oral poliovirus (which is also contraindicated for household contacts), smallpox (vaccinia), varicella, yellow fever, adenovirus, live oral typhoid (Ty21a), BCG, and intranasal influenza vaccine. In addition, exposure to persons who have chickenpox or herpes zoster should be avoided until the lesions have crusted over and no new lesions are appearing. Vaccinations using inactivated or killed microorganisms, components, and recombinant moieties are safe for transplant recipients. These include hepatitis A and hepatitis B, intramuscular influenza A and B, pneumococcal, *Haemophilus influenzae* b, inactivated poliovirus vaccine, diphtheria-pertussis-tetanus (DPT), and *Neisseria meningitidis*.

In general, vaccination should be avoided in the first 6 months after transplantation because of the potential for stimulating the immune response, with a higher chance of graft dysfunction and rejection. In addition, vaccinations within the first 6 months after transplantation are often ineffective because of heavy immunosuppression. For prevention of infection in adult travelers after solid organ transplantation, readers are referred to reference 17. Recommended vaccinations before and after transplantation are listed in Figure 101.8.

Recommended Immunizations Before and After Transplantation

Vaccine	Pre	Post
Measles–mumps–rubella	X	–
Diphtheria–tetanus-pertussis	X	Diphtheria and tetanus[a]
Varicella	X	Controversial
Poliovirus	X	Inactivated polio virus vaccine[b]
Haemophilus influenzae b	X	X
Influenza	X	X[c]
Pneumococcus	X	X[d]
Hepatitis B	X	X[e]
Hepatitis A	X	X[f]
Human papillomavirus (HPV)	X[g]	–

Figure 101.8 Recommended immunizations before and after transplantation. [a]Booster every 10 years. [b]For travelers to endemic areas (i.e., some parts of Asia, Africa). [c]Annually. [d]Every 3 to 5 years. [e]Monitor titers. [f]For travelers to endemic areas. [g]Nonpregnant female transplant candidates aged 9 to 26 years.

TRANSPLANT-ASSOCIATED MALIGNANT NEOPLASMS

Recipients of organ transplants are at increased risk for development of neoplasms compared with the general population. Similar to post-transplantation infectious complications, the time to occurrence of different types of malignant neoplasms after transplantation appears to follow a timetable pattern. The Israel Penn International Transplant Tumor Registry data on the time of appearance of different neoplasms after solid organ transplantation are shown in Figure 101.9. PTLD generally occurs early after transplantation; skin cancers occur with increasing frequency with time. The intensity and duration of immunosuppression as well as the ability of these agents to promote replication of various oncogenic viruses are important risk factors. The associations between human papillomaviruses and cervical and vulvar carcinoma, EBV and PTLD, HBV and HCV and hepatocellular carcinoma, and HHV-8 and Kaposi's sarcoma are well established. Figure 101.10 provides a summary

Time of Appearance of Neoplasms After Transplantation and Initiation of Immunosuppression	
Type of Cancer	**Median (months)**
Lymphomas	12
Kaposi's sarcoma	13
Carcinomas (excluding Kaposi's)	41
Carcinomas of cervix	46
Hepatobiliary carcinomas	68
Skin cancers	69
Carcinoma of vulva or perineum	114
All cancers	46

Figure 101.9 Time of appearance of neoplasms after transplantation and initiation of immunosuppression.

Meta-Analysis Standardized Incidence Ratios for Cancers Related to Infections in Transplant Recipients	
Cancers	**Meta-Analysis SIRs**
EBV-related cancers	
Hodgkin's lymphoma	3.89 (2.42–6.26)
Non-Hodgkins lymphoma	8.07 (6.40–10.2)
HHV–8–related cancers	
Kaposi 's sarcoma	208.0 (114–369)
HBV/HCV-related cancers	
Liver	2.13 (1.16–3.91)
HPV-related cancers	
Cervix uteri	2.13 (1.37–3.30)
Vulva and vagina	22.8 (15.8–32.7)
Penis	15.8 (5.79–34.4)
Anus	4.85 (1.36–17.3)
Oral cavity and pharynx	3.23 (2.40–4.35)
Non-melanocytic–related skin	28.6 (9.39–87.2)

Figure 101.10 Meta-analysis standardized incidence ratios (SIRs) for cancers related to infections in transplant recipients. EBV, Epstein-Barr virus; HBV, hepatitis B virus; HCV, hepatitis C virus; HHV, human herpesvirus; HPV, human papillomavirus. *(Modified from reference 18.)*

of the incidence of cancers related to infections in transplant recipients.[18]

An analysis of the USRDS database[19] documented that the cancer rates for most common cancers, such as colon, lung, prostate, stomach, esophagus, pancreas, ovary, and breast, are nearly twofold higher after kidney transplantation compared with the general population. Although registry studies have limitations, all transplant recipients should adhere to standard cancer surveillance appropriate for age (Fig. 101.11).[20] In patients with a history of pre-transplantation malignant neoplasms, close monitoring for recurrences in the post-transplantation period is mandatory. The highest recurrence rates have been observed with multiple myeloma (67%), non-melanoma skin cancers (53%), bladder carcinomas (29%), sarcomas (29%), symptomatic renal cell carcinomas (27%), and breast carcinomas (23%).[21] In an analysis of registry data involving 90 patients with a history of pretransplantation prostate adenocarcinoma (77 renal, 10 heart, and 3 liver transplant recipients), prostate cancer recurrences were found to relate to the stage of disease at initial diagnosis.[22] Tumor recurrence rates were 14%, 16%, and 33% for stage I, stage II, and stage III diseases, respectively. Hence, a longer waiting time may be necessary for more advanced disease. Suggested guidelines for tumor-free waiting periods for common pretransplantation malignant neoplasms are shown in Figure 101.12.

Post-Transplantation Lymphoproliferative Disorder

PTLD is the most common post-transplantation malignant neoplasm in children; in adults, it is the second most common malignant neoplasm after skin cancer. PTLD has been reported to occur in 1% to 5% of renal transplant recipients.

The majority of PTLD is non-Hodgkin's lymphoma of B-cell origin, and more than 80% to 90% are linked to EBV infection. Based on the World Health Organization classification, PTLD can be divided into three distinct morphologic groups: (1) diffuse B-cell hyperplasia, (2) polymorphic PTLD (usually monoclonal), and (3) monomorphic PTLD that includes high-grade invasive lymphoma of B- or T-lymphocyte centroblasts. Diffuse B-cell hyperplasia is usually seen in children and young adults and commonly occurs within the first year after transplantation. Polymorphic PTLD represents the most common type of PTLD in both children and adults and may occur at any time after transplantation. In contrast, monomorphic B-cell PTLD is often seen several years after transplantation and may resemble non-Hodgkin's lymphoma in the general population. In a retrospective analysis of registry data for 402 recipients of kidney transplants, PTLD occurred at a median of 18 months (range, 1 to 310 months) after transplantation.

PTLD may present with constitutional symptoms such as fevers, night sweats, and weight loss or localized symptoms of the respiratory tract (infection or mass, including tonsillar or even gingival involvement), gastrointestinal tract (diarrhea, pain, perforation, bleeding, mass), or central nervous system (CNS) (headache, seizure, confusion). In contrast to lymphomas in the general population, in which lymph nodes are almost always involved, lymph node involvement is absent in more than 80% of patients with PTLD.

Risk factors for PTLD include primary EBV infection, younger age, antecedent history of CMV disease, and use of antilymphocyte antibody (e.g., antithymocyte globulin, OKT3). A history of pretransplantation malignant disease and fewer HLA matches are associated with an increased risk of PTLD. Cyclosporine and tacrolimus may enhance the development of EBV-associated PTLD by directly promoting the survival of EBV-infected B cells, presumably through the inhibition of EBV-transformed cells from apoptosis.[23]

Reduction or discontinuation of immunosuppressive therapy, particularly antilymphocyte antibody, cyclosporine, tacrolimus, or MMF, is recommended as first-line treatment; prednisone is increased to 10 to 15 mg daily to prevent allograft rejection. Sirolimus has a strong antiproliferative effect on PTLD-derived B-cell lines,[24] but whether sirolimus may limit B-cell lymphoma growth while simultaneously providing immunosuppression to prevent graft rejection awaits studies. Acyclovir or ganciclovir therapy and reduction in immunosuppression are beneficial and may be curative in benign polyclonal B-cell proliferation. The

Preventive Care Recommendations for Cancer Surveillance in Renal Transplant Recipients

Screening For	Starting at Age	Preventive Care	Screening Frequency
Colorectal cancer	Average risk: 50 years	Colonoscopy or FOBT + Flex sig[1]	Colonoscopy: every 10 years FOBT[1]: every year Flex sig[1]: every 5 years
	Increased risk: 40 years	Colonoscopy	Every 5 years if a parent or sibling had colorectal cancer at <60 years of age
		or	At 10 years younger than the youngest family member with cancer
		or	Every 10 years if the relative was 60 years
		or	Consider referral to medical genetics if two or more first degree relatives had colorectal cancer
Skin cancer[1]	Monthly self examination of skin, total-body skin examination every 6 to 12 months by qualified physicians and dermatologists[2]		
Females			
Breast cancer	50–69[1] years	Breast examination and screening mammography	Every 1 or 2 years
	40–49[1] years	Breast examination and screening mammography	Every 1 or 2 years (no evidence for or against for this age group)
	Before age 30 years (if mother or sister had breast cancer)		
Cervical cancer	Once sexually active	Pap smear and pelvic examination	Every year
Males			
Prostate cancer	50 years	Digital rectal examination	Every year
	40[3] years	PSA testing	Frequency for testing is not established

Figure 101.11 Preventive care recommendations for cancer surveillance in renal transplant recipients. [1]As recommended by the American Transplant Society and the European Best Practice Guidelines on renal transplantation. [2]The American College of Preventive Medicine recommends regular screening for high-risk individuals but none for low-risk individuals. [3]Recommended for African Americans, family history of prostate cancer, patients receiving chronic immunosuppression for organ transplantation. FOBT, fecal occult blood testing; Flex sig, flexible sigmoidoscopy; PSA, prostate-specific antigen. *(Sources: The 2001 Cleveland Clinic Foundation Cancer Surveillance Task Force and reference 20.)*

role of antiviral therapy in B-cell monoclonal malignant transformation is less well defined; 50% to 90% mortality has been reported despite antiviral therapy. Surgical resection with or without adjunctive local irradiation has been suggested for localized disease. Local irradiation has been advocated as the treatment of choice for PTLD involving the central nervous system.

In lesions not amenable to surgery or more aggressive monoclonal types of PTLD, chemotherapy has been used with favorable results compared with reduction in immunosuppression alone. The most frequently used regimens are CHOP (cyclophosphamide, doxorubicin [Adriamycin], vincristine, and prednisone) and VAPEC-B (doxorubicin, etoposide, cyclophosphamide, methotrexate, bleomycin, and vincristine). Other reported promising novel therapies include ProMACE-CytaBOM (prednisone orally, doxorubicin, cyclophosphamide, etoposide-cytarabine, bleomycin, vincristine [Oncovin], methotrexate).[25] Adverse effects of chemotherapy include high mortality rates from sepsis and treatment-related toxicities. Rituximab, a chimeric monoclonal antibody with murine variable regions targeting the CD20 antigen and human IgG1-κ constant regions, has antitumor activity against CD20-expressing B-cell lymphomas. Early experiences with rituximab (two to six weekly doses of 375 mg/m^2) in patients with PTLD (in conjunction with reduction in immunosuppression) have shown promising results. Complete remission rates of 30% to 60% have been reported.[24] Although the response rates appear to vary substantially among patients and centers, rituximab in conjunction with reduction in immunosuppression is evolving as the treatment of choice for CD20$^+$ PTLD. The role of cytokine-based therapy, such as interferon alfa and anti–IL-6, remains poorly defined[25]; increased risk of allograft rejection is seen with anti–IL-6 treatment. Sirolimus, an immunosuppressant with antiproliferative properties, has been demonstrated to prevent proliferation of B-cell (but not T-cell) PTLD-derived tumor cell lines *in vitro* and *in vivo*.[26] Limited data from nine European transplant centers have shown tumor regression in 15 of 19 patients with PTLD who underwent minimization or withdrawal of CNIs and sirolimus conversion.[27]

Factors that adversely affect survival include multiple- versus single-site involvement, increasing age, B-cell predominance, use of antilymphocyte globulin or antithymocyte globulin and OKT3, and “early” versus “late” onset (within 6 to 12 months versus more than 12 months). In recipients of renal transplants with PTLD restricted to the allograft alone, transplant nephrectomy may improve survival.

Suggested Tumor-Free Waiting Periods for Commonly Encountered Pretransplantation Malignant Neoplasms

Cancer Type	Waiting Period
Renal	
Incidental, asymptomatic	None
Large, infiltrating	At least 2 years
Wilms' tumor	At least 2 years
Bladder	
In situ	None
Invasive	At least 2 years
Uterus	
In situ cervical	None
Invasive cervical	5 years
Uterine body	At least 2 years
Breast†	At least 5 years
Colorectal‡	At least 5 years
Prostate	At least 2 years
Lymphoma	At least 2 years
Lung cancer	At least 2 years
Skin	
Melanoma§	At least 5 years
Squamous cell	Surveillance
Basal cell	None

Figure 101.12 Suggested guidelines for tumor-free waiting periods for commonly encountered pretransplantation malignant neoplasms. Consultation service is available through the Israel Penn International Transplant Registry website, *www.ipittr.org*. †Early *in situ* (e.g., ductal carcinoma *in situ*) may require only a 2-year wait. Individuals with advanced breast cancer (stage III or IV) should be advised against transplantation. ‡In patients with localized disease (Dukes' stage A or B1), a 2- to 5-year waiting period may be sufficient. §*In situ* melanoma may require a shorter waiting period of 2 years (dermatology consultation is probably warranted).

Skin Cancers

Skin cancers are the most common *de novo* post-transplantation tumors in the adult transplant population and may occur 20 to 30 years earlier in immunosuppressed patients compared with the general population. The incidence of skin cancers is 20 times higher in sun-exposed areas and 7 times higher in non–sun-exposed areas. The use of sirolimus, an inhibitor of mammalian target of rapamycin (mTOR)–induced signaling, may delay the onset or reduce the incidence of post-transplantation skin and non-skin malignant neoplasms (discussed under management of post-transplantation malignant neoplasms).[28,29]

Risk factors for skin cancer include light skin color, intensity of sun exposure (ultraviolet light exposure), genetic factors, and duration of follow-up after transplantation. In addition, immunosuppression in combination with enhanced sunlight exposure may induce malignant changes in papilloma-induced warts.

Management of Immunosuppressive Therapy in Post-Transplantation Malignant Neoplasms

There is no consensus on the management of immunosuppressive therapy in patients with post-transplantation malignant neoplasms. It has been proposed by experts in the field that immunosuppression dose reduction or withdrawal may permit recovery of the immune system and control the progression of life-threatening malignant neoplasms. The former allows intact immune surveillance against malignant cells. Nonetheless, this approach is not without its attendant risk of graft rejection and graft loss. Furthermore, little is known as to how much and to what extent immunosuppression reduction or withdrawal might alter the natural history of established post-transplantation malignant neoplasms. In our opinion, CNI to sirolimus switch or CNI minimization in conjunction with sirolimus may be a viable therapeutic option (the antitumoral effect of sirolimus is discussed later). In patients with metastatic cancer, manipulation of immunosuppression is probably futile, and the risk of rejection and graft loss necessitating a return to dialysis is likely to outweigh the benefit.

Studies suggest that immunosuppressive agents have different effects on cancer risk after transplantation. The carcinogenic effects of OKT3, antithymocyte globulin, cyclosporine, tacrolimus, and azathioprine have been well documented. In contrast to azathioprine, MMF has been shown to have antiproliferative effects and has been suggested to protect against post-transplantation malignant neoplasms.[30,31] Analysis of more than 17,000 adult patients with preexisting DM indicated a significantly higher incidence of malignant transformation in azathioprine-treated than in MMF-treated patients (3.7% versus 2.2%; $P < .01$).[31] However, whether MMF is protective of post-transplantation malignant neoplasia remains speculative.

Both preclinical and clinical studies have demonstrated that mTOR inhibitors such as sirolimus and everolimus have antiproliferative and antitumor effects. Early studies in renal transplant recipients demonstrated a lower incidence of skin cancer with sirolimus-based therapy without cyclosporine *or* sirolimus maintenance therapy after early cyclosporine withdrawal compared with those who remained on cyclosporine and sirolimus combination therapy. It has been suggested that the protective effect of sirolimus against skin cancer is due to its inhibition of several ultraviolet light–induced mechanisms involved in skin carcinogenesis. The 5-year malignancy data of the Rapamune Maintenance Regimen trial demonstrated a lower incidence of both skin and non-skin cancers at 5 years after transplantation in recipients receiving sirolimus-based therapy and cyclosporine withdrawal at month 3 compared with those receiving sirolimus and cyclosporine combination therapy.[29] Sirolimus therapy has also been reported to result in successful clinical and histologic remission of Kaposi's sarcoma in renal transplant recipients.[32] Although sirolimus appears to provide satisfactory outcomes in certain cancers after transplantation, its use in the management of malignant disease after solid organ transplantation remains to be defined and should be tailored to each individual patient.

REFERENCES

1. Snyder JJ, Israni AK, Peng Y, et al. Rates of first infection following kidney transplantation in the United States. *Kidney Int.* 2009;75:317-326.
2. Fishman JA, Rubin RH. Infection in organ transplant recipients. *N Engl J Med.* 1998;338:1741-1751.
3. Fischer SA. Emerging virus in transplantation: There is more to infection after transplant than CMV and EBV. *Transplantation.* 2008;86:1327-1339.
4. Lipshutz G, Dow A, Pham PC, et al. CMV otitis. A rare presentation in an adult transplant recipient. *Transplantation.* 2008;85:1870-1871.

5. Fishman JA, Davis JA. Infection in renal transplant recipient. In: Morris PJ, Knechtle SJ, eds. *Kidney Transplantation*. 6th ed. Philadelphia: Saunders Elsevier; 2008:492-507.
6. Pham PT, Pham PC, Lipshutz G, Wilkinson AH. New onset diabetes mellitus after transplantation. *Endocrinol Metab Clin North Am*. 2007; 36:873-890.
7. Lowance D, Neumayer HH, Legendre CM, et al. Valacyclovir for the prevention of cytomegalovirus disease after renal transplantation. International Valacyclovir Cytomegalovirus Prophylaxis Transplantation Study Group. *N Engl J Med*. 1999;340:1462-1470.
8. Ozaki KS, Camara NOS, Nogueira E, et al. The use of sirolimus in ganciclovir-resistant cytomegalovirus infections in renal transplant recipients. *Clin Transplant*. 2007;21:675-680.
9. Canadian Society of Transplantation Consensus Workshop on Cytomegalovirus Management in Solid Organ Transplantation Final Report. *Am J Transplant*. 2005;5:218-227.
10. Drachenberg CB, Papadimitriou JC, Hirsch HH, et al. Histological patterns of polyomavirus nephropathy: Correlation with graft outcome and viral load. *Am J Transplant*. 2004;4:2082-2092.
11. Luke PP, Scantlebury VP, Jordan ML, et al. Reversal of steroid- and anti-lymphocyte antibody–resistant rejection using intravenous immunoglobulin (IVIG) in renal transplant recipients. *Transplantation*. 2001;72:419-422.
12. Riska H, Gronhagen-Riska C, Ahonen J. Tuberculosis and renal transplantation. *Transplant Proc*. 1987;19:4096-4097.
13. Munksgaard B. Mycobacterium tuberculosis. *Am J Transplant*. 2004;4(Suppl 10):37-41.
14. Hedelman JH, Goral S. Gastrointestinal complications of transplant immunosuppression. *J Am Soc Nephrol*. 2002;13:277-287.
15. Ponticelli C, Passerini P. Gastrointestinal complications in renal transplant recipients. *Transplant Int*. 2005;18:643-650.
16. Flohr T, Bonatti H, Frierson H, et al. Herpes simplex virus hepatitis after renal transplantation [letter]. *Transpl Infect Dis*. 2008;10:377-378.
17. Kotton CN, Ryan ET, Fishman JA. Prevention of infection in adults travelers after solid organ transplantation. *Am J Transplant*. 2005;5: 8-14.
18. Grulich AE, van Leeuwen MT, Falster MO. Incidence of cancers in people with HIV/AIDS compared with immunosuppressed transplant recipients: A meta-analysis. *Lancet*. 2007;370:59-67.
19. Kasiske BL, Snyder JJ, Gilbertson DT, Wang C. Cancer after kidney transplantation in the United States. *Am J Transplant*. 2004;4:905-913.
20. Wong G, Chapman JR, Craig JC. Cancer screening in renal transplant recipients: What is the evidence? Clin *J Am Soc Nephrol*. 2008;3: S87-S100.
21. Penn I. Evaluation of transplant candidates with pre-existing malignancies. *Ann Transplant*. 1997;2:14-17.
22. Woodle ES, Gupta M, Buell JF, et al. Prostate cancer prior to solid organ transplantation: The Israel Penn International Transplant Tumor Registry experience. *Transplant Proc*. 2005;37:958-959.
23. Beatty PR, Krams SM, Esquivel CO, et al. Effect of cyclosporine and tacrolimus on the growth of Esptein-Barr virus–transformed B-cell lines. *Transplantation*. 1998;65:1248-1255.
24. Nepomuceno RR, Balatoni CE, Natkunam Y, et al. Rapamycin inhibits the interleukin 10 transduction pathway and the growth of Epstein-Barr virus B cell lymphomas. *Cancer Res*. 2003;63:4472-4480.
25. Swinnen LJ, LeBlanc M, Grogan TM, et al. Prospective study of sequential reduction in immunosuppression, interferon alpha-2, and chemotherapy for posttransplant lymphoproliferative disorder. *Transplantation*. 2008;86:215-222.
26. Mentzer SJ, Perrine SP, Faller DV. The immunosuppressive macrolide RAD inhibits growth of human Epstein-Barr-virus-transformed B lymphocytes in vitro and in vivo: A potential approach to prevention and treatment of posttransplant lymphoproliferative disorders. *Proc Natl Acad Sci USA*. 2000;94:4285.
27. Pascual J. Post-transplant lymphoproliferative disorder—the potential of proliferation signal inhibitors. *Nephrol Dial Transplant*. 2007;22(Suppl 35):i27-i35.
28. Euvrard S, Ulrich C, Lefrancois N. Immunosuppressants and skin cancers in transplant patients: Focus on rapamycin. *Dermatol Surg*. 2004;30:628-633.
29. Campistol JM, Eric J, Oberbauer R, et al. Sirolimus therapy after early cyclosporine withdrawal reduces the risk for cancer in adult renal transplantation. *J Am Soc Nephrol*. 2006;17:581-589.
30. Penn I. The changing pattern of posttransplant malignancies. *Transplant Proc*. 1991;23:1101-1103.
31. Kauffman HM, Cherikh WS, McBride MA, et al. Post-transplant de novo malignancies in renal transplant recipients: The past and the present. *Transplant Int*. 2006;19:607-620.
32. Wong G, Chapman JR. Cancers after renal transplantation. *Transplant Rev (Orlando)*. 2008;22:141-149.

CHAPTER 102

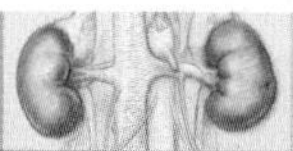

Medical Management of the Kidney Transplant Recipient: Cardiovascular Disease and Other Issues

Phuong-Thu T. Pham, Gabriel M. Danovitch, Son V. Pham

Although renal transplantation improves both survival and quality of life of the patient compared with dialysis, various medical issues can arise in the transplant recipient. This chapter provides an approach to the medical management of transplant-related complications. Infections and malignant neoplasms are discussed in Chapter 101.

CARDIOVASCULAR DISEASE

Death with a functioning graft is one of the major causes of late graft loss, with cardiovascular (CV) disease being the most frequent cause. Compared with the general population, CV mortality in transplant recipients is increased by nearly 10-fold among patients within the age range of 35 to 44 years and at least doubled among those between the ages of 55 and 64 years. Although renal transplantation ameliorates some CV risk by restoring renal function, it introduces new CV risks, including impaired glucose tolerance or diabetes mellitus, hypertension, and dyslipidemia that are derived, in part, from immunosuppressive medications. Renal transplant recipients have both conventional and unconventional CV risk factors (Fig. 102.1).[1,2]

Conventional Cardiovascular Disease Risk Factors

Post-transplantation Hypertension

Hypertension is a risk factor for both CV disease and kidney graft failure. The Collaborative Transplant Study (CTS) registry has documented a graded risk for graft failure with increasing levels of systolic and diastolic blood pressure.[3] Whether aggressive lowering of blood pressure retards the progression of graft failure similar to the delayed progression of renal disease in the general population with chronic kidney disease (CKD) remains to be studied. Hypertension is common after transplantation and is present in 50% to 90% of renal transplant recipients.[4,5] The wide range in the frequency may reflect the variable definitions of hypertension, donor source, immunosuppressive medications, time after transplantation, and level of graft function. Systolic blood pressure is highest immediately after transplantation and declines during the first year.[4] In the CTS registry, only 8% of transplant recipients had a systolic blood pressure below 120 mm Hg at 1 year; 33% had a blood pressure in the prehypertension range; 39% had stage 1 hypertension; and 20% had stage 2 hypertension despite antihypertensive therapy.[3] Preexisting hypertension, tacrolimus and to a greater degree cyclosporine, corticosteroids, quality of donor organ, delayed graft function, chronic allograft nephropathy, high body mass index (BMI) or excess weight gain, acute rejection episodes independent of creatinine clearance, recurrent or *de novo* glomerulonephritis, and transplant renal artery stenosis have all been implicated in post-transplantation hypertension. In rare cases, excess renin output from the native kidneys has also been suggested to contribute to post-transplantation hypertension.[4] In renal transplant recipients with severe hypertension refractory to medical therapy, bilateral native nephrectomy has been reported to improve blood pressure control.[6]

Management of post-transplantation hypertension should include attempts to identify and to treat the underlying etiology, lifestyle modifications (see Chapter 34), and treatment of associated CV risk factors. The initial target blood pressure goal is below 130/80 mm Hg, and in those with proteinuria, below 125/75 mm Hg. Although there is a lack of controlled clinical trials related to selection of antihypertensive agent, we recommend β-blockers in the perioperative setting as they have been shown to reduce ischemic heart disease events in high-risk candidates. In the early post-transplantation period, nondihydropyridine calcium channel blockers (CCBs) and diuretics are frequently used, the former for their beneficial effect on intraglomerular hemodynamics and the latter for their ability to eliminate salt and water in patients who are volume expanded postoperatively.

Angiotensin-converting enzyme (ACE) inhibitors and angiotensin receptor blockers (ARBs) have been found to block calcineurin toxicity in experimental models and are protective in patients with CKD. Although these effects are desirable, they can cause acute changes in renal function as well as hyperkalemia and hence are usually not started until renal function is stable. A meta-analysis of 21 randomized controlled trials (N = 1549 patients) demonstrated that ACE inhibitors and ARBs reduce proteinuria in transplant recipients, but they also reduce hematocrit (−3.5%; 95% CI −6.1 to −0.95) and glomerular filtration rate (GFR; −5.8 ml/min; 95% CI −10.6 to −0.99); there were insufficient data to determine a benefit on patient or graft survival.[7] Serum potassium and creatinine concentrations must be closely monitored; a rising serum creatinine concentration of more than 30% above baseline should also prompt clinicians to consider transplant renal artery stenosis. Finally, dihydropyridine CCBs were once used extensively because they counter calcineurin vasoconstriction. However, an unexpected association has been reported between the use of dihydropyridine CCBs and an increased risk for ischemic heart disease.[8] Dihydropyridine CCBs are also known to block renal autoregulation in CKD, in which they can increase proteinuria and may accelerate renal disease progression, especially in those not taking ACE inhibitors or ARBs.[1-2,9,10] Dihydropyridine CCBs should therefore be

Cardiovascular Risk Factors in Transplant Recipients			
Conventional		Unconventional	
Modifiable	Nonmodifiable	Modifiable (+/- potentially modifiable)	Nonmodifiable
Hypertension	Family history	Anemia	Prior acute rejection episodes
Dyslipidemia	Diabetes mellitus	Proteinuria	Preexisting CAC
Obesity	Male gender	Hyperhomocysteinemia	Deceased vs. living donor
Smoking	Age	Inflammatory cytokines ↑ C-reactive protein CMV infection* Hyperuricemia Impaired allograft function† Left ventricular hypertrophy‡ CD4 lymphopenia§ Low albumin	Pretransplantation splenectomy

Figure 102.1 Cardiovascular risk factors in transplant recipients. *Strict adherence to cytomegalovirus (CMV) prophylaxis protocol/CMV surveillance in high-risk candidates. †Calcineurin inhibitor minimization or withdrawal at the discretion of the clinician (variable results/difficult-to-modify risk factor). ‡Optimize blood pressure control; use angiotensin-converting enzyme inhibitors, angiotensin receptor AT_1 blockers. §Assess risks and benefits of T cell–depleting antibody treatment. Further studies are needed. CAC, coronary artery calcification.

Potential Advantages and Disadvantages of Different Classes of Antihypertensive Agents[1]		
Classes of drugs	Advantages	Disadvantages
β-Blockers	Perioperative use ↓ ischemic heart disease events	↑ Risk of symptomatic bradycardia when used with nondihydropyridine CCB Blunting of hypoglycemic awareness
CCB	↓ CNI-induced renal vasoconstriction[2] ↑ CNI level (may permit CNI dose reduction by up to 40%)[3]	Monotherapy with dihydropyridine CCB should be used with caution[4]
Diuretics	Beneficial in patients who are volume expanded postoperatively	Hyperuricemia, gout
ACE Inhibitor/ARB	↓ Proteinuria Potential renal protective and cardioprotective effects Beneficial in patients with post-transplantation erythrocytosis	Potential worsening of anemia
Aldosterone receptor Blockers	May improve outcomes in heart failure	Severe hyperkalemia when used in combination with ACEI/ARB or in patients with poor kidney function
α-2-Blockers	Benign prostatic hypertrophy Neurogenic bladder	
Direct vasodilators		Tachycardia
Central α agonist		Depression

Figure 102.2 Potential advantages and disadvantages of different classes of antihypertensive agents. [1]In general, there is no absolute contraindication to the use of any antihypertensive agent in renal transplant recipients. [2]Both dihydropyridine and nondihydropyridine CCB. [3]Nondihydropyridine CCB. [4]See text. ACE inhibitor, angiotensin-converting enzyme inhibitors; ARB, angiotensin receptor blockers; CCB, calcium channel blockers; CNI, calcineurin inhibitors.

used as monotherapy with caution. Potential advantages and disadvantages of different classes of antihypertensive agents in renal transplant recipients are shown in Figure 102.2.

Post-transplantation Dyslipidemia

Dyslipidemia is common after transplantation, in part because of the hyperlipemic effect of corticosteroids, cyclosporine, tacrolimus, and sirolimus. Sirolimus and everolimus are associated with the worst lipid profiles, followed by cyclosporine and then tacrolimus. Other potential etiologic factors for post-transplantation dyslipidemia include age, diet, rapid weight gain, hyperinsulinemia, preexisting hypercholesterolemia, allograft dysfunction, proteinuria, and the use of β-blockers and diuretics.

Although hyperlipidemia often improves within the first 6 months after transplantation as the doses of immunosuppressive agents are reduced, total and low-density lipoprotein cholesterol goals as defined by the National Cholesterol Education Program (NCEP) guidelines *(http://www.nhlbi.nih.gov/about/ncep/index.htm)* are usually not achieved. Most patients require statins, which are not only lipid lowering but also protective against CV disease because of their additional effects of reducing circulating endothelin 1, C-reactive protein levels, systolic and diastolic blood pressure, and pulse pressure. However, the extent to which statins reduce C-reactive protein and ameliorate hemodynamic parameters remains to be studied.

The Assessment of Lescol in Renal Transplantation (ALERT) study demonstrated the efficacy of fluvastatin in reducing low-density lipoprotein cholesterol during a 5- to 6-year period. The incidence of major adverse cardiac events was also reduced with treatment, although this was not statistically significant. Additional analysis demonstrated a beneficial effect of early initiation of fluvastatin on CV outcome; patients who received statin therapy within the first 4 years after transplantation had a risk reduction of 64% compared with 19% for those who received therapy after 10 years. No statin effect on graft loss or doubling of serum creatinine was observed.[11,12] In another study, there was better graft function at 12 months after transplantation in recipients who received statins compared with those who did not receive statin therapy (difference in creatinine clearance of 6 ml/min; $P < .001$); in addition, less interstitial fibrosis was seen on protocol biopsies.[13]

Whereas statins appear beneficial in transplant recipients, the use of statins in the presence of calcineurin inhibitors, particularly cyclosporine, often results in several-fold increases in statin blood level and an increased risk for myopathy and rhabdomyolysis.[14]

Other lipid-lowering agents include fibric acid derivatives, nicotinic acid, bile acid sequestrants, and ezetimibe. Ezetimibe and statin combination therapy can significantly improve cholesterol control because of their complementary mechanisms of action. Ezetimibe blocks intestinal absorption of dietary cholesterol and related phytosterols, whereas statin inhibits hepatic cholesterol synthesis. Ezetimibe used alone or as adjunctive therapy with statin appears safe and effective in the treatment of dyslipidemia in renal transplant patients who are refractory to statin therapy.[15] In a single-center study, the addition of ezetimibe to statin therapy was shown to prevent the decline in renal function compared with controls.[16] Whether ezetimibe and statin combination therapy is superior to statin-alone therapy in CV disease risk factor reduction remains to be elucidated. To date, no significant drug-drug interaction between ezetimibe and calcineurin inhibitors or sirolimus has been reported.

Drug Therapy for Hypertriglyceridemia and Non–High-Density Lipoprotein Cholesterol Severe hypertriglyceridemia (triglyceride level >500 mg/dl) is seen more frequently since the introduction of sirolimus. Management includes sirolimus dose reduction, addition of a fibric acid derivative or nicotinic acid, and, in refractory cases, switching of sirolimus to mycophenolate mofetil (MMF) or tacrolimus. Of the most used fibric acid medications—bezafibrate, ciprofibrate, fenofibrate, and gemfibrozil—the first three can increase serum creatinine in cyclosporine-treated patients. Although all fibrates in combination with statins have been associated with creatine kinase elevations with or without overt rhabdomyolysis and myopathy, gemfibrozil may have a greater risk for causing myopathy compared with bezafibrate or fenofibrate.[14] Niacin monotherapy has not been reported to cause myopathy, but its combined use with lovastatin, pravastatin, or simvastatin may be associated with rhabdomyolysis. Bile acid sequestrants must be used with caution because of their potential interference with the absorption of other medications vital to renal transplant recipients. In addition, studies in the general population suggest that bile acid sequestrants may increase triglyceride levels. For a more complete list of drug-drug interaction of statins with other lipid-lowering agents, readers are referred to reference 14.

The 2004 National Kidney Foundation Work Group suggested that statin therapy be the first-line treatment of non–high-density lipoprotein cholesterol because of its well-established safety and efficacy in preventing CV disease in randomized trials in the general population. Fibrates are used for those intolerant of statin despite dose reduction or despite switching to another statin. Randomized controlled trials evaluating the safety and efficacy of statins and fibrates are still needed. For patients with fasting triglyceride levels of 1000 mg/dl (11.29 mmol/l) or higher, the Adult Treatment Panel III (ATP III) recommends a very low fat diet (<15% total calories), medium-chain triglycerides, and fish oils to replace some long-chain triglycerides. Suggested guidelines for treatment of dyslipidemia are summarized in Figure 102.3.

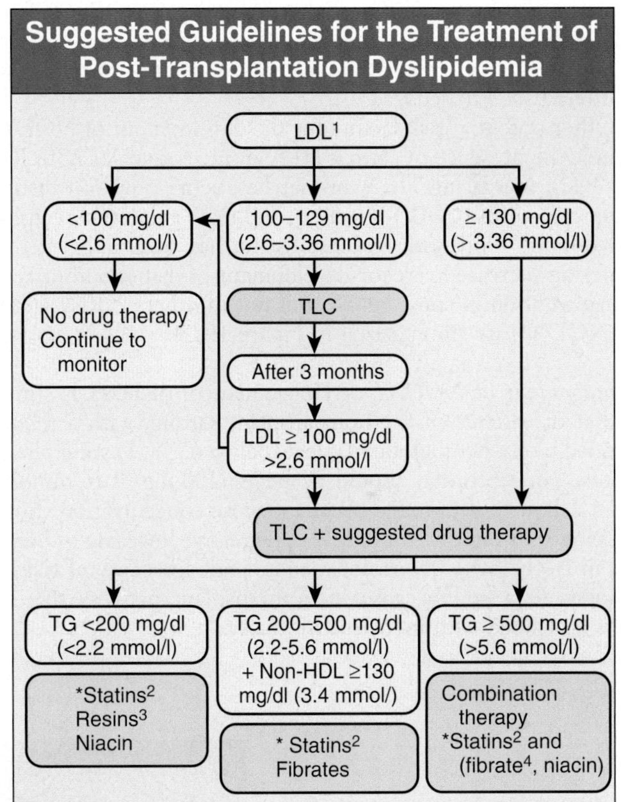

Figure 102.3 Suggested guidelines for the treatment of post-transplantation dyslipidemia. All transplant recipients should be regarded as coronary heart disease risk equivalent. Goals: low-density lipoprotein (LDL) <100 mg/dl (2.6 mmol/l) (optional <70 mg/dl) (1.8 mmol/l); triglyceride (TG) <200 mg/dl (2.2 mmol/l); high-density lipoprotein (HDL) >40 to 50 mg/dl (1.03-1.29 mmol/l).

*If LDL targets are not achieved with statin monotherapy, consider combination of statins plus cholesterol absorption inhibitors.[5] TLC, therapeutic lifestyle change (see text).

[1]LDL <70 mg/dl (1.8 mmol/l) has been suggested for very high risk patients (NCEP ATP III guidelines). [2]Statins are the most effective drugs and should be the agents of first choice. Start at low dose in patients receiving cyclosporine and tacrolimus. Monitor for myositis and transaminitis, particularly in those receiving combination therapy. [3]Bile acid sequestrants should probably not be taken at the same time as cyclosporine. [4]Extreme caution should be used with statin and fibrate combination therapy. [5]Consider cholesterol absorption inhibitors in patients intolerant of statins.

New-Onset Diabetes After Transplantation

New-onset diabetes after transplantation (NODAT) occurs in 4% to 25% of renal transplant recipients. The variation in reported incidence may be due to differences in definition, duration of follow-up, and the presence of both modifiable and nonmodifiable risks factors. Major risk factors include African American and Hispanic ethnicity (compared with Caucasians or Asians), obesity defined as BMI of 30 kg/m^2 or higher, age older than 40 to 45 years, family history of diabetes among first-degree relatives, impaired glucose tolerance before transplantation or presence of other components of the metabolic syndrome, recipients of deceased donor kidneys, and hepatitis C infection. Risk factors among immunosuppressive therapies include corticosteroids and the calcineurin inhibitors tacrolimus and, to a lesser extent, cyclosporine[16]; neither azathioprine nor MMF is diabetogenic. MMF may even mitigate the diabetogenic effect of tacrolimus, possibly by allowing clinicians to use lower doses.

Sirolimus is now recognized to be associated with reduced insulin sensitivity and a defect in the compensatory β-cell response. Sirolimus may be diabetogenic by impairing insulin-mediated suppression of hepatic glucose production, causing ectopic triglyceride deposition leading to insulin resistance, and by direct β-cell toxicity.[17]

Other potential risk factors for the development of NODAT include the presence of certain HLA antigens (such as A30, B27, and B42), increasing HLA mismatches, acute rejection history, cytomegalovirus (CMV) infection, and male gender of recipient and donor.[18] Polycystic kidney disease has been suggested to confer an increased risk for development of diabetes after renal transplantation in some studies but not in others.[18] Risk factors for NODAT are summarized in Figure 102.4.

Management of NODAT Management of diabetes is similar to that of patients in the nontransplant setting, with a recommended target hemoglobin A_{1c} level below 6.5%. Fasting plasma glucose concentration should be below 100 mg/dl (6 mmol/l), and a 2-hour postprandial plasma glucose concentration should be below 140 mg/dl (7.8 mmol/l). Aggressive lowering of hemoglobin A_{1c} below 6.0% is not recommended because of risks of hypoglycemia and because in nontransplant patients this has been associated with increased mortality.[19]

Overweight adults with impaired glucose tolerance should undergo lifestyle modifications including moderation of dietary sodium (<2400 mg of sodium a day) and saturated fat intake (<7% of calories from saturated fats, 2% to 3% of calories from *trans*-fatty acids), regular aerobic exercise, and weight reduction. Carbohydrate intake should be limited to 50% to 60% of calorie intake. The American Heart Association guidelines also suggested more than 25 g/day of dietary fiber and two servings of fish per week. Defining realistic goals, such as a target weight loss of 5% to 10% of total body weight, and a patient-centered approach to education may be invaluable in achieving success.

Modification of immunosuppression should be considered in high-risk patients. Corticosteroid dose reduction significantly improves glucose tolerance during the first year after transplantation. However, any dose reduction should be weighed against the risk of acute rejection. Conversion of tacrolimus to cyclosporine in patients who fail to achieve target glycemic control has yielded variable results.

Orally administered agents can be used either alone or in combination with insulin. Although oral agents are often effective, insulin therapy may be necessary in up to 40% of patients, particularly in the early post-transplantation period. The choice of pharmacologic therapy is based on the potential advantages and disadvantages associated with the different classes of oral agents. Metformin *(a biguanide derivative)* is preferred for overweight patients but is contraindicated in patients with impaired graft function (GFR <60 to 70 ml/min) as in this setting it can cause lactic acidosis. *Sulfonylurea derivatives* must be prescribed with care to patients with impaired graft function or to elderly patients because of the increased risk of hypoglycemia. In these patients, it is best to start with a low dose and to titrate upward every 1 to 2 weeks. The "non-sulfonylurea" *meglitinides* are insulin secretagogues with a mechanism of action similar to that of the sulfonylureas. They have a more rapid onset and shorter duration of action and seemingly lower risks of hypoglycemia. These agents are best suited for patients whose food intake is erratic, elderly patients, and patients with impaired graft function. They are best taken before meals, and the dose may be omitted if a meal is missed.

The *thiazolidinedione derivatives* (TZDs) are insulin sensitizers that may allow a reduction in insulin requirement. Potential adverse effects of these agents include weight gain, peripheral

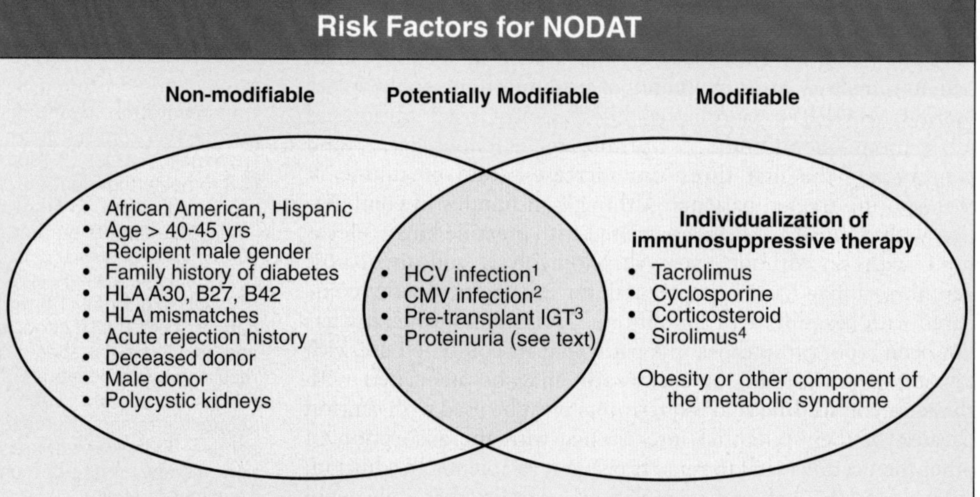

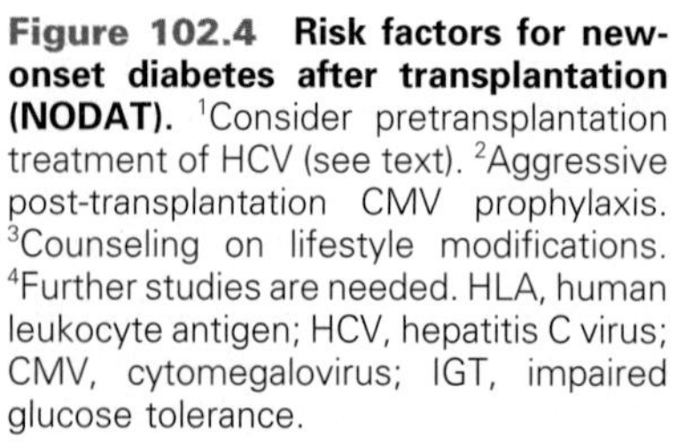

Figure 102.4 Risk factors for new-onset diabetes after transplantation (NODAT). [1]Consider pretransplantation treatment of HCV (see text). [2]Aggressive post-transplantation CMV prophylaxis. [3]Counseling on lifestyle modifications. [4]Further studies are needed. HLA, human leukocyte antigen; HCV, hepatitis C virus; CMV, cytomegalovirus; IGT, impaired glucose tolerance.

edema, anemia, pulmonary edema, and congestive heart failure. The incidence of peripheral edema is increased when TZDs are used in combination with insulin. More recently, during the A Diabetes Outcome Progression Trial (ADOPT) conducted to compare glycemic control in patients taking rosiglitazone, metformin, or glyburide, a higher incidence of fractures on the upper arm, hand, and foot among female patients treated with rosiglitazone was noted.[20,21] Subsequently, pioglitazone was also recognized to have similar increased risks of fractures in women but not in men, although further studies are needed.[21] The risk of fractures associated with the use of TZDs in the transplant setting is currently not known. Nonetheless, TZDs should be used with caution, particularly in female transplant recipients who are also receiving corticosteroids.

The incretin mimetics *glucagon-like peptide 1 analogues* (GLP-1) and incretin enhancers *dipeptidyl peptidase 4 inhibitors* (DPP-4) belong to a novel class of drugs that have been approved for use in type 2 diabetes. In contrast to insulin and most other glucose-lowering agents that cause weight gain and hypoglycemia, GLP-1 inhibitors and DPP-4 inhibitors have either a favorable or neutral effect on weight reduction and a lower risk of hypoglycemia. Exenatide is an incretin mimetic that stimulates insulin biosynthesis and secretion in a glucose-dependent manner and has been shown to lower both fasting and postprandial glucose concentrations. When it is added to sulfonylureas, thiazolidinediones, or metformin, it results in additional lowering of hemoglobin A_{1c} by approximately 0.5% to 1%. It also promotes weight loss through its effects on satiety and delayed gastric emptying. Sitagliptin and vildagliptin are DPP-4 inhibitors that act by enhancing the sensitivity of β cells to glucose, thereby enhancing glucose-dependent insulin secretion; they have also been shown to improve markers of β-cell function. Overall, this class of drugs has been shown to have neutral effects on weight.

Incretin-based therapy is an attractive treatment option for patients with NODAT because of its favorable effect on weight reduction/neutrality. Data on its safety and efficacy in renal transplant recipients are currently lacking. Caution should be exercised when these agents are used in the transplant setting, particularly with regard to drug-drug interactions. Vildagliptin should be avoided in patients with hepatic impairment, and the dose of sitagliptin should be adjusted for renal insufficiency.

The routine care of patients with post-transplantation diabetes mellitus should include an evaluation of hemoglobin A_{1c} level every 3 months and regular screening for diabetic complications, including microalbuminuria, retinopathy, and polyneuropathy with associated lower extremity ulcerations and infections. Fasting lipid profile should be measured annually. In transplant recipients with multiple CV risk factors, more frequent monitoring of lipid profile should be performed at the discretion of the clinicians. Figure 102.5 summarizes the suggested guidelines for the management of NODAT. Of note, hemoglobin A_{1c} cannot be accurately interpreted within the first 3 months after transplantation as anemia and impaired renal function can directly interfere with the A_{1c} assay. Recent blood transfusions or the use of dapsone may also alter hemoglobin A_{1c} levels.

Management of New-Onset Diabetes Mellitus After Transplantation

Dietary modification

- Dietitian referral
- For diabetic dyslipidemia: a diet low in saturated fats and cholesterol and high in complex carbohydrates and fiber is recommended.
- The AHA[1] guidelines suggest limiting cholesterol (<200 mg/day for those with diabetes mellitus); ≤ 7% of calories from saturated fats, 2% to 3% of calories from trans-fatty acids, and ≤ 2400 mg sodium/day. More than 25 g/day of dietary fiber and 2 servings of fish a week are also recommended.

Lifestyle modifications

- Exercise
- Weight reduction or avoidance of excessive weight gain
- Smoking cessation

Adjustment or modification in immunosuppressive medications[2]

- Rapid steroid taper, steroid-sparing or steroid avoidance protocols
- Tacrolimus to cyclosporine conversion

Pharmacologic therapy

- Acute, marked hyperglycemia (may require inpatient management)
- Intensive insulin therapy (consider insulin drip when glucose ≥400 mg/dl)
- Chronic hyperglycemia: treat to target Hb $A1_C$ ≥6.5%
- Oral glucose-lowering agent monotherapy or combination therapy[3] and/or insulin therapy
- Consider diabetologist referral if Hb $A1_C$ remains ≥9.0%

Monitoring of patients with NODAT

- Hemoglobin $A1_C$ every 3 months
- Screening for microalbuminuria
- Regular ophthalmologic examination
- Regular foot care
- Annual fasting lipid profile
- Aggressive treatment of dyslipidemia and hypertension

Figure 102.5 Management of new-onset diabetes mellitus after transplantation. [1]American Heart Association. [2]Clinicians must be familiar with the patient's immune history before manipulating immunosuppressive therapy. [3]The choice of a particular agent should be based on the characteristics of each individual patient (see text). *(Modified from reference 1.)*

Cigarette Smoking

As in the general population, cigarette smoking is associated with increased CV morbidity and mortality in renal transplant recipients.[22,23] Stopping smoking 5 years before transplantation reduced the risk of death by 29% (RR, 0.71; $P = .0304$).[23] Every effort should be made to encourage patients to stop smoking. A multifaceted approach including behavioral and pharmacologic strategies appears to be most effective.

Obesity

Obesity has a reported prevalence of 9.5% to 29% in transplant recipients. Studies in renal transplant recipients have shown that high BMI at transplantation is a significant independent predictor of congestive heart failure and atrial fibrillation.[24,25] The impact of BMI on cardiac-related death follows a U-shaped risk. In a large registry study, the adjusted risk of cardiac death increased at both low and high BMI compared with a reference group with a BMI of 22 to 24 (relative risk of 1.3 for BMI <20 and 1.4 for BMI >36).[26]

Management of post-transplantation obesity includes lifestyle and dietary modifications. Corticosteroid reduction or withdrawal must be balanced against the risk of graft rejection and graft loss. The use of pharmacologic agents for weight reduction in the post-transplantation period is currently not recommended because of unknown potential drug-drug interactions. There is a paucity of data on the safety and efficacy of post-transplantation gastric bypass surgery in ameliorating comorbid conditions such as hypertension, diabetes mellitus, and dyslipidemia. In a recent analysis of the U.S. Renal Data System (USRDS) database, mortality rates in patients undergoing gastric bypass after transplantation were higher compared with those without kidney disease who had undergone the same surgery. Although the difference in mortality rates was thought to be within "acceptable range" and attributed to poor healing associated with the use of immunosuppressive therapy, the routine recommendation of post-transplantation bariatric surgery awaits further studies.[27]

Unconventional Cardiovascular Disease Risk Factors

Proteinuria

Proteinuria has been reported in 9% to 40% of kidney transplant recipients with a functioning graft.[1] Controlled trials evaluating the beneficial effect of treating proteinuria in reducing CV risk in renal transplant recipients are lacking. Nonetheless, unless it is contraindicated, ACE inhibitors or ARBs should be considered in transplant recipients with microalbuminuria or overt proteinuria because of their well-established renoprotective, antiproteinuric, and cardioprotective effects. Whether the development of proteinuria associated with sirolimus adversely affects CV risks is currently unknown.

COMMON LABORATORY ABNORMALITIES

Anemia

Mild anemia is common in the early post-transplantation period when erythropoietin therapy is typically discontinued, but it generally improves within several weeks to months. Suggested etiologic factors for post-transplantation anemia include iron deficiency, folate deficiency, vitamin B_{12} deficiency, impaired graft function, acute rejection episodes, recent infection, and medications (such as azathioprine, MMF, sirolimus, and ACE inhibitors and ARBs). Anemia has also been reported to be more common in African American and female transplant recipients.

Profound iron deficiency should be treated with intravenous iron as tolerated. Erythropoietin and darbepoetin alfa are effective in the treatment of anemic renal transplant recipients. Refractory or severe anemia mandates a search for postoperative bleeding, particularly in those with a rapid fall in hematocrit. Other possibilities include tertiary hyperparathyroidism, underlying inflammatory conditions, and parvovirus B19 infection.

Erythropoietin-resistant anemia has been described in patients receiving sirolimus immunosuppression. In stable kidney transplant recipients, conversion from sirolimus to enteric-coated MMF may help resolve anemia in these patients.[28]

Leukopenia and Thrombocytopenia

Leukopenia and thrombocytopenia may be the result of myelosuppression due to medications including azathioprine, MMF, antilymphocyte antibody treatment, sirolimus, and trimethoprim-sulfamethoxazole. Withholding of the offending agent or dose reduction generally corrects these hematologic abnormalities. Severe leukopenia may be safely treated with granulocyte-stimulating factor. Thrombotic microangiopathy or CMV infection should be excluded. Parvovirus B19 infection may present with refractory anemia, pancytopenia, and thrombotic microangiopathy. More recently, an increase in the incidence of leukopenia was found in kidney and pancreas transplant recipients receiving alemtuzumab induction therapy.

Erythrocytosis

Post-transplantation erythrocytosis (PTE) occurs in 20% to 25% of transplant recipients within the first 2 years. Risk factors for PTE include the presence of native kidneys, male gender, excellent graft function and the absence of rejection episodes, high baseline hemoglobin concentration before transplantation, smoking, hypertension, and diabetes mellitus. Transplant renal artery stenosis is a risk factor for PTE in some but not all studies. Suggested pathogenic mechanisms include defective feedback regulation of erythropoietin metabolism, direct stimulation of erythroid precursors by angiotensin II, and abnormalities in circulating insulin-like growth factor 1 levels. Serum erythropoietin levels are inconsistently elevated.

Treatment is recommended for hemoglobin levels of 17 to 18 g/dl and higher or hematocrit levels of 52% to 55% and higher because of the associated risk of thromboembolic complications, hypertension, and headaches. Treatment with ACE inhibitors or ARBs is often sufficient, although phlebotomy may occasionally be necessary. A negative association between the use of sirolimus and PTE has been reported.[29] Whether sirolimus might prove to be beneficial in the prevention and treatment of PTE remains to be studied.

Hyperkalemia

Mild hyperkalemia is common in renal transplant recipients, particularly in the early post-transplantation period when relatively high doses of calcineurin inhibitor are given. It is often associated with mild hyperchloremic acidosis, a clinical presentation reminiscent of type 4 renal tubular acidosis. Suggested mechanisms of calcineurin inhibitor–induced hyperkalemia include hyporeninemic hypoaldosteronism, aldosterone resistance, and inhibition of cortical collecting duct potassium secretory channels. Cyclosporine decreases Na^+,K^+-ATPase activity in potassium secretory cells in the cortical and outer medullary collecting tubules, thereby decreasing intracellular potassium accumulation required for urinary secretion. In patients receiving cyclosporine or tacrolimus, a serum potassium level in the range of 5.2 to 5.5 mmol/l is typically seen and generally does not require treatment. Higher potassium levels, especially in the presence of concomitant use of drugs that may exacerbate hyperkalemia, such as ACE inhibitors, ARBs, and β-blockers, may require their discontinuation. Caution is needed when potassium-containing phosphorus supplements are prescribed. Although trimethoprim can cause hyperkalemia through an amiloride-like effect, the routine use of low-dose trimethoprim-sulfamethoxazole for prophylaxis is rarely the cause of severe or refractory hyperkalemia in renal transplant recipients. Finally, because efficient renal potassium secretion requires good urine flow, urinary obstruction must also be considered in the presence of hyperkalemia.

Treatment of hyperkalemia is discussed in Chapter 9. Sodium polystyrene sulfonate (Kayexalate) or calcium resonium enemas should be avoided in the immediate post-transplantation period to avoid colonic dilation and perforation.

Hypokalemia

Sirolimus may be associated with hypokalemia. Hypokalemia has been reported in 34% and potassium supplementation was required in 27% of patients treated with sirolimus.[30] Sirolimus-induced increased tubular secretion of potassium has been suggested as a possible mechanism.[31]

Hypophosphatemia

Hypophosphatemia is frequently encountered in the first months after transplantation, and when it is associated with hypercalcemia, it suggests post-transplantation hyperparathyroidism. In the absence of hypercalcemia, renal phosphate wasting syndrome or malnutrition should be considered.

Early after transplantation, hypophosphatemia may also be due to massive initial diuresis (particularly after living donor renal transplantation, when there is immediate graft function), defective renal phosphate reabsorption due to ischemic injury, glucosuria (due to hyperglycemia-induced osmotic diuresis), magnesium depletion, and corticosteroid use—the last by inhibiting proximal tubular reabsorption of phosphate. More recently, persistent increases in fibroblast growth factor 23 (FGF-23, a phosphatonin) in the post-transplantation period have been suggested to contribute to persistent hypophosphatemia.[32] FGF-23 enhances phosphate clearance and is elevated in CKD.

Treatment of hypophosphatemia is discussed in Chapter 10.

Hypercalcemia

Hypercalcemia is common after transplantation and is generally due to persistent secondary hyperparathyroidism. The concomitant presence of severe hypophosphatemia, particularly in patients with excellent graft function, may exacerbate hypercalcemia through stimulation of renal proximal tubular 1α-hydroxylase. Resolution of soft tissue calcifications, high-dose corticosteroid therapy, and immobilization are potential contributing factors. In about two thirds of cases, hypercalcemia resolves spontaneously within 6 to 12 months. However, spontaneous resolution occurs in less than half of those whose hypercalcemia existed before transplantation. Persistent hyperparathyroidism has generally been attributed to continued autonomous production of parathyroid hormone from nodular hyperplastic glands, reduced density of calcitriol receptors, and decreased expression of the membrane calcium sensor receptors that render cells more resistant to physiologic concentrations of calcitriol and calcium. The risk for development of persistent hyperparathyroidism is increased with the duration of dialysis and the severity of pretransplantation hyperparathyroidism. Severe hypercalcemia (>11.5 mg/dl [2.9 mmol/l]) or persistent hypercalcemia (≥12 months) requires further evaluation. Initial assessment should include an intact parathyroid hormone level. Imaging studies, including neck ultrasound or parathyroid technetium Tc 99m sestamibi scan, are required to determine if the clinically observed hyperparathyroidism arises from parathyroid adenoma, parathyroid gland hyperplasia, or hyperplastic nodular formation of the parathyroid glands.

Cinacalcet has been shown to reduce serum calcium in renal transplant recipients with hypercalcemic hyperparathyroidism. Parathyroidectomy is warranted in patients with tertiary hyperparathyroidism or persistent severe hypercalcemia for more than 6 to 12 months, symptomatic or progressive hypercalcemia, nephrolithiasis, persistent metabolic bone disease, calcium-related renal allograft dysfunction, or progressive vascular calcification and calciphylaxis.[33] Whether the advent of calcimimetics will reduce the need for parathyroidectomy remains to be studied.

Hypomagnesemia

Cyclosporine, tacrolimus, and sirolimus cause hypomagnesemia by inducing urinary magnesium wasting. Other factors that may contribute to post-transplantation hypomagnesemia include recovery from acute tubular necrosis, postobstructive polyuria, loop diuretic therapy, and renal tubular acidosis. Hypomagnesemia may be more common in diabetics. Serum magnesium concentration below 1.5 mg/dl (0.62 mmol/l) is common. Dietary magnesium intake is usually insufficient, and high-dose oral magnesium supplementation (e.g., 400 to 800 mg magnesium oxide three times a day) may be required. The intravenous administration of magnesium should be considered with severe hypomagnesemia (<1.0 mg/dl [0.41 mmol/l]), particularly in patients with coronary artery disease, in those with cardiac arrhythmias, and in those taking digitalis. Aggressive treatment of hypomagnesemia reduces cyclosporine-induced neurotoxicity and aids blood pressure control.

Abnormal Liver Function Test Results

Elevation of hepatic enzymes is common in the early post-transplantation period and is generally due to drug-related toxicity. Potential culprits include acyclovir, ganciclovir, trimethoprim-sulfamethoxazole, cyclosporine, tacrolimus, statins, and proton pump inhibitors. Cyclosporine and, less commonly, tacrolimus may cause transient, self-limited, dose-dependent elevations of transaminases and mild hyperbilirubinemia secondary to defective bile secretion. Elevated liver enzymes due to drug-related adverse effect usually improve or resolve after drug discontinuation or dose reduction.

Persistent or profound elevation in hepatic liver enzymes should prompt further evaluation to exclude infectious causes, including CMV, hepatitis B virus (HBV), and hepatitis C virus (HCV). In high-risk candidates for primary CMV infections (recipient seronegative, donor seropositive), it may occasionally be necessary to initiate CMV therapy pending laboratory results, particularly when there is a high index of clinical suspicion (fever, fatigue, malaise, gastroenteritis, leukopenia, or thrombocytopenia). Evidence of post-transplantation HBV reactivation (elevated alanine transaminase, histologic hepatitis, and serum DNA $>10^5$ copies/ml) should be treated with lamivudine. Some centers routinely initiate lamivudine prophylaxis in all HBsAg-positive candidates at the time of transplantation. Pretransplantation lamivudine prophylactic therapy is recommended in renal transplant candidates who have HBV DNA above 10^5 copies/ml and active liver disease, defined as an alanine transaminase value more than two times the upper limit of normal or biopsy-proven hepatic disease. Newer nucleoside analogs including entecavir and tenofovir have been recently recognized to provide improved viral suppression with lower emergence of resistance and toxicity and have become preferred first-line treatment options for patients with chronic hepatitis B. However, renal

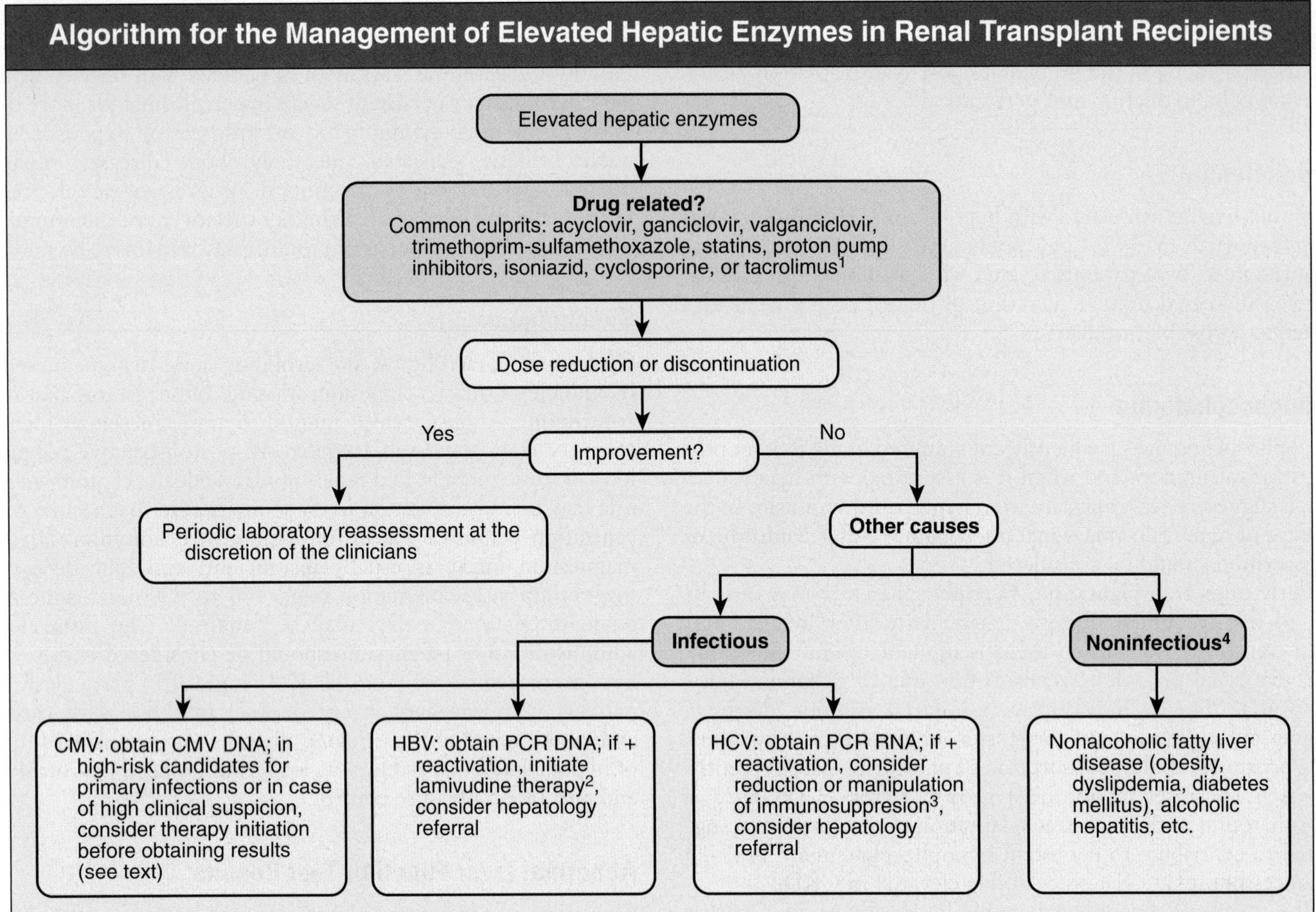

Figure 102.6 Algorithm for the management of elevated hepatic enzymes in renal transplant recipients. [1]Cyclosporine and less commonly tacrolimus may cause transient, self-limited, dose-dependent elevations of aminotransferase levels and mild hyperbilirubinemia secondary to defective bile secretion. [2]Some programs routinely commence lamivudine prophylactic therapy in all HBsAg-positive candidates at the time of transplantation. [3]There is currently no effective treatment of chronic hepatitis C in renal transplant recipients (see text). [4]Appropriate evaluation and management similar to nontransplant settings. CMV, cytomegalovirus; HBV, hepatitis B virus; HCV, hepatitis C virus; PCR, polymerase chain reaction.

dose adjustments and close monitoring of renal function with the use of tenofovir are advised due to its nephrotoxic potential.

There is currently no effective treatment of chronic hepatitis C in renal transplant recipients. Although treatment with interferon alfa may result in clearance of HCV RNA in 25% to 50% of cases, rapid relapse after drug withdrawal is nearly universal. More important, interferon alfa treatment has been shown to precipitate acute graft rejection and graft loss and is currently not recommended for renal transplant recipients with HCV infection. Management of HCV infection in this population of patients should probably rely on manipulation of immunosuppressive therapy. Experiences gained from liver transplantation indicate that corticosteroid therapy and antilymphocyte antibody treatment are associated with enhanced viral replication and more rapid progression to cirrhosis. On the basis of these observations, it is advisable to avoid antilymphocyte antibody induction therapy and to minimize corticosteroid dosage in transplant recipients with chronic HCV infection. Although early reports suggested that MMF may reduce HCV replication and delay recurrence in hepatitis C–positive liver transplant recipients, the antiviral properties of MMF and its impact on HCV replication and hepatitis C recurrence have not been consistently demonstrated in subsequent studies.

In vitro studies show that cyclosporine and mycophenolic acid (the active metabolite of MMF) are an effective combination for inhibition of HCV replication in the presence of interferon. In contrast, tacrolimus and methylprednisolone reduce rather than enhance the efficacy of interferon.[34] HCV-associated chronic hepatitis occurs in a significantly smaller number of patients treated with cyclosporine rather than tacrolimus. These studies suggest that cyclosporine may be superior to tacrolimus as an immunosuppressive agent in HCV-infected renal transplant recipients. An algorithm for the management of renal transplant recipients with elevated hepatic enzymes is shown in Figure 102.6.

BONE AND MINERAL METABOLISM AFTER TRANSPLANTATION

Post-transplantation Bone Disease

Post-transplantation bone disease is a common complication after kidney transplantation due to persistent renal osteodystrophy, the adverse effects of immunosuppression (mainly corticosteroids), persistent hyperparathyroidism, abnormalities in vitamin D metabolism, and reduced GFR. Corticosteroids directly inhibit osteoblastogenesis and induce apoptosis of osteoblasts and osteocytes. Corticosteroids also inhibit intestinal calcium absorption, enhance renal calcium excretion, and directly suppress gonadal hormone secretion. Low 25-hydroxyvitamin D levels after renal transplantation may also contribute to bone disease.

Other factors that have been suggested to contribute to post-transplantation bone loss include "normal" age-dependent osteoporosis, persistent metabolic acidosis, phosphate depletion, diabetes mellitus, hypogonadism, and smoking. Animal models suggest that cyclosporine and tacrolimus may also contribute to post-transplantation bone loss by stimulating bone resorption. The effects of calcineurin inhibitors in humans remains speculative, although increasing alkaline phosphatase and osteocalcin and increased osteoblastic and osteoclastic activities have been reported with cyclosporine treatment compared with azathioprine.

Osteoporosis

Post-transplantation decline in bone mineral density (BMD) is most pronounced in the first 6 months and correlates with higher corticosteroid exposure in the early post-transplantation period. The rate of bone loss varies from 3% to 10% and is most apparent at sites of cancellous bone, particularly the lumbar spine and axial skeleton. This early rapid decrease in BMD is usually followed by a slower rate of bone loss and reflects cumulative corticosteroid dose. Nonetheless, controversies exist as to whether bone loss continues to decline, stabilizes, or even reverses after the first year. A decrease in BMD averaging 1.7% per year in later post-transplantation years has been reported, whereas stabilization during the second year followed by an improvement of 1% to 2% per year thereafter was observed by others. Nevertheless, osteopenia and osteoporosis prevalence ranges from 31% to 41% 20 years after renal transplantation.

Evaluation of patients for bone loss or osteoporosis relies on the measurement of BMD by dual-energy x-ray absorptiometry (DEXA) scan. However, in the setting of combined osteoporosis and CKD, DEXA may be completely misleading. For instance, adynamic bone disease, mild hyperparathyroidism, and genuine osteoporosis may yield the same BMD, yet therapy is very different. Hence, BMD can only be interpreted in the clinical and laboratory setting, and bone biopsy should be performed if uncertainty arises.

Avascular Necrosis

Post-transplantation osteonecrosis (avascular necrosis) occurs with an incidence of 3% to 16% and most commonly affects the femoral head and neck. It usually occurs within the first few years after transplantation and may affect other joints, including the knees, shoulders, and, less commonly, ankles, elbows, and wrists. Early avascular necrosis of the femoral head commonly presents with hip or groin pain or referred knee pain. Symptoms may be aggravated by weight bearing but may also be paradoxically worse at night. Use of crutches to avoid weight bearing on the affected side is advisable. Core decompression, with or without bone grafting before the femoral head collapse, may relieve pain, but approximately 60% of cases require total arthroplasty. Osteotomy has also been used as a joint-sparing technique to treat osteonecrosis. Core decompression and osteotomy may have similar efficacy in early disease, but intertrochanteric osteotomy may be preferred for patients who have progressed to collapse of the femoral head by the time of diagnosis. Drastic corticosteroid dose reduction or discontinuation has little if any effect on altering the course of established avascular necrosis and may jeopardize graft function. Magnetic resonance imaging is the most sensitive technique for early detection; plain radiographs are of limited diagnostic value in the early stage. Predisposing factors for the development of avascular necrosis include greater exposure to intravenous corticosteroid pulse therapy, low bone mass, hyperparathyroidism, increasing dialysis duration, excessive weight gain, hyperlipidemia, microvascular thrombosis, and history of local trauma. Studies in renal transplant recipients maintained on a corticosteroid-free immunosuppressive regimen demonstrated low rates of avascular necrosis at 3-year follow-up.[35]

Prevention and Management of Post-transplantation Bone Disease

Management of post-transplantation bone disease has largely been based on studies involving postmenopausal osteoporosis and corticosteroid-induced osteopenia in nontransplant settings. Adequate calcium and vitamin D supplementation is generally recommended after transplantation to prevent rapid bone loss in the first post-transplantation year. Serum 25-hydroxyvitamin D levels should be obtained and levels kept above 30 ng/ml. In patients at increased risk for fracture, consideration should be given to rapid corticosteroid withdrawal or corticosteroid-free immunosuppressive protocols after the risks and benefits of acute rejection are weighed.

Bisphosphonates increase BMD in postmenopausal women and patients with corticosteroid-induced osteoporosis, particularly at the lumbar spine and trochanter. Although most studies to date suggest that bisphosphonates have a greater effect on increasing BMD than vitamin D analogues do, their efficacy in terms of fracture reduction compared with vitamin D analogues remains to be determined. In addition, because of the potential for bisphosphonates to oversuppress bone metabolism, their use in kidney transplant recipients with known adynamic bone disease remains unclear. Nonetheless, bisphosphonate therapy may be justifiable in potential high-risk candidates, including those with preexisting fractures or severe osteoporosis, patients with diabetes mellitus, postmenopausal women, and recipients of simultaneous pancreas-kidney transplants. The Kidney Disease: Improving Global Outcomes (KDIGO) guidelines suggest that consideration be given to bone biopsy before bisphosphonate therapy.

Other treatments are problematic. Calcitonin is considered relatively ineffective. Many older women and women with CKD also have deficiency in estrogen, and limited studies have shown that estrogen replacement therapy improves BMD in postmenopausal liver, lung, and bone marrow transplant recipients. Nonetheless, the CV risk associated with estrogen use may outweigh its benefits, and estrogen should be used with caution. Testosterone deficiency has also been implicated in the development of bone loss and fractures after transplantation. However, because testosterone may cause dyslipidemia, hepatic enzyme abnormalities, erythrocytosis, and prostatic hypertrophy, testosterone should probably be given only to men with true hypogonadism.

Gout

Hyperuricemia and gout are common among renal transplant recipients receiving cyclosporine-based immunosuppression, with a reported prevalence of 30% to 84% and 2% to 28%, respectively. Cyclosporine impairs renal excretion of uric acid secondary to decreases in GFR and increases net uric acid reabsorption by the proximal tubule. Potential contributing risk factors for the development of post-transplantation hyperuricemia and gouty arthritis include pretransplantation hyperuricemia, impaired graft function, obesity, and diuretic use.

Management of the acute gouty attack includes topical ice and rest of the inflamed joint. Pharmacologic treatments include colchicine, increased corticosteroid dose, and nonsteroidal anti-inflammatory agents (NSAIDs). The use of NSAIDs, however, should be avoided in patients with impaired graft function. Other treatment options have included intra-articular corticosteroids and parenteral adrenocorticotropic hormone (ACTH); ACTH is reserved for patients with multiple medical problems, such as impaired graft function, gastrointestinal bleeding, or gouty arthritis refractory to conventional therapy.

Management of chronic gout is directed at lowering of uric acid levels. Allopurinol should be started at a low dose (100 to 200 mg/day), particularly in the presence of impaired allograft function, because renal insufficiency predisposes to severe allopurinol toxicity due to retention of the metabolite oxypurinol. Allopurinol and azathioprine combination therapy should be avoided because of inhibition of azathioprine metabolism by allopurinol. In allopurinol-allergic patients, the new xanthine oxidase inhibitor febuxostat can be used. It is administered as 40 or 80 mg daily, and the dosing is not modified in renal failure.

Long-term prophylaxis may include reduction or discontinuation of diuretics, chronic low-dose allopurinol therapy, dietary modification, and consideration of alternative immunosuppressive therapy. Cyclosporine to tacrolimus switch has been reported to result in resolution of severe polyarticular gout refractory to conventional therapy. Small doses of colchicine at 0.6 mg daily may also prevent recurrent gouty attacks. However, colchicine should be used with caution, particularly in patients on statin therapy, due to the increased risk of myopathy. NSAIDS should be avoided in patients with impaired graft function.

OUTPATIENT CARE

We recommend that patients be seen two or three times a week for the first 2 weeks after transplantation, twice a week for the next 2 weeks, and weekly for the next month. After the first 2 months, the frequency of outpatient visits depends on the complexity of the patient's early postoperative course. Patients with stable graft function and an uneventful postoperative course can return to work or their regular daily activities 2 to 3 months after transplantation. Laboratory assessment during the first month after transplantation should include serum creatinine concentration and electrolyte values, fasting glucose level, liver enzymes, calcium and phosphorus levels, immunosuppressive drug levels, and complete blood count with platelets. Urine dipstick (and, if clinically indicated, urine culture and urine protein/creatinine ratio to monitor for disease recurrence, such as focal segmental glomerulosclerosis) should also be performed. After the first post-transplantation month, pertinent laboratory evaluation should be performed at the discretion of the clinician. After the first post-transplantation year, annual follow-up at a transplantation center is generally recommended.

REFERENCES

1. Pham PT, Pham PC, Danovitch GM. Cardiovascular disease posttransplant. *Semin Nephrol*. 2007;27:430-444.
2. Ojo AO. Cardiovascular complications after renal transplantation and their prevention. *Transplantation*. 2006;82:603-611.
3. Opelz G, Wujciak T, Ritz E, et al. Association of chronic kidney graft failure with recipient blood pressure. *Kidney Int*. 1998;53:217-222.
4. Kasiske BL, Anjum S, Shah R, et al. Hypertension after transplantation. *Am J Kidney Dis*. 2004;43:1071-1081.
5. Premasathian NC, Muehrer R, Brazy PC, et al. Blood pressure control in kidney transplantation. Therapeutic implications. *J Hum Hypertens*. 2004;18:871-877.
6. Fricke L, Doehn C, Steinhoff J, et al. Treatment of posttransplant hypertension by laparoscopic bilateral nephrectomy? *Transplantation*. 1998;65:1182-1187.
7. Hiremath S, Fergusson D, Doucette S, et al. Renin angiotensin system blockade in kidney transplantation: A systematic review of the evidence. *Am J Transplant*. 2007;7:2350-2360.
8. Kasiske BL, Chakkera H, Roel J. Explained and unexplained ischemic heart disease risk after renal transplantation. *J Am Soc Nephrol*. 2001;11:1735-1743.
9. Brenner BM, Cooper ME, de Zeeuw D, et al. Effects of losartan on renal and cardiovascular outcomes in patients with type 2 diabetes and nephropathy. *N Engl J Med*. 2001;345:861-869.
10. Agoda LY, Appel L, Bakris GL, et al. Effect of ramipril vs amlodipine on renal outcomes in hypertensive nephrosclerosis: A randomized controlled trial. *JAMA*. 2001;285:2719-2728.
11. Holdaas H, Fellstrom B, Jardin AG, et al. Beneficial effects of early initiation of lipid-lowering therapy following renal transplantation. *Nephrol Dial Transplant*. 2005;20:974-980.
12. Fellstrom B, Holdaas H, Jardine AG, et al. Effects of fluvastatin end points in the Assessment of Lescol in Renal Transplantation (ALERT) trial. *Kidney Int*. 2004;66:1549-1555.
13. Masterson R, Hweitson T, Leikis M, et al. Impact of statin treatment on 1-year functional and histologic renal allograft outcome. *Transplantation*. 2005;80:332-338.
14. Ballantyne CM, Corsini A, Davidson MH, et al. Risk for myopathy with statin therapy in high-risk patients. *Arch Intern Med*. 2003;163:553-564.
15. Chuang P, Langone AJ. Ezetimide reduces low-density lipoprotein cholesterol (LDL-C) in renal transplant patients resistant to HMG-CoA reductase inhibitors. *Am J Ther*. 2007;14:438-441.
16. Turk TR, Voropaeva E, Kohnle M, et al. Ezetimide treatment in hypercholesterolemic kidney transplant patients is safe and effective and reduces the decline of renal allograft function: A pilot study. *Nephrol Dial Transplant*. 2008;23:369-373.
17. Crutchlow MF, Bloom RD. Transplant-associated hyperglycemia: A new look at an old problem. *Clin J Am Soc Nephrol*. 2007;2:343-355.
18. Pham PT, Pham PC, Wilkinson AH. New onset diabetes mellitus after solid organ transplantation. *Endocrinol Metab Clin North Am*. 2007;36:873-890.
19. Gerstein HC, Miller ME, Bigger T, et al, for The Action to Control Cardiovascular Risk in Diabetes Study Group: Effects of intensive glucose lowering in type 2 diabetes. *N Engl J Med*. 2008;358:2545-2559.
20. Kahn SE, Haffner SM, Heise MA. Glycemic durability of rosiglitazone, metformin or glyburide monotherapy for the ADOPT study. *N Engl J Med*. 2006;355:2427-2443.
21. Hampton T. Diabetes drugs tied to fractures in women. *JAMA*. 2007;297:1645-1647.
22. Chuang P, Gibney EM, Chan L, et al. Predictors of cardiovascular events and associated mortality within two years of kidney transplantation. *Transplant Proc*. 2004;36:1387-1391.
23. Kasiske BL, Klinger D. Cigarette smoking in renal transplant recipients. *J Am Soc Nephrol*. 2000;11:753-759.
24. Abbott KC, Reynolds JC, Taylor AJ, et al. Hospitalized atrial fibrillation after renal transplantation in the United States. *Am J Transplant*. 2003;3:471-476.
25. Abbott KC, Yuan CM, Taylor AJ, et al. Early renal insufficiency and hospitalized heart disease after renal transplantation in the era of modern immunosuppression. *J Am Soc Nephrol*. 2003;14:2358-2365.
26. Lentine KL, Rocca-Rey LA, Bacchi G, et al. Obesity and cardiac risk after kidney transplantation: Experience at one center and comprehensive literature review. *Transplantation*. 2008;86:303-312.
27. Gore J. Obesity and renal transplantation: Is bariatric surgery the answer? Analysis and commentary. *Transplantation*. 2009;87:1115.
28. Augustine JJ, Rodriguez V, Padiyar A, et al. Reduction of erythropoietin resistance after conversion from sirolimus to enteric coated mycophenolate sodium. *Transplantation*. 2008;86:548-553.
29. Vlahakos DV, Marathias KP, Agroyannis B, Madias NE. Posttransplant erythrocytosis. *Kidney Int*. 2003;63;1187-1194.

30. Groth CG, Backman L, Morales JM, et al. Sirolimus (rapamycin)–based therapy in human renal transplantation. Similar efficacy and different toxicity compared with cyclosporine. *Transplantation.* 1999;67:1036-1042.
31. Morales JM, Andres A, Dominguez-Gil B, et al. Tubular function in patients with hypokalemia induced by sirolimus after renal transplantation. *Transplant Proc.* 2003;35(Suppl):154S-156S.
32. Kawarazaki H, Shibagaki Y, Shimizu H, et al. Persistent high level of fibroblast growth factor 23 as a cause of post-renal transplant hypophosphatemia. *Clin Exp Nephrol.* 2007;11:255-257.
33. Pham PC, Pham PT. Parathyroidectomy. In: Nissenson AR, Fine RN, eds. *Handbook of Dialysis Therapy*. 4th ed. Philadelphia: Saunders Elsevier; 2008:1024-1038.
34. Nanmoku K, Imaizumi R, Tojimbra T, et al. Effects of immunosuppressants on the progression of hepatitis C in hepatitis C virus–positive renal transplantation and the usefulness of interferon therapy. *Transplant Proc.* 2008;40:2382-2385.
35. Khwaja, Asolati M, Harmano J, et al. Outcome at 3 years with a prednisone-free maintenance regimen: A single center experience with 349 kidney transplant recipients. *Am J Transplant.* 2002;4:980-987.

CHAPTER 103

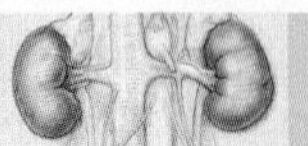

Chronic Allograft Injury

Moses D. Wavamunno, Philip J. O'Connell

DEFINITIONS

Advances in immunosuppression have resulted in a continuing reduction in acute rejection rates and improvement in short-term graft survival. However, this short-term improvement has had surprisingly little impact on long-term graft survival.[1] In the last 2 decades, 1-year renal allograft survival has increased from 50% to 94% in deceased donor kidney transplants and up to 97% in living related transplants. However, late graft loss continues to be the "Achilles' heel" of renal transplantation, with 5- and 10-year survival rates reported as 91% and 58% for deceased donor transplants and 90% and 77% for living donor recipients from U.S. registry data.[2] Australia and New Zealand registry data (ANZDATA) show that between 1991 and 1997, 1-year primary deceased donor graft survival improved from 85% to 91%, with only modest improvements in 5-year survival.[3]

A large proportion of late graft loss is preceded by chronic transplant dysfunction, a clinicopathologic syndrome characterized by slow progressive decline in graft function, proteinuria, hypertension, and histopathologic features of interstitial fibrosis and tubular atrophy. This was initially referred to as *chronic rejection*, a concept that emerged in the 1950s when arterial intimal fibrosis and glomerular abnormalities were seen in transplant recipients with late acute rejection episodes and circulating alloantibody,[4] and then severe recurrent rejection and late cellular rejection were noted as independent risk factors for graft failure.[5] For many years, it was believed that late allograft dysfunction was solely the result of an immune-mediated process.

The term *chronic allograft nephropathy*, introduced in 1991, was used to describe the same pathologic features as it had become increasingly clear that they are due to multiple different causes, of which the alloimmune response is but one.[6] More recently, there has been concern that chronic allograft nephropathy has been inappropriately considered a specific disease state rather than a term for nonspecific scarring. It was thought that the term inhibited the search for an accurate etiologic diagnosis, and hence it has been eliminated from the Banff classification of renal allograft pathology.[7] In recent years, there has been renewed emphasis on the importance of developing more specific etiologic diagnoses, such as chronic antibody-mediated rejection. However, this still leaves a large number of biopsies in which the injury is either multifactorial or unknown. This is now described in the Banff schema as *interstitial fibrosis/tubular atrophy with no evidence of specific etiology (IF/TA)* as a more specific description of the pathologic features. The new Banff schema is shown in Figure 103.1.

The problem with these terms is that they group together all causes rather than take into account the many factors important in the pathogenesis of the condition. These are discussed later but include, for example, prior donor disease, alloimmune factors, calcineurin inhibitor (CNI) nephrotoxicity, BK virus nephropathy, chronic hypertension, obstructive uropathy, and recurrent disease. In any individual patient, some or all of these features may play a role in the development of IF/TA and chronic transplant dysfunction.

EPIDEMIOLOGY

Chronic allograft injury is the leading cause of death-censored graft failure late after transplantation. Its incidence and prevalence are difficult to determine because the onset is often insidious and difficult to define, especially when not every patient undergoes a biopsy. However, in some studies, "protocol" biopsies have been obtained in all patients at predetermined intervals after transplantation. In these studies, evidence of IF/TA was found in 50% of protocol biopsies at 3 months and in 94% of protocol biopsies at 1 year after transplantation in recipients treated with CNIs.[8]

PATHOLOGY

The histologic changes characteristic of chronic allograft injury are wide ranging and vary according to the underlying causes present. They include glomerulosclerosis, fibrointimal thickening of large and medium-sized arteries, and interstitial fibrosis and tubular atrophy (Fig. 103.2).

Banff Classification of Chronic Renal Allograft Pathology

The Banff schema was developed in the early 1990s to standardize reporting of transplant pathology; it incorporated other classification systems then in use,[9,10] and with subsequent refinements, a scoring system for renal transplant pathology emerged. Lesions within individual anatomic compartments (vascular, glomerular, and interstitial) were classified as either acute or chronic and semiquantitatively scored by standardized definitions. Patterns of scored lesions, supported by specific pathologic features, were classified into a clinicopathologic diagnosis and graded. Chronic lesions representing sclerosing changes in the allograft were primarily defined by interstitial fibrosis and tubular atrophy and graded by severity and extent of tubulointerstitial damage into grade I (mild, 6% to 25% of cortex), grade II (moderate, 26% to 50%), and grade III (severe, >50% of cortical area). The schema also categorized other lesions, such as glomerulopathy, mesangial matrix increase, vascular fibrous intimal thickening, and arteriolar hyaline thickening. Patterns of scored lesions,

Banff Classification of Renal Allograft Pathology

1. Normal

2. Antibody mediated rejection
Documentation of circulating anti-donor, and C4d or allograft pathology
C4d deposition without morphologic evidence of active rejection (C4d+)
presence of circulating antidonor antibodies, no signs of acute or chronic T cell-mediated or antibody-mediated rejection
Acute antibody-mediated rejection
C4d+, presence of circulating antidonor antibodies, morphologic evidence of acute tissue injury, such as:
I. ATN-like minimal inflammation
II. Capillary and glomerular inflammation and/or thromboses
III. Arterial - v3
Chronic active antibody mediated rejection
C4d+, presence of circulating antidonor antibodies, morphologic evidence of tissue injury such as:
Glomerular double contours and/or peritubular capillary basement membrane multilayering and/or interstitial fibrosis/tubular atrophy and/or fibrous intimal thickening

3. Borderline changes
Suspicious for acute T-cell mediated rejection
No intimal arteritis but foci or tubulitis (t1, t2 or t3 with i0 or i1)

4. T cell mediated rejection
Acute T cell mediated rejection
Type
IA Interstitial infiltration and moderate tubulitis (i2 or i3 and t2)
IB Interstitial infiltration and severe tubulitis (i2 or i3 and t3)
IIA Mild to moderate intimal arteritis (v1)
IIB Severe intimal arteritis (v2)
III Transmural arteritis and/or fibrinoid change and/or smooth muscle necrosis
Chronic active T cell mediated rejection
"Chronic allograft arteriopathy"
Arterial fibrosis with mononuclear cell infiltration in fibrosis

5. Interstitial fibrosis and tubular atrophy, no specific etiology (formerly known as CAN)
Grade
I Mild interstitial fibrosis and tubular atrophy (<25% of cortical area)
II Moderate interstitial fibrosis and tubular atrophy (26%-50% of cortical area)
III Severe interstitial fibrosis and tubular atrophy (>50%) cortical area

6. Changes thought not due to rejecton - either acute or chronic (see fig. 103.8)

Figure 103.1 Banff classification of renal allograft pathology. (2007 update of original 1997 classification.) ATN, acute tubular necrosis; CAN, chronic allograft nephropathy.

supported by specific pathologic features, were then classified into a clinicopathologic diagnosis.[11,12]

It is now recognized that use of the nonspecific term *chronic allograft nephropathy* undermined recognition of morphologic features that could enable diagnosis of specific causes of chronic graft dysfunction.[7] Consequently, the schema has been modified (see Fig 103.1) to include various causes of chronic graft injury, such as:

- Chronic antibody-mediated rejection, described by basement membrane duplication in glomerular or peritubular capillaries in the presence of complement 4d deposition and antidonor HLA antibody.
- Chronic active T cell–mediated rejection, characterized by arterial intimal fibrosis with a mononuclear cell infiltrate.
- Interstitial fibrosis and tubular atrophy not otherwise specified.
- Nonimmune causes of injury, such as chronic CNI toxicity.

This classification provides a standardized and widely accepted framework for histologic analysis of renal allograft pathology. However, the pathology of a failing transplant represents a final common pathway of damage and injury from multiple overlaid mechanisms. In many cases, it can be impossible to assign a specific cause; indeed, multiple causes of interstitial fibrosis and tubular atrophy will often coexist within the same biopsy specimen.

Transplant Glomerulopathy

The term *transplant glomerulopathy* was coined in 1970 for glomerular abnormalities specific to renal allografts and distinct from recurrent or *de novo* glomerulonephritis (GN).[13] Transplant glomerulopathy is a characteristic element of chronic renal allograft pathology. Transplant glomerulopathy is characterized by duplication of glomerular capillary basement membrane, mesangial matrix expansion, and absence of immune deposits (Fig. 103.3). In addition, there is deposition of C4d in peritubular and glomerular capillaries (Fig. 103.4). Clinicopathologic studies suggest that transplant glomerulopathy is a manifestation of capillary injury occurring in conjunction with interstitial, peritubular capillary, and glomerular inflammation, although it may also occur independently of interstitial fibrosis, tubular atrophy, or transplant arteriopathy.[14] On electron microscopy, there is expansion of the subendothelial space with deposition of flocculent or fibrillary material, interposition of mesangial cell cytoplasm in the lamina densa, and mesangial matrix expansion (Fig.

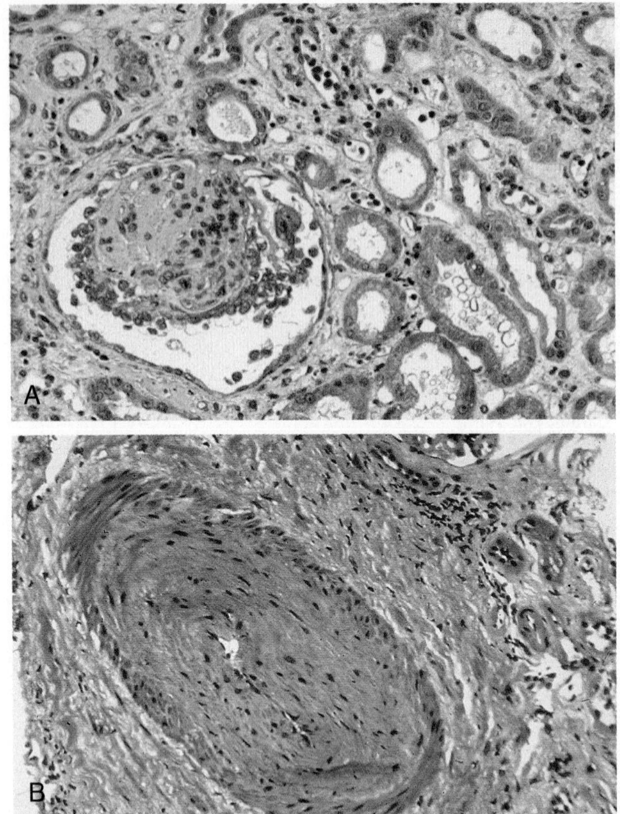

Figure 103.2 Histologic features of chronic allograft dysfunction and intestitial fibrosis/tubular atrophy with no evidence of specific etiology (IF/TA). A, Interstitial fibrosis and glomerulosclerosis. **B,** Fibro-intimal proliferation in an intrarenal artery.

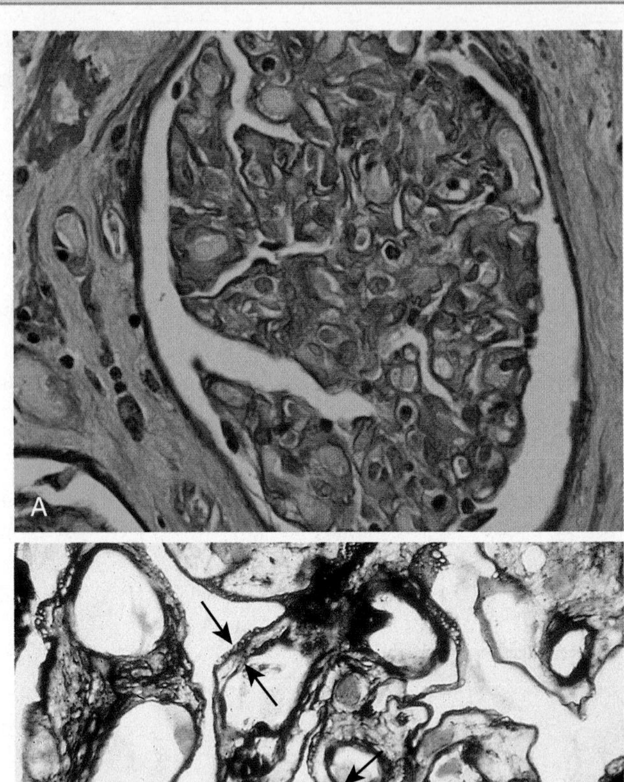

Figure 103.3 Transplant glomerulopathy: light microscopy. A, Note the mesangial expansion and thickening of the glomerular basement membranes (GBM). **B,** Note the GBM reduplication in capillary loops *(between arrows)*.

103.5). Ultrastructural abnormalities characteristic of endothelial activation occur long before glomerular basement membrane (GBM) duplication and graft dysfunction are evident, implying that endothelial injury is the initial insult that resulted in GBM remodeling (see Fig. 103.5).[15] An association between transplant glomerulopathy and peritubular capillary basement membrane duplication has been well described, suggesting that the process resulting in transplant glomerulopathy involves the entire glomerular and peritubular capillary beds.[16,17]

Role of Protocol Biopsies

Many studies of chronic graft pathology have relied on biopsies performed for graft dysfunction. These studies have inherent bias because the immediate cause of graft dysfunction may not reflect the complex interactions between various factors causing cumulative damage, making it difficult to identify contributions of the different etiologic factors.[8]

Our understanding of the pathophysiologic process of graft injury has improved with the use of surveillance or protocol biopsies as a monitoring tool for pathologic change. Protocol biopsies enable assessment of individual risk factors by detecting early pathologic abnormalities when renal function is stable and individual factors may be in operation; these abnormalities can then be used as surrogate markers for chronic injury. Several studies have shown that chronic pathologic changes detected by surveillance biopsies at 3 months after transplantation, when allograft function is stable, predict poor long-term graft survival,[18-20] whereas other studies have shown that subclinical rejection (defined as occurrence of histologic signs of acute rejection in patients with stable graft rejection) precedes long-term deterioration of graft function and that early intervention improves outcomes.[21] The use of surveillance biopsies in the research setting has given insight into the causes of renal allograft injury and their interactions.[22]

PATHOGENESIS

Factors associated with chronic graft injury are broadly categorized as nonimmune and immune. In most cases, the damage sustained by a renal graft is not the result of a single insult but rather the accumulated effect of multiple sequential or contemporaneous insults (Fig. 103.6) that are then modified by the kidney's limited healing response, which invariably involves fibrosis. This has led to the "cumulative damage" hypothesis that chronic allograft injury is the result of a series of time-dependent insults leading to nephron loss.[23] This loss of nephrons is progressive and accumulative and precedes glomerulosclerosis, a later event that follows increasing interstitial fibrosis and tubular atrophy.[8] In this model, both the site of insult and the subsequent injury are compartment specific. This association between injury and compartment-specific damage is summarized in Figure 103.7.

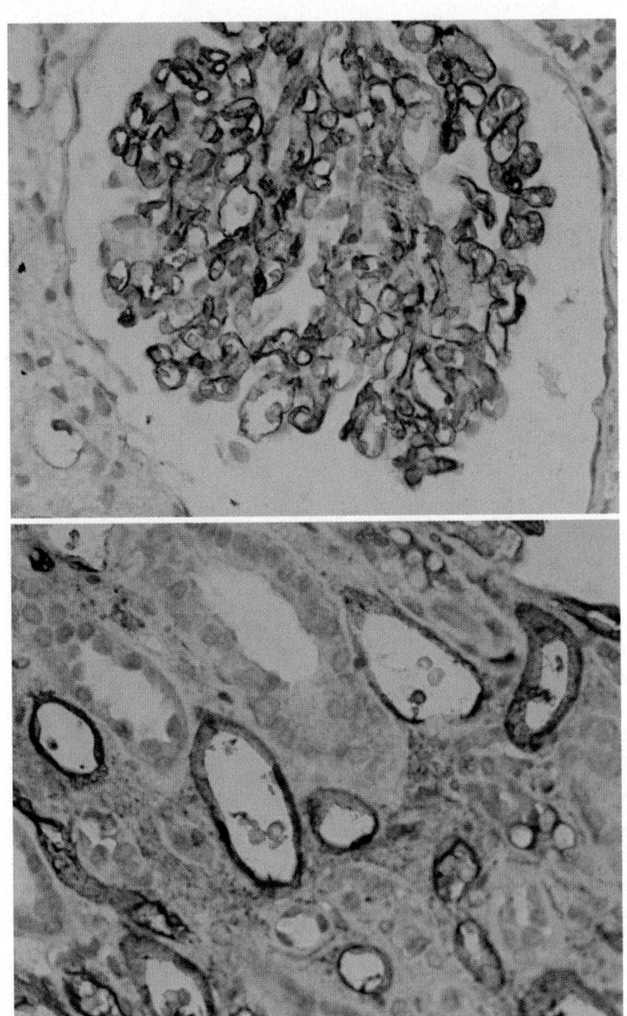

Figure 103.4 Transplant glomerulopathy: C4d immunoperoxidase staining in association with chronic antibody-mediated rejection. Staining of glomerular capillaries and circumferential staining of peritubular capillaries are typical.

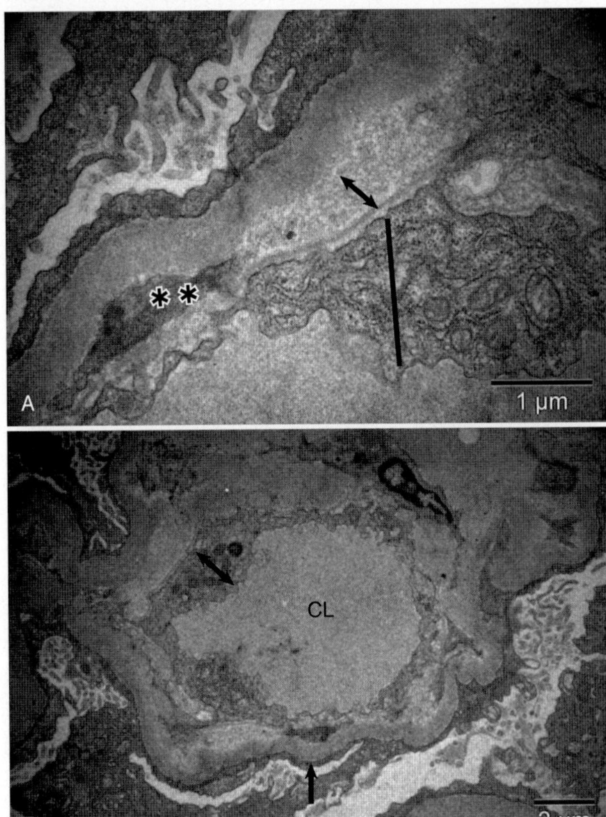

Figure 103.5 Transplant glomerulopathy: electron microscopy. A, Section of glomerular capillary loop (×24,000) demonstrating mesangial interposition *(asterisks)*, subendothelial expansion and new lamina densa *(double arrow)*, and endothelial hypertrophy *(line)*. **B,** A complete glomerular capillary loop (CL) with glomerular basement membrane (GBM) thickening *(single arrow)*, endothelial hypertrophy *(double arrow)*, expanded subendothelial space, mesangial interposition, and new lamina densa *(single arrow)*. Apparent GBM duplication is due to mesangial interposition and formation of new lamina densa.

IMMUNE-INDEPENDENT FACTORS

There are many nonimmune factors that over the life of the graft lead to IF/TA. These are described here and are summarized in Figure 103.8.

Ischemia and Reperfusion Injury

Graft survival is lower in recipients with longer ischemic times; this effect is present even after adjustment for other factors, such as transplant era, donor type, recipient age, and major histocompatibility complex (MHC) mismatches.[5,24,25] In protocol biopsies, acute tubular necrosis (ATN) is predictive of IF/TA[26] and has been identified as a cause of graft fibrosis at 3 and 12 months.[26,27] In a German study in which 258 patients underwent biopsy at 6, 12, and 26 weeks, longer cold ischemic time was a risk factor for the development of IF/TA at 26 weeks.[28] Ischemia-reperfusion injury may also be a factor in immune-mediated injury as ischemia and oxidative injury resulting from reperfusion are associated with activation of the adaptive immune response, antigen-presenting cells and Toll-like receptors (TCRs), and release of proinflammatory cytokines, which can lead to acute rejection and subsequent IF/TA.[29] In deceased donor transplantation, brain death amplifies this response. Brain death results in an "autonomic storm" with release of catecholamines and a sympathetic response, which results in cytokine release, endothelial cell activation, and amplification of the ischemia-reperfusion injury.[29]

Donor Age and Donor-Recipient Size Mismatching

Long-term graft survival is reduced in kidneys from older donors in both deceased donor and living donor transplants. This effect is attributed to a differential response to injury, impaired capacity to withstand stress, limited ability to repair structural damage, or amplification of external injury due to preexisting structural abnormalities. Reduced nephron mass resulting in glomerular hyperfiltration and hypertension with accelerated senescence is also a postulated mechanism.[30,31] The effect of kidney size mismatching is thought to be related to insufficient numbers of nephrons within the donor kidney, which in turn leads to compensatory hyperfiltration.[32] Although there are experimental data to support this hypothesis, the extent to which an inadequate number of nephrons contributes to chronic injury is unknown.

Risk Factors Associated with the Progression of Tubulointerstitial Damage and Renal Allograft Dysfunction
Donor Factors Deceased versus living donor Age Female sex Vascular disease Glomerular disease Brain death versus donation after cardiac death Nephron mass Ischemic time Delayed graft function
Recipient Factors African American race Older age Male sex Diabetes mellitus HLA matching Antidonor antibodies Hypertension, hyperlipidemia, diabetes, smoking Compliance with treatment
Graft function Serum creatinine at 1, 6, 12 months Change in serum creatinine between 6 and 12 months Change in GFR between 6 and 12 months GFR at 6 and 12 months
Evidence of graft injury Acute rejection, especially vascular rejection and late rejection CMV disease BK virus nephropathy Calcineurin nephrotoxicity Doppler ultrasound resistive index >0.80 Proteinuria >500 mg/24 h
Graft pathology in first year Subclinical rejection Nephrocalcinosis Arteriolar hyalinosis Interstitial fibrosis Tubular atrophy C4d binding Transplant glomerulopathy Recurrent or *de novo* glomerulonephritis

Figure 103.6 Risk factors associated with the progression of tubulointerstitial damage and renal allograft dysfunction. CMV, cytomegalovirus; GFR, glomerular filtration rate; HLA, human leukocyte antigen.

Tubulointerstitial Injury from BK Virus Nephropathy

BK virus is an endemic polyomavirus of high prevalence, low morbidity, long latency, and asymptomatic reactivation in immunocompetent individuals. It is seen increasingly in renal transplant recipients as more potent immunosuppression allows asymptomatic reactivation of primary infection and subsequent allograft dysfunction. BK virus nephropathy leads to IF/TA and needs to be considered in trying to identify the causes in an individual case.[33] The diagnosis and management of BK virus nephropathy are discussed further in Chapter 101.

Calcineurin Inhibitor Nephrotoxicity

CNI nephrotoxicity affects all histologic compartments of the transplanted kidney. Characteristic chronic CNI lesions include medial arteriolar hyalinosis, striped interstitial fibrosis, global glomerulosclerosis, and tubular microcalcification unrelated to other causes, such as tubular necrosis and hyperparathyroidism.[34-37] CNI-induced arteriolopathy is characterized by nodular hyaline deposits in the media of afferent arterioles sufficient to cause narrowing of the vascular lumen.[38,39] It is attributed to eosinophilic transformation and vacuolization of smooth muscle cells with subsequent necrosis. Arteriolar hyalinosis is the most reliable diagnostic marker of CNI nephrotoxicity. Confirmation of the diagnosis is made by exclusion of other causes, such as donor hyalinosis (which can be detected on the implantation biopsy specimen), diabetes, and hypertensive nephrosclerosis. Striped fibrosis is subjectively defined by a dense stripe of cortical fibrosis and atrophic tubules adjacent to normal cortex and is traditionally regarded as pathognomonic of CNI nephrotoxicity, but its appearance can be seen in any cause of fibrosis, especially if it is due to microvascular injury. It is likely that the associated arteriolopathy and narrowing of the lumen contribute to development of fibrosis and atrophy following watershed infarcts within areas of ischemia. Local hypoxia leads to formation of free oxygen radicals, which promote cellular death by apoptosis. In addition, upregulation of transforming growth factor β (TGF-β) is considered an important etiologic factor in CNI toxicity.[34]

Recurrent and *de novo* Glomerular Disease

Recurrent GN is diagnosed by exclusion of donor-transmitted disease and *de novo* GN. Its relative importance for graft loss increases as graft survival lengthens.[40] The clinical course and severity of recurrent glomerular disease often recapitulate the patient's native disease. Given that it is a relatively common occurrence and has implications for treatment and retransplantation, it should be looked for carefully in patients with a prior diagnosis of GN. Diagnosis and management of recurrent disease are discussed further in Chapter 104.

Deceased Donor Kidneys

Kidneys from living donors, regardless of their relationship with the recipients, survive longer than kidneys from deceased donors. Recipients of living donor kidneys have less late allograft failure and less histologic evidence of chronic allograft injury.[41] This increased survival of living donor kidneys is multifactorial. They have reduced ischemia time and lack the negative influence of deceased donor brain death, which causes an upregulation of cytokines and growth factors in the kidney and other organs. In general, they do not have preexisting donor disease; and because there is more time involved in planning, they are more likely to be selected so that they avoid non–complement-binding antidonor antibodies, which may not be detected on the traditional complement-dependent cytotoxicity assay.

Delayed Graft Function

Delayed graft function, usually defined by the need for dialysis in the first week after transplantation, is a risk factor for IF/TA.[26] There are also independent associations between delayed graft function and late graft failure and between delayed graft function and graft failure that is mediated by acute rejection. Major risk factors for delayed graft function are prolonged cold ischemia time, donor age older than 50 years, and peak panel reactive antibodies greater than 50%.[42] Ischemia and oxidative injury resulting from reperfusion of an ischemic kidney may cause an

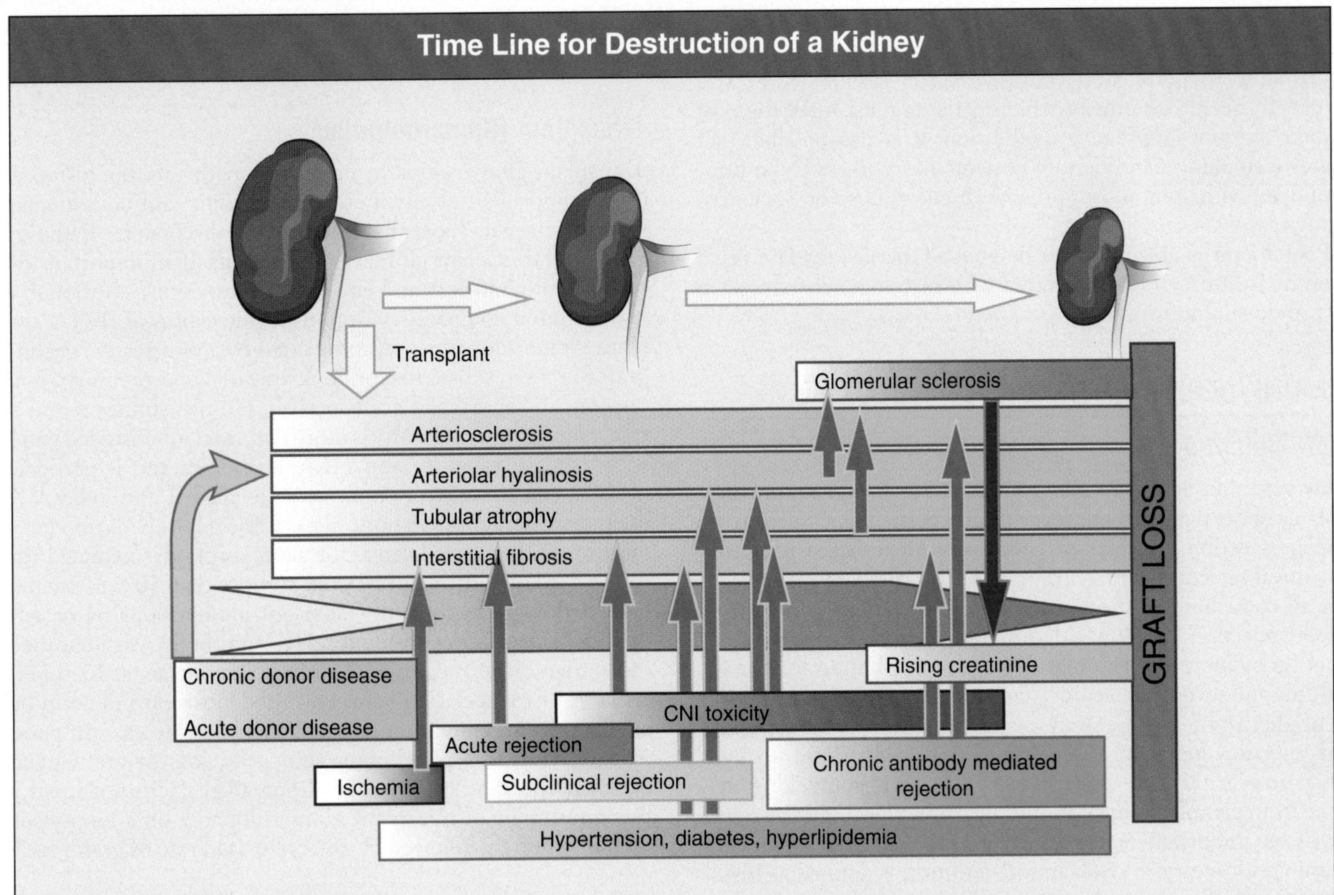

Figure 103.7 Chronic allograft dysfunction and compartment-specific pathologic changes. The individual factors causing chronic allograft dysfunction *(shown in the lower part of the figure)* are active at different stages in the life of a transplant kidney. There is evidence that each factor predominantly damages specific compartments of the kidney *(arrows)* causing pathologic changes which ultimately lead to graft loss. CNI, calcineurin inhibitor. *(Modified from reference 22.)*

Pathologic Features of Specific Chronic Diseases Other than Rejection that Can Lead to Interstitial Fibrosis/Tubular Atrophy

Cause	Pathology
Chronic hypertension	Arterial/fibrointimal thickening with reduplication of elastica, usually with small artery and arteriolar hyaline changes
Calcineurin inhibitor toxicity	Arteriolar hyalinosis with peripheral hyaline nodules and/or progressive increase in the absence of hypertension or diabetes Tubular cell injury with isometric vacuolization
Chronic obstruction	Marked tubular dilation; large Tamm-Horsfall protein casts with extravasation into interstitium and/or lymphatics
Bacterial pyelonephritis	Intratubular and peritubular neutrophils, lymphoid follicle formation
Viral infection	Viral inclusions on histology and immunohistology and/or electron microscopy

Figure 103.8 Pathologic features of specific chronic diseases that can lead to interstitial fibrosis/tubular atrophy (IF/TA). *(Modified from reference 7.)*

upregulation of MHC antigens or proinflammatory cytokines, predisposing to acute rejection.

Cardiovascular Risk Factors

The vasculopathy in chronic allograft injury resembles systemic vascular disease, raising the possibility that conventional cardiovascular disease (CVD) risk factors may be implicated. Hypertension occurs in more than 50% of transplant recipients. In a multicenter, retrospective study of 29,751 kidney transplant recipients with 7 years of follow-up, elevated systolic and diastolic blood pressure (BP) was associated with chronic graft failure in a multivariate analysis.[43] Hypertension is associated with IF/TA. Dyslipidemias, including raised levels of total cholesterol, low-density lipoprotein (LDL) cholesterol, and triglycerides, have been associated with late graft failure.[4] Cigarette smoking is associated with late renal allograft failure[44,45] either by a direct toxic effect on the allograft or more likely mediated by hypertension or other cardiovascular (CV) risk factors. In health systems in which patients must meet the cost of their immunosuppressive medication, it is also possible that cigarette smoking may identify patients more likely to be noncompliant with immunosuppressive medications for socioeconomic reasons.

Proteinuria is an important diagnostic marker for late renal allograft failure[44] and is associated with histologic changes seen in chronic allograft injury.[46]

IMMUNE-DEPENDENT FACTORS

Acute Rejection

Graft rejection leads to allograft damage, but its expression depends on its type, timing, severity, and persistence. Early acute cellular rejection, vascular or corticosteroid-resistant rejection, subclinical rejection, true chronic rejection, and late acute rejection all contribute to the burden of allograft injury. Interstitial cellular rejection is followed by interstitial fibrosis, and vascular rejection by increased vascular damage, contributing to injury.[47] Multiple and severe late acute T cell–mediated rejection episodes are predictive of chronic graft dysfunction more than early cellular rejection and acute vascular rejection, which have stronger associations with acute graft loss.[48,49] There is compelling evidence from protocol biopsy studies that subclinical cellular rejection is an important factor in early graft loss and subsequent chronic graft injury.[27,50] Subclinical rejection is defined as histologically proven acute rejection without concurrent renal dysfunction and is influenced by time after transplantation, prior acute rejection, HLA mismatch, and immunosuppression.[27] Interstitial lymphocyte infiltration may persist in some patients as true chronic cellular rejection, which is arbitrarily defined as subclinical rejection that persists beyond 1 year. Inflammatory mediators generate compartment-specific fibrosis, impaired graft function, and reduced survival.[27,51] Untreated subclinical rejection inflicts permanent tubulointerstitial damage and fibrosis and is associated with a poorer prognosis.[27] Prompt diagnosis, early treatment, and readjustment of baseline immunosuppression have been associated with improved outcomes.[50]

Chronic Antibody-Mediated Rejection

The contribution of donor-specific anti-HLA antibodies to allograft injury has been demonstrated in studies showing that presensitization and appearance of post-transplantation HLA antibodies are risk factors for early graft loss,[52,53] hyperacute rejection,[54] and a higher incidence of primary nonfunction and decreased graft survival.[55] Stenotic arterial lesions have been described in recipients with circulating antibodies and late graft loss.[56] Several studies have attempted to demonstrate a temporal relationship between appearance of antibodies and subsequent graft dysfunction.[57,58] The accepted diagnostic criteria for chronic antibody-mediated rejection include presence of circulating antidonor antibodies; diffuse positive C4d staining in the peritubular capillaries; and evidence of morphologic injury, which includes transplant glomerulopathy, peritubular capillary basement membrane multilayering, tubulointerstitial fibrosis, and arterial intimal fibrosis without duplication of lamina elastica interna (see Figs. 103.1 to 103.5). The time line for development of chronic antibody-mediated rejection includes appearance of antibody, deposition of complement, graft dysfunction, and subsequent pathologic abnormalities.[59]

Transplant Glomerulopathy

Transplant glomerulopathy and arteriopathy are the histopathologic abnormalities attributed to chronic antibody-mediated injury in renal allografts (see earlier discussion, Pathology). However, transplant glomerulopathy is itself an important cause of renal allograft loss and late graft dysfunction.[60] Although it is less common compared with nonspecific causes of IF/TA, transplant glomerulopathy is accompanied by a progressive decline in graft function, substantial or nephrotic-range proteinuria, hypertension, and shortened graft survival. Human studies report that transplant glomerulopathy is more common in sensitized patients with a broad range of anti-HLA antibodies and is particularly prevalent in those with donor-specific class II antibodies.[14] The incidence is highest if both class I and class II antibodies are present or there has been prior acute antibody-mediated rejection.[14] C4d deposition is reported in more than 50% of recipients with histologic features of transplant glomerulopathy or arteriopathy[52]; circulating antidonor HLA antibody was identified in more than 80% of cases with diffuse staining for C4d. There is also a strong association between C4d deposition and peritubular capillary multilamination of more than five layers.[52] In patients who develop transplant glomerulopathy, loss of graft function occurs before development of widespread glomerulosclerosis, and the appearance of transplant glomerulopathy on a biopsy specimen is generally followed by an accelerated rate of graft loss.[60]

Histologic Progression of Chronic Graft Injury

Our current understanding of the natural history and progression of chronic renal allograft injury comes from protocol biopsy studies evaluating the causes and correlates of chronic allograft dysfunction. A study of more than 900 protocol biopsies from recipients of simultaneous kidney-pancreas transplants has provided valuable insight into the relationships between graft fibrosis, arteriolar damage, and glomerular dysfunction.[8] This study showed that allograft injury occurred in two distinct phases: an early phase characterized by tubulointerstitial damage; and a late phase, which primarily involves the microvascular compartments (i.e., glomerular, peritubular, and interstitial capillary networks), leading to progressive interstitial fibrosis, tubular atrophy, and glomerulosclerosis. Causes of early tubulointerstitial injury include preexisting conditions in the donor kidney, such as warm and cold ischemia time and quality of donor organ preservation, as well as postimplantation events, such as early rejection, delayed graft function, and immunosuppressive toxicity. In contrast, graft injury in the late phase is primarily attributed to the effects of CNI toxicity and persistent and progressive subclinical inflammation.[61] This is summarized in Figure 103.7.

Mechanisms of Graft Injury

Graft dysfunction typically results from cumulative tissue injury arising from several pathogenic insults occurring in specific histologic compartments, modified by the kidney's healing response to the injury, alloimmunity, and immunosuppression. The starting condition of the transplanted kidney (which includes input organ quality and acute early events) and subsequent immune and nonimmune stressors contribute to loss of structural integrity of the graft and subsequent failure.[23]

Injury to any key component of a nephron results in functional failure of the whole unit. Individual nephrons fail because of glomerulosclerosis, transplant glomerulopathy, or loss of tubular components. Segmental glomerular injury leads to capsular adhesions, misdirection of ultrafiltrate, and reduction in overall functional efficiency.[62] Tubular malfunction is caused by localized apoptosis, tubular atrophy, or luminal obstruction from cellular debris leading to loss of tubular basement membrane (TBM) integrity and leakage.[63]

Chronic ischemia plays a major role in the initiation and perpetuation of glomerular and tubulointerstitial injury. Vascular narrowing due to glomerulosclerosis, CNI-induced arteriolar hyalinosis,[37] fibrointimal hyperplasia of small arteries, and cyclosporine-induced vasoconstriction cause ischemic injury, peritubular capillary loss,[47] and subsequent tubulointerstitial injury. An important aspect of graft injury is the process of tissue repair after injury. Repeated episodes of acute injury are followed by partial or incomplete resolution of inflammation, resulting in a vicious circle of inflammation, enhanced expression and recognition of alloreactive molecules, and further injury.[30] Evidence of an impaired healing process has been provided by studies that show an association between the presence of inflammatory cells within areas of fibrosis (activated fibrosis) and progressive damage, functional impairment, and reduced graft survival.[27] Variations in response to injury and impaired capacity to withstand stress because of increased donor age also contribute to limited ability to repair structural damage, causing further amplification of external insults by preexisting abnormalities and perpetuation of the vicious circle.

Differential Diagnosis of Chronic Allograft Dysfunction
Prerenal reversible hemodynamic dysfunction
Dehydration
Congestive cardiac failure
Nonsteroidal anti-inflammatory drugs
Antihypertensive medication
Graft renal artery stenosis
Intrinsic renal parenchymal disease
Acute rejection
Calcineurin inhibitor toxicity
Other nephrotoxic agents (e.g., lithium)
Recurrent renal disease
De novo glomerulonephritis
Drug-induced interstitial nephritis
Viral infections, CMV, polyomavirus
Bacterial pyelonephritis
Lymphomatous infiltrate
Late acute rejection, either iatrogenic or due to noncompliance
Obstructive renal disease
Ureteral stenosis
Prostatic hypertrophy
Other causes of bladder outlet obstruction (e.g., cancer, calculi)
Ureteral or bladder leak
Ureteral polyomavirus infection

Figure 103.9 Differential diagnosis of chronic allograft dysfunction. CMV, cytomegalovirus.

CLINICAL MANIFESTATIONS

Chronic allograft injury usually presents as a decline in glomerular filtration rate (GFR) or an increase in urine protein excretion. There are no specific clinical features of chronic allograft injury. All too often, it is first detected when it is already far advanced because clinical methods for detection of early declines in GFR are relatively insensitive. Serum creatinine remains the routine parameter for detection of changes in GFR in kidney transplant recipients. Whereas an acute rise in serum creatinine is a relatively sensitive albeit nonspecific indicator of acute allograft dysfunction from any cause, chronic changes in serum creatinine are not very sensitive for detection of chronic allograft dysfunction. Furthermore, patients with chronic allograft injury may have lower muscle mass, resulting in lower serum creatinine values than expected for the GFR. Estimation of GFR by the Nankivell formula or the Modification of Diet in Renal Disease (MDRD) formula may be helpful to supplement information from serial serum creatinine estimations. The value and limitations of measurement and estimation of GFR are discussed further in Chapter 3.

Proteinuria may also be the first manifestation of chronic allograft injury. Few studies have prospectively evaluated proteinuria as a tool for screening to detect chronic injury or other causes of allograft dysfunction. IF/TA is found in more than half of patients who undergo allograft biopsy for proteinuria and in 40% of those who have nephrotic-range proteinuria.[64] Transplant glomerulopathy is almost always accompanied by proteinuria. Except for proteinuria, the urinalysis is usually unremarkable in chronic allograft dysfunction. Clinical and histologic factors that are predictive of chronic allograft dysfunction are summarized in Figure 103.6.

DIFFERENTIAL DIAGNOSIS

Because the etiology of chronic allograft dysfunction is multifactorial, any specific diagnosis is made by combination of a biopsy with a review of the patient's past history to identify important etiologic factors, such as preexisting donor disease, prior rejection, and high-titer anti-HLA antibodies, as well as issues not related to alloimmunity, such as CNI toxicity, *de novo* GN, or recurrent renal disease. Chronic allograft dysfunction is common and can have many causes other than IF/TA. However, if it is left untreated, it can ultimately result in renal injury, which in turn will heal by scarring and interstitial fibrosis. The differential diagnosis of IF/TA is summarized in Figure 103.9.

Prerenal Causes

Prerenal causes of allograft dysfunction include reversible hemodynamic alterations that may occur from dehydration or congestive heart failure (CHF). Graft renal artery stenosis or stenosis of arteries proximal to the kidney allograft can cause a decline in kidney function. This is usually associated with difficult-to-control hypertension. Rarely, cholesterol emboli can present as a decrease in function late after transplantation.

Intrinsic Renal Causes

Acute rejection can occur late after transplantation and present as a gradual rise in serum creatinine with or without proteinuria. Late acute rejection is often the result of the patient's noncompliance with immunosuppressive medications. The diagnosis and management of acute deterioration of allograft function are discussed further in Chapters 99 and 100.

Viral infections, including cytomegalovirus (CMV) and polyomaviruses, especially BK virus, can also cause acute or chronic graft dysfunction. BK virus infection is suspected on finding BK virus in the serum or urine and confirmed by detecting virus in kidney tissue with either antibody staining or *in situ* hybridization. Histologic changes associated with BK virus nephropathy can resemble acute rejection, but renal tubular cell cytopathic changes are features that point to BK virus nephropathy. The presence of SV40 antigen, which can be detected routinely by immunohistochemistry, will differentiate between BK virus nephropathy and acute cellular rejection.

Allergic interstitial nephritis, often medication induced, and acute bacterial pyelonephritis are usually differentials for acute rather than for chronic allograft dysfunction.

Proteinuria, with or without a decline in kidney function, may be caused by *de novo* or recurrent glomerular diseases. The most common recurrent glomerular disease causing chronic allograft injury and graft loss is IgA nephropathy. Other recurrent diseases in the renal transplant are discussed in Chapter 104.

Postrenal Causes

Postrenal causes should also be considered. Although it is uncommon, ureteral obstruction can occur late after transplantation. Bladder dysfunction or prostatic hypertrophy can also cause allograft dysfunction and can lead to IF/TA.

TREATMENT

Strategies for the management of chronic allograft dysfunction rely on minimization of exposure to risk factors as there is no effective specific treatment. Current recommendations for the treatment of chronic allograft dysfunction are summarized in Figure 103.10.

Treatment Recommendations for Chronic Allograft Dysfunction
Minimize acute rejection Use adequate immunosuppression Monitor graft function and urine protein Investigate with biopsy for unexplained increases in serum creatinine, failure of serum creatinine to fall to acceptable levels, or proteinuria
Minimize subclinical rejection Use adequate immunosuppression Re-evaluate immunosuppression if subclinical rejection detected Consider use of protocol biopsies or have high index of suspicion
Minimize or eliminate CNI Consider low-dose tacrolimus with mycophenolate mofetil and prednisolone Consider substitution of CNI with mTOR inhibitor if clinically appropriate Consider withdrawal of CNI if immunologically very low risk (e.g., HLA–identical graft)
Control BP Aim for BP <130/80 mmHg Consider ACE inhibitor or ARB if proteinuria >500 mg/24 h
Treat other nonimmunologic risk factors Maintain LDL cholesterol <3.5 mmol/l Cessation of smoking Maintain compliance

Figure 103.10 Treatment recommendations for chronic allograft dysfunction. ACE, angiotensin-converting enzyme; ARB, angiotensin receptor blocker; BP, blood pressure; CNI, calcineurin inhibitor; HLA, human leukocyte antigen; LDL, low-density lipoprotein; mTOR, mammalian target of rapamycin.

Prevention

The use of young living donors and optimal HLA matching are helpful but often impossible in this era of long waiting times and donor shortage. Prolonged cold ischemic times should be avoided as much as possible to reduce the risk of delayed graft function. An effective strategy for minimization of IF/TA is early recognition and treatment of acute rejection. Effective immunosuppression that reduces the incidence and severity of acute cellular rejection is crucial as less alloimmune-mediated inflammation will result in less interstitial fibrosis and tubular atrophy. Surveillance biopsies have resulted in improved diagnosis and early treatment of subclinical acute rejection, a major cause of chronic injury. In units where protocol biopsies are not undertaken, there should be a high index of suspicion and a low threshold for performing diagnostic biopsies, especially in the first 6 months after transplantation. Prompt treatment of subclinical cellular rejection, when it is identified, has been shown to limit the degree of chronic damage at later time points.[50,65] Increased surveillance in high-risk patients, such as those receiving organs from older donors, may allow early intervention. If protocol biopsies are not being routinely performed, a biopsy should be undertaken if graft function fails to reach an acceptable baseline.

Maintenance Immunosuppression

Treatment of established IF/TA relies on modification of immunosuppression protocols, such as CNI avoidance or dose reduction. A meta-analysis suggested a beneficial effect of CNI withdrawal and replacement with mycophenolate mofetil (MMF) or sirolimus in minimizing CNI toxicity.[66] However, the recent CONVERT trial suggests that CNI avoidance and substitution with sirolimus after the development of IF/TA result in at best modest improvements in graft function.[67] Use of MMF with or without CNI reduction results in improved graft function and altered chronic transplant histology.[68,69] The SYMPHONY trial showed that low-dose tacrolimus in combination with MMF and prednisolone provided the best outcomes in patients with standard immunologic risk.[70] Patients without evidence of rejection may benefit from use of low-dose tacrolimus or, alternatively, avoidance of CNI altogether by substitution of an mammalian target of rapamycin (mTOR) inhibitor.

Apart from alterations in immunosuppression, effective management of comorbidities may help preserve kidney function. Efforts should be directed at BP control, treatment of hyperlipidemia, smoking cessation, and optimal glycemic control (management of these issues in transplant patients is discussed further in Chapter 102). Registry data suggest that prevention of smoking, reduction of serum cholesterol to less than 200 mg/dl (5.2 mmol/L), and lowering of BP to less than 130/80 mm Hg will improve long-term graft survival.

Proteinuria

Angiotensin-converting enzyme (ACE) inhibitors and angiotensin receptor blockers (ARBs) are used in native kidney disease to reduce proteinuria and to slow progression to renal failure; however, there are not yet any randomized controlled studies showing that they slow the rate of progression of chronic renal allograft injury. In fact, registry data suggest that the addition of ACE inhibitors or ARBs does not result in improved graft outcomes.[71] By contrast, a meta-analysis of trial data suggests that calcium channel blockers (CCBs) reduced graft loss and improved GFR, whereas the data regarding ACE inhibitors were inconclusive.[72]

REFERENCES

1. Meier-Kriesche HU, Schold JD, Srinivas TR, Kaplan B. Lack of improvement in renal allograft survival despite a marked decrease in acute rejection rates over the most recent era. *Am J Transplant.* 2004;4:378-383.
2. The US Organ Procurement and Transplantation Network and The Scientific Registry of Transplant Recipients 2003 Annual Report. *Am J Transplant.* 2004;4(Suppl 9):72-80.
3. Campbell S, Macdonald S, Excell L, Livinston B. Transplantation. Australia and New Zealand Dialysis and Transplant Registry: The 31st Annual Report. Adelaide Australia, 2008, pp 1-23.
4. Hume DM, Egdahl RH. Progressive destruction of renal homografts isolated from the regional lymphatics of the host. *Surgery.* 1955;38: 194-214.
5. Monaco AP, Burke JF Jr, Ferguson RM, et al. Current thinking on chronic renal allograft rejection: Issues, concerns, and recommendations from a 1997 roundtable discussion. *Am J Kidney Dis.* 1999;33: 150-160.
6. Paul LC. Chronic renal transplant loss. *Kidney Int.* 1995;47:1491-1499.
7. Solez K, Colvin RB, Racusen LC, et al. Banff '05 Meeting Report: Differential diagnosis of chronic allograft injury and elimination of chronic allograft nephropathy ("CAN"). *Am J Transplant.* 2007;7:518-526.
8. Nankivell BJ, Borrows RJ, Fung CL, et al. The natural history of chronic allograft nephropathy. *N Engl J Med.* 2003;349:2326-2333.
9. Isoniemi H, Taskinen E, Hayry P. Histological chronic allograft damage index accurately predicts chronic renal allograft rejection. *Transplantation.* 1994;58:1195-1198.
10. Colvin RB, Cohen AH, Saiontz C, et al. Evaluation of pathologic criteria for acute renal allograft rejection: Reproducibility, sensitivity, and clinical correlation. *J Am Soc Nephrol.* 1997;8:1930-1941.
11. Solez K, Axelsen RA, Benediktsson H, et al. International standardization of criteria for the histologic diagnosis of renal allograft rejection: The Banff working classification of kidney transplant pathology. *Kidney Int.* 1993;44:411-422.
12. Racusen LC, Solez K, Colvin RB, et al. The Banff 97 working classification of renal allograft pathology. *Kidney Int.* 1999;55:713-723.
13. Zollinger HU, Moppert J, Thiel G, Rohr HP. Morphology and pathogenesis of glomerulopathy in cadaver kidney allografts treated with antilymphocyte globulin. *Curr Top Pathol.* 1973;57:1-48.
14. Gloor JM, Sethi S, Stegall MD, et al. Transplant glomerulopathy: Subclinical incidence and association with alloantibody. *Am J Transplant.* 2007;7:2124-2132.
15. Wavamunno MD, O'Connell PJ, Vitalone M, et al. Transplant glomerulopathy: Ultrastructural abnormalities occur early in longitudinal analysis of protocol biopsies. *Am J Transplant.* 2007;7:2757-2768.
16. Ivanyi B. Transplant capillaropathy and transplant glomerulopathy: Ultrastructural markers of chronic renal allograft rejection. *Nephrol Dial Transplant.* 2003;18:655-660.
17. Regele H, Bohmig GA, Habicht A, et al. Capillary deposition of complement split product C4d in renal allografts is associated with basement membrane injury in peritubular and glomerular capillaries: A contribution of humoral immunity to chronic allograft rejection. *J Am Soc Nephrol.* 2002;13:2371-2380.
18. Seron D. Protocol biopsies as predictors of chronic allograft nephropathy. *Transplant Proc.* 2003;35:2131-2132.
19. Nickerson P, Jeffery J, Gough J, et al. Identification of clinical and histopathologic risk factors for diminished renal function 2 years post-transplant. *J Am Soc Nephrol.* 1998;9:482-487.
20. Nankivell BJ, Fenton-Lee CA, Kuypers DR, et al. Effect of histological damage on long-term kidney transplant outcome. *Transplantation.* 2001; 71:515-523.
21. Nankivell BJ, Kuypers DR, Fenton-Lee CA, et al. Histological injury and renal transplant outcome: The cumulative damage hypothesis. *Transplant Proc.* 2001;33:1149-1150.
22. Chapman JR, O'Connell PJ, Nankivell BJ. Chronic renal allograft dysfunction. *J Am Soc Nephrol.* 2005;16:3015-3026.
23. Nankivell BJ, Chapman JR. Chronic allograft nephropathy: Current concepts and future directions. *Transplantation.* 2006;81: 643-654.
24. Terasaki PI, Gjertson DW, Cecka JM, et al. Significance of the donor age effect on kidney transplants. *Clin Transplant.* 1997;11(Pt 1): 366-372.
25. Shoskes DA, Cecka JM. Deleterious effects of delayed graft function in cadaveric renal transplant recipients independent of acute rejection. *Transplantation.* 1998;66:1697-1701.
26. Kuypers DR, Chapman JR, O'Connell PJ, et al. Predictors of renal transplant histology at three months. *Transplantation.* 1999;67: 1222-1230.
27. Nankivell BJ, Borrows RJ, Fung CL, et al. Natural history, risk factors, and impact of subclinical rejection in kidney transplantation. *Transplantation.* 2004;78:242-249.
28. Schwarz A, Mengel M, Gwinner W, et al. Risk factors for chronic allograft nephropathy after renal transplantation: A protocol biopsy study. *Kidney Int.* 2005;67:341-348.
29. Kim IK, Bedi DS, Denecke C, et al. Impact of innate and adaptive immunity on rejection and tolerance. *Transplantation.* 2008;86: 889-894.
30. Halloran PF, Melk A, Barth C. Rethinking chronic allograft nephropathy: The concept of accelerated senescence. *J Am Soc Nephrol.* 1999;10: 167-181.
31. Melk A, Schmidt BM, Takeuchi O, et al. Expression of p16^{INK4a} and other cell cycle regulator and senescence associated genes in aging human kidney. *Kidney Int.* 2004;65:510-520.
32. Gourishankar S, Hunsicker LG, Jhangri GS, et al. The stability of the glomerular filtration rate after renal transplantation is improving. *J Am Soc Nephrol.* 2003;14:2387-2394.
33. Randhawa PS, Finkelstein S, Scantlebury V, et al. Human polyoma virus–associated interstitial nephritis in the allograft kidney. *Transplantation.* 1999;67:103-109.
34. Benigni A, Bruzzi I, Mister M, et al. Nature and mediators of renal lesions in kidney transplant patients given cyclosporine for more than one year. *Kidney Int.* 1999;55:674-685.
35. Mihatsch MJ, Thiel G, Ryffel B. Histopathology of cyclosporine nephrotoxicity. *Transplant Proc.* 1988;20(Suppl 3):759-771.
36. Waller JR, Nicholson ML. Molecular mechanisms of renal allograft fibrosis. *Br J Surg.* 2001;88:1429-1441.
37. Nankivell BJ, Borrows RJ, Fung CL, et al. Calcineurin inhibitor nephrotoxicity: Longitudinal assessment by protocol histology. *Transplantation.* 2004;78:557-565.
38. Antonovych TT, Sabnis SG, Austin HA, et al. Cyclosporine A–induced arteriolopathy. *Transplant Proc.* 1988;20(Suppl 3):951-958.
39. Austin HA 3rd, Palestine AG, Sabnis SG, et al. Evolution of ciclosporin nephrotoxicity in patients treated for autoimmune uveitis. *Am J Nephrol.* 1989;9:392-402.
40. Briganti EM, Russ GR, McNeil JJ, et al. Risk of renal allograft loss from recurrent glomerulonephritis. *N Engl J Med.* 2002;347:103-109.
41. Cosio FG, Grande JP, Larson TS, et al. Kidney allograft fibrosis and atrophy early after living donor transplantation. *Am J Transplant.* 2005;5:1130-1136.
42. McLaren AJ, Jassem W, Gray DW, et al. Delayed graft function: Risk factors and the relative effects of early function and acute rejection on long-term survival in cadaveric renal transplantation. *Clin Transplant.* 1999;13:266-272.
43. Opelz G, Wujciak T, Ritz E. Association of chronic kidney graft failure with recipient blood pressure. Collaborative Transplant Study. *Kidney Int.* 1998;53:217-222.
44. Matas AJ, Gillingham KJ, Humar A, et al. Immunologic and nonimmunologic factors: Different risks for cadaver and living donor transplantation. *Transplantation.* 2000;69:54-58.
45. Sung RS, Althoen M, Howell TA, et al. Excess risk of renal allograft loss associated with cigarette smoking. *Transplantation.* 2001;71: 1752-1757.
46. McLaren AJ, Fuggle SV, Welsh KI, et al. Chronic allograft failure in human renal transplantation: A multivariate risk factor analysis. *Ann Surg.* 2000;232:98-103.
47. Ishii Y, Sawada T, Kubota K, et al. Injury and progressive loss of peritubular capillaries in the development of chronic allograft nephropathy. *Kidney Int.* 2005;67:321-332.

48. Kasiske BL, Kalil RS, Lee HS, Rao KV. Histopathologic findings associated with a chronic, progressive decline in renal allograft function. *Kidney Int*. 1991;40:514-524.
49. Bellamy CO, Randhawa PS. Arteriolitis in renal transplant biopsies is associated with poor graft outcome. *Histopathology*. 2000;36:488-492.
50. Rush D, Nickerson P, Gough J, et al. Beneficial effects of treatment of early subclinical rejection: A randomized study. *J Am Soc Nephrol.* 1998;9:2129-2134.
51. Rush DN, Jeffery JR, Gough J. Sequential protocol biopsies in renal transplant patients. Clinico-pathological correlations using the Banff schema. *Transplantation*. 1995;59:511-514.
52. Mauiyyedi S, Pelle PD, Saidman S, et al. Chronic humoral rejection: Identification of antibody-mediated chronic renal allograft rejection by C4d deposits in peritubular capillaries. *J Am Soc Nephrol.* 2001;12: 574-582.
53. Regele H, Exner M, Watschinger B, et al. Endothelial C4d deposition is associated with inferior kidney allograft outcome independently of cellular rejection. *Nephrol Dial Transplant*. 2001;16:2058-2066.
54. Patel R, Terasaki PI. Significance of the positive crossmatch test in kidney transplantation. *N Engl J Med*. 1969;280:735-739.
55. Karpinski M, Rush D, Jeffery J, et al. Flow cytometric crossmatching in primary renal transplant recipients with a negative anti–human globulin enhanced cytotoxicity crossmatch. *J Am Soc Nephrol.* 2001;12: 2807-2814.
56. Jeannet M, Pinn VW, Flax MH, et al. Humoral antibodies in renal allotransplantation in man. *N Engl J Med*. 1970;282:111-117.
57. Terasaki PI, Ozawa M. Predicting kidney graft failure by HLA antibodies: A prospective trial. *Am J Transplant*. 2004;4:438-443.
58. Lee PC, Terasaki PI, Takemoto SK, et al. All chronic rejection failures of kidney transplants were preceded by the development of HLA antibodies. *Transplantation*. 2002;74:1192-1194.
59. Colvin RB, Smith RN. Antibody-mediated organ-allograft rejection. *Nat Rev Immunol*. 2005;5:807-817.
60. Suri DL, Tomlanovich SJ, Olson JL, Meyer TW. Transplant glomerulopathy as a cause of late graft loss. *Am J Kidney Dis*. 2000;35:674-680.
61. Nankivell BJ, Chapman JR. The significance of subclinical rejection and the value of protocol biopsies. *Am J Transplant*. 2006;6:2006-2012.
62. Kriz W, Hartmann I, Hosser H, et al. Tracer studies in the rat demonstrate misdirected filtration and peritubular filtrate spreading in nephrons with segmental glomerulosclerosis. *J Am Soc Nephrol.* 2001;12: 496-506.
63. Bonsib SM, Abul-Ezz SR, Ahmad I, et al. Acute rejection–associated tubular basement membrane defects and chronic allograft nephropathy. *Kidney Int*. 2000;58:2206-2214.
64. Yakupoglu U, Baranowska-Daca E, Rosen D, et al. Post-transplant nephrotic syndrome: A comprehensive clinicopathologic study. *Kidney Int*. 2004;65:2360-2370.
65. Kee TY, Chapman JR, O'Connell PJ, et al. Treatment of subclinical rejection diagnosed by protocol biopsy of kidney transplants. *Transplantation*. 2006;82:36-42.
66. Naesens M, Kuypers DR, Sarwal M. Calcineurin inhibitor nephrotoxicity. *Clin J Am Soc Nephrol*. 2009;4:481-508.
67. Schena FP, Pascoe MD, Alberu J, et al. Conversion from calcineurin inhibitors to sirolimus maintenance therapy in renal allograft recipients: 24-month efficacy and safety results from the CONVERT trial. *Transplantation*. 2009;87:233-242.
68. Nankivell BJ, Wavamunno MD, Borrows RJ, et al. Mycophenolate mofetil is associated with altered expression of chronic renal transplant histology. *Am J Transplant*. 2007;7:366-376.
69. Mengel M, Chapman JR, Cosio FG, et al. Protocol biopsies in renal transplantation: Insights into patient management and pathogenesis. *Am J Transplant*. 2007;7:512-517.
70. Ekberg H, Tedesco-Silva H, Demirbas A, et al. Reduced exposure to calcineurin inhibitors in renal transplantation. *N Engl J Med*. 2007;357: 2562-2575.
71. Opelz G, Zeier M, Laux G, et al. No improvement of patient or graft survival in transplant recipients treated with angiotensin-converting enzyme inhibitors or angiotensin II type 1 receptor blockers: A collaborative transplant study report. *J Am Soc Nephrol.* 2006;17:3257-3262.
72. Cross NB, Webster AC, Masson P, et al. Antihypertensives for kidney transplant recipients: Systematic review and meta-analysis of randomized controlled trials. *Transplantation*. 2009;88:7-18.

CHAPTER **104**

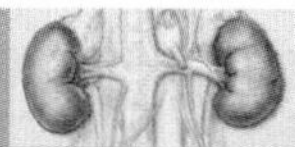

Recurrent Disease in Kidney Transplantation

Steven J. Chadban, Henri Vacher-Coponat

Kidney transplantation is a treatment, not a cure. Although transplantation may restore kidney function to the recipient, it does not necessarily remove the cause of the recipient's original kidney disease. Glomerulonephritis (GN) and diabetes are the two leading causes of end-stage renal disease (ESRD) worldwide and are the primary diseases afflicting the majority of patients considered for kidney transplantation. Both diseases may recur despite the different antigenic make-up of the new kidney and the altered states of recipient immunity and glucose metabolism due to immunosuppression.

The longer that a transplant remains *in situ*, the more likely it is to be affected by recurrence. As graft survival rates have increased during the past 30 years, mostly as a result of more effective antirejection therapies that prevent early graft loss, the incidence of recurrence has grown.[1] Within cohorts reassessed over time, an increase in the prevalence of recurrent disease with longer follow-up is also evident. An analysis of U.S. Renal Allograft Disease Registry data examining GN recurrence demonstrated a prevalence of 2.8% at 2 years, 9.8% at 5 years, and 18.5% at 8 years of follow-up after transplantation, and such patients were twice as likely to experience graft failure compared with those without recurrence.[2]

Recurrence has a powerful impact on transplant survival and one that is increasingly apparent with time after transplantation. In an analysis of data from the Australian registry (ANZDATA) including more than 1500 patients with biopsy-proven GN who received a kidney transplant, biopsy-proven recurrence was found to cause graft loss in 0.5% within 1 year after transplantation, 3.7% within 5 years, and 8.4% within 10 years (Fig. 104.1).[3] This study and several others have found recurrent disease to be the third most common cause of graft failure beyond the first year after transplantation, behind death with a functioning graft and chronic allograft nephropathy (CAN) but substantially ahead of acute rejection (see Fig. 104.1).[3]

This chapter reviews the pathogenesis, clinical features, diagnostic and management issues, and outcome data of relevance to clinicians and their patients in contemplating transplantation as a treatment of kidney failure caused by diseases with a propensity to recur.

De novo GN and new-onset diabetes after transplantation (NODAT) may also affect the transplanted kidney, although both are relatively uncommon. Both conditions may be difficult to distinguish from recurrence and indeed from CAN and are discussed under differential diagnosis. Like recurrent disease, both appear to increase in prevalence with time after transplantation. Given the high incidence of NODAT coupled with general increases in graft survival,[4] it is possible that *de novo* diabetic nephropathy in particular may become a significant clinical problem in the future. However, present data suggest that the major impact of NODAT in the first 10 years after transplantation is an increase in cardiovascular mortality with little impact on death-censored graft failure.[5]

DEFINITIONS

The diagnosis of recurrence almost invariably requires histologic demonstration of the same disease involving both the native and transplanted kidneys. In addition, the diagnosis of recurrence causing graft failure requires a clinical decision that recurrence was the dominant contributor to graft loss (other contributors may be present, such as CAN). A histologic diagnosis of the primary kidney disease is not obtained for all patients with ESRD, and the majority of transplant recipients do not undergo biopsy to look specifically for recurrent disease (which may require immunohistologic and electron microscopic examination of the biopsy specimen).[1] Coupled with the tendency of clinicians to make a clinical diagnosis of CAN and thereby to avoid biopsy in patients with declining graft function and proteinuria, the true incidence of disease recurrence is not known and is almost certainly underestimated by existing literature.

Additional factors cloud the available evidence. Many reports of disease recurrence are retrospective, single-center studies. Recall bias and incomplete documentation, changes in practice over time, and peculiarities of local patient populations and local practices may limit relevance to other populations. The most definitive reports have come from analyses of the large registry databases of Europe, the United States, and Australia. Registries capture data on large numbers of patients but are subject to bias. Factors that may introduce bias include unit participation rates; quantity and type of data collected; accuracy, uniformity, and consistency of reporting by units; and reliability of data entry. How recurrence is defined and diagnosed and which outcomes are measured are crucial. For example, IgA nephropathy (IgAN) recurred in 58% of cases in one series in which all recipients underwent biopsy[5] but in approximately 25% of cases in which biopsy was performed only when clinically indicated. When graft loss due to IgAN recurrence is the outcome measure, the risk decreases to approximately 10% at 10 years of follow-up.[3] Thus, definition of recurrence, outcome measures, study design, and source of data all need to be considered in assessing the published literature.

RECURRENT GLOMERULONEPHRITIS

Virtually all recognized forms of GN may recur after transplantation; however, the rate and consequences of recurrence vary

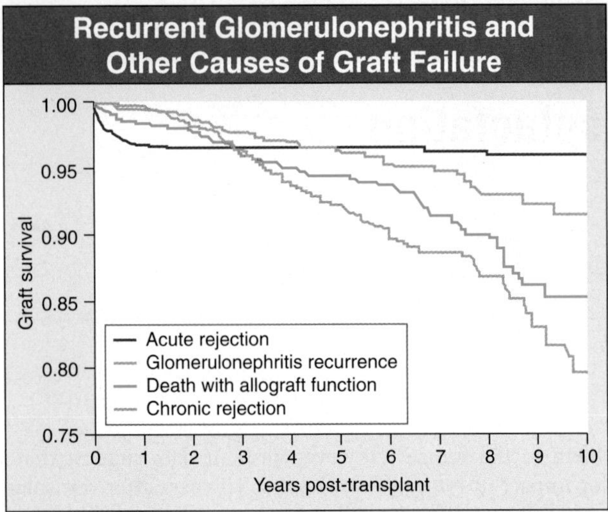

Figure 104.1 Recurrent glomerulonephritis and other causes of graft failure. Kaplan-Meier analysis of the relative contributions of acute rejection, glomerulonephritis recurrence, death, and chronic allograft nephropathy to graft loss during the first 10 years after transplantation among patients who underwent transplantation because of end-stage renal disease caused by glomerulonephritis. *(Modified with permission from reference 3.)*

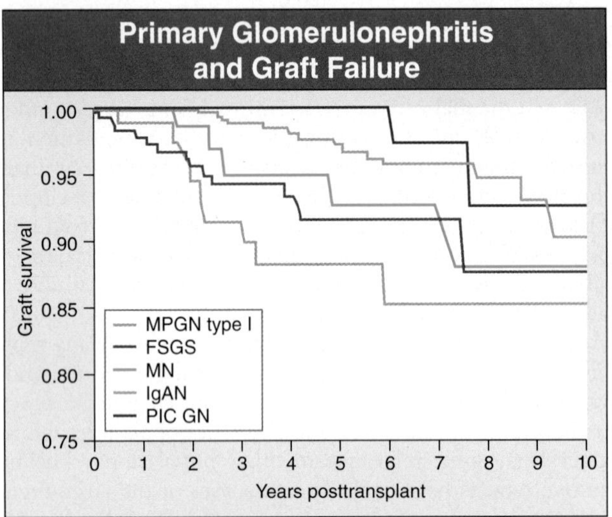

Figure 104.2 Primary glomerulonephritis and graft failure. Kaplan-Meier analysis of freedom from graft loss caused by recurrent glomerulonephritis during the first 10 years after kidney transplantation among patients with a primary diagnosis of glomerulonephritis. FSGS, focal and segmental glomerulosclerosis; IgAN, IgA nephropathy; MN, membranous nephropathy; MPGN, membranoproliferative glomerulonephritis; PIC GN, pauci-immune crescentic glomerulonephritis. *(Modified with permission from reference 3.)*

enormously. For example, anti–glomerular basement membrane (GBM) disease (Goodpasture's disease) recurs only rarely, but when it does, it is likely to cause rapid graft loss. In contrast, dense deposit disease (membranoproliferative GN type II, dense deposit disease) recurs in more than 80% of cases; however, the disease tends to be very slowly progressive, and graft survival beyond 10 years is typical. Numerically, recurrence of focal and segmental glomerulosclerosis (FSGS), IgAN, and membranous nephropathy (MN) are the most frequently encountered clinical problems (Fig. 104.2).

Factors in addition to the underlying type of GN may influence the risk of recurrence. Time of follow-up is clearly important and may be related to the duration of exposure of the graft to the nephritogenic factors responsible for GN.[1] In general, grafts that are lost early because of rejection are exposed relatively briefly and rarely develop recurrence. In contrast, those grafts that survive long term are exposed longer to nephritogenic factors and are more likely to develop recurrent GN. Consistent with this concept, recipients of HLA-identical transplants rarely suffer rejection, enjoy prolonged graft survival, but have a high rate of recurrent GN.[6] In one report of HLA-identical recipients, recurrent GN was present in 36% to 42% of those in whom biopsy was performed and resulted in 24% of graft losses, being the second most frequent cause of graft loss after death in this group.[6] Patients suffering first graft loss from recurrent GN are also at higher risk of recurrence and of graft loss due to recurrence in a subsequent graft.

The impact of choice of immunosuppressive agents may be significant; however, data in this area are sparse. Given that immune mechanisms contribute to the pathogenesis of most types of GN and that immunosuppression is effective in the treatment of several types, it is logical that immunosuppression in general probably decreases the incidence and severity of recurrence after transplantation. U.S. registry data (U.S. Renal Data System) on the impact of individual immunosuppressive agents on the incidence of recurrence failed to demonstrate superiority of any one agent over others.[7] Induction therapy may be one exception to this finding as a small, retrospective study found rabbit antithymocyte globulin to be associated with a lower risk of IgAN recurrence compared with either anti-CD25 antibodies or no induction.[8] *Post hoc* analyses of corticosteroid withdrawal trials suggest that this strategy does not lead to increased rates of recurrence.[9] Inclusion or addition of cyclophosphamide has been effective in the management of recurrent vasculitis affecting the graft.[10] Of major interest and concern is the tendency for patients maintained on (or particularly switched to) sirolimus to develop proteinuria and renal dysfunction. This effect appears to be more common among those with a primary diagnosis of GN, suggesting that sirolimus may either facilitate recurrence or, more likely, accelerate its impact on the graft.[11] Effects of individual agents are likely to be disease specific, and much needs to be learned in this area.

Strategies to reduce the risk of recurrence have been reported. Bilateral native nephrectomy as a means of eliminating persistent antigenic stimulation appears unhelpful; indeed, nephrectomized patients experienced a higher incidence of recurrence compared with those with native kidneys left *in situ* in one large single-center, retrospective study.[12] Induction of disease remission before transplantation and prolonged time on dialysis before transplantation, both aimed at permitting disease "burnout," do not appear to be effective except in the case of anti-GBM disease (Goodpasture's disease), in which a delay in transplantation until the patient has been serologically negative for at least 6 months virtually eliminates the risk of recurrence.[3] Avoidance of living related donation has been debated for years but overall appears not to have any impact on risk of recurrence.[13]

Clinical Features and Differential Diagnosis

As is the case with GN in native kidneys, proteinuria, hematuria, and deterioration in kidney function are the cardinal manifestations of recurrent GN. The pattern of renal and extrarenal manifestations is frequently similar to that of the native disease, except

Differential Diagnosis of Recurrent Glomerulonephritis

Diagnosis	Frequency and Timing	Clinical Features	Lab Features	Biopsy Features	Management
Recurrent glomerulonephritis	Common; variable timing, days to years	Proteinuria, hematuria, renal impairment, hypertension	Similar to primary glomerulonephritis; serology may be negative	Same as primary glomerulonephritis[4,5]	Disease specific
De novo glomerulonephritis	Uncommon; variable timing but typically later than recurrence	Proteinuria, hematuria, renal impairment	Type specific	Type specific[4,5,8]	Antiprogression strategies (see Chapter 69)
Chronic allograft nephropathy	Very common; increasing incidence with time	Hypertension, proteinuria, renal impairment Calcineurin inhibitor exposure		Tubulointerstitial fibrosis, arteriolar hyalinosis, transplant glomerulopathy	Minimize calcineurin inhibitor and antiprogression strategies (see Chapter 69)
Graft pyelonephritis	Uncommon Typically early after transplantation	Fever, pyuria, renal impairment	Positive blood or urine cultures	Neutrophil infiltration	Antibiotics
BK nephropathy	Uncommon; typically 1–5 yr after transplantation	Renal impairment, decoy cells in urine	Serum BK PCR positive	Tubulitis with tubular cell atypia and inclusions, normal glomeruli	Minimize immunosuppression and ? antiviral drugs
Acute rejection	Common; early	Renal impairment, oliguria	Nonspecific	Tubulitis ± vasculitis[15]	Increase immunosuppression
Renal tumor/PTLD	Uncommon, rare; early or late	Renal impairment, renal mass	Anemia, EBV positive	Atypical cells, mitoses, monoclonality	Minimize immunosuppression, ? chemotherapy

Figure 104.3 Differential diagnosis of recurrent glomerulonephritis. EBV, Epstein-Barr virus; PCR, polymerase chain reaction; PTLD, post-transplantation lymphoproliferative disease.

that in the opinion of the authors, the rate of progression may in general be slower. Extrarenal features of the primary condition may recur, such as thrombocytopenia and hemolysis in hemolytic-uremic syndrome and extrarenal vasculitis in recurrent Wegener's granulomatosis. Serology may be helpful in some cases, such as anti-GBM antibody detection in Goodpasture's disease, but it may be inconsistent in others, such as recurrent lupus nephritis.

The differential diagnosis of recurrent GN is clinically important as management may vary according to the diagnosis (Fig. 104.3). CAN and diabetic nephropathy, recurrent or *de novo*, may both present with progressive graft dysfunction, proteinuria, and hypertension and may therefore be clinically indistinguishable from recurrence. *De novo* GN should also be considered. Viral diseases of the kidney, particularly BK nephropathy, are an important alternative to consider as a reduction in immunosuppression and specific antiviral therapy may provide benefit. The need to exclude obstructive uropathy and tumors involving the graft warrants an ultrasound scan. Finally, recurrence may coexist with CAN or calcineurin inhibitor toxicity. Indeed, every condition that can lead to chronic graft dysfunction should be considered in the differential diagnosis of recurrence (see Fig. 104.3 and Chapter 103).

Histologic evidence of recurrence is required in all cases. Biopsy can provide the diagnosis, exclude alternative diagnoses that may require different approaches to treatment, and provide important prognostic information pertinent to the affected graft and also relevant to any future consideration of retransplantation. Full evaluation of the biopsy specimen by light microscopy, immunohistology, and electron microscopy is desirable and in many cases essential to confirm recurrence.[14] Light microscopy and immunohistology are necessary to differentiate recurrent from *de novo* GN, rejection, and calcineurin inhibitor toxicity. The presence of tubulitis should suggest acute rejection. CAN may produce chronic interstitial inflammation and transplant glomerulopathy, which may be indistinguishable from MPGN by light microscopy (Fig. 104.4; see also Chapter 103). The use of immunohistology to define the immunoglobulin and complement component content of immune deposits and electron microscopy to establish the structure of basement membrane and location of deposits may clarify the diagnosis.[14] Histologic appearances are typically no different from the patterns of GN in native kidneys and are illustrated in the relevant chapters of Section IV, Glomerular Disease. The risk of recurrence in common patterns of renal disease is summarized in Figure 104.5.

RECURRENCE OF SPECIFIC GLOMERULAR DISEASES

IgA Nephropathy and Henoch-Schönlein Purpura

IgAN is the most common form of GN leading to ESRD, and these patients are frequently transplant recipients. Histologic recurrence is frequent and increases with time; one study in which all recipients were subjected to protocol biopsy found recurrence in 58%.[15] Recurrence is difficult to predict. Patient characteristics, pretransplantation course, serum IgA glycosylation, and angiotensin-converting enzyme genotype have been found to have no predictive value.[1,15,16] Choice of immunosuppression after transplantation and post-transplantation course appear to have no impact,[7] although observational data suggest that induction with antithymocyte globulin may afford relative protection.[8] Living related donor transplantation has been associated with an increased risk of recurrence and graft loss in some

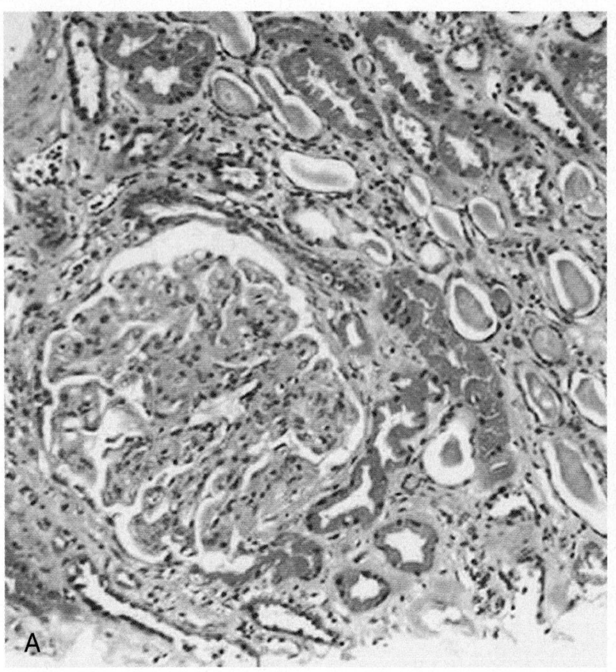

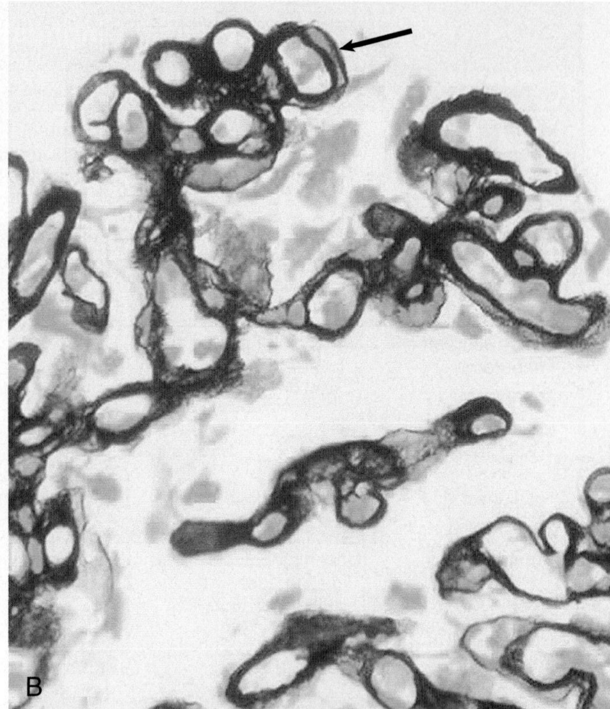

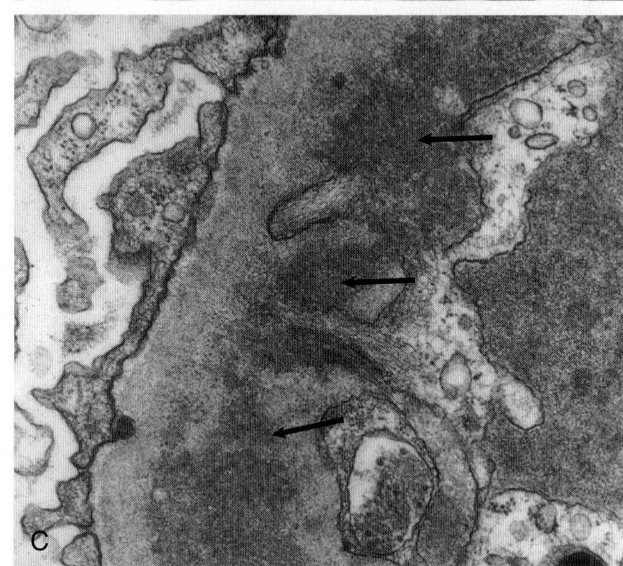

Figure 104.4 Transplant glomerulopathy and membranoproliferative glomerulonephritis (MPGN). Transplant biopsy specimen from a patient with end-stage renal disease due to biopsy-proven idiopathic MPGN type I who received a kidney transplant and had a progressive reduction in glomerular filtration rate with proteinuria of 1.5 g/day and hypertension. **A,** Light microscopy. Glomerular hypercellularity and lobulation on a background of chronic interstitial inflammation and fibrosis, with protein casts within dilated tubules. (Hematoxylin and eosin; magnification ×100.) **B,** Subendothelial deposits and basement membrane reduplication *(arrow)*. (Methenamine silver; magnification ×400.) **C,** Electron microscopy showing subendothelial electron-dense deposits (magnification ×7500) *(arrows)*. There were also prominent C3 deposits on immunofluorescence (not shown). Light microscopy was therefore suggestive of recurrent MPGN but was also consistent with associated transplant glomerulopathy. Immunofluorescence and electron microscopy (subendothelial deposits) confirmed recurrence of MPGN (compare Chapter 103, Figs. 103.3 to 103.5). *(**A** and **B** Courtesy Dr. Paul McKenzie, Royal Prince Alfred Hospital, Sydney, Australia)*

series but not in others[3] and does not justify the avoidance of living related donor transplantation in patients with IgAN.

The clinical expression of disease is variable and time dependent. Graft loss within the first 3 years after transplantation is uncommon (see Fig. 104.2), although it can be seen, particularly when there is extensive crescentic GN before transplantation or after previous graft loss due to recurrence.[16] The longer term outlook is not benign as progressive graft loss over time has been documented by all major studies. In one registry study that included 587 subjects with biopsy-proven IgAN, the risk of graft loss due to IgAN recurrence was approximately 10% within 10 years after transplantation.[3]

Recurrence of Henoch-Schönlein purpura (HSP) nephritis is less well characterized but appears to be similar to IgAN in all respects. The largest report that pooled patients from Belgium and Japan found recurrence in 35% and graft loss in 11% at 5 years of follow-up.[17]

Treatment of recurrent IgAN and HSP has not been systematically evaluated, and specific therapies, such as corticosteroids, mycophenolate mofetil (MMF), fish oil, and antiplatelet agents, cannot be recommended. The use of nonspecific measures to prolong kidney survival, such as tight blood pressure control, renin-angiotensin system (RAS) blockade, and avoidance of nephrotoxins, is appropriate.

Membranous Nephropathy

Data on recurrent MN are clouded by two key issues: the small number of subjects in reported series and the frequency of *de novo* MN after transplantation. *De novo* MN has been reported

Recurrent Diseases in Renal Transplants and Effects on Graft Survival

Disease	Clinical Recurrence Rate (%)	Graft Loss in Recurrent Disease (%)
Primary focal segmental glomerulosclerosis	20–50 (children), 10–15 (adults)	40–50
Membranoproliferative glomerulonephritis		
Type I	20–30	30–40
Type II	80	20, often late
Hemolytic-uremic syndrome (HUS)		
Classical D+ HUS	0–13	Uncommon
Atypical D− HUS	30–50	55–100
Familial HUS	57	Approaching 100
IgA nephropathy	30–40, increases with longer duration of follow-up (30%–60% histologic recurrence rate)	16–33
Henoch-Schönlein purpura	Rare (despite 50% histologic recurrence rate)	Rare
Membranous nephropathy	10–29 (histologic recurrence may be more common)	Up to 50
Systemic vasculitis, including Wegener's granulomatosis and microscopic polyangiitis	10–20	20–50
Anti-GBM disease (Goodpasture's disease)	<5	50
Systemic lupus erythematosus	1–30	Rare
Amyloidosis	25	10–20

Figure 104.5 Recurrent diseases in renal transplants and effects on graft survival.

in 2% to 15% of transplant recipients and tends to present more insidiously and later than recurrent MN.[18]

The largest series (pooled from centers in Belgium and France) reported a recurrence rate of 29% in 30 patients at 3 years after transplantation[18]; among those affected, graft loss was 38% at 5 years and 52% at 10 years of follow up. Recurrence is a significant clinical event causing proteinuria, nephrotic syndrome, and graft loss in 12% of recipients within 10 years after transplantation.[3] Clinical factors including pretransplantation disease course, duration of dialysis, HLA genotype, graft source, and immunosuppression are not predictive of risk. However, those with a previous graft loss due to recurrence are at high risk if they are retransplanted.[19]

Management of recurrent MN is based on anecdotal reports and extrapolation of data on the management of native kidney MN. Spontaneous remissions appear to be less common. The cumulative exposure to immunosuppressive therapy should be considered as these patients may be at increased risk of lymphoma. Live donor transplantation appears warranted for first grafts but, in the opinion of the authors, should probably be avoided for second grafts if the first was lost early because of recurrence.

Focal Segmental Glomerulosclerosis

Patients with renal failure due to FSGS incur a risk of recurrence of 20% to 30% for first transplants.[20,21] FSGS is a heterogeneous group of conditions. Those with familial or sporadic forms associated with mutation of slit diaphragm proteins such as podocin, those with FSGS secondary to vascular disease, and those with a very slow rate of progression are at substantially lower risk; whereas patients with an aggressive initial course (heavy proteinuria and renal failure within 3 years of onset), patients who are younger than 15 years, and patients with mesangial hypercellularity on biopsy or with recurrence in a previous graft are at greatest risk.[20,21] The rate of recurrence is more than 75% in subsequent grafts when the first graft was lost as a result of recurrence.[22] Living related donor transplantation has been implicated as a risk factor for recurrence; however, a major analysis of U.S. registry data (U.S. Renal Data System) refutes this notion.[13]

Recurrence occurs early, typically within the first month after transplantation, and is manifested initially by heavy proteinuria, followed by hypertension and graft dysfunction. Patients with recurrent disease appear more susceptible to acute rejection and acute kidney injury[23] as well as graft loss. Recurrence has been associated with early graft loss in up to 40% to 50% of cases[21]; however, the adoption of plasma exchange appears to have delayed graft loss in many cases and decreased the incidence of overall graft failure (see Fig. 104.2).[3]

A circulating 50-kd plasma protein that is bound to immunoglobulin appears to cause recurrent FSGS. The protein remains unidentified but is capable of inducing proteinuria when it is injected into rat kidneys.[24,25] Attempts to use the presence of the circulating "permeability factor" as a guide to the risk of recurrence have not produced a clinically useful test. Plasma exchange or immunoadsorption effectively removes the permeability factor because it is bound to immunoglobulin and as a result provides an effective therapy for many patients who develop recurrent FSGS.[24,25] Although it has not been subjected to a randomized, controlled, prospective trial, several series have reported disease remission in the majority of patients who receive treatment within 2 weeks of recurrence.[21,26] Potential for positive publication bias and the absence of randomized clinical trial evidence make prognostic information speculative; however, in the authors' assessment, response rates appear likely to exceed 50% when therapy is commenced within 2 weeks of the onset of clinically recurrent FSGS, with lower response rates anticipated when therapy is delayed. Given that graft survival appears to be significantly prolonged in cases that respond to therapy, a course of therapy is warranted in all cases unless clear

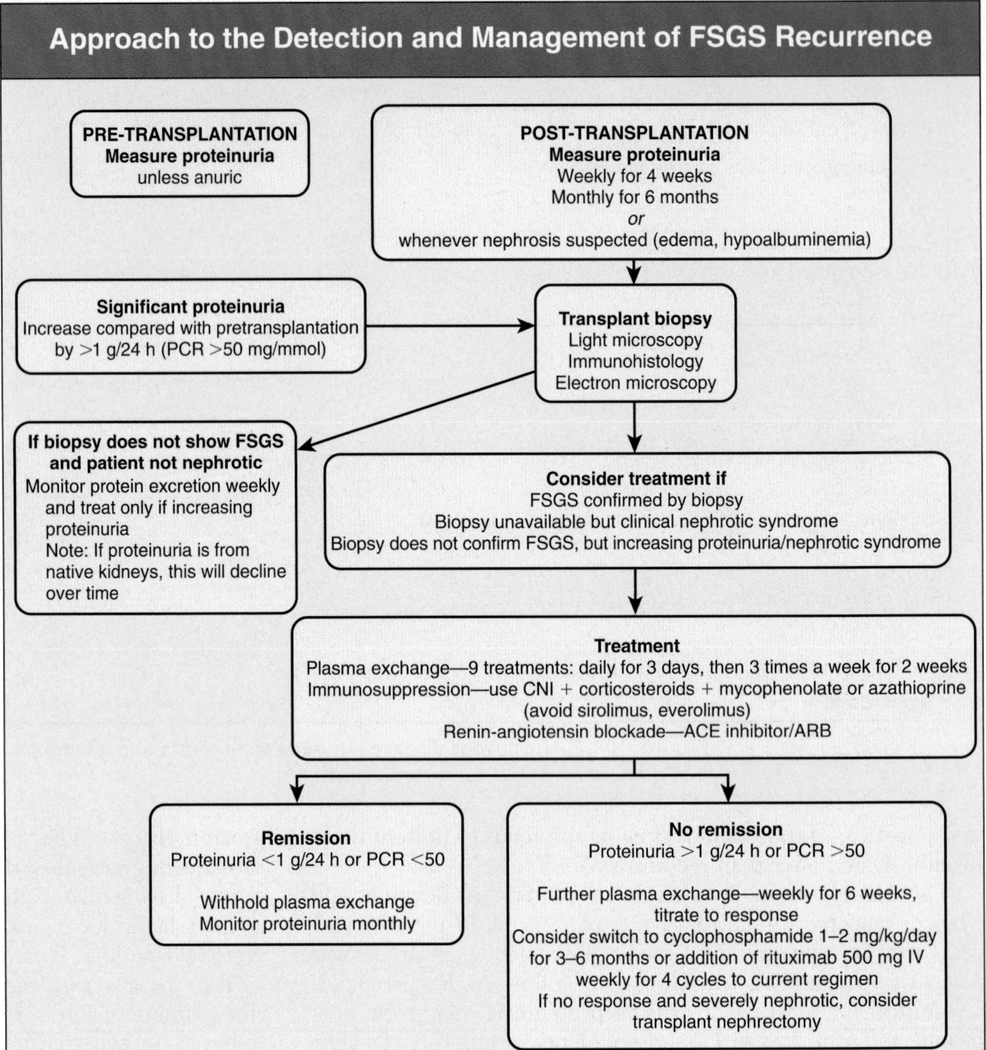

Figure 104.6 Approach to the detection and management of focal and segmental glomerulosclerosis (FSGS) recurrence. ACE, angiotensin-converting enzyme; ACR, albumin/creatinine ratio; ARB, angiotensin receptor blocker; CNI, calcineurin inhibitor. Authors' recommendation based on Davenport.[27]

contraindications to plasma exchange exist (see Chapter 95). A minority of patients with an incomplete response or relapse after cessation of initial therapy will require repeated or long-term plasma exchange[27] or concurrent treatment with secondary agents, such as rituximab or cyclophosphamide.[26,28] Pretransplantation plasma exchange has not been shown to be of benefit in the prevention of recurrence in the graft. The role of concomitant immunosuppressive therapy, in addition to that required to prevent acute rejection, is unclear, although in the opinion of the authors, it should be considered in cases in which stable remission induction is not achieved by plasma exchange alone. See Figure 104.6 for an approach to the management of recurrent FSGS.

Minimal change disease is a far less frequent cause of ESRD. Recurrence of disease after transplantation has been reported; however, it is difficult to be sure that the underlying disease was not FSGS.

Membranoproliferative Glomerulonephritis

Recurrent MPGN bears major clinical and histologic similarities to the subgroup of patients with CAN who have transplant glomerulopathy, and comprehensive assessment of transplant biopsy specimens (see Fig. 104.4 and compare with Figs. 103.3 to 103.5) as well as accurate diagnosis of the native kidney disease is crucial in making this distinction (see Fig. 104.3). MPGN is suggested by the presence of crescents on light microscopy, stronger staining for C3, and weaker staining for IgM on immunohistology and by the presence of subendothelial or intramembranous dense deposits on electron microscopy.[14] This distinction has important clinical implications, particularly as a recurrence carries a higher risk of subsequent recurrence should retransplantation be considered.

Membranoproliferative Glomerulonephritis Type I

This disorder appears to be mediated by glomerular deposition of immune complexes, triggered by exposure to endogenous or exogenous (e.g., hepatitis C virus [HCV]) antigens. As the antigens are not necessarily removed by transplantation, recurrence of disease is possible and is seen in 20% to 33% of graft recipients.[29] Graft loss has been reported in up to 40% of those with recurrence, and the risk of recurrence in subsequent grafts approaches 80%.[30] Significant geographic diversity in the risk of recurrence is evident, largely linked to the prevalence of HCV; much higher rates of graft loss due to recurrence are reported in areas where the majority of patients with MPGN are HCV positive, such as Spain,[29,31] compared with low HCV prevalence areas, such as Australia.[3] Patients receiving HLA-identical grafts appear to be at increased risk of recurrence in some series[29] but not in others.[3]

No form of treatment is proven, and the underlying cause of recurrent MPGN should be considered in each case. Prevention may be effective in HCV-associated MPGN, as interferon-based therapy appears to be effective for virus elimination if it is undertaken while the patient is on maintenance dialysis, and this provides substantial protection from HCV viremia and MPGN recurrence after subsequent transplantation.[31] By contrast, the use of interferon after transplantation may precipitate acute rejection and should be avoided. Other antivirals, such as ribavirin, are unlikely to be successful as monotherapy. Other forms of MPGN type I have been treated with immunosuppression or plasma exchange with success in single cases.

Dense Deposit Disease (Membranoproliferative Glomerulonephritis Type II)

This disease has been found to recur in 50% to 80% of grafts, typically presenting with proteinuria, hematuria, and slowly progressive loss of kidney function.[32] The disease course tends to be slow, and although graft loss due to recurrence is ultimately seen in approximately 20% of cases, this generally occurs beyond the first 10 years after transplantation.[3,32] Graft loss has been associated with male gender, crescents on biopsy, and heavy proteinuria.[32] No effective therapy is known, and although plasma exchange and immunosuppression have been described, these are not warranted in the opinion of the authors, and control of blood pressure and proteinuria with renin-angiotensin blockade is the preferred therapy. Given the emerging role of factor H mutations in dense deposit disease (see Chapter 21), plasma infusion or administration of recombinant factor H may prove useful in the future.

Membranoproliferative Glomerulonephritis Type III

Recurrence of this rare disease has been reported, resulting in graft loss in the longer term.[33]

Congenital Nephrotic Syndrome

Congenital nephrotic syndrome of the Finnish type has, in small case series, been reported to recur after transplantation and to cause graft loss; however, it is likely that the mechanism of kidney damage is quite different between primary and recurrent disease. In cases in which the primary disorder is caused by a mutation of the *NPHS1* gene that results in complete absence of nephrin, transplantation causes *de novo* exposure to nephrin in the transplanted kidney. Neoantigen exposure causes antibody development and deposition that damages the slit diaphragm and produces a type of MN with podocyte fusion on electron microscopy and a clinical picture of heavy proteinuria and ultimately graft failure.[34] Cyclophosphamide-based rescue therapy may be successful.[35]

ANCA-Associated Pauci-immune Vasculitis

A pooled analysis of all reported case series examining recurrence of antineutrophil cytoplasmic antibody (ANCA)–associated vasculitis, incorporating 127 patients, has largely clarified the behavior of this group of disorders after transplantation.[34] Disease recurrence was detected in 17% of cases after 4 to 89 months of follow-up, with renal involvement demonstrated in approximately 60% of these recurrences and graft losses reported in a minority of these. Clinical parameters were not useful in predicting those patients likely to suffer a relapse after transplantation. Pretransplantation disease course, duration of dialysis, ANCA titers at time of transplantation and during follow-up, c-ANCA or p-ANCA specificity, disease subtype (Wegener's granulomatosis, microscopic polyangiitis, or renal-limited vasculitis), and donor source had no significant impact on recurrence rate.[34]

The prevention and management of relapse have not been prospectively examined. In most reports, patients did not receive a transplant until they were in clinical remission; however, successful transplantation in the face of persisting ANCA positivity is well recognized. In the absence of evidence, the authors recommend that clinical remission be maintained for at least 6 months before transplantation to reduce the risk of recurrence and also to avoid the risks associated with transplantation in a debilitated patient, especially if ESRD has occurred soon after presentation with systemic vasculitis. Patients with renal relapses have generally been managed with cyclophosphamide-based regimens as used for renal vasculitis in native kidneys, reported to be successful in inducing a remission in 11 of 16 (69%) cases.[34] The negative impact of using cyclophosphamide to treat relapse has not been reported, but it would clearly include a significant increase in the risk of bladder cancer.

Kidney transplantation for ANCA-associated vasculitis is associated with a reduction in the frequency of disease relapse by approximately 50% compared with patients remaining on dialysis, and patient and graft survival after transplantation is similar to that of other transplant recipients.[34]

Goodpasture's Disease

Histologic recurrence of anti-GBM disease (Goodpasture's disease) is seen in 50% of patients who receive a transplant while circulating anti-GBM antibodies persist but rarely when patients undergo transplantation 6 months or more after the disappearance of anti-GBM antibodies. With delayed transplantation, the rate of clinical recurrence is very low, and since the implementation of this practice in Australia, no grafts were lost after transplantation in 47 cases observed for up to 10 years.[3] Rare episodes of recurrence should be treated as for native kidney disease with corticosteroids, cyclophosphamide, and aggressive plasma exchange (see Chapter 23).

Recurrent anti-GBM disease is distinct from *de novo* anti-GBM disease, which is seen in up to 15% of transplant recipients with Alport's syndrome who develop anti-GBM antibodies in response to neoantigen exposure (α chain of type IV collagen) through the transplant.[36] This is also discussed further in Chapter 23.

Lupus Nephritis

The reported recurrence rate of lupus nephritis (LN) has varied from 1% to 30%.[37,38] Recurrence has been reported early (days) and late (years) after transplantation, with a mean time to recurrence of 3.1 years in the largest series reported.[39] The clinical and histologic pattern of recurrence is variable, but it is typically more benign in histology and clinical expression than the patient's original disease. Whereas the majority of patients with ESRD caused by lupus have had diffuse proliferative (class III or class IV) disease, mesangial proliferative (class II) disease is the most commonly described lesion after transplantation, followed by class III and membranous (class V).[40] Duration of dialysis before transplantation and serologic activity do not predict recurrence, and antinuclear antibody titer and complement levels are unreliable markers of disease recurrence. There is no reliable relationship between recurrence of nephritis and activity of extrarenal lupus after transplantation.

The long-term outcome for lupus patients after transplantation is controversial but appears similar to that of the general post-transplantation population.[37] Whereas recurrence is an uncommon cause of graft loss within the first 10 years after transplantation, with no cases of graft loss reported from 86 recipients in one registry analysis,[3] late graft losses do occur. It is clear that lupus patients, particularly those with a lupus anticoagulant, are at increased risk of thrombotic events after transplantation, including graft thrombosis.[37]

Management of recurrent LN has not been systematically studied; however, the use of corticosteroids, cyclophosphamide, and plasma exchange has been reported, with variable results.[40] The impact of MMF, which is effective in management of diffuse proliferative LN in native kidneys, remains to be proven. Anticoagulation during the perioperative and early post-transplantation phases should be considered for those with a history of thrombosis or lupus anticoagulant positivity. Successful retransplantation has been reported after graft loss due to recurrence.[39]

Thrombotic Microangiopathy and Hemolytic-Uremic Syndrome

The diagnosis of recurrent thrombotic microangiopathy (TMA) or hemolytic-uremic syndrome (HUS) is complicated by the fact that *de novo* HUS is seen in 1% to 5% of kidney transplant recipients, most commonly in association with the use of calcineurin inhibitors (both tacrolimus and cyclosporine carry a similar risk), sirolimus, and OKT3 or with acute vascular rejection. Drug-induced *de novo* HUS is generally observed within 14 days of drug commencement.[41] A meta-analysis that examined 10 reports covering 159 grafts in 127 patients reported recurrence in 28% of cases, and this was strongly associated with a poor outcome; 1-year graft survival was 33% for those with recurrence versus 77% for those free from recurrence ($P <$ .001).[42] Recurrence risk is clearly associated with the type of HUS/TMA. Typical childhood postdiarrheal (D^+) HUS seldom recurs, whereas recurrence of atypical (D^-) HUS is frequent and, particularly in hereditary forms, may be associated with mutation of complement components or complement regulatory factors in up to 80% of cases. In a French pediatric series, atypical (D^-) HUS recurrence was observed in more 50% of cases, and of these, graft loss was seen in 80%.[41] Mutations in complement regulatory proteins I and H are associated with a risk of recurrence of approximately 80%, whereas HUS associated with membrane cofactor protein mutations recurs in only 20%. HUS associated with mutations of factors B and C3 has also been reported to recur after transplantation. Given the variation in risk of recurrence associated with mutations of different complement components, genotypic evaluation before transplantation is advisable in all cases of ESRD caused by atypical (D^-) HUS.[43] Recurrence is also associated with an older age at onset, rapid progression of the original disease, earlier transplantation, living related transplantation, and use of calcineurin inhibitors.[42] Recurrence is generally within the first 6 months after transplantation; however, late recurrences have been reported.[42] The clinical presentation may be gradual or abrupt, with thrombocytopenia, hemolysis, and progressive renal dysfunction.

Whereas *de novo* disease may respond to withdrawal of the inciting agent, management of recurrent disease is uncertain. The authors recommend withdrawal of any potential causative agent, such as calcineurin inhibitors, and if this is not effective after 48 hours, a trial of plasma exchange should be initiated with three half-plasma volume exchanges performed on 3 consecutive days using fresh frozen plasma for replacement. As an increased incidence of acute rejection has been reported in patients with recurrence,[44] inadequate immunosuppression after calcineurin inhibitor withdrawal should be avoided by a temporary increase in the dose of corticosteroids or mycophenolate. In cases of life-threatening thrombocytopenia or hemolysis, hematologic stability may be restored by transplant nephrectomy. When an underlying genetic complement regulatory protein defect is known, specific therapies are emerging, such as combined liver-kidney transplantation for factor H deficiency (see Chapter 28).[45] The prognosis of recurrent disease is poor. More than 50% of grafts are lost within the first year, and graft survival beyond 5 years is uncommon.[42] There is no evidence that calcineurin inhibitor avoidance is useful in preventing recurrence.

Scleroderma

An analysis of 86 patients reported to the United Network for Organ Sharing registry after receiving a kidney transplant for scleroderma demonstrated graft survival of 62% at 1 year and 47% at 5 years after transplantation; 24% of recipients died during the 10-year observation period.[46] The recurrence rate could not be accurately determined; however, recurrence was responsible for graft loss in 21% of cases in which the cause was identified, which is consistent with previously accepted recurrence rates. Risk factors for recurrence were not identified, and cyclosporine use did not appear to affect the recurrence rate.[46] The effect of transplantation on the extrarenal manifestations of scleroderma has not been well documented. The management of scleroderma after transplantation is unstudied; however, the use of RAS blockade after transplantation to treat hypertension would seem appropriate. Overall, the post-transplantation course of scleroderma appears to be similar to that of LN,[46] and renal transplantation appears to be an appropriate therapy for those with ESRD.

AMYLOID, LIGHT-CHAIN DISEASE, AND FIBRILLARY AND IMMUNOTACTOID GLOMERULOPATHIES

Amyloidosis

The risk and impact of recurrence for patients who undergo transplantation because of systemic amyloidosis are clearly dependent on its cause. Management of AL amyloid is primarily directed to treatment of the underlying plasma cell dyscrasia, most commonly by high-dose chemotherapy and bone marrow transplantation. AL amyloidosis will recur after transplantation if the malignant disease is not fully controlled but may be susceptible to further chemotherapy.

Secondary (AA) amyloidosis is typically a more insidious disease; renal failure is a relatively frequent complication, and renal transplantation is frequently effective. The risk of recurrence of AA amyloid depends on the ability to eradicate the underlying cause of chronic inflammation. Recurrence is unlikely in AA amyloid due to chronic infection if the infection can be eradicated before transplantation, whereas conditions such as rheumatoid arthritis may persist after transplantation and lead to recurrent amyloid in the graft. Patients with AA amyloid associated with familial Mediterranean fever, which can be managed after transplantation with colchicine, have recurrence in less than

5% of cases at 10 years after transplantation.[47] A Norwegian series of 62 transplants in patients with AA amyloid, mostly secondary to rheumatic diseases, demonstrated a recurrence rate of 10% at an average of 5 years of follow-up, causing graft loss in two cases only. Overall, patient and graft survival rates were 65% and 62%, respectively, at 5 years, with most losses due to infection.[48]

Light-Chain Nephropathy

Patients with light-chain nephropathy have occasionally received transplants, and recurrence is common; one case series reported recurrence in five of seven patients at a range of 2 to 45 months after transplantation. Those with recurrence developed proteinuria, hypertension, and progressive graft dysfunction. One of seven has enjoyed long-term graft function, and one died soon after transplantation because of myeloma.[49] Kidney transplantation is therefore generally inadvisable for patients with this disease, unless it is performed in conjunction with bone marrow transplantation as a means of curing the underlying disease.

Fibrillary and Immunotactoid Glomerulopathies

Fibrillary and immunotactoid glomerulopathies are known to recur in approximately 50% of those undergoing transplantation for these diseases. Although early graft loss due to recurrence has been reported, decline in graft function is most commonly slow and does not appear to have an impact on 5-year graft survival rates.[50]

RECURRENCE OF METABOLIC DISEASES AFFECTING THE KIDNEY TRANSPLANT

Diabetes Mellitus

Diabetes mellitus is the most common cause of ESRD in most parts of the world; however, these patients undergo transplantation less commonly than those with GN because of a higher prevalence and severity of cardiovascular comorbidity. Recurrence of diabetic nephropathy is well recognized both histologically and clinically, affecting at least 25% of recipients at an average follow-up of 6 years, with some cases diagnosed within 3 years of transplantation.[51] Histologic and clinical features are similar to those of native kidney diabetic nephropathy. The risk of graft loss due to recurrence has not been well documented but appears to be significantly less than with GN, probably because of the competing risk of death due to cardiovascular disease. New-onset diabetes after transplantation is also common and has been reported to cause nephropathy in the graft in a similar proportion of cases, also commonly manifested within 5 years of transplantation. The extent to which this contributes to graft loss also awaits clarification, although a recent analysis of registry data suggests that the impact on graft failure is insignificant in comparison to the impact on premature death with a functioning graft.[5]

Primary Hyperoxaluria

Primary hyperoxaluria (see Chapter 57) is a rare autosomal recessive disease caused by defective or absent hepatic production of alanine-glyoxylate aminotransferase, resulting in systemic accumulation of calcium oxalate (oxalosis). Kidneys and blood vessels in particular are affected. Kidney transplantation alone is frequently complicated by hyperoxaluria and consequent recurrence in the graft and ultimately graft loss (Fig. 104.7). By contrast, combined liver-kidney transplantation corrects the underlying metabolic deficit and permits long-term kidney graft survival. In an analysis of the U.S. Renal Data System that included 190 adults with oxalosis who went on to renal transplantation, 134 patients who received a kidney transplant alone experienced 48% 8-year death-censored graft survival. This was inferior to 56 patients who also received a liver (76%) and inferior to a control group with a primary diagnosis of GN (61%).[52] Aggressive removal of residual oxalate before transplantation by dialysis and after transplantation by pyridoxine supplementation and maintaining high urine volumes may also decrease the risk of graft damage.

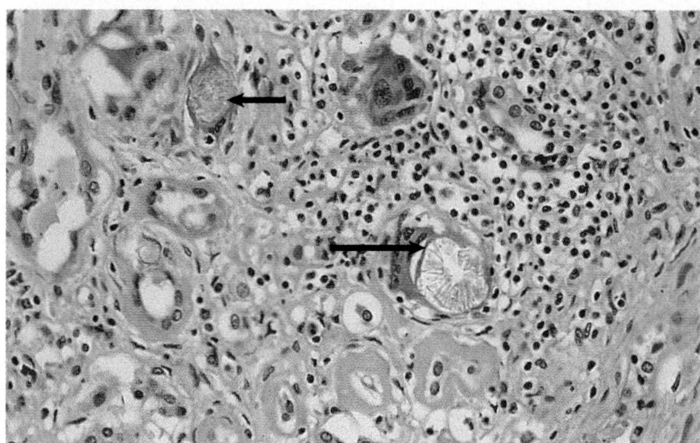

Figure 104.7 Recurrent primary hyperoxaluria. Light microscopy demonstrates oxalate crystals within the tubular lumen *(arrows)* with a secondary interstitial inflammatory infiltrate.

Fabry's Disease

Fabry's disease results from a defect in lysosomal α-galactosidase A enzyme, which results in tissue accumulation of trihexosylceramide, eventually causing ESRD (see Chapter 46). Recurrent Fabry's disease has been documented within the graft; however, graft survival does not appear to be affected. Treatment with recombinant α-galactosidase A, should this become widely available, is likely to reduce the risk of ESRD and also that of recurrence.

RECURRENCE OF VIRUS-ASSOCIATED NEPHROPATHIES AND TUMORS IN THE TRANSPLANTED KIDNEY

Virus-associated kidney diseases may recur after transplantation. Hepatitis B and C virus–associated MPGN and MN are known to recur; however, the risk of this can be substantially decreased by successful antiviral therapy before retransplantation (see Chapter 55).

Retransplantation has been reported in patients experiencing graft loss due to BK virus nephropathy. In the largest series, recurrence was documented in 1 of 10 transplant recipients at an average follow-up of 3 years.[53] Measures to decrease the risk of recurrence included delay in retransplantation by an average of 13 months and transplant nephroureterectomy in seven cases. Calcineurin inhibitor–based triple immunosuppressive therapy was used in all cases, and the one case of recurrence experienced stabilization of graft function after a reduction in immunosuppression.[53] Thus, retransplantation, ideally delayed until BK virus is not detectable in serum by polymerase chain reaction, appears to be safe and effective.

Patients who develop post-transplantation lymphoproliferative disease and incur graft loss due to direct infiltration or rejection after the withdrawal of immunosuppression may safely and successfully undergo retransplantation after a period of recovery. There was no evidence of recurrence reported in one series of five cases.[54]

REFERENCES

1. Chadban SJ. Glomerulonephritis recurrence in the renal graft. *J Am Soc Nephrol.* 2001;12:394-402.
2. Hariharan S, Adams MB, Brennan DC, Davis CL. Recurrent and de novo glomerular disease after renal transplantation: A report from Renal Allograft Disease Registry (RADR). *Transplantation.* 1999;68:635-641.
3. Briganti EM, Russ GR, McNeil J, et al. Risk of renal allograft loss from recurrent glomerulonephritis. *N Engl J Med.* 2002;347:103-109.
4. Hariharan S, Johnson CP, Breshahan BA, et al. Improved graft survival after renal transplantation in the United States, 1988 to 1996. *N Engl J Med.* 2000;342:605-612.
5. Cole EH, Johnston O, Rose CL, Gill JS. Impact of acute rejection and new-onset diabetes on long-term transplant graft and patient survival. *Clin J Am Soc Nephrol.* 2008;3:814-821.
6. Andresdottir MB, Hoitsma AJ, Assmann KJ, et al. The impact of recurrent glomerulonephritis on graft survival in recipients of human histocompatibility leucocyte antigen–identical living related donor grafts. *Transplantation.* 1999;68:623-627.
7. Mulay AV, Van Walraven C, Knoll GA. Impact of immunosuppressive medication on the risk of renal allograft failure due to recurrent glomerulonephritis. *Am J Transplant.* 2009;9:1-8.
8. Berthoux F, El Deeb S, Mariat C, et al. Antithymocyte globulin induction therapy and disease recurrence in renal transplant recipients with primary IgA nephropathy. *Transplantation.* 2008;85:1505-1507.
9. Ibrahim H, Rogers T, Casingal V, et al. Graft loss from recurrent glomerulonephritis is not increased with a rapid steroid discontinuation protocol. *Transplantation.* 2006;81:214-219.
10. Nachman PH, Segelmark M, Westman K, Hogan SL. Recurrent ANCA-associated small vessel vasculitis after transplantation: A pooled analysis. *Kidney Int.* 1999;56:1544-1550.
11. Ruiz JC, Campistol JM, Sanchez-Fructuso A, et al. Increase of proteinuria after conversion from calcineurin inhibitor to sirolimus-based treatment in kidney transplant patients with chronic allograft dysfunction. *Nephrol Dial Transplant.* 2006;21:3252-3257.
12. Odorico JS, Knechtle SJ, Rayhill SC, Pirsch JD. The influence of native nephrectomy on the incidence of recurrent disease following renal transplantation for primary glomerulonephritis. *Transplantation.* 1996;61:228-234.
13. Cibrik DM, Kaplan B, Campbell DA, Meier-Kriesche HU. Renal allograft survival in transplant recipients with focal segmental glomerulosclerosis. *Am J Transplant.* 2003;3:64-67.
14. Andresdottir MB, Assmann KJ, Koene RA, Wetzels JF. Immunohistological and ultrastructural differences between recurrent type I membranoproliferative glomerulonephritis and chronic transplant glomerulopathy. *Am J Kidney Dis.* 1998;32:582-588.
15. Odum J, Peh CA, Clarkson AR, et al. Recurrent mesangial IgA nephritis following renal transplantation. *Nephrol Dial Transplant.* 1994;9:309-312.
16. Ohmacht C, Kliem V, Burg M, Nashan B. Recurrent immunoglobulin A nephropathy after renal transplantation: A significant contributor to graft loss. *Transplantation.* 1997;64:1493-1496.
17. Meulders Q, Pirson Y, Cosyns JP, et al. Course of Henoch-Schönlein nephritis after renal transplantation. Report on 10 patients and review of the literature. *Transplantation.* 1994;58:1179-1186.
18. Schwarz A, Krause PH, Offerman G, Keller F. Impact of de novo membranous glomerulonephritis on the clinical course after kidney transplantation. *Transplantation.* 1994;58:650-654.
19. Cosyns JP, Couchoud C, Pouteil-Noble C, Squifflet JP. Recurrence of membranous nephropathy after renal transplantation: Probability, outcome and risk factors. *Clin Nephrol.* 1998;50:144-153.
20. Senggutuvan P, Cameron JS, Hartley RB, et al. Recurrence of focal segmental glomerulosclerosis in transplanted kidneys: Analysis of incidence and risk factors in 59 allografts. *Pediatr Nephrol.* 1990;4:21-28.
21. Artero M, Biava C, Amend W, et al. Recurrent focal glomerulosclerosis: Natural history and response to therapy. *Am J Med.* 1992;92:375-383.
22. Stephanian E, Matas AJ, Mauer SM, et al. Recurrence of disease in patients retransplanted for focal segmental glomerulosclerosis. *Transplantation.* 1992;53:755-757.
23. Kim EM, Striegel J, Kim Y, et al. Recurrence of steroid resistant nephrotic syndrome in kidney transplants is associated with increased acute renal failure and acute rejection. *Kidney Int.* 1994;45:1440-1445.
24. Savin VJ, Sharma R, Sharma M, et al. Circulating factor associated with increased glomerular permeability to albumin in recurrent focal segmental glomerulosclerosis. *N Engl J Med.* 1996;334:878-883.
25. Dantal J, Godfrin Y, Koll R, et al. Antihuman immunoglobulin affinity immunoadsorption strongly decreases proteinuria in patients with relapsing nephrotic syndrome. *J Am Soc Nephrol.* 1998;9:1709-1715.
26. Andresdottir MB, Ajubi N, Croockewit S, Assmann KJ. Recurrent focal glomerulosclerosis: Natural course and treatment with plasma exchange. *Nephrol Dial Transplant.* 1999;14:2650-2656.
27. Davenport RD. Apheresis treatment of recurrent focal segmental glomerulosclerosis after kidney transplantation: Re-analysis of published case-reports and case-series. *J Clin Apher.* 2001;16:175-178.
28. Hickson LJ, Gera M, Amer H, et al. Kidney transplantation for primary focal segmental glomerulosclerosis: Outcomes and response to therapy for recurrence. *Transplantation.* 2009;87:1232-1239.
29. Cruzado JM, Gil-Vernet S, Ercilla G, et al. Hepatitis C virus–associated membranoproliferative glomerulonephritis in renal allografts. *J Am Soc Nephrol.* 1996;7:2469-2475.
30. Andresdottir MB, Assmann KJ, Hoitsma AJ, Koene RA. Recurrence of type 1 membranoproliferative glomerulonephritis after renal transplantation: Analysis of the incidence, risk factors, and impact on graft survival. *Transplantation.* 1997;63:1628-1633.
31. Kamar N, Toupance O, Buchler M, et al. Evidence that clearance of hepatitis C virus RNA after alpha-interferon therapy in dialysis patients is sustained after renal transplantation. *J Am Soc Nephrol.* 2003;14:2092-2098.
32. Andresdottir MB, Assmann KJ, Hoitsma AJ. Renal transplantation in patients with dense deposit disease: Morphological characteristics of recurrent disease and clinical outcome. *Nephrol Dial Transplant.* 1999;14:1723-1731.
33. Morales JM, Martinez MA, Munoz de Bustillo E. Recurrent type III membranoproliferative glomerulonephritis after kidney transplantation. *Transplantation.* 1997;63:1186-1188.
34. Westman KWA, Bygren PG, Olsson H, Ranstam J. Relapse rate, renal survival and cancer morbidity in patients with Wegener's granulomatosis or microscopic polyangiitis with renal involvement. *J Am Soc Nephrol.* 1998;9:842-852.
35. Patrakka J, Ruotsalainen V, Reponen P, et al. Recurrence of nephrotic syndrome in kidney grafts of patients with congenital nephrotic syndrome of the Finnish type: Role of nephrin. *Transplantation.* 2002;73:394-403.
36. Gobel J, Olbricht CJ, Offner G, et al. Kidney transplantation in Alport's syndrome: Long-term outcome and allograft anti-GBM nephritis. *Clin Nephrol.* 1992;38:299-304.
37. Moroni G, Tantardini F, Gallelli B, et al. The long-term prognosis of renal transplantation in patients with lupus nephritis. *Am J Kidney Dis.* 2005;45:903-911.
38. Goral S, Ynares C, Shappell SB, et al. Recurrent lupus nephritis in renal transplant recipients revisited: It is not rare. *Transplantation.* 2003;75:651-656.
39. Goss JA, Cole BR, Jendrisk MD, et al. Renal transplantation for systemic lupus erythematosus and recurrent lupus nephritis: A single-centre experience and a review of the literature. *Transplantation.* 1991;52:805-810.
40. Stone JH, Millward CL, Olson JL, Amend WJ. Frequency of recurrent lupus nephritis among ninety-seven renal transplant patients during the cyclosporine era. *Arthritis Rheum.* 1998;41:678-686.
41. Le Quintrec M, Lionet A, Kamar N, et al. Complement mutation-associated de novo thrombotic microangiopathy following kidney transplantation. *Am J Transplant.* 2008;8:1694-1701.
42. Ducloux D, Rebibou JM, Semhoun-Ducloux S, Jamali M. Recurrence of hemolytic-uremic syndrome in renal transplant recipients: A meta-analysis. *Transplantation.* 1998;65:1405-1407.
43. www.renal.org/pages/pages/guidelines/other.php.
44. Artz MA, Steenbergen EJ, Hoitsma AJ, et al. Renal transplantation in patients with hemolytic uremic syndrome: High rate of recurrence and increased incidence of acute rejections. *Transplantation.* 2003;76:821-826.

45. Remuzzi G, Ruggenenti P, Codazzi D, et al. Combined kidney and liver transplantation for familial haemolytic uraemic syndrome. *Lancet*. 2002;359:1671-1672.
46. Chang YJ, Spiera H. Renal transplantation in scleroderma. *Medicine (Baltimore)*. 1999;78:382-385.
47. Sherif AM, Refaie AF, Sobh MA, et al. Long-term outcome of live donor kidney transplantation for renal amyloidosis. *Am J Kidney Dis*. 2003;42:370-375.
48. Hartmann A, Holdaas H, Fauchald P, et al. Fifteen years' experience with renal transplantation in systemic amyloidosis. *Transpl Int*. 1992;5:15-18.
49. Leung N, Lager DJ, Gertz MA, et al. Long-term outcome of renal transplantation in light-chain deposition disease. *Am J Kidney Dis*. 2004;43:147-153.
50. Pronovost PH, Brady HR, Gunning ME, Espinoza O. Clinical features, predictors of disease progression and results of renal transplantation in fibrillary/immunotactoid glomerulopathy. *Nephrol Dial Transplant*. 1996;11:837-842.
51. Bhalla V, Nast CC, Stollenwerk N, et al. Recurrent and de novo diabetic nephropathy in renal allografts. *Transplantation*. 2003;75:66-71.
52. Cibrik DM, Kaplan B, Arndorfer JA, Meier-Kriesche HU. Renal allograft survival in patients with oxalosis. *Transplantation*. 2002;74:707-710.
53. Ramos E, Vincenti F, Lu WX, et al. Retransplantation in patients with graft loss caused by polyoma virus nephropathy. *Transplantation*. 2004;77:131-133.
54. Birkeland SA, Hamilton-Dutoit S, Bendtzen K. Long-term follow-up of kidney transplant patients with posttransplant lymphoproliferative disorder: Duration of posttransplant lymphoproliferative disorder–induced operational graft tolerance, interleukin-18 course, and results of retransplantation. *Transplantation*. 2003;76:153-158.

CHAPTER 105

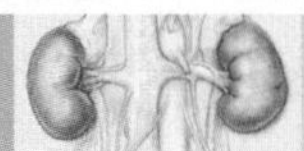

Outcomes of Renal Transplantation

Titte R. Srinivas, Jesse D. Schold, Herwig-Ulf Meier-Kriesche

Despite the increasing number of people worldwide living with a functioning kidney transplant, the waiting list for kidney transplants continues to grow. A transplant kidney is therefore a relatively scarce resource, making it critical that factors influencing transplant outcomes are well understood.

Data on transplant outcomes are derived from databases maintained by single transplant centers, cooperatives of single centers and industry-sponsored trials, and large multicenter registries. Large databases include the U.S. Renal Data System (USRDS),[1] the Scientific Registry of Transplant Recipients (SRTR),[2] the United Network for Organ Sharing (UNOS),[3] and the Collaborative Transplant Study (CTS); registries are also maintained by Canada, Australia, and New Zealand and the United Kingdom.[4,5] The USRDS and SRTR reports are based on mandatory reporting of outcomes for almost all transplant recipients in the United States. The CTS reports data submitted on a voluntary basis by participating centers in many countries. The SRTR and USRDS databases through cross-links to other databases contain well-validated data on dates of patient death and return to dialysis. However, the large registries typically lack clinically relevant data, such as immunosuppressive drug dosing, blood pressures, and serum lipids, whereas single-center observational studies and clinical trials frequently provide data on the impact of such variables on graft and patient survival.

"Hard outcomes" for renal allografts include graft and patient survival. "Soft outcomes" used as surrogates for graft survival include serum creatinine, proteinuria, rejection rates, and biopsy-derived pathologic features. Other important measures include days of hospitalization, quality of life, and patient satisfaction indices.

Randomized controlled trials of interventions, such as immunosuppressive regimens, are often impractical for comparison of effects on allograft survival.[5] It is difficult to design adequately powered trials to demonstrate statistically significant differences in graft or patient survival within the short periods of follow-up, given practical and financial constraints for the sample sizes needed in such trials.

UNDERSTANDING SURVIVAL MODELS

Survival analysis may also be referred to in other contexts as failure time analysis or time to event analysis. The events applicable for outcomes studies in transplantation include graft failure, return to dialysis or retransplantation, patient death, and time to acute rejection.[6,7]

Most analyses use the Kaplan-Meier method, which yields an *actuarial estimate* of graft survival. The assumptions underlying these models and the relevant terminology are summarized in Figure 105.1. Most national registries report graft survival as unadjusted or as being *adjusted* for age, gender, and end-stage renal disease (ESRD) diagnosis. This adjustment by multivariate techniques accounts for differences in baseline characteristics that may otherwise confound the results. Another relevant measure is the median graft survival, commonly referred to as the allograft *half-life*. This is distinct from the *conditioned half-life*, which is defined as the median graft survival among those who have already survived the first year after transplantation.[8] Graft survival may be reported as cumulative graft survival or its reciprocal, cumulative graft loss. When patient death is counted as a graft loss event, the results are reported as *overall graft loss (or survival)*. The most important causes of death with a functioning transplant are cardiovascular disease, infection, and malignant disease; the last two reflect the impact of the immunosuppressed state.[2] Death with a functioning transplant is an increasingly common cause of late graft loss with more older patients receiving kidney transplants.

Death with a functioning transplant when it is not counted as a graft loss is reported as *death-censored graft loss (survival)*. This allows study of factors affecting graft function independent of factors mediating mortality. An increased risk of mortality will be manifested as increased overall graft loss and relatively preserved death-censored graft loss. As a caveat, estimates of rates of death-censored graft loss may be biased by risk factors affecting both mortality and attrition of graft function, for example, diabetes mellitus and hypertension.

Graft loss is termed early graft loss in the first 12 post-transplantation months and late graft loss after the first 12 months.[9] Early graft loss is dominated by vascular technical failures, primary nonfunction, recipient death, or severe rejection. After 12 months, the rate of graft loss is lower and remains remarkably stable over time. The dominant causes of late graft loss include chronic rejection and multifactorial interstitial fibrosis and tubular atrophy (IF/TA, formerly designated chronic allograft nephropathy; see Chapter 103),[10] calcineurin inhibitor (CNI) nephrotoxicity, recurrent disease, and patient death. The predominant causes of patient mortality after 12 months are cardiovascular, infectious, and malignant diseases (Fig. 105.2). The principal causes of patient death in the first year are cardiovascular disease and infection (malignant disease is much less common).[9]

SURVIVAL ADVANTAGE FOR TRANSPLANTATION OVER DIALYSIS

Transplantation is accepted as conferring a durable survival benefit over dialysis, despite the inherent selection bias in that a transplant is a viable option only in the fittest dialysis patient.[11]

Assumptions and Key Features of Kaplan-Meier and Proportional Hazard Models
Survival analysis models *time to the event of interest*.
Not all possible events may have occurred by the end of the observation period; the only information available about some subjects is that they were free of the event of interest at the time of last follow-up (*censoring assumption*).
However, if the probability that a subject is censored is related to the probability of that subject suffering an event (*informative censoring*), then the application of censoring may be inappropriate (*noninformative censoring*).
A common descriptor of the survivorship of a cohort is the *hazard function*, which is commonly interpreted as the event rate at a particular point in time, conditional on surviving to that point in time.
There are different types of survival models that also are based on varying levels of assumptions. Kaplan-Meier plots do not require any distributional assumptions. Cox proportional hazard models do not specify a form for the underlying hazard but assume a proportional multiplicative effect of treatments and are also referred to as a semiparametric model.
Cox regression models can include multiple covariates but assume that the impact of these covariates does not change over time (*proportional hazards assumption*).
Differences in survival between two groups can be compared by using a variety of tests. For Kaplan-Meier plots, log-rank and Wilcoxon tests are most commonly used.
The *relative hazard* describes the ratio of time to outcome given a particular risk factor to time to outcome when the risk factor is not present.
Cox regression (proportional hazard model) is a multivariate method that allows an analysis of the relative contribution of numerous explanatory variables or potential cofounders to the variable of interest, time to event. Cox models assume that the relative hazard between grnups dos not change with time.

Figure 105.1 Survival analysis for kidney transplantation: assumptions and key features of Kaplan-Meier and proportional hazard models. *(Modified from references 6 and 7.)*

Common Causes of Kidney Transplant Failure	
Death with function	40%–45%
Failure of the transplant kidney	55%–60%
Chronic allograft nephropathy (chronic transplant glomerulopathy; 5%)	30%
Recurrent or *de novo* disease (including BK virus nephropathy)	10%
Miscellaneous and mixed picture (unknown, multifactorial, end-stage renal disease from medical illness)	10%
Technical and thrombosis	2%
Outright rejection	5%

Figure 105.2 Common causes of kidney transplant failure. *(U.S. Renal Data System from reference 9.)*

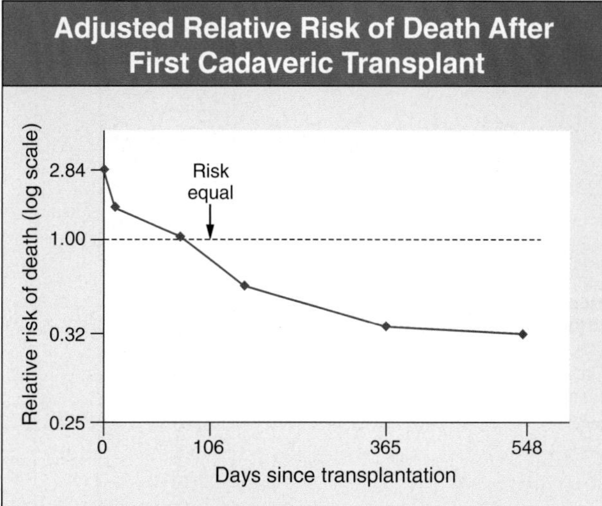

Figure 105.3 Adjusted relative risk of death among 23,275 recipients of a first cadaveric transplant. The reference group was the 46,164 patients on dialysis who were on the waiting list (relative risk 1.0). Values were adjusted for age, sex, race, cause of end-stage renal disease, year of placement on the waiting list, geographic region, and time from first treatment for end-stage renal disease to placement on the waiting list. *(U.S. Renal Data System with permission from reference 11.)*

The best comparator group is patients who have passed the initial evaluation for transplantation and are on a waiting list but not yet transplanted.

A study using the USRDS database showed that on average, after the first 106 post-transplantation days, the relative risk of death was higher for those patients on the waiting list who continued on dialysis.[11] This excess early mortality presumably reflected the medical and surgical risk associated with the transplant procedure *per se*. However, the time to equal risk of mortality observed in this study varied widely between 5 and 673 days after transplantation (Fig. 105.3). With up to 4 years of follow-up, transplantation was associated with a 68% lower risk of death. Transplantation particularly benefited diabetic recipients.[11]

The salutary effect of transplantation is likely to reflect reduction in cardiovascular mortality by successful transplantation. The better the function of the transplanted kidney, the lower the cardiovascular mortality (Fig. 105.4).[12]

Donor Source and Quality

Transplant kidneys are derived from living related or unrelated donors or deceased donors. Some deceased donor kidneys are retrieved after brain death but before cardiac death; others are retrieved after cardiac death (DCD). DCD kidneys form an increasingly valuable addition to the deceased donor pool. Donors are classified as being expanded criteria donors or standard criteria donors; this may be rather simplistic because there is a continuous spectrum of donor quality that has an impact on graft survival (Fig. 105.5).[13]

PATIENT AND GRAFT SURVIVAL IN KIDNEY TRANSPLANTATION

The data quoted in this section were obtained from the 2006 report of the SRTR for first and subsequent transplants (Fig. 105.6).[14] Living donor transplants have significantly better 1-, 3-,

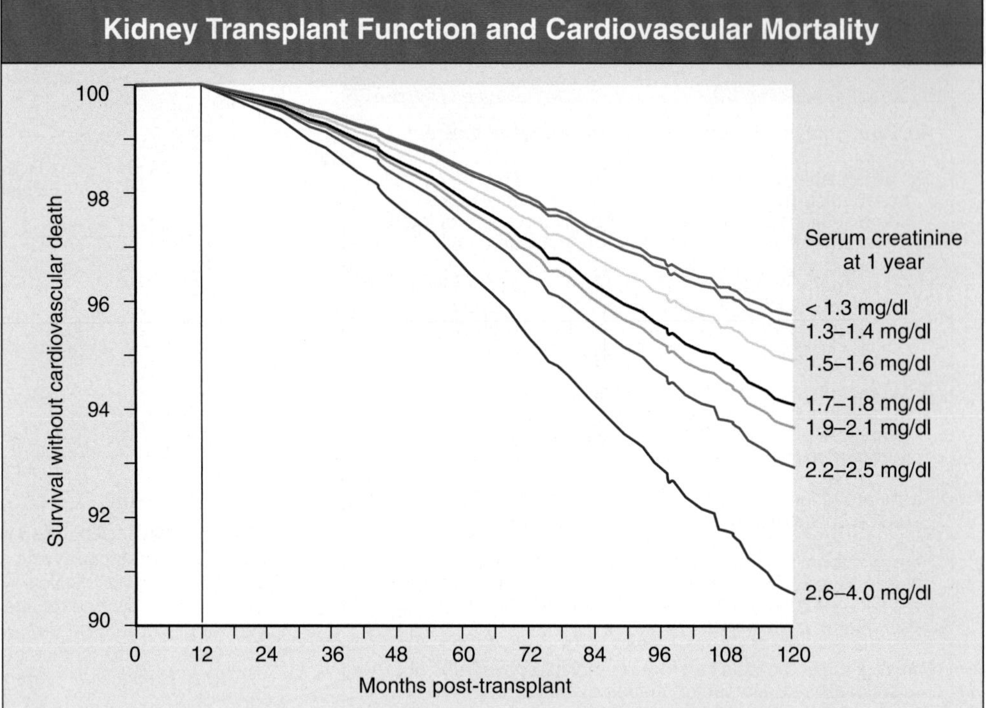

Figure 105.4 Kidney transplant function and cardiovascular mortality. Worse post-transplantation renal function is associated with higher risk of cardiovascular mortality. *(From reference 12.)*

Deceased Donor Nomenclature in Kidney Transplantation

Term	Definition
Expanded criteria donors (ECD)	For kidney, any deceased donor older than 60 years; or from a donor older than 50 years with two of the following: a history of hypertension, a terminal serum creatinine >1.5 mg/dl (132μmol/l), or death resulting from a cerebrovascular accident (stroke)
Donation after cardiac death (DCD)	Donation of any organ from a patient whose heart has irreversibly stopped beating; includes donors who also qualify as ECD under the kidney definition above
Standard criteria donors (SCD)	For kidney, a deceased donor who is neither ECD nor DCD. These donors have fewer risks associated with graft failure.

Figure 105.5 Deceased donor nomenclature in kidney transplantation.

and 5-year unadjusted graft survival compared with non–extended criteria deceased donor transplants, which in turn have graft survival superior to that of extended criteria deceased donor transplants.[14]

Patient survival data are higher than graft survival figures as most patients with failed grafts return to dialysis. Again, living donor transplantation has superior unadjusted patient survival rates at 1, 3, and 5 years compared with non–extended criteria deceased donor transplants, which in turn have graft survival superior to that of extended criteria deceased donor transplants.[14]

One-year graft survival has improved steadily during the past 25 years (Fig. 105.7).[15] First transplants consistently have better one-year survival than subsequent grafts, probably reflecting a superior immunologic risk profile.

LONG-TERM OUTCOMES IN RENAL TRANSPLANTATION

Graft Survival

There has been a steady improvement in long-term graft survival. This largely represents improving graft survival in higher risk patients, such as those undergoing retransplantation.[15] When first deceased donor transplants alone are assessed, recent improvements are less impressive.[16] Substantial improvements in graft survival have been reported by use of projected half-lives,[15] but these should be interpreted with caution as eventual actual outcomes may differ from actuarial estimates[16] Although there have been significant recent decreases in acute rejection rates during the first 2 years after transplantation,[16] this

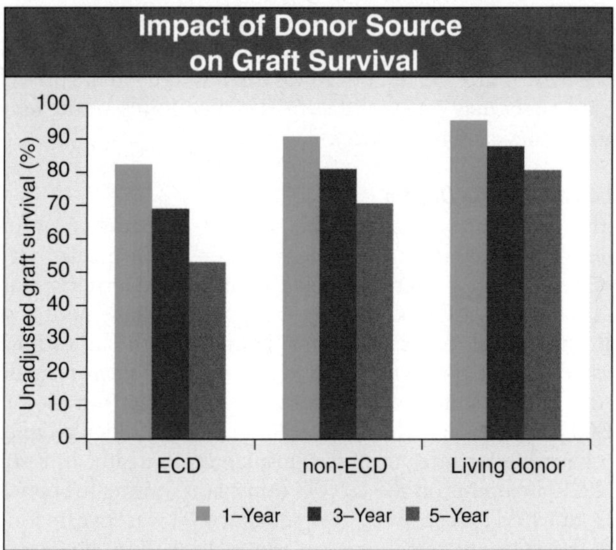

Figure 105.6 Impact of donor source on graft survival. The 1-, 3-, and 5-year unadjusted graft survival by donor source. ECD, expanded criteria donor. *(Modified from the 2006 SRTR Annual Report, reference 14.)*

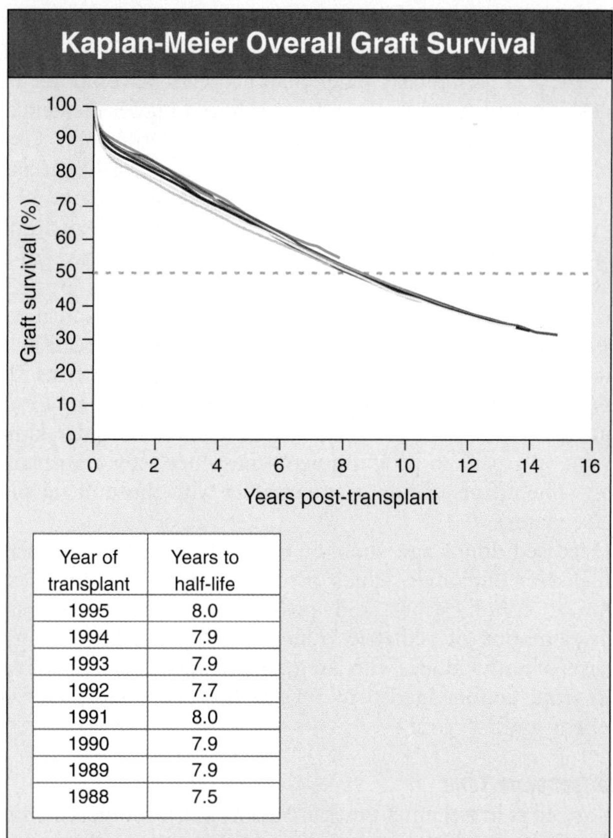

Year of transplant	Years to half-life
1995	8.0
1994	7.9
1993	7.9
1992	7.7
1991	8.0
1990	7.9
1989	7.9
1988	7.5

Figure 105.7 Kaplan-Meier overall graft survival by year of transplant: first deceased donor transplants, 1988-1995. The actuarial graft survival curves for each year from 1988 to 1995 are virtually superimposed with no significant difference in graft survival. Graft half-life varies from 7.5 to 8 years during the same period. *(From reference 6.)*

has not translated into improved long-term graft survival; indeed, death-censored graft survival has worsened. Moreover, in a greater proportion of acute rejection episodes, renal function did not return after treatment to pre-rejection baseline values, and this was associated with an incremental increase in the relative hazard for death-censored graft survival.[16,17] It may be that the more potent immunosuppression in current use allows the expression of only more severe episodes of acute rejection, so these episodes have less good outcomes. At the same time as there has been the use of increasingly intensive immunosuppression, there has also been an increasing recipient comorbidity, a decreasing donor quality (increasing numbers of older donors), and a disturbing rise in opportunistic infections such as polyomavirus (BK virus).

Beyond the first post-transplantation year, the principal causes of graft loss are patient death and multifactorial progressive fibrosis of the allograft, until recently termed chronic allograft nephropathy and now designated interstitial fibrosis/tubular atrophy (IF/TA), which is discussed further in Chapter 103.

Patient Survival

The predominant cause of death more than 1 year after transplantation remains cardiovascular disease, followed by infection and malignant disease. This is likely to reflect varying contributions from age, comorbidity, burden of immunosuppression, progressive allograft dysfunction, and side effects of immunosuppressive agents.

FACTORS AFFECTING RENAL ALLOGRAFT SURVIVAL

These can be considered as donor factors, recipient factors, or donor-recipient interactions.[18] From the point of view of clinical management and therapeutic interventions, another convenient way of discussing these factors is as alloimmune or nonalloimmune factors.

Donor Factors

The quality of the kidney immediately before transplantation has a major impact on long-term graft function.

Deceased Versus Living Donor

Donor source is one of the most important predictors of short- and long-term graft outcomes. In general, living donor grafts are associated with outcomes superior to those of deceased donor grafts. Not only does a living donor kidney contribute to superior long-term graft survival, it is also associated with a recipient survival benefit that is not fully understood. The advantage of living donor kidneys holds equally true for spousal and unrelated donors and appears to be in large part nonimmunologically mediated (at least non–HLA mediated).[19,20]

The better outcomes with living donors probably reflect several factors: the higher kidney quality provided by healthy living donors, the absence of brain death, the general benefits of elective as opposed to urgent surgery, the avoidance of ischemia-reperfusion injury, the higher nephron mass transplanted, and the effects of a shorter waiting time. The living donor transplant can be timed in such a way that the recipient is as fit as possible at the time of transplantation.[20] There may also be benefit attributable to better social support and emotional state and a greater sense of obligation to maintain medical compliance. However, in recent years, the age of living donors and recipients has continued to increase, both of which may have a negative impact on transplant outcomes in the future.

Donor Age

Deceased donor and living donor grafts from those older than 50 years, and particularly older than 65 years, have poorer outcomes. These results are thought to reflect a higher incidence of delayed graft function and of "nephron underdosing." Grafts from older donors have fewer functioning nephrons because of the involutory changes associated with the aging process and the age-related accumulation of hypertension and atherosclerosis. However, because of the organ donor shortage relative to the growing wait list, more organs from elderly donors are being used. The older the donor kidney (>18 years), the shorter the expected graft life.[21] This effect persists after correction for recipient characteristics that could produce similar effects. The older kidney has limited functional reserve to adapt to a range of insults. It has also been hypothesized that the older kidney may be on a path to programmed senescence after transplantation.[22] The effects of donor age interact with those of recipient age (see later).

Deceased donor age younger than 5 years is also associated with poorer outcomes, which probably reflects higher rates of technical complications and possibly nephron underdosing. Transplantation of pediatric kidneys *en bloc* (in which the graft consists of both kidneys with a segment of aorta and inferior vena cava) from donors aged 0 to 5 years has been associated with excellent graft survival.[23]

Cold Ischemia Time

Prolonged cold ischemia times are associated with incrementally higher risk of delayed graft function and poorer allograft survival, particularly when cold ischemia times exceed 24 hours (also see discussion on delayed graft function).[19,24]

Donor Nephron Mass

An imbalance between the metabolic/excretory demands of the recipient and the functional transplant mass has been postulated to play a causative role in the development and progression of chronic transplant dysfunction. Nephron underdosing is a possible consequence of perioperative ischemic damage and postoperative nephrotoxic drugs, or it may be an inherent consequence of a size or gender mismatch between donor kidney and recipient. It may lead to hyperfiltration, progressive glomerulosclerosis, and eventual graft failure. Kidneys from small donors transplanted into recipients of large body size would therefore have the highest risk of this problem.[25] There is limited support for this hypothesis from animal studies and retrospective human studies; in one relatively small single-center study, higher transplant kidney volumes in living donor transplantation correlated with better graft function.[26] There are no prospective studies of donor pairs with optimal matching of kidney size to recipient body size that might clarify this issue.

Donor Race

In the United States, the survival of deceased donor grafts obtained from African Americans is poorer than that of grafts from Caucasians. The reasons for this are unclear. It has been attributed to nephron underdosing, but it remains controversial whether African Americans have a decreased number of nephrons compared with Caucasians.[27]

Donor Gender

There is evidence that grafts from deceased female donors have slightly poorer survival, particularly in male recipients.[28] This probably reflects nephron underdosing. It is controversial whether there may also be a difference in the antigenic repertoire between female and male kidneys that could influence outcome. Because the donor gender effect was not observed in the pre-CNI era, the effect may reflect differential susceptibility of the female donor kidney to CNI toxicity.[29]

Expanded Criteria Donors

As the discrepancy between the number of patients awaiting kidney transplantation and the number of available organs increases, there is increasing use of expanded criteria donor (ECD) kidneys. ECD kidneys (see Fig. 105.5) have poorer survival than ideal deceased donor kidneys, with an estimated adjusted relative risk of failure greater than 1.7.[30] Factors mediating this effect include reduced baseline glomerular filtration rate of ECD kidneys and their preferential use for older recipients who have higher rates of post-transplantation death. In a study of 122,175 patients on the UNOS transplant waiting list between 1992 and 1997, mean ECD recipient survival was 5 years longer than for patients remaining on the waiting list, whereas the recipient of an ideal deceased donor kidney accrued a 13-year survival benefit. Diabetics obtained the greatest proportional survival benefit, and those with hypertensive renal disease incurred the greatest absolute gain in life-years.[31]

In the United States, UNOS has implemented policies that allow consenting patients to opt for both an ECD kidney and an "ideal" kidney. Those patients who decline listing for an ECD kidney could potentially incur the increased mortality associated with increased waiting time on dialysis. It is conceivable that the younger nondiabetic patient could wait longer on the list than an older diabetic recipient, who would gain the mortality benefit conferred by transplantation.[32] This survival benefit from the ECD transplant can be expected to be proportionately greater in regions with historically higher waiting times.[31]

With DCD kidneys, rates of delayed graft function and primary nonfunction are higher than with standard donors.[33] There is accumulating evidence, however, that long-term graft survival with DCD donors is similar to that with heart-beating deceased donors, although this probably reflects careful selection criteria.[34]

Recipient Factors

Recipient Age

In general, graft survival rates are poorer in those younger than 17 years and older than 65 years.[1] In the young, technical causes of graft loss, such as vessel thrombosis, aggressive rejection, and noncompliance with immunologic graft loss, are relatively more common. Conversely, death with a functioning graft is relatively rare in the young. In most developed countries, the mean age of the incident and prevalent ESRD population is increasing. Many of these patients have significant comorbidities, particularly cardiovascular disease and type 2 diabetes mellitus. Despite this, age *per se* is no longer regarded as a contraindication to transplantation, which still confers a survival advantage in the carefully selected elderly ESRD recipient.[11] It is critical to consider the effect of increasing waiting times on mortality in older patients with ESRD and their suitability for transplantation by the time they are actually offered a transplant. Recent SRTR data show that more than half of patients older than 60 years on the waiting list are expected to die before receiving a renal transplant.[35] This underscores the importance of stratifying transplant options for those on the waiting list based on age and comorbidity.

Whereas acute rejection is relatively infrequent in the elderly, there is less chance of a return to baseline function after treatment of an acute rejection episode. Death with a functioning graft is more common with increasing recipient age; however, death-censored graft loss also worsens with increasing age. Recipients aged 50 to 64 years accrue a 29% higher relative risk of graft loss compared with those aged 18 to 49 years, whereas those 65 years or older have a 67% higher relative risk for graft loss.[36] This effect of increasing age is independent of traditional determinants of graft survival, such as delayed graft function and acute rejection, and is independent of the immunosuppressive regimen employed. Increasing donor and recipient age is an independent risk factor for graft survival[37]; the best graft survival is obtained when a kidney from a young donor is transplanted into a young recipient, and the worst graft survival is obtained when kidneys from older donors are transplanted into older donors. The combination of advanced donor and recipient age may have a synergistic detrimental impact on graft survival, perhaps because of the dynamic interplay of an intrinsically senescent kidney transplanted into a senescent biologic milieu.

Death rates due to infection increase linearly with increasing recipient age in those on the transplant waiting list, and in the transplanted elderly patient, infectious mortality rises exponentially.[38] Overall mortality and cardiovascular mortality rise with increasing age, but the magnitude of this increased mortality is not greater in transplanted patients compared with those on the waiting list[38]; indeed, cardiovascular mortality is halved with successful transplantation in the elderly.[38] Death due to malignancy is also increased in elderly transplanted patients, perhaps reflecting the additive effects of pharmacologic immunosuppression to natural immune senescence. As yet, there are no reliable methods to measure delivery of effective immunosuppression that can assist further analysis of this issue.

Recipient Race

From the early days of transplantation in the United States, African American patients had inferior graft and patient survival rates. Proposed explanations have included heightened rejection risk, differing HLA polymorphisms compared with the predominantly Caucasian donor pool, differing pharmacokinetics of immunosuppressants, hypertension, noncompliance, and socioeconomic status. However, the difference between African Americans and Caucasians is becoming narrower with newer immunosuppressive regimens.[39,40] Despite the need for increasing immunosuppression to maintain freedom from acute rejection, African American transplant patients are at decreased risk for death due to infection, which may allow increased immunosuppression to be delivered relatively safely and possibly obviate some of the racial differences in graft survival that were seen in the past. Outcomes after living donor transplants are superior to those of deceased donor transplants in African Americans,[41] but living donation is relatively underused in African Americans and represents a potential target for intervention to improve transplant outcomes.

Socioeconomic factors associated with inability to pay for transplant medications (an issue in the United States and other countries in which universal health coverage does not exist), poorer access to high-quality medical care, and noncompliance may also play a role in mediating the interaction between race and outcomes. Interestingly, an analysis of the United Kingdom national database, a country in which there is universal health coverage, showed that graft survival was inferior in blacks compared with whites or Asians.[42] An Australian study suggested that inferior outcomes with transplantation in aboriginals may reflect a significant contribution of socioeconomic factors and differential access to care rather than a direct and exclusive contribution of race.[43]

Recipient Gender

SRTR data consistently demonstrate better graft survival in male recipients compared with female recipients of living donor kidneys.[44] An important difference is the higher degree of sensitization of female recipients to HLA antigens and possibly non–HLA antigens due to pregnancy and transfusions (which may be required for menstrual and pregnancy-related blood loss). Female recipients are at greater risk for acute rejection but show lower rates of progressive attrition of graft function.[45]

Recipient Sensitization Before and After Transplantation

Patients who are broadly sensitized (panel reactive antibody status >50%) at the time of transplantation have poorer early and late graft survival compared with nonsensitized recipients.[19] This decrement in early graft survival is mainly related to increased delayed graft function and acute rejection. Patients who are highly sensitized (most commonly as a result of previous transplants, pregnancy, and previous blood transfusions) are often given more intensive immunosuppression to reduce the risk of rejection, but this also exposes them to infectious and neoplastic risk. The donor-specific alloimmune response is a significant contributor to chronic transplant dysfunction and ultimately graft loss.[46] Although conditioning regimens incorporating plasma exchange and depleting antibodies or intravenous immune globulin can permit transplantation of highly sensitized individuals, the long-term outcomes of these transplants are still uncertain.[47]

Acute Rejection

Acute rejection remains the single greatest risk factor for chronic rejection and graft loss. Whereas acute rejection rates are decreasing, the association of acute rejection and chronic graft failure is increasing during the last 10 years.[48] The histologic grade of rejection, severity of renal functional impairment at the time of diagnosed rejection, timing of rejection episode, and completeness of response to antirejection treatment all have prognostic significance. Acute rejection episodes with return of allograft function to pre-rejection baseline levels are, however, associated with little impact on long-term allograft survival. Humoral rejection is typically more difficult to reverse and prejudices long-term graft survival to a greater extent than cell-mediated rejections do.[19]

Recipient Hepatitis C and Hepatitis B Positivity

Recipients who are hepatitis C virus (HCV) antibody positive at the time of transplantation have graft and patient survival inferior to that of those who are HCV negative. Higher mortality rates in this population are attributed mainly to infection and worsening liver disease.[49] Despite these limitations, transplantation of selected HCV-positive patients confers a survival benefit over remaining on the waiting list.[50,51]

The adverse effects of hepatitis B virus (HBV) surface antigen positivity on post-transplantation outcomes are much less pronounced in recent years, reflecting in part the availability of effective anti-HBV therapies.

Recipient Compliance

Poor compliance with the immunosuppressive regimen is known to increase the risk of acute rejection, particularly late acute rejection, and chronic transplant dysfunction. The exact magnitude of this problem is difficult to define. In a study of patients followed up to 5 years after transplantation, almost a quarter of the patients were identified as being noncompliant on the basis of direct questioning about missing medication doses, and this was associated with a large increase in risk of late acute rejection and poorer graft function.[52]

Obesity

Obesity (body mass index [BMI] >30 kg/m^2) constitutes an important risk factor for cardiovascular disease, hypertension, and diabetes mellitus in the general population. The effects of obesity on long-term graft and patient survival were examined in a study of 51,927 patients reported to the USRDS between 1988 and 1997.[53] There was an increased mortality at both low and high extremes of BMI.[53] This U-shaped relationship resembles that seen in the general population and also described the relationship between obesity and cardiovascular and infectious mortality. Furthermore, increasing BMI was associated with worsening death-censored graft survival.[54]

Transplantation does confer a survival advantage for the obese dialysis patient. This survival advantage holds true for both living and deceased donor transplantation.[55] However, weight loss among renal transplant candidates before the procedure did not have an impact on transplant outcomes in a retrospective study.[56]

Recipient Hypertension

Increasingly severe post-transplantation hypertension is associated with increasing risk of graft loss, and control of hypertension is associated with improved graft survival.[57] Unfortunately, there are only retrospective data that by themselves cannot establish a causal relationship between hypertension and graft loss. Based on extrapolations from studies in nontransplant populations, optimal treatment of hypertension (see Chapter 102) is a reasonable goal to minimize progression of renal dysfunction and the extrarenal complications associated with hypertension.

Recipient Dyslipidemia

Arteriolar fibrointimal hyperplasia is associated with chronic progressive attrition of graft function; this vascular lesion is morphologically reminiscent of atherosclerosis. In a small study, statin treatment was associated with better histologic appearances and better graft function at 1 year. Like treatment of hypertension, the use of lipid-lowering treatment after transplantation is based on evidence that largely represents extension of experiences from nontransplant populations. The treatment of dyslipidemia in transplant recipients is discussed in Chapter 102.

Recurrence of Primary Disease

Determining the incidence and prevalence of recurrent or *de novo* renal disease is not straightforward. In one of the best performed studies of transplant recipients whose cause of ESRD was glomerulonephritis, the cumulative incidence of graft loss at 10 years was 8.4%. In that population, recurrence of glomerulonephritis was the most important cause of graft loss, after chronic rejection and death.[58] It is likely that as graft survival improves with decreasing acute rejection rates, recurrent or *de novo* disease will become a more important cause of late graft loss, especially given the current trend toward minimizing maintenance immunosuppression. Recurrent disease in renal allografts is discussed further in Chapter 104.

Proteinuria

The degree of proteinuria correlates with poorer renal outcome in both native and transplant kidney disease.[59] Proteinuria may simply be a marker of renal damage, but there is speculation that proteinuria *per se* may accelerate graft loss in addition to other pathogenetic factors. Increasing evidence points to a link between humoral factors that mediate alloimmune glomerular damage leading to proteinuria. Sirolimus-based regimens have been implicated as a cause of proteinuria. CNI-based regimens may be associated with less proteinuria because of their effects on glomerular hemodynamics or superior immunologic protection. The role of angiotensin-converting enzyme inhibitors and angiotensin receptor blockers in slowing the progression of proteinuric renal diseases is discussed in Chapter 76.

Donor-Recipient Factors

Delayed Graft Function

Delayed graft function (DGF) is defined as failure of the renal transplant to function immediately, with the need for dialysis in the first post-transplantation week. DGF affects approximately 20% of deceased donor transplants. Slow graft function (SGF) is defined as serum creatinine concentration above 3.0 mg/dl (264 μmol/l) at 5 days after transplantation without requiring dialysis within 1 week of transplantation.[60] The main risk factors for DGF that are identifiable in the clinical setting include donor age or comorbidity, cold ischemia time, and warm ischemia time. DGF and SGF are likely to reflect the dynamic interplay of the status of the donor kidney (advanced donor age, donor history of hypertension) with peritransplantation injury (e.g., ischemia-reperfusion as a consequence of agonal events or during procurement followed by reperfusion) or cold preservation injury.[60] Warm ischemia time is also an important risk factor, although its exact contributions to the pathogenesis and maintenance of DGF are difficult to assess because of inaccurate reporting. Early single-center reports suggested that the negative impact of DGF on graft survival could be explained in part by a high incidence of acute rejection in cases with DGF.[61] In analyses of USRDS and UNOS data, DGF was independently associated with reduced short- and long-term graft survival.[62,63] In a small single-center study, DGF was associated with inferior renal function at 1 year.[64] ECD kidneys and DCD kidneys are more susceptible to DGF. Increasing cold ischemia time is associated with increased likelihood of DGF with DCD kidneys. Pulsatile machine perfusion of allografts (compared with static cold preservation) has been associated with fewer discards of ECD organs, lower DGF rates, and slight improvement in death-censored graft survival.[65] In a randomized clinical trial comparing machine perfusion with static cold preservation, machine perfusion was associated with a lower incidence of DGF, faster fall in serum creatinine concentration after transplantation, decreased duration of DGF, and better allograft survival at 1 year after transplantation.[66]

DGF and the use of pulsatile perfusion will continue to be of major clinical importance and will likely gain additional prominence with the larger numbers of ECD and DCD transplants that are now being performed.

HLA Matching

Better HLA matching still translates to superior graft survival, and this is the justification for the operation of national and international sharing systems for zero-mismatched renal kidneys, even though this practice prolongs cold ischemia times and increases DGF rate. However, with improved contemporary

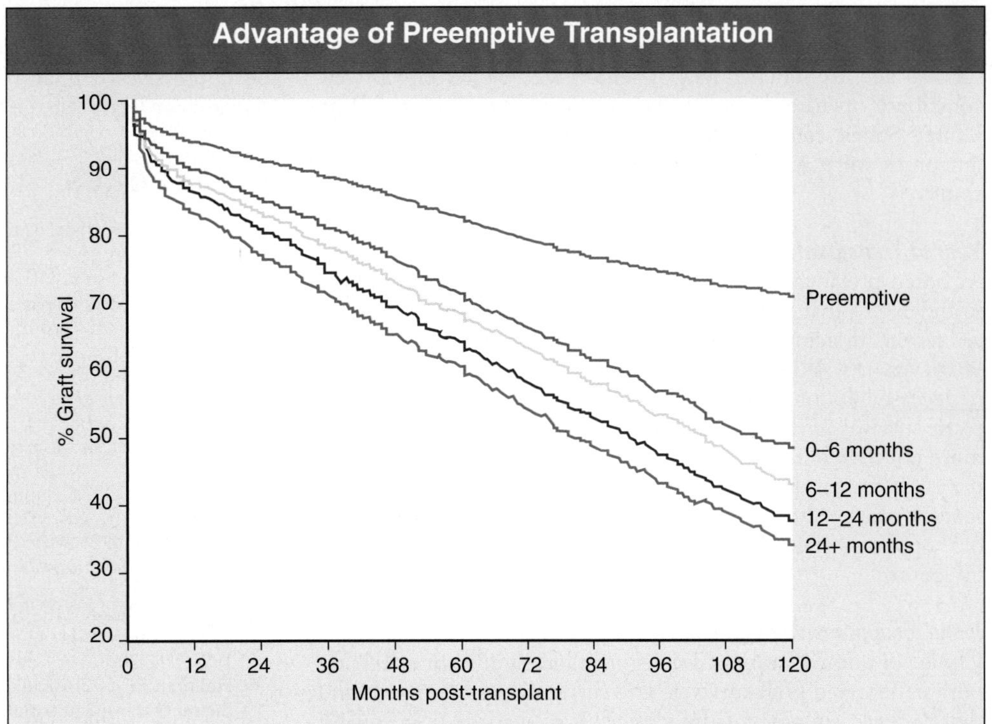

Figure 105.8 Advantage of preemptive transplantation. Preemptive transplants confer a survival advantage over transplants performed in patients who receive dialysis treatment before transplantation. Increasing pre-transplantation dialysis time translates to progressive decline in allograft survival. *(From reference 69.)*

immunosuppression, HLA matching has taken on less significance; for example, excellent graft survival has been noted in living donor transplants with use of unrelated donors, in which HLA mismatch is more the rule than the exception.[20]

Nevertheless, registry data confirm that the fewer HLA mismatches, the better the long-term graft survival, especially for donor-recipient pairs with zero mismatches.[67] The effect of HLA mismatches on graft survival persists after correction for acute rejection in multivariate analysis. Some studies have found a particularly negative effect of mismatch at the DR locus.[68] This relationship of HLA matching and long-term graft survival is a line of evidence for an immunologic element in IF/TA.[46] The effect of HLA matching is much less pronounced in living donor recipients. Recent analyses do suggest, however, that the better the HLA match, the lesser the sensitizing effect of graft loss. The overall body of evidence suggests that HLA matching continues to be an important determinant of long-term graft survival.

Waiting Time and Preemptive Transplantation

An analysis of USRDS data shows that a longer waiting time on dialysis is a significant risk factor for both death-censored graft survival and patient death with functioning graft after renal transplantation. Relative to preemptive transplantation, increasing waiting times incrementally increased both mortality risk and risk for death-censored graft survival after transplantation.[69]

In a retrospective cohort study of 8481 patients, preemptive transplantation was associated with a 52% reduction in the relative hazard for graft failure in the first year after transplantation, 82% in the second year, and 86% in the subsequent year compared with transplantation occurring after the start of dialysis.[70] Increasing duration of dialysis before transplantation significantly increased the risk for acute rejection within the first 6 months after transplantation.[70] Paired kidney studies can minimize the confounding effect of donor-related factors; in a paired kidney study involving 2405 pairs of kidneys, each kidney of each pair was transplanted into a recipient with differing times on ESRD.[71] Six antigen–matched kidneys were excluded from this study as a disproportionate number of these kidneys, through a national sharing program in the United States, were transplanted preemptively. Five-year and 10-year unadjusted graft survival and death-censored graft survival were significantly inferior in those subjects with more than 24 months of dialysis time versus those who incurred less than 6 months on dialysis (see Fig. 105.8).[69] These effects remained significant after adjustment for multiple factors that influence waiting time, such as high panel reactive antibody, advanced recipient age, and race. Part of the advantage of living donor compared with deceased donor transplantation may be explained by the effect of waiting time; a recipient of a deceased donor kidney with an ESRD time of less than 6 months may be expected to obtain graft survival roughly equivalent to that of living donor transplant recipients who wait for their transplant on dialysis for more than 2 years.[71]

The exact mechanisms for the benefits of preemptive transplantation are not clear, but alloreactivity is higher with increasing waiting time, an effect more pronounced in African Americans.[72]

The effect of time on dialysis is potentially modifiable in clinical practice. All patients with ESRD should be referred for transplantation in a timely manner, suitable candidates so identified should be listed as soon as possible, and preemptive transplantation before the start of dialysis should be the ideal goal.

Center Effect

Transplant outcomes vary widely between centers. This may reflect varying clinical expertise. However, mortality on the waiting list is the single biggest correlate of mortality after transplantation.[73] It is thus possible that centers with low waiting list mortality, either through selective listing of candidates or through other socioeconomic or geographic factors, may have lower post-transplantation mortality. It has been shown that centers with longest waiting times also have lower graft survival rates. Past performance and donor quality also significantly affect survival and are independent of center size. Center effects may contribute up to a 4-year difference in life expectancy. In the United States, centers with characteristics associated with good outcomes were distributed more or less uniformly across the country.[74]

Year of Transplant

As noted previously, long-term graft survival has not improved to the extent that might be expected on the basis of progressive reductions in acute rejection rates over the same time period.[17] However, it is slowly increasing, particularly among recipients of deceased donor kidneys. Factors influencing this gain in transplant survival have been attributed to varying contributions of more effective but not more toxic immunosuppressive regimens, better pretransplantation and post-transplantation general medical care, and more effective prevention and treatment of opportunistic infections (particularly cytomegalovirus infection).

Immunosuppressive Regimens

Choice of immunosuppressive regimen has significant effects on both patient and graft survival. The currently used regimens and the evidence supporting the clinician's choice are discussed in Chapter 100.

APPLYING OUTCOMES DATA IN PRACTICE

The clinician must use outcomes data derived from clinical trials or large observational studies to inform the care of individual patients. This is not straightforward; observational studies can only show associations, do not prove cause and effect, and do not necessarily imply that effects noted in aggregated studies translate automatically into expected outcomes in individual patients. The clinician should judiciously use data from both prospective and retrospectives studies in formulating the care of individual patients. However, the outcomes data discussed in this chapter lead to some broad principles for clinical practice.

Minimization of waiting time on dialysis or avoidance of dialysis altogether with preemptive transplantation is associated with the best outcomes. The best practice that can help optimize transplant outcomes is therefore early referral for transplantation and early identification of suitable living donors.

In the older recipient, careful attention must be directed to functional status, comorbidity, social support, and rehabilitation in the evaluation process, if the survival benefit of transplantation is to be maximized. Given the excess mortality of older people on the waiting list, identification of suitable living donors and consideration of methods to minimize waiting time, such as selective listing for ECD transplants and dual marginal kidneys, may be options to accrue the survival advantage of transplantation. The challenge is to balance equity, justice, and access so that the elderly transplant recipient receives an organ whose expected survival is optimal for the expected life span of the candidate.

Living donation should be maximized because it is associated with better transplant outcomes than with deceased donors, and this benefit is particularly prominent among some racial groups, including African Americans, who have otherwise inferior outcome with deceased donor transplantation than Caucasians do.

Other factors with major influence in graft and patient outcome are discussed elsewhere, including the choice of immunosuppressive regimen (Chapter 100) and maintenance of cardiovascular health in the transplant recipient (Chapter 102).

REFERENCES

1. United States Renal Data System. 2008 Annual Report. Available at: www.usrds.org.
2. Scientific Registry of Transplant Recipients. 2008 Annual Report. Available at: www.ustransplant.org.
3. United Network for Organ Sharing. 2008 Annual Report. Available at: www.unos.org.
4. Australia and New Zealand Dialysis and Transplant Registry; www.anzdata.org/au.
5. Kaplan B, Schold J, Meier-Kriesche HU. Overview of large database analysis in renal transplantation. *Am J Transplant*. 2003;3: 1052-1056.
6. Swinscow TDV, Campbell MJ. Survival analysis. In: Swinscow TDV, Campbell MJ, eds. *Statistics at Square One*. London: BMJ Books; 2002:126-134.
7. Katz MH. *Multivariable Analysis*. Cambridge: Cambridge University Press; 1999.
8. Opelz G, Mickey MR, Terasaki PI. Calculations on long-term graft and patient survival in human kidney transplantation. *Transplant Proc*. 1977;9:27-30.
9. Halloran PF, Gourishankar S, Vongwiwitana A, Weir MR. Approaching the renal transplant patient with deteriorating function: Progressive loss of function is not inevitable. In: Weir MR, ed. *Medical Management of Kidney Transplantation*. Philadelphia: Lippincott, Williams & Wilkins; 2005.
10. Solez K, Colvin RB, Racusen LC, et al. Banff 07 classification of renal allograft pathology: Updates and future directions. *Am J Transplant*. 2008;8:753-760.
11. Wolfe RA, Ashby VB, Milford EL, et al. Comparison of mortality in all patients on dialysis, patients on dialysis awaiting transplantation, and recipients of a first cadaveric transplant. *N Engl J Med*. 1999;341: 1725-1730.
12. Meier-Kriesche HU, Baliga R, Kaplan B. Decreased renal function is a strong risk factor for cardiovascular death after renal transplantation. *Transplantation*. 2003;75:1291-1295.
13. Schold JD, Kaplan B, Baliga RS, Meier-Kriesche HU. The broad spectrum of quality in deceased donor kidneys. *Am J Transplant*. 2005;5(pt 1):757-765.
14. Andreoni KA, Brayman KL, Guidinger MK, et al. Kidney and pancreas transplantation in the United States, 1996-2005. *Am J Transplant*. 2007;7(pt 2):1359-1375.
15. Hariharan S, Johnson CP, Bresnahan BA, et al. Improved graft survival after renal transplantation in the United States, 1988 to 1996. *N Engl J Med*. 2000;342:605-612.
16. Meier-Kriesche HU, Schold JD, Kaplan B. Long-term renal allograft survival: Have we made significant progress or is it time to rethink our analytic and therapeutic strategies? *Am J Transplant*. 2004;4: 1289-1295.
17. Meier-Kriesche HU, Schold JD, Srinivas TR, Kaplan B. Lack of improvement in renal allograft survival despite a marked decrease in acute rejection rates over the most recent era. *Am J Transplant*. 2004;4:378-383.
18. Magee CC, Chertow GM, Milford EL. Outcomes of renal transplantation. In: Feehally J, Floege J, Johnson RJ, eds. *Comprehensive Clinical Nephrology*. 3rd ed. Philadelphia: Mosby; 2007:1121-1129.
19. Kaplan B, Srinivas TR, Meier-Kriesche HU. Factors associated with long-term renal allograft survival. *Ther Drug Monit*. 2002;24:36-39.
20. Terasaki PI, Cecka JM, Gjertson DW, Takemoto S. High survival rates of kidney transplants from spousal and living unrelated donors. *N Engl J Med*. 1995;333:333-336.
21. Takemoto S, Terasaki PI. Donor age and recipient age. *Clin Transpl*. 1988;345-356.
22. Halloran PF, Melk A, Barth C. Rethinking chronic allograft nephropathy: The concept of accelerated senescence. *J Am Soc Nephrol*. 1999; 10:167-181.
23. Dharnidharka VR, Stevens G, Howard RJ. En-bloc kidney transplantation in the United states: An analysis of United Network of Organ Sharing (UNOS) data from 1987 to 2003. *Am J Transplant*. 2005;5: 1513-1517.

24. Salahudeen AK, Haider N, May W. Cold ischemia and the reduced long-term survival of cadaveric renal allografts. *Kidney Int.* 2004;65:713-718.
25. Brenner BM, Cohen RA, Milford EL. In renal transplantation, one size may not fit all. *J Am Soc Nephrol.* 1992;3:162-169.
26. Poggio ED, Hila S, Stephany B, et al. Donor kidney volume and outcomes following live donor kidney transplantation. *Am J Transplant.* 2006;6:616-624.
27. Hughson M, Farris AB 3rd, Douglas-Denton R, et al. Glomerular number and size in autopsy kidneys: The relationship to birth weight. *Kidney Int.* 2003;63:2113-2122.
28. Zeier M, Dohler B, Opelz G, Ritz E. The effect of donor gender on graft survival. *J Am Soc Nephrol.* 2002;13:2570-2576.
29. Neugarten J, Srinivas T, Tellis V, et al. The effect of donor gender on renal allograft survival. *J Am Soc Nephrol.* 1996;7:318-324.
30. Metzger RA, Delmonico FL, Feng S, et al. Expanded criteria donors for kidney transplantation. *Am J Transplant.* 2003;3(Suppl 4):114-125.
31. Ojo AO, Hanson JA, Meier-Kriesche H, et al. Survival in recipients of marginal cadaveric donor kidneys compared with other recipients and wait-listed transplant candidates. *J Am Soc Nephrol.* 2001;12:589-597.
32. Merion RM, Ashby VB, Wolfe RA, et al. Deceased-donor characteristics and the survival benefit of kidney transplantation. *JAMA.* 2005;294:2726-2733.
33. Cho YW, Terasaki PI, Cecka JM, Gjertson DW. Transplantation of kidneys from donors whose hearts have stopped beating. *N Engl J Med.* 1998;338:221-225.
34. Cooper JT, Chin LT, Krieger NR, et al. Donation after cardiac death: The University of Wisconsin experience with renal transplantation. *Am J Transplant.* 2004;4:1490-1494.
35. Schold J, Srinivas TR, Sehgal AR, Meier-Kriesche HU. Half of kidney transplant candidates who are older than 60 years now placed on the waiting list will die before receiving a deceased-donor transplant. *Clin J Am Soc Nephrol.* 2009;4:1239-1245.
36. Meier-Kriesche HU, Ojo AO, Cibrik DM, et al. Relationship of recipient age and development of chronic allograft failure. *Transplantation.* 2000;70:306-310.
37. Meier-Kriesche HU, Cibrik DM, Ojo AO, et al. Interaction between donor and recipient age in determining the risk of chronic renal allograft failure. *J Am Geriatr Soc.* 2002;50:14-17.
38. Meier-Kriesche HU, Ojo AO, Hanson JA, Kaplan B. Exponentially increased risk of infectious death in older renal transplant recipients. *Kidney Int.* 2001;59:1539-1543.
39. Meier-Kriesche HU, Ojo AO, Leichtman AB, et al. Effect of mycophenolate mofetil on long-term outcomes in African American renal transplant recipients. *J Am Soc Nephrol.* 2000;11:2366-2370.
40. Neylan JF. Effect of race and immunosuppression in renal transplantation: Three-year survival results from a US multicenter, randomized trial. FK506 Kidney Transplant Study Group. *Transplant Proc.* 1998;30:1355-1358.
41. Light JA, Barhyte DY, Lahman L. Kidney transplants in African Americans and non–African Americans: Equivalent outcomes with living but not deceased donors. *Transplant Proc.* 2005;37:699-700.
42. Rudge C, Johnson RJ, Fuggle SV, Forsythe JL. Renal transplantation in the United Kingdom for patients from ethnic minorities. *Transplantation.* 2007;83:1169-1173.
43. Cass A, Gillin AG, Horvath JS. End-stage renal disease in aboriginals in New South Wales: A very different picture to the Northern Territory. *Med J Aust.* 1999;171:407-410.
44. Kayler LK, Rasmussen CS, Dykstra DM, et al. Gender imbalance and outcomes in living donor renal transplantation in the United States. *Am J Transplant.* 2003;3:452-458.
45. Meier-Kriesche HU, Ojo AO, Leavey SF, et al. Gender differences in the risk for chronic renal allograft failure. *Transplantation.* 2001;71:429-432.
46. Terasaki PI. Humoral theory of transplantation. *Am J Transplant.* 2003;3:665-673.
47. Vo AA, Lukovsky M, Toyoda M, et al. Rituximab and intravenous immune globulin for desensitization during renal transplantation. *N Engl J Med.* 2008;359:242-251.
48. Meier-Kriesche HU, Ojo AO, Hanson JA, et al. Increased impact of acute rejection on chronic allograft failure in recent era. *Transplantation.* 2000;70:1098-1100.
49. Fabrizi F, Martin P, Dixit V, et al. Hepatitis C virus antibody status and survival after renal transplantation: Meta-analysis of observational studies. *Am J Transplant.* 2005;5:1452-1461.
50. Pereira BJ, Natov SN, Bouthot BA, et al. Effects of hepatitis C infection and renal transplantation on survival in end-stage renal disease. The New England Organ Bank Hepatitis C Study Group. *Kidney Int.* 1998;53:1374-1381.
51. Meier-Kriesche HU, Ojo AO, Hanson JA, Kaplan B. Hepatitis C antibody status and outcomes in renal transplant recipients. *Transplantation.* 2001;72:241-244.
52. Vlaminck H, Maes B, Evers G, et al. Prospective study on late consequences of subclinical non-compliance with immunosuppressive therapy in renal transplant patients. *Am J Transplant.* 2004;4:1509-1513.
53. Meier-Kriesche HU, Vaghela M, Thambuganipalle R, et al. The effect of body mass index on long-term renal allograft survival. *Transplantation.* 1999;68:1294-1297.
54. Meier-Kriesche HU, Arndorfer JA, Kaplan B. The impact of body mass index on renal transplant outcomes: A significant independent risk factor for graft failure and patient death. *Transplantation.* 2002;73:70-74.
55. Glanton CW, Kao TC, Cruess D, et al. Impact of renal transplantation on survival in end-stage renal disease patients with elevated body mass index. *Kidney Int.* 2003;63:647-653.
56. Schold JD, Srinivas TR, Guerra G, et al. A "weight-listing" paradox for candidates of renal transplantation? *Am J Transplant.* 2007;7:550-559.
57. Opelz G, Wujciak T, Ritz E. Association of chronic kidney graft failure with recipient blood pressure. Collaborative Transplant Study. *Kidney Int.* 1998;53:217-222.
58. Briganti EM, Russ GR, McNeil JJ, et al. Risk of renal allograft loss from recurrent glomerulonephritis. *N Engl J Med.* 2002;347:103-109.
59. Amer H, Fidler ME, Myslak M, et al. Proteinuria after kidney transplantation, relationship to allograft histology and survival. *Am J Transplant.* 2007;7:2748-2756.
60. Halloran PF, Hunsicker LG. Delayed graft function: State of the art, November 10-11, 2000. Summit meeting, Scottsdale, Arizona, USA. *Am J Transplant.* 2001;1:115-120.
61. Howard RJ, Pfaff WW, Brunson ME, et al. Increased incidence of rejection in patients with delayed graft function. *Clin Transplant.* 1994;8:527-531.
62. Shoskes DA, Cecka JM. Deleterious effects of delayed graft function in cadaveric renal transplant recipients independent of acute rejection. *Transplantation.* 1998;66:1697-1701.
63. Ojo AO, Wolfe RA, Held PJ, et al. Delayed graft function: Risk factors and implications for renal allograft survival. *Transplantation.* 1997;63:968-974.
64. Boom H, Mallat MJ, de Fijter JW, et al. Delayed graft function influences renal function, but not survival. *Kidney Int.* 2000;58:859-866.
65. Schold JD, Kaplan B, Howard RJ, et al. Are we frozen in time? Analysis of the utilization and efficacy of pulsatile perfusion in renal transplantation. *Am J Transplant.* 2005;5:1681-1688.
66. Moers C, Smits JM, Maathuis MH, et al. Machine perfusion or cold storage in deceased-donor kidney transplantation. *N Engl J Med.* 2009;360:7-19.
67. Held PJ, Kahan BD, Hunsicker LG, et al. The impact of HLA mismatches on the survival of first cadaveric kidney transplants. *N Engl J Med.* 1994;331:765-770.
68. Vereerstraeten P, Abramowicz D, De Pauw L, Kinnaert P. Experience with the Wujciak-Opelz allocation system in a single center: An increase in HLA-DR mismatching and in early occurring acute rejection episodes. *Transpl Int.* 1998;11:378-381.
69. Meier-Kriesche HU, Port FK, Ojo AO, et al. Effect of waiting time on renal transplant outcome. *Kidney Int.* 2000;58:1311-1317.
70. Mange KC, Joffe MM, Feldman HI. Effect of the use or nonuse of long-term dialysis on the subsequent survival of renal transplants from living donors. *N Engl J Med.* 2001;344:726-731.
71. Meier-Kriesche HU, Kaplan B. Waiting time on dialysis as the strongest modifiable risk factor for renal transplant outcomes: A paired donor kidney analysis. *Transplantation.* 2002;74:1377-1381.
72. Augustine JJ, Poggio ED, Clemente M, et al. Hemodialysis vintage, black ethnicity, and pretransplantation antidonor cellular immunity in kidney transplant recipients. *J Am Soc Nephrol.* 2007;18:1602-1606.
73. Schold JD, Srinivas TR, Howard RJ, et al. The association of candidate mortality rates with kidney transplant outcomes and center performance evaluations. *Transplantation.* 2008;85:1-6.
74. Schold JD, Harman JS, Chumbler NR, et al. The pivotal impact of center characteristics on survival of candidates listed for deceased donor kidney transplantation. *Med Care.* 2009;47:146-153.

CHAPTER 106

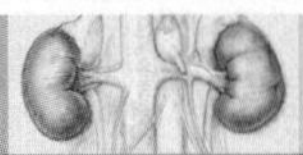

Pancreas and Islet Transplantation

Jonathan S. Fisher, M. Reza Mirbolooki, Jonathan R.T. Lakey, R. Paul Robertson, Christopher L. Marsh

Pancreas transplants are performed for the amelioration of insulin-requiring diabetes. Initially, pancreas transplants were performed only in those diabetic patients with chronic kidney disease who needed kidney transplants; these patients underwent simultaneous pancreas-kidney transplantation (SPK). Today, pancreas transplantation alone (PTA) or pancreas transplantation after living related or unrelated kidney transplantation (PAK) is increasingly common. SPK accounted for 67% of all pancreas transplants in 2006 (Fig. 106.1). The 2007 Annual Report of the Organ Procurement and Transplantation Network (OPTN) and the Scientific Registry of Transplant Recipients (SRTR) reveals that the number of pancreata recovered in the United States for 2006 increased by 53% compared with 1997, and there were approximately 4000 people in the United States waiting for pancreas transplants at the end of 2006.[1] Interestingly, there have been recent downward trends in numbers of patients registered for pancreas transplants. New SPK registrations rose from 1412 in 1997 to a high of 2007 in 2000 and declined to 1671 in 2006. Some of this reduction may be due to an increase in the number of patients receiving islet cell transplants. The relative roles of pancreas and islet cell transplantation remain controversial.

PATIENT SELECTION CRITERIA FOR PANCREAS OR ISLET TRANSPLANTATION

Indications for Transplantation

Indications for pancreas or islet transplantation include (1) insulin-dependent diabetes with associated diabetic complications (nephropathy, neuropathy, and retinopathy) and (2) diabetes with episodes of hypoglycemic unawareness.

A number of factors influence the choice between pancreas transplant and islet transplant. Because giving sufficient islets remains a limiting factor, islet transplants are more appropriate for patients with smaller insulin requirements, typically slender women. Larger patients (usually with higher insulin requirements) are more reliably served with whole-organ pancreas transplants. Islet transplantation is performed by a radiographic procedure and therefore is better suited for patients who cannot tolerate the surgical stress of whole-organ transplantation, such as older patients with severe coronary artery disease.

Pancreas or islet transplantations are not routinely performed for type 2 diabetes mellitus because the defect in type 2 diabetes is insulin resistance, not insulin deficiency. There may be a role for pancreas transplantation in type 2 diabetic patients who develop islet failure after years of insulin resistance.

Most of the pancreata for transplantation come from deceased donors. However, one approach to increasing the donor supply has involved living donor laparoscopic distal pancreatectomy with or without simultaneous laparoscopic nephrectomy.[2]

Should living kidney donor recipients be offered a PAK transplant? An analysis of the United Network for Organ Sharing (UNOS) database revealed no difference in survival of SPK recipients and living kidney donor recipients at up to 8 years of follow-up.[3] However, a European study showed an improved 10-year patient survival (83% in SPK versus 70% in kidney transplants alone) and noted a significantly lower progression of macrovascular disease (cerebrovascular, coronary, and peripheral vascular) with SPK transplants.[4] Therefore, the two-stage approach of PAK after a living donor kidney transplant should perhaps be offered to patients who have a living kidney donor and in whom the cardiovascular risk of the extended procedure required for SPK is considered too great.

The role of PTA transplants in those with preserved renal function has recently been questioned. A single-center study of 131 PTA recipients revealed that PTA is an independent risk factor for the development of renal failure, presumably because of the nephrotoxicity of long-term immunosuppression.[5] An analysis of the UNOS database demonstrated worse survival for those with diabetes and preserved kidney function receiving a PTA than for those who remained on the waiting list and received conventional therapy.[6] The recent SRTR data reveal 1-year patient survival rates similar for PAK, SPK, and PTA recipients (ranging from 95% to 97%). However, the 10-year patient survival rate was lowest for PAK recipients at 64% and similar for SPK and PTA recipients with rates of 70% and 71%. SPK transplants experienced the best pancreas graft survival rates, 86% at 1 year and 54% at 10 years. Graft survival rates for PAK and PTA recipients were similar to one another, with 1-year rates of 79% and 80%, respectively, and 10-year rates of 29% and 27%, respectively (Fig. 106.2).[1] Further close study is warranted, keeping in mind that a prospective, randomized trial of pancreas transplantation versus conservative therapy is not practical.

Medical Evaluation

The medical evaluation for the prospective pancreas transplant candidate is similar to that of the kidney-only recipient (see Chapter 98), although the cardiac workup is more extensive. The best candidates for transplantation are younger than 50 years and have a limited number of major complications of diabetes, such as hypoglycemic unawareness or diabetic neuropathy. Additional

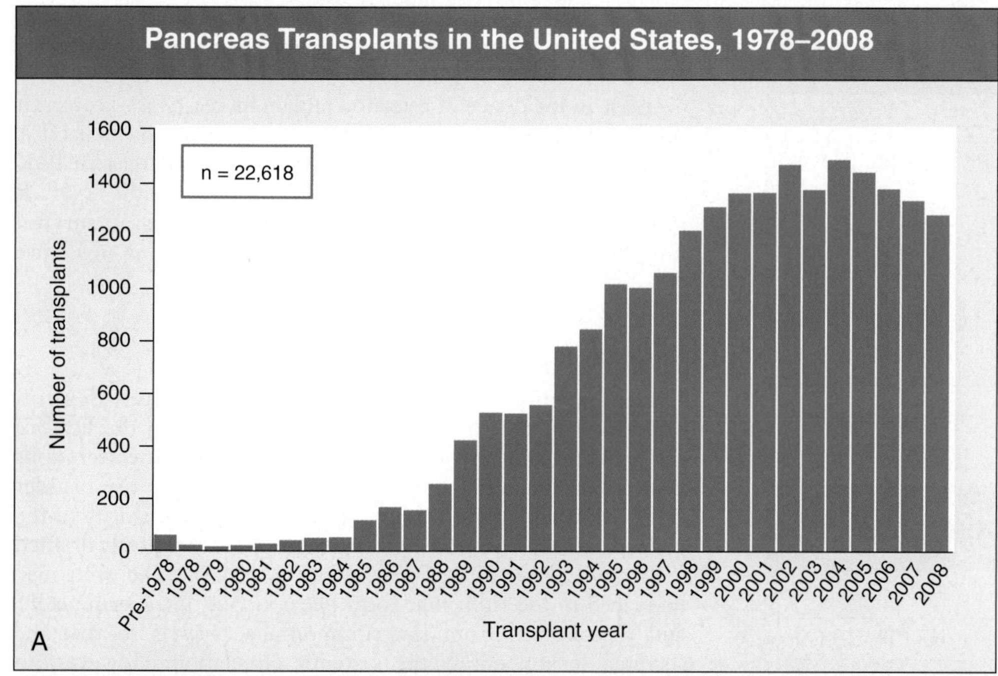

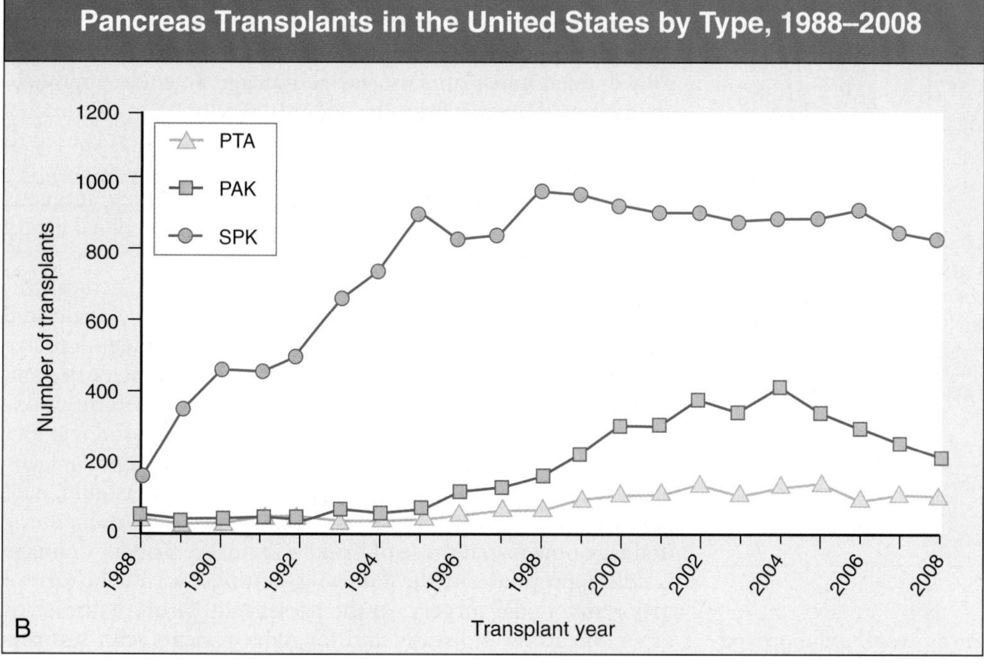

Figure 106.1 Pancreas transplantation. A, Number of recipients living in the United States with a functioning pancreas transplant at end of year, 1978-2008. **B,** Pancreas transplants by type in the United States, 1988-2008. PTA, pancreas transplantation alone; PAK, pancreas transplantation after living related or unrelated kidney transplantation; SPK, simultaneous pancreas-kidney transplantation. *(From reference 7.)*

complications, such as vascular disease, orthostatic hypotension, and severe gastroparesis, put patients at higher risk of post-transplantation complications, but none of these factors by themselves exclude a patient from transplantation. Cardiovascular status is the primary deciding factor for transplantation eligibility because the surgery, infections, risk of thrombotic complications, and, until recently, rejection are more severe in the pancreas transplant recipient, demanding that the cardiovascular system be strong enough to withstand multiple prolonged, hemodynamically stressful events. All patients require noninvasive cardiac stress evaluation because of the limited exercise capabilities of many patients. Cardiac catheterization is performed on the basis of the results of noninvasive testing or performed first for high-risk patients, typically those older than 45 years, those with diabetes duration of more than 25 years, smokers of more than 5 pack-years, and those with an abnormal electrocardiogram. Peripheral vascular disease is evaluated by clinical examination and by arterial duplex ultrasound. Patients with limb-threatening ischemia are typically poor pancreas transplant candidates. The medical evaluation for islet transplantation is similar to that for pancreas transplantation, but exclusion criteria are fewer because of lower surgical and inflammatory risks.

The last criteria for transplantation are that the donor and recipient match for ABO blood group and that the recipient sera are crossmatch negative against donor T cells by either the standard antiglobulin or flow cytometry crossmatch.

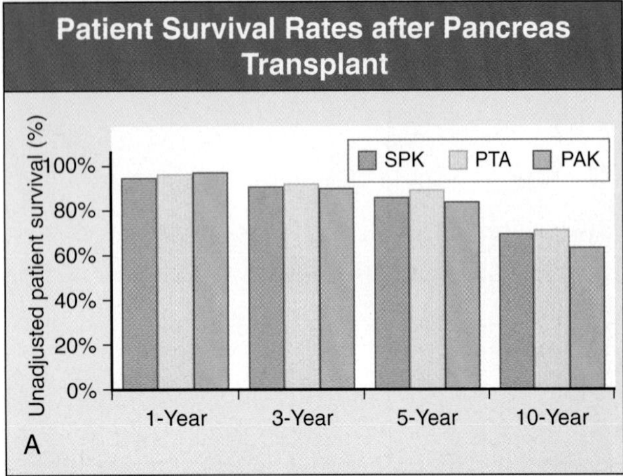

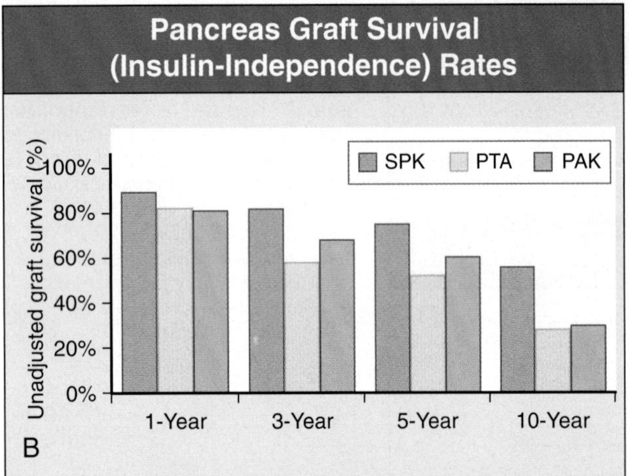

Figure 106.2 Patient and graft survival after pancreas transplantation. Unadjusted 1-, 3-, 5-, and 10-year pancreas patient and graft survival by type. **A,** Patient survival rates. **B,** Pancreas graft functional survival (insulin-independence) rates. PAK, pancreas transplantation after living related or unrelated kidney transplantation; PTA, pancreas transplantation alone; SPK, simultaneous pancreas-kidney transplantation. *(Redrawn from reference 1.)*

PANCREAS TRANSPLANTATION

Patient and Graft Survival

Pancreas graft survival rates have increased as a result of improved surgical techniques, improvement in the composition of the preservation fluid, and more effective immunosuppressive regimens, despite an increasing proportion of high-risk patients.

The most commonly used cold storage solution is the University of Wisconsin (UW) solution, which has increased early pancreas graft function and reduced the occurrence of preservation pancreatitis. A second cold storage solution, histidine-tryptophan-ketoglutarate (HTK), offers the advantages of better tissue perfusion due to lower viscosity, less reperfusion hyperkalemia, and significantly lower cost. However, studies have suggested a higher incidence of graft pancreatitis and an increased rate of graft loss with HTK, particularly with longer cold ischemic times.[8,9] Approaches using either a two-layer storage method with UW or an HTK solution and a second layer of highly oxygenated perfluorocarbon or the attachment of the pancreas to a low-pressure pulsatile perfusion system are being investigated.

The current gold standard immunosuppression for pancreas transplants is antibody induction therapy, tacrolimus, mycophenolate mofetil (MMF), and corticosteroids; this has led to a 40% decrease in incidence of rejection and an increase in 1-year graft survival to more than 90%.[9] UNOS registry data show that HLA matching has no effect on the outcome in SPK, whereas for PAK and PTA, a beneficial effect is seen by matching at the A and B loci.[10] The reported 1-, 3-, and 5-year patient and graft survival rates by use of these techniques and criteria are given in Figure 106.2.[1]

Surgical Procedure

Current practice is to transplant the whole pancreas with a cuff of duodenum, which preserves the blood supply of the head of the pancreas and provides a means to drain exocrine secretions into either the small bowel (enteric drainage) or the bladder (Figs. 106.3 and 106.4).[1] From 2004 to 2008, the majority of the pancreas transplants in the United States were enterically drained (SPK 85%, PAK 82%, PTA 78%; Fig. 106.5).[1] The graft may be placed in the right iliac fossa like a kidney, intraperitoneally, and vascularized from the common iliac vessels so that the secreted insulin enters the systemic circulation. However, an alternative is to construct the venous anastomosis to the superior mesenteric vein, allowing more physiologic insulin output through the portal circulation. Currently, 15% to 20% of enterically drained transplants use portal drainage. In either approach, an interposition graft from the donor (typically a Y graft containing common iliac with external and internal branches) is used to provide inflow from the recipient common iliac artery to the graft superior mesenteric and splenic arteries. Some surgeons have advocated reconnection of the graft gastroduodenal artery if the pancreaticoduodenal arcades are not intact.

Bladder drainage allows monitoring for rejection by measurement of urinary amylase and also avoids enterotomy-associated risks of infection and leak. The disadvantages of bladder drainage include susceptibility to dehydration, metabolic acidosis, and frequent bladder-related complications. Primary enteric drainage avoids these complications and is more physiologic but does not allow urinary amylase monitoring. With improved surgical techniques, increased use of real-time ultrasound, and percutaneous needle biopsy, the outcomes of portal enteric drainage now match those of bladder drainage. Bladder drainage is still appropriate in the following settings: with a history of major abdominal surgery; in the presence of Crohn's disease or other small bowel disease; and for older patients with less cardiovascular reserve, in whom a laparotomy may be avoided through a smaller lower quadrant retroperitoneal incision similar to that for a kidney transplant. Pancreas transplants with venous outflow to the superior mesenteric vein can be placed either anterior to the small bowel mesentery or in a retroperitoneal position behind the ascending colon, where the superior mesenteric vein is reached from the side. Surgical outcomes have not differed whether the venous drainage is systemic or portal. Although portal drainage is considered more physiologic and avoids hyperinsulinemia, these benefits are not well characterized.

Immunosuppression

Most centers use antibody induction therapy during the first 1 to 2 weeks after transplantation. OKT3 has largely been replaced by antithymocyte globulin (ATG).[11] Other centers use an

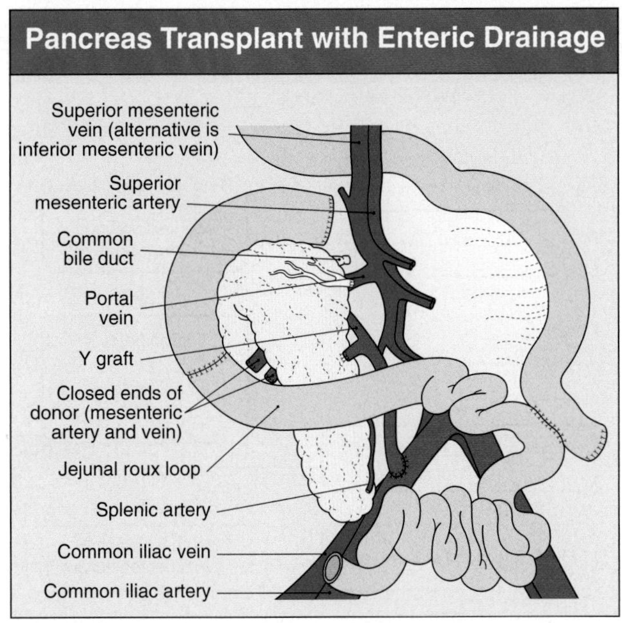

Figure 106.3 Pancreas transplant with enteric (portal) drainage.

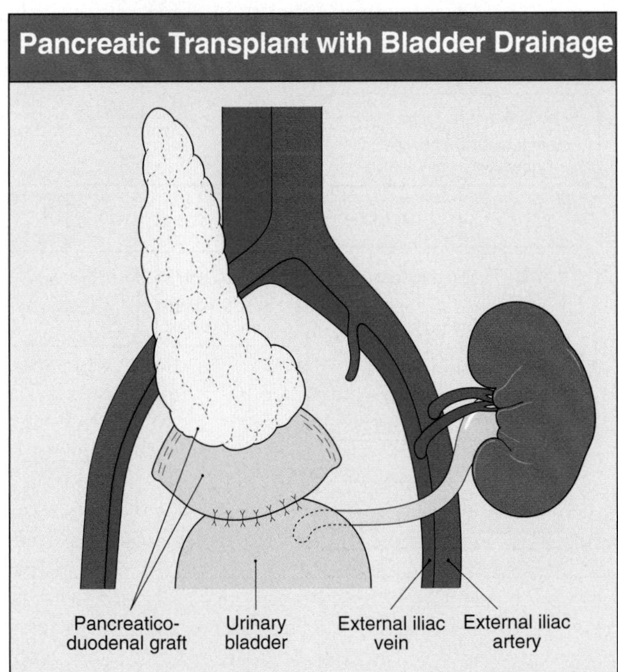

Figure 106.4 Pancreas transplant with bladder drainage. The pancreas may be placed in either the intraperitoneal or extraperitoneal position.

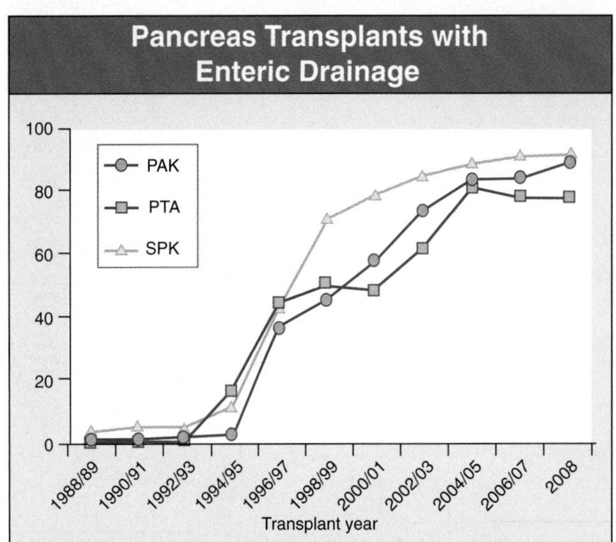

Figure 106.5 Pancreas transplant technique. Percentage of U.S. primary pancreas transplantations using enteric drainage, by recipient category and era, 1988-2008. There has been a shift toward enterically drained compared with bladder-drained pancreas transplantation. PAK, pancreas transplantation after living related or unrelated kidney transplantation; PTA, pancreas transplantation alone; SPK, simultaneous pancreas-kidney transplantation. *(Redrawn from reference 7.)*

interleukin-2 receptor antagonist (basiliximab, daclizumab) or, most recently, an anti-CD25 antibody (alemtuzumab).[12,13] Antibody-mediated rejection may be more common than acute cellular rejection in patients receiving alemtuzumab.[14] Most centers employ triple-drug maintenance immunosuppression with tacrolimus (or less commonly cyclosporine), MMF (or rarely azathioprine), and corticosteroids. There is increasing evidence of equivalent success with rapid corticosteroid elimination or corticosteroid avoidance protocols. Some centers replace the calcineurin inhibitor or MMF with sirolimus. With the more profound immunosuppressive induction produced by the newer antibodies (particularly alemtuzumab), there have been reports of immunosuppression protocols limited to a depleting antibody and a single additional agent.[13,15,16] Fortunately, cytomegalovirus (CMV) infection rates appear to be lower in corticosteroid-free regimens,[17] although there has been some increase in CMV infection in those receiving depleting antibody therapies.[12]

Graft Monitoring

The causes of pancreas graft dysfunction and the evaluation process are shown in Figures 106.6 to 106.8.

During the immediate perioperative phase, intravenous insulin is used to decrease the stress on the transplanted pancreas by maintaining serum glucose concentration around 100 to 120 mg/dl (5.5 to 6.6 mmol/l). Serum glucose values are not an early marker of pancreas dysfunction; elevations are observed only after significant parenchymal pancreatic damage has occurred. With bladder drainage, urinary amylase excretion is measured on 12-hour collections and reported as units per hour. During the first 1 to 2 weeks after transplantation, serum amylase may be elevated and urinary amylase decreased as a result of pancreatic preservation injury. Stable serum and urinary levels are usually attained within 2 weeks after transplantation. Thereafter, an elevated serum amylase or lipase concentration and a decreased urinary amylase concentration (typically by more than 20% of baseline) indicate possible graft injury, which must be evaluated. Both enterically drained and bladder-drained transplants may manifest elevated serum amylase and serum lipase concentrations, which are moderately sensitive markers of pancreas rejection. However, other conventional causes of pancreatitis can still occur. Elevated fasting glucose and 2-hour postprandial glucose levels are relatively late indicators and only indicate dysfunction without revealing cause.

Ultrasound examination of the pancreas transplant is performed frequently in the early post-transplantation period to rule

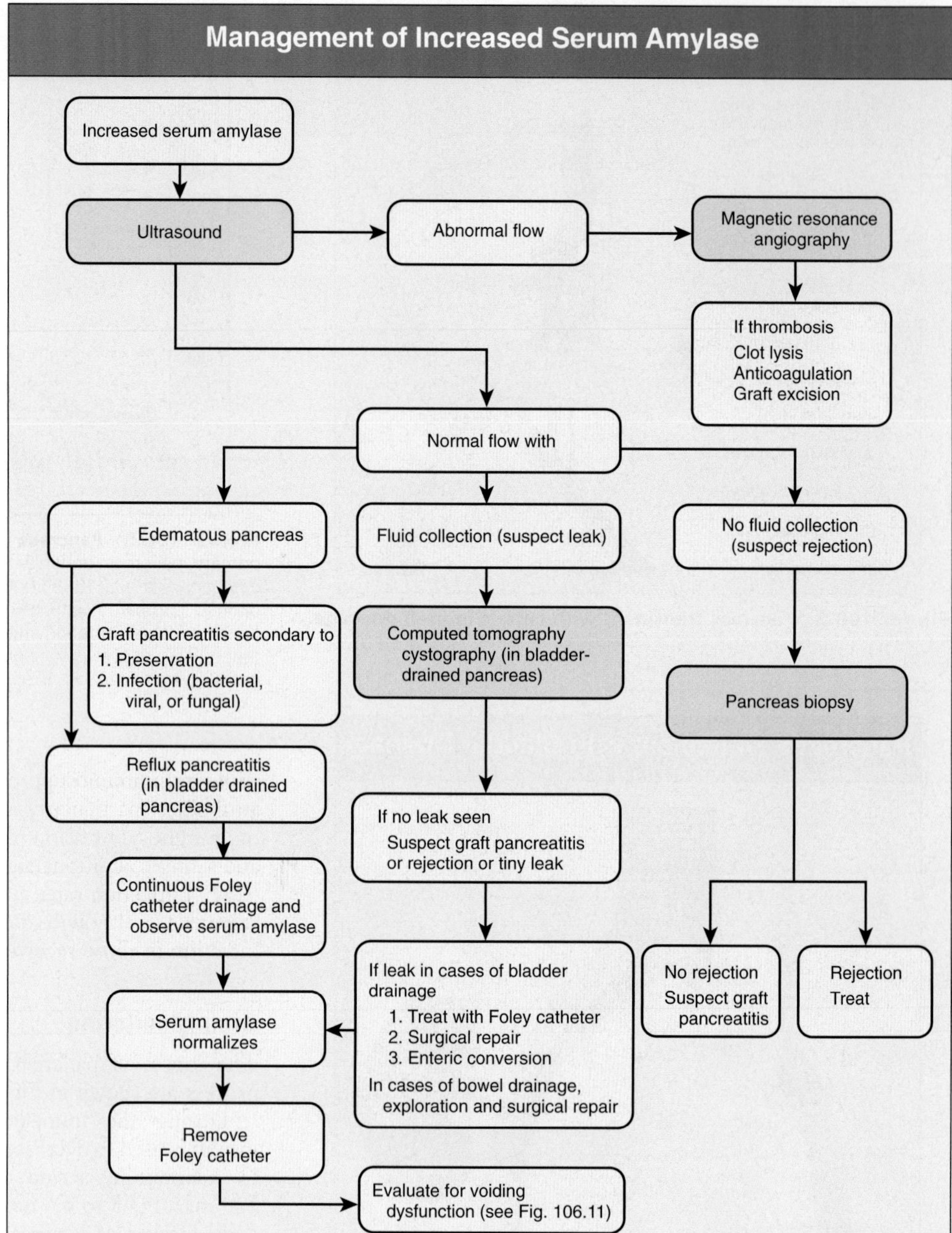

Figure 106.6 Management of increased serum amylase after pancreas transplantation.

out vascular thrombosis. If the pancreas cannot be well visualized by ultrasound scan, magnetic resonance imaging and angiography may be informative. Any inflammatory state can also yield images of an edematous gland; however, other than for vascular thrombosis, imaging generally cannot reveal the cause of the dysfunction.

Biopsy of the pancreas transplant remains the gold standard for diagnosis of acute or chronic rejection. A biopsy may be performed at certain time points by protocol or at times of graft dysfunction to identify rejection or other causes of pancreatic injury before irreversible tissue damage has occurred. The easiest approach is a percutaneous biopsy with ultrasound or computed tomography guidance. Cystoscopic biopsy through the duodenal cuff is used in bladder-drained transplants if the percutaneous technique is not possible because of difficult visualization or overlying bowel.[18] The most frequent complication of percutaneous biopsy is a perigraft hematoma or transient hematuria, but rarely seen are pancreatitis, arteriovenous fistula, abdominal hemorrhage, bowel perforation requiring exploration, and even graft loss.

Treatment of pancreas rejection is similar to that of kidney rejection and generally involves pulse intravenous corticosteroids or antilymphocyte antibodies (see Chapter 100).

Treatment response is achieved by following the return of serum amylase and lipase or urinary amylase to baseline values. Imaging can be used to show resolution of edema and inflammation. Repeated biopsy, usually at a 2-week interval, is required to show resolution of more moderate or severe rejections and to look for histologic signs of the development of chronic rejection.

Causes of Pancreas Graft Dysfunction
Rejection
Ductal obstruction
Vascular: arterial/venous thrombosis (partial/complete), arteriovenous fistula
Volume depletion
High calcineurin inhibitor levels
Graft pancreatitis (preservation, viral, bacterial, or fungal)
In cases of bladder drainage Reflux pancreatitis Urinary tract infection Anastomotic leak Bladder outflow obstruction
In cases of enteric drainage Anastomotic leak Bowel obstruction

Figure 106.7 Causes of pancreas graft dysfunction.

Evalution of Pancreas Graft Dysfunction

Assessment	Tests
Laboratory tests	Serum amylase, blood glucose human anodal trypsinogen, cyclosporine or tacrolimus levels, C-peptide In bladder-drained cases, urinary amylase and urine culture
Doppler ultrasound	Pancreatic blood flow, peripancreatic fluid collection, pancreatic ductal dilation In bladder-drained cases, evidence of bladder outlet obstruction
Computed tomography ± cystography	Looking for leak and collections; this is performed by cystography in bladder-drained cases

Figure 106.8 Evaluation of pancreas graft dysfunction.

Patients with isolated pancreas rejection have an increased risk for kidney graft loss, supporting the concordance of acute rejection in the majority of patients.[19] In SPK or PAK patients, when biopsy of the pancreas cannot be performed safely, a kidney transplant biopsy may be used as a surrogate indicator in conjunction with serum and urine tests.

Antimicrobial Prophylaxis

Antimicrobial prophylaxis is much like that for a kidney transplant alone. Trimethoprim-sulfamethoxazole is prescribed for the prevention of urinary tract infections and *Pneumocystis* infection. Oral clotrimazole or nystatin is used for the prevention of oral candidiasis; some centers use fluconazole for prophylaxis of *Candida* urinary tract infections and intra-abdominal fungal or yeast infections. Oral acyclovir is given to patients with a history of herpes simplex infection and to patients who are CMV negative and receive CMV-negative donor organs. Otherwise, valacyclovir or ganciclovir is given for 3 months after transplantation to all patients who are CMV positive or who receive CMV-positive organs. Patients treated for rejection are typically returned to any discontinued anti-infectious prophylaxis for 1 to 3 months after rejection therapy.

Metabolic Monitoring

In addition to monitoring of the serum and urinary concentrations of amylase and the serum concentration of lipase, serum creatinine, potassium, magnesium, and bicarbonate levels must be monitored. Magnesium wasting is common with calcineurin inhibitors and frequently requires oral supplementation. With bladder drainage, there is high urinary loss of bicarbonate in pancreatic exocrine secretions, which may require as much as 130 mmol/day of replacement. Without replacement, patients develop metabolic acidosis with nausea and vomiting, which may lead to volume depletion, hypotension (exacerbated by underlying autonomic neuropathy), and graft thrombosis. Oral sodium bicarbonate, typically 2 g four times daily, is needed. Fluid intake should be 2.5 to 3 l/day to accommodate pancreatic and renal fluid outputs. This intake may be difficult to achieve because abdominal bloating from diabetic gastroparesis is exacerbated by the large fluid intake and the gas released from sodium bicarbonate tablets. Patients who are unable to maintain adequate oral intake may require intravenous fluids including sodium bicarbonate. In patients who require intravenous repletion for longer than 1 month, consideration should be given to placement of a tunneled venous catheter or a buried central venous port for fluid administration.

Surgical Complications

Surgical complications of pancreas transplantation are shown in Figure 106.9. Superficial infections and deep-seated abscesses are commonly fungal. The source of fungal contamination is thought to be the duodenal segment. Therefore, topical antibiotic and antifungal solutions are used to irrigate the donor duodenum during procurement and implantation. Patients commonly receive 24 to 48 hours of postoperative antibiotics and fluconazole.

The causes of wound drainage are seroma, lymphocele, pancreatic fistula from either the tail or the anastomosis to the bladder or bowel, wound dehiscence, and preservation pancreatitis. Preservation pancreatitis may lead to wound drainage of whitish yellow, thick, noninfectious material formed from the enzymatic digestion of tissue, leading to fat necrosis and saponification. Wound drainage is seen more often with the extraperitoneal placement of the pancreas and also occurs when a pancreas from an obese donor is used. It is also associated with a mild increase in serum amylase concentration, low urinary amylase excretion, and variable changes in the serum glucose concentration.

Vascular complications occur in about 5% of patients and include arteriovenous fistulas due to surgery or biopsy, venous and arterial thrombosis, and rarely mycotic aneurysms. The pancreas is a low blood flow organ; vascular thrombosis rates were previously as high as 10%, but current rates are below 5%. Means of reducing the rate of thrombosis include minimization of warm and cold ischemia, procurement procedures involving a no-touch technique using the duodenum and spleen as handles, and postoperative antiplatelet activity with aspirin. In cases with longer cold ischemia times, a more edematous graft, or concern about low inflow or outflow, intravenous heparin is sometimes used for the first few postoperative days. Partial thrombosis

Surgical Complications Following Pancreas Transplantation

Type of Complication	Presentation	Diagnostic Findings and Testing	Treatment Options
Abscess	Fever, erythema of wound, wound drainage	Elevated white cell count (WBC), fluid collection on computed tomography (CT) scan, pus on aspiration	Open or percutaneous drainage
Graft pancreatitis	Pain over allograft, lower abdominal pain	Elevated serum amylase, enlarged pancreas allograft	Octreotide or somatostatin Foley catheter if bladder drained
Lymphocele	Mass on palpation, urgency if bladder compression	Fluid collection on CT scan, clear fluid on aspiration	Open or percutaneous drainage
Wound drainage	Pancreatic goo, no erythema	Culture, CT scan to rule out deep abscess	Local wound care
Dehiscence	Wound open		Wound care/surgical closure
Arterio venous fistula	Hematuria, abdominal bleeding	Doppler ultrasound, angiography	Embolization, surgical repair
Graft thrombosis	Elevated blood sugars Bloody urine if bladder drained	Low serum and urine amylase, sepsis-like syndrome, ultrasound or magnetic resonance imaging	If partial, thrombolytic therapy or anticoagulation (high risk of bleeding), graft pancreatectomy
Pancreatic fistula/leak (bowel drained)	Pain over allograft, sepsis, peritonitis, fever	Elevated WBC, fluid collection on CT scan	Surgical drainage and repair

Figure 106.9 Surgical complications following pancreas transplantation.

may resolve with thrombolytic therapy or anticoagulation. More extensive thrombosis requires urgent surgical intervention. Complete graft thrombosis, especially in the immediate postoperative period, mandates urgent graft removal to prevent sepsis syndrome or a more diffuse hypercoagulable state, leading to further vascular thrombotic complications such as myocardial infarction.

Nonsurgical Complications

Nausea and vomiting are common, and causes include gastroparesis, constipation, cholelithiasis or esophageal reflux developing from motility problems, and esophagitis with or without CMV disease. Antiemetics plus histamine H_2 blockers or proton pump inhibitors are usually effective therapy and are given for 2 to 3 months after transplantation. Persistent symptoms may require prokinetic agents (metoclopramide or erythromycin). Diarrhea can be caused by immunosuppressive medications, intrinsic gut motility problems, food intolerance, or CMV or other infection. Constipation is treated with increased fluid intake, dietary modification, increased activity, and regular low-dose schedule of stool softeners or laxatives.

Orthostatic hypotension may worsen after transplantation as a consequence of prolonged bed rest in the presence of diabetic autonomic neuropathy. Treatment may include a salt-loading diet, with a mineralocorticoid (fludrocortisone) or an α-adrenergic agonist (midodrine).[20]

Urologic Complications

Urologic complications are common after bladder drainage (Fig. 106.10).[21] Pretransplantation bladder dysfunction due to diabetic autonomic neuropathy causes a large-capacity bladder, decreased bladder sensation, increased residual urine volume, and decreased urinary flow rates. Bladder function is worsened by the autoaugmentation of the bladder by the added duodenal segment. Preoperative urodynamics are abnormal in up to 43% of patients but do not predict post-transplantation urologic complications such as reflux pancreatitis or infections.[22]

Urinalysis is difficult to interpret with the bladder-drained pancreas. The urine contains white cells from duodenal mucosal sloughing and may be leukocyte esterase positive without bacteriuria. Urine protein excretion is elevated to 1 to 3 g/day in most patients, composed of pancreatic enzymes, immunoglobulins, other globulins, albumin, and digested fragments of these proteins. Urinary albumin, if it is measurable in the presence of enzymatic degradation, may come from the transplanted or native kidneys.

Macroscopic hematuria occurs in up to 28% of bladder-drained pancreas recipients. Early hematuria is related to surgical trauma to the bladder or duodenal mucosa near the cystoduodenostomy site and usually clears with diuresis or bladder irrigation.[20] Continuous bladder irrigation requires caution because the cystoduodenostomy is vulnerable to rupture if the drainage catheter becomes obstructed. Late hematuria, beyond 2 to 4 weeks after transplantation, can arise from anastomotic bleeding, duodenal mucosal sloughing or ulceration, reflux pancreatitis, cystitis, graft thrombosis, rarely arteriovenous fistulas, and pseudoaneurysms. Evaluation should include ultrasound, urine culture, and cystoscopy. If the pancreas appears to be the source on cystoscopy, biopsy of the pancreas may be required to determine the exact cause.

Microscopic hematuria should be evaluated. Evidence is sought for recurrent disease, new renal disease, or genitourinary malignant neoplasms.

Urinary Tract Infections

Risk factors for urinary tract infection after pancreas transplantation include large bladder capacity, incomplete bladder emptying, high bladder urine pH (due to pancreatic bicarbonate), bladder and urethral mucosal irritation from activated pancreatic

Urologic Complications of Bladder-Drained Pancreas Transplants

Complication	Etiology	Presentation	Evaluation	Treatment Options
Urinary tract infection (UTI)	Diabetic bladder dysfunction (DBD)	Asymptomatic, or dysuria, fever, sepsis	Urine culture; check postvoid residual, if elevated urodynamics	Culture-specified antibiotics, prophylactic antibiotics Female: double and timed voiding, clean intermittent catheterization (CIC) Male: α-adrenoceptor blockers to aid bladder emptying, CIC, bladder neck/prostate incision. If treatment failure enteric conversion: Foley catheter drainage
Reflux pancreatitis	DBD	Asymptomatic or pain over pancreas allograft, elevated serum amylase	Check serum amylase, computed tomography (CT) cystogram to exclude leak or duct obstruction	If DBD: double and timed voiding, CIC, α-blockers to aid bladder emptying. If multiple and symptomatic episodes: bladder neck/ prostate incision or enteric diversion
Duodenal cystotomy leak	Ischemic injury to duodenal cuff, cytomegalovirus or other infection, rejection, DBD	Pain over allograft, or peritonitis, elevated serum amylase	Check serum amylase, elevated creatinine, leak on CT cystogram	Foley catheter drainage, if small If early, open surgical repair with resection and closure of layers, evaluate for DBD post recovery. If late, consider enteric conversion
Urethritis/dysuria syndrome, occasional urethral disruption	UTI or DBD causing activation of pancreatic enzymes with digestion of urethral mucosa	Dysuria, urinary retention, hematuria	Check postvoid residual, low-grade UTI; once recovered, evaluate for DBD	Foley catheter, analgesics, empirical treatment of UTI If multiple and symptomatic: enteric conversion

Figure 106.10 Urologic complications of bladder-drained pancreas transplants.

enzymes with the loss of mucosal barrier, prolonged bladder catheterization, and immunosuppression.[23] Most centers administer oral antibacterial and antifungal prophylaxis for up to 6 to 12 months or indefinitely after transplantation.

Urinary reflux pancreatitis, which causes pancreas graft dysfunction, may be associated with perigraft abdominal pain and fever. It is often a result of poor bladder function and requires drainage with a bladder catheter for 5 to 7 days and assessment of bladder dysfunction (Fig. 106.11).

A urethritis dysuria syndrome occurs in 2% to 8% of pancreas recipients with bladder drainage and is caused by uroepithelial exposure to the activated pancreatic proenzymes trypsinogen, chymotrypsinogen, and procarboxypeptidase. Pancreatic exocrine secretions consist of bicarbonate, amylase, lipase, and proenzymes, which are activated by the enterokinase in the graft duodenal brush border. Increased intravesical enzyme activation occurs with low-grade urinary infections and urinary stasis, and patients will develop voiding pain or penile, glandular, meatal, or vulval ulceration. Enzyme activation may be minimized by treatment of low-count bacteriuria, increase in fluid intake, and frequent voiding. If emptying does not improve with α-blockers, continuous Foley catheter drainage for 7 to 10 days has been effective.

Enteric Conversion

This is an option for most of the chronic urologic complications associated with bladder-drained pancreas transplantation. The indications are urethral disruption, recurrent urine leak, persistent bleeding, chronic urinary tract infection, dysuria, recurrent hypovolemia, and metabolic acidosis. The conversion rate varies from 8% to 14%. It is ideal to wait until 6 to 12 months after transplantation, when possible, to allow monitoring of urine amylase for early rejection episodes.

Late Complications

Late complications after pancreas transplantation typically fit into one of two patterns. There can be an acute presentation of graft rejection, not different from that seen in early graft dysfunction. The second pattern is more insidious; chronic inflammatory states from chronic rejection, ischemia, or infection may lead to gradual graft loss. Unfortunately, there is no practical test to measure small decrements in graft function in the way serum creatinine allows detection of kidney transplant dysfunction. Although it is lacking the necessary sensitivity, patients are typically asked to measure 2-hour postprandial glucose levels (which are more sensitive than fasting blood glucose levels) weekly and to report trends or sudden increases to the physician.

IMPACT OF PANCREAS TRANSPLANTATION ON DIABETIC COMPLICATIONS

Pancreas transplantation is performed to eliminate the need for exogenous insulin and the risk of severe hypoglycemic episodes and to stop or to reverse the consequences of hyperglycemia. Well-functioning pancreas transplants result in normal fasting blood glucose concentrations, normal glycated hemoglobin levels, and only slightly abnormal oral glucose tolerance testing.[24]

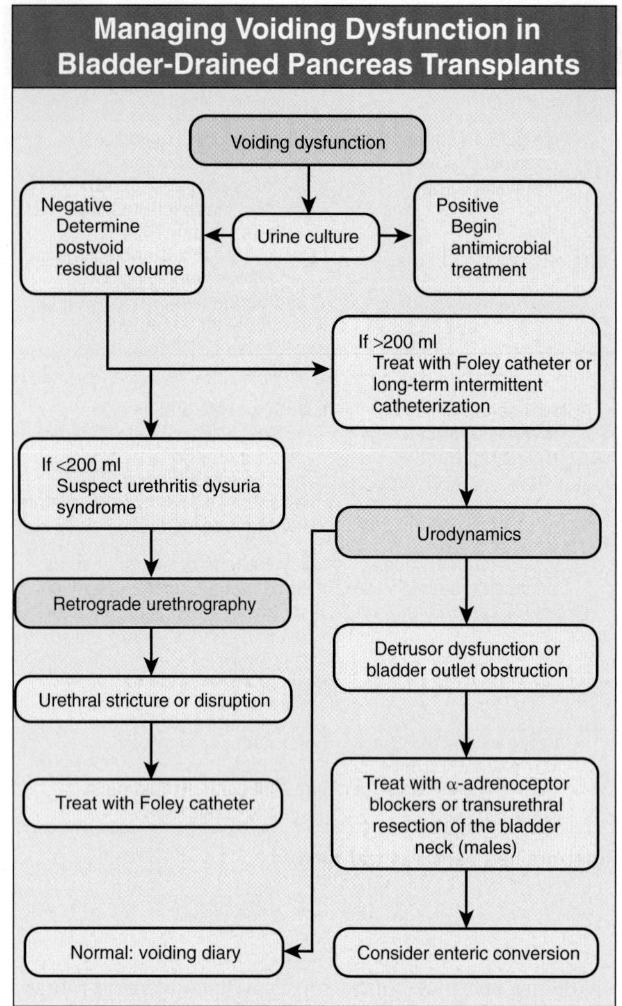

Figure 106.11 Management of post-transplantation voiding abnormalities. *(From reference 21.)*

Hypoglycemia

Although severe hypoglycemia is rare, mild hypoglycemia may develop in patients with a well-functioning pancreas graft once low baseline immunosuppression has been reached, especially in those patients who have regained little weight after transplantation and who are physically active. Postprandial hypoglycemic episodes are not always symptomatic. They are associated with high-carbohydrate meals, excessive intake of caffeine or alcohol, excessive exercise, and, in some patients with hypoglycemia, circulating anti-insulin antibodies. This is not often a significant clinical problem and is usually resolved by avoidance of carbohydrate-rich meals.

A major benefit of pancreas transplantation is restoration of glucagon secretory responses to hypoglycemia. In type 1 diabetics, the absence of functional β cells within the islet eliminates the normal physiologic response by which intra-islet insulin tonically dampens secretion of glucagon from α cells. Consequently, diabetic subjects are usually at risk of prolonged hypoglycemia secondary to injected insulin because there is failure of the normal counterregulatory action of glucagon on the liver to increase glycogenolysis. Despite the fact that the transplanted pancreas is placed ectopically and does not develop vagal control, the transplanted organ has normal glucagon responses to insulin-induced hypoglycemia and resultant counterregulation of hypoglycemia through increased hepatic glucose production. After pancreas transplantation, hypoglycemic awareness returns, as well as partial return of defective epinephrine secretion during insulin-induced hypoglycemia.

Hyperglycemia

Post-transplantation hyperglycemia may be caused by pancreas graft dysfunction, inadequate insulin release secondary to high tacrolimus or occasionally cyclosporine levels, resistance to insulin secondary to corticosteroids, weight gain, and inadequate physical activity. Although the use of tacrolimus has reduced pancreas graft rejection, it also decreases insulin gene transcription. If laboratory and imaging evaluations (see Fig. 106.8) are normal, hyperglycemia is the result of decreased insulin production or else of peripheral insulin resistance, which can be identified by measurement of glucose utilization rates and glucose/arginine-potentiated insulin secretion. In the absence of graft rejection, post-transplantation hyperglycemia should first be managed by dietary intervention and exercise. Insulin may be needed initially but can often be discontinued as oral hypoglycemic agents begin to take effect. Sulfonylureas are effective therapy. Hyperglycemia secondary to rejection is a late event and indicates irreversible graft damage. Because of the increased risk of rejection with manipulation of immunosuppression, minimizing the tacrolimus dose or changing to cyclosporine or sirolimus should not usually be considered until these measures have failed.

Microvascular Complications

Retinopathy

In a prospective funduscopic study of SPK patients during 45 months, there was a decreased need for post-transplantation laser therapy, and the diabetic retinopathy showed stabilization in 62%, improvement in 21%, and progression in 17%.[25] In the postoperative period, patients may develop neoproliferation and retinal hemorrhages if preoperative blood glucose control is very poor and blood glucose normalizes rapidly after transplantation. Patients remain at risk of retinal detachment because of scarring secondary to previous retinal damage. Cataracts are more common after transplantation.

Neuropathy

Sensory and motor nerve conduction velocities improve rapidly after pancreas transplantation and then stabilize.[26] Greater recovery is seen in nonobese, younger, shorter patients; in those with better initial action potential amplitudes; in those not receiving renal replacement therapy; and possibly in those receiving angiotensin-converting enzyme inhibitors or angiotensin receptor blockers.[27] The recovery of action potential amplitudes is gradual, continuing to improve up to 5 years beyond transplantation. Recovery is more complete in sensory than in motor nerves.

There is greater improvement in autonomic reactivity and gastric emptying in SPK recipients compared with diabetic kidney-only transplant recipients.[28] If autonomic symptoms are severe at the time of pancreas transplantation, improvement is unlikely.

Nephropathy

Early diabetic nephropathy is characterized by increased glomerular basement membrane thickness and an increase in mesangial volume. Renal transplant biopsy specimens from diabetics with SPK and kidney-only transplants within 2.5 years of transplantation show glomerular basement membrane thickness within the normal range. After 2.5 years from transplantation, 92% of renal biopsy specimens from the kidney-pancreas recipients have a normal glomerular basement membrane thickness compared with only 35% of the biopsy samples from the kidney-only recipients; relative mesangial volume was normal in 82% of the biopsy specimens from kidney-pancreas recipients compared with only 12% in the kidney-only recipients.[23] Thus, concurrent pancreas transplantation decreases the occurrence of the changes of diabetic nephropathy that may result in allograft loss.[29]

Vascular Disease

Successful kidney-pancreas transplantation results in a significant improvement in the control of hypertension compared with kidney transplant alone in type 1 diabetics.[30] Increase in peripheral vascular disease has been reported in kidney-pancreas transplant recipients compared with kidney-alone transplant recipients[31]; however, another study found the same prevalence of peripheral vascular disease after pancreas transplantation as occurred in diabetic kidney-only recipients who refused pancreas transplantation for nonmedical reasons and in nondiabetic kidney transplant recipients.[32] Encouragingly, one study showed that after a 10-year mean observation period, the progression of macrovascular diseases (cerebrovascular, coronary, and peripheral vascular) was significantly lower in recipients with a functioning SPK compared with a kidney transplant alone.[4]

A study using intravital microscopic evaluation of nail bed and conjunctival vasculature found improved vascularization (as assessed by a reduction in venular diameter, increased number of arterioles per unit area, and elevation of the perfusion capacity) only in kidney-pancreas recipients.[33]

Quality of Life and Social Issues

Pancreas transplantation is a very stressful event and can tax even the strongest of family relationships. Pretransplantation debilities (decreased vision, neuropathy, muscle weakness, orthostatic symptoms) can be exacerbated by the surgery and immunosuppressive medications. Patients who smoke or drink alcohol and are without family support do not survive as long after transplantation. However, kidney-pancreas transplant recipients with social support and well-functioning grafts report an increased global quality of life and frequently return to work, although the number returning to work is not much different from those receiving a kidney transplant alone.[34] In living donor simultaneous kidney-pancreas transplantation, preliminary results suggest a maintained level of quality of life for donors while recipients experience improvement.[35]

Pregnancy After Pancreas Transplantation

Within 1 year of transplantation, menstruation and ovulation return in most women of childbearing age. The United States National Transplantation Pregnancy Registry has reported 62 pregnancies in 40 SPK patients.[36] The outcomes were 50 live births, three therapeutic and 10 spontaneous abortions (one twin reduction), and one ectopic twin pregnancy. The newborn outcomes were prematurity (39 of 50), low birth weight (32 of 50), other neonatal complications (28 of 50), and neonatal death (1 of 50). Ten patients had rejections that resulted in grafts loss, and 58% of the patients required cesarean section. Hypertension, prematurity, preeclampsia, and growth retardation frequently complicated the pregnancies, even with good renal function. Gestational diabetes appeared in 3%.

All transplant recipient pregnancies require high-risk obstetric care. Consensus opinion is that pregnancy is safe by 1 year after transplantation under the following conditions: no rejection has occurred in the past year, graft function is stable, no active infections that could have a negative impact on the fetus (e.g., CMV infection) are present, and the patient is not taking any teratogenic medications.[37] MMF has been linked to structural malformations, and patients planning on conception should transition to another agent 6 weeks before trying to conceive.[38] Cyclosporine and tacrolimus levels often decline during pregnancy and require close monitoring to prevent rejection. Cesarean section is not mandatory; vaginal deliveries, however, must be observed for signs of allograft duodenal rupture. The average gestational period is 35 ± 2 weeks; the average birth weight is 2150 ± 680 g. There is no evidence that the children of transplant recipients are more likely to have abnormal development.

The management of other medical issues does not differ from that in kidney-only transplant recipients (see Chapters 101 and 102).

ISLET TRANSPLANTATION

Islet transplantation, with its reduced antigen load, technical simplicity, and low morbidity, has the potential to dramatically improve the quality of life of individuals with type 1 diabetes. The first series of islet allotransplantations in type 1 diabetic patients were reported in 1977.[39] There were then sporadic reports in the 1990s of insulin independence for extended periods after islet allotransplantation.[40,41] Autotransplantation studies then demonstrated that a critical mass of 300,000 IE (islet equivalents) could reestablish and maintain insulin independence beyond 2 years.[42] To date, the longest period of insulin independence after autotransplantation is more than 16 years.[43]

Islet After Kidney Transplantation

The initial allogeneic islet transplants in patients with type 1 diabetes were performed in the 1980s and 1990s in patients with end-stage renal disease as sequential islet after kidney (IAK) or simultaneous islet-kidney transplantation. Because the kidney transplant patients were already immunosuppressed, the IAK transplant procedure carried a minimal risk. However, there could be destabilization of the transplanted kidney and also islet dysfunction because most kidney transplant immunosuppression protocols included corticosteroids. Nevertheless, there were beneficial effects from improved glycemic control on both survival and function of transplanted kidneys.[44] Metabolic control (hemoglobin A_{1c} level and fasting glycemia) improved after IAK even in patients receiving low-dose corticosteroids. Adverse events included procedure-related pleural effusion and cholecystitis.[45]

Of the 237 well-documented allotransplants recorded in the Islet Transplant Registry from 1990 to 2000, less than 12% of recipients were insulin free at 1 year after transplantation. The reasons for this failure rate may include subtherapeutic islet implant mass, high rate of engraftment failure, islet damage in the liver (the site of implantation) by direct local toxic effects of the immunosuppressants, ineffective immunosuppression that fails to prevent rejection, recurrent autoimmune diabetes, and islet functional exhaustion. Four criteria were associated with insulin independence: (1) an islet implant mass of more than

6000 IE/kg, (2) a cold ischemia (preservation) time of less than 8 hours, (3) an induction therapy with polyclonal antibodies such as antilymphocyte globulin or thymoglobulin (ATG), and (4) the liver as the favored implantation site. Early immunosuppressive regimens were relatively ineffective in preventing allograft rejection compared with their effect on vascularized pancreas grafts. Most if not all immunosuppressive agents were associated with impaired β-cell function and reduced graft revascularization.

More success with insulin independence was reported in nonuremic type 1 diabetics transplanted with an average of 800,000 islets by use of the Edmonton protocol, a corticosteroid-free immunosuppression regimen of daclizumab, sirolimus, and low-dose tacrolimus. Although follow-up of this cohort has since confirmed long-term C-peptide production with therapy that is safe and well tolerated, insulin independence is maintained in only a minority.[45] There has since been an exponential increase in clinical islet transplant activity; more patients with type 1 diabetes have now received islet transplants in the past 5 years than in the entire preceding 30-year history of islet transplantation.

Technique of Islet Transplantation

The current technique of islet transplantation involves deceased donor pancreas procurement, organ preservation, enzymatic isolation of the islets, purification, and percutaneous injection of sterile islets into the liver through the portal vein by a catheter placed under radiographic guidance (Fig. 106.12). Although accessing of the portal vein percutaneously is relatively invasive, the entire procedure can be performed on an outpatient basis. Effective mechanical and physical methods to seal the catheter track reduce the risk of postprocedural bleeding.[46] Bleeding related to the procedure (23%), thrombus in segmental branches of the portal vein (8%), and punctured gallbladder (3%) are the most observed acute complications after islet transplantation.[47]

There is still a need for greater availability of transplantable islets as well as for improvement in islet engraftment and preservation. Although previous reports indicate that the two-layer method for pancreas preservation improves islet isolation outcome, our recent data show no beneficial effect of the two-

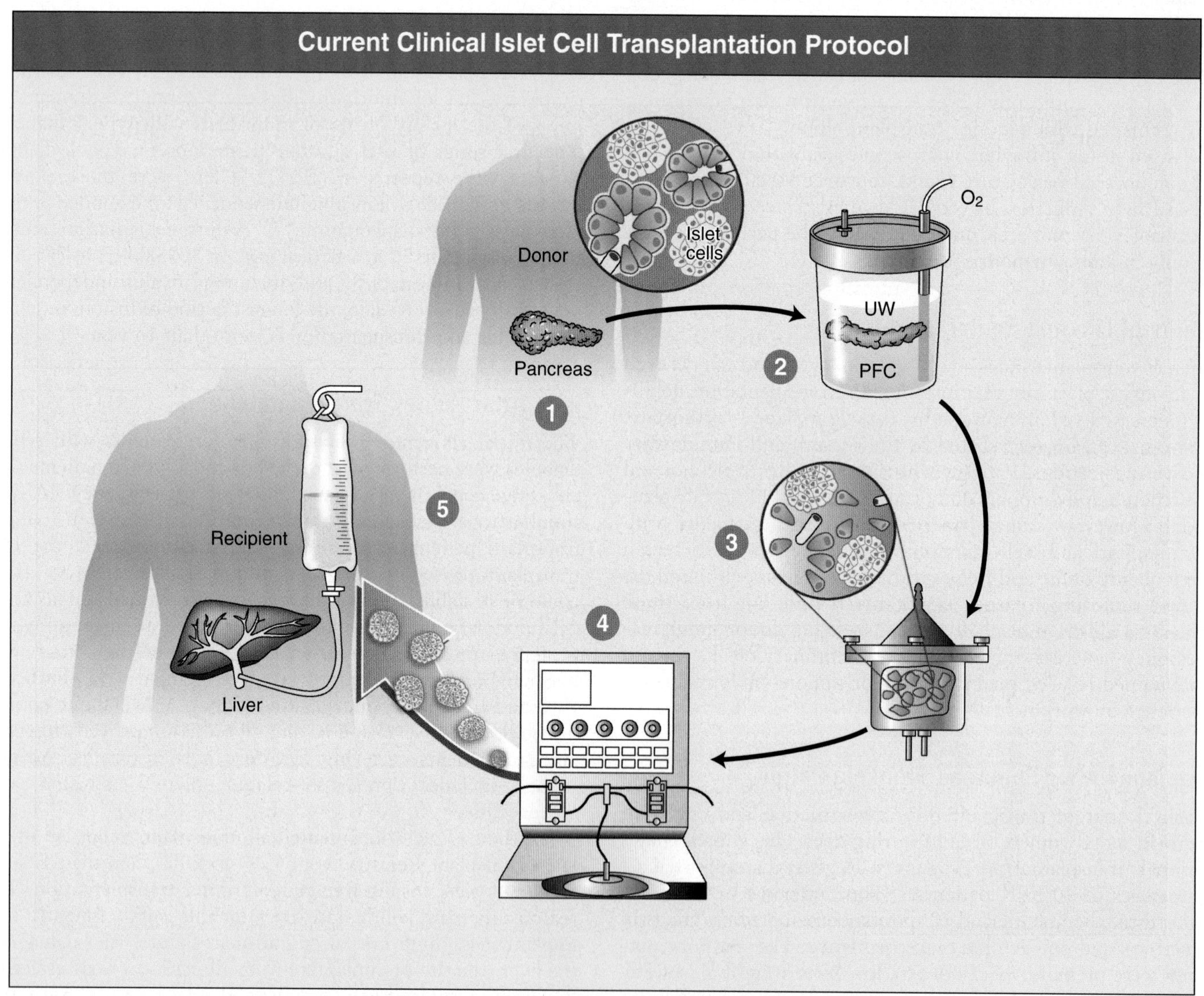

Figure 106.12 Current clinical islet cell transplantation protocol. The retrieved donor pancreas (1) is preserved (2) with a two-layer storage method using University of Wisconsin solution (UW) over a layer of highly oxygenated perfluorocarbon (PFC). The pancreas is distended with collagenase and placed in a digestion chamber (3). The disrupted exocrine and endocrine elements are purified by centrifugation (4), and the islet preparation free from exocrine elements is transplanted by intrahepatic portal vein infusion (5). *(Modified from reference 48.)*

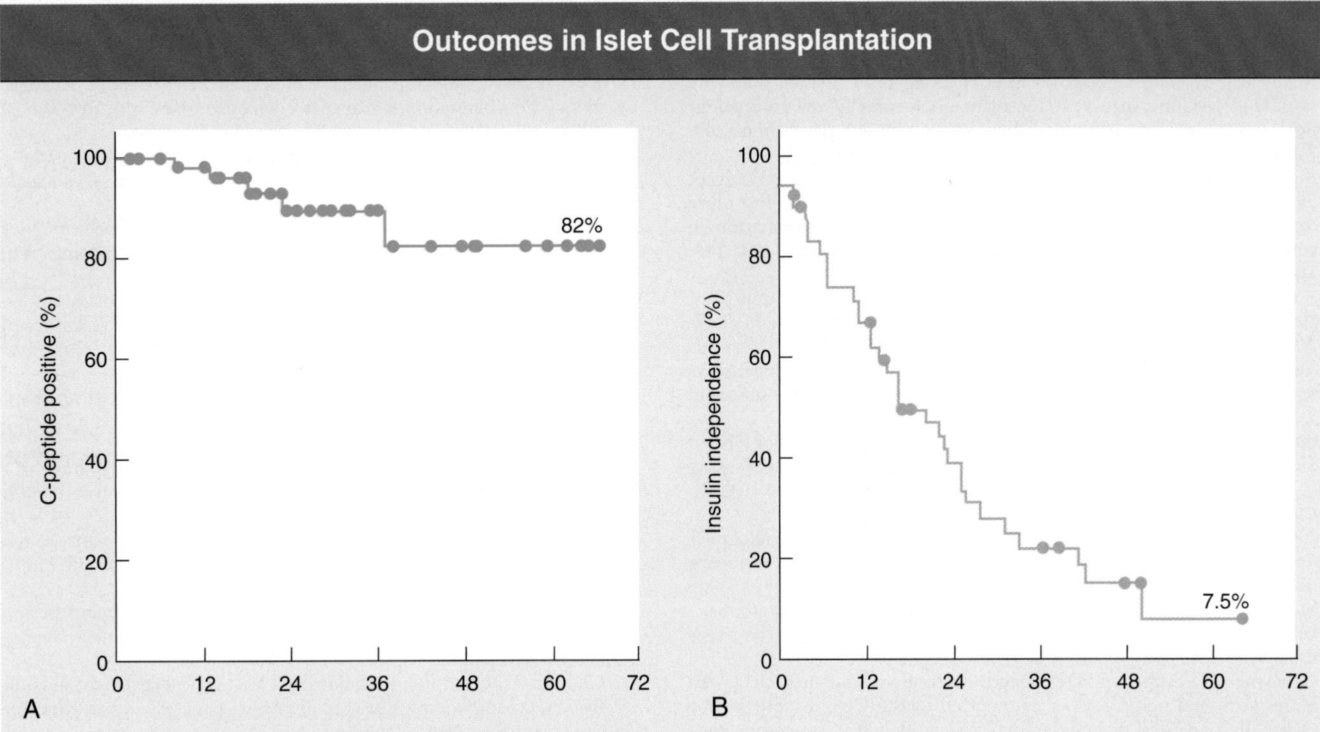

Figure 106.13 Outcomes in islet cell transplantation. A, Persistence of C-peptide secretion over time. The curves are dated from the time of the final transplant. **B,** Persistence of insulin independence over time. *(From reference 44.)*

layer method on islet isolation and transplantation outcomes.[46] Islet culture for 24 to 48 hours in antioxidant-enriched medium has improved the quality of islet preparations and facilitated the shipment of islets between centers.[47]

Medical Complications

There are also complications of islet transplantation that are not directly related to the procedure itself.[44] Changes consistent with fatty liver are reported in 22% of subjects who had magnetic resonance imaging after transplantation. Mouth ulcers occur in 90% of subjects, usually responding to simple antiseptic measures or topical triamcinolone ointment together with a reduction in the dose of sirolimus. Diarrhea (60%) and acne (52%) are frequent. Forty-three percent of recipients complained of edema, severe enough in 12% to necessitate a change in the immunosuppressive regimen. Weight loss is common.

Glycemic Control and Insulin Independence

Successful islet transplantation establishes normal hemoglobin A_{1c} levels, although the fasting glucose concentration tends to be slightly elevated, and there is often impaired glucose tolerance. Another difference between successful pancreas and islet transplants is that placement of islets within the liver results in failure of the α-cell response to hypoglycemia, even though there is responsiveness to intravenous arginine. In a recent analysis, 82% of 118 islet recipients in three North American centers were insulin free at 1 year.[47] However, in a 5-year follow-up in Edmonton,[41] only 7.5% maintained insulin independence, although 82% had detectable C-peptide (Fig. 106.13). The median duration of insulin independence was 15 months.

Immunosuppressive Regimens

Tacrolimus, cyclosporine, and corticosteroids are diabetogenic through increased peripheral insulin resistance or by direct islet cell toxicity. Oral administration increases portal venous drug concentrations and the possibility of significant injury to intrahepatic islet grafts. Most programs use corticosteroid-free and calcineurin inhibitor–sparing protocols for islet or kidney recipients with different combinations of MMF and sirolimus. MMF reduces early pancreas rejection rates. Insulin independence has now been achieved with islet grafts derived from non–heart-beating donors and after sequential kidney-islet transplantations using sirolimus-based therapy. Islet engraftment can also be improved with use of a calcineurin inhibitor–free regimen with profound T-cell depletion.[44] Anti–T cell therapy using ATG or OKT3 may be associated with a cytokine storm, which is toxic to islets, and newer induction agents (anti–interleukin-2 receptor blockers) may be particularly useful to minimize cytokine release.

A number of new immunosuppressive agents that offer the potential for more islet-friendly approaches are now entering clinical trials. These include combinations of biologic agents, such as ATG, rituximab, and alemtuzumab; novel anti–T cell biologic agents, some of which offer the prospect of inducing tolerance based on animal studies; and agents that produce costimulatory blockade.

REFERENCES

1. The 2007 Annual Report of the U.S. Organ Procurement and Transplantation Network and the Scientific Registry of Transplant Recipients: Transplant Data 1997-2006. Rockville, Md: Health Resources and Services Administration, Healthcare Systems Bureau, Division of Transplantation, chapter IV.

2. Tan M, Kandaswamy R, Sutherland DE, Gruessner RW. Laparoscopic donor distal pancreatectomy for living donor pancreas and pancreas-kidney transplantation. *Am J Transplant.* 2005;5:1966-1970.
3. Reddy KS, Stabelin D, Taranto S, et al. Long-term survival following simultaneous kidney-pancreas transplantation versus kidney transplantation alone in patients with type 1 diabetes mellitus and renal failure. *Am J Kidney Dis.* 2003;41:464-470.
4. Biesenbach G, Konigsrainer A, Gross C, Margreiter R. Progression of macrovascular diseases is reduced in type 1 diabetic patients after more than 5 years successful combined pancreas-kidney transplantation in comparison to kidney transplantation alone. *Transpl Int.* 2005;189: 1054-1060.
5. Scalea JR, Butler CC, Munivenkatappa BR, et al. Pancreas transplant alone as an independent risk factor for the development of renal failure: A retrospective study. *Transplantation.* 2008;86:1789-1794.
6. Venstrom JM, McBride MA, Rother KI, et al. Survival after pancreas transplantation in patients with diabetes and preserved kidney function. *JAMA.* 2003;290:2817-2823.
7. Gruessner AC, Sutherland DE. Pancreas transplant outcomes for United States [US] cases as reported to the United Network for Organ Sharing [UNOS] and the International Pancreas Transplant Registry [IPTR]. *Clin Transpl.* 2008;45-56.
8. Alonso D, Dunn TB, Rigley T, et al. Increased pancreatitis in allografts flushed with histidine-tryptophan-ketoglutarate solution: A cautionary tale. *Am J Transplant.* 2008;8:1942-1945.
9. Stewart ZA, Cameron AM, Singer AL, et al. Histidine-tryptophan-ketoglutarate (HTK) is associated with reduced graft survival in pancreas transplantation. *Am J Transplant.* 2008;8:1-5.
10. Gruessner AC, Sutherland DE. Pancreas transplant outcomes for United States (US) and non-US cases as reported to the United Network for Organ Sharing (UNOS) and the International Pancreas Transplant Registry (IPTR) as of June 2004. *Clin Transpl.* 2005;19:433-455.
11. Demartines N, Schiesser M, Clavien PA. An evidence-based analysis of simultaneous pancreas-kidney and pancreas transplantation alone. *Am J Transplant.* 2005;5:2668-2697.
12. Burke GW 3rd, Kaufman DB, Millis JM, et al. Prospective randomized trial of the effect of antibody induction in simultaneous pancreas and kidney transplantation: Three-year results. *Transplantation.* 2004;77: 1269-1275.
13. Kaufman DB, Levinthal JR, Gallon LG, et al. Alemtuzumab induction and prednisone-free maintenance immunotherapy in simultaneous pancreas-kidney transplantation comparison with rabbit antithymocyte globulin induction—long-term results. *Am J Transplant.* 2006;6: 331-339.
14. Pacual J, Pirsch JD, Odorico JS, et al. Alemtuzumab induction and antibody-mediated kidney rejection after simultaneous pancreas-kidney transplantation. *Transplantation.* 2009;87:125-132.
15. Gruessner RW, Kandaswamy R, Humar A, et al. Calcineurin inhibitor- and steroid-free immunosuppression in pancreas-kidney and solitary pancreas transplantation. *Transplantation.* 2005;79:1184-1189.
16. Thai NL. Khan A, Tom K, et al. Alemtuzumab induction and tacrolimus monotherapy in pancreas transplantation: One- and two-year outcomes. *Transplantation.* 2006;82:1621-1624.
17. Axelrod D, Leventhal JR, Gallon LG, et al. Reduction of CMV disease with steroid-free immunosuppression in simultaneous pancreas-kidney transplant recipients. *Am J Transplant.* 2005;5:1423-1429.
18. Perkins JD, Engen DE, Munn ST, et al. The value of cystoscopically-directed biopsy in human pancreaticoduodenal transplantation. *Clin Transpl.* 1989;3:306-315.
19. Kaplan B, West-Thielke P, Herren H, et al. Reported isolated pancreas rejection is associated with poor kidney outcomes in recipients of a simultaneous pancreas kidney transplant. *Transplantation.* 2008;9: 1229-1233.
20. Hurst GC, Somerville KT, Alloway RR, et al. Preliminary experience with midodrine in kidney/pancreas transplant patients with orthostatic hypotension. *Clin Transpl.* 2000;14:42-47.
21. Kuhr CS, Bakthavatsalam R, Marsh CL. Urologic aspects of kidney-pancreas transplantation. *Urol Clin North Am.* 2001;28:751-758.
22. Taylor RJ, Mays SD, Grothe TJ, Stratta RJ. Correlation of preoperative urodynamic findings to postoperative complications following pancreas transplantation. *J Urol.* 1993;150:1185-1188.
23. Smets YF, van der Pijl JW, van Dissel JT, et al. Infectious disease complications of simultaneous pancreas kidney transplantation. *Nephrol Dial Transplant.* 1997;12:764-771.
24. Robertson RP, Sutherland DE, Kendall DM, et al. Metabolic characterization of long term successful pancreas transplants in type I diabetes. *J Invest Med.* 1996;44:549-555.
25. Koznarova R, Saudek F, Sosna T, et al. Beneficial effect of pancreas and kidney transplantation on advanced diabetic retinopathy. *Cell Transplant.* 2000;9:903-908.
26. Allen RD, Al Harbi IS, Morris JG, et al. Diabetic neuropathy after pancreas transplantation: Determinants of recovery. *Transplantation.* 1997;63:830-838.
27. Hariharan S, Smith RD, Viero R, First MR: Diabetic neuropathy after renal transplantation. Clinical and pathologic features. *Transplantation.* 1996;62:632-635.
28. Hathaway DK, Abell T, Cardoso S, et al. Improvement in autonomic and gastric function following pancreas-kidney versus kidney-alone transplantation and the correlation with quality of life. *Transplantation.* 1994;57:816-822.
29. Fioretto P, Steffes MW, Sutherland DER, et al. Reversal of lesions of diabetic nephropathy after pancreas transplantation. *N Engl J Med.* 1998;339:69-75.
30. Elliot MD, Kapoor A, Parker MA, et al. Improvement in hypertension in patients with diabetes mellitus after kidney/pancreas transplantation. *Circulation.* 2001;104:563-569.
31. Morrissey PE, Shaffer D, Monaco AP, et al. Peripheral vascular disease after kidney-pancreas transplantation in diabetic patients with end-stage renal disease. *Arch Surg.* 1997;132:358-361.
32. Kausz A, Brunzell J, Marcovina S, et al. Lipid profile and peripheral vascular disease among diabetic patients receiving kidney-pancreas or kidney transplants. *J Am Soc Nephrol.* 1998;9:A680.
33. Cheung AT, Chen PC, Leshchinsky TV, et al. Improvement in conjunctival microangiopathy after simultaneous pancreas-kidney transplants. *Transplant Proc.* 1997;29:660-661.
34. Adang EM, Engel GL, van Hooff JP, Kootstra G. Comparison before and after transplantation of pancreas-kidney and pancreas-kidney with loss of pancreas: A prospective, controlled quality of life study. *Transplantation.* 1996;62:754-758.
35. Sukuzi A, Kenmochi T, Maruyama M, et al. Evaluation of quality of life after simultaneous pancreas and kidney transplantation from living donors using Short Form 36. *Transplant Proc.* 2008;40:2565-2567.
36. Armenti VT, Radomski JS, Moritz MJ, et al. Report from the National Transplantation Pregnancy Registry (NTPR): Outcome of pregnancy after transplantation. *Clin Transpl.* 2005;69-83.
37. Josephson MA, McKay DB. Considerations in the medical management of pregnancy in transplant recipients. *Adv Chronic Kidney Dis.* 2007;14: 156-157.
38. EBPG Expert Group on Renal Transplantation. European best practice guidelines for renal transplantation. Section IV. 10: Long-term management of the transplant recipient—pregnancy in renal transplant recipients. *Nephrol Dial Transplant.* 2002;17(Suppl 4):50.
39. Najarian JS, Sutherland DE, Matas AJ, et al. Human islet transplantation: A preliminary report. *Transplant Proc.* 1977;9:233-236.
40. Warnock GL, Kneteman NM, Ryan E, et al. Normoglycaemia after transplantation of freshly isolated and cryopreserved pancreatic islets in type 1 (insulin-dependent) diabetes mellitus. *Diabetologia.* 1991;34: 55-58.
41. Shapiro AM, Lakey JR, Ryan EA, et al. Islet transplantation in seven patients with type 1 diabetes mellitus using a glucocorticoid-free immunosuppressive regimen. *N Engl J Med.* 2000;343:230-238.
42. Farney AC, Hering BJ, Nelson L, et al. No late failures of intraportal human islet autografts beyond 2 years. *Transplant Proc.* 1998;30:420.
43. Robertson RP. Islet transplantation as a treatment for diabetes—a work in progress. *N Engl J Med.* 2004;350:694-705.
44. Ryan EA, Paty BW, Senior PA, et al. Five-year follow-up after clinical islet transplantation. *Diabetes.* 2005;54:2060-2069.
45. Cure P, Pileggi A, Froud T, et al. Improved metabolic control and quality of life in seven patients with type 1 diabetes following islet after kidney transplantation. *Transplantation.* 2008;85:801-812.
46. Owen RJ, Ryan EA, O'Kelly K, et al. Percutaneous transhepatic pancreatic islet cell transplantation in type 1 diabetes mellitus: Radiologic aspects. *Radiology.* 2003;229:165-170.
47. Shapiro AM, Ricordi C. Unraveling the secrets of single donor success in islet transplantation. *Am J Transplant.* 2004;4:295-298.
48. Mirbolooki M, Shapiro AMJ, Lakey JRT. A perspective on clinical islet transplantation: past, present and developments for future. *Immun Endoc Metab Agents Med Chem.* 2006;6:191-208.

CHAPTER 107

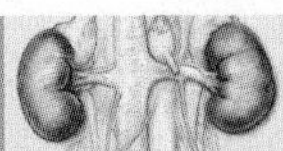

Kidney Disease in Liver, Cardiac, Lung, and Hematopoietic Cell Transplantation

Colm C. Magee

There is growing recognition that kidney disease can complicate all forms of solid organ nonrenal transplantation.[1] Kidney disease can occur in the immediate pretransplantation period, in the early postoperative period, or during the long term. In general, it is associated with longer hospitalization, higher morbidity, higher mortality, and more expense. Although there are organ-specific factors (such as the high prevalence of hepatitis C virus infection in liver transplant recipients) that have an impact on the incidence and severity of kidney disease, some useful generalizations can be made.

GENERIC ISSUES OF KIDNEY DISEASE IN NONRENAL SOLID ORGAN TRANSPLANTATION

Use of Serum Creatinine and Derived Equations to Measure Glomerular Filtration Rate

Transplant candidates and recipients often have low muscle mass and low creatinine generation. Hence, a mildly elevated serum creatinine concentration may "hide" severe kidney disease. This is particularly relevant in the pretransplantation patient with liver failure.[2] Such patients should have glomerular filtration rate (GFR) estimated by creatinine clearance (which will tend to overestimate) or preferably by iothalamate clearance (where it is available). Of the various serum creatinine–based equations to estimate GFR, the Modification of Diet in Renal Disease (MDRD) equation appears to correlate best with "true" post-transplantation GFR; however, even this equation has limited accuracy in all forms of solid organ transplantation.[2]

Nephrotoxicity of Calcineurin Inhibitors

The introduction of the calcineurin inhibitor (CNI) cyclosporine in the 1980s revolutionized the field of organ transplantation and dramatically improved the survival of nonrenal allografts. More than 30 years later, the CNIs cyclosporine and tacrolimus remain a cornerstone of immunosuppression in recipients of nonrenal allografts.[1] However, there is little doubt that CNIs contribute significantly to both acute kidney injury (AKI) and chronic kidney disease (CKD) in these recipients. There is speculation that CNI nephrotoxicity is more severe in nonrenal than in renal transplantation because (1) dosing and blood concentrations of CNIs tend to be higher in nonrenal transplantation and (2) the lack of normal innervation of the transplanted kidney may protect it from early CNI injury. CNIs also exacerbate post-transplantation hypertension and diabetes mellitus, which cause renal damage in the long term.

Acute CNI nephrotoxicity is thought to be mainly a prerenal syndrome due to vasoconstriction of the afferent glomerular arteriole (see also Chapter 97). Tubular damage and microvascular disease may occur in more severe cases. In the early post-transplantation period, AKI is usually multifactorial, and it is difficult to quantify the degree to which CNI toxicity is contributing to the problem. In practice, doses of CNIs are often temporarily reduced in the setting of AKI. CNI-induced thrombotic microangiopathy (TMA) is rare in nonrenal transplant recipients. Chronic CNI nephrotoxicity is probably due to prolonged renal ischemia and other effects, such as direct stimulation of renal fibrogenesis. Typically, the patient is hypertensive, and there is a steady fall in GFR, most marked in the first 6 to 12 months after transplantation (Fig. 107.1).[3] Dipstick urinalysis shows minimal or no hematuria and minimal or mild proteinuria. Urine protein-creatinine ratio or 24-hour urine collections confirm low-grade proteinuria. Renal histology shows interstitial fibrosis, arteriolar hyalinosis, arteriosclerosis, and secondary focal glomerulosclerosis. There may also be features of chronic TMA. In practice, renal biopsies are rarely performed unless there are clinical features suggestive of a renal disorder other than CNI toxicity.

Not surprisingly, the presumed high prevalence of chronic CNI nephrotoxicity has generated interest in low-dose or zero-dose CNI protocols. Just as in renal transplantation, these typically involve use of mycophenolate mofetil (MMF) or sirolimus.[1,4] However, there is still understandable reluctance to pursue such protocols because CNIs are considered such effective immunosuppressive agents, and an alternative organ replacement therapy analogous to dialysis is not available for other organ transplant recipients if severe rejection occurs. MMF has the advantage of being non-nephrotoxic; sirolimus has the disadvantages of potentiating the nephrotoxicity of cyclosporine and sometimes inducing proteinuria. Similar nephrotoxic interactions have been reported between everolimus and cyclosporine.[5] CNI-sparing strategies are discussed in more detail later.

Another strategy is to use tacrolimus as the *de novo* CNI or to switch from cyclosporine to tacrolimus if there is evidence of nephrotoxicity (cyclosporine is still commonly prescribed as the *de novo* CNI in heart and lung transplantation). The rationale is that tacrolimus provides equivalent or even better immunosuppression at doses and concentrations that are less nephrotoxic than cyclosporine. Furthermore, tacrolimus is associated with less hypertension and hyperlipidemia (which might exacerbate CKD) than cyclosporine. Conversely, it is associated with more post-transplantation diabetes mellitus. One study of healthy volunteers showed that tacrolimus (at trough concentrations of 5 to

15 ng/ml) had less effect on blood pressure and GFR than cyclosporine (at trough concentrations of 100 to 200 ng/ml),[6] but such studies in nonrenal transplant recipients have yielded conflicting results.

The utility of calcium channel blockers in ameliorating CNI nephrotoxicity in renal transplantation remains controversial, and there is limited evidence of such benefit in nonrenal transplantation. Experimental studies suggest that agents that block the renin-angiotensin system (RAS) may provide protection against the arteriolar hyalinosis and tubulointerstitial injury associated with chronic CNI use. The benefits on renal function of dosing cyclosporine based on C_2 (serum levels 2 hours after dosing) rather than C_0 (trough) concentrations remain unproven.

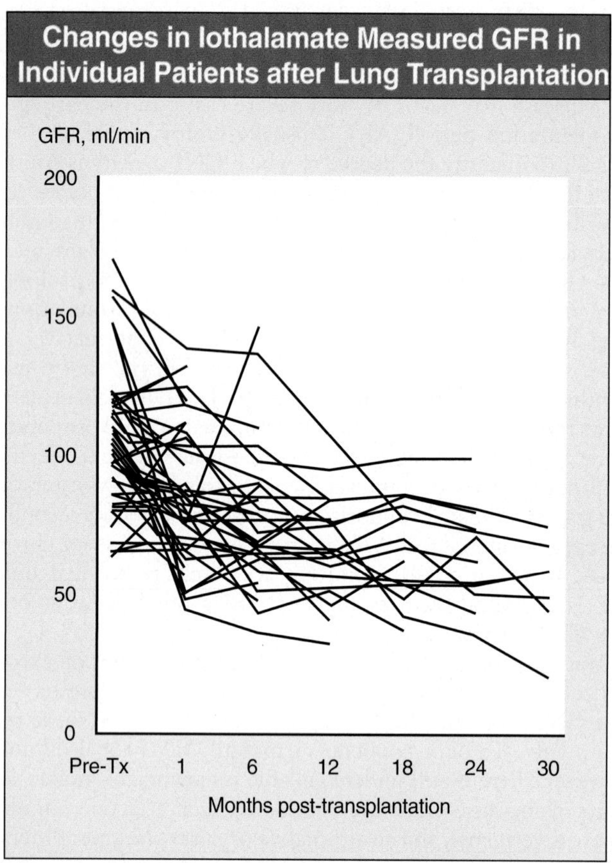

Figure 107.1 Changes in iothalamate measured GFR in individual patients after lung transplantation. Note the variation in GFR before transplantation and the large fall in many patients within the first 6 months. *(Modified from reference 3.)*

Acute Kidney Injury in the Immediate Pretransplantation Period

Not surprisingly, AKI can occur in the days to weeks immediately before liver, heart, or (less commonly) lung transplantation. Typically, the etiology of AKI is either prerenal (e.g., renal hypoperfusion or hepatorenal syndrome) or intrarenal (ischemic or toxic acute tubular necrosis) or a combination of both. AKI may develop on a background of CKD. A mildly elevated serum creatinine concentration may mask a significant fall in GFR in malnourished patients with severe organ failure.

Rates of reported AKI vary widely; rates may be modified by varying definitions of AKI, organ-specific risks of AKI, and center variability in the type of patients listed for transplantation. Management of AKI focuses on treatment of the underlying cause and provision of dialytic support according to standard criteria. Because the patients are critically ill, continuous renal replacement therapy (CRRT) may be preferred to intermittent hemodialysis, but there are no randomized controlled trials showing improved outcomes with this modality in this setting.

When severe or prolonged AKI occurs before planned transplantation, estimation of the degree of reversibility becomes very important, as presumed irreversible severe kidney injury is generally a contraindication to transplantation or shifts the management toward simultaneous dual organ (e.g., liver and kidney) transplantation. This is an area of ongoing debate in liver and, to a lesser extent, cardiac transplantation and is discussed in detail later. The general advantages and disadvantages of simultaneous dual organ transplantation are shown in Figure 107.2.

Although kidney biopsy might be useful in determining the degree of reversibility, in practice it is not commonly performed. This reflects the technical difficulties in performing the procedure in critically ill patients, particularly because of the high risk of coagulopathy, and the catastrophic consequences if a biopsy were complicated by a major bleed.

Acute Kidney Injury in the Early Post-transplantation Period

AKI is also common in the days to weeks after transplantation. This reflects several factors: pretransplantation renal function may have been compromised, the transplanted organ may have poor initial function, high doses of CNIs and other nephrotoxic agents may be prescribed, and the invasive surgery and high-dose immunosuppression predispose to severe infection (Fig. 107.3). AKI is associated with higher mortality in the early postoperative period.[7,8] This is likely to reflect both the association of AKI with other severe complications and also its direct effects on mortality. In those who survive, AKI is associated with increased risk

Advantages and Disadvantages of Simultaneous Kidney and Other Solid Organ Transplantation

Advantages	Disadvantages
Potentially provides much better renal function over the short and long term	Surgery more technically complex and prolonged Not needed when the AKI is reversible
Single donor - potential for lower cumulative dose of immunosuppression (as opposed to kidney transplantation later)	Deprives patients with 'definite' ESRD of a kidney transplant

Figure 107.2 Advantages and disadvantages of simultaneous kidney and other solid organ transplantation. AKI, acute kidney injury; ESRD, end-stage renal disease.

Causes of AKI After Solid Organ Transplantation

Prerenal	Intrarenal (ATN)	Postrenal
Hypovolemic shock (e.g. aggressive diuresis)	Prolonged shock	Rare
Cardiogenic shock (e.g. severe cardiac allograft dysfunction)	Cyclosporine/tacrolimus	
Distributive shock (e.g. sepsis)	Aminoglycosides, Amphotericin	
Cyclosporine/tacrolimus	IV Contrast Hydroxyethylstarch, IV Ig	

Figure 107.3 Causes of AKI after solid organ transplantation. ATN, acute tubular necrosis; IV Ig, intravenous immune globulin.

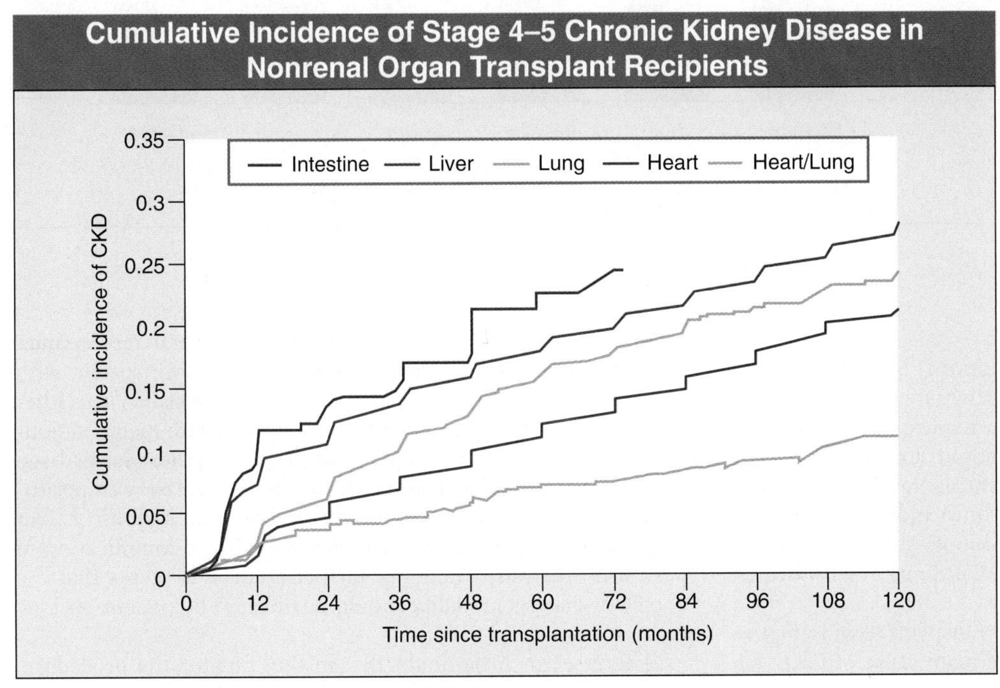

Figure 107.4 Cumulative incidence of CKD (eGFR <30 ml/min per 1.73 m²) after transplantation of various solid organs. *(Modified from reference 9.)*

for development of CKD.[9] Prevention or minimization of post-transplantation AKI involves careful selection of patients for transplantation, meticulous perioperative care, and avoidance of nephrotoxic agents.

Management of established AKI focuses on treatment of the underlying cause and provision of dialytic support according to standard criteria. Intermittent hemodialysis and CRRT are both used. Delayed introduction or reduced dosing of CNIs is sometimes employed, usually under the cover of induction antibody immunosuppression. How much this strategy improves renal function remains unclear.

Chronic Kidney Disease

With the higher number of solid organ transplants being performed worldwide and the longer survival of recipients, the absolute number of recipients with CKD has increased. In the largest and most comprehensive study to date, the cumulative incidence of post-transplantation CKD (defined as eGFR <30 ml/min per 1.73 m^2) at 5 years varied from 7% to 21% (Fig. 107.4).[9] By multivariate analysis, the following pretransplantation variables increased the risk for development of CKD: increasing age, female gender, white or black (as opposed to Asian) ethnicity, lower GFR, diabetes mellitus, hypertension, hepatitis C virus infection, and need for dialysis. The following post-transplantation variables were also implicated: postoperative AKI and initial use of cyclosporine (as opposed to tacrolimus).[9] These risk factors have been confirmed in other studies.

Many studies have also confirmed that whatever the transplanted organ, development of CKD, and especially of end-stage renal disease (ESRD), portends a poor prognosis (Fig. 107.5). Recipients with CKD have a relative risk of death of 4.6 compared with those without CKD.[9] The risk is highest in those with ESRD, but even in those not on dialysis, the relative risk of death was doubled.[9] Although it has not been well studied, CKD in this setting is presumably associated with the same complications as in nontransplant recipients, including anemia, hypertension, fluid overload, and bone and mineral disorders. Indeed, these complications might be more severe in nonrenal transplant recipients because of other risk factors. For example, antiproliferative immunosuppressants exacerbate anemia and corticosteroids exacerbate metabolic bone disease.

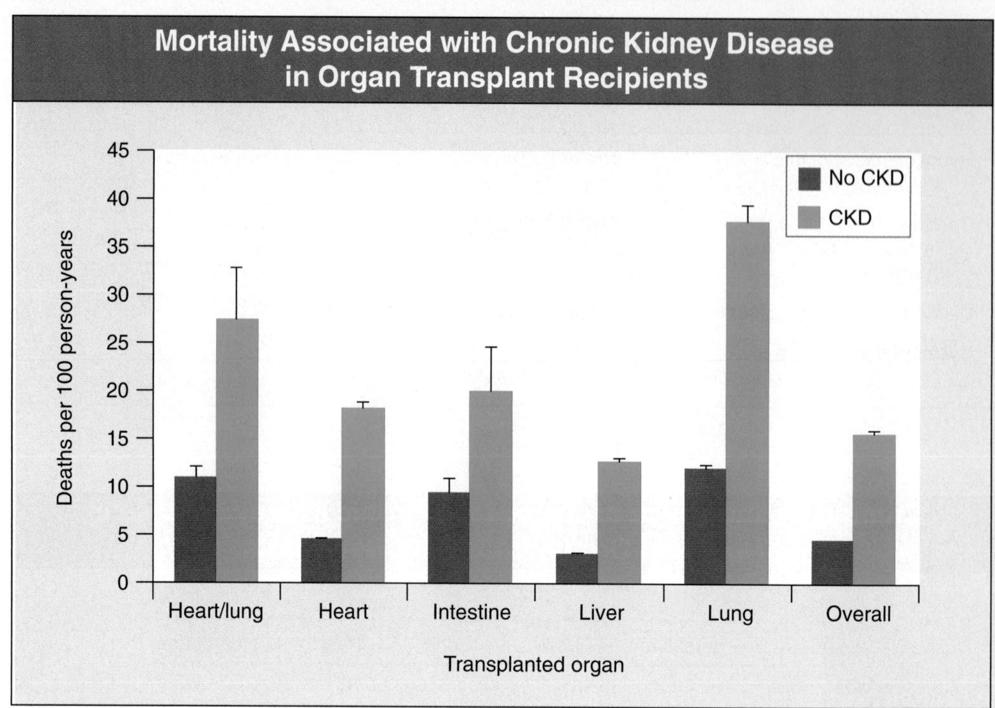

Figure 107.5 Mortality associated with stage 4 and stage 5 CKD in organ transplant recipients. *(Data from Scientific Registry of Transplant Recipients.)*

Management of Chronic Kidney Disease

The MDRD equation (despite its limitations) is useful in identifying CKD in these patients. In all patients with rising serum creatinine or falling GFR, referral to a nephrologist should be considered. The initial evaluation should include thorough review of renal function in the peritransplantation period and exposure to nephrotoxins. If urinalysis shows moderate or severe proteinuria or hematuria or both, renal biopsy should be considered; it can be highly informative in identifying renal diseases other than CNI nephrotoxicity.[10-12]

Close consultation with the primary transplant team is important. When CNI toxicity is deemed the main cause of CKD (as it is in the majority of cases), reduction in CNI dosage for patients at *low immunologic risk* should be considered. To maintain adequate immunosuppression, if the patient is receiving azathioprine, a change to MMF should be considered; if the patient is already receiving MMF, the dose should probably be increased. An alternative strategy is to substitute sirolimus for the CNI; this should not be done in the early post-transplantation period because of the adverse effects of sirolimus on wound healing. Finally, some have advocated switching of cyclosporine to low-dose tacrolimus, although the supporting data are less compelling. The majority of studies of CNI reduction or cessation in these settings are small and have limited follow-up.

The general management of CKD has not been well studied in nonrenal transplant recipients, but it seems reasonable to employ the same strategies used in the nontransplant CKD population. Thus, hypertension, anemia, and hyperparathyroidism should be managed according to standard guidelines. Although there is experimental evidence that angiotensin-converting enzyme (ACE) inhibitors might have important antifibrotic effects in nonrenal transplant CKD, there are no trials showing improved renal outcomes with ACE inhibitors or angiotensin receptor blockers compared with other antihypertensive agents. In practice, lifestyle modification and several antihypertensive drugs are usually required to achieve target blood pressure.

In those with severe CKD, planning for renal replacement therapy should begin early. The majority are treated with hemodialysis rather than with peritoneal dialysis. With either modality, mortality is much higher compared with matched nontransplant controls.[13,14] For example, outcomes have been reported in 21 cardiac transplant recipients treated with peritoneal dialysis; peritonitis was more common than in controls, but no patient was reported to have died of a direct complication of peritoneal dialysis.[13] Pending further studies, it seems that the choice of dialysis modality should be dictated by patient-specific factors.

There seems little doubt that in those fit for the procedure, sequential kidney transplantation is the best form of renal replacement therapy. Because patients are already transplanted, the addition of the renal allograft does not imply a huge increase in immunosuppression (typically, this is increased only in the perioperative period). When it is feasible, a preemptive live donor transplant is probably the best option. Initial mortality is higher in nonrenal transplant recipients receiving a kidney transplant as opposed to staying on the waiting list (reflecting the complications of surgery and more immunosuppression), but mortality during the medium and long term is much lower.[9]

Prevention of Chronic Kidney Disease

The rate of development and progression of CKD can probably be reduced by minimizing post-transplantation AKI (see earlier) and by rigorous control of hypertension during the long-term. Clearly, safe and effective non-CNI or low-dose CNI protocols would be an important advance in preventing severe CKD. Studies using induction antibody with corticosteroids, MMF, and low-dose tacrolimus are encouraging in this regard.[15,16]

BK Virus Nephropathy

This is a much-feared complication of kidney transplantation. Fortunately, although BK viruria is occasionally noted after liver, heart, or lung transplantation, the absolute risk of BK viremia and BK virus nephropathy remains low. This probably reflects the lack of a "second hit" to the native kidneys, such as HLA mismatching or inflammation. Nevertheless, BK virus nephropathy should be considered in the differential diagnosis of "unexplained" renal dysfunction after solid organ transplantation, especially because more intensive maintenance immunosuppressive protocols involving combined MMF and tacrolimus are being increasingly used.

Acute Kidney Injury in the Late Post-transplantation Period

Severe AKI occasionally occurs late after transplantation. The major causes are shown in Figure 107.3. Severe rhabdomyolysis has been reported, usually when statins are prescribed with cyclosporine and an inhibitor of the cytochrome P-450 system, such as diltiazem or the azoles. Treatment of late AKI is of the underlying cause plus the usual supportive measures.

KIDNEY DISEASE IN LIVER TRANSPLANTATION

AKI is common before liver transplantation. Indeed, use of the MELD (Model for End-stage Liver Disease) scoring system (which measures severity of hepatic dysfunction and risk of death) to guide allocation of deceased donor liver allografts in the United States means that a raised serum creatinine concentration increases the chances of the patient being offered a liver transplant.[17] The most common causes of AKI before transplantation are hepatorenal syndrome (see Chapter 72) and acute tubular necrosis or both. Prolonged hepatorenal syndrome may cause acute tubular necrosis. Glomerulonephritis is relatively common (cirrhosis is associated with IgA nephropathy and hepatitis C with membranoproliferative glomerulonephritis) but is rarely the cause of severe pretransplantation kidney disease. If renal replacement therapy is required, CRRT is often preferred, in part because it is thought to have less effect than intermittent dialysis on intracranial pressure.

Post-transplantation AKI is also common and is usually multifactorial.[8] In one recent series, 37% of liver transplants were complicated by some degree of AKI, 19% requiring renal replacement therapy.[8] Requirement for renal replacement therapy was associated with higher 30-day and 1-year mortality. Pretransplantation AKI associated with hepatorenal syndrome often but not always improves if the transplant is successful.

Although relatively low doses of CNIs are traditionally used in liver transplantation (because rejection is less of a concern than in other solid organ transplants), CKD remains common and is associated with higher mortality (see Fig. 107.5).[9] Thus, although CNIs are the most important cause of CKD, other factors must play a role. These include the high prevalence of hepatitis C and hepatitis B viral infections (which predispose to glomerulonephritis) and the high prevalence of diabetes (which predisposes to a number of renal problems, including diabetic nephropathy and renal infection).

Protocols involving reduction or cessation of CNIs have shown promising results. Delayed introduction of tacrolimus, with the cover of interleukin-2 receptor blockade, was recently shown in liver transplantation to better preserve renal function while maintaining excellent allograft and patient outcomes.[16] *De novo* use of sirolimus is not recommended as there is some concern that it may be associated with hepatic artery thrombosis.

Recommended Indications for Simultaneous Liver-Kidney Transplant in Patients Listed for Liver Transplant
CKD with GFR ≤30 ml/min
AKI or HRS with creatinine ≥2 mg/dl (176 μmol/l) and dialysis ≥8 weeks
CKD with biopsy showing >30% glomerulosclerosis or 30% interstitial fibrosis

Figure 107.6 Recommended indications for simultaneous liver-kidney transplantation in patients listed for liver transplantation. AKI, acute kidney injury; CKD, chronic kidney disease; GFR, glomerular filtration rate; HRS, hepatorenal syndrome. *(Modified from reference 17.)*

The number and percentage of simultaneous liver-kidney transplants have increased greatly in the United Stated during the last 10 years. In 1998, for example, there were 98; in 2008, there were 376 (approximately 6% of total liver transplants).[18] The principal reason is that the MELD system heavily weights higher serum creatinine concentration and prioritizes patients with renal dysfunction. Although patients with severe pretransplantation kidney disease do benefit from a combined transplant procedure, there is concern that too many simultaneous liver-kidney transplants are being performed and that current practice is depriving "real" ESRD patients of deceased donor kidney transplants.[19] The main issue, of course, is deciding which patients are likely to have meaningful renal recovery after liver transplant alone. Complicating factors in this setting are the known poor accuracy of serum creatinine (and equations based on it) in estimating GFR and concerns about the high risk of renal biopsy. Single-center studies suggest that use of a combination of clinical and histologic criteria allows effective prediction of which patients will benefit most from simultaneous liver-kidney transplantation.[20,21] These centers used iothalamate clearance to measure GFR in patients with suspected AKI. Renal biopsy was performed by the percutaneous or transjugular method and had a moderate rate of complications[20,21]; some believe that it adds little discriminating value.[22] A recent consensus conference has provided recommendations as to who should receive simultaneous liver-kidney transplants (Fig. 107.6).[17]

KIDNEY DISEASE IN CARDIAC TRANSPLANTATION

Preoperative AKI is common. In the largest reported study, 1% of heart transplant recipients required renal replacement therapy before transplantation.[9] The main cause of AKI is renal hypoperfusion due to severe congestive heart failure (type II cardiorenal syndrome; see Chapter 71). Ventricular assist devices are sometimes used as a bridge to cardiac transplantation and can improve renal function in this setting. Interestingly, there is emerging evidence that venous congestion is independently associated with the presence of AKI, although whether therapies based on reducing central venous pressure improve renal outcomes remains to be proven. In some cases, there may also be a component of chronic kidney injury due to renovascular disease or hypertension or atheroembolism.

Postoperative AKI is also common. In addition to the causes shown in Figure 107.3, factors that may be important after cardiac transplant surgery are prolonged aortic cross-clamping, large fluid volume shifts, and prolonged allograft ventricular dysfunction.

CKD is now well recognized as an important and common complication during the medium and long term (see Fig. 107.4). The cumulative incidence of stage 4 or stage 5 CKD in cardiac transplant recipients has been reported as 11% at 5 years, lower than in bowel, liver, or lung transplant recipients.[9] However, others have reported actuarial rates of ESRD as high as 20% after 10 years.[23] The principal cause of CKD after cardiac transplantation is CNI toxicity. Several studies have shown that early or late renal dysfunction is a risk factor for death after cardiac transplantation; furthermore, cardiac transplant recipients on dialysis have poorer survival compared with other ESRD patients.[14,24]

A number of studies have assessed reduction or cessation of CNIs in patients with significant CKD after cardiac transplantation. The majority are small and single center and have shown improvement in GFR with no adverse effects on the allograft.[25-28] However, these studies are of patients at low immunologic risk and do not have long-term follow-up. Indeed, one recent report warned of high rates of rejection after patients were switched to a corticosteroid plus MMF protocol.[29] Another pilot study showed concerning outcomes with a *de novo* CNI-free protocol,[30] which cannot at present be recommended.

As in liver transplantation, the question of whether the patient is best served by heart-alone or simultaneous heart and kidney transplantation sometimes arises. The concern here, again, is the reversibility of renal failure. The absolute number of such dual transplants remains low but is steadily increasing in the United States (62 in 2008, equivalent to about 1% of total heart transplants). Single-center reports have shown mixed results. One recent registry analysis found that simultaneous heart and kidney (as opposed to heart-alone) transplantation benefited only low-risk cases among those with eGFR below 33 ml/min.[31] Consensus guidelines have not yet been developed. At this time, it seems reasonable to limit the combined transplants to cases with severity of kidney disease similar to that shown in Figure 107.6.

KIDNEY DISEASE IN LUNG TRANSPLANTATION

Preoperative AKI is less common and severe, as evidenced by the fact that only 0.1% of lung transplant recipients are reported to require dialysis before transplantation.[9] CKD may be present before transplantation, however, because of diabetes mellitus or high exposure to aminoglycosides (mainly in patients with cystic fibrosis).

AKI after lung transplantation is common; in one series, 56% of patients had at least a doubling of serum creatinine in the first 2 weeks after transplantation.[7] AKI can occur for the usual reasons shown in Figure 107.3, but a number of factors specific to lung transplantation may be important. First, aggressive diuresis is often prescribed to minimize any pulmonary edema in the allograft.[7] Second, nephrotoxic antimicrobial agents, such as aminoglycosides and amphotericin, are sometimes required to treat resistant or severe infections.[7,12] Acute oxalate nephropathy leading to irreversible renal failure was recently described in two lung transplant recipients.[11] The pathogenesis is thought to involve gut hyperabsorption of oxalate because of impaired fatty acid absorption and altered gut flora. Although it is probably rare, this "new disease" emphasizes the importance of maintaining a broad differential diagnosis for any kidney disease occurring after solid organ transplantation and the utility of performing a renal biopsy when the clinical presentation is unusual.

As with other forms of post-transplantation CKD, the most common cause is CNI toxicity.[12] CNI dosing tends to be higher because of the increased risk of rejection in lung transplantation. A small number of studies have reported improvements in GFR when doses of CNIs were reduced, but more data are needed before this can be routinely recommended. If CNI reduction is attempted, it seems prudent to use MMF rather than sirolimus as additional immunosuppression in view of the risk of pneumonitis with sirolimus. *De novo* use of sirolimus is not recommended as it may cause breakdown of the bronchial anastomosis.

Interestingly, patients with pulmonary hypertension appear to have a lower GFR immediately before transplantation than do those with other diagnoses but exhibit a less severe fall in GFR after transplantation.[3] This probably reflects the adverse effects of pulmonary hypertension on renal perfusion and reversal of these effects after successful lung transplantation. Simultaneous lung-kidney transplantation is rarely performed.[18]

KIDNEY DISEASE IN HEMATOPOIETIC CELL TRANSPLANTATION

The general purpose of hematopoietic cell transplantation (HCT) is to allow administration of otherwise lethal (and ideally curative) doses of chemoradiotherapy, followed by engraftment of stem or progenitor cells for marrow recovery. Most commonly, HCT is used to treat hematologic malignant neoplasms, but other indications now include certain nonhematologic malignant neoplasms, severe genetic disorders (such as immunodeficiencies), and severe autoimmune diseases.[32] Stem and progenitor cells may be harvested from bone marrow, peripheral blood, or umbilical cord blood. Conventional *myeloablative* HCT uses intensive conditioning regimens involving high-dose chemotherapy and radiotherapy to ablate cancer cells and bone marrow; the hematopoietic system is then reconstituted by infusion and engraftment of stem cells. In allogeneic myeloablative HCT, non-self stem cells are used; in autologous myeloablative HCT, the patient's own cells are used. The toxicities of myeloablative regimens generally exclude older and sicker patients. *Nonmyeloablative* conditioning regimens have been developed to allow allogeneic HCT in such patients. These so-called "mini-allo" or "reduced conditioning" transplants involve less toxic conditioning; eradication of disease is mediated in part by allogeneic immunologic mechanisms, the "graft-versus-tumor" effect. In both forms of allogeneic HCT, acute and chronic graft-versus-host disease (GVHD) can be problematic; CNIs are typically prescribed to prevent and to treat this complication. The three main target organs of GVHD are the liver, gastrointestinal tract, and skin.

Tens of thousands of HCTs are performed worldwide every year.[32] It is now recognized that AKI and CKD are common complications of HCT and are associated with higher early and late mortality.[33] The types of HCT and their associated renal complications are shown in Figure 107.7.

Acute Kidney Injury After Hematopoietic Cell Transplantation

AKI is common after HCT, but its incidence and severity depend on the type of HCT (and on the definition of AKI used in reported series). It is common after myeloablative allogeneic HCT, reflecting the propensity of this regimen to cause profound immunosuppression (with associated risk of severe sepsis)

The Three Types of Haemopoietic Cell Transplantation and Their Associated Renal Complications

	Myeloablative allogeneic	Myeloablative autologous	Nonmyeloablative allogeneic
Diseases treated	Many leukemias, NHL, myelodysplastic syndromes	Lymphomas, multiple myeloma	As for myeloablative allogeneic
Used in patients> 60 years	Rarely	Sometimes	Commonly
Cormorbidities permissible before HCT	Minimal	Minimal	Some
Intensity of conditioning regimen	High	High	Low
GVHD after HCT	Common	None	Common
CNIs used routinely	Yes	No	Yes
Incidence of AKI	Very common; sometimes severe	Common	Common; rarely severe
Causes of AKI	VOD, shock syndromes, nephrotoxic drugs, CNIs	Shock syndromes, nephrotoxic drugs; occasionally VOD	CNIs
Incidence of CKD	Common	Common (but less severe than myeloablative allogenic)	Mild forms probably common
Causes of CKD	Irrersible AKI, Renal TMA, CNIs, ?GVHD	Irreversible AKI	Pretransplant mild CKD, irreversible AKI, CNIs, ?GVHD

Figure 107.7 The three types of hematopoietic cell transplantation and their associated renal complications. AKI, acute kidney injury; CKD, chronic kidney disease; CNIs, calcineurin inhibitors; GVHD, graft-versus-host disease; NHL, non-Hodgkin's lymphoma; TMA, thrombotic microangiopathy; VOD, veno-occlusive disease.

Causes of Kidney Disease According to Time After HCT

Immediate	Early (AKI in first 3 months)	Late
Tumor lysis syndrome	*Prerenal*	Thrombotic Microangiopathy*
Marrow/stem cell infusion toxicity	Hypovolemia	CNI toxicity
	Hepatorenal syndrome CNI toxicity	Irreversible AKI Membranous nephropathy/other glomerular diseases
	Intrarenal Ischemic toxic ATN (shock syndromes, aminoglycosides, amphotericin)	Recurrence of original disease which then affects kidneys (e.g. myeloma)*
	Postrenal Hemorrhagic cystitis	?GVHD

Figure 107.8 Causes of kidney disease according to time after HCT. *Can cause AKI also. AKI, acute kidney injury; ATN, acute tubular necrosis; CNI, calcineurin inhibitor; GVHD, graft-versus-host disease; HCT, hematopoietic cell transplantation. *(Modified from reference 36.)*

and liver damage (with associated risk of hepatorenal syndrome; see later); furthermore, CNIs are routinely prescribed for the first 100 days after transplantation. Severe AKI is least common after nonmyeloablative HCT (even though patients are older and sometimes sicker), reflecting the shorter period of pancytopenia and rarity of veno-occlusive disease of the liver as a post-transplantation complication; in fact, the principal cause of AKI is probably CNI toxicity.[34] Severe AKI necessitating dialysis is relatively rare.[34] Myeloablative autologous HCT has an intermediate incidence of AKI. Whatever the form of HCT, if dialysis is required for severe AKI, the overall prognosis is usually very poor (early mortality >70%).[35]

It is helpful to consider the causes of AKI according to the time period after HCT (Fig. 107.8).[36] Tumor lysis syndrome is now rare because the tumor burden at the time of HCT is rarely high and appropriate prophylaxis is widely used.[37] Marrow/stem cell infusion toxicity has been described after autologous HCT and is probably mediated by toxic cell breakdown products and DMSO, a cryopreservative used in the storage of autologous stem cells. DMSO can induce hemolysis of red blood cells and ultimately pigment nephropathy. Advances in cryopreservation and administration have made this complication rare.

Within the first few weeks of myeloablative HCT, when the conditioning regimen has caused pancytopenia, mucositis of the gastrointestinal tract, and liver damage, recipients are at high risk of many forms of AKI.[37] These include prerenal syndromes due to hepatorenal syndrome (see later) and hypovolemia (induced by vomiting and diarrhea or bleeding). Neutropenia predisposes to septic shock. Exposure to nephrotoxic agents, such as amphotericin, aminoglycosides, intravenous contrast agents, and CNIs, is relatively common and may also precipitate acute tubular necrosis. Obstructive uropathy is much rarer but can be due to severe hemorrhagic cystitis or fungal infection of the collecting system. Causes of hemorrhagic cystitis include high-dose cyclophosphamide and viral infection (by adenovirus or BK virus). BK virus nephropathy and adenovirus nephropathy have been described but appear to be rare.

Veno-occlusive Disease of the Liver

This is also known as hepatic sinusoidal obstructive syndrome and is one of the most common causes of severe AKI after myeloablative HCT, particularly allogeneic myeloablative HCT (see Figs. 107.7 and 107.8). The pathophysiologic mechanism is thought to involve radiotherapy- and chemotherapy-induced damage to the endothelium of hepatic venules with subsequent venular thrombosis and sinusoidal and portal hypertension.[37] Risk factors for development of veno-occlusive disease (VOD) include allogeneic HCT, older age, female gender, preexisting liver disease, use of cyclophosphamide or busulfan in the conditioning regimen, and exposure to methotrexate, progesterone, or antimicrobial drugs.[35]

Clinically, VOD is manifested as a form of hepatorenal syndrome. Frequently, there is a precipitating factor such as sepsis.[37] VOD generally appears during the first 30 days after HCT. The initial symptoms and signs are weight gain, edema, and ascites, then right upper quadrant abdominal pain and tenderness, jaundice, and abnormal liver function test results. Falling urine output, low urine sodium, and rising serum creatinine then follow.[37] The severity of disease varies. In mild to moderate cases, sodium and fluid restriction, diuresis, and analgesia may be required, and the syndrome eventually resolves. Severe VOD complicated by liver and renal failure (and frequently respiratory failure) carries a mortality approaching 100%.

The differential diagnosis includes acute GVHD of the liver, sepsis, drug-induced cholestasis, gallstone disease, and hepatotoxic effects of parenteral nutrition. The diagnosis of VOD is usually based on the typical clinical and laboratory features. On occasion, liver biopsy is needed to confirm the diagnosis.

Current preventive strategies for VOD include avoidance of precipitating factors when possible and use of ursodeoxycholate or low-dose heparin. Thrombolytics have been tested for treatment of severe VOD; not surprisingly, severe bleeding limits their use. The most encouraging therapy to date is defibrotide, a single-stranded oligonucleotide with antithrombotic and fibrinolytic effects on microvascular endothelium, but with apparently few systemic adverse effects.[38] Defibrotide is also showing encouraging results as a preventive agent.

Management of Acute Kidney Injury After Hematopoietic Cell Transplantation

Evaluation of the patient should be as for any patient with hospital-acquired AKI but with particular focus on the possible contribution of hepatorenal syndrome to the clinical picture. The patient's cancer diagnosis, conditioning regimen, and type of HCT should be carefully reviewed. When it is possible, further exposure to nephrotoxic drugs should be minimized (e.g., effective alternatives to amphotericin are now often available). If CNI trough concentrations are high, then reduction in dose should be considered. No randomized controlled trials have compared intermittent hemodialysis with CRRT in this setting. Whatever the modality used, the prognosis in those who develop severe AKI after HCT is poor. Continuous therapies do offer some potential advantages. In the setting of hepatorenal syndrome, there is some evidence that they are associated with less increase in intracranial pressure. In addition, the daily obligate fluid intake in these patients is frequently massive, and fluid balance is most easily controlled by a continuous dialysis technique. Vascular access can be problematic because of thrombocytopenia and neutropenia predisposing to bleeding and infection, respectively.

Chronic Kidney Disease After Hematopoietic Cell Transplantation

CKD is an important long-term complication of HCT, particularly allogeneic HCT.[33] Reported rates vary widely; in one recent review, the incidence in those surviving at least 100 days after HCT was 17%.[39] As recipients of HCT are living longer, CKD may become more prevalent, similar to the situation in solid organ transplants described earlier.

GVHD is thought not to affect the kidneys directly. However, there is evidence that GVHD or its accompanying inflammatory state may cause glomerular disease (see later); some believe that it may play a role in the pathogenesis of CKD also.[40]

The causes of CKD are shown in Figure 107.8.

Thrombotic Microangiopathy

Subacute or chronic renal TMA is probably the most common cause of CKD (particularly severe CKD) after HCT,[33] although this is disputed by some.[40] It typically is first manifested 4 to 12 months after HCT. Characteristic clinical features are slowly rising serum creatinine concentration, hypertension, and disproportionate anemia (see also Chapter 28). Dipstick urinalysis shows variable proteinuria and hematuria. Some cases have a much more fulminant presentation, however (e.g., as a severe nephritic syndrome). Careful review of previous laboratory test results will often show evidence of a low-grade TMA: intermittent or persistent elevation in plasma lactate dehydrogenase, low serum haptoglobin, low platelets, low hemoglobin, and sometimes schistocytosis. Renal imaging is usually unremarkable. Kidney biopsy is rarely required unless the presentation is atypical as the biopsy findings are unlikely to significantly alter management, and the biopsy carries increased risks in patients with thrombocytopenia and other morbidities. Histopathology typically shows microthrombi in arterioles and glomerular capillaries, mesangiolysis, glomerular basement membrane duplication, and tubular injury with interstitial fibrosis (Fig. 107.9).[37]

The main cause of TMA after HCT is thought to be direct damage to the renal endothelium, and possibly the tubulointerstitium, by the chemoradiotherapy conditioning regimen (particularly the radiotherapy component).[33,37] Renal tissue has much slower turnover than mucosal cells do and thus manifests chemoradiotherapy damage much later. Other factors, such as infection, GVHD, CNIs, and activation of the RAS, may play a facilitating role (Fig. 107.10).[36]

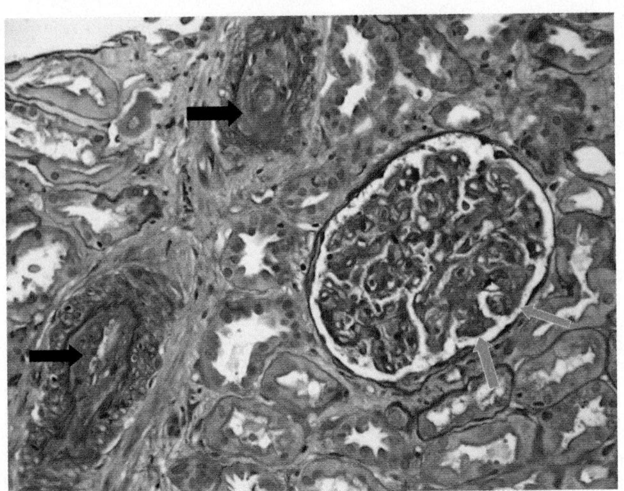

Figure 107.9 Thrombotic microangiopathy after allogeneic HCT. Renal biopsy specimen from a patient who had undergone allogeneic HCT and developed subacute renal failure 12 months later. Periodic acid–Schiff staining shows near-occlusion of two small arteries by subintimal connective tissue and swollen endothelium *(black arrows)*. The glomerulus shows thickened capillary walls with "double contours" and segmental occlusion and collapse of capillaries *(orange arrows)*. *(Courtesy Dr. H. Rennke, Harvard Medical School, Boston, USA.)*

Treatment of renal TMA after HCT is mainly supportive. Prevention involves renal shielding (from irradiation damage) and avoidance of other nephrotoxic agents at the time of conditioning. One small trial showed a trend toward better renal outcomes with captopril as opposed to placebo in patients who had undergone total body irradiation and HCT.[41]

Calcineurin Inhibitor and Sirolimus Nephrotoxicity

CNIs are routinely prescribed after allogeneic HCT to prevent and to treat GVHD. Long-term use of CNIs very likely contributes to CKD, as described before in solid organ transplantation.[42] However, as CNIs are often stopped after 3 to 6 months (unless there is ongoing GVHD), their contribution to CKD is generally thought to be limited. The contribution of CNIs to chronic renal TMA is unclear. There is a high incidence of TMA when sirolimus is added to CNI therapy, but fortunately this is often reversible.[43]

Glomerular Disease

Nephrotic syndrome has been described after both allogeneic and autologous HCT. In allogeneic HCT, it appears to be strongly associated with the presence of GVHD and to respond

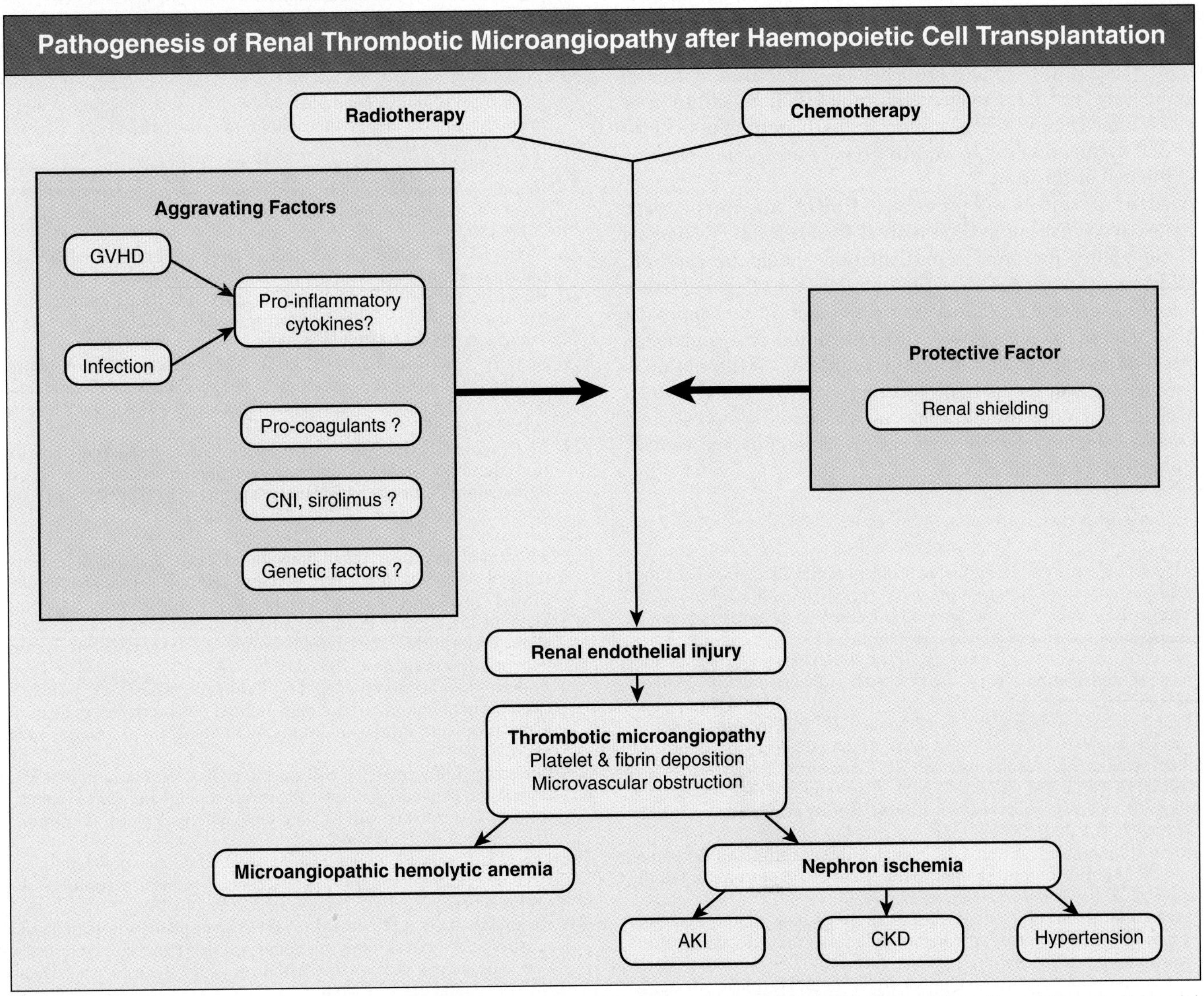

Pathogenesis of Renal Thrombotic Microangiopathy after Haemopoietic Cell Transplantation

Radiotherapy
Chemotherapy
Aggravating Factors
GVHD
Infection
Pro-inflammatory cytokines?
Pro-coagulants ?
CNI, sirolimus ?
Genetic factors ?
Protective Factor
Renal shielding
Renal endothelial injury
Thrombotic microangiopathy
Platelet & fibrin deposition
Microvascular obstruction
Microangiopathic hemolytic anemia
Nephron ischemia
AKI
CKD
Hypertension

Figure 107.10 Proposed pathogenesis of renal thrombotic microangiopathy after haemopoietic cell transplantation. AKI, acute kidney injury; CKD, chronic kidney disease; CNI, calcineurin inhibitor; GVHD, graft-versus-host disease; TMA, thrombotic microangiopathy. *(Modified from reference 36.)*

to more immunosuppression. *De novo* membranous nephropathy is the most common biopsy finding; minimal change disease has also been reported. The original hematologic disease (such as myeloma) may also recur with renal involvement.

Management of Hematopoietic Cell Transplantation–Related Chronic Kidney Disease

Careful review of the patient's pre- and post-HCT history is essential. Attention should be paid to the following: type of HCT and conditioning regimen (in particular, whether total body irradiation was used and at what dose) and degree of exposure to nephrotoxins. The examination frequently shows hypertension, hypervolemia, and skin GVHD. Blood test results should be reviewed carefully and tests repeated to assess for TMA; the laboratory features of TMA are often intermittent and not florid. Urine dipstick findings of hematuria and moderate proteinuria are suggestive of renal TMA but of course are not specific to this condition. Renal ultrasound is often used to exclude postrenal causes, but other imaging studies are usually unnecessary. As discussed before, kidney biopsy is rarely indicated.

General treatment should be as recommended for any patient with CKD. Aggressive control of hypertension is warranted. For the patient with TMA, plasma exchange does not appear to be beneficial.[37,44] RAS blockade slows progression in animal models of radiation nephropathy and is recommended for this reason and also for its beneficial effects in hypertensive proteinuric CKD.[33] CNI doses should probably be minimized if this is thought "safe" for the management of the HCT. Substitution of CNIs by interleukin-2 receptor blockers in the setting of GVHD and renal dysfunction might improve renal function but remains experimental at this time.[45]

A subset of patients will progress to ESRD, and overall, these patients have worse survival on dialysis than non-HCT controls do.[46] Suitability for renal transplantation should be carefully judged on a case-by-case basis. On occasion, the allogeneic stem cell donor can donate a kidney; a great benefit of this approach is that a state of tolerance to the allograft should exist, and hence minimal or no immunosuppression is required.[47] If this option is not available and the patient receives a conventional kidney transplant, low-dose immunosuppression should be prescribed as HCT recipients may not have normal immunity and remain at higher risk of infection.[47]

REFERENCES

1. Magee C, Pascual M. The growing problem of chronic renal failure after transplantation of a nonrenal organ. *N Engl J Med*. 2003;349:994-996.
2. Poggio ED, Batty DS, Flechner SM. Evaluation of renal function in transplantation. *Transplantation*. 2007;84:131-136.
3. Navis G, Broekroelofs J, Mannes GP, et al. Renal hemodynamics after lung transplantation. A prospective study. *Transplantation*. 1996;61:1600-1605.
4. Flechner SM, Kobashigawa J, Klintmalm G. Calcineurin inhibitor–sparing regimens in solid organ transplantation: Focus on improving renal function and nephrotoxicity. *Clin Transplant*. 2008;22:1-15.
5. Eisen HJ, Tuzcu EM, Dorent R, et al. Everolimus for the prevention of allograft rejection and vasculopathy in cardiac-transplant recipients. *N Engl J Med*. 2003;349:847-858.
6. Klein IH, Abrahams A, van Ede T, et al. Different effects of tacrolimus and cyclosporine on renal hemodynamics and blood pressure in healthy subjects. *Transplantation*. 2002;73:732-736.
7. Rocha PN, Rocha AT, Palmer SM, et al. Acute renal failure after lung transplantation: Incidence, predictors and impact on perioperative morbidity and mortality. *Am J Transplant*. 2005;5:1469-1476.
8. O'Riordan A, Wong V, McQuillan R, et al. Acute renal disease, as defined by the RIFLE criteria, post-liver transplantation. *Am J Transplant*. 2007;7:168-176.
9. Ojo AO, Held PJ, Port FK, et al. Chronic renal failure after transplantation of a nonrenal organ. *N Engl J Med*. 2003;349:931-940.
10. Pillebout E, Nochy D, Hill G, et al. Renal histopathological lesions after orthotopic liver transplantation (OLT). *Am J Transplant*. 2005;5:1120-1129.
11. Lefaucheur C, Hill GS, Amrein C, et al. Acute oxalate nephropathy: A new etiology for acute renal failure following nonrenal solid organ transplantation. *Am J Transplant*. 2006;6:2516-2521.
12. Lefaucheur C, Nochy D, Amrein C, et al. Renal histopathological lesions after lung transplantation in patients with cystic fibrosis. *Am J Transplant*. 2008;8:1901-1910.
13. Jayasena SD, Riaz A, Lewis CM, et al. Outcome in patients with end-stage renal disease following heart or heart-lung transplantation receiving peritoneal dialysis. *Nephrol Dial Transplant*. 2001;16:1681-1685.
14. Villar E, Boissonnat P, Sebbag L, et al. Poor prognosis of heart transplant patients with end-stage renal failure. *Nephrol Dial Transplant*. 2007;22:1383-1389.
15. Kobashigawa JA, Miller LW, Russell SD, et al. Tacrolimus with mycophenolate mofetil (MMF) or sirolimus vs. cyclosporine with MMF in cardiac transplant patients: 1-year report. *Am J Transplant*. 2006;6:1377-1386.
16. Neuberger JM, Mamelok RD, Neuhaus P, et al. Delayed introduction of reduced-dose tacrolimus, and renal function in liver transplantation: The "ReSpECT" study. *Am J Transplant*. 2009;9:327-336.
17. Eason JD, Gonwa TA, Davis CL, et al. Proceedings of Consensus Conference on Simultaneous Liver Kidney Transplantation (SLK). *Am J Transplant*. 2008;8:2243-2251.
18. Organ Procurement and Transplantation Network (OPTN): Multiple Organ Transplants in the USA, 2009.
19. Locke JE, Warren DS, Singer AL, et al. Declining outcomes in simultaneous liver-kidney transplantation in the MELD era: Ineffective usage of renal allografts. *Transplantation*. 2008;85:935-942.
20. Tanriover B, Mejia A, Weinstein J, et al. Analysis of kidney function and biopsy results in liver failure patients with renal dysfunction: A new look to combined liver kidney allocation in the post-MELD era. *Transplantation*. 2008;86:1548-1553.
21. Wadei HM, Geiger XJ, Cortese C, et al. Kidney allocation to liver transplant candidates with renal failure of undetermined etiology: Role of percutaneous renal biopsy. *Am J Transplant*. 2008;8:2618-2626.
22. Bloom RD, Reese PP. Chronic kidney disease after nonrenal solid-organ transplantation. *J Am Soc Nephrol*. 2007;18:3031-3041.
23. Rubel JR, Milford EL, McKay DB, Jarcho JA. Renal insufficiency and end-stage renal disease in the heart transplant population. *J Heart Lung Transplant*. 2004;23:289-300.
24. Alam A, Badovinac K, Ivis F, et al. The outcome of heart transplant recipients following the development of end-stage renal disease: Analysis of the Canadian Organ Replacement Register (CORR). *Am J Transplant*. 2007;7:461-465.
25. Angermann CE, Stork S, Costard-Jackle A, et al. Reduction of cyclosporine after introduction of mycophenolate mofetil improves chronic renal dysfunction in heart transplant recipients—the IMPROVED multi-centre study. *Eur Heart J*. 2004;25:1626-1634.
26. Gleissner CA, Doesch A, Ehlermann P, et al. Cyclosporine withdrawal improves renal function in heart transplant patients on reduced-dose cyclosporine therapy. *Am J Transplant*. 2006;6:2750-2758.
27. Hamour IM, Lyster HS, Burke MM, et al. Mycophenolate mofetil may allow cyclosporine and steroid sparing in de novo heart transplant patients. *Transplantation*. 2007;83:570-576.
28. Bestetti R, Theodoropoulos TA, Burdmann EA, et al. Switch from calcineurin inhibitors to sirolimus-induced renal recovery in heart transplant recipients in the midterm follow-up. *Transplantation*. 2006;81:692-696.
29. Groetzner J, Kaczmarek I, Schirmer J, et al. Calcineurin inhibitor withdrawal and conversion to mycophenolate mofetil and steroids in cardiac transplant recipients with chronic renal failure: A word of caution. *Clin Transplant*. 2008;22:587-593.
30. Leet AS, Bergin PJ, Richardson M, et al. Outcomes following de novo CNI-free immunosuppression after heart transplantation: A single-center experience. *Am J Transplant*. 2009;9:140-148.
31. Russo MJ, Rana A, Chen JM, et al. Pretransplantation patient characteristics and survival following combined heart and kidney transplantation: An analysis of the United Network for Organ Sharing Database. *Arch Surg*. 2009;144:241-246.
32. CIBMTR 2008 Progress Report: Center for International Blood and Marrow Transplant Research, 2009.

33. Cohen EP. Renal failure after bone-marrow transplantation. *Lancet.* 2001;357:6-7.
34. Parikh CR, Sandmaier BM, Storb RF, et al. Acute renal failure after nonmyeloablative hematopoietic cell transplantation. *J Am Soc Nephrol.* 2004;15:1868-1876.
35. Parikh CR, Coca SG. Acute renal failure in hematopoietic cell transplantation. *Kidney Int.* 2006;69:430-435.
36. Humphreys BD, Soiffer RJ, Magee CC. Renal failure associated with cancer and its treatment: An update. *J Am Soc Nephrol.* 2005;16:151-161.
37. Zager RA. Acute renal failure in the setting of bone marrow transplantation. *Kidney Int.* 1994;46:1443-1458.
38. Richardson PG, Murakami C, Jin Z, et al. Multi-institutional use of defibrotide in 88 patients after stem cell transplantation with severe veno-occlusive disease and multisystem organ failure: Response without significant toxicity in a high-risk population and factors predictive of outcome. *Blood.* 2002;100:4337-4343.
39. Ellis MJ, Parikh CR, Inrig JK, et al. Chronic kidney disease after hematopoietic cell transplantation: A systematic review. *Am J Transplant.* 2008;8:2378-2390.
40. Hingorani S. Chronic kidney disease in long-term survivors of hematopoietic cell transplantation: Epidemiology, pathogenesis, and treatment. *J Am Soc Nephrol.* 2006;17:1995-2005.
41. Cohen EP, Irving AA, Drobyski WR, et al. Captopril to mitigate chronic renal failure after hematopoietic stem cell transplantation: A randomized controlled trial. *Int J Radiat Oncol Biol Phys.* 2008;70:1546-1551.
42. Dieterle A, Gratwohl A, Nizze H, et al. Chronic cyclosporine-associated nephrotoxicity in bone marrow transplant patients. *Transplantation.* 1990;49:1093-1100.
43. Cutler C, Henry NL, Magee C, et al. Sirolimus and thrombotic microangiopathy after allogeneic hematopoietic stem cell transplantation. *Biol Blood Marrow Transplant.* 2005;11:551-557.
44. George JN, Li X, McMinn JR, et al. Thrombotic thrombocytopenic purpura–hemolytic uremic syndrome following allogeneic HPC transplantation: A diagnostic dilemma. *Transfusion.* 2004;44:294-304.
45. Wolff D, Wilhelm S, Hahn J, et al. Replacement of calcineurin inhibitors with daclizumab in patients with transplantation-associated microangiopathy or renal insufficiency associated with graft-versus-host disease. *Bone Marrow Transplant.* 2006;38:445-451.
46. Cohen EP, Piering WF, Kabler-Babbitt C, Moulder JE. End-stage renal disease (ESRD) after bone marrow transplantation: Poor survival compared to other causes of ESRD. *Nephron.* 1998;79:408-412.
47. Butcher JA, Hariharan S, Adams MB, et al. Renal transplantation for end-stage renal disease following bone marrow transplantation: A report of six cases, with and without immunosuppression. *Clin Transplant.* 1999;13:330-335.

INDEX

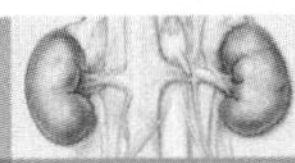

D

J

K

L

M

N

Q

R

T